evolve learning system

ELSEVIER

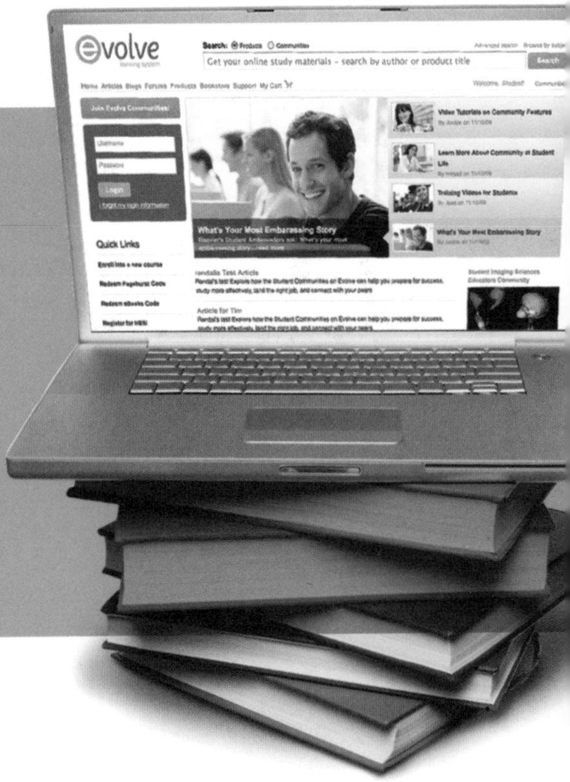

YOU'VE JUST PURCHASED MORE THAN A TEXTBOOK

ACTIVATE THE COMPLETE LEARNING EXPERIENCE THAT COMES WITH YOUR BOOK BY REGISTERING AT

http://evolve.elsevier.com/Canada/Perry/maternal/

Register today and gain access to:

- Anatomy Reviews
- Animations
- Answers to Critical Thinking Exercises
- Assessment Videos
- Audio Glossary
- Audio Summaries
- Care Plan Constructor
- Case Studies
- Childbirth Videos
- Critical Thinking Exercises
- Developmental/Sensory Assessment
- Dietary Reference Intakes
- Growth Measurements
- Nursing Skills
- Patterns of Inheritance
- Resources
- Review Questions
- Translation of FACES Pain Rating Scale

REGISTER TODAY!

MATERNAL CHILD NURSING CARE IN CANADA

SHANNON E. PERRY, RN, CNS, PhD, FAAN
Professor Emerita, School of Nursing
San Francisco State University
San Francisco, California

MARILYN J. HOCKENBERRY, PhD, RN-CS, PNP, FAAN
Director, Center for Research and Evidence-Based Practice
Nurse Scientist, Texas Children's Hospital;
Director of Nurse Practitioners
Texas Children's Cancer Center;
Professor, Department of Pediatrics
Baylor College of Medicine
Houston, Texas

DEITRA LEONARD LOWDERMILK, RNC, PhD, FAAN
Clinical Professor Emerita, School of Nursing
University of North Carolina at Chapel Hill
Chapel Hill, North Carolina

DAVID WILSON, MS, RNC
Faculty, School of Nursing
Langston University;
Staff, Pediatric Emergency Center
Saint Francis Hospital
Tulsa, Oklahoma

LISA KEENAN-LINDSAY, RN, MN, LCCE, PNC(C)
Professor, School of Health Sciences
Seneca College of Applied Arts and Technology
Toronto, Ontario

CHERYL A. SAMS, RN, BScN, MSN
Professor, School of Health Sciences
Seneca College of Applied Arts and Technology
Toronto, Ontario

First Edition

ELSEVIER

MOSBY
ELSEVIER

Adapted from Maternal Child Nursing Care, Fourth Edition, edited by Shannon E. Perry, Marilyn J. Hockenberry, Deitra Leonard Lowdermilk, and David Wilson.

Library and Archives Canada Cataloguing in Publication

Maternal child nursing care in Canada / Shannon E. Perry ... [et al.]. – 1st ed.
Includes bibliographical references and index.
ISBN 978-1-926648-28-6
1. Maternity nursing. 2. Pediatric nursing. I. Perry, Shannon E.
RG951.M38 2012 618.92′00231 C2011-907097-9
ISBN-13: 978-1-926648-28-6

Vice President, Publishing: Ann Millar
Developmental Editor: Jennifer Hermes
Managing Developmental Editor: Martina van de Velde
Publishing Services Manager: Deborah Vogel
Project Manager: Brandilyn Tidwell
Copy Editor: Jerrolyn Hurlbutt
Cover Design: Jessica Williams
Interior Design: Jessica Williams
Typesetting and Assembly: Toppan BestSet
Printing and Binding: Transcontinental

Elsevier Canada
905 King Street West, 4th Floor, Toronto, ON, Canada M6K 3G9
Phone: 1-866-896-3331
Fax: 1-866-359-9534

Printed in Canada

4 5 6 17 16 15

Contents

Part 1 Perinatal Nursing

UNIT 1 INTRODUCTION TO PERINATAL NURSING, 2

Chapter 1 Contemporary Perinatal Nursing in Canada, 2
Perinatal Nursing, 2
The History and Context of Health Care in Canada, 3
- Maternity Services in Canada, 3
- Millennium Development Goals: A Global Challenge, 5

Collaborative Woman- and Family-Centred Care, 6
- Family-Centred Maternity and Newborn Care, 6
- Woman-Centred Care, 6
- Multidisciplinary Collaborative Maternity Care, 7
- Integrative Healing, 7

Perinatal Health Indicators: The Canadian Perinatal Surveillance System, 7
- Trends in Fertility and Birth Rate, 8
- Multiple Birth Rate, 8
- Low Birth Weight and Preterm Birth, 8
- Breastfeeding Rates in Canada, 8
- Health Service Indicators: Rate of Inductions and Caesarean Delivery, 8

The Canadian Maternity Experiences Survey, 9
- Pregnancy, 9
- Labour and Birth, 9
- Postpartum, 9

Specialization and Evidence-Informed Nursing Practice, 9
- Cochrane Pregnancy and Childbirth Database, 10
- Joanna Briggs Institute, 10

Current Issues Affecting Perinatal Nursing Practice, 10
- Promoting Health and Normal Birth, 10
- The Place of Birth and "High-Tech" Care, 11
- Baby Friendly Initiative in Canada, 11
- Patient Safety and Risk Management, 11
- Community-Based Care, 11
- Involving Communities and Promoting Healthy Living, 12
- Health Literacy, 12
- A Global Perspective, 12

Ethical Issues in Perinatal Nursing, 13
Research in Perinatal Nursing, 13
- Ethical Guidelines for Nursing Research, 14

Addressing Current Challenges and Envisioning the Future, 14

Chapter 2 The Family and Culture, 16
The Family in Cultural and Community Context, 16
- The Family in Society, 16
- Family Organization and Structure, 16
- Family Dynamics, 17

Family Nursing, 17
- Family Assessment, 18
- Theories as Guides to Understanding and Working With Families, 18
- Family Systems Theory, 18
- The Calgary Family Assessment Model, 19
- Family Nursing as Relational Inquiry, 20

Cultural Factors Related to Family Health, 21
- Cultural Context of the Family, 21
- Cultural Diversity and Childbearing Families, 21

Providing Culturally Competent Perinatal Nursing Care, 22
- Cultural Awareness, 22
- Valuing Diversity and Avoiding Stereotyping, 22
- Communication, 22
- Personal Space, 24
- Time Orientation, 24
- Family Roles, 25
- Cultural Practices and Nursing Interventions, 25
- Integrating Cultural Competence With the Nursing Care Plan, 27
- Nursing Care Management, 27

Chapter 3 Community Care, 28
Community Health Promotion, 29
- Levels of Preventive Care, 29

Assessing the Community, 30
- Data Collection and Sources of Community Health Data, 30

Vulnerable Populations in the Community, 32
- Women, 33
- Implications for Nursing, 35

Home Care in the Community, 35
- Communication and Technology Applications, 35
- Maternal–Child Services in the Community, 36
- Nursing Care Management, 37
- Nursing Considerations, 38

Safety Issues for the Home Visiting Nurse, 40
- Personal Safety, 40

UNIT 2 WOMEN'S HEALTH, 42

Chapter 4 Health Promotion, 42
Reasons for Entering the Health Care System, 42
- Well-Woman Care, 42
- Fertility Control and Infertility, 42
- Preconception Counselling and Care, 43
- Pregnancy, 43
- Menstrual Problems, 43
- Perimenopause and Menopause, 44

Barriers to Receiving Health Care, 44
- Financial Issues, 44
- Cultural Issues, 44
- Gender Issues, 45
- Social and Cultural Factors, 45
- Health Risks in the Childbearing Years, 45
- Nutrition, 49
- Physical Fitness and Exercise, 51
- Stress, 51
- Sexual Practices, 53
- Medical Conditions, 54
- Gynecological Conditions, 54

Female Genital Mutilation, 54
Environmental and Workplace Hazards, 54
Anticipatory Guidance for Health Promotion and Illness Prevention, 55
Substance Use Cessation, 55
Health Screening Schedule, 56
Health Risk Prevention, 56
Health Protection, 56
Intimate Partner Violence, 58

Chapter 5 Health Assessment, 63
Female Reproductive System, 63
External Structures, 63
Internal Structures, 64
The Bony Pelvis, 66
Breasts, 67
Health Assessment, 68
Interview, 69
Women With Special Needs, 70
History, 73
Physical Examination, 74
Laboratory and Diagnostic Procedures, 79

Chapter 6 Reproductive Health, 81
Menstruation, 81
Menarche and Puberty, 81
Menstrual Cycle, 82
Prostaglandins, 84
Climacteric and Menopause, 84
Menstrual Cycle Concerns, 84
Amenorrhea, 84
Cyclic Perimenstrual Pain and Discomfort, 85
Alterations in Cyclic Bleeding, 91
Abnormal Uterine Bleeding, 92
Perimenopause and Menopause, 94
Infections, 95
Sexually Transmitted Infections, 95
Sexually Transmitted Bacterial Infections, 98
Sexually Transmitted Viral Infections, 101
Vaginal Infections, 108
Infection Control, 111
Problems of the Breast, 111
Fibrocystic Changes, 111
Fibroadenomas, 113
Lipomas, 113
Nipple Discharge, 113
Mammary Duct Ectasia, 113
Intraductal Papilloma, 114
Malignant Conditions of the Breast, 114

Chapter 7 Infertility, Contraception, and Abortion, 126
Infertility, 126
Incidence, 126
Factors Associated With Infertility, 126
Nursing Care Management, 127
Plan of Care and Implementation, 130
Contraception, 135
Nursing Care Management, 135
Methods of Contraception, 136
Abortion, 152
First-Trimester Abortion, 153
Second-Trimester Abortion, 154
Emotional Considerations, 154

UNIT 3 PREGNANCY, 157

Chapter 8 Preconception, Genetics, Conception, and Fetal Development, 157
Preconception, 157
Genetics, 157
Relevance of Genetics to Nursing, 158
Genetic History-Taking and Counselling Services, 159
The Human Genome Project, 161
Clinical Genetics, 162
Patterns of Genetic Transmission, 166
Nongenetic Factors Influencing Development, 167
Conception, 168
Cell Division, 168
Gametogenesis, 168
Conception, 168
Fertilization, 170
Implantation, 171
The Embryo and Fetus, 171
Primary Germ Layers, 172
Development of the Embryo, 172
Membranes, 172
Amniotic Fluid, 173
Yolk Sac, 173
Umbilical Cord, 173
Placenta, 174
Fetal Maturation, 176
Multifetal Pregnancy, 180

Chapter 9 Anatomy and Physiology of Pregnancy, 186
Obstetrical Terminology, 186
Pregnancy Tests, 187
Adaptations to Pregnancy, 188
Signs of Pregnancy, 188
Reproductive System and Breasts, 188
General Body Systems, 193

Chapter 10 Nursing Care During Pregnancy, 205
Confirmation of Pregnancy, 206
Signs and Symptoms, 206
Estimating Date of Birth, 206
Adaptation to Pregnancy, 206
Maternal Adaptation, 206
Paternal Adaptation, 208
Sibling Adaptation, 210
Grandparent Adaptation, 210
Nursing Care Management, 210
Reason for Seeking Care, 213
Current Pregnancy, 213
Obstetrical and Gynecological History, 213
Medical History, 214
Nutritional History, 215
History of Use of Drugs and Herbal Preparations, 215
Family History, 215
Social, Experiential, and Occupational History, 215
History of Physical or Sexual Abuse, 215
Review of Systems, 216
Physical Examination, 216
Laboratory Tests, 216
Follow-Up Visits, 218
Nursing Care Management, 222
Variations in Prenatal Care, 236

Perinatal Care Choices, 241
Options for Care Providers, 241
Childbirth and Perinatal Education, 243

Chapter 11 Maternal and Fetal Nutrition, 250
Nutrient Needs Before Conception, 250
Nutrient Needs During Pregnancy, 251
Energy Needs, 251
Protein, 256
Fluids, 256
Minerals, Vitamins, and Electrolytes, 257
Other Nutritional Issues During Pregnancy, 262
Nursing Care Management, 263
Nutrient Needs During Lactation, 270

Chapter 12 Pregnancy Risk Factors and Assessment: Maternal and Fetal, 273
Definition and Scope of the Problem, 273
Determinants of Health as Risk Factors, 274
Regionalization of Health Care Services, 274
Maternal Health Problems, 274
Mental Health Concerns, 274
Intimate Partner Violence During Pregnancy, 276
Fetal and Neonatal Health Problems, 277
Antepartum Testing in the First and Second Trimester, 277
Biochemical Assessment, 281
Third-Trimester Assessment for Fetal Well-Being, 285
Nursing Role in Antenatal Assessment for Risk, 291
Psychological Considerations, 291

Chapter 13 Pregnancy at Risk: Gestational Conditions, 294
Hypertension in Pregnancy, 294
Significance and Incidence, 294
Morbidity and Mortality, 295
Definition of Hypertensive Disorder of Pregnancy (HDP), 295
Classification, 295
The Link Between Hypertension and the Development of Pre-Eclampsia, 296
Nursing Care Management, 300
Gestational Diabetes Mellitus (GDM), 308
Maternal and Fetal Risks, 308
Screening for Gestational Diabetes Mellitus, 308
Interventions, 309
Hyperemesis Gravidarum, 310
Etiology, 310
Clinical Manifestations, 311
Collaborative Care, 311
Hemorrhagic Disorders, 312
Early Pregnancy Bleeding, 312
Premature Dilation of Cervix, 316
Ectopic Pregnancy, 318
Gestational Trophoblastic Disease, 320
Late Pregnancy Bleeding, 321
Nonobstetrical Surgery During Pregnancy, 330
Appendicitis, 330
Intestinal Obstruction, 330
Gynecological Problems, 331
Nursing Care Management, 331
Trauma During Pregnancy, 331
Significance, 331
Maternal Physiological Characteristics, 332
Fetal Physiological Characteristics, 333
Mechanisms of Trauma, 333
Nursing Care Management, 334

Chapter 14 Pregnancy at Risk: Pre-Existing Conditions, 338
Metabolic Disorders, 339
Diabetes Mellitus, 339
Nursing Care Management, 342
Thyroid Disorders, 350
Cardiovascular Disorders, 352
Congenital Heart Disease, 353
Acquired Heart Disease, 355
Contraindications to Pregnancy, 356
Nursing Care Management, 356
Cardiopulmonary Resuscitation of the Pregnant Woman, 362
Anemia, 362
Iron Deficiency Anemia, 364
Folic Acid Deficiency Anemia, 364
Sickle Cell Hemoglobinopathy, 364
Thalassemia, 364
Pulmonary Disorders, 365
Asthma, 365
Cystic Fibrosis, 366
Gastrointestinal Disorders, 367
Cholelithiasis and Cholecystitis, 367
Inflammatory Bowel Disease, 367
Integumentary Disorders, 367
Neurological Disorders, 368
Epilepsy, 368
Restless Legs Syndrome, 368
Multiple Sclerosis, 369
Bell's Palsy, 369
Autoimmune Disorders, 369
Systemic Lupus Erythematosus, 369
Myasthenia Gravis, 369
Obesity, 370
Antepartum Risks, 370
Intrapartum and Postpartum Risks, 370
Nursing Care Management, 370
Human Immunodeficiency Virus and Acquired Immunodeficiency Syndrome, 371
Preconception Counselling, 371
Pregnancy Risks, 371
Nursing Care Management, 372
Substance Use, 373
Barriers to Treatment, 373
Legal Considerations, 373
Nursing Care Management, 373

UNIT 4 CHILDBIRTH, 378

Chapter 15 Labour and Birth Processes, 378
Factors Affecting Labour, 378
Passenger, 378
Passageway, 380
Powers, 385
Position of the Labouring Woman, 386
Process of Labour, 388
Signs Preceding Labour, 388
Onset of Labour, 388
Stages of Labour, 388
Mechanism of Labour, 389

Physiological Adaptation to Labour, 391
Fetal Adaptation, 391
Maternal Adaptation, 391

Chapter 16 Comfort Measures for Labour, 394
Discomfort During Labour and Birth, 394
Neurological Origins, 394
Perception of Pain, 395
Expression of Pain, 395
Factors Influencing Pain Response, 395
Assessing Coping During Labour, 398
Nonpharmacological Management of Discomfort, 398
Childbirth Preparation Methods, 400
Nonpharmacological Comfort Strategies, 402
Pharmacological Management of Discomfort, 407
Sedatives, 407
Analgesia and Anaesthesia, 407
Nursing Care Management, 416

Chapter 17 Fetal Health Surveillance During Labour, 423
Fetal Health Surveillance, 423
Basis for Monitoring, 423
Fetal Response, 423
Uterine Activity, 424
Fetal Assessment, 424
Monitoring Techniques, 424
Intermittent Auscultation, 425
Electronic Fetal Monitoring, 426
Admission Fetal Monitor Strips, 430
Fetal Heart Rate Patterns, 430
Baseline Fetal Heart Rate, 430
Fetal Heart Rate Variability, 431
Periodic and Episodic Changes in Fetal Heart Rate, 431
Nursing Care Management, 435
Electronic Fetal Monitoring Pattern Recognition, 435

Chapter 18 Nursing Care During Labour and Birth, 442
First Stage of Labour, 442
Nursing Care Management, 442
Assessment of Labour, 444
Second Stage of Labour, 468
Duration of Second Stage, 470
Nursing Care Management, 470
Maternal Position, 471
Bearing-Down Efforts, 472
Fetal Heart Rate and Pattern, 473
Support of the Partner, 473
Supplies, Instruments, and Equipment, 474
Birth in a Delivery Room or Birthing Room, 474
Water Birth, 475
Mechanism of Birth: Vertex Presentation, 475
Use of Fundal Pressure, 476
Management of Infant Born in Meconium-Stained Fluid, 476
Perineal Trauma Related to Childbirth, 476
Emergency Childbirth, 478
Third Stage of Labour, 478
Umbilical Cord Blood Banking, 481
Maternal Physical Status, 481
Immediate Assessment and Care of the Newborn, 481
Fourth Stage of Labour, 483
Postanaesthesia Recovery, 485
Family–Newborn Relationships, 485

Chapter 19 Labour and Birth at Risk, 488
Preterm Labour and Birth, 488
Preterm Birth Versus Low Birth Weight, 488
Nursing Care Management, 490
Preterm Prelabour Rupture of Membranes (PPROM), 497
Nursing Care Management: Home Versus Hospital, 497
Dystocia, 498
Dysfunctional Labour, 498
Alterations in Pelvic Structure, 499
Fetal Causes, 499
Position of the Woman, 502
Psychological Responses, 502
Nursing Care Management, 503
Abnormal Labour Patterns, 503
Trial of Labour, 505
Postterm Pregnancy, Labour, and Birth, 505
Maternal and Fetal Risks, 505
Nursing Care Management, 505
Induction of Labour, 506
Augmentation of Labour, 511
Assisted and Operative Births, 511
Forceps-Assisted Birth, 511
Vacuum-Assisted Birth, 512
Caesarean Birth, 513
Vaginal Birth After Caesarean (VBAC), 519
Obstetrical Emergencies, 520
Shoulder Dystocia, 520
Prolapsed Umbilical Cord, 521
Rupture of the Uterus, 522
Amniotic Fluid Embolism (Anaphylactoid Syndrome of Pregnancy), 523

UNIT 5 POSTPARTUM PERIOD, 526

Chapter 20 Maternal Physiological Changes, 526
Reproductive System and Associated Structures, 526
Uterus, 526
Cervix, 528
Vagina and Perineum, 528
Abdomen, 528
Endocrine System, 529
Placental Hormones, 529
Pituitary Hormones and Ovarian Function, 529
Urinary System, 529
Urine Components, 529
Postpartal Diuresis, 529
Urethra and Bladder, 530
Gastrointestinal System, 530
Appetite, 530
Bowel Evacuation, 530
Breasts, 530
Breastfeeding Mothers, 530
Nonbreastfeeding Mothers, 530
Cardiovascular System, 530
Blood Volume, 530
Cardiac Output, 531
Varicosities, 531

Neurological System, 531
Musculoskeletal System, 532
Integumentary System, 532
Immune System, 532

Chapter 21 Nursing Care During the Fourth Trimester, 534
Transfer From the Recovery Area, 534
Postpartum Care, 535
Criteria for Discharge, 535
Nursing Care Management—Physical Needs, 536
Nursing Care Management—Psychosocial Needs, 548
Nursing Care Management—Discharge Teaching, 552

Chapter 22 Transition to Parenthood, 556
Parental Attachment, Bonding, and Acquaintance, 556
Assessment of Attachment Behaviours, 558
Parent–Infant Contact, 558
Communication Between Parent and Infant, 560
The Senses, 560
Entrainment, 561
Biorhythmicity, 561
Reciprocity, Synchrony, and Habituation, 561
Parental Role After Childbirth, 562
Transition to Parenthood, 562
Parental Tasks and Responsibilities, 563
Becoming a Mother, 563
Resuming Sexual Intimacy, 564
Postpartum Adjustment in the Lesbian Couple, 564
Becoming a Father, 565
Infant–Parent Adjustment, 566
Rhythm, 566
Behavioural Repertoires, 566
Responsivity, 566
Diversity in Transitions to Parenthood, 567
Age, 567
Social Support, 569
Culture, 569
Socioeconomic Conditions, 570
Personal Aspirations, 570
Parental Sensory Impairment, 570
Visually Impaired Parent, 570
Hearing-Impaired Parent, 571
Sibling Adaptation, 571
Grandparent Adaptation, 573
Nursing Care Management, 574

Chapter 23 Postpartum Complications, 577
Postpartum Hemorrhage, 577
Definition and Incidence, 577
Etiology and Risk Factors, 578
Nursing Care Management, 580
Hemorrhagic (Hypovolemic) Shock, 581
Coagulopathies, 584
Idiopathic Thrombocytopenic Purpura (ITP), 584
von Willebrand Disease, 584
Disseminated Intravascular Coagulation, 584
Thromboembolic Disease, 585
Incidence and Etiology, 585
Clinical Manifestations, 585
Medical Management, 585
Postpartum Infections, 586
Endometritis, 586
Wound Infections, 586
Urinary Tract Infections, 587
Mastitis, 587
Nursing Care Management, 587
Sequelae of Childbirth Trauma, 588
Uterine Displacement and Prolapse, 589
Cystocele and Rectocele, 589
Urinary Incontinence, 590
Genital Fistulas, 590
Nursing Care Management, 591
Postpartum Psychological Complications, 593
Postpartum Mood Disorders, 593
Nursing Care Management, 596
Loss and Grief, 599
Grief Responses, 599
Family Aspects of Grief, 601
Nursing Care Management, 602
Maternal Death, 607

UNIT 6 NEWBORN, 609

Chapter 24 Physiological Adaptations of the Newborn, 609
Transition to Extrauterine Life, 609
Physiological Adjustments, 609
Physical Assessment, 625
General Appearance, 636
Vital Signs, 636
Baseline Measurements of Physical Growth, 637
Neurological Assessment, 637
Behavioural Characteristics, 637
Sleep–Wake States, 638
Other Factors Influencing Behaviour of Newborns, 638
Sensory Behaviours, 639
Response to Environmental Stimuli, 640

Chapter 25 Nursing Care of the Newborn, 642
Birth Through the First 2 Hours, 642
Nursing Care Management, 642
From 2 Hours After Birth Until Discharge, 648
Nursing Care Management, 648
Common Newborn Problems, 651
Physical Injuries, 651
Physiological Problems, 652
Laboratory and Diagnostic Tests, 655
Collection of Specimens, 655
Supporting Parents in the Care of Their Infant, 660
Social Interactions, 660
Infant Feeding, 660
Therapeutic and Surgical Procedures, 661
Intramuscular Injection, 661
Therapy for Hyperbilirubinemia, 661
Circumcision, 663
Discharge Planning and Teaching, 667
Temperature, 667
Respirations, 667
Feeding Schedules, 667

Elimination, 667
Prevention of Sudden Infant Death Syndrome, 667
Safety and Holding, 668
Rashes, 668
Clothing, 669
Safety: Use of Car Seat, 669
Non-Nutritive Sucking, 670
Bathing, Cord Care, and Skin Care, 670
Infant Follow-Up Care, 671
Immunizations, 672

Chapter 26 Newborn Nutrition and Feeding, 676
Recommended Infant Nutrition, 676
Benefits of Breastfeeding, 676
Contraindications to Breastfeeding, 677
Choosing an Infant Feeding Method, 677
Nutrient Needs, 679
Overview of Lactation, 680
Breast Anatomy, 680
Milk Production, 681
Unique Properties of Human Milk, 682
Nursing Care Management: The Breastfeeding Mother and Infant, 683
Role of the Nurse in Promoting Successful Lactation, 698
Baby-Friendly Hospital Initiative, 699
Formula-Feeding, 700
Rationale for Formula-Feeding, 700
Parent Education, 700

Chapter 27 Infants With Gestational Age–Related Problems, 707
The Preterm Infant, 707
Late Preterm Infant, 708
Nursing Care Management, 710
Parental Adaptation to the Preterm Infant, 711
Growth and Development Potential, 726
Complications of Prematurity, 728
The Postterm Infant, 733
Meconium Aspiration Syndrome, 733
Persistent Pulmonary Hypertension of the Newborn, 733
Other Problems Related to Gestation, 734
Small-for-Gestational-Age Infants and Intrauterine Growth Restriction, 734
Large-for-Gestational-Age Infants, 735
Infants of Diabetic Mothers, 735
Discharge Planning and Transport, 737
Discharge Planning, 737
Transport to a Regional Centre, 738
Transport From a Regional Centre, 739

Chapter 28 The Newborn at Risk: Acquired and Congenital Problems, 743
Birth Trauma, 743
Nursing Care Management, 744
Neonatal Infections, 746
Sepsis, 746
Nursing Care Management, 747
Perinatally Acquired Infections, 749
Substance Use, 756
Alcohol, 757
Tobacco, 759
Marijuana, 760
Cocaine, 760
Phencyclidine ("Angel Dust"), 761
Heroin, 761
Methadone, 761
Methamphetamine, 761
Phenobarbital, 762
Caffeine, 762
Nursing Care Management, 762
Hemolytic Disorders, 765
Hemolytic Disease of the Newborn, 765
Nursing Care Management, 767
Congenital Anomalies, 768
Central Nervous System Anomalies, 768
Cardiovascular System Anomalies, 770
Respiratory System Anomalies, 770
Gastrointestinal System Anomalies, 772
Musculoskeletal System Anomalies, 775
Genitourinary System Anomalies, 776
Nursing Care Management, 778

Part 2 Pediatric Nursing

UNIT 7 CHILDREN, THEIR FAMILIES, AND THE NURSE, 786

Chapter 29 Contemporary Pediatric Nursing in Canada, 786
Health Care for Children, 786
Health Promotion, 787
Nutrition, 788
Dental Care, 788
Immunizations, 788
Childhood Health Problems, 788
Obesity and Type 2 Diabetes, 788
Childhood Injuries, 789
Violence, 791
Substance Use, 791
Mental Health Problems, 792
Mortality, 792
Infant Mortality, 792
Morbidity, 793
Childhood Morbidity, 793
The Art of Pediatric Nursing, 793
Philosophy of Care, 793
Family-Centred Care, 793
Atraumatic Care, 794
Role of the Pediatric Nurse, 794
Therapeutic Relationship, 794
Family Advocacy and Caring, 794
Disease Prevention and Health Promotion, 795
Health Teaching, 795
Support and Counselling, 795
Coordination and Collaboration, 795
Ethical Decision Making, 796
Research, 796
Critical Thinking and the Process of Nursing Children and Families, 796
Critical Thinking, 796
Evidence-Informed Practice, 796
Nursing Process, 797
Health Care Planning, 797
Future Trends, 798

Chapter 30 Community-Based Nursing Care of the Child and Family, 801
Nursing in the Community, 801
Roles and Functions, 802
  Demography, 802
  Epidemiology, 802
  Economics, 804
Community Nursing Process, 804
  Community Needs Assessment and Diagnosis, 804
  Community Planning, 805
  Community Intervention, 806
  Community Evaluation, 806

Chapter 31 Family Influences on Child Health Promotion, 808
General Concepts, 808
  Definition of Family, 808
  Family Nursing Interventions, 808
Family Roles, Relationships, and Strengths, 809
  Parental Roles, 809
  Role Learning, 809
Parenting, 813
  Motivation for Parenthood, 813
  Preparation for Parenthood, 813
  Transition to Parenthood, 813
  Parenting Behaviours, 814
  Limit Setting and Discipline, 814
Special Parenting Situations, 817
  Parenting the Adopted Child, 817
  Parenting and Divorce, 819
  Lone Parenting, 821
  Same-Sex Marriages and Parenting, 821
  Parenting in Reconstituted Families, 821
  Parenting in Dual-Earner Families, 821
  Foster Parenting, 822
  Accommodating Contemporary Parenting Situations, 822

Chapter 32 Social, Cultural, and Religious Influences on Child Health Promotion, 824
Social Determinants of Health, 824
  Key Social-Determinant Influences, 824
  The Child and Family in North America, 829
Cultural, Ethnic, and Religious Influences on Health Care, 831
  Susceptibility to Health Problems, 831
  Cultural Customs, 831
  Health Beliefs and Practices, 835
  Religious Beliefs, 837
  Importance of Culture and Religion to Nursing, 837

Chapter 33 Developmental Influences on Child Health Promotion, 844
Growth and Development, 844
  Foundations of Growth and Development, 844
  Biological Growth and Physical Development, 846
  Physiological Changes, 849
  Temperament, 849
Development of Personality and Mental Function, 850
  Theoretical Foundations of Personality Development, 850
  Theoretical Foundations of Mental Development, 852
  Development of Self-Concept, 855
Role of Play in Development, 856
  Classification of Play, 856
  Content of Play, 856
  Social Character of Play, 857
  Functions of Play, 858
  Toys, 858
Selected Factors That Influence Development, 859
  Heredity, 859
  Neuroendocrine Factors, 859
  Nutrition, 859
  Interpersonal Relationships, 861
  Socioeconomic Level, 862
  Disease, 862
  Environmental Hazards, 862
  Stress in Childhood, 863
  Influence of Mass Media, 864

UNIT 8 ASSESSMENT OF THE CHILD AND FAMILY, 869

Chapter 34 Communication, History, Physical, and Developmental Assessment, 869
Guidelines for Communication and Interviewing, 869
  Establishing a Setting for Communication, 869
  Computer Privacy and Applications in Nursing, 870
  Telephone Triage and Counselling, 870
Communicating With Families, 871
  Communicating With Parents, 871
  Communicating With Children, 873
  Communication Techniques, 876
History Taking, 876
  Performing a Health History, 876
Nutritional Assessment, 886
  Dietary Intake, 886
  Clinical Examination, 887
  Evaluation of Nutritional Assessment, 890
General Approaches Toward Examining the Child, 890
  Sequence of the Examination, 890
  Preparation of the Child, 890
Physical Examination, 892
  Growth Measurements, 893
  Physiological Measurements, 897
  General Appearance, 905
  Skin, 905
  Lymph Nodes, 906
  Head and Neck, 907
  Eyes, 907
  Ears, 912
  Nose, 915
  Mouth and Throat, 916
  Chest, 917
  Lungs, 919
  Heart, 920
  Abdomen, 922
  Genitalia, 924
  Anus, 926
  Back and Extremities, 926
  Neurological Assessment, 928
Developmental Assessment, 928
  Nipissing District Developmental Screen, 929

Chapter 35 Pain Assessment and Management, 934
Pain Assessment, 934
Behavioural Measures, 934
Physiological Measures, 934
Self-Report Measures, 935
Multidimensional Measures, 936
Pain Assessment in Specific Populations, 938
Pain in Neonates, 938
Children With Communication and Cognitive Impairment, 939
Cultural Issues in Pain Assessment, 939
Children With Chronic Illness and Complex Pain, 939
Pain Management, 940
Nonpharmacological Management, 940
Complementary Pain Medicine, 942
Pharmacological Management, 943

UNIT 9 HEALTH PROMOTION AND SPECIAL HEALTH PROBLEMS, 958

Chapter 36 The Infant and Family, 958
Promoting Optimum Growth and Development, 958
Biological Development, 958
Psychosocial Development, 963
Cognitive Development, 964
Development of Body Image, 965
Social Development, 966
Temperament, 968
Coping With Concerns Related to Normal Growth and Development, 970
Promoting Optimum Health During Infancy, 978
Nutrition, 978
Sleep and Activity, 981
Dental Health, 983
Immunizations, 983
Injury Prevention, 993
Anticipatory Guidance—Care of Families, 1003
Special Health Problems, 1003
Feeding Difficulties, 1003
Regurgitation and "Spitting Up", 1003
Colic (Paroxysmal Abdominal Pain), 1003
Growth Failure (Failure to Thrive), 1005
Disorders of Unknown Etiology, 1008
Sudden Infant Death Syndrome, 1008
Positional Plagiocephaly, 1011
Apnea and Apparent Life-Threatening Events, 1012

Chapter 37 The Toddler and Family, 1020
Promoting Optimum Growth and Development, 1020
Biological Development, 1020
Psychosocial Development, 1022
Cognitive Development, 1024
Development of Gender Identity, 1026
Social Development, 1027
Coping With Concerns Related to Normal Growth and Development, 1029
Promoting Optimum Health During Toddlerhood, 1032
Nutrition, 1032
Sleep and Activity, 1034
Dental Health, 1034
Injury Prevention, 1037

Chapter 38 The Preschooler and Family, 1049
Promoting Optimum Growth and Development, 1049
Biological Development, 1049
Psychosocial Development, 1052
Cognitive Development, 1052
Moral Development, 1053
Spiritual Development, 1053
Development of Body Image, 1053
Development of Sexuality, 1053
Social Development, 1053
Coping With Concerns Related to Normal Growth and Development, 1055
Promoting Optimum Health During Preschool Years, 1059
Nutrition, 1059
Sleep and Activity, 1060
Dental Health, 1060
Injury Prevention, 1061
Anticipatory Guidance—Care of Families, 1061
Infectious Disorders, 1062
Communicable Diseases, 1062
Encopresis, 1072
Child Maltreatment, 1072
Child Neglect, 1072
Physical Abuse, 1072
Sexual Abuse, 1073

Chapter 39 The School-Age Child and Family, 1083
Promoting Optimum Growth and Development, 1083
Biological Development, 1084
Psychosocial Development, 1085
Cognitive Development (Piaget), 1087
Moral Development (Kohlberg), 1088
Spiritual Development, 1089
Social Development, 1089
Developing a Self-Concept, 1092
Coping With Concerns Related to Normal Growth and Development, 1093
Promoting Optimum Health During the School Years, 1096
Nutrition, 1096
Sleep and Rest, 1096
Exercise and Activity, 1097
Dental Health, 1098
Sex Education, 1099
School Health, 1100
Injury Prevention, 1100
Special Health Problems, 1101
Health Problems Related to Sports Participation, 1101
Overuse Syndromes, 1103
Nurse's Role in Sports for Children and Adolescents, 1104
Altered Growth and Maturation, 1104
Tall or Short Stature, 1104
Sex Chromosome Abnormalities, 1105
Disorders With Behavioural Components, 1106
Attention-Deficit/Hyperactivity Disorder and Learning Disability, 1106
Enuresis, 1107
Post-Traumatic Stress Disorder, 1108
School Phobia, 1108
Recurrent Abdominal Pain, 1109
Eating Disorders, 1109

Conversion Reaction, 1109
Childhood Depression, 1110
Social Media, 1110

Chapter 40 The Adolescent and Family, 1113
Promoting Optimum Growth and Development, 1113
Biological Development, 1113
Psychosocial Development, 1117
Cognitive Development (Piaget), 1119
Moral Development (Kohlberg), 1119
Spiritual Development, 1119
Social Development, 1119
Adolescent Sexuality, 1122
Development of Self-Concept and Body Image, 1123
Promoting Optimum Health During Adolescence, 1124
Immunizations, 1125
Nutrition, 1125
Sleep and Rest, 1127
Exercise and Activity, 1127
Dental Health, 1127
Personal Care, 1127
Mental Health, 1129
Stress Reduction, 1129
Sexual Health, 1130
Injury Prevention, 1131
Anticipatory Guidance—Care of Families, 1133
Special Health Problems, 1133
Disorders Related to the Reproductive System, 1133
Amenorrhea, 1133
Dysmenorrhea, 1134
Vaginitis, 1135
Disorders of the Male Reproductive System, 1135
Gynecomastia, 1135
Eating Disorders, 1136
Obesity, 1136
Anorexia Nervosa and Bulimia Nervosa, 1141
Serious Health Problems With a Behavioural Component, 1144
Tobacco, 1144
Substance Use, 1146
Suicide, 1149

UNIT 10 SPECIAL NEEDS, ILLNESS, AND HOSPITALIZATION, 1156

Chapter 41 Chronic Illness, Disability, and End-of-Life Care, 1156
Perspectives on the Care of Children With Special Needs, 1156
Scope of the Problem, 1156
Trends in Care, 1157
The Family of the Child With Special Needs, 1159
Impact of the Child's Chronic Illness or Disability, 1159
Coping With Ongoing Stress and Periodic Crises, 1161
Assisting Family Members in Managing Their Feelings, 1162
Establishing a Support System, 1164
The Child With Special Needs, 1164
Developmental Aspects, 1164
Coping Mechanisms, 1164
Responses to Parental Behaviour, 1165
Type of Illness or Disability, 1166
Nursing Care of the Family and Child With Special Needs, 1166
Assessment, 1166
Provide Support at the Time of Diagnosis, 1166
Support the Family's Coping Methods, 1167
Educate About the Disorder and General Health Care, 1169
Promote Normal Development, 1170
Establish Realistic Future Goals, 1174
Perspectives on the Care of Children at the End of Life, 1174
Principles of Palliative Care, 1174
Decision Making at the End of Life, 1175
Treatment Options for Terminally Ill Children, 1176
Nursing Care of the Child and Family at the End of Life, 1179
Fear of Pain and Suffering, 1179
Fear of Dying Alone or of Not Being Present When the Child Dies, 1181
Fear of Actual Death, 1181
Organ or Tissue Donation and Autopsy, 1182
Grief and Mourning, 1183
Nurses' Reactions to Caring for Dying Children, 1184

Chapter 42 Cognitive and Sensory Impairment, 1189
Cognitive Impairment, 1189
General Concepts, 1189
Nursing Care of Children With Impaired Cognitive Function, 1190
Down Syndrome, 1195
Fragile X Syndrome, 1198
Sensory Impairment, 1199
Hearing Impairment, 1199
Visual Impairment, 1203
Deaf-Blind Children, 1209
Retinoblastoma, 1209
Autism Spectrum Disorders, 1210

Chapter 43 Family-Centred Home Care, 1216
General Concepts of Home Care, 1216
Definition, 1216
Home Care Trends and Needs, 1217
Effective Home Care, 1218
Discharge Planning and Selection of a Home Care Agency, 1219
Care Coordination (Case Management), 1220
Role of the Nurse, Training, and Standards of Care, 1221
Family-Centred Home Care, 1222
Respect for Diversity, 1223
Parent–Professional Collaboration, 1224
The Nursing Process, 1224
Promotion of Optimum Development, Self-Care, and Education, 1227
Safety Issues in the Home, 1228
Family-to-Family Support, 1229

Chapter 44 Reaction to Illness and Hospitalization, 1232
Stressors of Hospitalization and Children's Reactions, 1232
Separation Anxiety, 1232
Loss of Control, 1234
Effects of Hospitalization on the Child, 1236

Stressors and Reactions of the Family of the Hospitalized Child, 1237
Parental Reactions, 1237
Sibling Reactions, 1237
Altered Family Roles, 1237
Nursing Care of the Hospitalized Child, 1238
Preparation for Hospitalization, 1238
Nursing Interventions, 1242
Nursing Care of the Family, 1250
Support Family Members, 1250
Provide Information, 1250
Encourage Parent Participation, 1251
Prepare for Discharge and Home Care, 1252
Care of the Child and Family in Special Hospital Situations, 1253
Ambulatory or Outpatient Setting, 1253
Isolation, 1253
Emergency Admission, 1254
Critical Care Unit, 1256

Chapter 45 Pediatric Variations of Nursing Interventions, 1259
General Concepts Related to Pediatric Procedures, 1259
Informed Consent, 1259
Preparation for Diagnostic and Therapeutic Procedures, 1260
Surgical Procedures, 1265
Adherence to the Medical Treatment Plan, 1269
General Hygiene and Care, 1270
Maintaining Healthy Skin, 1270
Bathing, 1271
Oral Hygiene, 1271
Hair Care, 1272
Feeding the Sick Child, 1272
Controlling Elevated Temperatures, 1272
Family Teaching and Home Care, 1274
Safety, 1274
Strangulation Prevention, 1275
Environmental Factors, 1275
Infection Control, 1277
Transporting Infants and Children, 1278
Restraining Methods and Therapeutic Holding, 1279
Positioning for Procedures, 1281
Collection of Specimens, 1282
Urine Specimens, 1282
Stool Specimens, 1285
Blood Specimens, 1285
Respiratory Secretion Specimens, 1286
Administration of Medication, 1286
Determination of Medication Dosage, 1286
Oral Administration, 1288
Intramuscular Administration, 1289
Subcutaneous and Intradermal Administration, 1293
Intravenous Administration, 1293
Nasogastric, Orogastric, or Gastrostomy Administration, 1295
Rectal Administration, 1296
Optic, Otic, and Nasal Administration, 1296
Family Teaching and Home Care, 1297
Maintaining Fluid Balance, 1298
Measurement of Intake and Output, 1298
Parenteral Fluid Therapy, 1299
Procedures for Maintaining Respiratory Function, 1302
Inhalation Therapy, 1302
Bronchial (Postural) Drainage, 1304
Artificial Ventilation, 1304
Procedures Related to Alternative Feeding Techniques, 1308
Gavage Feeding, 1308
Gastrostomy Feeding, 1309
Nasoduodenal and Nasojejunal Tubes, 1310
Total Parenteral Nutrition, 1312
Family Teaching and Home Care, 1312
Procedures Related to Elimination, 1312
Enema, 1312
Ostomies, 1312
Family Teaching and Home Care, 1313

UNIT 11 HEALTH PROBLEMS OF CHILDREN, 1316

Chapter 46 Respiratory Dysfunction, 1316
Respiratory Infection, 1316
General Aspects of Respiratory Infections, 1316
Upper Respiratory Tract Infections, 1320
Nasopharyngitis, 1320
Acute Streptococcal Pharyngitis, 1321
Tonsillitis, 1322
Influenza, 1324
Otitis Media, 1325
Infectious Mononucleosis, 1328
Croup Syndromes, 1329
Acute Epiglottitis, 1329
Acute Laryngitis, 1330
Acute Laryngotracheobronchitis, 1331
Acute Spasmodic Laryngitis, 1332
Bacterial Tracheitis, 1332
Lower Respiratory Tract Infections, 1332
Bronchitis, 1332
Respiratory Syncytial Virus and Bronchiolitis, 1333
Other Respiratory Tract Infections, 1337
Pertussis (Whooping Cough), 1337
Tuberculosis, 1337
Severe Acute Respiratory Syndrome, 1340
Pulmonary Dysfunction Caused by Noninfectious Irritants, 1341
Foreign Body Aspiration, 1341
Aspiration Pneumonia, 1341
Acute Respiratory Distress Syndrome/Acute Lung Injury, 1342
Smoke Inhalation Injury, 1343
Environmental Tobacco Smoke Exposure, 1344
Long-Term Respiratory Dysfunction, 1344
Asthma, 1344
Cystic Fibrosis, 1356
Obstructive Sleep-Disordered Breathing, 1364
Respiratory Emergency, 1364
Respiratory Failure, 1364
Cardiopulmonary Resuscitation, 1365
Airway Obstruction, 1368

Chapter 47 Gastrointestinal Dysfunction, 1374
Nutritional Disturbances, 1374
Vitamin Imbalances, 1374
Complementary and Alternative Medicine, 1375

Mineral Imbalances, 1375
Vegetarian Diets, 1380
Nursing Care Management, 1380
The Dietary Reference Intakes, 1380
Protein-Energy Malnutrition, 1384
Food Sensitivity, 1384
Gastrointestinal Dysfunction, 1389
Dehydration, 1389
Disorders of Motility, 1392
Diarrhea, 1392
Constipation, 1399
Hirschsprung Disease, 1401
Vomiting, 1403
Gastroesophageal Reflux, 1403
Intestinal Parasitic Diseases, 1405
General Nursing Care Management, 1405
Giardiasis, 1405
Enterobiasis (Pinworms), 1407
Inflammatory Disorders, 1408
Acute Appendicitis, 1408
Meckel's Diverticulum, 1409
Inflammatory Bowel Disease, 1410
Peptic Ulcer Disease, 1414
Hepatic Disorders, 1416
Acute Hepatitis, 1416
Cirrhosis, 1419
Biliary Atresia, 1420
Structural Defects, 1421
Cleft Lip or Cleft Palate, 1421
Esophageal Atresia With Tracheoesophageal Fistula, 1425
Hernias, 1427
Obstructive Disorders, 1427
Hypertrophic Pyloric Stenosis, 1427
Intussusception, 1430
Malrotation and Volvulus, 1431
Anorectal Malformations, 1431
Malabsorption Syndromes, 1433
Celiac Disease, 1433
Short-Bowel Syndrome, 1434
Ingestion of Injurious Agents, 1435
Principles of Emergency Treatment, 1436
Heavy Metal Poisoning, 1440
Lead Poisoning, 1441

Chapter 48 Cardiovascular Dysfunction, 1451
Cardiovascular Dysfunction, 1451
History and Physical Examination, 1451
Diagnostic Evaluation, 1452
Nursing Care Management, 1453
Congenital Heart Disease, 1454
Circulatory Changes at Birth, 1455
Altered Hemodynamics, 1455
Classification of Defects, 1456
Clinical Consequences of Congenital Heart Disease, 1462
Heart Failure, 1462
Hypoxemia, 1474
Nursing Care of the Family and Child With Congenital Heart Disease, 1476
Help the Family Adjust to the Disorder, 1477
Educate the Family About the Disorder, 1477
Help the Family Manage the Illness at Home, 1478
Prepare the Child and Family for Invasive Procedures, 1478
Provide Postoperative Care, 1479
Plan for Discharge and Home Care, 1481
Acquired Cardiovascular Disorders, 1481
Bacterial (Infective) Endocarditis, 1481
Rheumatic Fever, 1483
Hyperlipidemia (Hypercholesterolemia), 1484
Cardiac Dysrhythmias, 1485
Pulmonary Hypertension, 1487
Cardiomyopathy, 1487
Heart Transplantation, 1488
Vascular Dysfunction, 1489
Systemic Hypertension, 1489
Kawasaki Disease (Mucocutaneous Lymph Node Syndrome), 1490
Anaphylaxis, 1494
Septic Shock, 1495

Chapter 49 Hematological or Immunological Dysfunction, 1500
Hematological and Immunological Dysfunction, 1500
Red Blood Cell Disorders, 1500
Anemia, 1500
Iron Deficiency Anemia, 1503
Sickle Cell Anemia, 1505
β-Thalassemia (Cooley Anemia), 1510
Aplastic Anemia, 1511
Defects In Hemostasis, 1512
Hemophilia, 1513
Idiopathic Thrombocytopenic Purpura, 1515
Disseminated Intravascular Coagulation, 1516
Epistaxis (Nosebleeding), 1517
Neoplastic Disorders, 1517
Leukemias, 1517
Lymphomas, 1524
Hodgkin's Disease, 1525
Non-Hodgkin's Lymphoma, 1526
Immunological Deficiency Disorders, 1526
HIV Infection and Acquired Immunodeficiency Syndrome, 1526
Severe Combined Immunodeficiency Disease, 1530
Wiskott-Aldrich Syndrome, 1530
Technological Management of Hematological and Immunological Disorders, 1530
Blood Transfusion Therapy, 1530
Hematopoietic Stem Cell (Bone Marrow) Transplantation, 1532
Apheresis, 1533

Chapter 50 Genitourinary Dysfunction, 1537
Genitourinary Dysfunction, 1537
Clinical Manifestations, 1537
Genitourinary Tract Disorders and Defects, 1541
Urinary Tract Infection, 1541
Obstructive Uropathy, 1545
External Defects, 1545
Glomerular Disease, 1547
Nephrotic Syndrome, 1547
Acute Glomerulonephritis, 1549
Miscellaneous Renal Disorders, 1551
Hemolytic Uremic Syndrome, 1551
Wilms' Tumour, 1552

Renal Failure, 1553
Acute Renal Failure, 1553
Chronic Renal Failure, 1555
Technological Management of Renal Failure, 1559
Dialysis, 1559
Transplantation, 1560

Chapter 51 Cerebral Dysfunction, 1562
Assessment of Cerebral Function, 1562
General Aspects, 1562
Increased Intracranial Pressure, 1563
Altered States of Consciousness, 1563
Neurological Examination, 1564
Special Diagnostic Procedures, 1567
Nursing Care of the Unconscious Child, 1569
Respiratory Management, 1570
Intracranial Pressure Monitoring, 1570
Nutrition and Hydration, 1571
Medications, 1572
Thermoregulation, 1572
Elimination, 1572
Hygienic Care, 1572
Positioning and Exercise, 1572
Stimulation, 1573
Family Support, 1573
Cerebral Trauma, 1573
Head Injury, 1573
Submersion Injuries, 1581
Nervous System Tumours, 1583
Brain Tumours, 1583
Neuroblastoma, 1585
Intracranial Infections, 1586
Bacterial Meningitis, 1586
Nonbacterial (Aseptic) Meningitis, 1589
Encephalitis, 1590
Rabies, 1591
Reye's Syndrome, 1591
Seizure Disorders, 1592
Epilepsy, 1593
Febrile Seizures, 1603
Cerebral Malformations, 1604
Cranial Deformities, 1604
Hydrocephalus, 1604

Chapter 52 Endocrine Dysfunction, 1611
Disorders of Pituitary Function, 1611
Hypopituitarism, 1611
Pituitary Hyperfunction, 1613
Precocious Puberty, 1614
Diabetes Insipidus, 1615
Syndrome of Inappropriate Antidiuretic Hormone, 1616
Disorders of Thyroid Function, 1616
Juvenile Hypothyroidism, 1617
Goitre, 1617
Lymphocytic Thyroiditis, 1617
Hyperthyroidism, 1618
Disorders of Parathyroid Function, 1620
Hypoparathyroidism, 1620
Hyperparathyroidism, 1621
Disorders of Adrenal Function, 1622
Acute Adrenocortical Insufficiency, 1622
Chronic Adrenocortical Insufficiency (Addison's Disease), 1623
Cushing's Syndrome, 1624
Congenital Adrenal Hyperplasia, 1625
Pheochromocytoma, 1626
Disorders of Pancreatic Hormone Secretion, 1627
Diabetes Mellitus Type 1, 1627
Diabetes Mellitus Type 2, 1639

Chapter 53 Integumentary Dysfunction, 1642
Integumentary Dysfunction, 1642
Skin Lesions, 1642
Wounds, 1643
General Therapeutic Management, 1646
Home Care and Family Support, 1651
Infections of the Skin, 1651
Bacterial Infections, 1651
Viral Infections, 1651
Dermatophytoses (Fungal Infections), 1653
Systemic Mycotic (Fungal) Infections, 1655
Skin Disorders Related to Chemical or Physical Contacts, 1655
Contact Dermatitis, 1655
Poison Ivy, Oak, and Sumac, 1655
Medication Reactions, 1657
Skin Disorders Related To Animal Contacts, 1657
Scabies, 1658
Pediculosis Capitis, 1659
Bed Bugs, 1661
Rickettsial Diseases, 1661
Lyme Disease, 1661
Pet and Wild Animal Bites, 1663
Human Bites, 1664
Cat-Scratch Disease, 1664
Skin Disorders Associated With Specific Age Groups, 1664
Diaper Dermatitis, 1664
Atopic Dermatitis (Eczema), 1665
Seborrheic Dermatitis, 1667
Acne, 1668
Thermal Injury, 1669
Burns, 1669
Sunburn, 1681
Cold Injury, 1682

Chapter 54 Musculoskeletal or Articular Dysfunction, 1684
The Immobilized Child, 1684
Physiological Effects of Immobilization, 1684
Psychological Effects of Immobilization, 1686
Effect on Families, 1687
Traumatic Injury, 1688
Soft-Tissue Injury, 1688
Fractures, 1690
The Child in a Cast, 1692
The Cast, 1693
The Child in Traction, 1695
Distraction, 1697
Amputation, 1698
Congenital Defects, 1699
Developmental Dysplasia of the Hip, 1699
Congenital Clubfoot, 1701
Metatarsus Adductus (Varus), 1703
Skeletal Limb Deficiency, 1703
Osteogenesis Imperfecta, 1704

Acquired Defects, 1705
Legg-Calvé-Perthes Disease, 1705
Slipped Capital Femoral Epiphysis, 1706
Kyphosis and Lordosis, 1707
Idiopathic Scoliosis, 1708
Infections of Bones and Joints, 1710
Osteomyelitis, 1710
Septic Arthritis, 1712
Skeletal Tuberculosis, 1712
Bone and Soft-Tissue Tumour, 1712
General Concepts: Bone Tumour, 1712
Osteosarcoma, 1713
Ewing's Sarcoma (Primitive Neuroectodermal Tumour), 1714
Rhabdomyosarcoma, 1715
Disorders of Joints, 1716
Juvenile Idiopathic Arthritis (Juvenile Rheumatoid Arthritis), 1716
Systemic Lupus Erythematosus, 1719

Chapter 55 Neuromuscular or Muscular Dysfunction, 1724
Congenital Neuromuscular or Muscular Disorders, 1724
Cerebral Palsy, 1724
Spina Bifida (Myelomeningocele), 1732
Spinal Muscular Atrophy, 1738
Infantile Spinal Muscular Atrophy (Werdnig-Hoffmann Disease), 1738
Juvenile Spinal Muscular Atrophy (Kugelberg-Welander Disease), 1740
Muscular Dystrophies, 1740
Duchenne (Pseudohypertrophic) Muscular Dystrophy, 1740
Acquired Neuromuscular Disorders, 1743
Guillain-Barré Syndrome (Infectious Polyneuritis), 1743
Tetanus, 1745
Botulism, 1746
Spinal Cord Injuries, 1748

APPENDIXES, 1753
A Relationship of Drugs to Breast Milk and Effect on Infant, 1753
B Developmental and Sensory Assessment, 1757
C Growth Measurements, 1759
D Common Laboratory Tests, 1764
E Pediatric Vital Signs and Parameters, 1773

About the Authors

Shannon E. Perry is Professor Emerita, School of Nursing, San Francisco State University. She received her diploma in nursing from St. Joseph Hospital School of Nursing, Bloomington, Illinois; a Baccalaureate in Nursing from Marquette University; an MSN from the University of Colorado Medical Center; and a PhD in Educational Psychology from Arizona State University. She completed a 2-year postdoctoral fellowship in perinatal nursing at the University of California, San Francisco, as a Robert Wood Johnson Clinical Nurse Scholar. Dr. Perry has had clinical experience as a staff nurse, head nurse, and supervisor in surgical nursing, obstetrics, pediatrics, gynecology, and neonatal nursing. She has served as expert witness and legal consultant. She has taught in schools of nursing in several states and was Interim Director and Director of the School of Nursing and Director of the Child and Adolescent Development Baccalaureate Program at SFSU. She was Marquette University College of Nursing Alumna of the Year in 1999 and the University of Colorado School of Nursing Distinguished Alumna of the Year in 2000, and she received the San Francisco State University Alumni Association Emeritus Faculty Award in 2005.

She is a Fellow in the American Academy of Nursing, a nursing consultant to the International Education Research Foundation, and co-chair of INESA, the International Nursing Education Services and Accreditation.

Dr. Perry's experience in international nursing includes teaching international nursing courses in the United Kingdom, Ireland, Italy, Thailand, Ghana, and China and participating in health missions in Ghana, Kenya, and Honduras. For her "exemplary contributions to nursing, public service, and selfless commitment and passion in shaping the future of international health," she received the President's Award from the Global Caring Nurses Foundation, Inc., in 2008.

Marilyn J. Hockenberry is Professor of Pediatrics in the Hematology/Oncology Division at Baylor College of Medicine. She is the Director of the Center for Research and Evidence-Based Practice for Texas Children's Hospital in Houston, Texas, and the Director of the Pediatric Nurse Practitioner Program in the Texas Children's Cancer Center. Her research focuses on symptom management and treatment-related side effects experienced by children who have cancer. Dr. Hockenberry's current studies are evaluating treatment-related fatigue, sleep-related disturbances, and neurocognitive deficits of leukemia treatment. She has authored over 50 articles and has served as the senior editor on the Wong nursing textbooks for the past 10 years.

Dr. Hockenberry completed her prenursing education at Mt. Vernon Nazarene College and received her Bachelors of Science from Capital University. She received her Masters of Science from Texas Woman's University and her doctorate of philosophy with distinction from the Medical College of Georgia. She is a Fellow of the American Academy of Nursing.

Deitra Leonard Lowdermilk is Clinical Professor Emerita, School of Nursing, University of North Carolina at Chapel Hill. She received her BSN from East Carolina University and her MEd and PhD in Education from UNC CH. She is certified in In-Patient Obstetrics by the National Certification Corporation. She is a Fellow in the American Academy of Nursing. In addition to being a nurse educator for over 34 years, Dr. Lowdermilk has clinical experience as a public health nurse and as a staff nurse in labor and delivery, postpartum, and newborn units, and she has worked in gynecological surgery and cancer care units.

Dr. Lowdermilk has been recognized for her expertise in nursing education. She has repeatedly been selected as Classroom and Clinical Teacher of the Year by graduating seniors. She was a recipient of the Educator of the Year Award from both the District IV Association of Women's Health, Obstetric and Neonatal Nurses (AWHONN) and the North Carolina Nurses Association. She also received the 2005 AWHONN Excellence in Education Award.

She is active in AWHONN, having served as Chair of the North Carolina Section of AWHONN, and has served as chair and member of various committees in AWHONN at the national, district, state, and local levels. She has served as guest editor for the *Journal of Obstetric, Gynecologic, and Neonatal Nursing* and served on editorial boards for other publications.

Dr. Lowdermilk's most significant contribution to nursing has been to promote excellence in nursing practice and education in women's health through integration of knowledge into practice. In 2005 she received the first Distinguished Alumni Award from East Carolina University School of Nursing for her exemplary contributions to the nursing profession in the area of maternal-child care and the community.

David Wilson is a graduate of Dallas Baptist College (now University) (BSN) and Texas Woman's University (MSN). He has more than 20 years of neonatal intensive care experience in Texas and Oklahoma. During his nursing career, David has worked in a number of positions including staff nurse, neonatal educator, outreach educator, nutrition support coordinator, and BLS and Neonatal Resuscitation Program instructor. David was involved in medical missions in Costa Rica and Colombia for 2 years. David has also been nursing faculty at several universities, either on a full-time or adjunct basis for 15 years. Writing for nursing publications is an endeavor he has enjoyed for many years. He has authored several articles pertaining to neonatal and pediatric nursing, has served as a reviewer for two nursing journals, and has been an author and contributor with Mosby/Elsevier since 1993. David is currently a staff nurse in the Children's Hospital Pediatric Emergency Center at Saint Francis Hospital in Tulsa, Oklahoma, and serves as nursing faculty for Langston University, Tulsa, Oklahoma.

We remember **Donna Lee Wong**, PhD, RN, PNP, CPN, FAAN, who passed away on May 4, 2008, following complications of leukemia. Donna was the original co-author of this book. She co-developed the Wong-Baker FACES Pain Rating Scale, which is used worldwide to assess pain in children and adults and has been used in extensive research on pain.

For those of us who had the honor of knowing this remarkable individual, she is most remembered for her outstanding generosity and concern for others. Donna taught us that nursing is about providing the best care possible and that our patients will be the better for it. She led by example, always looking for ways to improve care for pediatric patients. Donna Wong was an example for all of us who strive for excellence in our nursing profession. We hold her dear to our hearts and will continue to work to carry on her outstanding legacy. She will never be forgotten.

Lisa J. Keenan-Lindsay graduated from the University of Toronto for both her undergraduate and graduate degree. She worked in the area of pediatrics for the first several years of her career, mainly working in a pediatric intensive care unit at the Hospital for Sick Children. She has worked in the maternal-newborn area for over 20 years, holding a variety of positions, including staff nurse in labour and birth, and educator for a maternal-newborn department. Currently Lisa is a professor of nursing at Seneca College in the York University Collaborative BScN program. She has been involved in all aspects of nursing education including curriculum development and incorporation of simulation into the curriculum.

Lisa was an active member of AWHONN Canada for many years as a member of the section executive. She is now a board member for the newly formed Canadian Association of Perinatal, Women's Health Nurses (CAPWHN). She has previously been involved with the Society of Obstetricians and Gynaecologists of Canada (SOGC) as an RN member for the Maternal-Fetal Medicine Committee for many years and co-authored many SOGC Clinical Practice Guidelines. Lisa has also been a Lamaze certified childbirth educator for many years and continues to practice in this role in her community. Lisa is passionate about normalizing birth and works tirelessly at spreading the word in this endeavour.

Cheryl A. Sams is a graduate of Ryerson University (BScN) and D'Youville College (MSN). She has worked at the Hospital for Sick Children in Toronto since she graduated from nursing school. At Sick Kids, she has held many positions, including staff nurse, clinical educator, manager, director, and clinical nurse specialist. Cheryl has held many teaching positions at Ryerson University in the Post RN Program and the Nurse Practitioner Program. She has also taught at the University of Toronto in the BScN program. Currently Cheryl teaches at Seneca College in the York University Collaborative BScN program.

As an author, Cheryl enjoys contributing to the nursing body of literature. She has contributed chapters to the Canadian publication of Lewis et al.'s *Medical-Surgical Nursing* and Potter and Perry's *Fundamentals of Nursing*. She was one of the editors for *Mosby's Comprehensive Review for the Canadian RN Exam*.

Canadian Contributors

Janet D.C. Andrews, BScN, RN, MN
Nursing Specialist-Education
Obstetrics, Gynecology and Ophthamology
Saint Michael's Hospital
Toronto, Ontario
Chapters 22, 23

Debbie Aylward, RN, BScN, MScN
Perinatal Coordinator
Champlain Maternal Newborn Regional Program [CMNRP]
Ottawa, Ontario
Chapters 27, 28

Melanie Basso, RN, MSN, PNC(C)
Senior Practice Leader-Perinatal
B.C. Women's Hospital and Health Centre
Vancouver, British Columbia
Chapters 13, 14

Katherine A. Bertoni, BScN, MN, NP-PHC, CDE
Adult Diabetes Care and Research Program
McMaster University Medical Centre
Hamilton, Ontario
Chapters 43, 49

Bettina Braj, RN, BScN, MEd
Professor, School of Health Science
Seneca College
King City, Ontario
Chapter 50

Karen M. Breen-Reid, RN, MN
Advanced Nursing Practice Educator
The Hospital for Sick Children;
Adjunct Lecturer, Lawrence S. Bloomberg Faculty of Nursing
University of Toronto
Toronto, Ontario;
Part-time Lecturer, School of Nursing, University of Ghana
Legon, Accra, Ghana
Chapters 36, 41

Judy Lee Buchan, RN, BScN
Supervisor, Family Health
Reproductive Health Program
Health Services
Brampton, Ontario
Chapter 3

Nancy Caprara, RN, BScN, MN
Professor, School of Health Science
Seneca College
Toronto, Ontario
Chapter 31

Cheryl Dika, RN, MN, NP
Instructor/Nurse Practitioner
University of Manitoba
Winnipeg, Manitoba
Chapter 30

Sharon Dore, RN, MEd, MScN, PhD
Advance Practice Nurse, Clinical Nurse Specialist Obstetrics and Gynecology
Hamilton Health Sciences
Associate Clinical Professor, Department of Obstetrics and Gynecology and School of Nursing
McMaster University
Hamilton, Ontario
Chapter 17

Kerry Lynn Durnford, RN, MN
Instructor, Health and Human Services Program
Aurora College
Yellowknife, Northwest Territories
Chapter 4

Helen Edwards, RN, BA, MN
Director, Clinical Informatics and Technology Assisted Programs
Hospital for Sick Children
Toronto, Ontario
Chapter 32

Leanne Garratt, RN, BScN, MScN
Professor, School of Health Sciences
Seneca College
King City, Ontario
Chapter 35

Anne Hogarth, RN, BScN(C)
Professor, School of Health Sciences
Seneca College
Toronto, Ontario
Chapters 47, 48

Karen MacKinnon, RN, MScN, PhD
Assistant Professor, School of Nursing
University of Victoria
Victoria, British Columbia
Chapters 1, 2

Joan MacNeil, RN, BScN, MHSc, PhD
Assistant Professor, School of Nursing
University of Victoria
Victoria, British Columbia
Chapter 2

Rosella V. McCarthy, RN MSN CCCNP(C)
Clinical Nurse Specialist, Critical Care Program
B.C.'s Children's Hospital
Vancouver, British Columbia
Chapters 39, 40

Gladys McPherson, RN, PhD
Assistant Professor, School of Nursing
University of British Columbia
Vancouver, British Columbia
Chapters 39, 40

Annette Pejic, RN, BScN, MScN
Professor, School of Health Sciences
Seneca College
Toronto, Ontario
Chapters 42, 44, 51

Shelly Petruskavich, RN, MN, PNC(C)
Clinical Educator, Birthing Suites & Mother Baby Unit
Mississauga, Ontario
Chapters 18, 19

Nancy Watts, RN, MN, PNC(C)
Clinical Nurse Specialist
Perinatal and Women's Health,
London Health Sciences Centre
London, Ontario
Chapters 10, 15

Maureen White, RN, MN, IBCLC, PNC(C)
Assistant Professor, School of Nursing
Dalhousie University
Halifax, Nova Scotia
Chapter 26

Jo'Anne Yearley, RN, BSN, MN, PNC(C)
University College Professor
Vancouver Island University
Nanaimo, British Columbia
Chapters 20, 21

Contributors to the U.S. 4th Edition

CONTRIBUTING EDITOR

Patrick F. Barrera, BS
Assistant Director, Evidence-Based Clinical Decision Support
Center for Research and Evidence-Based Practice
Texas Children's Hospital
Houston, Texas

CONTRIBUTORS

Suzanne McMurtry Baird, MSN, RN
Assistant Professor, School of Nursing
Vanderbilt University
Nashville, Tennessee

Pat Mahaffee Gingrich, RN-C, MSN, WHNP
Clinical Assistant Professor, School of Nursing
University of North Carolina at Chapel Hill
Chapel Hill, North Carolina

Edward L. Lowdermilk, BS, RPh
Clinical Pharmacist
Piedmont Health Services
Siler City, North Carolina

Reviewers

Andrea Bridge, RN, BN, MScPH
Assistant Professor, School of Nursing
Mount Royal University
Calgary, Alberta

Sai Choon Choo, RN, BSN, MEd
Faculty of Health Sciences
Douglas College
New Westminster, British Columbia

Shelley L. Cobbett, RN, BN, GnT, MN, EdD
Adjunct Assistant Professor, School of Nursing
Dalhousie University
Halifax, Nova Scotia

Marianne Cochrane, RN, MN
Professor; Co-Director, Bachelor of Science in Nursing
Faculty of Health Sciences
University of Ontario Institute of Technology (UOIT)
Oshawa, Ontario

Manjit Dhanoa-Yasi, RN, BScN, MN
Lecturer, Lawrence Bloomberg Faculty of Nursing
University of Toronto
Toronto, Ontario

Debbie Fraser, MN, RNC-NIC
Associate Professor, Advanced Nurse Practitioner Program
Centre for Nursing and Health Studies
Athabasca University
Athabasca, Alberta

Neghesti G. Gebru, RN, MN
Assistant Professor, School of Nursing
Laurentian University
Sudbury, Ontario

Denise Hawthorne, RN, BSN, MA
Faculty of Health Sciences
Douglas College
New Westminster, British Columbia

Karen Hewson, BSN, MN
Assistant Professor, College of Nursing
University of Saskatchewan
Saskatoon, Saskatchewan

Marilyn Jacobs, RN, MN
Lecturer, School of Nursing
Memorial University
St. John's, Newfoundland

Stephanie Langford, RN, BScN, MEd
Teaching Associate and Clinical Coordinator
School of Nursing
University of Ottawa
Ottawa, Ontario

Mary Anne Moloney, BScN, MN
Professor, Faculty of Health & Human Sciences
Vancouver Island University
Nanaimo, British Columbia

Dave Patterson, RN, BN
Sessional Instructor, Faculty of Nursing
University of Calgary
Calgary, Alberta

Norma Ponzoni, MScN, MEd
Lecturer, School of Nursing
McGill University
Montreal, Quebec

Carla Shapiro, RN, MN
Instructor, Faculty of Nursing
University of Manitoba
Winnipeg, Manitoba

Preface

This first edition of *Maternal Child Nursing Care in Canada* combines essential maternity and pediatric nursing information into one text. The text focuses on the care of women during their reproductive years and the care of children from birth through adolescence. The promotion of wellness and the care for women experiencing common health concerns throughout the lifespan and care of the childbearing woman is addressed, as well as the health care of children and child development in the context of the family. The text provides a family-centred care approach that recognizes the importance of collaboration with families when providing care. This first edition of *Maternal Child Nursing Care in Canada* is designed to address the changing needs of Canadian women during their childbearing years and those of children during their developing years.

Maternal Child Nursing Care in Canada was developed to provide students with the knowledge and skills they need to become competent critical thinkers and to attain the sensitivity needed to become caring nurses. This first edition reflects the Canadian health care system, the importance of family-centred care, and the cultural diversity throughout the country. It includes the most accurate, current, and clinically relevant information available.

Approach

Professional nursing practice continues to evolve and adapt to society's changing health priorities. The rapidly changing health care delivery system offers new opportunities for nurses to alter the practice of maternity and pediatric nursing and to improve the way in which care is given. Increasingly, nursing care must be artfully constructed using research to inform the care provided. It is incumbent on nurses to use the most up-to-date and scientifically supported information on which to base their care. To assist nurses in providing this type of care, Evidence-Informed Practice boxes with implications for practice are included throughout the text.

Consumers of maternity and pediatric care vary in age, ethnicity, culture, language, social status, marital status, and sexual orientation. They seek care from a variety of health care providers in numerous health care settings, including the home. To meet the needs of these consumers, clinical education must offer students a variety of health care experiences in settings that include hospitals and birth centres, homes, clinics, private physicians' offices, shelters for the homeless or for women and children who require protection, and other community-based settings.

Nursing Care Management has been used as an organizing framework for discussion of nursing care in the chapters. This approach demonstrates how nursing must collaborate with other health care disciplines to provide the most comprehensive care possible to women and children. Nursing Process boxes include assessments, nursing diagnoses, expected outcomes, nursing care implementation, and evaluation of nursing care; these boxes are incorporated throughout the chapters. Nursing Care Plans reinforce the problem-solving approach to patient care. Throughout the discussion of assessment and care, warning signs and emergency situations are also highlighted to alert the nurse to signs of potential problems.

Patient education is an essential component of nursing care of women and children. The chapters on women's health promotion and screening emphasize teaching for self-care to promote wellness and to encourage preventive care. The chapter on transition to parenthood focuses on teaching to new families and infants at home. Special boxes highlight community care throughout the text. Family-Centred Teaching boxes incorporate family considerations important to care of women and children. Issues concerning grandparents, siblings, and different family constellations are also addressed. In the pediatric chapters, these boxes focus on the special learning needs of families caring for their child. Legal Tips are integrated throughout the maternity section to emphasize these issues as they relate to the care of women and infants.

This first edition features a contemporary design with logical, easy-to-follow headings and an attractive four-colour design that highlights important content and increases visual appeal. Hundreds of colour photographs and drawings throughout the text, many of them new, illustrate important concepts and techniques to further enhance comprehension. To help students learn essential information quickly and efficiently, we have included numerous features that prioritize, condense, simplify, and emphasize important aspects of nursing care. In addition, students are encouraged to apply critical thinking in real-life scenarios presented in the Critical Thinking Exercises.

Special Features

- **Electronic Resources** providing additional information related to chapter content are placed at the beginning of each chapter and highlighted throughout the text.
- **Learning Objectives** focus students' attention on the important content to be mastered.
- **Critical Thinking Exercises** present students with real-life situations and encourage them to make appropriate clinical judgments. Answer guidelines are provided on the book's Evolve site.
- **Evidence-Informed Practice** boxes are incorporated throughout the book. Findings that confirm effective practices or that identify practices with unknown, ineffective, or harmful effects are identified by an icon in the margin ().
- **Nursing Process** boxes help students to easily identify information on some major diseases and conditions.
- **Home Care** boxes emphasize patient and family self-care and provide information to help students transfer learning from the hospital to the home setting.

- **Cultural Awareness** boxes describe beliefs and practices about pregnancy, childbirth, parenting, and women's health concerns.
- **Family-Centred Teaching** boxes highlight the needs of families that should be addressed when family-centered care is provided.
- **Community Focus** boxes emphasize community issues, provide resources and guidance, and illustrate nursing care in a variety of settings.
- **Nursing Care Plans** are provided for all commonly encountered situations and disorders. Nursing diagnoses are included, as are rationales for nursing interventions that might not be immediately evident to students.
- **Patient Teaching** boxes assist students to help patients and families become involved in their own care with optimal outcomes.
- **Alternative and Complementary Therapies** are discussed for many pregnancy-related issues and are identified in the text by an icon in the margin ().
- **Atraumatic Care** boxes emphasize the importance of providing competent care while minimizing undue physical and psychological distress for the child and family.
- **Emergency** boxes alert students to the signs and symptoms of various emergency situations and provide interventions for immediate implementation.
- **Nursing Alerts** call the reader's attention to critical information that could lead to deteriorating or emergency situations.
- **Guidelines** boxes provide students with examples of various approaches to implementing care.
- **Medication Guide** boxes include key information about medications used in maternity and newborn care, including their indications, adverse effects, and nursing considerations.
- **Legal Tips** are integrated throughout Part 1 to provide students with relevant information to deal with important legal areas in the context of maternity nursing.
- **Key Points**, located at the end of each chapter, help the reader summarize major points, make connections, and synthesize information. The Key Points are also available in a downloadable audio format and can be found on this book's Evolve site.
- **Resources**, including Web sites and contact information for organizations and educational resources available for the topics discussed, are listed throughout.
- A highly detailed, cross-referenced **index** allows readers to quickly access needed information.

Teaching and Learning Package

Several ancillaries to this text have been developed for instructors and students to use in classroom and clinical settings.

Evolve. Evolve is an innovative Web site that provides a wealth of content, resources, and state-of-the-art information on maternity and pediatric nursing. Evolve's wide array of information includes course resources for instructors (Instructor's Manual, Test Bank, Image Collection, PowerPoint slides) and learning resources for students (Case Studies, Examination-style Review Questions, Nursing Skills, Assessment Videos, Animations, Nursing Care Plans, and more).

Instructor's Electronic Resource. The innovative electronic resources for the instructor (available online) contain the following components:

- *Instructor's Manual* contains learning objectives, chapter outlines and accompanying teaching strategies, learning activities, and curriculum guides for courses of varying lengths.
- *Electronic Test Bank* in ExamView format contains more than 1500 examination-style test items. An answer key with page references to the text and with rationales is included.
- *Electronic Image Collection*, containing more than 500 full-colour illustrations and photographs from the text, helps instructors develop presentations and explain key concepts.
- *PowerPoint Slides*, with lecture outlines for each chapter of the text, assist in presenting materials in the classroom.

Virtual Clinical Excursions: CD and Workbook Companion. A CD-ROM and workbook have been developed as a virtual clinical experience to expand student opportunities for critical thinking. This package guides the student through a computer-generated virtual clinical environment and helps the user apply textbook content to virtual patients in that environment. Case studies are presented that allow students to use this textbook as a reference to assess, diagnose, plan, implement, and evaluate "real" patients using clinical scenarios. The state-of-the-art technologies reflected on this CD-ROM demonstrate cutting-edge learning opportunities for students and facilitate knowledge retention of the information found in the textbook. The clinical simulations and workbook represent the next generation of research-based learning tools that promote critical thinking and meaningful learning

Acknowledgments

I would like to offer thanks to the many perinatal contributors from across the country who worked diligently to provide this text with a uniquely Canadian perspective. I would also like to extend a very special thank you to my husband, John Lindsay, and children Katie, Emily, and Jack Lindsay who encourage me to achieve my goals and without whose support this book would not have been completed.

Lisa Keenan-Lindsay

I would like to thank the many pediatric experts who have not only contributed to the "peds" part of this text but also made major contributions to the field of pediatric nursing in Canada. You make a difference every day to children and their families. I would also like to thank my husband, Stuart Sams, and my family for cheering me on.

Cheryl Sams

A special thank you goes to Jennifer Hermes, Jerrolyn Hurlbutt, Ann Millar, Brandilyn Tidwell, Martina van de Velde, and the rest of the group at Elsevier for all of their exceptional support and encouragement throughout the development of this book.

Lisa and Cheryl

Part 1

Perinatal Nursing

Unit 1 Introduction to Perinatal Nursing

Unit 2 Women's Health

Unit 3 Pregnancy

Unit 4 Childbirth

Unit 5 Postpartum Period

Unit 6 Newborn

Unit 1

1 Contemporary Perinatal Nursing in Canada

Learning Objectives

On completion of this chapter, the reader will be able to:

- Describe the scope of perinatal nursing in Canada today.
- Describe the history and context for maternity or perinatal care in Canada.
- Explore philosophical approaches and discuss guiding principles for working with childbearing women and their families.
- Examine current trends in perinatal health and compare epidemiological data among groups and populations.
- Explore women's experiences with childbearing and consider their feedback about perinatal health services.
- Consider how the social determinants of health influence the health of women and newborns, and explore approaches needed to address health inequities.
- Explore current issues affecting perinatal nursing practice and envision creative alternatives.

Electronic Resources

Additional information related to the content in Chapter 1 can be found on

evolve the companion Web site at

http://evolve.elsevier.com/Canada/Perry/maternal/

- Examination Review Questions

The focus of the first part of this book is maternity or perinatal nursing. Part 1 also has a section on women's health during the reproductive years. Chapter 1 presents a general overview of issues and trends related to the health and health care of women, newborns, and families during the childbearing year.

The second part of the book, which begins with Chapter 29, addresses the issues and trends related to the health care of children.

Perinatal Nursing

Perinatal nursing is a recognized specialty in Canada. Perinatal nurses work collaboratively with childbearing women and their families throughout the childbearing year, from preconception through pregnancy and childbirth, and over the postpartum transition period. Perinatal nurses promote the physical, emotional, social, and spiritual well-being of the whole family and work to address health inequities that influence health outcomes (Box 1-1).

Perinatal nurses care for childbearing women and families in many settings, including the hospital, the home, and a variety of ambulatory and community settings. Perinatal nurses also work collaboratively with other health and social care providers, such as physicians, midwives, nutritionists, doulas, and social workers, to name a few. Perinatal nursing intersects with neonatal nursing, where nurses with additional education provide intensive care for high-risk neonates, and with women's health nurses (including nurse practitioners) who may be involved in providing preconception, prenatal, and postpartum care.

Additional information about perinatal nursing, including professional standards and certification, can be obtained from the Canadian Association of Perinatal and Women's Health Nurses (CAPWHN, formerly known as the Association of Women's Health, Obstetric and Neonatal Nurses [AWHONN] Canada).

Nurses caring for women have helped make the health care system more responsive to women's needs. Nurses have developed strategies to improve the well-being of women and their newborns and have led efforts to develop and implement clinical practice guidelines that draw on current evidence or research. Through professional associations, nurses can have a voice in setting standards and influencing health policy by

BOX 1-1 Values and Guiding Principles for Perinatal Nursing in Canada

1. Caring: Perinatal nurses foster caring relationships with women and families, provide a physical and emotional presence and continuity of care, promote family health and development, and assist women and their families when they face childbearing challenges.
2. Health and Well-being: Perinatal nurses promote health and well-being by assisting women and their families to develop the knowledge and skills they need to achieve their optimal level of well-being in situations of developmental transitions, illness, or injury or in the process of dying.
3. Informed Decision Making: Perinatal nurses have a holistic view of women and families and respect their capacity to set goals and make decisions. Women and families have the right to make informed choices that are congruent with their own beliefs and values.
4. Dignity: Perinatal nurses are privileged to share the intimacy of the childbearing experience with women and their families. Knowing that women will have lasting memories of this important developmental process, they strive to positively influence the childbearing experience.
5. Confidentiality: Perinatal nurses recognize the importance of privacy, confidentiality, and maintaining the trust of women and their families.
6. Justice: Perinatal nurses uphold principles of justice by safeguarding human rights, equity, and fairness as they work with childbearing women, families, and newborns.
7. Accountability: Perinatal nurses act with integrity and in a manner consistent with their professional responsibilities and standards of practice.
8. Quality Practice Environments: Perinatal nurses advocate for safe, supportive, and respectful work environments.

(Adapted from AWHONN [2009]. *Standards for professional perinatal nursing practice and certification in Canada.* [2nd ed.]. Washington, DC: Author. Retrieved from http://www.capwhn.ca.)

actively participating in the education of the public and that of local, provincial, and federal legislators (e.g., http://www.capwhn.ca; http://www.cna-nurses.ca; http://www.awhonn.org). Some nurses hold elected office and influence health policy directly.

The History and Context of Health Care in Canada

Since the Lalonde Report was released in 1974, Canada has been a global leader in health promotion. In 1986, Canada hosted the first international conference on health promotion, which resulted in the Ottawa Charter. Three challenges for Canadians were identified: reducing health inequities, increasing prevention, and enhancing people's capacities to live with chronic disease and disability. The Charter also acknowledged the need for intersectoral collaboration, or looking beyond health, to include other sectors (e.g., income security, employment, education, housing, and transportation) (Public Health Agency of Canada [PHAC], 1986). In the late 1990s, interest expanded to creating evidence-informed programs that address all the determinants of health.

With the HIV/AIDS epidemic, increasing rates of tuberculosis and other infectious diseases, the threat of bioterrorism, and the severe acute respiratory syndrome (SARS) epidemic, Canadians were reminded of the importance of immunizations and public health measures. In 2004, the federal government created the Public Health Agency of Canada (PHAC). While the PHAC initially focused on population health and health promotion, the emergence of avian influenza shifted the focus toward planning for a pandemic.

Health services in Canada are organized provincially, and Medicare, Canada's government-funded health insurance program, provides universal medical and hospital services for all Canadians. The principles of the Canada Health Act include public administration, comprehensive "medically necessary" care, universality, portability, and accessibility. Home care, extended care, pharmaceuticals, and dental care are not currently covered under Medicare provisions. Thus, to some extent, the Medicare program shapes the health services offered to Canadians. In an effort to control health care costs, interest has grown in restructuring health services and developing community-based programs and preventive health services.

Maternity Services in Canada

Maternal and newborn services have evolved from our colonial and Aboriginal roots to the current system of regionalized perinatal and neonatal care (Box 1-2). Canada and the United States are unique internationally in that they have a very low percentage of well-woman care provided by midwives. Most perinatal care in Canada is provided by physicians, with obstetricians providing increasing percentages of perinatal care. Most births in Canada take place in hospitals, some with birth centres; home births account for a very small proportion of births (PHAC, 2009).

The delivery of maternity care within each community, province, and territory contains unique elements as each level of government tries to balance human resources, funding, and liability concerns with regulatory, educational, political, and demographic issues. Inequities in access to good-quality maternity care have developed particularly in rural, remote, inner-city, and First Nations, Métis, and Inuit communities, compared with access to such care in other Canadian communities. Many health inequities also result from conditions of vulnerability, known as the social determinants of health (Box 1-3), with poverty having the most significant influence on maternal child health (Pauly, MacKinnon, & Varcoe, 2009).

Both the Canadian Perinatal Health Report (Canadian Perinatal Surveillance System [CPSS], 2008) and the Maternity Experiences Survey (PHAC, 2009) note that poor women (women living below the low income cut-off), Aboriginal women, and young women with less education consistently have the poorest perinatal outcomes. Limited maternal education, young maternal age, poverty, and the lack of prenatal care appear to be associated with higher **infant mortality rates**. Poor nutrition, smoking and alcohol use, and overall poor

BOX 1-2 Historic Milestones in the Care of Mothers and Infants

1847—Ether used in Scotland for an internal podalic version (first reported use of obstetric anesthesia)
1848—Soeurs de Misericorde (Montreal) provide maternity care for unwed mothers
1861—Ignaz Semmelwies writes *The Cause, Concept, and Prophylaxis of Childbed Fever*
1892—A law is passed making it illegal to sell or advertise contraceptives in Canada
1897—Victoria Order of Nurses (VON) established to improve maternal and infant health and to train nurses.
1908—Childbirth classes started and prenatal care provided by outpost and public health nurses working in cities, small towns, and rural communities
1911—First milk bank in the United States established in Boston; by the 1970s there were 20 human milk banks across Canada that received donated breast milk
1912—Medical Council of Canada formed and makes midwifery illegal in most locations
1916—Margaret Sanger establishes the first American birth control clinic in Brooklyn, NY
1920—Midwifery legalized in the colony of Newfoundland
1923—First U.S. hospital centre for premature infant care established in Chicago
1933—Sodium pentothal used as anesthesia for childbirth; *Natural Childbirth* published by Grantly Dick-Read
1934—Dionne quintuplets born in Ontario and survive partly due to donated breast milk
1935—Sulphonamides introduced as cure for puerperal fever; Parents Information Bureau opened in Ontario to provide contraceptive information
1940—*Canadian Mother and Child* book first published and distributed free to Canadian mothers
1941—Penicillin used as treatment for infection
1944—Society of Obstetricians and Gynaecologists of Canada (SOGC) formed
1953—Apgar scoring system of neonatal assessment published by Virginia Apgar
1956—Oxygen determined to cause retrolental fibroplasia (now known as retinopathy of prematurity)
1957—Hospital Insurance and Diagnostic Services Act passed in Canada
1958—First fetal electrocardiogram from the maternal abdomen reported (first commercial electronic fetal monitor produced in the late 1960s); first clinical use of ultrasound to examine the fetus reported
1959—Agnes Higgins joins the Montreal Diet Dispensary and later develops an approach for improving nutrition for disadvantaged pregnant women (Higgins method); cytological studies demonstrate that Down syndrome is associated with a particular form of nondisjunction (trisomy 21)
1960—American Society for Psychoprophylaxis in Obstetrics (ASPO/Lamaze) and the International Childbirth Education Association (ICEA) formed; birth control pill introduced for "menstrual regulation" since contraceptives could not be legally prescribed in Canada; condoms available behind the counter in most pharmacies
1962—Thalidomide found to cause birth defects
1967—Rho(D) immune globulin produced for treatment of Rh incompatibility; Reva Rubin publishes article on maternal role attainment
1968—The *Medical Care Act* passed and provinces begin to implement health insurance plans; rubella vaccine available
1969—Nurses Association of the American College of Obstetricians and Gynecologists (NAACOG) founded in the United States; some Canadian nurses joined this organization; contraception decriminalized in Canada
1974—LaLonde Report recommends more attention to health promotion and disease prevention
1975—The *Pregnant Patient's Bill of Rights* published by ICEA
1976—First home pregnancy kits approved
1978—First test-tube baby born in Britain; outpost nursing program at Memorial University, Newfoundland includes a 10-month nurse-midwifery program
1980—Canadian Obstetrical Gynaecological and Neonatal Nurses (COGNN) formed as a special interest group within NAACOG
1986—Ottawa Charter for Health Promotion recommends more attention to health determinants; midwifery education program in Povungnituk, Quebec begins preparing Inuit midwives
1987—Safe Motherhood Initiative launched by the World Health Organization and other international agencies
1988—Abortion decriminalized in Canada; SOGC launches International Women's Health Program
1991—Canadian Paediatric Society recommends that a minimum of one person skilled in Neonatal Resuscitation be present at every delivery
1993—Midwifery Education program launched in Ontario; human embryos cloned in the United States; first Canadian statement on reducing the risk of SIDS released by Health Canada
1994—Midwifery legalized in Ontario; zidovudine guidelines published to reduce mother-to-fetus transmission of HIV
1995—Canadian Perinatal Surveillance System (CPSS) launched
1998—Mandatory folic acid fortification of all breads and cereals sold in Canada
1998—COGNN becomes AWHONN Canada (Association of Women's Health, Obstetric and Neonatal Nurses of Canada) and proposes to have perinatal nursing recognized as a specialty by the Canadian Nurses Association
1999—First emergency contraceptive pill for pregnancy prevention (Plan B) approved; midwifery legalized in Quebec with midwives practising in birth centres
2000—National guidelines for family-centred maternal and newborn care published; first Canadian Nurses Association Perinatal Nursing Certification exam; Canadian Association of Midwives (CAM) formed
2001—Joint Statement on Shaken Baby Syndrome released by Health Canada
2005—The Canadian Association of Neonatal Nurses (CANN) formed
2006—Human papillomavirus (HPV) vaccine first available
2008—Joint Policy Statement on Normal Birth released by SOGC; emergency contraception (Plan B) available over the counter in pharmacies
2009—*What Mothers Say: The Maternity Experiences Survey* published by the Public Health Agency of Canada
2010—One breast milk bank in Vancouver remains, although others are in development; midwifery recognized as a legal and regulated profession in many Canadian provinces and territories; SOGC releases policy statement "Returning Birth to Aboriginal, Rural, and Remote Communities"
2011—AWHONN Canada becomes the Canadian Association of Perinatal and Women's Health Nurses (CAPWHN)

BOX 1-3 Key Determinants of Health

1. Income and social status
2. Social support networks
3. Education and literacy
4. Employment and working conditions
5. Social environments
6. Physical environments
7. Personal health practices and coping skills
8. Healthy child development
9. Biology and genetic endowment
10. Health services
11. Gender
12. Culture

(Source: Public Health Agency of Canada. [2010]. *What determines health: Key determinants*. Retrieved from http://www.phac-aspc.gc.ca/ph-sp/determinants/index-eng.php#determinants.)

maternal health or chronic conditions such as hypertension are also important contributors. To address the factors associated with infant mortality, there needs to be a shift from the current emphasis on highly technological medical interventions toward a focus on health promotion and preventive care for low-income families and women experiencing conditions of vulnerability (see Box 1-3).

Women and their families are also affected by geography and the social resources and programs available in their communities. For instance, rural, remote, and Aboriginal communities may have well-developed social networks but have less access to specialized health services. Maternity services, an important part of primary health care services, are often more difficult to provide in rural and remote locations.

The explosion in technology in health care has contributed to escalating health care costs. New and more sophisticated tools are available for perinatal care, including electronic fetal health surveillance and more invasive pain relief measures. Most recently, rapid changes in **genetic** screening technologies have affected the ways in which women and their families experience pregnancy and health decision making. At the same time, expanded use of the Internet has had an exponential effect on the availability of health information for childbearing families and has increased awareness of the need for health literacy.

Health information technology is also having a profound impact on the ways in which health services are delivered. For instance, *telemedicine,* an umbrella term for the use of communication technologies and electronic information to provide or support health care when participants are separated by distance, enables specialists, including nurses, to provide health care and consultation when distance separates them from those needing care. While this technology can increase access to health services for people living in geographically isolated communities, nurses must use caution and evaluate the effects of such emerging technologies.

Another factor that affects the delivery and quality of maternal care is that fact that the Canadian childbearing population is diverse in terms of **culture**, **ethnicity**, race, socioeconomic status, and age. In 2006, 20% of people living in Canada were born outside the country (Statistics Canada, 2006). Statistics Canada predicts that by 2017, between 19 and 23% percent of Canadians will identify themselves as belonging to a visible minority. Chinese and South Asians make up the largest visible minority group, with "Blacks" and "Arabs" following. It is estimated that by 2017, as many as 50% of the people living in Toronto and Vancouver will identify as visible minorities (Statistics Canada, 2006).

Also in 2006, Aboriginal people in Canada, which includes First Nations, Métis, and Inuit, surpassed the 1 million mark, reaching 1,172,790. Importantly for maternity care provision between 1996 and 2006, the Aboriginal population increased by 45%, compared with 8% for the non-Aboriginal population. Although the populations in many Canadian towns and cities are aging, in some First Nations, Métis, and Inuit communities more than 40% of the residents are under 25 years of age (Statistics Canada, 2010).

Significant disparity exists in health outcomes among people of various racial and ethnic groups in Canada. For example, First Nations, Métis, and Inuit families and women living in poverty consistently have poorer perinatal and neonatal health outcomes. People also have different health needs, practices, and health service preferences related to their ethnic or cultural backgrounds. They may have dietary preferences and health practices that are not understood by caregivers. To meet the health care needs of a culturally diverse society, nurses must provide culturally safe and responsive care (see Chapter 2).

Millennium Development Goals: A Global Challenge

The Millennium Development Goals (MDGs) are 8 goals to be achieved by 2015 that respond to the world's main development challenges. The MDGs are drawn from the actions and targets contained in the Millennium Declaration that was adopted by 189 nations and signed by 147 heads of state and governments during the United Nations Millennium Summit in September 2000 (http://www.un.org/millenniumgoals/goals.html). Goals 3 through 5 of the MDGs relate specifically to women and children (Box 1-4). In 2010, the Canadian government promised to assist developing countries in

BOX 1-4 The United Nations Millennium Development Goals

Goal 1—Eradicate extreme poverty and hunger
Goal 2—Achieve universal primary education
Goal 3—Promote gender equality and empower women
Goal 4—Reduce child mortality
Goal 5—Improve maternal health
Goal 6—Combat HIV/AIDS*, malaria, and other diseases
Goal 7—Ensure environmental sustainability
Goal 8—Develop a global partnership for development

(Source: United Nations [2011]. *Millennium development goals: 2011 progress chart*. Retrieved from http://www.un.org/millenniumgoals/pdf/%282011E%29_MDReport2011_ProgressChart.pdf.)

**AIDS*, acquired immunodeficiency syndrome; *HIV*, human immunodeficiency virus.

addressing health inequities that affect mothers and infants and signed the Muskoka Accord (Canadian International Development Agency, 2010).

Collaborative Woman- and Family-Centred Care

Collaborative woman- and family-centred maternity care is the overarching framework identified in the conceptual model for perinatal nursing in Canada (AWHONN, 2009). This dynamic and complex process of providing safe, skilled, and individualized care is affected by women's beliefs and values, by the context for care, and by the availability of skilled maternity care providers.

Family-Centred Maternity and Newborn Care

Perinatal nurses made a significant contribution to the development of the national guidelines Family-Centred Maternity and Newborn Care Guidelines (Health Canada, 2000). This important document includes guiding principles and strategies for facilitating change to implement these evidence-informed guidelines (Box 1-5).

With family-centred care, fathers, partners, grandparents, siblings, and friends are supported to be present for labour and birth, including Caesarean births. Fathers may participate by "catching the baby" or cutting the umbilical cord (Fig. 1-1). **Doulas** (trained and experienced female labour attendants) may provide a continuous, one-on-one caring presence throughout the labour and birth. Newborn infants remain with the mother and are encouraged to breastfeed immediately after birth. Parents also participate in the care of their infants in neonatal intensive care units.

Woman-Centred Care

Woman-centred care is grounded in the assumption that women know their own bodies and are experts in their own health (Box 1-6). Women are also frequently both organizers

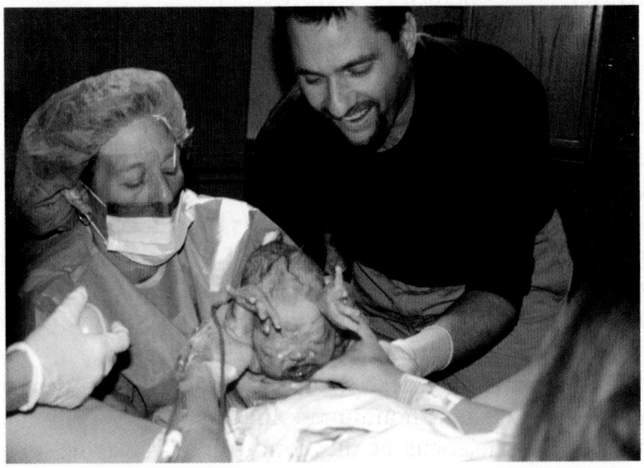

Fig. 1-1 Father "catching" newborn son. Mother is reaching down to help birth the baby. *(Courtesy Darren and Julie Nelson, Loveland, CO.)*

BOX 1-5 Guiding Principles of Family-Centred Maternity and Newborn Care

1. Birth is a celebration—a normal, healthy process.
2. Pregnancy and birth are unique for each woman.
3. The central objective of care for women, babies, and families is to maximize the probability of a healthy woman giving birth to a healthy baby.
4. Family-centred maternity and newborn care is based on research evidence.
5. Relationships between women, their families, and health care providers are based on mutual respect and trust.
6. Women are cared for within the context of their families (and their communities).
7. In order to make informed choices, women and their families need knowledge about their care.
8. Women have autonomy in decision making. Through respect and informed choice, women are empowered to take responsibility.
9. Health care providers have a powerful effect on women who are giving birth and on their families.
10. Family-centred care welcomes a variety of health care providers.
11. Technology is used appropriately in family-centred maternity and newborn care.
12. Quality of care includes a number of indicators.
13. Language is important (and needs to be inclusive, respectful, and empowering).

(Source: Family-Centred Maternity and Newborn Care: National Guidelines. Public Health Agency of Canada, 2000. Reproduced with permission from the Minister of Health, 2012.)

BOX 1-6 12 Elements of the Framework for Woman-Centred Health

Processes to Engage and Empower Women

1. Empowerment
2. Involvement and participation of women
3. Respect and safety
4. Collaborative work environments

Gender Differences That Affect Women's Health and Access to Health Care

5. Patterns or preferences in obtaining care
6. Forms of communication and interaction
7. Need for information
8. Decision-making processes

Support Structures and Approaches

9. Gender-inclusive approach to data
10. Gendered research and evaluation
11. Gender-sensitive training

Health Determinants and Systemic Inequalities

12. Intersecting oppressions and social justice concerns

(Adapted from Cory, J. [March 2007]. *Women-centred care: A curriculum for health care providers.* Vancouver BC: BC Women's Hospital and Health Centre. Retrieved from http://www.whrn.ca/documents/aaCurriculumforWomenCentredCareFinal.pdf.)

and providers of family caregiving. Woman-centred care also recognizes that women's childbearing experiences vary, respects the many differences among women, and acknowledges that gender is an important determinant of health.

Multidisciplinary Collaborative Maternity Care

A philosophy of respectful and collaborative work relationships between all different care providers underpins the framework for perinatal nursing in Canada. Nurses work with physicians, midwives, and doulas to provide appropriate care for families undergoing the childbirth experience. As contributors to the Multidisciplinary Collaborative Primary Maternity Care Project (MCP^2), which was funded in the context of a worsening shortage of maternity care providers, perinatal nurses helped to develop models and guidelines for multidisciplinary teams of professionals who work with childbearing women and their families (MCP^2, 2006). This project also resulted in identification of the need for a pan-Canadian framework for sustainable family-centred maternal and newborn care (Society of Obstetricians and Gynaecologists of Canada [SOGC], 2008).

Integrative Healing

Integrative healing encompasses complementary and alternative therapies that are sometimes used in combination with conventional Western modalities of treatment. Many popular alternative healing modalities offer human-centred care based on philosophies that honour the individual's beliefs, values, and desires. The focus of these modalities is on the whole person, not just on a disease complex. Women often find that integrative modalities are more consistent with their own belief systems and allow for more autonomy in health care decisions. Complementary and alternative therapies are identified throughout the text with an icon.

Perinatal Health Indicators: The Canadian Perinatal Surveillance System

The Canadian Perinatal Surveillance System (CPSS) was developed in 1995 to monitor maternal and infant health across Canada. The CPSS collects data from a number of sources (for example, vital statistics and the Canadian Institute for Health Information [CIHI]), analyzes and interprets the data, and writes papers and reports to be used as the basis for health policy and action. The CPSS has identified more than 50 health indicators and ranked many of these indicators for importance on the basis of current research evidence and knowledge about the determinants of health and impact of health outcomes.

The CPSS plays an important role in monitoring the quality of epidemiological (population) data available to assist with health and social service planning. Through data collection it has been determined that not every province has the same birth registration practices. The CPSS has thus been working with some data collection agencies to improve the quality of the data collected so that provincial and international comparisons are more meaningful.

Nurses need to be aware that there are important differences in definitions for health indicators. An example is infant mortality rates, which have been identified as one of the best indicators of a nation's health status (CPSS, 2008). However, the infant mortality rate is a complex health indicator that is dependent on how "live births" are defined and registered and on how fetal and neonatal deaths are recorded. For example, Canada and the United States have adopted the World Health Organization (WHO) definition of live birth to include all products of conception that show signs of life at birth, without reference to birth weight or gestational age of the **fetus**. Many European countries have adopted different definitions; for example, in Sweden live births are considered to be at least 27 weeks' gestation and fetal deaths (stillbirths) are not recorded before 28 weeks' gestation. In Canada there has been a recent trend to include as "live births" more neonates born at less than 500 grams and 20 weeks' gestation, which may result in Canada and the United States comparing poorly with many European countries (CPSS, 2008).

This variation in birth registration practices also happens within Canada. A recent review revealed that Alberta had the highest rate of registering these very small fetuses as live births. The effect of these various definitions on health practices and health systems is an excellent research question that has yet to be addressed.

Under-reporting is equally problematic, as estimates of infant mortality among First Nations, Métis, and Inuit populations in Canada have demonstrated. The CPSS also compares national rates to the results of research studies in which the investigators had more control over the quality of data collection. In this way, CPSS investigators were able to illustrate how mortality statistics for First Nations, Inuit, and Métis populations underestimate the problem of infant mortality because of low registration of births at the borderline of viability. Box 1-7 defines maternal and infant health indicators commonly used for reporting in Canada.

BOX 1-7 Common Perinatal Health Indicators

Birth rate—Number of live births in one year per 1000 population

Fertility rate—Number of births per 1000 women between the ages of 15 and 44 (inclusive), calculated on a yearly basis

Infant mortality rate—Number of deaths of infants under one year of age per 1000 live births

Maternal mortality rate—Number of maternal deaths from births and complications of pregnancy, childbirth, and puerperium (the first 42 days after termination of the pregnancy) per 100,000 live births

Neonatal mortality rate—Number of deaths of infants under 28 days of age per 1000 live births

Perinatal mortality rate—Number of stillbirths and number of neonatal deaths per 1000 live births

Stillbirth—An infant who at birth demonstrates no signs of life, such as breathing, heartbeat, or voluntary muscle movements

One way that the CPSS tries to improve data collection is by monitoring both birth and death registrations. Investigators found that in all provinces of Canada, except Ontario, the birth registrations of almost all infants who died were identified. They are working with the province of Ontario to improve Ontario's birth registration practices and have analyzed Ontario data separately in an appendix of the CPSS 2008 report.

The 2008 edition of the CPSS report includes 29 perinatal health indicators for which there is currently sufficient national data available. The report is organized in two sections. Section A reports on determinants of maternal, fetal, and infant health and includes health behaviours and practices (e.g., rates of maternal smoking and alcohol consumption during pregnancy) and health service indicators (e.g., labour induction and Caesarean rates). Section B includes maternal health outcomes (e.g., maternal mortality and rates of ectopic pregnancy) and fetal and infant health outcomes (e.g., **preterm** and **postterm** birth rates, multiple birth rates, and the prevalence of congenital anomalies).

One of the success stories included in the report is the decreasing rate of neural tube defects (including spina bifida and anencephaly) since 1995 following the introduction of folic acid supplementation for childbearing women. Increasing maternal obesity, preterm birth, and Caesarean rates are highlighted as areas of concern. The report also indicates that maternal alcohol consumption in pregnancy is under-reported (CPSS, 2008).

Trends in Fertility and Birth Rate

Fertility trends and birth rates reflect women's needs for health services. In recent years, more women living in Canada have delayed childbearing until they are 35 years of age or older. Women who conceive at older ages are more likely to experience chronic illnesses, placental problems, and multiple pregnancy, and their fetuses are more likely to have chromosomal abnormalities (e.g., Down syndrome). However, older women also tend to be better educated, have higher income levels (less poverty), and seek early prenatal care.

The rate of live births to teenage women in Canada has been steadily decreasing since 1996 (down 37% to 2006) (McKay and Barrett, 2010). Health problems associated with teen pregnancy include anemia and poor weight gain and twice the risk of delivering a preterm or low–birth weight baby (see Chapter 4). Teenage pregnancy can also influence the likelihood that women may not complete high school, which may result in underemployment and poverty. There are significant geographic variations in adolescent fertility rates, from the lowest in Quebec (3.1%) to the highest in Nunavut (24.4%), reflecting significant cultural differences and access to abortion services (CPSS, 2008).

Multiple Birth Rate

Multiple birth rates in Canada have increased, reflecting older maternal age at conception and the greater use of **assisted reproductive technologies** such as in vitro fertilization (IVF) (see Chapter 7). Multiple pregnancy results in health problems for both women (anemia, pre-eclampsia, Caesarean delivery) and their babies (preterm birth, low birth weight, perinatal death). There is growing evidence that decreasing the number of **embryos** may help decrease the poor health outcomes associated with higher order (more than twins) multiple pregnancies.

Low Birth Weight and Preterm Birth

The proportion of preterm infants (born before 37 completed weeks' gestation) has increased from 7.0% in 1995 to 8.2% in 2004. In industrialized nations, 60 to 80% of deaths to infants born without congenital anomalies are the result of preterm birth. Preterm birth is also associated with cerebral palsy and other long-term health problems. In 2004 there was significant regional variation in preterm birth rates, ranging from a low of 7.4% in Saskatchewan to a high of 12.2% in Nunavut (CPSS, 2008).

Babies born both small (<10th percentile for sex-specific standardized birth weights) and large (>90th percentile) for gestational age experience significant health problems (see Chapter 27). Maternal cigarette smoking accounts for about 30 to 40% of small-for-gestational-age (SGA) babies born in industrialized countries, where malnutrition is not a predominant factor. Large-for-gestational-age (LGA) babies and their mothers are more likely to experience birth trauma (shoulder dystocia, nerve injuries, and **postpartum** hemorrhage). Maternal diabetes is an important risk factor. LGA babies are more common in First Nations, Métis, and Inuit women (see Chapter 14).

Breastfeeding Rates in Canada

Breastfeeding is recognized internationally as the optimal method of infant feeding, with six months of exclusive breastfeeding currently recommended (Canadian Paediatric Society [CPS], 2009; WHO 2001). Breastfeeding initiation rates have been increasing steadily in Canada, with regional variation ranging from 62% in Newfoundland and Labrador to almost 98% in the Yukon. However, only about 18% of Canadian women continue to breastfeed exclusively for 6 months or longer (CPSS, 2008) (see Chapter 26).

Health Service Indicators: Rate of Inductions and Caesarean Delivery

The CPSS also monitors a number of health service indicators, including rates of labour induction and Caesarean delivery. Labour may be medically or surgically induced for a variety of reasons, including obstetrical complications or postterm pregnancy (see Chapter 19). Although generally considered safe, labour induction is associated with both maternal and fetal complications. Recent changes in the management of post term pregnancy have resulted in increased induction rates in Canada, although there are regional and provincial variations.

The proportion of women delivering by Caesarean section has increased steadily from 17.6% in 1995 to more than 25% 10 years later (CPSS, 2008). Most of this increase is due to a higher rate of primary (first-time) Caesarean sections, although the vaginal birth after Caesarean (VBAC) rate also decreased over the same time period. This trend is concerning, as evidence documents a higher risk of significant maternal morbidity (e.g., infection, thromboembolism, hysterectomy) for women who have a **Caesarean birth**.

The Canadian Maternity Experiences Survey

The Canadian Maternity Experiences Survey was designed by the CPSS and included more than 300 questions asked of 6421 women from across Canada. The stratified sample was drawn from women who lived with an infant as identified in the 2006 Canadian census. Women were interviewed by telephone for 45 minutes when their baby was between 5 and 14 months of age. An attempt was made to include young; First Nations, Métis, and Inuit; and immigrant women in the survey. The survey covered topics related to the experiences of pregnancy, childbirth, and the postpartum period and could be considered a snapshot in time and a rich source for the identification of concerns for further study. This report provides detailed information on many issues of concern for nurses (e.g., alcohol use, prenatal class attendance, social support, and stress). The report is available to download from the Public Health Agency of Canada Web site (see Additional Resources at the end of this chapter). The following sections highlight some of the most pertinent findings.

Pregnancy

Women were asked about the timing of their pregnancy. About half of the women indicated that it was "just right," whereas other women said that they would have liked to conceive earlier (23.4%), later (20%), or not at all (7.1%). Most women received prenatal care from an obstetrician (58%) or family physician (34%); fewer women received prenatal care from a midwife (6.1%) or nurse practitioner (0.6%). Most women (95%) initiated prenatal care in the first trimester and about two thirds of primiparous women attended prenatal classes (CPSS, 2008).

Most women (90%) took folic acid supplements in the first 3 months of pregnancy but more than 22% did not know that taking folic acid before pregnancy can help prevent some birth defects. More than one third of women had a high body mass index before pregnancy, with almost 14% of these women being in the obese category. Many women stopped smoking during pregnancy, but almost half of the women who had quit had resumed smoking at the time of the interview. Over 10% of women reported drinking any alcohol in pregnancy and 1% reported use of street drugs (this was likely underreported). The proportion of women who reported experiencing physical or sexual abuse in the previous 2 years was almost 11% (CPSS, 2008).

Labour and Birth

Almost 98% of births for women interviewed took place in hospital. A small number of births occurred at home (1.2%) or in birthing centres (0.8%). More than 25% of women travelled to another community to give birth, with 2.5% travelling more than 100 km. Almost 70% of women were cared for by an obstetrician during labour, while less than 15% had a family physician. Nurses and midwives were identified as primary care providers during childbirth for the remaining women.

About 74% of the women interviewed gave birth vaginally, with the rest giving birth by Caesarean section. Few women (8%) requested a Caesarean birth from their health care provider at any point during their pregnancy. Most women had their partners with them during labour, and some women had an additional birth companion. **Epidural** or spinal anaesthesia was the most frequent pain medication used (reported by 57% of women). More than 70% of women held their baby within 5 minutes of delivery (CPSS, 2008).

Postpartum

About one third of women who had a vaginal birth stayed in hospital less than 2 days. Women stayed slightly longer after Caesarean delivery. Most women (90%) initiated breastfeeding, but by 6 months "exclusive breastfeeding" had dropped to 14%, with another 54% of women reporting "any breastfeeding." Breastfeeding rates were higher in western than in eastern Canada. Most women were contacted by a health care provider (usually a nurse) after giving birth, but many did not speak with anyone until 7 days postpartum. Most women reported that they had enough information about infant and maternal care but seemed to be less informed about concerns related to the transition to parenthood.

Specialization and Evidence-Informed Nursing Practice

The increasing complexity of care required by women and their newborn has contributed to the growth of specialized knowledge and skills needed by nurses working with childbearing women and their families. This specialized knowledge is gained through experience, advanced degrees, and certification programs. In Canada, perinatal nurses can be recognized for their expertise through the Canadian Nurses Association (CNA) Certification program.

Advanced practice nurses, such as clinical nurse specialists, provide care for women with complex childbearing challenges, while midwives and nurse practitioners may provide primary care throughout a woman's life, including during pregnancy. Lactation consultants, many of whom are nurses, provide services on the postpartum unit, on an outpatient basis, or in the woman's home. Perinatal nurses work collaboratively with public health nurses, neonatal intensive care unit (NICU) nurses, and an increasing array of maternity and health care providers.

Evidence-informed practice, or providing nursing care that is guided by evidence gained through many forms of research, is increasingly emphasized in the nursing profession. Although not all practice can be evidence-informed, perinatal nurses must use the best available information to guide their interactions and interventions. The Association of Women's Health, Obstetric and Neonatal Nurses' (AWHONN) (http://www.awhonn.org) *Standards for Professional Perinatal Nursing Practice and Certification in Canada* (2009) includes an evidence-informed approach to practice. Discussion of nursing care and evidence-informed nursing boxes throughout this text provide many examples (see Evidence-Informed Practice box).

AWHONN has conducted six research-based practice projects (Box 1-8). These projects (available at http://www.awhonn.org) were conducted in several states and provinces

EVIDENCE-INFORMED PRACTICE Searching for and Evaluating the Evidence

Throughout this text you will see Evidence-Informed Practice boxes. These boxes provide examples of how a nurse might conduct an inquiry into an identified practice question. Curiosity, access to a virtual or real library, and research critique skills are needed for the nurse to be confident that his or her practice is informed by a sound foundation of evidence.

Nurses construct their practice informed by research from many different sources. Categorizing evidence by "levels" is being replaced with embracing multiple ways of knowing that includes personal knowledge. Experienced perinatal nurses have practice knowledge that they need to share with other nurses through publication. Indigenous ways of knowing are increasingly being recognized, and women are being acknowledged as experts in their own experiences of childbearing and family caregiving (MacKinnon, 2006). Qualitative research has added to our understanding of women's and family members' childbearing experiences.

In systematic reviews of quantitative research, such as those in the Cochrane Database, the research team uses a methodology to identify all studies relevant to a particular question. If the data are similar enough, they can be pooled into a meta-analysis. If the evidence is strong, some analyses will form the basis for recommendations for practice and guide further inquiry. Meta-synthesis of some forms of qualitative research is also being developed. Recommendations for best practice stand on the shoulders of the systematic analysts, who in turn stand on the many shoulders of primary researchers.

Provided the professional organization is well respected and the process is rigorous, clinical practice guidelines and consensus statements reflect the current state of knowledge. In Canada, the Society of Obstetricians and Gynaecologists of Canada (SOGC) has developed many clinical practice guidelines that will be of interest to perinatal nurses. These guidelines are available free of charge on their Web site (http://www.sogc.org). Perinatal units can adapt these recommendations to their specific institutions, enabling nurses to become more informed about current evidence and provide more effective care for childbearing families. However, perinatal nurses need to also develop an inquiring mind and questioning attitude toward all forms of current evidence. In this way, the knowledge base required for perinatal nursing will continue to grow and develop.

and staff nurses were involved in their implementation. For example, the Late Preterm Infant Initiative began in 2005 in response to the confusion that surrounded the care of infants who do not qualify for neonatal intensive care admission yet require extra vigilance in their care. By using guidelines and published reports, nurses can develop protocols and procedures based on published research and incorporate evidence into their own practice.

Cochrane Pregnancy and Childbirth Database

The Cochrane Pregnancy and Childbirth Database was first planned in 1976 with a small grant from the World Health Organization to Dr. Iain Chalmers and colleagues at Oxford University. In 1993 the Cochrane Collaboration was formed, and the Oxford Database of Perinatal Trials became known as the Cochrane Pregnancy and Childbirth Database. The Cochrane Collaboration oversees up-to-date, systematic reviews of randomized controlled trials and disseminates these reviews. The premise of the project is that these types of studies provide reliable evidence about the effects of maternity care.

BOX 1-8 Association of Women's Health, Obstetric and Neonatal Nurses Research-Based Practice Projects

- Transition of the preterm infant to an open crib
- Management of women in the second stage of labour
- Continence for women
- Neonatal skin care
- Cyclic pelvic pain and discomfort management
- Late preterm infant initiative

(Source: Retrieved from www.awhonn.org/awhonn/content.do?name=03_JournalsPubsResearch/3G_ResearchBasedPracticeProjects.htm.)

The evidence from these studies should encourage practitioners to implement useful measures and abandon those that are useless or harmful. Studies are ranked in six categories:

1. Beneficial forms of care
2. Forms of care that are likely to be beneficial
3. Forms of care with a trade-off between beneficial and adverse effects
4. Forms of care with unknown effectiveness
5. Forms of care that are unlikely to be beneficial
6. Forms of care that are likely to be ineffective or harmful

Practices that have been reviewed by the Collaboration are identified with a symbol throughout this text.

Joanna Briggs Institute

Founded in 1995 as an initiative of the Royal Adelaide Hospital and the University of Adelaide in Australia, the Joanna Briggs Institute (JBI) uses a collaborative approach for evaluating evidence from a range of sources (http://www.joannabriggs.edu.au). The JBI has formed collaborations with a variety of universities and hospitals around the world, including Canada. It provides another source for perinatal nurses to access information to support evidence-informed practice.

Current Issues Affecting Perinatal Nursing Practice

Promoting Health and Normal Birth

A guiding principle of the Family-Centred Maternity and Newborn Care national guidelines is that birth is a normal healthy process (see Box 1-5). Women must be viewed holistically and in the context in which they live. Their physical, mental, and social environment must be considered because these interdependent factors influence health and illness. Even the language that health care providers use to describe women and their problems needs to be examined. For example, practitioners may describe women as having an "incompetent cervix," as "failing to progress," or having an "arrest" of labour. They may describe a fetus as having intrauterine growth "retardation." They also may "allow" women a "trial" of labour. The use of these phrases implies failure or inadequacy on the part of the woman or fetus, and more positive language should be incorporated into the practitioner's vocabulary.

The Place of Birth and "High-Tech" Care

Advances in scientific knowledge and the identification of a large number of "high-risk" pregnancies have contributed to a health care system that emphasizes "high-tech" care. Maternity care has extended to include preconception counselling, more and better scientific techniques to monitor the mother and fetus, more definitive tests for genetic abnormalities and for identifying hypoxia and acidosis during labour, and neonatal intensive care units. Many women who labour in hospital settings are monitored electronically despite the lack of evidence that supports this practice.

Since childbirth is a normal life process, people are starting to question whether the hospital provides the best environment to support this important event in the life of a family. Birthing centres and home birth are options currently available to few Canadian women. Midwives are being integrated into the Canadian health care systems but remain in short supply. As experts in normal childbirth, midwives may be able to provide some balance to medicalized hospital practices.

Midwifery

Midwives play a significant role in the delivery of maternal child care. Although midwives have been in existence for years, it was only recently that midwives have been legislated in Canada and integrated into the health care system. Since the early 1990s when midwifery legislation was first passed, most provinces and territories have gradually implemented midwifery-oriented health policy, including legalization of the profession, standardization of training, and fees being remunerated through their respective provincial insurance plans. In 2008, 6% of women were cared for by midwives for their maternal care (PHAC, 2009). The Canadian Association of Midwives (CAM) is the national voice for midwifery in Canada. Midwives in Canada have their own regulations and education apart from nursing education. There are three primary principles of midwifery care: continuity of care, informed choice, and choice of birth place (Box 1-9).

BOX 1-9 Principles of Midwifery Care

Continuity of Care: Midwives typically work in small groups and are on call for 24 hours. Women and their families have the opportunity to get to know their midwife or midwives well before the baby is born and have a familiar caregiver with them for their entire pregnancy. Usually two midwives attend the birth and share the care throughout the pregnancy, labour, and birth and after delivery for six weeks.

Informed Choice: Midwives support women to play an active role in their own care throughout pregnancy and birth. During scheduled visits, the midwife provides comprehensive information so that women and their families can make informed choices about all aspects of their care. Midwives recognize and support the mother as the main decision-maker. Under the care of a midwife, women may have the choice of giving birth in hospital or out of hospital.

Choice of Birthplace: Midwives are trained to attend births both at home or in hospital and will help women choose the safest place for them. A midwife's training prepares her to be responsible for decisions about labour, delivery, postpartum, and newborn care both at home or in hospital. A midwife works closely with other community midwives, doctors, and nurses to maintain a high standard of care.

(Adapted from Ontario Ministry of Health and Long-term Care. [2011]. *Midwifery in Ontario*. Retrieved from http://www.health.gov.on.ca/english/public/program/midwife/midwife_mn.html.)

Baby Friendly Initiative in Canada

The Breastfeeding Committee for Canada (BCC) identified the WHO/UNICEF Baby Friendly Initiative (BFI) as a primary strategy for the protection, promotion, and support of breastfeeding. The WHO/UNICEF guidelines for the BFI propose that each country identify a BFI National Authority to facilitate the assessment and monitoring of the progress of BFI. The Breastfeeding Committee for Canada is the national authority for the BFI in Canada.

The BFI protects, promotes, and supports breastfeeding through the Ten Steps to Successful Breast-Feeding developed by UNICEF and the World Health Organization (see Box 26-2). Presently, just over 30 hospitals, birthing centres, and community health departments in Canada have received the Baby Friendly Designation (see discussion in Chapter 26).

Patient Safety and Risk Management

Adverse events are implicated in up to 23,750 deaths per year in Canada (French, 2006). Since the Institute of Medicine in the United States released its report in 1999, there has been a concerted effort to analyze causes of errors and develop strategies to avoid them. In 2001, the Royal College of Physicians and Surgeons of Canada held a one-day forum on patient safety that was attended by health care professionals and government officials. The National Steering Committee on Patient Safety (NSCPS) resulted from this meeting. In 2002, the NSCPS proposed a national integrated strategy for improving patient safety in Canadian health care, recommending the establishment of a Canadian Patient Safety Institute (CPSI) (Box 1-10). The CPSI facilitates collaboration among governments and care providers to enhance patient safety and provides a number of useful resources, including a root-cause analysis framework (CPSI, 2006) and competencies needed for patient safety (CPSI, 2009).

Community-Based Care

Discharge of a mother and baby within 24 hours of birth has created a growing need for follow-up and home care. Perinatal

BOX 1-10 Goals of the Canadian Patient Safety Institute (CPSI)

The CPSI will strive to be a leader for patient safety in the nation by:

- Fostering a system where knowledge and information about optimal patient safety practices are shared
- Influencing the necessary cultural shifts and championing changes in systems to improve patient safety
- Collaborating with stakeholders in an ongoing dialogue to support improvements in patient safety

(Source: The Canadian Patient Safety Institute. Retrieved from http://www.patientsafetyinstitute.ca/English/About/Pages/faqs.aspx#q4.)

nurses need to assess the resources that childbearing women have to support them during the postpartum period at home. In many cultures, women are cared for by extended family members so that their primary responsibility is to breastfeed and recover from childbirth. In our independent North American culture, women may need to be encouraged to ask for help. At times, perinatal nurses may need to advocate for a delay of hospital discharge until the needed supports are put in place. Collaboration with public health nurses and other community care providers is necessary to enable parents to make a safe transition from hospital to home (see Chapter 3). Enhancement of postpartum support services with the addition of homemakers, breastfeeding support services, and doulas may be needed to promote the health of Canadian families.

Some women who experience pregnancy complications are now cared for in the home by **antepartum** home care nurses. Portable fetal monitors and other forms of technology previously available only in the hospital are used. This change has affected the organizational structure of care, the costs of care, and the skills required to provide nursing care. Nursing care has become more community based with nurses providing care for women and infants in homeless shelters and for adolescents in school-based clinics, and promoting health at community centres, churches, and shopping malls (see Community Focus box).

COMMUNITY FOCUS

Culturally Appropriate and Adequate Prenatal Care

Make an appointment to visit a community health centre that serves childbearing women. Who are the staff and what are their qualifications (e.g., registered nurses, practical nurses, nutritionists, social workers, childbirth educators, lactation consultants)? Is a laboratory available? What clientele (e.g., racial and ethnic groups) does the centre serve? Are some of the staff representative of those racial and ethnic groups? Is the staff bilingual? Are educational materials available in languages spoken by the women served by the clinic? Is the centre located near public transportation for ease of access? Is the setting "family friendly" (e.g., are there reading materials available? A play area for children? A restroom? A place to breastfeed?)? Would you be willing to seek care in the centre? What could improve the setting?

Involving Communities and Promoting Healthy Living

Health services need to build on women's strengths and address their needs. They also need to maximize the use of community resources, volunteers, and paraprofessionals. Health education is an important strategy for perinatal nurses when it is based on the particular woman's learning needs. Sometimes group education or prenatal care may help women develop a strong support network. Topics commonly addressed include nutrition on a budget, financial and stress management, smoking cessation, alcohol and drug treatment, violence, social networking, community resources, and parenting. The opportunity to share experiences with other women and validate feelings and concerns may be more important than formal education. Online communities and prenatal classes may supplement local resources.

Health Literacy

Health literacy involves a spectrum of abilities, ranging from reading an appointment slip to interpreting medication instructions. These skills must be assessed routinely to recognize a problem and accommodate patients with limited literacy skills. An excellent resource is *Teaching Patients with Low Literacy Skills*, second edition (Doak, Doak, & Root, 1996).

Individuals and groups for whom English is a second language often lack the skills necessary to seek medical care and navigate the health care system. As a result of the increasingly multicultural Canadian population, there is an urgent need to address health literacy as a component of culturally and linguistically competent care. Health care providers can contribute to health literacy by speaking slowly and using simple, common words; avoiding jargon; and assessing whether the patient understands the discussion. The skillful use of an interpreter or telephone interpretation service can help promote understanding and **informed consent**.

A Global Perspective

The fifth Millennium Development Goal (see Box 1-4) is to improve maternal health and reduce the **maternal mortality rate** by 75% between 1990 and 2015. Worldwide, approximately 1400 women die each day of problems related to pregnancy or childbirth, with hemorrhage being the leading cause of death. There are great disparities in the maternal mortality rate between developing and developed countries. In Canada the maternal mortality ratio (number of maternal deaths per 100,000 live births) was 5.5 in 2004 (CPSS, 2008), whereas the rate in developing countries was 450 (WHO, 2008). As well, 3.6 million newborn babies die because of largely preventable complications during pregnancy, childbirth, and the postnatal period (WHO & International Confederation of Midwives, 2007). Most of the 3.2 million children living with human immunodeficiency virus (HIV) or acquired immunodeficiency syndrome (AIDS) acquired the infection through perinatal transmission and live in Sub-Saharan Africa. This difference illustrates the inequities that exist between industrialized and resource-poor parts of the world. In an effort to address this inequity the World Health Organization and partners in nursing developed Strategic Directions for Nursing and Midwifery Services (Box 1-11).

BOX 1-11 Strategic Directions for Nursing and Midwifery Services

- Health and human resource planning
- Management of health personnel
- Evidence-informed practice
- Education
- Stewardship and regulation

(Source: Al-Gasseer, N., & Persaud, V. [2003]. Measuring progress in nursing and midwifery globally. *Journal of Nursing Scholarship, 35*[4], 309–315.)

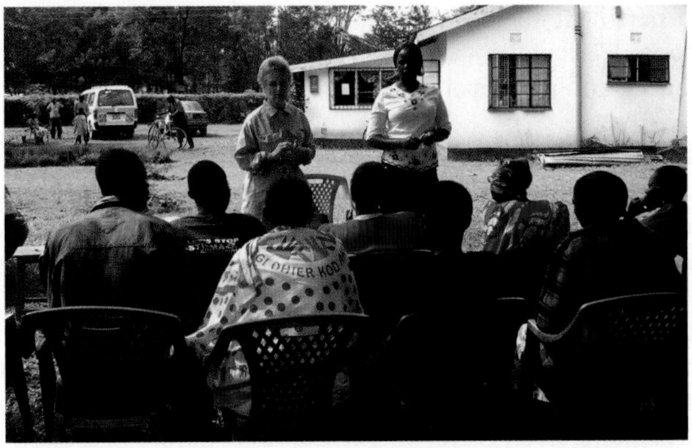

Fig. 1-2 Nurse teaching breast examination with the assistance of an interpreter to traditional birth attendants (TBAs) in a rural clinic in Kenya. (Both men and women serve as TBAs.) Women may detect lumps but usually do not seek care unless there is pain associated with the lump. *(Courtesy Shannon Perry, Phoenix, AZ.)*

If women have access to appropriate health care in the event of a complication, the maternal mortality rate will decrease. The infant mortality rate could also be decreased with relatively simple interventions. Keeping the newborn warm, exclusive breastfeeding, preventing malaria and tetanus, and enabling early recognition of illness and care seeking would have important results (SOGC, n.d.).

Another factor that can negatively affect maternal health is female genital mutilation, which is the removal of part or all of the female external genitalia for cultural or nontherapeutic reasons (WHO Study Group, 2006). Worldwide, many women undergo such procedures. With the growing number of immigrants from Africa and other countries where female genital mutilation is practised, nurses will increasingly encounter women who have undergone the procedure. These women are significantly more likely to have adverse obstetric outcomes, resulting in 1 or 2 additional perinatal deaths per 100 births (WHO Study Group, 2006). The International Council of Nurses and other health professionals have spoken out against the procedures as harmful to women's health and a violation of human rights.

As the world becomes a smaller place because of travel and communication technologies, nurses and other health care providers are gaining a global perspective and participating in activities to improve the health and health care of people worldwide (Perry & Mander, 2005). Nurses participate in medical outreach; provide obstetric, surgical, ophthalmological, orthopaedic, or other services; attend international meetings; conduct research; and provide international consultation (Fig. 1-2). International student and faculty exchanges occur. More articles about health and health care in various countries are appearing in nursing journals.

The Global Health eLearning Centre (http://www.globalhealthlearning.org) of the U.S. Agency of International Development (USAID) currently has 22 free online courses that are useful for nurses and other health care providers who plan to work in developing countries. Of these 22 courses, 14 pertain to the health of women and infants.

Ethical Issues in Perinatal Nursing

Ethical concerns and debates have multiplied with the increased use of technology and with scientific advances. For example, with reproductive technology, pregnancy is now possible in women who thought they would never bear children, including some who are menopausal or postmenopausal. Should scarce resources be devoted to achieving pregnancies in older women? Is giving birth to a child at an older age worth the risks involved? Should older parents be encouraged to conceive a baby when they may not live to see the child reach adulthood? Should a woman who is HIV positive have access to assisted reproduction services? Who should pay for reproductive technologies such as the use of induced ovulation and in vitro fertilization?

Questions about informed consent and allocation of resources must be addressed with innovations such as intrauterine fetal surgery, fetoscopy, therapeutic insemination, genetic engineering, stem cell research, surrogate childbearing, surgery for **infertility**, "test-tube" babies, fetal research, and treatment of very preterm babies. The introduction of long-acting contraceptives has created moral choices and policy dilemmas for health care providers and legislators (e.g., whether some women [substance users or women who are HIV positive] should be required to take the contraceptives). With the potential for great good that can come from fetal tissue transplantation, what research is ethical? What are the rights of the embryo? Should cloning of humans be permitted? Discussion and debate about these issues will continue for many years. Nurses and women, as well as scientists, physicians, attorneys, lawmakers, ethicists, and clergy, must be involved in the discussions.

Research in Perinatal Nursing

Research plays a vital role in building perinatal nursing science. Research can illuminate women's childbearing experiences, demonstrate that nursing care makes a difference, and identify areas for further study. For example, although prenatal care is associated with healthier infants, no one knows exactly which interventions produce this outcome. Many possible areas of research exist in maternity and women's health care. The clinician can identify areas for further research that are pertinent to the health and health care of women and infants. Perinatal nurses should promote the use of research funding and participate in research projects.

Ethical Guidelines for Nursing Research

Research with childbearing women and their families may create ethical dilemmas for the nurse. For example, participating in research may cause additional stress for a woman concerned about outcomes of genetic testing or for one who is waiting for an invasive procedure. Obtaining amniotic fluid samples or performing cordocentesis poses risks to the fetus (see Chapter 12). Nurses must protect the rights of human participants in all research. For example, nurses may need to collect data on or care for patients who are participating in clinical trials. The nurse should ensure that the participants are fully informed and aware of their rights as participants. The nurse may be involved in determining whether the benefits of research outweigh the risks to the mother and the fetus and needs to ensure that all research conducted has been approved by the appropriate research **ethics** board.

Addressing Current Challenges and Envisioning the Future

The challenges currently being faced by perinatal and women's health nurses need to be addressed creatively with a focus on the future and on promoting optional health and growth, enhancing childbearing experiences for Canadian (and all) women and their families (Box 1-12).

BOX 1-12 Goals for Perinatal Nursing: Looking Ahead to the Future

1. Recognizing the importance of childbearing for family health promotion and building collaborative relationships with women as family caregivers. Nurses will increasingly need to build upon strengths when working with women who experience childbearing challenges due to conditions of vulnerability.
2. Decreasing health service costs by expanding alternatives to highly technological hospital-based care, such as midwifery services, nurse practitioner–led health clinics, and alternative birth places, including birthing centres and women's homes
3. Expanding multiprofessional teams, with nurses being more involved in helping women access appropriate health services (screening and referral services)
4. Recognizing the contributions of traditional and integrative healers who support the belief systems and enhance health practices of childbearing women and their families
5. Re-examining patient safety so that the important role that nurses play in keeping patients safe, particularly in the hospital setting, is recognized
6. Promoting normal birth within highly technological birth environments for women and newborns who require this level of care
7. Promoting a culture of breastfeeding that also recognizes that breastfeeding may not be the best infant feeding option for all childbearing women
8. Disrupting existing power structures and practices by recognizing perinatal nurses' knowledge and skills and by building respectful, collaborative interprofessional health care teams
9. Recognizing the challenges experienced by both childbearing women and maternity care providers who live and work in rural, remote, First Nations, Métis and Inuit, and inner-city communities
10. Address health inequities by creating health policy and services that focus on both the resources needed for health (see Box 1-3, Key Determinants of Health) and access to health services
11. Utilizing electronic technologies to provide enhanced continuing professional education and build communities of practice where knowledge exchange is supported

Key Points

- Perinatal nursing focuses on caring for women and their families throughout the childbearing year.
- Perinatal nurses can play an active role in shaping health policy and health systems to be responsive to the needs of Canadian women.
- Childbirth practices have changed to become more woman- and family-centred and include more alternatives in provider, birth place, and care.
- Preterm birth, maternal obesity, and high Caesarean birth rates are current challenges in Canada.
- Integrative healing combines modern technology with ancient healing practices and encompasses the whole body, mind, and spirit.
- Women living in rural, remote, and Aboriginal communities and in poverty in inner cities experience significant health challenges.
- Of the determinants of health, poverty remains the most important factor resulting in conditions of vulnerability such as homelessness.
- Globally, women are still dying in childbirth, and infant mortality remains high.
- Perinatal nursing practice is increasingly informed by research.
- Collaborative multidisciplinary maternity care based on mutual respect and trust is one strategy for addressing the critical shortages of maternity care providers.
- Ethical concerns have multiplied with the increasing use of technology and scientific advances.

Audio Chapter Summaries

Access an Audio Summary of these Key Points on evolve

References

Association of Women's Health, Obstetric and Neonatal Nurses (AWHONN). (2009). *Standards for professional perinatal nursing practice and certification in Canada* (2nd ed.). Washington, DC: Author.

Canadian International Development Agency. (2010). *The Muskoka Initiative: The G-8 commitment.* Retrieved from http://www.acdi-cida.gc.ca/acdi-cida/ACDI-CIDA.nsf/eng/FRA-127113657-MH7#a1.

Canadian Paediatric Society. (2009). *Exclusive breastfeeding should continue to six months.* Retrieved from http://www.cps.ca/english/statements/n/breastfeedingmar05.htm.

Canadian Patient Safety Institute (CPSI). (2006). *Canadian root case analysis framework.* Retrieved from http://www.patientsafetyinstitute.ca/English/toolsResources/rca/Documents/March%202006%20RCA%20Workbook.pdf.

Canadian Patient Safety Institute. (CPSI). (2009). *Enhancing patient safety across the health professions.* Retrieved from http://www.patientsafetyinstitute.ca/English/education/safetyCompetencies/Documents/Safety%20Competencies.pdf.

Canadian Perinatal Surveillance System. (2008). *Canadian perinatal health report: 2008 edition.* Retrieved from http://www.phac-aspc.gc.ca/publicat/2008/cphr-rspc/index-eng.php.

Doak, C. C., Doak, L. G., & Root, J. H. (1996). *Teaching patients with low literacy skills* (2nd ed.). Philadelphia: Lippincott.

French, J. (2006). Medical errors and patient safety in health care. *Canadian Journal of Medical Radiation Technology, 37*(4), 9–13.

Health Canada. (2000). *Family-centred maternity and newborn care: National guidelines.* Ottawa: Author.

MacKinnon, K. (2006). Living with the threat of preterm labour: Women's work of keeping the baby in. *Journal of Obstetrical Gynecologic & Neonatal Nursing, 35*(6), 700–708.

McKay, A., & Barrett, M. (2010). Trends in teen pregnancy rates from 1996–2006: A comparison of Canada, Sweden, U.S.A., and England/Wales. *Canadian Journal of Human Sexuality, 19*(1/2), 43–52.

Multidisciplinary Collaborative Primary Maternity Care Project (MCP^2). (2006). *Final report.* Retrieved from http://www.mcp2.ca/english/studies_reports.asp.

Pauly, B., MacKinnon, K., & Varcoe, C. (2009). Revisiting "Who gets care?": Health equity as an arena for nursing action. *Advances in Nursing Science, 32*(2), 118–127.

Perry, S. E., & Mander, R. (2005). A global frame of reference: Learning from everyone, everywhere. *Nursing Education & Perspectives, 26*(3), 148–151.

Public Health Agency of Canada (PHAC). (1986). *Ottawa charter for health promotion.* Ottawa: Author. Retrieved from http://www.phac-aspc.gc.ca/ph-sp/docs/charter-chartre/pdf/charter.pdf.

Public Health Agency of Canada. (2009). *What mothers say: The Canadian maternity experiences survey.* Ottawa: Author. Retrieved from http://www.phac-aspc.gc.ca/rhs-ssg/survey-eng.php.

Society of Obstetricians and Gynaecologists of Canada (SOGC). (2008). *A national birthing initiative for Canada.* Retrieved from http://www.sogc.org/projects/birthing-itrategy_e.asp.

Society of Obstetricians and Gynaecologists of Canada. (n.d.). *Safe motherhood and newborn health.* Retrieved from http://iwhp.sogc.org/index.php?page=inetvu-mobile-solutions&hl=en_US.

Statistics Canada. (2006). *Canada's ethnocultural mosaic, 2006 census.* Catalogue no. 97-562-X. Ottawa: Author. Retrieved from http://www12.statcan.ca/english/census06/analysis/ethnicorigin/pdf/97-562-XIE2006001.pdf.

Statistics Canada. (2010). *2006 Aboriginal population profile for Victoria.* Ottawa: Author. Catalogue no. 89-638-X no. 2010004. Retrieved from http://www.statcan.gc.ca/pub/89-638-x/2010004/article/11086-eng.pdf.

WHO Study Group on Female Genital Mutilation and Obstetric Outcome; Banks, E., et al. (2006). Female genital mutilation and obstetric outcome: WHO collaborative prospective study in six African countries. *Lancet, 367*(9525), 1835–1841.

World Health Organization. (2001). *The optimal duration of exclusive breastfeeding: Report of an expert consultation.* Retrieved from http://www.who.int/nutrition/publications/optimal_duration_of_exc_bfeeding_report_eng.pdf.

World Health Organization. (2008). *Fact sheet: Maternal mortality.* Retrieved from http://www.who.int/making_pregnancy_safer/events/2008/mdg5/factsheet_maternal_mortality.pdf.

World Health Organization and International Confederation of Midwives. (2007). *Promoting the health of mothers and newborns during birth and the postnatal period.* Geneva, Switzerland: World Health Organization Press.

Additional Resources

Canadian Association of Perinatal and Women's Health Nurses (CAPWHN): http://www.capwhn.ca

Canadian Nurses Association Certification Process: http://www.cna-nurses.ca/cna/nursing/certification/default_e.aspx

Canadian Perinatal Surveillance System: http://www.phac-aspc.gc.ca/rhs-ssg/index-eng.php

Global Health eLearning Centre: http://www.globalhealthlearning.org

Health Canada Family-Centred Maternity and Newborn Care: National Guidelines: http://www.phac-aspc.gc.ca/hp-ps/dca-dea/publications/fcm-smp/index-eng.php

Joanna Briggs Institute: http://joannabriggs.edu.au/

Public Health Agency of Canada Determinants of Health: http://www.phac-aspc.gc.ca/ph-sp/determinants/index-eng.php#determinants

Society of Obstetricians and Gynaecologists of Canada: http://www.sogc.org

Unit 1

2 The Family and Culture

Learning Objectives

On completion of this chapter, the reader will be able to:

- Explore and describe the variety of family forms encountered by perinatal nurses in Canada today.
- Use the collaborative woman- and family-centred health framework to identify factors influencing family health.
- Explore and describe theories developed as guides to family nursing in Canada.
- Describe how different lenses contribute to our understanding of family health promotion.
- Explore and discuss how culture, broadly defined, influences the experiences of childbearing women and their families.
- Describe what is meant by cultural competence and reflect on how this will influence nursing practice.
- Explore ways to provide culturally responsive perinatal nursing care.

Electronic Resources

Additional information related to the content in Chapter 2 can be found on

evolve the companion Web site at

http://evolve.elsevier.com/Canada/Perry/maternal/

- Examination Review Questions

The Family in Cultural and Community Context

In perinatal nursing, ***family*** is defined by the woman and her social support network. Childbearing women in Canada today are supported and nurtured by family members and friends. Conversely, many of these same women are also the primary caregivers and health gatekeepers for family members, including their partners, children, and parents, and sometimes for friends or other relatives. In this chapter we will explore a variety of family forms cross-culturally, including Aboriginal and immigrant families, gay and lesbian families, adoptive families, and families whose childbearing is aided by reproductive technologies. The current emphasis in working with families is on collaboration, capacity building, and health promotion.

The Family in Society

The social context for the family can be viewed in relation to social and demographic trends that define the population as a whole. The Canadian childbearing population has become increasingly diverse in terms of culture, ethnicity, socioeconomic status, and age. Currently, the majority of women of childbearing age are employed outside the home. More women are delaying childbearing until an older age. Many families are also isolated from the support of extended families (Health Canada, 2000). This diversity is projected to increase in the future.

Of particular concern in Canada are immigrant and refugee women. It is difficult to assess the vulnerability of newcomer parents, as each situation is different and the specific events related to immigration become the determinants of health. The main issues faced by immigrant and refugee women are isolation from society, differing cultural values and beliefs, and the inability of large numbers of immigrant and refugee women to speak English or French. All of these factors will influence a woman's access to health care.

Each family sets up boundaries between itself and society. People are conscious of the difference between "family members" and "outsiders," or people without kinship status. Some families isolate themselves from the outside community; others have a wide community network that they can turn to in times of stress. Although boundaries exist for every family, family members set up channels through which they interact with society.

Family Organization and Structure

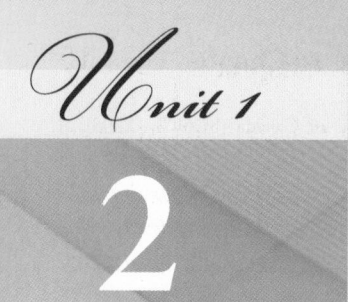

The woman defines her family and support system; she chooses who is included and excluded. Her definition of family may include one person or many different people. These may be the baby's father, siblings, and grandparents; the woman's partner (male or female); the baby's aunts and uncles; the woman's friends; and so on. Family-centred care treats the family as the unit of care delivery (Health Canada, 2000).

The **nuclear family** has long represented the traditional North American family in which male and female partners and their children live as an independent unit sharing roles, responsibilities, and economic resources (Fig. 2-1). In contemporary society, this nuclear family structure actually represents a relatively small number of families. The binuclear family is an alternate form of the traditional nuclear family arrangement resulting from divorce. Children of remarried parents then become members of both the maternal and paternal nuclear households. In joint custody, the court assigns divorcing parents equal rights to and responsibilities for the minor child or children.

Reconstituted or blended families (i.e., those formed as the result of divorce and remarriage) consist of unrelated family members (stepparents, stepchildren, and stepsiblings) who join together to create a new household.

Many nuclear families have other relatives living in the same household. These extended family members may be grandparents, aunts or uncles, or other people related by blood (Fig. 2-2). For some groups such as First Nations, Métis, and Inuit women, the family network is an important resource for promoting health and healing.

Lone-parent families comprise an unmarried biological or adoptive parent who may or may not be living with other adults. The lone-parent family may result from the loss of a spouse by death, divorce, separation, or desertion; from either a planned or unintended pregnancy; or from the adoption of a child by an unmarried woman or man. This family structure has become a common and acceptable choice in society, with Statistics Canada (2007) reporting that 26% of families with children are headed by a lone parent. Of the over 1.4 million lone-parent families, 20% are headed by men. This rate is growing twice as fast as that for women. However, this gender difference is significant because female-headed lone-parent families are more likely to have lower incomes and to experience poverty than male lone-parent families.

In Canada, the number of common-law families is increasing and now makes up 15.5% of families, whereas 20 years ago they made up only 7.2% (Statistics Canada, 2007). There are also an increasing number of lesbian and gay families who live together with or without children. Children in these families may be the offspring of previous heterosexual unions, conceived by one member of a lesbian couple through therapeutic insemination, or adopted.

Family Dynamics

Ideally, the family uses its resources to provide a safe, intimate, and nurturing environment that supports the biopsychosocial development of family members. The family provides for the nurturing of the newborn and the gradual socialization of the growing child. Children form their earliest and closest relationships with their parents or parenting persons; these affiliations continue throughout a lifetime. For better or worse, parent–child relationships influence self-worth and the ability to form later relationships. The family also influences the child's perceptions of the outside world. The family provides the growing child with an identity that possesses both a past and a sense of the future. Cultural beliefs, values, and rituals are passed from one generation to the next through the family.

Over time, the family develops protocols for problem solving, particularly those regarding important decisions such as having a baby, buying a house, or sending children to university. The criteria used in making decisions are based on family values and attitudes about the appropriateness of the behaviour and the moral, social, political, and economic events of society. The power to make critical decisions is given to a family member through tradition or negotiation. All families have strengths and the potential for growth. It is important for the nurse to identify those strengths and potential in order to facilitate the growth of the family (Black & Lobo, 2008).

Family Nursing

Use of the collaborative woman- and family-centred framework for perinatal nursing (Association of Women's Health, Obstetric and Neonatal Nurses [AWHONN], 2009) has brought greater understanding of how families need to be included in maternity care (see Box 1-1). Perinatal nurses'

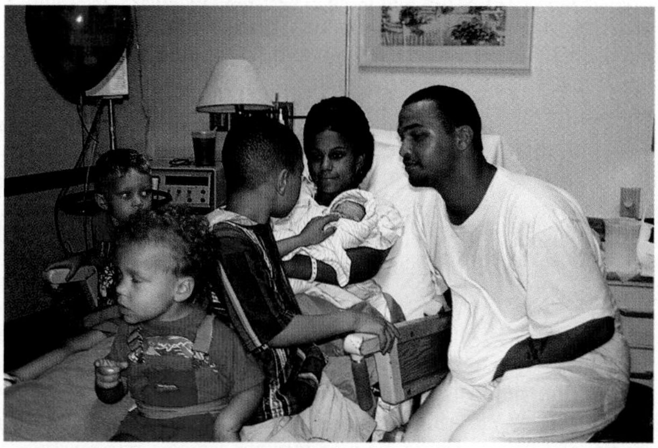

Fig. 2-1 Nuclear family. *(Marjorie Pyle, RNC, Lifecircle, Costa Mesa, CA.)*

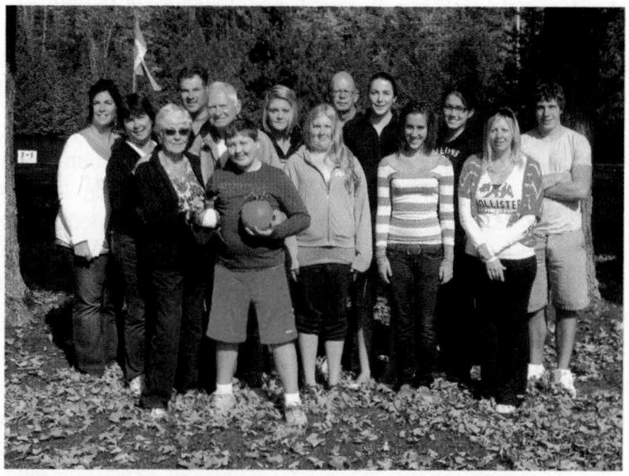

Fig. 2-2 Extended family. *(Courtesy Lisa Keenan-Lindsay.)*

commitment to working in partnership with families can enhance the health and well-being of the whole family. Thus nurses must become competent in working collaboratively with families in a variety of contexts and settings. Relationships between women, their families, and health care providers are based on mutual respect and trust. Such mutual respect and collaborative partnerships will help women give birth safely with power and dignity in a way that promotes the health of the whole family. As well, it is crucial that the woman and her family respect and trust nurses and other health care providers who will be providing care for her during times of vulnerability and change or transition (Health Canada, 2000).

The core concepts of woman- and family-centered care include the need for respect and safety, involvement and participation, information sharing and collaboration, and active involvement in decision-making processes (Cory, 2007). When treating the woman and family with respect and dignity, health care providers listen to and honour their perspectives and choices. They share information with families in ways that are positive, useful, timely, complete, and accurate. The family is supported in participating in their care and decision making at the level of their choice. Collaboration with women and their families in the development, implementation, and evaluation of policy and programs, facility design, professional education, and delivery of care by all involved is essential for providing family-centered care (Johnson et al., 2008).

Family Assessment

When selecting a family assessment framework, an appropriate model for a perinatal nurse is one that is health promoting rather than an illness-care model. The family can be assisted in fostering a healthy pregnancy, childbirth, and integration of the newborn into the family. Women experiencing perinatal health challenges or conditions of vulnerability (e.g., poverty) have additional needs that the nurse may need to address while also promoting the health of the childbearing family.

Theories as Guides to Understanding and Working With Families

A family theory can be used to describe families and how the family unit responds to events both within and outside the family. Each family theory makes certain assumptions about the family and has inherent strengths and limitations. Most nurses use a combination of theories in their work with families. A brief discussion of three theories used by nurses when working with families will be presented in the following sections, beginning with family systems theory. A brief synopsis of several other theories useful in working with families is included in Table 2-1.

Family Systems Theory

Among the caring disciplines, a systems approach to understanding the family has been used for many years. Many systems concepts are central to the delivery of holistic nursing care. These include recognition that changes occurring in one member affect the entire family and an appreciation that nurses who work with families also enter into a systemic relationship with them. This is especially true for nurses who provide perinatal nursing care in the community. Understanding how family members influence and interact with one another can help the nurse develop empathy with and respect for family strengths and different ways of functioning.

When applied to families, systems theory allows nurses to "view the family as a unit and thus focus on observing the interaction among family members rather than studying family members individually" (Wright & Leahey, 2005).

Table 2-1 Theories and Models Relevant to Family Nursing Practice

THEORY	SYNOPSIS OF THEORY
Family Life Cycle (Developmental) Theory (Carter & McGoldrick, 1999)	Families move through stages. The family life cycle is the context in which to examine the identity and development of the individual. Relationships among family members go through transitions. Although families have roles and functions, a family's main value is in relationships that are irreplaceable. The family involves different structures and cultures organized in various ways. Developmental stresses may disrupt the life cycle process.
Family Stress Theory (Boss, 2002)	This theory is concerned with ways families react to stressful events. Family stress can be studied within the internal and external contexts in which the family is living. The internal context involves elements that a family can change or control such as family structure, psychological defences, and philosophical values and beliefs. The external context consists of the time and place in which a particular family finds itself and over which the family has no control such as the culture of the larger society, the time in history, the economic state of society, the maturity of the individuals involved, the success of the family in coping with stressors, and genetic inheritance.
McGill Model of Nursing (Allen, 1997)	This model of situation-responsive nursing has a strength-based focus in clinical practice with families rather than a deficit approach. It identifies family strengths and resources, provides feedback about strengths, and assists the family to develop and elicit strengths and use resources. The McGill, or developmental health model, is particularly relevant for working with childbearing families, as pregnancy can be considered a "teachable moment" for promoting the health of the entire family.
The Collaborative Partnership approach (Gottlieb & Feeley, 2006)	This model builds upon the McGill Model of nursing and more fully develops a collaborative partnership approach to family nursing. A collaborative partnership is defined as "the pursuit of person-centred goals through a dynamic process that requires the active participation and agreement of all partners." Features of a collaborative partnership include mutual identification of and agreement on goals, sharing expertise and power, being respectful, accepting, and nonjudgemental and being open to learning together, learning to live with ambiguity, and being reflective and self-aware.

Within a systems framework, the individual takes on several roles as a unique and important person in his or her own system and as part of one or more subsystems within the larger family. For example, an individual may belong to one of several subsystems, such as a child subsystem or a parental subsystem. When considering more than one generation of a family, a married woman may belong to a parental subsystem in her own home and to a subsystem of children in relation to her own parents.

Wright and Leahy (2005) outlined the key characteristics of family systems theory:

- A family system is part of a larger suprasystem and is composed of many subsystems.
- The family as a whole is greater than the sum of its parts.
- A change in one family member affects all family members.
- The family is able to create a balance between change and stability.
- Family members' behaviours are best understood from a view of circular rather than linear causality.

Family systems theory encourages nurses to view individual family members as part of a larger family system that is influenced by and influencing others. Application of these concepts can guide assessment of and interventions for the family. For example, the childbearing family interacts as a system with many elements in the environmental suprasystem, including the health care community. The extent to which this suprasystem influences the family in matters such as prenatal care, childbirth education, and infant care depends on the permeability of the family's boundaries. A relatively closed family may want instructions only from others within the family, whereas a relatively open family may be more receptive to instructions from health care providers.

The Calgary Family Assessment Model

The Calgary Family Assessment Model (CFAM) is an example of a model that uses systems theory as well as other theories. Wright and Leahy (2005) described the CFAM as "an integrated, multidimensional framework based on the systems, cybernetics, communication, and change theoretical foundations and influenced by postmodernism and biology of cognition." The CFAM consists of three major categories: structural, developmental, and functional. There are several subcategories within each category. The three assessment categories and the many subcategories can be conceptualized as a branching diagram (Fig. 2-3). These categories and subcategories can be used to guide the assessment that will provide data to help the nurse better understand the family and formulate a plan of care.

A *family genogram*, which is a family tree format depicting relationships of family members over at least three generations (Fig. 2-4), provides valuable information about a family and can be placed in the nursing care plan for easy access by care providers. An *ecomap*, a graphic portrayal of social relationships of the patient and family, may also help the nurse understand the social environment of the family and identify support systems available to them (Fig. 2-5) (Rempel, Neufeld, & Kushner, 2007). Software is available to generate genograms and ecomaps (http://www.interpersonaluniverse.net).

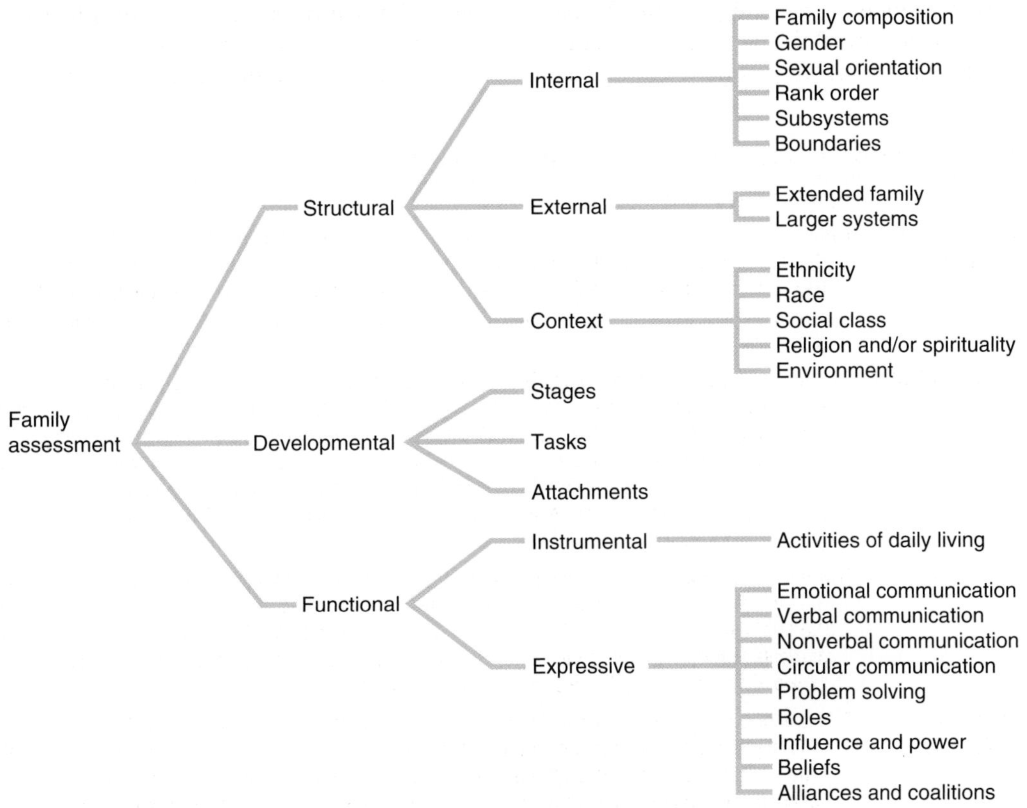

Fig. 2-3 Branching diagram of Calgary Family Assessment Model (CFAM). *(From Wright, L. [2005].* Nurses and families. *[4th ed.]. Philadelphia: FA Davis, with permission.)*

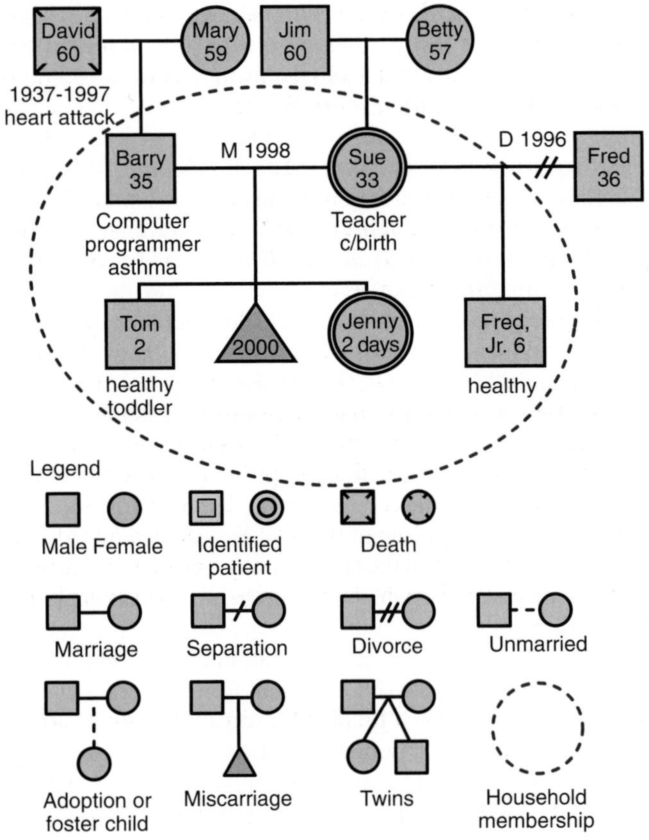

Fig. 2-4 Example of a family genogram.

Family Nursing as Relational Inquiry

Relational nursing challenges nursing practices based on structured assessment frameworks and proposes that nurses need to be "in relation" with women and family members, taking cues from the family and collaboratively identifying capacity and adversity patterns and building knowledge together for health promotion (Doane & Varcoe, 2005). It recognizes that families are socially located in historical, cultural, and environmental contexts and that these factors have a significant impact on family members' experiences of health and childbearing. Relational nursing moves beyond a health service provision approach toward one that recognizes the determinants of health and is more congruent with health promotion (Box 2-1).

This approach is understood as a process of inquiry, and it is this structure or process that forms the framework for thoughtful, interpretive, critical, and spiritual inquiry. Nurses learn together with women and family members about what matters most to them, about family strengths and health challenges, and about how to work toward better health for the childbearing woman, her baby, and her family.

This approach also considers the family from four lenses or perspectives: (1) a phenomenological lens, (2) a sociopolitical lens, (3) a spiritual lens, and (4) a socioenvironmental health promotion perspective. The phenomenological lens cues the nurse to learn more about the woman's and family members' experiences of health, childbearing, and illness. How did her mother experience pregnancy and childbirth? What is meaningful and significant to the family? The sociopolitical lens attends to power and gender, class, **ethnic**, racial, and professional relationships. The spiritual lens reminds us that

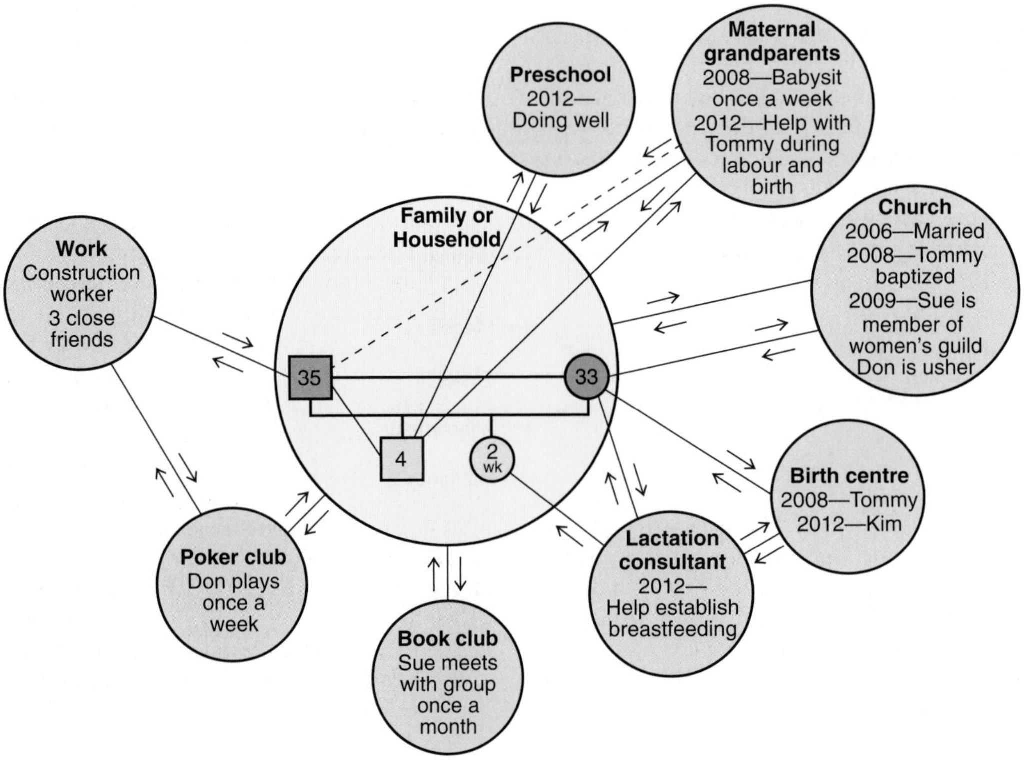

Fig. 2-5 Example of an ecomap. An ecomap describes social relationships and depicts available supports.

BOX 2-1 Relational Nursing Practice: Assessing and Intervening Processes

1. Entering into relation: Getting "in sync" with a family
2. Being in collaborative relation: Working together to assess and intervene
3. Inquiring into family health and healing experiences: What is meaningful and significant to the family?
4. Following the lead of families: Beginning from an unknowing stance, for example, one of curiosity and acceptance of diversity
5. Listening to and for: Listening by using the four lenses or perspectives described above.
6. Self-observation: Reflecting on how you are "in relation" with this particular family right now
7. Letting be and change: Creating the opportunity for the family to discover their own patterns, capacities, challenges, and contextual constraints as a foundation for change
8. Collaborative knowledge development: Drawing on both family and nursing knowledge
9. Pattern recognition: Identifying underlining patterns of experience that influence health and well-being and possibilities for change
10. Naming and supporting capacity: Building upon family strengths
11. Emancipatory action: Naming health inequities and working together to address structural inequalities (social justice lens)

(Adapted from Doane, G., & Varcoe, C. [2005]. *Family nursing as relational inquiry* [p. 228]. Philadelphia: Lippincott, Williams & Wilkins.)

childbearing has particular personal, cultural, and religious meanings and significance. A socioenvironmental perspective on health promotion is an understanding of health and health promotion that focuses on the family in their environmental context. It reminds perinatal nurses that nursing assessment and intervention are primarily about supporting women's and family choices and the capacity to live healthy, meaningful lives within their particular personal, physical or material, and social context.

Cultural Factors Related to Family Health

Cultural Context of the Family

Culture refers to the learned, shared, and transmitted values, beliefs, norms, and lifeways of a particular group that guides their thinking, decisions, and actions in patterned ways (Leininger, 1991). The culture of an individual is influenced by religion, environment, and historical events and plays a powerful role in the individual's behaviour and patterns of human interaction. Culture is not static; it is an ongoing process that influences people throughout their entire lives, from birth to death.

Cultural knowledge includes beliefs and values about each facet of life and is passed from one generation to the next. Cultural beliefs and traditions relate to food, language, religion, art, health and healing practices, kinship relationships, and all other aspects of community, family, and individual life. Culture also has been shown to have a direct effect on health behaviours. Values, attitudes, and beliefs that are culturally acquired may influence perceptions of illness as well as health care–seeking behaviour and responses to treatment. The impact of these influences must be assessed by health care professionals when providing health care and negotiating effective intervention strategies.

Many subcultures may be found within each culture. *Subculture* refers to a group existing within a larger cultural system that retains its own characteristics. A subculture may be an ethnic group or a group organized in other ways (such as a particular adolescent subculture). Each subculture holds rich and complex traditions, including health and social practices that have proven effective over time. These traditions vary from group to group. In a multicultural society, many groups can influence traditions and practices. As cultural groups come in contact with each other, varying degrees of acculturation may occur.

Multiculturalism in Canada

In 1971, Canada adopted multiculturalism as an official policy which confirmed the following:

- The value and dignity of all Canadians, regardless of their racial or ethnic origins, their language, or their religious affiliations
- The rights of First Nations, Métis, and Inuit peoples
- The status of Canada's two official languages: French and English

The Canadian government promotes multiculturalism by encouraging Canadians to participate in all aspects of life. Regardless of their cultural background, everyone can partake in social, cultural, economic, and political affairs. Everyone is equal and has a right to be heard. All people have the right to preserve their own ethnicity and faith in Canada.

Acculturation

Acculturation refers to changes that occur within one group or among several groups when people from different cultures come in contact with one another. People may retain some of their own culture while adopting some of the cultural practices of the dominant society. This familiarization among cultural groups results in some overt similarities in dress, lifestyle, and some mannerisms. Language patterns, food choices, and health practices in particular manifest differently among cultural groups. While acculturation can occur in Canada, the diversity and multiculturalism of people is still valued.

During times of family transitions such as childbearing or during crisis or illness, a woman may rely on old cultural patterns even after she has become acculturated in many ways. This is consistent with family developmental theory, which states that during times of stress, people revert to practices and behaviours that are most comfortable and familiar.

Cultural Diversity and Childbearing Families

Cultural diversity is increasing in Canada, and perinatal nurses will likely be working with families whose social class, sexual orientation, ethnicity, and cultural backgrounds differ from their own. At the same time, women interact with a variety of maternity care providers over the childbearing year, including physicians, nurses, midwives, labour companions or **doulas** (a person who provides support during labour), childbirth educators, and various others who help with physical or social needs. Culturally congruent care can only occur when the individual's and family's cultural values, expressions, or patterns regarding care are known and used appropriately and in meaningful ways by health care providers.

Collaborative woman- and family-centred maternity and newborn care is based on respect for pregnancy as a state of health and for childbirth as a normal physiological process. Among many cultures, birth is viewed as a completely normal process that can be managed with a minimum of involvement from health practitioners. The central objective of care for women, babies, and families is to maximize the probability of a healthy woman giving birth to a healthy baby. Health care providers share this aim and recognize each woman as an individual. For some women and families, however, the pregnancy may be unplanned or unwanted, and complications or adverse circumstances may occur. The birth itself may be complicated and the outcome unexpected. In these situations, collaborative woman- and family-centred care is even more important for supporting the family's unique needs.

Providing Culturally Competent Perinatal Nursing Care

The Canadian Nurses Association (CNA) (2010) has defined cultural competence in nursing as "the application of knowledge, skills, attitudes or personal attributes required by nurses to maximize respectful relationships with diverse populations of clients and co-workers." Values that underpin the provision of culturally competent care include respect, valuing difference, inclusivity, equity, and a commitment to providing culturally safe nursing care (Registered Nurses Association of Ontario [RNAO], 2007). *Cultural safety* is a newer term that was first used in New Zealand. The CNA (2010) defines cultural safety as "both a process and an outcome whose goal is to promote greater [health] equity."

Nursing care is delivered in multiple cultural contexts. These contexts include the cultures of the family, the nurse, and the health care system, as well as the larger culture of the society in which health care is delivered. If any of these cultural groups is excluded from the nurse's assessment and consideration, nursing care may fail to achieve its goals and may be culturally insensitive or unsafe.

In addition to issues of preserving and promoting human dignity, the development of cultural competence is of equal importance in terms of health outcomes. Nurses who relate effectively with women and families are better able to promote health and address conditions of vulnerability.

To provide culturally competent care, the nurse must assess the beliefs, values, and practices of women and their families. Women and their families can be asked about their expectations so that nurses can learn collaboratively with the particular woman and her family. It is also important for nurses to understand and value diversity and avoid stereotyping women and their families. Nurses should also consider all aspects of culture, including communication, space, time orientation, and family roles, when working with childbearing families.

Cultural Awareness

Nurses need to ask women questions about their hopes and expectations regarding childbearing, about their capacities, and about their needs for nursing assistance. Nurses can ask women about their place of birth (e.g., the country, rural or urban), about the length of time they have been in Canada, and about family and friends or their support network. Box 2-2 includes suggested questions to ask women when exploring their cultural expectations about childbearing.

Valuing Diversity and Avoiding Stereotyping

Nurses working with childbearing families should take care to avoid making stereotypic assumptions about any person based on appearance, sociocultural, or spiritual affiliations. Nurses should exercise sensitivity in working with every family, being careful to assess the ways in which they apply their own mixture of cultural traditions. Nurses need to reflect on their own beliefs, values, and practices (Box 2-3).

Communication

Communication is often the most challenging obstacle for nurses working with patients from diverse cultural groups. Communication is not merely the exchange of words. Instead, it involves (1) understanding the individual's language, including subtle variations in meaning and distinctive dialects; (2) appreciation of individual differences in interpersonal style; and (3) accurate interpretation of the volume of speech, as well as the meanings of touch and gestures. For example, members of some cultural groups tend to speak more loudly, with great emotion, and with vigorous and animated gestures when they are excited; this is true whether their excitement is related to positive or negative events or emotions. Therefore, it is important for the nurse to avoid rushing to judgement

BOX 2-2 Questions to Ask to Explore Cultural Expectations About Childbearing

1. What do you and your family believe that you should do to remain healthy during pregnancy?
2. What are the things you can or cannot do to improve your health and the health of your baby?
3. Do you have any special dietary needs or foods that you cannot eat?
4. Do you have beliefs about pregnancy, birthing, and the postpartum period that I need to know about?
5. Do you or your family have concerns or fears about hospitalization for childbirth?
6. Whom do you want with you during your labour?
7. What actions are important for you and your family to take after the baby's birth?
8. What do you and your family expect from the nurse(s) caring for you?
9. How will family members participate in your pregnancy, childbirth, and parenting?

BOX 2-3 Personal Reflection for Nurses and Maternity Care Providers

Recognize the influence of your own ethnicity and culture and their effects on your life.
Recognize the diversity of needs and experiences of those you serve.
Obtain details based on personal information actually given by the woman or family members rather than making assumptions.
Use simple language when discussing procedures.
Explore what is acceptable and suited to the woman for her care.
Involve family members with the consent of the patient.
Work out a mutually acceptable schedule of caring for the woman or newborn.

(Adapted from Best Start Resource Centre. [2009]. *Giving birth in a new land: Strategies for service providers working with newcomers.* Toronto: Author. Retrieved from http://www.beststart.org/resources/rep_health/Newcomer_%20Guide_Final.pdf)

regarding a patient's intent when the patient is speaking, especially in a language not understood by the nurse. In these situations it is critical that the nurse avoid instantaneous responses that may well be based on an incorrect interpretation of the patient's gestures and meaning. Instead, the nurse should withhold an interpretation of what has been communicated until it is possible to clarify the patient's intent. The nurse needs to enlist the assistance of a person who can help verify with the patient the true intent and meaning of the communication (see Critical Thinking Exercise).

CRITICAL THINKING EXERCISE

Culturally Competent Care in the Emergency Department

Arisha, a 37-year-old woman, accompanied by her 16-year-old son, Mahesh, is admitted to the emergency department (ED) with profuse vaginal bleeding. Arisha's primary language is Hindi, and she speaks very little English; Mahesh is fluent in Hindi and English. No health care providers present in the ED speak Hindi. The nurse assigned to care for Arisha must obtain a health history and perform an assessment. She wants to provide culturally competent care for Arisha.

1. Evidence—Is there sufficient evidence to determine what culturally competent nursing care consists of?
2. Assumptions—What assumptions can be made about culturally competent care and the role language plays in providing that care?
   a. How the nurse, who speaks no Hindi, might effectively communicate with Arisha
   b. How the nurse can obtain a health history with questions about vaginal bleeding, sexual activity, and pregnancy if Mahesh is the only person available who speaks Hindi
   c. How the nurse can provide culturally competent teaching
   d. What teaching materials and resources are appropriate; what questions are appropriate to gain information about sexual activity and the possibility of pregnancy
3. What implications and priorities for nursing care can be drawn at this time?
4. Are there alternative perspectives to your conclusions? How can you learn more?

Use of Interpreters

Inconsistencies between the language of family members and that of providers presents a significant barrier to effective health care. Because of the diversity of cultures and languages within the Canadian population, health care agencies are increasingly seeking the services of interpreters (of oral communication from one language to another) or translators (of written words from one language to another) to bridge these gaps and fulfill their obligation to provide culturally and linguistically appropriate health care (Box 2-4).

Finding the best possible interpreter in these circumstances is critically important. A number of personal attributes and qualifications contribute to an interpreter's potential to be effective. Ideally, interpreters should have the same native language and be of the same religion or have the same country of origin as the patient. Interpreters should have specific health-related language skills and experience and help bridge the language and cultural barriers between the patient and the health care provider. The person interpreting should be mature enough to be trusted with private information. It is not appropriate to use a child or another family member to interpret health care information. However, because the nature of nursing care is not always predictable and because nursing care provided in a home or community setting does not always allow expert, experienced, or mature adult interpreters, ideal interpretive services are sometimes impossible to find when they are needed. In crisis or emergency situations or when family members are experiencing extreme stress or emotional upset, it may be necessary to use family members as interpreters. If this situation occurs, the nurse must ensure that the patient is in agreement and comfortable with using the available interpreter to assist. Another alternative that has become more available in many settings is to access professional interpreters over the telephone.

When using an interpreter, the nurse needs to respect the family by creating an atmosphere of respect and privacy. Questions should be addressed to the woman and not to the interpreter. Even though an interpreter will of necessity be exposed to sensitive and privileged information about the family, the nurse should take care to ensure that confidentiality is maintained. A quiet location free from interruptions is the ideal place for interpretive services to take place. In addition, culturally and linguistically appropriate educational materials that are easy to read, with appropriate text and graphics, should be available to assist the woman and her family in understanding health care information. When using interpretive services, the nurse demonstrates respect for the woman and helps her maintain a sense of dignity by taking care to do all of the following:

- Respect the woman's wishes
- Involve her in the decision about who will be the most appropriate person to interpret under the circumstances

BOX 2-4 Working With an Interpreter

Step 1: Before the Interview

A. Outline your statements and questions. List the key pieces of information you want or need to know.
B. Learn something about the culture so that you can converse informally with the interpreter.

Step 2: Meeting With the Interpreter

A. Introduce yourself to the interpreter and converse informally. This is the time to find out how well he or she speaks English. No matter how proficient or what age the interpreter is, be respectful. Some ways to show respect are to ask a cultural question to acknowledge that you can learn from the interpreter or learn one word or phrase from the interpreter.
B. Emphasize that you would like to encourage the patient to ask questions if they have any concerns and feel comfortable doing so because some cultures consider asking questions to be inappropriate.
C. Make sure that the interpreter is comfortable with the technical terms you need to use. If not, take some time to explain them.

Step 3: During the Interview

A. Ask your questions and explain your statements (see Step 1) directly to the mother and maintain eye contact with her.
B. Make sure that the interpreter understands which parts of the interview are most important. You usually have limited time with the interpreter, and you want to have adequate time at the end for patient questions.
C. Try to get a "feel" for how much is "getting through." No matter what the language is, if in relating information to the patient the interpreter uses far fewer or far more words than you do, "something else" is going on.
D. Stop every now and then and ask the interpreter, "How is it going?" You may not get a totally accurate answer, but you will have emphasized to the interpreter your strong desire to focus on the task at hand. If there are language problems, (1) speak slowly, (2) use gestures (e.g., fingers to count or point to body parts), and (3) use pictures.
E. Ask the interpreter to elicit questions. This may be difficult, but it is worth the effort.
F. Identify cultural issues that may conflict with your requests or instructions.
G. Use the interpreter to give insight into possibilities for solutions.

Step 4: After the Interview

A. Speak to the interpreter and try to get an idea of what went well and what could be improved. This will help you to be more effective with this or another interpreter.
B. Make notes on what you learned for your future reference or to help a colleague.

Remember:

Your interview is a *collaboration* between you and the interpreter. Listen as well as speak.

Notes

1. Be sensitive to cultural and situational differences (e.g., an interview with someone from urban Germany will likely be different from an interview with someone from a transitional refugee camp).
2. This is not the time to pioneer new gender relations. Be aware that in some cultures it is difficult for a woman to talk about some topics with a husband or a father present.

(Courtesy Elizabeth Whalley, PhD, San Francisco State University.)

- Provide as much privacy as possible
- Use culturally appropriate learning aids

Personal Space

Cultural traditions define the appropriate personal space for various social interactions. Although the need for personal space varies from person to person and with the situation, the actual physical dimensions of comfort zones differ from culture to culture. Actions such as touching, placing the woman in proximity to others, taking away personal possessions, and making decisions for the woman can decrease personal security and heighten anxiety. Conversely, respecting the need for distance allows the woman to maintain control over personal space and support personal autonomy, thereby increasing her sense of security. For example, many Asian groups have reserved attitudes about physical contact, and touching a woman may create anxiety when health care is delivered. Nurses must touch patients, but they frequently do so without any awareness of the emotional distress they may be causing patients. It is important to ask permission before touching the woman or her newborn or children.

Time Orientation

Time orientation is a fundamental way in which culture affects health behaviours. People in various cultural groups may be relatively more oriented to past, present, or future. Those who focus on the past strive to maintain tradition or the status quo and have little motivation for formulating future goals. In contrast, individuals who focus primarily on the present neither plan for the future nor consider the experiences of the past. These individuals do not necessarily adhere to strict schedules and are often described as "living for the moment" or "marching to the beat of their own drummer." Individuals oriented toward the future maintain a focus on achieving long-term goals.

The time orientation of the childbearing family may affect nursing care. For example, talking to a family about bringing the infant to the clinic for follow-up examinations (events in the future) may be difficult for the family that is focused on the present concerns of day-to-day survival. Because a family with a future-oriented sense of time plans far in advance and thinks about the long-term consequences of present actions, they may be more likely to return as scheduled for follow-up visits. Despite the differences in time orientation, each family may be equally concerned for the well-being of its newborn.

Family Roles

Family roles involve the expectations and behaviours associated with a member's position in the family (e.g., mother, father, grandparent). Social class and cultural norms also affect these roles, with distinct expectations for men and women clearly determined by social norms. For example, culture may influence whether a man actively participates in pregnancy and childbirth, yet maternity care practitioners working in the Western health care system expect fathers to be involved. This can create a significant conflict between the nurse and the role expectations of very traditional Arab families, who usually view the birthing experience as a female affair. The way that health care practitioners facilitate such a family's care moulds the family's experience and perception of the Western health care system.

Cultural Practices and Nursing Interventions

In perinatal nursing, the nurse supports and nurtures beliefs that promote health, including those related to physical or emotional adaptation to childbearing. However, if certain practices might be harmful, the nurse should carefully explore them with the woman and suggest modifications that reduce harm and promote family health.

Table 2-2 provides examples of some cultural beliefs and practices surrounding childbearing. Rather than identifying particular cultural or ethnic groups, this table has been organized in a way that invites exploration of traditional beliefs and health practices and offers some strategies for nurses. These strategies aim to help nurses and other maternity care providers view these practices from a patient-centred perspective, while taking into account Canadian practices and regulations.

In using Table 2-2 as a guide, nurses should exercise sensitivity in working with every family, being careful to assess the ways in which they adopt and adapt their own mixture of cultural traditions. Nurses are also reminded to reflect on the ways in which their own cultural practices (including the culture of nursing) may be interpreted by women and family members. Nurses may not agree with all cultural practices, but it is important to respect the woman's decisions. Perinatal nurses need to listen to the stories that women and family members tell them about their culture, their childbearing experiences, and their needs.

Table 2-2 Cultural Practices and Successful Strategies During Childbearing and Parenting

STAGE	STRATEGIES
Pregnancy	
• In some cultures, the announcement of the pregnancy may be done in a specific manner (e.g., by a father or by the parents of the woman).	• Find out from the woman what her wishes are around the announcement of the pregnancy and respect these wishes.
• Rituals may be performed to protect mother and child (e.g., reading from a sacred text, not going out at night, covering her head, wearing an amulet, giving to charity).	• Begin by asking each woman about beliefs and practices around health and acknowledge these without judging.
• Parents may not have the social support they would have had in their home country.	• Highlight the benefits of building social support prior to the birth to reduce the risk of postpartum mood disorders and to facilitate breastfeeding. Show the woman specific ways of doing this through community, cultural, and religious groups, for example.
• In many cultures, women learn what they will need for pregnancy and childbirth through their mothers, sisters, and aunts.	• With the woman's permission, allow her partner, family, friends, and elders to accompany her to prenatal classes. • Respect the possibility that the partner may choose not to attend prenatal classes and that a family member will attend instead. • During the prenatal class, offer opportunities for participants to discuss their values and rituals related to pregnancy and birth as various topics come up. • Assist the participants in developing a birth and breastfeeding plan in class. • Clarify when the woman should come to hospital and what she should bring. • Ensure that a supportive environment is created in the prenatal classes to help women build a social network.
• Language may be a barrier for some newcomers.	• If possible, use prenatal educators from linguistic communities similar to those of patients.
• Pregnancy information may be obtained from elders (e.g., mother, mother-in-law).	• Collaborate with elders, friends, and relatives to educate the woman about the benefits of consistent medical check-ups. • Provide culturally appropriate, medically sound information about pregnancy, childbirth, and infant care.
• Many prenatal tests and the concept of regular prenatal appointments may be unknown to the pregnant woman.	• Explain the importance of prenatal care. • Explain the relevance of tests and make sure they are understood.

Continued

Table 2-2 Cultural Practices and Successful Strategies During Childbearing and Parenting—Cont'd

STAGE	STRATEGIES
• Women may have uncertainties regarding breastfeeding.	• Ask open-ended questions about the woman's beliefs, knowledge, and concerns about breastfeeding and make sure this information is in her files if it might have an impact on breastfeeding after the baby is born. • Give the woman information about where she can get help after the baby is born (breastfeeding clinic, lactation consultant, public health nurses, or breastfeeding peer mentor).
• The hospital may be a very unfamiliar setting to many newcomers. In many countries, home births are the norm.	• As with all expectant parents, a tour of the hospital is important to increase comfort levels. • Educate the woman about the birthing process and Canadian practices to avoid issues that may arise at the time of delivery concerning medications, episiotomy, newborn care, etc. • Inform the woman about the possibility of using a midwife for a home birth or a doula as a birth assistant in the hospital.
• Some women may avoid certain foods in pregnancy.	• Discuss nutrition with the woman, focusing on promoting a healthy pregnancy. Ensure that her diet is not deficient.
Labour and Birth	
• Some women may deliver in silence and others may moan, groan, or scream.	• Respect cultural practices displayed by the woman during the birthing process. Ask her what she feels like doing.
• Women may squat or sit to assist in the birthing process.	• Encourage the woman to use the most comfortable position for her during the birthing process.
• Some women might avoid pain-relieving medications such as epidurals and spinal medication.	• Explain the procedures with diagrams and models. • Suggest nonintrusive alternatives (e.g. warm towel on the back). • Ensure that the woman provides informed consent.
Postpartum	
• There may be specific rituals performed to welcome the newborn.	• Accommodate the rituals, if possible, keeping in mind that these rituals may be particularly important for couples who are isolated from their extended families and removed from their culture.
• In many religions, the outcome of the delivery (e.g., disability, Down syndrome, birth defect) is seen to be determined by God.	• These potential outcomes should be discussed during pregnancy. • Explain the short- and long-term consequences of the situation and the support options available. • Provide the family time to deal with the situation.
• In some cultures, female genital mutilation is a routine practice, involving the stitching of the inner layers of the labia minor or majora, the removal of the clitoris or other parts of the genitalia, or both.	• Educate yourself about the practice of female genital mutilation and the care required during childbirth.
• Women may refuse a Caesarean section.	• During pregnancy, educate the woman and her partner about the need for the procedure and the consequences of refusal. • Ensure informed consent at birth.
• Women may prefer same-gender service providers.	• Incorporate patient preferences in health-related decisions where possible and appropriate. • During pregnancy, let the woman know that it may not be possible to accommodate her preferences, depending on the staff on duty when she is admitted to the hospital.
• Women may expect nurses to do everything related to newborn care.	• During the prenatal stage, educate the woman about the roles and responsibilities of health care providers and other service providers in postpartum care. Encourage the involvement of family members in caregiving after the birth.
• The baby may sleep with the mother in bed.	• Educate the parents about safe sleeping guidelines.
• Personal hygiene practices may vary widely depending on the culture. Some women may not bathe or wash their hair or may bathe only once a week.	• Try to understand cultural hygiene practices and be understanding of a woman's preferences. • Explain the signs and symptoms of infection and the importance of contacting a health care provider if this occurs.

(Adapted from Best Start Resource Centre. [2009]. *Giving birth in a new land: Strategies for service providers working with newcomers.* Toronto: Author. Retrieved from http://www.beststart.org/resources/rep_health/Newcomer_%20Guide_Final.pdf.)

Integrating Cultural Competence With the Nursing Care Plan

In many cultures family members make most of the decisions for women; therefore, the central relationship between the nurse and the woman is mediated by the family. The nurse must recognize the cultural importance of the family in supporting the patient, in guiding decision making, and in preserving cultural integrity in the health care interaction.

Nursing Care Management

Assessment

When nurses develop plans of care for women and their families who are culturally different from themselves or from the dominant culture of the community, they should be certain to include an assessment that addresses psychosocial issues related to that diversity. No nursing care plan is complete without attention to nursing diagnoses that address cultural diversity issues.

Nursing Diagnoses

- *Decreased verbal communication and increased potential for misunderstanding related to*
  - — inability to speak or understand language
- *Coping, family, compromised related to*
  - — inability to obtain culturally appropriate health care
- *Health-seeking behaviours related to*
  - — keeping prenatal appointments
- *Powerlessness, risk for, related to*
  - — limited access to care for family members

Expected Outcomes

Examples of expected outcomes for perinatal patients are that the woman and family will do the following:

- Express (through an interpreter if necessary) understanding of health information and treatments
- Use support systems to cope effectively with problems (e.g., pregnancy complications, newborn complications or treatments)
- Perform procedures accurately, as evidenced by return demonstration
- Access financial assistance for care (if necessary)

Plan of Care and Implementation

The nursing plan of care is developed in collaboration with the woman and family on the basis of their available resources and health care needs.

Evaluation

Evaluation is based on promoting the best possible health for the woman, baby, and family. The plan is revised as necessary.

Key Points

- Contemporary Canadian society recognizes, accepts, and values diverse family forms.
- The family is a social network that acts as an important support system for its members.
- Family theories provide nurses with useful guidelines for working with childbearing families.
- Poverty and environmental factors, family resources and support systems, health challenges and responses to stress, and cultural and religious beliefs and practices are important factors influencing the health of the whole family.
- The beliefs and values of a culture are embedded in its economic, religious, kinship, and political structures and are reproduced through health and social practices.
- To provide quality care to women in their childbearing years and beyond, nurses should be aware of the cultural beliefs, values, and practices important to particular families.
- Perinatal nurses need to listen to the stories that women and family members tell them about their culture, their childbearing experiences, their resources, and their needs.

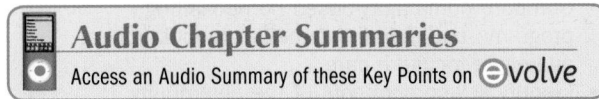

Audio Chapter Summaries

Access an Audio Summary of these Key Points on evolve

References

Allen, M. (1997). Comparative theories of the expanded role in nursing and implications for nursing practice: A working paper. *Nursing Papers*, *9*(2), 38–45.

Association of Women's Health, Obstetric and Neonatal Nurses (AWHONN). (2009). *Standards for professional perinatal nursing practice and certification in Canada* (2nd ed.). Washington, DC: Author.

Black, K., & Lobo, M. (2008). A conceptual review of family resilience factors. *Journal of Family Nursing*, *14*(1), 33–55. doi: 10.1177/1074840707312237

Boss, P. (2002). *Family stress management* (2nd ed.). Thousand Oaks, CA: Sage.

Canadian Nurses Association. (2010). *Position statement: Promoting cultural competence in nursing*. Ottawa: Author. Retrieved from http://www.cna-aiic.ca/CNA/documents/pdf/publications/PS114_Cultural_Competence_2010_e.pdf.

Carter, B., & McGoldrick, M. (1999). *The expanded family life cycle: Individual, family, and social perspectives* (3rd ed.). Boston: Allyn & Bacon.

Cory, J. (March 2007). *Women-centred care: A curriculum for health care providers*. Retrieved from http://www.bcwomens.ca/ForProfessionals/Resources/default.htm.

Doane, G., & Varcoe, C. (2005). *Family nursing as relational inquiry*. Philadelphia: Lippincott, Williams & Wilkins.

Gottlieb, L., & Feeley, N. (2006). *The collaborative partnership approach to care—A delicate balance*. Toronto: Mosby Elsevier.

Health Canada. (2000). *Family-centred maternity and newborn care: National guidelines*. Ottawa: Health Canada.

Johnson, C., et al. (2008). *Partnering with patients and families to design a patient- and family-centered health care system*. Bethesda, MD: Institute for Family-Centered Care.

Leininger, M. (1991). *Culture care diversity and universality: A theory of nursing*. New York: National League for Nursing.

Registered Nurses Association of Ontario (RNAO). (2007). *Embracing cultural diversity in health care: Developing cultural competence*. Toronto: Author.

Rempel, G., Neufeld, A., & Kushner, K. (2007). Interactive use of genograms and ecomaps in family caregiving research. *Journal of Family Nursing*, *13*(4), 403–419. doi: 10.1177/1074840707307917

Statistics Canada. (2007). *Canadian census*. Ottawa: Author.

Wright, L. M., & Leahey, M. (2005). *Nurses and families: A guide to family assessment and intervention* (4th ed.). Philadelphia: FA Davis.

Additional Resources

Best Start: http://www.beststart.org/

Canadian Nurses Association: http://www.cna-aiic.ca/CNA/default_e.aspx

Canadian Nurses Association & Aboriginal Nurses Association of Canada: Cultural Competence and Cultural Safety in Nursing Education: http://www.cna-nurses.ca/cna/documents/pdf/publications/First_Nations_Framework_e.pdf

Unit 1

3 Community Care

Learning Objectives

On completion of this chapter, the reader will be able to:

- Compare community-based home visiting programs and community health (population- or aggregate-focused) care.
- Identify key components of the community assessment process.
- List indicators of community health status and their relevance to perinatal health.
- Describe data sources and methods for obtaining information about community health status.
- Identify predisposing factors and characteristics of vulnerable populations within the context of the social determinants of health.
- Explore telephonic nursing care options in perinatal nursing in Canada.
- Describe how and when home care fits into the perinatal continuum of care.
- Discuss safety and infection control principles as they apply to the care of patients in their homes.
- Describe the nurse's role in maternal child home visiting.

Electronic Resources

Additional information related to the content in Chapter 3 can be found on

evolve the companion Web site at

http://evolve.elsevier.com/Canada/Perry/maternal/

- Examination Review Questions

Health care in Canada has evolved rapidly in recent years, with notable shifts in both the nature of health priorities and the ways in which health care is delivered to populations, families, and individuals. Today, greater emphasis is placed on health promotion and disease prevention than on the curative focus of past decades. This is in part a response to the skyrocketing costs of medical care and the realization that Canada's current health care system is unsustainable.

One major shift in health care delivery is the reduction in length of hospital stay, which reduces the overall cost to the Canadian health care system. Hospital stays after childbirth may be quite short, ranging from approximately 24 to 72 hours, depending on the type and nature of the delivery. By minimizing inpatient length of stay, nursing care has been transferred to home-based and community nursing care.

In Canada, maternal and early childhood survival rates are among the best in the world. This is in part due to relatively high levels of education and economic well-being and an effective health care system. With universal access to health services, most women in Canada receive high-quality care during their pregnancy. Also, an increasing number of women are engaging in healthy behaviours during pregnancy, and successful public health interventions, such as immunization and the folic acid fortification of foods, have been implemented (Canadian Perinatal Surveillance System [CPSS], 2008). However, there are emerging areas of concern, including increasing rates of maternal obesity, preterm birth, and Caesarean birth (see Chapter 1).

It is important to recognize that Canada does have vulnerable populations who face significant disparities. There are many women and children in this country who do not have ideal perinatal outcomes and who face significant health risks and considerable challenges. Rates of adverse pregnancy outcomes, including preterm birth and especially **intrauterine growth restriction,** generally rise with greater socioeconomic disadvantage. During pregnancy, women with low socioeconomic status are more likely to face stressful life events and chronic stressors and experience low gestational-weight gain. They are also less likely to initiate early prenatal care. All of these factors can translate into poor pregnancy outcomes. Poor fetal development is associated with many chronic diseases in later life (Wilkinson and Marmot, 2003). These disadvantaged groups also face a higher risk of maternal death (CPSS, 2008).

The high burden of illness responsible for premature loss of life arises in large part from the conditions in which people are born, grow, live, work, and age (World Health Organization [WHO], 2008). These social determinants of health (see Box 1-3) have a significant effect on health outcomes and influence a wide range of diseases. Compared to people with higher income, people with lower income have a shorter life expectancy, a higher risk of exposure to poor living and working conditions, and higher mortality rates. A higher income leads to better health—not only because it leads to the ability to buy adequate food, housing, and other necessities but also because it leads to more choices and a feeling of control over one's life (Townson, 1999).

Among vulnerable populations are the First Nations, Inuit, and Métis peoples, who face higher risks of adverse pregnancy and poor infant health outcomes. The CPSS (2008) reported that the increased infant death, preterm birth, and large-for-gestational-age rates among First Nations, Inuit, and Métis infants compared with those of non–First Nations infants were independent of neighbourhood socioeconomic status. Clearly, there are subpopulations living in Canada who experience significant health inequities. Other vulnerable populations include women with mental health issues, women working in the sex-trade industry, pregnant and parenting adolescents, as well as women whose newborn has been taken into custody by child protection services. The offspring of women belonging to these populations are also at increased risk for poor outcomes. Many of these poor outcomes are preventable through access to prenatal care and use of preventive health practices; clearly, comprehensive, community-based care that is culturally relevant and accessible for all mothers, infants, and families is needed. In the community, health care services range from individual care to group and community services and from primary prevention to tertiary care. Such services also include home visiting.

In community-based health care settings, both the aggregate (group of people who have shared characteristics) and the population become the focus of intervention. Health care providers are required to not only collaborate in order to determine health priorities for communities but also develop successful plans of care to be delivered in the health clinic, the community health centre, or the patient's home. Community-based health care, including public health services, is often under-resourced. Thus it is sometimes difficult to fully compensate for the gaps in health care service that currently exist.

Changing demands on the community-based nurse have evolved out of these societal, economic, and health-related trends. Acuity of illness of home-care patients is far greater than in the past, requiring the community nurse to become more adept in maternal assessment, direct care, and health teaching. Assessment of the neonate requires knowledge of parameters for measuring the health of a newborn within the first days of life. Skill in assisting with breastfeeding is essential. Knowledge of an ever-widening array of diverse family traditions, beliefs, and expectations related to childbearing has become even more critical for the nurse to effectively facilitate the transition involved when a family moves through the stages of incorporating a new member into their family.

Community and family cannot be considered separately as they are intertwined in many ways. Furthermore, as population demographics change, nurses are assuming greater roles in assessing community health status and providing health promotion and disease prevention interventions across the perinatal health continuum. In Chapter 2, an overview of family and cultural theory and assessment was presented. In this chapter, the integration of community and nursing care in the home is discussed within the context of family-centred nursing in relation to the Canadian Perinatal Health Surveillance Program. Methods of community assessment and the specific perinatal health needs of vulnerable populations are also discussed.

Community Health Promotion

Best practices in community-based health initiatives involve a thorough understanding of a community's health needs and priorities, environmental makeup, power relationships, and available resources as well as participation of community leaders. Empowerment of people, organizations, and communities who are working together is necessary for lasting change (Cottrell, Girvan, & McKenzie, 2006). A community-based framework helps to bring together multiple perspectives and diverse community resources to address a specific health priority.

The emphasis on community-based health promotion has grown in recent years with the recognition that many health issues require the collaborative efforts of a diverse community network to achieve public-health goals (Cottrell et al., 2006). These efforts are particularly relevant in relation to maternal–newborn health, which is affected by multiple public-health issues: maternal smoking and alcohol use, maternal obesity, teen pregnancy, substance abuse, and the consequences of inadequate prenatal care.

Levels of Preventive Care

Population-based care involves prevention activities focused on target needs that are identified in the community assessment process. These levels of prevention provide a framework for nursing interventions. *Primary prevention* involves health promotion and disease prevention activities to decrease the occurrence of illness and enhance general health and quality of life. Primary prevention precedes disease or dysfunction and encourages individuals to achieve the optimal level of health possible. Examples of primary prevention include health education and counselling about healthy lifestyle behaviours, including those related to nutrition and exercise. Other examples are immunizations, injury prevention through the use of seat belts and safety helmets, and environmental modifications to improve air quality. Educational programs that teach sex practices that reduce risk or that convey the dangers of smoking and drug use are also examples of primary prevention.

Secondary prevention is aimed at early detection of a disease and prompts treatment to either cure the disease or slow its progression and prevent subsequent disability (Maurer & Smith, 2005). Screening programs to detect disease while persons are asymptomatic are the most frequent forms of secondary prevention. Examples of this level of prevention are community blood pressure and cholesterol screenings that identify persons at high risk for heart attack and stroke and facilitate early treatment. Another example is a Pap (Papanicolaou) test, which is used to screen women in order to detect premalignant and malignant cells on the cervix opening. If this condition is treated early, cervical cancer can be successfully prevented or cured. The goal of secondary prevention is to shorten disease duration and severity, thus enabling an individual to return to normal function as quickly as possible.

Tertiary prevention follows the occurrence of a defect or disability and is aimed at preventing disability through restoration of optimal functioning. Persons who have developed disease are provided with treatment and rehabilitation to prevent complications and further deterioration. Examples of tertiary prevention are early treatment and management of diabetes to reduce problems, and rehabilitation of persons after a stroke.

Because most women are healthy during pregnancy, maternal–newborn nursing emphasizes primary and secondary prevention activities regardless of where care is provided. Tertiary prevention is frequently the focus for the ill pregnant patient at home or in the hospital.

Assessing the Community

Community assessment is a complex but well-defined process through which the unique characteristics of the populations and their special needs are identified in order to plan and evaluate health services for the community as a whole. The purpose of this process is to identify direct service and advocacy needs of the targeted aggregate or group and to improve health for the community. Engaging the community and key stakeholders in the process serves to increase buy-in and ultimately leads to better outcomes for the proposed services.

In community health assessment, data are collected, analyzed, and used to educate and mobilize communities, develop priorities, garner resources, and plan actions to improve the health of the public. Many models and frameworks of community assessment are available, but the actual process often depends on the extent and nature of the assessment to be performed, the time and resources available, and the way in which the information is intended to be used. For examples of community assessment tools, see the Additional Resources section at the end of the chapter.

The community-asset mapping approach provides an overview of community attributes and strengths that may facilitate long-term change and improved quality of life for community residents. Community capacity involves looking at a community's ability to address social and health problems or to develop knowledge, systems, and resources that contribute to a community's health status. These approaches help to direct the health promotion process by identifying community priorities and areas of needed change. The public health nurse or community health nurse may assist with community capacity building by working with the community to develop skills in accessing resources, developing social networks, and learning from the experience of others (Canadian Public Health Agency [CPHA], 2010).

Data Collection and Sources of Community Health Data

Data collection is often the most time-consuming phase of the community assessment process, but it provides an important definition and description of the community. Measures of community health include access to care, level of provider services available, and other social and economic factors. Consideration of individual, interpersonal, community, organizational, and policy level data and the interaction of these factors are important in providing a comprehensive framework for community health promotion. A community assessment model (Fig. 3-1) is often used to provide a comprehensive guide to data collection.

The most critical community indicators of perinatal health relate to the following: access to care, maternal mortality, infant mortality, low birth weight (LBW), stillbirths, first-trimester prenatal care, and rates for other screening tests (CPSS, 2008). Nurses may use these indicators as a reflection of access, quality, and continuity of health care in a community. For women and infants, access to a consistent source of health care is critical. Not having a regular medical doctor is associated with fewer health care visits with general practitioners and specialists who can play a role in screening and treating medical conditions early (Statistics Canada, 2010a). Over the past decade, the percentage of Canadians who report having a family doctor has declined slightly, although remote areas in Canada have the lowest numbers of people with family doctors. In 2008, only 38% of residents of the Northwest Territories said that they had a family doctor, whereas in Nunavut, less than 15% reported having a regular physician (Statistics Canada, 2010a). This is a significantly lower rate than that of the rest of the country, which ranges around 80%. When people do not have access to a primary health care provider they use walk-in clinics, hospital emergency departments, or community health centres.

Access to health care is also an important measure of community health. This indicator relates not only to the *availability* of health department services, hospitals, walk-in clinics, community health centres, or other sources of care but also to the accessibility of care. In many areas where facilities and providers are available, geographic and transportation barriers render the care inaccessible for certain populations. This is particularly true in rural areas or other remote locations. Other barriers to care should also be evaluated, including cultural and language barriers and lack of providers or specialty care. Local health departments provide varied levels and types of services, which are mandated by their respective provincial ministries of health. Depending on the level of funding received, they may or may not meet the needs of the populations they serve. For example, primary care services are limited in many areas, although health education is offered by most health departments.

Health departments at the municipal, regional, and provincial level are a valuable resource for annual reports of births

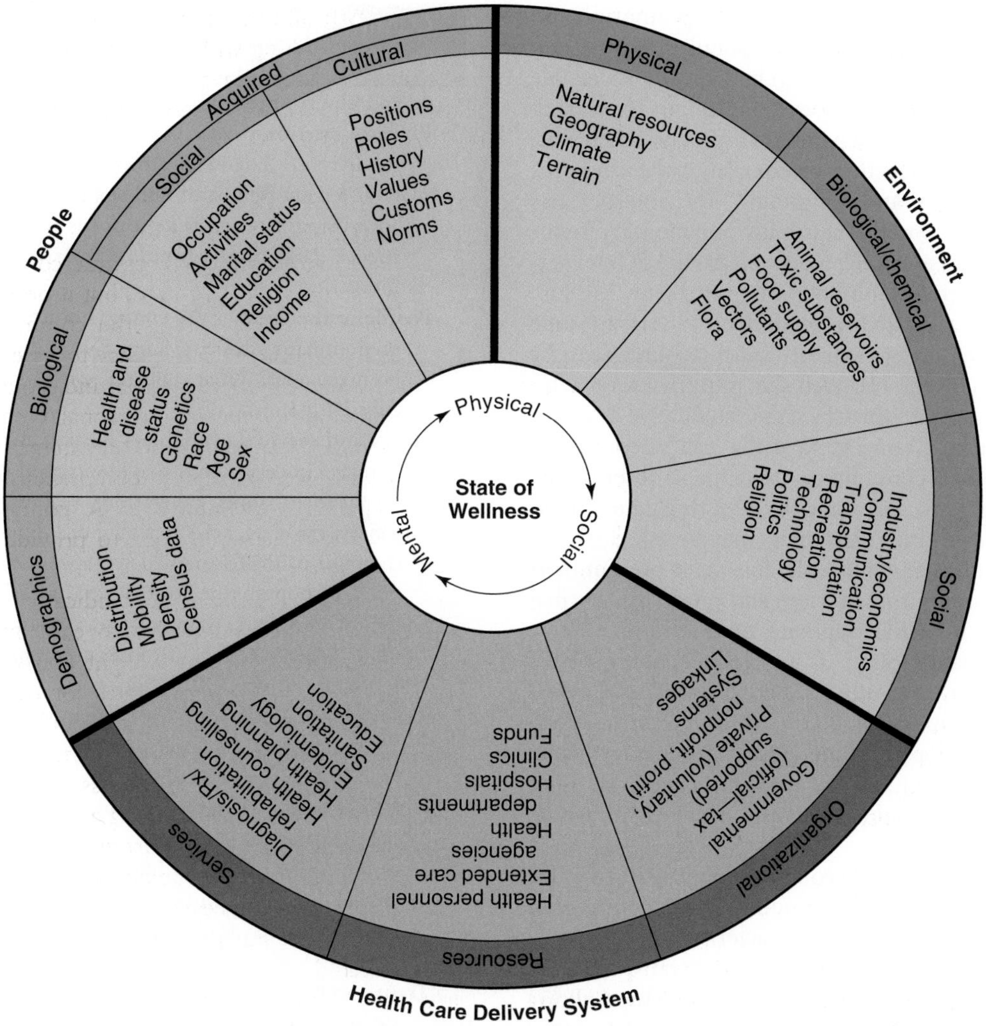

Fig. 3-1 Community health assessment wheel. *(From Clemen-Stone S. [2002]. Community assessment and diagnosis. In Clemen-Stone, S., McGuire, S., & Eigsti, D. [Eds]. [2002]. Comprehensive community health nursing: Family, aggregate, and community practice [6th ed.]. St. Louis: Mosby.)*

and deaths. Maternal and infant death rates are particularly important as they reflect health outcomes that may be preventable. Local health departments also compile extensive statistics about the birth complications, causes of death, and leading causes of morbidity and mortality for each age group. Local and provincial and territorial health data are compiled and reported through various agencies, including Health Canada (http://www.hc-sc.gc.ca), Statistics Canada (http://www.statcan.gc.ca), the Canadian Institute for Health Information (CIHI) (http://www.cihi.ca), and the Public Health Agency of Canada (PHAC) (http://www.phac-aspc.gc.ca). However, national data are only as accurate and reliable as the local data on which they are based; thus caution is needed in interpreting the data and applying them to specific population groups.

The Canadian government census provides data on population size, age ranges, sex, racial and ethnic distribution, socioeconomic status, educational level, employment, and housing characteristics. Summary data are available for most large metropolitan areas, arranged by postal code and census tract, which usually correspond to a neighbourhood comprising approximately 2000 to 8000 people. Assessment of individual census tracts within a community can help in identifying subpopulations or aggregates whose needs may differ from those of the larger community. For example, women at high risk for inadequate prenatal care according to age, race, and ethnic or cultural group may be readily identified, and outreach activities may be targeted appropriately.

Other sources of useful information are hospitals and voluntary health agencies. Community health resources include health care providers or administrators, government officials, religious leaders, and representatives of voluntary health agencies. Community or regional health councils exist in many areas, with oversight of specific health initiatives or programs for that region. These key informants often provide a unique perspective that may not be accessible through other sources. Community gatekeepers who are at the forefront of addressing the social and health care needs of the population are also critical links to population-specific health information.

The perinatal health nurse also may explore existing community health program reports, records of preventive health screenings, and other informal data. Established programs often provide reliable indicators of the health promotion and disease prevention characteristics of the population.

Professional publications are a rich and readily accessible source of information for all nurses. In addition to nursing and public health journals, behavioural and social science literature offers diverse perspectives on community health status for specific populations and subgroups. The Internet has increased the availability and accessibility of national, provincial, and local health data as well. However, the use of Internet-based resources for health information requires some caution, since data reliability and validity are difficult to verify. (Some guidelines for evaluation of Internet health resources can be found at the Health on the Net Web site: http://www.hon.ch.)

Data collection methods may be either qualitative or quantitative and may include visual surveys that can be completed by walking through a community, participant observation, interviews, focus groups, and analysis of existing data. Potential patients and health care consumers may be asked to participate in focus groups or community forums to present their views on needed community services and programs. Formal surveys conducted by mail, telephone, or face-to-face interviews can be a valuable source of information not available from national databases or other secondary sources. Several drawbacks exist with this method, however: surveys are generally expensive to develop and time-consuming to administer. In addition to the cost of such surveys, poor response rates often preclude a sufficiently representative response on which to base nursing interventions.

A walking survey is generally conducted by making a walk-through observation of the community (see Community Focus box), taking note of specific characteristics of the population, economic and social environment, transportation, health care services, and other resources. This method allows the nurse to collect subjective data and may facilitate other aspects of the assessment. Participant observation is another useful assessment method, in which the nurse actively participates in the community to understand the community more fully and to validate observations.

Finally, as part of the assessment process, nurses working in multiethnic and multicultural groups need an in-depth assessment of culturally based health behaviours.

Analysis and synthesis of data obtained during the assessment process help in generating a comprehensive picture of the community's health status, needs, and problem areas as well as its strengths and resources for addressing these concerns. The goals of this process are to assign priorities to community health needs and to develop a plan of action for correcting them. A comparison of community health data with provincial and national statistics may be useful in the identification of appropriate target populations and interventions to improve health outcomes.

COMMUNITY FOCUS

Community Walk-Through

As you observe the community, take note of the following:

Physical environment—Older neighbourhood or newer subdivision? Sidewalks, streets, and buildings in good or poor repair? Billboards and signs? What are they advertising? Are lawns kept up? Is there garbage in the streets? Parks or playgrounds? Parking lots? Empty lots? Industries?

People in the area—Old, young, homeless, children, predominant ethnicity, language? Is the population homogeneous? What signs do you see of different cultural groups?

Stores and services available—Restaurants: chain, local, ethnic? Grocery stores: neighbourhood or chain? Department stores, gas stations, real estate or insurance offices, travel agencies, pawn shops, liquor stores, discount or thrift stores, newspaper stands? Can people walk to shopping or do they need a car?

Social—Clubs, bars, fraternal organizations (e.g., Lion's Club, Canadian Legion), museums, community recreation centres?

Religious—Churches, synagogues, mosques? What denominations? Do you see evidence of their use other than on religious or holy days?

Health services—Drug stores, doctors' offices, clinics, dentists, mental health services, veterinarians, urgent care facilities, walk-in clinics, hospitals, shelters, nursing homes, home health agencies, public health services, local laboratory, traditional healers, (e.g., herbalists, palmists)?

Transportation—Cars, bus, taxi, subway, light rail, sidewalks, bicycle paths, access for disabled persons?

Education—Schools, before-school and after-school programs, child care, libraries, bookstores? What is the reputation of the school?

Government—What is the governance structure? Is there a mayor? City council? Are meetings open to the public? Are there signs of political activity (e.g., posters, campaign signs)?

Safety—How safe is the community? What is the crime rate? What types of crimes are committed? Are police visible? Is there a fire station? Are people comfortable walking in their neighbourhood after dark?

Evaluation of the community based on your observations—What is your impression of the community? Is the environment pleasing? Are services and transportation adequate? How difficult is it for residents to obtain needed services (i.e., how far do they have to travel)? Would you want to live in this community? Why or why not?

Vulnerable Populations in the Community

An assessment of population health includes a consideration of indicators related to diverse groups and **cultures**, particularly disenfranchised or "vulnerable" community members. Vulnerability in terms of health status and health outcomes may take many forms, including sociocultural, economic, and environmental risk factors that contribute to disparities in health. Health disparities are conditions that disproportionately affect certain racial, **ethnic**, or other groups. Low-income

Canadians are more likely to die earlier and to suffer more illnesses than Canadians with higher incomes, regardless of age, sex, race, and place of residence (Public Health Agency of Canada [PHAC], 2003). However, new immigrants often find themselves either underemployed or unemployed because of discrimination, complications around accreditation of foreign degrees, and social isolation.

Women

Women comprise 50.4% of the Canadian population (Statistics Canada, 2010b). Generally, women in Canada report good health, except those in areas where vulnerable populations are concentrated. Women's health experiences differ within and between social groups. For example, immigrant women; First Nations, Inuit, and Métis women; women in remote and rural areas; women with disabilities; women living with mental illness; women living in low-income situations; and lesbian, bisexual, and transgendered women have differential access to health services and differing health care needs (Statistics Canada, 2010b). Many women belonging to these vulnerable population groups struggle to find health care practitioners who are knowledgeable and respectful of their unique needs and who provide care that is culturally and socially sensitive.

One of the primary factors compromising women's health is lack of access to acceptable-quality health care. The barriers to care may take many forms: lack of health insurance if they are a recent immigrant, living in a medically underserved area, or an inability to obtain needed services, particularly basic services such as prenatal care. For example, some rural and remote areas have few physicians and midwives; women may have to travel hundreds of miles for this kind of care. Women often have lower incomes and less education than men and thus are considered at risk. Infant mortality is nearly two times higher for mothers without a high school education than for mothers with such education.

Immigrants and Refugees

Along with profound resilience and determination, refugees and immigrants have brought rich diversity to Canada in several important dimensions, including cultural heritage and customs, economic productivity, and enhanced national vitality. At the same time, multiple challenges accompany the dramatic influx of individuals and families from other countries.

Over the last decade there has been a steady increase in the number of immigrants moving to Canada. In 2001, 19% of all women living in Canada were born outside the country. Between 1991 and 2001, 1 million women arrived in Canada, constituting 34% of all foreign-born females (58% of the newcomer population were from Asia, including the Middle East; 7% were from Africa; 5% were from the Caribbean; and 6% were from Latin America). Approximately 74% of the newcomer population were visible minorities (Statistics Canada, 2006).

Immigrant women's rate of participation in the labour force is considerably lower than that of immigrant men and Canadian-born women. Women who are very recent immigrants—those who have been in the country five years or less—have the lowest employment rate, 49.1%. Women who have been in the country from five to ten years, and those who have been in Canada more than 10 years—called "established immigrants"—fare better, with employment rates of 56.3% and 50.3%, respectively (Statistics Canada, 2010b). Women born in Canada also have a lower employment rate then men born in Canada (Statistics Canada, 2010b).

Refugee status imposes a particular type of vulnerability on affected individuals and groups. Of primary significance are the precipitating factors by which people are displaced suddenly or forced to leave their country of origin: persecution, civil unrest, or war. Families are forced from their own homes to seek residence and employment elsewhere. Often these groups are extremely impoverished and face extreme physical and emotional stress when they arrive in Canada.

In general, refugees are more likely to live in poverty than are immigrants. Over time, health disparities that adversely affect health and well-being actually decline for the immigrant population as they become part of Canadian society. Many of the conditions or illnesses that immigrants and refugees acquire contribute to the persistence of disparities in their maternal and neonatal health outcomes.

Immigrants typically arrive in Canada with better health than that of the Canadian-born population. This is because immigrants are screened on medical and other health-related criteria before they are admitted to the country. However, as time passes, this "healthy immigrant effect" tends to diminish as their health status converges with that of the host population. Some medical problems may arise as immigrants age, as well as when they integrate and adopt behaviours that have negative health impacts. Other health problems may arise from the stress of immigration itself, which involves finding suitable employment and establishing a new social support network (Ng, Wilkins, Gendron, & Berthelot, 2005).

Some immigrant and refugee women may also have higher rates of chronic disease, including diabetes and acquired immune deficiency syndrome (AIDS). Women with underlying health conditions are at especially high risk for poor obstetric outcomes for themselves and their infants. They have high rates of preterm labour and gestational hypertension and often have intrauterine growth restriction, resulting in the birth of infants who are small for gestational age. These are the patients for whom the community health nurse may be providing care, and their needs are complex, demanding high levels of expertise and skill.

Adolescent Girls

While the adolescent population in Canada is generally considered healthy, this group of women is often vulnerable because of their high-risk behaviours. Adolescent girls, especially those from low-income or disrupted families, are more likely to engage in early sexual activity and other high-risk behaviours, with both immediate and long-term health consequences. The teenage pregnancy rate declined almost 37% in Canada from 1996 to 2006, compared to a drop of 25% in the United States (Dryburgh, 2007). Young women who are feeling optimistic about their futures tend to delay childbearing. Declining teen pregnancy rates for Canada in general are indicative of better sexual and reproductive health among young women. This decline in teen pregnancy can be attributed largely to more sexually active young people using reliable contraception such as condoms and birth control pills (Dryburgh, 2007). The incidence of **sexually transmitted infections** (STIs), primarily chlamydia and gonorrhea, is on the rise in Canada, with the highest rates occurring in adolescents and young adult females (PHAC, 2010) (see Chapter 6).

Adolescent health is another broad target area for community health promotion efforts, including health education and policy initiatives. Because adolescents often fail to perceive their own vulnerability, they need help navigating a complex environment and dealing with risk behaviours through preventive strategies that enhance decision making and increase protective factors.

Older Women

Women aged 65 and over constitute one of the fastest growing segments of the female population in Canada. In 2004, there were an estimated 2.3 million senior women, up 26% from 1991 and 72% from 1981. The growth rate in the number of older adult women has been twice that for women under the age of 65 over the course of the past couple of decades (Statistics Canada, 2006). In addition, women now predominate in the ranks of Canadian older adults, in large part because the life expectancy of women has risen more rapidly than that of men during most of the last century (Statistics Canada, 2006).

While most older women report that their overall health is relatively good, almost all have a chronic health condition as diagnosed by a health care professional. Arthritis or rheumatism and high blood pressure are the most common chronic health problems reported by older women. However, there are a great deal of preventive interventions that are effective in delaying or controlling age-related changes. Improving self-management activities such as diet and exercise are important health promotion elements for this population.

The share of the female population accounted for by older adult women is expected to continue to rise during the next several decades. Statistics Canada has projected that by 2016, 18% of all women will be aged 65 and over and by 2041, 27% of all women will be seniors. As well, the fact that women make up such a disproportionate share of the very oldest segments of the population has major implications. They tend to be the most vulnerable to serious health problems and the most likely to experience socioeconomic difficulties (Statistics Canada, 2006).

Homeless Women

Homelessness among women is an increasing social and health issue in Canada. Homeless women comprise a growing population that is at high risk for chronic and infectious diseases and premature death (Plumb, 2000). While both homeless women and men experience similar health problems, homeless women have distinct characteristics, vulnerabilities, and treatment needs. For instance, they may have a history of physical, sexual, or emotional abuse (Ontario Women's Health Council, 2002). Homeless women may also be pregnant or have young children in their custody. Some of the health issues of particular significance to this group of women include access to birth control, prenatal care, breast and cervical cancer screening, and sexually transmitted infections. Homeless women are also disproportionately represented among those with mental health problems and substance use disorders (Ontario Women's Health Council, 2002). Poverty is the primary cause of homelessness. Low-income rates are more prevalent among certain subgroups of women. First Nations, Métis and Inuit, and visible-minority women are nearly twice as likely as non–visible-minority women in Canada to have low incomes. Compared to two-parent families, lone mothers are almost five times more likely to have incomes that fall below the low income cut-off (LICOs) (Ontario Women's Health Council, 2002).

While homeless women are a heterogeneous group, they do share a number of similar features that may contribute to their overall poor health status. These include low income, unemployment, low levels of education, insufficient material resources, fear and mistrust of the health care system and of health care providers, and limited social support. Canada urgently needs to find new and innovative strategies that will address the barriers to health care that homeless women face both in cities and in more remote rural areas (Ontario Women's Health Council, 2002).

Although little is known about pregnancy in this population, about 20% of women do become pregnant while homeless. Pregnancy is linked to a whole host of health issues for homeless women. The homeless woman is at risk for pregnancy complications because of a lack of prenatal care, poor nutrition, stress, and exposure to violence. Homeless women face multiple barriers to prenatal care, including lack of transportation, distance to travel for care, and not having a health care provider. The unsafe environment and high-risk lifestyles often result in adverse perinatal outcomes.

Individuals With Low Literacy

Individuals and groups for whom English is a second language often lack the skills necessary to seek medical care and function adequately in the health care setting. Communication barriers may affect access to care, particularly in such areas as making appointments, applying for services, and obtaining transportation.

Health literacy involves a spectrum of abilities, ranging from reading an appointment slip to interpreting medication instructions. There is growing evidence of the effects of low health literacy on adult health status (http://www.hsph.harvard.edu/healthliteracy). Low health literacy may also be an independent contributor to a disproportionate disease burden among disadvantaged populations. Disparities in preventive care, early screening for cancer, and use of health care services, particularly among minority women, have also been linked to language barriers (Jacobs et al., 2005).

As Canada continues to become increasingly multicultural, nurses will be required to interact with non–English-speaking groups or those with limited health literacy. Consequently, health literacy must be viewed as a component of culturally and linguistically competent care. These skills must be assessed routinely in order to recognize a problem and accommodate patients with limited literacy skills.

Implications for Nursing

Working in the community or in the home with the full spectrum of family organizational styles, vulnerable populations, and cultural groups presents challenges for the nurse. Whether nursing care is focused on women and their newborns or on treatment and prevention of other health conditions in women, such as communicable diseases and STIs, nurses must exhibit a high degree of professionalism. Cultural sensitivity, compassion, and a critical awareness of family dynamics and social stressors that affect health-related decision making are critical components in developing an effective plan of care.

Successful health promotion among immigrant families depends on the resources, benefits, and policies that ensure their healthy development and successful social adjustment. Culturally competent health care and involvement of the immigrant community in health care programs are recommended strategies for improving the access to and effectiveness of health care for this population.

Nurses working with homeless women and families are challenged to locate these patients on a regular basis and to establish a therapeutic relationship with them. Health care providers may lack sufficient knowledge and sensitivity around the circumstances and special needs of this population and may inadvertently provide ineffective care. Many homeless women delay seeking health care or avoid it altogether because of having previous negative encounters with and lack of trust in health care providers (Ontario Women's Health Council, 2002).

Case management is recommended for coordinating the services and disciplines that may be involved in meeting the complex needs of these families. Whenever possible, general screening and preventive services must be provided when the woman seeks treatment as this may be the only opportunity to provide health information and intervention. Building on existing coping strategies and strengths, the health care provider can help the woman and her family to reconnect with a social support system. Nurses also have an important role in advocating for funding to support homeless health services and to improve access to preventive care for all homeless populations.

Home Care in the Community

In the current health care system, home care is an important component of health care delivery along the perinatal continuum of care (Fig. 3-2). The growing demand for home care is based on several factors:

- Interest in family birthing alternatives
- Shortened hospital stays
- New technologies that facilitate home-based assessments and treatments

As health care costs continue to rise, Canada is faced with the challenge of providing safe and effective perinatal care that is innovative and cost-effective and meets the expectations of an increasingly more demanding and educated public. With the shorter length of hospital stay after delivery, women and their babies are often discharged home before they are successfully breastfeeding, before they have mastered basic baby care activities, and without sufficient supports at home. Public health departments and community agencies across the country must try to meet the needs of these new families.

Communication and Technology Applications

As maternity care continues to consist of frequent and brief contacts with health care providers during the prenatal and **postpartum** periods, services that link maternity patients throughout the perinatal continuum of care have assumed greater importance. These services include telephonic nursing assessments, discharge planning, specialized education programs, parent support groups, home visiting programs, and nurse advice lines. Most health departments across the country offer phone lines to provide parents with support and education about pregnancy, breastfeeding, and parenting.

Telephonic nursing care through services such as nurse advice lines and telephonic nursing assessments is a valuable

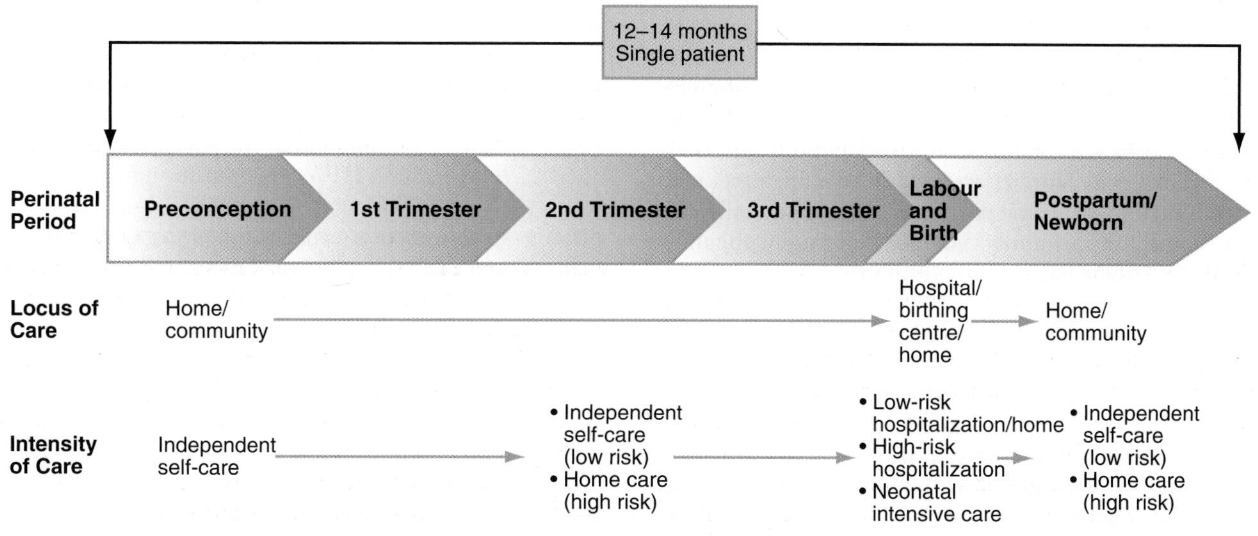

Fig. 3-2 Perinatal continuum of care.

means of managing health care problems and bridging the gaps between acute, outpatient, and home care services. Nursing care that occurs by telephone is interactive and responsive to immediate health care questions about particular health care needs. Warm lines are telephone lines offered as a community service to provide new parents with support, encouragement, and basic parenting education. Telephonic nursing assessments, or nurse consultation, assessment, and health education that take place during a telephone conversation, can be added to the plan of care if the patient requires a referral to a home visiting program. Telephonic nursing assessments are commonly used after a postpartum home care visit to follow up with a patient to assess if there has been an improvement or change in condition. This might include reassessing a woman's knowledge about the signs and symptoms of adequate hydration in breastfeeding or inquiring how the breastfeeding is going with a sleepy baby.

Maternal–Child Services in the Community

In Canada, public health and community health nurses provide most of the home visiting for childbearing families. Public-health early-child home visiting programs have been delivered free of charge for many years in every province and territory in Canada. All programs are voluntary, and parents can decide whether they want to participate in the program. Referrals are received from many sources: perinatal nurses, obstetricians, family doctors, midwives, childbirth educators, and individual parents. Individual health departments may provide an array of other services for the childbearing family. These may include childbirth education classes, breastfeeding clinics, mom and baby groups, postnatal mood disorder support services, and immunization clinics. Ideally, the public health nurse will begin to visit the family prior to the birth of the new baby to facilitate teaching about pregnancy, childbirth, and the transition to parenting. The nurse can assist families in preparation for childbirth and in arranging other community support services if needed.

Across the country, each home visiting program is slightly different. Many home visiting programs offer telephone support as well as home visiting, whereas others only provide service after the birth of the baby. In this case, the public health nurse will call the patient after she is home from the hospital to answer any urgent questions she might have and to do an assessment of how the new mother and baby are doing. If the program has sufficient funding to visit all new mothers, the nurse will arrange a time to visit mom and baby. Otherwise, only those families assessed to be at high risk will be offered a home visit. Some programs offer additional visiting by lay home visitors (family visitors), who work with families on a more frequent basis to provide more in-depth teaching and support.

These programs have received renewed attention because of their impact on healthy child development outcomes. In order to identify the provincial/territorial similarities and differences in home visiting programs in Canada and to illuminate the evidence that early child home visiting improves the health equity and health outcomes of children and their families, the National Collaborating Centre for the Determinants of Health (NCCDH) conducted a comprehensive, pan-Canadian environmental scan of these programs. A detailed description of the many different programs and services offered in each province and territory can be found at http://www.nccdh.ca/supportfiles/TK_KeyFactsGlossaryJune25_v6.pdf.

The range of services offered by these home visiting programs may include some or all of the following:

- Pregnancy teaching and childbirth preparation
- Taking care of the pregnant woman during pregnancy and after the baby is born
- Preparing for the baby
- Breastfeeding information and support
- Assessment and care of the newborn and mother
- Anticipatory guidance for parents
- Resources in the community
- Transitioning to solid foods
- What to expect as the child grows and develops
- How to keep children safe

Home visiting has many advantages for the new mother. She is able to stay at home and rest, and vulnerable neonates are not exposed to the weather or external sources of infection. She receives one-to-one supportive teaching and counselling free of charge and tailored specifically to her needs. The advantage for the nurse is that he or she can observe and interact with family members in their most natural and secure environment. Adequacy of resources and safety factors can be assessed. Teaching can be tailored to the actual home conditions, and other family members can be included. Some home visiting programs follow families until the babies are three years of age.

Childbirth Education Classes

Most health departments across the country offer some form of prenatal education for the public. This is often the first exposure a family has to the health department. Given that one of the key mandates of public health is to promote, protect, and preserve the health of the population, pregnancy is a very opportune time to engage families. Each health unit tailors their childbirth education program to meet the needs of their own community, subject to available funds.

Childbirth education classes provide important information for childbearing families. The prenatal curriculum may include many topics (Box 3-1).

Although traditional face-to-face classes are often the preferred mode of learning, many couples are unable to commit to attending regular classes because of conflicting work schedules and long commutes. Other couples prefer to obtain their

BOX 3-1 Childbirth Education Topics

- Physical and emotional changes during pregnancy
- Breastfeeding
- Nutrition during pregnancy
- Working during pregnancy
- Breathing and relaxation
- Labour and birth
- Becoming a dad
- Transition to parenting and new baby care

prenatal information online. To meet the needs of today's childbearing families, many health departments have begun to offer eLearning prenatal classes. This is an excellent way of reaching pregnant women and their partners who would not have attended face-to-face prenatal classes.

Prenatal classes may be offered by other providers within the community (see Community Focus box). Hospitals often offer classes for the patients delivering at their facility. There is usually a cost associated with these and other private classes. Many health departments offer free or fee-reduced classes.

Nursing Care Management

Home Visiting

The public health or community health nurse will review the home visiting referral, screening tool results, record of birth, available clinical data, demographic information, and any other relevant information and then set up the visit with the patient. During the telephone call to arrange a mutually convenient visiting time, the nurse will determine the goals of the visit. The nurse needs to review relevant policies and procedures, professional literature about any potential diagnosis, and community resources as part of the previsit preparation work (Box 3-2).

Before going on a home visit, the nurse will contact the woman in order to make necessary arrangements and obtain detailed instructions on the location of the home. In addition to establishing a convenient time to visit and the exact directions, through the initial contact by telephone the nurse is also setting the stage for the first home visit.

COMMUNITY FOCUS

Availability of Maternal Child Services in Your Community

To understand what services are available in your community, a good place to start is the Internet. Use the Internet to identify where the closest health department is located. Research what services are offered to childbearing families.

- How many other agencies provide services for childbearing families? Are they located in the area? What services do they offer?
- Are there registered nurses employed there? If not, what are the credentials of the people providing the services? Are there midwives and doulas also available?
- Is service provided in more than just English? If so, in what languages? Are interpreters available if needed?
- Do the agencies ever accept referrals for patients who cannot pay? Are there any bursaries or provisions made for families who cannot pay?
- Is there a maternal child home visiting program available in the community?

Based on the information you have gathered, are there adequate and appropriate services for pregnant women and their families in your area? If not, is there a postpartum care clinic where new mothers can access support for breastfeeding, hearing and dental screening, immunizations, well-baby care, and other related services?

During this contact, the nurse should identify himself or herself by name, title, and agency. He or she can then begin to build rapport with the patient. The nurse will convey the purpose of the home visits, if necessary. The nurse should briefly explain what will occur during the visit and approximately how long the visit will last. The woman should be asked to restrain any pets that may be present during the visit.

First Home Visit

Making the first home visit can be stressful for the nurse and the woman. The home visiting nurse is faced with an unknown environment controlled by the woman and her family. The woman and her family can also experience feelings about the unknown, such as anxiety about the way the nurse will treat them or what the nurse will do during the visit. The challenge for the public health or community health nurse is to establish a nurse–patient relationship and provide the prescribed services within the time provided for the initial home visit. One of the most important roles of the home nurse is modelling health-related behaviours for the patient and others who are in the home during the visit.

During the first visit, after introductions have been made, the nurse will complete extensive assessment documentation with the patient. If the nurse needs to consult with the patient's physician or other health care providers, a consent form will need to be signed by the patient. All patients have the right to participate actively in their plan of care. Explanation of these patient rights and responsibilities should begin the discussion about the nurse and patient roles during this initial visit.

Assessment

The primary goals of the assessment phase are to develop a trusting relationship and collect data by various methods to obtain a comprehensive patient profile (see Nursing Process box). It may not be feasible or appropriate to collect in-depth information about all areas of assessment during the first visit. However, in many instances the nurse may be limited to one visit and must obtain information pertinent to the current situation in that hour.

Establishing a trusting relationship begins with the previsit telephone call. An interview style that reflects sensitivity, conveys a nonjudgemental, accepting attitude, and shows respect for the woman's rights facilitates the development of that trusting relationship. A skillful interviewer avoids barriers to communication, such as false reassurance, advice-giving, excessive talking, and showing approval or disapproval. This nurse–patient relationship will continue to develop over the course of the home visits.

The nurse is a guest in the woman's home and should show respect for her and her belongings. Some adaptation of the home visit schedule may need to be made if numerous distractions interrupt a visit, such as caring for the needs of small children. The nurse may ask to have the volume of the television reduced or suggest moving to another room where it is more quiet and private.

Plan of Care and Implementation

The nursing plan of care is developed in collaboration with the patient, based on the health care and learning needs of the individual. Home visiting nurses work from a standard care plan and make adjustments in order to meet the needs of each

BOX 3-2 Protocol for Maternal–Child Home Visits

Previsit Interventions

1. Contact the family to arrange details for a home visit.
   a. Identify self, credentials, and role of the public health or community health nurse.
   b. Review the purpose of the home visit.
   c. Schedule a convenient time for the visit.
   d. Confirm address and route to the family home.
2. Review and clarify appropriate data.
   a. Review all available assessment data for the mother and fetus or infant (i.e., referral forms, hospital discharge summaries, family-identified learning needs).
   b. Review records of any previous nursing contacts.
   c. Contact other professional caregivers as necessary to clarify data (e.g., physician, midwife, nurse, referring source).
3. Identify community resources and teaching materials that are appropriate to meet needs already identified.
4. Plan the visit and prepare any resources required for the visit.

In-Home Interventions: Establishing a Relationship

1. Reintroduce self and establish purpose of the visit for the mother, infant, and family; offer the family an opportunity to clarify their expectations of contact.
2. Spend a brief time socially interacting with the family to become acquainted and establish a trusting relationship.

In-Home Interventions: Working With the Family

1. Conduct a systematic assessment of the mother and fetus or newborn to determine physiological adjustment and any existing complications.
2. Throughout the visit, collect data to assess the emotional adjustment of individual family members to pregnancy or birth and to lifestyle changes. Note evidence of family–newborn bonding and sibling rivalry; note relationships among the mother, father, children, and grandparents.
3. Determine adequacy of the support system.
   a. To what extent does someone help with cooking, cleaning, and other home management tasks?
   b. To what extent is help being provided in caring for the newborn and any other children?
   c. Are support persons encouraging the new mother to care for herself and get adequate rest?
4. Throughout the visit, observe the home environment for adequacy of resources:
   a. Space: privacy, safe play of children, sleeping
   b. Overall cleanliness and state of repair
   c. Number of steps the pregnant woman or new mother must climb
   d. Adequacy of cooking arrangements
   e. Adequacy of refrigeration and other food storage areas
   f. Adequacy of bathing, toilet, and laundry facilities
   g. Arrangements in home for newborn: sleeping, bathing, formula preparation (if needed), layette items, and diapers
5. Throughout the visit, observe the home environment for overall state of repair and existence of safety hazards:
   a. Storage of medications, household cleaners, and other substances hazardous to children
   b. Presence of peeling paint on furniture, walls, or pipes
   c. Factors that contribute to falls, such as dim lighting, broken steps, scatter rugs
   d. Presence of vermin
   e. Use of crib or playpen that fails to meet safety guidelines
   f. Existence of emergency plan in case of fire; fire alarm or extinguisher
6. Provide care to the mother, newborn, or both as per program protocol.
7. Provide teaching on the basis of previously identified needs.
8. Refer the family to appropriate community agencies or resources, such as telephone contact information lines and community support groups.
9. Ascertain that the woman knows potential problems to watch for and whom to call if they occur.

In-Home Interventions: Ending the Visit

1. Summarize the activities and main points of the visit.
2. Clarify future expectations, including scheduling of the next visit.
3. Review the teaching plan and highlight important points.
4. Provide information about reaching the nurse or public health department if needed before the next scheduled visit.

Postvisit Interventions

1. Document the visit thoroughly, using the required agency forms.
2. Initiate the plan of care on which the next encounter with the woman or family will be based.
3. Communicate appropriately to other staff assigned to care for the family. This may include follow-up with the family physician or other health care providers, if warranted.

individual patient. The frequency of the skilled nursing visit may vary with the individual plan of care, and often a family visitor or lay home visitor will be recommended if additional support is suggested.

Nursing Considerations

The provision of education during a home visit is a key component of the visit. This may include information about any specific high-risk condition(s), implications for pregnancy outcome, and measures for self-monitoring if the patient is pregnant. Verbal explanations should be supplemented with clearly written instructions if the patient has difficulty remembering or if there is a language barrier. Many written resources are available in multiple languages to facilitate the transfer of information and knowledge. General information to promote well-being, such as information about nutrition and common discomforts of pregnancy, should also be included if the visit is a prenatal visit.

The need for preparation for childbirth can be addressed by using books or DVDs and can be supplemented by

NURSING PROCESS: HOME VISIT

Assessment

The major areas of the assessment are demographics, medical history, general health history, medication history, sociocultural assessment, home and community environment, and physical assessment. Some of this information can be obtained from patient records sent to the health department from the hospital or from the previsit telephone assessment.

Social assessment includes information regarding the number in the family and the roles of each household member, which family members or individuals have taken on the roles of caregivers, and the woman's social support network (Box 3-3).

Nursing Diagnoses

Nursing diagnoses for maternal child care patients derived from data collected at the first home visit may include the following:

Lack of knowledge related to
- management of therapeutic regimen (e.g., post-Caesarean section, type 1 diabetes)
- newborn care and feeding
- jaundice

Compromised family coping related to
- newborn crying and irritability
- new immigrant status

Parenting difficulties related to
- maternal immaturity and lack of family support

Lack of diversional activity related to
- confinement at home

Planning

Examples of expected outcomes for maternal child patients include that the woman and family will do the following:

- Express understanding of learning
- Report decreased anxiety about performing basic care for the baby (diapering, breastfeeding, bathing)
- Use support systems to cope effectively with any problems (e.g., pregnancy complications, newborn complications or treatments)
- Perform procedures accurately, as evidenced by return demonstration
- Express decreased role strain

Interventions

Interventions are described in the text on pp. 37–40.

Evaluation

Evaluation is a continuous process through which the nurse must reassess the women's and family's condition or situation and any response to the interventions in relation to expected outcomes of care. In collaboration with the woman and family, the nurse then revises the nursing diagnoses and plan of care as necessary to meet mutually determined goals.

BOX 3-3 Psychosocial Assessment

Language

Identify the primary language spoken in the home.
Assess whether there are any language barriers to receiving support.

Community Resources and Access to Care

Identify primary and secondary means of transportation.
Identify community agencies that the family currently uses for health care and support.
Assess cultural and psychosocial barriers to receiving care.

Social Support

Determine the people living with the pregnant or postpartum woman.
Identify who assists with household chores.
Identify who assists with child care and parenting activities.
Identify who the pregnant or postpartum woman turns to with problems or during a crisis.

Interpersonal Relationship

Identify the way in which decisions are made in the family.
Identify the family's perception of the need for home visiting.
Identify roles of adults in caring for family members.

Caregiver

Identify the primary caregiver for the mother and baby.
Identify other caregivers and their roles.
Assess the caregiver's knowledge of newborn care and the purpose of home visits.
Identify potential strain from the caregiver role.
Identify the level of satisfaction with the caregiver role.

Stress and Coping

Identify what the woman perceives as lifestyle changes and their impact on her and her family.
Identify the changes that she and her family have made to adjust to the pregnancy or to birth of the newborn.

individual teaching at home. Coping with required bed rest or other limitations of activity is a problem for many women with high-risk pregnancies. The nurse may share strategies that others have used, offer help with time management, and provide information about additional support services. Teaching about infant care or the special needs of the **preterm infant** may be appropriate during the prenatal period.

Clear documentation of assessments, problems identified, treatments and interventions performed, and patient's responses are important. Nursing documentation should reflect an objective description of the nursing assessment data collected at each visit and the associated outcomes. Once the home visiting outcomes are achieved or the patient is discharged from the program, documentation should include information about the patient's status at the time of discharge, progress toward attaining health care goals, and plans for any follow-up care.

Appropriate care should be taken to complete the necessary home health care records accurately and in a timely manner. Documentation guidelines are agency specific but may include writing or dictating notes or using eDocumentation shortly after the visit.

Safety Issues for the Home Visiting Nurse

Nurse safety and infection control are two important aspects specific to home care. The nurse should be fully aware of the home environment and the neighbourhood in which the home care will be provided. Unlike hospitals, in which the environment is more predictable and controlled, the patient's neighbourhood and home have the potential for uncertainty. Home visiting nurses should take necessary safety precautions and avoid dangerous situations.

Personal strategies recommended for nurses visiting families with a history of violence or substance use include (1) self-awareness, (2) environmental assessment, (3) using listening and observation skills with patients to be aware of behavioural changes that indicate aggression or lack of impulse control, (4) planning for dealing with aggressive behaviour (i.e., allowing personal space and taking a nonaggressive stance), (5) making visits in pairs, and (6) having access to a cell phone at all times.

Personal Safety

The home care nurse must be aware of personal safety behaviours before going on a home visit. Dress should be casual but professional in appearance, with a first-name-only identification tag. Limited jewellery should be worn. Valuable personal items such as an expensive purse or coat should not be worn on a visit. Carrying an extra set of car keys in the nursing home care bag saves time and frustration if the nurse becomes locked out of the automobile. Automobile keys spread between the fingers with sharp ends outward can be used as a weapon if necessary. The same common-sense behaviours and precautions that guide a person's behaviour when alone in any setting should be followed by home visiting nurses.

The health department should have a copy of the nurse's home visiting itinerary, including contact telephone numbers if a patient does not have a telephone and information on the nurse's car (make, model, colour, and licence plate number). Many nurses carry agency-provided pagers or cell phones that allow the department to contact the nurse throughout the day in order to give information about patient updates or schedule changes. A cell phone is also useful for notifying patients when the nurse is delayed.

The automobile used for home visits, whether a personal or an agency-owned vehicle, should have regular preventive maintenance checks, an adequate fuel level, and road safety items stored in the trunk. Items to carry in the vehicle include maps, emergency telephone numbers, a flashlight, a first-aid kit, flares, a blanket, and equipment for inclement weather conditions. When making a visit to a patient in a more remote rural setting, other travel considerations may be needed, including taking additional supplies to the patient.

Home visiting nurses should park and lock their cars in a safe place that is visible from the street and the patient's home and away from hidden alleys. While driving to the patient's home, the nurse should assess the neighbourhood for safety, especially if it is unfamiliar. All valuable items should be stored out of sight before leaving the office. While walking to the patient's home, nurses should avoid groups of strangers hanging out in doorways or alleys and avoid entering into vacant buildings or entering a yard that has an unrestrained dog. The home or building should not be entered if the nurse has any safety concerns. All health departments have policies to follow for such situations.

Patient's Home

Once inside the woman's home, the nurse may encounter unsafe situations, such as the presence of weapons, abusive behaviour, or health hazards. Each potentially hazardous situation must be dealt with according to agency policies and procedures. If abuse or neglect is reasonably suspected, the home care nurse should follow the department's and the province's regulations for reporting and documenting the situation. Nurses should maintain their own safety first and act accordingly throughout the visit.

Infection Control

The importance of infection control does not diminish because nursing care is being provided in the patient's home. Patients are not likely to become infected because of their home environment, but the nurse may become exposed to an infectious disease.

Hand washing remains the single most important infection-control procedure, and the caregiver is in a position to educate the family about the importance of this practice in preventing disease. Hands should be washed before and after each patient contact; wearing gloves does not eliminate the necessity for hand washing. If running water or clean facilities are unavailable, hands can be cleaned with a self-drying antiseptic solution. Public health nurses do not usually provide hands-on care to the patient unless it is for breastfeeding support. Specific nursing care varies across the country from province to province. Most hands-on care for interventions like dressing changes or wound care would be provided by a home care nurse and not by a community or public health nurse.

Key Points

- A *community* is defined as a locality-based entity composed of systems of societal institutions, informal groups, and aggregates that are interdependent and whose function is to meet a wide variety of collective needs.

- Most changes aimed at improving community health involve partnerships between community residents and health care workers.
- Methods of collecting data useful to the nurse working in the community include walking surveys, analysis of existing data, informant interviews, and participant observation.
- Vulnerable populations are groups that are at higher risk for developing physical, mental, or social health problems.
- Social and economic factors affect the scope of perinatal nursing practice.
- Telephonic nurse advice lines and telephonic nursing assessments are low-cost health care services that facilitate continuous patient education, support, and health care decision making, even though health care is delivered in multiple sites.
- Nurses who provide care in the community incorporate knowledge from community health nursing, acute care nursing, family therapy, health promotion, and patient education.
- Home visiting can be provided for women and infants throughout the perinatal period, beginning during the prenatal period and ending when the child is ready to enter school.
- Home visiting nurses should incorporate personal safety and infection control practices in the nursing plan of care.

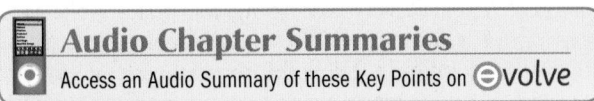

Audio Chapter Summaries

Access an Audio Summary of these Key Points on evolve

References

Canadian Perinatal Surveillance System. (2008). *Canadian perinatal health report: 2008 edition.* Retrieved from http://www.phac-aspc.gc.ca/dca-dea/publications/fcmc00-eng.php.

Canadian Public Health Agency. (2010). *Public health–community health nursing practice in Canada: Roles and activities* (4th ed.). Ottawa: Author. Retrieved from http://www.cpha.ca/uploads/pubs/3-1bk04214.pdf.

Cottrell, R., Girvan, J., & McKenzie, J. (2006). *Health promotion and education* (3rd ed.). San Francisco: Pearson Benjamin Cummings.

Dryburgh, H. (2007). Teenage pregnancy. *Health Reports, 12*(1). (Statistics Canada, Catalogue 82-003). Retrieved from http://www.statcan.gc.ca/kits-trousses/preg-gross/preg-gross-eng.htm.

Health Canada. (2000). *Family-centred maternity and newborn care: National guidelines.* Ottawa: Author.

Jacobs, E., et al. (2005). Limited English proficiency and cervical cancer screening in a multiethnic population. *American Journal of Public Health, 95*(8), 1410–1416.

Maurer, F., & Smith, C. (2005). *Community public health nursing practice: Health for families and populations* (3rd ed.). St. Louis: Saunders.

Ng, E., Wilkins, R., Gendron, F., & Berthelot, J. (2005). *Dynamics of immigrants' health in Canada: Evidence from the national population health survey.* Ottawa, Canada: Statistics Canada. Retrieved from http://www.statcan.gc.ca/pub/82-618-m/82-618-m2005002-eng.htm.

Ontario Women's Health Council. (2002). *The health status of homeless women: An inventory of issues.* Retrieved from http://www.ontla.on.ca/library/repository/mon/6000/10315600.pdf.

Plumb, J. D. (2000). Homelessness: Reducing health disparities. *Canadian Medical Association Journal, 163*(2), 172–173.

Public Health Agency of Canada. (2003). *What makes Canadians healthy or unhealthy?* Ottawa: Author. Retrieved from http://www.phac-aspc.gc.ca/ph-sp/determinants/determinants-eng.php#unhealthy.

Public Health Agency of Canada. (2010). *Report on sexually transmitted infection in Canada: 2008.* Ottawa: Author. Retrieved from http://www.phac-aspc.gc.ca/std-mts/report/sti-its2008/PDF/10-047-STI_report_eng-r1.pdf.

Statistics Canada. (2006). *Women in Canada: A gender-based statistical report* (5th ed.). Ottawa: Author (Cat No: 89-503-XIE). Retrieved from http://www.statcan.gc.ca/pub/89-503-x/89-503-x2005001-eng.pdf.

Statistics Canada. (2010a). *Having a regular medical doctor 2008.* Ottawa: Author. Retrieved from http://www.statcan.gc.ca/pub/82-625-x/2010001/article/11102-eng.htm.

Statistics Canada. (2010b). *Women in Canada: A gender-based statistical report* (6th ed.). Ottawa: Author (Cat No: 89-503-XWE). Retrieved from http://www.statcan.gc.ca/bsolc/olc-cel/olc-cel?lang=eng&catno=89-503-X.

Townson, M. (1999). *Health and wealth: How social and economic factors affect our well-being.* Ottawa: The Canadian Centre for Policy Alternatives.

Wilkinson, R., & Marmot, M. (2003). *Social determinants of health: The solid facts* (2nd ed.). Denmark: WHO Library Cataloguing in Publication Data. Retrieved http://www.euro.who.int/__data/assets/pdf_file/0005/98438/e81384.pdf.

World Health Organization. (2008). *Commission on the social determinants of health: Closing the gap in a generation. Health equity through action on the social determinants of health.* Geneva: Author. Retrieved http://whqlibdoc.who.int/publications/2008/9789241563703_eng.pdf.

Additional Resources

Community Assessment Tools

AssessNow: http://www.assessnow.info/resources/models-of-community-health-assessment

What Is a Community Assessment: http://content.calgary.ca/CCA/City+Hall/Business+Units/Community+and+Neighbourhood+Services/Publications+Guides+and+Directories/Community+Assessment+Handbook/What+is+a+Community+Assessment.htm

Unit 2

4 Health Promotion

Learning Objectives

On completion of this chapter, the reader will be able to:

- Identify reasons for women entering the health care delivery system.
- Analyze the determinants of health that may affect a woman's decision to seek and follow through with health care.
- Analyze conditions and characteristics that increase health risks for women.
- Evaluate programs of anticipatory guidance that promote health and the prevention of disease.
- Outline health-screening schedules for women in the childbearing years.
- Identify community resources to combat violence against women.
- Explain the cycle of violence and its use in assessment of and intervention for women who are victims of violence.
- Discuss the incidence of intimate partner violence in pregnant women.

Electronic Resources

Additional information related to the content in Chapter 4 can be found on

evolve the companion Web site at

http://evolve.elsevier.com/Canada/Perry/maternal/

- Examination Review Questions
- Critical Thinking Exercise—Women's Health and Safety

Reasons for Entering the Health Care System

Many women initially enter the health care system because of some reproductive system–related situation such as pregnancy, irregular menses, a desire for **contraception**, or an episodic illness, for example, a vaginal **infection**. Once the woman is in the system, it is important that health care providers recognize the importance of health promotion and preventive health maintenance and offer these services across the lifespan of women. This chapter addresses barriers to seeking health care and contains an overview of conditions and circumstances that increase health risks for women across the lifespan. Anticipatory guidance suggestions, such as nutrition and stress management, are included. Intimate partner violence (IPV) is also discussed.

Well-Woman Care

Current trends in the health care of women have shifted its scope from a reproductive focus to a holistic approach to women's health care, which goes beyond simple reproductive needs and includes a woman's health needs throughout her lifetime. This restructuring places women's health within the primary health care delivery system. Women's health assessment and screening focus on a multisystem evaluation emphasizing the maintenance and enhancement of wellness.

Many women first enter the health care delivery system for a Papanicolaou (Pap) test or for contraception. Visits to the nurse may be their only contact with the system unless they become ill. Some women postpone examination until a specific need arises, such as pregnancy, infertility, pain, abnormal bleeding, or vaginal discharge.

Health care needs vary with **culture**, religion, age, and personal differences. The changing responsibilities and roles of women, their socioeconomic status, and their personal lifestyles also contribute to differences in the health and behaviour of women. Employment outside the home, physical disability, single parenthood, and sexual orientation also can affect women's ability to seek and receive health care in clinical settings. As women age, many continue to address their primary health care needs within their established gynecological care setting; therefore, well-women's health care should include a complete history, physical examination, age-appropriate screening, and health promotion.

Fertility Control and Infertility

In 2006, more than half of women interviewed indicated that their pregnancies occurred at the right time; 23.4% wished they could have conceived earlier, 20% wished they could have conceived later, and 7.1% of women had unintended pregnancies (Public Health Agency of Canada [PHAC], 2009). Education is key to encouraging women to make family planning choices based on preference and actual benefit-to-risk ratios. Health care providers can influence the woman's motivation and ability to use contraception correctly.

The concept of health promotion applies to contraception, as can be seen in Box 4-1. The nurse can provide information regarding the need for child spacing, methods of family planning that are consistent with religious and personal preferences, noncontraceptive benefits of certain methods, the appropriate use of methods selected, and the protection of future fertility, when so desired (see Chapter 7 for further discussion of contraception).

Women enter the health care system also because of their desire to become pregnant. Approximately 8.5 to 16% of reproductive-age couples have problems with infertility (Medical Advisory Secretariat, 2006). Many couples delay starting their families until they are in their 30s or 40s, thus there is a greater period of time for them to be exposed to situations that may affect fertility negatively (including age-related infertility for the woman). In addition, **sexually transmitted infections** (STIs), which can predispose to decreased fertility, are becoming more common, and many women and men are in workplaces and home settings where they may be exposed to reproductive environmental hazards.

Infertility can cause emotional pain for many couples. The inability to produce a child sometimes results in feelings of failure and places inordinate **stress** on the couple's relationship. Much time, money, and emotional investment can be used for testing and treatment in efforts to build a family.

Steps toward prevention of infertility should be undertaken as part of ongoing routine health care. Such information is especially appropriate in preconception counselling. Primary care providers can undertake initial evaluation and provide counselling before couples are referred to specialists. For additional information about infertility, see Chapter 7.

Preconception Counselling and Care

With preconception health promotion, women and their partners are provided with information that is needed to make decisions about their reproductive future. This information can guide couples on how to identify and manage risk factors in their lives and in their environment. It can also be used to identify healthy behaviours that promote the well-being of the woman and her potential **fetus**.

Activities that promote health in mothers and babies must be initiated before the period of critical fetal organ development, which is between 17 and 56 days after fertilization. By the end of the eighth week after conception and certainly by the end of the first trimester, any major structural anomalies in the fetus are already present. Because many women do not realize that they are pregnant and do not seek prenatal care until well into the first trimester, the rapidly growing fetus may have already been exposed to many types of intrauterine environmental hazards during this most vulnerable developmental phase. Thus, preconception health care should occur well in advance of an actual pregnancy.

Preconception care is important for women who have had a problem with a previous pregnancy (e.g., miscarriage or preterm birth). Although causes are not always identifiable, in many cases problems can be identified and treated and do not recur in subsequent pregnancies.

Preconception care is also important in order to minimize fetal malformations. For example, the children of women who have type 1 diabetes mellitus have significantly more **congenital** anomalies than do children of mothers without diabetes. The rate of malformation is greatly reduced when the insulin-dependent woman with diabetes has excellent blood glucose control when she becomes pregnant and maintains euglycemia (normal blood sugar) throughout the period of organ development in the fetus.

There are many examples that illustrate the effects of maternal age or illnesses: agents such as drugs, viruses, and chemicals that produce anomalies in the fetus (teratogenic agents); genetically inherited diseases; or other conditions that might be harmful to the woman should a pregnancy occur. In many instances, counselling can provide assistance with behaviour modification before damage is done, or the woman can make an informed decision about her willingness to accept potential hazards (for more information, see Chapter 8).

The Public Health Agency of Canada (PHAC) has identified three areas in which preconception and pregnancy care can be improved to ensure good health outcomes for mothers and babies (Box 4-2).

BOX 4-1 Contraceptive Health Promotion

- Quality maternity care improves perinatal outcomes and health in general of the mother and her children.
- Achieving the desired family size enables a better sharing of all resources, with increases in education, health care, and other positive societal parameters.
- Contraceptives may positively affect future health. For example, use of condoms may prevent acquisition of human immunodeficiency virus infection; combined oral contraceptives may provide some protection against later development of cancer of the ovary and endometrium; and barrier methods decrease transmission of sexually transmitted infections, which can develop into pelvic inflammatory disease with resultant infertility or sterility and thus affect future childbearing capacity.

Pregnancy

A woman's entry into health care is often associated with pregnancy, for either confirmation of it or actual care. Early entry into prenatal care (i.e., within the first 12 weeks) enables identification of the woman at risk and initiation of measures to promote a healthy outcome. Major goals of prenatal care are listed in Box 4-3 and should be addressed in the first visit. Extensive discussion of pregnancy is found in Unit 3.

Menstrual Problems

Irregularities or problems with the menstrual period are among the most common concerns of women and often cause them to seek help from a health care provider. Common

BOX 4-2 Prenatal and Pregnancy Interventions to Improve Maternal and Newborn Health

1. Smoking during pregnancy and exposure of a child to environmental tobacco smoke are known risks to health. **Smoking cessation programs during pregnancy** are effective in increasing quit rates and decreasing intrauterine growth restriction and preterm birth.
2. **Screening and counselling of women who drink alcohol during pregnancy** has been shown to reduce consumption of alcohol and reduce adverse effects on the child.
3. **Use of vitamin supplements containing folic acid** prior to pregnancy and during the first trimester could prevent up to 70% of cases of neural tube defects such as spina bifida and anencephaly.

(From the Public Health Agency of Canada [2005]. *Make Every Mother and Child Count. Report on Maternal and Child Health in Canada.* Public Health Agency of Canada, 2005. Reproduced with the permission of the Minister of Health, 2011.)

BOX 4-3 Major Goals of Prenatal Care

Establish a therapeutic relationship and collaborate with the mother to do the following:

- Define health status of mother and fetus.
- Determine the gestational age of the fetus and monitor fetal development.
- Identify the woman at risk for complications and minimize the risk whenever possible.
- Provide appropriate education and counselling.

menstrual disorders include amenorrhea, dysmenorrhea, premenstrual syndrome, endometriosis, and menorrhagia or metrorrhagia. Simple explanation and counselling may handle the concern; however, history and examination must be completed, as well as laboratory or diagnostic tests, if indicated. Questions should never be considered inconsequential, and age-specific reading materials are recommended, especially for teenagers. See Chapter 6 for an in-depth discussion of menstrual problems.

Perimenopause and Menopause

Perimenopause is the interval between regular cycles of ovulation occurring and menopause (permanent infertility). The body responds to this natural transition in a number of ways, most of which are caused by the decrease in estrogen. Most women seeking health care during the perimenopausal period do so because of irregular bleeding. Others are concerned about vasomotor symptoms (hot flashes and flushes). Although fertility is greatly reduced during this period, women are urged to maintain some method of birth control because pregnancies still can occur. All women need to receive factual information, have myths dispelled, and undergo a thorough examination. During menopause they should have periodic health screenings.

Barriers to Receiving Health Care

The health of Canadians cannot be evaluated without consideration of the determinants of health (see Box 1-3). The Public Health Agency of Canada recognizes the following determinants of health: income and social status, social support networks, education and literacy, employment and working conditions, social environments, physical environments, personal health practices and coping skills, and healthy child development (Canadian Nurses Association [CNA], 2009; PHAC, 2010).

Financial Issues

Poverty is a significant health issue for Canadian women. It is estimated that more than 3.5 million Canadians live in poverty (Canada Without Poverty, 2009).

In Canada, disparity among races and socioeconomic classes affects many facets of life, including health. First Nations, Métis, and Inuit people in Canada are twice as likely as non-Aboriginal people to live in a home in need of major repair, are 90 times more likely to have no piped water, and are 5 times more likely to have no bathroom facilities (Adelson, 2005). Infant mortality rates for First Nations, Métis, and Inuit people in Canada have ranged from 1.7 to over 4 times national Canadian rates, and Aboriginal children under the age of 6 are less likely to access health care than are non-Aboriginal Canadian children (Smylie, Fell, & Ohlsson, 2010). Many First Nations, Métis, and Inuit women also have to leave their community during the last month of their pregnancy until delivery of their child in a hospital setting, creating significant disruption for the family and community. Some claim that this policy was created for the safety of women and their children during childbirth, while others call for a review of this policy using a postcolonial lens (Moffitt & Vollman, 2006).

Much of the existing health care system continues to be oriented toward treatment of acute or episodic conditions, although greater emphasis is being placed on health promotion. The Canadian Nurses Association has made efforts to encourage federal, provincial, and territorial governments to direct health care dollars toward health promotion with a focus on upstream thinking and preventing illness (CNA, 2009).

Cultural Issues

As our nation becomes more racially, ethnically, and culturally diverse, the health of minority groups has become a major issue. A variety of reasons are given to explain some of the differences in accessing care when financial barriers are adjusted. Some women experience racial discrimination or disrespectful, disillusioning, or discouraging encounters with community service providers such as social services and health care providers. A lack of cross-cultural communication also presents problems. Desired health outcomes are best achieved when the health care provider has knowledge of and understanding about the culture, language, values, priorities, and health beliefs of those in minority groups. Conversely, members of the group should understand the health goals to be achieved and the methods proposed to do so. Language differences can produce profound barriers between patients and providers. Even with an interpreter, misinformation can occur on both sides of the communication.

Providers must consider culturally based differences that could affect the treatment of diverse groups of women, and the women themselves must share practices and beliefs that could influence their responses or their willingness to comply. For example, women in some cultures value modesty to such an extent that they are reluctant to disrobe and as a result avoid physical examination unless it is absolutely necessary. Other women rely on their husbands to make major decisions, including those affecting the woman's health. Religious beliefs may dictate a plan of care, as with birth control measures or blood transfusions. Some cultural groups prefer traditional medicine, homeopathy, or prayer to Western medicine; others use a combination of some or all practices. A history of residential school abuse in Canada has had a tremendous impact on the definition of health for First Nations, Métis, and Inuit people. Even in areas where health programs are well established, individuals may not access programs because of a legacy of mistrust of institutions. Recognition of postcolonial factors that affect First Nations, Inuit, and Métis people is essential in the establishment of culturally safe policy and programs (Richmond, 2007).

Community collaboration is needed to ensure that health programs and policies are created in a culturally safe manner and that services will meet the needs of and be used by women and their families (see Chapter 3). It is not enough for health services to merely exist; they must be familiar and accessible to Canadians. This is especially important in the immigrant population, who may be struggling to navigate the Canadian health care system (Grewal, Bhagat, & Balneaves, 2008).

Gender Issues

Gender affects provider–patient communication and may influence access to health care in general. The most obvious gender consideration is that between men and women. Researchers have reported significant male–female differences in receipt of major diagnostic and therapeutic interventions, especially those for cardiac and kidney problems. Women tend to use primary care services more often than men and, some investigators believe, use them more effectively. The gender of the provider also plays a role; studies have shown that female patients have Pap tests and mammograms more consistently if they are seen by female providers.

Sexual orientation may produce another barrier to adequate health care. Some women may not disclose their sexual orientation to health care providers because they feel they may be at risk for hostility, inadequate health care, or breach of confidentiality. In many health care settings heterosexuality is assumed, and the setting may be one in which the woman does not feel welcome (magazines, brochures, and the environment reflect heterosexual couples, or the health care provider shows discomfort interacting with the woman). Lesbians may hold beliefs that are incorrect (e.g., that they have **immunity** to **human immunodeficiency virus** [HIV], STIs, and certain cancers [e.g., cervical]). The perceived lack of risk can result in a lack of medical care, as well as in health care providers giving incorrect advice or not providing appropriate cancer screening for these women. Not all gynecological cancers are related to sexual activity; women who have never had children may be more at risk for breast, ovarian, and endometrial cancer. Their risk for heart disease, cancer of the lung, and colon cancer is not different from that of heterosexual women. To offset stereotypes, it is necessary for providers to develop an approach that does not assume that all patients are heterosexual.

It is also important to address gender identity concerns and questions, particularly those posed by adolescents. A useful resource, *Questions and Answers: Gender Identity in Schools* (http://www.phac-aspc.gc.ca/publicat/qagis-qrise/index-eng.php), can help nurses to address some of these concerns.

Social and Cultural Factors

Differences exist among people from different socioeconomic levels and ethnic groups in terms of risk for illness and distribution of disease and death. Some diseases are more common among people of a specific ethnicity (e.g., sickle cell anemia in Blacks, Tay-Sachs disease in Ashkenazi Jews, adult lactase deficiency in Chinese, β-thalassemia in Mediterranean peoples, and cystic fibrosis in Northern Europeans). Cultural and religious influences can also increase health risks because the woman and her family may have life and societal values and a view of health and illness that dictate practices different from those expected in the Judeo-Christian Western model. Such practices may include food taboos or frequencies, methods of hygiene, effects of climate, care-seeking behaviours, willingness to undergo screening and diagnostic procedures, and value conflicts.

Socioeconomic status affects birth outcomes. The rates of perinatal and maternal deaths, preterm births, and low-birth-weight babies are considerably higher in disadvantaged populations (Martin et al., 2008). Social consequences for poor women as single parents are great because many mothers with few skills are caught in the bind of insufficient income to afford child care. Social isolation, especially among immigrant women, prevents women from accessing the support they need during pregnancy (Reitmanova & Gustafson, 2008). Multiple roles for women in general produce overload, conflict, and stress, resulting in higher risks for psychological illness.

Health Risks in the Childbearing Years

Maintaining optimal health is a goal for all women. Essential components of staying healthy are the identification of unrecognized problems and potential risks and the education and health promotion needed to reduce them. This is especially important for women in their childbearing years because conditions that increase a woman's health risks may not only compromise her well-being but also be associated with negative outcomes for both the mother and baby in the event of a pregnancy. An overview of conditions and circumstances that increase health risks in the childbearing years follows.

Age

Adolescents

As a female progresses through developmental ages and stages, she is faced with conditions that are age-related. All teens undergo progressive development of sex characteristics.

They experience the developmental tasks of **adolescence** such as establishing identity, developing sexual preference, separating from their family, and establishing career goals. Some of these situations can produce great stress for the adolescent, thus the health care provider should treat her very carefully. Female teenagers who enter the health care system usually do so for screening (Pap tests start at age 18 or when sexually active) or because of a problem, such as episodic illness or accidents. Gynecological problems are often associated with menses (either bleeding irregularities or dysmenorrhea), vaginitis or leukorrhea, STIs, contraception, or pregnancy. The adolescent may also be at risk for use of street drugs, eating disorders, and depression.

Most young women begin having sex in the mid- to late teens; for those who do not, the likelihood of having intercourse increases steadily with age. A sexually active teen who does not use contraception has a 90% chance of pregnancy within 1 year. Effective educational programs about sex and family life are imperative to control the rate of teen pregnancy and STIs. Most Canadian public schools have a sexual health and education component in their curriculum (Box 4-4; see Community Focus box).

BOX 4-4 Characteristics of Successful Sex and Family-Life Programs

- Focus clearly on reducing one or more sexual behaviours that lead to unintended pregnancy.
- Maintain age-appropriate and culturally relevant behavioural goals, teaching methods, and materials that coincide with the sexual-experience level of the participants.
- Use theoretical approaches that have demonstrated effectiveness at reducing other health-related risky behaviours. Such approaches include social learning theory, social inoculation theory, and cognitive behavioural theory.
- Allow sufficient time for presentation of information and completion of activities.
- Involve the participants to personalize the information being presented.
- Provide basic and scientifically accurate information about the risks of engaging in sexual intercourse without protection and about ways to avoid participating in unprotected sexual intercourse.
- Address social pressures (i.e., peers and media) to engage in sexual activity.
- Model communication, negotiation, and refusal skills.
- Select teachers or peer leaders who are committed to the program and provide training to help them facilitate the program.
- Give and continually reinforce a clear message of delaying intercourse, protected intercourse, or both.
- Link programs to other school and community interventions.

(Source: The American College of Obstetricians and Gynecologists Committee on Adolescent Health Care. [2007]. *Strategies for adolescent pregnancy prevention*. Washington, DC: Author; Society of Obstetricians and Gynecologists of Canada [2004]. *School-based and school-linked sexual health education and promotion in Canada*. Retrieved from http://www.sogc.org/guidelines/public/146E-PS-June2004.pdf.)

Teenage Pregnancy. The rate of teenage pregnancy in Canada has decreased almost 37% from 1996 to 2006. When teenage pregnancy does occur, it often introduces additional stress into an already stressful developmental period (McKay & Barrett, 2010). The emotional level of such teens is commonly characterized by impulsiveness and self-centred behaviour, and they often place primary importance on the beliefs and actions of their peers. In attempts to establish a personal and independent identity, many teens do not realize the consequences of their behaviour; their thinking processes do not include planning for the future. From a public health perspective, the rate of teenage pregnancy is significant because teen pregnancy is more common among disadvantaged teenagers and may be a predictor of other social, educational, and employment barriers in later life (Ministry of Health and Long-Term Care [MHLTC], 2009).

Teenagers usually lack the financial and social resources to support a pregnancy and may not have the maturity to avoid teratogens or to have prenatal care and instruction or follow-up care. Pregnant teens have a greater risk of developing health problems such as anemia, hypertension, eclampsia, and depressive disorders as well as of delivering newborns that are preterm or have low birth weight (MHLTC, 2009). Children of teen mothers may be at risk for abuse or neglect because of the teen's inadequate knowledge of child growth and development and of parenting. Implementation of specialized adolescent programs in schools, communities, and health care systems is demonstrating continued success in reducing the birth rate among teenagers.

Young and Middle Adulthood

Women ages 20 to 40 may be "juggling" family, home, and career responsibilities, with resulting increases in stress-related conditions. Health maintenance includes not only pelvic and breast screening but also promotion of a healthy lifestyle (i.e., good nutrition, regular exercise, no smoking, moderate or no alcohol consumption, sufficient rest, stress reduction, and referral for medical conditions and other specific problems). Common conditions requiring well-woman care include vaginitis, urinary tract infections, menstrual variations, obesity, sexual and relationship issues, and pregnancy.

COMMUNITY FOCUS

Sex Education, Violence Prevention, Sexual Abuse, and Rape Awareness in the Schools

Contact a public health nurse who works in a school. Find out what type of sex education, violence prevention, sexual abuse, and rape awareness is available at the school. Collaborate with the nurse and students to display a poster and pamphlets that provide accurate information about the extent of violence and what preventive measures the students might take. There may be a local violence against women coalition that can be consulted; alternatively, you can use Internet resources to design your display.

Some suggested resources include http://www.sexualityandu.ca and the Public Health Agency of Canada's *Canadian Guidelines for Sexual Health Education*, at http://www.phac.ca.

Parenthood After Age 35

The woman older than 35 years does not have a different physical response to a pregnancy per se but rather has had health status changes as a result of time and the aging process. These changes may be responsible for age-related pregnancy conditions. For example, a woman with type 2 diabetes may not have had expression of diabetes at age 22 years but may have full-blown disease when she is 38 years old. Other chronic or debilitating diseases or conditions increase in severity with time, and these in turn may predispose to increased risks during pregnancy. Of significance to women in this age group is the risk for certain genetic anomalies (e.g., Down syndrome). The opportunity for genetic counselling should be available to all (see Chapter 8).

Late Reproductive Age

Women of later reproductive age often experience change and a reordering of personal priorities. In general, the goals of education, career, marriage, and family have been achieved; now the woman has more time and opportunity for new interests and activities. Divorce rates are high at this age, and children leaving home may produce an "empty nest syndrome," resulting in increased levels of depression. Chronic diseases also become more apparent. Most problems for the well woman are associated with perimenopause (e.g., bleeding irregularities and vasomotor symptoms). Health maintenance screening continues to be of importance because some conditions such as breast disease or ovarian cancer occur more often during this stage.

Substance Use

Use of illicit drugs and inappropriate use of prescription drugs continue to increase and are found in all ages, races, and ethnic groups and at all socioeconomic levels. **Addiction** to substances is seen as a biopsychosocial disease, with several factors leading to risk. These include biogenetic predisposition, lack of resilience to stressful life experiences, and poor social support. Although women are less likely than men to abuse drugs, the rate of women who abuse drugs has risen significantly. Women who overuse substances have increased risk for development of their own health problems, and their offspring have increased risk for potential problems, including interference with optimal growth and development, and addiction. Nurses must be aware of the potential impact of **substance use** and how to detect it, as many women who have addiction issues may not readily access health care or disclose about their addictions.

Cigarette Smoking and Caffeine Consumption

Tobacco use is the leading cause of preventable death and illness. Smoking is linked to cardiovascular heart disease, various types of cancers (especially lung and cervical), chronic lung disease, and negative pregnancy outcomes. Tobacco contains nicotine, which is an addictive substance that creates physical and psychological dependence. Smoking rates have declined overall in Canada in recent years: in 2001, 24% of women smoked; the rate decreased to 18% in 2009 (Statistics Canada, 2010). Smoking rates vary across Canada, with the highest rates existing in the three territories. Twenty-three percent of women age 20 to 34 smoke (Statistics Canada, 2010). These are the major childbearing years, with significant consequences for pregnancy and the fetus. Smoking in pregnancy is known to cause a decrease in placental perfusion and is one cause of low birth weight in infants.

Cigarette smoking impairs fertility in both women and men, may reduce the age for menopause, and increases the risk for **osteoporosis** after menopause. Passive, or second-hand, smoke (environmental tobacco smoke) contains similar hazards and presents additional problems for the smoker and harm for the nonsmoker.

Caffeine is found in society's most popular drinks: coffee, tea, soft drinks, and energy drinks. It is a stimulant that can affect mood and interrupt body functions by producing anxiety and sleep interruptions. Heart arrhythmias may be made worse by caffeine, and there can be interactions with certain medications such as lithium. Birth defects have not been related to caffeine consumption; however, high intake has been related to a slight decrease in birth weight and may also increase the risk of miscarriage. Pregnant women should limit their consumption of caffeine to less than 300 mg/day, or a little more than two 8-oz cups (Health Canada, 2010). It is important for the nurse to educate the woman on the various sources of caffeine as it is found in a variety of food and drink products.

Alcohol Consumption

The amount and frequency of alcohol consumption among young Canadian women is alarming. Fifteen percent of young women (ages 18–19) and 11% of women (ages 20–24) report frequent drinking in excess of Canadian guidelines (Canadian Centre on Substance Abuse, 2004). Women who drink excessively are often depressed, have more motor vehicle injuries, and have a higher incidence of attempted suicide than do women in the general population. They are also at risk for alcohol-related liver damage. Early case finding and treatment are important in **alcoholism** for both the ill individual and family members.

Prenatal exposure to alcohol at high risk levels can have multiple, permanent cognitive and physical effects on the fetus (Society of Obstetricians and Gynecologists of Canada [SOGC], 2010a). Alcohol use during pregnancy can cause miscarriage, intrauterine growth restriction, low birth weight, premature birth, and physical malformations (Henderson, Gray, & Brockleburst, 2007) and is the leading cause of developmental disability in Canadian children (PHAC, 2005). In addition, women may experience nutritional deficiencies, pancreatitis, alcoholic hepatitis, deficient milk ejection (let-down), and cirrhosis (Cunningham et al., 2010).

Prescription Medication Use

Women are more likely than men to be prescribed mood-altering medications (Canadian Centre on Substance Abuse, 2008). Such medications can bring relief from undesirable conditions such as insomnia, anxiety, depression, and pain. Because the medications have mind-altering capacity, misuse can produce psychological and physical dependency in the same manner as illicit drugs. Risk-to-benefit ratios should be considered when such medications are used for more than a very short period of time.

Depression is the most common mental health problem in women. Many kinds of medications are used to treat depression. All of these psychotherapeutic medications can have some effect on the fetus and must be monitored very carefully.

Illicit Drug Use

Marijuana

Marijuana is a substance derived from the cannabis plant. It is usually rolled into a cigarette and smoked, but it also may be mixed into food and eaten. Marijuana produces an altered state of awareness, relaxation, euphoria, and reduced inhibition (Austin & Boyd, 2008). Some argue that prolonged use may lead to apathy, lack of energy, loss of desire to work or be productive, diminished concentration, poor personal hygiene, and preoccupation with marijuana—the amotivational syndrome—though research on this issue is inconclusive (Austin & Boyd, 2008).

Marijuana readily crosses the placenta and causes increased carbon monoxide levels in the mother's blood, which reduces the oxygen supply to the fetus. Research findings regarding the effects of marijuana on pregnancy are inconsistent; however, it may cause fetal abnormalities (Keegan, Parva, Finnegan, Gerson, & Belden, 2010).

Cocaine

Cocaine is a powerful central nervous system stimulant that is addictive because of the tremendous sense of euphoria that it creates. It can be snorted, smoked, or injected. **Crack,** or rock cocaine, is a form of the drug that is exceedingly potent and even more highly addictive. (Some say that an individual is "hooked" after the first use or at least after two or three "hits.") After ingestion of cocaine, an intensely pleasurable high results that is followed by an uncomfortable low; this increases the urge to repeat the drug.

Vancouver's Downtown Eastside is a community with some of the lowest incomes and greatest substance use issues in Canada. Research in this area reveals that crack cocaine use has increased in the past 10 years (The VANDU Women CARE Team, 2009). Predisposing factors and problems associated with cocaine use in pregnancy are polydrug use; poor nutrition; poverty; STIs; hepatitis B infection; dysfunctional family systems; employment difficulties; stress; anger; poor self-esteem; and previous or present physical, emotional, and sexual abuse. The clinical manifestations of cocaine use include tachycardia, pupillary dilation, and hypertension.

Cocaine affects all of the major body systems. Among other complications, it produces cardiovascular stress that can lead to heart attack or stroke, liver disease, central nervous system stimulation that can cause seizures, and even perforation of the nasal septum. Needle-borne diseases such as hepatitis B and acquired immunodeficiency syndrome (AIDS) are common among cocaine users. If the user is pregnant, there is an increased incidence of miscarriage, preterm labour, small-for-gestational-age babies, abruption of placenta, and stillbirth. Anomalies have been reported.

One of the promising treatments for cocaine use in pregnancy is acupuncture. A component of traditional Chinese medicine, acupuncture is used to redirect energy flow (chi) within the body, reduce cravings, and enhance well-being. The pace and location of the flow of chi can be influenced by the insertion of needles at certain points along the meridians to facilitate harmony (Otto, 2003). Evidence from controlled studies of the effectiveness of acupuncture alone or in combination with other therapies has been inconsistent (Vickers, Wilson, & Kleynen, 2002). Further investigation of this therapy is needed.

Opiates

The opiates include opium, heroin, meperidine, morphine, codeine, and **methadone**. Heroin is one of the most commonly used drugs of this class. It is usually taken by intravenous injection but can be smoked or "snorted." The signs and symptoms of heroin use are euphoria, relaxation, relief from pain, "nodding out" (apathy, detachment from reality, impaired judgement, and drowsiness), constricted pupils, nausea, constipation, slurred speech, and respiratory depression.

The incidence of heroin use among pregnant women is unknown; however, women with a dependency on heroin may use multiple drugs. Possible effects on pregnancy include preeclampsia, intrauterine growth restriction, miscarriage, premature rupture of membranes, infections, breech presentation, and preterm labour. Possible effects on the mother include poor nourishment with subsequent vitamin, iron, and folic acid deficiencies; medical complications from frequent use of dirty needles; STIs; and hypertension (Stuart & Laraia, 2005).

The recommended treatment is methadone maintenance combined with psychotherapy. This well-documented approach improves outcomes for both the woman and her fetus (Jambert-Gray, Lucas, & Hall, 2009; Stuart & Laraia, 2005). The other approach is slow medical withdrawal with methadone, but the safety of this second approach is questionable. In pregnancy, methadone is metabolized more rapidly, leading to withdrawal symptoms in less than 24 hours in many women. Withdrawal symptoms can include fetal hyperactivity and, if severe, preterm labour or fetal death (Jambert-Gray et al., 2009). Women may resort to heroin to alleviate the uncomfortable symptoms.

Methamphetamine

Use of methamphetamine in Canada is increasing (Department of Justice Canada, 2007). Relatively cheap, this highly addictive stimulant is hooking more and more people across the socioeconomic spectrum. This product is often mixed with other illicit drugs, including ecstasy; therefore, users may not even be aware when they are exposing themselves to this dangerous drug (Department of Justice Canada, 2007). Methamphetamine makes many users feel hypersexual and uninhibited and thus leads to more sex and less protection from pregnancy. It has been difficult to ascertain the extent of the effect of methamphetamine use on neonates as prenatal exposure typically correlates with poor prenatal care, which affects available research (Cruickshank & Dyer, 2009).The active metabolite of methamphetamine is amphetamine, a central nervous system stimulant known as both "speed" and "meth." The crystalline form of methamphetamine is known as "ice." When smoked, it produces a potent, long-lasting high (Cruickshank & Dyer, 2009). The active ingredient is pseudoephedrine and can be prepared using supplies typically purchased at a local pharmacy or department store; thus the potential for abuse is tremendous.

Clinical manifestations of methamphetamine use are euphoria, abrupt awakening, increased energy, talkativeness, elation, agitation, hyperactivity, irritability, grandiosity, diaphoresis, weight loss, insomnia, hypertension, increased temperature, ectopic heartbeat, urinary retention, constipation, dry mouth, paranoid delusions, and violent behaviour. Psychosis, hypertension, permanent neurological damage, and death may occur as a result of overdose (Cruickshank & Dyer, 2009). Most of the effects of **amphetamines** are similar to those of cocaine.

Although fewer maternal and neonatal complications have been attributed to this class of substances than to cocaine, the rates of preterm births and intrauterine growth restriction with smaller head circumference are higher in methamphetamine-exposed pregnant women than in pregnant women who use other substances.

Phencyclidine

Phencyclidine (PCP) is a synthetic drug known by various names ("peace pill," "elephant," "angel dust," "hog"). Its use is more prevalent among ethnic minorities and in people between the ages of 18 and 40. Its effects are unpredictable and include hostility, aggressiveness, and other bizarre behaviour (Stuart & Laraia, 2005). Signs and symptoms of PCP use include confusion, disorientation, euphoria, hallucinations, paranoia, grandiosity, agitation, a tendency toward violence, and antisocial behaviour; the severity of these symptoms depends on the dose. Clinical manifestations include red, dry skin; dilated pupils; nystagmus; ataxia; hypertension; rigidity; and seizures (Stuart & Laraia, 2005). Because some effects mimic the signs and symptoms of schizophrenia, a user may be admitted to a psychiatric unit.

The major concerns regarding PCP use in pregnant women are its association with polydrug abuse and the neurobehavioural effects on the neonate.

Other Illicit Drugs

A number of other street drugs pose risks to users. A few are derived from organic materials, but more and more are produced synthetically in laboratories. Sedatives such as "downers," "yellow jackets," or "red devils" are used to come off "highs." Hallucinogens alter perception and body function. PCP ("angel dust") and LSD produce vivid changes in sensation, often with agitation, euphoria, paranoia, and a tendency toward antisocial behaviour. Their use may lead to flashbacks, chronic psychosis, and violent behaviour. Hallucinogens taken during pregnancy may have negative neurobehavioural effects on the newborn.

Many prescription and nonprescription medications may also be transferred to the newborn via breast milk, and the potential impact must be discussed with breastfeeding women who use them (see Appendix A).

Nutrition

Good nutrition is essential for optimal health. A well-balanced diet helps prevent illness and also is used to treat certain health problems. Conversely, poor eating habits, eating disorders, and obesity are linked to disease and debility. *Eating Well With Canada's Food Guide* provides a variety of educational tools for patients and health care providers to promote health and reduce risks for chronic diseases through diet and physical activity. The Canadian Heart and Stroke Foundation also has a number of nutrition resources.

Nutritional Deficiencies

Overt disease caused by a lack of certain nutrients is rarely seen in Canada. However, insufficient amounts or imbalances of nutrients do pose problems for individuals and families. Overweight or underweight status, malabsorption, listlessness, fatigue, frequent colds and other minor infections, constipation, dull hair and nails, and dental caries are examples of problems that could be related to poor nutrition and indicate the need for further nutritional assessment. Poor nutrition, especially that related to obesity and high fat and cholesterol intake, may lead to more serious conditions and contribute to heart disease, **malignant** neoplasms, cerebrovascular diseases, and diabetes, many of the leading causes of morbidity and mortality in Canada.

Obesity

Obesity rates for Canadian women of childbearing age are between 11% and 21%, and rates are continuing to increase, especially among adolescents (SOGC, 2010b). The likelihood of being overweight is greater among families living in low socioeconomic neighbourhoods, where the social environment is often less conducive to physical activity because of lack of safety and lack of available resources and opportunities (Oliver & Hayes, 2005).

There has been some controversy over whether the body mass index (BMI) remains an effective diagnostic tool of assessing for obesity or if waist circumference offers us more clinically relevant information. Both BMI (Table 4-1) and waist circumference (Box 4-5) appear to have their value in assessing the patient for risk of obesity, central obesity, and cardiovascular disease. BMI is defined as a measure of an adult's weight in relation to his or her height, specifically the adult's weight in kilograms divided by the square of his or her height in metres.

Table 4-1 Ideal Body Weight With Body Mass Index and Risk

	BMI RANGE	RISK OF DEVELOPING HEALTH PROBLEMS
Underweight	<18.5	Increased
Normal weight	18.5–24.9	Least
Overweight	25.0–29.9	Increased
Obese Class I (mild)	30.0–34.9	High
Obese Class II (moderate)	35-39.9	Very high
Obese Class III (morbid)	>40	Extremely high

(Adapted from World Health Organization. [2000]. *Obesity: Preventing and managing the global epidemic.* Geneva: Author. Retrieved from http://whqlibdoc.who.int/trs/WHO_TRS_894.pdf.)
BMI, body mass index.

BOX 4-5 Waist Circumference

Measure your waist with clothing removed from abdomen. Place a measuring tape around waist, just above the hip bones.

Waist = ___________ centimeters.

Assess your health risk.

High Risk

A WC measurement of 88 cm or more for women is associated with an increased risk of developing health problems such as type 2 diabetes, coronary heart disease, and high blood pressure. As the cut-off points are approximate, a WC just below this measurement should also be taken seriously. The risk of developing health problems increases as WC measurement increases above the cut-off points.

WC, waist circumference.

(Source: Office of Nutrition Health and Policy. Health Canada [2002]. *Are you an apple or a pear? What's your waist to hip ratio?* Ottawa: Author. Retrieved from http://www.hc-sc.gc.ca/fn-an/nutrition/weights-poids/vitalit/apple_pear-pomme_poire-eng.php.)

Overweight and obesity are known risk factors for premature death, diabetes, heart disease, stroke, hypertension, dyslipidemia, and some cancers (breast and colon) (Canadian Cancer Society, 2010). In addition, obesity is associated with high cholesterol, menstrual irregularities, hirsutism (excess body and facial hair), stress incontinence, depression, complications of pregnancy, increased surgical risk, and shortened lifespan. Obese pregnant women are at risk for spontaneous **abortion**, hypertension, difficulties with fetal monitoring, and gestational diabetes as well as for intrapartum complications such as **macrosomia** and shoulder dystocia, Caesarean section, and thromboembolism (Smith, Hulsey & Goodnight, 2008; SOCG, 2010b) (see Chapter 14).

Other Considerations

Other dietary extremes also can produce risk. For example, insufficient amounts of calcium can lead to osteoporosis, too much sodium can aggravate hypertension, and megadoses of vitamins can cause adverse effects in several body systems. Fad weight-loss programs and yo-yo dieting (repeated weight gain and weight loss) result in nutritional imbalances and, in some instances, medical problems. Such diets and programs are not appropriate for weight maintenance. Adolescent pregnancy produces special nutritional requirements because the metabolic needs of pregnancy are superimposed on the teen's own needs for growth and maturation at a time when eating habits are usually less than ideal.

Anorexia Nervosa

Some women have a distorted view of their bodies and, no matter what their weight, perceive themselves to be much too heavy. As a result, they undertake strict and severe diets and rigorous extreme exercise. This chronic eating disorder is known as **anorexia nervosa**. Women can carry this condition to the point of starvation, with resulting endocrine and metabolic abnormalities. If it is not corrected, significant complications of arrhythmias, amenorrhea, cardiomyopathy, and congestive heart failure occur and in the extreme can lead to death. The condition commonly begins during adolescence in young women who have some degree of personality disorder. They gradually lose weight over several months, have amenorrhea (see Chapter 6), and are abnormally concerned with body image. A coexisting depression usually accompanies **anorexia**.

Society continues to put added pressure on women and young girls to be thin; in one survey 37% of young girls in grade 9 and 40% in grade 10 felt they were overweight (PHAC, 2008). Significant associations have also been found between Canadian women at risk for eating disorders and lifetime use of illicit drugs (Gadalla & Piran, 2007). A thorough history and assessment by the nurse, especially for the woman at risk, is paramount to preventing alterations in health.

There are no specific tests to diagnose anorexia nervosa. A medical history, physical examination, and screening tests help identify women at risk for eating disorders. Several tools are available to use in primary care settings. The SCOFF questionnaire is easy to administer and can help the nurse decide whether an eating disorder is likely and if the woman needs further assessment and may need psychiatric and medical intervention (Johnston et al., 2007; Parker, Lyons, & Bonner, 2005) (Box 4-6).

Bulimia Nervosa

Bulimia refers to secret, uncontrolled binge eating alternating with methods to prevent weight gain: self-induced vomiting, laxatives or diuretics, strict diets, fasting, and rigorous exercise. During a binge episode, large numbers of calories are consumed, usually consisting of sweets and "junk foods." Binges occur at least twice per week. Bulimia usually begins in early adulthood (ages 18 to 25) and is found primarily in females. Complications can include dehydration and electrolyte imbalance, gastrointestinal abnormalities, and cardiac arrhythmias. Bulimia is somewhat similar to anorexia in that it is an eating disorder and usually involves some degree of depression. Unlike those with anorexia, individuals with bulimia may feel shame or disgust about their disorder and tend to seek help earlier. The SCOFF screening assessment also can be used (see Box 4-6).

BOX 4-6 Screening for Eating Disorders: SCOFF Questions

Each question scores 1 point. A score of 2 or more indicates that the person may have anorexia nervosa or bulimia.

1. Do you make yourself **S**ick because you feel too full?
2. Do you worry about loss of **C**ontrol over the amount you eat?
3. Have you recently lost more than 6 kg in a 3-month period?
4. Do you think you are too **F**at even if others think you are too thin?
5. Does **F**ood dominate your life?

(Source: Hautala, L., et al. [2008]. Adolescents with fluctuating symptoms of eating disorders: A one-year prospective study. *Journal of Advanced Nursing, 6*, 674–680.)

Physical Fitness and Exercise

Exercise contributes to good health by lowering risks for a variety of conditions that are influenced by obesity and a sedentary lifestyle. It is effective in the prevention of cardiovascular disease and in the management of chronic conditions such as hypertension, arthritis, diabetes, respiratory disorders, and osteoporosis (Fig. 4-1). Exercise also contributes to stress reduction and weight maintenance. Women report that engaging in regular exercise improves their body image and self-esteem and acts as a mood enhancer. Aerobic exercise produces cardiovascular involvement because increasing amounts of oxygen are delivered to working muscles. Anaerobic exercise such as weight training improves individual muscle mass without stress on the cardiovascular system. Because women are concerned about both cardiovascular and bone health, weight-bearing aerobic exercises such as walking, running, racket sports, and dancing are preferred. However, excessive or strenuous exercise can lead to **hormone** imbalances, resulting in amenorrhea and its consequences. Physical injury is also a potential risk.

Kegel exercise, or pelvic muscle exercise, is used to strengthen the muscles that support the pelvic floor. It is unknown whether this method of pelvic strengthening alone will maintain pelvic strength in the long term; however, consistent use on a daily basis has shown short-term improvements in stress incontinence (Mason, Roe, Wong, Davies, & Bamber, 2010). Instructions for this exercise are in the Patient Teaching box.

Physical activity and exercise counselling for persons of all ages should be available at schools, work sites, and primary care settings. Specific recommendations include 30 to 60 minutes of moderate activity most days of the week for adults and 60 to 90 minutes most days of the week for children and adolescents (Heart and Stroke Foundation, 2010). Few Canadians exercise this often, and physical inactivity increases with age, especially during adolescence and early adulthood. Even small increases in activity can be beneficial. During pregnancy, an ongoing exercise regimen can be continued but should be decreased in intensity and duration (Fig. 4-2). Sedentary women should begin with low-intensity and low-impact workouts (see Evidence-Informed Practice box).

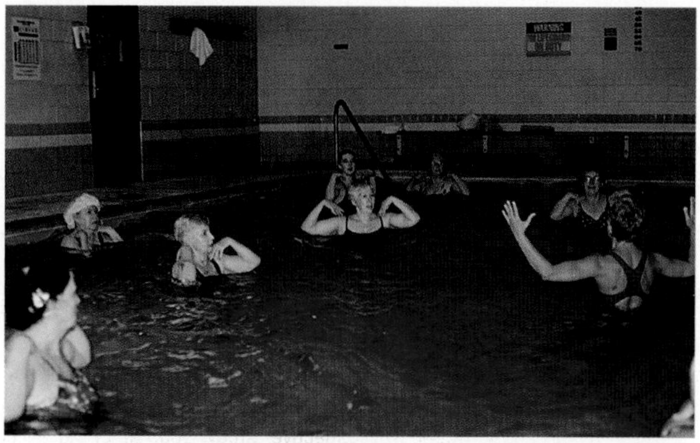

Fig. 4-1 Water aerobics improves cardiovascular function. *(Courtesy Jonas McCoy, Raleigh, NC.)*

Stress

The modern woman faces increasing levels of stress and, as a result, is prone to a variety of stress-induced illnesses. Stress often occurs because of conflict among multiple roles—for example, job and financial responsibilities can conflict with parenting and duties at home. To add to this burden, women

PATIENT TEACHING Kegel Exercise

Description and Rationale

Kegel exercise, or pelvic muscle exercise, is a technique used to strengthen the muscles that support the pelvic floor. This exercise involves regularly tightening (contracting) and relaxing the muscles that support the bladder and urethra. By strengthening these pelvic muscles, a woman can prevent or reduce accidental urine loss.

Technique

The woman needs to learn how to target the muscles for training and how to contract them correctly. One suggestion for teaching is to have the woman pretend she is trying to stop the flow of urine in midstream or to have her think about how her vagina is able to contract around and move up the length of the penis during intercourse.

The woman should avoid straining or bearing-down motions while performing the exercise. She should be taught to avoid straining down by exhaling gently and keeping her mouth open each time she contracts her pelvic muscles.

Specific Instructions

- Each contraction should be as intense as possible without contracting the abdomen, thighs, or buttocks.
- Contractions should be held for at least ten seconds. The woman may have to start with as little as two seconds per contraction until her muscles get stronger.
- She should rest for ten seconds or more between contractions so that the muscles have time to recover and each contraction can be as strong as she can make it.
- She should feel the pulling up and over the three muscle layers so that the contraction reaches the highest level of her pelvis.

Other Suggestions for Implementation

- At first the woman should set aside about 15 minutes a day to do the Kegel exercises.
- She may want to put up reminders such as notes on her bathroom mirror, her refrigerator, her TV, or a calendar to do the exercises.
- Positive results can be achieved by performing 30 a day.
- The best position for learning how to do Kegel exercises is to lie supine with the knees bent. Another position to use is on the hands and knees. Once the woman learns the proper technique, she can perform the exercises in other positions such as standing or sitting.

(Sources: Sampselle, C. M. [2000]. Behavioural interventions for urinary incontinence in women: Evidence for practice. *Journal of Midwifery & Women's Health, 45*(2), 94–103; Sampselle, C. M., et al. [1997]. Continence for women: Evidence-based practice. *Journal of Obstetric & Gynecologic Neonatal Nursing, 26*[4], 375–385.)

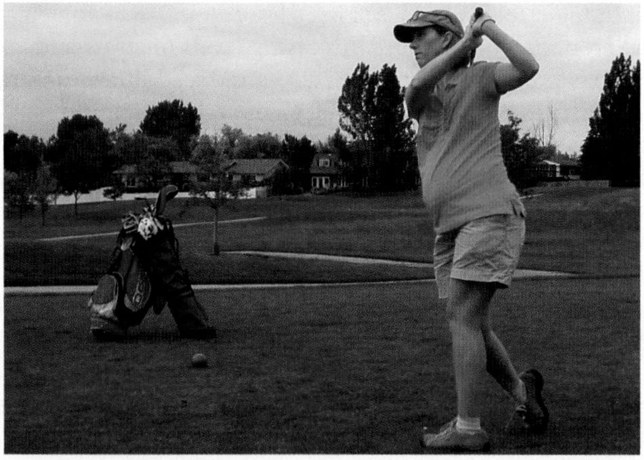

Fig. 4-2 Participation in physical activity is possible and important during pregnancy. A woman at 30 weeks of gestation enjoys a game of golf. *(Courtesy Julie Perry Nelson, Loveland, CO.)*

are socialized to be caregivers, which is emotionally draining in itself. They also may find themselves in positions of minimal power that do not allow them to have control over their everyday environments. Some stress is normal and contributes to positive outcomes. Many women thrive in busy surroundings. However, excessive or high levels of ongoing stress trigger physical reactions such as rapid heart rate, elevated blood pressure, slowed digestion, release of additional neurotransmitters and hormones, muscle tenseness, and a weakened immune system. Consequently, constant stress can contribute to clinical illnesses such as exacerbations of arthritis or asthma, frequent colds or infections, gastrointestinal upsets, cardiovascular problems, and infertility. Box 4-7 lists symptoms that may be related to chronic or extreme stress. Psychological symptoms such as anxiety, irritability, eating disorders, depression, insomnia, and substance use have also been associated with stress.

EVIDENCE-INFORMED PRACTICE Exercise and Work in Pregnancy

—Pat Gingrich

Ask the Question

What sorts of work and leisure activities are safe for pregnant women?

Search for Evidence

Search Strategies

Professional organization guidelines, meta-analyses, systematic reviews, randomized controlled trials, nonrandomized prospective studies, and retrospective studies since 2006

Databases Searched

CINAHL, Cochrane, Medline, National Guideline Clearinghouse, TRIP Database Plus, and the Web sites for SOGC, ACOG, AWHONN, and CDC

Critically Analyze the Evidence

Historically, health care providers worried that exercise during pregnancy might lead to poor uteroplacental perfusion or increased inflammatory response, resulting in low birth weight, gestational hypertension, or prematurity. These concerns led to restrictions on activity. However, exercise has been shown to have many physiological and psychological benefits. For example, in a randomized clinical trial of women with prior pre-eclampsia, walking and stretching promoted antioxidants and decreased recurrence of gestational hypertension (Yeo, 2009).

In a review of scientific literature on exercise in pregnancy, Gavard and Artal (2008) found that healthy women benefited from exercising, with no difference in birth weights or gestational age at birth when compared to sedentary women. Moderate leisure and work activity conferred a protective effect against pre-eclampsia and gestational diabetes, especially if the exercise predated the pregnancy. Even vigorous exercise such as running, bicycling, lap swimming, or racquetball did not make any difference in the outcomes of birth weight or gestational age. For a small group of very intense exercisers, birth weight decreased 200 to 400 g, which may reflect insufficient calories. Even previously sedentary women can initiate exercise during pregnancy, with no change in mean gestational age (Barakat, Stirling, & Lucia, 2008).

Occupational activities of prolonged hours, shift work, lifting, standing, and heavy physical work are not statistically associated with the outcomes of preterm birth, low birth weight, or gestational hypertension according to a systematic review by Bonzini, Coggon, and Palmer (2007). However, the authors caution that these activities do not confer any protective benefits and recommend decreasing work hours, standing time, and physical labour in the third trimester.

Implications for Practice

The nurse can encourage healthy pregnant and nonpregnant women to incorporate moderate exercise such as brisk walking for 30 minutes a day most days of the week. Benefits of regular exercise in pregnancy include weight control, psychological well-being, and a protective effect against gestational hypertension and diabetes. The benefits are greater if the woman begins exercise before pregnancy, but even sedentary women can safely start to exercise during pregnancy. There is no evidence that moderate cardiovascular exercise leads to prematurity or low birth weight.

Strenuous exercisers or women whose jobs require heavy labour, prolonged hours, and shift work may need to consider modifying their activity in late pregnancy. This might be of particular interest to pregnant nurses, whose jobs can involve long hours and physical labour.

References

Barakat, R., Stirling, J. R., & Lucia, A. (2008). Does exercise training during pregnancy affect gestational age? A randomised, controlled trial. *British Journal of Sports Medicine, 42*(8), 674–678.

Bonzini, M., Coggon, D., & Palmer, K. T. (2007). Risk of prematurity, low birth weight, and pre-eclampsia in relation to working hours and physical activities: A systematic review. *Occupational & Environmental Medicine, 67*, 228–243.

Gavard, J. A., & Artal, R. (2008). Effect of exercise on pregnancy outcome. *Clinics in Obstetrics & Gynecology, 51*(2), 467–480.

Yeo, S. (2009). Adherence to walking or stretching, and risk of preeclampsia in sedentary pregnant women. *Research in Nursing and Health, 32*, 379–390.

BOX 4-7 Stress Symptoms

Feelings of irritability, sadness or guilt
Change in sleep patterns
Change in weight or appetite
Difficulty in concentrating or making decisions
Negative thinking
Loss of interest in, enjoyment of, or energy for something you used to enjoy
Restlessness

(Adapted from Health Canada [2007]. *Mental health—coping with stress.* In collaboration with the Public Health Agency of Canada (PHAC). Reproduced with the permission of the Minister of Health, 2011.)

Stress Management

Because it is neither possible nor desirable to avoid all stress, women must learn how to manage it. The nurse should assess each woman for signs of stress, using therapeutic communication skills to determine risk factors and the woman's ability to function.

Some women must be referred for counselling or other mental health therapy. Referral to other members of the professional team such a social worker may also be needed. Women are twice as likely as men to suffer from depression, anxiety, or panic attacks. Nurses must be alert to the symptoms of serious mental disorders such as depression and anxiety and make referrals to mental health practitioners when necessary. Women experiencing major life changes such as separation and divorce, bereavement, serious illness, and unemployment need special attention.

Many centres offer support groups to help women prevent or manage stress. Social support and good coping skills can improve a woman's self-esteem and give her a sense of mastery. Anticipatory guidance for developmental or expected situational crises can help her plan strategies for dealing with potentially stressful events. Role-playing, relaxation techniques, biofeedback, meditation, desensitization, healing touch, imagery, assertiveness training, yoga, diet, exercise, and weight control are all techniques that nurses can include in their repertoire of helping skills.

Psychological Health

Adolescent girls and women are at increased risk for depression, and many cases go unrecognized and undiagnosed (Canadian Women's Health Network [CWHN], 2006). Depression due to the effects of hormonal and physiological changes during early pregnancy may not be detected (Kelly, Russon, & Katon, 2001). Nurses must also be alert for signs of depression in the antenatal period. A variety of tools are available for assessment of antenatal and postpartum depression, including the Edinburgh postnatal depression scale (Bowen & Muhajarine, 2006). Assessment of mental health is key to achieving overall health of the woman and her family. (See Chapter 12 for more discussion on this topic.)

Sexual Practices

Potential risks related to sexual activity include undesired pregnancy and STIs. The risks are particularly high for adolescents and young adults who engage in sexual intercourse at earlier ages. Adolescents report many reasons for wanting to be sexually active: peer pressure, desire to love and be loved, experimentation, to enhance self-esteem, and to have fun. However, many teens do not have the decision-making or values-clarification skills needed to take this important step. They may also lack knowledge about contraception and STIs. Many do not believe that becoming pregnant or getting an STI will happen to them. An important role for the nurse is to ensure that youth have the correct information. The Media Awareness Network has created a lesson plan that can be used to facilitate young people's acquisition of this knowledge. See http://www.media-awareness.ca/english/resources/educational/lessons/elementary/internet/sex_health_ed.cfm for more information.

Although some STIs can be cured with antibiotics, many cause significant problems. Possible sequelae include **infertility**, ectopic pregnancy, neonatal morbidity and mortality, genital cancers, AIDS, and even death. The incidence of STIs is increasing rapidly and reaching epidemic proportions. Choice of contraception has an impact on the risk of contracting an STI. No method of contraception offers complete protection. (See Chapter 6 for a detailed discussion of STIs, and see Chapter 7 for a discussion of contraception.)

STI and HIV Prevention Counselling

Prevention of STIs is predicated on the reduction of high-risk behaviours, through educating toward behavioural change. Behaviours that predispose to contracting an STI include having multiple and casual sexual partners and carrying out unsafe sexual practices. Specific self-management measures to prevent STIs are listed in Box 4-8. The overuse of alcohol and drugs is also a high-risk behavior as it results in impaired judgement and thoughtless acts. Behavioural changes must come from within; therefore, the nurse must provide sufficient information for the individual or group to "buy into" the need for change. Education is a powerful tool in health promotion and prevention of STIs and pregnancy. However, it works best

BOX 4-8 STI and HIV Prevention

- Prevention of STIs and HIV is possible only if there is no oral, genital, or rectal exchange of body fluids or if a person is in a long-term, mutually monogamous relationship with an uninfected partner.
- Correct use of latex condoms, although greatly reducing risk, is not exclusively protective.
- Sexual partners should be selected with great care.
- Partners should be asked about history of STIs.
- A new condom should be used for each act of sexual intercourse.
- Abstinence from sexual intercourse is encouraged for persons who are being treated for an STI or whose partners are being treated.
- Abstinence is also recommended if under the influence of drugs or alcohol.

(Adapted from SexualityandU: http://www.sexualityandu.ca.)
STI, sexually transmitted infection; *HIV,* human immunodeficiency virus.

when delivered in a way that takes into account the language, culture, and lifestyle of the intended listener.

Medical Conditions

Most women of reproductive age are relatively healthy. Heart disease; lung, breast, colon, and other nongynecological cancers; chronic lung disease; and diabetes are all concerns for adult women because they are among the leading causes of death in women. Certain medical conditions present during pregnancy can have deleterious effects on both the woman and the fetus. Of particular concern are risks from all forms of diabetes, urinary tract disorders, thyroid disease, hypertensive disorders of pregnancy, cardiac disease, and seizure disorders. Effects on the fetus vary and include intrauterine growth restriction, macrosomia, anemia, prematurity, immaturity, and stillbirth. Effects on the woman also can be severe. These conditions are discussed in later chapters.

Gynecological Conditions

Women are at risk throughout their reproductive years for pelvic inflammatory disease, endometriosis, STIs and other vaginal infections, uterine fibroids, uterine deformities such as bicornuate uterus, ovarian cysts, interstitial cystitis, and urinary incontinence related to pelvic relaxation. These gynecological conditions may contribute negatively to pregnancy by causing infertility, miscarriage, preterm labour (see Chapter 6), and fetal and neonatal problems. Gynecological cancers also affect women's health, although the risk for most cancers is low in pregnancy. Risk factors depend on the type of cancer. The impact of developing a gynecological problem or cancer on women and their families is shaped by a number of factors, including the specific type of problem or cancer, the implications of the diagnosis for the woman and her family, and the timing of the occurrence in the woman's and the family's lives.

Female Genital Mutilation

Female genital mutilation (FGM) is practised in more than 45 countries, most of which are in Africa. As individuals from these countries arrive in Canada, nurses will see patients who have had such procedures performed (see Cultural Awareness box).

CULTURAL AWARENESS

Female Genital Mutilation (FGM)

It is estimated that 100 to 140 million girls and women have undergone female genital mutilation (FGM) (female circumcision, female genital cutting, "cutting"). FGM occurs in women of many different ethnic, cultural, and religious backgrounds. The procedure involves the removal of part or all of the female external genitalia. The procedure may involve removal of the entire clitoris and labia minora. In some instances, the labia majora may be stitched together over the urethral and vaginal openings (infibulation).

Although FGM is usually performed during childhood, some communities circumcise infants or older females. The practice is recognized internationally as a violation of human rights, and many countries have policies and legislation to ban it. The World Health Organization is working to eliminate FGM. Canada and the U.S. federal government have criminalized the practice.

The extent of the FGM site affects the seriousness of complications. Common complications include bleeding, pain, local scarring, keloid or cyst formation, and infection. Impaired drainage of urine and menstrual blood may lead to chronic pelvic infections, pelvic and back pain, and chronic urinary tract infections. On occasion the girl will die from complications. Some women may require surgery before vaginal examination, intercourse, or childbirth if the vaginal opening is obstructed. Caesarean birth may be necessary.

Nurses are providing care to a growing number of women who have emigrated from the Middle East, Asia, and Africa, where FGM is common. Nurses must be sensitive to the unique needs of these patients, especially if these women have concerns about maintaining or restoring the intactness of the FGM site after childbirth.

(Sources: Center for Reproductive Rights [2008]. *Female genital mutilation (FGM). Legal prohibitions worldwide.* Retrieved from http://reproductiverights.org/en/document/female-genital-mutilation-fgm-legal-prohibitions-worldwide; World Health Organization. [2008]. *Eliminating female genital mutilation: An interagency statement UNAIDS, UNDP, UNECA, UNESCO, UNFPA, UNHCHR, UNHCR, UNICEF, UNIFEM, WHO.* Geneva: World Health Organization.)

Environmental and Workplace Hazards

A safe environment is a key determinant of health. Environmental hazards in the home, the workplace, and the community can contribute to poor health at all ages. Categories and examples of health-damaging hazards include the following: (1) pathogenic agents (viruses, bacteria, fungi, parasites); (2) natural and synthetic chemicals (natural toxins from animals, insects, and plants; consumer and industrial products such as pesticides and hydrocarbon gases; medical and diagnostic devices; tobacco; fuels; and drug and alcohol use); (3) radiation (radon, heat waves, sound waves); (4) food substances (added components that are not necessary for nutrition); and (5) physical objects (moving vehicles, machinery, weapons, water, and building materials). Canadians rate waste management, water quality, and air quality as the most important environmental issues facing their communities (Community Foundations of Canada, 2010).

Environmental hazards can affect fertility, fetal development, live birth, and the child's future mental and physical development. Children are at special risk for poisoning from lead found in paint and soil. The Canadian government is calling for strict guidelines regarding the amount of lead in children's toys, a regulation nonexistent in the rest of the world. Everyone is at risk from air pollutants such as tobacco smoke, carbon monoxide, smog, suspended particles (dust, ash, and asbestos), and cleaning solvents, as well as from noise pollution, pesticides, chemical additives, and poor preparation of food. Workers also face safety and health risks caused by ergonomically poor work stations and stress. It is important that risk assessments continue to be in effect to identify and understand environmental public health problems.

Safe drinking water is a basic determinant of health (Pike-Macdonald, Best, Twomey, Bennett, & Blakeley, 2007).

A significant number of communities are placed under a boil water advisory each year in Canada. While some advisories are preventative of a possible risk, others are based on actual risk. For example, community members in the First Nations community of Kashechewan, in Northern Ontario, called attention to this determinant of health and social justice issue in 2005 when a number of individuals became sick from contaminated water, resulting in an evacuation of almost half of the community. Working with communities to advocate for safe drinking water, lobby for proper sanitation and consistently high quality controls, and educate the public about how to maintain health in the face of a boil water advisory is a key role of the nurse.

Anticipatory Guidance for Health Promotion and Illness Prevention

Over the last several decades women have made tremendous strides in education, careers, policy making, and overall participation in today's complex society. There have been costs for these advances, however; although women are living longer, they may not be living better. As a result, the health care system needs to include greater attention to the health consequences for women. Women also must be active participants in their own health promotion and illness prevention (see Community Focus box).

Nurses have a major opportunity and responsibility to help women understand risk factors and motivate them to adopt healthy lifestyles that prevent disease. Lifestyle factors that affect health—and over which the woman has some control—include diet; tobacco, alcohol, and substance use; exercise; sunlight exposure; stress management; and sexual practices. Other influences such as genetic and environmental factors may be beyond the woman's control, although some opportunities for prevention exist (e.g., through environmental legislative activism or genetic counselling services).

Knowledge alone is not enough to bring about healthy behaviours. The woman must be convinced that she has some control over her life and that healthy life habits, including periodic health examinations, are a sound investment. She must believe in the efficacy of prevention, early detection, and therapy and in her ability to perform self-management practices. Many people believe that they have little control over their health, or they become so immobilized by fear and anxiety in the face of life-threatening illnesses such as cancer that they delay seeking treatment. The nurse must explore the reality of each woman's perceptions about health behaviours and individualize teaching if it is to be effective.

COMMUNITY FOCUS

Anticipatory Guidance for Health Promotion

Janie, a 30-year-old Cree woman who lives on a reserve, comes to the clinic after attending a health fair in which she learned that her blood sugar is above normal, she is overweight, and her blood pressure is elevated. She informs the nurse that she doesn't want to end up like her grandmother who had to have her toes amputated as a result of diabetes. Prepare a plan that uses community resources to meet Janie's needs to reduce her blood sugar and blood pressure and lose weight.

- Ascertain her opinion about her health status.
- Explore the determinants of health as they relate to Janie's health.
- Identify any need for counselling on nutrition, exercise, and stress management.
- Are physicians or nurse practitioners available in the community?
- What health education programs are available in the community?
- Working with Janie, develop an exercise program for her.
- What community resources are available to her?

Substance Use Cessation

All women at all ages will receive substantial and immediate benefits from smoking cessation. However, this is not easy, and most people will attempt to stop several times before they accomplish their goal. Many are never able to do so.

New approaches are needed to increase cessation among smokers and to discourage smoking among young women, especially in adolescence and during pregnancy. Health care providers can have an impact on smoking behaviour and should attempt to motivate smokers to stop smoking (Box 4-9). Raising questions about social consequences (e.g., stained teeth and foul-smelling breath and clothes) is sometimes effective with young people.

Those who wish to stop smoking can be referred to a smoking cessation program in which individualized methods can be implemented. At the very least, individuals should be guided to self-help materials available from Health Canada, the Canadian Lung Association, and the Canadian Cancer Society. Best practice guidelines regarding smoking cessation are also available from the Registered Nurses Association of Ontario (RNAO). See Additional Resources at end of chapter. The Training Enhancement in Applied Cessation Counselling and Health (TEACH) is a program designed to assist health care providers in counselling others to quit smoking with the hope of also creating sustainable knowledge development and transfer. During pregnancy, women seem to be highly motivated to stop or at least to limit smoking to 10 or fewer cigarettes a day. Insult to the fetus can be reduced or even avoided if this is done by the end of the first trimester.

Alcohol and other drugs exact a staggering toll on society, in terms of not only personal health but also their association with poverty and homelessness, family disorganization, violence, crime, motor vehicle injuries, reduced productivity, and economic costs. The use of alcohol and other drugs increases the risk of victimization and date rape and of acquiring HIV through shared needles or sexual contact. Alcohol and substance use are the leading preventable causes of birth defects.

While the legal drinking age varies among the provinces and territories (age 18 or 19), stronger regulation of advertising as well as tougher laws and law enforcement for alcohol- and drug-related offenses are being implemented. All primary

BOX 4-9 Interventions for Smoking Cessation: The Five A's

Ask

What was her age when she started smoking?
How many cigarettes does she smoke a day? When was her last cigarette?
Has she tried to quit?
Does she want to quit?

Assess

What are her reasons for not being able to quit before, or what made her start again?
Does she have anyone who can help her?
Does anyone else smoke at home?
Does she have friends or family who have quit successfully?

Advise

Give her information about the effects of smoking on her future health, on the members of her household, and on any future pregnancies.

Assist

Provide support; give self-help materials.
Encourage her to set a quit date.
Refer to a smoking-cessation program or provide information about nicotine replacement products (not recommended during pregnancy) if she is interested.
Teach and encourage use of stress reduction activities.
Provide for follow-up with a phone call, letter, or clinic visit.

Arrange Follow-Up

Arrange to follow the woman to find out about smoking-cessation status.
Make a phone call around the time of her quit date. Assess her status at every visit.
Congratulate her on her success, or provide support for her if she relapses.
Referral to intensive treatment may be necessary.

(Sources: Registered Nurses Association of Ontario. [2007]. *Best Practice Guideline: Integrating smoking cessation into daily nursing practice.* Toronto: Author. Retrieved from http://www.rnao.org/Storage/71/6589_BPG_smokingcessation-rev-2007C.pdf.; American College of Obstetricians and Gynecologists Committee on Health Care for Underserved Women; ACOG Committee on Obstetric Practice. [2005]. ACOG Committee Opinion No. 316, October 2005, Smoking cessation during pregnancy. *Obstetrics & Gynecology, 106*[4], 883–888.)

care providers should screen for alcohol and other drug use, with an understanding of the obvious problem with relying on self-reporting of these behaviours. The use of over-the-counter medications by women should also be explored.

Counselling for women who appear to be drinking excessively or using drugs may include strategies to increase self-esteem and teaching of new coping skills to resist and maintain resistance to alcohol and substance use. Appropriate referrals should be made, with the health care provider arranging the contact and then following up to ensure that appointments are kept. General referral to sources of support should also be provided. Many organizations provide information and support for those who are chemically dependent, and have local branches or contacts that are listed in the telephone book.

Anticipatory guidance includes teaching about the health and safety risks of alcohol and mind-altering substances and discouraging drug experimentation among preteen and high school students, as the use of drugs at an early age tends to predict greater involvement later.

Health Screening Schedule

Periodic health screening includes history, physical examination, education, counselling, and selected diagnostic and laboratory tests. This regimen provides the basis for overall health promotion, prevention of illness, early diagnosis of problems, and referral for appropriate management. Such screening should be customized according to a woman's age and risk factors. In most instances it is completed in health care offices, clinics, or hospitals; however, portions of the screening are now being carried out at events such as community health fairs. An overview of health screening recommendations for women over 18 years of age is provided in Table 4-2. Consistent with information provided earlier in this chapter, it is important for the nurse to continually educate and counsel on diet, exercise, smoking cessation, alcohol moderation, help for substance use, and stress management.

Health Risk Prevention

Often simple safety factors are forgotten or perceived not to be important. Nonetheless, injuries continue to have a major impact on the health status of all age groups. Awareness of hazards and implementation of safety guidelines will reduce risks. The nurse should regularly reinforce practices that will protect the individual from injury (Box 4-10). It is imperative that individuals take necessary precautions and avoid dangerous situations.

Health Protection

Nurses can make a difference in stopping violence against women and preventing further injury. Educating women that abuse is a violation of their rights and facilitating their access to protective and legal services constitute first steps. Encouragement for health care institutions to implement appropriate domestic violence screening programs is also of great value.

BOX 4-10 Safety Guidelines to Reduce Risk

- Wear seat belts at all times in a moving vehicle.
- Wear safety helmets when riding a motorcycle or bicycle.
- Follow driving rules of the road.
- Have working smoke alarms in place throughout the home and workplace; test them monthly.
- Avoid secondhand smoke.
- Reduce noise pollution or safeguard against hearing loss.
- Protect skin from ultraviolet light via sunscreen and clothing.
- Handle and store firearms appropriately.
- Practice water safety.

Table 4-2 Health Screening Recommendations for Women Age 18 Years and Older

INTERVENTION	RECOMMENDATION
Physical Examination	
Blood pressure	Every visit, but at least every 2 years
Height and weight	Every visit, but at least every 2 years
Pelvic examination	Recommended annually for any woman who has ever been sexually active
Skin examination	Family history of skin cancer or increased exposure to sunlight after age 40; every 3 years between ages 20 and 40; monthly self-examinations also recommended
Oral cavity examination	Mouth lesion or exposure to tobacco or excessive alcohol
Breast Examination	
Clinical examination*	Ages 40 to 49—at least every 2 years
	Ages 50 to 69—at least every 2 years
	Over 70—speak with health care provider
High risk	Annually after age 18 with history of premenopausal breast cancer in first-degree relative
Laboratory and Diagnostic Tests	
Blood cholesterol (fasting lipoprotein analysis)†	Yearly if over age of 50 and postmenopausal; preexisting heart disease, stroke, diabetes, hypertension; waist greater than 88 cm (35 inches); family history of heart disease or stroke
Papanicolaou (Pap) test*	Every 1 to 3 years once becoming sexually active and every 1 to 3 years thereafter even if not sexually active
Mammography‡	Ages 40 to 49—speak with health care provider about risk
	Ages 50 to 59—every 2 years
	Over age of 70—speak with health care provider about risk
Colon cancer screening	Fecal occult blood test every 2 years after age 50; more often if family history of colon cancer or polyps; screening colonoscopy at age 50
Bone mineral density testing§	Over age 65 for everyone; earlier if risk factors (family history of osteoporosis, early menopause)
Risk Groups	
Fasting blood sugar‖	Screen every 3 years in individuals ≥40 years of age
Hearing screen	Annually with exposure to excessive noise or when loss is suspected
Sexually transmitted infection screen	As needed with multiple sexual partners
Tuberculin skin test	Annually with exposure to persons with tuberculosis or in risk categories for close contact with the disease
Vision¶	5 years with diagnosis of type 1 diabetes then annual screening; at time of diagnosis of type II diabetes and then every 1 to 2 years
Immunizations**	
Diphtheria, tetanus, acellular pertussis, and inactivated polio virus vaccine (DTaP-IPV)	Booster every 10 years after primary series (given as infant)
Measles, mumps, rubella	Given once if no evidence of immunity (initial series given as infant)
Human papillomavirus (HPV)	3 doses for young girls ages 9 to 13. The recommended schedule is 3 doses at 0, 2, and 6 months, with a minimum interval of 1 month between the first 2 doses.
Hepatitis B††	Three doses: the second dose should be administered at least 1 month after the first dose, and the third at least 2 months after the second dose. Provinces and territories differ as to when the first dose is given.
Influenza	Annually after age 65 or in risk categories such as chronic diseases, immunosuppression, renal dysfunction

*Canadian Cancer Society (2010). Retrieved from http://www.cancer.ca/Canada-wide/Prevention/Getting%20checked.aspx?sc_lang=en.
†Canadian Heart and Stroke Foundation (2008). Retrieved from http://www.heartandstroke.ab.ca/site/c.lqIRL1PJJtH/b.3650911/k.5ACC/High_Blood_Cholesterol.htm?src=home.
‡Note: There is no consensus regarding mammograms for women between 40 and 49 years of age. Women are urged to discuss circumstances with their health care provider.
§Osteoporosis Canada (2002). Retrieved from http://www.osteoporosis.ca/index.php/ci_id/7000/la_id/1.htm.
‖Canadian Diabetes Association (2008). *Clinical practice guidelines for the prevention and management of diabetes in Canada*. Retrieved from http://www.diabetes.ca/files/cpg2008/cpg-2008.pdf.
¶National Coalition for Vision Health (2007). *Foundations for a Canadian vision health strategy*. Retrieved from http://www.visionhealth.ca/projects/documents/Foundations-For-A-Canadian-Vision-Health-Strategy.pdf.
**Immunization schedules vary among provinces and territories. See local public health agency for specific schedules.
††Some provinces and territories start the first hepatitis B injection after the newborn is 24 hours old, some at 2 months, and some not until age 13. Check individual provincial and territorial immunization schedules.

Many national and local organizations provide information and assistance for women in abusive situations. All nurses who work in women's health care should become familiar with local services and legal options for women.

Intimate Partner Violence

Intimate partner violence (IPV) is the most common form of violence experienced by women worldwide, with a reported incidence of 1 out of every 6 women having been a victim of domestic violence. In Canada, IPV is a significant social problem that affects many women and men each year and costs millions of dollars in annual medical costs. The risk of violence is particularly high for First Nations, Métis, and Inuit women; violence against these women has been linked to poor mental health, substance use, and sexually risky behaviour (Saylors & Daliparthy, 2006). It is estimated that approximately 1 in 3 Canadian women have experienced violence in their lives (Canadian Women's Foundation, 2011). Canadian Aboriginal people are three times as likely to be victims of violence (Department of Justice Canada, 2010). Several factors present in First Nations, Métis, and Inuit communities have been linked to this risk factor, including higher rates of unemployment, cohabitation, and alcohol use and greater family size (Brownridge, 2008). Of the over 20,000 women in shelters in 2006, over 70% of them brought their children with them to the shelter (Statistics Canada, 2009).

Although IPV is the preferred term, wife-battering, spouse abuse, and domestic or family violence are all terms that may be applied to a pattern of assaultive and coercive behaviours inflicted by a partner in a marriage or other significant, intimate relationship. Relationship violence rarely consists of a single episode; rather, is a pattern that may start with intimidation or threats (Fig. 4-3) and progress to more aggressive physical and sexual acts, resulting in injury to the woman (Box 4-11). Common elements of IPV are as follows: repeated use of abusive tactics that may increase in severity and frequency over time; a combination of physical violence and psychological attacks and controlling behaviours that create fear and compliance and inflict harm; behaviour aimed at controlling the woman; and use of tactics to increase dependence on the spouse and increase entrapment (SOGC, 2005) (see Critical Thinking Exercise).

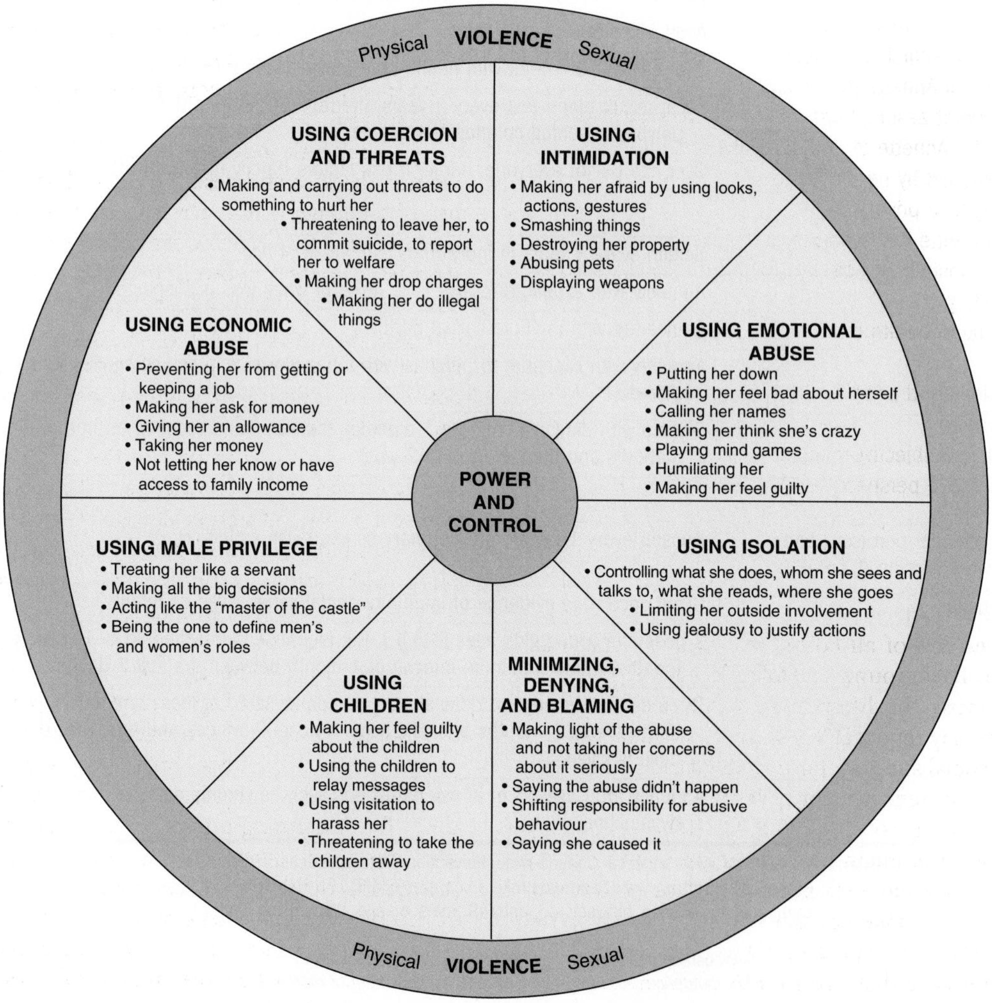

Fig. 4-3 Model of how power and control issues perpetuate battering. *(From Duluth Domestic Abuse Intervention Project. [1986].* Power and control: Tactics of men who batter. *Duluth, MN: Author.)*

BOX 4-11 Signs of Intimate Partner Violence

- Overuse of health services
- Vague, nonspecific complaints
- Missed appointments
- Unexplainable injuries
- Untreated serious injuries
- Injuries not matching the description
- Intimate partner never leaving the patient's side
- Intimate partner insisting on telling the story of the injury

(Source: Krieger, C. L. [2008]. Intimate partner violence: A review for nurses. *Nursing for Women's Health, 12*[3], 224–234.)

CRITICAL THINKING EXERCISE

Intimate Partner Violence

Annette is a 35-year-old married woman who comes to the clinic for complaints of abdominal pain and headaches. The nurse notices that Annette has bruises on her left cheek, forearms, and upper back. When the nurse asks about the cause of the bruises, Annette says that "she ran into a door." It is obvious to the nurse that the injuries could not have been caused by running into a door. What is the nurse's responsibility in this instance?

1. Evidence—Is there sufficient evidence to draw conclusions about the rights of Annette to privacy?
2. Assumptions—What assumptions can be made about the following risks for Annette of disclosing the fact that her injuries were caused by her husband?
   a. Annette's right to privacy
   b. Safety for Annette if she discloses domestic violence
   c. Nurse's responsibility to discuss domestic violence and offer a safety plan
   d. Determinants of health that may be a factor in this situation
3. What implications and priorities for nursing care can be drawn at this time?
4. Does the evidence objectively support your conclusion?
5. Are there alternative perspectives to your conclusion?

Cultural Considerations

Women of all races and of all ethnic, educational, religious, and socioeconomic backgrounds are affected by IPV. While all forms of abuse across the lifespan may be underreported, immigrant women may report IPV less than Canadian women because of lack of social support, poor understanding of rights and the health care system, fear of deportation, and cultural beliefs from their home country (SOGC, 2005). Reporting rates may not reflect the magnitude of the problem as many women do not disclose violence because of fear, embarrassment, or not having been asked by those from whom they seek help. Poor and uneducated women tend to be disproportionately represented because they are seen in emergency departments, they are financially more dependent, they have fewer resources and support systems, and they may have fewer problem-solving skills.

Table 4-3 lists some myths and facts about abuse and battering.

Cycle of Violence

Violence is neither random nor constant; rather, it occurs in repeated cycles. A three-phase cyclic pattern to the violent behaviour starts with a period of increasing tension leading to the violence. The abuse consists of slaps, punches to the face and head, kicking, stomping, punching, choking, pushing, breaking of bones, burns from irons, and mutilation from knives and guns. The honeymoon phase is characterized by a period of calm and remorse in which the male partner displays kind, loving behaviour and pleas for forgiveness. This honeymoon phase lasts until stress or other factors cause conflict and tension to mount again toward another episode of battering. Over time, the tension and battering phases last longer, and the calm phase becomes shorter until there is no honeymoon phase.

All women entering the health care system should be assessed for potential abuse. At least the following questions should be asked (SOGC, 2005):

- "Have you been hit, kicked, punched or otherwise hurt by someone within the past year?"
- "Do you feel safe in your current relationship?"
- "Have you ever been forced to have sex or engage in sexual activities against your will?"

These questions give a woman permission to disclose sensitive information.

A therapeutic relationship and skillful interviewing help women disclose and describe their abuse (Box 4-12). Skillful use of language is important when talking with women. For example, the term *victim* connotes powerlessness and hopelessness; a more empowering term is *survivor*. Women who have identified their abuse may appear passive, hostile, anxious, depressed, or hysterical because they may think they are at the mercy of the man's temper or that he is "out of control." In addition, they may be embarrassed, afraid, angry, sad, and shocked.

The most significant part of the intervention is to ensure that the woman has knowledge of the resources available to her and a plan of action should she stay with the violent partner. First, the nurse should provide services and telephone numbers of a hotline and of a women's shelter or other safe haven. The woman can be offered a telephone to call the shelter if this is an option she chooses. If she chooses to go back to the abuser, a safety plan includes necessities for a quick escape: a bag packed with personal items for an overnight stay (can be hidden or left with a neighbour), money or a chequebook, an extra set of car keys, and any legal documents for identification. Legal options such as those for restraining orders or arrest of the perpetrator also are important aspects of the safety plan (Box 4-13). A restraining order can be obtained 24 hours a day from the police department. Shelters also can be helpful with assistance in obtaining orders of protection. If the woman chooses not to act in the middle of a violent episode, she may use the hotline or shelter for some counselling when the threat of harm is no longer present. Of critical importance is a coordinated approach to maintain the safety of

evolve Critical Thinking Exercise—Women's Health and Safety

Table 4-3 Myths and Facts About Intimate Partner Violence

MYTHS	FACTS
Battering occurs in a small percentage of the population.	One fourth of all women experience violence by an intimate partner.
Being pregnant protects the woman from battering.	From 1.5 to 17% of all pregnant women are victims of violence during pregnancy. Violence frequently begins or escalates in frequency and intensity during pregnancy. Pregnancy may be the result of forced sex or of the man's control of contraception.
Battering occurs only in "problem" or lower-class families.	Intimate partner violence can occur in any family. Although lower-income families have a higher reported incidence of battering, it also occurs in middle- and upper-income families. Incidence is not accurately known because of the tendency of middle- and upper-income families to hide their battering.
Battered women like to be beaten and deliberately provoke the attack. They are masochistic.	Women are terrified of their assailants and go to great lengths to avoid a confrontation. In some cases, the woman may provoke her partner to release tension that, if left unchecked, might lead to a more severe beating and possible death.
Only men with psychological problems abuse women.	Many offenders are successful professionals. Research indicates that only a small number of abusers have psychological problems.
Only people who come from abusive families end up in abusive relationships.	Most women report that their partners were the first person to beat them.
Alcohol and drug use cause battering.	Although alcohol may be involved in abusive incidents, it is not the cause. Many offenders use alcohol as an excuse for the violence and shift the blame to the alcohol.
Women would leave the relationship if the abuse were really that bad.	Women who stay in the relationship do so out of fear and financial dependence. Shelters have long waiting lists.
Batterers and battered women cannot change.	Counselling may effectively help both the offenders and victims of violence.

(Sources: Caetano, R., Schafer, J., & Cunradi, C.B. [2001]. Alcohol-related intimate partner violence among white, black, and Hispanic couples in the United States. *Alcohol and Violence, 25*[1], 58–65; Society of Obstetricians and Gynecologists of Canada [2005]. SOGC clinical practice guideline: Intimate partner violence consensus statement. *Journal of Obstetrics and Gynaecology Canada, 27*[4], 365–388. Retrieved from http://www.sogc.org/guidelines/public/157E-CPG-April2005.pdf.)

BOX 4-12 What Not to Say to a Woman Who Has Been Subjected to Violence and What You Can Say and Do

What Not to Say

1. Do not ask "why." This question "revictimizes" and blames the victim.
2. Do not talk negatively about the abuser to the victim. She may become defensive and stop talking.
3. Do not talk directly to the abuser about your suspicions of abuse. The abuser will assume the victim told you, and the victim risks retaliation.

What to Say

1. "I'm afraid for your safety (and the safety of your children)."
2. "I believe you."
3. "It is progressive and will only get worse."
4. "You deserve better than this. You deserve to be treated with respect."
5. "You are not alone."
6. "It is a crime."
7. "I'm here for you."

What to Do

1. Empower the woman.
2. Sit down with her.
3. Assure her of total privacy and confidentiality (but only if you can).
4. Use your best listening and relational practice skills.
5. Call 911 or call local police and report any incident of imminent danger.
6. Give the woman the telephone number of the nearest women's shelter.

BOX 4-13 Safety Strategies

Survivors of intimate partner violence should try to maintain the following safety strategies:

- Always be aware of surroundings.
- Minimize time in kitchens, bathrooms, and closets when the abuser is near.
- Shop and bank at different places.
- Drive to work multiple ways.
- Get a protection order.
- Never lunch alone.
- Cancel joint credit cards and old bank accounts with abuser.
- Provide a picture of the abuser to security at workplace.
- Be escorted by workplace security to the car or transportation.
- When in danger, go to a place of safety and call 911 or local emergency response/police.
- Change locks on the house if the abuser has moved out.
- Get an unlisted telephone number.
- Block caller ID.

(Source: Krieger, C. L. [2008]. Intimate partner violence: A review for nurses. *Nursing & Women's Health, 12*[3], 224–234.)

women, access to health care, and nonjudgemental professionals (Cory & Dechief, 2007).

Prevention

Nurses can make a difference in stopping the violence and preventing further injury. Educating women that abuse is a violation of their rights and facilitating their access to protective and legal services is an important first step. Other helpful measures for nurses to take to discourage the risk of abusive relationships are promoting assertiveness and self-defence courses; suggesting support and self-help groups that encourage positive self-regard, confidence, and empowerment; and recommending educational and skills-development classes that will enhance independence and the ability to take care of oneself (Pennell & Francis, 2005). Classes for English-language learners may be particularly helpful to immigrant women. Nurses can offer information on local classes.

Key Points

- Many determinants of health, including culture and socioeconomic status, as well as personal circumstances, the uniqueness of the individual, and the stage of development, influence a person's recognition of need for care, the degree to which they will or will not access care, and the response to the health care system and therapy.
- Women have many reasons for accessing the health care system: well-woman care, fertility prevention, infertility, and pregnancy.
- Preconception counselling allows identification and possible remediation of potentially harmful personal and social conditions, medical and psychological conditions, environmental conditions, and barriers to care before pregnancy occurs.
- Conditions that increase a woman's health risks also increase risks for her offspring.
- Periodic health screening provides the basis for overall health promotion, prevention of illness, early diagnosis of problems, and referral for management.
- Health promotion and prevention of illness can help women to actualize their health potential by increasing motivation, providing information, and suggesting how to access specific resources.
- IPV against women is a major social and health care problem in Canada and includes physical, sexual, emotional, psychological, and economic abuse and affects all races and all socioeconomic, educational, and religious groups.

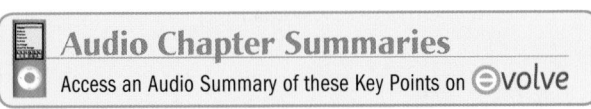

Audio Chapter Summaries
Access an Audio Summary of these Key Points on evolve

References

Adelson, N. (2005). The embodiment of inequity: Health disparities in Aboriginal Canada. *Canadian Journal of Public Health, 96,* S45–S61.

Austin, W., & Boyd, M. A. (2008). *Psychiatric nursing for Canadian practice.* New York: Lippincott.

Bowen, A., & Muhajarine, N. (2006). Antenatal depression. *Canadian Nurse, 102*(9), 27–30.

Brownridge, D. A. (2008). Understanding the elevated risk of partner violence against Aboriginal women: A comparison of two nationally representative surveys of Canada. *Journal of Family Violence, 23,* 353–367. doi: 10.1007/s10896-008-9160-0

Canada Without Poverty. (2009). *What is Canada's poverty rate?* Ottawa: Author.

Canadian Cancer Society. (2010). *Prevention.* Retrieved from http://www.cancer.ca/Canada-wide/Prevention.aspx?sc_lang=en.

Canadian Centre on Substance Abuse. (2004). *Canadian Addiction Survey.* Retrieved from http://www.ccsa.ca/eng/priorities/research/canadianaddiction/pages/default.aspx.

Canadian Centre on Substance Abuse. (2008). *Women overview.* Retrieved from http://www.ccsa.ca/Eng/Topics/Populations/Women/Pages/WomenOverview.aspx.

Canadian Nurses Association. (2009). *Position statement: Determinants of health.* Ottawa: Author.

Canadian Women's Foundation. (2011). *Report on violence against women, mental health and substance use.* Retrieved from http://www.bcwomens.ca/NR/rdonlyres/C1AA97BC-FAAB-40E9-972D-F377EE729080/50353/BCSTHCWFReport_Final_2011.pdf.

Canadian Women's Health Network. (2006). *Women and depression.* Retrieved from http://www.cwhn.ca/PDF/womenMentalHealth.pdf.

Community Foundations of Canada. (2010). *National public opinion survey: Local environment and sustainability.* Retrieved from http://www.vitalsignscanada.ca/nr-2010-public-opinion-survey-e.html#envqual.

Cory, J., & Dechief, L. (2007). *SHE framework: Safety and health enhancement for women experiencing abuse: A toolkit for health care providers and planners.* Retrieved from http://www.bcwomens.ca/NR/rdonlyres/FEDC2FC3-D01A-4F80-9D11-5A2FED19AEF4/37000/SHE_Framework_May20091.pdf.

Cunningham, F., et al. (2010). *Williams obstetrics* (23rd ed.). New York: McGraw Hill.

Cruickshank, C. C., & Dyer, K. R. (2009). A review of the clinical pharmacology of methamphetamine. *Addiction, 104,* 1085–1099. doi:10.1111/j.360-0443.2009.02564.x

Department of Justice Canada. (2007, July). *Methamphetamine report for Federal-Provincial-Territorial ministers responsible for justice.* Retrieved from http://www.justice.gc.ca/eng/dept-min/pub/meth/p2.html#a1_1.

Department of Justice Canada. (2010). *Aboriginal victimization in Canada: A summary of the literature.* Retrieved from http://www.justice.gc.ca/eng/pi/rs/rep-rap/rd-rr/rd3-rr3/p3.html.

Gadalla, T., & Piran, N. (2007). Eating disorders and substance abuse in Canadian men and women: A national study. *Eating Disorders, 15,* 189–203. doi: 10.1080/10640260701323458

Grewal, S. K., Bhagat, R., & Balneaves, L. G. (2008). Perinatal beliefs and practices of immigrant Punjabi women living in Canada. *Journal of Gynecologic and Neonatal Nursing, 37,* 290–300. doi: 10.1111/j.1552-6909.2008.00234.x

Health Canada (2010). *Healthy living: Caffeine.* Retrieved from http://www.hc-sc.gc.ca/hl-vs/iyh-vsv/food-aliment/caffeine-eng.php.

Heart and Stroke Foundation (2010). *Basic principles of physical activity.* Retrieved from http://www.heartandstroke.ab.ca/site/c.lqIRL1PJJtH/b.3651131/k.4EF0/Healthy_Living__Physical_Activity.htm.

Henderson, J., Gray, R., & Brockleburst, P. (2007). Systematic review of effects of low-moderate prenatal alcohol exposure on pregnancy outcome. *British Journal of Obstetrics and Gynaecology, 114,* 243–252.

Jambert-Gray, R., Lucas, K., & Hall, V. (2009) Methadone-treated mothers: Pregnancy and breastfeeding. *British Journal of Midwifery, 17,* 654–657.

Johnston, O., et al. (2007). Feasibility and acceptability of screening for eating disorders in primary care. *Family Practice, 24*(5), 511–517.

Keegan, J., Parva, M., Finnegan, M., Gerson, A., & Belden, M. (2010). Addiction in pregnancy. *Journal of Addictive diseases, 29,* 175–191.

Kelly, R. H., Russon, J., & Katon, W. (2001). Somatic complaints among pregnant women cared for in obstetrics: Normal pregnancy or depressive and anxiety symptom amplification revisited? *General Hospital Psychiatry, 23*(3), 107–113.

Martin, J. A., et al. (2008). Annual summary of vital statistics: 2006. *Pediatrics, 121,* 788–801.

Mason, L., Roe, B., Wong, H., Davies, J., & Bamber, J. (2010). Role of antenatal floor muscle exercises. *Journal of Clinical Nursing, 19,* 2777–2786.

McKay, A., & Barrett, M. (2010). Trends in teen pregnancy rates from 1996 to 2006: A comparison of Canada, Sweden, U.S.A., and England/Wales. *Canadian Journal of Human Sexuality, 19*(1/2), 43–52.

Medical Advisory Secretariat (2006). *In vitro fertilization and multiple pregnancies.* Toronto: Ontario Health Technology Advisory Committee; 2006. Retrieved from http://www.health.gov.on.ca/english/providers/program/ohtac/tech/reviews/pdf/rev_ivf_101906.pdf.

Ministry of Health and Long-term Care. (2009). *Initial report on public health.* Government of Ontario: Author. Retrieved from http://www.health.gov.on.ca/english/public/pub/pubhealth/init_report/pdfs/initial_rep_on_public_health_rep_20090821.pdf.

Moffitt, P. M., & Vollman, A. R. (2006). At what cost to health? Tlicho women's medical travel for childbirth. *Contemporary Nurse, 22,* 228–239. doi: 10.5172/conu.2006.22.2.228

Oliver, L. N., & Hayes, M. V. (2005). Neighbourhood socio-economic status and the prevalence of overweight Canadian children. *Canadian Journal of Public Health, 96,* 415–420.

Otto, K. (2003). Acupuncture and substance abuse: A synopsis with indications for further research. *American Journal of Addiction, 12*(1), 43–51.

Parker, S., Lyons, J., & Bonner, J. (2005). Eating disorders in graduate students: Exploring the SCOFF questionnaire as a simple screening tool. *Journal of American College Health, 52*(2), 103–107.

Pennell, J., & Francis, S. (2005). Safety conferencing: Toward a coordinated and inclusive response to safeguard women and children. *Violence Against Women, 11*(5), 666–692.

Pike-Macdonald, S., Best, D.G., Twomey, C., Bennett, L., & Blakeley, J. (2007). Promoting safe drinking water. *Canadian Nurse, 103,* 14–19.

Public Health Agency of Canada. (2005). *Fetal alcohol spectrum disorder (FASD): A framework for action.* Retrieved from http://www.phac-aspc.gc.ca/publicat/fasd-fw-etcaf-ca/index-eng.php.

Public Health Agency of Canada (2008). *Healthy settings for young people in Canada.* Retrieved from http://www.phac-aspc.gc.ca/hp-ps/dca-dea/publications/yjc/pdf/youth-jeunes-eng.pdf.

Public Health Agency of Canada (2009). *What mothers say: The Canadian maternity experiences survey.* Retrieved from http://www.phac-aspc.gc.ca/rhs-ssg/survey-eng.php.

Public Health Agency of Canada. (2010). *What determines health?* Retrieved from http://www.phac-aspc.gc.ca/ph-sp/determinants/index-eng.php.

Reitmanova, S., & Gustafson, D. L. (2008). "They can't understand it": Maternity health and care needs of immigrant Muslim women in St. John's, Newfoundland. *Maternal Child Health Journal, 12,* 101–111. doi: 10.1007/s10995-007-0213-4

Richmond, C. A. M. (2007, August). Narratives of social support and health in Aboriginal communities. *Canadian Journal of Public Health, 98,* 347–351.

Saylors, K., & Daliparthy, N. (2006). Violence against native women in substance abuse treatment. *American Indian and Alaskan Native Mental Health Research, 13,* 32–51.

Smith, S. A., Hulsey, T. & Goodnight, W. (2008). Effects of obesity on pregnancy. *Journal of Obstetric, Gynecologic, and Neonatal Nursing, 37,* 176–184. doi:10.111/j.1552-6909.200/8.00222.x

Smylie, J., Fell, D., Ohlsson, A., and The Joint Working Group on First Nations, Indian, Inuit, and Métis Infant Mortality of the Canadian Perinatal Surveillance System. (2010). Review of Aboriginal infant mortality rates in Canada: Striking and persistent Aboriginal/non-Aboriginal inequities. *Canadian Journal of Public Health, 101,* 143–148.

Society of Obstetricians and Gynaecologists of Canada. (2005). SOGC clinical practice guideline: Intimate partner violence consensus statement. *Journal of Obstetrics and Gynaecology Canada, 27*(4), 365–388. Retrieved from http://www.sogc.org/guidelines/public/157E-CPG-April2005.pdf.

Society of Obstetricians and Gynaecologists of Canada. (2010a). Alcohol use and pregnancy: Consensus clinical guidelines. *Journal of Obstetrics and Gynaecology Canada, 32*(8), Suppl 3. Retrieved from http://www.sogc.org/guidelines/documents/gui245CPG1008E.pdf.

Society of Obstetricians and Gynecologists of Canada. (2010b). SOGC Clinical practice guideline: Obesity in pregnancy. *Journal of Obstetrics and Gynaecology Canada, 32*(2), 165–173. Retrieved from http://www.sogc.org/guidelines/documents/gui239ECPG1002.pdf.

Statistics Canada (2009). *Family violence in Canada: A statistical profile.* Retrieved from http://www.statcan.gc.ca/pub/85-224-x/85-224-x2009000-eng.htm.

Statistics Canada. (2010). *Canadian community health survey.* Retrieved from http://www.statcan.gc.ca/cgi-bin/imdb/p2SV.pl?Function=getSurvey&SDDS=3226&lang=en&db=imdb&adm=8&dis=2.

Stuart, G. W., & Laraia, M. T. (2005). *Principles and practice of psychiatric nursing* (8th ed.). St. Louis, MO: Elsevier Mosby.

The VANDU Women CARE Team (2009, February). *"Me, I'm living it": The primary health experiences of women who use drugs in Vancouver's downtown eastside.* Retrieved from http://www.bccewh.bc.ca/publications-resources/documents/MeImLivingit.pdf.

Vickers, A., Wilson, P., & Kleynen, J. (2002). Effectiveness bulletin: Acupuncture. *Quality & Safety in Health Care, 11*(1), 92–97.

Additional Resources

Canadian Cancer Society: Smokers' Helpline: http://www.cancer.ca/Canada-wide/Support%20Services/CW-Smokers%20%20Helplines.aspx?sc_lang=en

Families Controlling and Eliminating Tobacco: Couples and smoking–What you need to know when you are pregnant (A resource for women): http://facet.ubc.ca/booklet/ (A resource for fathers): http://facet.ubc.ca/Downloads/DadsQuitSmoking.pdf

Health Canada: Quit Smoking: http://www.hc-sc.gc.ca/hc-ps/tobac-tabac/quit-cesser/index-eng.php

Registered Nurses' Association of Ontario Best Practice Guideline: Women Abuse: Screening, Identification and Initial Response: http://rnao.ca/sites/rnao-ca/files/Guideline__Supplement_PDF.pdf

Registered Nurses' Association of Ontario Best Practice Guideline: Woman Abuse Screening, Identification and Initial Response: http://rnao.ca/sites/rnao-ca/files/Guideline__Supplement_PDF.pdf

Registered Nurses' Association of Ontario Best Practice Guideline: Integrating Smoking Cessation Into Daily Nursing Practice: http://www.rnao.org/Storage/71/6589_BPG_smokingcessation-rev-2007C.pdf

The Lung Association: Smoking and Tobacco: http://www.lung.ca/protect-protegez/tobacco-tabagisme_e.php

Unit 2

5 Health Assessment

Learning Objectives

On completion of this chapter, the reader will be able to:

- Identify the structures and functions of the female reproductive system.
- Describe how to provide culturally competent care while completing a health assessment.
- Investigate how the history and physical examination can be adapted for women with special needs.
- Identify indications of intimate partner violence, appropriate screening, and referral to community agencies.
- Describe components of taking a woman's history and performing a physical examination.
- Identify the correct procedure for assisting with and collecting Papanicolaou test specimens.
- Review patient teaching of breast examination.

Electronic Resources

Additional information related to the content in Chapter 5 can be found on

evolve the companion Website at

http://evolve.elsevier.com/Canada/Perry/maternal/

- Examination Review Questions
- Anatomy Review—Adult Female Pelvis
- Anatomy Review—External Female Genitalia
- Anatomy Review—Female Pelvic Organs
- Animation—Breasts
- Animation—External Female Genitalia
- Animation—Female Reproductive Ducts
- Animation—Ovaries
- Animation—Ovarian Cycle
- Case Study—Health Assessment
- Skill—Breast Self-Examination

The purpose of this chapter is to review female anatomy and physiology as well as gynecological health assessment.

Female Reproductive System

The female reproductive system consists of external structures that are visible from the pubis to the perineum and internal structures that are located in the pelvic cavity as well as the breasts. The external and internal female reproductive structures develop and mature in response to estrogen and progesterone. This process starts in fetal life and continues through **puberty** and the childbearing years. Reproductive structures atrophy with age or in response to a decrease in ovarian hormone production. A complex nerve and blood supply supports the functions of these structures. There is great variation among women in the appearance of the external genitalia. **Heredity**, age, race, and the number of children a woman has borne influence the size, shape, and colour of her external organs.

External Structures

The external genital organs, or vulva, include all structures visible externally from the pubis to the perineum. These include the mons pubis, labia majora, labia minora, clitoris, vestibular glands, vaginal vestibule, vaginal orifice, and urethral opening. The external genital organs are illustrated in Fig. 5-1.

The *mons pubis* is a fatty pad that lies over the anterior surface of the symphysis pubis. In the postpubertal female the mons is covered with coarse, curly hair. The *labia majora* are two rounded folds of fatty tissue covered with skin that extend downward and backward from the mons pubis. The *labia* are highly vascular structures that develop hair on the outer surfaces after puberty. They protect the inner vulvar structures. The *labia minora* are two flat, reddish folds of tissue visible when the labia majora are separated. There are no hair follicles on the labia minora, but many sebaceous follicles and a few sweat glands are present. The interior of the labia minora is composed of connective tissue and smooth muscle and is supplied with extremely sensitive nerve endings. Anteriorly the labia minora fuse to form the prepuce (the hoodlike covering of the clitoris) and the frenulum (the fold of tissue under the clitoris). The labia minora join to form a thin, flat tissue, called the *fourchette,* underneath the vaginal opening at midline. The *clitoris,* located underneath the prepuce, is a small structure composed of erectile tissue with numerous sensory nerve endings. During sexual arousal the clitoris increases in size.

The *vaginal vestibule* is an almond-shaped area enclosed by the labia minora that contains openings to the urethra, Skene glands, vagina, and Bartholin glands. The urethra is not a reproductive organ but is discussed here because of its location. It usually is found about 2.5 cm below the clitoris. Skene glands are located on each side of the urethra and produce mucus, which aids in lubrication of the vagina. The vaginal opening is in the lower portion of the vestibule and varies in

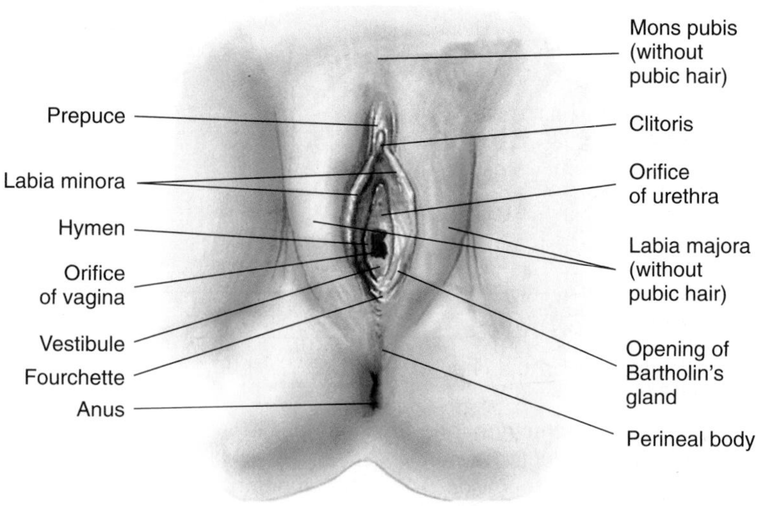

Fig. 5-1 External female genitalia.

evolve Anatomy Review—External Female Genitalia

evolve Animation—External Female Genitalia

evolve Anatomy Review—Female Pelvic Organs

shape and size. The *hymen*, a connective tissue membrane that surrounds the vaginal opening, can be perforated during strenuous exercise, insertion of tampons, masturbation, and vaginal intercourse. Bartholin glands lie under the constrictor muscles of the vagina and are located posteriorly on the sides of the vaginal opening, although the ductal openings usually are not visible. During sexual arousal, the glands secrete clear mucus to lubricate the vaginal introitus.

The area between the fourchette and the anus is the *perineum*, a skin-covered muscular area that covers the pelvic structures. The perineum forms the base of the perineal body, a wedge-shaped mass that serves as an anchor for the muscles, fascia, and ligaments of the pelvis. The muscles and ligaments form a sling that supports the pelvic organs.

Internal Structures

The internal structures include the vagina, uterus, uterine tubes, and ovaries.

The *vagina* is a fibromuscular, collapsible, tubular structure that lies between the bladder and rectum and extends from the vulva to the uterus. During the reproductive years, the mucosal lining is arranged in transverse folds called **rugae**. These rugae allow the vagina to expand during childbirth. Estrogen deprivation that occurs after childbirth, during lactation, and at **menopause** causes dryness and thinning of the vaginal walls and smoothing of the rugae. The vagina, particularly the lower segment, has few sensory nerve endings. Vaginal secretions are slightly acidic (pH 4 to 5) so that vaginal susceptibility to **infections** is limited. The vagina serves as a passageway for menstrual flow, as a female organ of copulation, and as a part of the birth canal for vaginal childbirth. The uterine cervix projects into a blind vault at the upper end of the vagina. There are anterior, posterior, and lateral pockets called **fornices** (singular: fornix) that surround the cervix. The internal pelvic organs can be palpated through the thin walls of these fornices.

The *uterus* is a muscular organ shaped like an upside-down pear that sits midline in the pelvic cavity between the bladder and rectum and above the vagina. Four pairs of ligaments support the uterus: cardinal, uterosacral, round, and broad. Single anterior and posterior ligaments also support the uterus. The *cul-de-sac of Douglas* is a deep pouch, or recess, posterior to the cervix formed by the posterior ligament.

The uterus is divided into two major parts, an upper triangular portion called the *corpus* and a lower cylindric portion called the *cervix* (Fig. 5-2). The **fundus** is the dome-shaped top of the uterus and is the site at which the uterine tubes enter the uterus. The *isthmus*, or lower uterine segment, is a short, constricted portion that separates the corpus from the cervix.

The uterus is the site of reception, implantation, retention, and nutrition of the fertilized ovum and later of the fetus during pregnancy and expels the fetus during childbirth. It is also responsible for cyclic menstruation.

The uterine wall is made up of three layers: the **endometrium**, the myometrium, and part of the peritoneum. The *endometrium* is a highly vascular lining made up of three layers, the outer two of which are shed during menstruation. The *myometrium* is made up of layers of smooth muscles that extend in three different directions (longitudinal, transverse, and oblique) (Fig. 5-3). Longitudinal fibres of the outer myometrial layer are found mostly in the fundus, and this arrangement assists in the expelling of the fetus during the birth process. The middle layer contains fibres from all three directions, which form a figure-eight pattern encircling large blood vessels. These fibres assist in ligating blood vessels after childbirth and controlling blood loss. Most of the circular fibres of the inner myometrial layer are around the site where the uterine tubes enter the uterus and around the internal cervical os (opening). These fibres help keep the cervix closed during pregnancy and prevent menstrual blood from flowing back into the uterine tubes during menstruation.

The cervix is made up of mostly fibrous connective tissues and elastic tissue, making it possible for the cervix to stretch during vaginal childbirth. The opening between the uterine cavity and the canal that connects the uterine cavity to the vagina (endocervical canal) is the *internal os*. The narrowed opening between the endocervix and the vagina is the *external os*, a small circular opening in women who have never been pregnant. The cervix feels firm (like the end of a nose) with a dimple in the centre that marks the external os.

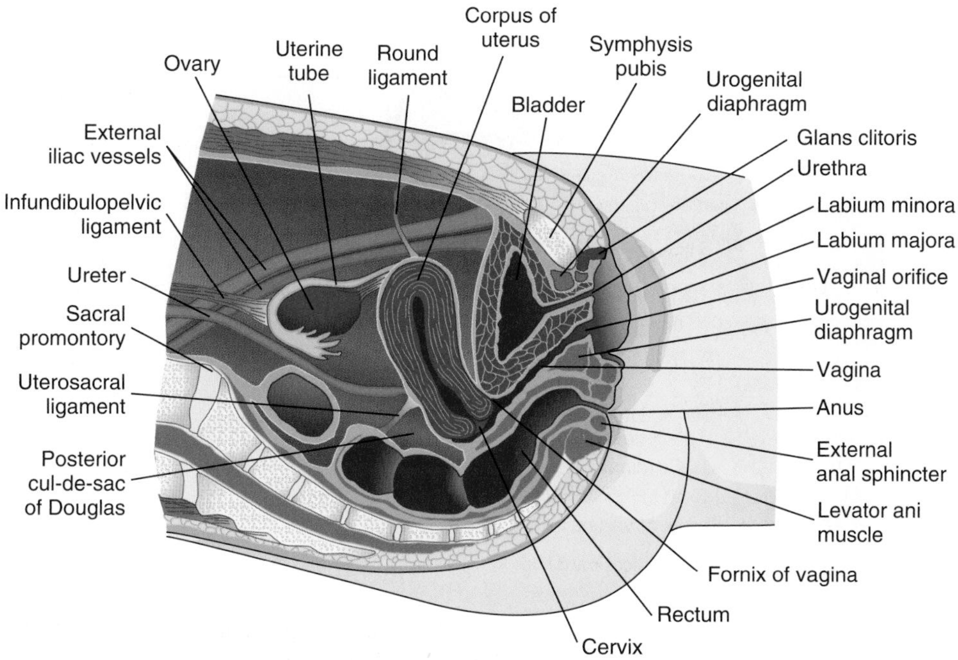

Fig. 5-2 Midsagittal view of female pelvic organs with woman lying supine.

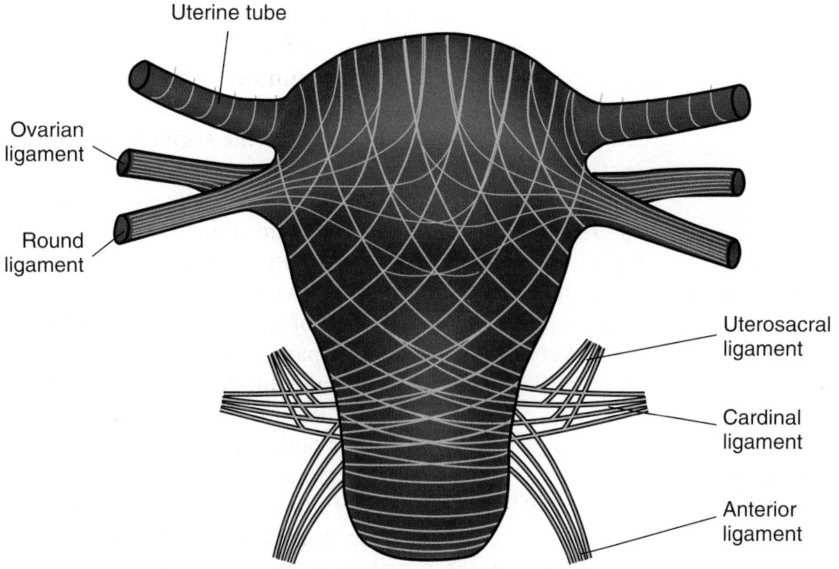

Fig. 5-3 Schematic arrangement of directions of muscle fibres. Note that uterine muscle fibres are continuous with supportive ligaments of the uterus.

The outer cervix is covered with a layer of squamous epithelium. The mucosa of the cervical canal is covered with columnar epithelium and contains numerous glands that secrete mucus in response to ovarian **hormones**. The squamocolumnar junction, where the two types of cells meet, is usually located just inside the cervical os. This junction also is called the *transformation zone* and is the most common site for neoplastic changes. Cells from this site are scraped for the Papanicolaou (Pap) test (see later discussion).

The *uterine tubes* (fallopian tubes) attach to the uterine fundus. The tubes are supported by the broad ligaments and range from 8 to 14 cm in length. The tubes are divided into four sections: the interstitial portion is closest to the uterus; the isthmus and the ampulla are the middle portions; and the infundibulum is closest to the ovary (Fig. 5-4). The uterine tubes provide a passage between the ovaries and the uterus for the movement of the ovum. The infundibulum has fimbriated (fringed) ends, which pull the ovum into the tube. The ovum is pushed along the tubes to the uterus by rhythmic contractions of muscles of the tubes and by the current produced by the movement of the **cilia** that line the tubes. The ovum is usually fertilized by the sperm in the ampulla portion of one of the tubes.

The *ovaries* are almond-shaped organs located on each side of the uterus below and behind the uterine tubes. During the reproductive years, they are approximately 3 cm long, 2 cm wide, and 1 cm thick; they diminish in size after menopause. Before **menarche** each ovary has a smooth surface; after menarche they are nodular because of repeated ruptures of follicles at ovulation. The two functions of the ovaries are ovulation and hormone production. **Ovulation** is the release of a mature ovum from the ovary at intervals (usually monthly). Estrogen, progesterone, and androgen are the hormones produced by the ovaries.

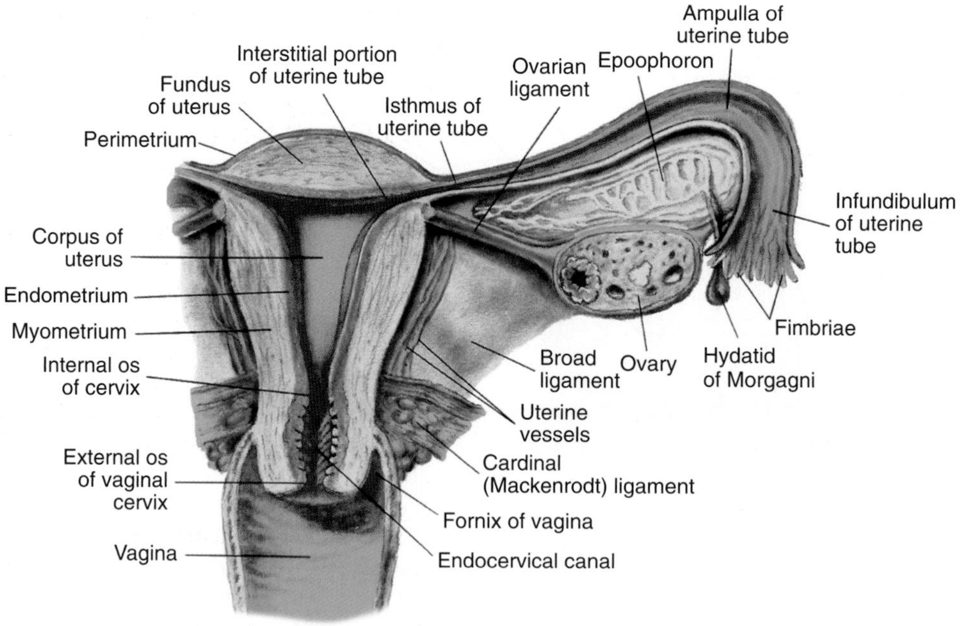

Fig. 5-4 Cross-section of uterus, fallopian tubes, ovaries, and upper vagina.

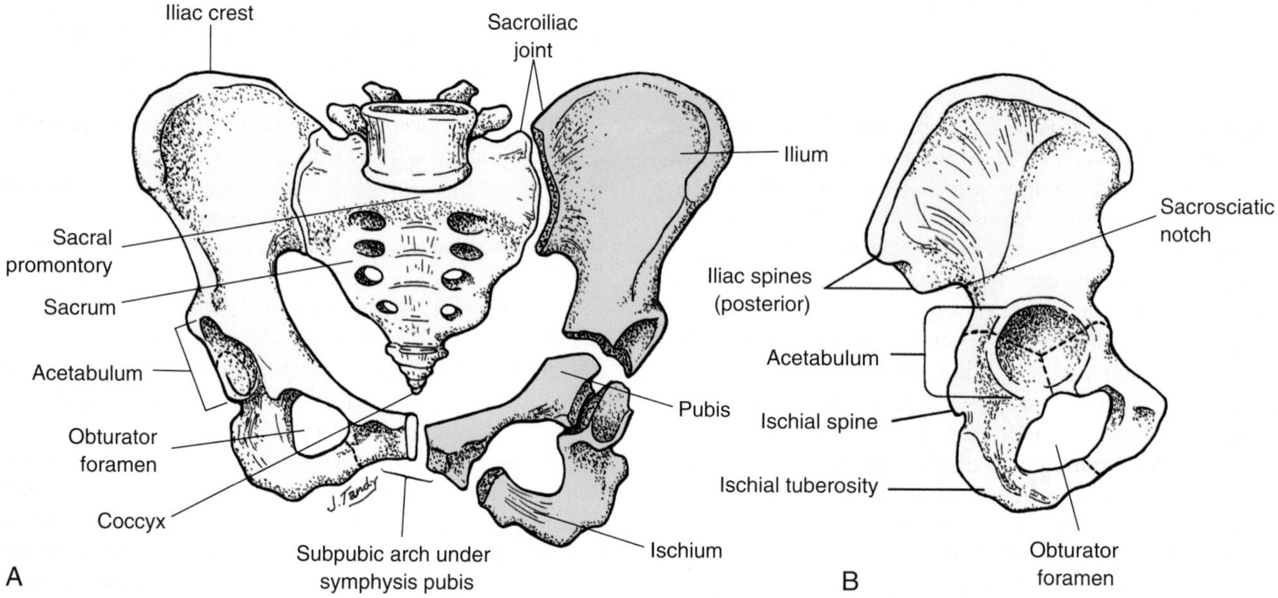

Fig. 5-5 Adult female pelvis. **A:** Anterior view. **B:** External view of innominate bone (fused).

The Bony Pelvis

The bony pelvis serves three primary purposes: protection of the pelvic structures, accommodation of the growing fetus during pregnancy, and anchorage of the pelvic support structures. The two innominate (hip) bones (consisting of ilium, ischium, and pubis), the sacrum, and the coccyx make up the four bones of the pelvis (Fig. 5-5). Cartilage and ligaments form the symphysis pubis, sacrococcygeal joint, and two sacroiliac joints that separate the pelvic bones.

The pelvis is divided into two parts: the false pelvis and the true pelvis (Fig. 5-6). The *false pelvis* is the upper portion above the pelvic brim or inlet. The *true pelvis* is the lower curved bony canal, which includes the inlet, the cavity, and the outlet through which the fetus passes during vaginal birth. The upper portion of the outlet is at the level of the ischial spines, and the lower portion is at the level of the ischial tuberosities and the pubic arch (see Fig. 5-5). Variations that occur in the size and shape of the pelvis are usually related to

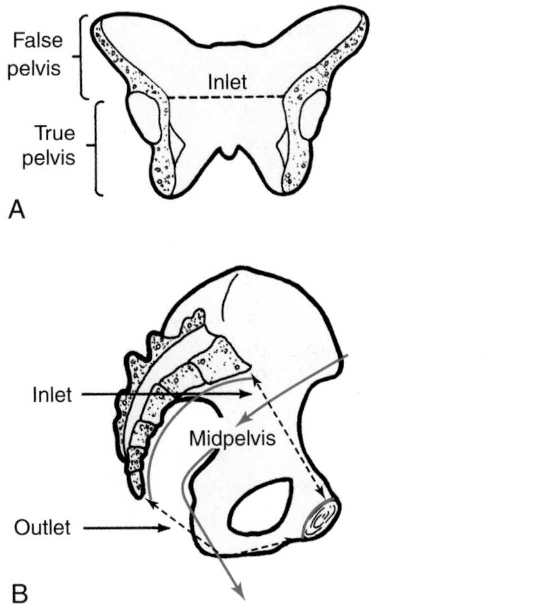

Fig. 5-6 Female pelvis. **A:** The cavity of false pelvis is shallow. **B:** The cavity of true pelvis is an irregularly curved canal *(arrows)*.

age, race, and sex. Pelvic ossification is complete at about 20 years of age.

Breasts

The *breasts* are paired mammary glands located between the second and sixth ribs (Fig. 5-7). About two thirds of the breast overlies the pectoralis major muscle, between the sternum and midaxillary line, with an extension to the axilla referred to as the *tail of Spence*. The lower one third of the breast overlies the serratus anterior muscle. The breasts are attached to the muscles by connective tissue or fascia.

The breasts of the healthy, mature woman are approximately equal in size and shape but often are not absolutely symmetric. The size and shape vary with the woman's age, heredity, and nutrition. However, the contour should be smooth with no retractions, dimpling, or masses. Estrogen stimulates growth of the breast by inducing fat deposition in the breasts, development of stromal tissue (i.e., increase in its amount and elasticity), and growth of the extensive ductile system. Estrogen also increases the vascularity of breast tissue.

Once ovulation begins in puberty, progesterone levels increase. The increase in progesterone causes maturation of mammary gland tissue, specifically the lobules and acinar structures. During **adolescence** fat deposition and growth of fibrous tissue contribute to the increase in the size of the glands. Full development of the breasts is not achieved until after the end of the first pregnancy or in the early period of lactation.

Each mammary gland is made up of 15 to 20 lobes radiating from the nipple and connected to the nipple by lactiferous ducts. Each lobe contains ductules and lobules. *Lobules* are grapelike clusters of secretory acini cells (often called *alveoli*). An *acinus* is a saclike terminal part of a compound gland emptying through a narrow lumen or duct. There are between 10 and 100 alveoli in each lobe. The alveoli are lined with epithelial cells that secrete colostrum and milk. Alveoli are surrounded by myoepithelial cells, which contract to expel milk through the ductules that merge into lactiferous ducts.

The ducts converge with 4 to 18 openings in a single nipple (mammary papilla), surrounded by an areola. The areola is more deeply pigmented than the skin of the breast. The rough appearance is caused by Montgomery's tubercles (combined milk and sebaceous glands) that are directly beneath the skin. These glands lubricate and protect the nipples and areolae during pregnancy and lactation and may provide sensory stimulation to guide the infant to the nipple. The nipple and areola contain smooth muscles which, when they contract, stiffen the nipple, making it easier for the breastfeeding infant to latch on to. Except during pregnancy and lactation, there is usually no discharge of fluid from the nipple.

evolve Animation—Breasts

The glandular structures and ducts are surrounded by protective fatty tissue and are separated and supported by fibrous suspensory Cooper's ligaments. *Cooper's ligaments* provide support to the mammary glands while permitting their mobility on the chest wall (see Fig. 5-7).

The vascular supply to the mammary gland is abundant. In the nonpregnant state, there is no obvious vascular pattern in the skin. The normal skin is smooth without tightness or shininess. The skin covering the breasts contains an extensive superficial lymphatic network that serves the entire chest wall and is continuous with the superficial lymphatic vessels of the neck and abdomen. The lymphatic vessels form a rich network in the deeper portions of the breasts. The primary deep lymphatic pathway drains laterally toward the axillae.

Besides their function of lactation, breasts function as organs for sexual arousal in the mature adult.

The breasts change in size and nodularity in response to cyclic ovarian changes throughout reproductive life. Increasing levels of both estrogen and progesterone in the 3 to 4 days before menstruation increase the vascularity of the breasts, induce growth of the ducts and acini, and promote water retention. The epithelial cells lining the ducts proliferate in number, the ducts dilate, and the lobules distend. The acini become enlarged and secretory, and lipid (fat) is deposited within their epithelial cell lining. As a result, breast swelling, tenderness, and discomfort are common symptoms just before the onset of menstruation. After menstruation, cellular proliferation begins to regress, acini begin to decrease in size, and retained water is lost. After breasts have undergone changes numerous times in response to the ovarian cycle, the proliferation and involution (regression) are not uniform throughout the breast. In time, after repeated hormonal stimulation, small persistent areas of nodulations may develop. This normal physiological change must be remembered when breast tissue is examined. Nodules may develop just before and during menstruation, when the breast is most active. The physiological alterations in breast size and activity reach their minimum level about 5 to 7 days after menstruation stops. Breast self-examination (BSE) is best carried out during this phase of the menstrual cycle.

Routine monthly BSE, which is the systematic **palpation** of breasts to detect signs of breast cancer or other changes, is no

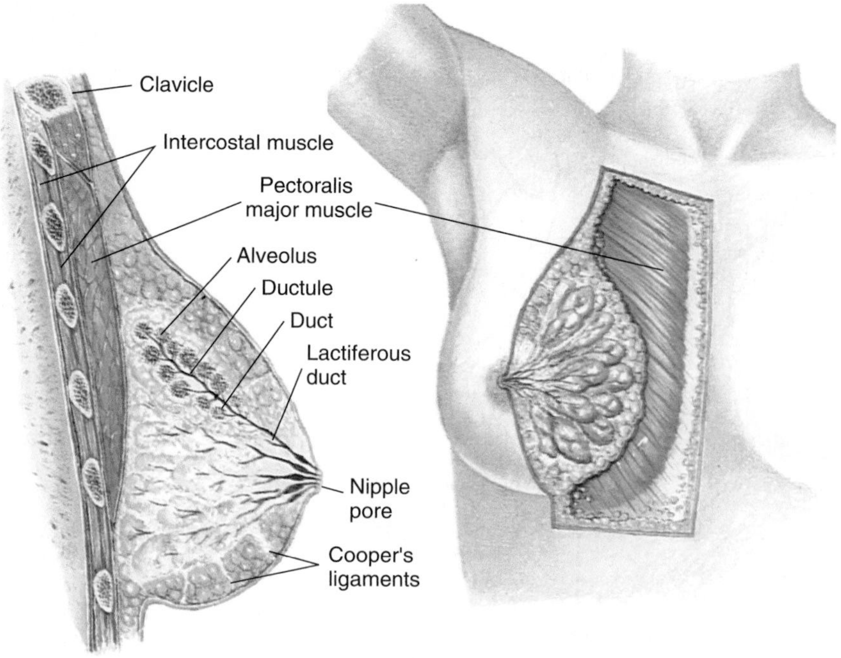

Fig. 5-7 Anatomy of the breast, showing position and major structures. *(From Seidel, H. M., et al. [2006].* Mosby's guide to physical examination *[6th ed., p. 493]. St. Louis: Mosby.)*

Table 5-1 Female Reproductive Physical Assessment Across the Life Cycle

	ADOLESCENT	ADULT	POSTMENOPAUSAL
Breasts	Tender when developing; buds appear; small, firm; one side may grow faster; areola diameter increases; nipples more erect	Grow to full shape in early adulthood; nipples and areola become darker	Become stringy, irregular, pendulous, and nodular; borders less well delineated; may shrink and become flatter, elongated, and less elastic; ligaments weaken; nipples positioned lower
Vagina	Vagina lengthens; epithelial layers thicken; secretions become acidic	Growth complete by age 20	Introitus constricts; vagina narrows, shortens, loses rugation; mucosa is pale, thin, and dry; walls may lose structural integrity
Uterus	Musculature and vasculature increase; lining thickens	Growth complete by age 20	Size decreases; endometrial lining thins
Ovaries	Increase in size and weight; menarche occurs between 8 and 16 years of age; ovulation occurs monthly	Growth complete by age 20	Size decreases to 1 to 2 cm; follicles disappear; surface convolutes; ovarian function ceases between 40 and 55 years of age
Labia majora	Become more prominent; hair develops	Growth complete by age 20	Labia become smaller and flatter; pubic hair becomes sparse and grey
Labia minora	Become more vascular	Growth complete by age 20	Become shinier and drier
Uterine tubes	Increase in size	Growth complete by age 20	Decrease in size

longer recommended by the Society of Obstetricians and Gynaecologists of Canada (SOGC) (2006) and the Canadian Cancer Society (2010a). Evidence-informed practice has changed because research analysis has shown that that BSE has not decreased mortality from breast cancer and has increased the number of **benign** biopsies. Women do need to know how their breasts feel and look and to watch for changes, but not on a regular schedule. Women who choose the BSE method need to be skilled and fully informed and include a yearly health professional breast assessment and routine **mammograms** (see Chapter 6 for further discussion). For women who want to perform BSE, the instructions are given in the Guidelines box. Table 5-1 compares the variations in physical assessment related to age difference in women.

Health Assessment

Trends in women's health have expanded its scope beyond a reproductive focus to include a holistic approach to health care across the lifespan and place women's health within primary care. Women's health assessment and screening focus on a systems evaluation that begins with a careful history and physical examination. During assessment and evaluation, the

Guidelines How to Do a Breast Self-Examination

- Lie down and place your right arm behind your head.
- Use the finger pads of the three middle fingers on your left hand to feel for lumps in the right breast. Use overlapping dime-sized circular motions of the finger pads to feel the breast tissue.

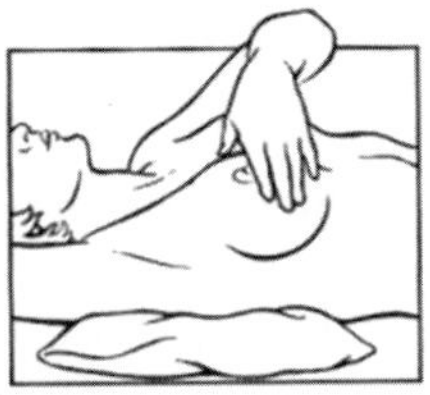

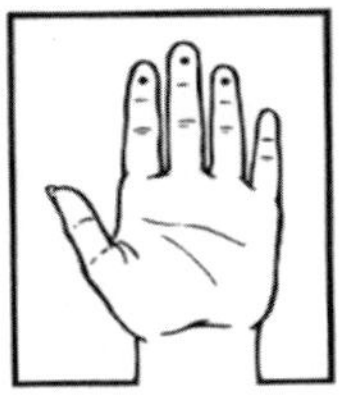

- Use three different levels of pressure to feel all the breast tissue. Light pressure is needed to feel the tissue closest to the skin; medium pressure to feel a little deeper; and firm pressure to feel the tissue closest to the chest and ribs. It is normal to feel a firm ridge in the lower curve of each breast, but you should tell your doctor if you feel anything else out of the ordinary. If you are not sure how hard to press, talk with your health care provider. Use each pressure level to feel the breast tissue before moving on to the next spot.
- Move around the breast in an up-and-down pattern, starting at an imaginary line drawn straight down your side from the underarm and moving across the breast to the middle of the chest bone (sternum or breastbone). Be sure to check the entire breast area going down until you feel only ribs and up to the neck or collarbone (clavicle).

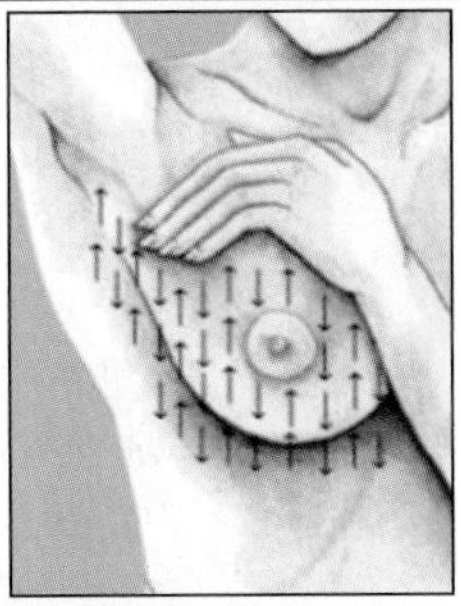

Breast Self-Examination
Examine up to the collarbone, out to armpit, in to middle of chest, and down to bottom of rib cage

- Repeat examination on the left breast, putting your left arm behind your head and using the finger pads of your right hand to do the examination.
- While standing in front of a mirror with your hands pressing firmly down on your hips, look at your breasts for any changes of size, shape, contour, or dimpling, or redness or scaliness of the nipple or breast skin. (The pressing down on the hips position contracts the chest wall muscles and enhances any breast changes.)
- Examine each underarm while sitting up or standing and with your arm only slightly raised so you can easily feel in this area. Raising your arm straight up tightens the tissue in this area and makes it harder to examine.

(From American Cancer Society. [2012]. *How to examine your breasts*. Retrieved from http://www.cancer.org/Cancer/BreastCancer/DetailedGuide/breast-cancer-detection.)

woman's responsibility for self-management, health promotion, and enhancement of wellness is emphasized.

Often it is a nurse who takes the history, orders diagnostic tests, interprets test results, makes referrals, coordinates care, and directs attention to problems requiring medical intervention. Advanced practice nurses who have specialized in women's health, such as nurse practitioners and clinical nurse specialists, perform complete physical examinations, including gynecological examinations.

Culturally competent nursing care should be delivered with an awareness of cultural diversity while respecting the unique qualities of each woman (Canadian Nurses Association [CNA], 2010). Such care cannot be provided in the absence of self-awareness. Nurses must acknowledge their own values, beliefs, and communication styles in order to understand what they contribute to cross-cultural communication. Increasingly, Canada is becoming more diverse in terms of racial, **ethnic**, linguistic, and religious backgrounds. The Registered Nurses Association of Ontario (RNAO) has developed Best Practice Guidelines to assist nurses in delivering culturally competent care. The key competency values include the following: inclusivity, respect, valuing differences, equity, and commitment (RNAO, 2007) (see Chapter 2).

Interview

Contact with the woman usually begins with an interview. This interview should be conducted in a private, comfortable, and relaxed setting (Fig. 5-8). The nurse is seated and makes sure that the woman is comfortable. The woman is addressed by her title and name (e.g., Mrs. Khan) and asked how she prefers to be addressed. Then the nurse introduces herself or himself using name and title. It is important to phrase questions in a sensitive and nonjudgemental manner. Body language should match verbal communication. The nurse needs to be aware of a woman's vulnerability and assure her of strict confidentiality. For many women, fear, anxiety, and modesty make the examination a dreaded and stressful experience. Many women are uninformed, misguided by myths, or afraid that they will appear ignorant by asking questions about sexual or reproductive functioning. The woman should be assured that no question is irrelevant.

The **history** begins with an open-ended question, such as "What brings you into the office (or clinic or hospital) today?" and is furthered by other prompts such as "Anything else?" and "Tell me about it." Additional ways of encouraging women to share information include the following:

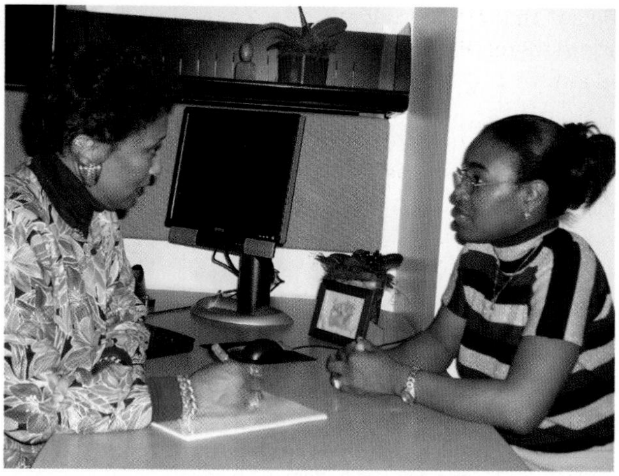

Fig. 5-8 Nurse interviews patient as part of annual physical examination. *(Courtesy Skip Davis, San Francisco, CA.)*

Facilitation—Using a word or posture that communicates interest, such as leaning forward, making eye contact, or saying "Mm-hmmm" or "Go on"

Reflection—Repeating a word or phrase that the woman has used

Clarification—Asking the woman what is meant by a stated word or phrase

Empathic responses—Acknowledging the feelings of a woman by statements such as "That must have been frightening"

Confrontation—Identifying something about the woman's behaviour or feelings not expressed verbally or apparently inconsistent with her history

Interpretation—Putting into words what you infer about the woman's feelings or about the meaning of her symptoms, events, or other matters

Direct questions may be necessary to elicit specific details. These should be worded in language that is understandable to the woman and expressed neutrally so that the woman will not be led into a specific response. The nurse should ask about one item at a time and proceed from the general to the specific (Seidel et al., 2006).

Cultural Considerations and Communication Variations

Recognizing signs and symptoms of disease and deciding to seek treatment are influenced by cultural perceptions. **Culture** evolves over time and is a system of symbols that are learned, shared, and passed on through generations of a social group. *Cultural competence* is the application of knowledge, skills, attitudes, and personal attributes required by nurses to provide care to diverse populations in a respectful manner (CNA, 2010). It is more than simply acquiring knowledge about another ethnic group. It is essential that a nurse have respect for the rich and unique qualities that cultural diversity brings to individuals. In recognizing the value of these differences, the nurse can modify the plan of care to meet the needs of each woman. The woman needs to be trusted that she is the expert on her life, culture, and experiences. If the nurse asks with respect and a genuine desire to learn, the woman will tell the nurse how to care for her. Modifications may be necessary for the physical examination. In many cultures a woman examiner is preferred. In some cultures it may be considered inappropriate for the woman to disrobe completely for the physical examination.

Communication may be hindered by different beliefs, even when the nurse and woman speak the same language. Examples of communication variations are listed in the Cultural Awareness box.

Women With Special Needs

Women With Disabilities

Women with emotional or physical disorders have special needs. Women who have vision, hearing, emotional, or physical disabilities should be respected and involved in the assessment and physical examination to the full extent of their capabilities. The nurse should communicate openly, directly, and with sensitivity. It is often helpful to learn about the disability directly from the woman, while maintaining eye contact. Family and significant others should be relied on only when absolutely necessary. The assessment and physical examination can be adapted to each woman's individual needs.

Communication with a woman who is hearing impaired can be accomplished without difficulty. Many of these women can read lips, write, or both. The interviewer who speaks and enunciates each word slowly and in full view may be easily understood. It is important that the interviewer not stand in front of a light source as this can make it more difficult for the woman to lip read. If a woman is not comfortable with lip

CULTURAL AWARENESS

Communication Variations

Conversational style and pacing—Silence may show respect or acknowledgement that the listener has heard. In cultures in which a direct "no" is considered rude, silence may mean no. Repetition or loudness may mean emphasis or anger.

Personal space—Cultural conceptions of personal space differ. For example, based on one's culture, someone may be perceived as being distant for backing off when approached or aggressive for standing too close.

Eye contact—Eye contact varies among cultures, from intense to fleeting. Consistent with the effort to refrain from invading personal space, avoiding direct eye contact may be a sign of respect.

Touch—The norms about how people should touch each other vary among cultures. In some cultures, physical contact with the same sex (embracing, walking hand in hand) is more appropriate than that with an unrelated person of the opposite sex.

Time orientation—In some cultures, involvement with people is more valued than being "on time." In other cultures, life is scheduled and paced according to clock time, which is valued over personal time.

(Source: Mattson, S. [2000]. Striving for cultural competence: Providing care for the changing face of the U.S. *AWHONN Lifelines*, 4[3], 48–52.)

reading, she may use an interpreter. In this case, it is important to continue to address the woman directly, avoiding the temptation to speak directly with the interpreter.

The visually impaired woman needs to be oriented toward the examination room and may have her guide dog with her. As with all patients, the visually impaired woman needs a full explanation of what the examination entails before proceeding. Before touching her, the nurse should explain, "Now I am going to take your blood pressure. I am going to place the cuff on your right arm." The woman can be asked if she would like to touch each of the items that will be used in the examination, to reduce her anxiety.

Many women and especially those with physical disabilities cannot comfortably lie in the lithotomy position for the pelvic examination. Several alternative positions may be used, including a lateral (side-lying) position, a V-shaped position, a diamond-shaped position, and an M-shaped position (Fig. 5-9). The woman can be asked what has worked best for her previously. If she has never had a pelvic examination or has never had a comfortable pelvic examination, the nurse should proceed slowly by showing her a picture of various positions and asking her which one she prefers. The nurse's support and reassurance can help the woman to relax, which will make the examination go more smoothly.

Women at Risk for Abuse

Nurses should screen all women who are entering the health care system for abuse. Abuse is a life-threatening public health problem that affects millions of women and their children. Prior to asking about abuse, all women should understand the reason for the questions being asked. A good way to present this is, "Because abuse happens to many women, we ask everyone about exposure to violence" (Perinatal Services BC, 2003). The risk for intimate partner violence (IPV) increases during pregnancy and after separation or divorce. Help for the woman may depend on the sensitivity with which the nurse screens for abuse, the discovery of abuse, and subsequent intervention. The nurse must be familiar with the laws governing abuse in the province in which she or he practises.

Pocket cards listing emergency numbers (abuse counselling, legal protection, and emergency shelter) may be obtained from local police departments, women's shelters, or emergency departments. It is helpful to have these on hand in the setting where screening is done. An abuse assessment screen (Fig. 5-10) can be used as part of the interview or written history. If a male partner is present, he should be encouraged to leave the room because the woman may not disclose experiences of abuse in his presence, or he may try to answer questions for her to protect himself. The same procedure applies for partners of lesbians or the adult children of older women.

Fear, guilt, and embarrassment may keep many women from giving information about family violence. Clues in the history and evidence of injuries on physical examination should elicit a high index of suspicion. The areas most commonly injured in women are the head, neck, chest, abdomen, breasts, and upper extremities. Burns and bruises in patterns

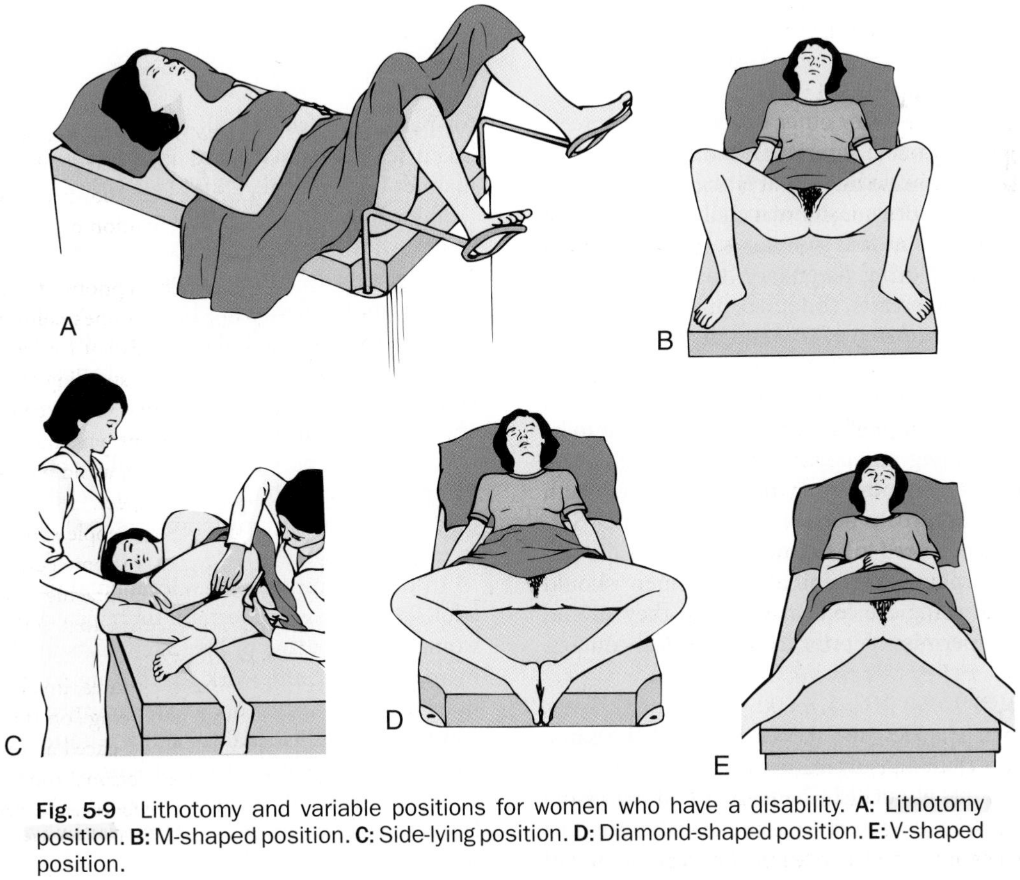

Fig. 5-9 Lithotomy and variable positions for women who have a disability. **A:** Lithotomy position. **B:** M-shaped position. **C:** Side-lying position. **D:** Diamond-shaped position. **E:** V-shaped position.

ABUSE ASSESSMENT SCREEN

1. Have you ever been emotionally or physically abused by your partner or someone important to you?

YES ☐ NO ☐

2. Within the last year, have you been hit, slapped, kicked, or otherwise physically hurt by someone?

YES ☐ NO ☐

If YES, by whom?________________

Number of times ________________

Mark the area of injury on body map.

3. Within the last year, has anyone forced you to have sexual activities?

YES ☐ NO ☐

If YES, who? ________________

Number of times ________________

4. Are you afraid of your partner or anyone you listed above?

YES ☐ NO ☐

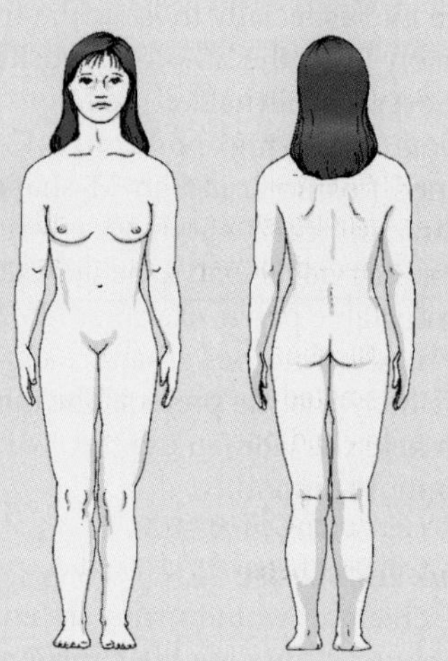

Fig. 5-10 Abuse assessment screen. *(Adapted from the Nursing Research Consortium on Violence and Abuse [1991].)*

resembling hands, belts, cords, or other weapons may be seen, as well as multiple traumatic injuries. Attention should be given to women who repeatedly seek treatment for somatic complaints such as headaches; insomnia; choking sensations; hyperventilation; gastrointestinal symptoms; and pain in the chest, back, or pelvis. During pregnancy, the nurse should assess for injuries to the breasts, abdomen, and genitalia. See Chapter 4 for further discussion of IPV and the care provided to women.

Abusive relationships are often about power and control of the abuser over the woman (see Fig. 4-3). It is important to be aware of this when doing any physical examination, as any perception of power and control over the woman by a health care provider may exacerbate her condition (Perinatal Services BC, 2003). Women need to be shown respect and allowed control during the physical examination. Women should always be addressed using eye contact first, and they should always be asked for permission prior to any physical contact.

Adolescents (Ages 13 to 19)

As a young woman matures, she should be asked the same questions that are included in any history. Particular attention should be paid to hints about risky behaviours, eating disorders, and depression. Sexual activity is addressed after rapport has been established. It is best to talk to a teen with the parent (or partner or friend) out of the room. Questions should be asked with sensitivity and in a gentle and nonjudgemental manner (Seidel et al., 2006) (see Critical Thinking Exercise).

Injury prevention should be a part of the counselling at routine health examinations, with special attention paid to use of seat belts, helmets, and firearms; recreational hazards; and sports involvement. The use of drugs and alcohol and the non-use of seat belts increase the risk of motor vehicle injuries, which account for the greatest proportion of accidental deaths in women. Information about contraceptives and sexually transmitted infection (STI) prevention may be needed for teens who are sexually active (see Chapter 6). Female athletes should have their weight assessed to ensure that they maintain an appropriate body mass index (BMI) (see Chapter 4).

In order to provide developmentally appropriate care for adolescents, it is important to review the major tasks for women in this stage of life. Such tasks include values assessment; education and work goal setting; formation of peer relationships that focus on love, commitment, and becoming comfortable with sexuality; and separation from parents. The teenager is egocentric as she progresses rapidly through emotional and physical change. Her feelings of invulnerability may lead to misconceptions such as the belief that unprotected sexual intercourse will not lead to pregnancy.

CRITICAL THINKING EXERCISE

Caring for an Adolescent Having Her First Pelvic Examination

Nita, a 16-year-old adolescent, who has recently had sex for the first time with her boyfriend, comes to the clinic for information about birth control. Before prescribing any contraceptives, the nurse practitioner suggests that she perform a pelvic examination. Nita says she has never had one and has heard that they hurt and are "a terrible experience."

1. Evidence—Is there sufficient evidence to draw conclusions about the possibility of performing a pain-free pelvic examination on Nita?
2. Assumptions—What assumptions about the following factors can be made about performing a pelvic examination on an adolescent?
   a. Need for confidentiality; the need for a valid consent
   b. The nurse's usual assessment procedure
   c. Equipment needed for pelvic examination of a young girl or woman
   d. Necessary education about sexuality and prevention of sexually transmitted infections and pregnancy
3. What implications and priorities for nursing care can be drawn at this time?
4. Does the evidence objectively support your conclusion?
5. Are there alternative perspectives to your conclusion?

History

At a woman's first visit, she is often expected to fill out a form with biographical and historical data before meeting with the examiner. This form aids the health care provider in completing the history during the interview. Most forms include information about the following categories:

- Biographical data
- Reason for seeking care
- Present health or history of present illness
- Past health
- Family history
- Screening for abuse
- Review of systems
- Functional assessment (activities of daily living)

The following section describes a complete health history based on the above categories.

Biographical data: Name, age, race, sex, marital status, occupation, religion, and ethnicity

Reason for seeking care: A response to the question, "What problem or symptom brought you here today?" If the woman lists more than one reason, focus on the one she thinks is most important.

Present health: Current health status is described with attention to the following:

- Use of safety measures: seat belts, bicycle helmets, designated driver
- Exercise and leisure activities: regularity
- Sleep patterns: length and quality
- Sexuality: Is she sexually active? With men, women, or both? STI and pregnancy prevention practices?
- Diet, including beverages: 24-hour dietary recall; caffeine: coffee, tea, cola, energy drinks, and chocolate intake
- Nicotine, alcohol, illicit or recreational drug use: type, amount, frequency, duration, and reactions
- Environmental and chemical hazards: home, school, work, and leisure setting; exposure to extreme heat or cold, noise, industrial toxins such as asbestos or lead, pesticides, radiation, cat feces, or cigarette smoke

History of present illness: A chronological narrative that includes onset of the problem, the setting in which it developed, its manifestations, and any treatments received is recorded. The woman's state of health before the onset of the present problem is determined. If the problem is long-standing, the reason for seeking attention at this time is elicited. The principal symptoms should be described with respect to the following:

- Location
- Quality or character
- Quantity or severity
- Timing (onset, duration, frequency)
- Factors that aggravate or relieve
- Associated factors
- Woman's perception of the meaning of the symptom

Past health:

- Infectious diseases: for example, measles, mumps, rubella, whooping cough, chickenpox, rheumatic fever, scarlet fever, diphtheria, polio, tuberculosis (TB), hepatitis
- Chronic disease and system disorders: arthritis, cancer, diabetes, heart, lung, kidney, seizures, thyroid, stroke, ulcers, sickle cell anemia
- Adult injuries, accidents
- Hospitalizations, operations, blood transfusions
- Obstetrical history
- Mental health concerns: previous history of depression, anxiety, bipolar; has this been treated?
- Allergies: medications, previous transfusion reactions, environmental allergies
- Immunizations: diphtheria; pertussis; tetanus; polio; measles, mumps, rubella; hepatitis B; varicella; influenza; pneumococcal vaccine; last TB skin test
- Last date of screening tests: Pap test, mammogram; stool for occult blood; sigmoidoscopy/colonoscopy; hematocrit; hemoglobin; rubella titre; urinalysis; cholesterol test; electrocardiogram; vision, dental, hearing examinations
- Current medications: name, dose, frequency, duration, reason for taking, and compliance with prescription medications; home remedies, over-the-counter medications, vitamin and mineral or herbal supplements used over a 24-hour period

Family history: Information about age and health of family members may be presented in narrative form or as a family tree or genogram: age, health or death of parents, siblings, spouse, and children. Check for history of diabetes; heart disease; hypertension; stroke; respiratory, renal, or thyroid problems; cancer; bleeding disorders; hepatitis; allergies; asthma; arthritis; TB; epilepsy; mental illness; human immunodeficiency virus (HIV); or other disorders.

Screen for abuse: Has she ever been hit, kicked, slapped, or forced to have sex against her wishes? Has she been verbally or emotionally abused? (See Fig. 5-10). Does she have a history of childhood sexual abuse? If yes, has she received counselling or does she need referral?

Review of systems: It is probable that all questions in each system will not be included every time a history is taken. Some questions regarding each system should be included in every history. The essential areas to be explored are listed in the following head-to-toe sequence. If a woman gives a positive response to a question about an essential area, more detailed questions should be asked.

- General: weight change, fatigue, weakness, fever, chills, or night sweats
- Skin: skin, hair, and nail changes; itching, bruising, bleeding, rashes, sores, lumps, or moles
- Lymph nodes: enlargement, inflammation, pain, suppuration (pus), or drainage
- Head: trauma, vertigo (dizziness), convulsive disorder, syncope (fainting); headache: location, frequency, pain type, nausea/vomiting, or visual symptoms present
- Eyes: glasses, contact lenses, blurriness, tearing, itching, photophobia, diplopia, inflammation, trauma, cataracts, glaucoma, or acute visual loss
- Ears: hearing loss, tinnitus (ringing), vertigo, discharge, pain, fullness, recurrent infections, or mastoiditis
- Nose and sinuses: trauma, rhinitis, nasal discharge, epistaxis, obstruction, sneezing, itching, allergy, or smelling impairment
- Mouth, throat, and neck: hoarseness, voice changes, soreness, ulcers, bleeding gums, goiter, swelling, or enlarged nodes
- Breasts: masses, pain, lumps, dimpling, nipple discharge, fibrocystic changes, or implants; breast examination practice
- Respiratory: shortness of breath, wheezing, cough, sputum, hemoptysis, pneumonia, pleurisy, asthma, bronchitis, emphysema, or TB; date of last chest X-ray.
- Cardiovascular: hypertension, rheumatic fever, murmurs, angina, palpitations, dyspnea, tachycardia, orthopnea, **edema**, chest pain, cough, cyanosis, cold extremities, ascites, *intermittent claudication* (leg pain caused by poor circulation to the leg muscles), phlebitis, or skin-colour changes
- Gastrointestinal: appetite, nausea, vomiting, indigestion, dysphagia, abdominal pain, ulcers, *hematochezia* (bleeding with stools), *melena* (black, tarry stools), bowel-habit changes, diarrhea, constipation, bowel-movement frequency, food intolerance, hemorrhoids, jaundice, or hepatitis; sigmoidoscopy, colonoscopy, barium enema, **ultrasound**
- Genitourinary: frequency, hesitancy, urgency, polyuria, **dysuria**, hematuria, nocturia, incontinence, stones, infection, or urethral discharge; menstrual history (e.g., age at menarche, length and flow of menses, last menstrual period, dysmenorrhea, intermenstrual bleeding, age at menopause or signs of menopause), **dyspareunia**, discharge, sores, itching
- Sexual health: sexual activity: with men, women, or both; contraceptive use; STIs
- Peripheral vascular: coldness, numbness and tingling, leg edema, claudication, varicose veins, thromboses, or emboli
- Endocrine: heat or cold intolerance, dry skin, excessive sweating, polyuria, polydipsia, polyphagia, thyroid problems, diabetes, or secondary sex characteristic changes
- Hematological: anemia, easy bruising, bleeding, **petechiae**, purpura, or transfusions
- Musculoskeletal: muscle weakness, pain, joint stiffness, scoliosis, lordosis, kyphosis, range-of-motion instability, redness, swelling, arthritis, or gout
- Neurological: loss of sensation, numbness, tingling, tremors, weakness, vertigo, paralysis, fainting, twitching, blackouts, seizures, convulsions, loss of consciousness or memory
- Mental status: moodiness, depression, anxiety, obsessions, delusions, illusions, or hallucinations

Functional assessment: Ability to care for self

Physical Examination

In preparation for the physical examination, the woman should be instructed on undressing and given a gown to wear during the examination. She is usually given the opportunity to undress privately. Objective data are recorded by system or location. A general statement of overall health status is a good way to start. Findings are described in detail.

- General appearance: age, race, sex, state of health, posture, height, weight, development, hygiene, affect, alertness, orientation, and communication skills
- Vital signs: temperature, pulse, respiration, blood pressure
- Skin: colour; integrity; texture; hydration; temperature; edema; excessive perspiration; unusual odour; presence and description of lesions; hair texture and distribution; nail configuration, colour, texture, and condition; presence of nail clubbing
- Head: size, shape, trauma, masses, scars, rashes, or scaling; facial symmetry; presence of edema or puffiness
- Eyes: pupil size, shape, reactivity, conjunctival injection, scleral icterus, fundal papilledema, hemorrhage, lids, extraocular movements, visual fields and acuity
- Ears: shape and symmetry, tenderness, discharge, external canal, and tympanic membranes; hearing—Weber should be midline (loudness of sound equal in both ears) and Rinne negative (no conductive or sensorineural hearing loss); should be able to hear whisper at 1 metre
- Nose: symmetry, tenderness, discharge, mucosa, turbinate inflammation, frontal or maxillary sinus tenderness; discrimination of odours
- Mouth and throat: hygiene; condition of teeth; dentures; appearance of lips, tongue, buccal and oral mucosa; erythema; edema; exudate; tonsillar enlargement; palate; uvula; gag reflex; ulcers
- Neck: mobility, masses, range of motion, trachea deviation, thyroid size, carotid bruits
- Lymphatic: cervical, intraclavicular, axillary, trochlear, or inguinal adenopathy; size, shape, tenderness, and consistency

- Breasts: skin changes, dimpling, symmetry, scars, tenderness, discharge, or masses; characteristics of nipples and areolae
- Heart: rate, rhythm, murmurs, rubs, gallops, clicks, heaves, or precordial movements
- Peripheral vascular: jugular vein distention, bruits, edema, swelling, vein distention, or tenderness of extremities
- Lungs: chest symmetry with respirations, wheezes, crackles, rhonchi, vocal fremitus, whispered pectoriloquy, percussion, and diaphragmatic excursion; breath sounds equal and clear bilaterally
- Abdomen: shape, scars, bowel sounds, consistency, tenderness, rebound, masses, guarding, organomegaly, liver span, percussion (tympany, shifting, dullness), or costovertebral angle tenderness
- Extremities: edema, ulceration, tenderness, varicosities, erythema, tremor, or deformity
- Genitourinary: external genitalia, perineum, vaginal mucosa, cervix; inflammation, tenderness, discharge, bleeding, ulcers, nodules, or masses; internal vaginal support; bimanual and rectovaginal palpation of cervix, uterus, and **adnexa**
- Rectal: sphincter tone, masses, hemorrhoids, rectal wall contour, tenderness, and stool for occult blood
- Musculoskeletal: posture, symmetry of muscle mass, muscle atrophy, weakness, appearance of joints, tenderness or crepitus, joint range of motion, instability, redness, swelling, or spine deviation
- Neurological: mental status, orientation, memory, mood, speech clarity and comprehension, cranial nerves II to XII, sensation, strength, deep tendon and superficial reflexes, gait, balance, and coordination with rapid alternating motions

BOX 5-1 Procedure: Assisting With Pelvic Examination (see Fig. 5-12)

1. Wash your hands. Assemble equipment.
2. Ask woman to empty her bladder before the examination (obtain clean-catch urine specimen as needed).
3. Assist with relaxation techniques. Have the woman place her hands on her chest at about the level of the diaphragm, breathe deeply and slowly (in through her nose and out through her O-shaped mouth), concentrate on the rhythm of breathing, and relax all body muscles with each exhalation (Barkauskas, Baumann, & Darling-Fisher, 2002).
4. Encourage the woman to become involved with the examination if she shows interest. For example, a mirror can be placed so that she can see the area being examined.
5. Assess for and treat signs of problems such as supine hypotension.
6. Warm the speculum in warm water if a prewarmed one is not available.
7. Instruct the woman to bear down when the speculum is being inserted.
8. Apply gloves and assist the examiner with collection of specimens for cytological examination such as a Pap test. After handling specimens, remove gloves and wash your hands.
9. Lubricate the examiner's fingers with water or water-soluble lubricant before bimanual examination.
10. Assist the woman to a sitting position upon completion of the examination.
11. Provide tissues to wipe lubricant from perineum.
12. Provide privacy for the woman while she is dressing.

Pelvic Examination

Many women fear the gynecological portion of the physical examination. The nurse can be instrumental in allaying these fears by providing information and assisting the woman to express her feelings to the examiner (Box 5-1).

The woman should be assisted into the lithotomy position for the pelvic examination. If the woman is not comfortable in this position then alternate positions may be used (see Fig. 5-9). When she is in the lithotomy position, the woman's hips and knees are flexed, with buttocks at the edge of the table, and her feet are supported by heel or knee stirrups.

Some women prefer to keep their shoes or socks on, especially if the stirrups are not padded. Many women express feelings of vulnerability and strangeness when in the lithotomy position. During the procedure, the nurse can assist the woman with relaxation techniques (see Box 5-1). Breathing techniques can be particularly helpful for the adolescent and for the woman whose introitus may be especially tight or for whom the experience is new or may provoke tension. Some women relax when they are encouraged to become involved with the examination by having a mirror placed so that they can view the area being examined. This type of participation helps with health teaching as well. Distraction is another technique that can be used effectively (e.g., placing interesting pictures on the ceiling over the head of the table).

Many women find it distressing to attempt to converse in the lithotomy position. Most women appreciate an explanation of the procedure as it unfolds, as well as coaching for the type of sensations they may expect. Generally, however, women prefer not to have to respond to questions until they are again upright and at eye level with the examiner. Being asked questions during the procedure, especially if they cannot see their questioner's eyes, may make some women tense.

A teenager's first speculum examination is the most important one because she will develop perceptions that will remain with her for future examinations. What the examination entails should be discussed with the teen while she is dressed. Models or illustrations can be used to show exactly what will happen. All of the necessary equipment should be assembled so that there are no interruptions (Fig. 5-11). Pediatric specula that are 1 to 1.5 cm wide can be inserted with minimal discomfort. If the teen is sexually active, a small adult speculum may be used.

External Inspection

The examiner wears gloves and sits at the foot of the table for the **inspection** of the external genitals and the speculum

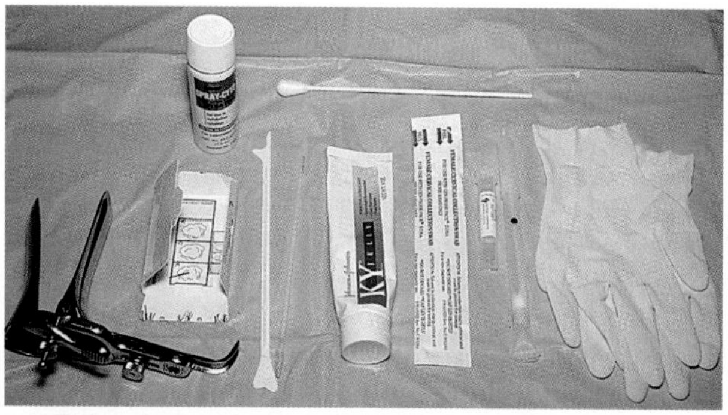

Fig. 5-11 Equipment used for pelvic examination. *(Courtesy Michael S. Clement, MD, Mesa, AZ.)*

examination. In good lighting, external genitals are inspected for sexual maturity, clitoris, labia, perineum, and lesions indicative of STIs. After childbirth or other trauma there may be healed scars.

External Palpation

Before touching the woman, the examiner should explain what is going to be done and what the woman should expect to feel (e.g., pressure). The examiner may touch the woman in a less sensitive area such as the inner thigh to alert her that the genital examination is beginning. This gesture may put the woman more at ease. The labia are spread apart to expose the structures in the vestibule: urinary meatus, Skene glands, vaginal orifice, and Bartholin glands (Fig. 5-12). To assess the Skene glands, the examiner inserts one finger into the vagina and "milks" the area of the urethra. Any exudate from the urethra or the Skene glands is cultured. Masses and erythema of either structure are assessed further. Ordinarily the openings to the Skene glands are not visible; prominent openings may be seen if the glands are infected (e.g., with gonorrhea). During the examination, the examiner needs to keep in mind the data from the review of systems, such as history of burning on urination.

The vaginal orifice is then examined. Hymenal tags are normal findings. With one finger still in the vagina, the examiner repositions the index finger near the posterior part of the orifice. With the thumb outside the posterior part of the labia majora, the examiner compresses the area of Bartholin glands located at the 8 o'clock and 4 o'clock positions and looks for swelling, discharge, and pain.

The support of the anterior and posterior vaginal wall is also assessed. The examiner spreads the labia with the index and middle finger and then will ask the woman to strain down. Any bulge from the anterior wall (urethrocele or **cystocele**) or posterior wall (**rectocele**) is noted and compared with the history, such as difficulty starting the stream of urine or constipation.

The perineum (area between the vagina and anus) is assessed for scars from old lacerations or **episiotomies**, thinning, fistulas, masses, lesions, and inflammation. The anus is assessed for hemorrhoids, hemorrhoidal tags, and integrity of the anal sphincter. The anal area is also assessed for lesions, masses, abscesses, and tumours. If there is a history of STI, the examiner may want to obtain a culture specimen from the anal canal at this time. Throughout the genital examination, the

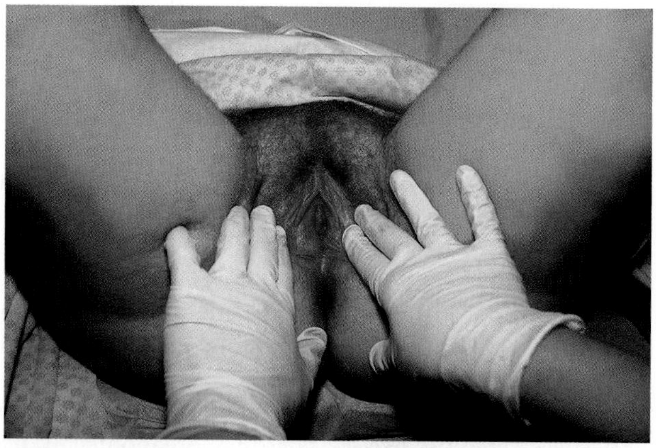

Fig. 5-12 External examination. Separation of the labia. *(From Wilson, S. F, & Giddens, J. F. [2009]. Health assessment for nursing practice [4th ed.]. St. Louis: Mosby.)*

BOX 5-2 Diethylstilbestrol—Yesterday and Today

Between 1938 and 1971, 5 to 10 million pregnant women who had previously experienced a miscarriage or premature birth received diethylstilbestrol (DES) to improve their chances of having a successful pregnancy. In 1971, researchers discovered that prenatal exposure to DES increases the risk of clear cell adenocarcinoma of the cervix and vagina. At that time the U.S. Food and Drug Administration issued a warning and advised physicians to stop prescribing DES. Currently researchers are discovering more adverse effects of exposure to DES. The women who received DES while pregnant have a moderate increase in the risk of breast cancer. DES daughters have an increased risk of pregnancy complications, infertility, and structural differences of the reproductive tract such as a T-shaped uterus. DES sons have an increased risk of noncancerous epididymal cysts. There are no known effects on granddaughters of women who received DES, but grandsons are 20 times more likely than those in the general population to have hypospadias.

(Source: Ferris, R. S., Sofer, D., & Zolor, J. S. [2003]. A drug of the past still haunts some. *American Journal of Nursing, 103*[8], 20.)

examiner should note any odour, which may indicate infection or poor hygiene.

Internal Examination

A vaginal speculum is used to view the vaginal vault and cervix. A vaginal speculum consists of two blades and a handle, and specula come in a variety of types and styles. The speculum is gently placed into the vagina and inserted to the back of the vaginal vault. The blades are opened to reveal the cervix and are locked into the open position (Fig. 5-13, A to D). The cervix is inspected for position and appearance of the os: colour, lesions, bleeding, and discharge. Cervical findings that are not within normal limits include ulcerations, masses, inflammation, and excessive protrusion into the vaginal vault. Anomalies such as a cockscomb (a protrusion over the cervix that looks like a rooster's comb), a hooded or collared cervix (seen in diethylstilbestrol daughters [Box 5-2]), or polyps should be noted.

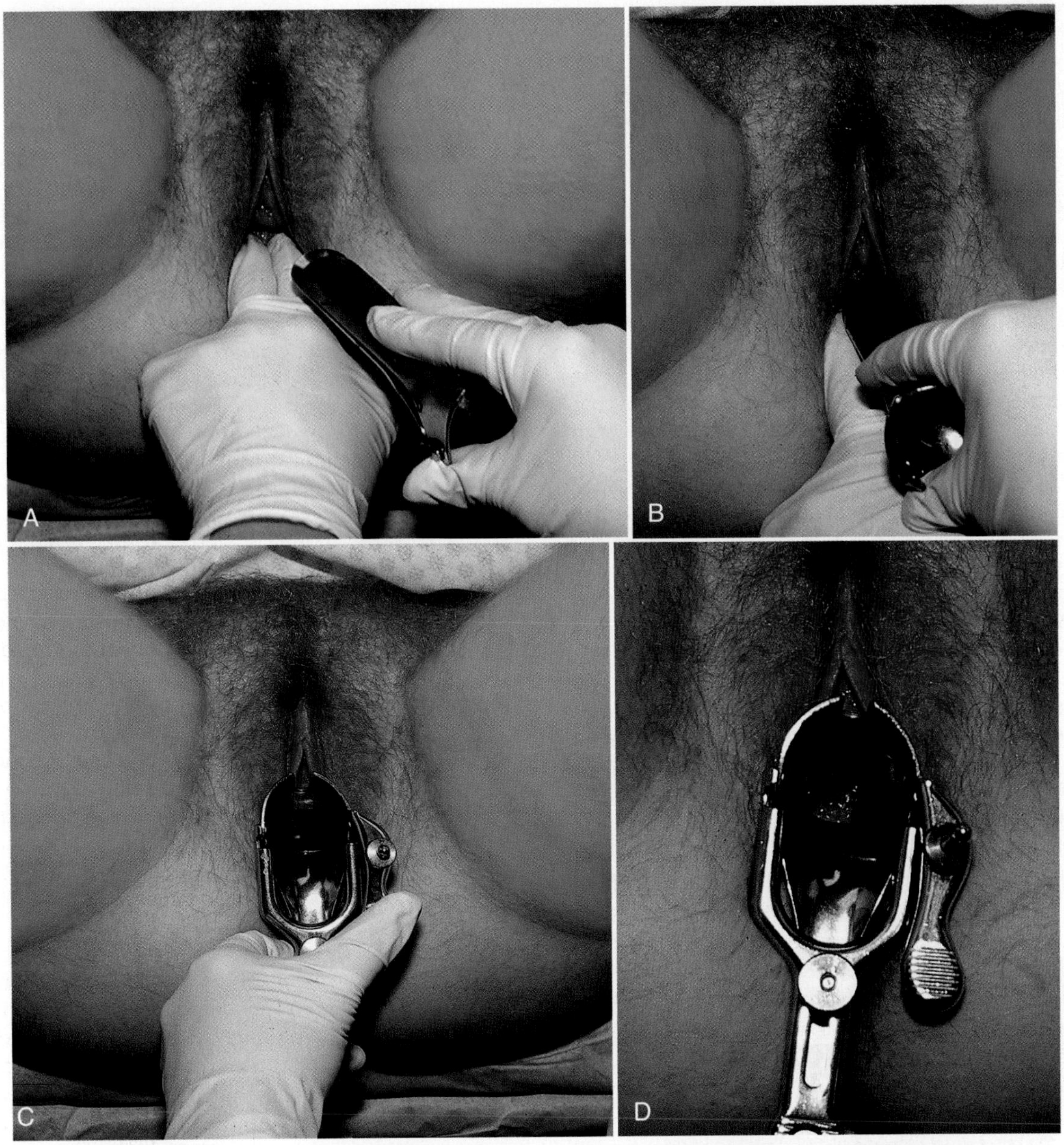

Fig. 5-13 Insertion of speculum for vaginal examination. **A:** Opening of the introitus. **B:** Oblique insertion of the speculum. **C:** Final insertion of the speculum. **D:** Opening of the speculum blades. *(From Wilson, S. F., & Giddens, J. F. [2009].* Health assessment for nursing practice *[4th ed., p. 435]. St. Louis: Mosby.)*

Collection of Specimens

The collection of specimens for cytological examination is an important part of the gynecological examination. Infection can be diagnosed by examination of specimens collected during the pelvic examination. These infections include candidiasis, trichomoniasis, bacterial vaginosis, group B streptococcus, gonorrhea, chlamydia, and herpes simplex virus. Once the diagnoses have been made, treatment can be instituted (see discussion in Chapter 6).

Papanicolaou Test. Carcinogenic conditions, whether potential or actual, can be determined by examination of cells from the cervix collected during the pelvic examination (i.e., a Pap test) (Box 5-3 and Fig. 5-14). Pap tests should be initiated within 3 years of initial vaginal sexual activity. Women with abnormal Pap results need more frequent testing. Pap screening can be discontinued in a woman who is 70 years old and has three to four negative smears in the past 10 years (Cancer Care Ontario, 2007).

Vaginal Wall Examination

After the specimens are obtained, the vagina is viewed when the speculum is rotated. The speculum blades are unlocked and partially closed. As the speculum is withdrawn it is rotated; the vaginal walls are inspected for colour, lesions, rugae, fistulas, and bulging.

Bimanual Palpation

The examiner stands for this part of the examination. A small amount of lubricant is placed on the first and second

BOX 5-3 Procedure: Papanicolaou Test

1. In preparation, make sure that the woman has not douched, used vaginal medications, or had sexual intercourse for at least 24 hours before the procedure. Reschedule the test if the woman is menstruating. Midcycle is the best time to test.
2. Assist the woman into a position that is most comfortable for her (usually lithotomy). A speculum is then inserted into the vagina.
3. Explain to the woman the purpose of the test and what sensations she will feel as the specimen is obtained (e.g., pressure but not pain).
4. The cytological specimen is obtained before any digital examination of the vagina is made or endocervical bacteriological specimens are taken with cotton swabbing of the cervix.
5. The Papanicolaou (Pap) test is done by using an endocervical sampling device (Cytobrush, Cervex-Brush, papette, or broom) (see Fig. 5-14). If the two-sample method of obtaining cells is used, the cytobrush is inserted into the canal and rotated 90 to 180 degrees, followed by a gentle smear of the entire transformation zone using a spatula. Broom devices are inserted and rotated 360 degrees 5 times. They obtain endocervical and ectocervical samples at the same time. If the patient has had a hysterectomy, the vaginal cuff is sampled. Areas that appear abnormal on visualization require colposcopy and biopsy. If using a one-slide technique, the spatula sample is smeared first. This is followed by applying the cytobrush sample (rolling the brush in the opposite direction from which it was obtained), which is less subject to drying artifact; the slide is then sprayed with preservative within 5 seconds.
6. The ThinPrep Pap Test is an improved method of preserving cells that reduces blood, mucus, and inflammation. The Pap specimen is obtained in the manner described previously, and the collection device (brush, spatula, or broom) is simply rinsed in a vial of preserving solution that is provided by the laboratory. The sealed vial with solution is sent off to the appropriate laboratory. A special processing device filters the contents, and a thin layer of cervical cells is deposited on a slide, which is then examined microscopically. Initial reports state that specimen adequacy is improved by 50% and detection of low-grade and more severe lesions is improved by 65%. The PapNet test is similar to the ThinPrep test.
7. Label the slides with the woman's name and site. Include on the form to accompany the slides the woman's name, age, last menstrual period, and parity and the reason for taking the cytological specimens.
8. Send specimens to the pathology laboratory promptly for staining, evaluation, and a written report, with special reference to abnormal elements, including cancer cells.
9. Advise the woman that repeat tests may be necessary if the specimen is not adequate.
10. Instruct the woman about routine checkups for cervical and vaginal cancer. The Canadian Cancer Society (2010b) advises that women over 18 years of age and those under 18 who are sexually active have the test every 1 to 3 years, depending on the previous test results.
11. Record the examination date on the woman's record.

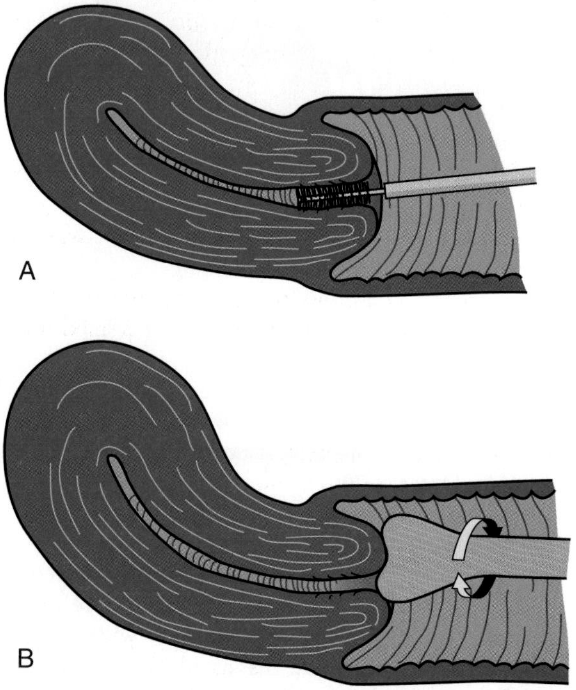

Fig. 5-14 Pap test. **A:** Collecting cells from the endocervix using a cytobrush. **B:** Obtaining cells from the transformation zone using a wooden spatula. *(From Katz, V. L., et al. [2007]. Comprehensive gynecology [5th ed.]. Philadelphia: Mosby.)*

fingers of the gloved hand for the internal examination. To avoid tissue trauma and contamination, the thumb is abducted, and the ring and little fingers are flexed into the palm (Fig. 5-15).

The vagina is palpated for distensibility, lesions, and tenderness. The cervix is examined for position, shape, consistency, motility, and lesions. The fornix around the cervix is palpated.

The other hand is placed on the abdomen halfway between the umbilicus and symphysis pubis and exerts pressure downward toward the pelvic hand. Upward pressure from the pelvic hand traps reproductive structures for assessment by palpation. The uterus is assessed for position, size, shape, consistency, regularity, motility, masses, and tenderness.

With the abdominal hand moving to the right lower quadrant and the fingers of the pelvic hand in the right lateral fornix, the fallopian tubes and ovaries are assessed for position, size, tenderness, and masses. The examination is repeated on the woman's left side.

Just before the intravaginal fingers are withdrawn, the woman is asked to tighten her vagina around the fingers as much as she can. If the muscle response is weak, the woman is assessed for her knowledge about Kegel exercises.

Rectovaginal Palpation

To prevent contamination of the rectum from organisms in the vagina, it is necessary to change gloves, add fresh lubricant,

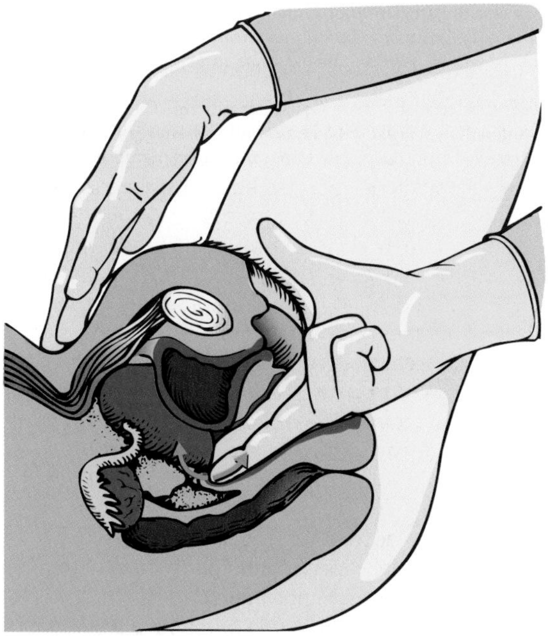

Fig. 5-15 Bimanual palpation of the uterus.

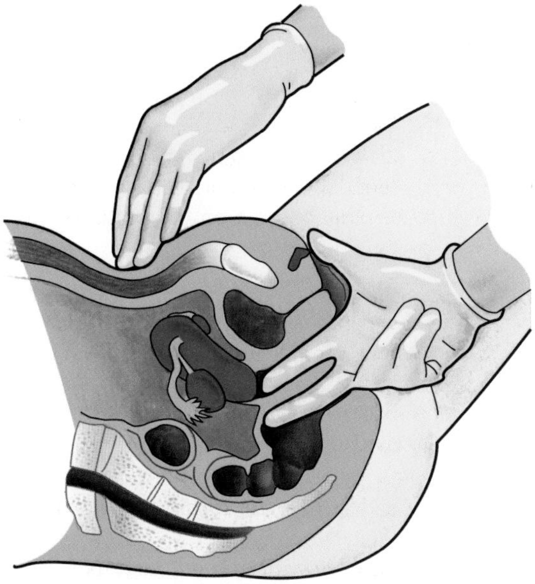

Fig. 5-16 Rectovaginal examination. *(From Seidel, H. M., et al. [2006].* Mosby's guide to physical examination *[6th ed., p. 609]. St. Louis: Mosby.)*

and then reinsert the index finger into the vagina and the middle finger into the rectum (Fig. 5-16). Insertion is facilitated if the woman strains down. The manoeuvres of the abdominovaginal examination are repeated. The rectovaginal examination enables assessment of the rectovaginal septum, the posterior surface of the uterus, and the region behind the cervix and the adnexa. The vaginal finger is removed and folded into the palm, leaving the middle finger free to rotate 360 degrees. The rectum is palpated for rectal tenderness and masses.

After the rectal examination is completed, the woman should be assisted into a sitting position, given tissues or wipes to cleanse herself, and afforded privacy to dress. The examiner returns after the woman is dressed, to discuss findings and the plan of care.

Pelvic Examination After Hysterectomy. The pelvic examination is done in much the same way as is done on a woman with a uterus. Vaginal screening using the Pap test is not recommended in women who have had a total hysterectomy with removal of the cervix for benign disease (Cancer Care Ontario, 2007). Because of the epidemic of human papillomavirus, which causes vaginal intraepithelial neoplasia, sampling of the vaginal cuff and vaginal walls after hysterectomy may still be practised, with schedules varying from every year to every 2 to 3 years.

Laboratory and Diagnostic Procedures

The following laboratory and diagnostic procedures are ordered at the discretion of the clinician, considering the patient and family history: hemoglobin, glycosalated hemoglobin ($HgbA_{1C}$), fasting blood glucose, total blood cholesterol, lipid profile, urinalysis, syphilis serology (Venereal Disease Research Laboratories [VDRL] or rapid plasma reagent [RPR]) and other screening tests for STIs, mammogram, tuberculosis skin testing, hearing, visual acuity, electrocardiogram, chest radiograph, pulmonary function, fecal occult blood, flexible sigmoidoscopy, and bone mineral density (dual energy X-ray absorptiometry [DEXA] scan). Results of these tests may be reported in person, by phone call, or by letter. Tests for HIV, hepatitis B, and drug screening may be offered with informed consent in high-risk populations. These test results are usually reported in person.

Key Points

- Health promotion and illness prevention help women to actualize their health potential by increasing motivation, providing information, and suggesting how to access specific resources.
- Periodic health screening, including history, physical examination, and diagnostic and laboratory tests, provides the basis for overall health promotion, prevention of illness, early diagnosis of problems, and referral for management.
- Health screening needs to be performed in a way that is culturally sensitive.
- Routine screening mammography and annual breast examinations by skilled practitioners are recommended for early detection of breast cancer.

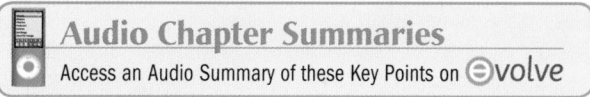

Audio Chapter Summaries

Access an Audio Summary of these Key Points on evolve

References

Barkauskas, V. H., Baumann, L. C., & Darling-Fisher, C. S. (2002). *Health and physical assessment* (3rd ed.). St. Louis: Mosby.

Canadian Cancer Society. (2010a). *Breast cancer. How to reduce your risk.* Retrieved from http://www.cancer.ca/~/media/CCS/Canada%20wide/Files%20List/English%20files%20heading/Library%20PDFs%20-%20English/Breast%20Cancer%20How%20to%20reduce%20your%20risk_Eng_july%202010.ashx.

Canadian Cancer Society. (2010b). *Cervical cancer.* Retrieved from http://www.cancer.ca/Canada-wide/Prevention/Getting%20checked/Cervical%20cancer%20NEW.aspx?sc_lang=en.

Canadian Nurses Association. (2010). *Canadian Nurses Association position statement: Promoting cultural competence in nursing.* Ottawa: Author. Retrieved from http://www.cna-aiic.ca/CNA/documents/pdf/publications/PS114_Cultural_Competence_2010_e.pdf.

Cancer Care Ontario. (2007). Ontario cervical cancer screening clinical practice guidelines. *Journal of Obstetrics and Gynaecology Canada, 29*(4), 344–353.

Perinatal Services BC. (2003). *Intimate partner violence during the perinatal period.* Vancouver, BC: Author. Retrieved from http://www.perinatalservicesbc.ca//sites/bcrcp/files/Guidelines/Obstetrics/IPVJuly2003Final.pdf.

Registered Nurses Association of Ontario. (2007). *Embracing cultural diversity in health care: Developing cultural competence.* Toronto: Author.

Seidel, H. M., et al. (2006). *Mosby's guide to physical examination* (6th ed.). St. Louis: Mosby.

Society of Obstetricians and Gynaecologists of Canada. (2006). Breast self-examination. *Journal of Obstetrics and Gynaecology Canada, 28*(8), 728–730. Retrieved from http://www.sogc.org/guidelines/documents/181E-CO-August2006.pdf.

Unit 2

6 Reproductive Health

Learning Objectives

On completion of this chapter, the reader will be able to:

- Differentiate the menstrual cycle in relation to hormonal, ovarian, and endometrial responses.
- Develop a nursing care plan for the woman with primary dysmenorrhea.
- Outline patient teaching about premenstrual syndrome.
- Relate the pathophysiology of endometriosis to associated symptoms.
- Evaluate the use of alternative therapies for menstrual disorders.
- Describe treatment for menopause symptoms.
- Describe prevention and treatment of sexually transmitted infections in women.
- Summarize the care of women with selected viral infections (i.e., human immunodeficiency virus and hepatitis B virus).
- Differentiate signs, symptoms, and management of selected vaginal infections.
- Review principles of infection control for human immunodeficiency virus and blood-borne pathogens.
- Discuss the pathophysiology and emotional effects of selected benign breast conditions and malignant neoplasms of the breasts that are found in women.

Electronic Resources

Additional information related to the content in Chapter 6 can be found on

evolve the companion Web site at

http://evolve.elsevier.com/Canada/Perry/maternal/

- Examination Review Questions
- Animation—Female Reproductive Ducts
- Animation—Menstrual Cycle: Uterine
- Animation—Ovaries
- Animation—Ovulation
- Animation—Pelvic Inflammatory Disease
- Case Study—Breast Cancer

Health issues may occur at any point in a woman's life, especially during the reproductive years. Many factors, including anatomic abnormalities, physiological imbalances, and lifestyle, can affect the menstrual cycle. The average woman may have some concerns related to her menstrual and gynecological health at some point in her life and may experience bleeding, pain, discharge, or infections associated with her reproductive organs or functions. This chapter provides information on the menstrual cycle, common menstrual problems, sexually transmitted infections, and selected other infections that can affect reproductive functions. Benign breast conditions are also discussed. Breast cancer is addressed in this chapter because it is the most common reproductive cancer occurring in women.

Menstruation

Menarche and Puberty

Although young girls secrete small, rather constant amounts of estrogen, a marked increase in secretion occurs between 8 and 11 years of age. The term **menarche** denotes first menstruation. **Puberty** is a broader term that denotes the entire transitional stage between childhood and sexual maturity. Increasing amounts and variations in gonadotropin and estrogen secretion develop into a cyclic pattern at least a year before menarche. In North America this occurs in most girls at about 13 years of age.

Initially, menstrual periods are irregular, unpredictable, painless, and anovulatory (no ovum is released from the ovary). After 1 or more years, a hypothalamic–**pituitary** rhythm develops, and the ovary produces adequate cyclic estrogen to make a mature ovum. Ovulatory (ovum released from the ovary) periods tend to be regular, monitored by progesterone.

Although pregnancy can occur in exceptional cases of true precocious puberty, most pregnancies in young girls occur after the normally timed menarche. All young adolescents of both sexes would benefit from knowing that pregnancy can occur at any time after the onset of menses.

Menstrual Cycle

Menstruation is the periodic uterine bleeding that begins approximately 14 days after **ovulation**. It is controlled by a feedback system of three cycles: endometrial, hypothalamic–pituitary, and ovarian. The average length of a menstrual cycle is 28 days, but variations are normal. The first day of bleeding is designated as day 1 of the menstrual cycle, or menses (Fig. 6-1). The average duration of menstrual flow is 5 days (with a range of 3 to 6 days), and the average blood loss is 50 mL (with a range of 20 to 80 mL), but these vary greatly.

For about 50% of women, menstrual blood does not appear to clot. The menstrual blood clots within the uterus, but the clot usually liquefies before being discharged from the uterus. Uterine discharge includes mucus and epithelial cells in addition to blood.

The menstrual cycle is a complex interplay of events that occur simultaneously in the **endometrium**, the **hypothalamus**, the pituitary glands, and the ovaries. The menstrual cycle prepares the uterus for pregnancy. When pregnancy does not occur, menstruation follows. A woman's age, physical and emotional status, and environment influence the regularity of her menstrual cycles.

Endometrial Cycle

The four phases of the endometrial cycle are (1) the menstrual phase, (2) the proliferative phase, (3) the secretory phase, and (4) the ischemic phase (see Fig. 6-1). During the menstrual phase shedding of the functional two-thirds of the endometrium (the compact and spongy layers) is initiated by periodic vasoconstriction in the upper layers of the endometrium. The basal layer is always retained, and regeneration begins near the end of the cycle from cells derived from the remaining glandular remnants or stromal cells in this layer.

The proliferative phase is a period of rapid growth lasting from about the fifth day to the time of ovulation. The endometrial surface is completely restored in approximately 4 days, or slightly before bleeding ceases. From this point on, an 8-fold to 10-fold thickening occurs, with a levelling off of growth at ovulation. The proliferative phase depends on estrogen stimulation derived from ovarian follicles.

The secretory phase extends from the day of ovulation to about 3 days before the next menstrual period. After ovulation, larger amounts of progesterone are produced. An edematous, vascular, functional endometrium is now apparent. At the end of the secretory phase, the fully matured secretory endometrium reaches the thickness of heavy, soft velvet. It becomes luxuriant with blood and glandular secretions, a suitable protective and nutritive bed for a fertilized ovum.

Implantation of the fertilized ovum generally occurs about 7 to 10 days after ovulation. With the rapid decrease in progesterone and estrogen levels, the spiral arteries go into spasm. During the ischemic phase, the blood supply to the functional endometrium is blocked, and necrosis develops. The functional layer separates from the basal layer, and menstrual bleeding begins, marking day 1 of the next cycle (see Fig. 6-1).

Hypothalamic–Pituitary Cycle

Toward the end of the normal menstrual cycle, blood levels of estrogen and progesterone decrease. Low blood levels of these ovarian **hormones** stimulate the hypothalamus to secrete gonadotropin-releasing hormone (GnRH). In turn, GnRH stimulates anterior pituitary secretion of follicle-stimulating hormone (FSH). FSH stimulates development of ovarian **graafian follicles** and their production of estrogen. Estrogen levels begin to decrease, and hypothalamic GnRH triggers the anterior pituitary to release luteinizing hormone (LH). A marked surge of LH and a smaller peak of estrogen (day 12; see Fig. 6-1) precede the expulsion of the ovum from the graafian follicle by about 24 to 36 hours. LH peaks at about day 13 or 14 of a 28-day cycle. If fertilization and implantation of the ovum have not occurred by this time, regression of the corpus luteum follows. Levels of progesterone and estrogen decline, menstruation occurs, and the hypothalamus is once again stimulated to secrete GnRH. This process is called the *hypothalamic–pituitary cycle*.

Ovarian Cycle

The primitive graafian follicles contain immature oocytes (primordial ova). Before ovulation, from 1 to 30 follicles begin to mature in each ovary under the influence of FSH and estrogen. The preovulatory surge of LH affects a selected follicle. The oocyte matures, ovulation occurs, and the empty follicle begins its transformation into the corpus luteum. This follicular phase (preovulatory phase) (see Fig. 6-1) of the ovarian cycle varies in length from woman to woman. Almost all variations in ovarian cycle length are the result of variations in the length of the follicular phase. On rare occasions (i.e., 1 in 100 menstrual cycles) more than one follicle is selected, and more than one oocyte matures and undergoes ovulation.

After ovulation, estrogen levels drop. For 90% of women only a small amount of withdrawal bleeding occurs, and it goes unnoticed. In 10% of women there is sufficient bleeding for it to be visible, resulting in what is termed *midcycle bleeding*.

The luteal phase begins immediately after ovulation and ends with the start of menstruation. This postovulatory phase of the ovarian cycle usually requires 14 days (range 13 to 15 days). The corpus luteum reaches its peak of functional activity 8 days after ovulation, secreting the steroids estrogen and progesterone. Coincident with this time of peak luteal functioning, the fertilized ovum is implanted in the endometrium. If no implantation occurs, the corpus luteum regresses, and steroid levels drop. Two weeks after ovulation, if fertilization and implantation do not occur, the functional layer of the uterine endometrium is shed through menstruation.

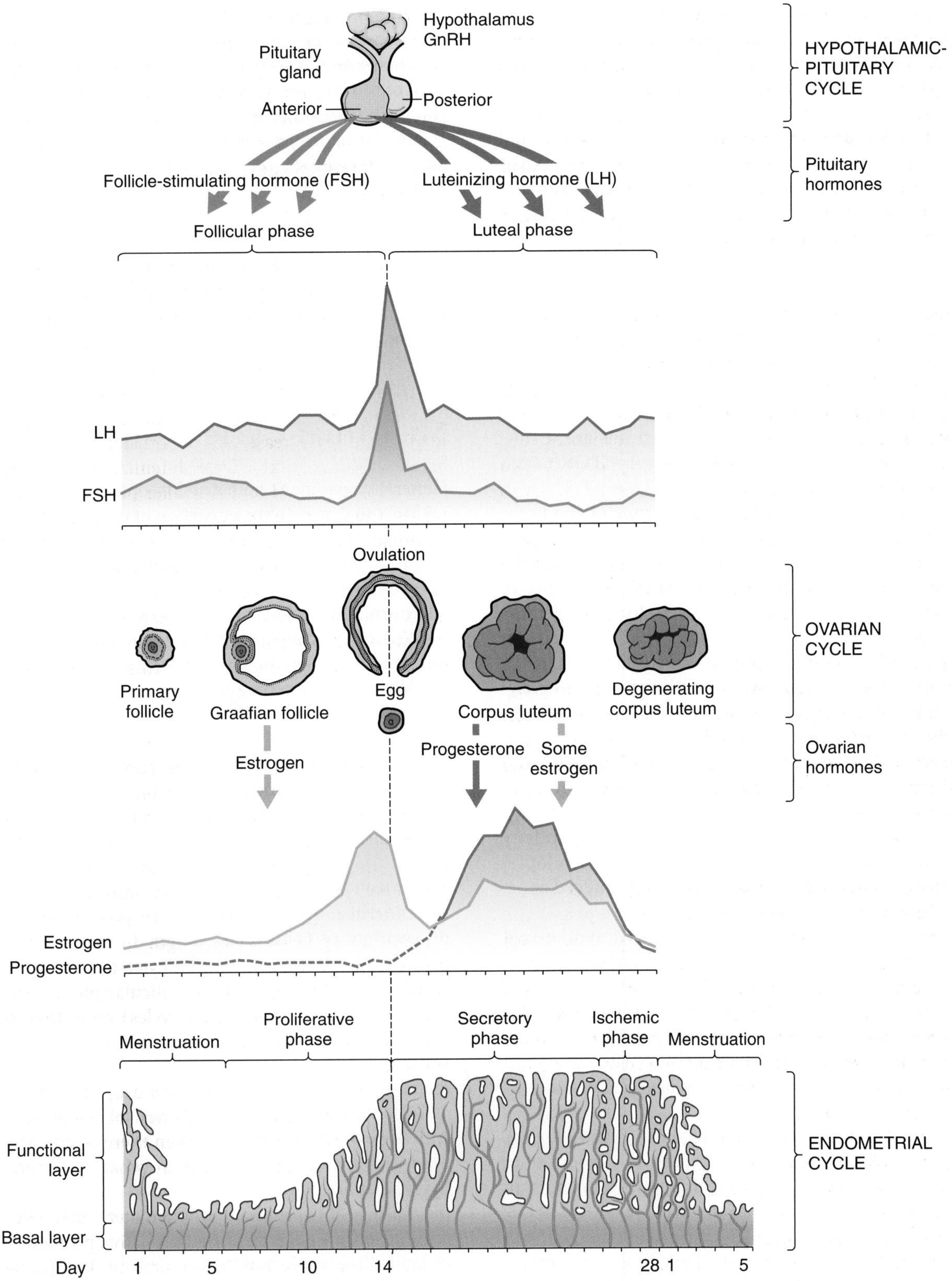

Fig. 6-1 Menstrual cycle: hypothalamic–pituitary, ovarian, and endometrial. *GnRH*, gonadotropin-releasing hormone.

evolve Animation—Ovarian Torsion

evolve Animation—Menstrual Cycle: Uterine

evolve Animation—Ovulation

Other Cyclic Changes

When the hypothalamic–pituitary–ovarian axis functions properly, other tissues undergo predictable responses. Before ovulation, the woman's basal body temperature is often less than 37°C; after ovulation, with increasing progesterone levels, her basal body temperature rises. Changes in the cervix and cervical mucus follow a generally predictable pattern. Preovulatory and postovulatory mucus is viscous (thick) so that sperm penetration is discouraged. At the time of ovulation, cervical mucus is thin and clear. It looks, feels, and stretches like egg white. This stretchable quality is termed **spinnbarkeit**. Some women have localized lower abdominal pain, called *mittelschmerz*, that coincides with ovulation. Some spotting may occur.

Prostaglandins

Prostaglandins (PGs) are oxygenated fatty acids classified as hormones. The different kinds of prostaglandins are distinguished by letters (PGE and PGF), numbers (PGE_2), and letters of the Greek alphabet ($PGF_{2\alpha}$).

Prostaglandins are produced in most organs of the body, including the uterus. Menstrual blood is a potent prostaglandin source. Prostaglandins are metabolized quickly by most tissues. They are biologically active in minute amounts in the cardiovascular, gastrointestinal, respiratory, urogenital, and nervous systems. They also exert a marked effect on metabolism, particularly on glycolysis. Prostaglandins play an important role in many physiological, pathological, and pharmacological reactions. $PGF_{2\alpha}$, PGE_4, and PGE_2 are most commonly used in reproductive medicine.

Prostaglandins affect smooth muscle contractility and modulation of hormonal activity. Indirect evidence indicates that prostaglandins have an effect on ovulation, fertility, changes in the cervix and cervical mucus that affect receptivity to sperm, tubal and uterine motility, sloughing of endometrium (menstruation), onset of miscarriage and induced abortion, and onset of labour (term and preterm).

After exerting their biological actions, newly synthesized prostaglandins are rapidly metabolized by tissues in such organs as the lungs, kidneys, and liver.

Prostaglandins may play a key role in ovulation. If prostaglandin levels do not rise along with the surge of LH, the ovum remains trapped within the graafian follicle. After ovulation prostaglandins may influence production of estrogen and progesterone by the corpus luteum.

The introduction of prostaglandins into the vagina or the uterine cavity (from ejaculated semen) increases the motility of uterine musculature, which may assist the transport of sperm through the uterus and into the oviduct.

Prostaglandins produced by the woman cause regression of the corpus luteum and regression and sloughing of the endometrium, resulting in menstruation. Prostaglandins increase myometrial response to oxytocic stimulation, enhance uterine contractions, and cause cervical dilation. They may be a factor in the initiation of labour, the maintenance of labour, or both. They may also be involved in dysmenorrhea (see discussion later in chapter) and pre-eclampsia and eclampsia (see Chapter 13).

Climacteric and Menopause

The **climacteric** is a transitional phase during which ovarian function and hormone production decline. This phase spans the years from the onset of premenopausal ovarian decline to the postmenopausal time when symptoms stop. **Menopause** (from the Latin *mensis*, month, and Greek *pauses*, to cease) can be dated with certainty only 1 year after menstruation ceases. The average age at natural menopause is 51.4 years, with an age range of 35 to 60 years. Perimenopause is a period preceding menopause that lasts about 4 years. During this time ovarian function declines. Ova slowly diminish, and menstrual cycles may be anovulatory, resulting in irregular bleeding. The ovary stops producing estrogen, and eventually menses no longer occur.

Menstrual Cycle Concerns

Generally, a woman's menstrual frequency stabilizes at 28 days within 1 to 2 years after puberty with a range of 26 to 34 days. Although no woman's cycle is exactly the same length every month, the typical month-to-month variation in an individual's cycle is usually plus or minus 2 days. However, greater but still normal variations are commonly noted.

Women typically have menstrual cycles for about 40 years. Once a cyclic, predictable pattern of monthly bleeding is established, women may worry about any deviation from that pattern or from what they have been told is normal for all menstruating women. A woman may be concerned about her ability to conceive and bear children or believe that she is not really a woman without monthly evidence. A sign such as amenorrhea or excess menstrual bleeding can be a source of severe distress and concern for a woman.

Amenorrhea

Amenorrhea, the absence of menstrual flow, is a clinical sign of a variety of conditions. Generally the following circumstances should be evaluated: (1) the absence of both menarche and secondary sexual characteristics by age 14 years; (2) the absence of menses by age 16, regardless of normal growth and development (primary amenorrhea); or (3) a 3- to 6-month cessation of menses after a period of menstruation (secondary amenorrhea).

Amenorrhea is most commonly the result of pregnancy. Although amenorrhea is not a disease, it is often a sign of disease. It may occur from any defect or interruption in the hypothalamic–pituitary–ovarian–uterine axis (see Fig 6-1). It may also result from anatomical abnormalities, other endocrine disorders such as hypothyroidism or hyperthyroidism, chronic diseases such as type 1 diabetes, medications such as phenytoin (Dilantin), illicit drug use (opiates, marijuana, cocaine), eating disorders, strenuous exercise, emotional stress, and oral contraceptive use.

Assessment of amenorrhea begins with a thorough history and physical examination. An important initial step is to be sure that the woman is not pregnant. Specific components of the assessment process depend on a patient's age—adolescent, young adult, or perimenopausal—and whether she has previously menstruated.

Hypogonadotropic Amenorrhea

Hypogonadotropic amenorrhea reflects a problem in the central hypothalamic–pituitary axis. In rare instances a pituitary lesion or genetic inability to produce FSH and LH is at fault. Once pregnancy has been ruled out by a β-human chorionic gonadotropin (hCG) pregnancy test, diagnostic tests may include FSH level, thyroid-stimulating hormone (TSH) and prolactin levels, radiographic or computed tomography scan of the pituitary gland, and a progestational challenge (Bielak & Harris, 2010).

Hypogonadotropic amenorrhea often results from hypothalamic suppression as a result of stress (in the home, school, or workplace) or a sudden and severe weight loss, eating disorders, strenuous exercise, or mental illness. Research on the interaction between nervous system or neurotransmitter functions and hormone regulation throughout the body has demonstrated a biological basis for the relation of stress to physiological processes. Women who are more than 20% underweight for height or who have had rapid weight loss may report amenorrhea, as may women with eating disorders such as **anorexia nervosa**. Amenorrhea is one of the classic signs of anorexia nervosa. The interrelation of disordered eating, amenorrhea, and premature osteoporosis has been described as the female athlete triad (http://www.bodysense.ca/files/pdfs/BS-FemaleAthleteTriad-E.pdf). A loss of calcium from the bone, comparable to that seen in postmenopausal women, may occur with this type of amenorrhea.

Exercise-associated amenorrhea can occur in women undergoing vigorous physical and athletic training and is thought to be associated with many factors, including body composition (height, weight, and percentage of body fat); type, intensity, and frequency of exercise; nutritional status; and presence of emotional or physical stressors. Women who participate in sports emphasizing low body weight are at greatest risk, including the following:

- Sports in which performance is subjectively scored (e.g., dance, gymnastics)
- Endurance sports favouring participants with low body weight (e.g., distance running, cycling)
- Sports in which body contour–revealing clothing is worn (e.g., swimming, diving, volleyball)
- Sports with weight categories for participation (e.g., rowing, martial arts)
- Sports in which prepubertal body shape favours success (e.g., gymnastics, figure skating)

Management

When amenorrhea is caused by hypothalamic disturbances, the nurse is an ideal health professional to assist women with this condition. Many of the causes are potentially reversible (e.g., stress, weight loss for nonorganic reasons) through counselling and education, which are primary interventions and appropriate nursing roles. When a stressor known to predispose a woman to hypothalamic amenorrhea is identified, initial management involves addressing the stressor. Together, the woman and nurse plan how the woman can decrease or discontinue medications known to affect menstruation, correct weight loss, deal more effectively with psychological stress, address emotional distress, and alter exercise routine.

The nurse can work with the woman to help her identify, cope with, and eliminate sources of stress in her life. Deep-breathing exercises and relaxation techniques are simple yet effective stress-reduction measures. Referral for biofeedback or massage therapy also may be useful. In some instances, referrals for psychotherapy may be indicated.

If a woman's exercise program is thought to contribute to her amenorrhea, several options exist for management. She may decide to decrease the intensity or duration of her training or to gain 2 to 3% in body weight. Accepting this alternative may be difficult for a person who is committed to a strenuous exercise regimen. The woman and nurse may have several sessions before the woman elects to try exercise reduction. Many young female athletes may not understand the consequences of low bone density or osteoporosis; nurses can point out the connection between low bone density and stress fractures. The nurse and woman should also investigate other factors that may be contributing to the amenorrhea and develop plans for altering lifestyle and decreasing stress.

A daily calcium intake of 1500 mg is recommended for women experiencing amenorrhea associated with the female athlete triad. Some researchers have found that oral contraceptives have a positive effect on bone density in amenorrheic premenopausal women (Liu & Lebrun, 2006).

Cyclic Perimenstrual Pain and Discomfort

Cyclic perimenstrual pain and discomfort (CPPD) is a concept developed by a nurse science team for a research project for the Association of Women's Health, Obstetric and Neonatal Nurses (AWHONN, 2003; Collins, Sharp et al., 2002). This concept includes dysmenorrhea, premenstrual syndrome (PMS), and premenstrual dysphoric disorder (PMDD), as well as symptom clusters that occur before and after the menstrual flow starts. CPPD is a health problem that can have a significant impact on a woman's quality of life. The following discussion focuses on the three main conditions of CPPD.

Dysmenorrhea

Dysmenorrhea, or pain during or shortly before menstruation, is one of the most common gynecological problems in women of all ages. Most adolescents have dysmenorrhea in the first 3 years after menarche. Young adult women ages 17 to 24 are most likely to report painful menses. Dysmenorrhea improves in most women after a full-term pregnancy (Fritz & Speroff, 2010). Between 30 and 40% of women report some level of discomfort associated with menses, and 7 to 15% report severe dysmenorrhea. However, the amount of disruption caused in women's lives is difficult to determine. It has been estimated that up to 10% of women with dysmenorrhea have pain severe enough to interfere with their functioning for 1 to 3 days a month. Menstrual problems, including dysmenorrhea, are more common in women who smoke and who are obese. Symptoms usually begin with menstruation, although some women have discomfort several hours before onset of flow. The range and severity of symptoms differ from woman to woman and from cycle to cycle in the same woman. Symptoms of dysmenorrhea may last several hours or several days. Pain is usually located in the suprapubic area or lower abdomen. Women describe the pain as sharp, cramping, or gripping or as a steady dull ache; pain may radiate to the lower back or upper thighs. Traditionally dysmenorrhea is differentiated as primary or secondary.

Primary Dysmenorrhea

Primary dysmenorrhea, a condition associated with abnormally increased uterine activity, is caused by myometrium contractions induced by prostaglandins (PGs) in the second half of the menstrual cycle. During the luteal phase and subsequent menstrual flow, $PGF_{2\alpha}$ is secreted. The uterine muscle of both normal and dysmenorrheic women is sensitive to prostaglandins; however, the amount of prostaglandin produced is the major differentiating factor (Fritz & Speroff, 2010). Excessive release of $PGF_{2\alpha}$ increases the amplitude and frequency of uterine contractions and causes vasospasm of the uterine arterioles, resulting in ischemia and cyclic lower abdominal cramps. Systemic responses to $PGF_{2\alpha}$ include backache, weakness, sweating, gastrointestinal symptoms (**anorexia**, nausea, vomiting, and diarrhea), and central nervous system symptoms (dizziness, syncope, headache, and poor concentration). Pain begins at the onset of menstrual flow and lasts from 8 to 48 hours. The release of most prostaglandins during menstruation occurs in the first 48 hours, which coincides with the greatest intensity of symptoms.

Primary dysmenorrhea is not caused by underlying pathology. Rather, it is the occurrence of a physiological alteration in some women. Primary dysmenorrhea usually appears within 6 to 12 months after menarche when ovulation is established. Anovulatory bleeding, common in the first few months or years after menarche, is painless. Because both estrogen and progesterone are necessary for primary dysmenorrhea to occur, it is experienced only with ovulatory cycles. This problem is most common in women in their late teens and early twenties; the incidence declines with age.

Management. Management of primary dysmenorrhea depends on the severity of the problem and an individual woman's response to various treatments. Women with symptoms of primary dysmenorrhea may not seek medical assistance and frequently do not make use of the prescription therapies that are available, as they may consider severe and incapacitating pain as inevitable (Society of Obstetricians and Gynaecologists of Canada [SOGC], 2005). Education and support are important components of nursing care. Because menstruation is so closely linked to reproduction and sexuality, menstrual problems such as dysmenorrhea can have a negative influence on sexuality and self-worth. Nurses can correct myths and misinformation about menstruation and dysmenorrhea by providing facts about what is normal.

Exercise helps relieve menstrual discomfort, through increased vasodilation and subsequent decreased ischemia; release of endogenous opiates, specifically β-endorphins; suppression of prostaglandins; and shunting of blood flow away from the viscera, resulting in less pelvic congestion. A specific exercise that nurses can suggest to their patients is pelvic rocking.

In addition to maintaining good nutrition at all times, specific dietary changes may be helpful in decreasing some of the systemic symptoms associated with dysmenorrhea. Decreased salt and refined-sugar intake in the 7 to 10 days before expected menses may reduce fluid retention. Increasing water intake may serve as a natural diuretic. Including natural diuretics such as asparagus, cranberry juice, peaches, parsley, and watermelon in the diet may help reduce edema and related discomforts. Decreasing red-meat intake and switching to a low-fat diet may also help to minimize dysmenorrheal symptoms.

Medications used to treat primary dysmenorrhea in women not desiring contraception include prostaglandin synthesis inhibitors, primarily nonsteroidal anti-inflammatory drugs (NSAIDs) (Table 6-1). NSAIDs are effective if begun 2 to 3 days before menses or with the first sign of bleeding. This regimen decreases the possibility of a woman taking these medications early in pregnancy (Fritz & Speroff, 2010). Often if one NSAID is ineffective, a different one will be effective. All NSAIDs have potential gastrointestinal side effects, including nausea, vomiting, and indigestion. All women taking NSAIDs should be warned to report dark-coloured stools, which may be an indication of gastrointestinal bleeding. Women with a history of aspirin sensitivity or allergy should avoid all NSAIDs. Approximately 80% of dysmenorrheic women obtain relief with prostaglandin inhibitors.

Over-the-counter (OTC) preparations indicated for primary dysmenorrhea contain the same active ingredients (e.g., ibuprofen or naproxen sodium) as those in prescription preparations. However, the labelled recommended dose may be subtherapeutic. Preparations containing acetaminophen are even less effective because acetaminophen does not have the antiprostaglandin properties of NSAIDs.

Oral contraceptive pills (OCPs) are a reasonable choice for women who may want to use contraception. The benefits of OCP use are attributed to decreased prostaglandin synthesis associated with an atrophic decidualized endometrium (Fritz & Speroff, 2010). No single OCP has been shown to be superior to another for the relief of primary dysmenorrhea. OCPs are a particularly good choice for therapy because they combine contraception with a positive effect on dysmenorrhea, menstrual flow, and menstrual irregularities. Since OCPs have adverse effects, women may not wish to use them for dysmenorrhea. OCPs may be contraindicated for some women. (See Chapter 7 for a complete discussion of OCPs.) Depot medroxyprogesterone acetate (DMPA) works by suppressing ovulation, which results in relief of dysmenorrhea symptoms. Levonorgestrel intrauterine system (Mirena) is an **intrauterine device (IUD)** that releases progestin inside the uterine cavity, causing a local effect on the endometrium, and can be considered for use with primary dysmenorrhea.

If dysmenorrhea is not relieved by one of the NSAIDs or OCPs, further investigation into the cause of the symptoms is necessary. Conditions associated with dysmenorrhea include Müllerian duct anomalies, **endometriosis**, and pelvic inflammatory disease (PID).

Often more than one alternative for alleviating menstrual discomfort and dysmenorrhea can be offered. Women can then try various options and decide which ones work best for

Table 6-1 Medications Used to Treat Dysmenorrhea

MEDICATION	EFFECTIVENESS	COMMON ADVERSE EFFECTS	COMMENTS
Ibuprofen (Motrin, Advil)	Most effective	Nausea, dyspepsia, rash pruritus, headache, drowsiness	If GI upset occurs, take with food, milk, or antacids; avoid alcoholic beverages; do not take with aspirin
Naproxen	Effective	See Ibuprofen	See Ibuprofen
Mefenamic acid (Ponston, Mefenamic)	Effective	Severe diarrhea, nausea and vomiting	Very potent and effective prostaglandin-synthesis inhibitor Antagonizes already formed prostaglandins Increased incidence of adverse GI effects
Aspirin	Somewhat effective	See Ibuprofen	If GI upset occurs, take with food, milk; avoid alcoholic beverages
Meloxicam (Mobicox)	Effective	Dizziness, drowsiness	Better GI tolerability; avoid other NSAIDs, aspirin, or acetaminophen
Diclofenac (Voltarin)	Effective	Nausea, diarrhea, constipation, abdominal distress, dyspepsia, flatulence	Enteric coated: immediate release
Acetaminophen	Less effective	Good GI tolerance Can cause liver damage with 3 or more alcoholic drinks/day	Does not have anti-prostaglandin property of NSAIDs

(Source: Society of Obstetricians and Gynaecologists of Canada. [2005]. Primary dysmenorrhea consensus guideline. *Journal of Obstetrics and Gynaecology Canada, 27*[12], 1117–1130. Printed with permission of the SOGC.)

Note: Risk with all NSAIDs is gastrointestinal ulceration, possible bleeding, and prolonged bleeding time. Incidence of adverse effects is dose related. Reported incidence, 3 to 9%. Do not give if patient has hemophilia or bleeding ulcers; do not give if patient has had an allergic or anaphylactic reaction to aspirin or another NSAID; do not give if patient is taking anticoagulant medication.

GI, gastrointestinal; *NSAID*, nonsteroidal anti-inflammatory drug.

them. Heat (heating pad or hot bath) minimizes cramping by increasing vasodilation and muscle relaxation and minimizing uterine ischemia. Massaging the lower back can reduce pain by relaxing paravertebral muscles and increasing pelvic blood supply. Soft rhythmic rubbing of the abdomen (effleurage) may be useful because it provides distraction and an alternative focal point. High-frequency transcutaneous electrical nerve stimulation (TENS) has been found to increase pain relief in women with dysmenorrhea. TENS involves the use of electrodes to stimulate the skin and decrease pain perception (see Fig. 16-7) (SOGC, 2005).

Complementary and alternative medicine (CAM) therapies have become increasingly popular. Therapies such as acupuncture, acupressure, biofeedback, desensitization, hypnosis, guided imagery, meditation, massage, reiki, relaxation exercises, and therapeutic touch have been used to treat pelvic pain (Dehlin & Schuiling, 2013; Proctor & Farquhar, 2004). Other CAM that may be useful in the treatment of primary dysmenorrhea include vitamin B_1, vitamin E, fish oil/vitamin B_{12} combination, magnesium, vitamin B_6, Toki-shakuyaku-san, and Neptune krill oil (SOGC, 2005). Herbal preparations including Chinese herbal medicine have long been used for management of menstrual problems, including dysmenorrhea (Table 6-2). However, it is essential that women understand that these therapies are not without potential toxicity and may cause drug interactions.

NURSING ALERT Nurses must routinely ask women about the use of herbal and other alternative therapies and document their use.

Secondary Dysmenorrhea

Secondary dysmenorrhea is menstrual pain that develops later in life than primary dysmenorrhea, typically after age 25. It is associated with an underlying pelvic pathology such as adenomyosis, endometriosis, PID, endometrial polyps, or submucous or interstitial myomas (fibroids). Women with secondary dysmenorrhea often have other symptoms that may suggest the underlying cause. For example, heavy menstrual flow with dysmenorrhea suggests a diagnosis of leiomyomata, adenomyosis, or endometrial polyps. Pain associated with endometriosis often begins a few days before menses but can be present at ovulation and continue through the first days of menses or start after menstrual flow has begun. In contrast to primary dysmenorrhea, the pain of secondary dysmenorrhea is often characterized by dull, lower abdominal aching that radiates to the back or thighs. Often women experience feelings of bloating or pelvic fullness. In addition to a physical examination with a careful pelvic examination, diagnosis may be assisted by ultrasound examination, **dilation and curettage (D&C)**, endometrial biopsy, or laparoscopy.

Treatment is directed toward removal of the underlying pathology. Many of the measures described for pain relief of primary dysmenorrhea are also helpful for women with secondary dysmenorrhea. Surgical options may be used to decrease the pain in women when other medical alternatives have been refused or were unsuccessful, and hysterectomy can be considered when all other options have failed and fertility is no longer a consideration (SOGC, 2005).

Premenstrual Syndrome

PMS is a complex, poorly understood condition that includes a number of cyclic symptoms occurring in the luteal phase of the menstrual cycle. About 85% of women experience mood or somatic symptoms or both that coincide with their menstrual cycles. Between 5 and 14% of women report symptoms severe enough to be disabling. All age groups are affected, with women

Table 6-2 Herbal Medicinals Taken Orally for Menstrual Disorders

SYMPTOMS/ INDICATIONS	HERBAL	ACTION	CONTRAINDICATIONS	ADVERSE REACTIONS	DRUG INTERACTIONS
Menstrual cramping	Black haw	Uterine antispasmodic; β_2-agonist activity	None known	None known	None known
	Ginger	Anti-inflammatory			
Premenstrual discomfort (anxiety, tension, depression), dysmenorrhea	Black cohosh root	Estrogen-like LH suppressant, binds to estrogen receptors	Pregnancy Caution: breastfeeding, liver disorder	Gastric irritation, CNS side effects at high doses	None known
Tension, breast pain	Bugleweed	Antigonadotropic, antithyrotropic, decreased prolactin levels	Thyroid disease	Thyroid enlargement with prolonged high dose	Interferes with diagnostic radioactive isotopes
Mastodynia, premenstrual discomfort, menstrual cycle irregularities	Chaste tree fruit	Decreased prolactin levels	None known	Itching, urticaria	Possible antagonism of dopaminergic antagonists
Dysmenorrhea	Potentilla	Increased tonus and contraction frequency in uterus	Pregnancy and lactation	Gastric irritation	None known
	Dong quai	Stimulates and relaxes uterus; anti-inflammatory; possibly analgesic activity	Phototoxicity Liver and renal damage in animal studies Abortifacient	Pregnancy	Coumarin components may increase risk of bleeding
Menorrhea and metrorrhagia	Shepherd's purse	Increased uterine contractions	None known	None known	None known

(Sources: Bascom, A. [2002]. *Incorporating herbal medicine into clinical practice.* Philadelphia: FA Davis; Dog, L. [2000]. *An integrative approach to dysmenorrhea.* Corrales, NM: Integrative Medicine Education Association; Dog, L. [2001]. *Endocrinology and women's issues.* Third Annual Conference on Clinical Relevance of Medicinal Herbs and Nutritional Supplements in the Management of Major Medical Problems, September 21–23, 2001; Health Canada [2007]. *Black cohosh.* Retrieved from http://www.hc-sc.gc.ca/dhp-mps/alt_formats/hpfb-dgpsa/pdf/prodnatur/mono_cohosh-grappes-eng.pdf; Schellenberg, R. [2001]. Treatment for the premenstrual syndrome with *Agnus castus* fruit extract: Prospective, randomized, placebo controlled study. *British Medical Journal, 322*[7279], 134–137; Stevinson, C., & Ernst, E. [2001]. Complementary/alternative therapies for premenstrual syndrome: A systemic review of random controlled trials. *American Journal of Obstetrics and Gynecology, 185*[1], 227–235.)
CNS, central nervous system; *LH,* luteinizing hormone.

in their 20s and 30s most frequently reporting symptoms. Ovarian function is necessary for the condition to occur. PMS does not occur before puberty, after menopause, or during pregnancy (see Critical Thinking Exercise). The condition is not dependent on the presence of monthly menses; women who have had a hysterectomy without bilateral salpingo-oophorectomy (BSO) still can have cyclic symptoms.

It is difficult to establish a universal definition of PMS because so many symptoms have been associated with the condition. However, Fritz and Speroff (2010) suggest that the simplest definition is a common-sense one: "The cyclic appearance of one or more of a large constellation of symptoms just prior to menses, occurring to such a degree that lifestyle or work is affected, followed by a period of time entirely free of symptoms." PMS symptoms include distressing physical, mood, and behavioural experiences.

Premenstrual Dysphoric Disorder

PMDD is a diagnostic term for a smaller percentage of women who suffer from severe PMS with an emphasis on mood symptoms (American Psychiatric Association [APA], 2010). Commonly, symptoms occur in the final 7 to 10 days of the menstrual cycle. Symptoms reported include abdominal bloating, anxiety, tension, breast tenderness, crying episodes, depression, fatigue and lack of energy, irritability, difficulty

CRITICAL THINKING EXERCISE

Premenstrual Syndrome in Adolescents

Brandy, a 17-year-old high school student, has been diagnosed with premenstrual syndrome (PMS). The week before her menses, she is irritable, cries easily, becomes angry over little things, has breast and abdominal discomfort, and in general, "feels terrible." She tells the nurse in the health centre that her friends get mad at her when she just wants to be left alone and that she has trouble concentrating in class. She asks the nurse for ways to deal with her PMS. What advice can the nurse give Brandy?

1. Evidence—Is there an evidence base for practical suggestions for dealing with PMS?
2. Assumptions—What assumptions can be made about the following aspects of PMS?
   a. Physical symptoms
   b. Psychological factors
   c. Behavioural changes
   d. Effective therapies
3. What implications and priorities for nursing care can be drawn at this time?
4. Does the evidence objectively support your conclusion?
5. Are there alternative perspectives to your conclusion?

concentrating, appetite changes, thirst, and swelling of the extremities (Fritz & Speroff, 2010). The most common symptoms are those associated with mood disturbances.

A diagnosis of PMS is made only when the following criteria are met (AWHONN, 2003; Taylor, Schuiling, & Sharp, 2013):

- Symptoms occur in the luteal phase and resolve within a few days of onset of menses.
- A symptom-free period occurs in the follicular phase.
- Symptoms are recurrent.
- Symptoms have a negative impact on some aspect of a woman's life.
- Other diagnoses that better explain the symptoms have been excluded.

For a diagnosis of PMDD, the following criteria must be met:

- Five or more affective and physical symptoms are present in the week before menses and absent in the follicular phase of the menstrual cycle.
- At least one of the symptoms is irritability, depressed mood, anxiety, or emotional lability.
- Symptoms interfere markedly with work, school, usual social activity, or interpersonal relationships.
- Symptoms are not caused by an exacerbation of another condition or disorder.

These criteria must be confirmed by prospective daily ratings for at least two menstrual cycles (APA, 2010).

The etiology of PMS and PMDD is not clear, but there is general agreement that they are distinct psychiatric and medical syndromes rather than an exacerbation of an underlying psychiatric disorder. They do not occur if there is no ovarian function. A number of biological and neuroendocrine etiologies have been suggested; however, none have been substantiated conclusively as the causative factor. It is likely that biological, psychosocial, and sociocultural factors contribute to PMS and PMDD (Fritz & Speroff, 2010; Taylor et al., 2013). There are several risk factors for PMDD: personal history of a major mood disorder; family history of mood disorder; premenstrual depression; premenstrual mood changes; past history of sexual abuse; and past, present, or current domestic violence. Readers are encouraged to explore current feminist, medical, and social science literature for more information on PMS.

Management

There is little agreement on management of PMS. A careful, detailed history and daily log of symptoms and mood fluctuations spanning several cycles may give direction to a plan of management. Any changes that assist a woman with PMS to exert control over her life have a positive impact.

Education is an important component of the management of PMS. Nurses can advise women that self-help modalities often result in significant symptom improvement. Women have found a number of complementary and alternative therapies to be useful in managing the symptoms of PMS. Diet and exercise changes are a useful way to begin and provide symptom relief for some women. Nurses can suggest that patients not smoke and limit their consumption of refined sugar (less than 75 mL/day), salt (less than 3 g/day), red meat (less than 90 mL/day), alcohol (less than 30 mL/day), and caffeinated beverages.

Women can be encouraged to include whole grains, legumes, seeds, nuts, vegetables, fruits, and vegetable oils in their diet. Use of natural diuretics (see the section on dysmenorrhea management earlier in this chapter) may help reduce fluid retention. Nutritional supplements may assist in symptom relief. Calcium (1200 mg/day), magnesium (300 to 400 mg/day), and vitamin E (100 to 150 mg/day) have been shown to be moderately effective in relieving symptoms, to have few adverse effects, and to be safe. For some women, daily supplements of evening primrose oil decrease premenstrual mood symptoms, breast pain, and fluid retention. The safety of this herb is well established; however, approximately 2% of those taking evening primrose oil may have stomach distress, nausea, or headaches. Other herbal therapies have long been used to treat PMS; specific suggestions are found in Table 6-2.

Regular exercise (aerobic exercise three to four times a week), especially in the luteal phase, is widely recommended for relief of PMS symptoms. A monthly program that varies in intensity and type of exercise according to PMS symptoms is best. Women who exercise regularly seem to have less premenstrual anxiety than do nonathletic women. It is thought that aerobic exercise increases β-endorphin levels to offset symptoms of depression and elevate mood. Yoga, acupuncture, hypnosis, chiropractic therapy, and massage therapy have all been reported to have a beneficial effect on women with PMS.

Counselling in the form of support groups or individual or couple counselling may be helpful. Stress-reduction techniques may also assist with symptom management. If these strategies do not provide significant symptom relief in 1 to 2 months, medication is often begun. Many medications have been used in treatment of PMS, but no single medication alleviates all PMS symptoms.

Medications often used in the treatment of PMS include diuretics, prostaglandin inhibitors (NSAIDs), progesterone, and OCPs. Serotonergic-activating agents, including the selective serotonin reuptake inhibitors (SSRIs) fluoxetine (Prozac), sertraline (Zoloft), paroxetine (Paxil), and citalopram (Celexa), have been shown to decrease severe premenstrual symptoms, including depression (Brown, O'Brien, Marjoribanks, & Wyatt, 2009). Common adverse effects are headaches, sleep disturbances, dizziness, weight gain, dry mouth, and decreased libido.

Endometriosis

Endometriosis is characterized by the presence and growth of endometrial tissue outside of the uterus. The tissue may be implanted on the ovaries; anterior and posterior cul-de-sac; broad, uterosacral, and round ligaments; rectovaginal septum; sigmoid colon; appendix; pelvic peritoneum; cervix; and inguinal area (Fig. 6-2). Endometrial lesions have been found in the vagina and surgical scars, as well as on the vulva, perineum, and bladder. Lesions have also been found on sites far from the pelvic area, such as the thoracic cavity, gallbladder, and heart. A cystic lesion of endometriosis found in the ovary is sometimes described as a chocolate cyst because of the dark colouring of the contents of the cyst caused by the presence of old blood.

Endometrial tissue contains glands and stoma and responds to cyclic hormone stimulation in the same way that the uterine

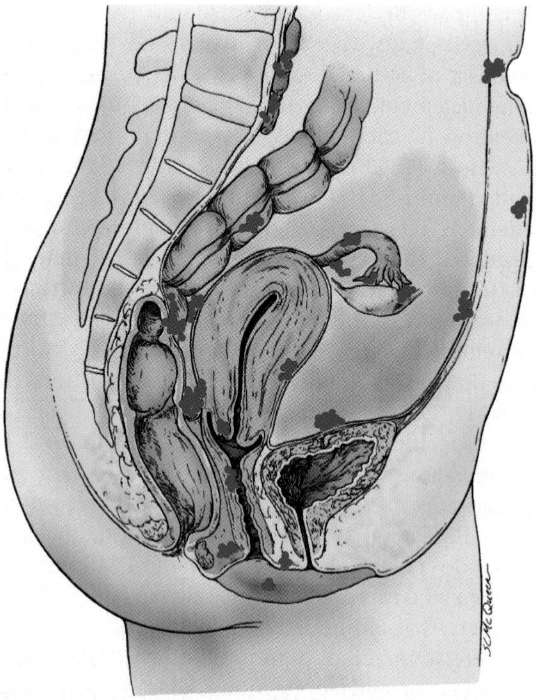

Fig. 6-2 Common sites of endometriosis. *(From Katz, V. L., et al. [2007]. Comprehensive gynecology [5th ed.]. Philadelphia: Mosby.)*

endometrium does but often out of phase with it. The endometrial tissue grows during the proliferative and secretory phases of the cycle. During or immediately after menstruation, the tissue bleeds, resulting in an inflammatory response with subsequent fibrosis and adhesions to adjacent organs.

The overall incidence of endometriosis is 3 to 10% in reproductive-age women, 20 to 40% in infertile women, and 5 to 20% in women with persistent pelvic pain (Fritz & Speroff, 2010). Although the condition usually develops in the third or fourth decade of life, endometriosis has been found in adolescents, with disabling pelvic pain or abnormal vaginal bleeding. Endometriosis may worsen with repeated cycles, or it may remain asymptomatic and undiagnosed, eventually disappearing after menopause. However, endometriosis has been reported to occur in about 5% of postmenopausal women receiving menopausal hormone therapy. The condition appears equally in women of all cultures and it occurs across all socioeconomic levels. There appears to be a familial tendency to develop endometriosis; the condition is six to seven times more prevalent in women who have a first-degree relative with endometriosis than in the general population (Fritz & Speroff, 2010).

Several theories regarding the cause of endometriosis have been suggested. However, the etiology and pathology of this condition continue to be poorly understood. One of the most widely accepted theories is transplantation or retrograde menstruation. According to this theory, endometrial tissue is refluxed through the uterine tubes during menstruation into the peritoneal cavity, where it implants on the ovaries and other organs. Retrograde menstruation has been documented in a number of surgical studies and is estimated to occur in 90% of menstruating women. For most women, endometrial tissue outside the uterus is destroyed before it can implant or seed in the peritoneal cavity or elsewhere. Endometriosis may develop in only 10 to 15% of women because of differences in the functioning of an individual's immune system. It also may reflect differences in genetic makeup or environmental challenges (Fritz & Speroff, 2010).

Symptoms ranging from nonexistent to incapacitating vary among women. The severity of symptoms can change over time and may not reflect the extent of the disease. The major symptoms of endometriosis are pelvic pain, dysmenorrhea, and dyspareunia (painful intercourse). Women may also have persistent noncyclic pelvic pain, pelvic heaviness, or pain radiating into the thighs. Many women report bowel symptoms such as diarrhea, pain with defecation, and constipation caused by avoiding defecation because of the pain. Less common symptoms include abnormal bleeding (hypermenorrhea, menorrhagia, or premenstrual staining) and pain during exercise, as a result of adhesions. Women who have endometriosis may also have other conditions, such as chronic fatigue syndrome, fibromyalgia, endocrine disorders, and autoimmune disorders (Conversations with Colleagues, 2002–2003). Impaired fertility may result from adhesions around the uterus that pull the uterus into a fixed, retroverted position. Adhesions around the uterine tubes may block the fimbriated ends or prevent the spontaneous movement that carries the ovum to the uterus.

Management

Treatment is based on the severity of symptoms and the goals of the woman. Women must be assessed for the level of pain they experience, their pain coping strategies, and the impact of the pain on their life. Women without pain who do not want to become pregnant need no treatment. In women with mild pain who may desire a future pregnancy, treatment may be limited to use of NSAIDs during menstruation (see earlier discussion of these medications).

Suppression of endogenous estrogen production and subsequent endometrial lesion growth is the cornerstone of management of the disease. Two main classes of medications are used to suppress endogenous estrogen levels: GnRH agonists and androgen derivatives. GnRH agonist therapy (leuprolide [Lupron, Eligard] or nafarelin [Synarel]) acts by suppressing pituitary gonadotropin secretion. FSH and LH stimulation of the ovary declines markedly, and ovarian function decreases significantly. A medically induced menopause develops, resulting in anovulation and amenorrhea. Shrinkage of already established endometrial tissue, significant pain relief, and interruption in further lesion development follow. The hypoestrogenism results in hot flashes in almost all women. Trabecular bone loss is common, although most loss is reversible within 12 to 18 months after the medication is stopped.

Both leuprolide (3.75 mg intramuscular injection given once a month) and nafarelin (200 mg administered twice daily by nasal spray) are effective and well tolerated. Both medications reduce endometrial lesions and pelvic pain associated with endometriosis and have post-treatment pregnancy rates similar to that of danazol (Cyclomen) therapy (Fritz & Speroff, 2010). Common adverse effects of these medications are those of natural menopause—hot flashes and vaginal dryness. Occasionally, women report headaches and muscle aches.

Treatment is usually limited to 6 months in order to minimize bone loss. Although unlikely, it is possible for a woman to become pregnant while taking a GnRH agonist. Because the potential teratogenicity of this medication is unclear, women should use a barrier contraceptive during treatment.

Danazol, a mildly androgenic synthetic steroid, suppresses FSH and LH secretion, thus producing anovulation and hypogonadotropism. This results in decreased secretion of estrogen and progesterone and regression of endometrial tissue. Danazol can produce adverse effects severe enough to cause a woman to discontinue the medication. Adverse effects include masculinizing traits in the woman (weight gain, edema, decreased breast size, oily skin, hirsutism, and deepening of the voice), all of which often disappear when treatment is discontinued. Other adverse effects are amenorrhea, hot flashes, vaginal dryness, insomnia, and decreased libido. Migraine headaches, dizziness, fatigue, and depression are also reported. Danazol treatment has been reported to adversely affect lipids, with a decrease in high-density lipoprotein levels and an increase in low-density lipoprotein levels. Danazol should never be prescribed when pregnancy is suspected, and barrier contraception should be used with it because ovulation may not be suppressed. Danazol can produce pseudohermaphroditism in female fetuses. The medication is contraindicated in women with liver disease and should be used with caution in women with cardiac and renal disease.

Women who have early symptomatic disease and who can postpone pregnancy may be treated with continuous OCPs that have a low estrogen-to-progestin ratio to shrink endometrial tissue. Any low-dose OCPs can be used if taken for 15 weeks, followed by 1 week of withdrawal. This therapy is associated with minimal adverse effects and can be taken for extended periods.

Continuous combined hormone therapy (OCPs, estrogen/progestin patch, estrogen/progestin vaginal ring) for menstrual suppression and administration of NSAIDs are the usual treatment for adolescents under the age of 16 who have endometriosis. GnRH agonists are usually not used, as the resultant hypoestrogenic state can affect bone mineralization (ACOG Committee on Adolescent Health Care, 2005; SOGC, 2005).

Surgical intervention is often needed for severe, acute, or incapacitating symptoms. Decisions regarding the extent and type of surgery are influenced by a woman's age, her desire for children, and location of the disease. For women who do not want to preserve their ability to have children, the only definite cure is total abdominal hysterectomy with bilateral salpingo-oopherectomy (TAH with BSO). In women who are in their childbearing years and who want children and in whom the disease does not prevent bearing children, reproductive capacity should be retained through careful removal by surgery or laser therapy of all endometrial tissue possible, with retention of ovarian function.

Regardless of the type of treatment (short of TAH with BSO), endometriosis recurs in approximately 40% of women. Thus, for many women, endometriosis is a chronic disease with conditions such as persistent pain or **infertility**. Counselling and education are critical components of nursing care for women with endometriosis. Women need an honest discussion of treatment options, with potential risks and benefits of each option reviewed. Because pelvic pain is a subjective, personal experience that can be frightening, support is important. Sexual dysfunction resulting from dyspareunia is common and may necessitate referral for counselling. Support groups for women with endometriosis may be found in some locations. The Infertility Awareness Association of Canada (http://www.iaac.ca), an organization for infertile couples, or the Canadian Women's Health Network (http://www.cwhn.ca) may also be helpful. The nursing care discussed in the previous section on dysmenorrhea is appropriate for managing persistent pelvic pain and dysmenorrhea experienced by women with endometriosis.

Alterations in Cyclic Bleeding

Women often have changes in the amount, duration, interval, or regularity of menstrual cycle bleeding. Often women worry about menstruation that is short or small in amount or occurs too frequently.

Oligomenorrhea and Hypomenorrhea

The term *oligomenorrhea* is often used to describe decreased menstruation—in amount, time, or both. However, *oligomenorrhea* more correctly refers to infrequent menstrual periods characterized by intervals of 40 to 45 days or longer, and *hypomenorrhea* to scanty bleeding at normal intervals. The causes of oligomenorrhea are often abnormalities of hypothalamic, pituitary, or ovarian function. Oligomenorrhea also can be physiological or part of a woman's normal pattern for the first few years after menarche or for several years before menopause.

Treatment is aimed at reversing the underlying cause, if possible. Hormone therapy using progestins, with or without estrogens, also may be used to prevent complications of unopposed estrogen production (endometrial hyperplasia or carcinoma) or of absent estrogen (vaginal dryness, hot flashes or flushes, osteoporosis).

Women with menstruation characterized by prolonged intervals between cycles need education and counselling. The cause of the condition and the rationale for a specific treatment should be discussed, as should advantages and disadvantages of hormone therapy. If a woman chooses medical intervention, she should be provided with written instructions, taught how to take the medications, and made aware of adverse effects of any medications. Teaching and counselling should emphasize the importance of the woman keeping careful records of her vaginal bleeding.

Metrorrhagia

Metrorrhagia, or intermenstrual bleeding, refers to any episode of bleeding, whether spotting, menses, or hemorrhage, that occurs at a time other than the normal menses. *Mittelstaining,* a small amount of bleeding or spotting that occurs at the time of ovulation (14 days before onset of the next menses), is considered normal.

Women taking OCPs may have midcycle bleeding or spotting. (See Chapter 7 for a discussion of the side effects of OCPs.) If the OCP does not sufficiently maintain a hypoplastic endometrium, the endometrium will begin to shed, usually in small amounts at a time, a process termed *breakthrough bleeding*. Breakthrough bleeding is most common in the first three cycles of OCPs. The reduced potency of OCPs (resulting in increased safety) has decreased the amount of available hormones, making it more important that blood levels be kept constant. Taking the pill at exactly the same time each day may alleviate the woman's problem. If the spotting continues, a different formulation that increases either the estrogen or progestin component of the pill can be tried.

Progestin-only contraceptive methods (oral and injectable) also may cause midcycle bleeding, especially in the first several cycles. Women should be advised of this and counselled to report continuation of breakthrough bleeding after the first three to six cycles to their health care provider.

Women with an IUD may have spotting between their periods and a heavier menstrual flow.

The causes of intermenstrual bleeding are varied (Box 6-1). It is important that the nurse always consider the possibility that any woman who has not undergone menopause and who seeks care for intermenstrual bleeding is or has recently been pregnant.

Treatment of intermenstrual bleeding depends on the cause and may include reassurance and education concerning mittlestaining, observation of three menstrual cycles for presumed functional ovarian cyst, adjustment of an OCP, removal of foreign bodies, and treatment for vaginal infections. More complex treatment may consist of removal of polyps; evaluation and treatment of an abnormal Papanicolaou (Pap) test, including **colposcopy,** biopsy, cautery, cryosurgery, or conization; and surgery, chemotherapy, or radiation treatment for malignancy. Important nursing roles include reassurance, counselling, education, and support.

Menorrhagia

Menorrhagia (hypermenorrhea) is defined as excessive menstrual bleeding in either duration or amount. A single episode of heavy bleeding may occur, or a woman may have regular flooding as a pattern in which she changes tampons or pads every few hours for several days. The causes of heavy menstrual bleeding are many, including hormonal disturbances, systemic disease, **benign** and malignant neoplasms, infection, and contraception (IUDs).

NURSING ALERT If the woman herself considers the amount or duration of bleeding to be excessive, the problem should be investigated.

Hemoglobin and hematocrit provide objective indicators to actual blood loss and should always be assessed.

A single episode of heavy bleeding may signal an early pregnancy loss. This type of bleeding is often thought to be a period that is heavier than usual, perhaps delayed, and is associated with abdominal pain or pelvic discomfort. When early pregnancy loss is suspected, a hematocrit and serum β-hCG pregnancy test should be done.

Uterine leiomyomas (fibroids or myomas) are a common cause of menorrhagia. *Fibroids* are benign tumours of the smooth muscle of the uterus, the etiology of which is unknown. They are estrogen sensitive and commonly develop during the reproductive years and shrink after menopause. Other uterine growths ranging from endometrial polyps to adenocarcinoma and endometrial cancer are other common causes of both heavy menstrual and intermenstrual bleeding.

Treatment for menorrhagia depends on the cause of the bleeding. Treatment options include medical and surgical management. Most fibroids can be monitored by frequent examinations to judge growth, if any, and correction of anemia, if present. Women with menorrhagia should be warned not to use aspirin because of its tendency to increase bleeding. Medical treatment is directed toward temporarily reducing symptoms, shrinking the myoma, and reducing its blood supply. This reduction is often accomplished with the use of a GnRH agonist.

If the woman wishes to retain childbearing potential, a myomectomy may be done. Myomectomy, or removal of the tumours only, is particularly difficult if multiple myomas must be removed. If the woman does not want to preserve her childbearing function or if she has severe symptoms (severe anemia, severe pain, considerable disruption of lifestyle), hysterectomy or endometrial ablation (laser surgery or electrocoagulation) may be done. Based on the assumption that control of arterial blood flow to the fibroid will control symptoms, uterine artery embolization has been reported to result in reduced menorrhagia, less dysmenorrhea, and reduced pelvic pressure and urinary symptoms. This method of treatment is used for women who have completed their childbearing since there is a risk for loss of fertility.

BOX 6-1 Causes of Intermenstrual Bleeding

Reproductive Disorder
- Functional ovarian cyst
- Cervical erosion infection
- Leiomyoma
- Polyps, uterine or endocervical
- Trauma
- Foreign body
- Malignancy of reproductive tract

Pregnancy Issues
- Pregnancy: implantation
- Miscarriage
- Ectopic pregnancy
- Molar pregnancy
- Retained placenta: miscarriage or induced abortion
- Retained placenta: birth

Infections
- Endometritis
- Sexually transmitted infections

Abnormal Uterine Bleeding

Abnormal uterine bleeding (AUB) is any form of uterine bleeding that is irregular in amount, duration, or timing and is not related to regular menstrual bleeding. Box 6-2 lists possible causes of AUB. Although often used interchangeably, the

BOX 6-2 Possible Causes of Abnormal Uterine Bleeding

Pregnancy-Related Conditions
Threatened or spontaneous miscarriage
Retained products of conception after elective abortion
Ectopic pregnancy
Placenta previa/placenta abruptio
Trophoblastic disease

Lower Reproductive Tract Infections
Cervicitis
Endometritis
Myometritis
Salpingitis

Benign Anatomical Abnormalities
Adenomyosis
Leiomyomata
Polyps of the cervix or endometrium
Neoplasms
Endometrial hyperplasia
Cancer of cervix and endometrium
Hormonally active tumours (rare)
Vaginal tumours (rare)

Malignant Lesions
Cervical squamous cell carcinoma
Endometrial adenocarcinoma
Estrogen-producing ovarian tumours
Testosterone-producing ovarian tumours
Leiomyosarcoma

Trauma
Genital injury (accidental, coital trauma, sexual abuse)
Foreign body
Lacerations

Systemic Conditions
Adrenal hyperplasia and Cushing's disease
Blood dyscrasias
Coagulopathies
Hypothalamic suppression (from stress, weight loss, excessive exercise)
Polycystic ovary disease
Thyroid disease
Pituitary adenoma or hyperprolactinemia
Severe organ disease (renal or liver failure)

Iatrogenic Causes
Medications with estrogenic activity
Anticoagulants
Exogenous hormone use (oral contraceptives, menopausal hormone therapy)
Selective serotonin reuptake inhibitors
Tamoxifen
Intrauterine devices
Herbal preparation (e.g., ginseng)

(Source: Albers, J. R., Hull, S. K., & Wesley, R. M. [2004]. Abnormal uterine bleeding. *American Family Physician, 69*, 1915–1926; 1931–1932.)

terms *AUB* and *dysfunctional uterine bleeding (DUB)* are not synonymous. DUB is a subset of AUB and is diagnosed by ruling out pregnancy, systemic conditions, genital tract pathology, and **iatrogenic** causes (Albers, Hull, & Wesley, 2004). DUB is most frequently caused by anovulation. When there is no LH surge or if the corpus luteum does not produce sufficient progesterone to support the endometrium, it will begin to involute and shed. This most often occurs at the extremes of a woman's reproductive years—when the menstrual cycle is just becoming established at menarche or when it draws to a close at menopause. DUB also can be found with any condition that gives rise to chronic anovulation associated with continuous estrogen production. Such conditions include obesity, hyperthyroidism and hypothyroidism, polycystic ovarian syndrome, and any of the endocrine conditions discussed in the sections on amenorrhea and oligomenorrhea.

Women also may unknowingly use medications that have an impact on the endometrium (e.g., ginseng, an herbal root, has been associated with estrogen activity and abnormal bleeding). A diagnosis of DUB is made only after all other causes of abnormal menstrual bleeding have been ruled out (Albers et al., 2004).

Management

When uterine bleeding is severe and a woman's hemoglobin level is less than 80 g/L (hematocrit <0.23), the woman may be hospitalized and given conjugated estrogens (Premarin), 25 mg, intravenously. The dose may be repeated until bleeding stops or slows significantly (usually within 1 to 5 hours [Dodd & Sinert, 2007]). If bleeding continues after instituting intravenous estrogen, it can be tamponaded by inserting a pediatric Foley catheter into the cervical os and inflating it. The balloon is filled with saline until the bleeding stops. If blood exits through the catheter, the catheter should be clamped. The balloon may be left in place for 12 to 24 hours (Dodd & Sinert, 2007).

If the bleeding has not stopped in 12 to 24 hours, D&C may be done to control severe bleeding and hemorrhage. An endometrial biopsy may be carried out at the same time in order to evaluate endometrial tissue or rule out endometrial cancer. After this treatment, oral conjugated estrogen is given for 21 days. During the last 7 to 10 days of this estrogen regimen, progesterone (e.g., medroxyprogesterone [Provera]) is added. Alternatively, a combined OCP is given for 21 days after intravenous therapy.

Once the acute phase has passed, the woman is maintained on cyclic, low-dose OCPs for 3 to 6 months. Such long-term treatment will help prevent recurrence of the pattern of DUB and hemorrhage. If the woman wants contraception, she should continue to take OCPs. If the woman has no need for contraception, the treatment may be stopped to assess her bleeding pattern. If her menses does not resume, a progestin regimen may be prescribed after ruling out pregnancy. This is done to prevent persistent anovulation with chronic unopposed endogenous estrogen hyperstimulation of the endometrium, which can result in eventual atypical tissue changes.

If the recurrent, heavy bleeding is not controlled by hormone therapy or D&C, ablation of the endometrium through laser treatment may be performed. Nursing roles include informing patients of their options, counselling and education as indicated, and referring to the appropriate specialists and health care services (see Nursing Process box).

Perimenopause and Menopause

A natural part of aging, *menopause* is considered the point at which a woman has not had a menstrual period for 12 months. The average age for menopause to occur is 51.4 years, with an age range of 35 to 60 years. *Perimenopause* is the period of time prior to this when a woman experiences physical and emotional changes; this lasts an average of 5 years. During this time, ovarian function declines. Ova slowly diminish, and menstrual cycles may be anovulatory, resulting in irregular bleeding. The ovary stops producing estrogen, and eventually menses no longer occur. Any woman with postmenopausal bleeding always needs to be investigated for cancer.

Menopause symptoms may vary from mild to intense. The common symptoms that women report include vasomotor instability (hot flashes, night sweats), depression, anxiety, irritability, vaginal dryness, atrophic vaginitis, decreased **libido,** fatigue, aches and pains, and insomnia.

Some women will find that vasomotor symptoms decrease when they make lifestyle modifications: eating well, maintaining a healthy weight, exercising, and reducing core body temperature (dressing in layers and drinking cold fluids), as well as by limiting consumption of triggers (alcohol, caffeine, and nicotine) (SOGC, 2009). Stress management (relaxation, yoga, meditation) may also help with some psychological symptoms.

The use of black cohosh and foods that contain phytoestrogens may improve menopausal symptoms, including hot flashes. Isoflavone (found in soy), vitamin E, St. John's wort, and valerian may also be used (SOGC, 2006). Natural health products are classified as drugs; thus women should be asked about the use of any complementary therapies in order to decrease the risk of interactions with any medications. At present, the use of these therapies may be useful for some women, although research on the use of complementary and alternative therapy is limited, and women should be advised that alternative measures should be used with caution (SOGC, 2009).

Hormonal replacement therapy (HRT) is also used to decrease menopausal symptoms. Some women do not qualify for the use of these medications because of risk factors. There has been some increased risk of breast cancer, ovarian cancer, thromboembolism, and heart disease identified with estrogen/progesterone therapy, and estrogen-only therapy has shown an increased rate of strokes (SOGC, 2009). Women for whom HRT is contraindicated or not desired may use nonhormonal therapies. These include certain antidepressant medications, gabapentin, clonidine, and bellergal, which may provide some relief from hot flashes. These medications have their own adverse effects (SOGC, 2009).

Every woman will go through the transition of menopause differently. Women need an understanding health care provider who can explain what is normal and provide support. An excellent resource for information for women is found at http://www.menopauseandu.ca.

NURSING PROCESS: THE WOMAN WITH A MENSTRUAL DISORDER

Assessment

Take a careful menstrual, obstetric, sexual, and contraceptive history.

Explore the woman's perceptions of her condition, cultural or ethnic influences, experiences with other caregivers, lifestyle, and patterns of coping.

Evaluate the amount of pain or bleeding experienced and its effect on daily activities.

Note home remedies and prescriptions to relieve discomfort.

A symptom diary, in which the woman records emotions, behaviours, physical symptoms, diet, and exercise and rest patterns, is a useful diagnostic tool.

Nursing Diagnoses

Difficulty with individual or family coping related to
–insufficient knowledge of the cause of the disorder
–emotional and physiological effects of the disorder

Lack of knowledge related to
–self-management
–available therapy for the disorder

Risk for disturbed body image related to
–menstrual disorder
–sexual dysfunction

Acute pain related to
–menstrual disorder

Planning

Expected outcomes are that the woman will do the following:

- Communicate understanding of reproductive anatomy, etiology of her disorder, medication regimen, and diary use
- Develop personal goals that benefit her emotionally and physically
- Choose appropriate therapeutic measures for her menstrual problems
- Develop strategies to adapt successfully to the condition if cure is not possible

Interventions

Medical interventions are discussed on pp. 84-93

- Express concern for and acceptance of the woman's symptoms as valid.
- Correlate data from the daily diary about emotional status, subjective feelings, and physical state with physiological changes.
- The clinician facilitates insights and suggests therapeutic options. The woman (or couple) makes choices considered best for her (or them).
- Support groups are an important resource.

Evaluation

The nurse can be assured that care has been effective when the woman reports improvement in the quality of her life, skill in self-management, and a positive self-concept and body image.

Infections

Sexually Transmitted Infections

Sexually transmitted infections (STIs) comprise more than 25 infectious organisms that cause infections or infectious disease syndromes, transmitted primarily by close, intimate contact (Box 6-3). The term *STIs* has replaced *sexually transmitted diseases (STDs)* as it also includes infections that may be asymptomatic; we use only STIs in this text. Caused by a wide spectrum of bacteria, viruses, protozoa, and ectoparasites (organisms that live on the outside of the body, such as a louse), STIs continue to be a significant and increasing public health concern in Canada, with rates of the three nationally reportable bacterial STIs (chlamydia, gonorrhea, and syphilis) increasing, especially among women aged 15 to 24. The World Health Organization (WHO) has developed a global strategy for the prevention and control of STIs because of the health and economic burden of STIs (WHO, 2007) (see Community Focus box). The most common STIs in women are chlamydia, human papillomavirus (HPV), gonorrhea, herpes simplex virus (HSV) type 2, syphilis, and human **immunodeficiency** virus (HIV) infection. Neonatal effects of STIs are discussed in Chapter 28.

Prevention

Preventing infection (primary prevention) is the most effective way of reducing the adverse consequences of STIs for women and for society. With the advent of serious and potentially lethal STIs that are either not readily cured or incurable, primary prevention becomes critical. Prompt diagnosis and treatment of current infections (secondary prevention) can prevent personal complications and transmission to others.

Preventing the spread of STIs requires that women at risk for transmitting or acquiring infections change their behaviour. A critical first step is for the nurse to include questions about a woman's sexual history, sexual risk behaviours, and drug-related risky behaviours as a part of her assessment (Box 6-4). Effective techniques in providing prevention counselling include using open-ended questions, using understandable language, and reassuring the woman that treatment will be provided regardless of ability to pay, language spoken, or lifestyle (Public Health Agency of Canada [PHAC], 2010a). Prevention messages should include descriptions of specific actions to be taken to avoid acquiring or transmitting STIs (e.g., refraining from sexual activity if STI-related symptoms are present) and should be tailored to the individual woman, with attention given to her specific risk factors (see Patient Teaching box).

To be motivated to take preventive actions, a woman must believe that acquiring a disease will be serious for her and that she is at risk for infection. Most individuals tend to underestimate their personal risk of infection in a given situation.

BOX 6-3 Sexually Transmitted Infections

Bacteria

Chlamydia Nationally reportable
Gonorrhea Nationally reportable
Syphilis Nationally reportable (if infectious)
Chancroid
Lymphogranuloma venereum
Genital mycoplasmas

Viruses

Human immunodeficiency virus Nationally reportable
Herpes simplex virus, types 1 and 2
Cytomegalovirus
Viral hepatitis A and B
Human papillomavirus

Protozoa

Trichomoniasis

Parasites

Pediculosis (may or may not be sexually transmitted)
Scabies (may or may not be sexually transmitted)

COMMUNITY FOCUS

Sexually Transmitted Infections

While in the clinic, interview a nurse about sexually transmitted infections commonly seen in the clinic.

- What are the most common infections seen in the clinic?
- Has the incidence of infections changed over the last 5 years? Which infections have increased and which have decreased in incidence during that time?
- Are adolescents seen in the clinic? Is there a special clinic for adolescents?
- How much independence does the nurse have in diagnosing and treating the sexually transmitted infections?
- What patient teaching guidelines are available in the clinic? Are the guidelines available in languages other than English?

PATIENT TEACHING Prevention of Genital Tract Infections in Women

- Practise genital hygiene.
- Choose underwear or hosiery with a cotton crotch.
- Avoid tight-fitting clothing (especially tight jeans).
- Select cloth car seat covers instead of vinyl.
- Limit the time spent in damp exercise clothes (especially swimsuits, leotards, and tights).
- Limit exposure to bath salts or bubble bath.
- Avoid coloured or scented toilet tissue.
- If sensitive, discontinue use of feminine hygiene deodorant sprays.
- Use condoms.
- Void before and after intercourse.
- Decrease dietary sugar.
- Drink yeast-active milk and eat yogourt (with lactobacilli).
- Do not douche.

BOX 6-4 Assessing Risk Behaviours for Human Immunodeficiency Virus and Other Sexually Transmitted Infections

Information should be requested in a nonjudgemental manner, using language that is understandable.

Answer the following questions for all the times in your life from 1977* to the present.

Relationship

Do you have a regular sexual partner?
If yes, how long have you been with this person?
Do you have any concerns about your relationship?
If yes, what are they? (e.g., violence, abuse, coercion)

Sexual Risk Behaviour

When was your last sexual contact? Was that contact with your regular partner or with a different partner?
Have you ever had an oral, vaginal, or anal sexual experience with another person?
With how many different people? 1? 2 or 3? 4 to 10? More than 10?
How many different sexual partners have you had in the past 2 months? In the past year? Have your partners been men, women, or both?
Have any of your sexual encounters been with people from a country other than Canada? If yes, where and when?
How do you meet your sexual partners (when travelling, in a bathhouse, on the Internet?)
Do you use male condoms? Female condoms? Other barriers? All the time, some of the time, never?
What influences your choice to use protection or not?
Rate your risk for STI (no risk, low risk, medium risk, or high risk). Why do you choose this rating?

STI History

Have you ever

- thought that a sex partner put you at risk for AIDS or an STI (intravenous drug user, bisexual)?
- been tested for an STI or HIV? If yes, what was your last screening date?
- had an STI (herpes, gonorrhea, genital warts, chlamydia)? If yes, what and when?

When was your last sexual contact of concern?
If symptomatic, how long have you had the symptoms that you are experiencing?

Reproductive Health History

Do you, your partner, or both use contraception? If yes, what?
Have you ever

- had any reproductive health problems? If yes, when? What?
- had an abnormal Pap test? If yes, when?
- been pregnant? If yes, how many times? What was the outcome (number of live births, abortions, miscarriages)?

Substance Use

Do you use alcohol? Drugs? If yes, how often and what type?
Have you ever

- injected drugs using shared equipment, including street drugs or steroids? When was the last sharing date?
- had sex with a person who uses and shares equipment?
- had sex while stoned, high, or too drunk to remember the details?

Blood-Related Risks

Have you ever

- had a blood transfusion?
- had sex with a person who had a blood transfusion?
- had sex with a person with hemophilia?
- received donor semen, egg, or transplanted organ or tissue?
- had tattoos or piercings? If yes, were they done with sterile equipment (i.e. professionally)?

Psychosocial History

Have you ever

- traded sex for money, drugs, or shelter?
- paid for sex? If yes, what is the frequency, duration, and last event?
- been forced to have sex? If yes, when and by whom?
- been sexually abused? Ever been physically or mentally abused? If yes, when and by whom?

Do you have a home? If no, where do you sleep?

(Adapted from Marrazzo, J. M., Guest, F., & Cates, W. [2007]. Reproductive tract infections, including HIV and other sexually transmitted infections. In R. Hatcher, et al. *Contraceptive technology* [19th ed.]. New York: Ardent Media; Public Health Agency of Canada [2010]. *Canadian guidelines on sexually transmitted infections* [Catalogue No. HP40-1/2010E-PDF]. Ottawa: Author. Retrieved from http://www.phac-aspc.gc.ca/std-mts/sti-its/pdf/sti-its-eng.pdf [page 7–8].)

*Relates to risk of HIV—infection not known to exist in humans until this time.
AIDS, acquired immunodeficiency syndrome; *HIV,* human immunodeficiency virus; *STI,* sexually transmitted infection.

Thus, many women may not perceive themselves as being at risk for contracting an STI, and telling them that they should carry **condoms** may not be well received. Although levels of awareness of STIs are generally high, widespread misconceptions or specific gaps in knowledge also exist. Therefore, nurses have a responsibility to ensure that their patients have accurate, complete knowledge about transmission and symptoms of STIs and the behaviours that place them at risk for contracting an infection.

Primary preventive measures are individual activities aimed at avoiding infection. Risk-free options include complete abstinence from sexual activities that transmit semen, blood, or other body fluids or that allow for skin-to-skin contact (PHAC, 2010a). Involvement in a mutually monogamous relationship with an uninfected partner also eliminates risk of contracting STIs. When neither of these options is realistic for a woman, the nurse must focus on other, more feasible measures.

STI Prevention Strategies

An essential component of primary prevention is counselling the woman about sexual practices so that she can avoid acquiring or transmitting STIs. These practices include attaining knowledge of her partner, reducing her number of partners, practising low-risk sex, and avoiding the exchange of body fluids.

Reducing the number of partners and avoiding partners who have had many previous sexual partners decreases a woman's chances of contracting an STI. Discussing each new partner's previous sexual history and exposure to STIs will augment other efforts to reduce risk; however, sexual partners are not always truthful about their sexual history. Women must be cautioned that measures for avoiding transmission of infections are always advisable, even when partners insist otherwise. Critically important is whether male partners will accept wearing condoms. Women should be cautioned against making decisions about a partner's sexual and other behaviours based on appearances and unfounded assumptions, such as the following (Marrazzo, Guest, & Cates, 2007):

- Single people have many partners and risky practices.
- Older people have few partners and infrequent sexual encounters.
- Sexually experienced people know how to avoid transmitting infections.
- Married people are heterosexual, low risk, and monogamous.
- People who look healthy are healthy.
- People with good jobs do not use drugs.

Sexually active persons also may benefit from carefully examining a partner for lesions, sores, ulcerations, rashes, redness, discharge, swelling, and odour before initiating sexual activity.

Women should be taught low-risk sexual practices, as well as which sexual practices to avoid (see Box 4-8). Sexual fantasizing is safe, as are caressing, hugging, body rubbing, and massage. Mutual masturbation is low risk as long as there is no contact with a partner's semen or vaginal secretions. All sexual activities are safe when both partners are monogamous, trustworthy, and known (by testing) to be free of disease. Women need to be encouraged to think about the risk of STIs and to consider pre-sex testing before they become sexually active with a new partner so they can be proactive in prevention of the risk of transmission. Women also need to discuss limiting alcohol or drug intake prior to sexual activity as these can impact decision-making and negotiation skills (PHAC, 2010a).

The physical barrier promoted for the prevention of sexual transmission of HIV and other STIs is the condom (male and female). The nurse should teach women to use a condom with every sexual encounter; to use latex or plastic male condoms rather than natural skin condoms for STI protection; to use a condom with a current expiration date; to use each one only once; and to handle it carefully to avoid damaging it with fingernails, teeth, or other sharp objects. Condoms should be stored away from high heat. Although it is not ideal, women may choose to safely carry condoms in wallets, shoes, or inside a bra. Women can be taught the differences among condoms: price ranges, sizes, and where they can be purchased. Explicit instructions for how to apply a male condom are included in Box 7-8.

The female condom—a lubricated polyurethane sheath with a ring on each end that is inserted into the vagina—has been shown in laboratory studies to be an effective mechanical barrier to viruses, including HIV. Studies suggest that the female condom is at least as effective as male condoms in preventing transmission of STIs (Hoffman et al., 2004). What is important and should be stressed by nurses is the consistent use of condoms for every act of sexual intimacy when there is the possibility of transmission of disease. Women need to be encouraged to discuss concerns with their partner (Box 6-5).

There is concern about the potential for cervicovaginal epithelial disruption with nonoxynol-9 (N-9)–based spermicides. Frequent use of spermicides containing N-9 has been associated with genital lesions and may increase HIV transmission; thus condoms lubricated with N-9 are not recommended (PHAC, 2010a).

Certain sexual practices should be avoided in order to reduce one's risk of infection. Abstinence from any sexual activities that could result in exchange of infective body fluids helps decrease risk. Anal–genital intercourse, anal–oral contact, and anal–digital activity are high-risk sexual behaviours and should be avoided. Because enteric infections are transmitted by oral–fecal contact, avoidance of oral–anal activities, "rimming" (licking the anal area), and digital–anal activities should reduce the likelihood of infection. Vaginal intercourse should never follow anal contact unless a condom has been used and then removed and replaced with a new condom.

BOX 6-5 Strategies to Enhance a Woman's Negotiation and Communication Skills Regarding Condom Use

- Suggest that the woman talk with her partner about condom use at a time not during sexual activity.
- Role play possible partner reactions with the woman and her alternative responses.
- For a woman who appears particularly uncomfortable, ask her to rehearse how she might approach the topic of condom use.
- Women may feel more comfortable and in control of the situation if they sort out their feelings and fears before talking with their partners. Reassure the woman that it is natural to be uncomfortable and that the hardest part is getting started.
- Suggest that the woman clarify for herself what she will and will not do sexually.
- Suggest that the woman begin the conversation by saying, "I need to talk with you about something that is important to both of us. It's hard for me, and I feel embarrassed, but I think we need to talk about ways to reduce risk when we have sex."
- The partner may need time to think about what he has heard.
- If the partner resists risk-reducing sexual behaviours, the woman may wish to reconsider the relationship.

Sexual transmission occurs through direct skin or mucous membrane contact with infectious lesions or body fluids. Because mucosal linings are delicate and subject to considerable mechanical trauma during intercourse, small abrasions often may occur, facilitating entry of infectious agents into the bloodstream. The rectal epithelium is especially easy to traumatize with penetration. Sexual practices that increase the likelihood of tissue damage or bleeding, such as fisting (inserting a fist into the rectum or vagina), should be avoided. Deep kissing when lips, gums, or other tissues are raw or broken also should be avoided.

Sexually Transmitted Bacterial Infections

Chlamydia

Chlamydia trachomatis is a reportable STI in Canada. Rates of chlamydia in Canada and elsewhere have been steadily increasing; between 1998 and 2007 the rate of chlamydia in females increased by 60% (PHAC, 2009). These infections are often silent and highly destructive. Their sequelae and complications can be very serious. In women, chlamydial infections are difficult to diagnose; the symptoms, if present, are nonspecific.

Early identification of *C. trachomatis* is important because untreated infection often leads to acute salpingitis or PID. PID is the most serious complication of chlamydial infections, and past chlamydial infections are associated with an increased risk of ectopic pregnancy and tubal factor infertility. Chlamydial infection of the cervix causes inflammation that results in microscopic cervical ulcerations. These ulcerations may increase the risk of acquiring HIV infection.

The highest rate is in youth and adults aged 15 to 24; this age group accounts for approximately two-thirds of all cases (PHAC, 2010a). Risky behaviours, such as having sex with multiple partners and failure to use barrier methods of birth control, increase a woman's risk of chlamydial infection. Lower socioeconomic status may be a risk factor as some individuals in this group may not seek any or adequate treatment.

Screening and Diagnosis

In addition to obtaining information about the presence of risk factors (see Box 6-4), the nurse should inquire about the presence of any symptoms. The Public Health Agency of Canada (PHAC) recommends screening all sexually active women under the age of 25 (PHAC, 2010a).

Although chlamydia infections are usually asymptomatic, some women may experience spotting or postcoital bleeding, mucoid or purulent cervical discharge, or **dysuria**. Bleeding results from inflammation and erosion of the cervical columnar epithelium. Women taking OCPs may have breakthrough bleeding.

Diagnosis of chlamydia is by culture (which is expensive and labour intensive), enzyme immunoassay (which is less expensive but has less sensitivity), and nucleic acid amplification (which is expensive but has about 90% sensitivity). Special culture media and proper handling of specimens are important. Thus the nurse should always know what is required in the individual practice site.

Management

The recommendations for the treatment of urethral, cervical, and rectal chlamydial infections are doxycycline (100 mg orally twice a day for 7 days) or azithromycin (1 g orally in a single dose) (PHAC, 2010a). Azithromycin is often prescribed when compliance may be a problem because only one dose is needed; however, expense is a concern with this medication. If the woman is pregnant, erythromycin (500 mg orally four times a day for 7 days) or amoxicillin (500 mg orally three times a day for 7 days) is used. Women who have a chlamydial infection and are also infected with HIV should be treated with the same regimen as that used for those who are not infected with HIV.

Because chlamydia is often asymptomatic, the woman should be cautioned to take all medication prescribed. Women treated with recommended or alternative regimens do not need to be retested unless symptoms continue. It is recommended that pregnant women be retested 3 weeks after completing the medication, although the validity of this practice has not been established (PHAC, 2010a). All sexual partners who have had contact with the index case within 60 days prior to symptom onset must be tested and treated (PHAC, 2010a). Chlamydia is a reportable disease to the local health authority in all provinces and territories. Local public health authorities are able to help notify contacts.

Gonorrhea

Gonorrhea is probably the oldest communicable disease in Canada. The reported incidence of gonorrhea has more than doubled from 1997 to 2006, with females between 15 and 19 years of age being most affected (PHAC, 2009). The incidence of medication-resistant cases of gonorrhea, in particular penicillinase-producing *Neisseria gonorrhoeae*, is increasing dramatically in North America.

Gonorrhea is caused by the aerobic, gram-negative diplococci *N. gonorrhoeae*. It is transmitted almost exclusively by sexual contact. The principal means of transmission is genital-to-genital contact during sexual activity; however, it is also spread by oral–genital and anal–genital contact. There is also evidence that infection may spread in females from vagina to rectum. Although the organism has been recovered from inanimate objects artificially inoculated with the bacteria, there is no evidence that natural transmission occurs this way.

Women are often asymptomatic, with one third of infections in adolescent women going unnoticed. When symptoms are present, they are often less specific than the symptoms in men. Women may have a purulent endocervical discharge, but discharge is usually minimal or absent.

Menstrual irregularities may be the initial symptom, or women may complain of pain: persistent or acute severe pelvic or lower abdominal pain, or longer, more painful menses. Infrequently dysuria, vague abdominal pain, or low backache often prompts a woman to seek care. Gonococcal rectal infection may occur in women after anal intercourse; 10 to 30% of urogenital infections are accompanied by rectal infection. Individuals with rectal gonorrhea may be completely asymptomatic or, conversely, have severe symptoms with profuse purulent anal discharge, rectal pain, and blood in the stool. Rectal itching, fullness, pressure, and pain are also common symptoms, as is diarrhea. A diffuse vaginitis with vulvitis is the most common form of gonococcal infection in prepubertal girls. There may be few signs of infection; or vaginal discharge, dysuria, and swollen, reddened labia may be present.

Screening and Diagnosis

Because gonococcal infections in women are often asymptomatic, the PHAC recommends screening all women at risk for gonorrhea (PHAC, 2010a). Gonococcal infection cannot be diagnosed reliably by clinical signs and symptoms alone. Individuals may have "classic" symptoms, vague symptoms that may be attributed to a number of conditions, or no symptoms at all. Cultures should be obtained from the endocervix, the rectum, and, when indicated, the pharynx. Because coinfection is common, any woman suspected of having gonorrhea should have a chlamydial culture and serological test for syphilis unless one has been done within the past 2 months.

Management

Management of gonorrhea is straightforward, and with appropriate antibiotic therapy the cure is usually rapid. Single-dose efficacy is a major consideration in selecting an antibiotic regimen for women with gonorrhea. Another important consideration is the high proportion (45%) of women with coexisting chlamydial infections. The treatment of choice for uncomplicated urethral, endocervical, and rectal infections in pregnant and nonpregnant women is cefixime (400 mg orally once) or ceftriaxone (125 mg intramuscularly once). The PHAC recommends concomitant treatment for chlamydia unless a chlamydia test is negative, because coinfection is common (PHAC, 2010a). All women with both gonorrhea and syphilis should also be treated for syphilis according to PHAC guidelines (see discussion of syphilis later in this chapter).

Gonorrhea is highly communicable. Recent (past 60 days) sexual partners must be notified and should be examined, cultured, and treated with appropriate regimens. Most treatment failures result from reinfection. The woman needs to be informed of this, as well as of the consequences of reinfection in terms of chronicity, complications, and potential infertility. Women should be counselled to use condoms. All women with gonorrhea should be offered confidential counselling and testing for HIV infection.

LEGAL TIP Gonorrhea, chlamydia, infectious syphilis, and HIV are reportable communicable diseases in all provinces and territories. Health care providers are legally responsible for reporting all cases of these STIs to local public health authorities. Women should be informed that the case will be reported, told why it will be reported, and informed of the possibility of being contacted by a health department epidemiologist.

Syphilis

Syphilis, one of the earliest described STIs, is caused by *Treponema pallidum*, a motile spirochete. Transmission is thought to be by entry through microscopic abrasions in the subcutaneous tissue, which can occur during sexual intercourse. The disease can also be transmitted through kissing, biting, or oral–genital sex. Transplacental transmission may occur at any time during pregnancy; the degree of risk is related to the quantity of spirochetes in the maternal bloodstream.

The rate of infectious syphilis in Canada in 2008 was 4.2 per 100,000, an increase of 568% since 1999 (PHAC, 2010b). Much of the increase in cases was observed in men having sex with men, although the rates are higher in the Aboriginal populations in British Columbia, Alberta and Yukon (PHAC, 2010b).

Syphilis is a complex disease that can lead to serious systemic disease and even death when untreated. Infection manifests itself in distinct stages with different symptoms and clinical manifestations. Primary syphilis is characterized by a primary lesion, the chancre, which appears 5 to 90 days after infection. This lesion often begins as a painless papule at the site of inoculation and then erodes to form a nontender, shallow, indurated, clean ulcer several millimetres to centimetres in size (Fig. 6-3). Secondary syphilis occurs 6 weeks to 6 months after the appearance of the chancre. It is characterized by a widespread, symmetrical, maculopapular rash on the palms and soles and generalized lymphadenopathy. The infected individual also may experience fever, headache, and malaise.

Condylomata lata (broad, painless, pink-gray, wartlike infectious lesions) may develop on the vulva, perineum, or anus. If the woman is untreated, she enters a latent phase that is asymptomatic for most individuals. Left untreated, about one third of these women will develop tertiary syphilis. Neurological, cardiovascular, musculoskeletal, or multiorgan system complications can develop in the third stage.

Screening and Diagnosis

All women who are diagnosed with another STI or with HIV should be screened for syphilis. Diagnosis depends on

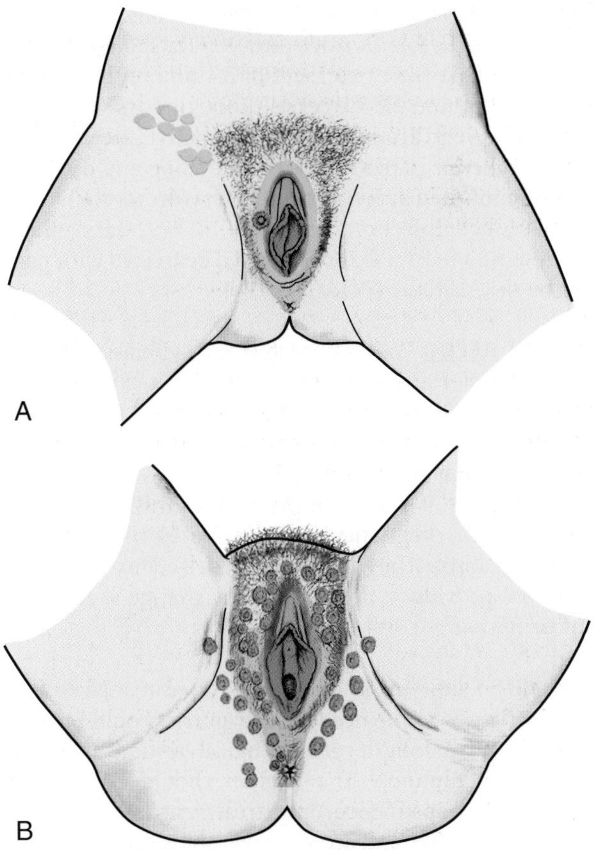

Fig. 6-3 Syphilis. **A:** Primary stage: chancre with inguinal adenopathy. **B:** Secondary stage: condylomata lata.

microscopic examination of primary and secondary lesion tissue and serology during latency and late infection. A test for antibodies may not be reactive in the presence of active infection because it takes time for the body's immune system to develop antibodies to any antigens. Up to one third of people in early primary syphilis may have nonreactive serological tests. Two types of serological tests are used: nontreponemal and treponemal. Nontreponemal antibody tests such as VDRL (Venereal Disease Research Laboratories) and RPR (rapid plasma reagin) are used as screening tests. False-positive results are not unusual, particularly when conditions such as acute infection, autoimmune disorders, malignancy, pregnancy, and drug **addiction** exist, and after immunization or vaccination. The treponemal tests, fluorescent treponemal antibody absorbed and microhemagglutination assays for antibody to *T. pallidum*, are used to confirm positive results. Test results in patients with early primary or incubating syphilis may be negative. Seroconversion usually takes place 6 to 8 weeks after exposure; thus testing should be repeated in 1 to 2 months when a suggestive genital lesion exists.

Tests (e.g., wet preps and cultures) for concomitant STIs (e.g., chlamydia and gonorrhea) should be done and HIV testing offered if indicated.

evolve Animation—Pelvic Inflammatory Disease

Management

Penicillin is the preferred medication for treating patients with syphilis. It is the only proven therapy that has been widely used for patients with neurosyphilis, **congenital** syphilis, or syphilis during pregnancy. Intramuscular penicillin G benzathine (2.4 million units intramuscularly once) is used to treat primary, secondary, and early latent syphilis. Women with syphilis of longer than 1 year's duration (late latent or tertiary stages) require weekly treatment of 2.4 million units of penicillin G benzathine for 3 weeks. Although doxycycline, tetracycline, and erythromycin are alternative treatments for penicillin-allergic patients, both tetracycline and doxycycline are contraindicated in pregnancy, and erythromycin is unlikely to cure a fetal infection. Therefore, if necessary, pregnant women should receive skin testing and be treated with penicillin or be desensitized (PHAC, 2010a).

NURSING ALERT Patients treated for syphilis may experience a Jarisch–Herxheimer reaction. This is an acute febrile reaction often accompanied by headache, myalgias, and arthralgias that develop within the first 24 hours of treatment. The reaction may be treated symptomatically with analgesics and antipyretics. If treatment precipitates this reaction in the second half of pregnancy, women are at risk for preterm labour and birth. They should be advised to contact their health care provider if they notice any change in fetal movement or have any contractions.

Monthly follow-up is mandatory so that repeated treatment may be given, if needed. The nurse should emphasize the necessity of long-term serological testing even in the absence of symptoms. The woman should be advised to practice sexual abstinence until treatment is completed, all evidence of primary and secondary syphilis is gone, and serological evidence of a cure is demonstrated. Infectious syphilis is reportable in all provinces and territories to the PHAC. Noninfectious syphilis is reportable at the provincial/territorial level but not to the PHAC. All sexual or perinatal contacts must be notified and treated. Preventive measures should be discussed (PHAC, 2010a).

Pelvic Inflammatory Disease

Pelvic inflammatory disease (PID) is an infectious process that most commonly involves the uterine tubes, causing salpingitis; the uterus, causing endometritis; and, more rarely, the ovaries and peritoneal surfaces. Multiple organisms have been found to cause PID; most cases are associated with more than one organism. In the past, the most common causative agent was thought to be *N. gonorrhoeae*; however, *C. trachomatis* is now estimated to cause one half of all cases of PID. In addition to gonorrhea and chlamydia, a wide variety of anaerobic and aerobic bacteria cause PID. It encompasses a wide variety of pathological processes; the infection can be acute, subacute, or chronic and can have a wide range of symptoms.

Most PID results from the ascending spread of microorganisms from the vagina and endocervix to the upper genital tract. This spread most commonly happens at the end of or just after menses following reception of an infectious agent. During the menstrual period, several factors facilitate the development of an infection: the cervical os is slightly open, the cervical mucus barrier is absent, and menstrual blood is an excellent medium for growth. PID also may develop after a miscarriage or an induced **abortion**, pelvic surgery, or childbirth.

Risk factors for acquiring PID are those associated with the risk of contracting an STI, including young age, multiple partners, high rate of new partners, and a history of STIs. Women who use IUDs may be at increased risk for PID if they have more than one sexual partner or if the partner has other sexual partners because they are at higher risk for acquiring an STI. Most of this risk occurs in the first months after IUD insertion. PID tends to recur and is a significant public health problem in Canada. There are approximately 100,000 cases of PID annually in Canada, although many cases are unreported (PHAC, 2010a).

Women who have had PID are at increased risk for ectopic pregnancy, infertility, and persistent pelvic pain. After a single episode of PID, a woman's risk for ectopic pregnancy increases sevenfold compared with the risk for women who have never had PID. Other problems associated with PID include **dyspareunia**, pyosalpinx (pus in the uterine tubes), tubo-ovarian abscess, and pelvic adhesions.

The symptoms of PID vary, depending on whether the infection is acute, subacute, or chronic. However, pain is common to all clinical presentations. It may be dull, cramping, and intermittent (subacute) or severe, persistent, and incapacitating (acute). The woman with acute PID also may complain of intermenstrual bleeding. Physical examination reveals adnexal tenderness, with or without rebound, and exquisite tenderness with cervical movement (Chandelier sign). Pelvic tenderness is usually bilateral. There may or may not be a palpable adnexal swelling or thickening. A urethral or cervical discharge, often purulent in nature, may be present. A fever of 38.3°C or above is characteristic. Significant laboratory data include an elevated white blood cell count and a markedly elevated erythrocyte sedimentation rate. Fever and peritonitis are more characteristic of gonococcal PID; PID caused by other organisms is more likely to be "silent." Because PID caused by chlamydia is more commonly asymptomatic, it more often results in tubal obstruction from delayed diagnosis or inadequate treatment.

Screening and Diagnosis

A careful history is necessary to distinguish between PID and other conditions that cause abdominal pain, such as an ectopic pregnancy or appendicitis. A menstrual history is useful in establishing the relationship of onset of pain to menses and in identifying any variations from normal in the cycle. Other relevant history includes recent pelvic surgery, birth, induced abortion, or dilation of the cervix; purulent vaginal discharge; irregular bleeding; and a longer, heavier menstrual period. A sexual history will assist in identifying possible increased risk for STI exposure. Symptoms of an STI in a woman's partner(s) also should be noted.

Vital signs need to be obtained and a complete physical examination performed. Criteria for diagnosing PID include oral temperature greater than 38.3°C, abnormal cervical or vaginal discharge, elevated erythrocyte sedimentation rate, and laboratory documentation of cervical infection with *N. gonorrhoeae* or *C. trachomatis* (PHAC, 2010a). Physical findings of lower abdominal tenderness, bilateral adnexal tenderness, and cervical motion tenderness are important in making a clinical diagnosis of PID. Essential laboratory data are a complete blood count with differential, a pregnancy test (to rule out ectopic pregnancy), and cervical cultures for gonorrhea and chlamydia.

Management

Perhaps the most important nursing intervention is prevention counselling. Primary prevention includes education in how to avoid contracting STIs; secondary prevention involves preventing a lower genital tract infection from ascending to the upper genital tract. Early diagnosis and treatment is essential in order to maintain fertility. Instructing women in self-protective behaviours, such as practices to use to avoid contracting STIs and use of barrier methods, is critical. Women who use hormonal contraception or an IUD and those who have chosen tubal ligation and who are at risk for infection, must be reminded to use a condom with intercourse. Also important is the detection of asymptomatic gonorrheal and chlamydial infections through routine screening of women who practice risky behaviours or have specific risk factors, such as age. When an STI is diagnosed, partner notification is essential in order to prevent reinfection.

When and if women with PID are hospitalized varies according to their particular circumstances. The PHAC recommends hospitalization for parenteral antibiotic treatment in the following situations (PHAC, 2010a):

- Surgical emergencies such as appendicitis cannot be excluded.
- The woman has a tubo-ovarian abscess.
- The woman is pregnant.
- Severe illness precludes outpatient management.
- The woman is unable to tolerate or follow an outpatient oral regimen.
- The woman has failed to respond to oral outpatient therapy.
- The woman has severe illness, nausea and vomiting, or high fever.

Although treatment regimens vary with the infecting organism, generally a broad-spectrum antibiotic is used. Several antimicrobial regimens have proved to be effective, and no single therapeutic regimen of choice exists. The woman with acute PID should be on bed rest in a semi-Fowler's position. Comfort measures include **analgesics** for pain and all other nursing measures applicable to a patient confined to bed. Few pelvic examinations should be done during the acute phase of the disease. During the recovery phase, the woman should restrict her activity and make every effort to get adequate rest and a nutritionally sound diet. Follow-up laboratory work after treatment should include endocervical cultures for a test of cure.

Health education is central to effective management of PID. Nurses should explain the nature of the disease to women and encourage them to comply with all therapy and prevention recommendations, emphasizing the need to take all medication, even if symptoms disappear. Any potential problems (such as lack of money for prescriptions or lack of transportation to return for follow-up appointments) that would prevent a woman from completing a course of treatment should be identified. Also, referrals should be made for assistance as needed and the importance of follow-up visits stressed. Women should be counselled to refrain from sexual intercourse until their treatment is completed. Contraceptive counselling, including information on barrier methods such as condoms, the contraceptive sponge, and the diaphragm, should be provided. A woman with a history of PID should not use an IUD as her contraceptive method.

The woman with PID may be acutely ill or have long-term discomfort. Either or both take an emotional toll. Pain in itself is debilitating and is compounded by the infectious process. The potential or actual loss of reproductive capabilities can be devastating and can adversely affect the woman's concept of herself. Part of the nurse's role is to help the woman adjust her self-concept to fit reality and to accept alterations in a way that promotes health. Because PID is so closely tied to sexuality, **body image**, and self-concept, the woman diagnosed with it will need supportive care. Her feelings should be discussed and her partner(s) included in the discussion, when appropriate.

Sexually Transmitted Viral Infections

Human Papillomavirus

Human papillomavirus (HPV) infection, previously named genital or venereal warts, is an STI that was first described in 25 AD and is now the most common viral STI seen in ambulatory health care settings, affecting 550,000 Canadians annually (SOGC, 2007). It is estimated that 70% of the adult population will have at least one genital HPV infection over their lifetime (PHAC, 2008). HPV, a double-stranded DNA virus, has more than 40 serotypes that can be transmitted sexually, 5 of which are known to cause genital wart formation and 13 of which are currently thought to have oncogenic (tumour-causing) potential (PHAC, 2008; SOGC, 2007). HPV is the primary cause of cervical neoplasia (Canadian Cancer Society [CCS], 2009).

In women, HPV lesions (also called *Condylomata acuminata*) are most commonly seen in the posterior part of the introitus. Lesions also are found on the buttocks, vulva, vagina, anus, and cervix (Fig. 6-4). Typically the lesions are small (2 to 3 mm in diameter and 10 to 15 mm in height), soft, papillary swellings occurring singly or in clusters on the genital and anal–rectal region. Infections of long duration may appear as a cauliflower-like mass. In moist areas such as the vaginal introitus, the lesions may appear to have multiple fine, finger-like projections. Vaginal lesions are often multiple. Flat-topped papules, 1 to 4 mm in diameter, are seen most often on the cervix. Often these lesions are visualized only under magnification. Warts are usually flesh coloured or slightly darker on White women, black on Black women, and brownish on Asian women. The lesions are usually painless; but they may be uncomfortable, particularly when very large, inflamed, or ulcerated. Chronic vaginal discharge, pruritus, or dyspareunia can occur.

During pregnancy, a significant proportion of pre-existing HPV lesions enlarge greatly, a proliferation presumably resulting from the relative state of immunosuppression present during this period. Lesions may become so large during pregnancy that they affect urination, defecation, mobility, and fetal descent, although birth by Caesarean section is rarely necessary. **Caesarean birth** may be performed when extensive growths are present. Initial observation of large growths can be misleading, suggesting that the entire vagina is involved. However, all of the growth may derive from one stalk, and in such cases it may be possible to push the large mass to the side, allowing the baby to pass through.

Screening and Diagnosis

A woman with HPV lesions may complain of symptoms such as a profuse, irritating vaginal discharge, itching, dyspareunia, or postcoital bleeding. She also may report "bumps" on her vulva or labia. History of a known exposure is important; however, because of the potentially long latency period and the possibility of subclinical infections in men, the lack of a history of known exposure cannot be used to exclude a diagnosis of HPV infection.

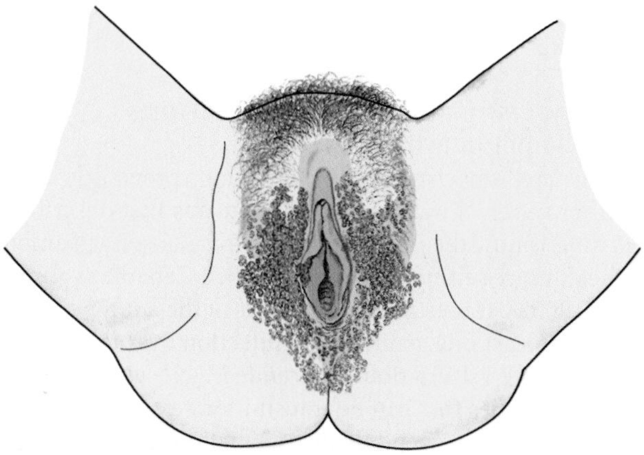

Fig. 6-4 Human papillomavirus (HPV) infection. Genital warts or condylomata acuminata.

Physical inspection of the vulva, perineum, anus, vagina, and cervix is essential whenever HPV lesions are suspected or seen in one area. Because speculum examination of the vagina may block some lesions, it is important to rotate the speculum blades until all areas are visualized. When lesions are visible, the characteristic appearance previously described is considered diagnostic. However, in many instances cervical lesions are not visible, and some vaginal or vulvar lesions also may be unobservable to the naked eye. Because of the potential spread of vulvar or vaginal lesions to the anus, gloves should be changed between vaginal and rectal examinations.

Viral screening and typing for HPV is available but not standard practice. History, evaluation of signs and symptoms, Pap test, and physical examination are used in making a diagnosis. The HPV-DNA test can be used in women over the age of 30 in combination with the Pap test to screen for types of HPV that are likely to cause cancer or in women with abnormal Pap test results (SOGC, 2007). The only definitive diagnostic test for presence of HPV is histological evaluation of a biopsy specimen.

HPV lesions must be differentiated from molluscum contagiosum and condylomata lata. Molluscum contagiosum lesions are half-domed, smooth, flesh-coloured–to–pearly white papules with depressed centres. Condylomata lata are a form of secondary syphilis and generally are flatter and wider than genital warts. A serological test for syphilis would confirm the diagnosis of secondary syphilis.

Management

Untreated warts may resolve on their own in young women since their immune systems may be strong enough to fight the HPV infection. Treatment of genital warts, if needed, is often difficult. No therapy has been shown to eradicate HPV. Therefore, the goal of treatment is removal of warts and relief of signs and symptoms, not the eradication of HPV (SOGC, 2007). The patient often must make multiple office visits; frequently many different treatment modalities will be used. Eradication of the virus is not considered conclusive even after there is no visible evidence of wart tissue because of the high incidence of recurrence.

Treatment of genital warts should be guided by preference of the woman, available resources, and experience of the health care provider. No one of the treatments is superior to all other treatments, and no one treatment is ideal for all warts (PHAC, 2008). Imiquimod and podofilox/podophyllotoxin 0.5% are treatments that can be self-applied. Podophyllin, bi- or trichloracetic acid (TCA), cryotherapy, excision, and laser ablation are all office-based treatments. Because the lesions can proliferate and become friable during pregnancy, many experts recommend their removal using cryotherapy, ablative treatments, or TCA (PHAC, 2008).

Women who have discomfort associated with genital warts may find that bathing with an oatmeal solution and drying the area with cool air from a hair dryer provides some relief. Keeping the area clean and dry also decreases the growth of the warts. Cotton underwear and loose-fitting clothes that decrease friction and irritation may lessen discomfort. Women should be advised to maintain a healthy lifestyle to aid the immune system and be counselled regarding diet, rest, stress reduction, and exercise.

Patient counselling should address how the virus is transmitted and stress that no immunity is conferred with infection and that reacquisition of the infection is likely with repeated contact. Women need to know that partners should be checked even if they are asymptomatic. Because HPV is highly contagious, the majority of women's partners will be infected and should be treated. All sexually active women with multiple partners or a history of HPV should be encouraged to use latex condoms and a vaginal spermicide for intercourse to decrease acquisition or transmission of condylomata.

Instructions for all medications and treatments must be detailed. Women should be informed before treatment of the possibility of post-treatment pain associated with specific therapies. The importance of thorough treatment of concurrent vaginitis or STI should be emphasized. The link between cervical cancer and HPV infections and the need for close follow-up should be discussed. Annual health examinations are recommended to assess disease recurrence and to screen for cervical cancer. Women should be counselled to have regular Pap screening as recommended for women without genital warts. The presence of genital warts is not an indication for a change in Pap test frequency or for cervical colposcopy (SOGC, 2007).

Women with HPV infection may radically alter their sexual practices both from fear of transmission to and from a partner and from genital discomfort associated with treatment, which may have a negative impact on their sexual relationships. Unless the partner accepts and understands the necessary precautions, it may be difficult for the woman to follow the treatment regimen. The nurse can offer to discuss feelings that the woman may have. When indicated, joint counselling can be suggested.

Prevention

Preventive strategies that have been suggested include abstinence from all sexual activity, staying in a long-term monogamous relationship, the use of condoms, and prophylactic vaccination (SOGC, 2007). A vaccine against HPV was approved by Health Canada in 2006 and is recommended for females ages 9 to 26. The vaccine protects against the two most common oncogenic HPV types (16 and 18), which cause approximately 70% of cases of cervical cancer, and the two common low-risk types (6 and 11) that cause approximately 90% of anogenital warts (SOGC, 2007). The HPV vaccine is highly effective and is given in three doses over a 6-month period (months 0, 2, and 6). All provinces and territories in Canada have implemented publically funded HPV vaccine programs with the goal of reducing the risk of cervical cancer (PHAC, 2010c). The Aboriginal community of Nunavut could benefit from targeted prevention measures, as the incidence of high-risk HPV in these women is twice that in the other provinces and territories (Healey et al., 2001).

Herpes Simplex Virus

Unknown until the middle of the twentieth century, herpes simplex virus (HSV) infection is now widespread in Canada, especially in women. HSV infection results in painful, recurrent ulcers. It is caused by two different antigen subtypes of HSV: HSV type 1 (HSV-1) and HSV type 2 (HSV-2). HSV-2 is usually transmitted sexually and HSV-1, nonsexually. Although HSV-1 is more commonly associated with gingivostomatitis and oral labial ulcers (fever blisters) and HSV-2 with genital lesions, neither type is exclusively associated with the respective sites.

Although HSV infection is not a reportable disease in Canada, it is estimated that 50,000 new cases of HSV occur annually (Money et al., 2008). Recurrent HSV infections are much more common. Most persons infected with HSV-2 have not been diagnosed, and most infections are transmitted by persons unaware that they are infected.

An initial HSV genital infection is characterized by multiple painful lesions, fever, chills, malaise, and severe dysuria and may last 2 to 3 weeks. Women generally have a more severe clinical course than men do. Women with primary genital herpes have many lesions that progress from macules to papules; they then progress to form vesicles, pustules, and ulcers that crust and heal without scarring (Fig. 6-5). These ulcers are extremely tender, and primary infections may be bilateral. Women also may have itching, inguinal tenderness, and lymphadenopathy. Severe vulvar edema may develop, and women may have difficulty sitting. HSV cervicitis is common with initial HSV-2 infections. The cervix may appear normal or be friable, reddened, ulcerated, or necrotic. A heavy, watery-to-purulent vaginal discharge is common. Extragenital lesions may be present because of autoinoculation. Urinary retention and dysuria may occur secondary to autonomic involvement of the sacral nerve root.

Women with recurrent episodes of HSV infections commonly have only local symptoms that are usually less severe than those associated with the initial infection. Systemic symptoms are usually absent, although the characteristic prodromal genital tingling is common. Recurrent lesions are unilateral, are less severe, and usually last 5 to 7 days. Lesions begin as vesicles and progress rapidly to ulcers. Few women with recurrent disease have cervicitis.

An association between cervical cancer and HSV-2 has been observed. It is theorized that genital herpes is a marker for high-risk sexual behaviours associated with other STIs, including HPV. Women must be encouraged to have annual Pap tests and gynecological examinations.

Screening and Diagnosis

A diagnosis of herpes is facilitated by a careful history. A history of exposure to an infected person is important,

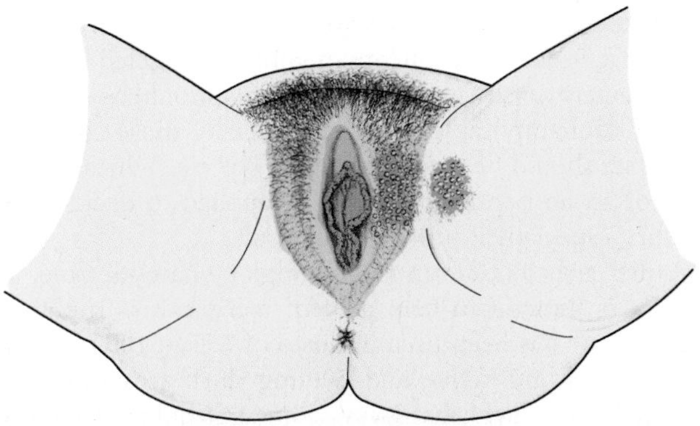

Fig. 6-5 Herpes genitalis.

although infection from an asymptomatic individual is possible. A history of having viral symptoms such as malaise, headache, fever, or myalgia suggests herpes infection. Local symptoms such as vulvar pain, dysuria, itching, or burning at the site of infection and painful genital lesions that heal spontaneously are also highly suggestive of HSV infections. The nurse should ask about history of a primary infection, prodromal symptoms, vaginal discharge, and dyspareunia.

During the physical examination, the nurse should assess for inguinal and generalized lymphadenopathy and elevated temperature. The entire vulvar, perineal, vaginal, and cervical areas should be carefully inspected for vesicles or ulcerated or crusted areas. A speculum examination may be very difficult for the woman because of the extreme tenderness often associated with herpes infections. Although a diagnosis of herpes infection may be suspected from the history and physical examination, it is confirmed by laboratory studies. A viral culture is obtained by swabbing exudate during the vesicular stage of the disease. In primary HSV infection viral shedding is prolonged, and HSV is more easily isolated.

Management

Genital herpes is a chronic and recurring disease for which there is no known cure. Management is directed toward specific treatment during primary and recurrent infections, prevention, self-help measures, and psychological support.

Systemic antiviral medications partially control the symptoms and signs of HSV infections when used for the primary or recurrent episodes or when used as daily suppressive therapy. These medications also decrease the transmission of the infection; however, these medications do not eradicate the infection, nor do they alter subsequent risk, frequency, or recurrences after the medication is stopped. Three antiviral medications provide clinical benefit: acyclovir, valacyclovir, and famciclovir. Safety and efficacy have been clearly shown in persons taking acyclovir daily for up to 3 years.

Cleaning lesions twice a day with saline helps prevent secondary infection. Measures that may increase comfort for women when lesions are active include warm sitz baths with baking soda; keeping lesions dry by using cool air from a hair dryer or by patting dry with a soft towel; wearing cotton underwear and loose clothing; using drying aids such as hydrogen peroxide, Burow's solution, or oatmeal baths; applying cool, wet, black tea bags to lesions; and applying compresses with an infusion of cloves or peppermint oil and clove oil to lesions.

Oral analgesics such as aspirin or ibuprofen may be used to relieve pain and systemic symptoms associated with initial infections. Because the mucous membranes affected by herpes are extremely sensitive, any topical agents should be used with caution. Nonantiviral ointments, especially those containing cortisone, should be avoided. A thin layer of lidocaine ointment or an antiseptic spray may be applied to decrease discomfort, especially if walking is difficult.

A diet rich in vitamin C, B-complex vitamins, zinc, and calcium is thought to help prevent recurrences. The amino acid L-lysine has been used in doses of 750 to 1000 mg daily while lesions are active and 500 mg during asymptomatic periods. It is thought that L-lysine has an inhibitory effect on the multiplication of the HSV.

Counselling and education are critical components of the nursing care of women with herpes infections. Information regarding the etiology, signs and symptoms, transmission, and treatment should be provided. The nurse should explain that each woman is unique in her response to herpes and emphasize the variability of symptoms. Women should be helped to understand when viral shedding and, thus, transmission to a partner are most likely. They should be counselled to refrain from sexual contact from the onset of prodrome until the complete healing of lesions.

Some authorities recommend consistent use of condoms for all persons with genital herpes. Condoms may not prevent transmission, particularly male-to-female transmission; however, this does not mean that the partners should avoid all intimacy. Women can be encouraged to maintain close contact with their partners while avoiding contact with lesions. Women should be taught how to look for herpetic lesions using a mirror and good light source and a wet cloth or finger covered with a finger cot to rub lightly over the labia. The nurse should ensure that women understand that when lesions are active, they should not share intimate articles (e.g., washcloths or wet towels) that come into contact with the lesions. Only plain soap and water are needed to clean hands that have come in contact with herpetic lesions; isolation is neither necessary nor appropriate.

The nurse should explain the role of precipitating factors in the reactivation of the latent virus and recurrent episodes. Stress, menstruation, trauma, febrile illnesses, chronic illness, and ultraviolet light have all been found to trigger genital herpes. Women may wish to keep a diary to identify stressors that seem to be associated with recurrent herpes attacks so that they can then avoid these stressors when possible. The role of exercise in reducing stress can be discussed. Referral for stress-reduction therapy, yoga, or meditation classes may be indicated. Avoiding excessive heat, sun, and hot baths and using a lubricant during sexual intercourse to reduce friction may also be helpful. Women in their childbearing years should be counselled about the risk of herpes infection during pregnancy. They should be instructed to use condoms if there is any risk of contracting an STI from a sexual partner. If they become pregnant while taking acyclovir, the risk of birth defects does not appear to be higher than that for the general population; however, continued use should be based on whether the benefits for the woman outweigh the possible risks to the fetus. Acyclovir does enter breast milk, but the amount of medication ingested during breastfeeding is very low and is usually not a health concern (Organization of Teratology Information Services, 2003).

The emotional impact of contracting herpes can be considerable. No cure is available, and most women experience recurrences. At diagnosis many emotions may surface—helplessness, anger, denial, guilt, anxiety, shame, or inadequacy. Women need the opportunity to discuss their feelings and may need help in learning to live with the disease. A woman can be encouraged to think of herself as someone who is healthy and merely inconvenienced from time to time. Herpes can affect a woman's sexuality, her sexual practices, and her current and future relationships. She may need help in discussing her HSV status with her partner or with future partners.

Viral Hepatitis

Five different viruses (hepatitis viruses A, B, C, D, and E) account for almost all cases of viral hepatitis in humans. Hepatitis viruses A, B, and C are discussed here. Hepatitis D and E viruses, common among users of intravenous drugs and recipients of multiple blood transfusions, are not included in this discussion.

Hepatitis A

Hepatitis A virus (HAV) infection is acquired primarily through a fecal–oral route by ingestion of contaminated food, particularly milk, shellfish, or polluted water, or person-to-person contact. Hepatitis A, like other enteric infections, can be transmitted during sexual activity. People who are at risk for developing HAV include food workers who are exposed to contaminated food or water, injection drug users, people who live or work in developing countries or visit them, incarcerated individuals, and household contacts of individuals with HAV. HAV infection is characterized by flu-like symptoms with malaise, fatigue, anorexia, nausea, pruritus, fever, and upper right quadrant pain. Serological testing to detect the immunoglobulin M (IgM) antibody is done to confirm acute infections. The IgM antibody is detectable 5 to 10 days after exposure and can remain positive for up to 6 months. Because HAV infection is self-limited and does not result in chronic infection or chronic liver disease, treatment is usually supportive. Women who become dehydrated from nausea and vomiting or who have fulminating hepatitis A may need to be hospitalized. Medications that might cause liver damage or that are metabolized in the liver (e.g., acetaminophen, ethyl alcohol) should be avoided. A well-balanced diet is recommended. Hepatitis A vaccine is recommended for women at high risk for exposure to HAV. The vaccine is also safe for pregnant women. (PHAC, 2006).

Hepatitis B

Hepatitis B virus (HBV) infection is an STI and is the virus most threatening to the fetus and neonate. It is caused by a large DNA virus and is associated with three antigens and their antibodies: hepatitis B surface antigen (HBsAg), HBV antigen (HBeAg), HBV core antigen (HBcAg), antibody to HBsAg (anti-HBs), antibody to HBeAg (anti-HBe), and antibody to HBcAg (anti-HBc). Screening for active or chronic disease or disease immunity is based on testing for these antigens and their antibodies.

Populations at the greatest risk for HBV include women who have a history of acute or chronic liver disease, work or receive treatment in a dialysis unit, or have household or sexual contact with a hemodialysis patient. Women who work or live in institutions for the mentally challenged are considered to be at risk, as are women with a history of multiple blood transfusions. Health care workers and public safety workers exposed to blood in the workplace are at risk. Behaviours such as having multiple sexual partners and a history of intravenous drug use increase the risk of contracting HBV infections.

HBsAg has been found in blood, saliva, sweat, tears, vaginal secretions, and semen. Drug users who share needles are at risk for HBV, as are health care workers who are exposed to blood and needlesticks. Perinatal transmission most often occurs in infants of mothers who have acute hepatitis infection late in the third trimester or during the intrapartum or postpartum periods. Such transmission is due to exposure to HBsAg-positive vaginal secretions, blood, amniotic fluid, saliva, and breast milk. HBV has also been transmitted through artificial insemination. Although HBV can be transmitted via blood transfusion, the incidence of such infections has decreased significantly since the testing of blood for HBsAg became routine.

HBV infection is a disease of the liver. In the adult, the course of the infection can be fulminating and the outcome fatal. Symptoms of HBV infection are similar to those of hepatitis A: arthralgias, arthritis, lassitude, anorexia, nausea, vomiting, headache, fever, and mild abdominal pain. Later the woman may have clay-coloured stools, dark urine, increased abdominal pain, and jaundice. Between 5 and 10% of individuals with HBV have persistent HBsAg and become chronic hepatitis B carriers.

Screening and Diagnosis. All women at high risk for contracting HBV should be screened on a regular basis. Since screening only individuals at high risk may not identify up to 50% of HBsAg-positive women, screening for the presence of HBsAg is recommended in all pregnant women at the first prenatal visit (PHAC, 2008).

Testing for HBV is complex. Patients with acute hepatitis B generally have detectable serum HBsAg levels in the late incubation phase of the disease, 2 to 5 weeks before symptoms appear. Anti-HBs with a negative HBsAg test signals immunity. Anti-HBs with a positive antigen denotes a chronic carrier state. During this time, the disease can be transmitted. During the recovery phase the patient may continue to be infectious, even though HBsAg cannot be detected. This is called the "window phase" and is identified by anti-HBc in the absence of anti-HBs. Women should be prepared for repeated testing because HBV screening tests may also be used to monitor progression of the disease.

Components of the history to be obtained when hepatitis B is suspected include inquiry about the symptoms of the disease and the risk factors outlined earlier. Physical examination includes inspection of the skin for rashes, inspection of the skin and conjunctiva for jaundice, and palpation of the liver for enlargement and tenderness. Weight loss, fever, and general debilitation should be noted. If the HBsAg is positive, further laboratory studies may be ordered (anti-HBe, anti-HBc, serum glutamic-oxaloacetic transaminase, alkaline phosphatase, and liver panel).

Prevention. Primary prevention of HBV should be the focus for treatment. Primary prevention should include counselling and education regarding risk behaviours, harm reduction strategies (needle exchange programs) and hepatitis B vaccination (pre-exposure). Since the early 1990s, all provinces and territories have had either a universal school-based hepatitis B vaccination program aimed at children aged 9 to 13 or an infant vaccination program (PHAC, 2006). Hepatitis B vaccine should also be offered to high-risk groups (Box 6-6). The vaccine is given in a series of three (four if rapid protection is needed) doses over a 6-month period, with the first two doses given at least 1 month apart. For adults the vaccine is given in the deltoid muscle.

Secondary prevention is the administration of hepatitis B immune globulin (HBIG). This should be offered to

BOX 6-6 High-Risk Groups for Hepatitis B

- Children from HBV-endemic areas who may be exposed to HBV via extended family or the community
- Populations or communities in which HBV is highly endemic
- Residents and staff of institutions for the mentally or developmentally challenged
- Sex workers
- Hemodialysis patients
- Household and sexual contacts of acute HBV cases and HBV carriers
- Pregnant women
- Injection drug users
- Staff and inmates of correctional facilities
- Travellers to HBV-endemic areas
- Those who have recently acquired an STI
- Those whose regular sex partner is HBsAg positive
- Those with multiple sex partners
- Those with occupational risk (e.g., health care workers and emergency service workers who may be exposed to blood, blood products, or body fluids that may contain the virus)
- Children in childcare settings in which there is an HBV-infected child
- People who are HIV positive
- Sexual partners of any of those listed above

(Source: Public Health Agency of Canada [2006]. *Canadian immunization guide* [7th ed.]. Reproduced with the permission of the Minister of Health, 2011.)

HBV, hepatitis B virus; *HBsAg*, hepatitis B surface antigen; *HIV*, human immunodeficiency virus.

individuals, including pregnant women who have percutaneous (needlestick) or mucosal exposure, up to 7 days after exposure and to sexual contacts within 14 days of exposure (ideally within 48 hours), followed by hepatitis B vaccine. For infants born to HBV-infected mothers, the first dose of hepatitis B vaccine should be administered within 12 hours of birth and HBIG given immediately after birth (efficacy decreases sharply after 48 hours) (PHAC, 2008).

Management. There is no specific treatment for hepatitis B. Recovery is usually spontaneous in 3 to 16 weeks. Pregnancies complicated by acute viral hepatitis are managed on an outpatient basis. Women should be advised to increase bed rest; eat a high-protein, low-fat diet; and increase their fluid intake. They should avoid alcohol and medications metabolized in the liver.

Patient education includes explanation of the meaning of hepatitis B infection, including transmission, state of infectivity, and sequelae. The nurse should also explain the need for immunoprophylaxis for household members and sexual contacts. To decrease transmission of the virus, women with hepatitis B or who test positive for HBV should be advised to maintain a high level of personal hygiene (e.g., wash hands after using the toilet; carefully dispose of tampons, pads, and bandages in plastic bags; not share razor blades, toothbrushes, needles, or manicure implements; have her male partner use a condom if he is unvaccinated and without hepatitis; avoid sharing saliva through kissing or through sharing of silverware or dishes; and wipe up blood spills immediately with soap and water). Patients should inform all health care providers of their carrier state. Postpartum women should be reassured that breastfeeding is not contraindicated if the infant receives prophylaxis after birth and is currently on the immunization schedule.

Hepatitis C

Hepatitis C (HCV) is an important cause of chronic liver disease and is becoming a major public health problem worldwide (Boucher et al., 2000). In Canada it is estimated that approximately 250,000 people are infected with hepatitis C (Sherman et al., 2007). The most common risk factor is a history of intravenous drug use. Other risk factors include STIs such as hepatitis B and HIV, multiple sexual partners, tattoos and body piercing, and a history of blood transfusions. Hepatitis C is readily transmitted through exposure to blood.

Most patients with HCV are asymptomatic or have general flu-like symptoms similar to those of hepatitis A. HCV infection is confirmed by the presence of anti-C antibody during laboratory testing. Routine HCV testing is recommended for women who have ever injected drugs; women who received a blood transfusion before July 1992; children of HCV-positive women; health care, emergency, medical, and public safety workers; and women with chronic liver disease (Pinnette et al., 2009). Counselling and testing should be offered to pregnant women with known risk factors.

Interferon alfa-2b and ribavirin for 6 to 12 months are the main treatment for HCV infection, although the effectiveness of this treatment varies. Treatment for drug use is an important adjunct for many persons with HCV (Sherman et al., 2007).

Currently, there is no vaccine to prevent hepatitis C. Transmission of HCV through breastfeeding has not been reported, although women with cracked, bleeding nipples are advised to stop breastfeeding until the nipples heal.

Human Immunodeficiency Virus

Although HIV has traditionally been thought of as a disease affecting gay men, heterosexual transmission is now the most common means of transmission in women. An estimated 25% of cases of HIV are among women, an increase from 10% in 1995 (PHAC, 2008). Although the incidence of HIV has decreased among the general population, the rate among First Nations, Métis, and Inuit populations has been increasing (PHAC, 2010b).

Transmission of HIV, a retrovirus, occurs primarily through exchange of body fluids (semen, blood, or vaginal secretions). Severe depression of the cellular immune system associated with HIV infection characterizes acquired immunodeficiency syndrome (AIDS). For both men and women the most commonly reported opportunistic diseases are *Pneumocystis carinii* pneumonia, candida esophagitis, and wasting syndrome. Other viral infections such as HSV and cytomegalovirus infections seem to be more prevalent in women than in men. PID may be more severe in HIV-infected women, and rates of HPV and cervical dysplasia may be higher. The clinical course of HPV infection in women with HIV infection is accelerated, and recurrence is more frequent.

Once HIV enters the body, seroconversion to HIV positivity usually occurs within 6 to 12 weeks. Although HIV seroconversion may be totally asymptomatic, it usually is accompanied by a viremic, influenza-like response. Symptoms include fever, headache, night sweats, malaise, generalized lymphadenopathy, myalgias, nausea, diarrhea, weight loss, sore throat, and rash.

Laboratory studies may reveal leukopenia, thrombocytopenia, anemia, and an elevated erythrocyte sedimentation rate. HIV has a strong affinity for surface-marker proteins on T lymphocytes. This affinity leads to significant T-cell destruction. Both clinical and epidemiological studies have shown that declining CD4 levels are strongly associated with increased incidence of AIDS-related diseases and death in many different groups of HIV-infected persons.

Transmission of the virus from mother to fetus can occur throughout the perinatal period. Exposure may occur to the fetus through the maternal circulation as early as the first trimester of pregnancy, to the infant during labour and birth by inoculation or ingestion of maternal blood and other infected fluids, or to the infant through breast milk (Lawrence & Lawrence, 2011; Riordan & Wambach, 2010).

Screening and Diagnosis

Screening for HIV as well as teaching and counselling on risk factors, indications for being tested, and testing are major roles for nurses caring for women today, as up to 30% of people living with HIV are unaware of their HIV status (PHAC, 2008). A number of behaviours place women at risk for HIV infection. These include intravenous drug use, high-risk sex practices, multiple sex partners, and a previous history of multiple STIs. HIV infection is usually diagnosed by using HIV-1 and HIV-2 antibody tests. Antibody testing is done first with a sensitive screening test such as the enzyme immunoassay. Reactive screening tests must be confirmed by an additional test such as the Western blot or an immunofluorescence assay. If a positive antibody test is confirmed by a supplemental test, it means that a woman is infected with HIV and is capable of infecting others. HIV antibodies are detectable in at least 95% of patients within 3 months after infection. Although a negative antibody test usually indicates that a person is not infected, antibody tests cannot exclude recent infection. Because the HIV antibody crosses the placenta, a definite diagnosis of HIV in children younger than 18 months is based on laboratory evidence of HIV in blood or tissues by culture, nucleic acid, or antigen detection (Centers for Disease Control and Prevention, Workowski, & Berman, 2010).

Counselling for HIV Testing

Counselling before and after HIV testing is standard nursing practice. It is a nurse's responsibility to assess a woman's understanding of the information such a test would provide and to ensure that the patient thoroughly understands the emotional, legal, and medical implications of a positive or negative test before she is ready to take an HIV test. One's life is profoundly altered by knowledge of HIV seropositivity, as a unique stigma is often associated with HIV infection. This stigma extends to those who are asymptomatic but seropositive.

Unless rapid testing is done, there is generally a 1- to 3-week waiting period after testing for HIV; this can be a very anxious time for the woman. It is helpful if the nurse informs her that this time period between blood drawing and test results is routine. Test results must always be communicated in person, and women should be informed in advance that this is the procedure. Whenever possible, the person who provided the pretest counselling should also be the one to tell the woman her test results. The nurse should make sure that the woman understands what a positive test result means and review the reliability of the test results.

Some women when informed of negative results may increase their practice of risk behaviours because they equate negativity with immunity. Others may believe that negative means "bad" and positive means "good." The woman's reaction to a negative test should be explored by asking, "How do you feel?" Counselling sessions for women with an HIV-negative result are another opportunity to provide education. Emphasis can be placed on ways in which a woman can remain HIV-free. She should be reminded that if she has been exposed to HIV in the past 6 months, she should be retested, and that she should have ongoing testing if she continues practising high-risk behaviours.

Pregnancy and HIV

Pregnancy is not encouraged for women who are HIV positive. Preconception counselling is recommended; contraceptive counselling should be offered to HIV-positive women who do not desire pregnancy. HIV-infected women should be informed specifically about the risks for perinatal infection. Current evidence indicates that 25 to 30% of infants born to untreated HIV-infected women are infected with HIV, whereas the transmission rate in treated women is less than 2%. The most important aspect to decreasing the rate of perinatal transmission is the identification of HIV in pregnant women. Routine HIV screening should be done for all pregnant women and is discussed in Chapter 10.

Perinatal transmission of HIV has decreased by 67% since 1994 because of a three-part regimen consisting of (1) the administration of antiretroviral prophylaxis (zidovudine [ZDV]) to women during pregnancy, (2) intravenous ZDV during labour, and (3) ZDV to the newborn infant for 6 weeks. Subsequent studies using antiretroviral therapy (ART) demonstrated a reduction of perinatal transmission to less than 2% of births in women with HIV. The major side effect of ZDV is bone marrow suppression; thus periodic hematocrit, white blood cell count, and platelet count assessments should be performed.

Women who are HIV positive should also be vaccinated against hepatitis B, pneumococcal infection, *Haemophilus influenzae* type B, and viral influenza. To support any pregnant woman's immune system, appropriate counselling is provided about optimal nutrition, sleep, rest, exercise, and stress reduction. Use of condoms is encouraged in order to minimize further exposure to HIV if her partner is the source.

The rate of transmission of HIV during breastfeeding is 9% (Coutsoudis et al., 2004). Thus, in Canada, where safe and affordable substitutes are available, HIV-infected women should be counselled not to breastfeed (Canadian Paediatric Society [CPS], 2008). Giving nevirapine once daily to breastfeeding infants from days 8 to 42 of life helps the infants remain HIV negative. It is used more in developing countries where safe water and affordable feeding substitutes are not available (National Institute of Child Health and Human Development, 2008). There is risk of liver toxicity in women with CD4 counts greater than 250 cells/mm^3, thus nevirapine should be used with caution.

Caesarean birth performed before rupture of membranes and onset of labour has been shown to be of benefit for preventing vertical transmission of HIV in women who did not have antiretroviral therapy or received only ZDV in pregnancy. The benefits of Caesarean birth for women who received combination therapy are less clear (Centers for Disease Control and Prevention [CDC], 2006). Complications after Caesarean birth are more common in HIV-positive women than in uninfected women.

Management

During the initial contact with an HIV-infected woman, the nurse should establish what the woman knows about HIV infection and that she is being cared for by a medical practitioner or a facility with expertise in caring for persons with HIV infections, including AIDS. Psychological referral also may be indicated. Resources such as counselling for financial assistance, grief counselling, and legal advocacy may be appropriate. All women who are drug users should be referred to a **substance use** program. A major focus of counselling is prevention of transmission of HIV to partners.

Nurses counselling seropositive women who wish to receive contraceptive information may recommend (1) oral contraceptives and latex condoms, or (2) tubal sterilization or vasectomy and latex condoms. The IUD is not appropriate for the HIV-infected woman because of the increased risk of infection. Female condoms or abstinence can be recommended to women whose partners refuse to use condoms.

Routine gynecological care for HIV-positive women should include a pelvic examination every 6 months. Careful Pap screening is essential because of the greatly increased incidence of abnormal findings. In addition, HIV-positive women should be screened for syphilis, gonorrhea, chlamydia, and other vaginal infections.

No cure is available for HIV infection. Rare and unusual diseases are characteristic of HIV infection. Opportunistic infections and concurrent diseases should be managed vigorously with treatment specific to the infection or disease.

Discussion of the medical care of HIV-positive women and women with AIDS is beyond the scope of this chapter. The reader is referred to the U.S. Centers for Disease Control and Prevention (CDC) (http://www.cdc.gov) and Web sites such as Canadian AIDS Treatment Information Exchange (http://www.catie.ca) for current information and recommendations.

Vaginal Infections

Vaginal discharge and itching of the vulva and vagina are among the most common reasons a woman seeks help from a health care provider. Women cite discomfort from vaginal discharge more than any other gynecological symptom. Women who have adequate endogenous or exogenous estrogen will have vaginal secretions. Vaginal discharge resulting from infection must be distinguished from normal secretions. Normal vaginal secretions (or leukorrhea) are clear to cloudy in appearance. The discharge may turn yellow after drying; is slightly slimy; is nonirritating; and has a mild, inoffensive odour. Normal vaginal secretions are acidic, with a pH range of 4 to 5. The amount of leukorrhea differs with phases of the menstrual cycle, with greater amounts occurring at ovulation and just before menses. Leukorrhea is also increased during pregnancy. Normal vaginal secretions contain lactobacilli and epithelial cells.

Vaginitis, or abnormal vaginal discharge, is an infection caused by a microorganism. The most common vaginal infections are bacterial vaginosis (BV), candidiasis, and trichomoniasis. *Vulvovaginitis*, inflammation of the vulva and vagina, may be caused by vaginal infection; copious leukorrhea, which can cause maceration of tissues; and chemical irritants, allergens, and foreign bodies, which may produce inflammatory reactions.

Bacterial Vaginosis

BV, formerly called nonspecific vaginitis, *Haemophilus vaginitis*, or *Gardnerella*, is the most common type of vaginitis. BV is associated with preterm labour and birth. The exact etiology of BV is unknown and it is not usually considered an STI. It is a syndrome in which normal H_2O_2–producing lactobacilli are replaced with high concentrations of anaerobic bacteria (*Gardnerella* and *Mobiluncus*). With the proliferation of anaerobes, the level of vaginal amines is raised, and the normal acidic pH of the vagina is altered. Epithelial cells slough, and numerous bacteria attach to their surfaces (clue cells). When the amines are volatilized, the characteristic odour of BV occurs.

Screening and Diagnosis

A careful history may help distinguish BV from other vaginal infections if the woman is symptomatic. Women with previous occurrence of similar symptoms, diagnosis, and treatment should be queried because women with BV often have been treated incorrectly due to misdiagnosis.

Most women with BV complain of a characteristic "fishy odour" in the vaginal area, although not all note it. The odour may be noticed by the woman or her partner after heterosexual intercourse because semen releases the vaginal amines. When present, the BV discharge is usually profuse; thin; and white, grey, or milky in appearance. Some women also may experience mild irritation or pruritus.

Microscopic examination of vaginal secretions is always done (Table 6-3). Both normal saline and 10% potassium hydroxide (KOH) smears should be made. The presence of clue cells confirmed by wet smear is highly diagnostic because the phenomenon is specific to BV (PHAC, 2008). Vaginal secretions should be tested for pH and amine odour. Nitrazine paper is sensitive enough to detect a pH of 4.5 or greater. The fishy odour of BV will be released when KOH is added to vaginal secretions on the lip of the withdrawn speculum.

Management

Treatment of BV with oral metronidazole (Flagyl) is most effective (PHAC, 2008). Metronidazole is an antiprotozoal and antibacterial agent. Adverse effects of metronidazole are numerous and include a sharp, unpleasant metallic taste in the mouth; furry tongue; central nervous system reactions; and urinary tract disturbances. When oral metronidazole is taken,

Table 6-3 Wet Smear Tests for Vaginal Infections

INFECTION	TEST	POSITIVE FINDINGS
Trichomoniasis	Saline wet smear (vaginal secretions mixed with normal saline on a glass slide)	Presence of many white blood cell protozoa
Candidiasis	Potassium hydroxide (KOH) prep (vaginal secretions mixed with KOH on a glass slide)	Presence of hyphae and pseudohyphae (buds and branches of yeast cells)
Bacterial vaginosis	Normal saline smear	Presence of clue cells (vaginal epithelial cells coated with bacteria)
	Whiff test (vaginal secretions mixed with KOH)	Release of fishy odour

the patient is advised not to drink alcoholic beverages or she may experience severe adverse effects of abdominal distress, nausea, vomiting, and headache. Gastrointestinal symptoms are common whether alcohol is consumed or not. Treatment of sexual partners is not recommended because sexual transmission of BV has not been proven.

Several adverse outcomes are associated with BV during pregnancy: preterm labour and birth, premature rupture of the membranes, intra-amniotic infection, and postpartum endometritis. Therefore, pregnant women should be treated to relieve vaginal symptoms and the signs of infection. Consideration should also be given to evaluation and treatment of asymptomatic women at high risk for preterm birth (Yudin et al., 2008).

Metronidazole is contraindicated if the woman is breastfeeding because high concentrations have been found in infants. If it is necessary to prescribe metronidazole for the lactating woman, she can suspend breastfeeding temporarily (pump and discard milk to maintain supply) and resume it 48 to 72 hours after taking the last dose.

Candidiasis

Vulvovaginal candidiasis (VVC), or yeast infection, is the second most common type of vaginal infection in Canada. It is estimated that approximately 75% of women will have at least one episode of VVC in their lifetime (PHAC, 2008). Although vaginal candidiasis infections are common in healthy women, those seen in women with HIV infection are often more severe and persistent. Genital candidiasis lesions may be painful, and coalescing ulcerations necessitate continuous, prophylactic therapy.

The most common organism is *Candida albicans*. It is estimated that 80 to 95% of yeast infections in women are caused by this organism. However, in the past 10 years the incidence of non–*C. albicans* infections has increased steadily. Women with chronic or recurrent infections often are infected with a higher percentage of non–*C. albicans* species than are women with their first infection or those who have few recurrences.

Numerous factors have been identified as predisposing a woman to yeast infections. These include antibiotic therapy, particularly broad-spectrum antibiotics such as ampicillin, tetracycline, cephalosporins, and metronidazole; diabetes, especially when uncontrolled; pregnancy; obesity; diets high in refined sugars or artificial sweeteners; use of corticosteroids and exogenous hormones; and immunosuppressed states. Clinical observations and research have suggested that tight-fitting clothing and underwear or pantyhose made of nonabsorbent materials create an environment in which a vaginal fungus can grow (see Patient Teaching box).

The most common symptom of yeast infection is vulvar and possibly vaginal pruritus. The itching may be mild or intense, may interfere with rest and activities, and may occur during or after intercourse. Some women report a feeling of dryness. Others may have painful urination as the urine flows over the vulva. The latter usually occurs in women who have excoriations resulting from scratching. Most often the discharge is thick, white, lumpy, and cottage cheese–like. The discharge may be found in patches on the vaginal walls, cervix, and labia. Commonly the vulva is red and swollen, as are the labial folds, vagina, and cervix. Although there is no odour characteristic of yeast infections, sometimes a yeasty or musty smell is noted.

PATIENT TEACHING Yeast Infection—Inadequate Patient Education

Marcella, an 82-year-old widow, had a precancerous lesion excised from her forehead and was placed on a broad-spectrum antibiotic for 1 week. She later presented to the clinic with profuse, white vaginal discharge; severe itching; and excoriation on her labia, in her groin, and extending onto her buttocks and lower abdomen. When she expressed hesitance in talking to the physician, the nurse assured her that she would be with her during the examination. Marcella said that wasn't the problem. When the nurse examined Marcella, she said that her problem looked like a yeast infection and asked Marcella if she had been taking antibiotics. The nurse explained that yeast infections are common when taking antibiotics. The physician verified the diagnosis and prescribed Monistat. On further discussion, the nurse determined that Marcella had thought that she picked up a sexually transmitted infection (STI) when she used a public restroom and was ashamed and embarrassed to discuss her problem, so had not told anyone or sought treatment earlier. When Marcella returned home and told her daughter that she had seen a physician, her daughter stated, "You have a yeast infection." When Marcella asked how she knew that, the daughter said that her friend and her daughter both had developed yeast infections when on antibiotics.

This situation could have been avoided if the physician who prescribed the antibiotic or the nurse had told Marcella that yeast infections are common when antibiotics are taken or if Marcella had discussed the condition with her daughter. Marcella can be counselled to discuss problems and seek care in the early stages of a problem, even when discussing the condition may be embarrassing. Had she discussed this with her daughter, treatment could have been started much sooner, and Marcella would have avoided the distress she experienced. Marcella also needs some teaching about the transmission of STIs.

Screening and Diagnosis

In addition to noting the woman's symptoms, their onset, and their course, the history is a valuable screening tool for identifying predisposing risk factors. Physical examination should include a thorough inspection of the vulva and vagina. A speculum examination is always done. Commonly, saline and KOH wet smear and vaginal pH are obtained (see Table 6-3). Vaginal pH is normal with a yeast infection; if the pH is greater than 4.5, trichomoniasis or BV should be suspected. The characteristic pseudohypha (bud or branching of a fungus) may be seen on a wet smear done with normal saline; however, they may be confused with other cells and artifacts.

Management

A number of antifungal preparations are available for the treatment of *C. albicans*. Fluconazole in a single dose can be prescribed, and other medications (e.g., miconazole [Monistat] and clotrimazole [Canesten]) are available as OTC agents. Fluconazole is contraindicated in pregnancy. The first time a woman suspects that she has a yeast infection she should see a health care provider for confirmation of the diagnosis and treatment recommendation. If she has another infection, she may wish to purchase an OTC preparation and self-treat. Treatments should begin to work in 2 to 3 days. If she elects to do this, she should always be counselled to seek care for numerous recurrent or chronic yeast infections. If vaginal discharge is extremely thick and copious, vaginal **débridement** with a cotton swab followed by application of vaginal medication may be effective.

Women who have extensive irritation, swelling, and discomfort of the labia and vulva may find sitz baths helpful in decreasing inflammation and increasing comfort. Adding Aveeno powder to the bath may also increase the woman's comfort. Not wearing underpants to bed may help decrease symptoms and prevent recurrences. Completion of the full course of treatment prescribed is essential to removing the pathogen. Medication should be continued even during menstruation. Women should be counselled not to use tampons during menses because the medication will be absorbed by the tampon. If possible, intercourse should be avoided during treatment; if this is not feasible, the woman's partner should use a condom to prevent introduction of more organisms. Suggested measures to prevent genital tract infections are in the Patient Teaching box on p. 95.

Trichomoniasis

Trichomoniasis is a cause of up to 25% of all vaginal infections and is almost always a sexually transmitted infection. Trichomoniasis is caused by *Trichomonas vaginalis*, an anaerobic, one-celled protozoan with characteristic flagella. Although trichomoniasis may be asymptomatic, commonly women have yellowish-to-greenish, frothy, mucopurulent, copious, and malodourous discharge. Inflammation of the vulva, vagina, or both may be present, and the woman may complain of irritation and pruritus. Dysuria and dyspareunia are often present. Typically the discharge worsens during and after menstruation. Often the cervix and vaginal walls demonstrate the characteristic "strawberry spots" or tiny **petechiae**, and the cervix may bleed on contact. In severe infections the vaginal walls, cervix, and, occasionally, the vulva may be acutely inflamed.

Screening and Diagnosis

In addition to obtaining a history of current symptoms, a careful sexual history should be obtained. Any history of similar symptoms and the treatments used should be noted. The nurse should determine whether the patient's partner or partners were treated and if she has had subsequent sexual relations with new partners.

A speculum examination is always done, even though it may be very uncomfortable for the woman; relaxation techniques and breathing exercises may help the woman with the procedure. Any of the classic signs may or may not be present on physical examination. The typical one-celled flagellate trichomonads are easily distinguished on a normal saline wet prep. Trichomoniasis also may be identified on Pap tests. Because trichomoniasis is an STI, once diagnosis is confirmed, appropriate laboratory studies for other STIs should be carried out.

Management

The recommended treatment is metronidazole (Flagyl), 2 g orally in a single dose (PHAC, 2008). Although the male partner is usually asymptomatic, it is recommended that he receive treatment also because he often harbors the trichomonads in the urethra or prostate. It is important that nurses discuss the importance of partner treatment with patients because it is likely that the infection will recur if partners are not treated. Women need to be taught that they should not drink alcohol during and for 24 hours after therapy as there is a risk of a disulfuram (antabuse) reaction (PHAC, 2008). Symptoms of this reaction include dizziness, headache, shortness of breath, palpitation, and nausea and vomiting.

Women with trichomoniasis need to understand the sexual transmission of this disease. The patient must know that the organism may be present without observable symptoms, perhaps for several months, and that it is not possible to determine when she became infected. Women should be informed of the necessity for treating all sexual partners and given suggestions about how to raise the issue with their partner(s) (see Home Care box).

HOME CARE

Sexually Transmitted Infections

- Take your medication as directed.
- Use comfort measures for symptom relief as suggested by your health care provider.
- Keep your appointment for repeat cultures or checkups after your treatment to make sure that your infection is cured.
- Advise your sexual partner(s) to be tested and treated, if necessary.
- Abstain from sexual intercourse until your treatment is completed or for as long as you are advised by your health care provider.
- Use practices to prevent infection when sexual intercourse is resumed.
- Call your health care provider immediately if you notice bumps, sores, rashes, or discharges.
- Keep all future appointments with your health care provider, even if things appear normal.

Infection Control

Infection-control measures are essential for protecting care providers and preventing hospital-acquired infection of patients, regardless of the infectious agent. The risk for occupational transmission varies with the disease. Even when the risk is low, as with HIV, the existence of any risk warrants reasonable precautions. Routine precautions (precautions to use in care of all persons for infection control) are listed in Box 6-7.

Problems of the Breast

Approximately 50% of women have a breast problem at some point in their adult lives. The most common sign of a breast problem is a palpable mass. Most of these lumps are benign, although finding them may produce anxiety for the woman, who may fear she has cancer. With the exception of skin cancer, cancer of the breast is the most frequently diagnosed cancer in women in Canada (CCS, 2010). The development of breast cancer can have a far-reaching impact on the woman and her family. Beyond the obvious physiological alterations, the woman also may experience threats to her self-concept and her ability to cope. The condition and its treatments can affect a woman's concept of herself as a sexual being. A woman's family is also challenged in the way they respond to her diagnosis. When breast cancer occurs during or after pregnancy, it adds to the complexity of both physical and emotional responses to childbearing.

Fibrocystic Changes

The most common benign breast problem is fibrocystic change. Fibrocystic change is not a disease but a condition found in varying degrees in healthy women's breasts. Fibrocystic changes

BOX 6-7 Routine Precautions

Assume that every person is potentially infected or colonized with an organism that could be transmitted in the health care setting, and apply the following infection control practices during the delivery of health care.

Hand Hygiene

During the delivery of health care, avoid unnecessary touching of surfaces in close proximity to the patient to prevent both contamination of clean hands from environmental surfaces and transmission of pathogens from contaminated hands to surfaces. When hands are visibly dirty, contaminated with proteinaceous material, or visibly soiled with blood or body fluids, wash them with either a nonantimicrobial soap and water or an antimicrobial soap and water. If hands are not visibly soiled or after removing visible material with nonantimicrobial soap and water, decontaminate them. The preferred method of hand hygiene is with an alcohol-based hand rub. Alternatively, hands may be washed with an antimicrobial soap and water. Perform hand hygiene: (a) before having direct contact with patients or environment; (b) before an aseptic procedure; (c) after exposure risk to body fluid; (d) when leaving the room after touching the patient or any objects in the patient's environment; and (e) after removing gloves. Wash hands with nonantimicrobial soap and water or with antimicrobial soap and water if contact with spores (e.g., *Clostridium difficile* or *Bacillus anthracis*) is likely to have occurred. The physical action of washing and rinsing hands under such circumstances is recommended because alcohols, chlorhexidine, iodophors, and other antiseptic agents have poor activity against spores. Do not wear artificial fingernails or extenders if duties include direct contact with patients at high risk for infection and associated adverse outcomes (e.g., NICUs, ICUs, or operating rooms). Develop an organizational policy for the wearing of non-natural nails by health care personnel who have direct contact with patients outside of the groups previously specified.

Personal Protective Equipment

Observe the following principles of use:

- Wear personal protective equipment (PPE) when the nature of the anticipated patient interaction indicates that contact with blood or body fluids may occur. Prevent contamination of clothing and skin during the process of removing PPE. Before leaving the patient's room or cubicle, remove and discard PPE and perform hand hygiene.
- **Gloves**—Wear gloves when it can be reasonably anticipated that contact with blood or other potentially infectious materials, mucous membranes, nonintact skin, or potentially contaminated intact skin (e.g., of a patient incontinent of stool or urine) could occur. Wear gloves with fit and durability appropriate to the task. Wear disposable medical examination gloves when providing direct patient care and cleaning the environment or medical equipment. Remove gloves after contact with a patient, the surrounding environment (including medical equipment), or both, using proper technique to prevent hand contamination. Do not wear the same pair of gloves for the care of more than one patient. Do not wash gloves for the purpose of reuse since this practice has been associated with transmission of pathogens. Change gloves during patient care if the hands will move from a contaminated body site (e.g., perineal area) to a clean body site (e.g., face). Perform hand hygiene after removing gloves.
- **Gowns**—Wear a gown that is appropriate to the task to protect skin and prevent soiling or contamination of clothing during procedures and patient care activities when contact with blood, body fluids, secretions, or excretions is anticipated. Wear a gown for direct patient contact if the patient has uncontained secretions or excretions. Remove gown and perform hand hygiene before leaving the patient's environment. Do not reuse

Continued

BOX 6-7 Routine Precautions—cont'd

gowns, even for repeated contacts with the same patient. Routine donning of gowns on entrance into a high-risk unit (e.g., CCU, NICU, HSCT unit) is not indicated.

- **Mouth, nose, and eye protection**—Use PPE to protect the mucous membranes of the eyes, nose, and mouth during procedures and patient care activities that are likely to generate splashes or sprays of blood, body fluids, secretions, and excretions. Select masks, goggles, face shields, and combinations of each according to the need anticipated by the task performed. During aerosol-generating procedures (e.g., bronchoscopy, suctioning of the respiratory tract [if not using in-line suction catheters], endotracheal intubation) in patients who are not suspected of being infected with an agent for which respiratory protection is otherwise recommended (e.g., *Mycobacterium* tuberculosis, SARS, or hemorrhagic fever viruses), wear one of the following: a face shield that fully covers the front and sides of the face, a mask with attached shield, or a mask and goggles (in addition to gloves and gown).

Respiratory Hygiene and Cough Etiquette

Educate health care personnel on the importance of source-control measures to contain respiratory secretions to prevent droplet and fomite transmission of respiratory pathogens, especially during seasonal outbreaks of viral respiratory tract infections (e.g., influenza, RSV, adenovirus, parainfluenza virus) in communities. Implement the following measures to contain respiratory secretions in patients and accompanying individuals who have signs and symptoms of a respiratory infection, beginning at the point of initial encounter in a health care setting (e.g., triage, reception and waiting areas in emergency departments, outpatient clinics, and physician offices). Post signs at entrances and in strategic places (e.g., elevators, cafeterias) within ambulatory and inpatient settings with instructions to patients and other persons with symptoms of a respiratory infection to cough or sneeze into their sleeve and perform hand hygiene after hands have been in contact with respiratory secretions. Provide tissues and no-touch receptacles (e.g., foot-pedal operated lid or open, plastic-lined wastebasket) for disposal of tissues. Provide resources and instructions for performing hand hygiene in or near waiting areas in ambulatory and inpatient settings; provide conveniently located dispensers of alcohol-based hand rubs and, where sinks are available, supplies for hand hygiene. During periods of increased prevalence of respiratory infections in the community (e.g., increased number of patients seeking care for a respiratory infection), offer masks to coughing patients and other symptomatic persons (e.g., persons who accompany ill patients) on entry into the facility or medical office and encourage them to maintain special separation, ideally a distance of at least 1 metre, from others in common waiting areas. Some facilities may find it logistically easier to institute this recommendation year-round as a standard of practice.

Safe Injection Practices

The following recommendations apply to the use of needles, the use of cannulas that replace needles, and, where applicable, intravenous delivery systems. Use aseptic technique to avoid contamination of sterile injection equipment. Do not administer medications from a syringe to multiple patients, even if the needle or cannula on the syringe is changed. Needles, cannulas, and syringes are sterile, single-use items; they should not be reused for another patient or to access a medication or solution that might be used for a subsequent patient. Use fluid infusion and administration sets (i.e., intravenous bags, tubing, and connectors) for one patient only and dispose appropriately after use. Consider a syringe or needle/cannula contaminated once it has been used to enter or connect to a patient's intravenous infusion bag or administration set. Use single-dose vials for parenteral medications whenever possible. Do not administer medications from single-dose vials or ampules to multiple patients or combine leftover contents for later use. If multidose vials must be used, both the needle or cannula and syringe used to access the multidose vial must be sterile. Do not keep multidose vials in the immediate patient treatment area and store them in accordance with the manufacturer's recommendations; discard them if sterility is compromised or questionable.

Infection Control Practices for Special Lumbar Puncture Procedures

Wear a surgical mask when placing a catheter or injecting material into the spinal canal or subdural space (i.e., during myelograms, lumbar puncture, and spinal or epidural anesthesia).

(Source: Centers for Disease Control and Prevention. [2007]. *Standard precautions. Excerpted from Guideline for isolation precautions: Preventing transmission of infectious agents in healthcare settings 2007.* Updated October 12, 2007. Retrieved from http://www.cdc.gov/hicpac/2007IP/2007isolationPrecautions.html.)

HSCT, hematopoietic stem cell transplant; *ICU,* intensive care unit; *NICU,* neonatal intensive care unit; *RSV,* respiratory syncytial virus; *SARS,* severe acute respiratory syndrome.

are palpable thickenings in the breast that are usually associated with pain and tenderness. The pain and tenderness fluctuate with the menstrual cycle and can become progressively worse until menopause. The histological findings associated with fibrocystic changes are considered part of the spectrum of normal involutional patterns of the breast; thus the changes are not a disease.

Etiology

Fibrocystic changes tend to appear most commonly in women in their 20s and 30s. No known etiological agent is responsible for benign breast disease, although an imbalance of estrogen and progesterone may be responsible. One theory is that estrogen excess and progesterone deficiency in the luteal phase of the menstrual cycle may cause changes in breast tissue. Risk factors associated with benign breast disease include **nulliparity**, low parity, late menopause, and estrogen therapy.

Clinical Manifestations and Diagnosis

The usual clinical presentation of fibrocystic change is lumpiness in both breasts; single simple cysts may also occur. Symptoms usually develop about a week before menstruation begins and subside about a week after menstruation ends. They include dull, heavy pain and a sense of fullness and tenderness that increases premenstrually. The woman with fibrocystic change may form cysts that manifest as painful enlarging lumps in her breasts. Cysts are common in premenopausal women who are not receiving estrogen therapy. The cysts are soft on palpation, well differentiated, and movable. Deeper cysts, especially aggregations of cysts, are indistinguishable by palpation from carcinomas, which are malignant growths that infiltrate surrounding tissue.

A first step in the workup of a breast lump is an ultrasound to determine if it is fluid filled or solid. Fluid-filled cysts are aspirated, and the woman is monitored on a routine basis for development of other cysts. If the lump is solid, a mammogram is obtained if the woman is older than 35 years. Fine-needle aspiration (FNA) is then performed, regardless of the woman's age, to determine the nature of the lump. In some cases a core biopsy may be needed after FNA to harvest adequate amounts of tissue for pathological examination.

Management

Treatment for fibrocystic change is usually conservative, with diuretics and restriction of salt and fluid. Vitamin E supplements also have been recommended, although megadose therapy should be avoided. Even though no research support has been found, some advocate eliminating dimethylxanthines such as caffeine. Some women report relief of symptoms by avoiding smoking and not consuming alcohol. Recommended pain-relief measures include taking analgesics or NSAIDs such as ibuprofen, wearing a supportive bra, and applying heat to the breasts. Some women report relief while taking oral contraceptives, but others report worsening of symptoms. Women may need to try several approaches for a number of months before improvement is noted. Surgical removal of nodules is attempted only in select cases. For multiple nodules, the surgical approach involves multiple incisions and tissue manipulation and may not prevent the development of more nodules.

Fibroadenomas

The next most common benign condition of the breast is fibroadenoma. Fibroadenomas occur in women from puberty through menopause. Masses are solid, encapsulated, and nontender and are most often found in the upper outer quadrant of the breast.

The cause of fibroadenomas is unknown. Fibroadenomas are characterized by discrete, usually solitary lumps less than 3 cm in diameter. Occasionally the woman with a fibroadenoma experiences tenderness in the tumour during the menstrual cycle. Fibroadenomas increase in size during pregnancy and shrink as the woman ages. Fibroadenomas do not increase in size in response to the menstrual cycle (in contrast to fibrocystic cysts). The mass tends to remain the same size or increase in size slowly over time.

Diagnosis is made by a review of the history and physical examination. A mammogram, ultrasound examination, or magnetic resonance imaging may be used to determine the type of lesion. FNA may be used to determine the underlying disorder. Surgical excision may be necessary if the lump is suspicious for malignancy or if the symptoms are severe. Fibroadenomas do not respond to either dietary changes or hormone therapy. Periodic observation of masses by professional physical examination or mammogram may be all that is necessary for masses not needing surgical intervention.

Lipomas

A *lipoma* is a tumour composed of fat that is soft and has discrete borders. The cause of lipoma is unknown. Lipomas are often found in women over 45 years of age, usually on the chest wall and breast. They are characterized as palpable soft masses that are mobile and nontender. Mammograms can be used to make a diagnosis; biopsy usually is not needed. Lipomas can be surgically excised if removal is desired.

Nipple Discharge

Nipple discharge is a common occurrence that concerns many women. Although most nipple discharge is physiological, each woman who has this problem must be evaluated carefully. A small percentage of women are found to have a serious endocrine disorder or malignancy. Bilateral serous discharge expressed during nipple stimulation can be considered a normal finding. Patient education and reassurance are indicated.

Galactorrhea is another form of breast discharge not related to malignancy. Galactorrhea manifests as a bilaterally spontaneous, milky, sticky discharge. It is a normal finding in pregnancy. It can also occur as the result of elevated prolactin levels, which in turn may occur as a result of a thyroid disorder, pituitary tumour, or chest wall surgery or trauma. A complete medication history is essential because certain medications can precipitate galactorrhea (e.g., OCPs and neuroleptic medications).

The optimal time to draw blood to determine a prolactin level is between 8 and 10 AM. Ideally prolactin levels should not be determined directly after a breast examination, sexual activity, or exercise session. Diagnostic tests that may be indicated include prolactin levels, microscopic analysis of the discharge, a thyroid profile, a pregnancy test, and a mammogram.

Mammary Duct Ectasia

Mammary duct ectasia is an inflammation of the ducts behind the nipple. The cause of mammary duct ectasia is unknown. It occurs most often in perimenopausal women and is characterized by a nipple discharge that is thick, sticky, and white, brown, green, or purple. Often the woman will experience a burning pain, itching, or a palpable mass behind the nipple.

The diagnostic workup includes a mammogram and aspiration and culture of fluid. Duct ectasia is usually self-limiting, requiring only reassurance of the woman. An infection in the inflamed area can occur and requires antibiotic therapy. Incision and drainage is necessary if an abscess develops. Treatment also may include a local excision of the affected duct(s) if the woman has no future plans to breastfeed.

Intraductal Papilloma

Intraductal papilloma is a rare benign condition that develops in the terminal nipple ducts. The cause is unknown. It usually occurs in women between 30 and 50 years of age. Usually too small to be palpated (less than 0.5 cm), this papilloma causes serous, serosanguineous, or bloody nipple discharge. The discharge is unilateral and spontaneous. After the possibility of malignancy is eliminated, the affected segments of the ducts and breasts are surgically excised.

Table 6-4 compares common manifestations of benign breast masses.

Care Management

Assessment should include a careful history and physical examination. The history should focus on risk factors for breast diseases, events related to the breast mass, and health-maintenance practices. Risk factors for breast cancer are discussed later in this chapter. Information related to the breast mass should include how, when, and by whom the mass was discovered. The nurse should document the following patient information: pain, whether symptoms increase with menses, dietary habits, smoking habits, and the use of oral contraceptives. The woman's emotional status, including her stress level, fears, and concerns, and her ability to cope should also be assessed.

Physical examination may include assessment of the breasts for symmetry, masses (size, number, consistency, and mobility), and nipple discharge.

Nursing actions might include the following:

- Discuss the intervals for and facets of breast screening, including professional examination and mammography. Women with breast implants may need special views of the breast and precautions taken to avoid rupture of the implant during mammography.
- Provide written educational materials in the woman's primary language.
- Encourage expression of fears and concerns about treatment and prognosis.
- Provide specific information regarding the woman's condition and treatment, including dietary changes, medication therapy, comfort measures, stress management, and surgery.
- Describe pain-relieving strategies in detail and collaborate with the primary health care provider to ensure effective pain control.
- Encourage discussion of feelings about body image.

Malignant Conditions of the Breast

Mortality rates from breast cancer have declined since 1990. Nonetheless, 1 in 9 Canadian women will develop breast cancer in her lifetime, and 1 out of every 25 is expected to die from it (CCS, 2010).

Etiology

Although the exact cause of breast cancer continues to elude investigators, certain factors that increase a women's risk for developing a malignancy have been identified. These factors are listed in Box 6-8.

The most important predictor of risk for breast cancer is age; a woman's risk increases as her age increases. Most of the other risk factors involve the effects of the menstrual–reproductive cycle (probably the effect of estrogen or progesterone) on the development of breast cancer. Fewer menstrual cycles and early childbearing appear to have a protective effect. Although most breast cancers are not related to genetic factors, the identification of the *BRCA1* and *BRCA2* genes demonstrated the role of **heredity** and genetic **mutations** in this disease. Only about 5 to 10% of breast cancers are caused by a specific inherited mutation that confers a high risk of developing breast cancer.

Ethical Considerations of Genetic Testing

Although knowing whether one is hereditarily predisposed to breast cancer may have benefits, the extent to which an individual can benefit from this information remains unclear. Confirming one's mutation status may provide a sense of control in life plans or it may create high levels of anxiety

Table 6-4 Comparison of Common Manifestations of Benign Breast Masses

FIBROCYSTIC CHANGES	FIBROADENOMA	LIPOMA	INTRADUCTAL PAPILLOMA	MAMMARY DUCT ECTASIA
Multiple lumps	Single lump	Single lump	Single or multiple	Mass behind nipple
Nodular	Well delineated	Well delineated	Not well delineated	Not well delineated
Palpable	Palpable	Palpable	Nonpalpable	Palpable
Movable	Movable	Movable	Nonmobile	Nonmobile
Round, smooth	Round, lobular	Round, lobular	Small, ball-like	Irregular
Firm or soft	Firm	Soft	Firm or soft	Firm
Tenderness influenced by menstrual cycle	Usually asymptomatic	Nontender	Usually nontender	Painful, burning, itching
Bilateral	Unilateral	Unilateral	Unilateral	Unilateral
May or may not have nipple discharge	No nipple discharge	No nipple discharge	Serous or bloody nipple discharge	Thick, sticky nipple discharge

BOX 6-8 Risk Factors for Breast Cancer*

- Age
- Previous history of breast cancer
- Family history of breast cancer, especially a mother or sister or daughter diagnosed before menopause or if mutations on *BRCA1* or *BRCA2* genes are present
- Previous history of ovarian, endometrial, colon, or thyroid cancer
- Family history of ovarian cancer
- Early menarche (before age 12 years)
- Late menopause (after age 55 years)
- Nulliparity or first pregnancy after age 30 years
- Use of estrogen plus progestin replacement therapy
- Daily alcohol use
- Obesity after menopause
- Previous history of benign breast disease with epithelial hyperplasia or dense breast tissue
- Radiation treatment to the chest area (for example, to treat Hodgkin lymphona), especially before age 30
- Race (White women have the highest incidence)
- High socioeconomic status
- Sedentary lifestyle
- History of birth control use

(Source: Canadian Cancer Society [2010]. *Causes of breast cancer*. Retrieved from http://www.cancer.ca/Canadawide/About%20cancer/Types%20of%20cancer/Causes%20of%20breast%20cancer.aspx?sc_lang=en.)

*Risk factors are cumulative (i.e., the more risk factors present, the greater the likelihood of breast cancer occurring).

and distress. Genetic testing can alter decisions regarding family and intimate relationships, childbearing, body image, and quality of life. Regardless of whether results are positive or negative for *BRCA1* and *BRCA2* mutations, the results can have a highly negative impact on women's lives. Women at increased risk for breast cancer need comprehensive information about the benefits and limitations of genetic testing to ensure that informed decisions about genetic testing can be made. Because decisions regarding genetic testing, genetic counselling, and breast cancer risk assessment are highly individualized, health care providers should be careful in making any generalizations about women at risk for breast cancer.

Some known and suspected environmental risk factors include exposure to organochlorine pesticides and other synthetic chemicals, hormonal factors (both exogenous and endogenous), diet, tobacco and alcohol use, radiation, and magnetic fields. However, definitive links between these factors and breast cancer have not been established.

Clinical outcomes of the Women's Health Initiative randomized controlled trial to assess the risks and benefits of estrogen and progestin in healthy postmenopausal women were released in May 2002. The safety monitoring board recommended that the trial be stopped because the overall health risks exceeded the benefits. These risks included 290 cases of breast cancer in the study group of about 8500 women (Writing Group for the Women's Health Initiative Investigators, 2002). Further evidence indicated that combined estrogen and progestin increased the risk of breast cancer as well as the risk of heart disease, stroke, blood clots, and urinary incontinence more than estrogen alone among healthy users (National Cancer Institute [NCI], 2007).

Women considering HRT should be cautious and consult with their health care providers to determine their suitability for it. Maintaining a normal weight, eating a diet rich in fruits and vegetables and low in fat, limiting intake of alcohol, not smoking, and getting regular exercise seem to exert a protective effect against the development of breast cancer (NCI, 2007).

Information about breast cancer risks can be confusing, and women can overestimate or underestimate their risks. The Breast Cancer Risk Assessment Tool can be used by women and health professionals to calculate risk. This tool was developed and verified by the National Cancer Institute (NCI) to predict the risk of breast cancer in 5 years and over the lifetime (to age 90 years) of a woman. The tool is available on the Internet at the NCI Web site (http://www.cancer.gov/bcrisktool/).

An accurate estimation of risk for breast cancer is needed so that women may be given rational management recommendations. During breast cancer risk counselling, facts should be presented to women by their health care provider in a supportive, nondirective way, without personal opinions or preferences. Discussion should also include treatment options and prognosis of breast cancer, as well as risks and benefits of alternative methods of prevention and early diagnosis. A woman's recognition of having increased breast cancer risk can carry psychological consequences such as anxiety, guilt, depression, and reduced **self-esteem**. Enormous guilt may be experienced by high-risk women who pass specific genetic mutations on to their children. Psychological intervention should be considered to assist individuals in coping with these significant adverse sequelae (Sakorafas, 2003).

Chemoprevention

Researchers from the NCI and other groups have investigated the role of tamoxifen and raloxifene, both of which protect bone health, in the prevention of breast cancer (NCI, 2006). Both tamoxifen and raloxifene reduce by 50% the risk of invasive breast cancer in postmenopausal women who are at risk for the disease. Raloxifene may be an ideal choice for the woman at high risk for both osteoporosis and breast cancer. Tamoxifen also reduces the recurrence of breast cancer in women with prior breast malignancies. Patients should be made aware of the risk of occasional serious adverse effects before taking tamoxifen (NCI, 2006) (see later discussion).

Pathophysiology

Breast cancer occurs when there are genetic alterations in the DNA of breast epithelial cells. Many types of breast cancer exist. Genetic alterations, either inherited or spontaneous, are found in the epithelial cells, compromising ductal or lobular tissue. Researchers are investigating which oncogenes (potentially cancer-inducing genes) may cause breast cancer or change its growth pattern and how the process can be stopped.

Breast cancer begins in the epithelial cells lining the mammary ducts of the breast. The rate of breast cancer growth depends on the effect of estrogen and progesterone. These cancers can be either invasive (infiltrating) or noninvasive (in situ). Invasive or infiltrating breast cancers can grow into the wall of the mammary duct and into the surrounding tissues. The most frequently occurring cancer of the breast is invasive ductal carcinoma. Ductal carcinoma originates in the lactiferous ducts and invades surrounding breast structures. The tumour is usually unilateral, not well delineated, solid, nonmobile, and nontender. Lobular carcinoma originates in the lobules of the breasts. It is usually bilateral and nonpalpable. Nipple carcinoma (Paget's disease) originates in the nipple. It usually occurs with invasive ductal carcinoma and can cause bleeding, oozing, and crusting of the nipple.

Breast cancer can invade surrounding tissues in such a way that the primary tumour has tentacle-like projections. This invasive growth pattern can result in the irregular tumour border felt on palpation. As the tumour grows, fibrosis develops around it and can shorten Cooper's ligaments. When Cooper's ligaments are shortened, the result is the characteristic **peau d'orange** (orange peel–like) skin changes and edema associated with some breast cancers. If the breast cancer invades the lymphatic channels, tumours can develop in the regional lymph nodes, often occupying the axillary lymph nodes. The tumour may invade the outer layers of skin, creating ulcerations.

Metastasis results from seeding of the breast cancer cells into the blood and lymph systems, leading to tumour development in the bones, lungs, brain, and liver.

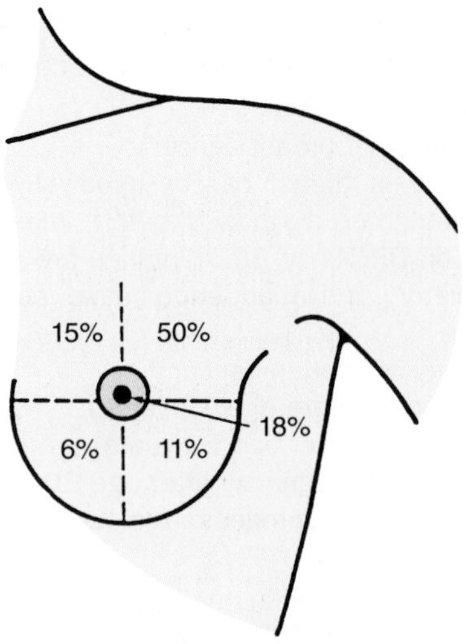

Fig. 6-6 Relative location of malignant lesions of the breast.

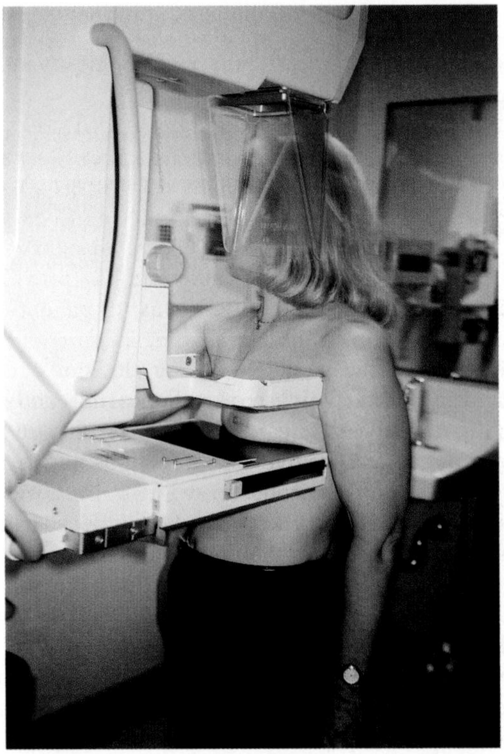

Fig. 6-7 Mammography. *(Courtesy Shannon Perry, Phoenix, AZ.)*

Clinical Manifestations and Diagnosis

Breast cancer in its earliest form can be detected on a mammogram before it can be felt by the woman or her health care provider. However, approximately 90% of all breast lumps are detected by the woman. Of these, only 20 to 25% are malignant. It is important that women know what is normal for their own breasts by examining them periodically. While routine breast self examination (BSE) is not recommended, for women who would like to perform BSE, the method is provided on p. 69 (see Chapter 5), More than half of all lumps are discovered in the upper outer quadrant of the breast (Fig. 6-6). The most common initial sign is a lump or thickening of the breast. The lump may feel hard and fixed or soft and spongy. It may have well-defined or irregular borders. It may be fixed to the skin, thereby causing dimpling to occur. A bloody or clear unilateral nipple discharge may be present.

Unilateral and spontaneous discharge (without nipple manipulation) is associated with mastitis, intraductal papilloma, and cancer. The discharge is usually intermittent and persistent and may be clear, serous, green-grey, purulent, serosanguineous, or sanguineous. Women with these findings need a complete diagnostic workup to determine the actual cause of their signs.

As a general principle, any unilateral breast sign or symptom (i.e., mass, discharge, pain, or itching) is a more ominous finding than a bilateral sign or symptom. However, all findings should be carefully followed up to avoid missing a serious diagnosis such as cancer. Any delay in treatment can adversely affect the woman's subsequent prognosis and treatment options.

Early detection and diagnosis reduce the mortality rate because the cancer is found when it is smaller, lesions are more localized, and there tends to be a lower percentage of positive nodes. Therefore, it is imperative that protocols for assessment and diagnosis be established. Regular clinical examination by a qualified health care provider and screening mammography (X-ray filming of the breast) (Fig. 6-7) can aid in the early detection of breast cancers. Table 6-5 lists the current recommendations of the Canadian Cancer Society for breast cancer screening.

Table 6-5 Screening Guidelines for Breast Cancer: Detection in Asymptomatic Women Recommended by the Canadian Cancer Society

AGE (YEARS)	EXAMINATION	FREQUENCY
40–49	Clinical breast examination by a trained health care provider. Talk to doctor about risk of breast cancer, along with the benefits and risks of mammography	Every 2 years
50–69	Clinical breast examination by a trained health care provider.	At least every 2 years
	Mammography	Every 2 years
70 or older	Talk to doctor about how often testing should be done	

(Source: Canadian Cancer Society [2010]. *Breast cancer.* Retrieved from http://www.cancer.ca/Canada-wide/Prevention/Getting%20checked/Breast%20cancer%20NEW.aspx?sc_lang=en)

Note: Screening mammography and clinical breast examinations are the most reliable methods of finding breast cancer.

Major obstacles to breast cancer screening include older age; knowledge, attitudinal, and behavioural barriers (e.g., fear, ignorance, lack of motivation); and organizational barriers (e.g., scheduling problems, lack of availability of mammography services, lack of physician referral). Strategies that may be helpful to health care providers in improving screening for breast cancer include related education and encouragement of older women; continuing education of providers; use of reminder systems in office practice; use of patient-directed literature; and interventions that reward, support, and prompt desired screening behaviours.

Cultural factors may influence a woman's decision to participate in breast cancer screening. Knowledge of these factors and use of culturally sensitive tailored messages and materials that appeal to the unique concerns, beliefs, and reading abilities of identified groups of women who do not participate in breast screening may assist the nurse in helping women overcome barriers to seeking care (see Cultural Awareness box).

A variety of technologies are used in breast cancer screening (Box 6-9).

When a suspicious finding on a mammogram is noted or when a lump is detected, diagnosis is confirmed by means of FNA, core needle biopsy, or needle localization biopsy. Needle localization biopsy requires the collaborative efforts of the radiologist and the surgeon. This often requires that the procedure take place in two different settings (radiology and surgery). Patients need specific information about the procedures, duration, and possible outcomes.

Cytological analysis of cells from aspirated breast tissue is extremely useful as an adjunct to the clinical evaluation of a palpable mass. If the mass resolves after aspiration, malignancy is unlikely. However, if the mass remains after aspiration, it should be biopsied because there is a greater chance of cancer being present.

Laboratory diagnosis of breast cancer and possible cancer metastasis includes complete blood count, liver enzyme levels, serum calcium level, and alkaline phosphatase level. Elevated liver enzyme levels indicate possible liver metastasis, and increased serum calcium and alkaline phosphatase levels may indicate bone metastasis.

CULTURAL AWARENESS

Breast Screening Practices

Certain minority women tend to have low compliance rates in the use of early screening methods for breast cancer. Many factors play a role in influencing the screening practices of these women. Asian women cited unawareness of mammography tests, gender and modesty concerns unique to their cultural beliefs, and fear resulting from a sense of vulnerability to breast cancer.

Interventions that will encourage minority women to participate in early breast cancer screening practices begin with the development of culturally sensitive community education programs designed to help women overcome barriers to reaching optimal levels of health. Programs should be designed to educate small groups of woman about risk factors of breast cancer, prevention strategies, and early detection methods. Recruitment of women may be communicated through fliers in neighborhoods, women's groups, churches, clubs, and organizations. Use of incentives to reward participation may be helpful. Nurses and guest speakers of similar ethnicity to that of the attending group who are breast cancer survivors would be valuable in providing meaningful information and support and past, present, and future perspectives to the educational content.

(Source: Office of Minority Health, U.S. Department of Health and Human Services, Office of Public Health and Science. [2009]. *Breast cancer. A resource guide for minority women.* Retrieved from http://minorityhealth.hhs.gov/assets/pdf/checked/1/Breast_Cancer_2009.pdf.)

BOX 6-9 Technologies for Breast Cancer Screening

Screen-film mammography—Gold standard for breast cancer screening

Full-field digital mammography—Identifies breast cancers missed by screen-film mammography

Computer-aided detection and diagnosis (CAD)—Digitizes screen-film mammograms and analyzes them for abnormalities

Ultrasound—Valuable adjunct to mammography; helpful in distinguishing between fluid-filled and solid masses; useful in performing image-guided biopsies

Magnetic resonance imaging (MRI)—Screening adjunct to mammography and ultrasound

evolve Case Study—Breast Cancer

Prognosis

Major advances in understanding the biology of cancer have occurred in the past 10 years. Many studies support the theory that breast cancer is a systemic disease; micrometastasis could be present at the initial presentation with or without nodal involvement. The area in which affected lymph nodes are located is also prognostic. The involvement of axillary lymph nodes worsens the prognosis of breast cancer. However, nodal involvement and tumour size remain the most significant prognostic criteria for long-term survival (Fig. 6-8).

Other biological factors that are helpful in predicting response to therapy or survival include estrogen receptor assay, progesterone receptor assay, tumour ploidy (the amount of DNA in a tumour cell compared with that in a normal cell), S-phase index or growth rate (the percentage of cells in the S phase of cellular division, calculated by flow cytometric determinations of the S-phase fraction), and histological or nuclear grade. Estrogen and progesterone receptors are proteins in the cell cytoplasm and surface of some breast cancer cells. When these receptors are present, they bind to estrogen or progesterone, and binding promotes growth of the cancer cell. A breast cancer can have estrogen receptors (ERs), progesterone receptors (PRs), or both types. Knowledge of the ER status of the cancer is valuable in predicting which patients will respond to HRT.

Human epidermal growth factor receptor 2 (HER2), which is associated with cell growth, is overexpressed in 30% of all breast cancers and is associated with loss of cell regulation and uncontrolled cell proliferation. Thus, a positive HER2 status is associated with aggressive tumours, poor prognosis, and resistance to some chemotherapeutic drugs.

Medical Management

Medical management of breast cancer includes surgery, breast reconstruction, radiation therapy, adjuvant hormone therapy, and chemotherapy.

Surgery

The most frequently recommended surgical approaches are lumpectomy and modified radical mastectomy (Fig. 6-9). Breast conserving surgery known as a lumpectomy involves the removal of the breast tumour, a small amount of surrounding tissue, and a sampling of axillary lymph nodes, leaving the pectoralis major muscle intact. Lumpectomy offers survival equivalent to that with modified radical mastectomy.

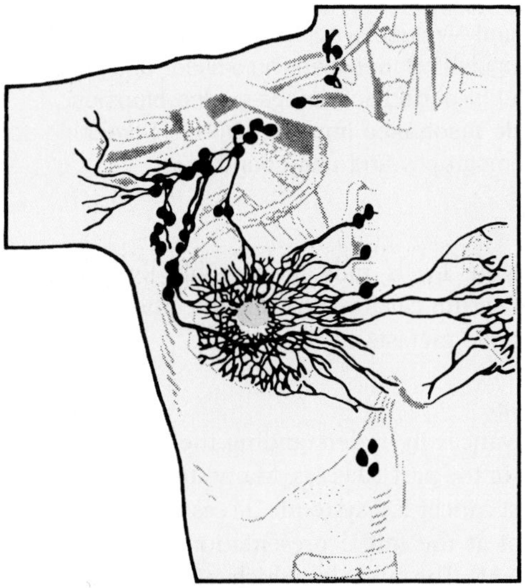

Fig. 6-8 Lymphatic spread of breast cancer.

Total mastectomy (see Fig. 6-9, A) (also called simple mastectomy) is the removal of all breast tissue, nipple, and areola; the axillary nodes and pectoral muscles are not removed. Modified radical mastectomy (see Fig. 6-9, B) is the removal of the entire breast and a sample of axillary lymph nodes, sparing the pectoral muscles. A radical mastectomy (see Fig. 6-9, C), although rarely performed, removes the entire breast, axillary nodes, and the pectoral muscles. The type of surgery that is done depends on the size of the tumour and its location.

Mastectomy is used for the treatment of early-stage breast cancer when (1) there are multiple tumours in different parts of the breast, (2) tumour removal alone would produce a cosmetically unacceptable result, (3) the breast had been radiated previously, (4) the woman is in the first or second trimester of pregnancy, (5) there are persistent positive margins after reasonable surgery, and (6) there is a possible history of collagen-vascular disease. Women who are found to have metastatic breast cancer at the time of diagnosis usually do not have a mastectomy because it does not offer increased chances of survival.

Axillary dissection is performed as a standard part of breast cancer treatment to obtain prognostic information and maintain local control in the axilla, and it is helpful in determining the need for adjunctive systemic treatment by indicating whether nodes are positive for metastatic cells. Lymphatic mapping and sentinel node biopsy is a minimally invasive technique that identifies women with axillary node involvement. The sentinel node is the first node that receives lymphatic drainage from the tumour and is identified by injecting vital blue dye or radioactive dye in the area surrounding the tumour. A small incision in the axilla allows for identification of the blue-stained lymphatic channel leading to the blue sentinel node, either visually or by gamma probe. This node then can be removed and examined for the presence of tumour cells, instead of performing an entire axillary dissection. Clinical trials have reported identification of the sentinel node in more than 95% of cases, with false-negative rates for predicting axillary nodal metastases of less than 5%.

Women who have these surgeries experience cosmetic changes. Change in shape (because of lumpectomy) or loss of a breast results in a change in body image, which can cause significant alterations in perceptions of femininity and in sexual image and interest.

Breast Reconstruction

The goals of surgical breast reconstruction are achievement of symmetry and preservation of body image. Surgical reconstruction can be done immediately or at a later date. Immediate reconstruction at the time of mastectomy does not change survival rates or interfere with therapy or the treatment of recurrent disease. Women choose surgical reconstruction for the following reasons: the need to feel complete again, to avoid using an external prosthesis, to achieve symmetry, to decrease self-consciousness about appearance, and to enhance femininity.

Autologous flap reconstruction involves the use of the woman's own tissue to create a breast. Types of autologous flaps are the latissimus dorsi flap, the transverse rectus abdominis myocutaneous (TRAM) flap, and the deep interior

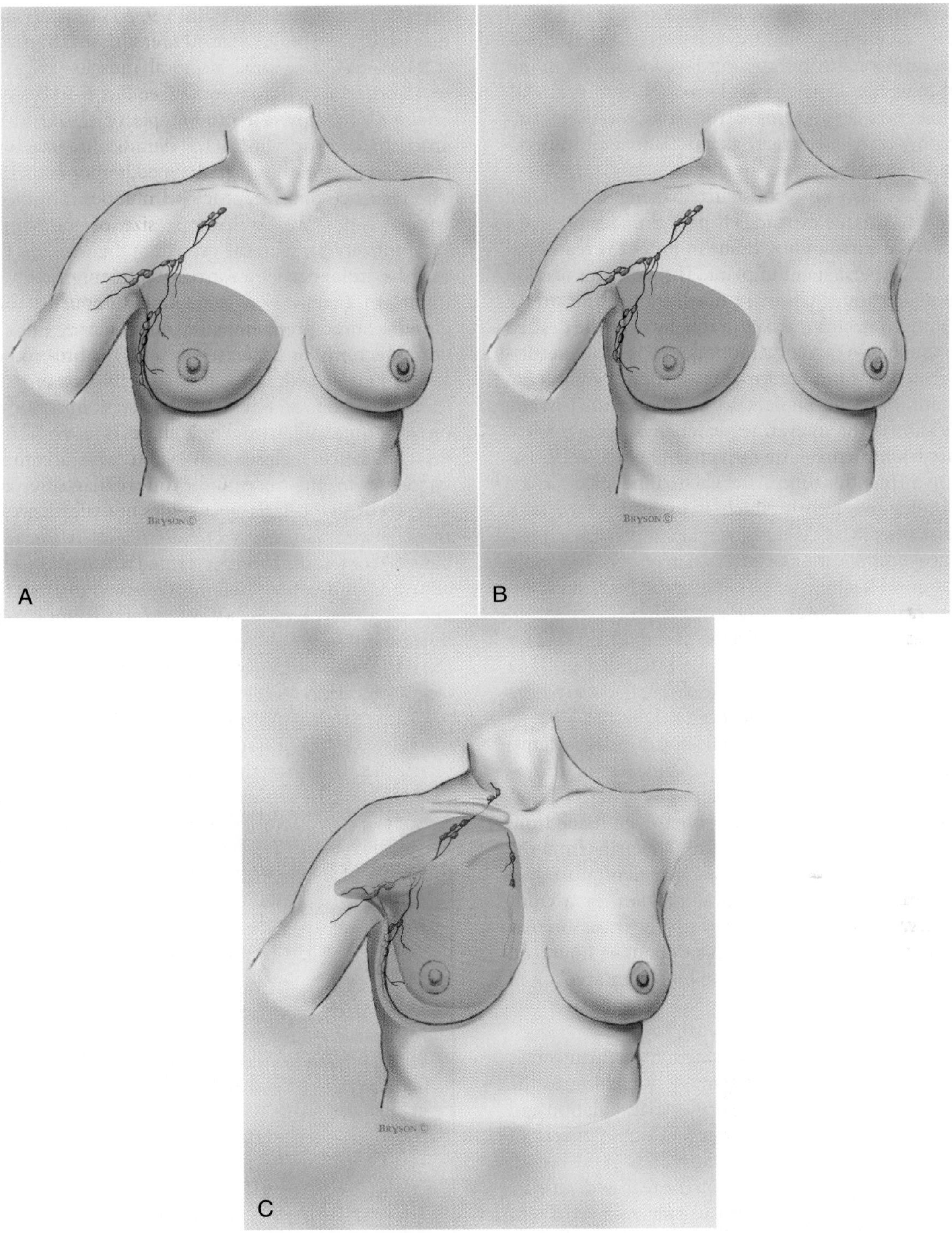

Fig. 6-9 Surgical alternatives for breast cancer. Pink highlighted area indicates tissue removed at mastectomy. **A**: Total (simple) mastectomy. **B**: Modified radical mastectomy. **C**: Radical mastectomy. *(Courtesy of http://www.breastcancer.org/treatment/surgery/mastectomy/what_is.jsp.)*

epigastric perforator flap. The latissimus dorsi and TRAM flaps are most common. After the reconstruction is done, postoperative care specific to the procedure focuses on monitoring of the skin flap for signs of decreased capillary refill, hematoma, infection, and necrosis. This is followed by standard mastectomy activity restrictions and patient education.

Breast Implants

The breast may also be reconstructed using saline-filled tissue expanders. A tissue expander is placed under the chest tissue to stretch the surrounding tissue in order to create adequate space for the permanent implant. Through an injection port, the tissue expander is slowly filled with saline over a period of months to stretch the skin gradually until the desired symmetry is attained. Ongoing emotional support is needed for women who choose this option because they often become impatient waiting for the implant to be totally filled or are self-conscious about the uneven appearance of their breasts. Use of cotton padding to equalize the appearance of the breasts may be helpful during this time. After each saline injection the woman has mild discomfort, which is easily relieved with ibuprofen or naproxen. As with all implantation procedures, risks of surgical complications such as hematoma, infection, and delayed wound healing are possible, as are capsular contractions from or leakage of the implant.

In 2006, Health Canada approved the use of silicone gel for implants (Health Canada, 2006). Women interested in these implants should be informed of all associated risks before making a decision to undergo the procedure.

After the woman has recovered from initial reconstructive surgery, she may choose to have nipple and areolar reconstruction. Nipple reconstruction is achieved by using an autologous skin graft to construct a nipple, either from tissue from the remaining nipple or from a donor site. Tiny flaps from the new breast itself also may be used. This outpatient procedure requires local anaesthesia, intravenous sedation, or a combination of both, depending on how much sensation has returned to the breast. The procedure lasts about an hour, and 4 weeks later tattooing may be used to create an areola and match the colour of the natural nipple.

Radiation

The standard therapy for early-stage breast cancer is lumpectomy followed by radiation therapy. Radiation to the breast destroys tumour cells remaining after manipulation and handling of the tumour during surgery. Adverse effects of radiation therapy include swelling and heaviness in the breast, sunburn-like skin changes in the treated area, and fatigue. Changes to the breast tissue and skin usually resolve in 6 to 12 months. Radiation therapy in the area of the axilla can cause lymphedema of the ipsilateral arm. Close medical follow-up is important after conservative surgery and radiation, and should be adjusted according to individual need (Grunfeld, Dhesy-Thind, & Levine, 2005).

Adjuvant Therapy

Chemotherapy administered soon after initial diagnosis and surgical removal of the tumour is referred to as *adjuvant chemotherapy*. Adjuvant chemotherapy (chemotherapy and endocrine therapy) is used to either eradicate or impede the growth of micrometastatic (microscopic cell metastasis) disease. Adjuvant chemotherapy significantly reduces the risks for recurrence and mortality in patients with node-positive disease.

Hormone Therapy

In order to determine whether a woman is a candidate for hormone therapy, a receptor assay is performed. After the entire tumour or a portion is removed by biopsy or excision, cancer cells are examined by a pathologist for ERs and PRs. The presence of a receptor on the cell wall indicates that the woman is positive for that type of hormone receptor. If these receptors are present, the growth of the woman's breast cancer may be influenced by estrogen, progesterone, or both. It is unknown exactly how these hormones affect breast cancer growth. Some premenopausal women may undergo bilateral oophorectomy to decrease the supply of hormones available for tumour growth.

Tamoxifen is an oral anti-estrogen medication that mimics progesterone and estrogen. It attaches to the hormone receptors on cancer cells and prevents natural hormones from attaching to the receptors. When tamoxifen fits into the receptors, the cell is unable to grow. Adjuvant hormone therapy with tamoxifen is recommended for all postmenopausal women with breast cancer. In this group of women, adjuvant tamoxifen therapy improves disease-free survival and, in some cases, length of survival. Women treated with hormone therapy should receive therapy for at least 5 years (National Comprehensive Cancer Network [NCCN], 2010). (see Medication Guide).

MEDICATION GUIDE

Tamoxifen (Nolvadex, Tamofen)

Action

Anti-estrogenic effects; attaches to hormone receptors on cancer cells and prevents natural hormones from attaching to the receptors

Indications

For treatment of metastatic breast cancer, treatment of breast cancer in postmenopausal women after breast cancer surgery and radiation therapy, to reduce the incidence of breast cancer in women at high risk

Dosage

20 to 40 mg orally daily. Dosages greater than 20 mg should be given in divided doses (AM and PM).

Adverse Reactions

Common side effects include hot flashes, nausea, vomiting, vaginal bleeding or discharge, menstrual irregularities, and rash. Hair loss is an uncommon effect. Serious side effects include deep vein thrombosis, increased risk of endometrial cancer, and stroke.

Nursing Considerations

The medication may be taken on an empty stomach or with food. Missed doses should be taken as soon as possible, but taking two doses at once is not recommended. A barrier or nonhormonal form of contraception is recommended in premenopausal women because tamoxifen may be harmful to the fetus.

Raloxifene is an oral selective ER modulator. It is used to prevent osteoporosis in postmenopausal women. Raloxifene works as well as tamoxifen in reducing breast cancer risk in women with a high risk for breast cancer. There is less risk of thromboembolic events, uterine cancer, and cataracts in women who take raloxifene than in those who take tamoxifen (see Medication Guide).

Aromatase inhibitors markedly suppress plasma estrogen levels in postmenopausal women by inhibiting or inactivating aromatase, the enzyme responsible for synthesizing estrogens from androgenic substrates. Aromatase inhibitors such as anastrozole, letrozole, and exemestane have been shown to be effective agents in hormone therapy for breast cancer. Clinical trials have indicated that letrozole is better than tamoxifen in treating advanced disease in postmenopausal women and that anastrozole is at least as good. In early-stage breast cancer, adjuvant therapy with anastrozole appears to be superior to adjuvant therapy with tamoxifen in reducing recurrence in postmenopausal women. The aromatase inhibitors appear to be well tolerated, with a lower incidence of adverse effects than that for tamoxifen. The adverse effects of aromatase inhibitors include hot flashes, vaginal dryness, musculoskeletal pain, and headache.

Chemotherapy

Chemotherapy with multiple drug combinations is used in the treatment of recurrent and advanced breast cancer, with positive results. Combination regimens and sequential single agents may be used (NCCN, 2010). Some chemotherapeutic drugs provide additional treatment options for women with metastatic breast cancer.

Because chemotherapy drugs are designed to kill rapidly reproducing cells, normal body cells that rapidly reproduce (red and white blood cells, gastric mucosa, and hair) also can be affected during treatment. Thus chemotherapy can cause leukopenia, neutropenia, thrombocytopenia, anemia, gastrointestinal side effects (nausea, vomiting, anorexia, mucositis), and partial or full hair loss.

Chemotherapy treatments are usually given in ambulatory care settings once or twice per month. During the **informed consent** process, before the treatment is selected, the woman and her family members should be educated about the names of the medications, routes of administration, treatment schedule, timing and ordering of medications, length of time of administration, reimbursed and unreimbursed costs of therapy, potential adverse effects, management of adverse effects, possible changes in body image (e.g., full or partial hair loss), recovery time after treatment (necessitating lost work time), and need for a caregiver to transport the woman to treatment and care for her afterward.

Depending on the medications used, the treatments may include intravenous, subcutaneous, and oral medications. Often a long-term central venous catheter is inserted when the women will be receiving chemotherapy for an extended period or when she will receive medications that may damage the vein. Presence of a central venous catheter, hair loss, loss of part or all of her breast, menopause, and possible infertility all have the potential to cause a change in body image and to increase emotional distress for the woman with breast cancer.

Breast cancer treatment often causes changes in reproductive function. The postmenopausal woman may have to cope with hair loss and other unpleasant adverse effects from chemotherapy as well as loss of part or all of her breast. The premenopausal woman may experience these changes along with symptoms of menopause and possible infertility. The young woman with breast cancer may become devastated by an early and abrupt menopause and the possibility of jeopardized reproductive function. These factors can seriously affect the young woman's quality of life.

Chemotherapy drugs are mutagenic and teratogenic. Any woman who is of childbearing age and receiving chemotherapy, even though no longer menstruating, must use a contraceptive. Birth control pills are not recommended because they contain hormones that may assist in the growth of cancer. A contraceptive method can be chosen with the assistance of the gynecologist and the medical oncologist, and it must be used before chemotherapy begins and continue to be used until the medical oncologist and gynecologist believe it is safe to discontinue use.

With the advance in monoclonal antibody technology, it is now possible to test for residual disease with a serum tumour marker, CA 15-3, if it is secreted by the patient's tumour. From 75 to 80% of women with breast cancer secrete this tumour marker. If the level of CA 15-3 is elevated at the time of diagnosis, circulating levels of CA 15-3 can be checked periodically through the treatment course to measure response. This technology is used to determine effectiveness

MEDICATION GUIDE

Raloxifene Hydrochloride (Evista)

Action

A selective estrogen receptor modulator, serving as an agonist and antagonist to estrogen receptor sites

Indications

Treatment and prevention of osteoporosis, reduction in the risk of invasive breast cancer in postmenopausal women with osteoporosis, reduction of risk of invasive breast cancer in postmenopausal women at high risk for invasive breast cancer

Dosage

60 mg orally daily

Adverse Reactions

Common adverse effects include hot flashes, nausea, vomiting, peripheral edema arthralgia, and sweating. Serious and life-threatening adverse effects can occur from the existing condition. Raloxifene is contraindicated in women with an active or past history of venous thromboembolism.

Nursing Considerations

The medication may be taken on an empty stomach or with food. Missed doses should be taken as soon as possible, but taking two doses at once is not recommended. Counsel the woman to contact her primary health care provider if leg pain or a feeling of warmth in the lower legs, swelling of the hands and feet, sudden chest pain or shortness of breath, or sudden changes in vision occur. Calcium, 1500 mg plus vitamin D 400 to 800 units daily, is recommended.

of therapy for cancer without the need for second-look diagnostic surgery.

Care Management

Before surgery, women need to be assessed for psychological preparation and specific teaching needs. General preoperative teaching and care are given, including expectations regarding physical appearance, pain management, equipment to be used (e.g., intravenous therapy, drains), and emotional support. The emotional reaction to the diagnosis of cancer is always intense, and the many disruptions caused by the disease challenge the woman's and family's ability to cope. A visit from a woman who has had a similar experience may be beneficial both before and after surgery. The woman should be reminded that when she awakens after surgery, her arm on the affected side will feel tight.

Postoperative nursing care focuses on recovery. After recovery from anesthesia, the woman is returned to her room. Special precautions must be observed to prevent or minimize lymphedema of the affected arm.

NURSING ALERT When vital signs are taken, never apply the blood pressure cuff on the affected arm.

The affected arm is elevated with pillows above the level of the right atrium. Blood is not drawn from this arm, and it is not used for intravenous therapy. Early arm movement should be encouraged. Any increase in the circumference of that arm needs to be reported immediately.

Nursing care of the wound involves observation for signs of hemorrhage (dressing, drainage tubes, and Hemovac or Jackson-Pratt drainage reservoirs are emptied at least every 8 hours and more frequently as needed), shock, and infection. Dressings are reinforced as necessary. The woman is asked to turn (alternating between unaffected side and back), cough (while the nurse or the woman applies support to the chest), and deep breathe every 2 hours. Breath sounds are auscultated every 4 hours. Active range-of-motion exercise of legs should be encouraged. Parenteral fluids need to be given until adequate oral intake is possible. Emotional support should be continued.

The woman is given self-management instructions and usually discharged to home after 24 hours or more, depending on the type of procedure done (see Home Care box). Lumpectomy is an outpatient procedure, and the patient usually returns home a few hours after surgery. A woman is discharged 24 to 48 hours after modified radical mastectomy. A referral for home nursing care can be made if the woman needs assistance caring for her incision. Through CancerConnection, a breast cancer survivor who has been trained in how to offer information can offer telephone support (see Community Focus box). The resources offered may include a list of sources for prostheses and lingerie. The woman should be encouraged to do arm exercises at least twice a day (see Patient Teaching box).

Exercise is increased as tolerated and stopped at the point of pain. Initially the woman will alternately clench and extend her fingers and then progress to wrist and elbow exercises, gradually abducting her arm and raising it to and over her head. She should be encouraged to exercise through assistance

HOME CARE

After a Mastectomy

- Wash your hands well before and after touching the incision area or drains.
- Empty surgical drains twice a day and as needed, recording the date, time, drain site (if more than one drain is present), and amount of drainage in millilitres in a diary you will take to each surgical checkup until your drains are removed. (Before discharge you may receive a graduated container for emptying drains and measuring drainage.)
- Avoid driving, lifting more than 5 kg, or reaching above your head until given permission by your surgeon.
- Take medications for pain as soon as pain begins.
- Perform arm exercises as directed.
- Call your physician if inflammation of the incision or swelling of the incision or the arm occurs.
- Avoid tight clothing, tight jewellery, and other causes of decreased circulation in the affected arm.
- Until drains are removed, wear loose-fitting underwear (camisole or half-slip) and clothes, pinning surgical drains inside clothing. (You will be taught how to do this safely.)
- After drains are removed and surgical sites are healing and still tender, wear a mastectomy bra or camisole with a cotton-filled, muslin temporary prosthesis. Temporary prostheses of this type are often available through the Canadian Cancer Society.
- Avoid depilatory creams; strong deodorants; and shaving of the affected chest area, axilla, and arm.
- Sponge bathe until drains are removed.
- Return to the surgeon's office for incision check, drain inspection, and possible drain removal as directed.
- Contact the Canadian Cancer Society for assistance in obtaining an external prosthesis and lingerie when dressings, drains, and staples are removed and wound is healing and nontender.
- Contact your insurance company for information about coverage of the prosthesis and wig, if needed. Obtain prescriptions for a prosthesis and wig to submit with receipts of purchase for these items to the insurance company. If insurance does not pay for these items, contact the hospital or agency social worker or provincial Cancer Society for assistance.
- Encourage your mother, sisters, and daughters (if applicable) to have annual professional breast examinations and mammography (if appropriate).
- Keep follow-up visits for professional examination, a mammogram, and testing to detect recurrent breast cancer.
- Expect decreased sensation and tingling at incision sites and in the affected arm for weeks to months after surgery.
- Resume sexual activities as desired.

COMMUNITY FOCUS

Canadian Cancer Society

Check the Internet for the Canadian Cancer Society's Web site (http://www.cancer.ca) for their peer supports and services. Identify the services provided by the program and the requirements to become a volunteer. Visit the women's clinic in a local community health agency. Are materials about the different programs visible in the waiting areas? Talk to one of the nurses who work in the clinic (make an appointment for this conversation). What does she know about CancerConnection? Does she refer her patients to this program? What is her evaluation of the program? Has she met any of the volunteers? Do her patients have positive things to say about the program?

with her care—washing her face, brushing her teeth, and eating with her hand and arm on the affected side. Physiotherapy may be prescribed to improve strength and mobility of the affected arm.

Concerns about appearance after breast surgery may affect the woman's self-concept. Before surgery, the woman and her partner need to receive information about the woman's postoperative appearance. Some women may not want to view their surgical site, but it is important to give them the opportunity to do so and to provide emotional support at that time. Both the woman and her partner need to be able to discuss feelings and concerns about accepting the changes. Information about community resources and support groups such as CancerConnection may be beneficial. An invaluable resource is the Canadian Cancer Society, which provides via the

PATIENT TEACHING Exercises After Breast Surgery

It is important to talk to your doctor before starting any exercises. A physical or occupational therapist can help design an exercise program for you.

Exercises in Lying Position

These exercises should be performed on a bed or the floor while lying on your back with your knees and hips bent, feet flat.

Wand Exercise

This exercise helps increase the forward motion of the shoulders. You will need a broom handle, yardstick, or other similar object to perform this exercise.

- Hold the wand in both hands with palms facing up.
- Lift the wand up over your head (as far as you can), using your unaffected arm to help lift the wand, until you feel a stretch in your affected arm.
- Hold for 5 seconds.
- Lower arms and repeat five to seven times.

Elbow Winging

This exercise helps increase the mobility of the front of your chest and shoulder. It may take several weeks of regular exercise before your elbows will get close to the bed (or floor).

- Clasp your hands behind your neck with your elbows pointing toward the ceiling.
- Move your elbows apart and down toward the bed (or floor).
- Repeat five to seven times.

Exercises in Sitting Position

Shoulder Blade Stretch

This exercise helps increase the mobility of the shoulder blades.

- Sit in a chair very close to a table with your back against the chair back.
- Place the unaffected arm on the table with your elbow bent and palm down. Do not move this arm during the exercise.
- Place the affected arm on the table, palm down with your elbow straight.
- Without moving your trunk, slide the affected arm toward the opposite side of the table. You should feel your shoulder blade move as you do this.
- Relax your arm and repeat five to seven times.

Shoulder Blade Squeeze

This exercise also helps increase the mobility of the shoulder blade.

- Facing straight ahead, sit in a chair in front of a mirror without resting on the back of the chair.
- Arms should be at your sides with elbows bent.
- Squeeze shoulder blades together, bringing your elbows behind you. Keep your shoulders level as you do this exercise. Do not lift your shoulders up toward your ears.
- Return to the starting position and repeat five to seven times.

Side Bending

This exercise helps increase the mobility of the trunk and body.

- Clasp your hands together in front of you and lift your arms slowly over your head, straightening your arms.
- When your arms are over your head, bend your trunk to the right while bending at the waist and keeping your arms overhead.
- Return to the starting position and bend to the left.
- Repeat five to seven times.

Exercises in Standing Position

Chest Wall Stretch

This exercise helps stretch the chest wall.

- Stand facing a corner with your toes approximately 20 to 25 cm from the corner.
- Bend your elbows and place your forearms on the wall, one on each side of the corner. Your elbows should be as close to shoulder height as possible.
- Keep your arms and feet in position and move your chest toward the corner. You will feel a stretch across your chest and shoulders.
- Return to starting position and repeat five to seven times.

Shoulder Stretch

This exercise helps increase the mobility in the shoulder.

- Stand facing the wall with your toes approximately 20 to 25 cm from the wall.
- Place your hands on the wall. Use your fingers to "climb the wall," reaching as high as you can until you feel a stretch.
- Return to starting position and repeat five to seven times.

(Source: American Cancer Society. [2008]. *Exercises after breast surgery*. Retrieved from www.cancer.org/docroot/CRI/content/CRI_2_6x_Exercises_After_Breast_Surgery.asp?sitearea=CRI&viewmode=print&.)

Internet specific, up-to-date recommendations on breast cancer treatments.

Before discharge, considerable time should be spent counselling the woman and her family about the aspects of self-management. Printed instructions should be given to the woman and her family (see Nursing Care Plan: The Woman with Breast Cancer on the Evolve Web site).

Key Points

- Normal feedback regulation of the menstrual cycle depends on an intact hypothalamic–pituitary–gonadal mechanism.
- The myometrium of the uterus is uniquely designed to expel the fetus and promote hemostasis after birth.
- Menstrual disorders diminish the quality of life for affected women and their families.
- PMS is a disorder that begins in the luteal phase of the menstrual cycle and ends with the onset of menses.
- Endometriosis is characterized by secondary amenorrhea, dyspareunia, abnormal uterine bleeding, and infertility.
- Alternative therapies are beneficial in relieving some discomforts associated with menstrual disorders.
- Menopause is a healthy transition that has different symptoms and may require different treatments.
- Key strategies for preventing STIs are the practice of and education in safer sex behaviours.
- STIs are responsible for substantial mortality and morbidity, great personal suffering, and a heavy economic burden in Canada.
- Pregnancy confers no immunity against infection; both mother and fetus must be considered when a pregnant woman contracts an infection.
- Approximately 50% of women experience a breast problem at some point in their adult lives; the risk of a Canadian woman developing breast cancer is 1 in 9.
- Annual clinical breast examinations by a health care provider and routine screening mammograms are recommended for early detection of breast cancer.
- Treatment for breast cancer includes surgery, radiation, and chemotherapy.

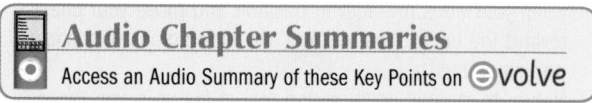

Audio Chapter Summaries

Access an Audio Summary of these Key Points on evolve

References

Albers, J. R., Hull, S. K., & Wesley, R. M. (2004). Abnormal uterine bleeding. *American Family Physician, 69*, 1915–1926, 1931–1932.

American College of Obstetricians and Gynecologists Committee on Adolescent Health Care. (2005). Endometriosis in adolescents. ACOG Committee Opinion No. 310. *Obstetrics and Gynecology, 105*(4), 921–927.

American Psychiatric Association. (2010). *Diagnostic and statistical manual of mental disorders* (5th ed., Development). Washington, DC: American Psychiatric Association Press. Retrieved from http://www.dsm5.org/ProposedRevisions/Pages/proposedrevision.aspx?rid=484

Association of Women's Health, Obstetric and Neonatal Nurses (AWHONN). (2003). *Evidence-based clinical practice guideline: Nursing management for cyclic perimenstrual pain and discomfort.* Washington, DC: Author.

Bielak, K. M., & Harris, G. S. (2010). *Amenorrhea.* Updated April 8, 2010. Retrieved from http://www.emedicine.com/ped/topic2779.htm.

Boucher, M., Gruslin, A., et al. (2000). SOGC clinical practice guideline: The reproductive care of women living with hepatitis C infection. *Journal of Obstetrics and Gynaecology Canada, 22*(10), 820–844. Retrieved from http://www.sogc.org/guidelines/public/96E-CPG-October2000.pdf.

Brown, J., O'Brien, P. M., Marjoribanks, J., & Wyatt, K. (2009). Selective serotonin reuptake inhibitors for premenstrual syndrome. *Cochrane Database of Systematic Reviews, 2009,* Issue 2. Art. No. CD001396. doi: 10.1002/14651858.CD001396.pub2. Retrieved from http://onlinelibrary.wiley.com/o/cochrane/clsysrev/articles/CD001396/pdf_abstract_fs.html.

Canadian Cancer Society. (2009). *Causes of cervical cancer.* Toronto: Author. Retrieved from http://www.cancer.ca/Canada-wide/About%20cancer/Types%20of%20cancer/Causes%20of%20cervical%20cancer.aspx?sc_lang=en.

Canadian Cancer Society. (2010). *Breast cancer statistics.* Toronto: Author. Retrieved from http://www.cancer.ca/Canada-wide/About%20cancer/Cancer%20statistics/Stats%20at%20a%20glance/Breast%20cancer.aspx?sc_lang=en.

Canadian Paediatric Society. (2008). Position statement: Testing for HIV infection in pregnancy. *Paediatric Child Health, 13*(3), 221–224.

Centers for Disease Control and Prevention. (2006). Achievements in public health: Reduction in perinatal transmission of HIV infection—United States, 1985–2005. *MMWR: Morbidity & Mortality Weekly Report, 55*(21), 592–597.

Centers for Disease Control and Prevention, Workowski, K. A., & Berman, S. M. (2010). *Sexually transmitted diseases treatment guidelines, 2010.* Retrieved from http://www.cdc.gov/std/treatment/2010/default.htm.

Collins Sharp, B., et al. (2002). Cyclic perimenstrual pain and discomfort: The scientific basis for practice. *Journal of Obstetric, Gynecologic, and Neonatal Nursing, 31*(6), 637–649.

Conversations with Colleagues. (2002–2003). Endometriosis sufferers risk other diseases. *AWHONN Lifelines, 6*(6), 502–504.

Coutsoudis, A., Dabis, F., Fawzi, W., Gaillard, P., Haverkamp, G., et al.; Breastfeeding and HIV International Transmission Study Group. (2004). Late postnatal transmission of HIV-1 in breast-fed children: An individual patient data meta-analysis. *Journal of Infectious Diseases, 189*, 2154–2166.

Dehlin, L., & Schuiling, K. (2013). Chronic pelvic pain. In K. Schuiling & F. Likis (Eds.), *Women's gynecologic health.* Burlington, MA: Jones & Bartlett.

Dodd, N., & Sinert, R. (2007). *Dysfunctional uterine bleeding.* Updated September 16, 2010. Retrieved from http://emedicine.medscape.com/article/257007-overview.

Fritz, M., & Speroff, L. (2010). *Clinical gynecologic endocrinology and infertility* (8th ed.). Philadelphia: Lippincott Williams & Wilkins.

Grunfeld, E., Dhesy-Thind, S., & Levine, M. (2005). Clinical practice guidelines for the care and treatment of breast cancer: Follow-up after treatment for breast cancer (2005 update). *Canadian Medical Association Journal, 172*(10), 1319–1320.

Healey, S. M., Aronson, K. J., Mao, Y., Schlecht, N. F., Mery, L. S., Ferenczy, A., et al. (2001). Oncogenic human papillomavirus infection and cervical lesions in aboriginal women of Nunavut, Canada. *Sexually Transmitted Diseases, 28*, 694–700.

Health Canada. (2006). *Summary basis of decision (SBD) Inamed style 410 Silicone-filled breast implants.* Ottawa: Health Products and Food Branch, Government of Canada. Retrieved from http://www.hc-sc.gc.ca/dhp-mps/prodpharma/sbd-smd/phase1-decision/md-im/sbd_smd_2006_inamed410_88573-eng.php.

Hoffman, S., et al. (2004). The future of the female condom. *Perspectives on Sexual and Reproductive Health, 36*(3), 120–126.

Lawrence, R.A., & Lawrence, R.M. (2011). *Breastfeeding: A guide for the medical profession* (7th ed.). Philadelphia: Mosby.

Liu, S., & Lebrun, C. (2006). Effect of oral contraceptives and hormone replacement therapy on bone mineral density in premenopausal and perimenopausal women: A systematic review. *British Journal of Sports Medicine, 40*(1), 11–24.

Marrazzo, J. M., Guest, F., & Cates, W. (2007). Reproductive tract infections, including HIV and other sexually transmitted infections. In R. Hatcher et al. (Eds.), *Contraceptive technology* (19th ed.). New York: Ardent Media.

Money, D., & Steben, M., et al. (2008). SOGC clinical practice guideline: Genital herpes: Gynaecological aspects. *Journal of Obstetrics and Gynaecology Canada, 30*(4), 347–353. Retrieved from http://www.sogc.org/guidelines/documents/gui207CPG0804_000.pdf.

National Cancer Institute. (2006). Results of the study of tamoxifen and raloxifene (STAR) released: Osteoporosis drug raloxifene shown to be as effective as tamoxifen in preventing invasive breast cancer. *National Cancer Institute News*, April 17, 2006. Retrieved from http://www.cancer.gov/newscenter.

National Cancer Institute. (2007). *Menopausal hormone replacement therapy use and cancer: Questions and answers: Fact sheet*. Retrieved from http://www.cancer.gov/cancertopics/factsheet/Risk/menopausal-hormones.

National Comprehensive Cancer Network. (2010). *Breast cancer: NCCN guidelines for patients*. Retrieved from http://www.nccn.com/images/patient-guidelines/pdf/breast.pdf.

National Institute of Child Health and Human Development. (2008). *Extended nevirapine regimens reduce HIV transmission and death in breastfed infants of HIV-infected mothers*. Retrieved from http://www.nichd.nih.gov/news/releases/swen_pepi_020608.cfm.

Organization of Teratology Information Services. (2003). *Acyclovir (Zovirax)/valacyclovir (Valtrex) in pregnancy*. Retrieved from http://www.OTISpregnancy.org.

Pinnette, G. D., et al. (2009). *Primary care management of chronic hepatitis C: Professional desk reference*. Retrieved from http://www.phac-aspc.gc.ca/hepc/pubs/pdf/hepc_guide-eng.pdf.

Proctor, M., & Farquhar, C. (2004). Dysmenorrhoea. *Clinical Evidence, 12*, 2524–2547.

Public Health Agency of Canada. (2006). *Canadian immunization guide* (7th ed.) (Cat. No. HP40-3/2006E). Ottawa: Author. Retrieved from http://www.phac-aspc.gc.ca/publicat/cig-gci/pdf/cig-gci-2006_e.pdf.

Public Health Agency of Canada. (2008). *Canadian guidelines on sexually transmitted infections*. Ottawa: Author. Retrieved from http://www.phac-aspc.gc.ca/std-mts/sti-its/guide-lignesdir-eng.php.

Public Health Agency of Canada. (2009). *Brief report on sexually transmitted infections in Canada: 2007* (Cat. No. HP37-10/2007E-PDF). Ottawa: Author. Retrieved from http://www.phac-aspc.gc.ca/publicat/2009/sti-its/pdf/sti_brief-its_bref_2009-eng.pdf.

Public Health Agency of Canada. (2010a). *Canadian guidelines on sexually transmitted infections* (Cat. No. HP40-1/2010E). Ottawa: Author. Retrieved from http://www.phac-aspc.gc.ca/std-mts/sti-its/guide-lignesdir-eng.php.

Public Health Agency of Canada. (2010b). *Report on sexually transmitted infection in Canada: 2008*. Ottawa: Author. Retrieved from http://www.phac-aspc.gc.ca/std-mts/report/sti-its2008/PDF/10-047-STI_report_eng-r1.pdf.

Public Health Agency of Canada. (2010c). *The facts on the safety and effectiveness of the HPV vaccine*. Retrieved from http://www.phac-aspc.gc.ca/std-mts/hpv-vph/fact-faits-vacc-eng.php.

Riordan, J., & Wambach, K. (2010). *Breastfeeding and human lactation* (4th ed.). Boston: Jones & Bartlett.

Sakorafas, G. (2003). The management of women at high risk for breast cancer: Risk estimation and prevention strategies. *Cancer Treatment Reviews, 29*(2), 79–89.

Sherman, M., Shafran, S., Burak, K., Doucette, K., Wong, W., et al. (2007). Management of chronic hepatitis C: Canadian consensus guidelines. *Canadian Journal of Gastroenterology, 21*(Suppl C), 25C–34C.

Society of Obstetricians and Gynaecologists of Canada. (2005). SOGC clinical practice guideline: Primary dysmenorrhoea consensus guideline. *Journal of Obstetrics and Gynaecology Canada, 27*(12), 1117–1130. Retrieved from http://www.sogc.org/guidelines/public/169E-CPG-December2005.pdf.

Society of Obstetricians and Gynaecologists of Canada. (2006). Canadian consensus conference update on menopause, 2006 update. *Journal of Obstetrics and Gynaecology Canada, 28*(Special edition), S1–S112.

Society of Obstetricians and Gynaecologists of Canada. (2007). SOGC clinical practice guideline: Canadian consensus guideline on human papillomavirus. *Journal of Obstetrics and Gynaecology Canada, 29*(8), Supplement 3. Retrieved from http://www.sogc.org/guidelines/documents/gui196CPG0708revised.pdf.

Society of Obstetricians and Gynaecologist of Canada. (2009). SOGC clinical practice guideline: Menopause and osteoporosis update 2009. *Journal of Obstetrics and Gynaecology Canada, 31*(1), Suppl 1, S1–S46. Retrieved from http://www.sogc.org/guidelines/documents/menopause_JOGC-Jan_09.pdf.

Taylor, D., Schuiling, K., & Sharp, B. (2013). Menstrual cycle pain and discomforts. In K. Schuiling & F. Likis (Eds.), *Women's gynecologic health* (2nd ed.). Burlington. MA: Jones & Bartlett.

World Health Organization. (2007). *Global strategy for the prevention and control of sexually transmitted infections: 2006–2015: Breaking the chain of transmission*. Geneva: Author. Retrieved from http://whqlibdoc.who.int/publications/2007/9789241563475_eng.pdf.

Writing Group for the Women's Health Initiative Investigators. (2002). Risks and benefits of estrogen plus progestin in healthy postmenopausal women: Principal results from the Women's Health Initiative randomized controlled trial. *Journal of the American Medical Association, 288*(3), 366–368.

Yudin, M., Money, D.; Infectious Diseases Committee. (2008). SOGC Clinical Practice Guideline: Screening and management of bacterial vaginosis in pregnancy. *Journal of Obstetrics and Gynaecology Canada, 30*(8), 702–708. Retrieved from http://www.sogc.org/guidelines/documents/gui211CPG0808.pdf.

Additional Resources

Bodysense: http://www.bodysense.ca/
Breast Cancer Risk Assessment Tool: http://www.cancer.gov/bcrisktool/
Canadian Cancer Society: http://www.cancer.ca/
Canadian Women's Health Network: http://www.cwhn.ca/
Infertility Awareness Association of Canada: http://www.iaac.ca/
Menopauseandu.ca: http://www.Menopauseandu.ca
Sexualityandu.ca: http://www.Sexualityandu.ca

Unit 2

7 Infertility, Contraception, and Abortion

Learning Objectives

On completion of this chapter, the reader will be able to:

- List common causes of infertility.
- Discuss the psychological impact of infertility.
- Describe common diagnoses and treatments for infertility.
- Compare reproductive alternatives for couples experiencing infertility.
- State the advantages and disadvantages of methods of contraception.
- Explain common nursing interventions that facilitate contraceptive use.
- Describe the techniques used for medical and surgical interruption of pregnancy.
- Recognize ethical, legal, cultural, and religious considerations of infertility, contraception, and elective abortion.

Electronic Resources

Additional information related to the content in Chapter 7 can be found on

evolve the companion Web site at http://evolve.elsevier.com/Canada/Perry/maternal/

- Examination Review Questions
- Critical Thinking Exercise—Patient Teaching: Contraception

This chapter addresses infertility, associated tests, and common therapies; contraception; and abortion. Available alternatives and psychosocial implications are discussed.

Infertility

Incidence

Infertility is a serious medical concern that affects quality of life and is a problem for 8.5 to 16% of reproductive-age couples (Medical Advisory Secretariat, 2006). Infertility implies subfertility, a prolonged time to conceive, in contrast to sterility, or the inability to conceive. Normally a fertile couple has approximately a 20% chance of conception in each ovulatory cycle. Primary infertility applies to a woman who has never been pregnant. Secondary infertility applies to a woman who has been pregnant in the past.

The prevalence of infertility is relatively stable among the overall population. It increases with the age of the woman, particularly in those older than 40 years of age. Probable causes of infertility include the trend toward delaying pregnancy until later in life, when fertility decreases naturally and the prevalence of diseases such as endometriosis and ovulatory dysfunction increases. It is debated whether an actual increase in male infertility has occurred or it is more readily identified because of improvements in diagnosis.

Diagnosis and treatment of infertility require considerable physical, emotional, psychological, and financial investment over an extended period of time. Men and women often perceive infertility differently. Women generally experience more stress from undergoing tests and treatments, place greater importance on having children, are more accepting of indicated treatments, and want children more than men (Sherrod, 2004). Views of fertility and infertility also vary by culture (see Cultural Awareness box).

Feelings connected with infertility are many and complex. The origins of some of these feelings are myths, superstitions, misinformation, or magical thinking about the causes of infertility. Other feelings arise from the need to undergo many tests and examinations and from a perception of being "different" from others. The attitude, sensitivity, and caring nature of those who are involved in the assessment and treatment of infertility lay the foundation for the couple's ability to cope with the many tests and treatments they must undergo. Team members must respect individuals' and couples' desires in choosing to stop treatment and to select other alternatives such as remaining childless or pursuing adoption. The Infertility Awareness Association of Canada (http://www.iaac.ca) is an organization that provides support, advocacy, and education about infertility for the infertility community as well as for health care providers.

Factors Associated With Infertility

Many factors, those affecting both males and females, contribute to normal fertility. A normally developed reproductive tract in both the male and the female partner is essential.

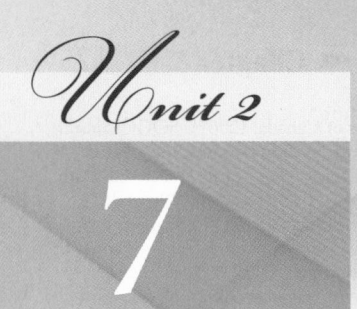

CULTURAL AWARENESS

Fertility and Infertility

Worldwide, cultures continue to use symbols and rites that celebrate fertility. One fertility rite that persists today is the custom of throwing rice at the bride and groom. Other fertility symbols and rites include passing out congratulatory cigars, candy, or pencils by a new father, and baby showers held in anticipation of a child's birth. In many cultures, the responsibility for infertility is usually blamed on the woman. A woman's inability to conceive may be caused by her sins, evil spirits, or the fact that she is an inadequate person. The virility of a man in some cultures remains in question until he demonstrates his ability to reproduce by having at least one child (D'Avanzo, 2008).

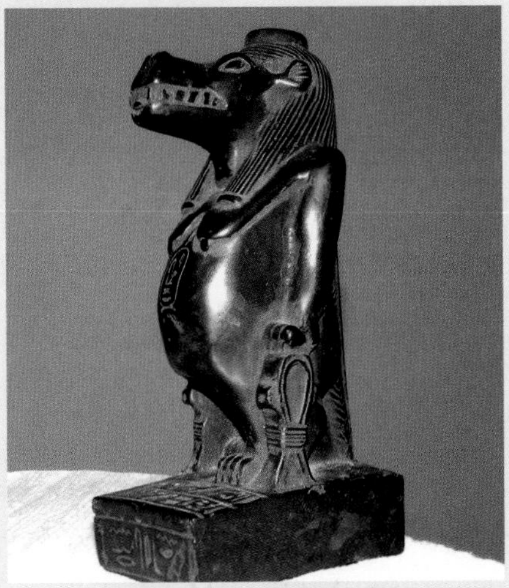

Taweret, goddess of fertility, Egypt. *(Courtesy Julie Perry Nelson, Phoenix, AZ.)*

BOX 7-1 Factors Affecting Female Fertility

Ovarian Factors

Developmental anomalies

Anovulation—primary
- Pituitary or hypothalamic hormone disorder
- Adrenal gland disorder
- Congenital adrenal hyperplasia

Anovulation—secondary
- Disruption of hypothalamic–pituitary–ovarian axis
- Amenorrhea after discontinuing oral contraceptive pills
- Premature ovarian failure
- Polycystic ovarian syndrome

Increased prolactin levels

Tubal/Peritoneal Factors

Developmental anomalies
Reduced tubal motility
Inflammation within the tube
Tubal adhesions
Endometriosis

Uterine Factors

Developmental anomalies
Endometrial and myometrial tumours
Asherman syndrome (uterine adhesions or scar tissue)

Vaginal–Cervical Factors

Vaginal–cervical infections
Cervical mucus inadequate
Isoimmunization (development of sperm antibodies)

Other Factors

Nutritional deficiencies (i.e., anemia)
Thyroid dysfunction
Obesity
Idiopathic condition

Normal functioning of an intact hypothalamic–pituitary–gonadal axis supports gametogenesis (the formation of sperm and ova). The lifespans of the sperm and the ovum are short. Although sperm remain viable in the female's reproductive tract for 48 hours or longer, probably only a few retain fertilization potential for more than 24 hours. Ova remain viable for about 24 hours, but the optimal time for fertilization may be no more than 1 to 2 hours (Cunningham et al., 2010); thus timing of intercourse becomes critical. The couple should be taught about the menstrual cycle and the way to detect ovulation (see the discussion later in the chapter).

An alteration in one or more of these structures, functions, or processes results in some degree of impaired fertility. Causes of impaired fertility can lie with either the male or female. In general, about 20% of couples will have unexplained or **idiopathic** causes of infertility. Among the 80% of couples who have an identifiable cause of infertility, about 40% are related to factors in the female partner, 40% are related to factors in the male partner, and 20% are related to factors in both partners (Lobo, 2007; Nelson & Marshall, 2008). Boxes 7-1 and 7-2 list factors affecting female and male infertility.

Nursing Care Management

The nurse assists in the assessment of the infertile couple (see Nursing Process box). Some of the data needed to investigate impaired fertility are of a sensitive, personal nature. The couple may view the obtaining of such data as an invasion of privacy. The tests and examinations are occasionally painful and intrusive and can take the romance out of lovemaking. Couples need a high level of motivation to endure the investigation.

Because multiple factors involving both partners are common, the investigation of impaired fertility is conducted systematically and simultaneously for both the male and the female partner. Both partners must be interested in finding a solution to the problem. The medical investigation requires time (3 to 4 months) and may be of considerable financial expense (Box 7-3). It may cause emotional distress and strain on the couple's relationship.

Assessment of Female Infertility

Investigation of impaired fertility begins for the woman with a complete **history** and physical examination. A complete

NURSING PROCESS: INFERTILITY

Assessment

Obtain data relevant to fertility through interview and physical examination.

Identify whether infertility is primary or secondary.

Note religious, cultural, and ethnic data because these may place restrictions on tests and treatments.

Obtain results from diagnostic tests.

Nursing Diagnoses

Disturbed body image or risk for situational low self-esteem related to

– impaired fertility

Decisional conflict related to

– therapies for impaired fertility
– alternatives to therapy (e.g., childfree living or adoption)

Sexual dysfunction related to

– loss of libido secondary to medically imposed restrictions

Social isolation related to

– impaired fertility, its investigation, and its management

Planning

Expected outcomes include that the woman or family will do the following:

- Communicate understanding of the anatomy and physiology of the reproductive system
- Communicate understanding of treatment for any abnormalities identified through various tests and examinations and be able to make an informed decision about treatment
- Resolve guilt feelings and not need to focus blame
- Conceive or, failing to conceive, decide on an alternative acceptable to both of them (childfree living or adoption)

Interventions

Teach, counsel, and reinforce information about tests and test results.

Assist the couple to

- Express and discuss feelings.
- Separate concepts of success and failure of treatment for infertility from personal success and failure.
- Recognize infertility as a loss and resolve these feelings even if treatment is successful.

Explore support systems of the couple:

- Persons available to assist
- Relationship to couple
- Ages, availability
- Available cultural or religious support

Refer for mental health counselling, as necessary.

Evaluation

Evaluation of the effectiveness of care of the couple experiencing impaired fertility is based on the previously stated outcomes.

BOX 7-2 Factors Affecting Male Fertility

Structural or Hormonal Disorders

Undescended testes
Hypospadias
Varicocele
Obstructive lesions of the epididymis and vas deferens
Low testosterone levels
Hypopituitarism
Endocrine disorders
Testicular damage caused by mumps
Retrograde ejaculation

Substance Use

Changes in sperm from cigarette smoking or use of heroin, marijuana, amyl nitrate, butyl nitrate, ethyl chloride, or methaqualone
Decrease in libido from use of heroin, methadone, selective serotonin reuptake inhibitors, or barbiturates
Impotence from use of alcohol or antihypertensive medications

Other Factors

Sexually transmitted infections
Exposure to workplace hazards such as radiation or toxic substances
Exposure of scrotum to high temperatures
Nutritional deficiencies
Antisperm antibodies
Idiopathic conditions

BOX 7-3 Insurance Coverage for Infertility

All provinces in Canada cover the cost of diagnostic testing and some medical and surgical treatment of infertility through provincial insurance plans. As of 2010, Québec is the only province to include in vitro fertilization in this funding. Québec will now pay for three cycles of in vitro treatments. The Canadian Fertility and Andrology Society has publicly supported Québec's decision and strongly advocates for both regulation and public funding of in vitro fertilization. Private insurance plans may pay for some aspects of treatment. Patients need information about what they can expect from their private insurers and are encouraged to contact companies to obtain more complete information.

general physical examination is followed by a specific assessment of the reproductive tract. Laboratory data, including routine urine and blood tests, are collected.

A woman may have an abnormal uterus and tubes (Fig. 7-1) as a result of in utero exposure to diethylstilbestrol (see Box 5-2). Any history of infection of the genitourinary system should be noted. Bimanual examination of internal organs may reveal lack of mobility of the uterus or abnormal contours of the uterus and adnexa.

Diagnostic Testing

The basic infertility survey of the female involves evaluation of the cervix, uterus, tubes, and peritoneum; detection of

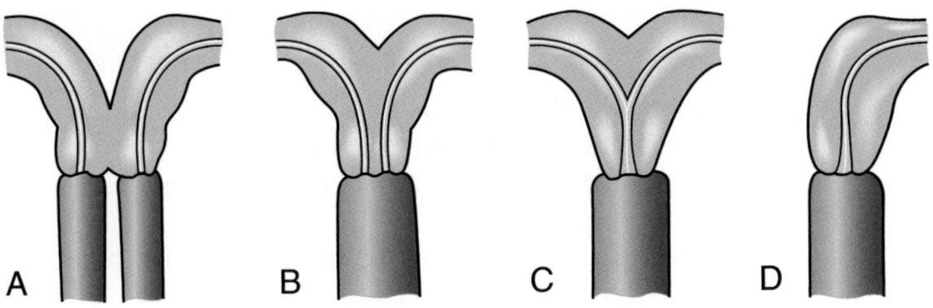

Fig. 7-1 Abnormal uterus. **A:** Complete bicornuate uterus with vagina divided by a septum. **B:** Complete bicornuate uterus with normal vagina. **C:** Partial bicornuate uterus with normal vagina. **D:** Unicornuate uterus.

Table 7-1 Tests for Impaired Fertility

TEST OR EXAMINATION	TIMING (MENSTRUAL CYCLE DAYS)	RATIONALE
Hysterosalpingogram	7-10	Late follicular, early proliferative phase; will not disrupt a fertilized ovum; may open uterine tubes before time of ovulation
Postcoital test	1-2 days before ovulation	Ovulatory late proliferative phase; look for normal motile sperm in cervical mucus
Sperm immobilization antigen-antibody reaction	Variable, ovulation	Immunological test to determine sperm and cervical mucus interaction
Assessment of cervical mucus	Variable, ovulation	Cervical mucus should have low viscosity, high spinnbarkeit
Ultrasound diagnosis of follicular collapse	Ovulation	Collapsed follicle is seen after ovulation
Serum assay of plasma progesterone	20-25	Midluteal midsecretory phase; check adequacy of corpus luteal production of progesterone
Basal body temperature	Chart entire cycle	Elevation occurs in response to progesterone, documents ovulation
Endometrial biopsy	21-27	Late luteal, late secretory phase; check endometrial response to progesterone and adequacy of luteal phase
Sperm penetration assay	After 2 days but ≤1 week of abstinence	Evaluation of ability of sperm to penetrate an egg

ovulation; hormone analysis; assessment of immunological compatibility; and evaluation of psychogenic factors (Table 7-1). Ultrasound (timed—during the luteal phase), endometrial biopsy, hysterosalpingography (x-ray examination of the uterine cavity and tubes after instillation of radiopaque contrast material through the cervix), and laparoscopy (to detect and possibly treat problems such as endometriosis or adhesions in the peritoneal cavity) may be performed. The nurse can alleviate some of the anxiety associated with testing by explaining the timing and rationale for each test. Test findings favourable to fertility are summarized in Box 7-4.

Couples should be cautioned that everything can be normal and conception still may not occur. Unexplained infertility accounts for 20% of cases (American Society for Reproductive Medicine [ASRM], 2008). Conversely, even poor test results do not mean that pregnancy will not occur.

Assessment of Male Infertility

The systematic investigation of infertility in the male patient begins with a thorough history and physical examination. Assessment of the male patient proceeds in a manner similar to that of the female patient, starting with noninvasive tests.

Semen Analysis

The basic test for male infertility is semen analysis. A complete semen analysis, study of the effects of cervical mucus on sperm forward motility and survival, and evaluation of the sperm's ability to penetrate an ovum provide basic information. Sperm counts vary from day to day and depend on emotional and physical status and sexual activity. Therefore, a single analysis may be inconclusive. A minimum of two analyses must be performed several weeks apart to assess male fertility.

Semen is collected by ejaculation into a clean container or a plastic sheath that does not contain a spermicidal agent. The specimen is usually collected by masturbation following 2 to 5 days of abstinence from **ejaculation**. The semen is examined at the collection site or taken to the laboratory in a sealed container within 2 hours of ejaculation. Exposure to excessive heat or cold should be avoided. Commonly accepted values for semen characteristics are given in Box 7-5. If results are in the fertile range, no further sperm evaluation is necessary. If results are not within this range, the test is repeated. If subsequent results are still in the subfertile range, further evaluation is needed to identify the problem.

Hormone analyses are done for testosterone, gonadotropin, follicle-stimulating hormone (FSH), and luteinizing hormone (LH). The sperm penetration assay and other alternative tests can be used to evaluate the ability of sperm to penetrate an egg. Testicular biopsy may be warranted. Scrotal ultrasound is used to examine the testes for presence of **varicoceles** and to identify abnormalities in the scrotum and spermatic cord. Transrectal ultrasound is used to evaluate the ejaculatory ducts, seminal vesicles, and vas deferens.

BOX 7-4 Summary of Findings Favourable to Fertility

1. Follicular development, ovulation, and luteal development are supportive of pregnancy:
   a. Basal body temperature (presumptive evidence of ovulatory cycles) is biphasic, with temperature elevation that persists for 12 to 14 days before menstruation (see Fig. 7-8).
   b. Cervical mucus characteristics change appropriately during phases of the menstrual cycle (see discussion later in the chapter).
   c. Laparoscopic visualization of pelvic organs verifies follicular and luteal development.
2. The luteal phase is supportive of pregnancy:
   a. Levels of plasma progesterone are adequate.
   b. Findings from endometrial biopsy samples are consistent with day of cycle.
3. Cervical factors are receptive to sperm during expected time of ovulation:
   a. Cervical os is open.
   b. Cervical mucus is clear, watery, abundant, and slippery and demonstrates good spinnbarkeit and arborization (fern pattern).
   c. Cervical examination does not reveal lesions or infections.
   d. Postcoital test findings are satisfactory (adequate number of live, motile, normal sperm present in cervical mucus).
   e. No immunity to sperm is demonstrated.
4. The uterus and uterine tubes are supportive of pregnancy:
   a. Uterine and tubal patency are documented by (1) spillage of dye into the peritoneal cavity; and (2) outlines of uterine and tubal cavities of adequate size and shape, with no abnormalities.
   b. Laparoscopic examination verifies normal development of internal genitals and absence of adhesions, infections, endometriosis, and other lesions.
5. The male partner's reproductive structures are normal:
   a. There is no evidence of developmental anomalies of penis (hypospadius), testicular atrophy, or varicocele (varicose veins on the spermatic vein in the groin).
   b. There is no evidence of infection in the prostate, seminal vesicles, and urethra.
   c. Testes are more than 4 cm in largest diameter.
6. Semen is supportive of pregnancy:
   a. Sperm (number per millilitre) are adequate in ejaculate.
   b. Most sperm show normal morphology.
   c. Most sperm are motile, forward moving.
   d. No autoimmunity exists.
   e. Seminal fluid is normal.

Assessment of the Couple

Postcoital Test

The postcoital test (PCT) is one method used to test for adequacy of coital technique, cervical mucus, sperm, and degree of sperm penetration through cervical mucus. The test is performed within several hours after ejaculation of semen into the vagina. A specimen of cervical mucus is obtained from the cervical os and examined under a microscope. The quality of mucus and the number of forward-moving sperm are noted. A PCT with good mucus and motile sperm is associated with fertility.

BOX 7-5 Semen Analysis

Semen volume 2.5 mL
Sperm concentration/density ≥20 million/mL
Normal morphology ≥30%; normal shaped heads >14%
Motility
- Number of active cells as percentage of total number of cells ≥50%
- Quality of movement of sperm (rated 0–4) ≥2

Liquefaction <20 minutes

(Source: RESOLVE. [2008]. *The semen analysis*. Retrieved from http://www.resolve.org/diagnosis-management/infertility-diagnosis/the-semen-analysis.html.)

Intercourse is synchronized with the expected time of ovulation (as determined from evaluation of basal body temperature [BBT], cervical mucus changes, and usual length of menstrual cycle or use of LH detection kit to determine LH surge). Intercourse should occur only in the absence of vaginal infection. Couples may experience some difficulty abstaining from intercourse for 2 to 4 days before expected ovulation and then having intercourse with ejaculation on schedule. Sex on demand may strain the couple's interpersonal relationship. A problem may arise if the expected day of ovulation occurs when facilities or the physician is unavailable (such as over a weekend or holiday).

Plan of Care and Implementation

Psychosocial

Infertility is recognized as a major life stressor that can affect **self-esteem**; relations with the spouse, family, and friends; and careers. Psychological responses to the diagnosis of infertility may tax a couple's capacity for giving and receiving physical and sexual closeness. The prescriptions and proscriptions for achieving conception may add tension to a couple's sexual functioning. Couples may report decreased desire for intercourse, orgasmic dysfunction, or midcycle **erectile disorders**. Treatment for infertility is complex and stressful, and 30% of couples quit treatment before becoming pregnant, because of the associated psychological distress (Boivin, Griffiths, & Venetis, 2011). Some women may feel that their stress levels will affect whether treatment is successful; however, Boivin et al. (2011) showed that emotional distress was unlikely to be a cause of infertility treatment failure. Couples need support and encouragement to express their concerns about infertility treatment.

In order to deal comfortably with a couple's sexuality, nurses must be comfortable with their own sexuality so that they can better help couples understand why the private act of lovemaking needs to be shared with health care providers. Nurses need up-to-date factual knowledge about human sexual practices and must be accepting of the preferences and activities of others, without being judgemental. They must be skilled in interviewing and in therapeutic use of self, sensitive to the nonverbal cues of others, and knowledgeable about each couple's sociocultural and religious beliefs (see Critical Thinking Exercise).

The woman or couple facing infertility may exhibit behaviours of the grieving process that are associated with other types of loss. The loss of one's genetic continuity with the generations to come can lead to a loss of self-esteem, a sense of inadequacy as a woman or a man, a loss of control over one's destiny, and a reduced sense of self. Infertile individuals can have impaired self-concept and experience greater dissatisfaction with their marriage. Not all people will have all these reactions, nor can it be predicted how long any reaction will last for any one individual.

If the couple conceives, their concerns and problems with infertility may not be over. Many couples are overjoyed with the pregnancy; however, some are not. Some couples rearrange their lives, sense of self, and personal goals based on accepting their infertile state. The couple may think that those who worked with them to identify and treat impaired fertility expect them to be happy with the pregnancy. They may be shocked to find that they feel resentment because the pregnancy, once a cherished dream, now necessitates another change in goals, aspirations, and identities. The normal ambivalence toward pregnancy may be perceived as reneging on the original choice to become parents. The couple might choose to abort the pregnancy at this time. Other couples worry about miscarriage. If the couple wishes to continue with the pregnancy, they will need the care that other expectant couples need.

If the couple does not conceive, they are assessed regarding their desire to be referred for help with adoption, therapeutic intrauterine insemination, other reproductive alternatives, or choosing a child-free state. The couple may find helpful a list of agencies, support groups, and other resources in their community, such as the Infertility Awareness Association of Canada (http://www.iaac.ca) and the Infertility Network (http://www.infertilitynetwork.org).

CRITICAL THINKING EXERCISE

Infertility Workup

Crista is 31 years old and is a registered nurse working in the operating room at a local hospital. Anthony is 34 years old and is a fireman. They have been trying to become pregnant for the past 8 years. They have come for an infertility workup and are wondering about the possibility of in vitro fertilization. The nurse does the initial intake interview and some counselling. Crista and Anthony express discouragement, disillusionment, and anxiety. They have many questions about the probability of achieving pregnancy after this length of time.

1. Evidence—Is there sufficient evidence to draw conclusions about the probability of achieving pregnancy?
2. Assumptions—What assumptions can be made about a couple experiencing infertility? What are the costs of infertility treatment?
3. What implications and priorities for nursing care can be drawn at this time?
4. Does the evidence objectively support your conclusion?
5. Are there alternative perspectives to your conclusion?

Nonmedical

Simple changes in lifestyle may be effective in the treatment of subfertile men. Only water-soluble lubricants should be used during intercourse because many commonly used lubricants contain **spermicides** or have spermicidal properties. High scrotal temperatures may be caused by daily hot tub baths or saunas that keep the testes at temperatures too high for efficient spermatogenesis.

Treatment is available for women who have immunological reactions to sperm. The use of **condoms** during genital intercourse for 6 to 12 months will reduce female antibody production in most women who have elevated antisperm antibody titers. After the serum reaction subsides, condoms are used at all times except at the expected time of ovulation. Approximately one third of couples with this problem conceive by following this course of action.

Changes in nutrition and habits may increase fertility for both men and women. For example, a well-balanced diet, exercise, decreased alcohol intake, abstinence from smoking or using drugs, and stress management may be effective. Women who are obese should be counselled to try to reach a healthy weight, which may improve their ability to conceive.

Herbal Alternative Measures

Most herbal remedies have not been proven clinically to promote fertility or to be safe in early pregnancy and should be taken by the woman only as prescribed by a physician or midwife who has expertise in herbology. Relaxation, osteopathy, stress management (e.g., aromatherapy, yoga), and nutritional and exercise counselling have been reported to increase pregnancy rates in some women. Herbal remedies that promote fertility in general include red clover flowers, nettle leaves, dong quai, and false unicorn root (Weed, 1986). Vitamin E, calcium, and magnesium may promote fertility and conception. Vitamins E and C, glutathione, and coenzyme Q_{10} are antioxidants that have proven beneficial effects for male infertility (Sheweita, Tilmisany, Al-Sawaf, 2005). Herbs to avoid while trying to conceive include licorice root, yarrow, wormwood, ephedra, fennel, goldenseal, lavender, juniper, flaxseed, pennyroyal, passionflower, wild cherry, cascara, sage, thyme, and periwinkle.

Medical

Pharmacological therapy for female infertility is often directed at treating ovulatory dysfunction by either stimulating or enhancing ovulation so that more oocytes mature. These medications include clomiphene citrate, human menopausal gonadotropin (HMG), FSH, recombinant FSH (rFSH), and human chorionic gonadotropin. Gonadotropin-releasing hormone (GnRH) agonists and progesterones are also used.

These medications are extremely potent and require daily monitoring with ovarian ultrasound and monitoring of estradiol levels to prevent hyperstimulation. The incidence of multiple pregnancies with the use of these medications is greater than 25%. When failure to ovulate is caused by hypothalamic–pituitary dysfunction or failure to respond to clomiphene,

GnRH may be used. Thyroid-stimulating hormone (Synthroid) is indicated if the woman has hypothyroidism.

The woman with low estrogen levels may be a candidate for conjugated estrogens and medroxyprogesterone. A hypoestrogenic condition may result from a high stress level or from a decreased percentage of body fat as a result of an eating disorder (e.g., anorexia nervosa) or excessive exercise. Hydroxyprogesterone supplementation with vaginal suppositories or intramuscular injection is used to treat luteal phase defects. In the presence of adrenal hyperplasia, prednisone, a glucocorticoid, is taken orally. Treatment of **endometriosis** may include danazol, progesterone, combined oral contraceptives, or GnRH agonists. Infections are treated with appropriate antimicrobial formulations.

Polycystic ovarian syndrome (PCOS) is the cause of some infertility, a condition that includes at least two of the following criteria: oligo-ovulation or anovulation, hyperandrogenism, and polycystic ovaries on ultrasound assessment. Fifty percent of these women are often obese, and weight loss, exercise, and lifestyle modifications often restore ovulatory cycles and should be the first method of treatment. Clomiphene citrate with or without metformin has also been shown to increase ovulation and pregnancy rates. Gonadotropins should be considered second-line therapy for fertility in anovulatory women with PCOS. The treatment requires ultrasound and laboratory monitoring. High cost and the risk of multiple pregnancy and of ovarian hyperstimulation syndrome are drawbacks of the treatment (Vause et al., 2010).

Drug therapy may be indicated for male infertility. Problems with the thyroid or adrenal glands are corrected with appropriate medications. Infections are identified and treated with antimicrobials. FSH, HMG, and clomiphene may be used to stimulate spermatogenesis in men with hypogonadism.

The primary care provider is responsible for fully informing patients about the prescribed medications. However, the nurse must be ready to answer patients' questions and to confirm their understanding of the drug, its administration, potential adverse effects, and expected outcomes. Because information varies with each drug, the nurse must consult the medication package inserts, pharmacology references, the physician, and the pharmacist, as necessary.

Surgical

A number of surgical procedures can be used for problems causing female infertility. Ovarian tumors must be excised. Whenever possible, functional ovarian tissue is left intact. Scar tissue adhesions caused by chronic infections may cover much or all of the ovary. These adhesions usually necessitate surgery to free and expose the ovary so that ovulation can occur.

Hysterosalpingography is useful for identification of tubal obstruction and for the release of blockage (Fig. 7-2). During laparoscopy, delicate adhesions may be divided and removed, and endometrial implants may be destroyed by electrocoagulation or laser (Fig. 7-3). Laparotomy and even microsurgery may be required for extensive repair of the damaged tube. Prognosis depends on the degree to which tubal patency and function can be restored.

Reconstructive surgery (e.g., the unification operation for **bicornuate uterus**) often improves a woman's ability to conceive and carry the fetus to term. Surgical removal of tumours or fibroids involving the endometrium or uterus often improves the woman's chance of conceiving and maintaining the pregnancy to viability. Women who undergo surgical treatment of uterine tumours or maldevelopment and go on to have a successful pregnancy may require birth by Caesarean section near term gestation because the enlarging uterus may rupture as a result of weakness in the area of reconstructive surgery.

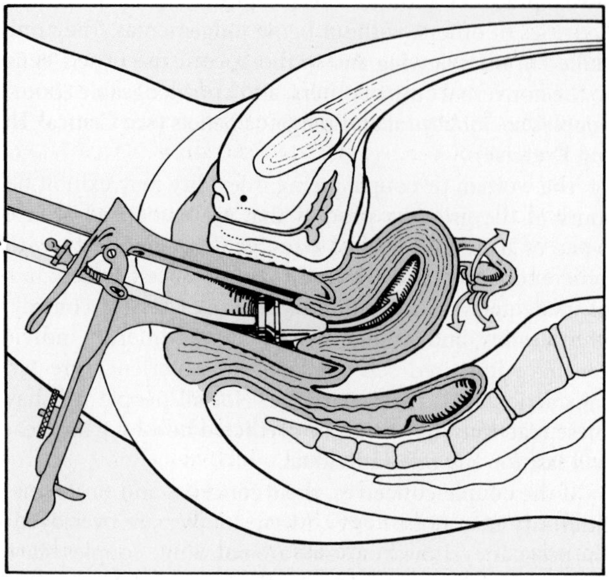

Fig. 7-2 Hysterosalpingography. Note that the contrast medium flows through the intrauterine cannula and out through the uterine tubes.

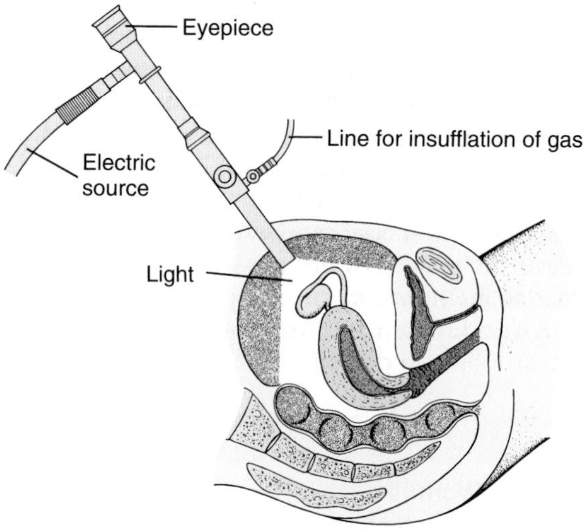

Fig. 7-3 Laparoscopy.

Chronic inflammation and infection can be eliminated by radial chemocautery (destruction of tissue with chemicals) or thermocautery (destruction of tissue with heat, usually electrical) of the cervix, cryosurgery (destruction of tissue by application of extreme cold, usually liquid nitrogen), or conization (excision of a cone-shaped piece of tissue from the endocervix). When the cervix has been deeply cauterized or frozen or when extensive conization has been performed, extreme limitation of mucus production by the cervix may result. Therefore, the absence of a mucus bridge from the vagina to the uterus can make sperm migration difficult or impossible. Therapeutic intrauterine insemination may be necessary for the sperm to be carried directly through the internal os of the cervix.

Surgical procedures may also be used for problems causing male infertility. Surgical repair of varicocele has been relatively successful in increasing sperm count but not fertility rates. Microsurgery to reanastomose (restore tubal continuity) the sperm ducts after vasectomy can restore fertility.

Assisted Reproductive Technologies

Although there have been remarkable developments in reproductive medicine, assisted reproductive technologies (ARTs) account for less than 1% of all Canadian births (Canadian Fertility and Andrology Society [CFAS], 2009; Statistics Canada, 2009). ARTs are associated with many ethical and legal issues (Box 7-6). The Assisted Human Reproduction Act sets legislation for all aspects of ART in Canada. The act prohibits human cloning and other unacceptable activities, while protecting the health and safety of people who use ART (Government of Canada, 2004). Nurses can provide relevant information to couples so that they have an accurate understanding of their chances for a successful pregnancy and live birth and can make an informed decision. Couples need to be counselled about the risks of multiple births, to facilitate informed decision making regarding the number of embryos to transfer (Min et al., 2006). The implications of having a multiple birth need to be explored, including the risk of preterm birth, possible admission to special care nurseries, and increased morbidity for multiples. Nurses also can provide anticipatory guidance about the moral and ethical dilemmas regarding the use of ARTs. Some of the ARTs for treatment of infertility include in vitro fertilization–embryo transfer (IVF-ET), gamete intrafallopian transfer (GIFT) (Fig. 7-4), zygote intrafallopian transfer (ZIFT), ovum transfer (oocyte donation), embryo adoption, embryo hosting and surrogate parenting, and therapeutic donor insemination (TDI). Table 7-2 describes these procedures and the possible indications for ARTs. Other options include intracytoplasmic sperm injection, assisted hatching, and adoption.

LEGAL TIP Cryopreservation of Human Embryos. Couples who have excess embryos frozen for later transfer must be fully informed before consenting to the procedure in order to make decisions about the disposal of embryos in the event of death, divorce, or the decision at a later time that the couple no longer wants the embryos.

Complications

Most pregnancies achieved through ART are uncomplicated and result in the birth of healthy children, although a higher number of ART pregnancies are associated with

BOX 7-6 Issues to Be Addressed by Infertile Couples Before Using Assisted Reproductive Technologies

- Risks of multiple gestation
- Possible need for multifetal reduction
- Possible need for donor oocytes, sperm, or embryos or for gestational carrier (surrogate mother)
- Whether or how to disclose facts of conception to offspring
- Freezing embryos for later use
- Possible risks of long-term effects of medications and treatment on women, children, and families
- Cost of treatment (emotional, monetary, and time)

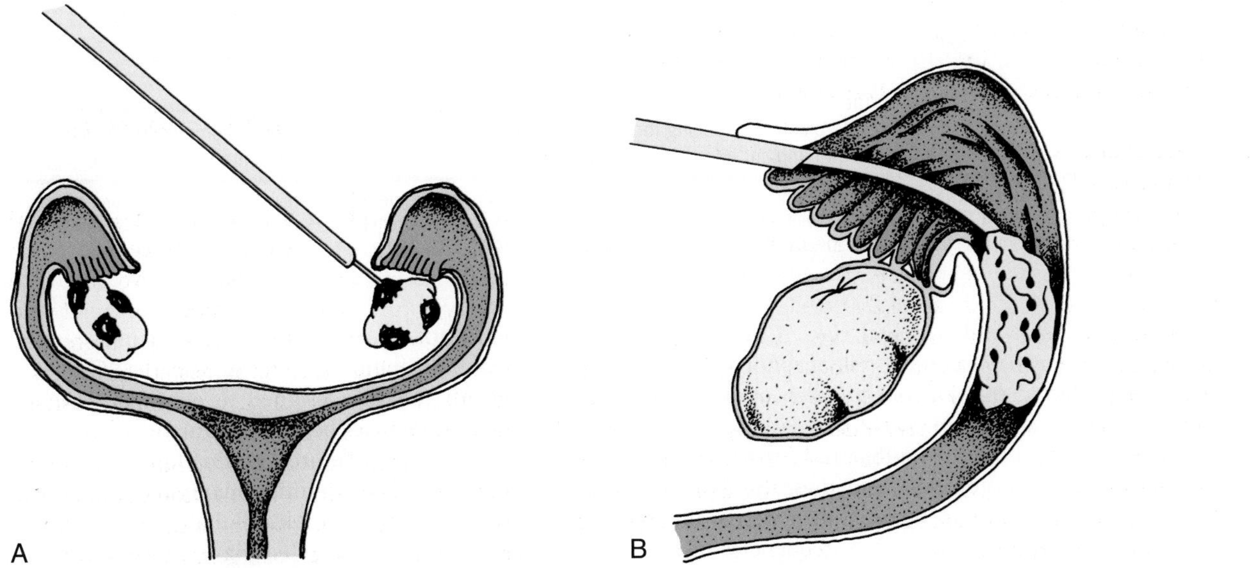

Fig. 7-4 Gamete intrafallopian transfer (GIFT). **A:** Through laparoscopy a ripe follicle is located, and fluid containing the egg is removed. **B:** The sperm and egg are placed separately in the uterine tube, where fertilization occurs.

Table 7-2 Assisted Reproductive Technologies

PROCEDURE	DEFINITION	INDICATIONS
In vitro fertilization–embryo transfer (IVF-ET)	A woman's eggs are collected from her ovaries, fertilized in the laboratory with sperm, and transferred to her uterus after normal embryo development has occurred.	Tubal disease or blockage; severe male infertility; endometriosis; unexplained infertility; cervical factor; immunological infertility
Gamete intrafallopian transfer (GIFT)	Oocytes are retrieved from the ovary, placed in a catheter with washed motile sperm, and immediately transferred into the fimbriated end of the uterine tube. Fertilization occurs in the uterine tube.	Same as for IVF-ET, except there must be normal tubal anatomy, patency, and absence of previous tubal disease in at least one uterine tube
IVF-ET and GIFT with donor sperm	This process is the same as that described previously except in cases where the husband's fertility is severely compromised and donor sperm can be used; if donor sperm are used, the wife must have indications for IVF and GIFT.	Severe male infertility; azoospermia; indications for IVF-ET or GIFT
Zygote intrafallopian transfer (ZIFT)	This process is similar to IVF-ET; after in vitro fertilization the ova are placed in one uterine tube during the zygote stage.	Same as for GIFT
Donor oocyte	Eggs are donated by an IVF procedure, and the donated eggs are inseminated. The embryos are transferred into the recipient's uterus, which is hormonally prepared with estrogen–progesterone therapy.	Early menopause; surgical removal of ovaries; congenitally absent ovaries; autosomal or sex-linked disorders; lack of fertilization in repeated IVF attempts because of subtle oocyte abnormalities or defects in oocyte–spermatozoa interaction; woman over 40 who may not want to risk chromosomal deficiency in her own eggs
Donor embryo (embryo adoption)	A donated embryo is transferred to the uterus of an infertile woman at the appropriate time (normal or induced) of the menstrual cycle.	Infertility not resolved by less aggressive forms of therapy; absence of ovaries; male partner is azoospermic or severely compromised
Gestational carrier (embryo host); surrogate mother	A couple undertakes an IVF cycle, and the embryo(s) is transferred to another woman's uterus (the carrier), who has contracted with the couple to carry the baby to term. The carrier has no genetic investment in the child. **Surrogate motherhood** is a process by which a woman is inseminated with semen from the infertile woman's partner and then carries the baby until birth.	Congenital absence or surgical removal of uterus; a reproductively impaired uterus, myomas, uterine adhesions, or other congenital abnormalities; a medical condition that might be life threatening during pregnancy, such as diabetes, immunological problems, or severe heart, kidney, or liver disease It is illegal in Canada to pay someone to be a surrogate.
Therapeutic donor insemination (TDI)	Donor sperm are used to inseminate the female partner.	Male partner is azoospermic or has a very low sperm count; couple has a genetic defect; male partner has antisperm antibodies; lesbian couple
Intracytoplasmic sperm injection	One sperm cell is selected to be injected directly into the egg to achieve fertilization. It is used with IVF.	Same as TDI
Assisted hatching	The zona pellucida is penetrated chemically or manually to create an opening for the dividing embryo to hatch and implant into the uterine wall.	Recurrent miscarriages; to improve implantation rate in women with previously unsuccessful IVF attempts; advanced age

(Data from American Society for Reproductive Medicine. [2008]. *Frequently asked questions about infertility*. Retrieved from www.asrm.org/awards/index.aspx?id=3012; Government of Canada. [2004]. *Assisted human reproduction act.* Ottawa: Minister of Justice. Retrieved from http://laws.justice.gc.ca/PDF/Statute/A/A-13.4.pdf; Van Voorhis, B. J. [2006]. Outcomes from assisted reproductive technology. *Obstetrics & Gynecology, 107*[1], 183–200.)

increased perinatal and neonatal risks. Children conceived through ART may have a higher risk of abnormalities than do children conceived spontaneously (Allen et al., 2006). Multiple gestations are more likely and are associated with increased risks for both the mother and fetuses. Ectopic pregnancies do occur more often, and these carry a significant maternal risk. There is no increase in maternal or perinatal complications with TDI; the same frequencies of anomalies (about 5%) and obstetric complications (between 5 and 10%) that accompany natural insemination (through sexual intercourse) also apply to TDI.

Preimplantation Genetic Diagnosis

Preimplantation genetic diagnosis (PGD) is a form of early genetic testing designed to eliminate embryos with serious genetic diseases before implantation through one of the ARTs and to avoid future termination of pregnancy for genetic reasons. Through micromanipulation, a single cell can be removed from a multicellular embryo for genetic study (i.e., embryo biopsy) (Georgia Reproductive Specialists, 2007; Kearnes et al., 2005). PGD is used clinically in over 20 centres around the world. Couples must be counselled about their options and choices and the implications of their choices when genetic analysis is considered. For example, the transfer of only embryos that are free from abnormalities can increase the implantation rate and decrease the miscarriage rate and may increase the likelihood of the birth of a healthy infant (Kearnes et al, 2005).

Adoption

Couples may choose to build their family by adopting children who are not their own biologically. With increased availability of birth control and abortion and an increase in single mothers who choose to keep their babies, the availability of White infants for adoption is extremely limited. Minority infants, infants with special needs, older children, and foreign adoptions are other options (Fig. 7-5). Many couples choosing adoption must invest significant time, emotional energy, and sometimes money into the process. Foreign adoptions can take years to complete and couples need to be aware of what the process involves.

Couples who decide to adopt a child have decided that being a parent is more important than the actual process of birthing the child. The birth process is a very small aspect of having a baby and becoming a parent. So much emphasis is placed on being pregnant and having a child composed of one's own genetic makeup that the focus of the reason to have a child gets obscured.

Contraception

Contraception is the intentional prevention of pregnancy during sexual intercourse. *Birth control* is the device or practice used to decrease the risk of conceiving, or bearing, offspring. *Family planning* is the conscious decision regarding when to conceive or to avoid pregnancy throughout the reproductive years. With the wide assortment of birth control options available, it is possible for a woman to use several different contraceptive methods at various stages throughout her fertile years. Nurses interact with the woman to compare and contrast available options, reliability, relative cost, protection from sexually transmitted infections (STIs), the individual's comfort level, and the partner's willingness to use a particular birth control method. Those who use contraception can still be at risk for pregnancy if their choice of contraceptive method is not perfect or is used incorrectly. Providing adequate instruction about how to use a contraceptive method, when to use a back-up method, and when to use emergency contraception can decrease the risk of unintended pregnancy.

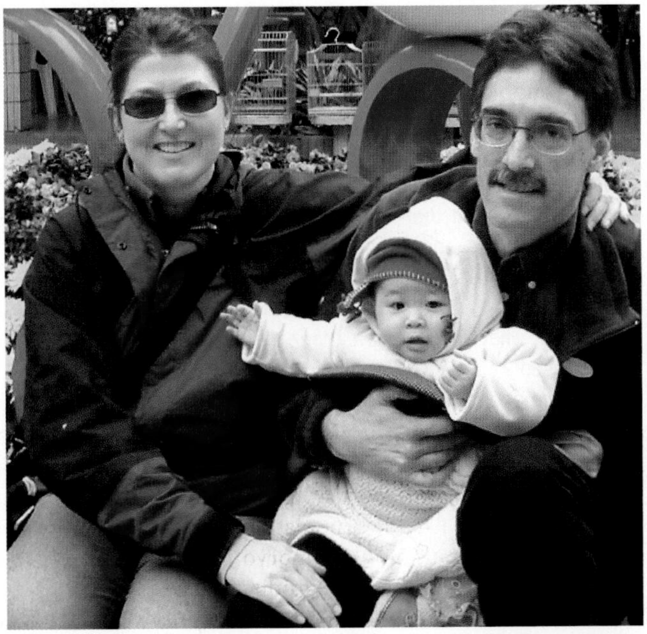

Fig. 7-5 After two miscarriages, this couple chose adoption. *(Courtesy Shannon Perry, Phoenix, AZ.)*

Nursing Care Management

A multidisciplinary approach may help in assisting a woman to choose and correctly use an appropriate contraceptive method (see Nursing Process box). Nurses, midwives, nurse practitioners, and other advanced practice nurses and physicians have the knowledge and expertise to assist a woman in making decisions about contraception that will satisfy the woman's personal, social, cultural, and interpersonal needs. These needs include appropriate spacing of pregnancies (see Evidence-Informed Practice box).

Unbiased patient teaching is fundamental to initiating and maintaining any form of contraception. The nurse needs to counter myths with facts, clarify misinformation, and fill in gaps of knowledge. The ideal contraceptive should be safe, easily available, economical, acceptable, simple to use, and promptly reversible. Although no method may ever achieve all of these objectives, significant advances in the development of new contraceptive technologies have occurred over the past 30 years.

Contraceptive failure rate refers to the percentage of contraceptive users expected to have an unplanned pregnancy during the first year even when they use a method consistently and correctly. Contraceptive effectiveness varies from couple to couple and depends on both the properties of the method and the characteristics of the user (Box 7-7). Failure rates decrease over time, either because a user gains experience with and uses a method more appropriately or because the less effective users stop using the method.

BOX 7-7 Factors Affecting Contraceptive Method Effectiveness

- Frequency of intercourse
- Motivation to prevent pregnancy
- Understanding of how to use the method
- Adherence to and consistent use of method—related to the method: cost, accessibility, ease of use, convenient, few or no side effects
- Provision of short-term or long-term protection
- Likelihood of pregnancy for the individual woman

NURSING PROCESS: CONTRACEPTION

Assessment

Obtain a history (including menstrual, contraceptive, and obstetric).
Perform a physical examination (including pelvic examination).
Complete laboratory tests.
Determine the woman's knowledge about contraception and her sexual partner's commitment to any particular method.
Obtain data about the frequency of coitus, number of sexual partners, level of contraceptive involvement, and her or her partner's objections to any specific method(s).
Assess the woman's level of comfort and willingness to touch her genitals and cervical mucus.
Identify myths and determine religious and cultural factors.
Carefully note the woman's verbal and nonverbal responses to hearing about the various available methods. An individual's reproductive life plan must be considered.

Nursing Diagnoses

Decisional conflict related to
- contraceptive alternatives
- partner's willingness to agree on a contraceptive method

Risk for infection related to
- unprotected sexual intercourse
- use of contraceptive method
- broken skin or mucous membrane secondary to surgery, intrauterine device insertion, or hormonal implant

Spiritual distress related to
- discrepancy between religious or cultural beliefs and choice of contraception

Planning

Expected outcomes are that the woman will do the following:
- Communicate understanding about contraceptive methods
- State comfort and satisfaction with the method chosen
- Use the contraceptive method correctly and consistently
- Experience no adverse sequelae as a result of the chosen method of contraception
- Prevent unplanned pregnancy or plan a pregnancy

Interventions

Informed consent is a vital component in the education of the woman concerning contraception or sterilization.
The nurse has the responsibility of documenting information provided and the woman's understanding of that information.
Counter myths with facts, clarify misinformation, and fill in gaps of knowledge (see pp. 136–152).

Evaluation

The nurse can be reasonably assured that care was effective when the patient-centred expected outcomes have been achieved: the woman and her partner learn about the various methods of contraception, the couple achieves pregnancy only when planned, and they have no adverse sequelae as a result of the chosen method of contraception.

Safety of a method depends on the woman's medical history. Barrier methods offer some protection from STIs, and oral contraceptives may lower the incidence of ovarian and endometrial cancer but have a slightly increased risk of thromboembolic problems.

Methods of Contraception

The following discussion of contraceptive methods provides the nurse with information needed for patient teaching. After implementing the appropriate teaching for contraceptive use, the nurse will supervise return demonstrations and practice to assess patient understanding (see Critical Thinking Exercise). The woman is given written instructions and telephone numbers for questions. If the woman has difficulty understanding written instructions, she (and her partner, if available) should be offered graphic material and a telephone number to call, as necessary, or an opportunity to return for further instruction.

Coitus Interruptus

Coitus interruptus (withdrawal) involves the male partner withdrawing his penis from the woman's vagina before he

evolve Critical Thinking Exercise—Patient Teaching: Contraception

CRITICAL THINKING EXERCISE

Contraception for Adolescents

Marie is a 16-year-old First Nations young woman who comes to the Nursing Station, on the reserve, seeking contraception. She has recently become sexually active and tells the nurse that she is concerned that her mother will find out. She also has many questions about the type of contraception to use. She seeks the nurse's advice to help in her decision making.

1. Evidence—Is there sufficient evidence to draw conclusions about what advice to give Marie? What is the age of consent?
2. Assumptions—What assumptions can be made about contraception for adolescents (types, legal issues, and implications of culture on choice)?
3. What implications and priorities for nursing care can be drawn at this time?
4. Does the evidence objectively support your conclusion?
5. Are there alternative perspectives to your conclusion?

EVIDENCE-INFORMED PRACTICE Optimal Birth Spacing

—*Pat Gingrich*

Ask the Question

What interval between pregnancies is optimal for maternal and neonatal health?

Search for Evidence

Search Strategies

Professional organization guidelines, meta-analyses, systematic reviews, randomized controlled trials, nonrandomized prospective studies, and retrospective studies since 2006

Databases Searched

CINAHL, Cochrane, Medline, National Guideline Clearinghouse, TRIP Database Plus, and the Web sites for the Association for Women's Health, Obstetric and Neonatal Nurses (AWHONN), Centers for Disease Prevention and Control (CDC), Family Health International, Planned Parenthood, and World Health Organization (WHO)

Critically Analyze the Evidence

In a systematic review of 22 eligible studies (Dewey & Cohen, 2007), the interpregnancy interval (IPI) was defined as the time between the end of one pregnancy and the beginning of the next. In some countries, a longer IPI was associated with a significantly lower risk of child malnutrition. The risk of stunting (height-for-age greater than 2 standard deviations [SD] below the normal range) is decreased if the IPI is 36 months or more. In a Canadian cohort of 98,330 women, being unmarried increases the risk for small-for-gestational-age status in an IPI of less than 12 months (Auger et al., 2008).

Dewey and Cohen (2007) further speculated that breastfeeding may place additional nutritional pressure on the women. Eight studies showed no link between the recuperative interval (the time between weaning and subsequent pregnancy) and maternal weight or body mass index. Four studies they reviewed showed no relationship between IPI and maternal micronutrients, most notably anemia.

In another systematic review of 22 eligible studies (Conde-Agudelo, Rosas-Bermúdez, & Kafury-Goeta, 2007), a longer IPI was associated with an increased risk for pre-eclampsia, especially after 5 years. Some speculate that, as that much time passes, the woman's immune system becomes resensitized to foreign protein, much like that of a nulliparous woman. Similarly, women who experienced labour dystocia showed a decreased risk of dystocia in subsequent labours, but that protective effect faded as the IPI lengthened. Short IPI (less than 18 months) was associated with bleeding (placenta previa and abruption), premature rupture of membranes, endometritis, and maternal mortality. Women attempting trial of labour after undergoing Caesarean section were more at risk for uterine rupture and blood transfusion with a short IPI, especially if the IPI was less than 6 months.

A study in India of 80,164 women demonstrated that births spaced 36 to 59 months apart resulted in fewer stillbirths and neonatal deaths than with either shorter or longer birth intervals (Williams et al., 2008).

In a prospective comparative study of 562 births, Rodrigues and Barros (2008) demonstrated that an IPI of less than 6 months increased the risk for early preterm birth (less than 34 weeks of gestation) but had no effect on late preterm birth (34 to 37 weeks of gestation). Similarly, in a population-based cohort study of 156,330 women, DeFranco et al. (2007) found an increasing risk of preterm birth as the IPI decreased.

Implications for Practice

There is strong evidence that avoiding pregnancy for at least a year after birth, especially after a Caesarean birth, contributes to maternal and neonatal health. Single marital status, a marker for psychosocial stressors, may heighten the negative effects on fetal growth when the IPI is less than 12 months. Optimal interpregnancy interval will enable the woman's body to fully recover from the previous pregnancy and birth to provide adequate nutrition to herself and a subsequent fetus, while retaining the protective effects against recurrent dystocia and pre-eclampsia. An IPI of 18 to 36 months seems to meet these criteria.

Implications for Contraception

Such a window of time might comfortably include such highly effective methods as an intrauterine device, Depo-Provera for the first year, and combined hormonal contraceptives after weaning.

References

Auger, N., et al. (2008). The joint influence of marital status, interpregnancy interval, and neighborhood on small for gestational age birth: A retrospective cohort study. *BMC Pregnancy and Childbirth, 28*(8), 7.

Conde-Agudelo, A., Rosas-Bermúdez, A., & Kafury-Goeta, A. C. (2007). Effects of birth spacing on maternal health: A systematic review. *American Journal of Obstetrics and Gynecology, 196*(4), 297–308.

DeFranco, E. A., et al. (2007). A short interpregnancy interval is a risk factor for preterm birth and recurrence. *American Journal of Obstetrics and Gynecology, 197*(3), 264.e1–6.

Dewey, K. G., & Cohen, R. J. (2007). Does birth spacing affect maternal or child nutritional status? A systematic literature review. *Maternal and Child Nutrition, 3*(3), 151–173.

Rodrigues, T., & Barros, H. (2008). Short interpregnancy interval and risk of spontaneous preterm delivery. *European Journal of Obstetrics and Gynecology and Reproductive Biology, 136*(2), 184–188.

Williams, E. K., et al. (2008). Birth interval and risk of stillbirth or neonatal death: Findings from rural north India. *Journal of Tropical Pediatrics, 54*(5), 321–327.

ejaculates. Although coitus interruptus has been criticized as being an ineffective method of contraception, it is a good choice for couples who do not have another contraceptive available. Effectiveness is similar to barrier methods and depends on the man's ability to withdraw his penis before ejaculation. The percentage of women who will experience an unintended pregnancy within the first year of typical use (failure rate) of withdrawal is about 19% (Sexualityandu, 2010a). Coitus interruptus does not protect against STIs or human immunodeficiency virus (HIV) infection.

Natural Birth Control Methods

With natural birth control methods, women learn how to determine the beginning and the end of the fertile period of their menstrual cycle. Fertility awareness methods (FAMs) of contraception refer to a natural birth control method outside of a religious framework that supports the use of barrier methods (condom, diaphragm, and spermicide), emergency contraception, and abortion. **Natural family planning (NFP)** typically refers to natural birth control that is taught and practised within a religious framework, most commonly

Catholic-centred organizations. It does not support the use of barrier methods, emergency contraception, or abortion. When women who want to use FAM/NFP are educated about the menstrual cycle, three phases are identified:

1. Infertile phase: before ovulation
2. Fertile phase: about 5 to 7 days around the middle of the cycle, including several days before and during ovulation and the day afterward
3. Infertile phase: after ovulation

The human ovum must be fertilized no later than 16 to 24 hours after ovulation. While motile sperm have been recovered from the uterus and the oviducts as long as 7 days after **coitus**, their ability to fertilize the ovum probably lasts no longer than 24 to 48 hours. Pregnancy is unlikely to occur if a couple abstains from intercourse for 4 days before and 3 or 4 days after ovulation (fertile period). Unprotected intercourse on the other days of the cycle (safe period) should not result in pregnancy.

Although ovulation can be unpredictable in many women, teaching the woman about how she can directly observe her fertility patterns is an empowering tool. There are many categories of natural birth control methods. To prevent pregnancy, each one uses a combination of charts, records, calculations, tools, observations, and either abstinence (NFP) or barrier methods of birth control during the fertile period in the menstrual cycle. The charts and calculations associated with these methods can also be used to increase the likelihood of detecting the optimal timing of intercourse to achieve conception.

Advantages of these methods include low-to-no cost, absence of chemicals and hormones, and lack of alteration in the menstrual flow pattern. Disadvantages of FAM/NFP include adherence to strict record keeping, 3 to 6 cycles to learn, unintentional interference from external influences that may alter the woman's core body temperature and vaginal secretions, decreased effectiveness in women with irregular cycles (particularly adolescents who have not established regular ovulatory patterns), decreased spontaneity of coitus, and attending time-consuming training sessions by qualified instructors. The effectiveness of natural birth control methods depends on the users' adherence to the plan. For the typical user, who may not follow all the rules, the effectiveness of FAM/NFP is 75 to 88% (Sexualityandu, 2010a). Natural birth control methods do not protect against STIs or HIV infection. FAM/NFP methods involve several techniques to identify high-risk, fertile days. The following discussion includes the most common techniques, as well as some promising techniques for the future.

Calendar Rhythm Method

Practice of the calendar rhythm method is based on the number of days in each cycle, counting from the first day of menses. The fertile period is determined after accurately recording the length of menstrual cycles for 6 months. The beginning of the fertile period is estimated by subtracting 18 days from the length of the shortest cycle. The end of the fertile period is determined by subtracting 11 days from the length of the longest cycle. If the shortest cycle is 24 days and the longest is 30 days, application of the formula to calculate the fertile period is as follows:

Shortest cycle, 24 − 18 = day 6
Longest cycle, 30 − 11 = day 19

To avoid conception, the couple would abstain during the fertile period, days 6 through 19.

If the woman has very regular cycles of 28 days each, the formula indicates the fertile days to be as follows:

Shortest cycle, 28 − 18 = day 10
Longest cycle, 28 − 11 = day 17

To avoid conception, the couple would abstain from days 10 through 17 because ovulation occurs on day 14 ± 2 days. A major drawback of the calendar method is that one is trying to predict future events with past data. The unpredictability of the menstrual cycle is also not taken into consideration. The calendar rhythm method alone is not recommended as a reliable method of birth control and is most useful as an adjunct to the basal body temperature (BBT) or cervical mucus method.

Standard Days Method

The standard days method (SDM) is essentially a modified form of the calendar rhythm method that has a "fixed" number of days of fertility for each cycle (i.e., days 8 to 19). A CycleBeads necklace (i.e., a colour-coded string of beads) can be purchased as a tool to track fertility (Fig. 7-6). Day 1 of the menstrual flow is counted as the first day to begin the counting. Women who use this device are taught to avoid unprotected intercourse on days 8 to 19 (white beads on CycleBeads necklace). Although this method is useful to women whose cycles are 26 to 32 days long, it is unreliable for those who have longer or shorter cycles (CycleBeads, 2007). This is the least effective natural birth control method and is not generally recommended (Sexualityandu, 2010a).

Basal Body Temperature (BBT) Method

The **basal body temperature (BBT)** is the lowest body temperature of a healthy person, taken immediately after waking and before getting out of bed. The BBT usually varies from 36.2° to 36.3°C during menses and for approximately 5 to 7 days afterward (Fig. 7-7).

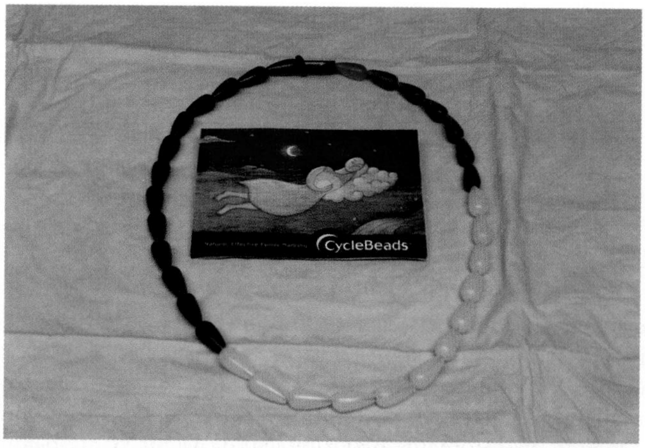

Fig. 7-6 CycleBeads. Red bead marks the first day of the menstrual cycle. White beads mark days that are likely to be fertile days; therefore, unprotected intercourse should be avoided. Brown beads are days when pregnancy is unlikely and unprotected intercourse is permitted. *(Courtesy Dee Lowdermilk, Chapel Hill, NC.)*

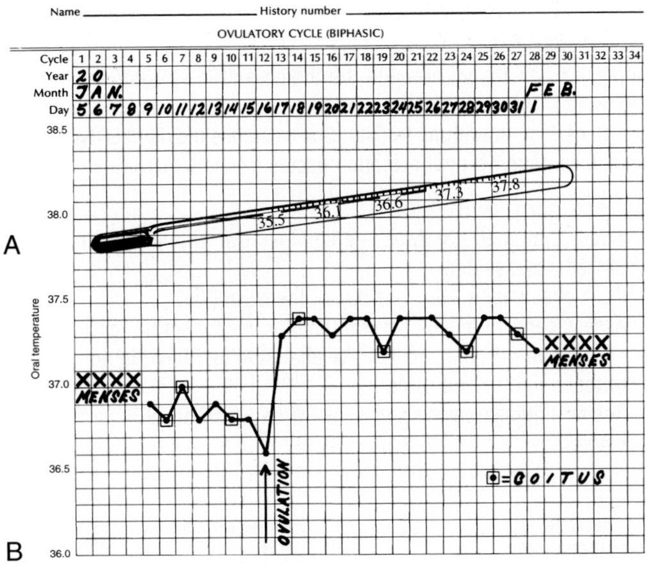

Fig. 7-7 **A:** Special thermometer for recording basal body temperature, marked in tenths to enable the person to read more easily. **B:** Basal temperature record shows decrease and sharp increase at time of ovulation. Biphasic curve indicates ovulatory cycle.

About the time of ovulation, a slight drop in temperature (approximately 0.5°C) may occur in some women, but others may have no decrease at all. After ovulation, in concert with the increasing progesterone levels of the early luteal phase of the cycle, the BBT increases slightly (approximately 0.4° to 0.8°C). The temperature remains on an elevated plateau until 2 to 4 days before menstruation. Then it decreases to the low levels recorded during the previous cycle unless pregnancy has occurred. In that event, the temperature remains elevated. If ovulation fails to occur, the pattern of lower body temperature continues throughout the cycle.

To use this method, the fertile period is defined as the day of first temperature drop, or first elevation, through 3 consecutive days of elevated temperature. Abstinence begins the first day of menstrual bleeding and lasts through 3 consecutive days of sustained temperature rise (at least 0.2°C). The decrease and subsequent increase in temperature are referred to as the *thermal shift*. When the entire month's temperatures are recorded on a graph, the pattern described is more apparent. It is more difficult to perceive day-to-day variations without the entire picture (see Guidelines box). Infection, fatigue, less than 3 hours of sleep per night, awakening late, and anxiety may cause temperature fluctuations and alter the expected pattern. If a new BBT thermometer is purchased, this fact is noted on the chart because the readings may vary slightly. Jet lag, alcohol taken the evening before, or sleeping in a heated waterbed must also be noted on the chart because each affects the BBT. Therefore, the BBT alone is not a reliable method of predicting ovulation.

Cervical Mucus Ovulation-Detection Method

The cervical mucus ovulation-detection method (Billings method; Creighton model ovulation method) requires that the woman recognize and interpret the cyclic changes in the amount and consistency of cervical mucus that characterize her own unique pattern of changes. The cervical mucus that accompanies ovulation is necessary for viability and motility of sperm. Without adequate cervical mucus, coitus does not result in conception. To learn the cycle, women check the quantity and character of mucus on the vulva or introitus with their fingers or with tissue paper each day for several months. To ensure an accurate assessment of changes, the cervical mucus should be free from semen, contraceptive gels or foams, and blood or discharge from vaginal infections for at least one full cycle. Other factors that create difficulty in identifying mucus changes include douches and vaginal deodorants, being in the sexually aroused state (which thins the mucus), and taking medications such as antihistamines, which dry the mucus. Intercourse is considered safe without restriction beginning on the fourth day after the last day of wet, clear, slippery mucus (postovulation).

Some women find this method unacceptable if they are uncomfortable touching their genitals. Regardless of whether a woman wants to use this method for contraception, it is to her advantage to learn to recognize mucus characteristics at ovulation (see Guidelines box). Self-evaluation of cervical mucus can be highly accurate and useful diagnostically for any of the following purposes:

- To alert the couple to the re-establishment of ovulation while breastfeeding and after discontinuation of oral contraception
- To note anovulatory cycles at any time and at the beginning of menopause
- To assist couples in planning a pregnancy

Symptothermal Method

The symptothermal method is the most reliable natural birth control method. This method combines the BBT and cervical mucus methods with awareness of secondary, cycle phase–related symptoms. The woman gains fertility awareness as she learns the psychological and physiological symptoms that mark the phases of her cycle. Secondary symptoms include increased libido, midcycle spotting, mittelschmerz, pelvic fullness or tenderness, and vulvar fullness.

GUIDELINES Basal Body Temperature

- Discuss basal body temperature (BBT) with the woman.
- Show the woman a diagram depicting the phases of the menstrual cycle.
- Discuss the hormones in the woman's body that are responsible for her menstrual cycle and ovulation.
- Show the woman a sample BBT graph (see Fig. 7-7) and the biphasic line seen in ovulatory cycles.
- Show the woman the BBT thermometer and how it is calibrated.
- Provide a demonstration of how to take an oral temperature.
- Encourage the woman to demonstrate taking and reading the thermometer and graphing the temperature while the nurse watches.
- Encourage the woman to start a log to keep track of any other activity that might interfere with her true BBT.

GUIDELINES Cervical Mucus Characteristics

Setting the Stage

- Show charts of the menstrual cycle along with changes in the cervical mucus.
- Have the woman practise with raw egg white.
- Supply her with a basal body temperature (BBT) log and graph if she does not already have one.
- Explain that the assessment of cervical mucus characteristics is best when mucus is not mixed with semen, contraceptive jellies or foams, or discharge from infections.

Content Related to Cervical Mucus

- Explain to the woman (or couple) how cervical mucus changes throughout the menstrual cycle.

Right before ovulation the thick mucus becomes more watery, thin and clear. It feels like a lubricant and can be stretched approximately 12 cm between the thumb and forefinger (similar to egg white); this is called *spinnbarkeit*. This characteristic indicates the period of maximum fertility. Sperm deposited in this type of mucus can survive until ovulation occurs.

Assessment Technique

- Stress that good handwashing is imperative to begin and end all self-assessment.
- Start observation from last day of menstrual flow.
- Assess cervical mucus several times a day for several cycles. Mucus can be obtained from vaginal introitus; there is no need to reach into vagina to cervix.
- Record findings on the same record on which her BBT is entered.

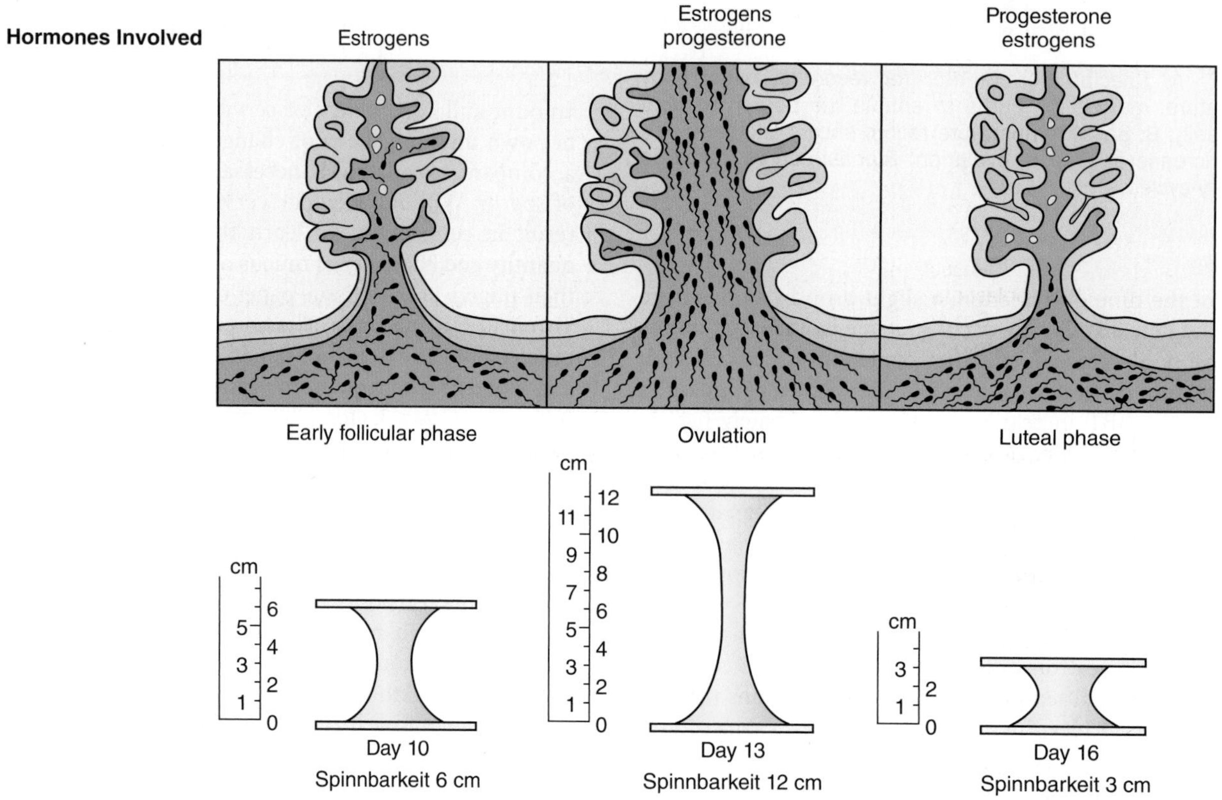

Cervical changes are a third sign that may be used to determine fertility. The woman is taught to palpate her cervix to assess for changes indicating ovulation: the cervical os dilates slightly, the cervix softens and rises in the vagina, and cervical mucus is copious and slippery. The woman notes days on which coitus, changes in routine, and illness have occurred (Fig. 7-8). Calendar calculations and cervical mucus changes are used to estimate the onset of the fertile period; changes in cervical mucus or the BBT are used to estimate its end.

If a woman's cycle does not follow a regular pattern, the use of natural birth control methods may be more difficult. In general, FAM/NFP methods are not recommended for women with the following difficulties: irregular cycles, inability to interpret the fertility signs correctly, or persistent infections that affect the signs of fertility (Sexualityandu, 2010a).

Home Predictor Test Kits for Ovulation

All the methods previously discussed are indicative of ovulation but do not prove its occurrence or exact timing. The urine predictor test for ovulation is a major addition to the NFP/FAM methods to help women who want to plan the time of their pregnancies and for those who are trying to conceive (Fig. 7-9). The urine predictor test for ovulation detects the sudden surge of LH that occurs approximately 12 to 24 hours before ovulation. Unlike BBT, the test is not affected by illness, emotional upset, or physical activity. For home use, a test kit contains sufficient material for several days' testing during

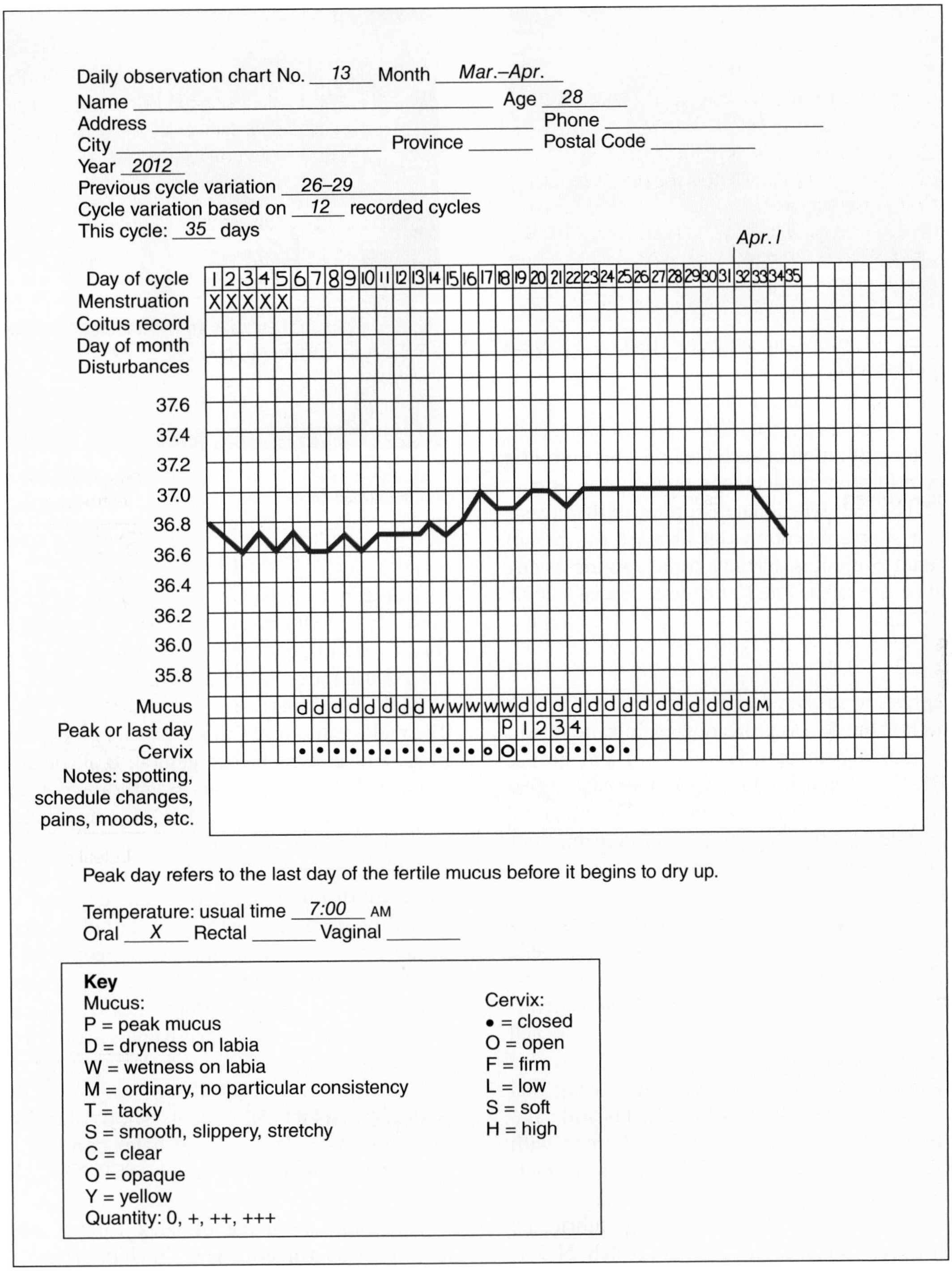

Fig. 7-8 Example of completed symptothermal chart.

each cycle. A positive response indicating an LH surge is noted by a colour change that is easy to read. Directions for use of urine predictor test kits vary with the manufacturer. Saliva predictor tests for ovulation use dried, nonfoamy saliva as a tool to show fertility patterns. More research is needed to determine the efficacy of use of these tests for pregnancy prevention.

Breastfeeding: Lactational Amenorrhea Method

The lactational amenorrhea method (LAM) can be a highly effective, temporary method of birth control. It is more popular in underdeveloped countries and traditional societies where breastfeeding is used to prolong birth intervals.

When the infant suckles at the mother's breast, a surge of prolactin hormone is released, which inhibits estrogen production and suppresses ovulation and the return of menses. LAM works best if the mother is exclusively or almost exclusively breastfeeding, if the woman has not had a menstrual flow since giving birth, and if the infant is under 6 months of age. Effectiveness is enhanced by frequent feedings at intervals of less than 4 hours during the day and no more than 6 hours

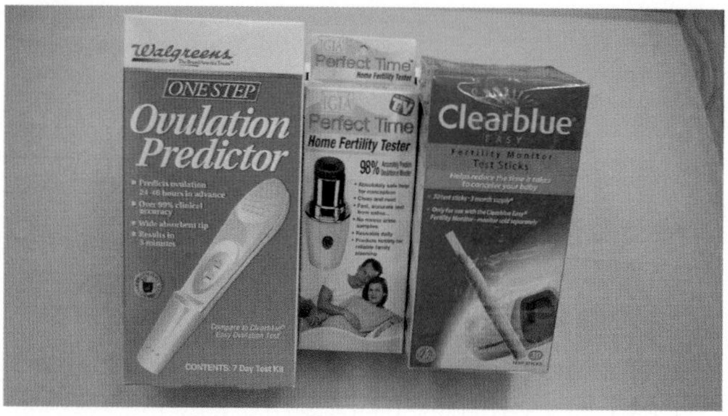

Fig. 7-9 Examples of ovulation predictor tests. *(Courtesy Shannon Perry, Phoenix, AZ.)*

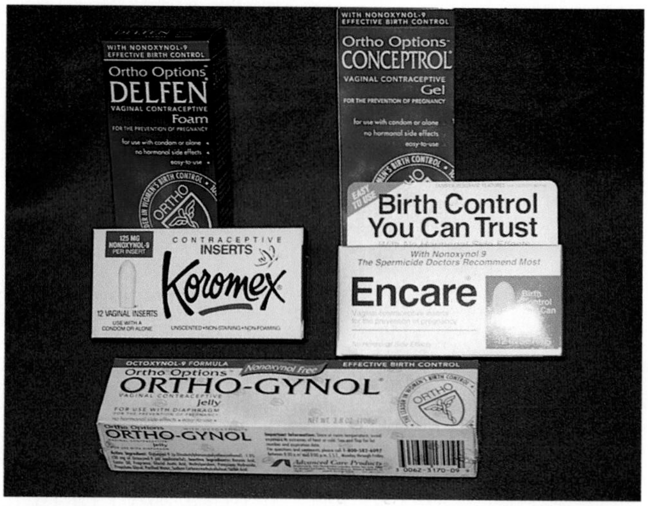

Fig. 7-10 Spermicides. *(Courtesy Marjorie Pyle, RNC, Life Circle, Costa Mesa, CA.)*

during the night, long duration of each feeding, and no bottle supplementation or limited supplementation by spoon or cup. The woman should be counselled that disruption of the breastfeeding pattern or supplementation can increase the risk of pregnancy and after 6 months, fertility could resume at any time. The typical failure rate is 2% (Kennedy & Trussell, 2007; Sexualityandu, 2010a).

Barrier Methods

Barrier contraceptives have gained in popularity not only as a contraceptive method but also as protection against the spread of STIs such as human papilloma virus (HPV) and herpes simplex virus (HSV). Some male condoms and female vaginal methods provide a physical barrier to several STIs, and some male condoms provide protection against HIV. **Spermicides** serve as chemical barriers against the sperm.

Spermicides

Spermicides such as nonoxynol-9 (N-9) work by reducing the sperm's mobility; the chemicals attack the sperm flagella and body, thereby preventing the sperm from reaching the cervical os. N-9, the most commonly used spermicidal chemical in Canada, is a surfactant that destroys the sperm cell membrane; however, data now suggest that frequent use (more than two times a day) of N-9 or use as a lubricant during anal intercourse may increase the transmission of STIs and HIV and can cause lesions (Sexualityandu, 2010b). Women with high-risk behaviours that increase their likelihood of contracting HIV and other STIs are advised to avoid the use of spermicidal products containing N-9, including lubricated condoms, diaphragms, and cervical caps to which N-9 is added (Sexualityandu, 2010b; Society of Obstetricians and Gynaecologists Canada [SOGC], 2004).

Intravaginal spermicides are marketed and sold without prescriptions as aerosol foams, tablets, suppositories, creams, films, and gels (Fig. 7-10). Preloaded, single-dose applicators small enough to be carried in a small purse are available. Effectiveness of spermicides depends on consistent and accurate use. Not more than 1 hour before sexual intercourse, the spermicide should be inserted high into the vagina so that it makes contact with the cervix. Spermicide must be reapplied for each additional act of intercourse, even if a barrier method is used. Studies have shown varying effectiveness rates for spermicidal use alone. Spermicide can also be used as a form of emergency contraception if inserted immediately after an accident with another contraceptive method. The failure rate for the use of spermicide is 21% for typical use and 6% for perfect use (Sexualityandu, 2010b).

Male Condoms

The male condom is a thin, stretchable sheath that covers the penis and is used before genital, oral, or anal contact. It is removed when the penis is withdrawn from the partner's orifice after ejaculation (Fig. 7-11, A). Condoms lubricated with N-9 are not recommended for preventing STIs or HIV (Health Canada, 2010a). Latex condoms break down with oil-based lubricants (e.g., petroleum jelly and suntan oil) and should be used only with water-based or silicone lubricants. Because of the growing number of people with latex allergies, condom manufacturers have begun using polyurethane, which is thinner and stronger than latex. Research is being conducted to determine the effectiveness of polyurethane condoms in protecting against STIs and HIV.

NURSING ALERT All patients should be questioned about the potential for latex allergy. Latex condom use is contraindicated for patients with latex sensitivity.

Condoms are made of latex rubber, which provides a barrier to sperm and STIs (including HIV); polyurethane (strong, thin plastic); or natural membranes (animal tissue). In addition to providing a physical barrier for sperm, nonspermicidal latex condoms also provide a barrier for STIs (particularly gonorrhea, chlamydia, and trichomonas) and HIV transmission. A small percentage of condoms are made from lamb cecum (natural skin). Natural skin condoms do not provide the same protection against STIs and HIV infection as that of latex condoms. Natural skin condoms contain small pores that could allow passage of viruses such as hepatitis B, HSV, and HIV.

A functional difference in condom shape is the presence or absence of a sperm reservoir tip. To enhance vaginal stimulation, some condoms are contoured and rippled or have ribbed

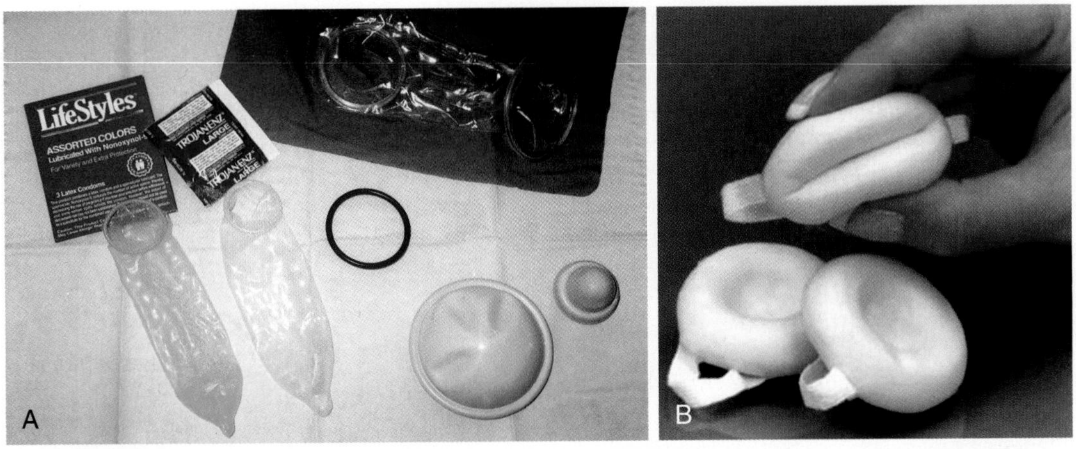

Fig. 7-11 A: Mechanical barriers. Clockwise from top: female condom, cervical cap, diaphragm, types of male condoms, vaginal ring (hormonal) (centre). B: Contraceptive sponge. *(A, Courtesy Donna Rowe, University of North Carolina Student Health, Chapel Hill, NC. B, Courtesy Allendale Pharmaceuticals, Inc., Allendale, NJ.)*

or roughened surfaces. Thinner construction increases heat transmission and sensitivity; a variety of colours increases their acceptability and attractiveness. A wet jelly or dry powder lubricates some condoms. Spermicide is added to the interior or exterior surfaces of some condoms. Typical failure rate for the first year of use of the male condom is 15%.

NURSING ALERT It is a false assumption that everyone knows how to use condoms. To prevent unintended pregnancy and the spread of STIs, it is essential that condoms be used correctly. Proper instruction in use must be provided (Box 7-8). All types of condoms must be discarded after each single use. They are available without prescription.

Female Condoms

The female condom is a vaginal sheath made of polyurethane and has flexible rings at both ends (see Fig. 7-11, A). The closed end of the pouch is inserted into the vagina and anchored around the cervix; the open ring covers the labia. Women whose partners will not wear a male condom can use this as a protective mechanical barrier. Rewetting drops or oil- or water-based lubricants can be used to help decrease the distracting noise that is produced while penile thrusting occurs. The female condom is available in one size, is intended for single use only, and is sold over the counter. Disadvantages include difficulty for some women to insert them correctly and the cost per use. The female condom can also be inserted into the anus of both men and women for anal intercourse. When used this way, the inner ring of the condom is inserted into the rectum and the outside ring rests on the anus. Male condoms should not be used concurrently because the friction from both sheaths can increase the likelihood of either or both tearing (Canadian Federation for Sexual Health [CFSH], 2008a). Used perfectly, the failure rate is 5% (Sexualityandu, 2010b).

Diaphragm

The contraceptive **diaphragm** is a shallow, dome-shaped, latex or silicone device with a flexible rim that covers the cervix (see Fig. 7-11, A). The diaphragm is a mechanical barrier to the meeting of sperm with the ovum. By holding spermicide in place against the cervix for the 6 hours it takes to destroy the sperm, the diaphragm also provides a chemical barrier to pregnancy. Diaphragms are available in a wide range of diameters (50 to 95 mm) and differ in the inner construction of the circular rim. The types of rims are coil spring, arcing spring, and wide-seal rim. The diaphragm should be the largest size the woman can wear without being aware of its presence. It is 80 to 94% effective depending on how well the diaphragm is used (CFSH, 2009).

Nursing Considerations. The woman using a diaphragm needs an annual gynecological examination to assess the fit of the diaphragm. The device should be replaced every 2 years and may need to be refitted after a 20% weight loss or gain, term birth, or second-trimester miscarriage and after any abdominal or pelvic surgery (Planned Parenthood, 2008). Because various types of diaphragms are on the market, the nurse should use the package insert when teaching the woman how to use and care for the diaphragm (see Home Care box).

Disadvantages of diaphragm use include the reluctance of some women to insert and remove the diaphragm. Although it can be inserted up to 6 hours before intercourse, a cold diaphragm and a cold gel temporarily reduce vaginal response to sexual stimulation if insertion of the diaphragm occurs immediately before intercourse. Some women or couples object to the messiness of the spermicide. These annoyances of diaphragm use, along with failure to insert the device once foreplay has begun, are the most common reasons for failures of this method. Side effects may include irritation of tissues related to contact with spermicides. The diaphragm is not a good option for women with poor vaginal muscle tone or recurrent urinary tract infections.

For proper placement, the diaphragm must rest behind the pubic symphysis and completely cover the cervix. To decrease the chance of exerting urethral pressure, the woman should be reminded to empty her bladder before diaphragm insertion and immediately after intercourse.

Diaphragms are contraindicated for women with pelvic relaxation (uterine prolapse) or a large **cystocele**. **Toxic shock**

BOX 7-8 Male Condoms

Mechanism of Action

The sheath is applied over the erect penis before insertion or loss of pre-ejaculatory drops of semen. Used correctly, condoms prevent sperm from entering the cervix. Spermicide-coated condoms cause ejaculated sperm to be immobilized rapidly, thus increasing contraceptive effectiveness.

Failure Rate

- Typical users, 15%
- Correct and consistent users, 3%

Advantages

- Safe
- No side effects
- Readily available
- Premalignant changes in cervix can be prevented or ameliorated in women whose partners use condoms
- Method of male nonsurgical contraception

Disadvantages

- Lovemaking must be interrupted to apply sheath.
- Sensation may be altered.
- If used improperly, spillage of sperm can result in pregnancy.
- Condoms occasionally may tear during intercourse.

STI Protection

If a condom is used throughout the act of intercourse and there is no unprotected contact with female genitals, a latex rubber condom, which is impermeable to viruses, can act as a protective measure against sexually transmitted infections.

Nursing Considerations

Teach the man or woman or both to do the following:

- Use a new condom (check expiration date) for each act of sexual intercourse or other acts between partners that involve contact with the penis.
- Place the condom after the penis is erect and before intimate contact.
- Place the condom on the head of the penis (A) and unroll it all the way to the base (B).
- Leave an empty space at the tip (A); remove any air remaining in the tip by gently pressing air out toward the base of the penis.

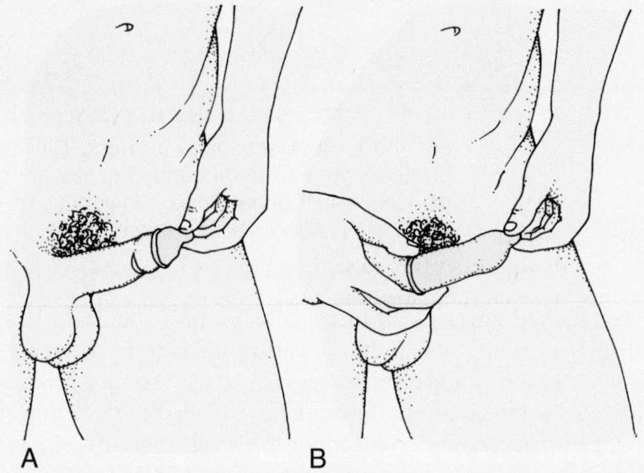

- If a lubricant is desired, use water-based products such as K-Y lubricating jelly. Do not use petroleum-based products because they can cause the condom to break.
- After ejaculation, carefully withdraw the still-erect penis from the vagina, holding onto the condom rim; remove and discard the condom.
- Store unused condoms in a cool, dry place.
- Do not use condoms that are sticky, brittle, or obviously damaged.

syndrome (TSS), although reported in very small numbers, can occur in association with the use of the contraceptive diaphragm and cervical caps. The nurse should instruct the woman about ways to reduce her risk for TSS. These measures include prompt removal 6 to 8 hours after intercourse, not using the diaphragm or cervical caps during menses, and learning and watching for danger signs of TSS.

NURSING ALERT The nurse should alert the woman who uses a diaphragm or cervical cap as a contraceptive method for signs of TSS. The most common signs include a sunburn type of rash, diarrhea, dizziness, faintness, weakness, sore throat, aching muscles and joints, sudden high fever, and vomiting.

Cervical Cap

The **cervical cap** is made of silicone rubber and has a soft dome and firm brim (see Fig. 7-11, A). The cap fits snugly around the base of the cervix close to the junction of the cervix and vaginal fornices. It is recommended that the cap remain in place no less than 6 hours and not more than 48 hours at a time. It is left in place at least 6 hours after the last act of intercourse. The seal provides a physical barrier to sperm. The extended period of wear may be an added convenience for women.

Instructions for the actual insertion and use of the cervical cap closely resemble the instructions for use of the contraceptive diaphragm. Some of the differences are that the cervical cap can be inserted hours before sexual intercourse and remain in for 48 hours but spermicide needs to be applied with each sexual encounter.

Nursing Considerations. The angle of the uterus, the vaginal muscle tone, and the shape of the cervix may interfere with the ease of fitting and use of the cervical cap. Correct fitting requires time, effort, and skill of both the woman and the clinician (see Home Care box). The woman must check the position of the cap before and after each act of intercourse.

Because of the potential risk of TSS associated with the use of the cervical cap, another form of birth control is recommended for use during menstrual bleeding and up to at least 6 weeks postpartum. The cap should be refitted after any

HOME CARE

Use and Care of the Diaphragm

Positions for Insertion of Diaphragm

Squatting

- Squatting is the most commonly used position, and most women find it satisfactory.

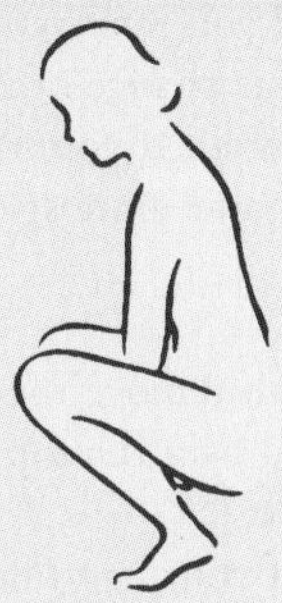

Leg-Up Method

- Another position is to raise the left foot (if right hand is used for insertion) on a low stool and, while in a bending position, insert the diaphragm.

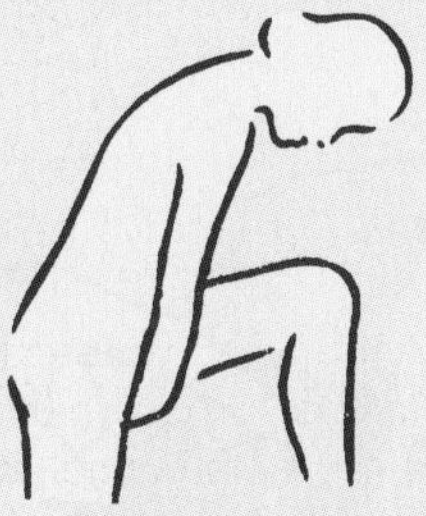

Chair Method

- Another practical method for diaphragm insertion is to sit far forward on the edge of a chair.

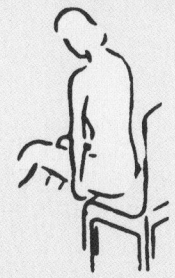

Reclining

- You may prefer to insert the diaphragm while in a semi-reclining position in bed.

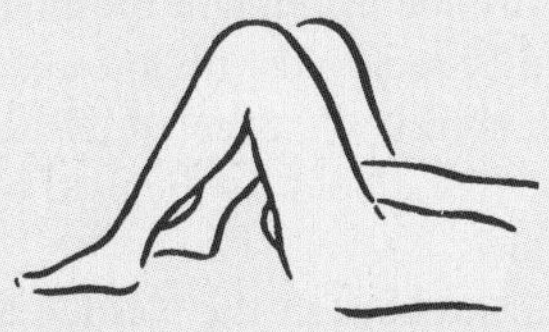

Inspection of Diaphragm

Your diaphragm must be inspected carefully before each use. The best way to do this is to do the following:

- Hold the diaphragm up to a light source. Carefully stretch the diaphragm at the area of the rim, on all sides, to make sure that there are no holes. Remember, it is possible to puncture the diaphragm with sharp fingernails.
- Another way to check for pinholes is to carefully fill the diaphragm with water. If there is any problem, it will be seen immediately.
- If your diaphragm is puckered, especially near the rim, this could mean thin spots.
- The diaphragm should not be used if you see any of these; consult your health care provider.

Preparation of Diaphragm

- Rinse off cornstarch. Your diaphragm must always be used with a spermicidal lubricant to be effective. Pregnancy cannot be prevented effectively by using the diaphragm alone.
- Always empty your bladder before inserting the diaphragm. Place about 10 mL (2 tsp) of contraceptive jelly or contraceptive cream on the side of the diaphragm that will rest against the cervix (or whichever way you have been instructed). Spread it around to coat the surface and the rim. This aids in insertion and offers a more complete seal. Many women also spread some jelly or cream on the other side of the diaphragm.

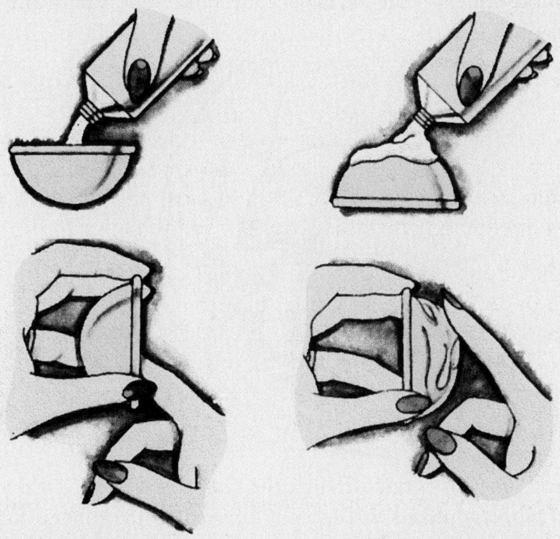

Insertion of Diaphragm

- The diaphragm can be inserted as long as 6 hours before intercourse. Hold the diaphragm between your thumb and fingers. The dome can either be up or down, as directed by your health care provider. Place your index finger on the outer rim of the compressed diaphragm.

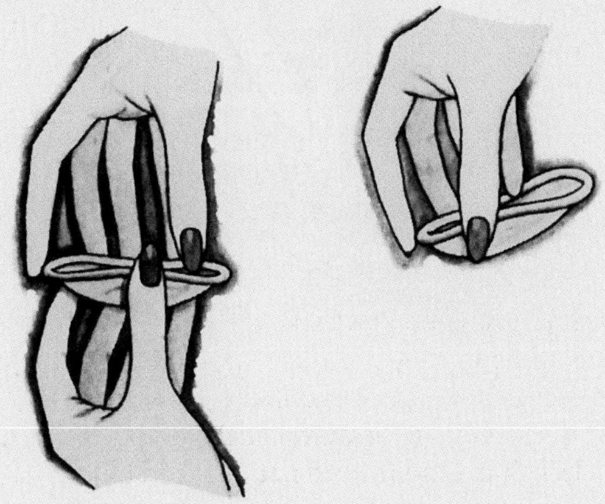

Continued

HOME CARE

Use and Care of the Diaphragm—cont'd

- Use the fingers of the other hand to spread the labia (lips of the vagina). This will assist in guiding the diaphragm into place.
- Insert the diaphragm into the vagina. Direct it inward and downward as far as it will go to the space behind and below the cervix.

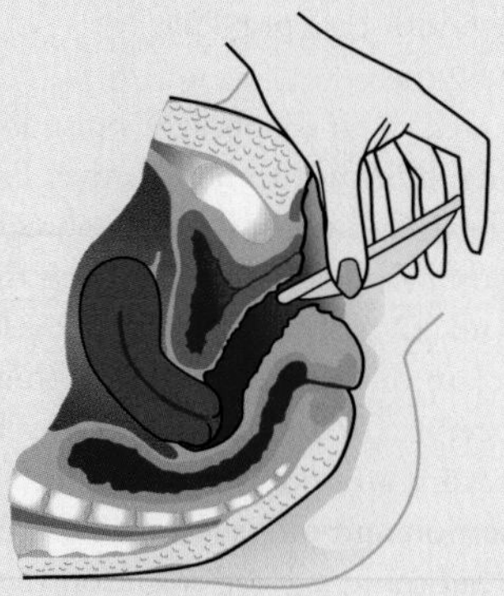

- Tuck the front of the rim of the diaphragm behind the pubic bone so that the rubber hugs the front wall of the vagina.

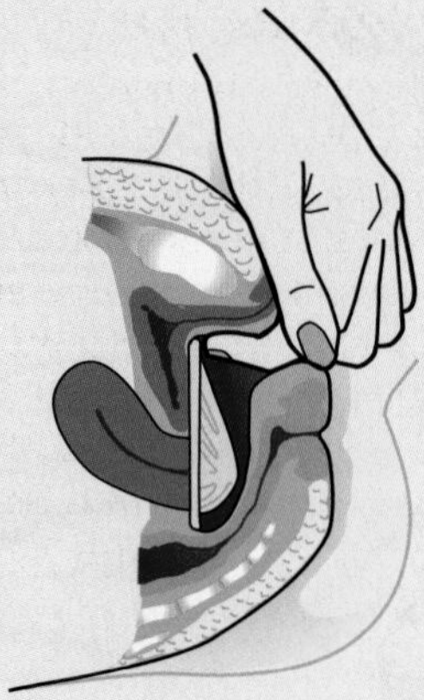

- Feel for your cervix through the diaphragm to be certain it is properly placed and securely covered by the rubber dome.

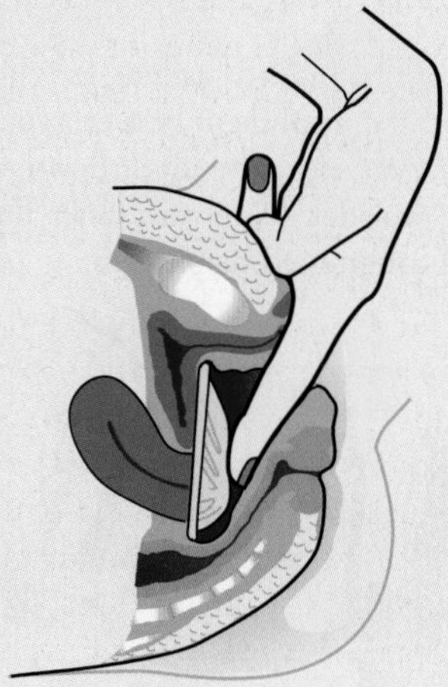

General Information

- Regardless of the time of the month, you must use your diaphragm every time intercourse takes place. Your diaphragm must be left in place for at least 6 hours after the last intercourse. If you remove your diaphragm before the 6-hour period, your chance of becoming pregnant could be greatly increased. If you have repeated acts of intercourse, you must add more spermicide for each act of intercourse.

Removal of Diaphragm

- The only proper way to remove the diaphragm is to insert your forefinger up and over the top side of the diaphragm and slightly to the side.
- Next turn the palm of your hand downward and backward, hooking the forefinger firmly on top of the inside of the upper rim of the diaphragm, breaking the suction.
- Pull the diaphragm down and out. This avoids the possibility of tearing it with the fingernails. You should not remove the diaphragm by trying to catch the rim from below the dome.

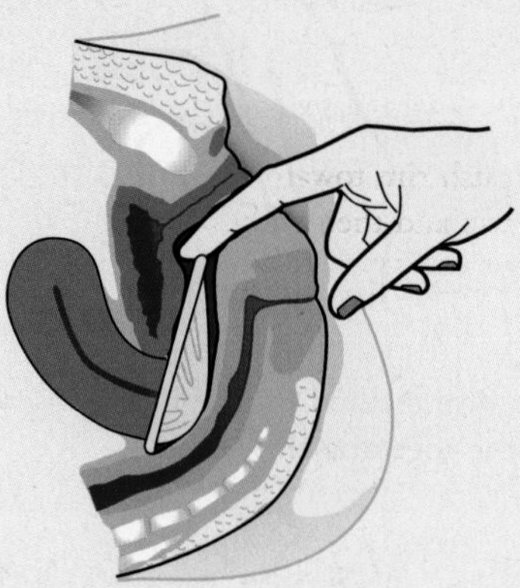

Care of Diaphragm

- When using a vaginal diaphragm, avoid using oil-based products such as certain body lubricants, mineral oil, baby oil, vaginal lubricants, or vaginitis preparations. These products can weaken the rubber.
- A little care means longer wear for your diaphragm. After each use, wash the diaphragm in warm water and mild soap. Do not use detergent soaps, cold-cream soaps, deodorant soaps, or soaps containing oil products because they can weaken the rubber.
- After washing, dry the diaphragm thoroughly. All water and moisture should be removed with a towel. Dust the diaphragm with cornstarch. Scented talc, body powder, baby powder, and the like should not be used because they can weaken the rubber.
- Place the diaphragm back in the plastic case for storage. Do not store it near a radiator or heat source or exposed to light for an extended period.

HOME CARE

Use of the Cervical Cap

- Push cap up into the vagina until it covers cervix.

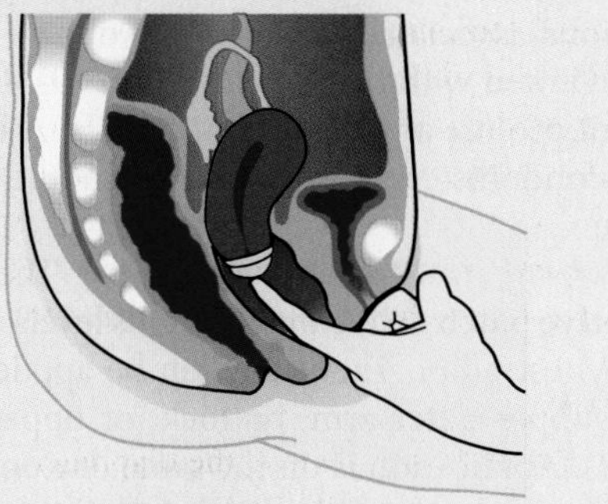

- Press rim against the cervix to create a seal.

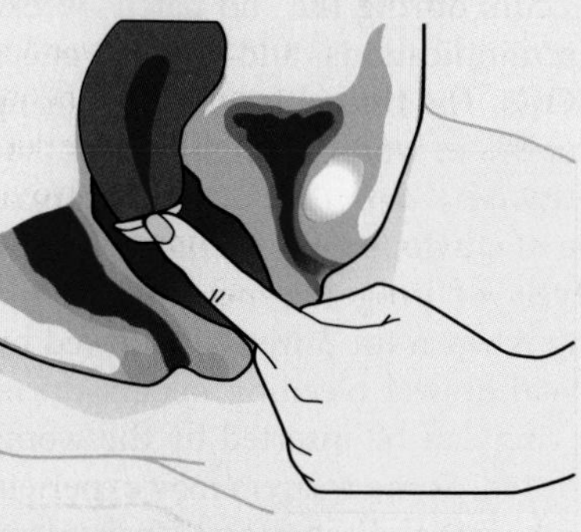

- To remove, push rim toward right or left hip to loosen from the cervix and then withdraw.

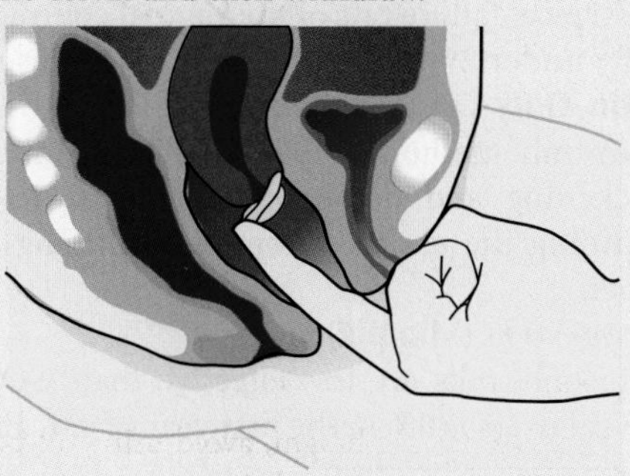

- The woman can assume several positions to insert the cervical cap. See the four positions shown for inserting the diaphragm.

gynecological surgery or birth and after major weight loss or gain. Otherwise, the size should be checked at least once a year.

Women who are not good candidates for wearing the cervical cap include those with abnormal Pap test results, those who cannot be fitted properly with the existing cap sizes or who find the insertion and removal of the device too difficult, those with a history of TSS or with vaginal or cervical infections, and those who experience allergic responses to the cap or to spermicide. There is a difference in effectiveness for women who have already given birth and women who have not. Failure rate for typical use for nulliparous women is 20%. For women who have had previous children, the failure rate for typical use is 40% (Sexualityandu, 2010b).

Table 7-3 Hormonal Contraception

COMPOSITION	ROUTE OF ADMINISTRATION	DURATION OF EFFECT
Combination estrogen and progestin (synthetic estrogens and progestins in varying doses and formulations)	Oral	24 hours; extended cycle—12 weeks
	Transdermal patch	7 days
	Vaginal ring insertion	3 weeks
Progestin only		
Norethindrone, norgestrel	Oral	24 hours
Medroxyprogesterone acetate	Intramuscular or subcutaneous injection	3 months
Levonorgestrel	Intrauterine system	5 years

Contraceptive Sponge

The vaginal sponge is a small, round, polyurethane sponge that contains N-9 spermicide (see Fig. 7-11, B). It is designed to fit over the cervix (one size fits all). The side that is placed next to the cervix is concave for better fit. The opposite side has a woven polyester loop to be used for removal of the sponge. The sponge must be moistened with water before it is inserted into the vagina to cover the cervix. It provides protection for up to 24 hours and for repeated instances of sexual intercourse. The sponge should be left in place for at least 6 hours after the last act of intercourse. Wearing it longer than 24 to 30 hours may put the woman at risk for TSS. The typical failure rate in the first year of use is 40% for parous women and 20% for nulliparous women.

Hormonal Methods

There are many different types of hormonal contraceptive formulations available in Canada. General classes are described in Table 7-3. Because of the wide variety of preparations available, the woman and nurse must read the package insert for information about specific products prescribed. Formulations include combined estrogen–progestin steroidal medications or progestational agents. The formulations are administered orally, transdermally, vaginally, or by injection.

Combined Estrogen–Progestin Contraceptives

Oral Contraceptives. The normal menstrual cycle is maintained by a feedback mechanism. FSH and LH are secreted in response to fluctuating levels of ovarian estrogen and progesterone. Regular ingestion of combined oral contraceptive pills (COCs) suppresses the action of the hypothalamus and anterior pituitary, leading to insufficient secretion of FSH and LH; therefore, follicles do not mature, and ovulation is inhibited.

Other contraceptive effects are induced by the combined steroids. Maturation of the endometrium is altered, making it a less favourable site for implantation. COCs also have a direct effect on the endometrium so that, from 1 to 4 days after the last COC is taken, the endometrium sloughs and bleeds as a result of hormone withdrawal. The withdrawal bleeding is usually less profuse than that of normal menstruation and may last only 2 to 3 days. Some women have no bleeding at all. The cervical mucus remains thick from the effect of the progestin. Cervical mucus under the effect of progesterone does not provide as suitable an environment for sperm penetration as does the thin, watery mucus at ovulation.

Monophasic pills provide fixed dosages of estrogen and progestin. They alter the amount of progestin and sometimes the amount of estrogen within each cycle. These preparations reduce the total dosage of hormones in a single cycle without sacrificing contraceptive efficacy. To maintain adequate hormone levels for contraception and enhance compliance, COCs should be taken at the same time each day. Taken exactly as directed, COCs prevent ovulation, and pregnancy cannot occur. The overall effectiveness rate is almost 100%.

Because taking the pill does not relate directly to the sexual act, its acceptability may be increased. Improvement in sexual response may occur once the possibility of pregnancy is not an issue. For some women it is convenient to know when to expect the next menstrual flow.

Contraindications for COC use include a history of thromboembolic disorders, cerebrovascular or coronary artery disease, breast cancer, estrogen-dependent tumours, pregnancy, impaired liver function, liver tumour, lactation less than 6 weeks postpartum, smoking if older than 35 years (more than 15 cigarettes a day), headaches with focal neurological symptoms, surgery with prolonged immobilization or any surgery on the legs, hypertension (160/100), and diabetes mellitus (of more than 20 years' duration) with vascular disease. The risk of venous thromboembolism is rare although slightly increased over that of women who do not use COCs; women should have individualized risk assessments to determine who might benefit from another type of contraception (Reid et al., 2010).

The effectiveness of oral contraceptives is decreased when the following medications are taken simultaneously:

- Anticonvulsants such as barbiturates, oxycarbazepine, phenytoin, phenobarbital, carbamazepine, primidone, and topiramate
- Systemic antifungals such as griseofulvin
- Antituberculosis drugs such as rifampicin and rifabutin
- Anti-HIV protease inhibitors such as nelfinavir and amprenavir

After discontinuing oral contraception, fertility usually returns quickly, but fertility rates are slightly lower the first 3 to 12 months after discontinuation.

Oral contraceptives have been shown to have benefits that are not related to birth control, including regulation and reduction of both menstrual bleeding and dysmenorrhea, and treatment of premenstrual syndrome, menstrual migraines, acne, and hirsutism. There are also some long-term benefits, such as reduced rates of endometrial, ovarian, and colorectal cancer (Reid et al., 2010).

Nursing Considerations. Many different preparations of oral hormonal contraceptives are available. Because of the wide variations, each woman must be clear about the unique dosage regimen for the preparation prescribed for her and follow directions on the package insert. Directions for care after missing one or two tablets vary (Fig. 7-12). Women need to be instructed to consider emergency contraception or back-up contraception, depending on when during the month the pills are missed and how many pills are missed. Signs of potential complications associated with the use of oral contraceptives must be reviewed with the woman (Box 7-9). Oral contraceptives do not protect a woman against STIs. A barrier method such as condoms and spermicide should be used for protection.

Transdermal Contraceptive System. The **transdermal contraceptive patch** delivers continuous levels of progesterone and ethynyl estradiol. The patch can be applied to the lower abdomen, upper outer arm, buttock, or upper torso (except the breasts). Application is on the same day once a week for 3 weeks, followed by a week without the patch. Withdrawal bleeding occurs during the "no patch" week. Mechanisms of action, contraindications, and adverse effects are similar to those of COCs. The typical failure rate during the first year of use is under 3% in women weighing less than 90 kg.

Contraceptive Vaginal Ring. The **contraceptive vaginal ring** (made of ethylene vinyl acetate copolymer) delivers continuous levels of progesterone and ethynyl estradiol. One vaginal ring is worn for 3 weeks, followed by a week without the ring. Withdrawal bleeding occurs during the "no ring" week. The ring can be inserted by the woman and does not have to be fitted. Some wearers may experience vaginitis, leukorrhea, and vaginal discomfort. Mechanisms of action, contraindications, and adverse effects are similar to those of COCs. The typical failure rate of the vaginal contraceptive ring is reportedly under 2% during the first year of use.

Progestin-Only Contraception

Progestin-only methods impair fertility by inhibiting ovulation, thickening and decreasing the amount of cervical mucus, thinning the endometrium, and altering cilia in the uterine tubes.

Oral Progestins (Minipill)

Progestin-only pills are less effective than COCs. Failure rate for typical users is 8% in the first year of use. Effectiveness

BOX 7-9 Signs of Potential Complications: Oral Contraceptives

The woman should be alerted to immediately stop taking the pill and report the following symptoms to the health care provider. The word ACHES helps in remembering this list:

A—Abdominal pain: may indicate a problem with the liver or gallbladder

C—Chest pain or shortness of breath: may indicate possible clot problem within lungs or heart

H—Headaches (sudden or persistent): may be caused by cardiovascular accident or hypertension

E—Eye problems: may indicate vascular accident or hypertension

S—Severe leg pain: may indicate a thromboembolic process

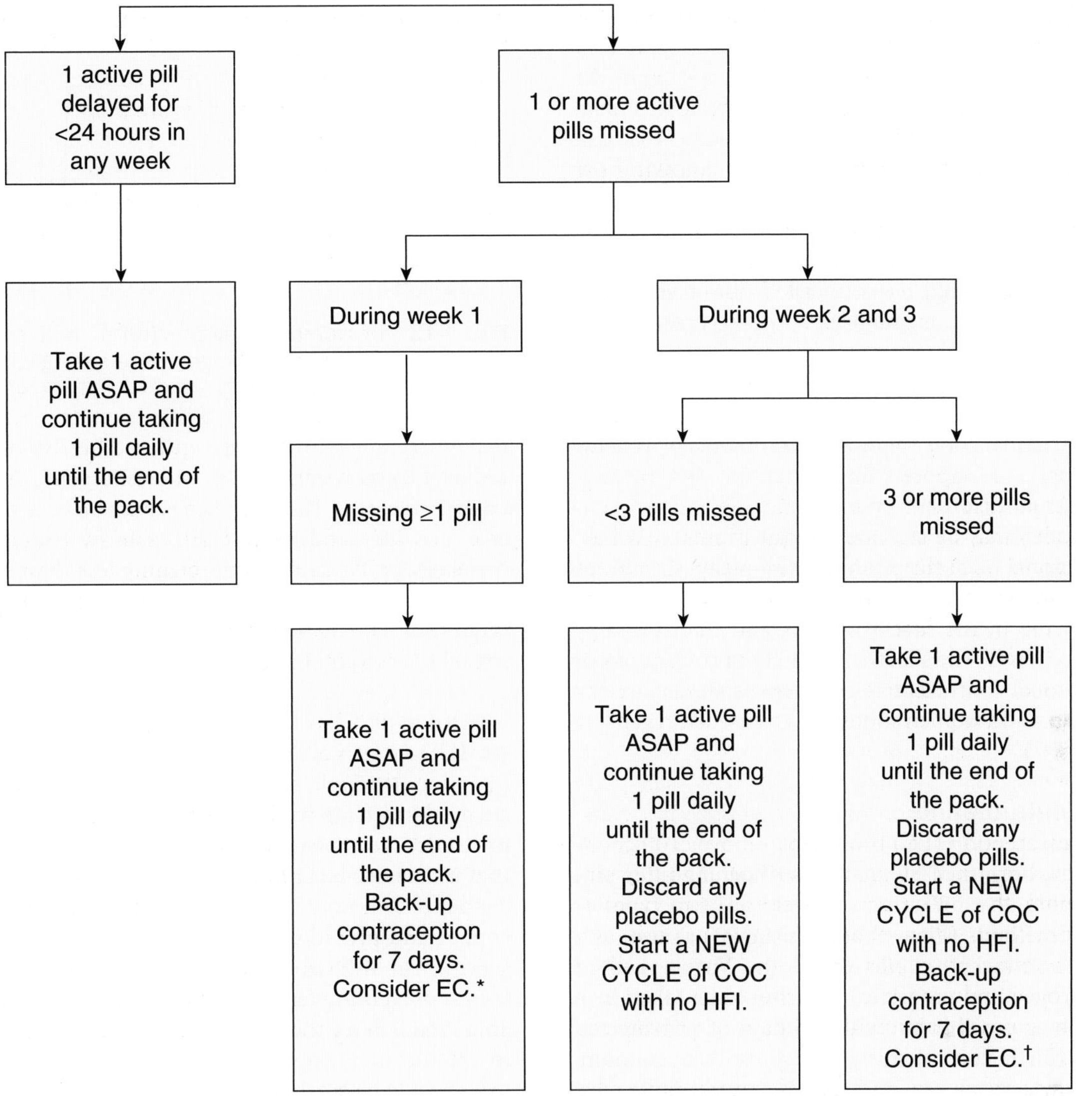

*If unprotected intercourse within the last 5 days.
†If repeated or prolonged omission.

Fig. 7-12 Flowchart for missed contraceptive pills. *ASAP*, as soon as possible; this may mean that 2 pills are taken on that day. *COC*, combined oral contraceptive; *EC*, emergency contraception; *HFI*, hormone free interval. *(Courtesy Society of Obstetricians and Gynaecologists of Canada [2008]. SOGC clinical practice guideline: Missed hormonal contraceptives: New recommendations.* Journal of Obstetrics and Gynaecology Canada, *30[11], 1050–1061. Retrieved from http://www.sogc.org/guidelines/documents/gui219ECO0811.pdf. Printed with permission from the SOGC.)*

is increased if minipills are taken correctly. Because minipills contain such a low dose of progestin, the minipill must be taken at the same time every day. Users often complain of irregular vaginal bleeding.

Injectable Progestins. Depot medroxyprogesterone acetate (DMPA; Depo-Provera) is given subcutaneously or intramuscularly in the deltoid or gluteus maximus muscle. DMPA should be initiated during the first 5 days of the menstrual cycle and administered every 11 to 13 weeks.

NURSING ALERT When administering an injection of progestin (e.g., Depo-Provera), the site should not be massaged after the injection because this action can hasten the absorption and shorten the period of effectiveness.

Advantages of DMPA include a contraceptive effectiveness comparable to that of COCs, long-lasting effects, requirement of injections only four times a year, and the unlikelihood of lactation being impaired. Adverse effects at the end of a year include decreased bone mineral density, weight gain, lipid changes, increased risk of venous thrombosis and thromboembolism, irregular vaginal spotting, decreased libido, and breast changes. Other disadvantages include no protection against STIs. Return to fertility may be delayed as long as up to

18 months after discontinuing DMPA. Typical failure rate is 3% in the first year of use.

NURSING ALERT Women who use DMPA may lose significant bone mineral density with increasing duration of use. It is unknown if this effect is reversible. It is unknown if use of DMPA during adolescence or early adulthood, a critical period of bone accretion, will reduce peak bone mass and increase the risk of osteoporotic fracture in later life. Women who receive DMPA should be counselled about vitamin D and calcium intake as well as exercise in order to protect bone health.

Continuous and Extended Hormonal Contraception

Continuous hormonal contraception, with no breaks, is being used increasingly to suppress menstruation, for medical reasons (menstrual disorders—see Chapter 6) and women's preferences (vacations, sports, and special events). Women who use hormonal contraception continuously should be counselled about expected bleeding patterns. Bleeding or spotting is normal in the first 3 months and then bleeding significantly decreases. The short-term safety of continuous or extended hormonal contraceptive regimens is similar to that of cyclic regimens and women should be counselled regarding this (SOGC, 2007).

Emergency Contraception

Emergency contraception (EC) is available in over 100 countries. In Canada, hormonal EC methods (morning-after pill) are available without a prescription. There are two types of progestin-only methods (Plan B® and NorLevo®) as well as a series of four contraceptive pills called the Yuzpe method (combined estrogen and progestin). EC should be taken by a woman as soon as possible but within 5 days of unprotected intercourse or birth control mishap (e.g., broken condom, dislodged ring or cervical cap, missed oral contraceptive pills, late for injection) to prevent unintended pregnancy (CFSH, 2008b). If taken before ovulation, EC prevents ovulation by inhibiting follicular development. If taken after ovulation occurs, there is little effect on ovarian hormone production or the endometrium. To minimize the adverse effect of nausea that occurs with high doses of estrogen and progestin, the woman can be advised to take an over-the-counter antiemetic 1 hour before each dose. If the woman vomits within 1 hour after taking the medication she will need to repeat the dose. Women with contraindications for estrogen use should use progestin-only EC. No medical contraindications for EC exist, except pregnancy and undiagnosed abnormal vaginal bleeding (Stewart, Trussell, & Van Look, 2007). If the woman does not begin menstruation within 21 days after taking the pills, she should be evaluated for pregnancy (CFSH, 2008b). EC is ineffective if the woman is pregnant as the pills do not disturb an implanted pregnancy. Risk of pregnancy is reduced by as much as 75% and 89% if the woman takes EC pills (Stewart et al., 2007).

Intrauterine devices (IUDs) containing copper (Fig. 7-13, A) provide another EC option. The IUD should be inserted within 7 days of unprotected intercourse (CFSH, 2008b). This method is suggested only for women who wish to have the benefit of long-term contraception. The risk of pregnancy is reduced by as much as 99% with emergency insertion of the copper-releasing IUD. An IUD must be inserted by a health care provider and is only available by prescription, which makes it less accessible than hormonal EC methods.

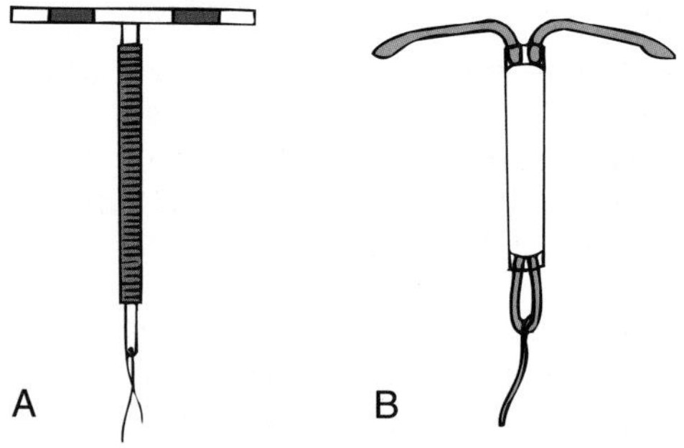

Fig. 7-13 Intrauterine devices (IUDs) and systems (IUSs). **A:** Copper T IUD. **B:** Levonorgestrel-releasing IUS.

Contraceptive counselling should be provided to all women requesting EC, including a discussion of modification of risky sexual behaviours to prevent STIs and unwanted pregnancy.

Intrauterine Contraceptive Devices

An IUD is a small T-shaped device with bendable arms for insertion through the cervix into the uterine cavity. Two strings hang from the base of the stem through the cervix and protrude into the vagina for the woman to feel, for assurance that the device has not been dislodged (see Fig. 7-13, A). The copper IUD is made of radiopaque polyethylene and fine solid copper and provides up to 5 years of protection. The copper serves primarily as a spermicide and inflames the endometrium, preventing fertilization. Sometimes women experience an increase in bleeding and cramping within the first year after insertion, but nonsteroidal anti-inflammatory drugs (NSAIDs) can provide pain relief. The typical failure rate in the first year of use of the copper IUD is 0.8% (CFSH, 2008c).

The IUD offers constant contraception without the need to remember to take pills each day or engage in other manipulation before or between coital acts. As long as the woman is not pregnant, an IUD can be placed at any time during the menstrual cycle. An IUD may be inserted shortly after childbirth or first-trimester abortion. Contraceptive effects are reversible. When pregnancy is desired, the IUD may be removed by the health care provider.

Disadvantages of IUD use include increased risk of pelvic inflammatory disease in the first 20 days after insertion and risk of bacterial vaginosis and uterine perforation. The IUD offers no protection against STIs or HIV.

Intrauterine Systems

The levonorgestrel intrauterine system (IUS) (Mirena) (see Fig. 7-13, B) releases levonorgestrel from its vertical reservoir. Effective for up to 5 years, it impairs sperm motility, irritates the lining of the uterus, and has some anovulatory effects (Grimes, 2007). Uterine cramping and uterine bleeding are usually decreased with this device, although irregular spotting is common in the first few months following insertion. The risk of uterine perforation is a rare complication of the use of

Mirena. This risk is increased in women after pregnancy, during lactation, and with abnormal uterine anatomy (Health Canada, 2010b). Women need to be counselled about this risk and to identify signs of possible uterine rupture (lower abdominal pain and bleeding). The typical failure rate in the first year of use is 0.2% (Trussell, 2007).

Nursing Considerations

The woman should be taught to check for the presence of the IUD/IUS thread after menstruation to rule out expulsion of the device. If pregnancy occurs with the IUD/IUS in place, the system should be removed immediately in the first trimester if the strings are visible. Later in pregnancy, ultrasound examination should be used to localize the IUD/IUS and to rule out placenta previa. Retention of the IUD/IUS during pregnancy increases the risk of septic miscarriage and ectopic pregnancy (Grimes, 2007). Some women allergic to copper develop a rash, necessitating removal of the copper-bearing IUD. Signs of potential complications are listed in Box 7-10.

Sterilization

Sterilization refers to surgical procedures intended to render the person infertile. Most procedures involve the occlusion of the passageways for the ova and sperm (Fig. 7-14, A). For the woman, the oviducts (uterine tubes) are occluded; for the man, the sperm ducts (vas deferens) are occluded. Only surgical removal of the ovaries (oophorectomy) or uterus (hysterectomy) or both result in absolute sterility for the woman. All other sterilization procedures have a small but definite failure rate (i.e., pregnancy may result).

Female Sterilization

Female sterilization (bilateral **tubal ligation**) may be done immediately after giving birth (within 24 to 48 hours), concomitantly with abortion, or as an interval procedure (during any phase of the menstrual cycle). Half of all female sterilization procedures are performed immediately after a pregnancy. Sterilization procedures can be done safely on an outpatient basis. Failure rate for methods of female sterilization vary by the method and the woman's age, but the average is 0.5% (CFSH, 2007).

Tubal Occlusion. A laparoscopic approach or a minilaparotomy may be used for tubal ligation (Fig. 7-15), tubal electrocoagulation, or the application of bands or clips. Electrocoagulation and ligation are considered to be permanent methods. Use of the bands or clips has the theoretical advantage of possible removal and return of tubal patency (see Patient Teaching box).

BOX 7-10 Signs of Potential Complications: Intrauterine Devices or Intrauterine Systems

Signs of potential complications related to intrauterine devices can be remembered using the PAINS mnemonic:

P—Period late, abnormal spotting or bleeding
A—Abdominal pain, pain with intercourse
I—Infection exposure, abnormal vaginal discharge
N—Not feeling well, fever, or chills
S—String missing; shorter or longer

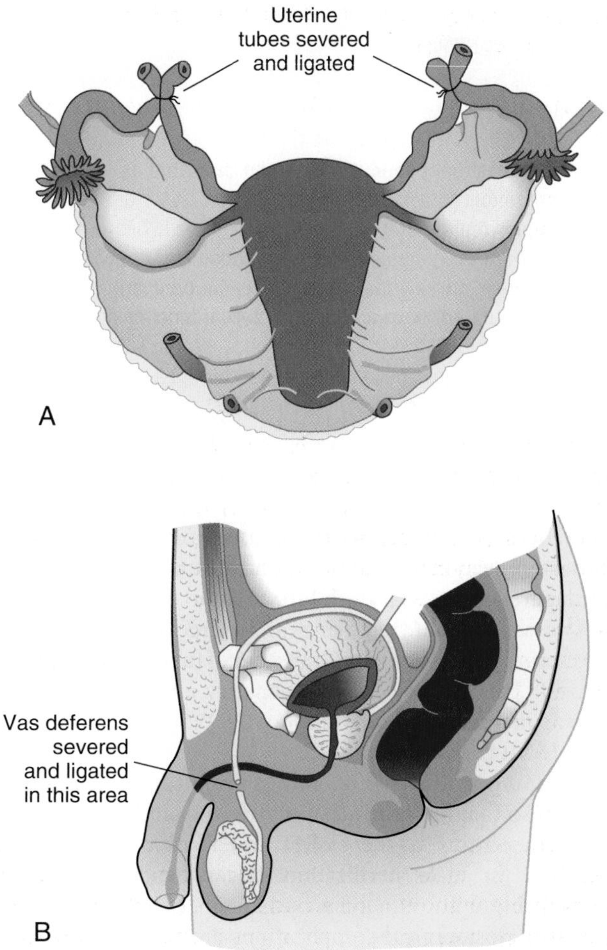

Fig. 7-14 Sterilization. **A:** Uterine tubes ligated and severed (tubal ligation). **B:** Sperm duct ligated and severed (vasectomy).

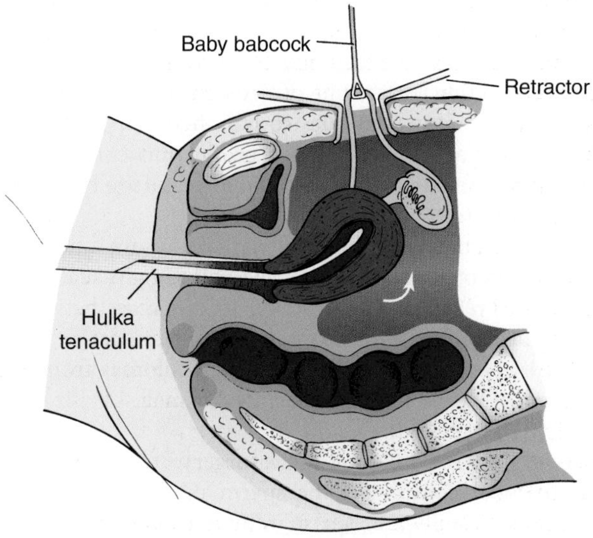

Fig. 7-15 Use of minilaparotomy to gain access to uterine tubes for occlusion procedures. Tenaculum is used to lift uterus upward (*arrow*) toward incision.

PATIENT TEACHING What to Expect After Tubal Ligation

- You should expect no change in hormones and their influence.
- Your menstrual period will be about the same as before the sterilization.
- You may feel pain at ovulation.
- The ovum disintegrates within the abdominal cavity.
- It is highly unlikely that you will become pregnant.
- You should not have a change in sexual functioning; you may enjoy sexual relations more because you will not be concerned about becoming pregnant.
- Sterilization offers no protection against sexually transmitted infections. Therefore, you may need to use condoms.

Tubal Reconstruction. Restoration of tubal continuity (reanastomosis) and function is technically feasible except after laparoscopic tubal electrocoagulation. Sterilization reversal is costly, difficult (requiring microsurgery), and uncertain. The success rate varies with the extent of tubal destruction and removal. The risk of ectopic pregnancy after tubal reanastomosis is increased by 2 to 12.5%.

Male Sterilization

Vasectomy is the sealing, tying, or cutting of a man's vas deferens so that the sperm cannot travel from the testes to the penis. Vasectomy is the easiest and most commonly used operation for male sterilization. It can be done with local anaesthesia on an outpatient basis. Pain, bleeding, infection, and other postsurgical complications are considered the disadvantages to the surgical procedure.

Two methods are used for scrotal entry: conventional and no-scalpel vasectomy. The surgeon identifies and immobilizes the vas deferens through the scrotum. Then the vas is ligated or cauterized (see Fig. 7-14, B). Surgeons vary in their techniques to occlude the vas deferens: ligation with sutures, division, cautery, application of clips, excision of a segment of the vas, fascial interposition, or some combination of these methods.

Vasectomy has no effect on potency (ability to achieve and maintain erection) or volume of ejaculate. Endocrine production of testosterone continues so that secondary sex characteristics are not affected. Sperm production continues, but sperm are unable to leave the epididymis and are lysed by the immune system.

Complications after bilateral vasectomy are uncommon and usually not serious. They include bleeding (usually external), suture reaction, and reaction to the anaesthetic agent. Men occasionally may develop a hematoma, infection, or epididymitis. Less common are painful granulomas from accumulation of sperm. The failure rate for male sterilization is 0.15% (CFSH, 2008d).

Tubal Reconstruction. Microsurgery to reanastomose (restore tubal continuity) the sperm ducts can be accomplished successfully (i.e., sperm in the ejaculate) in more than 90% of cases; however, the fertility rate is only about 50%. The rate of success decreases as the time since the procedure increases. The vasectomy may result in permanent changes in the testes that leave men unable to father children. The changes are those ordinarily seen only in older men (e.g., interstitial fibrosis [scar tissue between the seminiferous tubules]). Some men develop antibodies against their own sperm (autoimmunization).

Laws and Regulations

All provinces have strict regulations for informed consent. Health care providers must ensure that while obtaining informed consent there is an explanation of benefits and risks and options and determination of whether the person is competent to understand the information. Explanation must be made in the person's own language, or an interpreter must be provided to ensure that the person understands all information. Although the partner's consent is not required by law, the woman is encouraged to discuss the situation with her partner. Sterilization of minors or mentally incompetent individuals is illegal.

Nursing Considerations

The nurse plays an important role in assisting people with decision making so that all requirements for informed consent are met. The nurse also provides information about alternatives to sterilization such as contraception.

Information must be given about what is entailed in the various procedures, how much discomfort or pain can be expected, and what type of care is needed. Many individuals fear sterilization procedures because of the imagined effect on their sexual life. They need reassurance concerning the hormonal and psychological basis for sexual function and that uterine tube occlusion or vasectomy has no biological sequelae in terms of sexual adequacy.

Preoperative care includes health assessment, which includes a psychological assessment, physical examination, and laboratory tests. The nurse needs to confirm the woman's understanding of printed instructions. Ambivalence and extreme fear of the procedure should be reported to the physician.

Postoperative care depends on the procedure performed (e.g., laparoscopy, laparotomy for tubal occlusion, or vasectomy). General care includes recovery after anaesthesia, vital signs, fluid–electrolyte balance (intake and output, laboratory values), prevention or early identification and treatment of infection or hemorrhage, control of discomfort, and assessment of emotional response to the procedure and recovery.

Discharge planning depends on the type of procedure performed. In general, the patient is given written instructions about observing for and reporting symptoms and signs of complications, the type of recovery to be expected, and the date and time for a follow-up appointment.

Abortion

Induced abortion is the purposeful interruption of a pregnancy before 20 weeks of gestation. (Miscarriage is discussed in Chapter 13.) Many factors contribute to a woman's decision to have an abortion. Indications include (1) preservation of the life or health of the mother, (2) genetic disorders of the fetus, (3) rape or incest, and (4) the pregnant woman's request. The control of birth, given that it concerns human sexuality and the question of life and death, is one of the most emotional components of health care.

Abortion in Canada is safe and legal. The laws for abortion in Canada have changed over the last 35 years, from being very restricted before 1969 to unrestricted in 1988. Today, Canada is one of the only countries in the world without abortion regulation. Abortion is available throughout pregnancy, although more than 90% are performed in the first trimester and only 2% to 3% are performed after 16 weeks. Hospitals maintained by Roman Catholics and some of those maintained by strict fundamentalists forbid abortion (and often sterilization) despite legal challenges. Women on Prince Edward Island must travel to another province to obtain an abortion.

Rates of biological complications after abortions, such as ectopic pregnancy, infection, or hemorrhage, tend to be low if the woman aborts during the first trimester. Psychological sequelae of induced abortion are uncommon and may be related to circumstances and support systems surrounding the pregnant woman, such as the attitudes reflected by friends, family, and health care workers. The woman facing an abortion is pregnant and will exhibit the emotional responses shared by all pregnant women, including the possibility of postbirth depression.

Nurses and other health care providers often struggle with the same values and moral convictions as those of the pregnant woman. The conflicts and doubts of the nurse can be readily communicated to women who are already anxious. Regardless of personal views on abortion, nurses who provide care to women seeking abortion have an ethical responsibility to counsel women about their options and to make appropriate referrals.

LEGAL TIP Nurses' Rights and Responsibilities Related to Abortion. If nurses are requested to provide care that is against their religious or moral beliefs, they must continue to provide safe, compassionate, competent, ethical care until alternative arrangements can be made. If a nurse anticipates a conflict of conscience, the nurse has an obligation to notify his or her employer so that alternative arrangements can be made. Declaring a conflict with conscience or "conscientious objection" is a serious matter that must be addressed. Nurses' rights and responsibilities related to caring for abortion patients should be protected through policies that describe how the institution will accommodate the nurse's ethical or moral beliefs and what the nurse should do to avoid patient abandonment in such situations. Nurses should know what policies are in place in their institutions and encourage such policies to be *written.*

(Source: Canadian Nurses Association. [2008]. *Code of ethics for registered nurses*. Ottawa: Author. Retrieved from http://www.cna-aiic.ca/CNA/documents/pdf/publications/Code_of_Ethics_2008_e.pdf.)

Counselling about abortion includes helping the woman identify how she perceives the pregnancy and providing information about the choices available (i.e., having an abortion or carrying the pregnancy to term and then either keeping the infant or placing the baby for adoption) and about the types of abortion procedures (see Critical Thinking Exercise).

CRITICAL THINKING EXERCISE

Termination of Pregnancy

Angelica is a 19-year-old single woman whose contraceptive failed. She is 6 weeks pregnant and is seeking termination of the pregnancy. She has many questions for the nurse in the family planning clinic: What procedure is most likely to be chosen at this gestation? What are the risks associated with the procedure? Should her boyfriend be involved in the decision to terminate the pregnancy?

1. Evidence—Is there sufficient evidence to draw conclusions about what information the nurse should provide Angelica?
2. Assumptions—What assumptions can be made about Angelica's reaction to termination of the pregnancy?
   a. Psychological and emotional reactions and sequelae
   b. Physical response
   c. Future childbearing
   d. Relationship with her boyfriend
3. What implications and priorities for nursing care can be drawn at this time?
4. Does the evidence objectively support your conclusion?
5. Are there alternative perspectives to your conclusion?

First-Trimester Abortion

Methods for performing early elective abortion (less than 10 weeks of gestation) include surgical (aspiration) and medical methods (mifepristone with prostaglandin and methotrexate with misoprostol).

Surgical (Aspiration) Abortion

Aspiration (vacuum or suction curettage) is the most common procedure in the first trimester. Aspiration abortion is usually performed under local anaesthesia in a physician's office, a clinic, or a hospital. The ideal time for performing this procedure is 8 to 12 weeks after the last menstrual period. The suction procedure for performing an early elective abortion usually requires less than 5 minutes.

A bimanual examination is done before the procedure to assess uterine size and position. A speculum is inserted, and the cervix is anaesthetized with a local anaesthetic agent. The cervix is dilated, if necessary, and a cannula connected to suction is inserted into the uterine cavity. The products of conception are evacuated from the uterus.

During the procedure, the woman should be kept informed about what to expect next (e.g., menstrual-like cramping and sounds of the suction machine). The nurse needs to assess the woman's vital signs. The aspirated uterine contents must be carefully inspected to ascertain whether all fetal parts and adequate placental tissue have been evacuated. After the abortion, the woman can rest on the table until she is ready to stand. She will then remain in the recovery area or waiting room for 1 to 3 hours in case any excessive cramping or bleeding occurs; then she is discharged.

Bleeding after the operation is normally about the equivalent of a heavy menstrual period, and cramps are rarely severe. Excessive vaginal bleeding and infection such as endometritis or salpingitis are the most common complications of induced abortion. Retained products of conception are the primary cause of vaginal bleeding. Evacuation of the uterus, uterine massage, and administration of oxytocin or methylergonovine may be necessary. Prophylactic antibiotics to decrease the risk of infection are recommended (Davis, 2006). Postabortion pain can be relieved with NSAIDs such as ibuprofen.

Nursing Interventions

Instructions following a surgical abortion differ among health care providers (e.g., tampons should not be used for at least 3 days or should be avoided for up to 3 weeks, and resumption of sexual intercourse may be permitted within 1 week or discouraged for 2 weeks). The woman may shower daily. She should be instructed to watch for excessive bleeding and other signs of complications (Box 7-11) and to avoid douches of any type. The woman may expect her menstrual period to resume 4 to 6 weeks after the day of the procedure. The nurse should offer information about the birth control method the woman prefers, if this has not been done during the counselling interview that usually precedes the decision to have an abortion. The woman must be strongly encouraged to return for her follow-up visit so that complications can be detected and an acceptable contraceptive method prescribed. A pregnancy test may also be performed to determine if the pregnancy has been terminated successfully.

Medical Abortion

Medical abortions are available in Canada for up to 9 weeks after the last menstrual period and should be considered in women who will be diligent with follow-up. Methotrexate and misoprostol are the drugs used in the current regimens to induce early abortion.

Methotrexate is a cytotoxic drug that causes early abortion by blocking folic acid in fetal cells so they cannot divide. Misoprostol (Cytotec) is a prostaglandin analog that acts directly on the cervix to soften and dilate it and on the uterine muscle to stimulate contractions. Methotrexate can be given intramuscularly or orally (usually mixed with orange juice). Vaginal placement of misoprostol follows in 3 to 7 days. Women commonly have nausea, vomiting, and cramping after the misoprostol insertion. The woman needs to return for a follow-up visit to confirm that the abortion is complete. If abortion does not occur, misoprostol is repeated, or vacuum aspiration is performed. Misoprostol can also be used alone.

BOX 7-11 Complications From Induced Abortion

Call your health care provider if you have any of the following signs:

- Fever greater than 38°C
- Chills
- Bleeding greater than two saturated pads in 2 hours or heavy bleeding lasting a few days
- Foul-smelling vaginal discharge
- Severe abdominal pain, cramping, or backache
- Abdominal tenderness (when pressure applied)
- No return of menstrual period within 6 weeks

(Source: Paul, M., & Stewart, F. [2007]. Abortion. In R. Hatcher, et al. [Eds.], *Contraceptive technology* [19th ed.]. New York: Ardent Media.)

Misoprostol 800 mcg is placed high in the vagina every 24 to 48 hours for up to three applications. Blood work at 7 days confirms whether this regimen was successful.

With any medical abortion regimen, the woman usually will experience bleeding and cramping. Adverse effects of the medications include nausea, vomiting, diarrhea, headache, dizziness, fever, and chills. These are attributed to misoprostol and usually subside in a few hours after administration.

Second-Trimester Abortion

Second-trimester abortion is associated with more complications than are first-trimester abortions. Medical induction and dilation and evacuation (D&E) are both safe and effective methods for terminations in the second trimester. However, D&E is considered superior between 14 and 18 weeks' gestation (Davis, 2006). Induction of uterine contractions can also be used.

Dilation and Evacuation

D&E can be performed at any point up to 20 weeks of gestation. The cervix requires more dilation because the products of conception are larger. Often laminaria are inserted into the cervix several hours or several days before the procedure to assist in dilating the cervix. Misoprostol may also be applied to the cervix. The procedure is similar to that of vaginal aspiration, except that a larger cannula is used and other instruments may be needed to remove the fetus and placenta. Nursing care includes monitoring vital signs, providing emotional support, administering analgesics, and postoperative monitoring. Disadvantages of D&E include possible long-term harmful effects on the cervix.

Medical Induction

Prior to medical induction, women may require cervical ripening with osmotic dilators, prostaglandins, or the insertion of a balloon catheter. Intra-amniotic injections of hypertonic solutions (e.g., saline) injected directly into the uterus and uterotonic agents (e.g., prostoglandin) are effective. Extra-amniotic prostaglandin can also be used. Labour may also be induced using carboprost intramuscularly, concentrated oxytocin infusion, or misoprostol (orally or vaginally). The particular method that is used should be based on the expertise of the health care provider and the wishes of the woman (Davis, 2006).

Emotional Considerations

The woman considering an abortion will need help in exploring the meaning of the various alternatives and consequences to herself and her significant others. It is often difficult for a woman to express her true feelings (e.g., what abortion means to her now and in the future and what support or regret her friends and peers may demonstrate). A calm, matter-of-fact approach from the nurse can be helpful. Clarifying, restating, and reflecting statements; open-ended questions; and feedback are communication techniques that can be used to maintain a realistic focus on the situation and bring the woman's problems into the open. If family or friends cannot be involved, scheduling time for nursing personnel to give the necessary support is an essential component of the care plan.

Information about alternatives to abortion such as referral to adoption agencies or to support services if the woman chooses to keep her baby should be provided. If a decision is made to have an abortion, the woman must be assured of continued support. Information about what is entailed in various procedures, how much discomfort or pain can be expected, and what type of care is needed must be given. The various feelings, including depression, guilt, regret, and relief, that the woman might experience after the abortion should be discussed. Information about community resources for post-abortion counselling may be needed.

Studies have indicated that after the abortion, most women report relief, but some have temporary distress or mixed emotions. Evidence of long-term depression after elective abortion has been inconclusive. Guilt and anxiety may occur more with young women, women with poor social support, multiparous women, and women with a history of psychiatric illness. Women having second-trimester abortions may have more emotional distress than women having abortions in the first trimester. Because symptoms can vary among women who have had abortions, nurses must assess women for grief reactions and facilitate the grieving process through active listening and nonjudgemental support and care.

Key Points

- Infertility is the inability to conceive and carry a fetus to term gestation at a time the couple has chosen to do so.
- Infertility affects about 8 to 16% of otherwise healthy adults. It increases in women older than 35 years.
- In Canada about one third of infertility is related to female causes, one third is related to male causes, and 20% of the causes are unexplained.
- Common etiological factors of infertility include decreased sperm production, ovulation disorders, polycystic ovary syndrome, tubal occlusion, and endometriosis.
- Reproductive alternatives for family building include IVF-ET, GIFT, ZIFT, oocyte donation, embryo donation, TDI, **surrogate motherhood,** and adoption.
- Infertility treatment can involve emotional and monetary costs for those involved.
- A variety of contraceptive methods with various effectiveness rates, advantages, and disadvantages are available.
- Women and their partners should choose the contraceptive method(s) best suited to them.
- Effective contraceptives are available through both prescription and nonprescription sources.
- Proper concurrent use of spermicides and latex condoms provides protection against STIs.
- Tubal ligations and vasectomies are permanent sterilization methods.
- Induced abortion performed in the first trimester is safer and less complex than an abortion performed in the second trimester.
- The most common complications of induced abortion include infection, retained products of conception, and excessive vaginal bleeding.

Audio Chapter Summaries

Access an Audio Summary of these Key Points on evolve

References

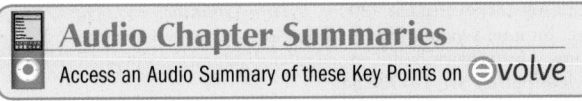

Allen, V. M., Wilson, R. D., et al. (2006). Joint SOGC/CFAS Guideline: Pregnancy outcomes after assisted reproductive technology. *Journal of Obstetrics and Gynaecology Canada, 28*(3), 220–233. Retrieved from http://www.sogc.org/guidelines/public/173E-JCPG-March2006.pdf.

American Society for Reproductive Medicine (ASRM) (2008). *Frequently asked questions about infertility.* Retrieved from http://www.asrm.org/awards/index.aspx?id=3012.

Boivin, J., Griffiths, E., & Venetis, C. A. (2011). Emotional distress in infertile women and failure of assisted reproductive technologies: meta-analysis of prospective psychosocial studies. *British Medical Journal, 342,* d223. doi: 10.1136/bmj.d223

Canadian Federation for Sexual Health (2007). *Tubal ligation.* Retrieved from http://www.cfsh.ca/Your_Sexual_Health/Contraception-and-Safer-Sex/Contraception-and-Birth-Control/tubal-ligation.aspx.

Canadian Federation for Sexual Health (2008a). *Female condom.* Retrieved from http://www.cfsh.ca/Your_Sexual_Health/Contraception-and-Safer-Sex/Contraception-and-Birth-Control/Female-Condom.aspx.

Canadian Federation for Sexual Health (2008b). *Emergency contraception.* Retrieved from http://www.cfsh.ca/Your_Sexual_Health/Contraception-and-Safer-Sex/Emergency-Contraception/.

Canadian Federation for Sexual Health (2008c). *IUD.* Retrieved from http://www.cfsh.ca/Your_Sexual_Health/Contraception-and-Safer-Sex/Contraception-and-Birth-Control/IUD.aspx.

Canadian Federation for Sexual Health (2008d). *Vasectomy.* Retrieved from http://www.cfsh.ca/Your_Sexual_Health/Contraception-and-Safer-Sex/Contraception-and-Birth-Control/Vasectomy.aspx.

Canadian Federation for Sexual Health (2009). *Diaphragm.* Retrieved from http://www.cfsh.ca/Your_Sexual_Health/Contraception-and-Safer-Sex/Contraception-and-Birth-Control/Diaphragm.aspx.

Canadian Fertility and Andrology Society (2009). *Human assisted reproduction 2009 live birth rates for Canada.* Montreal: Author. Retrieved from http://www.cfas.ca/index.php?option=com_content&view=article&id=924%3Ahuman-assisted-reproduction-2009-live-birth-rates-for-canada&catid=929%3Apress-releases&Itemid=460.

Cunningham, F. G., et al. (2010). *Williams obstetrics* (23rd ed.). New York: McGraw-Hill.

CycleBeads. (2007). *Frequently asked questions.* Retrieved from http://www.cyclebeads.com/FAQ/.

Davis, V. (2006). SOGC Clinical Practice Guideline: Induced abortion guidelines. *Journal of Obstetrics and Gynaecology Canada, 28*(11), 1014–1027. Retrieved from http://www.sogc.org/guidelines/documents/gui184E0611.pdf.

D'Avanzo, C. E. (2008). *Pocket guide to cultural health assessment* (4th ed.). St. Louis: Mosby.

Georgia Reproductive Specialists. (2007). *Micromanipulation.* Retrieved from http://www.ivf.com/icsi.html.

Government of Canada. (2004). *Assisted human reproduction act.* Ottawa: Minister of Justice. Retrieved from http://laws.justice.gc.ca/PDF/Statute/A/A-13.4.pdf.

Grimes, D. (2007). Intrauterine devices (IUDs). In R. Hatcher, et al. (Eds.), *Contraceptive technology* (19th ed.). New York: Ardent Media.

Health Canada. (2010a). *It's your health: Condoms* (Catalogue #H13-7/75-2010E-PDF). Ottawa: Author. Retrieved from http://www.hc-sc.gc.ca/hl-vs/iyh-vsv/prod/condom-eng.php#ro.

Health Canada. (2010b). *Public communication. Health Canada endorsed important safety information on Mirena.* Retrieved from http://www.hc-sc.gc.ca/dhp-mps/medeff/advisories-avis/public/_2010/mirena_pc-cp-eng.php.

Kearnes, W., et al. (2005). Preimplantation genetic diagnosis and screening. *Seminars in Reproduction Medicine, 23*(4), 336–347.

Kennedy, K., & Trussell, J. (2007). Postpartum contraception and lactation. In R. Hatcher, et al. (Eds.), *Contraceptive technology* (19th ed.). New York: Ardent Media.

Lobo, R. (2007). Infertility: Etiology, diagnostic evaluation, management, prognosis. In V. L. Katz, et al. (Eds.), *Comprehensive gynecology* (5th ed.). St. Louis: Mosby.

Medical Advisory Secretariat. (2006). *In vitro fertilization and multiple pregnancies*. Toronto: Ontario Health Technology Advisory Committee. Retrieved from http://www.health.gov.on.ca/english/providers/program/ohtac/tech/reviews/pdf/rev_ivf_101906.pdf.

Min, J. K., Claman, P., Hughes, E., et al. (2006). SOGC/CFAS Guideline: Guidelines for the number of embryos to transfer following in vitro fertilization. *Journal of Obstetrics and Gynaecology Canada, 28*(9), 799–813. Retrieved from http://www.sogc.org/guidelines/documents/182E-CPG-Septembre2006.pdf.

Nelson, A., & Marshall, J. (2008). Impaired fertility. In R. Hatcher, et al. (Eds.), *Contraceptive technology* (19th ed.). New York: Ardent Media.

Planned Parenthood. (2008). *Diaphragms*. Updated May 15, 2008. Retrieved from http://www.plannedparenthood.org.

Reid, R., et al. (2010). SOGC Clinical Practice Guideline: Oral contraceptives and the risk of venous thromboembolism: an update. *Journal of Obstetrics and Gynaecology Canada, 32*(12), 1192–1197. Retrieved from http://www.sogc.org/guidelines/documents/gui252CPG1012E.pdf.

SexualityandU. (2010a). *Natural methods*. Retrieved from http://sexualityandu.ca/birth-control/birth_control_methods_contraception/natural_methods.

SexualityandU. (2010b). *Non-hormonal methods*. Retrieved from http://sexualityandu.ca/birth-control/birth_control_methods_contraception/non-hormonal-methods.

Sherrod, R. A. (2004). Understanding the emotional aspects of infertility: Implications for nursing practice. *Journal of Psychosocial Nursing and Mental Health Services, 42*(3), 40–49.

Sheweita, S., Tilmisany, A., & Al-Sawaf, H. (2005). Mechanisms of male infertility: Role of antioxidants. *Current Drug Metabolism, 6*(5), 495–501.

Society of Obstetricians and Gynaecologists of Canada. (2004). Clinical Practice Guideline: Canadian contraception consensus. *Journal of Obstetrics and Gynaecology Canada, 26*(4), 347–387. Retrieved from http://www.sogc.org/guidelines/public/143E-CPG3-April2004.pdf.

Society of Obstetricians and Gynaecologists of Canada. (2007). Canadian consensus guideline on continuous and extended hormonal contraception 2007. *Journal of Obstetrics and Gynaecology Canada, 27*(7), Supplement 2, S1–S32. Retrieved from http://www.sogc.org/guidelines/documents/gui195CPG0707_000.pdf.

Statistics Canada. (2009). *Births 2007.* (Cat. No. 84F0210X.) Ottawa: Author. Retrieved from http://www.statcan.gc.ca/pub/84f0210x/84f0210x2007000-eng.pdf.

Stewart, F., Trussell, J., & Van Look, P. (2007). Emergency contraception. In R. Hatcher, et al. (Eds.), *Contraceptive technology* (19th ed.). New York: Ardent Media.

Trussell, J. (2007). The essentials of contraception: Efficacy, safety, and personal considerations. In R. Hatcher, et al. (Eds.), *Contraceptive technology* (19th ed.). New York: Ardent Media.

Vause, T. D., Cheung, A. P., Sierra, S., Claman, P., Graham, J., et al. (2010). SOGC Clinical Practice Guideline: Ovulation induction in polycystic ovary syndrome. *Journal of Obstetrics and Gynaecology Canada, 32*(5), 495–502. Retrieved from http://sogc.org/guidelines/documents/gui242CPG1005E.pdf.

Weed, S. (1986). *Wise woman herbal for the childbearing year*. Woodstock, NY: Ash Tree Publishing.

Additional Resources

Assisted Human Reproduction Canada: http://www.ahrc-pac.gc.ca
Canadian Federation of Sexual Health: http://www.cfsh.ca
Infertility Awareness Association of Canada: http://www.iaac.ca
National Infertility Association: http://www.Resolve.org
SexualityandU: http://www.sexualityandu.ca

Unit 3

Preconception, Genetics, Conception, and Fetal Development

8

Learning Objectives

On completion of this chapter, the reader will be able to:

- Discuss the importance of preconception counselling.
- Explain the key concepts of basic human genetics.
- Describe expanded roles for nurses in genetics and genetic counselling.
- Examine ethical dimensions of genetic screening.
- Summarize the process of fertilization.
- Describe the development, structure, and functions of the placenta.
- Describe the composition and functions of the amniotic fluid.
- Identify three organs or tissues arising from each of the three primary germ layers.
- Summarize the significant changes in growth and development of the embryo and fetus.
- Identify the potential effects of teratogens during vulnerable periods of embryonic and fetal development.

Electronic Resources

Additional information related to the content in Chapter 8 can be found on

evolve the companion Web site at

http://evolve.elsevier.com/Canada/Perry/maternal/

- Examination Review Questions
- Animation—Fertilization and Implantation
- Animation—First Trimester, Fetal Development
- Animation—Male Accessory Sex Glands
- Animation—Male External Genitalia
- Animation—Male Reproductive Ducts
- Animation—Maternal and Fetal Circulation
- Animation—Oogenesis and Meiosis
- Animation—Pathway of Ovum
- Animation—Pathway of Sperm
- Animation—Second Trimester, Fetal Development
- Animation—Spermatogenesis
- Animation—Spermatozoa
- Animation—Testes
- Animation—Third Trimester, Fetal Development
- Critical Reference—Patterns of Inheritance
- Critical Thinking Exercise—Genetic Counselling

This chapter discusses the importance of preconception care and presents a brief discussion of **genetics** and the role of the nurse in genetics. It also provides an overview of the processes of fertilization and development of the normal embryo and fetus.

Preconception

If women receive appropriate care prior to pregnancy, there will be improved health outcomes for both mothers and newborns. Preconception care involves identifying and modifying risk factors in women in order to improve their health. Risk factors may include medical, behavioural, and social factors, many of which may be modifiable.

The American College of Obstetricians and Gynecologists (ACOG, 2005) suggests that all women should be asked the question, "Are you considering pregnancy or could you possibly become pregnant?" If women state that they are considering pregnancy, then care can be focused to ensure optimum health. Women should have an evaluation of their overall health and of opportunities for improving their health, and they should receive education about the effects of social, environmental, nutritional, occupational, behavioural, and genetic factors during pregnancy. Also, women at high risk for an adverse pregnancy outcome should be identified (Wilson et al., 2011). Such evaluation also involves identifying undiagnosed, untreated, or poorly controlled medical conditions. The goal of preconception health care is to optimize the health of every woman (Wilson et al., 2011). The components of preconception care, such as health promotion, risk assessment, and interventions, are outlined in Box 8-1.

Genetics

Genetic counselling is an important aspect of preconception and prenatal care. Recent advances in molecular biology and genomics have revolutionized the field of health care by providing the tools needed to determine the hereditary component of many diseases and improve our ability to predict susceptibility to disease, onset and progression of disease, and

BOX 8-1 Components of Preconception Care

Health Promotion: General Teaching

Nutrition
Healthy diet, including folic acid
Optimum weight
Exercise and rest
Avoidance of substance use (tobacco, alcohol, "recreational" drugs)
Use of risk-reducing sex practices
Attending to family and social needs

Risk Factor Assessment

Medical history
- Immune status (e.g., rubella, hepatitis B, varicella)
- Family history (e.g., genetic disorders)
- Illnesses (e.g., infections)
- Current use of medications (prescription, nonprescription)

Reproductive history
- Contraceptive
- Obstetric

Psychosocial history
- Spouse or partner and family situation, including intimate partner violence
- Availability of family or other support systems
- Readiness for pregnancy (e.g., age, life goals, stress)

Financial resources
Environmental (home, workplace) conditions
- Safety hazards
- Toxic chemicals
- Radiation

Interventions

Anticipatory guidance and teaching
Treatment of medical conditions and results
- Medications
- Cessation of or reduction in substance use
- Immunizations (e.g., rubella, tuberculosis, hepatitis)

Nutrition, diet, and weight management
Exercise
Referral for genetic counselling
Referral to and use of
- Family planning services
- Family and social needs management

response to medications (Guttmacher & Collins, 2005; Loescher & Merkle, 2005; Seo & Ginsburg, 2005). With this increase in genetic knowledge, there has been a gradual shift from *genetics* (the study of single genes and their effects) to *genomics* (the study of the functions and interactions of all the genes in the genome) (Lea, 2008).

The demand for genetic services, especially genetic testing, has never been greater. Genetics is recognized as a contributing factor in virtually all human illnesses. In maternity care, genetics issues occur before, during, and after pregnancy. With growing public interest in genetics, increasing commercial pressures, and Internet opportunities for individuals, families, and communities to participate in the direction and design of their genetic health care, genetic services are rapidly becoming an integral part of routine health care (Rubinstein & Roy, 2005).

For most genetic conditions therapeutic or preventive measures do not exist or are very limited. Consequently, the most useful means of reducing the incidence of these disorders is by preventing their transmission. It is standard practice to assess all pregnant women for heritable disorders to identify potential problems. The incidence of chromosome aberrations is estimated to be 0.5 to 0.6% in newborns. Approximately 62% of miscarriages and 5 to 7% of stillbirths and perinatal deaths are caused by chromosomal abnormalities (Hamilton & Wynshaw-Boris, 2009; Lashley, 2007).

Genetic disorders affect people of all ages, from all socioeconomic levels, and from all racial and ethnic backgrounds. They affect not only individuals but also families, communities, and society. Advances in genetic testing and genetically based treatments have altered the care provided to affected individuals. Improvements in diagnostic capability have resulted in earlier diagnosis and enabled individuals who previously would have died in childhood to survive into adulthood (Lashley, 2007). The genetic aberrations that lead to a disorder are present at birth but may not be manifested for many years, or possibly never manifested.

Some disorders appear more often in ethnic groups. Examples include Tay-Sachs disease in Ashkenazi Jews, French Canadians of the Eastern St. Lawrence River valley area of Québec, Cajuns from Louisiana, and the Amish in Pennsylvania; β-thalassemia in Mediterranean, Middle Eastern, Central Asian, Indian, and Far Eastern groups and in those of African heritage; sickle cell anemia in people who are Black; α-thalassemia in those from Southeast Asia, South China, the Philippine Islands, Thailand, Greece, and Cyprus; lactase deficiency in adult Chinese and Thailanders; neural tube defects in those from Ireland, Scotland, and Wales; phenylketonuria (PKU) in the Irish, Scots, Scandinavians, Icelanders, and Poles; cystic fibrosis (CF) in Whites, Ashkenazi Jews, and Latin Americans; and Niemann-Pick disease, type A, in Ashkenazi Jews (Hamilton & Wynshaw-Boris, 2009; Wapner, Jenkins, & Khalek, 2009).

Relevance of Genetics to Nursing

Genetic disorders span every clinical practice specialty and site, including school, clinic, office, hospital, mental health agency, and community health settings. Because the potential impact on families and the community is significant (Box 8-2), genetics must be integrated into nursing education and practice. Genetic information, technology, and testing must be incorporated into health care services.

Expanded or new roles for nurses with expertise in genetics and genomics are developing in many areas of maternity and women's health nursing. These areas include but are not limited to preconception counselling and preimplantation diagnosis for patients at risk for the transmission of a genetic disorder; prenatal screening and testing; prenatal care for women with psychiatric disorders that have a genetic component, such as bipolar disorder and schizophrenia; newborn screening and testing; the care of families who have lost a fetus or a child affected by a genetic condition; the identification

BOX 8-2 Potential Impact of Genetic Disease on Family and Community

- Financial cost to family
- Decrease in planned family size
- Loss of geographic mobility
- Decreased opportunities for siblings
- Loss of family integrity
- Loss of career opportunities and job flexibility
- Social isolation
- Lifestyle alterations
- Reduction in contributions to their community by families
- Disruption of husband–wife or partner relationship
- Threatened family self-concept
- Coping with intolerant public attitudes
- Psychological effects
- Stresses and uncertainty of treatment
- Physical health problems
- Loss of dreams and aspirations
- Cost to society of institutionalization or home or community care
- Cost to society because of additional problems and needs of other family members
- Cost of long-term care
- Housing and living arrangement changes

(From Lashley, F. [2007]. *Essentials of clinical genetics in nursing practice,* New York: Springer.)

BOX 8-3 Nursing Skills Used In Genetic Counselling

- Taking detailed family histories
- Developing treatment plans
- Providing treatments
- Counselling clients
- Working with families
- Teaching risk reduction and health promotion
- Making referrals
- Providing follow-up
- Working in multidisciplinary teams

(Source: Canadian Nurses Association [2005]. *Nursing and genetics: Are you ready?* Ottawa: Author. Retrieved from http://www.cna-aiic.ca/CNA/documents/pdf/publications/NN_Genetics_05_e.pdf.)

COMMUNITY FOCUS

Resources for Families With Children With Genetic Disorders

Select an organization that is specific to a genetic disorder (e.g., neurofibromatosis, Marfan syndrome, Down syndrome). Access the Web site for the organization. What services and resources are available for families? Are these services and resources free, or must the family pay for them? Is there a branch of the organization available in your city? If there is no branch of the organization available in your city, where could families go for information and assistance? For your selected genetic disorder, prepare a list of resources for families with a child with the disorder.

and care of children with genetic conditions, and their families; and the care of women with genetic conditions who require specialized care during pregnancy, such as women with congenital heart disease, CF, Marfan syndrome (http://www.marfan.org), or factor V Leiden.

Although diagnosis and treatment of genetic disorders requires medical skills, nurses use their nursing skills as they assume important roles in counselling people about genetically transmitted or genetically influenced conditions (Box 8-3). Most diseases have a genetic component, and nurses are usually the ones who provide follow-up care and maintain contact with the patients. Community health nurses can identify groups within populations that are at high risk for illness and provide care to individuals, families, and groups. They are a vital link in follow-up for newborns who may need newborn screening.

Referral to appropriate agencies is an essential part of the follow-up management. Many organizations and foundations (e.g., the Canadian Cystic Fibrosis Foundation and Muscular Dystrophy Canada) help provide services and equipment for affected children. There are also numerous parent groups in which the family can share experiences and derive mutual support from other families with similar problems.

Probably the most important of all nursing functions is providing emotional support to the family during all aspects of the counselling process. Feelings that arise under the real or imagined threat posed by a genetic disorder are as varied as the people being counselled. Responses may include a variety of stress reactions such as apathy, denial, anger, hostility, fear, embarrassment, grief, and loss of self-esteem.

The United States and United Kingdom have advanced education for genetic nursing, with well-developed curriculum and specialization certification. Presently, there is no genetics education available in Canada for nurses, although researchers are pursuing the development of genetic education and professional development activities in general and of advanced practice nursing in genetics (Canadian Nurses Association [CNA], 2005).

evolve Critical Thinking Exercise—Genetic Counseling

Genetic History-Taking and Counselling Services

It is standard practice in perinatal care to determine whether a heritable disorder exists in a couple or in anyone in either of their families. The goal of screening is to detect or define risk for disease in low-risk populations and to identify those for whom diagnostic testing may be appropriate. A nurse can obtain a genetic history using a questionnaire or checklist such as the one in Fig. 8-1.

Genetic counselling that follows may occur in the office, or referral to a geneticist may be necessary. Health professionals should become familiar with people who provide genetic counselling and the places that offer counselling services in their area of practice (see Community Focus box).

Risk Factors for Genetic Disorders

Answer the following questions about risk factors. If you answer "yes" to any of them, you may be at increased risk for having a baby with a genetic disorder.

______Will you be age 35 years or older when your baby is due?

______Will the baby's father be age 50 years or older when your baby is due?

______If you or the baby's father are of Mediterranean or Asian descent, do either of you or anyone in your families have thalassemia?

______Is there a family history of neural tube defects?

______Have you or the baby's father ever had a child with a neural tube defect?

______Is there a family history of congenital heart defects?

______Is there a family history of Down syndrome?

______Have you or the baby's father ever had a child with Down syndrome?

______If you or the baby's father are of Eastern European Jewish, French Canadian, or Cajun descent, is there a family history of Tay-Sachs disease?

______If you or your partner are of Eastern European Jewish descent, is there a family history of Canavan disease or any other genetic disorders?

______If you or your partner are of African descent, is there a family history of sickle cell disease or sickle cell trait?

______Is there a family history of hemophilia?

______Is there a family history of muscular dystrophy?

______Is there a family history of cystic fibrosis?

______Is there a family history of Huntington's disease?

______Does anyone in your family or the family of the baby's father have cystic fibrosis?

______Is anyone in your family or the baby's father's family developmentally disabled?

______If so, was that person tested for fragile X syndrome?

______Do you, the baby's father, anyone in your families, or any of your children have any other genetic diseases, chromosomal disorders, or birth defects?

______Do you have a metabolic disorder such as diabetes or phenylketonuria?

______Do you have a history of pregnancy issues (miscarriage or stillbirth)?

Fig. 8-1 Questionnaire for identifying couples having increased risk for offspring with genetic disorders. *(Courtesy American College of Obstetricians and Gynecologists [2010].* Your pregnancy and childbirth: month to month *[5th ed]. Washington, DC: ACOG.)*

Individuals and families seek out or are referred for genetic counselling for a wide variety of reasons and at all stages of their lives. Some seek preconception or prenatal information; others are referred after the birth of a child with a birth defect or a suspected genetic condition; still others seek information because they have a family history of a genetic condition. Regardless of the setting or the individual and family's stage of life, genetic counselling should be offered and available to all individuals and families who have questions about genetics and their health.

Estimation of Risk

Most families with a history of genetic disease want an answer to the following question: What is the chance that our future children will have this disease? Because the answer to this question may have profound implications for individual family members and the family as a whole, health care providers must be able to answer this question as accurately as they can in a timely manner.

If a couple has not yet had children but is known to be at risk for having children with a genetic disease, they will be given an occurrence risk. Once the mating of a couple has produced one or more children with a genetic disease, the couple will be given a recurrence risk. Both occurrence and recurrence risks are determined by the mode of inheritance for the genetic disease in question. For genetic diseases caused by a factor that segregates during cell division (genes and chromosomes), risk can be estimated with a high degree of accuracy by application of the Mendelian principles (http://www.ncbi.nlm.nih.gov/entrez/query.fcgi?db=OMIM) (see Community Focus box).

In an autosomal dominant disorder, both the occurrence and recurrence risk is 50%, or 1 in 2, that a subsequent offspring will be affected. The recurrence risk for autosomal recessive disorders is 25%, or 1 in 4. For X-linked disorders, recurrence is related to the sex of the child. **Translocation** chromosomes have a high risk of recurrence.

The risk of recurrence for multifactorial conditions can be estimated empirically. An empiric risk is based not on genetics theory but rather on experience and observation of the disorder in other families. Recurrence risks are determined by applying the frequency of a similar disorder in other families to the case under consideration.

Disorders in which a subsequent pregnancy would carry no more risk than there is for pregnancy alone (estimated at 1 in 30) include those resulting from isolated incidences not likely to be present in another pregnancy. These disorders include maternal infections (e.g., rubella and toxoplasmosis), maternal ingestion of drugs, most chromosomal abnormalities, and a disorder determined to be the result of a fresh mutation.

Interpretation of Risk

The guiding principle for genetics counsellors has traditionally been the principle of nondirectiveness. According to the principle of nondirectiveness, the individual who is providing genetics counselling respects the right of the individual or family being counselled to make autonomous decisions. Counsellors using a nondirective approach avoid making recommendations, and they try to communicate genetics information in an unbiased manner. The first step in providing nondirective counselling is becoming aware of one's own values and beliefs. Another important step is recognizing how one's values and beliefs can influence or interfere with the communication of genetics information.

The counsellor provides appropriate information about the nature of the disorder, the extent of the risks in the specific case, the probable consequences, and (if appropriate) alternative options available; however, the final decision to become pregnant or to continue a pregnancy must be left to the family. An important nursing role is reinforcing the information that the families are given and continuing to interpret this information on their level of understanding.

COMMUNITY FOCUS

Internet Resources on Genetics

Identify two Web sites for resources on genetics for parents from a search of the Internet. Access the sites.

- Compare and contrast the appearance, readability, and information contained in the sites.
- To whom would you recommend these sites?
- Is the information contained culturally relevant?
- What information would parents need?
- How could you as a nurse use this information?

An important concept that must be emphasized to families is that *each pregnancy is an independent event.* For example, in monogenic disorders in which the risk factor is 1 in 4 that the child will be affected, the risk remains the same no matter how many affected children are already in the family. Families may make the erroneous assumption that the presence of one affected child ensures that the next three will be free of the disorder. However, "chance has no memory." The risk is 1 in 4 for each pregnancy. In a family with a child who has a disorder with multifactorial causes, however, the risk increases with each subsequent child born with the disorder.

The Human Genome Project

The Human Genome Project was a publicly funded international effort coordinated by the National Institutes of Health and the U.S. Department of Energy (http://www.doegenomes.org). When the Human Genome Project was initiated in 1990, the ultimate goal of the project was to map the human genome (the complete set of genetic instructions in the nucleus of each human cell) by 2005. In April 2003, a complete version of the human genome was announced (http://www.genome.gov/11006929).

Two key findings from initial efforts to sequence and analyze the human genome are that (1) all humans are 99.9% identical at the DNA level, and (2) approximately 20,000 to 25,000 genes (pieces or sequences of DNA that contain information needed to make proteins) make up the human genome. This is a much smaller number than the 80,000 to 150,000 estimated by scientists. A new explanation for human complexity, given the relatively small number of genes, is that humans use their genes more efficiently. Humans are able to do much more with their genes than other species. Instead of producing only one protein per gene, most human genes produce at least three proteins.

Initial efforts to sequence and analyze the human genome have proven invaluable in the identification of genes involved in disease and in the development of genetic tests. Hundreds of genes involved in diseases such as Huntington's disease (HD), breast cancer, colon cancer, Alzheimer's disease, achondroplasia, and CF have been identified. The number of commercially available genetic tests continues to increase and can be found at GeneTests (http://www.genetests.org).

Genetic Testing

Genetic testing involves the analysis of human DNA, ribonucleic acid (RNA), chromosomes (threadlike packages of genes and other DNA in the nucleus of a cell), or proteins to detect abnormalities related to an inherited condition. Genetic tests can be used to examine directly the DNA and RNA that make up a gene (direct or molecular testing), look at markers that are coinherited with a gene that causes a genetic condition (linkage analysis), examine the protein products of genes (biochemical testing), or examine chromosomes (**cytogenetic** testing).

Most of the genetic tests now being offered in clinical practice are tests for single-gene disorders in patients with clinical symptoms or who have a family history of a genetic disease. Some of these genetic tests are prenatal tests, or tests used to identify the genetic status of a pregnancy at risk for a genetic condition. Current prenatal testing options include first-trimester screening (nuchal translucency combined with biological markers), integrated prenatal screening (a blood test combined with ultrasound examination to see if a pregnant woman is at increased risk for carrying a fetus with a neural tube defect or a chromosome abnormality, such as Down syndrome), and invasive procedures (amniocentesis and chorionic villus sampling) (see discussion in Chapter 12). Other tests are carrier screening tests, which are used to identify individuals who have a gene mutation for a genetic condition but do not show symptoms of the condition because it is a condition that is inherited in an autosomal recessive form (e.g., CF, sickle cell disease, Tay-Sachs disease).

Another type of genetic testing is predictive testing, which is used to clarify the genetic status of asymptomatic family members. The two types of predictive testing are presymptomatic and predispositional. Mutation analysis for HD, a neurodegenerative disorder, is an example of presymptomatic testing. If the gene mutation for HD is present, symptoms of HD are certain to appear if the individual lives long enough. Testing for a *BRCA1* gene mutation to determine breast cancer susceptibility is an example of predispositional testing. Predispositional testing differs from presymptomatic testing in that a positive result (indicating that a *BRCA1* mutation is present) does not indicate a 100% risk of developing the condition (breast cancer).

In addition to using genetic tests to test for single-gene disorders, they are being used for population-based screening (e.g., province-mandated newborn screening for PKU and other inborn errors of metabolism [IEMs]).

Factors Influencing the Decision to Undergo Genetic Testing

Decisions about genetic testing are shaped, and in many instances constrained, by factors such as social norms and where care is received. Most pregnant women in Canada now have at least one ultrasound examination and undergo some type of multiple-marker screening, and a growing number undergo other types of prenatal testing. The range of prenatal testing options available to a pregnant woman and her family may vary significantly, based on where the pregnant woman receives prenatal care. Certain types of prenatal testing may not be available in smaller communities and rural settings (e.g., chorionic villus sampling and fluorescent in situ hybridization analysis). In addition, certain types of genetic testing may not be offered in conservative medical communities (e.g., preimplantation diagnosis).

There are ethical dimensions to making the decision to be tested. The decision to undergo testing is seldom an autonomous one based solely on the needs and preferences of the individual being tested. Instead, it is often a decision based on feelings of responsibility and commitment to others (Van Riper, 2005; Van Riper & McKinnon, 2004). For example, a woman who has a family history of CF may decide to have genetic testing, but then decisions must be made about the outcome of the pregnancy depending on the results of the testing.

Gene Therapy (Gene Transfer)

The aim of gene therapy is to correct defective genes that are responsible for disease development. The most common technique is to insert a normal gene in a location within the genome to replace a gene that is nonfunctional (http://www.ornl.gov/sci/techresources/Human_Genome/medicine/genetherapy.shtml). In the early 1990s, there was a great deal of optimism about the possibility of using genetic information to provide quick solutions to a long list of health problems. Although the early optimism about gene therapy was probably never fully justified, it is likely that the development of safer and more effective methods for gene delivery will ensure a significant role for gene therapy in the treatment of some diseases. Major challenges include targeting the right gene to the right location in the right cells, expressing the transferred gene at the right time, and minimizing adverse reactions. No human gene therapy product has yet been approved by Health Canada. Current research includes treatment for inherited blindness, lung cancer tumours, melanoma, myeloid disorders, deafness, sickle cell disease, and other blood disorders.

Ethical, Legal, and Social Implications

Because of widespread concern about misuse of the information gained through genetics research, 5% of the Human Genome Project budget was designated for the study of the ethical, legal, and social implications (ELSIs) of human genome research. During the past decade, issues of high priority for this program have been privacy and fairness in the use and interpretation of genetic information; clinical integration of new genetic technologies; issues surrounding genetics research, such as possible discrimination and stigmatization; and education for professionals and the general public about genetics, genetics health care, and the ELSIs of human genome research. These programs address the potential that genetic information may be used to discriminate against individuals or for eugenic purposes. Informed consent is very difficult to ensure when some of the outcomes, benefits, and risks of genetic testing remain unknown. Continued awareness of and vigilance against such misuse of information is the collective responsibility of health care providers, ethicists, and society. Some ethical considerations include the following: What is normal or a disability and who decides? Are disabilities diseases that need to be prevented or cured? Who will have access to these expensive therapies? Who will pay for them?

Clinical Genetics

Genetic Transmission

Human development is a complicated process that depends on the systematic unraveling of instructions found in the genetic material of the egg and the sperm. Development from conception to birth of a normal, healthy baby occurs without incident in most cases; however, occasionally some anomaly in the genetic code of the embryo creates a birth defect or disorder. The science of genetics seeks to explain the underlying causes of congenital disorders (disorders present at birth) and the patterns in which inherited disorders are passed from generation to generation.

Genes and Chromosomes

The hereditary material carried in the nucleus of each somatic (body) cell determines an individual's physical characteristics. This material, called *DNA*, forms threadlike strands known as *chromosomes*. Each chromosome is composed of many smaller segments of DNA referred to as *genes*. Genes or combinations of genes contain coded information that determines an individual's unique characteristics. The code consists of the specific linear order of the molecules that combine to form the strands of DNA. Genes control both the types of proteins that are made and the rate at which they are produced. Genes never act in isolation; they always interact with other genes and the environment.

All normal human **somatic cells** contain 46 chromosomes arranged as 23 pairs of homologous (matched) chromosomes; one chromosome of each pair is inherited from each parent. There are 22 pairs of **autosomes**, which control most traits in the body, and one pair of sex chromosomes, which determines sex and some other traits. The larger female chromosome is called the X; the smaller male chromosome is the Y. Generally the presence of a Y chromosome causes an embryo to develop as a male; in the absence of a Y chromosome, the individual develops as a female. Thus, in a normal female, the homologous pair of sex chromosomes is XX, and in a normal male, the homologous pair is XY.

Homologous chromosomes (except the X and Y chromosomes in males) have the same number and arrangement of genes. In other words, if an autosome has a gene for hair colour, its partner also has a gene for hair colour—in the same location on the chromosome. Although both genes code for hair colour, they may not code for the same hair colour. Genes at corresponding loci on homologous chromosomes that code for different forms or variations of the same trait are called **alleles.** An individual with two copies of the same allele for a given trait is said to be **homozygous** for that trait. With two different alleles the person is **heterozygous** for the trait.

The term **genotype** typically is used to refer to the genetic makeup of an individual in the context of discussing a specific gene pair, but at times *genotype* is used to refer to an individual's entire genetic makeup or all the genes that the individual can pass on to future generations. **Phenotype** refers to the observable expression of an individual's genotype, such as physical features, a biochemical or molecular trait, and even a psychological trait. A trait or disorder is considered *dominant* if it is expressed or phenotypically apparent when only one copy of the gene is present. It is considered *recessive* if it is expressed only when two copies of the gene are present.

As more is learned about genetics, the concepts of dominance and recessivity have become more complex, especially in X-linked disorders (Lashley, 2007). For example, traits considered to be recessive may be expressed even when only one copy of a gene located on the X chromosome is present. This occurs frequently in males because males have only one X chromosome; thus they have only one copy of the genes located on the X chromosome. Whichever gene is present on the one X chromosome determines which trait is expressed. Conversely, females have two X chromosomes; thus they have two copies of the genes located on the X chromosome. However, in any female somatic cell only one X chromosome is functioning (otherwise there would be inequality in gene dosage between males and females). This process, known as X-inactivation, or the Lyon hypothesis, is generally a random occurrence (i.e., there is a 50:50 chance of the maternal X or the paternal X being inactivated). Occasionally, the percentage of cells that have the X with an abnormal or mutant gene is very high. This helps explain why hemophilia, an X-linked recessive disorder, can clinically manifest itself in a female known to be a heterozygous carrier (a female who has only one copy of the gene mutation). It also helps explain why traditional methods of carrier detection are less effective for X-linked recessive disorders; the possible range for enzyme activity values can vary greatly, depending on which X chromosome is inactivated.

Chromosome Abnormalities

Chromosome abnormalities are a major cause of reproductive loss, congenital problems, and gynecological disorders and account for approximately 4 to 7% of perinatal deaths and 0.5 to 1% of infants born with multiple anomalies. Errors resulting in chromosome abnormalities can occur in **mitosis** or **meiosis**. These errors can occur in either the autosomes or the sex chromosomes. Even without the presence of obvious structural malformations, small deviations in chromosomes can cause problems in fetal development.

The pictorial analysis of the number, form, and size of an individual's chromosomes is known as a **karyotype**. Cells from any nucleated, replicating body tissue (not red blood cells, nerves, or muscles) can be used. The most commonly used tissues are white blood cells and fetal cells in amniotic fluid. The cells are grown in a culture and arrested when they are in metaphase and then dropped onto a slide. This breaks the cell membranes and spreads the chromosomes, making them easier to visualize. The cells are stained with special stains (e.g., Giemsa stain) that create striping or "banding" patterns. These patterns aid in the analysis because they are consistent from person to person. Once the chromosome spreads are photographed or scanned by a computer, they are cut out and arranged in a specific numeric order according to their length and shape. They are numbered from largest to smallest, 1 to 22, and the sex chromosomes are designated by the letter X or Y. Each chromosome is divided into two "arms" designated by p (short arm) and q (long arm). A female karyotype is designated as 46, XX, and a male karyotype is designated as 46, XY. Fig. 8-2 illustrates the chromosomes in a body cell and a karyotype. Karyotypes can be used to determine the sex of a child and the presence of any gross chromosomal abnormalities.

Autosome Abnormalities

Autosome abnormalities involve differences in the number or structure of autosome chromosomes (pairs 1 to 22) resulting from unequal distribution of the genetic material during **gamete** (egg and sperm) formation.

Abnormalities of Chromosome Number. *Euploidy* is the term used to denote the correct number of chromosomes. Deviations from the correct number of chromosomes, or the **diploid** number (2 N, 46 chromosomes), can be one of two types: (1) **polyploidy**, in which the deviation is an exact multiple of the haploid number of chromosomes, or one chromosome set (23 chromosomes); or (2) *aneuploidy*, in which the numeric deviation is not an exact multiple of the haploid set (Lashley, 2007). A triploid (3 N) cell is an example of a

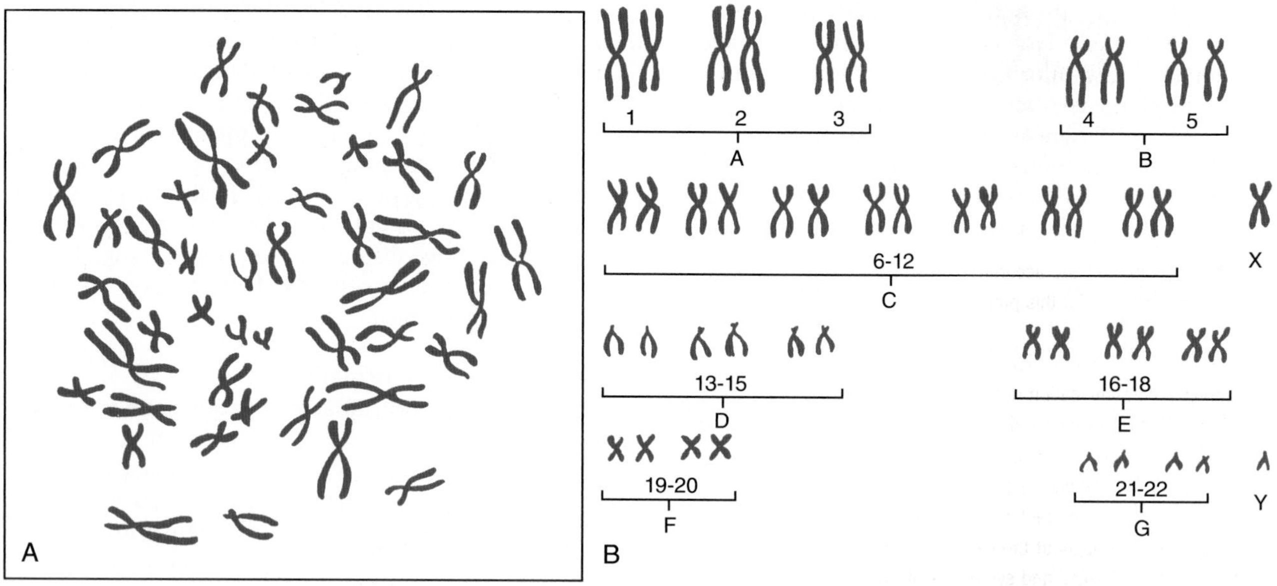

Fig. 8-2 Chromosomes during cell division. **A:** Example of photomicrograph. **B:** Chromosomes arranged in karyotype; female and male sex-determining chromosomes.

polyploidy. It has 69 chromosomes. A tetraploid (4 N) cell, also an example of a polyploidy, has 92 chromosomes.

Aneuploidy is the most commonly identified chromosome abnormality in humans. It occurs in at least 5% of all clinically recognized pregnancies, and it is the leading known cause of pregnancy loss. Aneuploidy also is the leading genetic cause of developmental disability. The two most common aneuploid conditions are monosomies and trisomies. A **monosomy** is the product of the union between a normal gamete and a gamete that is missing a chromosome. Monosomic individuals only have 45 chromosomes in each of their cells. The product of the union of a normal gamete with a gamete containing an extra chromosome is a *trisomy*. Trisomies are more common than monosomies. Trisomic individuals have 47 chromosomes in each of their cells.

Limited data are available concerning the origin of monosomies because when an embryo is missing an autosomal chromosome, the embryo never survives. Although a great deal of variation exists among trisomies with regard to the parent and stage of origin of the extra chromosome, most trisomies are maternal meiosis I errors. This means that most trisomies are caused by nondisjunction during the first meiotic division (i.e., one pair of chromosomes fails to separate). One of the resulting cells contains two chromosomes, and the other contains none.

The most common trisomal abnormality is Down syndrome, or trisomy 21 (47,XX+21, female with Down syndrome; or 47,XY+21, male with Down syndrome). Although the risk of having a child with Down syndrome increases with maternal age (incidence is approximately 1 in 1200 for a 25-year-old woman; 1 in 350 for a 35-year-old woman; and 1 in 30 for a 45-year-old woman), children with Down syndrome can be born to mothers of any age. Eighty percent of children with Down syndrome are born to mothers younger than 35 years (National Down Syndrome Society, 2010a, 2010b). Since the average age of mothers when they give birth to children with Down syndrome is about 27 years, the Society of Obstetricians and Gynaecologists of Canada (2007) recommends that all pregnant women be offered prenatal screening for Down syndrome and not just women over 35. The risk of a mother having a second child with Down syndrome is about 1% when the cause of the Down syndrome is trisomy 21 (see Nursing Care Plan) (see also Fig. 42-6 and discussion in Chapter 42).

Other autosomal trisomies that have been identified are trisomy 18 (Edwards syndrome) and trisomy 13 (Patau's syndrome). Infants with trisomy 18 and trisomy 13 are usually severely to profoundly developmentally delayed. Although both conditions have a very poor prognosis, with the vast majority of affected infants dying within the first few days of life, a significant percentage of these infants survive the first 6 months to 1 year of life; some children with trisomy 18 and trisomy 13 have lived beyond 10 years of age.

Nondisjunction can also occur during mitosis. If this occurs early in development when cell lines are forming, the individual has a mixture of cells, some with a normal number of chromosomes and others either missing a chromosome or containing an extra chromosome. This condition is known as *mosaicism*. Mosaicism in autosomes is most commonly seen as another form of Down syndrome. Approximately 1 to 2% of individuals with Down syndrome have mosaic Down syndrome.

Abnormalities of Chromosome Structure. Structural abnormalities can occur in any chromosome. Types of structural abnormalities include translocation, duplication, deletion, microdeletion, and inversion. Translocation occurs when there is an exchange of chromosome material between two chromosomes. Exposure to certain drugs, viruses, and radiation can cause translocations, but often they arise for no apparent reason. Thus, instead of two normal pairs of chromosomes, the individual has one normal chromosome of each pair and a third chromosome that is a fusion of the other two

NURSING CARE PLAN ● The Family With a Diagnosis of a Fetus With Down Syndrome at 18 Weeks' Gestation

Nursing Diagnosis: Risk for interrupted family processes related to diagnosis of fetus with an inherited disorder

Expected Outcome

The couple will communicate accurate information about Down syndrome and the implications for this pregnancy as well as for future pregnancies.

Nursing Interventions/Rationales

Use therapeutic communication during discussions with the couple *to provide opportunity for expression of concern.*

Assess knowledge base of couple regarding information about Down syndrome and inheritance patterns *to correct any misconceptions and establish basis for teaching plan.*

Provide information throughout the genetics evaluation regarding risk status and clinical signs and symptoms of Down syndrome *to give couple a realistic picture of neonate's defects and assist with decision making for future pregnancies.*

Refer to support groups, social services, or counselling *to assist with family cohesive actions and decision making.*

Refer to child development specialist *to provide family with realistic expectations regarding cognitive and behavioural differences of child with Down syndrome.*

Nursing Diagnosis: Situational low self-esteem related to diagnosis of inherited disorder as evidenced by parents' statements of guilt and shame

Expected Outcome

The parents will express an increased number of positive statements regarding the upcoming birth of their child with Down syndrome.

Nursing Interventions/Rationales

Assist parents in listing strengths and coping strategies that have been helpful in past situations *to use appropriate strategies during this situational crisis.*

Encourage expression of feelings using therapeutic communication *to provide clarification and emotional support.*

Clarify and provide information regarding Down syndrome *to decrease feelings of guilt and gradually increase feelings of positive self-esteem.*

Refer for further counselling as needed *to provide more in-depth and ongoing support.*

Nursing Diagnosis: Risk for impaired parenting related to birth of neonate with Down syndrome

Expected Outcome

Parents demonstrate competent skills in parenting a child with Down syndrome and willingness to care for neonate.

Nursing Interventions/Rationales

Discuss and role play with parents ways of informing family and friends of diagnosis *to promote positive aspects of infant and decrease potential isolation from social interactions.*

Provide anticipatory guidance about what to expect as infant develops *to help family to be prepared for behavioural problems or mental deficits.*

Nursing Diagnosis: Spiritual distress related to situational crisis of fetus diagnosed with Down syndrome

Expected Outcome

Parents seek appropriate support persons (e.g., family members, priest, minister, rabbi) for assistance.

Nursing Interventions/Rationales

Listen for cues indicative of parents' feelings ("Why did God do this to us?") *to identify messages indicating spiritual distress.*

Acknowledge parents' spiritual concerns and encourage expression of feelings *to help build a therapeutic relationship.*

Facilitate visits from clergy and provide privacy during visits *to demonstrate respect for parents' relationship with clergy.*

Encourage parents to discuss concerns with clergy *to use expert spiritual care resources to help the parents.*

Facilitate interaction with family members and other support persons *to encourage expressions of concern and seek comfort.*

Nursing Diagnosis: Risk for social isolation related to full-time caretaking responsibilities for a neonate with Down syndrome

Expected Outcome

Parents will describe a plan to use resources to prevent social isolation.

Nursing Interventions/Rationales

Provide opportunity for parents to express feelings about caring for a neonate with Down syndrome *to facilitate effective communication and trust.*

Discuss with parents their expectations about caring for the neonate *to identify potential areas of concern.*

Assist parents in identifying potential caregiving resources *to permit parents to return to a routine at home.*

Refer to support groups of parents of children with Down syndrome *to enlist support, understanding, and strategies for coping.*

chromosomes. As long as all genetic material is retained in the cell, the individual is unaffected but is a carrier of a balanced translocation.

If a gamete receives the two normal chromosomes or the fused chromosome, the resulting offspring will be clinically normal. If the gamete receives one of the two normal chromosomes and the fused version, the resulting offspring will have an extra copy of one of the chromosomes. This condition is called an *unbalanced translocation* and often has serious clinical effects.

Whenever a portion of a chromosome is deleted from one chromosome and added to another, the gamete produced may have either extra copies of genes or too few copies. The clinical effects produced may be mild or severe, depending on the amount of genetic material involved. Two of the more common conditions are the deletion of the short arm of chromosome 5 (cri du chat syndrome) and the deletion of the long arm of chromosome 18.

Sex Chromosome Abnormalities

Several sex chromosome abnormalities are caused by nondisjunction during gametogenesis in either parent. The most common deviation in females is Turner's syndrome, or monosomy X (45,X). The affected female exhibits juvenile external genitalia with undeveloped ovaries. She is usually short in stature with webbing of the neck and lymphedema of her hands and feet. Intelligence may be impaired. Most affected embryos miscarry spontaneously.

The most common deviation in males is Klinefelter's syndrome, or trisomy XXY. The affected male has poorly developed secondary sexual characteristics and small testes. He is infertile, usually tall, and effeminate and may be slow to learn. Males who have mosaic Klinefelter's syndrome may be fertile.

Patterns of Genetic Transmission

Heritable characteristics are those that can be passed on to offspring. The patterns by which genetic material is transmitted to the next generation are affected by the number of genes involved in the expression of the trait. Many phenotypic characteristics result from two or more genes on different chromosomes acting together (referred to as *multifactorial inheritance*); others are controlled by a single gene (*unifactorial inheritance*). Specialists in genetics (e.g., geneticists, genetics counselors, and nurses with advanced expertise in genetics) predict the probability of the presence of an abnormal gene from the known occurrence of the trait in the individual's family and the known patterns by which the trait is inherited.

Multifactorial Inheritance

Most common congenital malformations result from multifactorial inheritance, a combination of genetic and environmental factors. Examples are cleft lip, cleft palate, congenital heart disease, neural tube defects, and pyloric stenosis. Each malformation may range from mild to severe, depending on the number of genes for the defect present or the amount of environmental influence. A **neural tube defect** may range from spina bifida, a bony defect in the lumbar region of the vertebrae with little or no neurological impairment, to anencephaly, the absence of brain development, which is always fatal. Some malformations occur more often in one sex. For example, pyloric stenosis and cleft lip are more common in males, and cleft palate is more common in females.

Unifactorial Inheritance

If a single gene controls a particular trait, disorder, or defect, its pattern of inheritance is referred to as *unifactorial Mendelian* or *single-gene inheritance*. The number of single-gene disorders far exceeds the number of chromosomal abnormalities. Potential patterns of inheritance for single-gene disorders include autosomal dominant, autosomal recessive, and X-linked dominant and recessive modes of inheritance (Fig. 8-3).

Autosomal Dominant Inheritance

Autosomal dominant inheritance disorders are those in which only one copy of a variant allele is needed for phenotypic expression. The variant allele may appear as a result of a *mutation*, a spontaneous and permanent change in the normal gene structure. In this case, the disorder occurs for the first time in the family. Usually an affected individual comes from multiple generations having the disorder (see Fig. 8-3, B and C). There is a vertical pattern of inheritance (there is no skipping of generations; if an individual has an autosomal dominant disorder such as HD, so must one of his or her parents). Males and females are affected equally.

Autosomal dominant disorders are not always expressed with the same severity of symptoms. For example, a woman who has an autosomal dominant disorder may show few symptoms and may not become aware of her diagnosis until after she gives birth to a severely affected child. The predicting

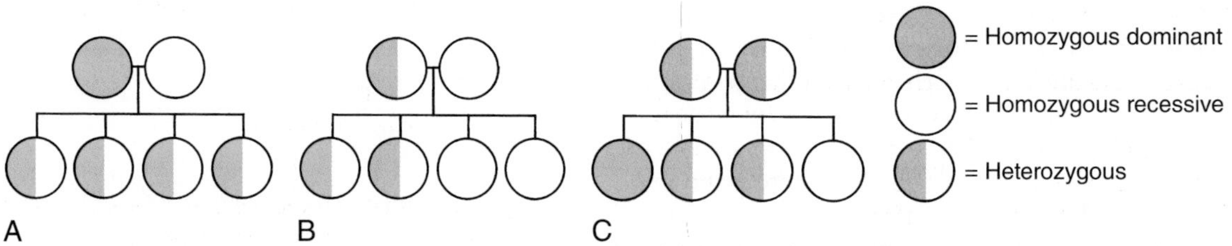

Fig. 8-3 Possible offspring in three types of matings. **A:** Homozygous-dominant parent and homozygous-recessive parent. Children: all heterozygous, displaying dominant trait. **B:** Heterozygous parent and homozygous-recessive parent. Children: 50% heterozygous, displaying dominant trait; 50% homozygous, displaying recessive trait. **C:** Both parents heterozygous. Children: 25% homozygous, displaying dominant trait; 25% homozygous, displaying recessive trait; 50% heterozygous, displaying dominant trait.

of whether an offspring will have a minor or severe abnormality is not possible. Examples of autosomal dominant disorders are Marfan syndrome, neurofibromatosis, myotonic dystrophy, Stickler's syndrome, Treacher Collins syndrome, and achondroplasia (dwarfism).

Autosomal Recessive Inheritance

Autosomal recessive inheritance disorders are those in which both genes of a pair must be abnormal for the disorder to be expressed. Heterozygous individuals have only one variant allele and are unaffected clinically because their normal gene overshadows the variant allele. They are known as *carriers* of the recessive trait. Because these recessive traits are inherited by generations of the same family, an increased incidence of the disorder occurs in consanguineous matings (closely related parents). For the trait to be expressed, two carriers must each contribute a variant allele to the offspring (see Fig. 8-3, C). The chance of the trait occurring in each child is 25%. A clinically normal offspring may be a carrier of the gene. Autosomal recessive disorders have a horizontal pattern of inheritance rather than the vertical pattern seen with autosomal dominant disorders (i.e., autosomal recessive disorders are usually observed in one or more siblings but not in earlier generations). Males and females are equally affected. Most inborn errors of metabolism (IEMs), such as PKU, galactosemia, maple syrup urine disease, Tay-Sachs disease, sickle cell anemia, and CF, are autosomal recessive inherited disorders.

Inborn Errors of Metabolism. More than 350 IEMs have been recognized (Jorde et al., 2010). Individually, IEMs are relatively rare, but collectively they are common (1 in 5000 live births). IEMs occur when a gene mutation reduces the efficiency of encoded enzymes to a level at which normal metabolism cannot occur. Defective enzyme action interrupts the normal series of chemical reactions from the affected point onward. The result may be an accumulation of a damaging product, such as phenylalanine in PKU, or the absence of a necessary product, such as the lack of melanin in albinism caused by lack of tyrosinase. Diagnostic and carrier testing are available for a growing number of IEMs. In addition, many provinces in Canada have started screening for specific IEMs as part of their expanded newborn screening programs using tandem mass spectrometry. However, many of the deaths caused by IEMs are the result of enzyme variants not currently screened for in many of the newborn screening programs (Jorde et al., 2010). (See Table 25-3 for screening tests for IEMs.) (See discussion of IEMs in Chapter 25.)

X-Linked Dominant Inheritance

X-linked dominant inheritance disorders occur in males and heterozygous females; but because of X inactivation, affected females are usually less severely affected than affected males, and they are more likely to transmit the variant allele to their offspring (Lashley, 2007). Heterozygous females have a 50% chance of transmitting the variant allele to each offspring. The variant allele is often lethal in affected males because, unlike affected females, they have no normal gene. Mating of an affected male and an unaffected female is uncommon as a result of the tendency for the variant allele to be lethal in affected males. Relatively few X-linked dominant disorders have been identified. Two examples are vitamin D–resistant rickets and fragile X syndrome. (See discussion in Chapter 42.)

X-Linked Recessive Inheritance

Abnormal genes for X-linked recessive inheritance disorders are carried on the X chromosome. Females may be heterozygous or homozygous for traits carried on the X chromosome because they have two X chromosomes. Males are hemizygous because they have only one X chromosome carrying genes, with no alleles on the Y chromosome. Therefore, X-linked recessive disorders are most often manifested in the male, with the abnormal gene on his single X chromosome. Hemophilia, colour blindness, and Duchenne muscular dystrophy are all X-linked recessive disorders.

The male receives the disease-associated allele from his carrier mother on her affected X chromosome. Female carriers (those heterozygous for the trait) have a 50% probability of transmitting the disease-associated allele to each offspring. An affected male can pass the disease-associated allele to his daughters but not to his sons. The daughters will be carriers of the trait if they receive a normal gene on the X chromosome from their mother. They will be affected only if they receive a disease-associated allele on the X chromosome from both their mother and their father.

Nongenetic Factors Influencing Development

Not all **congenital** disorders are inherited. *Congenital* means that the condition was present at birth. Some congenital malformations may be the result of **teratogens** (i.e., environmental substances or exposures that result in functional or structural disability). In contrast to other forms of developmental disabilities, disabilities caused by teratogens are in theory totally preventable. Known human teratogens are drugs and chemicals, infections, exposure to radiation, and certain maternal conditions such as diabetes and PKU (Box 8-4). A teratogen has the greatest effect on the organs and

BOX 8-4 Etiology of Human Malformations

Environmental

Maternal conditions—Alcoholism, diabetes, endocrinopathies, phenylketonuria, smoking, nutritional problems
Infectious agents—Rubella, toxoplasmosis, syphilis, herpes simplex, cytomegalic inclusion disease, varicella, Venezuelan equine encephalitis
Mechanical problems (deformations)—Amniotic band constrictions, umbilical cord constraint, disparity in uterine size and uterine contents
Chemicals, drugs, radiation, hyperthermia

Genetic

Single-gene disorders
Chromosomal abnormalities

Unknown

Polygenic or multifactorial (gene–environment interactions)
"Spontaneous" errors of development
Other unknowns

(Modified from Hudgins, L., & Cassidy, S. B. [2006]. Congenital anomalies. In R. J. Martin, A. A. Fanaroff, & M. C. Walsh (Eds.), *Fanaroff and Martin's neonatal-perinatal medicine: Diseases of the fetus and infant* [8th ed.]. St. Louis: Mosby.)

evolve Animation—Spermatogenesis

evolve Animation—Spermatozoa

evolve Animation—Pathway of Sperm

evolve Animation—Pathway of Ovum

parts of an embryo during its periods of rapid differentiation. This occurs during the embryonic period, specifically from days 15 to 60. During the first 2 weeks of development, teratogens either have no effect on the embryo or have effects so severe that they cause miscarriage. Brain growth and development continue during the fetal period, and teratogens can severely affect mental development throughout gestation (Fig. 8-4).

In addition to genetic makeup and the influence of teratogens, the adequacy of maternal nutrition influences development. The embryo and fetus must obtain the nutrients they need from the mother's diet; they cannot tap the maternal reserves. Malnutrition during pregnancy produces low-birth-weight newborns who are susceptible to infection and other conditions. Malnutrition also affects brain development during the latter half of gestation and may result in learning disabilities in the child. Inadequate folic acid is associated with neural tube defects.

Conception

Cell Division

Cells are reproduced by two different methods: mitosis and meiosis. In *mitosis*, the body cells replicate to yield two cells with the same genetic makeup as the parent cell. First the cell makes a copy of its DNA, and then it divides. Each daughter cell receives one copy of the genetic material. Mitotic division facilitates growth and development or cell replacement.

Meiosis, the process by which germ cells divide and decrease their chromosome number by half, produces gametes (eggs and sperm). Each homologous pair of chromosomes contains one chromosome received from the mother and one from the father; thus meiosis results in cells that contain 1 of each of the 23 pairs of chromosomes. Because these germ cells contain 23 single chromosomes, half of the genetic material of a normal somatic cell, they are called *haploid*. When the female gamete (egg or ovum) and the male gamete (spermatozoon) unite to form the zygote, the diploid number of human chromosomes (46, or 23 pairs) is restored.

The process of DNA replication and cell division in meiosis allows different alleles (genes on corresponding loci that code for variations of the same trait) for genes to be distributed at random by each parent and then rearranged on the paired chromosomes. The chromosomes then separate and proceed to different gametes. Because the two parents have genotypes derived from four different grandparents, many combinations of genes on each chromosome are possible. This random mixing of alleles accounts for the variation of traits seen in the offspring of the same two parents.

Gametogenesis

Oogenesis, the process of egg (ovum) formation, begins during fetal life of the female. All the cells that may undergo meiosis in a woman's lifetime are contained in her ovaries at birth. The majority of the estimated 2 million primary oocytes (the cells that undergo the first meiotic division) degenerate spontaneously. Only 400 to 500 ova will mature during the approximately 35 years of a woman's reproductive life. The primary oocytes begin the first meiotic division (i.e., they replicate their DNA) during fetal life but remain suspended at this stage until puberty (Fig. 8-5, A). Then, usually monthly, one primary oocyte matures and completes the first meiotic division, yielding two unequal cells: the secondary oocyte and a small polar body. Both contain 22 autosomes and one X sex chromosome.

At ovulation, the second meiotic division begins. However, the ovum does not complete the second meiotic division unless fertilization occurs. At fertilization, a second polar body and the **zygote** (the united egg and sperm) are produced (see Fig. 8-5, C). The three polar bodies degenerate. If fertilization does not occur, the ovum also degenerates.

When a male reaches puberty, his testes begin the process of **spermatogenesis**. The cells that undergo meiosis in the male are called *spermatocytes*. The primary spermatocyte, which undergoes the first meiotic division, contains the diploid number of chromosomes. The cell has already copied its DNA before division; thus four alleles for each gene are present. Because the copies are bound together (i.e., one allele plus its copy on each chromosome), the cell is still considered diploid.

During the first meiotic division, two haploid secondary spermatocytes are formed. Each secondary spermatocyte contains 22 autosomes and one sex chromosome; one contains the X chromosome (plus its copy), and the other the Y chromosome (plus its copy). During the second meiotic division, the male produces two gametes with an X chromosome and two gametes with a Y chromosome, all of which will develop into viable sperm (see Fig. 8-5, B).

Conception

Conception, defined as the union of a single egg and sperm, marks the beginning of a pregnancy. Conception occurs not as an isolated event but as part of a sequential process. This sequential process includes gamete (egg and sperm) formation, ovulation (release of the egg), union of the gametes (which results in an embryo), and implantation in the uterus.

Ovum

Meiosis occurs in the female in the ovarian follicles and produces an egg, or ovum. Each month one ovum matures with a host of surrounding supportive cells. At ovulation, the ovum is released from the ruptured ovarian follicle. High estrogen levels increase the motility of the uterine tubes so that their cilia are able to capture the ovum and propel it through the tube toward the uterine cavity. An ovum cannot move by itself.

Two protective layers surround the ovum (Fig. 8-6). The inner layer is a thick, acellular layer called the *zona pellucida*. The outer layer, called the *corona radiata*, is composed of elongated cells.

Ova are considered fertile for approximately 24 hours after ovulation. If unfertilized by a sperm, the ovum degenerates and is resorbed.

Sperm

Ejaculation during sexual intercourse normally propels about a teaspoon of semen containing as many as 200 to 500 million

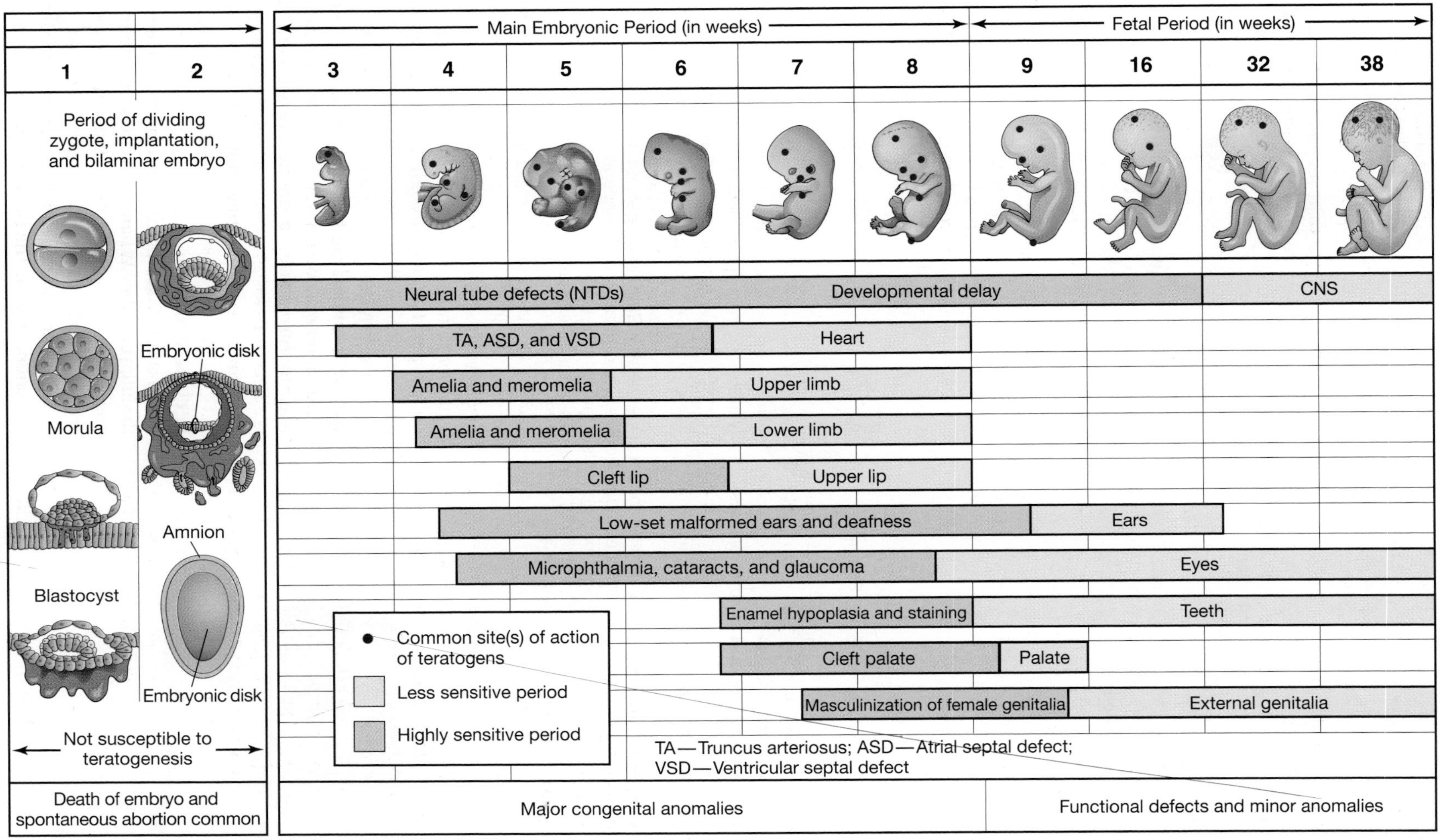

Fig. 8-4 Sensitive, or critical, periods in human development. *Dark colour* denotes highly sensitive periods; *light colour* indicates stages that are less sensitive to teratogens. *(From Moore, K. L., & Persaud, T. V. N. [2008].* Before we are born: Essentials of embryology and birth defects *[7th ed., p. 313]. Philadelphia: Saunders.)*

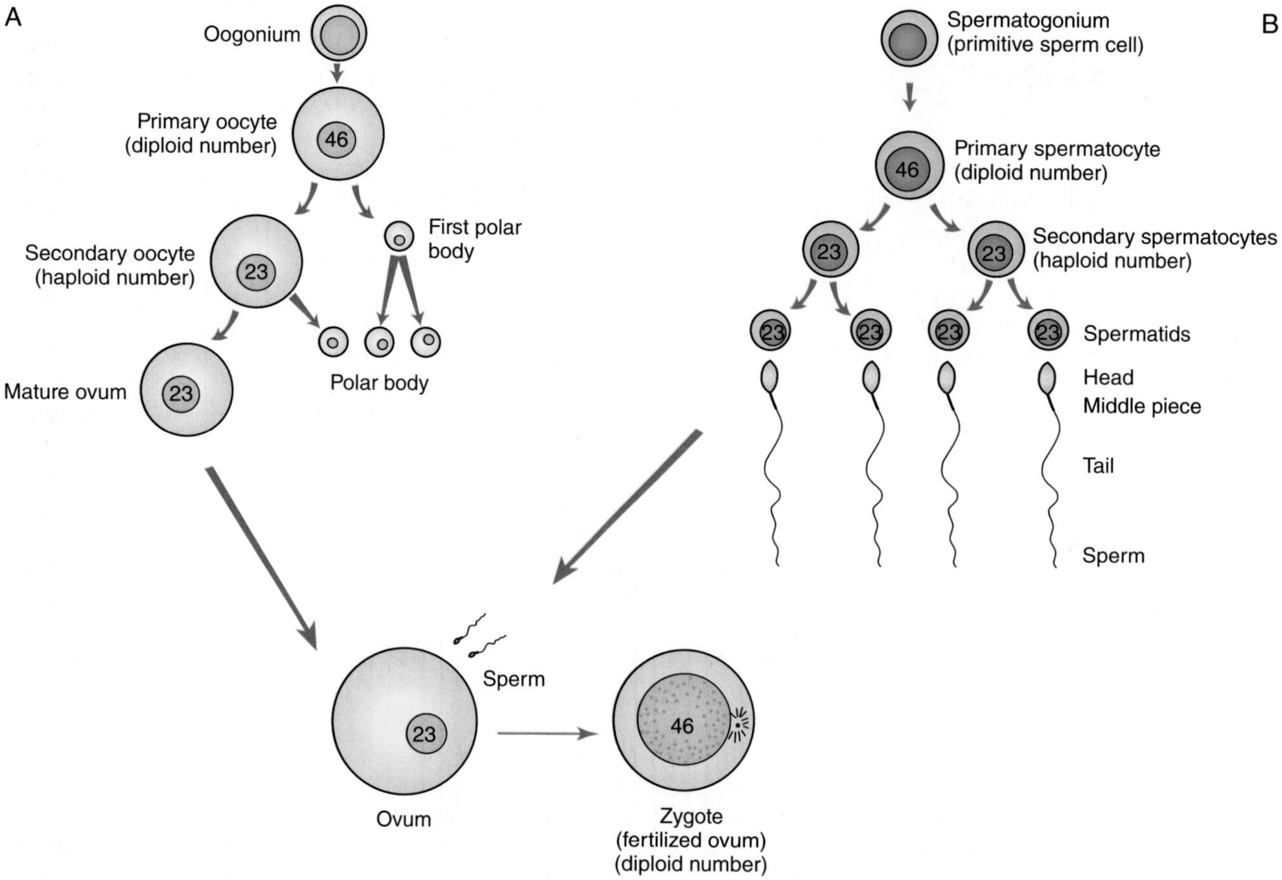

Fig. 8-5 Gametogenesis and fertilization. **A:** Oogenesis. Gametogenesis in the female produces one mature ovum and three polar bodies. Note relative difference in overall size between ovum and sperm. **B:** Spermatogenesis. Gametogenesis in the male produces four mature gametes, the sperm. **C:** Fertilization results in the single-cell zygote and restoration of the diploid number of chromosomes.

evolve Animation–Testes

evolve Animation–Oogenesis and Meiosis

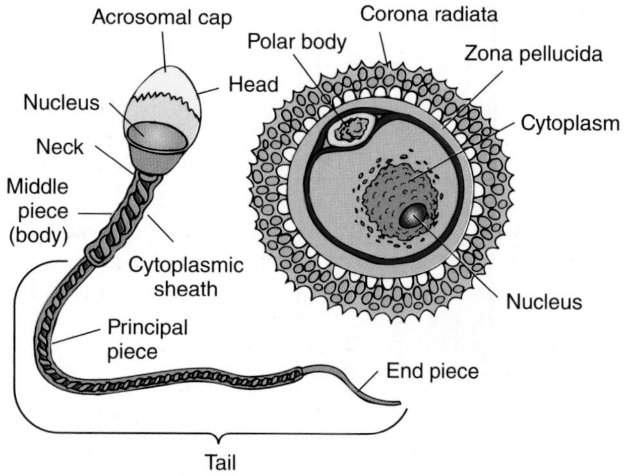

Fig. 8-6 Sperm and ovum.

sperm into the vagina. The sperm swim by means of the flagellar movement of their tails. Some sperm can reach the site of fertilization within 5 minutes, but average transit time is 4 to 6 hours. Sperm remain viable within the woman's reproductive system for an average of 2 to 3 days. Most sperm are lost in the vagina, within the cervical mucus, or in the endometrium or they enter the tube that contains no ovum.

As sperm travel through the female reproductive tract, enzymes are produced to aid in their capacitation. *Capacitation* is a physiological change that removes the protective coating from the heads of the sperm. Small perforations then form in the acrosome (a cap on the sperm) and allow enzymes (e.g., hyaluronidase) to escape (see Fig. 8-6). These enzymes are necessary for the sperm to penetrate the protective layers of the ovum before fertilization.

Fertilization

Fertilization takes place in the ampulla (the outer third) of the uterine tube. When a sperm successfully penetrates the membrane surrounding the ovum, both sperm and ovum are enclosed within the membrane, and the membrane becomes impenetrable to other sperm; this process is termed the *zona reaction*. The second meiotic division of the secondary oocyte is then completed, and the ovum nucleus becomes the female pronucleus. The head of the sperm enlarges to become the male pronucleus, and the tail degenerates. The nuclei fuse, and the chromosomes combine, restoring the diploid number (46) (Fig. 8-7). Fertilization, the formation

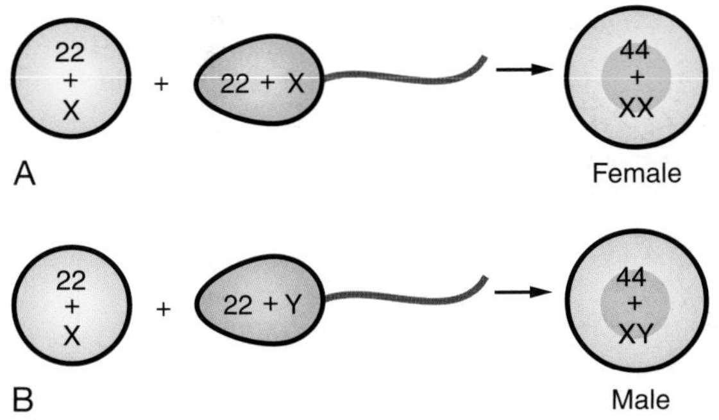

Fig. 8-7 Fertilization. **A:** Ovum fertilized by X-bearing sperm to form female zygote. **B:** Ovum fertilized by Y-bearing sperm to form male zygote.

of the zygote (the first cell of the new individual), has been achieved.

Mitotic cellular replication, called *cleavage*, begins as the zygote travels the length of the uterine tube into the uterus. This voyage takes 3 to 4 days. Because the fertilized egg divides rapidly with no increase in size, successively smaller cells, called *blastomeres*, are formed with each division. A 16-cell morula, a solid ball of cells, is produced within 3 days and is still surrounded by the protective zona pellucida (Fig. 8-8, A). Further development occurs as the morula floats freely within the uterus. Fluid passes through the zona pellucida into the intercellular spaces between the blastomeres, separating them into two parts: the trophoblast (which gives rise to the placenta) and the embryoblast (which gives rise to the embryo). A cavity forms within the cell mass as the spaces come together, forming a structure called the *blastocyst cavity*. When the cavity becomes recognizable, the whole structure of the developing embryo is known as the *blastocyst*. Stem cells are derived from the inner cell mass of the blastocyst. The outer layer of cells surrounding the cavity is the *trophoblast*.

Implantation

The zona pellucida degenerates; the trophoblast cells displace endometrial cells at the implantation site; and the blastocyst embeds in the endometrium, usually in the anterior or posterior fundal region. Between 6 and 10 days after fertilization, the trophoblast secretes enzymes that enable it to burrow into the endometrium until the entire blastocyst is covered. This is known as *implantation*. Endometrial blood vessels erode, and some women have implantation bleeding (slight spotting and bleeding during the time of the first missed menstrual period). Chorionic villi, fingerlike projections, develop out of the trophoblast and extend into the blood-filled spaces of the endometrium. These villi are vascular processes that obtain oxygen and nutrients from the maternal bloodstream and dispose of carbon dioxide and waste products into the maternal blood.

After implantation, the endometrium is called the **decidua**. The portion directly under the blastocyst, where the chorionic villi tap into the maternal blood vessels, is the *decidua basalis*. The portion covering the blastocyst is the *decidua capsularis*, and the portion lining the rest of the uterus is the *decidua vera* (Fig. 8-9).

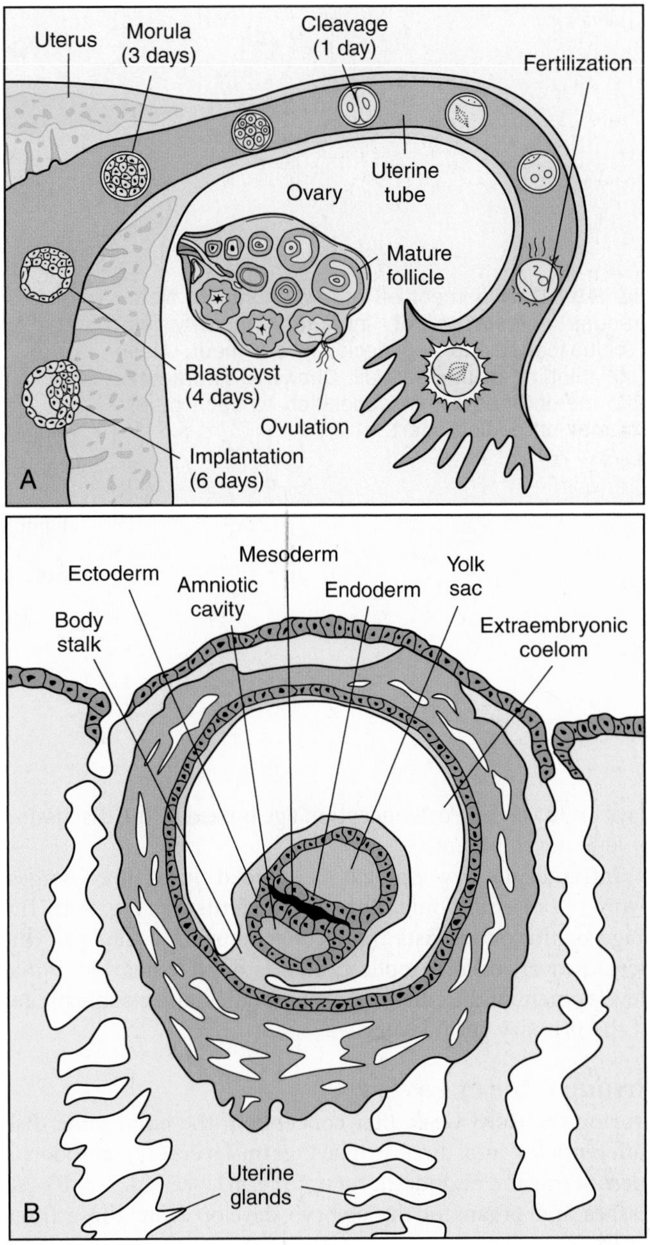

Fig. 8-8 **A:** First weeks of human development. Follicular development in ovary, ovulation, fertilization, and transport of early embryo down uterine tube and into uterus, where implantation occurs. **B:** Blastocyst embedded in endometrium. Germ layers forming. *(**A**, From Carlson, B. [2005].* Human embryology and developmental biology *[3rd ed.]. St. Louis: Mosby. **B**, Adapted from Langley, L., et al. [1980].* Dynamic human anatomy and physiology *[5th ed.]. New York: McGraw-Hill.)*

evolve Animation—Male Reproductive Ducts

evolve Animation—Fertilization and Implantation

The Embryo and Fetus

Pregnancy lasts approximately 10 lunar months, 9 calendar months, 40 weeks, or 280 days. Length of pregnancy is computed from the first day of the last menstrual period (LMP) until the day of birth. However, conception occurs approximately 2 weeks after the first day of the LMP. Thus the post-conception age of the fetus is 2 weeks less, for a total of 266

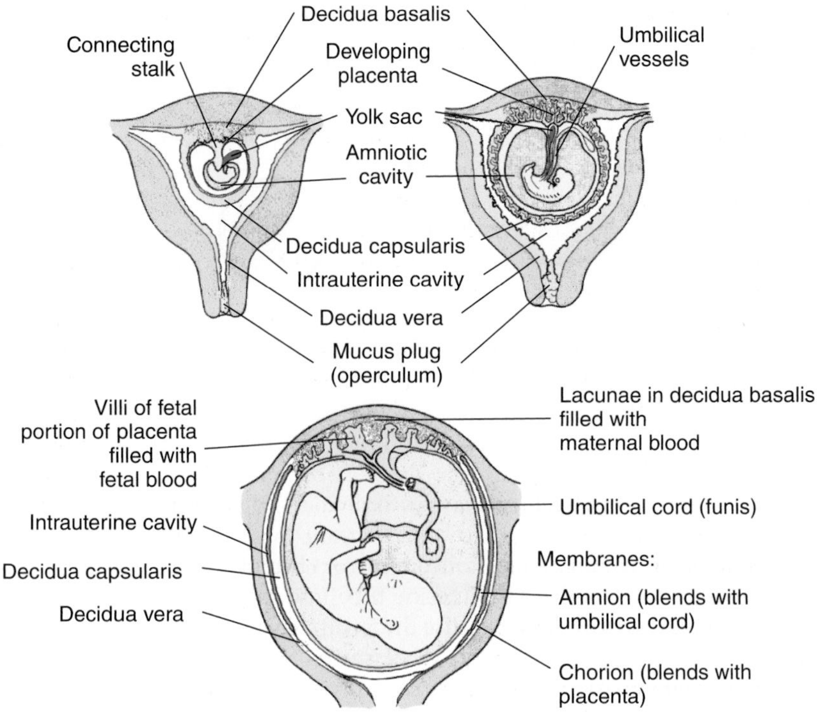

Fig. 8-9 Development of fetal membranes. Note gradual obliteration of intrauterine cavity as decidua capsularis and decidua vera meet. Also note thinning of uterine wall. Chorionic and amnionic membranes are in apposition to each other but may be peeled apart.

days or 38 weeks. Postconception age is used in the discussion of fetal development.

Intrauterine development is divided into three stages: ovum or pre-embryonic, **embryo**, and **fetus** (see Fig. 8-4). The stage of the ovum lasts from conception until day 14. This period covers cellular replication, blastocyst formation, initial development of the embryonic membranes, and establishment of the primary germ layers.

Primary Germ Layers

During the third week after conception, the embryonic disk differentiates into three primary germ layers: the ectoderm, mesoderm, and endoderm (or entoderm) (see Fig. 8-8, B). All tissues and organs of the embryo develop from these three layers.

The *ectoderm*, the upper layer of the embryonic disk, gives rise to the epidermis, glands (anterior pituitary, cutaneous, and mammary), nails and hair, central and peripheral nervous systems, lens of the eye, tooth enamel, and floor of the amniotic cavity.

The *mesoderm*, the middle layer, develops into the bones and teeth, muscles (skeletal, smooth, and cardiac), dermis and connective tissue, cardiovascular system and spleen, and urogenital system.

The *endoderm*, the lower layer, gives rise to the epithelium lining the respiratory and digestive tracts, including the oropharynx, liver and pancreas, urethra, bladder, and vagina. The endoderm forms the roof of the yolk sac.

Development of the Embryo

The stage of the embryo lasts from day 15 until approximately 8 weeks after conception, when the embryo measures approximately 3 cm from crown to rump. The embryonic stage is the most critical time in the development of the organ systems and the main external features. Developing areas with rapid cell division are the most vulnerable to malformation caused by environmental teratogens. At the end of the eighth week, all organ systems and external structures are present, and the embryo is unmistakably human (see Fig. 8-4, and Visible Embryo, at http://www.visembryo.com, for a pictorial view of normal and abnormal development).

Membranes

At the time of implantation, two fetal membranes that will surround the developing embryo begin to form. The *chorion* develops from the trophoblast and contains the chorionic villi on its surface. The villi burrow into the decidua basalis and increase in size and complexity as the vascular processes develop into the placenta. The chorion becomes the covering of the fetal side of the placenta. It contains the major umbilical blood vessels that branch out over the surface of the placenta. As the embryo grows, the decidua capsularis stretches. The chorionic villi on this side atrophy and degenerate, leaving a smooth chorionic membrane.

The inner cell membrane, the *amnion*, develops from the interior cells of the blastocyst. The cavity that develops between this inner cell mass and the outer layer of cells (trophoblast) is the *amniotic cavity* (see Fig. 8-8, B). As it grows larger, the amnion forms on the side opposite the developing blastocyst (see Fig. 8-8, B, and Fig. 8-9). The developing embryo draws the amnion around itself to form a fluid-filled sac. The amnion becomes the covering of the umbilical cord and covers the chorion on the fetal surface of the placenta. As the embryo grows larger, the amnion enlarges to accommodate the embryo then fetus and the surrounding amniotic fluid. The amnion eventually comes in contact with the chorion surrounding the fetus (see Critical Thinking Exercise).

Amniotic Fluid

At first the amniotic cavity derives its fluid by diffusion from the maternal blood. The amount of fluid increases weekly; 800 to 1200 mL of transparent liquid is normally present at term. The volume of amniotic fluid changes constantly. The fetus swallows fluid, and fluid flows into and out of the fetal lungs. The fetus urinates into the fluid, greatly increasing its volume.

The amniotic fluid serves many functions for the embryo and fetus. Amniotic fluid helps maintain a constant body temperature. It serves as a source of oral fluid and as a repository for waste. It cushions the fetus from trauma by blunting and dispersing outside forces. It allows freedom of movement for musculoskeletal development. The fluid keeps the embryo from tangling with the membranes, facilitating symmetric growth of the fetus. If the embryo does become tangled with the membranes, amputations of extremities or other deformities can occur from constricting amniotic bands.

The volume of amniotic fluid is an important factor in assessing fetal well-being. Having less than 300 mL of amniotic fluid (**oligohydramnios**) is associated with fetal renal abnormalities. Having more than 2 L of amniotic fluid *(polyhydramnios)* is associated with gastrointestinal and other malformations.

Amniotic fluid contains albumin, urea, uric acid, creatinine, lecithin, sphingomyelin, bilirubin, fructose, fat, leukocytes, proteins, epithelial cells, enzymes, and lanugo hair.

CRITICAL THINKING EXERCISE

Ultrasound Dating of Pregnancy

Sandra believes she is 8 weeks pregnant, but her family physician believes she is closer to 12 weeks of gestation. Sandra has come to the clinic for an ultrasound examination for dating. She has many questions for the nurse: How can they tell what gestation she is? What would the fetus look like at this time if she is 8 weeks' gestation? If she is 12 weeks' gestation? What fetal structures would be apparent on ultrasound if she is 8 weeks pregnant? If she is 12 weeks pregnant? Would any structural anomalies be apparent at 8 weeks? At 12 weeks? Why is it important to date a pregnancy accurately? What information should the nurse provide Sandra?

1. Evidence—Is there sufficient evidence to draw conclusions about what information the nurse should provide to Sandra?
2. Assumptions—What assumptions can be made about the following factors?
   a. Sandra's motivation to learn about fetal development
   b. Sandra's understanding of fetal development
   c. Sandra's knowledge about ultrasound examinations
   d. Why dating the pregnancy is important
3. What implications and priorities for nursing care can be drawn at this time?
4. Does the evidence objectively support your conclusion?
5. Are there alternative perspectives to your conclusion?

Study of fetal cells in amniotic fluid through amniocentesis yields much information about the fetus. Genetic studies (karyotyping) provide knowledge about the sex and the number and structure of chromosomes. Other studies such as the **lecithin/sphingomyelin (L/S) ratio** determine the health or maturity of the fetus (see Chapter 12).

Yolk Sac

At the same time the amniotic cavity and amnion are forming, another blastocyst cavity forms on the other side of the developing embryonic disk (see Fig. 8-8, B). This cavity becomes surrounded by a membrane, forming the yolk sac. The yolk sac aids in transferring maternal nutrients and oxygen, which have diffused through the chorion, to the embryo. Blood vessels form to aid transport. Blood cells and plasma are manufactured in the yolk sac during the second and third weeks while uteroplacental circulation is being established and forming primitive blood cells until hematopoietic activity begins. At the end of the third week, the primitive heart begins to beat and circulate the blood through the embryo, connecting stalk, chorion, and yolk sac.

The folding in of the embryo during the fourth week results in incorporation of part of the yolk sac into the body of the embryo as the primitive digestive system. Primordial germ cells arise in the yolk sac and move into the embryo. The shrinking remains of the yolk sac degenerate (see Fig. 8-8, B), and by the fifth or sixth week the remnant has separated from the embryo.

Umbilical Cord

By day 14 after conception, the embryonic disk, amniotic sac, and yolk sac are attached to the chorionic villi by the connecting stalk. During the third week, the blood vessels develop to supply the embryo with maternal nutrients and oxygen. During the fifth week, the embryo has curved inward on itself from both ends, bringing the connecting stalk to the ventral side of the embryo. The connecting stalk becomes compressed from both sides by the amnion and forms the narrower umbilical cord (see Fig. 8-9). Two arteries carry blood from the embryo to the chorionic villi, and one vein returns blood to the embryo. Approximately 1% of umbilical cords contain only two vessels: one artery and one vein. This occurrence is sometimes associated with congenital malformations.

The cord rapidly increases in length. At term the cord is 2 cm in diameter and ranges from 30 to 90 cm in length (with an average of 55 cm). It twists spirally on itself and loops around the embryo and fetus. A true knot is rare, but false knots occur as folds or kinks in the cord and may jeopardize circulation to the fetus. Connective tissue called *Wharton's jelly* prevents compression of the blood vessels and ensures continued nourishment of the embryo and fetus. Compression can occur if the cord lies between the fetal head and the pelvis or is twisted around the fetal body. When the cord is wrapped around the fetal neck, it is called a **nuchal cord**.

Because the placenta develops from the chorionic villi, the umbilical cord is usually located centrally. The blood vessels are arrayed out from the centre to all parts of the placenta (Fig. 8-10, B). A peripheral location is less common and is known as a *battledore placenta* (see Fig. 13-14, B).

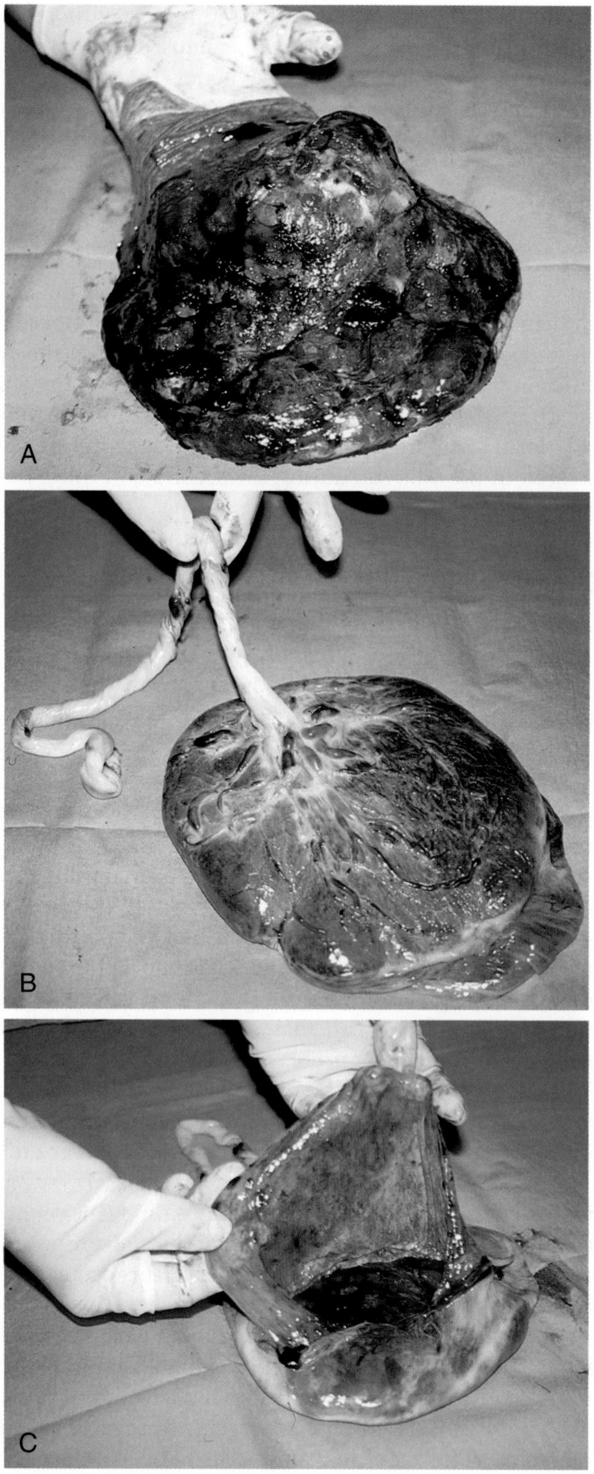

Fig. 8-10 Full-term placenta. **A:** Maternal (or uterine) surface, showing cotyledons and grooves. **B:** Fetal (or amniotic) surface, showing blood vessels running under amnion and converging to form umbilical vessels at attachment of umbilical cord. **C:** Amnion and smooth chorion are arranged to show that they are (1) fused and (2) continuous with margins of placenta. *(Courtesy Marjorie Pyle, RNC, Lifecircle, Costa Mesa, CA.)*

Placenta

Structure

The placenta begins to form at implantation. During the third week after conception, the trophoblast cells of the chorionic villi continue to invade the decidua basalis. As the uterine capillaries are tapped, the endometrial spiral arteries fill with maternal blood. The chorionic villi grow into the spaces with two layers of cells: the outer syncytium and the inner cytotrophoblast. A third layer develops into anchoring septa, dividing the projecting decidua into separate areas called *cotyledons*. In each of the 15 to 20 cotyledons the chorionic villi branch out, and a complex system of fetal blood vessels forms. Each cotyledon is a functional unit. The whole structure is the placenta (see Fig. 8-10).

The maternal–placental–embryonic circulation is in place by day 17, when the embryonic heart starts beating. By the end of the third week, embryonic blood is circulating between the embryo and the chorionic villi. In the intervillous spaces, maternal blood supplies oxygen and nutrients to the embryonic capillaries in the villi (Fig. 8-11). Waste products and carbon dioxide diffuse into the maternal blood.

The placenta functions as a means of metabolic exchange. Exchange is minimal at this time because the two cell layers of the villous membrane are too thick. Permeability increases as the cytotrophoblast thins and disappears; by the fifth month only the single layer of syncytium is left between the maternal blood and the fetal capillaries. The syncytium is the functional layer of the placenta. By the eighth week, genetic testing may be done on a sample of chorionic villi obtained by aspiration biopsy; however, limb defects have been associated with chorionic villi sampling done before 10 weeks (see Chapter 12). The structure of the placenta is complete by the twelfth week. The placenta continues to grow wider until 20 weeks, when it covers about half of the uterine surface. It then continues to grow thicker. The branching villi continue to develop within the body of the placenta, increasing the functional surface area.

Functions

One of the early functions of the placenta is as an endocrine gland that produces four hormones necessary to maintain the pregnancy and support the embryo and fetus. The hormones are produced in the syncytium.

The protein hormone human chorionic gonadotropin (hCG) can be detected in the maternal serum by 8 to 10 days after fertilization, shortly after implantation. This hormone is the basis for pregnancy tests. The hCG preserves the function of the ovarian corpus luteum, ensuring a continued supply of estrogen and progesterone needed to maintain the pregnancy. Miscarriage occurs if the corpus luteum stops functioning before the placenta can produce sufficient estrogen and progesterone. The hCG reaches its maximum level at 50 to 70 days and then begins to decrease.

The other protein hormone produced by the placenta is human chorionic somatomammotropin (hCS) or human placental lactogen (hPL). This substance is similar to a growth hormone and stimulates maternal metabolism to supply needed nutrients for fetal growth. This hormone increases the resistance to insulin, facilitates glucose transport across the

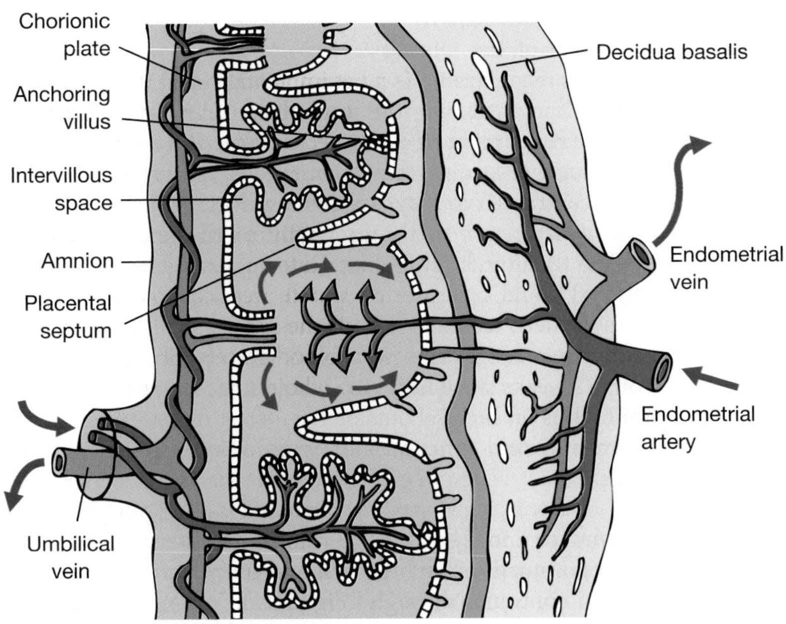

Fig. 8-11 Schematic drawing of the placenta illustrating how it supplies oxygen and nutrition to the embryo and removes its waste products. Deoxygenated blood leaves the fetus through the umbilical arteries and enters the placenta, where it is oxygenated. Oxygenated blood leaves the placenta through the umbilical vein, which enters the fetus via the umbilical cord.

placental membrane, and stimulates maternal breast development to prepare for lactation.

The placenta eventually produces more of the steroid hormone progesterone than the corpus luteum does during the first few months of pregnancy. Progesterone maintains the endometrium, decreases the contractility of the uterus, and stimulates development of breast alveoli and maternal metabolism.

By 7 weeks after fertilization, the placenta is producing most of the maternal estrogens, which are steroid hormones. The major estrogen secreted by the placenta is estriol, whereas the ovaries produce mostly estradiol. Measuring estriol levels is a clinical assay for placental functioning. Estrogen stimulates uterine growth and uteroplacental blood flow. It causes a proliferation of the breast glandular tissue and stimulates myometrial contractility. Placental estrogen production increases greatly toward the end of pregnancy. One theory for the cause of the onset of labour is the decrease in circulating levels of progesterone and the increased levels of estrogen.

The metabolic functions of the placenta are respiration, nutrition, excretion, and storage. Oxygen diffuses from the maternal blood across the placental membrane into the fetal blood, and carbon dioxide diffuses in the opposite direction. In this way, the placenta functions as a lung for the fetus.

Carbohydrates, proteins, calcium, and iron are stored in the placenta for ready access to meet fetal needs. Water, inorganic salts, carbohydrates, proteins, fats, and vitamins pass from the maternal blood supply across the placental membrane into the fetal blood, supplying nutrition. Water and most electrolytes with a molecular weight less than 500 readily diffuse through the membrane. Hydrostatic and osmotic pressures aid in the flow of water and some solutions. Facilitated and active transport assist in the transfer of glucose, amino acids, calcium, iron, and substances with higher molecular weights. Amino acids and calcium are transported against the concentration gradient between the maternal blood and fetal blood.

The fetal concentration of glucose is lower than the glucose level in the maternal blood because of its rapid metabolism by the fetus. This fetal requirement demands larger concentrations of glucose than simple diffusion can provide. Therefore, maternal glucose moves into the fetal circulation by active transport.

Pinocytosis is a mechanism used for transferring large molecules such as albumin and gamma (γ) globulins across the placental membrane. This mechanism conveys the maternal immunoglobulins that provide early passive immunity to the fetus.

Metabolic waste products of the fetus cross the placental membrane from the fetal blood into the maternal blood. The maternal kidneys then excrete them. Many viruses can cross the placental membrane and infect the fetus. Some bacteria and protozoa first infect the placenta and then infect the fetus. Drugs can also cross the placental membrane and may harm the fetus. Caffeine, alcohol, nicotine, carbon monoxide and other toxic substances in cigarette smoke, and prescription and recreational drugs (such as marijuana and cocaine) readily cross the placenta (Box 8-5).

Although no direct link exists between the fetal blood in the vessels of the chorionic villi and the maternal blood in the intervillous spaces, only one cell layer separates them. Breaks occasionally occur in the placental membrane. Fetal erythrocytes then leak into the maternal circulation, and the mother may develop antibodies to the fetal red blood cells. This is often the way the Rh-negative mother becomes sensitized to the erythrocytes of her Rh-positive fetus. (See the discussion of isoimmunization in Chapter 28.)

Although the placenta and fetus are analogous to living tissue transplants, they are not destroyed by the host mother. Either the placental hormones suppress the immunological response or the tissue evokes no response.

Placental function depends on the maternal blood pressure supplying the circulation. Maternal arterial blood, under pressure in the small uterine spiral arteries, spurts into the

BOX 8-5 Developmentally Toxic Exposures in Humans

- Androgens
- Angiotensin-converting enzyme inhibitors
- Carbamazepine
- Cigarette smoking
- Cocaine
- Coumarin anticoagulants
- Cytomegalovirus
- Diethylstilbestrol
- Ethanol
- Hyperthermia
- Iodides
- Ionizing radiation (more than 10 rads)
- Isotretinoin
- Lead
- Lithium
- Methimazole
- Methyl mercury
- Parvovirus B19
- Penicillamine
- Phenytoin
- Radioiodine
- Rubella
- Syphilis
- Tetracycline
- Thalidomide
- Toxoplasmosis
- Trimethadione
- Valproic acid
- Varicella

intervillous spaces (see Fig. 8-11). As long as rich arterial blood continues to be supplied, pressure is exerted on the blood already in the intervillous spaces, pushing it toward drainage by the low-pressure uterine veins. At term gestation, 10% of the maternal cardiac output goes to the uterus.

If there is interference with the circulation to the placenta, the placenta cannot supply the embryo or fetus. Vasoconstriction such as that caused by hypertension or cocaine use diminishes uterine blood flow. Decreased maternal blood pressure or decreased cardiac output also diminishes uterine blood flow.

When a woman lies on her back with the pressure of the uterus compressing the vena cava, blood return to the right atrium is diminished. (See Fig. 18-3 and the discussion of supine hypotension in Chapter 10.) Excessive maternal exercise that diverts blood to the muscles away from the uterus compromises placental circulation. Optimal circulation is achieved when the woman is lying at rest on her side. Decreased uterine circulation may lead to intrauterine growth restriction of the fetus and infants who are small for gestational age.

Uterine contractions seem to enhance the movement of blood through the intervillous spaces, aiding placental circulation. However, prolonged contractions or too-short intervals between contractions during labour can reduce the blood flow to the placenta (see Chapter 17).

Fetal Maturation

The stage of the fetus lasts from 9 weeks (when the fetus becomes recognizable as a human being) until the pregnancy ends. Changes during the fetal period are not as dramatic because refinement of structure and function is taking place. The fetus is less vulnerable to teratogens, except for those that affect central nervous system functioning.

Viability refers to the capability of the fetus to survive outside the uterus. In the past, the earliest age at which fetal survival could be expected was 28 weeks after conception. With modern technology and advances in maternal and neonatal care, viability is now possible at 20 weeks after conception (22 weeks since LMP; fetal weight of 500 g or more). The limitations on survival outside the uterus are based on central nervous system function and oxygenation capability of the lungs.

Respiratory System

The respiratory system begins development during embryonic life and continues through fetal life and into childhood. The development of the respiratory tract begins in week 4 and continues through week 17 with formation of the larynx, trachea, bronchi, and lung buds. Between 16 and 24 weeks, the bronchi and terminal bronchioles enlarge, and vascular structures and primitive alveoli are formed. Between 24 weeks and term birth, more alveoli form. Specialized alveolar cells, type I and type II cells, secrete pulmonary surfactants to line the interior of the alveoli. After 32 weeks sufficient surfactant is present in developed alveoli to provide infants with a good chance of survival.

Pulmonary Surfactants

The detection of the presence of pulmonary **surfactants**, surface-active phospholipids, in amniotic fluid has been used to determine the degree of fetal lung maturity, or the ability of the lungs to function after birth. Lecithin (L) is the most critical alveolar surfactant required for postnatal lung expansion. It is detectable at approximately 21 weeks and increases in amount after week 24. Another pulmonary phospholipid, sphingomyelin (S), remains constant in amount. Thus the measure of lecithin in relation to sphingomyelin, or the L/S ratio, is used to determine fetal lung maturity. When the L/S ratio reaches 2:1, the infant's lungs are considered to be mature. This occurs at approximately 35 weeks of gestation.

Certain maternal conditions that cause decreased maternal placental blood flow, such as maternal hypertension, placental dysfunction, infection, or corticosteroid use, accelerate lung maturity. This apparently is caused by the resulting fetal hypoxia, which stresses the fetus and increases the blood levels of corticosteroids that accelerate alveolar and surfactant development.

Conditions such as gestational diabetes and chronic glomerulonephritis can delay fetal lung maturity. The use of intrabronchial synthetic surfactant in the treatment of respiratory distress syndrome in the newborn has greatly improved the chances of survival for preterm infants (see Chapter 27).

Fetal respiratory movements have been seen on ultrasound examination as early as week 11. These fetal respiratory movements may aid in development of the chest wall muscles and regulate lung fluid volume. The fetal lungs produce fluid that expands the air spaces in the lungs. The fluid drains into the amniotic fluid or is swallowed by the fetus.

Before birth, secretion of lung fluid decreases. The normal birth process squeezes out approximately one third of the fluid. Infants of Caesarean births do not benefit from this squeezing process; thus they may have more respiratory difficulty at birth. The fluid remaining in the lungs at birth is usually resorbed into the infant's bloodstream within 2 hours of birth.

Fetal Circulatory System

The cardiovascular system is the first organ system to function in the developing human. Blood vessel and blood cell formation begin in the third week and supply the embryo with oxygen and nutrients from the mother. By the end of the third week, the tubular heart begins to beat, and the primitive cardiovascular system links the embryo, connecting stalk, chorion, and yolk sac. During the fourth and fifth weeks, the heart develops into a four-chambered organ. By the end of the embryonic stage, the heart is developmentally complete.

The fetal lungs do not function for respiratory gas exchange; thus a special circulatory pathway, the ductus arteriosus, bypasses the lungs. Oxygen-rich blood from the placenta flows rapidly through the umbilical vein into the fetal abdomen (Fig. 8-12). When the umbilical vein reaches the liver, it divides into two branches. One branch circulates some oxygenated blood through the liver. Most of the blood passes through the ductus venosus into the inferior vena cava. There it mixes with the deoxygenated blood from the fetal legs and abdomen on its way to the right atrium. Most of this blood passes straight through the right atrium and through the foramen ovale, an opening into the left atrium. There it mixes with the small amount of deoxygenated blood returning from the fetal lungs through the pulmonary veins.

The blood flows into the left ventricle and is squeezed out into the aorta, where the arteries supplying the heart, head, neck, and arms receive most of the oxygen-rich blood. This pattern of supplying the highest levels of oxygen and nutrients to the head, neck, and arms enhances the cephalocaudal (head-to-rump) development of the embryo and fetus.

Deoxygenated blood returning from the head and arms enters the right atrium through the superior vena cava. This blood is directed downward into the right ventricle, where it is squeezed into the pulmonary artery. A small amount of blood circulates through the resistant lung tissue, but the majority follows the path with less resistance through the

evolve Animation—Maternal and Fetal Circulation

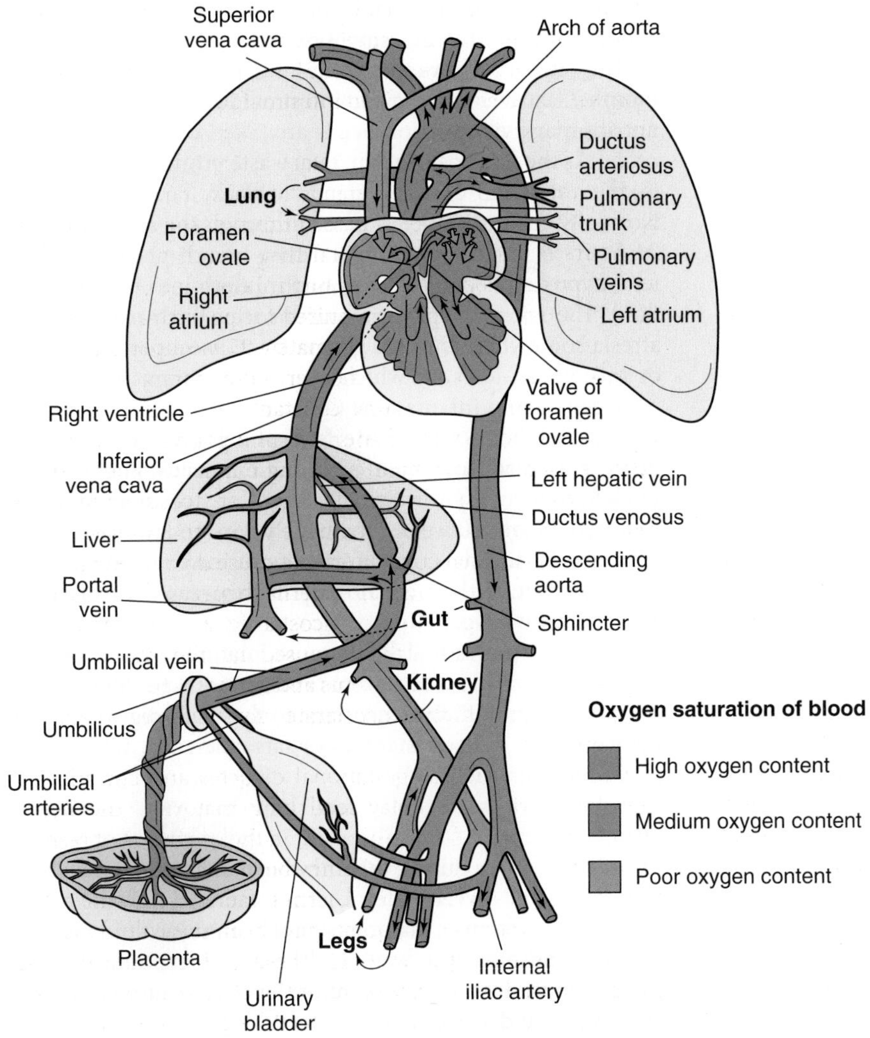

Fig. 8-12 Schematic illustration of fetal circulation. The *colours* indicate the oxygen saturation of the blood, and the *arrows* show the course of the blood from the placenta to the heart. The organs are not drawn to scale. Observe that three shunts permit most of the blood to bypass the liver and lungs: (1) ductus venosus, (2) foramen ovale, and (3) ductus arteriosus. The poorly oxygenated blood returns to the placenta for oxygen and nutrients through the umbilical arteries. *(From Moore, K. L., & Persaud, T. V. N. [2008]. Before we are born: Essentials of embryology and birth defects [7th ed., p. 221]. Philadelphia: Saunders.)*

ductus arteriosus into the aorta, distal to the point of exit of the arteries supplying the head and arms with oxygenated blood. The oxygen-poor blood flows through the abdominal aorta into the internal iliac arteries, where the umbilical arteries direct most of it back through the umbilical cord to the placenta. There the blood gives up its wastes and carbon dioxide in exchange for nutrients and oxygen. The blood remaining in the iliac arteries flows through the fetal abdomen and legs, ultimately returning through the inferior vena cava to the heart.

The following three special characteristics enable the fetus to obtain sufficient oxygen from the maternal blood:

1. Fetal hemoglobin carries 20 to 30% more oxygen than maternal hemoglobin.
2. The hemoglobin concentration of the fetus is about 50% greater than that of the mother.
3. The fetal heart rate is 110 to 160 beats per minute, making the cardiac output per unit of body weight higher than that of an adult.

Hematopoietic System

Hematopoiesis, the formation of blood, occurs in the yolk sac (see Fig. 8-8, B), beginning in the third week. Hematopoietic stem cells seed the fetal liver during the fifth week, and hematopoiesis begins there during the sixth week. This accounts for the relatively large size of the liver between the seventh and ninth weeks. Stem cells seed the fetal bone marrow, spleen and thymus, and lymph nodes between weeks 8 and 11.

The antigenic factors that determine blood type are present in the erythrocytes soon after the sixth week. For this reason, the Rh-negative woman is at risk for isoimmunization in any pregnancy that lasts longer than 6 weeks after fertilization.

Hepatic System

The liver and biliary tract develop from the foregut during the fourth week of gestation. The embryonic liver is prominent, occupying most of the abdominal cavity. Bile, a constituent of meconium, begins to form in the twelfth week.

Glycogen is stored in the fetal liver beginning at week 9 or 10. At term, glycogen stores are twice those of the adult. Glycogen is the major source of energy for the fetus and for the neonate stressed by in utero hypoxia, extrauterine loss of the maternal glucose supply, the work of breathing, or cold stress.

Iron is also stored in the fetal liver. If maternal intake is sufficient, the fetus can store enough iron to last for 5 months after birth.

During fetal life the liver does not have to conjugate bilirubin for excretion because the unconjugated bilirubin is cleared by the placenta. Therefore, the glucuronyl transferase enzyme needed for conjugation is present in the fetal liver in amounts less than those required after birth. This predisposes the neonate, especially the preterm infant, to hyperbilirubinemia.

Coagulation factors II, VII, IX, and X cannot be synthesized in the fetal liver because of the lack of vitamin K synthesis in the sterile fetal gut. This coagulation deficiency persists after birth for several days and is the rationale for the prophylactic administration of vitamin K to the newborn.

Gastrointestinal System

During the fourth week, the shape of the embryo changes from being almost straight to a C shape as both ends fold in toward the ventral surface. A portion of the yolk sac is incorporated into the body from head to tail as the primitive gut (digestive system).

The foregut produces the pharynx, part of the lower respiratory tract, the esophagus, the stomach, the first half of the duodenum, the liver, the pancreas, and the gallbladder. These structures evolve during the fifth and sixth weeks. Malformations that can occur in these areas include esophageal atresia, hypertrophic pyloric stenosis, duodenal stenosis or atresia, and biliary atresia.

The midgut becomes the distal half of the duodenum, the jejunum and ileum, the cecum and appendix, and the proximal half of the colon. The midgut loop projects into the umbilical cord between weeks 5 and 10. A malformation, omphalocele, results if the midgut fails to return to the abdominal cavity, causing the intestines to protrude from the umbilicus. Meckel diverticulum is the most common malformation of the midgut. It occurs when a remnant of the yolk stalk that has failed to degenerate attaches to the ileum, leaving a blind sac.

The hindgut develops into the distal half of the colon, the rectum and parts of the anal canal, the urinary bladder, and the urethra. Anorectal malformations are the most common abnormalities of the digestive system.

The fetus swallows amniotic fluid beginning in the fifth month. Gastric emptying and intestinal peristalsis occur. Fetal nutrition and elimination needs are taken care of by the placenta. As the fetus nears term, fetal waste products accumulate in the intestines as dark green–to-black, tarry meconium. Normally this substance is passed through the rectum within 24 hours of birth. Sometimes with a breech presentation or fetal hypoxia, meconium is passed in utero into the amniotic fluid. The failure to pass meconium after birth may indicate atresia somewhere in the digestive tract; an imperforate anus; or meconium ileus, in which a firm meconium plug blocks passage (seen in infants with CF).

The metabolic rate of the fetus is relatively low, but the infant has great growth and development needs. Beginning in week 9, the fetus synthesizes glycogen for storage in the liver. Between 26 and 30 weeks, the fetus begins to lay down stores of brown fat in preparation for extrauterine cold stress. Thermoregulation in the neonate requires increased metabolism and adequate oxygenation.

The gastrointestinal system is mature by 36 weeks. Digestive enzymes (except pancreatic amylase and lipase) are present in sufficient quantity to facilitate digestion. The neonate cannot digest starches or fats efficiently. Little saliva is produced.

Renal System

The kidneys form during the fifth week and begin to function approximately 4 weeks later. Urine is excreted into the amniotic fluid and forms a major part of the amniotic fluid volume. Oligohydramnios is indicative of renal dysfunction. Because the placenta acts as the organ of excretion and maintains fetal water and electrolyte balance, the fetus does not need functioning kidneys while in utero. However, at birth the kidneys are required immediately for excretory and acid–base regulatory functions.

A fetal renal malformation can be diagnosed in utero. Corrective or palliative fetal surgery may treat the malformation successfully, or plans can be made for treatment immediately after birth.

At term the fetus has fully developed kidneys. However, the glomerular filtration rate is low, and the kidneys lack the ability to concentrate urine. This makes the newborn more susceptible to both overhydration and dehydration.

Most newborns void within 24 hours of birth. With the loss of the swallowed amniotic fluid and the metabolism of nutrients provided by the placenta, voidings for the first days of life are scant until fluid intake increases.

Neurological System

The nervous system originates from the ectoderm during the third week after fertilization. The open neural tube forms during the fourth week. It initially closes at what will be the junction of the brain and spinal cord, leaving both ends open. The embryo folds in on itself lengthwise at this time, forming a head fold in the neural tube at this junction. The cranial end of the neural tube closes, then the caudal end closes. During week 5, different growth rates cause more flexures in the neural tube, delineating three brain areas: the forebrain, midbrain, and hindbrain.

The forebrain develops into the eyes (cranial nerve II) and cerebral hemispheres. The development of all areas of the cerebral cortex continues throughout fetal life and into childhood. The olfactory system (cranial nerve I) and thalamus also develop from the forebrain. Cranial nerves III and IV (oculomotor and trochlear) form from the midbrain. The hindbrain forms the medulla, the pons, the cerebellum, and the remainder of the cranial nerves. Brain waves can be recorded on an electroencephalogram by week 8.

The spinal cord develops from the long end of the neural tube. Another ectodermal structure, the neural crest, develops into the peripheral nervous system. By the eighth week, nerve fibres traverse throughout the body. By week 11 or 12, the fetus makes respiratory movements, moves all extremities, and changes position in utero. The fetus can suck his or her thumb, swim in the amniotic fluid pool, and turn somersaults and sometimes ties a knot in the umbilical cord. Sometime between 16 and 20 weeks, when the movements are strong enough to be perceived by the mother as "the baby moving," quickening has occurred. The perception of movement occurs earlier in the multipara than in the primipara. The mother also becomes aware of the sleep and wake cycles of the fetus.

Sensory Awareness

Purposeful movements of the fetus have been demonstrated in response to a firm touch transmitted through the mother's abdomen. Because it can feel, the fetus requires anaesthesia when invasive procedures are done.

Fetuses respond to sound by 24 weeks. Different types of music evoke different movements. The fetus can be soothed by the sound of the mother's voice. The fetus becomes accustomed (habituates) to noises heard repeatedly. Hearing is fully developed at birth.

The fetus is able to distinguish taste. By the fifth month, when the fetus is swallowing amniotic fluid, a sweetener added to the fluid causes the fetus to swallow faster. The fetus also reacts to temperature changes. A cold solution placed into the amniotic fluid can cause fetal hiccups.

The fetus can see. Eyes have both rods and cones in the retina by the seventh month. A bright light shone on the mother's abdomen in late pregnancy causes abrupt fetal movements. During sleep time rapid eye movements have been observed similar to those occurring in children and adults while dreaming.

At term the fetal brain is approximately one-fourth the size of an adult brain. Neurological development continues. Stressors on the fetus and neonate (e.g., chronic poor nutrition or hypoxia, drugs, environmental toxins, trauma, disease) cause damage to the central nervous system long after the vulnerable embryonic time for malformations in other organ systems. Neurological insult can result in cerebral palsy, neuromuscular impairment, developmental delay, and learning disabilities.

evolve Animation—Male External Genitalia

Endocrine System

The thyroid gland develops along with structures in the head and neck during the third and fourth weeks. The secretion of thyroxine begins during the eighth week. Maternal thyroxine does not readily cross the placenta; therefore, the fetus that does not produce thyroid hormones will be born with congenital hypothyroidism. If untreated, hypothyroidism can result in severe developmental delay. Screening for hypothyroidism is included in the newborn screening done after birth.

The adrenal cortex is formed during the sixth week and produces hormones by the eighth or ninth week. As term approaches, the fetus produces more cortisol. This is believed to aid in initiation of labour by decreasing the maternal progesterone and stimulating production of prostaglandins.

evolve Animation—Male Accessory Sex Glands

The pancreas forms from the foregut during the fifth through eighth weeks. The islets of Langerhans develop during the twelfth week. Insulin is produced by week 20. In infants of mothers with uncontrolled diabetes, maternal hyperglycemia produces fetal hyperglycemia, stimulating hyperinsulinemia and islet cell hyperplasia. This results in a macrosomatic (large-size) fetus. The hyperinsulinemia also blocks lung maturation, placing the neonate at risk for respiratory distress and hypoglycemia when the maternal glucose source is lost at birth. Control of the maternal glucose level before and during pregnancy minimizes problems for the fetus and infant.

Reproductive System

Sex differentiation begins in the embryo during the seventh week. Female and male external genitalia are indistinguishable until after the ninth week. Distinguishing characteristics appear around the ninth week and are fully differentiated by the twelfth week. When a Y chromosome is present, testes are formed. By the end of the embryonic period, testosterone is being secreted and causes formation of the male genitalia. By week 28, the testes begin descending into the scrotum. After birth, low levels of testosterone continue to be secreted until the pubertal surge.

The female, with two X chromosomes, forms ovaries and female external genitalia. By the sixteenth week, oogenesis has been established. At birth, the ovaries contain the female's lifetime supply of ova. Most female hormone production is delayed until puberty. However, the fetal endometrium responds to maternal hormones, and withdrawal bleeding or vaginal discharge **(pseudomenstruation)** may occur at birth when these hormones are lost. The high level of maternal estrogen also stimulates mammary engorgement and secretion of fluid ("witch's milk") in newborn infants of both sexes.

Musculoskeletal System

evolve Animation—First Trimester, Fetal Development

Bones and muscles develop from somites which are masses of mesoderm by the fourth week of embryonic development. At that time, the cardiac muscle is already beating. The mesoderm next to the neural tube forms the vertebral column and ribs. The parts of the vertebral column grow toward each other to enclose the developing spinal cord. *Ossification*, or bone formation, begins. If there is a defect in the bony fusion, various forms of spina bifida may occur. A large defect affecting several vertebrae may allow the membranes and spinal cord to pouch out from the back, producing neurological deficits and skeletal deformity.

The flat bones of the skull develop during the embryonic period, and ossification continues throughout childhood. At birth, connective tissue sutures exist where the bones of the skull meet. The areas where more than two bones meet (called **fontanels**) are especially prominent. The sutures and fontanels allow the bones of the skull to mould, or move during birth, enabling the head to pass through the birth canal.

evolve Animation—Second Trimester, Fetal Development

The bones of the shoulders, arms, hips, and legs appear in the sixth week as a continuous skeleton with no joints. Differentiation occurs, producing separate bones and joints. Ossification continues through childhood to allow growth. Beginning in the seventh week muscles contract spontaneously. Arm and leg movements are visible on ultrasound examination, although the mother does not perceive them until sometime between 16 and 20 weeks.

Integumentary System

The epidermis begins as a single layer of cells derived from the ectoderm at 4 weeks. By the seventh week, there are two layers of cells. The cells of the superficial layer are sloughed and become mixed with the sebaceous gland secretions to form the white, cheesy **vernix caseosa**, the material that protects the skin of the fetus. The vernix is thick at 24 weeks but becomes scant by term.

evolve Animation—Third Trimester, Fetal Development

The basal layer of the epidermis is the germinal layer, which replaces lost cells. Until 17 weeks, the skin is thin and wrinkled, with blood vessels visible underneath. The skin thickens, and all layers are present at term. After 32 weeks, as subcutaneous fat is deposited under the dermis, the skin becomes less wrinkled and red in appearance.

By 16 weeks, the epidermal ridges are present on the palms of the hands, the fingers, the bottom of the feet, and the toes. These handprints and footprints are unique to that infant.

Hairs form from hair bulbs in the epidermis that project into the dermis. Cells in the hair bulb keratinize to form the hair shaft. As the cells at the base of the hair shaft proliferate, the hair grows to the surface of the epithelium. Very fine hairs, called **lanugo**, appear first at 12 weeks on the eyebrows and upper lip. By week 20 they cover the entire body. At this time, the eyelashes, eyebrows, and scalp hair are beginning to grow. By week 28, the scalp hair is longer than the lanugo, which thins and may disappear by term gestation.

Fingernails and toenails develop from thickened epidermis at the tips of the digits beginning during the tenth week. They grow slowly. Fingernails usually reach the fingertips by 32 weeks, and toenails reach toe tips by 36 weeks.

Immunological System

During the third trimester, albumin and globulin are present in the fetus. The only immunoglobulin (Ig) that crosses the placenta, IgG, provides passive acquired immunity to specific bacterial toxins. The fetus produces IgM by the end of the first trimester. This is produced in response to blood group antigens, gram-negative enteric organisms, and some viruses. IgA is not produced by the fetus; however, **colostrum**, the precursor to breast milk, contains large amounts of IgA and can provide passive immunity to the neonate who is breastfed.

The normal term neonate can fight infection but not as effectively as an older child. The preterm infant is at much greater risk for infection.

Table 8-1 summarizes embryonic and fetal development.

Multifetal Pregnancy

Twins

The incidence of twinning is 1 in 43 pregnancies (Benirschke, 2009). The rate of multiple birth has risen from 2.2% in 1995 to 3.0% in 2004 (Public Health Agency of Canada [PHAC], 2008). This is partly attributed to delayed childbearing. The use of ovulation-enhancing drugs and IVF if more than one embryo is implanted are also factors.

Dizygotic Twins

When two mature ova are produced in one ovarian cycle, both have the potential to be fertilized by separate sperm. This results in two zygotes, or dizygotic twins (Fig. 8-13). There are always two amnions, two chorions, and two placentas that may be fused together. These dizygotic or fraternal twins may be the same sex or different sexes and are genetically no more alike than siblings born at different times. Dizygotic twinning occurs most often in families with a history of twinning. Dizygotic twinning increases in frequency with maternal age up to 35 years, with parity, and with the use of fertility drugs.

Monozygotic Twins

Identical or monozygotic twins develop from one fertilized ovum, which then divides (Fig. 8-14). They are the same sex and have the same genotype. If division occurs soon after fertilization, two embryos, two amnions, two chorions, and two placentas that may be fused will develop. Most often division occurs between 4 and 8 days after fertilization; there are two embryos, two amnions, one chorion, and one placenta. Rarely division occurs after the eighth day following fertilization. In this case, there are two embryos within a common amnion and a common chorion with one placenta. This often causes circulatory problems because the umbilical cords may tangle together, and one or both fetuses may die. If division occurs very late, cleavage may not be complete, and conjoined, or "Siamese," twins could result (see Fig. 8-14, C). Monozygotic twinning occurs in approximately 1 of 250 births

Table 8-1 Milestones in Human Development Before Birth Since Last Menstrual Period

4 WEEKS	8 WEEKS	12 WEEKS
External Appearance		
Body flexed, C-shaped; arm and leg buds present; head at right angles to body	Body fairly well formed; nose flat, eyes far apart; digits well formed; head elevating; tail almost disappeared; eyes, ears, nose, and mouth recognizable	Nails appearing; resembles a human; head erect but disproportionately large; skin pink, delicate
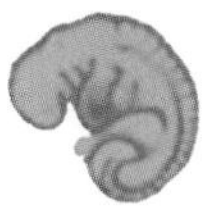	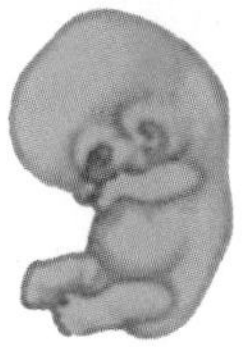	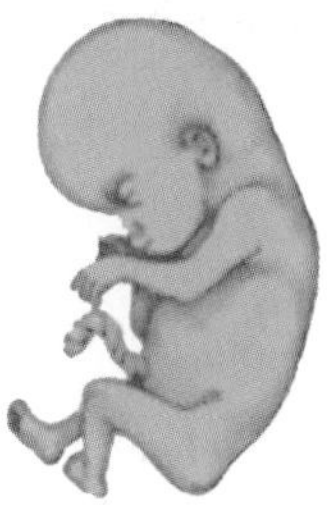
Crown-to-Rump Measurement; Weight		
0.4–0.5 cm; 0.4 g	2.5–3 cm; 2 g	6–9 cm; 19 g
Gastrointestinal System		
Stomach at midline and fusiform; conspicuous liver; esophagus short; intestine a short tube	Intestinal villi developing; small intestines coil within umbilical cord; palatal folds present; liver very large	Bile secreted; palatal fusion complete; intestines have withdrawn from cord and assume characteristic positions
Musculoskeletal System		
All somites present	First indication of ossification—occiput, mandible, and humerus; fetus capable of some movement; definitive muscles of trunk, limbs, and head well represented	Some bones well outlined, ossification spreading; upper cervical to lower sacral arches and bodies ossify; smooth muscle layers indicated in hollow viscera
Circulatory System		
Heart develops, double chambers visible, begins to beat; aortic arch and major veins completed	Main blood vessels assume final plan; enucleated red cells predominate in blood	Blood forming in marrow
Respiratory System		
Primary lung buds appear	Pleural and pericardial cavities forming; branching bronchioles; nostrils closed by epithelial plugs	Lungs acquire definite shape; vocal cords appear
Renal System		
Rudimentary ureteral buds appear	Earliest secretory tubules differentiating; bladder-urethra separates from rectum	Kidney able to secrete urine; bladder expands as a sac
Nervous System		
Well-marked midbrain flexure; no hindbrain or cervical flexures; neural groove closed	Cerebral cortex begins to acquire typical cells; differentiation of cerebral cortex, meninges, ventricular foramina, cerebrospinal fluid circulation; spinal cord extends entire length of spine	Brain structural configuration almost complete; cord shows cervical and lumbar enlargements; fourth ventricle foramina are developed; sucking present
Sensory Organs		
Eye and ear appearing as optic vessel and otocyst	Primordial choroid plexuses develop; ventricles large relative to cortex; development progressing; eyes converging rapidly; internal ear developing	Earliest taste buds indicated; characteristic organization of eye attained
Genital System		
Genital ridge appears (fifth week)	Testes and ovaries distinguishable; external genitalia sexless but begin to differentiate	Sex recognizable; internal and external sex organs specific

Continued

Table 8-1 Milestones in Human Development Before Birth Since Last Menstrual Period—cont'd

	16 WEEKS	20 WEEKS	24 WEEKS
External Appearance	Head still dominant; face looks human; eyes, ears, and nose approach typical appearance on gross examination; arm/leg ratio proportionate; scalp hair appears	Vernix caseosa appears; lanugo appears; legs lengthen considerably; sebaceous glands appear	Body lean but fairly well proportioned; skin red and wrinkled; vernix caseosa present; sweat glands forming
	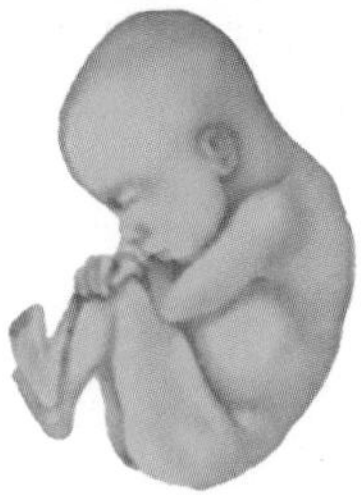	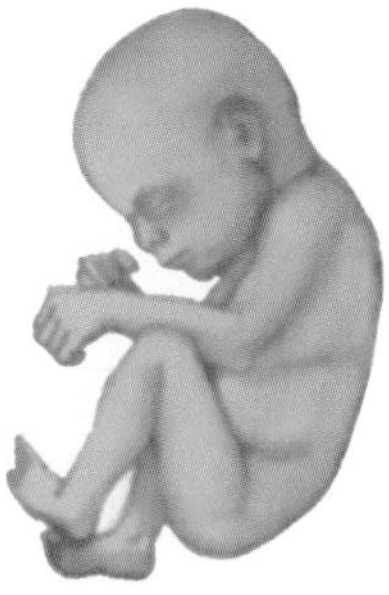	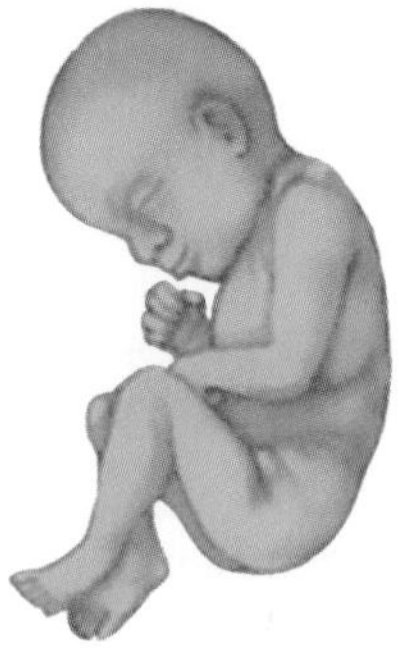
Crown-to-Rump Measurement; Weight	11.5–13.5 cm; 100 g	16–18.5 cm; 300 g	23 cm; 600 g
Gastrointestinal System	Meconium in bowel; some enzyme secretion; anus open	Enamel and dentine depositing; ascending colon recognizable	
Musculoskeletal System	Most bones distinctly indicated throughout body; joint cavities appear; muscular movements can be detected	Sternum ossifies; fetal movements strong enough for mother to feel	
Circulatory System	Heart muscle well developed; blood formation active in spleen		Blood formation increases in bone marrow and decreases in liver
Respiratory System	Elastic fibres appear in lungs; terminal and respiratory bronchioles appear	Nostrils reopen; primitive respiratory-like movements begin	Alveolar ducts and sacs present; lecithin begins to appear in amniotic fluid (wk 26–27)
Renal System	Kidney in position; attains typical shape and plan		
Nervous System	Cerebral lobes delineated; cerebellum assumes some prominence	Brain grossly formed; cord myelination begins; spinal cord ends at level of first sacral vertebra (S-1)	Cerebral cortex layered typically; neuronal proliferation in cerebral cortex ends
Sensory Organs	General sense organs differentiated	Nose and ears ossify	Can hear
Genital System	Testes in position for descent into scrotum: vagina open		Testes at inguinal ring in descent to scrotum

Table 8-1 Milestones in Human Development Before Birth Since Last Menstrual Period—cont'd

28 WEEKS	30-31 WEEKS	36 AND 40 WEEKS
External Appearance		
Lean body, less wrinkled and red; nails appear	Subcutaneous fat beginning to collect; more rounded appearance; skin pink and smooth; has assumed birth position 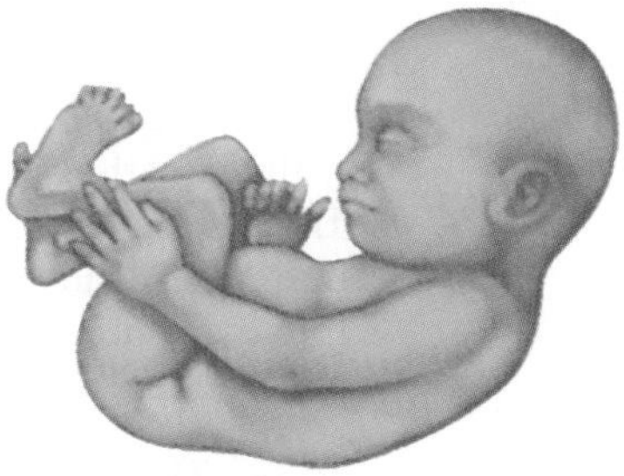	36 wk–Skin pink, body rounded; general lanugo disappearing; body usually plump 40 wk–Skin smooth and pink; scant vernix caseosa; moderate-to-profuse hair; lanugo on shoulders and upper body only; nasal and alar cartilage apparent
Crown-to-Rump Measurement; Weight		
27 cm; 1100 g	31 cm; 1800-2100 g	36 wk–35 cm; 2200-2900 g 40 wk–40 cm; 3200 g
Musculoskeletal System		
Astragalus (talus, ankle bone) ossifies; weak, fleeting movements; minimum tone	Middle fourth phalanxes ossify; permanent teeth primordia seen; can turn head to side	36 wk–Distal femoral ossification centres present; sustained, definite movements; fair tone; can turn and elevate head 40 wk–Active, sustained movement; good tone; may lift head
Respiratory System		
Lecithin forming on alveolar surfaces	L/S ratio = 1.2 : 1	36 wk–L/S ratio = 2 : 1 40 wk–Pulmonary branching only two-thirds complete
Renal System		
		36 wk–Formation of new nephrons ceases
Nervous System		
Appearance of cerebral fissures, convolutions rapidly appearing; indefinite sleep-wake cycle; cry weak or absent; weak suck reflex		36 wk–End of spinal cord at level of third lumbar vertebra (L3); definite sleep-wake cycle 40 wk–Myelination of brain begins; patterned sleep-wake cycle with alert periods; cries when hungry or uncomfortable; strong suck reflex
Sensory Organs		
Eyelids reopen; retinal layers completed, light receptive; pupils capable of reacting to light	Sense of taste present; aware of sounds outside mother's body	
Genital System		
	Testes descending to scrotum	40 wk–Testes in scrotum; labia majora well developed

L/S, lecithin/sphingomyelin.

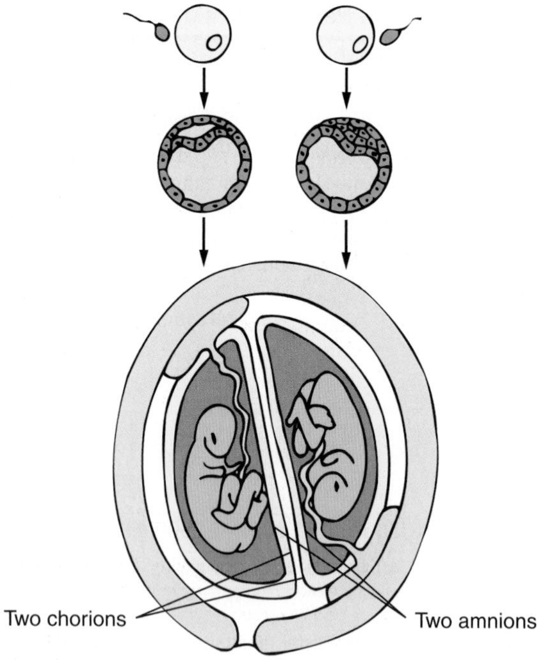

Fig. 8-13 Formation of dizygotic twins. There is fertilization of two ova, two implantations, two placentas, two chorions, and two amnions.

(Benirschke, 2009). There is no association with race, heredity, maternal age, or parity. Fertility drugs also increase the incidence of monozygotic twinning.

Other Multifetal Pregnancies

The occurrence of **multifetal pregnancies** with three or more fetuses has increased with the use of fertility drugs and IVF. Triplets occur in about 1 of 1341 pregnancies (Benirschke, 2009). They can occur from the division of one zygote into two, with one of the two dividing again, producing identical triplets. Triplets can also be produced from two zygotes, one dividing into a set of identical twins and the second zygote a single fraternal sibling, or from three zygotes. Quadruplets, quintuplets, sextuplets, and so on have similar possible derivations.

Key Points

- Preconception counselling is important to improve the health of all women and to ensure healthy pregnancy outcomes.
- Genetic disease affects people of all ages, from all socioeconomic levels, and from all racial and ethnic backgrounds.
- Genetic disorders span every clinical practice specialty.
- Nurses have a role to play in genetic counselling.

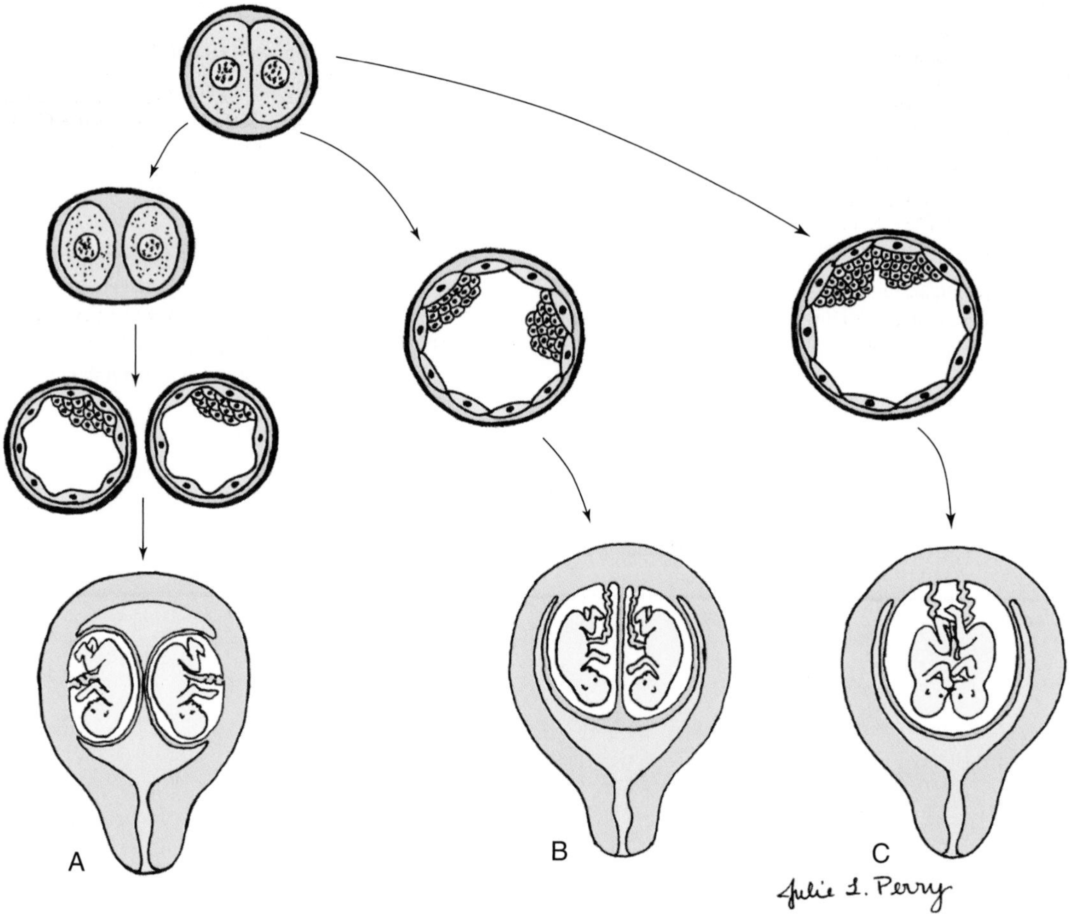

Fig. 8-14 Formation of monozygotic twins. A: One fertilization: blastomeres separate, resulting in two implantations, two placentas, and two sets of membranes. B: One blastomere with two inner cell masses, one fused placenta, one chorion, and separate amnions. C: One blastomere with incomplete separation of cell mass, resulting in conjoined twins.

- Genes are the basic units of heredity responsible for all human characteristics. They comprise 23 pairs of chromosomes: 22 pairs of autosomes and one pair of sex chromosomes.
- Genetic disorders follow Mendelian inheritance patterns of dominance and segregation and an independent assortment of normal genetic transmission.
- Multifactorial inheritance includes both genetic and environmental contributions.
- Human gestation is approximately 280 days after the LMP or 266 days after conception.
- Fertilization occurs in the uterine tube within 24 hours of ovulation. The zygote undergoes mitotic divisions, creating a 16-cell morula.
- Critical periods occur in human development during which the embryo or fetus is vulnerable to environmental teratogens.

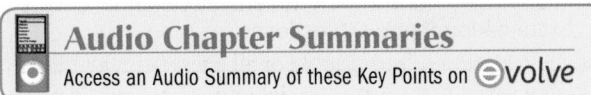

Audio Chapter Summaries
Access an Audio Summary of these Key Points on evolve

References

American College of Obstetricians and Gynecologists Preconception Care Work Group. (2005). *The importance of preconception care in the continuum of women's health care.* ACOG Committee Opinion, No. 313;2005.

Benirschke, K. (2009). Multiple gestation. The biology of twinning. In R. K. Creasy, et al. (Eds.), *Creasy & Resnik's maternal-fetal medicine: Principles and practice* (6th ed.). Philadelphia: Saunders.

Canadian Nurses Association (CNA). (2005). *Nursing and genetics: Are you ready?* Ottawa: Author. Retrieved from http://www.cna-aiic.ca/CNA/documents/pdf/publications/NN_Genetics_05_e.pdf.

Guttmacher, A., & Collins, F. (2005). Realizing the promise of genomics in biomedical research. *Journal of the American Medical Association, 294*(11), 1399–1402.

Hamilton, B. A., & Wynshaw-Boris, A. (2009). Basic genetics and patterns of inheritance. In R. K. Creasy, et al. (Eds.), *Creasy & Resnik's maternal-fetal medicine: Principles and practice* (6th ed.). Philadelphia: Saunders.

Jorde, L., et al. (2010). *Medical genetics* (4th ed.). St. Louis: Mosby.

Lashley, F. (2007). *Essentials of clinical genetics in nursing practice.* New York: Springer.

Lea, D. (2008). Genetic and genomic healthcare: Ethical issues of importance to nurses. *Online Journal of Issues in Nursing, 13*(1), Manuscript No. 4, 2008. Retrieved from http://www.nursingworld.org/MainMenuCategories/ANAMarketplace/ANAPeriodicals/OJIN/TableofContents/vol132008/No1Jan08/GeneticandGenomicHealthcare.aspx.

Loescher, L., & Merkle, C. (2005). The interface of genomic technologies and nursing. *Journal of Nursing Scholarship, 37*(2), 111–119.

National Down Syndrome Society. (2010a). *Down syndrome fact sheet.* Retrieved from www.ndss.org/index.php?option=com_content&view=article&id=54&Itemid=74.

National Down Syndrome Society. (2010b). *About down syndrome. Incidences and maternal age.* Retrieved from www.ndss.org/index.php?option=com_content&view=article&id=61&Itemid=78.

Public Health Agency of Canada (2008). *Canadian perinatal health report, 2008 edition* (Cat. No. HP10-12/2008E). Ottawa: Author. Retrieved from http://www.phac-aspc.gc.ca/publicat/2008/cphr-rspc/pdf/cphr-rspc08-eng.pdf.

Rubinstein, W., & Roy, H. (2005). Practicing medicine at the front lines of the genomic revolution. *Archives of Internal Medicine, 165*(16), 1815–1817.

Seo, D., & Ginsburg, G. (2005). Genomic medicine: Bringing biomarkers to clinical medicine. *Current Opinion in Chemical Biology, 9*(4), 381–386.

Society of Obstetricians and Gynaecologists of Canada. (2007). Prenatal screening for fetal aneuploidy. *Journal of Obstetrics and Gynaecology Canada, 29*(20), 146–161. Retrieved from http://www.sogc.org/guidelines/documents/187E-CPG-February2007.pdf.

Van Riper, M. (2005). Genetic testing and the family. *Journal of Midwifery and Women's Health, 50*(3), 227–233.

Van Riper, M., & McKinnon, W. (2004). Genetic testing for breast and ovarian cancer susceptibility: A family experience. *Journal of Midwifery and Women's Health, 43*(3), 210–219.

Wapner, R. J., Jenkins, T. M., & Khalek, N. (2009). Prenatal diagnosis of congenital disorders. In R. K. Creasy, et al. (Eds.), *Creasy & Resnik's maternal-fetal medicine: Principles and practice* (6th ed.). Philadelphia: Saunders.

Wilson, R.D., et al. (2011). SOGC Clinical Practice Guideline: Genetic considerations for a women's pre-conception evaluation. *Journal of Obstetrics and Gynaecology Canada, 33*(1), 57–64.

Additional Resources

Canadian Association of Genetic Counsellors: https://cagc-accg.ca/
Canadian Down Syndrome Society: http://www.cdss.ca

Unit 3

9 Anatomy and Physiology of Pregnancy

Learning Objectives

On completion of this chapter, the reader will be able to:

- Determine gravidity and parity using the five digit system.
- Describe the various types of pregnancy tests, including timing and interpretation of results.
- Explain the expected maternal anatomical and physiological adaptations to pregnancy.
- Differentiate among presumptive, probable, and positive signs of pregnancy.
- Identify maternal hormones produced during pregnancy, their target organs, and their major effects on pregnancy.
- Compare the characteristics of the abdomen, vulva, and cervix of the nullipara and multipara.

Electronic Resources

Additional information related to the content in Chapter 9 can be found on

evolve the companion Web site at

http://evolve.elsevier.com/Canada/Perry/maternal/

- Animation—First Trimester, Fetal Development
- Animation—Second Trimester, Fetal Development
- Animation—Third Trimester, Fetal Development
- Examination Review Questions

The goal of maternity care is a healthy pregnancy with a physically safe and emotionally satisfying outcome for mother, infant, and family. Consistent health care and surveillance are important to achieve this goal. However, many maternal adaptations are unfamiliar to pregnant women and their families. Helping the pregnant woman to recognize the relationship between her physical status and the plan for her care can enable her to make good decisions and encourages her to participate in her care.

Obstetrical Terminology

An understanding of the following terms used to describe pregnancy and the pregnant woman (Cunningham et al., 2010) is essential to the study of maternity care:

Gravida—A woman who is pregnant

Gravidity—Pregnancy

Multigravida—A woman who has had two or more pregnancies

Multipara—A woman who has completed two or more pregnancies to 20 weeks of gestation or more

Nulligravida—A woman who has never been pregnant

Nullipara—A woman who has not completed a pregnancy with a fetus or fetuses beyond 20 weeks of gestation

Parity—The number of pregnancies in which the fetus or fetuses have reached 20 weeks of gestation, not the number of fetuses (e.g., twins) born. Parity is not affected by whether the fetus is born alive or is stillborn (i.e., showing no signs of life at birth).

Postdate or postterm—Pregnancy that goes beyond 41 completed weeks of pregnancy (Crane et al., 2001)

Preterm—A pregnancy that has reached 20 weeks of gestation but before completion of 37 weeks of gestation

Primigravida—A woman who is pregnant for the first time

Primipara—A woman who has completed one pregnancy with a fetus or fetuses who have reached 20 weeks of gestation

Term—A pregnancy from the beginning of week 37 of gestation to the end of week 41 of gestation

Viability—Capacity to live outside the uterus, occurring about 22 to 25 weeks of gestation

Information about obstetrical history is gathered during history-taking interviews. Obtaining and documenting this information accurately is important in planning care for the pregnant woman.

The five digit system, separated by hyphens, provides information about the woman's obstetrical history. The first digit represents gravidity (number of all pregnancies); the second digit represents the total number of term births (at 37 or more weeks' gestation); the third indicates the number of preterm births (after 20 weeks to 37 weeks' gestation); the fourth identifies the number of abortions (miscarriage or elective termination of pregnancy); and the fifth is the number of children currently living. The number of births is the actual number of children born during each pregnancy. The acronym GTPAL (gravidity, term, preterm, abortions, living children) may be helpful in remembering this system of notation. For example, if a woman who is pregnant only once gives birth at week 35 and the infant survives, the

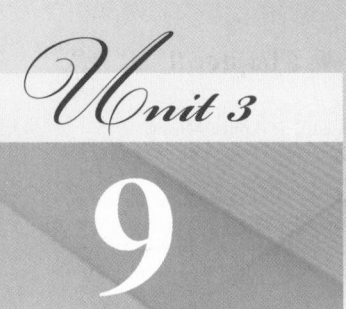

Table 9-1 Examples of Obstetrical History Information

	Five-Digit System				
	G	T	P	A	L
CONDITION	GRAVIDITY	TERM BIRTH	PRETERM BIRTHS	ABORTIONS AND MISCARRIAGES	LIVING CHILDREN
Kathy is pregnant for the first time.	1	0	0	0	0
She carries the pregnancy to term, and the neonate survives.	1	1	0	0	1
She is pregnant again.	2	1	0	0	1
Her second pregnancy ends in miscarriage at 10 wk.	2	1	0	1	1
During her third pregnancy she gives birth at 36 wk to twins.	3	1	2	1	3

abbreviation that represents this information is "1-0-1-0-1." During her next pregnancy the abbreviation would be "2-0-1-0-1." Additional examples are given in Table 9-1. Another system that is sometimes used is gravidity/parity. The first digit (G) indicates the number of pregnancies the woman has had, and the parity (P) indicates the number of pregnancies that have reached 20 weeks' gestation. This system can be confusing and does not provide enough information about the woman, so it should not be used.

Pregnancy Tests

Early detection of pregnancy encourages early initiation of care. Human chorionic gonadotropin (hCG) is the earliest biological marker for pregnancy. Pregnancy tests are based on the recognition of hCG or a beta (β) subunit of hCG. Production of β-hCG begins as early as the day of implantation and can be detected as early as 7 to 10 days after conception (Blackburn, 2007). The level of hCG rises until it peaks at about 60 to 70 days of gestation and then declines until about 80 days of gestation. It remains stable until about 30 weeks and then gradually increases until term. Higher than normal levels of hCG may indicate ectopic pregnancy, abnormal gestation (e.g., fetus with Down syndrome), or multiple gestation; an abnormally slow increase or a decrease in hCG levels may indicate impending miscarriage (Cunningham et al., 2010).

Serum and urine pregnancy tests are performed in clinics, offices, women's health centres, public health unit clinics, and laboratory settings. Urine pregnancy tests may be performed at home (see Community Focus box). Both serum and urine tests can provide accurate results. A 7- to 10-mL sample of venous blood is collected for serum testing. Most urine tests require a first-voided morning urine specimen because it contains levels of hCG approximately the same as those in serum. Random urine samples usually have lower levels. Urine tests are less expensive and provide more immediate results than serum tests.

Many different pregnancy tests are available (Fig. 9-1). The wide variety of tests precludes discussion of each. The nurse should read the manufacturer's directions for the test that is used.

Enzyme-linked immunosorbent assay (ELISA) testing is the most popular method of testing for pregnancy. It uses a specific monoclonal antibody (anti-hCG) with enzymes that bond with hCG in urine. ELISA technology is the basis for most over-the-counter home pregnancy tests. With these one-step tests the woman usually applies urine to a strip or absorbent-tipped applicator and reads the results. The test kits come with directions for collection of the specimen, the testing procedure, and reading of results. A positive test result is indicated by a simple colour change reaction or a digital reading. Most manufacturers of the kits provide a toll-free telephone number to call if users have concerns and questions about test

COMMUNITY FOCUS

Home Pregnancy Test Kits

Visit a pharmacy in your neighbourhood. How many different types of pregnancy home test kits are available in the pharmacy? Read the labels on three different types of pregnancy home test kits. Do the kits include material for more than one test? Are the directions printed in more than one language? After reading the directions, do you have questions about how to perform the test or how to interpret the results? If so, what does that say about the likelihood that the tests will be used correctly?

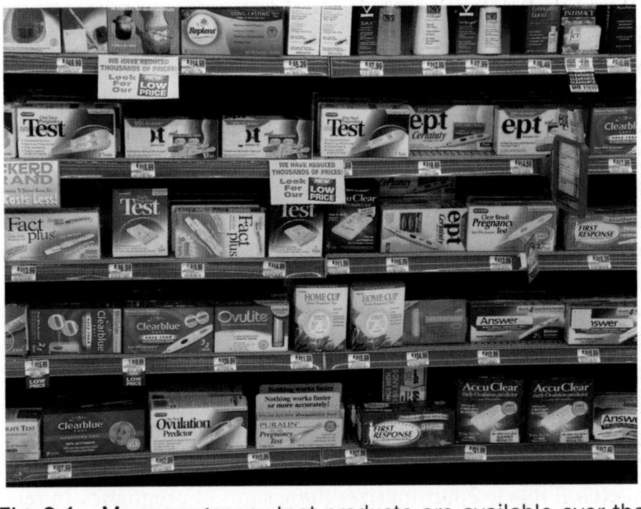

Fig. 9-1 Many pregnancy test products are available over the counter. *(Courtesy Dee Lowdermilk, Chapel Hill, NC.)*

procedures or results. The most common error in performing home pregnancy tests is doing the test too early in pregnancy (Pagana & Pagana, 2006).

Interpreting the results of pregnancy tests requires some judgement. The type of pregnancy test and its degree of sensitivity (the ability to detect low levels of a substance) and specificity (the ability to discern the absence of a substance) must be considered in conjunction with the woman's history. This includes the date of her last normal menstrual period, her usual cycle length, and results of previous pregnancy tests. It is important to know if the woman is taking any medications or is a substance user. Medications such as anticonvulsants and tranquilizers can cause false-positive results, whereas diuretics and promethazine can cause false-negative results (Pagana & Pagana, 2006). Improper collection of the specimen, hormone-producing tumours, and laboratory errors can also cause inaccurate results.

Women who use a home pregnancy test should be advised about the variations in accuracy reporting and to use caution when interpreting results. Whenever there is any question, further evaluation or retesting may be appropriate.

Adaptations to Pregnancy

Maternal physiological adaptations are attributed to the hormones of pregnancy and to mechanical pressures arising from the enlarging uterus and other tissues. These adaptations protect the woman's normal physiological functioning, meet the metabolic demands that pregnancy imposes on her body, and provide a nurturing environment for fetal development and growth (see Critical Thinking Exercise). Although pregnancy is a normal phenomenon, problems can occur.

Signs of Pregnancy

Some physiological adaptations are recognized as the signs and symptoms of pregnancy. Three commonly used categories of these signs and symptoms are (1) presumptive—those subjective changes felt by the woman (e.g., amenorrhea, fatigue, breast changes); (2) probable—those objective changes observed by an examiner (e.g., Hegar sign, ballottement, pregnancy tests); and (3) positive—those signs attributed only to the presence of the fetus (e.g., hearing fetal heart tones, visualizing the fetus, palpating fetal movements). Occasionally, these signs may mean something else besides the presence of a fetus. Table 9-2 summarizes these signs of pregnancy in relation to when they might occur and gives other possible causes for their occurrence.

Reproductive System and Breasts

Uterus

Changes in Size, Shape, and Position

High levels of estrogen and progesterone stimulate phenomenal uterine growth in the first trimester. Early uterine enlargement results from increased vascularity and dilation of blood vessels, hyperplasia (production of new muscle fibres and fibroelastic tissue) and hypertrophy (enlargement of preexisting muscle fibres and fibroelastic tissue), and development of the decidua. By 7 weeks of gestation the uterus is the size of a large hen's egg; by 10 weeks it is the size of an orange (twice its nonpregnant size); and by 12 weeks it is the size of a grapefruit. After the third month, uterine enlargement is primarily the result of mechanical pressure of the growing fetus.

As the uterus enlarges, it also changes in shape and position. At conception the uterus is shaped like an upside-down pear. During the second trimester, as the muscular walls strengthen and become more elastic, the uterus becomes spherical or globular. Later, as the fetus lengthens, the uterus becomes larger and more ovoid and rises out of the pelvis into the abdominal cavity.

The pregnancy may "show" after the fourteenth week, although this may depend on the woman's height and weight. Abdominal enlargement may be less apparent in the nullipara with good abdominal muscle tone (Fig. 9-2). Posture also

CRITICAL THINKING EXERCISE

Awareness of Physiological Changes of Pregnancy

Marlys is pregnant with her first child, and Janice is pregnant with her third child. They are both at approximately 18 weeks of gestation and have come to a prenatal appointment. While they are in the waiting room, you overhear Marlys asking Janice about some "old wives' tales" that she has heard:

- If she raises her arms above her head, the cord will wrap around the baby's neck.
- Putting a knife under the bed while she is labouring will "cut" the pain.
- If she dangles a needle in front of her abdomen, she will be able to tell if the baby is a boy or a girl.
- A rapid fetal heartbeat means that the baby will be a girl.

Marlys says that she has not felt her baby move yet, whereas Janice says that she has been feeling fetal movement for over 2 weeks. Marlys also has questions about some of the changes in her body that she has experienced or expects to experience. Janice bases her responses on her own experience. Based on the conversation you have overheard, you identify a need to spend some time with Marlys and Janice discussing physiological changes of pregnancy.

1. Evidence—Is there sufficient evidence to draw conclusions about the normal physiological changes in pregnancy in primigravidas and multiparas that the nurse should discuss with Marlys and Janice?
2. Assumptions—Describe an underlying assumption about each of the following topics:
   a. Differences in the normal physiological changes in pregnancy between primigravidas and multiparas
   b. Reversibility of these physiological changes in pregnancy
   c. Information provided by the health care provider
   d. Deviations from normal in the physiological changes of pregnancy
3. What implications and priorities for nursing care can be drawn at this time?
4. Does the evidence objectively support your conclusion?
5. Are there alternative perspectives to your conclusion?

Table 9-2 Signs of Pregnancy

TIME OF OCCURRENCE (GESTATIONAL AGE)	SIGN	OTHER POSSIBLE CAUSE
Presumptive		
3-4 wk	Breast changes	Premenstrual changes, oral contraceptives
4 wk	Amenorrhea	Stress, vigorous exercise, early menopause, endocrine problems, malnutrition
4-14 wk	Nausea, vomiting	Gastrointestinal virus, gastroenteritis
6-12 wk	Urinary frequency	Infection, pelvic tumours
12 wk	Fatigue	Stress, illness
16-20 wk	Quickening	Gas, peristalsis
Probable		
5 wk	Goodell's sign	Pelvic congestion
6-8 wk	Chadwick's sign	Pelvic congestion
6-12 wk	Hegar's sign	Pelvic congestion
4-12 wk	Positive pregnancy test (serum)	Hydatidiform mole, choriocarcinoma
6-12 wk	Positive pregnancy test (urine)	False-positive result may be caused by pelvic infection, tumours
16 wk	Braxton Hicks or prelabour contractions	Myomas, other tumours
16-28 wk	Ballottement	Tumours, cervical polyps
Positive		
5-6 wk	Visualization of fetus by real-time ultrasound examination	No other causes
6 wk	Fetal heart tones detected by ultrasound examination	No other causes
16 wk	Visualization of fetus by radiographic study	No other causes
8-17 wk	Fetal heart tones detected by Doppler ultrasound stethoscope	No other causes
17-19 wk	Fetal heart tones detected by fetal stethoscope	No other causes
19-22 wk	Fetal movements palpated	No other causes
Late pregnancy	Fetal movements visible	No other causes

influences the type and degree of abdominal enlargement that occurs. In normal pregnancies, the uterus enlarges at a predictable rate.

As the uterus grows, it may be palpated above the symphysis pubis sometime between the twelfth and fourteenth weeks of pregnancy (Fig. 9-3). The uterus rises gradually to the level of the umbilicus at 20 to 22 weeks of gestation and nearly reaches the xiphoid process at term. Between weeks 38 and 40, fundal height decreases as the fetus begins to descend and engage in the pelvis (lightening) (see Fig. 9-3, dashed line). Generally, lightening occurs in the nullipara anytime in the last 4 weeks before the onset of labour and in the multipara at the start of labour.

Uterine enlargement is determined by measuring fundal height (see Fig. 10-7). This measurement is commonly used to estimate the duration of pregnancy. However, variation in the position of the fundus or the fetus, variations in the amount of amniotic fluid present, the presence of more than one fetus, maternal obesity, and variation in examiner technique can reduce the accuracy of this estimation.

Generally, the uterus rotates to the right as it elevates, probably because of the presence of the rectosigmoid colon on the left side. However, the extensive hypertrophy (enlargement) of the round ligaments keeps the uterus in the midline. Eventually, the growing uterus touches the anterior abdominal wall and displaces the intestines to either side of the abdomen (Fig. 9-4). When a pregnant woman is standing, most of her uterus rests against the anterior abdominal wall; this can alter her centre of gravity.

At approximately 6 weeks of gestation, softening and compressibility of the lower uterine segment (uterine isthmus) occurs (Hegar's sign) (Fig. 9-5). This results in exaggerated uterine anteflexion during the first 3 months of pregnancy. In this position, the uterine fundus presses on the urinary bladder, causing the woman to have urinary frequency.

Changes in Contractility

Soon after the fourth month of pregnancy, uterine contractions can be felt through the abdominal wall. These contractions, referred to as **Braxton Hicks contractions**, are irregular and painless contractions that occur intermittently throughout pregnancy. These contractions facilitate uterine blood flow through the intervillous spaces of the placenta and promote oxygen delivery to the fetus. Although Braxton Hicks contractions are not painful, some women are surprised by them and over time may find them to be annoying. After the twenty-eighth week, these contractions become more definite,

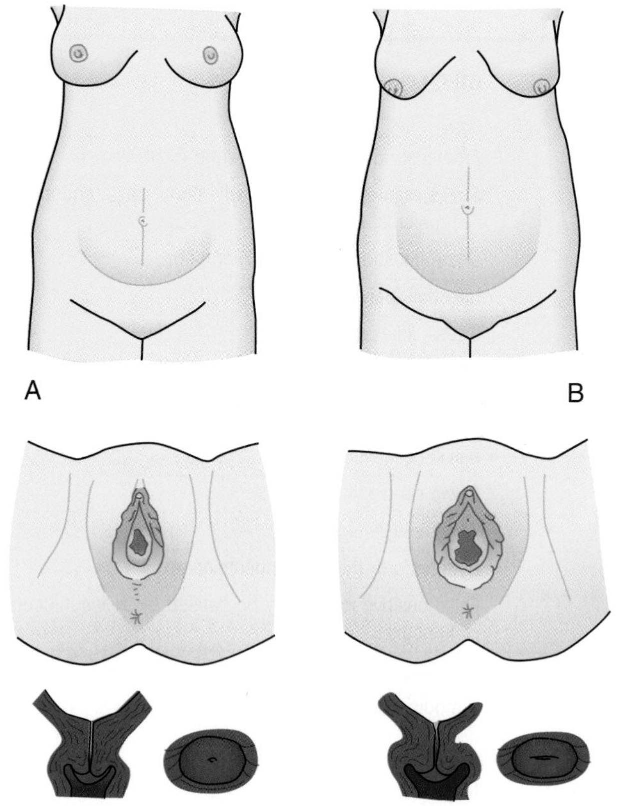

Fig. 9-2 Comparison of abdomen, vulva, and cervix in A, nullipara, and B, multipara, at the same stage of pregnancy.

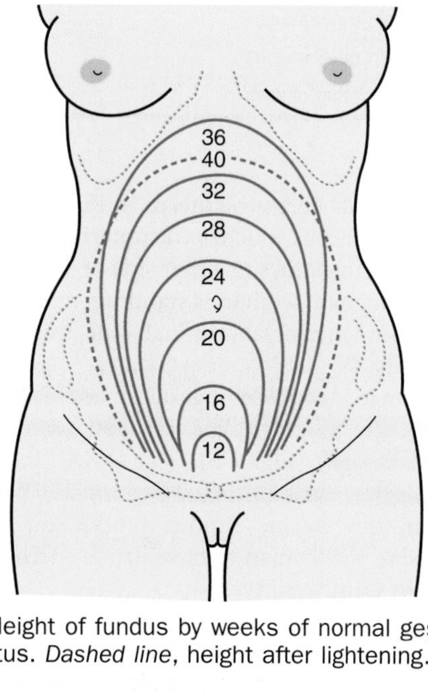

Fig. 9-3 Height of fundus by weeks of normal gestation with a single fetus. *Dashed line*, height after lightening.

but they usually cease with walking or exercise. Braxton Hicks contractions can be mistaken for true labour; however, they do not increase in intensity or duration or cause cervical dilation. Conversely, premature labour contractions can be mistaken for Braxton Hicks contractions and thus lead to a delay in seeking treatment.

Uteroplacental Blood Flow

Placental perfusion depends on the maternal blood flow to the uterus. Blood flow increases rapidly as the uterus increases in size. Although uterine blood flow increases twentyfold, the fetoplacental unit grows even more rapidly. Consequently, more oxygen is extracted from the uterine blood during the latter part of pregnancy (Cunningham et al., 2010). In a normal term pregnancy, one sixth of the total maternal blood volume is within the uterine vascular system. The rate of blood flow through the uterus averages 500 mL/min, and oxygen consumption of the gravid uterus increases to meet fetal needs. Three factors known to decrease uterine blood flow are low maternal arterial pressure, contractions of the uterus, and maternal supine position. Estrogen stimulation may increase uterine blood flow. Doppler ultrasound examination can be used to measure uterine blood flow velocity, especially in pregnancies at risk due to conditions associated with decreased placental perfusion such as hypertension, intrauterine growth restriction, diabetes mellitus, and multiple gestation (Blackburn, 2007) (see Fig. 12-14).

Using an ultrasound device or a fetal stethoscope, the examiner may hear the uterine souffle or bruit, a rushing or blowing sound of maternal blood flowing through uterine arteries to the placenta that is synchronous with the maternal pulse. The funic souffle, which is synchronous with the fetal heart rate and is caused by fetal blood coursing through the umbilical cord, may also be heard, as well as the actual heartbeat of the fetus.

Cervical Changes

In a normal, unscarred cervix, a softening of the cervical tip may be observed about the beginning of the sixth week. This probable sign of pregnancy, **Goodell's sign**, is brought about by increased vascularity, slight hypertrophy, and hyperplasia (increase in number of cells). The muscle and its collagen-rich connective tissue become loose, edematous, highly elastic, and increased in volume. The glands near the external os proliferate beneath the stratified squamous epithelium, giving the cervix the velvety appearance characteristic of pregnancy. Friability is increased and can result in slight bleeding after vaginal examination or after coitus with deep penetration.

Pregnancy can also cause the squamocolumnar junction, the site for obtaining cells for cervical cancer screening, to be located away from the cervix. Because of these changes, evaluation of abnormal Papanicolaou (Pap) tests during pregnancy can be complicated. However, careful assessment of all pregnant women is important because approximately 3% of all cervical cancers are diagnosed during pregnancy (Copeland & Landon, 2007).

The cervix of the nullipara is rounded. Lacerations of the cervix almost always occur during the birth process. After childbirth, with or without lacerations, the cervix becomes more oval in the horizontal plane, and the external os appears as a transverse slit (see Fig. 9-2).

Changes Related to the Presence of the Fetus

Passive movement of the unengaged fetus is called *ballottement* and can be identified generally between the sixteenth and eighteenth week. Ballottement is a technique of palpating a floating structure by bouncing it gently and feeling it

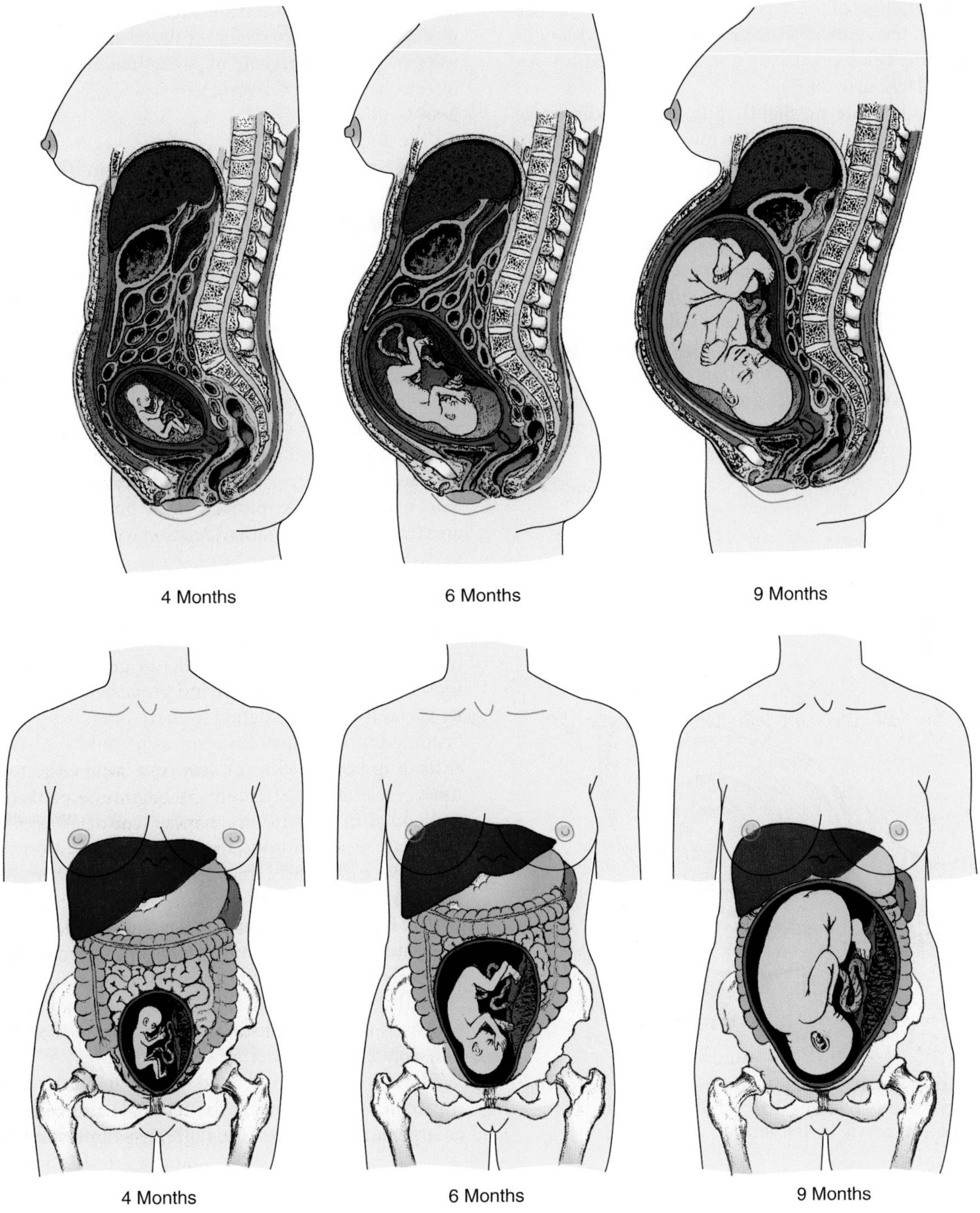

Fig. 9-4 Displacement of internal abdominal structures and diaphragm by the enlarging uterus at 4, 6, and 9 months of gestation.

rebound. To palpate the fetus, the examiner places a finger within the vagina and taps gently upward, causing the fetus to rise. The fetus then sinks, and a gentle tap is felt on the finger (Fig. 9-6).

The first recognition of fetal movements, or "feeling life," may occur as early as the fourteenth week in the multiparous woman. The nulliparous woman may not notice these sensations until the eighteenth week or later. **Quickening** is commonly described as a flutter and is difficult to distinguish from peristalsis. Fetal movements gradually increase in intensity and frequency. The week in which quickening occurs provides a tentative clue in dating the duration of gestation.

Vagina and Vulva

Pregnancy hormones prepare the vagina for stretching during labour and birth by causing the vaginal mucosa to thicken, connective tissue to loosen, smooth muscle to hypertrophy, and the vaginal vault to lengthen. Increased vascularity results in a violet-bluish colour of the vaginal mucosa and cervix. The deepened colour, termed **Chadwick's sign**, may be evident as early as the sixth week but is easily noted by the eighth week of pregnancy (Blackburn, 2007).

Leukorrhea is a white or slightly grey mucoid discharge with a faint musty odour. This copious mucoid fluid occurs in response to cervical stimulation by estrogen and progesterone. The fluid is whitish because of the presence of many exfoliated vaginal epithelial cells caused by the hyperplasia of normal pregnancy. This vaginal discharge is never pruritic or blood stained. The mucus fills the endocervical canal, resulting in the formation of the mucous plug (operculum) (Fig. 9-7). The operculum acts as a barrier against bacterial invasion.

During pregnancy, the pH of vaginal secretions is more acidic, ranging from about 3.5 to about 6.0 (normal is 4.0 to 7.0), because of increased production of lactic acid (Cunningham et al., 2010). Although this acidic environment provides more protection against some organisms, the glycogen-rich environment of the vagina makes the pregnant woman more vulnerable to other infections, especially yeast infections, such as *Candida albicans* (Duff, Sweet, & Edwards, 2009).

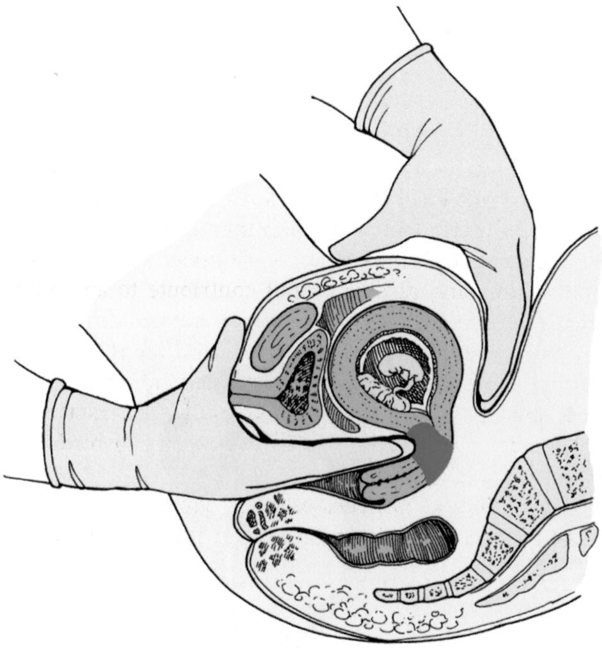

Fig. 9-5 Hegar's sign. Bimanual examination for assessing compressibility and softening of isthmus (lower uterine segment) while the cervix is still firm.

The increased vascularity of the vagina and other pelvic viscera results in a marked increase in sensitivity. This increased sensitivity may lead to a high degree of sexual interest and arousal, especially during the second trimester of pregnancy. The increased congestion, plus the relaxed walls of the blood vessels and the heavy uterus, may result in edema and varicosities of the vulva. The edema and varicosities usually resolve during the postpartum period.

External structures of the perineum are enlarged during pregnancy because of an increase in vasculature, hypertrophy of the perineal body, and deposition of fat (Fig. 9-8). The labia majora of nullipara women approximate (come together) and obscure the vaginal introitus; those of the parous woman separate and gape after childbirth and perineal or vaginal injury. See Fig. 9-2 for a comparison of the perineum of the nullipara and that of the multipara in relation to the pregnant abdomen, vulva, and cervix.

Breasts

Fullness, heightened sensitivity, tingling, and heaviness of the breasts begin in the early weeks of gestation in response to increased levels of estrogen and progesterone. Breast sensitivity varies from mild tingling to sharp pain. Nipples and areolae become more pigmented; secondary pinkish areolae develop, extending beyond the primary areolae; and nipples become more erectile. Hypertrophy of the sebaceous (oil) glands embedded in the primary areolae, called *Montgomery tubercles*, may be seen around the nipples. These sebaceous glands may have a protective role in that they keep the nipples lubricated for breastfeeding.

The richer blood supply causes the vessels beneath the skin to dilate. Once barely noticeable, the blood vessels become visible, often appearing in an intertwining blue network beneath the surface of the skin. Venous congestion in the breasts is more obvious in primigravidas. **Striae gravidarum** may appear at the outer aspects of the breasts.

During the second and third trimesters, growth of the mammary glands accounts for the progressive breast enlargement (Fig. 9-9). The high levels of luteal and placental

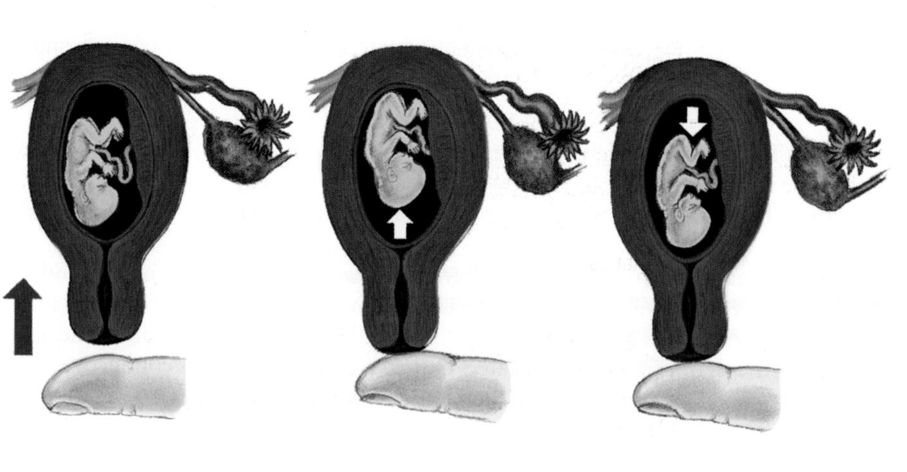

Fig. 9-6 Internal ballottement (18 weeks).

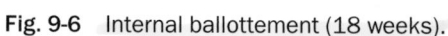

hormones in pregnancy promote proliferation of the lactiferous ducts and lobule-alveolar tissue so that palpation of the breasts reveals a generalized, coarse nodularity. Glandular tissue displaces connective tissue, and as a result the tissue becomes softer and looser.

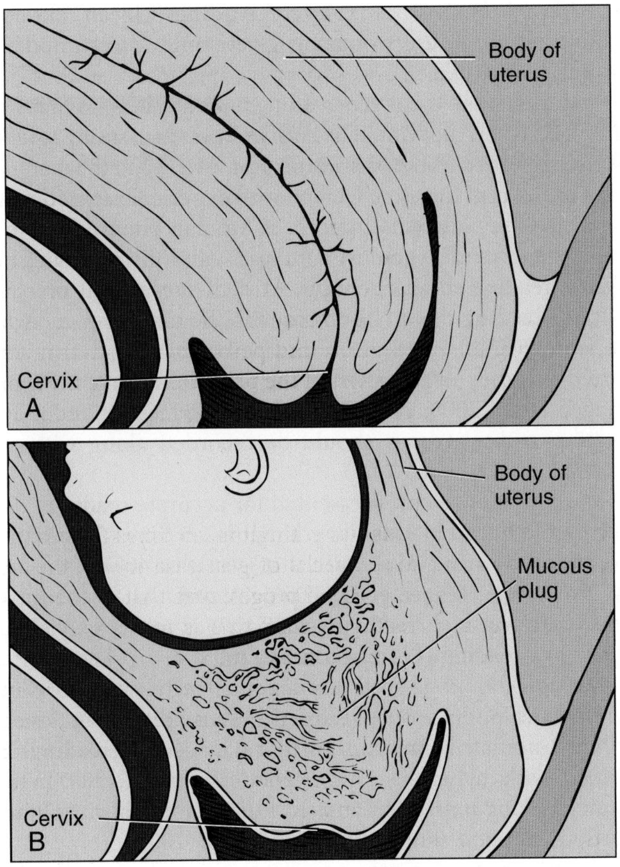

Fig. 9-7 A: Cervix in nonpregnant woman. **B:** Cervix during pregnancy.

Although development of the mammary glands is functionally complete by midpregnancy, **lactation** is inhibited until a decrease in estrogen level occurs after birth. A thin, clear, viscous secretory material (precolostrum) can be found in the acini cells by the third month of gestation. **Colostrum**, the creamy, white-to-yellowish-to-orange premilk fluid, may be expressed from the nipples as early as 16 weeks of gestation, although some women never secrete this until after birth (Blackburn, 2007). See Chapter 26 for a discussion of lactation.

General Body Systems

Cardiovascular System

Maternal adjustments to pregnancy involve extensive anatomical and physiological changes in the cardiovascular system. Cardiovascular adaptations protect the woman's normal physiological functioning, meet the metabolic demands pregnancy imposes on her body, and provide for fetal developmental and growth needs.

Slight cardiac hypertrophy (enlargement) is probably secondary to increased blood volume and cardiac output that occurs in pregnancy. The heart returns to its normal size after childbirth. As the diaphragm is displaced upward by the enlarging uterus, the heart is elevated upward and rotated forward to the left (Fig. 9-10). The apical impulse, a point of maximal intensity, is shifted upward and laterally about 1 to 1.5 cm. The degree of shift depends on the duration of pregnancy and the size and position of the uterus.

The changes in heart size and position and the increases in blood volume and cardiac output contribute to auscultatory changes common in pregnancy. There is more audible splitting of S_1 and S_2, and S_3 may be readily heard after 20 weeks of gestation. In addition, systolic and diastolic murmurs may be heard over the pulmonic area. These changes are transient and disappear in most women shortly after they give birth (Cunningham et al., 2010).

Between 14 and 20 weeks of gestation, the pulse increases about 10 to 15 beats per minute, and this persists to term.

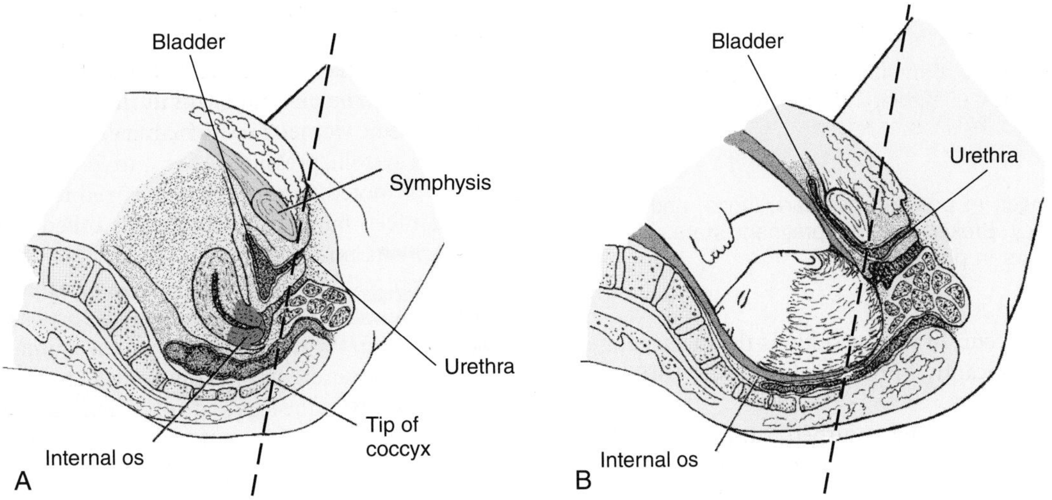

Fig. 9-8 A: Pelvic floor in a nonpregnant woman. **B:** Pelvic floor during labour. Note marked hypertrophy and hyperplasia below dotted line joining tip of coccyx and inferior margin of symphysis. Note elongation of bladder and urethra as a result of compression. Fat deposits are increased.

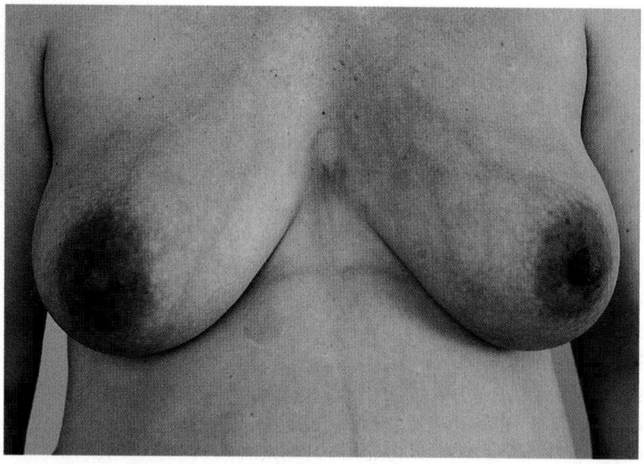

Fig. 9-9 Enlarged breasts in pregnancy with venous network and darkened areolae and nipples. *(From Seidel, H. M., et al. [2006].* Mosby's guide to physical examination *[6th ed., p. 513]. St. Louis: Mosby.)*

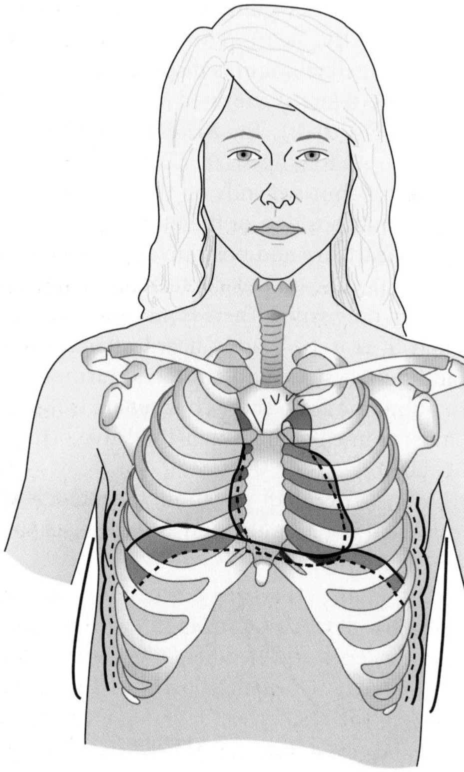

Fig. 9-10 Changes in position of heart, lungs, and thoracic cage in pregnancy. *Broken line*, nonpregnant state; *solid line*, change that occurs in pregnancy.

Palpitations may occur. In twin gestations the maternal heart rate increases significantly in the third trimester (Blackburn, 2007).

The cardiac rhythm may be disturbed. The pregnant woman may experience sinus arrhythmia, premature atrial contractions, and premature ventricular systole. In the healthy woman with no underlying heart disease, no therapy is needed. Women with pre-existing heart disease need close medical and obstetrical supervision during pregnancy (see Chapter 14).

Blood Pressure

Arterial blood pressure (brachial artery) varies with age; activity level; presence of health problems, pain, or both; circadian rhythm; and use of alcohol, tobacco, or other substances. Additional factors to consider during pregnancy include maternal anxiety, maternal position, and type of blood pressure apparatus (Pickering et al., 2005).

Maternal anxiety can elevate readings. If an elevated reading is found, the woman is given time to rest, and the reading is repeated.

Maternal position affects readings. Brachial blood pressure is highest when the woman is sitting; lowest when she is lying in the lateral recumbent position; and intermediate when she is supine, except for some women who experience hypotensive syndrome (see later discussion). A woman should have her blood pressure measured in both arms, and the arm with the highest reading should be used. At each subsequent prenatal visit, the reading should be obtained in the same arm and with the woman in a seated position with her back and arm supported and her upper arm at the level of the right atrium (Magee et al., 2008; Pickering et al., 2005; Sibai, 2007). The position and arm used should be recorded along with the reading.

The proper-size cuff is essential for accurate readings. The cuff should have a bladder length that is 1.5 times the circumference of the arm and a width that is at least 40% of the arm circumference (Magee et al., 2008). A cuff that is too small yields a falsely high reading; a cuff that is too large yields a falsely low reading (Pickering et al., 2005).

Caution should be used when comparing auscultatory and oscillatory blood pressure readings because discrepancies can occur. Automated monitors will give inaccurate readings in women with hypertensive conditions (Gordon, 2007). If a woman's blood pressure is above 140/90, a manual cuff should be used, for accurate results (Magee et al., 2008).

Systolic blood pressure usually remains the same as the prepregnancy level but may decrease slightly as pregnancy advances. Diastolic blood pressure begins to decrease in the first trimester, continues to drop until 24 to 32 weeks, and gradually increases and returns to prepregnancy levels by term (Blackburn, 2007).

Some degree of compression of the vena cava occurs in all women who lie on their backs during the second half of pregnancy. Some women experience a fall of more than 30 mm Hg in their systolic pressure. After 4 to 5 minutes a reflex bradycardia is noted, cardiac output is reduced by half, and the woman feels faint. This condition is called *supine hypotensive syndrome* (Cunningham et al., 2010).

Compression of the iliac veins and inferior vena cava by the uterus causes increased venous pressure and reduced blood flow in the legs, except when the woman is in the lateral position. These alterations contribute to the dependent edema, varicose veins in the legs and vulva, and hemorrhoids that may develop in the latter part of term pregnancy (Fig. 9-11).

Blood Volume and Composition

The degree of blood volume expansion varies considerably. Blood volume increases by approximately 1500 mL, or 40 to 50% above nonpregnancy levels (Cunningham et al., 2009). This increase consists of 1000 mL of plasma plus 450 mL of

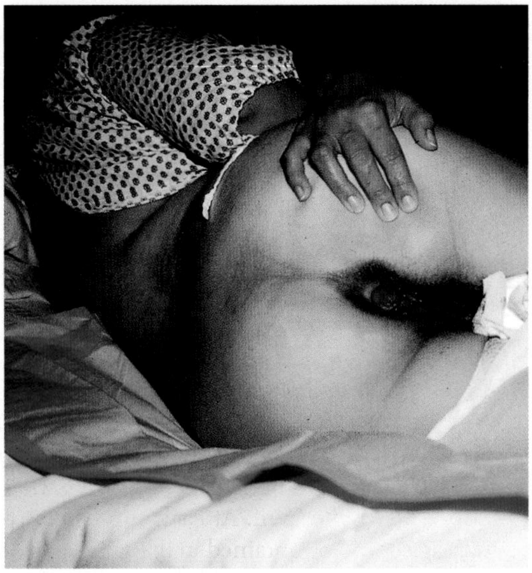

Fig. 9-11 Hemorrhoids. *(Courtesy Marjorie Pyle, RNC, Lifecircle, Costa Mesa, CA.)*

red blood cells (RBCs). The increase in volume starts at weeks 10 to 12, peaks at weeks 32 to 34, and decreases slightly at week 40. The volume in a multiple gestation increases above that for a single fetus (Blackburn, 2007). Increased blood volume is a protective mechanism. It is essential for meeting the blood volume needs of the hypertrophied vascular system of the enlarged uterus, for adequately hydrating fetal and maternal tissues when the woman assumes an erect or supine position, and for providing a fluid reserve to compensate for blood loss during birth and the puerperium. Peripheral vasodilation allows for a normal blood pressure despite the increased blood volume in pregnancy.

During pregnancy, there is an accelerated production of RBCs (normal, 4.0 to 5.2×10^{12}/L). The percentage of increase depends on the amount of iron available. The RBC mass increases by 20 to 30% (Blackburn, 2007).

Because the plasma increase is greater than the increase in RBC production, there is a decrease in normal hemoglobin values (120 to 160 g/L blood) and hematocrit values (0.37 to 0.47). This state of hemodilution is referred to as *physiological anemia*. The decrease is more noticeable during the second trimester, when rapid expansion of blood volume occurs faster than RBC production. If the hemoglobin value drops to 110 g/L or less or if the hematocrit decreases to 0.32 or less, the woman is considered anemic (Samuels, 2007).

The total white blood cell count increases during the second trimester and peaks during the third trimester. This increase is primarily in the granulocytes; the lymphocyte count stays about the same throughout pregnancy. See Table 9-3 for laboratory values during pregnancy.

Cardiac Output

Cardiac output increases from 30 to 50% over the nonpregnant rate by week 32 of pregnancy; it declines to about a 20% increase at 40 weeks of gestation. This elevated cardiac output is largely a result of increased stroke volume and heart rate and occurs in response to increased tissue demands for oxygen (Blackburn, 2007).

Cardiac output in late pregnancy is appreciably higher when the woman is in the lateral recumbent position than when she is supine. In the supine position, the large, heavy uterus often impedes venous return to the heart and affects blood pressure. Cardiac output increases with any exertion such as labour and birth. Table 9-4 summarizes cardiovascular changes in pregnancy.

Circulation and Coagulation Times

The circulation time decreases slightly by week 32. It returns to near normal by term. There is a greater tendency for blood to coagulate (clot) during pregnancy because of increases in various clotting factors (i.e., factors VII, VIII, IX, and X, and fibrinogen). This tendency, combined with the fact that fibrinolytic activity (the splitting up or dissolving of a clot) is depressed during pregnancy and the postpartum period, provides a protective function to decrease the chance of bleeding but also makes the woman more vulnerable to thrombosis, especially after Caesarean birth.

Respiratory System

Structural and ventilatory adaptations occur during pregnancy to provide for maternal and fetal needs. Maternal oxygen requirements increase in response to the acceleration in metabolic rate and the need to add to the tissue mass in the uterus and breasts. In addition, the fetus requires oxygen and a way to eliminate carbon dioxide.

Elevated levels of estrogen cause the ligaments of the rib cage to relax, permitting increased chest expansion (see Fig. 9-10). The transverse diameter of the thoracic cage increases by about 2 cm and the circumference by 6 cm (Cunningham et al., 2010). The costal angle increases, and the lower rib cage appears to flare out. The chest may not return to its prepregnant state after birth (Seidel et al., 2006).

The diaphragm is displaced by as much as 4 cm during pregnancy. With advancing pregnancy, chest breathing replaces abdominal breathing, and it becomes less possible for the diaphragm to descend with inspiration. Thoracic breathing is primarily accomplished by the diaphragm rather than by the costal muscles (Blackburn, 2007).

The upper respiratory tract becomes more vascular in response to elevated levels of estrogen. As the capillaries become engorged, edema and hyperemia develop within the nose, pharynx, larynx, trachea, and bronchi. This congestion within the tissues of the respiratory tract gives rise to several conditions commonly seen during pregnancy, including nasal and sinus stuffiness, epistaxis (nosebleed), changes in the voice, and marked inflammatory response to even a mild upper respiratory infection.

Increased vascularity of the upper respiratory tract also can cause the tympanic membranes and eustachian tubes to swell, giving rise to symptoms of impaired hearing, earaches, or a sense of fullness in the ears.

Pulmonary Function

Respiratory changes in pregnancy are related to the elevation of the diaphragm and changes in the chest wall. Changes in the respiratory centre result in a lowered threshold for carbon dioxide. The actions of progesterone and estrogen are presumed to be responsible for the increased sensitivity of the respiratory centre to carbon dioxide (see Table 9-5 for

Table 9-3 Laboratory Values for Pregnant and Nonpregnant Women

VALUES	NONPREGNANT	PREGNANT
Hematological		
Complete Blood Count		
Hemoglobin, g/L	120–160*	>110
Hematocrit	0.37–0.47	>0.32
RBC volume, per millilitre	1400	1650
Plasma volume, per millilitre	2400	40–60% increase
RBC count $\times 10^{12}$/L	4.0–5.4	5–6.25
White blood cells, $\times 10^{9}$/L	4–10	5–15
Neutrophils, %	62–68	60–85
Lymphocytes, %	20–40	15–40
Erythrocyte sedimentation rate, mm/hr	<30	Elevated in second and third trimesters
Mean corpuscular hemoglobin concentration (MCHC) g/L packed RBCs	320–360	No change
Mean corpuscular hemoglobin (MCH), pg/cell	27–34	No change
Mean corpuscular volume per mm^3	80–95	No change
*Blood Coagulation and Fibrinolytic Activity**		
Factor VII	65–140	Increases in pregnancy, returns to normal in early puerperium
Factor VIII	55–145	Increases during pregnancy and immediately after birth
Factor IX	60–140	Same as factor VII
Factor X	45–155	Same as factor VII
Factor XI	65–135	Decreases in pregnancy
Factor XII	50–150	Same as factor VII
Prothrombin time, sec	11–12.5	Decreases slightly in pregnancy
Partial thromboplastin time (PTT), sec	60–70	Decreases slightly in pregnancy and decreases during second and third stage of labour (indicates clotting at placental site)
Bleeding time, min	1–9 (Ivy method)	No appreciable change
Platelets, $\times 10^{9}$/L	130–400	No significant change until 3–5 days after birth and then increases rapidly (may predispose woman to thrombosis) and gradually returns to normal
Fibrinolytic activity		Decreases in pregnancy and then abruptly returns to normal (protection against thromboembolism)
Fibrinogen, g/L	2–4	Levels increase late in pregnancy
Mineral/Vitamin Concentrations		
Vitamin B_{12}, folic acid, ascorbic acid	Normal	Moderate decrease
Serum Proteins		
Total, g/L	60–83	55–75
Albumin, g/L	35–50	Slight increase
Globulin, total, g/L	23–34	30–40
Blood Glucose		
Fasting, mmol/L	<5.3	Decreases
2-hr postprandial, mmol/L	<8.9	75 gram glucose challenge test: <5.3 initially, <10.6 at 1 hr and <8.9 at 2 hr (if 2 out of 3 are higher than normal, would be diagnosed as abnormal)
Acid–Base Values in Arterial Blood		
PO_2, mm Hg	80–100	104–108 (increased)
PCO_2, mm Hg	35–45	27–32 (decreased)
Sodium bicarbonate (HCO_3), mmol/L	21–28	18–31 (decreased)
Blood pH	7.35–7.45	7.40–7.45 (slightly increased, more alkaline)

Table 9-3 Laboratory Values for Pregnant and Nonpregnant Women—cont'd

VALUES	NONPREGNANT	PREGNANT
Hepatic		
Bilirubin, total, mcmol/L	5.1–17	Unchanged
Serum cholesterol, mmol/L	<5.2	Increases at 16–32 wk of pregnancy; remains at this level until after birth
Serum alkaline phosphatase, U/L	35–120	Increases from wk 12 of pregnancy to 6 wk after birth
Serum albumin, g/L	35–50	Increases slightly
Renal		
Bladder capacity, mL	1300	1500
Renal plasma flow, mL/min	490–700	Increases by 25–30%
Glomerular filtration rate, mL/min	88–128	Increases by 30–50%
Blood urea nitrogen, mmol/L	3.6–7.1	Decreases
Serum creatinine, mcmol/L	50–90	Decreases
Serum uric acid, mmol/L	0.16–0.43	Decreases but returns to prepregnancy level by end of pregnancy
Urine glucose	Negative	Present in 20% of pregnant women
Intravenous pyelogram	Normal	Slight-to-moderate hydroureter and hydronephrosis; right kidney larger than left kidney

(Sources: Blackburn, S. [2007]. *Maternal, fetal, & neonatal physiology: A clinical perspective* [3rd ed.]. St. Louis: Saunders; Canadian Diabetic Association [2008]. CDA 2008 clinical practice guidelines for the prevention and management of diabetes in Canada, *Canadian Journal of Diabetes, 32*[1]; Fischbach, F. [2002]. *A manual of laboratory and diagnostic tests* [7th ed.]. Philadelphia: Lippincott, Williams & Wilkins; Gordon, M. [2007]. Maternal physiology in pregnancy. In S. G. Gabbe, J. R. Niebyl, & J. L. Simpson [Eds.], *Obstetrics: Normal and problem pregnancies* [5th ed.]. New York: Churchill Livingstone; Pagana, K. D., & Pagana, T. J. [2006]. *Mosby's manual of diagnostic and laboratory tests* [3rd ed.]. St. Louis: Mosby; Samuels, P. [2007]. Hematology complications of pregnancy. In S. G. Gabbe, J. R. Niebyl, & J. L. Simpson [Eds.], *Obstetrics: Normal and problem pregnancies* [5th ed.]. Philadelphia: Churchill Livingstone.)
*Pregnancy represents a hypercoagulable state.
Note: Abbreviations should not be used in practice.
RBC, red blood cell.

Table 9-4 Cardiovascular Changes in Pregnancy

PARAMETER	CHANGE
Heart rate	Increases 10–15 beats/min
Blood pressure	
Systolic	Slight or no decrease from prepregnancy levels
Diastolic	Slight decrease to midpregnancy (24–32 wk) and gradual return to prepregnancy levels by end of pregnancy
Blood volume	Increases by 1500 mL or 40–50% above prepregnancy level
Red blood cell mass	Increases 17%
Hemoglobin	Decreases
Hematocrit	Decreases
White blood cell count	Increases in second and third trimesters
Cardiac output	Increases 30–50%

Table 9-5 Respiratory Changes in Pregnancy

PARAMETER	CHANGE
Respiratory rate	Unchanged or slightly increased
Tidal volume	Increased 30–40%
Vital capacity	Unchanged
Inspiratory capacity	Increased
Expiratory volume	Decreased
Total lung capacity	Unchanged to slightly decreased
Oxygen consumption	Increased 20–40%

(Source: Gordon, M. [2007]. Maternal physiology. In S. G. Gabbe, J. R. Niebyl, & J. L. Simpson [Eds.], *Obstetrics: Normal and problem pregnancies* [5th ed.]. Philadelphia: Churchill Livingstone.)

respiratory changes in pregnancy). Although pulmonary function is not impaired by pregnancy, diseases of the respiratory tract may be more serious during this time (Cunningham et al., 2009). One important factor related to this may be the increase in oxygen requirements.

Basal Metabolic Rate

The basal metabolic rate (BMR) increases during pregnancy. This increase varies considerably, depending on the prepregnancy nutritional status of the woman and on fetal growth (Blackburn, 2007). The BMR returns to nonpregnant levels by 5 to 6 days after birth. The elevation in BMR reflects increased oxygen demands of the uterine–placental–fetal unit and greater oxygen consumption because of increased maternal cardiac work. Peripheral vasodilation and acceleration of sweat gland activity help dissipate the excess heat resulting from the increased BMR during pregnancy. Pregnant women may experience heat intolerance. Lassitude and fatigability after only slight exertion are experienced by many women in early pregnancy. These feelings, along with a greater need for sleep, may persist and may be caused in part by the increased metabolic activity.

Acid–Base Balance

By about the tenth week of pregnancy, there is a decrease of about 5 mm Hg in the partial pressure of carbon dioxide (PCO_2). Progesterone may be responsible for increasing the sensitivity of the respiratory centre receptors so that tidal volume increases and PCO_2 decreases, the base excess (HCO_3, or bicarbonate) decreases, and pH increases slightly. These alterations in acid–base balance indicate that pregnancy is a state of respiratory alkalosis compensated by mild metabolic acidosis (Gordon, 2007). These changes also facilitate the transport of CO_2 from the fetus and O_2 release from the mother to the fetus (Table 9-5).

Renal System

The kidneys are responsible for maintaining electrolyte and acid–base balance, regulating extracellular fluid volume, excreting waste products, and conserving essential nutrients.

Anatomical Changes

Changes in renal structure result from hormonal activity (estrogen and progesterone), pressure from an enlarging uterus, and an increase in blood volume. As early as the tenth week of pregnancy, the renal pelvis and the ureters dilate. Dilation of the ureters is more pronounced above the pelvic brim, in part because they are compressed between the uterus and the pelvic brim. In most women the ureters below the pelvic brim are of normal size. The smooth-muscle walls of the ureters undergo hyperplasia and hypertrophy and muscle tone relaxation. The ureters elongate, become tortuous, and form single or double curves. In the latter part of pregnancy, the renal pelvis and ureter dilate more on the right side than on the left because the heavy uterus is displaced to the right by the sigmoid colon.

Because of these changes, a larger volume of urine is held in the pelvis and ureters, and urine flow rate is slowed. Urinary stasis or stagnation has several consequences:

- There is a lag between the time urine is formed and when it reaches the bladder. Therefore, clearance test results may reflect substances contained in glomerular filtrate several hours before.
- Stagnated urine is an excellent medium for the growth of microorganisms. In addition, the urine of pregnant women contains more nutrients, including glucose, that increase the pH (making the urine more alkaline). This makes pregnant women more susceptible to urinary tract infection.

Bladder irritability, nocturia, and urinary frequency and urgency (without dysuria) are commonly reported in early pregnancy. These bladder symptoms may return near term, especially after lightening occurs.

Urinary frequency results initially from increased bladder sensitivity and later from compression of the bladder (see Fig. 9-8). In the second trimester, the bladder is pulled up out of the true pelvis into the abdomen. The urethra lengthens to 7.5 cm as the bladder is displaced upward. The pelvic congestion that occurs in pregnancy is reflected in hyperemia of the bladder and urethra. This increased vascularity causes the bladder mucosa to be traumatized and bleed easily. Bladder tone may decrease, which increases the bladder capacity to 1500 mL. At the same time, the bladder is compressed by the enlarging uterus, resulting in the urge to void even if the bladder contains only a small amount of urine.

Functional Changes

In normal pregnancy, renal function is altered considerably. Glomerular filtration rate (GFR) and renal plasma flow increase early in pregnancy (Cunningham et al., 2009). These changes are caused by pregnancy hormones; an increase in blood volume; and the woman's posture, physical activity, and nutritional intake. The woman's kidneys must manage the increased metabolic and circulatory demands of the maternal body and also the excretion of fetal waste products.

Renal function is most efficient when the woman lies in the lateral recumbent position and is least efficient when the woman assumes a supine position. A side-lying position increases renal perfusion, which increases urine output and decreases edema. When the pregnant woman is lying supine, the heavy uterus compresses the vena cava and the aorta, and cardiac output decreases. As a result, blood flow to the brain and heart is continued at the expense of other organs, including the kidneys and uterus.

Fluid and Electrolyte Balance

Selective renal tubular resorption maintains sodium and water balance, regardless of changes in dietary intake and losses through sweat, vomitus, or diarrhea. Extra sodium is normally retained during pregnancy to meet fetal needs. To prevent excessive sodium depletion, the maternal kidneys undergo a significant adaptation by increasing tubular resorption. Because of the need for increased maternal intravascular and extracellular fluid volume, additional sodium is needed to expand fluid volume and maintain an isotonic state. As efficient as the renal system is, it can be overstressed by excessive dietary sodium intake or restriction or by the use of diuretics. Severe hypovolemia and reduced placental perfusion are two consequences of using diuretics during pregnancy.

The capacity of the kidneys to excrete water is more efficient during the early weeks than later in pregnancy. As a result, some women feel thirsty in early pregnancy because of the greater amount of water loss. The pooling of fluid in the legs in the latter part of pregnancy decreases renal blood flow and GFR. This pooling is sometimes referred to as physiological or dependent edema and requires no treatment. The normal diuretic response to the water load is triggered when the woman lies down, preferably on her side, and the pooled fluid re-enters general circulation.

Normally, the kidney resorbs almost all the glucose and other nutrients from the plasma filtrate. However, in pregnant women, tubular resorption of glucose is impaired so that **glycosuria** occurs at varying times and to varying degrees. Normal values range from 0 to 7.0 mmol/L, meaning that during any day, the urine is sometimes positive and sometimes negative for glucose. In nonpregnant women, blood glucose levels must be at 8.0 to 10 mmol/L or greater before glucose is "spilled" into the urine (not resorbed). During pregnancy, glucosuria occurs when maternal glucose levels are lower than 7.0 mmol/L. The reason why glucose, as well as other nutrients such as amino acids, is wasted during pregnancy is not understood, nor has the exact mechanism been discovered. Although glucosuria may be found in normal pregnancies (2+ levels may be seen with increased anxiety states), the possibility of diabetes mellitus and gestational diabetes must be kept in mind.

Proteinuria does not usually occur in normal pregnancy except during labour or after birth (Cunningham et al., 2009). However, the increased amounts of amino acids that must be filtered may exceed the capacity of the renal tubules to absorb them, and small amounts of protein may be lost in the urine. The amount of protein excreted is not an indication of the severity of renal disease, nor does an increase in protein excretion in a pregnant woman with known renal disease necessarily indicate a progression in her disease. However, a pregnant woman with hypertension and proteinuria must be evaluated carefully because she may be at greater risk for an adverse pregnancy outcome (Gordon, 2007) (Table 9-6).

Table 9-6 Renal Changes in Pregnancy

PARAMETER	CHANGE
Bladder capacity	Increased
Glomerular filtration rate	Increased 30–50%
Renal plasma flow	Increased 30%
Blood urea nitrogen	Decreased
Creatinine	Decreased
Glucose (in urine)	Present in 20% of pregnant women

Integumentary System

Alterations in hormone balance and mechanical stretching are responsible for several changes in the integumentary system during pregnancy. Hyperpigmentation is stimulated by the anterior pituitary hormone melanotropin, which is increased during pregnancy. Darkening of the nipples, areolae, axillae, and vulva occurs at about the sixteenth week of gestation. Facial melasma (also called *chloasma* or *mask of pregnancy*) is a blotchy, brownish hyperpigmentation of the skin over the cheeks, nose, and forehead, especially in pregnant women with dark complexions. Chloasma appears in 50 to 70% of pregnant women, beginning after the sixteenth week and increasing gradually until term. The sun intensifies this pigmentation in susceptible women. Chloasma caused by normal pregnancy usually fades after birth.

The *linea nigra* (Fig. 9-12) is a pigmented line extending from the symphysis pubis to the top of the fundus in the midline. This line is known as the linea alba before hormone-induced pigmentation. In primigravidas the extension of the linea nigra, beginning in the third month, keeps pace with the rising height of the fundus; in multigravidas the entire line often appears earlier than the third month. Not all pregnant women develop lineae nigra, and some women notice hair growth along the line with or without the change in pigmentation.

Striae gravidarum, or stretch marks (seen over the lower abdomen in Fig. 9-12), appear in 50 to 90% of pregnant women during the second half of pregnancy. These may be caused by the action of adrenocorticosteroids. Striae reflect separation within the underlying connective (collagen) tissue of the skin. These slightly depressed streaks tend to occur over areas of maximum stretch (the abdomen, thighs, and breasts). The stretching sometimes causes a sensation that resembles itching. The tendency to develop striae may be familial. After birth they usually fade, although they never disappear completely. The colour of striae varies, depending on the pregnant woman's skin colour. The striae appear pinkish on a woman with light skin and are lighter than the surrounding skin in dark-skinned women. In the multipara, in addition to the striae of the present pregnancy, glistening silvery lines (in light-skinned women) or purplish lines (in dark-skinned women) are commonly seen. These represent the scars of striae from previous pregnancies.

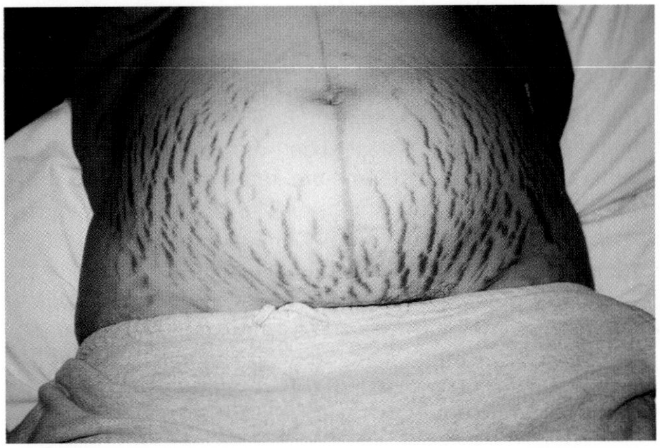

Fig. 9-12 Striae gravidarum and linea nigra in a dark-skinned person. *(Courtesy Shannon Perry, Phoenix, AZ.)*

Angiomas are commonly referred to as *vascular spiders*. These tiny, star-shaped or branched, slightly raised, and pulsating end-arterioles are usually found on the neck, thorax, face, and arms. They occur as a result of elevated levels of circulating estrogens. The spiders are bluish in colour and do not blanch with pressure. Vascular spiders appear during the second to fifth month of pregnancy in about 65% of White women and 10% of Black women. The spiders usually disappear after birth (Blackburn, 2007).

Pinkish-red diffusely mottled or well-defined blotches are seen over the palmar surfaces of the hands in about 60% of White women and 35% of Black women during pregnancy (Blackburn, 2007). These colour changes, called *palmar erythema,* are related primarily to increased estrogen levels (Box 9-1).

Some dermatological conditions have been identified as unique to pregnancy or as having an increased incidence during pregnancy. Mild pruritus (pruritus gravidarum) is a relatively common dermatological symptom during pregnancy. The goal of management is to relieve the itching. Topical steroids and emollients are the usual treatment. The problem usually resolves during the postpartum period (Papoutsis & Kroupouzos, 2007). Systemic diseases can also cause pruritus, but these causes are uncommon or rare (Cappell, 2007) (Box 9-2). Pre-existing skin diseases may complicate pregnancy or be improved.

BOX 9-1 Ethnic Considerations for Skin Assessment During Pregnancy

Integumentary system changes vary greatly among women of different racial backgrounds. For example, vascular spiders and palmar erythema are seen more often in White women than in Black women. Areolar pigmentation varies by race: Black women have the darkest areolae, White women have the lightest, and Asian and First Nations, Inuit, and Métis women have intermediate pigmentation. When performing physical assessments, the colour of the woman's skin should be noted, along with any changes that may be attributed to pregnancy.

BOX 9-2 Prevalence of Dermatological Disorders of Pregnancy

Pruritic urticarial papules and plaques of pregnancy (PUPPP)—1:130 to 1:300
Prurigo of pregnancy (PP)—1:300 to 1:450
Herpes gestationis (HG)—1:50,000
Pruritic folliculitis of pregnancy (PFP)—Very rare; about 30 cases

(Source: Papoutsis, J., & Kroupouzos, G. [2007]. Dermatologic disorders. In S. G. Gabbe, J. R. Niebyl, & J. L. Simpson [Eds.], *Obstetrics: Normal and problem pregnancies* [5th ed.]. Philadelphia: Churchill Livingstone.)

NURSING ALERT Women with severe acne taking isotretinoin (Accutane) should avoid pregnancy while receiving the treatment because it is teratogenic and associated with major fetal malformations.

Gum hypertrophy may occur during pregnancy. An *epulis* (gingival granuloma gravidarum) is a red, raised nodule on the gums that bleeds easily. This lesion may develop around the third month and usually continues to enlarge as pregnancy progresses. It is usually managed by avoiding trauma to the gums (e.g., using a soft toothbrush). An epulis usually regresses spontaneously after birth.

Nail growth may be accelerated. Some women may notice thinning and softening of the nails. Oily skin and acne vulgaris may occur during pregnancy. In some women the skin clears and looks radiant. *Hirsutism*, the excessive growth of hair or growth of hair in unusual places, is commonly reported. An increase in fine hair growth may occur but tends to disappear after pregnancy. However, growth of coarse or bristly hair does not usually disappear after pregnancy. The rate of scalp hair loss slows during pregnancy; increased hair loss may be noted in the postpartum period.

Increased blood supply to the skin leads to increased perspiration. Women feel hotter during pregnancy, possibly related to a progesterone-induced increase in body temperature and the increased BMR.

Musculoskeletal System

The gradually changing body and increasing weight of the pregnant woman usually cause noticeable changes in her posture (Fig. 9-13) and in the way she walks. The great abdominal distention gives the pelvis a forward tilt, decreased abdominal muscle tone, and increased weight bearing. The woman's centre of gravity shifts forward, requiring a realignment of the spinal curvatures. An increase in the normal lumbosacral curve (lordosis) develops, and a compensatory curvature in the cervicodorsal region (exaggerated anterior flexion of the head) develops to help her maintain balance. Aching, numbness, and weakness of the upper extremities may result. Large breasts and a stoop-shouldered stance further accentuate the lumbar and dorsal curves. Walking is more difficult; the waddling gait of the pregnant woman is well known. The ligamentous and muscular structures of the middle and lower spine may be severely stressed. These and related changes often cause musculoskeletal discomfort, especially in older women or those with a back disorder or a faulty sense of balance.

Slight relaxation and increased mobility of the pelvic joints are normal during pregnancy. This is secondary to the exaggerated elasticity and softening of connective and collagen tissue caused by increased circulating steroid sex hormones, especially estrogen. Relaxin, an ovarian hormone, assists in this relaxation and softening. These adaptations permit enlargement of pelvic dimensions to facilitate labour and birth. The degree of relaxation varies, but considerable separation of the symphysis pubis and the instability of the sacroiliac joints may cause pain and difficulty in walking. Obesity or multifetal pregnancy tends to increase the pelvic instability. Peripheral joint laxity also increases as pregnancy progresses; the cause for this is not known (Cunningham et al., 2009).

The muscles of the abdominal wall stretch and ultimately lose some tone. During the third trimester, the rectus abdominis muscles may separate (Fig. 9-14), allowing abdominal contents to protrude at the midline. The umbilicus flattens or protrudes. After birth, the muscles gradually regain tone. However, separation of the muscles (diastasis recti abdominis) may persist.

Neurological System

Little is known about specific alterations in function of the neurological system during pregnancy, aside from hypothalamic–pituitary neurohormonal changes. Specific physiological alterations resulting from pregnancy may cause the following neurological or neuromuscular symptoms:

- Sensory changes in the legs occur as a result of compression of pelvic nerves or vascular stasis caused by enlargement of the uterus.
- Pain from dorsolumbar lordosis is due to traction on nerves or compression of nerve roots.
- Carpal tunnel syndrome occurs from edema of the peripheral nerves during the third trimester (Samuels & Niebyl, 2007). The edema compresses the median nerve beneath the carpal ligament of the wrist. Smoking and alcohol consumption can impair the microcirculation and may worsen the symptoms. The syndrome is characterized by paresthesia (abnormal sensation such as burning or tingling caused by a disorder of the sensory

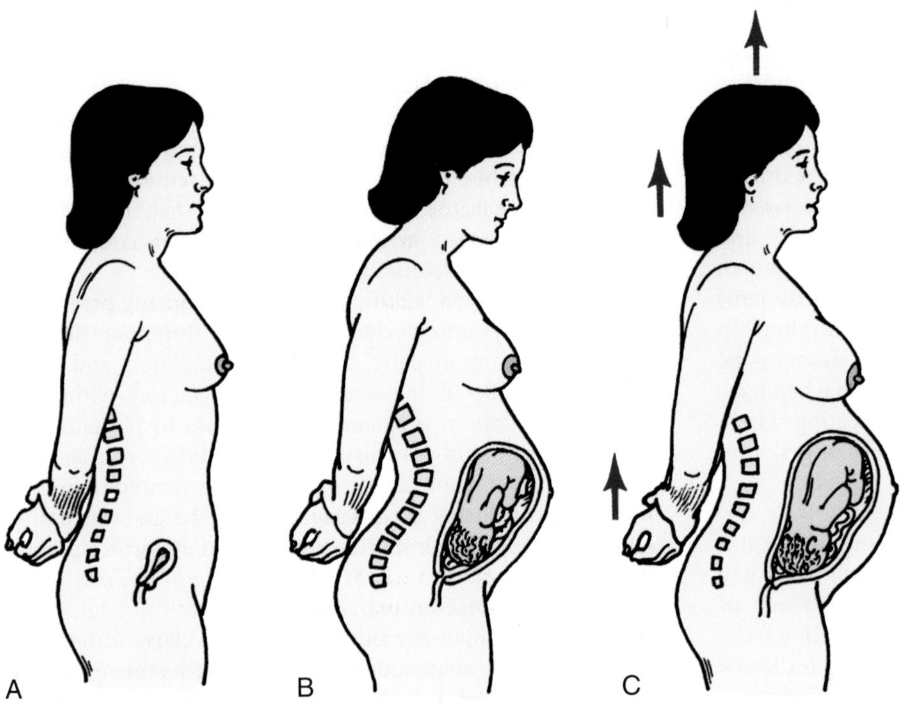

Fig. 9-13 Postural changes during pregnancy. **A:** Nonpregnant. **B:** Incorrect posture during pregnancy. **C:** Correct posture during pregnancy.

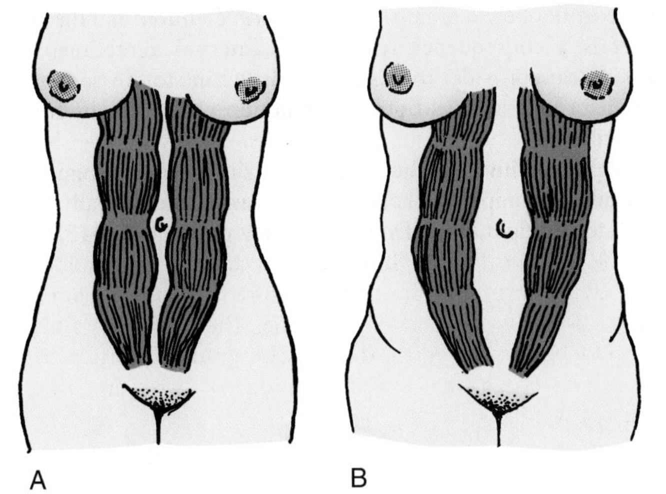

Fig. 9-14 Possible change in rectus abdominis muscles during pregnancy. **A:** Normal position in nonpregnant woman. **B:** Diastasis recti abdominis in pregnant women.

nervous system) and pain in the hand, radiating to the elbow. The dominant hand is usually affected most, although as many as 80% of women report symptoms in both hands. Symptoms usually regress after pregnancy. Some patients may require surgical treatment (Samuels & Niebyl, 2007).

- Acroesthesia (numbness and tingling of the hands) is caused by the stoop-shouldered stance (see Fig. 9-13, B) assumed by some women during pregnancy. The condition is associated with traction on segments of the brachial plexus.
- Tension headache is common when anxiety or uncertainty complicates gestation. However, vision problems such as refractive errors, sinusitis, or migraine may also be responsible for headaches.
- "Light-headedness," faintness, and even syncope (fainting) are common during early pregnancy. Vasomotor instability, postural hypotension, or hypoglycemia may be responsible.
- Hypocalcemia may cause neuromuscular problems such as muscle cramps or tetany.

Gastrointestinal System

Appetite

During pregnancy, the woman's appetite and food intake fluctuate. Early in pregnancy, some women have nausea with or without vomiting (morning sickness), possibly in response to increasing levels of hCG and altered carbohydrate metabolism (Gordon, 2007). Morning sickness or nausea and vomiting of pregnancy (NVP) appear at about 4 to 6 weeks of gestation and usually subside by the end of the third month (first trimester) of pregnancy. Severity varies from mild distaste for certain foods to more severe vomiting. The condition may be triggered by the sight or odour of various foods. By the end of the second trimester, the appetite increases in response to increasing metabolic needs. Rarely does NVP have harmful effects on the embryo, the fetus, or the woman. Whenever the vomiting is severe or persists beyond the first trimester or when it is accompanied by fever, pain, or weight loss, further evaluation is necessary, and medical intervention is likely.

Women may have changes in their sense of taste, leading to cravings and changes in dietary intake. Some women have nonfood cravings (**pica**) such as for ice, clay, and laundry starch. Usually the subjects of these cravings, if consumed in small amounts, are not harmful to the pregnancy if the woman has adequate nutrition with appropriate weight gain; however, if the woman eats large quantities of nonfood items, this can interfere with her appetite and she may not get appropriate nutrition (Gordon, 2007).

Mouth

The gums become hyperemic, spongy, and swollen during pregnancy. They tend to bleed easily because the increasing levels of estrogen cause selective increased vascularity and connective tissue proliferation (a nonspecific gingivitis). Epulis (discussed in the section on the integumentary system) may develop at the gum line. Some pregnant women complain of ptyalism (excessive salivation), which may be caused by the decrease in unconscious swallowing by the woman when nauseated or from stimulation of salivary glands by eating starch. This normally subsides between 12 and 14 weeks of gestation (Cunningham et al., 2009; Russell & Mayberry, 2008).

Teeth

The pregnant woman requires about 1300 mg of calcium and approximately the same amount of phosphorus every day during pregnancy. This is an increase of about 300 mg of each of these elements over nonpregnant needs. With a well-balanced diet, these requirements are satisfied. Serious dietary deficiency may deplete the mother's bony stores of these elements, but tooth calcium is stable and not available to the fetus (Russell & Mayberry, 2008). Gingivitis and poor dental hygiene may contribute to dental **caries**, which can lead to the loss of a tooth and during pregnancy may be a risk factor for preterm birth, low birth weight, and pre-eclampsia (Russell & Mayberry, 2008).

Esophagus, Stomach, and Intestines

Herniation of the upper portion of the stomach (hiatal hernia) occurs in 15 to 20% of pregnant women after the seventh or eighth month. This condition results from upward displacement of the stomach, which causes a widening of the hiatus of the diaphragm. It occurs more often in multiparas and older or obese women.

Increased estrogen production causes decreased secretion of hydrochloric acid. Therefore, peptic ulcer formation or flare-up of existing peptic ulcers is uncommon during pregnancy and may improve (Gordon, 2007).

Increased progesterone production causes decreased tone and motility of smooth muscles, resulting in esophageal regurgitation, slower emptying time of the stomach, and reverse peristalsis. As a result, the woman may experience "acid indigestion" or heartburn (pyrosis) beginning as early as the first trimester and intensifying through the third trimester.

In response to increased needs during pregnancy, iron is absorbed more readily in the small intestine. Even when the woman is deficient in iron, it will continue to be absorbed in sufficient amounts for the fetus to have a normal hemoglobin level.

Increased progesterone may result in an increase in water absorption from the colon and may cause constipation. Constipation can also result from hypoperistalsis (sluggishness of the bowel), food choices, lack of fluids, iron supplementation, decreased activity level, abdominal distention by the pregnant uterus, and displacement and compression of the intestines. If the pregnant woman has hemorrhoids (see Fig. 9-11) and is constipated, the hemorrhoids can evert or bleed during straining at stool.

Gallbladder and Liver

The gallbladder is often distended because of its decreased muscle tone during pregnancy. Increased emptying time and thickening of bile caused by prolonged retention are typical changes. These features, together with slight hypercholesterolemia from increased progesterone levels, may account for the development of gallstones during pregnancy.

Hepatic function is difficult to appraise during pregnancy. However, only minor changes in liver function develop. Occasionally, intrahepatic cholestasis (retention and accumulation of bile in the liver caused by factors within the liver) occurs late in pregnancy in response to placental steroids. It may result in pruritus gravidarum (severe itching) with or without jaundice. These distressing symptoms are difficult to treat during pregnancy and may be associated with fetal risk. However, symptoms subside after birth (Cappell, 2007).

Abdominal Discomfort

Intra-abdominal alterations that can cause discomfort include pelvic heaviness or pressure, round ligament tension, flatulence, distention and bowel cramping, and uterine contractions. In addition to displacement of intestines, pressure from the expanding uterus causes an increase in venous pressure in the pelvic organs. Although most abdominal discomfort is a consequence of normal maternal alterations, the health care provider must be constantly alert to the possibility of disorders such as bowel obstruction or an inflammatory process.

Appendicitis may be difficult to diagnose in pregnancy because the appendix is displaced upward and laterally, high and to the right, away from McBurney point (Fig. 9-15).

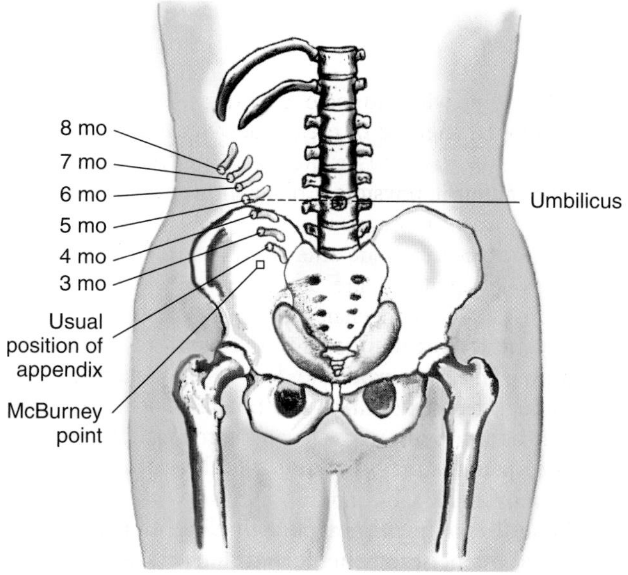

Fig. 9-15 Change in position of appendix in pregnancy. Note McBurney point.

Table 9-7 Hormones and Effects of Changes During Pregnancy

HORMONE	SOURCE	EFFECTS OF CHANGES DURING PREGNANCY
Human chorionic gonadotropin	Fertilized ovum and chorionic villi	Maintains corpus luteum production of estrogen and progesterone until placenta takes over the function
Progesterone	Corpus luteum until 14 wk of gestation, then the placenta	Suppresses secretion of FSH and LH by the anterior pituitary; maintains pregnancy by relaxing smooth muscles, decreasing uterine contractility; causes fat to deposit in subcutaneous tissues over the maternal abdomen, back, and upper thighs; decreases mother's ability to use insulin
Estrogen	Corpus luteum until 14 wk of gestation, then the placenta	Suppresses secretion of FSH and LH by the anterior pituitary; causes fat to deposit in subcutaneous tissues over the maternal abdomen, back, and upper thighs; promotes enlargement of genitals, uterus, and breasts; increases vascularity; relaxes pelvic ligaments and joints; interferes with folic acid metabolism; increases the level of total body proteins; promotes retention of sodium and water; decreases secretion of hydrochloric acid and pepsin; decreases mother's ability to use insulin
Serum prolactin	Anterior pituitary	Responsible for initial lactation
Oxytocin	Posterior pituitary	Stimulates uterine contractions; stimulates the let-down or milk-ejection reflex
Human chorionic somatomammotropin (previously called human placental lactogen)	Placenta	Acts as a growth hormone; contributes to breast development; decreases maternal metabolism of glucose; increases the amount of fatty acids for metabolic needs
Thyroxine-binding globulin, thyroxine, triiodothyronine	Thyroid	Causes moderate enlargement of the thyroid gland but woman remains euthyroid; possibly plays role in early neural development of the fetus
Parathyroid	Parathyroid	Controls calcium and magnesium metabolism
Insulin	Pancreas	Decreases production of insulin to protect fetus and its need for glucose
Cortisol	Adrenal glands	Stimulates production of insulin; increases peripheral resistance to insulin
Aldosterone	Adrenal glands	Stimulates resorption of excess sodium from the renal tubules

FSH, follicle-stimulating hormone; *LH,* luteinizing hormone.

Endocrine System

Profound endocrine changes are essential for pregnancy maintenance, normal fetal growth, and postpartum recovery. Hormones, their sources, and their effects on the pregnancy are presented in Table 9-7.

Key Points

- ELISA testing, with monoclonal antibody technology, is the most popular method of pregnancy testing and is the basis for most over-the-counter home pregnancy tests.
- The biochemical, physiological, and anatomical adaptations that occur during pregnancy are profound and revert back to the nonpregnant state after birth and lactation.
- Maternal adaptations are attributed to the hormones of pregnancy and to mechanical pressures arising from the enlarging uterus and other tissues.
- Adaptations to pregnancy protect the woman's normal physiological functioning, meet the metabolic demands that pregnancy imposes, and provide for fetal developmental and growth needs.
- Presumptive, probable, and positive signs of pregnancy aid in the diagnosis of pregnancy; only positive signs (identification of a fetal heart tone, verification of fetal movements, and visualization of the fetus) can establish the diagnosis of pregnancy.
- Although the pH of the pregnant woman's vaginal secretions is more acidic than in the nonpregnant state, she is more vulnerable to some vaginal infections, especially yeast infections.
- Increased vascularity and sensitivity of the vagina and other pelvic viscera may lead to a high degree of sexual interest and arousal.
- Some adaptations to pregnancy result in discomforts such as fatigue, urinary frequency, nausea, constipation, and breast sensitivity.
- Balance and coordination are affected by changes in joints and in the woman's centre of gravity as pregnancy progresses.

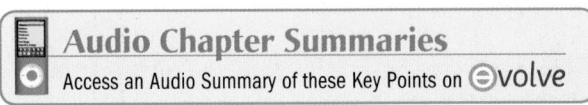

Audio Chapter Summaries

Access an Audio Summary of these Key Points on evolve

References

Beebe, K. (2005). The perplexing parity puzzle. *AWHONN Lifelines, 9*(5), 394–399.

Blackburn, S. (2007). *Maternal, fetal, & neonatal physiology: A clinical perspective* (3rd ed.). St. Louis: Saunders.

Cappell, M. (2007). Hepatic and gastrointestinal diseases. In S. G. Gabbe, J. R. Niebyl, & J. L. Simpson (Eds.), *Obstetrics: Normal and problem pregnancies* (5th ed.). Philadelphia: Churchill Livingstone.

Copeland, L., & Landon, M. (2007). Malignant diseases and pregnancy. In S. G. Gabbe, J. R. Niebyl, & J. L. Simpson, (Eds.), *Obstetrics: Normal and problem pregnancies* (5th ed.). Philadelphia: Churchill Livingstone.

Crane, J., et al. (2001). SOGC Clinical Practice Guideline: Induction of labour at term. *Journal of Obstetrics and Gynaecology Canada, 23*(8), 717–728. Retrieved from http://www.sogc.org/guidelines/public/107E-CPG-August2001.pdf.

Cunningham, F., et al. (2010). *Williams obstetrics* (23rd ed.). New York: McGraw Hill.

Duff, W., Sweet, R., & Edwards, R. K. (2009). Maternal and fetal infections. In R. K. Creasy, et al. (Eds.), *Creasy & Resnik's maternal-fetal medicine: Principles and practice* (6th ed.). Philadelphia: Saunders.

Gordon, M. (2007). Maternal physiology. In S. G. Gabbe, J. R. Niebyl, & J. L. Simpson (Eds.), *Obstetrics: Normal and problem pregnancies* (5th ed.). Philadelphia: Churchill Livingstone.

Magee, L., et al. (2008). SOGC Clinical Practice Guideline: Diagnosis, evaluation and management of the hypertensive disorders of pregnancy. *Journal of Obstetrics and Gynaecology Canada, 30*(3), Suppl 1, Retrieved from http://www.sogc.org/guidelines/documents/gui206CPG0803_001.pdf.

Pagana, K. D., & Pagana, T. J. (2006). *Mosby's diagnostic and laboratory test reference* (7th ed.). St. Louis: Mosby.

Papoutsis, J., & Kroupouzos, G. (2007). Dermatologic disorders. In S. G. Gabbe, J. R. Niebyl, & J. L. Simpson (Eds.), *Obstetrics: Normal and problem pregnancies* (5th ed.). Philadelphia: Churchill Livingstone.

Pickering, T., et al. (2005). Recommendations for blood pressure measurement in humans and experimental animals. Part 1: Blood pressure measurement in humans: statement for professionals from the Subcommittee of Professional and Public Education of the American Heart Association Council on High Blood Pressure Research. *Hypertension, 45*(1), 142–161.

Russell, S., & Mayberry, L. (2008). Pregnancy and oral health. *American Journal of Maternal Child Nursing, 33*(1), 32–37.

Samuels, P. (2007). Hematology complications of pregnancy. In S. G. Gabbe, J. R. Niebyl, & J. L. Simpson (Eds.), *Obstetrics: Normal and problem pregnancies* (5th ed.). Philadelphia: Churchill Livingstone.

Samuels, P., & Niebyl, J. (2007). Neurologic disorders. In S. G. Gabbe, J. R. Niebyl, & J. L. Simpson (Eds.), *Obstetrics: Normal and problem pregnancies* (5th ed.). Philadelphia: Churchill Livingstone.

Seidel, H., et al. (2006). *Mosby's guide to physical examination* (6th ed.). St. Louis: Mosby.

Sibai, B. (2007). Hypertension. In S. G. Gabbe, J. R. Niebyl, & J. L. Simpson (Eds.), *Obstetrics: Normal and problem pregnancies* (5th ed.). Philadelphia: Churchill Livingstone.

Unit 3

Nursing Care During Pregnancy

10

Learning Objectives

On completion of this chapter, the reader will be able to:

- Describe the processes of confirming pregnancy and estimating the date of birth.
- Summarize the physical, psychosocial, and behavioural changes that usually occur as the mother and other family members adapt to pregnancy.
- Discuss the benefits of prenatal care and problems of accessibility for some women.
- Outline the patterns of health care to assess maternal and fetal health status at the initial visit and follow-up visits during pregnancy.
- Identify the typical nursing assessments, diagnoses, interventions, and methods of evaluation in providing care for the pregnant woman.
- Discuss education needed by pregnant women to understand physical discomforts related to pregnancy and to recognize the signs and symptoms of potential complications.
- Explain the impact of culture, age, parity, and number of fetuses on the response of the family to the pregnancy and on the prenatal care provided.
- Compare different care-provider options for childbirth care.
- Determine the scope of childbirth education in the community.

Electronic Resources

Additional information related to the content in Chapter 10 can be found on

evolve the companion Web site at http://evolve.elsevier.com/Canada/Perry/maternal/

- Examination Review Questions
- Assessment Video—Chest Wall, Breast, Abdomen/Fundal Height, Fetal Lie, Presentation, Position, Fetal Heart Rate
- Case Study—First Trimester
- Case Study—Second Trimester
- Case Study—Third Trimester
- Critical Thinking Exercise—Adolescent Pregnancy
- Critical Thinking Exercise—Discomforts of Pregnancy

The prenatal period is a time of physical and psychological preparation for birth and parenthood. Becoming a parent is one of the maturational milestones of adult life. It is a time of intense learning for parents and those close to them. The prenatal period provides a unique opportunity for nurses and other members of the health care team to have an influence on family health. During this period, essentially healthy women seek regular care and guidance. The perinatal nurse's health promotion interventions can affect the well-being of the woman, her unborn child, and the rest of her family for many years.

Regular prenatal visits, ideally beginning soon after the first missed menstrual period, offer opportunities to ensure the health of the expectant mother and her infant. Prenatal health care involves the diagnosis and treatment of pre-existing maternal disorders and those that may develop during the pregnancy. Care is designed to monitor the growth and development of the fetus and identify abnormalities that may interfere with the course of normal pregnancy. The woman and her family can seek support to reduce stress and learn parenting skills.

Pregnancy lasts 9 calendar months. However, health care providers use the concept of lunar months, which last 28 days (or 4 weeks), to describe the duration of pregnancy or gestational age. Thus normal pregnancy lasts about 10 lunar months, that is, 40 weeks, or 280 days. Pregnancy is divided into three 3-month periods, or **trimesters**. The first trimester covers weeks 1 through 13; the second, weeks 14 through 26; and the third, weeks 27 through term gestation (38 to 40 weeks). The focus of this chapter is on meeting the health needs of the expectant family over the course of pregnancy, which is known as the *prenatal period*.

Confirmation of Pregnancy

Women may suspect pregnancy when they miss a menstrual period. Many women come to the first visit after a positive home pregnancy test. However, the clinical diagnosis of pregnancy before the second missed period may be difficult in some women. Factors such as physical variations, lack of relaxation, obesity, or tumours may confound even the experienced examiner. However, accuracy is important because emotional, social, or medical consequences related to an inaccurate diagnosis, either positive or negative, can be extremely serious. A correct date for the first day of the last (normal) menstrual period (LMP), the date of intercourse, and a **basal body temperature (BBT)** record may be of great value in the accurate determination of pregnancy (see Chapter 7).

Signs and Symptoms

Great variability is possible in the subjective and objective symptoms of pregnancy. Therefore, the diagnosis of pregnancy may be uncertain for a time. It is based on signs and symptoms that are reported during history taking or found during physical examination. These signs and symptoms are classified as presumptive, probable, or positive (see Table 9-2, p. 189).

Estimating Date of Birth

When pregnancy is confirmed, the woman's first question usually is when she will give birth. This date is called the **estimated date of birth** (EDB). Because the exact date of conception is usually unknown, several formulas have been suggested for calculating the EDB. None of these guides is infallible, but Nägele's rule is reasonably accurate and is the method usually used.

Nägele's rule is as follows: after determining the first day of the LMP, subtract 3 months, add 7 days and 1 year; or alternatively, add 7 days to the LMP and count forward 9 months. For example, if the first day of the LMP was September 10, 2012, the EDB is June 17, 2013.

Nägele's rule assumes that the woman has a 28-day menstrual cycle and that the pregnancy occurred on the fourteenth day of the cycle. An adjustment is in order if the cycle is longer or shorter than 28 days. Only about 5% of pregnant women give birth spontaneously on the EDB as determined by Nägele's rule. Most women give birth during the period extending from 7 days before to 7 days after the EDB.

Adaptation to Pregnancy

Pregnancy affects all family members, and each family member must adapt to the pregnancy and interpret its meaning in light of his or her own needs. This process of family adaptation to pregnancy takes place within a cultural environment influenced by societal trends. Dramatic changes have occurred in Western society in recent years, and the perinatal nurse must be prepared to support not only traditional families but also lone-parent families, reconstituted families, dual-career families, and nontraditional families.

Much of the investigation of family dynamics in pregnancy by scholars in the United States and Canada has been done with White, middle-class nuclear families; thus findings may not apply to families who do not fit the traditional North American model. For example, terms such as *spouse*, *husband*, and *wife* are used consistently in family literature but may not fit the configuration of a given family in the nurse's care. Adaptation of terms is appropriate to avoid offence to the family and embarrassment to the nurse. The term *partner* is often an appropriate alternative.

Maternal Adaptation

Women of all ages use the months of pregnancy to adapt to the maternal role, a complex process of social and cognitive learning. Pregnancy functions as a rite of passage and indicates that maturity has been reached. In the 1960s, Reva Rubin (1984) began studying maternal role adaptation. She described the developmental tasks of pregnancy as follows:

- Accepting the pregnancy
- Identifying the role of mother
- Reordering the relationships between her mother and herself and between herself and her partner
- Establishing a relationship with the unborn child
- Preparing for the birth experience

Pregnancy can be stressful but also rewarding as the woman prepares for a new level of caring and responsibility. Her self-concept changes in readiness for parenthood as she anticipates her new role. She moves gradually from being self-contained and independent to being committed to a lifelong concern for another human being. The partner's emotional support is an important factor in the successful accomplishment of these developmental tasks. Single women with limited support may have difficulty making this adaptation.

Accepting the Pregnancy

The first step in adapting to the maternal role is accepting the idea of pregnancy and assimilating the pregnant state into the woman's way of life. Mercer (1995) described this process as "cognitive restructuring."

The degree of acceptance is reflected in the woman's emotional responses. Initially, many women are dismayed at finding themselves pregnant, especially if the pregnancy is unplanned. Eventual acceptance of pregnancy parallels the growing acceptance of the reality of a child. Nonacceptance of the pregnancy should not be equated with rejection of the child. A woman may dislike being pregnant but feel love for the child to be born.

Women who are happy and pleased about their pregnancy usually have high self-esteem and tend to be confident about outcomes for themselves, their babies, and other family members. Despite a general feeling of well-being, many pregnant women are surprised to experience emotional lability (i.e., rapid and unpredictable changes in mood). These swings in emotions and increased sensitivity to others are disconcerting to the expectant mother and those around her. Increased irritability, explosions of tears and anger, and feelings of great joy and cheerfulness alternate, apparently with little or no provocation. Profound hormonal changes that are part of the maternal response to pregnancy may be responsible for these mood changes.

Most women have ambivalent feelings during pregnancy, regardless of whether the pregnancy was intended. **Ambivalence**—having conflicting feelings at the same time—is considered a normal response for people preparing for a new role. For example, during pregnancy, women may feel great pleasure that they are fulfilling a lifelong dream, but they also may feel great regret that life as they now know it is ending.

Even women who are pleased to be pregnant may experience feelings of hostility toward the pregnancy or the unborn child from time to time. Intense feelings of ambivalence that persist through the third trimester may indicate an unresolved conflict with the motherhood role (Mercer, 1995). After the birth of a healthy child, memories of these ambivalent feelings usually are dismissed. If the child is born with a defect, a woman may look back at the times when she did not want the pregnancy and feel intense guilt. She may believe that her ambivalence caused the birth defect. She will need reassurance that her feelings were not responsible for the problem.

Identifying With the Mother Role

The process of identifying with the mother role begins early in each woman's life, when she is being mothered as a child. Her social group's perception of what constitutes the feminine role can subsequently influence her in choosing between motherhood and a career, being married or single, being independent rather than interdependent, or being able to manage multiple roles. Practice roles such as playing with dolls, baby-sitting, and taking care of siblings may increase her understanding of what being a mother entails.

Many women have always wanted a baby; they like children, and look forward to motherhood. Their high motivation to become a parent promotes acceptance of pregnancy and eventual prenatal and parental adaptation. Other women apparently have not considered in any detail what motherhood means to them. During pregnancy, conflicts such as not wanting the pregnancy and child-related or career-related decisions need to be resolved.

Reordering Personal Relationships

Close relationships held by the pregnant woman undergo change as she prepares emotionally for the new role of mother. As family members learn their new roles, periods of tension and conflict may occur. Promoting effective communication patterns between the expectant mother and her own mother and between the expectant mother and her partner are common nursing interventions during the prenatal visits.

The woman's relationship with her mother is significant in adapting to pregnancy and motherhood. Important components in the pregnant woman's relationship with her mother are the mother's availability (past and present), her reactions to her daughter's pregnancy, respect for her daughter's autonomy, and the willingness to reminisce (Mercer, 1995).

The mother's reaction to her daughter's pregnancy signifies her acceptance of the grandchild and of her daughter. If the mother is supportive, the daughter has an opportunity to discuss pregnancy and labour and her feelings of joy or ambivalence with a knowledgeable and accepting woman (Fig. 10-1). Reminiscing about the pregnant woman's early childhood and sharing the grandmother-to-be's account of her childbirth experience can help the daughter anticipate and prepare for labour and birth.

Although the woman's relationship with her mother is significant in considering her adaptation in pregnancy, the most important person to the pregnant woman is usually the father of her child. A woman who is nurtured by her partner during pregnancy has fewer emotional and physical symptoms, fewer labour and childbirth complications, and an easier postpartum adjustment. Women express two major needs within this relationship during pregnancy: feeling loved and valued, and having the child accepted by the partner.

The marital or committed relationship is not static but evolves over time. The addition of a child changes forever the nature of the bond between partners. This can be a time when couples grow closer and the pregnancy has a maturing effect on the partners' relationship as they assume new roles and discover new aspects of one another. Partners who trust and support each other are able to share mutual dependency needs (Mercer, 1995).

Sexual expression during pregnancy is highly individual; some women may find their interest in sex increases, and for some women it decreases. The sexual relationship is affected by physical, emotional, and interactional factors, including myths about sex during pregnancy, sexual dysfunction, and physical changes in the woman. Myths about body functions and fantasies about the influence of the fetus as a third party in lovemaking are commonly expressed. An individual may also inaccurately attribute anomalies, developmental disability, and other injuries to the fetus and mother to sexual

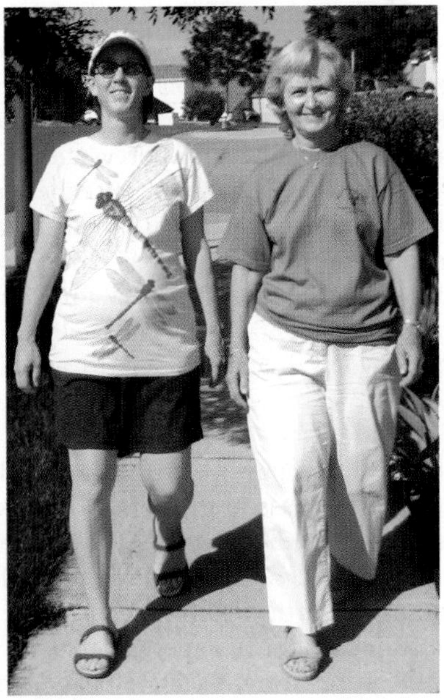

Fig. 10-1 A pregnant woman and her mother enjoy a walk together. *(Courtesy Shannon Perry, Phoenix, AZ.)*

relations during pregnancy. Some couples fear that the woman's genitals will be drastically changed by the birth process. Couples may not express their concerns to the health care provider because of embarrassment or because they do not want to appear foolish. (See discussion later in this chapter on p. 234.)

Establishing a Relationship With the Fetus

Emotional attachment—feelings of being tied by affection or love—begins during the prenatal period as women use fantasizing and daydreaming to prepare themselves for motherhood (Rubin, 1975). They think of themselves as mothers and imagine maternal qualities they would like to possess. Expectant parents desire to be warm, loving, and close to their child. They try to anticipate changes that the child will bring in their lives and wonder how they will react to noise, disorder, reduced freedom, and caregiving activities. The mother–child relationship progresses through pregnancy as a developmental process that unfolds in three phases.

In phase 1, the woman accepts the biological fact of pregnancy. She needs to be able to state, "I am pregnant." In phase 2, the woman accepts the growing fetus as distinct from herself and as a person to nurture. She can now say, "I am going to have a baby." Attachment by a mother to her child is enhanced by experiencing a planned pregnancy, and it increases when ultrasound examination and **quickening** confirm the reality of the fetus. During phase 3, the woman prepares realistically for the birth and parenting of the child. She expresses the thought, "I am going to be a mother," and defines the nature and characteristics of the child. For example, she may speculate about the child's sex (if she has not had an ultrasound examination that confirms the sex) and personality traits based on patterns of fetal activity.

Although the mother alone experiences the child within, both parents and siblings believe the unborn child responds in a very individualized, personal manner. Family members may interact with the unborn child by talking to the fetus and stroking the mother's abdomen, especially when the fetus shifts position. They may sing to, play music for, or read to the fetus. The fetus may have a nickname used by family members.

Parents may occasionally show or voice disappointment over the sex of the child. The parents may experience grief and a sense of loss at birth as they release their fantasized image of the child and begin to accept the real child. However, these negative responses are usually temporary. Providing an accepting environment for parental reactions facilitates the parent's ability to move beyond disappointment to acceptance.

Preparing for Childbirth

Many women actively prepare for birth. They read books, view films, attend parenting classes, and talk to other women. They seek the caregiver with whom they feel most comfortable for advice, monitoring, and caring. The multipara has her own history of labour and birth, which influences her approach to preparation for this childbirth experience.

Anxiety can arise from the mother's concern about safe passage for herself and her child during the birth process (Mercer, 1995; Rubin, 1975). This concern may not be expressed overtly but rather through the making of plans for care of the new baby and other children in case "anything should happen." The nurse needs to listen for such cues of the mother's concern. These feelings persist despite statistical evidence about the safe outcome of pregnancy for mothers and their infants. Many women fear the pain of childbirth or fear mutilation because they do not understand anatomy and the birth process. Education by the perinatal nurse can alleviate many of these fears.

Toward the end of the third trimester, breathing is difficult and fetal movements become vigorous enough to disturb the mother's sleep. The discomforts of pregnancy can become troublesome and it is more difficult to perform everyday activities and assume a comfortable position for sleep and rest. A strong desire to see the end of pregnancy, to be over and done with it, makes women at this stage ready to move on to childbirth.

Paternal Adaptation

For most men, pregnancy can be a time of preparation for the parental role, with intense learning (see Family-Centred Teaching box).

FAMILY-CENTRED TEACHING

Paternal Adaptation

A man's emotional responses to becoming a father, his concerns, and his informational needs change during the course of pregnancy. Three styles of involvement provide examples of different ways men can experience pregnancy (May, 1980, 1982). Men may be involved in pregnancy as an observer (i.e., avoiding direct involvement in activities such as parent education classes and decisions about breastfeeding). Others are more expressive and display a strong emotional response to pregnancy and a desire to be a full partner in the project. Some expectant fathers experience the couvade syndrome and have pregnancy-like symptoms such as nausea and other gastrointestinal complaints, fatigue, and other physical discomforts. Other fathers adopt the instrumental style, seeing tasks they can perform in their role as manager of the pregnancy. They feel responsible for the outcome of the pregnancy and are protective and supportive of their partner.

The father's beliefs and feelings about the ideal mother and father and his cultural expectation of appropriate behaviour during pregnancy affect his response to his partner's need for him. One man may engage in nurturing behaviour; another may feel lonely and alienated as the woman becomes physically and emotionally engrossed in the unborn child. The man may seek comfort and understanding outside the home or become interested in a new hobby or involved with his work. Some men view pregnancy as proof of their masculinity and their dominant role. To others, pregnancy has no meaning in terms of responsibility to either mother or child. However, for most men, pregnancy is a time of preparation for the parental role, fantasy, great pleasure, and intense learning.

Accepting the Pregnancy

The ways in which fathers adjust to the parental role have been the subject of considerable research. In older societies, the man enacted the ritual couvades; that is, he behaved in specific ways and respected taboos associated with pregnancy and giving birth. In this way, the man's new status was recognized and endorsed. During the past 30 years, changing cultural and professional attitudes have encouraged fathers' participation in the childbirth experience (Fig. 10-2). There are still many cultures in which childbirth is considered a female domain and men are not encouraged to be part of the process. It is important that the nurse be aware and understanding of different cultural expectations.

Identifying With the Father Role

Each man brings to pregnancy attitudes that affect the way in which he adjusts to the pregnancy and parental role. His memories of the fathering he received from his own father, the experiences he has had with child care, and the perceptions of the male and father roles within his social group guide his selection of the tasks and responsibilities he will assume. Some men are highly motivated to nurture and love a child. They may be excited and pleased about the anticipated role of father. Others may be more detached or even hostile to the idea of fatherhood.

Reordering Personal Relationships

The partner's main role in pregnancy is to nurture and respond to the pregnant woman's feelings of vulnerability. The partner also must deal with the reality of the pregnancy. The partner's support indicates involvement in the pregnancy and preparation for attachment to the child.

Some aspects of a partner's behaviour indicate rivalry. Direct rivalry with the fetus may be evident, especially during sexual activity. Men may protest that fetal movements prevent sexual gratification or that the fetus is watching them during sexual activity. Feelings of rivalry may be unconscious and not verbalized but expressed in subtle behaviours.

The woman's increased introspection may cause her partner to feel uneasy as she becomes preoccupied with thoughts of the child and of motherhood, with her growing dependence on her physician or midwife, and with her re-evaluation of the couple's relationship.

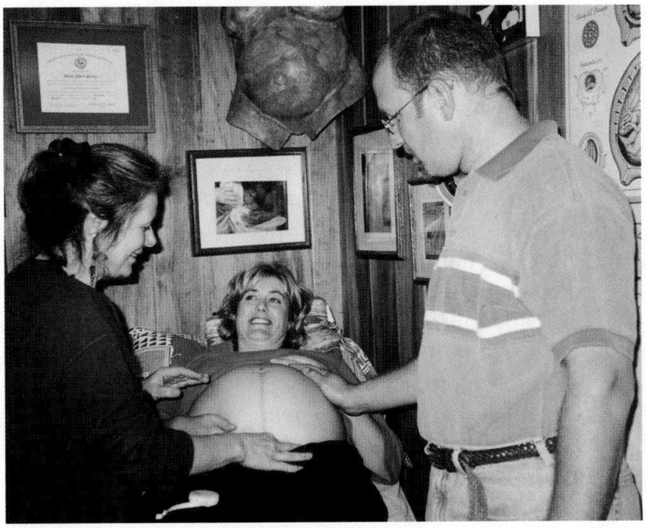

Fig. 10-2 Father participating in prenatal visit. The nurse instructs him in palpating fundus. *(Courtesy Shannon Perry, Phoenix, AZ.)*

Establishing a Relationship With the Fetus

The father–child attachment can be as strong as the mother–child relationship, and fathers can be as competent as mothers in nurturing their infants. The father–child attachment also begins in pregnancy. A father may rub or kiss the maternal abdomen; try to listen, talk, or sing to the fetus; or play with the fetus as he notes fetal movement. Calling the unborn child by name or nickname helps to confirm the reality of pregnancy and promote attachment.

Men prepare for fatherhood in many of the same ways that women prepare for motherhood (i.e., by reading and fantasizing about the baby). Daydreaming about their role as father is common in the last weeks before the birth; men rarely describe their thoughts unless they are reassured that such daydreams are normal. They may adjust work commitments or plan vacations so that they can spend time with their new family.

Nurses can help fathers identify concerns and prepare for the role of being a father by asking questions such as the following:

- What does the word *father* mean to you?
- How do you see yourself as a father?
- What do you expect the baby to look and act like?
- Have you thought about the baby's crying? Changing diapers? Burping the baby? Being awakened at night? Sharing your partner with the baby?

The father may not wish to answer such questions when he is asked but may need time to think them through or discuss them with his partner.

As the birth day approaches, fathers have more questions about fetal and newborn behaviours. Some fathers are shocked or amazed at the small size of the clothes and furniture for the baby. The nurse can tell the father about the unborn child's ability to respond to light, sound, and touch and encourage him to feel and talk to the fetus. Discussions with new fathers, as in childbirth classes, may be welcomed.

Preparing for Childbirth

The days and weeks immediately before the expected day of birth are characterized by anticipation and anxiety. Boredom and restlessness are common as the couple focuses on the birth process; however, during the last 2 months of pregnancy many expectant fathers experience a surge of creative energy at home and on the job. They can become dissatisfied with their present living space. If possible, they tend to act on the need to alter the environment (e.g., remodelling, painting). This activity can be overt evidence of their sharing in the childbearing experience. They are able to channel the anxiety and other feelings experienced during the final weeks before birth into productive activities. This behaviour earns recognition and compliments from friends, relatives, and their partners.

Often a father's major concerns include getting the mother to a medical facility in time for the birth and not appearing ignorant. Many men want to be able to recognize labour and determine when it is appropriate to leave for the hospital or call the physician or midwife. They fantasize different situations and plan what they will do in response to them; they may rehearse taking various routes to the hospital, timing each route at different times of the day.

Some prospective fathers have questions about the birthing suite's furniture, nursing staff, and location, as well as the availability of the physician and anaesthesiologist. Others want to know what is expected of them when their partners are in labour. A tour of the hospital may help alleviate some of these concerns. The man may have fears concerning safe passage of his partner and about the mutilation or death of his partner or child. It is important that he express these fears; otherwise he cannot help his mate deal with her unspoken or overt apprehension.

With the exception of childbirth preparation classes, a man has few opportunities to learn ways to be an involved and active partner in this rite of passage into parenthood (see Family-Centred Teaching box). The tensions and apprehensions of the unprepared, unsupportive father are readily transmitted to the mother and may increase her fears.

The same fears, questions, and concerns may affect birth partners who are not the biological fathers. Birth partners need to be kept informed, supported, and included in all activities in which the mother desires their participation. The nurse can do much to promote pregnancy and birth as a family experience.

Sibling Adaptation

Sharing the spotlight with a new brother or sister may be the first major crisis for a child. The older child often experiences a sense of loss or feels jealous at being "replaced" by the new baby. Some of the factors that influence the child's response are age, the parents' attitudes, the father's role, the length of separation from the mother, the hospital's visitation policy, and how the child has been prepared for the change.

The mother with other children must devote time and energy to reorganizing her relationships with these children. She needs to prepare siblings for the birth of the baby (Box 10-1). She can begin the process of **role transition** in the family by including the children in the pregnancy and being sympathetic to older children's concerns about losing their places in the family hierarchy (Fig. 10-3). No child willingly gives up a familiar position.

Classes to prepare children for the birth of a new brother or sister are available in many communities (Fig. 10-4) (see Family-Centred Teaching box).

Grandparent Adaptation

Expectant grandparenthood can represent a maturational milestone for the parent of an expectant parent. Some grandparents describe having a grandchild as the best thing that ever happened to them; they can enjoy the child without assuming responsibility for the child's care (Fig. 10-5). For other grandparents, when the mother is a young adolescent or for other reasons, such as a mother's substance use, the grandchild may mean assuming care and raising another child when they thought childrearing was over.

To be truly family oriented, maternity care must include the grandparent in the implementation of the nursing process with the whole childbearing family. A class for grandparents is one method of incorporating the grandparents into the family system and encouraging communication between the generations (see Family-Centred Teaching box).

FAMILY-CENTRED TEACHING

Maternal–Paternal–Fetal Relationship

Emotional attachment to the child begins during the prenatal period. Parents fantasize and daydream to prepare for parenthood. Early in pregnancy the woman accepts the biological fact of pregnancy and incorporates the idea of a child into her body and self-image. When the fetus is viewed on ultrasound, it becomes more real. During the second trimester, there is growing awareness of the child as a separate being. When she accepts the reality of the child, the woman becomes more introspective. She seems to withdraw and concentrate her interest on the unborn child. Her partner may feel left out, and other children in the family may become more demanding in efforts to redirect the mother's attention to themselves.

The fantasy child may have familial characteristics and superior abilities; its appearance may be that of a 3- or 4-month-old infant. Both parents and siblings believe the unborn child responds in an individualized, personal manner. Some families become involved by choosing the child's name and anticipating the child's sex if it is not already known. Some families select the child's name as early as the first month of pregnancy. Family tradition, religious customs, and continuation of one's own name or names of relatives and friends are important in the selection process. Family members may interact a great deal with the unborn child by trying to listen to, talk to, and play with the fetus and stroking or kissing the mother's abdomen, especially when the fetus moves.

Nurses must continue to seek to understand and foster attitudes and behaviours that promote early attachment and reduce the risk of negative long-term effects such as child neglect and abuse. More research relating psychological variables to prenatal attachment and maternal–paternal–fetal interaction with maternal–paternal–child interaction is needed, including research with lesbian couples and unpartnered women. Tools to measure maternal–fetal attachment are the Maternal–Fetal Attachment Scale* and the Prenatal Attachment Inventory.†

*Cranley, M. S. (1981). Development of a tool for the measurement of maternal attachment during pregnancy. *Nursing Research, 30*(5), 281–284.

†Müller, M. E. (1993). Development of the prenatal attachment inventory. *Western Journal of Nursing Research, 15*(2), 199–211.

Nursing Care Management

The purpose of prenatal care is to identify existing risk factors and other deviations from normal so that pregnancy outcomes

BOX 10-1 Tips for Sibling Preparation

Prenatal

Adjust the timing and content of information about an anticipated infant to the age and understanding of the older child.

Take your child on a prenatal visit. Let the child listen to the fetal heartbeat and feel the baby move.

Involve the child in preparations for the baby, such as helping to decorate the baby's room.

Move the child to a bed (if still sleeping in a crib) at least 2 months before the baby is due or wait until a few months after the birth.

Read books, show videos, or take child to sibling preparation classes, including a hospital tour.

Answer your child's questions about the coming birth and what babies are like, as well as any other questions.

Take your child to the homes of friends who have babies so that the child has realistic expectations of what babies are like.

During the Hospital Stay

Have someone bring the child to the hospital to visit you and the baby (unless you plan to have the child attend the birth).

Don't force interactions between the child and the baby. Often the child will be more interested in seeing you and being reassured of your love.

Help the child explore the infant by showing how and where to touch the baby.

Give the child a gift (from you or from you, the father, and the baby).

Going Home

Leave the child at home with a relative or baby-sitter.

Have someone else carry the baby from the car so that you can hug the child first.

Adjustment After the Baby Is Home

Arrange for a special time with the child alone with each parent.

Don't exclude the child during infant feeding times. The child can sit with you and the baby and feed a doll or drink juice or milk with you or sit quietly with a game.

Prepare small gifts for the child so that, when the baby gets gifts, the sibling won't feel left out. The child can also help open the baby gifts.

Praise the child for acting age appropriately (so that being a baby does not seem better than being older).

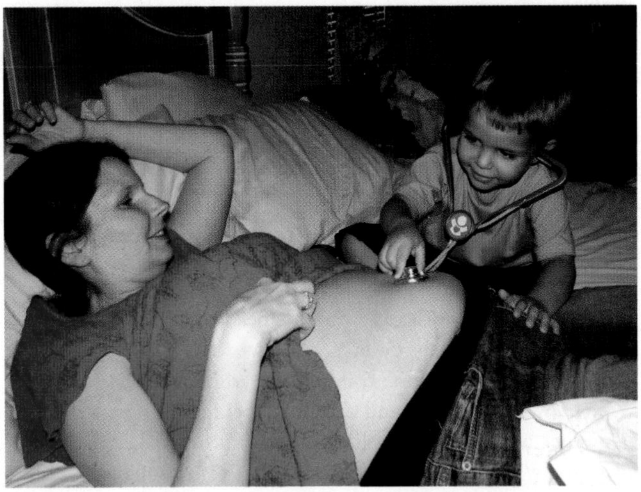

Fig. 10-3 A 4-year-old likes to examine the pregnant abdomen of his mother. *(Courtesy Kara George, Phoenix, AZ.)*

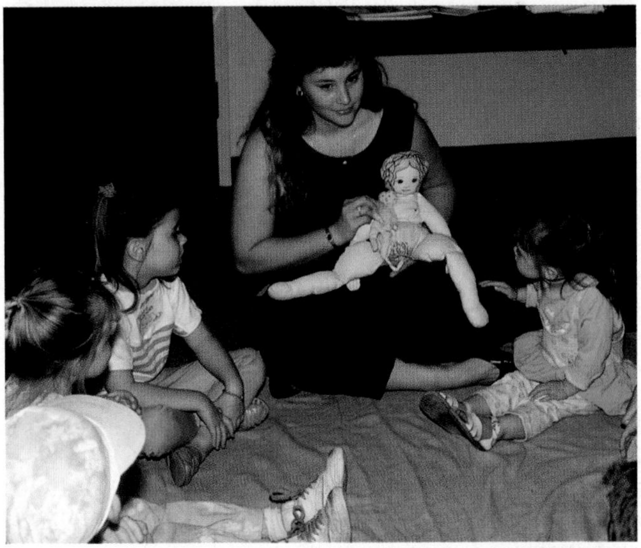

Fig. 10-4 A sibling class of preschoolers learns about childbirth and infant care using dolls. *(Courtesy Marjorie Pyle, RNC, Lifecircle, Costa Mesa, CA.)*

can be enhanced (Johnson, Gregory, & Niebyl, 2007). Major emphasis is placed on preventive aspects of care, primarily to encourage the pregnant woman to practise optimal self-management and report unusual changes early so that problems can be minimized or prevented. In holistic care, nurses provide information and guidance about not only the physical changes but also the psychosocial impact of pregnancy on the woman and members of her family. Therefore, the goals of prenatal nursing care are to foster a safe birth for the infant and mother and to promote satisfaction of the mother and family with the pregnancy and birth experience.

In Canada in 2006, 95% of pregnant women received care in the first trimester (Public Health Agency of Canada [PHAC], 2009). Prenatal care is sought routinely by women of middle or high socioeconomic status. Lack of culturally sensitive care providers and barriers in communication caused by differences in language may interfere with access to care. Immigrant women from cultures in which prenatal care is not emphasized may not know to seek routine prenatal care. Thus birth outcomes in these populations are less positive, with higher rates of maternal and fetal or newborn complications. In particular, newborns with low birth weight (LBW) (less than 2500 g) and infant mortality have been associated with inadequate prenatal care.

Barriers to obtaining health care during pregnancy include inadequate numbers of health care providers, unpleasant

FAMILY-CENTRED TEACHING

Sibling Adaptation to Pregnancy and Birth

Sibling responses to pregnancy vary with age and dependency needs. The 1-year-old infant seems largely unaware of the process, but the 2-year-old child notices the change in the mother's appearance and may comment, "Mommy's fat." The 2-year-old child's need for sameness in the environment makes the child aware of any change. Toddlers may exhibit more clinging behaviour and revert to dependent behaviours in toilet training or eating. Parents need to be reassured that this is a normal behaviour.

By age 3 or 4 years, children like to be told the story of their own beginning and accept its being compared to the present pregnancy. They like to listen to heartbeats and feel the baby moving in utero (see Fig. 10-3). Sometimes they worry about how the baby is being fed and what it wears.

School-age children take a more clinical interest in their mother's pregnancy. They may want to know in more detail, "How did the baby get in there?" and "How will it get out?" Children in this age group notice pregnant women in stores, churches, and schools and sometimes seem shy if they need to approach a pregnant woman directly. On the whole, they look forward to the new baby, see themselves as "mothers" or "fathers," and enjoy buying baby supplies and readying a place for the baby. Because they still think in concrete terms and base judgements on the here and now, they respond positively to their mother's current good health.

Early and middle adolescents preoccupied with the establishment of their own sexual identity may have difficulty accepting the overwhelming evidence of the sexual activity of their parents. They reason that if they are too young for such activity, certainly their parents are too old. They seem to take on a critical parental role and may ask, "What will people think?" or "How can you let yourself get so fat?" Many pregnant women with teenage children confess that their teenagers are the most difficult factor in their current pregnancy.

Late adolescents do not appear to be unduly disturbed. They realize that they soon will be gone from home. Parents usually report that they are comforting and act more like other adults than children.

FAMILY-CENTRED TEACHING

Grandparent Adaptation to Pregnancy and Birth

Every pregnancy affects all family relationships. For expectant grandparents a first pregnancy in a child is undeniable evidence that they are growing older. Many think of a grandparent as old, white haired, and becoming feeble of mind and body; however, some people face grandparenthood while still in their thirties or forties. A mother-to-be announcing her pregnancy to her mother may be greeted by a negative response that indicates she is not ready to be a grandmother. Both daughter and mother may be startled and hurt by the response.

Some expectant grandparents not only are nonsupportive but also use subtle means to decrease the self-esteem of the young parents-to-be. Mothers may talk about their terrible pregnancies; fathers may discuss the endless cost of rearing children; and mothers-in-law may complain that their sons are neglecting them because their concern is now directed toward the pregnant daughters-in-law.

However, most grandparents are delighted with the prospect of a new baby in the family. It reawakens their feelings of their own youth, the excitement of giving birth, and their delight in the behaviour of the parents-to-be when they were infants. They set up a memory store of their child's first smiles, first words, and first steps that can be used later for "claiming" the newborn as a member of the family. Their satisfaction and that of the parents comes with the realization that continuity between past and present is guaranteed.

The grandparent is the historian who transmits the family history, a resource person who shares knowledge based on experience, a role model, and a support person. The grandparent's presence and support can strengthen family systems by widening the circle of support and nurturance. Other sources of information cannot replace the unique contribution that grandparents make.

Many women report that their pregnancies bridged the final gap between them and their own mothers. The estrangement that began in adolescence disappears as the now-pregnant daughter experiences joys, concerns, and anxieties similar to those her mother felt before her.

clinic facilities or procedures, inconvenient clinic hours, distance from health care facilities, lack of transportation, fragmentation of services, inadequate finances, and personal attitudes. The availability and accessibility of prenatal care may be improved by increasing the use of advanced practice nurses in collaborative practice with physicians or midwives. The effectiveness of a regular schedule of home visiting by nurses during pregnancy also has been validated.

The current model for providing prenatal care has been used for more than a century. The initial visit usually occurs in the first trimester, with monthly visits occurring through week 28 of pregnancy. Thereafter, visits are scheduled every 2 weeks until week 36 and then every week until birth. This model is currently being questioned, and in some practices there is a growing tendency to have fewer visits with women who are at low risk for complications. Health care providers are challenged to create a system of prenatal care that has minimal barriers along with a focus on individualized care (Box 10-2). A prenatal history form is the best way to document information obtained (see Nursing Process box).

The therapeutic relationship between the nurse and the woman is established during the initial assessment interview (Fig. 10-6). It is a time for planned, purposeful communication that focuses on specific content. The data collected are of two types: the woman's subjective appraisal of her health status and the nurse's objective observations. The nurse observes the woman's affect, posture, body language, skin colour, and other physical and emotional signs.

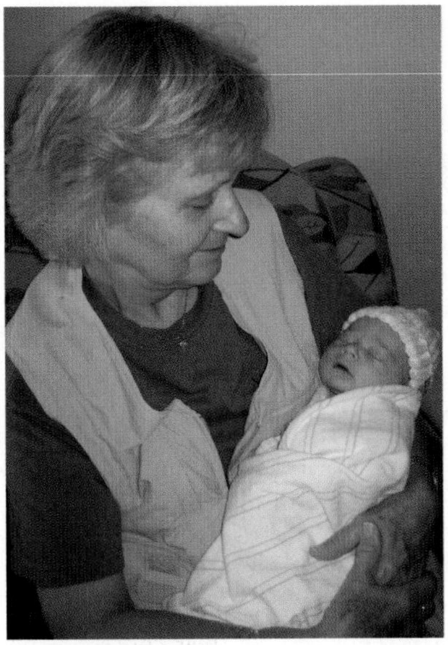

Fig. 10-5 A grandmother relaxes with her grandson. *(Courtesy Shannon Perry, Phoenix, AZ.)*

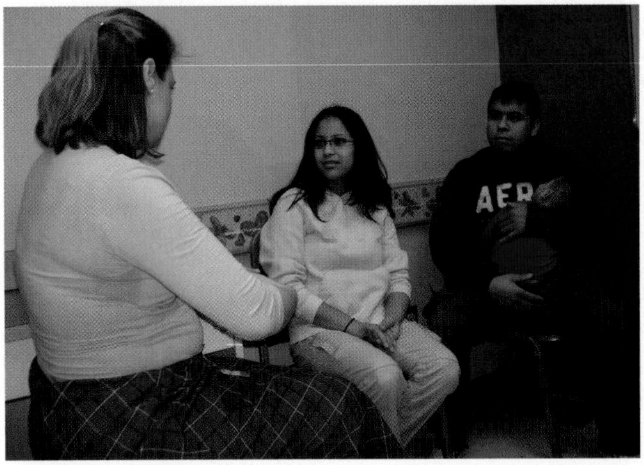

Fig. 10-6 Prenatal interview. *(Courtesy Dee Lowdermilk, Chapel Hill, NC.)*

BOX 10-2 Centring Pregnancy Approach

In response to the decreasing number of maternity care providers, there has been a call to develop new models of prenatal care. Rising (1998), a certified nurse-midwife, developed an innovative approach that emphasizes the assessment of risk, education, and support in a group setting, using a holistic and comprehensive focus. In this centreing pregnancy (CP) approach, women have over 20 contact hours with a health care provider during pregnancy and after delivery. Eight to 12 women are placed in gestational age cohort groups; group sessions begin at 12 to 16 weeks of gestation and end with an early postpartum meeting (Carlson & Lowe, 2006).

Before groups begin, each woman has an individual assessment, physical examination, and history. At the beginning of the group meeting women measure their own blood pressure, weigh themselves, test their own urine with dipsticks, and record the results. Fundal height and the fetal heart rate are assessed individually and privately. Individual follow-up is scheduled as needed (Carlson & Lowe, 2006).

The South Community Birth Program (SCBP) in Vancouver, British Columbia uses a Centreing Pregnancy approach. Low-risk pregnant women in the underserved community of South Vancouver receive collaborative, multidisciplinary care from family physicians, midwives, community health nurses, and doulas. This is the first such multidisciplinary program of its kind in Canada in which midwives and family physicians share the care of patients (http://www.scbp.ca/).

Results assessing the effectiveness of this approach have been promising; in a study of adolescents, the incidence of low birth weight was reduced, and rates of breastfeeding were increased (Grady & Bloom, 2004). Other studies of CP are ongoing.

Often the pregnant woman is accompanied by one or more family members. The nurse needs to build a relationship with these people as part of the social context of the patient. With her permission, those accompanying the woman can be included in the initial prenatal interview, and the observations and information about the woman's family form part of the database. For example, if the woman is accompanied by small children, the nurse can ask about her plans for child care during the time of labour and birth. Special needs are noted at this time (e.g., wheelchair access, assistance in getting on and off the examining table, and cognitive deficits).

Reason for Seeking Care

Although pregnant women are scheduled for "routine" prenatal visits, they often come to the health care provider seeking information or reassurance about a particular concern. When the woman is asked a broad, open-ended question, such as "How have you been feeling?", she may reveal problems that could otherwise be overlooked. The woman's chief concerns should be recorded in her own words to alert other personnel to the priority of needs identified by her. At the initial visit, a typical desire is for information about what is normal in the course of pregnancy.

Current Pregnancy

The presumptive signs of pregnancy may be of great concern to the woman. A review of symptoms she is experiencing and how she is coping with them helps establish a database for developing a plan of care. Some early teaching may be provided at this time.

Obstetrical and Gynecological History

Data are gathered on the woman's age at menarche; menstrual history; contraceptive history; the nature of any infertility or gynecological conditions; history of any sexually transmitted infections (STIs); her sexual history; and a detailed history of all her pregnancies, including the present one, and their outcomes. The date of the last Papanicolaou (Pap) test and the result are noted. The date of her LMP is obtained to establish the EDB.

NURSING PROCESS: NURSING CARE DURING PREGNANCY

Assessment

The assessment process begins at the initial prenatal visit and is continued throughout the pregnancy.

- History (comprehensive health history, obstetrical and gynecological history, family history; physical abuse)
- Interview (psychosocial profile; mental status; risk assessment; symptoms she is experiencing)
- Physical examination (review of body systems; vital signs, weight; pelvic examination; fetal heart rate)
- Review of laboratory tests

Nursing Diagnoses

Nursing diagnoses that may be appropriate in the prenatal period include the following:

Anxiety related to
- physical discomforts of pregnancy
- previous history of anxiety/depression
- ambivalent and labile emotions
- changes in family dynamics
- fetal well-being
- ability to manage anticipated labour

Interrupted family processes related to
- changing roles and responsibilities
- inadequate understanding of physical and emotional changes in pregnancy
- increased concern about labour

Decreased knowledge regarding self-care measures for
- posture and body mechanics
- rest and relaxation
- personal hygiene
- activity and exercise
- safety

Disturbed sleep pattern related to
- discomforts of late pregnancy
- anxiety about approaching labour

Planning

Prenatal care ideally is a multidisciplinary activity in which nurses work with physicians or midwives, nutritionists, social workers, and others. Collaboration among these individuals is necessary to provide holistic care that meets the needs of individual women.

Examples of expected outcomes of prenatal care are that the pregnant woman will achieve the following:

- Indicate decreased anxiety about the health of her fetus and herself
- Describe improved family dynamics
- Show appropriate weight gain patterns
- Report signs and symptoms of complications
- Describe appropriate measures taken to relieve physical discomforts
- Develop a realistic birth plan

Interventions

The nurse–patient relationship is critical in setting the tone for further interaction.

- Listen with an attentive expression, use touch, and maintain eye contact.
- Recognize the woman's feelings and her right to express these feelings.
- Be perceptive in identifying unvoiced needs; ask for a patient-generated solution and a subsequent report of its effectiveness.
- Teach for self-management (see text).
- Supportive care involves developing, augmenting, or changing the mechanisms used by women and their families in coping with stress.
- The woman must be a willing partner in a purely voluntary relationship. The relationship can be refused or terminated at any time by the pregnant woman or her family.

Evaluation

Evaluation of the effectiveness of care of the woman during pregnancy is based on the previously stated outcomes.

Medical History

The medical history includes medical or surgical conditions that may affect the pregnancy or that may be affected by the pregnancy. For example, a pregnant woman who has diabetes or epilepsy requires special care. Because women may be anxious during the initial interview, the nurse's reference to cues such as a MedicAlert bracelet can prompt the woman to explain allergies; chronic diseases; or medications being taken, such as cortisone, insulin, or anticonvulsants.

The nature of previous surgical procedures should also be described. If a woman has had uterine surgery or extensive repair of the pelvic floor, a Caesarean birth may be necessary; appendectomy rules out appendicitis as a cause of right lower quadrant pain in pregnancy. Spinal surgery may contraindicate the use of spinal or epidural anaesthesia, and breast augmentation or reduction procedures may impact the breastfeeding experience. Any injury involving the pelvis should be noted.

Often women who have chronic or disabling conditions forget to mention them during the initial assessment because they have adapted to them. Special shoes or a limp may indicate the existence of a pelvic structural defect, an important consideration in pregnant women. The nurse should watch for these special characteristics and sensitively inquire about them, thus obtaining individualized data that will provide the basis for a comprehensive nursing care plan. Observations are a vital component of the interview process because they prompt the nurse and the woman to focus on the specific needs of the woman and her family.

A detailed mental health history also needs to be completed. Whether the woman or any family member has a previous history of depression or any other mental health issues should be noted. It is important to identify these issues early in pregnancy so that prompt assessment and treatment can be implemented if concerns arise. A history of mental health concerns increases the risk for the development of further issues during pregnancy and in the postpartum period.

Nutritional History

The nutritional status of a pregnant woman has a direct effect on the growth and development of the fetus. A dietary assessment can reveal special diet practices, food allergies, eating behaviours, the practice of **pica**, and other factors related to her nutritional status (see Box 11-4). Pregnant women are usually motivated to learn about good nutrition and respond well to nutritional advice generated by this assessment. Cultural influences on diet and food selection should also be considered (see Chapter 11).

History of Use of Drugs and Herbal Preparations

A woman's past and present use of drugs, both legal (over-the-counter [OTC], prescription, and herbal medications; caffeine; alcohol; nicotine) and illegal (e.g., marijuana, cocaine, heroin) must be assessed because many substances cross the placenta and can harm the developing fetus. Today increased numbers of individuals, including pregnant women, are using herbal preparations. Thus it is important for health care providers to question women about their use of herbal preparations and to document their responses.

Periodic urine toxicology screening tests are often recommended during pregnancy for women who have a history of illegal substance use, if consent is given by the woman (see Legal Tip).

LEGAL TIP Screening for Drug Use. Hospitals must obtain informed consent from a pregnant woman before she can be tested for drug use (Kehringer, 2003).

Family History

The family history provides information about the woman's immediate family, including parents, siblings, and children. These data help identify familial or genetic disorders or conditions that could affect the present health status of the woman or her fetus.

Social, Experiential, and Occupational History

Situational factors such as the family's ethnic and cultural background and socioeconomic status are assessed during the history taking. The following information may be obtained over several encounters. The woman's perception of this pregnancy is explored by asking her such questions as the following: Is this pregnancy wanted or not, planned or not? Is the woman or couple pleased or displeased, accepting or nonaccepting? What problems related to finances, career, or living accommodations may arise as a result of the pregnancy? The family support system is determined by asking her such questions as the following: What primary support is available to her? Are changes needed to promote adequate support? What are the existing relationships among mother, father or partner, siblings, and in-laws? What preparations are being made for her care and that of dependent family members during labour and for the care of the infant after birth? Is financial, educational, or other support needed from the community? What are the woman's ideas about childbearing, her expectations of the infant's behaviour, and her outlook on life and the female role?

Other questions that should be asked include the following: What does the woman think it will be like to have a baby in the home? How is her life going to change by having a baby? What plans are interrupted by having a baby at this time? During interviews throughout the pregnancy, the nurse should remain alert for the appearance of potential parenting problems such as depression, lack of family support, and inadequate living conditions. The nurse must assess the woman's attitude toward health care, particularly during childbearing; her expectations of health care providers; and her view of the relationship between herself and the nurse.

Coping mechanisms and patterns of interacting should also be identified. Early in the pregnancy, the nurse should determine the woman's knowledge of pregnancy, maternal changes, fetal growth, self-management, and care of the newborn, including feeding. Before planning for nursing care, the nurse needs information about the woman's decision-making abilities and living habits (e.g., exercise, sleep, diet, diversional interests, personal hygiene, clothing). Common stressors during childbearing include the baby's welfare, the labour and birth process, the behaviours of the newborn, the relationship with the baby's father and her family, changes in body image, and physical symptoms.

Attitudes concerning the range of acceptable sexual behaviours during pregnancy are also explored. Questions such as the following could be asked: What has your family (partner, friends) told you about sex during pregnancy? The woman's sexual self-concept is given emphasis by asking questions such as the following: How do you feel about the changes in your appearance? How does your partner feel about your body now? How do you feel about wearing maternity clothes?

Women should be questioned regarding their occupation, past and present, since this may adversely affect maternal and fetal health. For some women, heavy lifting and exposure to chemicals and radiation may be part of their daily work, and these activities can negatively affect the pregnancy. For others, long hours of sitting at a desk working on a computer can contribute to carpal tunnel syndrome or circulatory stasis in the legs.

History of Physical or Sexual Abuse

All women should be assessed for a history or risk of physical or sexual abuse, particularly because the likelihood of intimate partner violence (IPV) increases during pregnancy (see Chapter 4 for a detailed discussion). A history of childhood sexual abuse also needs to be assessed, as this can have implications on the woman's labour experience. Although visual cues from the woman's appearance or behaviour may suggest the possibility of abuse, no one profile of the woman who experiences IPV exists. Identification of abuse and immediate clinical intervention that includes information about safety can result in behaviour that may prevent future abuse and increase the safety and well-being of the woman and her infant. During pregnancy, the target body parts change during abusive episodes. Women report physical blows directed to the head, breasts, abdomen, and genitalia. Sexual assault is common.

IPV and pregnancy in teenagers constitutes a particularly difficult situation. Adolescents may be trapped in the abusive relationship because of their inexperience. Many professionals and the adolescents themselves ignore the violence because it may not be believable, because relationships are transient, and because the jealous and controlling behaviour is interpreted as love and devotion. Routine screening for abuse and sexual assault is recommended for pregnant adolescents.

Review of Systems

During this portion of the interview, the woman is asked to identify and describe pre-existing or concurrent problems in any of the body systems, and her mental status is assessed. The woman is questioned about physical symptoms she has experienced, such as shortness of breath or pain. Pregnancy affects and is affected by all body systems; therefore, information on the present status of body systems is important in planning care. For each sign or symptom described, the following additional data should be obtained: body location, quality, quantity, chronology, aggravating or alleviating factors, and associated manifestations (onset, character, and course) (Seidel et al., 2006).

Physical Examination

The initial physical examination provides the baseline for assessing subsequent changes. The examiner should determine the woman's needs for basic information regarding reproductive anatomy and provide this information, along with a demonstration of the equipment that may be used during the examination and an explanation of the procedure itself. The interaction requires an unhurried, sensitive, and gentle approach with a matter-of-fact attitude.

The physical examination begins with assessment of vital signs, including blood pressure (BP), height, and weight (for calculation of body mass index [BMI]). The bladder should be empty before pelvic examination is done. A urine specimen can be obtained to test for protein, glucose, or leukocytes or for other tests.

Each examiner develops a routine for proceeding with the physical examination; most choose the head-to-toe progression. Heart and lung sounds are evaluated, and extremities examined. The skin is assessed for changes in pigmentation, rashes, and edema. Distribution, amount, and quality of body hair are of particular importance because the findings reflect nutritional status, endocrine function, and attention to hygiene. The thyroid gland is assessed carefully, as are the breasts and abdomen. The height of the **fundus** is noted if the first examination occurs after the first trimester of pregnancy. See Chapter 5 for a detailed description of the physical examination.

evolve Case Study—First Trimester

Pelvic Examination During Pregnancy

During pregnancy, the pelvic examination is done in the same way as it is during a routine examination on a nonpregnant woman (see Chapter 5). A Pap test may be done initially, and cytological specimens are collected to test for gonorrhea, chlamydia, human papillomavirus (HPV), and herpes simplex virus (HSV) (see Chapter 6). Whenever a pelvic examination is performed, the tone of the pelvic musculature and the woman's knowledge of Kegel exercises are assessed (see Chapter 4, Patient Teaching box). Particular attention is paid to the size of the uterus because this is an indication of the duration of gestation. The nurse present during the examination can coach the woman at this time in breathing and relaxation techniques as needed. One vaginal examination during pregnancy is recommended; another is usually not done unless indicated for medical reasons.

While the pregnant woman is in the lithotomy position, the nurse must watch for supine hypotension (decrease in blood pressure) caused by the weight of the uterus pressing on the vena cava and aorta. Symptoms of supine hypotension include pallor, dizziness, faintness, breathlessness, tachycardia, nausea, clammy skin, and sweating. The woman should be positioned on her side until symptoms resolve and vital signs stabilize (see Emergency Box). The vaginal examination can be done with the woman in lateral position.

Laboratory Tests

The data yielded through laboratory examination of specimens obtained during the examination add important information about the symptoms of pregnancy and the woman's health status.

Specimens are collected at the initial visit so that any abnormal findings can be treated. Blood is drawn for a variety of tests (Table 10-1). A sickle cell screen is recommended for women of African, Asian, or Middle Eastern descent. The folate level is measured when indicated. In addition, pregnant women and fathers with a family history of cystic fibrosis may elect to have blood drawn for testing to ascertain if they are a cystic fibrosis carrier (Fries, Bashford, & Nunes, 2006). Urine is tested for glucose (diabetes), protein (pre-eclampsia), and nitrites and leukocytes (urinary tract infection). Urine specimens are usually tested by dipstick. Culture and sensitivity tests are

EMERGENCY

Supine Hypotension

Signs and Symptoms

Pallor
Dizziness, faintness, breathlessness
Tachycardia
Nausea
Clammy (damp, cool) skin; sweating

Intervention

Position woman on her side until her signs and symptoms subside and vital signs stabilize within normal limits.

Table 10-1 Laboratory Tests in Prenatal Period

LABORATORY TEST	PURPOSE
Hemoglobin, hematocrit/WBC, differential	Detects anemia/detects infection
Hemoglobin electrophoresis	Identifies women with hemoglobinopathies (e.g., sickle cell anemia, β-thalassemia)
Blood type, Rh, and irregular antibody	Identifies fetuses at risk for developing erythroblastosis fetalis or hyperbilirubinemia in neonatal period
Rubella, chicken pox and parvovirus B19 titre	Determines immunity to rubella, chicken pox and parvovirus
Tuberculin skin testing; chest film after 20 wk of gestation in women with reactive tuberculin tests	Screens for exposure to tuberculosis
Urinalysis, including microscopic examination of urinary sediment; pH, specific gravity, colour, glucose, albumin, protein, RBCs, WBCs, casts, acetone; hCG	Identifies women with unsuspected diabetes mellitus, renal disease, hypertensive disease of pregnancy; infection; occult hematuria
Urine culture	Identifies women with asymptomatic bacteriuria
Renal function tests: BUN, creatinine, electrolytes, creatinine clearance, total protein excretion	Evaluates level of possible renal compromise in women with a history of diabetes, hypertension, or renal disease
Papanicolaou test	Screens for cervical intraepithelial neoplasia, herpes simplex type 2, and HPV
Vaginal or rectal smear for *Neisseria gonorrhoeae*, *Chlamydia*, HPV, GBS	Screens high-risk population for asymptomatic infection; GBS done at 35–37 wk
RPR/VDRL/FTA-ABS	Identifies women with untreated syphilis
HIV antibody,* hepatitis B surface antigen, toxoplasmosis	Screens for infection
1-hr glucose tolerance	Screens for gestational diabetes; done at initial visit for women with risk factors; recommended to be done at 28 wk for all pregnant women
2-hr glucose tolerance	Screens for diabetes in women with elevated glucose level after 1-hr test; must have two elevated readings for diagnosis
Cardiac evaluation: ECG, chest x-ray film, and echocardiogram	Evaluates cardiac function in women with a history of hypertension or cardiac disease

*With patient permission.
BUN, blood urea nitrogen; *ECG*, electrocardiogram; *FTA-ABS*, fluorescent treponemal antibody absorption test; *GBS*, group B streptococcus; *hCG*, human chorionic gonadotropin; *HIV*, human immunodeficiency virus; *HPV*, human papilloma virus; *RBC*, red blood cell; *RPR*, rapid plasma reagin; *VDRL*, Venereal Disease Research Laboratories; *WBC*, white blood cell.

ordered as necessary. A purified protein derivative tuberculin test may be administered to assess exposure to tuberculosis.

STI Screening in Pregnancy

All pregnant women should have screening for STIs done early in pregnancy. Cervical cultures for chlamydia and gonorrhea should be done at the first prenatal visit. All women should be tested for hepatitis B virus (HBV) and syphilis at the first prenatal visit, and if they are considered to be high risk (see Box 6-6), blood testing should be repeated later in pregnancy or on admission for labour and birth (PHAC, 2008b) (see Chapter 6).

HIV in Pregnancy

Testing for antibodies to the human immunodeficiency virus (HIV) is strongly recommended for all pregnant women (Keenan-Lindsay et al., 2006) (Box 10-3). Transmission of HIV from mother to fetus can occur throughout the perinatal period. Exposure may occur to the fetus through the maternal circulation as early as the first trimester of pregnancy, to the infant during labour and birth by inoculation or ingestion of maternal blood and other infected fluids, or to the infant through breast milk (Lawrence & Lawrence, 2011; Riordan & Wambach, 2010).

The incidence of perinatal transmission from an untreated HIV-positive mother to her fetus ranges from 25 to 35%. Zidovudine decreases perinatal transmission and the risk of infant death. Elective Caesarean birth may reduce the risk of transmission from the mother to child. Thus testing has the potential to identify HIV-positive women who can then be treated and to reduce the risk of transmission from mother to child to 2%.

Barriers to routine prenatal testing may be the requirement for lengthy HIV prevention counselling and documentation of **informed consent** for HIV testing. For pregnant women, testing rates are higher when opt-out testing is used than when opt-in strategies with requirements for written documentation of informed consent for HIV testing are used (Keenan-Lindsay et al., 2006).

Health Canada has approved methods of rapid testing for HIV. The tests have accuracy rates of 98 to 99%. If the results are reactive, further testing is done (PHAC, 2007). Some labour units are using rapid HIV testing in women who have unknown HIV status on admission.

Maternity nurses should be advocates for the fetus while accepting the pregnant woman's decision regarding testing, treatment, or both for HIV. Health care providers have an obligation to ensure that pregnant women are well informed

BOX 10-3 HIV Screening for Pregnant Women and Their Infants

HIV Screening in Pregnancy

All pregnant women in Canada should be offered HIV screening, with appropriate counselling. Targeted testing of women thought to be at higher risk will fail to identify all HIV-positive women, as some women do not perceive themselves to be at risk, nor do their health care providers. HIV testing must be voluntary and free from coercion. No woman should be tested without her knowledge. Some provinces have universal screening in which all women are screened with notification (opt-out approach) unless the woman declines (Alberta, Newfoundland & Labrador, North West Territories & Nunavut). Most provinces have a policy of encouraging women to have the screening done (opt-in approach).

The use of mandatory screening may affect the ability to make an informed choice and could lead some women to avoid antenatal care. Testing must be offered appropriately so that women will understand the importance of screening.

Pregnant women should receive oral or written information that includes an explanation of HIV infection, a description of interventions that can reduce HIV transmission from mother to infant, and the meaning of positive and negative test results. They should be offered an opportunity to ask questions and to decline testing. Women should also be reassured that all testing is done in confidence.

No additional process or written documentation of informed consent beyond that required for other routine prenatal tests should be required for HIV testing.

If a patient declines an HIV test, this decision should be documented in the medical record.

Timing of HIV Testing

Women should be tested as early as possible in pregnancy.

Rapid Testing During Labour

Any woman with undocumented HIV status at the time of labour should be screened with a rapid HIV test unless she declines (opt-out screening). Reasons for declining a rapid test should be explored.

Immediate initiation of appropriate antiretroviral prophylaxis should be recommended to women on the basis of a reactive rapid test result without waiting for the result of a confirmatory test.

Postpartum/Newborn Testing

When a woman's HIV status is still unknown at the time of birth, she should be screened with a rapid HIV test immediately after giving birth unless she declines (opt-out screening).

When the mother's HIV status is unknown, rapid testing of the newborn as soon as possible after birth is recommended so that antiretroviral prophylaxis can be offered to HIV-exposed infants. Women should be informed that identifying HIV antibodies in the newborn indicates that the mother is infected.

The benefits of neonatal antiretroviral prophylaxis are best realized when it is initiated within 12 hours after birth.

(Sources: Branson, B. M., et al. [2006]. Revised recommendations for HIV testing of adults, adolescents, and pregnant women in health-care settings. *Morbidity & Mortality Weekly Report, 55*[RR-14], 1–17; Keenan-Lindsay, L., et al. [2006]. SOGC clinical practice guideline: HIV screening in pregnancy. *Journal of Obstetrics and Gynaecology Canada, 28*[12], 1103–1107.)

about HIV symptoms, testing, and methods of decreasing maternal–fetal transmission. However, mandatory HIV screening involves ethical issues related to privacy, discrimination, social stigma, and reproductive risks to the pregnant woman.

Follow-Up Visits

Monthly visits are scheduled routinely during the first and second trimesters, although additional appointments may be made as the need arises. However, during the third trimester, the possibility for complications increases, and closer monitoring is warranted. Starting with week 28, visits are scheduled every 2 weeks until week 36 and then every week until birth unless the health care provider individualizes the schedule. Individual needs, complications, and risks of the pregnant woman may warrant visits more or less often. The pattern of interviewing the woman first and then assessing physical changes and performing laboratory tests is maintained.

Interview

Follow-up visits are less intensive than the initial prenatal visit. At each of these follow-up visits, the woman is asked to summarize relevant events that have occurred since the previous visit. She is asked about her general emotional and physiological well-being, any concerns or problems, and questions she may have. Personal and family needs are identified and explored.

A woman's emotional state can affect her and her family's general well-being. Thus the nurse needs to ask whether the woman has had any mood swings, reactions to changes in her body image, bad dreams, or worries. Positive feelings (her own and those of her family) are also noted. The reactions of family members to the pregnancy and the woman's progression through the developmental tasks of pregnancy are also assessed and recorded.

During the third trimester, current family situations and their effect on the woman are assessed (e.g., the response of partner, siblings, and grandparents to the pregnancy and the coming child). The nurse needs to assess the parents' understanding of the following: the warning signs that indicate emergencies such as bleeding and abdominal pain, the signs of preterm and term labour, the labour process and anxieties about labour, fetal development, and methods to assess fetal well-being. The nurse should ascertain whether the woman is planning to attend childbirth preparation classes and what she knows about the control of discomfort during labour.

A review of the woman's physical systems is appropriate at each visit, and any suggestive signs or symptoms are assessed in depth. Discomforts reflecting adaptations to pregnancy are identified. Special inquiries should be made about possible infections (e.g., genitourinary tract, respiratory tract). The woman's knowledge of and success with self-management measures are assessed, as well as outcomes of prescribed therapy.

Physical Examination

Re-evaluation is a constant aspect of a pregnant woman's care. Each woman reacts differently to pregnancy. As a result, careful monitoring of the pregnancy and her reactions to care is vital. Physiological changes are documented as the pregnancy progresses and are reviewed for possible deviations from normal progress.

At each visit, physical parameters are measured. BP is taken at every visit using the same arm and with the woman seated. Her weight is measured, and the appropriateness of the weight gain is evaluated in relation to her BMI. Urine may be checked by dipstick. The presence and degree of edema are noted. For examination of the abdomen, the woman lies on her back with her arms by her side and head supported by a pillow. The bladder should be empty. Abdominal inspection is followed by measurement of the height of the fundus (Fig. 10-7). While the woman lies on her back, the nurse should be alert for the occurrence of supine hypotension (see Emergency box).

The findings revealed during the interview and physical examination reflect the status of maternal adaptations. When any of the findings is suspicious, an in-depth examination needs to be performed. For example, careful interpretation of BP is important in the risk-factor analysis of all pregnant women. A rise in systolic blood pressure (SBP) of 30 mm Hg or more over the baseline pressure or a rise in the diastolic blood pressure (DBP) of 15 mm Hg over the baseline pressure is also a significant finding, regardless of the absolute values, and should be closely monitored. A SBP of 140 mm Hg or more and a DBP of 90 mm Hg or more, based on the average of at least two measurements, suggest the presence of hypertension (Society of Obstetricians and Gynaecologists of Canada [SOGC], 2008). See Chapter 13 for an in-depth discussion of problems associated with hypertension.

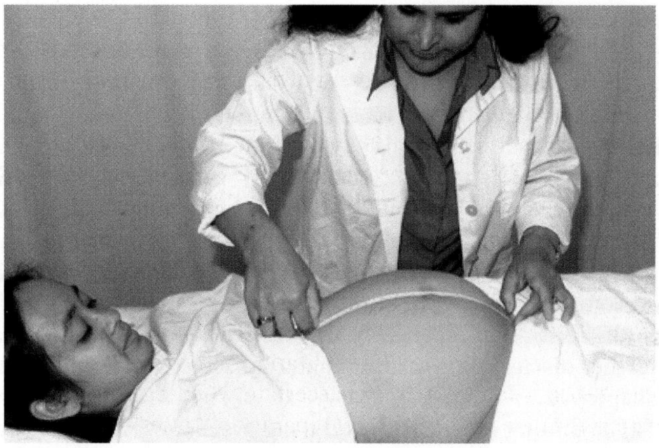

Fig. 10-7 Measurement of fundal height from symphysis to top of fundus. Note position of hands and measuring tape. *(Courtesy Chris Rozales, San Francisco, CA.)*

The pregnant woman is monitored continuously for a range of signs and symptoms that indicate potential complications in addition to hypertension. For example, persistent and excessive vomiting and ketonuria may indicate the development of hyperemesis gravidarum. Uterine cramping and vaginal bleeding are signs of threatened miscarriage. Chills and fever are symptoms of infection. Discharge from the vagina may be amniotic fluid or associated with infection (Box 10-4).

Fetal Assessment

Toward the end of the first trimester, before the uterus is an abdominal organ, the fetal heart rate (FHR) can be heard with an ultrasound fetoscope or an ultrasound stethoscope. To hear the FHR, the instrument is placed in the midline just above the symphysis pubis and firm pressure is applied. The woman and her family should be offered the opportunity to listen to the fetal heart. The health status of the fetus is assessed at each visit for the remainder of the pregnancy.

Fundal Height

During the second trimester, the uterus becomes an abdominal organ. The *fundal height*, or measurement of the height of the uterus above the symphysis pubis, is used as one indicator of fetal growth. The measurement also provides a gross estimate of the duration of pregnancy. During the second and third trimesters (weeks 18 to 30), the height of the fundus in centimetres is approximately the same as the number of weeks of gestation if the woman's bladder is empty at the time of measurement (Cunningham et al., 2010). Measurement of fundal height may aid in the identification of high risk factors. A stable or decreased fundal height may indicate the presence of **intrauterine growth restriction** (IUGR); an excessive increase could indicate the presence of multifetal gestation (more than one fetus) or hydramnios.

A paper tape is typically used to measure fundal height. To increase the reliability of the measurement, the same person examines the pregnant woman at each of her prenatal visits; often this is not possible. All clinicians who examine a particular pregnant woman should be consistent in their measurement technique. (see Fig. 10-7).

Gestational Age

Fetal gestational age is determined from the menstrual history, contraceptive history, pregnancy test results, and the following findings obtained from the clinical evaluation:

- First uterine evaluation: date, size
- Fetal heart first heard: date, method (Doppler stethoscope, fetoscope)
- Date of quickening
- Current fundal height, estimated fetal weight
- Current week of gestation by history of LMP or ultrasound examination (or both)
- Ultrasound examination: date, week of gestation, biparietal diameter
- Reliability of dates

Quickening ("feeling life") refers to the mother's first perception of fetal movement. It usually occurs between weeks 16 and 20 of gestation and is initially experienced as a fluttering sensation. The mother's report should be recorded. Multiparas often perceive fetal movement earlier than primigravidas; sometimes this may occur as early as 14 weeks.

BOX 10-4 Signs of Potential Complications During the First, Second, and Third Trimesters

First Trimester

Signs and Symptoms	Possible Causes
Severe vomiting	Hyperemesis gravidarum
Chills, fever	Infection
Burning on urination	Infection
Diarrhea	Infection
Abdominal cramping; vaginal bleeding	Miscarriage, ectopic pregnancy

Second and Third Trimesters

Signs and Symptoms	Possible Causes
Persistent, severe vomiting	Hyperemesis gravidarum, hypertension, pre-eclampsia
Sudden discharge of fluid from vagina before 37 weeks	Premature rupture of membranes
Vaginal bleeding, severe abdominal pain	Miscarriage, placenta previa, abruptio placentae
Chills, fever, burning on urination, diarrhea	Infection
Severe backache or flank pain	Kidney infection or stones; preterm labour
Change in fetal movements: absence of fetal movements after quickening, any unusual change in pattern or amount	Fetal jeopardy or intrauterine fetal death
Uterine contractions; pressure; cramping before 37 weeks	Preterm labour
Visual disturbances: blurring, double vision, or spots	Hypertensive conditions, pre-eclampsia
Swelling of face or fingers and over sacrum	Hypertensive conditions, pre-eclampsia
Headaches: severe, frequent, or continuous	Hypertensive conditions, pre-eclampsia
Muscular irritability or convulsions	Hypertensive conditions, pre-eclampsia
Epigastric or abdominal pain (perceived as severe stomach ache)	Hypertensive conditions, pre-eclampsia, abruptio placentae
Glycosuria, positive glucose tolerance test reaction	Gestational diabetes mellitus

Routine ultrasound examination in early pregnancy has been recommended for fetal screening (see Chapter 12). This ultrasound may be used to establish the duration of pregnancy if the woman cannot give a precise date for her LMP or if the size of the uterus does not conform to the EDB as calculated by Nägele's rule. Ultrasound also provides information about the well-being of the fetus. However, the routine use of ultrasound examination has not been found to substantively improve fetal outcome .

Health Status

The assessment of fetal health status includes consideration of fetal movement. The mother is instructed to note the extent and timing of fetal movements and report immediately if the pattern changes or movement ceases. Regular movement has been found to be a reliable indicator of fetal health (Liston et al., 2007) (see Chapter 12).

The fetal heart rate (FHR) is checked on routine visits once it has been heard (Fig. 10-8). Early in the second trimester, the heartbeat may be heard with the Doppler stethoscope (see Fig. 10-8, B). To detect the heartbeat before the fetal position can be palpated by Leopold manoeuvres (see Fig. 18-4), the scope is moved around the abdomen until the heartbeat is heard. Each nurse develops a set pattern for searching the abdomen for the heartbeat (e.g., starting in the midline about 2 to 3 cm above the symphysis, followed by the left lower quadrant). The heartbeat is counted for 1 minute, and the quality and rhythm are noted. Later in the second trimester, the FHR can be determined with the fetoscope or Pinard fetoscope (see Fig. 10-8, A and C). A normal rate and rhythm are other good indicators of fetal health. Once the heartbeat is noted, its absence is cause for immediate investigation.

Intensive investigation of fetal health status is initiated if any maternal or fetal complications arise (e.g., maternal hypertension, IUGR, premature rupture of membranes [PROM], irregular or absent FHR, absence of fetal movements after quickening). Careful, precise, and concise recording of patient responses and laboratory results contributes to the continuous supervision vital to ensuring the well-being of the mother and fetus.

Laboratory Tests

The number of routine laboratory tests done during follow-up visits in pregnancy is limited. A clean-catch urine specimen is obtained to test for levels of glucose, protein, nitrites, and leukocytes at each visit. Urine specimens for culture and sensitivity, and blood samples are obtained only if signs and symptoms warrant.

The multiple marker test, or triple screen test, is used to detect Down syndrome and other chromosome abnormalities. Done between 16 and 18 weeks of gestation, it measures maternal serum alpha fetoprotein (MSAFP), human chorionic gonadotropin (hCG), and unconjugated estriol (Wapner, Jenkins, & Khalek, 2009). Combining these three markers with maternal age allows a high detection rate for Down syndrome. High levels are associated with neural tube defects, and abnormally low levels may be associated with Down syndrome or other trisomies (SOGC, 2007). Further discussion regarding maternal screening testing is in Chapter 12.

The finding of risk factors during pregnancy may indicate the need to repeat some tests at other times. For example, exposure to tuberculosis would necessitate repeat testing. Other blood tests are repeated as necessary.

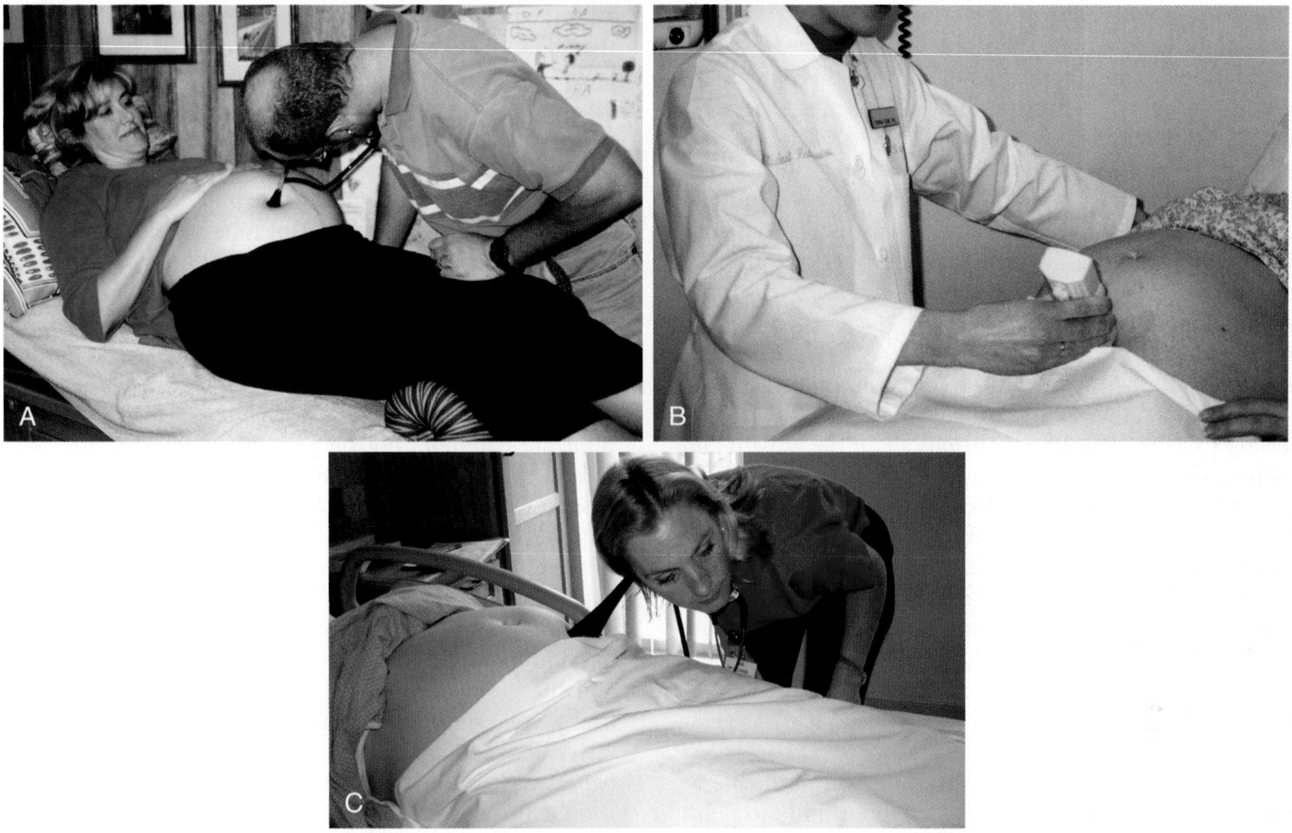

Fig. 10-8 Detecting fetal heartbeat. **A:** Father can listen to the fetal heart with a fetoscope (first detectable at 18 to 20 weeks with a fetoscope). **B:** Doppler ultrasound stethoscope (fetal heartbeat detectable at 12 weeks). **C:** Pinard stethoscope. Note: Hands should not touch the stethoscope while the nurse is listening. *(**A**, Courtesy Shannon Perry, Phoenix, AZ. **B**, Courtesy Dee Lowdermilk, Chapel Hill, NC. **C**, Courtesy Julie Perry Nelson, Loveland, CO.)*

STIs in Pregnancy. STIs are common in pregnancy and may have negative effects on the mother and fetus. Testing for STIs should be repeated late in the third trimester (36 weeks) if the woman was previously positive or if she is younger than age 25, has a new sex partner, or has multiple sex partners (PHAC, 2010). Pregnant women should be asked whether they or their partner(s) have had genital lesions (HSV). Any suspicious or recurrent lesions found during pregnancy should be cultured to document HSV.

Gonococcal infections in pregnancy potentially affect both the mother and infant. Women with cervical gonorrhea may develop salpingitis in the first trimester. Perinatal complications of gonococcal infection include premature rupture of membranes, preterm birth, **chorioamnionitis**, neonatal sepsis, IUGR, and maternal postpartum sepsis. Amniotic infection syndrome—manifested by placental, fetal, and umbilical cord inflammation following premature rupture of the membranes—may result from gonorrheal infection during pregnancy.

During pregnancy, maternal infection with HSV-2 can have adverse effects on both the mother and fetus. Viremia occurs during the primary infection, and congenital infection is possible although rare. Primary infections during the first trimester have been associated with increased miscarriage rates. During pregnancy, the use of acyclovir and valacyclovir after 36 weeks' gestation may reduce the recurrence rate and thus the need for a Caesarean birth; the use of medication has not been shown to reduce the risk of maternal–child transmission (Money et al., 2008; PHAC, 2008a). Because neonatal HSV infection is such a devastating disease, prevention is critical.

Group B Streptococcus (GBS). It is recommended that all women be screened at 36 to 37 weeks of gestation for GBS using a rectovaginal culture. GBS may be considered a normal vaginal flora in a woman who is not pregnant. It is present in 9 to 23% of healthy pregnant women. However, GBS infection is associated with poor pregnancy outcomes. GBS infections are an important factor in perinatal and neonatal morbidity and mortality, usually resulting from vertical transmission from the birth canal of the infected mother to the infant during birth.

Other Tests

Other diagnostic tests are available to assess the health status of both the pregnant woman and the fetus. For example, ultrasound may be performed to determine the status of the pregnancy. Fetal nuchal translucency screening uses ultrasound measurement of fluid in the nape of the fetal neck between 10 and 14 weeks of gestation to identify possible fetal abnormalities (see Fig. 12-1). Chorionic villus sampling or amniocentesis may be needed to evaluate the fetus for genetic disorders or gestational maturity. These and other tests used to determine health risks for the mother and infant are described in Chapter 12.

Nursing Care Management

Because of the large number of health care providers involved in care of the expectant mother, unintentional gaps or overlaps in care may occur. To better coordinate prenatal care services for childbearing families, a care path can be used to improve consistency of care and reduce costs. It can also guide health care providers in carrying out the appropriate assessments and interventions in a timely way. Use of care paths also can contribute to improved satisfaction of families with the prenatal care provided, and members of the health care team may function more efficiently and effectively.

Education About Maternal and Fetal Changes

The expectant mother needs information on many topics. Expectant parents typically are curious about the growth and development of the fetus, the consequent changes that occur in the mother's body, and how to cope with changes. Mothers may be more tolerant of the discomforts related to the continuing pregnancy if they understand the underlying causes. The nurse who is observant, listens, and knows typical concerns of expectant parents can anticipate what questions will be asked and prompt mothers and their partners to discuss what is on their minds. The nurse can also offer printed literature to supplement the individualized teaching that he or she provides; women often avidly read books and pamphlets related to their own experience. When nurses read the literature before distributing it, they have an opportunity to point out areas that may not correspond with local health care practices. To be most effective, the material must reflect the pregnant woman's or couple's ethnicity, culture, and literacy level and the agency's resources. It is important to include family members in health education. As more individuals use the computer for information, the pregnant woman or couple may have questions from their Internet reviews. Nurses can share recommended Web sites from reliable sources.

Patients who receive conflicting advice or instruction are likely to grow frustrated with members of the health care team and the care provided. Several topics that may cause concern in pregnant women are discussed in the following sections.

Nutrition

Good nutrition is important in the maintenance of maternal health during pregnancy and in the provision of adequate nutrients for embryonic and fetal development. Assessing a woman's nutritional status and weight gain and providing information on nutrition are part of the nurse's responsibilities in providing prenatal care. Teaching may include discussion about foods high in iron, encouragement to take prenatal vitamins, and recommendations to limit caffeine intake. In some settings, a registered dietitian conducts classes for pregnant women on the topics of nutritional status and nutrition during pregnancy or interviews them to assess their knowledge of these topics. Nurses can refer women to a registered dietitian if a need is revealed during the nursing assessment. (For detailed information on maternal and fetal nutritional needs and related nursing care, see Chapter 11.)

Personal Hygiene

During pregnancy, the sebaceous (sweat) glands are highly active because of hormonal influences, and women often perspire freely. They may be reassured that the increase is normal and that their previous patterns of perspiration will return after the postpartum period. Baths and warm showers can be therapeutic because they relax tense, tired muscles; help counter insomnia; and make the pregnant woman feel fresh. Tub bathing is permitted even in late pregnancy because little water enters the vagina unless under pressure. However, the temperature of the water should not be higher than 39°C as this will increase the woman's core body temperature and can cause postural hypotension. Hot tubs should also be avoided for this reason. Tub bathing after rupture of the membranes needs to be carefully monitored and may be contraindicated in some women.

Prevention of Urinary Tract Infection

Because of physiological changes that occur in the renal system during pregnancy (see Chapter 9), urinary tract infections are common, but they may be asymptomatic. Women should be instructed to inform their health care provider if blood or pain occurs with urination. These infections pose a risk to the mother and fetus, mainly through increasing rates of preterm labour; thus their prevention or early treatment is essential.

The nurse can assess the woman's understanding and use of good hand-washing techniques before and after urinating and the importance of wiping the perineum from front to back. Soft, absorbent toilet tissue, preferably white and unscented, should be used; harsh, scented, or printed toilet paper may cause irritation. Bubble bath or other bath oils should be avoided because these can irritate the urethra. Women should wear underpants and panty hose with a cotton crotch and avoid wearing tight-fitting slacks or jeans for long periods. Anything that allows a buildup of heat and moisture in the genital area can foster the growth of bacteria.

Some women do not consume enough fluid and food. After ascertaining the woman's food preferences, the nurse should advise the woman to drink at least 2 L (eight glasses) of liquid a day to maintain an adequate fluid intake that ensures frequent urination. Pregnant women should not limit fluids in an effort to reduce the frequency of urination. Women need to know that if urine looks dark (concentrated), they must increase their fluid intake. The consumption of yogourt and acidophilus milk can help prevent urinary tract and vaginal infections. Although drinking cranberry juice is often recommended, there is conflicting evidence regarding its effectiveness and the effective dose needed to prevent urinary tract infections.

The nurse should review healthy urination practices with the woman. Women should be told not to ignore the urge to urinate, because holding urine lengthens the time bacteria are in the bladder and allows them to multiply. Women should plan ahead when faced with situations that may normally require them to delay urination (e.g., a long car ride). They should always urinate before going to bed at night. Bacteria also can be introduced during intercourse. Therefore, women are advised to urinate before and after intercourse and to then drink a large glass of water to promote additional urination.

Kegel Exercises

Kegel exercises—deliberate contraction and relaxation of the pubococcygeus muscle—strengthen the muscles around the reproductive organs and improve muscle tone. Many women are not aware of the muscles of the pelvic floor until it is pointed out that these are the muscles used during urination and sexual intercourse and that they can be consciously controlled. The pelvic floor muscles encircle the vaginal outlet, and they need to be exercised. An exercised muscle can stretch and contract readily at birth. Practising pelvic muscle exercise during pregnancy also results in fewer complaints of urinary incontinence in late pregnancy and postpartum (see Chapter 4, Patient Teaching box).

Preparation for Breastfeeding the Newborn

Pregnant women are usually eager to discuss their plans for feeding the newborn. Breast milk is the food of choice, in part because breastfeeding is associated with a decreased incidence in perinatal morbidity and mortality. The Canadian Paediatric Society recommends exclusive breastfeeding for at least 6 months with continuation to 2 years or beyond. However, a deep-seated aversion to breastfeeding by the mother, the mother's need for certain medications, and certain medical complications such as active tuberculosis and newly diagnosed breast cancer are contraindications to breastfeeding. Although hepatitis B antigen has not been shown to be transmitted through breast milk, as an added precaution it is recommended that infants born to hepatitis B antigen–positive women receive hepatitis B vaccine and hepatitis B immune globulin shortly after birth. Nursing is discouraged in women who are HIV positive and live in developed countries, because of the risk of HIV transmission (Lawrence & Lawrence, 2011). Women who live in developing countries may be encouraged to exclusively breastfeed their infant, as the risk of obtaining HIV is less than the risk of severe gastroenteritis that may cause death.

A woman's decision about the method of infant feeding is made before pregnancy; thus it is essential to educate women of childbearing age about the benefits of breastfeeding. The woman and her partner are encouraged to decide what method of feeding is suitable for them; however, the benefits of breastfeeding should be emphasized. Once the couple has been given information about the advantages and disadvantages of breastfeeding and bottle-feeding, they can make an informed choice. Health care providers should support these decisions and provide any needed assistance.

Women with inverted nipples may need special consideration if they are planning to breastfeed, although research has shown that no treatment prenatally was the best treatment (Lawrence & Lawrence, 2011). The pinch test is done to determine whether the nipple is everted or inverted (Fig. 10-9). To perform the pinch test, the woman places her thumb and forefinger on her areola and presses inward gently. This action will cause her nipple either to stand erect or to invert. Most nipples will stand erect.

Exercises to break the adhesions that cause the nipple to invert do not work and may in fact cause uterine contractions (Lawrence & Lawrence, 2011). The use of breast shells, small plastic devices that fit over the nipple, by women with flat or inverted nipples is sometimes recommended but only with careful follow-up (Fig. 10-10). Breast shells exert a continuous, gentle pressure around the areola that pushes the nipple through a central opening in the inner shield. It is probably better to wait until the first few days after birth to assess for flat nipples (Lawrence & Lawrence, 2011).

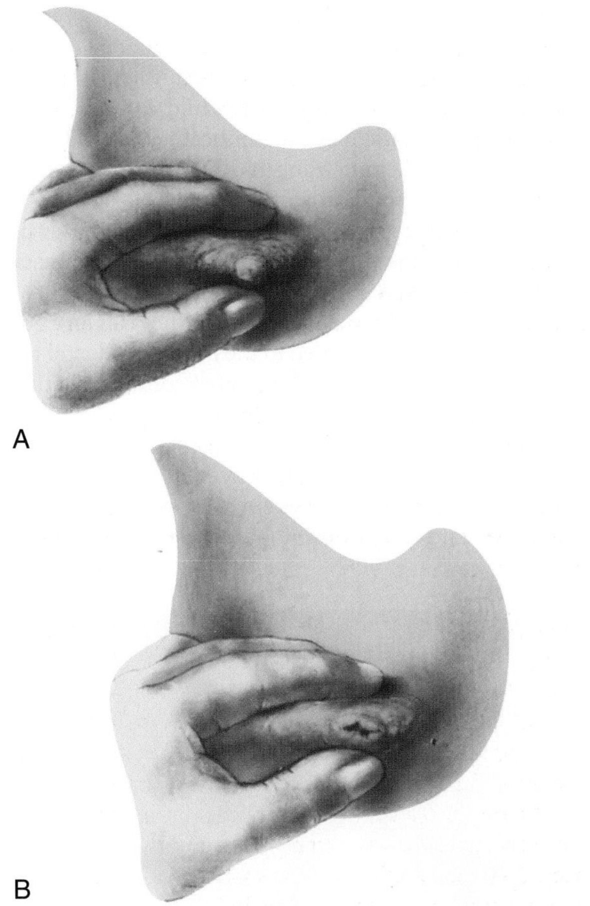

Fig. 10-9 Pinch test. **A:** Normal nipple everts with gentle pressure. **B:** Inverted nipple inverts with gentle pressure. *(Modified from Lawrence, R. A., & Lawrence, R. M. [2011].* Breastfeeding: A guide for the medical profession *[7th ed., p. 241]. St. Louis: Mosby.)*

The woman should be taught to cleanse the nipples with warm water to prevent blocking of the ducts with dried colostrum. Soap, ointments, alcohol, and tinctures should not be applied because they remove protective oils that keep nipples supple. The use of these substances may cause the nipple to crack during early lactation (Lawrence & Lawrence, 2011).

The woman who plans to breastfeed should purchase a nursing bra that will accommodate her increased breast size during the last few months of pregnancy and during lactation. If her breasts are very heavy or if the woman feels uncomfortable with the weight unsupported, the bra can be worn day and night. Some pregnant women may leak **colostrum** during the pregnancy and some may not. Whether this occurs does not relate to how much breast milk a mother will produce after the birth of the baby.

Dental Health

Dental care during pregnancy is especially important because nausea during pregnancy may lead to poor oral hygiene and allow dental **caries** to develop. Fluoride toothpaste should be used daily. Inflammation and infection of the gingival and periodontal tissues may occur. There is some evidence linking periodontal infections and preterm birth,

LBW (Lopez, 2005), and an increased risk for pre-eclampsia (Boggess et al., 2003).

Because calcium and phosphorus in the teeth are fixed in enamel, the old adage "for every child a tooth" is not true. There is no scientific evidence indicating that filling teeth or even dental extraction using local or nitrous oxide–oxygen anaesthesia causes miscarriage or premature labour. However, antibacterial therapy should be considered for sepsis, especially in pregnant women who have had rheumatic heart disease or nephritis. Emergency dental surgery is not contraindicated during pregnancy; however, the risks and benefits of surgery need to be explained to the mother. If dental treatment is necessary, the woman will be most comfortable during the second trimester.

Physical Activity

Physical activity promotes a feeling of well-being in the pregnant woman. It improves circulation, promotes relaxation and rest, and counteracts boredom, as it does in the nonpregnant woman. Women should be advised that adverse pregnancy or neonatal outcomes are not increased for exercising women (Davies et al., 2003). Detailed exercise tips for pregnancy are presented in the Home Care box on next page.

Exercises that help relieve the low back pain that often arises during the second trimester because of the increased weight of the fetus are demonstrated in Fig. 10-11.

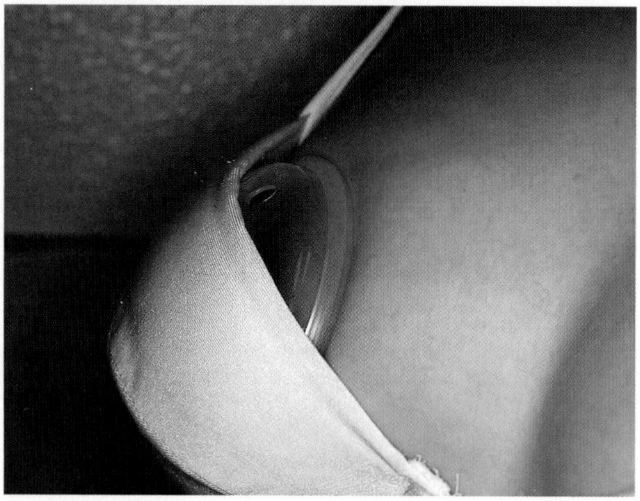

Fig. 10-10 Breast shell in place inside bra to evert nipple. *(Courtesy Michael S. Clement, MD, Mesa, AZ.)*

Posture and Body Mechanics

Skeletal, musculature, and hormonal changes (relaxin) in pregnancy can predispose the woman to backache and possible injury. As pregnancy progresses, the pregnant woman's centre of gravity changes, pelvic joints soften and relax, and stress is placed on abdominal musculature. Poor posture and body mechanics contribute to the discomfort and potential for injury (see Patient Teaching box). To minimize these problems, women can learn good body posture and body mechanics (Fig. 10-12). The activities described in the Home Care box, p. 226, can also promote greater physical comfort.

Rest and Relaxation

The pregnant woman is encouraged to plan regular rest periods, particularly as pregnancy advances. The side-lying position is recommended to promote uterine perfusion and fetoplacental oxygenation by eliminating pressure on the ascending vena cava and descending aorta, which can lead to supine hypotension (Fig. 10-13). Lying on the left side allows for the most blood flow through the uterus, although women should be taught that it acceptable to rest on either side. The mother should also be shown the way to rise slowly from a side-lying position, to prevent placing strain on the back and minimize the orthostatic hypotension caused by changes in position common in the latter part of pregnancy. To stretch and rest back muscles at home or at work, the woman can do the following exercises:

- While standing behind a chair, the woman supports and balances herself using the back of the chair (Fig. 10-14). She squats for 30 seconds and then stands for 15 seconds. She should repeat this six times, in several sets per day, as needed.

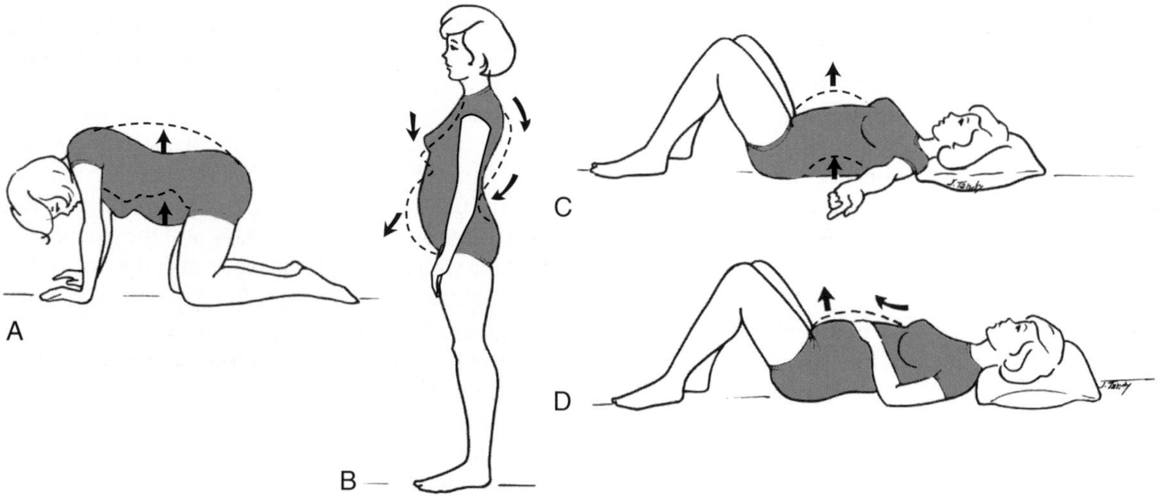

Fig. 10-11 Exercises to relieve back pain. **A** to **C**: Pelvic rocking relieves low backache (excellent for relief of menstrual cramps as well). **D**: Abdominal breathing aids relaxation and lifts the abdominal wall off the uterus.

HOME CARE

Exercise Tips for Pregnant Women

Participate in Aerobic and Strength-Conditioning Exercises

- You can do this as part of a healthy lifestyle during pregnancy as long as you are not considered high risk. When starting an aerobic exercise program, previously sedentary women should begin with 15 minutes of continuous exercise three times a week, increasing gradually to 30-minute sessions four times a week.

Maintain a Good Fitness Level Throughout Pregnancy

- Do this in moderation; do not try to reach peak fitness or train for an athletic competition. Elite athletes who continue to train during pregnancy require supervision by an obstetrical care provider with knowledge of the impact of strenuous exercise on maternal and fetal outcomes.

Perform Warm-Up and Stretching Exercises

- These exercises prepare your joints for more strenuous exercise and lessen the likelihood of strain or injury to your joints. After the fourth month of gestation, you should not perform exercises flat on your back.

Monitor the Intensity of Exercise

- You should be able to converse easily while exercising. If you cannot, you need to slow down.

Include a Cool-Down Period

- You need some mild activity involving your legs after an exercise period to help bring your respiration, heart, and metabolic rates back to normal and prevent the pooling of blood in the exercised muscles.

Choose Activities That Will Minimize the Risk of Loss of Balance and Fetal Trauma

Avoid Risky Activities

- Activities such as surfing, mountain climbing, skydiving, and racquetball require precise balance and coordination and thus may be dangerous. Avoid activities that require holding your breath and bearing down (Valsalva manoeuvre). Jerky, bouncy motions also should be avoided.
- Avoid downhill snow skiing, because the centre of gravity changes and there is risk of falls; contact sports such as ice hockey, soccer, and basketball; and scuba diving, because the pressure from the water could put the baby at risk for decompression sickness.

Avoid Becoming Overheated for Extended Periods of Time

- It is best not to exercise for more than 35 minutes, especially in hot, humid weather. As your body temperature rises, the heat is transmitted to your fetus.

Do Not Use Hot Tubs and Saunas

Drink Two or Three 250-mL Glasses of Water After You Exercise

- After you exercise you need to replace the body fluids lost through perspiration. While exercising, drink water whenever you feel the need.

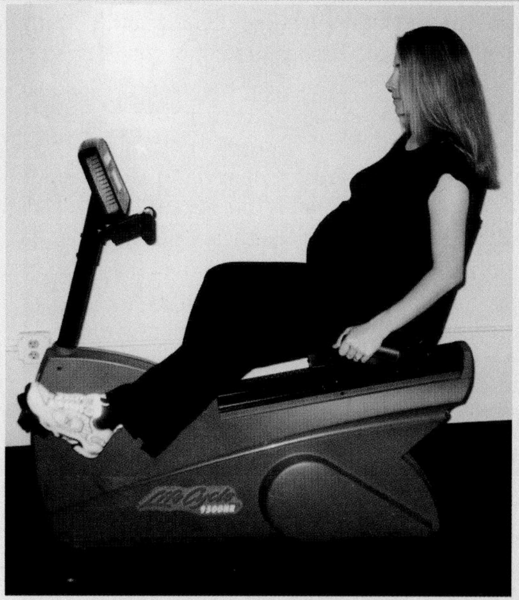

Riding a recumbent bicycle provides exercise while supplying back support. *(Courtesy Shannon Perry, Phoenix, AZ.)*

Take Your Time

- This is not the time to be competitive or train for activities requiring speed or long endurance.

Wear a Supportive Bra

- Your increased breast weight may cause changes in posture and put pressure on the ulnar nerve.

Wear Supportive Shoes

- As your uterus grows, your centre of gravity shifts, and you compensate for this by arching your back. These natural changes may make you feel off balance and more likely to fall.

Stop Exercising Immediately Upon Experiencing Warning Signs

- If you experience shortness of breath, chest pain, dizziness, painful uterine contraction, vaginal bleeding, or leakage of amniotic fluid, you should stop exercising immediately and consult your health care provider.

(Sources: American Congress of Obstetricians and Gynecologists [ACOG]. [2003]. Exercise during pregnancy, ACOG Education Pamphlet; Baby Center Australia [n.d.]. *Exercises recommended throughout pregnancy*. Retrieved from http://www.babycenter.com.au/pregnancy/fitness/recommendedexercises; *Exercise during pregnancy: Signs of danger*. Retrieved from http://www.babycenter.com.au/pregnancy/fitness/dangersigns/; *Fitness and exercise in pregnancy*. Retrieved from http://www.babycenter.com.au/pregnancy/fitness; Davies, G. A., et al. [2003]. SOGC/CSEP joint clinical practice guideline: Exercise in pregnancy and the postpartum period. *Journal of Obstetrics and Gynaecology Canada, 25*[6], 516–522.)

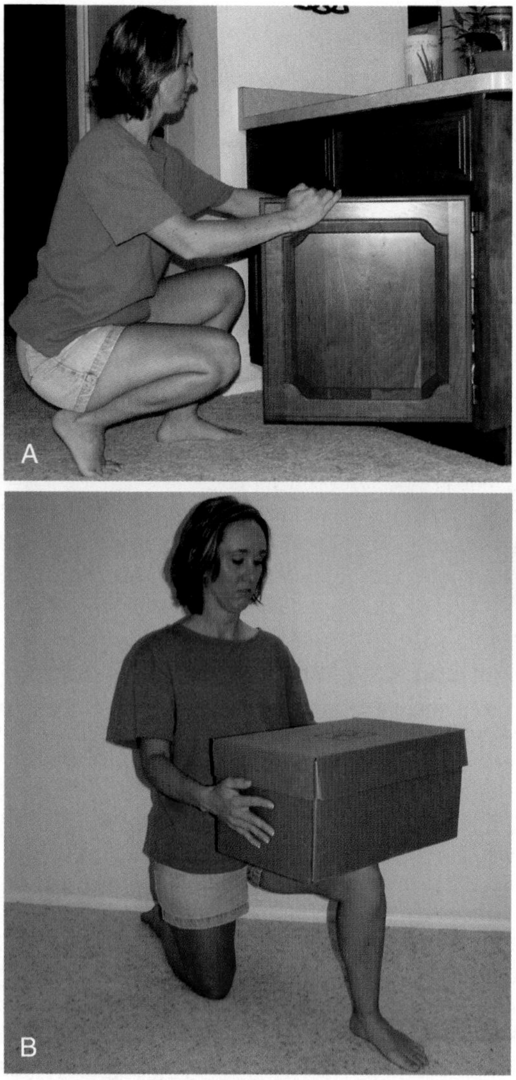

Fig. 10-12 Correct body mechanics. A: Squatting. B: Lifting. *(Courtesy Julie Perry Nelson, Loveland, CO.)*

HOME CARE

Posture and Body Mechanics

To Prevent or Relieve Backache

- Do pelvic tilt:
  - Pelvic tilt (rock) on hands and knees (see Fig. 10-11, A) and while sitting in straight-back chair.
  - Pelvic tilt (rock) in standing position against a wall or lying on floor (see Fig. 10-11, B and C).
  - Perform abdominal muscle contractions during pelvic tilt while standing, lying, or sitting to help strengthen rectus abdominis muscle (see Fig. 10-11, D).
  - Use good body mechanics.
  - Use hot water bottle or ice packs intermittently on back to relieve discomfort.
  - Use leg muscles to reach objects on or near floor. Bend at the knees, not the back. Knees are bent to lower body to squatting position. Keep feet shoulder width apart to provide a solid base to maintain balance (see Fig. 10-12, A).
  - Lift with the legs. To lift a heavy object (e.g., young child), place one foot slightly in front of the other and keep it flat as you lower yourself onto one knee. Lift the weight, holding it close to your body and never higher than the chest. To stand up or sit down, place one leg slightly behind the other as you raise or lower yourself (see Fig. 10-12, B).

To Restrict the Lumbar Curve

- For prolonged standing (e.g., ironing or because of employment), place one foot on low footstool or box; change positions often.
- Move car seat forward so that knees are bent and higher than hips. If needed, use a small pillow to support low back area.
- Sit in chairs low enough to allow both feet to be placed on floor, preferably with knees higher than hips.

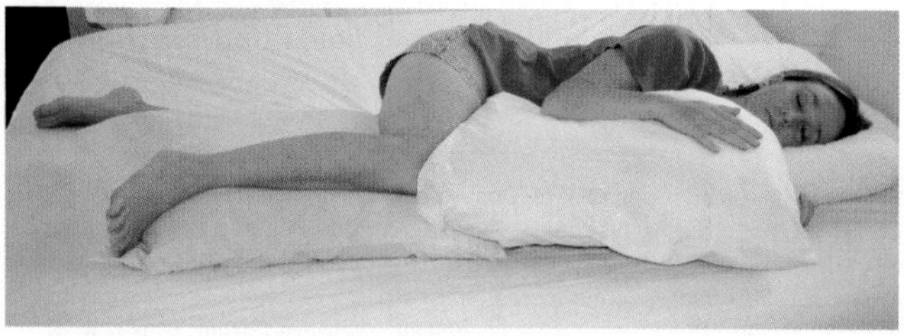

Fig. 10-13 Side-lying position for rest and relaxation. *(Courtesy Julie Perry Nelson, Loveland, CO.)*

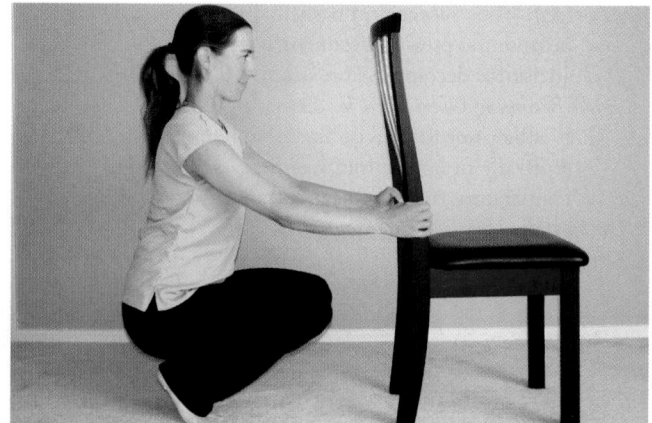

Fig. 10-14 Squatting for muscle relaxation and strengthening and for keeping leg and hip joints flexible. *(Courtesy Julie Perry Nelson, Loveland, CO.)*

- While sitting in a chair, the woman lowers her head to her knees for 30 seconds and then raises her head. She should repeat this six times, several times per day, as needed.

Conscious relaxation is the process of releasing tension from the mind and body through deliberate effort and practice. The ability to relax consciously and intentionally can be beneficial for the following reasons:

- To relieve the normal discomforts related to pregnancy
- To reduce stress and diminish pain perception during the childbearing cycle
- To heighten self-awareness and trust in one's own ability to control responses and functions
- To help cope with stress in everyday life situations, whether the woman is pregnant or not

The techniques for conscious relaxation are numerous and varied. The guidelines given in Box 10-5 can be used by anyone.

Employment

Employment of pregnant women usually has no adverse effects on pregnancy outcomes. Job discrimination that is based solely on pregnancy is illegal. However, some job environments pose potential risk to the fetus (e.g., dry cleaning plants, chemical laboratories, and parking garages). Excessive fatigue is usually the deciding factor in the termination of employment. Strategies to improve safety during pregnancy are described in the Patient Teaching box.

Women in sedentary jobs need to walk around at intervals to counter the sluggish circulation in the legs. They should neither sit nor stand in one position for long periods of time. They should avoid crossing their legs at the knees because this can foster the development of varices and thrombophlebitis. Standing for long periods also increases the risk of preterm labour. The pregnant woman's chair should provide adequate back support. Use of a footstool can prevent pressure on veins, relieve strain on varicosities, minimize swelling of feet, and prevent backache.

Clothing

Some women continue to wear their usual clothes during pregnancy as long as they fit and feel comfortable. If maternity clothing is needed, outfits may be purchased new or found in good condition at thrift shops or garage sales. Comfortable, loose clothing is best. Tight bras and belts, stretch pants, garters, tight-top knee socks, body shapers, and other constrictive clothing should be avoided because tight clothing over the perineum encourages vaginitis and miliaria (heat rash), and impaired circulation in the legs can cause varicosities.

Maternity bras are constructed to accommodate the increased breast weight, chest circumference, and size of breast tail tissue (under the arm). These bras have drop-flaps over the nipples to facilitate breastfeeding. A good bra can help prevent neck ache and backache.

Maternity support hose give considerable comfort and promote greater venous emptying in women with large varicose veins. Ideally, support stockings should be put on before the woman gets out of bed in the morning. Figure 10-15 demonstrates a position for resting the legs and reducing swelling.

BOX 10-5 Conscious Relaxation Tips

Preparation—Loosen clothing, assume a comfortable sitting or side-lying position with all parts of body well supported with pillows. The use of soothing music is optional.

Beginning—Allow yourself to feel warm and comfortable. Inhale and exhale slowly and imagine peaceful relaxation coming over each part of the body, starting with the neck and working down to the toes. People who learn conscious relaxation often speak of feeling relaxed even if some discomfort is present.

Maintenance—Use imagery (fantasy or daydream) to maintain the state of relaxation. Using active imagery, imagine yourself moving or doing some activity and experiencing its sensations. Using passive imagery, imagine yourself watching a scene such as a lovely sunset.

Awakening—Return to the wakeful state gradually. Slowly begin to take in stimuli from the surrounding environment.

Further retention and development of the skill—Practise regularly for some periods each day (e.g., at the same hour for 10 to 15 minutes each day to feel refreshed, revitalized, and invigorated).

PATIENT TEACHING Safety During Pregnancy

Changes in the body caused by pregnancy include relaxation of joints, alteration to the centre of gravity, faintness, and discomforts. Problems with coordination and balance are common. Therefore, the woman should follow these guidelines:

- Use good body mechanics.
- Use safety features on tools and vehicles (safety seat belts, shoulder harnesses, headrests, goggles, helmets) as specified.
- Avoid activities requiring coordination, balance, and concentration.
- Take rest periods; reschedule daily activities to meet rest and relaxation needs.

Embryonic and fetal development are vulnerable to environmental teratogens. Many potentially dangerous chemicals are present in the home, yard, and workplace: cleaning agents, paints, sprays, herbicides, and pesticides. The soil and water supply may be unsafe. Therefore, the woman should follow these guidelines:

- Read all labels for ingredients and proper use of product.
- Ensure adequate ventilation with clean air.
- Dispose of wastes appropriately.
- Wear gloves when handling chemicals.
- Change job assignments or workplace as necessary.
- Avoid high altitudes (not in pressurized aircraft), which could jeopardize oxygen intake.

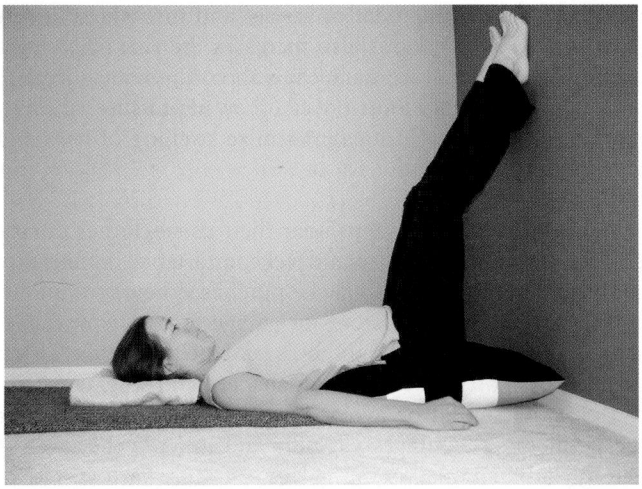

Fig. 10-15 Position for resting legs and reducing edema and varicosities. Encourage the woman with vulvar varicosities to include a pillow under her hips. *(Courtesy Julie Perry Nelson, Loveland, CO.)*

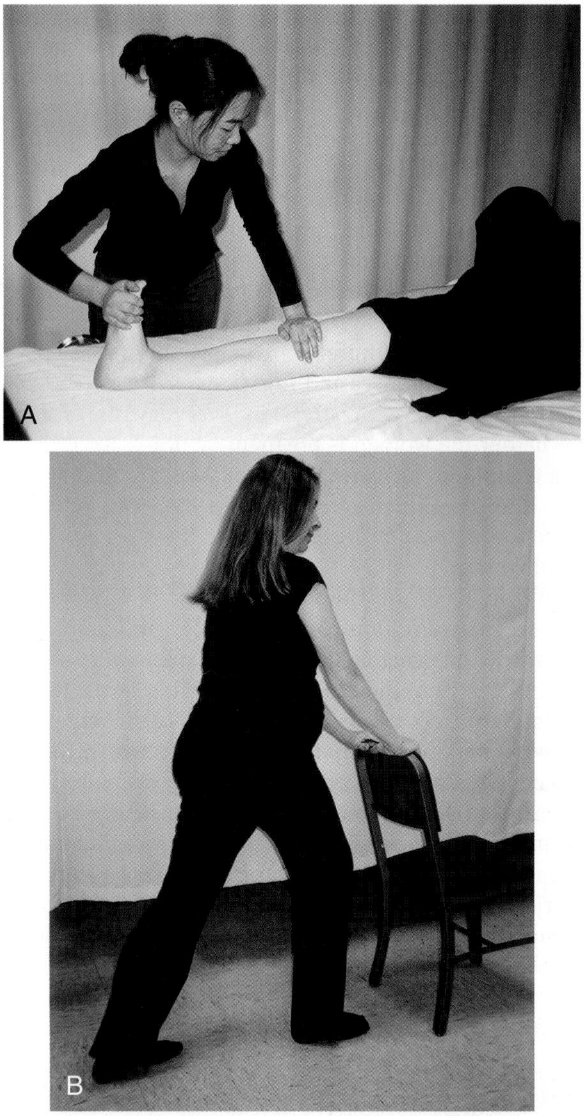

Fig. 10-16 Relief of muscle spasm (leg cramps). **A:** Another person dorsiflexes foot with the knee extended. **B:** Woman stands and leans forward, thereby dorsiflexing foot of the affected leg. *(Courtesy Shannon Perry, Phoenix, AZ.)*

Comfortable shoes that provide firm support and promote good posture and balance are advisable. Very high heels and platform shoes are not recommended because of the woman's changed centre of gravity, which can cause her to lose her balance. In addition, the woman's pelvis tilts forward in the third trimester, increasing her lumbar curve. The resulting leg aches and cramps will be aggravated by shoes that do not provide good support. Figure 10-16 shows exercises to relieve leg cramps.

Travel

Travel is not contraindicated for low-risk pregnant women. Women with high-risk pregnancies are advised to avoid long-distance travel after fetal viability has been reached, to avert the economic and psychological consequences of giving birth to a preterm infant far from home. Travel to areas where medical care is poor, water is untreated, and malaria is prevalent should be avoided if possible. Women who contemplate foreign travel should be aware that some provincial health insurance plans may not cover all expenses for birth in a foreign setting or even hospitalization for preterm labour. In addition, vaccinations for foreign travel may be contraindicated during pregnancy.

Pregnant women who travel for long distances should schedule periods of activity and rest. While sitting, the woman can practise deep breathing, foot circling, and alternately contracting and relaxing different muscle groups. She should avoid becoming fatigued. Although travel in itself is not a cause of adverse outcomes such as miscarriage or preterm labour, certain precautions are recommended when travelling in a car. For example, when riding in a car, the pregnant woman should wear seatbelts and stop and walk every hour.

Maternal death as a result of injury is the most common cause of fetal death. The next most common cause is placental separation (abruptio placentae) that occurs because body contours change in reaction to the force of a collision. The uterus as a muscular organ can adapt its shape to that of the body, but the placenta is not resilient. At the impact of collision, placental separation can occur. The lap belt should be worn low across the hip bones and as snug as is comfortable (Fig. 10-17). The shoulder harness should be worn above the gravid uterus and below the neck to prevent chafing. The pregnant woman should sit upright. The headrest should be used to avoid whiplash injury.

Air travel in large commercial jets usually poses little risk to the pregnant woman, but policies regarding flight by pregnant women vary from airline to airline. The pregnant woman is advised to inquire about restrictions or recommendations from her carrier. Most health care providers allow air travel up to 36 weeks of gestation in women without medical or

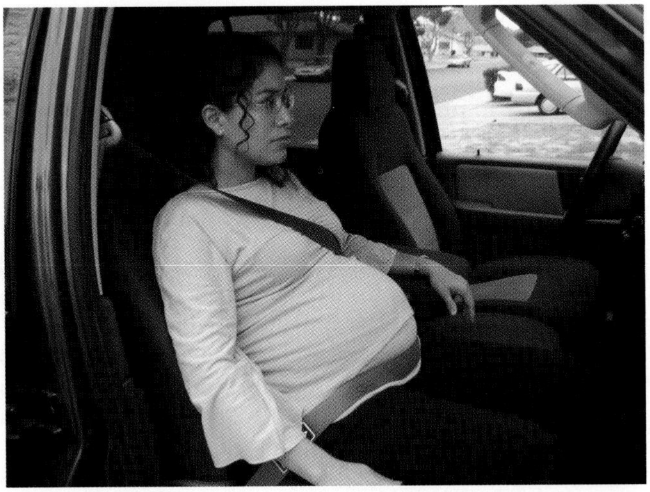

Fig. 10-17 Proper use of seat belt and headrest. *(Courtesy Brian and Mayannyn Sallee, Las Vegas, NV.)*

pregnancy complications. Magnetometers (metal detectors) used at airport security checkpoints are not harmful to the fetus. The 8% humidity at which cabins are maintained in commercial airlines may result in some water loss; hydration (with water) should be maintained under these conditions. Sitting in the cramped seat of an airliner for prolonged periods may increase the risk of superficial and deep thrombophlebitis. A pregnant woman is encouraged to take a 15-minute walk around the aircraft during each hour of travel to minimize this risk (see the Patient Teaching box earlier in this chapter). However, women who are pilots, flight attendants, or frequent flyers expose themselves to in-flight radiation that exceeds recommended levels (Barish, 2004). It is recommended that pregnant women not fly more than 200 hours during their pregnancy (Health Canada, 2007). Resources from Health Canada, Radiation Protection Bureau can assist the health care provider in determining safe levels for women at high risk for radiation exposure.

Medications and Herbal Preparations

Although much has been learned in recent years about fetal drug toxicity, the possible teratogenicity of many medications, both prescription and OTC, is still unknown. This is especially true for new medications and combinations of medications. Moreover, certain subclinical errors or deficiencies in intermediate metabolism in the fetus may cause an otherwise harmless medication to be converted into a hazardous one. The greatest danger of medication-caused developmental defects in the fetus extends from the time of fertilization through the first trimester, a time when the woman may not realize she is pregnant. Self-treatment must be discouraged. The use of all medications, including OTC medications, herbs, and vitamins, should be limited, and a careful record kept of all therapeutic and nontherapeutic agents used. If women have questions regarding certain medications, they can be directed to http://www.motherisk.org/women/index.jsp.

Immunizations

Some concern has been raised over the safety of various immunization practices during pregnancy. Immunization with live or attenuated live viruses is contraindicated during pregnancy because of potential teratogenicity. Live virus vaccines include those for measles (rubeola and rubella), chicken pox, mumps, and the Sabin (oral) poliomyelitis vaccine (no longer used in the Canada). Vaccines consisting of killed viruses that may be administered during pregnancy include tetanus, diphtheria, recombinant hepatitis B, rabies vaccines, and most influenza vaccines. Pregnant women are strongly encouraged to receive yearly flu shots as it has been found that they are at higher risk for complications from influenza.

Alcohol, Cigarette Smoke, Caffeine, and Drugs

A safe level of alcohol consumption during pregnancy has not yet been established. Although the consumption of occasional alcoholic beverages may not be harmful to the mother or her developing embryo or fetus, complete abstinence is strongly advised (SOGC, 2010). Maternal **alcoholism** is associated with high rates of miscarriage and fetal alcohol spectrum disorder (FASD); the risk for miscarriage in the first trimester is dose related (three or more drinks per day). Growing evidence indicates that the pattern of drinking (frequency, timing, and duration), especially in the first trimester, is more predictive of fetal damage than is the amount. FASD includes fetal alcohol syndrome (FAS), partial fetal alcohol syndrome/disorder, and alcohol-related neurodevelopmental disabilities. An estimated 9 in every 1000 children are born with FASD (PHAC, 2005). Low birth weight, behavioural problems, and learning disabilities are some of the potential lifelong struggles facing individuals with FASD (see Chapter 28). Severe facial deformities of FASD occur at day 20 of conception when women may not even suspect that they are pregnant.

The Society of Obstetricians and Gynaecologists of Canada (SOGC) (2010) recommends that each pregnant woman be screened for alcohol use during pregnancy. Using a harm reduction approach, they recommend that screening involve a thorough history, motivational interviewing, specific questionnaires, and diagnostic testing, bearing in mind that the woman has a right to refuse laboratory testing.

The SOGC (2010) states that one or two interview questions about alcohol use is an effective way to screen women and identify women who require further education or intervention. Questions may include the following:

- When was the last time you had a drink?
- Do you ever enjoy a drink or two?
- Do you sometimes drink beer, wine, or other alcoholic beverages?
- Do you ever use alcohol?
- In the past month or two, have you ever enjoyed a drink or two?

If a woman indicates that she does not consume alcohol, then positive reinforcement is beneficial. Research has shown that brief interventions can be very useful in helping a pregnant woman who drinks low to moderate amounts of alcohol to reduce her alcohol intake during pregnancy. If a woman identifies that she requires further intervention, a more in-depth assessment of drinking practices is necessary (SOGC, 2010). Several tools that are useful for this include the TWEAK, T-ACE, and CRAFFT tools, described in the SOGC

Clinical Practice Guideline: Alcohol Use and Pregnancy Clinical Consensus Guidelines (http://www.sogc.org/guidelines/documents/gui245CPG1008E.pdf).

Cigarette smoking or continued exposure to secondhand smoke (even if the mother does not smoke) is associated with IUGR and an increase in perinatal and infant morbidity and mortality. Smoking is associated with an increased frequency of preterm labour, PROM, abruptio placentae, placenta previa, and fetal death, possibly resulting from decreased placental perfusion (Niebyl & Simpson, 2007). Smoking-cessation activities should be incorporated into routine prenatal care.

In Canada, 10% of women reported smoking daily or occasionally during the last three months of pregnancy although this varied greatly by province (PHAC, 2009). All women who smoke should be strongly encouraged to quit or at least reduce the number of cigarettes they smoke (see Critical Thinking Exercise). Pregnant women need to be told about the negative effects of secondhand smoke on the fetus and encouraged to avoid such environments. Efforts focused on preventing girls and women from beginning to smoke should be intensified.

Most studies of human pregnancy have revealed no association between caffeine consumption and birth defects or LBW (Weng, Odouli, & Li, 2008). However, some studies have documented an increased risk for miscarriage with caffeine intake greater than 300 mg/day or fetal growth restriction with caffeine intake greater than 223 mg/day. Therefore, because other effects are unknown, pregnant women are advised to limit their caffeine intake to no more than 2 cups of coffee or cola per day (Health Canada, 2010).

Regarding use of street drugs, 6.7% of Canadian women reported using such drugs in the 3 months before pregnancy, with women ages 15 to 24 years having the highest incidence of use (PHAC, 2009). It is important to note that this statistic is likely to be much higher because of the risk of underreporting by women. Any drug or environmental agent that enters the pregnant woman's bloodstream has the potential to cross the placenta and harm the fetus. Marijuana, heroin, and cocaine are common examples of such substances. Although substance use in pregnancy is a major public health concern and comprehensive care of drug-addicted women improves maternal and neonatal outcomes, few facilities are available for treatment of these women.

evolve Critical Thinking Exercise—Discomforts of Pregnancy

evolve Case Study—Third Trimester

Normal Discomforts

Pregnant women are confronted with symptoms that would be considered abnormal in the nonpregnant state. Women pregnant for the first time have an increased need for explanations of the causes of the discomforts and advice on ways to relieve the discomforts. The discomforts are fairly specific to each trimester of pregnancy. Table 10-2 provides information about the physiology, prevention, and self-management of discomforts experienced during the three trimesters. Box 10-6 lists alternative therapies used in pregnancy. Nurses can do much to allay a first-time mother's anxiety about such symptoms by telling her about them in advance, using terminology that the woman (or couple) can understand. When the woman understands the rationale for treatment, she is more likely to participate in her care. Interventions should be individualized, with attention given to the woman's lifestyle and culture.

NURSING ALERT Although complementary and alternative therapies may benefit the woman during pregnancy, some practices should be avoided because they may cause miscarriage or preterm labour. It is important to ask the woman what therapies she may be using.

Recognizing Potential Complications

One of the most important responsibilities of care providers is to alert the pregnant woman to signs and symptoms that indicate a potential complication of pregnancy. The woman needs to know how and to whom such warning signs should be reported (see Box 10-4). It is difficult to remember specifics when stressed by a disturbing symptom. Therefore, it is

CRITICAL THINKING EXERCISE

Smoking Cessation During Pregnancy

Doreen is a 25-year-old who is 8 weeks pregnant. At her first prenatal visit a history is taken; she reports that she smokes about half a pack of cigarettes a day. She says she knows that she should probably try to cut down, but she has been smoking since she was 15. She has tried to quit smoking before and has not been successful. How would you respond to her statement?

1. Evidence—Is there sufficient evidence to draw conclusions about what the nurse should say?
2. Assumptions—What assumptions can be made about the following issues?
   a. Effects of smoking on pregnancy
   b. Cessation interventions for pregnant women
3. What implications and priorities for nursing care can be made at this time?
4. Does the evidence objectively support your conclusion?
5. Are there alternative perspectives to your conclusion?

BOX 10-6 Alternative Therapies Used in Pregnancy

Touch and Energetic Therapies

Massage
Acupressure
Therapeutic touch
Healing touch

Mind–Body Healing

Imagery
Meditation, prayer, reflection
Biofeedback
Other modalities that may fall outside of nurse practice guidelines unless the nurse has completed additional training or certification:

- Herbs
- Homeopathy
- Traditional Chinese medicine

Table 10-2 Discomforts Related to Pregnancy

DISCOMFORT	PHYSIOLOGY	EDUCATION FOR SELF-MANAGEMENT
First Trimester		
Breast changes, new sensation; pain, tingling, tenderness	Hypertrophy of mammary glandular tissue and increased vascularization, pigmentation, and size and prominence of nipples and areolae caused by hormonal stimulation	Wear supportive maternity bras with pads to absorb discharge (may be worn at night); wash with warm water and keep dry; breast tenderness may interfere with sexual expression and foreplay but is temporary
Urgency and frequency of urination: often noted in third trimester as well	Vascular engorgement and altered bladder function caused by hormones; bladder capacity reduced by enlarging uterus and fetal presenting part	Empty bladder regularly; perform Kegel exercises; limit fluid intake before bedtime; wear perineal pad; report pain or burning sensation to primary health care provider
Languor and malaise; fatigue (early pregnancy, most commonly)	Unexplained; may be caused by increasing levels of estrogen, progesterone, and hCG or by elevated BBT; psychological response to pregnancy and its required physical/psychological adaptations	Rest as needed; eat well-balanced diet to prevent anemia
Nausea and vomiting, morning sickness—occurs in 50–75% of pregnant women; starts between first and second missed periods and lasts until about fourth missed period; may occur any time during day; fathers also may have symptoms	Cause is unknown; may result from hormonal changes, possibly hCG; may be partly emotional, reflecting pride in, ambivalence about, or rejection of pregnant state	Avoid empty or overloaded stomach; maintain good posture—give stomach ample room; stop smoking; eat dry carbohydrate on awakening; remain in bed until feeling subsides or alternate dry carbohydrate 1 hr with fluids such as hot herbal decaffeinated tea, milk, or clear coffee the next hour until feeling subsides; eat five to six small meals per day; avoid fried, odorous, spicy, greasy, or gas-forming foods; ginger supplementation, acupuncture, or acupressure may be beneficial (SOGC, 2002); consult primary health care provider if intractable vomiting occurs (medication may be prescribed)
Ptyalism (excessive salivation) may occur starting 2–3 wk after first missed period	Possibly caused by elevated estrogen levels; may be related to reluctance to swallow because of nausea	Use astringent mouthwash, chew gum, eat hard candy as comfort measures
Gingivitis and epulis (hyperemia, hypertrophy, bleeding, tenderness); condition disappears spontaneously 1–2 mo after birth: often noted throughout pregnancy	Increased vascularity and proliferation of connective tissue from estrogen stimulation	Eat well-balanced diet, with adequate protein and fresh fruits and vegetables; brush teeth gently and observe good dental hygiene; avoid infection; see dentist
Nasal stuffiness; epistaxis (nosebleed)	Hyperemia of mucous membranes related to high estrogen levels	Use humidifier; avoid trauma; normal saline nose drops or spray may be used
Leukorrhea: often noted throughout pregnancy	Hormonally stimulated cervix becomes hypertrophic and hyperactive, producing abundant amount of mucus	Not preventable; do not douche; wear perineal pads; perform hygienic practices such as wiping front to back; report to primary health care provider if accompanied by pruritus, foul odour, or change in character or colour
Psychosocial dynamics, mood swings, mixed feelings	Hormonal and metabolic adaptations; feelings about female role, sexuality, timing of pregnancy, and resultant changes in life and lifestyle	Participate in pregnancy support group; communicate concerns to partner, family, and others; request referral for supportive services if needed (financial assistance)
Second Trimester		
Pigmentation deepens, acne, oily skin	Melanocyte-stimulating hormone (from anterior pituitary)	Not preventable; it usually resolves during puerperium
Spider nevi (angiomas) appear over neck, thorax, face, and arms during second or third trimester	Focal networks of dilated arterioles (end-arteries) from increased concentration of estrogens	Not preventable; they fade slowly during late puerperium but rarely disappear completely
Palmar erythema occurs in 50% of pregnant women; may accompany spider nevi	Diffuse reddish mottling over palms and suffused skin over thenar eminences and fingertips; may be caused by genetic predisposition or hyperestrogenism	Not preventable; condition fades within 1 wk after giving birth

Continued

Table 10-2 Discomforts Related to Pregnancy—cont'd

DISCOMFORT	PHYSIOLOGY	EDUCATION FOR SELF-MANAGEMENT
Pruritus (noninflammatory)	Unknown cause; various types as follows: nonpapular; closely aggregated pruritic papules Increased excretory function of skin and stretching of skin possible factors	Keep fingernails short and clean; contact primary health care provider for diagnosis of cause Not preventable; symptomatic; can be managed with Keri baths, mild sedation, distraction, tepid baths with sodium bicarbonate or oatmeal added to water, lotions and oils, change of soaps or reduction in use of soap, loose clothing
Palpitations	Unknown; should not be accompanied by persistent cardiac irregularity	Not preventable; contact primary health care provider if accompanied by symptoms of cardiac decompensation
Supine hypotension (vena cava syndrome) and bradycardia	Induced by pressure of gravid uterus on ascending vena cava when woman is supine; reduces uteroplacental and renal perfusion	Assume side-lying position or semisitting posture, with knees slightly flexed (see also Emergency box, p. 216)
Faintness and, rarely, syncope (orthostatic hypotension): may persist throughout pregnancy	Vasomotor lability or postural hypotension from hormones; in late pregnancy may be caused by venous stasis in lower extremities	Exercise moderately (deep breathing, vigorous leg movements); avoid sudden changes in position* and warm crowded areas; move slowly and deliberately; keep environment cool; avoid hypoglycemia by eating five to six small meals per day; wear elastic hose; sit as necessary; if symptoms are serious, contact primary health care provider
Food cravings	Cause unknown; craving determined by culture or geographic area	Not preventable; satisfy craving unless it interferes with well-balanced diet; report unusual cravings to primary health care provider
Heartburn (pyrosis or acid indigestion): burning sensation, occasionally with burping and regurgitation of a little sour-tasting fluid	Progesterone slows GI tract motility and digestion, reverses peristalsis, relaxes cardiac sphincter, and delays emptying time of stomach; stomach displaced upward and compressed by enlarging uterus	Limit or avoid gas-producing or fatty foods and large meals; maintain good posture; drink hot herbal tea; primary health care provider may prescribe antacid between meals; contact primary health care provider for persistent symptoms
Constipation	GI tract motility slowed because of progesterone, resulting in increased reabsorption of water and drying of stool; intestines compressed by enlarging uterus; predisposition to constipation because of oral iron supplementation	Drink six glasses of water per day; include roughage in diet; exercise moderately; maintain regular schedule for bowel movements; use relaxation techniques and deep breathing; do not take stool softener, laxatives, mineral oil, other medications, or enemas without first consulting primary health care provider
Flatulence with bloating and belching	Reduced GI motility because of hormones, allowing time for bacterial action that produces gas; swallowing air	Chew foods slowly and thoroughly; avoid gas-producing foods, fatty foods, large meals; exercise, maintain regular bowel habits
Varicose veins (varicosities): may be associated with aching legs and tenderness; may be present in legs and vulva; hemorrhoids are varicosities in perianal area	Hereditary predisposition; relaxation of smooth muscle walls of veins because of hormones causing tortuous dilated veins in legs and pelvic vasocongestion; condition aggravated by enlarging uterus, gravity, and bearing down for bowel movements; thrombi from leg varices are rare but may be produced by hemorrhoids	Avoid obesity, lengthy standing or sitting, constrictive clothing, and constipation and bearing down with bowel movements; exercise moderately; rest with legs and hips elevated (see Fig. 10-15); wear support stockings; thrombosed hemorrhoid may be evacuated; relieve swelling and pain with warm sitz baths; apply astringent compresses locally
Headaches (through wk 26)	Emotional tension (more common than vascular migraine headache); eye strain (refractory errors); vascular engorgement and congestion of sinuses resulting from hormone stimulation	Conscious relaxation; contact primary health care provider for constant "splitting" headache to assess for pre-eclampsia
Carpal tunnel syndrome (involves thumb, second and third fingers, lateral side of little finger)	Compression of median nerve resulting from changes in surrounding tissues; pain, numbness, tingling, burning; loss of skilled movements (typing); dropping of objects	Not preventable; elevate affected arms; splinting of affected hand may help; regressive after pregnancy; surgery is curative
Periodic numbness, tingling of fingers (acrodysesthesia) occurs in 5% of pregnant women	Brachial plexus traction syndrome resulting from drooping of shoulders during pregnancy (occurs especially at night and early morning)	Maintain good posture; wear supportive maternity bra; condition will disappear if lifting and carrying baby does not aggravate it

Table 10-2 Discomforts Related to Pregnancy—cont'd

DISCOMFORT	PHYSIOLOGY	EDUCATION FOR SELF-MANAGEMENT
Round ligament pain (tenderness)	Stretching of ligament caused by enlarging uterus	Not preventable; rest, maintain good body mechanics to avoid overstretching ligament; relieve cramping by squatting or bringing knees to chest; sometimes heat helps
Joint pain, backache, and pelvic pressure; hypermobility of joints	Relaxation of symphyseal and sacroiliac joints because of hormones, resulting in unstable pelvis; exaggerated lumbar and cervicothoracic curves caused by change in centre of gravity resulting from enlarging abdomen	Maintain good posture and body mechanics; avoid fatigue; wear low-heeled shoes; abdominal supports may be useful; practise conscious relaxation; sleep on firm mattress; apply local heat or ice; get back rubs; do pelvic rock exercise (see Fig. 10-11); rest; condition disappears 6–8 wk after birth
Third Trimester		
Shortness of breath and dyspnea: occur in 60% of pregnant women	Expansion of diaphragm limited by enlarging uterus; diaphragm elevated about 4 cm; some relief after lightening	Maintain good posture; sleep with extra pillows; avoid overloading stomach; stop smoking; contact health care provider if symptoms worsen, to rule out anemia, emphysema, and asthma
Insomnia (later weeks of pregnancy)	Fetal movements, muscle cramping, urinary frequency, shortness of breath, or other discomforts	Reassurance, conscious relaxation, back massage or effleurage, support of body parts with pillows, and warm milk or warm shower before retiring are helpful
Psychosocial responses: mood swings, mixed feelings, increased anxiety	Hormonal and metabolic adaptations; feelings about impending labour, birth, and parenthood	Reassurance and support from significant other and nurse and improved communication with partner, family, and others are helpful
Perineal discomfort and pressure	Pressure from enlarging uterus, especially when standing or walking; multifetal gestation	Rest, conscious relaxation, and good posture are helpful; contact health care provider for assessment and treatment if pain is present
Leg cramps (gastrocnemius spasm), especially when reclining	Compression of nerves supplying lower extremities because of enlarging uterus; reduced level of diffusible serum calcium or elevation of serum phosphorus; aggravating factors: fatigue, poor peripheral circulation, pointing toes when stretching legs or when walking, drinking more than 1 L of milk per day	Dorsiflex foot until spasm relaxes; use massage if not reddened or increased temperature at site (see Fig. 10-16, A); stand on cold surface; supplement orally with calcium carbonate or calcium lactate tablets; aluminum hydroxide gel, 30 mL, with each meal removes phosphorus by absorbing it; avoid pointing toes
Ankle edema (nonpitting) to lower extremities	Edema aggravated by prolonged standing, sitting, poor posture, lack of exercise, constrictive clothing, or hot weather	Intake ample fluid for natural diuretic effect; put on support stockings before arising; rest periodically with legs and hips elevated (see Fig. 10-15); exercise moderately; contact health care provider if generalized edema develops; diuretics are contraindicated

*Caution woman to rise slowly and sit on edge of bed or to assume hands-and-knees posture before rising and to get up slowly after sitting or squatting.
BBT, basal body temperature; *GI,* gastrointestinal; *hCG,* human chorionic gonadotropin.

important that the woman and her family receive a printed form written at the appropriate literacy level listing the signs and symptoms that warrant an investigation and the phone numbers to call with questions or in an emergency.

The nurse must answer questions honestly as they arise during pregnancy. Pregnant women often have difficulty deciding when to report signs and symptoms. The mother should be encouraged to refer to the printed list of potential complications and to listen to her body. If she senses that something is wrong, she should call her care provider immediately. Several signs and symptoms must be discussed more extensively. These include vaginal bleeding, alteration in fetal movements, symptoms of pre-eclampsia, rupture of membranes, and preterm labour.

Recognizing Preterm Labour

Teaching each expectant mother to recognize preterm labour is necessary for early diagnosis and treatment. Preterm labour occurs after the twentieth week but before the thirty-seventh week of pregnancy. It consists of uterine contractions that, if untreated, cause the cervix to open earlier than normal, resulting in preterm birth.

Although the exact etiology of preterm labour is unknown, it is assumed to have multiple causes. An increased incidence of preterm birth is associated with sociodemographic factors such as poverty, low educational level, lack of social support, smoking, intimate partner violence, and stress. Other risk factors include a previous preterm labour (McPheeters et al., 2005), current multifetal gestation, and some uterine

HOME CARE

How to Recognize Preterm Labour

Because the onset of preterm labour is subtle and often hard to recognize, it is important to know how to feel your abdomen for uterine contractions. You can feel for contractions in the following way:

- While lying down, place your fingertips on the top of your uterus. A contraction is the periodic tightening or hardening of your uterus. If your uterus is contracting, you will actually feel your abdomen get tight or hard and then feel it relax or soften when the contraction is over.
- If you think you are having any signs and symptoms of preterm labour (see below), empty your bladder, drink 3 to 4 glasses of water for hydration, lie down tilted toward your side, and place a pillow at your back for support.
- Check for contractions for 1 hour. To tell how often contractions are occurring, check the minutes that elapse from the beginning of one contraction to the beginning of the next.
- It is not normal to have frequent uterine contractions (every 10 minutes or more often for 1 hour).
- Contractions of labour are regular, frequent, and hard. They also may be felt as a tightening of the abdomen, a menstrual-like cramp, or a backache (see Fig. 10-18). This type of contraction causes the cervix to efface and dilate.
- Call your doctor, midwife, or labour and birth unit or go to the hospital if any of the following signs occur:
  - You have uterine contractions every 10 minutes or more often for 1 hour *or*
  - You feel pelvic pressure that is not relieved
  - You have any bloody spotting or leaking of fluid from your vagina
- It is often difficult to identify preterm labour. Accurate diagnosis requires assessment by the health care provider, usually in the hospital or clinic.

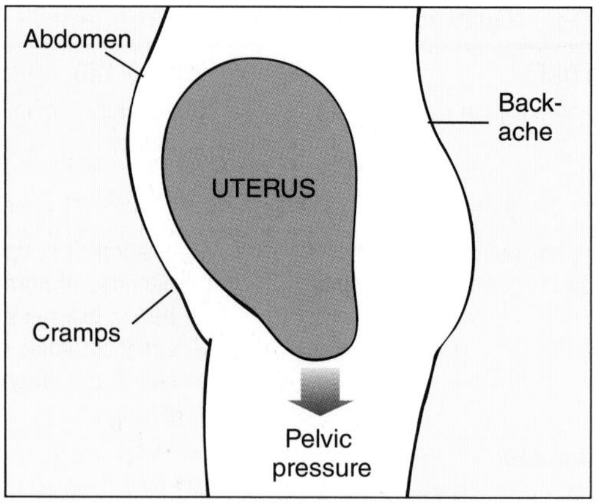

Fig. 10-18 Symptoms of preterm labour.

and cervical variations (March of Dimes Birth Defects Foundation, 2005).

If a woman knows the warning signs and symptoms of preterm labour and seeks care early enough, prevention of preterm birth may be possible. Warning signs and symptoms of preterm labour are given in the Home Care box. Figure 10-18 shows where in the body the signs and symptoms of preterm labour may be located.

Sex Counselling

Sex counselling of expectant couples includes countering misinformation, providing reassurance of normality, and suggesting alternative behaviours. The uniqueness of each couple is considered within a biopsychosocial framework (see Home Care box). Nurses can initiate discussion about sexual adaptations that must be made during pregnancy. They need a sound knowledge base about the physical, social, and emotional responses to sex during pregnancy. Not all perinatal nurses are comfortable dealing with the sexual concerns of their patients; nurses who are aware of their personal strengths and limitations in dealing with sexual content will be better prepared to make referrals, if necessary (Westheimer & Lopater, 2005).

As pregnancy progresses, changes in body shape, body image, and levels of discomfort influence both partners' desire for sexual expression. During the first trimester, the woman's sexual desire may decrease, especially if she has breast tenderness, nausea, fatigue, or sleepiness. As she progresses into the second trimester, her sense of well-being, combined with the increased pelvic congestion that occurs at this time, may increase her desire for sexual release. In the third trimester, somatic complaints and physical bulkiness may increase her physical discomfort and diminish her interest in sex.

Many women merely need "permission" to be sexually active during pregnancy. Other women need information about the physiological changes that occur during pregnancy and to have myths dispelled that are associated with sex during pregnancy. It may also be helpful for women to know about positions for intercourse that decrease pressure on the gravid abdomen (Westheimer & Lopater, 2005). All of these issues are within the purview of the perinatal nurse and should be an integral component of the health care provided.

Some couples need to be referred for sex or family therapy. Couples whose long-standing problems with sexual dysfunction are intensified by pregnancy are good candidates for sex therapy. When a sexual problem is a symptom of a more serious relationship problem, the couple may benefit from family therapy.

Countering Misinformation

Many myths and much of the misinformation related to sex and pregnancy are masked by seemingly unrelated issues. For example, a discussion about the baby's ability to hear and see in utero may be prompted by questions about the baby being an observer of lovemaking. The counsellor must be sensitive to the issues behind such questions when counselling in this highly charged emotional area.

HOME CARE

Sexuality in Pregnancy

- Be aware that maternal physiological changes such as breast enlargement, nausea, fatigue, abdominal changes, perineal enlargement, leukorrhea, pelvic vasocongestion, and orgasmic responses may affect sexuality and sexual expression.
- Discuss responses to pregnancy with your partner.
- Keep in mind that cultural prescriptions (do's) and proscriptions (don'ts) may affect your responses.
- Although your libido may be depressed during the first trimester, it often increases during the second and third trimesters.
- Discuss and explore the following with your partner:
  - Alternative behaviours (e.g., mutual masturbation, foot massage, cuddling).
  - Alternative positions (e.g., female superior, side-lying) for sexual intercourse.
- Intercourse is safe as long as it is not uncomfortable. There is no correlation between intercourse and miscarriage, but observe the following precautions:
  - Abstain from intercourse if you experience uterine cramping or vaginal bleeding; report event to your caregiver as soon as possible.
  - Abstain from intercourse (or any activity that results in orgasm) if you have a history of premature dilation of the cervix until the problem is corrected or if your membranes are ruptured.
- Continue to use risk reduction behaviours. Women at risk for acquiring or conveying sexually transmitted infections are encouraged to use condoms during sexual intercourse throughout pregnancy.

Suggesting Alternative Behaviours

Researchers have not demonstrated that, for the obstetrically and medically healthy woman, coitus and orgasm are contraindicated at any time during pregnancy (Cunningham et al., 2010). However, women with a history of more than one miscarriage; a threatened miscarriage in the first trimester; impending miscarriage in the second trimester; or premature rupture of membranes (PROM), bleeding, or abdominal pain during the third trimester should use caution regarding coitus and orgasm.

Solitary and mutual masturbation and oral–genital intercourse may be used by couples as alternatives to penile–vaginal intercourse. Partners who enjoy cunnilingus (oral stimulation of the clitoris or vagina) may feel "turned off" by the normal increase in amount and odour of vaginal discharge during pregnancy. Couples who practise cunnilingus should be cautioned against the blowing of air into the vagina, particularly during the last few weeks of pregnancy, when the cervix may be slightly open. An air embolism can occur if air is forced between the uterine wall and fetal membranes and enters the maternal vascular system through the placenta.

Showing the woman or couple illustrations of the possible variations of coital position can be helpful (Fig. 10-19). The female-superior, side-by-side, rear-entry, and facing-each-other positions are alternatives to the traditional male-superior position. The woman astride (superior position) allows her to control the angle and depth of penile penetration, as well as protect her breasts and abdomen. During the third trimester, the side-by-side position or any position that places less pressure on the pregnant abdomen and requires less energy may be preferred.

Multiparous women sometimes have significant breast tenderness in the first trimester. A coital position that avoids direct pressure on the woman's breasts and decreased breast fondling during love play can be recommended to such couples. The woman should also be reassured that this condition is normal and temporary.

Some women complain of lower abdominal cramping and backache after orgasm during the first and third trimesters. A back rub can often relieve some of the discomfort and provide a pleasant experience. A tonic uterine contraction, often lasting up to a minute, replaces the rhythmic contractions of orgasm during the third trimester. Changes in FHR without fetal distress have also been reported.

The objective of risk reduction is to provide prophylaxis against the acquisition and transmission of STIs (e.g., HSV, HPV, and HIV). Because these diseases may be transmitted to the woman and her fetus, the use of condoms is recommended throughout pregnancy if the woman is at risk for acquiring an STI.

Well-informed nurses who are comfortable with their own sexuality and the sex-counselling needs of expectant couples can offer information and advice in this valuable but often neglected area. They can establish an open environment in which couples can feel free to introduce their concerns about sexual adjustment and seek support and guidance. This intervention is as important for lesbian women and their partners as it is for women partnered with men.

Psychosocial Support

Esteem, affection, trust, concern, consideration of cultural and religious responses, and listening are all components of the emotional support that nurses can give to the pregnant woman and her family. The woman's satisfaction with her relationships and support, her feeling of competence, and her sense of being in control are all important issues to be addressed. A discussion of fetal responses to stimuli such as sound, light, maternal posture, and tension, as well as patterns of sleeping and waking, can be helpful. Other issues that can arise for the pregnant woman and couple include fear of pain, loss of control, and possible birth of the infant before reaching the hospital. Parental concerns about the responsibilities and tasks of parenthood; the safety of the mother and unborn child; siblings and their acceptance of the new baby; social and economic responsibilities; and possible conflicts in cultural, religious, or personal value systems should be addressed.

The father's or partner's commitment to the pregnancy, the couple's relationship, and their concerns about sexuality and

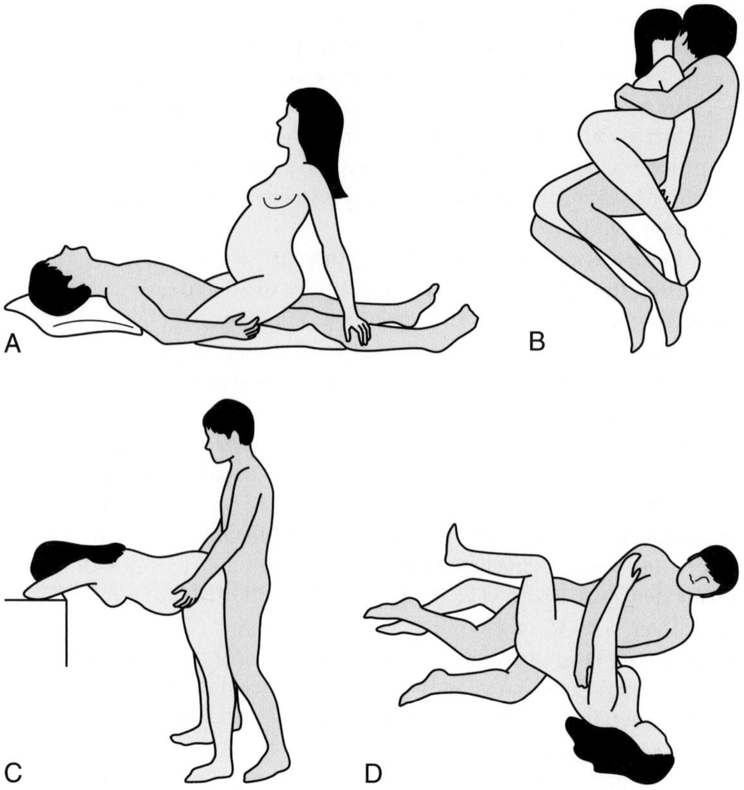

Fig. 10-19 Positions for sexual intercourse during pregnancy. **A:** Female superior. **B:** Side by side. **C:** Rear entry. **D:** Facing each other.

sexual expression can emerge as issues for many expectant parents.

By providing the prospective mother and father with opportunities to discuss their concerns and validating the normality of their responses, the perinatal nurse can meet their needs to some degree. Nurses must also recognize that men tend to feel more vulnerable during their partner's pregnancy. Female partners may also have these feelings. Anticipatory guidance and health promotion strategies can help partners cope with their concerns. Nursing intervention may help them to deal with such concerns either directly through counselling or indirectly through the education of the mothers. Health care providers can stimulate and encourage open dialogue between the couple.

All women should be assessed for depression and anxiety during pregnancy, and some provinces have adapted this into the routine care provided. The Edinburgh Postnatal Depression Scale (EPDS) has been found to be useful as a screening tool (see Fig. 22-6). If women are identified as having depression or anxiety during the pregnancy, it is important that they receive treatment. If left untreated, there can be serious implications to both the mother and child (BC Reproductive Care Program, 2003).

Variations in Prenatal Care

The course of prenatal care described thus far can seem to suggest that the experiences of childbearing women are similar and that nursing interventions are uniform across all populations. Although typical patterns of response to pregnancy are easily recognized and many aspects of prenatal care indeed are consistent, pregnant women enter the health care system with individual concerns and needs. The nurse's ability to assess unique needs and tailor interventions to the individual is the hallmark of expertise in providing care. Factors that influence prenatal care and a woman's response to it include culture, age, and number of fetuses.

Cultural Influences

Prenatal care as we know it is a phenomenon of Western medicine. In the biomedical model of care, women are encouraged to seek prenatal care as early as possible in their pregnancy by visiting a physician, midwife, office, or clinic. Such visits are routine and follow a systematic sequence, with the initial visit followed by monthly, then semimonthly, then weekly visits. Monitoring weight and BP; testing blood and urine; teaching specific information about diet, rest, and activity; and preparing for childbirth are common components of prenatal care. This model is not only unfamiliar but may seem strange to many groups. Thus different models for providing prenatal care for women should be explored.

Many cultural variations in prenatal care exist. Even if the prenatal care described is familiar to a woman, some practices may conflict with the beliefs and practices of a subculture group to which she belongs. Because of these and other factors such as lack of money, lack of transportation, and language barriers, women from diverse cultures may not keep prenatal appointments. The nurse may misinterpret their behaviour as appearing to be uncaring, lazy, or ignorant.

For many women, concern for modesty is a deterrent against seeking prenatal care. Some women consider exposing body parts, especially to a man, a major violation of their modesty. For many women, invasive procedures such as vaginal examination may be so threatening that they cannot be discussed even with their own husbands. Thus they prefer a female health care provider. Too often, health care providers assume that women lose this modesty during pregnancy and labour, but most women value and appreciate efforts to maintain their modesty.

In many cultural groups a physician is deemed appropriate only in times of illness. Because pregnancy is considered a normal process and the woman is in a state of health, the services of a physician are considered inappropriate. Western medicine's view of problems in pregnancy may differ from that of members of other cultural groups.

Cultural prescriptions tell women what to do, and cultural proscriptions establish taboos. The purposes of these practices are to prevent maternal illness caused by a pregnancy-induced imbalanced state and to protect the vulnerable fetus. Prescriptions and proscriptions regulate the woman's emotional response, clothing, physical activity and rest, sexual activity, and dietary practices. Exploration of the woman's beliefs, perceptions of the meaning of childbearing, and health care practices may help health care providers foster her self-actualization, promote attainment of the maternal role, and positively influence her relationship with her spouse.

To provide culturally sensitive care, the nurse must be knowledgeable about specific practices and customs. Although it is not possible to know all there is to know about every culture and subculture or the many lifestyles that exist, it is important to learn about the varied cultures in the setting in which a nurse practices. By exploring and becoming knowledgeable in the cultural beliefs and practices related to childbearing, the nurse can better support and nurture the beliefs that promote physical or emotional adaptation (Box 10-7). However, if potentially harmful beliefs or activities are identified, the nurse should sensitively provide education and propose modifications.

Besides proscriptions regarding food, other proscriptions involve forms of magic. For example, some Latin Americans believe pregnant women should not be allowed to witness an eclipse of the moon because it may cause a cleft palate in the infant. They also believe that exposure to an earthquake may precipitate preterm birth, miscarriage, or a breech presentation. In some cultures, a pregnant woman must not ridicule someone with an affliction for fear her child might be born with the same handicap. A mother should not hate a person lest her child resemble that person. Dental work should not be done during pregnancy because it may cause a baby to have a "harelip." A folk belief widely held in many cultures is that the pregnant woman should refrain from raising her arms above her head and from tying knots because such movements tie knots in the umbilical cord and may cause it to wrap around the baby's neck. Another belief is that placing a knife under the bed of a labouring woman will "cut" her pain.

Emotional Response

Virtually all cultures emphasize the importance of maintaining a socially harmonious and agreeable environment for the pregnant woman (see Community Focus box). A lifestyle with minimal stress is important in ensuring a successful outcome for the mother and baby. Harmony with other people must be fostered, and visits from extended family members may be required to demonstrate pleasant and noncontroversial relationships. If discord exists in a relationship, it is usually dealt with in culturally prescribed ways.

Physical Activity and Rest

Norms that regulate physical activity of mothers during pregnancy vary tremendously. Many groups, including First Nations, Métis, and Inuit as well as some Asian groups, encourage women to be active, to walk, and to engage in normal although not strenuous activities to ensure that the baby is healthy and not too large. Other groups such as Filipinos believe that any activity is dangerous, and others willingly take over the work of the pregnant woman. Some Filipinos believe that this inactivity protects the mother and child. The mother is encouraged simply to produce the succeeding generation. If health care providers do not know of this belief, they could misinterpret this behaviour as laziness

BOX 10-7 Antepartum Cultural Assessment

All cultures recognize pregnancy as a special transitional period and have particular customs and beliefs that dictate behaviour during this time. In the antepartum period, the nurse should assess the following:

- Beliefs of whether pregnancy is a state of illness or health
- Behavioural expectations of the mother and the health care provider
- Dietary prescriptions or restrictions (e.g., hot/cold balance theory, pica)
- Activity restrictions or prescriptions (e.g., use of massage)
- Availability of advice (e.g., from whom and at what time advice will be sought and when prenatal care will begin [if at all])
- Considerations of modesty

COMMUNITY FOCUS

Availability of Culturally Appropriate Childbirth Resources

Select a cultural group different from your own within your community and identify childbirth-related beliefs and practices that are unique to that group. Are there stores in the area that sell items that meet the needs of that group? Does the community centre have activities or classes that are directed toward that group? Are there outreach programs in the community that meet the cultural needs of the group? Are childbirth education programs available that provide essential information while incorporating cultural patterns? Are childbirth classes available in languages other than English? What written and online resources are available in the appropriate language and are they comprehensive? What could you, as a nurse, contribute to the community that would help meet the needs of that group?

or noncompliance with the desired prenatal health care regimen. It is important for the nurse to find out the way that each pregnant woman views activity and rest.

Sexual Activity

In most cultures, sexual activity is not prohibited until the end of pregnancy. Some Latin Americans view sexual activity as necessary to keep the birth canal lubricated. Conversely, some Vietnamese have definite proscriptions about sexual intercourse, requiring abstinence throughout the pregnancy because it is thought that sexual intercourse may harm the mother and the fetus.

Nutrition

Nutritional information given by Western health care providers may be a source of conflict for many cultural groups. Such a conflict commonly is not discovered by health care providers unless they understand the dietary beliefs and practices of the particular people for whom they are caring. For example, Muslims have strict regulations about the preparation of food; if meat cannot be prepared as prescribed, they may omit it from their diets. Many cultures permit pregnant women to eat only warm foods; for example, Latin Americans believe women who are pregnant should only eat hot food and postpartum women should eat cold food (see Chapter 11).

evolve Critical Thinking Exercise—Adolescent Pregnancy

Age Differences

The age of the childbearing couple may have a significant influence on their physical and psychosocial adaptation to pregnancy. Normal developmental processes that occur in both very young and older mothers are interrupted by pregnancy and require a different type of adaptation to pregnancy than that of the woman of typical childbearing age. Although the individuality of each pregnant woman is recognized, special needs of expectant mothers 15 years of age or younger or those 35 years of age or older are summarized here.

Adolescents

Teenage pregnancy rates have decreased in Canada. In 2004, the rate of adolescent females giving birth was 4.8%, down from 6.5% in 1995 (PHAC, 2008b). Many of these pregnancies are unintended. Pregnancy rates are higher among teens with lower educational levels and who are economically disadvantaged. Most of these young women are unmarried, and many are not ready for the emotional, psychosocial, and financial responsibilities of parenthood.

When adolescents become pregnant and decide to give birth, they are much less likely than older women to access adequate prenatal care, with many receiving no care at all. These young women also are more likely to smoke and less likely to gain adequate weight during pregnancy.

Delayed entry into prenatal care may be the result of late recognition of pregnancy, denial of pregnancy, or confusion about the services that are available. Such a delay in care may leave inadequate time before birth to attend to correctable problems. The very young pregnant adolescent is at higher risk for each of the confounding variables associated with poor pregnancy outcomes (e.g., socioeconomic factors) and for the conditions associated with a first pregnancy, regardless of age (e.g., gestational hypertension). However, when prenatal care is initiated early and consistently and confounding variables are controlled, very young pregnant adolescents are at no greater risk (nor are their infants) for an adverse outcome than older pregnant women. Thus the role of the nurse in reducing the risks and consequences of adolescent pregnancy is twofold: first, to encourage early and continued prenatal care; and second, to refer the adolescent, if necessary, for appropriate social support services, which can help reverse the effects of a negative socioeconomic environment (Fig. 10-20; see Nursing Care Plan).

Women Older Than 35 Years of Age

Two groups of older parents have emerged in the population of women having a child late in their childbearing years. One group consists of women who have many children and who have an additional child during the menopausal period. The other group consists of women who have deliberately delayed childbearing until their late thirties or early forties.

Multiparous Women. Multiparous women may have never used contraceptives because of personal choice or a lack of knowledge about contraceptives. They also may be women who have used contraceptives successfully during the childbearing years but, as menopause approached, ceased menstruating regularly or stopped using contraception and subsequently became pregnant. The older multiparous woman may believe that pregnancy separates her from her peer group and that her age is a hindrance to close associations with young mothers. Other parents welcome the unexpected infant as evidence of continuing maternal and paternal roles.

Nulliparous Women. The number of first-time pregnancies in women between ages 35 and 40 has increased significantly over the last two decades. Currently 11% of first births occur in women older than 35 years of age (Johnson et al., 2012). Reasons for delaying pregnancy include advanced education, career priorities, better contraceptive measures, and infertility. Women who have experienced infertility may have spent incredible time, expense, and emotional anguish trying to get pregnant (see Chapter 7).

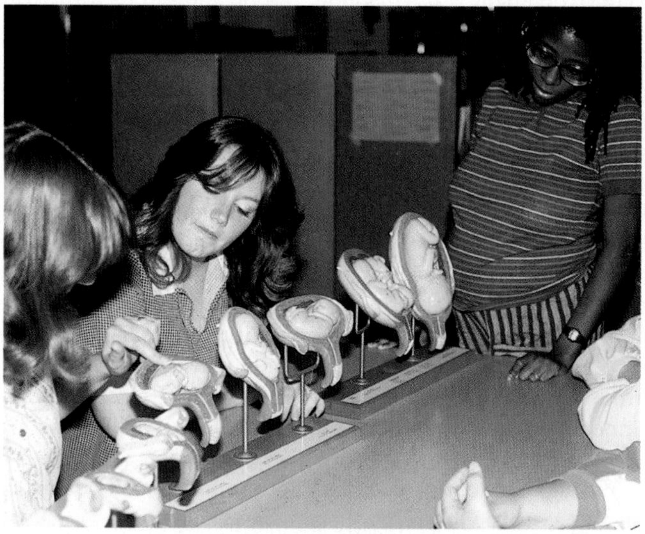

Fig. 10-20 Pregnant adolescents review fetal development. *(Courtesy Marjorie Pyle, RNC, Lifecircle, Costa Mesa, CA).*

NURSING CARE PLAN ● Adolescent Pregnancy

Nursing Diagnosis: Imbalanced nutrition: less than body requirements related to intake insufficient to meet metabolic needs of fetus and adolescent patient

Expected Outcomes

Patient will gain weight as prescribed by age, take prenatal vitamins/iron as prescribed, and maintain normal hematocrit and hemoglobin.

Nursing Interventions/Rationales

Assess current diet history/intake *to determine prescriptions for additions or changes in present dietary pattern.*

Compare prepregnancy weight with current weight *to determine if pattern is consistent with appropriate fetal growth and development.*

Provide information about food prescriptions for appropriate weight gain, considering preferences for "fast food" and peer influences, *to correct any misconceptions and increase chances for compliance with diet.*

Include the patient's immediate family or support system during instruction *to ensure that the person preparing family meals receives information.*

Nursing Diagnosis: Risk for injury, maternal or fetal, related to inadequate prenatal care and screening

Expected Outcomes

Patient will experience uncomplicated pregnancy and give birth to a healthy fetus at term.

Nursing Interventions/Rationales

Provide information, using therapeutic communication and confidentiality, *to establish relationship and build trust.*

Discuss the importance of ongoing prenatal care and possible risks to adolescent patient and fetus *to reinforce that ongoing assessment is crucial to the health and well-being of the patient and fetus, even if the patient feels well.* The adolescent patient is more at risk for certain complications that may be avoided or managed early if prenatal visits are maintained.

Discuss risks of alcohol, tobacco, and recreational drug use during pregnancy *to minimize risks to the patient and fetus, because adolescent patients have a higher substance use rate than the rest of the pregnant population.*

Assess for evidence of sexually transmitted infection (STI) and provide information regarding safer sexual practices *to minimize risk to the patient and fetus because an adolescent is more at risk for STIs.*

Screen for pre-eclampsia on an ongoing basis *to minimize risk because the adolescent population is more at risk for pre-eclampsia.*

Nursing Diagnosis: Social isolation related to body image changes of pregnant adolescent as evidenced by patient statements and concerns

Expected Outcomes

Patient will identify support systems and report decreased feelings of social isolation.

Nursing Interventions/Rationales

Establish a therapeutic relationship *to listen objectively and establish trust.*

Discuss with the patient changes in relationships that have occurred as a result of the pregnancy *to determine extent of isolation from family, peers, and father of the baby.*

Provide referrals and resources appropriate for developmental stage of the patient *to give information for patient support.*

Provide information on parenting classes, breastfeeding classes, and teen childbirth preparation classes (if available) *to give further information and group support, which lessens social isolation.*

Nursing Diagnosis: Interrupted family processes related to adolescent pregnancy

Expected Outcome

Patient will re-establish relationship with important family members.

Nursing Interventions/Rationales

Encourage communication with the mother *to clarify roles and relationships related to birth of the infant.*

Encourage communication with father of the baby (if she desires continued contact) *to ascertain level of support to be expected from the father.*

Refer to support group *to learn more effective problem-solving methods and reduce conflict within the family.*

Nursing Diagnosis: Disturbed body image related to situational crisis of pregnancy

Expected Outcome

Pregnant adolescent will make positive comments about her body image during the pregnancy.

Nursing Interventions/Rationales

Assess pregnant adolescent's perception of self related to pregnancy *to provide basis for further interventions.*

Give information on expected body changes that occur during pregnancy, *to provide a realistic view of these temporary changes.*

Provide opportunity to discuss personal feelings and concerns *to promote trust and support.*

Nursing Diagnosis: Risk for impaired parenting related to immaturity and lack of experience in new role of adolescent mother

Expected Outcome

Parents will demonstrate parenting roles with confidence.

Nursing Interventions/Rationales

Provide information on growth and development *to enhance knowledge so that the adolescent mother can have basis for caring for her infant.*

Refer to parenting classes *to enhance knowledge and obtain support for providing appropriate care to the newborn and infant.*

Initiate discussion of child care *to assist the adolescent in problem solving for future needs.*

Assess parenting abilities of the adolescent mother and father *to provide baseline for education.*

Provide information on parenting classes that are appropriate for parents' developmental stage *to give them an opportunity to share common feelings and concerns.*

Assist parents to identify pertinent support systems *to give assistance with parenting as needed.*

These women choose parenthood over a childfree lifestyle. They often are established in a career and a lifestyle with a partner that includes time for self-attention, the establishment of a home with accumulated possessions, and freedom to travel (Benzies et al., 2006). The dilemma of choice includes recognition that being a parent will have both positive and negative consequences. Couples need to discuss the consequences of childbearing and childrearing before committing themselves to this lifelong venture. Partners in this group seem to share the preparation for parenthood, the planning for a family-centred birth, and the desire to be loving and competent parents. However, the reality of child care may prove difficult for them.

During pregnancy, parents explore the possibilities and responsibilities of changing identities and new roles. They must prepare a safe and nurturing environment during pregnancy and after birth. They must integrate the child into an established family system and negotiate new roles (parent, sibling, and grandparent roles) for family members.

Adverse perinatal outcomes are more common in older primiparas than in younger women, even when they receive good prenatal care. Women 35 years of age and older are more likely than younger primiparas to have LBW infants, premature birth, IUGR, abruptio placentae, and multiple births (Johnson, 2012; Montan et al., 2007; PHAC, 2008b). The incidence of malpresentation also is more common in older primiparas, and they are more likely to have a Caesarean birth. The occurrence of these complications is quite stressful for the new parents, thus nursing interventions that provide information and psychosocial support in addition to care for physical needs are important.

Multifetal Pregnancy

A *multifetal pregnancy*, or pregnancy with more than one fetus, increases the risk for adverse outcomes for both the mother and fetuses. The maternal blood volume is increased, resulting in an increased strain on the maternal cardiovascular system. Anemia often develops because of a greater demand for iron by the fetuses. Marked uterine distention, increased pressure on the adjacent viscera and pelvic vasculature, and diastasis of the two rectus abdominis muscles may occur (see Fig. 9-14). Placenta previa develops more commonly in multifetal pregnancies because of the large size or placement of the placentas. Premature separation of the placenta may occur before the second and any subsequent fetuses are born.

Twin pregnancies often end prematurely. Spontaneous rupture of membranes before term is common. Congenital malformations are twice as common in monozygotic twins as in singletons, although there is no increase in the incidence of congenital anomalies in dizygotic twins. Two-vessel cords (i.e., cords with a single umbilical artery) occur more often in twins than in singletons; this abnormality is most common in monozygotic twins. The most serious problem for the fetus is the local shunting of blood between placentas (twin-to-twin transfusion); this causes the recipient twin to be larger and the donor twin to be small, pallid, dehydrated, malnourished, and hypovolemic. However, the larger twin may develop congenital heart failure during the first 24 hours after birth.

The clinical diagnosis of multifetal pregnancy is accurate in about 90% of cases. The likelihood of a multifetal pregnancy is increased if, during a careful assessment, any one or a combination of the following factors is noted:

- History of dizygotic twins in the female lineage
- Use of fertility drugs
- More rapid uterine growth for the number of weeks of gestation
- Hydramnios
- Palpation of more than the expected number of small or large parts
- Asynchronous fetal heartbeats or more than one fetal electrocardiographic tracing
- Ultrasonographic evidence of more than one fetus

The diagnosis of multifetal pregnancy can come as a shock to many expectant parents, and they may need additional support and education to help them cope with the changes they face. She should be counselled that maternal adaptations will probably be more uncomfortable and be provided with information about the possibility of a preterm birth.

If the presence of more than three fetuses is diagnosed, the parents may receive counselling regarding selective reduction of the fetuses to reduce the incidence of premature birth and improve the opportunities for the remaining fetuses to grow to term gestation (Cleary-Goldman, Chitkara, & Berkowitz, 2007). This situation poses an ethical dilemma for many couples, especially those who have worked hard to overcome problems with infertility and those who harbour strong values regarding the right to life. Nurse-initiated discussions to identify what resources could help the couple (e.g., a minister, priest, rabbi, or mental health counsellor) can make the decision-making process somewhat less traumatic.

Prenatal care given to women with multifetal pregnancies includes changes in the pattern of care and modifications in other aspects such as the amount of weight gained and the nutritional intake necessary. The prenatal visits of these mothers are scheduled at least every 2 weeks in the second trimester and weekly thereafter. The recommended weight gain in twin gestations is 16 to 20 kg (Cleary-Goldman, Chitkara, & Berkowitz, 2007). Iron and vitamin supplements are desirable. Since pre-eclampsia and eclampsia occur more commonly during multifetal pregnancies, the health care team needs to work aggressively to prevent, identify, and treat these complications of pregnancy.

The considerable uterine distention involved in a multifetal pregnancy can cause the backache commonly experienced by pregnant women to be even worse. Maternity support hose may be worn to control leg varicosities. Every multifetal pregnancy is at risk for preterm labour; thus these women need to receive education regarding the signs of preterm labour and more frequent monitoring (nonstress tests) (Elliott, 2007). Some practitioners recommend bed rest beginning at 20 weeks for women carrying multiple fetuses, to prevent preterm labour. Other practitioners question the value of prolonged bed rest. If bed rest is recommended, the mother needs to assume the lateral position in order to promote increased placental perfusion. If birth is delayed until after the thirty-sixth week, the risk of morbidity and mortality decreases for the neonates.

Multiple newborns will likely place a strain on finances, space, workload, and the mother's and family's coping abilities. Lifestyle changes may be necessary. Parents will need assistance in making realistic plans for the care of the babies (e.g., how to breastfeed and whether to raise them as "alike" or as separate individuals). Parents can be referred to national organizations such as Multiple Births Canada (http://www.multiplebirthscanada.org) and the La Leche League (http://www.lalecheleague.org) for further support.

Perinatal Care Choices

One of the principles of family-centred care is that a variety of health care providers are part of the childbearing experience (Health Canada, 2000). Women must feel they are respected and trusted within the care relationship. Women have the option to choose from a variety of health care providers and this may include physicians, nurses, midwives, doulas, childbirth educators and various others who may help with physical or social needs (Health Canada, 2000). Those caring for women during pregnancy, birth and the early parenting period must work together to provide appropriate care for women and their families.

The environment in which a woman gives birth is equally as influential as education about how to listen to and work with her body during childbirth. Women need to be provided information about choices and be encouraged to ask potential care providers the following questions, to ensure that they feel comfortable with the choices they make:

- Who can be with me during labour and birth?
- What happens during a normal labour and birth in your setting?
- How do you allow for differences in culture and beliefs?
- Can I walk and move around during labour? What position do you suggest for birth?
- What things do you normally do to a woman in labour?
- How do you help mothers stay as comfortable as they can be? Besides medications, how do you help relieve the pain of labour?
- What if my baby is born early or has special problems?
- What support do you have for breastfeeding mothers?

Options for Care Providers

Physician Care

In 2006, physicians (obstetricians and family practice physicians) attended approximately 84% of births (PHAC, 2009). Physicians see both low-risk and high-risk patients. Family practice physicians may need backup from obstetricians if a specialist is needed for a problem, such as Caesarean birth. Almost all physicians manage births in a hospital setting. A woman may see one doctor for her entire pregnancy and birth or, more commonly, she may be cared for in a group practice setting, seeing multiple physicians and having the physician who is on call present at the birth.

Midwives

Registered midwives in Canada are educated through a university program as a profession distinct from nursing. Throughout history, midwives have held a holistic view of childbirth. Midwives care for low-risk obstetrical patients. Care is often noninterventionist, and the woman and her family are encouraged to be active participants in the care. Women are often cared for by one or two midwives who provide care throughout the pregnancy, birth, and postpartum period. Many women appreciate the continuity of care that this model of care provides. Midwives refer patients with complications to physicians. Births may be managed in a hospital setting, in a birth centre, or at home.

Women who are seeing a midwife may have some of their visits with the midwife at their home. The midwife will typically have one prenatal visit and several postpartum visits at the patient's home. This reduces stress on the new mother, who may find it difficult in the first few weeks after birth to get out with the baby.

In Canada, midwives are regulated by the Canadian Association of Midwives, although currently, not all provinces and territories have legislation regarding the practice of midwives. Approximately 6% of all births in Canada are attended by a midwife (PHAC, 2009).

Doula

A **doula** is a trained and experienced professional who provides continuous physical, emotional, and informational support to the mother and her partner before, during, and just after birth, or provides emotional and practical support during the postpartum period, alongside other health care providers. There are birth doulas, who provide support during labour, and postpartum doulas, who provide assistance after the birth; both are part of the health care team (Health Canada, 2000). Doulas usually work on a fee-for-service basis, and many will offer a sliding scale for families who cannot afford to pay for their services. Doulas provide service at home as well as at the hospital, depending on the needs of the woman.

Currently, many couples employ a doula for labour support. A Cochrane synopsis of 15 trials involving 12,791 women found that "continuous labour support like that provided by doulas reduces a woman's likelihood of having pain medication, increases her satisfaction and chances for spontaneous birth, and has no known risks" (Hodnett et al., 2007).

A doula typically meets with the mother and her partner before labour to ascertain their expectations and desires for the birth experience. During labour and birth, the doula works collaboratively with other health care providers and the woman's support people and focuses on assisting the woman and the couple to achieve their goals. Postpartum doulas may assist with breastfeeding, teaching, and care of the mother or siblings. The postpartum doula's role is flexible, meeting the needs of the family to ensure that the mother is able to care for herself and the new baby.

Box 10-8 provides questions to ask when interviewing a prospective doula.

Birth Setting Choices

With careful thought, the concept of family, or woman-centred maternity care can be implemented in any setting. Currently, the three primary options for birth settings are the hospital,

BOX 10-8 Questions to Ask When Choosing a Doula

To discover the specific training, experience, and services offered by anyone who provides labour support, potential patients should ask the following questions of that person:

- What training have you had?
- Tell me about your experience with birth, personally and as a doula.
- What is your philosophy about childbirth and supporting women and their partners through labour?
- May we meet to discuss our birth plans and the role you will play in supporting me and my partner through childbirth?
- May we call you with questions or concerns before and after the birth?
- When do you try to join women in labour? Do you come to our home or meet us at the hospital?
- Do you meet with us after the birth to review the labour and answer questions?
- Do you work with one or more backup doulas for times when you are not available? May we meet them?
- What is your fee?

(From DONA International. [2008]. *DONA International position paper: The birth doula's contribution to modern maternity care.* Retrieved from www.dona.org/pdfs/position_papers/BIRTH%20Paper%204%20page.pdf.)

birth centre, and home, depending on the province in which a woman lives. Women consider several factors in choosing a setting for childbirth, including where the care provider has privileges and characteristics of the birthing unit. Approximately 98% of all births in Canada take place in a hospital setting (PHAC, 2009); the other 2% occur in homes or birthing centres. However, the types of labour and birth services vary greatly, from the traditional labour and delivery rooms with separate postpartum and newborn units to in-hospital birthing centres where all or almost all care takes place in a single unit.

Labour, Delivery, Recovery, Postpartum (Birthing) Rooms

Labour, delivery, and recovery (LDR) and labour, delivery, recovery, and postpartum (LDRP) rooms offer families a comfortable, private space for childbirth (Fig. 10-21). Women admitted to LDR units go through labour and give birth there and spend the first 1 to 2 hours postpartum there for immediate recovery, to have time with their families to bond with their newborns. After this period of recovery, the mothers and newborns are transferred to a postpartum unit and nursery or a mother–baby unit for the duration of their stay. Care is provided by different nursing staff (e.g., labour and delivery nurses, postpartum nurses, nursery nurses). In most hospitals in Canada, the same nurse provides care for both mothers and newborns (mother–baby or couplet care).

In LDRP units, total care is provided, from admission for labour through postpartum discharge, in the same room and usually by the same nursing staff. The woman and her family may stay in this unit for 6 to 48 hours after giving birth. The

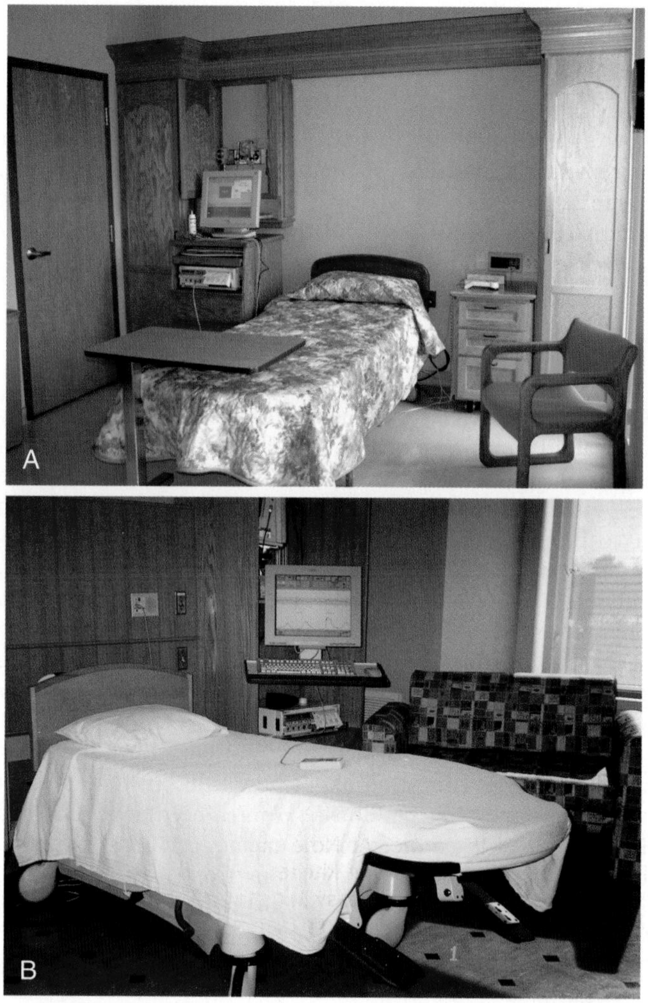

Fig. 10-21 **A:** Labour, delivery, and recovery unit. **B:** Labour, delivery, recovery, and postpartum unit. *(**A**, Courtesy Julie Perry Nelson, Loveland, CO. **B**, Courtesy Dee Lowdermilk, Chapel Hill, NC.)*

units are furnished in a homelike atmosphere, similar to LDR units, but have accommodations for family members to stay overnight (see Fig. 10-21, B).

Both LDR and LDRP units are equipped with fetal monitors, emergency resuscitation equipment for mother and newborn, and heated cribs or warming units for the newborn. Often this equipment is out of sight in cabinets or closets when it is not being used (see Fig. 10-21, A).

Birth Centres

Free-standing birth centres are usually built in locations separate from the hospital but may be located nearby, in case transfer of the woman or newborn is needed. These birth centres are intended to offer families a safe alternative to hospital or home birth. The centres are usually staffed by nurses, midwives, or physicians who also have privileges at the local hospital. Only women considered low risk are admitted for care.

Birth centres typically have homelike accommodations, including a double bed for the couple and a crib for the newborn (Fig. 10-22, A). Emergency equipment and medications are available but stored out of view. Private bathroom

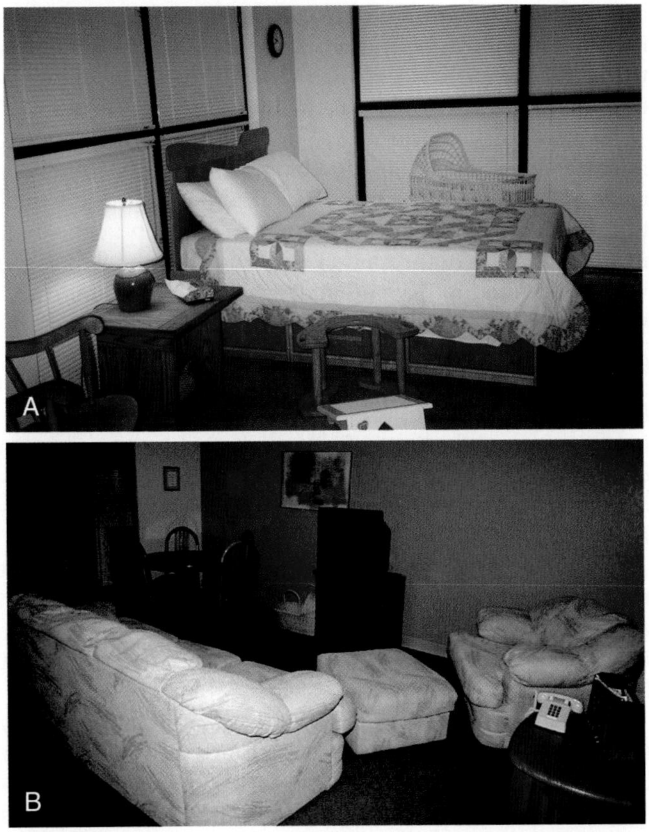

Fig. 10-22 Birth centre. **A:** Note double bed, baby crib, and birthing stool. **B:** Lounge and kitchen. *(**A**, Courtesy Dee Lowdermilk, Chapel Hill, NC. **B**, Courtesy Michael S. Clement, MD, Mesa, AZ. Photo location: Bethany Birth Centre, Phoenix, AZ.)*

facilities are incorporated into each birth unit. There may be an early labour lounge or a living room and small kitchen (see Fig. 10-22, B). The family is admitted to the birth centre for labour and birth and will remain there until discharge, which often takes place within 6 hours of the birth.

When births occur in a birth centre or a home setting, there needs to be a plan for transfer to hospital if this becomes necessary. Ambulance service and emergency procedures must be readily available.

Home Birth

Home birth has always been popular in certain countries such as Sweden and The Netherlands. In developing countries, hospitals or adequate facilities often are unavailable to most pregnant women, and home birth is a necessity. In Canada, home births account for approximately 1% of births and are usually attended by midwives (PHAC, 2009).

With a home birth, the family is in control of the experience, and the birth may be more physiologically natural in familiar surroundings (see Community Focus box). The mother may be more relaxed than she would be in the hospital environment. The family can assist in and be a part of the birth, and the mother–father or partner–infant (and sibling–infant) contact is immediate and sustained. Serious infection may be less likely (assuming aseptic principles are followed) because it is usual for people to be relatively immune to the bacteria in their own home.

> **COMMUNITY FOCUS**
>
> *Deciding About a Home Birth*
>
> Maxine, 37 years old and G1-T0-P0-A0-L0, is interested in having a home birth. She is currently 14 weeks pregnant, and her pregnancy is progressing normally. According to an ultrasound examination she has one fetus of appropriate size for gestational age with no detectable anomalies. She would like to pursue midwifery care with plans for a home birth. Explore the options for home birth in your province that are available for Maxine. What are the guidelines for midwifery care in your area? What patients are eligible for midwifery care? How many women have home births in your area and how many have hospital births? What provisions are needed for a home birth?

Over time, many studies have documented the safety of home births. Olsen and Jewell (1998) reported a meta-analysis of observational studies that found that planned home birth is safe, with fewer interventions than in planned hospital births. Most recently, the surveillance and risk assessment division in the Public Health Agency of Canada conducted a prospective cohort study involving certified professional midwives of 5418 births across the United States and Canada. Substantially lower rates of epidurals, episiotomies, forceps deliveries, vacuum extractions, and Caesarean births occurred among them, including the 12% of patients who were transferred to the hospital. No mothers died, and infant mortality was similar to rates of other low-risk home and hospital births. Thus, although home births are considered countercultural by some in Canada, there is no evidence base to discourage low-risk couples who desire a carefully planned out-of-the-hospital birth from having a home birth (Johnson & Daviss, 2005).

Childbirth and Perinatal Education

A goal of childbirth and perinatal education is to assist individuals and their family members to make informed, safe decisions about pregnancy, birth, and early parenthood. A specific focus is to convey the potential long-lasting, empowering effect that birth experiences have on women and the impact that early parenting experiences have on the development of children and the family. Perinatal education programs are an expansion of the earlier childbirth education movement, when only a set of classes in the third trimester of pregnancy was offered, to prepare parents for the birth of their child.

Today perinatal education programs consist of a menu of class series and activities from preconception through pregnancy, childbirth, and the early months of parenting. It takes a well-informed, articulate childbirth educator to teach consumer-oriented childbirth classes. Optimally, these classes help women trust their bodies and offer them a way to take full advantage of the opportunities presented by a prepared-for and well-supported childbirth experience.

For the new family, prior experience related to the pregnancy and the birth of others or in the care of younger siblings or relatives is increasingly uncommon, given the small size of many North American families. As a result, many individuals facing parenthood may have little information about what to expect and do not have the important skills necessary to deal effectively with pregnancy, childbirth, or parenthood. Perinatal education classes can partially fill this void.

Preconception education and care are designed to foster good decision-making regarding conception and health maintenance and promote healthy behaviours for the health of the woman and her potential fetus. Potential parents are encouraged to do the following:

- Establish lifestyle behaviours that maintain optimal health (e.g., eating a healthy diet, including sources of folic acid; getting enough rest and exercise; avoiding alcohol use, smoking, and other drugs)
- Prepare psychologically for pregnancy and the responsibilities that come with parenthood and build a support system to sustain the new family throughout the perinatal year
- Identify, minimize, or treat risk factors before conception (e.g., medical conditions, such as diabetes mellitus; substance use; use of medications for chronic illness; or infections, including STIs)
- Screen for health hazards in the workplace or home
- Obtain, when warranted, genetic counselling to identify carriers of inherited diseases (e.g., Tay-Sachs disease, sickle cell disease, or β-thalassemia)
- Compare the quality and philosophical bases of the perinatal care options available

The components of general preconception education, such as health promotion, risk assessment, and interventions, are outlined in Box 8-1.

All health-promoting education should be provided in a context that emphasizes the ability of a healthy body to adapt to the changes that accompany pregnancy. Without this context of health, routine care and testing for risks may foster a mindset in families that pregnancy is a pathological condition and not a healthy mind–body–spirit event.

Previous pregnancy and childbirth experiences are important elements that influence current learning needs. The woman's (and support person's) age, cultural background, personal philosophy in regard to childbirth, socioeconomic status, spiritual beliefs, and learning styles all need to be assessed when developing the best plan to help the woman meet her needs.

Most childbirth education classes are attended by the pregnant woman and her partner, although a friend, teenage daughter, or parent may be the designated support person. Classes may also be held for grandparents and siblings to prepare them for their attendance at birth or the arrival of the baby (see Fig. 10-4). Siblings often see a film about birth and learn ways they can help welcome the baby. They also learn to cope with changes, including a reduction in parental time and attention. Grandparents learn about current child-care practices and how to help their adult children in a supportive way to adapt to parenting.

Childbirth Education

When women are prepared for childbirth and are well supported, childbirth can present a unique and powerful opportunity for women to find their core strength in a manner that forever changes their self-perception. In providing the requisite childbirth education, it is important to remember that expectant parents and their families have different interests and information needs as the pregnancy progresses.

Early pregnancy ("early bird") classes provide fundamental information. Classes are developed around the following areas: (1) early fetal development, (2) physiological and emotional changes of pregnancy, (3) human sexuality, and (4) the nutritional needs of the mother and fetus. Environmental and workplace hazards may be addressed. Exercises, nutrition, warning signs, drug use, and self-medication are topics of interest and concern.

Midpregnancy classes emphasize the woman's participation in self-management. Classes provide information on preparing for newborn feeding; infant care; basic hygiene; common discomforts and simple, safe remedies; infant health; parenting; and updating and refining of the **birth plans** (see Evidence-Informed Practice box on breastfeeding education).

Late pregnancy classes address labour and birth. Different methods of coping with labour and birth have been developed and are often the basis for various prenatal classes. These include Lamaze, Bradley, and Dick-Read (see Chapter 16). A hospital tour may be included.

Throughout the series of classes, it is important to identify support systems that people can use during pregnancy and after birth. Such support systems help parents function independently and effectively. During all the classes, members should be encouraged to openly express their feelings and concerns about any aspect of pregnancy, birth, and parenting.

Fathers or partners often worry about their role in childbirth classes and during labour and birth, as well as about the safety of their partner and baby during the birth. Many partners elect to participate actively during labour and the birth of their child. However, as noted earlier, some men, because of personal or cultural views of the father role, neither want nor intend to participate. It is important that the partners agree on each other's roles.

Current Practices in Childbirth Education

A variety of approaches to childbirth education have evolved as childbirth educators attempt to meet learning needs. In addition to classes designed specifically for pregnant adolescents, their partners, or parents, classes exist for other groups with special learning needs. These include classes for first-time mothers over age 35, single women, adoptive parents, and parents of twins.

Refresher classes for parents with children not only review coping techniques for labour and birth and address any concerns from their previous birth but also help couples prepare for sibling reactions and adjustments to a new baby. Caesarean birth classes are offered for couples who have this kind of birth scheduled because of breech position or other risk factors. Other classes focus on vaginal birth after Caesarean (VBAC) as many women successfully give birth vaginally after previous Caesarean birth.

Because of the multicultural composition of the population in Canada, there is great diversity in attitudes, expectations, and behaviours judged appropriate during pregnancy and

EVIDENCE-INFORMED PRACTICE The Usefulness of Prenatal Breastfeeding Education —*Pat Gingrich*

Ask the Questions

Does prenatal education about breastfeeding promote the initiation of breastfeeding and continuation of exclusive breastfeeding for 3 and 6 months? If so, what prenatal education strategies are most effective?

Search for Evidence

Search Strategies

Professional organization guidelines, meta-analyses, systematic reviews, randomized controlled trials, nonrandomized prospective studies, and retrospective studies since 2006

Databases Searched

CINAHL; Cochrane; Medline; and the Web sites for the Association for Women's Health, Obstetric and Neonatal Nurses (AWHONN), Centers for Disease Prevention and Control (CDC), National Institute for Health and Clinical Excellence (NICE), and the Academy of Breastfeeding Medicine

Critically Analyze the Evidence

After reviewing scientific literature indicating that health care provider attitude and ongoing support have a significant impact on initiation and duration of exclusive breastfeeding, the Academy of Breastfeeding Medicine published a protocol calling for health care providers to discuss the benefits of breastfeeding, beginning with the first visit in the first trimester (Academy of Breastfeeding Medicine Protocol Committee, 2006). The guidelines encourage an ongoing conversation with the patient and her family about feeding plans, attitudes, and previous experiences. Both parents are encouraged to attend prenatal breastfeeding classes before making a decision. Educational materials should include written, nonformula-advertising materials and may also include visual aids, books, and videos.

A Cochrane Systematic Review of nine prenatal education trials totaling 2284 women found that the benefits and strategies of prenatal education are difficult to compare because of greatly differing interventions and outcome measures (Gagnon & Sandall, 2007). One particular challenge of studying this topic is the difficulty of randomizing women to the interventions or control, when randomization may contradict a woman's choice. The reviewers were not able to determine benefits or best strategies for prenatal education.

However, a subsequent randomized, controlled trial (RCT) of 450 healthy women in Singapore who were over 34 weeks of gestation demonstrated that breastfeeding initiation and duration were significantly improved if the women were given either a prenatal education session (video, individual instruction, and written materials) or two postnatal support sessions (individual instruction in hospital and at 2 weeks, with written materials) when compared to women receiving usual care (Su et al., 2007).

Group prenatal education sessions may also be both effective and efficient for the health care provider. In a more recent RCT of 1047 pregnant women, the participants randomized to receive weekly group educational and facilitated support sessions with their gestational peers from 18 weeks until term had significantly increased breastfeeding initiation, more prenatal knowledge, more readiness for labour and delivery, and increased satisfaction compared to women receiving usual treatment. There were no differences in costs, and birth weights remained similar. Interestingly, the women in the support group also had significantly fewer preterm births (Ickovics et al., 2007).

Implications for Practice

The literature and expert opinion confirm the value of prenatal education for initiation and duration of exclusive breastfeeding. Especially for the primipara or the woman lacking social support for breastfeeding, it makes sense for the health care provider to start the dialogue early in pregnancy or possibly before pregnancy and use each contact to further educate the expectant family on the many benefits of breastfeeding. There is enough information to recommend combinations of individual instruction and noncommercial written and multimedia material. Group education sessions may provide cost-effective use of the educator's time, along with added emotional and social support for participating families at similar gestational ages.

References

Academy of Breastfeeding Medicine Protocol Committee. (2006). ABM clinical protocol No. 14: Breastfeeding-friendly physician's office. Part 1: Optimizing care for infants and children. *Breastfeeding Medicine, 1*(2), 115–119.

Gagnon, A. J., & Sandall, J. (2007). Individual or group antenatal education for childbirth or parenthood, or both. In *The Cochrane Database of Systematic Reviews 2007,* Issue 3. Chichester, UK: John Wiley & Sons.

Ickovics, J. R., et al. (2007). Group prenatal care and perinatal outcomes: A randomized, controlled trial. *Obstetrics and Gynecology, 110*(2 Pt. 1), 330–339.

Su, L.-L., et al. (2007). Antenatal education and postnatal support strategies for improving rates of exclusive breastfeeding: Randomized controlled trial. *British Medical Journal, 335*(7620), 596.

early parenthood. No one approach can meet all needs. For example, classes for new immigrants are particularly effective when taught in their first language (e.g., Punjabi, Tagalog, Cantonese). For classes to be meaningful, parent educators must understand the value systems in other cultures and their influence on issues such as nutrition, exercise, valuing of early prenatal care, maternal weight gain, and infant feeding practices. Prenatal educators must establish rapport, be understood, and build on cultural practices, reinforcing the positive and promoting change only if a practice, such as pica, is directly harmful. For topics discussed during childbirth education class, see Box 3-1.

Components of Perinatal Education Programs

A variety of approaches to perinatal education that go beyond preparation for birth have evolved as educators attempt to meet the learning and support needs of expectant parents and to capitalize on their openness to learning. For example, prenatal and new-mother weekly exercise classes can offer both physiological and social support for a mixture of expectant and new mothers who may also elect to stay connected by e-mail for support between weekly classes. However, it is important that a focus on preparation for birth not become lost in all the topics that could be offered to expectant parents. Some of the additional topics mentioned below might fit well into a second-trimester class as part of an organized series for the perinatal year.

Birth Plans

The birth plan is a natural evolution of a contemporary wellness-oriented lifestyle in which patients assume a level of responsibility for their own health. The birth plan is a tool with which parents can explore their childbirth options and choose those that are most important to them. It can serve as a means of open communication between the pregnant woman and her partner and between the couple and health care providers. The plan must be viewed as tentative and based on a best-case scenario since the realities of what is feasible may change as the actual labour and birth unfold. The options of women with a high risk pregnancy or those in whom complications develop during labour may be more limited.

It is useful for the nurse in a prenatal practice setting to initiate a discussion of choices and birth planning during the first and second prenatal visits. An early introduction to the idea of a birth plan allows the couple time to think about events or situations that could make their childbearing experience more meaningful and those they would prefer to avoid.

Some maternity practices provide printed material describing available options and giving answers to commonly asked questions. Tours of the birth setting are offered by almost all birthing facilities. The nurse can provide couples with pertinent information and make them aware of the various options for care and the advantages and consequences of each so they can begin making informed decisions. Early plans can be modified as the couple learns more details in their childbirth class.

Some health care providers provide birth plan templates, and there are numerous interactive programs on the Internet that will assist couples in creating their birth plans. However, childbirth educators should screen any such programs before referring couples to them as some contain advertising that is contrary to promoting good health.

Topics for birth plan discussion and decision making are given in Box 10-9.

Pain Management

Fear of pain in labour is a key issue for pregnant women and the reason given by many for attending childbirth education classes. Numerous studies show that women who have received childbirth preparation later report no less pain but do report a greater ability to cope with the pain during labour and birth and increased birth satisfaction compared to unprepared women. Thus, although pain management strategies are an essential component of childbirth education, pain eradication is not the primary source of birth satisfaction. Control in childbirth (i.e., participation in decision making) has repeatedly been found to be the primary source of birth satisfaction. The advantages and disadvantages of all pain management strategies for coping with labour are discussed in Chapter 16.

BOX 10-9 Questions to Consider When Developing a Birth Plan

Partner's participation—Attend prenatal visits? Childbirth and parent education classes? Present during labour? During birth? During Caesarean birth?

Birth setting—Hospital delivery room or birthing room (if available)? A birthing centre? Home?

Labour management—Walk around during labour? Use a rocking chair? Use a shower? Use a tub if available? Intermittent or continuous use of an electronic fetal monitor? Have music or dimmed lighting? Have older children or other people present? Is telemetry monitoring available? Consider stimulation of labour? Pain management strategies?

Birth—Positions—Side-lying? On hands and knees, kneeling, or squatting? Use a birthing bed? Or delivery table? Will you be photographing, videotaping, or recording any of the labour or birth? Who would you like to be present—partner, older siblings, other family members, friends, or doula? What do you know about the use of forceps? Episiotomies? Will your partner want to cut the umbilical cord?

Immediately after birth—Do you want to hold the baby skin-to-skin right away? Breastfeed immediately?

Postpartum care—What kind of care do you anticipate—labour, delivery, recovery, postpartum room; mother–baby coupling? Would you like to attend classes, or do you prefer to get such information through one-on-one discussion, DVDs, or handouts? On which subjects?

Relaxation

Relaxation or reduction of body tension is a technique suggested by virtually all childbirth education organizations. Learning relaxation in childbirth education classes can help couples with the stresses of pregnancy, childbirth, and adjustment to parenting and can be a form of stress management throughout life. A review of research across many studies found that relaxation skill is reported to be the most effective nonpharmacological strategy for coping with the stress of labour. Ideally, relaxation is combined with activity such as walking, slow dancing, rocking, and position changes that help the baby rotate through the pelvis. Rhythmic motion stimulates mechanoreceptors in the brain, which decreases pain perception.

Imagery and Visualization

Imagery and visualization also are taught in classes during preparation for birth. Although research on their use in childbirth is scant, clinical reports suggest that imagery and visualization can be used to produce a sense of well-being during pregnancy, assist with cervical dilation, and decrease the experience of pain and tension during labour. A variety of skills taught in childbirth classes augment relaxation during pregnancy and labour. All can be taught as lifetime skills useful to the couple and can be used to teach their children to cope with the stresses of life.

Conscious Breathing

Breathing in a conscious, deliberate pattern is a visible technique and thus is frequently used in the media to characterize childbirth preparation. Relaxed individuals automatically slow their breathing; thus slowing one's breathing serves to increase one's relaxation. During labour, nursing support includes guiding couples in the application of breathing and relaxation methods and adapting methods to their particular needs.

Biofeedback

The use of observation in class (informal biofeedback) helps couples develop awareness of their bodies and learn strategies to change their responses to stress. During preparation for birth, formal biofeedback (in which machines prenatally detect skin temperature, blood flow, or muscle tension) can prepare women to perfect their relaxation response.

Energy Work, Massage, Music, and Acupressure

Energy work such as therapeutic touch or healing touch involves energy fields around the body and can be taught in class for use during labour to decrease anxiety and pain and increase relaxation. Certified practitioners in energy work are consulted throughout pregnancy and during childbirth by women who have access to such care.

Music promotes relaxation and has been known for centuries to be generally therapeutic. Acupressure, which consists of applying pressure to various pressure points, has been correlated with relief of dizziness, headaches, back pain, nausea, leg cramps, and labour pain. Massage has been shown in a randomized trial to decrease pain and anxiety during labour, and the husbands' participation in massage positively increases the experience for the woman.

Preparation for Caesarean Birth

Given that almost 26% of births in Canada are by Caesarean surgery, this is an important topic for birth preparation education. The expectant parents can be helped to know what they can do to avoid the necessity of a Caesarean birth. Caesarean birth rates vary widely by care provider and care setting. They may be more common in women who choose epidurals, in part because the mother's muscles do not effectively assist the infant in rotation through the pelvis; in part because, if given early, epidurals prolong labour; and in part because the mother has less urge to push. In a setting where nursing support during labour is low and the care provider rate of Caesarean birth is high, women should be aware that their chances of a Caesarean birth are increased.

Effort can be directed at preventing the need for a subsequent Caesarean birth or preparing for it when it is inevitable or highly likely. Women who have planned Caesarean births also need to feel that they have some control over their birth experience, and it is important that this is discussed with them. Women with a prior Caesarean birth can be encouraged to explore the possibility of a vaginal birth, although this is not the case for those who have a history of classic vertical or unknown uterine incisions or those with medical contraindication. In many communities there are VBAC support groups, physicians who are known to be supportive, and special childbirth classes for those attempting a VBAC. Mothers can be prepared for the differences in postpartum recovery after a Caesarean birth. Their hospital stay will be longer, their need for assistance at home will be greater, and they may need extra support to establish breastfeeding comfortably, compared to women who have a vaginal birth.

Childbirth Education Outcomes

The effects of childbirth education have consistently been shown to be in birth satisfaction, building confidence, and building relationships. Physiological outcomes are not demonstrated to be strongly influenced by educating expectant parents. One reason for this finding may be that research has not focused on this. Many researchers treat childbirth education as a direct influence on the birth without considering the mediating influence of care providers' philosophy and their usual type of care. If these were considered, a more accurate evaluation of the influence of childbirth education on birth outcomes might be obtained.

Pregnancy is a time when expectant parents anticipate change in their lives and are open to many types of education. This education can enhance their health and coping skills in pregnancy, childbirth, and early parenting. It also can influence how they relate to health care professionals over a lifetime, how they problem solve with each other, and how they launch their new family. It is an opportunity for nurses to engage in meaningful health promotion and the building of resilience and connection in families.

Key Points

- The prenatal period is a preparatory one, both physically and psychologically.
- Psychosocial aspects of care may affect pregnancy, childbirth, and the adjustment of the new family.
- The pregnant woman's readiness to learn is at a high level, making this an excellent time to help her expand her self-management skills.
- Maternal physical and familial adaptations to pregnancy generate needs that the nurse can anticipate and meet.
- Even with a normal pregnancy, the nurse must remain alert to hazards such as supine hypotension, warning signs and symptoms, and signs of a family having difficulty coping with the pregnancy
- Women need to have appropriate care and screening provided throughout the pregnancy to ensure a healthy outcome.
- Each pregnant woman needs to know how to recognize and report preterm labour.
- Parent–child, sibling–child, and grandparent–child relationships are affected by pregnancy.
- Cultural prescriptions and proscriptions influence responses to pregnancy and to the health care delivery system.
- Childbirth education promotes women to feel confident that their bodies are able to give birth and teaches coping strategies that enhance their ability to give birth.
- Childbirth education is a process designed to help parents make the transition from the role of expectant parents to the role and responsibilities of parents of a new baby.

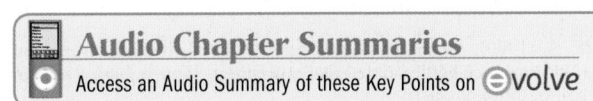

Audio Chapter Summaries

Access an Audio Summary of these Key Points on Evolve

References

Barish, R. (2004). In-flight radiation exposure during pregnancy. *Obstetrics and Gynecology, 103*(6), 1326–1330.

BC Reproductive Care Program. (2003). *Reproductive mental health guideline 3: Identification and assessment of reproductive mental illness during the preconception and perinatal periods.* Retrieved from http://www.perinatalservicesbc.ca//sites/bcrcp/files/Guidelines/Rmhg/Guideline3NewJan2003.pdf.

Benzies, K., et al. (2006). Factors influencing women's decisions about timing of motherhood. *Journal of Obstetric, Gynecologic, and Neonatal Nursing, 35*(5), 625–633.

Boggess, K., et al. (2003). Maternal periodontal disease is associated with an increased risk for preeclampsia. *Obstetrics and Gynecology, 101*(2), 227–231.

Carlson, N. S., & Lowe, N. K. (2006). Centering pregnancy: A new approach to prenatal care. *MCN: American Journal of Maternal Child Nursing, 31*(4), 218–223.

Cleary-Goldman, J., Chitkara, U., & Berkowitz, R. (2007). Multiple gestation. In S. G. Gabbe, J. R. Niebyl, & J. L. Simpson (Eds.), *Obstetrics: Normal and problem pregnancies* (5th ed.). Philadelphia: Churchill Livingstone.

Cunningham, F., et al. (2010). *Williams obstetrics* (23rd ed.). New York: McGraw Hill.

Davies, G. A., et al. (2003). Joint SOGC/CSEP clinical practice guideline. Exercise in pregnancy and the postpartum period. *Journal of Obstetrics and Gynaecology Canada, 25*(6), 516–522. Retrieved from http://www.sogc.org/guidelines/public/129E-JCPG-June2003.pdf.

Elliott, J. P. (2007). Preterm labour in twins and high-order multiples. *Clinics in Perinatology, 34*(4), 599–609.

Fries, M., Bashford, M., & Nunes, M. (2006). Implementing prenatal screening for cystic fibrosis in routine obstetric practice. *American Journal of Obstetrics and Gynecology, 192*(2), 527–534.

Grady, M., & Bloom, K. (2004). Pregnancy outcomes of adolescents enrolled in a Centering Pregnancy Program. *Journal of Midwifery and Women's Health, 49*(5), 412–420.

Health Canada. (2000). *Family-centred maternity and newborn care: National guidelines* (Cat. No. H39-527/2000E). Ottawa: Author.

Health Canada. (2007). *Cosmic radiation exposure and air travel.* Ottawa: Environmental and Workplace Health, Health Canada. Retrieved from http://www.hc-sc.gc.ca/ewh-semt/radiation/comsic-cosmique-eng.php.

Health Canada. (2010). *Health Canada reminds Canadians to manage caffeine consumption.* Ottawa: Government of Canada. Retrieved from http://www.hc-sc.gc.ca/ahc-asc/media/advisories-avis/_2010/2010_40-eng.php.

Hodnett, E., et al. (2007). Continuous support for women during childbirth. *Cochrane Database of Systematic Reviews,* Issue 3, CD003766.

Johnson, A., & Tough, S. (2012). SOGC committee opinion: Delayed childbearing. *Journal of Obstetrics and Gynaecology Canada, 34*(1), 80–93.

Johnson, K., & Daviss, B. (2005). Outcomes of planned home births and certified professional midwives: Large prospective study in North America. *British Medical Journal, 330*(7505), 1416.

Johnson, T. R., Gregory, K. D., & Niebyl, J. R. (2007). Preconception and prenatal care: Part of the continuum. In S. G. Gabbe, J. R. Niebyl, & J. L. Simpson (Eds.), *Obstetrics: Normal and problem pregnancies* (5th ed.). Philadelphia: Churchill Livingstone.

Keenan-Lindsay, L., et al. (2006). SOGC clinical practice guideline: HIV screening in pregnancy. *Journal of Obstetrics and Gynaecology Canada, 28*(12), 1103–1107. Retrieved from http://www.sogc.org/guidelines/documents/185E-CPG-December2006.pdf.

Kehringer, K. (2003). Informed consent: Hospitals must obtain informed consent prior to drug testing pregnant patients. *Journal of Law, Medicine and Ethics, 32*(3), 455–457.

Lawrence, R. A., & Lawrence, R. M. (2011). *Breastfeeding: A guide for the medical profession* (7th ed.). St. Louis: Mosby.

Liston, R., et al. (2007). SOGC clinical practice guideline: Fetal health surveillance: Antepartum and intrapartum consensus guideline. *Journal of Obstetrics and Gynaecology Canada, 29*(9), Suppl 4. Retrieved from http://www.sogc.org/guidelines/documents/gui197CPG0709r.pdf.

Lopez, R. (2005). Periodontal disease, preterm birth, and low birth weight. *Evidence-Based Dentistry, 6*(4), 90–91.

March of Dimes Birth Defects Foundation. (2005). *PeriStats: Born too soon and too small in the United States.* Retrieved from http://www.marchofdimes.com/peristats.

May, K. A. (1980). A typology of detachment and involvement styles adopted during pregnancy by first-time expectant fathers. *Western Journal of Nursing Research, 2*(2), 444–461.

May, K. A. (1982). Three phases of father involvement in pregnancy. *Nursing Research, 31*(6), 337–342.

McPheeters, M., et al. (2005). The epidemiology of threatened preterm labour: A prospective cohort study. *American Journal of Obstetrics and Gynecology, 192*(4), 1325–1330.

Mercer, R. (1995). *Becoming a mother.* New York: Springer.

Money, D., et al. (2008). SOGC clinical practice guideline: Guidelines for the management of herpes simplex virus in pregnancy. *Journal of Obstetrics and Gynaecology of Canada, 30*(6), 514–519. Retrieved from http://www.sogc.org/guidelines/documents/gui208CPG0806.pdf.

Montan, S. (2007). Increased risk in the elderly parturient. *Current Opinion in Obstetrics and Gynecology, 19*(2), 110–112.

Niebyl, J. R., & Simpson, J. L. (2007). Drugs and environmental agents in pregnancy and lactation: Embryology, teratology, epidemiology. In S. G. Gabbe, J. R. Niebyl, & J. L. Simpson (Eds.), *Obstetrics: Normal and problem pregnancies* (5th ed.). Philadelphia: Churchill Livingstone.

Olsen, O., & Jewell, M. (1998). Home versus hospital birth. *The Cochrane Database of Systematic Reviews,* Issue 3, CD000352.

Public Health Agency of Canada. (2005). *Fetal alcohol spectrum disorder (FASD): A framework for action.* Ottawa: Author. Retrieved from http://www.phac-aspc.gc.ca/publicat/fasd-fw-etcaf-ca/index-eng.php.

Public Health Agency of Canada. (2007). *Point-of-care HIV testing using simple/rapid HIV test kits: Guidance for health-care professionals.* Ottawa: Author. Retrieved from http://www.phac-aspc.gc.ca/publicat/ccdr-rmtc/07vol33/33s2/index-eng.php.

Public Health Agency of Canada. (2008a). *Canadian guidelines on sexually transmitted infections* (Cat. No. HP40-1/2010E-PDF). Ottawa: Author. Retrieved from http://www.phac-aspc.gc.ca/std-mts/sti-its/guide-lignesdir-eng.php.

Public Health Agency of Canada. (2008b). *Canadian perinatal report—2008 Edition* (Cat. No. HP10-12/2008E-PDF). Ottawa: Government of Canada. Retrieved from http://www.phac-aspc.gc.ca/publicat/2008/cphr-rspc/behaviours-comportements-eng.php.

Public Health Agency of Canada. (2009). *What mothers say: The Canadian maternity experiences survey* (Cat. No. HP5-74/2-2009E). Ottawa: Government of Canada.

Public Health Agency of Canada. (2010). *Canadian guidelines on sexually transmitted infections* (Cat. No. HP40-1/2010E). Ottawa: Author. Retrieved from http://www.phac-aspc.gc.ca/std-mts/sti-its/guide-lignesdir-eng.php.

Riordan, J., & Wambach, K. (2010). *Breastfeeding and human lactation* (4th ed.). Boston: Jones & Bartlett.

Rising, S. (1998). Centering pregnancy: An interdisciplinary model of empowerment. *Journal of Nurse-Midwifery, 43*(1), 46–54.

Rubin, R. (1975). Maternal tasks in pregnancy. *Maternal Child Nursing Journal, 4*(3), 143–153.

Rubin, R. (1984). *Maternity identity and the maternal experience.* New York: Springer.

Seidel, H. M., et al. (2006). *Mosby's guide to physical examination* (6th ed.). St. Louis: Mosby.

Society of Obstetricians and Gynaecologists of Canada. (2002). Clinical practice guideline: The management of nausea and vomiting of pregnancy. *Journal of Obstetrics and Gynaecology Canada, 24*(10), 817–823. Retrieved from http://www.sogc.org/guidelines/public/120E-CPG-October2002.pdf.

Society of Obstetricians and Gynaecologists of Canada. (2007). Clinical practice guideline: Screening for fetal aneuploidy. *Journal of Obstetrics and Gynaecology Canada, 29*(2), 146–161. Retrieved from http://sogc.org/guidelines/documents/187E-CPG-February2007.pdf.

Society of Obstetricians and Gynaecologists of Canada. (2008). SOGC clinical practice guideline: Diagnosis, evaluation and management of the hypertensive disorders of pregnancy. *Journal of Obstetrics and Gynaecology Canada, 30*(3), Suppl 1 (S1–S48). Retrieved from http://www.sogc.org/guidelines/documents/gui206CPG0803hypertensioncorrection.pdf.

Society of Obstetricians and Gynaecologists of Canada. (2010). SOGC clinical practice guideline: Alcohol use and pregnancy consensus clinical guideline. *Journal of Obstetrics and Gynaecology Canada, 32*(8), Suppl 3. Retrieved from http://www.sogc.org/guidelines/documents/gui245CPG1008E.pdf.

Wapner, R. J., Jenkins, T. M., & Khalek, N. (2009). Prenatal diagnosis of congenital disorders. In R. K. Creasy, et al. (Eds.), *Creasy & Resnik's maternal–fetal medicine: Principles and practice* (6th ed.). Philadelphia: Saunders.

Weng, X., Odouli, R., & Li, D. (2008). Maternal caffeine consumption during pregnancy and the risk of miscarriage: A prospective cohort study. *American Journal of Obstetrics and Gynecology, 198*(3), 279.e1–8.

Westheimer, R., & Lopater, S. (2005). *Human sexuality: A psychosocial perspective* (2nd ed.). Philadelphia: Lippincott Williams & Wilkins.

Additional Resources

Health Canada Radiation Protection Bureau: http://www.hc-sc.gc.ca/ahc-asc/branch-dirgen/hecs-dgsesc/sep-psm/rpb-br-eng.php

Motherisk: http://www.motherisk.org/women/index.jsp

Multiple Births Canada: http://www.multiplebirthscanada.org

Peel Region Health Department: Parenting in Peel

Just for Dads: http://www.peelregion.ca/health/family-health/just-for-dad/

Toddlers and Preschoolers: Jealousy and Sibling Rivalry: http://www.peelregion.ca/health/family-health/toddlers-and-preschoolers/behaviour/jealousy.htm

Perinatal Services BC (guidelines for care): http://www.perinatalservicesbc.ca/

http://www.perinatalservicesbc.ca//sites/bcrcp/files/resources/EPDS.pdf

Society of Obstetricians and Gynaecologists of Canada (SOGC): http://www.sogc.org

Unit 3

11 Maternal and Fetal Nutrition

Learning Objectives

On completion of this chapter, the reader will be able to:

- Explain recommended maternal weight gain during pregnancy.
- Compare the recommended level of intake of energy sources, protein, and key vitamins and minerals during pregnancy and lactation.
- Give examples of the food sources that provide the nutrients required for optimal maternal nutrition during pregnancy and lactation.
- Examine the role of nutrition supplements during pregnancy.
- List nutritional risk factors during pregnancy.
- Compare the dietary needs of adolescent and mature pregnant women.
- Analyze examples of eating patterns of women from different ethnic or cultural backgrounds and identify potential dietary problems.
- Assess nutritional status during pregnancy.

Electronic Resources

Additional information related to the content in Chapter 11 can be found on

evolve the companion Web site at

http://evolve.elsevier.com/Canada/Perry/maternal/

- Examination Review Questions
- Case Study—Nutrition During Pregnancy for the Overweight Woman
- Critical Thinking Exercise—Nutrition Education

As discussed earlier (see Box 1-3), the determinants of health are important social and individual factors that influence the health of Canadians. Many of the determinants of health have an impact on the quality and amount of dietary intake that women receive, which can ultimately influence pregnancy outcomes (Fig. 11-1). Maternal nutritional status is a significant factor because it is potentially alterable and because good nutrition before and during pregnancy can help prevent a variety of problems. Inadequate nutrition can lead to an increase in the number of **low-birth-weight** (LBW) **infants** (birth weight of 2500 g or less) and preterm infants that are born (Ramakrishnan, 2004). Neonatal and infant mortality and morbidity is increased for moderately LBW infants and is five times higher in infants born weighing more than 2500 g; the risk for **very-low-birth-weight** (VLBW) **infants** (less than 1500 g) is more than 100 times that of infants born weighing 2500 g or more (Canadian Institute for Health Information [CIHI], 2009; Public Health Agency of Canada [PHAC], 2008). Six percent of babies born in Canada weigh less than 2500 g at birth (CIHI, 2010). Thus it is essential that the importance of good nutrition be emphasized to all women of childbearing potential. Nutrition assessment, intervention, and evaluation must be an integral part of the nursing care given to all pregnant women.

Nutrient Needs Before Conception

A healthful diet before conception is the best way to ensure that adequate **nutrients** are available for the developing fetus. Folate or folic acid intake is of particular concern in the periconceptual period. Folate is the form in which this vitamin is found naturally in foods, and folic acid is the form used in the fortification of grain products and other foods and in vitamin supplements. Neural tube defects (failure in closure of the neural tube) are more common in infants of women with poor folic acid intake. In Canada, approximately 260 babies are born each year with a neural tube defect (Health Canada, 2005). Proper closure of the neural tube is required for normal formation of the spinal cord. The neural tube begins to close within the first month of gestation, often before the woman realizes that she is pregnant. It is estimated that the incidence of neural tube defects could be decreased by as much as 70% if all women had an adequate folate intake during the periconceptual period (Cornel, Smit, & de Jong-van den Berg, 2005). All women capable of becoming pregnant are advised to consume 0.4 to 1.0 mg of folic acid daily in fortified foods (ready-to-eat cereals and enriched grain products) or supplements and a diet rich in folate-containing foods, such as green leafy vegetables, whole grains, and fruits (Health Canada, 2011b) (Table 11-1).

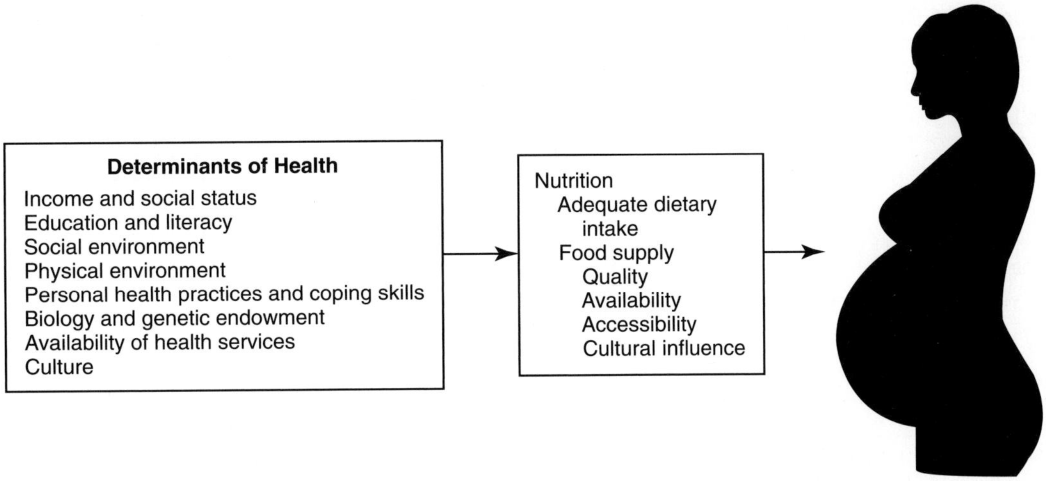

Fig. 11-1 Determinants of health that influence nutritional status.

Nutrient Needs During Pregnancy

Nutrient needs are determined, at least in part, by the stage of gestation. The amount of fetal growth varies during the different stages of pregnancy. During the first trimester, the synthesis of fetal tissues places relatively few demands on maternal nutrition. Therefore, during the first trimester, when the embryo or fetus is very small, the needs are only slightly increased over those before pregnancy. In contrast, the last trimester is a period of noticeable fetal growth when most of the fetal stores of energy sources and minerals are deposited. Thus, as fetal growth progresses during the second and third trimesters, the pregnant woman's need for some nutrients increases greatly.

The Institute of Medicine, in partnership with Health Canada, publishes recommendations for **Dietary Reference Intakes** (DRIs) for the people of Canada and the United States. The DRIs consist of **Recommended Dietary Allowances** (RDAs), Adequate Intakes (AIs), and Upper Limits (ULs) (i.e., guidelines for avoiding excessive intakes of nutrients that may be toxic if consumed in excess). DRIs are recommendations for daily nutritional intakes that meet the needs of almost all (97 to 98%) of the healthy members of the population. The DRIs include a wide variety of nutrients and food components; they are divided into age, sex, and life-stage categories (e.g., infancy, pregnancy, and lactation). They can be used as goals in planning the diets of individuals (Table 11-2).

Energy Needs

Energy (**kilocalories**, or kcal) needs are met by carbohydrate, fat, and protein in the diet. No specific recommendations exist for the amount of carbohydrate and fat in the diet of the pregnant women. However, intake of these nutrients should be adequate to support the recommended weight gain. Although protein can be used to supply energy, its primary role is to provide amino acids for the synthesis of new tissues (see discussion later in this chapter). The estimated energy expenditure for the first trimester is the same as in the prepregnant state; during the second **trimester** the RDA is 340 kcal greater than the prepregnancy needs, and during the third trimester it is 452 kcal more than the prepregnant needs (Institute of Medicine, 2009). Longitudinal assessment of weight gain during pregnancy is the best way to determine whether the kilocalorie intake is adequate; very underweight or active women may require more than the recommended increase in kilocalories to sustain the desired rate of weight gain.

Weight Gain

The optimal weight gain during pregnancy is not known precisely. However, it is known that the amount of weight gained by the mother during pregnancy has an important bearing on the course and outcome of pregnancy. When the mother is significantly underweight or overweight when pregnancy begins, or when weight gain during pregnancy is either too low or too high, both maternal and fetal risks are increased. Although adequate weight gain does not necessarily indicate that the diet is nutritionally adequate, it is associated with a reduced risk of giving birth to a **small-for-gestational-age** (SGA) **infant** or preterm infant. Severely underweight women are also more likely to have preterm labour and to give birth to LBW infants. Greater-than-expected weight gain during pregnancy may occur for many reasons, including multiple gestation, edema, pre-eclampsia, and overeating. Women who are obese (either before or during pregnancy) tend to have more complications in pregnancy (Watkins et al., 2003) (see Chapter 14). There is an increased likelihood of macrosomia and fetopelvic disproportion; **congenital** anomalies, operative birth; emergency Caesarean birth; postpartum hemorrhage; wound, genital tract, or urinary tract infection; birth trauma; and late fetal death.

The desirable weight gain during pregnancy varies among women. The primary factor to consider in making a weight gain recommendation is the appropriateness of the prepregnancy weight for the woman's height (Table 11-3). Ideally, all women would achieve their desirable body weight before conception.

Table 11-1 Sources of Dietary Folate

FOOD	1 FOOD GUIDE SERVING	MICROGRAMS* OF FOLATE AS DIETARY FOLATE EQUIVALENTS (mcg DFES)
Lentils and romano beans	175 mL	265–270
Black beans	175 mL	190
Okra	125 mL	140
White beans	175 mL	125
Asparagus and spinach, cooked	125 mL	120
Salad greens, such as Romaine lettuce, mustard greens, and endive	250 mL	80–110
Pinto beans, kidney beans, and chickpeas	175 mL	70–100
Pasta made with enriched wheat flour	125 mL	90
Avocado	½ fruit	80
Sunflower seeds, shelled	60 mL	80
Bagel made with enriched wheat flour	½ bagel (45 g)	60–75
Brussels sprouts, beets, and broccoli, cooked	125 mL	70
Bread made with enriched wheat flour or enriched corn meal	1 slice or ½ pita or ½ tortilla (35 g)	45–65
Spinach, raw	250 mL	60
Orange juice from concentrate	125 mL	60
Parsley	125 mL	50
Parsnips	125 mL	50
Peanuts, shelled	60 mL	45
Eggs	2 large	45
Corn	125 mL	40
Seaweed	125 mL	40
Orange	1 medium	40
Green peas	125 mL	40
Raspberries, strawberries, blackberries	125 mL	15–35
Enriched ready-to-eat cereal	30 g	10–35
Broccoli and cauliflower, raw	125 mL	30
Snow peas	125 mL	30
Pineapple juice	125 mL	30
Walnuts, almonds, and hazelnuts, shelled	60 mL	20–30
Baby carrots	125 mL	25
Kiwifruit	1 large	20
Clementine	1 fruit	20

(Source: Health Canada [2009]. *Prenatal nutrition guidelines for health professionals. Folate* [Cat. No. H164-109/2-2009E-PDF]. Ottawa: Author [pp. 4–5]. Retrieved from http://www.hc-sc.gc.ca/fn-an/pubs/nutrition/folate-eng.php.)
Amounts of folate are listed in food in mcg. The amount required daily is 0.4 to 1.0 mg.
*Amounts are approximate based on Canadian Nutrient File, Health Canada (2007). *Canadian nutrient file. Compilation of Canadian food composition data. Users' guide.*

A commonly used method of evaluating the appropriateness of weight for height is the body mass index (BMI) (see Table 4-1). The BMI is calculated by the following formula:

$$\text{BMI} = \text{Weight} \div \text{Height}^2$$

where the weight is in kilograms and height is in metres. Thus for a woman who weighed 51 kg before pregnancy and is 1.57 m tall:

$$\text{BMI} = 51\ \text{kg} \div (1.57\ \text{m})^2,\ \text{or}\ 20.7$$

Pattern of Weight Gain

Weight gain should take place throughout pregnancy. The risk of delivering an SGA infant is greater when the weight gain early in pregnancy has been poor. The likelihood of preterm birth is greater when the gains during the last half of pregnancy have been inadequate. These risks exist even when the total gain for the pregnancy is in the recommended range.

The optimal rate of weight gain depends on the stage of pregnancy. During the first and second trimesters, growth takes place primarily in maternal tissues; during the third

Table 11-2 Recommendations for Daily Intakes of Selected Nutrients During Pregnancy and Lactation

NUTRIENT (UNITS)	RECOMMENDATION FOR NONPREGNANT WOMAN	RECOMMENDATION FOR PREGNANCY*	RECOMMENDATION FOR LACTATION*	ROLE IN RELATION TO PREGNANCY AND LACTATION	FOOD SOURCES
Energy (kilocalories [kcal] or kilojoules [kJ]†)	Variable	First trimester, same as nonpregnant; second trimester, nonpregnant needs + 340 kcal (1423 kJ); third trimester, nonpregnant needs + 452 kcal (1891 kJ)	First 6 mo, nonpregnant needs + 330 kcal (1380 kJ); second 6 mo, nonpregnant needs + 400 kcal (1674 kJ)	Growth of fetal and maternal tissues; milk production	Carbohydrate, fat, and protein
Protein (g)	46	First trimester, second and third trimesters, nonpregnant needs + 25 g‡	Nonpregnant needs + 25 g	Synthesis of the products of conception; growth of maternal tissue and expansion of blood volume; secretion of milk protein during lactation	Meats, eggs, cheese, yogourt, legumes (dry beans and peas, peanuts), nuts, grains
Water (L)	2.7 total (2.2 in beverages)	3 total (2.3 in beverages)	3.8 total (3.1 in beverages)	Expansion of blood volume, excretion of wastes; milk secretion	Water and beverages made with water, milk, juices; all foods, especially frozen desserts, fruits, lettuce and other fresh vegetables
Fibre (g)	25	28	29	Promotes regular bowel elimination; reduces long-term risk of heart disease, diverticulosis, and diabetes	Whole grains, bran, vegetables, fruits, nuts and seeds
Minerals					
Calcium (mg)	1300/1000	1300/1000	1300/1000	Fetal and infant skeleton and tooth formation; maintenance of maternal bone and tooth mineralization	Milk, cheese, yogourt, sardines or other fish eaten with bones left in; deep green leafy vegetables except spinach or Swiss chard; calcium-set tofu, baked beans, tortillas
Iodine (mcg)	150	220	290	Increased maternal metabolic rate	Iodized salt, seafood, milk and milk products, commercial yeast breads, rolls, and doughnuts
Iron (mg)	15/18	27	9/10	Maternal hemoglobin formation; fetal liver iron storage	Liver, meats, whole grain or enriched breads and cereals, deep green leafy vegetables, legumes, dried fruits
Magnesium (mg)	360/310–320	400/350–360	360/310–320	Involved in energy and protein metabolism, tissue growth, muscle action	Nuts, legumes, cocoa, meats, whole grains
Zinc (mg)	8	12/11	14/12	Component of numerous enzyme systems; possibly important in preventing congenital malformations	Liver, shellfish, meats, whole grains, milk

Continued

Table 11-2 Recommendations for Daily Intakes of Selected Nutrients During Pregnancy and Lactation—cont'd

NUTRIENT (UNITS)	RECOMMENDATION FOR NONPREGNANT WOMAN	RECOMMENDATION FOR PREGNANCY*	RECOMMENDATION FOR LACTATION*	ROLE IN RELATION TO PREGNANCY AND LACTATION	FOOD SOURCES
Fat-Soluble Vitamins					
A (mcg)	700	750/770	1200/1300	Essential for cell development, tooth bud formation, bone growth	Deep green leafy vegetables, dark yellow vegetables, fruits, chili peppers, liver, fortified margarine and butter
D (mcg)	15 (600 IU)	15 (600 IU)	15 (600 IU)	Involved in absorption of calcium and phosphorus; improves mineralization	Fortified milk and margarine, egg yolk, butter, liver, seafood
E (mg)	15	15	19	Antioxidant (protects cell membranes from damage), especially important for preventing breakdown of RBCs	Vegetable oils, green leafy vegetables, whole grains, liver, nuts and seeds, cheese, fish
K (mcg)	75/90	75 (14- to 18-yr-old) 90 (19- to 50-yr-old)	75 (14- to 18-yr-old) 90 (19- to 50-yr-old)	Involved in synthesis of protein, blood coagulation, and bone metabolism	Green leafy vegetables, plant oils, margarine, soybeans, lentils
Water-Soluble Vitamins					
B_6 or pyridoxine (mg)	1.2/1.3	1.9	2	Involved in protein metabolism	Meats, liver, deep green vegetables, whole grains
B_{12} (mcg)	2.4	2.6	2.8	Production of nucleic acids and proteins; especially important in formation of RBCs and neural functioning	Milk and milk products, eggs, meats, liver, fortified soy milk
C (mg)	65/75	80/85	115/120	Tissue formation and integrity, formation of connective tissue; enhancement of iron absorption	Citrus fruits, strawberries, melons, broccoli, tomatoes, peppers, raw deep green leafy vegetables
Folate (mcg)	400	600	500	Prevention of neural tube defects, support for increased maternal RBC formation	Fortified ready-to-eat cereals and other grain products, green leafy vegetables, oranges, broccoli, asparagus, artichokes, liver

(Sources: Health Canada [2010]. *Dietary reference intakes tables.* Ottawa: Author. Retrieved from http://www.hc-sc.gc.ca/fn-an/nutrition/reference/table/index-eng.php; Institute of Medicine. [2004]. *Dietary reference intakes for energy, carbohydrate, fibre, fat, fatty acids, cholesterol, protein, and amino acids.* Washington, DC: National Academies Press; Institute of Medicine. [2004]. *Dietary reference intakes: Applications in dietary planning.* Washington, DC: National Academies Press; and Institute of Medicine. [2004]. *Dietary reference intakes for water, potassium, sodium, chloride, and sulfate.* Washington, DC: National Academies Press.)

*When two values appear, separated by a diagonal slash, the first is for females younger than 19 years, and the second is for those 19 to 50 years of age.

†The international metric unit of energy measurement is the joule (J). 1 kcal = 4.184 kJ.

‡Add an additional 25 g in twin pregnancies.

IU, international units; *RBC,* red blood cell.

Table 11-3 Recommended Rate of Weight Gain in Pregnancy*

PREPREGNANCY BMI CATEGORY	Mean† Rate of Weight Gain in Second and Third Trimester kg/WEEK	lb/WEEK	Recommended Range of Total Weight Gain kg	lb
BMI <18.5 Underweight	0.5	1.0	12.5–18	28–40
BMI 18.5–24.9 Normal weight	0.4	1.0	11.5–16	25–35
BMI 25.0–29.9 Overweight	0.3	0.6	7–11.5	15–25
BMI ≥30‡ Obese	0.2	0.5	5–9	11–20

(Source: Health Canada. [2009]. *Prenatal nutrition guidelines for health professionals. Maternal weight and weight gain in pregnancy.* Retrieved from http://www.hc-sc.gc.ca/fn-an/alt_formats/pdf/consultation/init/matern-weight-poids2009/draft-ebauche-eng.pdf.)
*Recommended rate of weight gain and total weight gain for singleton pregnancies according to prepregnancy BMI (adapted from Institute of Medicine, 2009).
†Rounded values.
‡A narrower range of weight gain may be advised for women with a prepregnancy BMI of 35 or greater. Individualized advice is recommended for these women.

trimester, growth occurs primarily in fetal tissues (see Table 11-3).

In multiple gestations, weight gain during the first half of pregnancy appears to be especially important (Luke, 2005). For the first trimester of twin gestation, a gain of 0.3 to 0.8 kg a week has been associated with positive outcomes. This general goal should be adjusted for prepregnancy weight (i.e., 0.6 to 0.8 kg weekly for underweight women and 0.3 to 0.6 kg weekly for obese women). Similarly, during mid-pregnancy in twin gestation, recommended weekly weight gains are 0.45 to 0.9 kg, with the lower value being for obese women and the higher one for underweight women. During late pregnancy, weekly gains of 0.3 to 0.6 kg are recommended for the woman pregnant with twins (Luke, 2005).

The recommended energy (kcal) intake corresponds to the recommended pattern of gain. For the first trimester there is no increment; an additional 340 kcal per day and 452 kcal per day over the prepregnant intake during the second and third trimester, respectively, are recommended. The amount of food providing the needed increase is not great. The additional calories can be obtained by eating 2 to 3 extra Canada Food Guide Servings from any of the food groups.

The reasons for an inadequate weight gain (less than 1 kg per month for normal-weight women or less than 0.5 kg per month for obese women during the last two trimesters) or excessive weight gain (more than 3 kg per month) should be evaluated thoroughly. Possible reasons for deviations from the expected rate of weight gain, besides inadequate or excessive dietary intake, include measurement or recording errors, differences in weight of clothing, time of day, and accumulation of fluids. An exceptionally high gain is likely to be caused by an accumulation of fluids; and a gain of more than 3 kg in a month, especially after the twentieth week of gestation, may indicate the development of pre-eclampsia.

Hazards of Restricting Adequate Weight Gain

An obsession with thinness and dieting pervades the North American culture. Figure-conscious women may find it difficult to make the transition from guarding against weight gain before pregnancy to valuing weight gain during pregnancy. In counselling these women, the nurse can emphasize both the positive effects of good nutrition and the adverse effects of maternal malnutrition (manifested by poor weight gain) on infant growth and development. This counselling should include information on the components of weight gain during pregnancy (Fig. 11-2) and the amount of this weight that will be lost at birth. Because lactation can help reduce maternal energy stores gradually, this could be an incentive for women to breastfeed their infants and thus be an opportunity for the nurse to promote breastfeeding.

Obesity and Pregnancy

In Canada, 15 to 18% of women of childbearing age are considered obese (Statistics Canada, 2011). Women who are obese have an increased risk of pregnancy disorders, including miscarriage, hypertensive disorders of pregnancy, and gestational diabetes, and an increased risk of fetal anomalies (2 times greater risk of neural tube defects), macrosomic fetus (>4000 g), and unexplained stillbirths. Labour complications include a 3 times greater risk of having a Caesarean section with more complications, including increased blood loss and wound infections (see Chapter 14) (Davies et al., 2010). However, pregnancy is not a time for weight reduction. Even overweight or obese pregnant women need to gain at least enough weight to equal the weight of the products of conception (fetus, placenta, and amniotic fluid). If overweight women limit their energy intake to prevent weight gain, they may also excessively limit their intake of important nutrients. Moreover, dietary restriction results in catabolism of fat stores,

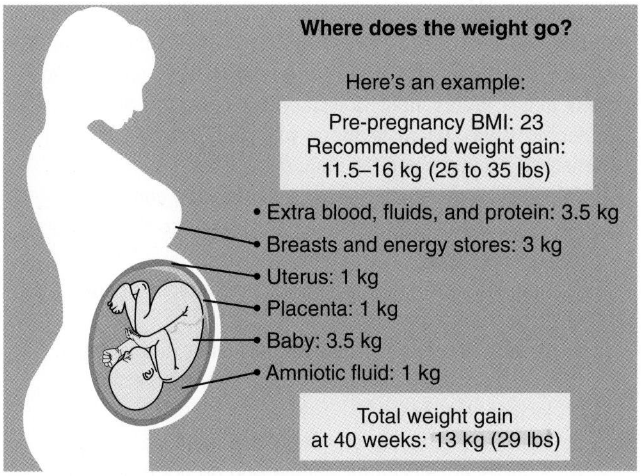

Fig. 11-2 Distribution of weight gain in pregnancy. The numbers represent an average; variation among women is great. The component with the greatest fluctuation is the weight increase attributed to extravascular fluids (edema) and maternal reserves of fat. *(Adapted from Health Canada. [2010].* Healthy weight gain during pregnancy. *Retrieved from http://www.hc-sc.gc.ca/fn-an/alt_formats/pdf/nutrition/prenatal/hwgdp-ppspg-eng.pdf.)*

which in turn augments the production of ketones. While the long-term effects of mild ketonemia during pregnancy are not known, ketonuria has been found to be correlated with preterm labour. It should be stressed to obese women (and to all pregnant women) that the quality of the food is important: nutrient-dense foods should be consumed and empty-calorie foods avoided (see Critical Thinking Exercise). Women who are overweight before pregnancy should be counselled to try to attain an ideal weight before becoming pregnant.

Weight gain is important, but excessive weight gain can be detrimental. Excessive weight gained during pregnancy may be difficult to lose after pregnancy, contributing to chronic overweight or obesity, an etiological factor in a host of chronic diseases, including hypertension, diabetes mellitus, and arteriosclerotic heart disease. The woman who gains 18 kg or more during pregnancy is especially at risk. When counselling the woman, it is best not to focus unduly on weight gain because this could result in feelings of stress and guilt in the woman who does not follow the preferred pattern of gain.

Food energy intake, and particularly intake of fat, may be high among low-income pregnant women, as this food is less expensive.

Health Canada's *Eating Well With Canada's Food Guide* sets recommendations for daily food intake for Canadians that are based on RDAs (see Table 11-2).

CRITICAL THINKING EXERCISE

Nutrition and the Overweight Pregnant Woman

Aysha, age 22, of Black and Asian descent is 3 months pregnant and comes to her initial appointment for diagnosis and care. Aysha appears to be overweight for her height (167 cm, 85 kg). To provide optimal care for her, you plan to calculate her pre-pregnancy body mass index. When her pregnancy is confirmed, you are asked to plan a diet with Aysha that meets the minimum daily requirements and allows for growth of the pregnancy. You know that it is important to include consideration of personal preferences and cultural factors in your plan. With Aysha, identify barriers to implementing the plan.

1. Evidence—Is there sufficient evidence to draw conclusions about an appropriate nutrition plan, taking into consideration personal preferences and cultural factors?
2. Assumptions—Describe underlying assumptions about each of the following issues:
   a. Dietary Reference Intakes for pregnancy and lactation
   b. Indicators of nutritional risk in pregnancy; possibility of lactose intolerance
   c. Daily food guide for pregnancy and lactation
   d. Sources of calcium for women who do not drink milk
3. What implications and priorities for nursing care can be drawn at this time?
4. What resources are available to assist Aysha and her family when planning meals?
5. Does the evidence objectively support your conclusion?
6. Are there alternative perspectives to your conclusion?

Protein

Protein, with its essential constituent nitrogen, is the nutrition element that is basic to growth. Adequate protein intake is essential to meet increasing physiological demands in pregnancy. These demands arise from the rapid growth of the fetus; the enlargement of the uterus and its supporting structures, the mammary glands, and the placenta; an increase in maternal circulating blood volume and subsequent demand for increased amounts of plasma protein to maintain colloidal osmotic pressure; and the formation of amniotic fluid.

Milk, meat, eggs, and cheese are complete-protein foods with a high biological value. Legumes (dried beans and peas), whole grains, and nuts are also valuable sources of protein. In addition, these protein-rich foods are a source of other nutrients such as calcium, iron, and B vitamins; plant sources of protein often provide needed dietary fibre. *Eating Well With Canada's Food Guide* recommends a daily food plan that would supply the quantities of protein needed (Table 11-4). It is recommended that pregnant women have at least 150 g of cooked fish per week, as fish contributes to a healthy pregnancy (Health Canada, 2009a).

When choosing fish, pregnant and nursing women should be especially careful to select those that are low in mercury. Larger fish that eat smaller fish are usually higher in mercury. See Nursing Alert.

NURSING ALERT High levels of mercury can harm the developing nervous system of the fetus or young child. Certain fish are especially high in mercury. Women who may become pregnant, women who are pregnant or nursing, and young children need to follow some precautions: limit consumption of fresh or frozen tuna, shark, swordfish, escolar, marlin, and orange roughy to 150 g/month, and eat as much as 75 g/week of a variety of commercially caught fish and shellfish low in mercury such as shrimp, salmon, pollock, catfish, and canned light tuna (but limit intake of albacore or "white" tuna and tuna steaks, which contain more mercury, to 300 g/week). Additional information about mercury levels in a variety of commercial fish is available at http://www.hc-sc.gc.ca/fn-an/securit/chem-chim/environ/mercur/cons-adv-etud-eng.php (Health Canada, 2011a).

Fluids

Essential during the exchange of nutrients and waste products across cell membranes, water is the main substance of cells, blood, lymph, amniotic fluid, and other vital body fluids. It also aids in maintaining body temperature. A good fluid intake promotes regular bowel function; constipation is sometimes a problem during pregnancy. The recommended daily intake is about 8 glasses (2 L) of fluid. Water, milk, and juices are good sources, although pregnant women should limit their intake of fruit juice, as they can be high in calories and therefore lead to extra weight gain. Foods in the diet should supply an additional 700 mL or more of fluid. Dehydration may increase the risk of cramping, contractions, and preterm labour.

Caffeine in moderate amounts has not been proven to cause adverse effects during pregnancy. However, women who consume more than 300 mg of caffeine daily (equivalent to a little more than 2 cups of coffee) may be at

Table 11-4 *Eating Well With Canada's Food Guide* Recommendations for Teenagers and Women (Aged 19–50)*

FOOD GROUP	SERVING SIZE	SUGGESTED NUMBER OF SERVINGS: TEENS	SUGGESTED NUMBER OF SERVINGS: WOMEN (AGED 19–50)
Grain Products			
Eat a variety and include half of servings as whole grains. Include whole-grain and enriched breads, cereals, pasta, and rice.	1 slice bread; ½ bun, bagel, or English muffin; 30 g ready-to-eat cereal; 125 mL (½ cup) cooked grains, 150 g hot cereal	6	6–7
Vegetables and Fruit			
Eat at least one dark green and one orange vegetable daily. Have vegetables and fruit more often than juice.	240 mL (1 cup) raw leafy greens; 125 mL (½ cup) of others, 125 mL (½ cup) fruit juice, 1 medium apple, orange, banana, peach, etc; 125 mL (½ cup) small or diced fruit	7	7-8
Milk and Alternatives			
Skim, 1%, 2%. Need 500 mL daily for adequate vitamin D	240 mL (1 cup) milk, 175 g yogourt; 50 g cheese	3-4	2
Meat and Alternatives			
Beans, lentils, tofu often Eat peanut butter or nuts rarely to avoid excessive fat intake. Limit egg intake to reduce cholesterol intake; trim fat from meat, and remove skin from poultry. Eat at least 2 servings of fish each week.	75 g or 125 mL meat, fish or poultry, 175 mL cooked beans, 2 eggs, 30 mL (2 tbsp) peanut butter	2	2
Other			
30–45 mL of unsaturated fat each day (canola, corn, flaxseed, olive, peanut, soybean, sunflower) Drink water regularly.			

(Source: Health Canada. [2007]. *Eating well with Canada's food guide* [Cat. No. H164-38/1-2007E]. Ottawa: Author [pp. 1–2]. Retrieved from http://www.hc-sc.gc.ca/fn-an/alt_formats/hpfb-dgpsa/pdf/food-guide-aliment/view_eatwell_vue_bienmang-eng.pdf. Reproduced with the permission of the Minister of Health, 2011.)
*Pregnant and lactating women should choose an extra 2 to 3 Food Guide Servings per day. This can be included in a meal or as a snack.

increased risk of miscarriage and giving birth to infants with IUGR. The ill effects of caffeine have been proposed to result from vasoconstriction of the blood vessels supplying the uterus or from interference with cell division in the developing fetus. Consequently, caffeine-containing products such as caffeinated coffee, tea, soft drinks, and cocoa beverages should be consumed only in limited quantities (300 mg daily). See the Evidence-Informed Practice box regarding safety of herbal teas.

Aspartame (NutraSweet, Equal), acesulfame potassium (Ace K, Sunett, Sweet One), and sucralose (Splenda), artificial sweeteners commonly used in low- or no-calorie beverages and low-calorie food products, have not been found to have adverse effects on the normal mother or fetus and thus are approved by Health Canada for use during pregnancy. Aspartame, which contains phenylalanine, should be avoided by pregnant women with phenylketonuria (PKU) (Table 11-5). Stevia (stevioside) is a sweetener that has not been approved by Health Canada.

Energy drinks claim to give people extra physical and mental energy. They are highly caffeinated beverages that also contain sugar, artificial sweeteners, amino acids, vitamins, and herbs. Energy drinks are not recommended for children or for pregnant or breastfeeding women (HealthLink BC, 2010).

Minerals, Vitamins, and Electrolytes

In general, the nutrient needs of pregnant women, except perhaps the need for folate and iron, can be met through dietary sources. Counselling about the importance of a varied diet rich in vitamins and minerals should be a part of every pregnant woman's early prenatal care and should be reinforced throughout pregnancy. Supplements of certain nutrients are recommended when the woman's diet is very nutritionally poor or when significant nutritional risk factors are present. Nutritional risk factors in pregnancy are listed in Box 11-1.

Iron

Iron is needed both to allow the transfer of adequate iron to the fetus and to permit expansion of the maternal red blood cell (RBC) mass. However, poor iron intake and absorption, which can result in iron deficiency anemia, is relatively common among women in the childbearing years. In Canada, anemia is a common condition in childbearing-aged women (approximately 25%) and in men and women with chronic gastrointestinal blood loss. It may be caused by low intake of iron, poor absorption of iron, or blood loss (Health Canada, 2009b). Iron-deficiency anemia is more prevalent in isolated First Nations communities and in teenage girls of South Asian descent (British Columbia Ministry of Health Services, 2004). Anemic women are poorly prepared to tolerate hemorrhage at the time of birth. In addition, women who have iron-deficiency anemia during early pregnancy are at increased risk of preterm birth and LBW infants. Iron deficiency during the third trimester apparently does not carry the same risk.

EVIDENCE-INFORMED PRACTICE Safety of Herbal Teas During Pregnancy

—Cheryl Sams

Ask the Question

Is it safe for pregnant women to drink herbal teas?

Search for Evidence

Search Strategies

Professional organization guidelines, meta-analyses, systematic reviews, randomized controlled trials, nonrandomized prospective studies, and retrospective studies since 2006

Databases Searched

CINAHL; Cochrane; Medline; and the Web sites for Health Canada, Motherisk, Public Health Agency of Canada, the Society of Obstetricians and Gynaecologists of Canada, and the Canadian Dietitian Association

Critically Analyze the Evidence

The Public Health Agency of Canada (PHAC) has guidelines that recommend the types of herbal teas that can be used when a woman is pregnant. The topic of herbal teas is an important issue for the pregnant mother. In North America, there is increasing interest in and trend toward using herbal and natural food products as well as complementary and alternative therapies. In addition, many pregnant women turn to herbal teas to avoid caffeine intake. It is important to recommend that all pregnant women consult with their health care providers before using herbal products.

Herbal tea (tisane or ptisan) is made with fruit or other herbs without *Carmelia sinesis*. Caution is needed with use because these teas can contain powerful medicinal-like ingredients. They can also contain other medicines or allergens or be poisonous or contaminated with toxins. The herbs can cause uterine stimulation or contractions or have a toxic effect on the fetus or mother. Interaction with medications can also be a problem.

There are gaps and limited clinical studies on the effect of herbs on pregnant women. Herbs or herbal teas vary greatly in concentration and in mix of ingredients. The Society of Obstetricians and Gynaecologists of Canada (SOGC) guidelines recommend two or three weak cups per day of raspberry leaf herbal tea: raspberry leaf is considered safe; ginger, citrus peel, rosehip, lemon balm, and peppermint can be used in moderate amounts. The following herbs should be avoided because safety has not been established: chamomiles, echinacea, evening primrose oil, ginkgo, St. John's wort, and tea tree oil. The following herbs are unsafe and need to be avoided: black cohosh, burdock, calendula, chaste tree, dong quai, feverfew, ginseng, hops, juniper, kava, licorice (as a herb), passionflower, valerian, uva-ursi, wild yam, and blue cohosh (PHAC, 2008; SOGC, 2011).

Implications for Practice

It is essential for all pregnant women to know the guidelines for safe use of herbs and herbal teas. Many women think that a natural product means that it is safe to use. It is difficult for the consumer to sift through the available information to determine what is evidence informed and what is not. Health Canada and the Public Health Agency of Canada are good sources and clearly outline the national guidelines for consumers.

References

Public Health Agency of Canada. (2008). *Caffeine in pregnancy*. Ottawa: Author. Retrieved from http://www.phac-aspc.gc.ca/hp-gs/know-savoir/caffeine-eng.php.

Society of Obstetricians and Gynaecologists of Canada. (2011). *Women's health information*. Ottawa: Author. Retrieved from http://www.sogc.org/health/pregnancy-herbal_e.asp.

BOX 11-1 Indicators of Nutritional Risk in Pregnancy

- Adolescence
- Frequent pregnancies: three within 2 years
- Poor fetal outcome in a previous pregnancy
- Poverty
- Poor diet habits with resistance to change
- Use of tobacco, alcohol, or drugs
- Weight at conception significantly under or over normal weight
- Problems with weight gain
- Any weight loss
- Weight gain of less than 1 kg/month after the first trimester
- Weight gain of more than 1 kg/week after the first trimester
- Multifetal pregnancy
- Low hemoglobin or hematocrit values (or both)

The RDA of iron during pregnancy is 27 mg/day. Health Canada recommends that all pregnant women take a daily multivitamin with 16 to 20 mg of iron (Health Canada, 2009b). Pregnant women who are **vegetarian** may need an increased amount of iron. This dose is well below the level of iron supplementation that has been linked to negative side effects (reduced zinc absorption and gastrointestinal symptoms) (Health Canada, 2009b). Iron supplements may be poorly tolerated during the nausea that is prevalent in the first trimester and may need to be started after week 12. Iron supplementation of women with iron deficiency can improve maternal hematological indices and appears to reduce the rate of LBW births. If maternal iron-deficiency anemia is present (preferably diagnosed by measurement of serum ferritin, a storage form of iron), increased dosages (60 to 120 mg daily) are recommended. Certain foods taken with an iron supplement can promote or inhibit absorption of iron from the supplement (e.g., tea or coffee close to meals). See the Patient Teaching box regarding iron supplementation. Even when a woman is taking an iron supplement, she should

Table 11-5 Use of Artificial Sweeteners During Pregnancy

SWEETENER	OTHER NAMES	COMPARISON TO SUGAR	FLAVOUR	SAFE DURING PREGNANCY AND LACTATION?	CALORIC VALUE	STABILITY	USES	OTHER
Acesulfame Potassium	Ace K, Sunette, Sweet One	200× sweeter, (300× sweeter when blended with aspartame)	Bitter or metallic aftertaste in large amounts	Yes	0	Heat stable	Baked goods, frozen desserts, sugar-free gelatin, pudding, and beverages	Mixing with other sweeteners reduces aftertaste
Aspartame	Equal, Nutrasweet	200× sweeter (300× sweeter when blended with Ace K)	Sugar-like sweetness with no bitter aftertaste	Yes, unless woman has Phenylketonuria (PKU)	4 kcal/g	Heat sensitive (breaks down and loses sweetness)	Soft drinks, gelatin, desserts, pudding mixes, breakfast cereal, beverages, gum, dairy products	Has the same calories as sugar but has a much sweeter taste. Less is needed for the same sweetness.
Cyclamate	Sugar Twin	30× sweeter	Slowly gets sweeter with lasting sweet flavour	No—has been linked to cancer and is banned in the U.S.	0	Heat stable	Variety of foods, beverages, cooking and baking	Health Canada doesn't allow its addition to foods. It is approved as a table-top sweetener, with proper labelling.
Saccharin	Sweet'n Low	300× sweeter	Bitter aftertaste in large amounts	No—saccharin can cross the placenta and may affect the fetus	0	Heat stable	Variety of foods, beverages, cooking and baking	Use only if advised by a physician. Caution: read labels, as it may be used as an ingredient.
Stevia	Sweet Leaf	Up to 300× sweeter	Varying reports; some report bitter or licorice aftertaste	No—stevia is an herb and hasn't been proven safe in pregnancy	0	Heat stable	Variety of foods, beverages, cooking and baking	Only sold as a dietary supplement in Canada. It cannot be added to foods. This may change in the future.
Sucralose	Splenda	600× sweeter	No bitter aftertaste	Yes	0	Heat stable	Baked goods, nonalcoholic drinks, gum, coffees/teas, frostings, fats/oils, frozen desserts, fruit juice, sweet sauce	Made from sugar itself
Sugar Alcohols	Polyols (Sorbitol, Manitol, Isomalt)	½ as sweet	Gives a cooling sensation in the mouth	Yes	~2 kcal/g	Heat stable	Manufactured for use in sugar-free candies, cookies, chewing gum, etc.	Does not cause cavities because it is not fermented by bacteria. May have a laxative effect.

(Source: Brant County Health Unit. [n.d]. *Artificial sweeteners and your pregnancy* [Pamphlet]. Brantford, ON: Author. Retrieved from http://www.bchu.org/pdf/Nutrition/Artificial_Sweeteners_2_page.pdf. Reprinted with permission from the Brant County Health Unit.)

PATIENT TEACHING
Iron Supplementation

- Vitamin C (in citrus fruits, tomatoes, melons, and strawberries) and heme iron (in meats) increase the absorption of iron supplement; therefore, include these in the diet often.
- Bran, tea, coffee, milk, oxalates (in spinach and Swiss chard), and egg yolk decrease iron absorption. Avoid consuming them at the same time as the supplement.
- Iron is absorbed best if it is taken when the stomach is empty (i.e., take it between meals with a beverage other than tea, coffee, or milk).
- Iron can be taken at bedtime if abdominal discomfort occurs when it is taken between meals.
- If an iron dose is missed, take it as soon as it is remembered if that is within 13 hours of the scheduled dose. Do not double up on the dose.
- Keep the supplement in a childproof container and out of the reach of any children in the household.
- The iron may cause stools to be black or dark green.
- Constipation is common with iron supplementation. A diet high in fibre with adequate fluid intake is recommended.

include good food sources of iron in her daily diet (see Table 11-2).

Counselling About Iron Supplementation

A variety of dietary factors can affect the completeness of absorption of an iron supplement. The Patient Teaching box summarizes important points regarding iron supplementation.

Calcium

There is no increase in the DRI of calcium during pregnancy and lactation over that recommended for the nonpregnant woman (see Table 11-2). The DRI (1000 mg daily for women 19 years and older and 1300 mg for those younger than 19 years) appears to provide sufficient calcium for fetal bone and tooth development to proceed while maintaining maternal bone mass.

Milk and yogourt are especially rich sources of calcium, providing approximately 300 mg per 240 mL. Nevertheless, many women either do not consume these foods or do not consume adequate amounts to provide the recommended intakes of calcium. One problem that can interfere with milk consumption is **lactose intolerance**, the inability to digest milk sugar (lactose) caused by the lack of the lactase enzyme in the small intestine. Lactose intolerance is relatively common in adults, particularly among Asians and First Nations, Métis, and Inuit. Milk consumption can cause abdominal cramping, bloating, and diarrhea in individuals with lactose intolerance, although many of these individuals can tolerate small amounts of milk without symptoms. Yogourt, sweet acidophilus milk, buttermilk, cheese, chocolate milk, and cocoa may be tolerated even when fresh fluid milk is not. Commercial lactase supplements (e.g., Lactaid) are widely available to consume

BOX 11-2 Calcium Sources for Women Who Do Not Drink Milk

Each of the following provides approximately the same amount of calcium as 240 mL (1 cup) of milk:

Fish
90 g can of sardines
150 g can of salmon (if bones are eaten)

Beans and Legumes
750 mL (3 cups) of cooked dried beans
625 mL (2½ cups) of refried beans
500 mL (2 cups) of baked beans with molasses
240 mL (1 cup) of tofu (calcium is added in processing)

Greens
240 mL (1 cup) of collards
365 mL (1½ cups) of kale or turnip greens

Baked Products
3 pieces of cornbread
3 English muffins
4 slices of French toast
2 waffles (15 cm in diameter)

Fruits
11 dried figs
270 mL (1⅛ cups) of orange juice with calcium added

Sauces
90 mL (3 oz) of pesto sauce
150 g (5 oz) of cheese sauce

with milk. Many supermarkets stock lactase-treated milk. The lactase in these products hydrolyzes, or digests, the lactose in milk, making it possible for lactose-intolerant people to drink milk.

In some cultures adults rarely drink milk. For example, Latin American people may use milk only as an additive in coffee. Pregnant women from these cultures may need to consume nondairy sources of calcium (Box 11-2). Vegetarian diets may also be deficient in calcium. If calcium intake appears low and the woman does not change her dietary habits despite counselling, a daily supplement containing 600 mg of elemental calcium may be needed. Calcium supplements may also be recommended when a pregnant woman experiences leg cramps caused by an imbalance in the calcium-to-phosphorus ratio. Bone meal supplements are not recommended in pregnancy (Box 11-3).

Magnesium

Magnesium is necessary for bone and tissue growth. Diets of women in the childbearing years are likely to be low in magnesium, and as many as half of pregnant and lactating women may have inadequate intake (Institute of Medicine, 2004). Adolescents and low-income women are especially at risk. Dairy products, nuts, whole grains, and green leafy vegetables are good sources of magnesium.

BOX 11-3 Complementary and Alternative Therapies

Bone meal, which is sometimes used as a calcium source by pregnant women, is frequently found to be contaminated with lead. Lead freely crosses the placenta; thus regular maternal intake of bone meal may result in high levels of lead in the fetus.

(Source: Shannon, M. [2003]. Severe lead poisoning in pregnancy. *Ambulatory Pediatrics, 3*[1], 37–39.)

Sodium

During pregnancy the need for sodium increases slightly, primarily because the body water is expanding (e.g., the expanding blood volume). Sodium is essential for maintaining body water balance. In the past, dietary sodium was routinely restricted in an effort to control the peripheral edema that commonly occurs during pregnancy. It is now recognized that moderate peripheral edema is normal in pregnancy, occurring as a response to the fluid-retaining effects of elevated levels of estrogen. Severe sodium restriction may make it difficult for pregnant women to achieve an adequate diet. Grain, milk, and meat products, which are good sources of nutrients needed during pregnancy, are significant sources of sodium. In addition, sodium restriction may stress the adrenal glands and the kidneys as they attempt to retain adequate sodium. In general, sodium restriction is necessary only if the woman has a medical condition such as renal or liver failure or hypertension that warrants such a restriction.

Excessive intake of sodium is discouraged during pregnancy, just as it is in nonpregnant women, because it may contribute to the development of hypertension in salt-sensitive individuals. An adequate sodium intake for pregnant and lactating women, as well as nonpregnant women in the childbearing years, is estimated to be 1.5 g/day, with a recommended upper limit of intake of 2.3 g/day (Institute of Medicine, 2004). Table salt (sodium chloride) is the richest source of sodium, with approximately 2.3 g of sodium contained in 6 g (1 tsp) of salt. Most canned foods contain added salt unless the label states otherwise. Large amounts of sodium are also found in many processed foods, including meats (e.g., smoked or cured meats, cold cuts, and corned beef), frozen entrées and meals, baked goods, mixes for casseroles or grain products, soups, and condiments. Products low in nutritive value and excessively high in sodium include pretzels, potato and other chips (except salt-free), pickles, ketchup, prepared mustard, steak and Worcestershire sauces, some soft drinks, and bouillon. A moderate sodium intake can usually be achieved by salting food lightly in cooking; adding no additional salt at the table; and avoiding low-nutrient, high-sodium foods.

Potassium

Diets including adequate intake of potassium are associated with a reduced risk of hypertension. Potassium has been identified as one of the nutrients most likely to be lacking in the diets of women of childbearing years (Institute of Medicine, 2004). A diet including 8 to 10 servings of unprocessed fruits and vegetables daily, along with moderate amounts of low-fat meats and dairy products, has been effective in reducing sodium intake while providing adequate amounts of potassium.

Zinc

Zinc is a constituent of numerous enzymes involved in major metabolic pathways. Zinc deficiency is associated with malformations of the central nervous system in infants. When large amounts of iron and folic acid are consumed, the absorption of zinc is inhibited, and serum zinc levels are reduced as a result. Because iron and folic acid supplements are commonly prescribed during pregnancy, pregnant women should be encouraged to consume recommended sources of zinc daily (see Table 11-2). Women with anemia who receive high-dose iron supplements also need supplements of zinc and copper.

Fluoride

There is no evidence that prenatal fluoride supplementation reduces the child's likelihood of tooth decay during the preschool years. No increase in fluoride intake over the nonpregnant RDAs is currently recommended during pregnancy (Institute of Medicine, 2004).

Fat-Soluble Vitamins

Fat-soluble vitamins—A, D, E, and K—are stored in the body tissues. These are of special concern during pregnancy because vitamin E intake is among the nutrients most likely to be lacking in the diets of women of childbearing age, and intake of vitamins A and D is also low in the diets of some women (Institute of Medicine, 2004). With chronic overdoses these vitamins can reach toxic levels. Because of the high potential for toxicity, pregnant women are advised to take fat-soluble vitamin supplements only as prescribed.

Adequate intake of vitamin A is needed so that sufficient amounts of the vitamin can be stored in the fetus. A well-chosen diet including adequate amounts of deep yellow and deep green vegetables and fruits such as leafy greens, broccoli, carrots, cantaloupe, and apricots provides sufficient amounts of carotenes that can be converted in the body to vitamin A. Congenital malformations have occurred in infants of mothers who took excessive amounts of preformed vitamin A (from supplements) during pregnancy; thus supplements are not recommended for pregnant women. Vitamin A analogs such as isotretinoin (Accutane), which are prescribed for the treatment of cystic acne, are of special concern. Isotretinoin use during early pregnancy has been associated with an increased incidence of heart malformations, facial abnormalities, cleft palate, hydrocephalus, and deafness and blindness in the infant, as well as an increased risk of miscarriage. Topical agents such as tretinoin (Atralin) do not appear to enter the circulation in any substantial amounts, but their safety in pregnancy has not been confirmed.

Vitamin D plays an important role in the absorption and metabolism of calcium. The main food sources of this vitamin are enriched or fortified foods such as milk and ready-to-eat cereals. Vitamin D is also produced in the skin by the action of ultraviolet light (in sunlight). Severe deficiency may lead to neonatal hypocalcemia and tetany, as well as to hypoplasia of the tooth enamel. Women with lactose intolerance and those who do not include milk in their diet for any reason are at risk for vitamin D deficiency. Other risk factors are dark skin; habitual use of clothing that covers most of the skin (e.g., Muslim women with extensive body covering); and living in northern latitudes where sunlight exposure is limited, especially during the winter. Use of recommended amounts of sunscreen with a sun protection factor (SPF) rating of 15 or greater reduces skin vitamin D production by as much as 99%, thus regular intake of fortified foods or a supplement may be needed.

Vitamin E is needed for protection against oxidative stress, and pregnancy is associated with increased oxidative stress. Indeed, oxidative stress has been proposed as an explanation for the etiology of pre-eclampsia (Allen, 2005). Vegetable oils and nuts are especially good sources of vitamin E, and whole grains and green leafy vegetables are moderate sources.

Vitamin K is involved in the synthesis of proteins needed for blood coagulation and bone metabolism. The RDA for women is 90 mcg/day. The classic sign of vitamin K deficiency is an increase in prothrombin time; severe cases result in hemorrhage. Food sources are green leafy vegetables, plant oils and margarine, and soybeans and lentils.

Water-Soluble Vitamins

Body stores of water-soluble vitamins are much smaller than those of fat-soluble vitamins. In contrast to fat-soluble vitamins, water-soluble vitamins are readily excreted in the urine. Therefore, recommended sources of these vitamins must be consumed frequently. Toxicity with overdose is less likely than with fat-soluble vitamins.

Folate or Folic Acid

Because of the increase in RBC production during pregnancy and the nutrition requirements of the rapidly growing cells in the fetus and placenta, pregnant women should consume about 50% more folic acid than that needed by nonpregnant women. Folic acid (0.4 mg daily) is most important preconception and during the first trimester. In Canada, all enriched grain products (which includes most white breads, flour, and pasta) must contain folic acid at a level of 0.15 mg/100 g of flour. This level of fortification is designed to supply approximately 0.1 mg of folic acid daily in the average Canadian diet and has significantly increased folic acid consumption in the population as a whole. All women of childbearing potential need careful counselling about including good sources of folate in their diets (see Table 11-1). Supplemental folic acid is usually prescribed to ensure that intake is adequate. Women who have borne a child with a neural tube defect, have diabetes or epilepsy, or are obese are advised to consume 4 mg of folic acid daily; a supplement is required for them to achieve this level of intake. Folic acid decreases the risk of other congenital anomalies, including congenital heart defects, urinary tract anomalies, oral facial clefts, and limb defects. All birth defects could be decreased by 50% with folic acid supplementation (Wilson et al., 2003).

Pyridoxine

Pyridoxine, or vitamin B_6, is involved in protein metabolism. Although levels of a pyridoxine-containing enzyme have been reported to be low in women with pre-eclampsia, there is no evidence that supplementation prevents or corrects the condition. No supplement is recommended routinely, but women with poor diets and those at nutritional risk (see Box 11-1) may need a supplement providing 2 mg/day. Pyridoxine has been effective in reducing the nausea and vomiting of early pregnancy in some trials.

Vitamin C

Vitamin C, or ascorbic acid, plays an important role in tissue formation and enhances the absorption of iron. The vitamin C needs of most women are readily met by a diet that includes at least one daily serving of citrus fruit or juice or another good source of the vitamin (see Table 11-2), but women who smoke need more. For women at nutritional risk, a supplement of 50 mg/day is recommended. However, if the mother takes excessive doses of this vitamin during pregnancy, a vitamin C deficiency may develop in the infant after birth.

Vitamin B_{12}

Vitamin B_{12} is involved in the production of nucleic acids and proteins; it is especially important in the formation of RBCs and neural functioning. It is found in milk and milk products, eggs, meats, liver, and fortified soy milk.

Multivitamin–Multimineral Supplements During Pregnancy

Food can and should be the normal vehicle to meet the additional needs imposed by pregnancy, except for iron. In addition, the recommended folate or folic acid intake may be difficult for some women to achieve. Some women habitually consume diets that are deficient in necessary nutrients and for whatever reason may be unable to change this intake. For this reason, the Society of Obstetricians and Gynaecologists of Canada (SOGC) recommends that all women who are planning a pregnancy take a multivitamin supplement that contains folic acid (Wilson et al., 2007). It is important that the pregnant woman understands that the use of a vitamin–mineral supplement does not lessen the need to consume a nutritious, well-balanced diet.

Other Nutritional Issues During Pregnancy

Pica and Food Cravings

Pica, the practice of consuming nonfood substances (e.g., clay, dirt, and laundry starch) or excessive amounts of foodstuffs low in nutritional value (e.g., cornstarch, ice or freezer frost, baking powder, and baking soda), is often influenced by the woman's cultural background (Fig. 11-3). Black women report practising pica more than other women, as do women from rural areas and women with a family history of pica (Corbett, Ryan, & Werenich, 2003). Regular and heavy consumption of low-nutrient products may cause more nutritious foods to be displaced from the diet, and the items consumed may interfere with the absorption of nutrients, especially minerals. As an example, cornstarch ingestion is popular among Black women. It is a source of "empty" calories; half a cup (64 g) provides 240 kcal (57 kJ) but almost no vitamins, minerals, or protein. Grotegut and colleagues (2006) reported a case of a 31-week gestation multigravida ingesting a box of baking soda (454 g of sodium

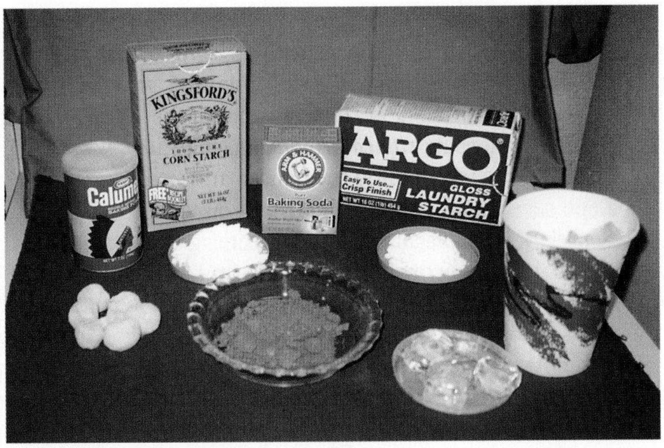

Fig. 11-3 Nonfood substances consumed in pica: red clay from Georgia, Nzu from Eastern Nigeria, baking powder, corn starch, baking soda, laundry starch, and ice. Some individuals practise poly-pica (consuming more than one of these substances). *(Courtesy Shannon Perry, Phoenix, AZ.)*

bicarbonate) each day, which resulted in severe hypokalemic metabolic alkalosis and rhabdomyolysis. More than one substance may be ingested (Ngozi, 2008). Women with pica have lower hemoglobin levels than those of women without pica.

Moreover, there is a risk that nonfood items are contaminated with heavy metals or other toxic substances. Among Mexican women, consumption of "tierra" includes both soil and pulverized Mexican pottery (Klitzman et al., 2002; Shannon, 2003). Lead contamination of soils and soil-based products has caused high levels of lead in both pregnant women and their newborns. The possibility of pica must be considered when pregnant women are found to be anemic, and the nurse should provide counselling about the health risks associated with pica (Corbett et al., 2003).

The existence of pica and details of the types and amounts of products ingested are likely to be discovered only by the sensitive interviewer who has developed a relationship of trust with the woman. It has been proposed that pica and food cravings (e.g., the urge to have ice cream, pickles, or pizza) during pregnancy are caused by an innate drive to consume nutrients missing from the diet. However, research has not supported this hypothesis.

Adolescent Pregnancy Needs

Many adolescent females have diets that provide less than the recommended intake of key nutrients, including energy, calcium, and iron. Pregnant adolescents and their infants are at increased risk of complications during pregnancy and parturition. Growth of the pelvis is delayed in comparison with growth in stature, which helps to explain why **cephalopelvic disproportion** and other mechanical problems associated with labour may be more common among young adolescents. Competition for nutrients between the growing adolescent and the fetus may also contribute to some of the poor outcomes apparent in teen pregnancies. Pregnant adolescents should be encouraged to choose a weight gain goal at the upper end of the range for their BMI.

Efforts to improve the nutritional health of pregnant adolescents focus on improving the nutrition knowledge, meal planning, and food selection and preparation skills of young women; promoting access to prenatal care; and developing nutrition interventions and educational programs that are effective with adolescents. It is also important to understand the factors that create barriers to change in the adolescent population.

Pre-Eclampsia

The cause of pre-eclampsia is not known. There has been speculation that the poor intake of several nutrients, including calcium, magnesium, vitamin B_6, and protein, might foster its development. There is no definitive evidence that nutrition deficiencies are causes or that nutrition supplements can help prevent it. At present, a diet adequate in the recommended nutrients (see Table 11-2) appears to be the best means of reducing the risk of pre-eclampsia.

Nursing Care Management

During pregnancy, nutrition plays a key role in achieving an optimal outcome for the mother and her unborn baby (see Nursing Process box). Motivation to learn about nutrition is usually higher during pregnancy as parents strive to "do what's right for the baby." Optimal nutrition cannot eliminate all problems that may arise during pregnancy, but it does establish a good foundation for supporting the needs of the mother and her unborn baby (see Community Focus box).

Diet History

A *diet history* is a description of the woman's usual food and beverage intake and factors affecting her nutritional status. These include such factors as medications being taken and adequacy of income to allow her to purchase the necessary foods.

Obstetrical and Gynecological Effects on Nutrition

Nutrition reserves may be depleted in the multiparous woman or one who has had frequent pregnancies (especially three pregnancies within 2 years). A history of preterm birth or the birth of an LBW or SGA infant may indicate inadequate dietary intake. Pre-eclampsia may also be a factor in poor maternal nutrition. Birth of a large-for-gestational-age infant may indicate the existence of maternal diabetes mellitus. Previous contraceptive methods also may affect reproductive health. Increased menstrual blood loss often occurs during the first 3 to 6 months after placement of an intrauterine contraceptive device. Consequently, the user may have low iron stores or even iron-deficiency anemia. Oral contraceptive agents are associated with decreased menstrual losses and increased iron stores. However, oral contraceptives may interfere with folic acid metabolism.

Medical History

Chronic maternal illnesses such as diabetes mellitus, renal disease, liver disease, cystic fibrosis, or other malabsorptive disorders; seizure disorders and the use of anticonvulsant agents; hypertension; and PKU may affect a woman's nutritional status and dietary needs. In women with illnesses

NURSING PROCESS: NUTRITION

Assessment

Assessment is based on a diet history obtained from an interview and review of the woman's health records, physical examination, and laboratory results. Ideally, a nutritional assessment is performed before conception so that any recommended changes in diet, lifestyle, and weight can be undertaken before the woman becomes pregnant.

Nursing Diagnoses

Imbalanced nutrition: less than body requirements related to
- inadequate information about nutrition needs and weight gain during pregnancy
- misperceptions regarding normal body changes during pregnancy and inappropriate fear of becoming fat
- inadequate income or skills in meal planning and preparation

Imbalanced nutrition: more than body requirements related to
- excessive intake of energy (calories) or decrease in activity during pregnancy
- use of unnecessary dietary supplements

Constipation related to
- decrease in gastrointestinal motility because of elevated progesterone levels
- compression of intestines by the enlarging uterus
- oral iron supplementation

Planning

Nutrition-related outcomes are that the woman will do the following:
- Achieve an appropriate weight gain during pregnancy, which takes into account such factors as prepregnancy weight, whether she is overweight or obese or underweight, and whether the pregnancy is single or multifetal
- Consume adequate nutrients from the diet and supplements to meet estimated needs
- Cope successfully with nutrition-related discomforts associated with pregnancy, such as morning sickness, pyrosis (heartburn), and constipation
- Avoid or reduce potentially harmful practices, such as smoking, alcohol consumption, and caffeine intake
- Return to prepregnancy weight (or an appropriate weight for height) within 6 months of giving birth

Interventions

- Acquaint the woman with nutrition needs during pregnancy and, if necessary, the characteristics of an adequate diet.
- Help her individualize her diet so that she achieves an adequate intake while conforming to her personal, cultural, financial, and health circumstances.
- Acquaint her with strategies for coping with the nutrition-related discomforts of pregnancy.
- Help her use nutrition supplements appropriately.
- Consult with and make referrals to other professionals or services as indicated.

Evaluation

- Compare the woman's weight gain with standardized grids showing recommended patterns.
- Compare the woman's diet with the plan in Table 11-4. It is essential that individual factors affecting nutrition needs and dietary intake be considered.
- Use data from physical examination and laboratory testing to confirm that nutritional status is adequate.

COMMUNITY FOCUS

Canada Prenatal Nutrition Program

The Canadian Prenatal Nutrition Program (CPNP) funds community groups to develop or enhance programs for vulnerable pregnant women. Through a community development approach, the CPNP aims to reduce the incidence of unhealthy birth weights, improve the health of both infant and mother, and encourage breastfeeding.

Look for a Canada Prenatal Nutrition Program in your area. Contact the program and, if possible, visit the clinic. What services are offered by the Program? Who are the clients that use this service? How difficult is it to access the services provided by the Program? Does the clinic employ a dietitian or nutritionist? Are there materials and services provided in a variety of languages? Identify strengths and weaknesses of nutrition education in that setting. How do women get access to the services provided by CPNP?

Canada Prenatal Nutrition Program (CPNP): http://www.phac-aspc.gc.ca/dca-dea/programs-mes/cpnp_main-eng.php

that have resulted in nutrition deficits or that require dietary treatment (e.g., diabetes mellitus, PKU), it is extremely important that nutritional care be started and that the condition be optimally controlled before conception. A registered dietitian can provide in-depth counselling for the woman who requires medical nutrition therapy during pregnancy and lactation.

Usual Maternal Diet

The woman's usual food and beverage intake, adequacy of income and other resources to meet her nutrition needs, dietary modifications, food allergies and intolerances, medications and nutrition supplements being taken, history of pica, and cultural dietary requirements should be ascertained. In addition, the presence and severity of nutrition-related discomforts of pregnancy such as morning sickness, constipation, and pyrosis (heartburn) should be determined. The nurse should be alert to any evidence of eating disorders such as **anorexia nervosa**, **bulimia**, or frequent and rigorous dieting before or during pregnancy.

The impact of food allergies and intolerances on nutritional status ranges from very important to almost nil. Lactose intolerance is of special concern in pregnant and lactating women because no other food group equals milk and milk products in terms of calcium content. If a woman has lactose intolerance, the interviewer should explore her intake of other calcium sources (see Box 11-2).

The assessment must include an evaluation of the woman's financial status and her knowledge of healthy dietary practices. The quality of the diet improves with increasing socioeconomic status and educational level. Poor women may not have access to adequate refrigeration and cooking facilities and may find it difficult to obtain nutritious food (see Fig. 11-1). Pregnancy rates are high among homeless women, and many of these women cannot or do not take advantage of services such as prenatal nutrition programs.

Box 11-4 provides a simple tool for obtaining diet history information. When potential problems are identified, they should be followed up with a careful interview.

Physical Examination

Anthropometric (body) measurements provide short- and long-term information on a woman's nutritional status and are thus essential to the assessment. At a minimum, the woman's height and weight must be determined at the time of her first prenatal visit, and her weight should be measured at each subsequent visit (see earlier discussion of BMI).

A careful physical examination can reveal objective signs of malnutrition (Table 11-6). However, it is important to note that some of these signs are nonspecific and that the physiological changes of pregnancy may complicate the interpretation of physical findings. For example, lower extremity edema often occurs in calorie and protein deficiency, but it may also be a normal finding in the third trimester of pregnancy. Interpretation of physical findings is made easier by taking a thorough health history and conducting laboratory testing, if indicated.

BOX 11-4 Food Intake Questionnaire

How many servings of the following did you eat or drink yesterday? If the way you ate yesterday wasn't the way you usually eat, choose a recent day that was typical for you.

Beer, wine, other alcoholic drinks ______
Tea ______
Coffee ______
Fruit drink ______
Water ______
Cheese ______
Macaroni and cheese ______
Other foods with cheese (such as lasagna, cheeseburgers) ______
Orange or grapefruit ______
Bananas ______
Peaches or apricots ______
Green salad ______
Spinach or greens ______
Green peas ______
Sweet potatoes ______
Carrots ______
Meat ______
Fish ______
Peanut butter ______
Dried beans or peas ______
Bacon or sausage ______
Bread ______
Rice ______
Spaghetti or other pasta ______
Tortillas ______
French fries ______
Cookies ______
Pie ______
Orange or grapefruit juice ______
Fruit juice other than orange or grapefruit ______
Soft drinks ______
Milk ______
Cereal with milk ______
Yogourt ______
Pizza ______
Melon (such as watermelon, cantaloupe, honeydew) ______
Berries (specify kind) ________
Apples ______
Other fruit ______
Broccoli ______
Green beans ______
Potatoes (other than fried) ______
Corn ______
Other vegetables ______
Chicken or turkey ______
Eggs ______
Nuts ______
Hot dogs ______
Cold cuts ______
Rolls ______
Cereal ______
Noodles ______
Chips ______
Cake ______
Doughnuts or pastries ______

Are you often bothered by any of the following? (Circle all that apply.)
Nausea Vomiting Heartburn Constipation

Are you on a special diet? No ______ Yes ______ If yes, what kind? ________

Do you try to limit the amount or kind of food you eat to control your weight? No ___ Yes ___

Do you avoid any foods for health or religious reasons? No ______ Yes ______ If yes, what foods? ________

Do you take any prescribed drugs or medications? No ______ Yes ______ If yes, what are they? ________

Do you take any over-the-counter medications (such as aspirin, cold medicines, Tylenol)? No ______ Yes ______ If yes, what are they? ________

Do you ever have trouble affording the food you need? No ______ Yes ______

Do you have any help getting the food you need? No ______ Yes ______ (If yes, circle all that apply.)
Prenatal Nutrition Program
School lunch or breakfast
Food from a food pantry, soup kitchen, or food bank

Table 11-6 Physical Assessment of Nutritional Status

SIGNS OF GOOD NUTRITION	SIGNS OF POOR NUTRITION
General Appearance	
Alert, responsive, energetic, good endurance	Listless, apathetic, cachectic, easily fatigued, looks tired
Muscles	
Well developed, firm, good tone, some fat under skin	Flaccid, poor tone, undeveloped, tender, "wasted" appearance
Nervous System Function	
Good attention span, not irritable or restless, normal reflexes, psychological stability	Inattentive, irritable, confused, burning and tingling of hands and feet, loss of position and vibratory sense, weakness and tenderness of muscles, decrease or loss of ankle and knee reflexes
Gastrointestinal Function	
Good appetite and digestion, normal regular elimination, no palpable organs or masses	Anorexia, indigestion, constipation or diarrhea, liver or spleen enlargement
Cardiovascular Function	
Normal heart rate and rhythm, no murmurs, normal blood pressure for age	Rapid heart rate, enlarged heart, abnormal rhythm, elevated blood pressure
Hair	
Shiny, lustrous, firm, not easily plucked, healthy scalp	Stringy, dull, brittle, dry, thin and sparse, depigmented, can be easily plucked
Skin (General)	
Smooth, slightly moist, good colour	Rough, dry, scaly, pale, pigmented, irritated, easily bruised, petechiae
Face and Neck	
Skin colour uniform, smooth, pink, healthy appearance; no enlargement of thyroid gland; lips not chapped or swollen	Scaly, swollen, skin dark over cheeks and under eyes; lumpiness or flakiness of skin around nose and mouth; thyroid enlarged; lips swollen; angular lesions or fissures at corners of mouth
Oral Cavity	
Reddish pink mucous membranes and gums; no swelling or bleeding of gums; tongue healthy pink or deep red in appearance, not swollen or smooth, surface papillae present; teeth bright and clean, no cavities, no pain, no discolouration	Gums spongy, bleed easily, inflamed or receding; tongue swollen, scarlet and raw, magenta colour, beefy, hyperemic and hypertrophic papillae, atrophic papillae; teeth with unfilled caries, absent teeth, worn surfaces, mottled
Eyes	
Bright, clear, shiny, no sores at corners of eyelids, membranes moist and healthy pink colour, no prominent blood vessels or mound of tissue (Bitot's spots) on sclera, no fatigue circles beneath	Eye membranes pale, redness of membrane, dryness, signs of infection, Bitot's spots, redness and fissuring of eyelid corners, dryness of eye membrane, dull appearance of cornea, soft cornea, blue sclera
Extremities	
No tenderness, weakness, or swelling; nails firm and pink	Edema, tender calves, tingling, weakness; nails spoon-shaped, brittle
Skeleton	
No malformations	Bowlegs, knock-knees, chest deformity at diaphragm, beaded ribs, prominent scapulas

Laboratory Testing. The only nutrition-related laboratory testing needed by most pregnant women is a hematocrit or hemoglobin measurement to screen for the presence of anemia. Because of the **physiological anemia of pregnancy**, the reference values for hemoglobin and hematocrit must be adjusted during pregnancy. The lower limit of the normal range for hemoglobin during pregnancy is 110 g/L (compared with 120 g/L in the nonpregnant state). The lower limit of the normal range for hematocrit is 0.32 (compared with 0.37 in the nonpregnant state). Cut-off values for anemia are higher in women who smoke or live at high altitudes because the decreased oxygen-carrying capacity of their RBCs causes them to produce more RBCs than other women.

A woman's history or physical findings may indicate the need for additional testing. These tests might include a complete blood cell count with a differential to identify megaloblastic or macrocytic anemia and measurement of levels of specific vitamins or minerals believed to be lacking in the diet.

For many women with uncomplicated pregnancies, the nurse can serve as the primary source of nutrition education during pregnancy. The registered dietitian who has specialized training in evaluating diets, planning nutrition needs during illness, recognizing ethnic and cultural food patterns, and translating nutrient needs into food patterns often serves as a consultant. Pregnant women with serious nutrition problems, those with intervening illnesses such as diabetes (either pre-existing or gestational), and any others requiring in-depth dietary counselling should be referred to the dietitian.

Nutrition Counselling

Nutrition teaching can take place in a one-on-one interview or in a group setting. In either case, teaching should emphasize the importance of choosing a varied diet using *Canada's Food Guide*, composed of readily available foods rather than specialized diet supplements. The importance of consuming adequate amounts from the milk, yogourt, and cheese group must be emphasized, especially for adolescents and women younger than 25 years of age who are still actively adding calcium to their skeletons; adolescents need at least 750 to 1000 mL (3 to 4 glasses of milk) from the milk group daily. Good nutrition practices (and avoidance of poor practices such as smoking and alcohol or drug use) are essential content for prenatal classes designed for women in early pregnancy.

Eating Well With Canada's Food Guide can be used as a guide to making daily food choices during pregnancy, just as it is during other stages of the life cycle. Additional individualized information and resources are available from Health Canada at http://www.hc-sc.gc.ca/fn-an/alt_formats/hpfb-dgpsa/pdf/food-guide-aliment/table_female-femme_preg-ence_age19-50-eng.pdf. On the Web site is an option for My Food Guide Servings Tracker (for Pregnancy or Lactation). *Eating Well With Canada's Food Guide* is translated into 10 different languages, including versions for First Nations, Inuit, and Métis. See the Additional Resources listed at the end of the chapter.

Safe Food Preparation

Pregnant women and their unborn or newborn children are at an increased risk for foodborne illnesses because they have a weaker immune system. For example, pregnant women are about 20 times more likely to get listeriosis than other healthy adults. Listeriosis is a rare but serious infection that is caused by consuming a type of bacterium called *Listeria monocytogenes* (commonly called *Listeria*) that is sometimes found in food, water, and soil. If a pregnant woman develops listeriosis during the first 3 months of her pregnancy, she may experience a miscarriage. Up to 2 weeks before a miscarriage, pregnant women may experience a mild flu-like illness with chills, fatigue, headache, as well as muscular and joint pain. Listeriosis later on in the pregnancy can result in a stillbirth or the birth of an acutely ill child (Health Canada, 2010).

For safe preparation of food and to decrease the risk of contacting *Listeria* or other foodborne illnesses, Health Canada (2010) recommends the following guidelines:

- Follow all food instructions on the label of the package.
- Clean and sanitize all food preparation surfaces, knives, and utensils with a kitchen sanitizer or using a 5 mL ratio of household bleach to 750 mL of water followed by a water rinse. This is particularly important when preparing raw fish meat.
- Clean all fruits and vegetables carefully before eating.
- Refrigerate any perishable or prepared foods at 4°C or below. The warmer the refrigerator, the higher the bacterial count will be. Keep leftovers for only 2 to 3 days and reheat to an internal temperature of 74°C.
- Defrost frozen foods in the refrigerator, in cold water, or in the microwave, but never defrost at room temperature.
- Wash and disinfect the refrigerator on a frequent basis, which decreases the risk of bacteria in food being transferred to uncontaminated food stuff.

Medical Nutrition Therapy

During pregnancy and lactation, the food plan for women with special medical nutrition therapy may have to be modified. The registered dietitian can instruct these women about their diets and assist them in meal planning. However, the nurse should understand the basic principles of the diet and be able to reinforce the diet teaching.

The nurse should be especially aware of the dietary modifications necessary for women with diabetes mellitus (either gestational or pre-existing). This disease is relatively common, and fetal morbidity and mortality occur more often in pregnancies complicated by **hyperglycemia** or **hypoglycemia** (see discussion of diabetes in Chapter 14). Every effort should be made to maintain blood glucose levels in the normal range throughout pregnancy. The food plan of the woman with diabetes usually includes four to six meals and snacks daily, with the daily carbohydrate intake distributed fairly evenly among the meals and snacks. The complex carbohydrates—fibres and starches—should be well represented in the diet. To maintain strict control of the blood glucose level, the pregnant woman with diabetes usually must monitor her own blood glucose daily.

Coping With Nutrition-Related Discomforts of Pregnancy

The most common nutrition-related discomforts of pregnancy are nausea and vomiting (or "morning sickness"), constipation, and pyrosis.

Nausea and Vomiting

Nausea and vomiting are most common during the first trimester, and although nausea and vomiting usually only cause only mild-to-moderate nutrition problems, they may be a source of substantial discomfort. Antiemetic medications, vitamin B_6, ginger, and pericardium 6 acupressure (Fig. 11-4) may be effective in reducing the severity of nausea (Borrelli et al., 2005; Jewell & Young, 2004). The pregnant woman may find the following suggestions helpful in alleviating the problems:

- Eat dry, starchy foods such as dry toast, Melba toast, or crackers on awakening in the morning and at other times when nausea occurs.
- Avoid consuming excessive amounts of fluids early in the day or when nauseated (but compensate by drinking fluids at other times).
- Avoid smoke, strong odours, alcohol, and caffeine.
- Eat small amounts frequently (every 2 to 3 hours) and avoid large meals that distend the stomach.
- Avoid skipping meals and thus becoming extremely hungry, which may worsen nausea. Have a snack such as

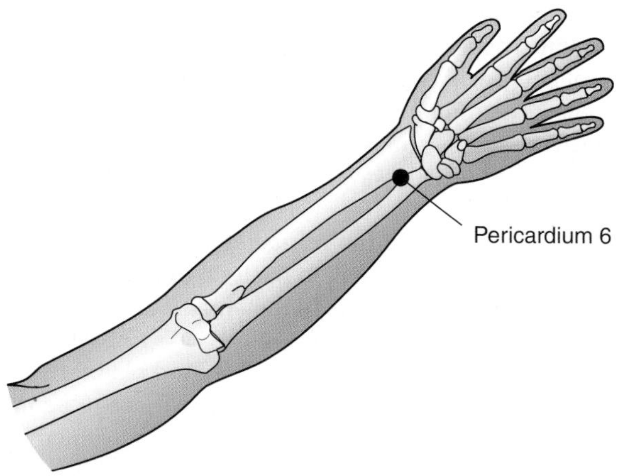

Fig. 11-4 Pericardium 6 (P6) acupressure/acupuncture point for nausea.

cereal with milk, a small sandwich, or yogourt before bedtime.
- Avoid sudden movements. Get out of bed slowly and eat soon after getting out of bed.
- Decrease intake of fried and other fatty foods. Good choices are starches such as pastas, rice, and breads, and low-fat, high-protein foods such as skinless broiled or baked poultry, cooked dry beans or peas, lean meats, and broiled or canned fish.
- Some women find that tart foods or drinks (e.g., lemonade) or salty foods (e.g., potato chips) are tolerated during periods of nausea. Smelling fresh-cut lemons may also be helpful.
- Breathe fresh air to help relieve nausea. Keep the environment well ventilated (e.g., open a window), go for a walk outside, or decrease cooking odours by using an exhaust fan.
- Eat foods served at cool temperatures and foods that give off little aroma.
- Try herbal teas such as those made with peppermint (see herbal teas listed earlier in the chapter, on p. 258) to decrease nausea.
- Avoid brushing teeth immediately after eating.

Hyperemesis gravidarium can be a life-threatening condition in which a woman has protracted vomiting, retching, severe dehydration, and weight loss requiring hospitalization. See Chapter 13, p. 310 for discussion on this condition.

Constipation

Improved bowel function generally results from increasing the intake of fibre (e.g., wheat bran and whole-wheat products, popcorn, and raw or lightly steamed vegetables) in the diet. Fibre helps retain water within the stool, creating a bulky stool that stimulates intestinal peristalsis. The recommendation for pregnant women for fibre is 28 g/day. An adequate fluid intake (at least 50 mL/kg/day) helps hydrate the fibre and increase the bulk of the stool. Warm or hot fluids may increase peristalsis more than cold fluids. Making a habit of regular exercise that uses large muscle groups (walking, swimming, cycling) also helps stimulate bowel motility. Laxatives should not be taken unless first discussed with their health care provider.

Pyrosis

Pyrosis, or heartburn, is usually caused by reflux of gastric contents into the esophagus. This condition can be minimized by eating small, frequent meals, rather than two or three larger meals, daily. Food should be chewed slowly. Because fluids increase the distention of the stomach, they should not be consumed with foods. The woman needs to be sure to drink adequate amounts between meals. Avoiding spicy, fried, or greasy foods may help alleviate the problem, as will avoidance of coffee, colas, alcohol, and smoking. Reflux can be exacerbated by lying down immediately after eating and wearing clothing that is tight across the abdomen. Occasionally, women may take antacids to help with heartburn. Not all antacids are safe; thus women should check with their health care provider prior to taking medication.

Cultural Influences

Consideration of a woman's cultural food preferences enhances the nurse's communication with the woman and provides a greater opportunity for following appropriate food requirements. Women in most cultures are encouraged to eat a diet typical for them. The nurse needs to be aware of what constitutes a typical diet for each cultural or ethnic group present in her patient population. However, because several variations may occur within one cultural group, a careful exploration of individual preferences is needed. Although ethnic and cultural food beliefs may seem at first glance to conflict with the dietary instruction provided by physicians, nurses, and dietitians, it is often possible for the empathic health care provider to identify cultural beliefs that are congruent with the modern understanding of pregnancy and fetal development. Many cultural food practices have some merit or the culture would not have survived. Food cravings during pregnancy are considered normal by many cultures, but the kinds of cravings often are culturally specific. Nutrition beliefs and the practices of selected cultural groups are summarized in Table 11-7.

Vegetarian Diets

Vegetarian diets represent another cultural effect on nutritional status. Foods basic to almost all vegetarian diets are vegetables, fruits, legumes, nuts, seeds, and grains, but with many variations. Semi-vegetarians, who are not true vegetarians, include fish, poultry, eggs, and dairy products in their diets but do not eat beef or pork. Such a diet can be completely adequate for pregnant women. Another type of vegetarians, **lacto-ovovegetarians**, consumes eggs and dairy products in addition to plant products. Iron and zinc intake may not be adequate in these women, but such diets can be otherwise nutritionally sound. Strict vegetarians, or **vegans**, consume only plant products. Because vitamin B_{12} is found only in foods of animal origin, this diet is deficient in vitamin B_{12}. As a result, strict vegetarians should take a supplement or regularly consume vitamin B_{12}–fortified foods (e.g., soy milk). Vitamin B_{12} deficiency can result in megaloblastic anemia, glossitis (inflamed red tongue), and neurological deficits in the mother. Infants born to affected mothers are likely to have megaloblastic anemia and exhibit neurodevelopmental delays. Iron, calcium, zinc, and vitamin B_6 intake may also be low in

Table 11-7 Characteristic Food Patterns of Selected Cultures

MILK GROUP	PROTEIN GROUP	FRUITS AND VEGETABLES	BREADS AND CEREALS	POSSIBLE DIETARY CONSIDERATIONS
First Nations, Métis, and Inuit				
Fresh milk Evaporated milk for cooking Ice cream Cream pie	Pork, beef, lamb, rabbit Fowl, fish, eggs Legumes Sunflower seeds Nuts: walnuts, acorn, pine, peanut butter Game meat	Green peas, beans Beets, turnips Green leafy and other vegetables Grapes, apples, bananas, other fresh fruits Roots Blueberries	Refined bread Whole wheat Cornmeal Rice Dry cereals "Fry" bread Tortillas Bannock	Obesity, diabetes, alcoholism, nutrition deficiencies expressed in dental problems and iron-deficiency anemia Inadequate amounts of all nutrients Excessive use of sugar Difficulty accessing fresh fruit and vegetables
Middle Eastern* (Armenian, Greek, Syrian, Turkish)				
Yogourt Little butter	Lamb Nuts Dried peas, beans, lentils Sesame seeds	Peppers, tomatoes, cabbage, grape leaves, cucumbers, squash Dried apricots, raisins, dates	Cracked wheat and dark bread	Many meats and vegetables fried Lack of fresh fruits Insufficient foods from milk group High consumption of sweets, lamb fat, and olive oil Halal diet
Chinese				
Soy milk†	Pork sausage‡ Eggs and pigeon eggs Fish Lamb, beef, goat Fowl: chicken, duck Nuts Legumes Soybean curd (tofu)	Many vegetables Radish leaves Bean, bamboo sprouts	Rice/rice flour products Cereals, noodles Wheat, corn, millet seed	Tendency of some immigrants to use large amounts of grease in cooking Limited use of milk and milk products Often low in protein, calories, or both Soy sauce (high sodium)
Filipino (Spanish-Chinese Influence)				
Flavoured milk Milk in coffee Cheese: gouda, cheddar	Pork, beef, goat, rabbit Chicken Fish Eggs, nuts, legumes	Many vegetables and fruits	Rice, cooked cereals Noodles: rice, wheat	Limited use of milk and milk products Tendency to prewash rice Tendency to have only small portions of protein foods
Italian				
Cheese Some ice cream	Meat Eggs Dried beans	Leafy vegetables Potatoes Eggplant, tomatoes, peppers Fruits	Pasta White breads, some whole wheat Farina Cereals	Prefer expensive imported cheeses; reluctant to substitute less expensive domestic varieties Tendency to overcook vegetables Limited use of whole grains High consumption of sweets Alcohol commonly consumed with larger meals Extensive use of olive oil Insufficient servings from milk group
Japanese (Isei, More Japanese Influence; Nisei, More Westernized)				
Increasing amounts being used by younger generations	Pork, beef, chicken Fish Eggs Legumes: soy, red, lima beans Tofu Nuts	Many vegetables and fruits Seaweed	Rice, rice cakes Wheat noodles Refined bread, noodles	Excessive sodium: pickles, salty crisp seaweed, MSG, and soy sauce Insufficient servings from milk group May use prewashed rice
Scandinavian (Danish, Finnish, Norwegian, Swedish)				
Cream Butter Cheeses	Wild game Fish (fresh or dried) Eggs	Berries Dried fruit Vegetables: coleslaw, roots	Whole wheat, rye, barley, sweets (cookies and sweet breads)	Insufficient fresh fruits and vegetables High consumption of sweets, pickled or salted meats, and fish

Continued

Table 11-7 Characteristic Food Patterns of Selected Cultures—cont'd

MILK GROUP	PROTEIN GROUP	FRUITS AND VEGETABLES	BREADS AND CEREALS	POSSIBLE DIETARY CONSIDERATIONS
Southeast Asian (Vietnamese, Cambodian)				
Generally not taken Coffee with condensed cow's milk Plain yogourt Ice cream (rare) Soybean milk	Fish (daily): fresh, dried, salted Poultry/egg, duck, chicken Pork Beef (seldom) Dry beans Tofu	Seasonal variety: fresh or preserved Green leafy vegetables Yams Corn	Rice: grains, flour, noodles French bread "Cellophane" (bean starch) noodles	Fresh milk products generally not consumed Poultry/eggs may be limited Meat considered "unclean" is avoided Preference for diet high in salt and pepper, as well as rice and pork High intake of MSG and soy sauce
South Asian (India, Pakistan, Sri Lanka, and Bangladesh)				
Condensed milk Yogourt	Meat—seldom Beef Lamb	Coconut milk Squash, peas, pumpkin, beans Mango, papaya, pomegranate	Naan Makki Roti Dhokai, Dosa Rice	Curry and highly spiced foods
Jewish: Orthodox*				
Milk† Cheese†	Meat (bloodless; Kosher prepared): beef, lamb, goat, deer, poultry (all types), no pork Fish with fins and scales only No crustaceans	Wide variety	Wide variety	High intake of sodium in meat products

*Religious holidays may involve fasting, which is believed to increase the likelihood of preterm labour. Fasting requirement may be waived during pregnancy.
†Lactose intolerance is relatively common in adults.
‡Lower in fat content than Western sausage.
MSG, monosodium L-glutamate.

women on this diet, and some strict vegetarians have excessively low caloric intakes. The protein intake should be assessed especially carefully because plant proteins tend to be incomplete in that they lack one or more amino acids required for growth and maintenance of body tissues. However, the daily consumption of a variety of different plant proteins—grains, dried beans and peas, nuts, and seeds—helps to provide all of the essential amino acids.

Nutrient Needs During Lactation

Nutrition needs during lactation are similar in many ways to those during pregnancy (see Table 11-2 and previous discussion on pregnancy). Needs for energy (kilocalories), protein, calcium, iodine, zinc, the B vitamins (thiamine, riboflavin, niacin, pyridoxine, and vitamin B_{12}), and vitamin C remain greater than nonpregnant needs. The recommendations for some of these (e.g., vitamin C, zinc, and protein) are slightly to moderately higher than during pregnancy. This allowance covers the amount of the nutrients released in the milk, as well as the needs of the mother for tissue maintenance. In the case of iron and folic acid, the recommendation during lactation is lower than that during pregnancy. Both of these nutrients are essential for RBC formation and thus for maintaining the increase in the blood volume that occurs during pregnancy. With the decrease in maternal blood volume to nonpregnant levels after birth, maternal iron and folic acid needs also decrease. Many lactating women have a delay in the return of menses; this conserves blood cells and also reduces iron and folic acid needs. It is especially important that the calcium intake be adequate; if it is not and the woman does not respond to nutrition counselling, a supplement of 600 mg of calcium per day may be needed.

The recommended energy intake for the first 6 months is an increase of 330 kcal more than the woman's nonpregnant intake. It is difficult to obtain adequate nutrients for maintenance of lactation if total caloric intake is less than 1800 kcal. Because of the deposition of energy stores, the woman who has gained the optimal amount of weight during pregnancy is heavier after birth than at the beginning of pregnancy. However, as a result of the caloric demands of lactation, the lactating mother usually experiences a gradual but steady weight loss. The woman who does not breastfeed loses weight gradually if she consumes a balanced diet that provides slightly less than her daily energy expenditure. A reasonable weight loss goal for nonlactating women is 0.5 to 1 kg per week; a loss of 1 kg per month is recommended for most lactating women who need to lose weight. On average, at 6 weeks after giving birth, women retain 3 to 7 kg of the weight gained during pregnancy, and two thirds of them weigh more than they did before pregnancy (Walker, Sterling, & Timmerman, 2005).

A woman who is overweight may be able to lose up to 2 kg per month without decreasing her milk supply. Those at risk for obesity and overweight need follow-up to ensure that they know how to make wise food choices, primarily from fruits, vegetables, whole grains, lean meats, and low-fat dairy products. An hour of moderately vigorous physical activity (e.g., walking, jogging, swimming, cycling, aerobic dance) most days of the week will improve the ability of the woman to lose weight gradually and maintain the weight loss.

Fluid intake must be adequate to maintain milk production; the mother's level of thirst is the best guide to the right amount. There is no need to consume more fluids than those needed to satisfy thirst.

Smoking, alcohol intake, and excessive caffeine intake should be avoided during lactation. Smoking can impair milk production, and it exposes the infant to the risk of passive smoking. It is speculated that the infant's psychomotor development may be affected by maternal alcohol use, and alcoholic beverages (two drinks per day) may impair the milk ejection reflex. Caffeine intake can lead to a reduced iron concentration in milk and consequently contribute to the development of anemia in the infant. The caffeine concentration in milk is only approximately 1% of the mother's plasma level, but caffeine seems to accumulate in the infant. Breastfed infants of mothers who drink large amounts of coffee or caffeine-containing soft drinks may be unusually active and wakeful.

Key Points

- A woman's nutritional status before, during, and after pregnancy contributes significantly to her well-being and that of her infant.
- Many physiological changes occurring during pregnancy and lactation influence the need for additional nutrients and the efficiency with which the body uses them.
- Both the total maternal weight gain and the pattern of weight gain are important determinants of the outcome of pregnancy.
- The appropriateness of the mother's prepregnancy weight for height (BMI) is a major determinant of her recommended weight gain during pregnancy.
- Nutritional risk factors include adolescent pregnancy, nicotine use, alcohol or drug use, faddish food habits, a low weight for height, and frequent pregnancies.
- Iron supplementation is recommended during pregnancy. Other supplements may be warranted when nutritional risk factors are present.
- The nurse and the woman are influenced by cultural and personal values and beliefs that the nurse needs to take into account during nutrition counselling.
- Pregnancy complications that may be nutrition related include anemia, gestational hypertension, gestational diabetes, and IUGR.
- Dietary adaptation can be an effective intervention for some of the common discomforts of pregnancy, including nausea and vomiting, constipation, and heartburn.

Audio Chapter Summaries

Access an Audio Summary of these Key Points on Evolve

References

Allen, L. (2005). Multiple micronutrients in pregnancy and lactation: An overview. *American Journal of Clinical Nutrition, 81*(5), 1206S–1212S.

Borrelli, F., et al. (2005). Effectiveness and safety of ginger in the treatment of pregnancy-induced nausea and vomiting. *Obstetrics and Gynecology, 105*(4), 849–856.

British Columbia Ministry of Health Services. (2004). *Investigation and management of iron deficiency*. Retrieved from http://www.bcguidelines.ca/gpac/pdf/irondef.pdf.

Canadian Institute for Health Information. (2009). *Too early, too small: A profile of small babies across Canada*. Ottawa: Author. Retrieved from http://secure.cihi.ca/cihiweb/products/too_early_too_small_en.pdf.

Canadian Institute for Health Information. (2010). *Highlights of the 2008–2009 selected indicators describing the birthing process in Canada*. Ottawa: Author. Retrieved from http://secure.cihi.ca/cihiweb/products/childbirth_highlights_2010_05_18_e.pdf.

Corbett, R., Ryan, C., & Weinrich, S. (2003). Pica in pregnancy: Does it affect pregnancy outcomes? *MCN: American Journal of Maternal Child Nursing, 28*(3), 183–189.

Cornel, M., Smit, D., & de Jong-van den Berg, L. (2005). Folic acid—The scientific debate as a base for public health policy. *Reproductive Toxicology, 20*(3), 411–415.

Davies, G. A., Maxwell, C., McLeod, L., Gagnon, R., Basso, M., et al. (2010). *SOGC Clinical Practice Guideline: Obesity in pregnancy*. Retrieved from http://www.sogc.org/guidelines/documents/gui239ECPG1002.pdf.

Grotegut, C. A., et al. (2006). Baking soda pica: A case of hypokalemic metabolic alkalosis and rhabdomyolysis in pregnancy. *Obstetrics and Gynecology, 107*(2, Pt. 2), 484–486.

Health Canada. (2005). *Folic acid and birth defects*. Retrieved from http://www.hc-sc.gc.ca/hl-vs/iyh-vsv/med/folic-folique-eng.php.

Health Canada. (2009a). *Prenatal nutrition guidelines for health professionals: Fish and omega 3 fatty acids* (Cat. No. H164-109/4-2009E-PDF). Ottawa: Author. Retrieved from http://www.hc-sc.gc.ca/fn-an/alt_formats/hpfb-dgpsa/pdf/pubs/omega3-eng.pdf.

Health Canada. (2009b). *Prenatal nutrition guidelines for health professionals: Iron contributes to a healthy pregnancy* (Cat. No. H164-109/1-2009E-PDF). Ottawa: Author. Retrieved from http://www.hc-sc.gc.ca/fn-an/pubs/nutrition/iron-fer-eng.php.

Health Canada. (2010). *Listeria and food safety* (Cat. No. H13-7/47-2010E-PDF). Ottawa: Author. Retrieved from http://www.hc-sc.gc.ca/hl-vs/iyh-vsv/food-aliment/listeria-eng.php.

Health Canada. (2011a). *Mercury in fish: Questions and answers*. Ottawa: Author. Retrieved from http://www.hc-sc.gc.ca/fn-an/securit/chem-chim/environ/mercur/merc_fish_qa-poisson_qr-eng.php.

Health Canada. (2011b). *Prenatal nutrition*. Ottawa: Author. Retrieved from http://www.hc-sc.gc.ca/fn-an/nutrition/prenatal/index-eng.php.

HealthLink BC. (2010). *Energy drinks*. Healthlink BC, File 109. Retrieved from http://www.healthlinkbc.ca/healthfiles/hfile109.stm.

Institute of Medicine. (2004). *Dietary reference intakes for water, potassium, sodium, chloride, and sulfate*. Washington, DC: National Academies Press.

Institute of Medicine. (2009). *Weight gain during pregnancy: Reexamining the guidelines*. Washington DC: National Academies Press.

Jewell, D., & Young, G. (2004). Interventions for nausea and vomiting in early pregnancy (Cochrane Review). In *The Cochrane Library, Issue 4*. Chichester, UK: John Wiley & Sons.

Klitzman, S., et al. (2002). Lead poisoning among pregnant women in New York City: Risk factors and screening practices. *Journal of Urban Health, 79*(2), 225–237.

Luke, B. (2005). Nutrition in multiple gestations. *Clinics in Perinatology, 32*(2), 403–429, vii.

Ngozi, P. O. (2008). Pica practices of pregnant women in Nairobi, Kenya. *East African Medical Journal, 85*(2), 72–79.

Public Health Agency of Canada. (2008). *Canadian perinatal health report*. Ottawa: Author. Retrieved from http://www.phac-aspc.gc.ca/publicat/2008/cphr-rspc/pdf/cphr-rspc08-eng.pdf.

Ramakrishnan, U. (2004). Nutrition and low birth weight: From research to practice. *American Journal of Clinical Nutrition, 79*, 17–21.

Shannon, M. (2003). Severe lead poisoning in pregnancy. *Ambulatory Pediatrics, 3*(1), 37–39.

Statistics Canada. (2011). *Overweight and obese adults (self-reported), 2010*, Ottawa: Author. Retrieved http://www.statcan.gc.ca/pub/82-625-x/2011001/article/11464-eng.htm.

Walker, L., Sterling, B., & Timmerman, G. (2005). Retention of pregnancy-related weight in the early postpartum period: Implications for women's health services. *Journal of Obstetric and Gynecologic Neonatal Nursing, 34*(4), 418–427.

Watkins, M. L., et al. (2003). Maternal obesity and risk for birth defects. *Pediatrics 111*, 1152–1158.

Wilson, R. D., et al. (2003). SOGC clinical practice guideline: The use of folic acid for the prevention of neural tube defects and other congenital anomalies. *Journal of Obstetricians and Gynaecologists of Canada, 25*(11), 959–965. Retrieved from http://www.sogc.org/guidelines/public/138E-CPG-November2003.pdf.

Wilson, R. D., et al. (2007). Joint SOGC-Motherisk clinical practice guideline: Pre-conceptional vitamin/folic acid supplementation 2007: The use of folic acid in combination with a multivitamin supplement. *Journal of Obstetricians and Gynaecologists of Canada, 29*(12), 1003–1013. Retrieved from http://www.sogc.org/guidelines/documents/guiJOGC201JCPG0712.pdf.

Additional Resources

Eating Well With Canada's Food Guide: Translated Versions of the Guide (10 different languages): http://www.hc-sc.gc.ca/fn-an/food-guide-aliment/order-commander/guide_trans-trad-eng.php

Eating Well With Canada's Food Guide__First Nations, Inuit and Métis: http://www.hc-sc.gc.ca/fn-an/pubs/fnim-pnim/index-eng.php

Eat Right Ontario: http://www.eatrightontario.ca/en/default.aspx

Unit 3

Pregnancy Risk Factors and Assessment: Maternal and Fetal

12

Learning Objectives

On completion of this chapter, the reader will be able to:

- Explore the scope of high-risk pregnancy.
- Identify the determinants of health that influence pregnancy outcomes.
- Examine risk factors identified through history taking, physical examination, and diagnostic techniques.
- Describe diagnostic techniques and implications of findings.
- Describe the nursing role in antepartum risk assessment.
- Discuss psychological considerations associated with a high-risk pregnancy diagnosis.

Electronic Resources

Additional information related to the content in Chapter 12 can be found on

evolve the companion Web site at

http://evolve.elsevier.com/Canada/Perry/maternal/

- Examination Review Questions

Although most pregnancies and births are considered low risk, there are still some births that are categorized as high risk due to maternal or fetal complications. Identification of the risks, together with appropriate and timely intervention during the perinatal period, can prevent morbidity and mortality among mothers and infants.

Using current Canadian demographic information, women and families can be identified as at risk on the basis of factors other than biophysical criteria. The increasing numbers of homeless and other pregnant women who have limited access to prenatal care during any stage of pregnancy and the behaviours and lifestyles that pose a risk to the health of the mother and fetus contribute to the increasing incidence of high-risk pregnancies. More women are presenting with mental health issues at any stage of their lives, including during pregnancy, and this can also contribute to increased risks. Difficulty accessing care may be related to language barriers, to arranging appropriate services, and to limited health care facilities being available in remote or rural communities.

Care of high-risk patients requires the collaborative efforts of various health care providers. In this chapter, care of the high-risk woman and the factors associated with a diagnosis of high risk are discussed. Diagnostic techniques used to monitor the maternal–fetal unit are also outlined. Finally, psychological considerations of care of the woman experiencing a high-risk pregnancy are addressed.

Definition and Scope of the Problem

A *high-risk pregnancy* is one in which the life or health of the mother or infant is jeopardized by a disorder coincident with or unique to pregnancy. For the mother, the high-risk status arbitrarily extends through the puerperium (4 to 6 weeks after childbirth). Postbirth maternal complications usually are resolved within 1 month of birth, but perinatal morbidity may continue for months or years.

High-risk pregnancy is a critical problem for modern medical and nursing care. The current social emphasis on the quality of life and the wanted child has resulted in a reduction of family size and the number of unwanted pregnancies. At the same time, technological advances have facilitated pregnancies in previously infertile couples. As a consequence, emphasis is on the safe birth of normal infants who can develop to their potential. Scientific and technological advances have allowed perinatal health care to reach a level far beyond that previously available.

The diagnosis of high risk imposes a situational crisis on the family. These crises include, for example, loss of pregnancy before the anticipated date; development of gestational diabetes mellitus, with its potential complications; or birth of a neonate who does not meet cultural, societal, or familial norms and expectations.

Determinants of Health as Risk Factors

There are many factors that contribute to high-risk pregnancies; an analysis of the determinants of health (see Box 1-3) provides a more comprehensive approach to providing care. Social and individual factors associated with high-risk childbearing include income and social status, social support networks, education, employment and working conditions, physical environment, personal health practices and coping skills, biology and genetics, availability of health services, and culture. Some personal health practices and lack of coping skills can place the mother and fetus at risk. Examples include substance use, failure to seek prenatal care, inadequate nutritional status, poor dental hygiene, and psychosocial stressors (Box 12-1).

The determinants of health are interrelated and cumulative in their effects on health outcomes. A comprehensive database for pregnancy risk assessment can help ensure that appropriate resources are available. In Canada, the Canadian Perinatal Surveillance System (CPSS) provides this database (see Chapter 1, p. 7). The CPSS reports on 29 maternal, fetal, and infant health determinants and outcomes. The view is that health status is influenced by a range of factors; thus it is important to monitor not only health outcomes but also factors—such as behaviours, physical and social environments, and health services—that may affect those outcomes.

Regionalization of Health Care Services

Early and ongoing risk assessment is a crucial component of perinatal care. Conditions associated with perinatal morbidity and mortality can be prevented or treated, or the patient can be referred to more skilled health care providers. Factors to consider when determining a patient's risk status include resources available locally to treat the condition, availability of appropriate facilities for transport if needed, and determination of the best match for the patient's needs.

It is neither feasible nor reasonable for each hospital to develop and maintain the full spectrum of services required for high-risk perinatal patients. Consequently, regionalization of health care has emerged. This system of coordinated care, in which facilities within a geographic region are organized to provide different levels of care, also applies to preconception and ambulatory prenatal care services (see Community Focus box).

COMMUNITY FOCUS

Resources for Parents Experiencing a High-Risk Pregnancy

Contact the nearest high-risk pregnancy unit to assess the resources available for parents (e.g., pamphlets, Web sites for high-risk pregnancies) and to learn what screening is recommended during pregnancy to identify problems. For what problems is the screening conducted? What information or resources are available in your community for the problems identified? How can women access the resources that are available? What geographic area does this unit serve? What determinants of health are influencing these women's lives? What is the role of the nurse in this unit?

Maternal Health Problems

The leading causes of maternal death attributable to pregnancy differ throughout the world. In general, three major causes have persisted for the last 50 years: hypertensive disorders, infection, and hemorrhage. In Canada today, the leading causes of maternal mortality are hypertensive disorders, pulmonary embolism, hemorrhage, and ectopic pregnancy. Factors that are strongly related to maternal death include age (younger than 20 years or 35 years or older), lack of prenatal care, and low education status. Specific pregnancy problems and risk factors are listed in Box 12-2.

The maternal mortality rate in Canada was 7.8 per 100,000 live births between 2008 and 2010 (Public Health Agency of Canada [PHAC], 2011). Although the overall number of maternal deaths is small, maternal mortality remains a significant problem because a high proportion of these deaths are preventable, primarily through improving access to and use of prenatal care services. Nurses can be instrumental in educating the public about the importance of obtaining early and regular care during pregnancy.

Mental Health Concerns

Mental health issues may become apparent during the antepartum period, as well women with pre-existing mental health issues are deciding to become pregnant. Bowen and Muhajarine (2006) found in a literature review that depression in mothers can have detrimental effects on infants including difficulty breastfeeding, difficult weight gain, increased stress related behaviours and sleep difficulty. Early education for prenatal patients and families about depression is an essential piece of health promotion. Interprofesional collaboration and appropriate referrals are important interventions for the nurse to initiate when concerns regarding depression are identified (Strass & Billay, 2008).

Perinatal Services British Columbia have developed guiding principles for the care of women with mental health issues (BC Reproductive Care Program, 2003). The guiding principles include the following:

- All women from a variety of backgrounds (social, economic, racial, cultural) are at risk for mental health issues.
- Providing services that preserve the mother–infant dyad is optimal.
- Care needs to be provided in a humane, supportive, caring environment so that women feel strengthened and supported while being treated. These women will often present in an acute state of distress, have fragile self-esteem, and experience multiple complex stressors.
- A collaborative team approach is optimal.
- Every effort should be made within communities to link services to provide support to women.

Newborns are sensitive to the emotional states of their mothers. If the mother is distressed or has a mental health issue, this can lead to difficulty bonding. Therefore, it is important that mothers be identified and treated during pregnancy or in the postpartum period. The use of a screening tool during pregnancy is helpful in identifying women at risk for mental health issues. Perinatal Services BC has a number of

BOX 12-1 Influence of Determinants of Health on Maternal and Newborn Outcomes

Biology and Genetic Factors

Genetic considerations—Genetic risks include heritable factors that originate within the mother or fetus and affect the development or functioning of either or both. Genetic factors may interfere with normal fetal or neonatal development, result in congenital anomalies, or create difficulties for the mother. These factors include altered genes, transmittable inherited disorders, chromosome anomalies, multiple pregnancy, large fetal size, and ABO incompatibility. A genetic risk assessment should be done to determine the family's heritable risk (see Chapter 8).

Demographic Characteristics

Availability of health care—The availability and quality of prenatal care vary greatly with geographic region. Women in metropolitan areas have more prenatal visits than women in remote and rural areas, who have fewer opportunities for specialized care because of the distance they have to travel and consequently have a higher incidence of maternal mortality. On average, women in an inner city may have less access to health care than women in affluent neighbourhoods as there may be more immigrants who do not know how to access the health care system who are living in the city.

Physical environments—There may be unsafe soil and water conditions and environmental exposure to pollutants. An example of this is in the First Nations reserve of Kashechewan in Ontario. In 2005, the water was contaminated and the community had to be moved until *E. coli* levels were reduced. Many First Nations, Métis, and Inuit communities have boil-water alerts to ensure that they are drinking safe water. Another example is the consumption of mercury-contaminated fish, which may pose health risks to a developing fetus.

Income and social status—Poverty underlies many other risk factors and leads to inadequate financial resources for food; poor general health; increased risk for medical complications of pregnancy; and greater prevalence of adverse environmental influences such as substandard living conditions, poor hygiene, and inadequate nutrition.

Education—Risk for adverse perinatal outcomes decreases as educational level increases. Education is an important determinant that influences many of the other determinants of health.

Social support networks—The increased mortality and morbidity rates for single women, including a greater risk for pre-eclampsia, are often related to inadequate prenatal care, lower socioeconomic status, lower level of education, and a younger childbearing age. Women with limited social support networks in the form of family or friends often have fewer resources to help them cope.

Culture—Infant mortality rates are higher among First Nations, Métis, and Inuit people. Ethnicity is also an indicator of other sociodemographic risk factors. There may be cultural beliefs that do not support the need for regular prenatal care.

Employment/working hazards—Occupational hazards can be grouped into chemical, physical, biological, and psychological hazards. The risk to the fetus depends on the timing of exposure, the dose, and fetal and maternal susceptibility. Women who work at highly demanding jobs or do shift work have higher pregnancy risks.

Personal Health Practices and Coping Skills

Substance use—Smoking is associated with intrauterine growth restriction and low birth weight; alcohol consumption has adverse effects on the fetus, resulting in fetal alcohol spectrum disorders, which include fetal alcohol syndrome, alcohol-related neurodevelopmental disorder, and alcohol-related birth defects; drugs can be teratogenic, cause metabolic disturbances, produce chemical effects, or cause depression or alteration of central nervous system function.

Lack of access to prenatal care—Failure to diagnose and treat complications early is a major risk factor arising from lack of access to care. This may be due to: depersonalization of the system, resulting in long waits, routine visits, variability in health care personnel, and unpleasant physical surroundings; lack of understanding of the need for early and continued care; and fear of the health care system and its providers. Language difficulties and lack of knowledge about care options for new immigrants may also make access to appropriate care difficult.

Nutritional status—Adequate nutrition, without which fetal growth and development cannot proceed normally, is one of the most important determinants of pregnancy outcome (see Fig. 11-1). Conditions that influence nutritional status include the following: young age; three pregnancies in the previous 2 years; tobacco, alcohol, or drug use; inadequate dietary intake because of chronic illness or food fads; and inadequate or excessive weight gain (see Chapter 11).

Dental hygiene—Periodontal disease increases the risk for preterm birth and low birth weight.

Psychosocial stressors—Childbearing triggers profound and complex physiological, psychological, and social changes, with evidence to suggest a relationship between emotional distress and birth complications. This risk factor includes conditions such as specific intrapsychic disturbances and addictive lifestyles; a history of child abuse or intimate partner violence (see discussion later); inadequate support systems; family disruption or dissolution; and maternal role changes or conflicts.

(Modified from Gilbert, E. S. [2007]. *Manual of high risk pregnancy and delivery* [4th ed.]. St. Louis: Mosby; Public Health Agency of Canada [2008]. *Canadian perinatal report—2008 Edition* [Cat. HP10-12/2008E-PDF]. Ottawa: Government of Canada. Retrieved from http://www.phac-aspc.gc.ca/publicat/2008/cphr-rspc/behaviours-comportements-eng.php.)

BOX 12-2 Specific Pregnancy Problems and Related Risk Factors

Preterm Labour
Age younger than 16 or older than 35 years
Low socioeconomic status
Maternal weight below 50 kg
Poor nutrition
Previous preterm birth
Incompetent cervix
Uterine anomalies
Smoking
Drug addiction and alcohol use
Multiple gestation
Abnormal fetal presentation
Preterm rupture of membranes
Placental abnormalities
Infection, including dental problems

Polyhydramnios
Diabetes mellitus
Multiple gestation
Fetal congenital abnormalities
Isoimmunization (Rh or ABO)
Nonimmune hydrops
Abnormal fetal presentation

Intrauterine Growth Restriction
Multiple gestation
Poor nutrition
Maternal cyanotic heart disease
Prior pregnancy with intrauterine growth restriction
Maternal collagen diseases
Pregestational hypertension
Gestational hypertension
Recurrent antepartum hemorrhage
Smoking
Maternal diabetes with vascular problems
Fetal infections
Fetal cardiovascular anomalies
Drug addiction and alcohol use
Fetal congenital anomalies
Hemoglobinopathies

Oligohydramnios
Renal agenesis (Potter's syndrome)
Prolonged rupture of membranes
Intrauterine growth restriction

Postterm Pregnancy
Placental sulphatase deficiency
Perinatal hypoxia, acidosis
Placental insufficiency

Chromosome Abnormalities
Maternal age 35 years or older at birth
Balanced translocation (maternal and paternal)

(From Gillen-Goldstein, J., et al. [2006]. Methods of assessment for pregnancy at risk. In A. H. DeCherney, L. Nathan, & M. Goodwin [Eds.], *Current diagnosis and treatment: Obstetrics and gynecology* [10th ed.]. New York: Lange Medical Books/McGraw-Hill.)

guidelines concerning reproductive mental health issues, including specific guidelines for screening and care for specific disorders (http://www.perinatalservicesbc.ca/Reproductive%20Mental%20Health%20Guidelines.htm).

Intimate Partner Violence During Pregnancy

Abuse during pregnancy increases the risk for abruptio placentae, preterm birth, low-birth-weight infants, and infections from forced sex. Women who are in abusive situations may delay seeking health care during pregnancy or may receive inconsistent care (BC Reproductive Care Program, 2003). It is important to assess women for intimate partner violence (IPV) to ensure that they receive appropriate health care.

During pregnancy, the perinatal nurse should assess for abuse at each prenatal visit and on admission to labour (see Box 4-11). Battering episodes initiate or increase during pregnancy for a variety of reasons: (1) the biopsychosocial stresses of pregnancy may strain the relationship beyond the couple's ability to cope, and frustration is followed by violence; (2) the man may be jealous of the fetus, resenting the intrusion into the couple's relationship and the woman's displacement of attention; (3) the man may be angry at the unborn child or the woman; and (4) the beating may be the man's conscious or subconscious attempt to end the pregnancy. After birth, the mother may be so physically and emotionally drained that she may have difficulty bonding with her infant. She may be at risk of becoming an abusive mother regardless of whether she remains in the abusive relationship.

Estimates of prevalence of violence in pregnancy vary, ranging from 5.7 to 6.6% to as high as 29% (PHAC, 2008b). Most women abused before pregnancy will be abused during the pregnancy, and the frequency and incidence may escalate. Abuse also may happen for the first time during pregnancy. Pregnant adolescents are abused at higher rates than are adult women; thus they should be considered at high risk. Violence during pregnancy in teenagers constitutes a particularly difficult situation. Adolescents may be more trapped in the abusive relationship than adult women because of their inexperience. They may ignore the violence because the jealous and controlling behaviour is interpreted as love and devotion. Because pregnancy in young adolescent girls may be the result of sexual abuse, feelings about the pregnancy should be assessed.

A pregnant woman may be accompanied by her husband to the antepartum appointment if she does not speak English and the husband does. Unless an interpreter is available, it is difficult to interview the woman alone; in addition, asking questions about abuse through an interpreter is more difficult unless the interpreter is a woman and can communicate the nurse's sensitivity and concern accurately. See Box 4-12 for a discussion of how to communicate with the woman who is being subjected to IPV.

Abuse is about control of one person over another (see Fig. 4-3). In health care situations, many women can feel this same type of power from health care providers. When providing care to the woman who is a victim of IPV, it is important to give her information that can enable her to make her own decisions and have control over her decisions.

Fetal and Neonatal Health Problems

The leading causes of neonatal morbidity and mortality are preterm and multiple birth rates. Other causes of neonatal death include disorders relating to low birth weight, respiratory distress syndrome, the effects of maternal complications, and sudden infant death. Despite universal health care, the infant death rate is higher if the mother is of poor socioeconomic status. Racial differences in the infant mortality rates continue to challenge public health experts. The rate of stillbirth and perinatal mortality is at least two times greater in First Nations, Métis, and Inuit populations (Canadian Institute of Health [CIHI], 2003). Increased rates of survival during the neonatal period have resulted largely from high-quality prenatal care and the improvement in perinatal services, including technological advances in neonatal intensive care and obstetrics.

Reducing infant mortality rates requires the removal of various barriers to care, including financial, educational, sociocultural, and logistical barriers, so that pregnant women can seek and receive appropriate health services. Commitment in this area is required at the national, provincial, and local levels. More research is needed to identify the extent to which the determinants of health, individually and collectively, affect perinatal morbidity and mortality. Ultimately, barriers to care must be removed and perinatal services modified to meet contemporary health care needs.

Antepartum Testing in the First and Second Trimester

The major expected outcome of antepartum testing is the detection of potential fetal compromise. Ideally, the technique used will identify fetal compromise before intrauterine asphyxia of the fetus occurs so that the health care provider can take measures to prevent or minimize adverse perinatal outcomes. No single test can provide this information. Assessment tests should be selected on the basis of their effectiveness, and the results must be interpreted in light of the complete clinical picture. The most reliable evidence for effectiveness is provided by randomized controlled trials. Nurses can be informed about the most recent research on fetal assessment by using an up-to-date systematic review, such as the Cochrane Database of Systematic Reviews (http://www.cochrane.org.au/libraryguide/guide_data.asp). Box 12-3 lists recommendations of care for fetal assessment screening that are based on evidence from this database.

BOX 12-3 Fetal Assessment Screening: Recommendations for Care

Beneficial Effects

- Doppler ultrasound use in pregnancy at high risk for fetal compromise

Effects Likely to Be Beneficial

- Ultrasound examination to resolve questions about fetal size, structure, or position
- Selective use of ultrasonography to estimate gestational age in first and early second trimesters
- Ultrasound use to confirm suspected multiple pregnancy
- Ultrasound use to assess amniotic fluid volume
- Early second-trimester amniocentesis for identification of chromosome abnormalities
- Transabdominal instead of transvaginal chorionic villus sampling

Trade-off Between Beneficial and Adverse Effects

- Formal systems of risk scoring
- Routine use of early ultrasonography
- Chorionic villus sampling versus amniocentesis for diagnosing chromosome abnormalities
- Serum alpha-fetoprotein screening for neural tube defects
- Triple screen test for Down syndrome and neural tube defects

Effectiveness Unknown

- Placental grading by means of ultrasonography to improve perinatal outcome
- Biophysical profile for fetal surveillance

Effects Unlikely to Be Beneficial

- Routine use of ultrasonography for fetal anthropometry (body measurements) in late pregnancy
- Routine fetal movement counts to improve perinatal outcome
- Use of Doppler ultrasound screening in all pregnancies
- Routine measurement of cervical length in prevention of preterm birth
- Measurement of placental hormones (estriol and human placental lactogen)

Effects Likely to Be Ineffective or Harmful

- Nipple stimulation test to improve perinatal outcome
- Nonselective nonstress test to improve perinatal outcome
- Contraction stress test to improve perinatal outcome

(Source: Enkin, M., et al. [2007]. *A guide to effective care in pregnancy and childbirth.* Oxford University Press. Retrieved from http://www.childbirthconnection.org/article.asp?ClickedLink=194&ck=10218&area=2.)

Prenatal Screening

First-trimester pregnancy screening for fetal aneuploidy (Down syndrome and trisomy 18) and second-trimester ultrasound examination to detect fetal anomalies should be offered to all pregnant women. Previously, women over the age of 35 were offered invasive testing, but this has been found to miss many cases of fetal anomalies. The Society of Obstetricians and Gynaecologists of Canada (SOGC) states that maternal age should be removed as an indication for invasive testing (SOGC, 2007), and with recent advances in maternal screening and ultrasound techniques, it is possible to offer all pregnant women a noninvasive method of screening. If the screening test is above a set cut-off level or if a woman is 40 years old at the time of the birth, invasive testing should be offered (amniocentesis or chorionic villus sampling; see discussion later in this chapter). There are regional differences across the country as to what screening tests are available, due to cost and the availability of trained ultrasound technicians. There are presently three options available for noninvasive screening.

First-Trimester Screening (FTS)

First-trimester screening (FTS) involves undergoing an ultrasound examination for nuchal translucency, combined with maternal serum biochemical markers. In *nuchal translucency* (NT) screening, ultrasound measurement of fluid in the nape of the fetal neck between 11 and 14 weeks of gestation is used to identify possible fetal abnormalities (Fig. 12-1). A finding of fluid collection that is greater than 2.5 mm is considered abnormal, whereas a measurement of 3 mm or greater is highly indicative of genetic disorders or physical anomalies.

First-trimester maternal serum biochemical markers are pregnancy-associated plasma protein-A (PAPP-A) and free beta-human chorionic gonadotropin (ß-hCG). PAPP-A is lower in Down syndrome pregnancies, and free ß-hCG is higher. FTS using all the criteria will detect 83% cases of Down syndrome, with a 5% false-positive rate (SOGC, 2007). If an FTS screening test is done, it is still recommended that women be screened for open neural tube defects (NTDs) at an 18- to 22-week ultrasound examination. A limitation of FTS is its lack of availability in some centres.

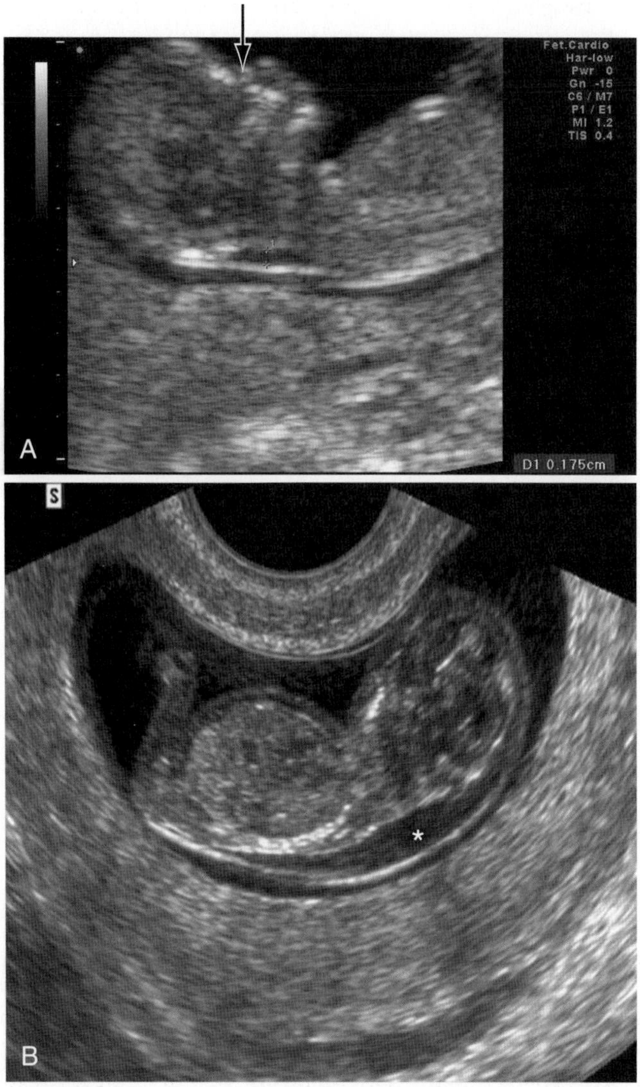

Fig. 12-1 Fetal nuchal translucency. **A:** Nuchal lucency (calipers) and nasal bone (arrow) in 12-week fetus. **B:** Increased nuchal translucency. Transvaginal ultrasound performed at 12 weeks demonstrates a sonolucent area (*asterisk*) over the posterior neck and upper thorax. *(From Martin, R. J., Fanaroff, A. A., & Walsh, M. C. [2006].* Fanaroff and Martin's neonatal–perinatal medicine: Diseases of the fetus and infant *[8th ed.]. Philadelphia: Mosby.)*

Second-Trimester Serum Screening

Maternal serum alpha fetoprotein (MSAFP) levels are used as a screening tool for NTD in pregnancy. Through this technique, approximately 80 to 85% of all open NTDs and open abdominal wall defects can be detected early in pregnancy.

AFP is produced by the fetal liver and is detectable in increasing quantities in the serum of pregnant women from 14 to 34 weeks. Although amniotic fluid AFP is diagnostic for NTD, MSAFP is a screening tool only and identifies candidates for the more definitive procedures of amniocentesis and ultrasound examination. MSAFP screening can be done with reasonable reliability any time between 15 and 22 weeks of gestation (16 to 18 weeks being ideal) (Wapner, Jenkins, & Khalek, 2009).

The cause of NTDs is not well understood, but 95% of all affected infants are born to women with no family history of similar anomalies (Wapner et al., 2009). The birth of one affected child increases the risk of NTD recurrence in future pregnancies (Manning, 2009).

Down syndrome—and probably other autosomal trisomies—is associated with lower-than-normal levels of MSAFP and amniotic fluid AFP. The triple-marker test is also performed at 16 to 18 weeks of gestation and uses the levels of three maternal serum markers: MSAFP, unconjugated estriol, and hCG, in combination with maternal age to calculate a new risk level. If a fetus has Down syndrome, the MSAFP and unconjugated estriol levels are low, and the hCG level is elevated. With these two additional screening tests, approximately 72% of fetuses with Down syndrome can be identified. Testing for dimeric inhibin-A (DIA) improves the detection rate to 75 to 80%, and this is part of a quad screen (SOGC, 2007). DIA is elevated in Down syndrome and other trisomies.

Integrated Prenatal Screening

The integrated prenatal screening (IPS) is a two-step process, which includes first- and second-trimester serum screening with or without NT. This screening method is superior to the other two methods, with a detection rate of 85%, a lower false-positive rate (1%), and thus a reduction in the number of invasive diagnostic procedures needed. IPS is based on the use of PAPP-A and NT in the first trimester and the quad screen in the second trimester; results are released when all the testing is completed. If NT is not available, PAPP-A is done in the first trimester and either triple or quad screening is done in the second trimester. This testing results in the detection of 83% of abnormalities (SOGC, 2007).

Ultrasound

Sound is a form of wave energy that causes small particles in a medium to oscillate. The frequency of sound, which refers to the number of peaks or waves that move over a given point per unit of time, is expressed in hertz (Hz). Sound with a frequency of 1 cycle, or 1 peak per second, has a frequency of 1 Hz. When directional beams of sound strike an object, an echo is returned. The time delay between the emission of the sound and the return of the echo and the direction of the echo are noted. From these data, the distance and location of an object can be calculated.

Ultrasound is sound frequency higher than that detectable by humans (greater than 20,000 Hz). Diagnostic ultrasound instruments operate within a frequency range of 2 to 10 kHz, which is below the range used by sonar and radar equipment. Ultrasound images are a reflection of the strength of the sending beam, the strength of the returning echo, and the density of the medium (e.g., muscle [uterus], bone, tissue [placenta], fluid, or blood) through which the beam is sent and returned.

Diagnostic ultrasonography is an important technique in antepartum fetal surveillance (Fig. 12-2). It provides critical information to health care providers regarding fetal activity and **gestational age,** normal versus abnormal fetal growth curves, visual assistance with which invasive tests may be

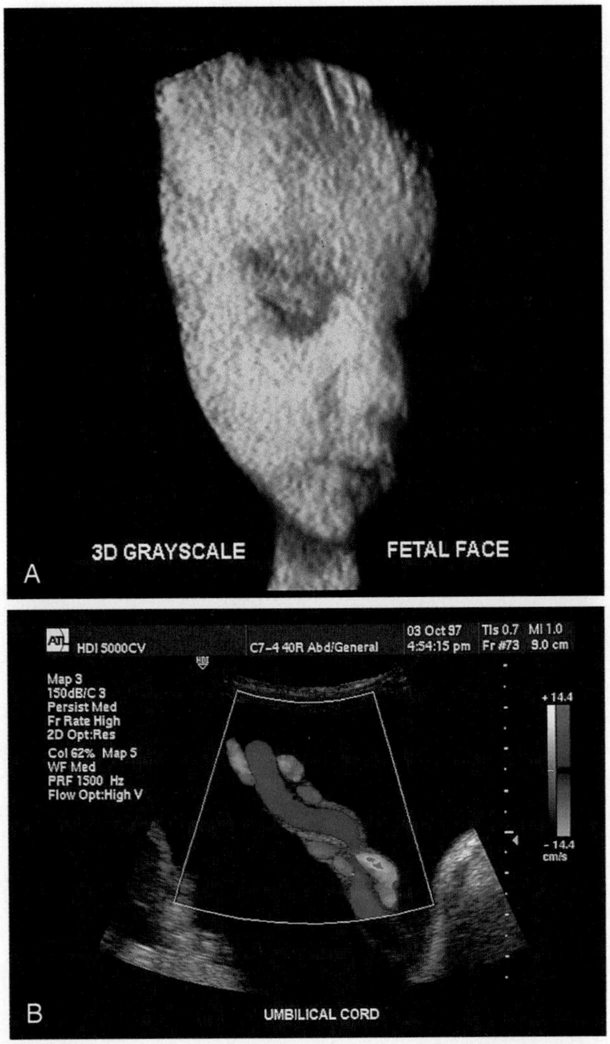

Fig. 12-2 Two views of the fetus during ultrasonography. **A:** Fetal face (20 weeks). **B:** Umbilical cord (26 weeks). *(Courtesy Advanced Technology Laboratories, Bothell, WA.)*

performed more safely, and fetal and placental anatomy early in pregnancy. Ultrasound examination done later during pregnancy assesses fetal well-being and will be discussed later in the chapter. Ultrasound examination can be done abdominally or transvaginally during pregnancy. Both methods produce a three-dimensional view from which a pictorial image is obtained. Abdominal ultrasonography is more useful after the first trimester when the pregnant uterus becomes an abdominal organ.

For the procedure, the woman is usually required to have a full bladder to push the uterus up in order to get a better image of the fetus. Transmission gel is applied to the abdomen before a transducer is moved over the skin to enhance transmission and reception of the sound waves. The woman is positioned with small pillows under her head and knees. The display panel is positioned so that the woman and her partner can observe the images on the screen if they so desire.

Transvaginal Ultrasound Examination

Transvaginal ultrasound examination, in which the probe is inserted into the vagina, allows pelvic anatomy to be evaluated in greater detail and allows intrauterine pregnancy to be diagnosed earlier. It is used in the first trimester to detect ectopic pregnancies, monitor the developing embryo, help identify abnormalities, and help establish gestational age. In some instances it may be used as an adjunct to abdominal scanning to evaluate preterm labour, by assessing the cervical length, in second- and third-trimester pregnancies. A transvaginal ultrasound examination is well tolerated by most patients because it alleviates the need for a full bladder. It is especially useful in obese patients whose thick abdominal layers cannot be penetrated adequately with an abdominal approach.

A transvaginal ultrasound examination may be performed either with the woman in a lithotomy position or with her pelvis elevated by towels, cushions, or a folded pillow. This pelvic tilt is optimal to image the pelvic structures. A protective cover such as a condom, the finger of a clean rubber surgical glove, or a special cover provided by the manufacturer is used to cover the probe. The probe is lubricated with a water-soluble gel and placed in the vagina either by the examiner or by the woman herself. During the examination, the position of the probe or the tilt of the examining table may be changed to view the complete pelvis. The procedure is not physically painful, although the woman will feel pressure as the probe is moved.

Indications for Use

Major indications for the use of obstetrical sonography are shown by trimester in Box 12-4. Ultrasonography can lead to earlier diagnoses, allowing therapy to be instituted early in pregnancy. This decreases the severity and duration of morbidity, both physical and emotional, for the family. For example, early diagnosis of a fetal anomaly gives the family choices such as (1) preparation for the care of an infant with a disorder, (2) intrauterine surgery or other therapy for the fetus, or (3) termination of the pregnancy. Ultrasonography can be used to assess gestational age, anatomy, and growth. In the third trimester, it can be used to assess for fetal well-being; this is discussed later in the chapter.

Fetal Heart Activity. Fetal heart activity can be demonstrated as early as 6 to 7 weeks by real-time echo scanners and at 10 to 12 weeks by Doppler mode. By 9 to 10 weeks, gestational trophoblastic disease can be diagnosed. Fetal death can be confirmed by lack of heart motion; the presence of fetal scalp edema, and maceration; and overlap of the cranial bones.

Gestational Age. Gestational dating by ultrasonography is indicated for conditions such as the following: (1) uncertain dates for the last normal menstrual period, (2) recent discontinuation of oral contraceptives, (3) bleeding during the first trimester, (4) uterine size that does not agree with dates, (5) integrated prenatal screening, and (6) other high-risk conditions.

During the first 20 weeks of gestation, ultrasonography provides an accurate assessment of gestational age because most normal fetuses grow at the same rate. With increased fetal age, the accuracy of gestational-age estimates using ultrasound decrease, as fetuses grow at different rates. Four methods of fetal age estimation are used: (1) determination of gestational sac dimensions (at about 8 weeks), (2) measurement of crown-rump length (between 5 and 10 weeks), (3) measurement of the biparietal diameter (BPD) (after 12 weeks), and (4) measurement of femur length (after 12 weeks) (Richards, 2007). Fetal BPD at 36 weeks should be approximately 8.7 cm. Term pregnancy and fetal maturity can be diagnosed with some confidence if the biparietal measurement by ultrasound is greater than 9.8 cm (Fig. 12-3), especially when this is combined with appropriate femur length measurement.

Fetal Growth. Fetal growth is determined by intrinsic growth potential and the environmental factors that may enhance or inhibit that growth. Conditions that indicate the need for ultrasound assessment of fetal growth include the following: (1) poor maternal weight gain or pattern of weight gain, (2) previous pregnancy with intrauterine growth restriction (IUGR), (3) chronic infections, (4) ingestion of drugs (tobacco, alcohol, over-the-counter medications, and street drugs), (5) maternal diabetes mellitus, (6) hypertension, (7) **multifetal pregnancy,** and (8) other medical or surgical complications.

Serial evaluations of BPD (see Fig. 12-3), head circumference (Fig. 12-4), limb length, and abdominal circumference

BOX 12-4 Major Uses of Ultrasonography During Pregnancy

First Trimester
- Confirm pregnancy
- Confirm viability
- Determine gestational age
- Rule out ectopic pregnancy
- Detect multiple gestation
- Visualization during chorionic villus sampling
- Detect maternal abnormalities such as bicornuate uterus, ovarian cysts, fibroids
- Detect presence and location of an intrauterine contraceptive device
- Assess nuchal translucency

Second Trimester
- Assess fetal anatomy
- Establish or confirm dates
- Confirm viability
- Detect polyhydramnios, oligohydramnios
- Detect congenital anomalies
- Detect intrauterine growth restriction (IUGR)
- Confirm placental placement
- Assess cervical length
- Visualization during amniocentesis

Third Trimester
- Confirm viability
- Detect macrosomia
- Detect congenital anomalies
- Detect IUGR
- Determine fetal position
- Detect placenta previa or abruptio placentae
- Visualization during amniocentesis, external version
- Biophysical profile
- Assess amniotic fluid volume
- Doppler flow studies
- Detect placental maturity

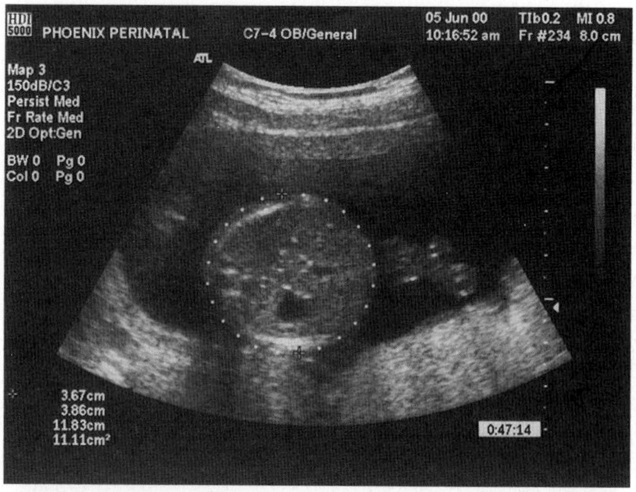

Fig. 12-3 Biparietal cephalometry on ultrasound scan. *(Courtesy Michael S. Clement, MD, Mesa, AZ.)*

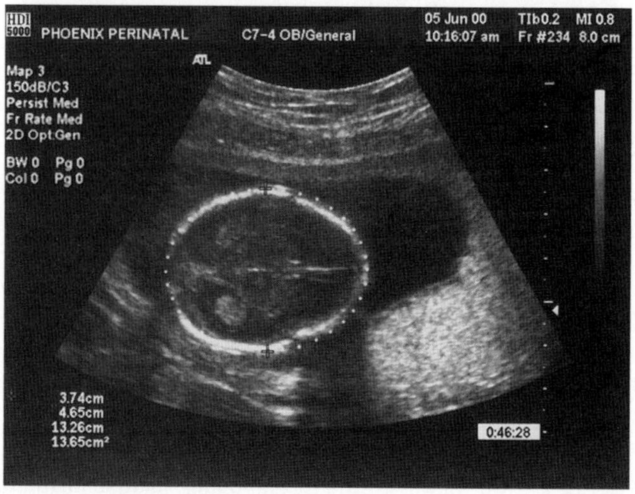

Fig. 12-4 Head circumference. *(Courtesy Michael S. Clement, MD, Mesa, AZ.)*

(Fig. 12-5) can differentiate among size discrepancy resulting from inaccurate dates, true IUGR, and macrosomia. IUGR may be symmetric (the fetus is small in all parameters) or asymmetric (head and body growth vary). Symmetric IUGR implies a chronic or long-standing insult and may be caused by low genetic growth potential, intrauterine infection, undernutrition, heavy smoking, or chromosome aberration. Asymmetric growth reflects an acute or late-occurring deprivation such as placental insufficiency resulting from hypertension, renal disease, or cardiovascular disease. Reduced fetal growth is still one of the most frequent conditions associated with stillbirth.

Macrosomic infants (those weighing 4000 g or more) are at increased risk for dystocia, traumatic injury, and asphyxia during birth. Macrosomia in the infant of a mother with diabetes is asymmetric and characterized by increases in fat and muscle in the abdomen and shoulders; head circumference remains normal. Macrosomia in an infant whose mother is obese without glucose intolerance results in symmetric changes (i.e., excessive growth of abdominal and head circumferences).

Routine assessment for fetal size has not been found to be beneficial and may increase the number of women hospitalized and requiring induction of labour without any increase in benefit (Enkin et al., 2000). Third-trimester ultrasonography for assessment of size should only be done in women who have identified risk factors.

Fetal Anatomy. Depending on the gestational age, the following structures can be identified on ultrasound scans: head (including ventricles and blood vessels), neck, spine, heart, stomach, small bowel, liver, kidneys, bladder, limbs, and umbilical cord. The SOGC recommends that all women be offered a routine second-trimester ultrasound examination between 18 and 22 weeks. Second-trimester ultrasonography should be used to screen for multiple fetuses, location of placenta, and gestational age, and a complete anatomical scan should be performed (Cargill et al., 2009). Ultrasonography can be used to confirm normal anatomy and detect major fetal malformations. The presence of an anomaly may influence where the birth takes place (e.g., a delivery room instead of a labour, delivery, and recovery room, or a subspecialty centre instead of a basic care centre) and the method of birth (vaginal versus Caesarean), to optimize neonatal outcomes.

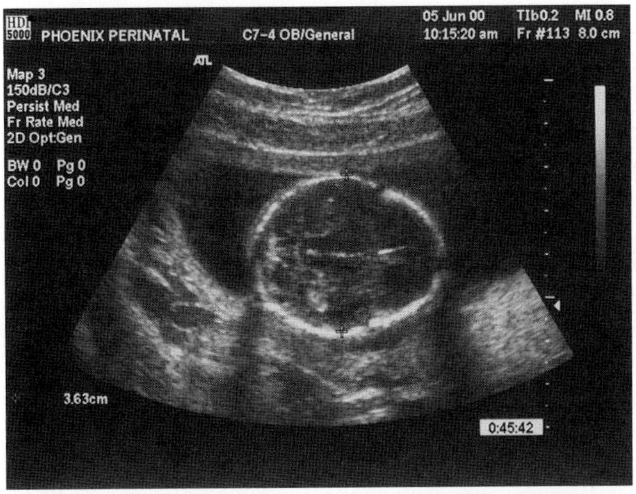

Fig. 12-5 Abdominal circumference. *(Courtesy Michael S. Clement, MD, Mesa, AZ.)*

Placental Position and Function. The pattern of uterine and placental growth and the fullness of the maternal bladder influence the apparent location of the placenta as viewed by ultrasonography. During the first trimester, differentiation between the endometrium and small placenta is difficult. By 14 to 16 weeks, the placenta is clearly defined, but its relationship to the internal cervical os can sometimes be altered dramatically by changing the degree of fullness of the maternal bladder. In approximately 15 to 20% of all pregnancies in which ultrasound scanning is performed during the second trimester, the placenta seems to be overlying the os, but at term the incidence of placenta previa is only 0.5%. Thus the diagnosis of placenta previa can seldom be confirmed before 27 weeks, primarily because of the elongation of the lower uterine segment as pregnancy advances.

Another use of ultrasonography is grading of placental maturation. Calcium deposits are of significance in postterm pregnancies because, as they increase, the available surface area that can be adequately bathed by maternal blood decreases. The point at which this results in fetal wastage and hypoxia cannot be determined precisely; however, effects usually are observable by 42 weeks and are progressive.

Nursing Role

The main role of nurses in obstetrical ultrasound examination is in counselling and educating women about ultrasound scans. Providing accurate information about the procedure is imperative to allay the mother's anxiety. Although ultrasound scanning has become a widely used diagnostic tool, recommendations for the procedure are based on expectations of a fetal problem and thus may cause concern. Women should be provided ample opportunity to ask questions and be reassured that the procedure is safe. In the 40 years that diagnostic ultrasonography has been used, no conclusive evidence of any harmful effects on humans has emerged. Although the possibility of unidentified biological effects exists, the benefits to the woman of prudent use of diagnostic ultrasound appear to outweigh any possible risk. The SOGC has made recommendations regarding nonmedical use of ultrasound (Box 12-5).

Biochemical Assessment

Biochemical assessment involves biological examination (e.g., chromosomes in exfoliated cells) and chemical determinations (e.g., lecithin/sphingomyelin [L/S] ratio and bilirubin level) (Table 12-1). Procedures used to obtain the specimens for study include amniocentesis, percutaneous umbilical blood sampling (PUBS), chorionic villus sampling (CVS), and maternal sampling.

Coombs' Test

Maternal blood is tested in the indirect Coombs' test, a screening test for Rh incompatibility; it is discussed in Chapter 28. If the maternal titer for Rh antibodies is greater than 1:8, amniocentesis for determination of bilirubin in amniotic fluid is indicated to determine the severity of fetal hemolytic anemia. The Coombs' test can also detect other antibodies that may place the fetus at risk for incompatibility with maternal antigens.

Amniocentesis

Amniocentesis is performed to obtain amniotic fluid, which contains fetal cells. Under direct ultrasound visualization, a needle is inserted transabdominally into the uterus, amniotic fluid is withdrawn into a syringe, and various assessments are performed (Fig. 12-6). Amniocentesis is possible after week 14 of pregnancy, when the uterus becomes an abdominal organ and sufficient amniotic fluid is available for testing (see Table 12-1). Indications for the procedure include prenatal diagnosis of genetic disorders or congenital anomalies (NTDs in particular), assessment of pulmonary maturity, and diagnosis of fetal hemolytic disease.

Complications in the mother and fetus occur in less than 1% of cases and include the following:

Maternal—Hemorrhage, fetomaternal hemorrhage with possible maternal Rh isoimmunization, infection, labour, abruptio placentae, inadvertent damage to the intestines or bladder, and amniotic fluid embolism. Given the possibility of fetomaternal hemorrhage, it is standard practice after an amniocentesis to administer immune globulin D (e.g., RhoGAM) to the woman who is Rh negative.

Fetal—Death, hemorrhage, infection (amnionitis), direct injury from the needle, miscarriage or preterm labour, and leakage of amniotic fluid.

Many of the complications have been minimized or eliminated by using ultrasound scanning to determine the exact position of the fetus, placenta, and pockets of amniotic fluid.

Indications for Use

Genetic Concerns. The incidence of genetic disorders is increased in women older than 35 years, those with a previous child with a chromosome abnormality, or those with a family history of chromosome anomalies. However, the SOGC states that screening based on maternal age should be abandoned, except for women over the age of 40 at the time of birth, and that all women should be offered noninvasive screening for Down syndrome or trisomy 18. Older women should have the option of going automatically to CVS/amniocentesis, as well as women who screen above a set risk cut-off level (SOGC, 2007).

BOX 12-5 Nonmedical Use of Ultrasonography During Pregnancy

There has been an increase in the use of ultrasonography for entertainment purposes or to determine fetal sex. These ultrasound scans are often done to provide keepsake videos. Although there is no determined risk of exposure to ultrasound, it does involve exposure to targeted energy that could cause subtle changes to fetal development. Therefore, the Society of Obstetricians and Gynaecologists of Canada and Health Canada recommend that ultrasonography not be done for nonmedical reasons. There is no governing body ensuring that operators are competent and that there is maintenance of technical safeguards with the use of nonmedical ultrasound. The amount of fetal energy exposure due to extended duration to ensure a suitable commercial product may not be monitored. With nonmedical ultrasound examination, there is also no obligation to report fetal concerns (Van den Hof, Bly, et al., 2007).

Table 12-1 Summary of Biochemical Monitoring Techniques

TEST	POSSIBLE FINDINGS	CLINICAL SIGNIFICANCE
Maternal Blood		
Coombs' test	Titer of 1:8 and rising	Significant Rh incompatibility
Amniotic Fluid Analysis		
Colour	Meconium	Possible hypoxia or asphyxia
Lung profile		
L/S ratio	>2:1	Fetal lung maturity
Phosphatidylglycerol	Present	Fetal lung maturity
Creatinine	>150 mcmol/L	Gestational age >36 wk
Bilirubin (ΔOD 450 nm)*	<0.015	Gestational age >36 wk, normal pregnancy
	High levels	Fetal hemolytic disease in Rh-isoimmunized pregnancies
Lipid cells	>10%	Gestational age >35 wk
Osmolality	Decline after 20-wk gestation	Advancing nonspecific gestational age
Genetic disorders Sex-linked Chromosomal Metabolic	Dependent on cultured cells for karyotype and enzymatic activity	Counselling possibly required

*The presence of bilirubin changes the colour of amniotic fluid. The change in optical density (ΔOD) is a measure of the amount of bilirubin in the amniotic fluid.
L/S, lecithin/sphingomyelin.

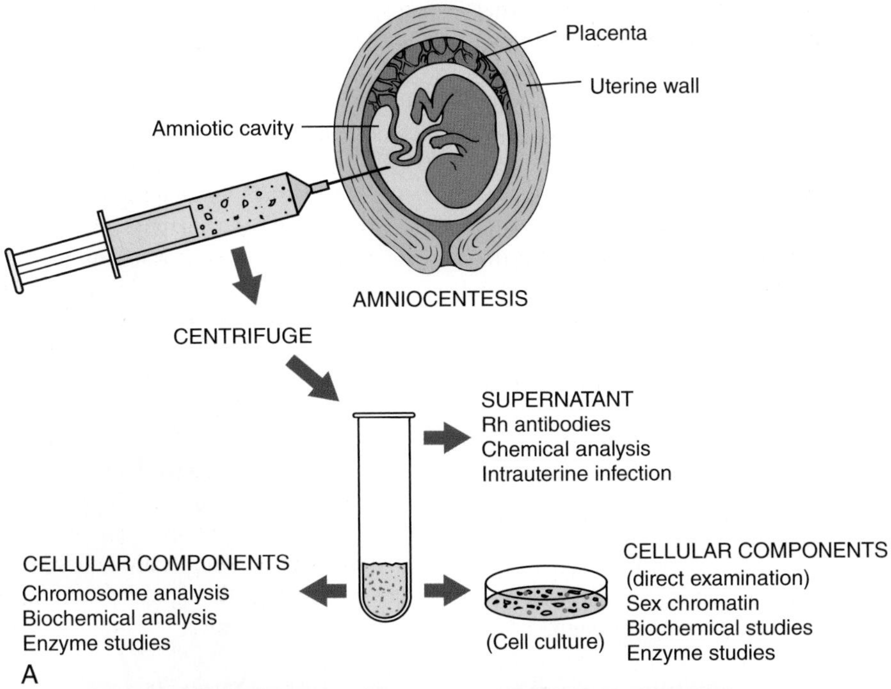

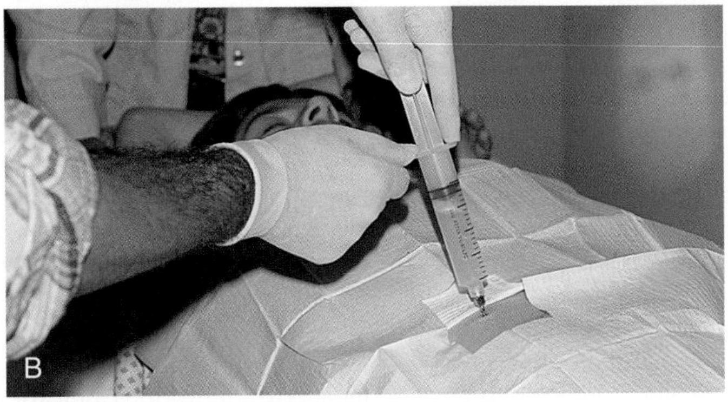

Fig. 12-6 **A:** Amniocentesis and laboratory use of amniotic fluid aspirant. **B:** Transabdominal amniocentesis. *(**B**, Courtesy Marjorie Pyle, RNC, Lifecircle, Costa Mesa, CA.)*

Fetal cells are cultured for **karyotyping** of chromosomes (see Chapter 8). Karyotyping is used to determine fetal sex, which is important if a sex-linked disorder (occurring almost always in a male fetus) is suspected.

Biochemical analysis of enzymes in amniotic fluid can be used to detect inborn errors of metabolism. For example, AFP levels in amniotic fluid are assessed as a follow-up for elevated levels in maternal serum. High AFP levels in amniotic fluid help confirm the diagnosis of an open NTD, such as spina bifida or anencephaly, or an open abdominal wall defect, such as omphalocele. The elevation results from the increased leakage of cerebrospinal fluid into the amniotic fluid through the closure defect. AFP levels also may be elevated in a normal multifetal pregnancy and with intestinal atresia, presumably caused by lack of fetal swallowing.

A concurrent test indicating the presence of acetylcholinesterase in amniotic fluid almost always indicates a fetal defect (Wapner et al., 2009). In such instances, follow-up ultrasound examination is recommended.

Fetal Maturity. Accurate assessment of fetal maturity is possible through examination of amniotic fluid or its exfoliated cellular contents. Table 12-1 lists laboratory studies that are used to demonstrate term pregnancy and fetal maturity. A quick means of determining an approximate L/S ratio is the shake test, foam test, or bubble stability test. Serial dilutions of fresh amniotic fluid are mixed with ethanol and shaken. After 15 minutes, the amount of bubbles present at different dilutions indicates the presence of surfactant.

Fetal Hemolytic Disease. Another indication for amniocentesis is the identification and follow-up of fetal hemolytic disease in cases of isoimmunization. The procedure is usually not done until the mother's serum antibody titer reaches 1:8 and is increasing. Currently, PUBS is the procedure of choice to evaluate and treat fetal hemolytic disease.

Meconium. The presence of meconium in the amniotic fluid is usually determined by visual inspection of the sample. The significance of meconium in the amniotic fluid varies, depending on when it is found.

Meconium in the amniotic fluid before early labour begins is not usually associated with an adverse fetal outcome. The finding may be the result of an acute and subsequently corrected fetal stress, chronic ongoing stress, or simply the physiological passage of meconium. Because there is some association between meconium in amniotic fluid in the third trimester and hypertensive conditions and postmaturity, the fetus should undergo further antepartum evaluation. Labour induction may be considered if the fetal status appears compromised (Resnik & Resnik, 2009).

Intrapartal meconium-stained amniotic fluid is an indication for more careful evaluation by electronic fetal monitoring (EFM) and perhaps fetal scalp blood sampling. However, the presence of meconium should not be the sole indicator for intervention.

Three possible reasons exist for the passage of meconium during the intrapartal period: (1) it is a normal physiological function that occurs with maturity (meconium passage is uncommon before weeks 23 to 24, but there is an increased incidence after 38 weeks); (2) it is the result of hypoxia-induced peristalsis and sphincter relaxation; and (3) it may be a sequel to umbilical cord compression–induced vagal stimulation in mature fetuses. Thick, fresh meconium passed for the first time in late labour, associated with nonremediable severe variable or late FHR decelerations, is an ominous sign.

Percutaneous Umbilical Blood Sampling

Direct access to the fetal circulation during the second and third trimesters is possible through **percutaneous umbilical blood sampling** (PUBS), or cordocentesis. PUBS is the most widely used method for fetal blood sampling and transfusion. It involves the insertion of a needle directly into the fetal umbilical vessel under ultrasound guidance. Ideally, the umbilical cord is punctured 1 to 2 cm from its insertion into the placenta (Fig. 12-7). At this point, the cord is well anchored and will not move, and the risk of maternal blood contamination (from the placenta) is slight. Generally 1 to 4 mL of blood is removed and tested immediately by means of the Kleihauer-Betke procedure to ensure that it is fetal blood. Indications for the use of PUBS include prenatal diagnosis of inherited blood disorders, karyotyping of malformed fetuses, detection of fetal infection, determination of the acid–base status of fetuses with IUGR, and assessment and treatment of isoimmunization and **thrombocytopenia** in the fetus (Wapner et al., 2009). Complications that can occur include leaking of blood from the puncture site, cord laceration, thromboembolism, preterm labour, premature rupture of membranes, and infection.

In fetuses at risk for isoimmune hemolytic anemia, PUBS enables precise identification of fetal blood type and red blood cell (RBC) count and may eliminate the need for further intervention. If the fetus is positive for the presence of maternal antibodies, a direct blood test can confirm the degree of anemia resulting from hemolysis. Intrauterine transfusion of severely anemic fetuses can be done 4 to 5 weeks earlier than through the intraperitoneal route.

Follow-up includes continuous fetal heart rate (FHR) monitoring for several minutes to 1 hour and a repeat ultrasound examination 1 hour later to ensure that no bleeding or hematoma formation has occurred.

Chorionic Villus Sampling

The combined advantages of earlier diagnosis and rapid results have made **chorionic villus sampling** (CVS) a popular

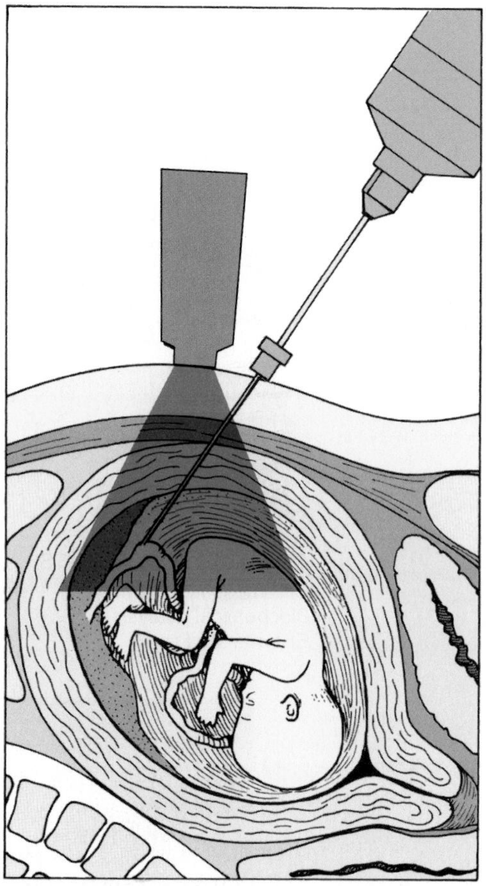

Fig. 12-7 Technique for percutaneous umbilical blood sampling guided by ultrasonography.

technique for genetic studies, although some risks to the fetus exist. Indications for CVS are similar to those for amniocentesis; however, second-trimester amniocentesis appears to be safer than CVS (Alfirevic, Sunberg, & Brigham, 2004; Wilson et al., 2005). The benefits of earlier diagnosis must be weighed against the increased risk of pregnancy loss and risk of anomalies.

The procedure is performed between 10 and 13 weeks of gestation and involves the removal of a small tissue specimen from the fetal portion of the placenta. Because chorionic villi originate in the zygote, that tissue reflects the genetic makeup of the fetus.

CVS can be accomplished either transcervically or transabdominally. In transcervical sampling, a sterile catheter is introduced into the cervix under continuous ultrasonographic guidance, and a small portion of the chorionic villi is aspirated with a syringe. The aspiration cannula and obturator must be placed at a suitable site, and rupture of the amniotic sac must be avoided.

If the abdominal approach is used, an 18-gauge spinal needle with stylet is inserted under sterile conditions through the abdominal wall into the chorion frondosum under ultrasound guidance. The stylet is then withdrawn, and the chorionic tissue is aspirated into a syringe (Fig. 12-8).

Complications of the procedure include vaginal spotting or bleeding immediately afterward (Box 12-6), miscarriage

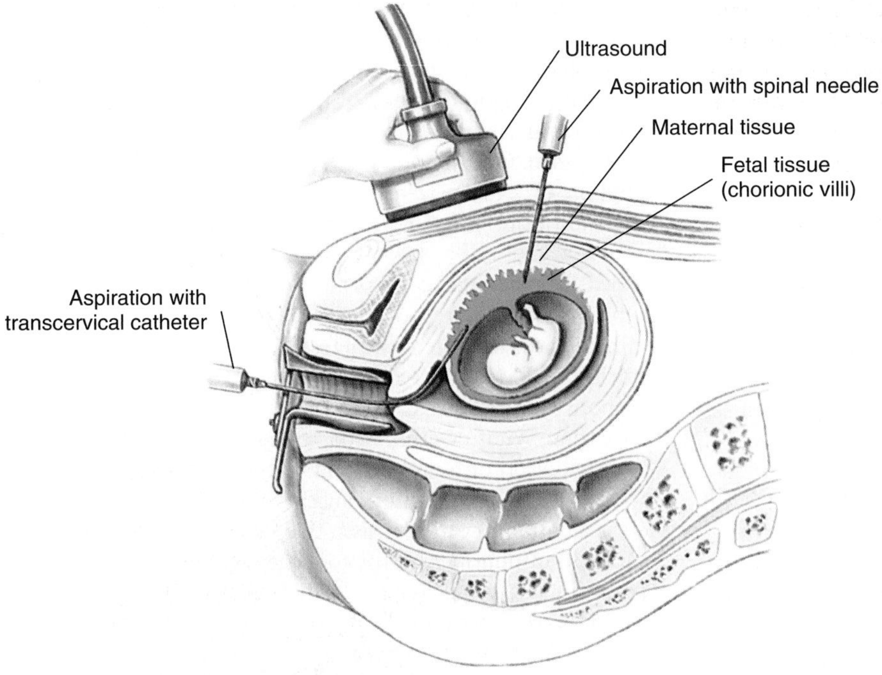

Fig. 12-8 Chorionic villi sampling (abdominal and transcervical methods). *(Courtesy Medical and Scientific Illustration, Crozet, VA.)*

BOX 12-6 Apt Test for Differentiation of Maternal and Fetal Blood

The Apt test is used to differentiate maternal and fetal blood when vaginal bleeding occurs during pregnancy or labour. It may be performed quickly by the following method: Add 0.5 mL of bloody fluid to 4.5 mL of distilled water and shake. Add 1 mL of 1% sodium hydroxide. Fetal and cord blood remains pink for 1 to 2 minutes. Maternal blood turns brown in 30 seconds. A Kleihauer-Betke procedure can be done in the laboratory to confirm the presence of fetal blood.

BOX 12-7 Fetal Rights

Amniocentesis, percutaneous umbilical blood sampling, and chorionic villus sampling are prenatal tests used for diagnosing fetal defects in pregnancy. They are invasive and carry risks to the mother and fetus. A consideration of elective abortion is linked to the performance of these tests because there is no treatment for genetically affected fetuses. Thus, the issue of fetal rights is a key ethical concern in prenatal testing for fetal defects.

(0.3%), rupture of membranes (0.1%), and chorioamnionitis (0.5%). Because of the possibility of fetomaternal hemorrhage, women who are Rh negative should receive immune globulin to avoid isoimmunization. An increased risk of limb anomalies (transverse digital anomalies) has been noted when CVS is done before 10 weeks of gestation (Box 12-7).

The use of amniocentesis and CVS is declining because of advances in noninvasive screening techniques. These techniques include measurement of nuchal translucency, maternal serum screening tests in the first and second trimesters, and ultrasonography in the second trimester (Benn et al., 2004; Wilson et al., 2005).

Ultrasound as Adjunct to Amniocentesis, Percutaneous Umbilical Blood Sampling, and Chorionic Villus Sampling

The safety of amniocentesis is increased when the exact position of the fetus, placenta, and pockets of amniotic fluid can be identified accurately. Ultrasound scanning has reduced the risks previously associated with amniocentesis, such as fetomaternal hemorrhage from a pierced placenta. PUBS and CVS are also guided by ultrasonography to accurately identify the cord and chorion frondosum (see Fig. 12-7).

Third-Trimester Assessment for Fetal Well-Being

Indications

Assessment during the first and second trimesters is directed primarily at the diagnosis of fetal anomalies. The goal of third-trimester testing is to determine whether the intrauterine environment continues to be supportive to the fetus. The testing is often used to determine the timing of childbirth for patients at risk for uteroplacental insufficiency. Gradual loss of placental function results first in inadequate nutrient delivery to the fetus, leading to IUGR. Subsequently, respiratory function is compromised, resulting in fetal hypoxia. Indications for increased fetal surveillance, including fetal movement counting, nonstress test (NST), contraction stress test (CST), biophysical profile (BPP), and other ultrasound tests, are listed in Box 12-8. There is presently no evidence to suggest the use of antenatal fetal testing in uncomplicated pregnancies less than 41 weeks (Liston et al., 2007).

BOX 12-8 Indications Associated With Increased Perinatal Morbidity/Mortality When Antenatal Fetal Surveillance May Be Beneficial

Previous Obstetrical History	
Maternal	Hypertensive disorder of pregnancy
	Placental abruption
Fetal	Intrauterine growth restriction
	Stillbirth
Current Pregnancy	
Maternal	Postterm pregnancy (>294 days, >42 weeks)
	Hypertensive disorders of pregnancy
	Pregestational diabetes
	Insulin requiring gestational diabetes
	Preterm premature rupture of membranes
	Chronic (stable) abruption
	Isoimmunization
	Abnormal maternal serum screen in absence of confirmed fetal anomaly
	Motor vehicle accident during pregnancy
	Vaginal bleeding
	Morbid obesity
	Advanced maternal age
	Assisted reproductive technologies
Fetal	Decreased fetal movement
	Intrauterine growth restriction
	Suspected oligohydramnios/polyhydramnios
	Multiple pregnancy
	Preterm labour

(Source: Liston, R., et al. [2007]. SOGC clinical practice guideline: Fetal health surveillance: Antepartum and intrapartum consensus guideline. *Journal of Obstetrics and Gynaecology Canada, 29*[9], Suppl 4, S1–S56. Retrieved from http://www.sogc.org/guidelines/documents/gui197CPG0709r.pdf.)

Fetal Movement Counting

Awareness of fetal activity by the mother is a simple yet valuable method for monitoring the condition of the fetus for all pregnant women, regardless of whether or not risk factors are present. All women should be taught to become aware of fetal movements in the third trimester and only if they perceive decreased movement or have risk factors they should begin daily monitoring/counting of fetal movements. Fetal movement counting (also called "kick counts") can be done at home, is simple to understand, is noninvasive, and usually does not interfere with a daily routine. Decreased fetal movement can be related to decreased placental perfusion and fetal acidemia.

Women should be taught the significance of the presence or absence of fetal movements, the procedure to use for counting, and when to notify their health care provider. The technique for fetal movement counting has the woman concentrating on the movements in a reclined (not supine) position. The recommended technique is to have women count six movements. If six movements are not felt in 2 hours, further evaluation of maternal and fetal status is required (Liston et al., 2007). This would initially include an NST or BPP (Fig. 12-9).

NURSING ALERT In assessing fetal movements it is important to remember that they are usually not present during the fetal sleep cycle; they may be temporarily reduced if the woman is taking depressant medication, drinking alcohol, or smoking a cigarette. They do not decrease as the woman nears term. Obesity and an anterior placenta decreases perception of fetal movement and, consequently, the ability of the mother to count fetal movements.

Fetal Responses to Hypoxia and Asphyxia

Observable fetal responses to hypoxia or asphyxia are the clinical basis for antepartum testing with electronic fetal monitoring (EFM). Hypoxia or asphyxia elicits a number of responses in the fetus. There is a redistribution of blood flow to certain vital organs. This series of responses including: redistribution of blood flow favouring vital organs, decreased total oxygen consumption, and a switch to anaerobic glycolysis is a temporary mechanism that enables the fetus to survive up to 30 minutes with limited oxygen supply without decompensation of vital organs. However, during more severe asphyxia or sustained hypoxemia, these compensatory responses are no longer maintained, and a decrease in the cardiac output, arterial blood pressure, and blood flow to the brain and heart occurs (Nageotte & Gilstrap, 2009), with characteristic FHR patterns reflecting these changes.

Variability

Considerable evidence supports the clinical belief that FHR variability indicates an intact nervous pathway through the cerebral cortex, midbrain, vagus nerve, and cardiac conduction system. With 98% accuracy in predicting fetal well-being, the presence of normal FHR variability is a reassuring indicator. Input from various areas of the brain decreases after cerebral asphyxia, leading to a decrease in variability after failure of the fetal hemodynamic compensatory mechanisms to maintain cerebral oxygenation (Nageotte & Gilstrap, 2009). As a rule, normal patterns with the NST or negative results with the CST are associated with favourable outcomes.

Nonstress Test

The **nonstress test** (NST) is the most widely applied technique for antepartum evaluation of the fetus, although there is poor evidence that NSTs decrease perinatal morbidity or mortality. The basis for the NST is that the normal fetus produces characteristic heart rate patterns in response to fetal movement. In the healthy fetus with an intact central nervous system, 90% of gross fetal body movements are associated with FHR accelerations. The acceleration with movement response may be blunted by hypoxia, acidosis, medications (analgesics, barbiturates, and β-blockers), fetal sleep, and some congenital anomalies (Tucker, Miller, & Miller, 2009).

The NST can be performed easily and quickly in an outpatient setting because it is noninvasive and has no known contraindications. Disadvantages centre around the high rate of false-positive results for atypical or abnormal tracings as a result of fetal sleep cycles, chronic tobacco smoking, medications, and fetal immaturity. The test is slightly less sensitive in detecting fetal compromise than the CST or BPP. No clinical contraindications exist for the NST, but results may be inconclusive if gestation is 26 weeks or less.

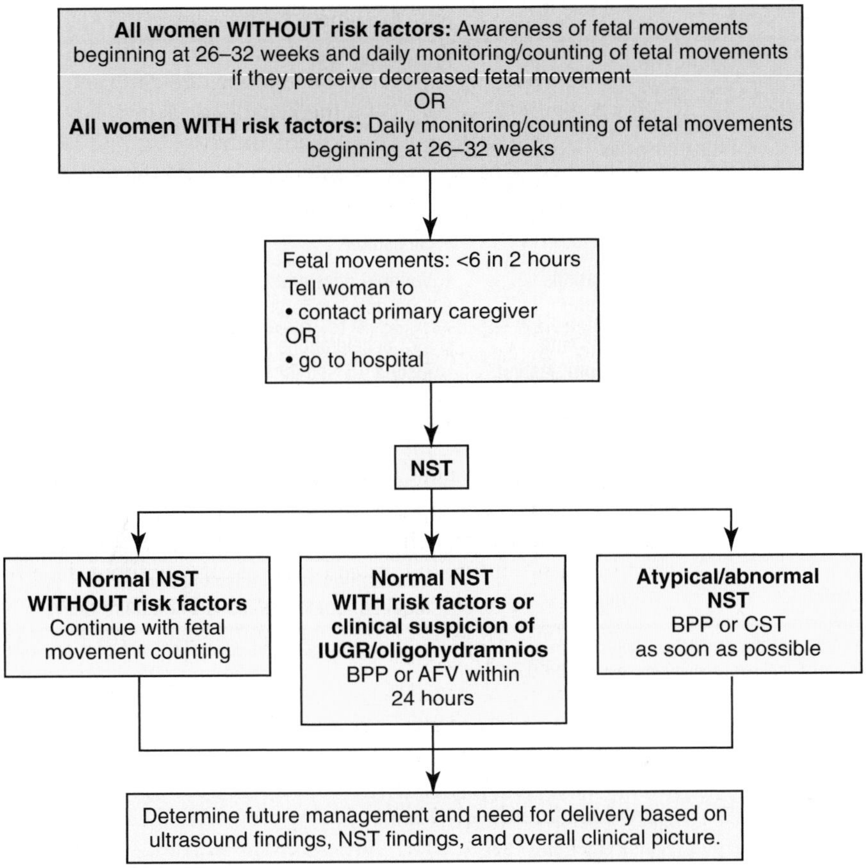

Fig. 12-9 Fetal movement algorithm. *AFV*, amniotic fluid volume; *BPP*, biophysical profile; *IUGR*, intrauterine growth restriction; *NST*, nonstress test. *(From Liston, R., et al. [2007]. SOGC clinical practice guideline: Fetal health surveillance: Antepartum and intrapartum consensus guideline.* Journal of Obstetricians and Gynaecologists of Canada, *29[9], Suppl 4, S1–S23. Retrieved from http://www.sogc.org/guidelines/documents/gui197CPG0709r.pdf.)*

Procedure

The woman should have an empty bladder and be seated in a reclining chair (or in a semi-Fowler position) with a slight left tilt, to optimize uterine perfusion and avoid supine hypotension. The FHR is recorded with a Doppler transducer, and a tocodynamometer is applied to detect uterine contractions or fetal movements. The tracing is observed for signs of fetal activity and a concurrent acceleration of FHR. If evidence of fetal movement is not apparent on the strip, the woman may be asked to depress a button on a handheld event marker connected to the monitor when she feels fetal movement. The movement is then noted on the tracing. Because almost all accelerations are accompanied by fetal movements, the movements need not be recorded for the test to be considered reactive. The test usually is completed in 20 minutes but should continue for up to 80 minutes if the response is not normal.

Administering glucose to the mother or stimulating the abdomen to encourage fetal movement is not recommended, as research has not proven either technique to be effective (Liston et al., 2007). Only **vibroacoustic stimulation** has had some impact on stimulating fetal movement, although it is not recommended because research has not concluded that this is safe or reliable (Liston et al., 2007).

Interpretation

Generally accepted criteria for a normal NST tracing for a fetus greater than 32 weeks' gestation are as follows (Fig. 12-10 and Table 12-2):

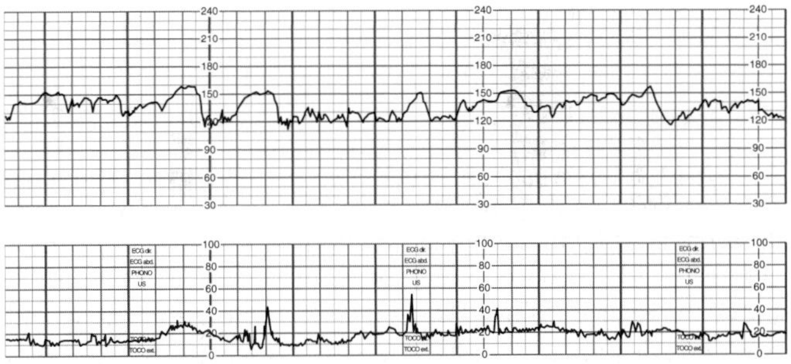

Fig. 12-10 Normal nonstress test. Fetal heart rate accelerations with fetal movement. *(From Tucker, S. M. [2004].* Pocket guide to fetal monitoring and assessment *[5th ed.]. St. Louis: Mosby.)*

- Two or more accelerations of 15 beats/minute (bpm) lasting for 15 seconds over a 20-minute period
- Normal baseline rate (110–160 bpm)
- Moderate variability (6–25 bpm)

An abnormal tracing persistently lacks accelerations after 80 minutes or contains significant abnormality of baseline heart rate or variability or shows evidence of significant deceleration (Fig. 12-11 and see Table 12-2). In this case, further assessments are needed with ultrasonography or BPP. In most cases, a normal NST is predictive of a good perinatal outcome for 1 week as long as there are no changes to the clinical picture, except in women with insulin-dependent diabetes or

Table 12-2 Antepartum Classification: Nonstress Test

PARAMETER	NORMAL NST	ATYPICAL NST	ABNORMAL NST
Baseline	• 110–160 bpm	• 110–160 bpm • >160 bpm <30 min • Rising baseline	• Bradycardia <100 bpm • Tachycardia >160 for >30 min • Erratic baseline
Variability	• 6–25 bpm (moderate) (see Fig 12-10) • ≦5 bpm (absent or minimal) for <40 min.	• ≦ (absent or minimal) for 40–80 min (see Fig. 12-11)	• ≦5 for ≧80 min • ≧25 bpm >10 min • Sinusoidal
Decelerations	• None or occasional variable <30 sec	• Variable decelerations 30–60 sec duration	• Variable decelerations >60 sec duration • Late decelerations
Accelerations term fetus	• ≧2 accelerations with acme of ≧15 bpm, lasting 15 sec <40 min of testing	• ≦2 accelerations with acme of ≧15 bpm, lasting 15 sec in 40–80 min	• ≦2 accelerations with acme of ≧15 bpm, lasting 15 sec in >80 min
Preterm fetus (<32 weeks)	• ≧2 accelerations with acme of ≧10 bpm, lasting 10 sec <40 min of testing	• ≦2 accelerations with acme of ≧10 bpm, lasting 10 sec in 40–80 min	• ≦2 accelerations with acme of ≧10 bpm, lasting 10 sec in >80 min
Action	Further assessment optional, based on total clinical picture	Further assessment required	URGENT ACTION REQUIRED An overall assessment of the situation and further investigation with ultrasonography or BPP is required. Some situations will require delivery.

(Source: Liston, R., et al. [2007]. SOGC clinical practice guideline: Fetal health surveillance: Antepartum and intrapartum consensus guideline. *Journal of Obstetrics and Gynaecology Canada, 29*[9], Suppl 4. Retrieved from http://www.sogc.org/guidelines/documents/gui197CPG0709r.pdf.)
bpm, beats per minute; *BPP*, biophysical profile; *NST*, nonstress test.

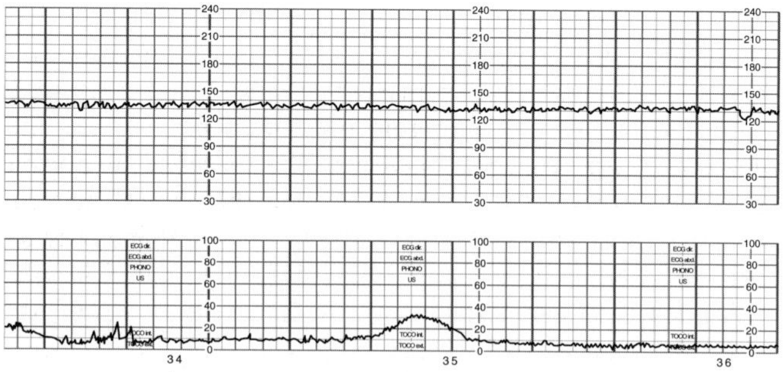

Fig. 12-11 Atypical or abnormal nonstress test (no fetal heart rate accelerations). *(From Tucker, S. M. [2004].* Pocket guide to fetal monitoring and assessment *[5th ed.]. St. Louis: Mosby.)*

postdates pregnancy. In these women, NSTs should be done twice weekly (Liston et al., 2007).

Contraction Stress Test

The **contraction stress test** (CST) was one of the first electronic methods to be developed for assessment of fetal well-being. Its purpose is to evaluate the response of the fetus to induced contractions and to thus identify poor placental function (Liston et al., 2007). Uterine contractions decrease uterine blood flow and placental perfusion. If this decrease is sufficient to produce hypoxia in the fetus, a deceleration in FHR results, beginning at the peak of the contraction and persisting after its conclusion (late deceleration). CSTs are used much less frequently now, as uteroplacental function can be assessed using BPP or vascular flow measurements.

NURSING ALERT In a healthy fetoplacental unit, uterine contractions usually do not produce late decelerations; when there is underlying uteroplacental insufficiency, contractions produce late decelerations.

Procedure

The woman is placed in a semi-Fowler position or sits in a reclining chair with a slight lateral tilt, to optimize uterine perfusion and avoid supine hypotension. She is monitored electronically with the fetal ultrasound transducer and uterine tocodynamometer. The tracing is observed for 10 to 20 minutes for baseline rate, variability, and the possible occurrence of spontaneous contractions. CST should not be done in the following situations: ruptured membranes, previous classic incision for Caesarean birth, preterm labour, placenta previa, and abruptio placentae. Multifetal pregnancy, previous preterm labour, hydramnios, more than 36 weeks of gestation, and incompetent cervix are relative contraindications for the CST.

The goal of a CST is to induce three contractions, each lasting 1 minute within a 10-minute period so that the fetal heart response to the contractions can be evaluated (Liston et al., 2007). The CST can be done using maternal nipple stimulation or with an oxytocin infusion. Negative results for a CST are associated with favourable results.

Nipple-Stimulated Contraction Test. Massaging the nipples causes a release of oxytocin from the posterior pituitary. The woman is instructed to stimulate one nipple through her clothing with the palmar surface of the fingers rapidly, but gently for 2 minutes, rest for 5 minutes, and repeat the cycles of massage and rest as necessary to achieve adequate uterine activity. Bilateral nipple stimulation may be considered when unable to achieve contractions while stimulating only one nipple. When adequate contractions or hyperstimulation occurs, stimulation should be stopped (Liston et al., 2007). Nipple stimulation has a shorter testing time than oxytocin infusion, although if nipple stimulation does not work, then oxytocin infusion should be considered.

Oxytocin-Stimulated Contraction Test. Exogenous oxytocin can also be used to stimulate uterine contractions. An intravenous (IV) infusion is started and an oxytocin infusion initiated through a piggyback port into the tubing of the main IV device. An infusion pump is used to ensure accurate dosage. The oxytocin infusion usually is begun at 0.5 to 1.0 mU/minute and increased by 1.0 mU/minute at 15- to 30-minute intervals until three uterine contractions of good quality are observed within a 10-minute period. Hyperstimulation is a risk, so slowly increasing the rate of oxytocin is recommended.

Interpretation

If a normal baseline fetal heart rate tracing and no late decelerations are observed with the contractions, the findings are considered to be negative (Fig. 12-12). A CST is positive if late decelerations occur with more than 50% of the induced contractions (Fig. 12-13 and Table 12-3).

After interpretation of the FHR pattern, the oxytocin infusion is discontinued, and the maintenance IV solution is infused until the uterine activity has returned to the prestimulation level. If the CST is negative, the IV device is removed, and the fetal monitor is disconnected. If the CST is positive, continued monitoring and further evaluation of fetal well-being are indicated. While the use of CSTs has decreased because it has been replaced by other technologies, one indication for the use of CST is to determine if a fetus that has other abnormal testing results could tolerate a vaginal birth instead of being delivered by Caeserean section. A fetus demonstrating an atypical or abnormal NST and a positive CST is less likely to tolerate labour (Liston et al., 2007).

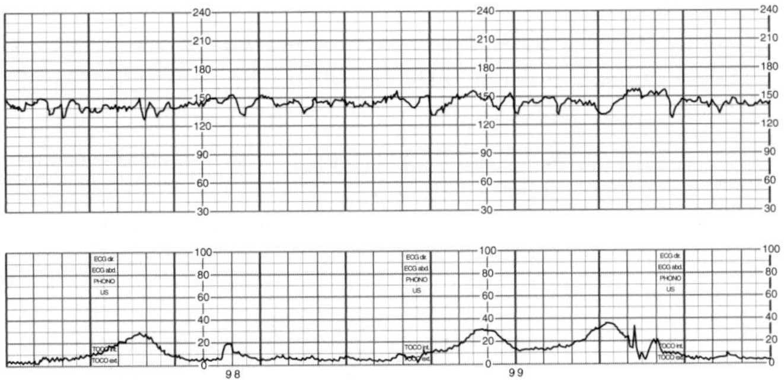

Fig. 12-12 Negative contraction stress test (normal external fetal heart rate tracing). *(From Tucker, S. M. [2004].* Pocket guide to fetal monitoring and assessment *[5th ed.]. St. Louis: Mosby.)*

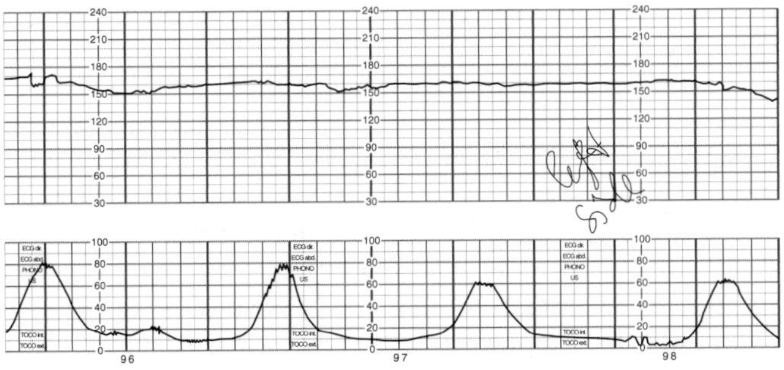

Fig. 12-13 Positive contraction stress test (abnormal late decelerations with uterine contractions). *(From Tucker, S. M. [2004].* Pocket guide to fetal monitoring and assessment *[5th ed.]. St. Louis: Mosby.)*

Ultrasound for Fetal Well-Being

Physiological parameters of the fetus that can be assessed with ultrasound scanning include amniotic fluid volume (AFV), vascular waveforms from the fetal circulation, heart motion, fetal breathing movements, fetal urine production, and fetal limb and head movements. Assessment of these parameters, singly or in combination, yields a fairly reliable picture of fetal well-being. The significance of these findings is discussed in the following sections.

Biophysical Profile (BPP)

Real-time ultrasound imaging permits detailed assessment of the physical and physiological characteristics of the developing fetus to such an extent that it is possible to examine the fetus in detail and to catalog normal and abnormal biophysical responses to stimuli. The BPP is a noninvasive dynamic assessment of a fetus that is based on the assessment of acute and chronic markers of fetal disease. The BPP assesses current fetal well-being by observing fetal breathing movements, fetal movements, fetal tone, and AFV.

The BPP may be considered a physical examination of the fetus, including determination of vital signs. The fetus responds to central hypoxia by alteration in movement, muscle tone, breathing, and heart rate patterns. The presence of normal fetal biophysical activities indicates that the central nervous system is functional; therefore, the fetus is not hypoxemic. BPP variables and scoring are detailed in Table 12-4. The BPP is done with or without an NST. If done with the NST, the score is out of 10, and if done without the NST, the score is out of 8.

The BPP is an evaluation of current fetal well-being (Liston et al., 2007). Fetal acidosis can be diagnosed early with an abnormal NST and absent fetal breathing movements. A BPP score of less than 6, or a score of 6 along with **oligohydramnios,** indicates that labour should be induced (see Table 12-4). The BPP identifies a pocket of amniotic fluid of less than 2 cm by 2 cm as oligiohydramnios. Fetal infection in women whose membranes rupture prematurely (at less than 37 weeks of gestation) can be diagnosed early by changes in biophysical activities that precede the clinical signs of infection and indicate the necessity for immediate birth. When the BPP score is normal and the risk of fetal death low, intervention is indicated only for obstetrical or maternal factors.

Amniotic Fluid Volume

Abnormalities in AFV are frequently associated with fetal disorders. Subjective determinants of oligohydramnios (decreased fluid) include the absence of fluid pockets in the uterine cavity and the impression of crowding of fetal small parts (arms and legs). This approach identifies a pocket depth of 2 to 8 cm as normal, 1 to 2 cm as marginal, and less than 1 cm as decreased. In the case of polyhydramnios (increased fluid), the criteria include multiple large pockets of fluid, the impression of a floating fetus, and free movement of fetal

Table 12-3 Interpretation of the Contraction Stress Test

INTERPRETATION	CLINICAL SIGNIFICANCE
Negative	
No late decelerations, with minimum of three uterine contractions within 10-min period (see Fig. 12-12)	Reassurance that the fetus is likely to survive labour should it occur within 1 wk; more frequent testing may be indicated by clinical situation
Positive	
Late decelerations occurring with at least half of contractions (see Fig. 12-13)	Management lies between use of other tools of fetal assessment, such as BPP, and termination of pregnancy; positive test result indicates that fetus is at increased risk for perinatal morbidity and mortality; physician may perform expeditious vaginal birth after successful induction or may proceed directly to Caesarean birth; decision to intervene determined by fetal monitoring and presence of FHR reactivity
Suspicious or Equivocal	
Prolonged, variable, or late decelerations occurring with less than 50% of the contractions	NST and CST should be repeated within 24 hr; if interpretable data cannot be achieved, other methods of fetal assessment must be used*
Equivocal–Hyperstimulatory	
Decelerations that are repetitive but not late in timing or pattern	Repeat test next day
Unsatisfactory	
Inadequate uterine contraction pattern or tracing too poor to interpret	Repeat test next day

(Source: Tucker, S. M., Miller, L. A., & Miller, D. A. [2009]. *Mosby's pocket guide to fetal monitoring; A multidisciplinary approach* [6th ed.]. St. Louis: Mosby.)
*Applies to results noted as suspicious, hyperstimulation, or unsatisfactory.
BPP, biophysical profile; *CST,* contraction stress test; *FHR,* fetal heart rate; *NST,* nonstress test.

Table 12-4 Biophysical Profile

VARIABLES	NORMAL (SCORE = 2)	ABNORMAL (SCORE = 0)
Fetal breathing movements	One or more episodes in 30 min, each lasting ≥30 sec	Episodes absent or no episode ≥30 sec in 30 min
Fetal movements	At least three trunk or limb movements in 30 min	Fewer than three episodes of body or limb movements in 30 min
Fetal tone	At least one episode of active extension with return to flexion of fetal limb or trunk; opening and closing of hand is considered normal tone	Absence of movement or slow extension/flexion
Amniotic fluid index	At least one cord and limb-free fluid pocket that is 2 cm by 2 cm in two measurements at right angles	No single pocket of fluid that is 2 cm by 2 cm
Nonstress test	May or may not be done	
Score		
Normal	8–10 (if amniotic fluid index is adequate)	
Equivocal test	6 (normal fluid)	Repeat testing within 24 hr
	6 (abnormal fluid)	Probable fetal asphyxia. Delivery of term fetus. In fetus <34 weeks, intensive surveillance may be used
Abnormal	<6	Associated with high probability of fetal asphyxia. Deliver for fetal indications

(Source: Liston, R., et al. [2007]. SOGC clinical practice guideline: Fetal health surveillance: Antepartum and intrapartum consensus guideline. *Journal of Obstetrics and Gynaecology Canada, 29*[9], Suppl 4. Retrieved from http://www.sogc.org/guidelines/documents/gui197CPG0709r.pdf.)

limbs (Harman, 2009, Liston et al., 2007). The diagnosis of polyhydramnios may be made when the largest pocket of fluid exceeds 8 cm in one vertical pocket.

The total AFV can be evaluated through a method in which the depths (in centimetres) of amniotic fluid in all four quadrants surrounding the maternal umbilicus are totalled, resulting in an amniotic fluid index (AFI). An AFI of less than 5 cm indicates oligohydramnios; 5 to 19 cm is considered a normal measurement; and a measurement greater than 20 cm reflects polyhydramnios (Gilbert, 2007). There is evidence that the use of AFI, rather than pocket size, increases intervention without improving outcomes (Liston et al., 2007).

Oligohydramnios is associated with rupture of the membranes and congenital anomalies (such as renal agenesis), IUGR, and fetal distress in labour. Polyhydramnios is associated with neural tube defects, obstruction of the fetal gastrointestinal tract, multiple fetuses, and fetal hydrops.

Doppler Blood Flow Analysis

One of the major advances in perinatal medicine is the ability to study blood flow noninvasively in the fetus and placenta with ultrasonography. Doppler blood flow analysis is a useful adjunct in the management of pregnancies at risk due to hypertension, IUGR, diabetes mellitus, multiple fetuses, or preterm labour.

When a sound wave is reflected from a moving target, there is a change in frequency of the reflected wave relative to the transmitted wave. This is called the *Doppler effect*. An ultrasound beam scattered by a group of RBCs is an example of this effect. The velocity of the RBCs can be determined by measuring the change in the frequency in the sound wave reflected off the cells.

The shifted frequencies can be displayed as a plot of velocity versus time, and the shape of these waveforms can be analyzed to give information about blood flow and resistance in a given circulation. Velocity waveforms from umbilical and uterine arteries, reported in systolic/diastolic (S/D) ratios, can be first detected at 15 weeks of pregnancy. Because of progressive decline in resistance in both the umbilical and the uterine arteries, this ratio decreases as pregnancy advances. Most fetuses achieve an S/D ratio of 3 or less by 30 weeks (Fig. 12-14). Persistent elevation of S/D ratios after 30 weeks is associated with IUGR, usually resulting from uteroplacental insufficiency. In postterm pregnancies evaluated by Doppler umbilical flow studies, an elevated S/D ratio indicates a poorly perfused placenta. Abnormal velocity study results are also seen with certain chromosome abnormalities (trisomy 13 and 18) and with lupus erythematosus in the mother. Exposure to nicotine from maternal smoking also increases the S/D ratio.

Nursing Role in Antenatal Assessment for Risk

The nurse's role is that of educator and support person when the woman is undergoing examinations such as ultrasonography, magnetic resonance imaging (MRI), CVS, PUBS, and amniocentesis. In some instances the nurse may assist the physician with the procedure. In many settings, nurses perform NSTs, CSTs, and BPPs; conduct an initial assessment; and begin necessary interventions for abnormal patterns. These nursing procedures are accomplished after additional education and training, under guidance of established protocols, and in collaboration with physicians. Patient teaching, which is an integral component of this role, involves preparing the woman for the procedure, interpreting the findings, and providing psychosocial support when needed.

Psychological Considerations

All women who undergo antenatal assessments are at risk for real and potential problems and may be anxious. In most instances, the tests are ordered because of suspected fetal compromise, deterioration of a maternal condition, or both. In the third trimester, pregnant women are most concerned about protecting themselves and their fetuses and consider themselves most vulnerable to outside influences. The label of "high risk" increases this sense of vulnerability.

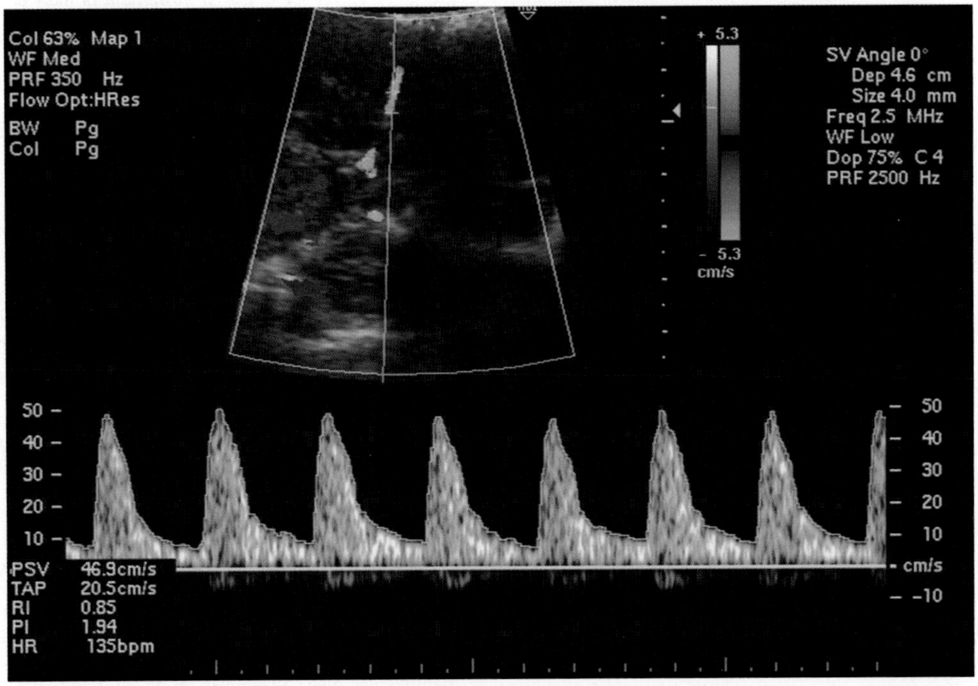

Fig. 12-14 Umbilical artery velocity waveform. *(From Callen, P. [2000].* Ultrasonography in obstetrics and gynecology *[4th ed.]. Philadelphia: Saunders.)*

COMMUNITY FOCUS

Support for At-Risk Pregnant Women

At-risk pregnant women experience many stressors. Social support can relieve some of the stress, including that during labour. Nurses, social workers, and midwives—as well as trained lay persons—have all provided labour support. Investigate in your setting whether such support is available for low-income women. Is there a doula program at the hospital where you did your maternity clinical rotation or in your city? Does the program provide this service on a sliding scale for low-income women? What is the background of the doulas in your setting or city? Where do the doulas receive training? Interview a woman who has used a doula. What were the positive and negative factors associated with having a doula during labour? Discuss your findings in a clinical conference.

When a woman is diagnosed with a high-risk pregnancy, she and her family may experience stress related to the diagnosis. The woman may exhibit various psychological responses, including anxiety, low self-esteem, guilt, frustration, and inability to function. The development of a high-risk pregnancy also can affect parental attachment, accomplishment of the tasks of pregnancy, and family adaptation to the pregnancy.

If the woman is fearful for her own well-being, she may continue to feel ambivalence about the pregnancy or not accept the reality of the pregnancy. She may not be able to complete preparations for the baby or go to childbirth classes if she is on bed rest or hospitalized. The family may become frustrated because they cannot engage in these activities that prepare them for parenthood. Nurses should assist women to pursue alternative modes of education if they are unable to attend regular childbirth classes.

Antepartum hospitalization is an added stressor for the high-risk pregnant woman and her family. The woman may be lonely because she is separated from her home and family. She may feel powerless and unable to make decisions for herself because her care is out of her control. Likewise, preparation for the birth process may be out of control of the woman and her family. Unexpected procedures and care for the woman or fetus may take priority over the usual birth plan and may not allow choices that would have been selected if the pregnancy had been normal.

The nurse can help the woman and her family regain control and balance in their lives by providing support and encouragement, information about the pregnancy problem and its management, and opportunities to make as many choices as possible about the woman's care (see Community Focus box).

Key Points

- A high-risk pregnancy is one in which the life or well-being of the mother or infant is jeopardized by a biophysical or psychosocial disorder coincident with or unique to pregnancy.
- The pregnancy, fetus, or neonate can be placed at risk through the influence of many of the determinants of health.
- Psychosocial perinatal warning indicators include characteristics of the parents, the fetus, the neonate, their support systems, and family circumstances.
- Intimate partner violence has a negative impact on pregnancy outcomes.
- There are ethnic disparities in maternal and perinatal mortality rates in Canada.
- The mortality rate decreases when risks are identified early and intensive care is applied.
- In the first and second trimester, antepartum testing is done to screen for fetal abnormalities, assess for gestational age, ensure appropriate growth, and assess placenta position.
- Biophysical assessment techniques include fetal movement counts and ultrasonography.
- Biochemical monitoring techniques include amniocentesis, PUBS, and CVS.
- Normal NSTs and negative CSTs suggest fetal well-being.
- Assessment tests may have some degree of risk for the mother and fetus and usually cause some anxiety for the woman and her family.

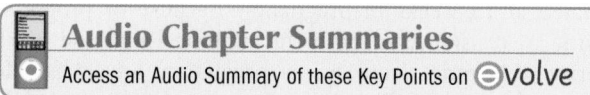

Audio Chapter Summaries

Access an Audio Summary of these Key Points on Evolve

References

Alfirevic, Z., Sunberg, S., & Brigham, S. (2004). Amniocentesis and chorionic villi sampling for prenatal diagnosis (Cochrane Review). In *The Cochrane Library, Issue 2*. Chichester, UK: John Wiley & Sons.

BC Reproductive Care Program. (2003). *Reproductive mental health guideline 1: Reproductive mental illness during the perinatal period—Principles and framework*. Vancouver, BC: Author. Retrieved from http://www.perinatalservicesbc.ca//sites/bcrcp/files/Guidelines/Rmhg/Guideline1PrinciplesJan2003.pdf.

Benn, P., et al. (2004). Changes in utilization of prenatal diagnosis. *Obstetrics and Gynecology, 103*(6), 1255–1260.

Bowen, A., & Muhajarine, N. (2006). Antenatal depression. *Canadian Nurse, 102*(9), 27–30.

Canadian Institute of Health. (2003). *Women's health surveillance report*. Ottawa: Author. Retrieved from http://secure.cihi.ca/cihiweb/products/CPHI_WomensHealth_e.pdf.

Cargill, Y., et al. (2009). SOGC clinical practice guideline: Content of a complete routine second trimester obstetrical ultrasound examination and report. *Journal of Obstetrics and Gynaecology Canada, 31*(3), 272–275. Retrieved from http://sogc.org/guidelines/documents/gui223CPG0903.pdf.

Enkin, M., et al. (2000). *A guide to effective care in pregnancy and childbirth* (3rd ed.). New York: Oxford University Press.

Gilbert, W. M. (2007). Amniotic fluid disorders. In S. G. Gabbe, J. R. Niebyl, & J. L. Simpson (Eds.), *Obstetrics: Normal and problem pregnancies* (5th ed.). Philadelphia: Churchill Livingstone.

Harman, C. R. (2009). Assessment of fetal health. In R. K. Creasy, et al. (Eds.), *Creasy & Resnik's maternal–fetal medicine: Principles and practice* (6th ed.). Philadelphia: Saunders.

Liston, R., et al. (2007). SOGC clinical practice guideline: Fetal health surveillance: Antepartum and intrapartum consensus guideline. *Journal of Obstetrics and Gynaecology Canada, 29*(9), Suppl 4. Retrieved from http://www.sogc.org/guidelines/documents/gui197CPG0709r.pdf.

Manning, F. (2009). Imaging in the diagnosis of fetal anomalies. In R. K. Creasy, et al. (Eds.), *Creasy & Resnik's maternal–fetal medicine: Principles and practice* (6th ed.). Philadelphia: Saunders.

Nageotte, M. P., & Gilstrap, L. C. (2009). Intrapartum fetal surveillance. In R. K. Creasy, et al. (Eds.), *Creasy & Resnik's maternal–fetal medicine: Principles and practice* (6th ed.). Philadelphia: Saunders.

Public Health Agency of Canada. (2008a). *Canadian perinatal report—2008 edition* (Cat. No. HP10-12/2008E-PDF). Ottawa: Government of Canada. Retrieved from http://www.phac-aspc.gc.ca/publicat/2008/cphr-rspc/behaviours-comportements-eng.php.

Public Health Agency of Canada. (2008b). *Healthy settings for young people in Canada*. Retrieved from http://www.phac-aspc.gc.ca/media/nr-rp/2008/2008_05bck-eng.php.

Public Health Agency of Canada. (2011). *Maternal mortality in Canada* (Cat. No. HP10-19/2011E-PDF). Ottawa: Government of Canada. Retrieved from http://www.phac-aspc.gc.ca/rhs-ssg/maternal-maternelle/mortality-mortalite/pdf/mortal-eng.pdf.

Resnik, J. L., & Resnik, R. (2009). Post-term pregnancy. In R. K. Creasy, et al. (Eds.), *Creasy & Resnik's maternal–fetal medicine: Principles and practice* (6th ed.). Philadelphia: Saunders.

Richards, D. S. (2007). Ultrasound for pregnancy dating, growth and diagnosis of fetal malformations. In S. G. Gabbe, J. R. Niebyl, & J. L. Simpson (Eds.), *Obstetrics: Normal and problem pregnancies* (5th ed.). Philadelphia: Churchill Livingstone.

Society of Obstetricians and Gynaecologists of Canada. (2007). Clinical Practice Guideline: Screening for fetal aneuploidy. *Journal of Obstetricians and Gynaecologists of Canada, 29*(2), 146–161. Retrieved from http://sogc.org/guidelines/documents/187E-CPG-February2007.pdf.

Strass, P., & Billay, E. (2008). A public health nursing initiative to promote antenatal health. *Canadian Nurse, 104*(2), 29–33.

Tucker, S. M., Miller, L. A., & Miller, D. A. (2009). *Mosby's pocket guide to fetal monitoring: A multidisciplinary approach* (6th ed.). St. Louis: Mosby.

Van den Hof, M. C., et al. (2007). Non-medical use of fetal ultrasound. *Journal of Obstetricians and Gynaecologists of Canada, 29*(4), 364–365. Retrieved from http://www.sogc.org/guidelines/documents/191E-PS-April2007.pdf.

Wapner, R. J., Jenkins, T. M., & Khalek, N. (2009). Prenatal diagnosis of congenital disorders. In R. K. Creasy, et al. (Eds.), *Creasy & Resnik's maternal–fetal medicine: Principles and practice* (6th ed.). Philadelphia: Saunders.

Wilson, R. D., et al. (2005). SOGC clinical practice guideline: Amended Canadian guideline for prenatal diagnosis (2005): Techniques for prenatal diagnosis. *Journal of Obstetrics and Gynaecology Canada, 27*(11), 1048–1054. Retrieved from http://www.sogc.org/guidelines/public/168E-CPG-November2005.pdf.

Additional Resources

Canadian Association of Genetic Counsellors: https://cagc-accg.ca/

Perinatal Services BC: http://www.perinatalservicesbc.ca/

Unit 3

13 Pregnancy at Risk: Gestational Conditions

Learning Objectives

On completion of this chapter, the reader will be able to:

- Differentiate between gestational hypertension and pre-existing hypertension.
- Describe the etiological theories and pathophysiology of pre-eclampsia.
- Compare care management of women with mild pre-eclampsia with care management of women with severe pre-eclampsia.
- Describe HELLP syndrome, including appropriate nursing actions.
- Understand the screening and care of a woman with gestational diabetes mellitus.
- Explain the effects of hyperemesis gravidarum on maternal and fetal well-being.
- Differentiate among causes, signs and symptoms, possible complications, and management of miscarriage, ectopic pregnancy, cervical insufficiency, and hydatidiform mole.
- Compare and contrast placenta previa and abruptio placentae in regard to signs and symptoms, complications, and management.
- Discuss the diagnosis and management of disseminated intravascular coagulation.
- Explain the basic principles of care for a pregnant woman undergoing abdominal surgery.
- Discuss implications of trauma on mother and fetus during pregnancy.
- Identify priorities in assessment and stabilization measures for the pregnant trauma victim.

Electronic Resources

Additional information related to the content in Chapter 13 can be found on

evolve the companion Web site at

http://evolve.elsevier.com/Canada/Perry/maternal/

- Examination Review Questions
- Case Study—Pre-eclampsia
- Critical Thinking Exercise—Pre-eclampsia
- Critical Thinking Exercise—Gestational Diabetes

Providing safe and effective care for a pregnant woman with high-risk conditions requires a multidisciplinary team working alongside the woman and her family. Each team member contributes unique knowledge and skills toward providing optimum outcomes for the mother and infant. This chapter discusses a wide range of disorders that can develop during pregnancy and place the woman and fetus at risk. Hypertension in pregnancy, gestational diabetes mellitus (GDM), hyperemesis gravidarum, hemorrhagic complications of early and late pregnancy, surgery during pregnancy, and trauma are discussed.

Hypertension in Pregnancy

Significance and Incidence

Hypertension is the most common medical problem encountered during pregnancy and will become more prevalent with the increase in obesity and older maternal age (Society of Obstetricians and Gynaecologists of Canada [SOGC], 2008). Approximately 1% of pregnancies are complicated by pre-existing hypertension, 5 to 6% of pregnancies are complicated by gestational hypertension without proteinuria, and a further 1 to 2% by pre-eclampsia (Allen, 2002; SOGC, 2008). Women at extremes of age—those who are younger than age 20 and older than age 40—have the highest rates of pregnancy-related hypertension. Rates of pre-existing hypertension in mothers ages 40 and older are eight times higher than for those under age 20 (29.2 compared to 3.7 per 1000 live births).

Morbidity and Mortality

Complications from significant hypertension are the leading cause of maternal morbidity and mortality and include renal and liver failure, HELLP syndrome (discussed later in this chapter), and cerebral edema with seizures (Mutter & Karumanchi, 2008). Maternal deaths associated with severe hypertension result primarily from complications of hepatic rupture, abruptio placentae, and eclampsia (characterized by seizures) (Roberts & Funai, 2009). Neonates of mothers with nonsevere gestational hypertension have lower morbidity and better neurodevelopmental outcomes than do neonates of mothers who were not hypertensive. However, the fetus of the eclamptic woman is at increased risk from abruptio placentae, preterm birth, intrauterine growth restriction (IUGR), and acute hypoxia. It is debated whether clinical care goals should focus on the prevention of pre-eclampsia rather than on the prevention of complications from severe pre-eclampsia. Therefore, to guide Canadian clinicians, the Society of Obstetricians and Gynaecologists of Canada (SOGC) (2008) has provided recommendations regarding both the prevention of pre-eclampsia and the prevention of its associated complications.

Definition of Hypertensive Disorder of Pregnancy (HDP)

Hypertension in pregnancy is defined as diastolic BP (dBP) of 90 mm Hg, as this level is associated with higher adverse perinatal outcomes. Women with a systolic BP (sBP) of 140 mm Hg should be followed closely and assessed for the development of diastolic hypertension. Previously, sBP was excluded from the definition of hypertension in pregnancy; however, even an intermittently elevated sBP is a risk marker for later development of gestational hypertension and thus should be followed closely with further investigation as appropriate. Findings of a high dBP must be repeatedly assessed to rule out "white coat" nervous hypertension and should be monitored over hours, days, or weeks to make a diagnosis of HDP. *Severe hypertension* is defined as a dBP of 110 mm Hg and a sBP of 160 mm Hg. This level of BP is associated with an increased risk of stroke in pregnancy (SOGC, 2008).

Classification

The classification system most commonly used in Canada is based on reports from the SOGC (2008) and the Canadian Hypertension Society (Moutquin et al., 1997). Hypertensive disorders of pregnancy should be classified as pre-existing or gestational hypertension.

Pre-existing hypertension is present before pregnancy or appears before 20 weeks of gestation. Gestational hypertension is the development of hypertension at or after 20 weeks. For both pre-existing and gestational hypertension, there are two subgroups: (1) with comorbid conditions and (2) with pre-eclampsia. The presence of three criteria is required to confirm this diagnosis: hypertension, **proteinuria**, and adverse conditions (SOGC, 2008) (Table 13-1). Edema and weight gain are no longer considered markers of pre-eclampsia, as neither is significantly associated with perinatal mortality and morbidity. The discussion here will focus mainly on gestational hypertension.

Pre-Existing Hypertension

Pre-existing hypertension is defined as hypertension present before the pregnancy or diagnosed before 20 weeks of gestation (Roberts & Funai, 2009; SOGC, 2008). Most women with pre-existing hypertension experience uncomplicated pregnancies; however, there is an increased risk of poor fetal growth and fetal demise. Preconception counselling is recommended for these women (American College of Obstetricians and Gynecologists [ACOG], 2002; SOGC, 2008).

Pre-Existing Hypertension With Superimposed Pre-Eclampsia

Approximately 25% of women with pre-existing hypertension develop pre-eclampsia or eclampsia. This disorder is associated with severe maternal and fetal complications. Pre-existing hypertension with superimposed pre-eclampsia is defined in the presence of the following findings:

- Hypertension before 20 weeks of gestation, with new-onset proteinuria
- Both hypertension and proteinuria before 20 weeks of gestation
- Sudden increase in proteinuria
- A sudden increase in BP in a woman whose hypertension was previously well controlled
- Thrombocytopenia
- Elevated liver enzymes

Table 13-1 Classification of Hypertensive Disorders of Pregnancy

PRIMARY DIAGNOSIS	DESCRIPTION/DEFINITION OF PRE-ECLAMPSIA
Pre-existing hypertension	Predates the pregnancy or appears before 20 weeks
A) with comorbid conditions	Resistant hypertension, or new or worsening proteinuria, or more adverse condition(s)
B) with pre-eclampsia (after 20 weeks' gestation)	
Gestational hypertension	Hypertension that appears after 20 weeks gestation
A) with comorbid conditions	Includes major cardiovascular risk factors, such as type I or II (but not gestational) diabetes, renal parenchymal or vascular disease, or cerebrovascular disease
B) with pre-eclampsia (after 20 weeks' gestation)	New proteinuria, or one or more adverse condition(s)

(Adapted from Society of Obstetricians and Gynaecologists of Canada. [2008]. SOGC clinical practice guideline: Diagnosis, evaluation and management of hypertensive disorders of pregnancy. *Journal of Obstetrics and Gynaecology Canada, 30*[3], Suppl 1, S1-S48. Retrieved from http://www.sogc.org/guidelines/documents/gui206CPG0803_001.pdf.)

The Link Between Hypertension and the Development of Pre-Eclampsia

Women with pre-existing hypertension have a 10 to 20% risk of developing pre-eclampsia. Women with pre-existing comorbidities, such as renal disease or type 1 diabetes, are also at increased risk. Women who develop hypertension prior to 34 weeks are also at increased risk of developing pre-eclampsia. Certain risk factors are associated with development of the condition, such as nulliparity, family history of pre-eclampsia, multiple gestation, obesity, and chronic medical disorders (Sibai, 2007). Some studies have shown an increased risk for pre-eclampsia in multiparous women with new partners for subsequent pregnancies (Sibai, 2007). There appears to be a paternal factor involved (i.e., men who fathered one pregnancy complicated by pre-eclampsia were nearly twice as likely to father a pre-eclamptic pregnancy in a different woman) (Sibai, 2007). Maternal markers for pre-eclampsia that indicate the need for vigilant maternal and fetal surveillance are listed in Table 13-2.

Pre-Eclampsia

Once the diagnosis of HDP has been made, women must be closely monitored for the development of pre-eclampsia, which often develops after the second **trimester** of pregnancy. *Pre-eclampsia* is a hypertensive disorder most commonly defined by new-onset proteinuria and, potentially, other end-organ dysfunction and may result in intrauterine fetal morbidity and mortality due to uteroplacental insufficiency and abruptio placentae. It is a multisystem, vasospastic disease process of reduced organ perfusion characterized by the presence of hypertension and proteinuria, with a clinical continuum from mild to severe (Table 13-3). It affects a myriad of maternal and fetal systems and if not controlled, results in poor perinatal outcomes.

The two key components to the diagnosis of mild pre-eclampsia are hypertension and new-onset proteinuria. Maternal symptoms that indicate a worsening or severe pre-eclampsia include visual disturbances, persistent headache, epigastric or right upper quadrant pain, and dyspnea. The presence of any of these symptoms alone does not indicate pre-eclampsia.

Fetal manifestations, which may occur independently or in conjunction with maternal symptoms, include oligohydramnios; IUGR; abnormal umbilical artery Doppler results indicating decreased blood flow to the fetus from a poorly functioning placenta; and stillbirth (SOGC, 2008).

Proteinuria

Proteinuria is defined as a concentration of 0.03 g/L or more in at least two random urine specimens collected at least 6 hours apart that have no evidence of urinary tract infection. In a 24-hour specimen, proteinuria is defined as a concentration of greater than 0.3 g/L per 24 hours (Box 13-1). The diagnosis of proteinuria should be based on the use of the urinary protein : creatinine ratio or 24-hour urine collection (Roberts & Funai, 2009; SOGC, 2008).

Pre-eclampsia contributes significantly to restrictions of fetal growth and the incidence of placental abruption. Impaired placental perfusion leads to early degenerative aging of the placenta. The rate of fetal complications is directly related to the severity of the disease (Sibai, 2007; SOGC, 2008).

Mild Pre-Eclampsia

Mild pre-eclampsia is defined as a combination of hypertension (sBP below 160 mm Hg and dBP below 110 mm Hg) and proteinuria, with no evidence of organ dysfunction (Roberts & Funai, 2009; Sibai, 2007). When there is an ongoing

Table 13-2 Risk Markers for Pre-Eclampsia

	First-Trimester Markers		*Second- or Third- Trimester Markers*
DEMOGRAPHICS	**PAST HISTORY**	**CURRENT PREGNANCY**	
	Previous pre-eclampsia Antiphospholipid antibodies Pre-existing medical condition(s) – pre-existing hypertension or initial diastolic BP ≥90 mm Hg – pre-existing renal disease – pre-existing diabetes mellitus	Multiple pregnancy	
Maternal age ≥40 years	Obesity (BMI ≥35 kg/m^2 Family history of pre-eclampsia	First ongoing pregnancy Interpregnancy interval ≥10 years Initial sBP ≥130 mm Hg or dBP ≥80 mm Hg needs to be at same level as Obesity	
Ethnicity: Nordic, Black, South Asian or Pacific Islander Lower socioeconomic status	Nonsmoking Thrombophilias (factor V Leiden/ protein S deficiency ↑ Pre-pregnancy triglycerides Family history of early-onset CV disease Cocaine and methamphetamine use	Interpregnancy interval <2 years Reproductive technologies New partner Gestational trophoblastic disease Excessive weight gain Infection during pregnancy	Elevated BP Abnormal maternal serum screening Abnormal uterine artery Doppler velocimetry Cardiac output >7.4 L/min Elevated uric acid Other laboratory markers

(Adapted from the Society of Obstetricians and Gynaecologists of Canada. [2008]. SOGC clinical practice guideline: Diagnosis, evaluation and management of hypertensive disorders of pregnancy. *Journal of Obstetrics and Gynaecology Canada, 30*[3], Suppl 1, S1-S48 [p. 19]. Retrieved from http://www.sogc.org/guidelines/documents/gui206CPG0803_001.pdf.)
BMI, body mass index; *BP*, blood pressure; *CV*, cardiovascular disease; *dBP*, diastolic blood pressure; *sBP*, systolic blood pressure.

Table 13-3 Differentiation Between Mild and Severe Pre-Eclampsia

	MILD PRE-ECLAMPSIA	SEVERE PRE-ECLAMPSIA
Maternal Effects		
Blood pressure (BP)	BP reading of ≥140/90 mm Hg × 2, >4-6 hr apart, no more than 1 wk apart	Rise to ≥160/110 mm Hg on two separate occasions
Mean arterial pressure	>105 mm Hg	>105 mm Hg
Proteinuria		
Quantitative 24-hr analysis	Proteinuria of >0.3 g in a 24-hr specimen or ≥30 mg/mmol urinary creatinine in a random urine sample	Proteinuria of >3–5 g in 24 hr
Qualitative dipstick	≥0.30 g/L on dipstick or 1+	2+ to 3+ protein on dipstick
Reflexes	May be normal	Hyper-reflexia >3+, possible ankle clonus
Urine output	Output matching intake, ≥30 mL/hr or <650 mL/24 hr	20 mL/hr or <400 mL–500 mL/24 hr
Headache	Absent/transient	Severe
Visual problems	Absent	Blurred, photophobia, blind spots on funduscopy
Irritability/changes in affect	Transient	Severe
Epigastric pain	Absent	Present
Serum creatinine	Normal	Elevated
Thrombocytopenia	Absent	Present
AST elevation	Normal or minimal	Marked
Fetal Effects		
Placental perfusion	Reduced	Decreased perfusion expressing as IUGR in fetus; FHR may show late decelerations in labour
Premature placental aging	Not apparent	At birth, placenta appearing smaller than normal for duration of pregnancy; premature aging apparent with numerous areas of ischemic necroses (white infarcts); numerous, intervillous fibrin deposition (red infarcts)

(Sources: American College of Obstetricians and Gynecologists. [2002]. *Diagnosis and management of preeclampsia and eclampsia* [ACOG practice bulletin number 33]. Washington, DC: Author; Report of the National High Blood Pressure Education Program Working Group on High Blood Pressure in Pregnancy. [2002]. Summary report. *American Journal of Obstetrics and Gynecology, 183*[1], S1–S22; Society of Obstetricians and Gynaecologists of Canada. [2008]. SOGC clinical practice guideline: Diagnosis, evaluation and management of hypertensive disorders of pregnancy. *Journal of Obstetrics and Gynaecology Canada, 30*[3], Suppl 1, S1–S48. Retrieved from http://www.sogc.org/guidelines/documents/gui206CPG0803_001.pdf.)

AST, aspartate aminotransferase; *FHR,* fetal heart rate; *IUGR,* intrauterine growth restriction.

BOX 13-1 Urine Protein Values

Protein readings are designated as follows:
- 0–negative
- Trace–trace
- +1–0.3 g/L
- +2–1.0 g/L
- +3–3.0 g/L
- +4–more than 10.0 g/L

suspicion of pre-eclampsia or of worsening pre-eclampsia, blood work and assessment for endothelial damage are indicated to monitor for the development of severe pre-eclampsia (see Table 13-3).

Severe Pre-Eclampsia

Severe pre-eclampsia is defined as having an sBP greater than 160 mm Hg or a dBP of at least 110 mm Hg and proteinuria of 3 to 5 g or more per 24-hour specimen (Sibai, 2007; SOGC, 2008). Other signs and symptoms associated with severe pre-eclampsia include the following: oliguria; cerebral disturbances such as altered level of consciousness, confusion, or headache; visual disturbances such as scotomata or blurred vision; hepatic involvement, including epigastric pain, right upper quadrant pain, impaired liver function, or elevated liver enzymes; thrombocytopenia with a platelet count less than 100×10^9/L; hemolytic anemia; pulmonary edema; and fetal growth restriction (see Table 13-3) (Roberts & Funai, 2009; Sibai, 2007; SOGC, 2008).

Eclampsia

Eclampsia, characterized by seizures, from profound cerebral effects of pre-eclampsia is the major maternal risk. As a rule, maternal and perinatal morbidity and mortality rates are highest when eclampsia is seen early in gestation (before 28 weeks), maternal age is greater than 25 years, the woman is a multigravida, and chronic hypertension or renal disease is present (Sibai, 2007). The fetus of the eclamptic woman is at increased risk for abruptio placentae, preterm birth, IUGR, and acute hypoxia.

The initial presentation of eclampsia varies, with one third of the women developing eclampsia during the pregnancy, one third during labour, and one third within 72 hours after giving birth (Emery, 2005).

The etiology of pre-eclampsia is theorized to include various possibilities: abnormal prostaglandin action, endothelial cell dysfunction, coagulation abnormalities, vasoconstrictor tone, and dietary deficiencies or excesses (Fig. 13-1). Immunological factors and genetic disposition may also play an important role (Sibai, 2007). Animal studies have suggested that abnormalities of the placenta are the cause of pre-eclampsia. The trophoblast cells of the placenta usually alter the spiral arteries in the uterus to accommodate increased blood flow. In pre-eclampsia, the vessels are abnormally thick walled and muscular and have higher resistance. The condition also results in a distinctive lesion called *acute atherosis*, and there is greater occurrence of placental infarcts. Placental perfusion is decreased, resulting in hypoxia; this in turn causes several pathophysiological abnormalities, especially endothelial damage. Many of these pathophysiological changes of pre-eclampsia occur before clinical symptoms develop (Sibai, 2007).

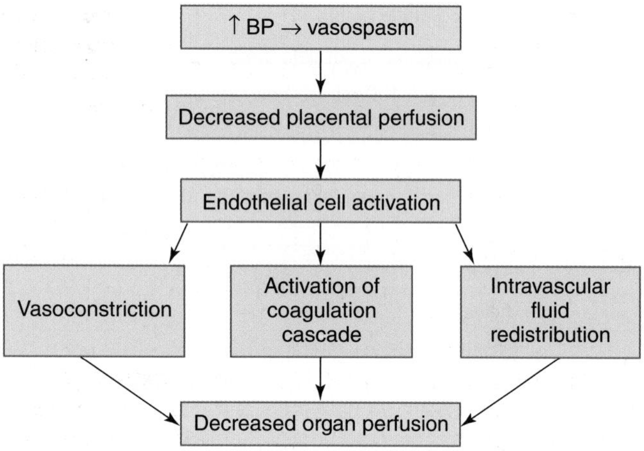

Fig. 13-1 Etiology of pre-eclampsia. *BP*, blood pressure.

Since the etiology of pre-eclampsia is unknown, various clinical trials have attempted to correct theoretical abnormalities present in pre-eclampsia as a means of preventing pre-eclampsia. Some methods used to prevent pre-eclampsia are listed in Box 13-2.

Pathophysiology

Pre-eclampsia progresses along a continuum from mild disease to severe pre-eclampsia, HELLP syndrome, or eclampsia. The pathophysiology of pre-eclampsia reflects alterations in the normal adaptations of pregnancy. Normal physiological adaptations to pregnancy include increased blood plasma volume, vasodilation, decreased systemic vascular resistance, elevated cardiac output, and decreased colloid osmotic pressure (Box 13-3). The main pathogenic factor is not an increase in BP but poor perfusion as a result of vasospasm. Arteriolar vasospasm diminishes the diameter of blood vessels, which impedes blood flow to all organs and increases BP (Roberts et al. & NHLBI Working Group on Research on Hypertension During Pregnancy, 2003; Roberts & Funai, 2009; SOGC, 2008) (see Community Focus box). Function in organs such as

BOX 13-2 Recommendations for Prevention of Pre-Eclampsia and Improvement of Pregnancy Outcomes in Women at Low Risk of Developing Pre-Eclampsia

Abstention from alcohol
Smoking cessation
Multivitamins containing folate (also to prevent neural tube defects)
- Calcium supplementation (at least 1 g/day orally)

Regular exercise
The following are NOT recommended for prevention of pre-eclampsia in low-risk women (due to insufficient evidence):
- Supplementation with magnesium or zinc
- Prostaglandin precursors such as fish and evening primrose oil
- High-protein and low-salt diet
- Calorie restriction for overweight women
- Low-dose aspirin (recommended for women at increased risk of pre-eclampsia)
- Vitamins C and E
- Thiazide diuretics
- Antihypertensive therapy (does not prevent pre-eclampsia)

(Adapted From Sibai, B. M. [2007]. Hypertension. In S. F. Gabbe, J. R. Niebyl, & J. L. Simpson [Eds.], *Obstetrics: Normal and problem pregnancies* [5th ed.]. Philadelphia: Churchill Livingstone; Society of Obstetricians and Gynaecologists of Canada. [2008]. SOGC clinical practice guideline: Diagnosis, evaluation and management of hypertensive disorders of pregnancy. *Journal of Obstetrics and Gynaecology Canada, 30*[3], Suppl 1, S1–S48. Retrieved from http://www.sogc.org/guidelines/documents/gui206CPG0803_001.pdf.)

BOX 13-3 Normal Physiological Adaptations to Pregnancy

Cardiovascular

↑ Blood volume; plasma volume expansion greater than red cell mass expansion, leading to physiological anemia of pregnancy
↓ Total peripheral resistance, decreases in blood pressure readings, and MAP
↑ Cardiac output resulting from increased blood volume; slight increase in heart rate to compensate for peripheral relaxation
↑ Oxygen consumption
Physiological edema related to ↓ plasma colloid osmotic pressure and ↑ venous capillary hydrostatic pressure

Hematological

↑ Clotting factors, predisposing to DIC and clotting
↓ Serum albumin resulting in decreases in colloid osmotic pressure, predisposing to pulmonary edema

Renal

↑ Renal plasma flow and glomerular filtration rate

Endocrine

↑ Estrogen production resulting in renin–angiotensin II–aldosterone secretion
↑ Progesterone production blocking aldosterone effect (slight ↓ Na)
↑ Vasodilator prostaglandins resulting in resistance to angiotensin II (slight ↓ blood pressure)

DIC, disseminated intravascular coagulation; *MAP,* mean arterial pressure.

the placenta, kidneys, liver, and brain is depressed by as much as 40 to 60%. The pathophysiological sequelae are shown in Fig. 13-2.

HELLP Syndrome

HELLP syndrome is a laboratory diagnosis for a variant of severe pre-eclampsia that is characterized by hemolysis (*H*), elevated liver enzymes (*EL*), and low platelets (*LPs*) (ACOG, 2002; Sibai, 2007; SOGC, 2008). To have a diagnosis of HELLP syndrome, the platelet count must be less than 100 × 10^9/L, and the liver enzyme levels (aspartate aminotransferase [AST] and alanine aminotransferase [ALT]) must be elevated. A unique form of coagulopathy (not disseminated intravascular coagulation [DIC]) occurs with HELLP syndrome. The platelet count is low, but coagulation factor assays, prothrombin time (PT), partial thromboplastin time (PTT), and bleeding time remain normal. In some instances, hemolysis does not occur, and the condition is termed ELLP (Sibai, 2007; Sibai, Dekker, & Kupferminc, 2005).

HELLP syndrome appears in approximately 20% of women with severe pre-eclampsia (ACOG, 2002; Emery, 2005). Most commonly, HELLP syndrome is seen in older, White, multiparous women. About 90% of women report a history of malaise for several days. Many women (65%) experience epigastric or right upper quadrant abdominal pain (possibly related to hepatic ischemia), and approximately half develop nausea and vomiting. Many women with HELLP syndrome may not have signs and symptoms of severe pre-eclampsia; many are normotensive and have no proteinuria. As a result, women with HELLP syndrome are often misdiagnosed with a variety of other medical or surgical disorders (Sibai, 2007).

Recognition of the clinical and laboratory findings associated with HELLP syndrome is important if early, aggressive therapy is to be initiated to prevent maternal and neonatal death. Complications reported with HELLP syndrome include renal failure, pulmonary edema, ruptured liver hematoma, DIC, and abruptio placentae (Sibai, 2007).

COMMUNITY FOCUS

The Woman With Pre-Eclampsia

Margie, a 25-year-old, G1 P0, single woman who is a school secretary, is seen in the clinic for her routine prenatal visit at 30 weeks of gestation. On examination, you note that she has gained 4 kg since her last clinic visit 2 weeks ago, her blood pressure is 150/94, and on a urine dipstick she has 1+ proteinuria.

- What is the likely diagnosis for Margie? What other signs and symptoms of this condition might you find? Develop a nursing care plan for Margie. What teaching about diet, rest, signs and symptoms to observe, and fetal assessment should be included in the plan?
- What community agencies or assistance is available to her? Develop a list of community resources for women in circumstances similar to Margie's.

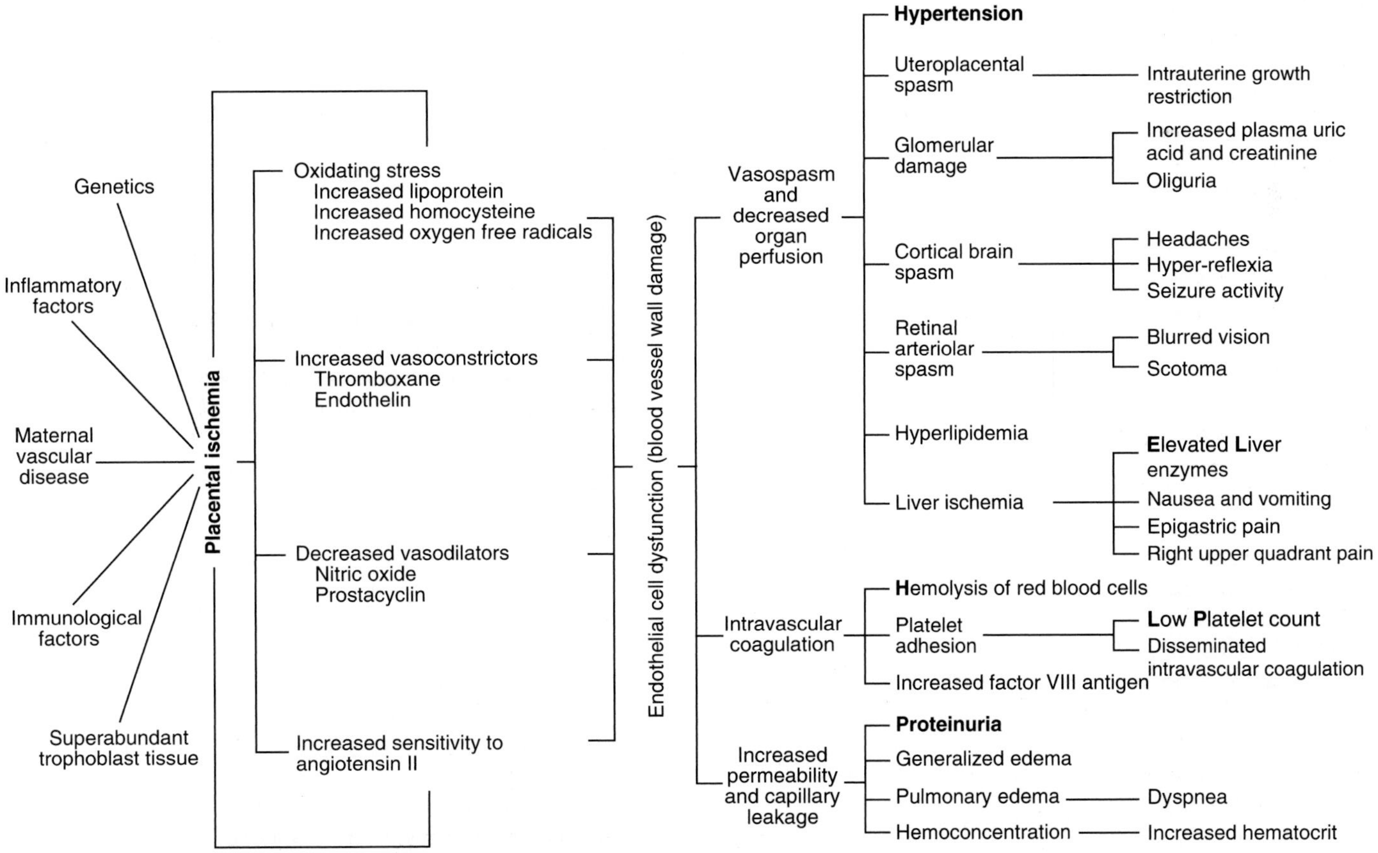

Fig. 13-2 Pathophysiology of pre-eclampsia. *(Adapted from Gilbert, E. S. [2007].* Manual of high risk pregnancy and delivery *[4th ed.]. St. Louis: Mosby.)*

Nursing Care Management

Hypertensive disorders of pregnancy can occur without warning or with the gradual development of symptoms (see Nursing Process box). The best prevention methods include early prenatal care for identification of women at risk and early detection of pre-eclampsia. The woman is assessed for maternal markers at her first prenatal visit (see Table 13-2).

Blood Pressure Assessment

Accurate and consistent assessment of BP is important for establishing a baseline and for monitoring subtle changes throughout the pregnancy. BP readings are affected by maternal position and measurement techniques, thus consistency must be ensured. Normally the dBP drops an average of 10 mm Hg below nonpregnant values by midgestation and

NURSING PROCESS: MILD PRE-ECLAMPSIA

Assessment

History

- Review medical history for diabetes mellitus, renal disease, and hypertension (comorbid conditions)
- Family history for hypertensive disorders, diabetes mellitus, and other chronic conditions
- Social history for marital status, cultural beliefs, activity level, and lifestyle behaviours (smoking; alcohol and drug use)

Interview

- Review of systems

Physical Examination

- BP
- Edema
- Deep tendon reflexes
- History or presence of headache, epigastric pain, visual disturbances
- Fetal heart rate and movement patterns
- Uterine tone and tenderness; vaginal bleeding

Review Laboratory Test Results

- CBC (including a platelet count)
- Clotting studies (including bleeding time, PT, PTT, and fibrinogen)
- Liver enzymes (LDH, AST, ALT)
- Chemistry panel (BUN, creatinine, glucose, uric acid)
- Type and screen, possible cross-match

Nursing Diagnoses

Nursing diagnoses for the woman with mild pre-eclampsia include the following:

Anxiety related to
- risk of complications from pre-eclampsia and its effect on the woman and her fetus

Ineffective individual/family coping related to
- the woman's restricted activity and concern over a complicated pregnancy
- the woman's inability to work outside the home
- the transfer of the woman to a tertiary centre for more intensive management

Powerlessness related to
- inability to prevent or control condition and outcomes

Ineffective tissue perfusion related to
- hypertension
- cyclic vasospasms
- cerebral edema
- hemorrhage
- risk of seizure

Risk for injury to fetus related to
- uteroplacental insufficiency and related intrauterine growth restriction
- preterm birth
- abruptio placentae

Nursing Diagnosis

Deficient diversional activity related to imposed bed rest

Expected Outcome

Patient will express diminished feelings of boredom.

Nursing Interventions/*Rationales*

Assist the woman to creatively explore personally meaningful activities that can be pursued from the bed *to ensure activities that have meaning, purpose, and value to the individual.*

Maintain emphasis on the woman's personal choices *to promote control and minimize imposition of routines by others.*

Evaluate what support and system resources are available in the environment *to assist in providing diversional activities.*

Explore ways for the woman to remain an active participant in home management and decision making *to promote her control.*

Engage support of family and friends in carrying out chosen activities and making necessary environmental alterations *to ensure success.*

Teach the woman about stress-management and relaxation techniques *to help manage tension of confinement.*

Planning

A multidisciplinary plan of care is developed together with the woman and her family.

Expected outcomes for care of patients with hypertensive disorders of pregnancy are that the woman will do the following:

- Recognize and immediately report abnormal signs and symptoms indicative of worsening condition
- Follow the medical regimen to minimize risk to herself and her fetus
- Identify and use available support systems
- Express her fears and concerns to cope with the condition and situation
- Develop no signs of eclampsia and its severely morbid complications
- Give birth to a healthy infant (preferably at or near term)
- Develop no adverse sequelae from her condition or its management

If the woman has mild pre-eclampsia (BP is stable, urine protein is less than 0.3 g/L in a 24-hour collection, and there is no evidence of end-organ dysfunction), she may be managed at home.

NURSING PROCESS: MILD PRE-ECLAMPSIA—cont'd

The maternal–fetal condition should be assessed at least two times per week. The woman may be asked to perform self-assessment daily, including recording of weight, urine dipstick testing, protein determinations, BP measurement, and fetal movement counting. She will be instructed to report immediately any subjective symptoms to her primary health care provider (see Home Care box) and to return to the high-risk clinic or physician's office for all appointments as scheduled.

Interventions (Home Care)

Assess maternal–fetal dyad at least 2 times/week.
Evaluate fetal growth by ultrasound every 2 weeks.
Teach counting of daily fetal movement counts from 26 weeks onward.
Perform nonstress test (NST) 2 times/week.
Recommend restricted activity levels.
Teach the woman how to cope with restricted activity.
Recommend diet as for normal pregnant women.
Review clinical signs to report (see Home Care box).
Involve the woman and her family in the plan of care.
Evaluate support systems.

Evaluation

Evaluation of the effectiveness of care of the woman with pre-eclampsia is based on the absence of complications for the mother and fetus or newborn.

ALT, alanine aminotransferase; *AST,* aspartate aminotransferase; *BP,* blood pressure; *BUN,* blood urea nitrogen; *CBC,* complete blood count; *FHR,* fetal heart rate; *LDH,* lactate dehydrogenase; *PT,* prothrombin time; *PTT,* partial thromboplastin time.

HOME CARE

Assessing and Reporting Clinical Signs of Pre-Eclampsia

Report Immediately Any Clinical Signs

- Report any increase in blood pressure, protein in urine, weight gain, or decreased fetal movement.*

Take Blood Pressure With Consistency

- Take blood pressure on the same arm with the woman in a sitting position each time for consistent and accurate readings. Support the arm on a table in a horizontal position at heart level.

Record Weight Daily

- Use the same scale, wearing the same clothes, at the same time each day, after voiding, and before breakfast for reliable daily recording of weight.

Dipstick Test Clean-Catch Urine Sample

- This is done to assess proteinuria; report frequency or burning on urination.

Assess Fetal Activity Daily

- Decreased activity (six or fewer movements in 2 hours) may indicate fetal compromise.

Keep Scheduled Prenatal Appointments

- Regular appointments need to be kept so that any changes in maternal or fetal condition can be detected immediately.

Keep a Daily Log or Diary

- Keep a log of assessments and bring it to prenatal visits.

*Thresholds for blood pressure, weight gain, fetal movement counts, and proteinuria are set by the physician or institutional protocol.

then slowly reaches nonpregnant levels in the third trimester. Evaluation of BP focuses on trends, not on a single reading (ACOG, 2002; Roberts & Funai, 2009). Box 13-4 presents recommendations for standardizing this procedure.

Other Assessments

Eyes

Although it is not a routine assessment during the prenatal period, evaluation of the fundus of the eye yields valuable data. An initial baseline finding of normal eye grounds assists in differentiating a pre-existing from a new disease process.

Deep Tendon Reflexes

Deep tendon reflexes (DTRs) are evaluated at baseline and throughout the pregnancy, to detect any changes. The biceps and patellar reflexes and ankle clonus are assessed and the findings recorded (Fig. 13-3 and Table 13-4). The evaluation of DTRs is especially important if the woman is being treated with magnesium sulphate. Absence of DTRs may be an indication of impending magnesium toxicity.

To elicit the biceps reflex, a downward blow is struck over the thumb, which is placed over the biceps tendon. Normal response is flexion of the arm at the elbow, described as a 2+ response (see Fig. 13-3, A, and Table 13-4).

The patellar reflex is elicited with the woman's legs hanging freely over the end of the examining table or with the woman lying on her side with the knee slightly flexed. A blow with a percussion hammer is dealt directly to the patellar tendon, inferior to the patella. Normal response is extension or kicking out of the leg, which is recorded as 2+ (see Fig. 13-3, B, and Table 13-4).

To assess for hyperactive reflexes (clonus) at the ankle joint, the examiner supports the leg with the knee flexed. With one hand, the examiner sharply dorsiflexes the foot, maintains the position for a moment, and then releases the foot (see Fig. 13-3, C). A normal (negative clonus) response is elicited when no rhythmic oscillations (jerks) are felt while the foot is held in dorsiflexion. When the foot is released, no oscillations are seen as the foot drops to the plantar-flexed position. An abnormal

BOX 13-4 Protocol for Blood Pressure Measurement

- Blood pressure (BP) should be measured with the woman in a sitting position with the arm at the level of the heart.
- Use the proper-size cuff (cuff should cover 1.5 times the circumference of the arm).
- Use Korotkoff phase V for the diastolic reading.
- If BP is consistently higher in one arm, the arm with the higher values should be used.
- Use manual sphygmomanometer, or an automated BP device that has been validated for use in pre-eclampsia.
- Women must be instructed in proper BP measurement if they are performing home BP monitoring.

(Adapted from Society of Obstetricians and Gynaecologists of Canada. [2008]. SOGC clinical practice guideline: Diagnosis, evaluation and management of hypertensive disorders of pregnancy. *Journal of Obstetrics and Gynaecology Canada, 30*[3], Suppl 1, S1–S48. Retrieved from http://www.sogc.org/guidelines/documents/gui206CPG0803_001.pdf.)

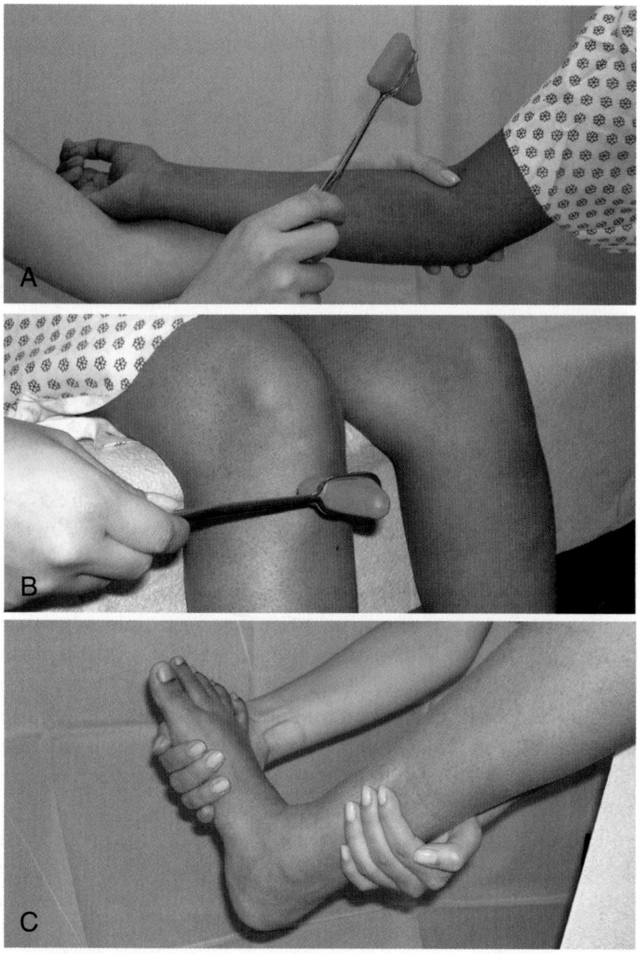

Fig. 13-3 Deep tendon reflexes. **A:** Biceps reflex. **B:** Patellar reflex with woman's legs hanging freely over end of examining table. **C:** Test for ankle clonus. *(Courtesy Shannon Perry, Phoenix, AZ.)*

Table 13-4 Assessing Deep Tendon Reflexes

GRADE	DEEP TENDON REFLEX RESPONSE
0	No response
1+	Sluggish or diminished
2+	Active or expected response
3+	More brisk than expected; slightly hyperactive
4+	Brisk, hyperactive, with intermittent or transient clonus

(From Seidel, H. M., et al. [2006]. *Mosby's guide to physical examination* [6th ed.]. St. Louis: Mosby.)

(positive clonus) response is indicated by rhythmic oscillations of one or more beats felt when the foot is in dorsiflexion and seen as the foot drops to the plantar-flexed position.

Signs and symptoms of progression of mild-to-severe pre-eclampsia, such as headaches, epigastric pain, and visual disturbances, should be noted. The signs of mild and severe pre-eclampsia are summarized in Table 13-3.

Fetal Health Surveillance

Uteroplacental perfusion can be decreased in women with pre-eclampsia. Fetal health surveillance, by means of such methods as the nonstress test (NST), contraction stress test (CST), biophysical profile (BPP), and serial ultrasonography, is used to assess fetal status. The fetal heart rate (FHR) is assessed for baseline rate, variability, and presence of accelerations. Abnormal baseline rate, decreased or absent variability, or late decelerations are indications of fetal intolerance to the intrauterine environment. Since the woman with pre-eclampsia is at risk for abruptio placentae, it is important to assess uterine tone and tenderness and check for the presence of vaginal bleeding. Doppler flow velocimetry studies can be used to evaluate uteroplacental perfusion (see Chapter 12).

NURSING ALERT Uterine tenderness along with increasing tone may be the earliest finding of an abruption. Idiopathic preterm contractions also may be an early sign.

An evaluation of fetal growth by ultrasound should be obtained at diagnosis and repeated every 2 weeks. Fetal movements are counted daily (see Chapter 12). Fetal compromise evidenced by slowed growth or an abnormal finding during testing may necessitate immediate delivery, depending on gestational age (labour induction or Caesarean birth) (ACOG, 2002; Roberts & Funai, 2009; Sibai, 2007).

Activity Restriction

Restricted activity with some bed rest in the lateral recumbent position is traditional therapy for pre-eclampsia and may improve uteroplacental blood flow. Complete bed rest for women with severe pre-eclampsia has been shown to be beneficial in decreasing BP and promoting fetal growth as well as improving in amniotic fluid levels. There is no evidence that bed rest improves pregnancy outcomes (Sibai, 2007). Adverse physiological outcomes related to bed rest include cardiovascular deconditioning; diuresis with accompanying fluid, electrolyte, and weight loss; muscle atrophy; and psychological stress (see Box 19-4). These changes may begin as early as the first day of bed rest and continue for the duration of therapy.

Thus, restricted activity with bathroom privileges is helpful for women with mild pre-eclampsia to help decrease negative effects (Maloni et al., 2004; Sibai, 2007).

Women with mild pre-eclampsia feel reasonably well, so boredom from the restriction is common (see Home Care box, Chapter 19, p. 494). Diversionary activities, visits from friends, telephone conversations, and creation of a comfortable and convenient environment are ways to cope with the boredom. Gentle exercise (e.g., range of motion, stretching, Kegel exercises, and pelvic tilts) is important in maintaining muscle tone, blood flow, regularity of bowel function, and a sense of well-being. Relaxation techniques can help reduce stress associated with the high-risk condition and prepare the woman for labour and the birth.

Diet

Diet and fluid recommendations are much the same as those for healthy pregnant women. Diets high in protein and low in salt are not recommended to prevent pre-eclampsia. The exception may be the woman with pre-existing hypertension that had been successfully controlled with a low-salt diet before the pregnancy. Adequate fluid intake helps maintain optimum fluid volume and aids in renal perfusion and bowel function (see Guidelines box).

For successful home care, the woman needs to be well educated about pre-eclampsia and motivated to follow the plan of care. All teaching should include the woman and her family; time must be allowed for assimilation of information, questions, and concerns. The woman's knowledge base is directly associated with her compliance with the prescribed treatment program. Methods for enhancing learning include visual aids, movies, handouts, and demonstrations with return demonstrations. The effects of illness, language, age, culture, beliefs, and support systems must also be considered.

Severe Pre-Eclampsia or HELLP Syndrome

Hospital Care

The woman with severe pre-eclampsia or HELLP syndrome should receive appropriate treatment in a tertiary care centre from a perinatology team, including maternal–fetal medicine specialists, high-risk obstetrical nurses, and an anaesthesiologist (see Nursing Care Plan). The need for tertiary care may result in the woman being transferred from her home community to a larger centre. The woman may be admitted to a high-risk antepartum or a labour and birth unit, depending on the hospital. If the woman's condition requires intensive monitoring, she will need to be in an obstetrical critical care unit or a medical intensive care unit for hemodynamic monitoring. If severe pre-eclampsia is diagnosed at less than 32 weeks, an initial observation period and conservative management may be attempted. When the gestational age is 32 to 36 weeks, labour may be induced. Vaginal birth is the preferred type of birth, and Caesarean birth should only be performed for obstetrical indications. In pregnancies of less than 32 weeks, antenatal corticosteroids will be given to promote fetal lung maturation. If the birth can be delayed for 48 hours, steroids such as betamethasone (see Medication Guide, p. 497) (12 mg intramuscularly 24 hours apart) may be given to the woman (Crane et al., 2003; SOGC, 2008).

Recognition of the clinical and laboratory findings of severe pre-eclampsia or HELLP syndrome is important in order to prevent maternal and perinatal mortality. The woman with severe pre-eclampsia or HELLP syndrome has multisystem involvement, and nursing care must focus on both the mother and fetus. Maternal and fetal surveillance, education of the woman and her family regarding the disease process, and supportive measures should be initiated. Assessments include review of the central nervous, cardiovascular, pulmonary, and renal systems. Weight is measured on admission and usually at the same time every day thereafter. Breath sounds are auscultated for crackles or diminished breath sounds, which may indicate pulmonary edema. An indwelling urinary catheter may be inserted to measure urinary output. An indwelling urinary catheter facilitates monitoring of renal function and effectiveness of therapy; however, the risk of urinary tract infection should be considered in the stable antepartum woman. Hemoglobin oxygen saturation can be assessed with a pulse oximeter. Baseline laboratory assessments include metabolic studies for liver enzyme (AST, ALT, lactate dehydrogenase [LDH]) determination, complete blood count (CBC) with platelets, coagulation profile to assess for DIC, and electrolyte studies to establish renal functioning (ACOG, 2002; Roberts & Funai, 2009; SOGC, 2008).

If there is uterine activity, vaginal examination may be done to check for cervical changes. Through abdominal palpation, uterine tonicity and fetal size, activity, and position can be determined. Assessments of fetal well-being (e.g., NST, BPP) should be ordered because of the potential for hypoxia related to uteroplacental insufficiency. Electronic monitoring to determine fetal status is initiated at least once a day with severe pre-eclampsia. The nurse's skill in implementing these techniques can be reassuring to the woman and her family. The woman's room should be close to staff and emergency medications, supplies, and equipment. Seizure precautions need to be taken (Box 13-5). Because of the risk for thromboembolism for the woman on bed rest, she may wear TED (anti-embolism) stockings, SCD (sequential compression device) boots, or both while in bed.

Intrapartum nursing care of the woman with severe pre-eclampsia or HELLP syndrome involves continuous maternal and fetal assessments as labour progresses. Invasive hemodynamic monitoring with a pulmonary artery catheter

GUIDELINES Nutrition for Women With Pre-Eclampsia

- Eat a nutritious, balanced diet according to Canada's Food Guide. Consult with a registered dietitian on the diet best suited for you as an individual.
- There is no sodium restriction; however, consider limiting excessively salty foods (pretzels, potato chips, pickles, sauerkraut).
- Eat foods with roughage (whole grains, raw fruits, and vegetables).
- Drink six to eight 250-mL glasses of water per day.
- Avoid alcohol and limit caffeine intake.

NURSING CARE PLAN ● Severe Pre-Eclampsia: Hospital Care

Nursing Diagnosis Risk for morbidity for mother and fetus related to hypertension, poor placental perfusion, and CNS irritability

Expected Outcomes

The woman will have decreased blood pressure (below 160/110), show diminished signs of CNS irritability (e.g., DTRs 2+, absence of clonus), and have no convulsions.

Nursing Interventions/*Rationales*

Establish baseline data (e.g., DTRs, clonus) *to use as basis for evaluating effectiveness of treatment.*

Administer IV magnesium sulphate per physician's orders *to decrease risk of convulsions.*

Monitor maternal vital signs, FHR, urine output, and DTRs and maintain IV flow rates at no greater than 80 mLs/hr. Have calcium gluconate available if needed *as antidote for magnesium sulphate toxicity (very rare).*

Maintain a quiet, darkened environment *to avoid stimuli that may precipitate seizure activity.*

Treat with antihypertensive medication as ordered *to prevent complications.*

Nursing Diagnosis Ineffective tissue perfusion related to pre-eclampsia secondary to arteriolar vasospasm

Expected Outcome

The woman will exhibit signs of increased vasodilation (diuresis, weight loss).

Nursing Interventions/*Rationales*

Establish baseline data (weight, degree of edema) *to use as a basis for evaluating the effectiveness of treatment.*

Administer antihypertensive medication as ordered *to prevent complications.*

Give IV magnesium sulphate per physician order *to reduce seizure risk, not to be given as an antihypertensive medication.*

Place woman on bed rest in a side-lying position *to maximize uteroplacental blood flow, reduce blood pressure, and promote diuresis.*

Monitor intake and output, edema, and weight *to assess for evidence of vasodilation and increased tissue perfusion.*

Nursing Diagnoses Risk for excess fluid volume related to poor kidney function and sodium retention secondary to administration of magnesium sulphate; risk for impaired gas exchange related to pulmonary edema secondary to increased vascular resistance; risk for decreased cardiac output related to use of antihypertensive medications; risk for injury to fetus related to uteroplacental insufficiency secondary to use of antihypertensive medications

Expected Outcomes

Patient will exhibit signs of normal fluid volume (balanced intake and output, normal serum creatinine levels, normal breath sounds), adequate oxygenation (normal respirations, fully oriented to person, time, and place), normal range of cardiac output (normal pulse rate and rhythm), and fetal well-being (adequate fetal movement, normal FHR).

Nursing Interventions/*Rationales*

Monitor woman for signs of third spacing of fluid volume (increased edema, decreased urine output, elevated serum creatinine level, weight gain, dyspnea, crackles) *to prevent complications.*

Monitor woman for signs of impaired gas exchange (increased respirations, dyspnea, altered blood gases, hypoxemia) *to prevent complications.*

Monitor woman for signs of decreased cardiac output (altered pulse rate and rhythm) *to prevent complications.*

Monitor fetus for signs of compromise (decreased fetal activity, abnormal EFM pattern) *to prevent complications.*

Record findings and report signs of increasing problems to physician *to enable timely interventions.*

CNS, central nervous system; *DTRs,* deep tendon reflexes; *EFM,* electronic fetal monitoring; *FHR,* fetal heart rate; *IV,* intravenous.

(Swan-Ganz catheter) may be required for accurate intravascular fluid volume measurement in the presence of pulmonary edema or acute renal failure (ACOG, 2002; Roberts & Funai, 2009).

Magnesium Sulphate

One important goal of care for the woman with pre-eclampsia is to prevent or control convulsions. Magnesium sulphate is the medication of choice in the prevention and treatment of convulsions caused by pre-eclampsia or eclampsia. It is administered as a secondary infusion ("piggyback") to the main intravenous (IV) line by volumetric infusion pump. An initial loading dose of 4 g diluted in at least 100 mL of IV fluid per protocol or physician's order is infused over 15 to 30 minutes. This dose is followed by a maintenance dosage of magnesium sulphate diluted in an IV solution per physician's order (e.g., 20 g of magnesium sulphate in 500 mL of normal saline) and administered by infusion pump at 1 g/hr (Gilbert, 2007). Data from the MAGPIE trial indicate that at this dose there is no need to draw serial serum magnesium levels (Duley et al., 2002). After the loading dose, there may be a transient lowering of the arterial BP secondary to relaxation of smooth muscle.

NURSING ALERT The woman's BP, pulse, and respiratory status should be monitored closely while the loading dose of magnesium sulphate is being administered intravenously and then every 15 to 30 minutes, depending on the stability of the woman's condition.

Magnesium sulphate is rarely given intramuscularly because the absorption rate cannot be controlled, injections are painful, and tissue necrosis can occur. The intramuscular (IM) route may be used, however, with some women who are being transported to a tertiary care centre. The IM dose is 4

BOX 13-5 Hospital Precautionary Measures for Seizures

Environment
- Quiet
- Nonstimulating
- Lighting subdued
- Seizure precautions (have magnesium sulphate available)
- Suction equipment tested and ready to use
- Oxygen administration equipment tested and ready to use

Call button within easy reach
Support for woman who may be separated from family and other children during her hospitalization
Emergency medication tray immediately accessible
- Antihypertensive medication (labetalol, nifedipine, hydralazine) immediately available
- Calcium gluconate immediately available (if receiving magnesium sulphate)

Emergency birth pack accessible

to 5 g given in the ventral gluteal (one on each side), for a total of 10 g (1% procaine may be ordered as an addition to the solution to reduce injection pain), and can be repeated at 4-hour intervals. Z-track technique should be used for the deep IM injection, followed by gentle massage at the site.

Magnesium sulphate interferes with the release of acetylcholine at the synapses, resulting in decreased neuromuscular irritability, depressed cardiac conduction, and decreased central nervous system (CNS) irritability. Because magnesium circulates free and unbound to protein and is excreted in the urine, accurate recordings of maternal urine output must be maintained.

Diuresis within 24 to 48 hours is an excellent prognostic sign; it is considered evidence that perfusion of the kidneys has improved as a result of relaxation of arteriolar spasm. With improved perfusion, fluid moves from interstitial spaces to the intravascular bed, and edema is reduced. Diuresis results in weight loss. Although diuresis generally indicates overall improvement, in the presence of worsening clinical status, it may indicate impending renal failure. As renal function declines and serum creatinine levels rise, renal filtration is compromised. In this situation, the woman can excrete large volumes of urine (greater than 200 mL/hr) but does not excrete magnesium sulphate.

Because magnesium sulphate is a CNS depressant, the nurse needs to assess for signs and symptoms of magnesium toxicity. This is rare with the 1 g/hr maintenance dose, and serum magnesium levels are only obtained when signs of toxicity are present. Early symptoms of toxicity include decreased DTRs, nausea, a feeling of warmth, flushing, muscle weakness, decreased reflexes, and slurred speech.

NURSING ALERT Loss of patellar reflexes, respiratory and muscular depression, oliguria, and a decreased level of consciousness are signs of magnesium toxicity. If magnesium toxicity is suspected, the infusion should be discontinued immediately. Calcium gluconate, the antidote for magnesium sulphate, may also be ordered (10 mL of a 10% solution, or 1 g) and given by slow IV push (usually by the physician) over at least 3 minutes to avoid undesirable reactions such as dysrhythmias, bradycardia, and ventricular fibrillation.

Magnesium sulphate does not seem to affect FHR variability in a healthy term fetus. Neonatal serum magnesium levels approximate those of the mother. Doses of magnesium sulphate that prevent maternal seizures have been determined to be safe for the fetus. Toxic levels in the newborn can cause depressed respirations and hyporeflexia at birth. It is important that the neonatal team attend the birth to provide resuscitation measures as needed. In a 2-year follow-up study, magnesium administration was not found to result in an excess of disability or death in mothers (Magpie Trial Follow-Up Study Collaborative Group, 2007b). At the 18-month follow-up, magnesium administration was not associated with a difference in disability or death in infants who had had in utero exposure to magnesium sulphate, compared with infants who had been exposed to a placebo (Magpie Trial Follow-Up Study Collaborative Group, 2007a).

NURSING ALERT Magnesium sulphate acts as a muscle relaxant and, when used during labour, may decrease the effectiveness of contractions. Women may need augmentation with oxytocin. The amount of oxytocin needs to be titrated individually to the woman who is receiving magnesium sulphate.

Control of Blood Pressure

Initiation of antihypertensive therapy reduces maternal morbidity and mortality rates associated with left ventricular failure and cerebral hemorrhage; therefore, antihypertensive medications may be ordered to lower BP. Antihypertensive therapy must not decrease the arterial pressure too much or too rapidly as it will impact uteroplacental perfusion. The target range for the diastolic pressure is between 85 and 105 mm Hg, and the systolic pressure between 130 and 155 mm Hg (SOGC, 2008).

Labetalol administered intravenously is the antihypertensive drug of choice for the treatment of hypertension. Nifedipine; methyldopa; other β-blockers such as acebutolol, metoprolol, pindolol, and propranolol; and hydralazine are also used (Table 13-5) (Roberts & Funai, 2009; Sibai, 2007; SOGC, 2008). The choice of medication used depends on the woman's response and physician preference.

NURSING ALERT When administering antihypertensive therapy, the nurse must remember that the medication effects depend on intravascular volume. Because pre-eclampsia is associated with contracted intravascular volume, initial doses should be given with caution and maternal response monitored closely.

Eclampsia

Eclampsia is usually preceded by various premonitory symptoms and signs, including headache, severe epigastric pain, and hyper-reflexia. However, convulsions can appear suddenly and without warning in a seemingly stable woman, with only minimum BP elevations (Sibai, 2007). Increased hypertension

Table 13-5 Pharmacological Control of Hypertension in Pregnancy

		Adverse Effects		
ACTION	TARGET TISSUE	MATERNAL	FETAL	NURSING ACTIONS
Hydralazine (Apresoline)				
Arteriolar vasodilator	Peripheral arterioles: to decrease muscle tone, decrease peripheral resistance; hypothalamus and medullary vasomotor centre for minor decrease in sympathetic tone	Headache, flushing, palpitation, tachycardia, some decrease in uteroplacental blood flow, increase in heart rate and cardiac output, increase in oxygen consumption, nausea and vomiting	Tachycardia; late decelerations and bradycardia if maternal diastolic pressure >90 mm Hg	Assess for effects of medications, alert woman (family) to expected effects of medications, assess blood pressure frequently because precipitous decrease can lead to shock and perhaps abruptio placentae; assess urinary output; maintain bed rest in a lateral position with side rails up; use with caution in presence of maternal tachycardia
Labetalol Hydrochloride				
β-Blocking agent causing vasodilation without significant change in cardiac output	Peripheral arterioles (see hydralazine)	Minimal: flushing, tremulousness; minimal change in pulse rate	Minimal, if any	See hydralazine; less likely to cause excessive hypotension and tachycardia; less rebound hypertension than hydralazine
Methyldopa (Aldomet)				
Maintenance therapy if needed: 250–500 mg orally every 8 hr (β_2-receptor agonist)	Postganglionic nerve endings: interferes with chemical neurotransmission to reduce peripheral vascular resistance, causes CNS sedation	Sleepiness, postural hypotension, constipation; rare: medication-induced fever in 1% of women and positive Coombs' test result in 20%	After 4 mo maternal therapy, positive Coombs' test result in infant	See hydralazine
Nifedipine				
Calcium channel blocker	Arterioles: to reduce systemic vascular resistance by relaxation of arterial smooth muscle	Headache, flushing; possible potentiation of effects on CNS if administered concurrently with magnesium sulphate, may interfere with labour	Minimal	See hydralazine; use caution if patient also getting magnesium sulphate

CNS, central nervous system.

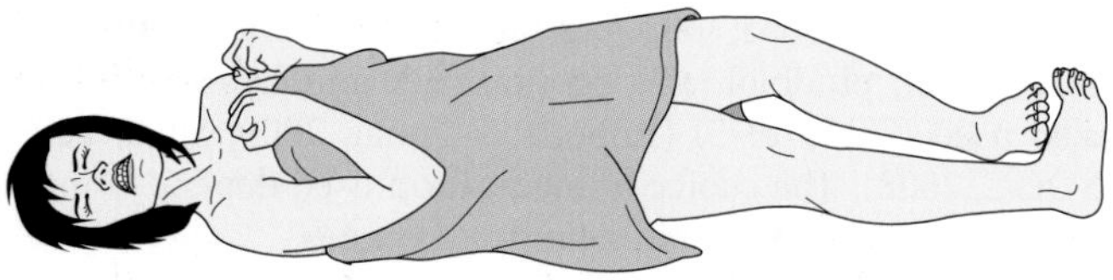

Fig. 13-4 Eclampsia (convulsion or seizure).

and tonic contraction of all body muscles (seen as arms flexed, hands clenched, legs inverted) precede the convulsions (Fig. 13-4). During this stage, muscles alternately relax and contract. Respirations are halted and then begin again with long, deep, stertorous inhalations.

Hypotension and then coma follow. Nystagmus and muscular twitching persist for a time. Disorientation and amnesia cloud the immediate recovery. Seizures may recur within minutes of the first convulsion, or the woman may never have another. During the convulsion, the pregnant woman and fetus are not receiving oxygen; thus eclamptic seizures produce a marked metabolic insult to both the woman and the fetus (Cunningham et al., 2010).

Immediate Care

The immediate goal of care during a convulsion is to ensure a patent airway (see Emergency box). Time, duration, and a description of the convulsions are recorded, and any urinary or fecal incontinence is noted. If possible, the fetus should be monitored for adverse effects; however, this task should not take precedence over other stabilizing care measures. Transient fetal bradycardia and decreased FHR variability are common. Administration of magnesium sulphate is recommended to prevent recurrent seizures. Phenytoin and benzodiazapines should not be used for eclampsia prophylaxis or treatment unless magnesium sulphate is contraindicated (SOGC, 2008).

EMERGENCY

Eclampsia

Tonic–Clonic Convulsion Signs

- Stage of invasion—2 to 3 seconds: eyes are fixed; twitching of facial muscles occurs
- Stage of contraction—15 to 20 seconds: eyes protrude and are bloodshot; all body muscles are in tonic contraction
- Stage of convulsion—Muscles relax and contract alternately (clonic); respirations are halted and then begin again with long, deep, stertorous inhalation; coma ensues

Intervention

- Keep airway patent: turn head to one side, place pillow under one shoulder or back if possible.
- Call for assistance.
- Protect woman from injury during seizure by having padded side rails raised and safely locked.
- Observe and record convulsion activity.

After Convulsion or Seizure

- Do not leave woman unattended until she is fully alert.
- Observe for postconvulsion coma, incontinence.
- Use suction as needed.
- Administer oxygen via face mask at 10 L/min.
- Start intravenous fluids and monitor intake.
- Give magnesium sulphate or anticonvulsant medication as ordered.
- Insert indwelling urinary catheter and monitor hourly output.
- Monitor blood pressure.
- Monitor fetal and uterine status.
- Expedite laboratory work as ordered to monitor kidney function, liver function, coagulation system, and medication levels.
- Provide hygiene and a quiet environment.
- Support woman and family and keep them informed.
- Be prepared to assist with birth when the woman is in stable condition.

A rapid assessment of uterine activity, cervical status, and fetal status should be performed after a convulsion. During the convulsion membranes can rupture, and the cervix can dilate because the uterus becomes hypercontractile and hypertonic; birth may be imminent. If birth is not imminent, once a woman's seizure activity and BP are controlled, a decision should be made regarding whether birth should take place. Since delivery is the definitive cure for the disease, the more serious the condition of the woman, the greater the need to proceed to the birth following the cessation of seizure activity. The means of birth (i.e., induction of labour vs. Caesarean birth) depends on maternal and fetal condition, fetal gestational age, presence of labour, and the cervical Bishop score. If fetal lungs are not mature and the birth can be delayed for 48 hours, steroids such as betamethasone can be given (Crane et al., 2003).

If the woman has been incontinent of urine and stool, or the membranes have ruptured during the convulsion, she will need assistance with hygiene and a change of gown. Oral care with a soft toothbrush may be of comfort.

NURSING ALERT Immediately after a seizure, the woman may be very confused and can be combative. Pad the side rails to prevent injury, and maintain a quiet, darkened environment. It may take several hours for the woman to regain her usual level of mental functioning. She should not be left alone. Provide emotional support to the family and discuss with them the seizure's management, rationale, and the woman's progress.

Laboratory tests should be ordered to assess for HELLP syndrome. Blood is typed and cross-matched for administration of packed red blood cells, as needed. The eclamptic woman is at high risk for abruptio placentae, with accompanying hemorrhage and shock. Other tests to perform include determination of electrolyte levels; liver function; and a complete hemogram and clotting profile, including platelet count and fibrin split product levels (to assess for DIC).

Aspiration is a leading cause of maternal morbidity and mortality after an eclamptic seizure. After initial stabilization and airway management, the nurse should anticipate orders for a chest x-ray film and possibly arterial blood gases to determine whether aspiration occurred.

Postpartum Nursing Care

The nursing care of the woman with hypertensive disease differs in a number of ways from that required in a normal postpartum period. After birth, the symptoms of pre-eclampsia or eclampsia resolve quickly, usually within 48 hours. However, hypertension may persist, and the woman should be monitored from days 3 to 6 after delivery. Resolution of the disease process is manifested by diuresis, which usually occurs within 24 hours after the birth. The hematopoietic and hepatic complications of HELLP syndrome may persist longer. Usually an abrupt decrease in platelet count occurs with a concomitant increase in LDH and AST levels after a trend toward normalization of values has begun. Generally, the laboratory abnormalities seen with HELLP syndrome resolve in 72 to 96 hours.

The woman will need careful assessment of her vital signs, intake and output, DTRs, level of consciousness, uterine tone, and lochia flow throughout the postpartum period. The magnesium sulphate infusion is continued 24 hours for seizure prophylaxis. Even if no convulsions occurred before the birth, they may occur during the postpartum period. The same assessments should continue until the medication is discontinued.

NURSING ALERT The woman is at risk for a boggy uterus and a large lochia flow as a result of the muscle-relaxant effects of magnesium sulphate therapy. Uterine tone and lochial flow must be monitored closely.

The pre-eclamptic woman is usually hemoconcentrated and unable to tolerate excessive postpartum blood loss. Oxytocin or prostaglandin products are used to control bleeding. Ergot products (e.g., ergonovine and methylergonovine) are contraindicated because they increase BP. The woman should be advised to report symptoms such as headaches and blurred vision. The nurse will need to assess affect, level of consciousness, BP, pulse, and respiratory status before an analgesic is given for headache. Magnesium sulphate potentiates the action of narcotics, CNS depressants, and calcium channel blockers; thus these medications must be administered with caution. The woman may need to be restarted on antihypertensive medication if her dBP exceeds 100 mm Hg at discharge.

Postpartum recovery may be prolonged as a result of the physiological consequences of prolonged bed rest. The nurse should accompany the woman when she ambulates after prolonged bed rest and assess for weakness, dizziness, shortness of breath, and muscle soreness. The woman will also need reassurance that the physiological effects of bed rest will reverse over time, when she resumes normal activity (Simpson & James, 2005). Postpartum thromboprophylaxis should be considered for the woman who has been on antenatal bed rest for more than 4 days or who has had a Caesarean section (SOGC, 2008).

The woman's and family's responses to labour or Caesarean section, the birth, and the newborn need to be monitored. Interactions and involvement in the care of the newborn can be encouraged as much as the woman and her family desire. If the pre-eclampsia was severe, the infant may be premature and in a special care nursery. The woman and her family may be worried about their infant's survival, and the day-to-day fluctuations in the infant's status can be emotionally draining (Simpson & James, 2005). In addition, the woman and her family need opportunities to discuss their emotional response to complications. The nurse can provide information concerning the prognosis. While pre-eclampsia and eclampsia do not necessarily recur in subsequent pregnancies (recurrence rate is approximately 30%), prenatal care is essential for assessment and early intervention. If the outcome for the mother or baby is unfavourable, the family should be assisted in coping with loss and grief.

evolve Critical Thinking Exercise—Gestational Diabetes

Gestational Diabetes Mellitus (GDM)

GDM is defined as hyperglycemia that is first recognized during pregnancy, usually during the second half of the pregnancy. In Canada, the prevalence of gestational diabetes is population-specific, varying from 3.7% in the non-Aboriginal population to up to 18% in the First Nations, Métis, and Inuit population (Dyck, Klomp, & Tan, 2002). Women with GDM are at significant risk of developing glucose intolerance later in life; about 50% will be diagnosed as having diabetes within 5 to 10 years. This is especially true of women whose GDM is diagnosed early in pregnancy and who also are obese. Classic risk factors for GDM include maternal age older than 30; obesity; family history of type 2 diabetes; and an obstetrical history of an infant weighing more than 4000 g or of hydramnios, unexplained stillbirth, miscarriage, or an infant with congenital anomalies. Other factors include hypertensive disorders, recurrent monilial vaginitis, and glucosuria on two consecutive visits to the clinic or office (Canadian Diabetes Association [CDA], 2008).

Fetal nutrient demands rise during the late second and third trimesters; maternal nutrient ingestion induces greater and more sustained levels of blood glucose. At the same time, maternal insulin resistance increases as a result of the insulin antagonistic effects of the placental hormones, cortisol and insulinase. Consequently, maternal insulin demands can rise as much as threefold. Most pregnant women are capable of increasing insulin production to compensate for the insulin resistance and maintain euglycemia. When the pancreas is unable to produce sufficient insulin or the insulin is not used effectively, GDM can result (Crowther, Hiller, McPhee, Jeffries, & Robinson, 2005).

Maternal and Fetal Risks

Compared with normal pregnant women, women with GDM have twice the risk of developing hypertensive disorders. They also have increased risk for fetal macrosomia, which can lead to increased rates of perineal lacerations, episiotomy, and Caesarean birth. In addition, fetal macrosomia may be associated with shoulder **dystocia** and birth trauma. GDM also places the neonate at increased risk for **hypoglycemia**, hypocalcemia, **hyperbilirubinemia**, **thrombocytopenia**, **polycythemia**, and respiratory distress syndrome (CDA, 2008).

The overall incidence of congenital anomalies among infants of women with GDM approaches that of the general population because GDM usually develops after week 20 of pregnancy—after the critical period of organogenesis (first trimester) has passed.

Screening for Gestational Diabetes Mellitus

The Canadian Diabetes Association (2008) recommends that all pregnant women be screened for the presence of GDM, although some practitioners still screen on the basis of risk factors. Assessment of relevant history, clinical risk factors, and laboratory screening of blood glucose levels (Fig. 13-5) should be performed. Women with multiple risk factors should be screened in the first trimester to identify **hyperglycemia** early. Low-risk women who are normal-weight women younger than 25 who have no family history of diabetes, are not members of an ethnic or a racial group known to have a high prevalence of the disease, and have no previous history of abnormal glucose tolerance or adverse obstetrical outcomes usually associated with GDM are often not screened (CDA, 2008). Women at high risk for developing GDM should be screened at the first prenatal visit and again at 24 to 28 weeks of gestation (CDA, 2008).

Recent changes in screening criteria for gestational diabetes have occurred as a result of the Hyperglycemia and Adverse Pregnancy Outcomes (HAPO) study (International Association of Diabetes and Pregnancy Study Group Consensus Panel, 2010), which examined maternal and neonatal outcomes in approximately 25,000 women with and without diabetes in pregnancy. The results of the study have informed clinicians' understanding of the relationship between increased plasma glucose and poor perinatal outcomes and have redefined the timing of testing for blood glucose as well as the test that is used. Testing of fasting plasma glucose (FPG) has been found to be easier and more convenient than the oral glucose tolerance test (OGTT).

Nursing diagnoses and expected outcomes of care for the woman with GDM are basically the same as those for women

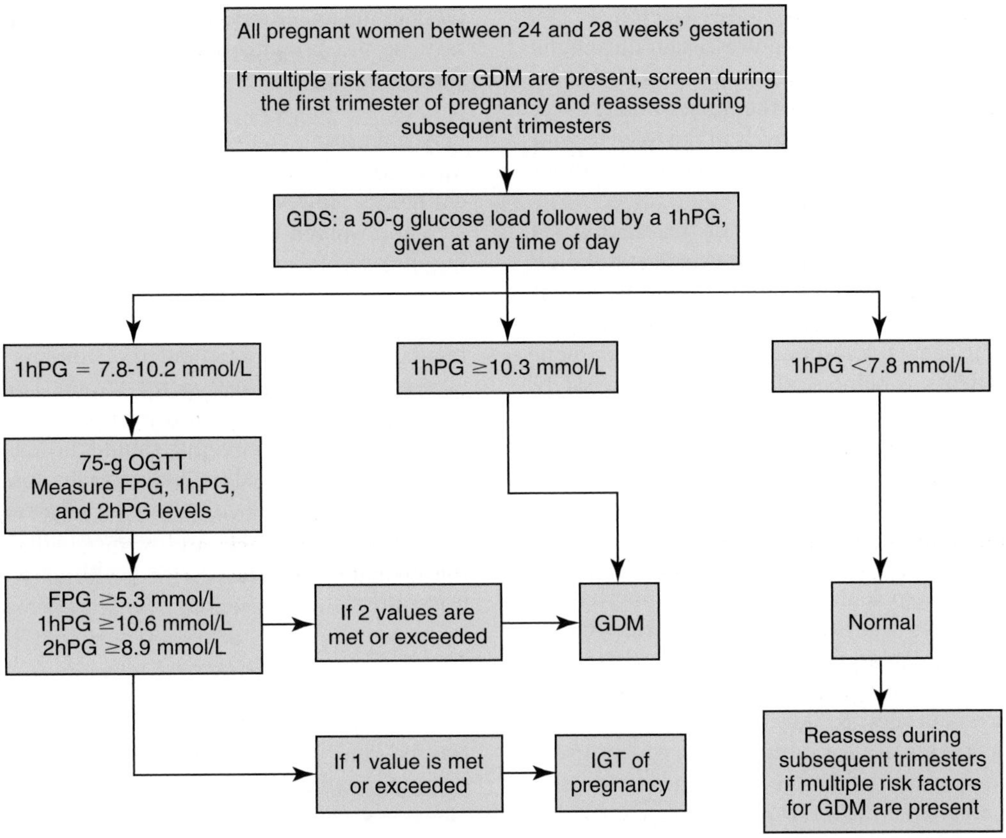

Fig. 13-5 Recommended screening and diagnosis for gestational diabetes. *FPG*, fasting plasma glucose; *GDM*, gestational diabetes mellitus; *GDS*, Gestational Diabetes Screen; *IGT*, impaired glucose test; *OGTT*, oral glucose tolerance test; *1hPG*, 1-hour plasma glucose; *2hPG*, 2-hour plasma glucose. *(From Canadian Diabetes Association. [2008]. Clinical practice guidelines for the prevention and management of diabetes in Canada.* Canadian Journal of Diabetes, *32[Suppl 1], S172.)*

with pregestational diabetes (see Chapter 14); however, the time frame for planning may be shortened with GDM because the diagnosis is usually made later in pregnancy.

Interventions

Antepartum

When the diagnosis of gestational diabetes is made, treatment begins immediately, allowing little or no time for the woman and her family to adjust to the diagnosis before they are expected to participate in the treatment plan. This is in contrast to the woman with pregestational diabetes, who may have had years to learn about the disease and adapt to dietary modifications, self-monitoring of glucose, and insulin administration. With each step of the treatment plan, the nurse and other health care providers should educate the woman and her family, providing detailed and comprehensive explanations to ensure understanding, participation, and compliance with the necessary interventions. Potential complications should be discussed and the need for maintenance of euglycemia throughout the remainder of the pregnancy reinforced. It may be reassuring for the woman and her family to know that GDM typically disappears when the pregnancy is over.

As with pregestational diabetes, the aim of therapy in women with GDM is meticulous blood glucose control. Fasting (preprandial) blood glucose levels should be between 3.8 and 5.2 mmol/L; 1 hour after meals (postprandial) they should be between 5.5 and 7.7 mmol/L; and 2-hour postprandial blood levels should be between 5.0 and 6.6 mmol/L (CDA, 2008).

Diet

Dietary modification is the mainstay of treatment for GDM. The woman with GDM is placed on a standard diabetic diet immediately upon diagnosis. Some authorities recommend fewer calories for overweight or morbidly obese women, believing that such a diet will cause less hyperglycemia and reduce the need for insulin (Landon, Catalano, & Gabbe, 2007). Dietary counselling by a nutritionist is recommended.

Exercise

Exercise in women with GDM appears to be safe. It helps lower blood glucose levels and may be instrumental in eliminating the need for insulin.

Monitoring Blood Glucose Levels

Regular blood glucose monitoring is necessary to determine if euglycemia can be maintained by diet and exercise. Women with GDM are encouraged to perform self-monitoring with blood glucose meters in order to adjust the management plan to achieve near-normal glycemia. Testing may be done at fasting, preprandial, and postprandial times, with values recorded in a log for review by the health care provider.

Insulin Therapy

Up to 20% of women with GDM require insulin during the pregnancy to maintain adequate blood glucose levels, despite compliance with the prescribed diet. The nurse should never assume that increased blood glucose levels in the woman with GDM have been caused by dietary indiscretion alone without first taking a thorough history.

Women who repeatedly exceed glucose thresholds for fasting and 2-hour postprandial values are usually started on insulin therapy. The woman and her family should be taught the necessary skills to manage insulin administration. The use of oral hypoglycemic agents, commonly used in the treatment of nonpregnant patients, is being studied to determine safety for use during pregnancy and the long-term effects of in utero exposure. Glyburide, a second-generation oral hypoglycemic agent, has been shown not to pass through the placenta. Langer and Conway (2000) compared the use of glyburide and insulin in women with GDM. They found similar improvement in maternal glucose levels in both groups. Furthermore, the incidence of fetal macrosomia and neonatal hypoglycemia in the two study groups was similar. Women with higher fasting and postprandial blood sugar values on their oral glucose tolerance test were found less likely to respond to glyburide (Conway, Gonzales, & Skiver, 2004). Even though oral hypoglycemic agents are becoming more widely used, more studies are recommended before they can be endorsed for general use in all women with GDM.

Fetal Surveillance

There is no standard recommendation for fetal surveillance in pregnancies complicated by GDM. Fetuses of women whose blood glucose levels are well controlled by diet are at low risk for fetal death or other fetal sequellae. Routine antepartum fetal testing on these women may not be done as long as their fasting and 2-hour postprandial blood glucose levels remain within normal limits and they have no other risk factors. Usually these women are allowed to progress to term and spontaneous labour without intervention. Once the woman reaches 40 weeks of gestation, fetal surveillance twice weekly is usually instituted (Liston et al., 2007).

Women with GDM whose blood glucose levels are not well controlled or who require insulin therapy, have hypertension, or have a history of previous stillbirth generally receive more intensive fetal biophysical monitoring. There is no standard recommendation regarding initiation of testing. Nonstress tests and biophysical profiles are often performed weekly, beginning from 32 to 36 weeks of gestation (Liston et al., 2007) (see Chapter 12).

Intrapartum

During labour and birth, blood glucose levels are monitored at least every hour to maintain levels at less than 8 mmol/L (CDA, 2008). Glucose levels within this range will decrease the severity of neonatal hypoglycemia. Women whose GDM has been managed on insulin can be controlled by a sliding scale of regular insulin that is titrated to blood sugars during labour. Even though IV fluids containing glucose may be given as maintenance fluids during birth, they should not be given as a bolus to the woman who has GDM. Assessment of routine uterine activity and FHR should be done. Although GDM is not an indication for Caesarean birth, it may be necessary in the presence of obstetrical complications such as macrosomia.

Postpartum

Most women with GDM return to normal glucose levels after childbirth. However, GDM is likely to recur in future pregnancies, and women with GDM are at significant risk of developing glucose intolerance later in life. Assessment for carbohydrate intolerance can be initiated 6 weeks to 6 months postpartum or after breastfeeding has stopped and should be repeated at regular intervals throughout the woman's life (CDA, 2008). Obesity is a major risk factor for the later development of diabetes. Thus women with a history of GDM, particularly those who are overweight, should be encouraged to make lifestyle changes that include weight loss and exercise in order to reduce this risk. Because offspring of women with GDM are at risk of developing obesity and diabetes in childhood or adolescence, regular health care for these children is essential.

Hyperemesis Gravidarum

Nausea and vomiting of pregnancy (NVP) is the most common medical condition in pregnancy, affecting 50 to 90% of women (Ebrahimi, Maltepe, Bournissen, & Koren, 2009; Mazzotti, Maltepe, Navioz, Magee, & Koren, 2000). It most commonly occurs between 4 and 9 weeks of gestation and usually lessens by the sixteenth week of pregnancy. In its extreme form, NVP may manifest as hyperemesis gravidarum (HG), a potentially life-threatening condition affecting 0.5 to 2% of pregnancies. It is characterized by protracted vomiting, retching, severe dehydration, and weight loss requiring hospitalization (Einarson, Maltepe, Boskovic, & Koren, 2007). HG usually begins during the first 10 weeks of pregnancy. It has been associated with women who are nulliparous, have increased body weight, have a history of migraines, or are pregnant with twins or hydatidiform mole (Kelly & Savides, 2009).

Although NVP may be classified as mild, moderate, or severe, the severity of nausea or vomiting may not adequately reflect the distress it causes. Vomiting may lead to dehydration, electrolyte imbalance, ketosis, and acetonuria (Kelly & Savides, 2009). Other causes of nausea and vomiting must be ruled out, including gastrointestinal, genitourinary, central nervous system, and toxic or metabolic problems (Firoz, Maltepe, & Einearson, 2010). In addition, an interrelated psychological component has been associated with hyperemesis and must be assessed (Cunningham et al., 2010; Kelly & Savides, 2009). The effects of HG on perinatal outcome vary with the severity of the disorder (Arseneault, et al., 2002).

Etiology

The etiology of HG is not well understood. Several theories have been proposed, although none of them adequately explains the disorder in all cases. HG may be related to high levels of estrogen or human chorionic gonadotropin (hCG) and associated with transient hyperthyroidism during pregnancy. Some research has found that women who have severe nausea and vomiting have a 1.5-fold increased chance of carrying a female infant, supporting the association between increased estrogen exposure and HG (Cunningham et al., 2010; Kelly & Savides, 2009). Esophageal reflux, reduced gastric motility, and decreased secretion of free hydrochloric acid may contribute to the disorder.

Psychological and social factors can also play a part in the development of HG. Ambivalence toward the pregnancy and increased stress may be associated with this condition (Cunningham et al., 2010; Kelly & Savides, 2009). Women may have to take time away from work, which affects their income and can produce feelings of anxiety (Arseneault, et al., 2002). Conflicting feelings about prospective motherhood, body changes, and lifestyle alterations—all normal reactions to pregnancy—may contribute to episodes of vomiting, particularly if these feelings are excessive or unresolved.

Clinical Manifestations

The woman with hyperemesis may have significant weight loss and symptoms of dehydration such as decreased BP, increased pulse rate, and poor skin turgor (Kelly & Savides, 2009). She is almost always unable to keep down even clear liquids taken by mouth. Laboratory tests may indicate electrolyte imbalances.

Collaborative Care

A thorough assessment to determine the severity of the problem must be completed by the nurse. In most cases, the woman should be examined in person, as the severity of illness is often difficult to determine over the telephone. The frequency, severity, and duration of episodes of nausea and vomiting must be determined. Other symptoms such as diarrhea, indigestion, and abdominal pain or distension should also be identified. Assessment of sleep patterns and disruption due to vomiting is important, as sleep deprivation may contribute to how the woman is coping (Ebrahimi et al., 2009). Prepregnancy weight and documented weight gain or loss during the pregnancy are important baseline data to collect. Any effective pharmacological and nonpharmacological interventions that the woman has used should be noted. The pharmacist and dietitian can play an important role in the care of a woman with hyperemesis.

A complete physical examination, including vital signs, should be performed, with attention to signs of fluid and electrolyte imbalance and nutritional status. A urine dipstick test for ketonuria should be obtained, as ketonuria can indicate the need for IV fluids for dehydration. Other laboratory tests that may be ordered include a urinalysis, CBC, electrolytes, renal and liver function tests, assessment of thyroid function, and bilirubin levels. These tests help rule out the presence of underlying diseases, such as pyelonephritis, pancreatitis, cholecystitis, hepatitis, and thyroid dysfunction (Arseneault, et al., 2002; Kelly & Savides, 2009).

Psychosocial assessment includes asking the woman about anxiety, fears, and concerns related to her own health and the effects on pregnancy outcome. Family members should be assessed for anxiety and in regard to their role in providing support for the woman.

Initial Care

Initially, the woman can manage her symptoms with clear liquids and small, frequent meals. The addition of a multivitamin, taken orally if tolerated, has been shown to improve a woman's status. Doxylamine succinate (Diclectin), an effective and safe treatment for nausea and vomiting in early pregnancy, is a commonly used outpatient medication. The use of alternative therapies such as ginger, acupuncture, and acupressure (see Fig. 11-4) has been shown to be beneficial to some women with nausea and vomiting (Matthews, Dowswell, Haas, Doyle, & O'Mathúna, 2010).

If the woman is unable to maintain clear liquids by mouth, she will require IV therapy for correction of fluid and electrolyte imbalances. In the past, women needing IV therapy were admitted to the hospital. Today they often are successfully managed on an outpatient basis or at home. Anti-emetic medications are introduced if nausea and vomiting are uncontrolled. Dimenhydrinate (Gravol) is given, with the addition of metoclopramide (Maxeran) if dimenhydrinate alone is not effective (Kelly & Savides, 2009). If these medications are not effective for controlling nausea and vomiting, the medication of choice is ondansetron (Zofran) (Cunningham et al., 2010). Methylprednisolone, which is a corticosteroid, may be used to treat refractory HG. Its use in early pregnancy has been associated with the development of cleft lip in fetuses, so it is often a later choice of medication (Arsenault, et al., 2002). For women with severe HG, consultation with gastrointestinal medicine or the administration of total parenteral nutrition (TPN) may need to be considered (Einarson et al., 2007). Some women also benefit from psychotherapy or stress-reduction techniques.

Interventions may include initiating and monitoring IV therapy; administering anti-emetics, antacids, or nutrition supplements; and monitoring the woman's response to interventions. The nurse needs to observe the woman for any signs of complications, such as metabolic acidosis, jaundice, or hemorrhage, and alert the primary care provider should these occur. Monitoring includes assessment of the woman's nausea, retching without vomiting, and vomiting, since the latter two symptoms, although related, are separate. A standardized assessment tool such as the Pregnancy-Unique Quantification of Emesis (PUQE) Scale allows objective quantification of the presence and severity of the nausea and vomiting and enables accurate monitoring (Table 13-6) (Davis, 2004; Ebrahimi et al., 2009). A PUQE score of 13 to 15 indicates severe symptoms; 7 to 12, moderate symptoms; and less than 6, mild symptoms. Treatment should be modified according to the score.

Accurate measurement of intake and output, including the amount of emesis, is an important aspect of nursing care. Oral hygiene while the woman is on nothing-by-mouth status and after episodes of vomiting helps allay associated discomfort. Assistance with positioning and providing a quiet, restful environment that is free from odours may give the woman some comfort. When the woman begins responding to therapy, limited amounts of oral fluids and bland foods such as crackers, toast, or baked chicken are given. The diet is progressed slowly as tolerated by the woman until she is able to consume a nutritionally sound diet. Because sleep disturbances may

Table 13-6 Pregnancy-Unique Quantification of Emesis Scale

Motherisk PUQE-24 Scoring System					
In the last 24 hours, for how long have you felt nauseated or sick to your stomach?	Not at all	1 hour or less	2–3 hours	4–6 hours	More than 6 hours
	(1)	(2)	(3)	(4)	(5)
In the last 24 hours, have you vomited or thrown up?	7 or more times	5–6 times	3–4 times	1–2 times	I did not throw up
	(5)	(4)	(3)	(2)	(1)
In the last 24 hours, how many times have you had retching or dry heaves without bringing anything up?	None	1–2 times	3–4 times	5–6 times	7 or more times
	(1)	(2)	(3)	(4)	(5)

PUQE 24 Score: ☐ Mild = ≤6 ☐ Moderate = 7–12 ☐ Severe = 13–15
(≤ = less than or equal to)
How many hours have you slept out of 24 hours? Why? ____________
On a scale of 0 to 10, how would you rate your well-being? ____________
0 (worst possible) - 10 (The best you felt before pregnancy)
Can you tell me what causes you to feel that way? ____________

(From Ebrahimi, N., Maltepe, C., Bournissen, F. G., & Koren, G. [2009]. Nausea and vomiting of pregnancy: Using the 24-hour Pregnancy-Unique Quantification of Emesis [PUQE-24] Scale. Motherisk Program, Hospital for Sick Children, Toronto. *Journal of Obstetrics and Gynaecology Canada, 31*[9], 803–807.)

accompany HG, adequate rest should be promoted. The nurse can assist in coordinating treatment measures and periods of visitation so that the woman has sufficient rest periods (see Nursing Care Plan).

Follow-Up Care

Most women are able to take nourishment by mouth after several days of treatment. They should be encouraged to eat small, frequent meals consisting of low-fat, high-protein foods; dry, bland foods; and cold foods, and to avoid greasy and highly seasoned foods (Davis, 2004; Sheehan, 2007). A snack before bedtime is also advised. They need to increase their dietary intake of potassium and magnesium. Herbal teas such as ginger, chamomile, and raspberry leaf may decrease nausea (Matthews et al., 2010). Taking fluids between meals rather than with them sometimes helps lessen nausea, as does drinking liquids from a cup with a lid and drinking tea or water with lemon slices (Davis, 2004; Sheehan, 2007). Many pregnant women find that cooking odours can be nauseating; having other family members cook may decrease nausea. Women should be counselled to contact their health care provider immediately if the nausea and vomiting recur, especially if accompanied by abdominal pain, dehydration, or weight loss greater than 2.3 kg in 1 week.

A few women will continue to experience intractable nausea and vomiting throughout pregnancy. Rarely, it is necessary to maintain a woman on enteral, or TPN, to provide adequate nutrition for the mother and fetus. Hospitalization is often required to provide ongoing assessment and care for the woman requiring TPN.

The woman with HG needs calm, compassionate, and sympathetic care, with recognition that the manifestations of hyperemesis can be physically and emotionally debilitating to the woman and stressful for her family. Irritability, tearfulness, and mood changes are often consistent with this disorder. Fetal well-being is a primary concern of the woman. The nurse can provide an environment conducive to discussion of concerns and assist the woman in identifying and mobilizing sources of support. The family should be included in the plan of care whenever possible. Their participation may help alleviate some of the emotional stress associated with this disorder.

Hemorrhagic Disorders

A multidisciplinary approach is warranted to optimize the outcome for both the mother and her fetus when there is bleeding during pregnancy. Maternal blood loss decreases vital oxygen-carrying capacity and places the woman at increased risk for **hypovolemia**, anemia, infection, preterm labour, and preterm birth (Gilbert, 2007). Oxygen delivery to the fetus is compromised. Fetal risks from maternal hemorrhage include blood loss or anemia, hypoxemia, hypoxia, anoxia, and preterm birth.

Hemorrhagic disorders in pregnancy are medical emergencies. The incidence and type of bleeding vary by trimester. In the first trimester, most bleeding is a result of miscarriage and ectopic pregnancy. Approximately 50% of bleeding in the third trimester is caused by placenta previa and abruptio placentae (Gilbert, 2007). Antepartum hemorrhage is a leading cause of maternal death, with ectopic pregnancy rupture, uterine rupture, and abruptio placentae being responsible for most maternal deaths.

With approximately 750 to 1000 mL/min (15% of maternal cardiac output) of blood flow to the uterine vasculature and placenta, disruption of vascular integrity has the potential for maternal exsanguination within 8 to 10 minutes. Prompt, expert teamwork on the part of the health care providers is essential to save the lives of the mother and infant.

Early Pregnancy Bleeding

Bleeding during early pregnancy is alarming to the woman and of concern to health care providers. The common bleeding disorders of early pregnancy include miscarriage, premature dilation of the cervix, ectopic pregnancy, and hydatidiform

NURSING CARE PLAN ● Hyperemesis Gravidarum

Nursing Diagnosis Imbalanced nutrition: less than body requirements related to nausea and persistent vomiting as evidenced by weight decrease as compared with prepregnant weight

Expected Outcomes

Woman will exhibit no further weight losses, and weight will stabilize.

Woman will tolerate regular diet with adequate nutrients for pregnancy with no further nausea and vomiting.

Nursing Interventions/*Rationales*

Ascertain woman's prepregnant weight and monitor her current weight and intake and output *to provide a database for care planning.*

Resume oral diet as tolerated and prescribed by caregiver *to provide oral nutrition at optimal time.*

Provide small, frequent bland meals as woman tolerates *to assess woman's response to limited oral intake.*

Administer anti-emetic and antacid medications as prescribed *to decrease or eliminate episodes of vomiting.*

Provide a quiet, restful environment *to decrease associated discomforts.*

Teach woman the importance of a low-fat, high-protein diet with fluids between meals *to provide optimal nutrition for fetal growth and keep nausea to a minimum.*

Refer to dietitian to develop optimal diet plan individualized to woman's current preferences, culture, and lifestyle *to encourage following the plan.*

Discuss with woman the importance of contacting her health care provider if intractable nausea and vomiting recur *to provide prompt treatment and avoid complications.*

Nursing Diagnosis Deficient fluid volume related to excessive vomiting as evidenced by fluid and electrolyte imbalance

Expected Outcome

Woman's fluid and electrolyte balance will be restored.

Nursing Interventions/*Rationales*

Assess and document skin turgor, condition of mucous membranes, vital signs, and urine specific gravity *to provide database for planning care.*

Obtain daily weight *to provide ongoing evaluation of care.*

Monitor laboratory values and report deviations from normal *to prevent complications.*

Maintain accurate intake and output record *to assess for evidence of fluid deficit.*

Initiate and maintain intravenous therapy carefully *to maintain fluid balance.*

Administer anti-emetics as prescribed *to inhibit nausea and vomiting.*

Begin oral fluids slowly and carefully *to increase tolerance and restore fluid balance.*

Nursing Diagnosis Anxiety related to effects of hyperemesis gravidarum on fetal well-being as evidenced by woman's statements of concern

Expected Outcome

Woman will exhibit decreased anxiety.

Nursing Interventions/*Rationales*

Use therapeutic communication to listen to the woman's concerns *to maintain a relationship and feeling of trust.*

Provide information regarding any potential risks to the fetus *to alleviate anxiety.*

Assist woman to identify personal strengths and previous coping mechanisms *to reinforce to woman the strengths and coping mechanisms that may help her during this illness.*

Help woman identify sources of support and mobilize support person or group of her choice *to provide support as needed.*

Engage social services as needed *for ongoing evaluation and assistance.*

mole (molar pregnancy). Women with advanced maternal age, smoking exposure, and prior preterm birth are more at risk for vaginal bleeding during pregnancy (Yang et al., 2005).

Miscarriage (Spontaneous Abortion)

A pregnancy that ends without medical or surgical method before 20 weeks of gestation or 500-g birth weight is defined as a *miscarriage* or *spontaneous abortion* (Cunningham et al., 2010).

The term *miscarriage* is used throughout this discussion because it is a more appropriate term to use with patients; abortion may be an insensitive term to use with families who are grieving a pregnancy loss. Therapeutic and elective abortion is discussed in Chapter 7.

Incidence and Etiology

Approximately 10 to 15% of all confirmed pregnancies end in miscarriage (Simpson & Jauniaux, 2007). However, the true rate of early pregnancy loss is close to 50% because of the high number of pregnancies that are not recognized in the 2 to 4 weeks after conception. Most of these pregnancy failures are due to **gamete** failure (e.g., sperm or oocyte dysfunction) (Petrozza & Berin, 2011). The risk of spontaneous abortion is increased in obese women (Davies et al., 2010).

An early miscarriage is one that occurs before 12 weeks of gestation. At least 50% of all clinically recognized pregnancy losses result from chromosome abnormalities (Griebel et al., 2005; Petrozza & Berin, 2011). More than 90% of miscarriages occur early, before 8 weeks, and only 2 to 3% occur after 8 weeks of gestation (Simpson & Jauniaux, 2007). Possible causes of early miscarriage include endocrine imbalance (as in women who have luteal-phase defects or insulin-dependent diabetes mellitus with high blood-glucose levels in the first trimester), immunological factors (e.g., antiphospholipid antibodies), infections (e.g., bacteriuria and *Chlamydia trachomatis*), systemic disorders (e.g., lupus erythematosus), and genetic factors (Gilbert, 2007; Simpson & Jauniaux, 2007).

A late miscarriage occurs between 12 and 20 weeks of gestation. It usually results from maternal causes such as advancing maternal age and parity, chronic infections, premature dilation of the cervix and other anomalies of the reproductive tract, chronic debilitating diseases, inadequate nutrition, and recreational drug use (Cunningham et al,. 2010). Little can be done to avoid genetic causes of pregnancy loss, but correction of maternal disorders, immunization against infectious diseases, adequate early prenatal care, and treatment of pregnancy complications can do much to prevent miscarriage.

Clinical Manifestations

Signs and symptoms of miscarriage depend on the duration of the pregnancy. The presence of uterine bleeding, uterine contractions, or back pain is an ominous sign in early pregnancy and must be considered a threatened miscarriage until proven otherwise.

If miscarriage occurs before the sixth week of pregnancy, the woman may report a heavy menstrual flow. Miscarriage that occurs between weeks 6 and 12 of pregnancy causes moderate discomfort and blood loss. A miscarriage that occurs after week 12 is typified by more severe pain, similar to that of labour, because the fetus must be expelled. The types of miscarriage include threatened, inevitable, incomplete, complete, and missed (Fig. 13-6). Diagnosis of the type of miscarriage is based on the signs and symptoms present (Table 13-7).

Symptoms of a *threatened miscarriage* (see Fig. 13-6, A) include spotting of blood with a closed cervical os. Mild uterine cramping may be present.

Inevitable (see Fig. 13-6, B) and *incomplete* (see Fig. 13-6, C) *miscarriages* involve a moderate-to-heavy amount of bleeding with an open cervical os. Tissue may be present with the bleeding. Mild-to-severe uterine cramping may be present. An inevitable miscarriage is often accompanied by rupture of membranes (ROM) and cervical dilation; passage of the products of conception occurs. An incomplete miscarriage involves the expulsion of the fetus with retention of the placenta (Cunningham et al., 2010; Gilbert, 2007).

In a *complete miscarriage* (see Fig. 13-6, D) all fetal tissue is passed, the cervix is closed, and there may be slight bleeding. Mild uterine cramping may be present.

The term *missed miscarriage* (see Fig. 13-6, E) refers to a pregnancy in which the fetus has died but the products of conception are retained in utero for up to several weeks. It may

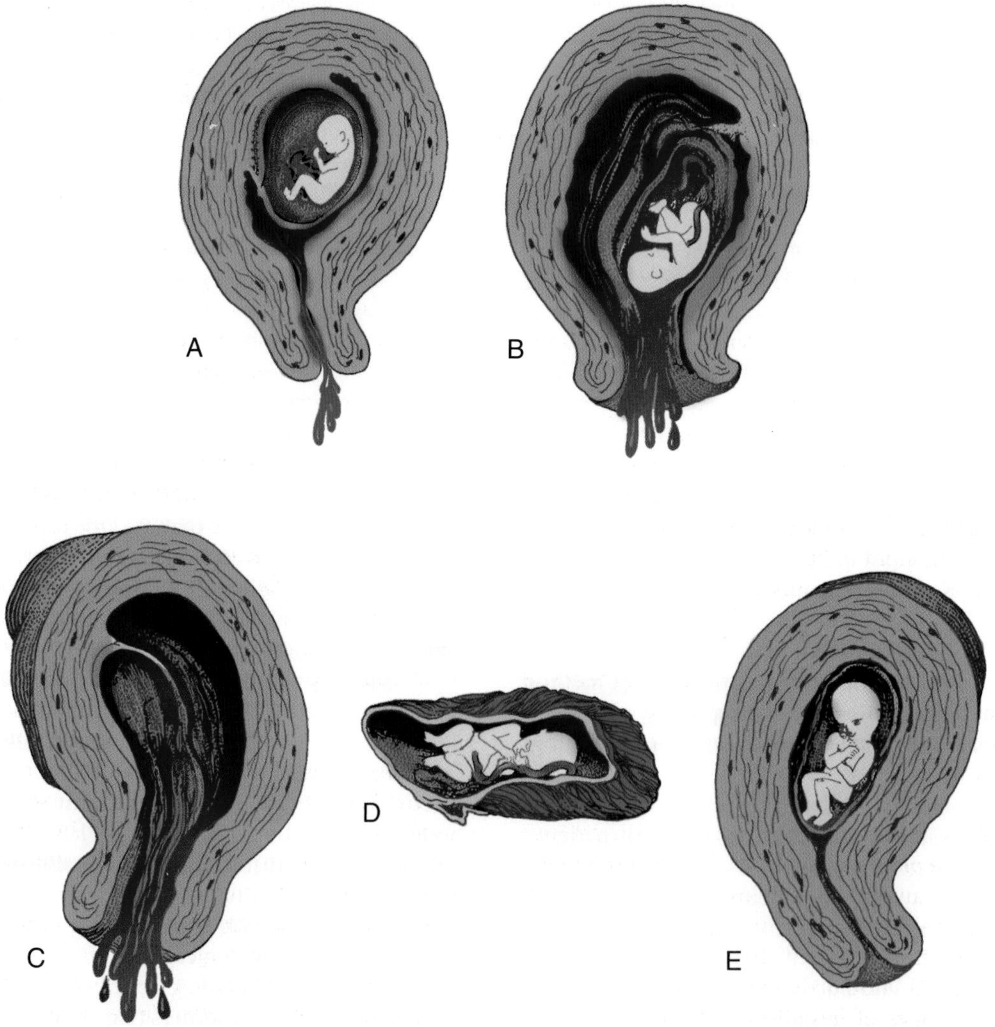

Fig. 13-6 Miscarriage. **A:** Threatened. **B:** Inevitable. **C:** Incomplete. **D:** Complete. **E:** Missed.

Table 13-7 Types of Miscarriage and Usual Management

TYPE OF MISCARRIAGE	AMOUNT OF BLEEDING	UTERINE CRAMPING	PASSAGE OF TISSUE	CERVICAL DILATION	MANAGEMENT
Threatened	Slight, spotting	Mild	No	No	Bed rest, sedation, and avoidance of stress and orgasm usually recommended; further treatment depends on woman's response to treatment
Inevitable	Moderate	Mild to severe	No	Yes	Prompt termination of pregnancy accomplished, usually by dilation and curettage
Incomplete	Heavy, profuse	Severe	Yes	Yes, with tissue in cervix	Prompt termination of pregnancy accomplished, usually by dilation and curettage
Complete	Slight	Mild	Yes	No	May not need further intervention if uterine contractions are adequate to prevent hemorrhage and there is no infection
Missed	None, spotting	None	No	No	If spontaneous evacuation of the uterus does not occur within 1 mo, pregnancy is terminated by method appropriate to duration of pregnancy; blood clotting factors are monitored until uterus is empty; possible DIC and incoagulability of blood with uncontrolled hemorrhage in cases of fetal death after the twelfth week if products of conception are retained for >5 wk
Septic	Varies, usually malodorous	Varies	Varies	Yes, usually	Immediate termination of pregnancy by method appropriate to duration of pregnancy; cervical culture and sensitivity studies done, and broad-spectrum antibiotic therapy (e.g., ampicillin) started; treatment for septic shock initiated if necessary
Recurrent	Varies	Varies	Yes	Yes, usually	Varies, depends on type; prophylactic cerclage may be done if premature cervical dilation is cause

(Adapted from Gilbert, E. S. [2007]. *Manual of high risk pregnancy and delivery* [4th ed.]. St. Louis: Mosby.)
DIC, disseminated intravascular coagulation.

be diagnosed by ultrasonic examination after the uterus stops increasing or even decreases in size. There may be no bleeding or cramping, and the cervical os remains closed.

Habitual miscarriage or recurrent spontaneous abortion is three or more consecutive pregnancy losses before 20 weeks of gestation. The etiology is often unclear but is thought to be multifactorial in nature (Pandey, Rani, & Agrawal, 2005). Women with a history of habitual miscarriage are at increased risk for preterm birth, placenta previa, and fetal anomalies in subsequent pregnancies (Cunningham et al., 2010). Vaginal bleeding, which may be slight to heavy, is usually malodorous. Surgical evacuation is required at this point.

Nursing Care Management

When a woman has vaginal bleeding early in pregnancy, a thorough assessment should be performed (Box 13-6). It is not uncommon for the woman and her family to be anxious and fearful about what may happen to her and to her pregnancy.

Various laboratory findings are characteristic of miscarriage. Evaluation of the placental hormone hCG is used in the diagnosis of pregnancy and pregnancy loss. The hormone can be detected in maternal plasma and urine 8 to 9 days after ovulation if the woman is pregnant. In early pregnancy the concentration of β-hCG should double every 1.4 to 2 days until about 60 or 70 days of gestation (Cunningham et al., 2010). Before 8 weeks of gestation, if miscarriage is suspected, two serum quantitative β-hCG levels are measured 48 hours apart. If a normal pregnancy is present, the β-hCG level doubles within that time. Ultrasonography can then be used to determine the presence of a viable gestational sac. With considerable or persistent blood loss anemia may develop. If infection is present, the white blood cell count is greater than 12×10^9/L. Sedimentation rate is not helpful for differential diagnostic purposes because an increased sedimentation rate occurs with pregnancy, anemia, or infection.

Medical–Surgical Management

Medical management of miscarriage (see Table 13-7) depends on the classification of the miscarriage and on signs and symptoms. Traditionally, threatened miscarriages have been managed with bed rest and supportive care. Follow-up treatment depends on whether the threatened miscarriage progresses to actual miscarriage or symptoms subside and the pregnancy remains intact. **Dilation and curettage (D&C)** is a surgical procedure in which the cervix is dilated and a curette inserted to remove uterine contents. A D&C is commonly used to treat inevitable and incomplete miscarriages. The nurse needs to reinforce explanations, answer any questions or concerns, and prepare the woman for surgery. Women require emotional support during this time of loss, especially if this was a wanted pregnancy.

Dilation and evacuation (D&E), performed after 16 weeks of gestation, consists of wide cervical dilation, followed by instrumental removal of the uterine contents.

BOX 13-6 Assessment of Bleeding in Pregnancy

Initial Database
Chief concern
Vital signs
Number of pregnancies, number of live births
Last menstrual period/estimated date of birth
Pregnancy history (previous and current)
Allergies
Nausea and vomiting
Pain (onset, quality, precipitating event, location)
Bleeding or coagulation problems
Level of consciousness
Emotional status and need for support

Early Pregnancy
Confirmation of pregnancy
Bleeding (bright or dark, intermittent or continuous)
Pain (type, intensity, persistence)
Vaginal discharge

Late Pregnancy
Estimated date of birth
Bleeding (quantity, associated pain)
Vaginal discharge
Amniotic membrane status
Uterine activity
Abdominal pain
Fetal status and viability

Before either surgical procedure is performed, a full history should be obtained, and general and pelvic examinations should be performed. General preoperative and postoperative care is appropriate for the woman requiring surgical intervention. Analgesia and anaesthesia appropriate to the procedure are used.

Outpatient management of first-trimester pregnancy loss may be accomplished with the use of misoprostol (a synthetic prostaglandin E_1 analog) intravaginally for up to 2 days (Moodliar, Bagratee, & Moodley, 2005; Yang et al., 2005) (see Chapter 19, p. 507). There has been no difference in short-term psychological outcomes between expectant and surgical management. If there is evidence of infection, unstable vital signs, or uncontrollable bleeding, a surgical evacuation is performed.

For late incomplete, inevitable, or missed miscarriages (16 to 20 weeks), misoprostol can be given orally or vaginally to induce labour and achieve vaginal delivery of the fetus(s). Prostaglandin (PGE_2) has been used for induction in this patient population; however, the extreme systemic adverse effects of this medication make it a less attractive option. IV oxytocin can also be used after 20 weeks' gestation when myometrial oxytocin binding sites have developed.

Nursing Care

Nursing care is individualized depending on the type of induction (see Chapter 19). Special care may be needed for management of adverse effects of PGE_2 suppositories, such as nausea, vomiting, and diarrhea. If the fetus(es) and placenta are not passed in their entirety, the woman may be prepared for manual or surgical evacuation of the uterus.

After evacuation of the uterus, 10 to 20 units of oxytocin in 1000 mL of fluid can be given to prevent hemorrhage. For excessive bleeding, ergot products such as ergonovine or a prostaglandin derivative such as carboprost tromethamine (hemabate) can be given to contract the uterus. Antibiotics are given as necessary. Analgesics such as ibuprofen may decrease discomfort from cramping. Blood transfusion may be required for shock or anemia. The woman who is Rh negative and has not developed isoimmunization is given an IM injection of Rh immune globulin (Rhogam) within 48 hours of the miscarriage.

Psychosocial aspects of care focus on what the pregnancy loss means to the woman and her family. Grief from perinatal loss is complex and is unique to each individual. Explanations of expected procedures, possible complications, and future implications for childbearing need to be provided. Culturally sensitive education regarding recognition of grief responses and how to manage these responses effectively may prevent adverse outcomes (Van & Meleis, 2003).

As with other fetal or neonatal loss, the woman should be offered the choice of spending time with the fetal remains. Depending on the gestational age of the fetus, hospital disposition of the remains may be offered. If the fetus is over 20 weeks gestation, the woman will need to make arrangements for burial of fetal remains. See Chapter 23 for further discussion on grief and loss.

NURSING ALERT Procedures for disposition of the fetal remains vary according to gestational age from province to province. The nurse should know what the required procedures are in his or her setting.

Home Care

The woman is usually discharged home after delivery or after a D&C when vital signs are stable, vaginal bleeding remains minimal, and she has recovered from anaesthesia. Discharge teaching emphasizes the need for rest. If significant blood loss has occurred, iron supplementation may be ordered. Teaching includes information about normal physical findings such as cramping and type and amount of bleeding, resumption of sexual activity, and family planning. Follow-up care is needed to assess the woman's physical and emotional recovery. Referrals to local support groups or counselling are provided as necessary (see Patient Teaching box).

Follow-up phone calls after a loss are important. The woman may appreciate a phone call on what would have been her due date. These calls provide opportunities for the woman to ask questions, seek advice, and receive information to help process her grief.

Premature Dilation of Cervix

Passive and painless dilation of the cervical os without labour or contractions of the uterus **(incompetent cervix)** may occur in the second trimester or early in the third trimester of pregnancy; miscarriage or preterm birth may result. Iams (2009) refers to this condition as "cervical insufficiency." Current researchers contend that cervical competence is variable and exists as a continuum that is determined in part by cervical length. Other factors include composition of the cervical

PATIENT TEACHING Discharge Teaching After Early Miscarriage

- Advise the woman to report any heavy, profuse, or bright red bleeding to her health care provider.
- Reassure the woman that a scant, dark discharge may persist for 1 to 2 weeks.
- To reduce the risk of infection, remind the woman not to put anything into the vagina for 2 weeks or until bleeding has stopped (e.g., no tampons, no vaginal intercourse). She should take antibiotics as prescribed.
- Advise the woman to eat foods high in iron and protein.
- Acknowledge that the woman has experienced a loss and that she may have mood swings and depression. Talking with her family and seeking support from friends will also help her to deal with her loss.
- Refer the woman to support groups, clergy, or professional counselling, as needed.
- Advise the woman that attempts at pregnancy should be postponed for at least 2 months to allow her body to recover.

(From Gilbert, E. S. [2007]. *Manual of high risk pregnancy and delivery* [4th ed.]. St. Louis: Mosby.)

tissue and the individual circumstances associated with the pregnancy in terms of maternal stress and lifestyle.

Etiology

Etiological factors include a history of cervical trauma, such as lacerations during childbirth or excessive cervical dilation for curettage or biopsy. Other causes are a congenitally short cervix and cervical or uterine anomalies. Reduced cervical competence is a clinical diagnosis based on history. Short labour and recurring loss of the pregnancy at progressively earlier gestational ages are characteristics of reduced cervical competence. Transvaginal ultrasound examination is used to diagnose this condition objectively. A short cervix (less than 25 mm in length) is indicative of reduced cervical competence. Often, but not always, the short cervix is accompanied by cervical funneling (beaking) or effacement of the internal cervical os (Iams & Romero, 2007; Rust et al., 2005).

Collaborative Care

Medical–Surgical Management

Conservative management consists of restricted activity, and hydration. Tocolytics are not required as the woman is not experiencing contractions. A cervical cerclage such as a Shirodkar or McDonald procedure may be performed. In the Shirodkar, maternal fascia lata is threaded submucosally in the cervix anteriorly and posteriorly and tied. In the McDonald cerclage, nonabsorbable ribbon (Mersilene) is placed around the cervix beneath the mucosa to constrict the internal os of the cervix (Fig. 13-7). A cerclage procedure can be classified according to time or whether it is elective (prophylactic), urgent, or emergent (Rust & Roberts, 2005).

Prophylactic cerclage is placed at diagnosis of the shortened or dilating cervix. The woman should refrain from intercourse, prolonged (i.e., more than 90 minutes) standing, and heavy lifting (Iams, 2009). She is monitored during the rest of her pregnancy with transvaginal ultrasound scans to assess for cervical shortening and funneling. The **cerclage** is electively removed (usually an office or a clinic procedure) when the woman reaches 35 to 37 weeks of gestation, or it may be left in place, and a Caesarean birth performed. Approximately 80 to 90% of pregnancies treated with cerclage result in live, viable births. A woman whose reduced cervical competence is diagnosed during the current pregnancy may undergo emergency cerclage placement. Risks of the procedure include premature rupture of membranes (PROM), preterm labour, and chorioamnionitis. Cerclage is rarely performed after 25 weeks of gestation (Iams, 2009).

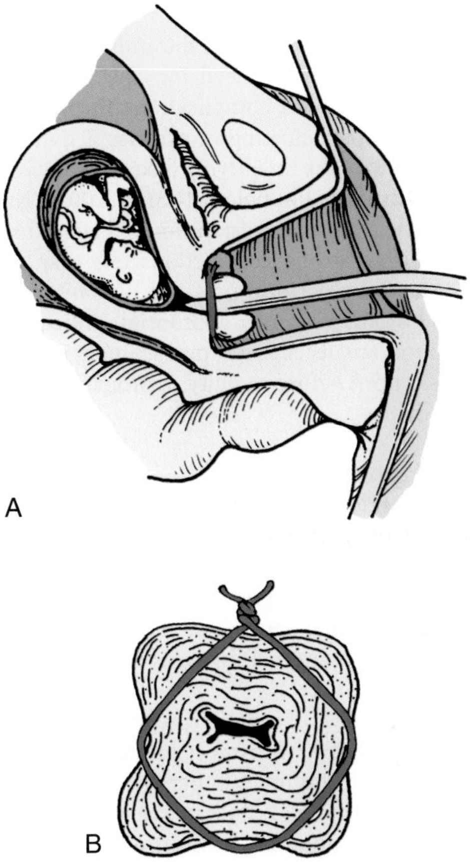

Fig. 13-7 **A:** Cerclage correction of recurrent premature dilation of cervix. **B:** Cross section of closed internal os.

Nursing Care

The nurse needs to assess the woman's feelings about her pregnancy and her understanding of the risk for preterm birth. The woman may feel guilty or feel she is to blame for the threat to her pregnancy. Therefore, it is important to evaluate the woman's support systems. She needs the support of her family, as well as that of health care providers.

If a cervical cerclage has been performed, the nurse will monitor the woman after surgery for the presence of uterine contractions, PROM, and signs of infection. Discharge teaching focuses on continued monitoring of these aspects at home. Home follow-up may be provided by nurses through antepartum home care programs.

Home Care

The woman must understand the importance of activity restriction at home and the need for close observation and supervision. Women with complications in pregnancies are discouraged from participating in exercise activities as exercise could exacerbate the underlying disorder (SOGC & Canadian Society of Exercise Physiology [CSEP], 2003). The woman should know the signs that warrant immediate transfer to the hospital, including strong contractions less than 5 minutes apart, PROM, severe perineal pressure, and an urge to push. If the fetus is born prematurely, appropriate anticipatory guidance and support are necessary. If management is unsuccessful and the fetus is born before viability, appropriate grief support should be provided.

Ectopic Pregnancy

Incidence and Etiology

An *ectopic pregnancy* is one in which the fertilized ovum is implanted outside the uterine cavity (Fig. 13-8). It accounts for 1:7000 to 1:30 000 of spontaneously conceived pregnancies (Morin, et al., 2005; Sepilian et al., 2011). The frequency is consistent across maternal age ranges and ethnic origins (Murray et al., 2005).

Approximately 95% of ectopic pregnancies occur in the uterine (fallopian) tube, with most located on the ampullar or largest portion of the tube. Other sites include the ovary (0.5%), abdominal cavity (1.5%), and cervix (0.3%) (Gilbert, 2007). Ectopic pregnancy is classified according to the site of implantation (e.g., tubal, ovarian). The uterus is the only organ capable of containing and sustaining a term pregnancy. However, 5 to 25% of abdominal pregnancies with birth by laparotomy may result in a living infant (Fig. 13-9). The risk of anomaly in these infants is as high as 40% (Gilbert, 2007).

Ectopic pregnancy is responsible for 9% of pregnancy-related deaths and is the leading cause of infertility (Sepilian et al., 2011). Women who have been treated surgically for ectopic pregnancy have a subsequent intrauterine pregnancy rate of 50 to 80%; the recurrent ectopic pregnancy rate is up to 10 to 25%. Women treated with methotrexate have an intrauterine pregnancy rate of 64%; the recurrent ectopic pregnancy rate is approximately 11% (Sepilian et al., 2011).

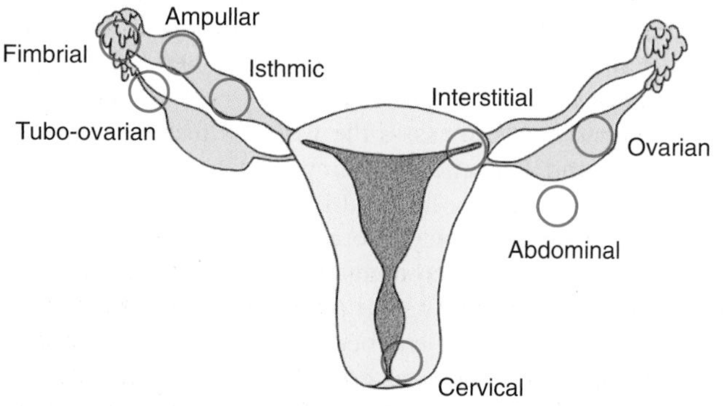

Fig. 13-8 Sites of implantation of ectopic pregnancies. Order of frequency of occurrence is ampullar, isthmic, interstitial, fimbrial, tubo-ovarian ligament, ovarian, abdominal cavity, and cervical (external os).

The reported incidence of ectopic pregnancy is rising as a result of improved diagnostic techniques, such as more sensitive β-hCG assays and the availability of transvaginal ultrasound (Morin, et al., 2005). An increased incidence of sexually transmitted infections (STIs), better treatment of pelvic inflammatory disease (which formerly would have caused sterility), increased numbers of tubal sterilizations, and surgical reversal of tubal sterilizations also have resulted in more ectopic pregnancies (Sepilian et al., 2011).

Clinical Manifestations

A missed menstrual period, adnexal fullness, and tenderness may suggest an unruptured tubal pregnancy. The tenderness can progress from a dull to colicky pain when the tube stretches. Pain may be unilateral, bilateral, or diffuse over the abdomen. Dark red or brown abnormal vaginal bleeding occurs in 50 to 80% of women. The normal doubling of serum levels of β-hCG over 48 hours supports a diagnosis of fetal viability but does not rule out ectopic pregnancy, and a rising β-hCG concentration that plateaus or does not reach 50% may suggest a failing or ectopic pregnancy. Falling levels confirm nonviability but do not rule out ectopic pregnancy (Murray et al., 2005). If the ectopic pregnancy ruptures, pain increases. It may be generalized, unilateral, or acute deep lower quadrant pain caused by blood irritating the peritoneum. Referred shoulder pain can occur from diaphragmatic irritation caused by blood in the peritoneal cavity. The woman may exhibit signs of shock related to the amount of bleeding in the abdominal cavity and not necessarily to obvious vaginal bleeding. An ecchymotic blueness around the umbilicus (Cullen sign), indicating hematoperitoneum, may develop in an undiagnosed, ruptured intra-abdominal ectopic pregnancy.

Collaborative Care

The differential diagnosis of ectopic pregnancy involves consideration of numerous disorders that share many signs and

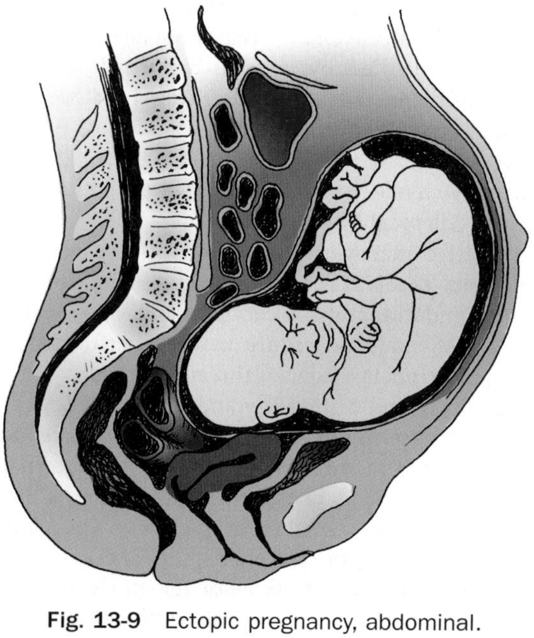

Fig. 13-9 Ectopic pregnancy, abdominal.

symptoms. Many of these women present to the emergency department experiencing first-trimester bleeding or pain. Miscarriage, ruptured corpus luteum cyst, appendicitis, salpingitis, ovarian cysts, torsion of the ovary, and urinary tract infection must be considered. The key to early detection of ectopic pregnancy is having a high index of suspicion for this condition. Any woman with complaints of abdominal pain, vaginal spotting or bleeding, and a positive pregnancy test should undergo screening for ectopic pregnancy.

Laboratory screening includes determination of serum progesterone and β-hCG levels. If either of these values is lower than would be expected for a normal pregnancy, the woman should be asked to return within 48 hours for serial measurements. Transvaginal ultrasonography is done to confirm intrauterine or tubal pregnancy (Morin, et al., 2005; Murray et al., 2005; Sepilian et al., 2011). Ultrasonographic identification of an intrauterine pregnancy (gestational sac plus yolk sac) rules out ectopic pregnancy in most women.

The woman should be assessed for the presence of active bleeding, which is associated with tubal rupture. If internal bleeding is present, the woman may have vertigo, shoulder pain, hypotension, and tachycardia. A vaginal examination should be performed only once, and then with great caution. Approximately half of women with tubal pregnancies have a palpable mass on examination. It is possible to rupture the mass during a bimanual examination; thus gentleness is critical.

Treatment Options

Ectopic pregnancy can resolve spontaneously by tubal abortion or regression of the pregnancy from the tube. However, about 90% of women with ectopic pregnancy and high serum β-hCG levels (greater than 2000 IU/L) require surgical intervention (Murray et al., 2005).

Surgical removal of the ectopic pregnancy by salpingotomy is possible before rupture. Ideally, the procedure is performed laparoscopically to improve maternal recovery, shorten hospitalization, and reduce morbidity from laparotomy (Murray et al., 2005).

Medical management of ectopic pregnancy is with administration of methotrexate, which is an antimetabolite and folic acid antagonist that destroys rapidly dividing cells. It may be used in a single-dose IM injection to treat unruptured pregnancies. It has been shown to produce results similar to those of surgical therapy in terms of high success rate, low complication rate, and good reproductive potential (Murray et al., 2005; Sepilian et al., 2011) (see Medication Guide).

NURSING ALERT Women receiving methotrexate should refrain from taking any analgesic stronger than acetaminophen. Stronger analgesics can mask symptoms of tubal rupture.

Advanced ectopic abdominal pregnancy requires laparotomy as soon as the woman has been stabilized for surgery. If the placenta of a second- or third-trimester abdominal pregnancy is attached to a vital organ such as the liver, separation and removal are usually not attempted because of risk of hemorrhage. The cord is cut flush with the placenta, and the abdomen is closed, leaving the placenta in place. Degeneration and absorption of the placenta usually occur without complication, although infection and intestinal obstruction may occur. Methotrexate may be given to dissolve the residual tissue (Gilbert, 2007; Murray et al., 2005).

MEDICATION GUIDE

Methotrexate

Action

Decreases action of dihydrofolic acid reductase enzyme, which stops growth of actively proliferating tissue such as a tumour or fetus; immunosuppressant

Indication

Ectopic pregnancy, rheumatic conditions, psoriasis, chemotherapy

Pretreatment Investigations

- CBC, blood group typing and antibody screen
- Liver and renal function tests
- Serum β-hCG levels
- Transvaginal ultrasound

Dose

- 50 mg/m^2 intramuscularly: may repeat in 1 week if decrease in β-hCG is less than 25%
- Administer Rh immune globulin 300 mcg, as needed

Adverse Reactions

Thrombocytopenia and other blood-related disorders, neurotoxicity, nausea and vomiting, fever, dizziness, diarrhea, pruritus

Nursing Considerations

Provide grief support for loss of pregnancy. Counsel woman to report increased abdominal pain, which could indicate tubal rupture. Follow-up care is needed until β-hCG levels are nondetectable. If methotrexate treatment fails, surgical intervention may be necessary.

Hospital Care

If surgery is planned for the woman with an ectopic pregnancy, general preoperative and postoperative care is appropriate. Vital signs (pulse, respirations, and BP) are assessed before surgery every 15 minutes or as needed, based on the severity of the bleeding and the woman's condition. Preoperative laboratory tests include determination of blood type and Rh factor, CBC, and serum quantitative β-hCG assay. Ultrasonography is used to confirm an extrauterine pregnancy. Blood replacement may be necessary. The nurse will verify the woman's Rh and antibody status and administer $Rh_o(D)$ immune globulin, if appropriate. The woman should be encouraged to express her feelings related to the loss. Referral to community resources may be appropriate.

Home Care

Some women can be treated on an outpatient basis if they meet certain criteria. Hemodynamically stable women with ectopic pregnancies are eligible for methotrexate therapy if the mass is unruptured and measures less than 3.5 cm in diameter by ultrasonography, there is no fetal cardiac activity noted on the ultrasound scan, the serum β-hCG level is less than 5000 IU/mL, there is no free fluid in the cul-de-sac (which indicates possible tubal rupture), and the woman is willing to comply with post-treatment monitoring (Murray et al., 2005;

Sepilian et al., 2011). Methotrexate therapy avoids surgery and is a safe and effective way of managing many cases of tubal pregnancy. The woman should be informed about how the medication works, what adverse effects are possible, whom to call if she has concerns or if problems develop, and the importance of follow-up care (see Patient Teaching box).

NURSING ALERT The woman receiving methotrexate therapy who drinks alcohol and takes vitamins containing folic acid (e.g., prenatal vitamins) increases her risk of having medication adverse effects or of exacerbating the ectopic rupture.

Future fertility should be discussed. Any woman who has had an ectopic pregnancy should be told to contact her health care provider as soon as she suspects that she might be pregnant, because of the increased risk for recurrent ectopic pregnancy. These women may need referral to grief or infertility support groups. In addition to the loss of the current pregnancy, they are faced with the possibility of future pregnancy losses and infertility.

Gestational Trophoblastic Disease

Gestational trophoblastic disease (GTD) includes disorders that arise from the placental trophoblast. It includes hydatidiform mole, invasive mole, and choriocarcinoma. *Gestational trophoblastic neoplasia* (GTN) refers to persistent trophoblastic tissue that is presumed to be malignant (Gilbert, 2007). Once almost invariably fatal, the treatment has progressed until today when GTN is the most curable gynecological malignancy.

Hydatidiform Mole

Hydatidiform mole (molar pregnancy) is a GTD. There are two distinct types: complete (or classic) mole and partial mole.

Incidence and Etiology

Hydatidiform mole occurs in 1 in 1000 pregnancies (Cohn, Ramaswamy, & Blum, 2009). The etiology is unknown, although there may be an ovular defect or nutrition deficiency. Women at higher risk for hydatidiform mole are those in their early teens or over age 40 or who have undergone ovulation stimulation with clomiphene (Clomid). The risk of developing a second mole is 1 to 2%.

Types

The complete mole results from fertilization of an egg, the nucleus of which has been lost or inactivated. The nucleus of a sperm (23,X) duplicates itself (resulting in the diploid number, 46,XX) because the ovum has no genetic material or the material is inactive. The mole resembles a bunch of white grapes (Fig. 13-10). The hydropic (fluid-filled) vesicles grow rapidly, causing the uterus to be larger than expected for the duration of the pregnancy. Usually the complete mole contains no fetus, placenta, amniotic membranes, or fluid. Maternal blood has no placenta to receive it; therefore, hemorrhage into the uterine cavity and vaginal bleeding occur. In about 20% of complete moles, progression toward choriocarcinoma occurs.

For a partial mole, chromosome studies often show a karyotype of 69,XXY; 69,XXX; or 69,XYY. This occurs as a result of two sperm fertilizing an apparently normal ovum. Partial moles often have embryonic or fetal parts and an amniotic sac. Congenital anomalies are usually present. The potential for malignant transformation is less than 6% (Copeland & Landon, 2007).

Clinical Manifestations

In the early stages, the clinical manifestations of a complete hydatidiform mole cannot be distinguished from normal pregnancy. Vaginal bleeding occurs in almost 95% of patients.

> **PATIENT TEACHING** Methotrexate for Ectopic Pregnancy
>
> - Keep all appointments (2 to 8 weeks).
> - Report any vaginal bleeding or abdominal pain.
> - Do not take any vitamins or folic acid.
> - Do not drink any alcohol.
> - Avoid prolonged sun exposure.
> - Avoid gas-forming foods.
> - Put nothing in the vagina (i.e., no tampons, douches, or intercourse). Do not take any analgesics stronger than acetaminophen.

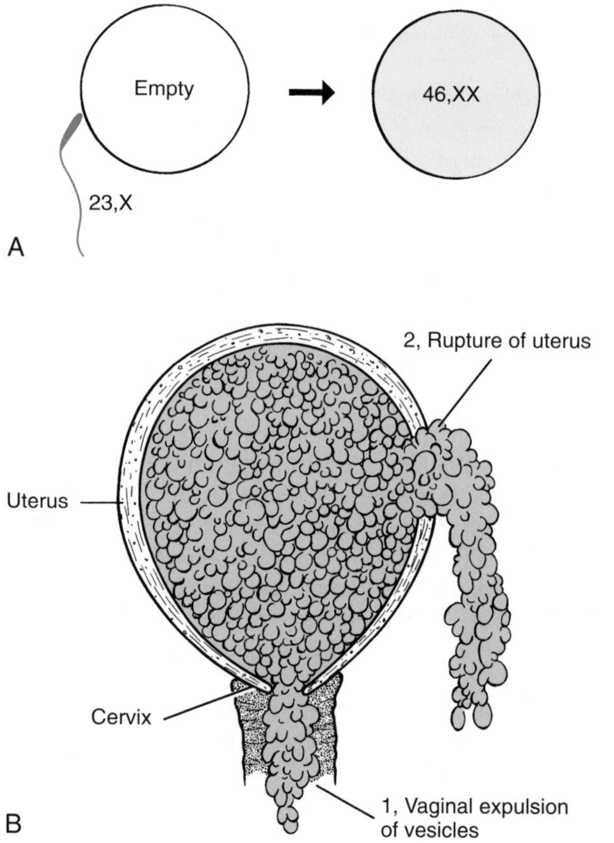

Fig. 13-10 **A:** Chromosome origin of complete mole. Single sperm (in colour) fertilizes an "empty" ovum. Reduplication of sperm's 23,X set gives completely homozygous diploid 46,XX. Similar process follows fertilization of empty ovum by two sperm with two independently drawn sets of 23,X or 23,Y; both karyotypes of 46,XX and 46,YY can therefore result. **B:** Uterine rupture with hydatidiform mole. *1,* Evacuation of mole through cervix. *2,* Rupture of uterus and spillage of mole into peritoneal cavity (rare).

The vaginal discharge may be dark brown (resembling prune juice) or bright red and either scant or profuse. It may continue for only a few days or intermittently for weeks. In early pregnancy, in about half of affected women the uterus is significantly larger than expected from menstrual dates.

Anemia from blood loss, excessive nausea and vomiting (hyperemesis gravidarum), and abdominal cramps caused by uterine distension are relatively common findings (Arseneault, et al., 2002). Pre-eclampsia occurs in about 15% of cases (usually between 9 and 12 weeks of gestation), but any symptoms of gestational hypertension before 24 weeks of gestation may suggest hydatidiform mole. Hyperthyroidism and pulmonary embolization of trophoblastic elements occur less commonly but are serious complications of hydatidiform mole. Partial mole causes few of these symptoms and may be mistaken for an incomplete or a missed miscarriage.

Collaborative Care

Medical–Surgical Management. Although most moles pass spontaneously, suction curettage offers a safe, rapid, and effective method of evacuating a hydatidiform mole, if necessary (Copeland & Landon, 2007). An alternative management plan for a woman who desires sterilization is hysterectomy. The use of **oxytocic** agents or prostaglandins is not recommended because of the increased risk of embolization of trophoblastic tissue (Copeland & Landon, 2007). Administration of Rh_o(D) immune globulin to women who are Rh negative is needed to prevent isoimmunization.

Nursing Care. Nursing assessments during prenatal visits should include observation for signs of molar pregnancy during the first 24 weeks. If hydatidiform mole is suspected, ultrasonography and serial β-hCG immunoassays are used to confirm the diagnosis. The sonographic pattern of a molar pregnancy is characterized by a diffuse snowstorm appearance. The β-hCG titre remains high or rises above the normal peak after the time it normally drops (i.e., 70 to 100 days).

The nurse needs to provide the woman and her family with information about the disease process, the necessity of a long course of follow-up, and the possible consequences of the disease. The nurse can help the woman understand and cope with pregnancy loss and recognize that the pregnancy was abnormal. The woman and her family should be encouraged to express their feelings, and information about support groups or counselling resources should be provided, if needed. The importance of contraceptive counselling and the need to postpone a subsequent pregnancy should also be conveyed.

NURSING ALERT To avoid confusing the signs of choriocarcinoma with the signs of pregnancy, pregnancy should be avoided for 1 year. Any contraceptive method, except the intrauterine device, is acceptable. Oral contraceptives are highly effective.

Home Care. Follow-up management includes frequent physical and pelvic examinations along with measurement of serum β-hCG until the level drops to normal and remains normal for 3 weeks. Monthly measurements are usually taken for a year (Gilbert, 2007). A rising titre and an enlarging uterus may indicate choriocarcinoma. Women with a complete hydatidiform molar pregnancy are at a 15 to 28% risk of requiring further management with chemotherapy for persistent trophoblastic disease (Wolfberg et al., 2005).

Gestational Trophoblastic Neoplasia

These types of tumours are classified as nonmetastatic, metastatic low risk, and metastatic high risk. After the evacuation of a hydatidiform molar pregnancy, approximately 20% of women are treated for malignancy. Almost 50% of these tumours occur after a hydatidiform mole. Approximately 30% follow an ectopic pregnancy or miscarriage, and 20% occur after an apparently normal birth at term. There is an almost 100% cure rate after nonmetastatic and low-risk metastatic GTN. Common sites of metastasis are the lungs, vagina, vulva/cervix, liver, and brain (Copeland & Landon, 2007). There is a 20% risk of maternal death after high-risk metastatic GTN.

Continued bleeding after evacuation of a hydatidiform mole is usually the most suggestive symptom of GTN. Other clinical signs include abdominal pain and uterine and ovarian enlargement. Signs of metastasis include pulmonary symptoms (e.g., dyspnea, cough). The diagnosis is usually confirmed by increasing or plateauing hCG levels after evacuation of a molar pregnancy. Once diagnosis is confirmed, other clinical studies (e.g., computed tomography scan of lungs and brain, chest x-ray, pelvic ultrasound, and liver scan) are done to determine the extent of the disease.

Single-agent chemotherapy is usually effective. Methotrexate has been the treatment of choice (see Medication Guide, p. 319). Hysterectomy with adjuvant chemotherapy is often the choice of treatment for nonmetastatic tumours in women who have completed their childbearing.

Therapy is continued until negative hCG levels are obtained. Follow-up after successful chemotherapy is by serum hCG levels obtained every month for a year (Gilbert, 2007). Physical examinations are done at least annually, and chest x-rays are done if indicated. Contraception is needed until the woman has been in remission for at least 6 months. Oral contraceptives are preferred, but barrier methods are acceptable if oral contraceptives are contraindicated. During a subsequent pregnancy, pelvic ultrasonography is recommended because the woman is at higher risk to develop another molar pregnancy. Serum hCG levels should be obtained 6 weeks after the birth.

Late Pregnancy Bleeding

Late pregnancy bleeding disorders include placenta previa, premature separation of placenta (**abruptio placentae**), and variations in the insertion of the cord and the placenta (Fig. 13-11). When a woman presents with bleeding in pregnancy, expedient assessment for and diagnosis of the cause of bleeding are essential to reduce the risk of maternal and perinatal morbidity and mortality.

Placenta Previa

Placenta previa is defined as a placenta implanted in the lower segment of the uterus, presenting ahead of the fetus. It occurs in 2.8/1000 singleton pregnancies and 3.9/1000 twin pregnancies and represents a significant clinical problem because the woman may require hospitalization for observation, she may require blood transfusion, and she is at risk for premature

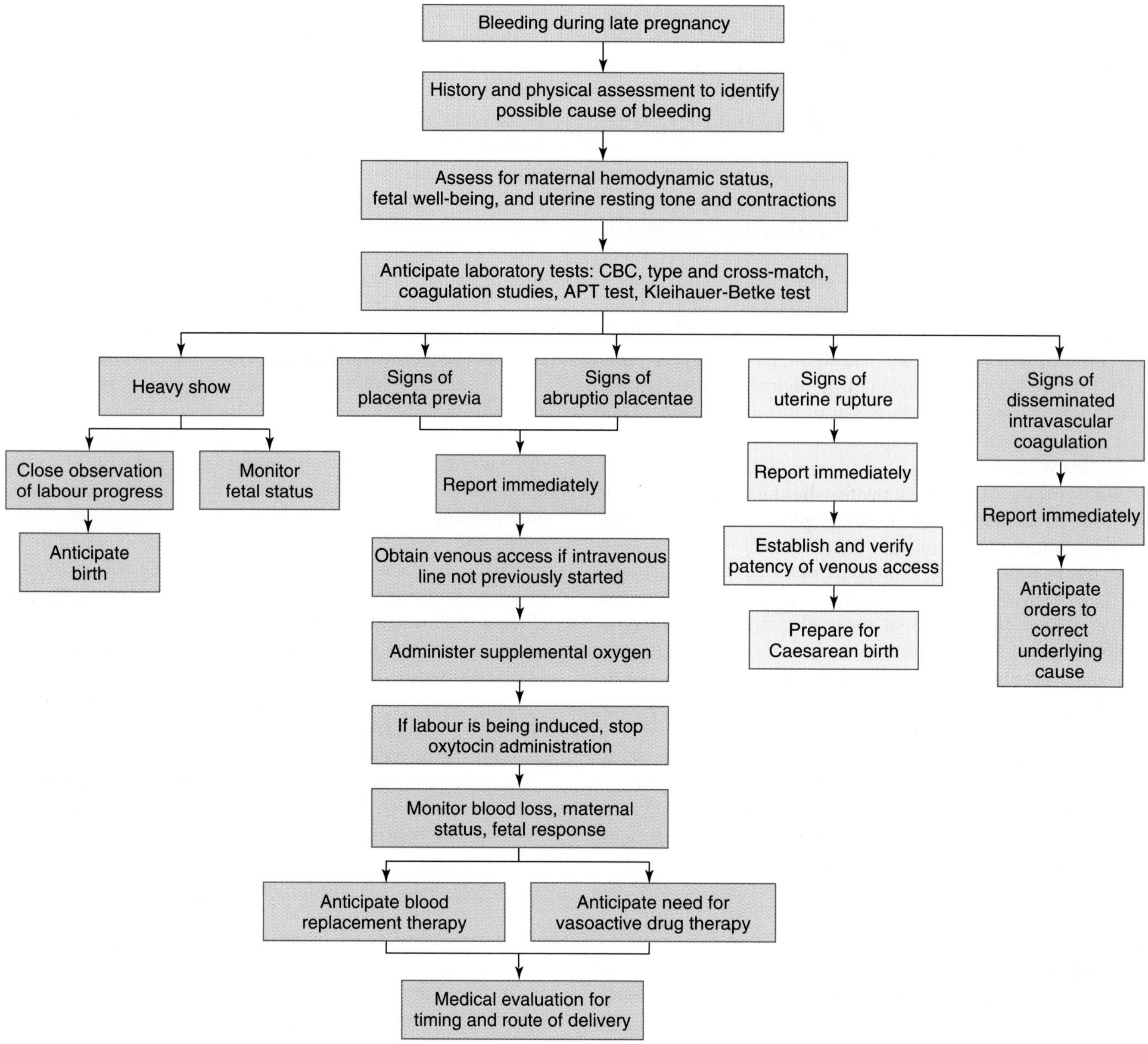

Fig. 13-11 Bleeding during late pregnancy. *CBC,* complete blood count.

delivery. In placenta previa, the placenta is implanted in the lower uterine segment near or over the internal cervical os. The degree to which the internal cervical os is covered by the placenta has traditionally been used to classify three types of placenta previa (Fig. 13-12). Placenta previa often is described as *complete, total,* or *central* if the internal os is entirely covered by the placenta. *Partial* placenta previa implies incomplete coverage of the internal os. *Marginal* placenta previa indicates that only an edge of the placenta extends to the internal os, but it may extend onto the os during dilation of the cervix during labour. The term *low-lying placenta* is used when the placenta is implanted in the lower uterine segment but does not reach the os.

Recent advances in sonographic diagnosis and a better understanding of the changing relationship of the internal cervical os and the placenta as pregnancy progresses have made these traditional definitions and classifications obsolete (Oppenheimer et al., 2007). Sonographers should report the actual distance from the placental edge to the internal cervical os by means of transvaginal sonography (TVS), using standard terminology of millimetres away from the os or millimetres of overlap. A placental edge exactly reaching the internal os is described as 0 mm. When the placental edge reaches or overlaps the internal cervical os on TVS between 18 and 24 weeks' gestation (incidence 2 to 4%), a follow-up examination for placental location in the third trimester is recommended. Overlap of more than 15 mm is associated with an increased likelihood of placenta previa at term (Oppenheimer et al., 2007). If the placenta implants in the lower uterine segment, a diagnosis of placenta previa may be made in the second trimester. However, as uterine growth continues throughout gestation, the placenta will usually migrate from the os toward the **fundus**, and the lower uterine segment will develop (Hull & Resnik, 2009; Oppenheimer

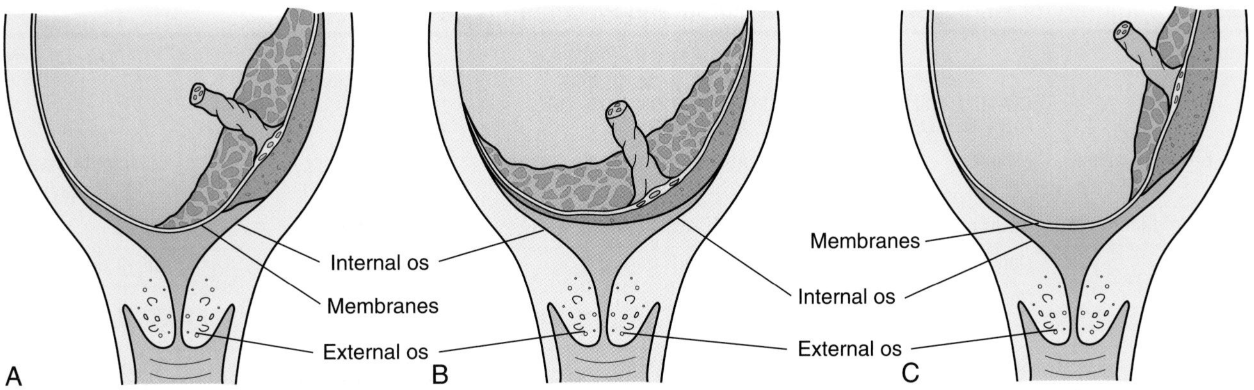

Fig. 13-12 Types of placenta previa. **A:** Low-lying placenta in second trimester. **B:** Placenta previa. **C:** Marginal placenta previa.

et al., 2007). The presence of placenta previa during the second trimester is a risk factor for the development of vasa previa. An alternative way to classify placenta previa is complete placenta previa (in the third trimester the placenta covers the internal os) and marginal placenta previa (the distance of the placenta is 2 to 3 cm from the internal os and does not cover it). When the exact relationship of the os to the placenta has not been determined or in cases of apparent placenta previa in the second trimester, the term *low-lying placenta* can be used (Hull & Resnik, 2009) (see Fig. 13-12).

Incidence and Etiology

The incidence of placenta previa is approximately 0.5% of births. The most important risk factors are previous placenta previa, previous Caesarean birth, and suction curettage for miscarriage or induced abortion, possibly related to endometrial scarring (see Critical Thinking Exercise). The association between prior Caesarean section, placenta previa, and placenta accreta (pathological adherence of the placenta) is well recognized. The incidence of placenta previa increases with the number of prior Caesarean sections, and the incidence of placenta previa seems to be on the rise because of the increasing rate of Caesarean sections. The risk also increases with multiple gestation (because of the larger placental area), multiparity, maternal age over 35 years, Black or Asian ethnicity, and smoking (Hull & Resnik, 2009).

Clinical Manifestations

Approximately 70% of women with placenta previa have painless uterine bleeding; 20% have vaginal bleeding associated with uterine activity. Previa should be suspected whenever vaginal bleeding occurs after 20 weeks of gestation. The bleeding is associated with the stretching and thinning of the lower uterine segment that occurs during the third trimester. Placental attachment is gradually disrupted, and bleeding occurs when the uterus is not able to contract adequately and stop blood flow from open vessels. The initial bleeding is usually a small amount of bright red loss and stops as clots form; however, it can recur at any time (Table 13-8).

Vital signs may be normal even with heavy blood loss because of the compensatory mechanisms of pregnancy, and up to 40% of blood volume can be lost without showing signs of shock. Clinical presentation and decreasing urinary output may be better indicators of acute blood loss than vital signs alone. FHR changes are not usually seen unless there is a major detachment of the placenta (Gilbert, 2007).

Abdominal examination usually reveals a soft, relaxed, nontender uterus with normal tone. If the fetus is lying longitudinally, the fundal height is usually greater than expected for gestational age because the low placenta hinders descent of the presenting fetal part. Leopold's manoeuvers may reveal a fetus in an oblique or breech position or lying transverse because of the abnormal site of placental implantation.

Maternal and Fetal Outcome

Complications associated with placenta previa include PROM, preterm labour and birth, surgery-related trauma to structures adjacent to the uterus, anaesthesia complications, blood transfusion reactions, overinfusion of fluids, abnormal placental attachments (e.g., placenta accreta), vasa previa, postpartum hemorrhage, anemia, thrombophlebitis, and infection.

CRITICAL THINKING EXERCISE

Placenta Previa

Marta is a 26-year-old woman, G6-T4-P0-A1-L4 at 26 weeks of gestation, who is seen in the emergency department with bright red vaginal bleeding. She is concerned about the bleeding and whether this means she will lose the baby.

1. Evidence—Is there sufficient evidence to draw conclusions about her diagnosis and preferred treatment?
2. Assumptions—What assumptions can be made about the following items?
   a. Possible diagnoses for Marta
   b. Physical assessment, laboratory tests, and diagnostic procedures that will be done to make a diagnosis
   c. The circumstances under which Marta would be transferred to the antepartum unit
   d. The circumstances under which Marta would be discharged home
3. What implications and priorities for nursing care can be drawn at this time?
4. Does the evidence objectively support your conclusion?
5. Are there alternative perspectives to your conclusion?

Table 13-8 Summary of Findings: Abruptio Placentae and Placenta Previa

	Abruptio Placentae			Placenta Previa
	CLASS 1: MILD SEPARATION (48% OF ALL CASES)	CLASS 2: MODERATE SEPARATION (27% OF ALL CASES)	CLASS 3: SEVERE SEPARATION (24% OF ALL CASES)	
Bleeding, external, vaginal	Minimal	Absent or moderate	Absent to heavy	Minimal to severe and life threatening
Total amount of blood loss	<500 mL	1000–1500 mL	>1500 mL	Varies
Colour of blood	Dark red	Dark red	Dark red	Bright red
Shock	Rare; none	Mild shock	Common, often sudden, profound	Uncommon
Coagulopathy	Rare; none	Occasional DIC	Frequent DIC	None
Uterine tonicity	Normal	Increased; may be localized to one region or diffuse over uterus; uterus fails to relax between contractions	Tetanic, persistent uterine contraction; boardlike uterus	Normal
Tenderness (pain)	Usually absent	Present (moderate to severe)	Agonizing, unremitting pain	Absent
Ultrasonographic Findings				
Location of placenta	Normal; upper uterine segment	Normal; upper uterine segment	Normal; upper uterine segment	Abnormal; lower uterine segment
Station of presenting part	Variable to engaged	Variable to engaged	Variable to engaged	High, not engaged
Fetal position	Usual distribution*	Usual distribution*	Usual distribution*	Commonly transverse, breech, or oblique
Other Findings				
Gestational or chronic hypertension	Usual distribution*	Commonly present	Commonly present	Usual distribution*
Fetal effects	Normal fetal heart rate pattern	Atypical fetal heart rate pattern	Abnormal fetal heart rate pattern; death can occur	Normal fetal heart rate pattern

(Adapted from Gaufberg, S. [2011]. Abruptio placentae. *eMedicine*. Retrieved from http://emedicine.medscape.com/article/795514-overview.)
*Usual distribution refers to the usual variations of incidence seen when there is no concurrent problem.
DIC, disseminated intravascular coagulation.

The greatest risk of fetal death is caused by preterm birth. Other fetal risks include malpresentation and congenital anomalies (Gilbert, 2007). Infants who are small for gestational age or have IUGR also have been associated with placenta previa. This association may be related to poor placental exchange or hypovolemia resulting from maternal blood loss and maternal anemia.

Nursing Care Management

The standard for the diagnosis of placenta previa is a transabdominal ultrasound examination (see Nursing Process box). It is accurate 93 to 97% of the time. Transvaginal ultrasound also is used for placental location, particularly when the exact relation of the lower placental margin to the internal os is not clearly seen with transabdominal examination (Hull & Resnik, 2009; Oppenheimer et al., 2007). If ultrasonographic scanning reveals a normally implanted placenta, a gentle speculum examination is performed to rule out local causes of bleeding (e.g., cervicitis, polyps, or carcinoma of the cervix), and a coagulation profile is obtained to rule out other causes of bleeding.

If expectant management is to be implemented, a vaginal speculum examination should be postponed until fetal viability is reached (preferably after 34 weeks of gestation). If a pelvic examination is needed before that time, it is possible that an immediate Caesarean birth may be required. The woman is taken to a delivery room or an operating room set up for Caesarean birth, because profound hemorrhage can occur during the examination. This type of vaginal examination, known as the *double-setup procedure*, is not often performed.

Hospital Care

Active Management. Acute care of a patient with a diagnosed placenta previa should be carried out in a labour and birth unit with continuous electronic monitoring of the fetus and uterine contractions. Maternal vital signs are assessed frequently for BP changes, increasing pulse rate, changes in level of consciousness, and oliguria. If the woman is at term (longer than or equal to 37 weeks of gestation) and in labour or bleeding persistently, immediate birth by Caesarean section is almost always indicated. The nurse should continuously assess maternal and fetal status while preparing the woman for surgery. In women with partial or marginal placenta previa (placental edge is greater than 2 mm from the cervical os) who have minimal bleeding, vaginal birth may be attempted (Oppenheimer et al., 2007).

Blood loss may not cease with the infant's birth. The large vascular channels in the lower uterine segment may continue to bleed because of the diminished muscle content in that

NURSING PROCESS: PLACENTA PREVIA

Assessment

A woman with third-trimester vaginal bleeding requires immediate evaluation. The assessment includes the following:

History

- Pregnancy (gravidity, parity, estimated date of birth)
- Course of pregnancy

Interview

- General status
- Bleeding (quantity, precipitating event, associated pain)

Physical Examination

- Vital signs
- Fetal status
- Presence of contractions or abdominal discomfort

Review Laboratory Test Results

- Complete blood count
- Blood type and Rh factor
- Coagulation profile
- Possible type and cross-match

Planning

Once placenta previa has been diagnosed, a management plan is developed on the basis of gestational age, amount of bleeding, and fetal condition. Expectant management (observation and bed rest) usually is implemented when the fetus is not mature. Outpatient management of placenta previa may be appropriate for stable women with home support, close proximity to a hospital, readily available transportation, and telephone communication (Oppenheimer et al., 2007).

Expected outcomes for the woman experiencing placenta previa may include that the woman will do the following:

- Communicate understanding of her condition and its management
- Identify and use available support systems
- Demonstrate compliance with prescribed activity limitations
- Develop no complications related to bleeding
- Give birth to a healthy term infant

Nursing Diagnoses

Potential nursing diagnoses for the woman with a placenta previa include the following:

Deficient fluid volume related to

- excessive blood loss secondary to placenta previa

Ineffective peripheral tissue perfusion related to

- hypovolemia and shunting of blood to central circulation

Anxiety/fear related to

- risk to the woman's life and risk of losing her baby

Anticipatory grieving related to

- actual or perceived threat to self, pregnancy, or infant

Interventions

Monitor

- Vital signs
- Fetal status
- Amount of bleeding
- Urine output
- Level of consciousness

Provide emotional support to the woman and her family.

Explain all procedures.

Administer medications as ordered.

Be prepared for an emergency Caesarean birth.

Notify the hospital chaplain or perinatal social workers to assist with support as indicated by the woman.

Evaluation

The expected outcomes of care are used to evaluate the care for the woman with placenta previa (see Nursing Care Plan).

region. The natural mechanism to control bleeding (i.e., the interlacing muscle bundles contracting around open vessels [the "living ligature" characteristic of the upper part of the uterus]) is absent in the lower part of the uterus. Postpartum hemorrhage may occur even if the fundus is contracted firmly.

Emotional support for the woman and her family is extremely important. The actively bleeding woman is concerned not only for her own well-being but for that of her fetus. All procedures should be explained, and a support person should be present. The woman should be encouraged to express her concerns and feelings. If the woman and her support person or family desire pastoral support, the nurse can notify the hospital chaplain service or provide information about other supportive resources.

Expectant Management. If the woman is less than 36 weeks of gestation and is not in labour, and the bleeding is mild or has stopped, expectant management (i.e., rest and close observation) is generally the treatment of choice to give the fetus time to mature in utero. The woman may remain in the hospital on bed rest with bathroom privileges and limited activity (up in a wheelchair for short periods of time) or be at home if bleeding is stable and the woman has support and lives in proximity to the hospital. Bleeding is assessed by checking the amount of bleeding on perineal pads, bed pads, and linens. Weighing of pads, although not often used, is one way to more accurately assess blood loss; 1 g is equal to 1 mL of blood.

Ultrasound examinations may be done every 2 weeks. Fetal surveillance may include NST or BPP once or twice weekly. Serial laboratory values are evaluated for decreasing hemoglobin and hematocrit levels and changes in coagulation values. Venous access with an IV infusion or heparin lock may be placed in case blood or blood component therapy is needed. Antepartum steroids (betamethasone) may be ordered to promote fetal lung maturity if the woman is at less than 34 weeks of gestation (Crane et al., 2003). No vaginal or rectal examinations are performed, and the woman is placed on pelvic rest (nothing in the vagina). Once she reaches 37 weeks of gestation and fetal lung maturity is documented, Caesarean birth can be scheduled.

The woman with placenta previa should always be considered a potential emergency because massive blood loss with resulting hypovolemic shock can occur quickly if bleeding resumes. The possibility always exists that she may require an emergency Caesarean section for birth. Placenta previa in a preterm gestation may be an indication for admission to a tertiary perinatal centre because many community hospitals are not equipped to perform emergency Caesarean births 24 hours per day, 7 days per week; nor can they provide neonatal intensive care.

Home Care

Criteria for home care management vary among primary perinatal providers and home care agencies and are usually determined on a case-by-case basis. To be considered for home care referral, the woman must be in stable condition with no evidence of active bleeding and must have the resources to be able to return to the hospital immediately if active bleeding resumes (Oppenheimer et al., 2007).

She must have close supervision by family or friends in the home. She should be taught how to assess fetal and uterine activity and bleeding and told to avoid intercourse, douching, and the use of enemas. She should limit her activities according to the advice of her physician and be advised to keep all appointments for fetal testing, laboratory assessments, and prenatal care (see Nursing Care Plan).

Placental Abruption (Premature Separation of Placenta)

Premature separation of the placenta before birth has a wide spectrum of clinical presentations and occurs in about 1% of pregnancies (Oyelese & Ananth, 2006). Premature separation of the placenta, or abruptio placentae, is the detachment of part or all of the placenta from its implantation site (Fig. 13-13). Separation occurs in the area of the decidua basalis after 20 weeks of pregnancy and before the birth of the baby.

Incidence and Etiology

Premature separation of the placenta is a serious event that accounts for significant maternal and fetal morbidity and mortality. Maternal hypertension is probably the most consistently identified risk factor for abruption. Cocaine use also is a risk factor as a result of cocaine-induced vasospasm leading to placental ischemia, reflex vasodilation, and disruption in the placental vasculature (Francois & Foley, 2007; MacDonald, Vermeulen, & Ray, 2007). Blunt external abdominal trauma, most often the result of motor vehicle accidents or maternal battering, is an increasingly significant cause of placental abruption (Francois & Foley, 2007). Maternal smoking significantly increases the risk of placental abruption. In the past, maternal age older than 35, parity, short umbilical cord, and folic acid deficiency were all thought to increase risk; however, more recent research has failed to confirm any of these as risk factors (Francois & Foley, 2007). Abruption is more likely to occur with polyhydramnios and in multiple gestation after birth of the first infant because of rapid uterine decompression. There is a significant (5 to 17%) recurrence risk for placental abruption. A woman who has had two previous premature separations has a recurrence risk of 25% in the next pregnancy (Francois & Foley, 2007).

Classification Systems

The most common classification of placental abruption is according to type and severity. This classification is summarized in Table 13-8.

Clinical Manifestations

The separation may be partial or complete, or only the margin of the placenta may be involved. Bleeding from the placental site may dissect (separate) the membranes from the decidua basalis and flow out through the vagina, it may remain concealed (retroplacental hemorrhage), or it may do both (see Fig. 13-13). Clinical symptoms vary with the degree of separation (see Table 13-8).

Minor degrees of placental abruption cause slight vaginal bleeding, vague abdominal pain, or false preterm labour (see Table 13-8). More extensive placental separation leads to acute fetal distress associated with maternal shock due to substantial revealed or concealed blood loss. Ultrasonography is commonly used at the bedside in a labour and delivery setting to exclude placenta previa in stable nonacute patients; it is rarely performed in unstable patients because the acute diagnosis is obvious (Walker, Whittle, Keating, & Kingdom, 2010).

Typically, vaginal bleeding, abdominal pain, "port wine"–stained amniotic fluid, uterine contractions or hypertonus, uterine tenderness, and abnormal FHR patterns or fetal death are seen with abruptio placentae. Although abdominal pain and uterine tenderness are characteristic of abruption, either finding may be absent in the presence of a silent abruption

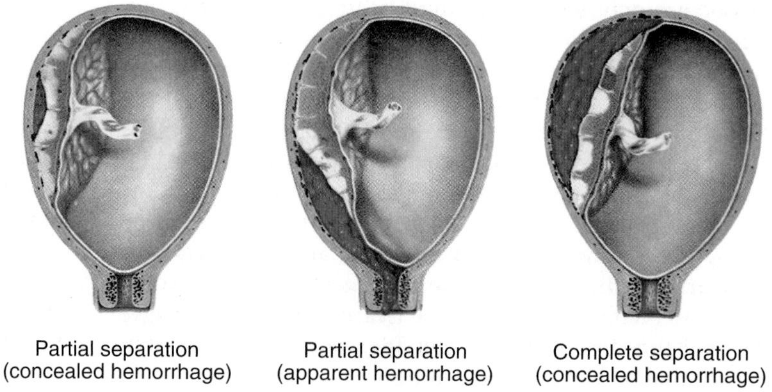

Fig. 13-13 Abruptio placentae. Premature separation of a normally implanted placenta.

NURSING CARE PLAN ● Placenta Previa

Nursing Diagnosis Decreased cardiac output related to bleeding secondary to placenta previa

Expected Outcome

Patient will exhibit signs of increased blood volume and restoration of cardiac output (i.e., normal pulse and blood pressure; normal heart and breath sounds; normal skin colour, tone, and turgor; normal capillary refill).

Nursing Interventions/*Rationales*

Assess uterus for tenderness and tone; assess bleeding rate, amount, colour, degree of bleeding, CBC values, and coagulation profile *to determine severity of situation.* Do not perform vaginal examination because it may stimulate further bleeding.

Establish baseline data for cardiac output (vital signs; heart and breath sounds; skin colour, tone, turgor; capillary refill; level of consciousness; urinary output; pulse oximetry) *to use as a basis for evaluating effectiveness of treatment.*

Initiate intravenous therapy or blood transfusions and medications per physician order *to restore blood volume and prevent organ compromise to mother and fetus.*

Place woman on bed rest *to decrease oxygen demands.*

Monitor vital signs, intake and output, hemodynamic status, and laboratory values *to evaluate treatment response.*

Provide emotional support to the woman and her family (e.g., explain procedures and their rationale; explain what is happening and what to expect; keep support person present) *to allay fears and give the family a sense of control.*

After stabilization, teach the woman home management, including bed rest, watching for spotting/bleeding, close follow-up with her health care provider, and preparation for immediate return to hospital, if needed, *to prevent or stem further complications.*

Nursing Diagnosis Risk for injury to fetus related to decreased uterine/placental perfusion secondary to bleeding

Expected Outcome

Woman will exhibit ongoing signs of fetal well-being (i.e., adequate fetal movement, normal fetal heart rate, normal NST, normal BPP).

Nursing Interventions/*Rationales*

Monitor fetus daily for signs of tachycardia, decreased movement, and atypical NST *to identify and treat changes in fetal status early.*

Obtain BPP per physician order *to assess for signs of chronic asphyxia.*

Advise woman to maintain maternal side-lying position *to prevent compression of aorta and vena cava.*

Nursing Diagnosis Risk for infection related to anemia and bleeding secondary to placenta previa

Expected Outcome

Woman will show no signs of intrauterine infection.

Nursing Interventions/*Rationales*

Monitor vital signs for elevated temperature, pulse, and decreased blood pressure; monitor laboratory results for elevated white blood cell count, differential shift; check for uterine tenderness and malodorous vaginal discharge *to detect early signs of infection resulting from exposure of placental tissue.*

Provide or teach perineal hygiene *to decrease the risk of ascending infection.*

Discuss the need to increase dietary iron and protein intake *to treat anemia.*

BPP, Biophysical profile; *CBC,* complete blood count; *NST,* nonstress test.

(Baird & Kennedy, 2008; Hull & Resnik, 2009). Bleeding may result in maternal hypovolemia (i.e., shock, oliguria, anuria) and coagulopathy. Mild-to-severe uterine hypertonicity is present. Pain is mild to severe and localized over one region of the uterus or diffuse over the uterus, with a "boardlike" abdomen (Baird & Kennedy, 2008).

Extensive myometrial bleeding damages the uterine muscle. If blood accumulates between the separated placenta and the uterine wall, it may produce a Couvelaire uterus: the uterus appears purplish and copper coloured, it is ecchymotic, and contractility is lost. Shock may occur and is out of proportion to blood loss. The Apt test result (for blood in amniotic fluid) is positive, hemoglobin and hematocrit levels decrease, and coagulation factor levels decrease. Clotting defects (e.g., DIC) develop in 10 to 30% of women, in most cases within 8 hours of hospital admission. A Kleihauer-Betke stain may be ordered to determine the presence of fetal-to-maternal bleeding (transplacental hemorrhage), although this test appears to be of no value in the general workup of patients with placental abruption (Hull & Resnik, 2009).

Maternal, Fetal, and Neonatal Outcomes

The maternal mortality rate approaches 1% in abruptio placentae; this condition remains one of the leading causes of maternal death. The mother's prognosis depends on the extent of placental detachment, overall blood loss, degree of DIC, and time between placental detachment and birth.

Maternal complications are associated with the abruption or its treatment. Hemorrhage, hypovolemic shock, hypofibrinogenemia, and thrombocytopenia are associated with severe abruption. Couvelaire uterus, DIC, and infection may occur. Renal failure and pituitary necrosis (Sheehan's syndrome) may result from ischemia. In rare cases, women who are Rh negative can become sensitized if fetal-to-maternal hemorrhage occurs and the fetal blood type is Rh positive.

Placental abruption accounts for about 12% of all perinatal deaths (Ananth, Berkowitz, Savitz, & Lapinski, 1999). Death occurs from fetal hypoxia, preterm birth, and IUGR. Risks of neurological deficits are increased (Hull & Resnik, 2009).

Collaborative Care

Abruptio placentae should be strongly suspected in the woman who has a sudden onset of intense, usually localized, uterine pain, with or without vaginal bleeding. Initial assessment is much the same as that for placenta previa. Physical examination usually reveals abdominal pain, uterine tenderness, and contractions. The fundal height may be measured over time, because increasing fundal height could indicate concealed bleeding. Approximately 60% of live fetuses exhibit abnormal signs on the electronic fetal heart monitor, such as loss of variability and late decelerations; uterine hyperstimulation and increased resting tone may also be noted on the monitor tracing (Francois & Foley, 2007).

Many women demonstrate coagulopathy, as evidenced by abnormal clotting studies (fibrinogen, platelet count, PT, PTT, fibrin split products). Ultrasound examination is used to rule out placenta previa; however, it is not always diagnostic for abruption (Walker et al., 2010). A retroplacental mass may be detected with ultrasonographic examination, but negative findings do not rule out a life-threatening abruption (Hull & Resnik, 2009).

Nursing diagnoses and expected outcomes are similar to those described for placenta previa.

Hospital Care. Treatment depends on the severity of blood loss and fetal maturity and status. If the abruption is mild, expectant management is implemented if the fetus is less than 36 weeks of gestation and not in distress. The woman is hospitalized and closely observed for signs of bleeding and labour. The fetal status is monitored with intermittent FHR monitoring and NST or BPP until fetal maturity is achieved. If the woman's condition deteriorates, immediate birth is indicated. Use of corticosteroids to accelerate fetal lung maturity is appropriately included in the plan of care for the woman managed expectantly (Crane et al., 2003; Hull & Resnik, 2009). Women who are Rh negative may be given $Rh_o(D)$ immune globulin if fetal-to-maternal hemorrhage occurs and the fetal blood is Rh positive.

If the mother is hemodynamically stable, a vaginal birth may be attempted if the fetus is alive and in no acute distress or if the fetus is dead. In the presence of fetal compromise, severe hemorrhage, coagulopathy, poor labour progress, or increasing uterine resting tone, a Caesarean birth is performed. At least one large-bore (16-gauge) IV line should be started. Maternal vital signs should be monitored frequently to observe for signs of declining hemodynamic status, such as increasing pulse rate and decreasing BP. Serial laboratory studies include hematocrit or hemoglobin determinations and clotting studies. Continuous electronic fetal monitoring is mandatory. An indwelling Foley catheter can be inserted for ongoing assessment of urine output, an excellent indirect measure of maternal organ perfusion.

Blood and fluid volume replacement will most likely be ordered, with the goals of maintaining the urine output at 30 mL/hr or more and the hematocrit at 0.30 or more. If these goals are not reached despite vigorous attempts at replacement, hemodynamic monitoring may be necessary. Fresh frozen plasma or cryoprecipitate may be given to maintain the fibrinogen level at a minimum of 2.95 to 4.41 mmol/L.

Vaginal birth may be feasible and is desirable especially in cases of fetal death. Caesarean birth should be reserved for cases of abnormal electronic fetal monitor (EFM) patterns or other obstetrical indications. Caesarean birth should not be attempted when the woman has severe and uncorrected coagulopathy because it may result in surgically uncontrollable bleeding.

Emotional support for the woman and her family is extremely important. If the woman is actively bleeding, she will be concerned not only for her own well-being but also for that of her fetus. All procedures should be explained, and a support person should be present.

Cord Insertion and Placental Variations

Placenta accreta is a serious complication of placenta previa. In this condition, trophoblastic invasion extends beyond the normal endometrial barrier. If the invasion extends into the myometrium, it is called *placenta increta. Placenta percreta* exists when the placental invasion extends beyond the uterine serosa (Hull & Resnik, 2009). Massive hemorrhage can occur with these conditions. Caesarean birth through a fundal incision, followed by total abdominal hysterectomy, may be indicated (Gagnon et al., 2009; Hull & Resnik, 2009).

Velamentous insertion of the cord and vasa previa are rare placental anomalies with a higher incidence in multiple gestation. Velamentous insertion of the cord occurs when the umbilical vessels begin to branch at the membranes and then course onto the placenta (Fig. 13-14, A). When the placenta is found to be low lying, further evaluation for placental cord insertion should be assessed (Gagnon et al., 2009). When some of the umbilical vessels cross the cervical os below the presenting part, vasa previa is diagnosed. ROM or traction on the cord may tear one or more of the fetal vessels. As a result, the fetus may rapidly bleed to death (Gagnon et al., 2009). Battledore (marginal) insertion of the cord (see Fig. 13-14, B) increases the risk of fetal hemorrhage, especially after marginal separation of the placenta.

Rarely, the placenta may be divided into two or more separate lobes, resulting in succenturiate placenta (see Fig. 13-14, C). Each lobe has a distinct circulation. The vessels collect at the periphery, and the main trunks eventually unite to form the vessels of the cord. Blood vessels joining the lobes may be supported only by the fetal membranes; therefore, they are in danger of tearing during labour, birth, or expulsion of the placenta. During expulsion of the placenta, one or more of the separate lobes may remain attached to the decidua basalis, preventing uterine contraction and increasing the risk of postpartum hemorrhage.

Clotting Disorders in Pregnancy

Normal Clotting

Normally, a delicate balance (homeostasis) is maintained between the opposing hemostatic and fibrinolytic systems. The hemostatic system is involved in the lifesaving process by stopping the flow of blood from injured vessels, in part through the formation of insoluble fibrin, which acts as a hemostatic platelet plug. The coagulation process involves an interaction of the coagulation factors in which each factor sequentially

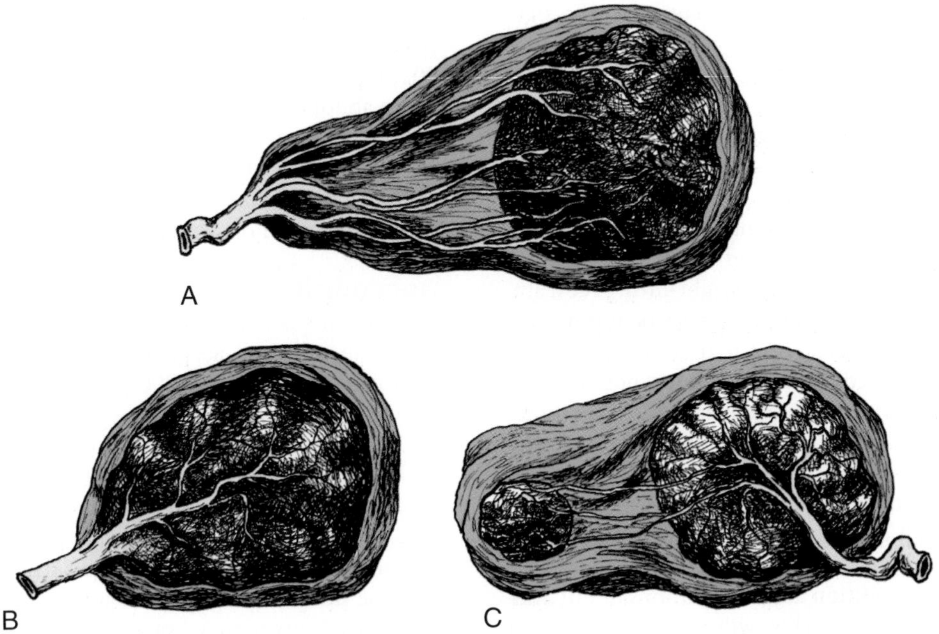

Fig. 13-14 Cord insertion and placental variations. **A:** Velamentous insertion of cord. **B:** Battledore placenta. **C:** Succenturiate placenta.

activates the factor next in line—the "cascade effect" sequence. The fibrinolytic system is the process by which the fibrin is split into fibrin degradation products and circulation is restored.

Clotting Problems

A history of abnormal bleeding, inheritance of unusual bleeding tendencies, or a report of significant aberrations of laboratory findings indicates a bleeding or clotting problem. For the pregnant woman, bleeding disorders are suspected if the woman has gestational hypertension, HELLP syndrome, retained dead fetus syndrome, amniotic fluid embolism, sepsis, or hemorrhage. Determination of hemostasis is made by testing the usual mechanisms for the control of bleeding, the function of platelets, and the necessary clotting factors. Most clotting disorders are more a concern in the immediate postpartum period. Recognition in the antepartal period may decrease hemorrhagic problems.

Disseminated Intravascular Coagulation (DIC)

DIC is a pathological form of clotting that is diffuse and consumes large amounts of clotting factors, causing widespread external or internal bleeding or both. DIC is an overactivation of the clotting cascade and the fibrinolytic system, resulting in the depletion of platelets and clotting factors. This results in the formation of multiple fibrin clots throughout the body's vasculature, even in the microcirculation. Blood cells are destroyed as they pass through these fibrin-choked vessels. Thus DIC results in a clinical picture of hemorrhage, anemia, and ischemia.

DIC is always a secondary diagnosis. In the obstetrical population, it is most often triggered by the release of large amounts of tissue thromboplastin; this occurs in abruptio placentae, retained dead fetus, and amniotic fluid embolus. Severe pre-eclampsia and sepsis are examples of conditions that can trigger DIC because of widespread damage to vascular integrity.

Medical Management. The diagnosis of DIC is based on clinical findings and laboratory markers. Physical examination reveals unusual bleeding. Spontaneous bleeding from the woman's gums or nose may be noted. Petechiae may appear around the BP cuff placed on her arm. Excessive bleeding may occur from the site of a slight trauma (e.g., venipuncture sites, IM or subcutaneous injection sites, or injury from insertion of urinary catheter). Maternal symptoms may include tachycardia and diaphoresis.

Laboratory tests reveal decreased hematocrit, hemoglobin, platelets, fibrinogen, antihemophilic factor, and prothrombin (the factors consumed during coagulation). Fibrinolysis is first increased but later severely depressed. Degradation of fibrin leads to the accumulation of fibrin split products in the blood. Fibrin split products have anticoagulant properties and thus prolong the PT. Bleeding time is normal, coagulation time shows no clot, clot retraction time shows no clot, and PTT is increased.

The primary management of DIC involves correction of the underlying cause, which may be treatment of existing infection, pre-eclampsia, or eclampsia, or removal of a placental abruption. Concomitantly, treatment is directed toward support of maternal physiological functioning and replacing essential factors faster than the body can consume them. IV fluids are given to replace volume lost through severe bleeding. Packed red blood cells are administered to maintain enough circulating red blood cells to ensure tissue oxygenation. Fresh frozen plasma or cryoprecipitate is given to replace fibrinogen and coagulation factors. Platelets may also be administered. Warming of fluids and blood prior to administration helps to keep the patient's body temperature within normal range, allowing oxygen use in the organs and tissues.

Nursing Care Management

The nurse caring for the pregnant woman at risk for DIC must be aware of risk factors. Careful and thorough assessment is required, with particular attention to the signs of bleeding (petechiae, oozing from injection sites, and hematuria). Because renal failure is one consequence of DIC, urinary output needs to be carefully monitored with an indwelling Foley catheter. The goal for urine output is 30 mL/hr or greater. Vital signs should be assessed frequently.

Supportive measures include keeping the pregnant woman in a side-lying tilt to maximize blood flow to the uterus. Oxygen may be administered through a tight-fitting rebreathing mask at 8 to 10 L/min or per hospital protocol or physician order. To provide oxygen delivery to the tissues, blood products are usually administered. If the woman has not yet given birth, fetal assessments by continuous electronic fetal monitoring should be carried out. DIC is usually corrected with birth, blood and volume replacement, and resolution of the cause and as coagulation abnormalities resolve.

The educational and emotional needs of the woman and her family must be recognized and supported. They need information about her condition and explanations of unfamiliar equipment and procedures. They will most likely be very anxious about the health of the mother and baby.

Von Willebrand's Disease

Von Willebrand's disease, a type of hemophilia, is probably the most common of all hereditary bleeding disorders. It results from a factor VIII deficiency and platelet dysfunction. It is transmitted as an incomplete autosomal dominant trait to both sexes. Although von Willebrand's disease is rare, it is one of the most common congenital clotting defects in North American women of childbearing age. Symptoms include a familial bleeding tendency, previous bleeding episodes, prolonged bleeding time (the most important test), factor VIII deficiency (mild to moderate), and bleeding from mucous membranes. Factor VIII increases during pregnancy, and this increase may be sufficient to offset danger from hemorrhage during childbirth.

Von Willebrand's disease is variable in its clinical course, severity, and laboratory values; thus it is possible for this condition to go undetected throughout pregnancy until bleeding problems develop after birth. A primary treatment for many women is desmopressin, which increases levels of plasma factor VIII and von Willebrand's factor (vWF) (Lockwood & Silver, 2009). If the woman is known to have von Willebrand's disease before labour, factor VIII levels should be monitored and factor VIII/vWF plasma concentrate given as needed to maintain activity at 50% of normal near-term gestation (Lockwood & Silver, 2009). Hemorrhage may occur 4 or 5 days after birth. The woman should remain in the hospital for several days after birth so she can be monitored for that complication.

Nonobstetrical Surgery During Pregnancy

As many as 2% of pregnant women will have surgery for nonobstetrical reasons (Kuczkowski, 2004). The need for abdominal surgery occurs as often among pregnant women as among nonpregnant women of comparable age. However, diagnosis of nonobstetrical complications is more difficult in the pregnant woman (Cohen-Kerem, Railton, Oren, Lishner, & Koren, 2005). An enlarged uterus and displaced internal organs may make abdominal palpation more difficult, may alter the position of an affected organ, or may change the usual signs associated with a particular disorder. The most common conditions necessitating abdominal surgery during pregnancy are appendicitis, intestinal obstruction, and gynecological problems.

Appendicitis

Appendicitis is the most common nongynecological cause of an acute surgical abdomen during pregnancy, occurring approximately once in 1500 pregnancies. The rate of premature labour induced by nonobstetrical surgical intervention is 3.5% and occurs more often following appendectomy than with any other type of surgery (Cohen-Kerem et al., 2005). Appendicitis occurs with approximately the same frequency during each trimester of pregnancy and in the postpartum period (Kelly & Savides, 2009). The diagnosis is often delayed because the usual signs and symptoms mimic some normal changes of pregnancy, such as nausea and vomiting and increased white blood cell count. As pregnancy progresses, the appendix is pushed upward and to the right from its usual anatomical location (see Fig. 9-15). Because of these changes, appendiceal rupture and peritonitis occur two to three times more often in pregnant women than in nonpregnant women (Kelly & Savides, 2009).

The woman with appendicitis most commonly has right lower quadrant pain, nausea and vomiting, and loss of appetite. Approximately half of these women will have muscle guarding. Moving the uterus tends to increase the pain. Temperature may be normal or mildly increased (to 38.3°C). Because of the physiological increase in white blood cells that occurs in pregnancy, laboratory findings are not helpful in the diagnosis (Kelly & Savides, 2009).

The diagnosis of appendicitis requires a high level of suspicion because the typical signs and symptoms are similar to those found in many other conditions, including pyelonephritis, round ligament pain, placental abruption, torsion of an ovarian cyst, cholecystitis, and preterm labour (Kelly & Savides, 2009).

Appendectomy before rupture usually does not require either antibiotic or tocolytic therapy. If surgery is delayed until after rupture, multiple antibiotics need to be ordered. Rupture is likely to result in preterm labour and necessitate the use of tocolytic agents.

Intestinal Obstruction

The second most common nonobstetrical abdominal emergency in pregnancy is intestinal obstruction. Any woman with a laparotomy scar is more likely to have an intestinal obstruction (adynamic ileus) during gestation. Adhesions as a result of previous surgery or pelvic inflammatory disease, an enlarging uterus, and displacement of the intestines are etiological factors.

Constipation; persistent cramplike, abdominal pain; vomiting; auscultatory rushes within the abdomen; and "laddering" of the intestinal shadows on x-ray films aid in the diagnosis of intestinal obstruction. Immediate surgical intervention is required for release of the obstruction. Pregnancy is rarely affected by the surgery, assuming the absence of complications such as peritonitis.

Gynecological Problems

Pregnancy predisposes a woman to ovarian problems, especially during the first trimester. Ovarian cysts and twisting of ovarian cysts or adnexal tissues may occur. Other problems include retained or enlarged cystic corpus luteum of pregnancy and bacterial invasion of reproductive or other intraperitoneal organs.

Laparotomy or laparoscopy may be required to discriminate between ovarian problems and early ectopic pregnancy, appendicitis, or an infectious process.

Nursing Care Management

Initial assessment of the pregnant woman requiring surgery focuses on her presenting signs and symptoms. A thorough history and physical examination should be performed. Laboratory testing includes, at a minimum, a CBC with differential and a urinalysis. FHR and activity and uterine activity should be monitored; constant vigilance is required in watching for symptoms of impending obstetrical complications. The extent of preoperative assessment is determined by the immediacy of surgical intervention and the specific condition that requires surgery.

Hospital Care

When surgery becomes necessary during pregnancy, the woman and her family will be concerned about the effects of the procedure and medication on fetal well-being and the course of pregnancy. An important part of preoperative nursing care is encouraging the woman to express her fears, concerns, and questions.

Preoperative care for a pregnant woman differs from that of a nonpregnant woman in one significant aspect: the presence of at least one other person—the fetus. Continuous FHR and uterine contraction monitoring may be performed if the fetus is considered viable. Procedures such as preparation of the operative site and time of insertion of IV lines and urinary retention catheters vary with the physician and the facility. However, in every instance there is total restriction of solid food and fluids or a clear specification of the type, amount, and time at which clear liquids may be taken before surgery. Some bowel preparation such as drinking clear liquids and taking laxatives may be required before surgery. Food by mouth is restricted for several hours before a scheduled procedure. If the woman experiences a prolonged nothing-by-mouth status, IV fluids with dextrose should be given. Even if she has had nothing by mouth—but more important, if surgery is unexpected—the woman is in danger of vomiting and aspirating, and special precautions are taken before the anaesthetic is administered (e.g., administering an antacid).

During surgery, perinatal nurses may collaborate with the surgical staff to meet the special needs of pregnant women. To improve fetal oxygenation, the woman should be positioned on the operating table with a lateral tilt, to avoid maternal compression of the vena cava. Continuous fetal and uterine monitoring during the procedure may be ordered because the risk of preterm labour is great. Depending on the surgical procedure, monitoring can be accomplished using sterile Aquasonic gel and a sterile sleeve for the transducer. Uterine contractions may be palpated manually. In the immediate recovery period, general observations and care pertinent to postoperative recovery should be initiated. Frequent assessments should be carried out for several hours after surgery. Whether the woman is cared for in the surgical postanaesthesia recovery area or in a labour and delivery unit, continuous fetal and uterine monitoring will likely be initiated or resumed because of the increased risk of preterm labour. **Tocolysis** may be necessary if preterm labour occurs.

Home Care

Plans for the woman's return home and for convalescent care should be completed as early as possible before discharge. The woman and other support persons must be taught signs of infection. Box 13-7 lists information that should be included in discharge teaching for the postoperative patient. The woman may also need referrals to various community agencies for evaluation of the home situation, child care, home health care, and financial or other assistance.

Trauma During Pregnancy

Trauma is a common complication during pregnancy and may be caused by vehicular crashes, falls, burns, industrial mishaps, violence, gunshot wounds, and other injuries in the home and community. Treatment of pregnant trauma victims is complicated because doctors and nurses who have expertise in the care of trauma victims do not have similar expertise in the care of pregnant women.

Significance

Approximately 6 to 7% of pregnancies are complicated by physical trauma, which accounts for 46% of maternal mortality (Chames & Pearlman, 2008). As pregnancy progresses, the risk of trauma increases, with more cases of trauma reported in the third trimester than earlier in gestation. Motor

BOX 13-7 Discharge Teaching for Home Care

- Care of incision site
- Diet and elimination related to gastrointestinal function
- Signs and symptoms of developing complications (wound infection, thrombophlebitis, pneumonia)
- Equipment needed and technique for assessing temperature
- Recommended schedule for resumption of activities of daily living
- Treatments and medications ordered
- List of resource persons and their telephone numbers
- Schedule of follow-up visits
- If birth has not occurred:
  - Assessment of fetal activity (kick counts)
  - Signs of preterm labour

vehicle crashes are the most common cause of trauma in pregnancy, accounting for 49%. Other common causes are falls, assaults, gunshot wounds, and burns. Approximately 50% of fetal deaths are associated with maternal trauma, and most of these are from motor vehicle crashes (Mattox & Goetzl, 2005). Maternal death caused by trauma is usually the result of head injury or hemorrhagic shock. Fetal death usually occurs as a sequelae to maternal death or as a result of placental abruption.

Acts of violence are a significant health problem for pregnant women. The risk of trauma caused by abuse is increased during pregnancy, and rates of recurrence are high. The reported incidence of physical abuse during pregnancy ranges from 4 to 8% (McFarlane, 2007). As many as 45% of women subject to intimate partner violence before pregnancy continue to be abused during the pregnancy. Women who are abused during pregnancy have a threefold risk of being murdered compared with nonpregnant abused women (McFarlane, 2007).

Trauma increases the incidence of miscarriage, preterm labour, abruptio placentae, and stillbirth (Mattox & Goetzl, 2005). The effect of trauma on pregnancy is influenced by the length of gestation, type and severity of the trauma, and degree of disruption of uterine and fetal physiological features. Fetal death as a result of trauma is more common than the occurrence of both maternal and fetal death (Shah & Kilcline, 2003). Less serious trauma is associated with numerous complications in pregnancy, including fetomaternal hemorrhage, abruptio placentae, intrauterine fetal death, and preterm labour and birth. Careful evaluation of mother and fetus after all types of trauma is imperative.

Multisystem trauma during pregnancy is usually the result of a serious motor vehicle crash, especially if the woman is not wearing a seat belt with a shoulder harness and is ejected from the vehicle. To improve chances of survival for both mother and fetus in a potential crash, pregnant women should wear properly positioned restraints at all times when in a motor vehicle (see Fig. 10-17). Failure to wear restraining devices occurred in 66% of cases in one study (Ikossi et al., 2005). Other researchers found that 95% of pregnant women surveyed either maintained or increased their seat belt use during pregnancy, and a large majority (73%) demonstrated correct usage. The perception that wearing a seat belt would protect them and their baby positively influenced their decision to wear a seat belt (McGwin et al., 2004).

Special considerations for the pregnant woman and her fetus are necessary when trauma occurs, because of the physiological alterations that accompany pregnancy and the presence of the fetus. Fetal survival depends on maternal survival; therefore, the pregnant woman must receive immediate stabilization and appropriate care for optimal fetal outcome.

Maternal Physiological Characteristics

Optimal care for the pregnant woman after trauma depends on having an understanding of the physiological state of pregnancy and its effects on trauma. The pregnant woman's body exhibits responses that are different from those of a nonpregnant person to the same traumatic insults. Because of the different responses to injury during pregnancy, management strategies must be adapted for appropriate resuscitation, fluid therapy, positioning, assessments, and most other interventions. Significant adaptations required for treatment of trauma in the pregnant woman are summarized in Table 13-9.

The uterus and bladder are confined to the bony pelvis during the first trimester of pregnancy and are at reduced risk for injury in cases of abdominal trauma. After pregnancy progresses beyond the fourteenth week, the uterus becomes an abdominal organ, and the risk for injury increases in cases of abdominal trauma. During the second and third trimesters, the distended bladder becomes an abdominal organ and is at increased risk for injury and rupture. Bowel injuries occur less often during pregnancy because of the protection provided by the enlarged uterus.

The elevated levels of progesterone that accompany pregnancy relax smooth muscle and profoundly affect the gastrointestinal tract. Gastrointestinal motility decreases, with a resultant increased time required for gastric emptying; the production of hydrochloric acid increases in the last trimester, and the gastroesophageal sphincter relaxes. Management of the unconscious pregnant woman's airway is of critical importance.

NURSING ALERT The unconscious pregnant woman is at increased risk for regurgitation of gastric contents and aspiration whenever her head is positioned lower than her stomach or if abdominal pressure is applied.

A pregnant woman has decreased tolerance for **hypoxia** and apnea because of her decreased functional residual capacity and increased renal loss of bicarbonate. **Acidosis** develops more quickly in the pregnant woman than in the nonpregnant state.

Cardiac output increases approximately 50% over prepregnancy values by 32 weeks of gestation and is positionally dependent in the third trimester. Because of compression of the inferior vena cava and descending aorta by the pregnant uterus, cardiac output decreases dramatically if the woman is placed in the supine position. Thus the supine position must be avoided, even in women with cervical spine injuries. It is of utmost importance that lateral uterine displacement be accomplished without any head movement. As soon as the neck is immobilized, the stretcher should be tilted laterally.

Circulating blood volume increases 50% during a singleton gestation, and pregnant women can tolerate a 1000-mL blood loss readily without demonstrating clinical signs. Hemodynamic instability that indicates the need for transfusion may not be apparent until blood loss nears 1200 to 1500 mL (Martin & Foley, 2009). Tachycardia and hypotension, typical of hypovolemic shock, may appear late in the pregnant trauma patient because of increased blood volume. Clinical signs of hemorrhage do not appear until after a 20 to 25% loss of circulating volume occurs, which will diminish uteroplacental perfusion. Although heart rate increases with pregnancy, a maternal heart rate greater than 100 beats/min should be considered abnormal. Continuous monitoring of oxygen saturation is advised, since desaturation may affect the oxygenation of the fetus and should be avoided.

Table 13-9 Maternal Physiological Adaptations During Pregnancy and in Relation to Trauma

SYSTEM	ALTERATION	CLINICAL RESPONSES
Respiratory	↑ Oxygen consumption	↑ Risk of acidosis
	↑ Tidal volume	↑ Risk of respiratory mismanagement
	↓ Functional residual capacity	
	Chronic compensated alkalosis ↓ $PaCO_2$ ↓ Serum bicarbonate	↓ Blood-buffering capacity
Cardiovascular	↑ Circulating volume, 1600 mL	Can lose 1000 mL of blood
	↑ Cardiac output	No signs of shock until blood loss >30% total blood volume
	↑ Heart rate	↓ Placental perfusion in supine position
	↓ Systemic vascular resistance	
	↓ Arterial blood pressure	
	Heart displaced upward to left	Point of maximal impulse, fourth intercostal space
Renal	↑ Renal plasma flow	
	Dilation of ureters and urethra	↑ Risk of stasis, infection
	Bladder displaced forward	↑ Risk of bladder trauma
Gastrointestinal	↓ Gastric motility	↑ Risk of aspiration
	↑ Hydrochloric acid production	
	↓ Competency of gastroesophageal sphincter	Passive regurgitation of stomach acids if head lower than stomach
Reproductive	↑ Blood flow to organs	Source of ↑ blood loss
	Uterine enlargement	Vena caval compression in supine position
Musculoskeletal	Displacement of abdominal viscera	↑ Risk of injury, altered rebound response
	Pelvic venous congestion	Altered pain referral
	Cartilage softened	↑ Risk of pelvic fracture Centre of gravity changed
	Fetal head in pelvis	↑ Risk of fetal injury
Hematological	↑ Clotting factors	↑ Risk of thrombus formation
	↓ Fibrinolytic activity	

Fetal Physiological Characteristics

Perfusion of the uterine arteries, which provide the primary blood supply to the uteroplacental unit, depends on adequate maternal arterial pressure because these vessels lack auto-regulation. Therefore, maternal hypotension decreases uterine and fetal perfusion. Maternal shock results in splanchnic and uterine artery vasoconstriction, which decreases blood flow and oxygen transport to the fetus. EFM tracings can assist in the evaluation of fetal status after trauma to assess for hypoxia and hypoperfusion, including tachycardia or bradycardia, decreased or absent baseline variability, and late decelerations.

Careful monitoring of fetal status assists greatly in maternal assessment because the fetal monitor tracing works as an "oximeter" of internal maternal well-being. Hypoperfusion can be present in the pregnant woman before the onset of clinical signs of shock. The EFM tracings may show the first signs of maternal compromise, such as when maternal heart rate, BP, and colour appear normal yet the EFM printout shows signs of fetal hypoxia (Tucker, Miller, & Miller, 2009).

Mechanisms of Trauma

Blunt Abdominal Trauma

Blunt abdominal trauma is most commonly the result of motor vehicle crashes but also may be the result of battering or falls. Maternal and fetal morbidity and mortality rates associated with motor vehicle crashes are directly correlated with whether the mother remains inside the vehicle or is ejected. Maternal death is usually the result of a head injury or exsanguination from a major vessel rupture. Serious retroperitoneal hemorrhage after lower abdominal and pelvic trauma is reported more frequently during pregnancy. Serious maternal abdominal injuries are usually the result of splenic rupture or liver and renal injury.

In the context of maternal survival of trauma, fetal death is usually the result of abruptio placentae. Placental separation is thought to be a result of deformation of the elastic myometrium around the relatively inelastic placenta. Shearing of the placental edge from the underlying decidua basalis ensues and is worsened by the increased intrauterine pressure caused by the impact. It is imperative that all pregnant victims be evaluated carefully for signs and symptoms of abruptio placentae after even minor blunt abdominal trauma.

Pelvic fracture can result from severe injury and produce bladder trauma or retroperitoneal bleeding with two-point displacement of pelvic bones. One point of displacement is common at the symphysis pubis, and the second point is posterior because of the structure of the pelvis. Careful evaluation for clinical signs of internal hemorrhage is indicated.

Direct fetal injury as a complication of blunt trauma during pregnancy most often involves the fetal skull and brain (Chames & Pearlman, 2008). Most commonly, this injury accompanies maternal pelvic fracture in late gestation after the fetal head becomes engaged. When the force of the impact is great enough to fracture the maternal pelvis, the fetus often sustains a skull fracture. Evaluation for fetal skull fracture or intracranial hemorrhage is then indicated.

Uterine rupture as a result of trauma is rare, occurring in only 0.6% of all reported cases of trauma during pregnancy.

Uterine rupture depends on numerous factors, including gestational age, the intensity of the impact, the presence of a predisposing factor such as a distended uterus caused by polyhydramnios or multiple gestation, or the presence of a uterine scar from previous uterine surgery (Cunningham et al., 2010; Gilbert, 2007). When uterine rupture occurs, the force responsible is usually a direct, high-energy blow. Fetal death is common with traumatic uterine rupture. However, maternal death occurs less than 10% of the time; when it does occur, it is usually the result of massive injuries sustained from an impact severe enough to rupture the uterus.

Thoracic Trauma

Thoracic trauma is reported to produce 25% of all trauma deaths. Pulmonary contusion results from nearly 75% of blunt thoracic trauma and is a potentially life-threatening condition. Pulmonary contusion can be difficult to recognize, especially if flail chest is also present or if there is no evidence of thoracic injury. It should be suspected in cases of thoracic injury, especially after blunt acceleration or deceleration trauma such as that occurring when a rapidly moving vehicle crashes into an immovable object.

Penetrating wounds into the chest can result in pneumothorax or hemothorax. This type of injury is usually caused by a vehicular crash that results in impalement by the steering column or a loose article in the vehicle that becomes a projectile with the force of impact. Stab wounds in the chest also may occur as a result of violence.

Nursing Care Management

Immediate Stabilization

Immediate priorities for stabilization of the pregnant woman after trauma should be identical to those of the nonpregnant trauma patient. Pregnancy should not result in any restriction of the usual diagnostic, pharmacological, or resuscitative procedures or manoeuvres. Fetal survival depends on maternal survival, and stabilization of the mother improves fetal chance of survival. The perinatal nurse is often called on to function collaboratively with emergency department or trauma unit staff members in providing care for the pregnant trauma victim.

NURSING ALERT Priorities of care for the pregnant woman after trauma must be to resuscitate the woman and stabilize her condition first and then consider fetal needs.

In cases of minor trauma, the woman is evaluated for vaginal bleeding, uterine irritability, abdominal tenderness, abdominal pain or cramps, and evidence of hypovolemia. A change in or absence of FHR or fetal activity, leakage of amniotic fluid, and presence of fetal cells in the maternal circulation (Kleihauer-Betke) are also included in the assessment.

Primary Survey

In cases of major trauma, the systematic evaluation begins with a primary survey and the initial ABCs of resuscitation:

Airway—Establish and maintain an airway.
Breathing—Ensure adequate breathing.
Circulation—Maintain an adequate circulatory volume.

Increased oxygen needs during gestation necessitate a rapid response. The presence of a cervical spine injury is always assumed.

NURSING ALERT Hyperextension of the neck should be avoided; instead, jaw thrust is used to establish an airway for the trauma victim.

Once an airway is established, assessment should focus on adequacy of oxygenation. The chest wall should be observed for movement. If breathing is absent, ventilations and endotracheal intubation are initiated. Supplemental oxygen should be administered with a tight-fitting, nonrebreathing face mask at 10 to 12 L/min to attempt to normalize maternal arterial oxygen tension ($Pa{O_2}$ 104 to 108 mm Hg) and hemoglobin saturation greater than 95% to optimize maternal and fetal status. The chest wall should be assessed for a penetrating chest wound or flail chest. Breathing with a flail chest will be rapid and laboured; chest wall movements will be uncoordinated and asymmetric; crepitus from bony fragments may be palpated.

Rapid placement of two large-bore (14- to 16-gauge) IV lines is necessary in most seriously injured patients. It is important to place the lines while veins are still distended. Cardiac arrest during the immediate stabilization period is usually the result of profound hypovolemia, necessitating massive fluid resuscitation. Infusion of crystalloids such as Ringer's solution or normal saline solution should be given as a 3:1 ratio (i.e., 3 mL of crystalloid replacement to 1 mL of the estimated blood loss is given over the first 30 to 60 minutes of acute resuscitation). Because of the 50% increase in blood volume during pregnancy, published formulas for nonpregnant adults that are used for estimating crystalloid and blood replacement to counter blood loss must be adjusted upward for pregnancy.

Replacement of red blood cells and other blood components should be anticipated and blood drawn for type, crossmatch, CBC, and platelet count. Infusion of type-specific packed red blood cells is usually necessary to improve fetal oxygenation status and to replace blood lost. During an extreme emergency, type O Rh-negative blood may be administered without matching.

If possible, vasopressor medications to restore maternal arterial BP should be avoided until volume replacement is administered. Although vasopressor agents result in decreased perfusion to the uterus, they should be given and not withheld if needed for successful resuscitation of the mother.

After 20 weeks of gestation, venous return to the heart is best accomplished by positioning the uterus to one side to eliminate the weight of the uterus compressing the inferior vena cava or the descending aorta. This facilitates efforts to establish the forward flow of blood through resuscitation and stabilization. If a lateral position is not possible because of resuscitative efforts or cervical spine immobilization, the uterus can be manually deflected to the left, or a wedge can be inserted underneath the right side of the backboard or stretcher.

Signs of bleeding may be more difficult to recognize in the pregnant woman because a 30 to 35% loss of maternal blood volume may produce only a minimal change in maternal mean arterial pressure. Hypovolemia can be detrimental for the fetus because the vascular bed of the uterus is a low-resistance system that depends on adequate maternal cardiac output and arterial pressure to maintain uterine and fetal perfusion. Maternal hypovolemia can be fatal for the fetus.

Establishing a baseline neurological status (level of consciousness, pupil size, and reactivity) is essential. The Glasgow Coma Scale is commonly used at the scene of the accident to help determine the extent of the head injury.

Secondary Survey

After immediate resuscitation and successful stabilization measures, a more detailed secondary survey of the mother and fetus should be accomplished. A complete physical assessment to include all body systems is performed.

The maternal abdomen should be evaluated carefully because a large percentage of serious injuries involve the uterus, intraperitoneal structures, and retroperitoneum. The pregnant woman's stomach is assumed to be full. A nasogastric tube can be used to empty the stomach to help prevent acid aspiration syndrome. An empty stomach facilitates respiratory efforts. The uterus should be evaluated for evidence of gross deformity, tenderness, irritability, or contractions.

The greatest clinical concern after a vehicular crash is abruptio placentae, because as many as 40% of these women will have an abruption (Mattox & Goetzl, 2005). Assessments should focus on recognition of this complication, with careful evaluation of fetal monitor tracings, uterine tenderness, labour, or vaginal bleeding. Ultrasound examination may be performed to determine gestational age, viability of fetus, and placental location. However, ultrasound studies cannot exclude abruptio placentae.

Peritoneal lavage for the pregnant woman after blunt abdominal trauma has proven to be a safe procedure and can be helpful in the early diagnosis of intraperitoneal injury or hemorrhage. Under direct visualization, the peritoneum is incised, and a peritoneal dialysis catheter is positioned. If aspiration yields free-flowing blood, the test is considered positive, and a laparotomy should be performed. This procedure is not necessary before laparotomy if intraperitoneal bleeding is clinically apparent. Indications for peritoneal lavage include abdominal symptoms or signs suggestive of intraperitoneal bleeding, alteration in mental status, unexplained shock, and severe multiple injuries (Cunningham et al., 2010).

If trauma is the result of a penetrating wound, the woman should be completely undressed and carefully examined for all entrance and exit wounds. Exploratory laparotomy is necessary after a gunshot wound to explore the abdominal cavity for organ damage and to repair any damage present, with careful examination of all organs, the entire bowel, and posterior vessels. If uterine injury is determined, the risks and benefits of Caesarean birth are quickly evaluated. A Caesarean birth is desirable if the fetus is alive and near term and may be necessary for the preterm fetus because of the high incidence of fetal injury in these cases. The fetus usually tolerates surgery and anaesthesia if adequate uterine perfusion and oxygenation are maintained. Tetanus prophylaxis guidelines are not changed by pregnancy.

Electronic Fetal Monitoring

Continuous electronic fetal monitoring may show early signs of abruptio placentae, including a change in baseline rate, loss of accelerations, and the presence of late decelerations. If the estimated gestational age is 24 weeks or greater, fetal monitoring should be initiated soon after the woman is stable because abruptio placentae usually becomes apparent shortly after the injury. Fetal monitoring should be continued and further evaluation initiated if any of these signs occur. Palpation is required to evaluate the intensity of contractions and the uterine resting tone. It is important to palpate between contractions to verify that the uterus is well relaxed. If the uterus does not relax between contractions, abruptio placentae could be present. Occasional uterine contractions are the most common finding with trauma during pregnancy, occurring in 40% of cases and resolving in 90% of cases with no adverse fetal outcome. The intensity and frequency of contractions are predictive of complications such as placental abruption and preterm labour. Elevated basal uterine tone also raises suspicion for traumatic placental abruption. Abruptio placentae occurring after trauma may be delayed for up to 48 hours after the incident.

In addition to helping to stabilize the woman, the nurse can provide emotional support for her and her family. If the trauma is the result of a motor vehicle accident, other family members may also have been critically injured or killed. The nurse should collaborate with other staff to make sure that questions are answered and consistent information given. Grief support may be necessary.

Discharge Planning

Following minor trauma, the woman may be discharged home, after several hours of evaluation. Her vital signs should be stable, with no evidence of bleeding at the time of discharge. The fetal tracing should be normal before monitoring is discontinued and the woman is discharged. Education for the woman and her family is very important. She should be instructed to contact her health care provider immediately if changes in fetal movement or signs and symptoms indicative of preterm labour, PROM, or placental abruption develop. If the trauma occurred as a result of domestic violence, the woman may need information about the abuse cycle; referral to a crisis centre, law enforcement agency, or counselling centre; and help in forming a safety plan (see Chapter 4, p. 56).

Perimortem Caesarean Birth

In the presence of multisystem trauma, perimortem Caesarean birth may be indicated. Removal of the stressor of pregnancy early in the process of resuscitation can increase the chance for maternal survival. Fetal survival is unlikely if Caesarean birth is accomplished more than 20 minutes after maternal death. Therefore, to facilitate resuscitative efforts, consideration may be given to Caesarean birth for maternal benefit after 5 minutes of resuscitative efforts that produce no response in the mother (Martin & Foley, 2009).

Key Points

- Hypertensive disorders of pregnancy are a leading cause of maternal and perinatal morbidity and mortality worldwide.

- The cause of pre-eclampsia is unknown, and there are no known reliable tests for predicting women at risk for developing pre-eclampsia/eclampsia.
- Pre-eclampsia/eclampsia is a multisystem disease, and the pathological changes are present long before clinical manifestations, such as hypertension, are evident.
- Once pre-eclampsia becomes clinically evident, therapeutic interventions may slow the progression of the disease, allowing the pregnancy to continue, but the underlying pathology continues.
- HELLP syndrome, which is a complication of pre-eclampsia/eclampsia, is considered life threatening.
- Magnesium sulphate, the anticonvulsant of choice for preventing or controlling eclamptic seizures, requires careful monitoring of reflexes, respirations, and renal function; its antidote, calcium gluconate, should be at the bedside.
- Intent of emergency interventions for eclampsia is to prevent self-injury, enhance oxygenation, reduce aspiration risk, and establish control with magnesium sulphate.
- Diagnosis of gestational diabetes mellitus is important to ensure glycemic control for women and thus improve perinatal outcomes.
- Ectopic pregnancy is a significant cause of maternal morbidity and mortality, even in developed countries.
- Abruptio placentae and placenta previa are differentiated by type of bleeding, uterine tonicity, and presence or absence of pain.
- Clotting disorders are associated with many obstetrical complications.
- The physiological adaptations of pregnancy mask warning signs and changes in vital signs during early shock state.
- Preoperative care for a pregnant woman differs from that for a nonpregnant woman in one significant aspect: the presence of the fetus.
- Trauma from accidents is the most common cause of death in women of childbearing age.
- Fetal survival depends on maternal survival. After trauma occurs, the first priority is resuscitation and stabilization of the mother before consideration of fetal status.
- Minor trauma is associated with major complications for the pregnancy, including abruptio placentae, fetomaternal hemorrhage, preterm labour and birth, and fetal death.

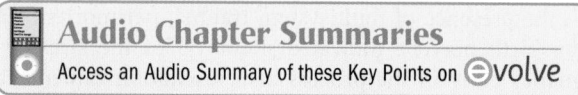

Audio Chapter Summaries

Access an Audio Summary of these Key Points on Evolve

References

Allen, V. M. (2002). *The effect of hypertensive disorders in pregnancy on perinatal outcomes: A population-based cohort study.* Ottawa: National Library of Canada.

American College of Obstetricians and Gynecologists. (2002). ACOG practice bulletin. Diagnosis and management of preeclampsia and eclampsia. Number 33. *International Journal of Gynaecology and Obstetrics, 77*(1), 67–75.

Ananth, C., Berkowitz, G., Savitz, D., & Lapinski, R. (1999). Placental abruption and adverse perinatal outcomes. *Journal of the American Medical Association, 282,* 1646–1651.

Arseneault, M., et al, (2002). SOGC clinical practice guideline: The management of nausea and vomiting of pregnancy. *Journal of Obstetrics and Gynaecology Canada, 24*(10), 817–823.

Baird, S. M., & Kennedy, B. B. (2008). Obstetric emergencies. In B. B. Kennedy, D. J. Ruth, & E. J. Martin (Eds.), *Intrapartum management modules: A perinatal education program.* Philadelphia: Wolters-Kluwer.

Canadian Diabetes Association. (2008). Clinical practice guidelines for the prevention and management of diabetes in Canada. *Canadian Journal of Diabetes, 32*(Suppl 1), S1–S201.

Chames, M. C., & Pearlman, M. D. (2008). Trauma during pregnancy: Outcomes and clinical management. *Clinics in Obstetrics and Gynecology, 51*(2), 398–408.

Cohen-Kerem, R., Railton, C., Oren, D., Lishner, M., & Koren, G. (2005). Pregnancy outcome following non-obstetric surgical intervention. *American Journal of Surgery, 190*(3), 476–473.

Cohn, D., Ramaswamy, B., & Blum, K. (2009). Malignancy and pregnancy. In R. K. Creasy, et al. (Eds), *Creasy & Resnik's maternal–fetal medicine: Principles and practice* (6th ed.). Philadelphia: Saunders.

Conway, D., Gonzales, O., & Skiver, D. (2004). Use of glyburide for the treatment of gestational diabetes: The San Antonio experience. *Journal of Maternal and Fetal Medicine, 15,* 51–55.

Copeland, L., & Landon, M. (2007). Malignant diseases in pregnancy. In S. G. Gabbe, J. R. Niebyl, & J. L. Simpson (Eds.), *Obstetrics: Normal and problem pregnancies* (5th ed.). New York: Churchill Livingstone.

Crane, J., et al. (2003). SOGC committee opinion: Antenatal corticosteroid therapy for fetal maturation. *Journal of Obstetrics and Gynaecology Canada, 25*(8), 45–48. Retrieved from http://www.sogc.org/guidelines/public/122e-co-janvier2003.pdf.

Crowther, C., Hiller, J., McPhee, A., Jeffries, W., & Robinson, J. (2005). Effect of treatment of gestational diabetes on pregnancy outcomes. *New England Journal of Medicine, 352,* 2477–2486.

Cunningham, F., et al. (2010). *Williams obstetrics* (23rd ed.). New York: McGraw Hill.

Davies, G., et al. (2010). SOGC clinical practice guideline: Obesity in pregnancy. *Journal of Obstetrics and Gynaecology Canada, 32*(2), 165–173.

Davis, M. (2004). Nausea and vomiting of pregnancy: An evidence-based review. *Journal of Perinatal and Neonatal Nursing, 18*(4), 312–328.

Duley, L., et al. (2002). Do women with pre-eclampsia, and their babies, benefit from magnesium sulphate? The Magpie Trial: A randomised placebo-controlled trial. *Lancet, 359,* 1877–1890.

Dyck, R., Klomp, H., & Tan, L. (2002). A comparison of rates, risk factors and outcomes of gestational diabetes between Aboriginal and non-Aboriginal women in the Saskatoon Health District. *Diabetes Care, 25,* 487–493.

Ebrahimi, N., Maltepe, C., Bournissen, F. G., & Koren, G. (2009). Nausea and vomiting of pregnancy: Using the 24-hour pregnancy-unique quantification of emesis (PUQE-24) Scale. *Journal of Obstetrics and Gynaecology Canada, 31*(9), 803–807.

Einarson, A., Maltepe, C., Boskovic, R., & Koren, G. (2007). Treatment of nausea and vomiting in pregnancy: An updated algorithm. *Canadian Family Physician, 53,* 2109–2111.

Emery, S. (2005). Hypertensive disorders of pregnancy: Over-diagnosis is appropriate. *Cleveland Clinic Journal of Medicine, 72*(4), 345–352.

Firoz, T., Maltepe, C., & Einarson, A. (2010). Nausea and vomiting in pregnancy is not always nausea and vomiting of pregnancy. *Journal of Obstetrics and Gynaecology Canada, 10,* 970–972.

Francois, K. E., & Foley, M. R. (2007). Antepartum and postpartum hemorrhage. In S. G. Gabbe, J. R. Niebyl, & J. L. Simpson (Eds.), *Obstetrics: Normal and problem pregnancies* (5th ed.). New York: Churchill Livingstone.

Gagnon, R., et al. (2009). SOGC clinical practice guideline: Guidelines for the management of vasa previa. *Journal of Obstetrics and Gynaecology Canada, 31*(8), 748–753. Retrieved from http://www.sogc.org/guidelines/documents/gui231CPG0908.pdf.

Gilbert, E. S. (2007). *Manual of high risk pregnancy and delivery* (4th ed.). St. Louis: Mosby.

Griebel, C., et al. (2005). Management of spontaneous abortion. *American Family Physician, 72*(7), 1243–1250.

Hull, A. D., & Resnik, R. (2009). Placenta previa, placenta accrete, abruptio placentae, and vasa previa. In R. K. Creasy, et al. (Eds.), *Creasy & Resnik's maternal–fetal medicine: Principles and practice* (6th ed.). Philadelphia: Saunders.

Iams, J. D. (2009). Cervical insufficiency. In R. K. Creasy, et al. (Eds.), *Creasy & Resnik's maternal–fetal medicine: Principles and practice* (6th ed.). Philadelphia: Saunders.

Iams, J. D., & Romero, R. (2007). Preterm birth. In S. G. Gabbe, J. R. Niebyl, & J. L. Simpson (Eds.), *Obstetrics: Normal and problem pregnancies* (5th ed.). New York: Churchill Livingstone.

Ikossi, D., et al. (2005). Profile of mothers at risk: An analysis of injury and pregnancy loss in 1,195 trauma patients. *Journal of the American College of Surgeons, 200*(1), 49–56.

International Association of Diabetes and Pregnancy Study Groups Consensus Panel. (2010). International Association of Diabetes and Pregnancy Study Group recommendations on the diagnosis and classification of hyperglycemia in pregnancy. *Diabetes Care, 33*, 676–691.

Kelly, T. F., & Savides, T. J. (2009). Gastrointestinal disease in pregnancy. In R. K. Creasy, et al. (Eds.), *Creasy & Resnik's maternal–fetal medicine: Principles and practice* (6th ed.). Philadelphia: Saunders.

Kuczkowski, K. M. (2004). Nonobstetric surgery during pregnancy: What are the risks of anesthesia? *Obstetrical and Gynecological Survey, 59*(1), 52–56.

Landon, M. B., Catalano, P. M., & Gabbe, S. G. (2007). Diabetes mellitus. In S. G. Gabbe, J. R. Niebyl, & J. L. Simpson (Eds.), *Obstetrics: Normal and problem pregnancies* (5th ed.). New York: Churchill Livingstone.

Langer, O., & Conway, D. (2000). Levels of glycemia and perinatal outcomes in pregestational diabetes. *Journal of Maternal Fetal–Medicine, 9*, 35–41.

Liston, R., et al. (2007). SOGC clinical practice guideline: Fetal health surveillance: Antepartum and intrapartum consensus guideline. *Journal of Obstetrics and Gynaecology Canada, 29*(9), Suppl 4. Retrieved from http://www.sogc.org/guidelines/documents/gui197CPG0709r.pdf.

Lockwood, C. J., & Silver, R. M. (2009). Coagulation disorders in pregnancy. In R. K. Creasy, et al. (Eds.), *Creasy & Resnik's maternal–fetal medicine: Principles and practice* (6th ed.). Philadelphia: Saunders.

MacDonald, S., Vermeulen, M., & Ray, J. (2007). Risk of fetal death associated with maternal drug dependence and placental abruption: A population-based study. *Journal of Obstetrics and Gynaecology Canada, 29*(7), 556–559.

Magpie Trial Follow-Up Study Collaborative Group. (2007a). The Magpie Trial: A randomised trial comparing magnesium sulphate with placebo for pre-eclampsia. Outcome for children at 18 months. *British Journal of Obstetrics and Gynaecology, 114*(3), 289–299.

Magpie Trial Follow-Up Study Collaborative Group. (2007b). The Magpie Trial: A randomised trial comparing magnesium sulphate with placebo for pre-eclampsia. Outcome for women at 2 years. *British Journal of Obstetrics and Gynaecology, 114*(3), 300–309.

Maloni, J. A., et al. (2004). Antepartum bed rest: Maternal weight change and infant birth weight. *Biological Research for Nursing, 5*(3), 177–186.

Martin, S. R., & Foley, M. R. (2009). Intensive care monitoring of the critically ill pregnant patient. In R. K. Creasy, et al. (Eds.), *Creasy & Resnik's maternal–fetal medicine: Principles and practice* (6th ed.). Philadelphia: Saunders.

Matthews, A., Dowswell, T., Haas, D. M., Doyle, M., & O'Mathúna, D. P. (2010). Interventions for nausea and vomiting in early pregnancy. *Cochrane Database of Systematic Reviews*, Issue 9, Art. No. CD007575. doi: 10.1002/14651858.CD007575.pub2

Mattox, K., & Goetzl, L. (2005). Trauma in pregnancy. *Critical Care Medicine, 33*(10S), S385–S389.

Mazzotta, P., Maltepe, C., Navioz, Y., Magee, L. A., & Koren, G. (2000). Attitudes, management and consequences of nausea and vomiting of pregnancy in the United States and Canada. *International Journal of Gynaecology and Obstetrics, 70*, 359–365.

McFarlane, J. (2007). Pregnancy following partner rape. What we know and what we need to know. *Trauma, Violence & Abuse, 8*(2), 127–134.

McGwin, G., et al. (2004). Knowledge, beliefs, and practices concerning seat belt use during pregnancy. *Journal of Trauma, 56*(3), 670–675.

Moodliar, S., Bagratee, J., & Moodley, J. (2005). Medical versus surgical evacuation of first-trimester spontaneous abortion. *International Journal of Gynaecology and Obstetrics, 91*(1), 21–26.

Morin, L., et al. (2005). SOGC clinical practice guideline: Ultrasound evaluation of first trimester pregnancy complications. *Journal of Obstetrics and Gynaecology Canada, 27*(6), 581–585. Retrieved from http://www.sogc.org/guidelines/public/161e-cpg-june2005.pdf.

Moutquin, J. M., et al. (1997). Report of the Canadian Hypertension Society Consensus Conference: Nonpharmacologic management and prevention of hypertensive disorders in pregnancy. *Canadian Medical Association Journal, 157*, 907–919.

Murray, H., et al. (2005). Diagnosis and treatment of ectopic pregnancy. *Canadian Medical Association Journal, 173*(8), 905–912.

Mutter, W. P., & Karumanchi, S. A. (2008). Molecular mechanisms of pre-eclampsia. *Microvascular Research, 75*(1), 1–8.

Oppenheimer, L., et al. (2007). SOGC clinical practice guideline: Diagnosis and management of placenta previa. *Journal of Obstetrics and Gynaecology Canada, 29*(3), 261–273. Retrieved from http://www.sogc.org/guidelines/documents/189e-cpg-march2007.pdf.

Oyelese, Y., & Ananth, C. V. (2006). Placental abruption. *Obstetrics and Gynecology, 108*, 1005–1016.

Pandey, M., Rani, R., & Agrawal, S. (2005). An update in recurrent spontaneous abortion. *Archives of Gynecology and Obstetrics, 272*(2), 95–108.

Petrozza, J., & Berin, I. (2011). Recurrent early pregnancy loss. *eMedicine*. Retrieved from http://emedicine.medscape.com/article/260495-overview.

Roberts, J., & Funai, E. F. (2009). Pregnancy-related hypertension. In R. K. Creasy, et al. (Eds.), *Creasy & Resnik's maternal–fetal medicine: Principles and practice* (6th ed.). Philadelphia: Saunders.

Roberts, J., et al. & NHLBI Working Group on Research on Hypertension During Pregnancy. (2003). Summary of the NHLBI Working Group on Research on Hypertension During Pregnancy. *Hypertension, 41*(3), 437–445.

Rust, O., et al. (2005). Does the presence of a funnel increase the risk of adverse perinatal outcome in a patient with a short cervix? *American Journal of Obstetrics and Gynecology, 192*(4), 1060–1066.

Rust, O., & Roberts, W. (2005). Does cerclage prevent preterm birth? *Obstetric and Gynecology Clinics of North America, 32*(3), 441–456.

Sepilian, V. P., et al. (2011). Ectopic pregnancy. *eMedicine*, March 8, 2011. Retrieved from http://www.emedicine.com/med/topic3212.htm.

Shah, A., & Kilcline, B. (2003). Trauma in pregnancy. *Emergency Medical Clinics of North America, 21*(3), 615–629.

Sheehan, P. (2007). Hyperemesis gravidarum: Assessment and management. *Australian Family Physician. 36*(9), 698–701.

Sibai, B. (2007). Hypertension in pregnancy. In S. G. Gabbe, J. R. Niebyl, & J. L. Simpson (Eds.), *Obstetrics: Normal and problem pregnancies* (5th ed.). New York: Churchill Livingstone.

Sibai, B., Dekker, G., & Kupferminc, M. (2005). Pre-eclampsia. *Lancet, 365*(9461), 785–799.

Simpson, J. L., & Jauniaux, E. R. M. (2007). Pregnancy loss. In S. G. Gabbe, J. R. Niebyl, & J. L. Simpson (Eds.), *Obstetrics: Normal and problem pregnancies* (5th ed.). New York: Churchill Livingstone.

Simpson, K., & James, D. (2005). *Postpartum care*. White Plains, NY: March of Dimes.

Society of Obstetricians and Gynaecologists of Canada. (2008). SOGC clinical practice guideline: Diagnosis, evaluation and management of the hypertensive disorders of pregnancy. *Journal of Obstetrics and Gynaecology Canada, 30*(3), Suppl 1, S1–S48. Retrieved from http://www.sogc.org/guidelines/documents/gui206CPG0803_001.pdf.

Society of Obstetricians and Gynaecologists of Canada and Canadian Society of Exercise Physiology. (2003). SOGC clinical practice guideline: Exercise in pregnancy and the postpartum period. *Journal of Obstetrics and Gynaecology Canada, 25*(6), 516–522. Retrieved from http://www.sogc.org/guidelines/public/129E-JCPG-June2003.pdf.

Tucker, S. M., Miller, L. A., & Miller, D. A. (2009). *Pocket guide to fetal monitoring: A multidisciplinary approach* (6th ed.). St. Louis: Mosby.

Van, P., & Meleis, A. I. (2003). Coping with grief after involuntary pregnancy loss: Perspectives of African American women. *Journal of Obstetric, Gynecologic & Neonatal Nursing, 32*(1), 28–39.

Walker, M., Whittle, W., Keating, S., & Kingdom, J. (2010). Sonographic diagnosis of chronic abruption. *Journal of Obstetrics and Gynaecology Canada, 32*(11), 1056–1058.

Wolfberg, A., et al. (2005). Postevacuation hCG levels and risk of gestational trophoblastic neoplasia in women with complete molar pregnancy. *Obstetrics and Gynecology, 106*(3), 548–552.

Yang, J., et al. (2005). Predictors of vaginal bleeding during the first two trimesters of pregnancy. *Paediatric and Perinatal Epidemiology, 19*(4), 276–283.

Unit 3

14 Pregnancy at Risk: Pre-Existing Conditions

Learning Objectives

On completion of this chapter, the reader will be able to:

- Differentiate the types of diabetes mellitus and their respective risk factors in pregnancy.
- Compare insulin requirements during pregnancy, the postpartum period, and lactation.
- Identify maternal and fetal risks and possible complications associated with diabetes in pregnancy.
- Develop a plan of care for the pregnant woman with pregestational diabetes.
- Understand the management of hyperthyroidism and hypothyroidism in a pregnant woman.
- Differentiate the management of various cardiovascular disorders in pregnant women.
- Discuss the different types of anemia and their effects during pregnancy.
- Describe the care of pregnant women with pulmonary disorders.
- Discuss the effects of gastrointestinal disorders on pregnancy.
- Review the effects of neurological disorders on pregnancy.
- Describe the care of women whose pregnancies are complicated by autoimmune disorders.
- Explain the effects on and the management of pregnant women with human immunodeficiency virus.
- Describe the care of the bariatric pregnant woman.
- Discuss the care of pregnant women who have issues related to substance use.

Electronic Resources

Additional information related to the content in Chapter 14 can be found on

evolve the companion Web site at

http://evolve.elsevier.com/Canada/Perry/maternal/

- Examination Review questions
- Case Study—Class III Cardiac Disorder
- Case Study—Pregestational Diabetes

For most women, pregnancy is a normal and healthy life event. However, for some women pregnancy can be a time of significant risk due to the presence of a chronic illness. Women actively participate in self-management of their illness along with the multidisciplinary team to best manage the changes in pregnancy to promote the best pregnancy outcomes.

The goal of the health care team is to work with women to promote as normal a pregnancy experience as possible, while supporting the unique maternal and fetal needs prompted by the existence of chronic conditions. Nurses are key members of the health care team who guide and support the woman and her family in achieving optimal outcomes for both her and her fetus.

This chapter focuses on nursing care for women with metabolic disorders, including diabetes mellitus and thyroid disorders; cardiovascular disorders; selected disorders of the respiratory, gastrointestinal, integumentary, and central nervous systems; and **autoimmune disorders**. Key elements of care for women with substance use issues, human immunodeficiency virus (HIV) infection, and obesity are also discussed.

Metabolic Disorders

Diabetes Mellitus

Advances in knowledge about the effects of pregnancy on diabetes care have improved the outcomes for women. Diabetic women who are pregnant have the greatest success when they work together with a multidisciplinary team involving the obstetrician, internist or endocrinologist, pediatrician, nurse, and dietitian. These women require education regarding the effects that pregnancy can have on their diabetes management in order to prevent complications. Women with type 1 and type 2 diabetes need to be on a schedule of frequent prenatal visits to support their knowledge about necessary changes to their diet and the importance of more frequent self-monitoring of blood glucose levels. They also need more frequent laboratory evaluation and more intensive fetal surveillance, and occasionally they may need hospitalization to achieve optimal pregnancy outcomes.

Recent studies have shown that the perinatal mortality rate for women with well-controlled diabetes, excluding major congenital malformations, is about the same as that for any other pregnancy (Landon, Catalano, & Gabbe, 2007). This is due to improvements in the understanding and management of strict maternal glucose control before conception and throughout the pregnancy. Before becoming pregnant, women with diabetes are strongly encouraged to have preconception counselling to optimize glycemic control, assess for presence of complications, review medications, and begin folate supplementation (Canadian Diabetes Association [CDA], 2008).

Nurses who provide care to pregnant women with diabetes must fully understand both the normal physiological responses to pregnancy, as well as the physiological effects and psychosocial implications of diabetes, to accurately assess the needs of the individual woman, help her plan for her care, and intervene when appropriate.

Pathogenesis

Diabetes mellitus is a group of metabolic diseases characterized by **hyperglycemia** resulting from defects in insulin secretion, insulin action, or both (Expert Committee on the Diagnosis and Classification of Diabetes Mellitus, 2003). *Insulin*, produced by β-cells in the islets of Langerhans of the pancreas, regulates blood glucose levels by enabling glucose to enter adipose and muscle cells, where it is used for energy. Insulin stimulates protein synthesis and the storage of free fatty acids. When insulin is insufficient or ineffective in promoting glucose uptake by the muscle and adipose cells, glucose accumulates in the bloodstream, resulting in hyperglycemia. Hyperglycemia causes hyperosmolarity of the blood, which attracts intracellular fluid into the vascular system, resulting in cellular dehydration and expanded blood volume. Consequently, the kidneys function to excrete large volumes of urine (*polyuria*) in an attempt to regulate excess vascular volume and excrete the unused glucose (**glycosuria**). Polyuria and cellular dehydration cause excessive thirst (*polydipsia*).

The body compensates for its inability to convert carbohydrate (glucose) into energy by burning proteins (muscle) and fats. The end products of this metabolism are **ketones** and fatty acids, which in excess quantity produce ketoacidosis and acetonuria. Weight loss occurs because of the breakdown of fat and muscle tissue. This tissue breakdown causes a state of starvation that compels the individual to eat excessive amounts of food (*polyphagia*).

Over time, diabetes that is not well controlled causes significant changes in both the microvascular and macrovascular circulations. These structural changes affect a variety of organ systems—primarily the heart, eyes, kidneys, and nerves. Complications resulting from diabetes include premature atherosclerosis, retinopathy, nephropathy, and neuropathy.

Classification

Diabetes during pregnancy is currently classified into two categories: pregestational and gestational diabetes. *Pregestational diabetes* is the label often given to type 1 or type 2 diabetes that existed before pregnancy.

People with type 1 diabetes have an absolute insulin deficiency caused by pancreatic islet β-cell destruction, which makes them prone to ketoacidosis. Type 1 diabetes is theorized to be caused by an autoimmune process, but the cause is primarily unknown (Expert Committee on the Diagnosis and Classification of Diabetes Mellitus, 2003).

Type 2 diabetes is the most prevalent form of the disease and affects individuals who have insulin resistance and relative (rather than absolute) insulin deficiency. Individuals may have type 2 diabetes for many years prior to diagnosis because hyperglycemia develops gradually and often is not severe enough for the person to recognize the classic signs of polyuria, polydipsia, and polyphagia. Many people who develop type 2 diabetes are obese or have an increased amount of body fat distributed primarily in the abdominal area. Other risk factors include aging, a sedentary lifestyle, hypertension, and prior gestational diabetes. Type 2 diabetes often has a strong family genetic predisposition (Expert Committee on the Diagnosis and Classification of Diabetes Mellitus, 2003).

Gestational diabetes mellitus (GDM) is the classification for women who have carbohydrate intolerance that is discovered during pregnancy. GDM is any degree of glucose intolerance with its onset or first recognition during pregnancy. This definition applies regardless of whether insulin is used for treatment or whether the diabetes persists after pregnancy. It does not exclude the possibility that glucose intolerance preceded the pregnancy. Women who experience gestational diabetes should be assessed for the presence of underlying disease 6 weeks to 6 months after the pregnancy ends (CDA, 2008) (see Chapter 13 for further discussion).

Metabolic Changes Associated With Pregnancy

Normal pregnancy is characterized by complex alterations in maternal glucose metabolism, insulin production, and metabolic homeostasis. During normal pregnancy, adjustments in maternal metabolism allow for adequate nutrition for both the mother and the developing fetus. Glucose, the primary fuel used by the fetus, is transported across the placenta through the process of carrier-mediated facilitated diffusion. This means that the glucose levels in the fetus are directly proportional to maternal levels. Although glucose crosses the placenta, insulin does not. By the tenth week of gestation, the evolve Case Study—Pregestational Diabetes

embryo or fetus secretes its own insulin at levels adequate to use the glucose obtained from the mother. Thus, as maternal glucose levels rise, fetal glucose levels are increased, resulting in increased fetal insulin secretion.

During the first **trimester** and early second trimester of pregnancy, the pregnant woman's metabolic status is significantly influenced by the rising levels of estrogen and progesterone. These hormones stimulate the β-cells in the pancreas to increase insulin production, which promotes increased peripheral use of glucose and decreased blood glucose, with fasting levels reduced by approximately 10% (Fig. 14-1, A). There is a concomitant increase in tissue glycogen stores and a decrease in hepatic glucose production, which together further encourage lower fasting glucose levels. As a result of these normal metabolic changes of pregnancy, women with type 1 and type 2 diabetes are prone to **hypoglycemia** (low blood glucose) during the first trimester.

During the later part of the second trimester and the third trimester, pregnancy exerts a **diabetogenic** effect on the maternal metabolic status. Because of the major hormonal changes, there is decreased tolerance to glucose, increased insulin resistance, decreased hepatic glycogen stores, and increased hepatic production of glucose. Increasing levels of human chorionic somatomammotropin, estrogen, progesterone, prolactin, cortisol, and insulinase increase insulin resistance through their actions as insulin antagonists. Insulin resistance is a glucose-sparing mechanism that ensures an abundant supply of glucose for the fetus. Maternal insulin requirements gradually increase from about 18 to 24 weeks of gestation to about 36 weeks of gestation, usually doubling by the end of pregnancy. During the last few weeks of pregnancy, women need to be reassured that their diabetes is not becoming worse with the increase in insulin and told that insulin requirements usually level off after 36 weeks' gestation until labour begins (see Fig. 14-1, B and C).

At birth, expulsion of the placenta prompts an abrupt decrease in levels of circulating placental hormones, cortisol, and insulinase (see Fig. 14-1, D). Maternal tissues quickly regain their prepregnancy sensitivity to insulin. For the non-breastfeeding mother, the prepregnancy insulin–carbohydrate balance usually returns in about 7 to 10 days (see Fig. 14-1, E). Lactation uses maternal glucose; thus the breastfeeding mother's insulin requirements remain low as long as she is nursing (see Fig. 14-1, E). On completion of weaning, the mother's prepregnancy insulin requirement is re-established (see Fig. 14-1, F).

Pregestational Diabetes Mellitus

Pregestational diabetes (type 1 and type 2) presents in approximately 0.5% of pregnancies, with type 2 now the more common diagnosis in childbearing-age women (Schaefer-Graf, Buchanan, Xiang, & Kjos, 2002). Fetal risks for women with type 1 and type 2 diabetes are similar; however, recent literature suggests that adverse pregnancy outcomes for women with type 2 diabetes are increasing and may be worse than those of their type 1 counterparts (Clausen, Mathiesen, & Ekborm, 2005). The increasing prevalence of type 2 diabetes in the pregnant population may be a contributing factor. Women with type 1 diabetes are more likely to have the vascular, retinal, or renal complications because their duration of illness is usually longer than that of women with type 2 diabetes. Almost all women with type 2 diabetes require insulin during pregnancy.

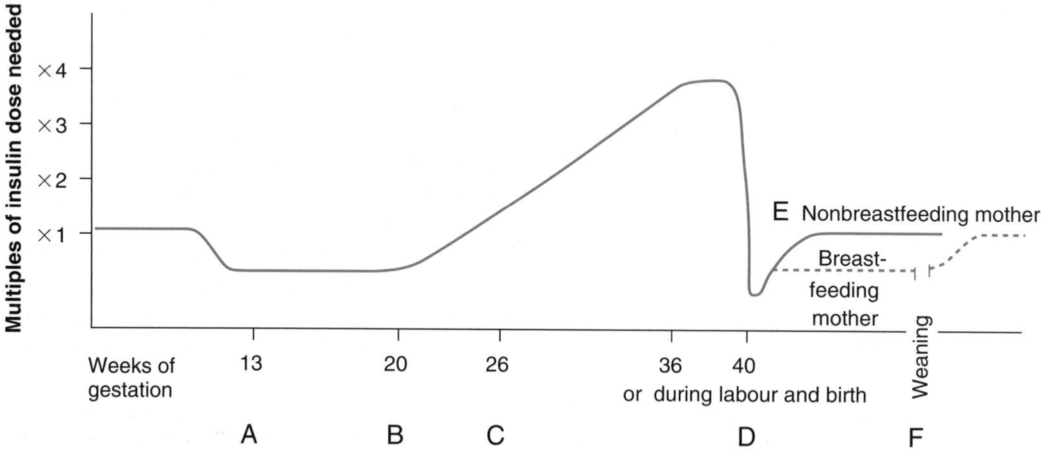

Fig. 14-1 Changing insulin needs during pregnancy. **A:** First trimester/early second trimester: Insulin need is reduced because of increased insulin production by the pancreas and increased peripheral sensitivity to insulin; nausea, vomiting, and decreased food intake by mother and glucose transfer to the embryo or fetus contribute to hypoglycemia. **B:** Late second trimester: Insulin need increases as placental hormones, cortisol, and insulinase act as insulin antagonists, decreasing the effectiveness of insulin. **C:** Third trimester: Insulin requirements gradually increase until about 36 weeks of gestation. **D:** Day of birth: Maternal insulin requirements drop drastically to approach prepregnancy levels. **E:** Breastfeeding mother maintains lower insulin requirements, as much as 25% less than prepregnancy; insulin need of nonbreastfeeding mother returns to prepregnancy levels in 7 to 10 days. **F:** At weaning of breastfeeding infant, mother's insulin need returns to prepregnancy levels.

Preconception Counselling

Preconception counselling is recommended by the Canadian Diabetes Association (CDA) and the Society of Obstetricians and Gynaecologists of Canada (SOGC) for all women of reproductive age with diabetes in order to support improved pregnancy outcomes (Allen et al., 2007; CDA, 2008). Preconception care to evaluate the woman's health status, plan the optimal time for pregnancy, improve self-management of optimal glycemic control before conception, and stabilize any vascular complications of diabetes (retinopathy, nephropathy, neuropathy, and cardiovascular disease) is ideal. However, it is estimated that fewer than 50% of women with type 1 diabetes plan their pregnancies and seek preconceptual counselling, and this figure is even lower for women with type 2 diabetes (CDA, 2008). Preconception counselling is particularly important because strict metabolic control before conception and in the early weeks of gestation during organogenesis is instrumental in decreasing the risk of congenital anomalies and spontaneous abortion (Box 14-1).

Preconception counselling should also include information regarding medications being used for glycemic control. While the use of oral antidiabetic medications is not recommended by the Canadian Diabetes Association, continued research is being conducted to determine their efficacy and safety before and during pregnancy. Some physicians may recommend that oral hypoglycemic agents be discontinued in the preconception period in women with type 2 diabetes. These women are started on insulin before pregnancy when the pregnancy is planned or as soon as the pregnancy is diagnosed when it is unplanned (CDA, 2008; Cunningham et al., 2010).

The woman's partner should be included in preconception counselling to improve the support for the woman and understanding of potential complications of pregnancy as a result of diabetes. The couple also should be informed of the anticipated alterations in the management of diabetes during pregnancy and the need for a multidisciplinary team approach to pregnancy care. Financial implications of the diabetic pregnancy and other demands related to frequent maternal and fetal surveillance should be discussed. Contraception is an important aspect of preconception counselling to assist the couple in planning the timing of pregnancy.

BOX 14-1 Goals for Self-Monitored Glucose Levels in Preconceptional Period

Recommended glycemic targets for preconception and during pregnancy:

Prepregnancy A_{1C}	<7%*
Pregnancy A_{1C}	≤6.0%

A_{1C} = glycosylated hemoglobin: With prolonged hyperglycemia, some of the hemoglobin remains saturated with glucose for the life of the red blood cell. Therefore, a test for glycosylated hemoglobin provides a measurement of glycemic control over time, specifically over the previous 8 to 12 weeks.

*Ideally, A_{1C} ≤6.0% if this can be safely achieved. In some women, particularly those with type 1 diabetes, higher targets may be necessary to avoid excessive hypoglycemia. Regular measurements of glycosylated hemoglobin provide data for altering the treatment plan and lead to improvement of glycemic control. A hemoglobin A_{1C} of 6 to 7% is the desired goal, which correlates to an average glucose of 5.5 to 7.7 mmol/L (CDA, 2008).

Maternal Risks and Complications

While morbidity and mortality rates have improved significantly for the pregnant woman with diabetes, risk remains for the development of significant complications during pregnancy. Assessment of risk is best done by evaluating the woman's blood glucose control and determining the length of time since diagnosis of the woman's diabetes and whether existing diabetic complications are present. Women with poor glycemic control, longer durations of diabetes, and presence of complications typically have less than optimal pregnancy outcomes, such as perinatal mortality, congenital malformations, hypertension, preterm delivery, **large-for-gestational-age infants**, Caesarean delivery, and neonatal morbidities (CDA, 2008).

Women with pregestational diabetes who have poor glycemic control (defined as a **glycosylated hemoglobin** value greater than 7.0% around the time of conception and in the early weeks of pregnancy) have a twofold increased incidence of early pregnancy loss (28%) (Langer & Conway, 2000). Women with good glycemic control before conception and in the first trimester are no more likely to have a miscarriage than women without diabetes (CDA, 2008).

Poor glycemic control later in pregnancy increases the rate of fetal **macrosomia** (excessive growth; defined as a birth weight greater than 4000 to 4500 g). Macrosomia occurs in up to 50% of pregnancies in women with gestational diabetes and in 40% of type 1 and type 2 diabetic pregnancies (Landon et al., 2007). These large infants tend to have a disproportionate increase in shoulder and trunk size; consequently, the risk of shoulder dystocia is greater in these babies than in other macrosomic infants. Thus women with type 1 and type 2 diabetes face an increased likelihood of Caesarean birth (because of failure to progress or failure of descent) or operative vaginal birth (use of forceps or vacuum extraction).

Hypertensive disorders such as pre-eclampsia or eclampsia occur much more frequently in women with pregestational diabetes, particularly in those who have renal dysfunction. Preterm labour or birth is also more likely to occur, especially with more severe hypertension, chronically elevated glucose levels, and presence of genital or urinary tract infections. For these reasons, the risk for induced preterm birth is greater in women with poorly controlled pregestational diabetes (Landon et al., 2007).

Women with type 1 and type 2 diabetes should have regular testing of their eyes for retinopathy. Regular assessments by an ophthalmologist who has knowledge of diabetes is recommended preconception, during the first trimester of pregnancy, as needed within the pregnancy, and again within 1 year postpartum (CDA, 2008). Women may develop retinopathy due to poor glycemic control and are at increased risk with comorbidities such as hypertension or renal disease (CDA, 2008). Women with existing mild-to-moderate retinopathy who become pregnant but maintain good glycemic control are not felt to be at increased risk of worsening retinopathy (CDA, 2008).

Women with diabetes who are contemplating a pregnancy should be screened for the presence of chronic kidney disease. During pregnancy, monitoring of renal function should occur using the albumin-to-creatinine ratio (ACR) and the estimated glomerular filtration rate (eGFR) (CDA, 2008). Kidney disease and microalbuminemia can be associated with poor outcomes for the mother and fetus. Pregnant women with diabetes should also be monitored for serum creatinine levels to assess for kidney status throughout the pregnancy so that deterioration in kidney function can be detected (CDA, 2008).

The most common concern in pregnancy is the loss of hypoglycemic awareness. This is more common in long-standing diabetes and creates safety concerns for the mother, especially at times when concentration is required, such as driving a car. Hypoglycemic awareness may or may not return postpregnancy.

Polyhydramnios, amniotic fluid in excess of 2000 mL occurs about 10 times more often in diabetic pregnancies than in nondiabetic pregnancies. The etiology for polyhydramnios has been theorized as increased amniotic glucose concentration or fetal hyperglycemia and polyuria; however, it is still unknown (Cunningham et al., 2010). Overdistension of the uterus caused by polyhydramnios increases the possibility of compression of maternal abdominal blood vessels (vena cava and aorta), causing supine hypotension. Women are also at risk for premature rupture of the membranes, cord prolapse, preterm labour, and postpartum hemorrhage with the presence of polyhydramnios.

Infections are more common and more serious in pregnant women with diabetes. Disorders of carbohydrate metabolism alter the body's normal resistance to infection. The inflammatory response, **leukocyte** function, and vaginal pH are all affected. Vaginal infections, particularly monilial vaginitis, are more common, as are urinary tract infections. Infection in the pregnant woman with diabetes may be critical, causing increased insulin resistance, which may result in hyper- or hypoglycemic reactions. Postpartum infection may also occur among women who have poorly controlled blood glucose.

Ketoacidosis, or accumulation of ketones in the blood resulting from hyperglycemia and leading to metabolic acidosis, is rare in women with type 2 diabetes. Women with type 1 diabetes may experience diabetic ketoacidosis (DKA) during the second and third trimesters when the diabetogenic effect of pregnancy is the greatest. Women at risk for preterm labour may be at increased risk for DKA from administration of steroids or some **tocolytic** medications. DKA may also occur because of the over- or underadministration of insulin. It may occur with blood glucose levels barely exceeding 11 mmol/L because of an increase in the body's resistance to insulin in pregnancy; nonpregnant thresholds are higher, at 16.7 to 19.5 mmol/L. In response to stress factors such as infection or illness, hyperglycemia occurs, with a resulting increase in hepatic glucose production and decreased peripheral glucose use. The presence of nausea, vomiting, and fever can lead to ketoacidosis. Stress hormones, which can impair insulin action and further contribute to insulin deficiency, are released. Fatty acids are mobilized from fat stores into the circulation. As they are oxidized, ketone bodies are released into the peripheral circulation. The woman's buffering system is unable to compensate, and metabolic acidosis develops. The excessive blood glucose and ketone bodies result in osmotic diuresis, with subsequent loss of fluid and electrolytes, volume depletion, and cellular dehydration. Prompt treatment of DKA is necessary to avoid maternal coma or death. Ketoacidosis at any time during pregnancy can lead to intrauterine fetal death and may stimulate preterm labour. The fetal mortality rate is approximately 50% with maternal ketoacidosis (Cunningham et al., 2010).

The risk of hypoglycemia is also increased. Early in pregnancy, when hepatic production of glucose is diminished and peripheral use of glucose is enhanced, hypoglycemia occurs frequently, often during sleep. Later in pregnancy, hypoglycemia may also result as insulin doses are adjusted to maintain **euglycemia** (a normal blood glucose level). Women with a prepregnancy history of severe hypoglycemia are at increased risk for severe hypoglycemia during gestation. Hypoglycemic episodes do not appear to have significant deleterious effects on fetal well-being. The long-term fetal effects of severe maternal hypoglycemia are as yet uncertain.

Fetal and Neonatal Risks and Complications

Despite the improvements in care of pregnant women with diabetes, sudden and unexplained stillbirth is still a significant risk (Landon et al., 2007). Congenital anomalies are the other major cause of perinatal deaths in pregnancies complicated by diabetes. The incidence of major congenital anomalies in infants born to women with diabetes is 6 to 10%, a twofold to fourfold increase over that of the general population (Reece & Homko, 2007). Central nervous system (CNS) defects (e.g., anencephaly, open spina bifida) are increased tenfold (Reece & Homko, 2007). Cardiac defects, especially ventricular septal defects (VSDs) and transposition of the great vessels, are increased fivefold (Landon et al., 2007). Caudal regression (also called caudal dysplasia or sacral agenesis) is a fetal anomaly found 200 to 400 times more often in pregnancies of mothers with diabetes (Landon et al., 2007).

Asymmetrical macrosomia refers to accelerated fetal trunk size in relation to the fetal head. The abdominal circumference is both greater than the ninetieth percentile for gestational age and 2 weeks larger when compared to head size. This discrepancy in growth is typically diagnosed with ultrasound examination. The implication of asymmetrical macrosomia is that there is an increased risk of birth trauma due to shoulder dystocia.

Other problems that cause significant neonatal morbidity include hypoglycemia, **respiratory distress syndrome**, **polycythemia,** and **hyperbilirubinemia** (Cunningham et al., 2010; Landon et al., 2007). See Chapter 27 for further discussion of neonatal risks associated with maternal diabetes.

Nursing Care Management

Nurses play a key role in helping women who are already diabetic understand how pregnancy may affect their management of diabetes (see Nursing Process box). Women require an individualized plan of care that builds on their in-depth knowledge of their own disease management to achieve euglycemia and prevent complications. The initial prenatal visit is the optimal time to assess the woman's knowledge regarding diabetes and pregnancy, review potential maternal and fetal complications, and begin the initial plan of care with the woman and her family. Subsequent visits are important for monitoring a woman's progress and identifying further learning needs. Teaching should include family members.

Antepartum Care

The presence of risk factors for the mother and her fetus means that the woman with diabetes is monitored more frequently than a woman with a low-risk pregnancy. Most pregnant women with diabetes are managed on an outpatient basis.

Achieving and maintaining euglycemia (normal blood glucose level; also called *normogylcemia*) with blood glucose levels in the range of 3.4 to 6.7 mmol/L (Table 14-1) is the primary goal of medical therapy for the pregnant woman with diabetes. Euglycemia is achieved through a combination of diet, insulin, exercise, and blood glucose determinations. A

NURSING PROCESS: PREGESTATIONAL DIABETES

Assessment

When a pregnant woman with diabetes initiates prenatal care, a thorough evaluation of her health status is completed. The assessment includes the following elements:

History

Routine prenatal and health history
Onset and type of diabetes
Degree of glycemic control before pregnancy

Interview

Learning needs:
- How the pregnancy will change the management of diabetes
- Potential maternal and fetal complications
- Plan of care, including self-management of glycemic control

Emotional status:
- Coping with pregnancy in the context of pre-existing diabetes
- Mental health status (e.g., depression)
- Dealing with "high-risk" status
- Fear of maternal and fetal complications, including fear of loss of pregnancy
- Fear of her ability to manage the changes necessary to maintain a safe and healthy pregnancy

Support system:
- Identifying significant persons and their roles
- Assessing reactions to the pregnancy and the management plan
- Reviewing maternal involvement in the treatment regimen
- Reviewing socioeconomic factors
- Assessing financial resources for increased use of diabetic equipment

Physical Examination

Current health status
Routine prenatal examination
Effects of diabetes on pregnancy
- Baseline electrocardiogram to assess cardiovascular status
- Blood-pressure monitoring to assess increased risk for pre-eclampsia
- Weight gain
- Fundal height: abnormal increase in size for dates may indicate hydramnios or fetal macrosomia

Presence of chronic complications: nephropathy, retinopathy, neuropathy, cardiovascular disease

Laboratory Tests

Glycosylated hemoglobin (A_{1C}) (glycemic control over time)
Baseline renal function with a serum protein/creatinine ratio (PCR) and a urine albumin/creatinine ratio (ACR)
Urinalysis and culture: initial prenatal visit and throughout the pregnancy (urinary tract infections are common in diabetic pregnancy)
Urine (ketones)
Thyroid function tests (see later discussion of thyroid disorders)

Nursing Diagnoses

Nursing diagnoses for the woman with pregestational diabetes include the following:

Need for knowledge related to
- pregnancy effects on diabetes management
- potential effects on pregnant woman and fetus

Anxiety, fear related to
- coping with a high-risk pregnancy
- effects of diabetes and its potential sequelae on the pregnant woman and the fetus

Risk for injury to fetus related to
- unexplained stillbirth
- birth trauma/shoulder dystocia

Risk for injury to mother related to
- improper insulin adjustment and administration
- effects of hypoglycemia and hyperglycemia
- possibility of Caesarean or operative vaginal birth
- potential for postpartum infection

Planning

An individualized plan of care is developed with the woman in collaboration with the multidisciplinary care team.

Expected outcomes of care include that the woman will participate in self-management to do the following:
- Articulate the plan of care during pregnancy
- Achieve and maintain glycemic control
- Indicate effective coping
- Experience no complications (maternal morbidity or mortality)
- Give birth to a healthy infant at term

Interventions

Antepartum

Attend routine prenatal visits every 1 to 2 weeks in the first and second trimesters and one to two times per week in the third trimester.
Receive education related to
- Need for increased frequency of glucose monitoring
- Importance of a daily maintenance of tight glucose control

Continued

NURSING PROCESS: PREGESTATIONAL DIABETES—cont'd

- Importance of good foot care and general skin care
- Diet alterations to support healthy growing fetus: nutrition counselling by registered dietitian
- Insulin therapy and how insulin requirement will change throughout the pregnancy
- Exercise/activity as designed by the physiotherapist and discussed with the primary health care provider (when other complications of pregnancy, such as bleeding, are not present)

Antenatal fetal surveillance, including

- Ultrasound (to determine gestational age and fetal growth; estimate fetal weight; detect hydramnios, macrosomia, and anomalies)
- Integrated pregnancy screen (IPS), which consists of three parts (see Chapter 12):
  - Step 1 is a blood test between 10 and 14 weeks for PAPPA.*
  - Step 2 is an ultrasound examination between 11 and 14 weeks for nuchal translucency and trisomy 21.
  - Step 3 is a quadruple marker screen (between 15 and 20 weeks).
- Fetal echocardiography (to detect cardiac anomalies)
- Doppler studies of the umbilical artery (to detect placental compromise)
- Fetal movement counts (daily after 26 weeks) (see Chapter 12)
- Nonstress tests (NST) (to evaluate fetal well-being)

Intrapartum

Conduct close monitoring to prevent complications (dehydration, hypoglycemia, hyperglycemia).

Determine blood glucose every 2 hours until active labour occurs, then hourly until delivery.

Insulin needs in labour are determined on a sliding scale, as insulin needs in pregnancy are not predictive of insulin needs in labour.

Test urine for ketones on an hourly basis in active labour.

Monitor fetal heart rate continuously to observe for fetal distress.

Observe for signs of shoulder dystocia.

Ensure that a neonatal care provider is present at birth.

Postpartum

Measure fasting blood glucose the morning after birth.

Monitor blood glucose levels and adjust insulin dosage as appropriate.

Observe for complications (pre-eclampsia, hemorrhage, postpartum infection).

Educate the diabetic mother on the benefits of breastfeeding for her and her newborn.

Provide family planning education.

Encourage a healthy balance between diet, insulin, and activity.

Evaluation

Effective care of the pregnant woman with pregestational diabetes is multifactorial and is evaluated by both the woman and her health care team. The best possible outcome for the diabetic woman and her new baby is the goal of diabetic management.

*PAPPA (pregnancy-associated plasma protein A) is one of several screening blood tests primarily used to assess the developing baby's risk for Down syndrome. The test is commonly done between 8 and 14 weeks of pregnancy. PAPPA is a protein that is generally present at lower than normal levels in babies with Down syndrome (trisomy 21) or intrauterine growth restriction and who are at increased risk for premature delivery.

Table 14-1 Target Blood Glucose Levels During Pregnancy

During Pregnancy	
Fasting and preprandial PG	3.8–5.2 mmol/L
1 hr postprandial PG	5.5–7.7 mmol/L
2 hr postprandial PG	5.0–6.6 mmol/L

(From Canadian Diabetes Association. [2008]. Clinical practice guidelines for the prevention and management of diabetes in Canada. *Canadian Journal of Diabetes, 32*[Suppl 1], S1–S201.)
PG, plasma glucose.

primary goal of nursing is to provide the woman with information on the changes to her diabetes management due to pregnancy, to help her achieve and maintain excellent blood glucose control.

Achieving euglycemia requires self-management by the woman and her family to make the necessary lifestyle adjustments, which can sometimes seem overwhelming. Maintaining tight blood glucose control is the primary goal of treatment; the woman needs to be realistic about her schedule of diet, exercise and activity, and insulin administration in order to achieve this goal. Blood glucose is measured frequently to determine how well the major components of therapy (diet, insulin, and exercise) are working together to control blood glucose levels.

Because the woman with diabetes is at risk for infections, eye problems, and neurological changes, foot care and general skin care are important. A daily bath should include good perineal and foot care. Lotions, creams, or oils can be applied to dry skin. The woman should avoid wearing tight clothing. She should always wear shoes or slippers that fit properly, preferably with socks or stockings. Feet should be inspected regularly, toenails should be cut straight across, and professional help should be sought for any foot problems. The woman needs to avoid extremes of temperature.

The woman should wear an identification bracelet at all times and carry her glucose meter, insulin, syringes or pens, and food to treat hypoglycemia, such as a fast-acting glucose along with a protein and a starch (see Community Focus box). The woman should be informed of how to report problems such as nausea, vomiting, and infections and should know how to reach her health care provider at all times (see Guidelines box).

COMMUNITY FOCUS
Accessibility of Diabetes Supplies

It is very important that health care providers be aware of the realities of the cost and availability of diabetes equipment. Visit the local pharmacy and examine the diabetes equipment and supplies that are available. Locate glucose meters, urine test strips, insulin syringes, and insulin pens. How much does each of these items cost? Read the directions for use of each item. How easy are the instructions to follow? Could a woman with low literacy skills read and understand them? Do the directions have illustrations? Are the directions available in more than one language (e.g., French) in addition to English? Does the pharmacy have someone who can teach women? How will this information be helpful in patient teaching?

GUIDELINES Treatment for Hypoglycemia

The goal of treating hypoglycemia is to identify and treat low blood glucose as it happens by using an effective fast-acting glucose to bring the blood sugar level back quickly without causing rebound hyperglycemia. The CDA (2008) guideline for treatment of hypoglycemia suggests that 15 g of glucose is required to raise blood sugar about 2.1 mmol/L in a 20-minute period.

- Be familiar with the signs and symptoms of hypoglycemia (nervousness, headache, shaking, irritability, personality change, hunger, blurred vision, sweaty skin, tingling of mouth or extremities).
- Check blood glucose level immediately when hypoglycemic symptoms occur.
- If blood glucose is below 3.4 mmol/L, immediately eat or drink something that contains 10 to 15 g of simple carbohydrate. Examples are as follows:
  - 175 mL (3/4 c) unsweetened fruit juice or regular soda
  - 15 mL (1 tbsp) or 3 packets of table sugar dissolved in water
  - 5 to 6 Life Savers candies
  - 15 mL (1 tbsp) honey
  - 15 g glucose in glucose tablet form
- Rest for 15 minutes; then recheck blood glucose.
- If glucose level is still <3.4 mmol/L, eat or drink another serving of one of the "glucose boosters" listed here.
- Wait 15 minutes, then recheck blood glucose. If it is still <3.4 mmol/L, notify a health care provider immediately.

(Source: Canadian Diabetes Association. [2008]. Clinical practice guidelines for the prevention and management of diabetes in Canada. *Canadian Journal of Diabetes, 32*[Suppl 1], S1–S201.)

Diet

The woman with type 1 or type 2 diabetes has usually had previous nutrition counselling regarding the management of diabetes. The pregnant woman needs to learn to incorporate changes into dietary planning, as pregnancy precipitates special nutrition concerns and needs. Nutrition counselling is primarily provided by a registered dietitian.

HOME CARE
Dietary Management of Diabetic Pregnancy

Follow the Prescribed Diet Plan

- Practice healthy eating for pregnancy based on *Eating Well With Canada's Food Guide*
- Divide daily food intake between three meals and two to four snacks, depending on individual lifestyle, hunger, blood glucose, ketones, insulin regime, and pregnancy-related factors, such as nausea, vomiting, heartburn, and constipation.
- Eat a substantial bedtime snack to prevent a severe drop in blood glucose level during the night.
- Limit the intake of fats if weight gain occurs too rapidly.
- Take daily vitamins and iron as prescribed by the health care provider.
- Avoid foods high in refined sugar.
- Eat at a consistent time each day; never skip meals or snacks.
- Reduce the intake of saturated fat and cholesterol.
- Eat foods high in dietary fibre.
- Avoid alcohol and caffeine.

Dietary management during diabetic pregnancy must be based on blood (not urine) glucose levels. The diet is individualized to allow for increased fetal and metabolic requirements, with consideration of such factors as prepregnancy weight and dietary habits, overall health, ethnic background, lifestyle, stage of pregnancy, knowledge of nutrition, and insulin therapy. The dietary goals are to have weight gain consistent with a normal pregnancy, prevent ketoacidosis, and achieve euglycemia through consistency in carbohydrate intake.

Energy needs are usually calculated on the basis of 30 to 35 kilocalories per kilogram of ideal body weight, with the average diet including 2200 kilocalories (first trimester) to 2500 kilocalories (second and third trimesters). Total calories should be distributed among three meals and at least two snacks. Meals should be eaten on time and never skipped. Snacks must be carefully planned in accordance with insulin therapy to avoid fluctuations in blood glucose levels. A large bedtime snack of at least 25 g of carbohydrate with some protein is recommended in order to help prevent hypoglycemia and starvation ketosis during the night.

The ratio of carbohydrates, protein, and fat is important for meeting the metabolic needs of the woman and the fetus. Approximately 40 to 50% of the total calories should be from carbohydrates, with a minimum of 250 g per day. Simple carbohydrates are limited; complex carbohydrates that are high in fibre content are recommended because the starch and protein in such foods help regulate the blood glucose level by more sustained glucose release. Protein intake should constitute 20% of the total calories; 30 to 40% of the daily caloric intake should come from fat, with no more than 10% being saturated fats (see Home Care box). Weight gain for most women should be about 12 kg during the pregnancy (Gilbert, 2007).

Exercise

Although exercise enhances the utilization of glucose and decreases insulin need in nonpregnant women with diabetes, there is limited data regarding exercise during pregnancy.

Evaluation of current activity levels is done in early pregnancy to help develop a personalized activity plan for the whole pregnancy. The primary health care provider, along with a physiotherapist, will monitor and adjust activity levels to prevent complications. Blood glucose levels are also closely monitored to appropriately adjust insulin intake. For women with vasculopathy, only mild exercise is recommended because exercise causes a redistribution of blood flow, which increases the potential for ischemic injury to the placenta and already compromised organs. Women with vasculopathy typically depend completely on exogenous insulin and are at greater risk for wide fluctuations in blood glucose levels and ketoacidosis, which can be worsened by exercise.

Exercise need not be vigorous to be beneficial: 15 to 30 minutes of walking four to six times a week is satisfactory for most pregnant women. Other exercises that may be recommended include non–weight-bearing activities such as arm ergometry or use of a recumbent bicycle. Musculoskeletal concerns are addressed to enable women to actively participate in their own well-being (see also Home Care box: Exercise Tips for Pregnant Women, in Chapter 10).

The best time for exercise is after meals, when the blood glucose level is rising. To monitor the effect of insulin on blood glucose levels, the woman can measure blood glucose before, during, and after exercise.

Monitoring Blood Glucose Levels

Blood glucose testing at home is the most important tool available to the woman for assessing her degree of glycemic control. In addition, this monitoring provides feedback on how well her insulin-dose treatment is working The data obtained facilitate interaction with the health care team in maintaining glycemic control and maximizing pregnancy outcomes (see Home Care box).

A thorough assessment of a diabetic woman's knowledge and skill related to blood glucose testing is essential to ensuring accurate monitoring of glucose levels during pregnancy. The nurse needs to work with the woman performing blood glucose monitoring in order to assess her accuracy and comfort with the glucose-monitoring system. It is helpful to include the family in the assessment and in subsequent instruction. Glucometers have a built-in memory to store glucose readings; however, the woman must also keep written records of her daily glucose levels. She should bring her written records, her meter containing stored test results, or both with her to each appointment. The woman should check the accuracy of her meter regularly. Health care providers can assist in this process by comparing the woman's results on her machine with the results of a laboratory test done at the same time on a capillary whole-blood sample.

Blood glucose levels are routinely measured at various times throughout the day, such as before breakfast, lunch, and dinner; 2 hours after meals; at bedtime; and in the middle of the night. The primary health care provider or endocrinologist determines the frequency and timing of routine blood glucose assessments for each individual woman.

NURSING ALERT Hyperglycemia may occur in the 2-hour postprandial values because blood glucose levels peak about 2 hours after a meal.

HOME CARE

Testing Blood Glucose Level

1. Gather supplies, check expiration date, and read instructions on testing materials. Prepare glucose reflectance meter for use according to manufacturer's directions.
2. Wash hands in warm water (warmth increases circulation).
3. Select site on side of any finger (all fingers should be used in rotation).
4. Pierce site with lancet (may use automatic, spring-loaded, puncturing device). Cleaning the site with alcohol is not necessary.
5. Drop hand down to side; with the other hand, gently squeeze finger from hand to fingertip.
6. Allow blood to drop onto testing strip. Be sure to cover the entire reagent area.
7. Determine blood glucose value using the glucose reflectance meter, following manufacturer's instructions.
8. Record results.
9. Repeat as instructed by health care provider and as needed for signs of hypoglycemia or hyperglycemia.

(Source: Canadian Diabetes Care Guide. [2010]. *Monitoring blood glucose*. Retrieved from http://www.diabetescareguide.com.)

Special circumstances may require more frequent testing. Women are instructed to check glucose levels at any sign of hypoglycemia or hyperglycemia. When there is any readjustment in insulin dosage or diet, more frequent measurement of blood glucose is warranted. If nausea, vomiting, or diarrhea occurs or if any illness is present, the woman will have to monitor her blood glucose levels more closely.

Target levels of blood glucose during pregnancy are lower than nonpregnant values. Acceptable fasting levels are generally between 3.8 and 5.2 mmol/L, and 2-hour postprandial levels should be less than 6.7 mmol/L (see Table 14-1) (CDA, 2008). The woman should be told to report episodes of hypoglycemia (less than 3.2 mmol/L) and hyperglycemia (greater than 11 mmol/L) to her health care provider immediately so that adjustments in diet or insulin therapy can be made.

Pregnant women with diabetes are much more likely to develop hypoglycemia than hyperglycemia because the goal of therapy is to maintain the blood glucose in a narrow, low-normal range of 3.8 to 5.2 mmol/L. Although a blood glucose level greater than 6.7 mmol/L is considered too high for a pregnant woman, it will not produce the classic signs and symptoms of hyperglycemia. However, many women will have signs and symptoms of hypoglycemia with blood glucose levels below 3.8 mmol/L.

Most episodes of mild or moderate hypoglycemia can be treated with oral intake of 10 to 15 g of simple carbohydrates (see Guidelines box, p. 345). If severe hypoglycemia occurs in which the woman experiences a decrease in or loss of consciousness or an inability to swallow, she will require a parenteral injection of **glucagon** or intravenous (IV) glucose.

Because hypoglycemia can develop rapidly and impaired judgement can be associated with even moderate episodes, it is vital that family members, friends, and work colleagues be able to recognize signs and symptoms quickly and initiate proper treatment, if necessary.

Although hyperglycemia is less likely to occur, it is still a dangerous complication. Hyperglycemia can rapidly progress to DKA. Women and their family members should be alert for signs and symptoms of hyperglycemia, especially when infections or other illnesses occur (see Home Care box).

Insulin Therapy. All type 1 and almost all type 2 diabetic women will use insulin during pregnancy. Women who are type 2 diabetics who were on oral antidiabetic agents must switch to insulin, as currently these agents are not recommended in pregnancy by the CDA (2008) because of an increased risk of perinatal mortality and pre-eclampsia. Insulin therapy must be individualized and adjusted to ensure proper glucose metabolism of the mother and fetus. In the first trimester, little or no change occurs in prepregnancy insulin requirements; however, insulin dosage may need to be decreased because of hypoglycemia. During the second and third trimesters, because of insulin resistance, the dosage must be increased to maintain target glucose levels.

The goal of administration of exogenous insulin during pregnancy is to achieve diurnal glucose levels that are similar to those of a nondiabetic pregnant woman. The insulin regimen for a pregnant woman will differ from that which was effective in the nonpregnant state in combinations and timing of insulin injections (Landon et al., 2007). Thus, for the woman with type 1 pregestational diabetes who has typically been accustomed to one injection per day of intermediate-acting insulin, multiple daily injections of mixed insulin are a new experience. Many women with type 1 diabetes use insulin pumps. Women require education to adjust their insulin dosages according to pregnancy needs.

The woman with type 2 diabetes previously treated with oral hypoglycemics is faced with the task of learning to self-administer injections of insulin. The nurse can be instrumental in providing education and support regarding insulin administration and the adjustment of insulin dosage to maintain euglycemia (see Patient Teaching box).

Many types of insulin are currently available. Beef and pork insulin have largely been replaced by biosynthetic human insulin preparations (Humulin or Novolin), which are less likely to cause antibody formation. Patients with new onset of diabetes are almost always started on this type of insulin. Lispro (Humalog) is a rapid-acting insulin preparation that has an onset of action within 25 minutes of injection and peaks in 30 minutes to 1½ hours. Advantages of lispro include convenience; because it is injected immediately before mealtime, there is less hyperglycemia after meals and there are fewer hypoglycemic episodes. Lispro insulin has a total duration of action of 4 to 5 hours (Landon et al., 2007) (Table 14-2).

HOME CARE

What to Do When Illness Occurs

Continue to Take Insulin

- Be sure to take insulin even though appetite and food intake may be less than normal. (Insulin needs are increased with illness or infection.)

Contact Your Health Care Provider

- Call your health care provider and relay the following information:
  - Symptoms of illness (e.g., nausea, vomiting, diarrhea)
  - Fever
  - Most recent blood glucose level
  - Urine ketones
  - Time and amount of last insulin dose

Take Preventive Measures

- Increase oral intake of fluids to prevent dehydration.
- Rest as much as possible.

Seek Emergency Treatment if Needed

- If you are unable to reach your health care provider and blood glucose exceeds 11.0 mmol/L with urine ketones present, seek emergency treatment at the nearest health care facility. Do not attempt to self-treat.

PATIENT TEACHING Self-Administration of Insulin (for Women Who Have Not Used Insulin Previously)

Procedure for Mixing Intermediate-Acting (NPH) and Short-Acting (Regular) Insulin

1. Wash your hands thoroughly and gather supplies. Be sure that the insulin syringe corresponds to the concentration of insulin you are using.
2. Inspect the insulin bottle to be certain that it is the appropriate type, and check the expiration date.
3. Gently rotate (do not shake) the insulin vial to mix the insulin.
4. Wipe off rubber stopper of each vial with alcohol.
5. Draw into syringe the amount of air equal to total dose.
6. Inject air equal to NPH dose into NPH vial. Remove syringe from vial.
7. Inject air equal to regular insulin dose into regular insulin vial.
8. Invert regular insulin bottle and withdraw regular insulin dose.
9. Without adding more air to NPH vial, carefully withdraw NPH dose.

Procedure for Self-Injection of Insulin

1. Select proper injection site (remember to rotate sites).
2. The injection site should be clean. Use of alcohol is not necessary. If alcohol is used, let it dry before injecting.
3. Pinch the skin up to form a subcutaneous pocket and, holding the syringe like a pencil, puncture the skin at a 45- to 90-degree angle. If there is a great deal of fatty tissue at the site, spread the skin taut and inject the syringe at a 90-degree angle.
4. Slowly inject the insulin.
5. Withdraw the needle.
6. Record the insulin dose and time of injection.

Table 14-2 Insulin Types: Expected Time of Action

TYPE OF INSULIN	ONSET	PEAK	DURATION
Rapid-acting insulin (clear) • Lispro • Aspartglulisine	10–15 min	1–2 hr 1–1.5 hr	3.5–4.75 hr 3–5 hr
Short-acting insulin (clear) • Humulin-R • Novolin ge Toronto	30 min	2–3 hr	6.5 hr
Inhaled insulin	20–30 min	2 hr	6 hr
Intermediate-acting insulin (cloudy) • Humulin-N • Novolin ge NPH	1–3 hr	5–8 hr	Up to 18 hr
Long-acting basal insulin (clear) • Detemir (Levemir) • Glargine (Lantus)	90 min	Not applicable	Up to 24 hr 16–24 hr 24 hr
Premixed insulin • Humulin 30/70 • Novolin ge 30/70, 40/60, 50/50 • Biphasic insulin aspart (Novomix 30) • Insulin lispro/lispro protamine Humalog Mix25 and Mix50	Varies as to what insulin is in syringe	Varies	Varies

(From Canadian Diabetes Association. [2008]. Clinical practice guidelines for the prevention and management of diabetes in Canada. *Canadian Journal of Diabetes, 32* [Suppl 1], S1–S201, p. S47.)

Most women with diabetes manage their insulin with two to three injections per day. Usually, two thirds of the daily insulin dose, with longer-acting (NPH) and short-acting (regular or lispro) insulin combined in a 2:1 ratio, is given before breakfast. The remaining one third, again a combination of longer- and short-acting insulin, is administered in the evening before dinner. To reduce the risk of hypoglycemia during the night, separate injections are often administered, with short-acting insulin given before dinner, followed by longer-acting insulin at bedtime. An alternative insulin regimen that works well for some women is to administer short-acting insulin before each meal and longer-acting insulin at bedtime (Landon et al., 2007).

Although subcutaneous insulin injections are most commonly used, increasing numbers of pregnant women are using continuous insulin infusion systems. The insulin pump is designed to mimic more closely the function of the pancreas in secreting insulin (Fig. 14-2). This portable, battery-powered device is worn like a pager during most daily activities. The pump infuses regular insulin at a set basal rate and has the capacity to deliver up to four different basal rates in 24 hours. It also delivers bolus doses of insulin before meals to control postprandial blood glucose levels. A fine-gauge plastic catheter is inserted into subcutaneous tissue, usually in the abdomen, and attached to the pump syringe by connecting tubing. The subcutaneous catheter and connecting tubing are changed every 2 to 3 days. Although the insulin pump is convenient and generally provides good glycemic control, complications such as DKA, infection, or hypoglycemic coma can still develop. Use of the insulin pump requires a knowledgeable, motivated patient; skilled health care providers; and 24-hour availability of emergency assistance (Landon et al., 2007).

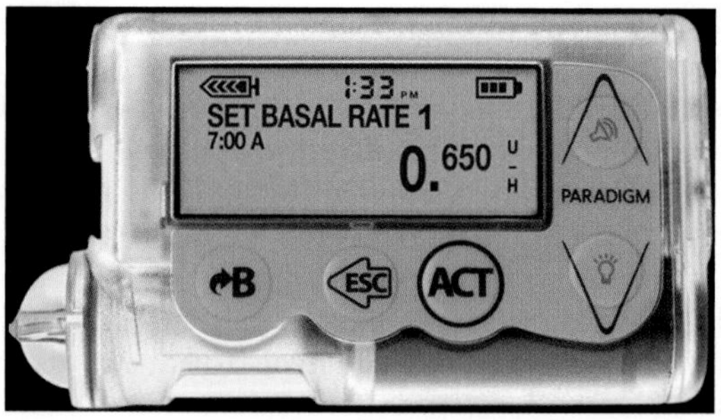

Fig. 14-2 Insulin pump shows basal rate for pregnant women with diabetes. *(MiniMed Paradigm® REAL-Time Revel™ Insulin Pump Manufactured by the Diabetes business unit of Medtronic, Inc.)*

Complications Requiring Hospitalization

Occasionally, diabetic women who are pregnant require hospitalization to regulate insulin dosage and stabilize glucose levels. Nursing care provided during hospitalization provides continuous support and education for regulating insulin therapy and blood glucose. Illness can lead to hyperglycemia and DKA and may require hospitalization, regardless of gestational age. Hospitalization during the third trimester for close maternal and fetal observation may be indicated for women whose diabetes is poorly controlled or who also have hypertension.

Determination of Birth Date and Mode of Delivery

The majority of diabetic pregnancies progress to term (38 to 40 weeks of gestation), as long as good metabolic control is maintained and all parameters of antepartum fetal surveillance remain within normal limits. Reasons to consider birth before term include poor metabolic control, worsening hypertensive disorders, fetal macrosomia, prior stillbirth, or fetal growth restriction and decreasing insulin requirements (Landon et al., 2007).

Induction of labour is often planned between 38 and 40 weeks, provided maternal glucose levels are well controlled. To confirm fetal lung maturity before birth, an amniocentesis may be performed in pregnancies of less than 39 weeks. For the pregnancy complicated by diabetes, fetal lung maturation is better predicted by the amniotic fluid phosphatidylglycerol than by the lecithin/sphingomyelin (L/S) ratio (see Chapter 12). If the fetal lungs are still immature, birth should be postponed as long as the results of fetal assessment remain normal. Induction of labour despite fetal lung maturity may be required on the basis of assessment of fetal compromise or if pre-eclampsia, deteriorating vision resulting from proliferative retinopathy, or worsening renal function develops. The involvement of the obstetrical team is critical to making the best decision for each individual woman.

A planned vaginal birth is the preferred mode of birth for women with pregestational diabetes. Caesarean birth should only be performed for obstetrical reasons, such as when antepartum testing suggests a compromised fetal status or estimated fetal weight is 4000 to 4500 g. Induction of labour is planned at term for the woman who has well-controlled blood glucose levels; however, practitioners must be alert to falling insulin requirements, which is an indication for delivery. If induction of labour does not result in active labour with cervical changes, a Caesarean birth may be necessary (Landon et al., 2007).

Intrapartum

During the intrapartum period, the woman with pregestational diabetes must be monitored closely to prevent complications related to dehydration, hypoglycemia, and hyperglycemia. Most women use large amounts of energy (kilocalories) to accomplish the work and manage the stress of labour and birth; however, this energy expenditure varies with the individual. Blood glucose levels and hydration must be controlled carefully during labour. An IV line is inserted for infusion of a maintenance fluid such as 5% dextrose in normal saline or lactated Ringer's solution. Insulin is administered by intermittent subcutaneous injection. In women who have difficulty regulating their blood glucose, a continuous insulin infusion may be required.

Blood glucose levels are assessed every hour in active labour. Fluids and insulin levels are adjusted to maintain blood glucose levels to less than 8 mmol/L. It is essential that these target glucose levels be maintained because hyperglycemia during labour can increase the likelihood of hypoglycemia in the neonate. During labour, continuous fetal heart monitoring is recommended for women who are taking insulin (Liston et al., 2007). Labouring women are encouraged to be mobile in labour; **telemetry** monitoring can be used to monitor the fetus remotely. Side-lying positions are preferred for the woman labouring in bed, to prevent supine hypotension due to a large fetus or polyhydramnios. Labour progresses without intervention, provided normal rates of cervical dilation, fetal descent, and fetal well-being are maintained. **Epidural** anaesthesia may be provided to women who require pain relief. Labour dystocia may occur because of a macrosomic infant or cephalopelvic disproportion, necessitating Caesarean birth. Labouring women with diabetes are monitored for diabetic complications, such as hyperglycemia, ketones in the urine, and ketoacidosis. During second-stage labour, the nurse should be alert for the possibility of shoulder dystocia if delivery of a macrosomic infant is attempted and should be prepared to assist with manoeuvres to free the fetal shoulder that is lodged behind the symphysis pubis (see Chapter 19, p. 520). Depending on the gestational age of the fetus at birth, a neonatologist or pediatrician may need to be present at the birth to provide neonatal care.

If a Caesarean birth is planned, it should be scheduled in the early morning to facilitate glycemic control. The morning dose of insulin is withheld, and the woman is given nothing by mouth. Regional anaesthesia (epidural or spinal) is recommended because hypoglycemia can be detected earlier if the woman is awake.

Postpartum

In the immediate postpartum period, insulin requirements decrease substantially because the major source of insulin resistance, the placenta, has been removed. Women with type 1 diabetes may require only one half the prenatal insulin dose on the first postpartum day, provided that they are eating a full diet. It takes several days after birth to re-establish carbohydrate homeostasis. Blood glucose levels are monitored in the postpartum period, and insulin dosage is adjusted accordingly. Blood glucose levels do not require such tight control after birth. Usually insulin is not given until the blood glucose level is greater than 11.0 mmol/L. Women with type 2 diabetes often require no insulin in the postpartum period and are able to maintain euglycemia through diet alone or with return to management with oral hypoglycemics.

Possible postpartum complications include pre-eclampsia or eclampsia, hemorrhage, and infection. Hemorrhage is a possibility if the mother's uterus was overdistended (by polyhydramnios or a macrosomic fetus) or overstimulated (by **oxytocin** induction). Postpartum infections such as endometritis are more likely to occur in a woman with diabetes.

Mothers are encouraged to breastfeed. In addition to the advantages of maternal satisfaction, breastfeeding has an antidiabetogenic effect. Insulin requirements may be half of prepregnancy levels because of the carbohydrate used in human milk production. Because glucose levels are lower, breastfeeding women are at increased risk for hypoglycemia, especially in the early postpartum period and after breastfeeding sessions.

The mother may have early breastfeeding difficulties. Poor metabolic control may delay lactogenesis and contribute to decreased milk production. Initial contact and opportunity to breastfeed the infant may be delayed because of institutional practices of separating mothers and babies post-Caesarean or placing infants of mothers with diabetes in neonatal intensive care units or special care nurseries for observation during the first few hours after birth. Support and assistance from nursing staff and lactation specialists can facilitate the mother's early experience with breastfeeding and encourage her to continue.

Infants who are exclusively breastfed are less likely to develop diabetes; exposure to artificial milk products before 8 days of age is an important risk factor for the disease. Breastfeeding has also been shown to reduce childhood obesity and may prevent the onset of type 2 diabetes (Schafer-Graf, Buchanan, Xiang, & Kjos, 2002).

Breastfeeding mothers with diabetes may be at increased risk for **mastitis** and yeast infections of the breast. Insulin dosage, which is decreased during lactation, must be readjusted at the time of weaning.

Family Planning and Contraception

The new mother needs information about family planning and contraception. While family planning is important for all women, it is essential for the woman with diabetes, to promote optimal outcomes in future pregnancies. Excellent glucose control at conception is crucial for all women with diabetes; therefore, the importance of conscientiously using a reliable contraceptive method until another pregnancy is desired should be stressed. No one best form of contraception exists for women with diabetes. Emphasis should be placed on consistent use of a reliable and effective birth control method. The risks and benefits of contraceptive methods should be discussed with the mother and her partner before discharge from the hospital.

The barrier methods are often recommended as safe, inexpensive options that have no inherent risks for women with diabetes (Landon et al., 2007). However, barrier methods are not as effective or convenient as some other forms of contraception.

The use of oral contraceptives is controversial because of the risk of thromboembolic events and myocardial infarction and the effect on carbohydrate metabolism. In women without vascular disease or other risk factors, combination low-dose oral contraceptives may be prescribed. Close monitoring of blood pressure and lipid levels is necessary to detect complications (Landon et al., 2007). Progestin-only oral contraceptives can be used because they minimally affect carbohydrate metabolism (Cunningham et al., 2010).

Some health care providers are reluctant to use intrauterine devices (IUDs) in women with diabetes because of concerns about infection. However, these women have used this method successfully.

Opinion is divided over the use of long-acting parenteral progestins such as Depo-Provera. Some authorities recommend their use, especially in women who may not be compliant with daily dosing of oral contraceptives or appropriate follow-up care. Others believe that these methods may adversely affect diabetic control (Landon et al., 2007).

The woman and her partner should be informed that the risks associated with pregnancy increase with the duration and severity of the diabetic condition and that pregnancy may contribute to vascular changes associated with diabetes. Thus the option of tubal ligation should be discussed with the woman who has completed her family or who has significant vasculopathy (see Nursing Care Plan).

Thyroid Disorders

Hyperthyroidism

Hyperthyroidism occurs in approximately 2 of every 1000 pregnancies (Mestman, 2007). In 90 to 95% of pregnant women it is caused by Graves' disease. Other rare but possible causes include functioning adenoma, toxic nodular goiter, excessive thyroid hormone intake, and thyroiditis (Inoue, Arata, Koren, & Ito, 2009; Mestman, 2007). Clinical manifestations of hyperthyroidism usually begin between 4 and 8 weeks of gestation and often involve severe nausea and vomiting. Because of the timing of the symptoms, hyperemesis gravidarum may be believed to be the diagnosis. Careful assessment by the primary care provider is necessary, including blood work that includes thyroid levels, to get an accurate diagnosis. Other symptoms that may be associated with an increased basal metabolic rate and increased sympathetic nervous system activity include fatigue, heat intolerance, warm skin, diaphoresis, emotional lability, tremulousness, tachycardia, and a wide pulse pressure. Because many of these symptoms are associated with pregnancy, hyperthyroidism can be difficult to diagnose. Signs that may help differentiate hyperthyroidism from normal pregnancy include unplanned weight loss, onycholysis (loose nails), and a pulse rate greater than 100 beats/min that does not decrease with the Valsalva manoeuvre. Laboratory assessment is important for determining elevated free thyroxine (T_4) levels and suppressed serum thyroid-stimulating hormone (TSH) levels. Hyperthyroidism is best diagnosed and treated prior to pregnancy. Moderate and severe hyperthyroidism can be detrimental during pregnancy, as untreated or inadequately treated women may have infants with low birth weight, intrauterine growth restriction (IUGR), prematurity, stillbirth, and hyper- or hypothyroidism (Mestman, 2007). Women with hyperthyroidism are at increased risk of developing severe pre-eclampsia, congestive heart failure, thyroid storm, miscarriage, placental abruption, and infection (Mestman, 2007).

The primary treatment of hyperthyroidism during pregnancy is with a medication called propylthiouracil (PTU). Patients generally show clinical improvement within 2 to 6 weeks of beginning therapy, but the medication requires 6 to 8 weeks to reach full effectiveness. During therapy, the woman's free T_4 levels are measured monthly; the results are used to taper the medication to the smallest effective dosage in order to prevent unnecessary fetal hypothyroidism (Mestman, 2007; Nader, 2009). PTU is well tolerated by most patients. Rare adverse effects include pruritus, skin rash, a metallic taste, nausea, bronchospasm, oral ulcerations, hepatitis, and a lupus-like syndrome (Mestman, 2007; Nader, 2009). The most severe adverse effect is agranulocytosis, which is more common in women over 40 years of age and in those taking high doses of PTU. Symptoms of agranulocytosis are fever, malaise, gingivitis, and sore throat, which should be reported immediately to the health care provider; the woman should stop taking the PTU. **Leukopenia** of a transient and benign nature may occur as a result of PTU therapy. PTU readily crosses the placenta and may induce fetal hypothyroidism and goiter (Mestman, 2007; Nader, 2009).

Methimazole, although widely prescribed for the treatment of hyperthyroidism in pregnancy in Europe, South America and Asia, is not commonly used in North America. Methimazole may be used to treat women who cannot tolerate taking propylthioruracil.

β-Adrenergic blockers such as propranolol may be used in women with severe hyperthyroidism symptoms. Long-term use is not recommended because of the potential for IUGR and altered response to anoxic stress, postnatal bradycardia, and hypoglycemia.

NURSING CARE PLAN ● Pregnancy Complicated by Pregestational Diabetes

Nursing Diagnosis: Need for knowledge related to change in diabetic management strategies

Expected Outcome

The woman will be able to communicate key information regarding changes to her diabetes management and have a new understanding of potential effects on herself and her fetus.

Nursing Interventions/*Rationales*

Assess the woman's current knowledge base regarding disease process, management changes, effects on pregnancy and fetus, and potential complications *to provide a starting place for further teaching.*

Review the pathophysiology of effects of diabetes on pregnancy and the fetus, the changes that occur throughout gestation, and potential complications *to promote patient understanding of information and support compliance with the treatment plan.*

Discuss diet and exercise changes as recommended by the endocrinologist, physiotherapist, and dietitian *to promote self-management.*

Review, if necessary, depending on learning needs, the signs and symptoms of complications of hypoglycemia and hyperglycemia and appropriate interventions *to promote prompt recognition of complications and self-management.*

Provide contact numbers for the health care team for prompt interventions and answers to questions on an ongoing basis *to promote patient and health team collaboration.*

Nursing Diagnosis: Risk for fetal morbidity related to elevated maternal glucose levels

Expected Outcome

Fetus will be born at term in a healthy state.

Nursing Interventions/*Rationales*

Assess woman's current control of diabetes *to identify risk for fetal death and congenital anomalies.*

Monitor fundal height during each prenatal visit *to identify appropriate fetal growth.*

Monitor for signs and symptoms of gestational hypertension to identify early manifestations *because pregnant women with diabetes are more at risk.*

Assess fetal movement and heart rate during each prenatal visit and perform twice-weekly nonstress tests during the last 4 weeks of pregnancy *to assess fetal well-being.*

Review procedure for blood glucose testing and insulin administration *to promote self-management.*

Nursing Diagnosis: Anxiety related to threat to maternal and fetal well-being as evidenced by the woman's verbal expressions of concern.

Expected Outcome

The woman identifies sources of anxiety and reports feeling less anxious.

Nursing Interventions/*Rationales*

Through therapeutic communication, foster an open relationship with the woman *to promote patient trust.*

Listen to the woman's feelings and concerns *to assess for any misconceptions or misinformation that may be contributing to anxiety.*

Review potential dangers by providing factual information *to correct any misconceptions or misinformation.*

Encourage the woman to share concerns with her health care team *to promote team collaboration in her care.*

Nursing Diagnosis: Risk for imbalanced nutrition: less than body requirements related to inability to ingest nutrients that are needed for a pregnancy complicated by diabetes

Expected Outcomes

The woman will communicate an understanding of dietary needs during pregnancy, gain weight that is consistent with a normal pregnancy, and maintain blood sugar levels between 3.4 and 6.7 mmol/L.

Nursing Interventions/*Rationales*

Assess caloric intake and dietary pattern *to evaluate the woman's understanding of and compliance with dietary regimen.*

Review the importance of regularity of meals and snacks *to promote compliance with the plan to achieve a healthy pregnancy.*

Review blood glucose monitoring, if necessary, *to determine if the woman is comfortable with monitoring.*

Weigh the woman at each prenatal visit *to assess weight gain.*

Refer to a dietitian for individualized counselling, if required, *to plan a diet that helps the woman to maintain normoglycemia and gain the appropriate amount of weight.*

Radioactive iodine must not be used in diagnosis or treatment of hyperthyroidism because it may compromise the fetal thyroid. If a mother taking hyperthyroid medication chooses to breastfeed, she needs to be aware that physiologically significant doses of the medication are passed to the infant through the breast milk. The infant's thyroid status should be monitored periodically so that newborn hypothyroidism can be prevented.

In severe cases, hyperthyroidism may be treated surgically with subtotal thyroidectomy during the second or third trimester. Because of the increased risk of miscarriage and preterm labour associated with major surgery, this treatment is usually reserved for women with severe disease, those for whom medication therapy proves toxic, and those who are unable to comply with the prescribed medical regimen. Postoperative hypothyroidism is common, occurring in at least 20% of women with hyperthyroidism.

NURSING ALERT A serious but uncommon complication of undiagnosed or partially treated hyperthyroidism is thyroid storm, which may occur in response to stresses such as infection, birth, or surgery. Symptoms of this rare condition include sudden fever, restlessness, tachycardia, vomiting, hypotension, or stupor. Congestive heart failure may also occur. Prompt treatment is essential to ensure a good maternal outcome; IV fluids and oxygen are administered along with high doses of PTU. Potassium iodide, antipyretics, glucocorticoids, and β-adrenergic blockers may also be given; sedation may be necessary for extreme restlessness (Mestman, 2007; Nader, 2009).

Hypothyroidism

Hypothyroidism during pregnancy is rare because women with this condition are often infertile, and failure of in vitro fertilization is more likely (Poppe, Velkeniers, & Glinoer, 2007). Hypothyroidism is usually the result of Hashimoto's disease (autoimmune thyroiditis), thyroid gland ablation by radiation, previous surgery, or antithyroid medications (Glinoer & Abalovich, 2007). Reduced thyroid function because of hypothalamic or pituitary failure is rare, with only a few reported cases. Iodine deficiency in women living in developed countries is also rare (Mestman, 2007; Nader, 2009), but in the rest of the world, the most common cause of thyroid problems is iodine deficiency, which affects more than 1.2 billion people (Glinoer and Abalovich, 2007). Pregnant women should be screened for the presence of hypothyroidism, as up to 2.2% of women had low levels of thyroid-stimulating hormone levels in one study (Allan et al., 2000).

Characteristic symptoms of hypothyroidism include maternal fatigue, weight gain, cold intolerance, constipation, cool and dry skin, coarsened hair, and muscle weakness. Laboratory findings during pregnancy include low or low–normal T_3 and T_4 levels and elevated levels of TSH.

Diagnosis and treatment of pregnant women with hypothyroidism is important, as pre-eclampsia, placental abruption, and stillbirth are significant risks when hypothyroidism remains unrecognized. Infants born to mothers with hypothyroidism may be of low birth weight and may be at risk for clinically relevant cognitive deficits if born premature. However, given the return of normal free thyroxine levels later in gestation, for the most part, these babies are healthy, without evidence of thyroid dysfunction.

Thyroid hormone supplements are used to treat hypothyroidism. In Canada, both levothyroxine (L-thyroxine [Synthroid]) and liothyronine (L-T_3) are most often prescribed during pregnancy (Nava-Campo, Soldin, & Koren, 2004). Levothyroxine is most often prescribed in pregnancy as it is considered safe and is not **teratogenic**.

As pregnancy progresses, the woman usually requires increased amounts of thyroid replacement hormone. Because of increased absorption in the small intestine, taking the medication on an empty stomach is recommended. Prenatal vitamins may inhibit absorption of thyroid replacements because of the presence of iron and calcium (Nava-Campo et al., 2004). Taking prenatal vitamins at least 4 hours after taking a thyroid replacement hormone is recommended. The aim of medication therapy is to maintain the woman's TSH level within the normal range for pregnant women. Dosage adjustments are made as necessary by measuring TSH levels periodically. Each dosage change should be followed 4 to 6 weeks later by determining the TSH level.

evolve Case Study—Class III Cardiac Disorder

NURSING ALERT Pregnant women should be told to take thyroid replacement hormone 4 hours before or after iron tablets because ferrous sulphate lowers the effectiveness of the medication (Cooper et al., 2007; Nava-Campo et al., 2004).

The fetus depends on maternal thyroid hormones until 12 weeks of gestation, when fetal production begins. Thus maternal hypothyroidism does not cause fetal hypothyroidism. However, maternal treatment of hypothyroidism may result in increased fetal levels of thyroid hormones. Careful monitoring of the neonate's thyroid status is important to detect any abnormalities.

Nursing Care

A pregnant woman with thyroid dysfunction requires education to ensure the best outcomes for herself and her fetus. This education should include information about the disorder and its potential impact on herself and her fetus, the medication regimen and possible adverse effects, the need for continuing medical supervision, and the importance of maintaining consistent levels of thyroid hormone. The family should be incorporated into the plan of care, to foster mutuality and support among the members.

The woman with hyperthyroidism may experience nervousness and hyperactivity concomitant with weakness and fatigue. Quiet diversional activities such as reading or crafts may help to channel her energy. Discomfort associated with hypersensitivity to heat (hyperthyroidism) or cold intolerance (hypothyroidism) can be minimized by wearing appropriate clothing, regulating environmental temperatures, and avoiding temperature extremes, when possible.

Nutrition counselling with a registered dietitian is an important component of management of symptoms. The woman with hyperthyroidism who has increased appetite and poor weight gain and the hypothyroid woman who has anorexia and lethargy need counselling to ensure adequate intake of nutritionally sound foods to meet both maternal and fetal needs.

Cardiovascular Disorders

The maternal cardiovascular system undergoes many changes that put a physiological strain on the heart during a normal pregnancy. The major cardiovascular changes that affect the patient with cardiac disease are increased intravascular volume; decreased systemic vascular resistance; increased heart rate and stroke volume; and increased cardiac output occur during pregnancy, labour, and birth. The normal heart compensates for the increased workload whereas the diseased heart is hemodynamically challenged. Cardiac decompensation (the inability of the heart to maintain sufficient cardiac output) may occur in the presence of myocardial or valvular disease.

Approximately 1% of pregnancies are complicated by cardiac heart disease (Davies & Herbert, 2007a). Hemodynamic changes during pregnancy, labour, and birth for the woman with cardiac disease can have a significant impact on cardiac output, increasing it up to 500 mL/min. The type of cardiac lesion present dictates the woman's mortality risk. Box 14-2 lists maternal cardiac disease risk groups.

The New York Heart Association (NYHA) classification of the functional capacity of patients with heart disease is a widely accepted standard and is as follows (Criteria Committee of the New York Heart Association, 1994):

Class I—Asymptomatic at normal levels of activity
Class II—Symptomatic with ordinary activity
Class III—Symptomatic with less than ordinary activity
Class IV—Symptomatic at rest

The NYHA classification system is a clear, practical guide for cardiac classification that can inform appropriate obstetrical care. Medical therapy is provided by a team approach that includes the woman, cardiologist, obstetrician, anaesthesia, and nurses. It is important to understand that the woman's functional classification may change over the course of the pregnancy because of the hemodynamic changes that occur in the cardiovascular system. There is a 45 to 50% increase in cardiac output compared with nonpregnancy resting values, with most of the increase occurring in the first trimester and the peaks being at around 25 to 32 weeks of gestation (Blanchard & Shabetai, 2009). The functional classification of the disease is determined at 3 months and again at 7 or 8 months of gestation. Pregnant women may progress from class I or II to III or IV during pregnancy.

The two broad categories of cardiac disease are **congenital** and acquired. The incidence of acquired disease (e.g., rheumatic heart disease) is decreasing in developed countries. Pregnant women with congenital cardiac disease are increasing in number because of advances in childhood treatment (Arafeh & Baird, 2006; Davies & Herbert, 2007b). Congenital heart disease is further separated into that with acyanotic lesions and disease with cyanotic lesions. These conditions are listed in Box 14-3 and then further discussed.

BOX 14-2 Maternal Cardiac Disease Risk Groups

Group 1 (Mortality Rate 1%)
Atrial and ventricular septal defects (uncomplicated)
Patent ductus arteriosus (uncomplicated)
Corrected tetralogy of Fallot
Pulmonic/tricuspid disease
Mitral stenosis
Porcine valve (NYHA class I and II)

Group II (Mortality Rate 5 to 15%)
Mitral stenosis with atrial fibrillation
Artificial heart valves
Mitral stenosis (NYHA class III and IV)
Uncorrected tetralogy of Fallot
Previous myocardial infarction
Marfan syndrome with normal aorta

Group III (Mortality Rate 25 to 50%)
Pulmonary hypertension
Coarctation of the aorta
Complicated Marfan syndrome with aortic involvement

(From Foley, M. R. [2004]. Cardiac disease. In G. A. Dildy, et al. [Eds.], *Critical care obstetrics* [4th ed.]. Malden, MA: Blackwell Science.)

Congenital Heart Disease

Congenital heart disease is classified as acyanotic or cyanotic. Women at increased risk for a cardiac event in pregnancy include those with a prior cardiac event or arrhythmia, NYHA functional class greater than II, or cyanosis, left heart obstruction, and systemic ventricular dysfunction.

Acyanotic Heart Lesions

Atrial and Ventricular Septal Defects

Atrial septal defects (ASD—an abnormal opening between the atria) and ventricular septal defects (VSD) (see Box 48-1) are the most common of the congenital heart lesions seen in pregnant women. These defects may go undetected because the woman usually is asymptomatic until pregnancy hemodynamic changes occur. The pregnant woman with an ASD or a VSD will most likely have an uncomplicated pregnancy unless the defect causes significant shunting and increased pulmonary vascular resistance. As a result of the increased plasma volume, some women may have right-sided heart failure or develop tachyarrhythmias as the pregnancy progresses.

Patent Ductus Arteriosus

This condition is rarely seen in adults, as most people with a patent ductus arteriosus (PDA) have it corrected as a newborn or as a child (see Box 48-1). Women with a corrected PDA do well in pregnancy and women with an uncorrected PDA who have a small to moderate size ductus and who have normal pulmonary arterial pressures are likely to experience

BOX 14-3 Cardiac Disorders in Pregnancy

Congenital Heart Disease
- Acyanotic congenital heart lesions
- Atrial and ventricular septal defects
- Patent ductus arteriosus
- Coarctation of the aorta
- Marfan syndrome
- Aortic stenosis
- Pulmonic stenosis

Cyanotic Congenital Heart Lesions
- Tetralogy of Fallot
- Ebstein's anomaly
- Eisenmenger's syndrome
- Primary pulmonary hypertension

Acquired Heart Disease
- Rheumatic heart disease
- Mitral stenosis
- Mitral regurgitation
- Aortic stenosis
- Aortic regurgitation

(Sources: Davies, G., & Herbert, W. [2007]. Heart disease in pregnancy 2: Congenital heart disease in pregnancy. *Journal of Obstetrics and Gynaecology Canada, 29*[5], 409–414. Retrieved from http://www.sogc.org/jogc/abstracts/full/200705_Obstetrics_2.pdf; Davies, G., & Herbert, W. [2007]. Heart disease in pregnancy 3: Acquired heart disease in pregnancy. *Journal of Obstetrics and Gynaecology Canada, 29*[6], 507–509. Retrieved from http://www.sogc.org/jogc/abstracts/full/200706_Obstetrics_2.pdf.)

few or no complications with pregnancy related to their cardiac defect (Davies & Herbert, 2007b). However, when there is more extensive left-to-right shunting, the hemodynamic changes in pregnancy can result in Eisenmenger's syndrome, which results in high morbidity and mortality for both the mother and fetus. Women in this situation are often encouraged to terminate the pregnancy.

Coarctation of the Aorta

The rare condition of uncorrected coarctation of the aorta (see Box 48-2) in pregnancy was once thought to be deadly for pregnant women; women were often counselled to terminate the pregnancy because of the severe risks to their own lives (Davies & Herbert, 2007b). However, these women have a very low mortality rate (0 to 3.5%), and pregnancy is well tolerated. Rupture or dissection of the aorta is a small risk that carries a high risk of mortality. In general, women with this cardiac disorder do well in pregnancy.

Marfan Syndrome

Marfan syndrome is an autosomal genetic condition characterized by generalized weakness of the connective tissue, resulting in joint deformity, ocular lens deformity, and weakness of the aortic wall and root (Arafeh & Baird, 2006). Mortality rates for women with Marfan syndrome have been reported as high as 50%; however, women with dilation of the aortic root of 40 mm or less have a mortality rate of less than 5% (Davies & Herbert, 2007b). Approximately 90% of these women have mitral valve prolapse, and 25% have aortic insufficiency with an increased risk of aortic dissection and rupture during pregnancy and birth. Excruciating chest pain and cardiac decompensation are the first signs of aortic rupture, which can occur primarily in the third trimester or the postpartum period. Therapy includes limiting of physical activity, prevention of hypertensive or hypotensive complications, and administration of β-blockers as needed. Aortic root measurements are taken early in pregnancy as a baseline and then at intervals to detect an increasing diameter. Preconception and genetic counselling are recommended to make women aware of the risks of pregnancy and that their newborns may inherit the syndrome (Easterling & Stout, 2007).

Mitral and Aortic Valve Stenosis

The concern regarding mitral and aortic valve lesions (see Box 48-2) in the pregnant women is the cardiac output fluctuations during pregnancy, labour, and birth. With many of these lesions only allowing a "fixed" cardiac output, pregnant women and their fetuses may have hemodynamic decompensation if cardiac output cannot meet the needs for tissue perfusion and oxygen transport. Mitral valve stenosis (narrowing of the opening of the mitral valve caused by stiffening of valve leaflets, thereby obstructing blood flow from the atrium to the ventricles) is the characteristic lesion often resulting from rheumatic heart disease (see discussion later in this chapter). As the mitral valve narrows, cardiac output decreases and **dyspnea** worsens, occurring first on exertion and eventually at rest. A tight stenosis plus the increase in blood volume and required cardiac output demands of normal pregnancy and birth may cause ventricular failure, pulmonary edema, and death (Blanchard & Shabetai, 2009). Women with aortic stenosis need to avoid hypovolemia during labour and birth, as this can result in significant falling in cardiac output. Strict control of postpartum blood loss is critical to improved outcomes for women after birth. Women with mild to moderate stenosis usually tolerate pregnancy well (Davies & Herbert, 2007b).

The pregnant woman with mitral or aortic stenosis typically is managed by reducing her activity, restricting dietary sodium, providing diuretic therapy, administering β-blocking medications to lower heart rate, and increasing bed rest. She should be monitored frequently for clinical symptoms and with routine echocardiograms to monitor atrial and ventricular size and heart valve function. For patients with NYHA class III or IV symptoms, balloon valvuloplasty may be considered. This procedure should be considered only when symptoms cannot be controlled by standard medical treatments. Balloon valvuloplasty is optimally performed after 20 weeks of gestation to decrease radiation risks to the fetus.

Pulmonic Stenosis

Women with severe pulmonic stenosis (see Box 48-2) are encouraged to have surgical correction before pregnancy in order to improve their outcomes of pregnancy (Davies & Herbert, 2007b). As with other cardiac disorders, women with mild-to-moderate disease do well in pregnancy; however, those with severe disease have a higher risk of right-sided heart failure, resulting in higher rates of pregnancy loss and poor maternal outcomes.

Cyanotic Congenital Heart Lesions

Tetralogy of Fallot

Tetralogy of Fallot includes several abnormalities caused by maldevelopment of the truncus arteriosus. The cardiac abnormalities include a ventral septal defect, pulmonary stenosis, overriding aorta, and right ventricular hypertrophy leading to a right-to-left shunt (see Box 48-3). Surgical correction of tetralogy of Fallot includes correction of the VSD and possibly the pulmonary stenosis. Women with corrected tetralogy of Fallot have a low mortality rate and have a positive pregnancy outcome. However, women with uncorrected tetralogy of Fallot have a high maternal risk (7%) and high rate of fetal loss (up to 22%) because of a decrease in systemic vascular resistance leading to left-to-right shunting (Blanchard & Shabetai, 2009; Davies & Herbert, 2007b). Medical management for women with uncorrected tetralogy of Fallot includes anticoagulant therapy, high-concentration oxygen administration, and invasive hemodynamic monitoring during labour and birth. As with all newborns born to mothers with congenital heart disease, they must be tested for the presence or absence of the cardiac lesion present in their mothers.

Eisenmenger's Syndrome

Eisenmenger's syndrome is a right-to-left or bidirectional shunting that can be at the atrial or ventricular level and is combined with elevated pulmonary vascular resistance (Easterling & Stout, 2007). The syndrome is associated with a mortality rate of approximately 50% during pregnancy or within the first month postpartum; thus pregnancy is contraindicated. If pregnancy occurs, termination may be recommended if the woman has significant pulmonary hypertension.

In women who continue pregnancy despite the risks, physical activity is strictly limited; prophylactic anticoagulation is considered (Easterling & Stout, 2007). Intensive care monitoring during labour and birth, guided by invasive hemodynamic parameters obtained with a pulmonary artery and arterial catheter and regional anaesthesia, is essential to optimize outcomes for the mother and fetus (Davies & Herbert, 2007b). A team approach involving a perinatologist, skilled critical care and perinatal nurses, and cardiology and anaesthesia care providers is essential.

Primary Pulmonary Hypertension

Mortality reports for women with primary pulmonary hypertension indicate that the mortality rate ranges between 30 and 56% (Davies & Herbert, 2007b). Because of the high risk to maternal health, pregnancy is contraindicated for women with primary pulmonary hypertension.

Acquired Heart Disease

Rheumatic Heart Disease

Rheumatic fever is increasingly uncommon in Canada. When it occurs, it usually develops suddenly, often several symptom-free weeks after an inadequately treated group A β-hemolytic streptococcal throat infection. Episodes of rheumatic fever create an autoimmune reaction in the heart tissue that leads to permanent damage of heart valves (usually the mitral valve and the aortic valve). The tricuspid and pulmonic valves may also be affected (Davies & Herbert, 2007c). This damage is referred to as rheumatic heart disease (RHD). RHD may be evident during acute rheumatic fever or discovered years later. Recurrences of rheumatic fever are common; each has the potential to increase the severity of heart damage. Heart murmurs resulting from stenosis, valvular insufficiency, or thickening of the walls of the heart characterize RHD. Abnormal pulse rate and rhythm and congestive heart failure are common. The American Heart Association (AHA) recommends prophylaxis to prevent infective endocarditis only in those patients who are at highest risk (Blanchard & Shabetai, 2009). Rheumatic fever can affect the aortic valve; although significant aortic stenosis in pregnant women is usually congenital. With this in mind, a fetal echocardiogram may be done to assess the fetus for the defect.

When the aortic valve orifice is less than one third of normal, limited cardiac output may occur, leading to increased left ventricular afterload, left ventricular hypertrophy, and failure. Pregnant women with any left-sided heart lesions are very sensitive to changes in intravascular volume. Intravascular volume balance is essential to preventing hypotension caused by hypovolemia and pulmonary edema caused by hypervolemia (Easterling & Stout, 2007)

Intrapartum care for women with severe disease includes invasive hemodynamic monitoring during labour and birth, with a goal toward maintaining adequate ventricular filling and cardiac output (Davies & Herbert, 2007c). Regional anaesthesia is needed to assist with decreasing tachycardia and control painful stress response. Careful monitoring in the postpartum period is essential in order to assess for postpartum adaptation to an increase in cardiac output. Management by skilled providers who are alert to the signs of cardiac decompensation is critical.

Mitral Valve Prolapse

Mitral valve prolapse (MVP) is a common, usually benign condition occurring in 1% of women (Blanchard & Shabetai, 2009). The mitral valve leaflets prolapse into the left atrium during ventricular systole, allowing some backflow of blood. Midsystolic click and late systolic murmur are hallmarks of this syndrome. Most cases are asymptomatic. A few women have atypical chest pain (sharp and located in the left side of the chest) that occurs at rest, is unrelated to exercise, and does not respond to nitrates. They may have anxiety, palpitations, dyspnea on exertion, and syncope. Specific treatment is usually not necessary except for symptomatic tachyarrhythmias. Pregnancy and its associated hemodynamic changes may change or alleviate the murmur and click of MVP, as well as its symptoms. Pregnancy is usually well tolerated; but, as with RHD, antibiotic prophylaxis may be given before invasive procedures for at-risk patients and for complicated vaginal births in patients with MVP.

Ischemic Heart Disease in Pregnancy

The incidence of coronary artery disease (CAD) in pregnancy is very low, approximately 1 in 10,000 births (Davies & Herbert, 2007d). Mortality rates for women with CAD are high, particularly in late pregnancy (Davies & Herbert, 2007d). Fetal loss is also high in this population. Diagnosis in pregnancy is difficult as this disease is often not suspected in the childbearing population. Risk factors include smoking, diabetes, and a family history of myocardial infarction before age 60 years, as well as chronic hypertension and lipid abnormalities (Davies & Herbert, 2007d). Practitioners need to be alert to symptoms of myocardial infarction in women with these risk factors. Diagnosis is confirmed with electrocardiogram (ECG) tracings and chest radiographs. Management is the same as in nonpregnant patients, preferably in a tertiary cardiac care setting. Women should not give birth within 2 weeks of myocardial infarction as the mortality rate has been shown to be up to 50% (Davies & Herbert, 2007d). Ongoing management of the pregnancy and close fetal surveillance will improve outcomes for this population.

Peripartum Cardiomyopathy

The criteria for the diagnosis of peripartum cardiomyopathy (PPCM) include development of congestive heart failure in the last month of pregnancy or within the first 5 postpartum months, lack of another cause for heart failure, and absence of heart disease before the last month of pregnancy (Easterling & Stout, 2007). Some data suggest that this definition could be expanded because the diagnosis of PPCM has been made at other times during gestation. The etiology of the disease is unknown; theories suggest genetic predisposition, autoimmunity, and viral infections.

PPCM is more common in older multiparous women, twin pregnancies, and women with pre-eclampsia (Davies & Herbert, 2007d; Grewal, Biswas, & Perloff, 2003). The incidence is 1 in 3000 to 4000 live births in North America, with the maternal mortality rate estimated to be in the range of 25 to 50%; the infant mortality rate is approximately 10% (Ramsey, Ramin, & Ramin, 2001). Maternal death is usually caused by thromboembolism, arrhythmia, or progressive heart failure.

Symptoms include breathlessness, dyspnea, cough, orthopnea, tachydysrhythmias, and edema, with radiological findings of cardiomegaly. The prognosis is good if cardiomegaly does not persist after 6 months postpartum. Women whose hearts remain enlarged after 6 months postpartum are highly likely to have PPCM in future pregnancies (Blanchard & Shabetai, 2009). Future pregnancy is contraindicated for women with persistent cardiomegaly or cardiac dysfunction (Davies & Herbert, 2007d).

Medical management of cardiomyopathy during pregnancy includes treatment similar to that for congestive heart failure and the potential for thromboembolism: diuretics, sodium restriction, afterload-reducing agents, anticoagulants, and digoxin. Angiotensin-converting enzyme inhibitors can be used only in the postpartum period because they are teratogenic agents and have been associated with severe fetal renal toxicity and stillbirth (Davies & Herbert, 2007d). The nursing care of women with PPCM is essentially the same as that for women with other types of cardiac problems.

Contraindications to Pregnancy

Contraindications to pregnancy in women with heart disease are listed in Box 14-4. The incidence of miscarriage is increased and preterm labour and birth are more prevalent in the pregnant woman with cardiac problems. In addition, IUGR is common, which may be the result of low oxygen pressure (Po_2) in the mother. The incidence of congenital heart lesions is increased in children of mothers with congenital heart disease; thus preconception counselling is important.

Nursing Care Management

Nursing care of the woman with a cardiovascular disorder combines routine peripartum care with care specific for the cardiac diagnosis and function (see Nursing Process box). Care of these women at low, medium, and high risk requires a multidisciplinary approach. The multidisciplinary team must work with the woman and her family in an environment that has the required resources to provide appropriate maternal hemodynamic monitoring. Table 14-3 lists the normal and abnormal cardiovascular signs during pregnancy.

The pregnant woman with cardiovascular disease will require some restriction of her activities. Bed rest during pregnancy affects all of the organ systems, but especially the cardiovascular and musculoskeletal systems. In addition, psychological adverse effects can be debilitating (Cunningham et al., 2010; Maloni, Brezinski-Tomasi, & Johnson, 2001). The

BOX 14-4 Contraindications to Pregnancy in a Woman With Heart Disease

- Dilated cardiomyopathy
- Primary pulmonary hypertension
- Eisenmenger's syndrome
- Marfan syndrome with aortic root dilation

(Source: Blanchard, D. G., & Shabetai, R. [2009]. Cardiac diseases. In R. K. Creasy, et al. [Eds.], *Creasy & Resnik's maternal–fetal medicine: Principles and practice* [6th ed.]. Philadelphia: Saunders.)

NURSING PROCESS: CARDIAC DISEASE

Assessment

The pregnant woman with cardiac disease requires detailed assessment throughout the perinatal period to ensure optimal maternal health, management of symptoms, and a healthy fetus. The high-risk pregnant woman's condition may be assessed as often as weekly.

Interview

The nurse elicits the following information from the woman:

Her personal medical history and that of her family
- Diseases of cardiovascular significance, including congenital heart disease, history of streptococcal infections, rheumatic fever, valvular disease, endocarditis, congestive heart failure, angina, or myocardial infarction

Factors that would increase stress on the heart (anemia, infection, and edema)

Adaptation to the physiological changes of pregnancy
- Review of the cardiovascular and pulmonary systems
- Presence of chest pain at rest or on exertion
- Edema of the face, hands, or feet; hypertension; heart murmurs; palpitations; paroxysmal nocturnal dyspnea; diaphoresis; and pallor or syncope
- Pulmonary symptoms such as cough, hemoptysis, shortness of breath, and orthopnea

Document all medications taken by the woman.

Assess for emotional stress that might further compromise cardiac status.

Physical Examination

Monitor the following:
- Presence and amount of edema
- Vital signs—must know baseline to assess for changes
- Discomforts of pregnancy
- Weight gain

Observe for signs of cardiac decompensation:
- Progressive generalized edema
- Crackles at base of lungs
- Pulse irregularity
- Shortness of breath

Review results of laboratory tests:
- Routine urinalysis and blood work (complete blood count and blood chemistry)
- Baseline 12-lead electrocardiogram (ECG) at the beginning of the pregnancy, and repeated as required
- Echocardiograms and pulse oximetry studies, as indicated
- Chest radiograph may be required as pregnancy progresses
- Fetal ultrasound examination, fetal movement count after 26 weeks' gestation, and nonstress tests (NST) (to determine fetal well-being)

Nursing Diagnoses

The following examples are some nursing diagnoses that may be formulated. As always, individualizing diagnoses is vital.

NURSING PROCESS: CARDIAC DISEASE—cont'd

Prenatal Period

Fear related to

- increased risk during perinatal period

Lack of knowledge related to

- cardiac condition as it relates to pregnancy
- requirements to alter self-management activities

Potential for activity intolerance related to

- cardiac condition

Risk for self-care deficit (bathing, grooming, and dressing) related to

- fatigue or activity intolerance
- need for bed rest

Impaired home maintenance related to

- woman's confinement to bed or limited activity level

Postpartum Period

Anxiety related to

- fear for infant's safety

Fear of dying related to

- perceived physiological inability to cope with stress of labour

Risk for impaired gas exchange related to

- cardiac condition

Risk for excess fluid volume related to

- extravascular fluid shifts

Ineffective breastfeeding related to

- fatigue from cardiac condition

Planning

Nursing care of the pregnant woman with a cardiovascular disorder combines routine perinatal care with care specific for the individual cardiac diagnosis and functional capacity of the woman. Such care requires a multidisciplinary approach, to optimize pregnancy outcomes and decrease pregnancy complications.

Expected outcomes might include that the pregnant woman (and family, if appropriate) will do the following:

- Express understanding of her specific cardiac disorder as it relates to pregnancy, management, and possible outcomes
- Describe her critical role in self-management, including medication intake, diet adjustments, and preparation for labour and birth
- Cope with emotional reactions to pregnancy and an infant at risk
- Adapt to the physiological stressors of pregnancy, labour, and birth
- Identify and use support systems
- Carry her fetus to viability or to term

Interventions

Review signs and symptoms of cardiac decompensation with the pregnant woman and her family.

Provide patient teaching.

The Woman With Class I or II Cardiac Disease

Requires 8 to 10 hours of sleep every day and should take 30-minute naps after meals.

Restrict activities (limit housework, shopping, and exercise) to the amount recommended for the functional classification of her heart disease.

The Woman With Class II Cardiac Disease

Avoid heavy exertion and stop any activity that causes even minor signs and symptoms of cardiac decompensation.

Admission to the hospital near term (or earlier if signs of cardiac overload or dysrhythmia develop) for evaluation and treatment.

The Pregnant Woman With Class III Cardiac Disease

Emphasize that bed rest for much of the day is necessary.

Treat infections promptly.

Provide nutrition counselling. Refer to a registered dietitian as necessary.

Administer cardiac medications as prescribed.

Monitor drug levels.

Monitor the woman's blood work.

Review results of tests for fetal maturity and well-being and placental sufficiency.

Reinforce the need for close medical supervision.

Evaluation

The nurse needs to use the previously stated expected outcomes as criteria to evaluate the care of the woman with cardiac disease.

community health nurse, social worker, and physiotherapist or occupational therapist are key resource people whose services may be incorporated into the plan of care.

Symptoms of cardiac decompensation may appear abruptly or gradually. Medical intervention must be instituted immediately to maintain optimal cardiac status. Dyspnea, palpitations, syncope, and edema commonly occur in pregnant women and can mask the symptoms of a developing or worsening cardiovascular disorder. A woman's sudden inability to perform activities that she previously was comfortable doing may indicate cardiovascular decompensation (Box 14-5).

Pregnancy outcomes vary as related to the severity of the cardiac condition present in the mother. The presence of cardiac disease may make the decision to become pregnant more difficult. Planned pregnancy should be discussed in preconception counselling with a skilled and knowledgeable provider. Unplanned pregnancy requires a full discussion with the woman to provide evidence-informed information about known pregnancy outcomes related to the various cardiac conditions. The woman's desire to continue the pregnancy must be explored. The nurse should review options for pregnancy termination with the woman if abortion is an

Table 14-3 Abnormal Cardiovascular Signs During Pregnancy

NORMAL	ABNORMAL
Signs	
Neck vein pulsation	Neck vein distension
Diffuse/displaced apical	Cardiomegaly; heave pulse
Split S_1, accentuated S_2	Loud P_2; wide split of S_2
Third heart sound	Summation gallop
Systolic murmur (1–2/6)	Loud systolic murmur (4–6/6)
Venous hum	Diastolic murmur
Sinus dysrhythmia	Sustained dysrhythmia
Peripheral edema	Clubbing/cyanosis

(Adapted from Mendelson, M. A. [1997]. Congenital cardiac disease and pregnancy. *Clinical Perinatology, 24*[2], 467–482.)

BOX 14-5 Signs of Potential Complications: Cardiac Decompensation

Pregnant Woman

Subjective Symptoms

Increasing fatigue or difficulty breathing or both with usual activities
Feeling of smothering
Frequent cough
Palpitations; feeling that her heart is racing
Swelling of face, feet, legs, fingers (e.g., rings do not fit anymore)

Nurse

Objective Signs

Irregular weak, rapid pulse (100 or more beats/min)
Progressive, generalized edema
Crackles at base of lungs after two inspirations and exhalations
Orthopnea; increasing dyspnea
Rapid respirations (25 or more breaths/min)
Moist, frequent cough
Increasing fatigue
Cyanosis of lips and nail beds

acceptable alternative. The woman's partner and family should be included in the discussion. Teaching sessions for the woman and her support people should be offered as indicated by their learning needs.

Plan of Care and Implementation

Nursing care for the pregnant woman with heart disease is focused on minimizing stress on the heart and ensuring that mother and fetus have a healthy outcome (see Nursing Care Plan). Cardiac stress is greatest between 28 and 32 weeks as the hemodynamic changes reach their maximum. The workload of the cardiovascular system is reduced by appropriate treatment of any coexisting emotional stress, hypertension, anemia, hyperthyroidism, or obesity.

PATIENT TEACHING The Pregnant Woman at Risk for Cardiac Decompensation

Assess for Risk and Understanding

- Assess the woman's lifestyle patterns, emotional status, and environment.
- Arrange for consultations as needed (e.g., dietitian, home care, child care, social work).
- Determine the woman's and her family's understanding of her heart disease and how the disease affects her pregnancy.
- Determine stressors in the woman's life. Assist the woman in identifying effective coping strategies.

Provide Instruction

- Instruct the woman to report signs of cardiac decompensation or congestive heart failure: generalized edema, distension of neck veins, dyspnea, pulmonary crackles, cough, palpitations, sudden weight gain.
- Instruct the woman to be watchful for signs of thromboembolism, such as redness, tenderness, pain, or swelling of the legs. Instruct her to seek medical help immediately if these symptoms occur.
- Instruct the woman to avoid constipation and thus straining with bowel movements (Valsalva manoeuvre) by taking in adequate fluids and fibre. A stool softener may be ordered.

Explore Self-Care and Resources

- Explore with the woman ways to obtain the needed rest throughout the day. Depending on the level of her cardiac disease, she may need to sleep 10 hours per night and rest for 30 minutes after meals (class I or II) or for most of the day (class III or IV).
- Help the woman make use of community resources, including support groups, as indicated.
- Emphasize the importance of keeping her prenatal visits.

(Sources: Arafeh, J. M., & Baird, S. M. [2006]. Cardiac disease in pregnancy. *Critical Care Nursing Quarterly, 29*, 32–52; Gilbert, E. S. [2007]. *Manual of high risk pregnancy and delivery* [4th ed.]. St. Louis: Elsevier.)

The woman needs a well-balanced diet with iron and folic acid supplementation, high protein, and adequate calories to gain weight. Iron supplements tend to cause constipation. She should increase her intake of fluids and fibre. A stool softener may be prescribed. It is important that the pregnant woman with cardiac disease avoid straining during defecation, thus causing the Valsalva manoeuvre (see Patient Teaching box). If sodium restriction is necessary, the amount should not be less than 2.5 g/day (Gilbert, 2007). The woman's intake of potassium should be monitored to prevent hypokalemia, especially if she is taking diuretics. A referral to a registered dietitian may be necessary.

Cardiac medications are prescribed as needed for the pregnant woman, with attention to fetal well-being. The hemodynamic changes that occur during pregnancy, such as increased plasma volume and increased renal clearance of drugs, can alter the amount of medication needed to establish and maintain a therapeutic drug level (Blanchard & Shabetai, 2009). Monitoring of the drug levels during the pregnancy is crucial

NURSING CARE PLAN ● The Pregnant Woman With Heart Disease

Nursing Diagnosis: Activity intolerance related to effects of pregnancy on the patient with cardiac disease

Expected Outcome

The woman will communicate a plan to change her lifestyle throughout pregnancy in order to avoid risk of cardiac decompensation.

Nursing Interventions/*Rationales*

Assist woman in identifying factors that decrease activity tolerance and explore the extent of limitations *to establish a baseline for evaluation.*

Help woman to develop an individualized program of activity and rest, taking into account the living and working environment, as well as the support of family and friends, *to maintain sufficient cardiac output.*

Teach woman to monitor physiological response to activity (i.e., pulse rate, respiratory rate) and reduce activity that causes fatigue or pain *to maintain sufficient cardiac output and prevent potential injury to the fetus.*

Enlist family and friends to assist woman in pacing activities and provide support in performing role functions and self-management activities that are too strenuous *to increase chances of adherence to activity restrictions.*

Suggest that the woman maintain an activity log that records activities, time, duration, intensity, and physiological response *to evaluate effectiveness of and compliance with the activity program.*

Discuss various quiet diversional activities that could be done by the woman *to decrease the potential for boredom during rest periods.*

Nursing Diagnosis: Risk for ineffective therapeutic regimen management related to woman's first pregnancy and perceived sense of wellness

Expected Outcome

The woman will participate in an effective therapeutic regimen for pregnancy complicated by heart disease.

Nursing Interventions/*Rationales*

Identify factors that could inhibit the woman from participating in a therapeutic regimen, such as insufficient knowledge about the effect of cardiac disease on pregnancy, *to promote early interventions such as teaching about the importance of rest.*

Teach the woman and family about factors such as lack of rest or not taking prescribed medications that could adversely affect the pregnancy *to provide information and promote a feeling of empowerment over the situation.*

Encourage expression of feelings about the disease and its potential effect on the pregnancy *to promote a sense of trust.*

Identify resources in the community *to provide a shared sense of common experiences.*

Encourage the woman to communicate her plan for carrying out the regimen of care *to evaluate the effects of teaching.*

Nursing Diagnosis: Decreased cardiac output related to increased circulatory volume secondary to pregnancy and cardiac disease

Expected Outcome

The woman will exhibit signs of adequate cardiac output (i.e., normal pulse and blood pressure; normal heart and breath sounds; normal skin colour, tone, and turgor; normal capillary refill; normal urine output; and no evidence of edema).

Nursing Interventions/*Rationales*

Reinforce the importance of activity–rest cycles *to prevent cardiac complications.*

Plan with the woman a schedule to visit her caregiver frequently *to provide adequate surveillance of high-risk pregnancy.*

Teach woman to lie in lateral position *to increase uteroplacental blood flow* and to elevate legs while sitting *to promote venous return.*

Monitor intake and output and check for edema *to assess for renal complications or venous return problems.*

Monitor fetal heart rate (FHR) and fetal activity and perform nonstress test (NST) as indicated *to assess fetal status and detect uteroplacental insufficiency.*

Nursing Diagnosis: Risk for ineffective tissue perfusion related to cardiac condition secondary to increased circulatory needs during pregnancy

Expected Outcomes

The woman will exhibit signs of hemodynamic stability (i.e., blood pressure, pulse, arterial blood gases [ABGs], and white blood cell [WBC] counts are within normal limits). The fetus will exhibit signs of well-being (i.e., fetal activity and FHR are within normal limits).

Nursing Interventions/*Rationales*

Monitor heart rate and rhythm, blood pressure, skin colour and temperature, WBC count, hemoglobin and hematocrit, and ABGs *to detect early signs of cardiac failure/hypoxia.*

Monitor fetal activity and FHR and perform NST as indicated *to assess fetal status and detect uteroplacental insufficiency.*

Teach woman how to detect and report early signs of cardiac decompensation *to prevent maternal and fetal complications.*

to maintain effective therapy for the woman while minimizing risk to the fetus. Research on the effects of cardiovascular medications on the fetus and pregnant woman has been limited. The nurse should review current pharmacological literature, especially when administering any medication to a pregnant woman (Table 14-4).

If anticoagulant therapy is required during pregnancy for conditions such as recurrent venous thrombosis, pulmonary embolus, RHD, prosthetic valves, or cyanotic congenital heart defects, low-molecular-weight heparin may be used because this large-molecule medication does not cross the placenta (Blanchard & Shabetai, 2009). The nurse must closely monitor the woman's blood work, including clotting factors. The woman may need to learn to self-administer heparin. She also requires specific nutrition education to avoid foods high in vitamin K, such as raw, dark green leafy vegetables, which

Table 14-4 Medications Used in Pregnancy for Cardiac Conditions

MEDICATION	SELECTED MATERNAL INDICATIONS	FDA PREGNANCY CATEGORY*	POSSIBLE ADVERSE FETAL EFFECTS
Cardiac Glycoside			
Digoxin, digitoxin	Arrhythmia	C	Maternal overdose can cause fetal toxicity and death
Anticoagulants			
Heparin	Thrombophlebitis Pulmonary hypertension	Does not cross the placenta	Heparin considered safe in pregnancy for the fetus
Warfarin	Same as heparin	X	Fetal anomalies, congenital malformations, hemorrhage; contraindicated in first trimester and at term
Diuretics			
Furosemide Thiazides	Hypertension	C	No known teratogenic effects; possible growth restriction; neonatal jaundice, thrombocytopenia, hemolytic anemia, hypoglycemia
β-Blockers			
Propranolol Metoprolol	Angina, hypertension, mitral valve prolapse, arrhythmia	C	During labour can cause bradycardia; after birth can cause hypoglycemia, hyperbilirubinemia
Vasodilators			
Hydralazine	Severe hypertension, pulmonary hypertension	C	Leukopenia and thrombocytopenia reported in newborns
Calcium Channel Blockers			
Nifedipine Verapamil	Angina, hypertension, arrhythmia (verapamil only)	C	Considered safe for use in pregnancy but no controlled human studies on fetal effects
Antiarrhythmics			
Quinidine Procainamide	Arrhythmia	C	Neonatal thrombocytopenia reported; quinidine preferred over procainamide

(Sources: Blanchard, D. G., & Shabetai, T. [2009]. Cardiac diseases. In R. K. Creasy, et al. [Eds.], *Creasy & Resnik's maternal–fetal medicine: Principles and practice* [6th ed.]. Philadelphia: Saunders; Arafeh, J. M., & Baird, S. M. [2006]. Cardiac disease in pregnancy. *Critical Care Nursing Quarterly, 29*[1], 32–52.)

*U.S. Food and Drug Administration (FDA) pregnancy categories: category A, controlled studies have not demonstrated a risk to the fetus; category C, animal studies have shown no adverse effects on the fetus, but there are no adequate studies in humans; potential benefits may be acceptable despite potential risks; category X, studies demonstrate fetal risk or abnormalities; risks outweigh potential benefits.

counteract the effects of the heparin. In addition, she will require a folic acid supplement.

Heart Surgery During Pregnancy

Ideally, a woman would have surgical correction of the cardiac lesion before pregnancy; however, pregnancy may be unplanned or the cardiac disease may be diagnosed for the first time during pregnancy. When medical therapy for a pregnant woman with cardiac disease is not sufficient to manage potentially life-threatening symptoms, cardiac surgery may be required. Early in the second trimester is the best time for surgery. The woman, fetus, and uterine activity must be monitored carefully during surgery. Closed cardiac surgery such as the release of a stenotic mitral valve can be achieved with little risk to the mother or fetus. Open heart surgery should be performed in a cardiac centre as it requires extracorporeal circulation. **Hypoxia** and fetal bradycardia must be assessed as they may occur as a result of low blood-flow rates. Periods of hypoxemia for the fetus can lead to neurological insult. An increase in flow rates on cardiopulmonary bypass may correct fetal bradycardia. Uterine contractions also increase in frequency before and during cardiopulmonary bypass and can be managed by medication.

LEGAL TIP Cardiac Emergencies. The management of cardiac emergencies such as maternal cardiopulmonary distress or arrest should be documented in policies, procedures, and protocols. Nursing scope of practice and independent nursing actions should be clearly identified.

Intrapartum

The woman with impaired cardiac function may have increased anxiety and fear of labour because giving birth places additional stressors on her already compromised cardiovascular system, which can result in a poor maternal outcome. General intrapartum management for cardiac disease focuses on strict fluid management, preventing hypotension and maternal tachycardia (>110 beats/min), and optimizing cardiac output (Arafeh & Baird, 2006).

Assessments include the routine assessments for all labouring women, as well as assessments for cardiac decompensation. In addition, arterial line placement and arterial blood gas evaluations may be needed to assess for adequate oxygenation. A pulmonary artery catheter (Swan-Ganz catheter) may be inserted to monitor hemodynamic status accurately during labour and birth. Electrocardiographic telemetry monitoring and continuous monitoring of blood pressure and pulse oximetry should be instituted for all women, and the fetus should be continuously monitored electronically (Arafeh & Baird, 2006).

NURSING ALERT A pulse rate of 110 beats/min or greater or a respiratory rate of 25 breaths/min or greater is a concern. Respiratory status should be checked frequently for developing dyspnea, coughing, or crackles at the base of the lungs. The colour and temperature of the skin should also be noted. Pale, cool, clammy skin may indicate cardiac shock.

Nursing care during labour and birth focuses on the promotion of cardiac function. Anxiety is minimized by maintaining a calm atmosphere in the labour and birth rooms. The nurse can provide anticipatory guidance by keeping the woman and her family informed of labour progress and events that will probably occur and by answering any questions they have. The woman's childbirth preparation method should be supported to the degree feasible for her cardiac condition. Nursing techniques that promote comfort, such as back massage, may be used.

Cardiac function is supported by keeping the woman's head and shoulders elevated and body parts resting on pillows. The side-lying position usually facilitates hemodynamics during labour. Discomfort is relieved with medication and supportive care. Epidural regional analgesia provides better pain relief than narcotics and causes fewer alterations in hemodynamics. Hypotension must be avoided.

The woman may require other types of medication (e.g., anticoagulants, prophylactic antibiotics). If evidence of cardiac decompensation appears, the physician may order furosemide (Lasix) for rapid diuresis and oxygen by intermittent positive pressure to decrease the development of pulmonary edema.

Spontaneous labour or planned induction of labour is the preferred method of birth for women with cardiac disease. If there are no obstetrical interventions, a planned, vaginal birth with the woman in a side-lying position to facilitate uterine perfusion is preferred. To prevent compression of popliteal veins and an increase in blood volume in the chest and trunk as a result of the effects of gravity, stirrups are not used. The second stage is carefully managed with passive second stage (allowing the fetal head to descend without pushing), prevention of the Valsalva manoeuvre (forced expiration against a closed airway, which, when released, causes blood to rush to the heart and overload the cardiac system), open glottis pushing, and consideration for operative vaginal delivery.

Vacuum extraction or outlet forceps may be used to decrease the length and workload of the heart in second-stage labour. Caesarean birth is not routinely recommended for women who have cardiovascular disease because there is a risk of dramatic fluid shifts, sustained hemodynamic changes, and increased blood loss. Bacterial endocarditis prophylaxis is not recommended, as the risk of bacteremia is low (Wilson et al., 2007).

Dilute IV oxytocin immediately after birth may be used to prevent hemorrhage. Ergot products should not be used because they tend to increase blood pressure. Fluid balance should be maintained and blood loss replaced. If tubal sterilization is desired, surgery is delayed at least several days to ensure homeostasis.

Postpartum

Monitoring for cardiac decompensation in the postpartum period is essential. The first 24 to 48 hours postpartum are the most hemodynamically difficult for the woman. During the immediate postpartum period, diuretic therapy may be required. Hemorrhage, infection, or both may worsen the cardiac condition. The woman with a cardiac disorder may continue to require a pulmonary artery catheter and arterial catheter to monitor volume status, cardiac output, blood pressure, and arterial blood gases.

NURSING ALERT The immediate postbirth period is hazardous for a woman whose heart function is compromised. Cardiac output increases rapidly as extravascular fluid is remobilized into the vascular compartment. At the moment of birth, intra-abdominal pressure is reduced drastically; pressure on veins is removed, the splanchnic vessels engorge, and blood flow to the heart is increased. When blood flow increases to the heart, a reflex bradycardia may result.

Care in the postpartum period needs to be tailored to the woman's functional capacity. Postpartum assessment of the woman with cardiac disease includes vital signs, oxygen saturation levels, lung and heart auscultation, edema, amount and character of bleeding, uterine tone and fundal height, urinary output, pain (especially chest pain), the activity–rest pattern, dietary intake, mother–infant interactions, and emotional state. The head of the bed should be elevated and the woman encouraged to lie on her side. Bed rest may be ordered, with or without bathroom privileges. Progressive ambulation may be permitted as tolerated. The nurse may help the woman meet her grooming and hygiene needs and other activities. Bowel movements without stress or strain for the woman are promoted with stool softeners, diet, and fluids.

The woman may need a family member to help in the care of the infant. While breastfeeding is encouraged for women with acquired and congenital heart disease, some women may not nurse their infants. The woman who chooses to breastfeed requires the support from her family and the nursing staff to assist in positioning herself or the infant for feeding. The infant should be brought to the mother and taken from her after the feeding to conserve her energy. Women who breastfeed may need less medication, especially fewer diuretics, for their cardiac condition. Because diuretics can cause neonatal diuresis that can lead to dehydration, lactating women must be monitored closely to determine if medication doses can be reduced and still be effective.

Women who are too ill to care for and feed their babies should be provided with opportunities to have the baby at the bedside so they can look at and touch the baby to establish an emotional bond. Having the baby skin-to-skin with the mother gives her a powerful opportunity to get to know her baby while expending little energy. If the mother is unable to hold her infant, the nurse or a family member can hold the infant at the mother's eye level and close enough for her to touch.

Discharge should be carefully planned with the woman and family. A clear plan to support the mother's need for a balance between rest and sleep periods along with activity must be discussed. The role of relatives, friends, and others in assisting with meal preparation and household duties as well as child care responsibilities must be addressed. The family may be referred to community resources (e.g., homemaking services) for additional support, as appropriate. The nurse should provide information to the couple about their re-establishing sexual relations and contraception needs or answer questions about tubal ligation or vasectomy. If tubal ligation is being considered as a method of contraception, the risks of surgery, especially for the woman with class III or IV heart disease, need to be explained. Women should be informed that oral contraceptives may be contraindicated because of the risk of thromboembolism. IUDs may put the woman at risk for infection, especially if she has a valve replacement. Injectable progestins are effective and safe (Easterling & Stout, 2007). Both the woman and her partner should discuss the options together in order to make the best choice for their individual situation.

Medical assessment and community health nurse follow-up is important after discharge to continue monitoring for cardiac decompensation, through the first few weeks after birth, due to hormone shifts that affect hemodynamics. Maternal cardiac output is usually stabilized by 2 weeks postpartum (Easterling & Stout, 2007).

Cardiopulmonary Resuscitation of the Pregnant Woman

Cardiac arrest in a pregnant woman is a rare event, most often related to events at the time of birth, such as amniotic fluid embolism, eclampsia, and drug toxicity. It can also occur as a result of complications of heart disease, such as congestive cardiomyopathy, aortic dissection, pulmonary embolism, or hemorrhage caused by a pregnancy-related pathological condition. Pre-existing disorders such as heart or pulmonary disease, hypertension, or autoimmune collagen vascular disease also increase this risk.

Various protocols exist for cardiopulmonary resuscitation (CPR) during pregnancy. The most widely used guide is the AHA advanced cardiac life support (ACLS) protocol (AHA, 2010). This protocol recommends standard CPR with the uterus displaced laterally, fluid-volume restoration, and defibrillation, if indicated. The decision for Caesarean birth should be made within 4 to 5 minutes of the mother's cardiac arrest. No matter what protocol is used, nurses and other health care providers must be prepared if CPR is to be successful.

In the event of cardiac arrest, standard resuscitative efforts with a few modifications are implemented. To prevent supine hypotension, the woman is placed on a flat, firm surface with the uterus displaced laterally either manually or with a wedge or rolled towel under her right hip or on her side supported by angled thighs of several rescuers or angled backs of several chairs (AHA, 2010). If a pregnant woman requires CPR outside a hospital setting, the focus of the new guidelines is C-A-B (*C*ompressions, *A*irway, *B*reathing). For untrained bystanders, the likelihood of providing CPR is greater if rescue breathing is not expected. Compressions should be provided at the depth of 5 centimetres at a rate of 100 times per minute (AHA, 2010).

Defibrillation with an automated external device (AED) is also key to increasing the chance of survival. If defibrillation is needed, the paddles, or AED pads must be placed one rib interspace higher than usual because the heart is slightly displaced by the enlarged uterus. If possible, the fetus should be monitored during the cardiac arrest. For pregnant women in hospital who require CPR, trained personnel need to tailor the sequence of rescue actions to the most likely cause of arrest. If a woman suddenly collapses, the health care provider should call for help and assess the woman for breathlessness and pulselessness prior to initiating CPR. By beginning immediate chest compressions, the delay is minimized in promoting circulation to the brain and key organs (see Emergency box).

Clearing an airway obstruction in a woman in the second or third trimester of pregnancy also requires a modification of the Heimlich manoeuvre (Fig. 14-3).

Complications that may be associated with CPR of a pregnant woman include laceration of the liver, rupture of the uterus, hemothorax, and hemoperitoneum. Fetal complications that may occur include cardiac dysrhythmia or asystole related to maternal defibrillation and medications, CNS depression related to antidysrhythmic medications and inadequate uteroplacental perfusion, and onset of preterm labour.

If resuscitation is successful, the woman and her fetus must receive careful monitoring. The woman remains at increased risk for recurrent pulmonary arrest and dysrhythmias (ventricular tachycardia, supraventricular tachycardia, and bradycardia). Therefore, her cardiovascular, pulmonary, and neurological status should be assessed continuously. Uterine activity and resting tone must be monitored. Fetal status and gestational age should be determined and used in decision making regarding continuation of the pregnancy or the timing and route of birth.

Anemia

Anemia is the most common medical disorder of pregnancy, affecting at least 20% of pregnant women. During pregnancy, women require more iron to support the increase in circulating blood volume. Anemia results in a reduction of the oxygen-carrying capacity of the blood, and the heart tries to compensate by increasing the cardiac output, which increases the workload of the heart. Women who have anemia of pregnancy with any other complication (e.g., pre-eclampsia) should be assessed for the possibility of further heart stress.

An indirect index of the oxygen-carrying capacity is the packed red blood cell volume, or hematocrit level. The normal hematocrit range in nonpregnant women is 0.37 to 0.47. Normal values for pregnant women with adequate iron stores may be as low as 0.32. This decreased level has been explained by the blood volume expansion of approximately 50% and total red blood cell mass expansion of approximately 25%. This hydremia (dilution of blood) is also called the **physiological anemia of pregnancy**.

Anemia in pregnancy is defined as a hemoglobin level of less than 100 g/L or a hematocrit of less than or equal to 0.32 (Langlois, Ford, & Chitayat, 2008). When a woman has anemia during pregnancy, the loss of blood at birth, even if minimal,

EMERGENCY

Cardiopulmonary Resuscitation of the Pregnant Woman in the Hospital

Determine unresponsiveness.
Activate emergency call system and get the emergency response cart.
Position woman on flat, firm surface with uterus displaced laterally with a wedge if possible (e.g., a rolled towel placed under her hip).

Circulation

Assess for the presence of a pulse by feeling carotid pulse for no longer than 10 seconds.
If there is no pulse, begin chest compressions at rate of a minimum of 100/min at a compression depth of at least 5 cm. Allow the chest to completely recoil after compression. Chest compressions may be performed slightly higher on the sternum if the uterus is enlarged enough to displace the diaphragm into a higher position.

Airway

Open airway with head tilt–chin lift manoeuvre.

Breathing

Assess for presence of breathing (look, listen, feel) for no longer than 8 seconds.
If the woman is not breathing, give 2 slow breaths; ensure that the chest rises with each breath.
Rescue breathing without chest compressions should be given at a rate of 10 to 12 breaths/min.
After four cycles of 30 compressions and 2 breaths, check her pulse for no longer than 10 seconds. The goal is to have the least interruption of chest compressions as possible. If pulse is not present, continue cardiopulmonary resuscitation.

Defibrillation

Use a defibrillator according to standard protocol to analyze heart rhythm, and deliver shock if indicated.

Birth

Consider perimortem Caesarean birth within 5 minutes if chest compressions are unsuccessful.

Relief of Foreign-Body Airway Obstruction

If the pregnant woman is unable to speak or cough, perform chest thrusts.
Stand behind the woman and place your arms under her armpits to encircle her chest. Press backward with quick thrusts until the foreign body is expelled (see Fig. 14-3).
If the woman becomes unresponsive, follow steps for victims who become unresponsive, but use chest thrusts instead of abdominal thrusts.

(Source: American Heart Association. [2010]. Guidelines for cardiopulmonary resuscitation and emergency cardiovascular care science. *Circulation, 122,* S639. Retrieved from http://circ.ahajournals.org/content/vol122/18_suppl_3/.)

is not well tolerated. She is at increased risk for requiring blood transfusions. Women with anemia have a higher incidence of puerperal complications such as infection than do pregnant women with normal hematological values. *Severe anemia*, defined as a hemoglobin level of less than 60 g/L, has been associated with decreased fetal oxygen levels that result in abnormal fetal heart rate patterns, decreased amniotic fluid volume, and fetal death.

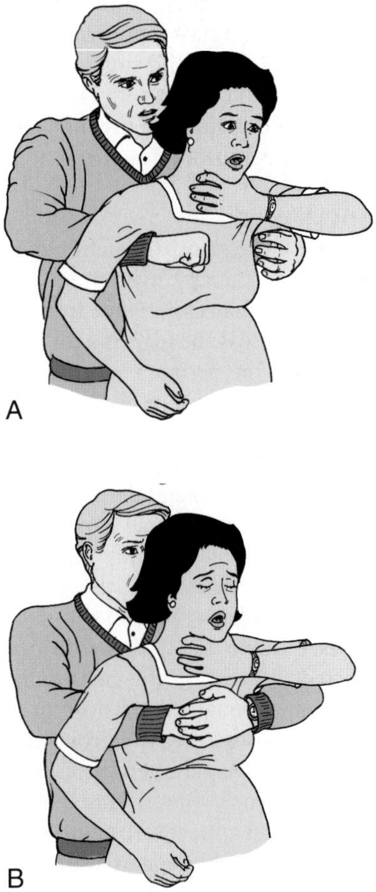

Fig. 14-3 Heimlich manoeuvre. Clearing airway obstruction in a woman in the late stages of pregnancy (can also be used in markedly obese person). **A:** Standing behind victim, place your arms under the woman's armpits and across the chest (between nipples). Place thumb side of your clenched fist against the middle of the sternum and place other hand over fist. **B:** Perform backward chest thrusts until foreign body is expelled or woman loses consciousness. If pregnant woman becomes unconscious because of foreign-body airway obstruction, place her on her back and kneel close to her side. (If possible, ensure that the uterus is displaced laterally by using, for example, a rolled blanket under her hip.) Open her mouth with tongue-jaw lift. If able to see obstruction, remove it if it can be done safely and attempt rescue breathing. If unable to ventilate, position hands as for chest compression. Deliver 30 chest compressions firmly, check mouth again for presence of obstruction, and attempt to provide rescue breathing. Continue sequence until the pregnant woman's airway is clear of obstruction or help has arrived to relieve you. If the woman is unconscious, give chest compressions as for a woman without a pulse.

Nursing care of the pregnant woman with anemia requires that the nurse be able to distinguish between the normal physiological anemia of pregnancy and the disease states. About 90% of cases of anemia in pregnancy are of the iron deficiency type. The remaining 10% embrace a considerable variety of acquired and hereditary anemias, including folic acid deficiency, sickle cell anemia, and thalassemia.

During prenatal visits, the nurse should take a diet history and provide dietary teaching as appropriate. Pregnancy may cause increased fatigue, stress, and financial difficulties for a woman with anemia as she copes with her activities of daily living. The nurse should assess the pregnant woman's needs and provide her with appropriate resources or referral.

Iron Deficiency Anemia

Pathological anemia of pregnancy is mainly the result of iron deficiency. Without iron therapy, even pregnant women who enjoy excellent nutrition may experience iron deficiency. Iron is actively transported across the placenta for fetal erythropoiesis. Ferritin levels are the primary screening tests used to diagnose iron deficiency anemia. A ferritin level of less than 25 mcg/L confirms the diagnosis.

If iron deficiency anemia is diagnosed, increased iron dosages are recommended (elemental iron, 60 to 120 mg/day). Diet alone cannot replace gestational iron losses. Inadequate nutrition without therapy will certainly mean iron deficiency anemia during late pregnancy and the puerperium. It is important to teach the pregnant woman about the significance of iron therapy (see Table 11-2). In addition, the woman should be instructed to decrease the gastrointestinal adverse effects of iron therapy through diet. Those pregnant women who cannot tolerate the prescribed oral iron because of nausea and vomiting should receive parenteral iron, such as an iron–dextran complex (Imferon). Blood transfusions should be considered for the woman with severe anemia to prevent fetal and maternal complications of decreased oxygen delivery.

Folic Acid Deficiency Anemia

Folic acid deficiency during conception and early pregnancy increases the incidence of neural tube defects, cleft lip, and cleft palate. Even in well-nourished women, it is common to have a folate deficiency. Poor diet, cooking with large volumes of water, or home canning of food (especially vegetables) may lead to folate deficiency. Malabsorption may play a part in the development of anemia caused by a lack of folic acid. Folic acid deficiency is common in multiple gestations. During pregnancy, the recommended daily intake is 0.4 mg per day of folic acid, although women who have a deficiency may need 1 mg or more per day (see Table 11-1).

Sickle Cell Hemoglobinopathy

Sickle cell hemoglobinopathy is a disease caused by the presence of abnormal hemoglobin in the blood. Sickle cell trait (SA hemoglobin pattern), sickling of the red blood cells but with a normal red blood cell lifespan, usually causes only mild clinical symptoms. Sickle cell anemia (sickle cell disease) is a recessive, hereditary, familial hemolytic anemia that affects those of African or Mediterranean ancestry. These individuals usually have abnormal hemoglobin types (SS or SC). People with sickle cell anemia have recurrent attacks (crises) of fever and pain in the abdomen or extremities. These attacks are attributed to vascular occlusion (from abnormal cells), causing tissue ischemia and acute and chronic organ dysfunction involving the spleen, brain, lungs, and kidneys. Pain and swelling of the extremities is common and occurs as a result of aseptic necrosis of the small carpal and tarsal bones. The hemolysis leads to chronic anemia and predisposes the woman to aplastic crises (Langlois et al., 2008). Crises are associated with normochromic anemia, jaundice, reticulocytosis, a positive sickle cell test, and demonstration of abnormal hemoglobin (usually SS or SC).

Almost 10% of Blacks in North America have the sickle cell trait, but fewer than 1% have sickle cell anemia. The anemia often is complicated by iron and folic acid deficiency.

Women with sickle cell trait usually do well in pregnancy, although they are at increased risk for urinary tract infections and hematuria and may be deficient in iron (Kilpatrick, 2009). If the woman has sickle cell anemia, the anemia that occurs in normal pregnancies may aggravate the condition and bring on more crises. Women in impending sickle cell crisis experience painful joints. Fetal complications include being small for gestational age, IUGR, and skeletal changes.

Pregnant women with sickle cell anemia can develop pyelonephritis, leg ulcers, bone abnormalities, strokes, cardiomyopathy, congestive heart failure, and pre-eclampsia. An aplastic crisis may result from serious infection. Red cell transfusions are the usual treatment for symptomatic patients; however, partial exchange transfusions or prophylactic transfusions are common as well and significantly reduce the number of painful crises (Kilpatrick, 2009). Caesarean birth is warranted only for obstetrical indications. Oral contraceptives are contraindicated because of the increased risk of thromboembolus.

Thalassemia

Thalassemia (Mediterranean or Cooley anemia) is a relatively common anemia in which an insufficient amount of globin is produced to fill the red blood cells. The condition eventually manifests itself in severe bone deformities caused by massive marrow tissue expansion. Thalassemia is a hereditary disorder that involves the abnormal synthesis of the alpha (α) or beta (β) chains of hemoglobin. β-Thalassemia is the more common variety in North America and is more common in individuals of Mediterranean, Middle Eastern, and Asian descent (Kilpatrick, 2009). The unbalanced synthesis of hemoglobin leads to premature red blood cell death, resulting in severe anemia. Thalassemia major is the homozygous form of the disorder; thalassemia minor is the heterozygous form. If both partners are found to be carriers of thalassemia or a Hb variant, or of a combination of thalassemia and a hemoglobin variant, they should be referred for genetic counselling. Ideally, this should be before conception, or as early as possible in the pregnancy. Additional molecular studies may be required to clarify the carrier status of the parents and thus the risk to the fetus (Langlois et al., 2008). Women with the thalassemia trait usually have an uncomplicated pregnancy.

Women with thalassemia major or minor often have infertility; thus there are few pregnancies in the literature from which to base key pregnancy management strategies. As many as 50% of these pregnancies have been complicated by stillbirth, IUGR, pre-eclampsia, or preterm birth (Langlois et al., 2008). Medical management consists of ongoing monitoring and transfusion therapy.

Women with thalassemia minor have a mild, persistent anemia; but the red blood cell level may be normal or even elevated. However, no systemic problems are caused by the anemia. Thalassemia minor must be distinguished from iron deficiency anemia.

Thalassemia-related anemia does not respond to iron therapy. Practitioners should avoid prolonged parenteral iron therapy as harmful, excessive iron storage can result. People with thalassemia minor have a normal lifespan despite a moderately reduced hemoglobin level.

Pulmonary Disorders

Dyspnea is common during pregnancy, occurring by most estimates in approximately 60% of women with exertion and fewer than 20% at rest. The symptom is so common that it usually is referred to as physiological dyspnea. Physiological dyspnea can occur early in pregnancy and does not interfere with daily activities. Although the gravid uterus is often blamed, hyperventilation due to increased progesterone levels probably is the most important mechanism. Distinguishing this physiological dyspnea from breathlessness caused by disorders complicating pregnancy or diseases that might coexist with pregnancy is key. The presence of other symptoms and signs of cardiopulmonary disease indicates a possible pathological nature of dyspnea, and the patient should be carefully evaluated.

A pregnant woman with a pulmonary disorder requires assessment, planning, and interventions specific to the disease process, in addition to the routine peripartum care. The perinatal nurse must be alert to pulmonary complications precipitated by the pregnancy.

Asthma

Bronchial asthma is an acute respiratory illness caused by allergens, irritants, marked changes in ambient temperature, certain medications (e.g., aspirin and β-blockers), or exercise. In many cases, the cause may be unknown. A history of positive allergen testing is common (75 to 85%) in people with asthma. In response to stimuli, there is widespread but reversible narrowing of the hyper-reactive airways, making it difficult to breathe. The clinical manifestations are some or all of the following: expiratory wheezing, productive cough, thick sputum, and dyspnea.

Approximately 4 to 8% of pregnant women have diagnosed asthma, making it the most common pulmonary disease in pregnancy (Koren, Sarkar, & Einarson, 2010; Whitty & Dombrowski, 2009). To classify the severity of asthma and determine management guidelines, the National Asthma Education and Prevention Program (NAEPP) Working Group on Asthma and Pregnancy published guidelines for classification, which can also guide practice in Canada. Pregnant women are classified as having mild intermittent, mild persistent, moderate persistent, and severe persistent asthma, based on exacerbation of symptoms, peak expiratory flow rate (PEFR), and forced expiratory volume in 1 second (FEV_1) (NAEPP, 2004) (Table 14-5). The effect of pregnancy on asthma is unpredictable. Approximately 33% of patients improve, 33% remain stable, and 33% worsen (Madappa & Sharma, 2010; Whitty & Dombrowski, 2009). Maternal morbidity is 2.3% with mild, 19.3% with moderate, and 26.9% with severe symptoms that required hospitalization (Whitty & Dombrowski, 2009). Physiological alterations induced by pregnancy do not make the pregnant woman more prone to

Table 14-5 Modified National Asthma Education and Prevention Program Asthma Severity Classification

CLASS	CRITERIA	TREATMENT
Mild intermittent	Symptoms ≤ twice/week or asymptomatic between exacerbations Nocturnal symptoms ≤ twice/month PEFR or FEV_1 ≥80%, variability ≤20%	No daily medications needed
Mild persistent	Symptoms > twice/week but not daily Nocturnal symptoms > twice/month PEFR or FEV_1 ≥80%, variability 20–30%	Preferred—Low-dose inhaled corticosteroid Alternative—Cromolyn (for rhinitus), leukotriene receptor antagonist (nonsteroidal) (determined to be safe in pregnancy*), or theophylline/aminophylline (serum level 5–12 mcg/mL)
Moderate persistent	Daily symptoms Nocturnal symptoms > once/week PEFR or FEV_1 >60–80% predicted, variability >30% Regular medications necessary to control symptoms	Preferred—Low-to-medium inhaled corticosteroid and salmeterol or medium dose inhaled corticosteroid Alternative—Low-to-medium dose inhaled corticosteroid and leukotriene receptor antagonist or low-to-medium dose inhaled corticosteroid and theophylline (serum level 27–66 mmol/L)
Severe	Continuous symptoms/frequent exacerbations Frequent nocturnal symptoms PEFR or FEV_1 ≤60% predicted, variability >30% Regular oral corticosteroids necessary to control symptoms	Preferred—High-dose inhaled corticosteroid and salmeterol and oral corticosteroid if needed Alternative—High-dose inhaled corticosteroid and theophylline (serum level 27–66 mmol/L) and oral corticosteroid if needed Albuterol 2–4 puffs as needed for PEFR or FEV_1 <80%, asthma exacerbations, or exposure to exercise or allergens; oral corticosteroid burst if inadequate response to albuterol, regardless of asthma severity

(From NAEPP Working Group. [2004]. *NAEPP Working Group report on managing asthma during pregnancy. Recommendations for pharmacologic treatment—2004 update* [NIH Publication No. 05-3279]. Bethesda, MD: National Lung, Heart, and Blood Institute.)

*Koren, G., Sarkar, M., & Einarson, A. (2010). The use of Montelukast in pregnancy. *Canadian Family Physician, 56*, 881–882.

FEV_1, forced expiratory volume in 1 second; *PEFR*, peak expiratory flow rate.

asthmatic attacks. Women often have few symptoms of asthma in the first trimester and the last weeks of pregnancy. Women with asthma in pregnancy have not been shown to have an increase in perinatal mortality, when the effects of smoking are removed (Breton et al., 2010). For women whose symptoms become severe in pregnancy, the challenging time is between 24 and 36 weeks of gestation (Burton & Reyes, 2001; Madappa & Sharma, 2010). An increase in congenital malformations was found in women who had acute asthma exacerbations in the first trimester of pregnancy (Blais & Forget, 2008).

The ultimate goal of therapy for asthma is to prevent hypoxic episodes in the mother and fetus through maintaining control of asthma symptoms and prevention of acute asthma exacerbations.The therapy has four objectives: (1) relieve the bronchospasm, (2) limit irritant stimuli, (3) decrease the pulmonary response to allergen exposure, and (4) limit the inflammatory response in the airways. These goals can be achieved in pregnancy by eliminating environmental triggers (e.g., dust mites, animal dander, pollen), adjusting medication therapy (e.g., bronchodilators and anti-inflammatory medications), and providing education to the pregnant woman. Respiratory infections should be treated with appropriate antibiotics, and mist or steam inhalation should be used to aid the expectoration of mucus. Acute episodes may require albuterol, steroids, aminophylline, β-adrenergic agents, and oxygen. Pharmacotherapy to control symptoms and treat airway inflammation is safer than exacerbations of symptoms during pregnancy. Patients should determine their PEFR with pulmonary function assessment before taking medications (Koren et al., 2010; Whitty & Dombrowski, 2009).

Asthma attacks can occur during labour; thus medications for asthma are continued in labour and postpartum. Pulse oximetry should be instituted to assess oxygenation levels during labour. Epidural analgesia reduces oxygen consumption and minute ventilation and is an effective strategy to help prevent complications in labour.

During the postpartum period, women who have asthma are at increased risk for hemorrhage. If excessive bleeding occurs, oxytocin is the recommended medication. Asthma medications are usually safe for administration during the postpartum period and lactation. The woman usually returns to her prepregnancy asthma status within 3 months after giving birth (Maddapa & Sharma, 2010).

Cystic Fibrosis

Cystic fibrosis is an autosomal recessive genetic disorder in which the exocrine glands produce excessive viscous secretions, causing problems with both respiratory and digestive functions. There is an increase in pulmonary capillary permeability, decrease of lung volume, and shunting, which results in arterial hypoxemia. Respiratory failure and early death (in the early 20s) may occur.

The gene for cystic fibrosis was identified in 1989. All infants born to mothers with cystic fibrosis are carriers of the gene. The disease occurs in 1 in 3300 White live births (Slack et al., 2006). If both potential parents are carriers of the cystic fibrosis gene, the SOGC recommends that cystic fibrosis carrier screening be offered to couples who are planning a pregnancy as the risk of inheriting the gene is 25% (Audibert et al., 2009; Wilson et al., 2002). Infertility appears to relate to changes in cervical mucus. Improvements in diagnosis and treatment have allowed an increasing number of women with cystic fibrosis to survive to adulthood. As a result of the advances in diagnostic capabilities and treatment, the median survival has increased from 14 years of age to 30 to 35 years of age. The median age of survival for women with pancreatic insufficiency is 27 years (Whitty & Dombrowski, 2009).

Pregnancy is tolerated well in women with good nutritional status, mild obstructive lung disease, and minimal impairment of lung function. In women with severe disease, the pregnancy is often complicated by chronic hypoxia and frequent pulmonary infections. Women with cystic fibrosis show a decrease in their residual lung volume during pregnancy, as do normal pregnant women, and are unable to maintain vital capacity. Presumably the pulmonary vasculature cannot accommodate the increased cardiac output of pregnancy. The results are decreased oxygen to the myocardium, decreased cardiac output, and increased hypoxia. A pregnant woman with less than 50% of expected vital capacity usually has a difficult pregnancy. Increased maternal and perinatal mortality rates are related to severe pulmonary infection. There is an increased incidence of preterm births, IUGR, and neonatal deaths in patients with cystic fibrosis. Predictors of adverse effects to the fetus and neonate are inadequate weight gain, dyspnea, and cyanosis.

In addition to the respiratory problems, pregnant women with cystic fibrosis have decreased insulin secretion and increased insulin resistance, resulting in a higher incidence for the development of gestational diabetes mellitus. A glucose tolerance test should be done at 20 weeks of gestation. Pancreatic insufficiency puts the woman at risk for malnutrition because she cannot meet the increased nutrition requirements of pregnancy. Fat-soluble vitamins should not be taken because of diminished absorption.

Weight and symptoms of malabsorption should be monitored at each prenatal visit, and pancreatic enzymes should be adjusted as necessary. Women with severe pancreatic insufficiency may require total parenteral nutrition (TPN). Routine respiratory management needs to be continued throughout the pregnancy. Hospitalization and antibiotic therapy are recommended when a pulmonary infection has been identified. Because cystic fibrosis places the pregnant woman at risk, nonstress testing should be initiated at 32 weeks.

During labour, monitoring for fluid and electrolyte balance is required to monitor for sodium loss and hypovolemia. Conversely, if the woman has any degree of cor pulmonale, fluid overload is a concern. Oxygen should be given freely during labour, and monitoring by pulse oximetry is recommended. Epidural or local anaesthesia is the preferred analgesic for birth. Vaginal birth is preferable; Caesarean birth should be reserved for the usual obstetrical indications.

Breastfeeding appears to be safe as long as the sodium content of the mother's milk is not abnormal. The milk is pumped and discarded until the sodium content has been determined. Milk samples should be tested periodically for sodium, chloride, and total fat, and the infant's growth pattern should be followed (Lawrence & Lawrence, 2011).

Gastrointestinal Disorders

Compromise of gastrointestinal function during pregnancy is a concern. Obvious physiological alterations, such as the greatly enlarged uterus, and less apparent changes, such as hormonal differences and hypochlorhydria (deficiency of hydrochloric acid in the stomach's gastric juice), require an understanding of proper diagnosis and treatment. Gallbladder disease and inflammatory bowel disease are two gastrointestinal disorders that may occur during pregnancy.

Cholelithiasis and Cholecystitis

Women are twice as likely to have cholelithiasis (presence of gallstones in the gallbladder) than men (Sun et al., 2009). It is hypothesized that estrogens cause increased cholesterol secretion and progesterone promotes biliary stasis. Pregnancy seems to make woman more vulnerable to gallstone formation. Decreased muscle tone allows gallbladder distension and thickening of the bile and prolongs emptying time. Increased progesterone levels result in a slight hypercholesterolemia. Nutrition counselling is important (see Home Care box).

Cholecystitis (inflammation of the gallbladder) may also occur during pregnancy, likely because increased pressure of the enlarged uterus interferes with the normal circulation and drainage of the gallbladder. Acute cholecystitis occurs most often in older women who have been pregnant several times and who have a history of previous attacks.

Women with acute cholecystitis usually have fatty food intolerance along with colicky abdominal pain radiating to the back or shoulder, nausea, and vomiting. Fever and an increased leukocyte count may also be present. Ultrasonography is often used to detect the presence of stones or dilation of the common bile duct.

Generally, gallbladder surgery should be postponed until the puerperium. Usually the woman can be treated with conservative medical therapy consisting of antibiotics, analgesics, IV fluids, bowel rest, and nasogastric suctioning (Chloptsios, Karanasiou, Ilias, Kavouras, & Stamatiou, 2007). TPN can be used in some cases as an alternative to surgery. Morphine should not be used as an analgesic because it may cause ductal spasm. The woman's condition should improve significantly within 48 hours of beginning treatment. Surgery may be necessary if the woman has repeated attacks of biliary colic, acute cholecystitis, obstructive **jaundice**, peritonitis, or pancreatitis. Laparoscopic cholecystectomy performed in the second trimester poses minimal risk to both the mother and fetus. (Williamson & Mackillop, 2009).

HOME CARE

Nutrition Counselling for the Pregnant Woman With Cholecystitis or Cholelithiasis

- Assess your diet for foods that cause discomfort and flatulence and omit foods that trigger episodes.
- Reduce dietary fat intake to 40 to 50 g/day.
- Limit protein to 10 to 12% of total calories.
- Choose foods so that most of the calories come from carbohydrates.
- Prepare food without adding fats or oils, as much as possible.
- Avoid fried foods.

Inflammatory Bowel Disease

Treatment of inflammatory bowel disease is the same for the pregnant woman as it is for the nonpregnant woman. Medications include prednisone and sulphasalazine. Vitamin and folic acid supplementation is especially important because of problems with malabsorption. Effects of inflammatory bowel disease on pregnancy are usually minimal. If the woman is severely debilitated, miscarriage, preterm birth, or fetal death can occur.

Integumentary Disorders

The skin surface may exhibit many physiological and pathological conditions during pregnancy. Dermatological disorders induced by pregnancy include **melasma** (chloasma), vascular "spiders," palmar **erythema**, and **striae gravidarum**. Skin problems generally aggravated by pregnancy are acne vulgaris (in the first trimester), erythema multiforme, herpetiform dermatitis (fever blisters and genital herpes), granuloma inguinale (Donovan bodies), condylomata acuminata (genital warts), neurofibromatosis (von Recklinghausen's disease), and pemphigus. Dermatological disorders usually improved by pregnancy include acne vulgaris (in the third trimester), seborrheic dermatitis (dandruff), and psoriasis. An unpredictable course during pregnancy may be expected in atopic dermatitis, lupus erythematosus, and herpes simplex. Disease processes during and soon after pregnancy may be extremely difficult to diagnose and treat.

NURSING ALERT Isotretinoin (Accutane), commonly prescribed for acne, is contraindicated in pregnancy because of its high teratogenicity; it must be avoided under all circumstances during pregnancy. Nursing mothers also should not use Accutane. The risk of birth defects among pregnant women is extremely high. These defects include hydrocephaly (enlargement of the fluid-filled spaces of the brain) and microcephaly (small head), heart defects, facial deformities such as cleft lip and missing ears, and developmental delays.

Pruritus is a common symptom in pregnancy-specific inflammatory skin diseases. The most common pregnancy-specific causes of pruritus are polymorphic eruption of pregnancy (also known as pruritic urticarial papules and plaques of pregnancy [PUPPP]) (Fig. 14-4), prurigo gestationis, and cholestasis of pregnancy. Symptoms usually appear in the third trimester and usually subside in the postpartum period. The abdomen is usually affected, but lesions can spread to the arms, thighs, back, and buttocks. Topical steroid therapy

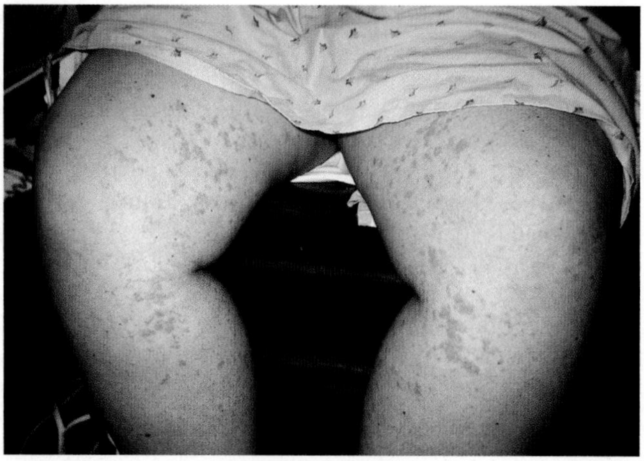

Fig. 14-4 Woman with pruritic urticarial papules and plaques of pregnancy (PUPPP). Lesions also are present on her arms, back, abdomen, and buttocks. *(Courtesy Shannon Perry, Phoenix, AZ.)*

usually provides relief, but some women may require systemic steroid therapy for severe symptoms (Papoutsis & Kroumpouzos, 2007).

Neurological Disorders

Pregnant woman with neurological disorders are becoming more prevalent with the improvement of medications for treatment of these disorders. However, unfortunately, many of these medications are potentially teratogenic to the fetus. The nurse should be aware of all medications the pregnant woman is taking to discuss the associated potential for producing congenital anomalies. As the pregnancy progresses, the woman's centre of gravity shifts and causes balance and gait changes, potentially changing her patterns of mobility during pregnancy. The woman should be advised of these expected changes and provided safety measures as appropriate. Family and community resources should be assessed to provide child care for the neurologically impaired woman as her ability to care for the baby on her own may be impaired.

Epilepsy

Epilepsy is a disorder of the brain, resulting in recurrent seizures; it is the most common neurological disorder accompanying pregnancy. The cause of epilepsy is not well understood; it may be related to developmental abnormalities or injury or have no identified cause. Seizures differ in presentation, ranging from absence seizures (brief losses of awareness without loss of consciousness) to tonic-clonic seizures (involving muscle rigidity, violent muscle contractions, and loss of consciousness). Both types of seizures are related to abnormal electrical activity in the brain. Women who have tonic-clonic seizures may experience them more frequently or have more severe complications during pregnancy, such as edema, **alkalosis**, fluid–electrolyte imbalance, cerebral hypoxia, hypoglycemia, and hypocalcemia. Seizures can also be triggered by hormonal changes, fatigue, or sleep deprivation.

NURSING ALERT Anticonvulsants may decrease the effectiveness of oral contraceptive agents, resulting in unplanned pregnancy.

Differentiating between epilepsy and eclampsia can pose a challenge for practitioners. Epilepsy and eclampsia can coexist. However, the presence of seizures with a normal plasma uric acid level; normal blood pressure; and lacking generalized edema, **proteinuria**, or both are more indicative of epilepsy.

The effects of pregnancy on epilepsy are unpredictable. Most women have no change in seizure activity during pregnancy, some have an increase, whereas others have a decrease in seizures.

Seizure control is the primary goal in treating pregnant women with epilepsy. Pregnant women must be educated about the risks associated with uncontrolled seizures. Changes to current anticonvulsant medications may have to be made to reduce the risks of teratogenicity. The benefits of effective seizure control versus the risk of uncontrolled seizures must be discussed on an individual basis.

If anticonvulsant therapy must be adjusted or introduced as a new therapy, the lowest effective dose must be used, and monotherapy is preferable to polytherapy. Babies born to mothers exposed to anticonvulsant medications are at increased risk of congenital malformations, cognitive impairment, and fetal death (Morrow et al., 2006). Congenital anomalies associated with anticonvulsant medications include cleft lip or palate, congenital heart disease, urogenital defects, and neural tube defects. Daily folic acid supplementation is required to replace depleted levels in mothers who take anticonvulsant medications.

Metabolic changes in pregnancy usually alter **pharmacokinetics**. In addition, nausea and vomiting may interfere with the ingestion and absorption of medication. A small risk of seizure activity exists during labour. If a woman experiences tonic-clonic seizures during pregnancy or labour, there is a threefold risk of abruptio placentae. Intravenous phenytoin can be administered as required. Serum levels of anticonvulsant medications should be checked within 48 hours of birth and at 1 to 2 weeks after birth because levels can change quickly and toxicity can develop.

During the neonatal period, infants can have a hemorrhagic disorder associated with anticonvulsant medication–induced vitamin K deficiency. Prophylaxis consists of maternal administration of vitamin K, 20 mg orally, daily during the last month of pregnancy and 1 mg intramuscularly to the newborn at birth. Neonates also should be monitored for drug withdrawal. All of the most prescribed anticonvulsant medications cross into breast milk; however, their use is not contraindicated with breastfeeding.

Restless Legs Syndrome

Restless legs syndrome (RLS) is a neurological disorder characterized by discomfort of the legs and an urge to move them, usually during rest or inactivity. The discomfort is relieved by movement, which causes disturbances in sleep patterns. It is generally idiopathic but is associated with anemia and pregnancy. The risk of having RLS is two to three times higher in pregnant women than in the general population (Djokanovic,

Garcia-Bournissend, & Koren, 2008; Manconi et al., 2004; Zucconi & Ferini-Strambi, 2004). Pre-existing RLS worsens during pregnancy, having the highest degree of severity in the third trimester, and disappears at the time of birth.

Multiple Sclerosis

Multiple sclerosis (MS), a patchy demyelinization of the spinal cord and CNS, may be a viral disorder. Women are affected twice as often as men, with the most common onset occurring during the childbearing years between ages 20 and 40. MS does not affect the normal course of pregnancy or birth (Aminoff, 2009).

Occasionally, MS may complicate pregnancy, but exacerbations and remissions are often unrelated to the pregnant state. Bed rest and steroids may be used to treat acute exacerbations. Nursing care of the pregnant woman with MS is similar to that of the pregnant woman with an uncomplicated pregnancy. Women with MS may have some decreased nerve function in the pelvic area, making it difficult to tell when labour begins. Although pregnancy is a remissive state for women with MS, the postpartum period is often the time when MS symptoms recur, sometimes with worsening symptoms.

Bell's Palsy

The incidence of Bell's palsy (idiopathic facial paralysis) in pregnancy is about 57 per 100,000 per year. The clinical manifestations include the sudden development of a unilateral facial weakness, often discovered first thing in the morning. In addition, taste on the anterior two thirds of the tongue may be lost, depending on the location of the lesion. Pain may occur in and around the ear. The incidence usually peaks during the third trimester and the puerperium. There is no relationship between the appearance of Bell's palsy and any complications of pregnancy.

No effects of maternal Bell's palsy have been observed in infants. Maternal outcome is generally good unless there is a complete block in nerve conduction. Steroids sometimes are prescribed for the condition, but they do not hasten recovery. In most affected women, 90% or more of facial function can be expected to return. Supportive care includes prevention of injury to the exposed cornea, facial muscle massage, careful chewing and manual removal of food from inside the affected cheek, and reassurance that return of total neurological function is likely.

Autoimmune Disorders

Autoimmune disorders make up a large group of diseases that disrupt the function of the immune system of the body. In these types of disorders, the body develops antibodies that attack its normally present antigens, causing tissue damage. Autoimmune disorders have a predilection for women in their reproductive years; therefore, associations with pregnancy are not uncommon. Pregnancy may affect the disease process. Some disorders adversely affect the course of pregnancy or are detrimental to the fetus. Autoimmune disorders of concern in pregnancy include systemic lupus erythematosus, myasthenia gravis, and rheumatoid arthritis.

Systemic Lupus Erythematosus

One of the most common serious disorders in women of childbearing age, systemic lupus erythematosus (SLE), is a chronic multisystem inflammatory disease characterized by autoimmune antibody production that affects the skin, joints, kidneys, lungs, CNS, and liver and other body organs. The exact cause is unknown, but viral infection and hormonal and genetic factors may be related. The prognosis is worse in women who are Asian, Indian, Black, or Latin American than in White women. Early symptoms such as fatigue, fever, skin rashes, weight loss, and arthralgias may be overlooked. Pericarditis is often the initial symptom. Eventually, all organs become involved. The condition is characterized by a series of exacerbations and remissions.

If the diagnosis has been established and the woman desires a child, she is advised to wait until she is in remission and cytotoxic medications (e.g., azathioprine, methotrexate, cyclophosphamide) have been stopped (Holmgren & Branch, 2007). An exacerbation of SLE during pregnancy or postpartum occurs in 15 to 60% of women (Holmgren & Branch, 2007).

SLE during pregnancy is associated with increased risk of spontaneous abortion, intrauterine fetal death, pre-eclampsia, IUGR, and preterm birth. Prognosis for both the mother and child are best when SLE is in remission for at least 6 months before the pregnancy and when the mother's underlying renal function is stable and normal or near normal. Lupus nephritis can get worse during pregnancy. Complications such as pre-eclampsia and HELLP syndrome may also occur.

Medical therapy is kept to a minimum in women who are in remission or who have a mild form of SLE. Anti-inflammatory medications such as prednisone and aspirin may be used. Immunosuppressive medications are not recommended during pregnancy but may be used in some situations when there is more risk with not treating SLE. Nursing care focuses on early recognition of signs of SLE exacerbation and pregnancy complications, education and support of the woman and her family, and assessment of fetal well-being.

While vaginal birth is preferred, Caesarean birth is common because of maternal and fetal complications. During labour, efforts are aimed at reducing the risk of infection, which is the leading cause of death in women with SLE.

During the postpartum period, the mother should rest as much as possible to prevent an exacerbation of SLE. Breastfeeding is encouraged unless the mother is taking immunosuppressive agents. Women with SLE should limit their number of pregnancies because of increased adverse perinatal outcomes and the guarded maternal prognosis (Holmgren & Branch, 2007). Family planning is important. Oral contraceptives with synthetic estrogens should not be used in women with active lupus nephritis.

Myasthenia Gravis

Myasthenia gravis (MG), an autoimmune motor (muscle) end-plate disorder that involves acetylcholine use, affects the motor function at the myoneural junction. Muscle weakness results, particularly in the eyes, face, tongue, neck, limbs, and respiratory muscles. Symptoms include easy fatigability; intermittent double vision (diplopia); upper eyelid drooping; and difficulty speaking, swallowing, and clearing secretions. In more serious cases, upper arm weakness and breathing difficulty are seen. The response of women with MG to pregnancy is unpredictable; remission, exacerbation, or remaining stable during pregnancy may occur.

NURSING ALERT If preterm labour occurs, magnesium sulphate, which interferes with neuromuscular transmission, is absolutely contraindicated.

Treatment is the same as for a nonpregnant woman. Usual medications include immunosuppressive medications and acetylcholinesterase inhibitors. Monitoring of blood glucose values is important because hyperglycemia may be the result of corticosteroid therapy. Thymectomy may result in remission of the disease but is best performed before or after pregnancy, if at all possible. Plasmapheresis or IV immunoglobulin therapy may be needed for severe weakness.

Women with MG usually tolerate labour well, but vacuum or forceps assistance for birth may be required because of muscle weakness. Oxytocin may be given to stimulate contractions. Narcotic analgesia should be avoided because it may precipitate respiratory depression. Regional analgesia is preferred. After birth, women must be carefully supervised because relapses often occur during the puerperium.

Approximately 10 to 15% of babies born to mothers with MG will develop neonatal myasthenia. Newborns must be assessed for symptoms of feeble cry, respiratory distress, and weak suck. These neonates may require ventilatory support. With proper management, complete recovery of the neonate should occur within 6 weeks (Aminoff, 2009).

Obesity

Obesity is a serious health concern that can have a profound impact on pregnancy. It is estimated that the number of obese and overweight women in Canada has risen from 9.7% in 1972 to 43.7% in 2010 (Statistics Canada, 2011). *Obesity* is defined using body mass index (BMI), which is defined as a measure of an adult's weight in kilograms divided by height in metres squared (kg/m^2) (see Table 4-1). Women with a BMI of 25 to 29.9 are considered overweight, whereas those with a BMI over 30 are considered obese. Overweight and obese women and their fetuses and infants are at increased risk of health complications. Pregnancy can exacerbate previous health issues or initiate new health complications during and after pregnancy. Comprehensive care of the bariatric patient is essential to ensure optimum outcomes for both mother and fetus.

Antepartum Risks

Obese women often have difficulty becoming pregnant and may require assisted reproductive technology. Once they are pregnant, women who are obese may have difficulty maintaining the pregnancy. There is an increased risk of spontaneous abortions, as well as increased recurrent pregnancy loss (Davies, Maxwell, & McLeod, 2010). Increased BMI also leads to an increased risk of stillbirth; women with a BMI greater than 40 having a three times greater rate of stillbirth after 28 weeks (Cedergren, 2004).

It is recommended that women who are overweight or obese attempt to obtain an ideal body weight before conception, to improve their own health as well as the pregnancy outcomes (Davies et al., 2010; Walters & Taylor, 2009/2010). Once the woman is pregnant, a weight loss program is not recommended and nutritional counselling may be required. Regular exercise during pregnancy appears to decrease the risks associated with obesity.

During pregnancy, obese women require increased surveillance and care. GDM screening should be done early in the pregnancy, as the risk for GDM and type 2 diabetes is increased in obese women (Davies et al., 2010). A dating ultrasound examination should be done because of irregular or anovulatory cycles, to confirm the estimated date of birth. During routine 18- to 22-week ultrasound examination, it can be difficult to visualize fetal structure and repeated ultrasound scans may be required to assess fetal anatomy. This assessment is important, as infants of obese mothers have in increased rate of birth defects, including neural tube, heart, ventral wall, and possibly orofacial defects (Davies et al., 2010). Obese women also have an increased risk of developing hypertension disorder of pregnancy. This risk increases as BMI increases (Davies et al., 2010).

Intrapartum and Postpartum Risks

Women who are obese also have increased risks during labour. There is an increased risk of shoulder dystocia, due to fetal macrosomia (see Chapter 19). If induction of labour is necessary, uterine contractility may be altered in obese women and higher doses of oxytocin may be required (Zhang, Bricker, Wray, & Quenby, 2007). The risk of Caesarean birth is increased in women who are obese; the risk is 20% for BMI less than 30 and 47.4% for BMI greater than 40 (Weiss et al., 2004). This increased risk could be due to a prolonged active phase of labour as well as cephalopelvic disproportion (CPD) or fetal **macrosomia**. Anaesthesia difficulties can also occur and are discussed in Chapter 16 (p. 420).

During the postpartum period, women may have more difficulty breastfeeding and will require extra support for positioning the newborn. Wound infections are increased as wound healing is delayed and dehiscence may occur. There is also an increased risk for venous thromboembolism and postpartum hemorrhage (PPH) (see Chapter 23, p. 586). The risk for PPH is increased because of decreased muscle tone, decreased physical activity, and the macrosomic fetus with a corresponding large placental implantation site.

Nursing Care Management

Caring for the bariatric woman during labour requires a caring, knowledgeable approach. Appropriate-sized equipment is required. A large manual blood pressure cuff is required as automated BP machines may not be accurate for BP assessment. It is important to have appropriate-sized beds, operating room tables, and stretchers and to know the weight limit on equipment. Bathrooms and shower stalls may require wider doors. It is also important to ensure that there is access to larger gowns, weigh scales, and epidural needles. Nurses need to use appropriate body mechanics when doing any lifting and to use mechanical lifts when necessary.

During labour, respiratory problems may occur, so it is necessary to monitor oxygen saturation levels along with performing thorough respiratory assessments. It may be difficult to palpate the fetus, so ultrasound examination may be necessary to confirm fetal position. Monitoring the fetus with electronic fetal monitoring may be difficult. When labour has progressed, it may be useful to use an internal scalp electrode to monitor the fetal heart rate and an intrauterine pressure catheter (see Chapter 17) to monitor the contractions (Davies et al., 2010). It is important to reposition the labouring woman frequently in order to provide maternal comfort and promote fetal descent.

The postpartum woman requires frequent assessments to monitor bleeding and vital signs. To decrease the risk of venous thromboembolism, it is important to encourage early ambulation with the use of graduated compression stockings when ambulating and TED stockings if on bed rest. Women may also require prophylactic heparin therapy.

Human Immunodeficiency Virus and Acquired Immunodeficiency Syndrome

Over the last 10 years, human immunodeficiency virus (HIV) infections have been increasing in Canadian women. The percentage of women newly diagnosed with HIV has increased to at least 25% of all new infections in Canada (Shrim, Garcia-Bournissen, Koren, & Farine, 2007). Young women are now one of the fastest growing populations of individuals with HIV infection. Women are more likely to have acquired the infection through heterosexual contact or IV drug use. Women from endemic countries, First Nations, Métis, and Inuit women, and women experiencing marginalization are at a higher risk for HIV infection. Violence, trauma, and being a young woman have all been found to contribute to a woman's vulnerability to HIV exposure, due to the inability to practise safer sex practices. The complication of prolonged HIV infection is acquired immunodeficiency syndrome (AIDS). Antiretroviral treatment (ART) works to decrease perinatal transmission rates along the progression of AIDS-related complications. This section addresses the management of the pregnant woman who is HIV positive. See Chapter 6 for more information about the diagnosis and management of nonpregnant women with HIV and Chapter 28 for a discussion of HIV infection in infants.

Preconception Counselling

At the present time in Canada, women who are HIV positive are having successful pregnancies, resulting in noninfected, healthy newborns (Burdge et al., 2003). The key to optimal perinatal outcomes for women is preconception pregnancy counselling and planning. Preconception pregnancy planning should include consultation with providers specialized in the area of HIV infections and pregnancy. This assessment should include a review of the woman's HIV history, current physical status, and prenatal and HIV-specific laboratory results. The other critical component of preconception counselling is to carefully review with the woman a plan on how to decrease the risk of transmission to the child as well as decrease the pregnancy, intrapartum, and postnatal risks.

Pregnancy Risks

Pregnant women who are HIV positive need to be engaged in ongoing specialized prenatal care that involves physicians, nurses, pharmacists, nutrition counsellors, social workers, and community support to ensure healthy outcomes for both the mother and infant. Care includes strict compliance with an antiretroviral medication regime, following through with regular HIV-specific blood-level monitoring (viral plasma levels and immunological functioning), and being well informed regarding labour, birth, and postpartum. Even if a diagnosis of HIV is made late in pregnancy or during the intrapartum period, it can be treated with antiretroviral medications, thus decreasing the risk of perinatal transmission.

HIV-positive women should be encouraged to seek prenatal care immediately if they suspect pregnancy in order to maximize chances for a positive outcome. Pregnancy itself does not appear to significantly accelerate the progression of HIV infection. One of the most overwhelming situations for a pregnant woman is when she is newly diagnosed with a positive HIV result. This situation requires intensive counselling and support for the women and often for her partner (see Critical Thinking Exercise).

Perinatal Transmission

Perinatal transmission may occur to the fetus through the maternal circulation as early as the first trimester of pregnancy, to the infant during labour and birth, or to the infant through breast milk. Factors that increase the likelihood of perinatal viral transmission are listed in Box 14-6.

Identification of the HIV-positive pregnant woman is especially important because antepartum and intrapartum antiviral medication therapy has been shown to greatly decrease the risk of viral transmission to the fetus. With optimal maternal child HIV-prevention treatment available throughout Canada, the percentage of infected newborns has decreased dramatically to less than 2% (Burdge et al., 2003). Without treatment, the HIV perinatal transmission rate can range between 25 and

BOX 14-6 Factors Increasing the Risk of Mother-to-Child Perinatal HIV Transmission

- Lack of maternal and infant treatment with antiretroviral medications and prevention
- Maternal plasma viral level greater than 1000 copies per millilitre
- Maternal vaginal infections during pregnancy
- Amniocentesis, chorionic villus sampling, or both
- Ruptured membranes
- Presence of chorioamnionitis
- Fetal scalp monitoring and venous scalp sampling
- Interventions such as forceps, vacuum, and external cephalic version
- Breastfeeding

CRITICAL THINKING EXERCISE

The Pregnant Woman Who Is HIV Positive

Betsy is being seen in the prenatal clinic at 34 weeks of gestation. She has been positive for the human immunodeficiency virus (HIV) for 2 years and has a past history of substance use, with a history of using intravenous cocaine and heroin for over 5 years. She has been substance free for the last 18 months. This is Betsy's first baby and it is an unplanned pregnancy. During your nursing assessment, she tells you that she was started on medication for her HIV when she was 3 months pregnant. Betsy does not seem to know the names of the pills she is taking and says she tries to remember to take them daily but sometimes misses some doses. As part of your care, you will be providing Betsy information about the importance of attending prenatal visits regularly, taking her antiretroviral medication daily, and having blood tests done monthly.

1. Evidence—Is there sufficient evidence to draw conclusions about the necessity of continued care, treatment, and support for Betsy and her infant?
2. Assumptions—What assumptions can be made about the following issues?
   a. The rationale and importance of compliance with Betsy's antiretroviral medication treatment, comprehensive prenatal care, and planning throughout her pregnancy
   b. Maternal and child HIV antiretroviral medication prophylaxis regime
   c. Risk factors for acquiring HIV infection that are in Betsy's history
   d. Review of perinatal HIV transmission prevention as you plan to provide care for Betsy and her infant
3. What implications and priorities for nursing care can be drawn at this time?
4. Does the evidence objectively support your conclusion?
5. Are there alternative perspectives to your conclusion?

40% (Shrim et al., 2007). Data show that almost all HIV-positive childhood diagnoses not attributed to mother-to-child transmission were in children from endemic countries (Centers for Disease Control and Prevention [CDC], 2007).

Obstetrical Complications

It is difficult to determine obstetrical risk in persons with HIV infection because so many confounding variables are often present. HIV-positive women may have lives complicated by such issues as substance use, mental health issues, poverty, poor nutrition, limited access to prenatal care, or concurrent sexually transmitted infection (STI). Many of these variables can account for a woman being at risk for preterm labour and birth, premature rupture of membranes, perinatal loss, and IUGR. The mode of birth for women who are HIV positive depends on the woman's plasma viral level and her status of labour upon admission. If a woman's plasma level is less than 1000 copies per millilitre and she has received ART, she can proceed with a vaginal birth. In women positive for HIV who are not receiving antiretrovirals and have a plasma load greater than 1000, an unknown plasma level, or antepartum bleeding, a Caesarean birth is recommended. The postpartum period for the woman infected with HIV may be notable for infection, hemorrhage, or both. Women without symptoms may have an unremarkable postpartum course; on the other hand, immunosuppressed women with symptoms may be at increased risk for postpartum urinary tract infections, vaginitis, postpartum endometritis, and poor wound healing. HIV-related **thrombocytopenia** may also increase the risk of hemorrhage.

Nursing Care Management

HIV counselling and testing is recommended for all pregnant women in Canada when they initially enter prenatal care. Women engaging in high-risk behaviour should be offered HIV testing at each trimester of their pregnancy. Not all HIV-positive women will be detected prenatally. Any woman whose HIV status is unknown at the time of labour or birth should be screened with a rapid HIV test, unless she declines (Keenan-Lindsay et al., 2006).

HIV-infected women should also be tested for other STIs, such as gonorrhea; syphilis; chlamydia; hepatitis B, C, and D; and herpes. Cytomegalovirus and toxoplasmosis antibody testing should be done because both infections can cause significant maternal and fetal complications and can be successfully treated with antimicrobial agents. Any history of vaccination and immune status should be documented, and chicken pox (varicella) and rubella titres should be determined. Women who are HIV positive should also be vaccinated against hepatitis B, pneumococcal infection, hemophilus B influenza, and viral influenza. A tuberculin skin test should be performed; a positive test necessitates a chest x-ray film to identify active pulmonary disease. A Papanicolaou (Pap) test should also be done.

All HIV-infected women should be treated with ART during pregnancy, regardless of the CD4 counts. ART should include three drugs from at least two classes of antiretroviral medications. The major adverse effect of these medications is bone marrow suppression. Periodic hematocrit, white blood cell count, and platelet count assessments should be performed. Women with CD4 counts of less than 200 cells/mm^3 should receive prophylactic treatment for *Pneumocystis carinii* pneumonia with daily trimethoprim-sulphamethoxazole. Any other opportunistic infections should be treated with medications specific for the infection; often dosages must be higher for women with HIV infection (Bernstein, 2007).

The woman who is HIV positive requires nutritional support and counselling. Weight gain or maintenance in pregnancy can be a challenge. Women need to be supported and counselled regarding safer sex practices to reduce risks for herself and her partner. Use of **condoms** and a **spermicide** is encouraged to minimize further exposure to HIV if her partner is positive.

The woman should be referred for drug rehabilitation, as necessary, to discontinue substance use. Use of alcohol, methamphetamines ("speed," "ice"), marijuana, cocaine, nitrites ("poppers," "snappers"), or other drugs compromises the body's immune system and increases the risks of AIDS and associated conditions. It also interferes with many medical and alternative therapies for AIDS. In addition, alcohol and other drugs affect the judgement of users, who may be more likely to engage in high-risk activities that increase their exposure to HIV.

IV zidovudine is administered to the HIV-positive woman during the intrapartum period. A loading dose is initiated on her admission in labour, followed by a continuous maintenance dosage throughout labour.

Every effort should be made during the birthing process to decrease the neonate's exposure to infected maternal blood and secretions if Caesarean birth is not scheduled and the woman goes into labour. If feasible, the membranes should be left intact until the birth. Increased duration of ruptured amniotic membranes has been associated with increased perinatal transmission. However, research has not shown these data to be statistically significant (Bernstein, 2007). If rupture of membranes occurs before labour, induction of uterine contractions with oxytocin may be appropriate. Fetal scalp electrode and scalp pH sampling should be avoided because these procedures may result in inoculation of the virus into the fetus. Operative vaginal delivery (forceps or vacuum extractor) and episiotomy should also be avoided, when possible (Bernstein, 2007).

Immediately after birth, infants should be wiped free of all body fluids. Prior to blood testing or any injections, the skin area should be cleansed well with soap and water. All staff working with the mother or infant must adhere to routine precautions for blood and other body fluids. The infant can be placed skin to skin with the mother after birth, but breastfeeding is discouraged because of the risk of transmission through breast milk. Oral zidovudine treatment for the infant is initiated within 6 hours of life and continues for up 6 weeks. In the postpartum period, it is critical that women who are HIV positive be assessed for postpartum infections. Women and their infants require close postpartum follow-up by providers specialized in HIV in the hospital and upon discharge. This will ensure that ART and maternal and infant blood work are maintained and monitored. A postpartum contraception discussion should be part of the nurse's and provider's discussion with the woman prior to discharge from the hospital.

Substance Use

Substance use among women in Canada is recognized as an increasing concern from both a health and a social perspective (Poole & Greaves, 2007). Women are using a variety of substances, the most common being alcohol, tobacco, and mood-altering and pain-relieving prescribed medications, as well as illicit drugs such as marijuana, cocaine, heroin, **crack**, crystal methamphetamine, and **opioids**. Women who use substances often have unplanned pregnancies. The effects of alcohol and illicit drugs on pregnant women and their unborn babies are well documented (Wisner et al., 2007). Alcohol and other drugs pass easily from a mother to her baby through the placenta. Smoking during pregnancy has serious health risks, including bleeding complications, miscarriage, stillbirth, prematurity, placenta previa, placental abruption, low birth weight, and sudden infant death syndrome (Wisner et al., 2007). Congenital abnormalities have occurred in infants of mothers who have taken drugs. The safest pregnancy is one in which the mother is totally drug and alcohol free, with one exception: for pregnant women addicted to heroin, methadone maintenance is safer for the fetus than acute opiate detoxification.

Substance use or *problematic use* can be defined by compulsive drug use and loss of control over use, resulting in physical, social, and psychological consequences. Symptoms of withdrawal and tolerance can be seen in women who use substances (Kissin et al., 2004).

Barriers to Treatment

Women who use substances and are pregnant often do not seek prenatal care for many reasons. The most notable of these are guilt, stigma, and shame, as well as the fear of losing custody of a child. Pregnant women who use substances commonly have little understanding of the ways in which these substances affect them, their pregnancies, and their infants. They often delay seeking prenatal care until labour begins. Traditionally, substance use treatment programs for women have not addressed issues that affect pregnant women, such as concurrent need for obstetrical care and child care for other children. Long waiting lists and lack of women-only recovery spaces present further barriers to treatment.

Legal Considerations

Nurses who care for women who use substances in pregnancy must use a nonjudgemental and women-centred approach. Women should be encouraged to attend prenatal care that is accessible for them and to participate in counselling and treatment. A flexible multidisciplinary team is invaluable when caring for women who are pregnant and using substances. It is critical to these women that they receive care and support based on a harm reduction model of care. Throughout Canada, every community needs to support policies that strengthen substance use prevention programs designed for young women and the provision of women-only treatment and recovery programs.

Drug Testing During Pregnancy

There is no legal requirement in Canada for a health care provider to test either the mother or the newborn for the presence of drugs, unless the provincial child agency requests this. However, nurses need to know the practices in the health region where they are working. In both hospitals and community health centres, it is best to consult with the facility's social workers regarding drug testing, following informed consent from the woman.

Nursing Care Management

The care of the woman who is pregnant and using substances should be based on self-disclosure of her present and past use, prenatal health history, physical findings, and laboratory results. Screening questions for alcohol, tobacco, prescribed and nonprescribed medications, and illicit substance use should be included in the overall assessment of all women, regardless of socioeconomic status, at their first prenatal visit. Women need to be assessed for a history of violence, abuse, and mental health concerns, as well as for other determinants of health, such as poverty and lack of housing and social supports that put women at risk and can increase their substance use.

It is critical for nurses and other providers to use a nonjudgemental interview and questioning technique when gathering substance-use information from women. Screening tools that have been developed and used in the past are not always accurate in the practice setting. Urine and toxicology testing are not recommended as a clinical screening tool for pregnant women. Testing of maternal hair and newborn meconium is also not recommended for clinical use. Maternal serum toxicology or urine testing is helpful to support a woman's self reporting of her current substance use status. When drug testing is ordered clinically or requested by the provincial child protection agency, informed consent from the woman is mandatory. When testing is ordered in the newborn, parental or guardian informed consent is also required.

Following the initial prenatal assessment, serial ultrasound studies should be performed to confirm gestational age. Some women may have had amenorrhea as a result of substance use or may not know when their last menstrual period occurred. There is an increased risk of stillbirth and of small-for-gestational-age infants as well as the potential for perinatal hypoxia. If concerns are detected, regular ultrasound examination and fetal surveillance with monitoring should be arranged.

In planning care for a pregnant woman who uses substances, the perinatal nurse must individualize her approach, taking the women's past history and expressed needs into consideration. Although the ideal long-term outcome is total abstinence, in Canada a harm reduction philosophy of care is practised, supporting a woman's desire to stop using as well as assisting her in reducing her risks. If the woman can only reduce her use of substances, support and care are still offered. A realistic goal may be to decrease substance use, and short-term outcomes will be necessary.

A multidisciplinary team model is essential when planning care for women who use substances. Major issues that must be addressed in treatment for these women that generally are not part of treatment for men are low self-esteem, stigmatization, high probability of sexual abuse and physical abuse, lack of social support, need for social services and child care, need for women's health services, and need for support and education in the mothering role. Housing or residential supervised communities may offer an ideal route toward stabilization in a safe environment. Recovery and treatment for women must demonstrate cultural sensitivity and recognition of diversity and ethnicity as an important part of her identity. Other needs of many of these women include relationship counselling, coping skills training, and vocational and legal assistance (Jos, Perlmutter, & Marshall, 2003).

Interventions with women who use substances need to begin with trust and communication. Women are often very receptive to learning how they can keep their growing fetus safe and healthy by stopping or reducing substance use. Women are often more receptive to making lifestyle changes during pregnancy than at any other time in their lives. The casual, experimental, or recreational drug user is often able to achieve and maintain abstinence from substances when she receives education, support, and continued monitoring throughout her pregnancy. Pregnancy presents a window of opportunity for motivating women to stop their use of substances.

Stabilization and treatment for women who use substances should be individualized for each woman, depending on the type of drug used and the frequency and amount of use.

Detoxification, short-term inpatient or outpatient treatment, long-term residential treatment, aftercare services, and self-help support groups are all possible options. Neonatal outcomes are improved among infants whose mothers received an integration of substance use treatment with prenatal care. In most communities in Canada, treatment options are limited for women, especially facilities that allow children to be with their mothers. Some women find organizations such as Alcoholics Anonymous or Narcotics Anonymous, based on the 12-step program, very helpful, and meetings can be found in almost every community. A caution for women using the 12-step program is that the program's emphasis is on powerlessness over addiction and avoidance of codependency, which some women might find disempowering and isolating.

Methadone maintenance treatment for pregnant women dependent on opiates is the current standard (Wisner et al., 2007). Methadone therapy, along with behavioural counselling, has been shown to decrease the use of opiates and other drugs, reduce high-risk activity, improve birth weight, and decrease the rates of pre-eclampsia and exposure to HIV. Disadvantages of methadone therapy include fetal heart rate changes (e.g., fewer accelerations, decreased rate and variability), a decrease in fetal breathing episodes, and neonatal abstinence syndrome (Wisner et al., 2007).

Cocaine use during pregnancy has increased dramatically in the last few years. A number of maternal and fetal complications accompany cocaine use, including placental abruption, stillbirth, prematurity, and small-for-gestational-age infants.

Because of the risks that women who use substances experience in their lives, exposure to STIs and HIV is increased. STI monitoring for gonorrhea and *Chlamydia* infection and antibody determinations for hepatitis B and HIV should be offered to substance-using women frequently. A chest x-ray film may be taken to assess for pulmonary problems such as hilar lymphadenopathy, pulmonary edema, bacterial pneumonia, and foreign-body emboli. A skin test to screen for tuberculosis may also be ordered.

Nurses must understand the reasons why women use substances, the barriers to stopping use, and their life experiences. Planning the best care for women who are pregnant and use substances must be based on a women-focused framework (Box 14-7). Mother–infant attachment should be promoted by identifying the woman's strengths and reinforcing positive maternal response and interactions.

Advice regarding breastfeeding must be individualized. Although all substances appear in breast milk, some in greater amounts than others, breastfeeding has many benefits. Breastfeeding should be delayed until the potential risks and benefits have been reviewed. Instructing and supporting women in hand expression, breast pumping, and then discarding of the expressed colostrum or breast milk is helpful for women wishing to breastfeed during this delay. Women should be

BOX 14-7 Perinatal Care for Women Who Use Substances

- Realize that the decision to stop using substances and engage in recovery can only be made by the woman herself.
- Understand that the nurse's role can be that of an advocate and facilitator for positive change in a woman's life.
- Educate yourself on the reasons why women use substances and the barriers to recovery in pregnancy. Know that violence, trauma, and mental health history contribute to a women's substance use and her ability to ask for help.
- Review the effects of perinatal substance use in pregnancy, intrapartum, and on the newborn infant.
- Women-centred and harm reduction practices are critical in caring for women who use substances. Respect, understanding, and choices should be key components in nursing care and planning.
- Familiarize yourself with community resources for women, including accessible health clinics and providers; housing services, both emergency and long term; counselling and mental health supports; and substance recovery and treatment centres. Contact numbers for community services should be available in the hospital and clinic for women and their providers.

encouraged to remain substance free if they are breastfeeding. Some women have no desire to breastfeed whereas others find it provides a strong motivation to achieve and maintain their substance-free status.

Before discharge, the woman needs to have an effective and resourceful discharge plan, which should be made with the assistance of nursing and other health care providers. If the woman is unable to provide care for her infant or has chosen not to care for her infant, the infant may be placed with her family or in foster care. Support and counselling for this mother is extremely beneficial, and planning for future visits with her infant is often helpful.

Most women who have a history of substance use will require assistance in planning for hospital discharge with their infant. Adequate and safe housing, food and formula provisions, transportation supports, and recovery and parenting supports are essential services for the woman to be successful as a new parent. The hospital or community social worker, along with the provincial child agency worker, will often be involved in assessing the woman's needs and in assisting the woman to ensure that supports and resources are put in place before discharge. Often family members or friends will be asked to become actively involved with the woman and her infant before discharge. The public or community health nurse will be asked to make home visits to assist and support the women and her infant. Postpartum doula support may also be helpful at this time. Community providers will encourage the women to follow up with them soon after discharge for regular postpartum visits for herself and her infant.

Key Points

- Careful monitoring of blood glucose levels, insulin administration, and dietary counselling are instrumental in creating a normal intrauterine environment for fetal growth and development in the pregnancy complicated by pre-existing diabetes mellitus.
- Poor maternal glycemic control before conception and in the first trimester of pregnancy may be responsible for fetal congenital malformations and maternal complications such as miscarriage, infection, pre-eclampsia, and dystocia (difficult labour) caused by macrosomia.
- Maternal insulin requirements increase as the pregnancy progresses and may quadruple by term as a result of insulin resistance created by placental hormones, insulinase, and cortisol.
- Thyroid dysfunction during pregnancy requires close monitoring of thyroid hormone levels to regulate therapy and prevent fetal insult.
- The stress of the normal maternal adaptations to pregnancy on a heart whose functions are already taxed may cause cardiac decompensation.
- In the case of cardiac arrest in a pregnant woman, the advanced cardiac life support (ACLS) guidelines should be implemented without modification.
- Anemia, the most common medical disorder of pregnancy, affects at least 20% of pregnant women.
- Women in their reproductive years show a predilection for autoimmune disorders (e.g., systemic lupus erythematosus and myasthenia gravis); therefore, these disorders may occur during pregnancy.
- Obesity in pregnancy is associated with more risk factors and requires increased surveillance.
- Perinatal administration of ART is recommended to decrease perinatal transmission of HIV from mother to child. HIV testing for all pregnant women is critical, and preconception counselling is best practice for women who are HIV positive.
- Women who use substances and are pregnant need a harm reduction care approach, with support from a variety of sources. These supports can come from partners, family, health care providers, and the community. Understanding why women use substances and the barriers to recovery will assist in a woman's success with stabilization and treatment.

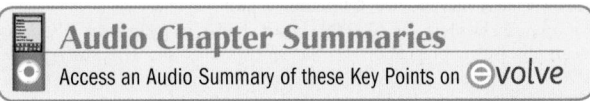

Audio Chapter Summaries

Access an Audio Summary of these Key Points on evolve

References

Allan, W., et al. (2000). Maternal thyroid deficiency and pregnancy complications: Implications for population screening. *Journal of Medical Screening, 7*, 127–130.

Allen, V., et al. (2007). SOGC clinical practice guideline: Teratogenicity associated with pre-existing and gestational diabetes. *Journal of Obstetrics and*

Gynaecology Canada, 29(11), 927–933. Retrieved from http://www.sogc.org/guidelines/documents/guiJOGC200CPG0711.pdf.

American Heart Association. (2010). American Heart Association Guidelines for cardiopulmonary resuscitation and emergency cardiovascular care science. Cardiac arrest in special situations. *Circulation, 112,* S 829–861. Retrieved from http://circ.ahajournals.org/cgi/content/full/122/18_suppl_3/S829.

Aminoff, M. J. (2009). Neurologic disorders. In R. K. Creasy, et al. (Eds.), *Creasy & Resnik's maternal–fetal medicine: Principles and practice* (6th ed.). Philadelphia: Saunders.

Arafeh, J. M., & Baird, S. M. (2006). Cardiac disease in pregnancy. *Critical Care Nursing Quarterly, 29*(1), 32–52.

Audibert, F., et al. (2009). SOGC technical update: Preimplantation genetic testing. *Journal of Obstetrics and Gynaecology Canada, 31*(8), 761–767. Retrieved from http://www.sogc.org/guidelines/documents/gui232TU0908.pdf.

Bernstein, H. (2007). Maternal and perinatal infection—viral. In S. G. Gabbe, J. R. Niebyl, & J. L. Simpson (Eds.), *Obstetrics: Normal and problem pregnancies* (5th ed.). New York: Churchill Livingstone.

Blais, L., & Forget, A. (2008). Asthma exacerbations during the first trimester of pregnancy and the risk of congenital malformations among asthmatic women. *Journal of Allergy and Clinical Immunology, 121*(6), 1379–1384.

Blanchard, D. G., & Shabetai, R. (2009). Cardiac diseases. In R. K. Creasy, et al. (Eds.), *Creasy & Resnik's maternal–fetal medicine: Principles and practice* (6th ed.). Philadelphia: Saunders.

Breton, M., et al. (2010). Risk of perinatal mortality associated with asthma during pregnancy: A 2-stage sampling cohort study. *Annals of Allergy, Asthma and Immunology, 105*(3), 211–217.

Burdge, D. R., et al. (2003). Canadian consensus guidelines for the management of pregnant HIV-positive women and their offspring. *Canadian Medical Association Journal, 168,* 1683–1688.

Burton, J., & Reyes, J. (2001). Breathe in, breathe out. Controlling asthma during pregnancy. *AWHONN Lifelines, 5*(1), 24–30.

Canadian Diabetes Association (CDA). (2008). Clinical practice guidelines for the prevention and management of diabetes in Canada. *Canadian Journal of Diabetes, 32*(Suppl 1), S1–S201.

Cedergren, M. (2004). Maternal morbid obesity and the risk of adverse pregnancy outcome. *Obstetrics and Gynecology, 103*(2), 219–224.

Centers for Disease Control and Prevention. (2007). *Reducing HIV transmission from mother to child: An opt-out approach to HIV screening.* Retrieved from www.cdc.gov/hiv/topics/perinatal/resources/factsheets/pdf/opt-out.pdf.

Chloptsios, C., Karanasiou, V., Ilias, G., Kavouras, N., & Stamatiou, K. (2007). Cholecystitis during pregnancy: A case report and brief review of the literature. *Clinical and Experimental Obstetrics and Gynecology, 34*(4), 250–251.

Clausen, T., Mathiesen, E., & Ekbom, P. (2005). Poor pregnancy outcome in women with type 2 diabetes. *Diabetes Care, 28,* 323–328.

Cooper, D. S., et al. (2007). The thyroid gland. In D. C. Gardner & D. Shoback (Eds.), *Greenspan's basic & clinical endocrinology* (8th ed.). New York: McGraw-Hill.

Criteria Committee of the New York Heart Association. (1994). *Nomenclature and criteria for diagnosis of diseases of the heart and great vessels* (9th ed.). Boston: Little, Brown.

Cunningham, F. G., et al. (2010). *Williams obstetrics* (23rd ed.). New York: McGraw Hill.

Davies, G., & Herbert, W. (2007a). Heart disease in pregnancy 1: Assessment and management of cardiac disease in pregnancy. *Journal of Obstetrics and Gynaecology Canada, 29*(4), 331–336. Retrieved from http://www.sogc.org/jogc/abstracts/full/200704_Obstetrics_2.pdf.

Davies, G., & Herbert, W. (2007b). Heart disease in pregnancy 2: Congenital heart disease in pregnancy. *Journal of Obstetrics and Gynaecology Canada, 29*(5), 409–414. Retrieved from http://www.sogc.org/jogc/abstracts/full/200705_Obstetrics_2.pdf.

Davies, G., & Herbert, W. (2007c). Heart disease in pregnancy 3: Acquired heart disease in pregnancy. *Journal of Obstetrics and Gynaecology Canada, 29*(6), 507–509. Retrieved from http://www.sogc.org/jogc/abstracts/full/200706_Obstetrics_2.pdf.

Davies, G., & Herbert, W. (2007d). Heart disease in pregnancy 4: Ischemic heart disease and cardiomyopathy in pregnancy. *Journal of Obstetrics and Gynaecology Canada, 29*(7), 575–579. Retrieved from http://www.sogc.org/jogc/abstracts/full/200707_Obstetrics_2.pdf.

Davies, G., et al. (2010). SOGC clinical practice guideline: Obesity in pregnancy. *Journal of Obstetrics and Gynaecology Canada, 32*(2), 165–173. Retrieved from http://www.sogc.org/guidelines/documents/gui239ECPG1002.pdf.

Djokanovic, N., Garcia-Bournissend, F., & Koren, G. (2008). Medications for restless legs syndrome in pregnancy. *Journal of Obstetrics and Gynaecology Canada, 30*(6), 505–507.

Easterling, T. R., & Stout, K. (2007). Heart disease. In S. G. Gabbe, J. R. Niebyl, & J. L. Simpson (Eds.), *Obstetrics: Normal and problem pregnancies* (5th ed.). New York: Churchill Livingstone.

Expert Committee on the Diagnosis and Classification of Diabetes Mellitus. (2003). Report of the Expert Committee. *Diabetes Care, 26*(Suppl 1), S5–S20.

Gilbert, E. S. (2007). *Manual of high risk pregnancy and delivery* (4th ed.). St. Louis: Mosby.

Glinoer, D., & Abalovich, M. (2007). Unresolved questions in managing hypothyroidism during pregnancy. *British Medical Journal, 335*(7614), 300–302.

Grewal, M., Biswas, M. K., & Perloff, D. (2003). Cardiac, hematologic, pulmonary, renal and urinary tract disorders in pregnancy. In A. H. DeCherney & L. Nathan (Eds.), *Current obstetric and gynecologic diagnosis and treatment* (9th ed.). New York: Lange Medical Books/McGraw-Hill.

Holmgren, C., & Branch, D. W. (2007). Collagen vascular diseases. In S. G. Gabbe, J. R. Niebyl, & J. L. Simpson (Eds.), *Obstetrics: Normal and problem pregnancies* (5th ed.). New York: Churchill Livingstone.

Inoue, M., Arata, N., Koren, G., & Ito, S. (2009). Hyperthyroidism during pregnancy. *Canadian Family Physician, 55,* 701–703.

Jos, P. H., Perlmutter, M., & Marshall, M. F. (2003). Substance abuse during pregnancy: Clinical and public health approaches. *Journal of Law, Medicine & Ethics, 31*(3), 340–350.

Keenan-Lindsay, L., et al. (2006). SOGC clinical practice guideline: HIV screening in pregnancy. *Journal of Obstetrics and Gynaecology Canada, 28*(12), 1103–1107. Retrieved from http://www.sogc.org/guidelines/documents/185E-CPG-December2006.pdf.

Kilpatrick, S. J. (2009). Anemia and pregnancy. In R. K. Creasy, et al. (Eds.), *Creasy & Resnik's maternal–fetal medicine: Principles and practice* (6th ed.). Philadelphia: Saunders.

Kissin, W. B., et al. (2004). Identifying pregnant women at risk for early attrition from substance abuse treatment. *Journal of Substance Abuse Treatment, 27,* 31–38.

Koren, G., Sarkar, M., & Einarson, A. (2010). The use of Montelukast in pregnancy. *Canadian Family Physician, 56,* 881–882.

Landon, M. B., Catalano, P. M., & Gabbe, S. G. (2007). Diabetes mellitus. In S. G. Gabbe, J. R. Niebyl, & J. L. Simpson (Eds.), *Obstetrics: Normal and problem pregnancies* (5th ed.). New York: Churchill Livingstone.

Langer, O., & Conway, D. (2000). Levels of glycemia and perinatal outcomes in pregestational diabetes. *Journal of Maternal-Fetal Medicine, 9,* 35–41.

Langlois, S., Ford, J., & Chitayat, D. (2008). SOGC clinical practice guideline: Carrier screening for thalassemia and hemoglobinopathies in Canada. *Journal of Obstetrics and Gynaecology Canada, 28*(4), 324–332. Retrieved from http://www.sogc.org/jogc/abstracts/200604_SOGCClinicalPracticeGuidelines_1.pdf.

Lawrence, R. A., & Lawrence, R. M. (2011). *Breastfeeding: A guide for the medical profession* (7th ed.). St. Louis: Mosby.

Liston, R., et al. (2007). SOGC clinical practice guideline: Fetal health surveillance: Antepartum and intrapartum consensus guideline. *Journal of Obstetrics and Gynaecology Canada, 29*(9), Suppl 4. Retrieved from http://www.sogc.org/guidelines/documents/gui197CPG0709r.pdf.

Madappa, T., & Sharma, S. (2010). Pulmonary disease and pregnancy. *eMedicine Pulmonology.* Retrieved from http://emedicine.medscape.com/article/303853-print.

Maloni, J. A., Brezinski-Tomasi, J. E., & Johnson, L. A. (2001). Antepartum bed rest: Effect upon the family. *Journal of Obstetric, Gynecologic & Neonatal Nursing, 30*(2), 67–77.

Manconi, M., et al. (2004). Pregnancy as a risk factor for restless legs syndrome. *Sleep Medicine, 5*(3), 305–308.

Mestman, J. H. (2007). Endocrine diseases in pregnancy. In S. G. Gabbe, J. R. Niebyl, & J. L. Simpson (Eds.), *Obstetrics: Normal and problem pregnancies* (5th ed.). New York: Churchill Livingstone.

Morrow, J., et al. (2006). Malformation risks of antiepileptic drugs in pregnancy: A prospective study from the UK Epilepsy and Pregnancy Register. *Journal of Neurology, Neurosurgery, and Psychiatry, 77*(2), 193–198.

Nader, S. (2009). Thyroid disease and pregnancy. In R. K. Creasy, et al. (Eds.), *Creasy & Resnik's maternal–fetal medicine: Principles and practice* (6th ed.). Philadelphia: Saunders.

National Asthma Education and Prevention Program (NAEPP) Working Group. (2004). *NAEPP Working Group report on managing asthma during pregnancy. Recommendations for pharmacologic treatment—2004 update* (NIH Publication No. 05-3279). Bethesda, MD: National Heart, Lung, and Blood

Institute. Retrieved from http://www.nhlbi.nih.gov/health/prof/lung/asthma/astpreg/astpreg_qr.pdf.

Nava-Campo, A., Soldin, A., & Koren, G. (2004). Hypothyroidism during pregnancy. *Canadian Family Physician, 50*, 549–551.

Papoutsis, J., & Kroumpouzos, G. (2007). Dermatologic disorders. In S. G. Gabbe, J. R. Niebyl, & J. L. Simpson (Eds.), *Obstetrics: Normal and problem pregnancies* (5th ed.). New York: Churchill Livingstone.

Poole, N., & Greaves, L. (2007). *Highs and lows: Canadian perspectives on women and substance use*. Toronto: Centre for Addiction and Mental Health.

Poppe, K., Velkeniers, B., & Glinoer, D. (2007). Thyroid disease and female reproduction. *Clinical Endocrinology, 66*, 309–321.

Ramsey, P. S., Ramin, K. D., & Ramin, S. M. (2001). Cardiac disease in pregnancy. *American Journal of Perinatology, 18*(5), 245–266.

Reece, E. A., & Homko, C. J. (2007). Prepregnancy care and the prevention of fetal malformations in the pregnancy complicated by diabetes. *Clinics in Obstetrics and Gynecology, 50*(4), 990–997.

Schaefer-Graf, U., Buchanan, T., Xiang, A., & Kjos, S. (2002). Clinical predictors for a high risk for the development of diabetes mellitus in the early puerperium in women with recent gestational diabetes mellitus. *American Journal of Obstetrics and Gynecology, 186*, 751–756.

Shrim, A., Garcia-Bournissen, F., Koren, G., & Farine, D. (2007). When pregnant women are not screened for HIV. *Canadian Family Physician, 53*, 1653–1655.

Slack, C., et al. (2006). Prenatal genetics: The evolution and future directions of screening and diagnosis. *Journal of Perinatal & Neonatal Nursing, 20*(1), 93–97.

Statistics Canada. (2011). *Health trends* (Statistics Canada Catalogue No. 82-213-XWE). Ottawa: Author. Retrieved from http://www12.statcan.gc.ca/health-sante/82-213/index.cfm?Lang=ENG.

Sun, H., et al. (2009). Gender and metabolic differences of gallstone diseases. *World Journal of Gastroenterology, 15*(15), 1886–1891.

Walters, M., & Taylor, J. (Dec, 2009/Jan 2010). Maternal obesity: Consequences and prevention strategies. *Nursing for Women's Health, 13*(6), 486–494.

Weiss, J. L., et al. (2004). FASTER Research Consortium. Obesity, obstetric complications and cesarean delivery rate—a population-based screening study. *American Journal of Obstetrics and Gynecology, 190*, 1091–1097.

Whitty, J. E., & Dombrowski, M. P. (2009). Respiratory diseases in pregnancy. In R. K. Creasy, et al. (Eds.), *Creasy & Resnik's maternal–fetal medicine: Principles and practice* (6th ed.). Philadelphia: Saunders.

Williamson, C., & Mackillop, L. (2009). Diseases of the liver, biliary system, and pancreas. In R. K. Creasy, et al. (Eds.), *Creasy & Resnik's maternal–fetal medicine: Principles and practice* (6th ed.). Philadelphia: Saunders.

Wilson, R. D., et al. (2002). SOGC Committee opinion: Cystic fibrosis carrier testing in pregnancy in Canada. *Journal of Obstetrics and Gynaecology Canada, 24*(8), 644–647. Retrieved from http://www.sogc.org/guidelines/public/118E-CO-August2002.pdf.

Wilson, W., et al. (2007). Prevention of infective endocarditis: Guidelines from the American Heart Association. *Circulation, 116*, 1736–1754.

Wisner, K. L., et al. (2007). Psychiatric disorders. In S. G. Gabbe, J. R. Niebyl, & J. L. Simpson (Eds.), *Obstetrics: Normal and problem pregnancies* (5th ed.). New York: Churchill Livingstone.

Zhang, J., Bricker, L., Wray, S., & Quenby, S. (2007). Poor uterine contractility in obese women. *British Journal of Obstetrics and Gynaecology, 114*, 343–348.

Zucconi, M., & Ferini-Strambi, L. (2004). Epidemiology and clinical findings of restless legs syndrome. *Sleep Medicine, 5*(3), 293–299.

Unit 4

15 Labour and Birth Processes

Learning Objectives

On completion of this chapter, the reader will be able to:

- Explain five factors that affect the labour process.
- Describe the anatomic structure of the bony pelvis.
- Recognize the normal measurements of the diameters of the pelvic inlet, cavity, and outlet.
- Explain the significance of the size and position of the fetal head during labour and birth.
- Summarize the cardinal movements of labour for a vertex presentation.
- Assess the maternal anatomical and physiological adaptations to labour.
- Describe fetal adaptations to labour.

Electronic Resources

Additional information related to the content in Chapter 15 can be found on

evolve the Companion Web site at

http://evolve.elsevier.com/Canada/Perry/maternal/

- Anatomy Review—Sutures and Fontanels
- Assessment Video Clips
- Examination Review Questions
- Critical Thinking Exercise—Fetal Presentation

During late pregnancy, the woman, her family, and the fetus prepare for the labour process. The fetus has grown and developed in preparation for extrauterine life. The woman has undergone various physiological adaptations during pregnancy that prepare her for birth and motherhood. Labour and birth represent the end of pregnancy, the beginning of extrauterine life for the newborn, and a change in the lives of the family members. This chapter discusses the factors affecting labour, the processes involved, the normal progression of events, and the adaptations made by both the woman and fetus.

Factors Affecting Labour

At least five factors affect the process of labour and birth. These are easily remembered as the five P's: passenger (fetus and placenta), passageway (birth canal), powers (contractions), **position** of the mother, and psychological response. The first four factors are presented here as the basis of understanding the physiological process of labour. The fifth factor is discussed in Chapter 18. Other factors that may be a part of the woman's labour experience may be important as well. VandeVusse (1999) identified external forces, including place of birth, preparation, type of provider (especially nurses), and procedures. Physiology (sensations) was identified as an internal force. These factors are discussed generally in Chapter 18 as they relate to nursing care during labour.

Passenger

The movement of the passenger, or fetus, through the birth canal is determined by several interacting factors: the size of the fetal head, fetal **presentation,** fetal **lie,** fetal attitude, and fetal position. Because the placenta also must pass through the birth canal, it can be considered a passenger along with the fetus; however, the placenta rarely impedes the process of labour in normal vaginal birth. An exception is the case of placenta previa (see Chapter 13).

Size of the Fetal Head

Because of its size and relative rigidity, the fetal head has a major effect on the birth process. The fetal skull is composed of two parietal bones, two temporal bones, the frontal bone, and the occipital bone (Fig. 15-1, A). These bones are united by membranous sutures: the sagittal, lambdoidal, coronal, and frontal (see Fig. 15-1, B). Membrane-filled spaces called *fontanels* are located where the sutures intersect. During labour, after the rupture of the membranes, palpation of the fontanels and sutures during vaginal examination reveals fetal presentation, position, and attitude.

The two most important fontanels are the anterior and posterior (see Fig. 15-1, B). The larger of these, the anterior fontanel, is diamond shaped, about 3 cm × 2 cm, and lies at the junction of the sagittal, coronal, and frontal sutures. It closes by 18 months after birth. The posterior fontanel lies at the junction of the sutures of the two parietal bones and the one occipital bone, is triangular, and is about 1 cm × 2 cm. It closes 6 to 8 weeks after birth.

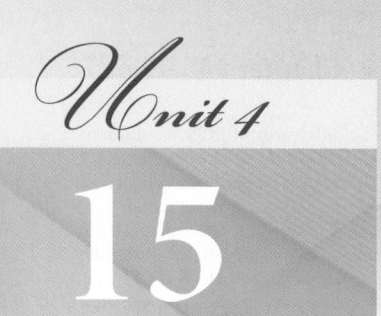

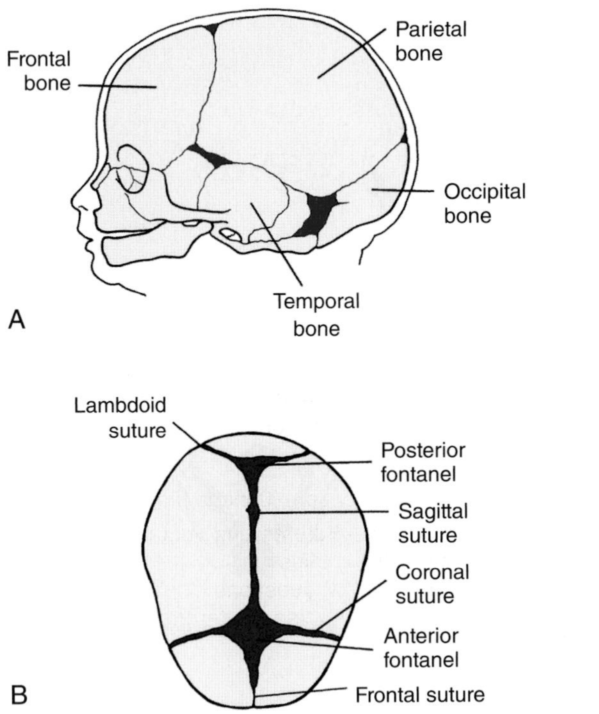

Fig. 15-1 Fetal head at term. **A:** Bones. **B:** Sutures and fontanels.

Sutures and fontanels make the skull flexible to accommodate the infant brain, which continues to grow for some time after birth. However, because the bones are not firmly united, slight overlapping of the bones, or moulding of the shape of the head, occurs during labour. This capacity of the bones to slide over one another also permits adaptation to the various diameters of the maternal pelvis. Moulding can be extensive, but the heads of most newborns assume their normal shape within 3 days after birth.

Although the size of the fetal shoulders may affect passage, their position can be altered relatively easily during labour so that one shoulder may occupy a lower level than the other. This creates a shoulder diameter that is smaller than the skull, facilitating passage through the birth canal. The circumference of the fetal hips is usually small enough not to create problems.

Fetal Presentation

Presentation refers to the part of the fetus that enters the pelvic inlet first and leads through the birth canal during labour at term. The three main presentations are *cephalic* (head first), occurring in 96% of births (Fig. 15-2); *breech* (buttocks or feet first), occurring in 3% of births (Fig. 15-3, A–C); and shoulder, seen in 1% of births (see Fig. 15-3, D). *Presenting part* refers to that part of the fetal body first felt by the examining finger during a vaginal examination. In a cephalic presentation, the presenting part is usually the occiput; in a breech presentation it is the sacrum; in the shoulder presentation it is the scapula. When the presenting part is the occiput, the presentation is noted as vertex (see Fig. 15-2). Factors that determine the presenting part include fetal lie, fetal attitude, and extension or flexion of the fetal head.

Fetal Lie

Lie is the relation of the long axis (spine) of the fetus to the long axis (spine) of the mother. The two primary lies are longitudinal, or vertical, in which the long axis of the fetus is parallel with the long axis of the mother (see Fig. 15-2); and transverse, horizontal, or oblique, in which the long axis of the fetus is at a right angle diagonal to the long axis of the mother (see Fig. 15-3, D). Longitudinal lies are either cephalic or breech presentations, depending on the fetal structure that first enters the mother's pelvis. Vaginal birth cannot occur when the fetus stays in a transverse lie. An oblique lie, one in which the long axis of the fetus is lying at an angle to the long axis of the mother, is less common and usually converts to a longitudinal or transverse lie during labour (Cunningham et al., 2010).

Fetal Attitude

Attitude is the relation of the fetal body parts to one another. The fetus assumes a characteristic posture (attitude) in utero partly because of the mode of fetal growth and partly because of the way the fetus conforms to the shape of the uterine cavity. Normally, the back of the fetus is rounded so that the chin is flexed on the chest, the thighs are flexed on the abdomen, and the legs are flexed at the knees. The arms are crossed over the thorax, and the umbilical cord lies between the arms and the legs. This attitude is termed *general flexion* (see Fig. 15-2).

Deviations from the normal attitude may cause challenges for the labour and birth process. For example, in a cephalic presentation, the fetal head may be extended or flexed in a manner that presents a head diameter that exceeds the limits of the maternal pelvis, leading to prolonged labour, forceps- or vacuum-assisted birth, or Caesarean birth (see Fig. 15-5, B and C).

Certain critical diameters of the fetal head are usually measured. The biparietal diameter, which is about 9.25 cm at term, is the largest transverse diameter and an important indicator of fetal head size (Fig. 15-4, B). In a well-flexed cephalic presentation, the biparietal diameter is the widest part of the head entering the pelvic inlet. Of the several anteroposterior diameters, the smallest and the most critical one is the suboccipitobregmatic diameter (about 9.5 cm at term). When the head is in complete flexion, this diameter allows the fetal head to pass through the true pelvis easily (Fig. 15-5, A). As the head is more extended, the anteroposterior diameter widens, and the head may not be able to enter the true pelvis (see Fig. 15-5, B and C).

evolve Critical Thinking Exercise–Fetal Presentation

Fetal Position

The presentation or presenting part indicates the portion of the fetus that overlies the pelvic inlet. *Position* is the relation of the presenting part (occiput, sacrum, mentum [chin], or sinciput [deflexed vertex]) to the four quadrants of the mother's pelvis (see Fig. 15-2). Position is denoted by a three-letter abbreviation. The first letter of the abbreviation denotes the location of the presenting part in the right (R) or left (L) side of the mother's pelvis. The middle letter stands for the specific presenting part of the fetus (O for occiput, S for sacrum, M for mentum [chin], and Sc for scapula [shoulder]).

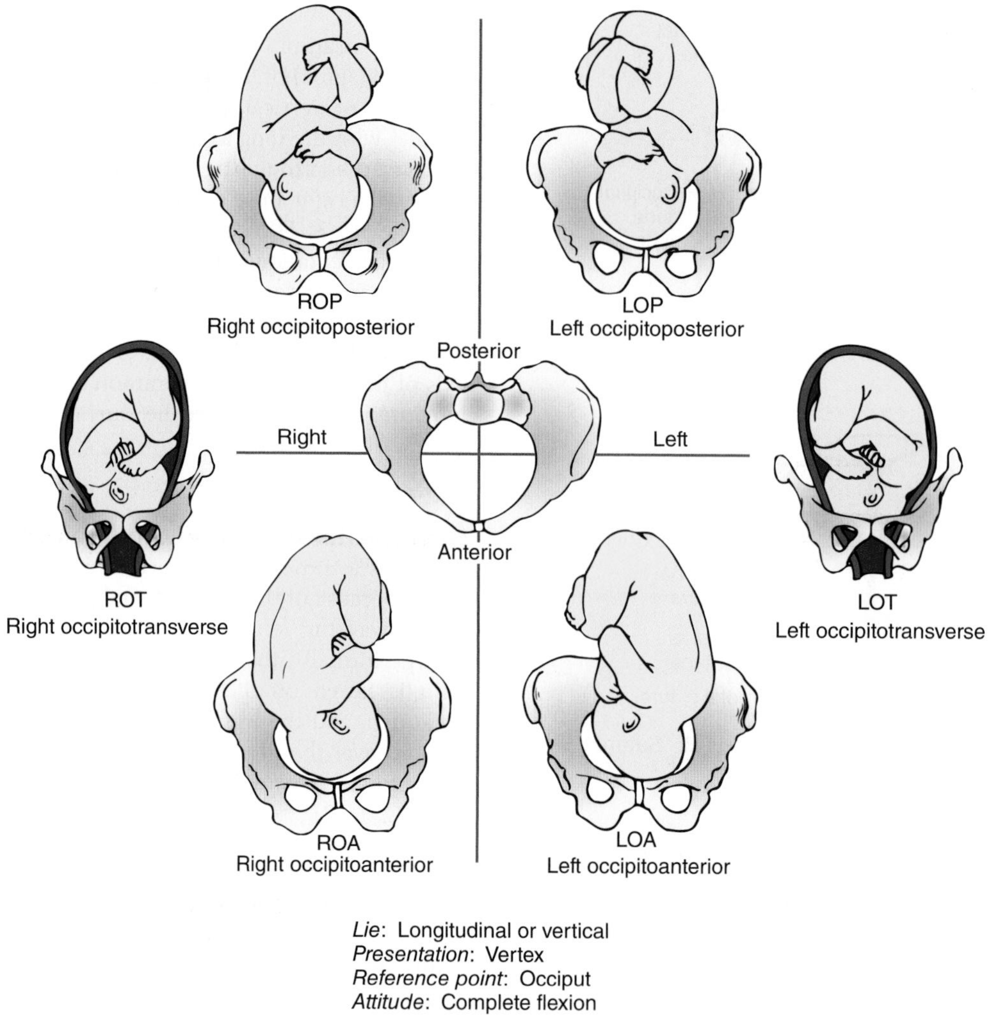

Fig. 15-2 Examples of fetal vertex (occiput) presentations in relation to front, back, or side of the maternal pelvis.

The third letter stands for the location of the presenting part in relation to the anterior (A), posterior (P), or transverse (T) portion of the maternal pelvis. For example, ROA means that the occiput is the presenting part and is located in the right anterior quadrant of the maternal pelvis (see Fig. 15-2). LSP means that the sacrum is the presenting part and is located in the left posterior quadrant of the maternal pelvis (see Fig. 15-3).

Station is the relation of the presenting part of the fetus to an imaginary line drawn between the maternal ischial spines and is a measure of the degree of descent of the presenting part of the fetus through the birth canal. The placement of the presenting part is measured in centimetres above or below the ischial spines (Fig. 15-6). For example, when the lowermost portion of the presenting part is 1 cm above the spines, it is noted as being minus (−) 1. At the level of the spines, the station is referred to as 0 (zero). When the presenting part is 1 cm below the spines, the station is said to be plus (+) 1. Birth is imminent when the presenting part is at +4 to +5 cm. The station of the presenting part should be determined when labour begins so that the rate of descent of the fetus during labour can be accurately determined.

Engagement is the term used to indicate that the largest transverse diameter of the presenting part (usually the biparietal diameter) has passed through the maternal pelvic brim or inlet into the true pelvis and usually corresponds to station 0. Engagement often occurs in the weeks just before labour begins in nulliparas and may occur before or during labour in multiparas. Engagement can be determined by abdominal or vaginal examination.

Passageway

The *passageway*, or birth canal, is composed of the mother's rigid bony pelvis and the soft tissues of the cervix, pelvic floor, vagina, and introitus (the external opening to the vagina). Although the soft tissues, particularly the muscular layers of the pelvic floor, contribute to vaginal birth of the fetus, the maternal pelvis plays a far greater role in the labour process because the fetus must successfully accommodate itself to this relatively rigid passageway.

Bony Pelvis

The anatomy of the bony pelvis is described in Chapter 5. The following discussion focuses on the importance of pelvic

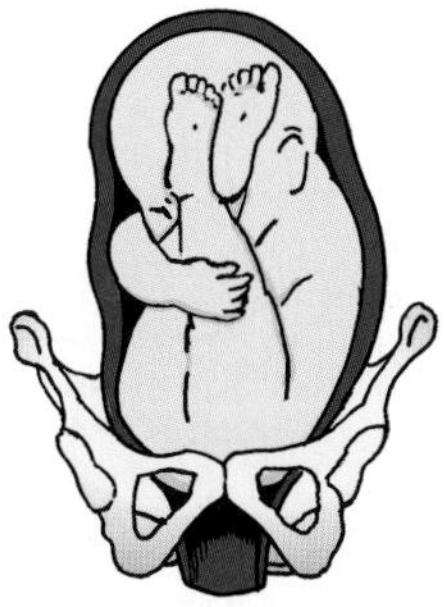

Frank breech

Lie: Longitudinal or vertical
Presentation: Breech (incomplete)
Presenting part: Sacrum
Attitude: Flexion, except for legs at knees

A

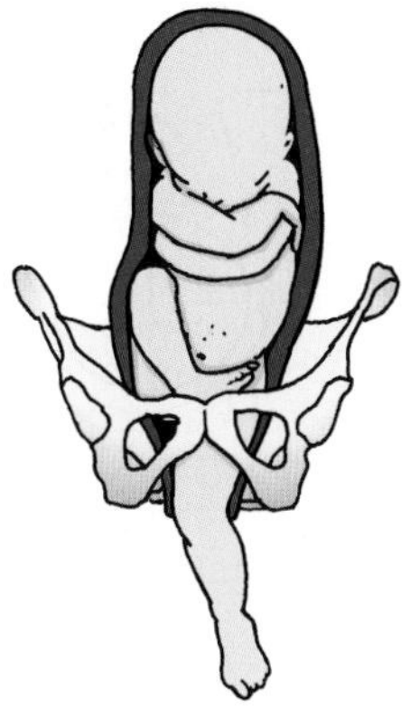

Single footling breech

Lie: Longitudinal or vertical
Presentation: Breech (incomplete)
Presenting part: Sacrum
Attitude: Flexion, except for one leg extended at hip and knee

B

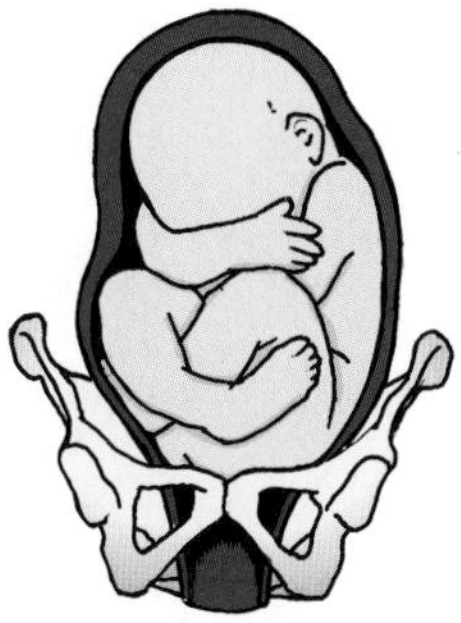

Complete breech

Lie: Longitudinal or vertical
Presentation: Breech (sacrum and feet presenting)
Presenting part: Sacrum (with feet)
Attitude: General flexion

C

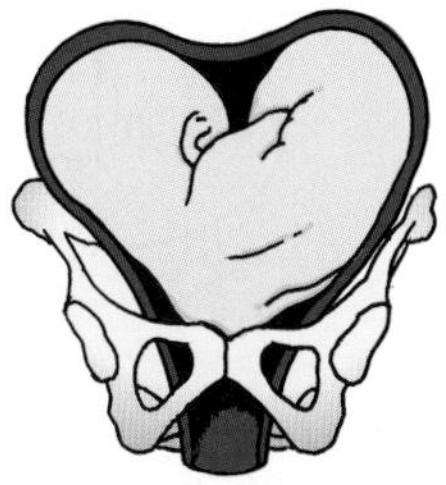

Shoulder presentation

Lie: Transverse or horizontal
Presentation: Shoulder
Presenting part: Scapula
Attitude: Flexion

D

Fig. 15-3 Fetal presentations. **A** to **C:** Breech (sacral) presentation. **D:** Shoulder presentation.

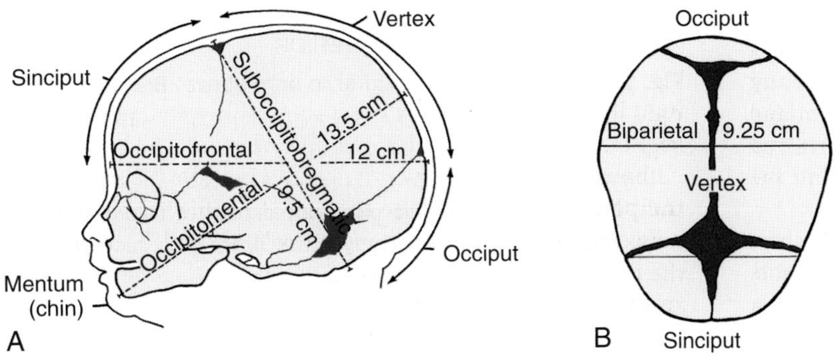

Fig. 15-4 Diameters of the fetal head at term. **A:** Cephalic presentations: occiput, vertex, and sinciput; and cephalic diameters: suboccipitobregmatic, occipitofrontal, and occipitomental. **B:** Biparietal diameter.

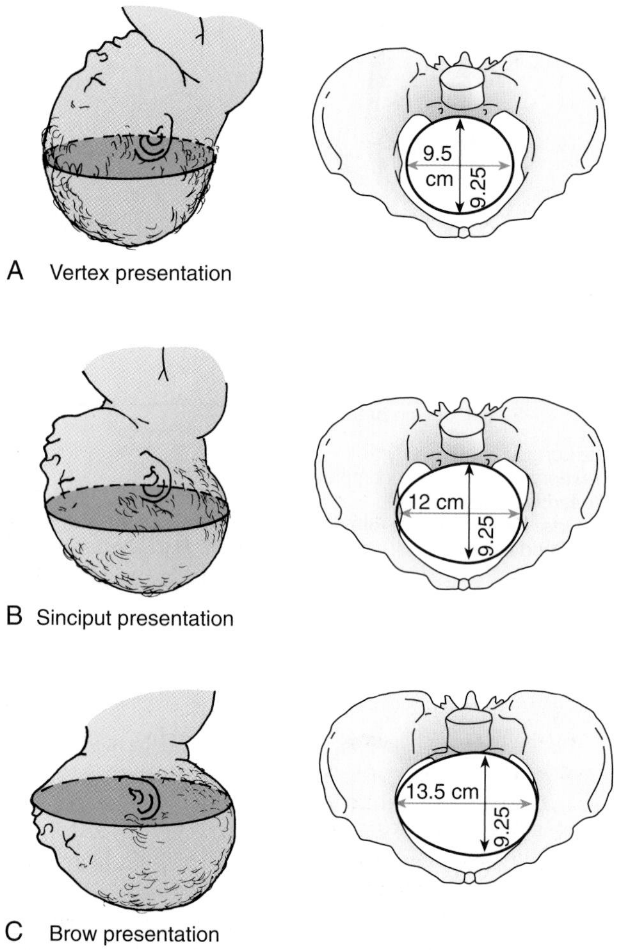

Fig. 15-5 Head entering pelvis. Biparietal diameter is indicated with shading (9.25 cm). **A:** Suboccipitobregmatic diameter: complete flexion of head on chest so that smallest diameter enters. **B:** Occipitofrontal diameter: moderate extension (military attitude) so that large diameter enters. **C:** Occipitomental diameter: marked extension (deflection) so that the largest diameter, which is too large to permit head to enter pelvis, is presenting.

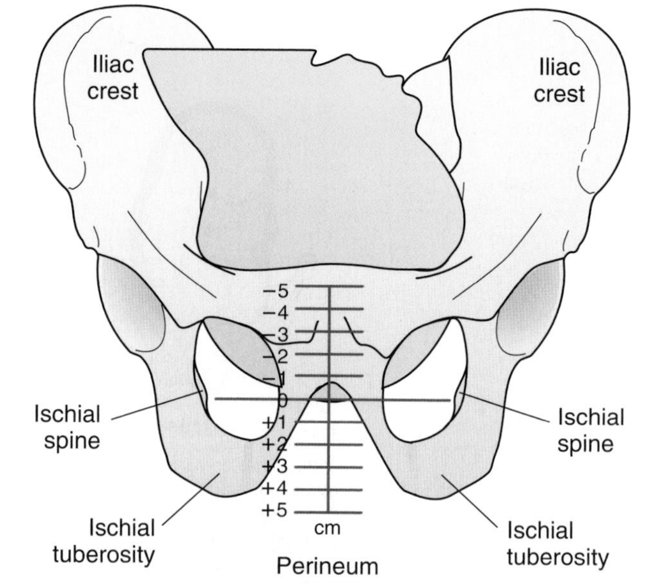

Fig. 15-6 Stations of presenting part, or degree of descent. The lowermost portion of the presenting part is at the level of the ischial spines, station 0.

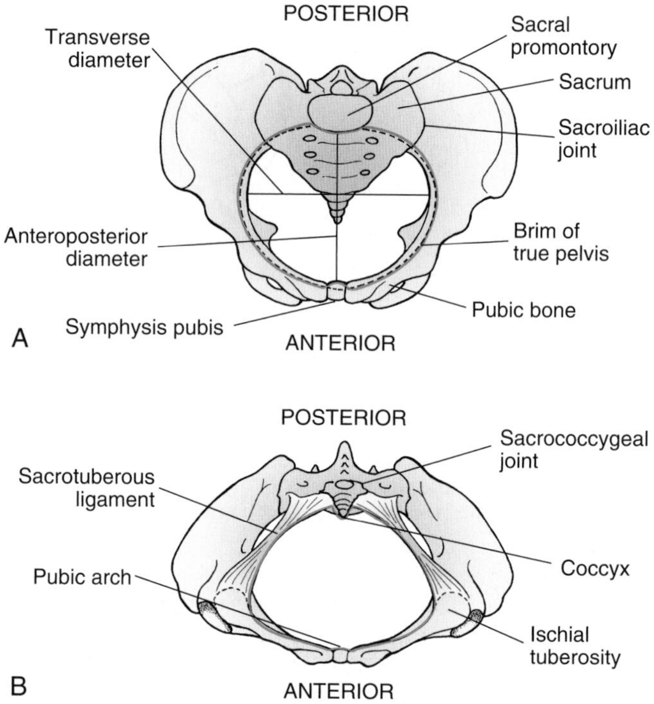

Fig. 15-7 Female pelvis. **A:** Pelvic brim above. **B:** Pelvic outlet from below.

configurations as they relate to the labour process. (It may be helpful to refer to Figs. 5-5 and 5-6.)

The *bony pelvis* is formed by the fusion of the ilium, ischium, pubis, and sacral bones. The four pelvic joints are the symphysis pubis, the right and left sacroiliac joints, and the sacrococcygeal joint (Fig. 15-7, B). The bony pelvis is separated by the brim, or inlet, into two parts: the false pelvis and the true pelvis. The *false pelvis* is the part above the brim and plays no part in childbearing. The *true pelvis*, the part involved in birth, is divided into three planes: the inlet, or brim; the midpelvis, or cavity; and the outlet.

The *pelvic inlet*, which is the upper border of the true pelvis, is formed anteriorly by the upper margins of the pubic bone, laterally by the iliopectineal lines along the innominate bones, and posteriorly by the anterior, upper margin of the sacrum and the sacral promontory.

The *pelvic cavity*, or midpelvis, is a curved passage with a short anterior wall and a much longer concave posterior wall. It is bounded by the posterior aspect of the symphysis pubis, the ischium, a portion of the ilium, the sacrum, and the coccyx.

The *pelvic outlet* is the lower border of the true pelvis. Viewed from below, it is ovoid; somewhat diamond shaped; and bounded by the pubic arch anteriorly, the ischial tuberosities laterally, and the tip of the coccyx posteriorly (see Fig. 15-7, B). In the latter part of pregnancy, the coccyx is movable

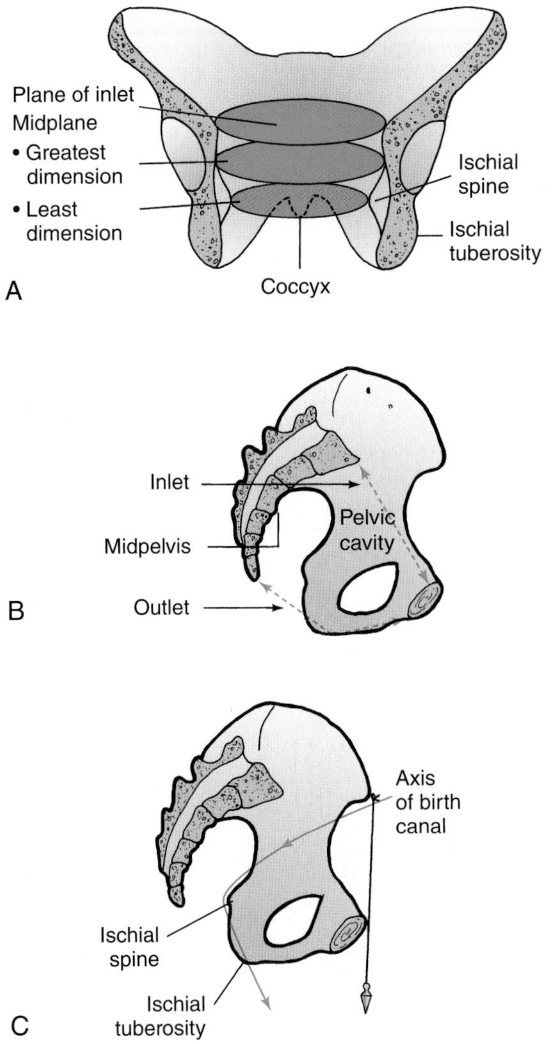

Fig. 15-8 Pelvic cavity. **A:** Inlet and midplane. Outlet not shown. **B:** Cavity of true pelvis. **C:** Note curve of sacrum and axis of birth canal.

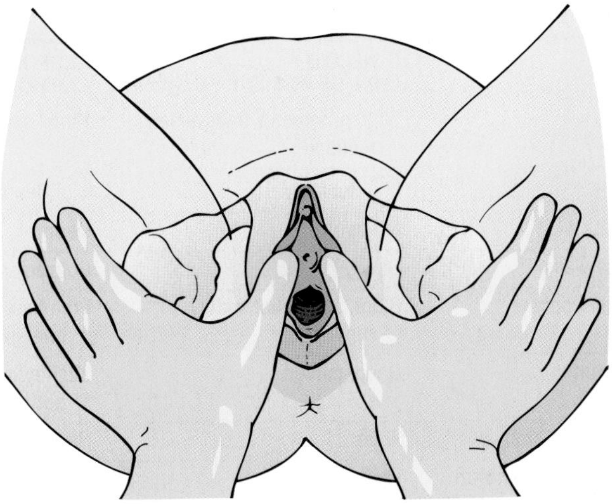

Fig. 15-9 Estimation of angle of subpubic arch. With both thumbs, examiner externally traces descending rami down to tuberosities. *(Redrawn from Barkauskas, V. H., Baumann, L. C., & Darling-Fisher, C. S. [2002].* Health and physical assessment *[3rd ed. p. 607]. St. Louis: Mosby.)*

(unless it has been broken in a fall and has fused to the sacrum during healing).

The pelvic cavity varies in size and shape at various levels. The diameters at the plane of the pelvic inlet, midpelvis, and outlet, plus the axis of the birth canal (Fig. 15-8), determine whether vaginal birth is possible and the manner by which the fetus may pass down the birth canal.

The subpubic angle, which determines the type of pubic arch, together with the length of the pubic rami and the intertuberous diameter, is of great importance. Because the fetus must first pass beneath the pubic arch, a narrow subpubic angle is less accommodating than a rounded wide arch. The method of measuring the subpubic arch is shown in Figure 15-9.

The four basic types of pelves are classified as follows:

1. Gynecoid (the classic female type)
2. Android (resembling the male pelvis)
3. Anthropoid (resembling the pelvis of anthropoid apes)
4. Platypelloid (the flat pelvis)

The gynecoid pelvis is the most common, with major gynecoid pelvic features present in 50% of all women. Anthropoid and android features are less common, and platypelloid pelvic features are the least common. Mixed types of pelves are more common than are pure types (Cunningham et al., 2010). Examples of pelvic variations and their effects on the mode of birth are given in Table 15-1.

Assessment of the bony pelvis can be performed during the first prenatal evaluation by the physician or midwife and need not be repeated if the pelvis is of adequate size and suitable shape. In the third trimester of pregnancy, the examination of the bony pelvis may be more thorough and the results more accurate because there is relaxation and increased mobility of the pelvic joints and ligaments as a result of hormonal influences. Widening of the joint of the symphysis pubis and the resulting instability may cause pain in any or all of the pelvic joints.

Because the examiner does not have direct access to the bony structures and because the bones are covered with varying amounts of soft tissue, estimates of size and shape are approximate. Precise bony pelvis measurements can be determined by use of computed tomography, ultrasonography, or x-ray films. However, radiographic examination is rarely done during pregnancy because of potential damage to the developing fetus.

Soft Tissues

The soft tissues of the passageway include the distensible lower uterine segment, cervix, pelvic floor muscles, vagina, and introitus. Before labour begins, the uterus is composed of the uterine body (corpus) and cervix (neck). After labour has begun, uterine contractions cause the uterine body to have a thick and muscular upper segment and a thin-walled, passive, muscular lower segment. A physiological retraction ring separates the two segments (Fig. 15-10). The lower uterine segment gradually distends to accommodate the intrauterine contents

Table 15-1 Comparison of Pelvic Types

	GYNECOID (50% OF WOMEN)	ANDROID (23% OF WOMEN)	ANTHROPOID (24% OF WOMEN)	PLATYPELLOID (3% OF WOMEN)
Brim	Slightly ovoid or transversely rounded	Heart shaped, angulated	Oval, wider anteroposteriorly	Flattened anteroposteriorly, wide transversely
	Round	Heart	Oval	Flat
Depth	Moderate	Deep	Deep	Shallow
Side walls	Straight	Convergent	Straight	Straight
Ischial spines	Blunt, somewhat widely separated	Prominent, narrow interspinous diameter	Prominent, often with narrow interspinous diameter	Blunt, widely separated
Sacrum	Deep, curved	Slightly curved, terminal portion often beaked	Slightly curved	Slightly curved
Subpubic arch	Wide	Narrow	Narrow	Wide
Usual mode of birth	Vaginal Spontaneous Occipitoanterior position	Caesarean Vaginal Difficult with forceps	Forceps/spontaneous Occipitoposterior or occipitoanterior position	Vaginal Spontaneous

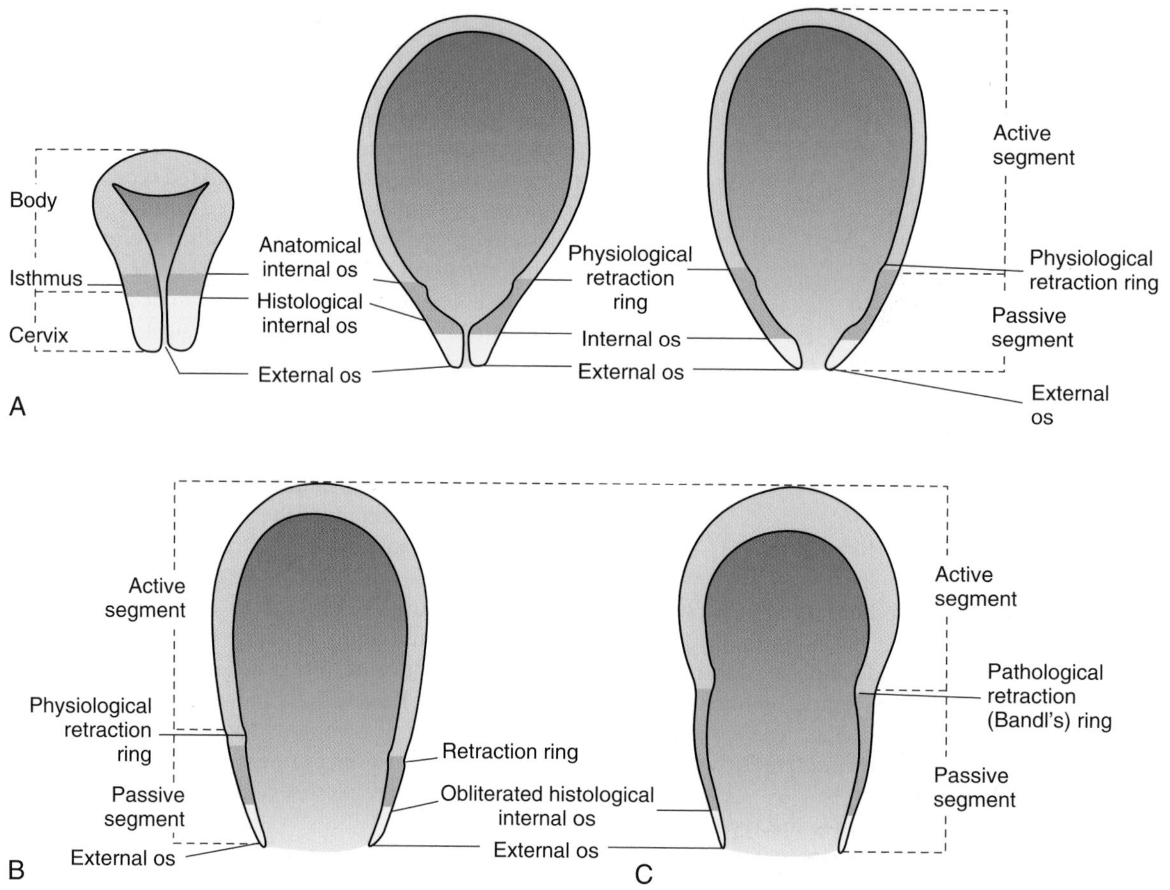

Fig. 15-10 Uterus in normal labour. **A:** In early first stage. **B:** In second stage. Passive segment is derived from lower uterine segment (isthmus) and cervix, and physiological retraction ring is derived from anatomical internal os. **C:** Uterus in abnormal labour in second-stage dystocia. Pathological retraction (Bandl's) ring that forms under abnormal conditions develops from the physiological ring.

as the wall of the upper segment thickens and its accommodating capacity is reduced. The contractions of the uterine body thus exert downward pressure on the fetus, pushing it against the cervix.

The cervix effaces (thins) and dilates (opens) sufficiently to allow the first fetal portion to descend into the vagina. As the fetus descends, the cervix is actually drawn upward and over this first portion.

The *pelvic floor* is a muscular layer that separates the pelvic cavity above from the perineal space below. This structure helps the fetus rotate anteriorly as it passes through the birth canal. As noted earlier, the soft tissues of the vagina develop throughout pregnancy until at term the vagina can dilate to accommodate the fetus and facilitate the birth of the fetus.

Powers

Involuntary and voluntary powers combine to expel the fetus and the placenta from the uterus. Involuntary uterine contractions, called the *primary powers*, signal the beginning of labour. Once the cervix has dilated, voluntary bearing-down efforts by the woman, called the *secondary powers*, augment the force of the involuntary contractions.

Primary Powers

The involuntary contractions originate at certain pacemaker points in the thickened muscle layers of the upper uterine segment. From the pacemaker points contractions move downward over the uterus in waves, separated by short rest periods. Terms used to describe these involuntary contractions include *frequency* (the time from the beginning of one contraction to the beginning of the next), *duration* (length of contraction), and *intensity* (strength of contraction).

The primary powers are responsible for the **effacement** and dilation of the cervix and descent of the fetus. *Effacement* of the cervix means the shortening and thinning of the cervix during the first stage of labour. The cervix, normally 2 to 3 cm long and about 1 cm thick, is obliterated or "taken up" by a shortening of the uterine muscle bundles during the thinning of the lower uterine segment that occurs in advancing labour. Only a thin edge of the cervix can be palpated when effacement is complete. Effacement generally is advanced in first-time term pregnancy before more than slight dilation occurs. In subsequent pregnancies, effacement and dilation of the cervix tend to progress together. The degree of effacement is expressed in percentages, from 0 to 100% (e.g., a cervix is 50% effaced) or in length in centimetres (Fig. 15-11, A to C).

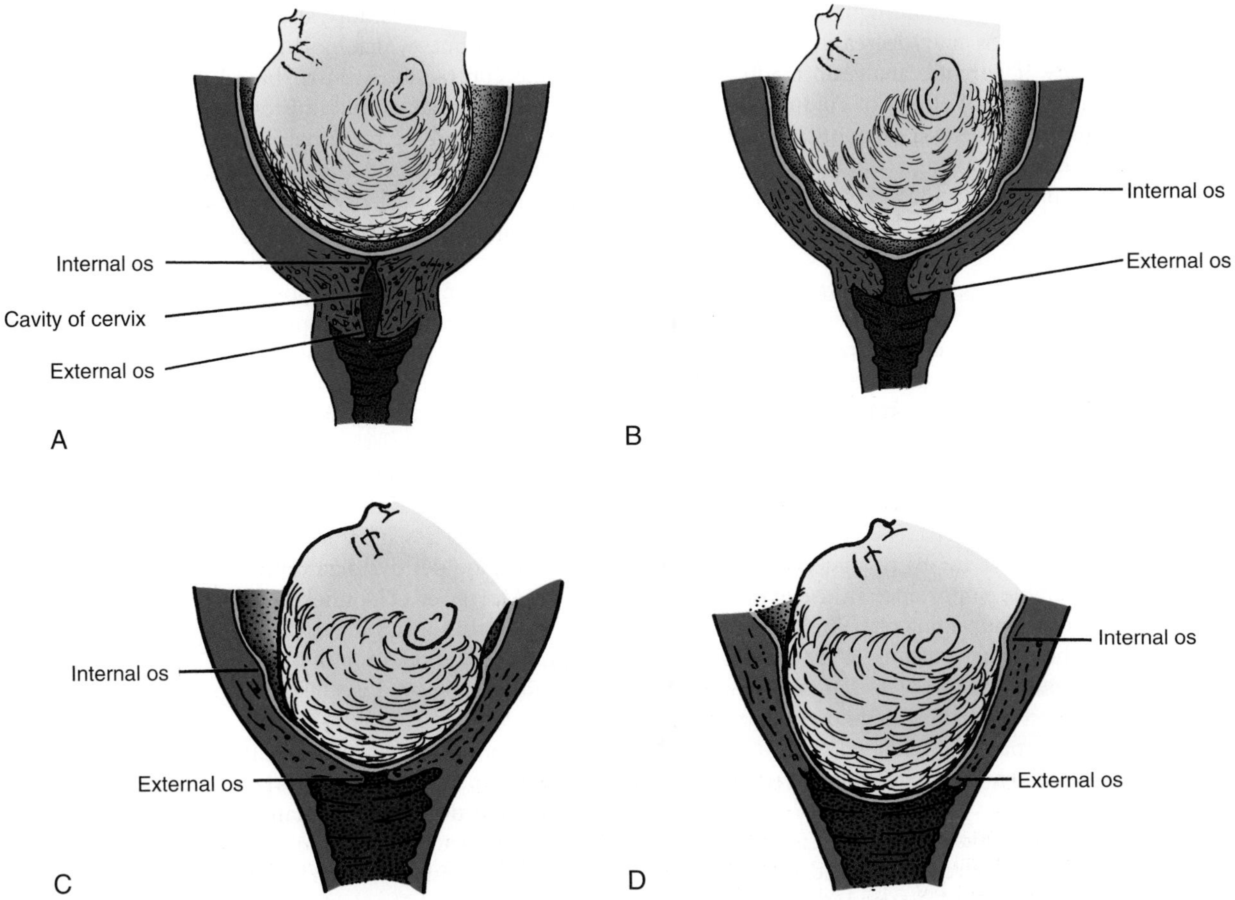

Fig. 15-11 Cervical effacement and dilation. Note how cervix is drawn up around presenting part (internal os). Membranes are intact, and head is not well applied to cervix. **A:** Before labour. **B:** Early effacement. **C:** Complete effacement (100%). Head is well applied to cervix. **D:** Complete dilation (10 cm). Cranial bones overlap somewhat, and membranes are still intact.

Dilation of the cervix is the enlargement or widening of the cervical opening and the cervical canal that occurs once labour has begun. The diameter of the cervix increases from less than 1 cm to full dilation (approximately 10 cm) to allow birth of a term fetus. When the cervix is fully effaced and dilated (and completely retracted), it can no longer be palpated (see Fig. 15-11, D). Full cervical dilation marks the end of the first stage of labour.

Dilation of the cervix occurs by the drawing upward of the musculofibrous components of the cervix, caused by strong uterine contractions. Pressure exerted by the amniotic fluid while the membranes are intact or by the force applied by the presenting part can promote cervical dilation. Scarring of the cervix as a result of prior infection or surgery may slow cervical dilation.

In the first and second stages of labour, increased intrauterine pressure caused by contractions exerts pressure on the descending fetus and the cervix. When the presenting part of the fetus reaches the perineal floor, mechanical stretching of the cervix occurs. Stretch receptors in the posterior vagina cause the release of endogenous oxytocin that triggers the maternal urge to bear down, or the Ferguson reflex.

Uterine contractions are usually independent of external forces. For example, labouring women who are paralyzed because of spinal cord lesions above T-12 have normal but painless uterine contractions (Cunningham et al., 2010). However, uterine contractions may decrease temporarily in frequency and intensity if narcotic analgesic medication is given early in labour. Studies of effects of epidural analgesia have demonstrated prolonged length of labour for nulliparas both in the active phase of first-stage labour and in second-stage labour (Salim et al., 2005; Schiessl et al., 2005).

Secondary Powers

As soon as the presenting part reaches the pelvic floor, the contractions change in character and become expulsive. The labouring woman experiences an involuntary urge to push. She uses secondary powers (bearing-down efforts) to aid in expulsion of the fetus as she contracts her diaphragm and abdominal muscles and pushes. These bearing-down efforts result in increased intra-abdominal pressure that compresses the uterus on all sides and adds to the power of the expulsive forces.

The secondary powers have no effect on cervical dilation, but they are of considerable importance in the expulsion of the infant from the uterus and vagina after the cervix is fully dilated. Studies have shown that pushing in the second stage is more effective and the woman is less fatigued when she begins to push only after she has the urge to do so rather than beginning to push when she is fully dilated without an urge to do so (Jacobson & Turner, 2008; Simpson & James, 2005; Yildirim & Beji, 2008).

When and how a woman pushes in the second stage is a much-debated topic. Studies have investigated the effects of spontaneous bearing-down efforts, directed pushing, delayed pushing, Valsalva manoeuvre (closed glottis and prolonged bearing down), and open-glottis pushing (Gupta, Hofmeyr, & Smyth, 2004; Simpson & James, 2005). Although no significant differences have been found in the duration of second-stage labour, adverse effects of certain types of pushing techniques have been reported. Fetal hypoxia and subsequent acidosis have been associated with prolonged breath holding and forceful pushing efforts (Simpson & James, 2005). Routine sustained strenuous bearing down results in increased pressure on the pelvic floor that is associated with pelvic floor and perineal trauma (Hanson, 2009; Schaffer et al., 2005). Continued study is needed to determine the effectiveness and appropriateness of strategies that nurses use to teach pushing techniques, the suitability and effectiveness of various pushing techniques related to atypical or abnormal fetal heart patterns, and the standards for length of pushing in terms of maternal and fetal outcomes (Gennaro, Mayberry, & Kafulafula, 2007).

Position of the Labouring Woman

Position affects the woman's anatomical and physiological adaptations to labour. Frequent changes in position relieve fatigue, increase comfort, and improve circulation. Therefore, a labouring woman should be encouraged to find positions that are most comfortable to her (Fig. 15-12, A).

An upright position (walking, sitting, kneeling, or squatting) offers a number of advantages. Gravity can promote the descent of the fetus. Uterine contractions are generally stronger and more efficient in effacing and dilating the cervix, resulting in shorter labour (Gupta et al., 2004).

An upright position also is beneficial to the mother's cardiac output, which normally increases during labour as uterine contractions return blood to the vascular bed. The increased cardiac output improves blood flow to the uteroplacental unit and the maternal kidneys. Cardiac output is compromised if the descending aorta and ascending vena cava are compressed during labour. Compression of these major vessels may result in supine hypotension that decreases placental perfusion (see the Emergency box in Chapter 10, p. 216). With the woman in an upright position, pressure on the maternal vessels is reduced, and compression is prevented. If the woman wishes to lie down, a lateral position is suggested (Blackburn, 2007). Upright positions for women who have epidural analgesia are associated with a reduced duration of labour (Roberts et al., 2005).

The "all fours" position (hands and knees) may be used to relieve backache if the fetus is in an occipitoposterior position and may assist in anterior rotation of the fetus and in cases of shoulder dystocia (Hunter, Hofmeyr, & Kulier, 2007; Jevitt, Morse, & O'Donnell, 2008). Initial research supports the use of this position even with epidural analgesia when the woman has good mobility, and it decreases the length of second stage as well as the need for assisted birth (Stremler et al., 2009).

Positioning for second-stage labour (see Fig. 15-12, B) may be determined by the woman's preference, but it is constrained by the condition of the woman or fetus, the environment, and the health care provider's confidence in assisting in a birth in a specific position. The predominant position in Canada is supine, followed by semi-sitting, with half of these women reporting use of stirrups for birth, even though research does not support this position (see Chapter 18) (Public Health Agency of Canada, 2009). Alternative positions and position changes that result in more births over an intact perineum are

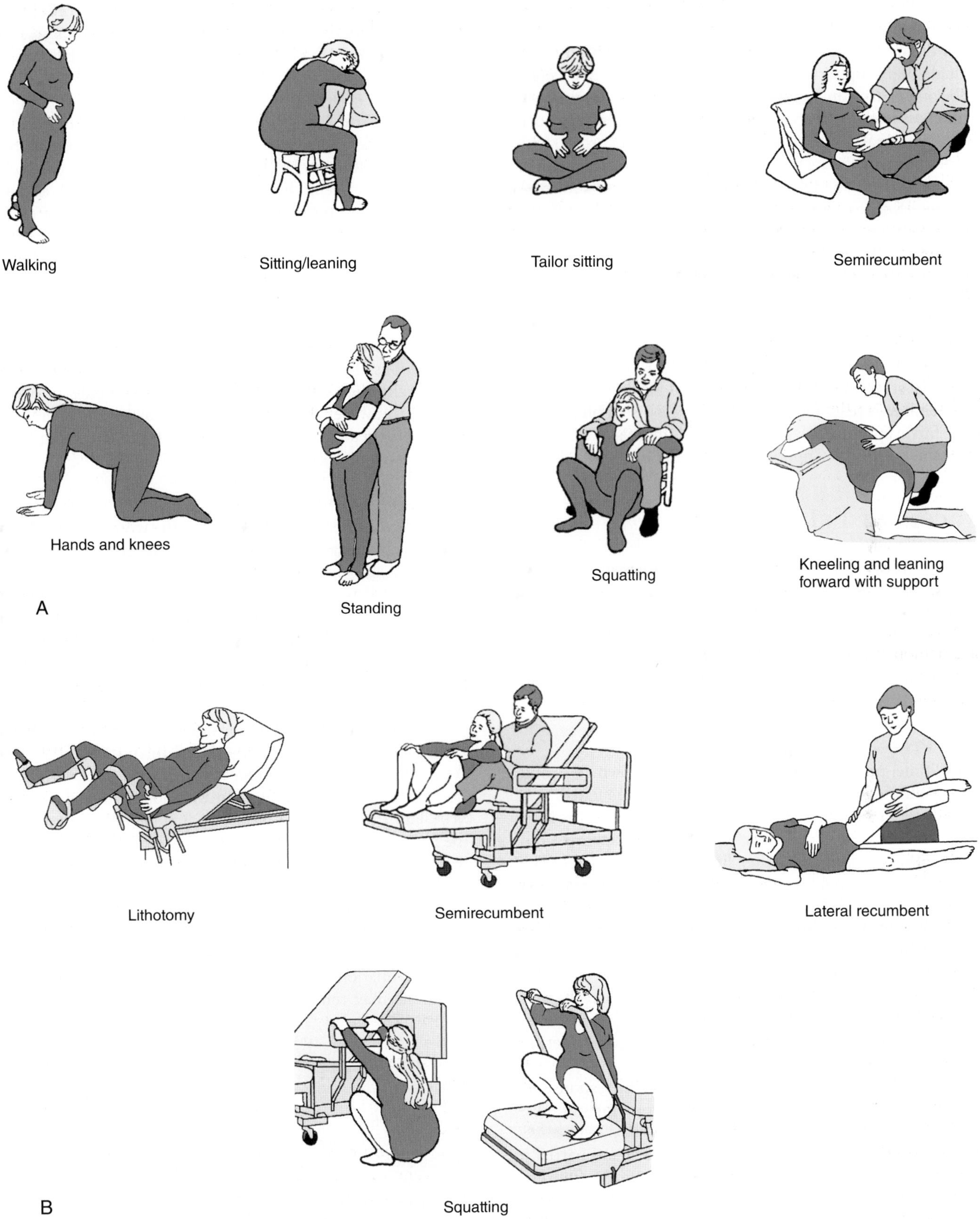
Walking
Sitting/leaning
Tailor sitting
Semirecumbent
Hands and knees
Standing
Squatting
Kneeling and leaning forward with support
A
Lithotomy
Semirecumbent
Lateral recumbent
B
Squatting

Fig. 15-12 Positions for labour and birth. **A:** Positions for labour. **B:** Positions for birth.

more commonly used by midwives and nurses (Jacobson & Turner, 2008).

A woman who pushes in a semirecumbent position needs adequate body support to push effectively because her weight will be on her sacrum, moving the coccyx forward and causing a reduction in the pelvic outlet. In a sitting or squatting position, abdominal muscles work in greater synchrony with uterine contractions during bearing-down efforts. Kneeling or squatting moves the uterus forward and aligns the fetus with the pelvic inlet and can facilitate the second stage of labour by increasing the pelvic outlet (Jacobson & Turner, 2008).

The lateral position can be used by the woman to help rotate a fetus that is in a posterior position. It also can be used when less force is needed for bearing down, such as when there is a need to control the speed of a precipitate birth (Simkin & Ancheta, 2000).

There is no evidence that any of these positions suggested for second-stage labour increases the need for the use of operative techniques (e.g., forceps- or vacuum-assisted birth, Caesarean birth, episiotomy), causes perineal trauma, or adversely affects the newborn (Gupta et al., 2004; Roberts et al., 2005).

Process of Labour

The term *labour* refers to the process of moving the fetus, placenta, and membranes out of the uterus and through the birth canal. Various changes take place in the woman's reproductive system in the days and weeks before labour begins. Labour itself can be discussed in terms of the mechanisms involved in the process and the stages the woman moves through.

Signs Preceding Labour

In first-time pregnancies, the uterus sinks downward and forward about 2 to 4 weeks before term, when the fetus's presenting part (usually the fetal head) descends into the true pelvis. This settling is called **lightening**, or "dropping," and usually happens gradually. After lightening, women breathe more easily, but usually more bladder pressure results from this shift, and consequently there is a return of urinary frequency. In a **multiparous** pregnancy, lightening may not take place until after uterine contractions are established and true labour is in progress.

The woman may complain of persistent low backache and sacroiliac distress as a result of relaxation of the pelvic joints. She may identify strong, frequent, but irregular uterine (**Braxton Hicks**) contractions.

The vaginal mucus becomes more profuse in response to the extreme congestion of the vaginal mucous membranes. Brownish or blood-tinged cervical mucus may be passed (bloody show). The cervix becomes soft (ripens) and partially effaced and may begin to dilate. The membranes may rupture spontaneously.

Other phenomena are common in the days preceding labour: (1) loss of 0.5 to 1.5 kg in weight, caused by water loss resulting from electrolyte shifts that in turn are produced by changes in estrogen and progesterone levels; and (2) a surge of energy. Women speak of having a burst of energy that they often use to clean the house and put everything in order. Less commonly, some women have diarrhea, nausea, vomiting, and indigestion. Box 15-1 lists signs that may precede labour.

Onset of Labour

The onset of true labour cannot be ascribed to a single cause. Many factors, including changes in the maternal uterus, cervix, and pituitary gland, are involved. Hormones produced by the normal fetal hypothalamus, pituitary, and adrenal cortex probably contribute to the onset of labour. Progressive uterine distention, increasing intrauterine pressure, and aging of the placenta seem to be associated with increasing myometrial irritability. This is a result of increased concentrations of estrogen and prostaglandins, as well as decreasing progesterone levels. The mutually coordinated effects of these factors result in the occurrence of strong, regular, rhythmic uterine contractions. The outcome of these factors working together is normally the birth of the fetus and the expulsion of the placenta; however, the means by which certain alterations trigger others and the ways in which proper checks and balances are maintained are not known.

Stages of Labour

Labour is considered "normal" when the woman is at or near term, no complications exist, a single fetus presents by vertex, and labour is completed within 18 hours. The course of normal labour, which is remarkably constant, consists of (1) regular progression of uterine contractions, (2) effacement and progressive dilation of the cervix, and (3) progress in descent of the presenting part. Four stages of labour are recognized. These stages are discussed in greater detail, along with nursing care for the labouring woman and family, in Chapter 18.

The first stage of labour is considered to last from the onset of regular uterine contractions to full dilation of the cervix. Commonly, the onset of labour is difficult to establish because the woman may be admitted to the labour unit just before birth, and the beginning of labour may be only an estimate. The first stage is much longer than the second and third combined. However, great variability is the rule, depending on the factors discussed previously in this chapter. Parity has a strong effect on the duration of first-stage labour (Gross, Drobnic, & Keirse, 2005). Full dilation may occur in less than 1 hour in some multiparous pregnancies. In first-time pregnancy, complete dilation of the cervix can take 18 hours or longer. Variations may reflect differences in the patient population

BOX 15-1 Signs Preceding Labour

- Lightening
- Return of urinary frequency
- Backache
- Stronger Braxton Hicks contractions
- Weight loss of 0.5 to 1.5 kg
- Surge of energy (also called nesting)
- Increased vaginal discharge; bloody show
- Cervical ripening
- Possible rupture of membranes

(e.g., risk status, age) or in clinical management of the labour and birth.

The first stage of labour is divided into three phases: a latent phase, an active phase, and a transition phase. During the latent phase, there is more progress in effacement of the cervix and little increase in descent. During the active and transition phases, there is more rapid dilation of the cervix and increased rate of descent of the presenting part. Maternal prepregnancy overweight and obesity can cause the active phase of labour to be longer than for women of normal weight (Liao, Buhimschi, & Norwitz, 2005). The active phase of labour may also be longer for Asian women (Debeic, Conell-Price, Evansmith, Shafer, & Flood, 2009).

The second stage of labour lasts from the time the cervix is fully dilated to the birth of the fetus. It takes an average of 20 minutes for a multiparous woman and 50 minutes for a **nulliparous** woman. A second stage of up to 2 hours has been considered within the normal range, but Cesaro (2004) found that a wider range of normal was still associated with no adverse effects on the mother or infant. Cheng, Hopkins, and Caughey (2004) found that a prolonged second stage was associated with increased rates of operative births and maternal morbidity. Epidural analgesia will likely prolong the second stage (Salim et al., 2005; Schiessl et al., 2005). Choosing different positions for the second stage, such as side-lying, squatting, or sitting, will shorten the second stage by increasing the efficacy of contractions, promoting uterine blood flow, and decreasing the likelihood of tears or episiotomies (Zwelling, 2010). Ethnicity may play a role in the length of second-stage labour. Greenberg and associates (2006) found that nulliparous Asian women had a longer second stage than that of nulliparous White women, whereas Black and Latin American women had shorter second stages of labour.

The third stage of labour lasts from the birth of the fetus until the placenta is delivered. The placenta normally separates with the third or fourth strong uterine contraction after the infant has been born. After it has separated, the placenta can be delivered with the next uterine contraction. Creating a warm environment, supporting skin-to-skin contact between mother and baby, and reducing fear and anxiety contribute to decreased catecholamine production and increased oxytocin production, which facilitate placental separation (Fry, 2007). The duration of the third stage may be as short as 3 to 5 minutes, although up to 1 hour is considered within normal limits. The risk of hemorrhage increases as the length of the third stage increases (Cunningham et al., 2010).

The fourth stage of labour arbitrarily lasts about 1 to 2 hours after birth of the placenta. It is the period of immediate recovery, when homeostasis is re-established. It is an important period of observation for complications, such as abnormal bleeding (see Chapter 23). The fourth stage of labour is also the time for bonding with the new baby and initiation of breastfeeding.

Mechanism of Labour

As already discussed, the female pelvis has varied contours and diameters at different levels, and the presenting part of the passenger is large in proportion to the passage. Therefore, for vaginal birth to occur, the fetus must adapt to the birth canal during the descent. The turns and other adjustments necessary in the human birth process are termed the *mechanism of labour* (Fig. 15-13). The seven cardinal movements of the mechanism of labour that occur in a vertex presentation are engagement, descent, flexion, internal rotation, extension, external rotation (restitution), and, finally, birth by expulsion. Although these movements are discussed separately, in actuality a combination of movements occurs simultaneously. For example, engagement involves both descent and flexion.

Engagement

When the biparietal diameter of the head passes the pelvic inlet, the head is said to be engaged in the pelvic inlet (see Fig. 15-13, A). In most nulliparous pregnancies, this occurs before the onset of active labour because the firmer abdominal muscles direct the presenting part into the pelvis. In multiparous pregnancies in which the abdominal musculature is more relaxed, the head often remains freely movable above the pelvic brim until labour is established.

Asynclitism

The head usually engages in the pelvis in a synclitic position (i.e., one that is parallel to the anteroposterior plane of the pelvis). Frequently, asynclitism occurs (the head is deflected anteriorly or posteriorly in the pelvis), which can facilitate descent because the head is being positioned to accommodate to the pelvic cavity (Fig. 15-14). Extreme asynclitism can cause cephalopelvic disproportion, even in a normal-size pelvis, because the head is positioned so that it cannot descend.

Descent

Descent refers to the progress of the presenting part through the pelvis. Descent depends on at least four forces: (1) pressure exerted by the amniotic fluid, (2) direct pressure exerted by the contracting fundus on the fetus, (3) force of the contraction of the maternal diaphragm and abdominal muscles in the second stage of labour, and (4) extension and straightening of the fetal body. The effects of these forces are modified by the size and shape of the maternal pelvic planes and the size of the fetal head and its capacity to mould.

The degree of descent is measured by the station of the presenting part (see Fig. 15-6). As mentioned earlier, little descent occurs during the latent phase of the first stage of labour. Descent accelerates in the active phase when the cervix has dilated to 5 to 7 cm. It is especially apparent when the membranes have ruptured.

In a first-time pregnancy, descent is usually slow but steady; in subsequent pregnancies, descent may be rapid. Progress in descent of the presenting part is determined by abdominal palpation and vaginal examination until the presenting part can be seen at the introitus.

Flexion

As soon as the descending head meets resistance from the cervix, pelvic wall, or pelvic floor, it normally flexes so that the chin is brought into closer contact with the fetal chest (see Fig. 15-13, B). Flexion permits the smaller suboccipitobregmatic diameter (9.5 cm) rather than the larger diameters to present to the outlet.

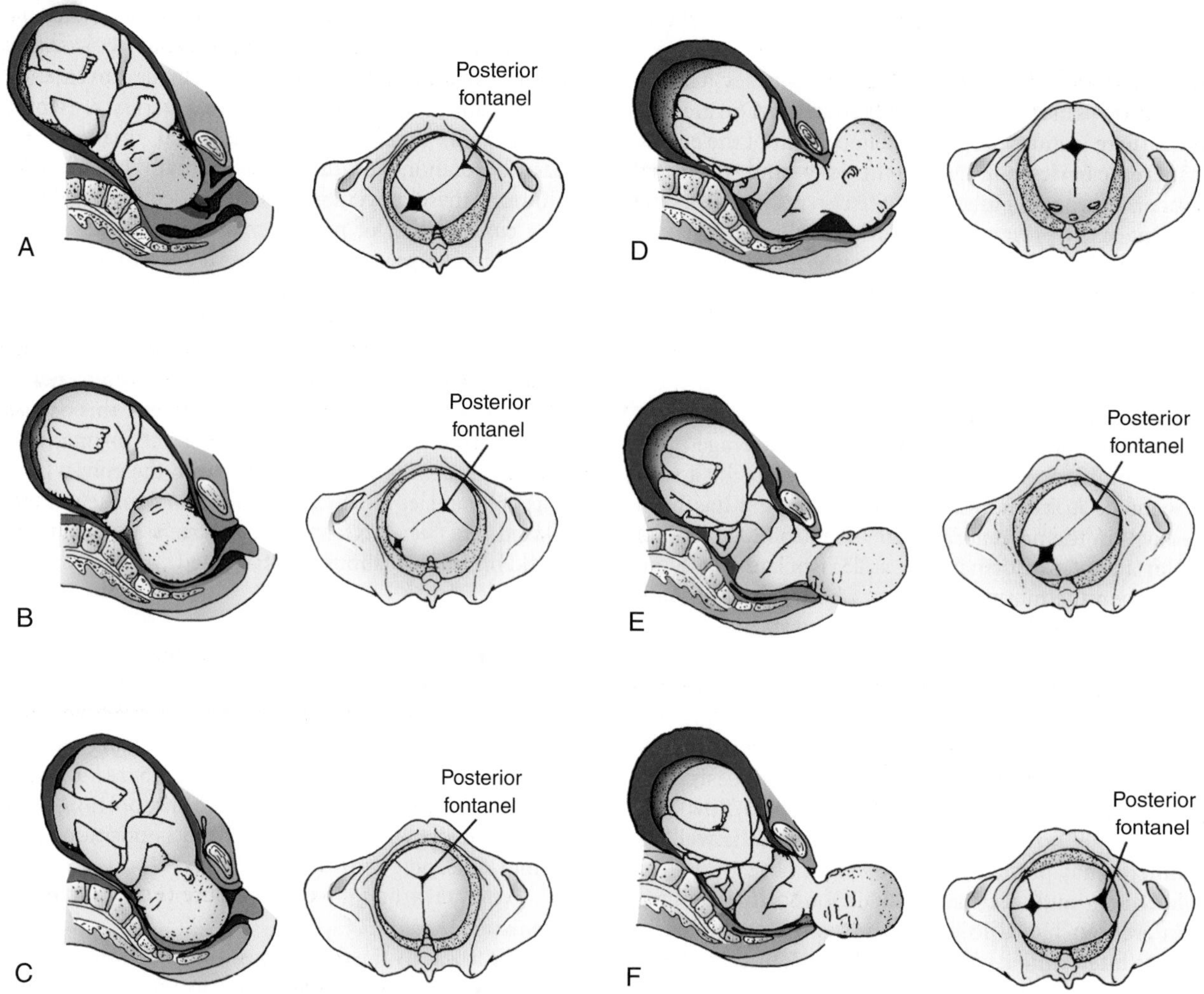

Fig. 15-13 Cardinal movements of the mechanism of labour. Left occipitoanterior position. **A:** Engagement and descent. **B:** Flexion. **C:** Internal rotation to occipitoanterior position. **D:** Extension. **E:** External rotation beginning (restitution). **F:** External rotation.

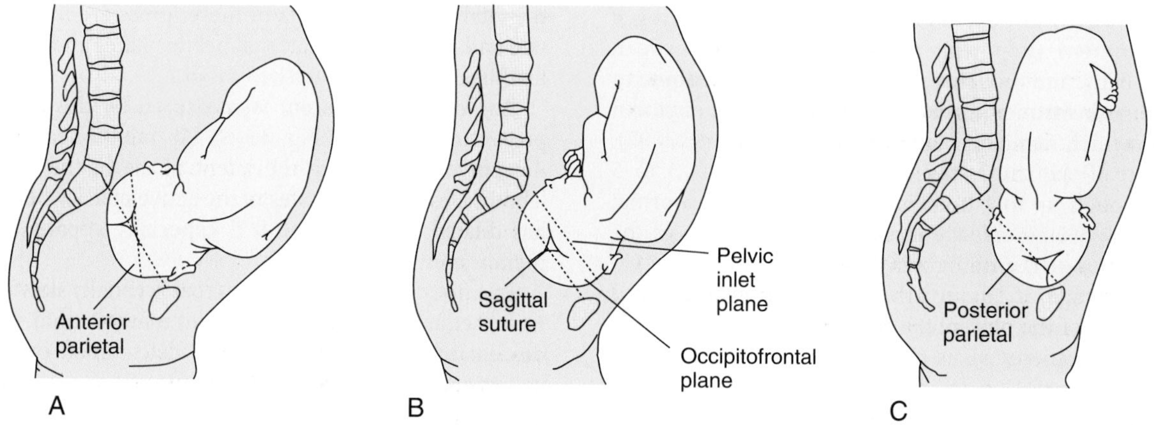

Fig. 15-14 Synclitism and asynclitism. **A:** Anterior asynclitism. **B:** Normal synclitism. **C:** Posterior asynclitism.

Internal Rotation

The maternal pelvic inlet is widest in the transverse diameter; therefore, the fetal head passes the inlet into the true pelvis in the occipitotransverse position. The outlet is widest in the anteroposterior diameter; in order for the fetus to exit, the head must rotate. Internal rotation begins at the level of the ischial spines but is not completed until the presenting part reaches the lower pelvis. As the occiput rotates anteriorly, the face rotates posteriorly. With each contraction the fetal head is guided by the bony pelvis and the muscles of the pelvic floor. Eventually, the occiput will be in the midline beneath the pubic arch. The head is almost always rotated by the time it reaches the pelvic floor (see Fig. 15-13, C). Both the levator ani muscles and the bony pelvis are important for achieving anterior rotation. A previous childbirth injury or regional anaesthesia may compromise the function of the levator sling.

Extension

When the fetal head reaches the perineum for birth, it is deflected anteriorly by the perineum. The occiput passes under the lower border of the symphysis pubis first, and then the head emerges by extension: first the occiput, then the face, and finally the chin (see Fig. 15-13, D).

Restitution and External Rotation

After the head is born, it rotates briefly to the position it occupied when it was engaged in the inlet. This movement is referred to as *restitution* (see Fig. 15-13, E). The 45-degree turn realigns the infant's head with her or his back and shoulders. The head can then be seen to rotate further. This external rotation occurs as the shoulders engage and descend in manoeuvres similar to those of the head (see Fig. 15-13, F). As noted earlier, the anterior shoulder descends first. When it reaches the outlet, it rotates to the midline and is delivered from under the pubic arch. The posterior shoulder is guided over the perineum until it is free of the vaginal introitus.

Expulsion

After birth of the shoulders, the head and shoulders are lifted up toward the mother's pubic bone, and the trunk of the baby is born by flexing it laterally in the direction of the symphysis pubis. When the baby has completely emerged, birth is complete, and the second stage of labour ends.

Physiological Adaptation to Labour

In addition to the maternal and fetal anatomical adaptations that occur during birth, physiological adaptations must occur. Accurate assessment of the labouring woman and fetus requires knowledge of these expected adaptations.

Fetal Adaptation

Several important physiological adaptations occur in the fetus. These changes occur in fetal heart rate (FHR), fetal circulation, respiratory movements, and other behaviours.

Fetal Health Surveillance (FHS)

FHS provides information about the condition of the fetus related to oxygenation. The average fetal heart rate (FHR) at term is 110 to 160 beats/min. Earlier in gestation the FHR is higher, with an average of approximately 160 beats/min at 20 weeks of gestation. The rate decreases progressively as the sympathetic nervous system in the fetus matures closer to term. However, temporary accelerations and slight early decelerations of the FHR can be expected in response to spontaneous fetal movement, vaginal examination, fundal pressure, uterine contractions, abdominal palpation, and fetal head compression. Stresses to the uterofetoplacental unit result in characteristic FHR patterns (see Chapter 17 for further discussion). Intermittent auscultation of the FHR during labour is recommended for low-risk women, with electronic monitoring used for women with identified risk factors in pregnancy or intrapartum (Lee et al., 2009; Liston et al., 2007).

Fetal Circulation

Fetal circulation can be affected by many factors, including maternal position, uterine contractions, blood pressure, and umbilical cord blood flow. Uterine contractions during labour tend to decrease circulation through the spiral arterioles and subsequent perfusion through the intervillous space. Most healthy fetuses are able to compensate for this stress and exposure to increased pressure while moving passively through the birth canal during labour. Usually, umbilical cord blood flow is undisturbed by uterine contractions or fetal position (Tucker, Miller, & Miller, 2009).

Fetal Respiration

Certain changes stimulate chemoreceptors in the aorta and carotid bodies to prepare the fetus for initiating respirations immediately after birth (Blackburn, 2007; Rosenberg, 2007). These changes include the following:

- Fetal lung fluid is cleared from the air passages as the infant passes through the birth canal during labour and (vaginal) birth.
- Fetal oxygen pressure (Po_2) decreases.
- Arterial carbon dioxide pressure (Pco_2) increases.
- Arterial pH decreases.
- Bicarbonate level decreases.
- Fetal respiratory movements decrease during labour.

Maternal Adaptation

As the woman progresses through the stages of labour, various body system adaptations cause the woman to exhibit both objective and subjective symptoms (Box 15-2).

Cardiovascular Changes

During each contraction, an average of 400 mL of blood is emptied from the uterus into the maternal vascular system. This increases cardiac output by about 12 to 31% in the first stage and about 50% in the second stage. The heart rate increases slightly (Gordon, 2007).

Changes in the woman's blood pressure also occur. Blood flow, which is reduced in the uterine artery by contractions, is redirected to peripheral vessels. As a result, peripheral resistance increases, and blood pressure increases (Gordon, 2007). During the first stage of labour, uterine contractions cause systolic readings to increase by approximately 10 mm Hg; therefore, assessing blood pressure between contractions provides more accurate readings. During the second stage, contractions may cause systolic pressures to increase by 30 mm Hg and diastolic readings to increase by 25 mm Hg, with both systolic and diastolic pressures remaining somewhat elevated between contractions (Gordon, 2007). Thus the woman already at risk for hypertension is at increased risk for complications such as cerebral hemorrhage.

BOX 15-2 Maternal Physiological Changes During Labour

- Cardiac output increases 12 to 31% in first stage; up to 50% in second stage.
- Heart rate increases slightly in first and second stages.
- Systolic blood pressure increases during uterine contractions in the first stage; systolic and diastolic pressures increase during uterine contractions in the second stage.
- White blood cell count increases.
- Respiratory rate increases.
- Temperature may be slightly elevated.
- Proteinuria (+1) may occur.
- Gastric motility and absorption of solid food is decreased; nausea and vomiting may occur during transition to second-stage labour.
- Blood glucose level decreases.

Supine hypotension (see Fig. 18-3, p. 452) occurs when the ascending vena cava and descending aorta are compressed. The labouring woman is at greater risk for supine hypotension if the uterus is particularly large because of multifetal pregnancy, hydramnios, or obesity or if the woman is dehydrated or hypovolemic. In addition, anxiety and pain, as well as some medications, can cause hypotension.

The woman should be discouraged from using the Valsalva manoeuvre (holding one's breath and tightening abdominal muscles) for pushing during the second stage. This activity increases intrathoracic pressure, reduces venous return, and increases venous pressure. The cardiac output and blood pressure increase, and the pulse slows temporarily. During the Valsalva manoeuvre, the fetus experiences a decreased oxygen saturation that is not seen with supported physiological pushing (Hanson, 2009). This can lead to fetal acidemia over time and decreased Apgar scores.

The white blood cell (WBC) count can increase (Blackburn, 2007). Although the mechanism leading to this increase in WBCs is unknown, it may be secondary to physical or emotional stress or to tissue trauma. Labour is strenuous, and physical exercise alone can increase the WBC count.

Some peripheral vascular changes occur, perhaps in response to cervical dilation or compression of maternal vessels by the fetus passing through the birth canal. Flushed cheeks, hot or cold feet, and eversion of hemorrhoids may result.

Respiratory Changes

Increased physical activity with greater oxygen consumption is reflected in an increase in the respiratory rate. Hyperventilation may cause respiratory alkalosis (an increase in pH), hypoxia, and hypocapnia (decrease in carbon dioxide). In the unmedicated woman in the second stage, oxygen consumption almost doubles. Anxiety also increases oxygen consumption.

Renal Changes

During labour, spontaneous voiding may be difficult for various reasons: tissue edema caused by pressure from the presenting part, discomfort, analgesia, and embarrassment. Proteinuria up to +1 is a normal finding because it can occur in response to the breakdown of muscle tissue from the physical work of labour.

Integumentary Changes

The integumentary system changes are evident, especially in the great distensibility (stretching) in the area of the vaginal introitus. The degree of distensibility varies with the individual. Despite this ability to stretch, even in the absence of episiotomy or lacerations, minute tears in the skin around the vaginal introitus occur.

Musculoskeletal Changes

The musculoskeletal system is stressed during labour. Diaphoresis, fatigue, proteinuria (+1), and possibly an increased temperature accompany the marked increase in muscle activity. Backache and joint ache (unrelated to fetal position) occur as a result of increased joint laxity at term. The labour process itself and the woman's pointing her toes can cause leg cramps.

Neurological Changes

Sensorial changes occur as the woman moves through phases of the first stage of labour and from one stage to the next. Initially, she may be euphoric. Euphoria gives way to increased seriousness, to amnesia between contractions during the second stage, and finally to elation or fatigue after giving birth. Endogenous endorphins (morphine-like chemicals produced naturally by the body) raise the pain threshold and produce sedation. In addition, physiological anaesthesia of perineal tissues, caused by pressure of the presenting part, decreases the perception of pain.

Gastrointestinal Changes

During labour, gastrointestinal motility and absorption of solid foods are decreased, and stomach-emptying time is slowed. Nausea and vomiting of undigested food eaten after onset of labour are common. Nausea and belching also occur as a reflex response to full cervical dilation. The woman may state that diarrhea accompanied the onset of labour, or the nurse may palpate the presence of hard or impacted stool in the rectum.

Endocrine Changes

The onset of labour may be triggered by decreasing levels of progesterone and increasing levels of estrogen, prostaglandins, and oxytocin. Metabolism increases, and blood glucose levels may decrease with the work of labour.

Accurate assessment of the mother and fetus during labour and birth depends on knowledge of these expected adaptations so that appropriate interventions can be implemented.

Key Points

- Labour and birth are affected by the five P's: passenger, passageway, powers, position of the woman, and psychological response.
- Because of its size and relative rigidity, the fetal head is a major factor in determining the course of birth.

- The diameters at the plane of the pelvic inlet, midpelvis, and outlet, plus the axis of the birth canal, determine whether vaginal birth is possible and the manner in which the fetus passes down the birth canal.
- Involuntary uterine contractions act to expel the fetus and placenta during the first stage of labour; these are augmented by voluntary bearing-down efforts during the second stage.
- The first stage of labour lasts from the time dilation begins to the time when the cervix is fully effaced and dilated. The second stage of labour lasts from the time of full dilation to the birth of the infant. The third stage of labour lasts from the infant's birth to the expulsion of the placenta. The fourth stage is approximately the first 2 hours after birth.
- The cardinal movements of the mechanism of labour are engagement, descent, flexion, internal rotation, extension, restitution and external rotation, and expulsion of the infant.
- Although the events precipitating the onset of labour are unknown, many factors, including changes in the maternal uterus, cervix, and pituitary gland, are thought to be involved.
- A healthy fetus with an adequate uterofetoplacental circulation will be able to compensate for the stress of uterine contractions.
- As the woman progresses through labour, various body systems adapt to the birth process.
- When pushing, the woman should be encouraged to use the open-glottis method rather than the closed-glottis method.

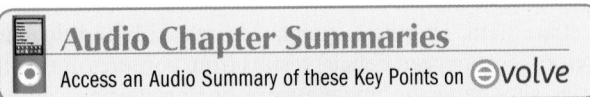

Audio Chapter Summaries

Access an Audio Summary of these Key Points on evolve

References

Blackburn, S. T. (2007). *Maternal, fetal, and neonatal physiology: A clinical perspective* (3rd ed.). St. Louis: Saunders.

Cesaro, S. (2004). Reevaluation of Friedman's labour curve: A pilot study. *Journal of Obstetric, Gynecologic & Neonatal Nursing, 33*(6), 713–722.

Cheng, Y., Hopkins, L., & Caughey, A. (2004). How long is too long: Does a prolonged second stage of labour in nulliparous women affect maternal and neonatal outcomes? *American Journal of Obstetrics and Gynecology, 191*(3), 933–938.

Cunningham, F., et al. (2010). *Williams obstetrics* (23rd ed.). New York: McGraw Hill.

Debiec, J., Conell-Price, J., Evansmith, J., Shafer, S., & Flood, P. (2009). Mathematical modeling of the pain and progress of the first stage of nulliparous labour. *Anesthesiology, 111*, 1093–1110.

Fry, J. (2007). Physiological third stage of labour: Support it or lose it. *British Journal of Midwifery, 15*(11), 693–695.

Gennaro, S., Mayberry, L., & Kafulafula, U. (2007). The evidence supporting nursing management of labour. *Journal of Obstetric, Gynecologic and Neonatal Nursing, 36*(6), 598–604.

Gordon, M. (2007). Maternal physiology. In S. G. Gabbe, J. R. Niebyl, & J. L. Simpson (Eds.), *Obstetrics: Normal and problem pregnancies* (5th ed.). New York: Churchill Livingstone.

Greenberg, M., et al. (2006). Are there ethnic differences in the length of labour? *American Journal of Obstetrics and Gynecology, 195*(3), 743–748.

Gross, M., Drobnic, S., & Keirse, M. (2005). Influence of fixed and time-dependent factors on duration of normal first stage labour. *Birth, 32*(1), 27–33.

Gupta, J. K., Hofmeyr, G. J., & Smyth, R. M. D. (2004). Position in the second stage of labour for women without epidural anaesthesia (Cochrane Review). *Cochrane Database of Systematic Reviews*, Issue 1. Art. No. CD002006. doi: 10.1002/14651858.CD002006.pub2

Hanson, L. (2009). Second stage labour care: Challenges in spontaneous bearing down. *Journal of Perinatal and Neonatal Nursing, 23*(1), 31–39.

Hunter, S., Hofmeyr, G. J., & Kulier, R. (2007). Hands and knees posture in late pregnancy or labour for fetal malposition (lateral or posterior). *Cochrane Database of Systematic Reviews*, Issue 4. Art. No. CD001063. doi: 10.1002/14651858.CD001063.pub3

Jacobson, P., & Turner, L. (2008). Management of the second stage of labour in women with epidural analgesia. *Journal of Midwifery & Women's Health, 53*(1), 82–85.

Jevitt, C. M., Morse, S., & O'Donnell, Y. S. (2008). Shoulder dystocia: Nursing prevention and posttrauma care. *Journal of Perinatal & Neonatal Nursing, 22*(1), 14–20.

Lee, L., et al. (2009). *Fundamentals of fetal health surveillance* (4th ed.). Vancouver BC: British Columbia Perinatal Health Program; produced by the Canadian Perinatal Programs Coalition.

Liao, J., Buhimschi, D., & Norwitz, E. (2005). Normal labour: Mechanism and duration. *Obstetric Gynecology Clinics of North America, 32*(2), 145–164.

Liston, R., et al. (2007). Fetal health surveillance: Antepartum and intrapartum consensus guideline. *Journal of Obstetrics and Gynaecology Canada 29*(9 Suppl 4), S1–S56, Retrieved from http://www.sogc.org/guidelines/documents/gui197CPG0709.pdf.

Public Health Agency of Canada. (2009). *What mothers say: The Canadian maternity experiences survey*. Ottawa: Author.

Roberts, C., et al. (2005). A meta-analysis of upright positions in the second stage to reduce instrumental deliveries in women with epidural analgesia. *Acta Obstetrica et Gynecologica Scandinavica, 84*(8), 794–798.

Rosenberg, A. (2007). The neonate. In S. G. Gabbe, J. R. Niebyl, & J. L. Simpson (Eds.), *Obstetrics: Normal and problem pregnancies* (5th ed.). New York: Churchill Livingstone.

Salim, R., et al. (2005). Continuous compared with intermittent epidural infusion on progress of labour and patient satisfaction. *Obstetrics and Gynecology, 106*(2), 301–306.

Schaffer, J., et al. (2005). A randomized trial of the effects of coached vs. uncoached maternal pushing during the second stage of labour on postpartum pelvic floor structure and function. *American Journal of Obstetrics and Gynecology, 192*(5), 1692–1696.

Schiessl, B., et al. (2005). Obstetrical parameters influencing the duration of second stage labour. *European Journal of Obstetric, Gynecological and Reproductive Biology, 118*(1), 17–20.

Simkin, P., & Ancheta, R. (2000). *The labour progress handbook: Early interventions to prevent and treat dystocia*. Oxford: Blackwell Science.

Simpson, K., & James, D. (2005). Effects of immediate versus delayed pushing during second-stage labour on fetal well-being: A randomized clinical trial. *Nursing Research, 54*(3), 149–157.

Stremler, R., et al. (2009). Hands and knees positioning during labour with epidural analagesia. *Journal of Obstetrical, Gynecological and Neonatal Nursing, 38*, 391–398.

Tucker, S., Miller, L., & Miller, D. (2009). *Mosby's pocket guide to fetal monitoring: A multidisciplinary approach* (6th ed.). St. Louis: Mosby.

VandeVusse, L. (1999). The essential forces of labour revisited: 13 Ps reported in women's stories. *MCN: American Journal of Maternal & Child Nursing, 24*(4), 176–184.

Yildirim, G., & Beji, N. (2008). Effects of pushing techniques in birth on mother and fetus: Randomized study. *Birth, 35*(1), 25–30.

Zwelling, E. (2010). Overcoming the challenges: Maternal movement and positioning to facilitate labour progress. *American Journal of Maternal/Child Nursing, 35*(2), 72–78.

Unit 4

16 Comfort Measures for Labour

Learning Objectives

On completion of this chapter, the reader will be able to:

- Compare various childbirth preparation methods.
- Identify nonpharmacological strategies to enhance relaxation and decrease discomfort during labour.
- Describe breathing and relaxation techniques used for each stage of labour.
- Discuss types of analgesia and anaesthesia used during labour.
- Compare pharmacological methods for relief of discomfort in different stages of labour and for different methods of birth.
- Describe nursing responsibilities appropriate for a woman receiving analgesia and anaesthesia during labour.

Electronic Resources

Additional information related to the content in Chapter 16 can be found on

evolve the companion Web site at

http://evolve.elsevier.com/Canada/Perry/maternal/

- Examination Review Questions
- Critical Thinking Exercise—Patient Receiving Epidural Block

Pain is an unpleasant, complex, highly individualized phenomenon with both sensory and emotional components. Pregnant women commonly worry about the pain they will experience during labour and birth and how they will react to and deal with that pain. Many physiological, psychosocial, and environmental factors influence the nature and degree of pain of a woman in labour and the manner in which she will respond to and cope with the pain (Lowe, 2002). A variety of childbirth preparation methods are available to help the woman or couple cope with the discomfort of labour. The methods selected depend on the situation, their availability, and the preferences of the woman.

The discomforts experienced during labour are discussed in this chapter, as are nonpharmacological and pharmacological interventions to relieve the discomfort during the different stages of labour. This information provides the basis for understanding the nurse's role in management of maternal discomfort during labour.

Discomfort During Labour and Birth

Neurological Origins

The pain and discomfort experienced during labour have two origins: visceral and somatic (Lowe, 2002). During the first stage of labour, uterine contractions cause cervical dilation and effacement. Uterine ischemia (decreased blood flow and therefore local oxygen deficit) results from compression of the arteries supplying the myometrium during uterine contractions. Pain impulses during the first stage of labour are transmitted through the T10 to T12 spinal nerve segment and accessory lower thoracic and upper lumbar sympathetic nerves. These nerves originate in the uterine body and cervix.

The pain from cervical changes, distension of the lower uterine segment, and uterine ischemia that predominates during the first stage of labour is *visceral* pain. It is located over the lower portion of the abdomen. Referred pain occurs when the pain that originates in the uterus radiates to the abdominal wall, lumbosacral area of the back, iliac crests, and gluteal area and down the thighs. The woman usually has discomfort only during contractions and is free of pain between contractions, although some women have continuous contraction-related low-back pain, even in the interval between contractions (Lowe, 2002; Trout, 2004).

During the second stage of labour, the stage of expulsion of the baby, the woman experiences *somatic* pain. This pain is often described as intense, sharp, burning, and well localized. Pain results from stretching and distension of perineal tissues and the pelvic floor to allow passage of the fetus, from distension and traction on the peritoneum and uterocervical supports during contractions, and from lacerations of soft tissue (e.g., cervix, vagina, perineum). Discomfort also can be produced by expulsive forces or pressure exerted by the presenting part on the bladder, bowel, or other sensitive pelvic structures. Pain impulses during the second stage of labour are carried from perineal tissues via the S2 to S4 spinal nerve segments and the parasympathetic system (Lowe, 2002).

Pain during the third stage of labour and the afterpains of the early postpartum period are uterine, similar to that experienced early in the first stage of labour. Areas of discomfort during labour are illustrated in Figure 16-1.

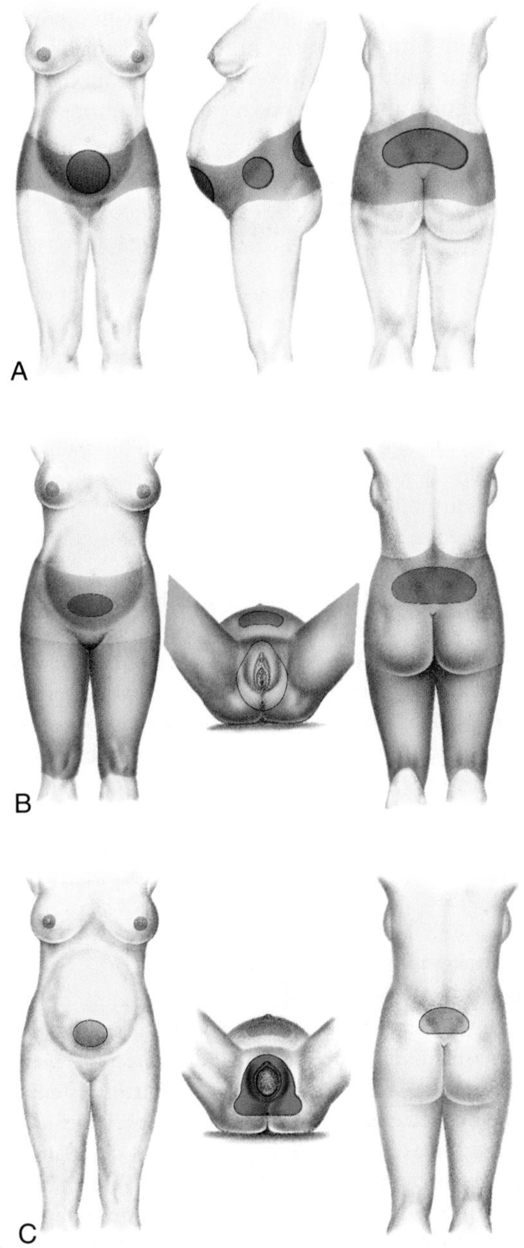

Fig. 16-1 Discomfort during labour. **A:** Distribution of labour pain during first stage. **B:** Distribution of labour pain during later phase of first stage and early phase of second stage. **C:** Distribution of labour pain during later phase of second stage and during birth. (Grey shading indicates areas of mild discomfort; light-coloured shading indicates areas of moderate discomfort; dark-coloured shading indicates areas of intense discomfort.)

Perception of Pain

Although the pain threshold is remarkably similar in all persons regardless of gender, social, ethnic, or cultural differences, these differences play a definite role in the person's perception of and behavioural responses to pain. The effects of factors such as culture, counterstimuli, and distraction in coping with pain are not fully understood. The meaning of pain and the verbal and nonverbal expressions given to pain are apparently learned from interactions within the primary social group. Cultural influences may impose unrealistic expectations. For instance, women from some cultural groups (e.g., Asian, Amish) believe it is shameful and counterproductive to scream or show pain and therefore avoid outward expressions when they are in pain (Trout, 2004).

Expression of Pain

Pain results in physiological effects and sensory and emotional (affective) responses. During childbirth, pain gives rise to identifiable physiological effects. Sympathetic nervous system activity is stimulated in response to intensifying pain, resulting in increased catecholamine levels. Blood pressure and heart rate increase. Maternal respiratory patterns change in response to an increase in oxygen consumption. Hyperventilation, sometimes accompanied by respiratory alkalosis, can occur as pain intensifies. Pallor and diaphoresis may be seen. Gastric acidity increases, and nausea and vomiting are common in the active phase of labour. Placental perfusion may decrease, and uterine activity may diminish, because of increased catecholamine levels, which shunt blood from the uterus to vital organs, potentially prolonging labour and affecting fetal well-being.

The sensory quality of visceral and somatic pain has been described as prickling, stabbing, burning, bursting, aching, heavy, pulling, throbbing, sharp, shooting, stinging, or cramping. The emotional (affective) quality of pain has been described as tiring, exhausting, annoying, sickening, and nauseating (Lowe, 2002).

Certain emotional (affective) expressions of suffering may be seen. Such changes include increasing anxiety with lessened perceptual field, writhing, crying, groaning, gesturing (hand clenching and wringing), and excessive muscular excitability throughout the body.

Factors Influencing Pain Response

Pain during childbirth is unique to each woman. How she perceives or interprets that pain is influenced by a variety of physiological, psychological, emotional, social, cultural, and environmental factors (Trout, 2004). Women who approach pain as a challenge for which they have sufficient resources to cope effectively are unlikely to equate pain with suffering. In contrast, women without sufficient self-confidence and coping strategies may feel threatened and view their pain experience as suffering (Lowe, 2002; Simkin & Bolding, 2004).

Pain is normally something most people try to avoid, but pain in labour needs to be presented as normal and having an important role in promoting labour. Women who learn to work with the pain may facilitate movement of the fetus through the birth canal. Actively responding to the pain by changing positions, rocking, or moaning may speed up the process of labour. The people supporting the woman in labour also need to understand the role of pain in normal labour and to feel comfortable watching the woman work with her pain.

Physiological Factors

A variety of physiological factors can affect the intensity of pain experienced by women during childbirth. Women with a history of dysmenorrhea may experience increased pain during childbirth as a result of higher prostaglandin levels. Back pain associated with menstruation also may increase the likelihood of contraction-related low-back pain. When upright positions are assumed during labour, they seem to result in decreased pain and an overall increase in comfort compared with that in the supine position. Women also report that being able to move freely to find a position of comfort is an important factor in reducing pain and muscle tension and in maintaining control during labour. The relation of fetal size to the dimensions of the maternal pelvis may also influence pain intensity (Lowe, 2002; Simkin & O'Hara, 2002).

Endorphins are endogenous opioids secreted by the pituitary gland that act on the central and peripheral nervous systems to reduce pain. β-Endorphin is the most potent of the endorphins. Although the physiological role of endorphins is not completely understood, it is thought that endorphin levels increase during pregnancy and birth in humans. Higher endorphin levels may increase the ability of women in labour to tolerate acute pain and may reduce their irritability and anxiety. Levels of β-endorphins are higher when a woman experiences a spontaneous, natural childbirth and levels are lower in medicated births.

Culture

The obstetrical population reflects the increasingly multicultural nature of Canadian society. As nurses care for women and families from a variety of cultural backgrounds, they must have knowledge and understanding of how culture mediates pain. Although all women expect to experience at least some pain and discomfort during childbirth, it is often their culture and religious belief system that determines how they will perceive, interpret, and respond to and manage the pain. For example, women with strong religious beliefs often accept pain as a necessary and inevitable part of bringing a new life into the world (Callister et al., 2003). First Nations, Métis, and Inuit women may endure pain quietly, whereas Latin American women may endure pain stoically because it is expected and esteemed but consider it acceptable to cry out. Chinese women often use soft voices and calm demeanors to cope with pain as a means of conserving energy during labour, whereas Mayan women may repeat a mantra and call out to the Lord to cope with pain and to enhance the labour process (Callister et al., 2003).

An understanding of the beliefs, values, expectations, and practices of various cultures will narrow the cultural gap and help the nurse to assess the labouring woman's experience of pain more accurately. This will in turn enable the nurse to provide culturally sensitive care by using appropriate pain-relief measures that preserve the woman's sense of control and self-confidence (see Cultural Awareness box) (see Table 18-1). It is important for the nurse to recognize that, although a woman's behaviour in response to pain may vary according to her cultural background, it may not accurately reflect the intensity of the pain she is experiencing. At the same time, each woman needs to be assessed as an individual, as each woman has a different experience of pain. The nurse must assess the woman for the physiological effects of pain and listen to the words the woman uses to describe the sensory and affective qualities of her pain (Lowe, 2002) (see Community Focus box).

Anxiety and Fear

Anxiety and fear are commonly associated with increased pain during labour. Mild anxiety is considered normal for a woman during labour and birth. However, excessive anxiety and fear cause catecholamine secretion, resulting in more pelvic pain

CULTURAL AWARENESS

Some Cultural Beliefs About Pain

The following are only examples of how women of different cultural backgrounds may react to pain. Because they are generalizations, the nurse must assess each woman experiencing pain that is related to childbirth.

Asian women may appear stoic and not exhibit reactions to pain, although it is acceptable to exhibit pain during childbirth. They consider it impolite to accept something when it is first offered; therefore, pain interventions may need to be offered more than once. Acupuncture may be used for pain relief.

Arab or Middle Eastern women may be vocal in response to labour pain. They may prefer medication for pain relief.

Latin American women may be stoic until late in labour, when they may become vocal and request pain relief.

First Nations women may use medications or remedies made from indigenous plants. They are often stoic in response to labour pain.

Women of African descent may express pain openly. Use of medication for pain relief varies.

COMMUNITY FOCUS

Culture and Pain

Talk to a man and a woman from a culture different from your own who have experienced childbirth. Ask her to describe her reactions to pain, how she sought relief of pain, the atmosphere of the childbirth setting, and the attitudes of the health care providers. Ask him if he was present for the birth and what his role in the birth was. How did his culture influence his role and reaction to childbirth? How did her culture influence her response to labour and the associated pain? What expressions of pain are "acceptable" in her culture? If he was present, how did he help her deal with the pain? What is the role of support persons in the labour process? Are the responses of the couple different from your responses to those same questions?

stimuli reaching the brain; this in turn magnifies pain perception (Lowe, 2002) (Fig. 16-2). As anxiety heightens, muscle tension increases, the effectiveness of the uterine contractions decreases, and pain intensifies; a cycle of increased fear and anxiety begins. Ultimately, this cycle will slow the progress of labour. The woman's "self-efficacy" or confidence in her ability to cope with pain will be diminished, potentially resulting in reduced effectiveness of pain-relief measures being used.

Previous Experience

Previous experience with pain and childbirth may affect a woman's description of her pain and her ability to cope with the pain. Childbirth may be a healthy young adult woman's first experience with significant pain; thus, she may not have developed effective pain coping strategies. She may describe the intensity of even early labour pain as pain "as bad as it can be." The nature of previous childbirth experiences also may affect a woman's responses to pain. For women who have had a difficult and painful previous birth experience, anxiety and fear from the past experience may lead to an increased perception of pain (see Critical Thinking Exercise). Conversely, a woman who has experienced a labour and birth in which the degree of pain matched her expectations and in which her coping skills were successful may have less anxiety and feel a sense of pride in her accomplishment (Trout, 2004). However, anxiety will increase if previous successful coping skills were ineffective during a more difficult labour.

Sensory pain for **nulliparous** women is often greater than that for **multiparous** women during early labour (dilation less than 5 cm) because their reproductive tract structures are less supple. During the transition phase of the first stage of labour and during the second stage of labour, multiparous women may experience greater sensory pain than nulliparous women because their more supple tissue increases the speed of fetal descent and thereby intensifies pain. The firmer tissue of nulliparous women results in a slower, more gradual descent. Affective pain is usually greater for nulliparous women throughout the first stage of labour but decreases for both nulliparous and multiparous women during the second stage of labour (Lowe, 2002).

Fatigue and sleep deprivation magnify pain. Most women have a decrease in quality of sleep over the last few days of pregnancy, and the spontaneous onset of labour occurs most often during the night (Beebe & Lee, 2007). Thus, many women have an increased perception of the intensity of pain during labour.

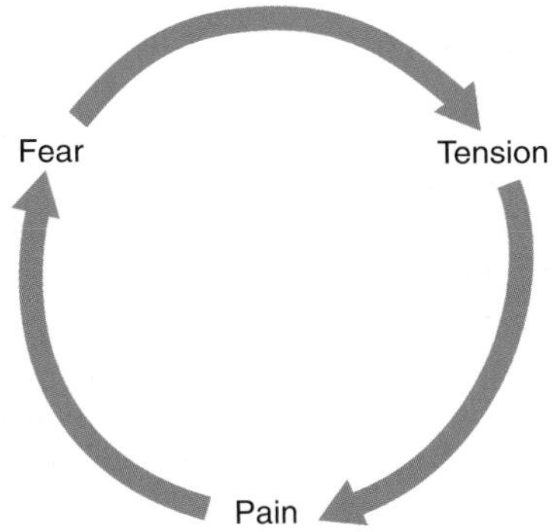

Fig. 16-2 Fear–tension–pain cycle.

Gate-Control Theory of Pain

Even particularly intense pain can at times be ignored. This is possible because certain nerve cell groupings within the spinal cord, brainstem, and cerebral cortex have the ability to modulate the pain impulse through a blocking mechanism. The gate-control theory of pain helps explain the way that hypnosis and the pain-relief techniques taught in childbirth preparation classes work to relieve the pain of labour. According to this theory, pain sensations travel along sensory nerve pathways to the brain, but only a limited number of sensations, or messages, can travel through these nerve pathways at one time. By using distraction techniques such as massage or stroking, music, focal points, and imagery, the capacity of nerve pathways to transmit pain is reduced or completely blocked. These distractions are thought to work by closing down a hypothetic gate in the spinal cord, thus preventing pain signals from reaching the brain. Perception of pain stimuli is thereby diminished.

In addition, when the woman in labour engages in neuromuscular and motor activity, such as changing positions and walking, activity within the spinal cord itself further modifies the transmission of pain. Cognitive work involving concentration on breathing and relaxation requires selective and directed cortical activity that activates and closes the gating mechanism as well. As labour intensifies, more complex cognitive techniques are required to maintain effectiveness. Therefore, the gate-control theory underscores the need for a supportive birth setting that allows the labouring woman to relax and use various higher mental activities.

CRITICAL THINKING EXERCISE

Anxiety in a Multipara in Active Labour

Jody was admitted in labour to a labour, birthing, and recovery (LBR) room 2 hours ago. She is 39 weeks of gestation in her second pregnancy. She is noticeably anxious and tells you that her first pregnancy ended at term but that the labour was "terrible. It was 22 hours long. I had an epidural but had to push and push to get the baby out." What interventions are appropriate?

1. Evidence—Is there sufficient evidence to draw conclusions about what intervention is needed?
2. Assumptions—Describe underlying assumptions about the following issues:
   a. Effects of anxiety on progress in labour
   b. Effect of parity on labour
   c. Effect of epidural analgesia on ability to push
   d. Education needed by Jody
3. What implications and priorities for nursing care can be made at this time?
4. Does the evidence objectively support your conclusions?
5. Are there alternative perspectives to your conclusions?

Supportive Care

Although the predominant medical approach to labour is that it is painful and the pain must be removed, an alternative view is that labour is a natural process; women can experience comfort and transcend the discomfort or pain to reach the joyful outcome of birth. Having needs and desires met engenders a feeling of comfort. Comfort may be viewed as strengthening. The most helpful interventions in enhancing comfort are using a caring nursing approach and providing supportive presence.

A woman's satisfaction with her childbirth experience is primarily influenced by the attitudes and behaviours of her caregivers, including the caregivers' ability to communicate and be helpful, supportive, accepting, and kind. In addition, her satisfaction is influenced by the degree to which she is able to stay in control of her labour and participate in decision making regarding it, including the pain-relief measures used.

The continuous supportive presence of a person (e.g., women with or without special training, including doulas, childbirth educators, family members, friends, nurses) who provides physical comfort, emotional support, ease of communication, and information and guidance to the woman in labour is a form of care that is beneficial to the woman and can improve labour outcomes. In the Canadian Maternity Experiences Survey, approximately 94% of women had a partner with them during labour, and most women were satisfied with the support they received from their companion (Public Health Agency of Canada [PHAC], 2009). Continuous support begun early in labour significantly relieves pain, improves outcomes, decreases interventions (e.g., use of pharmacological pain-relief measures) and complication rates (e.g., Caesarean rates and assisted vaginal birth) associated with labour, and enhances overall maternal satisfaction. Interestingly, a more positive effect was achieved when the continuous support was provided by a woman who was not part of the staff of the hospital (Enkin et al., 2000; Hodnett et al., 2007; Simkin & O'Hara, 2002). The Society of Obstetricians and Gynaecologists of Canada (SOGC) recommend that all women in labour receive continuous close support from an appropriately trained person (Liston et al., 2007).

Environment

According to Lowe (2002), environment should be viewed in terms of the persons present (e.g., how they communicate, their philosophy of care, practice policies, and quality of support) and the physical space in which the labour occurs. The quality of the environment can influence a woman's ability to cope with the pain of labour. Women prefer to be cared for by familiar caregivers in a comfortable, homelike setting (Hodnett, 2002). The environment should be safe and private, allowing a woman to feel free to be herself as she tries out different comfort measures. Stimuli, including light, noise, and temperature, should be adjusted according to the woman's preferences. There should be space for movement, and equipment should be readily available for a variety of nonpharmacological pain-relief measures such as birth balls, comfortable chairs, tubs, and showers. The familiarity of the environment can be enhanced by bringing items from home, such as pillows, objects for a focal point, music, and DVDs.

Assessing Coping During Labour

The observant nurse will look for cues to identify the woman's desired level of control in the management of pain and its relief. Commonly, it is not the amount of pain the woman experiences but whether she meets her goals for herself in coping with the pain that influences her perception of the birth experience as "good" or "bad."

The nurse should never assume that, because a woman is in labour, her pain must be uterine in origin. Because pain is a subjective phenomenon, the nurse must listen to the woman's description of her pain. A self-assessment tool such as a visual analog scale allows the woman to indicate on a line how severe or intense she perceives her pain to be. Pain is rated from "no pain" to "pain as bad as it can possibly be." Self-assessment is recommended to ensure that pain management is based on the subjective nature of the woman's pain rather than on the nurse's judgement of it. It is not unusual for a nurse to overestimate or underestimate the pain being experienced by a patient. When there are major cultural differences between the health care provider and the patient, inaccurate interpretation of pain intensity is more likely.

It is critical that the nurse take note of all pain characteristics, including location, intensity, quality, frequency, duration, and effectiveness of relief measures. While pain scales may be used with the labouring woman, their use may not always be appropriate as all women cope with pain differently. Some women may find questions about their level of pain confusing or annoying (Gulliver, Fisher, & Roberts, 2008). Nurses may assume that if a woman rates her pain level as high she requires medication, but some women may be able to manage high levels of pain during labour with the appropriate supportive care. Open-ended questions regarding how a woman is coping with labour may be more effective in ensuring that the woman's pain management needs are met. Gulliver et al. (2008) developed a tool that assists nurses in assessing how the mother is managing during labour as well as providing appropriate interventions depending on the assessment (Fig. 16-3). Use of the coping algorithm enables the nurse to provide care that is appropriate to that particular woman.

By completing a thorough assessment of the labouring woman, the nurse will be able to provide the appropriate pain-relief measures required by the woman. These measures may include nonpharmacological pain relief or the use of medication.

Nonpharmacological Management of Discomfort

Nonpharmacological measures are often simple, safe, and relatively inexpensive. They provide the woman with a sense of control over her childbirth as she makes choices about the measures that are best for her. During the prenatal period, the woman should explore a variety of nonpharmacological

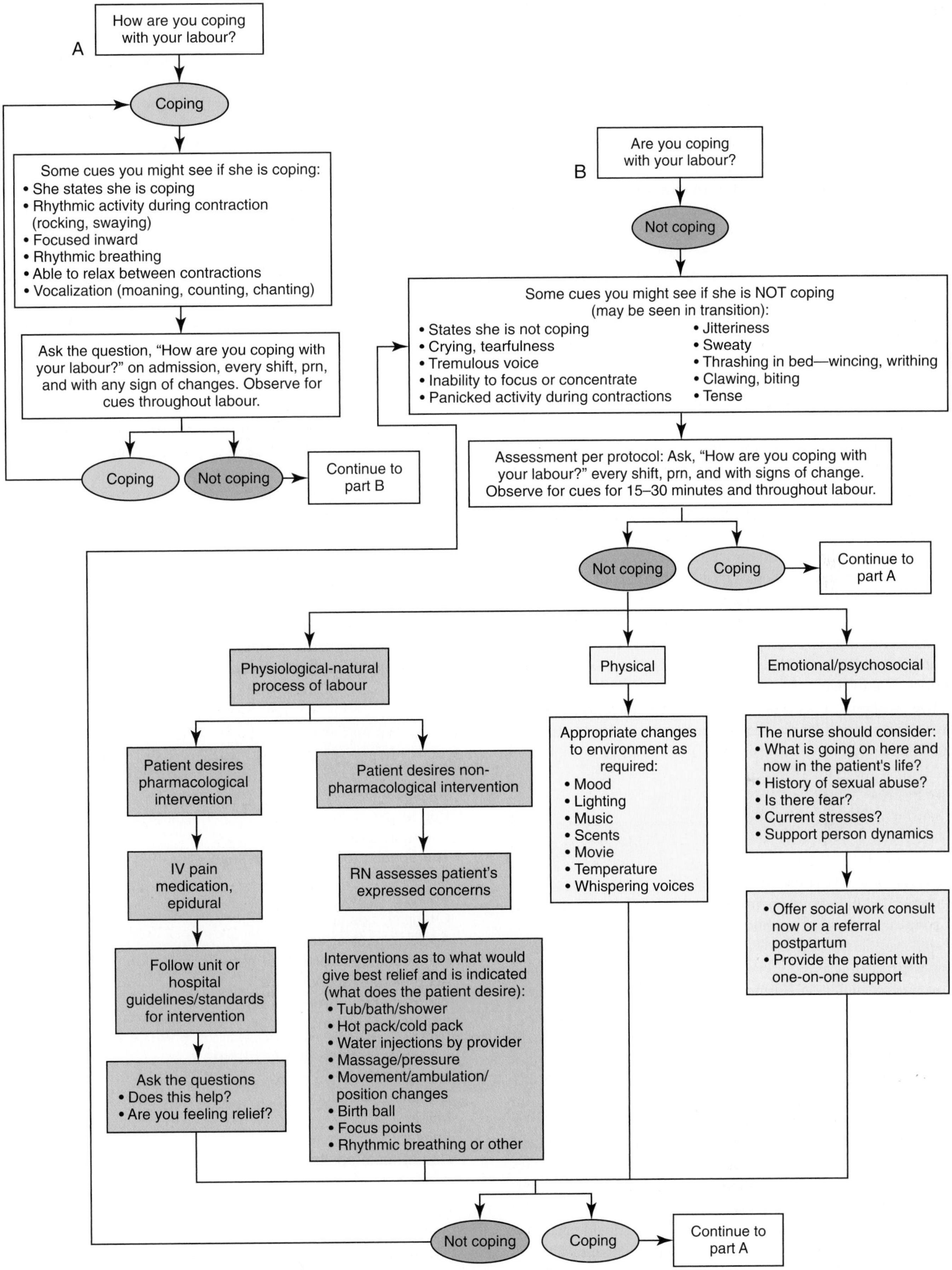

Fig. 16-3 Coping with labour algorithm. **A:** How to assess coping in labour. **B:** Strategies to help labouring women who are not coping. *(From Gulliver, B. G, Fisher, J., & Roberts, L. [2008]. A new way to assess pain in labouring women: Replacing the rating scale with a "coping" algorithm.* Nursing for Women's Health, 12*[5], 404–408.)*

measures. Techniques that she finds helpful in relieving stress and enhancing relaxation (e.g., music, meditation, massage, warm baths) also may be very effective as components of a plan for managing labour pain. The woman should be encouraged to communicate to her health care providers her preferences for relaxation and pain-relief measures and to actively participate in their implementation. She can prepare a **birth plan** that includes her preferences for pain-relief measures (see Box 10-9). Use of these measures requires the woman's active participation and support from her partner and caregivers.

The woman's perception of her behaviour during labour is of utmost importance in how she feels about her birth experience. If she has planned a nonmedicated birth but then needs and accepts medication, her self-esteem may falter. The nurse needs to provide verbal and nonverbal acceptance of her behaviour, as necessary, and reinforce this through discussion and reassurance after birth.

Many of the nonpharmacological methods for relief of discomfort are taught in different types of prenatal preparation classes, or the woman or couple may have read various books and magazine articles on the subject in advance (see Community Focus box). Many of these methods require practice for best results (e.g., hypnosis, patterned breathing and controlled relaxation techniques, biofeedback), although the nurse may use some of them successfully without the woman or couple having prior knowledge of them (e.g., slow-paced breathing, massage and touch, effleurage, counterpressure). Women should be encouraged to try a variety of methods and to seek alternatives if the measure being used is no longer effective (Box 16-1).

The analgesic effect of many nonpharmacological measures is comparable or even superior to opioids that are administered parenterally. Nonpharmacological measures are relatively inexpensive and safe with few, if any, major adverse reactions, and they can be used throughout labour.

COMMUNITY FOCUS

Resources for Alternative and Complementary Methods of Pain Relief

Survey your community for services that provide pregnant women with instruction in complementary or alternative nonpharmacological methods (e.g., biofeedback, aromatherapy, yoga, transcutaneous electrical nerve stimulation, massage, hypnosis) to relieve and cope with discomforts in pregnancy and pain during labour. Create a booklet that describes each of the methods. Include the following information in the booklet:

- A description of the methods and how they work
- Evidence available to validate effectiveness of the methods
- Internet addresses for the methods
- Agencies providing instruction in the methods; include contact information (address, telephone number), cost of the classes or service, and credentials of persons providing instruction
- At what point in pregnancy instruction should begin and the level of preparation and practice necessary for effective use

Childbirth Preparation Methods

Most health care providers recommend or offer childbirth preparation classes to expectant parents. Most proponents of prepared childbirth agree that the major causes of pain in labour are fear and tension (see Fig. 16-2). All childbirth methods attempt to reduce these factors and eliminate pain by increasing the woman's knowledge of the labour and birth process, enhancing her self-confidence and sense of control, preparing a support person, and training the woman in physical conditioning and relaxation breathing.

There are a few fine differences in prenatal education approaches, but in reality, few instructors adhere strictly to one particular method. Instead, they incorporate a variety of strategies aimed at increasing the woman's ability to cope with labour and minimize her need for medication.

Methods of Childbirth Education

Dick-Read Method

In the 1930s and 1940s, an English obstetrician, Dr. Grantly Dick-Read, wrote two publications (*Natural Childbirth*, 1933; *Childbirth Without Fear*, 1942) in which he theorized that pain in childbirth is socially conditioned and caused by a fear–tension–pain syndrome. In 1960, those who had been prepared for childbirth through his methods established the International Childbirth Education Association (ICEA). The

BOX 16-1 Nonpharmacological Strategies to Encourage Relaxation and Relieve Pain

Cutaneous Stimulation Strategies
Counterpressure
Effleurage (light massage)
Therapeutic touch and massage
Walking
Rocking
Changing positions
Applying heat or cold
Transcutaneous electrical nerve stimulation (TENS)
Acupressure/acupuncture
Water therapy (hydrotherapy)
Intradermal water block

Sensory Stimulation Strategies
Aromatherapy
Breathing techniques
Music
Imagery
Use of focal points

Cognitive Strategies
Childbirth education
Relaxation
Hypnosis
Biofeedback

Grantly Dick-Read method, referred to as Childbirth Without Fear, initially recommended deep abdominal breathing during early first-stage contractions, shallow breathing for later in the first stage, and sustained pushing with breath holding (Dick-Read, 1987). Women were taught to relax different muscle groups throughout the entire body, consciously and progressively, until a high degree of skill at relaxation was achieved. The aim was for the woman to relax completely between contractions and keep all muscles except the uterus relaxed during contractions.

HypnoBirthing

HypnoBirthing, the Mongan method, grew out of the work of Dr. Dick-Read, who taught that fear (of pain or birth) and tension (resulting from the fear) would lead to pain (HypnoBirthing, 2004; Mottershead, 2006). In HypnoBirthing, pregnant women (couples) learn how the birthing muscles work when the woman is in a state of relaxation. The aim is for the woman to be relaxed and in control. She will experience surges (contractions) while calm and relaxed, free of fear and tension. Testimonials from birthing women and their caregivers attest to the effectiveness of this technique, describing birth as rapid and pain free (HypnoBirthing, 2004).

Bradley Method

An early advocate of prepared childbirth was the Denver obstetrician, Robert Bradley, who wrote *Husband-Coached Childbirth* in 1965. He advocated what he called true "natural" childbirth, without any form of anaesthesia or analgesia and with a husband-coach present and specific breathing techniques for labour. The American Academy of Husband-Coached Childbirth was founded to make the Bradley method available and to prepare teachers (http://www.bradleybirth.com). In this method of partner-coached childbirth, breath control, abdominal breathing, and general body relaxation are used. Working in harmony with the body is emphasized (Bradley, 1981). Bradley's technique emphasizes environmental variables such as darkness, solitude, and quiet to make childbirth a more natural experience. Women using the Bradley method may appear to be sleeping during labour because they are in such a deep state of mental relaxation. Medication is discouraged.

Birthing From Within

Birthing From Within mentors (teachers) believe that childbirth is not a medical event but a profound rite of passage. Parents are taught the power of birthing-in-awareness. Mentors create a safe, nurturing class experience and help parents find their personal strength and wisdom. Birth is taught from four perspectives: mother, partner, baby, and culture. Parents are assisted in developing a pain-coping mindset. Birthing From Within advocates that parents deserve support for whatever birth option they choose. Partners provide the most help as loving partners and birth guardians, not as coaches (Birthing From Within, n.d.).

Childbirth and Postpartum Professional Association (CAPPA)

CAPPA is a nonprofit international organization, formed in 1998, that provides professional membership and training to antepartum doulas, childbirth educators, labour doulas, postpartum doulas, and lactation educators. They are proponents of evidence-informed practice in childbirth education. Their childbirth educators teach parents that childbirth is painful but that there are ways to deal with the pain. They generally recommend deep abdominal breathing in labour. Relaxation is vital to achievement of their goals for childbirth. Vocalization, position changes, walking, frequent urination, and hydrotherapy are useful techniques (CAPPA, 2008).

Lamaze Method

During the 1960s, the Lamaze method, originally known as the psychoprophylactic method (PPM), was introduced in the United States by Marjorie Karmel in her book, *Thank You, Dr. Lamaze*, published in 1959. The PPM offered new perspectives on preparing for childbirth, emphasizing control using the mind. The PPM combined controlled muscular relaxation and breathing techniques. Active relaxation was an integral part of the Lamaze method. The woman was taught to contract specific muscle groups (neuromuscular control) while relaxing the remainder of her body. She thus learned to relax the uninvolved muscles in her body while her uterus contracted. Instead of tensing during uterine contractions, women were conditioned to respond with relaxation and breathing patterns.

In 1960, the American Society for Psychoprophylaxis in Obstetrics (ASPO) was formed in New York and became a national organization to promote use of the Lamaze method and prepare teachers of the method. It continues to be an active organization, known since 1998 as Lamaze International and dedicated to advancing normal birth. Lamaze's Institute of Normal Birth publishes reviews of research related to normal birth. In the *Lamaze Guide to Giving Birth With Confidence*, the authors state that "Mothers do know how to give birth, simply; and doctors, hospitals, and technology have not made normal birth safer" (Lothian & Devries, 2005). They further state that women need to rediscover birth as a natural part of life, based on research that confirms that interfering in the normal birth process is harmful unless there is clear evidence that interference provides benefits.

Lamaze International's core values has become an ideal for many childbirth education organizations. It fits closely with the principles of perinatal care put forth by the World Health Organization (WHO, 1998) as well the Family-Centred Maternity and Newborn Care National Guidelines (Health Canada, 2000) (see Box 1-5), which state that care for normal pregnancy and birth should be removed from total control of doctors; be based on the use of appropriate technology (as opposed to overuse); and be evidence informed, regionalized, multidisciplinary, holistic, family centred, and culturally appropriate. Women should be involved in decision making, and their privacy, dignity, and confidentiality should be respected. They should feel empowered to make the choices that seem right for them.

The Lamaze Institute for Normal Birth (LINB) is an evidence-informed resource for new and expectant parents and childbirth professionals, whether they practice from a medical, nursing, or midwifery model of care. Its foundation comprises six care principles modified from the WHO recommendations (Box 16-2). These healthy birth practices are based on current research.

BOX 16-2 Lamaze Healthy Birth Practices

1. Let labour begin on its own.
2. Walk, move around, and change positions throughout labour.
3. Bring a loved one, friend, or doula for continuous support.
4. Avoid interventions that are not medically necessary.
5. Avoid giving birth on your back, and follow your body's surges to push.
6. Keep your baby with you—it's best for you, your baby, and breastfeeding.

(Source: Lamaze International [2012]. Retrieved from http://www.lamazeinternational.org/HealthyBirthPractices.)

Brief papers documenting the research supporting each of these care principles is available at http://www.lamaze.org. In addition, the LINB produces a free Internet-based newsletter that reviews recent studies that address some aspect of normal birth. Thus, all perinatal educators, perinatal care providers, and consumers can have ready access to current research on the subject of normal birth.

Evidence-Informed Childbirth Education

Many childbirth educators teach a plethora of techniques that originated in several different organizations or publications. An educator can assist a woman in developing her birth philosophy and inner knowledge and then provide her with an array of skills to choose from that can help her achieve the birth experience she wants.

There are many resources for evidence-informed care in pregnancy and childbirth (e.g., http://www.childbirthconnection.org, http://www.pregnancy.cochrane.org). How the childbirth educator uses this evidence in education programs depends on both the population that attends the classes and the care-provider practices in the community. In the role as advocate, the childbirth educator can let families know which care routines are ineffective or harmful and provide expectant parents ways to ask their care providers about their own routine practices. These discussions might affect their choice of care provision.

In 2008, a total of 6421 Canadian women were interviewed about their entire childbearing experience. While the majority of women reported a positive overall experience of labour and birth, the results suggested that a large percentage of mothers giving birth receive interventions that are not evidence informed (PHAC, 2009). For the childbirth educator, it takes skill, judgement, and tact to help consumers make choices about their desired care without undermining medical colleagues, particularly when local routine care frequently lacks an evidence base.

Childbirth Education Outcomes

Researchers studying childbirth education outcomes have not adopted a standard set of operational definitions of childbirth education or a theoretical framework that acknowledges that multiple factors, not childbirth education alone, have an impact on the outcomes. Research on the influence of childbirth education on biological birth outcomes has not accounted for the management mindset of those providing care during labour.

However, the research findings on positive childbirth education outcomes have been consistent over many decades. The effects of childbirth education have consistently been shown to increase birth satisfaction, build confidence, and build relationships. Research has not demonstrated that physiological outcomes are strongly influenced by educating expectant parents.

Pregnancy is a time when expectant parents anticipate change in their lives and are open to many types of education. This education can enhance their health and coping in pregnancy, childbirth, and early parenting. It also can influence how they relate to health professionals over a lifetime, problem solve with each other, and launch their new family. It is an opportunity for nurses to engage in meaningful health promotion and the building of resilience and connection in families.

Nonpharmacological Comfort Strategies

Relaxation

Relaxation or reduction of body tension is a technique suggested by virtually all childbirth education organizations. Learning relaxation in childbirth education classes can help couples with the stresses of pregnancy, childbirth, and adjustment to parenting and can be a form of stress management throughout life (Fig. 16-4). The research is clear that relaxation skill is the most effective nonpharmacological strategy for coping with the stress of labour.

Imagery and Visualization

Imagery and visualization are useful techniques in preparation for birth. Although research on their use is scant, clinical reports suggest that imagery and visualization can be used to produce a sense of well-being during pregnancy, assist with cervical dilation, and decrease the experience of pain and tension during labour. Imagery involves techniques such as imagining a walk through a restful garden or breathing in light, energy, and healing colour and breathing out worries and tension. Visualization of the baby coming down the birth

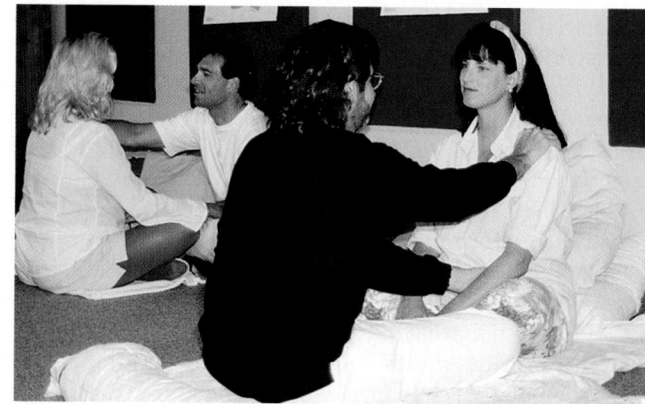

Fig. 16-4 Expectant parents learning relaxation techniques. *(Courtesy Marjorie Pyle, RNC, Lifecircle, Costa Mesa, CA.)*

canal during the second stage of labour can also be used effectively to enhance pushing efforts. A variety of skills taught in childbirth classes augment relaxation during pregnancy and labour. All of these can be taught as lifetime skills that are useful to the couple and that they can teach their children to cope with the stresses of life.

Music

Music, taped or live, enhances relaxation during labour, thereby reducing stress, anxiety, and the perception of pain. Women can prepare their musical preferences in advance and bring them to the hospital or birthing centre. Use of a headset or earphones may increase the effectiveness of the music because other sounds will be shut out. Live music provided at the bedside by a support person may also be very helpful in transmitting energy that decreases tension and elevates mood. Ocean waves and Baroque and New Age music have been shown to assist in relaxation.

Touch and Massage

Touch and massage have been an integral part of the traditional care process for women in labour. Touch can be as simple as holding the woman's hand, stroking her body, and embracing her. Head, hand, back, shoulder, and foot massage may be effective in reducing tension and enhancing comfort. Hand and foot massage may be especially relaxing in advanced labour when hyperesthesia limits a woman's tolerance for touch on other parts of her body.

Energy Work

Energy work such as therapeutic touch or healing touch involves manipulation of energy fields around the body and can be taught in class for use during labour to decrease anxiety and pain and increase relaxation. Certified practitioners in energy work can be consulted throughout pregnancy and during childbirth by women who have access to such care.

Conscious Breathing

Relaxed individuals automatically slow their breathing; conversely, slowing one's breathing serves to increase one's relaxation and hence may decrease the feeling of pain. Different approaches to childbirth preparation use varying breathing techniques to help the woman maintain control through contractions (Fig. 16-5 and Box 16-3). During labour, nursing support includes guiding couples in applying breathing and relaxation methods, adapting methods to their particular needs, and using pushing techniques for birth that avoid breath holding. Such techniques often involve moaning or making other noises as the woman pushes without holding her breath. There is no one right way to breathe; women are encouraged to find what works for them.

The woman and her support person must be aware of and watch for symptoms of respiratory alkalosis when rapid, shallow breathing results in hyperventilation: light-headedness, dizziness, tingling of fingers, or circumoral numbness. Such alkalosis may be eliminated by having the woman breathe into a paper bag held tightly around the mouth and nose. This enables her to rebreathe carbon dioxide and replace the bicarbonate ion. She can also breathe into her cupped hands if no bag is available.

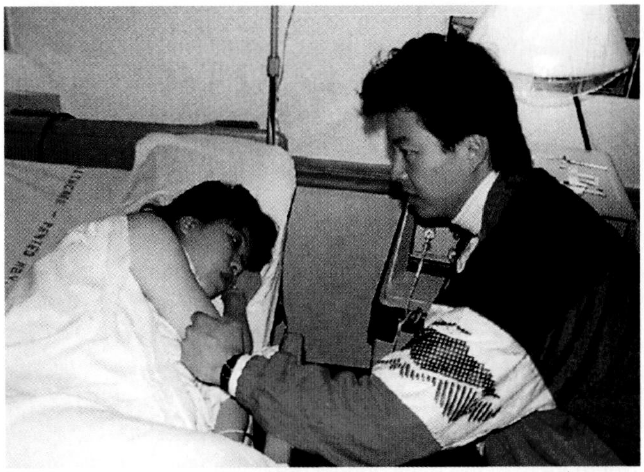

Fig. 16-5 Labouring woman using focusing and breathing techniques during contraction, with coaching from her partner. *(Courtesy Marjorie Pyle, RNC, Lifecircle, Costa Mesa, CA.)*

Effleurage and Counterpressure

Effleurage (light massage) and counterpressure bring relief to many women during the first stage of labour. *Effleurage* is a light stroking, usually of the abdomen, often in rhythm with breathing during contractions. It is used to distract the woman from contraction pain. The presence of monitor belts may make it difficult to perform effleurage on the abdomen; thus, a thigh or the chest may be used.

Counterpressure is steady pressure in the sacral area with the fist or heel of the hand, which may help the woman cope with the sensations of internal pressure and pain in the lower back.

Water Therapy (Hydrotherapy)

Bathing, showering, or jet hydrotherapy (whirlpool baths) using warm water are nonpharmacological measures that can be used to promote comfort and relaxation during labour, reduce fear of pain, and cope with pain (Maude & Foureur, 2007) (Fig. 16-6). Showers in early labour may provide relaxation and comfort. Sitting in a tub of body-temperature water has several immediate benefits. Buoyancy in the water results in general body relaxation and temporary relief from discomfort and pain. This reduces the woman's anxiety and enhances a feeling of well-being. Catecholamine production decreases. This triggers an increase in the levels of **oxytocin** (to stimulate uterine contractions) and endorphins (to reduce pain perception).

If the woman is experiencing "back labour" as a result of an occiput posterior or transverse position, she should be encouraged to assume the hands-and-knees or the side-lying position in the tub. Because this position decreases pain and increases relaxation and the production of oxytocin, the fetus can rotate spontaneously to the occiput anterior position.

In some settings, jet hydrotherapy may need to be approved by the woman's primary health care provider. The woman's

BOX 16-3 Paced Breathing Techniques

Cleansing Breath

Relaxed breath in through the nose and out the mouth, keeping shoulders relaxed

Used at the beginning and end of each contraction to enhance relaxation and as a signal to others

Slow-Paced Breathing (Approximately 6 to 10 breaths/min)

Not less than half the normal breathing rate using deep breaths into the abdomen

IN-2-3-4/OUT-2-3-4/IN-2-3-4/OUT-2-3-4

Modified-Paced Breathing (Approximately 32 to 40 breaths/min)

Not more than twice the normal breathing rate using shallow breathing into the upper chest. Can use the mouth or nose for breathing in and out

IN-OUT/IN-OUT/IN-OUT

Patterned-Paced Breathing (Same Rate as Modified-Paced Breathing But Using a Pattern)

Enhances concentration

3:1 Patterned breathing IN-OUT/IN-OUT/IN-OUT/IN-BLOW (repeat through contractions).

4:1 Patterned breathing IN-OUT/IN-OUT/IN-OUT/IN-OUT/IN-BLOW (repeat through contractions)

Pant-Blow Breathing (Same Rate as Modified-Paced Breathing)

Not more than twice the normal breathing rate (breaths/min × 2)

Upper chest, shallow breaths followed by relaxed exhales

The pant is an in breath and the blow is an out breath.

Pattern may vary: PANT-2-3-4-BLOW, or PANT-2-3-BLOW

Keep facial muscles relaxed.

Breathing During Second Stage—Pushing

Spontaneous Pushing

The urge to push is nearly involuntary. Many women hold their breath; remember to breathe.

Slow Exhalation Pushing (Open-Glottis Pushing)

Work with contraction; inhale and exhale slowly through pursed lips.

Grunting or making noise with exhalation keeps glottis open.

Directed Pushing (Closed-Glottis Pushing)

During contraction, the woman inhales and holds her breath while the support person counts to 6. She needs to exhale and inhale rapidly again, holding for another count of 6. Repeat until contraction is over.

(Adapted from BirthSource. [n.d.]. *Breathing.* Dayton, OH: Perinatal Education Associates. Retrieved from http://www.birthsource.com.)

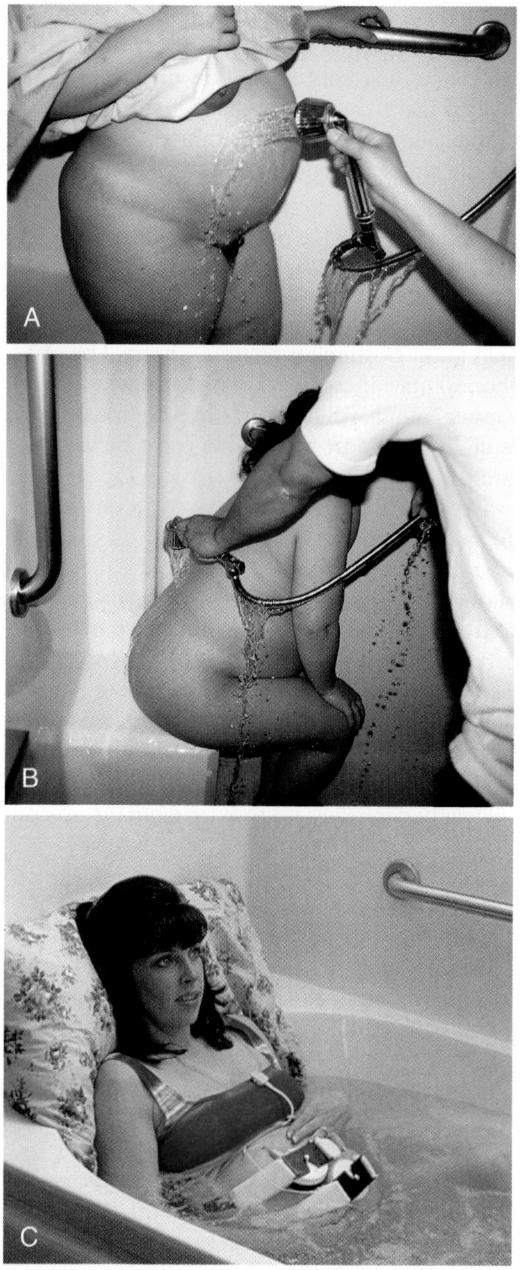

Fig. 16-6 Water therapy during labour. **A:** Use of shower during labour. **B:** Woman experiencing back labour relaxes as partner sprays warm water on her back. **C:** Woman relaxing in Jacuzzi. *(**A** and **B**, Courtesy Marjorie Pyle, RNC, Lifecircle, Costa Mesa, CA. **C**, Courtesy Spacelabs Medical, Redmond, WA.)*

vital signs must be within normal limits, and she should be in the active phase of the first stage of labour. If she is in the latent phase, her contractions may slow down. Fetal well-being must also be documented. Fetal heart rate (FHR) monitoring is done by doptone, fetoscope, or wireless external monitor device (see Fig. 16-6, C). Placement of internal electrodes is contraindicated for jet hydrotherapy. The woman's membranes may be intact or ruptured. If the membranes are ruptured, the fluid must be clear or only lightly stained with meconium.

There is no limit to the time that women can stay in the bath, and often they are encouraged to stay in it as long as desired. Most women use jet hydrotherapy for 30 to 60 minutes at a time. Repeated baths with occasional breaks may be more effective in relieving pain during long labours than unlimited amounts of time in the water. Water temperature should not exceed 37°C, to reduce the risk of hyperthermia. Monitoring of maternal temperature every hour and offering fluids will ensure that the labouring woman's temperature remains below 37.5°C (Perinatal Services, BC, 2007).

Transcutaneous Electrical Nerve Stimulation

Transcutaneous electrical nerve stimulation (TENS) involves the placement of two pairs of electrodes on either side of the woman's thoracic and sacral spine (Fig. 16-7). These electrodes provide continuous mild electrical current from a battery-operated device. During a contraction, the woman increases the stimulation from low to high intensity by turning control knobs on the device. High intensity should be maintained for at least 1 minute to facilitate release of endorphins. Women describe the resulting sensation as a tingling or buzzing and pain relief as good or very good. TENS is most useful for lower back pain during the early first stage of labour. There is limited evidence to suggest that TENS reduces pain in labour, but women should be provided the opportunity to use it if they wish (Dowswell et al., 2009). The nurse assists the woman in using TENS by explaining the device and its use, carefully placing and securing the electrodes, and closely evaluating its effectiveness (see Nursing Care Plan).

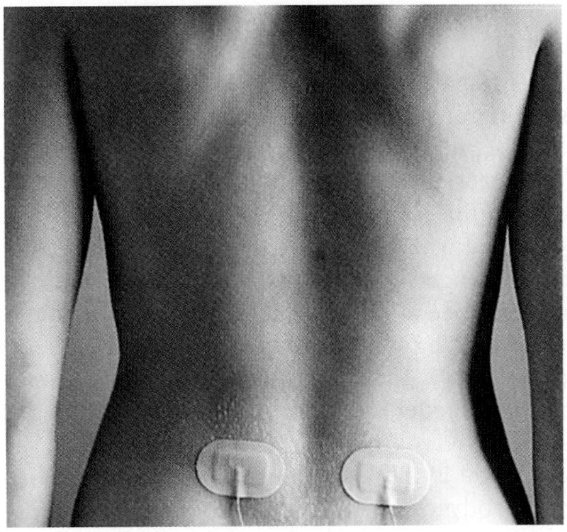

Fig. 16-7 Placement of transcutaneous electrical nerve stimulation (TENS) electrodes on back for relief of labour pain.

NURSING CARE PLAN • NONPHARMACOLOGICAL MANAGEMENT OF DISCOMFORT

Nursing Diagnosis: Anxiety related to ability to cope effectively with pain during labour

Expected Outcome

Woman will express decrease in anxiety and experience satisfaction with her labour and birth.

Nursing Interventions/*Rationales*

Assess whether the woman and significant other have attended childbirth classes, her knowledge of labour process, and her current level of anxiety *to plan supportive strategies.*

Assess the woman's plans for coping with labour *to enhance her feeling of control over the situation.*

Encourage the support person to remain with the woman in labour (if appropriate) *to provide support and increase probability of her response to comfort measures.*

Teach or review nonpharmacological techniques available to decrease anxiety and pain during labour (e.g., focusing and feedback, breathing techniques, effleurage, and sacral pressure) *to enhance chances of success in using these techniques.*

Explore other techniques that the woman or significant other may have learned in childbirth classes (e.g., hypnosis, yoga, acupressure, biofeedback, therapeutic touch, aromatherapy, imaging, music) *to provide the largest repertoire of coping strategies.*

Explore use of jet hydrotherapy if the woman meets use criteria (i.e., vital signs within normal limits, active phase of first-stage labour) *to aid relaxation and stimulate production of natural oxytocin.*

Explore use of transcutaneous nerve stimulation *to provide an increased perception of control over pain and an increase in release of endogenous opiates.*

Assist woman to change positions and to use pillows *to promote comfort and enhance labour.*

Assess bladder for distension and encourage voiding often (every 1 to 2 hours) *to avoid bladder distension and subsequent discomfort.*

Encourage rest between contractions *to minimize fatigue.*

Keep the woman and significant other informed about progress *to allay anxiety.*

Guide the couple through the labour stages and phases, helping them use and modify comfort techniques that are appropriate to each phase, *to ensure the greatest effectiveness of techniques used.*

Support the couple if pharmacological measures are requested to increase pain relief, explaining safety and effectiveness, *to reduce anxiety and maintain self-esteem and a sense of control over the labour process.*

Nursing Diagnosis: Health-seeking behaviour (labour) related to desire for a healthy outcome of labour and birth

Expected Outcome

Woman will participate in care planning for labour.

Nursing Interventions/*Rationales*

Discuss woman's birth plan and knowledge about the birth process *to collect data for the plan of care.*

Provide information about the labour process *to correct any misconceptions.*

Inform the woman about her labour status and fetus's well-being *to promote comfort and confidence.*

Discuss rationales for all interventions *to incorporate the woman into the plan of care.*

Incorporate nonpharmacological interventions into the plan of care *to increase the woman's sense of control during labour.*

Provide emotional support and ongoing positive feedback *to enhance positive coping mechanisms.*

Acupressure and Acupuncture

Acupressure techniques can be used in pregnancy and labour as well as postpartum to relieve pain and other discomforts. Pressure, heat, or cold is applied to acupuncture points termed *tsubos*. These points have an increased density of neuroreceptors and increased electrical conductivity. Acupressure is best applied over the skin without using lubricants. Pressure is usually applied with the heel of the hand, fist, or pads of the thumbs and fingers (Fig. 16-8). Synchronized breathing by the caregiver and the woman is suggested for greater effectiveness. Acupressure points are found on the neck; shoulders; hands; lower back, including sacral points; hips; area below the kneecaps; ankles; nails on the small toes; and soles of the feet.

Acupuncture is the insertion of fine needles into specific areas of the body to restore the flow of qi (energy) and decrease pain, which is thought to be obstructing the flow of energy. It should be done by a trained certified therapist. Current evidence indicates that acupuncture may be beneficial for relief of labour pain; however, further study is indicated (Florence & Palmer, 2003; Smith et al., 2006).

Application of Heat and Cold

Warmed blankets, warm compresses, heated rice bags, a warm bath or shower, or a moist heating pad can enhance relaxation and reduce pain during labour. Heat relieves muscle ischemia and increases blood flow to the area of discomfort. Heat application is effective for back pain caused by a posterior presentation or general backache from fatigue.

Cold application such as cool cloths or ice packs applied to the back, chest, and/or face during labour may be effective in increasing comfort when the woman feels warm. They may also be applied to areas of pain. Cold is often more effective for back pain caused by the posterior presentation. Cooling relieves pain by lowering the muscle temperature and relieving muscle spasms. A woman's culture may make the use of cold during labour unacceptable (Simkin & Bolding, 2004).

Cold will work for longer periods of time than heat, but heat and cold may be used alternately for a greater effect. Neither heat nor cold should be applied over ischemic or anaesthetized areas because tissues can be damaged. One or two layers of cloth should be placed between the skin and a hot or cold pack to prevent damage to the underlying integument (Simkin & Bolding, 2004).

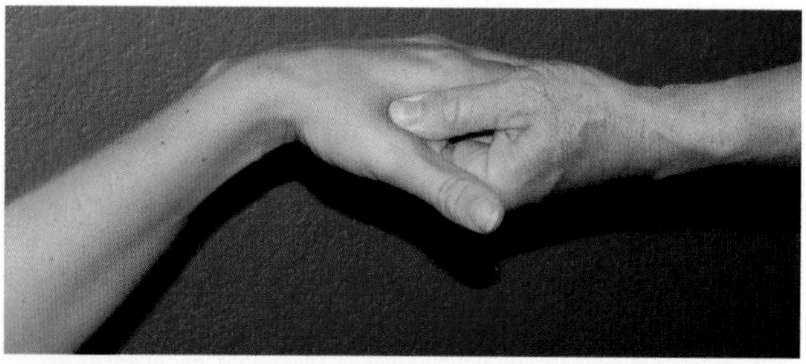

Fig. 16-8 Ho-Ku acupressure point (back of hand where thumb and index finger come together) used to enhance uterine contractions without increasing pain. *(Courtesy Julie Perry Nelson, Loveland, CO.)*

Hypnosis

Although hypnosis is not commonly used for pain management in Canada, it is associated with shorter labour, less analgesia, and higher 1-minute Apgar scores (VandeVusse et al., 2007). Current evidence suggests that hypnosis may relieve pain, increase the likelihood of vaginal birth, reduce the use of oxytocin, and enhance maternal satisfaction. Further research is required to confirm these potentially promising outcomes (Simkin & Bolding, 2004; Smith et al., 2006). Hypnosis techniques used for labour and birth place an emphasis on relaxation and diminishing fear, anxiety, and perception of pain (see earlier discussion of HypnoBirthing). The woman may be given direct suggestions about pain relief or indirect suggestions that she is experiencing diminished sensations. The woman receives posthypnotic suggestions such as "You will be able to push the baby out easily," to increase her confidence. To be successful, the woman must be educated extensively about hypnosis and practice the techniques during the prenatal period.

Biofeedback

Biofeedback is a relaxation technique that can be used for labour. It is based on the theory that, if a person can recognize physical signals, certain internal physiological events can be changed (i.e., whatever signs the woman has that are associated with her pain). For biofeedback to be effective, the woman must be educated during the prenatal period to become aware of her body and its responses and how to relax. The woman must learn how to use thinking and mental processes (e.g., focusing) to control body responses and functions. Informal biofeedback helps couples develop awareness of their bodies and learn strategies to change their responses to stress. If the woman responds to pain during a contraction with tightening of muscles, frowning, moaning, and breath holding, her partner can use verbal and touch feedback to help her relax. Formal biofeedback, which uses machines to detect skin temperature, blood flow, or muscle tension, also can prepare women to intensify their relaxation responses.

Aromatherapy

Aromatherapy uses oils distilled from plants, flowers, herbs, and trees to promote health and well-being and to treat illnesses. The use of herbal teas and vapours is reported to have positive effects in pregnancy and labour for some women. Lavender, clary sage, and bergamot promote relaxation and can be used by adding a few drops to a warm bath, to warm water used for soaking compresses applied to the body, to an aromatherapy lamp to vapourize a room, or to oil for a back massage. Drops of essential oils can also be put on a pillow or on a woman's brow or palms (Simkin & Bolding, 2004). Certain odours or scents can evoke pleasant memories and feelings of love and security. Before labour, the woman should choose the scents that she will use (Trout, 2004). Currently there is insufficient evidence to support the effectiveness of aromatherapy for pain relief in labour, although its use has elicited promising results (Smith et al., 2006).

NURSING ALERT Never apply the essential oils used for aromatherapy full strength directly to the skin. Most oils should be diluted in a vegetable oil base before use. Essential oils vary in terms of safe use during pregnancy. Inhaling vapours from the oils can lead to unpleasant adverse effects, including nausea or headaches.

Intradermal Sterile Water Block

An intradermal water block involves the injection of small amounts of **sterile** water (e.g., 0.05 to 0.1 mL) by using a fine needle (e.g., 25-gauge) into four locations on the lower back to relieve back pain (Fig. 16-9). It may be effective in early labour and in delaying the initiation of pharmacological pain-relief measures. Stinging will occur for about 20 to 30 seconds after injection, but back pain will be relieved for approximately 45 minutes to 2 hours. Effectiveness of this method may be related to the mechanisms of counterirritation (i.e., reducing localized pain in one area by irritating the skin in an area nearby), gate control, or an increase in the level of endogenous opioids (endorphins). When the effect wears off, the treatment can be repeated, or another method of pain relief can be used (Simkin & O'Hara, 2002).

Position Changes

All of the above comfort strategies should be combined with upright and gravity-enhancing positions, such as walking, slow dancing, and rocking. Rhythmic motion stimulates mechanoreceptors in the brain, which decreases pain perception and may enhance the labour process as it allows the fetus to move through the birth canal more easily. Labouring women will often find a position that feels right to them, although they should be encouraged to change their position every 20 to 30 minutes.

Pharmacological Management of Discomfort

When nonpharmacological pain-relief measures are no longer effective, the woman and her care provider may consider pharmacological measures for pain management. When pharmacological and nonpharmacological measures are used together, they increase the level of pain relief. Pharmacological measures can be implemented as labour becomes more active and discomfort and pain intensify, and when the woman decides that nonpharmacological methods are not working (see Fig. 16-3). Since 1981 more women have been taking advantage of pharmacological measures and fewer opt for no pharmacological support. The largest increase was noted in the use of **epidural** forms of analgesia (Bucklin et al., 2005).

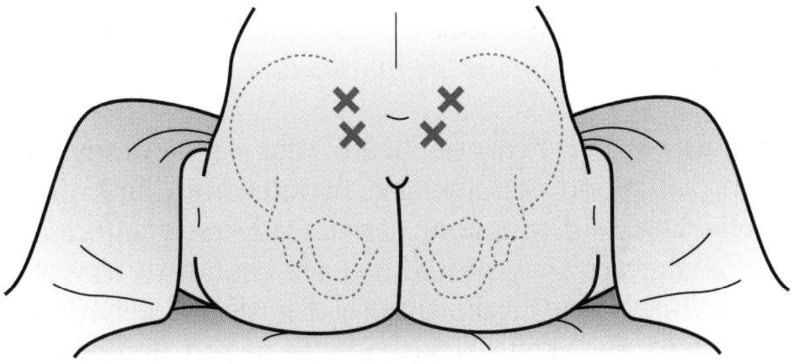

Fig. 16-9 Intradermal injections of 0.1 mL of sterile water in the treatment of women with back pain during labour. Sterile water is injected into four locations on the lower back, two over each posterior superior iliac spine (PSIS) and two 3 cm below and 1 cm medial to the PSIS. The injections should raise a bleb on the skin. Simultaneous injections administered by two clinicians decreases the pain of the injections. *(Courtesy Michael Norviel.)*

Sedatives

Sedatives relieve anxiety and induce sleep. They can be given to a woman when she is having a prolonged latent phase of labour or when there is a need to decrease anxiety or promote sleep. They can also be given to augment analgesics and reduce nausea when an opioid is used. Barbiturates such as secobarbital sodium (Seconal) can cause undesirable adverse effects, including respiratory and vasomotor depression that affects the woman and newborn. These effects are increased if a barbiturate is administered with another central nervous system (CNS) depressant such as an opioid analgesic. However, pain will be magnified if a barbiturate is given without an analgesic to women experiencing pain. Because of these disadvantages, barbiturates are seldom used.

Phenothiazines (e.g., promethazine [Phenergan], hydroxyzine [Atarax]) do not relieve pain but decrease anxiety and apprehension, increase sedation, and potentiate opioid analgesic effects. This potentiation effect causes the two drugs to work together more effectively so the opioid dose can be reduced. They can also be used to reduce the nausea and vomiting that often accompany opioid use. Metoclopramide (Maxeran) is an antiemetic that also can be used for this purpose.

Benzodiazepines (e.g., diazepam [Valium], lorazepam [Ativan]), when given with an opioid analgesic, seem to enhance pain relief and reduce nausea and vomiting, although the increased sedation experienced may be unacceptable to women in labour (Lehne, 2007).

Analgesia and Anaesthesia

The ideal obstetrical **analgesic** or **anaesthetic** provides adequate pain relief to women without increasing maternal or fetal risk or affecting the progress of labour. Nursing management of obstetrical analgesia and anaesthesia combines the nurse's expertise in maternity care with a knowledge and understanding of anatomy and physiology and of medications and their therapeutic effects, adverse reactions, and methods of administration.

The term *analgesia* refers to the alleviation of the sensation of pain or the raising of the threshold for pain perception without loss of consciousness.

Anaesthesia encompasses analgesia, amnesia, relaxation, and reflex activity. Anaesthesia abolishes pain perception by interrupting the nerve impulses to the brain. The loss of sensation may be partial or complete, sometimes with the loss of consciousness.

The type of analgesic or anaesthetic chosen is determined in part by the stage of labour and the method of birth planned (Box 16-4).

BOX 16-4 Pharmacological Control of Discomfort by Stage of Labour and Method of Birth

First Stage

Systemic analgesia
- Opioid agonist analgesics
- Opioid agonist–antagonist analgesics, co-drugs

Epidural (block) analgesia
Combined spinal–epidural (CSE) analgesia
Nitrous oxide

Second Stage

Nerve block analgesia/anaesthesia
- Local infiltration anaesthesia
- Pudendal block
- Spinal (block) anaesthesia
- Epidural (block) analgesia
- CSE analgesia

Nitrous oxide

Caesarean Birth

Spinal (block) anaesthesia
Epidural (block) anaesthesia
General anaesthesia

Systemic Analgesia

Systemic analgesia remains the major method of analgesia for the woman in labour when personnel trained in **regional analgesia** (i.e., epidural analgesia) are not available. It is a form of care with a trade-off between beneficial and adverse effects (Enkin et al., 2000). Systemic analgesics cross the blood–brain barrier to provide central analgesic effects. They also cross through the placenta. Once transferred to the fetus, analgesics cross the fetal blood–brain barrier more readily than the maternal blood–brain barrier. The duration of action will be longer in the fetus and newborn because the systemic analgesics used during labour have a significantly longer half-life in the fetus and newborn. Effects on the fetus and the newborn can be profound (e.g., respiratory depression, decreased alertness, delayed sucking), depending on the characteristics of the specific systemic analgesic used, the dosage given, and the route and timing of administration.

Intravenous (IV) administration is preferred to intramuscular (IM) administration because the onset of action of the medication is faster and more predictable; as a result, a higher level of pain relief usually occurs. IV patient-controlled analgesia is available in some locations for use during labour. With this method, the woman self-administers small doses of an opioid analgesic by using a pump programmed for dose and frequency. Overall, a lower total amount of analgesic is used, and maternal satisfaction is high. Classifications of analgesic medications used to relieve the pain of childbirth include opioid (narcotic) agonists and opioid (narcotic) agonist–antagonist compounds.

Choice of which medication to use often depends on preferences of the primary health care provider and the characteristics of the labouring woman. Types of systemic analgesics used may also vary from one obstetrical unit to another.

MEDICATION GUIDE

Opioid Agonist Analgesics: Hydromorphone Hydrochloride (Dilaudid)

Action

Opioid agonist analgesics stimulate mu and kappa opioid receptors to decrease transmission of pain impulses.

Indication

Moderate-to-severe labour pain; postoperative pain after Caesarean birth

Dosage and Route

Hydromorphone hydrochloride—1 mg IV every 3 hours as needed; 1 to 2 mg IM, may repeat in 3 to 6 hours if needed; or 3 to 4 mg, may repeat in 4 to 6 hours if needed

Adverse Effects

Nausea and vomiting, sedation, confusion, drowsiness, tachycardia or bradycardia, hypotension, dry mouth, pruritus, urinary retention, respiratory depression (woman and newborn), decreased fetal heart rate (FHR) variability, decreased uterine activity if given in early labour

Nursing Considerations

Assess maternal vital signs, degree of pain, FHR and pattern, and uterine activity before and after administration. Observe for respiratory depression, notifying primary health care provider if maternal respirations are 12 breaths/min or less. Encourage voiding every 2 hours and palpate for bladder distension. Administer with a phenothiazine or benzodiazepine, if ordered, to potentiate the analgesic effect, enhance sedation, and decrease nausea and vomiting. If birth occurs within 1 to 4 hours of dose, observe newborn for respiratory depression; have naloxone available as antidote. Implement safety measures as appropriate, including use of side rails and assistance with ambulation. Continue use of nonpharmacological pain-relief measures.

Opioid (Narcotic) Agonist Analgesics

Opioid agonist analgesics such as hydromorphone (Dilaudid), fentanyl (Sublimaze), and sufentanil citrate (Sufenta) are effective for the relief of severe, persistent, or recurrent pain. They have no amnesic effect but create a feeling of well-being or euphoria (see Medication Guide). These analgesics decrease gastric emptying and increase nausea and vomiting. Bladder and bowel elimination can be inhibited.

NURSING ALERT Because heart rate (e.g., bradycardia, tachycardia), blood pressure (e.g., hypotension), and respiratory effort (e.g., depression) can be adversely affected by opioid analgesics, they should be used cautiously in women with respiratory and cardiovascular disorders. Safety precautions should be taken because sedation and dizziness can occur after administration, increasing the risk for injury.

Women who receive opioids for their labour pain have less effective pain relief and are less satisfied with their pain management method than women whose pain is managed by using epidural analgesia. However, opioid use is associated with shorter labours, less oxytocin augmentation, and fewer instrumental vaginal births (e.g., forceps- or vacuum-assisted birth) than with epidural analgesia.

Meperidine hydrochloride (Demerol) used to be the most commonly used opioid agonist analgesic for women in labour, but it is no longer the preferred choice because other medications have fewer adverse effects. Its short half-life requires more frequent administration, increasing the risk for adverse reactions (e.g., dysphoria, irritability, seizures, tremors) related to the accumulation of a toxic metabolite (Lehne, 2007).

Fentanyl citrate (Sublimaze) and sufentanil citrate (Sufenta) are potent, short-acting opioid agonist analgesics (see Medication Guide). Sufentanil use is increasing because it has a more potent analgesic action than that of fentanyl when given via epidural. In addition, less sufentanil crosses the placenta, resulting in reduced fetal exposure. Onset of action after IV injection of either fentanyl or sufentanil occurs within 2 to 5 minutes; the action peaks in 3 to 5 minutes, and the duration of action is 30 to 60 minutes. More frequent dosing is required with fentanyl and sufentanil because of their relatively short duration of action. As a result, these opioids are most commonly administered **intrathecally** or via epidural, alone or in combination with a local anaesthetic agent (e.g., bupivacaine) (Lehne, 2007).

Opioid (Narcotic) Agonist–Antagonist Analgesics

An **agonist** is an agent that activates or stimulates a receptor to act; an **antagonist** is an agent that blocks a receptor or a medication designed to activate a receptor. Opioid agonist–antagonist compounds such as nalbuphine (Nubain) in the doses used during labour provide analgesia without causing respiratory depression in the mother or the neonate (see Medication Guide). This is less likely to cause nausea and vomiting, but sedation may be as great or greater when compared with pure opioid agonists. While both IM and IV routes are used for administration, the IV route is preferred. Nalbuphine is not suitable for women with an opioid dependence because the antagonist activity could precipitate withdrawal symptoms (abstinence syndrome) in both the mother and her newborn (Box 16-5).

Opioid (Narcotic) Antagonists

Opioids such as hydromorphone and fentanyl can cause excessive CNS depression in the mother and newborn. Current practice of giving lower doses of opioids intravenously has reduced the incidence and severity of opioid-induced CNS depression. Opioid antagonists such as naloxone (Narcan) can promptly reverse the CNS depressant effects, especially respiratory depression (see Medication Guide). In addition, the antagonist counters the effect of stress-induced levels of endorphins. An opioid antagonist is especially valuable if labour is more rapid than expected and birth is anticipated when the opioid is at its peak effect.

MEDICATION GUIDE

Fentanyl (Sublimaze) and Sufentanil (Sufenta)

Action

Opioid analgesics, rapid action with short duration (1 to 2 hours intramuscularly; 30 minutes to 1 hour intravenously)

Indication

For epidural or intrathecal analgesia, alone or in combination with a local anaesthetic

Dosage and Route

Fentanyl—50 to 100 mcg intramuscularly; 25 to 50 mcg intravenously

Epidural—fentanyl, 1 to 2 mcg with 0.125% bupivacaine at a rate of 8 to 10 mL/hr; sufentanil, 1 mcg with 0.125% bupivacaine at rate of 10 mL/hr

Adverse Effects

Dizziness, drowsiness, allergic reactions, rash, pruritus, respiratory depression, nausea and vomiting, urinary retention

Nursing Considerations

Assess for respiratory depression; naloxone should be available as antidote. Medication is administered by a physician.

BOX 16-5 Signs of Potential Complications—Maternal Opioid Abstinence Syndrome (Opioid/Narcotic Withdrawal)

- Yawning, rhinorrhea (runny nose), sweating, lacrimation (tearing), mydriasis (dilation of pupils)
- Anorexia
- Irritability, restlessness, generalized anxiety
- Tremors
- Chills and hot flashes
- Piloerection ("gooseflesh")
- Violent sneezing
- Weakness, fatigue, and drowsiness
- Nausea and vomiting
- Diarrhea, abdominal cramps
- Bone and muscle pain, muscle spasm, kicking movements

MEDICATION GUIDE

Opioid Agonist–Antagonist Analgesics: Nalbuphine (Nubain)

Action

Mixed agonist-antagonist analgesic; stimulates kappa opioid receptor and blocks mu opioid receptor

Indication

Labour pain; postoperative pain after Caesarean birth

Dosage and Route

10 mg intravenously; 10 to 20 mg intramuscularly q3-6h

Adverse Effects

Confusion, sedation, sweating; transient sinusoidal-like fetal heart rhythm; less respiratory depression, nausea, and vomiting

Nursing Considerations

See Medication Guide for hydromorphone hydrochloride (p. 408); may precipitate withdrawal symptoms in opioid-dependent women and their newborns. Nalbuphine IV may require a physician to administer, depending on hospital protocol.

MEDICATION GUIDE

Opioid Antagonist: Naloxone Hydrochloride (Narcan)

Action

Opioid antagonist that blocks both mu and kappa opioid receptors from the effects of opioid agonists

Indication

Reverses opioid-induced respiratory depression in woman or newborn; may be used to reverse pruritus from epidural opioids

Dosage and Route

Adult: Opioid overdose—0.4 to 2 mg intravenously, may repeat IV at 2- to 3-minute intervals up to 10 mg; if IV route unavailable, IM or SC administration may be used

Adult: Postoperative opioid depression—Initial dose 0.1 to 0.2 mg IV at 2- to 3-minute intervals up to three doses to desired degree of reversal obtained; may repeat dose in 1 to 2 hours if needed

Newborn: Opioid-induced depression—Initial dose is 0.1 mg/kg intravenously, intramuscularly, or subcutaneously; may be repeated at 2- to 3-minute intervals up to three doses until desired degree of reversal is obtained

Adverse Effects

Maternal hypotension and hypertension, tachycardia, hyperventilation, nausea and vomiting, sweating, and tremulousness

Nursing Considerations

The woman should delay breastfeeding until medication is out of her system; do not give to the mother or newborn if the woman is opioid dependent as it may cause abrupt withdrawal in the woman and newborn if given to the woman for reversal of respiratory depression caused by opioid analgesic; pain will return suddenly.

NURSING ALERT Although adults and newborns receive the same medication, the dosage is different for naloxone. It is important to ensure that the correct dose is given.

The antagonist may be given through the woman's IV line or it can be administered intramuscularly. The woman should be told the pain that was relieved with the use of the opioid analgesic will return with the administration of the opioid antagonist. Some authorities believe that unless maternal CNS depression is severe enough to affect her well-being and that of her fetus, the woman should not receive naloxone just before birth, in an attempt to prevent neonatal CNS depression. Placental transfer of naloxone is unpredictable; the newborn may not require treatment with an opioid antagonist; and the sudden return of severe pain could have adverse physiological and psychological effects on the mother (Lehne, 2007).

NURSING ALERT An opioid antagonist is contraindicated for an infant of an opioid-dependent woman because it may precipitate abstinence syndrome (withdrawal symptoms) (see Box 16-5).

An opioid antagonist can be given to the newborn as one part of the treatment for neonatal narcosis, which is a state of CNS depression in the newborn caused by an opioid. Prophylactic administration of naloxone is controversial. Affected infants may exhibit respiratory depression, hypotonia, lethargy, and a delay in temperature regulation. Risk for hypoxia, hypercarbia, and acidosis increases if neonatal narcosis is not treated promptly. Treatment involves ventilation, administration of oxygen, and gentle stimulation. Naloxone is administered, if still required, to reverse CNS depression. More than one dose of naloxone may be required because its half-life is shorter than the half-life of opioids. Alterations in neurological and behavioural responses may be evident for as long as 2 to 4 days after birth. Some depression of attention and social responsiveness can be evident for up to 6 weeks after birth. The significance of these neurobehavioural changes is unknown (Lehne, 2007).

Nerve Block Analgesia and Anaesthesia

A variety of local anaesthetic agents are used in obstetrics to produce regional analgesia (some pain relief and **motor block**) and anaesthesia (complete pain relief and motor block). Most of these agents are related chemically to cocaine and end with the suffix -caine. This helps to identify a local anaesthetic.

The principal pharmacological effect of local anaesthetics is the temporary interruption of the conduction of nerve impulses, notably pain. Examples of common agents are lidocaine (Xylocaine), bupivacaine (Marcaine), tetracaine (Pontocaine), and mepivacaine (Carbocaine, Isocaine). The solution strength of the local anaesthetic agent and the amount used depend on the type of nerve block being performed.

In rare instances, people are sensitive (allergic) to one or more local anaesthetics. Such a reaction may include respiratory depression, hypotension, and other serious adverse effects. Epinephrine, antihistamines, oxygen, and supportive measures should reverse these effects. Sensitivity may be identified by administering minute amounts of the medication to test for an allergic reaction.

Local Infiltration Anaesthesia

Local infiltration anaesthesia of perineal tissues is commonly used when an **episiotomy** is to be performed or when lacerations must be sutured after birth in a woman who does not have regional anaesthesia. Rapid anaesthesia is produced by injecting 10 to 20 mL of 1% lidocaine into the skin and then subcutaneously into the region to be anaesthetized. Epinephrine often is added to the solution to localize and intensify the anaesthesia in a limited region and to prevent excessive bleeding and systemic absorption by constricting local blood vessels. Repeated injections will prolong the anaesthesia as long as needed.

Pudendal Nerve Block

Pudendal nerve block, administered late in the second stage of labour, is useful if an episiotomy is to be performed or if forceps or a vacuum extractor is to be used to facilitate birth. It can also be administered during the third stage of labour if an episiotomy or lacerations have to be repaired. Its use has declined as a result of the increased use of epidural anaesthesia. Although it does not relieve pain from uterine contractions, it does relieve pain in the lower vagina, vulva, and perineum (Fig. 16-10, A). A pudendal nerve block must be administered 10 to 20 minutes before perineal anaesthesia is needed.

The pudendal nerve traverses the sacrosciatic notch just medial to the tip of the ischial spine on each side. Injection of an anaesthetic solution at or near these points anaesthetizes the pudendal nerves peripherally (Fig. 16-11). The transvaginal approach is generally used because it is less painful for the woman, has a higher rate of success in blocking pain, and tends to cause fewer fetal complications. Pudendal block does not change maternal hemodynamic or respiratory functions, vital signs, or FHR. However, the bearing-down reflex is lessened or lost completely.

Spinal Anaesthesia (Block)

In spinal anaesthesia (block) an anaesthetic solution containing a local anaesthetic alone or in combination with an opioid is injected through the third, fourth, or fifth lumbar interspace into the **subarachnoid space** (Fig. 16-12, A and B), where the anaesthetic solution mixes with cerebrospinal fluid (CSF). The use of this technique has increased for both elective and emergent Caesarean births and is more common than epidural anaesthesia for these types of births. Low spinal anaesthesia (block) may be used for vaginal birth, but it is not suitable for labour. Spinal anaesthesia (block) used for Caesarean birth provides anaesthesia from the nipple (T6) to the feet. If it is used for vaginal birth, the anaesthesia level is from the hips (T10) to the feet (see Fig. 16-12, C).

To initiate spinal anaesthesia (block), the woman needs to sit or to lie on her side (e.g., modified Sims position) with her back curved to widen the intervertebral space, to facilitate insertion of a small-gauge spinal needle and injection of the anaesthetic solution. The nurse needs to support the woman because she must remain still during placement of the spinal needle. The insertion is made between contractions. After the anaesthetic solution has been injected, the woman may be positioned upright to allow the heavier (hyperbaric) anaesthetic solution to flow downward, to obtain the lower level of anaesthesia suitable for a vaginal birth. She may be positioned supine with head and shoulders slightly elevated and the uterus displaced with a wedge under one of her hips, to obtain the higher level of anaesthesia desired for Caesarean birth (see Fig. 16-12, C). The anaesthetic effect usually begins 1 to 2 minutes after the anaesthetic solution is injected and lasts 1 to 3 hours, depending on the type of agent used.

Marked hypotension, impaired placental perfusion, and an ineffective breathing pattern may occur during any spinal anaesthesia. Before induction of the spinal anaesthetic (block), the woman's fluid balance should be assessed, and IV fluid is usually administered to decrease the potential for hypotension caused by sympathetic blockade (vasodilation with pooling of blood in the lower extremities decreases cardiac output). After induction of the anaesthetic, maternal blood pressure, pulse, and respirations and FHR must be checked and documented every 5 to 10 minutes. If signs of serious maternal hypotension (e.g., a drop in the baseline blood pressure of more than 20%) or abnormal fetal heart rate patterns (e.g., bradycardia, diminished variability, late decelerations) develop, emergency care must be given (see Emergency box).

Because the mother is not able to sense her contractions, she must be instructed when to bear down during a vaginal birth. Use of a combination of local anaesthetic agent and an opioid reduces the degree of motor function loss, thereby enhancing a woman's ability to push effectively. If the birth occurs in a delivery room (rather than a labour–delivery–recovery room), the woman will need assistance in the transfer to a recovery bed after expulsion of the placenta.

Advantages of spinal anaesthesia include ease of administration and absence of fetal hypoxia with maintenance of normotension. Maternal consciousness is maintained, excellent muscular relaxation is achieved, and blood loss is not excessive.

Disadvantages of spinal anaesthesia include medication reactions (e.g., **allergy**), hypotension, and an ineffective breathing pattern; cardiopulmonary resuscitation may be needed. When a spinal anaesthetic is given, the need for

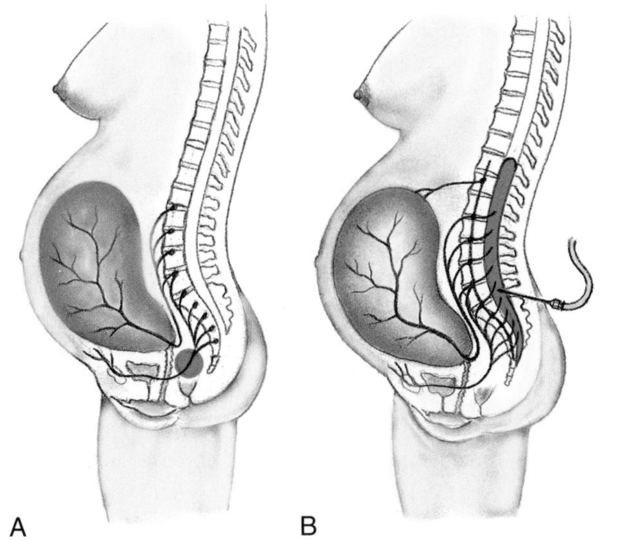

Fig. 16-10 Pain pathways and sites of pharmacological nerve blocks. **A:** Pudendal block; suitable during second and third stages of labour and for repair of episiotomy. **B:** Epidural block; suitable during all stages of labour and for repair of episiotomy.

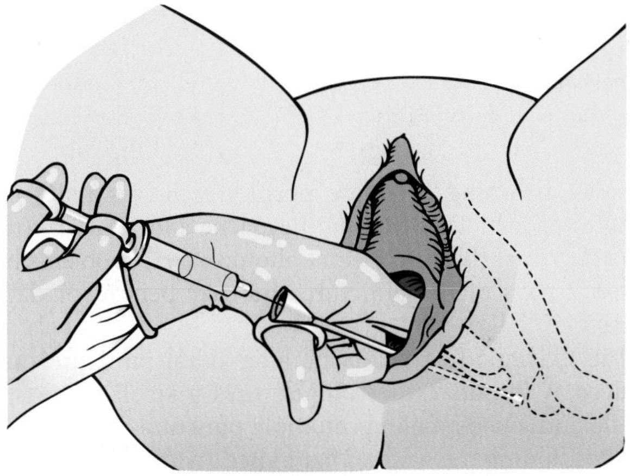

Fig. 16-11 Pudendal block. Use of needle guide ("Iowa trumpet") and Luer-Lok syringe to inject medication.

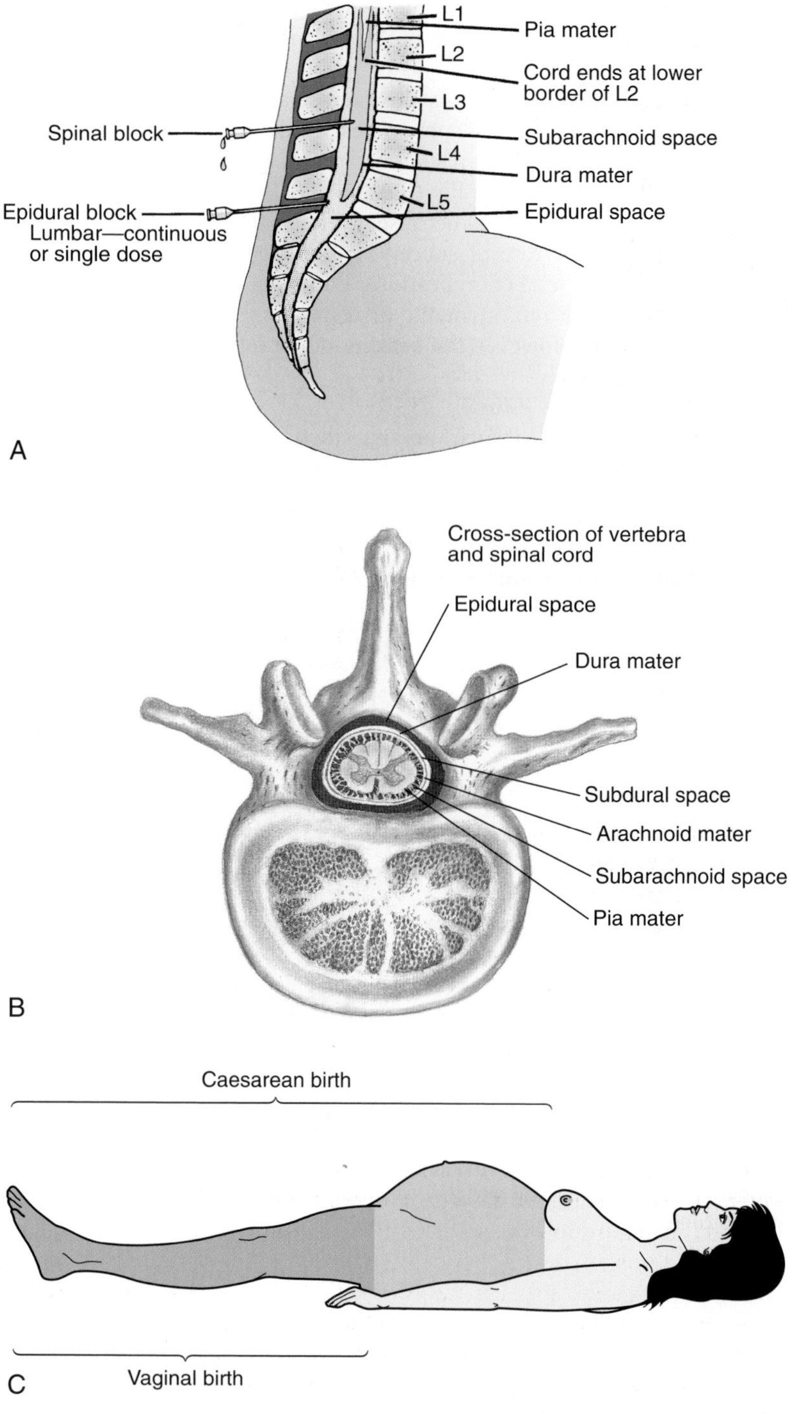

Fig. 16-12 **A:** Membranes and spaces of spinal cord and levels of sacral, lumbar, and thoracic nerves. **B:** Cross-section of vertebra and spinal cord. **C:** Levels of anaesthesia necessary for Caesarean and vaginal births.

operative delivery (i.e., episiotomy; forceps- or vacuum-assisted birth) tends to increase because voluntary expulsive efforts are reduced or eliminated. After birth, the incidence of bladder and uterine **atony** and postspinal headache is higher.

Postdural Puncture Headache. Leakage of CSF from the site of puncture of the dura mater (membranous covering of the spinal cord) is thought to be the major causative factor in postdural puncture headache (PDPH). Presumably, postural changes cause the diminished volume of CSF to exert traction on pain-sensitive CNS structures. Characteristically, assuming an upright position triggers or intensifies the headache, whereas assuming a supine position achieves relief in 30 minutes or less. The resulting headache and auditory (tinnitus) and visual (blurred vision, photophobia) problems begin within 2 days of the puncture and may persist for days or weeks.

The likelihood of headache after dural puncture can be reduced if the **anaesthesiologist** uses a small-gauge spinal needle and avoids making multiple punctures of the meninges. Positioning the woman flat in bed (with only a small, flat pillow for her head) for at least 8 hours after spinal anaesthesia also has been recommended to prevent headache, but no

EMERGENCY

Maternal Hypotension With Decreased Placental Perfusion

Signs/Symptoms

Maternal hypotension (20% drop from preblock level or less than 100 mm Hg systolic)
Fetal bradycardia
Decreased fetal heart rate variability

Interventions

Turn woman to lateral position or place pillow or wedge under hip (see Fig. 18-3, D) to deflect uterus.
Maintain intravenous infusion at rate specified, or increase as required per hospital protocol.
Administer oxygen by face mask at 10 to 12 L/min or per protocol.
Elevate woman's legs.
Notify physician, midwife, and anaesthesiologist.
Administer intravenous vasopressor (e.g., ephedrine) per protocol and physicians order.
Remain with the woman; continue to monitor maternal blood pressure and fetal heart rate every 5 minutes until her condition is stable or per primary health care provider's order.

definitive evidence shows that this measure is effective. Positioning the woman on her abdomen, a difficult if not impossible position after a Caesarean birth, is thought to decrease the loss of CSF through the puncture site. Hydration is purported to be of value in preventing and treating headache, but no compelling evidence supports its use (Cunningham et al., 2010). Initial treatment for PDPH usually includes oral analgesics; bed rest in a quiet, dimly lit or dark room; caffeine (oral liquids); and increased fluid intake.

An autologous epidural blood patch is the most rapid, reliable, and beneficial relief measure for PDPH. The woman's blood (i.e., 10 to 20 mL) is injected slowly into the lumbar epidural space, creating a clot that patches the tear or hole in the dura mater around the spinal cord. It is considered if the headache does not resolve spontaneously or after use of more conservative, noninvasive techniques (Fig. 16-13).

After the blood-patch procedure, the woman should be observed for alteration of vital signs, pallor, clammy skin, and leakage of CSF. A bandage and cold pack are placed on the puncture site, and the woman needs to rest in bed for approximately 1 hour. Discharge instructions include resting in bed for 24 to 48 hours, applying cold packs to the site as needed for comfort, avoiding analgesics that affect platelet aggregation (e.g., nonsteroidal anti-inflammatory drugs) for 2 days, drinking plenty of fluids, and observing for signs of infection at the site and neurological symptoms such as pain, numbness and tingling in legs, and difficulty with walking or elimination. The woman should be cautioned to avoid lifting, straining at stool, coughing, tub bathing, or swimming for at least 2 days.

Epidural Anaesthesia/Analgesia (Block)

Pain of uterine contractions and birth (vaginal and abdominal) can be relieved by injecting a suitable local anaesthetic agent (e.g., bupivacaine), an opioid analgesic (e.g., fentanyl, sufentanil), or both into the epidural (peridural) space. Injection is made between the fourth and fifth lumbar vertebrae for a lumbar epidural block (see Figs. 16-10, B, and 16-12, A). Depending on the type and amount of medication(s) used, an anaesthetic or analgesic effect will occur with varying degrees of motor impairment. The combination of an opioid with the local anaesthetic agent reduces the dose of anaesthetic required, thereby preserving a greater degree of motor function (McCool et al., 2004).

Lumbar epidural analgesia is the most effective pharmacological pain-relief method for labour currently available. As a result, it is the most commonly used method for relieving pain during labour in Canada. In 2006, just over one-half of Canadian women used epidural analgesia for their pain care during labour (PHAC, 2009) (Box 16-6). For relieving the discomfort of labour and vaginal birth, a block from T10 to S5 is required. For Caesarean birth, a block from at least T8 to S1 is essential

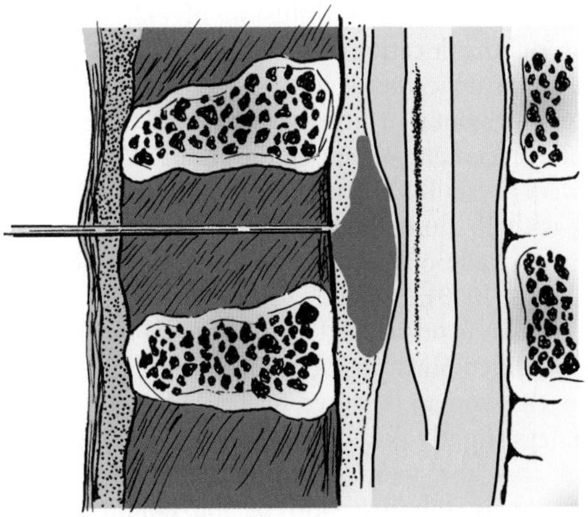

Fig. 16-13 Blood-patch therapy for spinal headache.

BOX 16-6 Do Women Have a Choice for Labour Analgesia?

"A technological birthing model that uses labour induction, epidural analgesia, continuous electronic fetal monitoring, and Cesarean delivery increasingly dominates labour and delivery wards in industrialized countries" (Leeman et al., 2003a). It is unknown whether the use of epidural analgesia by women in labour in Canada is a true preference or if it is selected because the only other choice is parenteral opioids. The rate of use of epidural analgesia is high in highly technological teaching hospitals. There is ample evidence of the benefits of the use of doulas and continuous support in labour, yet many women are not offered these options. Do women really have choices for pain management if they are not offered alternative pain strategies? Research is needed to discover which pain-relief methods women would choose if they were offered a wide range of options (Leeman et al., 2003b).

evolve Critical Thinking Exercise—Patient Receiving Epidural Block (see Fig. 16-12, C). The diffusion of epidural anaesthesia depends on the location of the catheter tip, the dose and volume of the anaesthetic agent used, and the woman's position (e.g., horizontal or head-up position).

Before placement of the epidural, an IV bolus of 500 to 1000 mL of crystalloids is usually given, although routine preloading with IV fluids before epidural analgesia is a form of care with a trade-off between beneficial and adverse effects (Enkin et al., 2000).

The woman is positioned as for a spinal block (i.e., sitting) or in a modified Sims position. For the modified lateral Sims position, the woman is placed on her side with her shoulders parallel, legs slightly flexed, and back arched (Fig. 16-14). It is essential that the woman maintain her position without moving during the insertion of the epidural catheter, to prevent misplacement, neurological injury, or hematoma formation. The nurse needs to remain at the woman's side and provide support during the procedure.

After the epidural has been placed, the woman should be positioned on her side, if possible, so that the uterus does not compress the ascending vena cava and descending aorta, which can impair venous return, reduce cardiac output, and decrease placental perfusion. Her position should be alternated from side to side at least every hour. Upright positions and ambulation may be encouraged, depending on the degree of motor impairment. Oxygen should be available to treat hypotension should it occur despite maintenance of hydration with IV fluid and displacement of the uterus to the side. Blood pressure should be monitored every 5 to 10 minutes for the first 30 minutes after insertion. Ephedrine (a vasopressor used to increase maternal blood pressure) and increased IV fluid infusion may be needed (see Emergency box). The FHR and progress in labour must be monitored because the woman in labour may not be aware of changes in strength of uterine contractions or of descent of the presenting part, although there is no evidence that supports the use of continuous electronic fetal monitoring. Intermittent auscultation is appropriate in many situations (Liston et al., 2007).

Several methods can be used for an epidural block. The most commonly used method is the continuous block, achieved by using a pump to infuse the anaesthetic solution through an indwelling plastic catheter. The least common method is an intermittent block, which is achieved by using repeated injections of anaesthetic solution. Patient-controlled epidural analgesia requires an indwelling catheter and a programmed pump that allows the woman to control the dosing. This method enhances a woman's sense of control over her labour and has been found to decrease the total amount of medication used.

The advantages of an epidural block include the following: the woman remains alert and is more comfortable and able to participate; good relaxation is achieved; airway reflexes remain

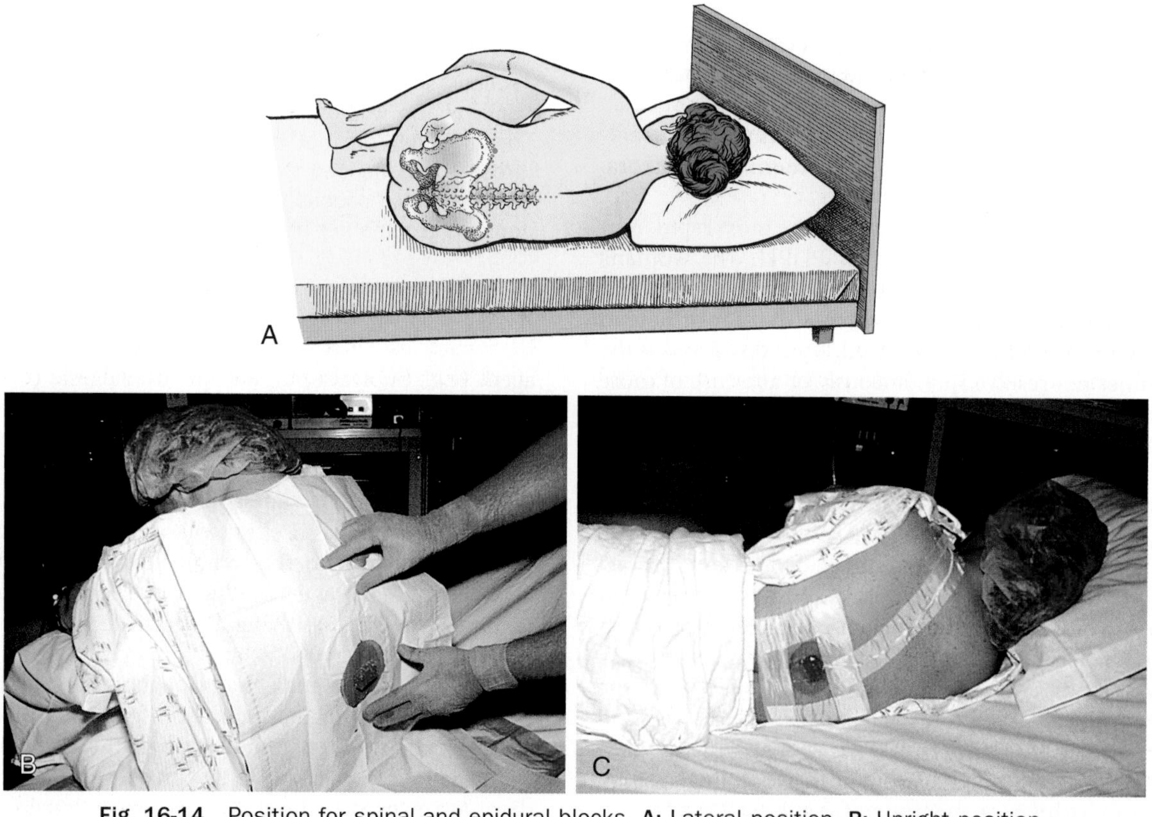

Fig. 16-14 Position for spinal and epidural blocks. **A:** Lateral position. **B:** Upright position. **C:** Catheter is taped to woman's back with port segment located near her shoulder. *(**B** and **C**, Courtesy Michael S. Clement, MD, Mesa, AZ.)*

intact; only partial motor paralysis develops; gastric emptying is not delayed; and blood loss is not excessive. Fetal complications are rare but may occur in the event of rapid absorption of the medication or marked maternal hypotension. The dose, volume, and type of medication(s) used can be modified to allow the woman to push; assume upright positions and walk; produce perineal anaesthesia; and permit forceps-assisted, vacuum-assisted, or Caesarean birth, if required (Cunningham et al., 2010).

The disadvantages of an epidural block are also numerous. Length of labour is longer; there are increased requirements for oxygen and oxytocin (Kukulu & Demirok, 2008). The woman's ability to move freely and maintain control of her labour is limited, related to the use of numerous medical interventions (e.g., an IV infusion, electronic monitoring, catheterization), the occurrence of orthostatic hypotension and dizziness, sedation, and weakness of the legs. CNS effects such as excitation, bizarre behaviour, tinnitus, disorientation, paresthesia, and convulsions can occur if a solution containing a local anaesthetic agent is accidentally injected into a blood vessel. Respiratory arrest can occur if the relatively high dosage used with an epidural block is accidentally injected into the subarachnoid space. Women who receive an epidural have an increased risk for hyperthermia (i.e., **intrapartum** temperature of 38°C or higher), especially when labour lasts longer that 12 hours. The temperature elevation most likely is related to thermoregulatory changes, although infection cannot be ruled out. The elevation in temperature can result in fetal tachycardia and neonatal workup for sepsis, regardless of whether signs of infection are present.

Severe hypotension (more than a 20% decrease in baseline blood pressure) as a result of sympathetic blockade can be an outcome of an epidural block (see Emergency box). It can result in a significant decrease in uteroplacental perfusion and oxygen delivery to the fetus (Anim-Somuah, Smyth, & Howell, 2005). Urinary retention and stress incontinence can occur in the immediate postpartum period. This temporary difficulty in urinary elimination could be related not only to the effects of the epidural block but also to the increased duration of labour and need for instrumental birth associated with the block. **Pruritus** (itching) is an adverse effect associated with the use of an opioid, including fentanyl and morphine. A relation between epidural analgesia and longer labour, increased incidence of fetal malposition, use of oxytocin, and forceps- or vacuum-assisted birth has been documented.

Research findings have been unable to demonstrate a significant increase in Caesarean birth associated with epidural analgesia (Anim-Somuah et al., 2005), although instrumental delivery rates are higher, as is the incidence of persistent occiput posterior positions. The adverse effects of epidurals can be minimized if administration occurs when the mother is in active labour (>4 cm dilated). Occasionally a PDPH can occur after accidental perforation of the dura mater during the administration of the epidural block. Because a larger needle is used for an epidural block, the risk for severe headache is higher as a result of greater CSF loss. For some women, the epidural block is not effective, and a second form of analgesia is required to establish effective pain relief. When women progress rapidly in labour, pain relief may not be obtained before birth occurs.

Combined Spinal–Epidural Analgesia

Use of opioids such as fentanyl and sufentanil to potentiate the effects of local anaesthetic agents reduces the amount of the local anaesthetic used, thereby reducing motor blockade. A combined spinal–epidural analgesia (CSEA) technique is an approach that can be used to block pain transmission without compromising motor ability (Kuczkowski, 2007). The opioid is injected into the subarachnoid space for rapid activation of the opioid receptors. A catheter is left in place in the epidural space to extend the duration of the analgesia by using a lower dose of a local anaesthetic agent alone or in combination with an opioid agonist analgesic. Although women can walk (hence the term *walking epidural*), they often choose not to do so because of sedation and fatigue, abnormal sensations in and weakness of the legs, and a feeling of insecurity. Often health care providers are reluctant to encourage or assist women to ambulate, for fear of injury. However, women can be assisted to change positions and use upright positions during labour and birth. Enhanced motor function facilitates more effective bearing-down efforts, thereby reducing the risk for forceps or vacuum-assisted birth (Mayberry et al., 2003; McCool et al., 2004).

CSEA may be associated with fetal bradycardia, necessitating close assessment of FHR and pattern. Since it involves both the puncture of the dura and the placement of a catheter in the epidural space, there is a higher risk for infection and PDPH.

Epidural and Intrathecal Opioids

Opioids also can be used alone, eliminating the effect of a local anaesthetic altogether. The use of epidural or intrathecal (spinal) opioids without the addition of a local anaesthetic agent during labour has several advantages. Opioids administered in this manner do not cause maternal hypotension or affect vital signs. The woman feels contractions but not pain. Her ability to bear down during the second stage of labour is preserved because the pushing reflex is not lost, and her motor power remains intact.

Fentanyl, sufentanil, or preservative-free morphine may be used. Fentanyl and sufentanil produce short-acting analgesia (i.e., 1.5 to 3.5 hours), and morphine may provide pain relief for 4 to 7 hours. Morphine may be combined with fentanyl or sufentanil. Short-acting opioids are often used in multiparous women, and morphine may be used in nulliparous women or women with a history of long labour. For most women, intrathecal opioids do not provide adequate analgesia for second-stage labour pain, episiotomy, or birth (Cunningham et al., 2010). Pudendal nerve blocks or local perineal infiltration anaesthesia may be necessary.

A more common indication for the administration of epidural or intrathecal analgesics is the relief of postoperative pain. For example, women who give birth by Caesarean section can receive fentanyl or morphine through a catheter. The catheter may then be removed; these women are usually free of pain for 24 hours. Occasionally, the catheter is left in place in the epidural space, in case another dose is needed.

Women who receive epidurally administered morphine after Caesarean birth are up soon after surgery with surprising ease and are able to care for their babies. Early ambulation and freedom from pain also facilitate bladder emptying, enhance peristalsis, and prevent clot formation in the lower extremities (e.g., thrombophlebitis). To those women who have had a previous Caesarean birth and experienced the usual postoperative pain, the effects of this approach seem miraculous. However, the mother may not understand why she may have pain after the opioid effect wears off.

Adverse effects of opioids administered by the epidural and intrathecal routes include nausea, vomiting, pruritus (itching), urinary retention, and delayed respiratory depression. These adverse effects are more common when morphine or fentanyl is administered. Antiemetics, antipruritics, and opioid antagonists are used to relieve these symptoms. For example, naloxone (Narcan), promethazine (Phenergan), or metoclopramide (Maxeran) may be administered. Hospital protocols should provide specific instructions for treatment of these adverse effects. Use of epidural opioids is not without risks. Respiratory depression is a serious concern; for this reason, the woman's respiratory rate should be assessed and documented every hour for 24 hours or per hospital protocol. Naloxone should be readily available for use if the respiratory rate decreases to less than 10 breaths/min or if the oxygen saturation rate decreases to less than 89%. Administration of oxygen by face mask may also be initiated, and the anaesthesia care provider should be notified.

Contraindications to Epidural Blocks. Contraindications to epidural analgesia or anaesthesia include the following:

- Acute antepartum hemorrhage—Acute hypovolemia leads to increased sympathetic tone to maintain the blood pressure; any anaesthetic technique that blocks the sympathetic fibres can produce significant hypotension that can endanger the mother and the baby.
- Anticoagulant therapy or bleeding disorder—If a woman is receiving anticoagulant therapy or has a bleeding disorder, injury to a blood vessel may cause the formation of a hematoma that may compress the cauda equina or the spinal cord and lead to serious CNS complications.
- Infection at the injection site—Infection can be spread through the peridural or subarachnoid spaces if the needle traverses an infected area.
- Allergy to the anaesthetic drug
- Maternal refusal or inability to cooperate
- Some types of maternal cardiac conditions

With an increase in the number of women who have body art and specifically low-back tattoos, there has been some concern over whether it is safe to give an epidural through a tattoo. The present recommendation is that an epidural should not be denied to someone with a low-back tattoo, although direct tattoo puncture should be avoided, if possible as there is potential for the epidural not to be effective (Mercier & Bonnet, 2009).

Effects of Epidural Block on Neonate. Debate persists concerning the effects of epidural anaesthesia and analgesia on the newborn's neurobehavioural responses. Findings from studies that examine associations between neurobehavioural outcome and epidural block are far from consistent. For example, studies comparing the neonatal neurobehavioural scores for infants born to mothers who did and mothers who did not receive epidural analgesia have shown little or no difference in the scores or have shown that the infants of mothers who received epidural anaesthesia did not score as well on neurobehavioural tests (Lieberman & O'Donoghue, 2002). Torvaldsen et al. (2006) found that women who received epidurals were less likely to fully breastfeed their newborns in the first few days after birth and discontinued breastfeeding earlier than women who did not receive epidurals. Women who receive epidural anaesthesia need adequate breastfeeding support after the birth.

Nitrous Oxide for Analgesia

Nitrous oxide mixed with oxygen can be inhaled in a low concentration (50% or less) to reduce but not eliminate pain during the first and second stages of labour. At the lower doses used for analgesia, the woman remains awake, and the danger of aspiration is avoided because the laryngeal reflexes are unaffected. It can be used in combination with other nonpharmacological and pharmacological measures for pain relief.

A face mask or mouthpiece is used to self-administer the gas. The woman should place the mask over her mouth and nose or insert the mouthpiece 30 seconds before the onset of a contraction (if regular) or as soon as a contraction begins (if irregular). When she inhales, a valve opens, and the gas is released. She should continue to inhale the gas slowly and deeply until the contraction starts to subside. When inhalation stops, the valve closes. Onset of action is 50 seconds; therefore, beginning the inhalation process 30 seconds before the onset of a contraction provides the best pain relief. During the interval between contractions, the woman should remove the device and breathe normally.

Most women who use nitrous oxide obtain adequate pain relief and are satisfied with the method. The nurse should observe the woman for nausea and vomiting, drowsiness, dizziness, hazy memory, and loss of consciousness. Loss of consciousness is more likely to occur if opioids are used with the nitrous oxide. The use of nitrous oxide does not appear to depress uterine contractions or cause adverse reactions in the fetus and newborn.

Nursing Care Management

The choice of pain relief depends on a combination of factors, including the woman's special needs and wishes, the availability of the desired method(s), the knowledge and expertise in nonpharmacological and pharmacological methods of the health care providers involved in the woman's care, and the phase and stage of labour (see Nursing Process box and Critical Thinking Exercise).

Informed Consent

The primary health care provider and anaesthesia care provider are responsible for informing women of the alternative methods of pharmacological pain relief available in the hospital. Nurses play a part in the informed consent process by clarifying and describing procedures and acting as the woman's advocate by asking the primary health care provider for further explanations.

NURSING PROCESS: PHARMACOLOGICAL PAIN RELIEF IN LABOUR

Assessment

The assessment of the woman, her fetus, and her labour is a joint effort of the nurse and the primary health care providers, who consult with the woman regarding their findings and recommendations. The assessment includes the following.

History

- Review prenatal record (parity, estimated date of birth, complications, medications)
- Allergies
- History of smoking; neurological and spinal disorders

Interview (by a Member of the Anaesthesia Care Team and the Nurse)

- Time of woman's last meal; type of food and fluid consumed
- Nature of existing respiratory condition (cold, allergy), allergies to medications, cleansing agents, or tape
- Childbirth preparation, knowledge and preferences for management of discomfort
- Type of analgesia or anaesthesia preferred (see Box 16-4)
- Herbal medications used
- Relevant events that have occurred since last contact with her primary health care provider
- If evidence of substance use, identify type of drug, last time drug taken, and method of administration

Physical Examination

- Character and status of labour and fetal response
- Maternal vital signs
- Fetal heart rate and pattern
- Uterine contractions
- Amniotic membranes and fluid
- Cervical effacement and dilation and station
- Length of labour and fatigue
- Hydration status (intake and output, mucous membranes, skin turgor, urine concentration)
- Bladder distension
- Signs of apprehension (fist clenching; restlessness)

Review of Results of Laboratory Tests

- Hemoglobin and hematocrit (anemia)
- Prothrombin time and platelet count (coagulopathy or bleeding disorder) (if ordered)
- White blood cell count and differential (infection) (if ordered)

Nursing Diagnoses

The following nursing diagnoses are relevant in the management of discomfort during labour and birth:

Acute pain related to

- processes of labour and birth

Risk for ineffective tissue perfusion related to

- effects of analgesia or anaesthesia
- maternal position

Anxiety or fear related to decreased knowledge base of

- procedure for nerve block analgesia
- expected sensation during nerve block analgesia

Risk for injury to fetus related to

- maternal hypotension
- maternal position (aortocaval compression)

Planning

A plan of care is developed for each woman to address her particular clinical and nursing problems. The nurse needs to collaborate with the primary health care provider, the anaesthesia care provider, and the labouring woman to select the aspects of care relevant to the woman and her family.

The expected outcomes for nursing care in the management of discomfort during labour and birth include the following:

- The woman will report the characteristics of her pain and discomfort and her level of coping.
- The woman will communicate understanding of her needs and rights with regard to pain-relief management that uses a variety of nonpharmacological and pharmacological methods reflecting her preferences.
- The woman will experience adequate pain relief without it adding to maternal risk (e.g., through the use of appropriate nonpharmacological methods and appropriate medication, including the appropriate dose, timing, and route of administration).
- The fetus will maintain well-being, and the neonate will adjust to extrauterine life without problems related to the management of maternal pain.

Interventions

Provide woman choice of pain management strategies and provide appropriate support.
Assist woman in use of nonpharmacological interventions.
Ensure informed consent to procedures and anaesthesia (see discussion below).
Administer pharmacological measures when requested by woman.
Prepare woman for procedures.
Monitor for sign of potential problems.
Protect woman and fetus from injury.
Monitor and record response to interventions.
Continue to provide supportive care.

Evaluation

Evaluation of the effectiveness of care of the woman needing management of discomfort during labour and birth is based on the previously stated outcomes.

CRITICAL THINKING EXERCISE

Pain Management

You are assigned to care for a 17-year-old, single, nulliparous woman in active labour who is thrashing about in her bed and requesting something for "this terrible pain." She did not attend childbirth preparation classes and is alone for labour. She has the PRN orders for pain that are routine on your unit. She can ambulate and has intermittent auscultation as appropriate for her stage of labour.

1. Evidence—Is there sufficient evidence to draw conclusions about what nonpharmacological and pharmacological pain-relief techniques can be instituted?
2. Assumptions—What assumptions can be made about the following issues?
   a. Reactions to pain of young, single woman who lacks support in labour
   b. Degree of pain relief expected by the woman
   c. Degree of pain relief expected by the nurse
   d. Nonpharmacological measures that are effective
3. What implications and priorities for nursing care can be drawn at this time?
4. Does the evidence objectively support your conclusion?
5. Are there alternative perspectives to your conclusion?

LEGAL TIP Informed Consent for Anaesthesia. The woman receives (in an understandable manner) all of the following:

- Explanation of the alternative methods of analgesia and anaesthesia available
- Description of anaesthetic and procedure for administration
- Description of the benefits, discomfort, risks, and consequences of the selected anaesthetic for the mother and the fetus
- Explanation of how complications can be treated
- Information that the anaesthetic is not always effective
- Indication that the woman may withdraw consent at any time
- Opportunity to have any questions answered
- Opportunity to explain in her own words components of the consent

Administration of Medication

Timing of Administration

Accurate monitoring of the progress of labour and assessment of the level of coping in the labouring woman assist the nurse in helping the woman decide when it is appropriate to start pharmacological control of discomfort. It is usually the nurse who notifies the primary health care provider when the woman needs pharmacological measures to relieve her discomfort. Knowledge of the medications used during childbirth is essential. The most effective route of administration is selected for each woman; then the medication is prepared and administered correctly.

Orders are often written for the administration of pain medication as needed by the woman and are based on the nurse's clinical judgement. Generally, pharmacological measures for pain relief are not implemented until labour has advanced to the active phase of the first stage of labour and the cervix is dilated approximately 4 to 5 cm, to avoid suppressing the progress of labour.

Preparation for Procedures

The nurse needs to review the methods of pain relief available to the woman (or validate her choices) and clarify information as necessary. The procedure and what will be asked of the woman (e.g., to maintain flexed position during insertion of epidural needle) must be explained. The woman can also benefit from knowing the route of administration of the medication, the degree of discomfort to expect from administration of the medication, the interval before the medication takes effect, and the expected pain relief from the medication. When an indwelling epidural catheter is to be threaded, the woman should be told that she may experience a momentary twinge down her leg, hip, or back and that this feeling is not a sign of injury.

A long needle is used for pudendal blocks (see Fig. 16-11). The sight of this needle may be frightening; the woman should be reassured that only the tip of the needle will be inserted.

Intravenous Route. The preferred route of administration of medications such as fentanyl and nalbuphine is through IV tubing administered into the port nearest the woman while the infusion of IV solution is stopped. The medication is given slowly in small doses at the beginning of a contraction and over three to five consecutive contractions. Because uterine blood vessels are constricted during contractions, the medication stays within the maternal vascular system for several seconds before the uterine blood vessels reopen. The IV infusion is then restarted slowly to prevent a bolus of medication from being administered. IV medications may be administered by a physician in some hospitals. With this method of injection, the amount of medication crossing the placenta to the fetus is minimized. The IV route has the following advantages:

- Onset of pain relief is rapid and more predictable.
- Pain relief is obtained with small doses of the drug.
- Duration of effect is more predictable.

Intramuscular Route. Although IM injections of analgesics are still used, they are not the preferred route of administration for the woman in labour. The advantages of using the IM route are its quick administration and no need to site an IV line.

Disadvantages of the IM route include the following:

- Onset of pain relief is delayed.
- Higher doses of medication are required.
- Medication is released at an unpredictable rate from the muscle tissue and is available for transfer across the placenta to the fetus.

IM injections given in the upper portion of the arm (deltoid site) seem to result in more rapid absorption and higher blood levels of the medication than do injections given in other sites. The deltoid is the preferred site if regional anaesthesia is planned later in labour because the autonomic blockage from the regional (e.g., epidural) anaesthesia causes blood flow to the gluteal region to be increased and accelerates absorption of the drug. The maternal plasma level of the drug necessary to bring pain relief usually is reached 45 minutes after IM injection, followed by a decline in plasma levels. The maternal drug levels (after IM injections) are unequal because of uneven distribution (maternal uptake) and metabolism.

Spinal/Epidural Nerve Blocks. An IV line needs to be established before induction of nerve blocks such as epidural and spinal blocks. Anaesthesia protocols often include the prophylactic administration of a bolus of IV fluid before epidural and spinal anaesthesia for blood volume expansion to prevent maternal hypotension. However, routine preloading with IV fluids before epidural analgesia involves a trade-off between beneficial and adverse effects (Enkin et al., 2000).

Lactated Ringer's and normal saline solutions are commonly used infusion solutions. Infusion solutions without dextrose are preferred, especially when the solution must be infused rapidly (e.g., to treat dehydration or maintain blood pressure) because solutions containing dextrose rapidly raise maternal blood glucose levels. The fetus responds to high blood glucose levels by increasing insulin production; fetal or neonatal hypoglycemia may result as the glucose is metabolized. In addition, dextrose changes osmotic pressure, so fluid is excreted from the kidneys more rapidly.

Because spinal nerve blocks can reduce bladder sensation, resulting in difficulty in voiding, the woman should empty her bladder before the induction of the block and should be encouraged to void at least every 2 hours thereafter. The nurse should palpate for bladder distension and measure urinary output to ensure that the bladder is being emptied completely. A distended bladder can inhibit uterine contractions and fetal descent, resulting in a slowing of the progress of labour. If a woman is unable to empty her bladder, a catheter may be necessary. An intermittent catheter is the preferred method, although occasionally an indwelling catheter may be considered. The status of the maternal–fetal unit and the progress of labour must be established before the block is performed. The nurse must assist the woman to assume and maintain the correct position for induction of epidural and spinal anaesthesia (see Fig. 16-14).

Signs of Potential Problems

The woman should be questioned about the use of herbal medications. There is potential for alternations in maternal hemodynamics (e.g., tachycardia, hypertension) and increased bleeding tendencies with herbal self-therapy (Kuczkowski, 2006).

Any medication can cause an allergic reaction that may be minor or as severe as anaphylaxis. Minor reactions can consist of a rash, rhinitis, fever, asthma, or pruritus. Management of the less acute allergic response is not an emergency. As part of the assessment for such allergic reactions, the nurse should monitor the woman's vital signs, respiratory status, cardiovascular status, platelet count, and white blood cell count. The woman should be observed for adverse effects of medications, especially drowsiness.

Severe allergic reactions may occur suddenly and lead to shock. The most dramatic form of anaphylaxis is sudden severe bronchospasm, vasospasm, severe hypotension, and death. Signs of anaphylaxis are largely caused by contraction of smooth muscles and may begin with irritability, extreme weakness, nausea, and vomiting. This may then lead to dyspnea, cyanosis, convulsions, and cardiac arrest. An acute allergic reaction—anaphylaxis—must be diagnosed and treated immediately. Treatment usually consists of 1:1000 epinephrine injected subcutaneously or intramuscularly, followed by parenteral administration of antihistamines. Supportive care is given to alleviate symptoms. The type of care is determined by the rapidly assessed cardiovascular and respiratory response of the woman to primary interventions. Cardiopulmonary resuscitation may be necessary. The nurse must also be alert to changes in fetal status: atypical or abnormal changes in FHR and pattern should be noted and reported to the primary health care provider.

Nursing Care and Safety

After a woman receives a spinal nerve block, she may not require massage and assistance with breathing but she will still need emotional support, reassurance, and information from the nurse. It is important to ensure that she receives reassurance and reminders that labour is still progressing. Having the woman feel the contractions with her hand will remind her of what is happening in her body. Some women may feel disappointed in themselves for requiring pain medication, and they need to be reassured regarding their decision.

Labouring women with a spinal block must be protected from injury by raising the side rails and placing a call bell within easy reach when the nurse is not in attendance. Oxygen and suction should be readily available at the bedside. The nurse must make sure that there is no prolonged pressure on an anaesthetized part (e.g., lying on one side with weight on one leg; tight bed linens on feet). If stirrups are used for birth, the nurse should pad them, adjust both stirrups to be at the same level and angle, and place both of the woman's legs into them while avoiding putting pressure on the popliteal angle.

To minimize the effects of an epidural, the woman should be assisted to remain as mobile as possible. When in bed, her position should be alternated from side to side a minimum of every hour to ensure adequate distribution of the anaesthetic solution, to maintain circulation to the uterus and placenta, and to facilitate descent of the fetus through the birth canal. The nurse can help the woman to assume upright positions such as sitting (e.g., modified throne position in which the woman sits on the bed with the bottom part lowered to place her feet below her body) (Fig. 16-15), the tug-of-war position (woman tugs on towel or sheet that is tied to the bar on the bed or held by the nurse), and squatting (by using the head of the bed or a squatting bar for support) (Fig. 16-16) in order to facilitate fetal descent and enhance bearing-down efforts (Gilder et al., 2002; Mayberry et al., 2003). Ambulation should

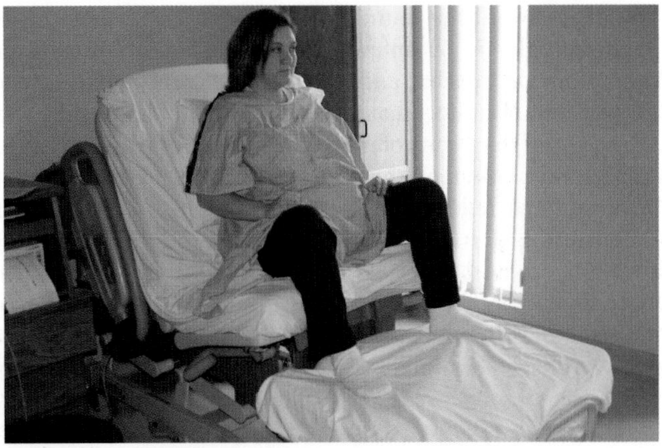

Fig. 16-15 Throne position. *(Courtesy Julie Perry Nelson, Loveland, CO.)*

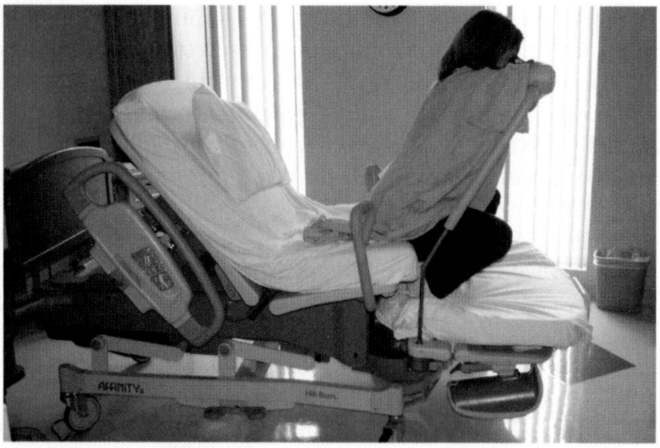

Fig. 16-16 Using squatting bar during labour. *(Courtesy Julie Perry Nelson, Loveland, CO.)*

be encouraged if the woman has received a "walking" epidural. Upright positions are important in the prevention of operative births (e.g., forceps- or vacuum-assisted birth). To prevent injury, the nurse must assess the level of motor function (e.g., three unassisted steps with accompaniment; standing and closing eyes, noting the degree of unsteadiness; ability to flex legs or rise from a supine position), level of sensation in the legs (e.g., degree of numbness), and level of sedation, before the woman is assisted out of bed and periodically thereafter (Mayberry et al., 2003). The woman should sit on the side of the bed before standing in order to determine whether orthostatic hypotension will occur. If she is not dizzy or light-headed, she can stand at the side of the bed and finally walk.

The second stage of labour is often prolonged in women who use epidural analgesia for pain management. Research evidence indicates that as long as the well-being of the mother and fetus is established, a period of "labouring down" to allow the fetus to descend and rotate with uterine contractions and the use of open-glottis pushing techniques when the fetus has reached a +1 station and is rotating to an anterior position are the best approaches to use for the management of second-stage labour (Mayberry, Clemmens, & De, 2002) (see Chapter 18 for a full discussion of second-stage labour management).

The nurse needs to monitor and record the woman's response to nonpharmacological pain-relief methods and medication(s). This includes the degree of pain relief, the level of apprehension, the return of sensations and perception of pain, and allergic or untoward reactions (e.g., hypotension, respiratory depression, and hypothermia). The nurse should continue to monitor maternal vital signs, blood pressure, strength and frequency of uterine contractions, changes in the cervix and station of the presenting part, presence of the bearing-down reflex, bladder filling, and state of hydration. Determining the fetal response after the administration of analgesia or anaesthesia is vital. The woman should be asked whether she (or the family) has any questions. The nurse needs to assess the woman's and her family's understanding of the need to ensure her safety (e.g., keeping side rails up, calling for assistance as needed).

The time that elapses between the administration of a narcotic and the baby's birth should be noted. Medication given to the newborn to reverse narcotic effects should also be recorded. After birth, the woman who has had spinal, epidural, or general anaesthesia needs to be assessed for return of sensory and motor function, in addition to the usual postpartum assessments.

Anaesthesia in the Obese Woman

Obesity is defined as a body mass index (BMI) of greater than 30 (see Table 4-1).

Maternal physiological changes are the product of hormonal influences and mechanical effects. In obese women, the weight of fat tissue and the subsequent added metabolic demands also affect maternal physiology. Both pregnancy and obesity cause blood volume and cardiac output to increase, and in the obese woman these levels expand in proportion to the amount of fat tissue. During labour and vaginal birth and in the immediate postpartum period, blood values and cardiac output in obese women can reach levels 80% greater than prelabour values. The enlarged uterus and abdominal fat mass also further increase the possibility of aortocaval compression.

The gastric emptying time is delayed, the tone of the cardiac sphincter is decreased, and the gastric contents are hyperacidic in all pregnant women. The obese woman is more likely to have a hiatal hernia and a marked increase in intragastric pressure and volume; therefore, these women are at great risk for regurgitation and aspiration.

Management of the obese woman during labour should focus on efforts to minimize oxygen consumption and maximize pulmonary function. Monitoring by pulse oximeter has been recommended. Epidural analgesia administered during the first stage of labour can bring about decreased demand on the metabolic and respiratory systems and improved oxygenation, because pain causes the catecholamine levels to increase, which in turn causes cardiac output to increase. Effective epidural analgesia retards this increase in catecholamine levels.

Epidural administration can be difficult in the obese woman; often multiple attempts are necessary to successfully place the epidural needle. It is often difficult to locate the midline and identify the epidural space. It is also difficult to position the woman; sitting is often the best position. More than one attempt to place the epidural is needed in approximately 75% of morbidly obese women (Davies et al., 2010). There is also the risk of the epidural catheter becoming dislodged (Saravanakumar, Rao, & Cooper, 2006). The use of epidurals may require significant staff resources; thus, their use may be limited in some settings (Davies et al., 2010).

IV opioids may be used during the first stage of labour; however, the doses and the effects must be monitored carefully because obese women are extremely sensitive to the respiratory depressant effects of opioids. Combined spinal epidural anaesthesia is an alternative to epidural anaesthesia. This option is now available in the morbidly obese pregnant woman because there is an appropriate long needle manufactured for this purpose (Kuczkowski, 2005).

In the obese woman who must give birth by Caesarean section, an epidural block is preferred over general anaesthesia. Problems associated with general anaesthesia in obese women include potential difficulties during intubation, a hypertensive effect of laryngoscopy and intubation, and aspiration and pulmonary complications. A spinal block may be used if there is insufficient time to induce an epidural block. Uterine displacement to prevent aortocaval compression is more difficult to achieve in the obese woman in the supine position needed for Caesarean birth. If the woman is extremely obese, a wedge may not be able to elevate one hip enough to prevent compression. In this case, it may be necessary to lift the abdominal fat pad off the abdomen manually until the peritoneal cavity has been entered.

Maternal Hypothermia After Analgesia and Anaesthesia

Hypothermia is defined as a core body temperature of less than 35°C. During labour and immediately after the birth, women are predisposed to hypothermia because of the combination of the vasodilation that normally occurs during pregnancy and the effects of the analgesia and anaesthesia.

Opioids, barbiturates, tranquilizers, and antiemetics are thought to affect thermoregulation by increasing vasodilation and radiant loss; epidural and spinal anaesthesia are thought to do so by inducing peripheral dilation. During labour, during vaginal or Caesarean birth, or immediately after birth, women may have shivering, hypotension, and respiratory distress. The hypothermia may result in cardiovascular, pulmonary, circulatory, hematological, neurological, or renal complications. The nurse can minimize these complications by making sure that the birthing areas are warm, wet drapes and towels are removed, women are covered with warm blankets after birth, and hypothermia is recognized early. Explaining these effects to the woman and her support people will help allay concerns.

Key Points

- The expected outcome of preparation for childbirth and parenting is that the woman and her partner have been provided with informed choices.
- Nonpharmacological pain and stress management strategies are valuable for managing labour discomfort on their own or in combination with pharmacological methods.
- Women need to be supported during labour by health care providers who feel comfortable assessing a woman's level of coping during labour and providing the appropriate support based on the woman's needs.
- The gate-control theory of pain and the stress response form the basis for many of the nonpharmacological methods of pain relief.
- The type of analgesic or anaesthetic to be used is determined by maternal and health care provider preference, the stage of labour, and the method of birth.
- Phenothiazines and benzodiazepines can be used during labour to decrease anxiety and apprehension, increase sedation, potentiate opioid analgesic effects, and reduce nausea and vomiting.
- Naloxone (Narcan) is an opioid (narcotic) antagonist that can reverse narcotic effects, especially respiratory depression.
- The use of opioid agonist–antagonist analgesics in women with pre-existing opioid dependence may cause symptoms of abstinence syndrome (opioid withdrawal).
- Pharmacological control of discomfort during labour requires collaboration among the health care providers and the woman in labour.
- The nurse must understand all comfort-related medications, their expected effects, potential adverse effects, and methods of administration.
- Maintenance of maternal fluid balance is essential during spinal and epidural nerve blocks.
- Maternal analgesia or anaesthesia potentially affects neonatal neurobehavioural response.
- Use of anaesthesia in women who are obese has increased risks.

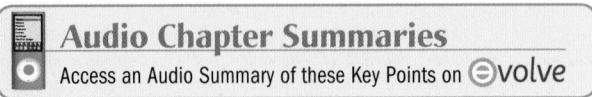

Audio Chapter Summaries

Access an Audio Summary of these Key Points on evolve

References

Anim-Somuah, M., Smyth, R., & Howell, C. (2005). Epidural versus no epidural or no analgesia in labour. *Cochrane Database of Systematic Reviews, Issue 4*. Chichester, UK: John Wiley & Sons.

Beebe, K. R., & Lee, K. (2007). Sleep disturbance in late pregnancy and early labour. *Journal of Perinatal & Neonatal Nursing, 21*(2), 103–108.

Birthing From Within. (n.d.). *Our mission.* Retrieved from http://www.birthingfromwithin.com.

Bradley, R. (1981). *Husband-coached childbirth* (3rd ed.). New York: Harper & Collins.

Bucklin, B., et al. (2005). Obstetric anesthesia workforce survey. *Anesthesiology, 103*(3), 645–653.

Callister, L. C., et al. (2003). The pain of childbirth: Perceptions of culturally diverse women. *Pain Management Nursing, 4*(4), 145–154.

Childbirth and Postpartum Professional Association (CAPPA). (2008). Retrieved from http://www.cappa.net.

Cunningham, F. G., et al. (2010). *Williams obstetrics* (23rd ed.). New York: McGraw Hill.

Davies, G. A., et al. (2010). SOGC clinical practice guideline: Obesity in pregnancy. *Journal of Obstetrics and Gynaecology Canada, 32*(2), 165–173. Retrieved from http://www.sogc.org/guidelines/documents/gui239ECPG1002.pdf.

Dick-Read, G. (1987). *Childbirth without fear* (5th ed.). New York: Harper & Collins.

Dowswell, T., et al. (2009). Transcutaneous electric nerve stimulation (TENS) for pain relief in labour. *Cochrane Database of Systematic Reviews, Issue 2.* Chichester, UK: John Wiley & Sons.

Enkin, M., et al. (2000). *A guide to effective care in pregnancy and childbirth* (3rd ed.). New York: Oxford University Press.

Florence, D. J., & Palmer, D. G. (2003). Therapeutic choices for the discomforts of labour. *Journal of Perinatal and Neonatal Nursing, 17*(4), 238–249.

Gilder, K., et al. (2002). Maternal positions in labour with epidural analgesia: Results from a multi-site survey. *AWHONN Lifelines, 6*(1), 40–45.

Gulliver, B. G., Fisher, J., & Roberts, L. (2008). A new way to assess pain in labouring women: Replacing the rating scale with a "coping" algorithm. *Nursing for Women's Health, 12*(5), 404–408.

Health Canada. (2000). *Family-centred maternity and newborn care: National guidelines* (Cat. No. H39-527/2000E ISBN 0-662-28702-9). Ottawa, ON: Author.

Hodnett, E. D. (2002). Pain and women's satisfaction with the experience of childbirth: A systematic review. *American Journal of Obstetrics and Gynecology, 186*(5 Suppl Nature), S160–S172.

Hodnett, E. D., et al. (2007). Continuous support for women during childbirth. *Cochrane Database of Systematic Reviews, Issue 3*. Chichester, UK: John Wiley & Sons.

HypnoBirthing. (2004). Retrieved from http://www.hypnosisforawakening.com.
Karmel, M. (1959). *Thank you, Dr. Lamaze*. New York: Dolphin Books.
Kuczkowski, K. M. (2005). Labour analgesia for the morbidly obese parturient: An old problem—new solution. *Archives of Gynecology and Obstetrics, 271*(4), 302–303.
Kuczkowski, K. M. (2006). Labour analgesia for the parturient with herbal medicine use: What does an obstetrician need to know? *Archives of Gynecology & Obstetrics, 274*(4), 233–239.
Kuczkowski, K. M. (2007). Labour pain and its management with the combined spinal-epidural analgesia: What does an obstetrician need to know? *Archives of Gynecology and Obstetrics, 275*(3), 183–185.
Kukulu, K., & Demirok, H. (2008). Effects of epidural anesthesia on labour progress. *Pain Management Nursing, 9*(1), 10–16.
Leeman, L., et al. (2003a). Editorial: Management of labour pain: Promoting patient choice. *American Family Physician, 68*(6), 1023–1026.
Leeman, L., et al. (2003b). The nature and management of labour pain. Part II. Pharmacologic pain relief. *American Family Physician, 68*(6), 1115–1120.
Lehne, R. A. (2007). *Pharmacology for nursing care* (6th ed.). Philadelphia: Saunders.
Lieberman, E., & O'Donoghue, C. (2002). Unintended effects of epidural anesthesia during labour: A systematic review. *American Journal of Obstetrics and Gynecology, 186*(5 Suppl Nature), S31–S68.
Liston, R., et al. (2007). Fetal health surveillance: Antepartum and intrapartum consensus guideline. *Journal of Obstetrics and Gynaecologists of Canada, 29*(9), s1–s56. Retrieved from http://www.sogc.org/guidelines/documents/gui197CPG0709.pdf.
Lothian, J., & Devries, C. (2005). *The official Lamaze guide: Giving birth with confidence*. New York: Meadowbrook Press.
Lowe, N. K. (2002). The nature of labour pain. *American Journal of Obstetrics and Gynecology, 186*(5 Suppl Nature), S16–S24.
Maude, R. M., & Foureur, M. J. (2007). It's beyond water; stories of women's experience of using water for labour and birth. *Women and Birth, 20*(1), 17–24.
Mayberry, L. J., Clemmens, D., & De, A. (2002). Epidural analgesia side effects, co-interventions, and care of women during childbirth: A systematic review. *American Journal of Obstetrics and Gynecology, 186*(5 Suppl Nature), S81–S93.
Mayberry, L. J., et al. (2003). Use of upright positioning with epidural analgesia: Findings from an observational study. *MCN: American Journal of Maternal Child Nursing, 28*(3), 152–159.
McCool, W. F., et al. (2004). Obstetric anesthesia: Changes and choices. *Journal of Midwifery and Women's Health, 49*(6), 505–513.
Mercier, F. J., & Bonnet, M. P. (2009). Tattooing and various piercing: Anaesthetic considerations. *Current Opinion in Anesthesiology, 22* (3), 436–441.
Mottershead, N. (2006). Hypnosis: Removing the labour from birth. *The Practising Midwife, 9*(3), 26–27.
Perinatal Services BC. (2007). *Pain management during labour*. Retrieved from http://www.perinatalservicesbc.ca//sites/bcrcp/files/Guidelines/Obstetrics/OB4PainManagement.pdf.
Public Health Agency of Canada. (2009). *What mothers say: The Canadian maternity experiences survey* (Cat. No. HP5-74/2-2009E-PDF). Ottawa, ON: Author. Retrieved from http://www.phac-aspc.gc.ca/rhs-ssg/pdf/survey-eng.pdf.
Saravanakumar, K., Rao, S., & Cooper, G. (2006). Obesity and obstetric anesthesia. *Anesthesia, 61*, 36–48.
Simkin, P., & Bolding, A. (2004). Update on nonpharmacologic approaches to relieve labour pain and prevent suffering. *Journal of Midwifery and Women's Health, 49*(6), 489–504.
Simkin, P. P., & O'Hara, M. (2002). Nonpharmacologic relief of pain during labour: Systematic reviews of five methods. *American Journal of Obstetrics and Gynecology, 186*(5 Suppl Nature), S131–S159.
Smith, C., et al. (2006). Complementary and alternative therapies for pain management in labour. *Cochrane Database of Systematic Reviews, Issue 4*. Chichester, UK: John Wiley & Sons.
Torvaldsen, S., Roberts, C. L., Simpson, J. M., Thompson, J. F., & Ellwood, D. A. (2006). Intrapartum epidural analgesia and breastfeeding: A prospective cohort study. *International Breastfeeding, 1*, 24. Retrieved from http://www.internationalbreastfeedingjournal.com/content/1/1/24.
Trout, K. (2004). The neuromatrix theory of pain: Implications for selected nonpharmacologic methods of pain relief for labour. *Journal of Midwifery and Women's Health, 49*(6), 482–488.
VandeVusse, L., et al. (2007). Hypnosis for childbirth: A retrospective comparative analysis of outcomes in one obstetrician's practice. *Journal of Midwifery and Women's Health, 50*(2), 109–119.
World Health Organization. (1998). *Workshop on perinatal care proceedings*. Venice, April 16–18. Geneva: Author.

Additional Resources

Childbirth and Postpartum Professional Association (CAPPA) Canada: http://www.cappacanada.ca/
Lamaze International: http://www.lamazeinternational.org
The International Childbirth Educators Association: http://www.icea.org/

Unit 4

17

Fetal Health Surveillance During Labour

Learning Objectives

On completion of this chapter, the reader will be able to:

- Explain baseline fetal heart rate (FHR), variability, rhythm, and periodic changes using intermittent auscultation (IA) or electronic fetal monitoring (EFM).
- Identify signs of normal, atypical, and abnormal FHR patterns.
- Compare FHR monitoring done by intermittent auscultation with electronic methods.
- Describe nursing measures that can be used to maintain FHR patterns within normal limits.
- Review the frequency and documentation of the monitoring process during labour.

Electronic Resources

Additional information related to the content in Chapter 17 can be found on

evolve the companion Web site at

http://evolve.elsevier.com/Canada/Perry/maternal/

- Critical Thinking Exercise—Fetal Monitoring

Fetal Health Surveillance

Clinical assessment of the fetal heart rate was initially described by the Swiss surgeon Mayer in 1818 (Association of Women's Health, Obstetric and Neonatal Nurses [AWHONN], 2009). With the advent of the fetoscope and stethoscope after the turn of the twentieth century, the listener could hear clearly enough to count the fetal heart rate (FHR). Electronic fetal monitoring (EFM) was introduced in the 1960s, used primarily with high-risk women in labour (Gray, 1983). Gray, a nurse from Halifax, published one of the first Canadian handbooks to guide nursing practice related to EFM. Most recently, the Society of Obstetricians and Gynaecologists of Canada (SOGC) has published the Canadian guidelines for antepartum and **intrapartum** fetal surveillance that are used in obstetrical practice throughout Canada (Liston et al., 2007). This chapter discusses the basis for fetal health surveillance during labour, the types of monitoring used, and nursing assessment and management of fetal heart rate status.

When EFM was first used clinically, it was anticipated that its use would decrease the rate of cerebral palsy (CP) and be more sensitive than auscultation by stethoscope in predicting and preventing fetal compromise (Garite, 2007). Consequently, the use of EFM rapidly expanded. However, research evidence has shown that EFM did not reduce the incidence of CP (Thacker, Stroup, & Change, 2006). Rising Caesarean birth rates have also been attributed to increased EFM use. The rate of Caesarean birth rates in Canada was 26.8% in 2009 (Canadian Institute for Health Information [CIHI], 2010), representing a 45% increase from the previous decade. While the SOGC recommends **intermittent auscultation** (IA) for healthy term women in spontaneous labour and reserves EFM for pregnancies at risk of adverse perinatal outcome, the predominant method of fetal surveillance during labour, as reported by Canadian women, remains EFM (Public Health Agency of Canada [PHAC], 2009).

Basis for Monitoring

Fetal Response

Because labour is a period of physiological stress for the fetus, frequent monitoring of fetal status is part of nursing care during labour. The fetal oxygen supply must be maintained during labour to prevent fetal compromise and promote newborn health after birth. Maternal factors, placental factors, and fetal factors may reduce the oxygen supply to the fetus; these are included in Box 17-1.

FHR and uterine activity (UA) must both be assessed together, and interpretation of the results should be based on the total clinical picture. Standards have been established for how frequently the FHR should be assessed, based on the clinical picture and the stage of labour. The SOGC recommends that the FHR be assessed hourly in the latent stage of labour or if a significant change occurs. In active labour, the FHR should be assessed every 15 to 30 minutes, and during active second stage, assessments are required every 5 minutes (Liston et al., 2007). In addition, the FHR should be assessed before and after rupture of membranes, administration of medications and anaesthesia, and more frequently when

BOX 17-1 Factors that May Affect Fetal Oxygenation in Labour

Maternal Factors

Decreased maternal arterial oxygen tension
- Respiratory disease
- Hypoventilation, seizure, trauma
- Smoking

Decreased maternal oxygen carrying capability
- Significant anemia (e.g., iron deficiency, hemoglobinopathies)
- Carboxyhemoglobin (smokers)

Decreased uterine blood flow
- Hypotension (e.g., blood loss, sepsis)
- Regional anaesthesia
- Maternal positioning

Chronic maternal conditions
- Vasculopathies (e.g., systemic lupus erythematosus, type I diabetes, chronic hypertension)
- Antiphospholipid syndrome

Uteroplacental Factors

Excessive uterine activity
- Hyperstimulation secondary to oxytocin, prostaglandins (PGE_2), or spontaneous labour
- Placental abruption

Uteroplacental dysfunction
- Placental abruption
- Placental infarction—dysfunction marked by IUGR, oligohydramnios, or abnormal Doppler studies
- Chorioamnionitis

Fetal Factors

Cord compression
- Oligohydramnios
- Cord prolapsed or entanglement

Decreased fetal oxygen carrying capability
- Significant anemia (e.g., isoimmunization, maternal–fetal bleed, ruptured vasa previa)
- Carboxygemoglobin (if mother is a smoker)

(From Liston, R., et al. [2007]. Fetal health surveillance: Antepartum and intrapartum consensus guideline. *Journal of Obstetrics and Gynaecologists of Canada, 29*[9], s1–s56, p. 25. Retrieved from http://www.sogc.org/guidelines/documents/gui197CPG0709.pdf.)

atypical or abnormal FHR patterns are identified. The perinatal nurse is responsible for having a readable EFM tracing.

Both the AWHONN (2009) and SOGC (Liston et al., 2007) recommend each facility have written guidelines regarding the appropriate use of each method of fetal surveillance and response to atypical and abnormal FHR. In clinical practice FHR patterns are described as normal with no intervention required (historically this was termed *reassuring*) or atypical or abnormal requiring intervention (historically termed *nonreassuring*) (Liston et al., 2007).

Uterine Activity

Uterine activity (UA) is assessed by palpation, a tocotransducer used for EFM, or an intrauterine pressure catheter (IUPC) (see discussion later in chapter). A normal UA pattern in labour is characterized by contractions occurring every 2 to 5 minutes and lasting less than 90 seconds, with a minimum of 30 seconds of rest period between contractions. Such contractions are moderate to strong in intensity as assessed by palpation. Uterine relaxation should be detected between contractions either by palpation or by an average intrauterine pressure of 15 mm Hg or less.

When assessing UA by palpation, the examiner should place his or her hand over the fundus. The contraction intensity is usually described as mild, moderate, or strong. The reference point for intensity is as follows:

Mild—Feels like the end of one's nose
Moderate—Feels as firm as one's chin
Strong—Feels as indentable as one's forehead

The contraction duration is measured in seconds, from the beginning to the end of the contraction. The frequency of contractions is measured in minutes, from the beginning of one contraction to the beginning of the next contraction. The examiner should keep his or her hand on the fundus after the contraction is over to evaluate uterine resting tone or relaxation between contractions. Normal resting tone between contractions is usually described as soft.

It is essential to document the UA in conjunction with the FHR assessment.

UA can be described as follows:

Normal—5 or fewer contractions in 10 minutes, averaged over a 30-minute window

Tachysystole—More than 5 contractions in 10 minutes, averaged over a 30-minute window
- Tachysystole should always be qualified by presence or absence of associated FHR decelerations.
- Tachysystole applies to both spontaneous or stimulated labour.
- The terms *hyperstimulation* and *hypercontractility* are not defined and should not be used (Macones et al., 2008).

Fetal Assessment

The goal of fetal surveillance is to identify possible fetal decompensation, allowing timely and effective interventions to prevent perinatal morbidity or mortality (Liston et al., 2007). Uterine activity is always assessed in association with fetal surveillance. Components of a normal intrapartum fetal surveillance assessment are given in Table 17-1. The types of fetal monitoring (IA and EFM) will be discussed later in the chapter.

Monitoring Techniques

The ideal method of fetal assessment during labour continues to be debated. Results from research studies indicate that IA of the FHR and EFM are associated with similar fetal outcomes in low-risk intrapartum patients (Gilbert, 2007). Furthermore, the use of EFM has been shown to increase the rate of intervention during labour, including Caesarean section, operative vaginal births, and greater use of anaesthesia. Given these findings, use of EFM is recommended for pregnancies at risk for adverse perinatal outcome but not for

Table 17-1 Normal Intrapartum Fetal Surveillance Findings

	IF USING IA	IF USING EFM
Baseline FHR	110–160 bpm	110–160 bpm
Rhythm	Regular (e.g., no skipped beats)	Not used with EFM
Variability	Not used with IA	Moderate (range of 6–25 bpm in FHR)
Deceleration	None heard	None or uncomplicated variables or early decelerations
Accelerations	May be heard	May be heard or seen

bpm, beats per minute; *EFM*, electronic fetal monitoring; *FHR*, fetal heart rate; *IA*, intermittent auscultation.

low-risk women (Liston et al., 2007). See Table 17-2 for antenatal and intrapartum conditions that are associated with adverse fetal outcome and might be considered high risk.

Despite the recommendation that EFM be used only for high-risk pregnancies, the use of EFM remains high, perhaps because of the following:

- Lack of nursing staff to provide one-to-one supportive care
- Caregiver skill and comfort with IA
- Belief that EFM will prevent all bad outcomes
- Caregiver belief that EFM record will prevent medical legal actions

Regardless of the method used, there should be discussion with the women about benefits, risks, and limitations of IA and EFM (Liston et al., 2007).

Intermittent Auscultation

With IA, fetal heart sounds are listened to at periodic intervals in order to assess the FHR. IA of the fetal heart can be performed with a Leff scope, a DeLee-Hillis fetoscope, a Pinard fetoscope (used commonly in countries outside North America) (see Fig. 10-8, C), or a doptone (a portable ultrasound fetoscope). If a Leff scope is used, the domed side should be opened to the connective tubing to the earpieces. The domed side is then applied to the maternal abdomen. The fetoscope is applied over the listener's head because bone conduction amplifies the fetal heart sounds for counting. The bell of the Pinard fetoscope is applied to the maternal abdomen while the nurse's ear is applied to the opposite end. The doptone transmits ultra-high-frequency sound waves reflecting movement of the fetal heart and converts these sounds into an electronic signal that can be counted (Fig. 17-1). The technique used for auscultation is described in Box 17-2.

NURSING ALERT Nurses may use the electronic transducer from the EFM to listen to the FHR using IA protocols; however, if the EFM is attached to an archived central monitoring system, it should not be used for IA.

If the FHR is assessed as normal, then IA will continue to be used. If an abnormal FHR is detected, the nurse should

Table 17-2 Antenatal and Intrapartum Conditions Associated With Increased Risk of Adverse Fetal Outcome

Anenatal		
Maternal		Hypertensive disorders of pregnancy
		Pre-existing diabetes mellitus/gestational diabetes
		Antepartum hemorrhage
		Maternal medical condition: cardiac, anemia, hyperthyroidism, vascular disease, and renal disease
		Maternal MVA/trauma
		Morbid obesity
Fetal		Intrauterine growth restriction (IUGR)
		Prematurity
		Oligohydramnios
		Abnormal umbilical artery Doppler velocimetry
		Isoimmunization
		Multiple pregnancy
		Breech presentation
Intrapartum		
Maternal		Vaginal bleeding in labour
		Intrauterine infection/chorioamnionitis
		Previous Caesarean birth
		Prolonged membrane rupture >24 hours at term
		Induced labour
		Hypertonic uterus
		Preterm labour
		Postterm labour (>42 weeks)
Fetal		Meconium staining of the amniotic fluid
		Abnormal fetal heart rate on auscultation

(From Liston, R., et al. [2007]. Fetal health surveillance: Antepartum and intrapartum consensus guideline. *Journal of Obstetrics and Gynaecologists of Canada, 29*[9], s1–s56. Retrieved from http://www.sogc.org/guidelines/documents/gui197CPG0709.pdf.)
MVA, motor vehicle accident.

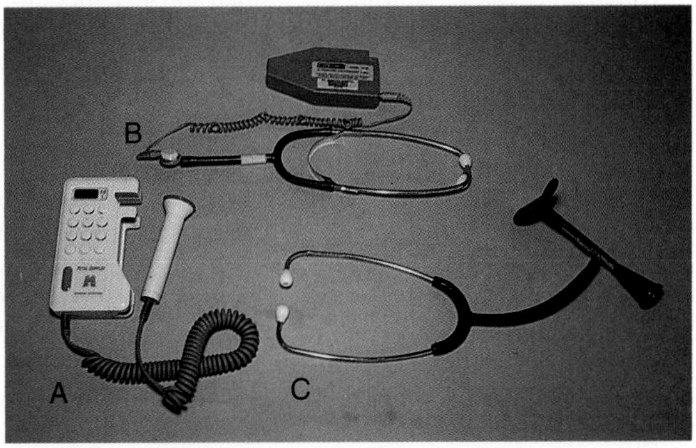

Fig. 17-1 **A:** Doptone. **B:** Ultrasound stethoscope. **C:** DeLee-Hillis fetoscope. *(Courtesy Michael S. Clement, MD, Mesa, AZ.)*

BOX 17-2 Intermittent Auscultation Procedure

Auscultation is performed as follows:

1. Perform Leopold's manoeuvres (see Fig. 18-4) by palpating the maternal abdomen to identify fetal presentation and position.
2. Place the listening device over the area of maximal intensity, usually the fetal back, to obtain the clearest and loudest sound. Apply ultrasound gel to Doppler ultrasound device if used.
3. Palpate the uterus for the absence of uterine activity (UA) so that the fetal heart rate (FHR) is assessed between contractions.
4. Assess the maternal radial pulse at the same time as listening to the FHR to differentiate it from the fetal rate.
5. Count the FHR for 60 seconds after contractions to identify the baseline rate. This rate can be assessed only between uterine contractions. The FHR obtained is recorded as a single number.
6. When listening to the FHR during labour, document the following:
   - Baseline FHR determined between contractions
   - Rhythm (regular or irregular)
   - Presence of increases (accelerations) or decreases (decelerations) of the FHR
   - Categorization of the FHR as normal or abnormal
7. Make a decision for ongoing care based on the findings (see Fig. 17-2).

evolve Critical Thinking Guidelines—Fetal Monitoring

auscultate after the next contraction, assess for maternal condition, and intervene according to the findings (Fig. 17-2). EFM may be initiated at this time, but it will depend on the findings and the total clinical picture.

NURSING ALERT It is always important to assess the maternal pulse at the same time as listening to the FHR with IA to ensure that it is different.

IA is easy to use, inexpensive, and less invasive than EFM. It is often more comfortable for the woman and gives her more freedom of movement. IA is recommended for healthy women at term in whom adverse perinatal outcomes are not expected (Liston et al., 2007).

Frequency of Intermittent Auscultation

The recommended frequency of IA depends on the stage of labour that the woman is in. Women in the latent phase of labour are often at home, so they do not need frequent assessments. If they are in the hospital, IA should be done at the time of assessment and every hour until there is a change in the woman's status. Once a woman is in active labour, IA is done every 15 to 30 minutes. During the active phase of the second stage of labour (when the woman is pushing), the frequency of IA increases to every 5 minutes (Liston et al., 2007).

NURSING ALERT When the FHR is auscultated and documented, it is inappropriate to use the descriptive terms associated with EFM (e.g., *moderate variability, variable deceleration*) because these terms are visual descriptions of the patterns produced on the monitor tracing. However, terms that are numerically defined, such as *bradycardia* and *tachycardia*, can also be used.

Every effort should be made to use the method of fetal assessment that the woman desires. However, auscultation of the FHR in accordance with the frequency recommended may sometimes be difficult in today's busy labour and birth units. When used as the primary method of fetal assessment, auscultation requires a 1:1 nurse-to-patient staffing ratio. If acuity and census change so that auscultation standards are no longer met, the nurse must discuss this with the labouring woman and may consider continuous EFM use until staffing can be arranged to meet the standards.

In some situations, IA can be challenging to use, particularly in morbidly obese women or if the fetus is very active or in a posterior position. The woman can become anxious if the examiner cannot readily count the fetal heartbeats. It often takes time for the inexperienced listener to locate the heartbeat and find the area of maximal intensity. To allay the mother's concerns, it is helpful to use a Doppler ultrasound device so that the mother can hear the sounds that the nurse hears. It is helpful to tell her that the nurse is "finding the spot where the sounds are loudest." If the examiner cannot locate the fetal heartbeat, assistance should be requested. In some cases, ultrasonography can be used to help locate the fetal heartbeat. Seeing the FHR on the ultrasound screen can be reassuring to the mother if there was initial difficulty in locating the best area for auscultation.

When using IA, UA is assessed by palpation (see p. 424). It is essential to document the uterine activity in conjunction with the FHR assessment. Labour flow records or computer charting systems that prompt notations of all assessments are useful for ensuring such comprehensive documentation.

Electronic Fetal Monitoring

The purpose of electronic FHR monitoring is the ongoing assessment of fetal oxygenation. While the goal of EFM is to detect fetal hypoxia and metabolic acidosis during labour and to provide timely intervention, as stated earlier, the use of EFM is associated with increased rates of Caesarean births and instrumental vaginal births, compared to rates with IA (see Evidence-Informed Practice box).

The two modes of EFM are (1) the external mode, which uses external **transducers** placed on the maternal abdomen to assess FHR and UA; and (2) the internal mode, which uses a spiral electrode applied to the fetal presenting part to assess the FHR and sometimes an IUPC to assess UA and pressure. The differences between the external and internal modes of EFM are summarized in Table 17-3.

External Monitoring

Separate transducers are used to monitor the FHR and UA (Fig. 17-3). The ultrasound transducer works by reflecting high-frequency sound waves off a moving interface: in this

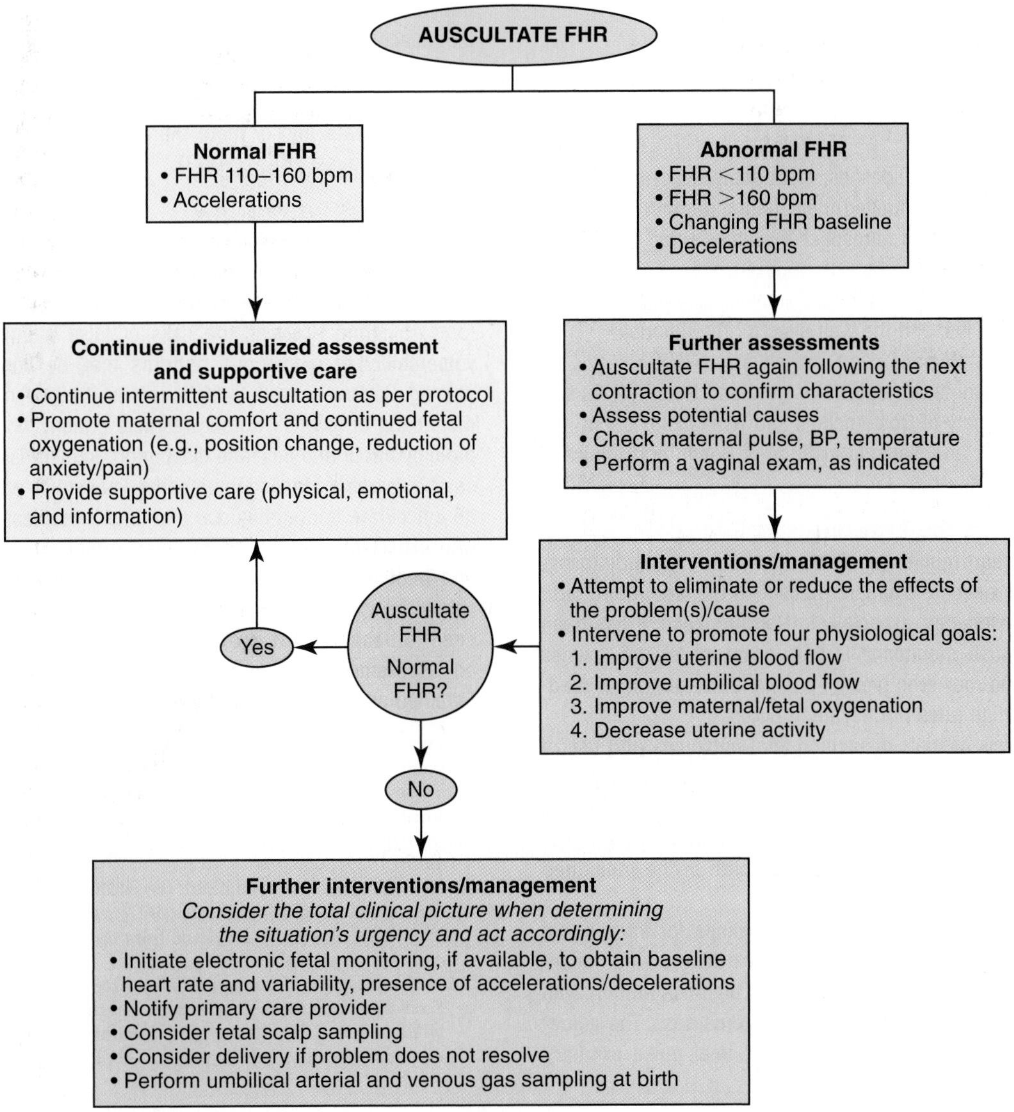

Fig. 17-2 Decision support tool for intermittent auscultation. *bpm*, beats per minute. *(From Liston, R., et al. [2007]. Fetal health surveillance: Antepartum and intrapartum consensus guideline.* Journal of Obstetrics and Gynaecologists of Canada, 29*[9], s1–s56, p. 30. Retrieved from* http://www.sogc.org/guidelines/documents/gui197CPG0709.pdf.*)*

Table 17-3 External and Internal Modes of Monitoring

EXTERNAL MODE	INTERNAL MODE
Fetal Heart Rate	
Ultrasound transducer: High-frequency sound waves reflect mechanical action of the fetal heart. It is noninvasive, does not require rupture of membranes or cervical dilation, and is used during both the antepartum and intrapartum periods.	*Spiral electrode:* This electrode converts the fetal ECG as obtained from the presenting part to the FHR via a cardiotachometer. This method can be used only when membranes are ruptured and the cervix is sufficiently dilated during the intrapartum period. The electrode penetrates into fetal presenting part by 1.5 mm and must be attached securely to ensure a good signal.
Uterine Activity	
Tocotransducer: This instrument monitors frequency and duration of contractions by means of a pressure-sensing device applied to the maternal abdomen. It is used during both the antepartum and intrapartum periods. Strength of the contraction must still be assessed by palpation as done with IA.	*Intrauterine pressure catheter (IUPC):* This instrument monitors the frequency, duration, and intensity of contractions. The two types of IUPCs are a fluid-filled system and a solid catheter that are introduced into the uterus. Both measure intrauterine pressure at the catheter tip and convert the pressure into millimeters of mercury on the uterine activity panel of the strip chart. Both can be used only when membranes are ruptured and the cervix is sufficiently dilated during the intrapartum period. The IUPC is rarely used in Canada.

ECG, electrocardiogram; *FHR*, fetal heart rate; *IA*, intermittent auscultation.

EVIDENCE-INFORMED PRACTICE Fetal Monitoring and the Machine That Goes "Beep" —*Pat Gingrich*

Ask the Question

What are the optimal methods of assessing fetal well-being during labour?

Search for Evidence

Search Strategies

Professional organization guidelines, meta-analyses, systematic reviews, randomized controlled trials, nonrandomized prospective studies, and retrospective studies since 2006

Databases Searched

CINAHL, Cochrane, Medline, National Guideline Clearinghouse, TRIP Database Plus, and the Web sites for the American Congress of Obstetricians and Gynecologists (ACOG), Association of Women's Health, Obstetric and Neonatal Nurses (AWHONN), Society of Obstetricians and Gynaecologists of Canada (SOGC), and National Institute of Health and Clinical Excellence (NICE)

Critically Analyze the Evidence

Electronic fetal heart monitoring (EFM; also known as cardiotocography [CTG]) has become standard practice in the labour and birth setting for many decades, especially in North America. It has been suggested that such monitoring is not necessary for the low-risk labour patient and may even present a risk of false abnormal readings, leading to high rates of Caesarean births.

A meta-analysis of trials measuring fetal outcomes and use of EFM showed that there was no significant change in Apgar scores for women who had EFM on admission for labour compared to women who were not monitored at admission. However, there was a statistically increased risk for Caesarean birth in the monitored women (Gourounti & Sandall, 2007).

The SOGC has issued professional guidelines for intrapartum care that do not recommend EFM for the low-risk labouring patient (Liston et al., 2007). EFM should be used for high-risk women, with fetal scalp blood pH testing if abnormal patterns arise. The guidelines do not recommend the routine use of fetal pulse oximetry. Similar clinical practice guidelines from NICE recommend intermittent auscultation (IA) at admission and during labour with a stethoscope or Doppler study. Use of continuous EFM should begin in the presence of meconium, bleeding, abnormal fetal heart rate (less than 110 beats/min or more than 160 beats/min), oxytocin use, or patient request (NICE, 2008).

Implications for Practice

Electronic fetal monitoring is here to stay, but it is only a tool. Women and providers have come to expect the constant feedback, and busy nurses have come to rely on the remote screens as they move from room to room. However, the risks of false alarms and the legal vulnerability of ambiguous patterns may be contributing to the soaring Caesarean rate, which carries its own risks. Continuous monitoring of low-risk women restricts patient mobility, which may prolong labour and increase discomfort. In high-risk situations, EFM can be valuable for picking up some fetal stress early but also may be inaccurate and ambiguous and cause needless anxiety. Women who expect routine monitoring need explanations about the risks and benefits of continuous monitoring versus those with IA and should be given informed choices. The health care team may also need to become more proficient and familiar with auscultation as an assessment tool, and they must consider the information obtained as one part of the total clinical picture.

References

Gourounti, K., & Sandall, J. (2007). Admission cardiotocography versus intermittent auscultation of fetal heart rate: Effects on neonatal Apgar score, on the rate of caesarean sections, and on the rate of instrumental delivery—a systematic review. *International Journal of Nursing Studies, 44*(6), 1029–1035.

Liston, R., et al. (2007). Fetal health surveillance: Antepartum and intrapartum consensus guideline. *Journal of Obstetrics and Gynaecology Canada, 29*(9 Suppl 4), s1–s56, Retrieved from http://www.sogc.org/guidelines/documents/gui197CPG0709.pdf.

National Institute for Health and Clinical Excellence (NICE). (2008). Intrapartal care: Care for healthy women and their babies during childbirth. NICE Clinical Guideline 55. London: Author. Retrieved from www.nice.org.uk/nicemedia/pdf/IPCNICEGuidance.pdf.

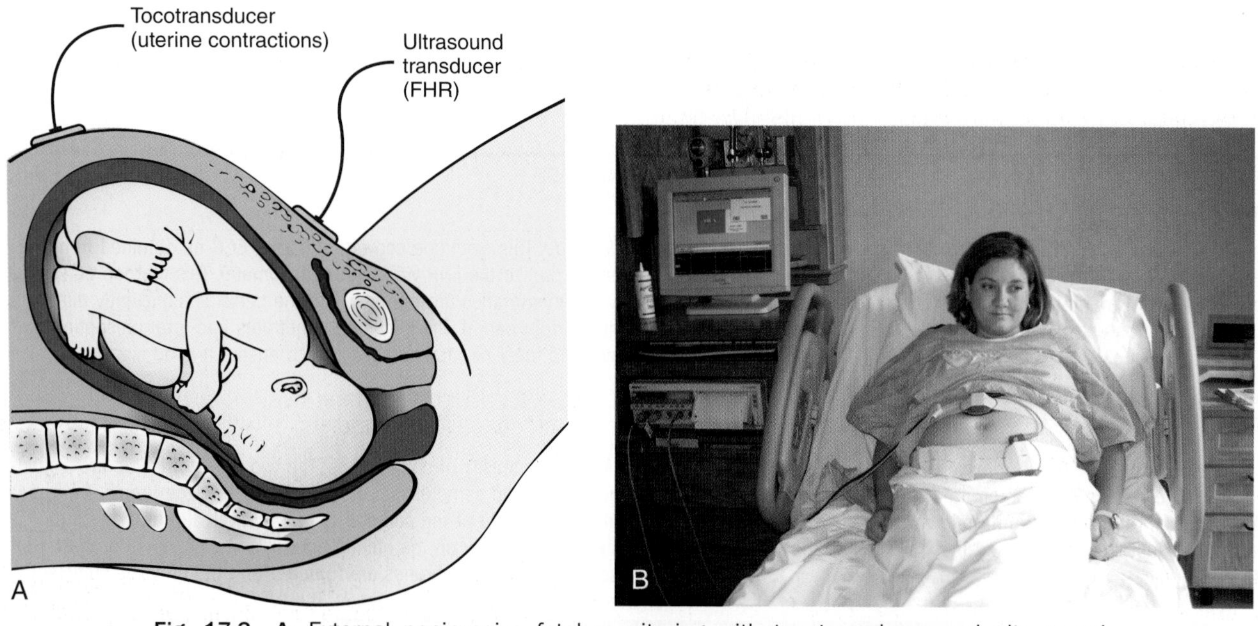

Fig. 17-3 **A:** External noninvasive fetal monitoring with tocotransducer and ultrasound transducer. FHR, fetal heart rate. **B:** Ultrasound transducer is placed below umbilicus over the area where fetal heart rate is best heard, and tocotransducer is placed on uterine fundus. *(B, Courtesy Julie Perry Nelson, Loveland, CO.)*

case, the fetal heart and valves. It is sometimes difficult to reproduce a continuous and precise record of the FHR because of artifacts introduced by fetal and maternal movement. Once the area of maximal intensity of the FHR has been located, conductive gel is applied to the surface of the ultrasound transducer, and the transducer is then positioned over this area. The FHR is printed on specially formatted monitor paper. The most common paper speed in Canada is 3 cm/min; however, some provinces use 1 or 2 cm/min. It is important to determine the paper speed prior to interpreting the EFM reading.

The tocotransducer (tocodynamometer) measures UA transabdominally. The device is placed over the fundus above the umbilicus. UA or fetal movements depress a pressure-sensitive surface on the side next to the abdomen. The tocotransducer can measure and record the frequency, regularity, and approximate duration of contractions but not their intensity. Because the tocotransducer of most electronic fetal monitors is designed for assessing UA in term pregnancy, it may not be sensitive enough to detect preterm UA. When monitoring the woman in preterm labour, remember that the fundus may be located below the level of the umbilicus. The nurse may need the woman to indicate when UA is occurring and must use palpation as an additional way of assessing contraction frequency and validating the monitor tracing. The strength of the contractions is always determined by palpation.

The external transducer is easily applied by the nurse. It must be repositioned at least every hour and as the woman or fetus changes position (see Fig. 17-3, B). To use it, the woman needs to assume a semisitting or lateral position. Use of an external transducer limits movement because it confines the woman to the bed or chair or within her room. Portable telemetry monitors allow observation of the FHR and UA patterns by means of centrally located electronic display stations. These portable units permit the woman to walk around during electronic monitoring.

Internal Monitoring

The technique of continuous internal monitoring may provide a more accurate appraisal of fetal well-being during labour than external monitoring because it is not interrupted by fetal or maternal movement (Fig. 17-4). For this type of monitoring, the membranes must be ruptured and the cervix sufficiently dilated (2 to 3 cm) to allow placement of the spiral electrode, IUPC, or both. Internal and external modes of monitoring may be combined (i.e., internal FHR with external UA or external FHR with internal UA) without difficulty. IUPC is not frequently used in Canada.

Internal monitoring of the FHR is accomplished by attaching a small spiral electrode to the presenting part; a continuous FHR will be displayed on the fetal monitor strip. To monitor UA internally, a solid IUPC is introduced into the uterine cavity. The solid catheter has a pressure-sensitive tip that measures changes in intrauterine pressure. As the catheter is compressed during a contraction, pressure is placed on the pressure transducer or strain gauge; this pressure is then converted into a pressure reading in millimeters of mercury. The average pressure for a strong contraction ranges from 50 to 60 mm Hg. The IUPC can measure the frequency, duration, and intensity of UCs as well as **uterine resting tone**.

The FHR and UA are displayed on the monitor paper with the FHR in the upper section and UA in the lower section. Figure 17-5 contrasts the internal and external modes of electronic monitoring. Note that each small square represents 10 seconds; each larger box of six squares equals 1 minute (when paper is moving through the monitor at the rate of 3 cm/min).

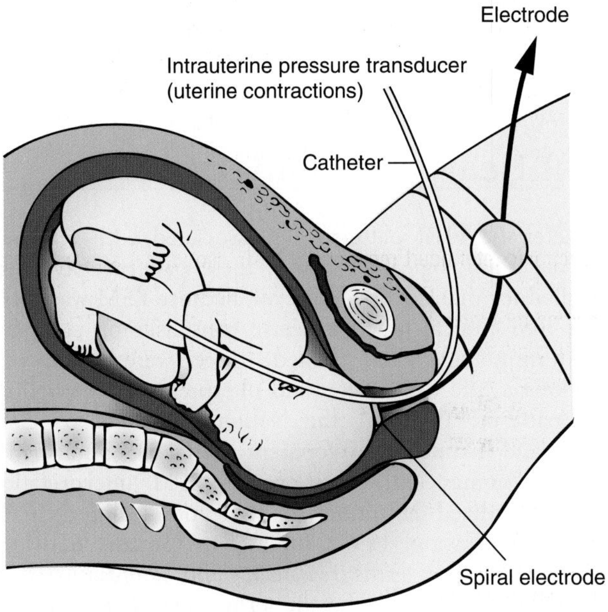

Fig. 17-4 Diagrammatic representation of internal invasive fetal monitoring with intrauterine pressure catheter and spiral electrode in place (membranes ruptured and cervix dilated).

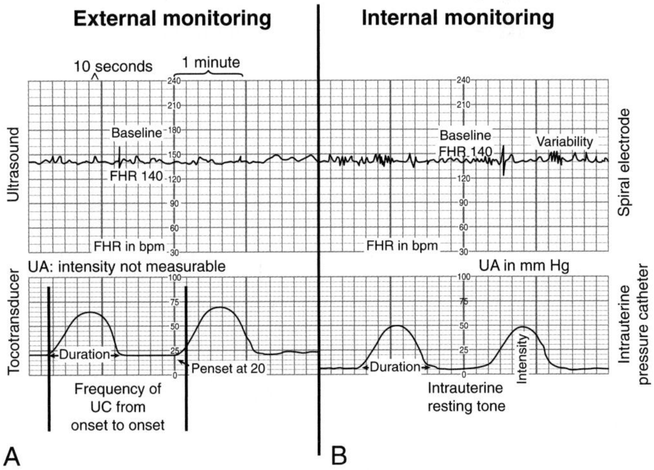

Fig. 17-5 Display of fetal heart rate and uterine activity on monitor paper. **A:** External mode with ultrasound and tocotransducer as signal source. **B:** Internal mode with spiral electrode and intrauterine catheter as signal source. Frequency of contractions is measured from the beginning of one contraction to the beginning of the next. *BPM,* beats per minute; *FHR,* fetal heart rate; *UA,* uterine activity; *UC,* uterine contractions. *(From Tucker, S. M., Miller, L. A., & Miller, D. A. [2009].* Mosby's pocket guide to fetal monitoring: A multidisciplinary approach *[6th ed.]. St. Louis: Mosby.)*

Admission Fetal Monitor Strips

There has been much debate over the routine use of admission electronic fetal monitor strips. Although it is common practice in many hospitals to perform a 20-minute monitor strip on admission, this is not supported by evidence or recommendations for low-risk women (Liston et al., 2007). The SOGC states that women who are at risk for adverse outcomes (see Table 17-2) should have admission fetal heart rate tracings, but for women with low risk there is no evidence showing any benefit. Admission fetal heart rate tracings should not be used to determine whether a woman is in labour. Palpation along with IA is an effective method to determine the status of labour and the fetus.

Fetal Heart Rate Patterns

Characteristic FHR patterns are associated with fetal and maternal physiological processes; these patterns have been identified for many years. However, because EFM was introduced into clinical practice before consensus on standardized terminology was reached, there were often wide variations in the description and interpretation of common FHR patterns. In 1997, the National Institute of Child Health and Human Development (NICHD) published a proposed nomenclature system for EFM interpretation, with standardized definitions for FHR monitoring (NICHD Planning Workshop, 1997). Initially in Canada, FHR was labelled using the terms *reassuring* and *nonreassuring*. In 2007, the SOGC introduced the terms *normal*, *atypical*, and *abnormal* for categorization of FHR patterns when using EFM (Table 17-4).

The FHR must be assessed systematically, including all key components (baseline FHR, variability, and accelerations or decelerations), and must include interpretation of uterine activity. Standard terminology should be used when describing the FHR tracing.

Baseline Fetal Heart Rate

The intrinsic rhythmicity of the fetal heart, the central nervous system (CNS), and the fetal autonomic nervous system controls the FHR. An increase in sympathetic response results in acceleration of the FHR, whereas stimulation of the parasympathetic system produces a slowing of the FHR. Usually, a balanced increase of sympathetic and parasympathetic response occurs during contractions, with no observable change in the baseline FHR.

Baseline FHR is the average rate during a 10-minute segment that excludes accelerations, decelerations, and periods of marked variability. There must be at least 2 minutes of baseline segments in a 10-minute segment (Macones et al., 2008). The normal range at term is 110 to 160 beats/min. It is rounded to increments of 5 beats/min and recorded as a range or as a single number (Liston et al., 2007).

Fetal *tachycardia* is a baseline FHR greater than 160 beats/min for 10 minutes or longer. Tachycardia is labelled either "atypical" or "abnormal," depending on the length of time it occurs (see Table 17-4). It can be considered an early sign of fetal hypoxemia, especially when associated with **late decelerations** and minimal or absent variability. Fetal tachycardia can result from maternal or fetal infection, such as prolonged rupture of membranes with amnionitis; from maternal hyperthyroidism or fetal anemia; from prolonged fetal activity; or in response to medications such as atropine or hydroxyzine (Atarax) or illicit drugs such as cocaine or methamphetamines. Table 17-5 discusses the significance of fetal tachycardia and the nursing implications.

Fetal *bradycardia* is a baseline FHR less than 110 beats/min for 10 minutes or longer. In the presence of possible fetal bradycardia, it is essential to confirm the maternal pulse to differentiate it from the fetal rate. True bradycardia occurs rarely and is not specifically related to fetal oxygenation. It is critical to distinguish true bradycardia from a prolonged deceleration, since the causes and management of these two conditions are very different. Bradycardia is often caused by some type of fetal

Table 17-4 Fetal Heart Rate Interpretation System When Using Electronic Fetal Monitoring

	NORMAL	ATYPICAL	ABNORMAL
Baseline (bpm)	• 110–160	• FHR 100–110 • FHR >160 for >30 min to <80 min • Rising baseline	• FHR <100 • FHR >160 for >80 min • Erratic baseline
Variability	• 6–25 bpm (moderate) • <5 bpm for <40 min	• ≤5 bpm for 40–80 min	• ≤5 bpm for >80 min • ≥25 bpm for >10 min • Sinusoidal
Decelerations	• None or occasional uncomplicated variables or early decelerations	• Repetitive (≥3) uncomplicated variable decelerations • Occasional late deceleration • Single prolonged deceleration >2 min but <3 min	• Repetitive (≥3) complicated variable decelerations • Late deceleration >50% of contractions • Single prolonged deceleration >3 min but <10 min
Accelerations	• Spontaneous accelerations present • Accelerations present with fetal scalp sampling	• Absence of acceleration with fetal scalp stimulation	• Usually absent

(From Liston, R., et al. [2007]. Fetal health surveillance: Antepartum and intrapartum consensus guideline. *Journal of Obstetrics and Gynaecologists of Canada, 29*[9 Suppl 4], s1–s56, Society of Obstetricians and Gynaecologists of Canada [SOGC] Clinical Practice Guideline 197. Ottawa, ON: Author. Retrieved from http://www.sogc.org/guidelines/documents/gui197CPG0709.pdf.)
bpm, beats per minute; *FHR*, fetal heart rate.

cardiac problem, such as structural defects involving the pacemakers or conduction system or fetal heart failure. Other causes of bradycardia include viral infections (cytomegalovirus), maternal hypoglycemia, and maternal hypothermia. The clinical significance of the bradycardia depends on the underlying cause and accompanying FHR patterns, including variability and the presence of accelerations or decelerations (Tucker, Miller, & Miller, 2009). Table 17-5 lists causes, clinical significance, and nursing interventions for bradycardia.

Fetal Heart Rate Variability

Baseline variability of the FHR can be described as fluctuations in the baseline FHR that are determined in a 10-minute window, excluding accelerations and decelerations. Fluctuations are irregular in amplitude and frequency and are visually quantified as the amplitude of the peak to trough in beats/min (AWHONN, 2009; Liston et al., 2007). Variability is classified as follows:

- Absent or undetectable variability (0 to 2 beats/min)
- Minimal variability (greater than undetectable but ≤5 beats/min)
- Moderate variability (6 to 25 beats/min)
- Marked variability (>25 beats/min) (Fig. 17-6)

The presence of moderate variability requires an intact medulla, a mature CNS, and an oxygenated brainstem (Lee et al., 2009). Diminished variability can result from fetal hypoxemia and acidosis and from certain medications that depress the CNS, including analgesics, opioids (morphine), barbiturates (secobarbital [Seconal]) and pentobarbital [Nembutal]), tranquilizers (diazepam [Valium]), ataractics (promethazine [Phenergan]), and general anaesthetics. Maternal smoking can also result in decreased FHR variability. In addition, a temporary decrease in variability can occur when the fetus is in a sleep state. These sleep states do not usually last longer than 30 minutes, although they can occasionally last up to 80 minutes. The interpretation of the FHR tracing should be within the context of the overall clinical picture. Table 17-6 contrasts key differences between increased and decreased variability.

A sinusoidal FHR pattern has a visually apparent, smooth, undulating sine wavelike pattern with a normal baseline FHR of 110 to 160. The cycle frequency is 3 to 5/min, which persists for 20 minutes or more. This uncommon pattern occurs when fetal hypoxia results from fetal anemia (hemoglobin <70 g/L) that may be due to Rh isoimmunization or fetal hemorrhage (e.g., abruptio placenta) (Lee et al., 2009).

Periodic and Episodic Changes in Fetal Heart Rate

Changes in FHR from the baseline are categorized as periodic or episodic. *Periodic* changes are those that occur with uterine contractions. *Episodic* changes are those that are not associated with contractions. These patterns include accelerations and decelerations (Macones et al., 2008).

Table 17-5 Fetal Tachycardia and Bradycardia and Nursing Implications

TACHYCARDIA	BRADYCARDIA
Definition	
FHR >160 beats/min lasting longer than 10 min	FHR <110 beats/min lasting longer than 10 min
Cause	
• Early fetal hypoxemia • Fetal cardiac arrhythmias and/or congenital anomalies • Maternal fever • Infection (including chorioamnionitis) • Parasympatholytic medications (atropine, hydroxyzine) • Maternal hyperthyroidism • Fetal anemia • Prolonged fetal activity • Drugs (caffeine, cocaine, methamphetamines)	• Fetal hypoxia/acidosis • AV dissociation (heart block)—may be related to maternal connective tissue disease (e.g., Lupus) • Structural defects • Viral infections (e.g., cytomegalovirus) • Medications • Maternal hypotension • Fetal heart failure • Maternal hypoglycemia • Maternal hypothermia • Maternal position
Clinical Significance	
Persistent tachycardia with no other FHR changes does not appear to be serious in terms of neonatal outcome (however, one needs to be aware of potential newborn sepsis if tachycardia is associated with maternal fever); tachycardia is an abnormal sign when associated with late decelerations, severe variable decelerations, or absence or minimal variability.	Baseline bradycardia alone is not specifically related to fetal oxygenation; the clinical significance of bradycardia depends on the underlying cause and the accompanying FHR patterns, including variability, accelerations, or decelerations.
Nursing Interventions	
• Confirm maternal vital signs • Notify the primary care provider and carry out health care provider's orders based on alleviating cause—this may include antipyretics, antibiotics, and cooling measures; fluid bolus • Intrauterine resuscitation if thought due to hypoxia (see Box 17-8)	• Confirm maternal pulse as different from FHR • Consider vaginal examination to rule out cord prolapsed • May consider scalp stimulation or scalp pH sampling • Other interventions, dependent on cause

AV, atrioventricular; *FHR*, fetal heart rate.

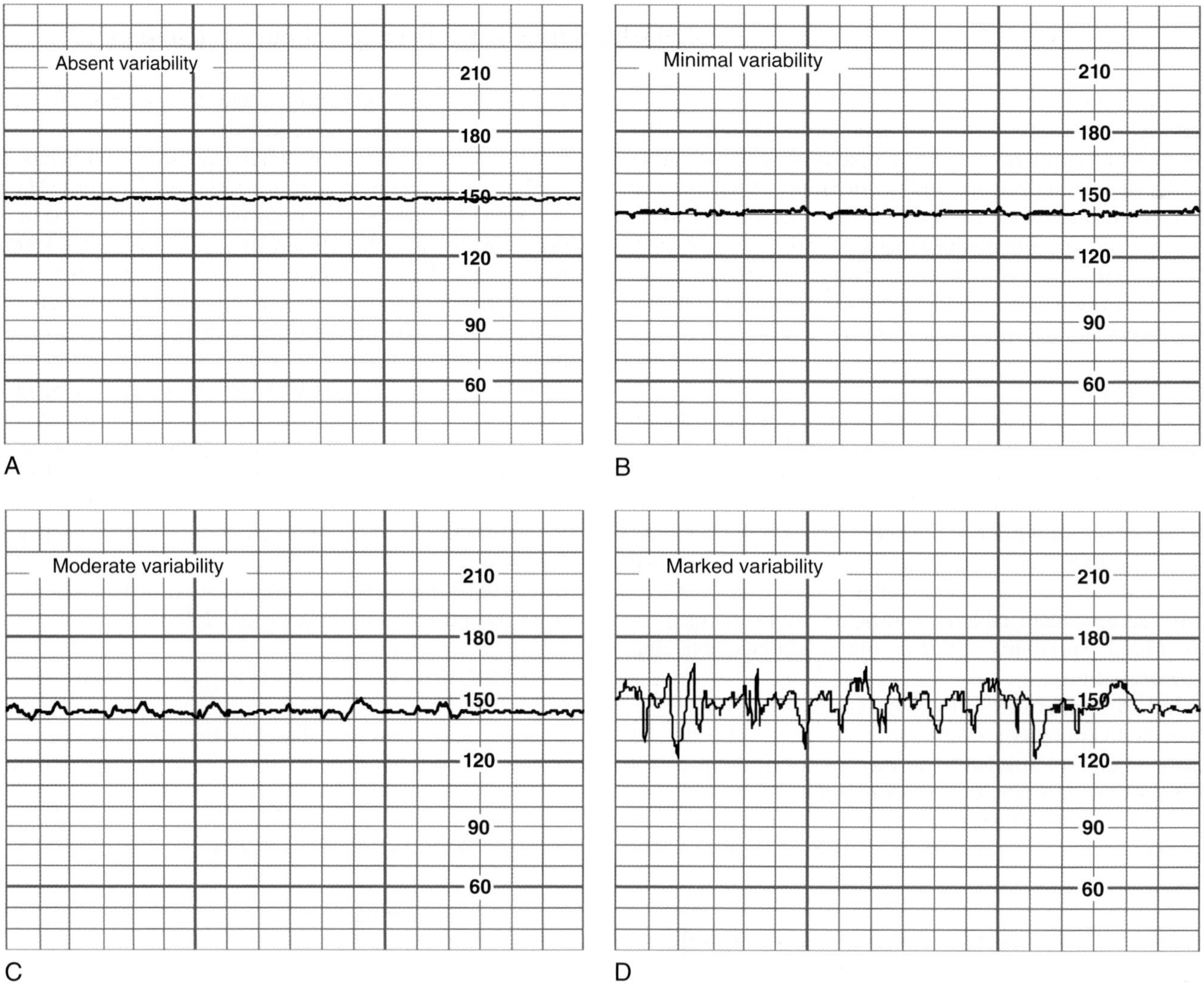

Fig. 17-6 Fetal heart rate variability. **A:** Absent or undetected. **B:** Minimal. **C:** Moderate. **D:** Marked. *(Modified from Tucker, S. M., Miller, L. A., & Miller, D. A. [2009].* Mosby's pocket guide to fetal monitoring: A multidisciplinary approach *[6th ed.]. St. Louis: Mosby.)*

Table 17-6 Variability: Increased and Decreased and Clinical Significance

INCREASED VARIABILITY	DECREASED VARIABILITY
Cause	
Early mild hypoxemia Hyper-oxygenation Fetal stimulation by the following: • Uterine palpation • Uterine contractions • Fetal activity • Maternal activity • Street drugs (e.g., cocaine and methamphetamines)	Hypoxia/acidosis CNS depressants Prematurity—less than 24 wk Maternal smoking Fetal sleep cycles Congenital abnormalities Fetal cardiac dysrhythmias
Clinical Significance	
Significance of marked variability not known; increased variability from a previous average variability is earliest FHR sign of mild hypoxemia	Benign when associated with periodic fetal sleep states, which last 20 to 30 min; if caused by drugs, variability usually increases as drugs are excreted; decreased variability is not reassuring and is considered a sign of potential fetal acidemia unless it has an identifiable temporary (e.g., fetal sleep) or correctable cause
Nursing Intervention	
Observe FHR tracing carefully for any nonreassuring patterns, including decreasing variability and late decelerations	Dependent on cause; intervention not warranted if associated with fetal sleep states or temporarily associated with CNS depressants; consider performing external stimulation of scalp during a vaginal examination to elicit acceleration of FHR or return to average variability; consider application of internal spiral electrode if needed for more accurate tracing; prepare for birth if so indicated by primary health care provider

CNS, central nervous system; *FHR,* fetal heart rate.

Accelerations

Acceleration of the FHR is defined as a visually apparent, abrupt increase in FHR above the baseline rate. *Abrupt* is defined as an increase from onset to peak of acceleration in less than 30 seconds (Liston et al., 2007) (Fig. 17-7). To be classed as an acceleration in a fetus >32 weeks' gestation, the increase must be 15 beats/min or greater above the baseline rate and last 15 seconds or more, with the return to baseline less than 2 minutes from the beginning of the acceleration. A *prolonged* acceleration is longer than 2 minutes but less than 10 minutes in length. Acceleration of the FHR for more than 10 minutes is considered a change in baseline rate. In fetuses <32 weeks' gestation, the definition of an acceleration is a peak of 10 beats/min or more above baseline for at least 10 seconds (Liston et al., 2007).

Accelerations can be periodic or episodic. They may occur in association with fetal movement or spontaneously. If accelerations do not occur spontaneously, they can be elicited by fetal scalp stimulation (Liston et al., 2007). Accelerations are considered a sign of fetal well-being. Their presence is highly predictive of a normal fetus with an intact oxygenated sympathetic nervous system (Lee et al., 2009). However, the lack of an acceleration with scalp stimulation does not predict fetal compromise (Liston et al., 2007). To perform fetal scalp stimulation, gently stroke the fetal scalp for 15 seconds during a vaginal exam but not during a contraction. Box 17-3 lists causes, clinical significance, and nursing interventions for accelerations.

Decelerations

Decelerations are classified as early, late, prolonged, and variable. FHR decelerations are described by their visual relation to the onset and end of a contraction and by their shape.

Early Decelerations

Early deceleration of the FHR is a visually apparent, usually symmetrical, gradual decrease and return to baseline FHR associated with UA (Fig. 17-8, A) (Lee et al., 2009). Generally, the onset, **nadir,** and recovery of the deceleration correspond to the beginning, peak, and end of the contraction. For this reason, early decelerations are sometimes referred to as the "mirror image" of a contraction.

Early decelerations are thought to be caused by transient fetal head compression and are considered a benign finding. They may also occur during vaginal examinations, as a result of fundal pressure, and during placement of a spiral electrode for internal fetal monitoring. When present, they usually occur during the first stage of labour, when the cervix is dilated 4 to 7 cm, but can also be seen during the second stage when the woman is pushing.

Because early decelerations are considered to be benign, interventions are not necessary. Early decelerations should be identified so that they can be distinguished from late or variable decelerations, which can be atypical or abnormal patterns and for which interventions are appropriate. Box 17-4 lists cause, clinical significance, and nursing interventions for early decelerations.

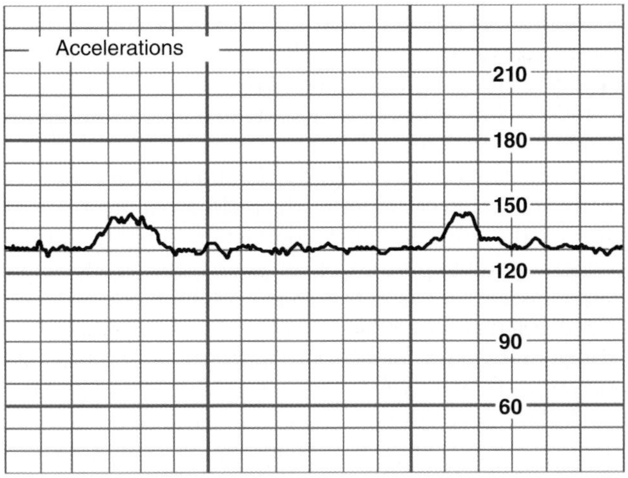

Fig. 17-7 Accelerations of fetal heart rate. *(From Tucker, S. M., Miller, L. A., & Miller, D. A. [2009].* Mosby's pocket guide to fetal monitoring: A multidisciplinary approach *[6th ed.]. St. Louis: Mosby.)*

BOX 17-3 Accelerations

Cause

- Spontaneous fetal movement
- Vaginal examination, including scalp stimulation or spiral electrode application
- Reaction to external sounds
- Breech presentation
- Occiput posterior position
- Uterine contractions
- Fundal pressure
- Abdominal palpation

Clinical Significance

Acceleration with fetal movement signifies fetal well-being, representing fetal alertness or arousal states.

Nursing Interventions

None required

BOX 17-4 Early Decelerations

Cause

Head compression resulting from the following:
- Uterine contractions
- Vaginal examination
- Fundal pressure
- Placement of internal spiral electrode
- Cephalopelvic disproportion (CPD); usually seen early in labour

Clinical Significance

Normal with no intervention and is not associated with fetal hypoxemia, acidemia, or low Apgar scores. If due to CPD, monitor labour progress.

Nursing Interventions

None required

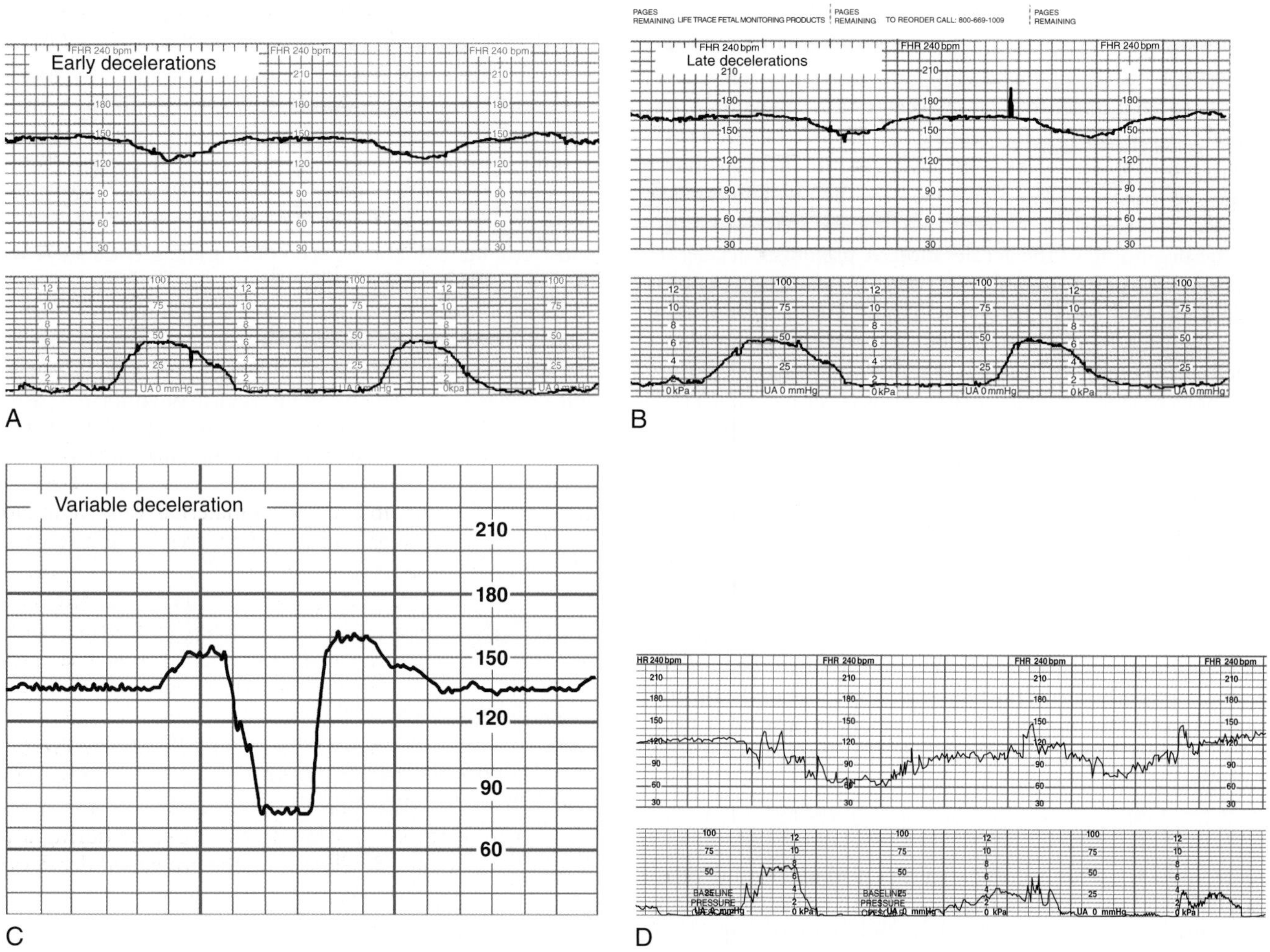

Fig. 17-8 Deceleration patterns. **A:** Early. **B:** Late. **C:** Variable. **D:** Prolonged. *(From Tucker, S. M., Miller, L. A., & Miller, D. A. [2009].* Mosby's pocket guide to fetal monitoring: A multidisciplinary approach *[6th ed.]. St. Louis: Mosby.)*

Late Decelerations

Late deceleration of the FHR is a visually apparent gradual decrease in and return to baseline FHR associated with uterine contractions (Liston et al., 2007). The deceleration begins after the contraction has started, and the lowest point of the deceleration occurs after the peak of the contraction. The deceleration usually does not return to baseline until after the contraction is over (see Fig. 17-8, B). Late decelerations reflect uteroplacental insufficiency, resulting in a lower fetal Po_2, which stimulates the fetal chemoreceptor to respond by stimulating the parasympathetic system. This sequence is visible following the peak of the contraction.

Persistent and repetitive late decelerations should be taken as an ominous sign when they are uncorrectable, especially if they are associated with decreased variability and tachycardia (Liston et al., 2007). A number of things can disrupt oxygen transfer to the fetus. The causes, clinical significance, and nursing interventions for late decelerations are described in Box 17-5.

Variable Decelerations

Variable decelerations are the most common type of deceleration. They are defined as a visual abrupt (<30 seconds) decrease in FHR below the baseline. The decrease is ≥15 beats/min, lasts at least 15 seconds, and returns to baseline in less than 2 minutes from the time of onset (see Fig. 17-8, C). They can occur during or between contractions (Lee et al., 2009).

Variable decelerations are most commonly found during the transition phase of the first stage of labour and during the second stage of labour as a result of umbilical cord compression or stretching during fetal descent (Garite, 2007). Box 17-6 lists causes, clinical significance, and nursing interventions for variable decelerations.

The appearance of variable decelerations differs from that of early and late decelerations, which closely approximate the shape of the corresponding contraction. Instead, variable decelerations often have a U, V, or W shape, characterized by a rapid descent and ascent to and from the nadir (or depth) of the deceleration (see Fig. 17-8, C).

Uncomplicated variables are spiky in appearance with rapid return to the baseline. They rarely alter the fetal pH and have little clinical significance. Complicated variables are more likely to affect fetal well-being, and the monitor strip is categorized as abnormal if at least three complicated variables occur. These decelerations can deplete the fetal reserve and lead to fetal hypoxemia. Complicated variable decelerations include the following:

BOX 17-5 Late Decelerations

Cause

Uteroplacental insufficiency caused by the following:

Acute Conditions
- Uterine tachysystole
- Maternal hypotension related to epidural or spinal anaesthesia, positioning
- Reduced maternal Po_2
- Acute placental disruption (i.e., abruption, previa)
- Intra-amniotic infection

Chronic Conditions
- Maternal comorbidities (e.g., diabetes, collagen disease, hypertension)
- Postmaturity
- Poor placental development/malformation

Clinical Significance

Atypical if pattern occurring occasionally; abnormal if occurring with >50% of contractions. Late decelerations are associated with fetal hypoxemia, acidemia, and low Apgar scores; they are considered ominous if persistent and uncorrected, especially when associated with fetal tachycardia and loss of variability.

Nursing Interventions

When occasional late decelerations are detected, change maternal position (lateral), check maternal vital signs, and continue to observe closely. When late decelerations are repetitive, intrauterine resuscitation needs to be initiated (see Box 17-8).

BOX 17-6 Variable Decelerations

Cause

Umbilical cord compression caused by the following:
- Maternal position with cord between fetus and maternal pelvis
- Cord around fetal neck, arm, leg, or other body part
- Short cord
- Knot in cord
- Prolapsed cord
- Decreased amniotic fluid

Clinical Significance

Variable decelerations occur in approximately 50% of all labours and are usually uncomplicated and correctable.

Nursing Interventions
- Change maternal position (side to side, knee chest).
- Also consider (particularly if complicated) intrauterine resuscitation (see Box 17-8).
- Notify primary care provider.
- Assist with vaginal or speculum examination to assess for possible cord prolapse.
- Assist with scalp stimulation, scalp pH, or amnioinfusion (see discussion later in chapter), if ordered.
- Alter pushing technique (e.g., open glottis, shorter pushes).
- Assist with birth (vaginal assisted or Caesarian) if pattern cannot be corrected.

- Deceleration to <70 beats/min lasting >60 seconds
- Loss of variability in the baseline FHR and in the trough of the deceleration
- Biphasic deceleration (W shape)
- Prolonged secondary accelerations or overshoot of 20 beats/min increase or lasting more than 20 seconds
- Slow return to baseline
- Continuation of baseline rate at lower level than that before deceleration
- Presence of fetal tachycardia or bradycardia

Prolonged Decelerations

A *prolonged deceleration* is a visually apparent decrease in FHR below the baseline 15 beats/min or more and lasting more than 2 minutes but less than 10 minutes (see Fig. 17-8, D). A deceleration lasting more than 10 minutes is considered a baseline change (Macones et al., 2008). Generally, the benign causes are pelvic examination, application of a spiral electrode, rapid fetal descent, and sustained maternal Valsalva manoeuvre. Other less benign causes are progressive severe variable decelerations, sudden umbilical cord prolapse, hypotension produced by spinal or epidural analgesia or anaesthesia, tetanic contraction, placental hemorrhage, **uterine rupture,** and maternal hypoxia, which may occur during a seizure.

When the deceleration lasts longer than 1 to 2 minutes, a loss of variability with rebound tachycardia usually occurs. Occasionally, a period of late decelerations follows. Prolonged decelerations usually are isolated events that end spontaneously. However, when a prolonged deceleration is seen late in the course of severe variable decelerations or during a prolonged series of late decelerations, the prolonged deceleration may occur just before fetal death.

NURSING ALERT Nurses should notify the primary care provider immediately and initiate appropriate intrauterine resuscitation when they see a prolonged deceleration.

Nursing Care Management

The primary goals of nursing care are to have healthy fetal and maternal outcomes. Knowledge of fetal status and standards for care determine the interventions implemented. All planning and interventions must take into account the total clinical picture and the resources that are available. The planning process includes meeting the needs of the woman and family, answering questions, and explaining nursing interventions (see Nursing Process box).

Although the use of EFM can be reassuring to many parents, it can be a source of anxiety to some. Therefore, the nurse needs to be particularly sensitive to the emotional, informational, and comfort needs of the woman in labour and those of her family and respond appropriately (Fig. 17-9 and Box 17-7).

Electronic Fetal Monitoring Pattern Recognition

Nurses need to evaluate essential components of an FHR tracing in order to determine whether immediate intervention is needed or whether there are indications to expedite birth.

NURSING PROCESS: FETAL MONITORING

Assessment

Maternal temperature, pulse, respiratory rate, blood pressure, position, comfort, voiding pattern, status of membranes, uterine contraction pattern, cervical effacement and dilation, and emotional status are assessed.

Fetal assessment includes fetal presentation, fetal position, fetal heart rate (FHR), and identification of FHR patterns. Frequency and type (intermittent auscultation [IA] or electronic fetal monitoring [EFM]) of FHR assessment should be done on the basis of stage of labour and total clinical picture.

A partogram can be used by the nurse to assess and document the components of the FHR based on the monitoring method being used.

All of the assessment information must be documented in the woman's medical record.

The EFM strip is evaluated to ensure that it is readable and can be interpreted.

Nursing Diagnoses

Possible nursing diagnoses include the following:

Decreased maternal cardiac output related to
- hypotension secondary to maternal position

Anxiety related to
- lack of knowledge concerning fetal monitoring during labour
- limited mobility or movement during monitoring
- fetal well-being

Impaired fetal gas exchange related to
- umbilical cord compression
- placental insufficiency

Acute pain related to
- use of belts to position transducers
- maternal position
- vaginal examinations associated with application of maternal or fetal internal monitoring equipment or fetal blood sampling

Risk for fetal injury related to
- unrecognized hypoxemia, hypoxia, or anoxia
- infection secondary to internal monitoring or scalp blood sampling

Planning

The care during labour given to women being monitored by IA or EFM should be the same. Both IA and EFM require knowledge of pathophysiology, equipment, and the skills to carry out the assessment. No one method is simpler than another. A care provider must be skilled in whatever method is being used.

Support given to women in labour is more important to them than the method of fetal monitoring that is being used (Garcia et al., 1985; Killen & Shy, 1989; Liston et al., 2007).

Expected outcomes for the pregnant woman and family and the fetus include the following:

- The woman will feel well supported during labour.
- The pregnant woman and family will communicate their understanding of the need for monitoring.
- The fetus will not have any hypoxemic, hypoxic, or anoxic episodes.
- Should fetal compromise occur, it will be identified promptly, appropriate nursing interventions such as intrauterine resuscitation will be initiated, and the primary health care provider will be notified.

Interventions

Provide continuous labour support.

Assess FHR patterns.

Implement independent nursing interventions.

Document observations and actions.

Observe established standards of care.

Report atypical or abnormal FHR patterns to the primary care provider.

Provide reassurance to the woman and her family.

Evaluation

Evaluation is a continuous process. The nurse can assume that care was effective when the outcomes for care have been achieved (see Nursing Care Plan).

These components are baseline rate, baseline variability, accelerations, decelerations, changes or trends in the FHR pattern over time, and uterine activity pattern (Tucker et al., 2009). Nurses evaluate these factors on the basis of the total clinical picture. They also must consider the estimated time interval until birth. Interventions are thus based on clinical judgement of a complex, integrated process (Simpson & James, 2005).

<u>LEGAL TIP</u> **Fetal Monitoring Standards.** Nurses who care for women during childbirth are legally responsible for maintaining an interpretable monitor strip, correctly interpreting FHR patterns, initiating appropriate nursing interventions based on those patterns, and documenting the outcomes of those interventions. Perinatal nurses are responsible for the timely notification of the primary care provider in the event of atypical or abnormal FHR patterns or contraction patterns (i.e., patterns that indicate the need for intervention or expedited birth). Perinatal nurses also are responsible for initiating the institutional chain of command should differences in opinion arise among health care providers about the interpretation of the FHR pattern and the intervention required.

Nursing Management of Atypical or Abnormal Patterns

Whenever one of the essential components of the FHR tracing is assessed as atypical or abnormal, corrective measures must be taken immediately. The purpose of these actions is to improve fetal oxygenation (Tucker et al., 2009). The term

NURSING CARE PLAN ● Fetal Monitoring During Labour

Nursing Diagnosis Maternal anxiety related to lack of knowledge about use of intermittent auscultation (IA) or electronic fetal monitoring (EFM)

Expected Outcomes
The woman will exhibit increased understanding about fetal monitoring and signs of reduced anxiety (i.e., absence of physical indicators, absence of perceived threat, and absence of feelings of dread).

Nursing Interventions/*Rationales*
Explain and demonstrate to the woman and labour support partner how the doptone, fetoscope, or electronic fetal monitor (internal or external) works in assessing fetal heart rate (FHR) and detecting and assessing quality of uterine contractions *to remove fear of unknown.*

When using the doptone or adjusting the monitor, explain to the couple what is being done and why, *because information increases understanding and allays anxiety.*

Explain that frequent position changes decrease discomfort; therefore, encourage frequent changes in position (other than supine) and explain any monitoring adjustments that are being made as a result *to reduce discomfort and allay anxiety.*

Nursing Diagnosis Risk for fetal injury related to inaccurate placement of transducers/electrodes, misinterpretation of results, or failure to use other assessment techniques to monitor fetal well-being

Expected Outcomes
Fetal well-being is adequately assessed, and any fetal compromise is identified immediately.

Nursing Interventions/*Rationales*
Carefully follow guidelines for selection of type of monitoring *to ensure that the proper types of monitoring devices are used.*

If EFM is required, check placement throughout monitoring process *to ensure that devices remain correctly placed.*

Regularly assess and record results of IA or EFM (FHR baseline, variability, decelerations, accelerations, uterine activity, contractions, uterine resting tone) *to provide consistent and timely evaluation of fetal well-being and progress of labour.*

Nursing Diagnosis Risk for maternal injury related to use of equipment, misinterpretation of uterine activity patterns, incorrect placement of external or internal monitors, or misinterpretation of contraction pattern

Expected Outcomes
Maternal well-being is assessed continuously, and any alterations are identified promptly.

Nursing Interventions/*Rationales*
Palpate uterine contractions *to identify strength.*

Periodically recheck placement and move every hour *to verify that all monitoring devices are accurately placed and to minimize discomfort.*

Use correct aseptic technique when assisting with insertion of internal monitors *to prevent infection.*

Nursing Diagnosis Risk for impaired physical mobility related to limited mobility with monitoring devices

Expected Outcome
The woman will be able to change positions and ambulate frequently.

Nursing Interventions/*Rationales*
Discontinue continuous electronic monitoring at intervals if there is a normal FHR pattern *to change position and increase mobility.*

Encourage the woman to change position (e.g., sit in chair or walk around the room) and reposition monitor as needed *to decrease complications of immobility.*

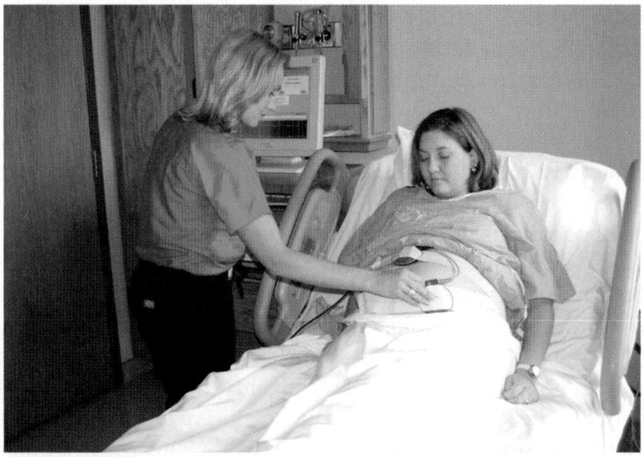

Fig. 17-9 Nurse explains electronic fetal monitoring as ultrasound transducer monitors the fetal heart rate. *(Courtesy Julie Perry Nelson, Loveland, CO.)*

intrauterine resuscitation is sometimes used to refer to the interventions initiated when an abnormal FHR pattern is noted. The purpose of these interventions is to improve uterine and intervillous space blood flow and increase maternal oxygenation and cardiac output (Simpson & James, 2005). Box 17-8 lists basic interventions to improve maternal and fetal oxygenation status.

Nurses must assign priorities to interventions in order to maximize the efficacy of the intrauterine resuscitation. The first priority is to open the maternal and fetal vascular systems; the second priority is to increase blood volume; and the third priority is to optimize oxygenation of the circulating blood volume.

Some interventions are specific to the FHR pattern. Nursing interventions appropriate for the management of tachycardia and bradycardia are given in Table 17-5, and those appropriate for the management of increased or decreased variability are given in Table 17-6. No specific nursing interventions are

BOX 17-7 Patient and Family Teaching When Intermittent Auscultation or Electronic Fetal Monitor Is Used

The following guidelines relate to patient teaching:

- Explain the purpose of monitoring to identify fetal well-being in labour.
- Explain each procedure.
- Provide the rationale for maternal position other than supine.
- Explain that fetal status can be assessed safely using intermittent auscultation (IA) or explain the need for electronic fetal monitoring (EFM) if there are risk factors for adverse perinatal outcome.
- If using EFM, explain that the lower tracing on the monitor strip paper shows uterine activity; the upper tracing shows the fetal heart rate (FHR).
- Reassure the woman and her partner that prepared childbirth techniques can be implemented without difficulty.
- Explain that breathing patterns based on the time and intensity of contractions can be enhanced by the observation of uterine activity on the monitor strip paper, which shows the onset of contractions.
- Using palpation, note peak of contraction; knowing that contraction will not get stronger and is half over is usually helpful. Note diminishing intensity.
- Reassure the woman and her partner that the use of internal monitoring does not restrict movement unless medically indicated. Portable telemetry monitors allow the FHR and uterine contraction patterns to be monitored and may increase ambulation during labour.
- Reassure the woman and her partner that the use of monitoring does not imply fetal jeopardy.

BOX 17-8 Management of Atypical or Abnormal Fetal Heart Rate Pattern

Intrauterine resuscitation
- Stop or decrease oxytocin.
- Change maternal position to left or right lateral.
- Improve hydration with IV fluid bolus.
- Perform vaginal examination to assess progress in labour or relieve pressure of presenting part off cord.
- Administer oxygen by mask at 8 to 10 L/min by tight face mask.
- Consider amnioinfusion (see discussion later in chapter) if variable decelerations are present.

Reduce maternal anxiety (to lessen catecholamine impact).

Coach woman to modify breathing or pushing techniques during second stage:
- Use open-glottis rather than Valsalva-style pushing.
- Use fewer pushing efforts during each contraction or make individual pushing efforts shorter.
- Push only with every second or third contraction.
- Push only with a perceived urge to push (with use of regional anaesthesia).

Notify primary health care provider.

(From Liston, R., Sawchuck, D., et al. [2007]. SOGC Clinical Practice Guideline: Fetal health surveillance: Antepartum and intrapartum consensus guideline. *Journal of Obstetrics and Gynaecologists of Canada, 29*[9 Suppl 4], s1–s56, p. 37. Retrieved from http://www.sogc.org/guidelines/documents/gui197CPG0709.pdf.)

required for the management of FHR acceleration or early deceleration (see Boxes 17-3 and 17-4). However, late and some types of variable FHR decelerations require aggressive intervention (see Boxes 17-5 and 17-6). The primary health care provider decides whether medical intervention should be instituted, what intervention is indicated, or whether immediate vaginal or Caesarean birth should be performed.

Additional Methods of Assessment and Intervention

Other methods of assessment and intervention are designed to be used in conjunction with IA or EFM in an effort to identify and intervene when there is an atypical or abnormal FHR pattern. These methods include fetal blood sampling, amnioinfusion, and tocolysis. Umbilical cord acid–base determination is an assessment technique that is a useful adjunct to the Apgar score in assessing the immediate condition of the newborn.

Fetal Scalp Blood Sampling

Fetal scalp blood sampling involves obtaining a capillary fetal blood sample in a fetus >34 weeks' gestation. It is obtained through a small incision in the fetal scalp taken through the dilated cervix. It is an adjunct to EFM when the pattern is difficult to interpret or is atypical or abnormal and birth is not imminent. The capillary sample is tested for pH. Results will guide the physician on whether to expedite delivery, reassess within 30 minutes, or allow labour to continue. If the pH is 7.20 or less, delivery is indicated because of the risk of fetal acidemia; pH greater than 7.20 requires further surveillance and reassessment in 30 minutes, especially if the atypical or abnormal EFM persists (Liston et al., 2007). There is some evidence that scalp lactate levels may also be used to determine fetal status. The blood may be easier to obtain as a very small sample of blood is required. The guideline for determination of fetal status is determined by the type of meter used, although lactate levels <4.2 probably indicate a healthy fetus; 4.2–4.8 requires continued monitoring and further testing in 30 minutes; >4.8 indicates immediate delivery is required (Wiberg-Itzel et al., 2008). Further research is necessary to determine the validity of scalp lactate.

Amnioinfusion

Amnioinfusion is infusion of room temperature isotonic fluid (usually normal saline or lactated Ringer's solution) into the uterine cavity through a double-lumen IUPC when the volume of amniotic fluid is low. Without the buffer of amniotic fluid, the umbilical cord can easily become compressed during contractions or fetal movement, diminishing the flow of blood between the fetus and placenta and resulting in variable decelerations and transient fetal hypoxemia. The purpose of amnioinfusion is to relieve intermittent umbilical cord compression by restoring the amniotic fluid volume to a normal or near-normal level (Tucker et al., 2009).

Women with an abnormally small amount of amniotic fluid (**oligohydramnios**) or no amniotic fluid (anhydramnios) are candidates for this procedure. Conditions that can result in oligohydramnios or anhydramnios are **uteroplacental insufficiency** and premature rupture of membranes.

In the past, amnioinfusion was also used to dilute moderate-to-thick meconium in an attempt to prevent meconium aspiration syndrome. However, a recent large research study found that amnioinfusion did not significantly reduce the incidence of meconium aspiration syndrome or perinatal death (Fraser et al., 2005). Therefore, routine amnioinfusion for meconium-stained amniotic fluid without the presence of variable decelerations is not recommended. Very few centres in Canada use amnioinfusion as a choice for treatment.

Nitroglycerine for Tachysystole

Nitroglycerine is used to relax the uterus in the presence of tachysystole with atypical or abnormal FHR. It can be administered by intravenous push or nasal spray. This therapy can be used as an adjunct to other interventions in the management of atypical or abnormal FHR patterns associated with increased UA. If there is no improvement, immediate surgical intervention for birth may be needed.

Umbilical Cord Acid–Base Determination

In assessing the immediate condition of the newborn after birth, a sample of cord blood is a useful adjunct to the Apgar score. The SOGC recommends that blood be withdrawn from the umbilical artery and vein and tested for pH, Pco_2, Po_2, and base excess (Liston et al., 2007). Umbilical arterial values reflect fetal condition and thus are considered by some as most relevant; umbilical venous blood values reflect placental function (Tucker et al., 2009). Umbilical cord gas measurements reflect the acid–base status of the newborn at birth, a measurement not reflected in the Apgar score (Table 17-7). If acidemia is present, the type—respiratory, metabolic, or mixed—is determined by analyzing the blood gas values (Table 17-8).

Patient and Family Teaching

Part of the perinatal nurse's role includes acting as a partner with the woman to achieve a high-quality birthing experience (see Community Focus box). In addition to providing teaching and support for the woman and her family regarding the labour and birth process, breathing techniques, use of equipment, and pain management techniques, the nurse should provide information on two factors that have an effect on fetal status: pushing and positioning.

Maternal Positioning

Maternal supine hypotensive syndrome is caused by the weight and pressure of the gravid uterus on the ascending vena cava when the woman is in a supine position. The supine position decreases venous return to the woman's heart and cardiac output and subsequently reduces her blood pressure. Low maternal blood pressure decreases intervillous space blood flow during uterine contractions and results in fetal hypoxemia. This is reflected on the fetal monitor as an atypical or abnormal FHR pattern, usually as late decelerations. The nurse should instruct the woman to avoid using the supine position, if possible. She should be encouraged to maintain an upright, side-lying, or semi-Fowler position with a lateral tilt to the uterus. Either the right or left lateral maternal position effectively enhances uteroplacental blood flow.

Discouraging the Valsalva Manoeuvre

The Valsalva manoeuvre can be described as the process of making a forceful bearing-down attempt while holding one's breath with a closed glottis and tightening the abdominal muscles. This process stimulates the parasympathetic division of the autonomic nervous system, producing a vagal response, and results in the decrease of maternal heart rate and blood pressure. Prolonged pushing in this manner can decrease placental blood flow, alter maternal and fetal oxygenation,

COMMUNITY FOCUS

Education About Electronic Fetal Monitoring

Interview childbirth educators from two different types of childbirth preparation classes regarding what they teach expectant parents about electronic fetal monitoring. Do the educators regard it to be "normal"? Do they discuss its advantages and disadvantages, or do they just describe it as a usual intervention? Do they discuss choice in labour (i.e., are parents able to select auscultation rather than electronic monitoring)? Intermittent rather than continuous monitoring? What implications does this information have for your practice as a labour and birth nurse?

Table 17-7 Approximate Normal Values for Cord Blood

CORD BLOOD	PH	Pco_2 (MM HG)	HCO_3 (MMOL/L)	BASE EXCESS (MMOL/L)
Artery	7.20-7.34	39.2-61.4	18.4-25.6	−5.5-0.1
Vein	7.28-7.40	32.8-48.6	18.9-23.9	−4.4-0.4

(From Liston, R., et al. [2007]. Fetal health surveillance: Antepartum and intrapartum consensus guideline. *Journal of Obstetrics and Gynaecology Canada* 29[9 Suppl 4], s1-s56. Retrieved from http://www.sogc.org/guidelines/documents/gui197CPG0709.pdf.)

Table 17-8 Types of Acidemia

	NORMAL	RESPIRATORY	METABOLIC	MIXED
pH	≥7.20	<7.20 (low)	<7.20 (low)	<7.20 (low)
PCO_2 (mm Hg)	40-60	>60 (high)	40-60 (normal)	>60 (high)
HCO_3 (mmol/L)	18-25	18-25 (normal)	<18 (low)	<18 (low)
Base excess (mmol/L)	−5.5-0	−5.5-0 (normal)	<−12 (low)	<−12

(Adapted from Tucker, S.M., Miller, L.A., & Miller, D.A. [2009]. *Mosby's pocket guide to fetal monitoring: A multidisciplinary approach* [6th ed.]. St Louis: Mosby.)

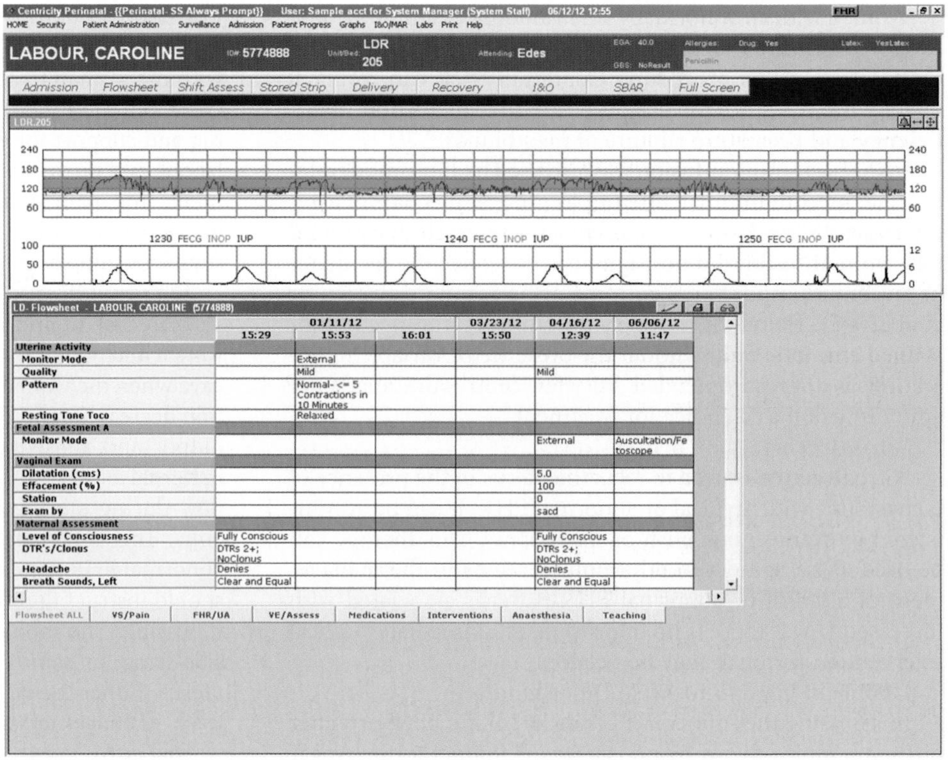

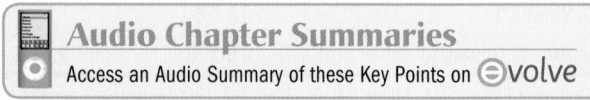

Fig. 17-10 With integration of the fetal monitor tracing into the electronic medical record, the nurse can view the fetal tracing while charting. *(Courtesy General Electric Healthcare Technologies, Barrington, IL.)*

decrease the fetal pH and Po_2, increase the fetal Pco_2, and increase the likelihood of fetal hypoxemia, as reflected in FHR pattern changes.

During the second stage of labour, when the woman needs to push, an alternative to breath holding with a closed glottis is to perform the open-mouth and open-glottis breathing-pushing technique. The nurse can instruct the woman to keep her mouth and glottis open and let air escape from the lungs during the pushing process. This may result in an audible grunting sound and will prevent the Valsalva manoeuvre (see Chapter 18, p. 473).

Documentation

Clear and complete documentation in the woman's medical record is essential. Each FHR and UA assessment must be documented in the woman's medical record. More and more hospitals are moving to use of the electronic medical record and computer charting. With computerized charting, each required component usually appears on the screen so that it will be addressed routinely. Often computerized charting includes forced choices that greatly increase the use of standardized FHR terminology by all members of the health care team. Electronic documentation also has space for comments on the EFM record, which is archived with the medical record (Fig. 17-10). As much as possible, duplicate documentation should be avoided. The nurse needs to follow the documentation standards for fetal surveillance as outlined by the hospital. Regardless of the documentation method, it is important that the time on the fetal monitor and the time the nurse uses to chart progress notes or other documentation are synchronous.

An important point in fetal surveillance documentation is that caregivers use proper descriptive terminology. It is important to avoid such terms as *asphyxia*, *hypoxia*, and *fetal distress*, as these terms are imprecise and nonspecific and lack standard definitions (Lee et al., 2009).

Key Points

- Fetal well-being during labour is gauged by the response of the FHR to UA.
- FHR characteristics include the baseline FHR, variability, accelerations, and decelerations.
- The monitoring of fetal well-being includes FHR assessment, watching for meconium-stained amniotic fluid, and assessment of maternal vital signs and UA.
- It is the responsibility of the nurse to assess FHR and patterns, implement independent nursing interventions, and report atypical and abnormal patterns to the primary care provider.
- The SOGC has established and published health care provider standards and guidelines for fetal heart monitoring.
- The emotional, informational, and comfort needs of the woman and her family must be addressed when the mother and her fetus are being monitored.
- Documentation is initiated and updated according to institutional protocol.

Audio Chapter Summaries

Access an Audio Summary of these Key Points on Evolve

Table 18-1 Sociocultural Basis of Pain Experience

WOMAN IN LABOUR	NURSE
Perception of Meaning	
Origin: Cultural concept of and personal experience with pain; for example: Pain in childbirth is inevitable, something to be endured. Pain in childbirth can be avoided completely. Pain in childbirth is punishment for sin. Pain in childbirth can be managed by the woman.	Origin: Cultural concept of and personal experience with pain; in addition, the nurse becomes accustomed to working with certain "expected" pain trajectories. For example, in obstetrics, pain is expected to increase as labour progresses, be intermittent, and have an end point; relief can be derived from medications once labour is well established and the fetus or newborn can cope with the amount and elimination of medications; relief can also come from the woman's knowledge, attitude, and support from the nurse, family, or friends.
Coping Mechanisms	
Woman may exhibit the following behaviours: She may be traditionally vocal or nonvocal; crying out or groaning or both may be part of her ritual response to pain. She may use counterstimulation to minimize pain (e.g., rubbing, applying heat, or applying counterpressure). She may use relaxation, distraction, or autosuggestion as pain-countering techniques. She may resist any use of "needles" as modes of administering pain-relief medications.	The nurse may respond as follows: Use self effectively (e.g., using tone of voice, closeness in space, and touch as media for conveying a message of interest and caring). Use avoidance, belittling, or other distracting actions as a protective device for self. Use pharmacological resources at hand judiciously. Use comfort measures. Take control for management of pain.
Expectations of Others	
The nurse may be seen as someone who will accept the woman's statement of pain and act as her advocate. Medical personnel may be expected to relieve the woman of all pain sensations. The nurse may be expected to be interested, gentle, kind, and accepting of behaviour exhibited.	Only certain verbal or nonverbal responses to pain may be accepted as appropriate responses. The couple that is prepared for childbirth may be expected to refuse medication and may wish to "do everything on their own." The woman's definition of pain may not be accepted (i.e., the woman may wish to experience pain and participate in controlling it or may not be able to accept any pain as reasonable).

abuse may fight the labour process by reacting in panic or anger toward care providers, take control of everyone and everything related to their childbirth, surrender by being submissive and dependent, or retreat by mentally dissociating themselves from the sensations of labour and birth (Hobbins, 2004; Simkin & Klaus, 2004).

The nurse can help these women to associate the sensations they are experiencing with the process of childbirth and not with their past abuse. The woman's sense of control should be maintained by explaining all procedures to her and why they are needed, validating her needs and paying close attention to her requests, proceeding at the woman's pace, accepting her often extreme reactions to labour, and protecting her privacy by limiting the exposure of her body and the number of people involved in her care. Caregivers must always approach a woman by making eye contact first before any physical contact is made. It is recommended that all labouring women be cared for in this manner because it is not unusual for a woman to choose not to reveal a history of sexual abuse (Hobbins, 2004; Simkin & Klaus, 2004).

Stress in Labour

The way in which women and their support person or family members approach labour is related to the manner in which they have been socialized to the childbearing process. Their reactions reflect their life experiences regarding childbirth—physical, social, cultural, and religious. Society communicates its expectations of acceptable and unacceptable maternal behaviours during labour and birth. These expectations may be used by some women as the basis for evaluating their own actions during childbirth. An idealized perception of labour and birth may be a source of guilt and a sense of failure if the woman finds the process less than joyous, especially when the pregnancy is unplanned or is the product of a shaky or terminated relationship. Often women have heard horror stories or seen friends or relatives go through labours that appear anything but easy. **Multiparous** women often base their expectations of the present labour on their previous childbirth experiences.

Feelings a woman has about her pregnancy and fears regarding childbirth should be discussed. This is especially important if the woman is a primigravida who has not attended childbirth classes or a multiparous woman who had a previous negative childbirth experience. Major fears and concerns relate to the process and effects of childbirth, maternal and fetal well-being, and the attitude and actions of the health care staff. Unresolved fears increase a woman's stress and can slow the process of labour as a result of the inhibiting effects of catecholamines associated with the stress response on uterine contractions.

Women in labour usually have a variety of concerns that they will voice if asked but rarely volunteer. It is important to ask the woman what she expects or to suggest that she ask her primary health care provider about an issue. The following are

BOX 18-2 Procedure: Tests for Rupture of Amniotic Membranes

Nitrazine Test for pH*

Explain procedure to the woman or couple.

Procedure

Wash hands.

Use nitrazine test paper, a dye-impregnated test paper for determining pH (differentiates amniotic fluid, which is slightly alkaline, from urine and purulent material [pus], which are acidic).

Wearing a sterile glove lubricated with water, place a piece of test paper at the cervical os.

or

Use a sterile, cotton-tipped applicator to dip deep into the vagina to pick up fluid; touch applicator to test paper. (Procedure may be done during speculum examination)

or

Use amniotic fluid indicator swabs (which have been impregnated with nitrazine).

Read Results

Membranes probably intact—Identifies vaginal and most body fluids that are acidic:

Yellow to olive green pH 5.0–6.0

Membranes probably ruptured—Identifies amniotic fluid that is alkaline:

Blue-green to deep blue pH 6.5–7.5

Realize that false test results are possible because of presence of bloody show, insufficient amniotic fluid, or semen.

Remove gloves and wash hands.

Document Results

Positive or negative

Test for Ferning or Fern Pattern*

Explain procedure to the woman or couple.

Wash hands, apply sterile gloves, obtain specimen of fluid (usually during sterile speculum examination).

Spread a drop of fluid from vagina on a clean glass slide with a sterile, cotton-tipped applicator.

Allow fluid to dry.

Examine slide under microscope. Observe for appearance of ferning (a frondlike crystalline pattern). (Do not confuse with cervical mucus test, when high levels of estrogen are responsible for causing the ferning.)

Observe for absence of ferning (alert staff to possibility that amount of specimen was inadequate or that specimen was urine, vaginal discharge, or blood).

Remove gloves and wash hands.

Document Results

Positive or negative

*In some settings, the specimen is collected by the nurse or primary health care provider and sent to the laboratory for interpretation of results.

as vomiting and aspiration into the respiratory tract can be a complication during an operative birth.

Any information not found in the antenatal record can be obtained during the admission assessment. Pertinent data include the **birth plan** (see Box 10-9), the choice of infant feeding method, the type of pain management requested, and the name of the newborn's health care provider. The patient profile should indicate the support person or family members desired during childbirth and their availability, and ethnic or cultural expectations and needs. The woman's use of alcohol, drugs, and tobacco before or during pregnancy should be determined.

The nurse should review the birth plan. If no written plan has been prepared, the nurse can help the woman formulate a birth plan by describing options available and find out the woman's wishes and preferences (see Box 10-9). The nurse needs to discuss with the woman the possibility that changes may be needed in her plan as labour progresses and assure her that information will be provided so that she can make informed decisions. The nurse can use the birth plan information to plan individualized care for the woman during labour.

The nurse should provide information about the agency's policies regarding photography and recording of the birth and under what circumstances they are allowed. Protection of privacy, safety, and infection control (e.g., where the person who is recording the event should stand) are major concerns for the parents-to-be and the agency. The woman's record should reflect that the birth was recorded.

Psychosocial Factors

The woman's general behaviour (and that of her partner) may provide clues to the type of supportive care she will need. However, the nurse should keep in mind that general appearance and behaviour may vary, depending on the stage and phase of labour (Table 18-1). Psychosocial factors to assess include the following:

Verbal interactions—Does the woman ask questions? Can she ask for what she needs? Does she talk to her support person(s)? Does she talk freely with the nurse or respond only to questions?

Body language—Is she relaxed or tense? What is her anxiety level? How does she react to being touched by the nurse or support person? Does she change positions or lie rigidly still? Does she avoid eye contact? Does she look tired? How much rest has she had during the past 24 hours?

Perceptual ability—Does she understand what the nurse says? Is there a language barrier? Are repeated explanations necessary because her anxiety level interferes with her ability to comprehend? Can she repeat what she has been told or demonstrate her understanding?

Discomfort level—To what degree does the woman describe what she is experiencing? How does she react to a contraction? Are any nonverbal pain messages seen? Does she complain to the nurse or her partner? Can she ask for comfort measures?

Women With a History of Sexual Abuse

Memories of sexual abuse can be triggered during labour by intrusive procedures such as vaginal examination; loss of control; feeling helpless and isolated in a strange environment; being unable to move freely as a result of being confined to bed and "restrained" by monitors, IV lines, and epidural catheters; being watched by students; and having intense sensations in the uterus and genital area, especially at the time when she must push the baby out. Women who are survivors of

The woman's past and present pregnancy histories should be carefully noted. These include gravidity; parity; and problems such as history of vaginal bleeding, pregestational or gestational hypertension, anemia, pregestational or gestational diabetes, infections (e.g., bacterial or sexually transmitted), and **immunodeficiency**.

If this is not the woman's first labour and birth experience, it is important to note the characteristics of her previous experiences. This information includes the duration of previous labours, the type of anaesthesia used, the kind of birth (e.g., spontaneous vaginal, forceps- or vacuum-assisted, or Caesarean birth), and the condition of the newborn. The woman's perception of her previous labour and birth experiences should be explored because it may influence her attitude toward her current experience.

It is important to confirm the expected date of birth (EDB). Other data in the antenatal record include patterns of maternal weight gain, physiological measurements such as maternal vital signs (blood pressure, temperature, pulse, respiration), fundal height, baseline fetal heart rate (FHR), and laboratory and diagnostic test results.

Laboratory test results include the woman's blood type and Rh factor, a complete or partial blood cell count (complete blood cell count [CBC], hemoglobin, and hematocrit), the 50-g glucose challenge test, determination of the rubella titre, serological tests (Venereal Disease Research Laboratories [VDRL] or rapid plasma reagin [RPR] test) for syphilis, hepatitis B surface antigen, culture for group B streptococci, screening for the human immunodeficiency virus (HIV), and urinalysis. Additional tests may include a tuberculosis screen with purified protein derivative (PPD) and a screen for sickle cell trait or other genetic disorders. Diagnostic tests include integrated prenatal screening (IPS), amniocentesis, nonstress test (NST), **biophysical profile**, and ultrasound examination.

Group B Streptococcus (GBS). GBS infection occurs in approximately 25% of women. Presence of GBS in the pregnant woman can increase the risk of transmission to the fetus. Neonatal GBS can be a devastating condition. Risk factors for neonatal GBS infection include positive prenatal culture for GBS in the current pregnancy; preterm birth of less than 37 weeks of gestation; **premature rupture of membranes** (PROM) for longer than 18 hours; **intrapartum** maternal fever higher than 38°C; and a positive history for early-onset neonatal GBS.

To decrease the risk of neonatal GBS infection, intravenous antibiotic prophylaxis (IAP) should be offered to all women who test positive. Also, if a culture is not available at onset of labour and if risk factors are present, IAP should be offered (Centers for Disease Control and Prevention [CDC], 2010). Since the introduction of universal screening for GBS (rectovaginal culture at 36 to 37 weeks), the rate of GBS infection in newborns has decreased by 70% (Money et al., 2004). IAP is not recommended before a Caesarean birth if labour or rupture of membranes has not occurred. The recommended treatment is penicillin G, 5 million units in an intravenous (IV) loading dose, and then 2.5 million units intravenously every 4 hours during labour. Ampicillin, 2 g IV loading dose, followed by 1 g intravenously every 4 hours, is an alternative therapy. Therefore, the woman who is GBS positive will usually have an IV line started shortly after admission to ensure that adequate antibiotics are administered.

Herpes Simplex Virus (HSV). Neonatal herpes simplex virus (HSV) infection can be a devastating disease, so women need to be screened for this during labour. Current recommendations include carefully examining and questioning all women about symptoms at the onset of labour (Money et al., 2008). If visible lesions are not present when labour begins, vaginal birth is acceptable. Caesarean birth within 4 hours after labour begins or membranes rupture is recommended if visible lesions are present. Infants who are born through an infected vagina should be carefully observed and have blood tested for the presence of HSV. Some experts recommend presumptive treatment of infants who were exposed to HSV during birth.

Interview

The woman's primary reason for coming to the hospital is determined in the interview. Her primary reason may be that she is certain she is in labour (contractions that are longer, stronger, closer together); her bag of waters (i.e., amniotic membranes) ruptured, with or without contractions; or she is unsure whether she is in labour.

Even the experienced mother may have difficulty determining the onset of labour. The woman should be asked to recall the events of the previous days and to describe the following:

- Time of onset of contractions and progress in terms of intensity, frequency, and duration
- Location and character of discomfort from the contractions (e.g., back pain, suprapubic discomfort)
- Persistence of contractions despite changes in maternal position and activity (e.g., walking or lying down)
- Presence and character of vaginal discharge or "show"
- Status of amniotic membranes such as gush or seepage of fluid (SROM [spontaneous rupture of membranes])

If there has been a discharge that may be amniotic fluid, the woman should be asked about the colour, odour, and amount and the time it was first noted. In many instances, a sterile speculum examination and a **nitrazine** (pH) or **fern test** can confirm that the membranes are ruptured (Box 18-2).

These descriptions can help the nurse assess the degree of progress in labour. Bloody or pink show is distinguished from bleeding in that it is pink and feels sticky because of its mucoid nature. It is scant to begin with and increases with effacement and dilation of the cervix. A woman may report a scant brownish discharge that can be attributed to cervical trauma resulting from vaginal examination or coitus within the previous 48 hours.

If general **anaesthesia** is required in an emergency, it is important to assess the woman's respiratory status. The nurse can determine this by asking the woman if she has a cold or related symptoms (e.g., stuffy nose, sore throat, or cough). The nurse should recheck the status of allergies. Some allergic responses cause swelling of mucous membranes of the respiratory tract, which could interfere with breathing and the administration of inhalation anaesthetics.

The nurse should record the type and time of the woman's last solid food and liquid intake before coming to the hospital, talking with friends can reduce the perception of early discomfort, help the time pass, and reduce anxiety.

The woman who lives a considerable distance from the hospital or who lacks adequate support and transportation may be admitted in early labour. The same measures used by the woman at home should be offered to the hospitalized woman in early labour.

Admission to Labour Unit

When the woman arrives at the labour unit, assessment is the top priority (Fig. 18-1). The nurse will first perform a screening assessment, using the techniques of interview and physical assessment, and review laboratory and diagnostic test findings to determine the health status of the woman and her fetus and the progress of her labour. The primary health care provider is then notified; if the woman is admitted, a detailed systems assessment is done (see Nursing Process).

When the woman is admitted, she usually is moved from a triage area to the room where she will labour and possibly give birth: the labour, delivery, and recovery (LDR) room; the labour, delivery, recovery, and postpartum (LDRP) room; or the labour room. Anyone coming in the room should be introduced; women often express concern about the number of people intruding on their labour experience, especially if the role of the person and purpose for his or her presence are not clearly identified.

The family-centred care approach views labour and birth as a normal, healthy life event with the woman and her support people being active participants (see Box 1-5). LDR or LDRP rooms are essential components of family-centred care, and the woman is encouraged to have anyone she wishes present for her support. After birth, the mother, baby, and support people are permitted to stay together to celebrate the arrival of a new family member.

The woman may be asked to undress and put on her own gown or a hospital gown. An admissions band is placed on the woman's wrist, as well as an **allergy** band (usually coloured), when relevant. Her personal belongings are put away safely or given to family members according to agency policy and her preference. Often, women who participate in prenatal education classes bring a birth bag with them that contains items to be used in labour. Tennis balls or rolling pins for counterpressure, a pillow for comfort and a reminder of home, music, an object for a focal point (e.g., meaningful picture, stuffed animal), and rice bags for warm packs may be included in her bag. This bag should be unpacked so that women will remember to use the comfort measures they brought with them.

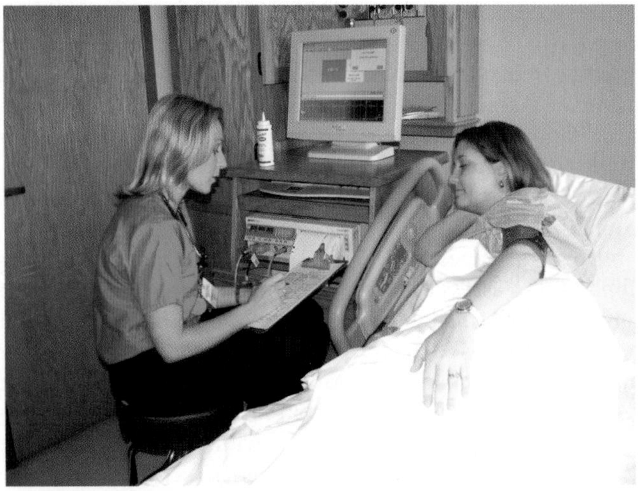

Fig. 18-1 Woman being admitted. *(Courtesy Julie Perry Nelson, Loveland, CO.)*

The nurse should orient the woman and her support people to the layout and operation of the unit and room. This includes the use of the call light and telephone system, the location of personal storage areas, and how to adjust lighting in the room and positions of the bed.

The nurse needs to reassure the woman that she is in competent, caring hands and that she and her partner can ask questions related to her care and the status of herself and her fetus at any time during labour. Any anxiety that the woman may have can be minimized by explaining terms commonly used during labour. Her interest, response, and prior experience will guide the depth of these explanations.

Admission Data

Hospital admission forms in either paper format or, more commonly today, computerized can provide guidelines for the acquisition of important assessment information when a woman in labour is being evaluated or admitted. Additional sources of data include the following: (1) antenatal record, (2) initial interview, (3) physical examination to determine baseline physiological parameters (e.g., vital signs), (4) laboratory and diagnostic test results, (5) expressed psychosocial and cultural factors, and (6) clinical evaluation of labour status.

Antenatal Data

The perinatal nurse reviews the antenatal record to identify the woman's individual needs and risks. Complete information regarding the woman's prenatal health status is essential to ensure the quality and safety of the care provided to her and to her fetus or newborn during labour and birth and in the postpartum period.

If the woman has not had any prenatal care or her antenatal record is unavailable, certain baseline information must be obtained. If she is having discomfort, the nurse should ask questions between contractions, when she can concentrate more fully on her responses. At times, the partner or support person(s) may need to be secondary sources of essential information.

It is important to know the woman's age so that the plan of care can be tailored to the needs of her age group. For example, a 14-year-old and a 40-year-old have different but specific needs, and their ages place them at risk for different problems. Height and weight relations are important to determine because a weight gain greater than that recommended may place the woman at a higher risk for Caesarean birth (Davies et al., 2010). This is especially true for women who are petite and have gained 16 kg or more. Other factors to consider are the woman's general health status, current medical conditions or allergies, respiratory status, and previous surgical procedures. Questioning about physical and substance use should form an integral part of the initial and ongoing assessment.

Assessment of Labour

Certain factors are assessed initially to determine whether the woman is in true labour and if she should come in for further assessment or admission to hospital (see Patient Teaching box). The pregnant woman may call her primary health care provider or come to the hospital while in false labour or early in the latent phase of the first stage of labour. She may feel discouraged, angry, or confused upon learning that the contractions that feel so strong and regular to her are not true contractions because they are not causing cervical dilation or are still not strong or frequent enough for hospital admission.

During the third trimester of pregnancy, women should be instructed about the stages of labour and the signs indicating its onset. They should be informed of the possibility that they will not be admitted to the hospital if they are 3 cm or less dilated. Later admission (i.e., during the active phase of labour at 4 cm or greater dilation) for low-risk women has been associated with an increased rate of spontaneous vaginal birth and fewer obstetrical interventions.

If the woman lives near the hospital and has adequate support and transportation, she may be asked to stay home or return home to allow labour to progress (i.e., until the contractions are more frequent and intense). The ideal setting for low-risk women in early labour is the familiar environment of her home. The nurse can use a telephone interview (Box 18-1) to assess the woman's status, give instructions regarding the optimal timing for admission, reinforce teaching of the signs that require immediate notification of the primary health care provider, and provide support and encouragement. The nurse should describe measures that the woman and her significant others can use to enhance the progress of labour, reduce anxiety, and maintain comfort. The woman should be informed that she can call back at any time to report concerns she may have or to ask questions. This is especially important for the **primigravida**, who may be very anxious and lack confidence in her ability to cope with labour.

A warm shower or bath can be relaxing for the woman in early labour. Soothing back, foot, and hand massages or a warm drink of preferred liquids such as tea or milk can help the woman rest and even sleep, especially if false or early labour is occurring at night. Diversional activities such as walking, reading, watching television, doing needlework, or

PATIENT TEACHING How to Distinguish True Labour From False Labour

True Labour

Contractions
- Occur regularly, becoming stronger, lasting longer, and occurring closer together
- Become more intense with walking
- Usually felt in lower back, radiating to lower portion of abdomen
- Continue despite use of comfort measures

Cervix (by vaginal examination done by health care provider)
- Shows progressive change (softening, effacement, and dilation, which may be signaled by the appearance of bloody show)
- Moves to an increasingly anterior position

False Labour

Contractions
- Occur irregularly or become regular only temporarily
- Often stop with walking or position change
- Can be felt in the back or abdomen above the navel
- Often can be stopped through the use of comfort measures

Cervix (by vaginal examination)
- May be soft, but there is no significant change in effacement or dilation or evidence of bloody show
- Is often in a posterior position

BOX 18-1 Telephone Interview With Woman in Latent Phase of Labour*

The perinatal nurse performs the following steps of the nursing process:

Assessment

Gathers data regarding the woman's status, including signs and symptoms indicative of true or false labour

Discusses instructions given by the woman's primary health care provider regarding when to come for admission

Planning and Implementation

Discusses with the woman whether she will come for labour assessment and admission or stay at home until contractions increase in duration, frequency, and intensity

Assures the woman that she is welcome to call the perinatal unit at any time to discuss her labour status

Answers questions the woman and her family may have about labour or provides instruction as needed

Suggests a variety of positions the woman can assume to maximally enhance uteroplacental and renal blood flow (e.g., side-lying position) and enhance the progress of labour (e.g., upright positions and ambulation)

Suggests diversional activities such as walking, reading, watching television, talking to friends

Suggests measures to maintain comfort such as a warm shower or a back or foot massage

Discusses the oral intake of foods and fluids appropriate for early labour (light meal and fluids)

Instructs the woman to come in immediately if membranes rupture (depending on instructions from health care provider), bleeding occurs, or fetal movements change or if she is having difficulty coping with the contractions

Evaluation

Evaluates whether instructions and information have been understood by the woman by asking her to communicate her understanding

Documentation

Documents all advice given over the telephone in the woman's record

*In some settings, nurses are no longer allowed to provide advice over the telephone but must refer the caller to her primary health care provider.

NURSING PROCESS: LABOUR

Assessment

Assessment begins at the first contact with the woman, whether by telephone or in person.
Review prenatal data from chart or patient.
Perform assessment, including Leopold's manoeuvres, uterine contractions, fetal heart rate, and status of cervix and membranes.
Review laboratory data.
Assess psychosocial factors.
Assess cultural factors.

Nursing Diagnoses

Nursing diagnoses appropriate for the woman in the first-stage labour include the following:

Anxiety related to
- negative experience with previous childbirth
- different cultural expectations
- lack of knowledge

Impaired urinary elimination related to
- reduced intake of oral fluids
- diminished sensation of bladder fullness associated with epidural anaesthesia/analgesia

Impaired fetal gas exchange related to
- maternal hypotension or hypertension
- intense uterine contractions
- compression of umbilical cord

Situational low self-esteem (maternal) related to
- inability to meet self-expectations of performance during childbirth
- loss of control during labour

Nursing diagnoses representing potential areas for concern during the second stage of labour include the following:

Risk for injury to mother and fetus related to
- persistent use of Valsalva manoeuvre

Situational low self-esteem related to
- lack of knowledge of normal, beneficial effects of vocalization during bearing-down efforts
- inability to carry out what she had planned for her birth experience

Ineffective coping related to
- coaching that contradicts woman's physiological urge to push

Anxiety related to
- lack of knowledge of perineal sensations associated with the urge to bear down

Examples of nursing diagnoses relevant to the third stage of labour include the following:

Risk for deficient fluid volume related to
- blood loss occurring following placental separation and expulsion
- inadequate contraction of the uterus

Anxiety related to
- lack of knowledge regarding birth of the placenta
- occurrence of perineal trauma and the need for repair

Fatigue related to
- energy expenditure associated with childbirth and the bearing-down efforts of the second stage

Planning

The nurse and woman set and prioritize expected outcomes that focus on the woman, the fetus, and the woman's support people.

Expected outcomes for the woman in labour are that the woman will accomplish the following:
- Continue normal progression of labour while the fetal heart rate and pattern remain normal and without signs of fetal compromise
- Maintain adequate hydration status through oral intake or intravenous (if required)
- Actively participate in the labour process
- Communicate discomfort and indicate the need for measures that help reduce discomfort and promote relaxation
- Accept comfort and support measures from support people and health care providers, as needed
- Sustain no injury to herself or the fetus during labour
- Expel the placenta with maternal blood loss of less than 500 mL or less than 1% of body weight
- Initiate, along with the partner and family, the processes of bonding and attachment with the newborn
- Express satisfaction with herself following labour

Interventions

Nursing care during first-stage labour includes both physical care and supportive care. Nursing interventions are described in the text (pp. 442–464) and in Table 18-4.

Evaluation

Evaluation is an ongoing process and is based on expected outcomes of care (see Nursing Care Plan, pp. 459–460).

woman often has lingering impressions of her childbirth experiences. Satisfaction with childbirth depends on the woman's ability to maintain a sense of control. Caregivers who encourage a woman to be actively involved in decision making and who are respectful, supportive, available, protective, encouraging, kind, patient, professional, calm, and comforting can help the woman remember her childbirth experiences in positive terms. A positive childbirth experience contributes to a woman's self-esteem and sense of accomplishment; this may in turn enhance the way she sees herself in her role as a mother. Frustrations that a woman feels about her childbirth experience stem from unmet expectations, loss of control, lack of knowledge, or the negative behaviours of some caregivers. A woman who perceives her childbirth to be unsatisfactory or traumatic could be at risk for postpartum depression and Caesarean birth for a subsequent pregnancy.

Unit 4

18 Nursing Care During Labour and Birth

Learning Objectives

On completion of this chapter, the reader will be able to:

- Review the factors included in the initial assessment of the woman in labour.
- Describe the ongoing assessment of maternal progress during the first, second, third, and fourth stages of labour.
- Recognize the physical and psychosocial findings that indicate maternal progress during labour.
- Describe fetal assessment during labour.
- Identify signs of developing complications during labour and birth.
- Develop a comprehensive plan of care for the woman and her significant others (support person[s], family) relevant to each stage of labour.
- Analyze the influence of cultural and religious beliefs and practices on the process of labour and birth.
- Evaluate research findings on the importance of support from the family, partner, doula, and nurse in facilitating maternal progress during labour and birth.
- Describe the role and responsibilities of the nurse in an emergency childbirth situation.
- Review the impact of perineal trauma on the woman's reproductive and sexual health.
- Discuss ways in which the nurse can use evidence-informed practices to enhance the quality of care that a woman receives during labour and birth.

Electronic Resources

Additional information related to the content in Chapter 18 can be found on

evolve **the companion Web site at**

http://evolve.elsevier.com/Canada/Perry/maternal/

- Examination Review Questions
- Animation—Vaginal Birth
- Assessment Video—Leopold's Manoeuvres
- Case Study—First Stage of Labour
- Case Study—Second/Third Stages of Labour
- Critical Thinking Exercise—Positioning During Labour
- Video—Childbirth (Vaginal)

The labour process is an exciting and anxious time for the woman and her significant others (e.g., support people, family). In a relatively short period, they experience one of the most profound changes in their lives.

For most women, labour begins with the first uterine contraction, continues with hours of work during cervical dilation and birth, and ends as the woman and her family begin the attachment process with the newborn. Nursing care management focuses on assessment and support of the woman and her support people and family throughout labour and birth, with the goal of ensuring the best possible outcome for all involved.

First Stage of Labour

Nursing Care Management

The first stage of labour begins with the onset of regular uterine contractions and ends with complete cervical **effacement** and dilation (see Nursing Process box). The first stage of labour consists of three phases: the latent phase (up to 3 cm of dilation), the active phase (4 to 7 cm of dilation), and the transition phase (8 to 10 cm of dilation).

Even though no two labours are identical, women who have given birth before often appear less anxious about the process, unless their previous experience was negative. A

References

Association of Women's Health, Obstetric and Neonatal Nurses (AWHONN). (2009). *Antepartum and intrapartum fetal heart rate monitoring: Clinical competencies and education guide* (5th ed.). Dubuque, IA: Kendall/Hunt.

Canadian Institute for Health Information (CIHI). (2010). *Health indicators.* Retrieved from http://www.cihi.ca/indicators.

Fraser, W. D., et al. (2005). Amnioinfusion Trial Group: Amnioinfusion for the prevention of the meconium aspiration syndrome. *New England Journal of Medicine, 353*(9), 909–917. doi: 10.1097/01.ogx.0000197831.56608.6e

Garcia, J., et al. (1985). Mother's views of continuous electonic fetal heart monitoring and intermittent auscultation in a randomized controlled trial. *Birth, 1985*, 79–85.

Garite, T. J. (2007). Intrapartum fetal evaluation. In S. Gabbe, J. Niebyl, & J. Simpson (Eds.), *Obstetrics: Normal and problem pregnancies* (5th ed.). Philadelphia: Churchill Livingstone.

Gilbert, E. S. (2007). *Manual of high risk pregnancy and delivery* (4th ed.). St. Louis: Mosby.

Gray, J. (1983). *Handbook of fetal heart rate monitoring.* Halifax, NS: Seaview Publishing.

Killen, M. G., & Shy, K. (1989). A randomized trial of electronic fetal monitoring in preterm labour. *Birth, 1989*, 7–12.

Lee, L., et al. (2009). *Fundamentals of fetal health surveillance* (4th ed.). Vancouver: British Columbia Perinatal Health Program.

Liston, R., et al. (2007). Fetal health surveillance: Antepartum and intrapartum consensus guideline. *Journal of Obstetrics and Gynaecology Canada, 29*(9 Suppl 4), s1–s56. Retrieved from http://www.sogc.org/guidelines/documents/gui197CPG0709.pdf.

Macones, G. A., et al. (2008). The 2008 National Institute of Child Health and Human Development Workshop Report on Electronic Fetal Monitoring: Update on definitions, interpretation, and research guidelines. *Journal of Obstetric, Gynecologic and Neonatal Nursing, 37*(5), 510–515. doi: 10.1097/AOG.0b013e3181841395

National Institute of Child Health and Human Development Research Planning Workshop. (1997). Electronic fetal heart rate monitoring: Research guidelines for interpretation. *American Journal of Obstetrics and Gynecology, 177*(6), 1385–1390.

Public Health Agency of Canada. (2009). *What mothers say: The Canadian maternity experiences survey* (Cat. No. HP5-74/2-2009E-PDF). Ottawa: Author.

Simpson, K., & James, D. (2005). Efficacy of intrauterine resuscitation techniques in improving fetal oxygen status during labour. *Obstetrics and Gynecology, 105*(6), 1362–1368. doi: 10.1097/01.AOG.0000164474.03350.7c

Thacker, S. B., Stroup, D., & Change, M. (2006). Continuous electronic heart rate monitoring for fetal assessment during labour [Cochrane review]. *Cochrane Database of Systematic Reviews* 2006(*3*). Chichester, UK: John Wiley & Sons. doi: 10,1002/14651858.CD000063.pub2.

Tucker, S. M., Miller, L. A., & Miller, D. A. (2009). *Mosby's pocket guide to fetal monitoring: A multidisciplinary approach* (6th ed.). St. Louis: Mosby.

Wiberg-Itzel, E., et al. (2008). Determination of pH or lactate in fetal scalp blood in management of intrapartum fetal distress: randomised controlled multicentre trial. *British Medical Journal, 336*(7656), 1284–1287.

Additional Resources

SOGC Fetal Health Surveillance: Antepartum and Intrapartum Consensus Guideline: http://www.sogc.org/guidelines/documents/gui197CPG0709.pdf

common concerns that women in labour have: Will my baby be all right? Will I be able to cope with labour? Will my labour be long? How will I act? Will I need medication? Will it work for me? Will my partner or someone be there to support me?

The nurse's responsibility to the woman in labour with regard to these concerns is to answer her questions or find out the answers, provide support for her and her support person and family, take care of her in partnership with the people the woman wants as her support team, and serve as their advocate. One of the most important aspects of nursing care for the labouring women is to develop a trusting relationship with the woman and her support people, as this will help the woman and her family to feel more comfortable expressing their feelings and concerns. Women can equate emotional support with information giving. Nurses are perceived as supportive when they explain things in detail by using positive terms and provide accurate information and specific directions. Women will feel empowered when they are given information they can understand and that reflects support of their efforts. This feeling of empowerment contributes to a positive perception of the birth experience. In contrast, a woman's level of anxiety and fear may increase when she does not understand what is being said.

The nurse needs to communicate to the woman that she is not expected to act in any particular way. Also, the woman's views and expectations regarding the nurse's role as caregiver should be determined. As labour progresses, the nurse–patient relationship will become increasingly important. Women need to trust in their own innate ability to give birth, and nurses need to support and protect each woman's efforts to achieve this outcome.

The partner, coach, and significant other(s) also experience stress during labour. The nurse can assist and support these individuals by identifying their needs and expectations and helping to make sure these are met. The nurse can ascertain what role the support person intends to fulfill and whether he or she is prepared for that role, by making observations and asking him or her questions such as the following: Has the couple attended childbirth classes? What role does this person expect to play? Is he or she nervous, anxious, aggressive, or hostile? Does he or she look hungry, tired, worried, or confused? Does he or she watch television, sleep, or stay out of the room instead of paying attention to the woman? Does he or she touch the woman? What is the character of the touch? The nurse should be sensitive to the needs of support people and provide teaching and support, as appropriate. Often the support that this person is able to give to the labouring woman is in direct proportion to the support he or she receives from nurses and other health care providers.

Cultural Factors

With Canada's increasingly diverse population, nurses need to be committed to providing culturally sensitive care and developing an appreciation of and respect for cultural diversity (Callister, 2005; Canadian Nurses Association [CNA], 2010). For the perinatal nurse, it is important to recognize a pregnant woman's ethnic (cultural) and religious values, beliefs, and practices in order to anticipate nursing interventions that should be included in a mutually acceptable plan of care that facilitates a feeling of safety and control. The woman should be encouraged to request caregiving behaviours and practices that are important to her. If a special request contradicts usual practices in that setting, the woman or nurse can ask the woman's primary health care provider to write an order to accommodate the special request. For example, in many cultures it is unacceptable to have a male caregiver examine a pregnant woman. Some health care providers will try to accommodate this request, if possible. In some cultures it is traditional to take the **placenta** home; in others, the woman is given only certain nourishments during labour. Some women believe that cutting her body, as with an episiotomy, allows her spirit to leave her body and that rupturing the membranes prolongs, not shortens, labour. It is important that the rationale for required care measures be carefully explained, particularly if they conflict with the woman's beliefs.

Cultural beliefs and values can influence a woman's reliance on her primary health care provider during labour and her desire to participate in making decisions about the care she receives (Callister, 2005). For instance, a Japanese woman in labour may assume the traditional role of a passive patient and may be reluctant to express her needs unless specifically asked to do so (Ito & Sharts-Hopko, 2002). First Nations, Métis, and Inuit women believe childbirth is a community event, one that places a high value on relationships, respect, and the collective perspective. With limited access to birthing centres, Aboriginal Canadians are often moved off reserve and away from their families in late pregnancy to await labour. This may cause a disruption of the balance and harmony that are critical for a positive birth experience.

Within cultures, women may learn the "right" way to behave in labour and thus react to the pain experienced in that way. These behaviours can range from total silence to moaning or screaming, but they are not in and of themselves a gauge of the degree of pain. A woman who moans with contractions may not be in as much physical pain as a woman who is silent but winces during contractions (see Table 18-1). For example, Chinese women may be stoic and quiet during labour and merely grimace during a contraction but not shout out. Rather than using pharmacological measures for pain relief, they may prefer the support of family members and nonpharmacological measures (Brathwaite & Williams, 2004; Cioffi, 2004). Chinese women who believe in the balance of yin and yang view childbirth as a source of heat loss from the body. Thus, providing hot fluids and a warm shower to these women during labour could be acceptable measures of restoring the heat that is being lost (Cioffi, 2004; D'Avanzo, 2008).

Some women believe that it is shameful to scream or cry out in pain if a man is present. If the woman's support person is her mother, she may perceive the need to "behave" more strongly than if her support person is the father of the baby. In general, the woman will perceive herself as failing or succeeding on the basis of her ability to adhere to these "standards" of behaviour. Conversely, a woman's behaviour in response to pain may influence the support received from significant others. In some cultures, women who lose control and cry out in pain may be scolded, whereas in other cultures, support people will be more helpful.

When assessing a woman's cultural and religious preferences, the nurse can ask questions regarding the following:

- The value and meaning placed on the childbirth experience
- The view of childbirth as a wellness or illness experience and as a private or social event
- Practices regarding diet, medications, activity, and emotional and physical support
- Appropriate maternal and paternal behaviours
- Birth companions—who they should be and what they should do
- Views regarding the newborn and newborn care immediately after birth

Culture and Father Participation

A companion is an important source of support, encouragement, and comfort to women during childbirth. The choice of a birth companion is influenced by the woman's cultural and religious background and by trends in the society in which she lives. For example, in Western societies, the partner is viewed as the ideal birth companion. Also, among the Laotian (Hmong), the father plays an important role in the birth. In some other cultures, however, the presence of a male in the labour and birth room is inappropriate (e.g., Mexican, Filipino, Chinese, Islamic, and Ethiopian) (D'Avanzo, 2008).

In many cultures, women share an affectional bond with their female relatives when it comes to home-related activities such as childbearing. The presence of another woman or women is highly desired at such occasions. Women who come from some of these cultures and who give birth in the hospital like to have at least one woman present for assistance. Vietnamese, Chinese, Indian, Syrian, and Orthodox Jewish women prefer a female companion during childbirth and are very concerned about their modesty. In addition to feeling shy, they cite the belief that female caregivers are more respectful and would provide a higher degree of comfort and psychosocial support (Bashour & Abdulsalam, 2005; D'Avanzo, 2008). Islamic women also are very modest (i.e., need to keep hair and body covered) and would not accept the presence of a man during childbirth, not even the father. In India, women are attended by other women and in rural areas by a local untrained midwife or dai. For couples from these cultures who immigrate to Canada, their roles may change. The nurse will need to talk with the woman and her support people to determine the roles that they wish to assume.

The Non–English-Speaking Woman in Labour

A woman's level of anxiety in labour rises when she does not understand what is happening to her or what is being said. Some misunderstanding may occur even when the language being spoken is the first language of the woman, and this may cause some stress, but the effect of misunderstanding on women who do not understand the language is much more dramatic. These women often feel a complete loss of control over their situation if there is no health care provider present who speaks their language. They can panic and withdraw or become physically abusive when someone tries to do something that they perceive might harm them or their baby. Sometimes a support person is able to serve as an interpreter. However, this must be done with caution because the interpreter may not be able to convey exactly what the nurse or others are saying or what the woman is saying, and this may raise the woman's stress level even more. It is important to identify the need for an interpreter early during antenatal care in order to ensure adequate time to coordinate the availability of this service when the patient arrives for labour assessment.

Ideally, a bilingual nurse will care for the woman. Alternatively, an employee or volunteer interpreter may be contacted for assistance. Preferably, the interpreter is from the woman's culture. For some women, a female interpreter may be more acceptable. If no one in the hospital is able to interpret, a translation service can be called so that an interpretation can take place over the telephone. Another alternative is for the labour and birth staff to prepare a set of cards with graphic depictions that illustrate common situations. These cards can be used to communicate with women who do not understand the language. Even when the nurse has limited ability to communicate orally with the woman, in most instances the nurse's efforts to communicate are meaningful and appreciated by the woman. Speaking slowly and avoiding complex words and medical terms can help a woman and her partner to better understand what is happening during labour and birth.

Physical Examination

The initial physical examination includes a general systems assessment; performance of Leopold's manoeuvres to determine fetal presentation, position, and point of maximal intensity (PMI) for auscultating the FHR; assessment of fetal status; assessment of uterine activity (UA); and vaginal examination to assess cervical effacement and dilation, fetal descent, and amniotic membranes and fluid. The findings of the admission physical examination serve as a baseline for assessing the woman's progress from that point.

It is important to obtain as many related pieces of information as possible before planning and implementing care. Women often focus on the nature of their contractions as the clearest indicator of how far advanced their labour is. However, the findings from the vaginal examination are more valid indicators of the phase of labour, especially for nulliparous women.

Expected maternal progress and minimum assessment guidelines during the first stage of labour are presented in Table 18-2. Routine precautions should be used for all assessment and care measures (Box 18-3). Hand hygiene (e.g., washing hands with soap or application of an alcohol-based antibacterial solution) before and after assessing the woman and providing care is a critical step in the prevention of infection transmission. The assessment findings need to be explained to the woman. Throughout labour, accurate documentation, following agency policy, should be done as soon as possible after a procedure has been performed (Fig. 18-2).

General Systems Assessment

A brief systems assessment should be performed. This includes assessment of the heart, lungs, and skin; an examination to determine the presence and extent of edema of the legs, face, and hands; and testing of deep tendon reflexes and for clonus if blood pressure is increased.

Vital Signs

Vital signs (temperature, pulse, respirations, and blood pressure) are assessed on admission, and initial values are used

Table 18-2 Expected Maternal Progress During First Stage of Labour

	*Phases Marked by Cervical Dilation**		
CRITERION	**0–3 CM (LATENT)**	**4–7 CM (ACTIVE)**	**8–10 CM (TRANSITION)**
Duration†	About 6–8 hr	About 3–6 hr	About 20–60 min
Contractions			
Strength	Mild to moderate	Moderate to strong	Strong to very strong
Rhythm	Irregular	More regular	Regular
Frequency	5–30 min apart	3–5 min apart	2–3 min apart
Duration	30–45 sec	40–70 sec	45–90 sec
Descent			
Station of presenting part	Nulliparous: 0 Multiparous: 0–2 cm	Varies: +1 to +2 cm Varies: +1 to +2 cm	Varies: +2 to +3 cm Varies: +2 to +3 cm
Show			
Colour	Brownish discharge, mucous plug, or pale pink mucus	Pink-to-bloody mucus	Bloody mucus
Amount	Scant	Scant to moderate	Copious
Behaviour and appearance‡	Excited; thoughts centre on self, labour, and baby; may be talkative or silent, calm or tense; some apprehension; pain controlled fairly well; alert, follows directions readily; open to instructions	Becomes more serious, doubtful of pain control, more apprehensive; desires companionship and encouragement; attention more inner directed; fatigue evidenced; malar (cheeks) flush; has some difficulty following directions	Pain described as moderate to severe; backache common; frustration, fear of loss of control, and irritability surface; vague in communications; amnesia between contractions; writhing with contractions; nausea and vomiting, especially if hyperventilating; hyperesthesia; perspiration of forehead and upper lips; shaking tremor of thighs; feeling of need to defecate, pressure on anus

*In the nullipara, effacement is often complete before dilation begins; in the multipara it occurs simultaneous with dilation.
†Duration of each phase is influenced by such factors as parity, maternal emotions, position, level of activity, fetal size, and presentation position. For example, the labour of a nullipara tends to last longer, on average, than the labour of a multipara. Women who ambulate and assume upright positions or change positions frequently during labour tend to experience a shorter first stage. Descent is often prolonged in breech presentations and occiput posterior positions.
‡Women who have epidural analgesia for pain relief may not demonstrate some of these behaviours.

BOX 18-3 Routine Precautions During Childbirth

Birth is a time when nurses and other health care providers are exposed to a great deal of maternal and newborn blood and body fluids. Observation of routine precautions is necessary to prevent the transmission of infection. Perinatal infections most often are transmitted through contact with body fluids. Routine precautions applicable to childbirth include the following:

The 4 Moments of hand hygiene are followed: (1) before initial patient/patient environment contact, (2) before aseptic procedure, (3) after body-fluid exposure risk, (4) after patient/patient environment contact.

Wear gloves (clean or sterile, as appropriate) when performing procedures that require contact with the woman's genitalia and body fluids, including bloody show (e.g., during vaginal examination, amniotomy, hygienic care of the perineum, insertion of an internal scalp electrode and intrauterine pressure monitor, and catheterization).

Wear cap, a mask that has a shield or protective eyewear, and shoe covers and cover gown during birth in an operating room. Gowns worn by the primary health care provider who is attending the birth should have a waterproof front.

Wear gloves when handling the newborn immediately after birth until the first bath is completed.

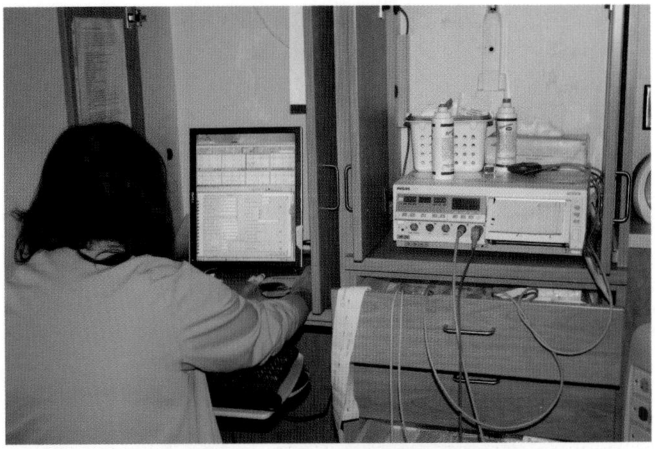

Fig. 18-2 Nurse documenting assessment findings on computer in a labour, delivery, recovery, postpartum room. *(Courtesy Shannon Perry, Phoenix, AZ.)*

for comparison with subsequent values. If blood pressure is elevated, it should be reassessed 30 minutes later, between contractions, after the woman has relaxed. To prevent supine hypotension and fetal distress, the woman should be encouraged to lie on her side and not supine (Fig. 18-3). Her temperature should be monitored so that signs of infection or fluid deficit (e.g., dehydration associated with inadequate intake of fluids) can be identified. The woman's intake and output should be measured at least every 8 hours. When indicated, urinary protein and ketone levels may be determined by using a dipstick.

evolve Assessment Video—Leopold's Manoeuvres

NURSING ALERT During labour, blood pressure should be assessed with an appropriate-sized sphygmomanometer and stethoscope for the most accurate results. Automatic devices that measure blood pressure have been found to overestimate the systolic pressure and underestimate the diastolic pressure. These devices further restrict freedom of movement and can also increase the discomfort of the woman as the cuff inflates and deflates on a regular basis. Maternal heart rate should be assessed by auscultation (i.e., apical rate) or palpation (i.e., radial pulse rate) rather than with a pulse oximeter (Simpson, 2005).

Leopold's Manoeuvres (Abdominal Palpation)

Leopold's manoeuvres are performed with the woman briefly lying on her back (Box 18-4 and Fig. 18-4). These manoeuvres help to identify the following: (1) number of fetuses; (2) presenting part, fetal lie, and fetal attitude; (3) degree of descent of the presenting part into the pelvis; and (4) expected location of the PMI of the FHR on the woman's abdomen.

Assessment of Fetal Heart Rate and Pattern

It is important for the nurse to understand the relationship between the location of the PMI of the FHR and fetal presentation, lie, and position. A risk for childbirth complications may be revealed by variations in these findings. The PMI of the FHR is the location on the maternal abdomen where the FHR is heard the loudest. It is usually directly over the fetal back. The PMI is also an aid in determining the fetal presentation and position (Fig. 18-5). In a vertex presentation, FHR is heard below the mother's umbilicus in either the right or left lower quadrant of the abdomen. In a breech presentation, the FHR is heard above the mother's umbilicus (see Fig. 18-5, A, and Fig. 18-6, C). As the fetus descends and rotates internally, the FHR is heard lower and closer to the midline of the maternal abdomen (see Fig. 18-6, B). The PMI of the fetus in the right occipitoanterior position moves to the midline just over the symphysis pubis

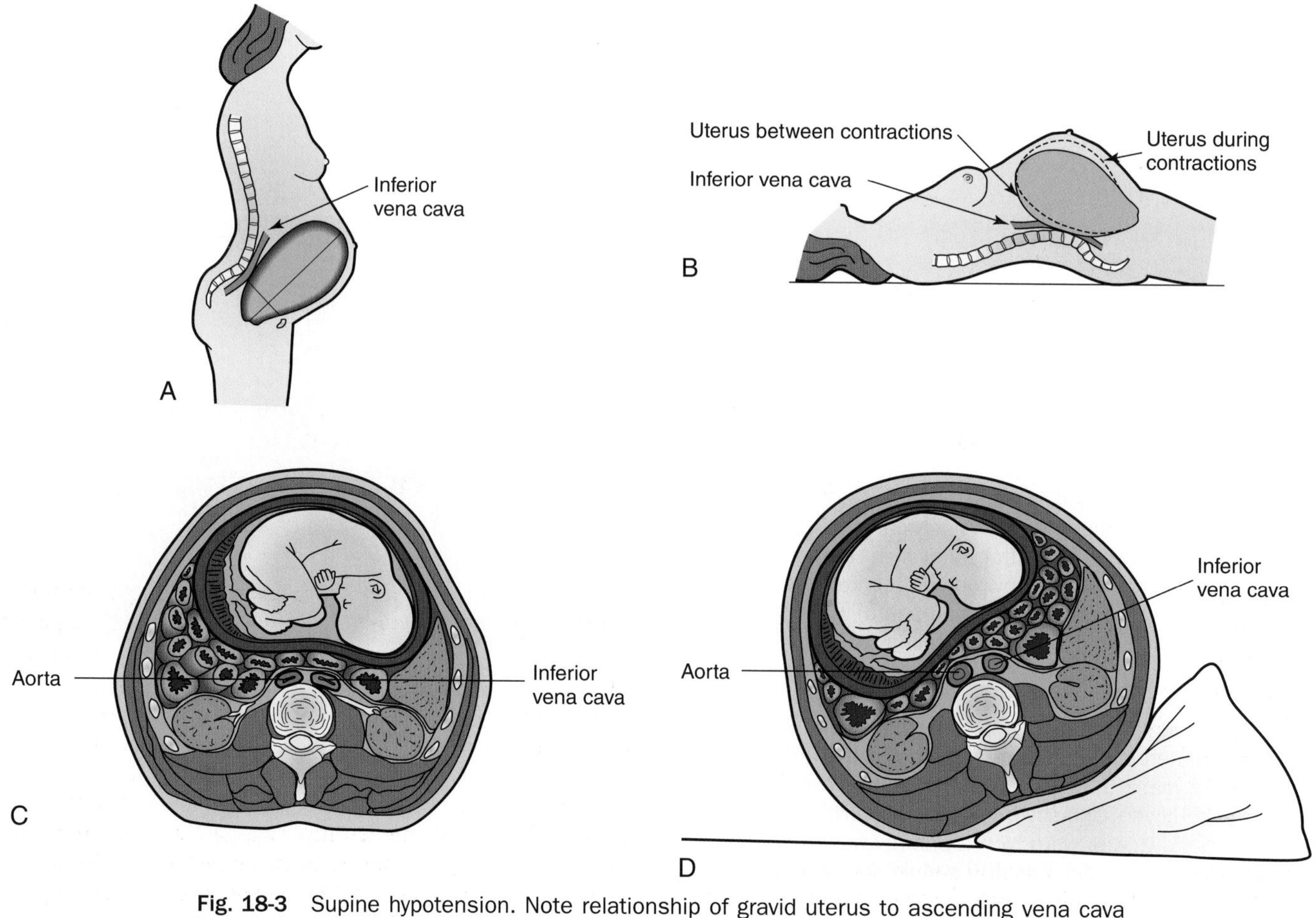

Fig. 18-3 Supine hypotension. Note relationship of gravid uterus to ascending vena cava in standing posture (**A**) and supine posture (**B**). Compression of aorta and inferior vena cava with woman in supine position (**C**). Relieved by use of a wedge pillow placed under woman's right side (**D**).

BOX 18-4 Procedure: Leopold's Manoeuvres and Determination of the Points of Maximal Intensity of the Fetal Heart Rate

Leopold's Manoeuvres

Wash hands.

Ask woman to empty bladder.

Position woman supine with one pillow under her head and her knees slightly flexed.

Place small rolled towels under woman's right or left hip to displace uterus off major blood vessels (prevents supine hypotensive syndrome; see Fig. 18-3, D).

If right-handed, stand on woman's right, facing her:

1. Identify fetal part that occupies the fundus. The head feels round, firm, freely movable, and palpable by ballottement; the breech feels less regular and softer. This manoeuvre is used to identify fetal lie (longitudinal or transverse) and presentation (cephalic or breech) (see Fig. 18-4, A).
2. Using the palmar surface of one hand, locate and palpate the smooth convex contour of the fetal back and the irregularities that identify the small parts (feet, hands, elbows). This manoeuvre helps identify fetal presentation (see Fig. 18-4, B).
3. With the right hand, determine which fetal part is presenting over the inlet to the true pelvis. Gently grasp the lower pole of the uterus between the thumb and fingers, pressing in slightly (see Fig. 18-4, C). If the head is presenting and not engaged, determine the attitude of the head (flexed or extended).
4. Turn to face the woman's feet. Using both hands, outline the fetal head (see Fig. 18-4, D) with the palmar surface of the fingertips. When the presenting part has descended deeply, only a small portion of it may be outlined. Palpation of the cephalic prominence helps identify the attitude of the head. If the cephalic prominence is bound on the same side as the small parts, this means that the head must be flexed and the vertex is presenting (see Fig. 18-4, D). If the cephalic prominence is on the same side as the back, this indicates that the presenting head is extended and the face is presenting (see Fig. 18-4, D).
5. Document fetal presentation, position, and lie and whether the presenting part is flexed or extended, engaged, or free floating. Use hospital's protocol for documentation (e.g., "Vtx, LOA, floating").

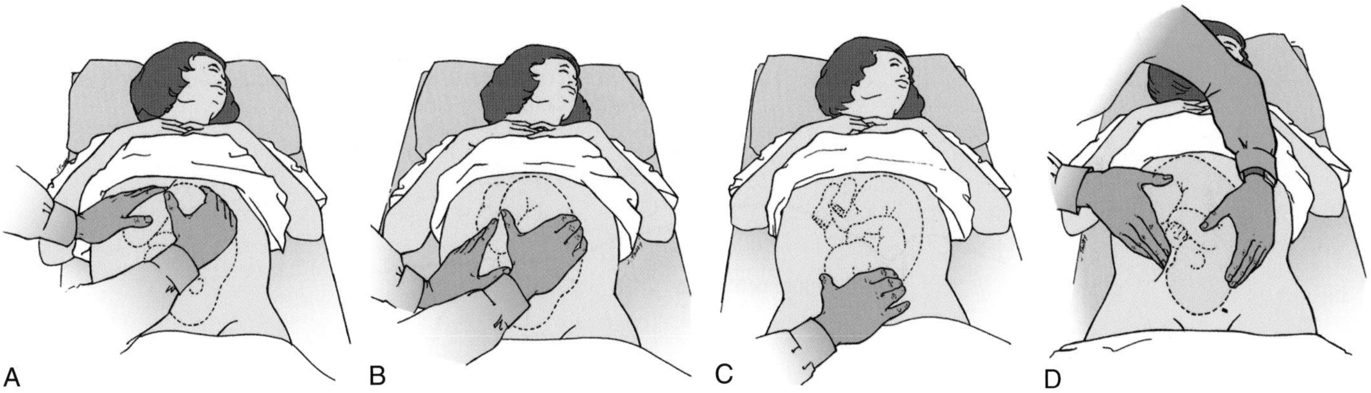

Fig. 18-4 Leopold's manoeuvres (see also Box 18-4).

(see Fig. 18-6, A and B). Just before birth, the fetal position is occipitoanterior, and the fetal back is directly above the symphysis pubis.

The FHR and pattern must also be assessed (1) immediately after ROM because this is the most common time for the umbilical cord to prolapse, (2) after any change in the contraction pattern or maternal status, and (3) before and after medicating the woman or performing a procedure.

Assessment of Uterine Activity (UA)

A general characteristic of effective labour is regular UA (i.e., contractions becoming more frequent and of increased duration); however, UA is not directly related to labour progress. Uterine contractions are the primary powers that act involuntarily to expel the fetus and placenta from the uterus. Several methods are used to evaluate the strength of uterine contractions: the woman's subjective description, palpation and timing of the contraction by a health care provider, and internal electronic monitoring.

Each contraction exhibits a wavelike pattern. It begins with a slow increment (the "building up" of a contraction from its onset) that gradually reaches an acme (the peak, with intrauterine pressure less than 80 mm Hg) and then diminishes rapidly (decrement, the "letting down" of the contraction). An interval of rest (intrauterine pressure less than 15 mm Hg) ends when the next contraction begins. The outward appearance of the woman's abdomen during and between contractions and the pattern of a typical uterine contraction are shown in Figure 18-7.

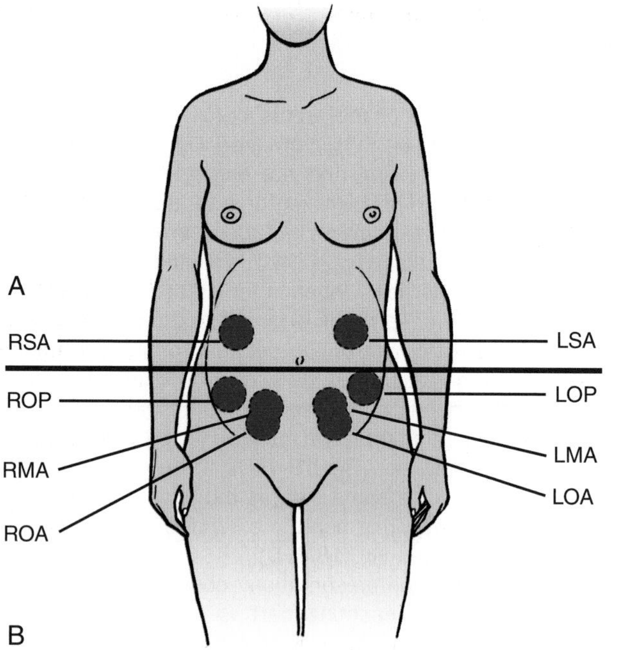

Fig. 18-5 Areas of maximal intensity of fetal heart rate for differing positions. *RSA*, right sacrum anterior; *ROP*, right occipitoposterior; *RMA*, right mentum anterior; *ROA*, right occipitoanterior; *LSA*, left sacrum anterior; *LOP*, left occipitoposterior; *LMA*, left mentum anterior; *LOA*, left occipitoanterior. **A:** Presentation is breech if fetal heart tones (FHTs) are heard above umbilicus. **B:** Presentation is vertex if FHTs are heard below umbilicus.

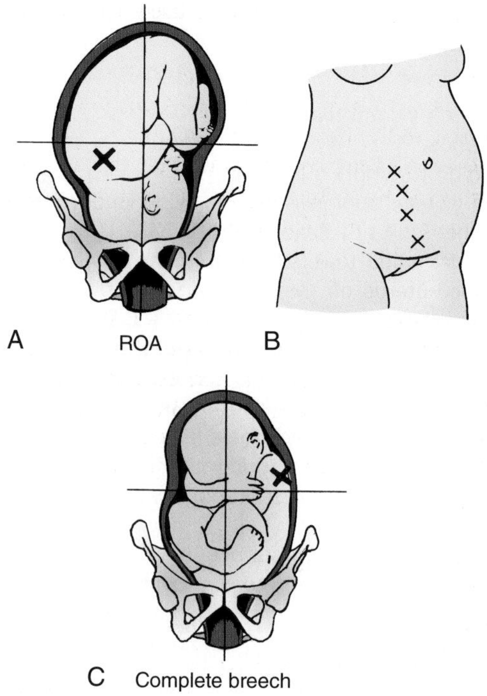

Lie: Vertical
Presentation: Breech (sacrum and feet presenting)
Reference point: Sacrum (with feet)
Attitude: General flexion

Fig. 18-6 Location of the fetal heart rate. **A:** With fetus in right occipitoanterior (ROA) position. **B:** Changes in location of point of maximal intensity of fetal heart tones as fetus undergoes internal rotation from ROA to OA position for birth. **C:** With fetus in left sacrum posterior position. *(**A** and **C**, Courtesy Ross Laboratories, Columbus, OH.)*

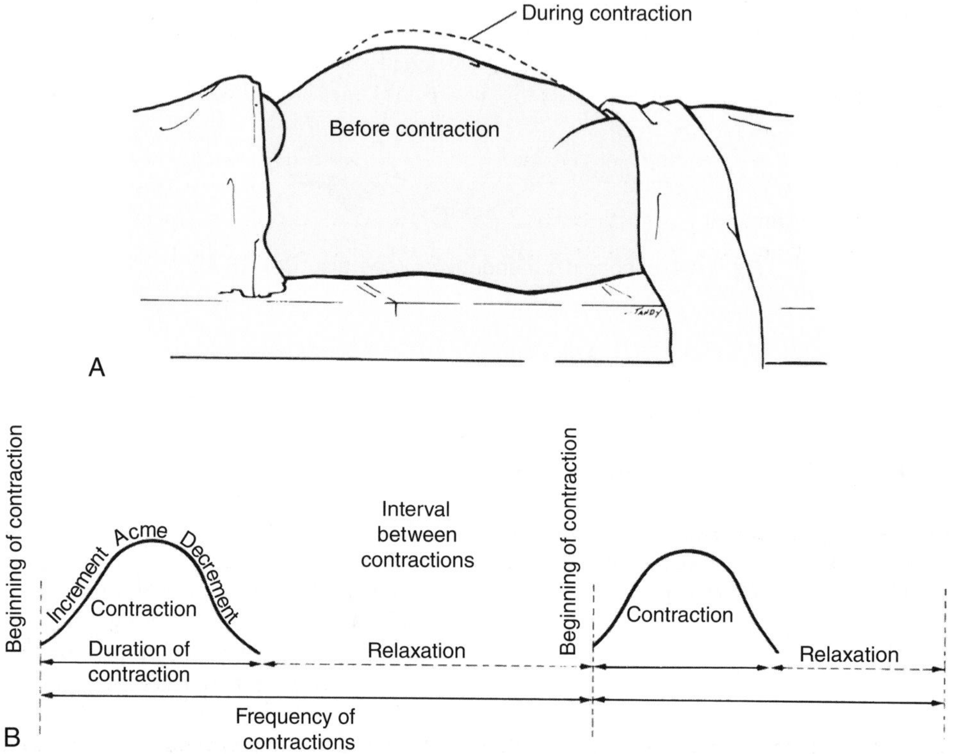

Fig. 18-7 Assessment of uterine contractions. **A:** Abdominal contour before and during uterine contractions. **B:** Wavelike pattern of contractile activity.

The following characteristics are used to describe a uterine contraction:

Frequency—How often uterine contractions occur; the time that elapses from the beginning of one contraction to the beginning of the next (in minutes)

Intensity—The strength of a contraction at its peak

Duration—The time that elapses between the onset and the end of a contraction (in seconds)

Resting tone—The tension in the uterine muscle between contractions

UA is assessed by palpation or by an external or internal electronic monitor. Frequency and duration can be measured by all three methods of uterine activity monitoring. Intensity can only be assessed using palpation or internal electronic monitoring. Palpation is subjective but along with the patient's report of the pain, is the best way to determine the intensity of uterine contractions. The following terms are used to describe what is felt on palpation:

Mild—Slightly tense fundus that is easy to indent with fingertips (feels like touching finger to tip of nose)

Moderate—Firm fundus that is difficult to indent with fingertips (feels like touching finger to chin)

Strong—Rigid, boardlike fundus that is almost impossible to indent with fingertips (feels like touching finger to forehead)

Women in labour tend to describe the pain of contractions in terms of their sensations in the lower abdomen or the back, which may be unrelated to the firmness of the uterine fundus. The amount of discomfort reported is a valid assessment of the pain the woman is experiencing.

On admission, a 20- to 30-minute baseline monitoring of uterine contractions and of the FHR pattern is recommended for women with risk factors for adverse perinatal outcomes (see Table 17-2) and is not recommended for healthy, term women in labour. Intermittent auscultation is the preferred method for healthy women after 36 weeks' (up to 41+3 weeks) gestation in spontaneous labour in the absence of risk factors (Liston et al., 2007; see Chapter 17 for more in-depth discussion).

The findings that are expected as labour progresses are summarized in Tables 18-2 and 18-5.

The nurse's responsibility in monitoring uterine contractions is to ascertain whether they are powerful and frequent enough to accomplish the work of expelling the fetus and the placenta.

NURSING ALERT If the characteristics of uterine activity (UA) are found to be abnormal, either exceeding or falling below what is considered acceptable in terms of the standard characteristics, the nurse should document the finding and report this finding to the primary health care provider.

Cervical Effacement, Dilation, Fetal Descent. UA must be considered in the context of its effect on cervical effacement and dilation and the degree of descent of the presenting part. The effect on the fetus must also be considered.

NURSING ALERT It is important for the nurse to recognize that active labour can last longer than the expected labour patterns. This finding should not be a cause for concern unless the fetus exhibits atypical or abnormal FHR patterns or the mother has a maternal fever.

Vaginal Examination

The vaginal examination reveals whether the woman is in true labour and enables the examiner to determine whether the membranes have ruptured (Fig. 18-8). Because this examination is often stressful and uncomfortable for the woman, it should be performed only when indicated by the status of the woman and her fetus. For example, a vaginal examination should be performed on admission, when significant change has occurred in UA, on maternal perception of perineal pressure or the urge to bear down, when membranes rupture, when the mother requests pain medication, or when variable decelerations of the FHR are noted (see Variable Decelerations, p. 434). A full explanation of the examination and support of the woman are important factors in reducing the stress and discomfort associated with the examination. Vaginal examinations can reveal the amount of dilatation and effacement as well as the station and presentation of the presenting part.

Laboratory and Diagnostic Tests

Analysis of Urine Specimen

A clean-catch urine specimen may be obtained to gather more data about the pregnant woman's health. It is a

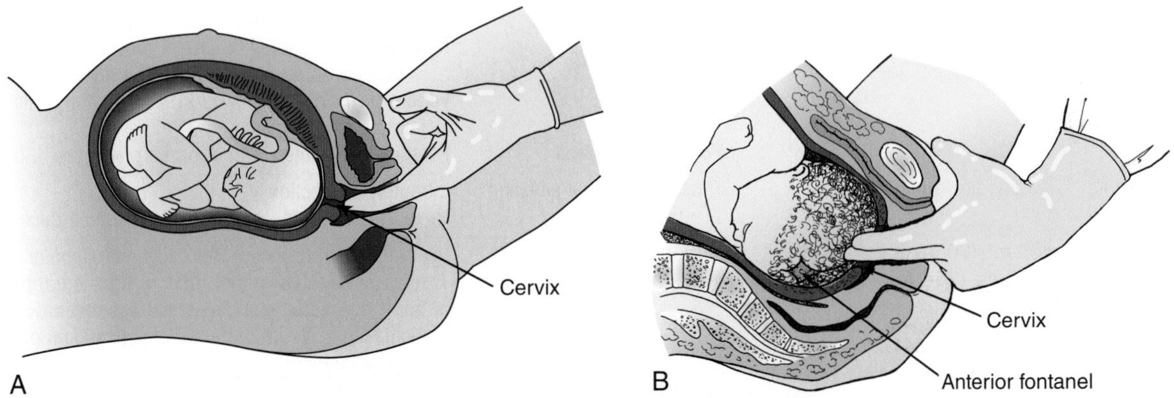

Fig. 18-8 Vaginal examination. **A:** Undilated, uneffaced cervix; membranes intact. **B:** Palpation of sagittal suture line. Cervix effaced and partially dilated.

convenient and simple procedure that can provide information about her hydration status (e.g., by specific gravity, colour, and amount), nutritional status (e.g., ketones), infection (e.g., leukocytes), or the status of possible complications such as pre-eclampsia (shown by finding protein in the urine). The results can be obtained quickly and help the nurse to determine appropriate interventions to implement.

Blood Tests

The blood tests performed vary with hospital protocol and according to the woman's health status. Blood can be obtained by a finger stick, venipuncture, or from the hub of a catheter used to start an IV line. More comprehensive assessments such as white blood cell count, red blood cell count, hemoglobin level, hematocrit, and platelet values are included in the CBC. A CBC may be ordered for women with a history of infection, anemia, hypertension, or other disorders.

If the woman's blood type has not been verified, blood is drawn to determine the type and Rh factor. If blood typing has already been done, the primary health care provider may choose not to repeat the test. If obvious signs of immunocompromise or substance use are present, other blood tests may be ordered, with consent of the woman.

Assessment of Amniotic Membranes and Fluid

Labour is initiated at term by SROM in approximately 8% of pregnant women. Almost 90% of women at term will go into spontaneous labour within 24 hours of spontaneous membrane rupture (More[OB], 2010). Membranes (the bag of waters) can also rupture spontaneously at any time during labour but most commonly in the transition phase of the first stage of labour.

NURSING ALERT The umbilical cord may prolapse when the membranes rupture. The FHR and pattern should be monitored closely for several minutes immediately after ROM to ascertain fetal well-being, and the findings should be documented.

Artificial ROM or **amniotomy** may be done to augment or induce labour or to facilitate placement of internal monitors when fetal status indicates the need for some form of direct assessment method (e.g., insertion of a fetal scalp electrode to the presenting part). (For the tests used to assess whether membranes have ruptured, see Box 18-2.) Assessment of amniotic fluid characteristics is described in Table 18-3.

Infection. After membranes rupture, microorganisms from the vagina can ascend into the amniotic sac, causing **chorioamnionitis** and placentitis to develop. For this reason, maternal temperature and vaginal discharge should be assessed frequently (every 1 to 2 hours) so that an infection developing after ROM can be identified early. However, even when membranes are intact, microorganisms may ascend and cause premature ROM. Careful assessment is critical; if an infection is suspected, appropriate antibiotics should be administered.

The nurse's responsibility is to report findings promptly to the woman and to the primary health care provider and to document them in the labour record. If abnormal findings are noted, continuous electronic monitoring is usually initiated and maintained for the duration of labour. The presence of meconium-stained amniotic fluid alerts the nurse to observe fetal status more closely. After birth, the newborn may be at high risk for alteration in respiratory status if meconium is aspirated into the lungs with the first breath.

Assessment findings serve as a baseline for evaluating the woman's progress during labour. Although some problems of labour are anticipated, others may appear unexpectedly during the clinical course of labour (Box 18-5).

Standards of Care

Standards of care guide the nurse in preparing for and implementing procedures with the expectant mother. Protocols for care based on standards include the following tasks:

1. Use an empathic approach when giving care:
   - Establish rapport with the woman and her significant others.
   - Respect the woman's individual needs and behaviours.
   - Be kind, caring, and competent when performing necessary procedures.
   - When explaining procedures, use words the woman can understand; repeat as necessary.

Table 18-3 Assessment of Amniotic Fluid

CHARACTERISTIC OF FLUID	NORMAL FINDING	DEVIATION FROM NORMAL FINDING	CAUSE OF DEVIATION FROM NORMAL
Colour	Pale, straw coloured; may contain white flecks of vernix caseosa, lanugo, scalp hair	Greenish-brown colour	Hypoxic episode in fetus; meconium in fluid
		Yellow-stained fluid	May be normal finding in breech presentation as pressure is exerted on fetal abdominal wall during descent Fetal hypoxia ≥36 hr before ROM; fetal hemolytic disease; intrauterine infection
		Port wine-coloured	Bleeding associated with abruptio placentae
Viscosity and odour	Watery; no strong odour	Thick, cloudy, foul-smelling	Intrauterine infection Large amount of meconium can make fluid thick
Amount (normally varies with gestational age)	400 mL (20 wk of gestation) 1000 mL (36–38 wk of gestation)	≥2000 mL (32–36 wk of gestation)	Hydramnios; associated with congenital anomalies of the fetus when fetus cannot drink or fluid is trapped in the body (e.g., fetal gastrointestinal obstruction or atresias); increased risk with maternal pregestational or gestational diabetes mellitus
		≤500 mL (32–36 wk of gestation)	Oligohydramnios; associated with incomplete or absent kidney; obstruction of urethra; infant cannot secrete or excrete urine

ROM, rupture of membranes.

BOX 18-5 Signs of Potential Labour Complications

- Contractions consistently lasting 90 seconds or more
- Contractions consistently occurring 2 minutes or less apart
- Intrauterine pressure of more than 75 mm Hg (determined by intrauterine pressure catheter monitoring) or resting tone of more than 15 mm Hg
- Fetal bradycardia, tachycardia, or persistently decreased variability (see Chapter 17)
- Irregular fetal heart rate; suspected fetal dysrhythmias
- Appearance of meconium-stained or bloody fluid from the vagina
- Arrest in progress of cervical dilation or effacement, descent of the fetus, or both
- Maternal temperature of 38°C or more
- Foul-smelling vaginal discharge
- Persistent bright-red or dark-red vaginal bleeding

  - Be aware that pain and discomfort are as the woman describes them.
  - Carry out appropriate comfort measures such as mouth and back care.
  - Include the support people in the care as desired by the woman and the support people.
  - Recognize that a woman's current childbirth experience and the actions of nurses and other health care providers can have a positive or negative effect on her future childbirth experiences.
2. Ensure that information on the woman's identification band is accurate (e.g., that the band is the appropriate colour for allergies).
3. Check the primary health care provider's orders.
4. Assess the orders for appropriateness and correctness (e.g., the dosage and route of administration of the analgesic to be administered to relieve discomfort).
5. Check all medications that are to be used.
6. Check the expiration date on any packs of supplies used for procedures.
7. Use routine precautions (see Box 18-3).
8. Document care according to hospital guidelines and communicate information to the primary health care provider when indicated.

Physical Nursing Care During Labour

Physical nursing care of the woman in labour is an essential component of her care. The various physical needs, requisite nursing actions, and rationale for care are presented in Table 18-4 and the Nursing Care Plan.

General Hygiene

Women in labour should be offered a shower or warm water bath, if available, to enhance the feeling of well-being and minimize the discomfort of contractions. Women should also be encouraged to wash their hands after voiding and to perform self-hygiene measures.

Nutrient and Fluid Intake

Oral Intake. Traditionally, the labouring woman was offered only clear liquids or ice chips or given nothing by mouth during the active phase of labour. This was to minimize the risk of anaesthesia complications and their sequelae should general anaesthesia be required in an emergency. These sequelae could include aspiration of gastric contents and resultant compromise in oxygen perfusion, which may endanger the lives of the mother and fetus. This practice is being challenged today because regional anaesthesia is used more often than general anaesthesia, even for emergency Caesarean births. Women are awake during regional anaesthesia and are able to participate in their own care and protect their airway.

Although gastric emptying is slowed as a result of labour, stress, and the use of narcotics or sedatives, fasting does not cause gastric contents to be eliminated and may even cause them to be more acidic. In addition, fasting is identified by many labouring women as a stressor with which they must cope and a source of frustration during labour related to a loss of control in meeting their own nourishment needs.

Adequate intake of fluids and calories is required to meet the energy demands and fluid losses associated with childbirth. The progress of labour slows, and ketosis develops if these demands are not met and fat is metabolized. Reduced energy for bearing-down efforts (pushing) increases the risk for a forceps- or vacuum-assisted birth. This is most likely to occur in women who begin to labour early in the morning after a night without caloric intake. Common practice is to allow clear liquids (e.g., water, tea, apple juice, clear sodas, gelatin, broth) during early labour, tapering off to ice chips and sips of water as labour progresses and becomes more active. However, when women are permitted to consume fluids and food freely, they typically regulate their own oral intake, eating light foods (e.g., eggs, yogourt, ice cream, dry toast and jelly, fruit) and drinking fluids during early labour and then tapering off to an intake of clear fluid and sips of water or ice chips as labour intensifies and the second stage approaches. Food and fluid consumed orally during labour can meet a labouring woman's hydration and energy demands and relieve stress (American College of Nurse-Midwives, 2008). Women who use nonpharmacological pain-relief measures and labour at home or in birthing centres are more likely to eat and drink during labour. In addition, the woman's sense of control and level of comfort are enhanced.

Withholding food and drink from women in labour is unlikely to be beneficial; offering oral fluids is demonstrably useful and should be encouraged (Enkin et al., 2000; Hofmeyr, 2005). Nurses should follow the orders of the woman's primary health care provider when offering the woman food or fluids during labour. However, as advocates, nurses can facilitate change by informing others of the current research findings that support the safety and effectiveness of the oral intake of food and fluid during labour and by initiating such research themselves.

Intravenous Intake. Fluids are administered intravenously to the labouring woman to maintain hydration when the woman is unable to ingest a sufficient amount of fluid orally or if she is receiving epidural or intrathecal analgesia. However, routine use of IV fluids during labour is a form of care that is unlikely to be beneficial and may be harmful (Enkin et al., 2000). In most cases, an electrolyte solution without glucose is adequate and does not introduce excess glucose into the bloodstream, which results in fetal **hyperglycemia** and fetal

Table 18-4 Physical Nursing Care During Labour

NEED	NURSING ACTIONS	RATIONALE
General Hygiene		
Showers/bed baths, Jacuzzi bath	Assess for progress in labour	Determines appropriateness of activity
	Supervise showers closely if woman is in true labour	Prevents injury from fall; labour may be accelerated
	Suggest allowing warm water to flow over back	Aids relaxation; increases comfort
Perineum	Cleanse frequently, especially after rupture of membranes and when show increases	Enhances comfort and reduces risk of infection
Oral hygiene	Offer toothbrush or mouthwash or wash the teeth with an ice-cold, wet washcloth as needed	Refreshes mouth; helps counteract dry, thirsty feeling
Hair	Brush, braid per woman's wishes	Improves morale; increases comfort
Handwashing	Offer washcloths before and after voiding and as needed	Maintains cleanliness; prevents infection
Face	Offer cool washcloth	Provides relief from diaphoresis; cools and refreshes
Gowns/linens	Change prn; fluff pillows	Improves comfort; enhances relaxation
Nutrient and Fluid Intake		
Oral	Offer fluids and solid foods, following orders of primary health care provider and desires of labouring woman	Provides hydration and calories; enhances positive emotional experience and maternal control
Intravenous (IV)	Establish and maintain IV line, if required, as ordered	Maintains hydration; provides venous access for medications if required
Elimination		
Voiding	Encourage voiding at least every 2 hr	A full bladder may impede descent of presenting part; overdistension may cause bladder atony and injury and postpartum voiding difficulty
Ambulatory woman	Encourage ambulation to bathroom if: • The presenting part is engaged • The woman is not drowsy from medication	Reinforces normal process of urination Precautionary measure to protect against prolapse of umbilical cord Precautionary measure to protect against injury
Woman on bed rest	Offer bedpan Allow tap water to run; pour warm water over vulva; give positive suggestion Provide privacy Put up side rails on bed Place call bell within reach Offer washcloth for hands Wash vulvar area	Prevents complications of bladder distension and ambulation Encourages voiding Shows respect for woman Prevents injury from fall Maintains cleanliness; prevents infection Maintains cleanliness; enhances comfort; prevents infection
Catheterization	Catheterize according to orders of primary health care provider or hospital protocol if measures to facilitate voiding are ineffective	Prevents complications of bladder distension
	Insert catheter between contractions	Minimizes discomfort
	Avoid force if obstacle to insertion is noted	"Obstacle" may be caused by compression of urethra by presenting part
Bowel elimination—sensation of rectal pressure	Help woman ambulate to bathroom or offer bedpan after careful assessment	Prevents misinterpretation of rectal pressure from the presenting part as need to defecate
	Perform vaginal examination	Determines degree of descent of presenting part
	Cleanse perineum immediately after passage of stool	Reduces risk of infection and sense of embarrassment

NURSING CARE PLAN ● Labour and Birth

Nursing Diagnosis: Potential anxiety related to labour and the birthing process

Expected Outcome

Woman exhibits decreased signs of anxiety.

Nursing Interventions/*Rationales*

Orient the woman and significant others to labour and birth unit and explain admission protocol *to allay initial feelings of anxiety.*

Assess the woman's knowledge, experience, and expectations of labour; note any signs or expressions of anxiety, nervousness, or fear *to establish a baseline for intervention.*

Discuss the expected progression of labour and describe what to expect during the process *to allay anxiety associated with the unknown.*

Actively involve the woman in care decisions during labour, interpret sights and sounds of environment (monitor sights and sounds, unit activities), and share information on progression of labour (vital signs, fetal heart rate, dilation, effacement) *to increase her sense of control and allay fears.*

Nursing Diagnosis: Acute pain related to increasing frequency and intensity of contractions

Expected Outcome

Woman exhibits signs of ability to cope with discomfort.

Nursing Interventions/*Rationales*

Assess woman's level of pain and strategies that she has used to cope with pain *to establish a baseline for intervention* (see Coping Scale, Fig. 16-3).

Encourage her significant other to remain as a support person during the labour process as able and appropriate *to assist with support and comfort measures.*

Instruct the woman and support person in use of specific techniques, such as conscious relaxation, focused breathing, effleurage, massage, and application of sacral pressure, *to increase relaxation, decrease intensity of contractions, and promote use of controlled thought and direction of energy* (see Chapter 16).

Provide comfort measures such as frequent mouth care *to prevent dry mouth*; application of a damp cloth to the forehead and changing of damp gown or bed covers *to relieve discomfort associated with diaphoresis*; and position changes *to reduce stiffness and enhance labour progress.*

Explain which analgesics and anaesthetics are available for use during labour and birth when requested *to provide knowledge to help the woman make decisions about pain control* (see Chapter 16).

Nursing Diagnosis: Risk for impaired urinary elimination related to sensory impairment secondary to labour

Expected Outcome

Bladder does not show signs of distension.

Nursing Interventions/*Rationales*

Palpate the bladder superior to the symphysis on a frequent basis *to detect a full bladder that occurs from increased fluid intake and inability to feel urge to void.*

Encourage frequent voiding (at least every 2 hours) and catheterize (intermittent) if necessary *to avoid bladder distension because it impedes progress of fetus down the birth canal and may result in trauma to the bladder.*

Assist the woman to the bathroom or commode to void, if appropriate, and provide privacy *to facilitate bladder emptying with an upright position (natural) and relaxation.*

Nursing Diagnosis: Risk for difficulty in coping that is related to birthing process

Expected Outcome

Woman actively participates in the second stage of labour with no evidence of injury to her or her fetus.

Nursing Interventions/*Rationales*

Monitor events of second-stage labour and birth, including physiological responses of the woman and fetus and emotional responses of the woman and partner, *to ensure maternal, partner, and fetal well-being.*

Provide ongoing feedback to the woman and partner *to allay anxiety and enhance participation.*

Continue to provide comfort measures and minimize distractions *to decrease discomfort and aid in focus on the birth process.*

Encourage the woman to experiment with various positions (every 20 to 30 minutes) *to assist downward movement of the fetus.*

Ensure that the woman takes deep, cleansing breaths before and after each contraction *to enhance gas exchange and oxygen transport to the fetus.*

Encourage the woman to push spontaneously when the urge to bear down is perceived during a contraction *to aid descent and rotation of the fetus.*

Encourage the woman to exhale, holding breath for short periods while bearing down, *to avoid holding breath and triggering a Valsalva manoeuvre, increasing intrathoracic and cardiovascular pressure, and decreasing perfusion of placental oxygen, placing the fetus at risk.*

Have the woman take deep breaths and relax between contractions *to reduce fatigue and increase effectiveness of pushing efforts.*

Have the mother pant as fetal head crowns *to control birth of the head.*

Explain to the woman and labour partner what is expected in the third stage of labour *to decrease anxiety.*

Have the woman maintain her position *to facilitate delivery of the placenta.*

Nursing Diagnosis: Fatigue related to energy expenditure required during labour and birth

Expected Outcome

Woman's energy levels are restored.

Nursing Interventions/*Rationales*

Educate the woman and her partner about the need for rest and help them plan strategies (e.g., limiting visitors, increasing role of support systems in performing functions associated with daily routines) that allow specific times for rest and sleep *to ensure that the woman can*

Continued

NURSING CARE PLAN ● Labour and Birth—cont'd

restore depleted energy levels in preparation for caring for a new infant.

Monitor the woman's fatigue level and the amount of rest received *to ensure restoration of energy.*

Nursing Diagnosis: Risk for deficient fluid volume related to decreased fluid intake and increased fluid loss during labour and birth

Expected Outcomes

Fluid balance is maintained, and there are no signs of dehydration.

Nursing Interventions/*Rationales*

Monitor fluid loss (i.e., blood, urine, perspiration) and vital signs; inspect skin turgor and mucous membranes for dryness *to evaluate hydration status.*

Administer oral or parenteral fluid per health care provider's orders *to maintain hydration.*

Monitor the fundus for firmness after placental separation *to ensure adequate contraction and prevent further blood loss.*

hyperinsulinism. After birth, the neonate's high level of insulin will then deplete his or her glucose stores, and **hypoglycemia** will result. If maternal ketosis occurs, the primary health care provider may order an IV solution containing a small amount of dextrose to provide the glucose needed to assist in fatty acid metabolism.

NURSING ALERT Nurses should carefully monitor the intake and output of labouring women receiving IV fluids because these women also face an increased danger of hypervolemia as a result of the fluid retention that occurs during pregnancy.

Elimination

Voiding. Voiding a minimum of every 2 hours should be encouraged. A distended bladder may impede descent of the presenting part, inhibit uterine contractions, and lead to decreased bladder tone or **atony** after birth. Women who receive epidural analgesia or anaesthesia are especially at risk for retention of urine, and the need to void should be assessed more frequently in them.

The woman should be assisted to the bathroom to void unless the primary health care provider has ordered bed rest. She may be unable to get up to use the bathroom in some situations—for example, when the woman is receiving epidural analgesia or anaesthesia, or it may be the nurse's judgement that ambulation would compromise the status of the labouring woman or her fetus. External monitoring can be interrupted for the woman to go to the bathroom for periods of up to 30 minutes if maternal–fetal condition is stable (Liston et al., 2007).

Catheterization. If the woman is unable to void, usually related to epidural anaesthesia, and her bladder is distended, she may need to be catheterized. Intermittent catheterization is preferred, to decrease the risk of infection. Most hospitals have protocols that rely on the nurse's judgement of the need for catheterization. Before performing the catheterization, the nurse should clean the vulva and perineum because vaginal show and amniotic fluid may be present.

Bowel Elimination. Most women do not have bowel movements during labour because of decreased intestinal motility. Stool that has formed in the large intestine often is moved downward toward the anorectal area by the pressure exerted by the fetal presenting part as it descends. In small numbers of women, this stool is expelled during second-stage pushing and birth. However, the passage of stool with bearing-down efforts may embarrass the woman, thereby reducing the effectiveness of these efforts. To prevent these problems, the nurse should immediately cleanse the perineal area to remove any stool, while at the same time reassuring the woman that the passage of stool at this time is a normal and expected event because the same muscles used to expel the baby also expel stool. Routine use of an enema to empty the rectum is considered to be harmful or ineffective and should be avoided (Enkin et al., 2000).

When the presenting part is deep in the pelvis, even in the absence of stool in the anorectal area, the woman may feel rectal pressure and think she needs to defecate. If the woman expresses the need to defecate, the nurse should perform a vaginal examination to assess cervical dilation and station. When a multiparous woman experiences the urge to defecate, this often means that birth will follow quickly.

Ambulation and Positioning

Freedom of maternal movement and choice of position through labour are forms of care likely to be beneficial for the labouring woman and should be encouraged (Enkin et al., 2000). The increased use of epidurals during childbirth accompanied by multiple medical interventions (e.g., monitors, IV infusions) and reduced motor control interfere with a woman's freedom of movement. If electronic fetal monitoring (EFM) is required, many birthing areas now use wireless fetal monitors (known as **telemetry**) to allow the woman to remain mobile while continuous monitoring of the fetus takes place.

The potential advantages of ambulation include enhanced uterine activity, decreased sensation of pain, distraction from the discomfort of labour, enhanced maternal control, and an opportunity for close interaction with the woman's partner and care provider as they help her walk. Ambulation is associated with a reduced rate of operative delivery (i.e., Caesarean birth, forceps- and vacuum-assisted birth) and less frequent use of **opioid** analgesics.

Walking, sitting, or standing during early labour is more comfortable than lying down and facilitates the progress of labour. Ambulation should be encouraged if the fetal presenting part is engaged after ROM and if the woman has not received medication for pain (Fig. 18-9). The woman may find

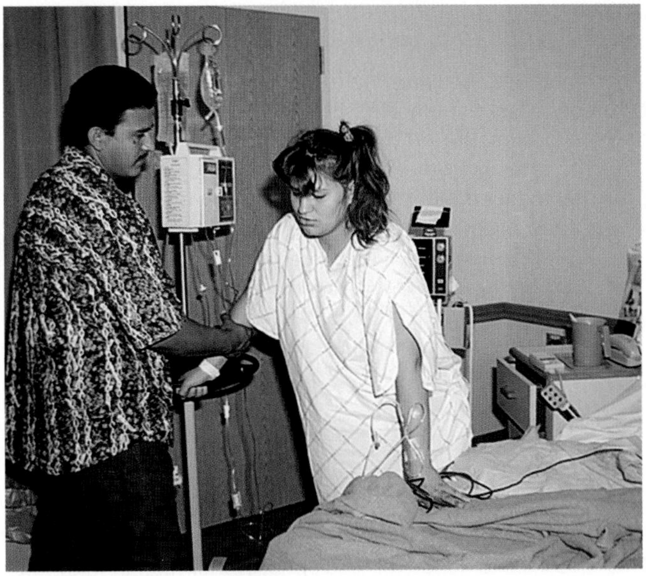

Fig. 18-9 Woman preparing to walk with partner. *(Courtesy Marjorie Pyle, RNC, Lifecircle, Costa Mesa, CA.)*

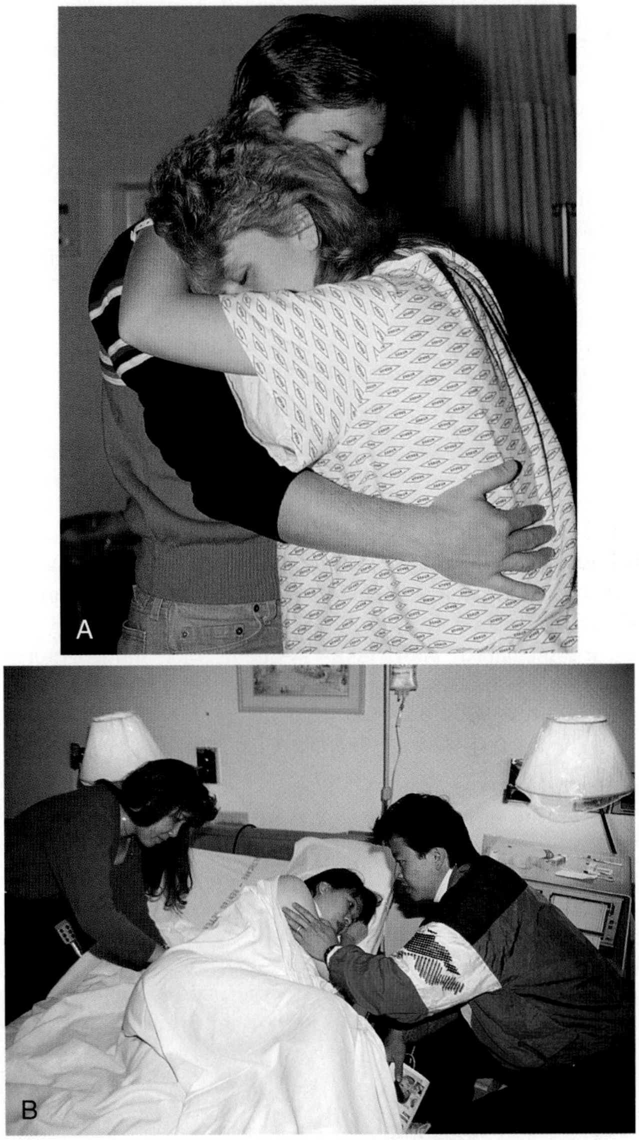

Fig. 18-10 **A:** Woman standing and leaning forward with support. **B:** Lateral position. Support person is applying sacral pressure while partner provides encouragement. *(Courtesy Marjorie Pyle, RNC, Lifecircle, Costa Mesa, CA.)*

it comfortable to stand and lean forward on her partner, doula, or nurse for support at times during labour (Fig. 18-10, A). At times, although rarely, ambulation is contraindicated because of maternal or fetal status.

When the woman lies in bed, she will usually change her position spontaneously as labour progresses. If she does not change position every 30 to 60 minutes, she should be assisted to do so. A variety of positions recommended for the labouring woman are described in Box 18-6. The side-lying (lateral) position promotes optimal uteroplacental and renal blood flow and increases oxygen saturation (see Fig. 18-10, B). If the woman wants to lie supine, the nurse may place a pillow under one hip as a wedge to prevent the uterus from compressing the aorta and vena cava. Sitting is not contraindicated unless it adversely affects fetal status, which can be determined by checking the FHR and pattern. If the fetus is in the occiput posterior position, it may be helpful to encourage the woman to squat during contractions because this position increases pelvic diameter, allowing the head to rotate to a more anterior position (Fig. 18-11, A). A hands-and-knees position during contractions is also recommended to facilitate the rotation of the fetal occiput from a posterior to an anterior position as gravity pulls the fetal back forward (see Fig. 18-11, B). See Box 18-7 for measures to assist a woman with a fetus that is in the occiput posterior position.

A birth ball (gymnastic ball, also used in physical therapy) can be used to support a woman's body as she assumes a variety of labour and birth positions (Fig. 18-12). The woman can sit on the ball while leaning over the bed, or she can lean over the ball to support her upper body and reduce stress on her arms and hands when she assumes a hands-and-knees position. Use of the birth ball can encourage pelvic mobility and pelvic and perineal relaxation when the woman sits on the firm yet pliable ball and rocks in rhythmic movements. Warm compresses applied to the perineum can maximize this relaxation effect. The birth ball should be large enough so that, when the woman sits, her knees are bent at a 90-degree angle and her feet are flat on the floor and approximately .75 m apart.

evolve Critical Thinking Exercises—Positioning During Labour

Supportive Care During Labour and Birth

Support during labour and birth involves emotional support, physical care and comfort measures, and provision of information. Effective support provided to women during labour can result in shorter labours, reduced rates of complications and surgical or obstetrical interventions (e.g., Caesarean births, labour augmentations and inductions, episiotomies, and forceps- and vacuum-assisted births), and enhanced self-esteem and satisfaction. Physical, emotional, and psychological support of the woman during labour and birth is a beneficial form of care demonstrated by clear research

BOX 18-6 Some Maternal Positions* During Labour and Birth

Semirecumbent Position

With the woman sitting with her upper body elevated to at least a 30-degree angle, place a wedge or small pillow under her hip to prevent vena caval compression and reduce the likelihood of supine hypotension (see Fig. 18-3, D).

- The greater the angle of elevation, the more gravity or pressure is exerted, which promotes fetal descent, the progress of contractions, and the widening of pelvic dimensions.
- It is sometimes more convenient for rendering care measures and for external fetal monitoring.

Lateral Position (see Fig. 18-10, B)

Have the woman alternate between left and right side-lying position, and provide abdominal and back support as needed for comfort.

- Removes pressure from the vena cava and back; enhances uteroplacental perfusion and relieves backache
- Makes it easier to perform back massage or counterpressure
- Associated with less frequent but more intense contractions
- May be used as a birthing position (see Fig. 18-14, A)
- Takes pressure off perineum

Upright Position

The gravity effect enhances the contraction cycle and fetal descent: the weight of the fetus places increasing pressure on the cervix; the cervix is pulled upward, facilitating effacement and dilation; impulses from the cervix to the pituitary gland increase, causing more oxytocin to be secreted; and contractions are intensified, thereby applying more forceful downward pressure on the fetus, but they are less painful.

- The fetus is aligned with the pelvis, and pelvic diameters are widened slightly.
- Effective upright positions include the following:
  - Ambulation (see Fig. 18-9)
  - Standing and leaning forward with support provided by coach, end of bed, back of chair, or birth ball; relieves backache and facilitates application of counterpressure or back massage (see Fig. 18-10 and Fig. 18-12)
  - Sitting up in bed, chair, birthing chair, on toilet or bedside commode
  - Squatting (see Fig. 18-11, A)

Hands-and-Knees Position

This position is ideal for occiput-posterior position of the presenting part (see Fig. 18-11, B; Box 18-7). Assume an "all-fours" position in bed or on a covered floor; this allows for pelvic rocking.

- Relieves backache characteristic of "back labour."
- Facilitates internal rotation of the fetus by increasing mobility of the coccyx, increasing the pelvic diameters, and using gravity to turn the fetal back and rotate the head.

*Assess the effect of each position on the labouring woman's comfort and anxiety level, progress of labour, and fetal heart rate and pattern. Alternate positions every 20 to 30 minutes.

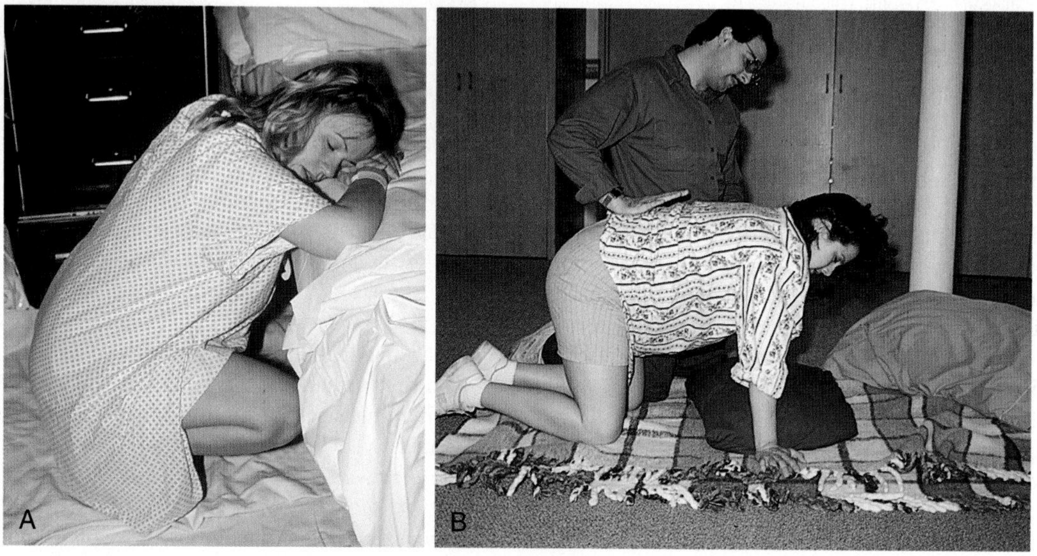

Fig. 18-11 Maternal positions for labour. **A:** Squatting. **B:** Woman in hands-and-knees position. *(Courtesy Marjorie Pyle, RNC, Lifecircle, Costa Mesa, CA.)*

evidence (see Evidence-Informed Practice box) (Enkin et al., 2000; MacKinnon, McIntyre, & Quance, 2005).

The labouring woman should feel safe in the birthing environment and feel free to be herself and use the comfort and relaxation measures she prefers. To enhance relaxation, bright overhead lights should be turned off when not needed. Noise and intrusions should be kept to a minimum. The temperature should be controlled to ensure the labouring woman's comfort. The room should be large enough to accommodate a comfortable chair for the woman's partner, the monitoring equipment, and hospital personnel. Couples can bring their own pillows to make the hospital surroundings more homelike and

BOX 18-7 Back Labour—Occiput Posterior Position

Measures to Reduce Back Pain During a Contraction

Counterpressure—Apply fist or heel of hand to sacral area

Heat or cold applications—Apply to sacral area

Double hip squeeze:

- Woman assumes a position with hip joints flexed, such as knee–chest position
- Partner, nurse, or doula places hands over gluteal muscles and presses with palms of hands up and inward toward centre of pelvis

Knee press:

- Woman assumes a sitting position with knees a few inches apart and feet flat on the floor or on a stool
- Partner, nurse, or doula cups a knee in each hand with heels of hands on top of tibia and then presses the knees straight back toward the woman's hips while leaning forward toward the woman

Measures to Facilitate Rotation of Fetal Head (May Also Relieve Back Pain)

Lateral abdominal stroking—Stroke abdomen in direction that fetal head should rotate

Hands-and-knees position (all-fours)—Can also be accomplished by kneeling while leaning forward over a birth ball, padded chair seat, bed, or over-the-bed table (see Fig. 18-11, B)

Squatting

Pelvic rocking

Stair climbing

Lateral position—Lie on side toward which the fetus should turn

Lunges—Widen pelvis on side toward which woman lunges

- Woman stands, facing forward, next to or alongside a chair so that she can lunge toward the side the fetal back is on or in the direction of the fetal occiput
- Woman places foot on seat of chair with toes pointed toward the back of the chair and then lunges
- Alternative position for lunge is kneeling

facilitate position changes. This type of an environment can help women view their childbirth experience as normal and not related to illness. Environmental modifications should reflect the preferences of the woman, including the number of visitors and availability of a telephone and music. Nurses should ensure that each woman labours in an optimal birth environment.

Labour Support by the Nurse

The nurse can alleviate a woman's anxiety by communicating clearly, explaining unfamiliar terms, providing information and explanations without her having to ask and at a level she understands, and preparing her for sensations she will experience and procedures that will follow. By encouraging the woman or couple to ask questions and by providing honest, understandable answers, the nurse can play a significant role in helping the woman achieve a satisfying birth experience.

Supportive, empathic nursing care for a woman in labour includes the following:

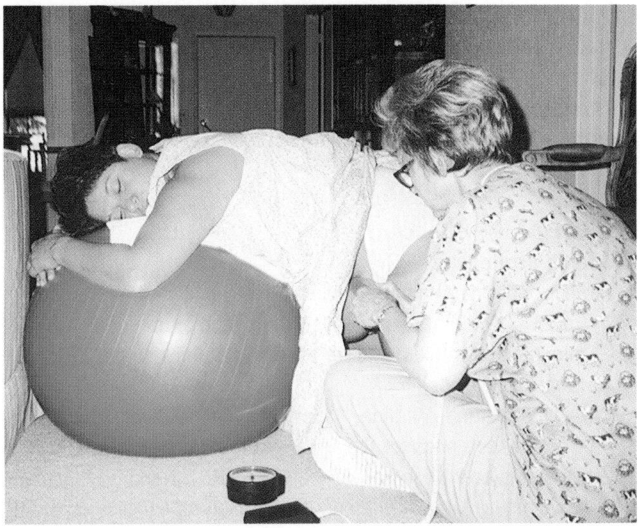

Fig. 18-12 Labouring woman using birth ball. *(Courtesy Polly Perez, Cutting Edge Press, Johnson, VT.)*

- Developing a trusting relationship with the woman and her support persons
- Helping the woman maintain control and participate to the extent she wishes in the birth of her infant
- Providing continuity of care that is nonjudgemental and respectful of her cultural and religious values and beliefs
- Meeting the woman's expected outcomes for her labour
- Listening to the woman's concerns and encouraging her to express her feelings
- Acting as the woman's advocate, supporting her decisions and respecting her choices as appropriate, and relating her wishes as needed to other health care providers
- Helping the woman conserve her energy and cope effectively with her pain and discomfort by using a variety of comfort measures that are acceptable to her
- Helping the woman manage her discomfort
- Acknowledging the woman's efforts during labour, including her strength and courage, as well as those of her partner, and providing positive reinforcement
- Protecting the woman's privacy and modesty
- Using touch and eye contact if appropriate

Couples who have attended childbirth education programs will know something about the labour process, coaching techniques, and comfort measures. The nurse should play a supportive role and keep the couple informed of the progress. Breathing and relaxation techniques and comfort measures described in Chapter 16 can be implemented.

Even when expectant parents have not attended childbirth education classes, the nurse can teach them simple breathing and relaxation techniques during the early phase of labour. In this case, the nurse may provide more of the coaching and supportive care, as some support persons may not feel able to fulfill this role.

Comfort measures vary with the situation (Fig. 18-13). The nurse can draw on the couple's repertoire of comfort measures and relaxation techniques learned during the pregnancy and through life experiences. Such measures include maintaining a comfortable, supportive atmosphere in the labour and birth

EVIDENCE-INFORMED PRACTICE The Benefits of Continuous Labour Support

—*Pat Gingrich*

Ask the Question

How does continuous labour support benefit labouring patients? Who should provide this support? Is this a nursing role?

Search for Evidence

Search Strategies

Professional organization guidelines, meta-analyses, systematic reviews, randomized controlled trials, nonrandomized prospective studies, and retrospective studies since 2006

Databases Searched

CINAHL, Cochrane, Medline, National Guideline Clearinghouse, and the Web sites for the Association of Women's Health, Obstetric and Neonatal Nurses (AWHONN), National Practice Guidelines, Lamaze International, Society of Obstetricians and Gynaecologists of Canada (SOGC), and World Health Organization (WHO)

Critically Analyze the Evidence

For millennia women have laboured in the company of other women—usually family or friends who have experienced birth themselves. In the last century, Western women in labour became more isolated in institutional, high-technology settings. Loss of dedicated labour support coincided with increasing technology, pain management, and operative births. Observers now question whether returning the human touch of birthing assistants could improve outcomes. Labour support could be provided by a trusted friend or doula not employed by the facility who offers the labouring women and her partner physical and emotional support, information, and advocacy but never medical advice. In 2007, the SOGC recommended that women in active labour receive continuous close labour support from an appropriately trained person (Liston et al., 2007).

A Cochrane systematic analysis reviewed 16 randomized, controlled trials involving 13,391 women from 11 countries. Taken as a whole, the studies demonstrated that continuous labour support leads to shorter labours, increased rates of vaginal birth, decreased use of analgesia, and increased satisfaction (Hodnett et al., 2007). These associations were especially true if the labour support was not an employee of the facility, the support was begun early in labour, and the setting did not typically use epidural analgesia.

In a randomized, controlled trial of 420 women, continuous labour support was associated with decreased rates of Caesarean and instrumental birth, decreased need for pain medication or regional analgesia, and 100% positive feelings about birth (McGrath & Kennell, 2008).

Finally, a retrospective study of 11,471 women found that doula support was associated with increased breastfeeding intention and initiation and fewer Caesarean births (Motti-Santiago et al., 2008). However, this study did not randomize; thus, the use of doulas and intention to breastfeed may represent prior related preferences of a certain population of women.

Implications for Practice

Nurses provide attentive care for labouring women, but their workload may preclude their continuous presence at the bedside. Partners might be well intentioned but may find the powerful reality of birth to be overwhelming. An experienced doula or birth attendant can keep the labouring woman calm and comfortable, which not only improves the experience emotionally but also reduces pain, release of stress hormones, and muscular tension, thereby facilitating vaginal birth. Doulas are not there to replace the nurse or partner but to provide support as needs arise and should be considered a valuable part of the care team. Institutions that see the measurable benefits of doulas are wise to value and encourage their contribution.

References

Hodnett, E. D., et al. (2007). Continuous support for women during childbirth. In *Cochrane Database of Systematic Reviews*, Issue 3. Chichester, UK: John Wiley & Sons.

Liston, R., et al. (2007). Fetal health surveillance: Antepartum and intrapartum consensus guideline. *Journal of Obstetrics and Gynaecology Canada*, *29*(9 Suppl 4), s1–s56, Retrieved from http://www.sogc.org/guidelines/documents/gui197CPG0709.pdf.

McGrath, S. K., & Kennell, J. N. (2008). A randomized controlled trial of continuous labour support: Effect on cesarean delivery rates. *Birth*, *35*(2), 92–97.

Motti-Santiago, J., et al. (2008). A hospital-based doula program and childbirth outcomes in an urban, multicultural setting. *Maternal and Child Health Journal*, *35*(3), 372–377.

area; using touch therapeutically (e.g., massage, heat or cold applied to the lower back in the event of back labour, a cool cloth applied to the forehead); providing nonpharmacological measures to relieve discomfort; administering analgesics when necessary; and, most of all, just being present (see Tables 18-1 and 18-5). See Chapter 16 for a full discussion of both pharmacological and nonpharmacological comfort measures.

While most women in labour respond positively to touch, permission should be obtained before using any measure involving touch. Back rubs and counterpressure may be offered, especially if the woman is experiencing back labour. A support person may be taught to exert counterpressure against the woman's sacrum (see Fig. 18-11, B). The back pain is caused by the occiput pressing on spinal nerves, and counterpressure lifts the occiput off these nerves, thereby providing some relief from pain. Once counterpressure is initiated, the woman will usually ask her partner to continue doing this for each following contraction. However, the partner will need to be relieved after a while because exerting counterpressure is hard work. Ice packs and heat also work to help relieve back labour; hand and foot massage can be soothing and relaxing. The nurse should always ask the mother if the massages are helpful.

Many women become more sensitive to touch (hyperesthesia) as labour progresses; this is a typical response during transition (see Table 18-2). They may tell their support person to leave them alone or to not touch them. The partner who is unprepared for this normal response may feel rejected and react by withdrawing active support. The nurse can reassure him or her that this response is a positive indication that the first stage is ending and the second stage is approaching. Women with increased sensitivity to touch may have a positive response when touched on surfaces of the body where hair does not grow, such as the forehead, the palms of the hands, and the soles of the feet.

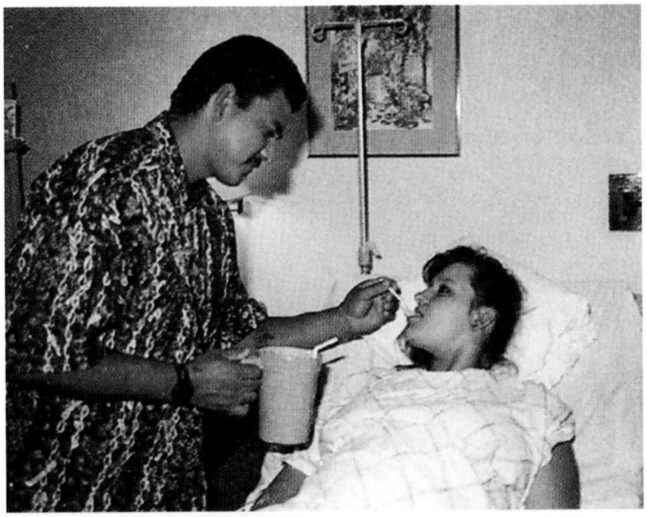

Fig. 18-13 Partner providing comfort measures. *(Courtesy Marjorie Pyle, RNC, Lifecircle, Costa Mesa, CA.)*

BOX 18-8 Guidelines for Supporting the Partner

- Orient the partner to the labour room and the unit; explain location of the cafeteria, toilet, and waiting room; visiting hours; and names and functions of personnel present.
- Inform the partner of sights and smells he or she can expect to encounter; encourage him or her to leave the room, if necessary.
- Respect the partner's or the couple's decision about the degree of his or her involvement. Offer the partner freedom to make decisions.
- Tell the partner when his or her presence has been helpful and continue to reinforce this throughout labour.
- Offer to teach the partner comfort measures.
- Inform the partner frequently of the progress of the labour and the woman's needs. Keep him or her informed about procedures to be performed.
- Prepare the partner for changes in the woman's behaviour and physical appearance.
- Remind him or her to eat; offer snacks and fluids if possible.
- Relieve the partner of the job of support person as necessary. Offer blankets if he or she is to sleep in a chair by the bedside.
- Acknowledge the stress experienced by each partner during labour and birth and identify normal responses.
- Attempt to modify or eliminate unsettling stimuli such as extra noise and extra light.

Labour Support by the Partner

The partner is often able to provide the comfort measures and touch that the labouring woman needs. When the woman becomes focused on her pain, sometimes the partner can persuade her to try nonpharmacological variations of comfort measures. In addition, the partner may be able to interpret the woman's needs and desires to staff members.

Throughout the past 30 years, childbirth preparation education has been widely available in Canada. Initially, the partner's ideal role was thought to be that of labour coach, and he or she was expected to actively help the woman cope with labour. However, this expectation may be unrealistic because some partners have concerns about their labour-coaching abilities. Because partners can participate in labour and birth in different ways, the nurse should encourage them to adopt the role most comfortable for them and for the woman rather than to assume an unnatural role. Participation in the birth is ego building: the partner can be of assistance and his or her presence is important.

The feelings of a first-time parent change as labour progresses. Although the partner may be calm at the onset of labour, feelings of fear and helplessness can begin to dominate as labour becomes more active and the partner realizes that labour is more work than he or she had anticipated. The first-time parent may feel excluded as birth preparations begin during the transition phase. Once the second stage begins and birth nears, the partner's focus will change from being on the woman to being on the baby who is about to be born (Table 18-5).

Ways in which the nurse can support the partner are detailed in Box 18-8. A well-informed partner can make an important contribution to the health and well-being of the mother and child, their family interrelationship, and the partner's self-esteem.

Labour Support by Doulas

Continuity of care has been cited by women as a critical component of a satisfying childbirth experience. This need can be met by a specially trained, experienced female labour attendant called a *doula*. The doula provides a continuous, one-on-one caring presence throughout the labour and birth process of the woman she is attending. This is a beneficial form of care (Enkin et al., 2000).

The primary role of the doula is to focus on the labouring woman and provide physical and emotional support by using soft, reassuring words; touching, stroking, and hugging; administering comfort measures to reduce pain and enhance relaxation; and walking with the woman, helping her to change positions, and encouraging her spontaneous bearing-down efforts. Doulas provide information and explain procedures and events. They advocate for the woman's right to participate actively in the management of her labour. These forms of caring help to reduce a woman's level of anxiety and fear, make her more confident and calm, and reduce the stress response that could inhibit the progress of labour.

The doula also supports the woman's partner, who often feels unqualified to be the sole labour support and may find it difficult to watch the woman when she is experiencing pain. The doula can encourage and praise the partner's efforts, create a partnership as caregivers, and provide respite care. Doulas also facilitate communication between the labouring woman and her partner and between the couple and the health care team (Simkin & Way, 2008).

Continuous supportive care that begins early in labour significantly reduces the Caesarean birth rate; duration of labour; use of oxytocin, analgesics, and forceps or vacuum-extractor; and requests for epidural anaesthesia (McGrath & Kennell, 2008). Labouring women also reported a higher level of satisfaction with their childbirth experience and greater success

Table 18-5 Woman's Responses and Support Person's Actions During First Stage of Labour

WOMAN'S RESPONSES	NURSE/SUPPORT PERSON'S ACTIONS*
Dilation of Cervix 0–3 cm (Latent) (Contractions: 30–45 sec Long, 5–30 min Apart, Mild to Moderate Intensity)	
Mood: alert, happy, excited, mild anxiety Labouring at home or settles into labour room if required; selects focal point Rests or sleeps if possible Uses breathing techniques if required Uses effleurage, focusing, and relaxation techniques	Provides encouragement, feedback for relaxation, companionship Helps to cope with contractions Provides distractions Encourages use of focusing techniques Helps to concentrate on breathing techniques if required Uses comfort measures Assists woman into comfortable position Informs woman of progress; explains procedures and routines Gives praise Offers fluids, ice chips as ordered
Dilation of Cervix 4–7 cm (Active) (Contractions: 40–70 sec Long, 3–5 Minutes Apart, Moderate to Strong in Intensity)	
Mood: seriously labour oriented, concentration and energy needed for contractions, alert, more demanding Continues relaxation, focusing techniques Uses breathing techniques if required Admitted to hospital if required by woman	Acts as buffer; limits assessment techniques to between contractions Assists with contractions Encourages woman as needed to help her maintain breathing techniques Uses comfort measures Assists with frequent position changes (q 30 min), emphasizing side-lying and upright positions Encourages voluntary relaxation of muscles of back, buttocks, thighs, and perineum; effleurage Applies counterpressure to sacrococcygeal area Encourages and praises Keeps woman aware of progress Assists with administration of analgesics if requested by woman (nurse only) Checks bladder; encourages her to void Gives oral care; offers fluids, ice chips as ordered
Dilation of Cervix 8–10 cm (Transition) (Contractions: 45–90 sec Long, 2–3 min Apart, Strong in Intensity)	
Mood: irritable, intense concentration, symptoms of transition (e.g., nausea, vomiting) Continues relaxation, needs greater concentration to do this Uses breathing techniques that are working for her Uses panting to overcome urge to push	Stays with woman; provides constant support Assists with contractions Reminds, reassures, and encourages woman to re-establish breathing pattern and concentration as needed Alerts woman to begin breathing pattern before contraction becomes too intense if she is sedated or drowsy Prompts panting respirations if woman begins to push prematurely Uses comfort measures Accepts woman's inability to comply with instructions Accepts irritable response to helping such as counterpressure Supports woman who has nausea and vomiting; gives oral care as needed; gives reassurance regarding signs of end of first stage Uses relaxation techniques (effleurage and voluntary relaxation) Keeps woman aware of progress

*Provided by nurses and support people.

with breastfeeding. Long-term benefits of doula care are reflected in more positive maternal feelings about their parenting ability and lower rates of postpartum mood disorders.

The roles of the nurse and the doula are complementary. They should work together as a team, recognizing and respecting the role each plays in supporting and caring for the woman and her partner during the childbirth process (Health Canada, 2000). The doula provides supportive nonmedical care measures, whereas the nurse provides this care and also focuses on monitoring the status of the maternal–fetal unit and implementing clinical care protocols, including pharmacological interventions, and documenting assessment findings, actions, and responses (Simkin & Way, 2008).

Labour Support by the Grandparents

When grandparents act as labour coaches, it is important to support them and treat them with respect. They may have ways to deal with pain that are based on their experience. They should be encouraged to help; one example of a supportive practice would be giving the woman herbal tea during labour. The nurse can act as a role model for parents by acknowledging the value of the grandparent's contributions to parental support and recognizing the difficulty that parents have in witnessing their child's discomfort or crisis, regardless of the age of that child. If they have never witnessed a birth, the nurse may need to provide explanations about what is happening. Many of the activities used to support partners also are appropriate for grandparents.

When possible, the nurse needs to offer the grandparents emotional support. A nurse can show such support by offering them liquid refreshments and initiating discussion with open-ended questions or statements such as "It is sometimes hard to watch a daughter in labour." Nursing actions that provide support for the grandparents can have a therapeutic effect on all members of the family. In turn, a strong, supportive family unit is important for the optimal growth and development of its newest member.

Siblings During Labour and Birth

The preparation of siblings for acceptance of the new child helps promote the attachment process. Such preparation and participation during pregnancy and labour may help the older children accept this change. The older child or children who know that they are important to the family become active participants. Rehearsal for the event before labour is essential.

The age and developmental level of children influence their responses to the addition of a new family member; therefore, preparation for the children to be present during labour is adjusted to meet each child's needs. The child younger than 2 years shows little interest in pregnancy and labour; for the older child, such preparation may reduce fears and misconceptions. Parents need to be prepared for labour and birth themselves and feel comfortable about the process and the presence of their children. Most parents have a "feel" for their children's maturational level and their physical and emotional ability to observe and cope with the events of the labour and birth process.

Preparation can include a description of the anticipated sights, events (e.g., ROM, monitors, IV infusions), smells, and sounds; a labour and birth demonstration; a tour of the birthing unit; and an opportunity to be around a real newborn. Children must learn that their mother will be working hard during labour and birth. She will not be able to talk to them during contractions. She may groan, scream, grunt, and pant at times and say things she would not say otherwise (e.g., "I can't take this anymore;" "Take this baby out of me"). They can be told that labour is uncomfortable but that their mother's body is made for the job.

Storybooks about the birth process can be read to or by children to prepare them for the event. Films are available for preparing preschool and school-age children to participate in the labour and birth experience. Most agencies require that a specific person be designated to watch over the children who are participating in their mother's childbirth experience, to provide them with support, explanations, diversions, and comfort as needed. Health care providers involved in attending women during birth must be comfortable with the presence of children and the unpredictability of their questions, comments, and behaviours.

Emergency Interventions

Emergency conditions that require immediate nursing intervention can arise with startling speed. Interventions for abnormal and atypical FHR, inadequate uterine relaxation, vaginal bleeding, infection, and prolapse of the cord are detailed in the Emergency box. For further information on abnormal FHR patterns, see Chapter 17.

EMERGENCY

Interventions for Emergencies

Signs	Interventions*
Atypical Fetal Heart Rate (FHR) Pattern	
Fetal bradycardia (FHR less than 110 beats/min for more than 10 min) >160 bpm for 30–80 min Rising baseline Variabilty <5 bpm for 40–80 min Decelerations • Repetitive (>3) uncomplicated variable decelerations • Occasional late decelerations • Single prolonged deceleration >2 min but <3 min No acceleration with fetal scalp stimulation	Notify primary health care provider.† Change woman to side-lying position. Discontinue oxytocin infusion if being infused. Increase intravenous (IV) fluid rate if fluid is being infused per protocol order. Administer oxygen at 8 to 10 L/min by tight face mask. Check maternal temperature for elevation. Start an IV line if one is not in place. Perform scalp stimulation and/or obtain fetal blood sample (>34 wk). Continue with close ongoing fetal surveillance.
Abnormal Fetal Heart Rate Pattern	
Fetal bradycardia (FHR less than 100 beats/min for more than 10 min) Fetal tachycardia (FHR above 160 beats/min for more than 80 min in term pregnancy) Erratic baseline Variability • ≤5 bpm for >80 min • >25 bpm for >10 min • Sinusodial Decelerations • Repetitive (≥3) complicated variable decelerations • Later decelerations in >50 of contractions • Single prolonged deceleration >3 min but <10 min Absence of FHR	Notify primary health care provider.† Change woman to side-lying position. Discontinue oxytocin infusion if being infused. Increase IV fluid rate if fluid is being infused per protocol order. Administer oxygen at 8 to 10 L/min by tight face mask. Check maternal temperature for elevation. Start an IV line if one is not in place. Administer amnioinfusion if ordered. Perform scalp stimulation and/or assist with obtaining fetal blood sample (>34 wk). Consider delivery.

Continued

EMERGENCY—cont'd

Interventions for Emergencies

Signs	Interventions*
Inadequate Uterine Relaxation	
Intrauterine pressure greater than 75 mm Hg (shown by intrauterine pressure catheter monitoring) Contractions consistently lasting more than 90 sec Contraction interval less than 2 min	Notify primary health care provider.† Discontinue oxytocin infusion if being infused. Change woman to side-lying position. Increase IV fluid rate if fluid is being infused. Administer oxygen at 8 to 10 L/min by tight face mask. Start an IV line if one is not in place. Palpate and evaluate contractions. Continue fetal surveillance. Give tocolytics (nitroglycerin: sublingual or IV push [by physician]) as ordered.
Vaginal Bleeding	
Vaginal bleeding (bright red, dark red, or in amount exceeding that expected during normal cervical dilation) Continuous vaginal bleeding with FHR changes Pain may or may not be present	Notify primary health care provider.† Continue fetal surveillance. Anticipate emergency (stat) Caesarean birth. Do NOT perform a vaginal examination.
Infection	
Foul-smelling amniotic fluid Maternal temperature above 38°C in presence of adequate hydration (straw-coloured urine) Fetal tachycardia greater than 160 beats/min for more than 10 min	Notify primary health care provider.† Institute cooling measures for labouring woman. Start an IV line if one is not in place. Assist with or perform collection of catheterized urine specimen and send to the laboratory for urinalysis and cultures.
Prolapse of Cord	
Fetal bradycardia with variable deceleration during uterine contraction Woman reports feeling the cord after membranes rupture Cord lies alongside or below the presenting part of the fetus; can be seen or felt in or protruding from the vagina Major predisposing factors: • Rupture of membranes with a gush • Loose fit of presenting part in lower uterine segment • Presenting part not yet engaged • Nonvertex position	Call for assistance. Have someone notify the primary health care provider immediately. Glove the examining hand quickly and insert two fingers into the vagina to the cervix; with one finger on either side of the cord or both fingers to one side, exert upward pressure against the presenting part to relieve compression of the cord. Place a rolled towel under the woman's hip. Place woman in extreme Trendelenburg or modified Sims' position or knee–chest position. Wrap the cord loosely in a sterile towel saturated with warm, sterile normal saline if the cord is protruding from the vagina. Administer oxygen at 8 to 10 L/min by face mask until birth is accomplished. Start IV fluids or increase existing drip rate. Continue to monitor FHR. Do not attempt to replace cord into cervix. Prepare for immediate birth (vaginal or Caesarean).

*Because emergency situations are often frightening events, it is important for the nurse to explain to the woman and her support person what is happening and how it is being managed.

†In most emergency situations, nurses take immediate action, following a protocol and standards of nursing practice. Another person can notify the primary health care provider, or this can be done by the nurse as soon as possible.

Second Stage of Labour

The second stage of labour is the stage in which the infant is born. This stage begins with full cervical dilation (10 cm) and complete effacement (100%) and ends with the baby's birth. The force exerted by uterine contractions, gravity, and maternal bearing-down efforts facilitates the spontaneous vaginal birth of a new baby.

The second stage comprises three phases: latent, descent, and transition phases. These phases are characterized by maternal verbal and nonverbal behaviours, uterine activity, the urge to bear down, and fetal descent (Table 18-6).

The *latent phase* is a period of rest and relative calm (i.e., "labouring down"). During this early phase, the fetus continues to descend passively through the birth canal and rotate to an anterior position as a result of ongoing uterine

Table 18-6 Expected Maternal Progress and Response During Second Stage of Labour and Action by Support Person

CRITERION	LATENT PHASE (AVERAGE DURATION, 10–30 MIN)	DESCENT PHASE (AVERAGE DURATION VARIES)*	TRANSITION PHASE (AVERAGE DURATION 5–15 MIN)
Contractions	Period of physiological lull for all criteria; period of peace and rest		
Magnitude (intensity)		Significant increase	Overwhelmingly strong; expulsive
Frequency		2–2.5 min	1–2 min
Duration		90 sec	90 sec
Descent, station	0 to +2	Increases and Ferguson reflex[†] activated, +2 to +4	Rapid, +4 to birth Fetal head visible in introitus
Show: colour and amount		Significant increase in dark-red bloody show	Bloody show accompanies birth of head
Spontaneous bearing-down efforts	Slight to absent, except during acme of strongest contractions	Increased urge to bear down	Greatly increased
Vocalization	Quiet; concern over progress	Grunting sounds or expiratory vocalization; announces contractions	Grunting sounds and expiratory vocalizations continue; may scream
Maternal behaviour	Experiences sense of relief that transition to second stage is finished Feels fatigued and sleepy Feels a sense of accomplishment and optimism, because the "worst is over" Feels in control	Senses increased urge to push Alters respiratory pattern: has short 4- to 5-sec breath holds with regular breaths in between five to seven times per contraction Makes grunting sounds or expiratory vocalizations Frequent repositioning	Shows decreased ability to listen or concentrate on anything but giving birth Describes ring of fire (burning sensation of acute pain as vagina stretches and fetal head crowns) Often shows excitement immediately after birth of head
Nurse or support person's actions[‡]	Encourages woman to "listen" to her body Continues support measures Suggests an upright position to encourage progression of descent if descent phase does not begin after 30 min	Encourages respiratory pattern of short breath holds Stresses normality and benefits of grunting sounds and expiratory vocalizations Encourages bearing-down efforts with urge to push Encourages or suggests maternal movement and position changes (upright, if descent is not occurring) Encourages woman to "listen" to her body regarding movement and position change if descent is occurring Discourages long breath holds Provides mirror to help woman see progress as she is pushing If birth is to occur in a delivery room, transfers woman to delivery room early to avoid rushing or, if permitted, offers her option of walking to delivery room Places woman in lateral recumbent position to slow descent if descent is too fast	Encourages slow, gentle pushing Explains that "blowing away the contraction" facilitates a slower birth of the head Provides mirror to help woman see the emerging fetal head (best to extend over two to three contractions) to help her understand the perinatal sensations or to feel the baby's head with her hand Coaches woman to relax mouth, throat, and neck to promote relaxation of pelvic floor Applies warm compress to perineum to promote relaxation

*Duration of descent phase can vary, depending on maternal parity, effectiveness of bearing-down effort, and presence of spinal or epidural anaesthesia/analgesia.
[†]Pressure of presenting part on stretch receptors of pelvic floor stimulates release of oxytocin from posterior pituitary, resulting in more intense uterine contractions.
[‡]Provided by nurses and support people.

evolve Case Study–Second/Third Stages of Labour

contractions. The woman is quiet and often relaxes with her eyes closed between contractions. The urge to bear down is not well established and is experienced only during the acme of a contraction or may not be experienced at all. Allowing a woman to rest during this phase and waiting until the urge to push intensifies reduces maternal fatigue, conserves energy for bearing-down efforts, and enables optimal maternal and fetal outcomes. Coaching a woman to push before her body signals readiness can result in a prolonged period of active pushing with limited-to-no progress. The woman can become dependent on her support person or nurses to tell her when and how to push. Women who have **epidural** analgesia may not feel the urge to bear down. They should be encouraged to wait to push until they have some sensation and may need coaching.

The *descent phase*, or phase of active pushing, is characterized by strong urges to bear down as the Ferguson reflex is activated by pressure of the presenting part on the stretch receptors of the pelvic floor. At this point, the fetal station is usually 1+, and the position is anterior. This stimulation causes the release of oxytocin from the posterior pituitary gland, which stimulates stronger, expulsive uterine contractions. During this phase, the woman becomes more focused on bearing-down efforts, which become rhythmic. She will change positions frequently to find a more comfortable pushing position. The woman often announces the onset of contractions and becomes more vocal as she bears down. The urge to bear down intensifies as descent progresses.

In the *transition phase*, the presenting part is on the perineum, and bearing-down efforts are most effective for promoting birth. The woman may be more verbal about the pain she is experiencing; she may scream or act out of control.

The nurse needs to encourage the woman to "listen" to and trust her body as she progresses through the phases of the second stage of labour (see Table 18-6). When a woman listens to her body to tell her when to bear down, her efforts become more effective, and she often feels more satisfied with her efforts to give birth to her baby.

If a woman is confined to bed, especially in a recumbent position, the rhythmic urge to bear down is delayed because gravity is not being used to press the presenting part against the pelvic floor. Women should be encouraged to use various positions for bearing down, such as side-lying, kneeling, squatting, sitting, or standing (Fig 18-14).

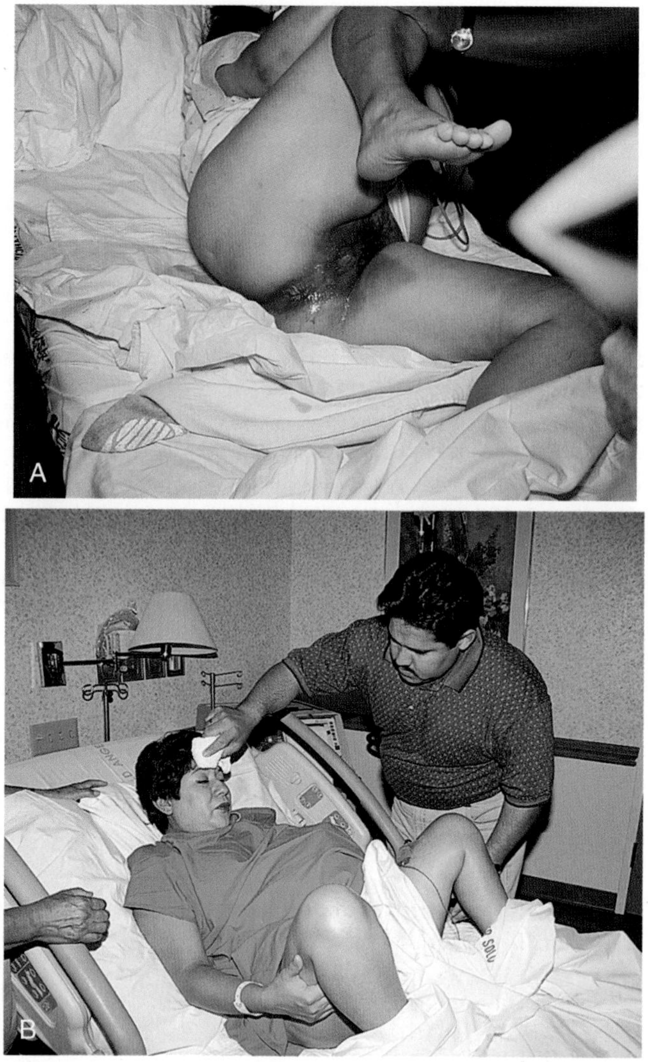

Fig. 18-14 **A:** Pushing, side-lying position, perineal bulging. **B:** Pushing, semisitting. Partner wiping woman's face with cool cloth between contractions. *(**A**, Courtesy Michael S. Clement, MD, Mesa, AZ. **B**, Courtesy Marjorie Pyle, RNC, Lifecircle, Costa Mesa, CA.)*

Duration of Second Stage

The duration of the second stage of labour is influenced by several factors, such as the effectiveness of the primary and secondary powers of labour; the type and amount of analgesia or anaesthesia being used; the physical and emotional condition, position, activity level, parity, and pelvic adequacy of the labouring woman; the size, presentation, and position of the fetus; and the nature and source of support the woman receives.

For many multiparous women, birth occurs within minutes of complete dilation, perhaps only one push later. Nulliparous women may push for 1 to 2 hours before giving birth. If the woman has been given epidural analgesia, pushing can last more than 2 hours. Epidural analgesia blocks or reduces the urge to bear down and limits the woman's ability to attain an upright position to push. By adjusting dosages to the lowest effective level, allowing the epidural to wear off at full dilation or after 1 hour of pushing, or using mixtures containing an opioid-agonist analgesic and a local anaesthetic, the woman can perceive more fully the urge to bear down, move more freely, and attain an upright position with assistance as a result of increased strength and sensation in her legs. This approach can enhance the ability to bear down effectively and achieve an uncomplicated vaginal birth. If the analgesia is allowed to wear off completely, the woman may have an increase in distress and the severity of pain. This results in an increase in sympathetic activity and the release of catecholamines. Catecholamines inhibit uterine contractions, potentially prolonging the second stage of labour. Allowing these women a "labouring down" period for fetal descent and rotation may result in a more positive outcome.

Commonly, a second stage of more than 2 hours may be considered prolonged in women without regional analgesia and is reported to the primary health care provider. By using assessment findings such as the FHR and pattern, the descent of the presenting part, the quality of the uterine contractions, and the status of the woman, premature intervention with episiotomy or forceps- or vacuum-assisted birth can be avoided. If the status of the maternal–fetal unit is normal and progress is continuing, interventions to end the second stage of labour are unwarranted. Less emphasis should be placed on a definite time limit for the second stage. The duration of active pushing has been found to be more relevant to the newborn's condition at birth than the duration of the second stage of labour itself.

Nursing Care Management

The only certain objective sign that the second stage of labour has begun is the inability to feel the cervix during vaginal examination, indicating that the cervix is fully dilated and effaced. The precise moment that this occurs is not easily determined because it depends on when a vaginal examination is performed to validate full dilation and effacement. This makes timing of the actual duration of the second stage difficult. Other signs that suggest the onset of the second stage include the following:

- Sudden appearance of sweat on upper lip
- An episode of vomiting
- Increased **bloody show**
- Shaking of extremities
- Increased restlessness; verbalization (e.g., "I can't go on")
- Involuntary bearing-down efforts

These signs commonly appear when the cervix reaches full dilation; however, women with an epidural block may not exhibit such signs. Other indicators for each phase of the second stage are given in Table 18-6.

Women can begin to experience an irresistible urge to bear down before full dilation. For some women, this occurs as early as 5 cm dilation. This is most often related to the station of the presenting part below the level of the ischial spines of the maternal pelvis. This occurrence creates a conflict between the woman, whose body is telling her to push, and her health care providers, who believe that pushing the fetal presenting part against an incompletely dilated cervix will result in cervical edema and lacerations and a slowing down of labour progress. The premature urge to bear down must be evaluated as a phase of labour progress, possibly indicating the onset of the second stage of labour. The timing when a woman pushes in relation to whether or not her cervix is fully dilated should be based on research evidence rather than on tradition or routine practice. It may be safe and effective for a woman to push with the urge to bear down at the acme of a contraction if her cervix is soft, retracting, and 8 cm or more dilated and if the fetus is at a 1+ station and rotating to an anterior position.

In the hospital, birth may occur in an LDR, LDRP, or delivery room. If the mother is to be transferred to the delivery room for birth, the nurse needs to make the transfer early enough to avoid rushing the woman. The birth area should be readied for the birth. Most North American hospitals have adopted the birthing practice of most non-Western societies in which labour and birth occur in the same room.

Maternal Position

There is no single correct position for childbirth. Labour is a dynamic, interactive process involving the woman's uterus, pelvis, and voluntary muscles. In addition, angles between the woman's pelvis and the baby constantly change as the fetus turns and flexes down the birth canal. The woman may want to assume various positions for childbirth, and she should be encouraged and helped to attain and maintain her positions of choice. Supine, semirecumbent, or lithotomy positions are still widely used in Western societies despite evidence that women prefer upright positions for their bearing-down efforts and birth.

Birth attendants play a major role in influencing a woman's choice of position for birth, with midwives tending to advocate the nonlithotomy positions for the second stage of labour. Upright positions for women with or without epidural anaesthesia facilitate birth and fetal descent and reduce the duration of the second stage of labour and the need for episiotomy, forceps, or vacuum extractor, in the following ways:

- Straighten the longitudinal axis of the birth canal and improve alignment of the fetus for passage through the pelvis
- Use gravity to direct the fetal head toward the pelvic inlet, thereby facilitating descent
- Enlarge pelvic dimensions and restrict the encroachment of the sacrum and coccyx into the pelvic inlet
- Increase uteroplacental circulation, resulting in more intense, efficient uterine contractions
- Enhance the woman's ability to bear down effectively, thereby minimizing maternal exhaustion

Squatting is highly effective in facilitating the descent and birth of the fetus. It is considered to be one of the best and most natural positions for the second stage of labour. Women should assume a modified, supported squat until the fetal head is engaged, at which time a deep squat can be used. A firm surface is required for this position, and the woman will need side support (see Fig. 18-11, A). In a birthing bed, a squatting bar is available that she can use to help support herself (see Fig. 16-16). A birth ball can help a woman maintain the squatting position. The fetus will be aligned with the birth canal, and pelvic and perineal relaxation are facilitated as she sits on the ball or holds it in front of her for support as she squats.

When a woman uses the supported standing position for bearing down, her weight is borne on both femoral heads, allowing the pressure in the acetabulum to increase the transverse diameter of the pelvic outlet by up to 1 cm. This can be helpful if descent of the head is delayed because the occiput has not rotated from the lateral (transverse diameter of pelvis) to the anterior position. Birthing or rocking chairs may be used to provide women with a good physiological position to enhance bearing-down efforts during childbirth, although some women feel restricted by a chair. The upright position provides a potential psychological advantage in that it allows the mother to see the birth as it occurs and maintain eye contact with the attendant. Most birthing chairs are designed so that, if an emergency occurs, the chair can be adjusted to the horizontal or the Trendelenburg position.

Oversized beanbag chairs and large floor pillows may be used for both labour and birth. They can mould around and support the mother in whatever position she selects. Birthing stools can be used to support the woman in an upright position similar to squatting. Women may want to sit on the toilet to push because they are concerned about stool incontinence during this stage. Sitting on the toilet is similar to squatting and is an ideal position for the primiparous woman to start the pushing stage. Women must be closely monitored and removed from the toilet before birth is imminent. Because sitting on chairs, stools, toilets, or commodes can increase perineal edema and blood loss, it is important to assist the woman to change her position frequently.

The side-lying position, with the upper part of the woman's leg held by the nurse or coach or placed on a pillow, is also an effective position for the second stage of labour (see Fig. 18-14, A). Women using the lateral position have more control over their bearing-down efforts. In addition, a slower, more controlled descent of the fetus results in a reduced risk of perineal trauma. Some women prefer a semisitting (semirecumbent) position. To maintain good uteroplacental circulation and enhance the woman's bearing-down efforts in this position, the woman's back and shoulders should be elevated to at least a 30-degree angle, and a wedge should be placed under one hip (see Fig. 18-14, B). The episiotomy rate for nulliparas has been found to be highest in this position.

The hands-and-knees position, along with pelvic rocking, is an effective position for birth because it enhances placental perfusion, helps rotate the fetus from a posterior to an anterior position, and may facilitate the birth of the shoulders, especially if the fetus is large (see Fig. 18-11, B). Perineal trauma may also be reduced. Women in the second stage of labour should be encouraged to change positions every 20 to 30 minutes if they are not making progress.

The birthing bed is commonly used today and can be set for different positions according to the woman's needs (Fig. 18-15). The woman can squat, kneel, sit, recline, or lie on her side, choosing the position most comfortable for her. At the same time there is exposure for examination, electrode placement, and birth. Squatting bars, over-the-bed tables, birth balls, and pillows can be used for support. The bed can be positioned for the administration of anaesthesia and is ideal for helping women receiving an epidural to assume different positions to facilitate birth. The bed can be used to transport the woman to the operating room if a Caesarean birth is necessary.

Bearing-Down Efforts

As the fetal head reaches the pelvic floor, most women experience the urge to bear down. Reflexively, the woman will begin to exert downward pressure by contracting her abdominal muscles while relaxing her pelvic floor. This bearing down is an involuntary response to the Ferguson reflex.

A strong expiratory grunt or groan (vocalization) often accompanies pushing when the woman exhales as she pushes. This natural vocalization by women during open-glottis bearing-down efforts should not be discouraged by nurses.

When assisting a woman to push, the nurse should encourage her to push as she feels like pushing (instinctive, spontaneous pushing) rather than giving a prolonged push on command (Yildirim & Beji, 2008). A woman can become confused and anxious when she is being told to do something in conflict with what her body is telling her. Using phrases such as "you are doing so well," "you are moving the baby down," and "follow what your body is telling you," rather than "Push, push, push," encourages a woman to feel confident in her body and what she is feeling (Sampselle et al., 2005).

Women usually begin to push naturally as the contractions increase in intensity and the Ferguson reflex strengthens. The nurse should monitor the woman's breathing so that she does not hold her breath for more than 5 to 7 seconds at a time and should remind her to ventilate her lungs fully by taking deep, cleansing breaths before and after each contraction. Bearing down while exhaling (open-glottis pushing) and taking breaths between bearing-down efforts help to maintain adequate oxygen levels for the mother and fetus, thereby enhancing fetal

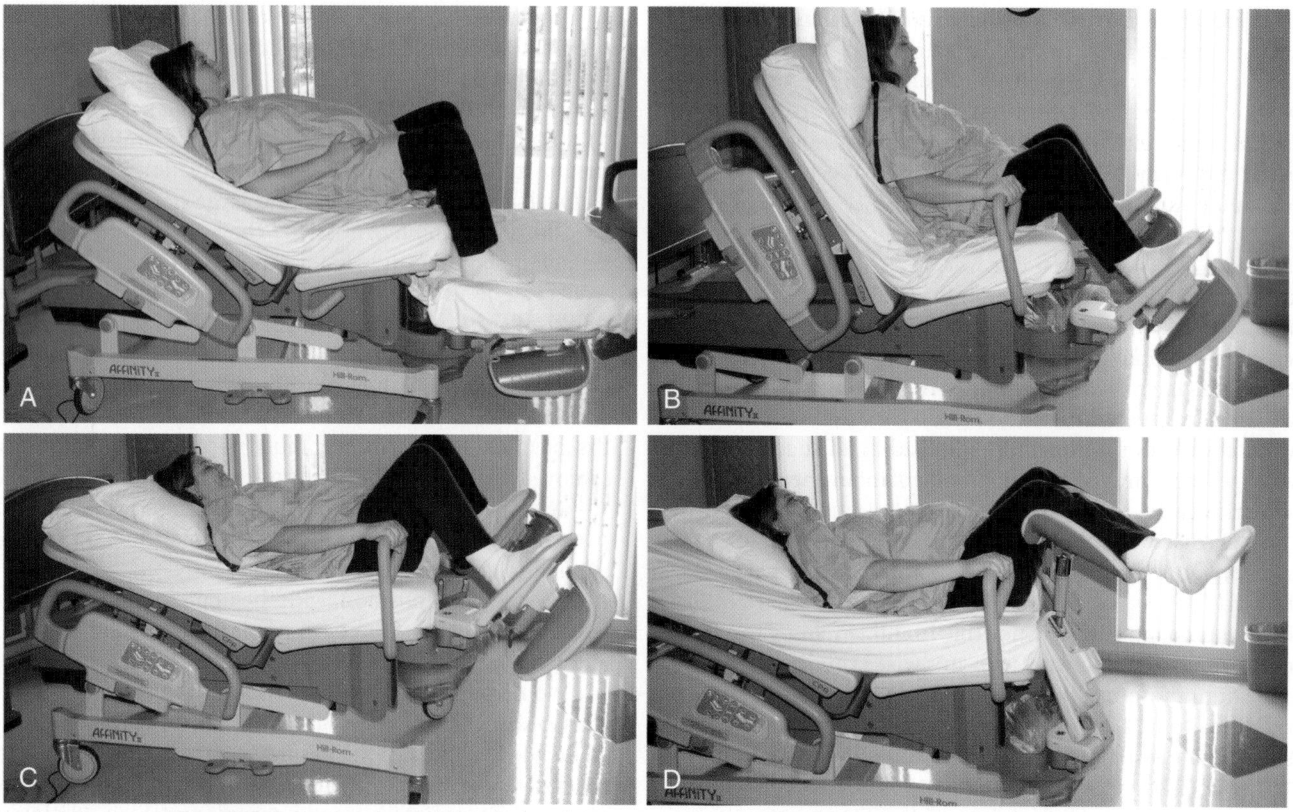

Fig. 18-15 The versatility of today's birthing bed makes it practical in many settings. **A:** Semirecumbent (modified throne position). **B:** High Fowlers (similar to sitting or squatting position). **C:** Lithotomy with foot rests. **D:** Lithotomy with stirrups. *(Courtesy Julie Perry Nelson, Loveland, CO.)*

well-being. Approximately five pushes occur during a contraction, with each push lasting about 5 seconds. Maternal benefits associated with spontaneous pushing include less perineal trauma, less maternal fatigue, and fewer forceps- or vacuum-assisted births. In addition, evidence indicates that the integrity of the pelvic floor is preserved, reducing the risk for future incontinence and pelvic organ prolapse (Sampselle et al., 2005; Simpson & James, 2005). Encouraging the mother to use a mirror to see the baby's head or to use her hand and feel the head often increases a mother's ability to push.

Prolonged breath holding or sustained, directed bearing down is still a common practice often beginning at 10 cm dilation and before the urge to bear down is perceived. The woman is coached to hold her breath, closing her glottis, and to push while the nurse or partner counts to 10. This method of bearing down triggers the Valsalva manoeuvre when the woman closes her glottis (closed-glottis pushing), thereby increasing intrathoracic and cardiovascular pressure, reducing cardiac output, and inhibiting perfusion of the uterus and the placenta. Breath holding for more than 5 to 7 seconds causes the perfusion of oxygen across the placenta to be diminished, resulting in fetal hypoxia (Simpson, 2005; Yildirim & Beji, 2008). This approach to bearing down is harmful or ineffective and should be discouraged (Enkin et al., 2000) (see Critical Thinking Exercise).

A woman may reach the second stage of labour and then experience a lack of readiness to complete the process and give birth to her child. She may have doubts about her readiness to be a mother or want to wait for her support person or primary health care provider to arrive. Fear, anxiety, or embarrassment regarding the unfamiliar or painful sensations and behaviours during pushing (e.g., sounds made, passage of stool) may be other inhibiting factors. Fear that the baby will be in danger once it emerges from the protective intrauterine environment may also be present. By recognizing that a woman may experience a need to hold back the birth of her baby, the nurse can address her concerns and effectively coach her through this stage of labour (see Table 18-6).

To ensure slow birth of the fetal head, the nurse should encourage the woman to control the urge to bear down, by coaching her to take panting breaths or exhale slowly through pursed lips as the baby's head crowns. At this point, the woman needs simple, clear directions from one person. Amnesia between contractions is often pronounced in the second stage, and the woman may have to be roused to cooperate in the bearing-down process.

NURSING ALERT A precipitous birth places a woman at risk for postpartum hemorrhage (PPH). Active management of the third stage of labour is indicated to prevent PPH in this situation.

Fetal Heart Rate and Pattern

Fetal heart rate assessment is done every 5 minutes during the second stage of labour. If atypical or abnormal patterns develop, prompt assessment or intervention must be initiated. The woman can be turned on her side to reduce the pressure of the uterus against the ascending vena cava and descending aorta (see Fig. 18-3), and oxygen can be administered at 8 to 10 L/min via a tight-fitting face mask (Tucker, Miller, & Miller, 2009). Often this is all that is required to restore a normal pattern. If the FHR and pattern do not become normal immediately, the primary health care provider should be notified quickly because medical intervention to hasten birth may be indicated (see Box 17-8).

CRITICAL THINKING EXERCISE

Spontaneous vs. Directed Bearing-Down Efforts

A controversy has arisen on the labour unit where you have your maternal–newborn clinical rotation. Some of the nurses and most of the obstetricians believe that women must be coached to begin pushing as soon as full dilation occurs to ensure that the second stage is not prolonged. The rest of the nurses and midwives and a few obstetricians believe that women know best when and how to push and encourage women in labour to follow what their bodies tell them. The nurse manager of the labour unit has encouraged those believing in spontaneous pushing to present a unit in-service to provide evidence showing that spontaneous pushing enhances the well-being of the maternal–fetal unit without a significant effect on the progress of the second stage of labour. What should the proponents of spontaneous pushing present at the unit in-service?

1. Evidence—Is there evidence that supports the benefits of spontaneous pushing?
2. Assumptions—What assumptions can be made about the following issues related to spontaneous pushing during the second stage of labour?
   a. Benefits of spontaneous pushing
   b. Risks associated with directed pushing
   c. Impact of timing on the onset of pushing during the second stage of labour
3. What influence does a woman's position have on the effectiveness of the pushing technique she uses?
4. Does the evidence support a recommended position to enhance the woman's bearing-down efforts?
5. Are there alternative perspectives to your conclusion?

LEGAL TIP Documentation. All observations (e.g., maternal vital signs, FHR and pattern, progress of labour) and nursing interventions, including patient response, should be documented concurrently with care. The course of labour and maternal–fetal response may change without warning. It is important that all documentation be clear (precise and legible), complete, and consistent, as well as compliant with institutional and professional standards.

Support of the Partner

During the second stage of labour, the woman needs continuous support and coaching (Table 18-6). Because the coaching process can be physically and emotionally tiring for support people, the nurse should offer them nourishment and fluids and encourage them to take short breaks. If birth occurs in an LDR or LDRP room, the partner may be allowed to wear street clothes or be required to wear a clean scrub outfit, cap, and mask (for the birth). The support person who attends the birth in a delivery room may be instructed to put on a cover gown or scrub clothes, mask, hat, and shoe covers as required by agency policy. The nurse should also specify support measures that can be used for the labouring woman and point out areas of the room in which the partner can move freely.

Supplies, Instruments, and Equipment

To prepare for birth in any setting, the birthing table is usually set up during the transition phase for nulliparous women and during the active phase for multiparous women.

The birthing supplies and instruments are arranged on a table or cart (Fig. 18-16). Principles of sterile technique are followed for gloving, identifying and opening sterile packages, adding sterile supplies to the table, unwrapping sterile instruments, and handing them to the primary health care provider. The crib or radiant warmer and equipment are readied for the support and stabilization of the infant, if required (Fig. 18-17).

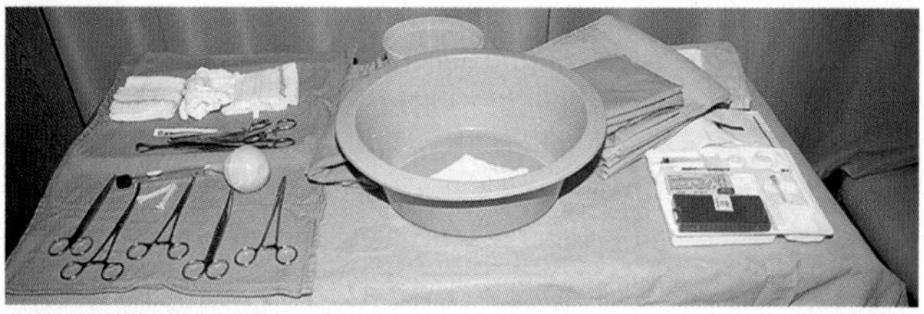

Fig. 18-16 Instrument table. *(Courtesy Marjorie Pyle, RNC, Lifecircle, Costa Mesa, CA.)*

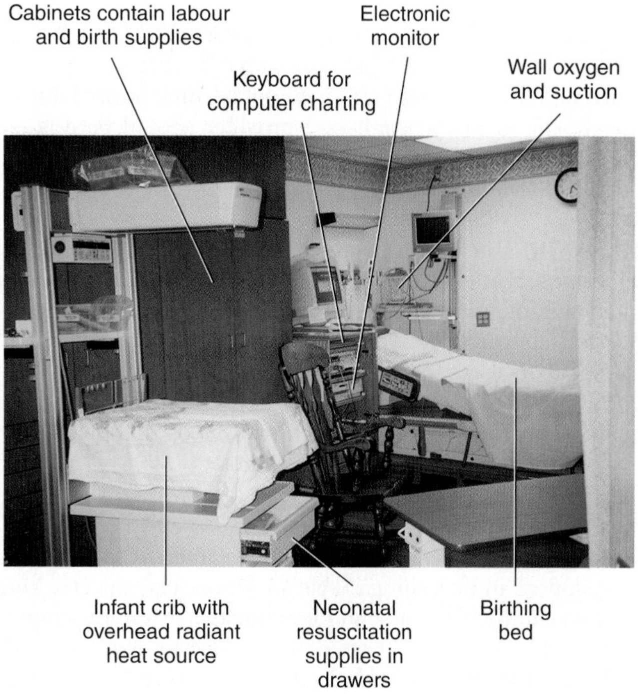

Fig. 18-17 Birthing room. *(Courtesy Dee Lowdermilk, Chapel Hill, NC.)*

The items used for birth may vary among different facilities; therefore, the procedure manual of each facility should be consulted to determine the protocols specific to that facility.

The nurse should estimate the time until the birth will occur and notify the primary health care provider if he or she is not in the patient's room.

Birth in a Delivery Room or Birthing Room

The woman will need assistance if she needs to move from the labour bed to the delivery table (Fig. 18-18). The various positions assumed for birth in a delivery room are the Sims' or lateral position, in which the attendant supports the upper part of the woman's leg, the dorsal position (supine position with one hip elevated), and the lithotomy position.

The lithotomy position has been the position most commonly used for birth in Western cultures, although this practice is changing slowly. The lithotomy position makes it more convenient for the primary health care provider to deal with complications that may arise. To place the woman in this position, her buttocks are brought to the edge of the table, and her legs are placed in stirrups. Care must be taken to pad the stirrups, raise and place both legs simultaneously, and adjust the shanks of the stirrups so that the calves of the legs are supported. There should be no pressure on the popliteal space. If the stirrups are not the same height, ligaments in the woman's back can be strained as she bears down, leading to considerable discomfort in the postpartum period. The lower portion of the table may be dropped down and rolled back under the table.

The routine use of a supine or lithotomy position for labour and birth has been identified as a clearly harmful or ineffective practice and should be discouraged (Enkin et al., 2000).

Other positions for birth include one in which the woman rests her feet on footrests while she holds onto a squatting bar or a side-lying position with the woman's upper leg supported by the coach, nurse, or squatting bar. The foot of the bed can be removed so that the primary health care provider attending the birth can gain better perineal access for delivering a large baby, using forceps or vacuum extractor, or performing an episiotomy, if necessary. Otherwise, the foot of the bed is left

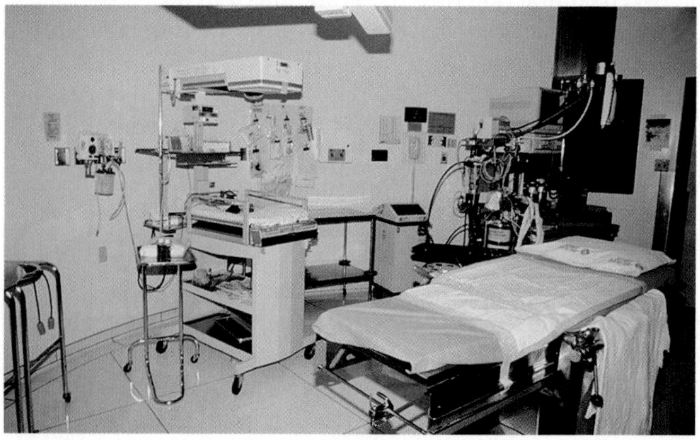

Fig. 18-18 Delivery room. *(Courtesy Michael S. Clement, MD, Mesa, AZ.)*

in place and lowered slightly to form a ledge that allows access for birth and serves as a place to lay the newborn (see Fig. 18-15, A).

The nurse needs to continue to coach and encourage the woman. The nurse should auscultate the FHR or evaluate the electronic monitor tracing every 5 minutes with active pushing and needs to keep the primary health care provider informed of the rate and pattern of the fetal heart. An oxytocic medication such as oxytocin can be prepared so that it is ready to administer after delivery of the anterior shoulder.

If the birth is in a delivery room, the primary health care provider may put on a cap, a mask that has a shield or protective eyewear, and shoe covers. Hands are scrubbed, a sterile gown (with waterproof front and sleeves) is donned, and gloves are put on. Nurses attending the birth may also need to wear caps, protective eyewear, masks, gowns, and gloves. The woman may then be draped with sterile drapes. Birth in an LDR or LDRP usually does not require this type of protective covering but wherever the birth occurs, routine precautions need to be observed (see Box 18-3).

The nurse can maintain contact with the parents by touching and verbally comforting them, explaining the reasons for care, and sharing in the parents' joy at the birth of their child.

Water Birth

There is evidence that immersion in water during first-stage labour can reduce pain and anxiety and does not appear to affect neonatal outcomes adversely. However, the effects of immersion during birth and in the third stage have not been determined by randomized, controlled trials that have a large enough sample to make a determination about maternal and neonatal outcomes.

If a woman wishes to have a water birth (Fig. 18-19), it usually occurs as part of a planned home birth with registered midwives, although may occasionally occur in hospitals. The infant can be placed in the mother's arms until the cord is cut.

Mechanism of Birth: Vertex Presentation

The three phases of spontaneous birth of a fetus in a vertex presentation are (1) birth of the head, (2) birth of the shoulders, and (3) birth of the body and extremities (see Chapter 15).

With voluntary bearing-down efforts, the head appears at the introitus (Fig. 18-20). **Crowning** occurs when the widest part of the head (the biparietal diameter) distends the vulva just before birth. The mother may state that she feels a burning sensation at this time as the perineum is stretched. The birth attendant may apply oil or lubricant to the perineum and stretch it as the head is crowning. Immediately before birth, the perineal musculature becomes greatly distended. If an episiotomy (incision into the perineum to enlarge the vaginal outlet) is necessary, it is done at this time. Local anaesthetic is often administered before the episiotomy.

The primary health care provider may use a hands-on approach to control the birth of the head, believing that guarding the perineum results in a gradual birth that will prevent fetal intracranial injury, protect maternal tissues, and reduce postpartum perineal pain. This approach involves (1) applying pressure against the rectum, drawing it downward to aid in flexing the head as the back of the neck catches under the

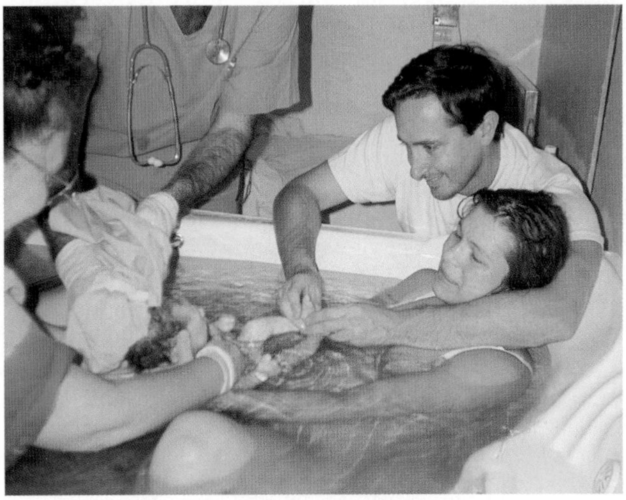

Fig. 18-19 Water birth. *(Courtesy Global Maternal/Child Health Association, Inc., Wilsonville, OR.)*

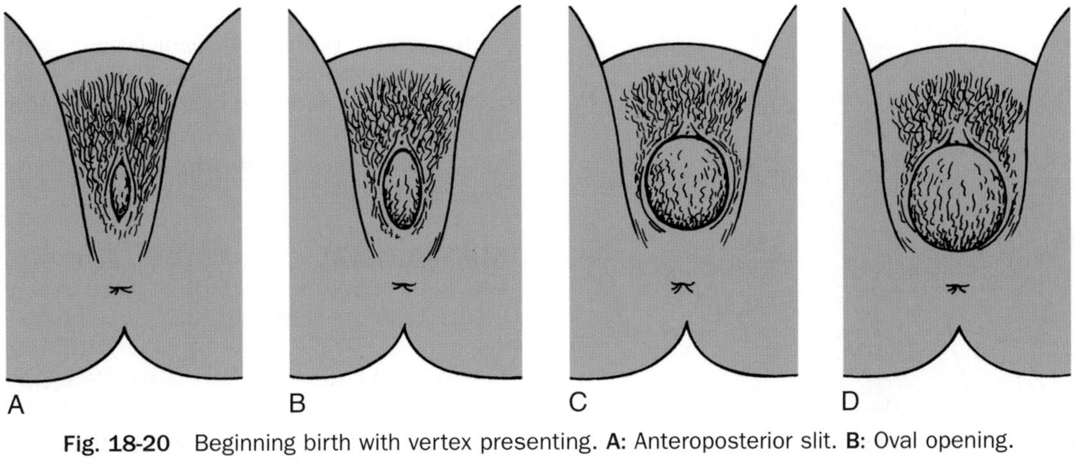

Fig. 18-20 Beginning birth with vertex presenting. **A:** Anteroposterior slit. **B:** Oval opening. **C:** Circular shape. **D:** Crowning.

symphysis pubis; (2) applying upward pressure from the coccygeal region (modified Ritgen manoeuvre) (Fig. 18-21) to extend the head during the actual birth, thereby protecting the musculature of the perineum; and (3) assisting the mother with voluntary control of the bearing-down efforts by coaching her to pant while letting uterine forces expel the fetus.

Some health care providers use a hands-poised (hands-off) approach when attending a birth. In this approach hands are prepared to place light pressure on the fetal head to prevent rapid expulsion. They are not placed on the perineum or used to assist with birth of the shoulders and body.

The hands-on and hands-poised approaches have similar results in terms of perineal trauma and condition of the newborn. However, perineal pain is slightly less 10 days after birth when the hands-on approach is used. Guarding the perineum is a form of care likely to be of benefit (Enkin et al., 2000).

The umbilical cord often encircles the neck (**nuchal cord**) but rarely so tightly as to cause hypoxia. After the head is born, gentle palpation is used to feel for the cord. If present, the cord should be slipped gently over the head. If the loop is tight or if there is a second loop, the cord is clamped twice, cut between the clamps, and unwound from around the neck before the birth is allowed to continue. Mucus, blood, or meconium in the nasal or oral passages may prevent the newborn from breathing. To eliminate this problem, moist gauze sponges may be used to wipe the nose and mouth.

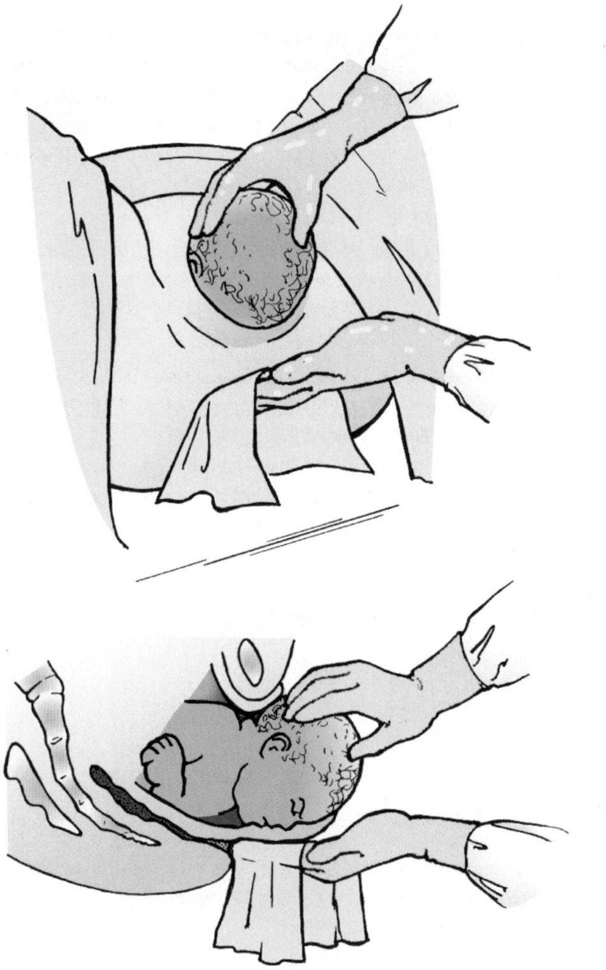

Fig. 18-21 Birth of head with modified Ritgen manoeuvre. Note control to prevent too-rapid birth of head.

Use of Fundal Pressure

Fundal pressure is the application of gentle, steady pressure against the fundus of the uterus to facilitate vaginal birth. Historically, it has been used when the administration of analgesia and anaesthesia decreased the woman's ability to push during the birth, for maternal exhaustion, or when second-stage fetal bradycardia or other abnormal FHR patterns were present. Use of fundal pressure by nurses is not advised because there is no standard technique available for this manoeuvre, and no current legal, professional, or regulatory standards exist for its use. Fundal pressure is contraindicated in shoulder dystocia and may result in injury to the fetus or newborn. The all-fours position (the Gaskin manoeuvre), suprapubic pressure, and maternal position changes are among the recommended interventions. There is very limited information about the use of fundal pressure to shorten second-stage labor in low-risk women.

Management of Infant Born in Meconium-Stained Fluid

Meconium staining of the amniotic fluid occurs when the fetus passes meconium at some time before birth. Meconium-stained fluid is green. The consistency of the fluid is described as either thin (light) or thick (particulate), depending on the amount of meconium present. Meconium-stained fluid can indicate an abnormal fetal status. However, many infants with meconium staining exhibit no signs of depression at birth. The major risk with meconium-stained fluid is the development of meconium aspiration syndrome (see Chapter 27).

The widely used practice of routinely suctioning meconium from the infant's airway after the head is born but before the shoulders are born is no longer recommended. Suctioning at this time was thought to be effective in reducing the incidence and severity of meconium aspiration in the neonate. Research does not support the efficacy of routine intrapartum suctioning to prevent meconium aspiration syndrome (Kattwinkel, 2011; Vain et al., 2004). The Canadian Pediatric Society (CPS) has published treatment recommendations for initial resuscitation of the newborn that include peripartum management of meconium (Canadian Neonatal Resuscitation Program Steering Committee [CNRPSC], 2007). The recommendation continues to include tracheal suctioning immediately after birth for meconium-stained nonvigorous infants but not for meconium-stained infants who are at term gestation and vigorous (CNRPSC, 2007).

NURSING ALERT Personnel skilled in neonatal resuscitation should be present for the birth of a meconium-stained infant (Miller, Fanaroff, & Martin, 2006).

Perineal Trauma Related to Childbirth

Lacerations

During every birth, some damage occurs to the soft tissues of the birth canal and adjacent structures. The tendency to sustain lacerations varies with each woman because the soft tissue in some women may be less distensible. Nulliparous women have tissues that are firmer and more resistant than those in multiparous women and thus have an increased risk for lacerations. Heredity may also be a factor. For example, the tissue of light-skinned women is not as readily distensible as that of darker-skinned women, and healing may be less efficient. The perineal skin and vaginal mucosa may appear intact, but numerous small lacerations in underlying muscle and its fascia may be obscured. Damage to pelvic supports usually is readily apparent and is repaired after birth. Some injuries to the supporting tissues, whether they were repaired or not, may lead to genitourinary and sexual problems later in life (e.g., pelvic relaxation, fistulas, uterine prolapse, **cystocele**, **rectocele**, **dyspareunia**, or urinary and bowel dysfunction).

Immediate repair promotes healing, limits residual damage, and decreases the possibility of infection. Immediately after birth, the cervix, vagina, and perineum should be inspected for damage. In addition, during the early postpartum period, the nurse and primary health care provider should continue to inspect the perineum carefully and evaluate lochia and symptoms to identify any previously missed injury.

Perineal Lacerations

If perineal lacerations are present, they usually occur when the fetal head is being born. The extent of the laceration is defined in terms of its depth:

First degree—Laceration extends through the skin and structures superficial to muscles.

Second degree—Laceration extends through muscles of perineal body.

Third degree—Laceration continues through anal sphincter muscle.

Fourth degree—Laceration also involves the anterior rectal wall.

Perineal injury is often accompanied by small lacerations on the medial surfaces of the labia minora below the pubic rami and to the sides of the urethra (periurethral) and clitoris. Lacerations in this highly vascular area often result in profuse bleeding. Such lacerations must be repaired with absorbable suture (Fig. 18-22).

Special attention must be paid to third- and fourth-degree lacerations so that the woman retains fecal continence. Measures should be taken to promote soft stools (e.g., roughage, fluid, activity, and stool softeners) in order to increase the woman's comfort and foster healing. Antimicrobial therapy may be used in some cases. Enemas and suppositories are contraindicated for these women. Simple perineal injuries usually heal without any significant problems, regardless of whether they were repaired. However, it is easier to repair a new perineal injury to prevent sequelae than it is to correct long-term damage.

Vaginal and Urethral Lacerations

Vaginal lacerations often occur in conjunction with perineal lacerations. Vaginal lacerations tend to extend up the lateral walls (sulci) and, if deep enough, involve the levator ani. Additional injury may occur high in the vaginal vault near the level of the ischial spines. Vaginal vault lacerations may be circular and may result from use of forceps to rotate the fetal head or from rapid fetal descent or precipitous birth.

Cervical Injuries

Cervical injuries occur when the cervix retracts over the advancing fetal head. These cervical lacerations occur at the lateral angles of the external os; most are shallow, and bleeding is minimal. More extensive lacerations may extend to the vaginal vault or beyond it into the lower uterine segment; serious bleeding may occur. Extensive lacerations may follow hasty attempts to enlarge the cervical opening artificially or to deliver the fetus before full cervical dilation is achieved. Injuries to the cervix can have adverse effects on future pregnancies and childbirths.

Episiotomy

An **episiotomy** is an incision made in the perineum to enlarge the vaginal outlet. There is clear evidence that routine or liberal performance of an episiotomy for birth is a form of care that is likely to be harmful or ineffective (Enkin et al., 2000; Hofmeyr, 2005). The Family-Centred Maternity and Newborn Care National Guidelines state that routine episiotomy should be abandoned (Health Canada, 2000). Episiotomy is performed more commonly in North America than in Europe; in Canada in 2007, 21% of women reported having an episiotomy (Public Health Agency of Canada [PHAC], 2009).

The side-lying position for birth causes less tension on the perineum, making possible a gradual stretching of the perineum with fewer indications for episiotomies. Currently, the practice in many settings is to manually support the perineum during birth and allow it to tear, rather than perform an episiotomy. Tears are often smaller than an episiotomy, are repaired easily or not at all, and heal quickly, usually with less pain. The pain and discomfort resulting from episiotomies can interfere with mother–infant interaction, breastfeeding, re-establishment of the sexual relationship with her partner,

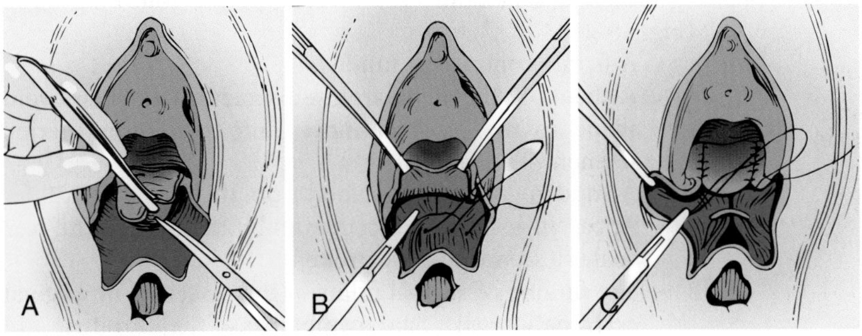

Fig. 18-22 Perineal lacerations. **A:** Bilateral sulcus tears, periurethral tear, and separation of anal sphincter. **B:** Exposure and approximation of levator ani structures. **C:** Approximation of torn bulbocavernous muscle.

and even emotional recovery after birth. The rate of episiotomies is lower when midwives rather than obstetricians attend births.

The type of episiotomy is designated by the site and direction of the incision (Fig. 18-23). Midline (median) episiotomy is used most commonly. It is effective, easily repaired, and generally the least painful. However, it is associated with a higher incidence of third- and fourth-degree lacerations. Sphincter tone is usually restored following primary healing and a good repair.

Mediolateral episiotomy is used in operative births when the need for posterior extension is likely. Although a fourth-degree laceration may be prevented, a third-degree laceration may occur. The blood loss is greater and the repair more difficult and painful than with midline episiotomies. It is more painful in the postpartum period, and the pain lasts longer.

Alternative measures for perineal management such as warm compresses and massage with a lubricant (e.g., prenatal and intrapartum) may have some effectiveness in reducing perineal trauma, as they may lessen the degree of perineal lacerations. Use of Kegel exercises in the prenatal and postpartum periods improves and restores the tone and strength of the perineal muscles. Health practices, including good nutrition and appropriate hygienic measures, help to maintain the integrity and suppleness of the perineal tissue, enhance healing, and prevent infection.

Female Genital Mutilation (FGM)

An increasing number of women are moving to Canada from countries where FGM is a common practice. FGM comprises all procedures that involve partial or total removal of the external female genitalia or other injury to the female genital organs for nonmedical reasons. This practice has been criminalized in Canada. FGM that seals or narrows the vaginal opening (infibulation) may lead to complications in childbirth, including prolonged or obstructed labour. Women may need the scar tissue surgically opened during childbirth, to facilitate safe passage of the fetus. For some women, the scarring may be so extensive that Caesarean birth is the only option.

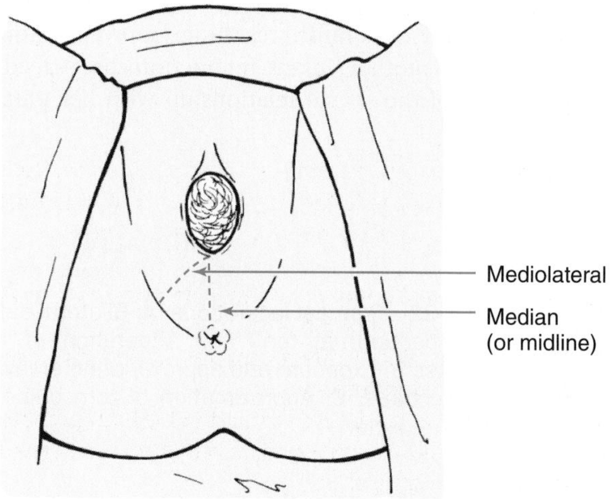

Fig. 18-23 Types of episiotomies.

In some provinces it is illegal for a care provider to reconstruct the infibulation, and they must only suture the area that was surgically incised (College of Physician and Surgeons of Ontario, 2004). Women may be concerned about this practice and need education before the birth regarding what will occur. After the birth they may need extra care for pain management and proper wound healing.

Emergency Childbirth

Even under the best of circumstances there probably will come a time when the perinatal nurse will be required to assist with the birth of an infant without medical assistance. Because it is neither possible nor desirable to prevent an impending birth, the perinatal nurse must be able to function independently and be skilled in the safe birth of a vertex fetus (Box 18-9).

A lateral Sims' position may be the position of choice for birth when (1) the birth is progressing rapidly and there is insufficient time for slow distension of the perineum; (2) the fetal head seems too large to pass through the introitus without laceration; or (3) the apparent size of the fetus is consistent with possible shoulder dystocia. In the lateral Sims' position less stress is placed on the perineum and better visualization of the perineum is possible as the upper leg is supported by the woman's partner or the nurse (see Fig. 18-14, A). In the event of shoulder dystocia, the lateral Sims' position increases the space needed for birth.

Third Stage of Labour

The third stage of labour lasts from the birth of the baby until the placenta is expelled. The goal in the management of the third stage of labour is the prompt separation and expulsion of the placenta in the easiest, safest manner. Before separation of the placenta, blood is collected from the umbilical cord. Cord blood is collected for arterial and venous cord gases as well as blood type, specifically if the mother is Rh negative.

The placenta is attached to the decidual layer of the thin endometrium of the basal plate by numerous fibrous anchor villi. After the birth of the fetus, strong uterine contractions cause the placental site to shrink markedly. This causes the anchor villi to break and the placenta to separate from its attachments. Normally, the first few strong contractions 5 to 7 minutes after the baby's birth cause the placenta to be sheared from the basal plate. A placenta cannot detach itself from a flaccid (relaxed) uterus because the placental site is not reduced in size.

Placental separation is indicated by the following signs (Fig. 18-24):

- A firmly contracting fundus
- A change in the uterus from a discoid to a globular ovoid shape as the placenta moves into the lower uterine segment
- A sudden gush of dark blood from the introitus
- Apparent lengthening of the umbilical cord as the placenta descends to the introitus
- The finding of vaginal fullness (the placenta) on vaginal examination or of fetal membranes at the introitus

BOX 18-9 Guidelines for Assistance at the Emergency Birth of a Fetus in the Vertex Presentation

1. The woman usually assumes the position most comfortable for her. A lateral position is often recommended.
2. Reassure the woman that birth is usually uncomplicated in these situations. Use eye-to-eye contact and a calm, relaxed manner. If someone else is available, such as the partner, that person could help support the woman in the position, assist with coaching, and compliment her on her efforts.
3. Wash your hands and put on gloves if available.
4. Place under woman's buttocks whatever clean material is available.
5. Avoid touching the vaginal area to decrease the possibility of infection.
6. As the head begins to crown, you should do the following:
   a. Perform an amniotomy (artificial rupture of membranes) if it is still intact.
   b. Instruct the woman to pant or pant-blow, thus minimizing the urge to push.
   c. Place the flat side of your hand on the exposed fetal head and apply gentle pressure toward the vagina to prevent the head from "popping out." The mother may participate by placing her hand under yours on the emerging head. Note: Rapid delivery of the fetal head must be prevented because a rapid change of pressure within the moulded fetal skull follows, which may result in dural or subdural tears and cause vaginal or perineal lacerations.
7. After the birth of the head, check for the umbilical cord. If the cord is around the baby's neck, try to slip it over the baby's head or pull it gently to get some slack so that you can slip it over the shoulders.
8. Wait until restitution (external rotation) occurs. After restitution, with one hand on each side of the baby's head, exert gentle pressure downward. Encourage the mother to give a small push so that the anterior shoulder emerges under the symphysis pubis and acts as a fulcrum; DO NOT PULL ON THE FETAL HEAD. Once the anterior shoulder is delivered, apply gentle pressure in the opposite direction to assist in the delivery of the posterior shoulder, which has passed over the sacrum and coccyx.
9. Be alert! Hold the baby securely because the rest of the body may emerge quickly. In an upward motion, complete the birth by cradling the baby's head and back in one hand and the buttocks in the other and place the baby skin to skin on the mother's abdomen.
10. Dry the baby quickly to prevent rapid heat loss, keep the baby skin-to-skin with the mother, and cover with warm blankets. Unless immediate resuscitation is required, there is no urgency to cut the cord. There is sufficient evidence that delayed cord clamping is beneficial for the baby, especially in the preterm population.
11. When ready, double-clamp and cut the cord. Collect arterial and venous cord gases as well as cord blood if the mother is Rh negative. Compliment her (them) on a job well done and on the baby, if appropriate.
12. Wait for the placenta to separate; do not tug on the cord. Note: Injudicious traction may tear the cord, separate the placenta, or invert the uterus. Signs of placental separation include a slight gush of dark blood from the introitus, lengthening of the cord, uterine fundus rising up in the abdomen, and change in the uterine contour from a discoid to globular shape.
13. Instruct the mother to push to deliver the separated placenta. Gently ease out the placental membranes using an up-and-down motion until the membranes are removed. Check the placenta for completeness and keep the placenta until it can be inspected by the primary health provider. If birth occurs outside a hospital setting, to minimize complications, do not cut the cord without proper clamps and a sterile cutting tool. Inspect the placenta for intactness. Place the baby on the placenta and wrap the two together for additional warmth.
14. Check the firmness of the uterus. Gently massage the fundus and demonstrate to the mother how she can massage her own fundus properly.
15. If supplies are available, clean the mother's perineal area and apply a peripad.
16. In addition to gentle massage of the fundus, the following measures can be taken to prevent or minimize hemorrhage:
   a. Put the baby to the mother's breast as soon as possible. Sucking or nuzzling and licking the nipple stimulates the release of oxytocin from the posterior pituitary. Note: If the baby does not or cannot nurse, manually stimulate the mother's nipples.
   b. Do not allow the mother's bladder to become distended. Assess the bladder for fullness and encourage her to void if fullness is found.
   c. Expel any clots from the mother's uterus.
17. Comfort or reassure the mother and her family or friends. Keep the baby skin-to-skin with mother and provide additional warmth to the mother. Give her fluids if available and tolerated.
18. If this is a multifetal birth, identify the infants in order of birth (using letters A, B, etc.).
19. Make notations regarding the following aspects of the birth:
   a. Fetal presentation and position
   b. Presence of cord around neck (nuchal cord) or other parts and number of times cord encircled part
   c. Colour, character, and amount of amniotic fluid if rupture of membranes occurs immediately before birth
   d. Time of birth
   e. Estimated time of determination of Apgar score (e.g., 1 and 5 minutes after birth), resuscitation efforts implemented, and ultimate condition of baby
   f. Sex of baby
   g. Time of placental expulsion and the appearance and completeness of the placenta
   h. Maternal condition: affect, amount of bleeding, and status of uterine tonicity
   i. Any unusual occurrences during the birth (e.g., maternal or paternal response, comments, or gestures in response to birth of baby).

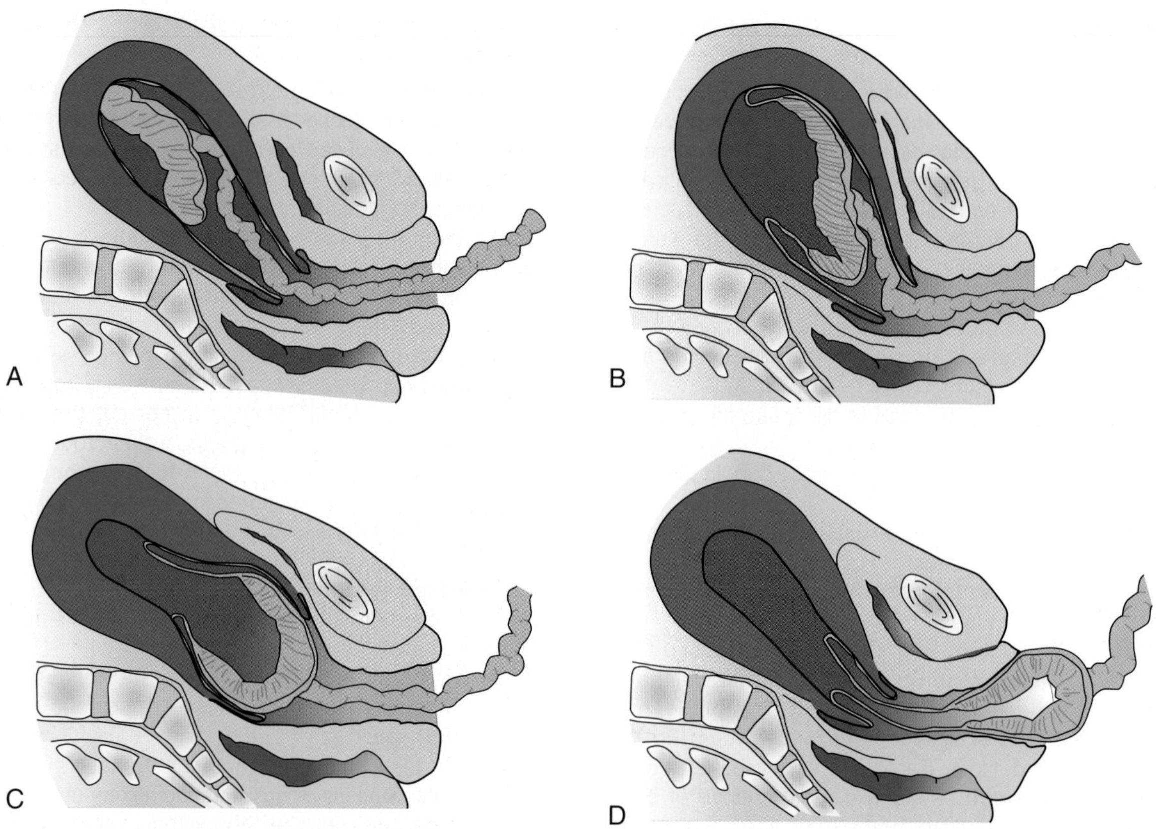

Fig. 18-24 Third stage of labour. **A:** Placenta begins the separation process in central portion with retroplacental bleeding. Uterus changes from discoid to globular shape. **B:** Placenta completes separation and enters lower uterine segment. Uterus is globular in shape. **C:** Placenta enters vagina, cord is seen to lengthen, and there may be increased bleeding. **D:** Expulsion (birth) of placenta and completion of third stage.

Depending on the preferences of the primary health care provider, an expectant or active approach may be used to manage the third stage of labour. Expectant management (watchful waiting) involves the natural, spontaneous separation and expulsion of the placenta by efforts of the mother, with clamping and cutting of the cord after pulsation ceases. It may involve the use of gravity or nipple stimulation to facilitate separation and expulsion, but no oxytocic (uterotonic) medications are given. A quiet, relaxed environment that supports close skin-to-skin contact between mother and newborn also promotes the release of endogenous oxytocin.

In active management, placental separation and expulsion are facilitated by administration of one or more oxytocic (uterotonic) medications after the birth of the anterior shoulder of the fetus, clamping and cutting of the umbilical cord immediately, and delivery of the placenta by application of controlled cord traction when signs of separation are noted. Research findings support the superiority of active management in terms of less blood loss and reduced risk of hemorrhage and other complications of the third stage of labour (Enkin et al., 2000; Leduc et al., 2009).

To assist in the delivery of the placenta, the woman is instructed to push when signs of separation have occurred. If possible, the placenta should be expelled by maternal effort during a uterine contraction. Alternate compression and elevation of the fundus plus minimal controlled traction on the umbilical cord may be used to facilitate delivery of the placenta and amniotic membranes. Oxytocics may be administered after the placenta is removed because they stimulate the uterus to contract, thereby helping to prevent hemorrhage.

Whether the placenta first appears by its shiny fetal surface (Schultze mechanism) or turns to show its dark roughened maternal surface (Duncan mechanism) is of no clinical importance. After the placenta and the amniotic membranes emerge, the primary health care provider will examine them for intactness to ensure that no portion remains in the uterine cavity (i.e., no fragments of the placenta or membranes are retained) (Fig. 18-25).

Some women and their families may have culturally based beliefs regarding the care of the placenta and the manner of its disposal after birth, viewing the care and disposal of the placenta as a way of protecting the newborn from bad luck and illness. Requests by the woman to take the placenta home and dispose of it according to her customs may be at odds with health care agency policies, especially those related to infection control and the disposal of biological wastes. Many cultures follow specific rules regarding the disposal of the placenta in terms of method (burning, drying, burying, or eating); site for disposal (in or near the home); and timing of disposal

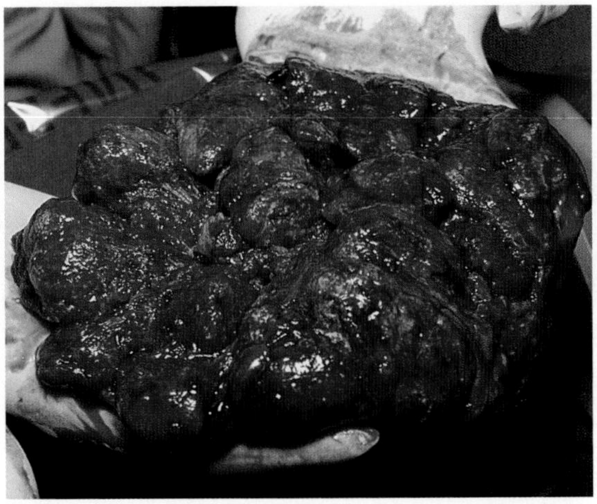

Fig. 18-25 Examination of the placenta. *(Courtesy Michael S. Clement, MD, Mesa, AZ.)*

(immediately after birth, time of day, or by astrological signs). Disposal rituals may vary according to the gender of the child and the length of time before another child is desired. If eaten, the placenta can be a means of restoring a woman's well-being after birth or ensuring quality breast milk. Health care providers can provide culturally sensitive health care by encouraging women and their families to express their wishes regarding the care and disposal of the placenta and by establishing a policy to fulfill these requests (D'Avanzo, 2008).

Umbilical Cord Blood Banking

Increasing numbers of couples are requesting that the blood from the umbilical cord be collected and subsequently banked. Umbilical cord blood is an excellent source of stem cells that may be used to treat certain cancers or blood diseases. In Canada, expectant parents have two options for cord blood banking: public or private banking. There are presently two public cord blood banks in the country: in Québec (only takes donations from certain hospitals in Québec) and in Alberta (only takes donations from Alberta and certain other cities). Private cord banking is available in many centres throughout the country, and arrangements are made prior to the birth of the newborn for collection. The cost of private banking can include an initial fee of between $1000 to $2000 with an additional yearly fee. The decision to bank cord blood is a personal decision made by parents, which must be made based on weighing the pros and cons.

Cord blood collection is done after the birth and before delivery of the placenta. Health care providers need to be aware of the proper method of collection to ensure that the maximum amount of blood is collected and that it is collected in a sterile manner. Delayed cord clamping may decrease the amount of blood collected; parents need to be aware of this so they can make informed choices about the care they want.

Maternal Physical Status

Physiological changes after birth are profound. The cardiac output increases rapidly as maternal circulation to the placenta ceases and the pooled blood from the lower extremities is mobilized. The pulse rate slows in response to the change in cardiac output and tends to remain slightly slower than before pregnancy for about 1 week.

Soon after the birth, the woman's blood pressure usually returns to prepregnancy levels. Several factors contribute to an elevated blood pressure at this time: the excitement of the second stage, certain medications, and the time of day (blood pressure is highest during the late afternoon). Analgesics and anaesthetics may also cause hypotension to develop in the hour after birth.

Signs of Potential Problems

The major risk for women during the third stage of labour is postpartum hemorrhage (see Chapter 23). While the primary health care provider completes the delivery of the placenta, the nurse observes the mother for signs of excessive blood loss, including alteration in vital signs, pallor, light-headedness, restlessness, decreased urinary output, and alteration in level of consciousness and orientation.

Because of the rapid cardiovascular changes taking place (e.g., the increased intracranial pressure during pushing and the rapid increase in cardiac output), the risks of rupture of a pre-existing cerebral aneurysm and formation of pulmonary emboli are greater than usual during this period. Another dangerous, unpredictable problem is amniotic fluid embolism (see Chapter 19).

Women with a history of cardiac disorders are at increased risk for cardiac decompensation and pulmonary edema as a result of circulatory changes associated with the birth of the fetus and expulsion of the placenta. The nurse should carefully assess the woman's respiratory pattern and effort, especially in the early postpartum period.

Care After Placental Delivery

The woman may feel some discomfort when the placenta is delivered and while the primary health care provider carries out the postbirth vaginal examination. The nurse can encourage her to use breathing and relaxation or distraction techniques to help her cope with the discomfort.

When the third stage is complete and any lacerations or episiotomy is sutured, the vulvar area is gently cleansed with warm water and a perineal pad or an ice pack is applied to the perineum. The birthing table or bed is repositioned, and the woman's legs are lowered simultaneously if she gave birth in the lithotomy position. Drapes are removed, and dry linen is placed under the woman's buttocks; she should be provided with a clean gown and a warm blanket. She should be assisted into her bed if she is to be transferred from the birthing area to the recovery area. The side rails should be raised during transfer. If the woman labours, gives birth, and recovers in the same bed and room, she should be refreshed following the protocol already described. Maternal and neonatal assessments for the fourth stage of labour need to be instituted. Box 18-10 summarizes the stages of normal vaginal childbirth.

Immediate Assessment and Care of the Newborn

The time of birth is the precise time when the entire body is out of the mother. This time must be noted on the record. If the condition of the newborn is not compromised, he or she evolve Video–Childbirth (Vaginal)

BOX 18-10 Normal Vaginal Childbirth

First Stage

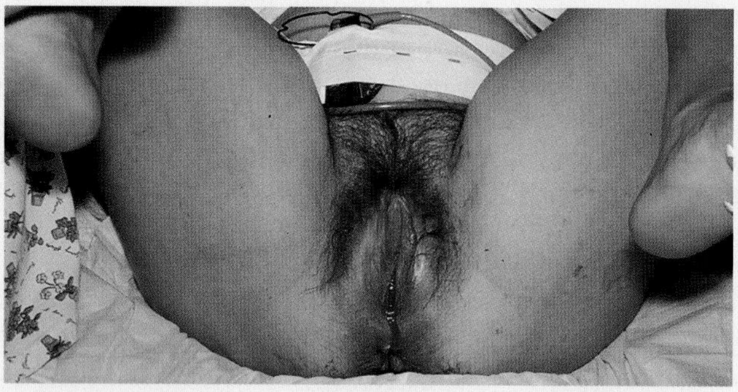

Anteroposterior slit; vertex visible during contraction.

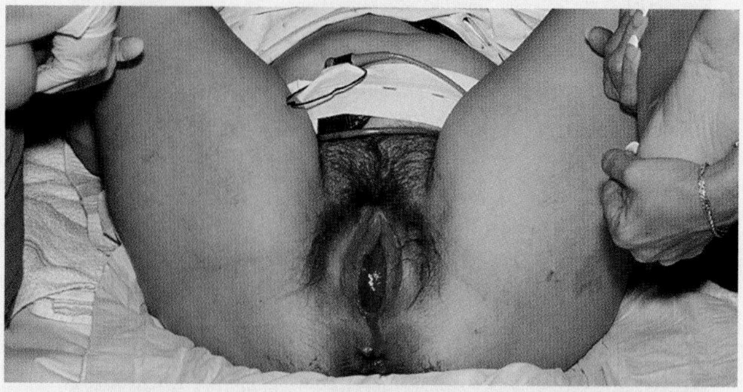

Oval opening; vertex presenting. Note: nurse (on left) is wearing gloves but support person (on right) is not.

Second Stage

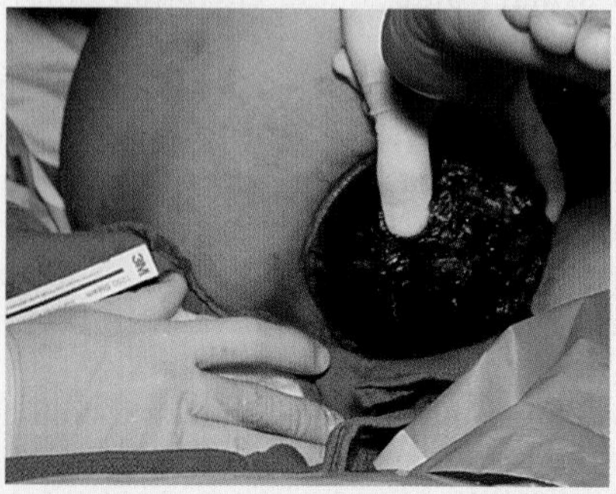

Crowning.

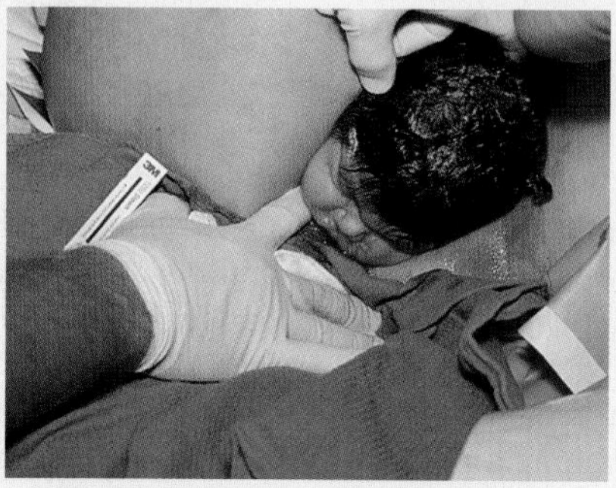

Primary care provider using Ritgen manoeuvre as head is born by extension.

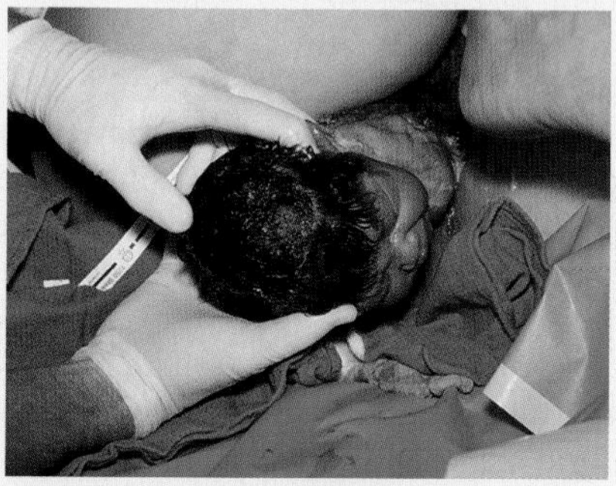

After checking for nuchal cord, the primary care provider supports head during external rotation and restitution.

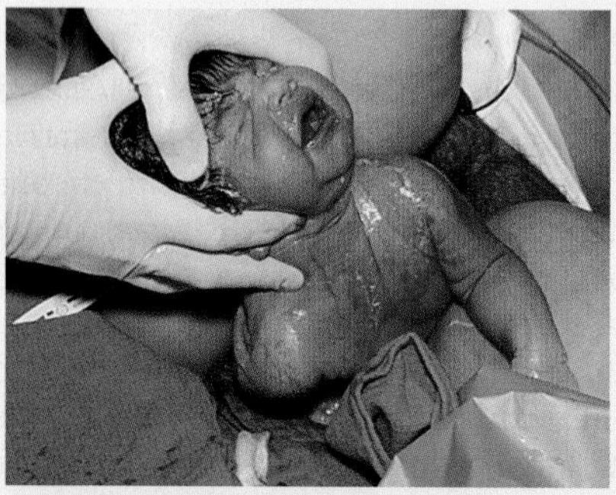

Birth of posterior shoulder.

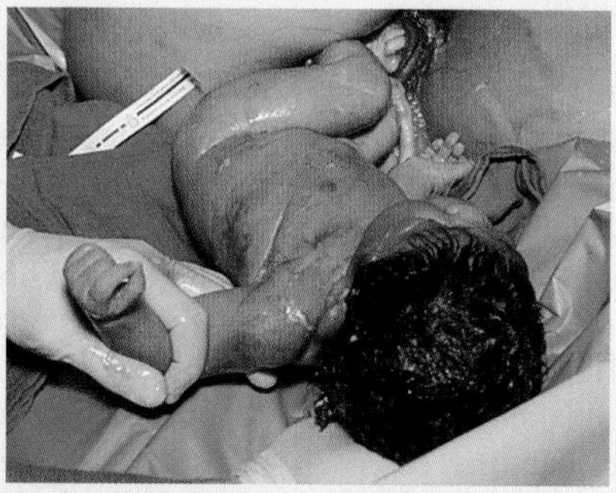

Birth of newborn by slow expulsion.

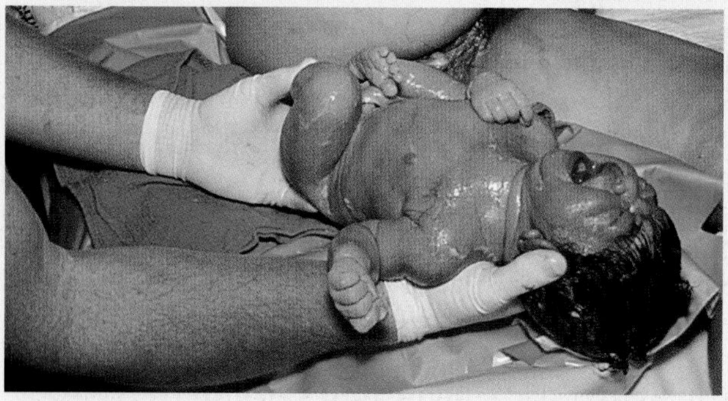

Second stage complete; note that newborn is not completely pink yet.

BOX 18-10 Normal Vaginal Childbirth—cont'd

Third Stage

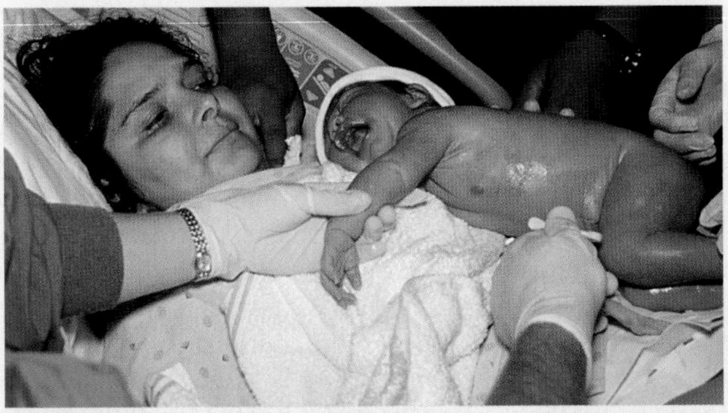

Newborn placed on mother's abdomen while cord is clamped and cut.

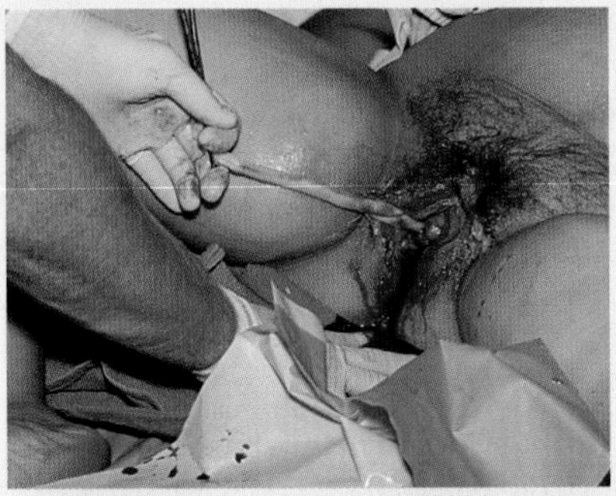

Note increased bleeding as placenta separates.

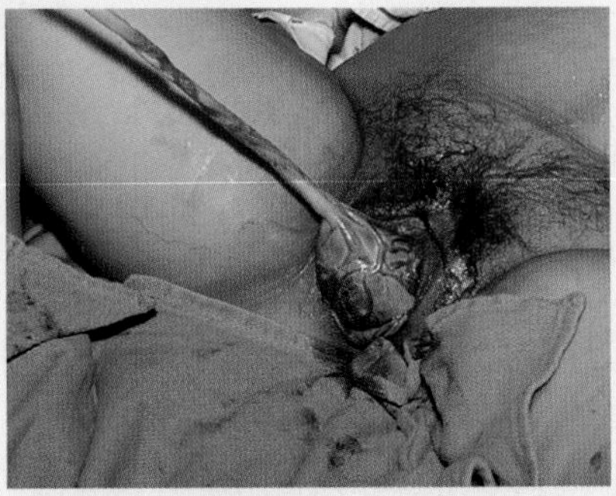

Expulsion of placenta.

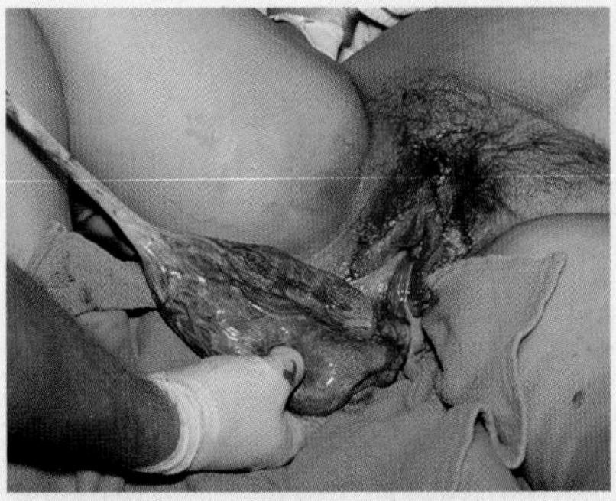

Expulsion is complete, marking the end of the third stage.

(Courtesy Michael S. Clement, MD, Mesa, AZ.)

evolve Animation—Vaginal Birth

should be dried and then placed skin to skin on the mother's abdomen immediately after birth and covered with a warm, dry blanket. The cord can be clamped at this time, and the primary health care provider may ask if the woman's partner would like to cut the cord. If so, the partner is given a sterile pair of scissors and instructed to cut the cord 1 inch (2.5 cm) above the clamp.

Recent evidence regarding timing of cord clamping shows that there is no difference in postpartum hemorrhage rates if the clamping is delayed; this practice increases iron stores in newborns at 6 months of age. There may be an increased risk of jaundice requiring phototherapy (McDonald & Middleton, 2008). Delayed cord clamping (1 to 3 minutes) should be considered for all newborns as iron deficiency has been associated with impaired development.

Care given immediately after the birth focuses on assessing and stabilizing the newborn. The nurse's primary responsibility at this time is the infant because the primary health care provider is involved with the delivery of the placenta and care of the mother. The nurse must watch the infant for signs of distress and initiate appropriate interventions should any appear.

Fourth Stage of Labour

The first 1 to 2 hours after birth, sometimes called the fourth stage of labour, is a crucial time for the mother and her newborn. Both are not only recovering from the physical process of birth but also becoming acquainted with each other and additional family members. During this time, maternal organs undergo their initial readjustment to the nonpregnant state, and the functions of body systems begin to stabilize. Meanwhile, the newborn continues the transition from intrauterine to extrauterine existence.

A brief assessment of the newborn can be performed while the baby is skin to skin on the mother. This includes checking the infant's airway and assigning the Apgar score; maintaining a patent airway; supporting respiratory effort; and preventing cold stress by drying the infant and maintaining uninterrupted skin-to-skin contact with the mother and covering the newborn with a warm blanket. A hat should be put on the newborn to keep the head warm. Newborns should only be brought to the radiant warmer if they require resuscitative measures.

When the baby is at the breast, the nurse has an opportunity to give the newborn a vitamin K injection. There is strong evidence to support the role of breastfeeding in reducing pain in the newborn during a painful procedure (see Chapter 25). After the baby has gone to the breast, the baby can be weighed and measured, eye prophylaxis administered, and an identification bracelet that corresponds to the mother's identification bracelet applied. Once these activities are done, the baby should be given back to the mother and placed skin to skin to support transition of the newborn. In some agencies, the mother's partner (or another person designated by the mother) is also given a corresponding identification bracelet.

The fourth stage of labour is an excellent time to begin breastfeeding because the infant is in an alert state and ready to nurse. Breastfeeding at this time also aids in the contraction of the uterus and the prevention of maternal hemorrhage. In some cultures, breastfeeding is not considered acceptable until the milk comes in. The benefits of early initiation of breastfeeding and the benefits of colostrum should be discussed with families at this time. In most centres the mother remains in the labour and birth area during this recovery time. If the woman is in an LDR room, the woman stays in the same room where she gave birth. In traditional settings, women are taken from the delivery room to a separate recovery area for observation.

Arrangements for care of the newborn vary during the fourth stage of labour. In most settings the baby remains with the mother, and the labour or birth nurse cares for both of them. In some institutions the baby is taken to the nursery for several hours of observation after an initial bonding period with the parents, although this is not done in many institutions (see Fig. 21-6).

If the recovery nurse has not previously cared for the new mother, his or her assessment begins with an oral report from the nurse who attended the woman during labour and birth and a review of the prenatal, labour, and birth records. Of primary importance are conditions that could predispose the mother to hemorrhage, such as precipitous labour, large baby, grand multiparity (having given birth many times), or induced labour. For healthy women, hemorrhage is probably the most dangerous potential complication.

During the first hour, physical assessments of the mother are frequent. All factors except temperature are assessed every 15 minutes for 1 hour. Temperature is assessed at the beginning and end of the recovery period. After the fourth 15-minute assessment, if all parameters have stabilized within the normal range, assessments are continued every 30 minutes in the second hour. Box 18-11 describes the physical assessment of the mother during the fourth stage of labour.

During the fourth stage of labour, many women experience intense tremors that resemble shivering from a chill. They are

BOX 18-11 Assessment During Fourth Stage of Labour

Before beginning the assessment, wash hands thoroughly, assemble necessary equipment, and explain the procedure to the patient.

Blood Pressure

Measure blood pressure per assessment schedule.

Pulse

Assess rate and regularity.

Temperature

Determine temperature.

Fundus

Put on clean examination gloves.

Position woman with knees flexed and head flat.

Just below the umbilicus, cup hand and press firmly into the abdomen. At the same time, stabilize the uterus at symphysis with the opposite hand.

If the fundus is firm (and bladder is empty), with uterus in midline, measure its position relative to the woman's umbilicus. Lay fingers flat on the abdomen under the umbilicus; measure how many centimetres (cm) fit between the umbilicus and top of the fundus. If the fundus is above the umbilicus, this is recorded as plus cm; if below, as minus cm. One fingerbreadth equals 1 cm.

If the fundus is not firm, massage it gently to contract and expel any clots before measuring distance from the umbilicus.

Place hands appropriately; massage gently only until firm.

Expel clots while keeping hands placed as in Fig. 21-3. With the upper hand, firmly apply pressure downward toward the vagina; observe perineum for amount and size of expelled clots.

Bladder

Assess distension by noting location and firmness of uterine fundus and observing and palpating the bladder. A distended bladder is seen as a suprapubic rounded bulge that is dull to percussion and fluctuates like a water-filled balloon. When the bladder is distended, the uterus is usually boggy in consistency, well above the umbilicus and to the woman's right side.

Assist the woman to void spontaneously. Measure amount of urine voided.

Catheterize as necessary.

Reassess after voiding or catheterization to make sure that the bladder is not palpable and the fundus is firm and in the midline.

Lochia

Observe lochia on perineal pads and on linen under the mother's buttocks. Determine amount and colour; note size and number of clots; note odour.

Observe perineum for source of bleeding (e.g., lacerations, episiotomy).

Perineum

Ask or assist woman to turn on her side and flex her upper leg on her hip.

Lift upper buttock.

Observe perineum in good lighting.

Assess laceration repair or episiotomy site repair for intactness, hematoma, edema, bruising, redness, and drainage.

Assess for presence of hemorrhoids.

Apply ice packs as needed.

commonly seen and are not related to infection. Several theories have been offered to explain these tremors or shivering: they may be the result of a sudden release of pressure on pelvic nerves after birth, a response to a fetus-to-mother transfusion that occurred during placental separation, a reaction to maternal adrenaline production during labour and birth, or a reaction to epidural anaesthesia. Warm blankets and reassurance that the chills or tremors are common and self-limiting and last only a short while are useful interventions.

The nutritional status of the woman needs to be assessed. Restriction of food and fluid intake and the loss of fluids (blood, perspiration, or emesis) during labour cause many women to express a strong desire to eat or drink soon after birth. In the absence of complications, a woman who has given birth vaginally; has recovered from the effects of the anaesthetic; and has stable vital signs, a firm uterus, and small-to-moderate lochial flow may have fluids and a regular diet, as desired.

Postanaesthesia Recovery

The woman who has given birth by Caesarean or who has received regional anaesthesia for a vaginal birth requires special attention during the recovery period. Obstetrical recovery areas are held to the same standard of care that would be expected of any other postanaesthesia recovery room. When caring for a woman recovering from anaesthesia, the nurse needs to to have available cardiopulmonary support and emergency supplies. Women who are recovering from anaesthesia require further assessments every 15 minutes, including activity, respirations, oxygen saturation, level of consciousness, and colour.

NURSING ALERT Regardless of her obstetrical status, no woman should be discharged from the recovery area until she has completely recovered from the effects of anaesthesia.

If the woman received general anaesthesia, she should be awake and alert and oriented to time, place, and person. Her respiratory rate should be within normal limits, and her oxygen saturation levels should be at least 95% as measured by a pulse oximeter. If the woman received epidural or spinal anaesthesia, she should be able to raise her legs, extended at the knees, off the bed; or flex her knees, place her feet flat on the bed, and raise her buttocks well off the bed. The numb or tingling, prickly sensation should be entirely gone from her legs. Women vary greatly in regard to length of time required to recover from regional anaesthesia. Often it takes several hours for these anaesthetic effects to disappear completely.

When fourth-stage recovery is complete, the woman will remain in her room if she is in an LDRP unit or will be transferred via wheelchair to a room on the postpartum unit if she gave birth in an LDR or delivery room. Women who are in LDRP rooms will stay in one room from admission until discharge. Often the same nurse will care for the family through all parts of her childbirth experience.

Family–Newborn Relationships

Most parents enjoy being able to handle, hold, explore, and examine the baby immediately after birth. Both parents can assist with the thorough drying of the infant. Skin-to-skin contact should be encouraged; holding the newborn next to the skin of either parent helps to maintain the baby's temperature.

The woman's reaction to the sight of her newborn may range from excited outbursts of laughing, talking, and even crying to apparent apathy. A polite smile and nod may be her only acknowledgment of the comments of nurses and the primary health care provider. Occasionally, the reaction is one of anger or indifference; the woman turns away from the baby, concentrates on her own pain, and may make hostile comments. These varied reactions can arise from pleasure, exhaustion, or deep disappointment. When evaluating parent–newborn interactions after birth, the nurse should also consider the cultural characteristics of the woman and her family and the expected behaviours of that culture. In some cultures, the birth of a male child is preferred, and women may grieve when a female child is born (D'Avanzo, 2008).

Whatever the reaction and its cause may be, the woman needs continued acceptance and support from all staff. Notation of the parents' reaction to the newborn should be made in the recovery record. Nurses can assess this reaction by asking themselves the following questions: How do the parents look? What do they say? What do they do? Further assessment of the parent–newborn relationship can be conducted as care is given during the period of recovery. This is especially important if warning signs (e.g., passive or hostile reactions to newborn, disappointment with sex or appearance of newborn, absence of eye contact, or limited interaction of parents with each other) were noted immediately after birth. The nurse may find it helpful to discuss with the woman's primary health care provider any warning signs that may have been noted.

Siblings often experience interest and excitement when the newborn appears. They can then be encouraged to touch or hold the baby (Fig. 18-26).

Parents usually respond to praise of their newborn. Many need to be reassured that the dusky appearance of the baby's extremities immediately after birth is normal until circulation is well established. If appropriate, the nurse should explain the reason for the moulding of the newborn's head. Information about hospital routine can be communicated. However, it is important for nurses to recognize that the cultural background of the parents may influence expectations of care and handling of their newborn immediately after birth. For example, some traditional Southeast Asians believe that the head should not be touched because it is the most sacred part of a person's body. They also believe that praise of the baby is dangerous because jealous spirits may cause the baby harm or take it away (D'Avanzo, 2008).

Determining a woman's satisfaction with and impressions of her childbirth experience is a critical component in the provision of high-quality maternal–newborn health care that meets the needs of women and families. Reviewing one's childbirth experience with someone who will listen, support, and explain has been found to reduce the degree of postpartum depression experienced by many women during the first week or so after birth.

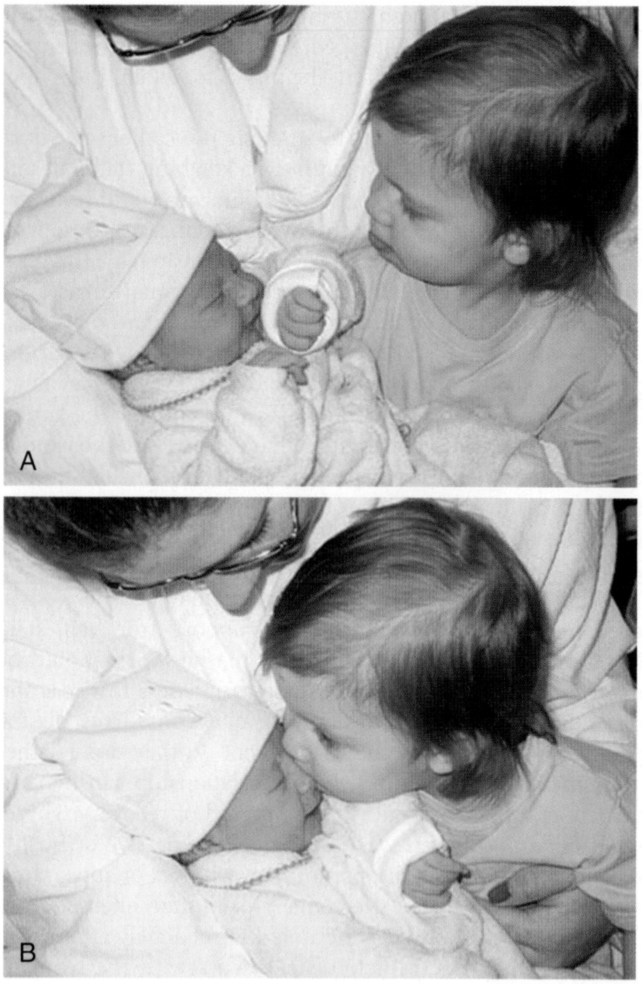

Fig. 18-26 Big sister being introduced to baby brother. **A:** Not sure who this new person is. **B:** A kiss says he is OK. *(Courtesy Rebekah Vogel, Ft. Collins, CO.)*

Key Points

- The onset of labour may be difficult to determine for both nulliparous and multiparous women.
- The familiar environment of the pregnant woman's home is most often the ideal place for a woman during the latent phase of the first stage of labour.
- The nurse assumes much of the responsibility for assessing the progress of labour and keeping the primary health care provider informed about progress in labour and deviations from expected findings.
- Regardless of the actual labour and birth experience, the woman's or couple's perception of the birth experience is most likely to be positive when events and performances are consistent with expectations, especially in terms of the woman maintaining control during labour and birth.
- The woman's level of anxiety may rise when she does not understand what is being said to her about her labour because of the medical terminology used or because of a language barrier.
- Coaching, emotional support, and comfort measures help the woman to use her energy constructively in relaxing and working with the contractions.
- The progress of labour is enhanced when a woman changes her position frequently during the first stage of labour.
- Doulas provide a continuous supportive presence during labour that can have a positive effect on the process of childbirth and its outcome.
- The cultural beliefs and practices of a woman and her significant others, including her partner, can have a profound influence on their approach to labour and birth.
- The quality of the nurse–patient relationship is a factor in the woman's ability to cope with the stressors of the labour process.
- Women with a history of sexual abuse often experience profound stress and anxiety during childbirth.
- Inability to palpate the cervix during vaginal examination indicates that complete effacement and full dilation have occurred and is the only certain, objective sign that the second stage has begun.
- When allowed to respond to the rhythmic nature of the second stage of labour, the woman normally changes body position, bears down spontaneously, and vocalizes (open-glottis pushing) when she perceives the urge to push (Ferguson reflex).
- Women should bear down several times during a contraction using the open-glottis pushing method; sustained closed-glottis pushing should be avoided because oxygen transport to the fetus will be inhibited.
- Objective signs indicate that the placenta has separated and is ready to be expelled; excessive traction (pulling) on the umbilical cord, before the placenta has separated, can result in maternal injury.
- Siblings present for labour and birth need preparation and support for the event.
- Most parents and families enjoy being able to handle, hold, explore, and examine the baby immediately after birth. Skin-to-skin contact between the mother or partner and baby should be encouraged.
- Women should be encouraged to initiate breastfeeding within 30 minutes of birth.
- Nurses should observe progress in the development of parent–child relationships and be alert for warning signs that may appear during the immediate postpartum period.
- Stimulation of the mothers' nipple manually or by the infant's suckling stimulates the release of oxytocin from the maternal posterior pituitary gland. Oxytocin stimulates the uterus to contract and thereby prevents hemorrhage.
- A woman who has just given birth benefits from reviewing her childbirth experience with the nurse who managed her care during the process of labour and birth.

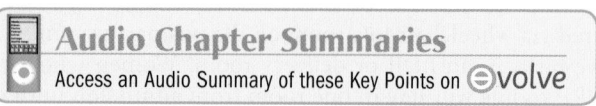

Audio Chapter Summaries
Access an Audio Summary of these Key Points on Evolve

References

American College of Nurse-Midwives. (2008). Providing oral nutrition to women in labour. *Journal of Midwifery and Women's Health, 53*(3), 276–283.

Bashour, H., & Abdulsalam, A. (2005). Syrian women's preferences for birth attendant and birth place. *Birth, 32*(1), 20–25.

Brathwaite, A., & Williams, C. (2004). Childbirth experiences of professional Chinese Canadian women. *Journal of Obstetric, Gynecologic and Neonatal Nursing, 33*(6), 748–755.

Callister, L. C. (2005). What has the literature taught us about culturally competent care of women and children? *MCN: American Journal of Maternal Child Nursing, 30*(6), 380–388.

Canadian Neonatal Resuscitation Program Steering Committee. (2007). *Addendum to the 2006 NRP provider textbook: Recommendations for specific treatment modifications in the Canadian context* (revised March 2007). Retrieved from http://www.cps.ca/NRP/addendum.pdf.

Canadian Nurses Association. (2010). *Position statement: Promoting cultural competence in nursing.* Ottawa, ON: Author. Retrieved from http://www.cna-aiic.ca/CNA/documents/pdf/publications/PS114_Cultural_Competence_2010_e.pdf.

Centers for Disease Control and Prevention. (2010). *2010 guidelines for the prevention of perinatal group B streptococcal disease.* Retrieved from http://www.cdc.gov/groupbstrep/guidelines/guidelines.html.

Cioffi, J. (2004). Caring for women from culturally diverse backgrounds: Midwives' experiences. *Journal of Midwifery and Women's Health, 49*(5), 437–442.

College of Physicians and Surgeons of Ontario. (2004). *Female circumcision, excision and infibulation.* Policy Number #2-01. Retrieved from http://www.cpso.on.ca/uploadedFiles/policies/policies/policyitems/female_circ.pdf.

D'Avanzo, C. E. (2008). *Mosby's pocket guide to cultural health assessment* (4th ed.). St. Louis: Mosby.

Davies, G., et al. (2010). SOGC clinical practice guideline: Obesity in pregnancy. *Journal of Obstetrics and Gynaecology Canada, 32*(2), 165–173. Retrieved from http://www.sogc.org/guidelines/documents/gui239ECPG1002.pdf.

Enkin, M., et al. (2000). *A guide to effective care in pregnancy and childbirth* (3rd ed.). New York: Oxford University Press.

Health Canada. (2000). *Family-centred maternity and newborn care: National guidelines.* Ottawa, ON: Health Canada.

Hobbins, D. (2004). Survivors of childhood sexual abuse: Implications for perinatal nursing. *Journal of Obstetric, Gynecologic and Neonatal Nursing, 33*(4), 485–497.

Hofmeyr, G. (2005). Evidence-based intrapartum care. *Best Practice and Research Clinical Obstetrics and Gynaecology, 19*(1), 103–115.

Ito, M., & Sharts-Hopko, N. (2002). Japanese women's experience of childbirth in the United States. *Health Care for Women International, 23*(6-7), 666–677.

Kattwinkel, J, (Ed.), (2011). *Textbook of neonatal resuscitation* (6th ed.). Elk Grove Village, IL: American Academy of Pediatrics and American Heart Association.

Leduc, D., et al. (2009). Active management of the third stage of labour: Prevention and treatment of postpartum hemorrhage. *Journal of Obstetrics and Gynaecology Canada, 31*(10), 980-993. Retrieved from: http://www.sogc.org/guidelines/documents/gui235CPG0910.pdf.

Liston, R., et al. (2007). Fetal health surveillance: Antepartum and intrapartum consensus guideline. *Journal of Obstetrics and Gynaecology Canada, 29*(9 Suppl 4), s1–s56. Retrieved from http://www.sogc.org/guidelines/documents/gui197CPG0709.pdf.

MacKinnon, K., McIntyre, M., & Quance, M. (2005). The meaning of the nurse's presence during childbirth. *Journal of Obstetric, Gynecologic and Neonatal Nursing, 34*(1), 28–36.

McDonald, S. J., & Middleton, P. (2008). Effect of timing of umbilical cord clamping of term infants on maternal and neonatal outcomes. *Cochrane Database of Systematic Reviews,* Issue 2. Art. No. CD004074. doi: 10.1002/14651858.CD004074.pub2

McGrath, S. K., & Kennell, J. H. (2008). A randomized controlled trial of continuous labour support for middle-class couples: Effect on cesarean delivery rates. *Birth, 35*(2), 92–97.

Miller, M., Fanaroff, A., & Martin, R. (2006). Respiratory disorders: Preterm and term infants. In R. Martin, A. Fanaroff, & M. Walsh (Eds.), *Fanaroff and Martin's neonatal-perinatal medicine: Diseases of the fetus and infant* (8th ed.). Philadelphia: Mosby.

Money, D., et al. (2004). SOGC clinical practice guideline: The prevention of early-onset neonatal group B streptococcal disease. *Journal of Obstetrics and Gynaecology Canada, 26*(9), 826–832. Retrieved from http://www.sogc.org/guidelines/public/149E-CPG-September2004.pdf.

Money, D., et al. (2008). SOGC clinical practice guideline: Guidelines for the management of herpes simplex virus in pregnancy. Retrieved from http://www.sogc.org/guidelines/documents/gui208CPG0806.pdf.

More, O. B. (2010). *Chapter: Management of labour.* Retrieved from http://www.moreob.com.

Public Health Agency of Canada. (2009). *What mothers say: The Canadian maternity experiences survey (Cat: HP5-74/2-2009E).* Ottawa, ON: Government of Canada.

Sampselle, C., et al. (2005). Provider support of spontaneous pushing during the second stage of labour. *Journal of Obstetric, Gynecologic and Neonatal Nursing, 34*(6), 695–702.

Simkin, P., & Klaus, P. (2004). *When survivors give birth.* Seattle, WA: Classic Day.

Simkin, P., & Way, K. (2008). Doulas of North America (DONA) International Position Paper: *The birth doula's contribution to modern maternity care.* Retrieved from http://www.dona.org/publications/position_paper_birth.php.

Simpson, K. (2005). The context and clinical evidence for common nursing practices during labour. *MCN: American Journal of Maternal Child Nursing, 30*(6), 356–363.

Simpson, K., & James, D. (2005). Effects of immediate versus delayed pushing during second-stage labour on fetal well-being: A randomized clinical trial. *Nursing Research, 54*(3), 149–157.

Tucker, S. M., Miller, L. A., & Miller, D. A. (2009). *Pocket guide to fetal monitoring and assessment* (6th ed.). St. Louis: Mosby.

Vain, N. E., et al. (2004). Oropharyngeal and nasopharyngeal suctioning of meconium-stained neonates before delivery of their shoulders: Multicentre, randomized controlled trial. *Lancet, 364*(9434), 597–602.

Yildirim, G., & Beji, N. K. (2008). Effects of pushing techniques in birth on mother and fetus: A randomized study. *Birth, 35*(1), 31–32.

Unit 4

19 Labour and Birth at Risk

Learning Objectives

On completion of this chapter, the reader will be able to:

- Differentiate between preterm birth and low birth weight.
- Identify risk factors for preterm labour and birth.
- Discuss current interventions to prevent preterm labour and birth.
- Discuss the use of tocolytics and antenatal glucocorticoids in preterm labour and birth.
- Evaluate the effects of prescribed bed rest on pregnant women and their families.
- Design a nursing care management plan for women with preterm premature rupture of the membranes.
- Summarize the nursing care management for a trial of labour, induction and augmentation of labour, forceps- and vacuum-assisted birth, Caesarean birth, and vaginal birth after a Caesarean birth.
- Describe the care of a woman experiencing postterm pregnancy.
- Discuss obstetrical emergencies and their appropriate management.

Electronic Resources

Additional information related to the content in Chapter 19 can be found on

evolve the companion Web site at

http://evolve.elsevier.com/Canada/Perry/maternal/

- Examination Review Questions
- Animation—Breech Birth
- Animation—Breech Examination
- Animation—Cord Prolapse
- Animation—Shoulder Dystocia
- Case Study—Postdate Pregnancy
- Case Study—Preterm Labour
- Video—Childbirth (Caesarean)

When complications arise during labour and birth, perinatal morbidity and mortality risks increase. Some complications may be anticipated, especially if the woman is identified as high risk during the antepartum period; others are unexpected or unforeseen. The woman, her family, and the health care team can feel devastated when things go wrong. Perinatal nurses must recognize these feelings if they are to provide effective support. It is crucial for nurses to understand the normal birth process in order to prevent and detect deviations from normal labour and birth and implement nursing measures when complications arise. Optimum care of the labouring woman, the fetus, and the family with complications is possible only when the perinatal nurse and other members of the obstetrical team use their knowledge and skills in a concerted effort to provide care. This chapter focuses on the problems of preterm labour and birth, dystocia, postterm pregnancy, and obstetrical emergencies.

Preterm Labour and Birth

Preterm labour is defined as cervical changes and regular uterine contractions occurring between 20 and 37 weeks of pregnancy. **Preterm birth** is any birth that occurs before the completion of 37 weeks of pregnancy. Preterm labour and preterm birth are the most serious complications of pregnancy because they lead to about 75% of all neonatal deaths. Preterm birth is second only to congenital anomalies as a cause of infant death. In 2008, the overall preterm birth rate for Canada was 7.9% while the rate of births that occur before the completion of 34 weeks of pregnancy was only 1 to 2% (Public Health Agency of Canada [PHAC], 2012; Statistics Canada, 2007).

Preterm Birth Versus Low Birth Weight

Although they have distinctly different meanings, the terms *preterm birth* or *prematurity* and *low birth weight* are often used interchangeably. Preterm birth describes length of gestation (i.e., less than 37 weeks regardless of the weight of the infant), whereas low birth weight describes only weight at the time of birth (i.e., 2500 g or less). Low birth weight is far easier to measure than preterm birth; thus, in many settings and publications, low birth weight has been used as a substitute term for preterm birth. However, preterm birth is a more dangerous health condition for an infant because length of time in the uterus correlates with immaturity of body systems. **Low-birth-weight infants** can be preterm but are not necessarily preterm. Pregnant women who are poorly nourished or have various complications of pregnancy that interfere with uteroplacental perfusion, such as gestational hypertension, may give birth to a baby at term who is low birth weight because of intrauterine growth restriction (IUGR). The number of women having newborns who were considered low birth weight was 7.8% in 2008 (PHAC, 2012).

The incidence of preterm birth in Canada is increasing, with rates higher among socially disadvantaged populations, single women, women with low levels of education, and women who receive late or no prenatal care. The preterm birth rate is higher among women younger than 18 years of age or older than 35 years (Lim, Butt, & Crane, 2011). **Multifetal pregnancy** from infertility treatment also is associated with an increase in preterm births.

Predicting Preterm Labour and Birth

The known risk factors for preterm birth are shown in Box 19-1. The risk factors most commonly associated with preterm labour and birth are a history of preterm birth and multiple gestation (see Critical Thinking Exercise). Using these risk factors, researchers have tried to determine which women might go into labour prematurely. However, no risk-scoring system has resulted in lowering the preterm birth rate in North America because at least 50% of all women who ultimately give birth prematurely have no identifiable risk factors (Martin et al., 2007).

Biochemical Marker

Fetal fibronectin (FFN) is a biochemical marker that may be used to predict who might experience preterm labour. FFN is a glycoprotein produced by the chorionic membranes with the purpose of providing adhesion between the chorion and deciduas. It is usually found in the cervix up to 22 weeks' gestation but not between 24 and 34 weeks unless there is cervical effacement and dilatation related to uterine contractions. During a vaginal examination; the presence of FFN is used to predict the likelihood of preterm labour in women who are at increased risk for this complication, including those with twin gestation (Blackburn, 2007). The value of detection of FFN in the management of women with preterm labour has been in determining the need for hospitalization or transfer to a tertiary centre if the FFN test is positive. If the test is negative, a plan for discharge can be developed with the woman if there are no other risk factors or complications. With a negative test, there is a greater than 95% likelihood that this woman will not go into labour in the next 14 days (Ontario Provincial Maternal–Newborn Advisory Committee [OPMNAC], 2008).

BOX 19-1 Risk Factors for Preterm Labour

Demographic Risks

Age (less than 15 years or more than 35 years)
Low socioeconomic status
Single women
Less than high school education

Biophysical Risks

Previous preterm labour or birth
Uterine anomalies or fibroids; uterine irritability
Cervical insufficiency, trauma, shortened length
Current pregnancy risks:

- Multifetal pregnancy
- Polyhydramnios
- Antepartum bleeding—Placental problems (e.g., placenta previa, abruptio placentae)
- Infections (e.g., pyelonephritis, recurrent urinary tract infections, asymptomatic bacteriuria, bacterial vaginosis, chorioamnionitis)
- Gestational hypertension
- Premature rupture of the membranes
- Fetal anomalies

Behavioural–Psychosocial Risks

Poor nutrition; weight loss or low weight gain
Smoking (more than 10 cigarettes a day)
Substance use (e.g., alcohol; illicit drugs, especially cocaine)
Inadequate prenatal care
Excessive physical activity (heavy physical work, prolonged standing, heavy lifting, young child care)
Excessive lifestyle stressors

(Sources: Gilbert, E. S. [2007]. *Manual of high risk pregnancy and delivery* [4th ed.]. St. Louis: Mosby; Iams, J. D., & Romero, R. [2007]. Preterm birth. In S. G. Gabbe, J. R. Niebyl, & J. L. Simpson [Eds.], *Obstetrics: Normal and problem pregnancies* [5th ed.]. New York: Churchill Livingstone; Varney, H. [2004]. *Varney's textbook for midwives* [4th ed.]. Sudbury, MA: Jones & Bartlett.)

CRITICAL THINKING EXERCISE

Preterm Labour

You are assigned to Yolanda, who is experiencing preterm labour at 28 weeks of gestation. She has a 2-year-old son at home. This is her third admission for preterm labour during this pregnancy. Her primary health care provider had told her she must remain hospitalized on bed rest until she reaches 37 weeks of gestation or until birth of the baby, whichever comes first. She tearfully asks you why she can't be at home on bed rest, who will help care for her son, and how she will manage to keep from going crazy staying in bed that long. How will you respond to her concerns?

1. Evidence—Is there sufficient evidence to draw conclusions about the benefits of bed rest to prevent preterm birth?
2. Assumptions—What assumptions can be made about the following issues?
   a. The impact her history might have on the medical and nursing care she receives during this pregnancy
   b. The pros and cons of home management versus hospital management for the prevention of preterm birth for this woman
   c. Ways to reduce the frustration and boredom that the woman will experience if she is restricted to bed rest for the next several weeks
   d. Resources available to assist with care of her 2-year-old son
3. What implications and priorities for nursing care can be drawn at this time?
4. Does the evidence objectively support your conclusion?
5. Are there alternative perspectives to your conclusion?

evolve Case Study—Preterm Labour

Endocervical Length

Another possible predictor of imminent preterm labour is endocervical length. Some studies have suggested that a shortened cervix precedes preterm labour and can be determined by ultrasound measurement. Women whose cervical length is more than 30 mm before 34 weeks of gestation are less likely to have a preterm birth than women whose cervical length is less than 30 mm (Iams, Romero, & Creasy, 2009). When a woman has a short cervix combined with a positive FFN result, her risk for spontaneous preterm birth is substantially higher than that for women positive for only one marker or none at all (Iams et al., 2009).

Causes of Preterm Labour and Birth

The cause of preterm labour may be unknown and is assumed to be multifactorial (Cunningham et al., 2010) (Box 19-2). **Infection** is thought to be a major etiological factor in some preterm labours, but trials of antibiotic therapy for all women at risk have not resulted in statistically significant reductions in preterm births (Iams et al., 2009). When cervical, bacterial, or urinary tract infections are present, the risk of preterm birth is increased. Thus, early continuous and comprehensive prenatal care, which can detect and treat infection, is essential in dealing with this aspect of preterm birth prevention.

BOX 19-2 Multifactorial Etiology of Preterm Labour and Birth

Maternal Behaviours

Smoking
Substance use (alcohol or illegal drugs)
Poor nutrition
Work/fatigue
Short interpregnancy interval
Sexual activity

Maternal Characteristics

Young or older age
Previous preterm birth
Short stature
Short cervix
Uterine anomalies
Diethylstilbestrol exposure
Prematurely dilated cervix
Low prepregnancy weight
Unmarried
Low socioeconomic status
Victim of intimate partner violence

Other Factors

Inadequate support systems
Stress
Uterine irritability
Multiple gestation
Late or no prenatal care
Preterm premature rupture of membranes
Anemia
Infection
Catecholamine release
Decreased progesterone production
Decidual cell disruption
Prostaglandin synthesis
Cytokine release

Recent evidence has demonstrated a possible link between periodontal infection and preterm labour and birth as a result of increased levels of prostaglandins released by the causative pathogens. Recommendations for all pregnant women include regular dental care before and during pregnancy, oral assessment as part of prenatal health care, and strict oral hygiene measures (e.g., brushing teeth, using dental floss, rinsing with baking soda and water after vomiting) (Wener & Lavigne, 2004).

Not all preterm births can or even should be prevented. Approximately 20 to 30% of all preterm births are indicated (i.e., babies are intentionally delivered prematurely because of pregnancy complications that put the life or health of the fetus or the mother in danger and not because of preterm labour). Another 30 to 40% are preceded by spontaneous rupture of membranes (preterm premature rupture of membranes [PPROM]) followed by labour and are not known to be preventable. Therefore, only about 40 to 50% of preterm births can possibly be prevented and are considered idiopathic preterm births (Alexander, 2007; Hollier, 2005).

Sociodemographic factors such as poverty, low educational level, lack of social support, smoking, little or no prenatal care, intimate partner violence, and stress are thought to contribute to the 50% of the preterm births that may be preventable (Iams et al., 2009). If prenatal care programs are to be effective in reducing the rate of preterm labour and birth, they must address these sociodemographic factors and develop strategies to attract all women to participate, including those at high risk for preterm labour.

Nursing Care Management

Preconception and prenatal care should be accessible to all women. This care should focus on performing ongoing holistic risk assessment, encouraging women to participate in health-promoting activity (e.g., good nutrition, exercise, stress management), and implementing appropriate medical and psychosocial interventions (see Nursing Process box).

Prevention

Prevention strategies that address risk factors associated with preterm labour and birth are less costly in human and financial terms than the high-tech and often lifelong care required by preterm infants and their families. Programs aimed at health promotion and disease prevention that encourage healthy lifestyles for the population in general and women of childbearing age in particular should be developed to prevent preterm labour and birth. One of the most important nursing interventions aimed at preventing preterm birth is the education of pregnant women about the early symptoms of preterm labour so that, if symptoms occur, the woman can be referred promptly to her care provider for more intensive care (Box 19-3) (Fritz & Smith, 2008). Patient education regarding symptoms of regular contractions or cramping between 20 and 37 weeks of gestation should involve informing the woman that these symptoms are not normal discomforts of pregnancy

NURSING PROCESS: PRETERM LABOUR

Assessment

Nursing assessment begins at the time of entry to prenatal care. It is essential that perinatal nurses teach pregnant women how to detect the early symptoms of preterm labour.

History

- Review antenatal record (parity, estimated date of birth, previous preterm pregnancies/births)
- Dental health
- Cervical, bacterial, or urinary tract infections
- Intimate partner violence

Interview

- Symptoms of preterm labour
- Activities that trigger symptoms (e.g., carrying heavy loads, heavy housework)
- Psychosocial and emotional status of the woman
- Impact of treatment on woman and her family

Physical Examination

- Ultrasound examination of cervical length
- Cervical status
- Evidence of rupture of membranes
- Uterine activity
- Fetal heart rate

Review of Results of Laboratory Tests

- Fetal fibronectin (if done)

Nursing Diagnoses

Nursing diagnoses relevant for women at risk for preterm birth include the following:

Lack of knowledge related to

- recognition of preterm labour symptoms

Impaired mobility related to

- prescribed bed rest

Risk for complicated grieving related to

- potential for birth of preterm infant

Planning

A plan of care is developed for each woman to address her particular clinical and nursing problems. The nurse collaborates with the primary health care provider and the woman to provide home or hospital care as appropriate.

Expected outcomes include that the woman will do the following:

- Learn the symptoms of preterm labour and be able to assess herself and her need for intervention
- Follow teaching suggestions and call her primary health care provider if symptoms occur
- Not experience preterm symptoms or, if she does, take appropriate action
- Maintain her pregnancy for at least 37 completed weeks
- Give birth to a healthy, full-term infant

Interventions

Teach woman early recognition of preterm labour symptoms.
Teach woman what to do if symptoms of preterm labour occur.
Support woman at home on bed rest.
Modify home environment for woman's convenience.
Monitor uterine activity.
Provide telephone support.
Administer tocolytics and antenatal glucocorticoids (see discussion later in chapter) as prescribed.
If preterm birth is inevitable, transfer woman to tertiary care centre.

Evaluation

Evaluation of the nursing care for a woman at risk for preterm labour is based on the expected outcomes of care (see Nursing Care Plan).

BOX 19-3 Signs and Symptoms of Preterm Labour

Uterine Activity

Uterine contractions more frequent than every 10 minutes, persisting for 1 hour or more
Uterine contractions painful or painless

Discomfort

Lower abdominal cramping similar to gas pains; may be accompanied by diarrhea
Dull, intermittent low back pain (below the waist)
Painful, menstrual-like cramps
Suprapubic pain or pressure
Pelvic pressure or heaviness
Urinary frequency

Vaginal Discharge

Change in character and amount of usual discharge: thicker (mucoid) or thinner (watery), bloody, brown or colourless, increased amount, odour
Rupture of amniotic membranes

and that contractions or cramping that does not go away, becomes regular in timing, or increases in intensity should prompt the woman to contact her primary health care provider. The Association of Women's Health, Obstetric and Neonatal Nurses (AWHONN) has developed a patient teaching tool to help identify risk factors for preterm labour and can be found at http://www.awhonn.org. Because no one can discriminate between **Braxton Hicks contractions** and the contractions of early preterm labour, Freda and Patterson (2001) suggest that the term *Braxton Hicks contractions* be eliminated from teaching about pregnancy expectations.

Some women will wait hours or days before contacting a health care provider after preterm labour symptoms have begun. Women may ignore the symptoms because of ignorance regarding their significance or a belief that the symptoms are expected during pregnancy. The symptoms may be attributed to other factors such as the flu, incontinence of urine, or working too hard. Some women become more vigilant, waiting to see if the symptoms subside, go away, or become worse. They may take action by seeking advice about

NURSING CARE PLAN ● Preterm Labour

Nursing Diagnosis: Lack of knowledge related to recognition of preterm labour

Expected Outcome

Woman and partner (if applicable) delineate the signs and symptoms of preterm labour.

Nursing Interventions/*Rationales*

Assess what the woman and partner know about abnormal signs and symptoms during pregnancy *to identify areas where knowledge is lacking.*

Discuss signs and symptoms that serve as warning signs of preterm labour *so that the woman or her partner has adequate information to identify problems early.*

Provide written supplemental materials that include a list of warning signs and instructions regarding what to do if any of the listed signs occur *so that the couple can reinforce and review learning and act swiftly and appropriately should a sign occur.*

Discuss and demonstrate how to assess and time the contractions *to provide needed skills to assess the signs of labour.*

Nursing Diagnosis: Risk for maternal/fetal injury related to recurrence of preterm labour

Expected Outcome

Woman demonstrates ability to assess self and fetus for signs of recurring labour; maternal–fetal well-being is maintained.

Nursing Interventions/*Rationales*

Teach the woman and partner how to monitor fetal and uterine contraction activity daily *to provide immediate evidence of a worsening condition.*

Have the woman or partner report rupture of membranes, vaginal bleeding, cramping, pelvic pressure, or low backache to an appropriate health care resource immediately *because such symptoms are signs of labour.*

Have the woman monitor her weight, diet, and fluid intake on a daily basis *to evaluate for potential problems.*

Have the woman use a side-lying position *to enhance placental perfusion.*

Teach the woman signs and symptoms of thrombophlebitis and encourage gentle exercise of lower extremities *because pregnancy and limited activity increase risk for clot formation.*

Inform the woman to abstain from sexual intercourse and nipple stimulation *because such activities may stimulate uterine contractions.*

Teach the woman to practice relaxation techniques *to decrease uterine tone and anxiety and stress.*

Takes tocolytic or other medications per physician's orders *to inhibit uterine contractions.*

Teach the woman and partner about medication adverse effects and have them report any of these medication side effects immediately *to prevent medication-induced complications.*

Have the family arrange for alternative strategies in carrying out the woman's usual roles and functions *to decrease stress and limit her temptations to increase activity.*

If small children are part of the household, encourage the family to make alternative arrangements for child care *to enhance the woman's compliance with bed rest protocol.*

Nursing Diagnosis: Anxiety related to preterm labour and potentially premature neonate

Expected Outcome

Feeling and symptoms of anxiety are reduced.

Nursing Interventions/*Rationales*

Provide a calm, soothing atmosphere and teach the family to provide emotional support *to facilitate coping.*

Encourage communication of fears *to decrease the intensity of emotional response.*

Involve the woman and family in the home management of her condition *to promote a greater sense of control.*

Help the woman identify and use appropriate coping strategies and support systems *to reduce fear and anxiety.*

Explore the use of desensitization strategies such as progressive muscle relaxation, visual imagery, or thought stopping *to reduce fear-related emotions and related physical symptoms.*

Nursing Diagnosis: Deficient diversional activity related to imposed bed rest

Expected Outcome

The woman will communicate diminished feelings of boredom.

Nursing Interventions/*Rationales*

Assist the woman to creatively explore personally meaningful activities that can be pursued from the bed *to ensure selection of activities that have meaning, purpose, and value to the individual.*

Maintain emphasis on personal choices of the woman *to promote control and minimize imposition of routines by others.*

Evaluate what support and system resources are available in the environment *to assist in providing diversional activities.*

Explore ways for the woman to remain an active participant in home management and decision making *to promote her sense of control.*

Engage support of family and friends in carrying out chosen activities and making necessary environmental alterations *to ensure success of relieving boredom.*

Encourage the woman to use the Internet to communicate with other women on bed rest *to obtain support and share feelings.*

Teach the woman about stress management and relaxation techniques *to help manage tension of confinement.*

what to do from family or friends, resting more, increasing fluid intake, taking a bath, or rubbing the back or abdomen. Persistence of symptoms and increasing severity will finally compel women to seek health care. Waiting too long to see a health care provider could result in inevitable preterm birth without the benefit of the administration of antenatal glucocorticoids (i.e., medication given to accelerate fetal lung maturity). (See discussion later on p. 496.) In this event, the neonate is born at higher risk for respiratory distress syndrome and intraventricular hemorrhage. Women who delay seeking care might give birth to an infant in a setting that is not equipped to care for a preterm neonate.

Early Recognition and Diagnosis

Early recognition of preterm labour is essential in order to successfully implement interventions such as **tocolytic** therapy and administration of antenatal glucocorticoids. The diagnosis of preterm labour is based on three major diagnostic criteria:

1. Gestational age between 20 and 37 weeks
2. Uterine activity (contractions)
3. Progressive cervical change (e.g., cervical effacement of 80% or cervical dilation of 2 cm or greater)

If the presence of FFN is used as another diagnostic criterion, a sample of cervical mucus for testing should be obtained before doing an examination for cervical changes because the lubricant used to examine the cervix can reduce the accuracy of the test for FFN.

The pregnant woman at 30 weeks of gestation with an irritable uterus but no documented cervical change is not in preterm labour. Misdiagnosis of preterm labour can lead to inappropriate use of pharmacological agents that can be dangerous to the health of the woman, the fetus, or both (Iams & Romero, 2007).

Lifestyle Modifications

Nurses caring for women with symptoms of preterm labour should question the women about whether they have symptoms when engaged in any of the following activities:

- Sexual activity
- Riding long distances in automobiles, trains, or buses
- Carrying heavy loads, such as laundry, groceries, or a small child
- Standing more than 50% of the time
- Heavy housework
- Climbing stairs
- Hard physical work
- Being unable to stop and rest when tired

If symptoms occur when the woman is engaged in any of these activities, the woman should reflect on what she was doing when the symptoms began and consider stopping those activities until 37 weeks of pregnancy, when preterm birth is no longer a risk. Counselling about lifestyle modifications should be individualized; only women who have symptoms of preterm labour when they are engaged in certain activities need to alter their lifestyles. There are no specific rules for which activities are safe for pregnant women and which are not. For example, sexual activity is not contraindicated during pregnancy. However, if symptoms of preterm labour occur after sexual activity, such activity may need to be curtailed until 37 weeks of gestation.

Bed Rest

Bed rest is a commonly used intervention for the prevention of preterm labour. Although frequently prescribed, bed rest is not a benign intervention, and there is no evidence in the literature to support the efficacy of this intervention in reducing preterm birth rates. It is a form of care of unknown effectiveness (Enkin et al., 2000; Sosa et al., 2004; Sprague et al., 2008). The deleterious effects of bed rest on women are well known (Box 19-4). Symptoms often are not resolved by 6 weeks postpartum (Maloni & Park, 2005).

The partner's constant worry about his or her partner and the baby and increased stress with the assumption of new roles and responsibilities when bed rest is prescribed have also been documented. Bed rest is costly for society; the estimated economic costs are based on lost wages, household help and child care expenses, and hospital costs. Prolongation of pregnancy does not necessarily occur despite the increased costs incurred.

Women on bed rest need support and encouragement, whether they are at home or hospitalized. Nurses can create support groups of hospitalized women on bed rest. Family, friends, and Internet resources, including chat rooms for women on bed rest at home, can be important sources of support for women and reduce the sense of isolation they can feel. Interacting with other women experiencing preterm labour and bed rest has been found to be highly therapeutic.

Health care providers must recognize the difficulty that women face when placed on bed rest. In caring for women

BOX 19-4 Adverse Effects of Bed Rest

Maternal Effects (Physical)
Weight loss; indigestion; loss of appetite
Muscle wasting, weakness; aching muscles
Potential for thrombus formation and thromboembolism
Bone demineralization and calcium loss
Decreased plasma volume and cardiac output
Increased clotting tendency; risk for thrombophlebitis
Alteration in bowel function
Sleep disturbance, fatigue
Prolonged postpartum recovery

Maternal Effects (Psychosocial)
Loss of control associated with role reversals
Dysphoria—Anxiety, depression, hostility, and anger
Guilt associated with difficulty complying with activity restriction and inability to meet role responsibilities
Boredom, loneliness
Emotional lability (mood swings); difficulty concentrating
Increased stress

Effects on Support System
Stress associated with role reversals, increased responsibilities, and disruption of family routines
Financial strain associated with loss of maternal income
Fear and anxiety regarding well-being of the mother and fetus

who try to do too much, nurses can explore with them the realities of their daily lives and work with them to set realistic guidelines for activity limitations that they will follow, thereby avoiding feelings of guilt associated with not being able to do more. This approach can help communicate to women that the nurse empathizes with the impact that bed rest has on their lives and the lives of their families (Sprague, 2004).

Home Care

The home care of the woman at risk for preterm birth is a challenge for the nurse, who must help the woman and her family deal with the many difficulties faced by families in which one member is incapacitated.

Regardless of the frequency of the visits, nursing care for the woman and family in the home demands organization and a sense of just how this family's life has been disrupted by the loss of activity of this essential family member. Families who are anxious about the health status of the mother and baby may need help learning how to organize time and space or restructure family routines so that the pregnant woman can remain a part of family activity while still maintaining bed rest. The nurse should also assist the family members in exploring their feelings about the anxieties of preterm labour and help them share their feelings with each other. The Home Care box and Family-Centred Teaching box detail activities for women on bed rest and for their children.

The woman's environment can be modified for convenience by using tables and storage units around her bed to keep essential items within reach (e.g., telephone, television, radio, CD player, computer with Internet access, snacks, books, magazines, newspapers, and items for hobbies) (Fig. 19-1). Ensuring that the bed or couch is near a window and the bathroom is also helpful. Covering the bed with an egg crate mattress can relieve discomfort. Women often find that preparing a daily schedule of meals, activities, and hygiene and grooming (e.g., shower, dressing in street clothes, applying

HOME CARE

Suggested Activities for Women on Bed Rest

- Set a routine for daily activities (e.g., getting dressed, moving from the bedroom to a "day bed-rest place," having social time, eating meals, self-monitoring fetal and uterine activity).
- Do passive exercises, as allowed.
- Review childbirth education information or have a childbirth class at home or on-line, if this can be arranged.
- Plan menus and make grocery shopping lists.
- Shop by phone or Internet.
- Read books about high-risk pregnancy or other topics.
- Keep a journal of the pregnancy.
- Keep a calendar of your progress.
- Reorganize files, recipes, household budget.
- Update address book.
- Do mending, sewing.
- Listen to audiotapes, watch videos or television.
- Do crossword puzzles, jigsaw puzzles, Sudoku, etc.
- Do craft projects; make something for the baby.
- Put pictures in photo albums.
- Call or e-mail a friend, family member, or support person each day.
- Treat yourself to a facial, manicure, neck massage, or other special treat when you need a lift.

(Sources: Gilbert, E. S. [2007]. *Manual of high risk pregnancy and delivery* [4th ed.]. St. Louis: Mosby; McCann, M. [2003]. *Days in waiting: A guide to surviving bedrest*. St. Paul, MN: deRuyter-Nelson Publications; Moondragon Birthing Services. [2009]. *Moondragon's pregnancy information: Coping with bedrest during pregnancy*. Retrieved from http://www.moondragon.org/pregnancy/bedrestcope.html; Tracy, A. [2001]. *The pregnancy bedrest book: A survival guide for expectant mothers and their families*. New York: Berkley Publishing Group.)

FAMILY-CENTRED TEACHING

Activities for Children of Women on Bed Rest

- Schedule brief play periods throughout the day.
- Keep a few favourite toys in a box or basket close to the bed or couch.
- Read to the child or children.
- Put puzzles together.
- Watch videos, play video games.
- Play cards or board games.
- Colour in colouring books.
- Cut out pictures from magazines and paste on cardboard.
- Play bed basketball with a soft (sponge) ball or rolled-up sock and a trash can or empty laundry basket.

(Sources: McCann, M. [2003]. *Days in waiting: A guide to surviving bed rest*. St. Paul, MN: deRuyter-Nelson Publications; Tracy, A. [2001]. *The pregnancy bedrest book: A survival guide for expectant mothers and their families*. New York: Berkley Publishing Group.)

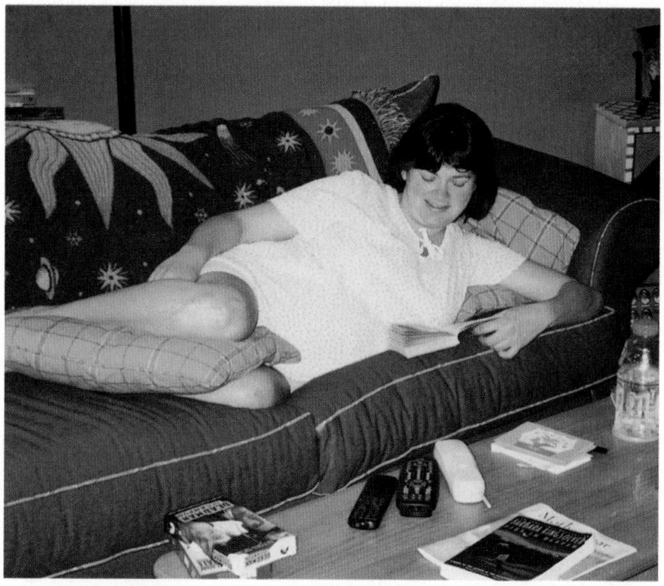

Fig. 19-1 Woman at home on restricted activity for preterm labour prevention. Note how she has arranged her daytime resting area so that needed items are close at hand. *(Courtesy Amy Turner, Cary, NC.)*

makeup) reduces boredom and helps them maintain control and normalcy. Limiting naps, eating smaller but more frequent meals, and performing gentle range-of-motion exercises can help reduce some of the detrimental effects of bed rest. It is essential that the woman and her family recognize that postpartum recovery will be slower as she works to regain strength and stamina.

Home Uterine Activity Monitoring

Home uterine monitoring systems were developed to provide uterine monitoring services in the home for women diagnosed with preterm labour. Nurses are usually an integral part of the systems developed by companies to educate the patients they serve. The use and effectiveness of home uterine activity monitoring (HUAM) continue to be controversial as research has shown that preterm birth rates have not decreased; instead, use of HUAM has led to more visits to birthing suites and increased obstetrical intervention and antepartum costs (Enkin et al., 2000).

Suppression of Uterine Activity

Tocolytics

Should preterm labour occur, women are usually admitted to the hospital for assessment; fetal monitoring; cervical and vaginal cultures; and assessment of cervical status, amniotic fluid leakage, and maternal temperature (an increase can be an early sign of chorioamnionitis). The initiation of tocolytic therapy might be considered at this time; however, once the pregnancy has progressed beyond 34 weeks of gestation, the benefits of prolonging the pregnancy do not justify its risk to the woman.

Tocolytic therapy, the administration of pharmaceutical agents that suppress uterine activity, has been studied since the late 1970s. At first it was thought that tocolytic therapy could prolong a threatened pregnancy indefinitely; research has demonstrated that a gain of 48 hours to several days is the best outcome that can be expected if the woman's cervix is less than 6 cm dilated. Once uterine contractions are suppressed, maintenance therapy may be implemented in an attempt to continue the suppression, or tocolytic treatment can be discontinued and resumed only if uterine contractions begin again. Research findings are complicated by selection of participants, some of whom may not be in preterm labour and would have delivered at term without treatment (Iams et al., 2009).

It is now thought that the best reason to use tocolytics is that they afford the opportunity to begin administering antenatal glucocorticoids to accelerate fetal lung maturity and reduce the severity of sequelae in infants born preterm (Iams & Romero, 2007). Their use also gains time for maternal transport to a facility with a neonatal intensive care unit.

NURSING ALERT To date, there are no medications approved by the Health Protection Branch of Health Canada to arrest preterm labour.

In Canada, the medications most commonly used for this purpose are indomethacin (Indocin), nifedipine (Procardia), and nitroglycerin. These medications are used on an "unlabeled" basis (i.e., medications known to be effective for a specific purpose although not specifically developed and tested for this purpose) (see Medication Guide). There are important contraindications to the use of all tocolytics (Box 19-5). Because these medications have the potential for serious adverse reactions in the mother and fetus, close nursing supervision during treatment is critical (Lehne, 2007) (Box 19-6).

Nifedipine, a calcium channel blocker, is a tocolytic agent that can suppress contractions. It works by inhibiting calcium from entering smooth muscle cells, thus reducing uterine contractions (Fritz & Smith, 2008; Iams & Romero, 2007). The mildness of maternal adverse effects and the ease of oral administration have increased its use. Maternal adverse effects relate primarily to hypotension that occurs with administration. Concerns regarding adverse fetal effects have been reduced. Safety is achieved by following recommended dosages and maintaining maternal blood pressure, thereby preserving

BOX 19-5 Contraindications to Tocolysis

Maternal

Severe pre-eclampsia or eclampsia
Active vaginal bleeding
Intrauterine infection (chorioamnionitis)
Cardiac disease
Medical or obstetrical condition that contraindicates continuation of pregnancy
Dilation greater than 6 cm

Fetal

Estimated gestational age greater than 34 weeks
Fetal death
Lethal fetal anomaly
Acute fetal distress
Chronic intrauterine growth restriction

BOX 19-6 Nursing Care for Women Receiving Tocolytic Therapy

- Explain the purpose and adverse effects of tocolytic therapy to the woman and her family.
- Position woman on her side to enhance placental perfusion and reduce pressure on the cervix.
- Monitor maternal vital signs, including lung sounds and respiratory effort, fetal heart rate and pattern, and labour status according to hospital protocol and professional standards.
- Assess mother and fetus for signs of adverse reactions related to the tocolytic being administered.
- Determine maternal fluid balance by measuring daily weight and intake and output.
- Provide psychosocial support and opportunities for women and family to express feelings and concerns.
- Offer comfort measures as required.
- Encourage diversional activities and relaxation techniques.

MEDICATION GUIDE

Tocolytic Therapy for Preterm Labour

Nifedipine (Adalat)*

Action

Calcium channel blocker; relaxes smooth muscles, including the uterus, by blocking calcium entry

Dosage and Route

Loading dose: 30 mg PO

Maintenance dosage: 10 to 20 mg PO q4–6h

Adverse Reactions

Maternal reactions include transient tachycardia, palpitations, hypotension, dizziness, headache, nervousness, peripheral edema, fatigue, nausea, and facial flushing. Fetal and newborn reactions are rare and are related to maternal hypotension, which would affect uteroplacental perfusion.

Nursing Considerations

Do not use sublingual route. Avoid use or use cautiously with antihypertensives because severe hypotension can result. Assess the woman and fetus according to agency protocol, being alert for adverse reactions.

Indomethacin*

Action

Prostaglandin synthetase inhibitor; relaxes uterine smooth muscle

Dosage and Route

Loading dose: 50 mg rectally or 50 to 100 mg orally; then 25 to 50 mg orally q6h for 48 hours

Adverse Reactions

Maternal reactions include nausea and vomiting, dyspepsia, pyrosis, dizziness, oligohydramnios, and reduced platelet aggregation increasing risk for hemorrhage. Fetal reactions involve constriction of ductus arteriosus progressing to premature closure. Neonatal reactions include bronchopulmonary dysplasia, respiratory distress syndrome, intracranial hemorrhage, necrotizing enterocolitis, and hyperbilirubinemia.

Nursing Considerations

Indomethacin is used if gestational age is less than 32 weeks. Administer for 48 hours or less. Do not use for women with bleeding potential (coagulopathy), peptic ulcer disease, or oligohydramnios. Assess the woman and fetus according to agency policy, being alert for adverse reactions. Determine amniotic fluid volume and function of ductus arteriosus before initiating therapy and within 48 hours of discontinuing therapy; assessment is critical if therapy continues for more than 48 hours. Administer with food or use rectal route to decrease gastrointestinal distress. Monitor for signs of postpartum hemorrhage.

Nitroglycerin*

Action

Vasodilating agent, relaxes vascular smooth muscle

Dosage and Route

Transdermal patch—Applied, and if patient's contractions persist after 1 hour, a second patch is applied. Keep both patches on and remove at 24 hours.

Adverse Reactions

Nitroglycerin can cause severe hypotension; thus, it should be used with caution in people who are volume depleted or who are already hypotensive. It can cause headaches that are usually transient. Tachycardia and postural hypotension can occur.

Nursing Considerations

Monitor vital signs closely to ensure vital signs remain at a normal level. Headaches can be treated with acetaminophen. Transdermal patch should be applied to non-hairy skin.

*Caution: Not approved by Health Canada for preterm labour (unlabeled use).

effective uteroplacental perfusion (Fritz & Smith, 2008; Iams & Romero, 2007).

Indomethacin, a nonsteroidal anti-inflammatory drug (NSAID), has been shown in some trials to suppress preterm labour by blocking the production of prostaglandins. Two prostaglandins are affected, prostacyclin and thromboxane. The decrease in prostacyclin suppresses uterine contractions, and the decrease in thromboxane suppresses platelet aggregation. However, both of these actions increase the risk for postpartum hemorrhage. Although NSAIDs pose the lowest risk for maternal adverse reactions, the severity of fetal adverse effects associated with their use for tocolysis makes them less commonly used than other classes of tocolytic medications. Risk for premature closure of the ductus arteriosus increases if treatment goes beyond 48 hours or if the gestational age of the fetus is 32 or more weeks. Therefore, limiting the use of indomethacin to a short duration of treatment (e.g., 2 to 3 days) or to women at less than 32 weeks of gestation is recommended (Fritz & Smith, 2008; Iams & Romero, 2007).

Nitroglycerin works to dilate blood vessels, predominantly those in venous vascular beds, as well as relax smooth muscles. An adverse effect of nitroglycerin is the decrease in blood pressure that it can cause. Women need to be monitored closely for postural hypotension and blood pressure that is too low to perfuse the fetus. Nitroglycerin appears to decrease the rate of preterm labour, although maternal adverse effects are greater (Smith et al., 2007). One nitroglycerin patch is applied and if contractions still persist after 1 hour, another patch is applied. Both patches should be removed at 24 hours.

Promotion of Fetal Lung Maturity

Antenatal Glucocorticoids

Antenatal glucocorticoids given as intramuscular injections to the mother accelerate fetal lung maturity. In addition, corticosteroid administration has been associated with a decrease in the incidence of neonatal intraventricular hemorrhage and necrotizing enterocolitis. All women between 24 and 34 weeks of gestation who are at risk of preterm delivery within 7 days should be considered candidates for antenatal treatment with a single course of corticosteroids (Crane et al., 2003; Roberts & Dalziel, 2006) unless there is a medical indication for immediate delivery, such as cord prolapse, chorioamnionitis, or abruptio placentae (National Institutes of Health, 2000). The regimen for administration of antenatal glucocorticoids is given in the Medication Guide.

NURSING ALERT Nurses need to know that any woman who is admitted to the hospital 24 to 34 weeks pregnant should receive antenatal glucocorticoids unless she has chorioamnionitis, active tuberculosis, or gastric ulcers. These

MEDICATION GUIDE

Antenatal Glucocorticoid Therapy With Betamethasone, Dexamethasone

Action*

This therapy stimulates fetal lung maturation by promoting release of enzymes that induce production or release of lung surfactant.

Indication

It is used to prevent or reduce the severity of respiratory distress syndrome in preterm infants between 24 and 34 weeks of gestation.

Dosage and Route

Betamethasone: 12 mg IM × 2 doses 24 hours apart
Dexamethasone: 6 mg IM × 4 doses 12 hours apart

Adverse Reactions

Maternal infection is possible, which may worsen maternal condition (diabetes, hypertension).

Nursing Considerations

Give deep intramuscular injection. Assess blood glucose levels and lung sounds. Do not give if woman has infection. Use in women with PPROM is not universally recommended.

IM, intramuscularly; *PPROM*, preterm premature rupture of membranes.
*Note: Health Canada has not approved these medications for this use (i.e., this is an unlabelled use for obstetrics).

FAMILY-CENTRED TEACHING

Impact of Preterm Birth

Parental concern for the well-being of the infant is apparent during and after labour. Perinatal staff need to provide support for the parents; however, false assurance of fetal health must be avoided. For some parents, the reality of the situation is not appreciated until they see their daughter or son in the intensive care unit. For those who experience fetal or neonatal death, the loss intensifies once the stress of labour and childbirth is over.

During the postpartum period, physical care of the mother is similar to that required after any vaginal birth. However, the family will be very anxious about the health and prognosis of the infant. Care of the preterm infant involves not only medical and nursing personnel but also parent participation. The nurse must be aware of the impact that a preterm birth may have on family dynamics. Parents must accept that the infant has special needs, and they must learn to meet those needs before discharge so that they have more realistic expectations when they are at home.

medications require a 24-hour period to become effective, with 48 hours needed for the full benefit; thus, timely administration is essential.

Management of Inevitable Preterm Birth

Labour that has progressed to a cervical dilation of 4 cm is likely to lead to inevitable preterm birth. Preterm births that occur in tertiary care centres lead to better neonatal and maternal outcomes. Therefore, women considered at risk for inevitable preterm birth should be transferred quickly to such a facility to ensure the best possible outcome. The first dose of antenatal corticosteroids should be given before transfer.

Although maternal transport may help to ensure a better health outcome for the mother and the baby, it may have a negative psychosocial impact. Women may be transported to tertiary care centres far from home, making visits by the family difficult and increasing the anxiety levels of both the woman and her family. Attention to the needs of the woman and her family before, during, and after the transport is essential to comprehensive nursing care for these families (see Family-Centred Teaching box).

Preterm Prelabour Rupture of Membranes (PPROM)

Prelabour rupture of membranes (PROM) is the rupture of the amniotic sac and leakage of amniotic fluid before the onset of labour. This can occur after 37 weeks of gestation (term PROM) or before 37 weeks gestation (PPROM). Term PROM occurs in 8% of pregnancies, while PPROM occurs in 2 to 3.5% of pregnancies but accounts for 33% of the cases of preterm birth (Lockwood, 2012). Although infection often precedes PPROM, its etiology remains unknown. Symptoms suggestive of PPROM are complaints of either a sudden gush of fluid or a slow leak of fluid from the vagina.

Infection and umbilical cord compression are serious adverse effects of PPROM, making the diagnosis a major complication of pregnancy. **Chorioamnionitis** is an intra-amniotic infection of the chorion and amnion that is potentially life threatening for the fetus and the woman. Most cases of intrauterine infection respond well to antibiotics, but sepsis can occur and can lead to maternal death. Fetal and neonatal complications from chorioamnionitis include congenital pneumonia, sepsis, and meningitis (Mercer, 2007). Even in the absence of infection, PPROM can precipitate cord prolapse or cause oligohydramnios, leading to cord compression and potentially life-threatening complications for the fetus.

Nursing Care Management: Home Versus Hospital

Since digital cervical examination before birth has been associated with neonatal infection and mortality, examinations should be avoided unless there is suspicion that birth is imminent. If cervical examination is required to determine dilation, a sterile speculum examination is recommended (Mercer, 2007). A visual pool of fluid in the posterior vaginal **fornix**, fluid passing from the cervical os, vaginal pH of greater than 6.0 to 6.5 (tested with nitrazine paper), or a positive **fern test** (microscopic arborized crystals) is used to determine if the discharge is amniotic fluid or urine (see Box 18-2). A woman with this diagnosis may be cared for at home, with more frequent visits to her primary health care provider (see Home Care box). Expectant management will continue as long as

HOME CARE

The Woman With Preterm Prelabour Rupture of Membranes

- Take your temperature and assess pulse every 4 hours when awake.
- Report temperature of more than 38°C.
- Remain on modified bed rest.
- Insert nothing in the vagina.
- Do not engage in sexual activity.
- Assess for uterine contractions.
- Do fetal movement counts daily.
- Do not take tub baths.
- Watch for foul-smelling vaginal discharge.
- Wipe front to back after urinating or having a bowel movement.
- Take antibiotics if prescribed.
- See primary health care provider as scheduled.

there are no signs of infection or concerns about the fetus. Nursing support of the woman and her family is critical at this time. The nurse should encourage expression of feelings and concerns, provide information, and make referrals as needed.

Frequent **biophysical profiles** (BPP) should be performed to determine fetal health status and estimate amniotic fluid volume (AFV) (see Chapter 12). The woman with PPROM also should be taught how to count fetal movements daily because a slowing of fetal movement has been shown to be a precursor to severe fetal compromise. Most women should feel six movements in 2 hours; if they do not, further antenatal testing (nonstress test [NST], BPP, or both) is required. Women should contact their caregivers or hospital as soon as possible (Liston et al., 2007). Antenatal glucocorticoids may be administered if chorioamnionitis is absent (Mercer, 2007).

Vigilance for signs of infection is a major part of the nursing care and patient education after PPROM. The woman must be taught how to keep her genital area clean and that nothing should be introduced into her vagina. Signs of infection (e.g., fever, foul-smelling vaginal discharge, maternal and fetal tachycardia) should be reported immediately to the primary health care provider. Prophylactic antibiotic therapy may be ordered in an effort to improve perinatal outcome by preventing infection (Mercer, 2007). However, in the absence of a positive group B streptococcus culture or signs of chorioamnionitis, the use of prophylactic antibiotics for PROM before labour at term or preterm is not recommended because of the possibility of resistant organisms if neonatal sepsis occurs (Mercer, 2007).

Dystocia

Dystocia is defined as abnormally slow progress of labour; it is caused by various conditions related to the five P's of labour (passenger, passageway, powers, position of the mother, and psychological response) (see Chapter 15). *Dystocia* is defined as greater than 4 hours of less than 0.5 cm per hour of cervical dilation in active labour or greater than 1 hour of active pushing with no descent of the presenting part (Society of Obstetricians and Gynaecologists of Canada [SOGC], 1995). Dystocia is a common reason for Caesarean birth (Gilbert, 2007). Dystocia can be caused by any of the following:

- Hypotonic, uncoordinated, or infrequent uterine contractions or ineffective maternal bearing-down efforts (the powers); the most common cause of dystocia
- Alterations in the pelvic structure (the passage way)
- Fetal causes, including abnormal **presentation** or position, anomalies, excessive size, and number of fetuses (the passenger)
- Maternal position during labour and birth
- Psychological responses of the mother to labour that are related to past experiences, preparation, culture and heritage, and support system

These five factors are interdependent. In assessing the woman for labour dystocia, the nurse must consider the ways in which they interact and influence labour progress. Dystocia should be suspected when there is an alteration in the characteristics of uterine contractions, a lack of progress in the rate of cervical dilation, or a lack of progress in fetal descent and expulsion.

Dysfunctional Labour

Dysfunctional labour is described as abnormal uterine contractions that prevent the normal progress of cervical dilation, effacement (primary powers), or descent (secondary powers). Gilbert (2007) lists several factors that are suspected to increase a woman's risk for uterine dystocia, including the following:

- Body build (e.g., 15 kg or more overweight; short stature)
- Uterine abnormalities (e.g., congenital malformations; overdistension, as with multiple gestation or hydramnios)
- Malpresentations and positions of the fetus
- **Cephalopelvic disproportion** (CPD)
- Overstimulation with **oxytocin**
- Maternal fatigue, dehydration and electrolyte imbalance, and fear
- Inappropriate timing of analgesic or anaesthetic administration

Dysfunction of uterine contractions can be further described as being *hypertonic* or *hypotonic.*

Hypertonic Uterine Dysfunction

The woman experiencing hypertonic uterine dysfunction, or primary dysfunctional labour, may be an anxious first-time mother who is having painful and frequent contractions that are ineffective in causing cervical dilation or effacement to progress. These contractions usually occur in the latent stage (cervical dilation of less than 4 cm) and are usually uncoordinated. The force of the contraction may be in the midsection of the uterus rather than in the fundus; therefore, the uterus is unable to apply downward pressure to push the presenting part against the cervix. The uterus may not relax completely between contractions (Gilbert, 2007).

Therapeutic rest, which is achieved with a warm bath or shower and the administration of analgesics such as morphine or nalbuphine (Nubain) to inhibit uterine contractions, reduce pain, and encourage sleep, is usually prescribed for the management of hypertonic uterine dysfunction (Gilbert, 2007). After a 4- to 6-hour rest, these women are likely to awaken in active labour with a normal uterine contraction pattern.

Hypotonic Uterine Dysfunction

The second and more common type of uterine dysfunction is hypotonic uterine dysfunction, or secondary uterine inertia. The woman initially makes normal progress into the active stage of labour, then the contractions become weak and inefficient or stop altogether (see Fig. 19-4, B). The uterus is easily indented, even at the peak of contractions. Intrauterine pressure during the contraction is insufficient for progress of cervical effacement and dilation (Gilbert, 2007). CPD and malposition are common causes of this type of uterine dysfunction.

Management usually consists of assessing the fetal heart rate (FHR) and pattern, characteristics of amniotic fluid if membranes are ruptured, and maternal well-being. If findings are normal, measures such as ambulation, hydrotherapy, stripping or rupture of membranes, nipple stimulation, and oxytocin infusion can be used to augment labour (see Nursing Care Plan).

Alterations in Pelvic Structure

Pelvic Dystocia

Pelvic dystocia can occur whenever there are contractures of the pelvic diameters that reduce the capacity of the bony pelvis, including the inlet, midpelvis, outlet, or any combination of these planes.

Disproportion of the pelvis is the least common cause of dystocia. Pelvic contractures may be caused by congenital abnormalities, maternal malnutrition, neoplasms, or lower spinal disorders. An immature pelvic size predisposes some adolescent mothers to pelvic dystocia. Pelvic deformities may also be the result of automobile or other accidents or trauma.

An inlet contracture is diagnosed when the diagonal conjugate is less than 11.5 cm. The incidence of face and shoulder presentation is increased. Because these presentations interfere with engagement and fetal descent, the risk of prolapse of the umbilical cord is increased. Inlet contracture is associated with maternal rickets and a flat pelvis. Weak uterine contractions may be noted during the first stage of labour in affected women.

Midplane contracture, the most common cause of pelvic dystocia, is diagnosed when the sum of the interischial spinous and posterior sagittal diameters of the midpelvis is 13.5 cm or less. Fetal descent is arrested (transverse arrest of the fetal head) because the head cannot rotate internally. These infants are usually born by Caesarean, but vacuum-assisted birth has been used safely when the cervix is fully dilated. Midforceps-assisted birth usually is not recommended because of the increased perinatal morbidity associated with this intervention.

Outlet contracture exists when the interischial diameter is 8 cm or less. It rarely occurs in the absence of midplane contracture. Women with outlet contracture have a long, narrow pubic arch and an android pelvis, which causes fetal descent to be arrested (see Table 15-1). Maternal complications include extensive perineal lacerations during vaginal birth because the fetal head is pushed posteriorly.

Soft Tissue Dystocia

Soft tissue dystocia results from obstruction of the birth passage by an anatomical abnormality other than that involving the bony pelvis. The obstruction may result from placenta previa that partially or completely obstructs the internal os of the cervix. Other causes such as leiomyomas (uterine fibroids) in the lower uterine segment, ovarian tumors, and a full bladder or rectum may prevent the fetus from entering the pelvis. Occasionally, cervical edema occurs during labour when the cervix is caught between the presenting part and the symphysis pubis or when the woman begins bearing-down efforts prematurely, inhibiting complete dilation. Sexually transmitted infections (e.g., human papillomavirus) can alter cervical tissue integrity and thus interfere with adequate effacement and dilation.

Bandl's ring, a pathological retraction ring that forms between the upper and lower uterine segments (see Fig. 15-10, C), is associated with prolonged rupture of membranes, protracted labour, and increased risk of **uterine rupture** (Cunningham et al., 2010).

Fetal Causes

Dystocia of fetal origin may be caused by anomalies, excessive fetal size and malpresentation, malposition, or multifetal pregnancy. Complications associated with dystocia of fetal origin include neonatal asphyxia, fetal injuries or fractures, and maternal vaginal lacerations. Although spontaneous vaginal birth is possible in these instances, a low-forceps or vacuum-assisted birth or Caesarean birth often is necessary.

Anomalies

Gross ascites, large tumors, and open neural tube defects such as myelomeningocele and hydrocephalus are fetal anomalies that can cause dystocia. The anomalies affect the relationship of the fetal anatomy to the maternal pelvic capacity, with the result that the fetus is unable to descend through the birth canal.

Cephalopelvic Disproportion

CPD, also called fetopelvic disproportion, is often related to excessive fetal size (i.e., 4000 g or more). When CPD is present, the fetus cannot fit through the maternal pelvis to be born vaginally. Excessive fetal size, or *macrosomia*, is associated with maternal diabetes mellitus, obesity, multiparity, or the large size of one or both parents. If the maternal pelvis is too small, abnormally shaped, or deformed, CPD may be of maternal origin. In this case, the fetus may be of average size or even smaller.

Malposition

The most common fetal malposition is persistent occipitoposterior position (i.e., right occipitoposterior or left occipitoposterior) (see Fig. 15-2), occurring in about 25% of all labours. Labour, especially the second stage, is prolonged; the woman typically complains of severe back pain from the pressure of

NURSING CARE PLAN ● Hypotonic Uterine Dysfunction With Protracted Active Phase

Nursing Diagnosis: Risk for injury to mother or fetus (or both) related to oxytocin augmentation secondary to labour dystocia

Expected Outcomes

Maternal–fetal well-being is maintained; labour progresses, and birth occurs.

Nursing Interventions/*Rationales*

Explain oxytocin protocol to the woman and her labour partner *to allay apprehension and enhance participation.*

Encourage the woman to void before beginning the protocol *to prevent discomfort and remove a barrier to labour progress.*

Apply the electronic fetal monitor per hospital protocol and obtain a 20-minute baseline strip *to ensure adequate assessment of fetal heart rate (FHR) and contractions.*

Administer the oxytocin per physician order using an (IV) infusion pump *to stimulate uterine activity and provide adequate control of the flow rate.*

Regulate the oxytocin per protocol (e.g., advancing the dosage in increments of 1 to 2 mU/min every 30 minutes) *to allow adequate evaluation of the woman's response to stimulation and prevent hyperstimulation and fetal hypoxia.*

Maintain oxytocin dosage and rate when contractions occur every 2 to 3 minutes with a duration of 40 to 90 seconds *to produce effective uterine stimulation without risk of hyperstimulation.*

Monitor maternal vital signs every 30 minutes *to assess for oxytocin-induced hypertension.*

Assess contractility pattern and fetal heart rate and pattern every 15 minutes *to assess uterine activity for possible hypertonicity or ineffective uterine response to oxytocin and to detect evidence of abnormal fetal heart rate pattern.*

Monitor intake and output (limit intake to 1000 mL/8 hr; output should be at least 120 mL/4 hr) *to assess for urinary retention and prevent water intoxication.*

Monitor cervical dilation, effacement, and station *to assess progress of labour.*

If hypertonicity with signs of an atypical or abnormal fetal status are detected, discontinue oxytocin immediately *to arrest the progress of hypertonicity*; turn woman on her side *to increase placental blood flow*; increase primary IV rate to 200 mL/hr (unless signs of water toxicity are present); administer oxygen via nonrebreather face mask *to enhance placental perfusion*; notify primary health care provider; and continuously monitor maternal vital signs and FHR *to provide ongoing assessment of maternal–fetal status.*

Nursing Diagnosis: Acute pain related to increasing frequency, regularity, intensity, and prolonged peak of contractions

Expected Outcome

The woman exhibits signs of increased comfort and coping with pain.

Nursing Interventions/Rationales

Prepare the woman and labour partner for the change in the nature of the contractions once the oxytocin drip is initiated *to prepare them and enable more effective coping.*

Review the use of specific techniques such as conscious relaxation, focused breathing, effleurage, massage, and application of sacral pressure *to increase relaxation, decrease intensity of pain of contractions, and promote use of controlled thought.*

Encourage the mother to change positions frequently (standing, sitting, side-lying, walking) *to decrease pain and enhance progress of labour.*

Provide comfort measures such as frequent mouth care to prevent dry mouth, application of damp cloth to forehead, and changing of damp gown or bed covers *to relieve discomfort of diaphoresis,* and of positioning *to reduce stiffness.*

Encourage conscious relaxation between contractions *to prevent fatigue, which contributes to increased perceptions of pain.*

Consult with the woman and labour partner about analgesics available for use during labour *to provide knowledge to help them make decisions about pain control.*

Nursing Diagnosis: Anxiety related to prolonged labour, increased pain, and fatigue

Expected Outcomes

Woman's anxiety is reduced; woman actively participates in the labour process.

Nursing Interventions/Rationales

Provide ongoing feedback to the woman and partner *to allay anxiety and enhance participation.*

Present care options when possible *to increase feelings of control.*

Continue to provide comfort measures to maintain a posture of support and caring and help the woman *to focus on the labour process.*

Encourage the woman and partner to continue to use mechanisms that promote effective labour (e.g., breathing, activity, positioning) *to keep the woman and partner actively involved in the labour process.*

the fetal head (occiput) pressing against her sacrum. Box 18-7 lists suggested measures to relieve back pain and promote rotation of the fetal occiput to an anterior position, which will facilitate birth (Gilbert, 2007).

Malpresentation

A malpresentation indicates that the fetus is presenting in a position other than vertex. Breech presentation is the most common form of malpresentation, occurring in approximately 3 to 4% of women at term. The four main types of breech presentation are frank breech (thighs flexed, knees extended), complete breech (thighs and knees flexed), and two types of incomplete breech—one in which the knee extends below the buttocks and the other in which the foot extends below the buttocks (Fig. 19-2). Breech presentations are associated with multifetal gestation, preterm birth, fetal and maternal anomalies, hydramnios, and oligohydramnios. Diagnosis is made by abdominal palpation (e.g., Leopold's manoeuvres; see Fig. 18-4) and vaginal examination and usually is confirmed by ultrasound scan (Lanni & Seeds, 2007).

During labour, fetal descent may be slow because the breech is not as good a dilating wedge as the fetal head; the labour itself is usually not prolonged. There is risk of prolapse of the umbilical cord if the membranes rupture in early labour. The aftercoming head can be trapped by an incompletely dilated cervix. The presence of meconium in amniotic fluid is not necessarily a sign of fetal compromise because it results from pressure on the fetal abdominal wall as it traverses the birth canal. The fetal heart tones of infants in a breech position are best heard at or above the maternal umbilicus.

Vaginal birth is accomplished by mechanisms of labour that manipulate the buttocks and lower extremities as they emerge from the birth canal. Piper forceps sometimes are used to deliver the aftercoming head. Late in pregnancy external cephalic **version** (ECV) may be tried to turn the fetus to a vertex presentation.

Although opinions vary, a Caesarean birth is commonly performed when the fetus is estimated to be larger than 3800 g or smaller than 1500 g, if this is a first pregnancy, if labour is ineffective, or if complications occur. Although Caesarean birth reduces the risks to the fetus, the maternal risks are increased. Women whose breech presentation occurs late in pregnancy need to be informed about the options for birth, including the risks associated with each option (Kotaska et al., 2009).

Face and brow presentations are uncommon and are associated with fetal anomalies, pelvic contractures, and CPD. Vaginal birth is possible if the fetus flexes to a vertex presentation, although forceps often are used. Caesarean birth is indicated if the presentation persists, if there is an abnormal FHR and pattern, or if labour stops progressing.

Caesarean birth is usually necessary for a fetus in a shoulder presentation (i.e., the fetus is in a transverse lie), although ECV may be attempted after 36 to 37 weeks of gestation in patients with intact membranes, no CPD, and no placenta previa (Thorp, 2009).

External Cephalic Version

ECV is used to attempt to turn the fetus artificially from a breech or shoulder presentation to a vertex presentation for birth. This is done by a physician. It may be attempted in a labour and birth setting after 36 weeks of gestation. ECV is accomplished by the exertion of gentle, constant pressure on the abdomen (Fig. 19-3). Before it is attempted, ultrasound scanning is done to determine the fetal position; locate the umbilical cord; rule out placenta previa; evaluate the adequacy of the maternal pelvis; and assess the amount of amniotic fluid, fetal age, and presence of any anomalies (Thorp, 2009). A nonstress test (NST) is performed to confirm fetal well-being, or the FHR and pattern are monitored for a period of time (20 minutes). Informed consent needs to be obtained. Contraindications to ECV include any contraindication to labour, uterine anomalies, previous classical Caesarean birth or other previous uterine surgery that would increase the risk of uterine rupture, CPD, antepartum hemorrhage, multifetal gestation, and oligohydramnios (Cunningham et al., 2010; Lanni & Seeds, 2007; MORE[OB], 2010). ECV performed at term to avoid breech birth is a beneficial form of care and may

evolve Animation—Breech Birth

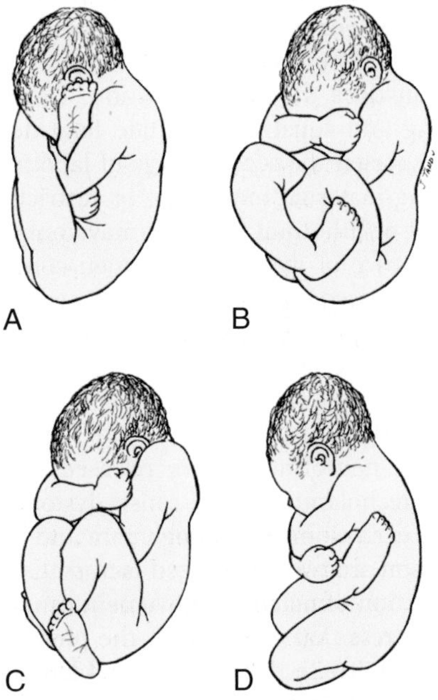

Fig. 19-2 Types of breech presentation. **A:** Frank breech: thighs are flexed on hips; knees are extended. **B:** Complete breech: thighs and knees are flexed. **C:** Incomplete breech: foot extends below the buttocks (footling). **D:** Incomplete breech: knee extends below the buttocks.

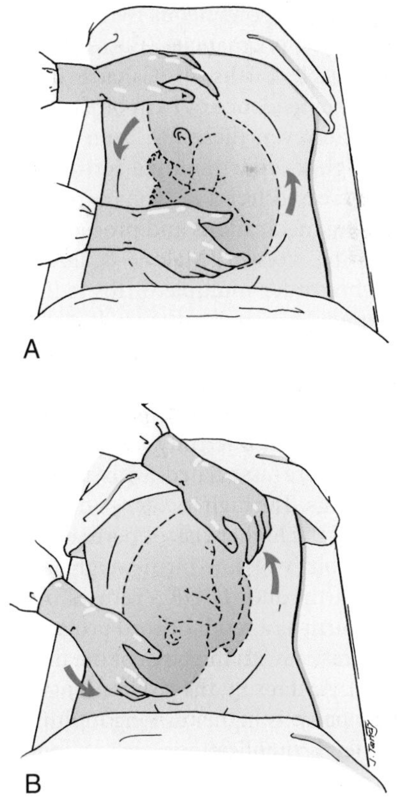

Fig. 19-3 External version of fetus from breech to vertex presentation. This must be achieved without force. **A:** Breech is pushed up out of pelvic inlet while head is pulled toward inlet. **B:** Head is pushed toward inlet while breech is pulled upward.

evolve Animation—Breech Examination

decrease the use of Caesarean section (Enkin et al., 2000; Hutton & Hofmeyr, 2006).

Before and during an attempted ECV, the nurse or physician monitors the FHR and pattern either with the external fetal monitor or by ultrasound scanning, especially for bradycardia and variable decelerations; checks maternal vital signs; and assesses the woman's level of comfort because the procedure may cause discomfort. ECV also poses risks of abruption, abnormal FHR patterns, rupture of membranes, and cord prolapse, and it is not always successful. After the procedure is completed, the nurse needs to continue to monitor maternal vital signs, uterine activity, and FHR pattern and assess for vaginal bleeding until the woman's condition is stable. Women who are Rh negative should receive Rh immune globulin because the manipulation can cause fetomaternal bleeding (Cunningham et al., 2010) (see Medication Guide, p. 548, Chapter 21).

Internal Version

With internal version, the fetus is turned by the care provider, who inserts a hand into the uterus and changes the presentation to cephalic (head) or podalic (foot). Internal version may be used in multifetal pregnancies to deliver the second fetus. The safety of this procedure has not been documented; maternal and fetal injuries are possible. The nurse's role is to monitor the status of the fetus and support the woman.

Multifetal Pregnancy

Multifetal pregnancy is the gestation of twins, triplets, quadruplets, or more infants. Spontaneous twin pregnancy occurs in approximately 1 in 90 pregnancies (Barrett & Bocking, 2000). The rate of multiple births in Canada in 2008 was 3% (PHAC, 2012). The incidence of twin births has been increasing since 1980; however, there has been a decreasing trend in triplet and higher-order multiple births since 1999. It is likely that the increased trend in twins is related to the use of fertility-enhancing medications and procedures and the older age of childbearing women (Malone & D'Alton, 2009). The decrease in higher-order multiple births is likely due to voluntary limits imposed in assisted reproduction centres on the number of embryos transferred and to multifetal pregnancy reduction (Malone & D'Alton, 2009). Women age 35 years and older are more likely than younger women to have a multifetal pregnancy with or without fertility-enhancing medications.

Multiple births are associated with more complications than are single births. The high incidence of fetal and newborn complications and the higher risk of perinatal death stem primarily from the birth of low-birth-weight infants resulting from preterm birth and IUGR. Fetuses may experience **hypoxia** during birth as a result of cord prolapse and the onset of placental separation with the birth of the first fetus (Malone & D'Alton, 2009). As a result, the risk for long-term problems, such as cerebral palsy, is higher among multiple births.

In addition, fetal complications such as congenital anomalies and abnormal presentations can lead to dystocia and an increased incidence of Caesarean birth. For example, in only half of all twin pregnancies do both fetuses present in the vertex presentation, the most favourable presentation for vaginal birth; in one third of pregnancies, one twin may present in the vertex presentation and one in breech.

The health status of the mother may be compromised by an increased risk for hypertension, anemia, and hemorrhage associated with uterine atony, abruptio placentae, and multiple or adherent placentas (Malone & D'Alton, 2009). Duration of the phases and stages of labour may vary from that experienced with singleton births.

Teamwork and planning are essential in the management of childbirth in multiple pregnancies, especially those of the higher-order multiples. The perinatal nurse plays a key role in coordinating the activities of many highly skilled health care providers. Early detection and effective care of maternal, fetal, and newborn complications associated with multiple births are essential to achieving a positive outcome for mothers and babies. Maternal positioning and active support are used to enhance labour progress and placental perfusion. Stimulation of labour with oxytocin, **epidural** anaesthesia, forceps and vacuum assistance, and internal or external cephalic version may be used to accomplish the vaginal birth of twins. Caesarean birth is most likely with higher-order multiple births. Each infant may have its own team of health care providers present at the birth. Emotional support that includes expression of feelings and full explanations of events as they occur and of the status of the mother and the fetuses and newborns is important for reducing the anxiety and stress that the mother and her family can experience. Web sites such as http://www.multiplebirthscanada.org and http://www.tripletconnection.org may be helpful for families having a multiple birth.

Position of the Woman

The functional relationships among the uterine contractions, the fetus, and the mother's pelvis are altered by the maternal position. The position can provide a mechanical advantage or disadvantage to the mechanisms of labour by altering the effects of gravity and the body part relations important to the progress of labour. For example, the hands-and-knees position facilitates rotation from a posterior occiput position more effectively than does the lateral position. Upright positions such as sitting and squatting facilitate fetal descent during pushing and shorten the second stage of labour (Terry et al., 2006). Limiting maternal movement or restricting labour to the recumbent or lithotomy position may compromise progress. The incidence of dystocia in women confined to these positions is increased, resulting in increased need for **augmentation of labour,** the use of forceps, and incidence of vacuum-assisted or Caesarean birth.

Psychological Responses

Hormones and neurotransmitters released in response to stress (e.g., catecholamines) can cause dystocia. Sources of stress vary for each woman, although pain and the absence of a support person are two recognized factors. Confinement to bed and restriction of maternal movement can be a source of psychological stress that compounds the physiological stress caused by immobility in the unmedicated labouring woman. When anxiety is excessive, it can inhibit normal cervical dilation and result in prolonged labour and increased pain perception. Anxiety also causes increased levels of stress-related hormones (e.g., β-endorphin, adrenocorticotropic hormone, cortisol, and epinephrine). These hormones act on the smooth muscles of the uterus; increased levels can cause dystocia by reducing uterine contractility. The continuous supportive presence of a nurse or doula may help to decrease the stress felt by the labouring woman.

Nursing Care Management

Women who have labour dystocia require nursing assessment to ensure maternal and fetal well-being. Electronic fetal monitoring should be used to assess for atypical or abnormal fetal heart rate patterns. Ultrasound scanning can identify potential dysfunctional labour problems related to the fetus (e.g., abnormal fetal position) or maternal pelvis. All of these assessments contribute to accurate identification of potential and actual nursing diagnoses related to dystocia and maternal–fetal compromise (see Nursing Process box).

Abnormal Labour Patterns

Six abnormal labour patterns were identified and classified by Friedman (1989) according to the nature of cervical dilation and fetal descent. The labour patterns seen in normal and abnormal labour are described in Table 19-1 and Fig. 19-4.

Table 19-1 Labour Patterns in Normal and Abnormal Labour

Normal Labour (See Fig. 19-4, A)

1. Dilation: continues
   a. Latent phase: <4 cm and low slope
   b. Active phase: >5 cm or high slope
   c. Deceleration phase: ≥9 cm
2. Descent: active at ≥9 cm dilation

Abnormal Labour (See Fig. 19-4, B)

PATTERN	NULLIPARAS	MULTIPARAS
Prolonged latent phase	>20 hr	>14 hr
Protracted active phase dilation	<1.2 cm/hr	<1.5 cm/hr
Secondary arrest: no change	≥2 hr	≥2 hr
Protracted descent	<1 cm/hr	<2 cm/hr
Arrest of descent	≥1 hr	≥½ hr
Failure of descent	No change during deceleration phase and second stage	
Precipitous labour	>5 cm/hr	10 cm/hr

NURSING PROCESS: DYSTOCIA

Assessment

Risk assessment is a continuous process for the labouring woman.

History

- Review prenatal record.

Interview

- Review findings obtained during initial interview at admission to labour unit.
- Psychological response to labour (anxiety or fear)
- Complication of pregnancy or labour in current or previous pregnancy and labour
- Assess whether the woman and family are fully informed about procedures.

Physical Examination

- Initial and ongoing physical assessment (maternal well-being; status of labour–dilation, effacement, station; fetal well-being–heart rate and pattern, presentation; status of membranes)
- Ultrasound scanning may be done to identify potential dysfunctional labour problems related to the fetus (e.g., abnormal fetal position) or maternal pelvis

Nursing Diagnoses

Nursing diagnoses that might be identified in women experiencing dystocia include the following:

Risk for maternal or fetal injury related to

- interventions implemented for dystocia

Powerlessness related to

- loss of control

Risk for infection related to

- preterm premature rupture of membranes
- operative procedures

Ineffective individual coping related to

- exhaustion
- inadequate support system

Planning

Nurses assume many caregiving roles when labour is complicated. They work collaboratively with other health care providers to provide care relevant to the woman and her family.

Expected outcomes for the woman who is experiencing dystocia include that the woman will do the following:

- Understand the causes and treatment of dysfunctional labour
- Use positive patterns of coping to maintain a positive self-concept
- Express relief of pain
- Experience labour and birth with minimal or no complications, such as infection, injury, or hemorrhage
- Give birth to a healthy infant who has not experienced an abnormal fetal status or birth injury

Interventions

Assist with or implement interventions for dystocia (e.g., positioning, version, augmentation of labour, cervical ripening).
Monitor fetal heart rate during procedures.
Monitor maternal vital signs.
Assess maternal level of comfort during painful procedures.
Provide explanations and support to the woman and her family.

Evaluation

Evaluation of the effectiveness of nursing care for a woman experiencing dystocia is based on the expected outcomes.

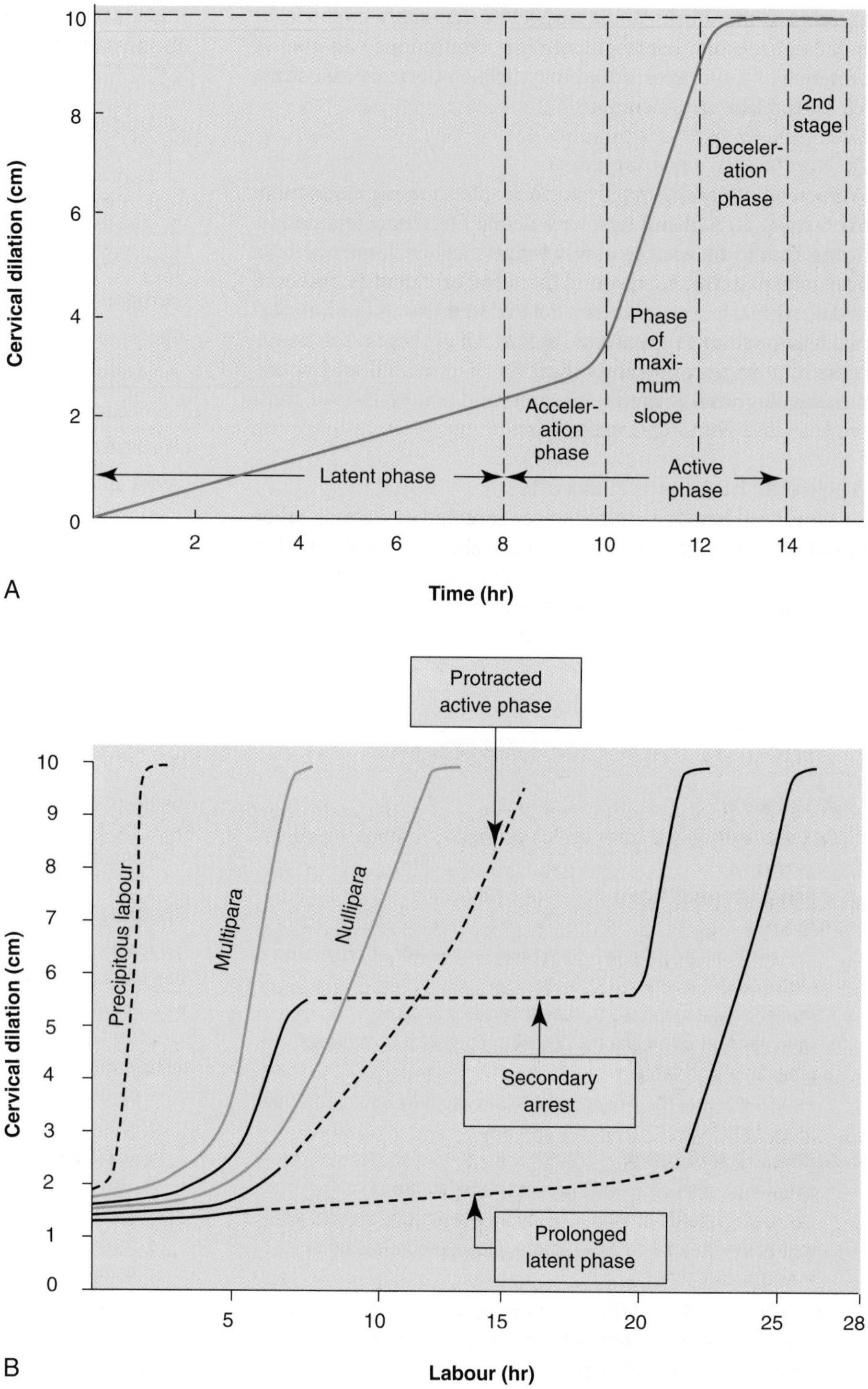

Fig. 19-4 Progress in labour. **A:** Depiction of a normal labour for a primigravida. **B:** Major types of deviation from normal progress of labour may be detected by noting dilation of cervix at various intervals after labour begins. Normal labour progression is depicted by red lines. If a woman exhibits an abnormal labour pattern, as depicted by *broken lines*, the primary health care provider should be notified.

These abnormal patterns may result from a variety of causes that include ineffective uterine contractions, pelvic contractures, CPD, abnormal fetal presentation or position, early use of analgesics, nerve block analgesia or anaesthesia, and anxiety and stress. Progress in either the first or second stage of labour can be protracted (prolonged) or arrested (stopped).

Abnormal progress can be identified by plotting cervical dilation and fetal descent on a labour graph (partogram) at various intervals after the onset of labour and comparing the resulting curve with the expected labour curve for a nulliparous or multiparous labour. Figure 19-4, A is a labour graph illustrating progress in a normal labour for a primigravida. Figure 19-4, B illustrates major types of deviation from the normal progress of labour. If a woman exhibits an abnormal labour pattern, the primary health care provider should be notified.

Health care providers must be careful when diagnosing a labour pattern as prolonged and when intervening on the basis of this diagnosis. Criteria defining the differences between false, latent, and active labour should be established. Evaluation of a woman's labour status in the hospital or unit admission areas is helpful in preventing the premature implementation of labour interventions such as administration of systemic opioid analgesics or induction of epidural analgesia or anaesthesia. If a woman is found to be in false or latent (early) labour, she can be sent home or remain in the admission area until labour becomes active. Women should not be admitted to the labour and birth unit until they are in active labour.

Precipitous Labour

Precipitous labour is defined as labour that lasts less than 3 hours from the onset of contractions to the time of birth. Precipitous labour may result from **hypertonic uterine contractions** that are tetanic in intensity. Maternal and fetal complications can occur as a result. Maternal complications can include uterine rupture, lacerations of the birth canal, and postpartum hemorrhage. Fetal complications can include hypoxia caused by decreased periods of uterine relaxation between contractions and intracranial hemorrhage related to rapid birth (Cunningham et al., 2010).

Women who have experienced precipitate labour often describe feelings of disbelief that their labour began so quickly, alarm that their labour progressed so rapidly, panic about the possibility that they would not make it to the hospital on time to give birth, and, finally, relief when they arrived at the hospital. In addition, women have expressed frustration when nurses would not believe them when they reported their readiness to push.

Trial of Labour

A *trial of labour* (TOL) is the observance of a woman and her fetus for a reasonable period of spontaneous active labour to assess the safety of vaginal birth for both. TOL may be initiated if the mother's pelvis is of questionable size or shape, if she wishes to have a vaginal birth after a previous Caesarean birth, or if the fetus is in an abnormal presentation. It is a form of care likely to be beneficial when implemented after a previous low-segment Caesarean birth. Fetal ultrasound examination may be done before a TOL to estimate fetal weight. The cervix must be ripe (soft and dilatable). During a TOL, the woman is evaluated for the occurrence of active labour, including adequate contractions, engagement and descent of the presenting part, and effacement and dilation of the cervix.

The perinatal nurse assesses maternal vital signs and FHR and pattern and should be alert for signs of potential complications. If complications develop, the nurse is responsible for initiating appropriate actions, including notifying the primary health care provider, and for evaluating and documenting the maternal and fetal responses to the interventions. Supporting and encouraging the woman and her partner and providing information on progress can reduce stress, enhance the labour process, and facilitate a successful outcome.

Postterm Pregnancy, Labour, and Birth

A *postterm* or *postdate pregnancy* is one that extends beyond the end of week 42 of gestation, or more than 294 days from the first day of the last menstrual period. The rate of postterm pregnancies in Canada has decreased, and in 2008 it was 0.62 per 100 live births (PHAC, 2012). Many pregnancies are misdiagnosed as prolonged. This can occur because (1) the pregnancy is inaccurately dated because the woman had an irregular menstrual cycle pattern, (2) an accurate date of the last menstrual period is unknown, or (3) entry into prenatal care was delayed or did not occur. Although the exact cause of postterm pregnancy is still unknown, a possible cause may be deficiency of placental estrogen and continued secretion of progesterone. Low levels of estrogen may result in a decrease in prostaglandin precursors and reduced formation of oxytocin receptors in the myometrium (Gilbert, 2007). A woman who experiences one postterm pregnancy is 50% more likely to experience it again in subsequent pregnancies (Divon, 2007).

Clinical manifestations of postterm pregnancy include maternal weight loss, decreased uterine size (because of decreased amniotic fluid), meconium in the amniotic fluid, and advanced bone maturation of the fetal skeleton with an exceptionally hard fetal skull (Gilbert, 2007).

Maternal and Fetal Risks

Maternal risks are often related to the birth of an excessively large infant. The woman is at increased risk for dysfunctional labour; birth canal trauma, including perineal lacerations and extension of episiotomy during vaginal birth; postpartum hemorrhage; and infection. Interventions such as **induction of labour** with prostaglandins or oxytocin, vacuum- or forceps-assisted birth, and Caesarean birth are more likely to be necessary. The woman also may experience fatigue and psychological reactions such as depression, frustration, and feelings of inadequacy as she passes her estimated date of birth (Gilbert, 2007).

Fetal risks appear to be twofold. The first is the possibility of prolonged labour, **shoulder dystocia,** birth trauma, and asphyxia from macrosomia, which is estimated to occur in approximately 25% of prolonged pregnancies (Divon, 2007). The second risk is the compromising effects on the fetus of an "aging" placenta. Placental function gradually decreases after 37 weeks of gestation. AFV declines to approximately 800 mL by 40 weeks of gestation and to about 400 mL by 42 weeks of gestation. The resulting **oligohydramnios** can lead to fetal hypoxia related to cord compression. If placental insufficiency is present, there is a high likelihood of an abnormal FHR pattern occurring during labour. Neonatal problems may include asphyxia, **meconium aspiration syndrome**, dysmaturity syndrome, hypoglycemia, polycythemia, and respiratory distress (Gilbert, 2007). An infant born after a postterm pregnancy needs to be further assessed for neurological, behavioural, intellectual, or developmental problems.

evolve Case Study—Postdate Pregnancy

Nursing Care Management

The management of postterm pregnancy is still controversial. The induction of labour at 41 to 42 weeks is suggested by some authorities as a means of reducing the rate of Caesarean birth and stillbirth or neonatal death. Others follow a more individualized approach, allowing the pregnancy to proceed to 43 weeks, as long as assessment of fetal well-being using a combination of tests is performed and the results of the tests are normal. Tests are usually performed on a weekly or twice-weekly basis (Divon, 2007).

Antepartum assessments for postterm pregnancy may include daily fetal movement counts, NSTs, AFV assessments, contraction stress tests, biophysical profiles (BPPs), and Doppler flow measurements (see Chapter 12). The woman and her family should be fully informed about the tests, including why they are being performed and the meaning of the results obtained in terms of the health of the mother and fetus.

An amniotic fluid index (AFI) of less than 5 has been associated with an increased risk of Caesarean birth for an abnormal fetal status and an Apgar score of less than 7 at 5 minutes. The BPP may be the best way of gauging fetal well-being because it combines nonstress testing with real-time ultrasound scanning to assess fetal movements, fetal breathing movements, and AFV. Ideally, the AFI should be greater than 8, with at least one pocket of amniotic fluid greater than 2 cm, and amniotic fluid should be present throughout the uterine cavity (Gilbert, 2007).

Cervical checks usually are performed weekly after 40 weeks of gestation to determine whether the condition of the cervix is favourable for induction. Vaginal secretions may be assessed for the amount of fetal fibronectin (FFN); a low concentration may predict increased risk for prolonged pregnancy, but results of studies have thus far been inconclusive (Divon, 2007; Gilbert, 2007).

During the postterm period, the woman should be encouraged to assess fetal activity daily, assess for signs of labour, and keep appointments with her primary health care provider (see Home Care box). The woman and her family should be encouraged to express their feelings about the prolonged pregnancy. They should be helped to realize that feelings of frustration, anger, impatience, and fear are normal. Emotional support is essential for the woman with a postterm pregnancy and her family.

If the woman's cervix is favourable, expectant management can be followed, but labour is usually induced with oxytocin. If the cervix is not favourable, fetal surveillance is continued, and a cervical ripening agent (e.g., prostaglandin E_2) may be administered, followed by oxytocin induction (Gilbert, 2007).

The fetus of a woman with a postterm pregnancy should be monitored electronically for a more accurate assessment of the fetal heart rate and pattern. Inadequate fluid volume leads to compression of the cord, which results in a transient fetal hypoxia that is reflected in variable or prolonged deceleration patterns. If oligohydramnios is present, **amnioinfusion** may be performed to restore AFV, to maintain a cushioning of the cord. However, performing an amnioinfusion prophylactically is likely to be ineffective or harmful (Enkin et al., 2000).

HOME CARE

Postterm Pregnancy

- Perform daily fetal movement counts.
- Assess for signs of labour.
- Call your primary health care provider if your membranes rupture or if you perceive a decrease in or no fetal movement.
- Keep appointments for fetal assessment tests or cervical checks.
- Come to the hospital soon after labour begins.

Although maternal–fetal risks related to amnioinfusion are rare, they can result from infection and overdistension of the uterine cavity with infused fluid and postpartum hemorrhage (Gilbert, 2007).

Induction of Labour

Induction of labour is the chemical or mechanical initiation of uterine contractions before their spontaneous onset for the purpose of bringing about the birth. In 2005, 21.8% of women who gave birth had their labours induced, and this rate has not changed considerably since 1996, when it was 20.7% (PHAC, 2008). Induction of labour is indicated when the risk to the mother, fetus, or both of continuing pregnancy exceeds the risk associated with labour and birth. The most common indication for induction is postdates. See Box 19-7 for situations when induction of labour may be considered.

There is evidence that elective induction increases the risk for Caesarean birth, especially for nulliparous women (Battista & Wing, 2007).

Success rates for induction of labour are higher when the cervix is favourable. A rating system such as the Bishop score (Table 19-2) can be used to evaluate the cervix for inducibility. For example, a score of 9 or more on this 13-point scale indicates that the cervix is soft, anterior, 50% or more effaced, and dilated 2 cm or more and that the presenting part is engaged. Induction of labour is likely to be more successful if the score is 6 or more (Gilbert, 2007).

BOX 19-7 Reasons to Consider Induction of Labour High Priority

- Severe pre-eclampsia
- Significant maternal disease not responding to treatment
- Significant but stable antepartum hemorrhage
- Chorioamnionitis
- Suspected fetal compromise
- Term prelabour rupture of membranes (PROM) with maternal group B streptococcus (GBS) colonization

Other Indications

- Postdates (41+ weeks)
- Diabetes mellitus
- Pre-eclampsia ≥37 weeks
- Alloimmune disease at or near term
- Intrauterine growth restriction
- PROM near or at term (GBS negative)
- Prevention of postterm pregnancy
- Intrauterine death (IUD) in current pregnancy
- Logistical problems (history of fast labour, distance from the hospital)
- IUD in prior pregnancy (to allay anxiety)

Unacceptable Indications

- Suspected fetal macrosomia
- Absence of fetal or maternal indication
- Caregiver or patient convenience

(Reference: MOREOB. [2010]. *Chapter: Induction of labour*. Retrieved from http://www.moreob.com.)

Cervical Ripening Methods

Both chemical and mechanical methods are used to induce labour. Intravenous (IV) oxytocin and amniotomy are the most common methods used in the Canada. Prostaglandins are increasingly used for inducing labour. The most effective protocol (e.g., dosage, frequency) to follow when using prostaglandins continues to be investigated.

Less commonly used methods include nipple stimulation (manual or with a breast pump), the ingestion of castor oil or herbal preparations, a soapsuds enema, stripping of membranes, and acupuncture (Thorp, 2009). Many folk beliefs exist regarding methods to induce labour. These methods include activity (e.g., walking, exercise, strenuous work, sexual intercourse), fasting, and increasing stress (e.g., frightening the woman). It is important for the nurse to know the practices a woman may believe in and follow because some of these methods can be harmful (e.g., strenuous activity).

Chemical Agents

Preparations of prostaglandin E_1 and prostaglandin E_2 can be used before induction to "ripen" (soften and thin) the cervix (see Medication Guide). This treatment usually results in a higher success rate for the induction of labour, lower dosages of oxytocin being given during the induction, and shorter induction times. In some cases women will go into labour after the application of prostaglandin, thereby eliminating the need to administer oxytocin to induce labour. Although prostaglandin E_1 (Misoprostol) is less expensive and more effective than oxytocin or prostaglandin E_2 for inducing labour and birth, it is associated with a higher risk for hyperstimulation of the uterus and should only be used for induction of labour with fetal demise (Crane et al., 2001; Thorp, 2009).

NURSING ALERT Prostaglandin E_1 (Misoprostol) is not approved for induction of labour by the Therapeutic Products Program of Health Canada. Misoprostol ripens the cervix, making it softer and causing it to begin to dilate and efface. A significant adverse effect is tachysystole with a potential for

Table 19-2 Bishop Score

	Score			
	0	1	2	3
Dilation (cm)	Closed	1-2	3-4	≥5
Effacement (%)	0-30	40-50	60-70	≥80
Station (cm)	−3	−2	−1, 0	+1, +2
Cervical consistency	Firm	Medium	Soft	
Cervix position	Posterior	Midposition	Anterior	

MEDICATION GUIDE

Cervical Ripening Using Prostaglandin E_2: Dinoprostone (Cervidil Insert; Prepidil Gel)

Action

Prostaglandin E_2 (PGE_2) ripens the cervix, making it softer and causing it to begin to dilate and efface; it stimulates uterine contractions.

Indications

PGE_2 is used for preinduction cervical ripening (to ripen cervix before oxytocin induction of labour when the Bishop score is 6 or less) and to induce labour or abortion (abortifacient agent).

Dosage and Route

Cervidil: Place Cervidil insert (10 mg dinoprostone gradually released over 12 hours) intravaginally into the posterior fornix. Remove after 12 hours or the onset of labour. Keep insert frozen until ready to use (no rewarming is needed). Uterine contractions usually begin in 5 to 7 hours. Induction may be initiated, if needed, 60 minutes after removal of the insert.

Prepidil: Insert Prepidil gel (2.5-mL syringe containing 0.5 mg of dinoprostone) into the cervical canal just below the internal cervical os or into the posterior fornix; a shield can be used to prevent insertion past the internal os. Repeat gel insertion in 6 hours as needed to a maximum of 1.5 mg in a 24-hour period. Bring gel to room temperature before administration. Do not force the warming process by using a warm water bath or other source of external heat such as microwave. Continue treatment until maximum dosage is administered or until an effective contraction pattern is established (three or more uterine contractions in 10 minutes), cervix ripens (Bishop score of 6 or more), or significant adverse reactions occur. Initiate oxytocin for induction of labour, if needed, within 6 to 12 hours after the last instillation of the gel.

Adverse Reactions

Potential adverse reactions include headache, nausea and vomiting, diarrhea, fever, hypotension, tachysystole (10 or more uterine contractions in 20 minutes with or without alteration of fetal heart rate or pattern), or fetal passage of meconium. Adverse reactions are more common with intracervical administration.

Nursing Considerations

Explain the procedure to the woman and her family. Ensure that an informed consent has been obtained per agency policy. Assess maternal-fetal unit before each insertion and during treatment, following agency protocol for frequency. Assess maternal vital signs and health status, fetal heart rate and pattern, and status of pregnancy, including indications for cervical ripening or induction of labour, signs of labour or impending labour, and the Bishop score. Recognize that an abnormal fetal heart rate pattern; maternal fever, infection, vaginal bleeding, or hypersensitivity; and regular, progressive uterine contractions and history of Caesarean birth or uterine scar contraindicate the use of dinoprostone. Use caution if the woman has a history of asthma; glaucoma; or renal, hepatic, or cardiovascular disorders. Have the woman void before insertion. Assist the woman to maintain a supine position with lateral tilt or a side-lying position for 60 minutes after insertion of gel or for 2 hours after placement of insert. Allow the woman to ambulate after a recommended period of bed rest and observation. Initiate oxytocin for induction of labour within 6 to 12 hours after last instillation of gel or at least 30 to 60 minutes after removal of the insert. Follow agency protocol for induction if ripening has occurred and labour has not begun. Document all assessment findings and administration procedures.

uterine rupture. It should only be used for induction of labour in women with fetal demise (second or third trimester).

Mechanical Methods

Mechanical dilators ripen the cervix by stimulating the release of endogenous prostaglandins from the fetal membranes and maternal decidua. Their use is associated with both beneficial and adverse effects (Enkin et al., 2000). Balloon catheters (e.g., Foley catheter) can be inserted into the intracervical canal to ripen and dilate the cervix and are often used in women attempting a trial of labour following a previous Caesarean birth. Hygroscopic dilators (substances that absorb fluid from surrounding tissues and enlarge) also can be used for cervical ripening. Laminaria tents (natural cervical dilators made from desiccated seaweed) and synthetic dilators containing magnesium sulphate (Lamicel) are inserted into the endocervix without rupturing the membranes. As they absorb fluid, they expand and cause cervical dilation. These dilators are left in place for 6 to 12 hours before being removed to assess cervical dilation. Fresh dilators are inserted if further cervical dilation is necessary. Synthetic dilators swell faster than natural dilators and become larger with less discomfort (Simpson, 2008). Nursing responsibilities for women who have dilators inserted include documentation of the number of dilators and sponges inserted during the procedure and the number removed and assessment for urinary retention, rupture of membranes, uterine tenderness/pain, contractions, vaginal bleeding, and abnormal fetal heart rate (Gilbert, 2007; Simpson, 2008).

Amniotomy

Amniotomy (i.e., artificial rupture of membranes) can be used to induce labour when the condition of the cervix is favourable (ripe) or to augment labour if progress begins to slow. Labour usually begins within 12 hours of the rupture; the duration of labour is decreased by up to 2 hours, especially if combined with oxytocin administration. If amniotomy does not stimulate labour, the resulting prolonged rupture may lead to infection. Other potential risks include umbilical cord prolapse and fetal injury. Once an amniotomy is performed, the woman is committed to giving birth. For this reason, amniotomy often is used in combination with oxytocin induction. Evidence from controlled trials clearly demonstrates that amniotomy combined with oxytocin for induction is more effective than either amniotomy or oxytocin alone and is a beneficial form of care (Enkin et al., 2000).

NURSING ALERT An amniotomy is performed by the primary health care provider (physician or midwife).

Before the procedure, the woman should be told what to expect; she should also be assured that the actual rupture of membranes is painless for her and the fetus, although she may experience some discomfort when the Amnihook is inserted through the vagina and cervix (Box 19-8).

The presenting part of the fetus should be engaged and well applied to the cervix to reduce the risk of cord prolapse. The woman should be free of active infection of the genital tract (e.g., herpes). The membranes are ruptured with an Amnihook and the amniotic fluid is allowed to drain slowly. The fluid is assessed for colour, odour, amount, and consistency (i.e., for the presence or absence of meconium or blood). The time of rupture should be recorded.

BOX 19-8 Procedure: Assisting With Amniotomy

Procedure

Explain to the woman what will be done.
Assess the woman for signs of infection, condition of cervix (e.g., ripeness, dilation), and station of the presenting part.
Assess fetal heart rate before procedure begins, to obtain a baseline reading.
Place several underpads under the woman's buttocks to absorb fluid.
Position the woman on a padded bed pan, fracture pan, or rolled-up towel to elevate her hips as needed.
Assist the health care provider who is performing the procedure by providing sterile gloves and lubricant for the vaginal examination.
Unwrap sterile package containing Amnihook or Allis clamp and pass instrument to the primary health care provider, who inserts it alongside the fingers and then hooks and tears the membranes.
Reassess fetal heart rate and pattern.
Assess colour, consistency, amount, and odour of fluid.
Assess the woman's temperature every 2 hours or per protocol.
Evaluate the woman for signs and symptoms of infection.

Documentation

Record the following:

- Indication for amniotomy
- Time of rupture
- Colour, odour, amount, consistency, and clarity of fluid
- Fetal heart rate and pattern before and after procedure
- Maternal status and how well procedure was tolerated

NURSING ALERT The FHR is assessed before and immediately after the amniotomy to detect any changes (transient tachycardia is common, but bradycardia and variable decelerations are not), which may indicate cord compression or prolapse.

The woman's temperature should be checked at least every 2 hours to rule out possible infection. If her temperature is 38°C or greater, the primary health care provider should be notified. The nurse needs to assess for other signs and symptoms of infection, such as maternal chills, fetal tachycardia, uterine tenderness on palpation, and foul-smelling vaginal drainage (Simpson, 2008). Comfort measures such as frequently changing the woman's underpads and perineal cleansing need to be implemented.

Oxytocin

Oxytocin is a hormone normally produced by the posterior pituitary gland; it stimulates uterine contractions. A synthetic version of this hormone may be used to either induce labour or augment (speed up) a labour that is progressing slowly because of inadequate uterine contractions. See Box 19-9 for indications and contraindications for oxytocin induction or augmentation.

Although certain maternal and fetal conditions are not contraindications to the use of oxytocin to stimulate labour, they do require special caution during its administration. These conditions include the following:

- Multifetal presentation
- Breech presentation
- Presenting part above the pelvic inlet
- Atypical FHR and pattern not requiring emergency birth
- Polyhydramnios
- Grand multiparity
- Previous Caesarean birth
- Maternal cardiac disease; hypertension

Oxytocin use can present hazards to the mother and the fetus. These hazards are primarily dose related; most problems are caused by high doses given rapidly. Maternal hazards include water intoxication and tumultuous labour with tetanic contractions, which may cause premature separation of the placenta, rupture of the uterus, lacerations of the cervix, or postpartum hemorrhage. These complications can lead to infection, hemorrhage, disseminated intravascular coagulation, or fetal compromise.

Tachysystole (more than 5 uterine contractions in a 10-minute period) may reduce the blood flow through the placenta and result in FHR changes (bradycardia, tachycardia, decreased or absent baseline variability, **late decelerations**) that may lead to fetal hypoxia. If the estimated date of birth is inaccurate, physical injury, neonatal hyperbilirubinemia, and prematurity are other hazards.

Informed consent to begin induction or augmentation of labour with oxytocin is the responsibility of the primary health care provider. Oxytocin is administered through a secondary IV line according to agency protocol and professional standards (Fig. 19-5 and Box 19-10). The nurse needs to titrate the oxytocin dose to achieve a regular uterine contraction pattern that causes cervical change. In the past, the aim of induction was to achieve a contraction pattern that simulates the active phase of labour as quickly as possible. However, research on uterine tolerance to oxytocin has now shown that lower physiological doses (e.g., initial dose of 0.5 to 1 mU/min with increments of 1 to 2 mU/min) given over a longer time period are as effective as previous protocols. A recommended dosage increment frequency is every 30 minutes, because 30 to 40 minutes is required for a steady state of oxytocin to be reached and for the full effect of a dosage increment to be reflected in more intense, frequent, and longer contractions. Such an approach reduces the amount of oxytocin required to achieve a spontaneous vaginal birth and decreases the risk for tachysystole, dysfunctional labour, operative vaginal birth, Caesarean birth, abnormal FHR patterns, and other adverse reactions such as water intoxication (Battista & Wing, 2007; Simpson, 2008).

Nursing Considerations

An evidence-informed written protocol for the preparation and administration of oxytocin should be established by the obstetrical department (physicians, midwives, nurses) in each institution. One procedure recommended for a woman who is eligible for induction of labour is discussed in Box 19-10.

BOX 19-9 Indications and Contraindications for Use of Oxytocin for Induction or Augmentation of Labour

The indications for oxytocin induction or augmentation of labour may include but are not limited to the following:

- Suspected fetal jeopardy (e.g., intrauterine growth restriction)
- Inadequate uterine contractions; dystocia
- Prelabour rupture of membranes
- Postterm pregnancy
- Chorioamnionitis
- Maternal medical problems (e.g., woman with severe Rh isoimmunization, inadequately controlled diabetes, chronic renal disease, or chronic pulmonary disease)
- Gestational hypertension (e.g., pre-eclampsia, eclampsia)
- Fetal death
- Multiparous women with history of precipitous labour or who live far from the hospital

The management of stimulation of labour is the same, regardless of indication. Because of the potential dangers associated with the injection of oxytocin in the prenatal and perinatal periods, there are contraindications to its use.

Contraindications to oxytocic stimulation of labour include but are not limited to the following:

- Cephalopelvic disproportion, prolapsed cord, transverse lie
- Abnormal fetal heart rate
- Placenta previa or vasa previa
- Prior classic uterine incision or uterine surgery
- Active genital herpes infection
- Invasive cancer of the cervix

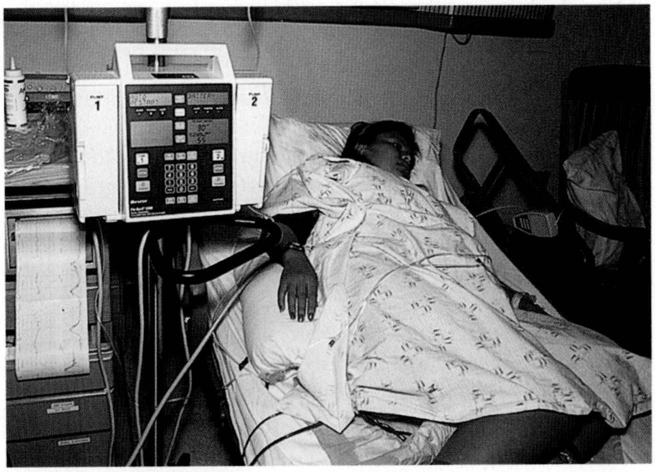

Fig. 19-5 Woman in side-lying position receiving oxytocin. *(Courtesy Michael S. Clement, MD, Mesa, AZ.)*

BOX 19-10 Protocol: Induction of Labour With Oxytocin

Patient/Family Teaching

Explain technique, rationale, and reactions to expect.
- Route and rate for administration of medication
- What "piggyback" is for
- Reasons for use—Induce labour, improve labour
- Importance of continuing labour support techniques, such as the use of the birth ball, rocking chair, etc.
- Reactions to expect concerning the nature of contractions—Intensity of contraction increases more rapidly, holds peak longer, and ends more quickly; contractions will come regularly and more often

Monitoring to anticipate:
- **Maternal**—Blood pressure, pulse, uterine contractions, uterine tone
- **Fetal**—Heart rate, activity/movements

Success to expect—Favourable outcome will depend on inducibility of cervix (e.g., Bishop score of >6)

Keep the woman and support person informed of progress.

Administration

Verify that the primary health care provider has discussed the indication and risks and benefits with the pregnant woman.

Verify that the indication for induction is documented.

Assess status of maternal–fetal unit (contractions, cervical status; monitor fetal heart rate [FHR] for at least 20 minutes before initiation of oxytocin infusion).

Position woman in a comfortable position that allows continuous surveillance of the fetal heart.

Prepare solution and administer with pump delivery system according to prescribed orders.
- Infusion pump and solution are set up (e.g., 20 units/500 mL lactated Ringer's solution or as per hospital protocol).
- Piggyback solution is connected to intravenous line at proximal port (port nearest point of venous insertion).
- Solution with oxytocin is flagged with medication label.
- Begin induction at 1 to 2 mU/min.
- Increase dosage 1 to 2 mU/min at intervals of 30 minutes until an adequate contraction pattern is established.
- Once labour is established, maintain or decrease oxytocin to a rate adequate for continued labour progress.
- Reassess if a dose of 20 mU/min is reached.

Maternal/Fetal Assessments

Monitor blood pressure, pulse, and respirations at least every 4 hours.

Monitor contraction pattern and uterine resting tone each time the FHR is evaluated and before every increment in dosage.

Assess intake and output; limit intravenous intake to 1000 mL/8 hr; output should be 120 mL or more every 4 hours.

Perform vaginal examination for effacement, dilation, and station, as indicated.

Monitor amniotic fluid for character and amount.

Monitor character and amount of bloody show and vaginal bleeding.

Monitor for nausea, vomiting, headache, and hypotension.

Assess fetal status using electronic fetal monitoring; evaluate tracing every 15 minutes during the active phase of labour, every 5 minutes during active pushing, and with each increment in dose.

Assess level of maternal discomfort and pain and the effectiveness of pain management.

Encourage change in position every 20 to 30 minutes; encourage walking or standing, if possible.

Observe emotional responses of the woman and her partner.

Reportable Conditions

Uterine tachysystole (with or without fetal heart rate changes)

Abnormal fetal heart rate and pattern (absent baseline variability and any of the following: [1] recurrent late decelerations, [2] recurrent variable decelerations, [3] bradycardia, and [4] prolonged decelerations)

Suspected uterine rupture

Inadequate uterine response at 20 mU/min

Emergency Measures

Discontinue use of oxytocin per hospital protocol and notify primary care provider immediately:
- Turn woman on her side.
- Give intravenous bolus of at least 500 mL lactated Ringer's solution.
- If there is an indeterminate or abnormal FHR pattern, consider giving the woman oxygen by nonrebreather face mask at 8 to 10 units/min or per protocol or primary health care provider's order.
- Prepare to administer nitroglycerine, if ordered, to decrease uterine activity.
- Continue monitoring fetal heart rate and pattern and uterine activity.

Documentation

Medication—Kind, amount, time of beginning, increasing dosage, maintaining dosage, and discontinuing medication

Reactions of mother and fetus:
- Uterine activity
- Progress of labour
- Fetal heart rate and pattern
- Maternal vital signs
- Nursing interventions and woman's response

Communication with physician or midwife

(Sources: American College of Obstetricians and Gynecologists. [1999/2006]. *Induction of labour*, ACOG Practice Bulletin No 20. Washington, DC: Author; Crane, J., et al. [2001]. SOGC clinical practice guideline: Induction of labour at term. *Journal of Obstetrics and Gynaecology Canada, 23*[8], 717–728. Retrieved from http://www.sogc.org/guidelines/public/107E-CPG-August2001.pdf.; Simpson, K. R. [2008]. *Cervical ripening and induction and augmentation of labour* [3rd ed.]. Washington, DC: Association of Women's Health, Obstetric and Neonatal Nurses.)

NURSING ALERT Oxytocin is decreased or discontinued and the health care provider notified if tachysystole resulting in an abnormal fetal heart rate or pattern occurs. Other nursing interventions, such as administering 10 L oxygen by nonrebreather mask, positioning the woman on her side, and administering an intravenous fluid bolus, are independent nursing interventions and are implemented immediately (see Emergency Measures in Box 19-10). Based on the status of the maternal–fetal unit, the primary health care provider may order the infusion to be restarted once the FHR and uterine activity return to acceptable levels. Depending on the FHR and pattern assessment and the length of time the infusion was discontinued, the oxytocin may be restarted at half the rate that resulted in tachysystole (e.g., discontinued for 10 to 20 minutes) or at the same rate as the initial rate (e.g., discontinued for more than 30 to 40 minutes) (Simpson, 2008) (see Nursing Care Plan: Hypotonic Uterine Dysfunction With Protracted Active Phase).

Augmentation of Labour

Augmentation of labour is the stimulation of uterine contractions after labour has started spontaneously but progress has been unsatisfactory. Augmentation is usually implemented for the management of hypotonic uterine dysfunction resulting in a slowing of labour (protracted active phase). Common augmentation methods include oxytocin infusion, amniotomy, and nipple stimulation. Noninvasive methods such as emptying the bladder, ambulation, position changes, relaxation measures, nourishment, hydration, and hydrotherapy can be attempted before invasive interventions are initiated. The procedures and nursing assessments are similar to those used for oxytocin induction of labour. Protocols for dosage and frequency of increments may vary (e.g., lower dosages may be needed to achieve spontaneous vaginal birth) (Gilbert, 2007; Simpson, 2008).

Some physicians advocate active management of labour in a primigravid woman (i.e., the augmentation of labour to establish efficient labour with aggressive use of oxytocin so that the woman gives birth within 12 hours of admission to the labour unit). The woman should be admitted only when labour is established (i.e., painful contractions, spontaneous rupture of membranes, complete effacement) (Kilpatrick & Garrison, 2007). Advocates of active management believe that intervening early (as soon as a nulliparous labour is not progressing at least 1 cm/hr) with amniotomy and the use of higher pharmacological oxytocin doses administered at frequent increment intervals (e.g., a starting dose of 6 mU/min with increases of 6 mU/min every 15 minutes to a maximum dosage of 40 mU/min) shortens labour and is associated with a lower incidence of Caesarean birth (Battista & Wing, 2007; Simpson, 2008). Active management of labour continues to be under study in North America to determine its effectiveness and its impact on perinatal morbidity and mortality rates. Thus far, results have been disappointing, especially in terms of reducing the rate of Caesarean births. The disappointing results have been attributed in part to a greater than one-to-one nurse/patient ratio and the high rate of epidural anaesthesia. It is considered to be a form of care of unknown effectiveness (Enkin et al., 2000; Gilbert, 2007).

Assisted and Operative Births

Forceps-Assisted Birth

A forceps-assisted vaginal birth is one in which an instrument with two curved blades is used to assist in the birth of the fetal head. The cephalic-like curve of the forceps commonly used is similar to the shape of the fetal head; a pelvic curve to the blades conforms to the curve of the pelvic axis. The blades are joined by a groove arrangement and prevent the forceps from compressing the fetal skull. Maternal indications for forceps-assisted birth include a maternal disease state that inhibits pushing efforts (e.g., cardiac disease) or the need to shorten the second stage.

Fetal indications include certain abnormal presentations, arrest of rotation, an abnormal fetal heart rate or pattern that necessitates birth, and delivery of an aftercoming head in a breech presentation. The use of forceps during childbirth has been decreasing; in 2001, the forcep-assisted delivery rate was 6.8% (Health Canada, 2003).

There are various definitions of forceps applications. Outlet forceps are used when the fetal scalp is visible on the perineum without manually separating the labia. Outlet forceps are used to shorten the second stage of labour (Fig. 19-6). *Low forceps* refers to the application of forceps to a fetal head that is at least at a +2 cm station. *Midforceps* is the application of forceps to the fetal head that is engaged (no higher than station 0) but above the +2 cm station. Midforcep-assisted birth is rare in Canada. In no instances should the forceps be applied to an unengaged presenting part.

Nursing Considerations

Prerequisites for the use of forceps must be met in order for the use to be successful (Box 19-11). The nurse will obtain the type of forceps requested by the physician (Fig. 19-7). The nurse may explain to the mother that the forceps blades fit like two tablespoons around an egg, with the blades coming over the baby's ears.

NURSING ALERT Because compression of the cord between the fetal head and the forceps causes a drop in FHR, the fetal heart rate and pattern are checked, reported, and recorded

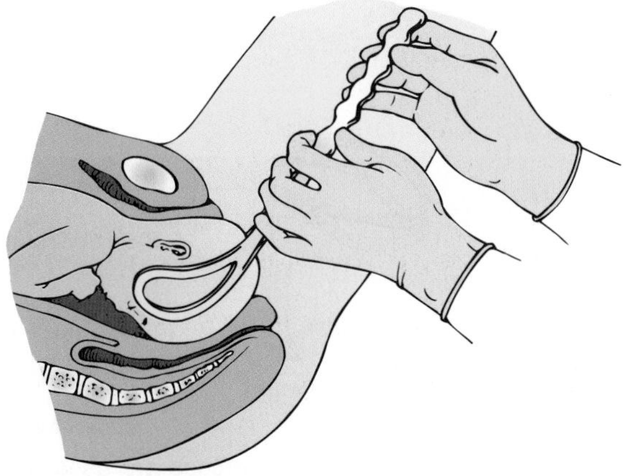

Fig. 19-6 Outlet forceps-assisted extraction of the head.

BOX 19-11 Prerequisites for Successful Forceps- or Vacuum-Assisted Birth

- Informed consent should be obtained by the physician before the procedure.
- The woman's cervix must be fully dilated to avoid lacerations and hemorrhage.
- The bladder should be empty.
- The vertex presenting part must be engaged and descended into a low station.
- Membranes must be ruptured so that the position of the fetal head can be determined and the forceps can firmly grasp the head during birth.
- Adequate maternal analgesia and appropriate support personnel need to be available.
- Absence of fetal conditions (i.e., bleeding disorders)
- Exact position of the head known
- Physician knowledge of the instruments, their use, and the complications that can arise
- Ongoing fetal and maternal assessment
- The maternal pelvis should be assessed and fetal weight estimated by the physician to determine adequacy for delivery.

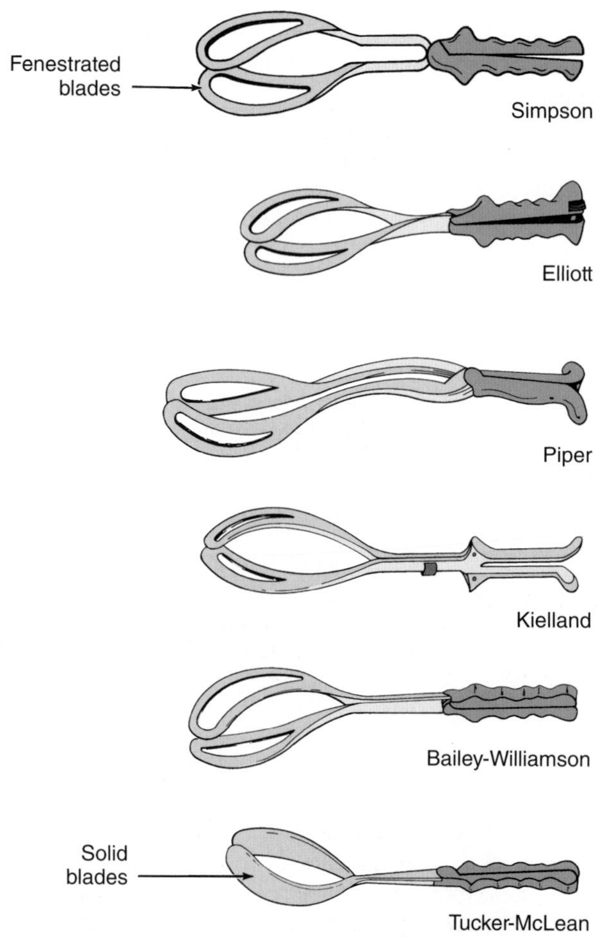

Fig. 19-7 Types of forceps. Piper forceps are used to assist delivery of the head in a breech birth.

before and after forceps are applied. If a decrease in FHR occurs, the physician can remove and reapply the forceps. Ordinarily, traction is applied during contractions.

After the birth, the mother should be assessed for vaginal and cervical lacerations (e.g., bleeding that occurs even with a contracted uterus); urine retention, which may result from bladder injuries or urethral injuries; and hematoma formation in the pelvic soft tissues, which may result from blood vessel damage. The infant should be assessed for bruising or abrasions at the site of the blade applications, facial palsy resulting from pressure of the blades on the facial nerve (cranial nerve VII), and subdural hematoma. Newborn and postpartum caregivers should be told that the birth was forceps assisted.

Vacuum-Assisted Birth

Vacuum-assisted birth, or vacuum extraction, is a birth method involving the attachment of a vacuum cup to the fetal head, using negative pressure to assist in the birth of the head. Indications for use are similar to those for outlet forceps. When an operative vaginal birth is required, vacuum assistance is preferred over forceps assistance (Cunningham et al., 2010).

When the birth is to be vacuum assisted, the woman is prepared for a vaginal birth in the lithotomy position to allow for sufficient traction. The cup is applied to the fetal head, and a caput develops inside the cup as the pressure is initiated (Fig. 19-8). Traction is applied by the physician to facilitate descent of the fetal head, and the woman is encouraged to push as suction is applied. The vacuum cup is released and removed after birth of the head. If vacuum extraction is not successful, a forceps-assisted or Caesarean birth is performed.

Risks to the newborn include **cephalhematoma**, scalp lacerations, and subdural hematoma. Fetal complications can be reduced by adhering strictly to the manufacturer's recommendations for method of application, degree of suction, and duration of application. Maternal complications are uncommon but can include perineal, vaginal, and cervical lacerations and soft tissue hematomas.

Nursing Considerations

The nurse's role for the woman who has a vacuum-assisted birth is one of support person and educator. The nurse can prepare the woman for birth and encourage her to remain active in the birth process by pushing during contractions. The FHR should be assessed frequently during the procedure. After birth, the newborn should be observed for signs of trauma at the application site and for cerebral irritation (e.g., poor sucking or listlessness). Documentation includes the number of applications, any "pop-offs," the number of pulls, and the maximum amount of suction used.

The newborn may be at risk for infection at the application site, hyperbilirubinemia and neonatal jaundice as bruising, a cephalhematoma, or subdural hematoma. Perinatal nurses should measure the head circumference following birth to monitor for subdural hematoma. The parents may need to be reassured that the caput succedaneum will begin to disappear in a few hours. Neonatal caregivers should be told that the birth was vacuum assisted.

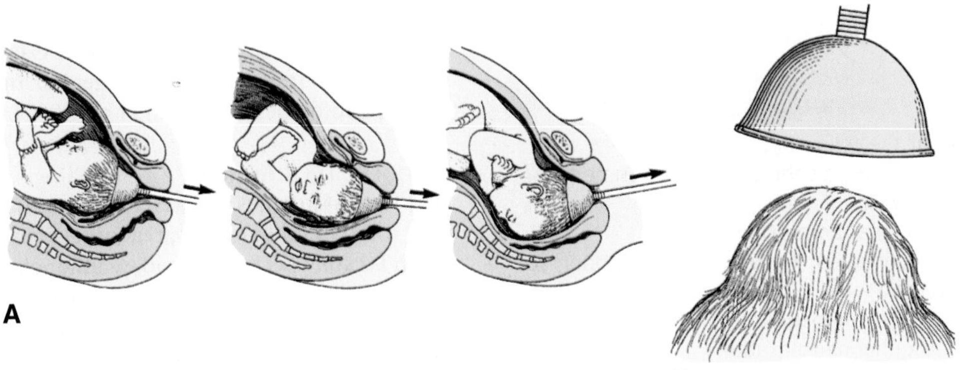

Fig. 19-8 Use of vacuum extraction to rotate fetal head and assist with descent. A: *Arrow* indicates direction of traction on the vacuum cup. B: Caput succedaneum formed by the vacuum cup.

Caesarean Birth

Caesarean birth is the birth of a fetus through a transabdominal incision of the uterus (Fig. 19-9). The purpose of Caesarean birth is to preserve the life or health of the mother, her fetus, or both; it may be the best choice when there is evidence of maternal or fetal complications. Incisions are made into the lower uterine segment rather than into the muscular body of the uterus and thus promote more effective healing. Since the advent of modern surgical methods and care and the use of antibiotics, maternal and fetal morbidity and mortality rates have decreased. Despite these advances, Caesarean birth still poses threats to the health of both the mother and her infant.

The incidence of Caesarean births increased from 17.6% in 1993 to 27.8 in 2009-2010 (Canadian Institute for Health Information [CIHI], 2007; PHAC, 2012). Factors cited in this increase include the increase in primary elective Caesarean births and a decline in the rate of vaginal birth after Caesarean **(VBAC)** (Martin et al., 2007). This decline may be the result of risks of VBAC (e.g., uterine rupture), legal pressures, conservative practice guidelines, and debate over the relative benefits and risks of Caesarean versus vaginal route for births.

Approaches for the management of labour and birth to reduce the rate of Caesarean births while increasing the rate of VBACs are presented in Box 19-12. These approaches involve the combined efforts of health care providers and pregnant women and their families. The labour management approach that most consistently reduces the risk for a Caesarean birth outcome is continuous, early-onset support of the labouring woman that is provided by another woman (e.g., doula, relative, friend, nurse, or midwife). When this woman is not a member of the labour unit staff and is thus able to spend all of her time providing physical and emotional support, the risk for Caesarean birth is further reduced (Hodnett et al., 2007).

The type of nursing care given also may influence the rate of Caesarean births. A labour management approach that uses one-to-one support and emphasizes ambulation, maternal position changes, relaxation measures, oral fluids and nutrition, hydrotherapy, and nonpharmacological pain relief can facilitate the progress of labour and reduce the incidence of dystocia.

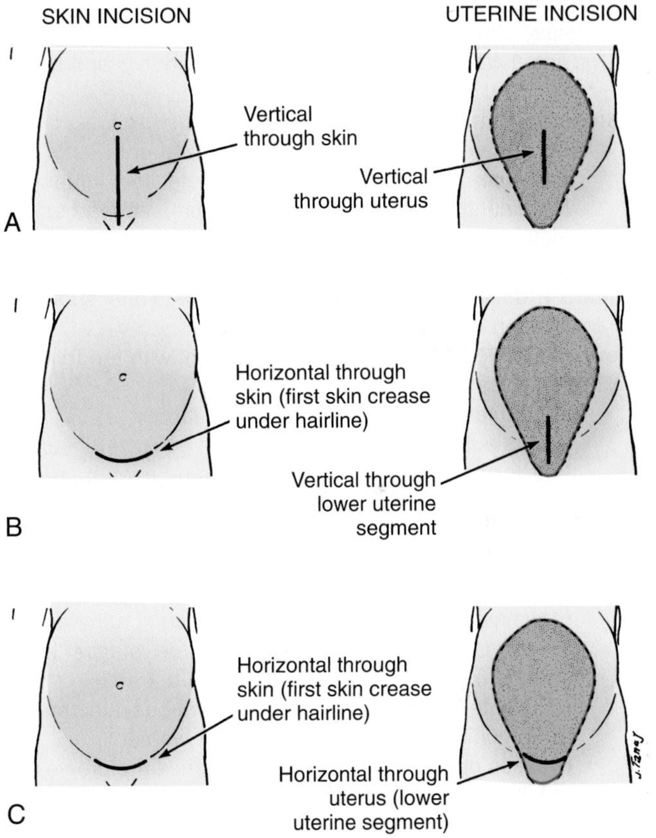

Fig. 19-9 Caesarean birth: skin and uterine incisions. A: Classic: vertical incisions of skin and uterus. B: Low cervical: horizontal incision of skin; vertical incision of uterus. C: Low cervical: horizontal incisions of skin and uterus.

Indications

There are few absolute indications for a Caesarean birth. Most are performed primarily for the benefit of the fetus. The indications most closely associated with Caesarean births include a consistently abnormal fetal heart rate pattern, CPD, malpresentations such as breech or shoulder, placental abnormalities (previa, abruptio), umbilical cord prolapse,

BOX 19-12 Selected Measures to Reduce Caesarean Birth Rate and Increase Rate of Vaginal Births After Caesarean

Educate women about the following:
- Advantages and safety of the home environment for early or latent labour
- Indicators for hospital admission
- Management techniques to use during labour to enhance progress
- Nonpharmacological measures to reduce pain and discomfort and enhance relaxation
- Safety and effectiveness of TOL and VBAC

Establish admission criteria for women in labour to:
- Distinguish clinical manifestations for false labour, latent/early labour, and active labour.
- Conduct admission assessments in a separate admissions area.
- Send women in false or early/latent labour home or keep them in the admissions area.
- Admit women in active labour to the labour and birth unit.

Use appropriate assessment techniques to:
- Determine status of the maternal–fetal unit.
- Establish an individualized rationale for initiating labour interventions such as epidural anaesthesia, induction/augmentation, amniotomy, and Caesarean birth.

Initiate a doula program that provides one-to-one support for women in labour.

Develop a philosophy of labour management with the following features:
- Schedules admission during active labour
- Avoids automatic interventions such as routine induction for spontaneous rupture of membranes at term or postterm pregnancy and Caesarean birth for breech presentation, twin gestation, genital herpes (unless active), or failure to progress
- Relies on assessment findings reflective of the status of the maternal–fetal unit rather than strict adherence to set ranges for the duration of the stages and phases of labour
- Uses intermittent rather than continuous electronic fetal monitoring of low-risk pregnant women
- Focuses on measures known to enhance the progress of labour, such as upright positions, frequent position changes, ambulation, oral nutrition and hydration, relaxation techniques, and hydrotherapy
- Emphasizes nonpharmacological measures to relieve pain
- Establishes criteria for elective Caesarean birth and TOL
- Encourages women who have had a previous Caesarean birth to participate in a TOL in order to attempt a vaginal birth

TOL, trial of labour; *VBAC*, vaginal birth after Caesarean.

dysfunctional labour pattern, and multiple gestation. Medical factors most closely associated with Caesarean birth include hypertensive disorders, active genital herpes, positive HIV status, and diabetes (Martin et al., 2007).

Surgical Techniques

The two main types of Caesarean operation are the classic and the lower-segment Caesarean incisions. Classic Caesarean birth is rarely performed today, although it may be used when rapid birth is necessary and in some cases of shoulder presentation, multiple gestation, and placenta previa. The incision is made vertically into the upper body of the uterus (see Fig. 19-9, A). Because the procedure is associated with a higher incidence of blood loss, pain after birth, infection, and uterine rupture in subsequent pregnancies than is lower-segment Caesarean birth, labour and vaginal birth after a classic Caesarean are contraindicated.

Lower-segment Caesarean birth can be achieved through a vertical or transverse incision into the uterus (see Fig. 19-9, B and C). The transverse incision is more popular because it is easier to perform, is associated with less blood loss and fewer postoperative infections, and is less likely to rupture in subsequent pregnancies (Cunningham et al., 2010).

Complications and Risks

Caesarean births are not without risk of complications for both the mother and fetus. Maternal complications include aspiration; pulmonary embolism; wound infection; wound dehiscence; thrombophlebitis; hemorrhage; urinary tract infection; injuries to bladder, ureters, or bowel; and complications related to anaesthesia. The fetus may be born prematurely if gestational age has not been accurately determined; fetal injuries can occur during the surgery (Landon, 2007).

Caesarean on Demand

The increase in Caesarean birth rates has become more complex as women request Caesarean births for reasons other than medical, obstetrical, or fetal indications. These reasons include the belief that the surgery will prevent future problems with pelvic support or sexual dysfunction and the convenience of planning a date when the father of the baby or support person is available. Some multiparous women may request a Caesarean after a previous traumatic vaginal birth caused by physical injury or psychological trauma (Gardner, 2003). The Society of Obstetricians and Gynaecologists of Canada (SOGC) does not promote Caesarean on demand and promotes natural childbirth but believes that the final decision as to the safest route for childbirth rests with the woman and her health care provider (SOGC, 2004). It is essential that women be fully informed about the risks and benefits of Caesarean birth when they consider requesting elective Caesarean birth.

Forced Caesarean Birth

A woman's refusal to undergo Caesarean birth for fetal reasons is often described as a maternal–fetal conflict. Health care providers are ethically obliged to protect the well-being of both the mother and the fetus; a decision for one affects the other. If a woman refuses a Caesarean birth that is recommended because of fetal jeopardy, health care providers must make every effort to find out why she is refusing and provide clear information to ensure that she is making an informed decision. If the woman continues to refuse surgery, the health care providers must decide if it is ethical to get a court order for the surgery; however, every effort should be made to avoid this legal step.

Scheduled Caesarean Birth

Caesarean birth is scheduled or planned if labour and vaginal birth is contraindicated (e.g., complete placenta previa, active genital herpes), if birth is necessary but labour is not inducible (e.g., hypertensive states that cause a poor intrauterine environment that threatens the fetus), or if this has been decided on by the physician and the woman (e.g., a repeat or elective Caesarean birth).

Women who are scheduled to have a Caesarean birth have time to prepare for it psychologically. However, the psychological responses of these women may vary. Those having a repeat Caesarean birth can have disturbing memories of the conditions preceding the initial surgical birth and their experiences in the postoperative recovery period. They can be concerned about the added burden of caring for an infant and perhaps other children while recovering from a surgical operation. Others can feel glad to have been relieved of the uncertainty about the date and time of birth and to be free from the pain of labour.

Unplanned Caesarean Birth

The psychosocial outcomes of unplanned or emergency Caesarean birth are usually more pronounced and negative in nature than the outcomes associated with a scheduled or planned Caesarean birth. Women and their families experience abrupt changes in their expectations for birth, postpartum care, and the care of the new baby at home. This may be a traumatic experience for all.

The woman usually approaches the procedure tired and discouraged after an ineffective and difficult labour. Fear can predominate as she worries about her own safety and well-being and that of her fetus. Because preoperative procedures must be done quickly and competently, the time available for explanation of the procedures and operation is often short. Maternal and family anxiety levels are high at this time, so much of what is said may be forgotten or misunderstood. These women need much supportive care.

After surgery, time must be spent reviewing the events preceding the operation and the operation itself to ensure that the woman understands what has happened and that gaps in her recollections are filled. This approach will help create more realistic memories of the childbirth experience, thereby having a more positive influence on future pregnancies and labours.

Prenatal Preparation

Whether a Caesarean birth is planned (scheduled) or unplanned (emergency or determined to be necessary during labour), the loss of the experience of giving birth to an infant in the traditional manner may have a negative effect on a woman's self-concept. She may feel frustration at losing control, disappointment, anger, and loss of self-esteem. These feelings are related to a change in body image and perceived inability to give birth as she had expected and hoped. Often women experience a delay in the ability to interact with their newborn after a Caesarean birth. They are less likely to breastfeed and may even have difficulty expressing positive feelings about their newborns for some time after birth. They often are less satisfied with their childbirth experience and report more fatigue and poor physical functioning during the first few weeks after discharge.

Success at mothering and in the recovery process can do much to restore the self-esteem of these women. Some women see the scar as mutilating, and worries about sexual attractiveness may surface. Some men are fearful of resuming intercourse because of the fear of hurting their partner. Parents may wonder if a Caesarean birth was absolutely necessary, and such feelings may surface even years later. A clear explanation should be given to the woman and her family regarding the necessity of the Caesarean birth. They should also be given opportunities to discuss the childbirth, in an effort to resolve concerns that may arise after the birth.

Concerned professionals and lay groups in the community have established organizations for Caesarean birth, to meet the needs of these women and their families. Such groups advocate that a discussion of Caesarean birth be included in all parenthood preparation classes. No woman can be guaranteed a vaginal birth, even if she is in good health and there is no indication of danger to the fetus before the onset of labour. For this reason, every woman needs to be aware of and prepared for this possibility.

Childbirth educators should teach about the similarities and differences between a Caesarean and vaginal birth. In support of the philosophy of family-centred birth, most hospitals have instituted policies that permit fathers and other partners and family members to share in these births as they do in vaginal ones. Women who have undergone Caesarean birth agree that the continued presence and support of their partners helped them respond positively to the entire experience.

In addition to preparing women for the possibility of Caesarean birth, childbirth educators should empower women to believe in their ability to give birth vaginally and to seek care measures during labour that will enhance the progress of their labours and reduce their risk for Caesarean birth.

Preoperative Care

Family-centred care is the goal for the woman who is to undergo Caesarean birth and her family. The preparation of the woman for Caesarean birth is the same as that for other elective or emergency surgery. The physician discusses with the woman and her family the need for the Caesarean birth and the prognosis for mother and infant. The anaesthesiologist assesses the woman's cardiopulmonary system and describes the options for anaesthesia. Informed consent is obtained for the procedure.

Blood and urine tests are usually done a day or two before a planned Caesarean birth or on admission to the labour unit. Laboratory tests, most commonly ordered to establish baseline data, include a complete blood cell count, blood typing, and possibly a urinalysis. Maternal vital signs and blood pressure and fetal heart rate and pattern continue to be assessed per hospital routine until the operation begins. Physical preoperative preparation usually includes inserting a retention (Foley) catheter to keep the bladder empty (this should be done after administration of anaesthetic, if possible) and administering prescribed preoperative medications. Because of the lower abdominal incision, the primary health care provider may order an abdominal-mons shave or a clipping of pubic hair. Clipping is the better option over shaving, to decrease the risk of infection. If general anaesthesia is to be used, an antacid is administered orally to neutralize gastric secretions in case of aspiration. Intravenous fluids are started to maintain hydration and provide an open line for the administration of medications, if needed.

Removal of dentures, nail polish, and jewellery may be optional, depending on hospital policies and type of anaesthesia used. If the woman wears glasses and is going to be awake, the nurse should make sure that her glasses accompany her to the operating room so she can see her infant. If the woman wears contact lenses, the nurse can find out whether they can be worn for the birth.

During preoperative preparation, the support person is encouraged to remain with the woman as much as possible to provide continuing emotional support (if this is culturally acceptable to the woman and support person). The nurse needs to provide essential information about the preoperative procedures during this time. Although the nursing actions may be carried out quickly if a Caesarean birth is unplanned, verbal communication, particularly explanations, is important. Silence can be frightening to the woman and her support person. The nurse's use of touch can communicate feelings of care and concern for the woman. The nurse can assess the woman's and her partner's perceptions about Caesarean birth. As the woman expresses her feelings, the nurse may identify possible self-concept concerns that may need to be addressed during the postpartum period. If there is time before the birth, the nurse can teach the woman about postoperative expectations and pain relief, turning, coughing, and deep-breathing measures.

Anaesthesia

Spinal, epidural (see Chapter 16, p. 413), and general anaesthetics are used for Caesarean births. Regional blocks (epidural and spinal) are popular because women want to be awake for and aware of the birth experience. However, the choice of anaesthetic depends on several factors. The mother's medical history or present condition, such as a spinal injury, hemorrhage, or coagulopathy, may rule out the use of regional anaesthesia. In the case of an emergency and the mother's or infant's life is at risk, general anaesthesia will most likely be used unless an epidural is already in place. The woman herself is a factor. She may not know all the options or may have fears about "a needle in her back" or of being awake and feeling pain. She needs to be fully informed about the risks and benefits of the different types of anaesthesia so that she can participate in the decision whenever there is a choice to be made.

General Anaesthesia

General anaesthesia is used infrequently for elective Caesarean birth. It may be necessary if there is a contraindication to spinal or epidural anaesthesia or if indications necessitate a rapid birth (vaginal or emergent Caesarean) without sufficient time to perform a block. In addition, being awake and aware during major surgery may be unacceptable for some women having a Caesarean birth.

If general anaesthesia is being considered, the nurse should give the woman nothing by mouth for 6 to 8 hours (per protocol) and see that an IV infusion is in place. If time allows, the nurse can premedicate the woman with a nonparticulate (clear) oral antacid (e.g., sodium citrate) to neutralize the acidic contents of the stomach. Aspiration of highly acidic gastric contents will damage lung tissue. Some anaesthetists also order the administration of a histamine blocker such as cimetidine to decrease production of gastric acid and metoclopramide (Maxeran) to increase gastric emptying. Before the anaesthesia is given, a wedge should be placed under one of the woman's hips to displace the uterus. Uterine displacement prevents aortocaval compression, which interferes with placental perfusion.

Thiopental, a short-acting barbiturate, is administered intravenously to render the woman unconscious; succinylcholine, a muscle relaxer, is then administered to facilitate passage of an endotracheal tube. The circulating nurse assists with applying cricoid pressure before intubation as the woman begins to lose consciousness. This manoeuvre blocks the esophagus and prevents aspiration should the woman vomit or regurgitate (Fig. 19-10). Pressure is released once the endotracheal tube is securely in place.

After the woman is intubated, nitrous oxide and oxygen in a 50:50 mixture are administered. A low concentration of a volatile halogenated agent (e.g., isoflurane) also may be administered to increase pain relief and reduce maternal awareness and recall. In higher concentrations isoflurane or methoxyflurane relaxes the uterus quickly and facilitates intrauterine manipulation, version, and extraction. However, at higher concentrations, these agents readily cross the placenta and can produce narcosis in the fetus and could

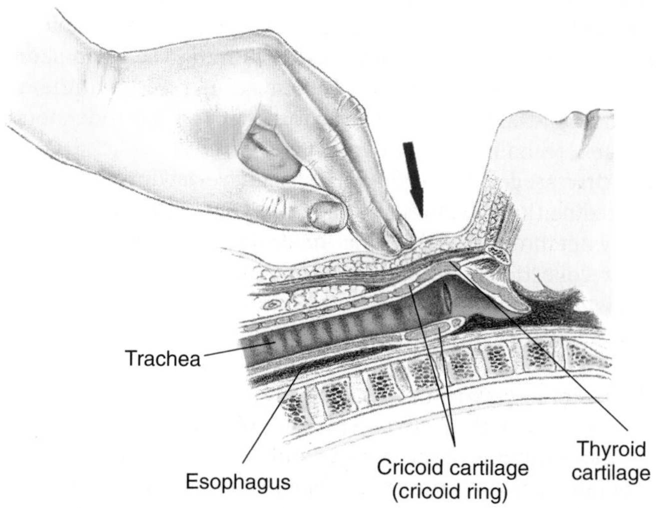

Fig. 19-10 Technique of applying pressure on cricoid cartilage to occlude esophagus to prevent pulmonary aspiration of gastric contents during induction of general anaesthesia.

reduce uterine tone after birth, increasing the risk for hemorrhage.

Intraoperative Care

Caesarean births occur in operating rooms in the surgical suite or in the labour and birth unit. Once the woman has been taken to the operating room, her care becomes the responsibility of the obstetrical team, surgeon, anaesthesiologist, and surgical nursing staff (Fig. 19-11). If possible, the partner, who is gowned appropriately, accompanies the mother to the surgical unit and remains close to her so that continued support and comfort can be provided. In an unplanned Caesarean birth, the nurse who cared for the woman during labour should be part of the nursing care team in the operating room, if possible.

The nurse who is circulating can assist with positioning the woman on the birth (surgical) table. It is important to position her so that the uterus is displaced laterally, to prevent compressing the inferior vena cava, which causes decreased placental perfusion. This is usually accomplished by placing a wedge under the hip. A Foley catheter is inserted into the bladder at this time if one is not already in place.

If the partner either is not allowed or chooses not to be present in the operative suite, the nurse can stay in communication with him or her and give progress reports whenever possible. If the mother is awake during the birth, the nurse or anaesthetist can tell her what is happening and provide support. The mother may be anxious about the sensations she is experiencing, such as the coldness of solutions used to prepare the abdomen and pressure or pulling during the actual birth of the infant. She also may be apprehensive because of the bright lights or the presence of unfamiliar equipment and masked and gowned personnel in the room. Explanations by the nurse can help decrease the woman's anxiety.

Care of the infant usually is delegated to a nurse or other care provider skilled in neonatal resuscitation. If risk factors are present, a pediatrician may also be present. A crib with resuscitation equipment is readied before surgery. Those responsible for care are expert not only in resuscitative techniques but also in the ability to detect normal and abnormal infant responses. After birth, if the infant's condition permits and the mother is awake, the baby may be placed skin to skin on the mother or her partner or can be given to the woman's partner to hold (Fig. 19-12). The infant whose condition is compromised is transported after initial stabilization to the nursery for observation and the implementation of appropriate interventions. In some institutions, the partner may accompany the infant; if not, personnel keep the family informed of the infant's progress, and parent–infant contacts are initiated as soon as possible.

If the family cannot (or does not want to) accompany the woman during surgery, they are directed to the surgical or obstetrical waiting room. The physician then reports on the condition of the mother and child to family members after the birth is completed. Family members may accompany the infant if he or she needs to be transferred to the nursery, giving them an opportunity to see and admire the new baby.

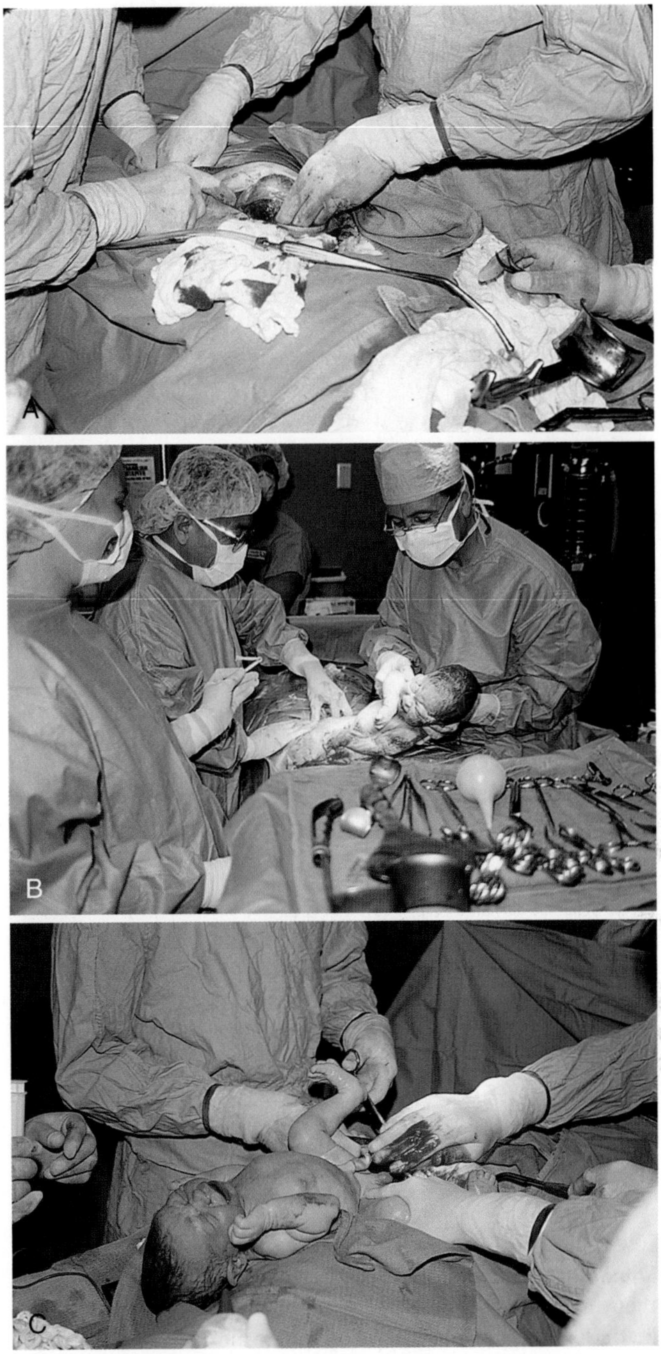

Fig. 19-11 Caesarean birth. **A:** "Bikini" incision has been made, the muscle layer is separated, the abdomen is entered, the uterus has been exposed and incised. Note small amount of bleeding. **B:** The neonate's birth through the uterine incision is nearly complete. **C:** A quick assessment is performed; note significant moulding of head resulting from cephalopelvic disproportion. *(Courtesy Marjorie Pyle, RNC, Lifecircle, Costa Mesa, CA.)*

NURSING ALERT Some mothers and parents want the privilege of informing family and friends of the sex of the infant (if it was not known before birth). Before responding to requests for such information from people waiting outside the birthing area, the nurse should check to see if the mother has given consent for such information to be released and to whom.

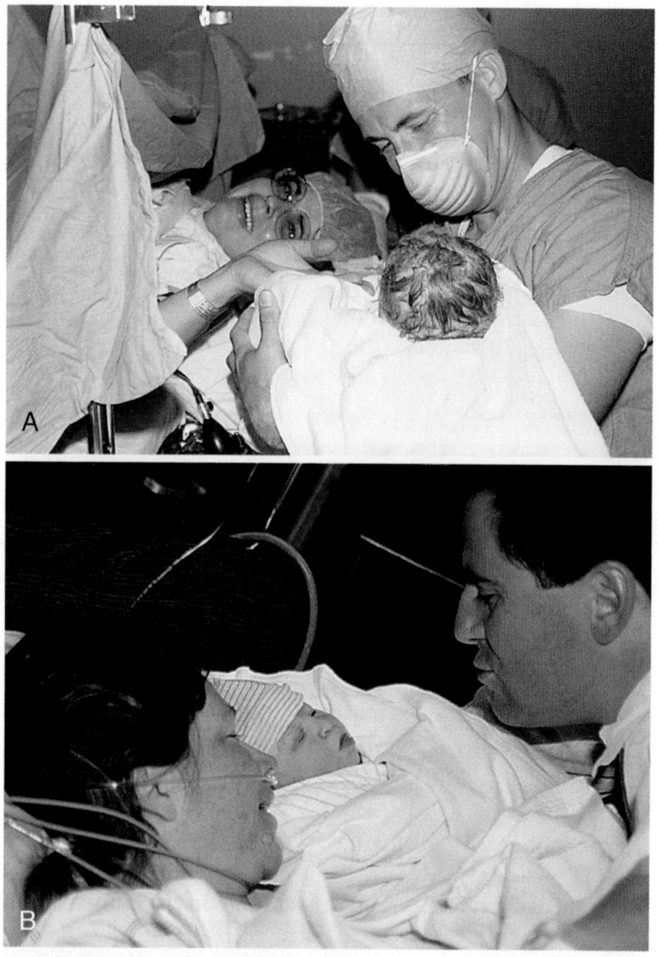

Fig. 19-12 **A:** Parents and their newborn. The physician manually removes the placenta; suctions the remaining amniotic fluid and blood from the uterine cavity; and closes the uterine incision, peritoneum, muscle layer, fatty tissue, and, finally, the skin while the new family shares some private time. **B:** Parents become better acquainted with their newborn while mother rests after surgery. *(Courtesy Marjorie Pyle, RNC, Lifecircle, Costa Mesa, CA.)*

Immediate Postoperative Care

Once surgery is completed, the mother is transferred to a recovery room or back to her labour room. After a Caesarean birth, women have both postoperative and postpartum needs that must be addressed. They are surgical patients, as well as new mothers. Nursing assessments in this immediate post-birth period follow agency protocol and include degree of recovery from the effects of anaesthesia, postoperative and postbirth status, and degree of pain. If general anaesthesia was administered, it is essential that a patent airway be maintained and that the woman be positioned to prevent possible aspiration until she is fully alert and responsive. Vital signs should be taken every 15 minutes for 1 to 2 hours or until stable. The condition of the incisional dressing, the fundus, and the amount of lochia need to be assessed, as well as IV intake and urine output through the Foley catheter. The woman should be helped to turn and do coughing, deep-breathing, and leg exercises. Medications to relieve pain can be administered as ordered.

Routine postpartum care is organized to facilitate parent–infant interaction as soon as possible and to answer the mother's questions. When appropriate, the nurse should assess the mother's readiness to see the baby, as well as her response to the anaesthesia and to the event that may have necessitated general anaesthesia (e.g., emergency Caesarean birth when vaginal birth was anticipated). If the baby is present, the mother and her partner should be given some time alone with him or her to facilitate bonding and attachment. Newborns should be placed skin to skin with the mothers as soon as possible, and breastfeeding can be initiated when the mother feels like trying, preferably within the first 30 to 60 minutes. If the woman is in a recovery area or her labour room, she usually is transferred to the postpartum unit after 1 to 2 hours or once her condition is stable and the effects of anaesthesia have worn off (i.e., she is alert, oriented, and able to feel and move extremities).

Postoperative or Postpartum Care

The attitude of the nurse and other health team members can influence the woman's perception of herself after a Caesarean birth. The caregivers should stress that the woman is a new mother first and a surgical patient second. This attitude helps the woman perceive herself as having the same problems and needs as those of other new mothers while at the same time requiring supportive postoperative care.

The woman's physiological concerns for the first few days may be dominated by pain at the incision site and pain resulting from intestinal gas—thus the need for pain relief. If epidural anaesthesia was used for the surgery, epidural opioids can be given in the immediate postoperative period to provide pain relief for approximately 24 hours. Otherwise, pain medications usually are given parenterally every 3 to 4 hours, or patient-controlled analgesia may be ordered. The most commonly used analgesics include opioids (e.g., hydromorphone) and NSAIDs (e.g., [naprosyn]). If opioids are used, an antiemetic (e.g., promethazine [Phenergan], ondansetron [Zofran]) is often ordered to be administered either as needed by the woman or around the clock as long as the opioid is used. Other comfort measures such as position changes, splinting the incision with pillows, and relaxation and breathing techniques may be implemented.

Ambulation and rocking in a rocking chair may relieve gas pains; avoiding consumption of gas-forming foods, the use of straws, and carbonated beverages may help minimize them (see Patient Teaching box).

Nurses must be alert to the woman's physiological needs, managing care to ensure adequate rest and pain relief. Mother–baby care (couplet care) for a Caesarean birth mother can be modified according to her physiological limitations as a surgical patient.

Daily care includes perineal care and routine hygienic care, including showering after the dressing has been removed (if showering is acceptable according to the woman's cultural beliefs and practices). The nurse needs to assess the woman's vital signs, incision, fundus, and lochia according to hospital policies, procedures, or protocols. Breath sounds, bowel sounds, circulatory status of lower extremities, and urinary and bowel elimination also are assessed. It is important to note maternal emotional status.

PATIENT TEACHING Postpartum Pain Relief After Caesarean Birth

Incisional Pain

- Splint incision with a pillow when moving or coughing.
- Use relaxation techniques such as music, breathing, and dim lights.

Intestinal Gas

- Walk as often as you can.
- Do not eat or drink gas-forming foods, carbonated beverages, or whole milk.
- Do not use straws for drinking fluids.
- Take antiflatulence medication if prescribed.
- Lie on your left side to expel gas.
- Rock in a rocking chair.

During the postpartum period, the nurse can provide care that meets the psychological and learning needs of mothers who have had Caesarean births. The nurse should explain postpartum procedures to help the woman participate in her recovery from surgery. Also, the nurse can help the woman plan care and visits from family and friends that allow for adequate rest periods. Information and assistance with infant care can facilitate adjustment to her role as a mother. The woman needs to be supported as she breastfeeds her baby, receiving individualized assistance to comfortably hold and position the baby at her breast. The side-lying position or football hold and the use of pillows to support the newborn can enhance comfort and facilitate successful breastfeeding.

Discharge after Caesarean birth is usually by the second or third postoperative day. The woman's predominant needs at home are for rest and sleep; relief of pain and discomfort; and assistance with household chores, infant care and feeding, and self-management. The nurse must provide discharge teaching to prepare the woman for self-management and newborn care in a limited time, while ensuring that the woman is comfortable and able to rest. The nurse should assess the woman's information needs and coordinate the health care team's efforts to meet them.

Discharge teaching and planning should include information about nutrition; measures to relieve pain and discomfort (see Patient Teaching box); exercise and specific activity restrictions; time management that includes periods of uninterrupted rest and sleep; hygiene, breast, and incision care; timing for resumption of sexual activity and contraception; signs of complications (see Home Care box); and infant care. The nurse should assess the woman's need for continued support or counselling to facilitate her emotional recovery from the birth. Her family and friends should be educated about her needs during the recovery process, and their assistance should be coordinated before discharge. Referrals to community agencies may be indicated to further promote the recovery process. A postdischarge program of telephone follow-up and home visits can facilitate the woman's full recovery after Caesarean birth.

HOME CARE

Signs of Postoperative Complications After Discharge

Report the following signs to your health care provider:

- Temperature exceeding 38°C
- Painful urination
- Lochia heavier than a normal period
- Foul-smelling lochia
- Wound separation
- Redness or oozing at the incision site
- Severe abdominal pain

Vaginal Birth After Caesarean (VBAC)

Indications for primary Caesarean birth such as dystocia, breech presentation, or abnormal FHR pattern often are non-recurring. Therefore, a woman who has had a Caesarean birth and subsequently becomes pregnant may not have any contraindications to labour and vaginal birth in that pregnancy and may attempt a VBAC.

Women who have had one previous Caesarean birth by low transverse incision, who have an adequate pelvis, and who have no other uterine scars or previous ruptures may attempt a TOL and VBAC. A physician must be available throughout active labour and be capable of performing an emergency Caesarean birth. TOL after Caesarean is relatively safe, but there is risk of uterine rupture through a lower uterine segment scar. Increased reports of uterine rupture in the United States and Canada raised concerns about the safety of VBAC. The incidence of uterine rupture appears to be related to the method of the second labour and birth (Thorp, 2009). The rate of uterine rupture was lowest with spontaneous vaginal birth and highest when labour was induced, especially if prostaglandins were used to ripen the cervix. Other risk factors include prior classic uterine incision extending into the fundus, single-layer rather than double-layer uterine closure, two or more previous Caesarean births, an interdelivery interval of 18 to 24 months or less, maternal age of 30 years or older, postpartum fever, and CPD. Women are most often the primary decision makers with regard to choice of birth method. During the antepartum period, the woman should be given information about VBAC and encouraged to choose it as an alternative to a repeat Caesarean, as long as no contraindications exist. VBAC support groups (e.g., http://www.vbac.com or http://www.ican-online.org) and prenatal classes can help prepare the woman psychologically for labour and vaginal birth.

TOL should occur in a hospital facility that has the equipment and personnel available to begin surgery within 30 minutes from the time a decision is made for Caesarean birth. Ideally, the woman is admitted to the labour and birth unit at the onset of spontaneous labour. In the active phase of labour, FHR and uterine activity are continuously monitored electronically, and IV access is established. Abnormal FHR patterns (e.g., prolonged decelerations, variable or late decelerations, and absent baseline variability) often precede rupture or signal its occurrence. The woman may also complain of abdominal, shoulder, or back pain, even with an epidural, and may exhibit signs of excessive blood loss. The physician should be immediately available during active labour.

There is conflicting evidence that administering oxytocin to induce or augment labour increases the risk of uterine rupture. If oxytocin is used for the TOL, caution and close monitoring of the labouring woman are urged. However, use of prostaglandins to ripen the cervix or induce labour is not recommended because they have been associated with an increased risk for uterine rupture (Landon, 2007).

Attention should be given to the woman's psychological and physical needs during the TOL. Anxiety increases the release of catecholamines and can inhibit the release of oxytocin, delaying the progress of labour and possibly leading to a repeat Caesarean birth. To alleviate anxiety, the nurse can encourage the woman to use breathing and relaxation techniques and change position to promote labour progress. The woman's partner can be encouraged to provide comfort measures and emotional support. Collaboration among the woman in labour, her partner, the nurse, and other health care providers often results in a successful VBAC. If a TOL does not proceed to vaginal birth, the woman will need support and encouragement to express her feelings about having another Caesarean birth. It is important that this outcome not be labelled a failed VBAC.

Obstetrical Emergencies

Shoulder Dystocia

evolve Animation—Shoulder Dystocia

Shoulder dystocia is an uncommon obstetrical emergency that increases the risk for fetal or neonatal and maternal morbidity and mortality during the attempt to deliver the fetus vaginally. It is estimated that 0.24 to 2% of all vaginal births are complicated by shoulder dystocia (Thorp, 2009). Shoulder dystocia is not predictable; many women who have risk factors will not develop the problem, whereas others with no apparent risk factors experience it.

Shoulder dystocia is a condition in which the head is born but the anterior shoulder cannot pass under the pubic arch. Fetopelvic disproportion caused by excessive fetal size (greater than 4000 g) or maternal pelvic abnormalities may be a cause of shoulder dystocia, although it can occur in the absence of any known risk factors.

The nurse should be observant for risk factors that could indicate the possibility of shoulder dystocia, including maternal obesity, previous birth of an infant weighing more than 4000 g, estimated fetal weight of more than 4000 g, diabetes mellitus, prolonged second stage of labour, prolonged transition phase of labour, previous instrumental midpelvic delivery, and previous shoulder dystocia. When the head emerges, it retracts against the perineum (turtle sign), and external rotation does not occur (Baird & Kennedy, 2008; Lanni & Seeds, 2007).

Risks to the fetus and newborn include birth injuries, asphyxia, brachial plexus damage, and fracture, especially of the humerus or clavicle. The mother's primary risk stems from excessive blood loss as a result of uterine atony or rupture, lacerations, extension of the episiotomy, or endometritis.

Nursing Care Management

Many manoeuvres, such as suprapubic pressure and maternal position changes, have been suggested and tried to free the anterior shoulder, although no one particular manoeuvre has been found to be most effective (Lanni & Seeds, 2007). Suprapubic pressure can be applied to the anterior shoulder using the Mazzanti or Rubin technique (Fig. 19-13) in an attempt to push the shoulder under the symphysis pubis.

In the McRoberts manoeuvre (Fig. 19-14), the woman's legs are flexed apart with her knees on her abdomen. This manoeuvre causes the sacrum to straighten, and the symphysis pubis rotates toward the mother's head; the angle of pelvic inclination is decreased, freeing the shoulder. Suprapubic pressure can be applied at this time. Having the woman move to a hands-and-knees position (the Gaskin manoeuvre), a

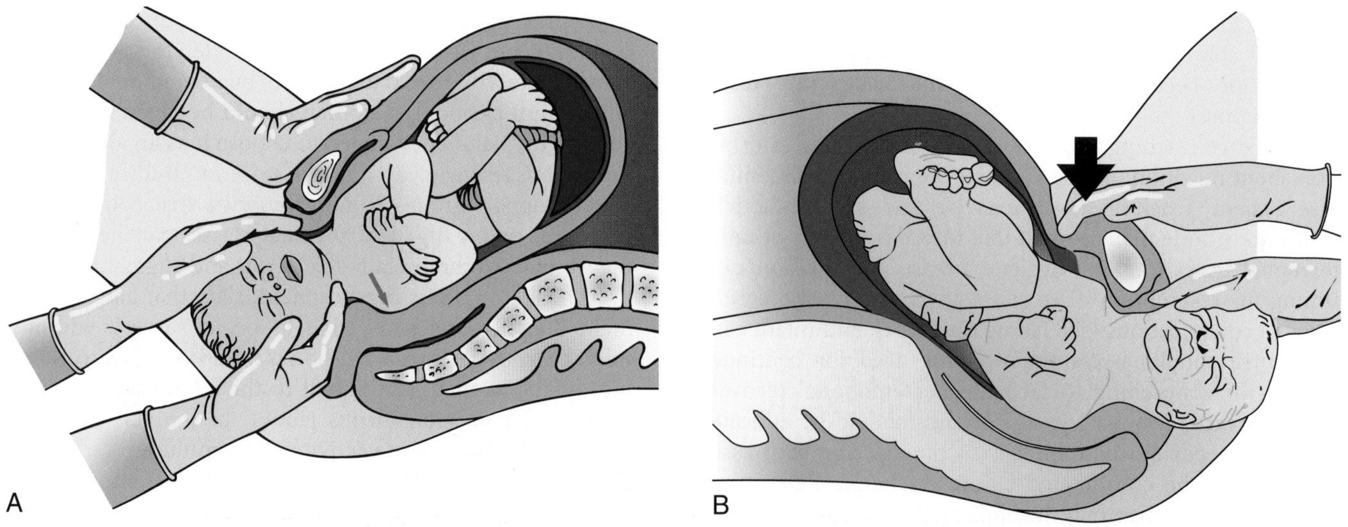

Fig. 19-13 Application of suprapubic pressure. **A:** Mazzanti technique: pressure is applied directly posteriorly and laterally above the symphysis pubis. **B:** Rubin technique: pressure is applied obliquely posteriorly against the anterior shoulder.

squatting position, or a lateral recumbent position also has been used to resolve cases of shoulder dystocia (Baird & Kennedy, 2008; Jevitt, 2005; Thorp, 2009). Fundal pressure is contraindicated as a method of relieving shoulder dystocia (see discussion, Chapter 18, p. 476).

When shoulder dystocia is diagnosed, the nurse needs to help the woman assume the position(s) that may facilitate birth of the shoulders, assist the primary health care provider with these manoeuvres, and monitor the fetal response. The nurse should also provide encouragement and support to reduce anxiety and fear.

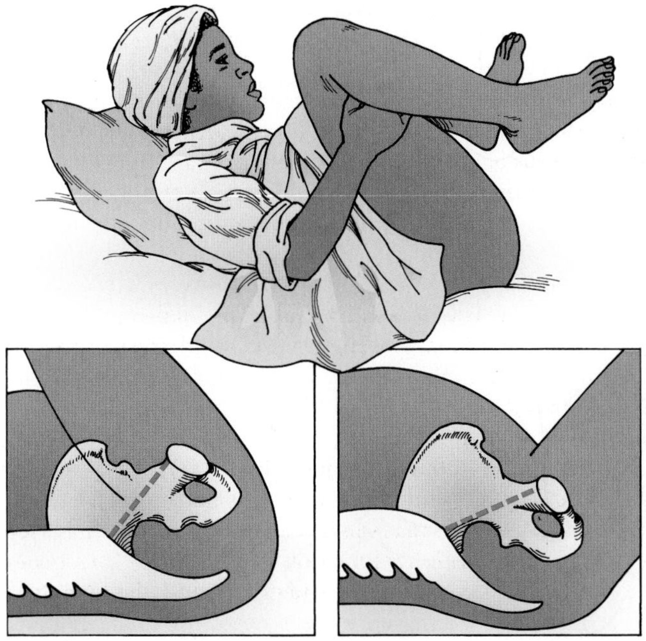

Fig. 19-14 McRoberts manoeuvre. *(Adapted from Lanni, S. M., & Seeds, J. W. [2007]. Malpresentations. In S. G. Gabbe, J. R. Niebyl, & J. L. Simpson [Eds.],* Obstetrics: Normal and problem pregnancies *[5th ed.]. New York: Churchill Livingstone.)*

Newborn assessment should include examination for fracture of the clavicle or humerus, brachial plexus injuries, and asphyxia. Maternal assessment should focus on early detection of hemorrhage and trauma to the soft tissue of the birth canal.

Prolapsed Umbilical Cord

evolve Animation—Prolapsed Umbilical Cord

Prolapse of the umbilical cord occurs when the cord lies below the presenting part of the fetus. Umbilical cord prolapse may be occult (hidden, not visible) at any time during labour, regardless of whether or not membranes are ruptured (Fig. 19-15, A and B). It is most common to see frank (visible) prolapse directly after rupture of membranes, when gravity washes the cord in front of the presenting part (see Fig. 19-15, C and D). Frank prolapse occurs in 0.1 to 0.6% of all births (Lin, 2006). Contributing factors are a long cord (longer than 100 cm), malpresentation (footling breech), transverse lie, or unengaged presenting part.

If the presenting part does not fit snugly into the lower uterine segment, as in polyhydramnios, when the membranes rupture, a sudden gush of amniotic fluid may cause the cord to be displaced downward. Similarly, the cord may prolapse during amniotomy if the presenting part is high. A small or preterm fetus may not fit snugly into the lower uterine segment; as a result, cord prolapse is more likely to occur.

Nursing Care Management

Prompt recognition of a **prolapsed cord** is important because fetal hypoxia resulting from prolonged cord compression (i.e., occlusion of blood flow to and from the fetus for more than 5 minutes) can occur and potentially lead to fetal hypoxia, newborn asphyxia, neurological brain injury, or death of the fetus. Pressure on the cord may be relieved by the examiner putting a sterile gloved hand into the vagina and holding the presenting part off of the umbilical cord (Fig. 19-16, A and B). The woman should be assisted into a position such as a modified Sims' (see Fig. 19-16, C), Trendelenburg, or knee–chest (see Fig. 19-16, D) position, in which gravity keeps the presenting part off the cord. If the cervix is fully dilated, a

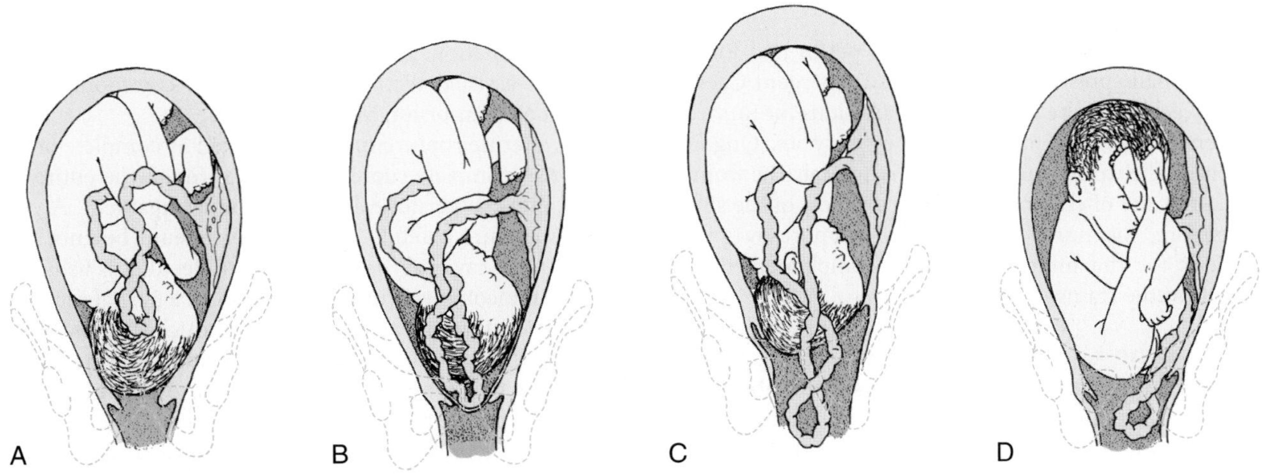

Fig. 19-15 Prolapse of umbilical cord. Note pressure of presenting part on umbilical cord, which endangers fetal circulation. **A:** Occult (hidden) prolapse of cord. **B:** Complete prolapse of cord. Note that membranes are intact. **C:** Cord presenting in front of fetal head may be seen in vagina. **D:** Frank breech presentation with prolapsed cord.

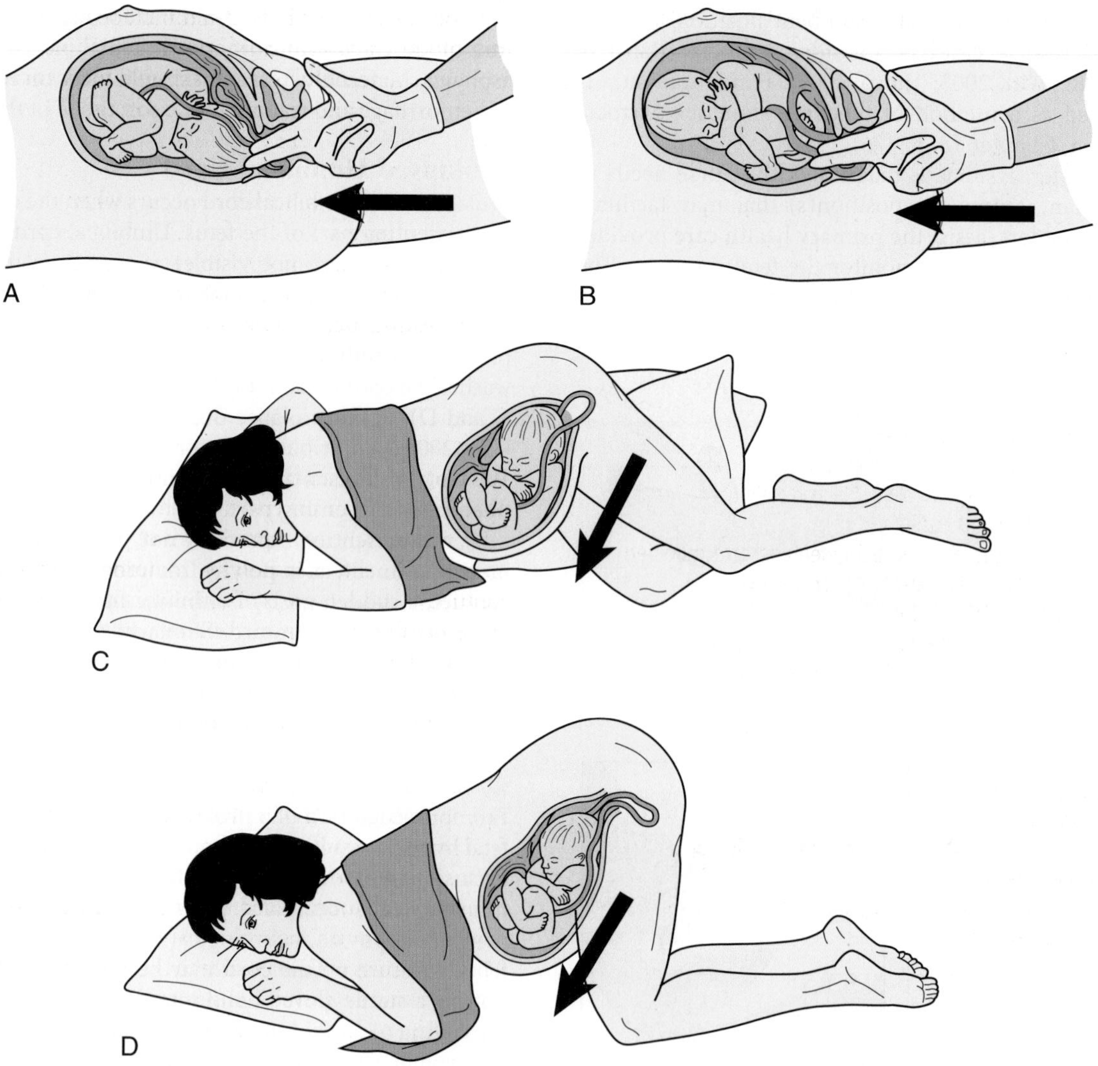

Fig. 19-16 *Arrows* indicate direction of pressure against presenting part to relieve compression of prolapsed umbilical cord. Pressure exerted by examiner's fingers in **A:** vertex presentation, and **B:** breech presentation. **C:** Gravity relieves pressure when woman is in modified Sims' position with hips elevated as high as possible with pillows. **D:** Knee–chest position.

forceps- or vacuum-assisted birth can be performed for the fetus in a cephalic presentation; otherwise, emergent Caesarean surgery is likely to be performed. Indications for immediate interventions are presented in the Emergency box. Ongoing assessment of the woman and her fetus is critical. The woman and her family are often aware of the seriousness of the situation; therefore, the nurse must provide support by giving explanations for the interventions being implemented and their effect on the status of the fetus.

Rupture of the Uterus

Rupture of the uterus is a rare but very serious obstetrical injury with an overall occurrence rate of approximately 1%. The most common cause of uterine rupture during pregnancy is the separation of a previous Caesarean birth scar. Other causes are uterine trauma (e.g., accidents, surgery), congenital uterine anomaly, intense spontaneous uterine contractions, labour stimulation (e.g., oxytocin, prostaglandin), an overdistended uterus (e.g., multifetal gestation), malpresentation, external or internal version, or a difficult forceps-assisted birth. It occurs more commonly in multigravidas than primigravidas.

A uterine rupture may be classified as complete or incomplete. A complete rupture extends through the entire uterine wall into the peritoneal cavity or broad ligament. An incomplete rupture extends into the peritoneum but not into the peritoneal cavity or broad ligament. Bleeding is usually internal. An incomplete rupture may also be a partial separation of an old Caesarean scar and may go unnoticed unless the woman has a subsequent Caesarean birth or other uterine surgery.

Signs and symptoms vary with the extent of the rupture and may be silent or dramatic. In an incomplete rupture, pain may not be present. The fetus is the most common indicator of uterine rupture, with electronic fetal monitor changes such as late or variable decelerations, decreased baseline variability, and an increased or decreased heart rate. The woman may experience vomiting, faintness, increased abdominal tenderness, and a lack of labour or fetal station progress.

EMERGENCY

Prolapsed Cord

Signs

Fetal bradycardia with variable deceleration occurs during uterine contraction.

The woman reports feeling the cord after membranes rupture.

The cord is seen or felt in or protruding from the vagina.

Interventions

Call for assistance.

Notify a physician with surgical privileges immediately.

Glove the examining hand quickly and insert two fingers into the vagina to the cervix. With one finger on either side of the cord or both fingers to one side, exert upward pressure against the presenting part to relieve compression of the cord (see Fig. 19-16, A and B). Place a rolled towel under the woman's right or left hip.

Place the woman in the extreme Trendelenburg or a modified Sims' position (see Fig. 19-16, C), or a knee-chest position (see Fig. 19-16, D).

If cord is protruding from the vagina, wrap it loosely in a sterile towel saturated with warm, sterile, normal saline solution.

Administer oxygen to the woman by mask at 8 to 10 L/min until birth is accomplished.

Start intravenous fluids or increase existing drip rate.

Continue to monitor fetal heart rate.

Explain to the woman and support person what is happening and the management plan.

Prepare for immediate vaginal birth if the cervix is fully dilated or for Caesarean birth if it is not.

Eventually, bleeding and the effects of blood loss will be noted, and the FHR may be lost. In a complete rupture the woman may complain of a sudden, sharp or "ripping" abdominal pain and may state that "something gave way." She may exhibit signs of hypovolemic shock caused by hemorrhage (i.e., hypotension; tachypnea; pallor; and cool, clammy skin). If the placenta separates, rapid fetal compromise will occur. If the fetus is expelled into the abdominal cavity, fetal parts may be palpable through the abdomen.

Nursing Care Management

Prevention is the best treatment. Women who have had a previous classic Caesarean birth are advised not to attempt vaginal birth in subsequent pregnancies. Women at risk for uterine rupture should be assessed closely during labour. Women whose labours are induced with oxytocin or prostaglandin (especially if their previous birth was Caesarean) should be monitored for signs of uterine hyperstimulation because this can precipitate uterine rupture. If hyperstimulation occurs, the oxytocin infusion is discontinued or decreased, and a tocolytic medication may be given to decrease the intensity of uterine contractions. After giving birth, women should be assessed for excessive bleeding, especially if the fundus is firm and signs of hemorrhagic shock are present.

If rupture occurs, the type of medical management depends on its severity. A small rupture may be managed with a laparotomy and birth of the infant, repair of the laceration, and blood transfusions, if needed. Hysterectomy and blood replacement are the usual treatments for a complete rupture.

The nurse's role may include starting IV fluids, transfusing blood products, administering oxygen, and assisting with preparation for immediate surgery. Supporting the woman's family and providing information about the treatment are important during this emergency. The maternal mortality rate in modern developed countries is 0 to 1% (Nahum & Pham, 2008). Providing information about spiritual support services or suggesting that the family contact their own support system may be warranted.

Amniotic Fluid Embolism (Anaphylactoid Syndrome of Pregnancy)

Amniotic fluid embolism (AFE) occurs when amniotic fluid, fetal cells, hair, or other debris enter the maternal circulation, triggering a rapid, complex series of pathophysiological events that lead to life-threatening maternal symptoms (Baird & Kennedy, 2008; Gilbert, 2007). This can occur because fluid can enter the maternal circulation any time there is an opening in the amniotic sac or maternal uterine veins accompanied by enough intrauterine pressure to force the amniotic fluid into the veins (e.g., if the placenta separates). Although uncommon (1 in 8000 to 30,000 pregnancies), this complication is the leading cause of maternal mortality. The maternal mortality rate is approximately 60 to 80% (Moore, 2008). A common first symptom is acute dyspnea, followed by severe hypotension (Moore, 2008; Schoening, 2006).

AFE cannot be predicted or prevented, and the cause for the reaction is unknown. A history of allergies is present in 41% of women with exposure to amniotic fluid (Moore, 2008). The condition is similar but not identical to anaphylactic shock; hence, a new diagnostic title, **anaphylactoid syndrome** of pregnancy, has been proposed.

Nursing Care Management

The immediate interventions for AFE are summarized in the Emergency box. Such medical management must be instituted immediately. Cardiopulmonary resuscitation is often needed. The woman is usually placed on mechanical ventilation, and rapid blood and volume replacement is initiated; coagulation defects are treated.

The nurse's immediate responsibility is to assist with the resuscitation efforts. The nurse should continuously monitor the fetus if the mother is undelivered and anticipate emergency Caesarean birth and neonatal resuscitation (Baird & Kennedy, 2008). If the woman survives, she is usually moved to a critical care unit where hemodynamic monitoring, blood replacement, and coagulopathy treatment are implemented. If cardiopulmonary arrest occurs, for optimal fetal survival a perimortem Caesarean birth should occur within 5 minutes.

Support of the woman's partner and family is needed; they will be anxious and distressed. Brief explanations of what is happening are important during the emergency and can be reinforced after the immediate crisis is over. If the woman dies and the infant survives, grieving, anger, and blame may interfere with parent–infant attachment (Perozzi & Englert, 2004). When both the mother and infant die, it is important that the

EMERGENCY

Amniotic Fluid Embolism (Anaphylactoid Syndrome of Pregnancy)

Signs

Respiratory distress
- Restlessness
- Dyspnea
- Cyanosis
- Pulmonary edema
- Respiratory arrest
- Circulatory collapse
- Hypotension
- Tachycardia
- Shock
- Cardiac arrest

Hemorrhage
- Coagulation failure: bleeding from incisions, venipuncture sites, trauma (lacerations); petechiae, ecchymoses, purpura
- Uterine atony

Tonic-clonic seizure activity

Interventions

Oxygenate.
- Administer oxygen by nonrebreather face mask (10 L/min) or resuscitation bag delivering 100% oxygen.
- Prepare for intubation and mechanical ventilation.
- Initiate or assist with cardiopulmonary resuscitation (see Chapter 14, p. 362). Tilt pregnant woman 30 degrees to side to displace uterus.
- Maintain cardiac output and replace fluid losses.
- Position woman on her side.
- Administer intravenous fluids.
- Administer blood: packed cells, fresh frozen plasma.
- Insert indwelling catheter and measure hourly urine output.

Correct coagulation failure.
Monitor fetal and maternal status.
Prepare for emergency birth.
Anticipate pulmonary artery and arterial catheter placement.
Prepare the mother and family for transfer to an intensive care environment or tertiary care centre after stabilization.
Provide emotional support to the woman, her partner, and her family.

family has the opportunity to spend time with them. Emotional support and involvement of the perinatal loss support team or other resource for grief counselling, including the pastoral care team (if desired by the family), are needed (see Box 23-7). Referral to grief and loss support groups is appropriate. The nursing staff also may need help in coping with emotions that result from a maternal death.

Key Points

- *Preterm labour* is defined as uterine contractions leading to cervical change occurring between 20 and 37 completed weeks of pregnancy; *preterm birth* is any birth that occurs before the completion of 37 weeks of pregnancy.
- The cause of preterm labour is unknown and is assumed to be multifactorial.
- Bed rest, a commonly prescribed intervention for preterm labour, has many deleterious adverse effects and has never been shown to decrease preterm birth rates.
- Preterm birth that occurs in a tertiary care centre leads to better neonatal and maternal outcomes.
- Vigilance for signs of infection is a major part of the care for women with PPROM.
- Dystocia results from differences in the normal relationships among any of the five factors affecting labour.
- Dysfunctional labour occurs as a result of hypertonic uterine dysfunction, hypotonic uterine dysfunction, or inadequate voluntary expulsive forces.
- The functional relationships among the uterine contractions, the fetus, and the mother's pelvis are altered by maternal positioning.
- Uterine contractility is increased by oxytocin and prostaglandin and decreased by tocolytic drugs.
- Cervical ripening using chemical or mechanical measures can increase the success of labour induction.
- Expectant parents benefit from learning about operative obstetrics (e.g., forceps- or vacuum-assisted birth, Caesarean birth) during the prenatal period.
- The basic purpose of Caesarean birth is to preserve the life and health of the mother and her fetus.
- Unless contraindicated, a vaginal birth may be possible after a previous Caesarean birth.
- Labour management that emphasizes one-to-one support of the labouring woman by another woman (doula, nurse, or midwife) can reduce the rate of Caesarean birth and increase the rate of VBACs.
- Postterm pregnancy may pose a risk to both the mother and the fetus.
- Obstetrical emergencies (e.g., shoulder dystocia, prolapsed cord, rupture of the uterus, and amniotic fluid embolism) occur rarely but require immediate intervention.
- The perinatal loss support team or other resource for grief counseling, including the pastoral care team, provides support for families experiencing death of the mother, the infant, or both.

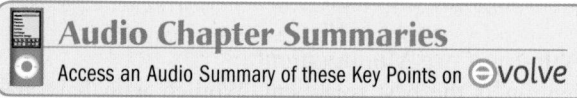

Audio Chapter Summaries

Access an Audio Summary of these Key Points on evolve

References

Alexander, G. R. (2007). Prematurity at birth: Determinants, consequences and geographic variation. In R. E. Behrman & A. S. Butler (Eds.), *Preterm birth: Causes, consequences, and prevention* (pp. 604–643). Washington, DC: National Academies Press.

Baird, S. M., & Kennedy, B. B. (2008). Intrapartum emergencies. In B. B. Kennedy, D. J. Ruth, & E. J. Martin (Eds.), *Intrapartum management modules: A perinatal education program* (4th ed.). Philadelphia: Wolters Kluwer.

Barrett, J., & Bocking, A. (2000). SOGC consensus statement: Management of twin pregnancies (part II). *Journal of Obstetrics and Gynaecology Canada, 22*(8), 607–610. Retrieved from http://www.sogc.org/guidelines/public/93E-CONS2-August2000.pdf.

Battista, L. R., & Wing, D. A. (2007). Abnormal labour and induction of labour. In S. G. Gabbe, J. R. Niebyl, & J. L. Simpson (Eds.), *Obstetrics: Normal and problem pregnancies* (5th ed.). New York: Churchill Livingstone.

Blackburn, S. T. (2007). *Maternal, fetal, and neonatal physiology: A clinical perspective* (3rd ed.). St. Louis: Saunders.

Canadian Institute for Health Information (2007). *Giving birth in Canada: Regional trends from 2001–2002 to 2005–2006*. Retrieved from https://secure.cihi.ca/free_products/Costs_Report_06_Eng.pdf.

Crane, J., et al. (2001). SOGC clinical practice guideline: Induction of labour at term. *Journal of Obstetrics and Gynaecology Canada, 23*(8), 717–728. Retrieved from http://www.sogc.org/guidelines/public/107E-CPG-August2001.pdf.

Crane, J., et al. (2003). Antenatal corticosteroid therapy for fetal maturation. *Journal of Obstetrics and Gynaecology Canada, 25*(1), 45–48. Retrieved from http://www.sogc.org/guidelines/public/122e-co-janvier2003.pdf.

Cunningham, F., et al. (2010). *Williams obstetrics* (23rd ed.). New York: McGraw Hill.

Divon, M. Y. (2007). Prolonged pregnancy. In S.G. Gabbe, J. R. Niebyl, & J. L. Simpson (Eds.), *Obstetrics: Normal and problem pregnancies* (5th ed.). New York: Churchill Livingstone.

Enkin, M., et al. (2000). *A guide to effective care in pregnancy and childbirth* (3rd ed.). New York: Oxford University Press.

Freda, M. C., & Patterson, E. (2001). *Preterm birth: Prevention and nursing management* (2nd ed.). March of Dimes Nursing Module. New York: March of Dimes.

Friedman, E. (1989). Normal and dysfunctional labour. In W. Cohen, et al. (Eds.), *Management of labour* (2nd ed.). Rockville, MD: Aspen.

Fritz, E. A., & Smith, N. W. (2008). Caring for the woman at risk for preterm labour or with premature rupture of membranes. In B. B. Kennedy, D. J. Ruth, & E. J. Martin (Eds.), *Intrapartum management modules: A perinatal education program* (4th ed.). Philadelphia: Wolters Kluwer.

Gardner, P. S. (2003). Previous traumatic birth: An impetus for requested cesarean birth. *Journal of Perinatal Education, 12*(1), 1–5.

Gilbert, E. S. (2007). *Manual of high risk pregnancy and delivery* (3rd ed.). St. Louis: Mosby.

Health Canada. (2003). *Canadian perinatal health report 2003 (Cat. No. H49-142/2003E)*. Ottawa, ON: Author. Retrieved from http://www.phac-aspc.gc.ca/publicat/cphr-rspc03/pdf/cphr-rspc03_e.pdf.

Hodnett, E., et al. (2007). *Continuous support for women during childbirth. Cochrane Database of Systematic Reviews, Issue 3*. Chichester, UK: John Wiley & Sons.

Hollier, L. M. (2005). Preventing preterm birth: What works, what doesn't. *Obstetrical and Gynecological Survey, 60*(2), 124–131.

Hutton, E.K., & Hofmeyr, G.J. (2006). External cephalic version for breech presentation before term. *Cochrane Database of Systematic Reviews 2006*, Issue 1. Art. No.: CD000084. DOI: 10.1002/14651858.CD000084.pub2.

Iams, J. D., & Romero, R. (2007). Preterm birth. In S. G. Gabbe, J. R. Niebyl, & J. L. Simpson (Eds.), *Obstetrics: Normal and problem pregnancies* (5th ed.). New York: Churchill Livingstone.

Iams, J. D., Romero, R., & Creasy, R. K. (2009). Preterm labour and birth. In R. K. Creasy, et al. (Eds.), *Creasy & Resnik's maternal–fetal medicine: Principles and practice* (6th ed.). Philadelphia: Saunders.

Jevitt, C. (2005). Shoulder dystocia: Etiology, common risk factors, and management. *Journal of Midwifery and Women's Health, 50*(6), 485–497.

Kilpatrick, S., & Garrison, E. (2007). Normal labour and delivery. In S. G. Gabbe, J. R. Niebyl, & J. L. Simpson (Eds.), *Obstetrics: Normal and problem pregnancies* (5th ed.). New York: Churchill Livingstone.

Kotaska, A., et al. (2009). SOGC clinical practice guideline: Vaginal delivery of breech presentation. *Journal of Obstetrics and Gynaecology Canada, 31(6)*, 557–566. Retrieved from http://www.sogc.org/guidelines/documents/gui226CPG0906.pdf.

Landon, M. B. (2007). Cesarean delivery. In S. G. Gabbe, J. R. Niebyl, & J. L. Simpson (Eds.), *Obstetrics: Normal and problem pregnancies* (5th ed.). New York: Churchill Livingstone.

Lanni, S. M., & Seeds, J. W. (2007). Malpresentations. In S. G. Gabbe, J. R. Niebyl, & J. L. Simpson (Eds.), *Obstetrics: Normal and problem pregnancies* (5th ed.). New York: Churchill Livingstone.

Lehne, R. (2007). *Pharmacology for nursing care* (6th ed.). Philadelphia: Saunders.

Lim, K., et al. (2011). SOGC clinical practice guideline: Ultrasonographic cervical length assessment in predicting preterm birth in singleton pregnancies. *Journal of Obstetrics and Gynaecology Canada, 33*(5), 486–499. Retrieved from http://www.sogc.org/guidelines/documents/gui257CPG1106E.pdf.

Lin, M. G. (2006). Umbilical cord prolapsed. *Obstetrical and Gynecological Survey, 61*(4), 269–277.

Liston, R., et al. (2007). Fetal health surveillance: Antepartum and intrapartum consensus guideline. *Journal of Obstetrics and Gynaecology Canada, 29*(9 Suppl 4), s1–s56. Retrieved from http://www.sogc.org/guidelines/documents/gui197CPG0709.pdf.

Lockwood, C. J. (2012). Overview of preterm labour and delivery. *UpToDate* [database online]. Retrieved from http://www.uptodate.com/contents/overview-of-preterm-labor-and-delivery.

Malone, F. D., & D'Alton, M. E. (2009). Multiple gestation. Clinical characteristics and management. In R. K. Creasy, et al. (Eds.), *Creasy & Resnik's maternal–fetal medicine: Principles and practice* (6th ed.). Philadelphia: Saunders.

Maloni, J., & Park, S. (2005). Postpartum symptoms after antepartum bedrest. *Journal of Obstetric, Gynecologic and Neonatal Nursing, 34*(2), 163–171.

Martin, J. A., et al. (2007). Births: Final data for 2005. *National Vital Statistics Report, 56*(6), 1–104.

Mercer, B. M. (2007). Premature rupture of membranes. In S. G. Gabbe, J. R. Niebyl, & J. L. Simpson (Eds.), *Obstetrics: Normal and problem pregnancies* (5th ed.). New York: Churchill Livingstone.

Moore, L. E. (2008). Amniotic fluid embolism. *eMedicine*. Retrieved from http://www.emedicine.com/med/topic122.htm.

MORE^{OB}. (2010). *Chapter: Assisted vaginal birth and vaginal breech birth*. Retrieved from http://www.moreob.com.

Nahum, G. G., & Pham, K. Q. (2008). Uterine rupture in pregnancy. *eMedicine*. Retrieved from http://www.emedicine.com/med/topic3746.htm.

National Institutes of Health. (2000). *Antenatal corticosteroids revisited: Consensus Development Conference Statement*. Bethesda, MD: Author. Retrieved from http://consensus.nih.gov.

Ontario Provincial Maternal–Newborn Advisory Committee. (2008). *Fetal fibronectin: Guideline for use in management of preterm labour*. Toronto: Author. Retrieved from http://www.pcmch.on.ca/FetalFibronectin.aspx.

Perozzi, K. J., & Englert, N. C. (2004). Amniotic fluid embolism: An obstetric emergency. *Critical Care Nurse, 24*(4), 54–61.

Public Health Agency of Canada. (2008). *Canadian perinatal health report, 2008 ed.* (Cat. No. HP10-12/2008E). Ottawa, ON: Health Canada. Retrieved from http://www.phac-aspc.gc.ca/publicat/2008/cphr-rspc/pdf/cphr-rspc08-eng.pdf.

Public Health Agency of Canada (2012). *Perinatal health indicators for Canada 2011*. (Cat. No. HP7-1/2011). Ottawa, ON: Author.

Roberts, D., & Dalziel, S.R. (2006). Antenatal corticosteroids for accelerating fetal lung maturation for women at risk of preterm birth. *Cochrane Database of Systematic Reviews 2006*, Issue 3. Art. No.: CD004454. DOI: 10.1002/14651858.CD004454.pub2.

Schoening, A. (2006). Amniotic fluid embolism: Historical perspectives and new possibilities. *MCN: American Journal of Maternal Child Nursing, 31*(2), 78–83.

Simpson, K. R. (2008). *Cervical ripening and induction and augmentation of labour* (3rd ed.). Washington, DC: Association of Women's Health, Obstetric, and Neonatal Nurses.

Smith, G. N., et al. (2007). Randomized double-blind placebo-controlled trial of transdermal nitroglycerin for preterm labour. *American Journal of Obstetrics and Gynecology, 196*(1), 37.e1–37.e8.

Society of Obstetricians and Gynaecologists of Canada. (1995). *Management of dystocia. Policy statement 40.* Ottawa: Author.

Society of Obstetricians and Gynaecologists of Canada. (2004). News: C-sections on demand—SOGC's position. *Birth, 31*(2), 154.

Sosa, C., et al. (2004). Bed rest in singleton pregnancies for preventing preterm birth. *Cochrane Database of Systematic Reviews, 1*, CD003581.

Sprague, A. (2004). The evolution of bed rest as a clinical intervention. *Journal of Obstetric, Gynecologic and Neonatal Nursing, 33*(5), 542–549.

Sprague, A. E., et al. (2008). Bed rest and activity restriction for women at risk for preterm birth: A survey of Canadian prenatal care providers. *Journal of Obstetrics and Gynaecology Canada, 30*(4), 317–326.

Statistics Canada. (2007). *Births 2007* (Cat. No. 84F0210X). Ottawa, ON: Author. Retrieved from http://www.statcan.gc.ca/pub/84f0210x/84f0210x2007000-eng.pdf.

Terry, R. R., et al. (2006). Postpartum outcomes in supine delivery by physicians vs. nonsupine delivery by midwives. *Journal of the American Osteopathic Association, 106*(4), 199–202.

Thorp, J. M. (2009). Clinical aspects of normal and abnormal labour. In R. K. Creasy, et al. (Eds.), *Creasy & Resnik's maternal–fetal medicine: Principles and practice* (6th ed.). Philadelphia: Saunders.

Wener, M., & Lavigne, S. (2004). Can periodontal disease lead to premature delivery? *AWHONN Lifelines, 8*(5), 422–431.

Unit 5

20 Maternal Physiological Changes

Learning Objectives

On completion of this chapter, the reader will be able to:

- Describe the anatomical and physiological changes that occur during the postpartum period.
- Identify characteristics of uterine involution and lochial flow and describe ways to measure them.
- List expected values for vital signs and blood pressure, deviations from normal findings, and probable causes of the deviations.

Electronic Resources

Additional information related to the content in Chapter 20 can be found on

evolve the companion Web site at

http://evolve.elsevier.com/Canada/Perry/maternal/

- Examination Review Questions

The postpartum period is the interval between the birth of the newborn and the return of the reproductive organs to their normal nonpregnant state. This period is sometimes referred to as the **puerperium**, or **fourth trimester** of pregnancy. Although the puerperium has traditionally been considered to last 6 weeks, this time frame varies among women. The physiological changes that occur during the reversal of the processes of pregnancy are distinctive, but they are normal. To provide care during the recovery period that is beneficial to the mother, her infant, and her family, the nurse must synthesize knowledge of maternal anatomy and physiology of the recovery period, the newborn's physical and behavioural characteristics, infant care activities, and the family response to the birth of the infant. This chapter focuses on anatomical and physiological changes that occur in the mother during the postpartum period.

Reproductive System and Associated Structures

Uterus

Involution Process

The return of the uterus to a nonpregnant state following birth is called **involution**. This process begins immediately after expulsion of the **placenta** with contraction of the uterine smooth muscle.

At the end of the third stage of labour the uterus is in the midline, approximately 2 cm below the level of the umbilicus, with the **fundus** resting on the sacral promontory. At this time, the uterus weighs approximately 1000 g.

Within 12 hours, the fundus may rise to approximately 1 cm above the umbilicus (Fig. 20-1). By 24 hours after birth, the uterus is about the same size as it was at 20 weeks of gestation. Involution progresses rapidly during the next few days. The fundus descends 1 to 2 cm every 24 hours. By the sixth **postpartum** day, the fundus is normally located halfway between the umbilicus and the symphysis pubis. The uterus should not be palpable abdominally after 2 weeks.

The uterus, which at full term weighs approximately 11 times its prepregnancy weight, involutes to approximately 500 g by 1 week after birth and to 350 g by 2 weeks after birth. At 6 weeks postpartum it weighs 50 to 60 g (see Fig. 20-1).

Increased estrogen and progesterone levels are responsible for stimulating the massive growth of the uterus during pregnancy. Prenatal uterine growth results from both *hyperplasia*, an increase in the number of muscle cells, and *hypertrophy*, an enlargement of the existing cells. After birth, the decrease in these **hormones** causes *autolysis*, the self-destruction of excess hypertrophied tissue. The additional cells laid down during pregnancy remain and account for the slight increase in uterine size after each pregnancy.

Subinvolution is the failure of the uterus to return to a nonpregnant state. The most common causes of subinvolution are retained placental fragments and **infection**.

Contractions

Postpartum hemostasis is achieved primarily by compression of intramyometrial blood vessels as the uterine muscle contracts rather than by platelet aggregation and clot formation. The hormone **oxytocin**, released from the **pituitary** gland, strengthens and coordinates these uterine contractions, which compress blood vessels and promote hemostasis. During the first 1 to 2 postpartum hours, uterine contractions may decrease in intensity and become uncoordinated. Because it is vital that the uterus remain firm and well contracted,

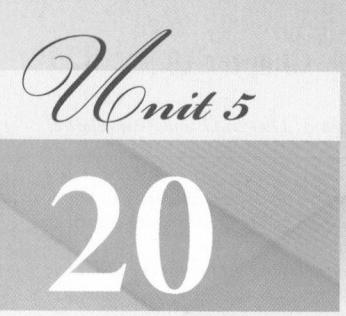

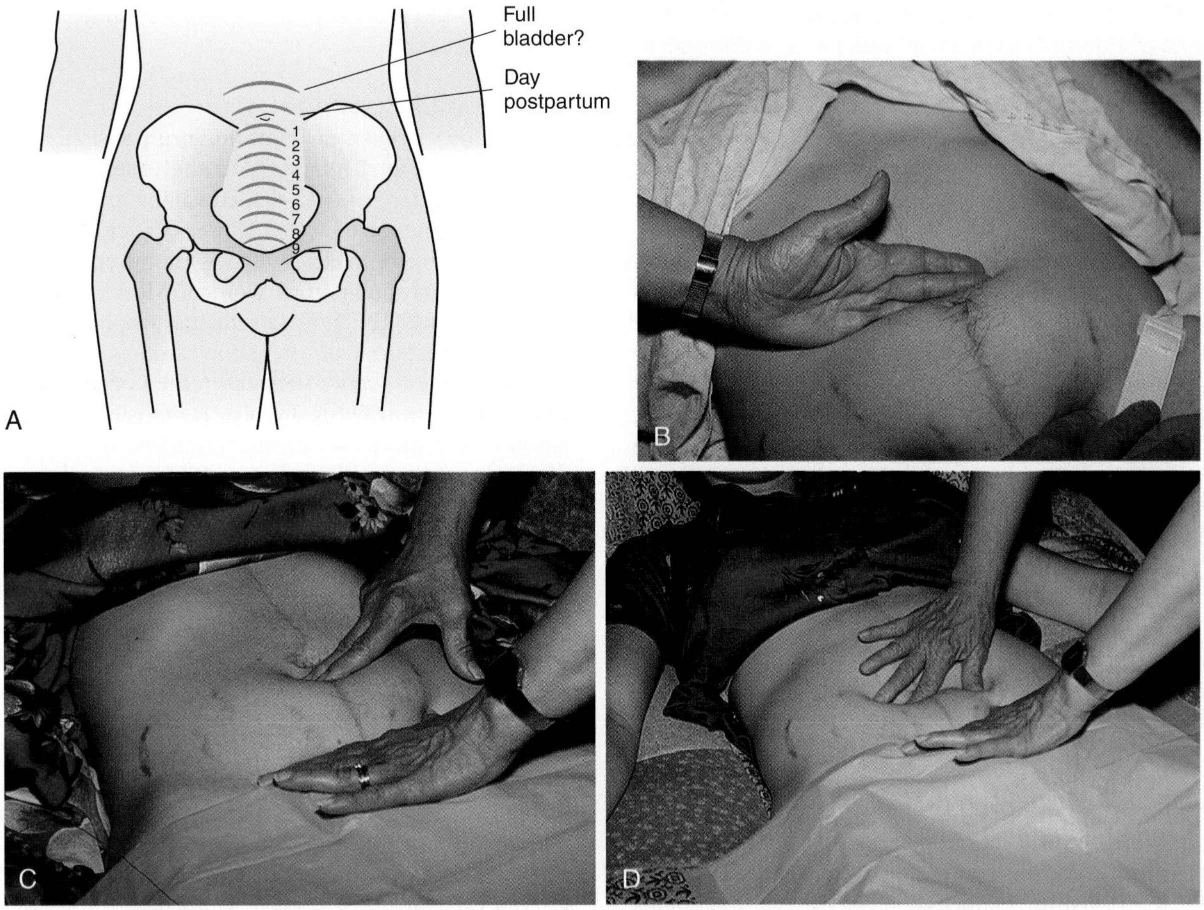

Fig. 20-1 Assessment of involution of uterus after childbirth. **A:** Normal progress, days 1 through 9. **B:** Size and position of uterus 2 hours after childbirth. **C:** Two days after childbirth. **D:** Four days after childbirth. *(B through D, Courtesy Marjorie Pyle, RNC, Lifecircle, Costa Mesa, CA.)*

exogenous oxytocin is usually administered intravenously or intramuscularly immediately after expulsion of the placenta. Women who plan to breastfeed may be encouraged to put the baby to breast immediately after birth because suckling stimulates oxytocin release.

Afterpains

In first-time mothers uterine tone is good, the fundus generally remains firm, and the woman usually perceives only mild uterine cramping. Periodic relaxation and vigorous contractions are more common in subsequent pregnancies and may cause uncomfortable cramping called **afterpains** (afterbirth pains), which persist throughout the early puerperium. Afterpains are more noticeable after births in which the uterus was overdistended (e.g., large baby, multifetal gestation, polyhydramnios). Breastfeeding and exogenous oxytocic medication usually intensify these afterpains because both stimulate uterine contractions.

Placental Site

Immediately after the placenta and membranes are expelled, vascular constriction and thromboses reduce the placental site to an irregular nodular and elevated area. Upward growth of the endometrium causes sloughing of necrotic tissue and prevents the scar formation characteristic of normal wound healing. This unique healing process enables the endometrium to resume its usual cycle of changes and permit implantation and placentation in future pregnancies. Endometrial regeneration is completed by postpartum day 16, except at the placental site. Regeneration at the placental site usually is not complete until 6 weeks after birth.

Lochia

Postbirth uterine discharge, commonly called **lochia**, initially is bright red (**lochia rubra**) and may contain small clots. For the first 2 hours after birth, the amount of uterine discharge should be about that of a heavy menstrual period. After that time, the lochia flow should steadily decrease.

Lochia rubra consists mainly of blood and decidual and trophoblastic debris. The flow pales, becoming pink or brown (**lochia serosa**) after 3 to 4 days. Lochia serosa consists of old blood, serum, leukocytes, and tissue debris. The median duration of lochia serosa discharge is 22 to 27 days (Katz, 2007). In most women about 10 days after childbirth the drainage becomes yellow to white (**lochia alba**). Lochia alba consists of leukocytes, decidua, epithelial cells, mucus, serum, and bacteria. It may continue for 2 to 6 weeks after the birth but may last longer and still be normal.

If the woman receives an oxytocic medication, regardless of the route of administration, the flow of lochia is often scant until the effects of the medication wear off. The amount of lochia is usually less after Caesarean births. Flow of lochia usually increases with ambulation and breastfeeding. Lochia tends to pool in the vagina when the woman is lying in bed; the woman then may experience a gush of blood when she stands. This gush should not be confused with hemorrhage.

Persistence of lochia rubra early in the postpartum period suggests continued bleeding as a result of retained fragments of the placenta or membranes. Recurrence of bleeding 7 to 14 days after birth is from the healing placental site. About 10 to 15% of women will still be having normal lochia serosa discharge at their 6-week postpartum examination (Katz, 2007). However, in most women, the continued flow of lochia serosa or lochia alba by 3 to 4 weeks after birth can indicate endometritis, particularly if fever, pain, or abdominal tenderness is associated with the discharge. Lochia should smell like normal menstrual flow; an offensive odour usually indicates infection.

Not all postpartal vaginal bleeding is lochia; vaginal bleeding after birth may be caused by unrepaired vaginal or cervical lacerations. Box 20-1 distinguishes between lochial and nonlochial bleeding.

Cervix

The cervix is soft immediately after birth. However, within 2 to 3 postpartum days it has shortened, become firm, and regained its form. The cervix up to the lower uterine segment remains edematous, thin, and fragile for several days after birth. The ectocervix (part of the cervix that protrudes into the vagina) appears bruised and has some small lacerations—optimal conditions for the development of infection. The cervical os, which dilated to 10 cm during labour, closes gradually. Two fingers may still be introduced into the cervical os for the first 4 to 6 days after birth; however, only the smallest curette can be introduced by the end of 2 weeks. The external cervical os never regains its prepregnant appearance; it is no longer shaped like a circle but appears as a jagged slit that is often described as a "fish mouth." **Lactation** delays the production of cervical and other estrogen-influenced mucus and mucosal characteristics.

BOX 20-1 Lochial and Nonlochial Bleeding

Lochial Bleeding

Lochia usually trickles from the vaginal opening. The steady flow is greater as the uterus contracts.

A gush of lochia may result as the uterus is massaged. If it is dark in colour, it has been pooled in the relaxed vagina, and the amount soon lessens to a trickle of bright red lochia (in the early puerperium).

Nonlochial Bleeding

If the bloody discharge spurts from the vagina, there may be cervical or vaginal tears in addition to the normal lochia.

If the amount of bleeding continues to be excessive and bright red, a tear may be the source.

Vagina and Perineum

Postpartum estrogen deprivation is responsible for the thinness of the vaginal mucosa and the absence of **rugae**. The greatly distended, smooth-walled vagina gradually returns to its prepregnancy size by 6 to 10 weeks after childbirth. Rugae reappear within 3 weeks, but they are never as prominent as they are in the nulliparous woman. Most rugae are permanently flattened. The mucosa remains atrophic in the lactating woman, at least until menstruation resumes. Thickening of the vaginal mucosa occurs with the return of ovarian function. Reduced estrogen levels are also responsible for a decreased amount of vaginal lubrication. Localized dryness and coital discomfort (**dyspareunia**) may persist until ovarian function returns and menstruation resumes. The use of a water-soluble lubricant to reduce discomfort during sexual intercourse is usually recommended.

Initially the introitus is erythematous and edematous, especially in the area of the **episiotomy** or laceration repair. It is barely distinguishable from that of a nulliparous woman if lacerations and an episiotomy have been carefully repaired, hematomas are prevented or treated early, and the woman practices good hygiene during the first 2 weeks after birth.

Most episiotomy or laceration repairs are visible only if the woman is lying on her side with her upper buttock raised or if she is placed in the lithotomy position. A good light source is essential for visualization of some repairs. An episiotomy or laceration heals the same way as any surgical incision. Signs of infection (pain, redness, warmth, swelling, or discharge) or loss of approximation (separation of the edges of the incision) may occur. Healing should occur within 2 to 3 weeks.

Hemorrhoids (anal varicosities) are commonly seen. Internal hemorrhoids may evert while the woman is pushing during birth. Women often experience associated symptoms such as itching, discomfort, and bright red bleeding upon defecation. Hemorrhoids usually decrease in size within 6 weeks of childbirth.

Pelvic Muscular Support

The supporting structure of the uterus and vagina may be injured during childbirth and may contribute to later gynecological problems. Supportive tissues of the pelvic floor that are torn or stretched during childbirth may require up to 6 months to regain tone. **Kegel exercises**, which help strengthen perineal muscles and encourage healing, are recommended after childbirth (see Patient Teaching box in Chapter 4, p. 51). *Pelvic relaxation* refers to the lengthening and weakening of the fascial supports of pelvic structures. These structures include the uterus, upper posterior vaginal wall, urethra, bladder, and rectum. Although relaxation can occur in any woman, it is commonly a direct but delayed complication of childbirth.

Abdomen

When the woman stands during the first days after birth, her abdomen protrudes and gives her a still-pregnant appearance. During the first 2 weeks after birth, the abdominal wall is relaxed (see Fig. 20-1). It takes about 6 weeks for the abdominal wall to return almost to its prepregnancy state (Fig. 20-2). The skin regains most of its previous elasticity, but some striae may persist. The return of muscle tone depends on previous tone, proper exercise, and the amount of adipose tissue. Occasionally, with or without overdistension because of a large fetus or multiple fetuses, the abdominal wall muscles separate, a condition termed **diastasis recti** abdominis (see Fig. 9-14, B). Persistence of this separation may be disturbing to the woman, but surgical correction rarely is necessary. With time, the separation becomes less apparent.

Endocrine System

Placental Hormones

Significant hormonal changes occur during the postpartal period. Expulsion of the placenta results in dramatic decreases of the hormones produced by that organ. Decreases in human chorionic somatomammotropin (also called human placental lactogen), estrogens, cortisol, and the placental enzyme insulinase reverse the diabetogenic effects of pregnancy, resulting in significantly lower blood sugar levels in the immediate puerperium. Mothers with type 1 diabetes will likely require much less insulin for several days after birth. Because these normal hormonal changes make the puerperium a transitional period for carbohydrate metabolism, it is more difficult to interpret glucose tolerance tests at this time.

Estrogen and progesterone levels drop markedly after expulsion of the placenta and reach their lowest levels 1 week after birth. Decreased estrogen levels are associated with breast engorgement and the diuresis of excess extracellular fluid accumulated during pregnancy. In nonlactating women, estrogen levels begin to increase by 2 weeks after birth and by postpartum day 17 are higher than in women who breastfeed (Katz, 2007).

Human chorionic gonadotropin disappears from maternal circulation in 14 days.

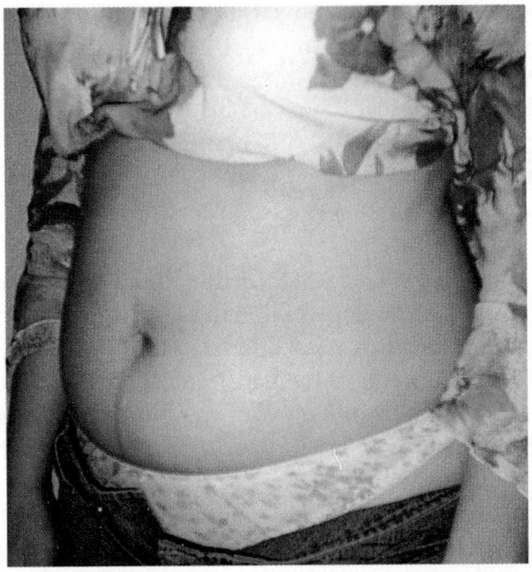

Fig. 20-2 Abdominal wall 6 weeks after vaginal birth is almost back to prepregnancy appearance. Note that the linea nigra is still visible. *(Courtesy Jodi Brackett, Phoenix, AZ.)*

Pituitary Hormones and Ovarian Function

Prolactin levels in blood rise progressively throughout pregnancy. In women who breastfeed, prolactin levels remain elevated and increase with each breastfeeding (Liu, 2009). Serum prolactin levels are influenced by the frequency of breastfeeding, the duration of each feeding, and the degree to which supplementary feedings are used. Individual differences in the strength of an infant's sucking stimulus probably also affect prolactin levels. In nonlactating women, prolactin levels decline after birth and reach the prepregnant range in 3 to 4 weeks (Liu, 2009).

Lactating and nonlactating women differ considerably in the timing of their first ovulation and when menstruation resumes. The persistence of elevated serum prolactin levels in breastfeeding women appears to be responsible for suppressing ovulation (Liu, 2009).

Ovulation occurs as early as 27 days after birth in nonlactating women, with a mean time of about 10 weeks. About 70% of nonbreastfeeding women resume menstruating by 12 weeks after birth. The mean time to ovulation in women who breastfeed is about 6 months (Katz, 2007). In lactating women, both the resumption of ovulation and the return of menses are determined in large part by breastfeeding patterns. Thus, discussion of contraceptive options early in the puerperium is necessary (see Chapter 7).

The first menstrual flow after childbirth is usually heavier than normal. Within three or four cycles the amount of menstrual flow returns to the woman's prepregnancy volume.

Urinary System

The hormonal changes of pregnancy (i.e., high steroid levels) contribute to an increase in renal function; diminishing steroid levels after childbirth may partly explain the reduced renal function that occurs during the puerperium. Kidney function returns to normal within 1 month after birth. About 6 weeks are required for the pregnancy-induced hypotonia and dilation of the ureters and renal pelves to return to the nonpregnant state (Katz, 2007). In a small percentage of women, dilation of the urinary tract may persist for 3 months or longer, increasing their chances of developing a urinary tract infection.

Urine Components

The renal **glycosuria** induced by pregnancy disappears, but lactosuria may occur in lactating women. The blood urea nitrogen increases during the puerperium as autolysis of the involuting uterus occurs. This breakdown of excess protein in the uterine muscle cells also results in a mild (+1) **proteinuria** for 1 to 2 days after childbirth in approximately 50% of women. Ketonuria may occur in women with an uncomplicated birth or after a prolonged labour with dehydration.

Postpartal Diuresis

Within 12 hours of birth, women begin to lose excess tissue fluid accumulated during pregnancy. Profuse diaphoresis often occurs, especially at night, for the first 2 or 3 days after childbirth. Postpartal diuresis, caused by decreased estrogen levels, removal of increased venous pressure in the lower extremities, and loss of the remaining pregnancy-induced increase in blood volume, also aids the body in ridding itself of excess fluid. Fluid loss through perspiration and increased urinary output accounts for a weight loss of approximately 2.25 kg during the puerperium.

Urethra and Bladder

Birth-induced trauma, increased bladder capacity following childbirth, and the effects of conduction anaesthesia (epidural or spinal) combine to cause a decreased urge to void. In addition, pelvic soreness caused by the forces of labour, vaginal lacerations, or the episiotomy reduces or alters the voiding reflex. Decreased voiding combined with postpartal diuresis may result in bladder distension.

Immediately after birth, excessive bleeding can occur if the bladder becomes distended because it pushes the uterus up and to the side and prevents it from contracting firmly. Later in the puerperium, overdistension can make the bladder more susceptible to infection and impede the resumption of normal voiding (Cunningham et al., 2010). With adequate emptying of the bladder, bladder tone is usually restored by 5 to 7 days after childbirth.

Gastrointestinal System

Appetite

The mother is often hungry shortly after birth and usually can tolerate a regular diet. Requests for extra portions of food and frequent snacks are not uncommon.

Bowel Evacuation

A spontaneous bowel evacuation may not occur for 2 to 3 days after childbirth. This delay can be explained by decreased muscle tone in the intestines during labour and the immediate puerperium, prelabour diarrhea, lack of food, or dehydration. The mother often anticipates discomfort during the bowel movement because of perineal tenderness as a result of episiotomy, lacerations, or hemorrhoids and may resist the urge to defecate. Women need to be encouraged to increase fluid and fibre intake to prevent constipation and discomfort. Regular bowel habits should be re-established when bowel tone returns.

Operative vaginal birth (forceps or vacuum use) and anal sphincter lacerations are associated with an increased risk of postpartum anal incontinence. If it occurs, anal incontinence is often temporary and may resolve within 6 months (Katz, 2007). Women should be taught during pregnancy about episiotomy and its possible sequelae. Pelvic floor (Kegel) exercises should be encouraged (see Patient Teaching box in Chapter 4, p. 51).

Breasts

Promptly after birth there is a decrease in the concentrations of hormones (i.e., estrogen, progesterone, human chorionic gonadotropin, prolactin, cortisol, and insulin) that stimulated breast development during pregnancy. The time it takes for these hormones to return to prepregnancy levels is determined in part by whether the mother breastfeeds her infant.

Breastfeeding Mothers

During the first 24 hours after birth, there is little, if any, change in the breast tissue. **Colostrum**, a clear, yellow fluid, may be expressed from the breasts. The breasts gradually become fuller and heavier as the colostrum transitions to milk by about 72 to 96 hours after birth; this is often referred to as the "milk coming in." The breasts may feel warm, firm, and somewhat tender. Bluish-white milk with a skim-milk appearance (true milk) can be expressed from the nipples. As milk glands and milk ducts fill with milk, breast tissue may feel somewhat nodular or lumpy. Unlike the lumps associated with fibrocystic breast disease or cancer (which can be palpated consistently in the same location), the nodularity associated with milk production tends to shift in position. Some women experience **engorgement**, but with frequent breastfeeding and proper care this is a temporary condition that typically lasts only 24 to 48 hours (see Chapter 26).

Nonbreastfeeding Mothers

The breasts generally feel nodular in contrast to the granular feel of breasts in nonpregnant women. The nodularity is bilateral and diffuse. Prolactin levels drop rapidly. Colostrum is present for the first few days after childbirth. **Palpation** of the breast on the second or third day as milk production begins may reveal tissue tenderness in some women. On the third or fourth postpartum day engorgement may occur. The breasts are distended (swollen), firm, tender, and warm to the touch (because of vasocongestion). Breast distension is caused primarily by the temporary congestion of veins and lymphatics rather than by an accumulation of milk. Milk is present but should not be expressed. Axillary breast tissue (the tail of Spence) and any accessory breast or nipple tissue along the milk line can be involved. Engorgement resolves spontaneously, and discomfort decreases usually within 24 to 36 hours. A breast binder or well-fitted supportive bra, ice packs, fresh cabbage leaves, or mild analgesics may be used to relieve discomfort. Nipple stimulation should be avoided. If suckling is never begun (or is discontinued), lactation ceases within a few days to a week.

Cardiovascular System

Blood Volume

Changes in blood volume after birth depend on several factors such as blood loss during childbirth and the amount of extravascular water (physiological **edema**) mobilized and excreted. Blood loss results in an immediate but limited decrease in total blood volume. Thereafter most of the blood volume increase during pregnancy (1000 to 1500 mL) is eliminated within the first 2 weeks after birth.

Pregnancy-induced hypervolemia (an increase in blood volume of at least 35% over prepregnancy values near term) (Katz, 2007) allows most women to tolerate considerable blood loss during childbirth. Many women lose approximately 500 mL of blood during vaginal birth of a single fetus and about twice this much during Caesarean birth (Monga, 2009) (see Critical Thinking Exercise).

Readjustments in the maternal vasculature after childbirth are dramatic and rapid. The woman's response to blood loss during the early puerperium differs from that in a nonpregnant woman. Three postpartum physiological changes protect the woman from excessive blood loss: (1) elimination of uteroplacental circulation reduces the size of the maternal vascular bed by 10 to 15%; (2) loss of placental endocrine function removes the stimulus for vasodilation; and (3) mobilization of extravascular water stored during pregnancy increases blood volume. Thus, **hypovolemic shock** usually does not occur in women who experience a normal blood loss during the puerperium.

Cardiac Output

Pulse rate, stroke volume, and cardiac output increase throughout pregnancy. Cardiac output remains increased for at least 48 hours after birth because of an increase in stroke volume. This increased stroke volume is caused by the return of blood to the maternal systemic venous circulation, a result of rapid decrease in uterine blood flow and mobilization of extravascular fluid (Monga, 2009). Stroke volume, cardiac output, end-diastolic volume, and systemic vascular resistance remain elevated over nonpregnant values for 12 weeks after birth and may not stabilize until 24 weeks after birth (Monga, 2009).

Vital Signs

Few alterations in vital signs are seen under normal circumstances. Heart rate and blood pressure return to nonpregnant levels within a few days (Katz, 2007) (Table 20-1). Respiratory function returns to nonpregnant levels by 6 to 8 weeks after birth. After the uterus is emptied, the diaphragm descends, the normal cardiac axis is restored, and the point of maximal impulse and the electrocardiogram are normalized.

CRITICAL THINKING EXERCISE

Maternal Postpartum Blood Loss and Fatigue

You are caring for four women on the postpartum unit, two of whom had vaginal births and two who had Caesarean births. Each of the women has complained about feeling tired and has expressed concern about the amount of blood she lost during birth. Before providing patient education related to fatigue after birth and blood loss, you review the nurses' notes, the intake and output records, and patient records for estimated blood loss and hemoglobin and hematocrit values.

1. Evidence—Is there sufficient evidence to draw conclusions about the relation between tiredness (fatigue) after birth and blood loss?
2. Assumptions—What assumptions can be made about the following factors?
   a. Comparison of amount of blood loss between women who give birth vaginally and by Caesarean
   b. Postpartum norms for hematocrit and hemoglobin for women who give birth vaginally and by Caesarean
   c. Causes of fatigue after birth
   d. Interventions to alleviate fatigue and replace blood lost at birth
3. What implications and priorities for nursing care can be drawn at this time?
4. Does the evidence objectively support your conclusion?
5. Are there alternative perspectives to your conclusion?

Blood Components

Hematocrit and Hemoglobin

During the first 72 hours after childbirth, there is a greater reduction of plasma volume than in the number of blood cells. This results in a rise in hematocrit and hemoglobin levels by the seventh day after birth. There is no increased red blood cell (RBC) destruction during the puerperium, but any excess will disappear gradually in accordance with the lifespan of the RBC. The exact time at which RBC volume returns to prepregnancy values is not known, but it is within normal limits when measured 8 weeks after childbirth (Katz, 2007).

White Blood Cell Count

Normal leukocytosis of pregnancy averages approximately 12×10^9/L. During the first 10 to 12 days after childbirth, values between 20 and 25×10^9/L are common. Neutrophils are the most numerous white blood cells. Leukocytosis, coupled with the normal increase in erythrocyte sedimentation rate, may obscure the diagnosis of acute infections at this time.

Coagulation Factors

Clotting factors and fibrinogen are normally increased during pregnancy and remain elevated in the immediate puerperium. When combined with vessel damage and immobility, this hypercoagulable state causes an increased risk of thromboembolism, especially after a Caesarean birth, although the risk is rare. Fibrinolytic activity also increases during the first few days after childbirth (Katz, 2007). Factors I, II, VIII, IX, and X decrease to nonpregnant levels within a few days. Fibrin split products, probably released from the placental site, can also be found in maternal blood.

Varicosities

Varicosities (varices) of the legs and around the anus (hemorrhoids) are common during pregnancy. All varices, even the less common vulvar varices, regress (empty) rapidly immediately after childbirth. Total or nearly total regression of varicosities is expected after childbirth.

Neurological System

Neurological changes during the puerperium are those that result from a reversal of maternal adaptations to pregnancy and those resulting from trauma during labour and childbirth.

Pregnancy-induced neurological discomforts disappear after birth. Elimination of physiological edema through the diuresis that follows childbirth relieves carpal tunnel syndrome by easing compression of the median nerve. The periodic numbness and tingling of fingers that afflict 5% of pregnant women usually disappear after the birth, unless lifting and carrying the baby aggravates the condition. Headache requires careful assessment. Postpartum headaches may be caused by various conditions, including gestational

Table 20-1 Vital Signs After Childbirth

NORMAL FINDINGS	DEVIATIONS FROM NORMAL FINDINGS AND PROBABLE CAUSES
Temperature	
During first 24 hours temperature may increase to 38°C as a result of dehydrating effects of labour. After 24 hours the woman should be afebrile.	A diagnosis of puerperal sepsis is suggested if an increase in maternal temperature to 38°C is noted after the first 24 hours after childbirth and recurs or persists for 2 days. Other possibilities are mastitis, endometritis, urinary tract infections, and other systemic infections.
Pulse	
Pulse, along with stroke volume and cardiac output, remains elevated for the first hour or so after childbirth. It then begins to decrease at an unknown rate to a nonpregnant rate.	A rapid pulse rate or one that is increasing may indicate hypovolemia as a result of hemorrhage or an increased temperature.
Respirations	
The respiratory rate should decrease to within the woman's normal prebirth range by 6–8 weeks after childbirth.	Hypoventilation may occur after an unusually high subarachnoid (spinal) block or epidural narcotic after a Caesarean birth.
Blood Pressure	
Blood pressure is altered slightly, if at all. Orthostatic hypotension, as indicated by feelings of faintness or dizziness immediately after standing up, can develop in the first 48 hours as a result of the splanchnic engorgement that may occur after birth.	A low or decreasing blood pressure may indicate the existence of hypovolemia secondary to hemorrhage; however, it is a late sign, and other symptoms of hemorrhage usually alert the staff. An increased reading may result from excessive use of vasopressor or oxytocic medications. Because gestational hypertension can persist into or occur first in the postpartum period, routine evaluation of blood pressure is needed. If a woman complains of headache, hypertension must be ruled out as a cause before analgesics are administered.

hypertension, stress, and leakage of cerebrospinal fluid into the extradural space during placement of the needle for administration of epidural or spinal anaesthesia (see Postdural Puncture Headache, p. 412). Depending on the cause and effectiveness of treatment, headaches last from 1 to 3 days to several weeks.

Musculoskeletal System

Adaptations of the mother's musculoskeletal system that occur during pregnancy are reversed in the puerperium. These adaptations include the relaxation and subsequent hypermobility of the joints and the change in the mother's centre of gravity in response to the enlarging uterus. The joints are completely stabilized by 6 to 8 weeks after birth. Although all other joints return to their normal prepregnancy state, those in the parous woman's feet do not. The new mother may notice a permanent increase in her shoe size.

Integumentary System

Chloasma of pregnancy usually disappears at the end of pregnancy. Hyperpigmentation of the areolae and linea nigra may not regress completely after childbirth. Some women will have permanent darker pigmentation of those areas. **Striae gravidarum** (stretch marks) on the breasts, abdomen, and thighs may fade but usually do not disappear.

Vascular abnormalities such as spider angiomas (nevi), palmar erythema, and epulis generally regress in response to the rapid decline in estrogens after the end of pregnancy. For some women, spider nevi persist indefinitely.

Hair growth slows during the postpartum period. Some women may experience hair loss because the amount of hair lost is temporarily more than the amount regrown. The abundance of fine hair seen during pregnancy usually disappears after giving birth; however, any coarse or bristly hair that appears during pregnancy usually remains. Fingernails return to their prepregnancy consistency and strength.

Profuse diaphoresis that occurs in the immediate postpartum period is the most noticeable change in the integumentary system; this is due to the loss of excess fluid in the body.

Immune System

No significant changes in the maternal immune system occur during the postpartum period. The mother's need for a rubella vaccination or for Rh_o(D) immune globulin for prevention of Rh isoimmunization should be determined (see Chapter 21, p. 547, for further discussion).

Key Points

- The uterus involutes rapidly after birth and returns to the true pelvis within 2 weeks and resumes normal size and position by 6 weeks.
- The rapid decrease in estrogen and progesterone levels after expulsion of the placenta is responsible for triggering

many of the anatomical and physiological changes in the puerperium.

- Assessment of lochia and fundal height is essential to monitor the progress of normal involution and to identify potential problems.
- The return of ovulation and menses is determined in part by whether the woman breastfeeds her infant.
- Few alterations in vital signs are seen after birth under normal circumstances.
- Hypercoagulability, vessel damage, and immobility predispose the woman to thromboembolism.
- Marked diuresis, decreased bladder sensitivity, and overdistension of the bladder can lead to problems with urinary elimination.
- Pregnancy-induced hypervolemia, combined with several postpartum physiological changes, allows the woman to tolerate considerable blood loss at birth.

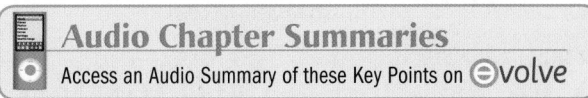

Audio Chapter Summaries

Access an Audio Summary of these Key Points on evolve

References

Cunningham, F., et al. (2010). *Williams obstetrics* (23rd ed.). New York: McGraw Hill.

Katz, V. (2007). Postpartum care. In S. G. Gabbe, J. R. Niebyl, & J. L. Simpson (Eds.), *Obstetrics: Normal and problem pregnancies* (5th ed.). New York: Churchill Livingstone.

Liu, J. H. (2009). Endocrinology of pregnancy. In R. K. Creasy, et al. (Eds.), *Creasy & Resnik's maternal–fetal medicine: Principles and practice* (6th ed.). Philadelphia: Saunders.

Monga, M. (2009). Maternal cardiovascular, respiratory, and renal adaptation to pregnancy. In R. K. Creasy et al. (Eds.), *Creasy & Resnik's maternal–fetal medicine: Principles and practice* (6th ed.). Philadelphia: Saunders.

Unit 5

21 Nursing Care During the Fourth Trimester

Learning Objectives

On completion of this chapter, the reader will be able to:

- Discuss postpartum care and discharge teaching.
- Summarize nursing interventions to prevent infection and excessive bleeding, promote normal bladder and bowel patterns, and care for the breasts of women who are breastfeeding or bottle-feeding.
- Identify common selection criteria for safe early postpartum discharge.
- Explain the influence of cultural expectations on postpartum adjustment.
- Describe the nurse's role in these postpartum follow-up strategies: home visits, telephone follow-up, warm lines and help lines, support groups, and referrals to community resources.

Electronic Resources

Additional information related to the content in Chapter 21 can be found on

evolve the companion Web site at http://evolve.elsevier.com/Canada/Perry/maternal/

- Examination Review Questions
- Case Study—Fourth Trimester
- Critical Thinking Exercise—Postpartum Complications
- Critical Thinking Exercise—Postpartum Home Care
- Critical Thinking Exercise—Priority Nursing Care: Postpartum Unit

The goal of nursing care in the immediate postpartum period is to assist women and their partners during their initial transition to parenting. In Canada, most women remain hospitalized no more than 1 or 2 days following a vaginal birth and less than 4 days following a Caesarean birth (Public Health Agency of Canada, 2009). Because there is so much important information to be shared with these women in a very short time, it is vital that their care be thoughtfully planned and provided. Care is focused on the woman's physiological recovery, her psychological well-being, and her ability to care for herself and her new baby. In addition, the nurse must consider the needs of other family members and include strategies in the plan of care to assist the family in adjusting to the new baby.

Transfer From the Recovery Area

After the initial recovery period also known as the fourth stage of labour (see Chapter 18, p. 483) has been completed, the woman may be transferred to a postpartum room in the same or another nursing unit. In facilities with labour-delivery-recovery-postpartum (LDRP) rooms, the woman labours, delivers, recovers, and spends the postpartum period in the same room, and the nurse who provides care during the recovery period may continue to care for the woman. Women who have received general or regional anaesthesia must be cleared for transfer from the recovery area by a member of the anaesthesia care team.

In preparing the transfer report, the recovery nurse uses information from the records of admission, birth record, and recovery. Information communicated to the postpartum nurse includes identity of the health care provider; gravidity and parity; age; anaesthetic used; any medications given; duration of labour and time of rupture of membranes; whether labour was induced or augmented; type of birth and repair; blood type and Rh status; group B streptococcus status; status of rubella **immunity**; syphilis and hepatitis serology test results (if positive); intravenous infusion of any fluids; physiological status since birth; description of **fundus**, **lochia**, bladder, and perineum; sex and weight of infant; time of birth; name of the newborn's care provider; chosen method of feeding; any abnormalities noted; and assessment of initial parent–infant interactions.

Most of this information is also documented for the nursing staff in the newborn nursery if the infant is transferred to that unit, although most newborns are cared for by the same nurse and in the same room as their mother (combined care). Most newborn nurseries in Canada are for infants that need more intensive nursing care. In addition, specific information should be provided regarding the infant's Apgar scores (see Chapter 25), weight, voiding, and stooling and whether the infant has been to the breast or formula fed. Nursing interventions that have been completed (e.g., eye prophylaxis and vitamin K injection) also must be recorded. Table 21-1 gives examples for documenting this information before the transfer of the woman from the recovery area.

Postpartum Care

The trend of shortened hospital stays is based largely on the view of childbirth as a healthy event and on efforts to reduce health care costs, coupled with consumer demands to have less medical intervention and more family-focused experiences (Box 21-1). Women who give birth may go home within a few hours, after the woman's and infant's conditions are stable and if the mother has appropriate support.

Criteria for Discharge

Early discharge can be a safe and satisfying option for women and their families when it is comprehensive and based on individual needs using a family-centred approach to care (Canadian Paediatric Society and Society of Obstetricians and Gynaecologists of Canada, 1996). Hospital stays do need to be long enough, however, to identify problems and ensure that the woman is sufficiently recovered and prepared to care for herself and the baby at home.

Table 21-1 Recovery Nurse's Report

ITEM	EXAMPLE OF DOCUMENTATION OF MOTHER	EXAMPLE OF DOCUMENTATION OF NEWBORN
Type of labour and birth; unusual observations, if any, of the placenta	Spontaneous or assisted (forceps, vacuum extraction) vaginal birth; vertex presentation; time of ROM	Spontaneous or assisted (forceps) vaginal birth; vertex presentation; time of ROM
GTPAL, age	G1-T0-P0-A0-L0, age 22 yr; 39 wk of gestation	G1-T0-P0-A0-L0, age 22 yr; 39 wk of gestation
Anaesthesia and analgesia used	None; epidural, low spinal, local	None; epidural, low spinal, local
Condition of perineum	Episiotomy; lacerations; intact	
Events since birth	Vital signs, BP, fundus, lochia, intake and output, medications (dosage, time of administration, and results); response to newborn; observation of family interactions, including siblings, if present	Vital signs, blood glucose level (if assessed), nursed at breast for ____ min Voided × 1; meconium stool × 1 Eye prophylaxis given Vitamin K injection given Held by siblings who are happy (or have other response to newborn)
Condition and sex of newborn; other information	Time of birth; weight; whether breastfeeding or bottle-feeding; sex of the baby	Time of birth; Apgar at 1 and 5 min; sex; weight; name of health care provider; breastfeeding or bottle feeding; mother's hepatitis B status and GBS status; whether mother received magnesium sulphate; time of last systemic analgesia
Relevant information from prenatal record	Need for rubella vaccination; presence of infections; hepatitis B status; HIV status; blood type; Rh status; GBS status and treatment if positive	Unremarkable pregnancy
Miscellaneous information: IV drip	If IV drip is infusing, rate of infusion, medications added (e.g., oxytocin), whether to keep open or discontinue after completion of bag that is hung	
Social factors	If woman is releasing baby for adoption, whether she wants to see baby, breastfeed, or allow visitors, or other preferences she may have	Baby up for adoption; to stay in NBN until discharge

BP, blood pressure; *GBS,* group B streptococcus; *HIV,* human immunodeficiency virus; *IV,* intravenous; *NBN,* newborn nursery; *ROM,* rupture of membranes.

BOX 21-1 Advantages and Disadvantages of Early Postpartum Discharge

Advantages

- Reinforces the concept of childbirth as a normal physiological event
- Allows shorter separations between mothers and other children
- Extends a couple's sense of control and participation beyond the birth itself
- Capitalizes on the security of the home environment during the stressors of early parenting
- Decreases unnecessary exposure to the pathogens in the hospital environment
- Allows beds on the maternity service to be used more effectively (i.e., quick turnover in patients or greater availability for patients with a complication)
- Allows more time for the mother, father or partner, infant, and other family members to bond
- Creates less disruption in the daily life of the family
- Promotes active involvement of the family and support persons in assisting the mother and newborn

Disadvantages

- Complications (maternal or newborn) may go unrecognized.
- Families may be or feel unprepared for the reality they face once the baby is at home.
- The mother is fatigued from the labour and childbirth process.
- The mother is experiencing postpartum pain or discomfort.
- The length of time for learning after the birth in the hospital setting is decreased.

It is essential that nurses consider the medical needs of the woman and her baby and provide care that is coordinated to meet those needs, with timely physiological interventions and treatment to prevent morbidity and hospital readmission. With predetermined criteria for identifying low risk in mothers and newborns (Box 21-2), the length of hospitalization can be based on medical need for care in an acute care setting or in consideration of ongoing care needed in the home environment (see Evidence-Informed Practice box). Community-based postpartum care programs are key to reducing readmission of newborns. Mothers should be contacted and, if needed, seen by a skilled caregiver within 24 to 48 hours after discharge to ensure that newborn health issues are identified (e.g., jaundice, dehydration).

Hospital-based maternity nurses continue to play invaluable roles as caregivers, teachers, and patient and family advocates in developing and implementing effective home care strategies. Postpartum order sets and maternal–newborn teaching checklists (Fig. 21-1) can be used to accomplish patient care and educational outcomes. With coordination, clinical care and education can be planned and provided throughout pregnancy, during the hospital stay, and in the home after discharge to ensure the family's continued well-being.

LEGAL TIP Early Discharge. Whether or not the woman and her family have chosen early discharge, the nurse and the primary health care provider are responsible for ensuring that the woman is not discharged before her condition has stabilized within normal limits.

Nursing Care Management—Physical Needs

The nursing plan of care includes both the postpartum woman and her infant, even if the nursery nurse retains primary responsibility for the infant (see Nursing Process box). In most hospitals in Canada, combined care (also called mother-baby care or single-room maternity care) is practiced. Nurses in these settings have been educated in both mother and infant care and function as primary nurses for the mother and infant.

BOX 21-2 Criteria for Discharge

Mother

Care of perineum is assured.

There are no intrapartum or postpartum complications that require ongoing treatment or observation.

The mother is mobile with adequate pain control.

Bladder and bowel functions are adequate (although she will probably not have had a bowel movement).

The mother has received Rh immune globulin, if appropriate.

The mother has demonstrated ability to feed the infant; i.e., the infant has demonstrated adequate latch.

Contraception advice has been provided.

The care provider for ongoing care has been identified and notified of discharge.

The community liaison nurse is aware of early discharge and has access to the patient's contact information for post-discharge follow-up.

The family is accessible for follow-up and the mother understands the necessity for and timing of newborn health checks.

If the home environment is not adequate, community resources are in place to support the new mother and infant.

The mother is aware of community resources and how and when to access these resources.

The mother has received Rubella immunization if she is not immune.

Infant

The infant is a term infant (37 to 42 weeks) with weight appropriate for gestational age.

There is normal cardiorespiratory adaptation to extrauterine life.

Temperature, respirations, and heart rate are within normal limits and stable. At least two successful feedings have been completed (normal sucking and swallowing).

Urination and stooling have occurred at least once.

There is no evidence of significant jaundice in the first 24 hours after the birth.

There is no evidence of sepsis.

There is no evidence of bleeding from circumcision for ≥2 hours (if procedure is performed prior to discharge).

Metabolic screening tests have been performed according to provincial policies; tests should be repeated at the follow-up visit if done before the infant is 24 hours old.

Newborn hearing screening test is completed prior to discharge; if not, alternative arrangements have been made for testing.

The mother is able to provide newborn care and recognizes signs of illness or concerns related to her newborn.

Arrangements have been made for assessment and evaluation of the mother and newborn within 48 hours of discharge, i.e., with a public health nurse, physician, or midwife.

The care provider responsible for continuing care is identified and arrangements have been made for a follow-up visit within 1 week of discharge.

Initial hepatitis B vaccine has been given or scheduled for the first follow-up visit if required by provincial legislation.

(Source: Canadian Paediatric Society and the Society of Obstetricians and Gynaecologists of Canada [1996]. Early discharge and length of stay for term birth. *Journal of Obstetrics and Gynaecology Canada, 18*, 1281–1285; Cargill, Y., et al. [2007]. SOGC policy statement: Postpartum maternal and newborn discharge. *Journal of Obstetrics and Gynaecology Canada, 29*[4], 357–359. Retrieved from http://www.sogc.org/guidelines/documents/190E-PS-April2007.pdf.)

EVIDENCE-INFORMED PRACTICE How Soon Is Too Soon? Early Discharge After Birth —*Pat Gingrich*

Ask the Question

What are the risks and benefits of early postpartum discharge for mother and baby? What do women want from their postpartum hospital experience?

Search for Evidence

Search Strategies

Professional organization guidelines, meta-analyses, systematic reviews, randomized controlled trials, nonrandomized prospective studies, and retrospective studies since 2006

Databases Searched

CINAHL; Cochrane; Medline; National Guideline Clearinghouse; TRIP Database Plus; and the Web sites for the Association of Women's Health, Obstetric and Neonatal Nurses (AWHONN), Society of Obstetricians and Gynaecologists of Canada (SOGC), and National Institute for Clinical Excellence (NICE)

Critically Analyze the Evidence

The optimum length of postpartum hospitalization has been debated for decades. After a period of shortened stays in the early 1990s, which critics dubbed "drive-through deliveries," research demonstrated an increase in infant problems and readmissions. Length of hospital stay after giving birth depends on many factors: the physical condition of the mother and baby, social support at home, patient education needs for self-care and infant care, and mental and emotional status of the mother.

Women who greatly prefer to go home will probably do better there. The professional recommendation by the National Institute for Health and Clinical Excellence (2011) supports early discharge at 24 hours after vaginal or Caesarean birth as long as there is neither fever nor complications and there will be close follow-up. According to a survey of 2583 Canadian women, effective follow-up such as an office or home visit or telephone contact with a health care provider within 72 hours of discharge significantly decreased infant readmissions and maternal postpartum depression (Goulet, D'Amour, & Pineault, 2007).

According to the professional guidelines published by the SOGC, the risk with early discharge is mainly to the infant, who may develop jaundice, infection, unrecognized heart or respiratory problems, or feeding problems (Cargill et al., 2007). The rate of emergency department visits and readmissions is higher for infants of young, primiparous, unmarried mothers.

Implications for Practice

In an ongoing population-based survey of 16,000 U.S. women, a qualitative analysis found some major themes for postpartum concerns of the women 2 to 9 months after birth: the need for social support, breastfeeding issues, newborn care, postpartum depression, and the perceived need to extend the hospital stay (Kanotra et al., 2007). Nurses have the most opportunity to assess the physical, psychological, and social well-being of their patients. Postpartum women deserve individualized patient education that includes comprehensive information and resources about infant care, breastfeeding, and postpartum depression. Educational information should be offered in many formats and include hands-on demonstrations. Written material should include 24-hour numbers to call for problems with infant care and breastfeeding and contact information for community parenting groups. All patients should go home with a realistic expectation of the social and financial support they will need. Finally, nurses can advocate for policies that support flexible lengths of hospital stays and programs recommended by the SOGC (i.e., early home visits, outpatient breastfeeding clinics, and early physician visits) (Cargill et al., 2007).

References

Cargill, Y., et al. (2007). SOGC clinical practice guideline: Postpartum maternal and newborn discharge. *Journal of Obstetrics and Gynaecology Canada, 29*(4), 357–359. Retrieved from http://www.sogc.org/guidelines/documents/190E-PS-April2007.pdf.

Goulet, L., D'Amour, D., & Pineault, R. (2007). Type and timing of services following postnatal discharge: Do they make a difference? *Womens Health, 45*(4), 19–39.

Kanotra, S., et al. (2007). Challenges faced by new mothers in the early postpartum period: An analysis of comment data from the 2000 Pregnancy Risk Assessment Monitoring System (PRAMS) survey. *Maternal and Child Health Journal, 11*(6), 549–558.

National Institute for Health and Clinical Excellence (2011). *Caesarean section, NICE Clinical Guideline 132*, London, NICE. Retrieved from http://www.nice.org.uk/nicemedia/live/13620/57163/57163.pdf.

Plan of Care and Implementation

Once the nursing diagnoses are formulated, the nurse will plan with the woman what nursing measures are appropriate and which ones are to be given priority. The nursing plan of care includes periodic assessments to detect deviations from normal physical changes, measures to relieve discomfort or pain, measures to prevent infection, and teaching and counselling designed to promote the woman's feelings of competence in self-management and baby care. Family members should be included in the teaching. The nurse needs to evaluate continuously and be ready to change the plan, if indicated. Almost all hospitals use standardized care plans or care maps as a base. The nurse's adaptation of the standardized plan to meet specific medical and nursing diagnoses results in individualized patient care (see Nursing Care Plan). Signs of potential problems that may be identified during the assessment process are listed in Box 21-3.

Nurses assume many roles while implementing the nursing plan of care. They provide direct physical care, teach mother and baby care, and provide **anticipatory guidance** and counselling. Perhaps most important, they nurture the woman by providing encouragement and support as she begins to assume the many tasks of motherhood. Nurses who take the time to "mother the mother" do much to increase feelings of self-confidence in new mothers.

The first step in providing individualized care is to confirm the woman's identity by checking her wristband. At the same time, the infant's identification number is matched with the corresponding band on the mother's wrist and, in some instances, the partner's wrist. The nurse should determine how the mother wishes to be addressed and note her preference in her record and in her nursing care plan.

The woman and her family should be oriented to their surroundings. Familiarity with the unit, routines, resources, and

POSTPARTUM TEACHING RECORD

(Teaching to include all white areas and shaded area, if applicable)

Trillium Health Centre

MOTHER'S ID # ________________

STAGE	BREASTFEEDING	BOTTLE FEEDING *(If breastfeeding only, not applicable)*	MOTHER CARE	INFANT CARE	INFANT SAFETY
ADMISSION (0-6 hours)	☐ Positions ☐ Latch/Breaking latch ☐ Sucking/Swallowing ☐ Frequency/Duration ☐ Cues, demand feeding ☐ Colostrum/Milk production ☐ Breast and nipple care RN's initials: _____/_____ Interpreted by: _________ ☐ Mom declined *	☐ Frequency, demand feeding ☐ Amount ☐ Positioning ☐ Burping RN's initials: _____/_____ Interpreted by: _________ ☐ Mom declined *	☐ Peri-care ☐ Lochia ☐ Care of episiotomy (if applicable) ☐ Afterpains/Pain management RN's initials: _____/_____ Interpreted by: _______ ☐ Mom declined *		☐ Bed sharing ☐ Sleep patterns/ Positions/SIDS ☐ Staff ID badge ☐ Mucus/Choking RN's initials: ___/___ Interpreted by: _____ ☐ Mom declined *
ONGOING (6-18 hours)	☐ Hand expression ☐ Signs that infant is getting enough ☐ Supplementation guidelines **If applicable:** ☐ Breast pump ☐ Cup feeding ☐ Lactation aid RN's initials: _____/_____ Interpreted by: _________ ☐ Mom declined *		***FOR C/S MOTHER:*** ☐ Care of incision ☐ Gas pains **If applicable:** ☐ Hemorrhoids ☐ Iron (iron-rich foods/ supplementation) RN's initials: _____/_____ Interpreted by: _______ ☐ Mom declined *	***Bathing:*** ☐ Diapering/Genitalia care ☐ Bathing, skin care ☐ Umbilicus ☐ Nail care ☐ Skin characteristics ☐ Crying/Soothing techniques ☐ Dressing infant RN's initials: ____/___ Interpreted by: ______ ☐ Mom declined *	☐ Voiding patterns ☐ Bowel patterns ☐ Jaundice ☐ Temperature taking ☐ Choking/ Spitting up RN's initials: ___/___ Interpreted by: _____ ☐ Mom declined *
DISCHARGE (18 hours until discharge)	☐ Engorgement ☐ Blocked ducts RN's initials: _____/_____ Interpreted by: _________ ☐ Mom declined *	☐ Breast care, Engorgement ☐ Bottle sterilization, Formula preparation, Types of formula RN's initials: _____/_____ Interpreted by: _________ ☐ Mom declined *	☐ Nutrition/Bowel care ☐ Vitamins—prenatal ☐ P/P adjustment—emotions, depression ☐ P/P warning signs (infection, hemorrhage) ☐ Pain management RN's initials:_____/____ Interpreted by: _______ ☐ Mom declined *		☐ Dehydration RN's initials: ____/___ Interpreted by: ______ ☐ Mom declined *
TEACHING REINFORCED	NOTES :*	NOTES :*	NOTES :*	NOTES :*	NOTES :*
INFORMATION AND PRINTED MATERIAL	☐ ***ADMISSION PACK:*** ▪ Breastfeeding Your Baby ▪ Breastfeeding Resources ▪ Breastfeeding Menu ▪ Newborn Screening ▪ Child Tax Credit ▪ Birth Registration ▪ Infant Health Card Information ▪ Community Resources	▪ Jaundice ▪ Can Your Baby Hear ▪ Car Seat Pamphlets ▪ Postpartum Exercises ▪ When Babies Cry ▪ Never Shake a Baby ▪ SIDS ▪ Health Info & Wellness Centre	☐ ***DISCHARGE PACK:*** • Copy of Maternal & Newborn D/C Summary • Postpartum DVD • Book – Great Beginnings • Baby Blanket		

Fig. 21-1 Mother and family learning checklist. *C/S*, Caesarean section; *P/P*, postpartum; *, nursing note written. *(Courtesy of Trillium Health Centre.)*

NURSING PROCESS: PHYSICAL NEEDS

Assessment

A focused physical assessment is performed on admission to the postpartum unit. If vital signs are within normal limits, assessment continues every 4 to 8 hours or as per unit protocol.

Interview (by postpartum nurse)
Mother's emotional status and energy level
Degree of physical discomfort, hunger, and thirst
Knowledge level concerning self-care and infant care

Physical Examination (BUBBLESS)

B = **Breasts** (firmness) and nipples (intact/erect)
U = **Uterine** fundus (location; consistency)
B = **Bladder** function (amount; frequency)
B = **Bowel** function (passing gas or bowel movement)
L = **Lochia** (amount; colour)
E = **Episiotomy or laceration** (perineum: discomfort; condition of repair [if done])
S = **Swelling** (legs: edema)
S = **(Ps)ychosocial Status** (see discussion later in chapter)
Intake and output if an intravenous infusion or a urinary catheter is in place
Dressing or incision if birth by Caesarean

Review of Results of Laboratory Tests

Postpartum hemoglobin and hematocrit (if ordered)
Rubella and Rh (if status is unknown)

Nursing Diagnoses

Examples of nursing diagnoses commonly established for the postpartum patient include the following:

Risk for deficient fluid volume (hemorrhage) related to
- uterine atony after childbirth

Urinary retention or constipation related to
- postchildbirth discomfort
- childbirth trauma to tissues
- decreased intake of fluids and solid foods (constipation only)

Acute pain related to
- uterine involution
- episiotomy or lacerations
- hemorrhoids
- engorged breasts

Disturbed sleep pattern related to
- discomforts of postpartum period
- long labour process
- infant care and hospital routine

Difficulty breastfeeding related to
- maternal discomfort
- infant positioning

Planning

The nursing plan of care includes both the postpartum woman and her infant. The organization of the mother's care must take the newborn into consideration. The day actually revolves around the baby's feeding and care times.

Expected outcomes for the postpartum period are based on the nursing diagnoses identified for the individual patient. Examples of common expected outcomes for physiological needs are that the woman will do the following:

- Remain free from infection
- Demonstrate normal involution and lochial characteristics
- Remain comfortable
- Demonstrate normal bladder and bowel patterns
- Demonstrate knowledge of breast care, whether breastfeeding or bottle-feeding
- Integrate the newborn into the family

Interventions

Provide direct care (e.g., administer analgesics, assist with ambulation, administer intravenous fluids, assist with personal hygiene, provide perineal care, change dressing).
Teach mother-baby care.
Provide anticipatory guidance and counselling.
Provide encouragement and support.
Teach mother to check the identity of anyone who cares for the baby.
Additional interventions are discussed in the text.

Evaluation

The nurse can be reasonably assured that care was effective when the expected outcomes of care for physical needs have been achieved.

BOX 21-3 Signs of Potential Physiological Complications

Temperature—More than 38°C after the first 24 hours
Pulse—Tachycardia or marked bradycardia
Blood pressure—Hypotension or hypertension
Energy level—Lethargy; extreme fatigue
Uterus—Deviated from the midline; boggy consistency; remains above the umbilicus after 24 hours
Lochia—Heavy, foul odour; bright red bleeding that is not lochia
Perineum—Pronounced edema; not intact; signs of infection; marked discomfort
Legs—Painful, reddened area; warmth on posterior aspect of calf
Breasts—Redness, heat, pain; cracked and fissured nipples; inverted nipples; palpable mass
Appetite—Lack of appetite
Elimination—Urine: inability to void, urgency, frequency, dysuria; bowel: constipation, diarrhea
Rest—Inability to rest or sleep

NURSING CARE PLAN • Postpartum Care—Vaginal Birth

Nursing Diagnosis: Risk for deficient fluid volume related to uterine atony/hemorrhage

Expected Outcomes

Fundus is firm, lochia is moderate, and there is no evidence of hemorrhage.

Nursing Interventions/*Rationales*

Monitor lochia (colour, amount, consistency) and count and weigh sanitary pads if lochia is heavy *to evaluate amount of bleeding.*

Monitor and palpate fundus for location and tone to determine status of uterus and dictate further interventions *because atonic uterus is the most common cause of postpartum hemorrhage.*

Monitor intake and output, assess for bladder fullness, and encourage voiding *because a full bladder interferes with involution of the uterus.*

Monitor vital signs (increased pulse and respirations, decreased blood pressure) and skin temperature and colour *to detect signs of hemorrhage/shock*.

Monitor postpartum hematology studies (if ordered) *to assess effects of blood loss.*

If fundus is boggy, apply gentle massage and assess tone response *to promote uterine contractions and increase uterine tone.* (Do not overstimulate because doing so can cause fundal relaxation.)

Express uterine clots *to promote uterine contraction*.

Explain to the woman the process of involution and teach her to assess and massage the fundus and report any persistent bogginess *to involve her in self-management and increase her sense of self-control.*

Administer oxytocic medications per health care provider's order and evaluate effectiveness *to promote continuing uterine contraction.*

Administer fluids, blood, blood products, or plasma expanders as ordered *to replace lost fluid and lost blood volume.*

Nursing Diagnosis: Acute pain related to postpartum physiological changes (hemorrhoids, episiotomy or laceration, breast engorgement, cracked/sore nipples)

Expected Outcome

Woman exhibits signs of decreased discomfort.

Nursing Interventions/*Rationales*

Assess location, type, and quality of pain *to direct intervention*.

Explain to woman the source and reasons for the pain, its expected duration, and treatments *to decrease anxiety and increase her sense of control.*

Administer prescribed pain medications *to provide pain relief.*

If pain is perineal (episiotomy, hemorrhoids), apply ice packs in the first 24 hours *to reduce edema and vulvar irritation and to reduce discomfort*; encourage sitz baths using cool water the first 24 hours *to reduce edema* and warm water thereafter *to promote circulation*; apply witch hazel compresses *to reduce edema*; teach woman to use prescribed perineal creams, sprays, or ointments *to depress response of peripheral nerves*; teach woman to tighten buttocks before sitting and to sit on flat, hard surfaces *to compress buttocks and reduce pressure on the perineum.* (Avoid donut and soft pillows because they separate the buttocks and decrease venous blood flow, increasing pain.)

If pain is from breasts and woman is breastfeeding, encourage use of a supportive bra *to increase comfort*; ascertain that infant has latched on correctly *to prevent nipple soreness*; vary infant position during feeding *to prevent nipple soreness.*

If breasts are engorged, have woman use cold compresses between feeding and warm compresses or take a warm shower before breastfeeding *to stimulate milk flow and relieve stasis.*

If nipples are sore, have woman air-dry nipples after feeding; apply expressed breastmilk or breast creams as prescribed *to soften nipples and relieve irritation, assess newborn latch.*

If pain is from breasts and the woman is not breastfeeding, encourage use of a tight supportive bra or breast binder, as well as application of ice packs or cold cabbage leaves *to reduce lactation and decrease heaviness.*

Nursing Diagnosis: Disturbed sleep pattern related to excitement, discomfort, and environmental interruptions

Expected Outcome

Woman sleeps for uninterrupted periods of time and feels rested after waking and has realistic expectations regarding the amount of sleep she will get when caring for a newborn.

Nursing Interventions/*Rationales*

Establish woman's routine sleep patterns and compare with current sleep pattern, exploring her expectations of the amount of sleep she will get as well as things that interfere with sleep *to determine the scope of the problem and direct interventions.*

Individualize nursing routines to fit woman's natural body rhythms (i.e., wake–sleep cycles); provide a sleep-promoting environment (i.e., darkness, quiet, adequate ventilation, appropriate room temperature); prepare woman for sleep using woman's usual routines (i.e., back rub, soothing music, warm milk); teach use of guided imagery and relaxation techniques *to promote optimum conditions for sleep.*

Avoid things or routines (i.e., caffeine, foods that induce heartburn, fluids, strenuous mental or physical activity) *that may interfere with sleep*.

Administer pain medication as prescribed *to enhance quality of sleep.*

Advise woman and her partner to limit visitors and activities *to avoid further taxation and fatigue*.

Teach woman to use infant's nap time as a time for her also *to nap and replenish energy and decrease fatigue.*

Nursing Diagnosis: Risk for impaired urinary elimination related to perineal trauma and effects of anaesthesia

Expected Outcomes

Woman will void within 6 to 8 hours after birth and empty bladder completely.

Nursing Interventions/*Rationales*

Assess position and character of uterine fundus and bladder *to ascertain if any further interventions are indicated because of displacement of the fundus or distension of the bladder.*

Measure intake and output *to assess any evidence of dehydration and subsequent decreased anticipated urine output.*

Encourage voiding by walking woman to the bathroom, running water over perineum, running water in sink, and providing privacy *to encourage voiding.*

Encourage oral intake *to replace any fluids lost during birth and to prevent dehydration.*

Catheterize as necessary with indwelling or straight method *to ensure bladder emptying and allow uterine involution.*

personnel reduces one potential source of anxiety: the unknown. The mother is reassured through knowing whom and how she can call for assistance and what she can expect in the way of supplies and services. If the woman's usual daily routine before admission differs from the routine of the facility, the nurse should work with the woman to develop a mutually acceptable routine.

While infant abduction from hospitals in Canada is rare, hospital staff should be alert and prepared for such an event. The mother should be taught to check the identity of any person who comes to remove the baby from her room. Hospital personnel wear picture identification badges. On some units all staff members wear matching scrubs or special badges. Other units use closed-circuit television, computer monitoring systems, or fingerprint identification pads. Patients and nurses must work together to ensure the safety of newborns in the hospital environment.

Prevention of Infection

One important means of preventing infection is maintenance of a clean environment. Bed linens should be changed as needed. Disposable pads should be changed frequently. Women should wear slippers when walking about to avoid contaminating the linens when they return to bed. Personnel must be conscientious about their **hand hygiene** to prevent cross-infection. Routine precautions must be practiced. Staff members with colds, coughs, or skin infections (e.g., a cold sore on the lips [herpes simplex virus type I]) must follow hospital protocol when in contact with postpartum patients. In many hospitals, staff with open herpetic lesions, strep throat, conjunctivitis, upper respiratory infections, or diarrhea are encouraged to avoid contact with mothers and infants by staying home until the condition is no longer contagious.

Proper care of the **episiotomy** site and any perineal lacerations prevents infection in the genitourinary area and aids the healing process. Educating the woman to wipe from front to back (urethra to anus) after voiding or defecating is a simple first step. In many hospitals, a squeeze bottle (peri bottle) filled with warm water or an antiseptic solution is used after each voiding to cleanse the perineal area (Box 21-4). The woman should change her perineal pad from front to back each time she voids or defecates and wash her hands thoroughly before and after doing so.

Prevention of Excessive Bleeding

The most frequent cause of excessive bleeding after childbirth is uterine **atony**, or failure of the uterine muscle to contract firmly. The two most important interventions for preventing excessive bleeding are maintaining good uterine tone and preventing bladder distension. If uterine atony occurs, the relaxed uterus distends with blood and clots, blood vessels in the placental site are not clamped off, and excessive bleeding results.

BOX 21-4 Interventions for Episiotomy, Lacerations, and Hemorrhoids

Explain both the procedure and rationale before implementation.

Cleansing

Teach the woman to:

- Wash hands before and after cleansing perineum and changing pads.
- Wash perineum with mild soap and warm water at least once daily.
- Cleanse from symphysis pubis to anal area.
- Apply peripad from front to back, protecting inner surface of pad from contamination.
- Wrap soiled pad and place in covered waste container.
- Change pad with each void or defecation or at least four times per day.
- Assess amount and character of lochia with each pad change.

Ice Pack (for First 24 Hours)

Apply a covered ice pack to perineum from front to back:

- During first 2 hours to decrease edema formation and to increase comfort
- After the first 2 hours following the birth to provide anaesthetic effect

Squeeze Bottle (Peri Bottle)

Demonstrate for woman and assist her; explain rationale.

Fill bottle with tap water warmed to approximately 38°C (comfortably warm on the wrist).

Instruct woman to position nozzle between her legs so that squirts of water reach perineum as she sits on toilet seat. Explain that it will take the whole bottle of water to cleanse the perineum.

Remind her to blot dry with toilet paper or clean wipes.

Remind her to avoid contamination from anal area.

Apply clean pad.

Sitz Bath: Disposable

Encourage woman to use at least twice a day for 20 minutes, if required.

Place call bell within easy reach.

Clamp tubing and fill bag with warm water.

Raise toilet seat and place bath in bowl with overflow opening directed toward back of toilet.

Place container above toilet bowl.

Attach tube into groove at front of bath.

Loosen tube clamp to regulate rate of flow; fill bath to about one-half full.

Teach woman to sit on sitz bath by first tightening gluteal muscles and keeping them tightened and then relaxing them after she is on the sitz bath.

Place dry towels within reach.

Ensure privacy.

Check woman in 15 minutes.

Topical Applications

Apply anaesthetic cream or spray: use sparingly three to four times per day, if required.

Offer witch hazel pads (Tucks) for after voiding or defecating; woman pats perineum dry from front to back and then applies witch hazel pads.

Excessive blood loss after childbirth can also be caused by vaginal or vulvar hematomas, unrepaired lacerations of the vagina or cervix, and retained placental fragments.

NURSING ALERT A perineal pad saturated in 15 minutes or less or pooling of blood under the buttocks is an indication of excessive blood loss requiring immediate assessment, intervention, and notification of the primary health care provider.

Accurate visual estimation of blood loss is an important nursing responsibility. Blood loss is usually described subjectively as scant, light, moderate, or heavy (profuse). Fig. 21-2 shows examples of perineal pad saturation corresponding to each of these descriptions.

Although postpartal blood loss may be estimated by observing the amount of staining on a perineal pad, it is difficult to judge the amount of lochial flow based only on observation of perineal pads. More objective estimates of blood loss include measuring serial hemoglobin or hematocrit values, weighing blood clots and items saturated with blood (1 g equals 1 mL), and establishing the millilitres it takes to saturate perineal pads being used.

Any estimation of lochial flow is inaccurate and incomplete without consideration of the time factor. The woman who saturates a perineal pad in 1 hour or less is bleeding much more heavily than the woman who saturates a perineal pad in 8 hours.

Nurses tend to overestimate rather than underestimate blood loss. Also, different brands of perineal pads vary in their saturation volume and soaking appearance. For example, blood placed on some brands tends to soak down into the pad, whereas on other brands it tends to spread outward. Nurses should determine saturation volume and soaking appearance for the perineal pad brands used in their institution to improve accuracy of blood loss estimation.

NURSING ALERT The nurse should always check under the mother's buttocks as well as on the perineal pad. Blood may flow between the buttocks onto the linens under the mother, although the amount on the perineal pad is slight; thus, excessive bleeding goes undetected.

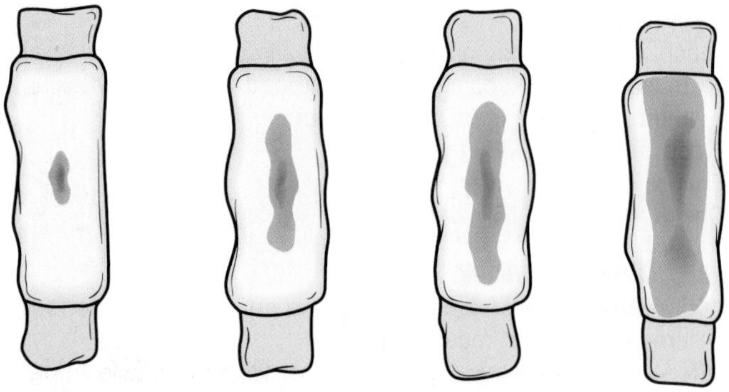

Fig. 21-2 Blood loss after birth is assessed by the extent of perineal pad saturation as (from left to right) scant; light; moderate; or heavy (one pad saturated within 2 hours).

Blood pressure is not a reliable indicator of impending **shock** from early hemorrhage. More sensitive means of identifying shock are provided by respirations, pulse, skin condition, and urinary output. The frequent physical assessments performed during the fourth stage of labour (see Box 18-11, p. 484) are designed to provide prompt identification of excessive bleeding (see Emergency box).

Maintenance of Uterine Tone

A major intervention to restore good tone is stimulation, by gently massaging the uterine fundus until firm (Fig. 21-3). Fundal massage can cause a temporary increase in the amount of vaginal bleeding seen as pooled blood leaves the uterus. Clots can be expelled. The uterus may remain boggy even after massage and expulsion of clots.

Fundal massage is a very uncomfortable procedure. Communicating the causes and dangers of uterine atony and the purpose of fundal massage to the woman can help her cooperate in the procedure. Teaching the woman to massage her own

EMERGENCY

Hypovolemic Shock

Signs and Symptoms

Persistent significant bleeding—perineal pad is soaked within 15 minutes; may not be accompanied by a change in vital signs or maternal colour or behavior.
Woman states she feels weak, light-headed, "funny," or "sick to my stomach" or "sees stars."
Woman begins to act anxious or exhibits air hunger.
Woman's skin turns ashen or greyish.
Skin feels cool and clammy.
Pulse rate increases.
Blood pressure declines.

Interventions

Notify primary health care provider.
If uterus is atonic, massage gently and expel clots to cause uterus to contract; compress uterus manually as needed, using two hands. Add oxytocic medication to IV drip as ordered.
Give oxygen by nonrebreather face mask or nasal prongs at 10 L/min.
Tilt woman to her side or elevate the right hip; elevate her legs to at least a 30-degree angle.
Provide additional or maintain existing IV infusion of lactated Ringer's solution or normal saline solution to restore circulatory volume.
Administer blood or blood products as ordered.
Monitor vital signs.
Insert an indwelling urinary catheter to monitor perfusion of kidneys.
Administer emergency medications as ordered.
Prepare for possible surgery or other emergency treatments or procedures.
Chart incident, medical and nursing interventions instituted, and results of treatments.

IV, intravenous.

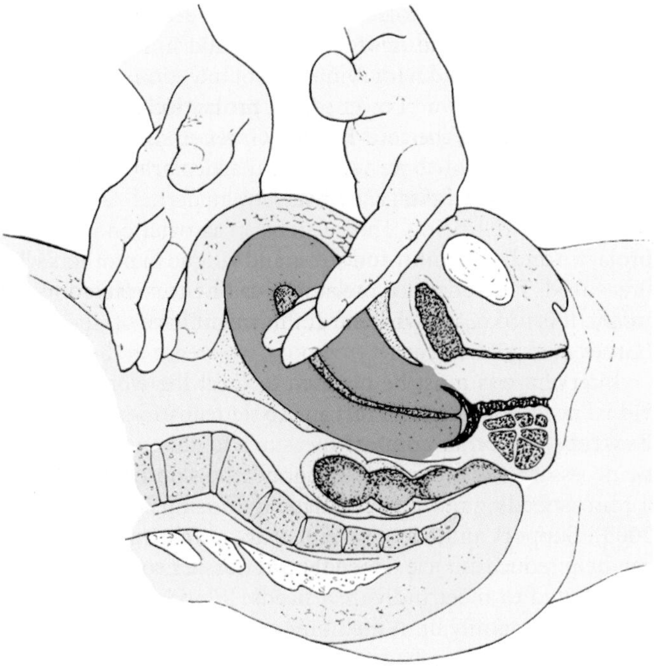

Fig. 21-3 Palpating and massaging fundus of uterus. Note that upper hand is cupped over fundus; lower hand dips in above symphysis pubis and supports the uterus while it is massaged gently.

fundus enables her to maintain some control and can decrease her anxiety.

Additional interventions likely to be used are administration of intravenous fluids and oxytocic medications (drugs that stimulate contraction of the uterine smooth muscle). See the Medication Guide (p. 583) for information about common oxytocic medications.

Prevention of Bladder Distension

A full bladder causes the uterus to be displaced above the umbilicus and usually to the right of the midline in the abdomen. It also prevents the uterus from contracting normally. Nursing interventions focus on helping the woman empty her bladder spontaneously as soon as possible. The first priority is to assist the woman to the bathroom or onto a bedpan if she is unable to ambulate. Having the woman listen to running water, placing her hands in warm water, or pouring water from a squeeze bottle over her perineum may stimulate voiding. Assisting the woman into the shower or sitz bath and encouraging her to void can be effective. Administering analgesics, if ordered, may be indicated because some women anticipate pain and thus fear voiding. If these measures are unsuccessful, a sterile catheter can be inserted to drain the urine.

Promotion of Comfort

Most women experience some degree of discomfort during the postpartum period. Common causes of discomfort include afterbirth pains (**afterpains**), episiotomy or perineal lacerations, hemorrhoids, and breast engorgement. The woman's description of the type and severity of her pain is the best guide in choosing an appropriate intervention. To confirm the location and extent of discomfort, the nurse needs to inspect and palpate areas of pain, as appropriate, for redness, swelling, discharge, and heat and observe for body tension, guarded movements, and facial tension. Blood pressure, pulse, and respirations may be elevated in response to acute pain. Diaphoresis may accompany severe pain. A lack of objective signs does not necessarily mean there is no pain because there may also be a cultural component to the expression of pain. Nursing interventions are intended to eliminate the pain sensation entirely or reduce it to a tolerable level that allows the woman to care for herself and her baby. Nurses may use both nonpharmacological and pharmacological interventions to promote comfort. Pain relief is enhanced by using more than one method or route.

Nonpharmacological Interventions

Warmth, distraction, deep breathing, imagery, therapeutic touch, relaxation, and interaction with the infant may decrease the discomfort associated with afterbirth pains. Simple interventions that can decrease the discomfort associated with an episiotomy or perineal lacerations include encouraging the woman to lie on her side whenever possible and to use a pillow when sitting. Other interventions include application of an ice pack (during first 24 hours); topical application (if ordered); cleansing with a squeeze bottle; and a cleansing shower, tub bath, or sitz bath. Many of these interventions, especially ice packs, sitz baths, and topical applications (such as witch hazel pads), are also effective for hemorrhoids. Box 21-4 gives more specific information about these interventions.

The discomfort associated with engorged breasts may be lessened by applying ice, heat, or cold cabbage leaves to the breasts and wearing a well-fitted support bra. Decisions about specific interventions for relieving engorgement are based on whether the woman chooses breastfeeding or bottle-feeding (see Chapter 26).

Pharmacological Interventions

Most health care providers routinely order a variety of analgesics to be administered as needed. These include both **opioid** (narcotic) and nonopioid (non-narcotic) (e.g., nonsteroidal anti-inflammatory drugs [NSAIDs]) choices, with their dosage and time frequency ranges. Topical application of antiseptic or anaesthetic ointments or sprays is a common pharmacological intervention for perineal pain. Patient-controlled analgesia pumps and epidural analgesia are technologies commonly used to provide pain relief after Caesarean birth.

NURSING ALERT The nurse should carefully monitor all women receiving opioids because respiratory depression and decreased intestinal motility are adverse effects. Breastfeeding mothers may be advised to restrict their use of codeine-based analgesics because of concerns of ultra-rapid metabolizing of codeine into morphine in some women. The high levels of morphine are transferred to the breastfeeding infant and may result in morphine overdose (U.S. Food and Drug Administration, 2007).

Many women want to participate in decisions about analgesia. If an analgesic is to be given, the nurse must, in conjunction with the mother, make a clinical judgement of the type, dosage, and frequency from the medications ordered. The woman should be informed of the prescribed analgesic and its common adverse effects; this teaching should be documented.

Breastfeeding mothers often have concerns about the effects of an analgesic on the infant. Although nearly all medications present in maternal circulation are also found in breast milk, many analgesics commonly used during the postpartum period are considered relatively safe for breastfeeding mothers. Often the timing of medications can be adjusted to minimize infant exposure. A mother may be given pain medication immediately after breastfeeding so that the interval between medication administration and the next nursing period is as long as possible. The decision to administer medications of any type to a breastfeeding mother must always be made by carefully weighing the woman's need against actual or potential risks to the infant.

If acceptable pain relief has not been obtained in 1 hour and there has been no change in the initial assessment, the nurse can contact the primary care provider for additional pain relief orders or further directions. Unrelieved pain results in fatigue, anxiety, and a worsening perception of the pain. It can also indicate the presence of a previously unidentified or untreated problem.

Promotion of Rest

The excitement and exhilaration experienced after the birth of the infant can make rest difficult. The new mother who is anxious about her ability to care for her infant or is uncomfortable may also have difficulty sleeping. The demands of the infant, the hospital environment and routines, and the frequent presence of visitors contribute to alterations in her sleep pattern (see Critical Thinking Exercise).

Fatigue is common in the postpartum period (Groër et al., 2005; Troy, 2003) and involves physiological components associated with long labours, Caesarean birth, anemia, and breastfeeding; psychological components related to depression and anxiety; and neuroendocrine and immune components. It is associated with symptoms of infection, postpartum stress, and depression. Lower serum **prolactin** levels are associated with depression and fatigue (Groër et al., 2005). Infant behaviour can contribute to fatigue, particularly for mothers of more difficult infants. Conversely, maternal fatigue can affect infant well-being. There can be an association with milk prolactin and melatonin and stress and fatigue in mothers who breastfeed. Prolactin and melatonin can be transferred to the infant. It is unknown what effect this might have on the infant (Groër et al., 2005).

Interventions must be planned to meet the woman's individual needs for sleep and rest and to set realistic expectations. Backrubs and other comfort measures to enhance sleep may be necessary for the first few nights. The side-lying position for breastfeeding minimizes fatigue in nursing mothers (Troy, 2003). Support and encouragement of mothering behaviours can help reduce anxiety. Hospital and nursing routines should be adjusted to meet individual needs. In addition, the nurse can help the family limit the number of visitors and provide a comfortable chair or bed for the partner. Because milk contains high levels of melatonin (which induces sleep) at night and is not detectable during the day, fatigued mothers who pump their milk might use morning milk to feed in the morning and evening milk to feed in the evening (Arendt, 2005; Groër et al., 2005).

CRITICAL THINKING EXERCISE

Fatigue and Rest After Childbirth

Patricia gave birth to her third baby; she has two children at home, ages 3 years and 18 months. Her husband travels frequently with his job. She is breastfeeding the baby without difficulty but is concerned about how she will care for all three of her children, stating, "I remember how tired I was after my last baby. I'm not sure I can manage with three children since my husband is gone so much. Do you have any suggestions to help me?"

1. Evidence—Is there sufficient evidence to draw conclusions about whether support would be helpful for Patricia?
2. Assumptions—What assumptions can be made about the following factors?
   a. The relation between breastfeeding and fatigue
   b. Support in the postpartum period
   c. The role of sleep and rest in relation to fatigue and depression
   d. Spacing of pregnancies and fatigue
3. What implications and priorities for nursing care can be drawn at this time?
4. Does the evidence objectively support your conclusion?
5. Are there alternative perspectives to your conclusion?

Promotion of Ambulation

Early ambulation is successful in reducing the incidence of thromboembolism and promoting the woman's more rapid recovery of strength. Free movement should be encouraged once anaesthesia wears off, unless an analgesic has been administered. After the initial recovery period is over, the mother should be encouraged to ambulate frequently.

The rapid decrease in intra-abdominal pressure after birth results in a dilation of blood vessels supplying the intestines (splanchnic engorgement) and causes blood to pool in the viscera. This condition contributes to the development of orthostatic hypotension and can occur when the woman who has recently given birth sits or stands, first ambulates, or takes a warm shower or sitz bath. The nurse must consider the baseline blood pressure; amount of blood loss; and type, amount, and timing of analgesic or anaesthetic medications administered when assisting a woman to ambulate.

NURSING ALERT Having a hospital staff member present the first time the woman gets out of bed after birth is important because she can feel weak, dizzy, faint, or light-headed.

Prevention of clot formation is important. Women who must remain in bed after giving birth are at increased risk for the development of a **thrombus**. They may have antiembolic stockings (TED hose) or a sequential compression device (SCD boots) ordered prophylactically. If a woman remains in bed longer than 8 hours (e.g., for postpartum magnesium sulphate therapy for pre-eclampsia), exercise to promote circulation in the legs is indicated, using the following routine:

- Alternate flexion and extension of feet.
- Rotate ankles in circular motion.

- Alternate flexion and extension of legs.
- Press back of knee to bed surface; relax.

If the woman is susceptible to thromboembolism, she should be encouraged to walk about actively and discouraged from sitting immobile in a chair. Women with increased risk for thromboembolism include: obesity (BMI>40), unexpected Cesarean birth, age over 35 years, and venous thromboembolism during pregnancy. These women should be offered low molecular weight heparin during the postpartum period. The length of time required for the prophylaxis ranges from 7 days to 8 weeks and depends on the number of risk factors (Royal College of Obstetricians and Gynaecologists, 2009). Sequential compression stockings may also be necessary to reduce the risk of thromboembolism postpartum.

Women with varicosities are advised to wear support hose. If a thrombus is suspected, as evidenced by warmth, redness, or tenderness in the suspected leg, the primary health care provider should be notified immediately; meanwhile the woman should be confined to bed with the affected limb elevated on pillows.

Promotion of Exercise

Most women who have just given birth are interested in regaining their nonpregnant figures. Postpartum exercise can begin soon after birth, although the woman should be encouraged to start with simple exercises and gradually progress to more strenuous ones. Fig. 21-4 illustrates a number of exercises appropriate for the new mother. Abdominal exercises are postponed until about 4 weeks after Caesarean birth.

Kegel exercises to strengthen muscle tone are extremely important, particularly after vaginal birth. Kegel exercises help women regain the muscle tone that is often lost as pelvic tissues are stretched and torn during pregnancy and birth. Women who maintain muscle strength may benefit years later by maintaining urinary continence.

It is essential that women learn to perform Kegel exercises correctly (see Patient Teaching box in Chapter 4, p. 51). Approximately one fourth of all women who learn Kegel exercises do them incorrectly and may increase their risk of incontinence. This may occur when women inadvertently bear down on the pelvic floor muscles, thrusting the perineum outward. The woman's technique can be assessed during the pelvic examination at her checkup by inserting two fingers intravaginally and checking whether the pelvic floor muscles correctly contract and relax.

Promotion of Nutrition

During the hospital stay, most women display a good appetite and eat well; nutritious snacks are usually welcomed. Women may request that family members bring to the hospital favourite or culturally appropriate foods (Fig. 21-5). Cultural dietary preferences must be respected. An example is that some Asian women will only eat hot food after birth and will avoid anything cold. This interest in food presents an ideal opportunity for nutrition counselling on dietary needs after pregnancy, such as for breastfeeding, preventing constipation and anemia, promoting weight loss, and promoting healing and well-being (see Chapter 11). Prenatal vitamins and iron supplements are often continued until 6 weeks after birth or until the ordered supply has been used.

Promotion of Normal Bladder Function

After giving birth, the mother should void spontaneously within 6 to 8 hours. The first several voidings should be measured to document adequate emptying of the bladder. A volume of at least 150 mL is expected for each voiding. Some women experience difficulty in emptying the bladder, possibly as a result of diminished bladder tone, edema from trauma, use of epidural or spinal anaesthetic, or fear of discomfort. Nursing interventions for inability to void and bladder distension are discussed on p. 543.

Promotion of Normal Bowel Function

Nursing interventions to promote normal bowel elimination include educating the woman about measures to avoid constipation, such as ensuring adequate roughage and fluid intake and promoting exercise. Alerting the woman to adverse effects of medications such as opioid analgesics (decreased gastrointestinal tract motility) may encourage her to implement measures to reduce the risk of constipation. Occasionally, stool softeners or laxatives may be necessary during the early postpartum period, especially if the woman has extensive perineal repairs. It is normal for a woman not to have a bowel movement for 2 to 3 days after birth, so many new mothers may be home before having a bowel movement.

Some mothers experience gas pains, especially if they had a Caesarean birth. Antigas medications may be ordered. Ambulation or rocking in a rocking chair may stimulate passage of flatus and relief of discomfort. Women with gas should avoid drinking carbonated beverages and avoid the use of straws.

Promotion of Breastfeeding

The first hour after childbirth is an excellent time to initiate breastfeeding. At this time, the infant is in an alert state and ready to nurse. Breastfeeding aids in the contraction of the uterus and prevention of maternal hemorrhage. This is an opportune time to instruct the mother in breastfeeding and assess the physical appearance of the breasts (see Community Focus box). Women will need continuous support throughout their hospitalization to ensure successful breastfeeding. (See Chapter 26 for further information on assisting the breastfeeding woman.)

Suppression of Lactation

Suppression of **lactation** is necessary when the woman has decided not to breastfeed or in the case of neonatal death. Wearing a well-fitted support bra or breast binder continuously for at least the first 72 hours after giving birth is important. Women should avoid breast stimulation, including running warm water over the breasts, newborn **suckling**, or pumping of the breasts. A few nonbreastfeeding mothers experience severe breast **engorgement** (swelling of breast tissue caused by increased blood and lymph supply to the breasts as the body produces milk, which occurs at about 72 to 96 hours after birth). If breast engorgement occurs, it usually can be managed satisfactorily with nonpharmacological interventions.

Ice packs to the breasts are helpful in decreasing the discomfort associated with engorgement. The woman should use a 15-minutes-on, 45-minutes-off schedule (to prevent the

evolve Critical Thinking Exercise—Postpartum Complications

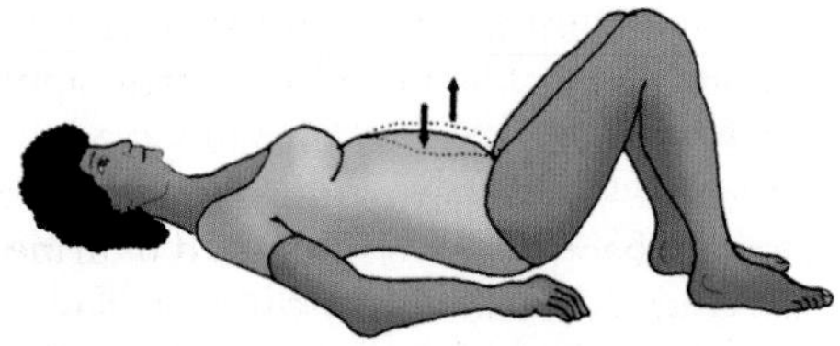

Abdominal Breathing. Lie on back with knees bent. Inhale deeply through nose. Keep ribs stationary and allow abdomen to expand upward. Exhale slowly but forcefully while contracting the abdominal muscles; hold for 3 to 5 seconds while exhaling. Relax.

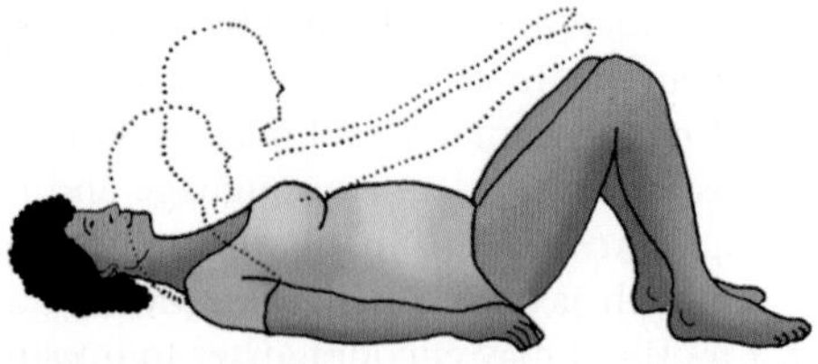

Reach for the Knees. Lie on back with knees bent. While inhaling, deeply lower chin onto chest. While exhaling, raise head and shoulders slowly and smoothly and reach for knees with arms outstretched. The body should rise only as far as the back will naturally bend while waist remains on floor or bed (about 6 to 8 inches). Slowly and smoothly lower head and shoulders back to starting position. Relax.

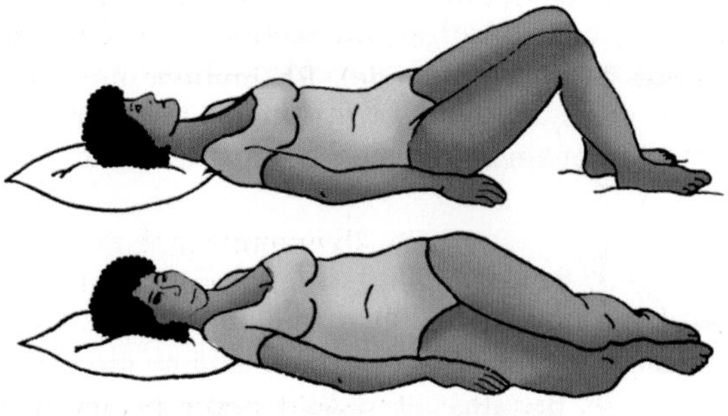

Double Knee Roll. Lie on back with knees bent. Keeping shoulders flat and feet stationary, slowly and smoothly roll knees over to the left to touch floor or bed. Maintaining a smooth motion, roll knees back over to the right until they touch floor or bed. Return to starting position and relax.

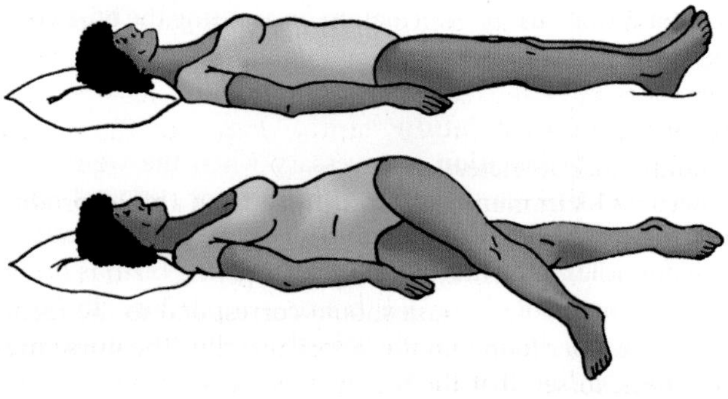

Leg Roll. Lie on back with legs straight. Keeping shoulders flat and legs straight, slowly and smoothly lift left leg and roll it over to touch the right side of floor or bed and return to starting position. Repeat, rolling right leg over to touch left side of floor or bed. Relax.

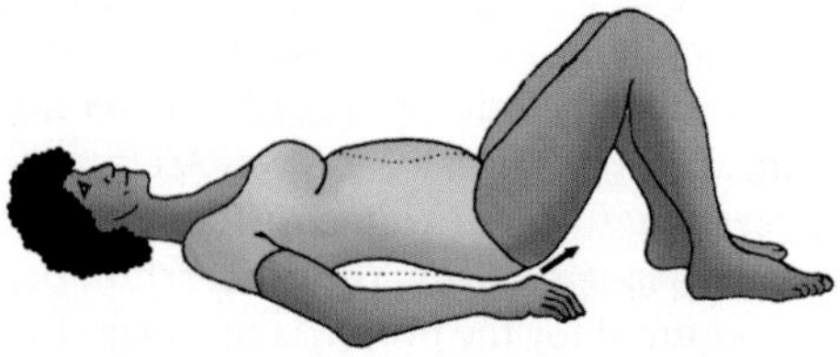

Combined Abdominal Breathing and Supine Pelvic Tilt (Pelvic Rock). Lie on back with knees bent. While inhaling deeply, roll pelvis back by flattening lower back on floor or bed. Exhale slowly but forcefully while contracting abdominal muscles and tightening buttocks. Hold for 3 to 5 seconds while exhaling. Relax.

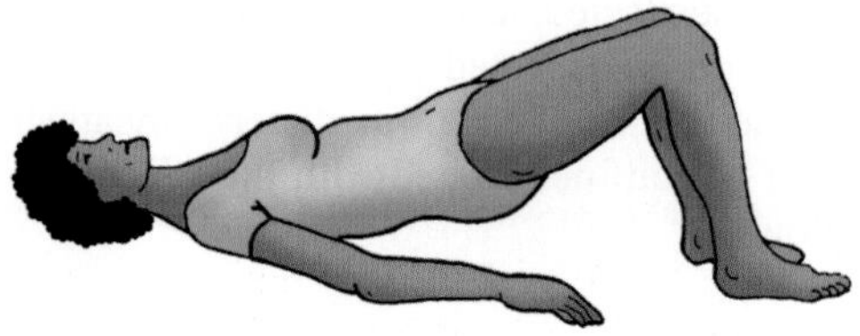

Buttocks Lift. Lie on back with arms at sides, knees bent, and feet flat. Slowly raise buttocks and arch back. Return slowly to starting position.

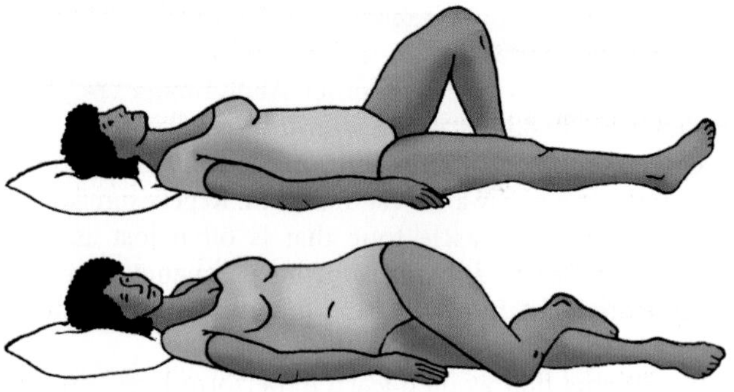

Single Knee Roll. Lie on back with right leg straight and left leg bent at the knee. Keeping shoulders flat, slowly and smoothly roll left knee over to the right to touch floor or bed and then back to starting position. Reverse position of legs. Roll right knee over to the left to touch floor or bed and return to starting position. Relax.

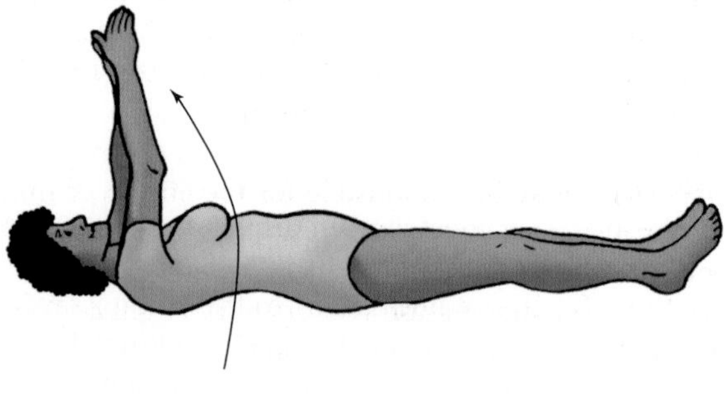

Arm Raises. Lie on back with arms extended at 90-degree angle from body. Raise arms so they are perpendicular and hands touch. Lower slowly.

Fig. 21-4 Postpartum exercise should begin as soon as possible. The woman should start with simple exercises and gradually progress to more strenuous ones.

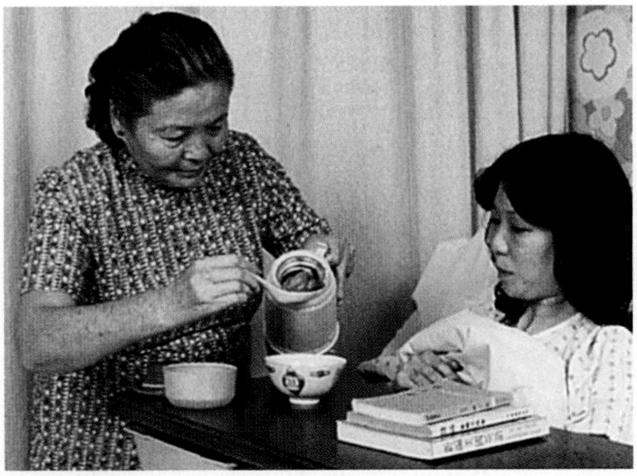

Fig. 21-5 Special foods are considered essential for recovery in Asian cultures. *(Courtesy Concept Media, Irvine, CA.)*

COMMUNITY FOCUS

Breastfeeding Support

Women breastfeed longer if they have support in their breastfeeding efforts. Nurses and lactation consultants provide support during inpatient stays after childbirth. Women can find support in the community in various groups. Social support interventions that include peer support are successful in increasing the duration of exclusive breastfeeding and satisfaction with breastfeeding. In discharge planning, nurses can refer breastfeeding mothers to community groups for support. Community health nurses can facilitate breastfeeding efforts through organizing or facilitating support groups. Mothers experienced in breastfeeding can facilitate these efforts.

Identify sources of breastfeeding support in your community. Are these resources free and available in various parts of the community? What form does the support take? Are there group classes? Is there individual consultation? Who provides the consultation? Make a list of the resources you identified and share the list with your clinical group.

rebound swelling that can occur if ice is used continuously), or she can place fresh, cold, washed cabbage leaves inside her bra. The leaves are replaced each time they wilt. Cabbage leaves have been used to treat swelling in other cultures for years (Mass, 2004). The exact mechanism of action is not known, but it is thought that naturally occurring plant estrogens or salicylates may be responsible for the effects. A mild analgesic may also be necessary to help the mother through this uncomfortable time. Medications that were once prescribed for lactation suppression (estrogen, estrogen and testosterone, and bromocriptine) are no longer used.

Health Promotion for Planning Future Pregnancies and Children

Rubella Vaccination

For women who have not had rubella or women who are serologically not immune (titre of 1 : 8 or enzyme immunoassay level less than 0.8), a subcutaneous injection of rubella vaccine is recommended in the immediate postpartum period to prevent the possibility of contracting rubella in future pregnancies. If women are vaccinated after birth, approximately 90% will seroconvert. The live attenuated rubella virus is not communicable; therefore, breastfeeding mothers can be vaccinated. However, because the virus is shed in urine and other body fluids, the vaccine should not be given if the mother or other household members are immunocompromised. Rubella vaccine is made from duck eggs; thus, women who have allergies to these eggs may develop a hypersensitivity reaction to the vaccine, for which they will need adrenaline. A transient arthralgia or rash is common in vaccinated women. Because the vaccine may be **teratogenic**, women must be informed about this fact.

LEGAL TIP **Rubella Vaccination.** Informed consent for rubella vaccination in the postpartum period includes information about possible adverse effects and the risk of teratogenic effects. Women must understand that they must practice **contraception** for 1 month after being vaccinated to avoid pregnancy.

Prevention of Rh Isoimmunization

Injection of Rh **immune globulin** (a solution of γ-globulin that contains Rh antibodies) within 72 hours after birth prevents sensitization in the Rh-negative woman who has had a fetomaternal transfusion of Rh-positive fetal red blood cells (RBCs) (see Medication Guide). Rh immune globulin promotes lysis of fetal Rh-positive blood cells before the mother forms her own antibodies against them.

NURSING ALERT After birth, Rh immune globulin is administered to all Rh-negative, antibody (Coombs' test)–negative women who give birth to Rh-positive infants. Rh immune globulin is administered to the mother intramuscularly or intravenously (RhoGAM). It should never be given to an infant.

The administration of 300 mcg of Rh immune globulin is usually sufficient to prevent maternal sensitization. However, if a large fetomaternal transfusion is suspected, the dosage needed should be determined by performing a Kleihauer-Betke test, which detects the amount of fetal blood in the maternal circulation. If more than 15 mL of fetal blood is present in maternal circulation, the dosage of Rh immune globulin must be increased.

Because Rh immune globulin is considered a blood product, precautions similar to those used for transfusing blood are necessary when it is given. The identification number on the woman's hospital wristband should correspond to the identification number found on the laboratory slip. The nurse must also check to see that the lot number of the laboratory slip corresponds to the lot number on the vial. Finally, the expiration date on the vial should be checked to ensure that it is a usable product.

Rh immune globulin suppresses the immune response. Therefore, the woman who receives both Rh immune globulin and rubella vaccine must be tested in 3 months to see if she has developed rubella immunity. If not, the woman will need another dose of rubella vaccine.

MEDICATION GUIDE

Rh Immune Globulin, RhoGAM

Action

Suppression of immune response in nonsensitized women with Rh-negative blood who receive Rh-positive blood cells because of fetomaternal hemorrhage, transfusion, or accident

Indications

Routine antepartum prevention at 26 to 28 weeks of gestation in women with Rh-negative blood; suppression of antibody formation after birth, miscarriage or pregnancy termination, abdominal trauma, ectopic pregnancy, amniocentesis, version, or chorionic villi sampling

Dosage/Route

Standard dose: 1 vial (300 mcg) IM in deltoid or ventrogluteal muscle

Microdose: 1 vial (50 mcg) IM in deltoid or ventrogluteal muscle

Rh_o(D) immune globulin can be given IM or IV

Adverse Effects

Myalgia, lethargy, localized tenderness and stiffness at injection site, mild and transient fever, malaise, headache, rarely nausea, vomiting, hypotension, tachycardia, and allergic response can occur.

Nursing Considerations

Give a standard dose to the mother at 28 weeks of gestation as prophylaxis or after an incident or exposure risk that occurs after 28 weeks of gestation (e.g., amniocentesis, second-trimester miscarriage or abortion, afterversion) and within 72 hours after birth if the baby is Rh positive.

Give a microdose for first-trimester miscarriage or abortion, ectopic pregnancy, or chorionic villi sampling.

Verify that the woman is Rh negative and has not been sensitized and, if postpartum, that the Coombs' test is negative and that baby is Rh positive. Provide explanation to the woman about the procedure, including the purpose, possible adverse effects, and the effect on future pregnancies. Have the woman sign a consent form if required by the agency. Verify correct dosage and confirm the lot number and woman's identity before giving the injection (verify with another registered nurse or by other procedure per agency policy); document administration per agency policy. Observe the patient for at least 20 minutes after administration for allergic response.

The medication is made from human plasma (a consideration if the woman is a Jehovah's Witness). Women receiving this medication must be informed about the risks and benefits, and the nurse needs to document this discussion and the patient's understanding before administering the medication. The risk of transmitting infectious agents, including viruses, cannot be completely eliminated.

IM, intramuscularly; *IV*, intravenously.

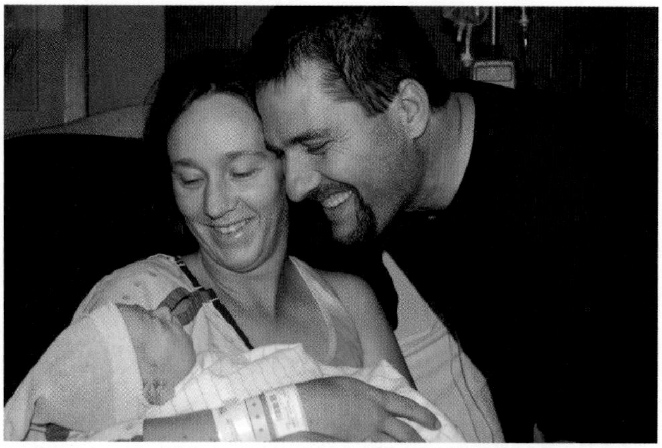

Fig. 21-6 Parents getting acquainted with their new son. *(Courtesy Julie and Darren Nelson, Loveland, CO.)*

Nursing Care Management—Psychosocial Needs

Meeting the psychosocial needs of new mothers involves assessing the parents' reactions to the birth experience, their feelings about themselves, and their interactions with the new baby (Fig. 21-6) and other family members. Specific interventions are then planned in order to increase the parents' knowledge and self-confidence as they assume the care and responsibility of the new baby and integrate this new member into their existing family structure. Such interventions need to complement parents' cultural expectations (see Nursing Process box and Chapter 22). While implementing the psychosocial plan of care for a postpartum woman, the nurse functions in the roles of teacher, encourager, and supporter, rather than doer. Topics that should be included in the psychosocial plan of care include promotion of parenting skills and adjustment of family members to the newborn infant (see Chapter 22).

Sometimes the findings of the psychosocial assessment indicate serious actual or potential problems that must be addressed. Box 21-5 lists several psychosocial needs that, at a minimum, warrant ongoing evaluation following hospital discharge. Women exhibiting these needs should be referred to appropriate community resources for assessment and management.

Cultural issues must be considered when planning care, as childbirth occurs within a sociocultural context. The nurse must take time to interact with the woman and her extended family in order to learn and understand which practices need to be followed regarding the new mother and her newborn infant. Recognizing the importance of family and community in relation to the woman and her infant is integral to providing culturally appropriate care.

Impact of the Birth Experience

Many women indicate a need to examine the birth process itself and look at their own behavior during labour in retrospect. Their partners may express similar desires. If their birth experience was quite different from that planned (e.g., induction, epidural anaesthesia, Caesarean birth), both partners may need to mourn the loss of their expectations before they can adjust to the reality of their actual birth experience. Inviting them to review the events and describe how they feel helps the nurse assess how well they understand what happened and how well they have been able to put their childbirth experience into perspective.

Maternal Self-Image

An important assessment concerns the woman's self-concept, body image, and sexuality. How this new mother feels about herself and her body during the **puerperium** may

NURSING PROCESS: PSYCHOSOCIAL NEEDS

Assessment

Assessment includes impact of birth experience, maternal self-image, mood, and parent–infant interactions.

Nursing Diagnoses

Nursing diagnoses related to psychosocial issues that are often established for the postpartum patient include the following:

Impaired verbal communication related to
- patient's hearing impairment
- language barriers

Impaired parenting related to
- long, difficult labour
- unmet expectations of labour and birth

Anxiety related to
- newness of parenting role, sibling rivalry, or response of grandparent

Risk for situational low self-esteem related to
- body image changes

Planning

The nursing plan of care includes the family and observations of relationships among family members.

Examples of common expected outcomes include that the woman (family) will do the following:
- Identify measures that promote a healthy personal adjustment in the postpartum period
- Maintain healthy family functioning based on cultural norms and personal expectations

Interventions

Provide support to learn parenting skills.
Provide encouragement and support.
See text discussion for additional interventions.

Evaluation

The nurse can be reasonably assured that care was effective if expected outcomes of care for psychosocial needs have been met.

BOX 21-5 Signs of Potential Psychosocial Complications

- Unable or unwilling to discuss labour and birth experience
- Refers to self as ugly and useless
- Excessively preoccupied with self (body image)
- Markedly depressed
- Lacks a support system
- Partner or other family members react negatively to baby
- Refuses to interact with or care for baby (e.g., does not name baby, does not want to hold or feed baby, is upset by vomiting and wet or dirty diapers) (cultural appropriateness of actions must be considered)
- Expresses disappointment over baby's sex
- Sees baby as messy or unattractive
- Baby reminds mother of family member or friend she doesn't like

affect her behavior and adaptation to parenting. The woman's self-concept and body image may also affect her sexuality. Overweight women can experience symptoms of depression and anxiety for several months postpartum.

Adaptation to Parenthood and Parent–Infant Interactions

The psychosocial assessment includes evaluating adaptation to parenthood as evidenced by the mother's and partner's reactions to and interactions with the new baby. Clues indicating successful adaptation begin to appear early in the postbirth period as parents react positively to the newborn infant and continue the process of establishing a relationship with their child.

Parents are adapting well to their new roles when they exhibit a realistic perception and acceptance of their newborn's needs and his or her limited abilities, immature social responses, and helplessness. Examples of positive parent–infant interactions include taking pleasure in the infant and the tasks done for and with him or her; understanding the infant's emotional states and providing comfort; and reading the infant's cues for new experiences and sensing his or her fatigue level (see Chapter 22).

Should these indicators be missing, the nurse must investigate further what is hindering the normal adaptation process. The nurse can ask several questions, such as "Do you feel sad often?" or "Do you have concerns about being a good parent?", that will help to determine if the woman is experiencing the normal "baby blues" or if there is a more serious underlying condition (i.e., postpartum **mood disorder**) (Jesse & Graham, 2005). See Chapter 23 for further discussion of postpartum mood disorders.

Postpartum Blues

The "pink" period surrounding the first day or two after birth, characterized by heightened joy and feelings of well-being, is often followed by a "blue" period. Approximately 50 to 80% of women of all ethnic and racial groups experience the postpartum blues or baby blues. During the blues, women are emotionally labile and often cry easily for no apparent reason. This lability seems to peak around the fifth day and subside by the tenth day. Other symptoms of postpartum blues include depression, a let-down feeling, restlessness, fatigue, insomnia, headache, anxiety, sadness, and anger. Postpartum blues are transient, mild, and time limited and do not require treatment other than reassurance (Kennerly & Gath, 1989). Biochemical, psychological, social, and cultural factors have been explored as possible causes of the postpartum blues; however, the etiology remains unknown.

Whatever the cause, the early postpartum period appears to be one of emotional and physical vulnerability for new mothers who may be psychologically overwhelmed by the reality of parental responsibilities. The mother may feel deprived of the supportive care she received from family members and friends during pregnancy. Some mothers regret the loss of the mother–unborn child relationship and mourn its passing. Still others have a let-down feeling when labour and birth are complete. Most women experience fatigue after childbirth, which is compounded by the around-the-clock demands of the new baby and can accentuate the feelings of depression. Postpartum depressive symptoms can have a negative effect on women's development of a maternal role. To help mothers cope with postpartum blues, nurses can suggest various strategies (see Patient Teaching box).

The Registered Nurses' Association of Ontario (RNAO) Best Practice Guideline: Interventions for Postpartum Depression recommends the use of the Edinburgh Postnatal Depression Scale (EPDS) as the screening tool of choice (RNAO, 2005). Inclusion of this tool on a discharge checklist can help mothers assess their level of blues and decide when to seek advice from their care provider (Fig. 21-7). The 10-question EPDS is an effective screening tool and easy to use, although use in non-English speaking women has not been validated. Women who score 13 or greater on the EPDS and those who have a history of depression or anxiety require more intensive postpartum follow-up (see Chapter 23).

Although the postpartum blues are usually mild and short-lived, approximately 10 to 15% of women experience a postpartum mood disorder (PPMD) (see Chapter 23). PPMD symptoms can range from mild to severe, with women having good and bad days. PPMD may also occur in fathers (Goodman, 2004). Both mothers and fathers should be screened for a PPMD. It can go undetected because new parents generally do not voluntarily admit to this kind of emotional distress out of embarrassment, guilt, or fear. Nurses must include teaching about how to differentiate symptoms of the blues and PPMD and urge parents to report depressive symptoms promptly if they occur (see Box 23-4).

Family Structure and Functioning

A woman's adjustment to her role as mother is affected greatly by her relationships with her partner, her mother and other relatives, and any other children (Fig. 21-8). Nurses can help ease the new mother's return home by identifying possible conflicts among family members and helping the woman plan strategies for dealing with these problems before discharge. Such a conflict could arise when couples have very different ideas about parenting. Dealing with the stresses of **sibling rivalry** and unsolicited grandparent advice can also affect the woman's transition to motherhood. Only by asking about other nuclear and extended family members can the nurse discover potential problems in such relationships and help plan workable solutions for them.

Impact of Cultural Diversity

The final component of a complete psychosocial assessment is the woman's cultural beliefs and values. Much of a woman's behavior during the postpartum period is strongly influenced by her cultural background. Nurses are likely to come into contact with women from many different countries and cultures. All cultures have developed safe and satisfying methods of caring for new mothers and babies. Only by understanding and respecting the values and beliefs of each woman can the nurse design a plan of care to meet individual needs (see Cultural Awareness box).

Cultural competence and cultural safety are prerequisites for nurses working in Canadian health care settings (Canadian Nurses Association [CNA], 2010). Canadian population statistics describe a projected increase in diversity within the Canadian population. Nurses must be prepared

PATIENT TEACHING Coping With Postpartum Blues

- Remember that the blues are normal.
- Get plenty of rest; nap when the baby does, if possible. Go to bed early and let friends know when to visit.
- Use relaxation techniques learned in childbirth classes (or ask the nurse to teach you and your partner some techniques).
- Do something for yourself. Take advantage of the time when your partner or family members care for the baby—soak in the tub or go for a walk.
- Plan a day out of the house—go to the mall with the baby, being sure to take a stroller or carriage, or go out to eat with friends without the baby. Many communities have churches or other agencies that provide child care programs, such as Mothers' Morning Out.
- Share your feelings with your partner. For example, talk about feeling tied down, if applicable; how the birth met your expectations; and things that will help you.
- If you are breastfeeding, give yourself and your baby time to learn.
- Monitor yourself closely for signs of depression, anxiety, and psychosis.
- Seek out and use community resources, such as La Leche League or community mental health centres.

CULTURAL AWARENESS
A Clash of Cultures

A Vietnamese woman who had been in Canada for 4 years was being cared for after childbirth. Instead of participating in the care of her infant, she refused to do so, remained in bed, wore a woolen cap, and appeared distressed and angry. The staff were puzzled and upset by her behaviour. One nurse decided to put into effect her newly learned concepts concerning cross-cultural nursing. She began by praising the woman's ability to speak English and, after eliciting a smile, remarked, "Every country has developed good ways to look after mothers and babies. Would you tell me about the care in Vietnam?" There was an immediate response. The woman explained that in her country women remained in bed for at least 10 days after birth and the biggest danger to their health was getting a cold. The baby was kept in the room with his mother, but either a grandmother or nurse took complete charge of the care.

With this information, the nurse was able to modify her plan of care to make it culturally relevant and thus more satisfying for the woman.

Edinburgh Postnatal Depression Scale (EPDS)

Name: ____________ Address: ____________

Your Date of Birth: ____________ Baby's Date of Birth: ____________ Phone: ____________

As you are pregnant or have recently had a baby, we would like to know how you are feeling. Please check the answer that comes closest to how you have felt IN THE PAST 7 DAYS, not just how you feel today.

Here is an example, already completed.

I have felt happy:

- ☐ Yes, all the time
- ☒ Yes, most of the time
- ☐ No, not very often
- ☐ No, not at all

(This would mean: "I have felt happy most of the time" during the past week.)

Please complete the other questions in the same way.

1. I have been able to laugh and see the funny side of things.
   - ☐ As much as I always could
   - ☐ Not quite so much now
   - ☐ Definitely not so much now
   - ☐ Not at all

2. I have looked forward with enjoyment to things.
   - ☐ As much as I ever did
   - ☐ Rather less than I used to
   - ☐ Definitely less than I used to
   - ☐ Hardly at all

*3. I have blamed myself unnecessarily when things went wrong.
   - ☐ Yes, most of the time
   - ☐ Yes, some of the time
   - ☐ Not very often
   - ☐ No, never

4. I have been anxious or worried for no good reason.
   - ☐ No, not at all
   - ☐ Hardly ever
   - ☐ Yes, sometimes
   - ☐ Yes, most of the time

*5. I have felt scared or panicky for no good reason.
   - ☐ Yes, quite alot
   - ☐ Yes, sometimes
   - ☐ No, not much
   - ☐ No, not at all

*6. Things have been getting on top of me.
   - ☐ Yes, most of the time I have not been able to cope at all
   - ☐ Yes, sometimes I have not been able to cope as well as usual
   - ☐ No, most of the time I have coped quite well
   - ☐ No, I have been coping as well as ever

*7. I have been so unhappy that I have had difficulty sleeping.
   - ☐ Yes, most of the time
   - ☐ Yes, sometimes
   - ☐ Not very often
   - ☐ No, not at all

*8. I have felt sad or miserable.
   - ☐ Yes, most of the time
   - ☐ Yes, quite often
   - ☐ Not very often
   - ☐ No, not at all

*9. I have been so unhappy that I have been crying.
   - ☐ Yes, most of the time
   - ☐ Yes, quite often
   - ☐ Only occasionally
   - ☐ No, never

*10. The thought of harming myself has occurred to me.
   - ☐ Yes, quite often
   - ☐ Sometimes
   - ☐ Hardly ever
   - ☐ Never

Administered/Reviewed by: ____________

SCORING

QUESTIONS 1, 2, & 4 (without an *)

Are scored 0, 1, 2 or 3 with top box scored as 0 and the bottom box scored as 3.

QUESTIONS 3, 5–10

(marked with an *)

Are reverse scored, with the top box scored as a 3 and the bottom box scored as 0.

Maximum score: 30

Possible Depression: 10 or greater

Always look at item 10 (suicidal thoughts)

Instructions for using the Edinburgh Postnatal Depression Scale:

1. The mother is asked to check the response that comes closest to how she has been feeling in the previous 7 days.
2. All the items must be completed.
3. Care should be taken to avoid the possibility of the mother discussing her answers with others. (Answers come from the mother or pregnant woman.)
4. The mother should complete the scale herself, unless she has limited English or has difficulty with reading.

Fig. 21-7 Edinburgh Postnatal Depression Scale (EPDS). *(Sources: Cox, J. L., Holden, J. M., & Sagovsky, R. [1987]. Detection of postnatal depression: Development of the 10-item Edinburgh Postnatal Depression Scale.* British Journal of Psychiatry, 150, *782–786; Wisner, K. L., Parry, B. L., & Piontek, C. M. [2002]. Postpartum depression.* New England Journal of Medicine, *347[3], 194–199.)*

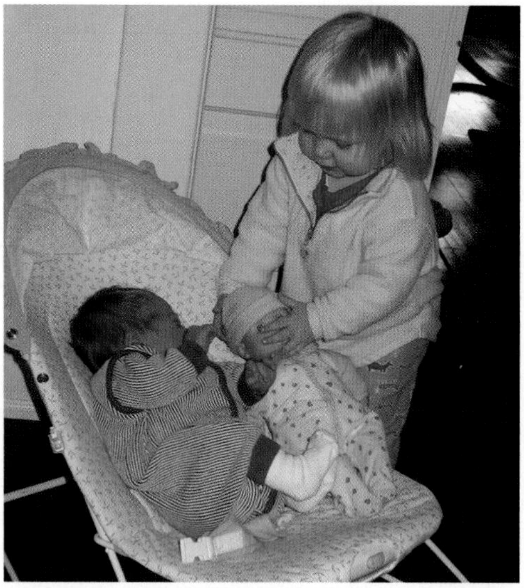

Fig. 21-8 Older sibling sharing her "baby" with her brother. *(Courtesy Wendy and Marwood Larson-Harris, Roanoke, VA.)*

to care for women and their families from diverse cultural backgrounds.

Many traditional health beliefs and practices exist among the different cultures within the North American population. Traditional health practices used to maintain health or avoid illnesses deal with the whole person (body, mind, and spirit). Women from various cultures may view health as a balance between opposing forces (e.g., cold vs. hot, yin vs. yang), being in harmony with nature, or just "feeling good." "The notion of 'balance' is fundamental to Aboriginal concepts of health" (Smylie et al., 2000) and may be expressed among First Nations, Métis, and Inuit women through distinct cultural practices in relation to labour, birth, and postpartum periods. Traditional practices among some cultures may include the observance of certain dietary restrictions, wearing certain clothing, or taboos for balancing the body; participation in certain activities such as sports and art for maintaining mental health; and use of silence, prayer, or meditation for developing spiritually. Some practices (e.g., using religious objects or eating garlic) are used to protect the person from illness and may involve avoiding people who are believed to create hexes and spells or who have an "evil eye." Restoration of health may involve a person accessing alternative and complementary health models (e.g., herbs, animal substances) or using a traditional healer. Rest, seclusion, dietary restraints, and ceremonies honouring the mother are all common traditional practices that are followed for the promotion of the health and well-being of the mother and baby. In Southeast Asia, pregnancy is considered to be a "hot" state, and childbirth results in a sudden loss of this state. Therefore, balance needs to be restored by increasing the return of the hot state, which is present physically or symbolically in hot food, hot water, and warm air. Women may wish to stay warm and avoid bathing, exercising, and hair washing for 7 to 30 days after childbirth. They may also prefer not to give their babies colostrum.

Another common belief is that the mother and baby remain in a weak and vulnerable state for a period of several weeks following birth. During this time, the mother may remain in a passive role, take no baths or showers, and stay in bed to prevent cold air from entering her body.

It is important that nurses consider all cultural aspects when planning care and not use their own cultural beliefs as the framework for that care. Although the beliefs and behaviours of other cultures may seem different or strange, they should be encouraged as long as the mother wants to conform to them and she and the baby have no ill effects. The nurse must determine whether a woman is using complementary medication during the postpartum period because active ingredients in some herbal remedies can have adverse physiological effects on the woman when ingested with prescribed medicines. Also, women who have immigrated to Western nations without their extended families may not have much help at home, making it difficult for them to observe these activity restrictions. Many young women who are first- or second-generation Canadians may follow their cultural traditions only when older family members are present or not at all.

Nursing Care Management—Discharge Teaching

Self-Management and Signs of Complications

Discharge planning begins at the time of admission to the unit and should be reflected in the plan of care developed for each woman. Because of the limited time available for teaching, nurses must target their teaching on expressed needs of the woman. Giving the woman a list of topics and asking her to indicate her teaching needs will help the nurse maximize teaching efforts and can increase the woman's retention of information.

Just before the time of discharge, the nurse should review the woman's chart to see that laboratory reports, medications, signatures, and other items are in order. Some hospitals use a checklist before the woman's discharge. The nurse should also verify that the infant is ready to be discharged.

No medication that would make the mother sleepy should be administered if she is the one who will be holding the baby on the way out of the hospital. In some instances, the woman is seated in a wheelchair and given the baby to hold. Some families leave unescorted and ambulatory, depending on hospital protocol. The woman's possessions are gathered and taken out with her and her family. The woman's and the baby's identification bands are carefully checked. In most hospitals, nurses must ensure that the parents are able to properly secure the baby in a car seat for the drive home (see Fig. 25-18).

Sexual Activity and Contraception

Feelings related to sexual adjustment after childbirth are often a cause of concern for new parents. Women who have recently given birth may be reluctant to resume sexual intercourse for fear of pain or worry that coitus could damage healing perineal tissue. Because many new parents are anxious for information but reluctant to bring up the subject, postpartum nurses should matter-of-factly include the topic of postpartum sexuality during their routine physical assessment. For example, while examining the episiotomy site the nurse can say, "I know you're sore right now, but it probably won't be long until you (or you and your partner) are ready to make love again. Do you have any questions about resuming sex?" This approach assures the woman and her partner that resuming sexual activity is a legitimate concern for new parents and indicates the nurse's willingness to answer questions and share information.

Many couples resume sexual activity before the traditional postpartum checkup 6 weeks after childbirth. Risk of hemorrhage and infection are minimal by approximately 2 weeks after birth. It is important that the nurse discuss the physical and psychological effects that giving birth can have on sexual activity (see Home Care box). Contraceptive options should be discussed with women (and their partners if present) before discharge so that they can make informed decisions about fertility management before resuming sexual activity. Waiting to discuss contraception at the 6-week checkup may be too late. It is possible, particularly in women who bottle-feed, for **ovulation** to occur as soon as 1 month after birth. A woman who engages in unprotected sex risks becoming pregnant.

HOME CARE

Resumption of Sexual Intercourse

- You can safely resume sexual intercourse by the second to fourth week after birth, when bleeding has stopped and the perineum is healed. For the first 6 weeks to 6 months, the vagina does not lubricate well, especially if you are breastfeeding.
- Your physiological reactions to sexual stimulation for the first 3 months after birth will be slower and less intense. The strength of the orgasm is reduced.
- A water-soluble gel, cocoa butter, or a contraceptive cream or jelly might be recommended for lubrication. If some vaginal tenderness is present, your partner can be instructed to insert one or more clean, lubricated fingers into the vagina and rotate them to help the vagina relax and identify possible areas of discomfort. A position in which you have control of the depth of the insertion of the penis also is useful. The side-by-side or female-on-top position may be more comfortable.
- The presence of the baby influences postbirth lovemaking. Parents hear every sound made by the baby; conversely, you may be concerned that the baby hears every sound you make. In either case, any phase of the sexual response cycle may be interrupted by hearing the baby cry or move, leaving both of you frustrated and unsatisfied. In addition, the amount of psychological energy you expended in child care activities may lead to fatigue. Newborns require a great deal of attention and time.
- Some women have reported feeling sexual stimulation and orgasms when breastfeeding their babies. Breastfeeding mothers often are interested in returning to sexual activity before nonbreastfeeding mothers are.
- You should be instructed to correctly perform the Kegel exercises to strengthen your pubococcygeal muscle. This muscle is associated with bowel and bladder function and vaginal feeling during intercourse.

Current contraceptive options are discussed in detail in Chapter 7. Women who are undecided about contraception at the time of discharge need information about using condoms with foam or creams until the first postpartum checkup.

Prescribed Medications

Women routinely continue to take their prenatal vitamins and iron during the postpartum period. It is especially important that women who are breastfeeding or discharged with a lower-than-normal hematocrit level take these medications as prescribed. Women with vaginal lacerations (third or fourth degree) or extensive episiotomies are usually prescribed stool softeners to take at home. Pain relief medications (analgesics or NSAIDs) may be prescribed, especially for women who had Caesarean birth. The nurse should make certain that the woman knows the route, dosage, frequency, and common adverse effects of all ordered medications.

Routine Mother and Baby Checkups

Women who have experienced uncomplicated vaginal births are still commonly scheduled for the traditional 6-week postpartum examination. Women who have had a Caesarean birth may be seen in the health care provider's office or clinic within 2 weeks after hospital discharge. The date and time for the follow-up appointment should be included in the discharge instructions. If an appointment is not made before the woman leaves the hospital, she should be encouraged to call the health care provider's office or clinic to schedule one.

Parents who have not already done so need to make plans for newborn follow-up at the time of discharge. Most offices and clinics like to see newborns for an initial examination within 48 to 72 hours after discharge. If an appointment for a specific date and time was not made for the infant before leaving the hospital, the parents should be encouraged to call the office or clinic right away.

Dealing With Visitors

A newborn in the family or neighborhood draws visitors. The nurse can help the parents explore ways in which they can assert their needs in such situations. When family or friends ask what they can do to help, the family can respond with "Please bring us a casserole or a meal" or "Could you please pick up some items at the grocery store?". The couple can work out a signal for alerting the partner that the new mother is becoming tired or uncomfortable and needs to have the partner invite the visitors into another part of the house. Some new mothers have found that if they remain in their robes and do not appear ready for company, visitors stay for a shorter time. A "Please Do Not Disturb" sign on the front door may be useful when the mother is resting.

Follow-Up After Discharge

Telephone Follow-Up

Many local health agencies have implemented postpartum telephone follow-up calls to their patients for assessment, health teaching, and identification of complications to effect timely intervention and referrals. Telephonic nursing assessments may also be used after a postpartum home care visit to reassess a woman's knowledge about the signs and symptoms of adequate intake by the breastfeeding infant or, after initiating home phototherapy, to assess the caregiver's knowledge regarding equipment complications.

Home Visits

Public health nurse visits to new mothers and babies can help bridge the gap between hospital care and routine visits to health care providers. Nurses are able to assess the mother, infant, and home environment; answer questions and provide education; and make referrals to community resources, if necessary. Home visits reduce the need for more expensive health care such as emergency department visits and rehospitalization. They can also help to improve the overall quality of care provided to infants and their parents. Ideally, immediate follow-up contact and home visits are available 7 days a week.

Community nursing care may not be available, even if needed, because of funding issues, but in most provinces mothers receive a phone call within the first week after discharge. Women who are assessed to be high risk may then receive a home visit from a public health nurse to assist with the new mother's concerns.

During the home visit, the nurse conducts an assessment of the mother and newborn to determine physiological adjustment, identify any existing complications, and answer any questions the mother has about herself or newborn care. Conducting the assessment in a separate room provides private time for the mother to ask questions on topics such as breast care, family planning, and constipation. The assessment should also include the mother's emotional adjustment and her knowledge of self-care and infant care (see Nursing Process box in Chapter 3, p. 39).

During the newborn assessment, the nurse can demonstrate and explain normal newborn behavior and capabilities and encourage the mother and family to ask questions or express concerns they may have.

Warm Lines

The **warm line** is another type of telephone link between the new family and concerned caregivers or experienced parent volunteers. A *warm line* is a helpline or consultation service, not a crisis intervention line. The warm line is appropriately used for dealing with less extreme concerns that can seem urgent at the time the call is placed but are not actual emergencies. Calls to warm lines commonly relate to infant feeding, prolonged crying, sibling rivalry, or postpartum mood disorder concerns. Warm-line services can extend beyond the **fourth trimester**. Families need to call when concerns arise and should be given telephone numbers for easy access to answers to their questions. Legal implications related to warm lines need to be addressed by each facility or agency before implementing this service.

Support Groups

The woman adjusting to motherhood sometimes seeks a special group experience. Postpartum women who have met earlier in prenatal clinics or on the hospital unit can begin to associate for mutual support. Members of childbirth preparation classes who attend a postpartum reunion can decide to extend their relationship during the fourth trimester.

A postpartum support group enables mothers and partners to share with and support each other as they adjust to parenting. Many new parents find it reassuring to discover that they are not alone in their feelings of confusion and uncertainty. An experienced parent can often impart concrete information to other members. Inexperienced parents can find themselves imitating the behavior of others in the group whom they perceive to be particularly capable.

Referral to Community Resources

In order to develop an effective referral system, it is important that the nurse have a clear understanding of the needs of the woman and family and of the organization and community resources available for meeting those needs. Locating and compiling information about available community services contributes to the development of a referral system. It is important for the nurse to develop his or her own resource file of local and national services that are frequently useful to postpartum families.

Key Points

- Postpartum care is modelled on the concept of health.
- Postpartum care will be influenced by knowledge of antepartum and intrapartum care.
- Cultural beliefs and practices affect the patient's response to the puerperium.
- The nursing care plan includes assessments to detect deviations from normal comfort measures for relieving discomfort or pain and safety measures for preventing infection.
- A postpartum assessment includes reviewing: breasts, uterus, bladder elimination, bowel elimination, amount and colour of lochia, condition of episiotomy or laceration, any swelling and psychological status
- Teaching and counselling measures are designed to promote the woman's feelings of competence in self-management and baby care.
- Common nursing interventions in the postpartum period include evaluating and treating the boggy uterus and the full urinary bladder; providing for nonpharmacological and pharmacological relief of pain and discomfort associated with the episiotomy, lacerations, afterbirth pains, or breastfeeding; and instituting measures to promote or suppress lactation.
- Meeting the psychosocial needs of new mothers involves taking into consideration the composition and functioning of the entire family as well as an understanding of different cultural beliefs and practices.
- Mothers may exhibit signs of postpartum blues (baby blues) or PPMD.
- Early postpartum discharge will continue as a result of consumer demand, medical necessity, discharge criteria for low-risk childbirth, and cost-containment measures.
- Postpartum teaching includes self-care needs, warning signs, exercise, and sexuality and resumption of sexual relations.
- Early discharge classes, telephone follow-up, home visits, warm lines, and support groups are effective means of facilitating physiological and psychological adjustments in the postpartum period.

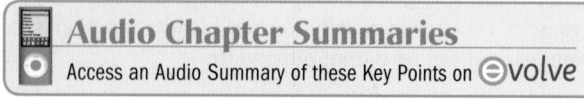

Audio Chapter Summaries
Access an Audio Summary of these Key Points on Evolve

References

Arendt, J. (2005). Melatonin: Characteristics, concerns, and prospect. *Journal of Biological Rhythms, 20*(4), 291–303.

Canadian Nurses Association. (2010). *Position statement: Cultural competence in nursing*. Ottawa, ON: Author.

Canadian Paediatric Society and Society of Obstetricians and Gynaecologists of Canada. (1996). Facilitating discharge home following a normal term birth. *Paediatric Child Health, 1*(2), 165–168.

Goodman, J. H. (2004). Paternal postpartum depression, its relationship to maternal postpartum depression, and implications for family health. *Journal of Advanced Nursing, 45*(1), 26–35.

Groër, M., et al. (2005). Neuroendocrine and immune relationships in postpartum fatigue. *MCN: American Journal of Maternal Child Nursing, 30*(2), 133–138.

Jesse, D., & Graham, M. (2005). Are you often sad and depressed? Brief measure to identify women at risk for depression in pregnancy. *MCN: American Journal of Maternal Child Nursing, 30*(1), 40–45.

Kennerly, H., & Gath, D. (1989) Maternity blues: Detection and measurement by questionnaire. *British Journal of Psychiatry, 155*, 356–373.

Mass, S. (2004). Breast pain: Engorgement, nipple pain and mastitis. *Clinics in Obstetrics and Gynecology, 47*(3), 676–682.

Public Health Agency of Canada. (2009). *What mothers say: The Canadian Maternity Experiences Survey*. Ottawa, ON: Author.

Registered Nurses' Association of Ontario (2005). *Interventions for postpartum depression*. Toronto: Author. Retrieved from http://www.rnao.org/Storage/11/600_BPG_Post_Partum_Depression.pdf.

Royal College of Obstetricians and Gynaecology. (2009). *Reducing the risk of thrombosis and embolism during pregnancy and the puerperium. Green-top guideline No. 37a*. London: Author. Retrieved from: http://www.rcog.org.uk/womens-health/clinical-guidance/reducing-risk-of-thrombosis-greentop37a.

Smylie, J., et al. (2000). SOGC policy statement: A guide for health professionals working with Aboriginal peoples. *Journal of Obstetrics and Gynaecology Canada 22*(12), 1070–1081. Retrieved from http://www.sogc.org/guidelines/public/100e-ps2-december2000.pdf.

Troy, N. (2003). Is the significance of postpartum fatigue being overlooked in the lives of women? *MCN: American Journal of Maternal Child Nursing, 28*(4), 252–257.

U.S. Food and Drug Administration (FDA). (2007). *Use of codeine products in nursing mothers—Questions and answers*. Retrieved from http://www.fda.gov/Drugs/DrugSafety/PostmarketDrugSafetyInformationforPatientsandProviders/ucm118113.htm.

Additional Resources

Edinburgh Postnatal Depression Scale: http://www.fresno.ucsf.edu/pediatrics/downloads/edinburghscale.pdf.

Perinatal Services BC: Postpartum Nursing Care Pathway: http://www.perinatalservicesbc.ca/NR/rdonlyres/EF4F92F4-5BFF-461E-8B0C-9E8B9EDCF2AD/0/ToolkitOBGuideline20PPNursingCarePathway.pdf.

Unit 5

22 Transition to Parenthood

Learning Objectives

On completion of this chapter, the reader will be able to:

- Identify parental and infant behaviours that facilitate parental attachment and those that inhibit it.
- Describe sensual responses that strengthen attachment.
- Examine the process of becoming a mother.
- Compare maternal and paternal adjustments to parenthood.
- Describe ways to facilitate parent–infant adjustment.
- Examine the effects of the following on parental response: parental age (i.e., adolescence and older than 35 years), social support, culture, socioeconomic conditions, personal aspirations, and sensory impairment.
- Describe sibling adjustment.
- Describe grandparent adaptation.

Electronic Resources

Additional information related to the content in Chapter 22 can be found on

evolve the companion Web site at http://evolve.elsevier.com/Canada/Perry/maternal/

- Examination Review Questions

Becoming a parent creates a period of change and instability for all men and women, whether they made a conscious decision to have children or the pregnancy was unplanned. This holds true whether parenthood is biological or adoptive and whether the parents are married couples; cohabiting couples; single mothers; single fathers; or gay, lesbian, or transgendered couples. Parenting can be described as a process of **role transition** that begins during pregnancy or while awaiting adoption. The transition is an ongoing process as the parent(s) and infant develop and change.

A thorough understanding of the process parents go through during their transition to parenthood guides the nurse in helping family members adapt. Family-centred care supports the family as the primary source of knowledge about what is best for them as they work in collaboration with health care providers to plan care (Srivastava, 2007). The parenting process requires cognitive and affective skills and knowledge, as well as motor skills. The infant's well-being and development depend on these components. This chapter reviews the transition to parenthood, including the parenting process and the adjustment of all those whom the mother calls family.

Parental Attachment, Bonding, and Acquaintance

The process by which a parent comes to love and accept a child and a child comes to love and accept a parent is referred to as **attachment**. Using the terms *attachment* and **bonding**, Klaus and Kennell (1976) originally proposed that the period shortly after birth is important to mother-to-infant attachment. They defined the phenomenon of bonding as a sensitive period in the first minutes and hours after birth, when mothers and fathers must have close contact with their infants for optimal later development. In 1982, they revised their theory of parent–infant bonding, modifying their claim of the critical nature of immediate contact with the infant after birth. They acknowledged the adaptability of human parents, stating that it took longer than minutes or hours for parents to form an emotional relationship with their infants. The terms *attachment* and *bonding* continue to be used interchangeably.

Women become attached to their fetus. Factors that influence maternal–fetal attachment include family support, psychological well-being, and having an ultrasound during pregnancy. Depression, substance use, and higher anxiety are associated with lower levels of attachment (Alhusen, 2008).

Attachment requires physical contact and early involvement between parent and infant to develop "the strong link" (Bialoskurski, Cox, & Hayes, 1999); through this activity the parent becomes acquainted with the infant, identifies the infant as an individual, and claims the infant as a member of the family. Attachment is facilitated by positive feedback (i.e., social, verbal, and nonverbal responses, whether real or perceived, that indicate acceptance of one partner by the other). Attachment occurs through a mutually satisfying experience. A mother commented on her son's grasp reflex, "I put my finger in his hand, and he grabbed right on. It's just a reflex, I know, but it felt good anyway."

The concept of attachment has been extended to include mutuality (i.e., the infant's behaviours and characteristics call forth a corresponding set of maternal behaviours and characteristics). The infant displays signalling behaviours such as crying, smiling, and cooing that initiate the contact and bring the caregiver to the child. These behaviours are followed by executive behaviours such as rooting, grasping, and postural adjustments that maintain the contact. The caregiver is attracted to an alert, responsive, cuddly infant and repelled by an irritable, apparently disinterested infant. Attachment occurs more readily with the infant whose temperament, social capabilities, appearance, and sex fit the parent's expectations. If the child does not meet these expectations, resolution of the parent's disappointment can delay the attachment process. A list of infant behaviours affecting parental attachment that continues to be a classic comprehensive reference is presented in Table 22-1. A corresponding list of parental behaviours that affect infant attachment is presented in Table 22-2.

An important part of attachment is acquaintance coupled with an understanding of the different sleep and awake states of the newborn. Parents use eye contact, touching, talking, and exploring to become acquainted with their infant during the immediate postpartum period. Adoptive parents undergo the same process when they first meet their new child. During this period, families engage in the *claiming process*, which is the identification of the new baby. The child is first identified in terms of likeness to other family members, then in terms of differences, and finally in terms of uniqueness. The unique newcomer is thus incorporated into the family. Parents scrutinize their infant carefully and point out characteristics that the child shares with other family members and that are indicative of a relationship between them. The claiming process is revealed by maternal comments such as the following: "David held him close and said, 'He's the image of his father,' but I found one part like me—his toes are shaped like mine."

Conversely, some mothers react negatively. They "claim" the infant in terms of the discomfort or pain the baby causes. The mother interprets the infant's normal responses as being negative toward her and reacts to her child with dislike or indifference. She does not hold the child close or touch the child to be comforting; for example, "The nurse put the baby into Marie's arms. She promptly laid him across her knees and glanced up at the television. 'Stay still until I finish watching—you've been enough trouble already.' "

Nurses play an important role in facilitating parental attachment. They can enhance positive parent–infant contacts by heightening parental awareness of an infant's responses, sleep–wake cycles, and their ability to communicate. As the parent attempts to become competent and loving in that role, nurses can bolster the parent's self-confidence and ego. Infants have different states that they move through, and nurses can point out the difference between quiet sleep and active sleep. More important, they can help parents to understand and respond appropriately to wakeful states. Nurses are in prime positions to identify actual and potential problems and to collaborate with other health care providers who will care for the parents after discharge. Nursing interventions related to the promotion of parent–infant attachment

Table 22-1 Infant Behaviours Affecting Parental Attachment

FACILITATING BEHAVIOURS	INHIBITING BEHAVIOURS
Visually alert; eye-to-eye contact; tracking or following of parent's face	Sleepy; eyes closed most of the time; gaze averted
Appealing facial appearance; randomness of body movements reflecting helplessness	Resemblance to person parent dislikes; hyperirritability or jerky body movements when touched
Smiles	Bland facial expression; infrequent smiles
Vocalization; crying only when hungry or wet	Crying for hours on end; colicky
Grasp reflex	Exaggerated motor reflex
Anticipatory approach behaviours for feedings; sucks well; feeds easily	Feeds poorly; regurgitates; vomits often
Enjoys being cuddled, held	Resists being held and cuddling by crying, stiffening body
Easily consolable	Inconsolable; unresponsive to parenting, caretaking tasks
Activity and regularity somewhat predictable	Unpredictable feeding and sleeping schedule
Attention span sufficient to focus on parents	Inability to attend to parent's face or offered stimulation
Differential crying, smiling, and vocalizing; recognizes and prefers parents	Shows no preference for parents over others
Approaches through locomotion	Unresponsive to parent's approaches
Clings to parent; puts arms around parent's neck	Seeks attention from any adult in room
Lifts arms to parents in greeting	Ignores parents

(From Gerson, E. [1973]. *Infant behavior in the first year of life.* New York: Raven Press.)

Table 22-2 Parental Behaviours Affecting Infant Attachment

FACILITATING BEHAVIOURS	INHIBITING BEHAVIOURS
Looks; gazes; takes in physical characteristics of infant; assumes en face position; eye contact	Turns away from infant; ignores infant's presence
Hovers; maintains proximity; directs attention to, points to infant	Avoids infant; does not seek proximity; refuses to hold infant when given opportunity
Identifies infant as unique individual	Identifies infant with someone parent dislikes; fails to discern any of infant's unique features
Claims infant as family member; names infant	Fails to place infant in family context or identify infant with family member; has difficulty naming
Touches; progresses from fingertip to fingers to palms to encompassing contact	Fails to move from fingertip touch to palmar contact and holding
Smiles at infant	Maintains bland countenance or frowns at infant
Talks to, coos, or sings to infant	Wakes infant when infant is sleeping; handles roughly; hurries feeding by moving nipple continuously
Expresses pride in infant	Expresses disappointment, displeasure in infant
Relates infant's behaviour to familiar events	Does not incorporate infant into daily life
Assigns meaning to infant's actions and sensitively interprets infant's needs	Makes no effort to interpret infant's actions or needs
Views infant's behaviours and appearance in positive light	Views infant's behaviour as exploiting, deliberately uncooperative; views appearance as distasteful, ugly

(From Mercer, R. [1983]. Parent–infant attachment. In L. Sonstegard, K. Kowalski, & B. Jennings [Eds.], *Women's health. Vol. 2: Childbearing*. New York: Grune & Stratton.)

are numerous and varied (Table 22-3). An excellent resource is the March of Dimes, at http://www.marchofdimes.com/nursing/modnemedia/othermedia/states.pdf.

Assessment of Attachment Behaviours

One of the most important areas of assessment is careful observation of behaviours thought to indicate the formation of emotional bonds between the newborn and family, especially the mother. Unlike physical assessment of the neonate, which has concrete guidelines to follow, assessment of parent–infant attachment requires much more skill in observation and interviewing. Rooming-in of mother and infant and liberal visiting privileges for the partner, siblings, and grandparents facilitate recognition of behaviours that demonstrate positive or negative attachment. An excellent opportunity exists during feeding. Guidelines for assessment of attachment behaviours are presented in Box 22-1.

During pregnancy and often even before conception occurs, parents develop an image of the "ideal" or "fantasy" infant. At birth, the fantasy infant becomes real. How closely the dream child resembles the real child influences the bonding process. Assessing such expectations during pregnancy and at the time of the infant's birth enables identification of discrepancies in the parents' view of the fantasy child and the real child.

The labour process significantly affects the immediate attachment of mothers to their newborn infants. Factors such as a long labour (Nystedt, Högberg, & Lundman, 2008), feeling tired or "drugged" after birth, and problems with breastfeeding can delay the development of initial positive feelings toward the newborn. Nurses providing breastfeeding support and referrals to groups such as La Leche League Canada (http://www.lllc.ca) or Postpartum Support International (http://postpartum.net) can be useful.

Parent–Infant Contact

Early Contact

Early close contact may facilitate the attachment process between parent and child. This does not mean that a delay will inhibit this process (humans are too resilient for that), but additional psychological energy may be needed to achieve the same effect. No scientific evidence has demonstrated that immediate contact after birth is essential for the human parent–child relationship.

Parents who desire but are unable to have early contact with their newborn (e.g., the infant was transferred to the neonatal intensive care nursery) can be reassured that such contact is not essential for optimal parent–infant interactions. Otherwise, adopted infants would not form the usual affectional ties with their parents. Nurses need to stress that the parent–infant relationship is a process that occurs over time.

Skin-to-Skin Contact

In a Cochrane review, early skin-to-skin contact (STS) had a positive effect on breastfeeding, breastfeeding duration, maternal affectionate love and touch during observed breastfeeding, and maternal attachment behaviour (Moore, Anderson, & Bergman, 2007). Better cardiorespiratory stability was observed in late-preterm infants with early STS; no negative short- or long-term effects were observed (Moore et al., 2007).

In a study examining the effects of kangaroo mother care (KMC) (STS) on mother–baby attachment in low-birth-weight infants, Gathwaia, Singh, and Balhara (2008) found that attachment scores were higher in the KMC group and that mothers were more involved in the caretaking of the baby.

In another study, when partners held their newborns skin to skin after a Caesarean birth, the infants cried less, were calmer, and became drowsy sooner than babies cared for in a cot (Erlandsson et al., 2007).

Table 22-3 Examples of Parent–Infant Attachment Interventions

INTERVENTION LABEL/DEFINITION	ACTIVITIES
Attachment Promotion	
Facilitation of development of parent–infant relationship	Provide skin-to-skin contact between mother or alternate caregiver immediately after birth by placing naked infant on chest, covered with a blanket to maintain temperature. Help parent(s) participate in infant care. Provide rooming-in in hospitals.
Environmental Management: Attachment Process	
Manipulation of patient's surroundings to facilitate development of parent–infant relationship	Create environment that fosters privacy. Individualize daily routine to meet parent's needs. Permit partner to sleep in room with mother. Develop policies that support family-centred maternity care.
Family Integrity Promotion: Childbearing Family	
Facilitation of growth of individuals or families who are adding infant to family unit	Prepare parent(s) for expected role changes involved in becoming a parent. Prepare parent(s) for responsibilities of parenthood. Prepare parents for the time demands of infant care, which adds about 40 hr/week to existing household demands. Monitor effects of newborn on family structure. Reinforce positive parenting behaviours.
Lactation Counselling	
Use of interactive helping process to assist in maintenance of successful breastfeeding	Correct misconceptions, misinformation, and inaccuracies about breastfeeding. Evaluate parent's understanding of infant's feeding cues (e.g., rooting, sucking, alertness). Determine frequency of feedings in relation to infant's needs. Demonstrate breast compression and discuss its advantages to increasing the milk supply.
Parent Education: Infant	
Instruction on nurturing and physical care needed during first year of life	Determine parent(s)'s knowledge, readiness, and ability to learn about infant care. Provide anticipatory guidance about developmental changes during first year of life. Teach parent(s) skills to care for newborn. Demonstrate ways in which parent(s) can stimulate infant's development. Discuss infant's capabilities for interaction. Demonstrate quieting techniques.
Risk Identification: Childbearing Family	
Identification of individual or family likely to experience difficulties in parenting and assigning priorities to strategies to prevent parenting problems	Determine developmental stage of parent(s). Review prenatal history for factors that predispose patient to complications. Ascertain understanding of English or other language used in community. Monitor behaviour that may indicate a problem with attachment. Plan for risk-reduction activities in collaboration with the individual or family.

(Adapted from Bulechek, G. M., Butcher, H. K., & Dochterman, J. M. [2008]. *Nursing interventions classification (NIC)* [5th ed.]. St. Louis: Mosby; Nomaguchi, K. M., & Milkie, M. A. [2003]. Costs and rewards of children: The effects of becoming a parent on adults' lives. *Journal of Marriage and Family, 65*, 356–374.)

BOX 22-1 Assessing Attachment Behaviours

- When the infant is brought to the parents, do they reach out for the infant and call him or her by name? (Recognize that in some cultures parents may not name the infant in the early newborn period.)
- Do the parents speak about the infant in terms of identification? For example, do they surmise whom the infant looks like or identify what appears special about their infant in comparison with other infants?
- When parents are holding the infant, what kind of body contact is there? Do parents feel at ease in changing the infant's position? Are fingertips or whole hands used? Do they avoid touching parts of the body or do they investigate and scrutinize body parts?
- When the infant is awake, what kinds of stimulation do the parents provide? Do they talk to the infant, to each other, or to no one? How do they look at the infant? Do they use direct visual contact, avoid eye contact, or look at other people or objects?
- How comfortable do the parents appear in terms of caring for the infant? Do they express any concern regarding their ability or disgust for certain activities, such as changing diapers?
- What types of affection do they demonstrate to the newborn (e.g., smiling, stroking, kissing, or rocking)?
- If the infant is fussy, what kinds of comforting techniques do the parents use (e.g., rocking, swaddling, talking, or stroking)?

Several and varied benefits of STS have been observed (see Chapter 26, p. 688). Nurses can facilitate this contact in most birth settings, whether the infant is preterm or term or birthed vaginally or by Caesarean, and with fathers or partners and mothers.

Extended Contact

Providing rooming-in facilities for the mother and her baby is common in most Canadian hospitals. The partner is encouraged to participate in the care of the infant, and siblings and grandparents are encouraged to visit and become acquainted with the infant. Partners are encouraged to take as active a role as they wish (Fig. 22-1). Extended contact with the infant should be available for all parents but especially for those at risk for parenting inadequacies, such as adolescents and low-income women. Any activity that optimizes family-centred care is worthy of serious consideration by postpartum nurses. Achieving Baby-Friendly status for a hospital is one means of promoting family-centred care. See more discussion on the Baby Friendly Hospital Initiative in Chapter 26.

Communication Between Parent and Infant

The parent–infant relationship is strengthened through the use of sensual responses and abilities by both partners in the interaction. The nurse should keep in mind that there may be cultural variations in these interactive behaviours.

The Senses

Touch

Touch, or the tactile sense, is used extensively by parents and other caregivers as a means of becoming acquainted with the newborn. Many mothers reach out for their infants as soon as they are born and the cord is cut. They lift them to their breasts, enfold them in their arms, and cradle them. Once the infant is close to them, they begin the exploration process with their fingertips, one of the most touch-sensitive areas of the body (Fig. 22-2). Within a short period of time, the caregiver uses the palm to caress the baby's trunk and eventually enfolds the infant. Gentle, stroking motions are used to soothe and quiet the infant. Patting or gently rubbing the infant's back is a comfort after feedings. Infants also pat the mother's breast as they nurse. Both seem to enjoy sharing each other's body warmth. There is a desire in parents to touch, pick up, and hold the infant. They often comment on the softness of the baby's skin and are aware of **milia** and rashes. As parents become increasingly sensitive to the infant's like or dislike of different types of touch, they draw closer to their baby.

Variations in touching behaviours have been noted in mothers from different cultural groups. For example, minimal touching and cuddling is a traditional Southeast Asian practice thought to protect the infant from evil spirits. By contrast, women in India and Bali have practiced infant massage, related to traditions and spiritual beliefs, since ancient times.

Eye Contact

Interest in having eye contact with the baby has been demonstrated repeatedly by parents. Some mothers remark that, once their babies have looked at them, they feel much closer to them. Parents spend much time getting their babies to open their eyes and look at them. In North American culture, eye contact appears to cement the development of a trusting relationship and is an important factor in human relationships at all ages (Fig. 22-3). In other cultures, eye-to-eye contact may be perceived differently (see Cultural Awareness box). For example, in Mexican culture, sustained direct eye contact is considered to be rude and immodest and even dangerous for some individuals. This danger may arise from the *mal ojo* (evil eye), resulting from excessive admiration. Women and children are thought to be more susceptible to the mal ojo (D'Avanzo, 2008).

As newborns become functionally able to sustain eye contact with their parents, time is spent in mutual gazing, often in the **en face** position. In this position, the parent's face

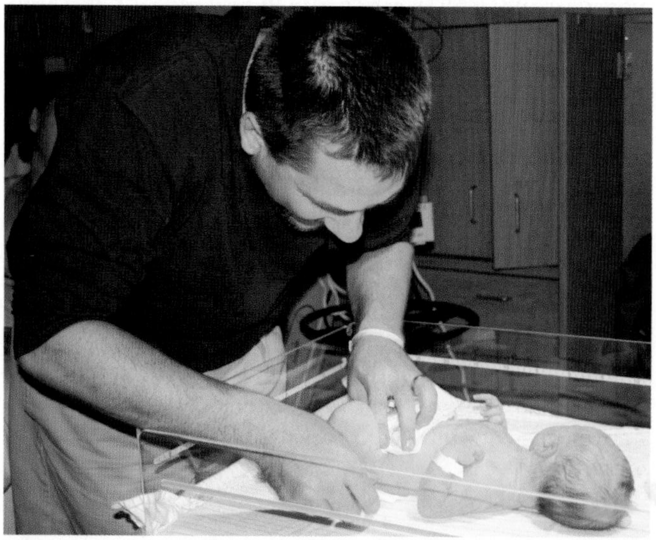

Fig. 22-1 Father changes diaper of his newborn son. *(Courtesy Darren Nelson, Loveland, CO.)*

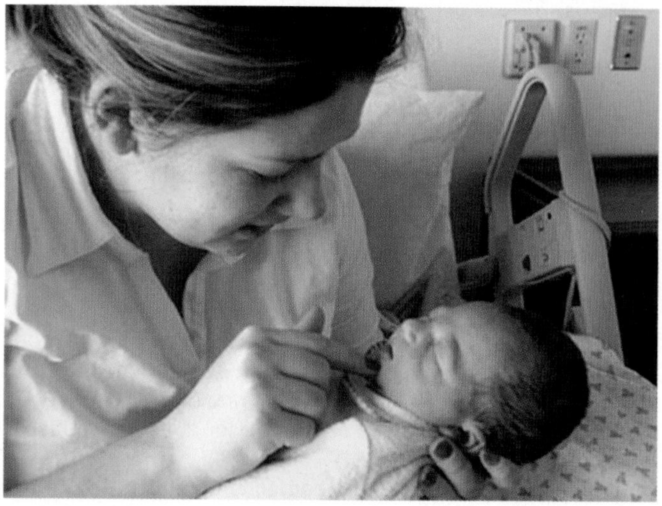

Fig. 22-2 Mother uses fingertip to explore infant. *(Courtesy Rebekah Vogel, Ft. Collins, CO.)*

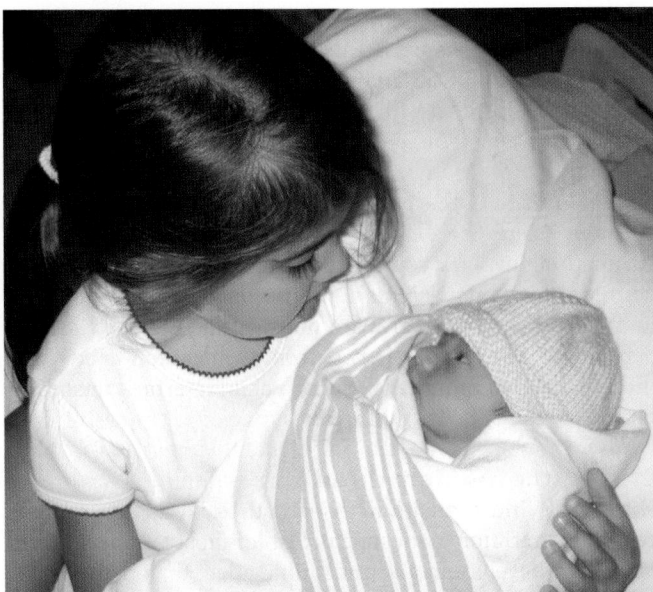

Fig. 22-3 Big sister in eye-to-eye contact with newborn brother. *(Courtesy Brian and Mayannyn Sallee, Las Vegas, NV.)*

CULTURAL AWARENESS

Fostering Bonding: Women of Varying Ethnic and Cultural Groups

Canadian women, families, and health care workers are made up of different races, socioeconomic backgrounds, sexual orientation, and ethnic groups. Childbearing practices and rituals may be incongruent with Anglo-Canadian standards. For example, Chinese families traditionally use extended family members to care for the newborn so that the mother can rest and recover, especially after a Caesarean birth. Some Asian and Latin American women do not initiate breastfeeding until their breast milk comes in. First Nations, Métis, and Inuit persons consciously place long silences in conversation for reflection and engage in minimal eye contact. It would be easy for Anglo-Canadian health care workers to perceive this as disrespect and indifference (Srivastava, 2007).

Nurses must become knowledgeable about childbearing beliefs and practices of diverse cultural and ethnic groups. They must also develop cultural sensitivity and use relevant cultural resources. The Registered Nurses' Association of Ontario has an excellent resource that recommends the development of cultural competency through knowledge as well as self-awareness and communication skills, to promote and embrace diversity. Because individual cultural variations exist within groups, nurses need to clarify with the patient and family members or friends the cultural norms that the patient follows. Incorrect judgements may be made about mother–infant bonding if nurses do not practice culturally sensitive care.

(Adapted from D'Avanzo, C. [2008]. *Mosby's pocket guide to cultural health assessment* [4th ed.]. St. Louis: Mosby; Registered Nurses' Association of Ontario. [2007]. *Embracing cultural diversity in health care: Developing cultural competence*. Toronto: Author. Retrieved from http://www.rnao.org/Storage/29/2336_BPG_Embracing_Cultural_Diversity.pdf; Srivastava, R. H. [2007]. *The healthcare professional's guide to cultural competence*. Toronto: Elsevier Canada.)

and the infant's face are approximately 20 cm apart and on the same plane.

Nursing and medical practices that encourage this interaction should be implemented. For example, immediately after birth, the infant should be placed naked, skin to skin, on the mother's abdomen or breasts, with the mother's and the infant's faces positioned so that they can easily make eye contact. Lights can be dimmed so that the infant's eyes will open. Instillation of prophylactic antibiotic ointment in the infant's eyes can be delayed until the infant and parents have had some time together in the first hour after birth.

Voice

The shared response of parents and infants to each other's voices is also remarkable. Parents wait tensely for the first cry. Once that cry has reassured them of the baby's health, they begin comforting behaviours. As the parents talk in high-pitched voices, the infant is alerted, stops crying temporarily, and turns toward them. This can be a wonderful bonding moment for fathers and partners.

The infant responds to higher-pitched voices and can distinguish the mother's voice from others soon after birth. Infants use their cries to signal hunger, pain, boredom, and fatigue. With experience, parents learn to distinguish such cries.

Odour

Another behaviour shared by parents and infants is a response to each other's odour. Mothers comment on the smell of their babies when first born and have noted that each infant has a unique odour. Infants learn rapidly to distinguish the odour of their mother's breast milk.

Entrainment

Newborns move in time with the structure of adult speech. They wave their arms, lift their heads, and kick their legs, seemingly "dancing in tune" to a parent's voice. Culturally determined rhythms of speech are ingrained in the infant long before spoken language is used to communicate. This shared rhythm also gives the parent positive feedback and establishes a positive setting for effective communication.

Biorhythmicity

The fetus is in tune with the mother's natural rhythms, such as heartbeats. After birth, a crying infant may be soothed by being held in a position where the mother's heartbeat can be heard or by hearing a recording of a heartbeat. One of the newborn's tasks is to establish a personal biorhythm, or to achieve biorhythmicity. Parents can help in this process by giving consistent loving care and using their infant's alert state to develop responsive behaviour and thereby increase social interactions and opportunities for learning (Fig. 22-4). The more quickly parents become competent in child care activities, the more quickly their psychological energy can be directed toward observing the communication cues that the infant gives them.

Reciprocity, Synchrony, and Habituation

Reciprocity is a type of body movement or behaviour that provides the observer with cues. The observer or receiver interprets the cues and responds to them. Reciprocity often takes several weeks to develop with a new baby. For example, when the newborn fusses and cries, the mother responds by picking up and cradling the infant; the baby becomes quiet and alert and establishes eye contact; and the mother verbalizes, sings, and coos while the baby maintains eye contact. As the baby habituates to the stimulus, the infant's responses stop, the baby then averts the eyes and yawns; and the mother decreases her active response (Fig. 22-5). If the parent continues to stimulate the infant, the baby may become fussy.

Synchrony refers to the fit between the infant's cues and the parent's response. When parent and infant have a synchronous interaction, it is mutually rewarding. Parents need time to interpret the infant's cues correctly. For example, after a certain time, the infant develops a specific cry in response to different situations, such as boredom, loneliness, hunger, and discomfort. The parent may need assistance in deciphering these cries, along with trial-and-error interventions, before synchrony develops.

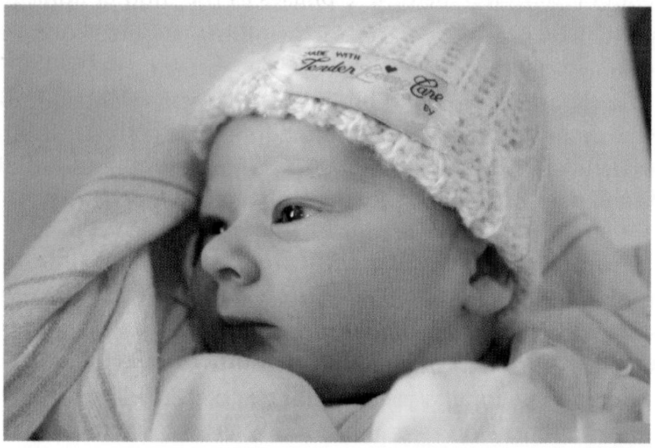

Fig. 22-4 Infant in alert state. *(Courtesy Julie and Darren Nelson, Loveland, CO.)*

Parental Role After Childbirth

Adaptation involves stabilizing tasks and coming to terms with commitments. Parents demonstrate growing competence in child care activities and are more attuned to their infant's behaviour. Typically, the period from the decision to conceive through the first months of having a child is termed the *transition to parenthood.*

Transition to Parenthood

Historically, the transition to parenthood was viewed as a crisis. The current perspective is that for most families parenthood is a developmental transition rather than a major life crisis. The transition to parenthood is described as a time of disorder and disequilibrium, as well as satisfaction, for mothers and their partners. Usual methods of coping often seem ineffective. Some parents can be so distressed that they are unable to be supportive of each other. Since men typically identify their spouses as their primary or only source of support, the transition can be harder for fathers, who feel deprived when the mothers, who are also experiencing stress, cannot provide their usual level of support. Strong emotions such as the helplessness, inadequacy, and anger that arise when dealing with a crying infant can catch many parents unprepared. On the other hand, parenthood allows adults to develop and display a selfless, warm, and caring side of themselves that may not be expressed in other adult roles.

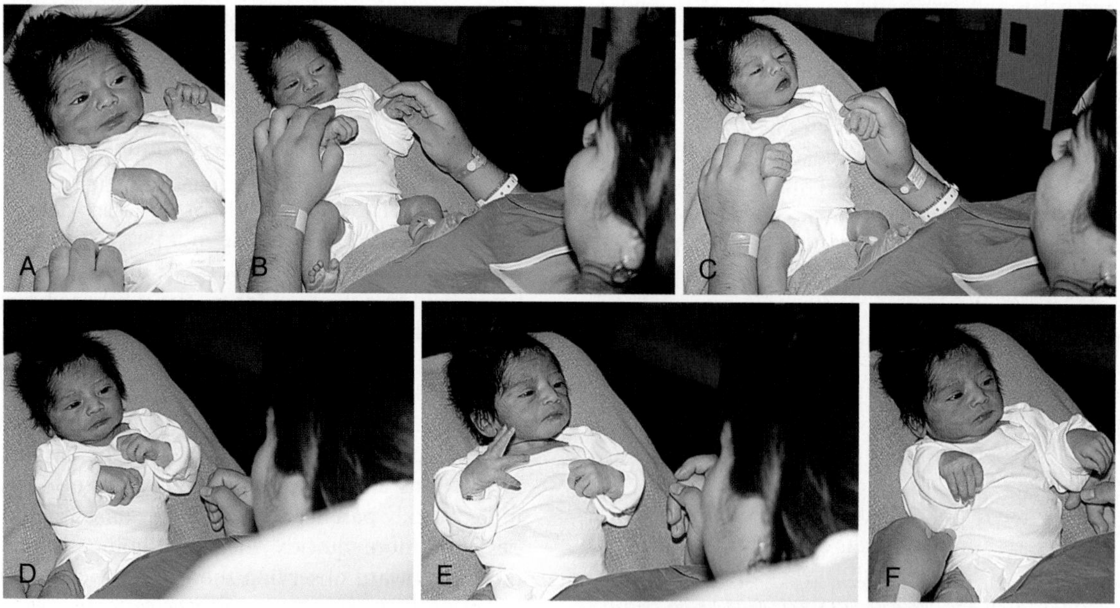

Fig. 22-5 Holding newborn in en face position, mother works to alert her daughter, 6 hours old. **A:** Infant is quiet and alert. **B:** Mother begins talking to daughter. **C:** Infant responds, opens mouth like her mother. **D:** Infant gazes at her mother. **E:** Infant waves hand. **F:** Infant glances away, resting. Hand relaxes. *(Courtesy Marjorie Pyle, RNC, Lifecircle, Costa Mesa, CA.)*

For most mothers and their partners, the transition to parenthood is viewed as an opportunity. Parents are stimulated to try new coping strategies as they work to master their new roles and reach new developmental levels. As they work through the transition, personal strength and resourcefulness are revealed.

Some parents have limited knowledge of what being a parent entails. These parents can benefit from more information on child care, changes in relationships, and differing views of parenting held by partners. Women have more support from female relatives and postnatal groups, whereas men often lack support mechanisms and have only health professionals and work colleagues for information and support (Deave & Johnson, 2008; Deave, Johnson, & Ingram, 2008).

Parental Tasks and Responsibilities

Parents need to reconcile the actual child with the fantasy and dream child. This means coming to terms with the infant's physical appearance, sex, innate temperament, and physical status. If the real child differs greatly from the fantasy child, parents may delay acceptance of the child. In some instances, they may never accept the child.

Some parents are startled by the normal appearance of the neonate—the size, colour, moulding of the head, Mongolian spots, or bowed appearance of the legs. Many fathers have commented that they thought the odd shape of the infant's head (moulding) meant that the infant would be mentally disabled.

Parents may know the sex of the infant before birth because of ultrasound assessments; for those who do not have this information, disappointment over the sex can take time to resolve. The parents can provide adequate physical care but find it difficult to be sincerely involved with the infant until this internal conflict has been resolved. As one mother remarked,

> I really wanted a boy. I know it is silly and irrational, but when they said, "She's a lovely little girl," I was so disappointed and angry—yes, angry—that I could hardly look at her. Oh, I looked after her okay, her feedings and baths and things, but I couldn't feel excited. To tell the truth, I felt like a monster not liking my child. Then one day she was lying there and she turned her head and looked right at me. I felt a flooding of love for her come over me, and we looked at each other a long time. It's okay now. I wouldn't change her for all the boys in the world.

Parents need to become adept in the care of the infant, including caregiving activities, noting the communication cues the infant gives to indicate needs and responding appropriately to those needs. Self-esteem grows with competence. Breastfeeding makes mothers feel they are contributing in a unique way to the welfare of the infant. The infant's response to parental care and attention can be interpreted as a comment on the quality of that care. Infant behaviours that parents interpret as positive responses to their care include being consoled easily, enjoying being cuddled, and making eye contact. Spitting up frequently after feedings, crying, and being unpredictable may be perceived as negative responses to parental care. Continuation of these infant responses that are viewed as negative can result in alienation of parent and infant, to the detriment of the infant.

Assistance, including advice by husbands, partners, mothers, mothers-in-law, and professional workers, can be seen as either supportive or an indication of how inept these others judge the new parents to be. Criticism, real or imagined, of the new parents' ability to provide adequate physical care, nutrition, or social stimulation for the infant can prove to be devastating. By providing encouragement and praise for parenting efforts, nurses can bolster the new parents' confidence.

Parents must establish a place for the newborn within the family group. Whether the infant is the firstborn or the last born, all family members must adjust their roles to accommodate the newcomer. The firstborn child needs support to accept a rival for parental affections. An older child needs help dealing with losing a favoured position in the family hierarchy. The parents are expected to negotiate these changes.

Becoming a Mother

Rubin (1961) identified three phases as the mother adjusts to her parental role. These phases are characterized by dependent behaviour, dependent–independent behaviour, and interdependent behaviour. The phases extend over the first several weeks (Table 22-4). Rubin's research was conducted when the length of stay in the hospital was for a longer period of time (3 to 5 or more days). With today's early discharge, women seem to move through the phases faster.

Mercer (2004) has suggested that the concept of maternal role attainment introduced by Rubin in 1967 be replaced with *becoming a mother* to signify the transformation and growth of the mother identity. Becoming a mother implies more than

Table 22-4 Phases of Maternal Postpartum Adjustment

PHASE	CHARACTERISTICS
Dependent: taking-in	First 24 hr (range of 1-2 days) Focus–Self and meeting of basic needs Reliance on others to meet needs for comfort, rest, closeness, and nourishment Excited and talkative Desire to review birth experience
Dependent-independent: taking hold	Starts second or third day; lasts 10 days to several weeks Focus–Care of baby and competent mothering Desire to take charge Nurturing and acceptance by others still important Eagerness to learn and practice–Optimal period for teaching by nurses Handling of physical discomforts and emotional changes Possible experience with blues
Interdependent: letting go	Focus–Forward movement of family as unit with interacting members Reassertion of relationship with partner Resumption of sexual intimacy Resolution of individual roles

(From Rubin, R. [1961]. Basic maternal behavior. *Nursing Outlook, 9*, 683–686.)

attaining a role; it includes learning new skills and increasing her confidence in herself as she meets new challenges in caring for her child or children.

The transition to motherhood requires adjustment for the mother and her family. There is disruption inherent in that adjustment, and some circumstances, such as problems in postpartum recovery or giving birth to a high-risk infant, add to the disruption (Nelson, 2003). Providing social support and enhancing maternal identity improve the ability of the mother to perceive and accurately interpret the signals of her infant and respond appropriately (Shin, Park, & Kim, 2006).

Nelson (2003) identified two social processes in maternal transition. The primary process is engagement, or making a commitment to being a mother, actively caring for her child, and experiencing his or her presence. The secondary process is experiencing herself as a mother, which leads to growth and transformation. During this process, she must learn how to mother and adapt to a changed relationship with her partner, family, and friends; she must examine herself in relation to the past and present and come to view herself as a mother; and she must make decisions regarding whether and when to return to work.

Not all mothers experience the transition to motherhood in the same way. For some women, becoming a mother entails multiple losses. For example, for some single women there may be a loss of the family of origin when they do not accept her decision to have the child and loss of a relationship with the father of the baby, with friends, and with their own sense of self. Women describe a loss of dreams, including loss of job, financial security, and a future profession (Keating-Lefler & Wilson, 2004). Accompanying these losses can be a loss of support.

Mercer (2004) has provided descriptors for the stages involved in establishing a maternal identity while becoming a mother: "(a) commitment, attachment, and preparation (pregnancy); (b) acquaintance, learning, and physical restoration (first 2 to 6 weeks following birth); (c) moving toward a new normal (2 weeks to 4 months); and (d) achievement of the maternal identity (around 4 months)." The time of achievement of the stages varies, and the stages may overlap. Achievement is influenced by mother and infant variables and the social environment (Mercer, 2004).

In addition to being familiar with the stages and general characteristics of becoming a mother, nurses must individualize their assessments and interventions. Mothers need to know that it is common to feel overwhelmed and insecure and to experience physical and mental fatigue in the first months of parenthood. Empathic listening and interactive dialogue are effective approaches to enhancing mother–infant interactions and assisting the parents in the transition (Mercer, 2006; Mercer & Walker, 2006). They need to be assured that this situation is temporary and that it will take 3 to 6 months to become comfortable in caregiving and in being a mother (Nelson, 2003). Maternal support by professionals should not end with hospital discharge but extend over the next 4 to 6 months. Nurses can advocate for the extension of such support services well into the postpartum period. More reality-based perinatal education programs are necessary to better prepare mothers and to decrease their anxiety.

Nurses can discuss, before and after birth, the usual postpartum concerns that mothers experience and can provide anticipatory guidance on coping strategies, such as resting when the infant sleeps and planning with an extended family member or friend to do the housework for the first week or two after the baby is born. In some provinces, once a mother is home, she will receive a phone call and, if needed, a visit from a public health nurse. Nurses should plan additional supportive counselling for first-time mothers inexperienced in child care, women whose careers had provided outside stimulation, women who lack friends or family members with whom to share delights and concerns, and adolescent mothers.

Resuming Sexual Intimacy

The couple may begin to engage in sexual intercourse during the second to fourth week after the baby is born, once lochia discharge has stopped. Some couples begin earlier, as soon as it can be accomplished without discomfort, depending on factors such as timing, amount of vaginal dryness, and breastfeeding status. Sexual intimacy enhances the adult aspect of the family, and the adult pair shares a closeness denied to other family members.

Changes in a woman's sexuality after childbirth are related to hormonal shifts, increased breast size, uneasiness with a body that has yet to return to a prepregnant size, chronic fatigue related to sleep deprivation, and physical exhaustion. Many new fathers speak of the alienation they experience when they observe the intimate mother–infant relationship, and some are frank in expressing feelings of jealousy toward the infant. The resumption of sexual intimacy seems to bring the parents' relationship back into focus.

Before and after birth, nurses should review with new parents their plans for other pregnancies and their preferences for contraception.

Postpartum Adjustment in the Lesbian Couple

Same-sex marriage has been legal in Canada since 2003. Little is known about postpartum role adjustment in the same-sex couple. Relationship satisfaction in first-time same-sex parent couples appears to be related to egalitarianism, commitment, sexual compatibility, and communication skills. The lesbian couple may have to adjust to the birth mother's decision for insemination by an anonymous sperm donor. Similar to heterosexual parent couples, most same-sex parent couples voice concern about less time and energy for their relationship after the arrival of the baby. Both partners consider themselves to be equal parents who share actively in childrearing. A primary concern of co-mothers and co-fathers is the legal vulnerability of same-sex families if the couple is not married.

Same-sex couples face strong social sanctions regarding pregnancy and parenting. Their families may not have resolved the initial dismay and guilt over learning of their child's homosexuality, or they may disagree with the couple's decision to conceive and be parents. Same-sex parents may encounter public ignorance and social and legal invisibility. With careful planning, their transition to parenthood will be successful. Education regarding equal parenting, sharing parenting at home, establishing a distinct parenting role within the family, and supporting each other's sense of identity as a parent can assist the same-sex couple in this transition. If family support is limited or absent, the nurse can help same-sex couples locate more supportive social groups.

Becoming a Father

Research on paternal adjustment to parenthood indicates that fathers go through predictable phases during their transition to parenthood (St. John, Cameron, & McVeigh, 2005). During this period, fathers experience intense emotions. Many fathers acknowledge that their expectations were of limited value once they were immersed in the reality of parenthood. Feelings that often accompany this reality are sadness, ambivalence, jealousy, frustration at not being able to participate in breastfeeding, and an overwhelming desire to be more involved. Most of these feelings are different from those that mothers report. Some fathers are pleasantly surprised at the ease and fun of parenting. In their transition to mastery, fathers take control and become more actively involved in the infant's life (Table 22-5).

First-time fathers tend to perceive the first 4 to 10 weeks of parenthood in much the same way that mothers do (i.e., as a period characterized by uncertainty, increased responsibility, disruption of sleep, and inability to control the time needed to care for the infant and re-establish the marital dyad). Fathers express concerns about receiving less attention from their partners relative to their relationship, the mother's lack of recognition of the father's desire to participate in decision making for the infant, and limited time for establishing a relationship with their infants. These concerns can precipitate feelings of jealousy of the infant. To help alleviate these feelings, the father should discuss his individual concerns and needs with his partner and become more involved with the infant.

Concerns of fathers are often not addressed adequately in prenatal or postnatal education. The father's relationship with the child is fostered by time alone with the child. Health professionals must address the father's needs to assist in his transition to parenthood (Premberg, Hellström, & Berg, 2008). An excellent resource for fathers is The New Fathers Guide from the Region of Peel Health Department (http://www.peelregion.ca/health/family-health/just-for-dad/index.htm).

Table 22-5 Development of a Father–Infant Relationship: Process Components

COMPONENT	CHARACTERISTICS
Making a commitment	Is willing to invest in and take responsibility for nurturing the relationship despite difficulties in parenting and other life demands Feels reality of commitment—At confirmation of pregnancy; during pregnancy and birth; when providing infant care; when infant responds to him Feels duty to nurture and protect because of helpless nature of infant Desires to get to know and be psychologically involved Is rewarded by infant smile, increased self-esteem, gaining a new dimension in life, finding the child within self
Becoming connected	First meeting with infant—Feels joy, elation, awe, and wonder Has sense of bond with the infant—May feel this at first meeting, when first touching or holding infant, or gradually during the first 2 months Turning point—Perceives infant as more responsive, predictable, and familiar
Making room for baby	Makes changes in work and in social and personal time, in relationship with wife or partner, and within self so that he is more physically and emotionally available to infant

Father–Infant Relationship

In North American culture, neonates have a powerful impact on their fathers, who can become intensely involved with their babies (Fig. 22-6). The term used for the father's absorption, preoccupation, and interest in the infant is **engrossment**. Characteristics of engrossment include some of the sensual responses relating to touch and eye-to-eye contact that were discussed earlier (see earlier section, The Senses, p. 560) and the father's keen awareness of features both unique and similar to himself that validate his claim to the infant. An outstanding response is one of strong attraction to the newborn. Fathers spend considerable time "communicating" with the infant and taking delight in the infant's response to them (Fig. 22-7). They can experience increased self-esteem and a sense of being proud, larger, more mature, and older after seeing their baby for the first time.

Fathers spend less time than mothers with infants, and their interactions with their infants tend to be characterized by stimulating social play rather than caretaking. The subtle and more obvious differences in stimulation from the mother and father provide a wider social experience for the infant.

Like mothers, fathers can benefit from nursing interventions during the postpartum period. Nurses can arrange

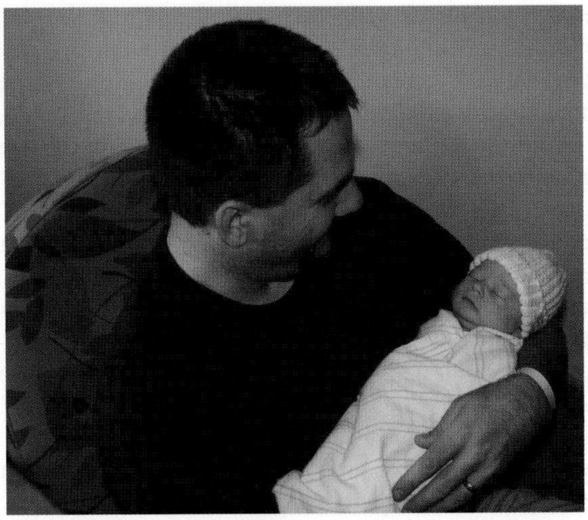

Fig. 22-6 Engrossment. Father absorbed in looking at his newborn son. *(Courtesy Darren Nelson, Loveland, CO.)*

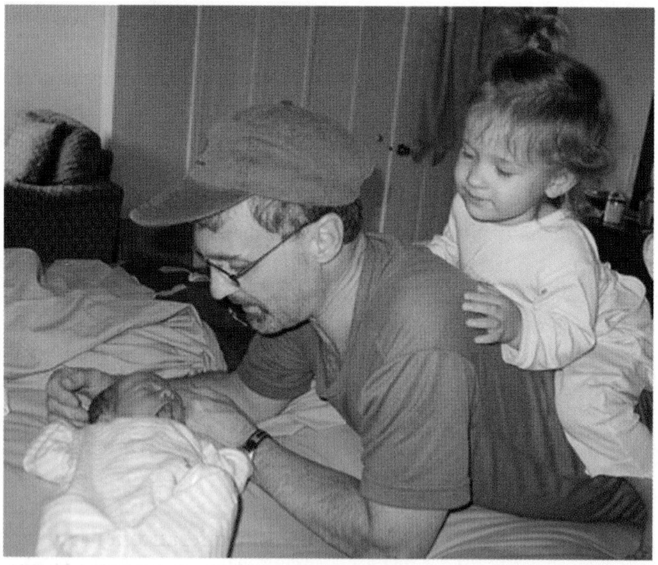

Fig. 22-7 Father interacting with newborn while sibling observes with interest. *(Courtesy Christine Brockett, Boulder, CO.)*

to teach infant care when the father is present and provide anticipatory guidance for fathers about the transition to parenthood. Separate prenatal and parenting classes and parenting support groups for fathers can provide them with an opportunity to discuss their concerns and have some of their needs met. Postpartum phone calls and home visits by a nurse should include time for assessment of the father's adjustment and needs.

Infant–Parent Adjustment

Newborns participate actively in shaping their parents' reaction to them. Behavioural characteristics of the infant influence parenting behaviours. The infant and parent each have unique rhythms, behaviours, and response styles that are brought to every interaction. Infant–parent interactions can be facilitated in at least three ways: (1) modulation of rhythm, (2) modification of behavioural repertoires, and (3) mutual responsivity. Nurses can teach parents about these three aspects of infant–parent interaction through discussions, written materials, and movies on infant capabilities. A creative approach is to record the parent–infant pair during an interaction and then use the individualized recording to discuss the pair's rhythm, behavioural repertoire, and responsivity.

Rhythm

To modulate rhythm, both parent and infant must be able to interact. Therefore, the infant must be in the alert state, one of the most difficult of the sleep–wake states to maintain. The alert state (see Fig. 22-4) occurs most often during a feeding or in face-to-face play. The parent must work hard to help the infant maintain the alert state long enough and often enough for interactions to take place. The en face position is usually assumed (see Fig. 22-5, D). Multiparous mothers in particular are very sensitive and responsive to the infant's feeding rhythms. Mothers learn to reserve stimulation for pauses in sucking activity and not to talk or smile excessively while the infant is sucking because the baby will stop feeding to interact with her. With maturity, the infant can sustain longer interactions by modulating activity rhythms (i.e., limb movement, sucking, gaze alternation, and habituation). Meanwhile, the parent becomes more attuned to the infant's rhythms and learns to modulate the rhythms, facilitating a rhythmic turn-taking interaction.

Behavioural Repertoires

Both the infant and the parent have a repertoire of behaviours they can use to facilitate interactions. Fathers and mothers engage in these behaviours, depending on the extent of their contact with the infant and their caregiving.

The infant's behavioural repertoire includes gazing, vocalizing, and facial expressions. The infant is able to focus and follow the human face from birth and to alternate the gaze voluntarily, looking away from the parent's face when understimulated or overstimulated (see Fig. 22-5, F). One of the key responses for the parents to learn is to be sensitive to the infant's capacity for attention and inattention. Developing this sensitivity is especially important when interacting with preterm infants.

Body gestures form a part of the infant's early language. Babies greet parents with waving hands (see Fig. 22-5, E) or a reaching out of hands. They can raise an eyebrow or soften their expression to elicit loving attention. Game playing can stimulate them to smile or laugh. Pouting or crying, arching of the back, and general squirming usually signal the end of an interaction.

The parents' repertoire includes various types of interactive behaviours, such as constantly looking at the infant and noting the infant's response. New parents often remark that they are exhausted from looking at the baby and smiling. Adults also "infantilize" their speech to help the infant listen. They do this by slowing the tempo, speaking loudly and rhythmically, and emphasizing key words. Phrases are repeated frequently. Infantilizing does not mean using baby talk, which involves distortion of sounds.

To communicate emotions to the infant, parents often use facial expressions such as slow and exaggerated looks of surprise, happiness, and confusion. Games such as "peek-a-boo" and imitation of the infant's behaviours are other means of interaction. For example, if the baby smiles, so does the parent; if the baby frowns, the parent responds in kind.

Responsivity

Contingent responses (responsivity) are those that occur within a specific time and are similar in form to a stimulus behaviour. The adult has the feeling of having an influence on the interaction. Infant behaviours such as smiling, cooing, and sustained eye contact, usually in en face position, are viewed as contingent responses. The infant's responses act as rewards to the initiator and encourage the adult to continue with the game when the infant responds positively. When the adult imitates the infant, the infant appears to enjoy it. A progression occurs in the types of behaviours that parents present for the baby to imitate; for example, in early interactions the parent will grimace rather than laugh, which is in keeping with the infant's developmental level. Such behaviours sustain interactions and promote harmony in the relationship.

Diversity in Transitions to Parenthood

The ways in which parents respond to the birth of their child are influenced by various factors, including age, social networks, culture, socioeconomic conditions, and personal aspirations for the future.

Age

Maternal age has a definite effect on the outcome of pregnancy. The mother and fetus are at highest risk when the mother is an adolescent or is more than 35 years old (see Critical Thinking Exercise).

The Adolescent Mother

Although it is biologically possible for the adolescent female to become a parent, her egocentricity and concrete thinking may interfere with her ability to parent effectively. The very young adolescent mother is inexperienced and unprepared to recognize the early signs of illness, potential danger, or household hazards. She may inadvertently neglect her child. In most instances, with adequate support and developmentally appropriate teaching, adolescents can learn effective parenting skills (Maputie, 2006).

The transition to parenthood may be difficult for adolescent parents. Coping with the developmental tasks of parenthood is often complicated by the unmet developmental needs and tasks of adolescence. Some young parents may experience difficulty accepting a changing self-image and adjusting to new roles related to the responsibilities of infant care. On the other hand, some adolescent parents may have higher self-concepts than their nonparenting peers.

As adolescent parents move through the transition to parenthood, they may feel "different" from their peers, excluded from "fun" activities, and prematurely forced to enter an adult social role. The conflict between their own desires and the infant's demands, in addition to the low tolerance for frustration that is typical of adolescence, further contribute to the normal psychosocial stress of childbirth (see Critical Thinking Exercise). Maintaining a relationship with the baby's father is beneficial for the teen mother and her infant.

Adolescent mothers provide warm and attentive physical care; however, they use less verbal interaction than do older parents, and adolescents tend to be less responsive and to interact less positively with their infants than older mothers. Interventions emphasizing verbal and nonverbal communication skills between mother and infant are important. Such intervention strategies must be concrete and specific because of the cognitive level of adolescents. In comparison with adult mothers, teenage mothers have a limited knowledge of child development. They tend to expect too much of their children too soon and often characterize their infants as being fussy. This limited knowledge may cause teenagers to respond to their infants inappropriately.

Many young mothers pattern their maternal role on what they themselves experienced. Therefore, nurses need to determine the kind of support that people close to the young mother are able and prepared to give and the kinds of community aid available to supplement this support. Many teenage mothers can identify a source of social support, with the predominant source being their own mothers.

Continued assessment of the new mother's parenting abilities during this postbirth period is essential. Ongoing support should be provided by involving the grandparents and other family members and through home visits and group sessions for discussion of infant care and parenting concerns. Outreach programs addressing self-management, parent–child interactions, and child injuries, in addition to programs that provide prompt and effective community intervention, can prevent serious problems from occurring. As the adolescent performs her mothering role within the framework of her family, she may need to address dependence and independence issues. The adolescent's family members also may need help adapting to their new roles.

CRITICAL THINKING EXERCISE

Postpartum Adjustment for the Adolescent and the Older Mother

You are a public health nurse and have had two patients referred to you. Carol is a 15-year-old first-time mother of a 5-day-old girl; she lives with her mother. The father of the baby, Robert, is 17 years old and attended childbirth classes with Carol. She is breastfeeding the baby but says that the baby sucks too slowly and takes too much time to eat. She said she thinks the baby should know enough to sleep longer at night. Robert would like to feed the baby some cereal since he heard that solid food will make a baby sleep longer at night.

Audrey is a 36-year-old attorney who has been practicing law for 7 years. She just gave birth to her first baby; she and her husband delayed parenting by choice until their careers were well established. She had an uneventful pregnancy, labour, and birth. During a telephone call 48 hours after discharge, when she was asked how things were going, Audrey burst into tears and said, "I didn't expect it to be like this! Nothing is going right."

1. Evidence—Is there sufficient evidence to draw conclusions about what teaching and care these new parents need?
2. Assumptions—What assumptions can be made about the following factors:
   a. The relationship of maternal age and postpartum adjustment
   b. The need for social support in the postnatal period
   c. The need for perinatal education
   d. Long-term prognosis for positive outcomes
3. What implications and priorities for nursing care can be drawn at this time?
4. Does the evidence objectively support your conclusion?
5. Are there alternative perspectives to your conclusion?

The Adolescent Father

The adolescent father and mother face immediate developmental crises, which include completing the developmental tasks of adolescence, making a transition to parenthood, and sometimes adapting to marriage. These transitions can be stressful. The nurse may initiate interaction with the adolescent father by asking him to be present when postpartum home visits are made and to accompany the mother and baby to well-baby checks at the clinic or health care provider's office. With the adolescent mother's agreement, the nurse may contact the father directly. Adolescent fathers need support to discuss their emotional responses to the pregnancy. The father's feelings of guilt, powerlessness, or bravado should be recognized because of their negative consequences for both the parents and the child. Counselling of adolescent fathers needs to be reality oriented. Topics such as finances, child care, parenting skills, and the father's role in the birth experience must be discussed. Teenage fathers also need to know about reproductive physiology, birth control options, and risk-reducing sex practices.

The adolescent father may continue to be involved in an ongoing relationship with the young mother and his baby. In many instances, he may also play an important role in making decisions about child care and raising the child. He may need help in developing realistic perceptions of his role as father to a child. He should be encouraged to use coping mechanisms that are not detrimental to the well-being of himself, his partner, or his child. The nurse can enlist support systems, parents, and professional agencies on his behalf.

Maternal Age Greater Than 35 Years

Women older than 35 years continue their childbearing either by choice or because of a lack or failure of contraception during the perimenopausal years. Some women have postponed pregnancy because of careers or other reasons, and some women of infertile couples finally become pregnant with the aid of technological advances (see Evidence-Informed Practice box).

Adjustment of older mothers to changes involved in becoming a parent and seeing themselves as competent is aided by support from their partners. Support from other family members and friends is also important for positive self-evaluation of parenting, a sense of well-being and satisfaction, and help in dealing with associated stress.

Changes in the sexual aspect of a relationship can create a stressor for new midlife parents. Mothers report that finding time and energy for a romantic rendezvous is more difficult,

EVIDENCE-INFORMED PRACTICE Having a Baby Later in Life

—Pat Gingrich

Ask the Question

What are the unique risks for advanced maternal age? Are there differences in expectations and nursing care for older primiparas than for younger new mothers?

Search for Evidence

Search Strategies

Professional organization guidelines, meta-analyses, systematic reviews, randomized controlled trials, nonrandomized prospective studies, and retrospective studies since 2006

Databases Searched

CINAHL, Cochrane, Medline, National Guideline Clearinghouse, TRIP Database Plus, and the Web sites for the Association of Women's Health, Obstetric and Neonatal Nursing (AWHONN), and Centers for Disease Control and Prevention (CDC)

Critically Analyze the Evidence

The childbearing years can span four decades of life. Many women are delaying childbirth well into their 30s or 40s. Older mothers are more likely to be educated and have a higher socioeconomic status but may lack some of the robust physical resilience of youth.

Advanced maternal age is a risk factor for not only trisomy 21 (Down syndrome) but also increased stillbirths, preterm births, and small-for-gestational-age and low-birth-weight infants, particularly in primigravidas over 40 (Delpisheh et al., 2008). A systematic review of 37 studies confirms that the risk of stillbirth increases significantly over age 35 (Huang et al., 2007).

Interestingly, even advanced age in the father may affect the offspring. A Danish study of 102,879 couples who gave birth between 1980 and 1996 demonstrated a significantly increased risk of mortality in offspring of fathers over age 45. The risk for mortality persisted into adulthood (Zhu et al., 2008).

Implications for Practice

Most older mothers have healthy and normal births. The nurse can ask open-ended questions about the baby and pregnancy to assess the psychosocial and emotional status of the patient. According to Suplee, Dawley, and Bloch (2007), older first-time mothers may have spent many years seeking pregnancy and may bring a "last-chance" focus to this new role. It is important for the nurse to facilitate realistic expectations in the parent regarding life changes. Some older women expect a trouble-free, controlled, "no-risk" birth and a quick return to normal. They may need reminders of the need for flexibility about the birth process and the realities of postpartum adjustment. Others may be insecure about their physical and mental abilities and may see themselves as "high-risk," requiring much care. The nurse can help the anxious mother focus on the normal and positive and encourage her to start envisioning holding her baby in her arms. Because many older first-time mothers may live far from family and have aging parents and their partners may work long hours, these mothers may not have an extensive social support system or realize how isolated they will feel. After birth, the nurse can provide the mother at home some resources about support groups and services and encourage networking among new mothers and play groups (Suplee et al., 2007).

References

Delpisheh, A., et al. (2008). Pregnancy late in life: A hospital-based study of birth outcomes. *Journal of Women's Health, 17*(6), 1–6. Retrieved from http://www.liebertonline.com/doi/abs/10.1089/jwh.2008.0514.

Huang, L., et al. (2007). Maternal age and risk of stillbirth: A systematic review. *Canadian Medical Association Journal, 178*(2), 165–172.

Suplee, P. D., Dawley, K., & Bloch, J. R. (2007). Tailoring peripartum nursing care for women of advanced maternal age. *Journal of Obstetric, Gynecologic and Neonatal Nursing, 36*(6), 616–623.

Zhu, J. L., et al. (2008). Paternal age and mortality in children. *European Journal of Epidemiology, 23*(7), 443–447.

largely because of the time it takes to care for an infant and the decreasing libido that normally accompanies getting older.

Work, career issues, and child care are major sources of conflict and stress for older mothers. Conflicts emerge over being disinterested in work, worrying about giving enough attention to work with the distractions of a new baby, and anticipating what it will be like to return to work.

Another major issue for older mothers with careers is the perception of loss of control. Mothers older than 35 are at a different stage in their careers than younger mothers, often having attained high levels of education, career, and income. The loss of control experienced when going from the consistency of a work role to the inconsistency of the parent role comes as a surprise to many. Helping the older mother have realistic expectations of herself and parenthood is essential.

New mothers who are also perimenopausal may find it hard to distinguish fatigue, loss of sleep, decreased libido, or other physiological symptoms as the causes of the change in their sex lives. Although many women view menopause as a natural stage of life, for midlife mothers this cessation of menstruation coincides with the state of parenthood. The changes of midlife and menopause can add more emotional and physical stress to older mothers' lives because of the time- and energy-consuming aspects of raising a young child.

Paternal Age Greater Than 35 Years

Older fathers describe their experience of midlife parenting as wonderful but not without drawbacks. What they see as positive aspects of parenthood in older years include increased love and commitment between the spouses, a reinforcement of why one married in the first place, a feeling of being complete, experiencing "the child" in oneself again, more financial stability than in younger years, and more freedom to focus on parenting rather than on career. A common theme expressed is sharing: sharing joy, sharing in raising the child, sharing as a family. The main drawback of midlife parenting is the change it makes in the relationship with their partner.

Social Support

Positive adaptation by new parents, including adolescent parents, is strongly related to social support during the transition to parenthood. Social support is multidimensional and includes the number of members in a person's social network, types of support, perceived general support, actual support received, and satisfaction with support available and received. The type and satisfaction of support appear to be more important than the total number of support network members.

Across cultural groups, families and friends of new parents form an important dimension of the parent's social network. Through seeking help within the social network, new mothers learn culturally valued practices and develop role competency.

Social networks provide a support system on which parents can rely for assistance, but they also can be a source of conflict. Sometimes a large network can cause problems because it results in conflicting advice coming from numerous people. Grandparents or in-laws are most appreciated when they assist with household responsibilities and do not intrude into the parents' privacy or judge them critically.

Because of the extent of restructuring and reorganization that occurs in a family with the birth of another child, the mother's moods and fatigue in the postpartum period can be helped more by situation-specific support from family and friends than by general support. General support addresses feeling loved, respected, and valued. Situation-specific support relates to practical concerns, such as physical needs and child care. For example, the practical support of a grandparent bathing the infant can help lessen a second-time mother's feelings of loss by providing her time to be with her firstborn child.

Culture

Cultural beliefs and practices are important determinants of health for the mother and infant and also influence parenting behaviours. Culture defines what is socially acceptable in terms of eye contact, touch, and space. Culture influences the interactions with the baby and the parent's or family's caregiving style. For example, providing for a period of rest and recuperation for the mother after birth is prominent in several cultures. Asian mothers are encouraged to remain at home with the baby at least 30 days after birth and are not supposed to engage in household chores, including care of the baby. Often, the grandmother takes over the baby's care immediately, even before discharge from the hospital (D'Avanzo, 2008). Jordanian mothers have a 40-day lying-in after birth during which their mothers or sisters care for the baby (D'Avanzo, 2008). Japanese mothers rest for the first 2 months after childbirth. Latin Americans may practice an intergenerational family ritual, *la cuarentena*. For 40 days after birth, the mother is expected to recuperate and get acquainted with her infant. Traditionally, this involves many restrictions concerning food (spicy or cold foods, fish, pork, and citrus are avoided; tortillas and chicken soup are encouraged); exercise; and activities, including sexual intercourse. Many women avoid bathing and washing their hair. The practice of *la cuarentena* incorporates individuals into the family, instills parental responsibility, and integrates the family during a critical life event (D'Avanzo, 2008).

The desire for and valuing of children is salient in all cultures. In Asian families, children are valued as a source of family strength and stability, are perceived as wealth, and are objects of parental love and affection. Infants almost always are given an affectionate cradle name that is used during the first years of life (e.g., a Filipino girl might be called "Bong-Bong" and a boy "Ling-Ling").

Differing cultural values can influence parents' interactions with health care providers. For example, Asians are taught to be humble and obedient; it is frowned upon to be outspoken. They are brought up to not question authority figures (such as a nurse), to avoid confrontation, and to respect the yin/yang balance in nature. Because of these learned values, an Asian mother might not confront the nurse about the length of time it has taken to receive the medication requested for her pain due to perineal laceration repair or a Caesarean incision.

Knowledge of cultural beliefs can help the nurse make more accurate assessments and diagnoses of observed parenting behaviours. For example, nurses may become concerned when they observe cultural practices that appear to reflect poor maternal–infant bonding. Algerian mothers may not unwrap and explore their infants as part of the acquaintance process because in Algeria babies are wrapped tightly in swaddling clothes to protect them physically and psychologically (D'Avanzo, 2008). The nurse may observe a Vietnamese woman who gives minimal care to her infant and refuses to cuddle or further interact with her baby. This apparent lack of interest in the newborn is this cultural group's attempt to ward off evil spirits and actually reflects an intense love and concern for the infant (Galanti, 2003). An Asian mother might be criticized for almost immediately relinquishing the care of the infant to the grandmother and not even attempting to hold her baby when it is brought to her room. However, in Asian extended families, members show their support for a new mother's rest and recuperation by assisting with the care of the baby. A mix of breastfeeding and bottle-feeding may be standard practice for Japanese mothers. This is out of concern for the mother's rest during the first 2 to 3 months and does not lead to any problems with lactation; breastfeeding is widespread and successful among Japanese women. Because all members of a cultural group do not necessarily adhere to traditional practices, it is important to validate which cultural practices are important to individual parents.

Cultural beliefs and values give perspective to the meaning of childbirth for a new mother. Nurses can provide an opportunity for a new mother to talk about her perception of the meaning of childbearing. In helping new families adjust to parenthood, nurses must provide culturally sensitive care by following principles that facilitate nursing practice within transcultural situations.

Socioeconomic Conditions

Socioeconomic conditions, a key determinant of health, often determine access to available resources. Parents whose economic condition is made worse with the birth of each child and who are unable to use an effective method of fertility management may find childbirth complicated by concern for their own health and a sense of helplessness. Mothers who are single, separated or divorced from their husbands, or without a partner, family, and friends for whatever reason may view the birth of a child with dread. Serious financial problems may override any desire for mothering the infant.

Homeless Women

Homeless women are a marginalized group who may require extensive nursing support. According to Little, Gorman, Dzendoletas, and Moravac (2007), a significant number of homeless youth (up to 27 years of age) are pregnant in major Canadian cities. Women come to live on the streets earlier than men and are more likely to have experienced sexual and physical abuse, mental health issues, and depression. Annually, approximately 350 infants are born in Toronto to mothers who are homeless (Little et al., 2007).

Care must be taken to encourage homeless pregnant women to seek prenatal care in order to reduce poor mother and baby outcomes. Caregiver attitudes, wait times, and transportation costs can be a deterrent to seeking prenatal care (Bloom et al., 2004). It is essential that parents develop therapeutic relationships with health care providers in order to increase the likelihood of these mothers trusting medical care for their children. Nurses must work diligently to develop these trusting relationships so that teaching can occur and so that the mother and nurse can work together to find suitable accommodation for these families.

Personal Aspirations

Parenthood may interfere with or block the plans of some women for personal freedom or advancement in their careers. Resentment about this loss may not have been resolved during the prenatal period; if it remains unresolved, it will spill over into caregiving activities. This may result in indifference toward and neglect of the infant or excessive concern and the setting of impossibly high standards for her own behaviour or the child's performance.

Nursing interventions include providing opportunities for mothers to express their feelings freely to an objective listener, discuss measures to permit personal growth, and learn about the care of their infant. Referring the woman to a support group of other mothers in the same situation may also be helpful.

Nurses also can be proactive in influencing changes in work policies related to maternity and paternity leaves, varying models of work sharing, and family-friendly work environments. Some corporations already structure their work sites to support new mothers (e.g., by providing on-site day care facilities and breastfeeding rooms).

Parental Sensory Impairment

In the early dialogue between the parent and child, each uses all senses—sight, hearing, touch, taste, and smell—to initiate and sustain the attachment process. A parent who has an impairment of one of the senses needs to maximize use of the remaining senses. These parents may need the assistance and support of a sighted or hearing person and other accommodations to their disability to help them become skilled parents. It is important for nurses and other health care providers to remember that these people are parents living with a disability and are not disabled parents. Most provinces now have legislation to ensure that people with disabilities have access to required resources.

Visually Impaired Parent

Visual impairment alone does not seem to have a negative effect on mothers' early parenting experiences. These mothers, just as sighted mothers, express the wonders of parenthood and encourage other visually impaired persons to become parents. Mothers with disabilities tend to value the importance of performing parenting tasks in the perceived culturally usual way.

Although visually impaired mothers initially feel pressure to conform to traditional, sighted ways of parenting, they soon adapt these ways and develop methods better suited to themselves. Activities that visually impaired mothers may do differently include preparation of the infant's nursery, clothes, and supplies. Mothers may put an entire clothing outfit together and hang it in the closet rather than keeping the items separately in drawers. They might develop a labelling system for the infant's clothing and put diapering, bathing, and other care supplies where these will be easy to locate with minimal searching. A strength that visually impaired parents have is a heightened sensitivity to other sensory outputs. A blind mother can tell when her infant is facing her because she can feel the baby's breath on her face.

One of the major difficulties that visually impaired parents experience is the skepticism, open or hidden, of health care providers. Visually impaired people sense reluctance on the part of others to acknowledge that they have a right to be parents. All too often, nurses and doctors lack the experience to deal with the childbearing and childrearing needs of visually impaired mothers and mothers with other disabilities (such as the hearing impaired, physically impaired, and mentally challenged). The nurse's best approach is to assess the mother's capabilities. From that basis the nurse can make plans to assist the woman, often in much the same way as for a mother with sight. Visually impaired mothers have made suggestions for providing care for women such as themselves during childbearing (Box 22-2). Such approaches by the nurse can help avoid a sense of increased vulnerability on the mother's part. Childbirth education resources and other materials are available in Braille.

Eye contact is considered important in North American culture. With a parent who is visually impaired, this critical factor in the parent–child attachment process is obviously missing. However, the visually impaired parent who may never have experienced this method of strengthening relationships does not miss it. The infant will need other sensory input from that parent. An infant looking into the eyes of a mother who is visually impaired may not be aware that the eyes are unseeing. Other people in the newborn's environment can participate in active eye contact to supply this need. However, a problem may arise if the visually impaired parent has an impassive facial expression. When her infant makes repeated unsuccessful attempts to engage in face play with the mother, he or she will abandon the behaviour with her and intensify it with the father or other persons in the household. Nurses can provide anticipatory guidance regarding this situation and help the mother learn to nod and smile while talking and cooing to the infant.

BOX 22-2 Nursing Approaches for Working With Blind and Visually Impaired Parents

Parents who are blind need the following:
- Verbal teaching by health care providers because printed maternity information is not accessible to blind people
- Explanations of routines
- To feel devices (e.g., monitors, pelvic models) and hear descriptions of the devices

Visually impaired parents need the following:
- An orientation to the hospital room that allows the parent to move about the room independently—for example, "Go to the left of the bed and trail the wall until you feel the first door. That is the bathroom."
- A chance to ask questions
- The opportunity to hold and touch the baby after birth

Nurses need:
- To demonstrate baby care by touch and follow with "Now let me see you do it."
- To give instructions such as "I'm going to give you the baby. The head is to your left side."

Hearing-Impaired Parent

The parent who has a hearing impairment faces another set of problems, particularly if the deafness dates from birth or early childhood. The mother and her partner are likely to have established an independent household. A number of devices that transform sound into light flashes are now marketed and can be fitted into the infant's room to permit immediate detection of crying. Even if the parent is not speech trained, vocalizing can serve as both a stimulus and a response to the infant's early vocalizing. Deaf parents can provide additional vocal training by use of recordings and television so that from birth the child is aware of the full range of the human voice. Young children acquire sign language readily, and the first sign used is as varied as the first word.

Hospitals and other institutions use various communication techniques and resources with the deaf, including having staff members or certified interpreters who are proficient in sign language. For example, providing written materials with demonstrations and having nurses stand where the parent can read their lips (if the parent practices lip reading) are two techniques that can be used. A creative approach is for the nursing unit to develop movies in which information on postpartum care, infant care, and parenting issues is signed by an interpreter and spoken by a nurse. A movie in which a nurse signs while speaking would be ideal. Many resources are available to the deaf parent also via the Internet.

Sibling Adaptation

Because the family is an interactive, open unit, the addition of a new family member affects everyone in the family. Siblings have to assume new positions within the family hierarchy (see Chapter 31, p. 810). The older child's goal is to maintain the lead position. Parents are faced with the task of caring for a new child while not neglecting the others. They need to distribute their attention in an equitable manner. When the newborn is born prematurely or has special needs, this can be difficult.

Reactions of siblings may result from temporary separation from the mother or changes in the mother's or father's behaviour. Positive behavioural changes of siblings include interest in and concern for the baby (see Fig. 22-3 and Fig. 22-8) and increased independence. Regression in toileting and sleep habits, aggression toward the baby, and increased seeking of attention and whining are examples of negative behaviours that are normal.

The parents' attitudes toward the arrival of the baby can set the stage for the other children's reactions (see Fig. 22-8). Because the baby absorbs the time and attention of the important people in the other children's lives, jealousy (**sibling rivalry**) is to be expected once the initial excitement of having

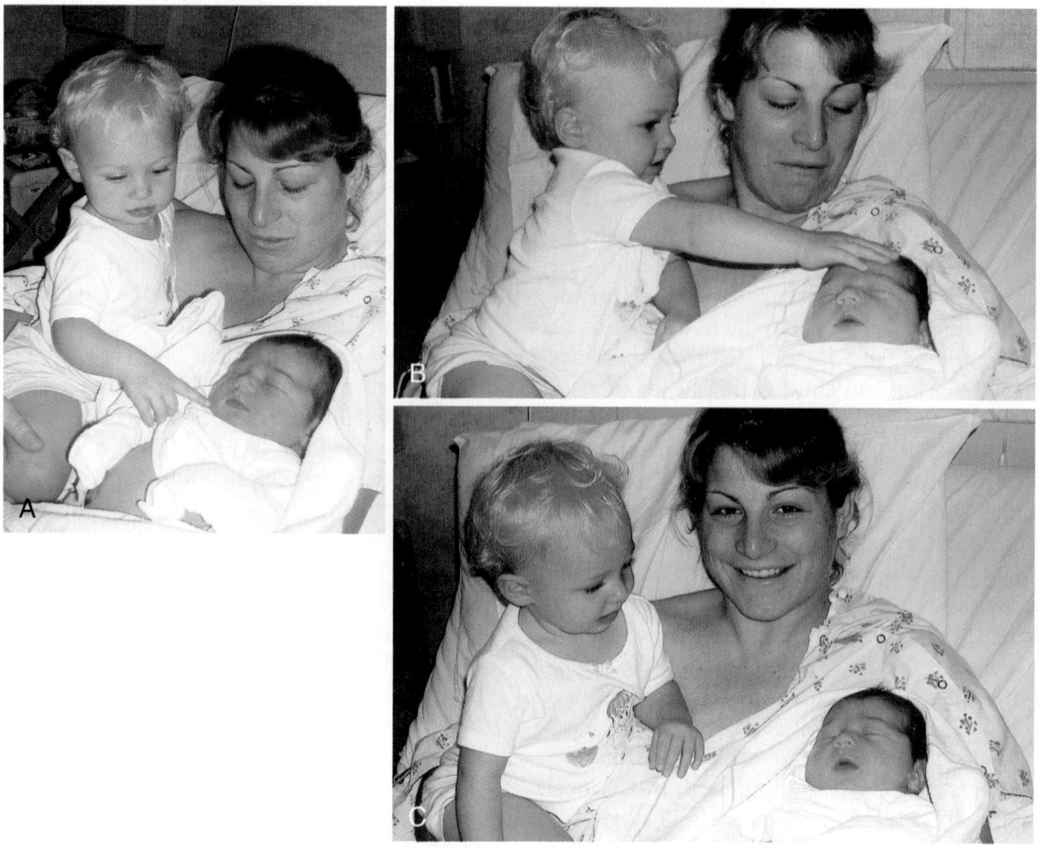

Fig. 22-8 First meeting. **A:** Sister touching new sibling with fingertip. **B:** Touching with whole hand. **C:** Smiles indicate acceptance. *(Courtesy Sara Kossuth, Los Angeles, CA.)*

a new baby in the home is over. However, sibling rivalry or negative behaviours in siblings may have been overemphasized in the past. Developmentally appropriate behaviours in siblings are similar before and after the baby arrives. Firstborn children seem to continue their usual routines and are more pleased with the newborns and more understanding of the baby's need for care than the parents predict. See the Region of Peel: Parenting in Peel Web site for more resources for parents on sibling rivalry (http://www.peelregion.ca/health/family-health/toddlers-and-preschoolers/behaviour/jealousy.htm).

Parents, especially mothers, spend much time and energy promoting sibling acceptance of a new baby. Participation in sibling preparation classes can make a difference in the ability of parents to cope with their behaviour. Older children are actively involved in preparing for the infant, and this involvement intensifies after the birth of the child. Parents have to manage their feelings of guilt that the older children are being deprived of parental time and attention. They have to monitor the behaviour of older children toward the more vulnerable infant and divert aggressive behaviour. Strategies that parents have used to facilitate siblings' acceptance of a new baby are presented in the Family-Centred Teaching box.

Siblings demonstrate acquaintance behaviours with the newborn. The acquaintance process depends on the information given to the child before the baby is born and on the child's cognitive development level. The initial behaviours of siblings with the newborn include looking at the infant and touching the head (see Fig. 22-8). The adjustment of older children to a newborn takes time, and children should be allowed to interact at their own pace rather than be forced to do so. To expect a young child to accept and love a rival for the parents' affection assumes an unrealistic level of maturity. Sibling love grows, as does other love (i.e., by being with another person and sharing experiences). This bond between siblings involves a secure base in which one child provides support for the other, is missed when absent, and is looked to for comfort and security.

Grandparent Adaptation

Grandparents experience a transition to grandparenthood. Intergenerational relationships shift, and grandparents must deal with changes in practices and attitudes toward childbirth, childrearing, and men's and women's roles at home and in the workplace (see Community Focus box). The degree to which grandparents understand and accept current practices can influence how supportive they are perceived to be by their adult children.

While they are adjusting to grandparenthood, most grandparents are experiencing normative middle- and old-age life

FAMILY-CENTRED TEACHING

Strategies for Facilitating Sibling Acceptance of a New Baby

- Take your firstborn child on a tour of your hospital room and point out similarities to his or her birth. "This is like the room I was in with you, and the baby is in the same kind of bassinet that you were in."
- Have a small gift from the baby to give to your older child each day.
- Give the older child a T-shirt that says, "I'm a big brother" (or "sister").
- Arrange for your children to be in the first group (grandparents, siblings) to see the newborn. Let them hold the baby in the hospital.
- Plan time for all children. "When I get home, I'll arrange my day so that I can finish the baby's care in the morning while Sam (first child) is at school. Maybe the baby will sleep part of the afternoon and I can spend some time with Sam."
- Fathers can spend time with the older sibling while mothers are taking care of the baby and vice versa. Siblings like to have time and attention from both parents.
- Give preschool and early school-age siblings a newborn doll as their baby to care for. Give the sibling a photograph of the new baby to take to school to show off his or her baby sibling. Older siblings may enjoy the responsibility of helping care for the newborn, such as learning how to change a diaper. One mother let her preschooler help burp the new baby by patting on the baby's back. She figured her son could pat the baby fairly firmly without harming him and at the same time let out some pent-up aggressive feelings.

COMMUNITY FOCUS

Helping Grandparents Bridge the Generation Gap

Interview a grandfather and grandmother about their experiences with childbirth and infant care. Prepare a "letter to new parents" (written from the grandparents' perspective), which can be included in prenatal kits distributed in childbirth preparation classes and made available to all family members on the postpartum unit. Include how the birth of their adult child occurred, how things are different now, what role the grandparent can play in helping the new parents adjust to home and child care, and what the grandparent might contribute to the family in memories.

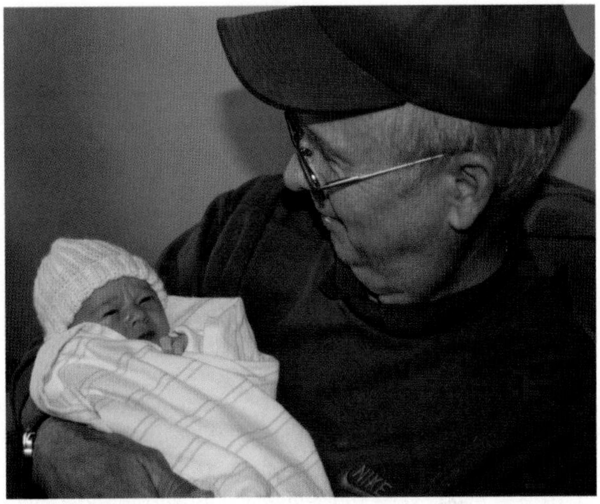

Fig. 22-9 Grandfather and new grandson get acquainted. *(Courtesy William Perry, Phoenix, AZ.)*

transitions, such as retirement and a move to smaller housing, and need support from their adult children. Some may feel regret about their limited involvement because of poor health or geographic distance. Maternal grandmothers, more so than the other three grandparents, may have high expectations of themselves that cause them to be self-critical.

The extent of involvement of grandparents in the care of the newborn depends on many factors (e.g., the willingness of the grandparents to become involved, their proximity, and ethnic and cultural expectations of their role) (Fig. 22-9). If the new parents live in Canada, Asian grandparents may be asked to come to Canada to care for the baby and mother after birth. Many Canadian-born paternal grandparents, in contrast to those in other cultures, consider themselves secondary to the maternal grandparents. Less seems expected of them, and they are initially less involved. Nevertheless, these grandparents are eager to help and express great pleasure in their son's fatherhood and his involvement with the baby (Fig. 22-10).

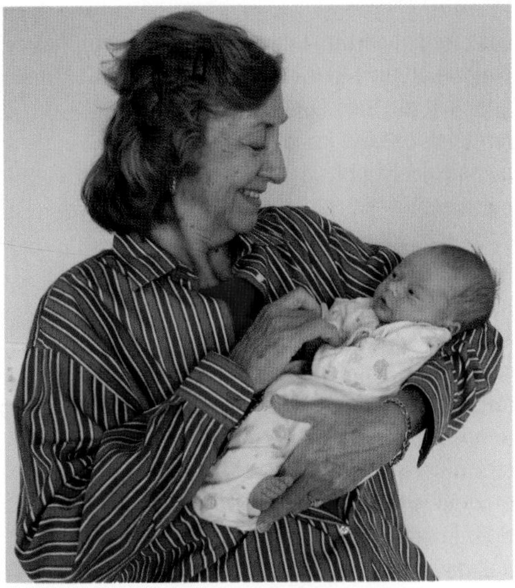

Fig. 22-10 Grandmother becoming acquainted with new grandson. *(Courtesy Diane Nelson, Las Vegas, NV.)*

For first-time parents, pregnancy and parenthood can reawaken old issues related to dependence versus independence. Some expectant parents may not plan on their parents' help immediately after the baby arrives. They want time "to be a family," inferring a couple–baby unit, not the intergenerational family network. Intergenerational help may be perceived as interference. However, contrary to their expectations, new parents do call on their parents for help, especially the maternal grandmother. Many grandparents are aware of their adult children's wishes for autonomy, respect these wishes, and remain available to help when asked.

Grandparents' classes can be used to bridge the generation gap and to help the grandparents understand their adult children's parenting concepts. The classes include information on up-to-date childbearing practices; family-centred care; infant care, feeding, and safety (car seats); and exploration of roles that grandparents can play in the family unit.

Increasing numbers of grandparents are providing permanent care to their grandchildren as a result of divorce, substance use, child abuse and neglect, teenage pregnancy, death, human immunodeficiency virus and acquired immunodeficiency syndrome, unemployment, and mental health problems. This emerging trend requires the nurse to evaluate the role of the grandparent in parenting the infant. Educational and financial considerations must be addressed and available support systems identified for these families.

Nursing Care Management

Numerous changes occur during the first weeks of parenthood. Nursing care management should be directed toward helping parents cope with infant care, role changes, altered lifestyle, and change in family structure resulting from the addition of a new baby (see Nursing Process box). Developing skill and confidence in caring for an infant can be anxiety provoking. Anticipatory guidance can help prevent a shock of reality in the transition from hospital or birthing centre to

NURSING PROCESS: TRANSITION TO PARENTHOOD

Assessment

Assessment should include a psychosocial assessment focusing on the following:

- Parent–infant attachment
- Adjustment to the parental role
- Sibling adjustment
- Social support
- Education needs
- Mother's and baby's physical adaptation

Early home visits are an excellent opportunity for the nurse to assess beginnings of positive or negative parenting behaviours and to provide positive reinforcement for loving and nurturing behaviours with the infant.

Parents who interact in inappropriate or abusive ways with their infants should be followed more closely, and an appropriate mental health practitioner or professional social worker should be notified.

Nursing Diagnoses

Readiness for enhanced family coping related to
- positive attitude and realistic expectations for newborn and adapting to parenthood
- nurturing behaviours with newborn
- communicating positive factors in lifestyle change

Risk for parenting difficulties related to
- decreased knowledge about infant care
- feelings of incompetence or lack of confidence
- unrealistic expectations of newborn or infant
- fatigue from interrupted sleep

Ineffective parental role performance related to
- role transition and role attainment
- unwanted pregnancy
- lack of resources to support parenting (e.g., no paid leave)

Risk for impaired parent–infant attachment related to
- difficult labour and birth
- postpartum complications
- neonatal complications and anomalies

Planning

A plan of care is formulated in collaboration with the family that incorporates their priorities and preferences to meet their specific needs.

Expected outcomes for effective transition to parenthood include that the parents will do the following:

- Demonstrate behaviours that reflect appreciation of sensory and behavioural capacities of the infant
- Communicate increasing confidence and competence in feeding, diapering, dressing, and sensory stimulation of the infant
- Identify deviations from normal health in the infant that should be brought to the immediate attention of the primary health care provider
- Relate effectively to the newborn's siblings and grandparents

Interventions

Provide anticipatory guidance on what to expect as the newborn grows and develops:
- Infant developmental milestones
- Sensory enrichment and infant stimulation

Provide interventions for promoting parent–infant attachment (see Table 22-3)

Provide suggestions for incorporating grandparents and siblings into interactions with newborn

Evaluation

Evaluation is based on the expected outcomes of care. The plan is revised as necessary.

NURSING CARE PLAN ● Home Care Follow-Up: Transition to Parenthood

Nursing Diagnosis: Disturbed sleep pattern related to infant demands and environmental interruptions

Expected Outcomes

Woman has realistic expectations regarding sleep and is able to sleep for uninterrupted periods and feels rested upon waking.

Nursing Interventions/*Rationales*

Discuss woman's routine and specify things that interfere with sleep *to determine the scope of the problem and direct interventions.*

Explore ways in which the woman and significant others can make the environment more conducive to sleep (e.g., privacy, darkness, quiet, back rubs, soothing music, warm milk); teach use of guided imagery and relaxation techniques *to promote optimal conditions for sleep.*

Eliminate things or routines (e.g., caffeine, foods that induce heartburn, strenuous mental or physical activity) *that may interfere with sleep.*

Advise the family to limit visitors and activities *to avoid further taxation and fatigue.*

Have the family plan specific times to care for the newborn to allow the mother time to sleep; have the mother learn to use infant nap time as a time for her to nap *to replenish energy and decrease fatigue.*

Nursing Diagnosis: Risk for financial difficulties related to addition of new family member, inadequate resources, or inadequate support systems

Expected Outcome

Appropriate resources are used.

Nursing Interventions/*Rationales*

Observe the home environment (e.g., available living space and sleeping arrangements; adequacy of facilities for food preparation and storage, hygiene, and toileting; overall state of repair; cleanliness; presence of safety hazards) *to determine adequacy and effective use of resources.*

Observe arrangements for the newborn such as sleeping space, care equipment, and supplies (bathing, changing, feeding, transportation) *to determine adequacy of resources.*

Identify and arrange referrals to needed social agencies (e.g., Canadian Prenatal Nutrition Program) *to address resource deficits (finances, supplies, equipment).*

Nursing Diagnosis: Risk for interrupted family processes related to inclusion of new family member

Expected Outcome

The infant is successfully assimilated into the family structure.

Nursing Interventions/*Rationales*

Explore with family the ways in which the birth and neonate have changed family structure and function *to evaluate functional and role adjustment.*

Observe family interaction with the newborn and note degree of bonding, evidence of sibling rivalry, and involvement in newborn care *to evaluate acceptance of newest family member.*

Clarify identified misinformation and misperceptions *to promote clear communication.*

Assist the family in exploring options for solutions to identified problems *to promote effective problem resolution.*

Support family efforts as they move toward adjusting and incorporating the new member *to reinforce new functions and roles.*

If needed, make referrals to appropriate social services or community agencies *to ensure ongoing support and care.*

home that might negate the parents' joy or cause them undue stress. For example, the nurse can teach parents a number of strategies that help quiet a fussy baby, prevent crying, and induce quiet attention or sleep (see Nursing Care Plan; see also Chapter 36).

Written information reinforcing education topics is helpful to provide to parents, as is a list of available community resources. Classes in the prenatal period or during the postpartum stay are helpful. Instructions for the first days at home should include at a minimum activities of daily living, dealing with visitors, and activity and rest.

Key Points

- The birth of a child necessitates changes in the existing interactional structure of a family.
- Attachment is the process by which the parent and infant come to love and accept each other.
- Attachment is strengthened through the use of sensual responses or interactions by both partners in the parent–infant interaction.
- In adjusting to the parental role, the mother moves from a dependent state **(taking-in)** to an interdependent state (letting go).
- Fathers experience emotions and adjustments during the transition to parenthood that are similar to and also distinctly different from those of mothers.
- Modulation of rhythm, modification of behavioural repertoires, and mutual responsivity facilitate infant–parent adjustment.
- Many factors (e.g., age, culture, socioeconomic level, and expectations of what the child will be like) influence adaptation to parenthood.
- Parents face a number of tasks related to sibling adjustment that require creative parental interventions.
- Grandparents can have a positive influence on the postpartum family.

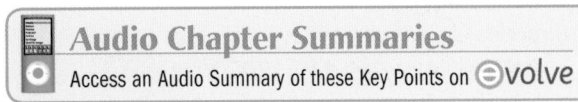

Audio Chapter Summaries

Access an Audio Summary of these Key Points on evolve

References

Alhusen, J. L. (2008). A literature update on maternal-fetal attachment. *Journal of Obstetric, Gynecologic and Neonatal Nursing, 37*(5), 315–328.

Bialoskurski, M., Cox, C. L., & Hayes, J. A. (1999). The nature of attachment in a neonatal intensive care unit. *Journal of Perinatal and Neonatal Nursing, 13*(1), 66–77.

Bloom, K. C., Bednarzuk, M. S., Devitt, D. L., Renault, R. A., Teaman, V., & Van Loock, D. M. (2004). Barriers to prenatal care for homeless pregnant women. *Journal of Obstetric, Gynecologic and Neonatal Nursing, 33,* 428–435.

D'Avanzo, C. (2008). *Mosby's pocket guide to cultural health assessment* (4th ed.). St. Louis: Mosby.

Deave, T., & Johnson, D. (2008). The transition to parenthood: What does it mean for fathers? *Journal of Advanced Nursing, 63*(6), 626–633.

Deave, T., Johnson, D., & Ingram, J. (2008). Transition to parenthood: The needs of parents in pregnancy and early parenthood. *BMC Pregnancy and Childbirth, 8,* 30. Retrieved from http://www.biomedcentral.com/1471-2393/8/30.

Erlandsson, K., et al. (2007). Skin-to-skin care with the father after cesarean birth and its effect on newborn crying and prefeeding behavior. *Birth, 34*(2), 105–114.

Galanti, G. (2003). *Caring for patients from different cultures* (3rd ed.). Philadelphia: University of Pennsylvania Press.

Gathwaia, G., Singh, B., & Balhara, B. (2008). KMC facilitates mother baby attachment in low birth weight infants. *Indian Journal of Pediatrics, 75*(1), 43–47.

Keating-Lefler, R., & Wilson, M. (2004). The experience of becoming a mother for single, unpartnered, Medicaid-eligible, first-time mothers. *Journal of Nursing Scholarship, 36*(1), 23–29.

Klaus, M., & Kennell, J. (1976). *Maternal-infant bonding.* St. Louis: Mosby.

Little, M., Gorman, A., Dzendoletas, D., & Moravac, C. (2007). Caring for the most vulnerable: A collaborative approach to supporting pregnant homeless youth. *Nursing for Women's Health, 11*(5), 458–466.

Maputie, M. S. (2006). Becoming a mother: Teenage mothers' experiences of first pregnancy. *Curationis, 29*(2), 87–95.

Mercer, R. T. (2004). Becoming a mother versus maternal role attainment. *Journal of Nursing Scholarship, 36*(3), 226–232.

Mercer, R. T. (2006). Nursing support of the process of becoming a mother. *Journal of Obstetric, Gynecologic and Neonatal Nursing, 35*(5), 649–651.

Mercer, R. T., & Walker, L. O. (2006). A review of nursing interventions to foster becoming a mother. *Journal of Obstetric, Gynecologic and Neonatal Nursing, 35*(5), 568–582.

Moore, E. R., Anderson, G. C., & Bergman, N. (2007). Early skin-to-skin contact for mothers and their healthy newborn infants. *Cochrane Database of Systemic Reviews, 18*(3), CD003519.

Nelson, A. (2003). Transition to motherhood. *Journal of Obstetric, Gynecologic and Neonatal Nursing, 32*(4), 465–477.

Nystedt, A., Högberg, U., & Lundman, B. (2008). Women's experiences of becoming a mother after prolonged labour. *Journal of Advanced Nursing, 63*(3), 250–258.

Premberg, A., Hellström, A. L., & Berg, H. (2008). Experiences of the first year as father. *Scandinavian Journal of Caring Sciences, 22*(1), 56–63.

Rubin, R. (1961). Basic maternal behaviour. *Nursing Outlook 9,* 683–686.

Shin, H., Park, Y. J., & Kim, M. J. (2006). Predictors of maternal sensitivity during the early postpartum period. *Journal of Advanced Nursing, 55*(4), 425–434.

Srivastava, R. H. (2007). *The healthcare professional's guide to clinical cultural competence.* Toronto: Elsevier.

St. John, W., Cameron, C., & McVeigh, C. (2005). Meeting the challenges of new fatherhood during the early weeks. *Journal of Obstetric, Gynecologic & Neonatal Nursing, 34*(2), 180–190.

Additional Resources

March of Dimes: Infant States: http://www.marchofdimes.com/nursing/modnemedia/othermedia/states.pdf

Parenting in Peel: http://www.peelregion.ca/health/family-health/

Unit 5

23

Postpartum Complications

Learning Objectives

On completion of this chapter, the reader will be able to:

- Identify causes, signs and symptoms, possible complications, and management of postpartum hemorrhage.
- Describe hemorrhagic shock as a complication of postpartum hemorrhage, as well as its management and the hazards of therapy.
- Identify causes, signs and symptoms, possible complications, and management of postpartum infection.
- Describe thromboembolic disorders, including incidence, etiology, signs and symptoms, and management of these disorders.
- Summarize the role of the nurse in the home setting in assessing potential problems and managing care of women with postpartum complications.
- Differentiate among postpartum emotional complications, including their incidence, risk factors, signs and symptoms, severity, and management.
- Describe emotional, behavioural, cognitive, and physical responses commonly experienced during the grieving process associated with perinatal loss.
- Identify specific nursing interventions to meet the special needs of parents and their families that are related to perinatal loss and grief.
- Differentiate between helpful and unhelpful responses in caring for parents experiencing loss and grief.

Electronic Resources

Additional information related to the content in Chapter 23 can be found on

evolve the companion Web site at

http://evolve.elsevier.com/Canada/Perry/maternal/

- Examination Review Questions
- Case Study—Postpartum Depression and Anxiety
- Critical Thinking Exercise—Postpartum Mood Disorder
- Critical Thinking Exercise—Neonatal Loss
- Nursing Care Plan—Fetal Death: 24 Weeks of Gestation

Providing safe and effective care of the woman and family experiencing postpartum physical and psychological complications, sequelae of childbirth trauma, or grief related to perinatal loss requires a collaborative effort from all members of the health care team. This chapter focuses on the postpartum complications of hemorrhage and infection, sequelae of childbirth trauma, psychological complications, and loss and grief.

Postpartum Hemorrhage

Definition and Incidence

Postpartum hemorrhage (PPH) is a leading cause of maternal morbidity and mortality worldwide. It remains a contributor to maternal morbidity in Canada (Public Health Agency of Canada [PHAC], 2004). PPH is a life-threatening event that can occur with little warning and is often unrecognized until the mother has profound symptoms. Traditionally, *postpartum hemorrhage* has been defined as the loss of 500 mL or more of blood after vaginal birth and 1000 mL or more after Caesarean birth. Either a 10% change in hematocrit between admission for labour and postpartum or the need for erythrocyte transfusion has also been used to define PPH (Francois & Foley, 2007). It has been classified as early or late with respect to the birth. Early, acute, or primary PPH occurs within 24 hours of the birth. According to More[OB] (2010), approximately 70% of immediate PPH is due to uterine atony. Late or secondary PPH occurs more than 24 hours but less than 6 weeks after the birth and is due to retained products, infection, or both (More[OB], 2010). Today's health care environment encourages shortened hospital stays after birth, which increases the potential for acute episodes of PPH to occur outside the traditional hospital or birth centre setting.

Etiology and Risk Factors

Excessive bleeding can be considered with reference to the stages of labour. From birth of the fetus until separation of the placenta, the character and quantity of blood passed may suggest excessive bleeding. For example, dark blood is probably of venous origin, perhaps from varices or superficial lacerations of the birth canal. Bright blood is arterial and may indicate deep lacerations of the cervix. Spurts of blood with clots may indicate partial placental separation. Failure of blood to clot or remain clotted indicates a pathological condition or coagulopathy, such as disseminated intravascular coagulation (DIC) (see later discussion, p. 584).

Excessive bleeding may occur during the period from the separation of the placenta to its expulsion or removal. Commonly, such bleeding is the result of incomplete placental separation, undue manipulation of the fundus, or excessive traction on the cord. After the placenta has been expelled or removed, persistent or excessive blood loss is often a result of atony of the uterus (i.e., failure to contract well or maintain contraction) or prolapse of the uterus into the vagina. Late PPH most commonly is the result of infection, subinvolution of the placental site, retained placental tissue, or coagulopathy (Francois & Foley, 2007). Risk factors for and causes of PPH are listed in Box 23-1.

BOX 23-1 Risk Factors and Causes of Postpartum Hemorrhage

Uterine atony
- Overdistended uterus—Large fetus, multiple fetuses, hydramnios, distension with clots
- Anaesthesia and analgesia—Conduction anaesthesia
- Previous history of uterine atony
- High parity
- Prolonged labour, oxytocin-induced labour
- Trauma during labour and birth—Forceps-assisted birth, vacuum-assisted birth, Caesarean birth

Lacerations of the birth canal
Retained placental fragments
Ruptured uterus
Inversion of the uterus
Placenta accreta, increta, percreta
Coagulation disorders
Placental abruption
Placenta previa
Manual removal of a retained placenta
Magnesium sulphate administration during labour or postpartum period
Chorioamnionitis
Uterine subinvolution

Uterine Atony

Uterine **atony** is marked hypotonia of the uterus. Normally, placental separation and expulsion are facilitated by contraction of the uterus, which also prevents hemorrhage from the placental site. The uterine corpus is in essence a basket weave of strong, interlacing smooth-muscle bundles through which many large maternal blood vessels pass (see Fig. 5-3). If the uterus is flaccid after detachment of all or part of the **placenta**, brisk venous bleeding occurs, and normal coagulation of the open vasculature is impaired and continues until the uterine muscle is contracted.

Uterine atony is the leading cause of early PPH, complicating approximately 1 in 20 births (Francois & Foley, 2007). It is associated with high parity, hydramnios, a **macrosomic** fetus, and multifetal gestation. In such conditions the uterus is "overstretched" and contracts poorly after birth. Other causes of atony include traumatic birth, use of halogenated anaesthesia (e.g., halothane) or magnesium sulphate, rapid or prolonged labour, **chorioamnionitis**, use of **oxytocin** for induction or augmentation of labour, and uterine atony in a previous pregnancy (Francois & Foley, 2007). According to More[OB] (2010), uterine atony may also be caused by retained blood clots, fibroids, and bladder distension.

Lacerations of the Genital Tract

Lacerations of the cervix, vagina, and perineum are also causes of PPH. Hemorrhage related to lacerations should be suspected if bleeding continues despite a firm, contracted uterine fundus. This bleeding can be a slow trickle, an oozing, or frank hemorrhage.

Factors that influence the causes and incidence of obstetrical lacerations of the lower genital tract include operative birth, precipitous birth, congenital abnormalities of the maternal soft parts, and contracted pelvis. Size, abnormal presentation, and position of the fetus; relative size of the presenting part and the birth canal; previous scarring from infection, injury, or surgery; and vulvar, perineal, and vaginal varicosities can also cause lacerations.

Extreme vascularity in the labia and periclitoral areas often results in profuse bleeding if laceration occurs. Hematomas may also be present.

Lacerations of the perineum are the most common of all injuries in the lower portion of the genital tract. These are classified as first, second, third, and fourth degree (see Chapter 18, pp. 476–477). An **episiotomy** may extend to become either a third- or fourth-degree laceration.

Prolonged pressure of the fetal head on the vaginal mucosa ultimately interferes with the circulation and may produce ischemic or pressure necrosis. The state of the tissues in combination with the type of birth may result in deep vaginal lacerations, with consequent predisposition to vaginal hematomas.

After the bleeding has been controlled, the care of the woman with lacerations of the perineum is similar to that for women with episiotomies (i.e., analgesia as needed for pain and hot or cold applications as necessary). Roughage in the diet and intake of fluids should be increased. Stool softeners may be used to assist the woman in re-establishing bowel habits without straining and putting stress on the suture lines.

NURSING ALERT To avoid injury to the suture line, a woman with third- or fourth-degree lacerations is not given rectal suppositories or enemas.

Hematomas

Pelvic **hematomas** (i.e., a collection of blood in the connective tissue) may be vulvar, vaginal, or retroperitoneal in origin. Vulvar hematomas are the most common. Pain is the most common symptom, and most vulvar hematomas are visible. Vaginal hematomas occur more commonly in association with a forceps-assisted birth, an episiotomy, or primigravidity (Francois & Foley, 2007).

Retroperitoneal hematomas are least common but are life threatening. They are caused by laceration of one of the vessels attached to the hypogastric artery, usually associated with rupture of a Caesarean scar during labour. During the postpartum period, if the woman reports a persistent perineal or rectal pain or a feeling of pressure in the vagina, a careful examination is made. However, a retroperitoneal hematoma may cause minimal pain, and the initial symptoms may be signs of shock (Francois & Foley, 2007).

Cervical lacerations usually occur at the lateral angles of the external os. Most are shallow, and bleeding is minimal. More extensive lacerations may extend into the vaginal vault or the lower uterine segment.

Hematomas are usually surgically evacuated. Once the bleeding has been controlled, usual postpartum care is provided with attention to pain relief, monitoring of the amount of bleeding, replacement of fluids, and review of laboratory results (hemoglobin and hematocrit).

Retained Placenta

Nonadherent Retained Placenta

Nonadherent retained placenta may result from partial separation of a normal placenta, entrapment of the partially or completely separated placenta by an hourglass constriction ring of the uterus, mismanagement of the third stage of labour, or abnormal adherence of the entire placenta or a portion of the placenta to the uterine wall. Placental retention because of poor separation is common in very preterm births (20 to 24 weeks of gestation).

Management of nonadherent retained placenta is by manual separation and removal by the primary health care provider. Supplementary anaesthesia is usually not needed for women who have had regional anaesthesia for birth. For other women, administration of light nitrous oxide and oxygen inhalation anaesthesia or intravenous (IV) thiopental facilitates intrauterine exploration and placental separation. After the removal, the woman is at continued risk for PPH and infection.

Adherent Retained Placenta

Abnormal adherence of the placenta occurs for unknown reasons, but it is thought to result from zygote implantation in an area of defective endometrium, so no zone of separation exists between the placenta and the decidua. The incidence of placenta accreta is increasing as a result of the rise in Caesarean birth rates (Oyelese & Smulian, 2006). Attempts to remove the placenta in the usual manner are unsuccessful, and laceration or perforation of the uterine wall may result, putting the woman at great risk for severe PPH and infection (Francois & Foley, 2007).

Unusual placental adherence may be partial or complete. The following degrees of attachment are recognized:

- **Placenta accreta**—Slight penetration of myometrium by placental trophoblast
- **Placenta increta**—Deep penetration of myometrium by placenta
- **Placenta percreta**—Perforation of uterus by placenta

Bleeding with complete or total placenta accreta may not occur unless separation of the placenta is attempted. With more extensive involvement, bleeding becomes profuse when delivery of the placenta is attempted. There is less blood loss if the diagnosis is made antenatally and no attempt is made to remove the placenta (Wong et al., 2008). Treatment includes blood component replacement therapy; hysterectomy may be indicated (Francois & Foley, 2007).

Inversion of the Uterus

Inversion (turning inside out) of the uterus after birth is a potentially life-threatening complication. The incidence of uterine inversion is approximately 1 in 2500 births (Francois & Foley, 2007) and may recur with a subsequent birth. Uterine inversion may be incomplete, complete, or prolapsed. Incomplete inversion cannot be seen but must be felt; a smooth mass can be palpated through the dilated cervix. In complete inversion the lining of the fundus crosses through the cervical os and forms a mass in the vagina. Prolapsed inversion of the uterus is obvious; a large, red, rounded mass (perhaps with the placenta attached) protrudes 20 to 30 cm outside the introitus.

Contributing factors to uterine inversion include fundal implantation of the placenta, vigorous fundal pressure, excessive traction applied to the cord, fetal macrosomia, tocolysis, prolonged labour, uterine atony, and abnormally adherent placental tissue (Francois & Foley, 2007). Uterine inversion occurs most often in multiparous women and with placenta accreta or increta. The primary presenting signs of uterine inversion are hemorrhage, shock, and pain. The uterus must be replaced into its proper position.

Prevention—always the easiest, cheapest, and most effective therapy—is especially appropriate for uterine inversion. The umbilical cord should not be pulled on unless the placenta has definitely separated.

Uterine inversion is an emergency situation requiring immediate recognition, maternal fluid resuscitation, replacement of the uterus within the pelvic cavity, and correction of associated clinical conditions. Tocolytics or halogenated anaesthetics may be given to relax the uterus before attempting replacement (Francois & Foley, 2007). Oxytocic agents are given after the uterus is repositioned; broad-spectrum antibiotics should be initiated. The woman's response to treatment should be observed closely in order to prevent shock or fluid overload. If the uterus has been repositioned manually, care must be taken to avoid aggressive fundal massage.

Subinvolution of the Uterus

Late postpartum bleeding may occur as a result of **subinvolution** of the uterus (delayed return of the enlarged uterus to normal size and function). Recognized causes of subinvolution include retained placental fragments and pelvic infection. Signs and symptoms include prolonged **lochial** discharge, irregular or excessive bleeding, and sometimes hemorrhage. A pelvic examination usually reveals a larger-than-normal uterus that may be boggy.

Treatment of subinvolution depends on the cause. Ergonovine 0.2 mg every 4 hours for 2 or 3 days and antibiotic therapy are the most common medications used. **Dilation and curettage** (D&C) may be needed to remove retained placental fragments or to debride the placental site.

Nursing Care Management

PPH may be sudden and even exsanguinating (see Nursing Process box). The nurse must be alert to the symptoms of hemorrhage and hypovolemic shock and be prepared to act quickly to minimize blood loss (Box 23-2). More[OB] (2010) recommends active management of the third stage of labour in order to prevent PPH, where possible. This involves administering oxytocin after the delivery of the anterior shoulder, considering delayed cord clamping, gentle cord traction, and immediate fundal massage after complete delivery. If it takes longer than 30 minutes to deliver the placenta, the risk of PPH increases six-fold (More[OB], 2010).

Late PPH develops at least 24 hours after birth or later in the postpartum period. The woman may be at home when the symptoms occur. Discharge teaching should emphasize the signs of normal involution, potential complications, and the importance of prompt assessment by a health care provider in the event of PPH.

Early recognition and diagnosis of PPH is critical to care management. The first step is to evaluate the contractility of the uterus. If the uterus is hypotonic, management is directed toward increasing contractility and minimizing blood loss.

The initial management of excessive postpartum bleeding is firm massage of the uterine fundus, expression of any clots in the uterus, eliminating bladder distension, 10 units of oxytocin intramuscularly or intravenously, and continuous IV infusion of 10 to 40 units of oxytocin in 1000 mL of Ringer's lactate or normal saline solution. If the uterus fails to respond to oxytocin, a dose of 0.2 mg ergonovine or .25 mg carboprost tromethamine (hemabate) may be given to produce sustained uterine contractions. Oral (400 to 800 mcg) and rectal (1000 mcg) misoprostol has also been administered, but there is no consensus about efficacy for management of PPH (Gülmezoglu et al., 2007; Magann & Lanneau, 2005). Doses must be administered in accordance with medical orders. See the Medication Guide for a comparison of medications used to manage PPH. In addition to the medications used to contract the uterus, rapid administration of crystalloid solutions, blood or blood products, or both are needed to restore the woman's intravascular volume (Francois & Foley, 2007).

BOX 23-2 Noninvasive Assessments of Cardiac Output in Postpartum Patients Who Are Bleeding

Palpation of pulses (rate, quality, equality)
- Arterial
- Blood pressure

Auscultation
- Heart sounds or murmurs
- Breath sounds

Inspection
- Skin colour, temperature, turgor
- Level of consciousness
- Capillary refill
- Urinary output
- Neck veins
- Pulse oximetry
- Mucous membranes

Presence or absence of anxiety, apprehension, restlessness, disorientation

NURSING ALERT Use of ergonovine or methylergonovine is contraindicated in the presence of hypertension or cardiovascular disease.

Hypotonic Uterus

Oxygen can be given to enhance oxygen delivery to the cells. A urinary catheter is usually inserted to ensure the bladder does not interfere with contraction of the uterus and to monitor urine output as a measure of intravascular volume. Laboratory studies usually include a complete blood count with platelet count, fibrinogen, fibrin split products, prothrombin time, and partial thromboplastin time. Blood type and antibody screen are done if not previously performed.

If bleeding persists, the physician or midwife may consider bimanual compression. This procedure involves inserting a fist into the vagina and pressing the knuckles against the anterior side of the uterus while placing the other hand on the abdomen and massaging the posterior uterus. If the uterus still does not become firm, the uterine cavity is explored manually for retained placental fragments. A uterine tamponade can be created using a uterine balloon which can be inserted vaginally and then inflated. If the preceding procedures are ineffective, surgical management may be the only alternative. Surgical management options include vessel ligation (i.e., uteroovarian, uterine, and hypogastric), selective arterial embolization, and hysterectomy (Francois & Foley, 2007).

Bleeding With a Contracted Uterus

If the uterus is firmly contracted and bleeding continues, the source of bleeding still needs to be identified and treated. Assessment may include visual or manual inspection of the perineum, vagina, cervix, or rectum and laboratory studies (e.g., hemoglobin, hematocrit, coagulation studies, and platelet count). Treatment depends on the source of the bleeding.

Herbal Remedies

Herbal remedies to control PPH have been used with some success in some settings. Some herbs have homeostatic actions, whereas others work as oxytocic agents to contract the uterus. Table 23-1 lists herbs that have been used and their actions. However, published evidence of the safety and efficacy of

NURSING PROCESS: POSTPARTUM HEMORRHAGE

Assessment

Review history for factors that predispose woman to postpartum hemorrhage (PPH).

Assess the following:

- Fundus for consistency and height
- Bleeding for colour and amount
- Perineum for signs of lacerations or hematomas
- Vital signs (VS) (VS may not be a reliable indicator of shock because of physiological adaptations of this period)
- Frequent VS checks may identify trends related to blood loss (tachycardia, tachypnea, decreasing blood pressure)
- Bladder for distension (distended bladder can displace uterus and prevent uterine contraction)
- Skin for warmth and dryness; nail beds for colour and capillary refill
- Laboratory studies (hemoglobin and hematocrit)

Nursing Diagnoses

Nursing diagnoses for women experiencing PPH include the following:

Deficient fluid volume related to

– excessive blood loss secondary to uterine atony, lacerations, or uterine inversion

Risk for injury (maternal) related to

– attempted manual removal of retained placenta
– administration of blood products
– operative procedures

Risk for parenting difficulties related to

– separation from infant secondary to treatment regimen

Ineffective peripheral tissue perfusion related to

– excessive blood loss and shunting of blood to central circulation

Planning

Early recognition and diagnosis of PPH is critical to care management. Care is planned in collaboration with the primary health care provider.

Expected outcomes for the woman experiencing PPH include that she will do the following:

- Maintain normal vital signs and laboratory values
- Develop no complications related to excessive bleeding
- Communicate understanding of her condition, its management, and discharge instructions
- Identify and use available support systems

Interventions

Massage fundus.

Empty bladder (catheterize if required); monitor urinary output.

Ensure intravenous access.

Administer oxytocin or other medications to stimulate uterine contraction per standing orders or protocols (see Medication Guide: Medications Used to Manage Postpartum Hemorrhage).

Notify primary health care provider.

Implement interventions to monitor or improve tissue perfusion (see Nursing Care Plan).

Provide fluid and blood replacement therapy as ordered.

Provide explanations to the woman and family about interventions being performed and the need to act quickly.

Provide discharge instructions:

- The woman may feel fatigue and exhaustion because of blood loss.
- Limit activities to conserve strength.
- Increase dietary iron and protein intake; iron supplements may be ordered.

Observe for delayed or insufficient lactation and postpartum depression.

Refer for home care or to community resources.

Evaluation

The nurse can be reasonably assured that care was effective to the extent that the expected outcomes have been achieved (see Nursing Care Plan).

herbal therapy is lacking. Evidence from well-controlled studies is needed before recommendation for practice should be made (Skidmore-Roth, 2010).

Hemorrhagic (Hypovolemic) Shock

Hemorrhage may result in hemorrhagic (hypovolemic) shock. Shock is an emergency situation in which the perfusion of body organs may become severely compromised; death may occur. Physiological compensatory mechanisms are activated in response to hemorrhage. The adrenal glands release catecholamines, causing arterioles and venules in the skin, lungs, gastrointestinal tract, liver, and kidneys to constrict. The available blood flow is diverted to the brain and heart and away from other organs, including the uterus. If shock is prolonged, the continued reduction in cellular oxygenation results in an accumulation of lactic acid and acidosis (from anaerobic glucose metabolism). Acidosis (lowered serum pH) causes arteriolar vasodilation; venule vasoconstriction persists. A circular pattern is established (i.e., decreased perfusion, increased tissue anoxia and acidosis, edema formation, and pooling of blood further decrease the perfusion). Cellular death occurs. See the Emergency box for assessments and interventions for hemorrhagic shock.

Medical Management

Vigorous treatment is necessary to prevent adverse sequelae. Management of hypovolemic shock involves restoring circulating blood volume and eliminating the cause of the hemorrhage (e.g., lacerations, uterine atony, or inversion). To restore circulating blood volume, a rapid IV infusion of crystalloid solution is given at a rate of 3 mL infused for every 1 mL of estimated blood loss (e.g., 3000 mL infused for 1000 mL of blood loss). Packed red blood cells (RBCs) are usually infused if the woman is still actively bleeding and no

NURSING CARE PLAN ● Postpartum Hemorrhage

Nursing Diagnosis: Deficient fluid volume related to postpartum hemorrhage

Expected Outcome

Woman will demonstrate fluid balance as evidenced by stable vital signs, prompt capillary refill time, and balanced intake and output.

Nursing Interventions/*Rationales*

Monitor vital signs, oxygen saturation, urine specific gravity, and capillary refill *to provide baseline data.*

Massage fundus as required *to decrease uterine atony.*

Measure and record amount and type of bleeding by weighing and counting saturated pads. If the woman is at home, teach her to count pads and save any clots or tissue. If the woman is admitted to hospital, save any clots and tissue for further examination *to estimate type and amount of blood loss for fluid replacement.*

Give explanation of all procedures *to reduce anxiety.*

Begin intravenous access with 18-gauge or larger needle for infusion of isotonic solution as ordered *to provide fluid or blood replacement.*

Administer medications as ordered, such as oxytocin, carboprost tromethamine (hemabate), misoprostil, or ergonovine, *to increase contractility of the uterus.*

Insert indwelling urinary catheter *to provide most accurate assessment of renal function and hypovolemia.*

Prepare for surgical intervention as needed *to stop the source of bleeding.*

Nursing Diagnosis: Ineffective tissue perfusion related to hypovolemia

Expected Outcome

Woman will have stable vital signs, oxygen saturation, arterial blood gases, and adequate hematocrit and hemoglobin.

Nursing Interventions/*Rationales*

Monitor vital signs, oxygen saturation, arterial blood gases, and hematocrit and hemoglobin *to assess for hypovolemic shock and decreased tissue perfusion.*

Assess for any changes in level of consciousness *to assess for evidence of hypoxia.*

Assess capillary refill, mucous membranes, and skin temperature *to note indicators of vasoconstriction.*

Give supplementary oxygen as ordered *to provide additional oxygenation to tissues.*

Use suction as needed, insert oral airway *to maintain clear, open airway for oxygenation.*

Monitor arterial blood gases *to provide information about acidosis or hypoxia.*

Administer sodium bicarbonate, if ordered, *to reverse metabolic acidosis.*

Nursing Diagnosis: Anxiety related to sudden change in health status

Expected Outcome

Woman will communicate that anxious feelings are diminished.

Nursing Interventions/*Rationales*

Using therapeutic communication, evaluate woman's understanding of events *to provide clarification of any misconceptions.*

Provide calm, competent attitude and environment *to aid in decreasing anxiety.*

Explain all procedures *to decrease anxiety about the unknown.*

Allow woman to express her feelings *to permit clarification of information and promote trust.*

Continue to assess vital signs or other clinical indicators of hypovolemic shock *to evaluate if psychological response of anxiety intensifies physiological indicators.*

Keep family informed of the mother's condition to enable them *to provide support.*

Table 23-1 Herbal Remedies for Postpartum Hemorrhage

HERBS	ACTION
Witch hazel	Homeostatic
Lady's mantle	Homeostatic
Blue cohosh	Oxytocic
Cotton root bark	Oxytocic
Motherwort	Promotes uterine contraction; vasoconstrictive
Shepherd's purse	Promotes uterine contraction
Alfalfa leaf	Increases availability of vitamin K; increases hemoglobin
Nettle	Increases availability of vitamin K; increases hemoglobin
Red raspberry leaves	Homeostatic; promotes uterine contraction

(Sources: Schirmer, G. [1998]. *Herbal medicine.* Bedford, TX: MED2000; Weed, S. [1986]. *Wise woman herbal for the childbearing years.* Woodstock, NY: Ash Tree.)

improvement in her condition is noted after the initial crystalloid infusion. Infusion of fresh frozen plasma may be needed if clotting factors and platelet counts are below normal values (Cunningham et al., 2010).

Nursing Interventions

While hemorrhagic shock can occur rapidly, the classic signs of shock may not appear until the postpartum woman has lost 30 to 40% of blood volume. The nurse must continue to reassess the woman's condition as evidenced by the degree of measurable and anticipated blood loss and mobilize appropriate resources.

Most interventions are instituted to improve or monitor tissue perfusion. The nurse must continue to monitor the woman's pulse and blood pressure. If invasive hemodynamic monitoring is ordered, the nurse may assist with placement of a central venous pressure (CVP) or pulmonary artery (Swan-Ganz) catheter. The nurse would then monitor CVP,

MEDICATION GUIDE

Medications Used to Manage Postpartum Hemorrhage

Oxytocin

Drug Action

Oxytocin promotes contraction of the uterus and decreases bleeding.

Adverse Effects

Adverse effects are infrequent and include water intoxication, and nausea and vomiting.

Contraindications

There are none for postpartum hemorrhage.

Dosage and Route

10 to 40 units/L diluted in lactated Ringer's solution or normal saline at 125 to 200 mU/min IV or 10 to 20 units IM

Nursing Considerations

Continue to monitor vaginal bleeding and uterine tone.

Methylergonovine; Ergonovine Maleate

Drug Action

These medications promote contraction of the uterus.

Adverse Effects

These include hypertension, nausea, vomiting, and headache.

Contraindications

These include hypertension and cardiac disease.

Dosage and Route

0.2 to 0.25 mg IV or IM

Nursing Considerations

Check blood pressure before giving dose and do not give it if blood pressure is more than 140/90 mm Hg; continue monitoring vaginal bleeding and uterine tone.

Carboprost Tromethamine (Hemabate)

Drug Action

Carboprost tromethamine promotes contraction of the uterus.

Adverse Effects

These include headache, nausea and vomiting, fever, tachycardia, hypertension, and diarrhea.

Contraindications

Asthma and hypersensitivity are contraindications.

Dosage and Route

0.25 mg IM or intramyometrially every 15 to 90 minutes, up to eight doses

Nursing Considerations

Continue to monitor vaginal bleeding and uterine tone.

Misoprostol (Cytotec)*

Drug Action

Misoprostol promotes contraction of the uterus.

Adverse Effects

These include headache, nausea and vomiting, and diarrhea.

Contraindications

Do not use misoprostol if there is a history of allergy to prostaglandins.

Dosage and Route

400 mcg orally (range 200 to 800 mcg) or 600 to 1000 mcg rectally

Nursing Considerations

Continue to monitor vaginal bleeding and uterine tone.

*Off-label use; research reports vary in conclusions about dosage and efficacy of use in comparison to other medications used to manage postpartum hemorrhage.
IM, intramuscularly; *IV,* intravenously.

EMERGENCY

Hemorrhagic Shock

Assessments	Characteristics
Respirations	Rapid and shallow
Pulse	Rapid, weak, irregular
Blood pressure	Decreasing (late sign)
Skin	Cool, pale, clammy
Urinary output	Decreasing
Level of consciousness	Lethargy → coma
Mental status	Anxiety → coma
Central venous pressure	Decreased

Interventions

Summon assistance and equipment.
Start intravenous infusion per standing orders.
Ensure patent airway; administer oxygen.
Continue to monitor status.

pulmonary artery pressure, or pulmonary artery wedge pressure as ordered.

Additional assessments to be made include evaluation of skin temperature, colour, and turgor and assessment of the woman's mucous membranes. If possible, breath sounds should be auscultated before fluid volume replacement, to provide a baseline for future assessment. Inspection for oozing at the sites of incisions or injections and assessment of the presence of petechiae or ecchymosis in areas not associated with surgery or trauma are critical in the evaluation for DIC (see later discussion, p. 584).

Oxygen is administered, preferably by a nonrebreathing face mask, at 10 to 12 L/min to maintain oxygen saturation. Oxygen saturation should be monitored with a **pulse oximeter**, although measurements may not always be accurate in a patient with hypovolemia or decreased perfusion. Level of consciousness is assessed frequently and provides additional indications of blood volume and oxygen saturation. In early stages of decreased blood flow, the woman may report "seeing stars" or feeling dizzy or nauseated. She may become restless and orthopneic. As cerebral hypoxia increases, she may become confused and react slowly to stimuli or not at all. Some women complain of headaches. An improved sensorium is an indicator of improved perfusion.

Continuous electrocardiographic monitoring may be indicated for the woman who is hypotensive or tachycardic, continues to bleed profusely, or is in shock. A Foley catheter with a urometer is inserted to allow hourly assessment of urine output. The most objective and least invasive assessment of adequate organ perfusion and oxygenation is a urine output of at least 30 mL/hr. Blood may be drawn and sent to the laboratory for studies that include hemoglobin and hematocrit levels, platelet count, and coagulation profile.

Fluid or Blood Replacement Therapy

Critical to successful management of the woman with a hemorrhagic complication is establishment of venous access, preferably with a large-bore IV catheter. The establishment of two IV lines facilitates fluid resuscitation. Vigorous fluid resuscitation includes the administration of crystalloids (lactated Ringer's, normal saline solution), colloids (albumin), blood, and blood components. Fluid resuscitation must be monitored carefully because fluid overload can occur. Intravascular fluid overload occurs most often with colloid therapy.

Transfusion reactions may follow administration of blood or blood components, including cryoprecipitates. Even in an emergency, each unit of fluid should be checked per hospital protocol. Complications of fluid or blood replacement therapy include hemolytic reactions, febrile reactions, allergic reactions, circulatory overloading, and air embolism.

LEGAL TIP **Standard of Care for Bleeding Emergencies.** The standard of care for obstetrical emergency situations such as PPH or hypovolemic shock is that provision should be made for the nurse to implement nursing actions independently. Policies, procedures, standing orders or protocols, and clinical guidelines should be established by each health care facility in which births occur and should be agreed on by health care providers involved in the care of obstetrical patients.

Coagulopathies

When bleeding is continuous and there is no identifiable source, a coagulopathy may be the cause. The woman's coagulation status must be assessed quickly and continuously. The nurse may draw and send blood to the laboratory for studies. Abnormal results depend on the cause and may include increased prothrombin time, increased partial thromboplastin time, decreased platelets, decreased fibrinogen level, increased fibrin degradation products, and prolonged bleeding time. Causes of coagulopathies may be pregnancy complications such as idiopathic or immune thrombocytopenic purpura (ITP), von Willebrand (vW) disease, or DIC.

Idiopathic Thrombocytopenic Purpura (ITP)

ITP is an autoimmune disorder in which antiplatelet antibodies decrease the lifespan of the platelets. **Thrombocytopenia**, capillary fragility, and increased bleeding time are diagnostic findings. ITP may cause severe hemorrhage after Caesarean birth or from cervical or vaginal lacerations. The incidence of postpartum uterine bleeding and vaginal hematomas is also increased.

Medical management focuses on control of platelet stability. If ITP was diagnosed during pregnancy, the woman likely was treated with corticosteroids or IV **immune globulin**. Platelet transfusions are usually given when there is significant bleeding. A splenectomy may be needed if the ITP does not respond to medical management.

von Willebrand Disease

von Willebrand disease, a type of hemophilia, is probably the most common of all hereditary bleeding disorders. Although vW disease is rare, it is among the most common congenital clotting defects in North American women of childbearing age. It results from a factor VIII deficiency and platelet dysfunction that is transmitted as an incomplete autosomal dominant trait to both sexes. Symptoms include a familial bleeding tendency, previous bleeding episodes, prolonged bleeding time (the most important test), factor VIII deficiency (mild to moderate), and bleeding from mucous membranes. Although factor VIII increases during pregnancy, there is still a risk for PPH as levels of vW factor begin to decrease (Lockwood & Silver, 2009).

The woman may be at risk for bleeding for up to 4 weeks after birth. The treatment of choice is administration of desmopressin, which promotes the release of vW factor and factor VIII. It can be given nasally, intravenously, or orally. Transfusion therapy with plasma products that have been treated for viruses and contain factor VIII and vW factor also may be used. Concentrates of antihemophiliac factor (Humate) may also be used (Lockwood & Silver, 2009; Samuels, 2007).

Disseminated Intravascular Coagulation

DIC is a pathological form of clotting that is diffuse and consumes large amounts of clotting factors, including platelets, fibrinogen, prothrombin, and factors V and VII. Widespread external bleeding, internal bleeding, or both can result. DIC also causes vascular occlusion of small vessels resulting from small clots forming in the microcirculation. In the obstetrical population, DIC may occur as a result of acute antepartum or PPH, abruptio placentae, amniotic fluid embolism, dead fetus syndrome (i.e., fetus dies but is retained in utero for at least 6 weeks), severe pre-eclampsia, sepsis, saline abortion, and acute fatty liver of pregnancy (Francois & Foley, 2007).

The diagnosis of DIC is made according to clinical findings and laboratory markers. Physical examination reveals unusual bleeding; spontaneous bleeding from the woman's gums or nose may be noted. **Petechiae** may appear around a blood pressure cuff placed on the woman's arm. Excessive bleeding may occur from the site of a slight trauma (e.g., venipuncture sites, intramuscular or subcutaneous injection sites, nicks from shaving of perineum or abdomen, and injury from insertion of a urinary catheter). Symptoms also may include tachycardia and diaphoresis. Laboratory tests reveal decreased levels of platelets, fibrinogen, proaccelerin, antihemophiliac factor, and prothrombin (the factors consumed during coagulation). Fibrinolysis is increased at first but is later severely depressed. Degradation of fibrin leads to the accumulation of fibrin split products in the blood; these have anticoagulant properties and prolong the prothrombin time. Bleeding time is normal, coagulation time shows no clot, clot-retraction time shows no clot, and partial thromboplastin time is increased. DIC must be distinguished from other clotting disorders before therapy is initiated.

Primary medical management in all cases of DIC involves correction of the underlying cause (e.g., removal of the dead fetus, treatment of existing infection or of pre-eclampsia or eclampsia, or removal of a placental abruption). Volume replacement, blood component therapy, optimization of oxygenation and perfusion status, and continued reassessment of laboratory parameters are the usual forms of treatment (Francois & Foley, 2007). Resolution of DIC usually begins with the birth of the neonate (Francois & Foley, 2007).

Nursing interventions include assessing for signs of bleeding, administering fluid or blood replacement as ordered, observing for signs of complications from the administration of blood and blood products, and protecting the woman from injury. Because renal failure is one consequence of DIC, urinary output is monitored, usually by insertion of an indwelling urinary catheter. Urinary output must be maintained at more than 30 mL/hr.

The woman and her family will be anxious or concerned about her condition and prognosis. The nurse should offer explanations about care and provide emotional support to them through this critical time.

Thromboembolic Disease

A thrombosis results from the formation of a blood clot or clots inside a blood vessel and is caused by inflammation (thrombophlebitis) or partial obstruction of the vessel. Three thromboembolic conditions are of concern in the postpartum period:

Superficial venous thrombosis—Involvement of the superficial saphenous venous system

Deep venous thrombosis—Involvement varies but can extend from the foot to the iliofemoral region

Pulmonary embolism—Complication of deep venous thrombosis occurring when part of a blood clot dislodges and is carried to the pulmonary artery, where it occludes the vessel and obstructs blood flow to the lungs

Incidence and Etiology

The incidence of venous thromboembolism (VTE) varies from about 1 in 1000 to 1 in 2000 pregnancies (Pettker & Lockwood, 2007). VTE can occur in each trimester of pregnancy and in the postpartum period. The incidence of VTE in the postpartum period has declined in the last 30 years because early ambulation after childbirth has become standard practice. The major causes of thromboembolic disease are venous stasis and hypercoagulation, both of which are present in pregnancy and continue into the postpartum period. Other risk factors include Caesarean birth, operative vaginal birth, history of venous thrombosis or varicosities, maternal age over 35, multiparity, and smoking (Pettker & Lockwood, 2007). The risk for VTE is increased in women who are obese. The Society of Obstetrician and Gynecologists of Canada (SOGC) recommends that each woman be evaluated for risk, and consideration for thromboprophylaxis should be individualized (Davies et al., 2010). Women who are at risk for VTE should have TED stockings applied soon after birth. If TED stockings do not fit, then a sequential compression device (SCD) should be used (Royal College of Obstetricians and Gynaecologists, 2009). Pulmonary embolism is the leading cause of maternal mortality in Canada (PHAC, 2004).

Clinical Manifestations

Superficial venous thrombosis is the most common form of postpartum thrombophlebitis. It is characterized by pain and tenderness in the lower extremity. Physical examination may reveal warmth; redness; and an enlarged, hardened vein over the site of the thrombosis. Deep vein thrombosis is more common in pregnancy and is characterized by unilateral leg pain, calf tenderness, and swelling. Physical examination may reveal redness and warmth, but women may also have a large clot with few symptoms. Signs and symptoms commonly seen include apprehension, cough, tachycardia, hemoptysis, elevated temperature, and pleuritic chest pain. Pulmonary embolism is characterized by **dyspnea** and **tachypnea**.

Physical examination is not a sensitive diagnostic indicator for thrombosis. Venography is the most accurate method for diagnosing deep venous thrombosis; however, it is an invasive procedure that exposes the woman and fetus to ionizing radiation and is associated with serious complications. Noninvasive diagnostic methods such as venous ultrasonography with or without colour Doppler are the most commonly used methods. Magnetic resonance imaging (MRI) and D-dimer assays may also be used (Pettker & Lockwood, 2007). Tachypnea and tachycardia are present with pulmonary embolism, and murmurs may be heard on cardiac auscultation. Echocardiographic abnormalities may be seen in right ventricular size or function (Pettker & Lockwood, 2007). Pregnancy limits the usefulness of arterial blood gases and oxygen saturation in diagnosis. A ventilation–perfusion scan, spiral computed tomography (CT) scan, magnetic resonance angiography, and pulmonary arteriogram may be used for diagnosis (Pettker & Lockwood, 2007).

Medical Management

Superficial venous thrombosis is treated with analgesia (nonsteroidal anti-inflammatory medications), rest with elevation of the affected leg, and graduated elastic compression stockings or pneumatic compression devices (Pettker & Lockwood, 2007). Heat may also be applied locally. Deep venous thrombosis is initially treated with anticoagulant therapy (usually continuous IV heparin), bed rest with the affected leg elevated, and analgesia. After the symptoms have decreased, the woman may be fitted with graduated elastic compression stockings to use when she is allowed to ambulate. IV heparin therapy continues for 5 to 7 days. Oral anticoagulant therapy (warfarin [Coumadin]) is started during this time and is continued for about 3 months. It is safe to use during lactation (see Medication Guide). Continuous IV heparin therapy is used for pulmonary embolism until symptoms have resolved. Intermittent subcutaneous heparin or oral anticoagulant therapy is usually continued for 6 months (Pettker & Lockwood, 2007).

In the hospital, nursing care of the woman with a thrombosis consists of continued assessments: inspection and palpation of the affected area; palpation of peripheral pulses; measurement and comparison of leg circumferences; inspection for signs of bleeding; monitoring for signs of pulmonary embolism, including chest pain, coughing, dyspnea, and tachypnea; and checking respiratory status for presence of crackles. Laboratory reports are monitored for prothrombin or partial thromboplastin times. The woman and her family

MEDICATION GUIDE

Warfarin Sodium (Coumadin)

Action

Warfarin blocks synthesis of clotting factors.

Indications

This medication is used for anticoagulation to prevent or treat blood clots.

Dosage

Oral dosing is dependent on blood tests.

Adverse Reactions

These include excessive bleeding, hemorrhage, rash, and gastrointestinal upset.

Nursing Considerations

Warfarin is contraindicated in pregnancy (can cause fetal death or birth defects). It is usually compatible with breastfeeding (Lawrence & Lawrence, 2011). Blood levels of the mother should be monitored. Inform woman to avoid alcohol, avoid cranberry products and large amounts of leafy green vegetables, and watch for bruising as it may be a sign of bleeding. They should avoid aspirin and nonsteroidal agents such as naproxen or ibuprofen. Warfarin may be taken with food or on empty stomach. Dose compliance is very important!

are assessed for their level of understanding about the diagnosis and their ability to cope during the unexpected extended period of recovery.

Interventions include explanations and education about the diagnosis and treatment. The woman will need assistance with personal care as long as she is on bed rest. The family should be encouraged to participate in her care if she and they wish. While the woman is on bed rest, she should be encouraged to change positions frequently but not to place the knees in a sharply flexed position that could cause pooling of blood in the lower extremities. She should also be cautioned not to rub the affected areas because rubbing could cause the clot to dislodge. Once the woman is allowed to ambulate, she should be taught how to prevent venous congestion by putting on the elastic stockings before getting out of bed.

Heparin and warfarin are administered as ordered. The physician should be notified if clotting times are outside the therapeutic level. If the woman is breastfeeding, she should be assured that neither heparin nor warfarin is excreted in significant quantities in breast milk. If the infant has been discharged, the family should be encouraged to bring the infant for feedings as permitted by hospital policy; the mother can also express milk to be sent home.

Pain can be managed with a variety of measures. Changing of positions, elevation of the leg, and application of moist heat may decrease discomfort. It may be necessary to administer analgesics and anti-inflammatory medications.

NURSING ALERT Medications containing aspirin are not given to women on anticoagulant therapy because aspirin inhibits synthesis of clotting factors and can lead to prolonged clotting time and increased risk of bleeding.

The woman is usually discharged home on oral anticoagulants and will need an explanation of the treatment schedule and possible adverse effects. If subcutaneous injections are to be given, the woman and her family must be taught how to administer the medication and about site rotation. They should also be given information about safe care practices to prevent bleeding and injury while she is on anticoagulant therapy, such as using a soft toothbrush and an electric razor. She will need information about follow-up with her health care provider for monitoring of clotting times and ensuring that the correct dosage of anticoagulant therapy is maintained. The woman should also use a reliable form of contraception if taking warfarin because warfarin is considered teratogenic (Pettker & Lockwood, 2007).

Postpartum Infections

Postpartum or puerperal infection is any clinical infection of the genital canal that occurs within 28 days after miscarriage, induced abortion, or childbirth. *Postpartum infection* is defined as the presence of a fever as well as an elevated white blood cell count. Puerperal infection is one of the major causes of morbidity and mortality throughout the world; however, in Canada, infection is a cause of readmission to hospital. Common postpartum infections include endometritis, wound infections, mastitis, urinary tract infections (UTIs), and respiratory tract infections.

The most common infecting organisms are the numerous streptococcal and anaerobic organisms. *Staphylococcus aureus*, gonococci, coliform bacteria, and clostridia are less common but serious pathogenic organisms that can cause puerperal infection. Postpartum infections are more common in women who are obese, have concurrent medical or immunosuppressive conditions or who had a Caesarean or other operative birth. Intrapartal factors such as prolonged rupture of membranes, prolonged labour, and internal maternal or fetal monitoring also increase the risk of infection (Duff, 2007). Factors that predispose the woman to postpartum infection are listed in Box 23-3.

Endometritis

Endometritis (infection of the lining of the uterus) is the most common postpartum infection. It usually begins as a localized infection at the placental site but can spread to the entire endometrium. Incidence is higher after Caesarean birth. Signs of endometritis include fever (usually greater than 38°C); increased pulse; chills; anorexia; nausea; fatigue and lethargy; pelvic pain; uterine tenderness; and foul-smelling, profuse lochia (Duff, 2007). Leukocytosis and a markedly increased RBC sedimentation rate are typical laboratory findings of postpartum infections. Anemia may also be present. Blood cultures or intracervical or intrauterine bacterial cultures (aerobic and anaerobic) should reveal the offending pathogens within 36 to 48 hours.

Wound Infections

Wound infections are common postpartum infections that often develop after the woman is at home. Sites of infection

BOX 23-3 Predisposing Factors for Postpartum Infection

Preconception or Antepartal Factors
- History of previous venous thrombosis, urinary tract infection, mastitis, pneumonia
- Diabetes mellitus
- Alcoholism
- Drug use
- Immunosuppression
- Anemia
- Malnutrition
- Obesity

Intrapartal Factors
- Caesarean birth
- Prolonged rupture of membranes
- Chorioamnionitis
- Prolonged labour
- Bladder catheterization
- Internal fetal or uterine pressure monitoring
- Multiple vaginal examinations after rupture of membranes
- Epidural anaesthesia
- Retained placental fragments
- Postpartum hemorrhage
- Episiotomy or lacerations
- Hematomas

include the Caesarean incision and repaired laceration or episiotomy site. Predisposing factors are similar to those for endometritis (see Box 23-3). Signs of wound infection include **erythema**, edema, warmth, tenderness, seropurulent drainage, and wound separation. Fever and pain may also be present. In order to decrease the risk of wound infections in women who have a Caesarean birth, the SOGC recommend that all women undergoing elective or emergency Caesarean section receive antibiotic prophylaxis. The timing of the antibiotic should be 15 to 30 minutes before the skin incision (Van Schalkwyk et al., 2010). Prophylactic antibiotics may also be considered for women who have third- and fourth-degree perineal injury, and the dose may be doubled for women who are morbidly obese (body mass index [BMI] > 35) (Van Schalkwyk et al., 2010).

Urinary Tract Infections

UTIs occur in 2 to 4% of postpartum women. Risk factors include urinary catheterization, frequent pelvic examinations, epidural anaesthesia, genital tract injury, history of UTI, and Caesarean birth. Signs and symptoms include **dysuria**, frequency and urgency, low-grade fever, urinary retention, hematuria, and pyuria. Costovertebral angle tenderness or flank pain may indicate upper UTI. The most common infecting organism is *Escherichia coli*, although other gram-negative aerobic bacilli also may cause UTIs (Duff, 2007).

Mastitis

Mastitis, or breast infection, affects 2 to 10% of women soon after childbirth, most of whom are first-time mothers who are breastfeeding. It occurs in fewer than 1% of nonbreastfeeding mothers (Newton, 2007). Mastitis is almost always unilateral and develops well after the flow of milk has been established (Fig. 23-1). The infecting organism generally is the hemolytic *S. aureus*. An infected nipple fissure usually is the initial lesion, followed by ductal system involvement. Inflammatory edema and engorgement of the breast soon obstruct the flow of milk in a lobe; regional, then generalized, mastitis follows. If treatment is not prompt, mastitis may progress to a breast abscess.

Symptoms rarely appear before the end of the first postpartum week and are more common in the second to fourth weeks. Chills, fever, malaise, and local breast tenderness are noted first. Localized breast tenderness, pain, swelling, redness, and axillary adenopathy may also occur. Antibiotics are prescribed. Lactation can be maintained by emptying the breasts every 2 to 4 hours by breastfeeding, manual expression, or a breast pump.

Nursing Care Management

Women with factors predisposing to postpartum infection (see Box 23-3) should be assessed carefully. Elevation of temperature, redness, and swelling are common signs. The woman may also complain of chills, fever, localized tenderness, or pain. Laboratory tests usually performed include a complete blood count, venous blood cultures, and uterine tissue cultures. Review of the woman's history and the laboratory results should be included in the assessment.

Nursing diagnoses for women experiencing postpartum infection include the following:

- Lack of knowledge related to
  - etiology, management, course of infection
  - transmission and prevention of infection
- Impaired tissue integrity related to
  - effects of infection process
- Acute pain related to
  - mastitis
  - puerperal infection
  - UTI

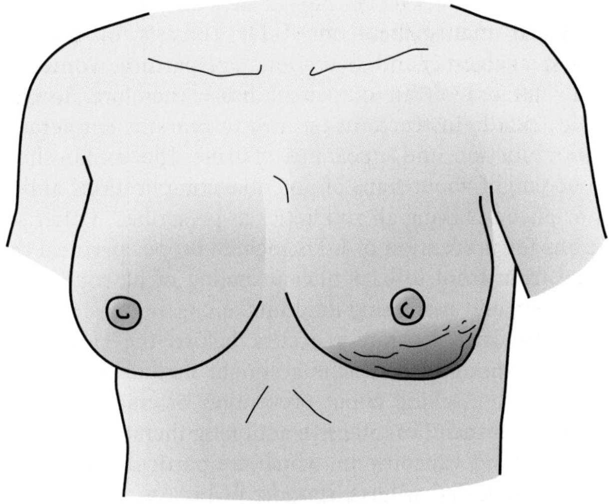

Fig. 23-1 Mastitis.

- Interrupted family processes related to
  - unexpected complication to expected postpartum recovery
  - pain
  - possible separation from newborn
  - interruption in process of realigning relationships after addition of the new family member
- Risk for impaired parenting related to
  - fear of spread of infection to newborn

The most effective and least expensive treatment of postpartum infection is prevention. Preventive measures include good prenatal nutrition to control anemia and intrapartal hemorrhage. Good maternal perineal hygiene with thorough hand hygiene is emphasized. Strict adherence to aseptic techniques by all health care personnel during childbirth and the postpartum period is very important.

Management of endometritis consists of IV broad-spectrum antibiotic therapy (cephalosporins, penicillins, or clindamycin and gentamicin) and supportive care, including hydration, rest, and pain relief. Antibiotic therapy is usually discontinued 24 hours after the woman is asymptomatic. Assessments of lochia, vital signs, and changes in the woman's condition should continue during treatment. Comfort measures depend on the symptoms and may include cool compresses, warm blankets, perineal care, and sitz baths. Teaching should include adverse effects of therapy, prevention of spread of infection, signs and symptoms of worsening condition, compliance with the treatment plan, and the need for follow-up care. Women may need to be assisted to maintain mother–infant interactions and breastfeeding.

Treatment of wound infections may combine antibiotic therapy with wound débridement. Wounds may be opened and drained. Nursing care includes frequent assessments of the wound and vital signs and wound care. Comfort measures include sitz baths, warm compresses, and perineal care. Teaching includes good hygiene techniques (e.g., changing perineal pads front to back, handwashing before and after perineal care), self-care measures, and signs of worsening conditions to report to the primary health care provider. The woman is usually discharged home for self-care or home nursing care after treatment is initiated in the inpatient setting.

Medical management for UTIs consists of antibiotic therapy, analgesia, and hydration. Postpartum women are usually treated on an outpatient basis; therefore, teaching should include instructions on how to monitor temperature, bladder function, and appearance of urine. The woman should also be taught about signs of potential complications and the importance of taking all antibiotics as prescribed. Other suggestions for prevention of UTIs include proper perineal care, wiping from front to back after urinating or having a bowel movement, and increasing fluid intake.

Because mastitis rarely occurs before the postpartum woman is discharged, teaching should include its warning signs and counselling about prevention of cracked nipples. Management includes intensive antibiotic therapy (e.g., cephalosporins and vancomycin, which are particularly useful in staphylococcal infections), support of breasts, local heat or cold, adequate hydration, and analgesics.

Almost all instances of acute mastitis can be avoided by using proper breastfeeding technique to prevent cracked nipples. Missed feedings, waiting too long between feedings, and abrupt weaning may lead to clogged nipples and mastitis. Cleanliness practiced by all who have contact with the newborn and new mother also reduces the incidence of mastitis. See also Chapter 26.

Postpartum women are usually discharged to home before 48 hours after birth. This is often before signs of infection are evident. Nurses in birth centres and hospital settings must be able to identify women at risk for postpartum infection and provide anticipatory teaching and counselling before discharge (see Community Focus box). After discharge, telephone follow-up, hot lines, support groups, lactation consultants, home visits by public health nurses, and teaching materials (movies, written materials) are all interventions that can be implemented to decrease the risk of postpartum infections.

Community nurses must be able to recognize signs and symptoms of postpartum infection so that the woman is alerted to contact her primary health care provider. These nurses must also be able to provide the appropriate nursing care for women who need follow-up home care.

Sequelae of Childbirth Trauma

Women are at risk for problems related to the reproductive system from the age of menarche through menopause and the older years. These problems, which include structural disorders of the uterus and vagina related to pelvic relaxation and urinary incontinence (UI), are often the delayed but direct result of childbearing.

With fetopelvic disproportion, prolonged labour, or a precipitous birth, structures of the vesical and vaginal walls are stretched and may be injured. The bladder neck and urethra may be compressed between the presenting part and the pubic bones or forced downward ahead of the presenting part. Since soft tissue damage usually occurs behind an intact vaginal epithelium, there is nothing visible to repair. Defects may also occur in women who have never been pregnant.

Structural disorders can have far-reaching effects for the woman and her family. Beyond the obvious physiological alterations, the woman can also experience threats to her self-concept and her ability to cope. A woman's concept of herself as a sexual being can be affected by the condition and its

COMMUNITY FOCUS

Prevention of Postpartum Infection

After giving birth, many women are discharged home before an infection can develop. Prepare a "Fact Sheet About Postpartum Infection" that could be distributed to postpartum women on discharge from the hospitals or birth centres in your community. Include signs and symptoms, and phone numbers and addresses of health care providers who could be contacted. Many Canadian communities have large populations who do not speak English, and this must be considered when teaching and or producing handout information.

treatments. Her family is also challenged in the way it responds to her diagnosis.

Uterine Displacement and Prolapse

Normally, the round ligaments hold the uterus in anteversion, and the uterosacral ligaments pull the cervix backward and upward. Uterine displacement is a variation of this normal placement. The most common type of displacement is posterior displacement, or retroversion, in which the uterus is tilted posteriorly and the cervix rotates anteriorly. Other variations include retroflexion and anteflexion (Fig. 23-2).

By 2 months postpartum, the ligaments should return to normal length, but in about one third of women the uterus remains retroverted. This condition is rarely symptomatic, but conception may be difficult because the cervix points toward the anterior vaginal wall and away from the posterior fornix, where seminal fluid pools after coitus. If symptoms occur, they may include pelvic and low back pain, exaggeration of premenstrual tension, and **dyspareunia**.

Uterine prolapse is a more serious type of displacement. Degrees of prolapse can vary from mild to complete. In complete prolapse, the cervix and body of the uterus protrude through the vagina, and the vagina is inverted (Fig. 23-3).

Uterine displacement and prolapse can be caused by congenital or acquired weakness of the pelvic support structures (often referred to as pelvic relaxation). In many cases, problems can be a delayed but direct result of childbearing. Although extensive damage may be noted and repaired shortly after birth, symptoms related to pelvic relaxation most often appear during the perimenopausal period, when the effects of ovarian hormones on pelvic tissues are lost and atrophic changes begin. Pelvic trauma, stress and strain, and the aging process are contributing causes. Other causes of pelvic relaxation include reproductive surgery and pelvic radiation.

Clinical Manifestations

Generally, symptoms of pelvic relaxation relate to the structure involved: urethra, bladder, uterus, vagina, cul-de-sac, or rectum. The most common complaints are pulling and dragging sensations, pressure, protrusions, fatigue, and low backache. Symptoms may be worse after prolonged standing or deep penile penetration during intercourse. Urinary incontinence may also occur.

Cystocele and Rectocele

Cystocele and rectocele often occur with uterine prolapse (although they can occur independently), causing the uterus to sag even further backward and downward into the vagina. **Cystocele** (Fig. 23-4, A) is the protrusion of the bladder downward into the vagina that develops when supporting structures in the vesicovaginal septum are injured. Anterior wall relaxation develops gradually over time as a result of congenital defects of support structures, childbearing, obesity, or advanced age. When the woman stands, the weakened anterior vaginal wall cannot support the weight of the urine in the bladder; the vesicovaginal septum is forced downward, the bladder is stretched, and its capacity is increased. With time, the cystocele enlarges until it protrudes into the vagina.

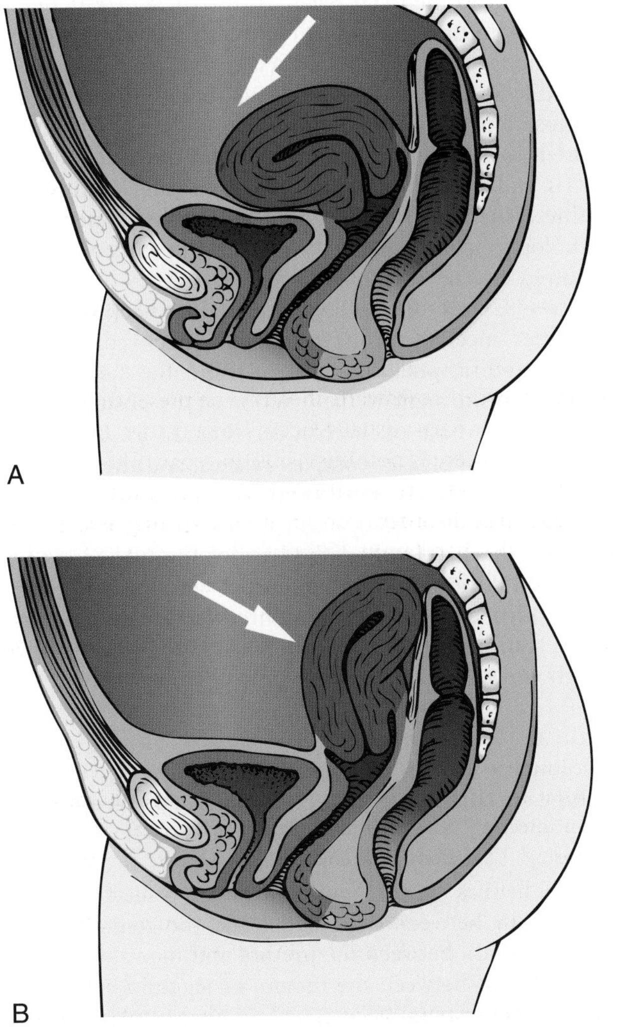

Fig. 23-2 Types of uterine displacement. **A:** Anterior displacement. **B:** Retroversion (backward displacement).

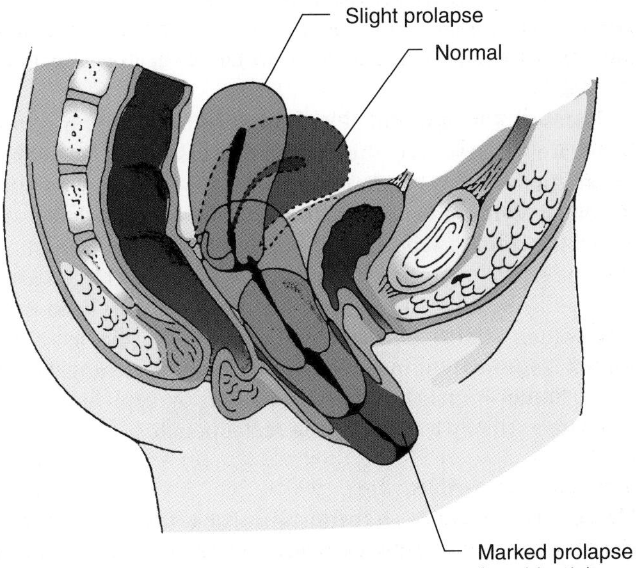

Fig. 23-3 Prolapse of uterus.

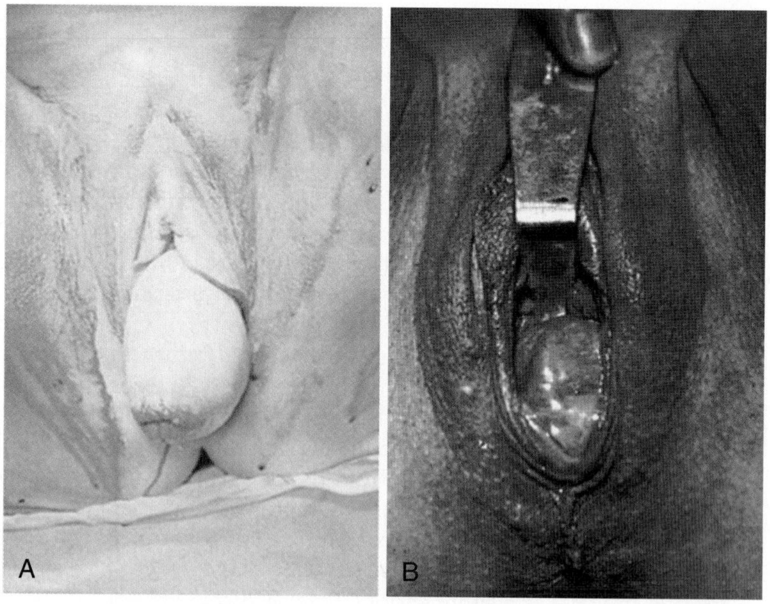

Fig. 23-4 Views of A: cystocele; B: rectocele. *(From Jarvis, C. [2008]. Physical assessment and health assessment [1st Canadian Edition]. Toronto: Saunders Canada.)*

Complete emptying of the bladder is difficult because the cystocele sags below the bladder neck. **Rectocele** is the herniation of the anterior rectal wall through the relaxed or ruptured vaginal fascia and rectovaginal septum; it appears as a large bulge that may be seen through the relaxed introitus (see Fig. 23-4, B).

Clinical Manifestations

Cystoceles and rectoceles often are asymptomatic. If symptoms of cystocele are present, they may include complaints of a bearing-down sensation or that "something is in my vagina." Other symptoms include urinary frequency, retention, incontinence, and possible recurrent cystitis and UTIs. On pelvic examination, there is a bulging of the anterior wall of the vagina when the woman is asked to bear down. Unless the bladder neck and urethra are damaged, urinary continence is unaffected. Women with large cystoceles complain of having to push upward on the sagging anterior vaginal wall in order to be able to void.

Rectoceles may be small and produce few symptoms, but some are so large that they protrude outside of the vagina when the woman stands. Symptoms are absent when the woman is lying down. A rectocele causes a disturbance in bowel function, a sensation of bearing down, or a sensation that the pelvic organs are falling out. With a very large rectocele it may be difficult to have a bowel movement. Each time the woman strains during bowel evacuation, the feces are forced against the thinned rectovaginal wall, stretching it even more. Some women facilitate evacuation by applying digital pressure vaginally to hold up the rectal pouch.

Urinary Incontinence

Urinary incontinence (UI) (uncontrollable leakage of urine) affects young and middle-age women; the prevalence increases as the woman ages. More than one third of women over the age of 60 have some form of UI (Mallett, 2005). Although nulliparous women can have UI, the incidence is higher in women who have given birth and also increases with parity. Conditions that disturb urinary control include stress UI, caused by sudden increases in intra-abdominal pressure, such as those following sneezing or coughing; urge incontinence, caused by disorders of the bladder and urethra, such as urethritis and urethral stricture, trigonitis, and cystitis; neuropathies, such as multiple sclerosis, diabetic neuritis, and pathological conditions of the spinal cord; and congenital and acquired urinary tract abnormalities.

Stress UI may follow injury to bladder neck structures. A sphincter mechanism at the bladder neck compresses the upper urethra, pulls it upward behind the symphysis, and forms an acute angle at the junction of the posterior urethral wall and the base of the bladder (Fig. 23-5). To empty the bladder, the sphincter complex relaxes, and the trigone contracts to open the internal urethral orifice and pull the contracting bladder wall upward, forcing urine out. The angle between the urethra and the base of the bladder is lost or increased if the supporting pubococcygeus muscle is injured; this change, coupled with a urethrocele, causes incontinence. Urine spurts out when the woman is asked to bear down or cough while she is in the lithotomy position.

Clinical Manifestations

Involuntary leaking of urine is the main sign. Episodes of leaking are common during coughing, laughing, and exercise.

Genital Fistulas

Genital fistulas are perforations between genital tract organs. Most occur between the bladder and the genital tract (e.g., vesicovaginal), between the urethra and the vagina (urethrovaginal), and between the rectum or sigmoid colon and the vagina (rectovaginal) (Fig. 23-6). Genital fistulas may also be a result of a congenital anomaly, gynecological surgery, obstetrical trauma, cancer, radiation therapy, gynecological trauma,

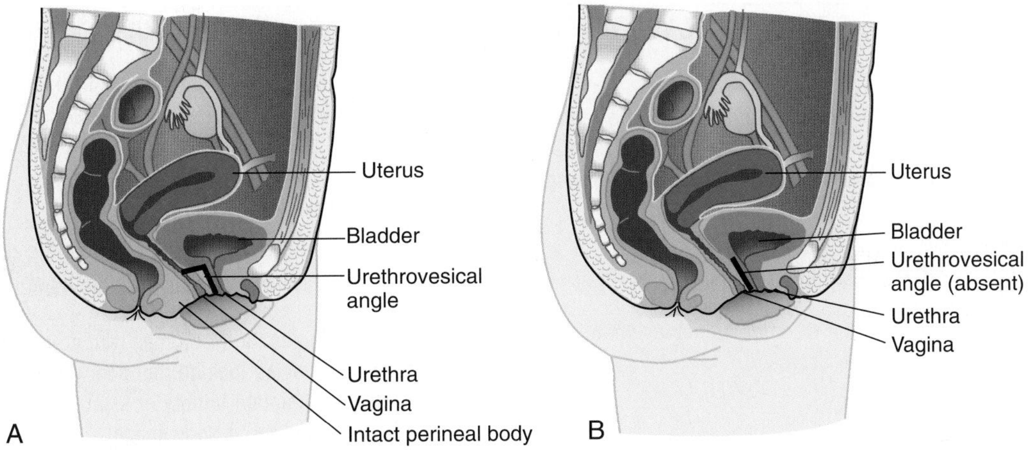

Fig. 23-5 Urethrovesical angle. **A:** Normal angle. **B:** Widening (absence) of angle.

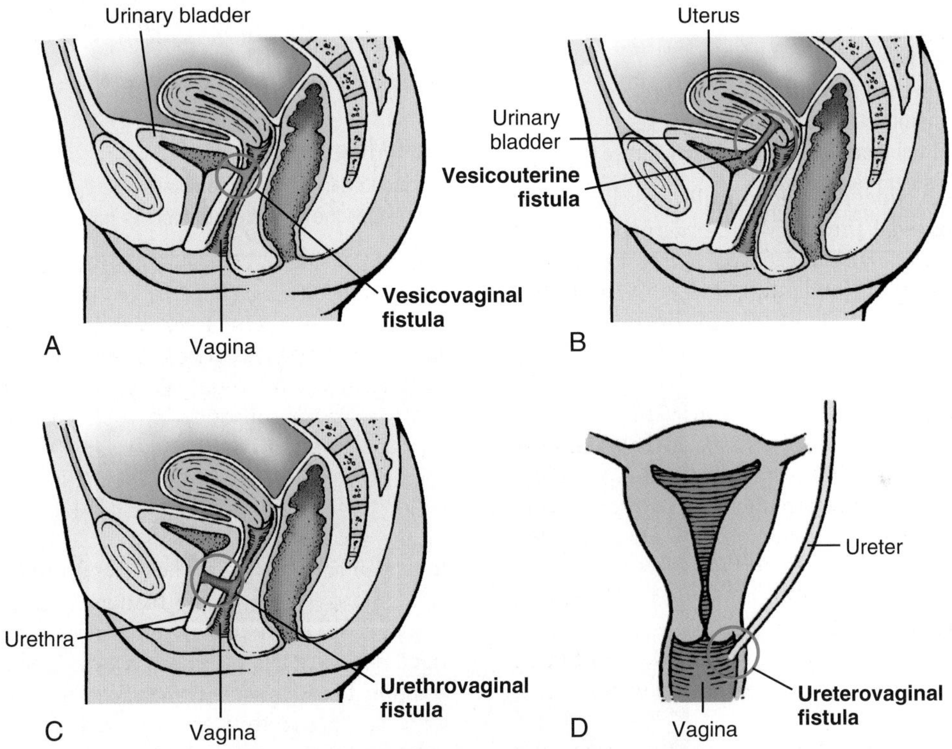

Fig. 23-6 Types of genitourinary fistulas. **A:** Vesicovaginal (bladder to vagina). **B:** Vesicouterine (bladder to uterus). **C:** Urethrovaginal (urethra to vagina). **D:** Ureterovaginal (ureter to vagina). Fistulas range in size from tiny and difficult to locate to large, disfiguring the base of the bladder. *(From Monahan, F. D., et al. [2007].* Phipps' medical-surgical nursing: Health and illness perspectives *[8th ed., p. 1696]. St. Louis: Mosby.)*

or infection (e.g., in the episiotomy). Fistulas are more common in women who have many children or have obstructed labours with minimal access to appropriate care, as in developing countries.

Clinical Manifestations

Signs and symptoms of vaginal fistulas depend on the site but may include the presence of urine, flatus, or feces in the vagina; odours of urine or feces in the vagina; and irritation of vaginal tissues.

Nursing Care Management

In general, nurses working with these women can provide information and self-care education to prevent problems before they occur, manage or reduce symptoms and promote comfort and hygiene if symptoms are already present, and recognize when further intervention is needed (see Nursing Process box). This information can be part of postpartum discharge teaching or provided at postpartum follow-up visits in clinics or physician or midwife offices, during postpartum home visits, or during gynecological health examinations. Information on

NURSING PROCESS: STRUCTURAL DISORDERS OF THE UTERUS AND VAGINA

Assessment

Assessment focuses primarily on the genitourinary tract, the reproductive organs, bowel elimination, and psychosocial and sexual factors. To support the appropriate medical diagnosis, the following measures are carried out:

- Health history is taken.
- Physical examination is performed.
- Laboratory tests are done.
- The woman's knowledge of the disorder, its management, and the possible prognosis is assessed.

Nursing Diagnoses

Possible nursing diagnoses for the patient with a structural disorder of the uterus or vagina include the following:

Constipation or diarrhea related to
- anatomical changes

Coping difficulties related to
- changes in body image

Dysfunctional family processes related to
- the woman's anatomical and functional changes

Social isolation, spiritual distress, disturbed body image, or situational low self-esteem related to
- changes in anatomy and function

Anxiety related to
- surgical procedure
- prognosis

Planning

The health care team works together to treat the disorders related to alterations in pelvic support and to help the woman manage her symptoms.

Expected outcomes for the woman with structural abnormalities of the uterus and vagina include that she will do the following:

- Regain and maintain urinary or fecal continence or both
- Cope with changes in body image
- Have satisfactory interpersonal relationships with her family and friends
- Have a reduction in anxiety related to her prognosis

Interventions

Various interventions are described in the text.

Evaluation

The nurse can be reasonably assured that care was effective to the extent that the expected outcomes have been achieved.

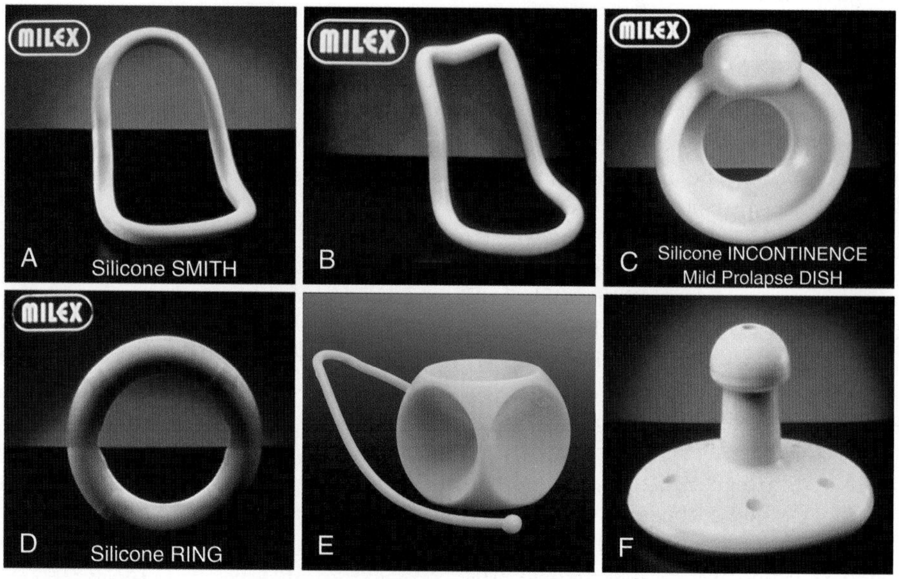

Fig. 23-7 Examples of pessaries. **A:** Smith. **B:** Hodge without support. **C:** Incontinence dish with support. **D:** Ring without support. **E:** Cube. **F:** Gellhorn. *(Courtesy Milex Products, Inc., a division of CooperSurgical, Trumbull, CT.)*

how to prevent or recognize problems can be a topic for workshops for women or health fairs in community settings.

Interventions for specific problems depend on the problem and the severity of the symptoms. If discomfort related to uterine displacement is a problem, several interventions can be implemented to treat uterine displacement. **Kegel exercises** can be performed several times a day to increase muscular strength (see Chapter 4, Patient Teaching box, p. 51). A knee–chest position performed for a few minutes several times a day can correct a mildly retroverted uterus. A pessary to support the uterus and hold it in the correct position may be inserted in the vagina (Fig. 23-7). Usually a pessary is used for only a short time because it can lead to pressure necrosis and vaginitis. Good hygiene is important; some women are taught to remove the pessary at night, cleanse it, and replace it in the morning. If the pessary is always left in place, regular douching with commercially prepared solutions or weak vinegar solutions (e.g., 15 mL to 1 L of water) to remove increased secretions and keep the vaginal pH at 4.0 to 4.5 is suggested. After a period of treatment, most women are free of symptoms and do not require the pessary. For these women, surgical correction is rarely indicated.

Treatment for uterine prolapse depends on the degree of prolapse. Pessaries may be useful in mild prolapse. Estrogen therapy also may be used in the older woman to improve tissue tone. If these conservative treatments do not correct the problem or there is a significant degree of prolapse, abdominal or vaginal hysterectomy is usually recommended.

Treatment for a cystocele includes use of a vaginal pessary or surgical repair. Pessaries may not be effective. The usual surgical procedure, done for large symptomatic cystoceles, is anterior repair (colporrhaphy), which involves a surgical shortening of pelvic muscles to provide better support for the bladder. An anterior repair is often combined with a vaginal hysterectomy.

Small rectoceles may not need treatment. The woman with mild symptoms may get relief from a high-fibre diet and adequate fluid intake, stool softeners, or mild laxatives. Vaginal pessaries usually are not effective. Large rectoceles that are causing significant symptoms are usually repaired surgically. A posterior repair (colporrhaphy) is the usual procedure. This surgery is performed vaginally and involves shortening the pelvic muscles to provide better support for the rectum. Anterior and posterior repairs may be performed at the same time and with vaginal hysterectomy.

Management of genital fistulas depends on the location. Surgical repair is the usual treatment; however, it may not be successful.

Nursing care of the woman with a cystocele, rectocele, or fistula requires great sensitivity because the woman's reactions are often intense. She may become withdrawn or hostile because of embarrassment about odours and soiling of her clothing that are beyond her control. Her sexuality is threatened; her partner may refuse sexual intimacy.

The nurse can tactfully suggest hygiene practices that reduce odour. Commercial deodorizing douches are available, or noncommercial solutions such as diluted chlorine (e.g., 5 mL of chlorine household bleach to 1 L of water) may be used. The chlorine solution is also useful for external perineal irrigation. Sitz baths and thorough washing of the genitalia with unscented, mild soap and warm water help. Sparse dusting with deodorizing powders can be useful.

If a rectovaginal fistula is present, enemas given before leaving the house may provide temporary relief from oozing of fecal material until corrective surgery is performed. Irritated skin and tissues may benefit from exposure to air or application of an emollient. Hygienic care is time consuming and may need to be repeated frequently throughout the day; protective pads or pants may need to be worn. All of these activities can be demoralizing to the woman and frustrating to her and her family.

Many of the nurse's efforts with these problems will be as part of a team working to prepare the woman for surgery. Preoperative teaching involves the primary nurse, operating room nurse, surgeon, and anaesthesiologist. Postoperative nursing care focuses on preventing infection and helping the woman avoid putting stress on the surgical site.

The nurse in the health promotion setting is usually most aware of the woman's living circumstances, physical limitations, and social problems and thus may be best suited to coordinate continuity of care after discharge.

Postpartum Psychological Complications

Mental health disorders in the postpartum period have implications for the mother, the newborn, and the entire family. Such conditions can interfere with attachment to the newborn and family integration, and some may threaten the safety and well-being of the mother, newborn, and other children. Fewer than 33% of women with postpartum mood disorders (PPMD) are detected by routine care (Coates, Schaefer, & Alexander, 2004). Because birth is usually thought to be a happy event, a new mother's emotional distress may puzzle and immobilize family and friends. When she most needs the caring attention of loved ones, they may either criticize or withdraw because of their own anxiety.

Postpartum Mood Disorders

Mood disorders are the predominant mental health disorder in the postpartum period. PPMD are mental health issues that affect the mother in the first year after the birth of the baby. This can include postpartum depression (PPD), postpartum anxiety, obsessive-compulsive disorder, and, rarely, psychosis. According to the Registered Nurses' Association of Ontario (RNAO) (2005), woman are significantly more likely to be admitted to a psychiatric hospital within the first 4 weeks postpartum than any other time in her life. Up to 75% of women experience a mild depression or "baby blues" after the birth of a child, although functioning of the woman is usually not impaired (RNAO, 2005) (see Chapter 21). However, up to 20% of women may experience PPMD. Baby blues and antepartum depression are predictors of depression (Kim et al., 2008; Reck et al., 2009; Watanabe et al., 2008). Some women have more serious depressions that can eventually incapacitate them to the point of being unable to care for themselves or their babies. Box 23-4 lists 13 risk factors for PPMD, with those having the greater effect listed first.

The cause of PPMD can be biological, psychological, situational, or multifactorial. It occurs in a variety of countries, although the manifestations may vary by culture. Also, cultures have varying beliefs and rituals that can affect the severity of PPMD (Bina, 2008; Goldbort, 2006).

Depressive symptoms may also be evident in fathers; 10% of fathers exhibit such symptoms. This depression interferes with positive enrichment activities with their children (Paulson, Dauber, & Leiferman, 2006).

PPMD may exert a moderate-to-large effect on the interaction of mothers and infants. Although a study in Taiwan showed that PPMD had no significant effect on infants' development (Wang et al., 2005), a study in the United Kingdom reported that infants of depressed mothers had significantly poorer weight gain (O'Brien et al., 2004). According to the RNAO (2005), PPMD can lead to infant attachment insecurity as well as emotional developmental delay.

BOX 23-4 Risk Factors for Postpartum Mood Disorders

1. Prenatal depression
2. Low self-esteem
3. Stress of child care
4. Prenatal anxiety
5. Life stress
6. Lack of social support
7. Marital relationship problems
8. History of depression
9. "Difficult" infant temperament
10. Postpartum blues
11. Single status
12. Low socioeconomic status
13. Unplanned or unwanted pregnancy

(Sources: Beck, C. [2001]. Predictors of postpartum depression: An update. *Nursing Research, 50*[5], 275–282; Beck, C. [2002]. Revision of the Postpartum Depression Predictors Inventory. *Journal of Obstetric, Gynecologic, and Neonatal Nursing, 31*[4], 394–402.)

Nurses should be strategically positioned to offer anticipatory guidance, assess the mental health of new mothers, offer therapeutic interventions, and make referrals when necessary (see Evidence-Informed Practice box). Failure to do so may result in tragic consequences. In the rarest of cases (postpartum psychosis), a disturbed mother may kill her infant, other family members, or herself (Lehmann, 2004).

The Diagnostic and Statistical Manual (DSM) of Mental Disorders contains the official guidelines for the assessment and diagnosis of psychiatric illness (American Psychiatric Association [APA], 2010); however, specific criteria for PPD are not listed. Instead, postpartum onset can be specified for any mood disorder either without psychotic features (i.e., PPD) or with psychotic features (i.e., postpartum psychosis) if the onset occurs within 4 weeks of childbirth (APA, 2010).

evolve Critical Thinking Exercise—Postpartum Mood Disorder

Postpartum Depression Without Psychotic Features

PPD is an intense and pervasive sadness with severe and labile mood swings; it is more serious and persistent than postpartum blues. Intense fears, anger, anxiety, and despondency that persist past the baby's first few weeks are not a normal part of postpartum blues. Occurring in approximately 10 to 15% of new mothers, these symptoms rarely disappear without outside help (Centers for Disease Control and Prevention [CDC], 2008; Paulson et al., 2006). Most of these mothers seek help only after reaching a "crisis point" (McCarthy & McMahon, 2008). The occurrence of this depression is higher among younger women and those with lower educational attainment (CDC, 2008). Mothers who have no one to talk to about their problems after giving birth tend to have a high rate of depression and a low rate of seeking help. This situation can be a concern for newly immigrated women who have difficulty with language and limited social support. Having established and supportive relationships facilitates seeking of care, as does outreach and follow-up (Sword et al., 2008).

The symptoms of postpartum major depression do not differ from those of nonpostpartum mood disorders except that the mother's ruminations of guilt and inadequacy feed her worries about being an incompetent and inadequate parent. There may be odd food cravings (often sweet desserts) and binges with abnormal appetite and weight gain. New mothers report an increased yearning for sleep, sleeping heavily but awakening instantly with any infant noise, and an inability to go back to sleep after infant feedings. Determining difficulty falling asleep is a relevant screening question to ascertain risk for depression (Goyal, Gay, & Lee, 2007).

A distinguishing feature of major depression is irritability. These episodes of irritability may flare up with little provocation and may sometimes escalate to violent outbursts or dissolve into uncontrollable sobbing. Many of these outbursts are directed against significant others ("He never helps me") or the baby ("She cries all the time, and I feel like hitting her"). Women with postpartum major depressive episodes often have severe anxiety, panic attacks, and spontaneous crying long after the usual duration of baby blues.

Many women feel especially guilty about having depressive feelings at a time when they believe they should be happy. They may be reluctant to discuss their symptoms or their negative feelings toward the infant. A prominent feature of depression is rejection of the infant, often caused by abnormal jealousy. The mother may be obsessed by the notion that the baby may take her place in her partner's affections. Attitudes toward the infant may include disinterest, annoyance with care demands, and blaming because of her lack of maternal feeling. The mother may appear awkward in her responses to the baby. Obsessive thoughts about harming the infant are very frightening to her. Often she does not share these thoughts because of embarrassment; when she does, other family members can become very frightened.

Medical Management

The natural course is one of gradual improvement over the 6 months after birth. However, supportive treatment alone is not efficacious for major depression. Pharmacological intervention is often required. Treatment options include antidepressants, antianxiety agents, and electroconvulsive therapy. Alternative therapies such as herbs, dietary supplements, massage, aromatherapy, and acupuncture may be helpful. Psychotherapy focuses on her fears and concerns regarding her new responsibilities and roles and monitoring for suicidal or homicidal thoughts. For some women, hospitalization is necessary.

Postpartum Depression With Psychotic Features

Postpartum psychosis is a syndrome most often characterized by depression (as described previously), delusions, and thoughts by the mother of harming either the infant or herself (Kaplan & Sadock, 2007).

A postpartum depression with psychotic features occurs in 1 to 2 per 1000 births (Kaplan & Sadock, 2007; RNAO, 2005). Once a woman has had one postpartum episode with psychotic features, there is a 30 to 50% likelihood of recurrence with each subsequent birth (APA, 2010).

Symptoms often begin within days after the birth, although the mean time to onset is 2 to 3 weeks and almost always

EVIDENCE-INFORMED PRACTICE Assessing for Postpartum Mood Disorder

—*Pat Gingrich*

Ask the Question

What is the best way to assess for postpartum mood disorder?

Search for Evidence

Search Strategies

Professional organization guidelines, meta-analyses, systematic reviews, randomized controlled trials, nonrandomized prospective studies, and retrospective studies since 2006

Databases Searched

CINAHL, Cochrane, Medline, National Guideline Clearinghouse, TRIP Database Plus, and the Web sites for the Association of Women's Health, Obstetric and Neonatal Nurses (AWHONN) and Society of Obstetricians and Gynaecologists of Canada (SOGC)

Critically Analyze the Evidence

Postpartum mood disorder (PPMD) is a serious and insidious disease that can rob a new family of valuable nurturing time. According to the Registered Nurses' Association of Ontario (RNAO) (2005), 13 to 20% of women experience some form of postpartum mood disorder. Risk factors for PPMD included young age and low socioeconomic status. PPMD information should be incorporated into existing programs for high-risk women, such as intimate partner violence services (Centers for Disease Control and Prevention [CDC], 2008).

A large prospective study of 40,000 Australian women found that risk factors for PPMD included previous history of depression, especially current or antenatal anxiety or depression, and low partner support (Milgrom et al., 2008). The authors recommend interventions targeted to women with current depression or anxiety and low social support.

Implications for Practice

The RNAO states that nurses should give individualized, flexible care; assess early and often, offering the Edinburgh Postnatal Depression Scale (EPDS), the most well-tested screening tool for patient self-test; intervene swiftly for a score greater than 13 on the EPDS or if there is any evidence of self-harm ideation on score item No. 10 or in their clinical judgement; and encourage peer support group participation (McQueen et al., 2008; RNAO, 2005) (see Fig. 21-7).

The Postpartum Social Support Questionnaire has shown preliminary promise as a valid and reliable screening tool (Hopkins & Campbell, 2008).

A systematic review of telephone support revealed that proactive telephone support decreases the symptoms of PPMD. Other postpartum benefits included prevention of smoking relapse and promotion of breastfeeding (Dennis & Kingston, 2008).

Nurses can also assist women by teaching them self-care, especially the symptoms and risk factors for PPMD; helping them to feel safe and empowered in discussing their mental and social health; and facilitating adequate social and partner support. Women and their families should be given written resources in their native language and emergency numbers to call. Last but not least, follow-up is a powerful tool for detection and deterrence of PPMD.

References

Centers for Disease Control and Prevention (2008). Prevalence of self-reported postpartum depression symptoms—17 states, 2004–2005. *MMWR: Morbidity and Mortality Weekly Report, 57*(14), 361–366.

Dennis, C. L., & Kingston, D. (2008). A systematic review of telephone support for women during pregnancy and the early postpartum period. *Journal of Obstetric, Gynecologic and Neonatal Nursing, 37*(3), 301–314.

Hopkins, J., & Campbell, S. B. (2008). Development and validation of a scale to assess social support in the postpartum period. *Archives in Women's Mental Health, 11*(1), 57–65.

McQueen, K., et al. (2008). Evidence-based recommendations for depressive symptoms in postpartum women. *Journal of Obstetric, Gynecologic and Neonatal Nursing, 37*(2), 127–136.

Milgrom, J., et al. (2008). Antenatal risk factors for postnatal depression: A large prospective study. *Journal of Affective Disorders, 108*(1-2), 147–157.

Registered Nurses' Association of Ontario (2005). *Interventions for postpartum depression.* Toronto: Author. Retrieved, from http://rnao.ca/sites/rnao-ca/files/Interventions_for_Postpartum_Depression.pdf.

within 8 weeks of birth (Kaplan & Sadock, 2007). Characteristically, the woman begins to complain of fatigue, insomnia, and retlessness and may have episodes of tearfulness and emotional lability. Complaints about the inability to move, or stand are also common. Suspiciousness, confusion, incoherence, irrational statements, and obsessive concerns about the baby's health and welfare may be present later (Kaplan & Sadock, 2007). Delusions may occur in 50% of all women, and hallucinations in about 25%. Auditory hallucinations that command the mother to kill the infant can also occur in severe cases. When delusions are present, they are often related to the infant. The mother may think the infant is possessed by the devil, has special powers, or is destined for a terrible fate (APA, 2010). Grossly disorganized behaviour may be manifested as a disinterest in the infant or an inability to provide care. Some insist that something is wrong with the baby or accuse nurses or family members of hurting or poisoning their child. Nurses are advised to be alert for mothers who are agitated, overactive, confused, complaining, or suspicious.

A specific illness included in depression with psychotic features is bipolar disorder (formerly called manic depressive illness). This mood disorder is preceded or accompanied by manic episodes characterized by elevated, expansive, or irritable moods. Clinical manifestations of a manic episode include at least three of the following symptoms that have been significantly present for at least 1 week: grandiosity, decreased need for sleep, pressured speech, flight of ideas, distractibility, psychomotor agitation, and excessive involvement in pleasurable activities without regard for negative consequences (APA, 2010). Because these women are hyperactive, they may not take the time to eat or sleep, which leads to inadequate nutrition, dehydration, and sleep deprivation. While in a manic state, mothers need constant supervision when caring for their infant. In most instances, they are too preoccupied to provide child care.

Medical Management

A favourable outcome is associated with a positive premorbid adjustment (before the onset of the disorder) and a supportive family network (Kaplan & Sadock, 2007). Because mood disorders are usually episodic, women may experience another episode of symptoms within a year or two of the birth. Postpartum psychosis is a psychiatric emergency, and the mother will probably need psychiatric hospitalization. Antipsychotics and mood stabilizers such as lithium are the treatments of choice (see Tables 23-2 and 23-3 for categories of risk during pregnancy). For mothers who are breastfeeding, some sources recommend that no pharmacological agents be prescribed (Kaplan & Sadock, 2007), whereas others advise caution while prescribing some agents (Schatzberg & Nemeroff, 2004). It is usually advantageous for the mother to have contact with her baby if she so desires, but visits must be closely supervised. Psychotherapy is indicated after the period of acute psychosis is past.

Nursing Care Management

Even though the prevalence of PPMD is fairly well established, women are unlikely to seek help from a mental health care provider (see Nursing Process box). Primary health care providers can usually recognize severe depression or postpartum psychosis but may miss milder forms; even if it is recognized, the woman may be treated inappropriately or subtherapeutically. Identification and treatment of maternal depression must be continued beyond the immediate postbirth period to prevent negative effects of maternal depression on the children of these mothers (Horwitz et al., 2007).

To recognize symptoms of PPMD as early as possible, the nurse should be an active listener and demonstrate a caring attitude. Nurses cannot depend on women to volunteer unsolicited information about their depression or ask for help. Examples of ways to initiate conversation include the following: "Now that you've had your baby, how are things going for you? Have you had to change many things in your life since having the baby?" and "How much time do you spend crying?"

If the nurse assesses that the new mother is depressed, she or he must ask if the mother has thought about hurting herself or the baby.

The Edinburgh Postnatal Depression Scale (EPDS) is a tool used for screening for PPMD (see Fig. 22-6). Women are asked to answer questions regarding how they have felt in the previous 7 days. The EDPS has 10 questions. Women who score greater than 13 and those who have a history of depression or anxiety require more intensive postpartum follow-up. Women who answer "yes" to the question about the thought of hurting themselves need immediate care.

NURSING ALERT Because mothers with depression with psychotic features may harm their infants, extra precaution is needed in assessment and intervention. The nurse needs to ask specifically if the mother has had thoughts about harming her baby.

On the Postpartum Unit

Nurses must discuss PPMD to prepare all new parents for potential problems in the postpartum period (see Patient Teaching box). Mothers are often discharged before the blues or depression occurs. The family must be able to recognize the symptoms and know where to go for help. Written materials that explain what the woman can do to prevent depression are useful.

Table 23-2 Mood Stabilizers

MOOD STABILIZERS	PREGNANCY RISK CATEGORY*	LACTATION RISK CATEGORY*
Carbamazepine (Tegretol)	D	L2
Clonazepam (Klonopin, Rivotril)	D	L3
Gabapentin	C	L3
Lamotrigine (Lamictal)	C	L3
Lithium carbonate (Carbolith, Lithane)	D	L4
Topiramate (Topamax)	C	L3
Valproic acid (Depakene, Epival ECT)	D	L2

*Hale, T. W. (2010). *Medications and mothers' milk* (14th ed.). Amarillo, TX: Hale.
C, animal studies show adverse effects on fetus but no controlled studies in pregnant women, or no studies available; *D,* positive evidence of human fetal risk; *L2,* medication studied in limited number of breastfeeding women with no adverse effects in infant, or evidence is remote; *L3,* no controlled studies, or studies show minimal nonthreatening effects; *L4,* possibly hazardous.

Table 23-3 Antipsychotic Medications

ANTIPSYCHOTIC MEDICATIONS	PREGNANCY RISK CATEGORY*	LACTATION RISK CATEGORY*
Traditional Antipsychotics		
Chlorpromazine hydrochloride	C	L3
Fluphenazine hydrochloride; fluphenazine deconate (Modecate Concentrate)	C	L3
Haloperidol deconate LA	C	L2
Perphenazine	C	L3
Thioridazine	C	L4
Trifluoperazine	Unknown	Unknown
Atypical Antipsychotics		
Aripiprazole (Abilify)	C	L3
Clozapine (Clozaril)	B	L3
Loxapine (Loxitane)	C	L4
Olanzapine (Zyprexa)	C	L2
Quetiapine (Seroquel)	C	L4
Risperidone (Risperdal)	C	L3
Ziprasidone (Zeldox)	C	L4

*Hale, T. W. (2010). *Medications and mothers' milk* (14th ed.). Amarillo, TX: Hale.
C, Animal studies show adverse effects on fetus but no controlled studies in pregnant women, or no studies available; *B,* Studies in pregnancy woman or animals show no fetal risk. The chance of fetal harm is remote but remains a possibility; *L2,* medication studied in limited number of breastfeeding women with no adverse effects in infant, or evidence is remote; *L3,* no controlled studies, or studies show minimal nonthreatening effects; *L4,* possibly hazardous.

NURSING PROCESS: POSTPARTUM MOOD DISORDER

Assessment

Observe for signs of depression.

Ask appropriate questions to determine moods, appetite, sleep, energy and fatigue levels, and ability to concentrate (see text for examples of questions to ask).

Use screening tools such as the Postpartum Depression Predictors Inventory–Revised (PDPI-R) (Beck, 2002) and the Edinburgh Postnatal Depression Scale (see Fig. 21-7).

If initial screening indicates that the woman may be depressed, refer her for formal screening, to determine the urgency of referral and type of provider.

Assess the woman's family for information and the need to express how they have been affected by the woman's emotional disorder.

Nursing Diagnoses

Possible nursing diagnoses for the woman experiencing postpartum mood disorder include the following:

Ineffective family coping related to
- increased care needs of mother and infant

Risk for impaired parenting related to
- inability of depressed mother to attach to and care for infant

Situational low self-esteem in the mother related to
- stresses associated with role changes

Risk for injury to newborn related to
- mother's depression (inattention to infant's needs for hygiene, nutrition, safety) and psychotropic medications via breast milk

Risk for violence (rare) toward self (mother) or children related to
- postpartum psychosis

Planning

Planning is focused on meeting the individual needs of the family to ensure safety, especially for the mother and infant and any other children, and facilitate functional family coping.

Specific measurable criteria can be developed on the basis of the following general outcomes:
- The mother will no longer be depressed.
- The mother's and infant's physical well-being will be maintained.
- The family will cope effectively.
- Family members will demonstrate continued healthy growth and development.
- The infant will be fully integrated into the family.

Interventions

Observe the mother carefully for signs of tearfulness; conduct further assessments as necessary.

Discuss postpartum mood disorders to prepare new parents for potential problems in the postpartum period.

If the postpartum nurse is concerned about the mother, request a mental health consult.

Provide routine instructions regarding postpartum mood disorders to the person who takes the woman home (i.e., "If you notice that your wife [or daughter] is upset or crying a lot, please call the postpartum care provider immediately. Don't wait for the routine postpartum appointment.").

Provide information about community resources for support.

Evaluation

The nurse can be assured that care has been effective if the physical well-being of the mother and infant is maintained, if the mother and family are able to cope effectively, and if each family member continues to show a healthy adaptation to the presence of the new member of the family.

PATIENT TEACHING Activities to Prevent Postpartum Depression

- Share knowledge about postpartum emotional problems with close family and friends.
- Take care of yourself: eat a balanced diet, exercise on a regular basis, and get enough sleep.
- Share your feelings with someone close to you; don't isolate yourself at home with the TV.
- Don't overcommit yourself or feel like you need to be a superwoman.
- Don't place unrealistic expectations on yourself.
- Don't be ashamed of having emotional problems after your baby is born. It happens to approximately 15% of women.

NURSING ALERT Because the newborn may be scheduled for a checkup before the mother's 6-week checkup, nurses in well-baby clinics or physician offices should be alert for signs of PPMD in new mothers and be knowledgeable about community referral resources.

In the Home and Community

Postpartum home visits can reduce the incidence of or complications from depression. A brief home visit or phone call at least once a week until the new mother returns for her postpartum visit may save the life of a mother and her infant; however, home visits may not be feasible or available. Some provinces have mandatory telephone follow-up of all new mothers after the birth, and women who are identified as high risk should receive more comprehensive follow-up. Supervision of the mother with emotional complications may become a prime concern. Because depression can greatly interfere with her mothering functions, family and friends may need to participate in the infant's care. This is a time for the extended family and friends to determine what they can do to help; the nurse can work with them to ensure adequate supervision and their understanding of the woman's mental illness (Linter & Gray, 2006).

When the woman has PPMD, a partner often reacts with confusion, shock, denial, and anger and feels neglected and blamed. The nurse can talk with the woman about how her condition is also hard for her partner and that he or she is probably very worried about her. Partners may withdraw or criticize when they are deeply worried about their partner. The nurse can provide nonjudgemental opportunities for the partner to express feelings and concerns, help the partner identify positive coping strategies, and be a source of encouragement for the partner to continue supporting the woman. Suggestions for partners of women with PPMD include helping around the house, setting limits with family and friends, going with her to doctor's appointments, educating himself or herself about PPMD, writing down concerns and questions to take to the doctor or therapist, and just being with her—sitting quietly, hugging her, and telling her that she is loved. Both the woman and her partner need an opportunity to express their needs, fears, thoughts, and feelings in a nonjudgemental environment.

Even if the woman is severely depressed, hospitalization can be avoided if adequate resources can be mobilized to ensure safety for both mother and infant. The community health nurse will need to make frequent phone calls or home visits for assessment and counselling. Community resources that may be helpful are temporary child care or foster care, homemaker service, meals on wheels, parenting guidance centres, mother's-day-out programs, and telephone support groups such The Pacific Post Partum Support Society (http://www.postpartum.org) and The Peel Postpartum Mood Disorder Program (http://www.pmdinpeel.ca).

Referral

Women with moderate-to-severe cases of PPMD should be referred to a mental health therapist such as an advanced-practice psychiatric nurse or psychiatrist for evaluation and therapy. Inpatient psychiatric hospitalization may be necessary. This decision is made when the safety of the mother or child is threatened.

Providing Safety

When depression is suspected, the nurse should ask the woman, "Have you thought about hurting yourself?" If delusional thinking about the baby is suspected, the nurse should ask, "Have you thought about hurting your baby?" Four criteria measure the seriousness of a suicidal plan: method, availability, specificity, and lethality. Has the woman specified a method? Is the method of choice available? How specific is the plan? If the method is concrete and detailed, with access to it right at hand, the suicide risk is increased. How lethal is the method? The most lethal method is shooting, with hanging being a close second. The least lethal method is slashing one's wrists. Medication overdose with tricyclic antidepressants (TCAs) causes death. Avoid use of TCAs in suicidal women because of the danger of overdose.

NURSING ALERT Suicidal thoughts or attempts are among the most serious symptoms of PPMD and require immediate assessment and intervention.

Psychiatric Hospitalization

Women with postpartum psychosis have a psychiatric emergency and must be referred immediately to a psychiatrist who is experienced in working with women with psychosis, can prescribe medication and other forms of therapy, and can assess the need for hospitalization.

LEGAL TIP **Commitment for Psychiatric Care.** If a woman with PPMD is experiencing active suicidal ideation or harmful delusions about the baby and is unwilling to seek treatment, legal intervention may be necessary to commit the woman to an inpatient setting for treatment.

Within the hospital setting, the reintroduction of the baby to the mother can occur at the mother's own pace. A schedule is set for increasing the number of hours during which the mother cares for the baby over several days, culminating in the infant staying overnight in the mother's room. This enables the mother to experience meeting the infant's needs and giving up sleep for the baby, a situation that is difficult for new mothers even under ideal conditions. The mother's readiness for discharge and caring for the baby should be assessed. Her interactions with her baby should also be carefully supervised and guided.

Nurses need to observe the mother for signs of bonding with the baby. Attachment behaviours are defined as eye-to-eye contact; physical contact that involves holding, touching, cuddling, and talking to the baby and calling the baby by name; and the initiation of appropriate care. A staff member should be assigned to keep the baby in sight at all times. Indirect teaching, praise, and encouragement are designed to bolster the mother's self-esteem and self-confidence.

Psychotropic Medications

If a woman is diagnosed with depression, antidepressant medications will often be used. If the woman is not breastfeeding, antidepressants can be prescribed without special precautions. In addition to TCAs, selective serotonin reuptake inhibitors and serotonin-norepinephrine reuptake inhibitors, monoamine oxidative inhibitors, and mood stabilizers, antipsychotic medications may be prescribed for nonbreastfeeding women.

Women taking mood stabilizers (see Table 23-2) must be taught about their many adverse effects, and those on lithium need to be told to have serum lithium levels drawn every 6 months. Women with severe psychiatric syndromes such as schizophrenia, bipolar disorder, or psychotic depression will probably require antipsychotic medications (see Table 23-3).

Patient education is important for those taking antipsychotic medications because most of these medications can cause sedation and orthostatic hypotension, both of which could interfere with the mother being able to safely care for her baby. The medications can also cause parasympathetic nervous system effects, such as constipation, dry mouth, blurred vision, tachycardia, urinary retention, weight gain, and agranulocytosis. Central nervous system effects may include akathisia, dystonias, Parkinsonism-like symptoms, tardive dyskinesia (irreversible), and neuroleptic malignant syndrome (potentially fatal).

The newer, atypical antipsychotic medications, such as aripiprazole, olanzapine, quetiapine, risperidone, and ziprasidone, are usually safer and have fewer adverse effects than the older, more traditional antipsychotics; however, their safety in breastfeeding women has not been established.

Psychotropic Medications and Lactation

A major clinical dilemma is the psychopharmacological treatment of women with a PPMD who want to breastfeed their infants. In the past, women were told to discontinue lactation. Current beliefs are that, although most medications will diffuse into breast milk, there are very few instances in which breastfeeding has to be discontinued (Pigarelli, Kraus, & Potter, 2005). Several factors influence the amount of drug an infant will receive through breastfeeding: the amount of milk produced, the composition of the milk (mature milk versus **colostrum**), the concentration of the medication, and the extent to which the breast was emptied during a previous feeding (Pigarelli et al., 2005). Infants also vary in their ability to absorb, metabolize, and excrete ingested medication. Premature infants may not have optimal liver function, and kidney function does not reach maturity until 2 to 4 months of age. Because all psychotropic medications pass through breast milk to the infant, the risks associated with the use of such medications must be weighed against the benefits associated with breastfeeding for both the mother and infant. None of these medications has been proven to be safe during lactation.

When breastfeeding women have emotional complications and need psychotropic medications, referral to a mental health provider who specializes in postpartum disorders is preferred. Depressed women need the nurse to reinforce the need to take antidepressants as ordered. Because antidepressants do not exert any effect for about 2 weeks and usually do not reach full effect for 4 to 6 weeks, many women discontinue taking the medication on their own. Patient and family teaching should reinforce the schedule for taking medications in conjunction with the infant's feeding schedule and the necessity to continue to take the medication until therapeutic effects occur.

Other Treatments for Postpartum Mood Disorders

Other treatments for PPMD include complementary and alternative therapies, such as those listed in Box 23-5, electroconvulsive therapy, and psychotherapy (group or individual). Alternative therapies may be used alone but often are used with other treatments for PPMD. Safety and efficacy studies of these alternative therapies are needed to ensure that care and advice are based on evidence.

BOX 23-5 Possible Alternative and Complementary Therapies for Postpartum Mood Disorders

Acupuncture
Acupressure
Aromatherapy
- Jasmine
- Ylang ylang
- Rose

Herbal
- Lavender tea

Healing touch or therapeutic touch
Massage
Relaxation techniques
Reflexology
Yoga

(Source: Weier, K., & Beal, M. [2004]. Complementary therapies and adjuncts in the treatment of postpartum depression. *Journal of Midwifery and Women's Health, 49*[2], 96–104.)

NURSING ALERT St. John's wort is often used to treat depression. It has not been proven safe for women who are breastfeeding.

Loss and Grief

Situational life crises can be superimposed on the experiences of childbearing. These may include infertility, premature labour or premature birth, a Caesarean birth, any perception of loss of control during the birthing experience, the birth of a boy when the parents wanted a girl or vice versa, the birth of a child with a handicap, a maternal death, or fetal or neonatal death (see Community Focus box). All of these situations have a common denominator: they are losses of what was hoped for, dreamed about, and planned.

From the perspective of health care providers, these crises vary in degree. However, from the perspective of the parents, the perceived loss may be the most terrible thing that has ever happened to them. At the birth, they are mourning instead of celebrating life.

Infant mortality rates continue to decrease in Canada, with a rate of 6.6 deaths per 1000 live births in 2008, the leading cause being prematurity (PHAC, 2012). Infants may die in the early postpartum period from prematurity, birth defects, and other acute illnesses. Thus, parents can experience grief before or during the childbearing experience.

The focus of this section is to prepare the nurse to provide sensitive, supportive, and therapeutic interventions to parents and families experiencing perinatal loss in a variety of settings. An overview of the grief process is presented as a guide for assessing and understanding the responses of bereaved women, men, and their families. Guidelines for intervention are given, and specific intervention approaches are discussed.

Grief Responses

Grief or bereavement has been described as a cluster of painful responses experienced by individuals coping with the death of

COMMUNITY FOCUS

Community Resources for Loss and Grief

Investigate what resources and support groups exist in your community to assist parents who have experienced a maternal death; birth of a "less-than-perfect" child; a Caesarean birth; or the death of a baby through miscarriage, stillbirth, or newborn death. Are resources available? Are there groups available for people with languages other than English? Are there enough of these resources to assist parents? How difficult was it for you to identify these resources? What could you do to make resources more known to bereaved parents and families?

someone with whom they had a close relationship, generally a relative or close friend (Lindemann, 1944). Many authors believe that there are overlapping phases in the grief process, but most do not believe that grief is experienced in "stages." Based on years of clinical work with bereaved parents and building on the conceptualization of others regarding grief following the death of a spouse, Miles (1984) developed a model of parental grief. Parental grief responses occur in three overlapping phases. There is an early period of acute distress and shock followed by a period of intense grief that includes emotional, cognitive, behavioural, and physical responses. The phase of reorganization is reached when parents return to their usual level of functioning in society, although the pain associated with the death remains. The duration of grief varies with the individual, but there is general agreement that grief is a long-term process that can extend for months and years. With a very close relationship such as with one's baby, some aspects of grief never truly end.

Acute Distress

The loss of a pregnancy or death of an infant is an acute and distressing experience for mothers and partners who planned for and expected a normal healthy infant as the outcome. The loss encompasses a loss of their identity as a mother or father and of their many dreams related to parenthood. The immediate reaction to news of a perinatal loss or infant death is a period of acute distress. Parents generally are in a state of shock and numbness. They may feel a sense of unreality, loss of innocence, and powerlessness, as though they were in a bad dream or in a fog or trancelike state. Disbelief and denial can occur. Sadness, devastation, depression, and intense outbursts of emotion and crying are common. In contrast, lack of affect, euphoria, and calmness may occur and may reflect numbness, denial, or a personal way of coping with stress.

Much of the attention during the time of a loss is on the mother; the partner is expected to be her main support. The response of partners may vary more than that of mothers and depends on the level of identification with the pregnancy. While partners may be more profoundly affected and grieve deeply for a perinatal loss, their feelings are often ignored.

Partners are distressed by the grief of the mother and often feel helpless at how to comfort her with the intense pain. Some partners may appear stoic and unemotional to maintain the societal expectation that they be "strong" for the mother and other family members. Because many men do not easily share their feelings or ask for help, special efforts may be needed to help them acknowledge these feelings and realize that they, too, have a right to support from others in their pain.

During this time of acute distress, parents face the first task of grief: accepting the reality of the loss. The pregnancy has ended, or the baby has died, and their lives have changed. Although parents are often required to make many decisions such as having an autopsy, naming the infant, and making funeral arrangements, normal functioning is impeded, and decisions are difficult to make. Grandparents, friends, clergy, or other relatives may be available to help the couple cope. However, it is important that the mother and her partner ultimately make the decisions that are right for them.

Intense Grief

The phase of intense grief encompasses many difficult emotions as the parents work through their pain and adjust to life without the wished-for child. In the early months after the loss, parents often experience feelings of loneliness, emptiness, and yearning. The mother may report that her arms ache to hold or nurse her baby and that she wakes to the sound of a baby crying. Both the mother and her partner may be preoccupied with thoughts about the wished-for child. Some parents cope with these feelings by avoiding memories and not talking about the baby, whereas others want to reminisce and discuss their loss over and over.

Deciding what to do about the nursery and baby clothes is particularly difficult during this period. Some women want the room taken down before they go home, whereas others want the room left intact until they have had time to grieve their loss. It is not unusual for a grandparent or other family member to want to rush home to take down the nursery, thinking that they would be sparing additional grief. In fact, their actions might only complicate the grief if the parents were not involved in the decision. The bereaved parents must go through these types of experiences in their own time frame so that healing can take place.

During this phase of intense grief, guilt may emerge from the deep feelings of helplessness in not somehow preventing the pregnancy loss or the death of the infant. Mothers are particularly vulnerable to feeling guilt because of their sense of responsibility for the well-being of the fetus and baby. With many perinatal losses, there is no clear cause of the event, leaving the woman to speculate about what she might have done or not done to bring about the loss. Guilt may be intense if the mother thinks she is being punished for some unrelated event, such as having had a prior induced abortion. Such self-blame is torture for mothers, and they need repeated emotional reassurance that they were not at fault.

Other common responses during this phase are anger, resentment, bitterness, and irritability. Anger may be focused on the health care team who failed to save the pregnancy or infant; toward a God who allowed the loss to occur; or toward family, friends, or peers when they do not provide the support the bereaved parents need and want. Some parents focus their resentment on parents who do not appreciate their children or neglect and abuse them. A sense of bitterness or generalized irritability rather than frank anger may be another response.

During the grief process, fear and anxiety can occur as a profound worry that something else bad might happen to another pregnancy. Some parents, especially mothers, are almost obsessed with the desire to become pregnant again; others struggle with whether they can cope with the possibility of another loss.

Deep sadness and depression can arise when the parent has full awareness of the loss. This often occurs several months after a perinatal loss and can continue for some time. Sadness and depression can be accompanied by disorganization and problems with cognitive processing, leading to behavioural changes such as difficulty in getting things done, an inability to concentrate, restlessness, confused thought processes, difficulty solving problems, and poor decision making. Disorganization and depression often cause difficulties in keeping up with work and family expectations. In addition, parents returning to work face issues such as handling well-meaning but painful comments or the silence of coworkers.

Physical symptoms of grief include fatigue, headaches, dizziness, and backaches. Parents are at risk for developing health problems such as colds or hypertension. It may be difficult to sleep; appetite may be depressed or voracious. Lack of sleep and inadequate nutrition and fluids can complicate other grief responses.

Grief responses are very personal, ongoing, and difficult to handle. Some parents may suppress or deny their feelings because of perceived societal indifference toward pregnancy loss and infant death. On the surface, suppression of feelings may be more socially acceptable. However, denying the pain of grief may lead to eventual physical and emotional distress or illness. Although bereaved parents have many ups and downs for many months and even years after a child's death, few parents actually become mentally ill or commit suicide. Knowing that these feelings are normal and that others have had similar feelings is helpful. The grief process during this phase is often difficult for partners. Some may continue to have difficulty sharing their feelings. A rift can occur if one parent, usually the mother, wants to talk about the loss and pain, and the other parent—often, but not always, the father—withdraws. Other signs of problems include reliance on alcohol and drugs, extramarital affairs, prolonged hours at work, and overinvolvement in activities outside the home as an escape.

Reorganization

From the time of the pregnancy loss or infant death, parents attempt to understand why this happened. This leads to a long and intense search for meaning. At first the "why" is focused on the cause of death, which is often never determined. Finding few good answers, parents next focus on "why me, why mine?" These questions can lead some parents into an existential search about the meaning of life and death. This search continues into the phase of reorganization and may lead to profound changes in the parents' view of the fragility of life.

Time helps to slowly ease the painful feelings of grief. Reorganization occurs when parents are better able to function at home and work, experience a return of self-esteem and confidence, can cope with new challenges, and have placed the loss in perspective. Reorganization begins to peak sometime after the first year, as parents begin to achieve the task of moving on with their lives. Enjoying the simple pleasures of life without feeling guilty, nurturing self and others, developing new interests, and re-establishing relationships are all signs of moving on. For some women and families, another pregnancy and the birth of a subsequent child are important steps in moving on with their lives; however, the term *recovery* is used because the grief related to perinatal loss can continue to varying degrees throughout life.

Parents who have suffered a pregnancy loss or infant death have shared that they will never forget the baby who died and they are not the same people as before the loss. The term *bittersweet grief* refers to the grief response that occurs with reminders of the loss. This typically happens on birthdays, death days, and anniversaries; at school events; during changes in the seasons; and during the time of the year when the loss occurred (Box 23-6). Grief feelings also can be triggered during subsequent pregnancies and after birth.

Resuming the couple's sexual relationship is an important aspect of recovery but can be very complicated. Many parents are comforted by the belief that their babies were conceived in love, lived in love, and died in love. Their love and intimacy created this child, and parents may believe that they may never experience joy and closeness again. Some couples may have an increased need for sexual activity in an attempt for closeness and healing, whereas others have a decreased desire for sexual intimacy.

Sexuality also brings with it decisions about a future pregnancy. Some couples are eager to have another child, although this child cannot replace the one who died and the grief will continue despite another pregnancy. Other parents have a deep fear of experiencing the pain of loss again, which can make the resumption of sexual activity difficult. These ambivalent feelings are normal, and couples can find themselves moving back and forth between the emotions of exhilaration and fear. The excitement that many other parents experience with a pregnancy is very different for previously bereaved parents. For some, this emotional distress can affect maternal attachment to the new baby. In one study, mothers who

BOX 23-6 Bittersweet Grief

To Jessica Mayo—on her eleventh birthday
Sunday, November 18, 1990
"The child who is born on the Sabbath day,
Is bonny and blithe and good and gay."
Sundays are special days,
...a day of rest, a day to play,
...a day to reflect on days past,
...a day to thank God for all that we bless.
I bless your memory.
I wish you were here.
On your eleventh birthday I still want to share,
...Your dreams of the future,
...Our memories past,
My baby's first cry,
My daughter's first laugh.
I was told you were an angel in heaven above.
Eleven years later, I'm an expert ...
At long-distance love.
On your third birthday I wrote my first poem
to you.
Eight years later, it's still true,
... no birthday cake,
no presents unwrapped ...
no pictures of you in your party hat.
But the candles are lit,
Never to go out.
For they burn forever in my heart.
Love, Mom
Kathie Rataj Mayo, 1990

(Used with permission of Gundersen Lutheran Medical Foundation, Inc., La Crosse, WI.)

became pregnant again within 6 months after a stillbirth had fewer depressive symptoms at a 3-year follow-up than those who did not have a subsequent pregnancy (Surkan et al., 2008).

Couples often mark the progress of the pregnancy in terms of fetal development, waiting anxiously until the number of weeks of the previous loss is passed. In some cases, the fear of repeated loss, especially after a stillbirth, is so great that induction of labour may be considered if the fetus is mature. Support groups are important in helping women through pregnancies after loss of a fetus or infant.

Family Aspects of Grief

Grandparents and Siblings

It is extremely important for the nurse taking care of these patients to keep in mind that they have an entire family to care for, including grandparents and siblings. Grandparents have hopes and dreams for a grandchild; these have been shattered. The grief of grandparents is often complicated by the fact that they are experiencing intense emotional pain by witnessing and feeling the immense grief of their own child. It is extremely difficult to watch their son or daughter experience unimaginable emotional trauma, with very few ways to comfort them and end their pain. As a result, the grief response may be complicated or delayed for grandparents. On occasion, some grandparents experience immense survivor guilt because they are alive and their grandchild has died.

The siblings of the expected infant also experience a profound loss. Most children have been prepared for having another child in the family, once the pregnancy is confirmed. These children's ages and stages of development must be considered in understanding how they view the event and experience the loss. A young child responds more to the response of his or her parents, picking up on the fact that they are behaving differently and are extremely sad. This can cause clinging, altered eating and sleeping patterns, or acting-out behaviours; and it is a time when parents have limited patience for responding to and meeting the needs of the child. Older children have a more complete understanding of the loss. School-age children may be frightened by the entire event, whereas teens may understand fully but feel awkward in responding.

Older siblings need to be included in grieving rituals, to the extent that the parents and the child feel comfortable. They may need to see the baby to realize the loss. Nurses need to have a basic understanding of how children view death and grief in order to reach out to siblings in an appropriate and sensitive manner. Nurses also need to help parents recognize and be sensitive to the grief of siblings, include them in family rituals, and keep the baby alive in the family memory.

evolve Critical Thinking Exercise–Neonatal Loss

Nursing Care Management

Nursing care of mothers and fathers experiencing a perinatal loss begins the first time they are faced with the potential loss of their pregnancy or death of their infant. Assessment is as important for families experiencing a miscarriage or ectopic pregnancy as it is for those experiencing stillbirth or neonatal loss. Supportive interventions are important at the time of the loss and after the parents have returned home.

Parents often cannot recall details of their experiences at the time of the child's death, but they may recall vividly a minor event that was perceived as particularly painful or particularly helpful. The interventions provided below are general ideas about what may be helpful to parents. However, care must be individualized to each parent and family. Cultural and spiritual beliefs and practices of individual parents and families must also be considered.

Communicating and Caring Techniques

Mothers, fathers, and extended families look to the medical and nursing staff for support and understanding during the time of loss. Therapeutic communication and counselling techniques help the mother, father, and other family members express their feelings and emotions, understand their responses to the loss, and make decisions.

The nurse should listen patiently while people tell their story of loss and grief. It may be necessary to ask questions that help people talk about their grief and the experiences surrounding the loss. However, grief responses in the initial days of crisis make it difficult for individuals to concentrate on what is being asked, think about what the question means, and respond to the question. The use of silence often gives the bereaved person the opportunity to collect thoughts and respond to questions. The nurse should resist the temptation to give advice or use clichés in offering support (Box 23-7).

Nurses need to become comfortable with their own feelings of grief and loss to effectively support and care for the bereaved. It is appropriate to express feelings with the bereaved families and share the moment with them. The nurse might use the following techniques in helping the family share and express their grief.

BOX 23-7 What to Say and What Not to Say to Bereaved Parents

What to Say

"I'm sad for you."
"How are you doing with all of this?"
"This must be hard for you."
"What can I do for you?"
"I'm sorry."
"I'm here, and I want to listen."

What Not to Say

"God had a purpose for her."
"Be thankful you have another child."
"The living must go on."
"I know how you feel."
"It's God's will."
"You have to keep on going for her sake."
"You're young; you can have others."
"We'll see you back here next year, and you'll be happier."
"Now you have an angel in heaven."
"This happened for the best."
"Better for this to happen now, before you knew the baby."
"There was something wrong with the baby anyway."

(Used with permission of Gundersen Lutheran Medical Foundation, Inc., La Crosse, WI.)

Help Mother, Father, and Other Family Members Actualize the Loss

When a loss or death occurs, the nurse should be sure that parents have been honestly told about the situation by their primary health care provider or others on the health care team. It is important for their nurse to be with the parents during this time. With early pregnancy loss, it is recommended that the term *miscarriage* be used consistently. With infant death, caregivers should use the words "dead" and "died," rather than "lost" or "gone" to assist the bereaved in accepting this reality. One way of actualizing the loss is to tell the parents the sex of the baby and give them the option of naming the fetus or help them name an infant who has died. Choosing a name helps make the baby a member of their family, so that the baby can be remembered in a special way.

NURSING ALERT A caution about naming is important to note. Naming is an individual decision that should never be imposed on parents. Beliefs and needs vary widely across individuals, cultures, and religions. Cultural taboos and rules in some religious faiths prohibit the naming of an infant who has died.

On the basis of vast clinical experience with parents, many professionals believe that seeing the dead fetus or baby helps parents face the reality of the loss, reduces painful fantasies, and offers an opportunity for closure. However, parents should never be made to feel that they should see or hold their baby when this is something that they do not really want. It is good policy for the nurse to first tell them about this option and then give them time to think about it. The nurse can ask a question such as "Some parents have found it helpful to see their baby. Would you like time to consider this?" Later the nurse can return and ask each parent individually what he or she has decided. Because the need or willingness to see the child also may vary between the mother and her partner, it is important to determine what each parent really wants. This should not be a joint decision made by one person or a decision made for the parents by grandparents or others.

In preparation for the visit with the baby, parents appreciate explanations about what to expect. A description of how their baby looks is important. For example, babies may have red, peeling skin like a bad sunburn, dark discolouration similar to bruises, moulding of the head that makes the head look soft and swollen, or birth defects. The nurse should make the baby look as normal as possible and remember that parents see their baby with different eyes from those of health care professionals. Bathing the baby, applying lotion to the baby's skin, combing hair, placing identification bracelets on the arm and leg, dressing the baby in a diaper and special outfit, sprinkling powder in the baby's blanket, and wrapping the baby in a pretty blanket conveys to the parents that their baby has been cared for in a special way. If the baby has been in the morgue, he or she can be placed underneath a warmer for 20 to 30 minutes and wrapped in a warm blanket before being brought to the parents. Cold cream rubbed over stiffened joints can help in positioning the baby. The use of powder and lotion stimulates the parent's senses and can help provide pleasant memories of their baby.

When bringing the baby to the parents, it is important to treat the baby as one would a live baby. Holding the baby close, touching a hand or cheek, using the baby's name, and talking with the parents about the special features of their baby convey that it is all right for them to do likewise. If a baby has a congenital anomaly, the nurse can desensitize the family by pointing out aspects of the baby that are normal. Nurses can help parents explore the baby's body as they desire. Parents often seek to identify family resemblance. A good question might be: "Who in your family does your baby resemble?"

Some families may like to have the opportunity to bathe and dress their baby. Although the skin may be fragile, parents can still apply lotion with cotton balls; sprinkle powder; tie ribbons; fasten the diaper; and place amulets, medallions, rosaries, or special toys or mementos in their baby's hands or next to their baby. Volunteer women in communities across the country often make special burial clothes to give parents at this difficult time. Parents may want to perform other parenting activities, such as combing the baby's hair, dressing the baby in a special outfit, wrapping the baby in a blanket, or placing the baby in a crib.

Parents need to be offered time alone with their baby if they wish. They also need to know when the nurse will return and how to call if they should need anything. If at all possible, the family should be placed in a private room, and the room should have a rocking chair for the parents to sit in when holding their baby. This offers the mother and father special time together with their baby and with other family members (Fig. 23-8). Marking the door to the room with a special card can be helpful in reminding staff that this family has experienced a loss (Fig. 23-9).

Sensitivity to parental needs in actualizing the loss and coping with the reality of the death is essential for their healing. Grandparents should be offered the same opportunities to hold, rock, swaddle, and love their grandchildren so that their grief is started in a healthy way.

Help Parents With Decision Making

At a time when parents are experiencing the great distress of a perinatal loss, and especially if the loss was of an infant, these parents have many decisions to make. Mothers, partners, and extended families look to the medical and nursing staff for guidance in knowing what decisions they must and can make and in understanding the options related to those decisions. It is a primary responsibility of the nurse to help them and to advocate for them because decisions made during the time of their loss will provide memories for a lifetime.

One decision might be related to conducting an autopsy. An autopsy can be very important in answering the question "why" if there is a chance that the cause of death can be determined. This information can be helpful in processing grief and perhaps in preventing another loss. Some parents may believe that their baby has been through enough and prefer not to have further information about the cause of death. Some religions prohibit autopsy or limit the choice to times when it may help prevent another loss. Options for the type of autopsy, such as excluding the head, should be made available to parents. Parents may need time to make this decision. There is no need to rush them unless there was evidence of contagious disease or maternal infection at the time of death.

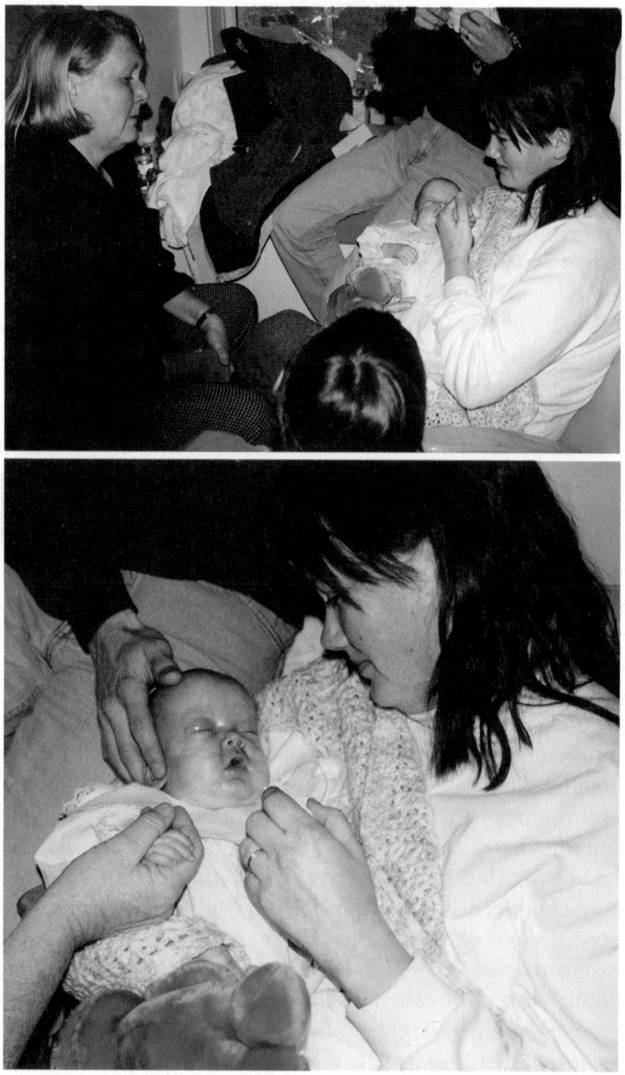

Fig. 23-8 Laura's family members say a special good-bye. *(Courtesy Amy and Ken Turner, Cary, NC.)*

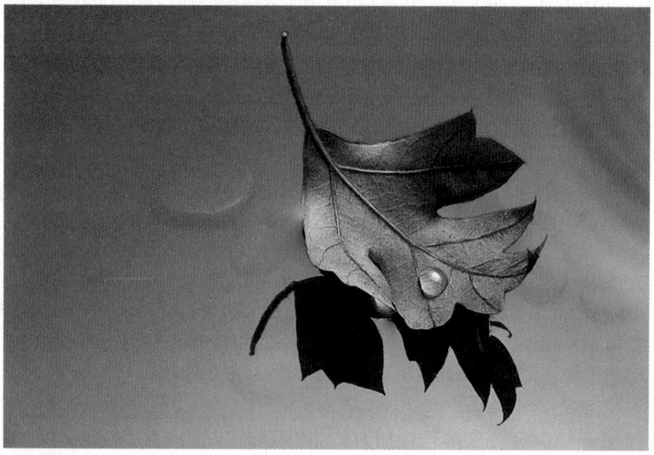

Fig. 23-9 Door card for room of mother who has experienced perinatal loss. *(Used with permission of Gundersen Lutheran Medical Foundation, Inc., La Crosse, WI.)*

Organ donation can be an aid to grieving and an opportunity for the family to see something positive associated with their experience. The most common donation is of corneas; donation of corneas from a baby can occur if the baby was born alive at 36 weeks of gestation or later.

Another important decision relates to spiritual rituals that may be helpful and important to parents. Support from clergy is an option that should be offered to all parents. Parents may wish to have their own pastor, priest, rabbi, or spiritual leader contacted; or they may wish to see the hospital's chaplain. They may choose to do neither. Clergy persons may offer the parents the opportunity for baptism, when appropriate. Other rituals that may be important include a blessing, a naming ceremony, anointing, ritual of the sick, memorial service, or prayer.

One of the major decisions that parents must make has to do with disposition of the body. Parents should be given information about the choices for the final disposition of their baby, regardless of gestational age. However, nurses must be aware of cultural and spiritual beliefs that may dictate the choices of parents, as well as the cost of burial, alternatives to burial, and provincial laws related to burial. A fetus younger than 20 weeks of gestation that weighs less than 500 g is considered a miscarriage; embryos, uterine tubes removed with an ectopic pregnancy, and tissue from a pregnancy obtained during a D&C are all considered tissue. Many hospitals will make arrangements for the cremation of these infants or tissue. The nurse should know the hospital's policies and procedures about burial and cremation and answer the parents' questions honestly. In Canada, if a fetus is greater than or equal to 20 weeks of gestational age or is born alive, it is the parents' responsibility to make the final arrangements for their baby.

LEGAL TIP **Laws Regarding Live Birth.** Laws in all provinces govern what constitutes a live birth. In most provinces, a live birth is considered to be any products of conception expelled from a woman that show any signs of life. Signs of life are considered to be any muscle irritability, respiratory effort, or heart rate, regardless of gestational age. All nurses should be knowledgeable about the provincial laws regarding what constitutes a live birth and the forms that must be completed and filed in the case of fetal death, stillbirth, or newborn death.

In making final arrangements for their baby, parents may want a special service. They may choose to have a service in the hospital chapel, visitation at a funeral home or their own home, a funeral service, or a graveside service. Parents can make any of these services as special, personal, and memorable as they like. They can choose special music, poetry, or prose written by themselves or others.

The timing for actions such as naming the baby, seeing and holding the baby, disposition of the body, and funeral arrangements should never be rushed. In some cases, the mother may be discharged home before these decisions are made. Then the family can think about them in the comfort of their home and contact the hospital in the following days to give their answers.

Help Bereaved to Acknowledge and Express Feelings

One of the most important goals of the nurse is to validate the experience and feelings of the parents by encouraging them to tell their stories and by listening with care. Because nurses tend to be very focused on the physical and emotional needs of the mother, it is especially important to ask the partner directly about his or her views of what happened and the feelings of loss.

Bereaved parents have many questions surrounding the event of their loss, and some questions can leave them feeling guilty. This is particularly true for mothers. Such questions include "What did I do?" "What caused this to happen?" "What do you think I should have, could have done?" Part of the grief process for bereaved parents is figuring out what happened, their role in the loss, why it happened to them, and why it happened to their baby. The nurse should recognize that these questions must be answered by the bereaved themselves; it is part of their healing. For example, a bereaved mother might ask, "Do you think that this was caused by painting the baby's room?" An appropriate response might be, "I understand you need to find an answer for why your baby died, but we really don't know why she died. What are some of the other things you have been thinking about?" Trying to give bereaved parents answers when there are no clear answers or trying to squelch their guilt feelings by telling them they should not feel guilty does not help them process their grief. In reality, many times there are no definite answers to the question of why this terrible thing has happened to them. However, factual information such as data about the frequency of miscarriages in pregnant women or the fact that there usually is no clear cause of a stillbirth can be helpful.

Feelings of anger, guilt, and sadness can occur immediately but often become more problematic in the early days and months after a loss. When a bereaved person expresses feelings of anger, it can be helpful to identify the feeling by simply saying, "You sound angry," or "You look angry." The nurse's willingness to sit down and listen to these surface feelings of anger can help the bereaved person move past them into the underlying feelings of powerlessness and helplessness in not being able to control the many aspects of the situation.

Normalize the Grief Process and Facilitate Positive Coping

While helping parents share their feelings of pain, it is critical to help them understand their grief responses and know that they are not alone in these painful responses. Most parents are not prepared for the raw feelings that they experience or the fact that these painful, complex feelings and related behavioural reactions continue for many weeks or months. Thus, reassuring them of the normality of their responses and preparing them for the length of their grief is important.

The nurse can help the parent be prepared for the emptiness, loneliness, and yearning; for the feelings of helplessness that can lead to anger, guilt, and fear; and for the disorganization, difficulty making decisions, and sadness and depression that are part of the grief process. Books and pamphlets about grief, if short and sensitive, can be given to parents to take home.

In the initial days after a loss, other useful strategies include follow-up phone calls, referrals to a perinatal grief support group, or providing a list of publications or Web sites intended for helping parents who have experienced a perinatal loss (e.g., http://www.bereavedfamilies.net/). However, as with any referral, the nurse should first read the materials or check out the Web sites or applicability.

To reduce relationship problems that can occur in grieving couples, it is particularly important to help them understand that they may respond and grieve in very different ways. The differences in grieving can lead to serious marital problems and be a risk factor for complicated bereavement. Remind the couple of the importance of being understanding and patient with each other.

Nurses can reinforce positive coping efforts and encourage attempts to resume normal activities; reinforce and encourage positive ways to hold onto memories of the pregnancy or baby while letting go; and help the parents organize a plan for daily activities, if needed. In particular, nurses should discourage overdependence on drugs and alcohol.

Meet the Physical Needs of the Postpartum Bereaved Mother

Coping with loss and grief after childbirth can be an overwhelming experience for the woman and her family. One particularly difficult aspect of the loss is the sound of crying babies and the happiness of other families on the unit who have given birth to healthy infants. The mother should be given the opportunity to decide if she wants to remain on the maternity unit or be moved to another hospital unit. She also should be helped to understand the pluses and minuses of each choice. Postpartum care and grief support may not be as good on another hospital unit where the staff are not experienced in postpartum and bereavement care.

The physical needs of a bereaved mother are the same as those of any woman who has given birth. The cruel reality for many bereaved mothers is that their milk can come in with no baby to nurse, their afterpains remind them of their emptiness, and gas pains feel as though a baby is still moving inside. The nurse should ensure that the mother receives appropriate medications to reduce these physical symptoms. Adequate rest, diet, and fluids must be offered to replenish her physical strength.

Mothers need postpartum care instructions on discharge. They also need ideas about how to cope with sleep problems, such as decreasing food or fluids that contain caffeine, limiting alcohol and nicotine consumption, exercising regularly, using strategies for rest, taking a warm bath or drinking warm milk before bedtime, doing relaxation exercises, listening to restful music, or a getting a massage. Furthermore, the couple needs to be encouraged and supported in maintaining their relationship and keeping open channels of communication. They also need to be prepared for some of the issues related to resuming sexual relations after perinatal loss.

Create Memories for Parents to Take Home

Parents may want tangible mementos of their baby to help them actualize the loss. Some may want to bring in a previously purchased baby book. Special memory books, cards, and information on grief and mourning are often available to give to parents (Fig. 23-10).

The nurse can provide information about the baby's weight, length, and head circumference to the family. Footprints and handprints can be taken and placed with the other information on a special card or in a memory or baby book.

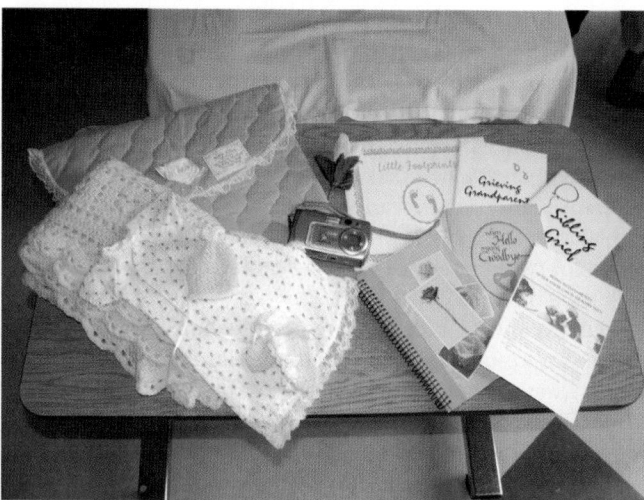

Fig. 23-10 Memory kit assembled at John C. Lincoln Hospital, Phoenix, AZ. Memory kits may include pictures of the infant, clothing, death certificate, footprints, ID bands, and ultrasound picture. *(Courtesy Julie Perry Nelson, Loveland, CO.)*

Sometimes it is difficult to obtain good handprints or footprints. Application of alcohol or acetone on the palms or soles can help the ink adhere to make the prints clearer, especially for small babies. When making prints, it is helpful to have a hard surface underneath the paper to be printed. The baby's heel or palm should be placed down first and the foot or hand rolled forward, keeping the toes or fingers extended. It may be helpful to have assistance in this procedure. If the print does not turn out, the nurse can trace around the baby's hands and feet, although this distorts the actual size. A form of plaster of Paris can also be used to make an imprint of the baby's hand or foot.

Parents often appreciate articles that were in contact with or used in caring for the baby. This might include the tape measure used to measure the baby, baby lotions, combs, clothing, hats, blankets, crib cards, and identification bands. The identification band helps the parents remember the size of the baby and personalizes the mementos. The nurse should ask parents if they wish to have these articles. A lock of hair may be another important keepsake. Parents must be asked for permission before cutting a lock of hair, which can be removed from the nape of the neck where it is not noticeable.

For some parents, pictures are the most important memento. Photographs are generally taken whenever there is an identifiable baby and when it is culturally acceptable to the family to take photos. It does not matter how tiny the baby is, what the baby looks like, or how long the baby has been dead. Pictures should include close-ups of the baby's face, hands, and feet and photos of the baby clothed and wrapped in a blanket and unclothed. If there are any congenital anomalies, close-ups of these also should be taken. Flowers, blocks, stuffed animals, or toys can be placed in the background to make the picture more special. Parents may want their pictures taken holding the baby. Keeping a camera nearby and taking pictures when parents are spending special time with their baby can provide special memories. Some parents may have their own camera or video camera and ask the nurse to record them as they bathe, dress, hold, or diaper their baby. An organization called Now I Lay Me Down to Sleep provides a professional photographer to take pictures for families at no cost. Their Web site can be consulted to determine if there is a photographer within the geographical location (http://www.nowilaymedowntosleep.org).

Cultural and Spiritual Needs of Parents

Many of the responses to perinatal loss and suggested interventions described in this section are based on middle-class European-American views. Although there may be no particular differences in individual, intrapersonal experiences of grief based on culture, ethnicity, or religions, there are complex differences in the meaning of children and parenthood, the role of women and men, the beliefs and knowledge about modern medicine, views about death, mourning rituals and traditions, and behavioural expressions of grief. Thus, nurses must be sensitive to the responses and needs of parents from various cultural backgrounds and religious groups. Nurses need to be aware of their own values and beliefs and acknowledge the importance of understanding and accepting the values and beliefs of others that are different or even in conflict with theirs. Further, it is critical to understand that the individual and unique responses of parents to a perinatal loss cannot be entirely predicted by their cultural or spiritual backgrounds. Each mother and partner must be approached first as an individual needing support during a profoundly difficult and distressing life experience.

Provide Postmortem Care

Preparation of the baby's body and transport to the morgue depend on the procedures and protocols developed by individual hospitals. Nurses should use a sensitive and respectful approach when taking the fetus or infant to the morgue. Postmortem care can be an emotional and sometimes difficult task for the nurse. However, nurses may find that providing postmortem care helps them find closure in their own grief related to a perinatal loss. This is particularly true for neonatal intensive care nurses who have cared for an infant for several hours, days, or weeks.

Documentation

Many hospitals have a checklist that is used in providing care, mobilizing members of the multidisciplinary health care team, communicating options that the family has chosen, and keeping track of all the details in meeting the needs of bereaved parents. The checklists may or may not be a permanent part of the chart. Documentation in the nursing notes of primary concerns, grief responses, health teaching, health care advice, and referrals of the mother or any other family members is essential to ensure continuity and consistency of care.

Provide Sensitive Care at and After Discharge

Leaving the hospital can be a devastating experience for the mother who has had a pregnancy loss, as not carrying a baby in her arms is a very empty and painful experience. It is especially difficult if others are seen leaving with babies; thus, the discharge of mothers and fathers who have suffered a perinatal loss should be done with great sensitivity to their feelings (i.e., they should not be discharged at a time when other mothers with live babies are leaving). Giving the mother a special flower to carry in her arms can be a thoughtful gesture.

The grief of the mother and her family does not end with discharge; it really begins once they return home, attend the funeral, and start to live their lives without their baby. There are numerous models for providing follow-up care to parents after discharge. Although there is no solid evidence from sound clinical trials regarding the benefit of these programs, nonexperimental studies and clinical evaluations suggest that these programs are helpful. Programs include hospital-based bereavement teams who provide support during hospitalization and follow-up contacts.

Phone calls after a loss may be helpful to some parents; however, it must be determined which parents do not want them. Follow-up calls let the parents know that someone still thinks and cares about them. The calls are made at predictably difficult times, such as the first week at home, 1 month to 6 weeks later, 4 to 6 months after the loss, and at the anniversary of the death. Families who have experienced a miscarriage, ectopic pregnancy, or death of a preterm baby may appreciate a phone call on the estimated date of birth. The calls provide an opportunity for parents to ask questions, share their feelings, seek advice, and receive information to help them process their grief.

A grief conference can be planned when parents return for an appointment with their doctor, nurses, and other health care providers. At the conference, the loss or death of the infant is discussed in detail, parents are given information about the baby's autopsy report and genetic studies, and they have opportunities to ask the questions that have arisen since their baby's death. Parents appreciate the opportunity to review the events of hospitalization, go over the baby's and mother's chart with their primary health care provider, and talk with those who cared for them and their baby during hospitalization. This is an important time to help parents understand the cause of the loss or accept the fact that the cause will forever be unknown. This gives health care providers the opportunity to assess how the family is coping with their loss and offer additional information and education on grief.

Some parents are very interested in finding a perinatal or parent grief support group. The opportunity to talk with others who have been through similar experiences, share memories of the pregnancy and the baby, and gain an understanding of the normality of the grief process generally have been found to be supportive. Over time, it may be the only place where bereaved parents can talk about the wished-for child and their grief. However, not all parents find such groups helpful.

When referring parents to a group, it is important to know something about the group and how it operates. For example, if a group has a religious base for their interventions, a nonreligious parent would not likely find the group to be helpful. If parents experiencing a perinatal loss are referred to a general parental grief group, they might feel overwhelmed with the grief of parents whose older children have died of cancer, suicide, or homicide. In addition, the grief of parents following a perinatal loss might be minimized by other parents. Thus, the needs of the parents must be matched with the focus of the group.

Maternal Death

In Canada it is rare for a woman to die in childbirth; the incidence of maternal deaths is one of the lowest in the world: in 2009 to 2010 it was 7.8 per 100,000 (PHAC, 2012). The partner and extended family who are faced with not only mourning the death of a wife and mother but also the death of the baby have a particularly difficult time. If the baby lives, the partner is faced with parenting a baby without a surviving mother. Death of a mother disrupts the family structure and leaves the partner with the care of a baby at a time when he or she is greatly distressed. Thus, the partner and extended family, especially other children and grandparents, need supportive grief counselling at the time of death and following discharge to be able to heal after such a devastating loss.

The nursing care of families at this time is similar to that already described. Options need to be offered, memories made, and mementos obtained and held for the family until they are ready for them. These families are at risk for developing complicated bereavement and altered parenting of the surviving baby and other children in the family. Referral to social services to help the family mobilize support systems and for counselling can help prevent potential problems before they develop and can be beneficial not only at the time of the loss but also in the future.

The emotional toll that a maternal death can take on the nursing and medical staff must also be addressed. Guilt, anger, fear, sadness, and depression are all common responses to a maternal death. The staff may want to review the situation surrounding the events, the medical record, and their responses in the forum of a mortality/morbidity review and a critical incident debriefing to help cope with the feelings and emotions that result from a maternal death. Attending memorial or funeral services may benefit staff and family. Follow-up conferences with a social worker or grief counsellor may be necessary.

Key Points

- PPH is the most common and most serious type of excessive obstetrical blood loss.
- Hemorrhagic (hypovolemic) shock is an emergency situation in which the perfusion of body organs may become severely compromised and death may ensue.
- Postpartum infection is a major cause of maternal morbidity and mortality throughout the world.
- Postpartum UTIs are common because of trauma experienced during labour.
- Breast infection affects about 1% of women soon after childbirth.
- Structural disorders of the uterus and vagina related to pelvic relaxation are often the delayed but direct result of childbearing.
- PPMD can influence maternal attachment to the newborn and must be identified and treated appropriately.
- An understanding of grief responses and the bereavement process is fundamental in implementation of the nursing process.

- Therapeutic communication and counselling techniques can help families identify their feelings and feel comfortable in expressing their grief.
- Follow-up after discharge is an essential component to providing care to families who have experienced a loss.
- Nurses need to be aware of their own feelings of grief and loss to provide a nonjudgemental environment of care and support for bereaved families.

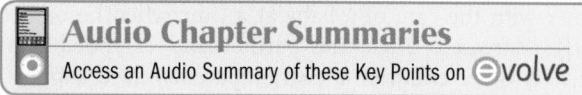

Audio Chapter Summaries

Access an Audio Summary of these Key Points on evolve

References

American Psychiatric Association (2010). *Diagnostic and statistical manual of mental disorders* (5th ed). Washington, DC: American Psychiatric Association Press. Retrieved from http://www.dsm5.org/proposedrevision/pages/proposedrevision.aspx?rid=146.

Beck, C. (2002). Revision of the Postpartum Depression Predictors Inventory. *Journal of Obstetric, Gynecologic and Neonatal Nursing, 31*(4), 394–402.

Bina, R. (2008). The impact of cultural factors upon postpartum depression: A literature review. *Health Care for Women International, 29*(6), 568–592.

Centers for Disease Control and Prevention (2008). Prevalence of self-reported postpartum depressive symptoms—17 states, 2004–2005. *MMWR: Morbidity and Mortality Weekly Report, 57*(14), 361–366.

Coates, A., Schaefer, C., & Alexander, J. (2004). Detection of postpartum depression and anxiety in a large health plan. *Journal of Behavioral Health Services and Research, 31*(2), 117–133.

Cunningham, et al. (2010). *Williams obstetrics* (23rd ed.). New York: McGraw Hill.

Davies, G., et al. (2010). SOGC clinical practice guideline: Obesity in pregnancy. *Journal of Obstetrics and Gynaecology Canada, 32*(2), 165–173.

Duff, P. (2007). Maternal and perinatal infection—bacterial. In S. G. Gabbe, J. R. Niebyl, & J. L. Simpson (Eds.), *Obstetrics: Normal and problem pregnancies* (5th ed.). New York: Churchill Livingstone.

Francois, K. E., & Foley, M. R. (2007). Antepartum and postpartum hemorrhage. In S. G. Gabbe, J. R. Niebyl, & J. L. Simpson (Eds.), *Obstetrics: Normal and problem pregnancies* (5th ed.). New York: Churchill Livingstone.

Goldbort, J. (2006). Transcultural analysis of postpartum depression. *MCN: American Journal of Maternal Child Nursing, 31*(2), 121–126.

Goyal, D., Gay, C. L., & Lee, K. A. (2007). Patterns of sleep disruption and depressive symptoms in new mothers. *Journal of Perinatal and Neonatal Nursing, 21*(2), 323–329.

Gülmezoglu, A., et al. (2007). Prostaglandins for prevention of postpartum haemorrhage. *Cochrane Database of Systematic Reviews 2007*, Issue 3.

Horwitz, S. M., et al. (2007). Prevalence, correlates, and persistence of maternal depression. *Journal of Women's Health, 16*(5), 678–691. doi: 10.1089/jwh.2006.0185

Kaplan, H., & Sadock, B. (2007). *Synopsis of psychiatry* (10th ed.). Baltimore: Williams & Wilkins.

Kim, Y. K., et al. (2008). Prediction of postpartum depression by sociodemographic, obstetric and psychological factors: A prospective study. *Psychiatry and Clinical Neurosciences, 62*(3), 331–340.

Lawrence, R. A., & Lawrence, R. M. (2011). *Breastfeeding: A guide for the medical profession* (7th ed.). St. Louis: Mosby.

Lehmann, C. (2004). House committee briefed on postpartum MH issues. *Psychiatric News, 39*(21), 26.

Lindemann, E. (1944). Symptomatology and management of acute grief. *American Journal of Psychiatry, 101*, 141–148.

Linter, N., & Gray, B. (2006). Childbearing and depression: What nurses need to know. *AWHONN Lifelines, 10*(1), 50–57.

Lockwood, C. J., & Silver, R. M. (2009). Coagulation disorders in pregnancy. In R. K. Creasy, et al. (Eds.), *Creasy & Resnik's maternal–fetal medicine: Principles and practice* (6th ed.). Philadelphia: Saunders.

Magann, E., & Lanneau, G. (2005). Third stage of labour. *Obstetric and Gynecology Clinics of North America, 32*(2), 323–332.

Mallett, V. T. (2005). Female urinary incontinence: What the epidemiologic data tell us. *International Journal of Fertility and Women's Medicine, 50*(1), 12–17.

McCarthy, M., & McMahon, C. (2008). Acceptance and experience of treatment for postnatal depression in a community mental health setting. *Health Care for Women International, 29*(6), 618–637.

Miles, M. (1984). Helping adults mourn the death of a child. In H. Wass & C. Corr (Eds.), *Children and death*. Washington, DC: Hemisphere Publishing.

More^{OB} (2010). *Postpartum hemorrhage*. Retrieved from http://www.Moreob.com.

Newton, E. R. (2007). Breast-feeding. In S. G. Gabbe, J. R. Niebyl, & J. L. Simpson (Eds.), *Obstetrics: Normal and problem pregnancies* (5th ed.). New York: Churchill Livingstone.

O'Brien, L., et al. (2004). Postnatal depression and faltering growth: A community study. *Pediatrics, 113*(5), 1242–1247.

Oyelese, Y., & Smulian, J. C. (2006). Placenta previa, placenta accreta, and vasa previa. *Obstetrics and Gynecology, 107*(4), 927–941.

Paulson, J. F., Dauber, S., & Leiferman, J. A. (2006). Individual and combined effects of postpartum depression in mothers and fathers on parenting behavior. *Pediatrics, 118*(2), 659–668.

Pettker, C. M., & Lockwood, C. J. (2007). Thromboembolic disorders. In S. G. Gabbe, J. R. Niebyl, & J. L. Simpson (Eds.), *Obstetrics: Normal and problem pregnancies* (5th ed.). New York: Churchill Livingstone.

Pigarelli, D., Kraus, C., & Potter, B. (2005). Pregnancy and lactation: Therapeutic considerations. In J. DiPiro, et al. (Eds.), *Pharmacotherapy: A pathophysiologic approach* (6th ed.). New York: McGraw-Hill.

Public Health Agency of Canada (2004). *Special report on maternal mortality and severe morbidity in Canada: Canadian Perinatal Surveillance System*. Ottawa, ON: Author. Retrieved from http://www.phac-aspc.gc.ca/rhs-ssg/srmm-rsmm/page1-eng.php.

Public Health Agency of Canada (2012). *Perinatal health indicators for Canada 2011*. (Cat. No. HP7-1/2011). Ottawa: Author.

Reck, C., et al. (2009). Maternity blues as a predictor of DSM-IV depression and anxiety disorders in the first three months' postpartum. *Journal of Affective Disorders, 113*(1-2), 77–87.

Registered Nurses' Association of Ontario (2005). *Interventions for postpartum depression*. Toronto: Author. Retrieved from http://rnao.ca/sites/rnao-ca/files/Interventions_for_Postpartum_Depression.pdf .

Royal College of Obstetricians and Gynaecologists (2009). *Reducing the risk of thrombosis and embolism during pregnancy and the puerperium. Green-top guideline No. 37a*. London: Author. Retrieved from: http://www.rcog.org.uk/womens-health/clinical-guidance/reducing-risk-of-thrombosis-greentop37a.

Samuels, P. (2007). Hematologic complications of pregnancy. In S. G. Gabbe, J. R. Niebyl, & J. L. Simpson (Eds.), *Obstetrics: Normal and problem pregnancies* (5th ed.). New York: Churchill Livingstone.

Schatzberg, A., & Nemeroff, C. (Eds.). (2004). *The American Psychiatric Publishing textbook of psychopharmacology* (3rd ed.). Washington, DC: American Psychiatric Publishing.

Skidmore-Roth, L. (2010). *Mosby's handbook of herbs and natural supplements* (4th ed.). St. Louis: Mosby.

Surkan, P. J., et al. (2008). Events after stillbirth in relation to maternal depressive symptoms: A brief report. *Birth, 35*(2), 153–157.

Sword, W., et al. (2008). Women's care-seeking experiences after referral for postpartum depression. *Qualitative Health Research, 18*(9), 1161–1173.

van Schalkwyk, J., et al. (2010). SOGC clinical practice guideline: Antibiotic prophylaxis in obstetric procedures. *Journal of Obstetrics and Gynaecology Canada, 32*(9), 878–884. Retrieved from http://www.sogc.org/guidelines/documents/gui247CPG1009E_000.pdf.

Wang, S., et al. (2005). Impact of postpartum depression on the mother–infant couple. *Birth, 32*(1), 39–44.

Watanabe, M., et al. (2008). Maternity blues as a predictor of postpartum depression: A prospective cohort study among Japanese women. *Journal of Psychosomatic Obstetrics and Gynaecology, 29*(3), 211–217.

Wong, H. S., et al. (2008). The maternal outcome in placenta accreta: The significance of antenatal diagnosis and non-separation of placenta at delivery. *New Zealand Medical Journal, 121*(1277), 30–38.

Unit 6

24 Physiological Adaptations of the Newborn

Learning Objectives

On completion of this chapter, the reader will be able to:

- Describe the changes in the biological system of the neonate during the transition to extrauterine life.
- Describe the sequence to follow in assessment of the newborn.
- Recognize deviations from normal physiological findings during examination of the newborn.
- Compare and contrast the four types of heat loss in a neonate and describe how to prevent heat loss.
- Describe the behavioural adaptations of the newborn, including periods of reactivity and sleep–wake states.
- Describe the sensory and perceptual functioning of the neonate.

Electronic Resources

Additional information related to the content in Chapter 24 can be found on

evolve the companion Web site at

http://evolve.elsevier.com/Canada/Perry/maternal/

- Examination Review Questions
- Anatomy Review—Changes in Circulation at Birth
- Anatomy Review—Sutures and Fontanels
- Assessment Video Clips
- Case Study—Newborn Health Problems
- Skill—Thermoregulation
- Video—Buttocks
- Video—Cremasteric Reflex
- Video—Legs (Symmetry, Length)
- Video—Male Breasts (Supine Position)
- Video—Moro Reflex
- Video—Neck (Posterior)
- Video—Plantar Grasp
- Video—Rooting and Sucking
- Video—Upper Extremities
- Video—Crying Female Neonate

The neonatal period includes the time from birth through the twenty-eighth day of life. By term gestation, the various anatomical and physiological systems of the fetus have reached a level of development and functioning that permits a separate existence from the mother. At birth, the newborn infant manifests behavioural competencies and a readiness for social interaction. These adaptations set the stage for future growth and development.

Transition to Extrauterine Life

Newborns undergo phases of relative instability during the first 6 to 8 hours after birth. These phases collectively are termed the *transition period* between intrauterine and extrauterine existence. The first phase of the transition period lasts up to 30 minutes after birth and is called the **first period of reactivity**. The newborn's heart rate increases rapidly to 160 to 180 beats/min but gradually falls by 30 minutes to a baseline rate between 100 and 160 beats/min. Respirations are irregular, with a rate between 60 and 80 breaths/min. Fine crackles may be present on **auscultation**; audible grunting, nasal flaring, and retractions of the chest may also be noted, but these should cease within the first hour of birth. The infant is alert and may have spontaneous startles, tremors, crying, and movement of the head from side to side. Bowel sounds are audible, and meconium may be passed.

After the first period of reactivity, the newborn either sleeps or has a marked decrease in motor activity. This period of unresponsiveness lasts from 60 to 100 minutes and is followed by a second period of reactivity.

The **second period of reactivity** occurs roughly between 4 and 8 hours after birth and lasts from 10 minutes to several hours. Brief periods of tachycardia and **tachypnea** occur, associated with increased muscle tone, skin colour changes, and mucus production. Meconium is commonly passed at this time. Most healthy newborns experience this transition regardless of type of birth; very preterm infants do not because of physiological immaturity.

Physiological Adjustments

Respiratory System

With the cutting of the umbilical cord, the infant undergoes rapid and complex physiological changes. The most critical and immediate adjustment is the establishment of respirations. With a vaginal birth, some lung fluid is squeezed from the newborn's trachea and lungs; in infants who are born by Caesarean birth, some lung fluid may be retained within the alveoli. With the first breath of air, the newborn begins a dynamic sequence of cardiopulmonary changes.

Initial breathing is probably the result of a reflex triggered by pressure changes, cool air temperature, noise, light, and other sensations related to the birth process. In addition, the **chemoreceptors** in the aorta and carotid bodies initiate neurological reflexes when arterial oxygen pressure (Po_2) falls, arterial carbon dioxide pressure (Pco_2) rises, and arterial pH falls. In most cases, an exaggerated respiratory reaction follows within 1 minute of birth, and the infant takes the first gasping breath and cries.

Once respirations are established, they are shallow and irregular, ranging from 30 to 60 breaths/min, with periods of periodic breathing that include pauses in respirations lasting less than 20 seconds. These episodes of periodic breathing occur most often during the active REM sleep cycle and decrease in frequency and duration with age. **Apneic spells** lasting 20 seconds or longer are an indication of a pathological process and should be carefully evaluated.

Signs of Respiratory Distress

Most term infants breathe spontaneously and continue to have normal respiratory patterns. Signs of respiratory distress may include nasal flaring, intercostal or subcostal retractions (i.e., drawing in of tissue between the ribs, or below the rib cage), or grunting with respirations. Suprasternal or subclavicular retractions with stridor or gasping most often represent an upper airway obstruction (Askin, 2009). Seesaw or paradoxical respirations (exaggerated rise in abdomen, with respiration, as chest falls) instead of abdominal respirations are abnormal and should be reported. A respiratory rate less than 30 or greater than 60 breaths/min with the infant at rest must be carefully evaluated. The respiratory rate can be negatively influenced (slowed, depressed, or absent) by analgesics or anaesthetics administered to the mother during birth. Apneic episodes may be related to a number of events (rapid increase in body temperature, hypothermia, hypoglycemia, and sepsis) that require careful evaluation. Tachypnea may result from inadequate clearance of lung fluid, or it may be an indication of newborn **respiratory distress syndrome**.

Maintaining Adequate Oxygen Supply

During the first hour of life the pulmonary lymphatics continue to remove large amounts of fluid. Removal of fluid is also a result of the pressure gradient from alveoli to interstitial tissue to blood capillary. Reduced vascular resistance accommodates this flow of lung fluid. Retention of lung fluid may interfere with the infant's ability to maintain adequate oxygenation, especially if other factors (e.g., meconium aspiration, congenital diaphragmatic hernia, esophageal atresia with fistula, **choanal atresia,** congenital cardiac defect, immature alveoli [absent or decreased]) compromise respiration.

The newborn's chest circumference is approximately 30 to 33 cm at birth. Auscultation of the chest of a newborn infant reveals loud, clear breath sounds that seem very near because there is less chest wall musculature. The ribs of the infant articulate with the spine at a horizontal rather than a downward slope; consequently, the rib cage cannot expand with inspiration as readily as an adult's. Because neonatal respiratory function is largely a matter of diaphragmatic contraction, abdominal breathing is characteristic of newborns. That is, the newborn infant's chest and abdomen rise simultaneously with inspiration, but because of the large size of the abdomen, chest movement is not as visible.

The outer walls of the alveoli are lined with **surfactant**, a protein manufactured in type II cells of the lungs. Lung expansion is largely dependent on chest wall contraction and adequate presence and secretion of surfactant. Surfactant lowers surface tension, thereby requiring less inspiratory pressure to keep the alveoli open with inspiration, and prevents total alveolar collapse on exhalation, thus maintaining alveolar stability. With absent or decreased surfactant, more pressure must be generated for inspiration, which may soon tire or exhaust preterm or sick term infants. Surfactant may be compared with soapy water on the surface of a group of inflated latex balloons: as air is let out of the balloons (exhalation phase), the soapy water prevents total collapse of the balloons, and, conversely, inflation of the balloons occurs readily because of decreased tension (friction) on their surfaces.

Cardiovascular System

The cardiovascular system changes significantly after birth. The infant's first breaths, combined with increased alveolar capillary distension, inflate the lungs and reduce pulmonary vascular resistance to pulmonary blood flow from the pulmonary arteries. Pulmonary artery pressure drops, and pressure in the right atrium declines. Increased pulmonary blood flow from the left side of the heart increases pressure in the left atrium, which causes a functional closure of the foramen ovale (see Chapter 48, p. 1455). During the first few days of life, crying may temporarily reverse the flow through the foramen ovale and lead to mild cyanosis.

In utero, fetal Po_2 is 27 mm Hg. After birth, when the Po_2 level in the arterial blood approximates 50 mm Hg, the ductus arteriosus constricts in response to increased oxygenation. Circulating hormone prostaglandin (PGE_2) levels also have an important role in closure of the ductus arteriosus. Later, the ductus arteriosus closes completely and becomes a ligament. With the clamping of the cord, the umbilical arteries, umbilical vein, and ductus venosus close and are converted into ligaments. The hypogastric arteries also occlude and become ligaments.

Heart Rate and Sounds

The heart rate averages 110 to 160 beats/min at birth, with variations noted during sleeping and waking states. Shortly after the first cry, the infant's heart rate may be as high as 175 to 180 beats/min. The range of the heart rate in the full-term newborn is 80 to 90 beats/min during sleep and up to 170 beats/min while awake. It is not unusual to find a heart rate of 180 beats/min when the infant cries. A heart rate that is either consistently high (more than 170 beats/min) or low (fewer than 80 beats/min) with the newborn at rest should be re-evaluated within an hour or when the infant's activity changes. Increased heart rate is often due to pyrexia and the newborn's temperature should be assessed.

The apical impulse (point of maximal impulse [PMI]) in the newborn is at the fourth intercostal space and to the left of the midclavicular line. The PMI is often visible and easily palpable because of the thin chest wall; this is also called *precordial activity*.

Apical pulse rates should be obtained on all infants. Auscultation should be for a full minute, preferably when the infant is asleep. An irregular heart rate in newborns is not uncommon in the first few hours of life. After this time, an irregular heart rate not attributed to changes in activity or respiratory pattern should be further evaluated.

Heart sounds during the neonatal period are of higher pitch, shorter duration, and greater intensity than during adult life. The first sound (S_1) is typically louder and duller than the second sound (S_2), which is sharp. The third and fourth heart sounds are not auscultated in newborns. Most heart murmurs heard during the neonatal period have no pathological significance, and more than half of the murmurs disappear by 6 months. However, the presence of a murmur and accompanying signs such as poor feeding, apnea, cyanosis, or pallor is considered abnormal and should be further investigated.

Blood Pressure

The newborn infant's average systolic blood pressure (BP) is 60 to 80 mm Hg and average diastolic BP is 40 to 50 mm Hg. The BP increases by the second day of life with minor variations noted during the first month of life. A drop in systolic BP (about 15 mm Hg) in the first hour of life is common. Crying and movement usually cause increases in the systolic BP. The measurement of BP is best accomplished with an oscillometric device while the infant is at rest. A correctly sized cuff must be used for accurate measurement of an infant's BP. Unless there is a specific indication, BP is not routinely measured in the healthy newborn. The practice of obtaining four extremity pressures in the early newborn period to detect coarctation of the aorta (COA) has been questioned (Razmus & Lewis, 2006) in light of evidence that COA defects do not manifest in the immediate postpartum period but more typically at approximately 12 to 14 days of age, a time when the ductus arteriosus closes (Taylor, 2005).

Blood Volume

Blood volume in the newborn is about 80 to 85 mL/kg of body weight. Immediately after birth, the total blood volume averages 300 mL, but this volume can increase by as much as 100 mL, depending on the length of time to cord clamping and cutting. The infant born prematurely has a relatively greater blood volume than the term newborn because the preterm infant has a proportionately greater plasma volume, not a greater red blood cell (RBC) mass.

Early or late clamping of the cord changes circulatory dynamics of the newborn. Late clamping expands the blood volume from the so-called placental transfusion of blood to the newborn. Recent data showed delayed cord clamping (no longer than 2 minutes after birth) in full-term neonates resulted in improved hematocrit, improved iron status, and a decrease in anemia; such benefits were observed over ages 2 to 6 months (Hutton & Hassan, 2007). In this study, **polycythemia** occurred with delayed clamping but was not harmful. Jaundice may occur, with an increased need for phototherapy (McDonald & Middleton, 2008).

Hematopoietic System

The hematopoietic system of the newborn exhibits certain variations from that of the adult. Levels of RBCs and leukocytes differ, but platelet levels are relatively the same.

Red Blood Cells and Hemoglobin

At birth, the average levels of RBCs and hemoglobin (fetal hemoglobin is predominant) are higher than those in the adult. Cord blood of the term newborn may have a hemoglobin concentration from 140 to 240 g/L (mean 170 g/L). The hematocrit ranges from 0.44 to 0.64 (mean 0.55). The RBC count is correspondingly elevated, ranging from 4.8 to 7.1 × 10^{12}/L. These values fall and reach the average levels of 110 to 170 g/L (hemoglobin), 4.2 to 5.2 × 10^{12}/L (RBC), and 0.28 to 0.42 (hematocrit), by the end of the first month. The blood values may be affected by delayed clamping of the cord, which results in a rise in hemoglobin, RBCs, and hematocrit. The source of the sample is a significant factor because capillary blood yields higher values than those of venous blood. The timing of the neonate's blood sample is also significant; the slight rise in RBCs after birth is followed by a substantial drop. At birth, the infant's blood contains an average of 70% fetal hemoglobin, but because of the shorter lifespan of the cells containing fetal hemoglobin, the percentage falls to 55% by 5 weeks and to 5% by 20 weeks. Iron stores generally are sufficient to sustain normal RBC production for 4 to 5 months in the term infant, at which time a physiological anemia that is usually transient may occur.

Leukocytes

Leukocytosis, with a white blood cell (WBC) count of approximately 18 × 10^9/L (range 9 to 30 × 10^9/L), is normal at birth. The number of WBCs increases to 23 to 24 × 10^9/L during the first day after birth. The initial high WBC count of the newborn decreases rapidly, and a stable level of 12 × 10^9/L is normally maintained during the neonatal period. Serious infection is not well tolerated by the newborn; leukocytes are slow to recognize foreign protein and to localize and fight infection early in life. Sepsis may be accompanied by a concomitant rise in granulocytes (neutrophilia); however, some infants may initially be seen with clinical signs of sepsis without a significant elevation in WBCs. In addition, events other than infection—prolonged crying, maternal hypertension, asymptomatic hypoglycemia, hemolytic disease, meconium aspiration syndrome, labour induction with oxytocin, surgery, difficult labour, high altitude, and maternal fever—may cause neutrophilia in the newborn (Weinberg & Powell, 2011).

Platelets

Platelet count ranges between 150 and 450 × 10^9/L and is essentially the same in newborns as in adults. A platelet level below 150 × 10^9/L is abnormal in a newborn (Blackburn, 2007). The levels of factors II, VII, IX, and X, found in the liver, are decreased during the first few days of life because the newborn cannot synthesize vitamin K. However, bleeding tendencies in the newborn are uncommon, and unless the vitamin K deficiency is great, clotting is sufficient to prevent hemorrhage.

Blood Groups

The infant's blood group is genetically determined and established early in fetal life. However, during the neonatal period, there is a gradual increase in the strength of the agglutinogens present in the RBC membrane. Cord blood samples may be used to identify the infant's blood type and Rh status.

Thermogenic System

Next to establishing respiration and adequate circulation, heat regulation is most critical to the newborn's survival. *Thermoregulation* is the maintenance of balance between heat loss and heat production. Newborns attempt to stabilize their core body temperatures within a narrow range. Hypothermia from excessive heat loss is a common and dangerous problem in neonates. The newborn's ability to produce heat (thermogenesis) often approaches that of the adult; however, the tendency toward rapid heat loss in a cold environment is increased in the newborn and poses a significant hazard to the infant during the transition to extrauterine life.

Thermogenesis

The shivering mechanism of heat production is not well developed in the newborn. **Nonshivering thermogenesis** is accomplished primarily by **brown fat**, which is unique to the newborn, and secondarily by increased metabolic activity in the brain, heart, and liver. Brown fat is located in superficial deposits in the interscapular region and axillae, as well as in deep deposits at the thoracic inlet, along the vertebral column, and around the kidneys. Brown fat has a richer vascular and nerve supply than ordinary fat. Heat produced by intense lipid metabolic activity in brown fat can warm the neonate by increasing heat production as much as 100%. Reserves of brown fat, usually present for several weeks after birth, are rapidly depleted with cold stress. The less mature the infant, the less reserve of this essential fat is available at birth.

Heat Loss

Heat loss in the newborn occurs by four modes (Fig. 24-1):

1. **Convection** is the flow of heat from the body surface to cooler ambient air. Because of heat loss by convection, the ambient temperature in the nursery is kept at approximately 24°C and newborns in open bassinets are wrapped to protect them from the cold. A cap may be worn to decrease heat loss from the infant's head.
2. **Radiation** is the loss of heat from the body surface to a cooler solid surface not in direct contact but in relative proximity. To prevent this type of loss, cribs and examining tables are placed away from outside windows and care is taken to avoid direct air drafts.
3. **Evaporation** is the loss of heat that occurs when a liquid is converted to a vapour. In the newborn, heat loss by evaporation occurs as a result of vaporization of moisture from the skin. This heat loss is intensified by failing to dry the newborn directly after birth or by drying the infant too slowly after a bath. The less mature the newborn, the more severe the evaporative heat loss. Evaporative heat loss, as a component of insensible water loss, is the most significant cause of heat loss in the first few days of life.
4. **Conduction** is the loss of heat from the body surface to cooler surfaces in direct contact. When admitted to the nursery, the newborn is placed in a warmed crib to minimize heat loss. The scales used for weighing the newborn should have a protective cover to minimize conductive heat loss.

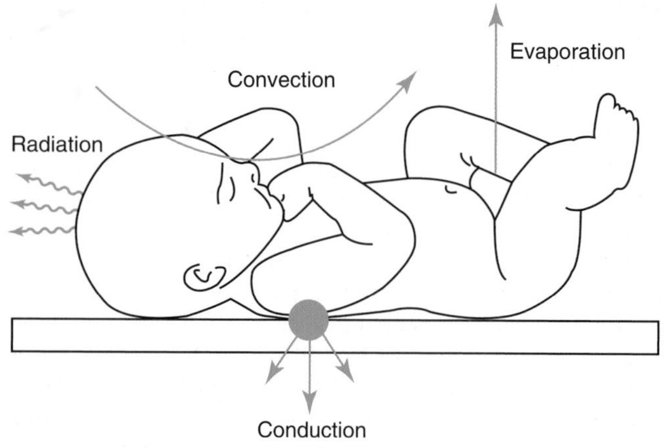

Fig. 24-1 Heat loss in the newborn occurs in four ways: convection, radiation, evaporation, and conduction. *(From WHO [1997].* Safe motherhood: thermal protection of the newborn, a practical guide *Retrieved from http://whqlibdoc.who.int/hq/1997/WHO_RHT_MSM_97.2.pdf.)*

Skin-to-Skin Contact

Loss of heat must be controlled to protect the infant. Control of such modes of heat loss is the basis of caregiving policies and techniques. One method for promoting maternal–newborn interaction is to place the naked healthy dried newborn next to the mother's skin and to cover both with a blanket; this is an alternative to separating mother and baby to put the newborn under a radiant warmer or wrapping the newborn in blankets. This skin-to-skin contact enhances newborn temperature control and interaction. Newborns that are placed skin to skin remain warmer than newborns who are held swaddled in their mother's arms. If the mother is unavailable, then the father or another significant person in the room could also put the newborn skin to skin (Dabrowski, 2007; Galligan, 2006).

Temperature Regulation

Anatomical and physiological differences among the newborn, child, and adult are notable. The newborn's ability to produce heat initially is less than that of an adult. Newborns have larger body surface to body weight (mass) ratios than those of children and adults. The newborn's flexed position helps guard against heat loss because it diminishes the amount of body surface exposed to the environment. Infants can also reduce the loss of internal heat through the body surface by constricting peripheral blood vessels.

Cold stress imposes metabolic and physiological problems on all infants, regardless of gestational age and condition. The respiratory rate increases in response to the increased need for oxygen. In the cold-stressed infant, oxygen consumption and energy are diverted from maintaining normal brain cell and cardiac function and growth to thermogenesis for survival. If the infant cannot maintain an adequate oxygen tension, vasoconstriction follows and jeopardizes pulmonary perfusion. As a consequence, the partial pressure of arterial oxygen (Pa_{O_2}) is decreased, and the blood pH drops. These changes may prompt a transient respiratory distress or may aggravate existing respiratory distress syndrome. Moreover, decreased pulmonary perfusion and oxygen tension may maintain or reopen the right-to-left shunt across the patent ductus arteriosus.

The basal metabolic rate increases with cold stress (Fig. 24-2). If cold stress is protracted, anaerobic glycolysis occurs,

evolve Skill—Thermoregulation

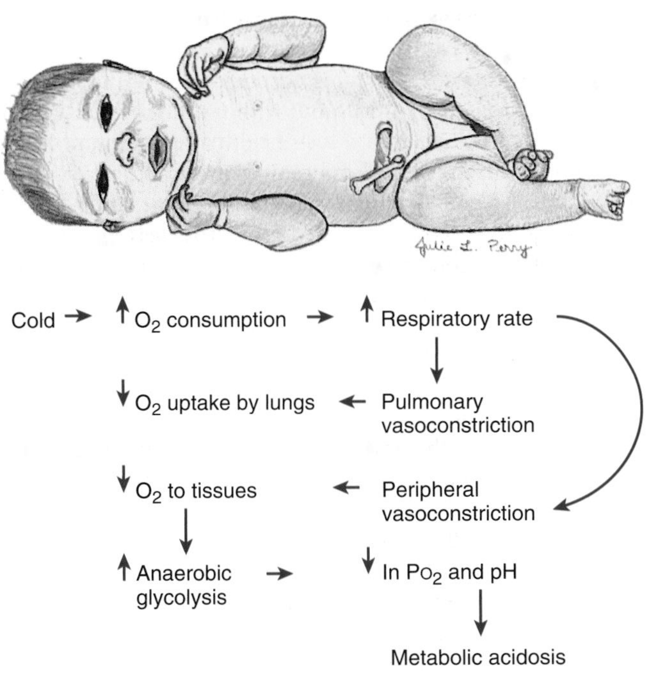

Fig. 24-2 Effects of cold stress. When an infant is stressed by cold, oxygen consumption increases and pulmonary and peripheral vasoconstriction occur, thereby decreasing oxygen uptake by the lungs and oxygen to the tissues; anaerobic glycolysis increases; and there is a decrease in Po_2 and pH, leading to metabolic acidosis.

resulting in increased production of acids. Metabolic acidosis develops, and if a defect in respiratory function is present, respiratory acidosis also develops. Excessive fatty acids may displace the bilirubin from the albumin-binding sites and exacerbate **hyperbilirubinemia**. Another metabolic consequence of cold stress is **hypoglycemia**. The process of anaerobic glycolysis utilizes approximately three to four times the amount of blood glucose, thereby depleting existing stores; if the infant is sufficiently stressed and low glucose stores are not replaced, hypoglycemia, which can be asymptomatic in the newborn, may ensue.

Hyperthermia develops more rapidly in the newborn than in the adult because of decreased ability to increase evaporative water losses from the skin. Although newborn infants have six times as many sweat glands per unit area as adults, in most newborns these glands do not function sufficiently to allow the infant to sweat. Serious overheating of the newborn can cause cerebral damage from dehydration or heat stroke and death.

Renal System

At term, the kidneys occupy a large portion of the posterior abdominal wall. The bladder lies close to the anterior abdominal wall and is an abdominal as well as a pelvic organ. In the newborn, almost all palpable masses in the abdomen are renal in origin.

At birth, a small quantity (approximately 40 mL) of urine is usually present in the bladder of a full-term infant. The frequency of voiding varies from 2 to 6 times per day during the first and second days of life and from 5 to 25 times during the subsequent 24 hours. About 6 to 8 voidings per day, at 1 week of age, of pale straw-coloured urine are indicative of adequate fluid intake. Generally, term infants void 15 to 60 mL of urine per kilogram per day.

Full-term newborns have limited capacity to concentrate urine; therefore, the specific gravity ranges from 1.001 to 1.020. The ability to concentrate urine fully is attained by about 3 months of age. After the first voiding, the infant's urine may appear cloudy (because of mucus content) and have a much higher specific gravity. This decreases as fluid intake increases. Normal urine during early infancy is usually straw coloured and almost odourless. Sometimes pink-tinged uric acid crystal stains appear on the diaper; these stains are normal.

Loss of fluid through urine, feces, lungs, increased metabolic rate, and limited fluid intake results in a 5 to 10% loss of the birth weight. This usually occurs over the first 3 to 5 days of life. If the mother is breastfeeding and her milk supply has not come in yet (which occurs by the third or fourth day after birth), the neonate is somewhat protected from dehydration by its increased extracellular fluid volume. The neonate should regain the birth weight within 10 to 14 days, depending on the feeding method (breast or bottle).

Because renal thresholds are low in the infant, bicarbonate concentration and buffering capacity are decreased. This may lead to acidosis and electrolyte imbalance.

Fluid and Electrolyte Balance

About 40% of the body weight of the newborn is extracellular fluid. Each day, the newborn takes in and excretes roughly 600 to 700 mL of water, which is 20% of the total body fluid, or 50% of the extracellular fluid. The glomerular filtration rate of a newborn is about 30 to 50% that of an adult. This results in a decreased ability to remove nitrogenous and other waste products from the blood. However, the newborn's ingested protein is almost totally metabolized for growth.

Sodium reabsorption is decreased as a result of a lowered sodium- and potassium-activated adenosine triphosphate activity. The decreased ability to excrete excessive sodium results in urine that is more hypotonic than plasma. There is a higher concentration of sodium, phosphates, chloride, and organic acids and a lower concentration of bicarbonate ions. The infant has a higher renal threshold for glucose.

Gastrointestinal System

The full-term newborn is capable of swallowing, digesting, metabolizing, and absorbing proteins and simple carbohydrates, and emulsifying fats. With the exception of pancreatic amylase, the characteristic enzymes and digestive juices are present even in low-birth-weight neonates.

In the adequately hydrated infant, the mucous membrane of the mouth is moist and pink; the hard and soft palates are intact. The presence of moderate to large amounts of mucus is common in the first few hours after birth. Small whitish areas (Epstein pearls) may be found on the gum margins and at the juncture of the hard and soft palate. The cheeks are full because of well-developed sucking pads. These, like the labial tubercles (sucking calluses) on the upper lip, disappear around the age of 12 months, when the sucking period is over.

evolve Case Study—Newborn Health Problems

Even though in utero sucking motions occur, as recorded by ultrasound, these motions are not coordinated with swallowing in any infant born before 32 to 33 weeks of gestation. Sucking behaviour is influenced by neuromuscular maturity, maternal medications received during labour and birth, and the type of initial feeding.

A special mechanism present in healthy term newborns coordinates the breathing, sucking, and swallowing reflexes necessary for oral feeding. Sucking in the newborn takes place in small bursts of three or four sucks at a time. The infant is unable to move food from the lips to the pharynx; therefore, placing the nipple (breast or bottle) well inside the baby's mouth is necessary. Peristaltic activity in the esophagus is uncoordinated in the first few days of life. It quickly becomes a coordinated pattern in healthy full-term infants, and they swallow easily.

Teeth begin developing in utero, with enamel formation continuing until about 10 years of age. Tooth development is influenced by neonatal or infant illnesses and medications, and by illnesses of or medications taken by the mother during pregnancy. The fluoride level in the water supply also influences tooth development. Occasionally an infant may be born with one or more teeth. Loose teeth should be removed because of risk of aspiration.

Bacteria are not present in the infant's gastrointestinal tract at birth. Soon after birth, oral and anal orifices permit entrance of bacteria and air. Generally, the highest bacterial concentration is found in the lower portion of the intestine, particularly in the large intestine. Normal colonic bacteria are established within the first week after birth, and normal intestinal flora help synthesize vitamin K, folate, and biotin. Bowel sounds can usually be heard shortly after birth.

Stomach capacity varies from 30 to 90 mL, depending on the infant's size. Emptying time for the stomach is highly variable. Several factors, such as time and volume of feedings or type and temperature of food, may affect the emptying time. The cardiac sphincter and nervous control of the stomach are immature, so some regurgitation may occur. Regurgitation during the first day or two of life can be decreased by avoiding overfeeding, by burping the infant, and by positioning the infant with the head slightly elevated.

Digestion

The infant's ability to digest carbohydrates, fats, and proteins is regulated by the presence of certain enzymes. Most of these are functional at birth. One exception is amylase, produced by the salivary glands after about 3 months and by the pancreas at about 6 months of age. This enzyme is necessary to convert starch into maltose and occurs in high amounts in colostrum. The other exception is lipase, which is also secreted by the pancreas; it is necessary for the digestion of fat. Thus, the normal newborn is capable of digesting simple carbohydrates and proteins but has a limited ability to digest fats.

Further digestion and absorption of nutrients occurs in the small intestine in the presence of pancreatic secretions, secretions from the liver through the common bile duct, and secretions from the duodenal portion of the small intestine.

Stools

At birth, the lower intestine is filled with meconium. Meconium is formed during fetal life from the amniotic fluid and its constituents, intestinal secretions (including bilirubin), and cells (shed from the mucosa). Meconium is greenish black and viscous and contains occult blood. The first meconium passed is usually sterile, but within hours all meconium passed contains bacteria. Most healthy term infants pass meconium within 12 to 24 hours of life, and almost all do so by 48 hours (Blackburn, 2007). The number of stools passed varies during the first week, being most numerous between the third and sixth days. Newborns fed early pass stools sooner. Progressive changes in the stooling pattern indicate a properly functioning gastrointestinal tract (Box 24-1 and Fig 24-3).

Hepatic System

The liver and gallbladder are formed by the fourth week of gestation. In the newborn, the liver can be palpated about 1 cm below the right costal margin because it is enlarged and occupies about 40% of the abdominal cavity. The infant's liver plays an important role in iron storage, carbohydrate metabolism, conjugation of bilirubin, and coagulation.

Iron Storage

The fetal liver, which serves as the site for production of hemoglobin after birth, begins storing iron in utero. The infant's iron store is proportional to total body hemoglobin content and length of gestation. At birth, the term neonate has an iron store sufficient to last 4 to 6 months; the preterm infant's iron stores are often lower and are depleted sooner.

Carbohydrate Metabolism

At birth, the newborn is cut off from its maternal glucose supply and, as a result, experiences an initial decrease in

BOX 24-1 Changes in Stooling Patterns of Newborns

Meconium

Meconium is the infant's first stool, composed of amniotic fluid and its constituents, intestinal secretions, shed mucosal cells, and possibly blood (ingested maternal blood or minor bleeding of alimentary tract vessels) (Fig. 24-3, A).

Passage of meconium should occur within the first 24 to 48 hours, although it may be delayed up to 7 days in very-low-birth-weight infants.

Transitional Stools

Transitional stools usually appear by the third day after initiation of feeding.

They are greenish brown to yellowish brown, are thin and less sticky than meconium, and may contain some milk curds (Fig. 24-3, B).

Milk Stool

Milk stool usually appears by the fourth day.

In breastfed infants, stools are yellow to golden, are pasty in consistency, and have a sweet-smelling odour (Fig. 24-3, C).

In formula-fed infants, stools are pale yellow to light brown, are firmer in consistency, and have an odour more characteristic of a normal stool.

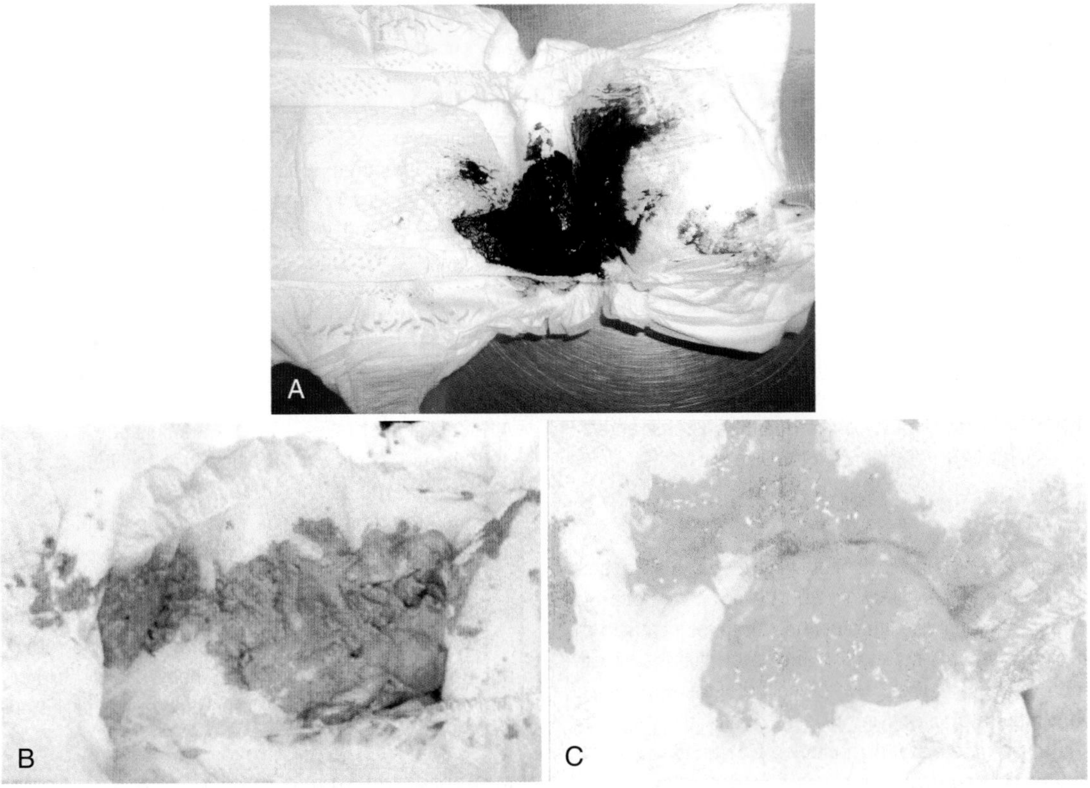

Fig. 24-3 Newborn stools. **A:** Meconium. **B:** Transition stool. **C:** Milk stool. *(**A**, Courtesy of Janet Andrews. **B, C**, Courtesy of Connie Livingstone.)*

serum glucose levels. The newborn's increased energy needs, decreased hepatic release of glucose from glycogen stores, increased RBC volume, and increased brain size may initially contribute to the rapid depletion of stored glycogen within the first 24 hours after birth. In most healthy term newborns, blood glucose levels stabilize at 2.5 to 3.0 mmol/L during the first several hours after birth; by the third day of life, the blood glucose levels should be approximately 3.0 to 3.5 mmol/L. The initiation of feedings assists in the stabilization of the newborn's blood glucose levels. Colostrum contains high amounts of glucose, thus also assisting in the stabilization of blood glucose levels in breastfed neonates (see Evidence-Informed Practice box).

Jaundice

Jaundice is the manifestation of the pigment **bilirubin** in the tissues of the body. Jaundice usually does not appear until the bilirubin level reaches 85 mcmol/L. Any visible jaundice within the first 24 hours of life or persistence of jaundice beyond 7 to 10 days requires further investigation into the cause, since this may represent an underlying pathological process (Fig. 24-4). See Chapter 25 for a further discussion of bilirubin metabolism and hyperbilirubinemia.

Coagulation

Coagulation factors, which are synthesized in the liver, are activated by vitamin K. The lack of intestinal bacteria needed to synthesize vitamin K results in transient blood coagulation deficiency between the second and fifth days of life. The administration of intramuscular vitamin K shortly after birth helps prevent clotting problems.

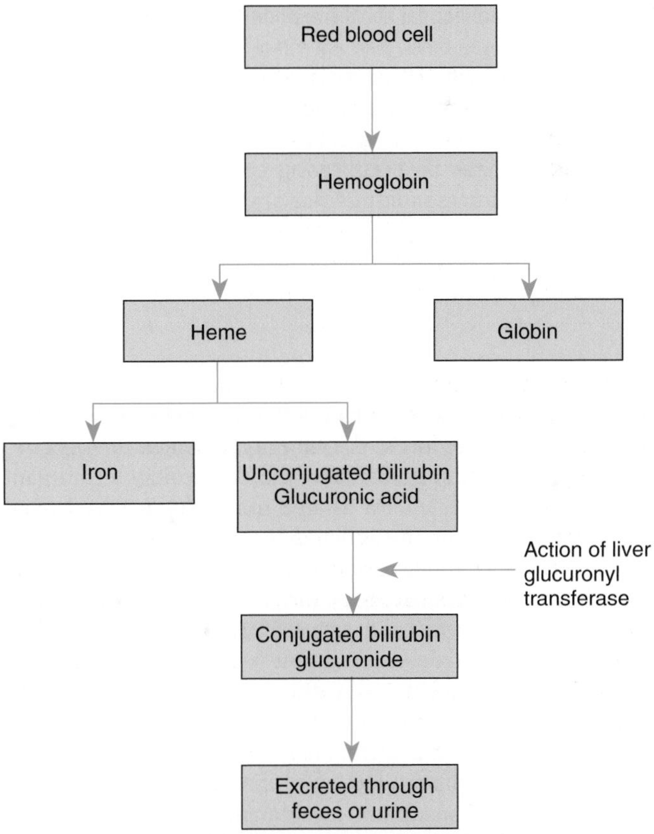

Fig. 24-4 Formation and excretion of bilirubin.

EVIDENCE-INFORMED PRACTICE Monitoring for Hypoglycemia

—Pat Gingrich

Ask the Question

What are the current recommendations for monitoring and treating neonatal hypoglycemia?

Search for Evidence

Search Strategies

Professional organization guidelines, meta-analyses, systematic reviews, randomized controlled trials, nonrandomized prospective studies, and retrospective studies since 2006

Databases Searched

CINAHL; Cochrane; Medline; National Guideline Clearinghouse; TRIP Database Plus; and Web sites for the Canadian Paediatric Society (CPS), Association of Women's Health, Obstetric and Neonatal Nursing (AWHONN), Centers for Disease Control (CDC), and World Health Organization (WHO)

Critically Analyze the Evidence

Hypoglycemia affects less than 1% of healthy newborns. Risk factors for hypoglycemia include weight below 2000 g or above 4000 g, small or large for gestational age, intrauterine growth restriction, less than 37 weeks of gestation, maternal diabetes or glucose imbalance, perinatal asphyxia, or sepsis. Hypoglycemia of the newborn is infrequently a symptom of underlying disease. Signs of hypoglycemia include irritability, jitteriness, high-pitched cry, pallor, sweating, lethargy, poor feeding, seizures, and respiratory difficulties.

A Best Practice Guideline from the Joanna Briggs Institute (2006) concluded that breastfeeding early and often, with thermoregulation through skin-to-skin contact, will normalize the glucose levels of most term, normal-weight infants during their first 48 hours. In 12 to 14% of normal healthy newborns, it is not unusual to have a blood glucose of less than 2.6 mmol/L in the first 3 days of life (CPS, 2004). The guidelines recommended against any supplemental glucose or water feedings or routine glucose monitoring, except in the case of obvious physical signs of hypoglycemia.

This emphasis on breastfeeding early (first hour) and often (10 to 12 feedings in first 24 hours) concurs with guidelines for breastfeeding by the Association of Women's Health, Obstetric and Neonatal Nurses (2007) and the Academy of Breastfeeding Medicine (Wight, Marinelli, & Academy of Breastfeeding Medicine Protocol Committee, 2006). The Academy's guidelines recommend breastfeeding every 1 to 2 hours and monitoring blood glucose level. If the blood glucose does not reach the goal of more than 2.2 mmol/L, consider administering glucose intravenously.

Implications for Practice

Skin-to-skin contact and early breastfeeding have proven benefits for early temperature and glucose stabilization of the newborn, as well as bonding during the newborn's first awake, interactive period. All nonessential tasks, such as administration of eye medications and vitamin K, should be delayed to facilitate this enriching time together. The nurse should be alert to the signs of hypoglycemia, which can appear late. For most infants without underlying pathological conditions, monitoring the glucose levels if signs of hypoglycemia are present and encouraging breastfeeding, rather than using supplemental formula or dextrose water, and skin-to-skin contact will correct the hypoglycemia within minutes or hours. Finally, the nurse can remember that every baby has his or her own normal range of glucose, which may run high or low in the normal range.

References

Association of Women's Health, Obstetric and Neonatal Nurses. (2007). *Breastfeeding support: Prenatal care through the first year* (2nd ed.), Evidence-Based Clinical Practice Guideline. Washington, DC: Author.

Canadian Paediatric Society. (2004). Screening guidelines for newborns at risk for low blood glucose. *Pediatrics and Child Health, 9*(10), 723–729.

Joanna Briggs Institute of Evidence Based Nursing. (2006). Management of asymptomatic hypoglycemia in healthy term neonates for nurses and midwives. *Best Practice, 10*(1), 1–4.

Wight, N., Marinelli, K. A., & Academy of Breastfeeding Medicine Protocol Committee. (2006). ABM clinical protocol #1: Guidelines for glucose monitoring and treatment of hypoglycemia in breastfed neonates. *Breastfeeding Medicine, 1*, 178–184.

Immune System

The cells that provide the infant with **immunity** are developed early in fetal life; however, they are not activated for weeks to months. For the first 3 months of life, the healthy term infant is somewhat protected by passive immunity received from the mother; however, this is dependent on the mother's previous exposure to antigens and her immunological response. The membrane-protective immunoglobulin A (IgA) is missing from the respiratory and urinary tracts and, unless the newborn is breastfed, is also absent from the gastrointestinal tract. The infant begins to synthesize IgG, and levels reach about 40% of adult levels by 1 year of age. Significant amounts of IgM are produced at birth, and adult levels are reached by 9 months of age. The production of IgA, IgD, and IgE is much more gradual, and maximum levels are not attained until early childhood. The infant who is breastfed receives significant passive immunity through the colostrum and breast milk.

Integumentary System

All skin structures are present at birth. The epidermis and dermis are bound loosely and are very thin. **Vernix caseosa** (a cheeselike whitish substance) is fused with the epidermis and serves as a protective covering. The infant's skin is sensitive and can be easily damaged. The term infant has erythematous (red) skin for a few hours after birth, after which it fades to its normal colour. The skin often appears blotchy or mottled, especially over the extremities. The hands and feet appear slightly cyanotic **(acrocyanosis);** this is caused by vasomotor instability and capillary stasis. Acrocyanosis is normal and appears intermittently over the first 7 to 10 days, especially with exposure to cold.

The healthy term infant usually has a plump appearance because of large amounts of subcutaneous tissue and extracellular water content. Subcutaneous fat accumulated during the last trimester acts as insulation. Fine **lanugo** hair may be noted

FAMILY-CENTRED TEACHING

Newborn Skin

A young couple with a healthy newborn girl calls the nurse because they are concerned about the small raised red dots on the baby's face and arms and that her skin is dry and flaky in certain places. The nurse assesses the newborn and concludes that the spots are not mosquito bites, as the family stated, but erythema toxicum. What further anticipatory guidance about normal newborn skin appearance could the nurse give the parents to reassure them that the newborn is healthy and normal?

FAMILY-CENTRED TEACHING

Swelling on the Scalp

A 2-day-old healthy newborn has a "bump" on the left side of the head. The mother is concerned that the baby may have somehow fallen out of the crib and injured the head. Nursing assessment findings are that the scalp swelling is raised and soft to the touch but does not cross cranial suture lines; there is no apparent bruising or discolouration. The neurological assessment reveals no significant findings, and the newborn's behaviour appears to be that of a healthy term infant. How could the nurse explain the condition and reassure the mother that her newborn has a common finding rather than an abnormal condition requiring immediate medical attention?

over the face, shoulders, and back. Edema of the face and **ecchymosis** (bruising) may be noted as a result of face presentation, forceps-assisted birth, or vacuum extraction (see Family-Centred Teaching box, Newborn Skin).

Creases can be found on the palms of the hands. The simian line, a single palmar crease, is often found in Asian infants or in infants with Down syndrome.

Caput Succedaneum

Caput succedaneum is a generalized, easily identifiable edematous area of the scalp, most commonly found on the occiput (Fig. 24-5, A). The sustained pressure of the presenting vertex against the cervix results in compression of local vessels, thereby slowing venous return. The slower venous return causes an increase in tissue fluids within the skin of the scalp, and an edematous swelling develops. This edematous swelling, present at birth, extends across the suture lines of the skull and disappears spontaneously within 3 to 4 days. Infants who are born with the assistance of vacuum extraction usually have a caput in the area where the cup was applied.

Cephalhematoma

Cephalhematoma is a collection of blood between a skull bone and its periosteum. Thus, a cephalhematoma does not cross a cranial suture line (see Fig. 24-5, C). Often caput succedaneum and cephalhematoma occur simultaneously.

Bleeding may occur with spontaneous birth from pressure against the maternal bony pelvis. Low forceps birth and difficult forceps rotation and extraction may also cause bleeding. This soft, fluctuating, irreducible fullness does not pulsate or bulge when the infant cries. It appears several hours or the day after birth and may not become apparent until a caput succedaneum is absorbed. A cephalhematoma is usually largest on the second or third day, by which time the bleeding stops (see Family-Centred Teaching box, Swelling on the Scalp). The fullness of a cephalhematoma spontaneously resolves in 3 to 6 weeks. It is not aspirated because infection may develop if the skin is punctured. As the hematoma resolves, hemolysis of RBCs occurs and jaundice may result. Hyperbilirubinemia and jaundice may occur from a cephalhematoma after the newborn is discharged home.

Subgaleal Hemorrhage

Subgaleal hemorrhage is bleeding into the subgaleal compartment (see Fig. 24-5, B). The subgaleal compartment is a potential space that contains loosely arranged connective tissue; it is located beneath the galea aponeurosis, the tendinous sheath that connects the frontal and occipital muscles and forms the inner surface of the scalp. The injury occurs as a result of forces that compress and then drag the head through the pelvic outlet (Paige & Moe, 2006). The use of the vacuum extractor at birth is associated with cases of subgaleal hemorrhage, neonatal morbidity, and death (Boo et al., 2005; Uchil & Arulkumaran, 2003). The bleeding extends beyond bone, often posteriorly into the neck, and continues after birth, with the potential for serious complications such as anemia or hypovolemic shock.

Early detection of the hemorrhage is vital; serial head circumference measurements and inspection of the back of the neck for increasing edema and a firm mass are an essential aspect of assessments of newborns who are delivered via a vacuum extractor. A boggy scalp, pallor, tachycardia, and increasing head circumference may also be early signs of a subgaleal hemorrhage (Doumouchtsis & Arulkumaran, 2006). Computed tomography (CT) or magnetic resonance imaging (MRI) is useful in confirming the diagnosis. Replacement of lost blood and clotting factors is required in acute cases of hemorrhage. Another possible early sign of subgaleal hemorrhage is a forward and lateral positioning of the newborn's ears because the hematoma extends posteriorly. Monitoring the infant for changes in level of consciousness and decreases in hematocrit is also key to early recognition and management. An increase in serum bilirubin levels may be seen as a result of the degradation of blood cells within the hematoma.

Sweat Glands

Sweat glands are present at birth but do not respond to increases in ambient or body temperature. Some fetal sebaceous gland hyperplasia and secretion of sebum result from the hormonal influences of pregnancy. Vernix caseosa is a product of the sebaceous glands. Removal of the vernix is followed by desquamation of the epidermis in most infants. Vernix has been shown to be an epidermal barrier with positive benefits for neonatal skin, such as decreasing the skin pH, decreasing skin erythema, and improving skin hydration; thus, it is recommended that vernix not be removed immediately after birth (Singh & Archana, 2008; Visscher et al., 2005). Distended, small, white sebaceous glands, noticeable on the newborn face, are known as **milia**.

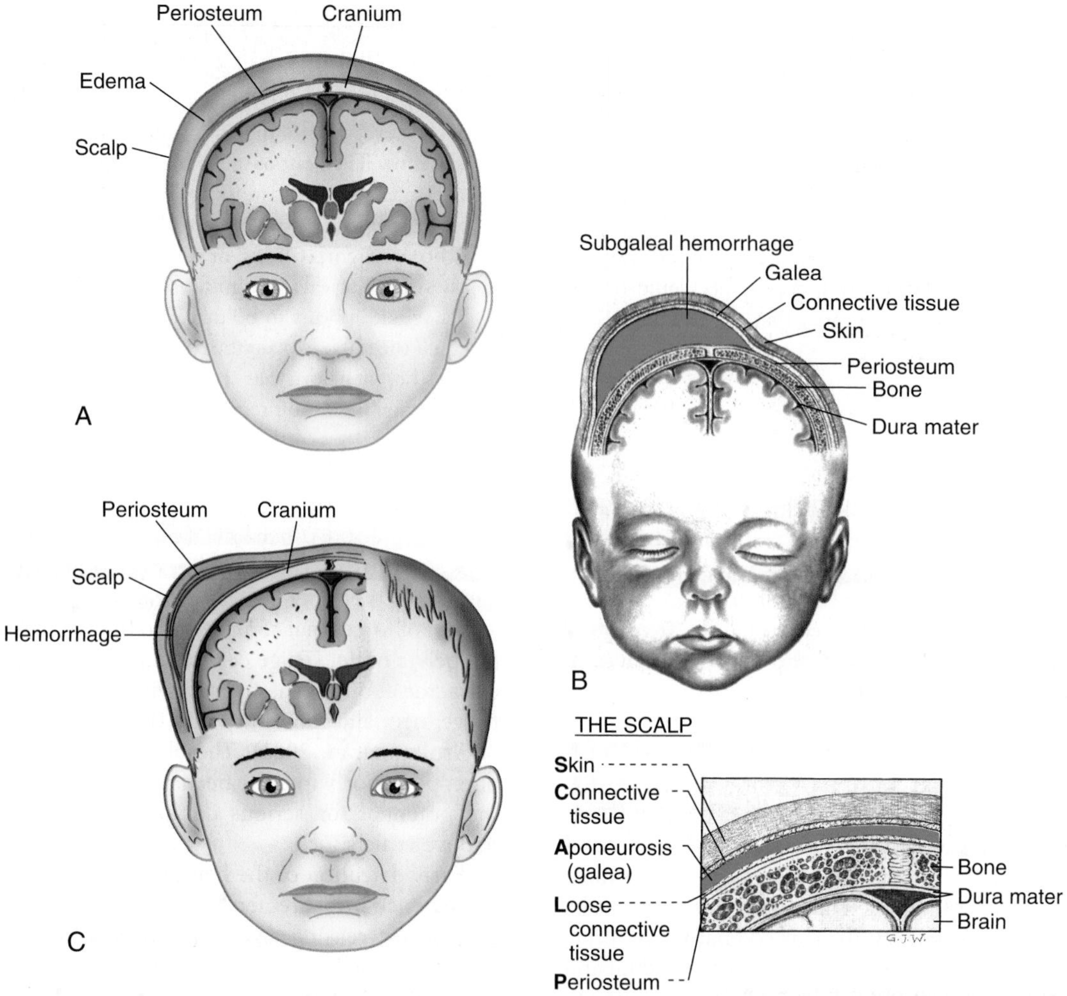

Fig. 24-5 **A:** Caput succedaneum. **B:** Subgaleal hemorrhage. **C:** Cephalhematoma. *(A and C, from Seidel, H. M., et al. [2006].* Mosby's guide to physical examination *[6th ed., p. 267]. St. Louis: Mosby.)*

Desquamation

Desquamation (peeling) of the skin of the term infant does not occur until a few days after birth. Large generalized areas of skin desquamation present at birth may be an indication of postmaturity.

Mongolian Spots

Mongolian spots, bluish black areas of pigmentation, may appear over any part of the exterior surface of the body, including the extremities. They are more commonly noted on the back and buttocks (Fig. 24-6). These pigmented areas are most frequently noted in newborns whose ethnic origins are in the Mediterranean area, Latin America, Asia, or Africa. They are more common in dark-skinned individuals but may occur in 5 to 13% of Whites as well (Blackburn, 2007). They fade gradually over months or years.

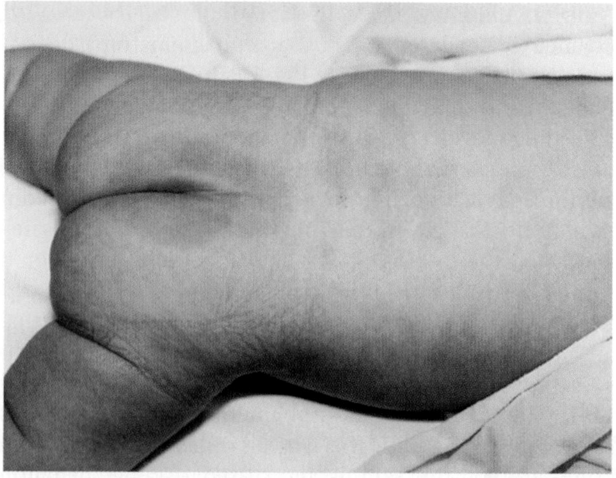

Fig. 24-6 Mongolian spot.

Nevi

Known as "stork bites," **telangiectatic nevi** are pink and easily blanched (Fig. 24-7, A). They appear on the upper eyelids, nose, upper lip, lower occiput bone, and nape of the neck. They have no clinical significance and fade between the first and second years of life.

A red mark, or **nevus vasculosus,** is a common type of capillary hemangioma. It consists of dilated, newly formed capillaries occupying the entire dermal and subdermal layers with associated connective tissue hypertrophy. The typical lesion is a raised, sharply demarcated, bright or dark red, rough-surfaced swelling. As the infant grows, the hemangioma may proliferate and become more vascular, often being

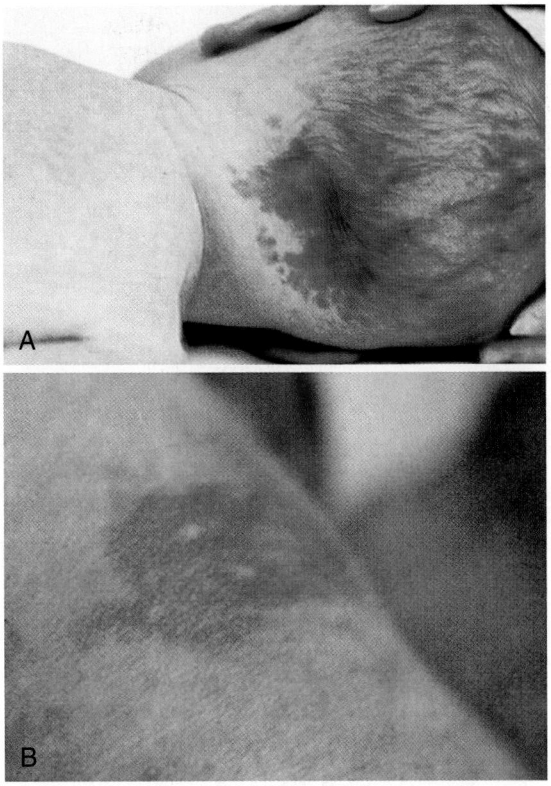

Fig. 24-7 **A:** Telangiectatic nevi (stork bite). **B:** Erythema toxicum. *(Courtesy Mead Johnson & Co., LLC.)*

referred to as a *capillary* or *strawberry hemangioma*. Lesions are usually single but may be multiple, with 75% occurring on the head. These lesions can remain until the child is of school age or sometimes even longer but can be removed successfully with pulsed dye laser therapy, interferon therapy, and prednisone administration. In some cases, subcutaneous injections of interferon alfa-2a or interferon alfa-2b may be required if prednisone therapy and the pulsed dye laser fail to control a problematic hemangioma.

A port-wine stain, or **nevus flammeus**, is usually observed at birth and is composed of a plexus of newly formed capillaries in the papillary layer of the corium. It is red to purple; varies in size, shape, and location; and is not elevated. True port-wine stains do not blanch on pressure or disappear. They are most commonly found on the face and neck.

Erythema Toxicum

Erythema toxicum, a transient rash, is also called *erythema neonatorum*, or *newborn rash*. It is found in term neonates during the first 3 weeks of age. It has lesions in different stages: erythematous macules, papules, and small vesicles (see Fig. 24-7, B). The lesions may appear suddenly anywhere on the body. The rash is thought to be an inflammatory response. Eosinophils, which help decrease inflammation, are found in the vesicles. Although the appearance is alarming, the rash has no clinical significance and requires no treatment.

Reproductive System

Female

At birth, the ovaries contain thousands of primitive germ cells. These represent the full complement of potential ova; no

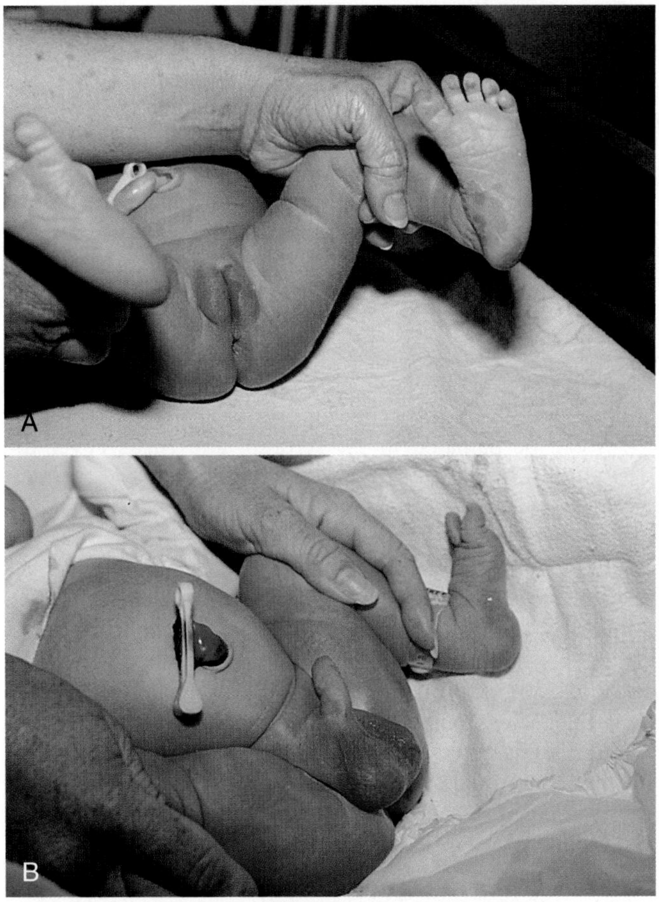

Fig. 24-8 External genitalia. **A:** Genitalia in female term infant. **B:** Genitalia in uncircumcised male infant. Rugae cover scrotum, indicating term gestation. *(Courtesy Marjorie Pyle, RNC, Lifecircle, Costa Mesa, CA.)*

oogonia form after birth in term infants. The ovarian cortex, which is made up primarily of primordial follicles, occupies a larger portion of the ovary in the female newborn than in the adult. From birth to sexual maturity, the number of ova decreases by approximately 90%.

An increase in estrogen during pregnancy, followed by a drop after birth, results in a mucoid vaginal discharge and some slight bloody spotting **(pseudomenstruation).** External genitalia (i.e., labia majora and minora) are usually edematous, with increased pigmentation. In term neonates, the labia majora and minora cover the vestibule (Fig. 24-8, A). In preterm infants, the clitoris is prominent and the labia majora are small and widely separated. Vaginal or hymenal tags are common findings and have no clinical significance. Vernix caseosa may be present between the labia and should not be forcibly removed during bathing.

If the girl was born in the breech position, the labia may be edematous and bruised. The edema and bruising resolve in a few days; no treatment is necessary.

Male

The testes (see Fig. 24-8, B) descend into the scrotum by birth in 90% of newborn boys and presence should be determined at the initial assessment. Although this percentage drops with preterm birth, by 1 year of age the incidence of undescended testes in all boys is less than 1%.

A tight **prepuce** (foreskin) is common in newborns. The urethral opening may be completely covered by the prepuce, which may not be retractable for 3 to 4 years. Smegma, a white cheesy substance, is commonly found under the foreskin. Small, white, firm cysts called *epithelial pearls* may be seen at the tip of the prepuce. In the preterm boy of less than 28 weeks of gestation, the testes remain within the abdominal cavity and the scrotum appears high and close to the body. By 28 to 36 weeks of gestation, the testes can be palpated in the inguinal canal and a few **rugae** appear on the scrotum. At 36 to 40 weeks of gestation, the testes are palpable in the upper scrotum and rugae appear on the anterior portion. After 40 weeks, the testes can be palpated in the scrotum and rugae cover the scrotal sac. The postterm neonate has deep rugae and a pendulous scrotum. The scrotum is usually more deeply pigmented than the rest of the skin, a difference that is especially apparent in darker-skinned infants. This pigmentation is a response to maternal estrogen. A hydrocele, caused by an accumulation of fluid around the testes, may be found. This can be transilluminated with a light and usually decreases in size without treatment.

If the male infant is born in a breech presentation, the scrotum is edematous and may be bruised (see Fig. 25-7). The swelling and discolouration subside within a few days.

evolve Video–Male Breasts (Supine Position)

Swelling of Breast Tissue

Swelling of the breast tissue in term infants of both sexes is caused by the hyperestrogenism of pregnancy. In a few infants a thin discharge (witch's milk) can be seen. This finding has no clinical significance, requires no treatment, and subsides within a few days as the maternal hormones are eliminated from the infant's body.

The nipples should be symmetrical on the chest. Breast tissue and areola size increase with gestation. The areola appears slightly elevated at 34 weeks of gestation. By 36 weeks, a breast bud of 1 to 2 mm is palpable; this increases to 12 mm by 42 weeks.

Skeletal System

evolve Anatomy Review–Sutures and Fontanels

The infant's skeletal system undergoes rapid development during the first year of life. At birth, more cartilage is present than ossified bone. Because of cephalocaudal (head-to-rump) development, the newborn looks somewhat out of proportion.

The head at term is one fourth of the total body length. The arms are slightly longer than the legs. In the newborn, the legs are one third of the total body length but only 15% of the total body weight. As growth proceeds, the midpoint in head-to-toe measurements gradually descends from the level of the umbilicus at birth to the level of the symphysis pubis at maturity.

The face appears small in relation to the skull. The skull appears large and heavy. Cranial size and shape can be distorted by moulding (the shaping of the fetal head through overlapping of the cranial bones to facilitate movement through the birth canal during labour) (Fig. 24-9).

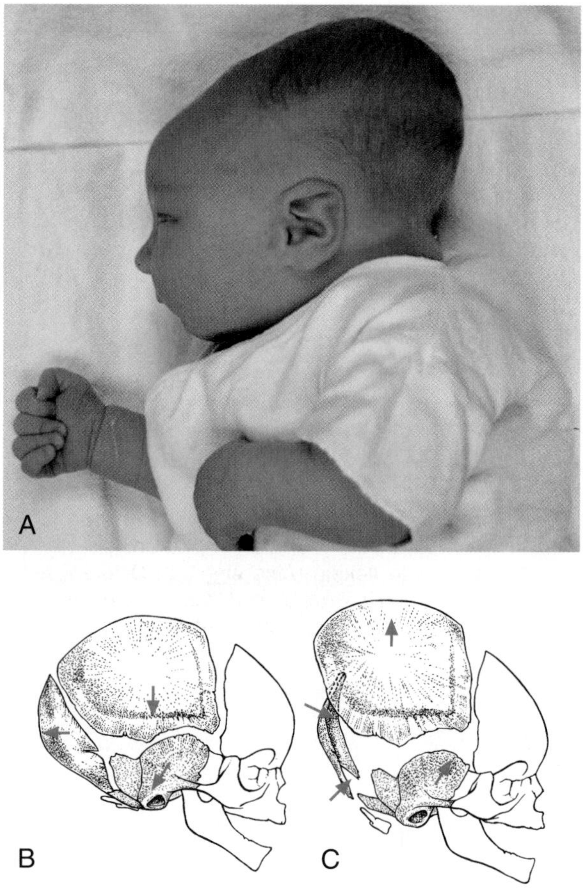

Fig. 24-9 Moulding. **A:** Significant moulding after vaginal birth. **B:** Schematic of bones with no moulding. **C:** Schematic of bones with moulding. *(**A**, Courtesy Kim Molloy, Knoxville, IA.)*

In some newborn infants, there is a significant separation of the knees when the ankles are held together, resulting in an appearance of bowlegs. At birth, there is no apparent arch to the foot. The extremities should be symmetrical and of equal length. Skin folds should be equal and symmetrical. The hips should be checked for dysplasia by a trained clinician using the Ortolani manoeuvre (Fig. 24-10). Fingers and toes should be equal in number and have nails. Extra digits **(polydactyly)** are sometimes found on the hands and feet. Fingers or toes may be fused **(syndactyly).** Creases can be found on the palms of the hands and cover the soles of the term newborn's feet. If the infant's presentation was breech, the knees may remain extended and the infant will maintain the in utero position for several weeks.

Two reflexes are elicited, the grasp and the Babinski reflex. To elicit the grasp reflex, touch the palms of the hands or soles of the feet near the base of the digits, causing flexion or grasping (Fig. 24-11). To elicit the Babinski reflex, stroke the outer sole of the foot upward from the heel across the ball of the foot, causing the big toe to dorsiflex and the other toes to hyperextend (Table 24-1 on p. 624).

The healthy newborn's spine appears straight and can be flexed easily. The vertebrae should appear straight and flat. The base of the spine should be free from a dimple. If a dimple is noted, further inspection is required to determine whether a sinus is present. A pilonidal dimple, especially with a sinus

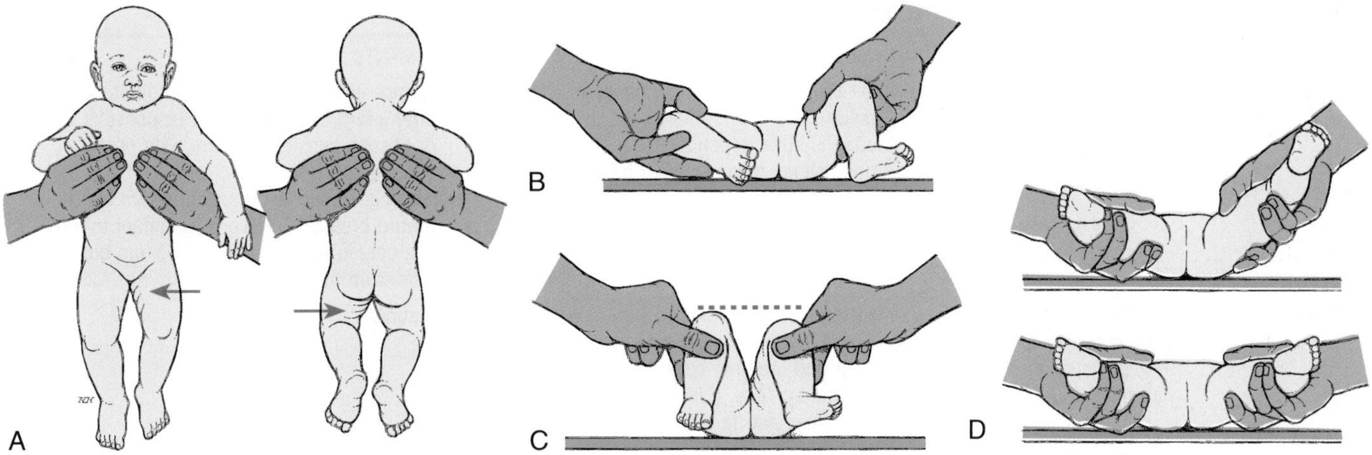

Fig. 24-10 Signs of developmental dysplasia of the hip. **A:** Asymmetry of gluteal and thigh folds with shortening of the thigh (Galeazzi sign). **B:** Limited hip abduction, as seen in flexion (Ortolani test). **C:** Apparent shortening of the femur, as indicated by the level of the knees in flexion (Allis sign). **D:** Ortolani test with femoral head moving in and out of acetabulum (in infants 1 to 2 months old). *(From Hockenberry, M. J., & Wilson, D. [2009].* Wong's essentials of pediatric nursing *[8th ed. p. 453]. St. Louis: Mosby.)*

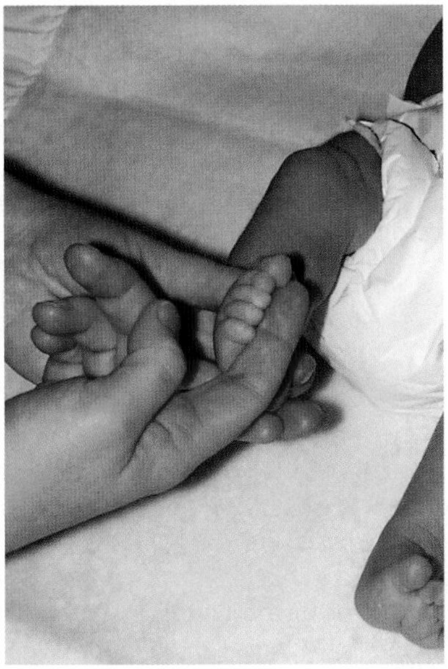

Fig. 24-11 Plantar grasp reflex. *(From Zitelli, B. J., & Davis, H. W. [2007].* Atlas of pediatric physical diagnosis *[5th ed.]. St. Louis: Mosby.)*

and a nevus pilosis (hairy nevus), may be associated with spina bifida.

Neuromuscular System

The neuromuscular system is almost completely developed at birth. The term newborn is a vital, responsive, and reactive being with a remarkable capacity for social interaction and self-organization.

Growth of the brain after birth follows a predictable pattern of rapid growth during infancy and early childhood; growth becomes more gradual during the remainder of the first decade and minimal during adolescence. The cerebellum ends its growth spurt, which began at about 30 gestational weeks, by the end of the first year.

evolve Video—Plantar Grasp

The brain requires glucose, as a source of energy, and a relatively large supply of oxygen for adequate metabolism. Such requirements signal a need for careful assessment of the infant's respiratory status. The necessity for glucose requires attentiveness to those neonates who are at risk for hypoglycemia (e.g., infants of diabetic mothers; infants who are **macrosomic** or small for gestational age; and newborns experiencing prolonged birth, hypoxia, or preterm birth).

Spontaneous motor activity may be seen as transient tremors of the mouth and chin, especially during crying episodes, and of the extremities, notably the arms and hands. Transient tremors are normal and can be observed in nearly every newborn. These tremors should not be present when the infant is quiet and should not persist beyond 1 month of age. Persistent tremors or tremors involving the entire body may indicate pathological conditions. Normal tremors, tremors of hypoglycemia, and central nervous system (CNS) disorders need to be differentiated so corrective care can be instituted as necessary.

Neuromuscular control in the newborn, although limited, can be noted. If newborns are placed face down on a firm surface, they will turn their heads to the side. They will attempt to hold their heads in line with their bodies if they are raised by their arms. Various reflexes serve to promote safety and adequate food intake.

Newborn Reflexes

The newborn infant has many primitive reflexes. The times at which these reflexes appear and disappear reflect the maturity and intactness of the developing nervous system. The most common reflexes found in the normal newborn are described in Table 24-1.

Text continued on page 625.

evolve Video–More Reflexes

evolve Video–Rooting and Sucking

Table 24-1 Assessment of Newborn Reflexes

REFLEX	ELICITING THE REFLEX	CHARACTERISTIC RESPONSE	COMMENTS
Rooting	Touch infant's lip, cheek, or corner of mouth with nipple or finger.	Infant turns head toward stimulus and opens mouth. Rooting is state dependent (e.g., if infant is in deep sleep, reflex may not be elicited).	Response is difficult if not impossible to elicit after infant has been fed; if response is weak or absent, consider preterm birth or neurological defect. Parental guidance: Avoid trying to turn head toward breast or nipple; allow infant to root; response disappears after 3-4* mo but may persist up to 1 yr.
Sucking	Elicit rooting reflex as above. Sucking may also be elicited by gently stroking tongue with nipple.	Infant opens mouth and begins to suck on nipple. A gloved finger may be used to elicit and evaluate suck. Sucking is state dependent (e.g., if infant is in deep sleep, reflex may not be elicited).	See above.
Swallowing	Feed infant; swallowing usually follows sucking and obtaining fluids.	Swallowing is usually coordinated with sucking and breathing and usually occurs without gagging, coughing, apnea, or vomiting.	If response is weak or absent, this may indicate preterm birth, effects of maternal analgesics, or illness that needs investigation. Sucking, swallowing, and breathing are often uncoordinated in preterm infant.
Grasp			
Palmar	Place finger in palm of hand.	Infant's fingers curl around examiner's fingers.	Palmar response lessens by 3-4 mo; parents enjoy this contact with infant.
Plantar (see Fig. 24-11)	Place finger at base of toes.	Toes curl downward.	Plantar response lessens by 8 mo.
Extrusion	Touch or depress tip of tongue.	Newborn forces tongue outward.	Response disappears about fourth to fifth month.
Glabellar (Myerson)	Tap over forehead, bridge of nose, or maxilla of newborn whose eyes are open.	Newborn blinks for first four or five taps.	Continued blinking with repeated taps is consistent with extrapyramidal signs.
Tonic neck or "fencing"	With infant in a supine neutral position, turn head to one side.	With infant facing left side, arm and leg on that side extend; the opposite arm and leg flex (turn head to right, and extremities assume opposite postures).	Responses in leg are more consistent. Complete response disappears by 3-4 mo; incomplete response may be seen until third or fourth year. After 6 wk, persistent response is a sign of an abnormality.

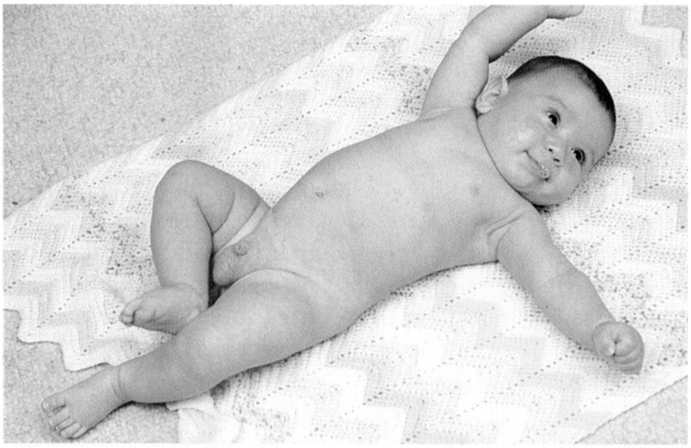

Classic pose in tonic neck reflex. *(Courtesy Marjorie Pyle, RNC, Lifecircle, Costa Mesa, CA.)*

Moro (or startle)	Hold infant in semisitting position, allowing head and trunk to fall backward (with support). Place infant supine on flat surface; make a loud, abrupt noise. This reflex is state dependent.	Symmetrical abduction and extension of arms are seen; fingers fan out and form a *C* with thumb and forefinger; slight tremor may be noted; arms are adducted in embracing motion and return to relaxed flexion and movement. A cry may accompany or follow motor movement. Legs may follow similar pattern of response. Preterm infants do not complete "embrace"; instead, their arms fall backward because of weakness.	Response is present at birth; complete response may be seen until 8 wk; body jerk only is seen between 8 and 18 wk; response is absent by 6 mo if neurological maturation is not delayed; response may be incomplete if infant is in deep sleep state; give parental guidance about normal response. Asymmetrical response may connote injury to brachial plexus, clavicle, or humerus. Persistent response after 6 mo indicates possible neurological abnormality, such as cerebral palsy.

*All durations for persistence of reflexes are based on time elapsed after 40 wk of gestation; that is, if newborn was born at 36 wk of gestation, add 1 mo to all time limits given.

Table 24-1 Assessment of Newborn Reflexes—cont'd

REFLEX	ELICITING THE REFLEX	CHARACTERISTIC RESPONSE	COMMENTS

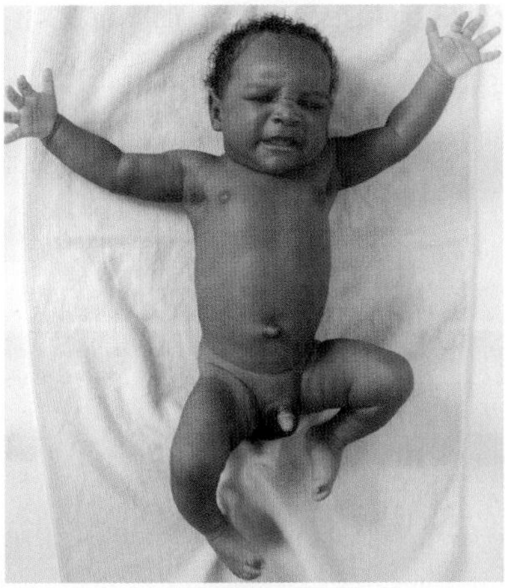

Moro reflex. *(Courtesy Paul Vincent Kuntz, Texas Children's Hospital, Houston.)*

REFLEX	ELICITING THE REFLEX	CHARACTERISTIC RESPONSE	COMMENTS
Stepping or "walking"	Hold infant vertically under arms or on trunk, allowing one foot to touch table surface.	Infant will simulate walking, alternating flexion and extension of feet; term infants walk on soles of their feet, and preterm infants walk on their toes.	Response is normally present for 3-4 wk.

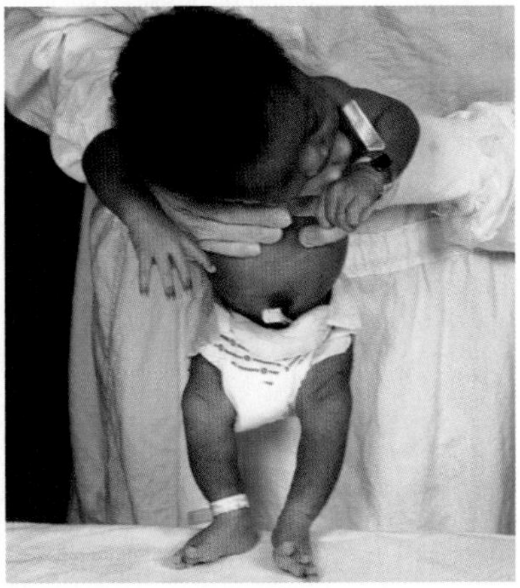

Stepping reflex. *(From Dickason, E. J., Silverman, B. L., & Kaplan, J. A. (1998).* Maternal-infant nursing care *(3rd ed.). St. Louis: Mosby.)*

REFLEX	ELICITING THE REFLEX	CHARACTERISTIC RESPONSE	COMMENTS
Crawling	Place newborn on abdomen.	Newborn makes crawling movements with arms and legs.	Response should disappear about 6 wk of age.

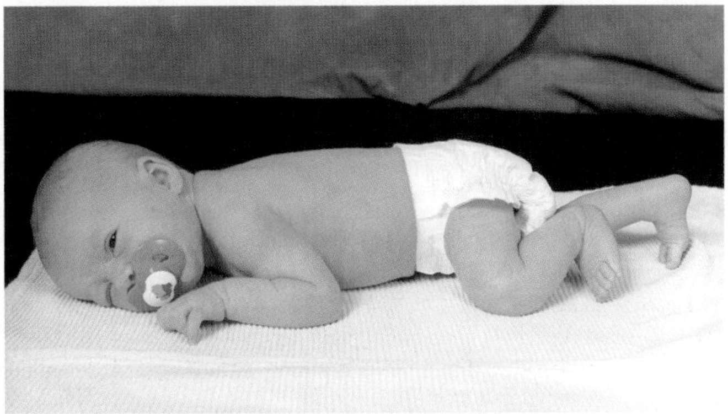

Crawling reflex. *(Courtesy Paul Vincent Kuntz, Houston, Texas Children's Hospital, Houston.)*

REFLEX	ELICITING THE REFLEX	CHARACTERISTIC RESPONSE	COMMENTS
Deep tendon	Use finger instead of percussion hammer to elicit patellar, or knee jerk, reflex; newborn must be relaxed.	Reflex jerk is present; even with newborn relaxed, nonselective overall reaction may occur.	

Continued

Table 24-1 Assessment of Newborn Reflexes—cont'd

REFLEX	ELICITING THE REFLEX	CHARACTERISTIC RESPONSE	COMMENTS
Crossed extension	With infant in supine position, examiner extends one leg of infant and presses down knee. Stimulation of sole of foot of fixated limb should cause free leg to flex, adduct, and extend as if attempting to push away stimulating agent.	Opposite leg flexes, adducts, and then extends.	This reflex should be present during newborn period.

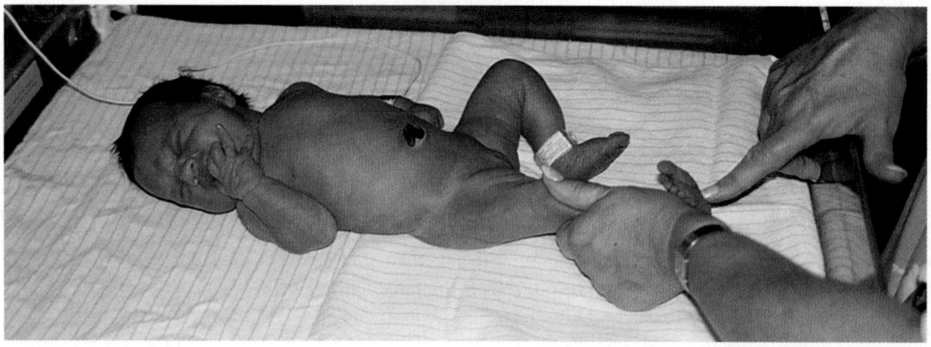

Crossed extension reflex. *(Courtesy Marjorie Pyle, RNC, Lifecircle, Costa Mesa, CA.)*

Babinski (plantar)	On sole of foot, beginning at heel, stroke upward along lateral aspect of sole, then move finger across ball of foot.	All toes hyperextend, with dorsiflexion of big toe—recorded as a positive sign.	Absence requires neurological evaluation, should disappear after 1 yr of age. Response depends on infant's general muscle tone, maturity, and condition.

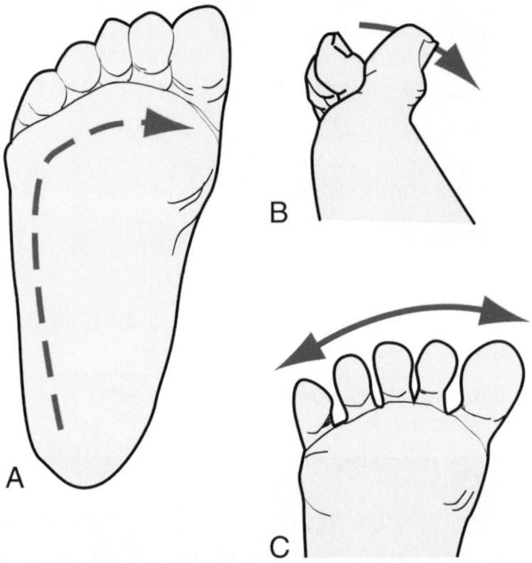

Babinski reflex. **A:** Direction of stroke. **B:** Dorsiflexion of big toe. **C:** Fanning of toes. *(From Hockenberry, M. J., & Wilson, D. [2007].* Wong's nursing care of infants and children *[8th ed.]. St. Louis: Mosby.)*

Pull-to-sit (traction response); postural tone	Pull infant up by wrists from supine position with head in midline.	Head comes forward with body with minimal lag; head falls forward when placed in sitting position.	Response disappears by fourth week.
Truncal incurvation (Galant)	Place infant prone on flat surface; run finger down back about 4-5 cm lateral to spine, first on one side and then down the other. Correct response involves infant flexing trunk and swinging pelvis toward stimulus.	Trunk is flexed and pelvis is swung toward stimulated side.	Absence suggests general depression of nervous system. With transverse lesions of cord, no response below the level of lesion is present. Response may vary but should be obtainable in all infants, including the preterm. If not seen in first few days, it is usually apparent by 5-6 days.

Table 24-1 Assessment of Newborn Reflexes—cont'd

REFLEX	ELICITING THE REFLEX	CHARACTERISTIC RESPONSE	COMMENTS

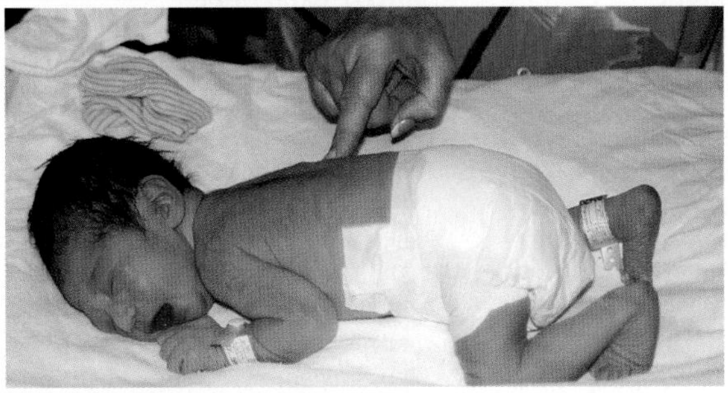

Trunk incurvation reflex. *(Courtesy Marjorie Pyle, RNC, Lifecircle, Costa Mesa, CA.)*

REFLEX	ELICITING THE REFLEX	CHARACTERISTIC RESPONSE	COMMENTS
Magnet	Place infant in supine position, partially flex both lower extremities, and apply light pressure with fingers to soles of feet. Normally, while examiner's fingers maintain contact with soles of feet, lower limbs extend.	Both lower limbs should extend against examiner's pressure.	Absence suggests damage to central nervous system. Weak reflex may be seen after breech presentation without extended legs or may indicate sciatic nerve stretch syndrome. Breech presentation with extended legs may evoke exaggerated response.

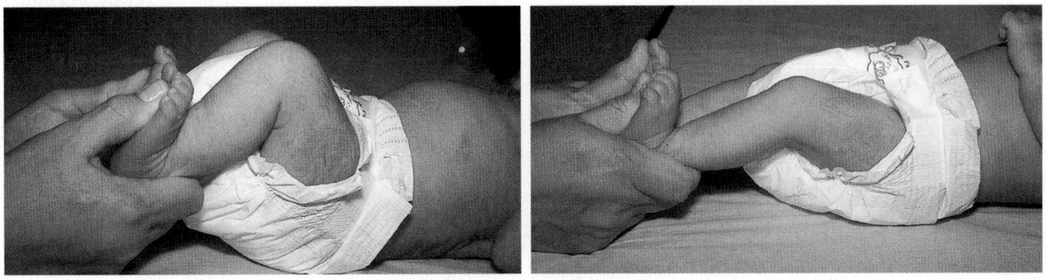

Magnet reflex. *(Courtesy Michael S. Clement, MD, Mesa, AZ.)*

REFLEX	ELICITING THE REFLEX	CHARACTERISTIC RESPONSE	COMMENTS
Additional newborn responses: yawn, stretch, burp, hiccup, sneeze	These are spontaneous behaviours.	They may be slightly depressed temporarily because of maternal analgesia or anaesthesia, fetal hypoxia, or infection.	Parental guidance: Most of these behaviours are pleasurable to parents. Parents need to be assured that behaviours are normal. Sneeze is usually a response to mucus in nose and not an indicator of a cold (upper respiratory tract infection). No treatment is needed for hiccups; sucking may help. In the preterm infant, these are signs of neurodevelopmental immaturity and physiological stress.

Physical Assessment

The assessment of the newborn should progress in a systematic manner, with evaluation and assessment of each system (e.g., respiratory and cardiovascular). It is recommended that assessment of features (e.g., observing general colour, tone, and posture; auscultating heart tones and breath sounds) that least disturbs the newborn be conducted first. The assessment can proceed in a head-to-toe manner. The findings provide a database for implementing the nursing process with newborns and for providing anticipatory guidance for the parents.

An immediate assessment of the newborn is carried out to evaluate the infant's transition to extrauterine life. The Apgar score (see Table 25-1), determined at 1 and 5 minutes, provides information that must be considered in the context of data from the total assessment.

A complete physical examination should be done within 24 hours after birth, after the newborn's temperature stabilizes or the infant has been placed under a radiant warmer. The area used for examination should be well lit, warm, and free from drafts. The infant is undressed as needed and placed on a firm, warmed, flat surface. It is important that the examination be done in such a way that the infant maintains adequate body temperature, as the impact of cold stress is significant (see Fig. 24-2). The physical assessment should begin with a review of the maternal history and prenatal and intrapartum records. This provides a background for recognition of any potential problems. This assessment also includes general appearance, behaviour, vital signs measurements, and maternal–infant interactions. Descriptions of any variations from normal and all abnormal findings should be included (Table 24-2). Ideally,

Text continued on page 636.

Table 24-2 Physical Assessment of Newborn Normal Findings

AREA ASSESSED AND APPRAISAL PROCEDURE	AVERAGE FINDINGS	NORMAL VARIATIONS	DEVIATIONS FROM NORMAL RANGE—POSSIBLE PROBLEMS (ETIOLOGY)
Posture			
Inspect newborn before disturbing for assessment. Refer to maternal chart for fetal presentation, position, and type of birth (vaginal, surgical), since newborn readily assumes in utero position.	Vertex: arms, legs in moderate flexion; fists clenched Resistance to having extremities extended for examination or measurement, crying possible when attempted Cessation of crying when allowed to resume curled-up fetal position (lateral) Normal spontaneous movement bilaterally asynchronous (legs flex and extend in alternating fashion) but equal extension in all extremities	Frank breech: legs straighter and stiff, newborn assuming intrauterine position in repose for a few days Prenatal pressure on limb or shoulder possibly causing temporary facial asymmetry or resistance to extension of extremities	Hypotonia, relaxed posture while awake (preterm or hypoxia in utero, maternal medications, neuromuscular disorder such as spinal muscular atrophy) Hypertonia (chemical dependence, central nervous system [CNS] disorder) Limitation of motion in any of extremities (see Skeletal System, p. 620)
Vital Signs			
Check heart rate and pulses Thorax (chest): Inspection Palpation Auscultation Apex: mitral valve Second interspace, left of sternum: pulmonic valve Second interspace, right of sternum: aortic valve Junction of xiphoid process and sternum: tricuspid valve	Visible pulsations in left midclavicular line, fifth intercostal space Apical pulse, fourth intercostal space, midclavicular region, 110–160 beats/min Quality: first sound (closure of mitral and tricuspid valves) and second sound (closure of aortic and pulmonic valves) sharp and clear	80–100 beats/min (sleeping) to 180 beats/min (crying); possibly irregular for brief periods, especially after crying Murmur, especially over base or at left sternal border in interspace 3–4 (foramen ovale anatomically closing at about 1 yr)	Tachycardia: persistent, ≥180 beats/min (respiratory distress syndrome [RDS], pneumonia, fever) Bradycardia: persistent, ≤80 beats/min (congenital heart block, maternal lupus) Murmur (possibly functional) Arrhythmias: irregular rate Sounds: Distant (pneumopericardium) Poor quality Extra (S_3, S_4) Heart on right side of chest (dextrocardia), often accompanied by reversal of intestines
Peripheral pulses: femoral, brachial, popliteal, posterior tibial	Peripheral pulses equal and strong		Weak or absent peripheral pulses (decreased cardiac output, thrombus, possible coarctation of aorta if weak on left and strong on right) Bounding
Obtain temperature Axillary: method of choice until 3 yr of age Temporal and intra-auricular thermometers: not proved effective in measuring newborn temperature	Axillary: 37°C Temperature stabilized by 6–8 hr of age	36.5°-37.2°C Heat loss from evaporation, conduction, convection, radiation (see Fig. 24-1)	Subnormal (preterm birth, infection, low environmental temperature, inadequate clothing, dehydration) Increased (infection, high environmental temperature, excessive clothing, proximity to heating unit or in direct sunshine, chemical dependence, dehydration) Temperature not stabilized by 6–8 hr after birth (if mother received magnesium sulphate, newborn less able to conserve heat by vasoconstriction; maternal analgesics possibly reducing thermal stability in newborn)

Table 24-2 Physical Assessment of Newborn Normal Findings—cont'd

AREA ASSESSED AND APPRAISAL PROCEDURE	AVERAGE FINDINGS	NORMAL VARIATIONS	DEVIATIONS FROM NORMAL RANGE—POSSIBLE PROBLEMS (ETIOLOGY)
Vital Signs—cont'd			
Observe and monitor respiratory rate and effort: Observe respirations when infant is at rest. Count respirations for a full minute. Listen for sounds with stethoscope and observe chest movement. Observe respiratory effort.	30–60 breaths/min Tendency to be shallow and irregular in rate, rhythm, and depth when infant is awake Crackles may be heard after birth No adventitious sounds audible on inspiration and expiration Breath sounds: bronchial: loud, clear	Short periodic breathing episodes and no evidence of respiratory distress or apnea (>20 seconds); periodic breathing First period (reactivity): 40–60 breaths/min Second period: 50–70 breaths/min Stabilization (1–2 days): 30–60 breaths/min Crackles (fine)	Apneic episodes: >20 sec (preterm infant: rapid warming or cooling of infant; CNS or blood glucose instability) Bradypnea: <25 breaths/min (maternal narcosis from analgesics or anaesthetics, birth trauma) Tachypnea: >60 breaths/min (RDS, transient tachypnea of the newborn, congenital diaphragmatic hernia) Breath sounds: Crackles (coarse), rhonchi, wheezing Expiratory grunt (narrowing of bronchi) Distress evidenced by nasal flaring, grunting, retractions, laboured breathing Stridor (upper airway occlusion)
Obtain blood pressure (BP) Check oscillometric monitor BP cuff: BP cuff width affects readings; use appropriately sized cuff and palpate brachial, popliteal, or posterior tibial pulse (depending on measurement site). Not routinely done in healthy newborns	At birth: Systolic: 60–80 mm Hg Diastolic: 40–50 mm Hg At 10 days: Systolic: 95–100 mm Hg Diastolic: 45–75 mm Hg	Variation with change in activity level: awake, crying, sleeping	Difference between upper and lower extremity pressures (coarctation of aorta) Hypotension (sepsis, hypovolemia) Hypertension (coarctation of aorta, renal involvement, thrombus)
Weight			
Put protective liner cloth or paper in place and adjust scale to 0 g. Weigh at same time each day. Protect newborn from heat loss.	Female: 3400 g Male: 3500 g Regaining of birth weight within first 2 wk	2500–4000 g Acceptable weight loss: 5 to 10% in first 3–5 days Second baby weighing more than first (on average)	Weight ≤2500 g (preterm, small for gestational age, rubella syndrome) Weight ≥4000 g (large for gestational age, maternal diabetes, heredity—normal for these parents) Weight loss 10–15% (growth failure, dehydration); assess breastfeeding success, latch-on

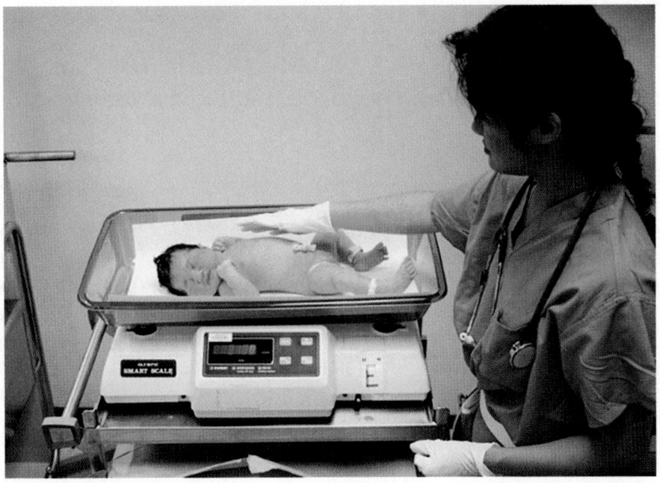

Weighing the infant. Note that a hand is held over the infant as a safety measure. The scale is covered to protect against cross-infection and heat loss. *(Courtesy Kim Molloy, Knoxville, IA.)*

Note: Weight, length, and head circumference should all be close to the same percentile for any child.

Continued

Table 24-2 Physical Assessment of Newborn Normal Findings—cont'd

AREA ASSESSED AND APPRAISAL PROCEDURE	AVERAGE FINDINGS	NORMAL VARIATIONS	DEVIATIONS FROM NORMAL RANGE—POSSIBLE PROBLEMS (ETIOLOGY)
Length			
Measure length from top of head to heel. Measuring is difficult in term infants because of moulding and incomplete extension of knees.	45-55 cm		<45 cm or >55 cm (chromosomal abnormality, heredity—normal for these parents); some syndromes result in shorter-than-average limb length (skeletal dysplasias, achondroplasia)

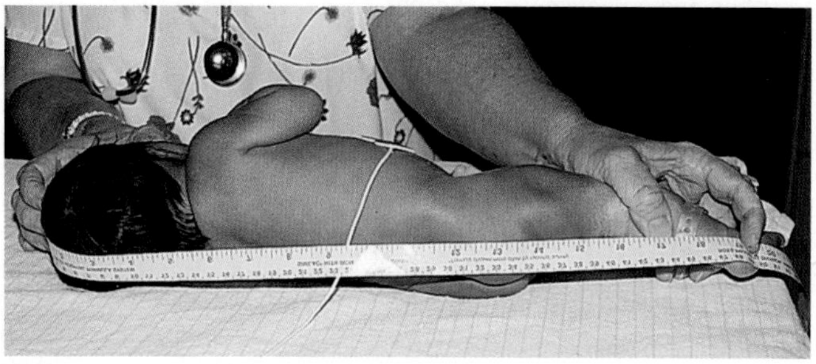

Length, crown to heel. To determine total length, include length of legs. If measurements are taken before the infant's initial bath, wear gloves. *(Courtesy Marjorie Pyle, RNC, Lifecircle, Costa Mesa, CA.)*

AREA ASSESSED AND APPRAISAL PROCEDURE	AVERAGE FINDINGS	NORMAL VARIATIONS	DEVIATIONS FROM NORMAL RANGE—POSSIBLE PROBLEMS (ETIOLOGY)
Head Circumference			
Measure head at greatest diameter: occipitofrontal circumference May need to remeasure on second or third day after resolution of moulding and caput succedaneum	33-35 cm Circumference of head and chest approximately the same for first 1 or 2 days after birth; chest circumference rarely measured on routine basis	32-36.8 cm	Microcephaly: head ≤32 cm (maternal rubella, toxoplasmosis, cytomegalovirus, fused cranial sutures [craniosynostosis]) Hydrocephaly: sutures widely separated, circumference ≥4 cm more than chest circumference (infection) Increased intracranial pressure (hemorrhage, space-occupying lesion)

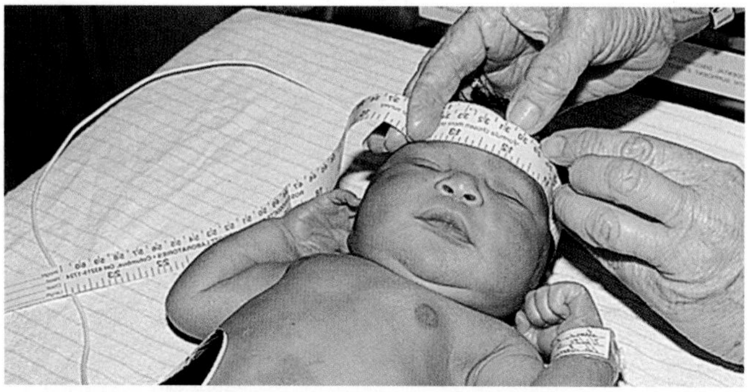

Circumference of head. *(Courtesy Marjorie Pyle, RNC, Lifecircle, Costa Mesa, CA.)*

AREA ASSESSED AND APPRAISAL PROCEDURE	AVERAGE FINDINGS	NORMAL VARIATIONS	DEVIATIONS FROM NORMAL RANGE—POSSIBLE PROBLEMS (ETIOLOGY)
Skin			
Check colour. Inspect and palpate: Inspect seminaked newborn in well-lit, warm area without drafts; natural daylight is best. Inspect newborn when quiet and alert.	Generally pink Varying with ethnic origin; skin pigmentation beginning to deepen right after birth in basal layer of epidermis Acrocyanosis common after birth	Mottling Harlequin sign Plethora Telangiectases ("stork bites" or capillary hemangiomas) (see Fig. 24-7, A) Erythema toxicum neonatorum ("newborn rash") (see Fig. 24-7, B) Milia	Dark red (preterm, polycythemia) Gray (hypotension, poor perfusion) Pallor (cardiovascular problem, CNS damage, blood dyscrasia, blood loss, twin-to-twin transfusion, infection) Cyanosis (hypothermia, infection, hypoglycemia, cardiopulmonary diseases, neurological, or respiratory malformations)
		Petechiae over presenting part	Generalized petechiae (clotting factor deficiency, infection)
		Ecchymoses from forceps in vertex births or over buttocks, genitalia, and legs in breech births	Generalized ecchymoses (hemorrhagic disease)

Note: Weight, length, and head circumference should all be close to the same percentile for any child.

Table 24-2 Physical Assessment of Newborn Normal Findings—cont'd

AREA ASSESSED AND APPRAISAL PROCEDURE	AVERAGE FINDINGS	NORMAL VARIATIONS	DEVIATIONS FROM NORMAL RANGE—POSSIBLE PROBLEMS (ETIOLOGY)
Skin—cont'd			
Observe for jaundice	None at birth	Physiological jaundice in up to 60% of term infants in first week of life	Jaundice within first 24 hr (increased hemolysis, Rh isoimmunization, ABO incompatibility)
Observe for birthmarks or bruises: Inspect and palpate for location, size, distribution, characteristics, and colour, if obstructing airway or oral cavity		Mongolian spot (see Fig. 24-6) in infants of African, Asian, or other ethnicities with darker-coloured skin	Capillary hemangiomas Nevus flammeus: port-wine stain Nevus vasculosus: strawberry hemangioma Cavernous hemangioma
Check skin condition: Inspect and palpate for intactness, smoothness, texture, edema, pressure points if ill or immobilized	Eyelid edema (result of eye prophylaxis) Opacity: few large blood vessels visible indistinctly over abdomen	Slightly thick; superficial cracking, peeling, especially of hands, feet No visible blood vessels, a few large vessels clearly visible over abdomen Some fingernail scratches	Edema on hands, feet; pitting over tibia; periorbital (overhydration; hydrops) Texture thin, smooth, or of medium thickness; rash or superficial peeling visible (preterm, postterm) Numerous vessels very visible over abdomen (preterm) Texture thick, parchmentlike; cracking, peeling (postterm) Skin tags, webbing Papules, pustules, vesicles, ulcers, maceration (impetigo, candidiasis, herpes, diaper rash)
Weigh infant as per routine. Inspect and palpate: Gently pinch skin between thumb and forefinger over abdomen and inner thigh to check for turgor. Note presence of subcutaneous fat deposits (adipose pads) over cheeks and buttocks.	After pinch is released, skin returns to original state immediately.	Normal weight loss after birth: up to 10% of birth weight Dehydration: loss of weight is best indicator Possibly puffy Variation in amount of subcutaneous fat	Loose, wrinkled skin (prematurity, postmaturity, dehydration: fold of skin persisting after release of pinch) Tense, tight, shiny skin (edema, extreme cold, shock, infection) Lack of subcutaneous fat, prominence of clavicle or ribs (preterm, malnutrition)
Observe vernix caseosa:	Whitish, cheesy, odourless	Usually more found in creases, folds	Absent or minimal (postterm) Abundant (preterm) Green colour (possible in utero release of meconium or presence of bilirubin) Odour (possible intrauterine infection)
Assess lanugo: Inspect for this fine, downy hair, amount and distribution.	Over shoulders, pinnae of ears, forehead	Variation in amount	Absent (postterm) Abundant (preterm, especially if lanugo abundant, long, and thick over back)
Head			
Palpate skin.	See Skin (this table)	Caput succedaneum, possibly showing some ecchymosis (see Fig. 24-5, A)	Cephalhematoma (see Fig. 24-5, C)
Inspect shape and size.	Making up one fourth of body length Moulding (see Fig. 24-9)	Slight asymmetry from intrauterine position Lack of moulding (preterm, breech presentation, Caesarean birth)	Severe moulding (birth trauma) Indentation (fracture from trauma)

Continued

Table 24-2 Physical Assessment of Newborn Normal Findings—cont'd

AREA ASSESSED AND APPRAISAL PROCEDURE	AVERAGE FINDINGS	NORMAL VARIATIONS	DEVIATIONS FROM NORMAL RANGE—POSSIBLE PROBLEMS (ETIOLOGY)
Head—cont'd			
Palpate, inspect, and note status of fontanels (open vs. closed).	Anterior fontanel 5-cm diamond, increasing as moulding resolves Posterior fontanel triangle, smaller than anterior	Variation in fontanel size with degree of moulding Difficulty in feeling fontanels possible because of moulding	Fontanels: Full, bulging (tumour, hemorrhage, infection) Large, flat, soft (malnutrition, hydrocephaly, delayed bone age, hypothyroidism) Depressed (dehydration)
Palpate sutures.	Palpable and separated sutures	Possible overlap of sutures with moulding	Sutures: Widely spaced (hydrocephaly) Premature closure (fused) (craniosynostosis)
Inspect pattern, distribution, and amount of hair; feel texture.	Silky, single strands lying flat; growth pattern toward face and neck	Variation in amount	Fine, woolly (preterm) Unusual swirls, patterns, or hairline; or coarse, brittle (endocrine or genetic disorders)
Eyes			
Check placement on face.	Eyes and space between eyes each one-third the distance from outer (left) to outer (right) canthus	Epicanthal folds (upward sloping): characteristic in some ethnicities	Epicanthal folds when present with other signs (chromosomal disorders such as Down, cri-du-chat syndromes)

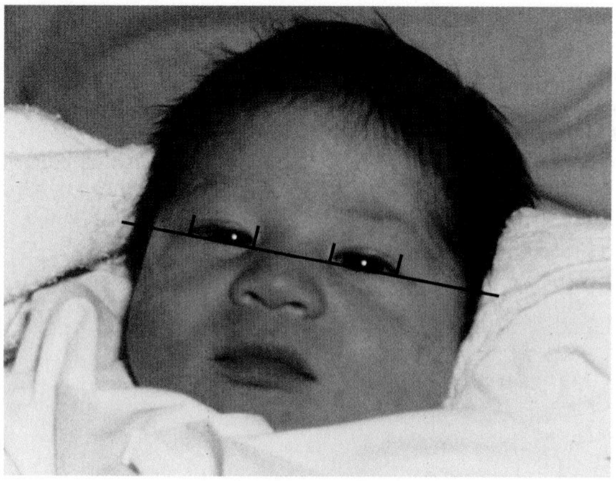

Eyes. In pseudostrabismus, inner epicanthal folds cause the eyes to appear misaligned; however, corneal light reflexes are perfectly symmetrical. Eyes are symmetrical in size and shape and are well placed.

AREA ASSESSED AND APPRAISAL PROCEDURE	AVERAGE FINDINGS	NORMAL VARIATIONS	DEVIATIONS FROM NORMAL RANGE—POSSIBLE PROBLEMS (ETIOLOGY)
Check for symmetry in size and shape.	Symmetrical in size, shape		
Check eyelids for size, movement, and blink.	Blink reflex	Edema if eye prophylaxis ointment instilled	
Assess for discharge.	None No tears	Occasional presence of some tears	Discharge: purulent (infection) Chemical conjunctivitis from eye medication is common—requires no treatment
Evaluate eyeballs for presence, size, and shape.	Both present and of equal size, both round, firm	Subconjunctival hemorrhage	Agenesis or absence of one or both eyeballs Lens opacity or absence of red reflex (congenital cataracts, possibly from rubella, retinoblastoma [cat's eye reflex]) Lesions: coloboma, absence of part of iris (congenital) Pink colour of iris (albinism) Jaundiced sclera (hyperbilirubinemia)

Table 24-2 Physical Assessment of Newborn Normal Findings—cont'd

AREA ASSESSED AND APPRAISAL PROCEDURE	AVERAGE FINDINGS	NORMAL VARIATIONS	DEVIATIONS FROM NORMAL RANGE—POSSIBLE PROBLEMS (ETIOLOGY)
Eyes—cont'd			
Check pupils	Present, equal in size, reactive to light		Pupils: unequal, constricted, dilated, fixed (intracranial pressure, medications, tumour)
Evaluate eyeball movement.	Random, jerky, uneven, focus possible briefly, following to midline	Transient strabismus or nystagmus until third or fourth month	Persistent strabismus Doll's eyes (increased intracranial pressure) Sunset (increased intracranial pressure)
Assess eyebrows: amount of hair, pattern	Distinct (not connected in midline)		Connection in midline (Cornelia de Lange syndrome)
Nose			
Observe shape, placement, patency, and configuration.	Midline Some mucus but no drainage Preferential nose breather Sneezing to clear nose	Slight deformity (flat or deviated to one side) from passage through birth canal	Copious drainage (rarely, congenital syphilis) Blockage–membranous or bone with cyanosis at rest and return of pink colour with crying (choanal atresia) Malformed (congenital syphilis, chromosomal disorder) Flaring of nares (respiratory distress)
Ears			
Observe size, placement on head, amount of cartilage, open auditory canal	Correct placement: line drawn through inner and outer canthi of eyes reaching to top notch of ears (at junction with scalp) Well-formed, firm cartilage	Size: small, large, floppy Darwin's tubercle (nodule on posterior helix)	Agenesis Lack of cartilage (preterm) Low placement (chromosomal disorder, cognitive impairment, kidney disorder) Preauricular tag or sinus Size: possibly overly prominent or protruding ears

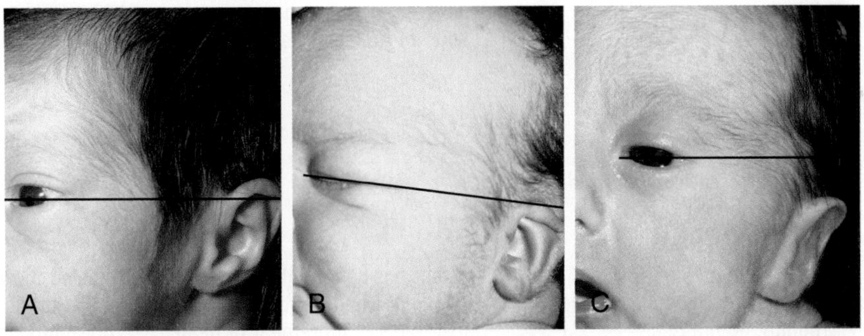

Placement of ears on the head in relation to a line drawn from the inner to the outer canthus of the eye. **A:** Normal position. **B:** Abnormally angled ear. **C:** True low-set ear. *(Courtesy Mead Johnson & Co., LLC.)*

AREA ASSESSED AND APPRAISAL PROCEDURE	AVERAGE FINDINGS	NORMAL VARIATIONS	DEVIATIONS FROM NORMAL RANGE—POSSIBLE PROBLEMS (ETIOLOGY)
Assess hearing. Perform newborn hearing screening to identify deficits (in some provinces).	Responds to voice and other sounds	State (e.g., alert, asleep) influencing response	Lack of response to loud noise should not imply deafness.
Face			
Observe overall appearance and symmetry of face.	Rounded and symmetrical; influenced by birth type or any moulding	Positional deformities associated with intrauterine positioning, cranial moulding	Asymmetrical facial features may be accompanied by other characteristics such as low-set ears, absence of outer ear, or other structural disorders (hereditary, chromosomal aberration)

Continued

Table 24-2 Physical Assessment of Newborn Normal Findings—cont'd

AREA ASSESSED AND APPRAISAL PROCEDURE	AVERAGE FINDINGS	NORMAL VARIATIONS	DEVIATIONS FROM NORMAL RANGE—POSSIBLE PROBLEMS (ETIOLOGY)
Mouth			
Inspect and palpate. Assess buccal mucosa: Dry or moist Pink Status intact Assess lips for colour, configuration, and movement.	Symmetry of lip movement	Transient circumoral cyanosis	Apparent anomalies in placement, size, shape (cleft lip and/or palate, gums) Cyanosis, circumoral pallor (respiratory distress, hypothermia) Asymmetry in movement of lips (seventh cranial nerve paralysis)
Check gums.	Pink gums	Inclusion cysts (Epstein pearls—Bohn nodules, whitish, hard nodules on gums or roof of mouth)	Teeth: predeciduous or deciduous (hereditary)
Assess tongue for colour, mobility, movement, and size.	Tongue not protruding; freely movable; symmetrical in shape, movement Sucking pads inside cheeks	Short lingual frenulum (tongue-tie)	Macroglossia (preterm, chromosomal disorder) Thrush: white plaques on cheeks or tongue that bleed if touched (*Candida albicans*)
Assess palate (soft, hard): Arch Uvula	Soft and hard palates intact Uvula in midline	Anatomical groove in palate to accommodate nipple, disappearance by 3–4 yr of age Epstein pearls	Cleft hard or soft palate
Assess chin.	Distinct chin		Micrognathia—recessed chin with prominent overbite (Pierre Robin sequence or other syndrome)
Evaluate saliva for amount and character.	Mouth moist, pink		Excessive salivation and choking or turning blue (esophageal atresia, tracheoesophageal fistula)
Check reflexes: Rooting, sucking, extrusion See Table 24-1.	Reflexes present	Reflex response dependent on state of wakefulness and hunger	Absent (preterm)
Neck			
Inspect and palpate for movement, flexibility, masses, and bruising.	Short, thick, surrounded by skin folds; no webbing		Webbing (Turner syndrome)
Check sternocleidomastoid muscles, movement and position of head.	Head held in midline (sternocleidomastoid muscles equal), no masses Freedom of movement from side to side and flexion and extension; no movement of chin past shoulder	Transient positional deformity apparent when newborn is at rest; passive movement of head possible	Restricted movement, holding of head at angle (torticollis [wryneck], opisthotonos) Absence of head control (preterm birth, Down syndrome, hypotonia [spinal muscular atrophy])
Assess trachea for position and thyroid gland.	Thyroid not palpable		Mass (enlarged thyroid, cystic hygroma) Distended veins (cardiopulmonary disorder) Skin tags
Chest			
Inspect and palpate: Shape	Almost circular, barrel shaped	Tip of sternum possibly prominent	Bulging of chest, unequal movement (pneumothorax, pneumomediastinum) Malformation (funnel chest—pectus excavatum)
Observe respiratory movements.	Symmetrical chest movements, chest and abdominal movements synchronized during respirations	Occasional retractions, especially when crying	Retractions with or without respiratory distress (preterm, RDS) Paradoxical breathing

evolve Video–Neck (Posterior)

Table 24-2 Physical Assessment of Newborn Normal Findings—cont'd

AREA ASSESSED AND APPRAISAL PROCEDURE	AVERAGE FINDINGS	NORMAL VARIATIONS	DEVIATIONS FROM NORMAL RANGE—POSSIBLE PROBLEMS (ETIOLOGY)
Chest—cont'd			
Evaluate clavicles.	Clavicles intact		Fracture of clavicle (trauma); crepitus
Assess ribs.	Rib cage symmetrical, intact; moves with respirations		Poor development of rib cage and musculature (preterm)
Assess nipples for size, placement, and number.	Nipples prominent, well formed, symmetrically placed		Nipples: Supernumerary, along nipple line Malpositioned or widely spaced
Observe breast tissue.	Breast nodule: approximately 6 mm in term infant	Breast nodule: 3–10 mm Secretion of witch's milk	Lack of breast tissue (preterm) Sounds: bowel sounds (see Abdomen, below)
Abdomen			
Inspect and palpate umbilical cord.	Two arteries, one vein Whitish gray Definite demarcation between cord and skin; no intestinal structures within cord Dry around base, drying Odourless Cord clamp may be in place	Reducible umbilical hernia	One artery (renal anomaly) Meconium stained (intrauterine distress) Bleeding or oozing around cord (hemorrhagic disease) Redness or drainage around cord (infection, possible persistence of urachus) Hernia: herniation of abdominal contents through cord opening (e.g., omphalocele); defect covered with thin, friable membrane, possibly extensive
Inspect size of abdomen and palpate contour.	Rounded, prominent, dome shaped because abdominal musculature not fully developed Liver possibly palpable 1–2 cm below right costal margin No other masses palpable No distension Few visible veins on abdominal surface	Some diastasis recti (separation) of abdominal musculature	Gastroschisis: herniation of abdominal contents to the side or above the cord; contents not covered by membranous tissue and may include liver Distension at birth (ruptured viscus, genitourinary masses or malformations: hydronephrosis, teratomas, abdominal tumours): Mild (overfeeding, high gastrointestinal tract obstruction) Marked (lower gastrointestinal tract obstruction, anorectal malformation, anal stenosis), often with bilious emesis Intermittent or transient (overfeeding) Partial intestinal obstruction (stenosis of bowel) Visible peristalsis (obstruction) Malrotation of bowel or adhesions Sepsis (infection)
Auscultate bowel sounds and note number, amount, and character of stools.	Sounds present within minutes after birth in healthy term infant Meconium stool passing within 24–48 hr after birth		Scaphoid, with bowel sounds in chest and severe respiratory distress (congenital diaphragmatic hernia)
Assess colour.		Linea nigra possibly apparent and caused by hormone influence during pregnancy	
Observe movement with respiration.	Respirations primarily diaphragmatic, abdominal and chest movement synchronous		Decreased or absent abdominal movement with breathing (phrenic nerve palsy, congenital diaphragmatic hernia)

Continued

Table 24-2 Physical Assessment of Newborn Normal Findings—cont'd

AREA ASSESSED AND APPRAISAL PROCEDURE	AVERAGE FINDINGS	NORMAL VARIATIONS	DEVIATIONS FROM NORMAL RANGE—POSSIBLE PROBLEMS (ETIOLOGY)
Genitalia			
Female (see Fig. 24-8, A)			
Inspect and palpate: General appearance Clitoris Labia majora Labia minora Discharge Vagina Urinary meatus	Female genitalia Usually edematous Usually edematous, covering labia minora in term newborns Possible protrusion over labia majora Smegma Open orifice Mucoid discharge Hymenal/vaginal tag Beneath clitoris, difficult to see	Increased pigmentation caused by pregnancy hormones Edema and ecchymosis after breech birth Blood-tinged discharge from pseudomenstruation caused by pregnancy hormones Some vernix caseosa between labia possible Rust-stained urine (uric acid crystals)	Ambiguous genitalia—wide variation (small phallus not well distinguished from enlarged clitoris) Virilized female—extremely large clitoris (congenital adrenal hyperplasia) Enlarged clitoris with urinary meatus on tip, absent scrotum, micropenis, fused labia Stenosed meatus Labia majora widely separated and labia minora prominent (preterm) Absence of vaginal orifice Fecal discharge (fistula) Bladder exstrophy (bladder outside abdominal cavity and turned inside out)
Male (see Fig. 24-8, B) Inspect and palpate:			
General appearance	Male genitalia	Increased size and pigmentation caused by pregnancy hormones Wide variation in size of genitalia	Ambiguous genitalia
Penis:			Micropenis
Urinary meatus appearance—should be at tip of penile shaft	Foreskin covers glans (if uncircumcised), meatus at tip of penis		Urinary meatus not on tip of glans penis (hypospadias, epispadias, foreskin may be retracted or absent); chordee (ventral curvature)
Prepuce (foreskin)—do not forcibly retract foreskin if uncircumcised	Prepuce covering glans penis and not retractable	Prepuce removed if circumcised	Round meatal opening
Scrotum: Rugae (wrinkles)	Large, edematous, pendulous in term infant; covered with rugae	Scrotal edema and ecchymosis if breech birth Hydrocele, small, noncommunicating	Scrotum smooth and testes undescended (preterm, cryptorchidism) Bifid scrotum Hydrocele Inguinal hernia
Testes	Palpable on each side	Bulge palpable in inguinal canal	Undescended (preterm)
Check reflexes: Cremasteric	Testes retracted, especially when newborn is chilled		
Check urination	Voiding within 24 hr, stream adequate, amount adequate Voiding 6-10 times/day by day 5-6	Rust-stained urine (uric acid crystals)	No void in first 24 hr Renal agenesis: Potter syndrome
Extremities			
Make a general check: Inspect and palpate: Degree of flexion Range of motion Symmetry of motion Muscle tone	Assuming of position maintained in utero Attitude of general flexion Full range of motion, spontaneous movements	Transient (positional) deformities	Limited motion (malformations) Poor muscle tone (preterm, maternal medications, CNS anomalies)

evolve Video—Cremasteric Reflex

Table 24-2 Physical Assessment of Newborn Normal Findings—cont'd

AREA ASSESSED AND APPRAISAL PROCEDURE	AVERAGE FINDINGS	NORMAL VARIATIONS	DEVIATIONS FROM NORMAL RANGE—POSSIBLE PROBLEMS (ETIOLOGY)
Extremeties—cont'd			
Observe arms and hands: Inspect and palpate: Colour Intactness Appropriate placement	Longer than legs in newborn period Contours and movements symmetrical	Slight tremors sometimes apparent Some acrocyanosis	Asymmetry of movement (fracture or crepitus, brachial nerve trauma, malformations) Asymmetry of contour (malformations, fracture) Amelia or phocomelia (teratogens) Palmar creases Simian line with short, incurved little fingers (Down syndrome)
Number of fingers	Five on each hand Fist often clenched with thumb under fingers		Webbing of fingers: syndactyly Absence or excess of fingers Strong, rigid flexion; persistent fists; positioning of fists in front of mouth constantly (CNS disorder) Yellowed nail beds (meconium staining)
Evaluate joints: Shoulder Elbow Wrist Fingers	Full range of motion, symmetrical contour		Increased tonicity, clonus, prolonged tremors (CNS disorder)
Check reflex: grasp (palmar and plantar)			
Observe legs and feet: Inspect and palpate: Colour Intactness Length in relation to arms and body and to each other	Appearance of bowing because lateral muscles more developed than medial muscles	Feet appearing to turn in but can be easily rotated externally, positional defects tending to correct while infant is crying Acrocyanosis	Amelia, phocomelia (chromosomal defect, teratogenic effect) Temperature of one leg differing from that of the other (circulatory deficiency, CNS disorder)
Number of toes	Five on each foot		Webbing, syndactyly (chromosomal defect) Absence or excess of digits (chromosomal defect, familial trait)
Femur Head of femur as legs are flexed and abducted, placement in acetabulum (see Fig. 24-10)	Intact femur		Femoral fracture (difficult breech birth) Developmental dysplasia of the hip
Major gluteal folds	Major gluteal folds even		Hip dysplasia
Soles of feet	Soles well lined (or wrinkled) over two thirds of foot in term infants Plantar fat pad giving flat-footed effect		Soles of feet: Few creases (preterm) Covered with creases (postterm) Congenital clubfoot
Evaluate joints: Hip Knee Ankle Toes	Full range of motion, symmetrical contour		Hypermobility of joints (Down syndrome)
Check reflexes (see Table 24-1)			Asymmetrical movement (trauma, CNS disorder)
Back			
Assess anatomy: Inspect and palpate: Spine, shoulders, scapulae, iliac crests	Spine straight and easily flexed Infant able to raise and support head momentarily when prone	Temporary minor positional deformities; correction with passive manipulation	Limitation of movement (fusion or deformity of vertebra)

Continued

evolve Video–Upper Extremities

evolve Video–Legs (Symmetry, Length)

Table 24-2 Physical Assessment of Newborn Normal Findings—cont'd

AREA ASSESSED AND APPRAISAL PROCEDURE	AVERAGE FINDINGS	NORMAL VARIATIONS	DEVIATIONS FROM NORMAL RANGE—POSSIBLE PROBLEMS (ETIOLOGY)
Back—cont'd			
Base of spine—pilonidal dimple or sinus	Shoulders, scapulae, and iliac crests lining up in same plane		Meningocele, myelomeningocele (spina bifida cystica) Pigmented nevus with tuft of hair, located anywhere along the spine, often associated with spina bifida occulta Sinus (opening to spinal cord)
Check reflexes (spinal related): Test trunk incurvation reflex (see Table 24-1).	Trunk flexed and pelvis swings to stimulated side	May not be apparent in first few days but is usually present in 5–6 days	If transverse lesion is present, no response below lesion; absence of response: CNS abnormality or CNS depression
Test magnet reflex.	Lower limbs extend as pressure applied to feet with legs in semiflexed position	Weak or exaggerated response with breech presentation	Absence suggestive of CNS damage or malformation
Anus			
Inspect and palpate: Placement Patency	One anus with good sphincter tone Passage of meconium within 24 hr after birth	Passage of meconium within 48 hr after birth	Imperforate anus without fistula Rectal atresia and stenosis Absence of anal opening; drainage of fecal material from vagina in female or urinary meatus in male (rectal fistula) or along perineal raphe (midline area between base of penis and anus) (anorectal malformation)
Test for sphincter response (active “wink” reflex).	Anal “wink” present, anal opening patent		
Stools			
Observe frequency, colour, and consistency.	Meconium followed by transitional and soft yellow stool (Fig. 24-3)		No stool (obstruction), dehydration Frequent watery stools (infection, phototherapy)

evolve Video—Buttocks

the assessment should take place in the presence of the parents; this provides the parents an opportunity to learn about the unique characteristics of their infant. Ongoing assessments of the newborn should be made and an evaluation performed before discharge.

General Appearance

The neonate's maturity level can be gauged by assessment of general appearance. Features to assess in the general survey include posture, activity, any overt signs of anomalies that may cause initial distress, presence of bruising or other consequences of birth, and state of alertness. The normal resting position of the neonate is one of general flexion (Fig. 24-12).

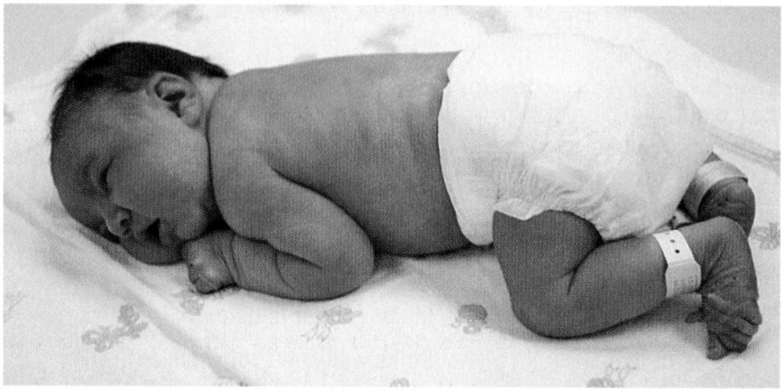

Fig. 24-12 Newborn in position of flexion in prone position while awake. *(From Hockenberry, M. J., et al. [2007].* Wong's nursing care of infants and children *[8th ed., p. 274]. St. Louis: Mosby.)*

Vital Signs

The temperature, heart rate, and respiratory rate are always obtained. BP is not normally assessed unless cardiac problems are suspected. An irregular, very slow, or very fast heart rate may indicate a need for further evaluation of circulatory status, including BP measurement.

Axillary temperature is a safe, accurate substitute for rectal temperature in the neonate. Electronic thermometers have expedited this task and provide a reading within 1 minute. Temporal artery, tympanic, and oral routes for measuring temperature in the newborn are not considered accurate (Asher & Northington, 2008). Taking an infant's temperature may cause the infant to cry and struggle against the placement of the thermometer in the axilla. Before taking the temperature, the examiner may determine the apical heart rate and respiratory rate while the infant is quiet and at rest. The normal axillary temperature averages 37°C with a range from 36.5° to 37.2°C.

The respiratory rate varies with the state of alertness and activity after birth. Respirations are abdominal and can be counted by observing or by lightly feeling the rise and fall of the abdomen while listening to air entry. Neonatal respirations are shallow and irregular. It is important to count the respirations for a full minute to obtain an accurate count as there can be episodes of periodic breathing during which respirations may cease for up to 20 seconds and then resume again. The examiner should also observe for symmetry of chest movement. The average respiratory rate is between 30 and 60 breaths/min or may be higher than 60 breaths/min if the newborn is very active or crying (see Table 24-2).

An apical pulse rate should be obtained on all newborns. Auscultation should be for a full minute, preferably when the infant is asleep or in a quiet alert state. The infant may need to be held and comforted during assessment. Heart rate may range from 80 to 170 beats/min shortly after birth and, when the infant's condition has stabilized, from 110 to 160 beats/min. Brachial and femoral pulses should be assessed for equality and strength.

If BP is measured, an oscillometric monitor calibrated for neonatal pressures is preferred. An appropriate-sized cuff (width-to-arm or calf ratio of 0.45 to 0.70, or approximately ½ to ¼) is essential for accuracy. Neonatal BP usually is highest immediately after birth and falls to a minimum by 3 hours after birth. It then begins to rise steadily and reaches a plateau between 4 and 6 days after birth. This measurement is usually equal to that of the immediate postbirth BP. The BP varies with the neonate's activity; accurate measurement is best obtained while the newborn is at rest. In an Australian study of 406 infants born at term (without maternal diabetes or hypertension; birth weight range, 2425 to 4990 g), median systolic and diastolic oscillometric BPs on the second day of life were 68 mm Hg (range, 46 to 91 mm Hg) and 43 mm Hg (range, 27 to 58 mm Hg), respectively (Kent et al., 2007). Median oscillometric BP increased slightly on the third and fourth days of life.

A baseline pulse oximetry measurement may be obtained along with palpation of peripheral pulses (brachial, femoral, pedal) before the infant's discharge from the birth institution, especially if there is concern for a congenital cardiac defect.

Baseline Measurements of Physical Growth

Baseline measurements are taken and recorded to help assess the progress and determine the growth patterns of the neonate. These may be recorded on growth charts. The following measurements are made when the neonate is assessed.

Weight

The newborn is usually weighed shortly after birth, in the labour and birthing area, in the mother's room, or on admission to the nursery. Care must be taken to ensure that the scales are balanced. The totally unclothed neonate is placed in the centre of the scale, which is usually covered with a disposable pad or cloth to prevent heat loss via conduction and prevent cross-infection. The nurse should place one hand over (but not touching) the neonate to prevent the infant from falling off the scale (see p. 627). Most newborns need to be weighed only at birth and at discharge, although newborns who are small for gestational age or who are not feeding well may require daily weighing. This should be done at the same time every day during the hospital stay. Birth weight of a term infant typically ranges from 2500 to 4000 g.

Head Circumference and Length

The head is measured at the widest part, which is the occipitofrontal diameter (see p. 628). The tape measure is placed around the head just above the infant's eyebrows. The term neonate's head circumference ranges from 32 to 36.8 cm.

The length may be difficult to obtain because of the flexed posture of the newborn (p. 628). The examiner places the newborn on a flat surface and extends the leg until the knee is flat against the surface. Placing the head against a perpendicular surface and extending the leg may assist with this measurement. In the term neonate, head-to-heel length ranges from 45 to 55 cm.

Neurological Assessment

The physical assessment includes a neurological assessment of newborn reflexes (see Table 24-1). This provides useful information about the infant's nervous system and state of neurological maturation. Many reflex behaviours (e.g., sucking and rooting) are important for proper development. Other reflexes such as gagging and sneezing act as primitive safety mechanisms. The assessment needs to be carried out as early as possible because abnormal signs present in the early neonatal period may require further investigation before the newborn is discharged home.

Behavioural Characteristics

The healthy newborn must accomplish behavioural and biological tasks to develop normally. Behavioural characteristics form the basis of the infant's social capabilities. Normal newborns differ in their activity levels, feeding and sleeping patterns, and responsiveness. Parents' reactions to their newborns are often determined by these differences. Showing parents the unique characteristics of their infant helps parents develop a more positive perception of the infant, with increased interaction between infant and parent.

Behavioural responses, as well as physical characteristics, change during the period of transition. The Brazelton Neonatal Behavioural Assessment Scale (BNBAS) can be used to systematically assess the infant's behaviour (Brazelton & Nugent, 1996). The BNBAS is an interactive examination that assesses the infant's response to 28 areas organized according to the clusters in Box 24-2. It is generally used as a research

BOX 24-2 Clusters of Neonatal Behaviours in Brazelton Neonatal Behavioural Assessment Scale

- Habituation—Ability to respond to and then inhibit responding to discrete stimulus (e.g., light, rattle, bell, pinprick) while asleep
- Orientation—Quality of alert states and ability to attend to visual and auditory stimuli while alert
- Motor performance—Quality of movement and tone
- Range of state—Measure of general arousal level or arousability of infant
- Regulation of state—How infant responds when aroused
- Autonomic stability—Signs of stress (e.g., tremors, startles, skin colour) related to homeostatic (self-regulator) adjustment of the nervous system
- Reflexes—Assessment of several neonatal reflexes

or diagnostic tool and requires special training for its implementation.

In addition to its use as an initial and ongoing tool to assess neurological and behavioural responses, the BNBAS can be used to assess initial parent–infant relationships and as a guide for parents to help them focus on their infant's individuality and develop a deeper attachment to their child. See Chapter 22 for further discussion of attachment.

Sleep–Wake States

Variations in the state of consciousness of infants are called sleep–wake states. The six states form a continuum from deep sleep to crying (Fig. 24-13). There are two sleep states (i.e., deep sleep and light sleep) and four wake states (i.e., drowsy, quiet alert, active alert, and crying) (Blackburn, 2007). Each state has specific characteristics and state-related behaviours. The optimum state of arousal is the quiet alert state. During this state, infants smile, vocalize, move in synchrony with speech, watch their parents' faces, and respond to people talking to them (see Family-Centred Teaching box). Infants respond to internal and external environmental factors by controlling sensory input and regulating the sleep–wake states; the ability to make smooth transitions between states is called *state modulation*. The ability to regulate sleep–wake states is essential in the infant's neurobehavioural development. The more immature the infant, the less he or she is able to cope with factors, external or internal, that affect the sleep–wake patterns.

Infants use purposeful behaviour to maintain the optimum arousal state, as follows: (1) actively withdrawing by increasing physical distance; (2) rejecting by pushing away with hands and feet; (3) decreasing sensitivity by falling asleep or breaking eye contact by turning their head; or (4) using signalling behaviours, such as fussing and crying. These behaviours enable infants to quiet themselves and reinstate readiness to interact.

> **FAMILY-CENTRED TEACHING**
>
> *Newborn Behaviour*
>
> A first-time single mother asks the nurse about her newborn's activity. She voices concern that the newborn cries when she changes his diaper. "He sleeps a lot and only wakes up to eat or when I change his diaper. Is that normal?" Develop a short parent teaching lesson to present newborn behaviour and care in relation to the following: sleep–wake states, newborn activities and relationship to crying behaviours in the first few days of life, and how to comfort and console the newborn.

The first 6 weeks of life involve a steady decrease in the proportion of active REM sleep to total sleep. A steady increase in the proportion of quiet sleep to total sleep also occurs. Periods of wakefulness increase. For the first few weeks, the wakeful periods seem dictated by hunger, but soon a need for socializing appears as well. The newborn sleeps approximately 16 to 18 hours a day, with periods of wakefulness gradually increasing. By the fourth week of life, some infants stay awake from one feeding to the next.

Other Factors Influencing Behaviour of Newborns

Gestational Age

The gestational age of the infant and level of CNS maturity affect the observed behaviour. In an infant with an immature

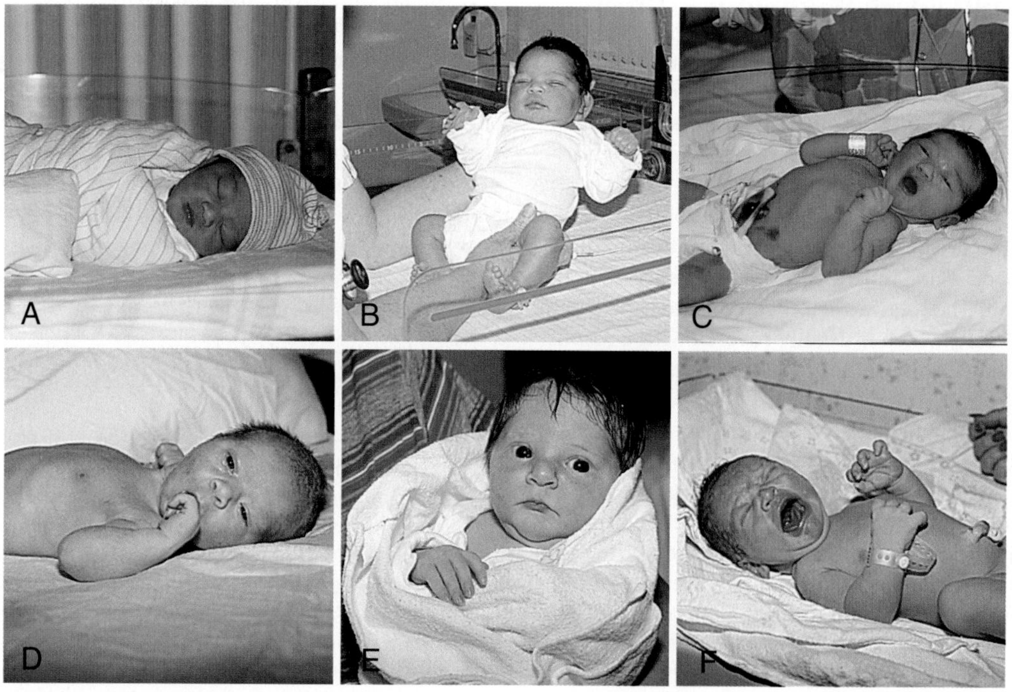

Fig. 24-13 Newborn sleep–wake states. **A:** Deep sleep. **B:** Light sleep. **C:** Drowsy. **D:** Quiet alert. **E:** Active alert. **F:** Crying. *(Courtesy Marjorie Pyle, RNC, Lifecircle, Costa Mesa, CA.)*

CNS (preterm), the entire body responds to a pinprick of the foot, although the response may not be observed by an untrained observer; the mature infant withdraws only the foot. CNS immaturity is reflected in reflex development, sleep–wake states, and ability (or inability) to regulate or modulate a smooth transition between different states. Preterm infants have brief periods of alertness but have difficulty maintaining the state without becoming overstimulated, which leads to autonomic instability unless intervention is implemented. Preterm or sick infants show signs of fatigue or physiological stress sooner than full-term healthy infants.

Time

The time elapsed since labour and birth affects infants' behaviour as they attempt to become organized initially. Time elapsed since the previous feeding and time of day may also influence infants' responses.

Stimuli

Environmental events and stimuli affect infants' behavioural responses. The newborn responds to animate and inanimate stimuli. Nurses in intensive care nurseries have observed that infants respond to loud noises, bright lights, monitor alarms, and tension in the unit. If a mother is tense and is nervous or uncomfortable while feeding her infant, the infant may sense her tension and demonstrate difficulty feeding.

Medication

Controversy surrounds the effects of maternal medication (e.g., analgesia and anaesthesia) during labour on infant behaviour. Some researchers note that infants of mothers given certain analgesic medications may continue to demonstrate poor state organization after the fifth day; medication effects have been noted as long as 30 days after birth. Other researchers maintain that the effect can be beneficial or nonexistent.

Sensory Behaviours

From birth, infants possess sensory capabilities that indicate a state of readiness for social interaction. Infants effectively use behavioural responses in establishing their first dialogues. These responses, coupled with the newborns' "baby appearance" (e.g., facial proportions of forehead and eyes larger than the lower part of the face) and their small size and helplessness, evoke feelings of wanting to hold and protect them and to interact with them.

Vision

At birth, the eye is structurally incomplete and the muscles are immature. The process of accommodation is not present at birth but improves over the first 3 months of life. The pupils react to light, the blink reflex is easily stimulated, and the corneal reflex is activated by light touch. Term newborns can see objects as far away as 0.7 metres. The clearest visual distance is 20 to 30 cm, which is about the distance the infant's face is from the mother's face as she breastfeeds or cuddles. Infants are sensitive to light; they will frown if a bright light is flashed in their eyes and will turn toward a soft, red light. If the room is darkened, they will open their eyes wide and look about. By 2 months of age, they can detect colour; but at 5 days of age and younger, they seem more attracted by black-and-white patterns.

Response to movement is noticeable. If a bright light is shown to newborns (even at 15 minutes of age), they will follow it visually; some will even turn their heads to do so. Because human eyes are bright, shiny objects, newborns will track their parents' eyes. Parents often comment on how exciting this behaviour is. The development of eye-to-eye contact is important for parent–infant attachment. Children of blind parents, and parents who have blind children, must circumvent this obstacle to form a relationship.

Visual acuity is surprising; even at 2 weeks of age, infants can distinguish patterns with stripes 3 mm apart. By 6 months their vision is as acute as that of an adult. They prefer to look at patterns rather than plain surfaces, even if the latter are brightly coloured. Infants prefer more complex patterns to simple ones. They prefer novelty (changes in pattern) by 2 months of age. The infant of a few weeks of age is thus capable of responding actively to an enriched environment.

Hearing

As soon as the amniotic fluid drains from the ears, the infant's hearing is similar to that of an adult. Loud sounds of about 90 decibels cause the infant to react with a startle reflex. The newborn responds to low-frequency sounds such as a heartbeat or lullaby by decreasing motor activity or stopping crying. High-frequency sound elicits an alerting response.

The infant responds readily to the mother's voice. Studies indicate a selective listening to maternal voice sounds and rhythms during intrauterine life that prepares newborns for recognition of and interaction with their primary caregivers—their mothers. Newborns are accustomed to hearing the regular rhythm of the mother's heartbeat. As a result, they respond by relaxing and ceasing to fuss and cry if a regular heartbeat simulator is placed in their cribs.

Hearing loss is a common major abnormality at birth; approximately 1 to 3 in 1000 normal term infants are profoundly deaf and another 3 in 1000 have serious hearing loss (Canadian Paediatric Society [CPS], 2008). To identify affected infants, the hearing of infants should be screened before discharge from the hospital because when hearing loss is detected, intervention can be initiated early in life (Fig. 24-14). In Canada, hearing screening is mandatory in some provinces but not required in all. If the newborn does not pass the screening test, further investigation is required. When hearing loss is detected, intervention can be started early.

Smell

Newborns react to strong odours, such as alcohol or vinegar, by turning their heads away. Breastfed infants are able to smell breast milk and can differentiate their mother from other lactating women by the smell (Lawrence & Lawrence, 2011).

Taste

The newborn can distinguish between tastes, and various types of solutions elicit differing facial expressions. A tasteless

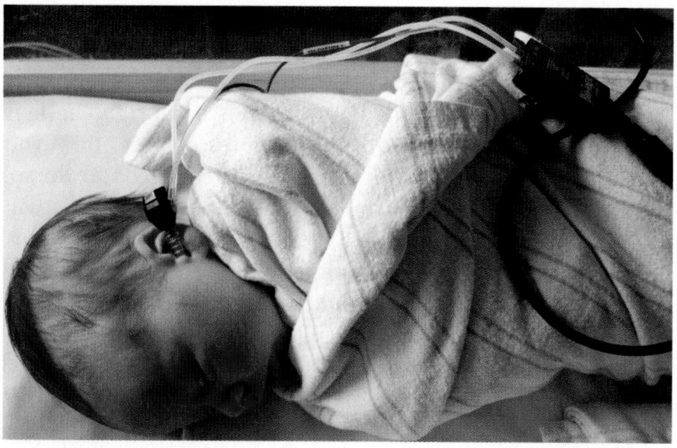

Fig. 24-14 Hearing screening. *(Courtesy Cheryl Briggs, RN, Annapolis, MD.)*

solution produces no response, a sweet solution elicits eager sucking, a sour solution causes puckering of the lips, and a bitter liquid produces a grimace.

Young infants are particularly oriented toward the use of their mouths, both for meeting their nutritional needs for rapid growth and for releasing tension through sucking. The early development of circumoral sensation, muscle activity, and taste would seem to be preparation for survival in the extrauterine environment.

Touch

The newborn is responsive to touch on all parts of the body. The face (especially the mouth), hands, and soles of the feet appear to be the most sensitive. Reflexes can be elicited by stroking the infant. The newborn's responses to touch suggest that this sensory system is well prepared to receive and process tactile messages. Touch and motion are essential to normal growth and development and infant massage is a way to increase tactile stimulation. However, each infant is unique, and variations can be seen in newborns' responses to touch. Birth trauma or stress, and depressant medications taken by the mother decrease the infant's sensitivity to touch or painful stimuli.

Response to Environmental Stimuli

Temperament

Classic studies have identified individual variations in the primary reaction pattern of newborns and described them as temperament. Newborns' style of behavioural response to stimuli is guided by temperament, affecting their sensory threshold, ability to habituate, and response to maternal behaviours. Newborns possess individual characteristics that affect selective responses to various stimuli present in the internal and external environments.

The three major patterns of behavioural style, or temperament, are as follows (Chess, 1969; Chess & Thomas, 1977):

1. The easy child, who demonstrates regularity in bodily functions, readily adapts to change, has a predominantly positive mood and moderate sensory threshold, and approaches new situations or objects with a moderate response.
2. The slow-to-warm-up child, who has a low activity level, withdraws on first exposure to new stimuli, is slow to adapt and low in intensity of response, and is somewhat negative in mood.
3. The difficult child, who is irregular in bodily functions, is intense in reactions, generally negative in mood, and resistant to change or new stimuli and often cries loudly for long periods.

Habituation

Habituation is a protective mechanism that allows the infant to become accustomed to environmental stimuli. Habituation is a psychological and physiological phenomenon in which the response to a constant or repetitive stimulus is decreased. In the term newborn, this can be demonstrated in several ways. Shining a bright light into a newborn's eyes will cause a startle or squinting the first two or three times. The third or fourth flash will elicit a diminished response, and by the fifth or sixth flash, the infant ceases to respond (Brazelton & Nugent, 1996). The same response pattern holds true for the sounds of a rattle or stroking the bottom of the foot.

The ability to habituate allows the healthy term newborn to select stimuli that promote continued learning about the social world, thus avoiding overload. The intrauterine environment appears to have programmed the newborn to be especially responsive to human voices, soft lights, soft sounds, and sweet tastes.

The newborn quickly learns the sounds in the home environment and is able to sleep in their midst. The selective responses of the newborn indicate cerebral organization capable of memory and making choices. The ability to habituate depends on the state of consciousness, hunger, fatigue, and temperament. These factors also affect consolability, cuddliness, irritability, and crying.

Consolability

Barr (1990) described variations in newborns' ability to console themselves or to be consoled. In the crying state, most newborns initiate one of several ways to reduce their distress. Hand-to-mouth movements are common, with or without sucking, as well as alerting to voices, noises, or visual stimuli.

Cuddliness

Cuddliness is especially important to parents because they often gauge their ability to care for the child by the child's responses to their actions. The degree to which newborns mould into the contours of the person holding them varies. Barr (1990) tested the effect of body contact and vestibular stimulation in both soothing babies and creating alertness. The vestibular stimulation of being picked up and moved had the greater effect.

Irritability

Some newborns cry longer and harder than others. For some, the sensory threshold seems low. They are readily upset by unusual noises, hunger, wetness, or new experiences and thus respond intensely. Others with a high sensory threshold require a great deal more stimulation and variation to reach the active, alert state.

Crying

Crying in an infant may signal hunger, discomfort, pain, desire for attention, or fussiness. Many parents can learn to distinguish among the cries, and this ability can increase their confidence as a parent. The duration of crying is also highly variable in each infant; newborns may cry for as little as 5 minutes or as much as 2 hours or more per day. The amount of crying peaks in the second month and then decreases. There is a diurnal rhythm of crying, with more crying occurring in the evening hours. High-pitched crying can indicate a neurological disorder and should be investigated. Colic is described as loud crying associated with abdominal cramping and is discussed in more detail in Chapter 36.

Parents need to learn that most crying is normal and a way for the newborn to communicate his or her needs. Some parents who are exhausted and overwhelmed can become frustrated with a baby who cries excessively. Parents need to be taught to recognize when they have reached their limit and that if this occurs, it is important to put the newborn in a safe place and take a few minutes away from the baby.

Key Points

- By full term, the newborn's various anatomical and physiological systems have reached a level of development and functioning that permits a physical existence apart from the mother.
- The appearance of jaundice during the first day of life or persistence of jaundice beyond 7 to 10 days may indicate a pathological process that requires further investigation.
- Heat loss in the healthy term newborn may exceed the capacity to produce heat; this can lead to metabolic and respiratory complications that threaten the newborn's well-being.
- Assessment of the newborn requires data from the prenatal, intrapartum, and postpartum periods.
- The newborn assessment should proceed systematically so that each system is thoroughly evaluated.
- Some reflex behaviours are important for the newborn's survival.
- Individual personalities and behavioural characteristics of infants play a major role in the ultimate relationship between infants and their parents.
- Each full-term newborn has a predisposed capacity to handle the multitude of stimuli in the external world.

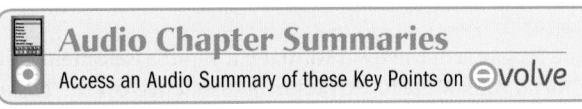

Audio Chapter Summaries

Access an Audio Summary of these Key Points on evolve

References

Asher, C., & Northington, L. K. (2008). Position statement for measurement of temperature/fever in children. *Journal of Pediatric Nursing, 23*(3), 234–235. doi:10.1016/j.pedn.2008.03.005

Askin, D. F. (2009). Chest and lungs assessment. In E. P. Tappero & M. E. Honeyfield (Eds.), *Physical assessment of the newborn* (4th ed.). Petaluma, CA: NICU Ink.

Barr, R. G. (1990). The normal crying curve: What do we really know? *Developmental Medicine and Child Neurology, 32*(4), 356–362.

Blackburn, S. T. (2007). *Maternal, fetal, and neonatal physiology: A clinical perspective* (3rd ed.). St. Louis: Saunders.

Boo, N. Y., et al. (2005). Risk factors associated with subaponeurotic haemorrhage in full-term infants exposed to vacuum extraction. *British Journal of Obstetrics and Gynaecology, 112*, 1516–1521. doi: 10.1111/j.1471-0528.2005.00732.x

Brazelton, T., & Nugent, J. (1996). *Neonatal behavioural assessment scale* (3rd ed.). London: MacKeith.

Canadian Paediatric Society. (2008). *Your baby's hearing*. Retrieved from http://www.caringforkids.cps.ca/pregnancybabies/BabyHearing.htm.

Chess, S. (1969). Individuality and baby care. *Developmental Medicine and Child Neurology, 11*(6), 749–754.

Chess, S., & Thomas, A. (1977). Temperament and the parent–child interaction. *Pediatric Annals, 6*(9), 574–582.

Dabrowski, G. A. (2007). Skin-to-skin contact: Giving birth back to mothers and babies. *Nursing for Women's Health, 11*(1), 65–71. doi: 10.1111/j.1751-486X.2007.00119.x

Doumouchtsis, S. K., & Arulkumaran, S. (2006). Head injuries after instrumental vaginal deliveries. *Current Opinion in Obstetrics and Gynecology, 18*(2), 129–134. doi:10.1016/j.clp.2007.11.006

Galligan, M. (2006). Skin-to-skin treatment of neonatal hypothermia. *MCN: American Journal of Maternal Child Nursing, 31*(5), 298–304.

Hutton, E. K., & Hassan, E. S. (2007). Late vs. early clamping of the umbilical cord in full-term neonates: Systematic review and meta-analysis of controlled trials. *Journal of the American Medical Association, 297*(11), 1241–1252. doi:10.1001/jama.297.11.1241

Kent, A. L., et al. (2007). Blood pressure in the first year of life in healthy infants born at term. *Pediatric Nephrology, 22*(10), 1743–1749. doi: 10.1007/s00467-007-0561-8

Lawrence, R. A., & Lawrence, R. M. (2011). *Breastfeeding: A guide for the medical profession* (7th ed.). St. Louis: Mosby.

McDonald, S. J., & Middleton, P. (2008). Effect of timing of umbilical cord clamping of term infants on maternal and neonatal outcomes. *Cochrane Database of Systematic Reviews*, Issue 2. Art. No. CD004074. doi: 10.1002/14651858.CD004074.pub2

Paige, P. L., & Moe, P. C. (2006). Neurologic disorders. In G. B. Merenstein & S. L. Gardner (Eds.), *Handbook of neonatal intensive care* (6th ed.). St. Louis: Mosby.

Razmus, I. J., & Lewis, L. (2006). Using four limb blood pressures as a screening tool in normal newborns. *Society of Pediatric Nurses News, 15*(6), 5–7.

Singh, G., & Archana, G. (2008). Unraveling the mystery of vernix caseosa. *Indian Journal of Dermatology, 53*(2), 54. doi: 10.4103/0019-5154.41645

Taylor, M. L. (2005). Coarctation of the aorta: Critical catch for newborn well-being. *Nurse Practitioner, 30*(12), 34–43.

Uchil, D., & Arulkumaran, S. (2003). Neonatal subgaleal hemorrhage and its relationship to delivery by vacuum extraction. *Obstetric and Gynecological Survey, 58*(10), 687–693.

Visscher, M. O., et al. (2005). Vernix caseosa in neonatal adaptation. *Journal of Perinatology, 25*(7), 440–446. doi:10.1038/sj.jp.7211305

Weinberg, J. A., & Powell, K. R. (2011). Laboratory aids for diagnosis of neonatal sepsis. In J. S. Remington, J. O. Klein, C. B. Wilson, V. Nizet, & Y. Maldonado (Eds.), *Infectious diseases of the fetus and newborn infant* (7th ed.). Philadelphia: Elsevier.

evolve Video—Crying Female Neonate

Unit 6

25 Nursing Care of the Newborn

Learning Objectives

On completion of this chapter, the reader will be able to:

- Identify the purpose and components of the Apgar score.
- Compare and contrast the characteristics of preterm, late preterm, term, and postterm neonates.
- Perform a gestational age assessment on a newborn.
- Explain what is meant by a safe environment.
- Discuss jaundice and phototherapy as well as the guidelines for teaching parents about this treatment.
- Explain purposes and methods of circumcision, the postoperative care of the circumcised infant, and parent teaching information regarding care of the circumcised or uncircumcised penis.
- Review procedures for performing a heel stick, collecting urine specimens, and assisting with venipuncture.
- Explain pain-management strategies for newborns.
- Review anticipatory guidance that nurses provide parents before discharge.

Electronic Resources

Additional information related to the content in Chapter 25 can be found on

evolve the companion Web site at

http://evolve.elsevier.com/Canada/Perry/maternal/

- Examination Review Questions
- Case Study—The Normal Newborn
- Critical Thinking Exercise—Circumcision
- Critical Thinking Exercise—Jaundice
- Skill—Changing a Diaper
- Skill—Infant Bathing
- Skill—Pain Assessment
- Skill—Swaddling
- Video—Circumcision
- Video—Crying Female Neonate

Although most infants make the necessary biopsychosocial adjustment to extrauterine existence without undue difficulty, their well-being depends on the care they receive from others. This chapter describes the assessment and care of the infant from immediately after birth until discharge.

Birth Through the First 2 Hours

Nursing Care Management

Care begins immediately after birth and focuses on assessing and stabilizing the newborn's condition. The nurse has primary responsibility for the infant during this period, since the physician or midwife is involved with the care of the mother. The nurse must be alert for any signs of distress and initiate appropriate interventions.

With the possibility of transmission of viruses such as hepatitis B virus and human immunodeficiency virus (HIV) via maternal blood and blood-stained amniotic fluid, the newborn must be considered a potential contamination source until proved otherwise. As part of routine precautions, nurses should wear gloves when handling the newborn until blood and amniotic fluid are removed by bathing; gloves should be worn for all diaper changes as well.

Assessment

Initial Assessment and Apgar Scoring

The first assessment of the newborn is performed immediately after birth using the Apgar score (Table 25-1) and a brief physical examination (Box 25-1). A more comprehensive physical examination may be completed within 24 hours of birth (see Table 24-2).

Apgar Score

The Apgar score is used to make a rapid assessment of the newborn's transition to extrauterine existence on the basis of five signs indicating his or her physiological state: (1) heart rate, based on **auscultation** with a stethoscope or **palpation** of the umbilical cord; (2) respiratory rate, based on observed movement or auscultation of respiratory efforts; (3) muscle tone, based on degree of flexion and movement of the extremities; (4) reflex irritability, based on response to stimulation; and (5) generalized skin colour, described as pallid, cyanotic, or pink (see Table 25-1). Evaluations are made at 1 and 5 minutes after birth and can be done by the nurse or birth

Table 25-1 Apgar Score

SIGN	SCORE 0	1	2
Heart rate	Absent	Slow (<100 beats/min)	≥100 beats/min
Respiratory rate	Absent	Slow (hypoventilation), weak cry	Good, crying
Muscle tone	Flaccid	Some flexion of extremities	Well flexed
Reflex irritability	No response	Grimace	Cry or active withdrawal
Colour	Blue, pale	Body pink, extremities blue	Completely pink

BOX 25-1 Initial Physical Assessment of Infant by Body System

Central Nervous System
- ☐ Infant moves all four extremities; flexion, muscle tone appropriate
- ☐ Symmetrical features, movement
- ☐ Moro, suck, rooting, and grasp reflexes present
- ☐ Anterior fontanel soft and flat

Cardiovascular System
- ☐ Heart auscultation, regular in rate and rhythm
- ☐ Transient acrocyanosis, otherwise pink in colour
- ☐ Pulses strong, equal bilaterally
- ☐ Capillary refill less than 3 seconds centrally and in peripheral tissues (not nail beds)

Respiratory System
- ☐ Lungs auscultated, clear bilaterally with minimal fine crackles shortly after birth
- ☐ Respiratory rate less than 60 breaths/min
- ☐ Respiratory effort nonlaboured
- ☐ Absence of nasal flaring, grunting, retractions

Genitourinary System
- ☐ Male: urethral opening at tip of penis, testes descended bilaterally; female: labia minora and majora intact, hymenal tag may be visible

Gastrointestinal System
- ☐ Abdomen soft, no visible distension
- ☐ Cord attached and clamped
- ☐ Anus patent

Eyes, Ears, Nose, and Throat
- ☐ Eyes clear
- ☐ Palates intact
- ☐ Nares patent
- ☐ Ears in place; correct alignment

Skin

Colour __ pink __ acrocyanotic
- ☐ Skin lesions or abrasions documented
- ☐ Birthmarks documented
- ☐ Caput/moulding
- ☐ Other

attendant. Scores of 0 to 3 indicate severe distress, scores of 4 to 6 indicate moderate difficulty, and scores of 7 to 10 indicate that the infant is having minimal or no difficulty adjusting to extrauterine life. The Apgar score is reassessed at 10 and 20 minutes if the score is less than 7 at 5 minutes. Apgar scores do not predict future neurological outcome but are useful for describing the newborn's transition to the extrauterine environment (see Family-Centred Teaching box). Should resuscitation be required, it should be initiated before the 1-minute Apgar score (American Academy of Pediatrics [AAP] & American College of Obstetricians and Gynecologists [ACOG], 2007).

FAMILY-CENTRED TEACHING

Significance of the Apgar Score

The Apgar score was developed to provide a systematic method of assessing an infant's condition at birth. Researchers have tried to correlate Apgar scores with various outcomes such as development, intelligence, and neurological development. In some instances, researchers have attempted to attribute causality to the Apgar score, that is, to suggest that the low Apgar score caused or predicted later problems. This is an inappropriate use of the Apgar score. Instead, the score should be used to ensure that infants are systematically observed at birth to ascertain the need for immediate care. A physician, midwife, or nurse may assign the score; however, to avoid the real or perceived appearance of bias, the person assisting with the birth should not assign the score. Lack of consistency in the assigned scores limits studies of the Apgar's long-term predictive value. Because infants often do not receive the maximum score of 10, parents need to know that scores of 7 to 10 are within normal limits. This useful tool needs to be used appropriately; health care providers, parents, and the public may need education to ensure appropriate use of the score.

(Data from Montgomery, K. [2000]. Apgar scores: Examining the long-term significance. *Journal of Perinatal Education, 9*[3], 5–9.)

Initial Physical Assessment

The initial physical assessment includes a brief review of systems (see Box 25-1):

External—Note skin colour, general activity, muscle tone, position; assess nasal patency by closing one nostril at a time while observing respirations; assess skin: peeling, lack of subcutaneous fat (preterm or postterm), temperature; note meconium staining of cord, skin, fingernails, or amniotic fluid (staining may indicate fetal release of meconium); note length of nails and development of creases on soles of feet.

Chest—Auscultate apical heart for rate and rhythm, heart tones, and presence of abnormal sounds; note character of respirations and presence of crackles or other adventitious sounds; note quality of breath sounds by auscultation and observation.

Abdomen—Verify characteristics of abdomen (rounded, flat, concave) and absence of anomalies; auscultate bowel sounds; note number of vessels in cord and general status of cord (e.g., thin, emaciated; thick, tortuous, presence of **hematoma**).

Neurological—Check muscle tone and assess Moro and suck reflexes; palpate anterior **fontanel**; note by palpation the presence and size of the fontanels and sutures.

Genitourinary—Note external sex characteristics and any abnormalities; check anal patency, presence of meconium; note passage of urine.

Other observations—Note gross structural malformation obvious at birth that may require immediate medical attention (e.g., omphalocele, meningocele).

The nurse responsible for the care of the newborn immediately after birth should verify that respirations have been established, dry the infant thoroughly, assess temperature, and place identical identification bracelets on the infant and the mother. In some settings, the partner or whoever the mother deems appropriate will also wear an identification bracelet. Immediately after birth, if the newborn has made the transition to extrauterine life satisfactorily, the infant should be placed on the mother's chest for skin-to-skin contact. This helps maintain the infant's optimum temperature and promotes parental bonding. The newborn should be placed on the mother's breast shortly after birth to begin the breastfeeding process (World Health Organzation [WHO], 2009). If the mother is not available, the newborn could be placed skin-to-skin with the father or partner (Fig. 25-1). Healthy newborns should remain with the parents throughout the hospital stay, although some infants who require extra care may be admitted to a nursery.

The initial examination of the newborn can occur while the nurse is drying the infant; preferably observations can be made while the infant is lying on the mother's chest or in her arms immediately after birth. Efforts should be directed toward minimizing interference in the initial parent–infant acquaintance process. If the infant is breathing effectively, is pink, and has no apparent life-threatening anomalies or risk factors requiring immediate attention, further examination should be delayed until after the newborn has spent at least 1 hour skin-to-skin with the mother and preferably after breastfeeding has been initiated (WHO, 2009). Routine procedures and the admission process should be carried out in the mother's room, although they may sometimes occur in a separate nursery.

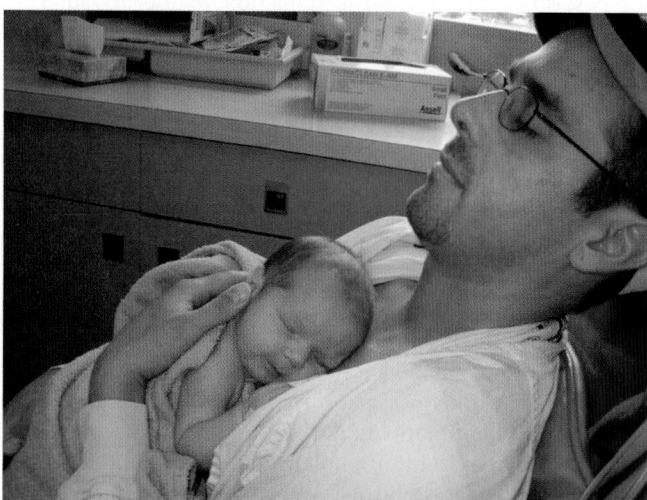

Fig. 25-1 Father and newborn skin-to-skin. *(Courtesy Fraser Health, Surrey, BC.)*

Today's childbirth practices are designed to promote family-centred care. Parents generally wish to share in the birth process and have early contact with their infant. Early contact between mother and newborn can be important in developing future relationships. It also has a positive effect on the duration of breastfeeding. There are physiological benefits of early mother–infant contact: **oxytocin** and **prolactin** levels rise in the mother, and suckling activity is activated in the infant. The process of developing active immunity begins as the infant ingests flora from the mother's **colostrum**.

The nursing process in the immediate care of the newborn and family is outlined in the Nursing Process box.

Implementation

Changes can occur rapidly in the newborn immediately after birth. Assessment must be followed by implementation of appropriate care.

Airway Maintenance

Generally, the normal term infant born vaginally has little difficulty clearing the airway. Most secretions are moved by gravity and brought by the cough reflex to the oropharynx to be drained or swallowed. The infant who has difficulty clearing mucus from the airway may initially be placed in a side-lying position (head stabilized, not in Trendelenburg position) until secretions are cleared and then placed supine. A side-lying position should only be used when parents are given an explanation for why this position is being used and that it will only be a temporary measure until the mucus has cleared.

If the infant has excess mucus in the respiratory tract, the mouth and nasal passages may be gently suctioned with a bulb syringe (Fig. 25-2). Routine chest percussion and suctioning of healthy term and near-term infants should be avoided; there is insufficient evidence to support anything other than gentle nasopharyngeal and oropharyngeal suctioning to clear secretions (Hagedorn, 2006). The infant who is choking on secretions should be supported with his or her head to the side. The mouth is suctioned first to prevent the infant from inhaling pharyngeal secretions by gasping, as newborns are obligatory nose breathers. The bulb is compressed and inserted into one side of the mouth. The centre of the infant's mouth should be avoided because this could stimulate the gag reflex. The nasal passages are suctioned one nostril at a time. Some type of suctioning equipment should be available for use in the newborn's room. Parents should be shown how to use a bulb syringe and asked to perform a return demonstration. The nurse should also listen to the infant's respirations and lung

NURSING PROCESS: NEWBORN CARE

Assessment

A brief initial assessment is performed to detect any problems that may impair an effective newborn transition. Once the infant has stabilized, and maternal-infant contact and breastfeeding have occurred, a more thorough examination may take place, including the gestational-age assessment.

Nursing Diagnoses

Nursing diagnoses are established after analysis of the findings of the physical assessment. Nursing diagnoses for the newborn include the following:

Ineffective airway clearance related to
- airway obstruction with mucus, blood, and amniotic fluid
- inability to clear mucus by cough and expectoration

Risk for imbalanced body temperature related to
- imbalance between body heat loss and heat production

Pain related to
- heel stick, circumcision, venipuncture

Readiness for enhanced parenting related to
- knowledge of newborn's social capabilities
- knowledge of newborn's dependency needs
- knowledge of biological characteristics of the newborn

Decreased role performance related to
- misinterpretation of newborn's behavioural cues
- inadequate knowledge about newborn's basic care needs (feeding, bathing, sleep-wake patterns, stooling and voiding patterns)

Risk for unstable blood glucose related to
- increased glucose utilization at birth
- decreased endogenous glucose supply

Neonatal jaundice related to
- increasing serum bilirubin levels
- inability to metabolize and excrete bilirubin
- increased hemolysis

Implementation and Interventions

A number of intervention strategies for the newborn infant are discussed on pp. 642–647.

Planning

Expected outcomes can apply to both the infant and the parents. Expected outcomes for the newborn during the immediate recovery period include that the infant will do the following:

- Maintain an effective breathing pattern
- Maintain effective thermoregulation
- Maintain adequate cardiac output, circulation, and tissue perfusion
- Remain free from infection
- Receive necessary nutrition for growth
- Receive bilirubin assessment and screening within the first few days of life to determine risk for increasing levels of serum bilirubin

Expected outcomes for the parents include that they will do the following:

- Attain knowledge, skill, and confidence relevant to infant care activities
- State understanding of biological and behavioural characteristics of the newborn
- Begin to integrate the newborn into the family

Evaluation

The nurse can be reasonably assured that care was effective to the extent that the expected outcomes for care have been achieved.

sounds with a stethoscope to determine whether there are crackles, rhonchi, or inspiratory stridor. Fine crackles may be auscultated for several hours after birth. If air movement is adequate, suctioning is rarely necessary. If required, a bulb syringe may be used to clear the mouth and nose. If the bulb syringe does not clear mucus interfering with respiratory effort, mechanical suction can be used. If the newborn has an obstruction that is not cleared with suctioning, further investigation is necessary to determine whether there is a mechanical defect (e.g., tracheoesophageal fistula, choanal atresia [see Chapter 28) causing the obstruction.

Deeper suctioning may be necessary to remove mucus from the infant's nasopharynx or posterior oropharynx; however, this should be performed only after an assessment of the risks involved. Proper catheter insertion and suctioning for 5 seconds or less per catheter insertion help prevent vagal stimulation and hypoxia. If wall suction is used, the pressure should be adjusted to less than 80 mm Hg. After the catheter is properly placed, suction is created by placing one's thumb

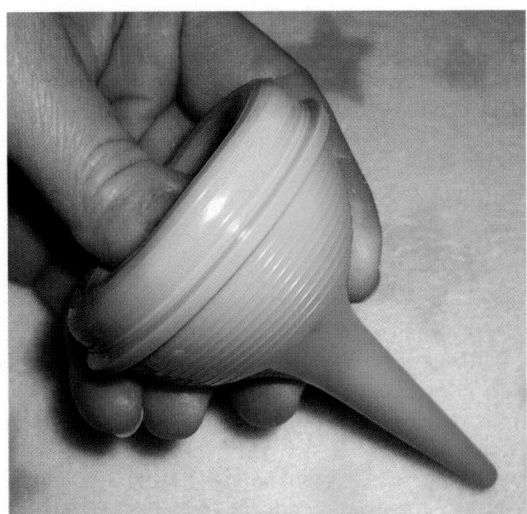

Fig. 25-2 Bulb syringe. The bulb must be compressed before insertion. *(Courtesy Cheryl Briggs, RN, Annapolis, MD.)*

over the control as the catheter is carefully rotated and gently withdrawn. This procedure may need to be repeated until the infant has a clear airway.

Maintaining an Adequate Oxygen Supply

Four conditions are essential for maintaining an adequate oxygen supply:

1. A clear airway
2. Effective establishment of respirations
3. Adequate circulation, adequate perfusion, and effective cardiac function
4. Adequate thermoregulation (exposure to cold stress increases oxygen and glucose needs). Signs of potential complications related to abnormal newborn breathing are listed in Box 25-2.

Body Temperature Maintenance

Effective neonatal care includes maintenance of an optimal thermal environment (see Thermoregulation, Chapter 24, p. 612). Cold stress increases the need for oxygen and may deplete **glucose** stores. The infant may react to exposure to cold by increasing the respiratory rate and may become cyanotic. The best way to stabilize the newborn's body temperature is to place the infant directly on the mother or partner's abdomen and covering the infant with a warm blanket (skin-to-skin contact) (see Fig. 25-1). Allowing **vernix caseosa** to remain on the infant's skin has not been associated with a decrease in axillary temperature in the first hour after birth (Visscher et al., 2005).

Newborns should not be separated from their mother, but if this is necessary because of a medical condition, the nurse should place the thoroughly dried newborn under a radiant warmer or in a warm incubator unit until the body temperature stabilizes. The infant's skin temperature is used as the point of control when using a warmer with a servocontrolled mechanism. The control panel usually is kept at between 36° and 37°C. This setting should maintain the healthy term infant's skin temperature at around 36.5° to 37°C. A thermistor probe (automatic sensor) is usually placed on the upper quadrant of the abdomen immediately below the right or left costal margin (never over a bone); a reflector adhesive patch may be used over the probe to provide adequate warming. This will ensure detection of minor temperature changes resulting from external environmental factors or neonatal factors (peripheral vasoconstriction, vasodilation, or increased metabolism) before a dramatic change in core body temperature develops. The servocontroller adjusts the warmer temperature to maintain the infant's skin temperature within the preset range. The sensor needs to be checked periodically to ensure that it is securely attached to the infant's skin. The newborn's axillary temperature should be checked every hour (or more often as needed) until his or her temperature stabilizes. The time required to stabilize and maintain body temperature varies; each newborn should be allowed to achieve thermal regulation as necessary, and care should be individualized.

During all procedures, heat loss must be avoided or minimized for the newborn. The initial bath should be postponed until the newborn's skin temperature is stable and can adjust to heat loss from a bath. For every infant, the exact and optimal timing of the bath varies and should be individualized according to the infant's ability to maintain a stable body temperature.

Even a healthy term infant can become hypothermic. Birth in a car on the way to the hospital, a cold birthing room, or inadequate drying and wrapping immediately after birth may cause the infant's temperature to fall below normal range (**hypothermia**). Warming the hypothermic newborn should be accomplished with care, as rapid warming may cause apnea and acidosis in an infant. The warming process needs to be monitored to progress slowly over a period of 2 to 4 hours.

Immediate Interventions

It is the nurse's responsibility to perform certain interventions fairly soon after birth to ensure the safety of the newborn. Such interventions may be delayed for an hour or two in order for uninterrupted maternal–infant bonding to occur.

Eye Prophylaxis

The instillation of a prophylactic agent in the eyes (Fig. 25-3) is recommended for all neonates and is mandatory by

BOX 25-2 Newborn Breathing: Signs of Distress

Bradypnea—Respirations (less than 30 breaths/min)
Tachypnea—Respirations (60 breaths/min or more)
Abnormal breath sounds—Crackles (fine crackles may be heard in first few hours after birth), wheezing, rhonchi, expiratory grunting, stridor, diminished or absent air movement
Respiratory distress—Nasal flaring, retractions (substernal or intercostals), laboured breathing, apnea lasting 20 seconds or longer

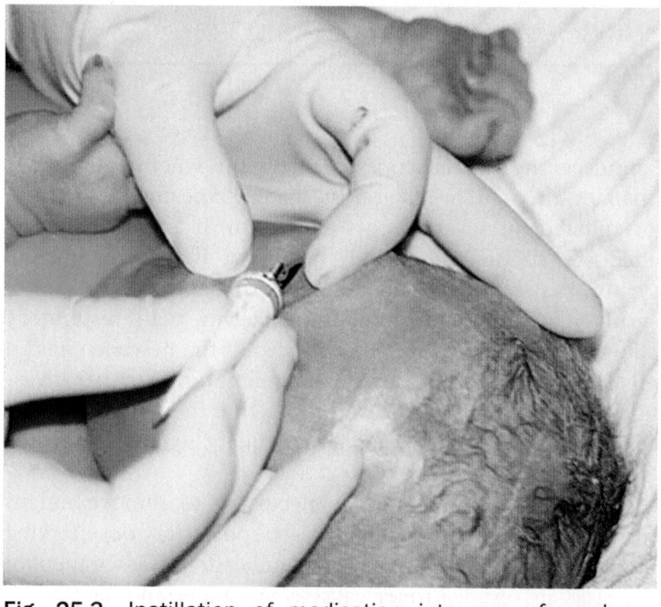

Fig. 25-3 Instillation of medication into eye of newborn. The thumb and forefinger are used to open the eye; medication is placed in the lower conjunctiva from the inner to the outer canthus. *(Courtesy Marjorie Pyle, RNC, Lifecircle, Costa Mesa, CA.)*

law in some provinces as a precaution against **ophthalmia neonatorum.** This is an inflammation of the eyes from gonorrheal or chlamydial infection, contracted by the newborn during passage through the mother's birth canal. In Canada, if the family objects to this treatment, the primary care provider may ask that the parents sign an informed refusal form, and their refusal will be noted in the neonate's record. The agent used for prophylaxis varies according to hospital protocols, but usual agents include forms of erythromycin or tetracycline. Instillation of eye prophylaxis may be delayed until 2 hours after birth to facilitate eye contact and parent–infant attachment and bonding (Health Canada, 2000) (see Medication Guide).

Vitamin K Prophylaxis

Administration of vitamin K intramuscularly is routine in the newborn period to prevent hemorrhagic disease of the newborn (HDNB). A single injection of 1.0 mg of vitamin K for babies greater than or equal to 1500 g and 0.5 mg for those less than 1500 g is given within 6 hours after birth (Canadian Paediatric Society & College of Family Physicians of Canada [CPS & CFPC], 2009). Oral vitamin K is not recommended, although if parents refuse an intramuscular injection, the recommendation is an oral dose of 2.0 mg vitamin K at the time of the first feeding. Parents should be advised of the importance of the baby receiving follow-up doses and be cautioned that their infants remain at an increased risk of late HDNB (including the potential for intracranial hemorrhage) using oral dosing (CPS & CFPC, 2009). Vitamin K is produced in the gastrointestinal tract by bacteria, starting soon after microorganisms are introduced. By day 8, normal newborns are able to produce their own vitamin K (see Medication Guide).

NURSING ALERT Vitamin K is never administered via the intravenous route for prevention of hemorrhagic disease of the newborn except in some cases of a preterm infant who has no muscle mass. In such cases, the medication should be diluted and given over 10 to 15 minutes with the infant being closely monitored with a cardiorespiratory monitor. Rapid bolus administration of vitamin K may cause cardiac arrest.

MEDICATION GUIDE

Eye Prophylaxis With Erythromycin Ophthalmic Ointment 0.5% and Tetracycline Ophthalmic Ointment 1%

Action

Erythromycin and tetracycline antibiotic ointments are both bacteriostatic and bactericidal. They provide prophylaxis against *Neisseria gonorrhoeae*.

Indication

These medications are used for the prevention of ophthalmia neonatorum in newborns of mothers who are infected with gonorrhea.

Neonatal Dosage

Apply a 1 to 2 cm ribbon of ointment to the lower conjunctival sac of each eye; the medicines may also be used in drop form.

Adverse Reactions

They may cause chemical conjunctivitis that lasts 24 to 48 hours; vision may be blurred temporarily.

Nursing Considerations

Administer within 1 to 2 hours of birth. Wear gloves. Cleanse eyes if necessary before administration. Open eyes by putting a thumb and finger at the corner of each lid and gently pressing on the periorbital ridges. Squeeze the tube and spread the ointment from the inner canthus of the eye to the outer canthus. Do not touch the tube to the eye. After 1 minute, excess ointment may be wiped off. Observe eyes for irritation. Explain treatment to parents.

Eye prophylaxis for ophthalmia neonatorum is required by law in some provinces in Canada.

MEDICATION GUIDE

Vitamin K: Phytonadione

Action

This intervention provides vitamin K; the newborn does not have the intestinal flora to produce this vitamin in the first week after birth. Vitamin K promotes formation of clotting factors (II, VII, IX, and X) in the liver.

Indication

Vitamin K is used for prevention and treatment of hemorrhagic disease in the newborn.

Neonatal Dosage

Administer a 1.0 mg dose of vitamin K for babies greater than or equal to 1500 g, and 0.5 mg dose for those less than 1500 g, intramuscularly within 6 hours of birth; the dose may be repeated if the newborn shows bleeding tendencies. The oral dose recommendation is 2.0 mg vitamin K at the time of the first feeding. Use of the parenteral form of vitamin K for oral administration is all that is currently available. This should be repeated at 2 to 4 weeks and 6 to 8 weeks of age. Parents should be advised of the importance of the baby receiving follow-up doses.

Adverse Reactions

Edema, erythema, and pain at the injection site may occur rarely; hemolysis, jaundice, and hyperbilirubinemia have been reported, particularly in preterm infants.

Nursing Considerations

Wash hands prior to donning gloves. If an oral dose is given, ensure that parents know the importance of follow-up and that the newborn is at increased risk for hemorrhagic disease of the newborn (HDNB).

Intramuscular Injection

Administer injection in the middle third of the vastus lateralis muscle using a 25-gauge, ⅝-inch (16-mm) to ⅞-inch (22-mm) needle. Inject into skin that has been cleaned, or allow alcohol (or other skin antiseptic) to dry on puncture site for 1 minute to remove organisms and prevent infection. Stabilize the leg firmly and grasp muscle between the thumb and fingers. Insert the needle at a 90-degree angle; aspirate and inject medication slowly if there is no blood return. After removing the needle, rub gently on the injection site with a dry gauze square to decrease the pain. Observe for signs of bleeding from the site. See Atraumatic Care box on newborn pain management (p. 658).

From 2 Hours After Birth Until Discharge

Nursing Care Management

Most hospitals have adopted variations of single-room maternity care (SRMC) or mother–baby (couplet) care. One nurse provides care for both the mother and the newborn. SRMC allows the infant to remain with the parents after the birth. Many of the procedures, such as assessment of weight and measurement, instillation of eye medication, administration of vitamin K, and physical assessment, may be carried out in the labour and birth unit. Nurses who work in an SRMC unit; a labour, delivery, and recovery (LDR) room; or a labour, delivery, recovery, and postpartum (LDRP) room must be educated in intrapartum, neonatal, and postpartum nursing care and competent in providing it. If the infant is transferred to the nursery, the infant's identification should be verified by the nurse receiving the infant, who places the baby in a warm environment and begins the admission process.

Assessment

Physical Assessment

A complete physical examination is performed within 24 hours, after the infant's condition has stabilized (see Guidelines box). See Chapter 24 for a detailed description of this examination.

Assessment of Gestational Age

Assessment of **gestational age** is important because perinatal morbidity and mortality rates are related to gestational age and birth weight. A frequently used method of determining gestational age is the simplified Assessment of Gestational Age scale by Ballard, Novak, and Driver (1979). The Ballard scale assesses six external physical and six neuromuscular signs. Each sign has a number score, and the cumulative score correlates with a maturity rating of 26 to 44 weeks of gestation.

The new simplified Ballard scale, a revision of the original scale, can be used with newborns as young as 20 weeks of gestation (Fig. 25-4, A). The tool has the same physical and neuromuscular sections but includes −1 scores that reflect signs of extremely preterm infants, such as fused eyelids; imperceptible breast tissue; sticky, friable, transparent skin; no **lanugo**; and square-window (flexion of wrist) angle of greater than 90 degrees. The examination of infants with a gestational age of 26 weeks or less should be performed at a postnatal age of less than 12 hours. For infants with a gestational age of at least 26 weeks, the examination can be performed up to 96 hours after birth; however, to ensure accuracy, it is recommended that the initial examination be performed within the first 48 hours of life. Neuromuscular adjustments after birth in extremely immature neonates require that a follow-up examination be performed to further validate neuromuscular criteria. The new Ballard scale overestimates gestational age by 2 to 4 days in infants younger than 37 weeks of gestation, especially at gestational ages of 32 to 37 weeks (Ballard et al., 1991). See Box 25-3 for specific tests used in gestational-age assessment.

GUIDELINES Physical Examination of the Newborn

Provide a normothermic and nonstimulating examination area.
Check that equipment and supplies are working properly and are accessible.
Undress only the body area to be examined to prevent heat loss.
Proceed in an orderly sequence (usually head to toe) with the following exceptions:
- Perform all procedures that require quiet first, such as observing position, skin colour, tone, and condition.
- Next auscultate the lungs, heart, and abdomen.
- Perform more disturbing procedures, such as testing reflexes, last.
- Measure head and length at the same time to compare results.

Proceed quickly to avoid stressing the infant.
Comfort the infant during and after examination; involve parent in the following:
- Talking softly to the infant
- Holding the infant's hands against chest
- Swaddling and holding the infant
- Giving the infant a gloved finger to suck

Classification of Newborns by Gestational Age and Birth Weight

Classification of infants at birth by both birth weight and gestational age is a more satisfactory method for predicting mortality risks and providing guidelines for management of the neonate than estimating gestational age or birth weight alone. The infant's birth weight, length, and head circumference are plotted on standardized graphs that identify normal values for gestational age (see Fig. 25-4, B, for weight chart, and Box 27-1).

Intrauterine growth curves developed by Battaglia and Lubchenco (1967) have been used since 1967 to classify infants according to birth weight and gestational age. Since that time, other intrauterine growth charts have emerged that reflect a more heterogeneous sample population than previously described (Cunningham et al., 2010). The primary intrauterine growth charts that provide national reference data include the work of Arbuckle, Wilkins, and Sherman (1993) and that of Kramer and colleagues (2001), which represent intrauterine growth among the Canadian population. Thomas and colleagues (2000) concluded that intrauterine growth measured by head circumference, birth weight, and length varies according to race and gender. In one study, Asian and Latin American newborns had lower mean birth weights, shorter mean lengths, and smaller mean head circumferences than those of White newborns (Madan et al., 2002). It is recommended that nurses access and use the most current intrauterine growth chart specific to the population being evaluated, especially when considering multiples such as twins. See http://www.stmichaelshospital.com/birthweights.php for birthweight curves that have been developed based on maternal ancestry.

The infant whose weight is appropriate for gestational age (AGA) (between the 10th and 90th percentiles) can be presumed to have grown at a normal rate regardless of the length of gestation—preterm, term, or postterm. The infant who is large for gestational age (LGA) (above the 90th percentile) can be presumed to have grown at an accelerated rate during fetal life; the small-for-gestational-age (SGA) infant (below the 10th percentile) can be presumed to have grown at a restricted rate during intrauterine life. When gestational age is determined according to the Ballard scale, the newborn will fall into one of the following nine possible categories for birth weight and gestational age: AGA—term, preterm, postterm; SGA—term, preterm, postterm; or LGA—term, preterm, postterm. Birth weight influences mortality: the lower the birth weight, the higher the mortality. The same is true for gestational age: the lower the gestational age, the higher the mortality (Stoll, 2007).

Late Preterm Infant

Much attention has been focused on infants who are considered "late preterm"; they are often the size and weight of term infants and may be treated as healthy newborns. Late preterm infants, born at 34 to 36-6/7weeks of gestation, have risk factors due to their physiological immaturity that require close attention by nurses working with them (Bakewell-Sachs, 2007; Engle et al., 2007). These risk factors include the tendency to develop respiratory distress, temperature instability, hypoglycemia, apnea, feeding difficulties, jaundice, and hyperbilirubinemia. Nurses must be cognizant of the risk factors for

ESTIMATION OF GESTATIONAL AGE BY MATURITY RATING

NEUROMUSCULAR MATURITY

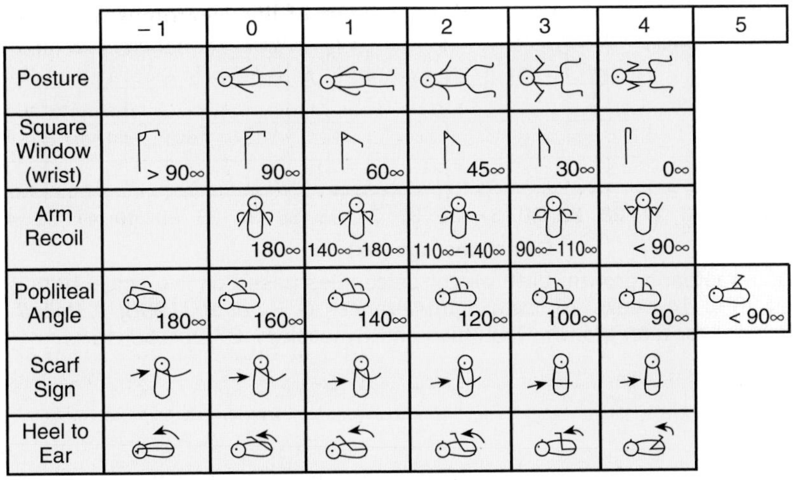

PHYSICAL MATURITY

Skin	Sticky friable transparent	Gelatinous red, translucent	Smooth pink, visible veins	Superficial peeling&/ or rash, few veins	Cracking pale areas rare veins	Parchment deep cracking no vessels	Leathery cracked wrinkled
Lanugo	None	Sparse	Abundant	Thinning	Bald areas	Mostly bald	
Plantar Surface	Heel-toe 40–50 mm:–1 <40 mm: –2	>50 mm no crease	Faint red marks	Anterior transverse crease only	Creases ant. 2/3	Creases over entire sole	
Breast	Imperceptible	Barely perceptible	Flat areola no bud	Stippled areola1–2 mm bud	Raised areola 3–4 mm bud	Full areola 5–10 mm bud	
Eye/Ear	Lids fused loosely: –1 tightly: –2	Lids open pinna flat stays folded	Slightly curved pinna; soft; slow recoil	Well-curved pinna; soft but ready recoil	Formed firm instant recoil	Thick cartilage ear stiff	
Genitals (male)	Scrotum flat, smooth	Scrotum empty faint rugae	Testes in upper canal rare rugae	Testes descending few rugae	Testes down good rugae	Testes pendulous deep rugae	
Genitals (female)	Clitoris prominent labia flat	Prominent clitoris small labia minora	Prominent clitoris enlarging minora	Majora minora equally prominent	Majora large minora small	Majora cover clitoris minora	

MATURITY RATING

Score	Weeks
–10	20
–5	22
0	24
5	26
10	28
15	30
20	32
25	34
30	36
35	38
40	40
45	42
50	44

A

Fig. 25-4 Estimation of gestational age. **A:** New Ballard scale for newborn maturity rating. Expanded scale includes extremely preterm infants and has been refined to improve accuracy in more mature infants. See Box 25-3 for explanation of assessments of neuromuscular maturity. *(A, From Ballard, J., et al. [1991].* New Ballard score, expanded to include extremely premature infants. *Journal of Pediatrics, 119[3], 417.)*

Continued

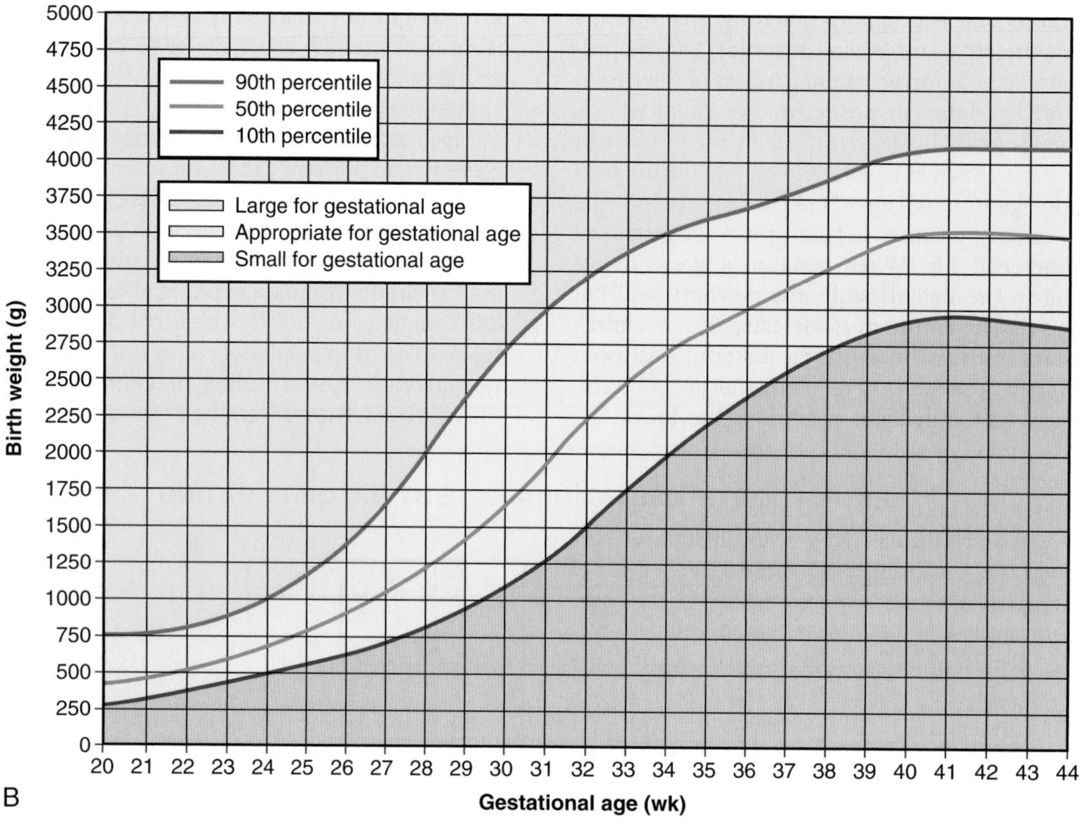

B

Fig. 25-4, cont'd B: Intrauterine growth: birth weight percentiles based on live single births at gestational ages 20 to 44 weeks. *(**B**, Data from Alexander, G. R., et al. [1996]. A United States national reference for fetal growth.* Obstetrics and Gynecology, *87[2], 163–168.)*

BOX 25-3 Techniques Used in Assessing Gestational Age

Posture

With infant quiet and in a supine position, observe degree of flexion in arms and legs. Muscle tone and degree of flexion increase with maturity. Full flexion of the arms and legs = score 4.*

Square Window

With thumb supporting back of arm below the wrist, apply gentle pressure with index and third fingers on dorsum of hand without rotating infant's wrist. Measure angle between base of thumb and forearm. Full flexion (hand lies flat on ventral surface of forearm) = score 4.

Arm Recoil

With infant supine, fully flex both forearms on upper arms and hold for 5 seconds; pull down on hands to fully extend and rapidly release arms. Observe rapidity and intensity of recoil to a state of flexion. A brisk return to full flexion = score 4.

Popliteal Angle

With infant supine and pelvis flat on a firm surface, flex lower leg on thigh and then flex thigh on abdomen. While holding knee with thumb and index finger, extend lower leg with index finger of the other hand. Measure degree of angle behind knee (popliteal angle). An angle of less than 90 degrees = score 5.

Scarf Sign

With infant supine, support head in midline with one hand; use the other hand to pull infant's arm across the shoulder so that infant's hand touches shoulder. Determine location of elbow in relation to midline. Elbow does not reach midline = score 4.

Heel to Ear

With infant supine and pelvis flat on a firm surface, pull foot as far as possible up toward ear on same side. Measure distance of foot from ear and degree of knee flexion (same as popliteal angle). Knees flexed with a popliteal angle of less than 10 degrees = score 4.

(From Hockenberry, M. J., & Wilson, D. [2011]. *Wong's nursing care of infants and children* [9th ed.]. St. Louis: Mosby.)

*See Fig. 25-4 for scale and interpretation of scores.

late preterm infants and continually watch for the development of problems related to the infant's immaturity. The late preterm infant's care is further addressed in Chapter 27 (p. 708).

Common Newborn Problems

Physical Injuries

Birth trauma includes any physical injury sustained by a newborn during labour and birth. Many injuries are minor and readily resolve in the neonatal period without treatment. Other types of trauma require some form of intervention. A few are serious enough to be fatal.

Several factors predispose an infant to birth trauma. Maternal factors include uterine dysfunction that leads to prolonged or precipitous labour, preterm or postterm labour, and **cephalopelvic disproportion**. Injury may result from **dystocia** caused by fetal macrosomia, multifetal gestation, abnormal or difficult presentation, and congenital anomalies. Intrapartum events that can result in scalp injury include the use of intrapartum monitoring of the fetal heart rate and fetal scalp blood sampling. Obstetrical birth techniques can also cause injury. These include forceps birth, vacuum extraction, external version and breech extraction, and Caesarean birth (see Skeletal Injuries, and Peripheral Nervous System Injuries, Chapter 28).

Soft-Tissue Injuries

Subconjunctival and retinal hemorrhages result from rupture of capillaries caused by increased pressure during birth. The hemorrhages clear within 5 days after birth and usually present no further problems. Parents need explanation and reassurance that these injuries are harmless.

Erythema, **ecchymoses**, petechiae, abrasions, lacerations, or edema of buttocks and extremities may be present. Localized discolouration may appear over presenting parts and may result from application of forceps or the vacuum extractor. Ecchymoses and edema may appear anywhere on the body. Petechiae, or pinpoint hemorrhagic areas, acquired during birth may extend over the upper trunk and face. These lesions are benign if they disappear within 2 or 3 days of birth and no new lesions appear. Ecchymoses and petechiae may be signs of a more serious disorder, such as thrombocytopenic purpura. To differentiate hemorrhagic areas from a skin rash or discolouration, apply pressure to the skin with two fingers. Petechiae and ecchymoses do not blanch because extravasated blood remains within the tissues, whereas skin rashes and discolourations do blanch.

Trauma secondary to dystocia occurs to the presenting fetal part. Forceps injury and bruising from the vacuum cup occur at the site of application of the instruments. In a forceps injury there is commonly a linear mark across both sides of the face that is in the shape of the blades of the forceps. The affected areas are kept clean to minimize risk of infection. These injuries usually resolve spontaneously within several days with no specific therapy. With the increased use of the vacuum extractor, the incidence of these lesions have been significantly reduced.

Bruises over the face may be the result of face presentation (Fig. 25-5). In a breech presentation, bruising and swelling may be seen over the buttocks or genitalia (Fig. 25-6). The skin over the entire head may be ecchymotic and covered with petechiae caused by a tight nuchal cord or a precipitous delivery.

Accidental lacerations may be inflicted with a scalpel during Caesarean birth. These cuts may occur on any part of the body but are most often found on the scalp, buttocks, and thighs. Usually they are superficial and only need to be kept

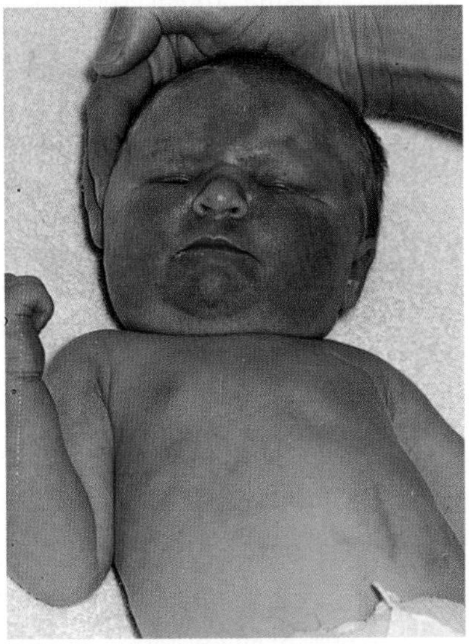

Fig. 25-5 Marked bruising on the entire face of an infant born vaginally after face presentation. Less severe ecchymoses were present on the extremities. Phototherapy was required for treatment of jaundice resulting from the breakdown of accumulated blood. *(From O'Doherty, N. [1986].* Neonatology: Micro atlas of the newborn. *Nutley, NJ: Hoffmann–La Roche.)*

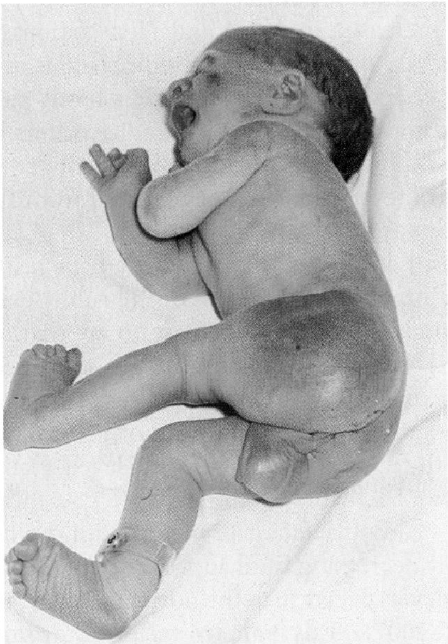

Fig. 25-6 Swelling of genitalia and bruising of the buttocks after a breech birth. *(From O'Doherty, N. [1986].* Neonatology: Micro atlas of the newborn. *Nutley, NJ: Hoffmann–La Roche.)*

clean. Butterfly adhesive strips will hold together the edges of more serious lacerations. Rarely, sutures are needed.

Physiological Problems

Conjugation of Bilirubin

Bilirubin is one of the products derived from the hemoglobin released with the breakdown of red blood cells (RBCs) and the myoglobin in muscle cells. The hemoglobin is broken down by the reticuloendothelial cells, converted to bilirubin, and released in an unconjugated form. Unconjugated (indirect) bilirubin is relatively insoluble and almost entirely bound to circulating albumin, a plasma protein. The unbound bilirubin can leave the vascular system and permeate other extravascular tissues (e.g., skin, sclera, and oral mucous membranes). The resulting yellow colouring is termed **jaundice**.

evolve Critical Thinking Exercise—Jaundice

In the liver, the unbound bilirubin is conjugated with glucuronide in the presence of the enzyme glucuronyl transferase. The conjugated form of bilirubin (direct bilirubin) is soluble and is excreted from liver cells as a constituent of bile. Along with other components of bile, direct bilirubin is excreted into the biliary tract system, which carries the bile into the duodenum. Bilirubin is converted to urobilinogen and stercobilinogen within the duodenum through the action of the bacterial flora. Urobilinogen is excreted in urine and feces; stercobilinogen is excreted in the feces (see Fig. 24-3). The total serum bilirubin (TSB) level is the sum of the levels of both conjugated and unconjugated bilirubin.

Physiological Jaundice

Approximately 50 to 60% of all full-term newborns are visibly jaundiced (yellow) by the second through fifth day of life. TSB levels less than 85 mcmol/L usually are not reflected in visible skin jaundice. Although the neonate has the functional capacity to convert bilirubin, physiological **hyperbilirubinemia** commonly occurs in infants, due to immature liver function. Physiological jaundice or neonatal hyperbilirubinemia occurs in 80% of preterm newborns. The incidence of physiological jaundice is increased in Asian and First Nations, Métis, and Inuit infants. Although neonatal jaundice is considered benign, bilirubin may accumulate to hazardous levels and lead to a pathological condition. Neonatal jaundice occurs because the newborn has a higher rate of bilirubin production than does an adult and the reabsorption of bilirubin from the neonatal small intestine is considerable.

Two phases of physiological jaundice have been identified in full-term infants. In the first phase, bilirubin levels of White and Black infants gradually increase to approximately 85 to 100 mcmol/L by 60 to 72 hours of life, then decrease to a plateau of 35 to 50 mcmol/L by the fifth day (Blackburn, 2007). In Asian infants, levels reach a peak of 170 to 240 mcmol/L around the third to fifth day of life; the levels gradually fall to 35 to 50 mcmol/L by the seventh to tenth day. Bilirubin levels maintain a steady plateau state in the second phase without increasing or decreasing until approximately 12 to 14 days, at which time levels decrease to the normal value of 17 mcmol/L (Blackburn, 2007). This pattern varies according to racial group, method of feeding (breast versus bottle), and gestational age. In preterm formula-fed infants, serum bilirubin levels may peak as high as 170 to 200 mcmol/L at 5 to 6 days of life and decrease slowly over a period of 2 to 4 weeks.

Some characteristics of physiological jaundice include the following:

- The infant is otherwise well in relation to cardiorespiratory status, neurological status, carbohydrate metabolism, feeding pattern, and elimination.
- In term infants, jaundice first appears after 24 hours and disappears by the end of the seventh day.
- In preterm infants, jaundice is first evident after 48 hours and disappears by the ninth or tenth day.
- The infant's predischarge TSB falls below the high-risk category (below 95th percentile) on the hour-specific nomogram (Fig. 25-7).
- The serum concentration of unconjugated bilirubin usually does not exceed 200 mcmol/L in term infants and 255 mcmol/L in preterm infants.
- Direct bilirubin does not exceed 17 to 26 mcmol/L.
- Indirect or unconjugated bilirubin concentration does not increase by more than 85 mcmol/L per day.

See Table 25-2 for the varying causes of neonatal indirect hyperbilirubinemia.

NURSING ALERT The appearance of jaundice during the first 24 hours of life or persistence beyond the ages previously delineated usually indicates a potential pathological process that requires further investigation.

In the newborn intestine, the enzyme β-glucuronidase is able to convert conjugated bilirubin into the unconjugated form, which is subsequently reabsorbed by the intestinal mucosa and transported to the liver. This process, known as enterohepatic circulation or enterohepatic shunting, is accentuated in the newborn and is thought to be a primary mechanism in physiological jaundice (Maisels, 2005). Feeding (1) stimulates peristalsis and produces more rapid passage of meconium, thus diminishing the amount of reabsorption of unconjugated bilirubin; and (2) introduces bacteria to aid in

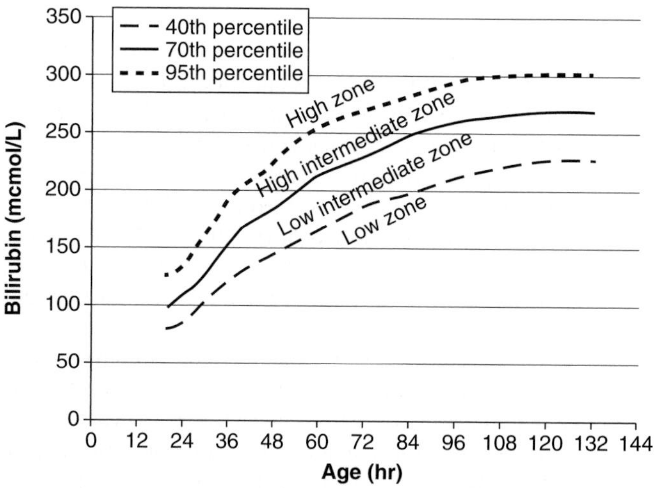

Fig. 25-7 Nomogram for evaluation of screening total serum bilirubin (TSB) concentration in term and late preterm infants, according to the TSB concentration obtained at a known postnatal age in hours. *(From American Academy of Pediatrics: Reproduced and adapted with permission from* Pediatrics *2004;114:297-316. © 2004 by the American Academy of Pediatrics.)*

Table 25-2 Causes of Neonatal Indirect Hyperbilirubinemia

BASIS	CAUSES
Increased Production of Bilirubin	
Increased hemoglobin destruction	Fetomaternal blood group incompatibility (Rh, ABO) Congenital red blood cell abnormalities Congenital enzyme deficiencies (G6PD, galactosemia) Sepsis Enclosed hemorrhage (cephalhematoma, bruising)
Increased amount of hemoglobin	Polycythemia (maternal–fetal or twin–twin transfusion, SGA) Delayed cord clamping
Increased enterohepatic circulation	Delayed passage of meconium, meconium ileus, or plug Fasting or delayed initiation of feeding Intestinal atresia or stenosis
Altered Hepatic Clearance of Bilirubin	
Alteration in uridine diphosphoglucuronyl transferase production or activity	Immaturity Metabolic or endocrine disorders (e.g., Criglar-Najjar syndrome, hypothyroidism, disorders of amino acid metabolism)
Alteration in hepatic function and perfusion (and thus conjugating ability)	Sepsis (also causes inflammation) Asphyxia, hypoxia, hypothermia, hypoglycemia Medications and hormones
Hepatic obstruction (associated with direct hyperbilirubinemia)	Congenital anomalies (biliary atresia, cystic fibrosis) Biliary stasis (hepatitis, sepsis) Excessive bilirubin load (often seen with severe hemolysis)

(From Blackburn, S. T. [2007]. *Maternal, fetal, and neonatal physiology: A clinical perspective* [3rd ed.]. St. Louis: Saunders.)
G6PD, glucose-6-phosphate dehydrogenase; *SGA*, small for gestational age.

the reduction of bilirubin to urobilinogen. Colostrum, a natural laxative, facilitates meconium evacuation.

Every newborn should be assessed for jaundice. To differentiate cutaneous jaundice from normal skin colour, the nurse needs to apply pressure with a finger over a bony area (e.g., nose, forehead, and sternum) for several seconds to empty all the capillaries in that spot. If jaundice is present, the blanched area will look yellow before the capillaries refill. The conjunctiva and buccal mucosa are also assessed, especially in darker-skinned infants. It is better to assess for jaundice in natural light because artificial lighting and the reflection from walls can distort the actual skin colour. Visual assessment of jaundice does not, however, provide an accurate assessment of the level of serum bilirubin, particularly in infants with darker skin colour; only 50% of babies with a TSB concentration greater than 128 mmol/L appear jaundiced (CPS, 2007).

Jaundice is generally first noticed in the head, especially the sclera and mucous membranes, and then progresses gradually to the thorax, abdomen, and extremities. The degree of jaundice is determined by serum bilirubin measurements. Normal values of unconjugated bilirubin are 3.4 to 24 mmol/L. The most common therapy used to treat a high serum bilirubin level or a rapidly increasing level is phototherapy.

It is important to note that the evaluation of jaundice is based not just on serum bilirubin and transcutaneous bilirubin levels but also on the timing of the appearance of clinical jaundice; gestational age at birth; age in hours since birth; family history, including maternal Rh factor; evidence of hemolysis; feeding method; infant's physiological status; and the progression of serial serum bilirubin levels.

Pathological jaundice is that level of serum bilirubin which, if left untreated, can result in sensorineural hearing loss; mild cognitive delays; and kernicterus, which is the deposition of bilirubin in the brain. With ever-changing medical terminology in the literature, there is less emphasis on pathological jaundice, more by omission than anything else. Nonetheless, one might consider any newborn jaundice as being physiological (see preceding discussion) unless proven otherwise, in which case the condition may be considered pathological.

Kernicterus describes the yellow staining of the brain cells that may result in bilirubin encephalopathy. The damage occurs when the serum concentration reaches toxic levels, regardless of cause. There is evidence that a fraction of unconjugated bilirubin crosses the blood–brain barrier in neonates with physiological hyperbilirubinemia. When certain pathological conditions exist in addition to elevated bilirubin levels, the blood–brain barrier has increased permeability to unconjugated bilirubin, creating the potential for irreversible damage. The exact level of serum bilirubin required to cause damage is not known. The signs of bilirubin encephalopathy are those of central nervous system depression or excitation. Prodromal symptoms consist of decreased activity, lethargy, irritability, hypotonia, and seizures. Those who survive may eventually show evidence of neurological damage, such as cognitive impairment, cerebral palsy, attention-deficit/hyperactivity disorder, delayed or abnormal motor movement (especially ataxia or athetosis), behaviour disorders, perceptual problems, or sensorineural hearing loss.

Noninvasive monitoring of bilirubin via cutaneous reflectance measurements (transcutaneous bilirubinometry [TcB]) allows for repetitive estimations of bilirubin; however, there are limitations to the use of TcB monitors: They are more accurate at lower TSB levels, are not accurate once phototherapy is initiated, and may be unreliable with changes in skin colour and thickness. TcB monitors may be used to screen clinically significant jaundice and decrease the need for serum bilirubin measurements (CPS, 2007). With shorter maternity stays, the value of transcutaneous bilirubin measurements as an assessment tool in follow-up home care has been demonstrated in a homogeneous population. However, because transcutaneous bilirubin measurements are affected by race, gestational age, and birth weight, their use in heterogeneous populations remains limited for diagnostic purposes (Engle et al., 2002). The use of hour-specific serum bilirubin levels to predict term newborns at risk for rapidly rising levels has become an official recommendation by the Canadian Paediatric Society for monitoring healthy neonates at 35 weeks of gestation or greater before discharge from the hospital (CPS, 2007). Use of a nomogram (see Fig. 25-7) with three levels (high, intermediate, or low risk) of rising TSB values assists in the determination of newborns that might need further evaluation after discharge. Universal bilirubin screening based on hour-specific TSB may be done at the same time as the routine newborn profile (phenylketonuria [PKU], galactosemia, and others) (CPS, 2007). The hour-specific bilirubin-risk nomogram is used to determine the infant's risk for development of hyperbilirubinemia requiring medical treatment or closer screening. Subsequent studies have demonstrated the accuracy of the nomogram in predicting infants with rapidly rising bilirubin levels requiring evaluation or treatment (Keren et al., 2008).

Risk factors that place infants in the high-risk category include gestational age less than 38 weeks, breastfeeding (exclusive or partial), a sibling who had significant jaundice, visible bruising, cephalohematoma, male sex, maternal age older than 25 years, ethnic background (Asian or European), and jaundice appearing before discharge (CPS, 2007). It is recommended that healthy infants (35 weeks or greater) receive assessment of bilirubin between 24 and 72 hours of life. If intervention is not required, further follow-up will depend on individual risk factors. If an infant is discharged before 24 hours of age, the infant needs further review within 24 hours by someone experienced in newborn care and with access to testing (CPS, 2007). The guidelines for monitoring and treating neonatal hyperbilirubinemia are discussed later in the chapter (see Community Focus box).

Jaundice Associated With Breastfeeding

Breastfeeding is associated with an increased incidence of jaundice. Two types have been identified; however, nomenclature may vary among experts. In addition, these types may overlap and may not be easily differentiated from each other (Blackburn, 2007). Breastfeeding-associated jaundice (early-onset jaundice) begins at 2 to 4 days of age and occurs in approximately 10 to 25% of breastfed newborns. The jaundice is related to the process of breastfeeding and probably results from decreased caloric and fluid intake by breastfed infants before the milk supply is well established, since fasting is associated with decreased hepatic clearance of bilirubin (Blackburn, 2007; Porter & Dennis, 2002). The presence of decreased caloric intake (less milk), weight loss of more than 5 to 7% in the first 5 days of life, increasing serum bilirubin (unconjugated) levels, decreased stooling, and increased jaundice is also sometimes referred to as *starvation jaundice* or *nonbreastfeeding jaundice*. To prevent this pattern, the following measures are suggested: initiation of breastfeeding within the first few hours of life, continuous rooming-in with the mother, breastfeeding 10 to 12 times per day, no supplements, recognition of and response to hunger cues, and breastfeeding support by a knowledgeable individual (CPS, 2007; Gartner & Herschel, 2001). Newborns with breastfeeding-associated jaundice are at greater risk for developing high bilirubin levels in the first week of life and must be closely monitored.

Breast milk jaundice (late-onset jaundice) may initially begin as the early-onset variety or may begin at age 4 to 6 days and occurs in 2 to 3% of breastfed infants. Rising levels of bilirubin peak during the second week and gradually diminish. Despite high levels of bilirubin that may persist for 3 to 12 weeks, these infants are well and have no signs of hemolysis or liver dysfunction. The jaundice may be caused by factors in the breast milk (pregnanediol, fatty acids, and β-glucuronidase) that either inhibit the conjugation or decrease the excretion of bilirubin. Less frequent stooling by breastfed infants may allow extended time for reabsorption of bilirubin from stools (Blackburn, 2007). (See Chapter 26 for a discussion of these conditions in relation to nutrition.)

> **COMMUNITY FOCUS**
>
> *Neonatal Jaundice*
>
> Prepare a poster presentation for community health care workers that addresses the Canadian Paediatric Society (2007) guidelines for monitoring jaundiced newborns in the first week of life according to the hour-specific risk nomogram. In the poster address the issue of monitoring breastfeeding progress and elimination in relation to neonatal jaundice.

Hypoglycemia

Hypoglycemia during the early newborn period of a term infant is often defined as a blood glucose concentration less than adequate to support adequate neurological, organ, and tissue function; however, the precise level at which this occurs in every neonate is not known. At birth, the maternal source of glucose is cut off with the clamping of the umbilical cord. Most healthy term newborns experience a transient decrease in glucose levels, with a subsequent mobilization of free fatty acids and ketones to help maintain adequate glucose levels (Blackburn, 2007). Insulin does not cross the placental barrier, thus predisposing some infants to low glucose levels as a result of increased insulin activity. Infants who are asphyxiated or have other physiological stress may experience hypoglycemia as a result of a decreased glycogen supply, inadequate **gluconeogenesis**, or overutilization of glycogen stored during fetal life.

Cornblath and colleagues (2000) have suggested an operational threshold at which interventions to increase serum glucose levels should be instituted to prevent serious effects. For the healthy full-term infant, born after an uneventful pregnancy and birth, recommendations are to monitor glucose levels only in the presence of risk factors (see discussion below) or clinical manifestations of hypoglycemia; in these infants a plasma glucose of less than 2.5 mmol/L requires intervention. Healthy full-term, breastfed newborns may not fit into this category because human milk appears to provide adequate substrate (Cornblath et al., 2000). Hoseth and colleagues (2000) evaluated blood glucose levels in healthy full-term, breastfed infants and found significant hypoglycemia in only 2 of the 223 infants during the first 4 days of life.

In infants who are at risk for altered metabolism as a result of maternal illness factors (diabetes, gestational hypertension) or newborn factors (perinatal hypoxia, infection, hypothermia, **polycythemia**, congenital malformations, hyperinsulinism, SGA, fetal hydrops), close observation and monitoring of blood glucose levels within 2 to 3 hours of birth is recommended. If the newborn has a blood glucose level below 2.0 mmol/L, intervention such as breastfeeding or bottle-feeding should be instituted. If levels remain low despite feeding, intravenous (IV) dextrose is warranted. In such infants, the treatment should be aimed at maintaining the blood glucose levels above 2.5 mmol/L (Cornblath et al., 2000). Blood glucose levels for infants with severe hyperinsulinism may need to be higher (3.3 mmol/L) to prevent serious effects. While hypoglycemia in preterm infants requires further study, it has been suggested that values be maintained above 2.6 mmol/L (Cornblath et al., 2000).

Researchers further recommend that emphasis be placed less on an absolute glucose value and more on promoting normoglycemia with interventions for less optimal values (Blackburn, 2007). Monitoring blood glucose in the asymptomatic healthy term neonate (not at risk) on a routine basis is not recommended (Cornblath et al., 2000; CPS, 2004).

Signs of hypoglycemia include jitteriness; irregular respiratory effort; cyanosis; apnea; weak, high-pitched cry; feeding difficulty; lethargy; twitching; eye rolling; and seizures. The signs may be transient but recurrent.

Hypoglycemia in the low-risk term infant is usually eliminated by feeding the infant a source of carbohydrate (i.e., preferably human milk) and putting the newborn skin-to-skin with a parent. Occasionally, the IV administration of glucose is required for infants with persistently high insulin levels or in those with depleted stores of glycogen.

Hypocalcemia

Hypocalcemia in infants is defined as serum calcium levels less than 2 mmol/L in the term infant, and slightly lower (1.75 mmol/L) in the preterm infant; ideally, ionized fraction levels reflect the biologically active form and levels range from 0.75 to 1.1 mmol/L depending on the measurement method (Blackburn, 2007). Hypocalcemia may occur in newborns of diabetic mothers, in those who experienced perinatal asphyxia or trauma, and in preterm infants. Early-onset hypocalcemia usually occurs within the first 24 to 48 hours after birth. Signs of hypocalcemia include jitteriness, tremors, twitching, high-pitched cry, irritability, apnea, and laryngospasm, although some infants may be asymptomatic (Blackburn, 2007).

Treatment for the condition includes early feeding of an appropriate source of calcium such as fortified human milk or a preterm infant formula. In some cases (e.g., the medically unstable, extremely-low-birth-weight infant), the administration of IV elemental calcium and phosphorus may be necessary.

Because jitteriness is a symptom of both hypoglycemia and hypocalcemia, the latter must be considered if therapy for hypoglycemia is ineffective.

Laboratory and Diagnostic Tests

Because newborns experience many transitional events in the first 28 days of life, laboratory samples are often gathered to determine adequate physiological adaptation and to identify disorders that may adversely affect the child's life beyond the neonatal period. Most laboratory tests for newborn screening may be obtained from the neonate with a heel puncture. Tests that may be performed include bilirubin levels, blood glucose, newborn screening tests (e.g., PKU, hypothyroidism [T_4], sickle cell disease, and galactosemia), and drug serum levels. Box 25-4 lists standard laboratory values in a term newborn.

Tandem mass spectrometry has the potential for identifying as many as 40 inborn errors of metabolism (IEMs). With tandem mass spectrometry, earlier identification of IEMs may prevent further developmental delays and morbidities in affected children (Ontario Newborn Screening Program, n.d.). Newborn screening is done between 24 and 48 hours of age, although if a newborn is discharged prior to 24 hours it is recommended that the blood work be done before discharge and then again within 2 weeks (Perinatal Services BC, 2010).

All provinces have programs for newborn screening, but the number of conditions screened for varies by province. Newborn screening is considered the standard of care and specific consent from the parents is not required, although parents can decline the testing. If this occurs, it is important to ensure that they understand the importance of screening. Information about which tests are performed in each province can be obtained from provincial and territorial health departments. Some of the major disorders for which infants are screened are described in Table 25-3.

Collection of Specimens

Ongoing evaluation and screening of the newborn often require obtaining blood by heel stick or venipuncture.

Heel Stick

Some blood specimens are drawn by laboratory technicians; however, nurses may be required to perform heel sticks to obtain blood for glucose monitoring or newborn screening. The same technique is needed to complete the metabolic screening form on Guthrie paper or to test for galactosemia and hypothyroidism or other IEMs (see Table 25-3).

It is often helpful to warm the heel before the sample is taken; application of heat for 5 to 10 minutes helps dilate the

BOX 25-4 Standard Laboratory Values in a Term Newborn*

Hemoglobin	166–175 g/L
Hematocrit	0.51–0.56
Glucose	2.5–3.6 mmol/L
Leukocytes (white blood cells)	10–26 × 10^9/L
Bilirubin, total serum	<34 mcmol/L
Blood Gases	
Arterial	pH 7.32–7.48
	Pco_2 26–42 mm Hg
	Po_2 60–70 mm Hg
Base excess	−10 to −2 mmol/L (whole blood)
Bicarbonate, serum	21–28 mmol/L (arterial)
Anion gap	7–16 mmol/L
Venous	pH 7.31–7.41
	Pco_2 40–50 mm Hg
	Po_2 40–50 mm Hg

(From Blackburn, S. T. [2007]. *Maternal, fetal, and neonatal physiology: A clinical perspective* [3rd ed.]. St. Louis: Saunders.)

*These values may change significantly in the first week of life.

Table 25-3 Newborn Screening Summary

DISORDER AND EVIDENCE	SYMPTOMS	SCREENING INCIDENCE	TREATMENT
PKU (classic) Elevated phenylalanine plasma concentrations	Severe cognitive impairment if early detection and treatment not started, eczema, seizures, behaviour disorders, decreased pigmentation, distinctive musty or mouselike odour	1:12,000 in Ontario*	Lifelong dietary management with low-phenylalanine diet; possible tyrosine supplementation
Congenital hypothyroidism (primary) Low T_4, elevated TSH	Asymptomatic at birth; mental and motor delays (although neonatal detection and treatment has decreased incidence of cognitive impairment); short stature; coarse, dry skin and hair; hoarse cry; constipation	1:3000 to 1:4000 live births in Ontario with some ethnic variation	Maintain l-thyroxine levels in upper half of normal range; periodic bone age testing to monitor growth
Galactosemia (transferase deficiency) Elevated galactose; low or absent fluorescence	Hypotonia, lethargy, vomiting, diarrhea, metabolic acidosis, *Escherichia coli* sepsis, liver dysfunction, cognitive impairment, jaundice, blindness, cataracts, long-term behavioural problems, neurological impairment	1:60,000	Eliminate galactose and lactose from the diet; use soy formulas in infancy; lactose-free solid foods
Maple syrup urine disease Elevated leucine	Poor feeding; lethargy; hypotonia; vomiting; ketoacidosis; seizures; sweet maple syrup odour in urine, cerumen, or sweat	1:200,000 in Ontario Higher in Mennonites and those of French Canadian ancestry	Branched-chain amino acid–free formula with added protein-based formula; thiamine supplement in some individuals; lifelong treatment and monitoring necessary
Homocystinuria Elevated methionine and homocysteine	Infancy: nonspecific growth failure; developmental delay; more commonly diagnosed around 3 yr Cognitive impairment, seizures, behavioural disorders, early-onset thromboses, dislocated lenses, tall lanky body habitus	1:200,000 to 1:300,000 babies in Ontario; more prevalent in Irish, Danish, German, and Australian populations (1:20,000 to 1:60,000)	Methionine-restricted diet; cysteine supplement; vitamin B_6 supplement if responsive
Congenital adrenal hyperplasia Elevated 17-hydroxyprogesterone; abnormal electrolytes	Hyponatremia, hyperkalemia, hypoglycemia, dehydration; weight loss; hypotension; shock in "salt wasting" type; female virilization; progressive virilization in both sexes	1:15,000 in Ontario	Reduce excessive corticotropins; replace glucocorticoids and mineralocorticoids; corrective surgery for ambiguous genitalia (intersex assignment is controversial)
Sickle cell/hemoglobin SC (thalassemias)	Repeated infections, growth failure, pallor, hemolytic anemia; sickle cell crisis	Sickle cell anemia more common in African, Mediterranean, Middle Eastern, and Asian communities: 1:400 individuals from Carribbeans and parts of Africa	Preventive care: treatment of meningococcal and pneumococcal infections; hydroxyurea (antisickling agent); prevent human parvovirus B19 infection (limits production of reticulocytes)
Biotinidase deficiency Deficient or absent activity of biotinidase on colorimetric assay	Myoclonic seizures, hypotonia, feeding difficulties, organic aciduria, fungal infections, ataxia, skin rash, hearing loss, alopecia, optic nerve atrophy, developmental delay, coma, and death	1:60,000 in Ontario	5–20 mg biotin daily; less with partial deficiency

(Data from Debaun, M.R., & Vichinsky, E. [2007]. Hemoglobinopathies. In Kliegman, R.M. et al. *Nelson textbook of pediatrics* [18th ed.]. Philadelphia: Saunders; LaFranchini, S. [2007]. Disorders of the thyroid gland. In Kliegman, R.M. et al. *Nelson textbook of pediatrics* [18th ed.]. Philadelphia: Saunders; Ontario Newborn Screening Program [n.d.] Retrieved from http://www.newbornscreening.on.ca/bins/content_page.asp?cid=7-21&lang=1; Rezvani, I. [2007]. Metabolic diseases. In Kliegman, R.M. et al. *Nelson textbook of pediatrics* [18th ed.]. Philadelphia: Saunders.)

PKU, phenylketonuria; *TSH,* thyroid-stimulating hormone.

*Not all provinces screen for all conditions, so screening incidences are listed as per Ontario, where statistics are monitored.

blood vessels in the area. A cloth soaked with warm water (not hot) and wrapped loosely around the foot provides effective warming (Fig. 25-8, A). Disposable heel warmers are available from a variety of companies; they should be used with care to prevent burns. Nurses should wear gloves when collecting any specimen. The nurse cleanses the area with an appropriate skin antiseptic, allows the area to dry, restrains the infant's foot with a free hand, and then punctures the site. A spring-loaded automatic puncture device causes less pain and requires fewer punctures than a manual lance blade; therefore, manual lance

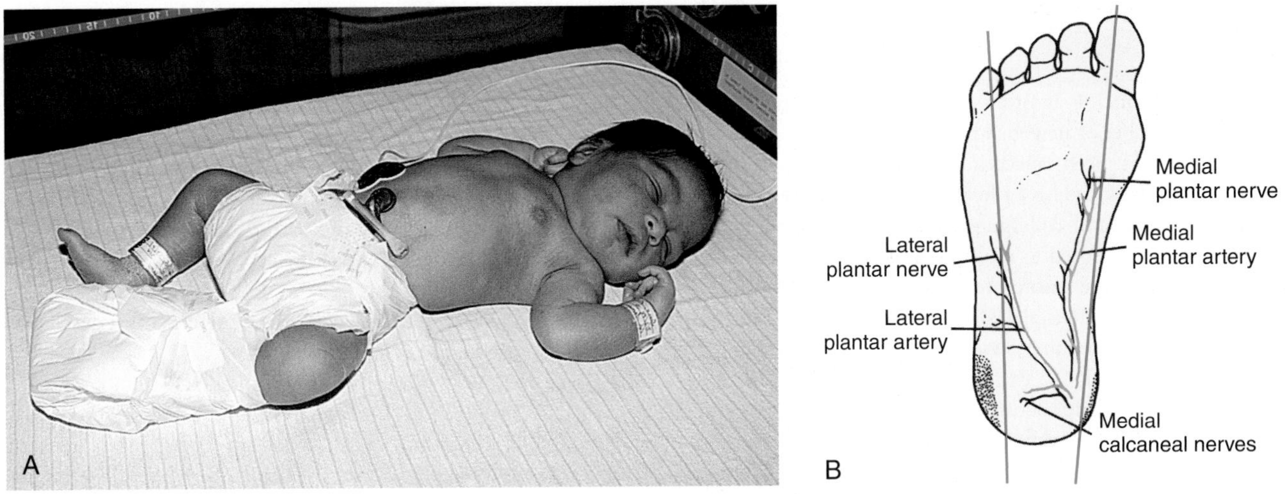

Fig. 25-8 Heel stick. **A:** Newborn with foot wrapped for warmth to increase blood flow to extremity before heel stick. **B:** Heel stick sites (shaded areas) on infant's foot for obtaining samples of capillary blood. *(A, Courtesy Marjorie Pyle, RNC, Lifecircle, Costa Mesa, CA.)*

blades should not be used on neonates. It is important to fill all of the circles on the metabolic screening form with blood.

The most serious complication of infant heel stick is necrotizing osteochondritis from lancet penetration of the bone (Meehan, 1998). To prevent this, the penetration should be made at the outer aspect of the heel and should be no deeper than 2.4 mm. To identify the appropriate puncture site, the nurse should draw an imaginary line running from between the fourth and fifth toes and parallel to the lateral aspect of the foot to the heel where the stick should be made; a second line can also be drawn from the great toe to the medial aspect of the heel (see Fig. 25-8, B). Repeated trauma to the walking surface of the heel can cause fibrosis and scarring that may lead to problems with walking later in life. After the specimen has been collected, pressure is applied with a dry gauze square. No further skin cleanser should be applied because this will cause the site to continue to bleed. The site is then covered with an adhesive bandage. The nurse needs to ensure proper disposal of equipment used, review the laboratory requisition for correct identification, and check the specimen for adequate labelling and routing.

A heel stick is traumatic for the infant and causes pain. To reassure the infant and to promote feelings of safety, the neonate should be cuddled and comforted when the procedure is complete, and appropriate pain management measures should be taken to minimize the pain (see Atraumatic Care box).

Venipuncture

Venous blood samples can be drawn from the antecubital, saphenous, superficial wrist, and, rarely, scalp veins. If an existing IV site is used to obtain a blood specimen, it is important to consider the type of infusion fluid; contamination of the blood with the fluid can alter results.

When venipuncture is required, positioning of the needle is extremely important. Although regular venipuncture needles may be used, some individuals prefer butterfly needles. A 25-gauge needle is adequate for blood sampling in neonates, with minimal hemolysis being observed when the proper procedure is followed. It is necessary to be patient during the procedure because the blood return from small veins is slow; consequently, the small needle must remain in place longer. A tourniquet is optional but may help increase blood flow with venipuncture. The mummy restraint commonly is used to help secure the infant (see Fig. 45-7).

evolve Skill–Pain Assessment

For blood gas studies, the blood sample container is packed in ice (to reduce blood cell metabolism) and taken immediately to the laboratory for analysis.

Pressure must be maintained over an arterial puncture with a dry gauze square for at least 3 to 5 minutes to prevent bleeding from the site. The nurse should observe the infant frequently for evidence of bleeding or hematoma at the puncture site for at least an hour after any venipuncture. The infant's tolerance of the procedure should be noted and recorded. The infant should be cuddled and comforted (e.g., rocked, given a pacifier) when the procedure is completed, and appropriate pain management measures should be taken to minimize the pain.

NURSING ALERT Only venous or capillary blood samples may be used for newborn screening and genetic studies; cord blood is not used for these samples.

Obtaining a Urine Specimen

Examination of urine is a valuable laboratory tool for infant assessment, but the way in which the specimen is collected may influence the results. The urine sample should be fresh and examined within 1 hour of collection.

A variety of urine collection bags are available (Fig. 25-9) (see also Fig. 45-10). These are clear plastic, single-use bags with adhesive material around the opening at the point of attachment.

To prepare the infant, the nurse removes the diaper and places the infant in a supine position. The genitalia, perineum, and surrounding skin are washed and thoroughly dried because the adhesive of the bag will not stick to moist,

ATRAUMATIC CARE

Heel Punctures

Repeated heel lancing is often necessary to obtain sufficient blood for a number of newborn blood tests, including newborn screening. It has been anecdotally observed that newborns appear to withdraw the heel when touched for subsequent heel punctures. Taddio and colleagues (2002) found that infants of diabetic mothers exposed to multiple heel punctures in the first 24 to 36 hours of life learned to anticipate pain and exhibited more intense pain responses. The use of automated lancet devices causes less pain and requires fewer punctures than manual lance blades (Blain-Lewis, 1992; Paes et al., 1993). Additional studies have shown that venipuncture performed by an experienced phlebotomist elicited fewer pain responses (as measured by the Premature Infant Pain Profile [PIPP]) from full-term newborns than did heel punctures (Shah & Ohlsson, 2001). The need for additional skin punctures was reduced with venipuncture. Although maternal anxiety was initially higher in the venipuncture group, mothers who observed the venipuncture reported seeing less pain response than mothers who observed heel punctures.

Oral sucrose and non-nutritive sucking have proved effective in decreasing the pain associated with heel punctures in preterm and full-term infants during the first week of life (Gibbins et al., 2002; Harrison, Johnston, & Loughnan, 2003; Stevens, Yamada, & Ohlsson, 2004); however, the exact dose range that proves effective varies among several studies (Stevens et al., 2004). In one study, infants experiencing venipuncture were given either oral sucrose (30%) and a skin placebo or the eutectic mixture of local anaesthetic (EMLA). Pain scores were measured with the PIPP, and infants receiving the oral sucrose solution exhibited fewer pain signs than those in the EMLA group (Gradin et al., 2002). Giving newborns 2 mL of oral sucrose solution (25% and 50%) significantly reduced crying time and heart rate after 3 minutes in comparison with controls (sterile water) during heel-stick sampling for serum bilirubin concentrations (Haouari et al., 1995). Newborns given 2 mL of concentrated oral sucrose solution showed a significant reduction in crying time and heart rate in comparison with controls (given sterile water) during heel-stick sampling and other painful stimuli (Stevens et al., 2004).

Evidence indicates that as little as 2 mL of a 24% oral sucrose solution is effective in decreasing pain in full-term and preterm infants. In addition, the best analgesic effect is achieved when sucrose is administered 2 minutes before the painful procedure, with a pacifier or syringe. In one study protocol in which oral sucrose was effective, 0.5 mL of 24% oral sucrose solution was administered 2 minutes before the heel puncture, during puncture, and 5 minutes after the heel puncture (Gibbins et al., 2002). Eriksson and Finnstrom (2004) found that repeated administration of a 30% sucrose solution before heel lance in healthy full-term infants did not decrease the pain-relieving effect of the glucose solution; the study's aim was to determine whether multiple oral glucose administrations would cause tolerance to glucose. Monitoring for adverse effects must accompany each administration (Noerr, 2001).

The mother's holding the infant in skin-to-skin contact significantly reduces the child's distress during the procedure (Blass & Watt, 1999; Gray, Watt, & Blass, 2000; Johnston et al., 2003). Breastfeeding during heel puncture in full-term newborns is effective in decreasing pain scores when compared with placebo or a 30% oral sucrose solution (Carbajal et al., 2003).

Applying the topical anaesthetic EMLA to reduce the pain of heel lance has produced mixed results in full-term and preterm infants (Fitzgerald, Millard, & McIntosh, 1989; Stevens et al., 1999; Taddio et al., 1998). Grunau and colleagues (2004) noted that placing preterm infants in a prone (vs. supine) position for heel stick did not decrease the pain response and that additional pain-relieving measures for this population are necessary.

Music was found to decrease the pain response to heel stick in a small group of preterm infants (Butt & Kisilevsky, 2000). A study comparing the effects of swaddling and containment on preterm infants undergoing heel stick failed to demonstrate significant differences between the two interventions (Huang et al., 2004).

These studies provide evidence of a number of effective ways to decrease the pain associated with heel puncture in full-term and preterm newborns. It is essential that nurses use all available resources to advocate for the prevention and management of neonatal pain during such procedures as heel puncture. Because the overall goal is to decrease the effect on infants of painful interventions such as heel stick, a combination of pharmacological and nonpharmacological interventions is recommended (American Academy of Pediatrics & Canadian Paediatric Society [AAP & CPA], 2006).

A number of commercially available oral sucrose solutions now exist. When these are not available, the pharmacy can mix an oral sucrose solution to ensure a clean product. An approximate 25% sucrose solution is made by mixing 5 mL of granulated (table) sugar with 20 mL sterile water; however, this method is the least desirable to prevent contamination of the solution and subsequent problems.

powdered, or oily skin surfaces. The protective paper is removed to expose the adhesive (see Fig. 25-9, A). For female infants, the perineum is stretched to flatten skin folds; then the adhesive area is pressed firmly to the skin all around the urinary meatus and vagina. (Note: Start with the narrow portion of the butterfly-shaped adhesive patch.) The nurse must be certain to start at the bridge of skin separating the rectum from the vagina and work upward (see Fig. 25-9, B). For male infants the penis (and scrotum, depending on the size of the collection device) is tucked through the opening of the collector before the nurse removes the protective paper from the adhesive; then the protective paper is removed, and the flaps are pressed firmly to the perineum, making certain that the entire adhesive coating is firmly attached to skin and

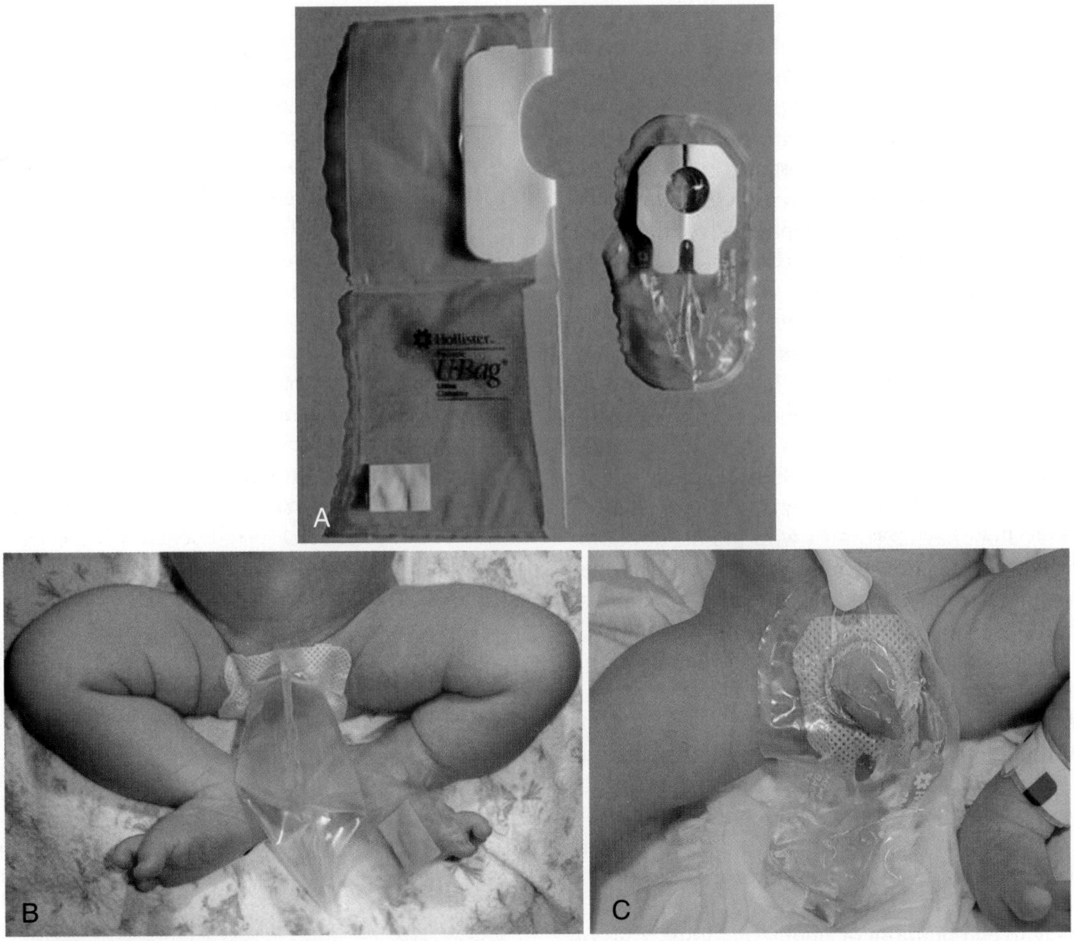

Fig. 25-9 Collection of urine specimen. **A:** Protective paper is removed from the adhesive surface. **B:** Applied to females. **C:** Applied to males. *(Courtesy Cheryl Briggs, RN, Annapolis, MD.)*

the edges of the opening do not pucker (see Fig. 25-9, C). This helps ensure a leak-proof seal and decreases the chance of contamination from stool. Cutting a slit in the diaper and pulling the bag through the slit may also help prevent leaking. The specimen can be aspirated with a syringe or drained directly from the bag.

Collection of a 24-hour specimen from an infant can be a challenge, sometimes requiring light restraint with elbow restraints. The 24-hour urine bag is applied in the manner just described, and the urine is placed in an appropriate receptacle. The infant's skin should be watched closely for signs of irritation and for lack of a proper seal.

For some types of urine testing, urine can be aspirated directly from the diaper by means of a syringe without a needle. If the diaper has absorbent gelling material that traps urine, a small gauze pad or cotton balls are placed inside the diaper and the urine is aspirated from the cotton or gauze.

Implementation

In the inpatient setting, priorities of care must be established and a systematic teaching plan for infant care devised. One way to achieve this is to use care paths. A care path may be developed that covers the changes expected in the infant during the first few days of life. Modifications in the care path to individualize newborn care may be necessary. The existing care path may also be used by nursing staff following care of the mother–newborn dyad at home in the first few weeks of life, to ensure that the infant receives appropriate care and screening, which was once provided in the acute care setting. When variations from the care path occur, further assessment and intervention may be necessary.

Protective Environment

The provision of a protective environment is basic to the care of the newborn. Hospital personnel develop their own policies and procedures for protecting the newborns under their care. Prescribed standards cover areas such as infection-control measures and safety factors.

Measures to Control Infection

Measures to control infection include adequate floor space for positioning bassinets at least 90 cm apart in all directions, hand-washing facilities, and areas for cleaning and storing equipment and supplies. Only those personnel directly involved in the care of mothers and infants are allowed in these areas, thereby reducing the opportunities for the introduction of pathogenic organisms.

NURSING ALERT Personnel are instructed to use good hand hygiene techniques. The most important single measure in the prevention of neonatal infection is hand hygiene. Hand hygiene must be carried out before initial patient–environment contact, before an aseptic procedure, after body fluid exposure, and after patient–environment contact. Hand hygiene must also occur after contact with potentially contaminated objects (e.g., computer keyboards, telephone, countertops). Inanimate objects should be cleaned with an appropriate bactericidal solution.

Health care workers must wear gloves when handling the infant before blood and amniotic fluid have been removed from the infant's skin, when drawing blood (e.g., heel stick), and during diaper changes.

Visitors and health care providers, including nurses, physicians, parents, siblings, and grandparents, are expected to wash their hands before having contact with infants or equipment. Individuals with infectious conditions, including upper respiratory tract or gastrointestinal tract infections and infectious skin conditions, should be excluded from contact with newborns or must take special precautions when working with infants.

Safety Factors

Although abduction is rare in Canada, health care institutions must be proactive in protecting newborns from abduction. Measures taken include placing matching identification bracelets on newborns and their parents and using identification bands with radiofrequency transmitters that set off an alarm if the bracelet is removed or if a certain threshold is crossed (doorway to exit building or floor). In addition, agencies must conduct periodic unit- and hospital-wide drills aimed at preventing newborn abductions. Personnel caring for newborns must be clearly identified by photo identification, and parents must be educated about measures to prevent abduction from the mother's room.

Supporting Parents in the Care of Their Infant

The caregiver's sensitivity to the infant's social responses is basic to the development of a mutually satisfying parent–child relationship (Leitch, 1999). Sensitivity increases over time as parents become more aware of their infant's social capabilities.

Social Interactions

The activities of daily care during the neonatal period present the best times for infant and family interactions (see Cultural Awareness box). While caring for their newborn, the mother and father can talk to the infant, play baby games, caress and cuddle the child, and perhaps use infant massage. In Figure 25-10, a mother, father, and infant are shown engaging in arousal, imitation of facial expression, and smiling. Too much stimulation should be avoided after feeding and before a sleep period. Older siblings' contact with a newborn is encouraged and supervised depending on the child's developmental level.

CULTURAL AWARENESS

Cultural Beliefs and Practices Regarding Newborns

Nurses working with childbearing families from cultures and ethnic groups other than their own must be aware of cultural beliefs and practices that are important to individual families. People with a strong sense of heritage may hold on to traditional health beliefs long after adopting other Canadian lifestyle practices. These health beliefs may involve practices regarding the newborn. For example, some Asians, Latin Americans, and Eastern Europeans delay breastfeeding because they believe that colostrum is "bad." Some Latin Americans and Africans place a belly band over the infant's navel. The birth of a male child is generally preferred by Asians and Indians, and some Asians and Haitians delay naming their infant. East Indians may want to put something sweet on the newborn's lips right after birth.

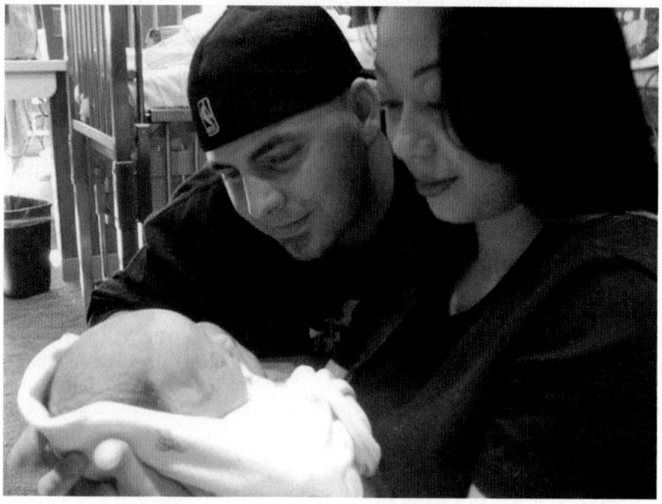

Fig. 25-10 Mother–father–baby interaction. *(From Hockenberry, M. J., & Wilson, D. [2007].* Wong's nursing care of infants and children *[8th ed., p. 371]. St. Louis: Mosby.)*

Infant Feeding

The infant should be put to breast ideally within the first hour after birth. Newborns are placed on demand feeding schedules and allowed to feed when they awaken and demonstrate typical hunger cues, regardless of the amount of time since the previous feeding. Ordinarily, mothers are encouraged to breastfeed their infants at least every 2 to 3 hours (bottle-feed every 3 to 4 hours) or on demand to ensure adequate fluid intake and weight gain. Breastfed babies nurse more often than bottle-fed babies because breast milk is digested faster than formulas made from cow's milk and the stomach empties sooner as a result. Breastfed newborns feed an average of 10 to 12 times per day. Water and dextrose water supplements are not recommended in the newborn period, since these have the tendency to decrease breastfeeding. There is no evidence to support dextrose or water feedings in newborns. For a thorough discussion of infant feeding, see Chapter 26.

Therapeutic and Surgical Procedures

Intramuscular Injection

As discussed previously, it is routine to administer a single dose of 0.5 to 1 mg of vitamin K intramuscularly (see Medication Guide earlier in this chapter).

Hepatitis B vaccination is recommended for infants at highest risk of contracting hepatitis B. This includes newborns born to women who have hepatitis B or whose hepatitis B status is unknown or if another family member who lives in the home has hepatitis B. If the infant is born to an infected mother or to a mother who is a chronic carrier, hepatitis B vaccine and hepatitis B **immune globulin** (HBIG) should be given within 12 hours of birth (see Medication Guides). In some provinces the hepatitis B vaccine is given at birth, whereas in others it is given before the child is a preteen. See the Public Health Agency of Canada Web site to see the schedule for different provinces (http://www.phac-aspc.gc.ca/im/ptimprog-progimpt/table-1-eng.php). The hepatitis B vaccine is given in one site and the HBIG in another. Parental consent must be obtained before administering these medications.

In most cases a 25-gauge, ⅝-inch (16-mm) to ⅞-inch (22-mm) needle should be used for the vitamin K and hepatitis B vaccine injections. Selection of the site for injection is important. Injections must be given in muscles large enough to accommodate the medication, and major nerves and blood vessels must be avoided. The muscles of newborns may not tolerate more than 0.5 mL per intramuscular injection. The preferred injection site for newborns is the vastus lateralis (Fig. 25-11). The dorsogluteal muscle is very small, poorly developed, and dangerously close to the sciatic nerve, which occupies a larger proportion of space in infants than in older children. Therefore, it is not recommended as an injection site in small children. The newborn's deltoid muscle has an inadequate amount of muscle for intramuscular administration. An important factor in preventing and minimizing local reaction to intramuscular injections is adequate deposition of the fluid (medication) deep within the muscle; muscle size, needle length, and amount of medication injected should be carefully considered.

For an injection, the neonate's leg should be stabilized (see Fig. 45-8 for containment method). The nurse should wear gloves and should cleanse the injection site with an appropriate skin antiseptic. The needle is inserted into the vastus lateralis at a 90-degree angle. The plunger of the syringe is gently withdrawn, and if no blood is aspirated, the medication is injected. If blood is aspirated, the needle is withdrawn and the injection is given in another site. The needle is withdrawn quickly and pressure is maintained at the site to minimize the pain.

The nurse should always comfort the infant after an injection and consider other pain management techniques while performing the task (see Atraumatic Care box on p. 658). Needles should never be recapped; they should be properly discarded in an appropriate safety container. It is important to record medication, date and time, amount, route, and site of injection on the newborn's medical record.

Therapy for Hyperbilirubinemia

The best therapy for hyperbilirubinemia is prevention. Because bilirubin is excreted in meconium, prevention can be

---

MEDICATION GUIDE

*Hepatitis B Vaccine (Recombivax HB, Engerix-B)**

Action

Hepatitis B vaccine induces protective anti-hepatitis B antibodies in 95 to 99% of healthy infants who receive the recommended three doses. The duration of protection of the vaccine is unknown.

Indication

Hepatitis B vaccine provides immunization against infection caused by all known subtypes of hepatitis B virus.

Neonatal Dosage

The usual dosage is Recombivax HB 5 mcg/0.5 mL or Engerix-B 10 mcg/0.5 mL at birth, 1 month, and 6 months. (See also Immunizations, Chapter 36.)

Adverse Reactions

Common adverse reactions are rash, fever, erythema, swelling, and pain at injection site.

Nursing Considerations

Parental consent must be obtained before administration. Wear gloves. See Medication Guide: Vitamin K (p. 647) for intramuscular administration. If the infant was born to a hepatitis B surface antigen (HBsAg)-positive mother, hepatitis B immune globulin (HBIG) should be given within 12 hours of birth in addition to the hepatitis B vaccine. Separate sites must be used. Document immunization administration on a vaccination card for parent(s) to have a record.

*Note: The combination vaccines containing hepatitis B are not recommended for the birth (first) dose.

MEDICATION GUIDE

Hepatitis B Immune Globulin

Action

Hepatitis B immune globulin (HBIG) provides a high titre of antibody to hepatitis B surface antigen (HBsAg).

Indication

The HBIG vaccine provides prophylaxis against infection in infants born to HBsAg-positive mothers.

Neonatal Dosage

Administer one 0.5 mL dose intramuscularly within 12 hours of birth.

Adverse Reactions

Hypersensitivity may occur.

Nursing Considerations

The vaccine must be given within 12 hours of birth. Wear gloves. See Medication Guide: Vitamin K (p. 647) for intramuscular administration. HBIG may be given at the same time as hepatitis B vaccine, but in a separate syringe and at a different site. Document immunization administration on a vaccination card for parent(s) to have a record.

facilitated by early frequent feeding, which stimulates passage of meconium. However, despite early passage of meconium, some term infants may have trouble conjugating the increased amount of bilirubin derived from disintegrating fetal RBCs. As a result, the serum levels of unconjugated bilirubin may rise beyond normal limits, causing hyperbilirubinemia. The goal of treatment of hyperbilirubinemia is to help reduce the newborn's serum levels of unconjugated bilirubin. There are two ways to reduce unconjugated bilirubin levels: phototherapy and exchange blood transfusion. Exchange transfusion is used to treat those infants whose levels of serum bilirubin are rising rapidly despite the use of intensive phototherapy (see discussion in Chapter 28, p. 768).

Phototherapy

During phototherapy, the infant is placed, seminude, approximately 45 to 50 cm on or under special phototherapy lights. The distance may vary based on unit protocol and type of light used. The most effective therapy is achieved with lights at 400 to 550 nanometers, and a blue-green light spectrum is the most efficient (Steffensrud, 2004). The lamp energy output should be monitored routinely during treatment with a photometer to ensure efficacy of therapy. Phototherapy is carried out until the infant's serum bilirubin level decreases to within an acceptable range. The decision to discontinue therapy is based on a definite downward trend in the serum bilirubin values.

Several precautions must be taken while the infant is undergoing phototherapy. The infant's eyes must be protected by an opaque mask to prevent overexposure to the light. The eye shield should cover the eyes completely but not occlude the nares. Before the mask is applied, the infant's eyes should be closed gently to prevent excoriation of the corneas. The mask should be removed periodically and during infant feedings so that the eyes can be checked and cleansed with water and the parents can have visual contact with the infant (Fig. 25-12, A and B, and Family-Centred Teaching box).

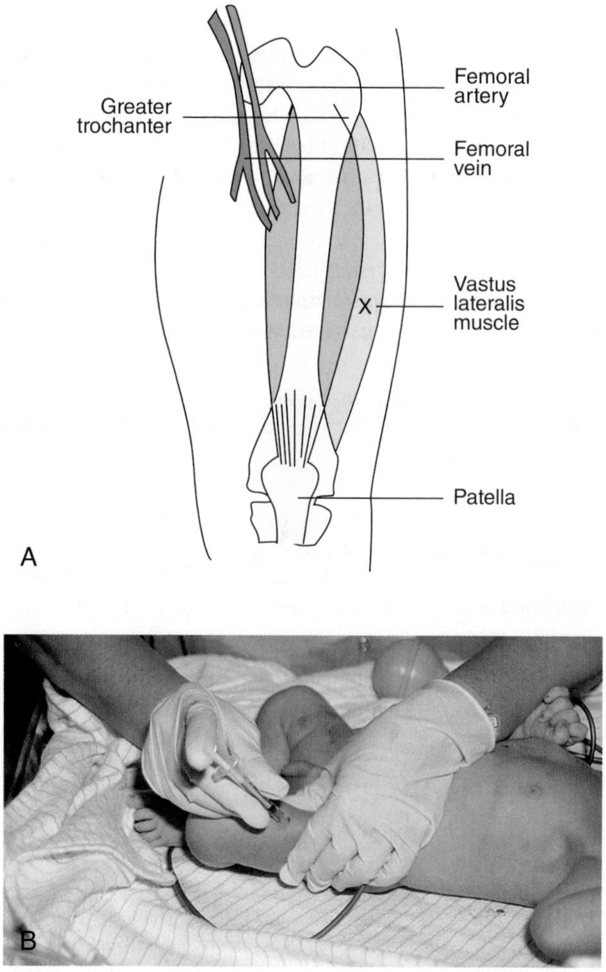

Fig. 25-11 Intramuscular injection. **A:** Acceptable intramuscular injection site (X) for newborn infant. **B:** Infant's leg being stabilized for intramuscular injection. The nurse is wearing gloves to give the injection. *(**B**, Courtesy Marjorie Pyle, RNC, Lifecircle, Costa Mesa, CA.)*

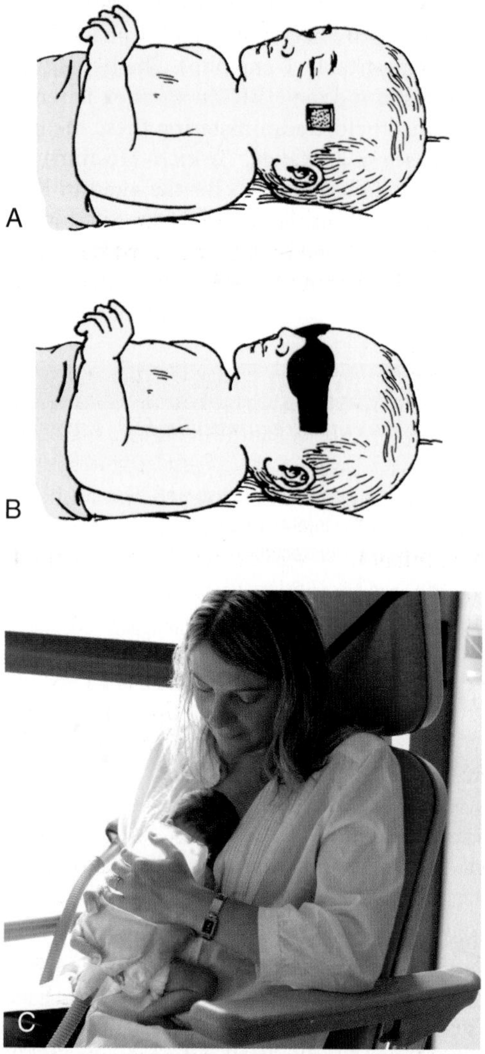

Fig. 25-12 Eye patches for newborns receiving phototherapy. **A:** Small Velcro patch stuck to both sides of head. **B:** Eye cover sticks to Velcro patch, which reduces movement of eye cover and facilitates removal for feedings. **C:** A mother can put newborn skin-to-skin without interrupting phototherapy when a fibreoptic blanket is used. *(**C**, Courtesy Mother and Childcare, Phillips Healthcare, Monroeville, PA.)*

FAMILY-CENTRED TEACHING

Phototherapy and Parent–Infant Interaction

The traditional use of phototherapy has evoked concerns regarding a number of psychobehavioural issues, including parent–infant separation, potential social isolation, decreased sensorineural stimulation, altered biological rhythms, altered feeding patterns, and activity changes. Parental anxiety is greatly increased, particularly at the sight of the newborn blindfolded and under special lights. The interruption of breastfeeding for phototherapy is a potential deterrent to successful maternal–infant attachment and interaction. Because research has demonstrated that bilirubin catabolism occurs primarily within the first few hours of the initiation of phototherapy, there is increased support for the removal of the infant from treatment for feeding and holding. Intermittent phototherapy may be just as effective as continuous therapy when used correctly. The benefits of stopping phototherapy for short periods so that parents can feed and hold the newborn should be carefully weighed by the health care team and the parents.

Often a "string bikini" made from a disposable face mask is used instead of a diaper. This allows optimal skin exposure, yet provides sufficient protection to the genitalia and bedding. Before its application, the metal strip must be removed from the mask to avoid burning the infant. Lotions and ointments should not be used during phototherapy because they absorb heat and can cause burns.

Phototherapy may cause changes in the infant's temperature depending partially on the bed used: bassinet, incubator, or radiant warmer. The infant's temperature should be closely monitored at least every 2 hours. Phototherapy lights may increase the rate of insensible water loss, making it possible for fluid loss and dehydration to occur. Therefore, it is important that the infant be adequately hydrated. Hydration maintenance in the healthy newborn is carried out with human milk or infant formula; there is no advantage or benefit to administering oral glucose or plain water because these do not promote excretion of bilirubin in stools and may in fact perpetuate enterohepatic circulation, thus delaying bilirubin excretion. Urine output may be decreased or unaltered; the urine may appear dark gold or brown.

The number and consistency of stools should be monitored. Bilirubin breakdown increases gastric motility, which results in loose stools that can cause skin excoriation and breakdown. The infant's buttocks must be cleaned after each stool to help maintain skin integrity. A fine maculopapular rash may appear during phototherapy, but this is transient. Because visualization of the infant's skin colour is difficult with blue light, appropriate cardiorespiratory monitoring should be implemented based on the infant's overall condition.

When a newborn requires phototherapy, it is important to try to maintain maternal–infant contact and, if possible, phototherapy should be initiated in the mother's room. A number of newer phototherapy products, including the Bilibed, use fluorescent light for phototherapy. With such systems the infant may be cared for at home. Alternative devices for phototherapy include a fluorescent bank of lights, halogen spotlights, LED (light-emitting diode) units, and a fibreoptic pad. When a fibreoptic pad is used, the newborn can remain in an open crib or in the mother's arms during treatment (see Fig. 25-12, C). In certain situations, the infant's bilirubin levels may be increasing rapidly and require intensive phototherapy; this involves the use of a combination of intensive conventional lights and fibreoptic or halogen lights to maximize bilirubin reduction. All aspects of phototherapy should be accurately recorded in the infant's medical record.

Parent Education

Serum levels of bilirubin in the newborn continue to rise until the fifth day of life. Many parents leave the hospital within 24 hours of birth, and some as early as 6 hours after birth. Therefore, parents must receive education regarding jaundice and its treatment. They should have written instructions for assessing the infant's condition and the name of a contact person to whom they should report their findings and concerns. Some regional health departments provide a home visit to evaluate the infant's condition and to monitor the mother's health as well.

evolve Critical Thinking Exercise–Circumcision

Circumcision

The reported rate of circumcision in Canada in 2007 was 32%; the rates are highest in Alberta (44%) and Ontario (43%) and below 10% in Northwest Territories and Nova Scotia (Public Health Agency of Canada [PHAC], 2009). Circumcision of male infants is usually performed within the first few weeks of life and may occur before the newborn is discharged from the hospital, or it may be done as an outpatient procedure. In 1996, the Canadian Paediatric Society (CPS) noted that, despite scientific evidence of potential medical benefits of circumcision, the data are not sufficient to recommend routine circumcision. The CPS further recommended that if circumcision is performed, analgesia should be used (CPS, 1996).

Circumcision is a matter of personal parental choice. Parents usually decide to have their newborn circumcised on the basis of one or more of the following factors: religious conviction, tradition, culture, social norms, or perceived hygiene. Regardless of the reason for the decision, parents should be given unbiased information and the opportunity to discuss the benefits and risks (see Community Focus box).

Procedure

Circumcision involves removal of the **prepuce** (foreskin) of the glans. The procedure is not usually done immediately after

COMMUNITY FOCUS

Newborn Circumcision

Prepare a poster presentation to provide parents information on newborn circumcision. Because circumcision is considered an optional surgical procedure, it may not be performed until after the infant is discharged home. Include in your display the advantages and disadvantages of circumcision, as well as the care of the uncircumcised penis in infants and young children.

birth because of the danger of cold stress and decreased clotting factors, but it may be performed in the hospital before the infant's discharge. Many circumcisions are done after the newborn is discharged from the hospital. The circumcision of a Jewish boy is performed on the eighth day after birth and is done at home in a ceremony called a *bris*, unless the infant is ill. The timing is logical from a physiological standpoint because clotting factors drop somewhat immediately after birth and do not return to prebirth levels until the end of the first week.

Feedings are usually withheld up to 2 to 3 hours before the circumcision to prevent vomiting and aspiration. To prepare the infant for the circumcision, he is positioned on a plastic restraint form (Fig. 25-13) or held by a staff member, and the penis is cleansed with soap and water or other prep solution such as povidone-iodine. The infant is draped to provide warmth and a sterile field, and the sterile equipment is readied for use.

Although some circumcision procedures require no special equipment or appliances (Fig. 25-14), numerous instruments have been designed for this purpose. Use of the Gomco clamp (Fig. 25-15) may make this an almost bloodless operation. The procedure itself takes only a few minutes to perform. After it is completed, a small petrolatum gauze dressing or a generous amount of petrolatum or A&D ointment may be applied to the penis for the first few days to prevent the diaper from adhering to the site. A PlastiBell is another method used for the circumcision. The advantages are that it applies constant direct pressure to prevent hemorrhage during the procedure and afterward protects against infection, keeps the site from sticking to the diaper, and prevents pain with urination. When using the plastic bell for circumcision, it is first fitted over the glans, the suture is tied around the rim of the bell, and excess prepuce is cut away. The plastic rim remains in place for about a week; it falls off after healing has taken place, usually within 5 to 7 days (Fig. 25-16). Petrolatum is not usually needed when the bell is used.

evolve Video–Circumcision

Procedural Pain Management

Circumcision is painful. The pain is manifested by both physiological and behavioural changes in the infant (see discussion that follows). Four types of **anaesthesia** and **analgesia** are used in newborns undergoing circumcision: ring block, dorsal penile nerve block (DPNB), topical anaesthetic such as **eutectic mixture of lidocaine and prilocaine (EMLA)** (prilocaine-lidocaine), and concentrated oral sucrose. Nonpharmacological methods such as non-nutritive sucking, containment, and swaddling may be used to enhance pain management (see Atraumatic Care box). The Cochrane Group exploring pain relief for neonatal circumcision found that DPNB was the most effective intervention for decreasing pain, and EMLA was also somewhat effective (Brady-Fryer, Wiebe, & Lander, 2004).

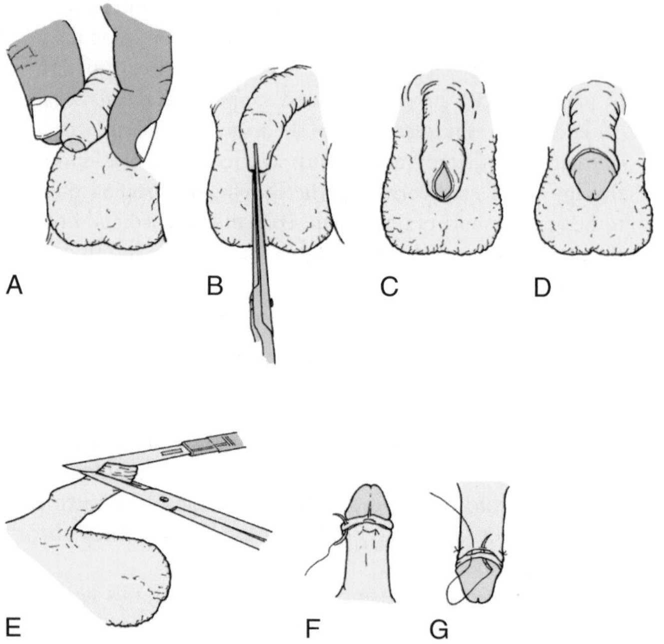

Fig. 25-14 Technique of circumcision. **A** to **D:** Prepuce is stripped and slit to facilitate its retraction behind glans penis. **E:** Prepuce is now clamped and excessive prepuce cut off. **F** and **G:** A very small needle with plain 2-0 or 3-0 catgut is used for suturing; some physicians prefer silk.

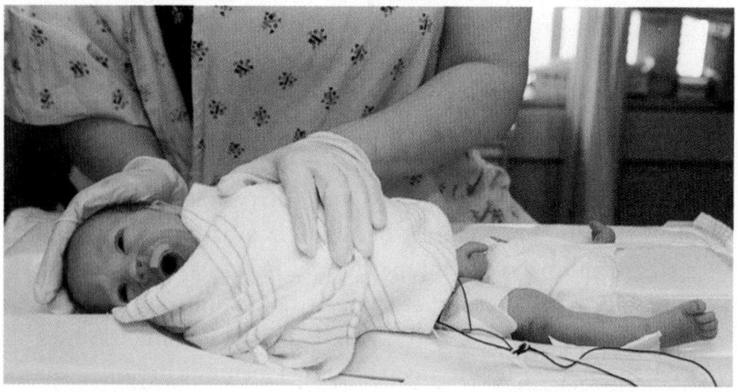

Fig. 25-13 Proper positioning of infant in Circumstraint. *(Courtesy Paul Vincent Kuntz, Texas Children's Hospital, Houston, TX.)*

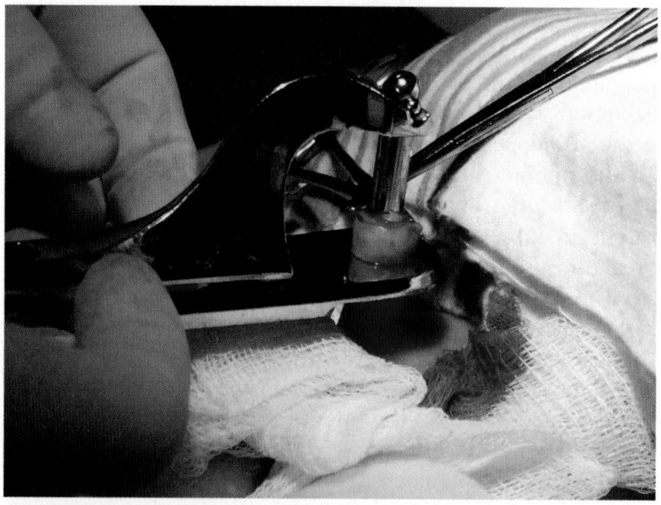

Fig. 25-15 Circumcision with Gomco clamp. Prepuce is drawn over cone and clamp is applied; hemostasis occurs, and then prepuce (over cone) is cut away. *(Courtesy Cheryl Briggs, RN, Annapolis, MD.)*

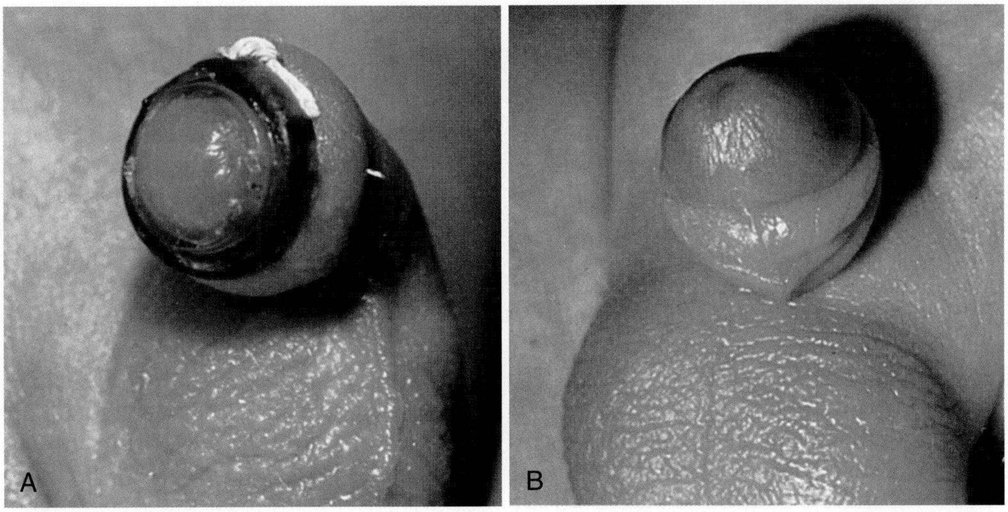

Fig. 25-16 Circumcision using Hollister PlastiBell. **A:** Suture around rim of PlastiBell controls bleeding. **B:** Plastic rim and suture drop off in 7 to 10 days. *(Owned by Briggs Healthcare, Waukegan, IL.)*

After the circumcision, the infant should be comforted until he is quieted. If the parents were not present during the procedure, the infant should be returned to them. Afterwards, the infant may be fussy for several hours and may have disturbed sleep–wake states and disorganized feeding behaviours. Oral acetaminophen may be administered before the procedure and every 4 hours thereafter (as ordered by the practitioner) for a maximum of five doses in 24 hours or a maximum of 75 mg/kg/day. For additional discussion of neonatal pain, see Chapter 35.

Care of the Newly Circumcised Infant

The nurse should check the infant hourly for the next 4 to 6 hours to make certain that no bleeding is occurring and that voiding is normal. If bleeding is noted from the circumcision, the nurse can apply gentle pressure to the site of bleeding with a folded sterile gauze pad or sprinkle powdered gel foam on it. If the bleeding is not easily controlled, a blood vessel may need to be ligated. In this event, one nurse notifies the physician and prepares the necessary equipment (i.e., circumcision tray and suture materials) while another nurse maintains intermittent pressure until the physician arrives. If the parents take the baby home before the end of the observation period, they must be taught the proper home care (see Patient Teaching box). Nursing actions should be planned and implemented to prevent infection. Prepackaged commercial wipes for cleaning the diaper area should not be used because they contain alcohol, which delays healing and causes discomfort. Instead, the nurse should wash the penis gently with water to remove urine and feces and, if necessary, apply fresh petrolatum around the glans after each diaper change.

The glans penis, normally dark red during healing, becomes covered with a yellow exudate within 24 hours. This is part of normal healing, not an infective process. No attempt should be made to remove the exudate, which persists for 2 to 3 days. Parents should be taught to fanfold the diaper so that it does not press on the circumcised area. They should be encouraged

PATIENT TEACHING Care of the Circumcised Newborn at Home

Wash hands before touching the newly circumcised penis.

Check for Bleeding
- Check circumcision for bleeding with each diaper change.
- If bleeding occurs, apply gentle pressure with a folded sterile gauze square. If bleeding does not stop with pressure, notify the primary health care provider.

Observe for Urination
- Check to see that the infant urinates after being circumcised.
- Infant should have wet diapers appropriate for age (see Home Care Box, p. 673).

Keep Area Clean
- Change diaper and inspect circumcision at least every 4 hours.
- Wash penis gently with warm water to remove urine and feces. Apply petrolatum liberally to the glans with each diaper change (omit petrolatum if PlastiBell was used).
- Use soap only after circumcision is healed (5 to 6 days).
- Sponge bath only until circumcision heals.
- Fanfold diaper to prevent pressure on the circumcised area.

Check for Infection
- Glans penis is dark red after circumcision, then becomes covered with yellow exudate in 24 hours. This is normal and will persist for 2 to 3 days. Do not attempt to remove it.
- Redness, swelling, or discharge indicates infection. Notify the primary health care provider if you think the circumcision area is infected.

Provide Comfort
- Circumcision is painful. Handle the area gently.
- Provide acetaminophen as required and ordered by health care provider.
- Provide extra holding, feeding, and opportunities for non-nutritive sucking for a day or two.

ATRAUMATIC CARE

*Guidelines for Pain Management During Neonatal Circumcision**

Pharmacological Interventions

Use of Topical Anaesthetic Only

One hour before the procedure, administer acetaminophen (e.g., Tylenol, 15 mg/kg) as ordered by the practitioner.

Place a thick layer (1 g) of an eutectic mixture of lidocaine and prilocaine (EMLA)† cream around the penis where the prepuce (foreskin) attaches to the glans. Avoid placing cream on the tip of the penis where it may come in contact with the urethral opening.

Cover the penis with a "finger cot" that is cut from a vinyl or latex glove, or a piece of plastic wrap, and secure the bottom of the covering with tape. Avoid using Tegaderm or large amounts of tape on the skin because removing the adhesive causes pain and can irritate the fragile skin.

If the infant urinates during the time EMLA is applied (1 hour) and a significant amount of EMLA is removed, reapply the cream and covering. The total application of EMLA should not exceed a surface area of 10 cm^2 (1¼ × 1¼ inches).

Remove cream with clean cloth or tissue. Blanching of skin is an expected reaction to EMLA's application under an occlusive dressing; erythema and some edema may occur also.

Two minutes before starting the procedure, give the infant a sucrose solution; 24% (weight/volume) sucrose solution is available commercially. Use this solution to coat the pacifier (recoat several times before and during the procedure) or use a cotton-tipped applicator that is dipped in the solution.

After the procedure, apply petrolatum or A&D ointment on a 5 × 5 cm dressing before diapering infant to prevent the wound from adhering to the dressing or diaper.

Administer acetaminophen as ordered by the practitioner 4 hours after the initial dose; give additional doses as needed but not to exceed five doses in 24 hours or a maximum dosage of 75 mg/kg/day.

Use of Dorsal Penile Nerve Block or Ring Block

One hour before the procedure administer acetaminophen as ordered by the practitioner.

One hour before the procedure, apply EMLA. For the dorsal penile nerve block (DPNB) apply EMLA to the prepuce as described previously and at the penile base. For the ring block apply EMLA to the prepuce as described previously and to the shaft of the penis. Use a topical anaesthetic in conjunction with the DPNB or ring block to avoid the pain of injecting the anaesthetic.

Use a 30-gauge needle to administer the lidocaine.‡ For the DPNB, 0.4 mL of the lidocaine is infiltrated at the 10:30 and 1:30 o'clock positions in Buck's fascia at the penile base. For the ring block, 0.4 mL of lidocaine is infiltrated subcutaneously on each side of the shaft of the penis below the prepuce.

For maximum anaesthesia, wait 5 minutes after injection of lidocaine. An alternative anaesthetic is chloroprocaine, which is as effective as lidocaine after 3 minutes.

Approximately 2 minutes before the circumcision, administer concentrated oral sucrose solution as described previously.

After the procedure, apply A&D ointment or petrolatum and administer acetaminophen as described previously.

Nonpharmacological Interventions

In addition to the preceding pharmacological interventions:

- If a Circumstraint board is used, pad with blankets or other thick, soft material such as lamb's wool. A more comfortable, padded, and physiological restraint that places the infant semireclining can also decrease distress (Stang et al., 1997).
- Provide the parents, caregiver, or another staff member with the option of holding the infant during the procedure or being present during the circumcision.
- Swaddle the upper body and legs to provide warmth and containment and to reduce movement.
- If the baby is not swaddled and is unclothed, use a radiant warmer to prevent hypothermia. Shield the infant's eyes from overhead lights.
- Prewarm any topical solutions to be used in sterile preparation of the surgical site by placing it in a warm blanket or towel.
- Play infant relaxation music§ before, during, and after the procedure; allow parents or other caregiver the option of choosing the music.
- After the procedure, remove restraints and swaddle the infant. Immediately have the parent, other caregiver, or nursing staff hold the infant. Continue to have the infant suck on a pacifier or offer feeding.

(Data from Broadman, L. M., et al. [1987]. Post-circumcision analgesia: A prospective evaluation of subcutaneous ring block of the penis. *Anesthesiology, 67*, 339–402; Howard, C. R., Howard, F. M., & Weitzman, M. L. [1994]. Acetaminophen analgesia in neonatal circumcision: The effect on pain. *Pediatrics, 93*[4], 641–646; Lander, J., et al. [1997]. Comparison of ring block, dorsal penile nerve block, and topical anesthesia for neonatal circumcision. *Journal of American Medical Association, 278*, 2157–2162; Mintz, M. R., & Grillo, R. [1989]. Dorsal penile nerve block for circumcision. *Clinical Pediatrics, 28*, 590–591; Serour, F., Mandelberg, A., & Mori, J. [1998]. Slow injection of local anesthetic will decrease pain during dorsal penile nerve block. *Acta Anaesthesiologica Scandinavica, 42*, 926–928; Spencer, D. M., et al. [1992]. Dorsal penile nerve block in neonatal circumcision: Chloroprocaine versus lidocaine. *American Journal of Perinatology, 9*[3], 214–218; Stang, H., et al. [1997]. Beyond dorsal penile nerve block: A more humane circumcision. *Pediatrics, 100*[2], e3; Stevens, B., et al. [1997]. The efficacy of sucrose for relieving procedural pain in neonates—a systematic review and meta-analysis. *Acta Paediatrica, 86*, 837–842; Taddio, A., et al. [1997]. Efficacy and safety of lidocaine-prilocaine cream [EMLA] for pain during circumcision. *New England Journal of Medicine, 336*[17], 1197–1201.)

*There is sufficient evidence and support for use of combined analgesia, nonpharmacological interventions (such as swaddling), and local anaesthesia during the procedure to provide holistic pain management (Anand & International Evidence-Based Group for Neonatal Pain, 2001; Geyer et al., 2002; Razmus, Dalton, & Wilson, 2004; Taddio et al., 2000).

†EMLA is approved for use in infants age 37 weeks of gestation. Although the package insert warns that patients taking acetaminophen are at greater risk for developing methemoglobinemia, there have been no reported cases of this complication in children taking acetaminophen and using EMLA. In fact, there is no evidence that acetaminophen induces methemoglobinemia in humans (Prescott, 1996). The only reported cases of methemoglobinemia from acetaminophen have been in cats and dogs (Hjelle & Grauer, 1986).

‡In one study the use of buffered lidocaine, which normally reduces stinging sensation of lidocaine, did not provide effective anaesthesia for DPNB (Stang et al., 1997). The study on slow injection of the anaesthetics lidocaine and bupivacaine compared 40 versus 80 seconds in patients aged 15 to 53 years (Serour, Mandelberg, & Mori, 1998).

§Suggested infant relaxation music: Heartbeat Lullabies by Terry Woodford. Available from Baby-Go-To-Sleep Center, Audio-Therapy Innovations, Inc., PO Box 550, Colorado Springs, CO 80901, 800-537-7748; http://www.babygotosleep.com.

to change the diaper at least every 4 hours to prevent it from sticking to the penis.

Discharge Planning and Teaching

Infant care activities can cause much anxiety for the new parent. Support from nursing staff members can be an important factor in determining whether new mothers seek and accept help in the future. All parents appreciate anticipatory guidance in the care of their infant. The nurse should not try to cover all the content at one time because the parents can be overwhelmed by too much information and become anxious. However, because new mothers go home quickly from the hospital, it is difficult for nurses to teach all the content that is necessary. It is important to start teaching on admission to the hospital. Public health nurses may visit families after birth and provide teaching, but this is not a standard across the country.

To set priorities for teaching, the nurse should follow parental cues. Learning needs should be identified before beginning to teach. Teaching regarding normal growth and development and the infant's changing needs (e.g., for personal interaction and stimulation, growth milestones, exercise, injury prevention, and social contacts), as well as the topics that follow, should be included during discharge planning with parents.

Temperature

The nurse should review the following topics:

- The causes of elevation in body temperature (e.g., overwrapping, cold stress with resultant vasoconstriction, or response to infection) and the body's response to extremes in environmental temperature
- Signs to be reported, such as high (all fevers in children under 2 months of age should be seen by a health care provider) or low temperatures with accompanying fussiness, lethargy, irritability, poor feeding, and crying
- Ways to promote normal body temperature, such as dressing the infant appropriately for the environmental air temperature and protecting the infant from exposure to direct sunlight, and how to assess whether the infant is hot or cold by feeling the back of the neck
- Use of warm wraps or extra blankets in cold weather
- Method for taking the newborn's axillary temperature

Respirations

The nurse should review the following points:

- Normal variations in the rate and rhythm
- Reflexes such as sneezing to clear the airway (this is normal and does not mean the newborn has a cold)
- Need to protect the infant from (1) exposure to people with upper respiratory tract infections and respiratory syncytial virus (see Chapter 46); (2) exposure to secondhand and thirdhand tobacco smoke; and (3) suffocation from loose bedding, water beds, and beanbag chairs; drowning (in bath water); entrapment under excessive bedding or in soft bedding; anything tied around the infant's neck; blind cords near cribs; and poorly constructed playpens, bassinets, or cribs
- Sleep position—on back when put to sleep
- A commonly aspirated substance is baby powder, which usually is a mixture of talc (hydrous magnesium silicate) and other silicates. Parents are advised to substitute a cornstarch preparation if they prefer to use a powder. The powder should be placed in the caregiver's hand and then applied to the skin, never sprinkled directly onto the skin.
- Symptoms of the common cold: nasal congestion and excessive drainage of mucus, coughing, sneezing, difficulty swallowing or breathing, decreased vigor in feeding, and low-grade fever.

Advise parents on measures to help the infant with a cold, such as the following:

- Feeding smaller amounts more often to prevent overtiring the infant
- Holding the baby in an upright position to feed
- For sleeping, raising the infant's head and chest by raising the mattress 30 degrees (do not use a pillow)
- Avoiding drafts; not overdressing the baby
- Using only medications prescribed by a physician (Over-the-counter "cold" remedy medications are not appropriate for use in infants and should be avoided [Sharfstein et al., 2007].)
- Using nasal saline drops in each nostril and suctioning well with a bulb syringe to remove secretions

Feeding Schedules

Feeding practices and schedules for newborns are discussed in Chapter 26.

Elimination

A review includes the following reminders:

- Colour of normal urine and number of voidings to expect each day (Home Care Box, p. 673)
- Changes to be expected in the colour of the stool (i.e., meconium to transitional to soft yellow or golden yellow) and the number of bowel evacuations, plus the odour of stools for breastfed or bottle-fed infants (see Box 24-1 and Fig. 24-3)
- Expected pattern of stools in formula-fed infants (i.e., as few as one stool every other day after the first few weeks of life)

Prevention of Sudden Infant Death Syndrome

The rate of sudden infant death syndrome (SIDS) in Canada is 1 in every 3000 babies; the rate is higher among First Nations, Métis, and Inuit infants (Canadian Paediatric Society [CPS], Canadian Foundation for Sudden Infant Deaths [CFSID], Canadian Institute for Child Health, Health Canada, Public Health Agency of Canada [PHAC], 2011). This guideline recommends placing the infant to sleep in the supine position to prevent SIDS. The prone position has been associated with an increased incidence of SIDS. Death rates from SIDS have decreased by more than 50% in Canada since the original "Back to Sleep" campaign was started in 1999 (CPS et al., 2011) (see Critical Thinking Exercise). Other recommendations for preventing SIDS include ensuring a smoke-free environment (before and after birth), providing a safe crib environment (no toys or loose bedding), room sharing for 6 months, avoiding instances of the infant being overheated, and no sleeping in waterbeds or on sofas (CPS et al.,

2011). Breastfeeding and pacifier use may also decrease the rate of SIDS.

Anatomically, the infant's shape—a barrel chest and flat, curveless spine—makes it easy for the infant to roll from the side to the prone position; thus, the side-lying position for sleep is not recommended. When the infant is awake, tummy time can be provided under parental supervision so that the infant may begin to develop appropriate muscle tone for eventual crawling; this tummy time is also effective in the prevention of a misshaped head (positional plagiocephaly). Newborns should be placed on their stomach several times per day for increasing lengths of time but always when they are awake and supervised by an adult (CPS et al., 2011).

Safety and Holding

Care must also be taken to prevent the infant from rolling off flat, unguarded surfaces. When an infant is on such a surface, the parent or nurse who must turn away from the infant even for a moment should always keep one hand placed securely on the infant. The infant should always be held securely with his or her head supported because newborns are unable to maintain an erect head posture for more than a few moments. Fig. 25-17 illustrates various positions for holding an infant with adequate support.

All personnel working with infants must have current infant **cardiopulmonary resuscitation** (CPR) certification. Many institutions offer infant CPR courses to parents before discharge (see also Figs. 46-13 and 46-14).

Rashes

Diaper Rash

The warm, moist atmosphere in the diaper area provides an optimal environment for *Candida albicans* growth; dermatitis appears in the perianal area, inguinal folds, and lower abdomen. The affected area is intensely erythematous with a sharply demarcated, scalloped edge, often with numerous satellite lesions that extend beyond the larger lesion. The usual source of infection is from handling by persons who do not

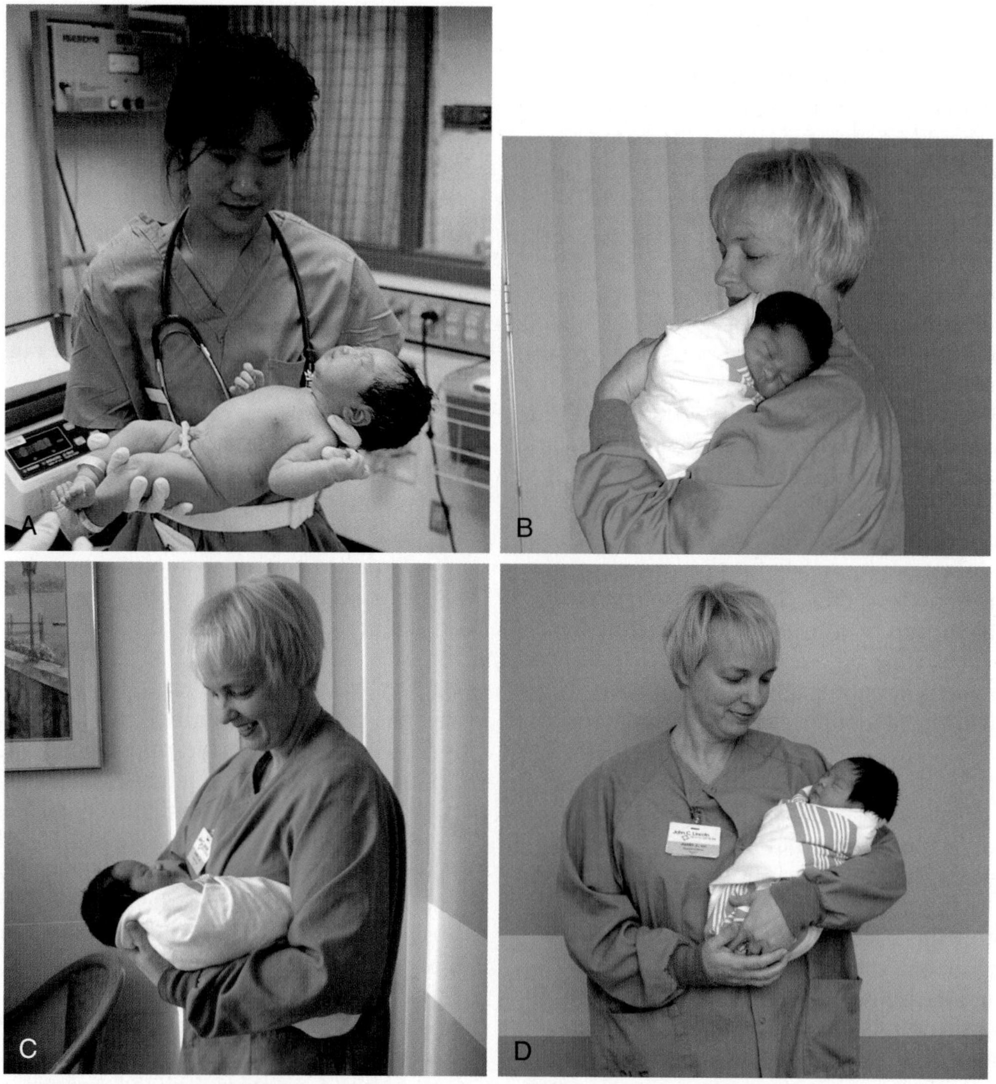

Fig. 25-17 Holding baby securely with support for the head. **A:** Holding infant while moving from one place to another. Baby is undressed to show posture. **B:** Holding baby upright in "burping" position. **C:** "Football" hold. **D:** Cradling hold. *(**A**, Courtesy Kim Molloy, Knoxville, IA. **B**, **C**, and **D**, Courtesy Julie Perry Nelson, Loveland, CO.)*

CRITICAL THINKING EXERCISE

Late Preterm Infant, Sudden Infant Death Syndrome, and Infant Sleep Position

Mary gave birth to a 35-week, 2250-g female infant. This is her third baby; the other children are 18 and 20 years old. Mary and Delilah are being discharged today. The nurse has given her instructions about feeding, stooling patterns, and jaundice but said nothing about sleeping position. Mary said that she has noticed that some of the nurses placed Delilah on her side; the mother further indicates that she worked in the nursery during college and, if babies were placed on their backs, they tended to spit up and turn blue. Mary has voiced concerns to the nurse about placing her new baby on her back to sleep at home. How should the nurse respond to Mary's concerns?

1. Evidence—Is there sufficient evidence to draw conclusions about the safety and efficacy of the supine position for sleep for the late preterm infant in reducing the incidence of sudden infant death syndrome (SIDS)?
2. Assumptions—What assumptions can be made about the following factors related to infant positioning?
   a. Role modelling by nurses
   b. Sleep position in the hospital versus sleep position at home
   c. Sleep position for late preterm versus term infants
3. What implications and priorities for nursing care can be drawn at this time?
4. Does the evidence objectively support your conclusion?
5. Are there alternative perspectives to your conclusion?

practice adequate hand hygiene. It may also appear 2 to 3 days after an oral infection (thrush).

Therapy consists of applications of an anticandidal ointment, such as clotrimazole or miconazole, with each diaper change. Sometimes the infant also is given an oral antifungal preparation such as nystatin or fluconazole to eliminate any gastrointestinal source of infection.

Washing and drying the wet and soiled area and changing the diaper immediately after voiding or stooling will prevent and help treat diaper rash. Parents can be taught to expose the buttocks to air to help dry up diaper rash. Because bacteria thrive in moist dark areas, exposing the skin to dry air decreases bacterial proliferation. A skin barrier ointment such as zinc oxide may be effective in preventing further excoriation, especially in the presence of loose stools or systemic gastrointestinal candidiasis; the latter will require treatment with a systemic antifungal medication.

Other Rashes

A rash on the cheeks may result from the infant's scratching with long unclipped fingernails or from rubbing the face against the crib sheets, particularly if regurgitated stomach contents are not washed off promptly. The newborn's skin begins a natural process of peeling and sloughing after birth. Dry skin may be treated with a neutral-pH lotion, but this should be used sparingly. Newborn rash, **erythema toxicum**, is a common finding (see Fig. 24-7, B, p. 619) and needs no treatment.

Clothing

Parents commonly ask how warmly they should dress their infant. A simple rule of thumb is to dress the child as they dress themselves, adding or subtracting clothes and wraps for the child as necessary. Feeling the temperature of the skin at the back of the infant's neck is often an indicator of whether the child is too hot or cold. A cotton shirt and diaper may be sufficient clothing for the young infant. A cap or bonnet is needed to protect the scalp and minimize heat loss if the weather is cool, or to protect against sunburn and shade the eyes if it is sunny and hot. Wrapping the infant snugly in a blanket maintains body temperature and promotes a feeling of security. Overdressing in warm temperatures can cause discomfort, as can underdressing in cold weather. Overdressing the infant has also been associated with SIDS. Parents are encouraged to dress the infant in flame-retardant clothing. Infant sunglasses are available to protect the eyes when outdoors.

Safety: Use of Car Seat

Infants should travel only in federally approved, rear-facing safety seats secured in the rear seat (Fig. 25-18). The safest area of the car is in the middle of the back seat. A car seat that faces the rear gives the best protection for the infant's disproportionately weak neck and heavy head. In this position, the force of a frontal crash is spread over the head, neck, and back; the back of the car seat supports the spine. Car seats have expiration dates on them as well as Canadian Standards Association stickers, and parents need to ensure the car seat they are using is safe. A car seat that has been in a previous car accident should not be used. See Additional Resources for more information on car seat installation.

NURSING ALERT Infants should use a rear-facing car seat from birth to 10 kg (22 lb), and the child must be able to walk unassisted. If the child meets these criteria and is under 1 year of age, they should remain in a rear-facing care seat. It is advisable to keep a child in a rear-facing car seat even after these criteria have been met.

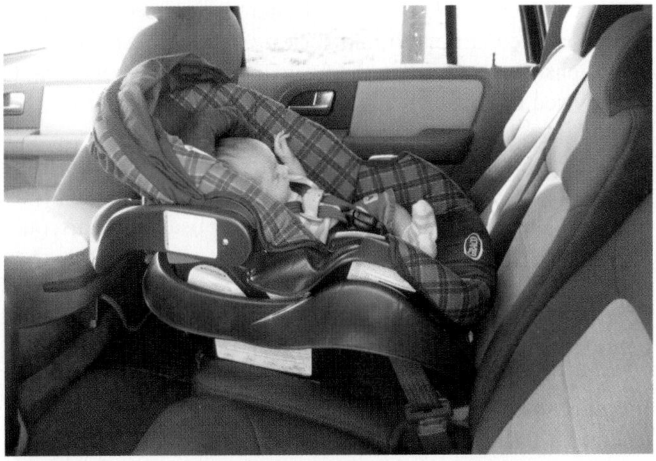

Fig. 25-18 Rear-facing infant seat in rear seat of car. Infant is placed in seat when going home from the hospital. *(Courtesy Brian and Mayannyn Sallee, Las Vegas, NV.)*

The car seat is secured using the vehicle seat belt; the infant is secured using the harness system in the car seat. If the infant must ride in the front seat, the air bag must be turned off to prevent injury from the air bag.

NURSING ALERT In cars equipped with air bags, rear-facing infant seats should not be placed in the front seat unless the air bag has been deactivated. Serious injury can occur if the air bag inflates because these types of infant seats fit closer to the dashboard than a passenger does.

Car Seat Testing

evolve Video—Crying Female Neonate

Infants born at less than 37 weeks of gestation and with birth weight less than 2500 g should be observed in a car seat for a period (a minimum of 90 to 120 minutes is recommended by the Canadian Paediatric Society) before discharge (CPS, 2000). The infant is monitored for apnea, bradycardia, and a decrease in oxygen saturation. See Community Focus (Chapter 27, p. 738) for procedure. It may be necessary to place blanket rolls on either side of the infant for support of the head and trunk. To prevent slumping, the back-to-crotch strap distance should be 14 cm (see Chapter 36, Motor Vehicle Injuries, for additional car restraint information). If the preterm infant fails the car seat test, a car bed may be used to provide safe transportation.

Non-Nutritive Sucking

Sucking is the infant's chief pleasure. However, sucking needs may not be satisfied by breastfeeding or bottle-feeding alone. In fact, sucking is such a strong need that infants who are deprived of sucking, such as those with a cleft lip, will suck on their tongues. Some newborns are born with sucking pads on their fingers that developed during in utero sucking. Several benefits of non-nutritive sucking have been demonstrated, such as an increased weight gain in preterm infants, increased ability to maintain an organized state, and decreased crying.

Problems arise when parents are concerned about the sucking of fingers, thumbs, or pacifiers and try to restrain this natural tendency. Before giving advice, nurses should investigate the parents' feelings and base the guidance they give on the information solicited. For example, some parents may see no problem with the use of a finger but may find the use of a pacifier objectionable. In general, there is no need to restrain either practice, unless thumb sucking persists past 4 years of age or past the time when the permanent teeth erupt. Parents are advised to consult with their health care provider on this topic.

The risk of SIDS is shown to be lower in infants who use a pacifier (CPS, 2003). The Canadian Foundation for the Study of Infant Deaths recommends that pacifier use not be discouraged, but if pacifiers are used in breastfeeding infants, they should not be introduced until after 1 month of age when breastfeeding is well established, to decrease the possibility of breastfeeding concerns (CPS et al., 2011).

A parent's excessive use of the pacifier to calm the child should also be explored, however. It is not unusual for parents to place a pacifier in the infant's mouth as soon as he or she begins to cry, thus reinforcing a pattern of distress-relief.

If parents choose to let their child use a pacifier, they need to be aware of certain safety considerations before purchasing one. A homemade or poorly designed pacifier can be dangerous because the entire object may be aspirated if it is small, or a portion may become lodged in the pharynx. Improvised pacifiers, such as those commonly made in hospitals from a padded nipple, also pose dangers because the nipple may separate from the plastic collar and be aspirated. Safe pacifiers are made of one piece that includes a shield or flange large enough to prevent entry into the mouth and a handle that can be grasped (Fig. 25-19).

Bathing, Cord Care, and Skin Care

Bathing serves a number of purposes. It provides opportunities for (1) completely cleansing the infant, (2) observing the infant's condition, (3) promoting comfort, and (4) parent–child–family socializing.

An important consideration in skin cleansing is preservation of the skin's acid mantle, which is formed from the uppermost horny layer of the epidermis, sweat, superficial fat, metabolic products, and external substances such as amniotic fluid and microorganisms. At birth, the skin has a pH of 6.4. Within 4 days, the pH of the newborn's skin surface falls to within the bacteriostatic range (pH less than 5) (Krebs, 1998). The use of a mild soap that is pH neutral is recommended, as alkaline soaps (such as Ivory) and oils, powders, and lotions may alter the acid mantle, thus providing a medium for bacterial growth. Some institutions recommend washing with plain water only for the first 4 days, although mild soap has been found to have minimal effect on skin bacterial colonization (Medves & O'Brien, 2001).

Although the sponging technique may be used, bathing the newborn by immersion results in less heat loss and less crying and is thus recommended even with the umbilical cord still intact. Immersion bathing is considered a safe alternative to sponge bathing provided the infant's condition is stable (no temperature instability, respiratory or cardiac illness) and he or she is dried off immediately afterward and kept warm (Association of Women's Health, Obstetric and Neonatal Nurses, 2007). A daily bath is not necessary for achieving cleanliness and may do more harm by disrupting the integrity of the newborn's skin; cleansing the perineum after a soiled diaper and daily cleansing of the face may suffice.

Until the initial bath is completed, hospital personnel must wear gloves to handle the newborn.

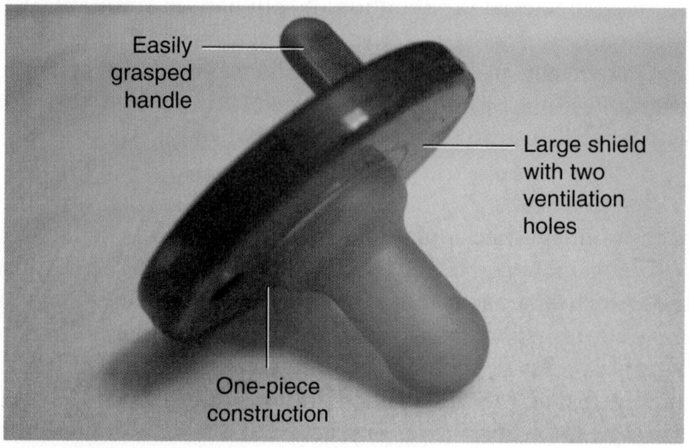

Fig. 25-19 Design of a safe pacifier. *(Courtesy Julie Perry Nelson, Loveland, CO.)*

Umbilical Cord Care

Care of the umbilical cord is an important aspect of nursing care and parent teaching. The goal of care is prevention and early detection of hemorrhage or infection. The umbilical cord stump is an excellent medium for bacterial growth and can easily become infected.

Hospital protocol determines the technique for routine cord care. Common methods include the use of no treatment, alcohol alone, soap and water, sterile water, povidone-iodine, triple dye or antimicrobial agents. The use of antiseptic agents has been shown to prolong cord drying and separation (Zupan, Garner, & Omari, 2004). Studies regarding bacterial growth and colonization according to the cleansing method used have produced varied results (Golombek, Brill, & Salice, 2002; Janssen et al., 2003). A Cochrane Review of 21 studies found no significant difference between cords treated with antiseptics compared with dry cord care or placebo; there were no reported systemic infections or deaths, and a trend toward reduced colonization was found in cords treated with antiseptics (Zupan et al., 2004). Recommendations for cord care by the Association of Women's Health, Obstetric and Neonatal Nurses (2007) include cleaning the cord initially with sterile water and subsequently cleaning the cord with water. The use of alcohol is associated with prolonged cord drying and separation (McConnell et al., 2004) and rarely used in Canada. Parents should be taught the method of cord care that is used by the institution.

The stump and base of the cord should be assessed for edema, erythema, and drainage with each diaper change. The stump deteriorates through the process of dry gangrene; thus, odour alone is not a positive indicator of omphalitis (infection of the umbilical stump).

The umbilical cord begins to dry, shrivel, and blacken by the second or third day of life depending in part on the cleansing method used. The umbilicus should be inspected often for signs of infection (e.g., foul odour, redness, and purulent discharge), granuloma (i.e., small, red, raw-appearing polyp where the umbilical cord separates), bleeding, and discharge. The cord clamp may be removed when the cord is dry, in about 24 to 36 hours, although this is not routine practice in all hospitals (Fig. 25-20). Some institutions send the newborn home with the clamp still in place and it will fall off when the cord falls off. It is important to ensure that if a cord clamp remover is used, it is disinfected between uses.

The cord normally falls off 10 to 14 days after birth but may remain attached for as long as 3 weeks. Parents should be instructed in appropriate home cord care (per practitioner or institution protocol) and the expected time of cord separation.

The Home Care box contains information regarding bathing, skin care, cord care, cutting nails, and dressing the infant.

Infant Follow-Up Care

With shorter hospital stays, the focus and site of infant care are changing. Home care may be provided either by a nurse

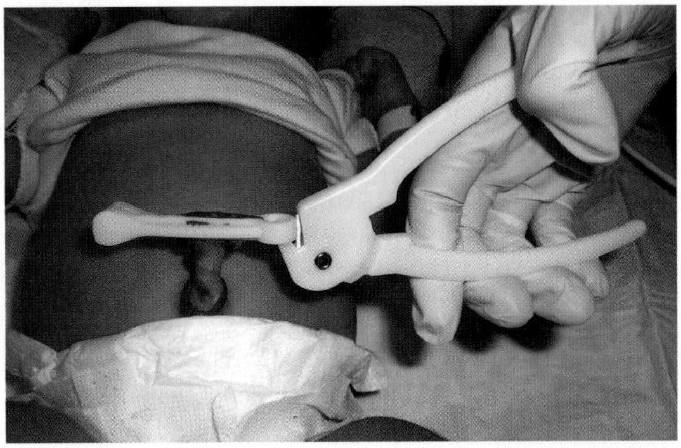

Fig. 25-20 Using special scissors, remove clamp after cord begins drying (about 24 hours). *(Courtesy Cheryl Briggs, RN, Annapolis, MD.)*

HOME CARE

Newborn Bath

Fit Baths Into the Family Schedule

- Give a bath at any time convenient to you, but not immediately after a feeding period because the increased handling may cause regurgitation.

Prevent Heat Loss

- The temperature of the room should be no cooler than 24°C, and the bathing area should be free of drafts.
- Control heat loss during the bath to conserve the infant's energy. Bathing the infant quickly, exposing only what is being washed, and thoroughly drying the infant are all important parts of the bathing technique.

Gather Supplies and Clothing Before Starting

- Clothing suitable for wearing indoors: diaper, shirt; stretch suit or nightgown optional
- Towels for drying infant and a clean washcloth
- Receiving blanket
- Tub or sink for water

Bathe the Baby

- Bring infant to the bathing area when all supplies are ready.
- Never leave the infant alone on the bath table or in bath water, not even for a second! If you have to leave, take the infant with you or put the infant back into the crib.
- Fill the tub to try to cover as much of the infant's body as you feel comfortable. Infants like to have as much of their body under water as possible.
- Test temperature of the water. It should feel pleasantly warm to the inner wrist (36.6° to 37.2°C). Do not hold infant under running water—water temperature may change, and the infant may be scalded or chilled rapidly.
- Use a mild, unscented, pH-neutral (5.5 to 7.0) soap or cleanser.
- Always work from clean to dirty. Start with the face, neck, and ears first. Do not use soap on the face. Cleanse the eyes from the inner canthus outward, using separate parts of a

Continued

HOME CARE

Newborn Bath—cont'd

clean washcloth for each eye. For the first 2 or 3 days, there may be a discharge resulting from the reaction of the conjunctiva to the ointment used as a prophylactic measure against infection. Any discharge should be considered abnormal and reported to the health care provider.

- Cleanse ears and nose with twists of moistened cotton or a corner of the washcloth. Do not use cotton-tipped swabs because they may cause injury.
- Creases under the chin and arms and in the groin may need daily cleansing. The crease under the chin may be exposed by elevating the infant's shoulders 5 cm and letting the head drop back.
- When washing the infant's hair, hold the baby in a football hold. Wash infant's hair before or after body to prevent heat loss from prolonged exposure to cold (scalp loses heat rapidly because of size). Wash the scalp with warm water and mild soap; dry thoroughly. Scalp desquamation, called *cradle cap*, often can be prevented by removing any scales with a fine-toothed comb or brush after washing. If the condition persists, notify the health care provider.
- Undress the baby and wash body, arms, and legs by placing in tub. Pat dry gently.

Prevent Skin Trauma

- The fragile skin can be injured by too vigorous cleansing.
- If stool or other debris has dried and caked on the skin, apply a thin layer of scent-free petroleum jelly or other commercial preparations to remove it. Do not attempt to rub it off, since abrasion may result.
- Being gentle, patting dry rather than rubbing, and using a mild soap without perfumes or colouring are recommended. Chemicals in the colouring and perfume can cause rashes on sensitive skin.

Care of the Cord

- With a washcloth, cleanse around base of the cord where it joins the skin. It is acceptable to submerge the cord under the water. Dry the cord thoroughly after the bath. Notify the health care provider of any discharge or skin inflammation around the cord.
- Because the cord skin essentially necroses (dies), there will be a slight odour until the cord falls off; however, any discharge or redness should be reported to the practitioner.
- The clamp may be removed before the newborn is discharged from the birth centre, although some centres leave the clamps on until the cord falls off.
- The diaper should be folded back from the cord to allow the cord to be dried by air and to prevent soiling from urine.
- When the cord drops off after 10 to 15 days, small drops of blood may be seen when the baby cries. This will heal by itself. It is not dangerous.

Care of Hands and Feet

- Wash and dry between the fingers and toes.
- Use caution cutting the nails—use blunt scissors, or a nail file. The nails have to grow out far enough from the skin so that the skin is not cut by mistake. Nails should be kept short so infants do not scratch themselves. Covering hands with mitts may frustrate infants who wants to suck on them, so it is better to keep nails short.

Cleanse Genitalia

- Cleanse the infant's genitalia daily and after voiding or defecating.
- For girls, the genitalia may be cleansed by separating the labia and gently washing from the pubic area to the anus.
- For uncircumcised boys, do not retract the foreskin. In most newborns, the inner layer of the foreskin adheres to the glans and the foreskin cannot be retracted. By age 3 years in 90% of boys, the foreskin can be retracted easily without causing pain or trauma. For others, the foreskin is not retractable until adolescence. As soon as the foreskin is partly retractable and the child is old enough, he can be taught self-care.
- Once healed, the circumcised penis does not require any special care other than cleansing with diaper changes.

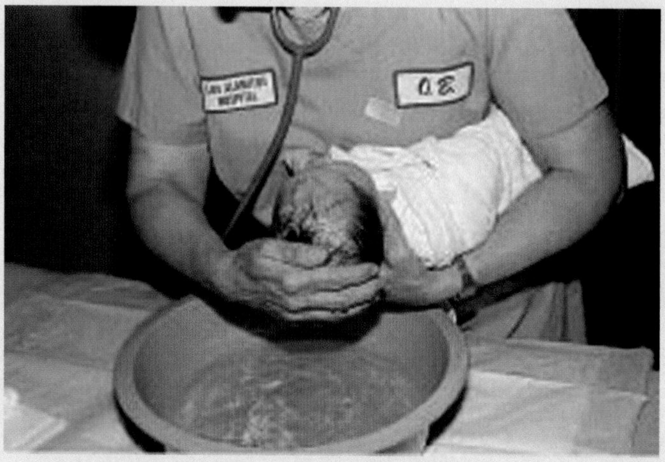

Wash hair with baby wrapped to prevent heat loss from wet scalp using the football hold. *(Courtesy Marjorie Pyle, RNC, Lifecircle, Costa Mesa, CA.)*

as part of the routine follow-up care of patients or through a visiting nurse or community health nurse referral service. For infants discharged early, newborn home care is essential.

Parents should plan for their child's routine follow-up health care at the following ages: within 2 or 3 days to check for status of jaundice, feeding, and elimination (see also Physiological Jaundice, p. 652, for follow-up guidelines); at 2 to 4 weeks of age; then every 2 months until 6 to 7 months of age; then every 3 months until 18 months; at 2 years; at 3 years; at preschool; and every 2 years thereafter.

Immunizations

The schedule for immunizations should be reviewed with the parents. See Chapter 36 for a complete discussion of infant immunizations.

HOME CARE

*Newborn Home Care**

- Wet diapers—One wet diaper for each day of life until fifth to sixth day; then 6 to 10 per day
- Breastfeeding—Successful latch-on and feeding 10 to 12 times a day (24-hour period). Audible swallowing should be evident.
- Formula feeding—Successfully, voiding as above, taking 60 to 90 mL (approximately) on demand or at least every 4 hours
- Circumcision—Wash with warm water only; yellow exudate forming, nonbleeding; no tub bath until healed
- Stools—At least one soft stool every 48 to 72 hours (bottle-feeding), or two or three per day (breastfeeding)
- Colour—Pink to ruddy when crying; pink centrally when at rest or asleep
- Activity—Four or five wakeful periods per day; alerts to environmental sounds and voices
- Jaundice—Physiological jaundice (not appearing in first 24 hours), feeding, voiding, and stooling as noted above. Notify practitioner of suspicion of pathological jaundice (appears within 24 hours of birth; ABO/Rh problem suspected), decreased activity, poor feeding, or dark orange skin colour persisting after the fifth day in light-skinned newborn. Obtain bilirubin levels before discharge and identify risk per hour-specific risk nomogram (see Fig. 25-7).
- Cord—Kept above diaper line; nonodourous; drying
- Breathing—Respiratory rate can be irregular and there should be no evidence of sternal retractions, grunting, or nasal flaring; temperature 36.5° to 37.2°C axillary
- Position of sleep—On back

(From Hockenberry, M. J., & Wilson, D. [2011]. *Wong's nursing care of infants and children* [9th ed.]. St. Louis: Mosby.)

*Any deviation from the above or suspicion of poor newborn adaptation should be reported to the practitioner at once.

Key Points

- Assessment of the newborn requires data from the prenatal, intrapartum, and postnatal periods.
- Knowledge of biological and behavioural characteristics is essential for guiding assessment and interpreting data.
- Providing a protective environment is a key responsibility of the nurse and includes such measures as careful identification procedures, protection from abduction, support of physiological functions, and measures to prevent infection.
- Maintenance of adequate ventilation includes ensuring an open airway and a body temperature within the normal range.
- Parent education is a major responsibility of the nurse and includes involvement of parents in all phases of the nursing process.
- The newborn has social as well as physical needs.
- Circumcision is an elective surgical procedure.
- Parents appreciate anticipatory guidance in the care of the newborn.

Audio Chapter Summaries

Access an Audio Summary of these Key Points on evolve

References

American Academy of Pediatrics and Canadian Paediatric Society. (2006). Prevention and management of pain in the neonate: An update. *Pediatrics, 118*(5), 2231–2241. Retrieved from http://aappolicy.aappublications.org/cgi/reprint/pediatrics;118/5/2231.pdf. doi:10.1542/peds.2006-2277

American Academy of Pediatrics, American College of Obstetricians and Gynecologists. (2007). *Guidelines for perinatal care* (6th ed.). Elk Grove Village, IL: Author.

Anand, K. J., & International Evidence-Based Group for Neonatal Pain. (2001). Consensus statement for the prevention and management of pain in the newborn. *Archives of Pediatric and Adolescent Medicine, 155*(2), 173–179.

Arbuckle, T., Wilkins, R., & Sherman, G. (1993). Birth weight percentiles by gestational age in Canada. *Obstetrics and Gynecology, 81*(1), 39–48.

Association of Women's Health, Obstetric and Neonatal Nurses. (2007). *Neonatal skin care: Evidence-based clinical practice guideline* (2nd ed.). Washington, DC: Author.

Bakewell-Sachs, S. (2007). Near-term/late preterm infants. *Newborn and Infant Nursing Reviews, 7*(2), 67–71. doi:10.1053/j.nainr.2007.05.001

Ballard, J., Novak, K., & Driver, M. (1979). A simplified score for assessment of fetal maturity of newly born infants. *Journal of Pediatrics, 95*(5 Pt 1), 769–774.

Ballard, J., et al. (1991). New Ballard score, expanded to include extremely premature infants. *Journal of Pediatrics, 119*(3), 417–423.

Battaglia, F. C., & Lubchenco, L. O. (1967). A practical classification of newborn infants by weight and gestational age. *Journal of Pediatrics, 71*(2), 159–161.

Blackburn, S. T. (2007). *Maternal, fetal, and neonatal physiology: A clinical perspective* (3rd ed.). St. Louis: Saunders.

Blain-Lewis, N. (1992). Comparative studies of bruising and healing after heelstick. *Neonatal Intensive Care, 5*(5), 18–21.

Blass, E. M., & Watt, L. B. (1999). Suckling- and sucrose-induced analgesia in human newborns. *Pain, 83*(3), 611–623.

Brady-Fryer, B., Wiebe, N., & Lander, J. A. (2004). Pain relief for newborn circumcision. *Cochrane Database Systematic Reviews, 2004*(3), CD004217.

Butt, M. L., & Kisilevsky, B. S. (2000). Music modulates behaviour of premature infants following heel lance. *Canadian Journal of Nursing Research, 31*(4), 17–39.

Canadian Paediatric Society. (1996). Neonatal circumcision revisited. *Canadian Medical Association Journal, 154*(6), 769–780. Retrieved from http://www.cps.ca/english/statements/fn/fn96-01.htm.

Canadian Paediatric Society. (2000). Assessment of babies for car seat safety before hospital discharge. *Paediatric Child Health, 5*(1), 53–56. Retrieved from http://www.cps.ca/english/statements/FN/fn00-02.htm.

Canadian Paediatric Society. (2003). Recommendations for the use of pacifiers. *Paediatrics and Child Health, 8*(8), 515–519. Reaffirmed February 2011. Retrieved from http://www.cps.ca/english/statements/cp/cp03-01.htm.

Canadian Paediatric Society. (2004). Screening guidelines for newborns at risk for low blood glucose. *Paediatric Child Health, 9*(10), 723–729. Retrieved from http://www.cps.ca/english/statements/FN/fn04-01.pdf.

Canadian Paediatric Society. (2007). Guidelines for detection, management and prevention of hyperbilirubinemia in term and late term newborn infants [35 or more weeks gestation]. *Paediatric Child Health, 12*(Suppl B), 1B–12B. Retrieved from http://www.cps.ca/english/statements/FN/FN07-02.pdf.

Canadian Paediatric Society, Canadian Foundation for Study of Infant Deaths, Canadian Institute for Child Health, Health Canada & Public Health Agency of Canada (2011). *Joint statement on safe sleep: Preventing sudden infant deaths in Canada.* Ottawa: PHAC. Retrieved from http://www.phac-aspc.gc.ca/hp-ps/dca-dea/stages-etapes/childhood-enfance_0-2/sids/pdf/jsss-ecss2011-eng.pdf.

Canadian Paediatric Society & College of Family Physicians of Canada. (2009). Routine administration of vitamin K to newborns. *Paediatric Childs Health, 2*(6), 429–431. Retrieved from http://www.cps.ca/english/statements/FN/fn97-01.htm.

Carbajal, R., et al. (2003). Analgesic effect of breast feeding in term neonates: Randomized controlled trial. *British Medical Journal, 326*(7379), 13.

Cornblath, M., et al. (2000). Controversies regarding operational definition of neonatal hypoglycemia: Suggested thresholds. *Pediatrics, 105*(5), 1141–1145.

Cunningham, F. G., et al. (2010). *Williams obstetrics* (23rd ed.). New York: McGraw-Hill.

Engle, W. A., et al. (2007). "Late-preterm" infants: A population at risk. *Pediatrics, 120*(6), 1390–1401. doi:10.1542/peds.2007-2952

Engle, W. D., et al. (2002). Assessment of a transcutaneous device in the evaluation of neonatal hyperbilirubinemia in a primarily Hispanic population. *Pediatrics, 110*(1 Pt 1), 61–67.

Eriksson, M., & Finnstrom, O. (2004). Can daily repeated doses of orally administered glucose induce tolerance when given for neonatal pain relief? *Acta Paediatrica, 93*(2), 246–249.

Fitzgerald, M., Millard, C., & McIntosh, N. (1989). Cutaneous hypersensitivity following peripheral tissue damage in newborn infants and its reversal with topical anaesthesia. *Pain, 3*(1), 31–36.

Gartner, L. M., & Herschel, M. (2001). The management of breastfeeding, part 2: Jaundice and breastfeeding. *Pediatric Clinics of North America, 48*(2), 389–400.

Geyer, J., et al. (2002). An evidence-based multidisciplinary protocol for neonatal circumcision pain management. *Journal of Obstetric, Gynecologic and Neonatal Nursing, 31*(4), 403–410.

Gibbins, S., et al. (2002). Efficacy and safety of sucrose for procedural pain relief in preterm and term neonates. *Nursing Research, 51*(6), 375–382.

Golombek, S. G., Brill, P. E., & Salice, A. L. (2002). Randomized trial of alcohol versus triple dye for umbilical cord care. *Clinical Pediatrics, 41*(6), 419–423.

Gradin, M., et al. (2002). Pain reduction at venipuncture in newborns: Oral glucose compared with local anesthetic cream. *Pediatrics, 110*(6), 1053–1057.

Gray, L., Watt, L., & Blass, E. M. (2000). Skin-to-skin contact is analgesic in healthy newborns. *Pediatrics, 105*(1), 110–111. Retrieved from http://www.pediatrics.org/cgi/content/full/105/1/e14.

Grunau, R. E., et al. (2004). Does prone or supine position influence pain responses in preterm infants at 32 weeks gestational age? *Clinical Journal of Pain, 20*(2), 76–82.

Hagedorn, M. E. (2006). Respiratory distress. In G. B. Merenstein & S. L. Gardner (Eds.), *Handbook of neonatal intensive care* (6th ed.). St. Louis: Mosby.

Haouari, N., et al. (1995). The analgesic effect of sucrose in full-term infants: A randomised controlled trial. *British Medical Journal, 310*(6993), 1498–1500.

Harrison, D., Johnston, L., & Loughnan, P. (2003). Oral sucrose for procedural pain in sick hospitalized infants: A randomized-controlled trial. *Journal of Paediatric and Child Health, 39*(8), 591–597.

Health Canada. (2000). *Family-centred maternity and newborn care: National guidelines* (Cat. H39-527/2000E). Ottawa: Ministry of Health.

Hjelle, J. J., & Grauer, G. F. (1986). Acetaminophen-induced toxicosis in dogs and cats. *Journal of the American Veterinary Medical Association, 188*(7), 742–749.

Hoseth, E., et al. (2000). Blood glucose levels in a population of healthy, breast fed, term infants of appropriate size for gestational age. *Archives of Diseases in Childhood: Fetal Neonatal Edition, 83*(2), F117–F119.

Huang, C. M., et al. (2004). Comparison of pain responses of premature infants to the heelstick between containment and swaddling. *Journal of Nursing Research, 12*(1), 31–40.

Janssen, P. A., et al. (2003). To dye or not to dye: A randomized, clinical trial of a triple dye/alcohol regimen versus dry cord care. *Pediatrics, 111*(1), 15–20.

Johnston, C. C., et al. (2003). Kangaroo care is effective in diminishing pain response in preterm neonates. *Archives of Pediatric and Adolescent Medicine, 157*(11), 1084–1088.

Keren, R., et al. (2008). A comparison of alternative risk-assessment strategies for predicting significant neonatal hyperbilirubinemia in term and near-term infants. *Pediatrics, 121*(1), e170–e179. doi:10.1542/peds.2006-3499

Kramer, M. S., et al. (2001). A new and improved population-based Canadian reference for birth weight for gestational age. *Pediatrics, 108*(2), e35, 462.

Krebs, T. (1998). Cord care: Is it necessary? *Mother and Baby Journal, 3*(2), 5–12, 18–20.

Leitch, D. (1999). Mother–infant interaction: Achieving synchrony. *Nursing Research, 48*(1), 55–58.

Madan, A., et al. (2002). Racial differences in birth weight of term infants in a northern California population. *Journal of Perinatology, 22*(3), 230–235.

Maisels, M. J. (2005). Jaundice. In M. G. MacDonald, M. D. Mullett, & M. M. Seshia (Eds.), *Neonatology: Pathophysiology and management of the newborn* (6th ed.). Philadelphia: Lippincott.

McConnell, T. P., et al. (2004). Trends in umbilical cord care: Scientific evidence for practice. *Newborn and Infant Nursing Reviews, 4*(4), 211–222.

Medves, J., & O'Brien, B. (2001). Does bathing newborns remove potentially harmful pathogens from the skin? *Birth: Issues in Perinatal Care, 28*(3), 161–165.

Meehan, R. (1998). Heelsticks in neonates for capillary blood sampling. *Neonatal Network, 17*(1), 17–24.

Noerr, B. (2001). Sucrose for neonatal procedural pain. *Neonatal Network, 20*(7), 63–67.

Ontario Newborn Screening Program. (n.d.). *Information for health care providers.* Retrieved from http://www.newbornscreening.on.ca/bins/content_page.asp?cid=7-272.

Paes, B., et al. (1993). A comparative study of heel-stick devices for infant blood collection. *American Journal of Diseases in Childhood, 147*(3), 346–348.

Perinatal Services BC. (2010). *Newborn screening.* Retrieved from http://www.perinatalservicesbc.ca/sites/bcrcp/files/Guidelines/Newborn/NBS_Guideline_9.pdf.

Porter, M. L., & Dennis, B. L. (2002). Hyperbilirubinemia in the term newborn. *American Family Physician, 65*(4), 599–606, 613–614.

Prescott, L. F. (1996). *Paracetamol (acetaminophen): A critical bibliographic review.* Bristol, UK: Taylor & Francis.

Public Health Agency of Canada. (2009). *What mothers say: The Canadian maternity experiences survey* (Cat No: HP5-74/2-2009E). Ottawa: Author.

Razmus, I. S., Dalton, M. E., & Wilson, D. (2004). Pain management for newborn circumcision. *Pediatric Nursing, 30*(5), 414–417, 427.

Serour, F., Mandelberg, A., & Mori, J. (1998). Slow injection of local anesthetic will decrease pain during dorsal penile nerve block. *Acta Anaesthesiologica Scandinavica, 42*(8), 926–928.

Shah, V., & Ohlsson, A. (2001). Venipuncture versus heel lance for blood sampling in term neonates. *Cochrane Database Systematic Reviews* (2), CD001452.

Sharfstein, J. M., et al. (2007). Over the counter but no longer under the radar: Pediatric cough and cold medications. *New England Journal of Medicine, 357*(23), 2321–2324.

Stang, H. J., et al. (1997). Beyond dorsal penile nerve block: a more humane circumcision. *Pediatrics, 100*(2), E3.

Steffensrud, S. (2004). Hyperbilirubinemia in term and near-term infants: kernicterus on the rise? *Newborn and Infant Nursing Reviews, 4*(4), 191–200.

Stevens, B., Yamada, J., & Ohlsson, A. (2004). Sucrose for analgesia in newborn infants undergoing painful procedures. *Cochrane Database Systematic Reviews* (3), CD001069.

Stevens, B., et al. (1999). Management of pain from heel lance with lidocaine-prilocaine (EMLA) cream: Is it safe and efficacious in preterm infants? *Journal of Development and Behavior in Pediatrics, 20*(4), 216–221.

Stoll, B. J. (2007). The fetus and the neonatal infant. In R. M. Kliegman, et al. (Eds.), *Nelson textbook of pediatrics* (18th ed.). Philadelphia: Saunders.

Taddio, A., et al. (1998). A systematic review of lidocaine-prilocaine cream (EMLA) in the treatment of acute pain in neonates. *Pediatrics, 101*(2), e1. Retrieved from http://www.pediatrics.org/cgi/content/full/101/2/e1.

Taddio, A., et al. (2000). Combined analgesia and local anesthesia to minimize pain during circumcision. *Archives in Pediatric and Adolescent Medicine, 154*(5), 620–623.

Taddio, A., et al. (2002). Conditioning and hyperalgesia in newborns exposed to repeated heel lances. *Journal of the American Medical Association, 288*(7), 857–861.

Thomas, P., et al. (2000). A new look at intrauterine growth and the impact of race, altitude, and gender. *Pediatrics, 106*(2), e21.

Visscher, M. O., et al. (2005). Vernix caseosa in neonatal adaptation. *Journal of Perinatology, 25*(7), 440–446. doi:10.1038/sj.jp.7211305

World Health Organization. (2009). *Infant and young child feeding: Model chapter for textbooks for medical students and allied health professionals.* Geneva: Switzerland. WHO Press. Retrieved from http://whqlibdoc.who.int/publications/2009/9789241597494_eng.pdf.

Zupan, J., Garner, P., & Omari, A.A. (2004). Topical umbilical cord care at birth. *Cochrane Database of Systematic Reviews* (3), CD001057 [Updated 2009].

Additional Resources

Canadian Foundation for the Study of Infant Deaths: http://www.sidscanada.org/

City of Brampton, Fire and Emergency Services: Is Your Child Safe and Secure? (Information on car seats): http://www.brampton.ca/en/residents/fire-emergency-services/Fire-Safety/Pages/Child-Safe-and-Secure.aspx

Ontario Newborn Screening: Fact Sheets for Parents (in many different languages): http://www.newbornscreening.on.ca/bins/content_page.asp?cid=6-14-210

Perinatal Services BC Newborn Guidelines: http://www.perinatalservicesbc.ca//sites/bcrcp/files/Guidelines/Newborn/

Public Health Agency of Canada: Safe Sleep for Your Baby: http://www.phac-aspc.gc.ca/hp-ps/dca-dea/stages-etapes/childhood-enfance_0-2/sids/index-eng.php

Transport Canada – Keep Kids Safe (Car seat information): http://www.tc.gc.ca/eng/roadsafety/safedrivers-childsafety-car-time-stages-1083.htm

Unit 6

26 Newborn Nutrition and Feeding

Learning Objectives

On completion of this chapter, the reader will be able to:

- Describe current recommendations for infant feeding.
- Discuss benefits of breastfeeding for infants, mothers, families, and society.
- Describe the nutritional needs of newborns.
- List newborn feeding readiness cues.
- Describe the anatomy and physiology of breastfeeding.
- Identify nursing interventions to facilitate and promote successful breastfeeding.
- List signs of adequate intake in the breastfed infant.
- Identify common concerns associated with breastfeeding and nursing interventions to help resolve them.
- Discuss patient teaching for the family who is formula-feeding their newborn.

Electronic Resources

Additional information related to the content in Chapter 26 can be found on

evolve the companion Web site at

http://evolve.elsevier.com/Canada/Perry/maternal/

- Examination Review Questions
- Case Study—Breastfeeding
- Critical Thinking Exercise—Breastfeeding
- Critical Thinking Exercise—Formula Preparation
- Skill—Infant Feeding

Good nutrition in infancy fosters optimal growth and development. Infant feeding is more than the provision of nutrition; it represents an opportunity for social and psychological interaction between parent and infant. It can also establish a basis for developing good eating habits and influence lifelong health habits. The health care of infants requires knowledge of their nutritional needs. This chapter focuses on meeting the nutritional needs for normal growth and development from birth to 6 months of age, with an emphasis on the neonatal period, when feeding practices and patterns are established. Both breastfeeding and formula-feeding are addressed.

Recommended Infant Nutrition

The World Health Organization (WHO), Health Canada, and Canadian Paediatric Society (CPS) recommend exclusive breastfeeding for the first 6 months of life for healthy, term infants (CPS, 2005; Health Canada, 2004a; WHO, 2010a). Breast milk is recognized as the optimal food for infants, and breastfeeding may continue for 2 years or longer. Nutrient-rich complementary foods, with particular attention to iron, should be introduced at 6 months. Breastfed babies should also receive a daily vitamin D supplement until their diet provides a reliable source or until they reach 1 year of age (Canadian Paediatric Society, Dieticians of Canada, & Health Canada, 2005). If weaned before 12 months, infants should receive iron-fortified infant formula.

Benefits of Breastfeeding

Human milk is designed specifically for human infants and is nutritionally superior to any alternative. Breast milk is considered a living tissue because it contains almost as many live cells as blood. It is bacteriologically safe and is always fresh. The nutrients in breast milk are more easily absorbed than those in formula.

Benefits of breastfeeding for the infant include the following:

- Breast milk enhances maturation of the gastrointestinal tract and contains immune factors that contribute to a lower incidence of gastroenteritis, neonatal necrotizing enterocolitis, lymphoma, childhood obesity, Crohn's disease, and celiac disease (CPS et al., 2005).
- Breastfed infants receive specific antibodies and cell-mediated immunological factors that help protect against otitis media, respiratory illnesses such as respiratory syncytial virus and pneumonia, urinary tract infections, bacteremia, and bacterial meningitis (CPS et al., 2005).
- There is a lower incidence of certain allergies among breastfed infants from families at high risk. Atopic

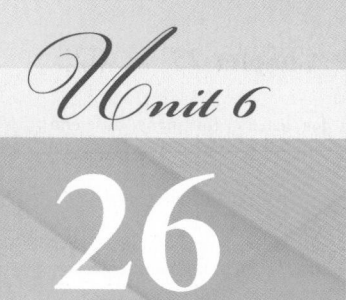

dermatitis is reduced by 42% among infants breastfed for at least 3 months (in children with a family history of atopy). Allergic manifestations occur at a greater rate and are more severe in formula-fed infants (Halken & Host, 1996; Ip et al., 2007).
- Breastfed infants are less likely to die from sudden infant death syndrome (SIDS) (CPS et al., 2005).
- Breast milk may have a protective effect against childhood lymphoma and type 1 and type 2 diabetes mellitus (Horta et al., 2007; Ip et al., 2007).
- Breast milk may enhance cognitive development for term and preterm infants (Kramer et al., 2008; Vohr et al., 2006).
- Breastfeeding appears to have an analgesic effect for infants undergoing painful procedures such as venipuncture and heel stick (Carbajal et al., 2003; Gray et al., 2002; Johnston et al., 2008).

Maternal benefits include the following:
- Women who have breastfed have a decreased risk of ovarian cancer, uterine cancer, rheumatoid arthritis, and breast cancer (Enger et al., 1998; Pikwer et al., 2009; Rosenblatt & Thomas, 1995).
- Breastfeeding promotes uterine involution and is associated with a decreased risk of postpartum hemorrhage (Lawrence & Lawrence, 2011).
- Mothers who are breastfeeding tend to return to their prepregnancy weight more quickly.
- Breastfeeding may provide some protection against the development of osteoporosis and risk for hip fractures (Eisman, 1998).
- Breastfeeding provides a unique bonding experience, increases maternal-role attainment, and may provide protection against postpartum depression when breastfeeding difficulties are appropriately addressed (Kendall-Tackett, 2007: Lawrence & Lawrence, 2011).

Benefits to families and society include the following:
- Breastfeeding is convenient; there are no bottles or other equipment to purchase, clean, or dispose of (a benefit to the community by not having to dispose of formula bottles and equipment used in manufacture).
- Breastfed babies are portable; when traveling, there are fewer supplies to take along.
- Parental absenteeism from work is decreased (Cohen, Mrteck, & Mrteck, 1995).
- Breastfeeding saves money. The cost of formula far exceeds the cost of extra food for the lactating mother. Because breastfed babies have a lower incidence of illness and infection, health care costs are lower for families and for federal and provincial governments.

Contraindications to Breastfeeding

Contraindications to breastfeeding include the following (CPS, 2006; Lawrence & Lawrence, 2011):
- Maternal cancer therapy or diagnostic and therapeutic radioactive isotopes
- Active tuberculosis not under treatment in the mother
- Human immunodeficiency virus (HIV) infection in the mother, in developed countries
- Maternal herpes simplex lesion on a breast
- Galactosemia (classic) in the infant
- Maternal substance use (e.g., cocaine, methamphetamines, marijuana)
- Maternal human T-cell leukemia virus type 1
- Some medications that may exert an untoward effect on the breastfeeding infant; use of these requires consultation of the practitioner and available references such as Hale (2010) or Motherisk (http://www.motherisk.org)

Conditions that are not considered contraindications to breastfeeding are as follows (CPS, 2006):
- Maternal infection with hepatitis C
- Hepatitis B surface antigen (HBsAg)—positive status
- Maternal fever
- Mothers who are cytomegalovirus (CMV) positive

Choosing an Infant Feeding Method

Women who elect to breastfeed usually do so because they are aware of the benefits to the infant. Many seek the unique bonding experience between mother and infant that is characteristic of breastfeeding. Support from the partner and family is a major factor in a mother's decision to breastfeed and in her ability to do so successfully. Ideally, prenatal preparation includes the woman's partner, who needs information about the benefits of breastfeeding and how he or she can participate in infant care and nurturing.

Prenatal breastfeeding classes are an excellent vehicle for relaying important information to expectant parents. Each encounter with an expectant mother is an opportunity to dispel myths, clarify misinformation, and address personal concerns. Connecting expectant mothers with women who are breastfeeding or who have successfully breastfed and are from similar backgrounds may be helpful. Peer counselling programs, such as those instituted by La Leche League, are beneficial, particularly in low-socioeconomic groups, where bottle-feeding is common. To provide effective support for the mother, health care providers must be knowledgeable about the benefits of breastfeeding, the basic process of breastfeeding, breastfeeding management, and interventions for common concerns (Box 26-1).

The percentage of women who initiate breastfeeding rose from 81.5% in 2001 to 87.0% in 2005, and the rate has been steady since then (Statistics Canada, 2009). In 2009, 87.5% of Canadian women breastfed their most recent baby, if only for a short time. Of those who started to breastfeed, 6.9% stopped after less than 1 week, and by 1 month, 21.4% had stopped. The rate of women who exclusively breastfed (no water, other liquids, or solid food) for 6 months or longer has increased from 21% in 2007 to 24.4% in 2009 (Statistics Canada, 2009). However, among those who continued to breastfeed, 53.9% continued for 6 months or longer; only 15.9% breastfed for more than a year (Statistics Canada, 2009). Although there are reports that breastfeeding is declining among First Nations, Métis, and Inuit families, in selected First Nations communities 43% of children were breastfed longer than 6 months (UNICEF, 2009). Breastfeeding patterns vary across Canada and across communities, with a trend toward higher initiation rates in the west and among women over 25 years of age (Public Health Agency of Canada [PHAC], 2009a). The proportion of women who initiate breastfeeding is increased if the

BOX 26-1 Guidelines for Breastfeeding Support

During pregnancy, perform an assessment that includes intent to breastfeed, breastfeeding history, access to breastfeeding support, a breast examination, and a medication use history.

Develop a prenatal care plan to prepare the woman for lactation.

Inform the mother and her family of the importance of early and frequent skin-to-skin contact after birth.

After birth, the nurse:

- Encourages the mother to position her baby skin-to-skin on the mother's chest as soon as possible and until after the first feeding unless medically contraindicated
- Assists with recognition of early feeding cues, latch-on, and positioning, as needed
- Reinforces the need for frequent feedings of breast milk (without supplementation)
- Gives discharge instructions emphasizing signs of successful breastfeeding
- Provides information about community resources for breastfeeding support
- Encourages breastfeeding, especially for preterm and low-birth-weight infants
- Reinforces the recommendation for exclusive breastfeeding for the first 6 months, with the introduction of complementary foods at 6 months and continued breastfeeding up to 2 years and beyond.

(Adapted from International Lactation Consultant Association. [2005]. *Clinical guidelines for the establishment of exclusive breastfeeding.* Retrieved from http://www.ilca.org/files/resources/ilca_publications/ClinicalGuidelines2005.pdf; Registered Nurses' Association of Ontario. [2003]. *Breastfeeding best practice guidelines for nurses.* Toronto: Author. Retrieved from http://www.rnao.org/Storage/11/564_BPG_Breastfeeding.pdf; Registered Nurses' Association of Ontario [2007]. *Breastfeeding best practice guidelines revision supplement.* Toronto: Author. Retrieved from http://rnao.ca/sites/rnao-ca/files/Breastfeeding_Best_Practice_Guidelines_for_Nurses.pdf.)

mother has higher education or the household income is higher (Millar & Maclean, 2005).

Cultural Influences on Infant Feeding

Cultural beliefs and practices are significant influences on infant feeding methods. For example, the tradition among First Nations, Métis, and Inuit people was for infants to be exclusively breastfed until they were able to digest other food sources. These traditional practices shifted to bottle-feeding in the 1950s when infant formula was introduced to the population. The incidence of breastfeeding among this population remains somewhat lower than that for the general population in Canada. Seventy-three percent of off-reserve First Nations, Métis, and Inuit children ages 3 years and under were breastfed compared to 82% of other children in Canada in the same age group, although there now appears to be a trend toward increased breastfeeding among Aboriginal populations (Reading et al., 2007). Among First Nations, Métis, and Inuit peoples are communities unique in culture, language, and history; thus, their breastfeeding practices and beliefs vary. For instance, among the Cree women of Northern Québec, breastfeeding is the norm and is considered good for the health of the baby. These women accept the traditional view that in order to make milk, they must eat very well and expect to have difficulty losing their pregnancy weight. The Cree concept of *miyupimaatisiiun*, or "being alive well," which places emphasis on quality of life rather than on aspects of the physical body, has been a starting point for community-based programs that support breastfeeding while addressing issues of obesity in this population (Vallianatos et al., 2006).

Many cultures typically do not give colostrum to newborns and only begin breastfeeding after the milk has "come in." This practice occurs among some Filipinos, Latin Americans, Vietnamese, Hmong, Koreans, and Nigerians. When breastfeeding is delayed until the milk is in, babies are given prelacteal food. In India, infants may be fed liquids such as honey, tea, water, or sugar water before the initiation of breastfeeding (Choudhry, 1997; McKenna, 2009). Other cultures begin breastfeeding immediately and offer the breast each time the infant cries.

Cultural attitudes regarding modesty and breastfeeding are important considerations in whether a woman breastfeeds her baby. Language barriers may also prevent successful breastfeeding and counselling.

Muslim and Jewish cultures value breastfeeding of infants. Muslim women also have the tradition of a 40-day rest period, during which the woman is relieved of housekeeping duties and other women help care for her. During this time, the mother may exclusively breastfeed; however, Muslim women typically terminate exclusive breastfeeding early in infancy (Chertok, Shoham-Vardi, & Hallak, 2004). For most Jewish women, breastfeeding is perceived as being important, but its practice is highly influenced by maternal education level, assimilated cultural values depending on geographic region of origin, and previous breastfeeding experience (Chertok et al., 2004).

In a survey on beliefs and practices regarding breastfeeding and infant feeding among women in Canada from Asian, Latin American, Portuguese, African, Caribbean, Russian, Central European, Eastern European, and Islamic cultures, key informants from all cultures stressed that parents wanted what is best for their children (Agnew, Gilmore, & Sullivan, 1997). This perspective provides a focus for nursing discussions on infant feeding. Nurses need to clarify individual parental expectations of infant feeding and collaborate with parents to meet their goals.

With the large percentage of immigrants in Canada, it is incumbent on nurses to consider the range of cultural values related to breastfeeding and the benefits of breastfeeding so that the mother can make an informed decision based on both knowledge and an approach that is personally acceptable. Breastfeeding support services need to be provided in a culturally sensitive manner and, where possible, in the family's mother tongue. One of the goals of the Canada Prenatal Nutrition Program (CPNP) is to provide long-term funding to community groups to develop or enhance programs for breastfeeding education and support (PHAC, 2008).

Sociocultural values may preclude the mother from receiving adequate information on breastfeeding; for example, if the family is strongly patriarchal and the father is the only

English-speaking person in the family and acts as translator, the necessary information being conveyed to the mother by the health care provider may not be correctly translated. Persons immigrating to North America often tend to acquire the local customs of their new home; although breastfeeding may have been common in their own country, they may abandon the practice in their new country, considering it "outdated" (Riordan & Gill-Hopple, 2001). This trend varies across Canada; for example, research conducted in Québec showed that infants of low-income women born outside of Canada are more likely to be breastfed than infants of Canadian-born low-income women (Simard et al., 2005).

Nutrient Needs

Energy

Infants require adequate caloric intake to provide energy for growth, digestion, physical activity, and maintenance of organ metabolic function. It is estimated that the average energy intake in a breastfeeding infant is 500 kcal/day (based on average milk intake of 0.78 L/day) (Institute of Medicine, 2005). For the first 3 months, the infant needs approximately 110 kcal/kg/day. From 3 months to 6 months, the requirement decreases to approximately 100 kcal/kg/day. This decreases slightly to 95 kcal/kg/day from 6 to 9 months, and increases to 100 kcal/kg/day from 9 months to 1 year.

Human milk provides approximately 20 kcal/30 mL; the greatest amount of energy is provided by the fat content of breast milk. Infant formulas are made to simulate the caloric content of human milk; standard formulas for healthy term infants contain 20 kcal/30 mL.

Carbohydrates

Because newborns have only small hepatic glycogen stores, carbohydrates should provide at least 40 to 45% of the total calories in the diet. Moreover, newborns may have limited ability for **gluconeogenesis** (formation of glucose from amino acids and other substrates) and ketogenesis (formation of ketone bodies from fat), which are mechanisms that provide alternative energy sources.

As the primary carbohydrate in human milk (approximately 75 g/L), lactose is the most abundant carbohydrate in the diet of infants up to 6 months of age. Lactose provides calories in an easily available form; its slow breakdown and absorption probably also increase calcium absorption. Corn syrup solids or glucose polymers are added to infant formulas to supplement the lactose in cow's milk and provide sufficient carbohydrates.

The Dietary Reference Intake Adequate Intake (DRI AI) for carbohydrate is 60 g/day in the first 6 months of life and 95 g/day for the next 6 months (Institute of Medicine, 2005).

Fat

For infants to acquire adequate calories from the limited amount of human milk or formula they are able to consume, at least 15% of the calories provided must come from fat (triglycerides). Fat is the major source of energy in the diet of the infant fed human milk. Fat in human milk is easier to digest and absorb than that in cow's milk because of the arrangement of the fatty acids on the glycerol molecule and because of the presence of the enzyme lipase. The DRI AI for fat is 31 g/day, which reflects the amount received by infants who are breastfed during the first 6 months of life (Institute of Medicine, 2005).

Modified cow's milk is used to make most infant formulas, but the milk fat is removed and replaced by another fat source, such as corn oil, that can be easily digested and absorbed by the infant. If whole milk or evaporated milk without added carbohydrate is fed to infants, the resulting fecal loss of fat (and therefore loss of energy) may be excessive because the milk moves through the infant's intestines too quickly for adequate absorption to take place. This can lead to poor weight gain. There is evidence that whole milk may also increase the infant's chances for developing allergies from exposure to cow's milk protein.

In addition to its energy contributions, fat also furnishes essential fatty acids (EFAs), which are required for growth and tissue maintenance. EFAs are components of cell membranes and precursors of some hormones. Inadequate intake of EFAs results in eczema and growth failure. The lack of EFAs in skim and low-fat milk is another reason why infants should not be fed these products.

In recent years, the discovery of long-chain polyunsaturated fatty acids (LCPUFA) in human milk has led to the addition of arachidonic acid (ARA) and docosahexaenoic acid (DHA) to formula, both of which are considered important in the infant's growth, neurodevelopment, and visual function (Fleith & Clandinin, 2005; Morin, 2004). Studies in full-term infants receiving supplements with DHA and ARA have produced mixed results regarding cognitive function and visual acuity (Heird, 2007; Simmer, Patole, & Rao, 2008). LCPUFAs are available from a variety of sources, including egg yolk lipid, phospholipids, and triglyceride. The evidence for supplementation of formula for preterm infants with LCPUFAs, however, has been more convincing, producing some transient improvement in visual acuity and general development (American Academy of Pediatrics, 2009).

Protein

The protein requirement per unit of body weight is greater in the newborn than at any other time of life. The protein content of human milk, which is lower than that of unmodified cow's milk, is ideal for the newborn. Human milk contains far more lactalbumin (or whey protein) in relation to casein than does cow's milk, and lactalbumin is more easily digested than casein. In addition, the amino acid composition of human milk is suited to the newborn's metabolic capabilities. For example, phenylalanine and methionine levels are low, and cystine and taurine levels are high. The protein in some commercial formulas is modified to increase the amount of lactalbumin and to decrease the relative proportion of casein to more closely approximate human milk. The concentration of protein in infant formula is 14.5 to 16 g/L (American Academy of Pediatrics, 2009). The DRI AI for protein is 1.52 g/kg/day (Institute of Medicine, 2005).

Water

The water requirement for healthy term infants is about 75 to 100 mL/kg/day (Heird, 2007). The DRI for water intake for the

0- to 6-month-old infant is 700 mL/24 hr; for the 7- to 12-month-old, the DRI requirement is 800 mL/24 hr. Neither breastfed nor formula-fed infants, even those living in hot climates, need to be fed supplemental water. Breast milk contains 87% water, which easily meets fluid requirements. Feeding water to infants may cause water toxicity with resulting hyponatremia and seizures. Infants have little room for fluctuation in fluid balance and should be monitored closely for fluid intake and water loss if certain illness factors exist. Infants lose water through excretion of urine and through insensible losses such as respiration. Most healthy infants take in an adequate amount of fluid daily in either breast milk or commercial formula. Conditions that may lead to a decrease in oral intake and subsequent fluid deficit include gastroenteritis (vomiting and diarrhea), poor intake due to illness (congestive heart failure), or conditions affecting the mechanical process of eating (e.g., thrush, viral stomatitis, ankyloglossia [tight lingual frenulum], or poor **latch-on** early in breastfeeding).

Juices are not necessary for proper nutrient intake. There is no evidence that juice intake provides better nutrients than human milk or fortified formula, but there are data indicating that excess juice consumption may replace essential elements, leading to nutritional deficits (CPS et al., 2005). Juices may also cause significant dental decay, especially when consumed from a bottle.

Vitamins

Human milk contains all the vitamins required for infant nutrition, with individual variations based on maternal diet and genetic differences. Vitamins are added to cow's milk formulas to approximate the levels in breast milk. Cow's milk contains adequate amounts of vitamin A and vitamin B complex; vitamin C (ascorbic acid) and vitamin E must be added.

Vitamin D is also added to commercial infant formulas. The vitamin D content of human milk is low; thus, vitamin D available to the infant during the first 6 months of life depends initially on the vitamin D status of the mother during pregnancy. After 6 months, vitamin D is obtained from the infant's diet and exposure to sunlight. Canadian recommendations regarding vitamin D supplementation are based on Canada's northern geographic latitude, current practices related to protection from the sun, prevalence of vitamin D deficiency rickets, and history of safe use of vitamin D supplementation. Health Canada recommends that all breastfed, healthy term infants in Canada receive a daily vitamin D supplement of 10 mcg (400 IU). Supplementation should begin at birth and continue until the infant's diet includes at least 10 mcg (400 IU) per day of vitamin D from other dietary sources or until the breastfed infant reaches 1 year of age (Health Canada, 2004b).

Vitamin K, required for blood coagulation, is produced by intestinal bacteria. However, the gut is relatively sterile at birth, and a few days are needed for intestinal flora to become established and produce vitamin K. To prevent hemorrhagic problems in the newborn, an injection of vitamin K is routinely given within the first 6 hours after birth, following initial stabilization of the baby and family–baby interaction (Canadian Paediatric Society & College of Family Physicians of Canada, 1997) (see Chapter 25, Medication Guide on vitamin K).

Minerals

The mineral content of commercial infant formula is designed to reflect that of breast milk. Whole cow's milk is much higher in mineral content than human milk, which makes it unsuitable for infants in the first year of life. Minerals are typically highest in human milk during the first few days after birth and decrease slightly throughout lactation.

The ratio of calcium to phosphorus in human milk is 2:1, a proportion optimal for bone mineralization. Although cow's milk is high in calcium, the calcium-to-phosphorus ratio is low, resulting in decreased resorption. Consequently, young infants (less than 12 months) fed whole cow's milk are at risk for hypocalcemia, tetany, and seizures. The calcium-to-phosphorus ratio in commercial infant formulas is between the ratios of human and cow's milk.

Milk of all types is low in iron; however, iron from human milk is better absorbed than that from cow's milk, iron-fortified formula, or infant cereals. Breastfed infants benefit from the high lactose and vitamin C levels in human milk, which facilitate iron absorption. The infant who is totally breastfed normally maintains adequate hemoglobin levels for at least the first 6 months of life. After that time, iron-fortified cereals and other iron-rich foods may be added to the diet. Infants weaned from the breast before 6 months of age and all formula-fed infants should receive an iron-fortified commercial infant formula until 12 months of age. Infants should not be given low-iron formula (CPS, 2007a).

The fluoride levels in human milk and in commercial formulas are low. This mineral, which is important in the prevention of dental **caries**, may cause staining of the permanent teeth (fluorosis) in excess amounts. Fluoride supplementation should be considered for any child over age 6 months whose drinking water is deficient in fluoride or if other factors put the child at high risk for developing dental caries (Canadian Dental Association [CDA], 2010; CPS, 2002).

Overview of Lactation

Breast Anatomy

Each female breast is composed of 4 to 18 segments (lobes) embedded in fat and connective tissue and well supplied with blood vessels, lymphatic tissue, and nerves (Fig. 26-1). Within each lobe are many alveoli (the milk-producing cells) surrounded by myoepithelial cells, which contract to send the milk forward into the ductules. Each ductule enlarges into lactiferous ducts, where the milk is stored until the let-down reflex triggers the myoepithelial cells to contract and eject the milk out though the nipple pores (Riordan & Wambach, 2009). Each nipple has pores from the ends of the ducts through which milk is transferred to the **suckling** infant. The ducts do not widen into sinuses behind the nipple as previously thought. The nipple tissue is erectile and surrounded by

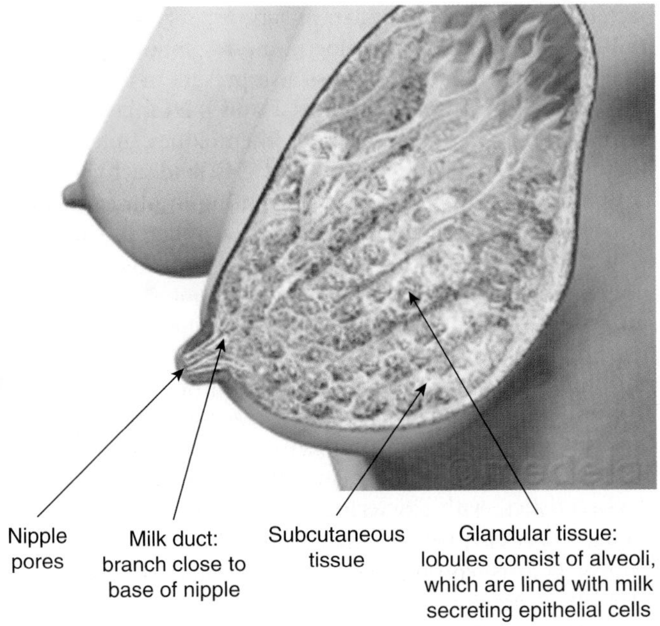

Fig. 26-1 Detailed structural features of human mammary gland. *(© 2006 Medela AG.)*

an area of darker pigmentation known as the areola. The nipple and areola are very elastic so that they can be drawn fully into the infant's mouth for deep latch-on (Lawrence & Lawrence, 2011).

Although nearly every woman can lactate, some mothers have insufficient glandular development to exclusively breastfeed their infants. Typically these women experienced few breast changes during either puberty or early pregnancy. In some cases, these women may still be able to breastfeed and offer supplemental nutrition to support optimal infant growth. Devices are available that enable mothers to offer supplements while the baby is at the breast (Fig. 26-2).

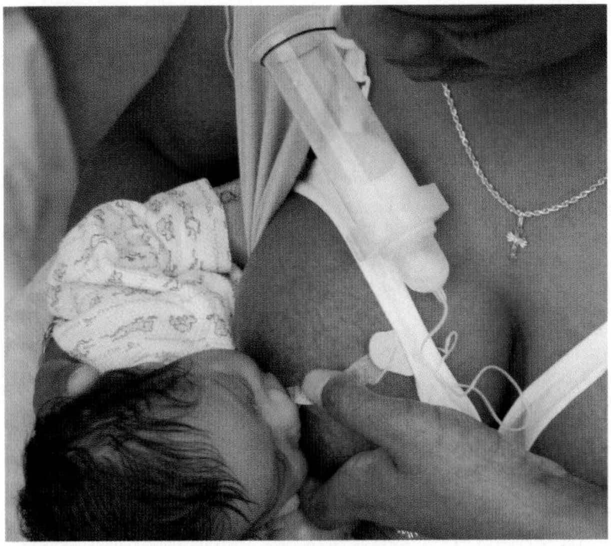

Fig. 26-2 Supplemental nursing system. *(© 2005 Medela, Inc.)*

Milk Production

After the mother gives birth, there is a precipitous fall in her estrogen and progesterone levels, triggering release of **prolactin** from the anterior pituitary. Prolactin prepares the breasts to secrete milk during pregnancy and to synthesize and secrete milk during lactation. Prolactin levels are highest during the first 10 days after birth; they gradually decline over time but remain above baseline levels for the duration of lactation. Prolactin is produced in response to infant suckling and emptying the breasts (lactating breasts are never completely empty; milk is constantly being produced by the alveoli as the infant feeds) (Fig. 26-3, A). Milk production is a supply-meets-demand system; that is, as milk is removed from the breast, more is produced. Limited transfer of milk during feedings can lead to a decrease in milk production.

Oxytocin is another hormone essential to lactation. As the nipple is stimulated by the suckling infant, the posterior pituitary is prompted by the **hypothalamus** to produce oxytocin. This hormone is responsible for the **milk ejection reflex** (MER), or let-down reflex (see Fig. 26-3, B). The myoepithelial cells surrounding the alveoli respond to oxytocin by contracting and sending the milk forward through the ducts to the nipple.

Oxytocin is the same hormone that stimulates uterine contractions during labour. Oxytocin contracts the mother's uterus after birth to control postpartum bleeding and to promote uterine involution. Thus, mothers who breastfeed are at decreased risk for postpartum hemorrhage. The uterine contractions that occur with breastfeeding can be painful during and after the feeding, particularly in multiparas, for 3 to 5 days after giving birth.

Prolactin and oxytocin have been referred to as the "mothering hormones" because they are known to affect the postpartum woman's emotions, as well as her physical state. Many women report feeling thirsty or relaxed during breastfeeding, probably as a result of these hormones.

The nipple erection reflex is an integral part of lactation. When the infant cries, suckles, or rubs against the breast, the nipple becomes erect. This assists in the propulsion of milk through the ducts to the nipple pores. Nipple size, shape, and ability to become erect vary with individuals. Some women have flat or inverted nipples that do not become erect with stimulation; however, these women are usually able to learn to breastfeed successfully. It is important that these infants are not offered bottles or pacifiers until breastfeeding is well established.

As a method to increase milk supply, some herbal products are presented as safe and effective alternatives to prescription or over-the-counter medications; certain herbal agents, the galactogogues, are reported to increase breast milk production. There are insufficient data to confirm or deny the assertion of increased milk production using galactogogues, and mothers are cautioned to seek advice from a practitioner to ensure that the herbal preparations will not harm the breastfeeding infant (Conover & Buehler, 2004).

evolve Case Study—Breastfeeding

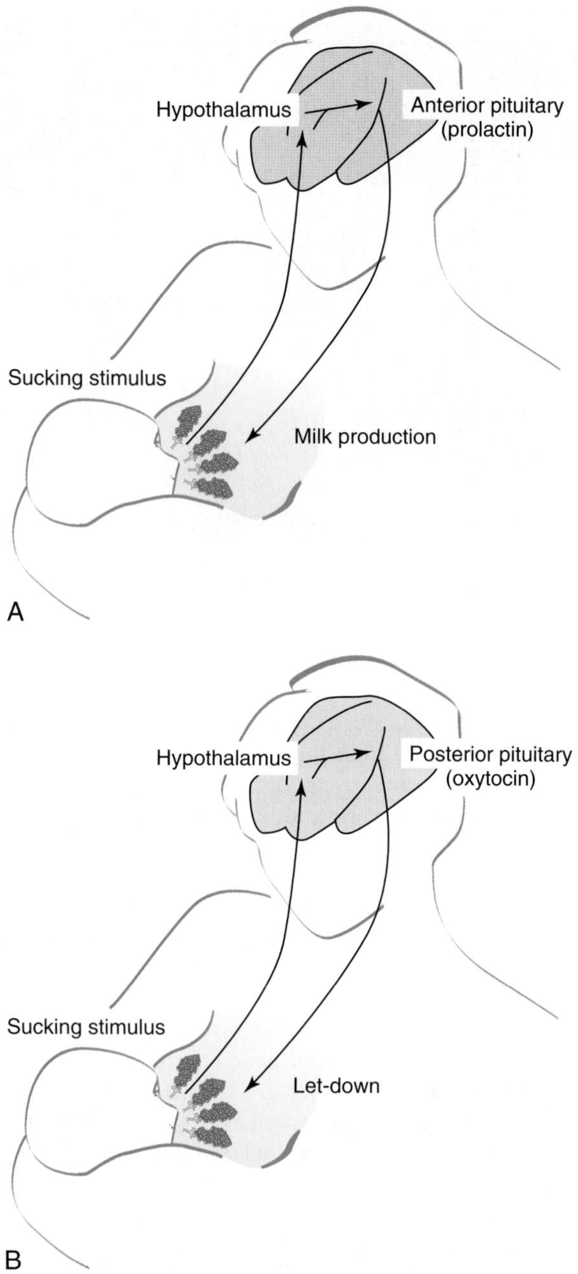

Fig. 26-3 Maternal breastfeeding reflexes. **A:** Milk production. **B:** Let-down.

Unique Properties of Human Milk

Human milk is a highly complex, species-specific fluid uniquely designed to meet the human infant's needs. It is specific to the needs of each newborn; for example, the milk of mothers of preterm infants differs in composition from that of mothers who give birth at term. Breast milk consists of a number of micronutrients that are *bioavailable*, meaning these nutrients are available in quantities and with qualities that make them easily digestible by the newborn's intestine and absorbed for energy and growth.

Human milk contains immunologically active components that provide some protection against a broad spectrum of bacterial, viral, and protozoan infections. Secretory **immune globulin** A (IgA) is the major immune globulin in human milk; IgG, IgM, IgD, and IgE are also present in human milk. In addition, human milk contains T and B **lymphocytes**, epidermal growth factor, cytokines, chemokines, interleukins, bifidus factor, complement (C3 and C4), and lactoferrin, all of which have specific roles in preventing localized and systemic bacterial and viral infections (Lawrence & Lawrence, 2011).

Human milk contains the two proteins, whey (lactalbumin) and casein (curd), in a ratio of approximately 60:40 (versus 80:20 in most cow's milk–based formula). This ratio in human milk makes it more digestible and produces the soft stools seen in breastfed infants. Human milk has a laxative effect; thus, constipation is uncommon in breastfed infants. The whey protein, and lactoferrin, in human milk has iron-binding characteristics with bacteriostatic capabilities, particularly against gram-positive and gram-negative aerobes, anaerobes, and yeasts. Giving iron to breastfed newborn infants interferes with this process and, in particular, promotes the growth of *E. coli* (Lawrence & Lawrence, 2011).

Digestive enzymes present in human milk include amylases, lipases, proteases, and ribonucleases, which enhance the digestion and absorption of various nutrients (Lawrence & Lawrence, 2011). The fat content of human milk is composed of lipids, triglycerides, and cholesterol; cholesterol is an essential element for brain growth. The function of these lipids is to allow optimum intestinal absorption of fatty acids and provide essential fatty acids and polyunsaturated fatty acids. Furthermore, lipids contribute approximately 50% of the total calories in human milk (Lawrence & Lawrence, 2011). Although the overall fat content in human milk is higher than in cow's milk–based formula, the infant uses it more efficiently. The primary source of carbohydrate in human milk is lactose, which is present in higher concentrations (68 g/L) than in cow's milk–based formula (49 g/L). Other carbohydrates found in human milk include glucose, galactose, and glucosamine. The carbohydrates not only serve as a large percentage of the total calories in human milk but also have a protective function; the oligosaccharides in human milk stimulate the growth of *Lactobacillus bifidus* and prevent bacteria from adhering to epithelial surfaces (Lawrence & Lawrence, 2011).

Human milk composition and volumes vary according to the stage of lactation. In lactogenesis stage I, beginning in pregnancy, the breasts are preparing for milk production. **Colostrum**, a clear, yellowish fluid, is present in the breasts of most women by week 22 of pregnancy (Hartmann et al., 2003). Colostrum is more concentrated than mature milk and is extremely rich in immune globulins. It has higher concentrations of protein, fat-soluble vitamins, and minerals, but less fat, than mature milk. The high protein level of colostrum facilitates binding of bilirubin, and the laxative action of colostrum promotes early passage of meconium. Colostrum gradually changes to **transitional milk**; this is referred to as "the **mature milk** coming in," or lactogenesis stage II. By the third to fifth day after birth, most women have experienced this onset of copious milk secretion. Breast milk continues to change in composition for approximately 10 days, when the mature milk is established in stage III of lactogenesis (Lawrence & Lawrence, 2011).

Composition of mature milk changes during each feeding. As the infant nurses, the fat content of breast milk increases. Initially there is a release of bluish white **foremilk** that is part skim milk (about 60% of the volume) and part whole milk (about 35% of the volume). It provides primarily lactose, protein, and water-soluble vitamins. The **hindmilk**, or cream (about 5%), is usually let down 10 to 20 minutes into the feeding, although it may occur sooner. It contains the denser calories from fat necessary for optimal growth and contentment between feedings. Because of this changing composition of human milk during each feeding, it is important to breastfeed the infant long enough to supply a balanced feeding. Milk production gradually increases, so that by the time the infant is 2 weeks old, the mother produces 720 to 900 mL of milk every 24 hours. Babies experience fairly predictable **growth spurts** (i.e., at about 10 days, 3 weeks, 6 weeks, 3 months, and 4 to 6 months), when more frequent feedings stimulate increased milk production. These more frequent feedings usually last 24 to 48 hours, and then the infants resume their usual feeding pattern.

Nursing Care Management: The Breastfeeding Mother and Infant

Assessment

Infant

The nurse must consider several factors to effectively assist the breastfeeding infant. Maturity level, any birth trauma or maternal risk factors, congenital defects or physical instability, and state of alertness all affect the infant's readiness and ability to breastfeed.

During feeding, the infant is assessed by direct observation for feeding cues, latch-on, position and alignment, and suckling and swallowing. A breastfeeding assessment tool known as LATCH was developed by Jensen, Wallace, and Kelsey in 1994. Subsequent research has demonstrated that early LATCH scores are linked to breastfeeding success at 6 weeks of age (Kumar et al., 2006; Mannel, 2011). The tool involves assessing for the following:

L (characteristics of latch-on)
A (degree of audible swallowing)
T (type of nipple)
C (maternal comfort)
H (holding skills)

Systematic assessment of these five aspects can assist the mother and nurse to focus on what is needed for extra support.

After the feeding, the infant is observed for behaviour such as contentment or sleepiness. Elimination patterns are noted: Within 24 hours after birth, at least one wet diaper and one stool; by day 3, three or four wet diapers and one or two stools that are beginning to change from meconium to yellow; after day 4 (and mother's mature milk has "come in"), six to eight wet diapers and at least three stools per 24 hours (see p. 689). Other factors to assess include the presence of jaundice, weight loss greater than 7%, and whether the infant has regained birth weight by 10 to 14 days of age. See Box 27-3 for calculation of weight loss. The feeding pattern should include cue-based feedings without time restrictions, on average at least 8 to 12 times per 24 hours (International Lactation Consultant Association [ILCA], 2005; Registered Nurses' Association of Ontario [RNAO], 2003) (see Critical Thinking Exercise).

Mother

The nurse should carefully assess the mother's knowledge of breastfeeding and her physical and psychological readiness to breastfeed. Factors to include are her previous experience with breastfeeding, knowledge about breastfeeding, cultural factors, physical features of the breasts or nipples or other possible physical limitations, psychological readiness (time since birth, mood, and energy level), and support of the mother's partner or other family members.

During the time in the hospital, the nurse can help the mother view each breastfeeding session as a "feeding lesson" or "practice session" that will foster maternal confidence and a satisfying breastfeeding experience for mother and infant. Assessment includes condition of nipples, transition to mature milk, breasts feeling lighter or softer after feeding, the mother feeling relaxed or sleepy after feeding, uterine cramping or increased lochia flow during and after a feeding, and the mother's appearance of comfort with breastfeeding techniques.

The nursing process in the care of the breastfeeding mother–infant pair is outlined in the Nursing Process box.

evolve Skill—Infant Feeding

CRITICAL THINKING EXERCISE

Neonatal Breastfeeding

Neide is a 27-year-old married woman from Costa Rica who recently moved to Canada and has a 5-day-old, 3288 g male infant. His birth weight was 3540 g. She is being seen in the clinic for a follow-up consultation on breastfeeding and jaundice. On examination the infant is alert, fussy, and visibly jaundiced. Neide admits that breastfeeding has not been going as well as planned and she is not certain the infant is receiving enough milk. She states, in tears, that all the baby does is cry and fuss when she places him to the breast, and she wants to try formula. She recalls that yesterday the baby had one or two greenish stools and three or four wet diapers.

1. Evidence—Is there sufficient evidence to draw conclusions about the effectiveness of the infant's breastfeeding pattern?
2. Assumptions—What assumptions can be made about the following factors?
   a. The infant's ability to latch-on
   b. Adequacy of breast milk intake
   c. The need for additional infant assessments
   d. The mother's desire to give the infant formula
   e. The mother's physical and emotional status
3. What implications and priorities for nursing care can be drawn at this time?
4. Does the evidence objectively support your conclusion?
5. Are there alternative perspectives to your conclusion?

NURSING PROCESS: BREASTFEEDING MOTHER–INFANT PAIR

Assessment

The assessment of the breastfeeding mother–newborn pair must include an assessment of infant feeding cues and the mother's physical and psychological readiness to breastfeed. Additional assessment guidelines are discussed on previous page.

Nursing Diagnoses

Nursing diagnoses for the breastfeeding woman and infant may include the following:

Effective breastfeeding related to
- mother's knowledge of breastfeeding techniques
- mother's appropriate response to infant's feeding cues for hunger and satiation
- mother's ability to facilitate exclusive and effective breastfeeding

Risk for ineffective breastfeeding related to
- limited knowledge of newborn's feeding cues, reflexes, and breastfeeding techniques
- lack of support by partner, family, or friends
- lack of maternal self-confidence; presence of anxiety, fear of failure
- poor infant suckling reflex
- difficulty waking sleepy newborn

Risk for imbalanced nutrition: less than body requirements related to
- increased caloric and nutrient needs for breastfeeding (mother)
- incorrect latch-on and inability to transfer milk (infant)

Risk for deficient fluid volume related to
- ineffective suckling (infant)
- delayed or infrequent feeding

Planning and Implementation

The expected outcomes include that the full-term infant will do the following:

- Give clear hunger cues (hands to mouth, rooting, licking, sucking)
- Latch on and feed effectively at least 8 to 12 times per day after the first 24 hours
- Have a weight loss of less than 7 to 10% and no further weight loss after day 3
- Begin to gain weight by day 5 and return to birth weight by 10 to 21 days
- Remain well hydrated (increase numbers of wet diapers by 1 each day of life until the fifth day, then 6 to 8 wet diapers and at least 3 to 4 bowel movements every 24 hours with no meconium stool after day 4)
- Gives satiation cues (e.g., comes off breast, falls asleep); sleeps or appears contented between feedings

Examples of expected outcomes for the mother include that she will do the following:

- Communicate and demonstrate understanding of breastfeeding techniques, including positioning and latch-on, signs of adequate feeding, responses to feeding cues and self-care
- Report no nipple discomfort with breastfeeding
- Express satisfaction with the breastfeeding experience
- Consume a nutritionally balanced diet with appropriate caloric and fluid intake to support breastfeeding

Nursing interventions for the breastfeeding mother-infant pair are discussed on pp. 683–700.

Evaluation

Evaluation is based on the expected outcomes, and the care plan is revised as needed, on the basis of evaluation.

Implementation

The ideal time to begin breastfeeding is within the first hour after birth, when the infant is in the quiet, alert state (WHO, 2010a).

In the early days after birth, interventions are focused on helping the mother and the newborn initiate breastfeeding and achieve some degree of success and satisfaction before discharge from the hospital. Interventions to promote breastfeeding progress from basics, such as interpreting cues, latch-on, and positioning, to signs of adequate feeding and self-care measures, such as prevention of engorgement. With early discharge from the hospital, it is increasingly important to assess the mother–infant dyad in relation to feeding ability. In some cases, either a home visit or a visit to a health care practitioner is appropriate within 48 to 72 hours after discharge to ensure that adequate latch-on is taking place and that the infant is progressing in feeding, elimination, and jaundice patterns. The visit is also an excellent opportunity to evaluate the mother's status, answer any questions about self-care or newborn care, and reinforce positive parenting and child care abilities.

Positioning

There are four basic positions for breastfeeding: football hold; cradle; cross-cradle, or across-the-lap; and side-lying position (Fig. 26-4). Initially it is best to use the position that most easily facilitates latch-on while allowing maximum comfort for the mother. The football hold is usually preferred by mothers who gave birth by Caesarean section or have larger breasts (Fig. 26-4, A). The cross-cradle, or across-the-lap, hold also works well for early feedings (Fig. 26-4, B). Cradling is the most common breastfeeding position for infants who have learned to latch on easily and feed effectively (Fig. 26-4, C). The side-lying position allows the mother to rest while breastfeeding and is often preferred by women experiencing perineal pain and swelling (Fig. 26-4, D). Before discharge from the hospital, the mother should be assisted in trying all of the positions so that she will feel confident in her ability to vary positions at home.

Before starting a feeding, the mother should be in a comfortable position and the baby should be awake and demonstrating hunger cues. Pillows may be used to provide support for her back and arms after the baby has latched comfortably. The infant is placed at the level of the breast and turned completely facing the mother so that the infant is "belly-to-belly," with the arms "hugging" the breast. When positioned skin-to-skin, many infants will find the nipple and latch spontaneously. Other infants may need some help. The newborn's nose should be pointing toward the mother's nipple, avoiding "centering" the mouth over the nipple. It is important that the mother support the newborn's neck and shoulders with her hand and not push on the occiput. The infant's body should be held in correct alignment (i.e., ears, shoulders, and hips are in a straight line) during latch-on and feeding.

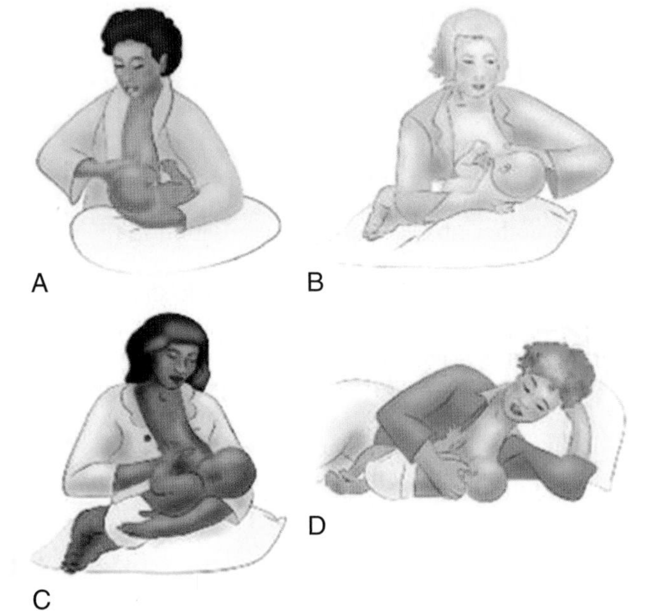

Fig. 26-4 Breastfeeding positions. **A:** Football hold. **B:** Cross-cradle. **C:** Cradling. **D:** Side-lying position. *(Courtesy Best Start Ontario.)*

Latch-On

In preparation for latch-on, it may be helpful for the mother to manually express a few drops of colostrum or milk to spread over the nipple. This lubricates the nipple and may entice the baby to open the mouth as the milk is tasted.

To facilitate latch-on, the mother may support her breast in one hand with the thumb on top and the fingers underneath at the back edge of the areola; this is called the *C hold* (Fig. 26-5, A). She may also compress the breast slightly so that an adequate amount of breast tissue is taken into the mouth with latch-on. Some mothers need to support the breast during feeding for at least the first few weeks until the infant can stay latched on easily.

The mother lightly touches the infant's upper lip with her nipple, stimulating the mouth to open (rooting reflex). When the mouth is open wide and the tongue is down, the mother brings the baby in close (Fig. 26-5, B), with the head slightly tilted so that the chin touches the breast first; if the infant does not move forward independently, she can quickly pull the infant onto the nipple (Fig. 26-5, C). She should bring the infant to the breast, not the breast to the infant. If the breast is pushed into the infant's mouth, the infant often closes the mouth too soon and does not latch on.

The amount of the areola in the newborn's mouth with latch-on depends on the size of the newborn's mouth and the size of the areola and nipple. In general, the infant's mouth should cover the nipple and areola, with more of the areola visible above the baby's upper lip than below the lower lip (Fig. 26-6).

When the newborn is latched on correctly, the chin should be pressed into the breast, and the cheeks and nose may be lightly touching the breast. The mother should not pull the nipple out of the mouth when trying to create a breathing space for the newborn's nose. Depressing the breast tissue around the newborn's nose is not necessary. If the mother is worried about the infant's breathing, she can raise the newborn's hips slightly to change the angle of the infant's head at the breast. If the newborn cannot breathe, reflexes will prompt the newborn to move the head and pull back to breathe.

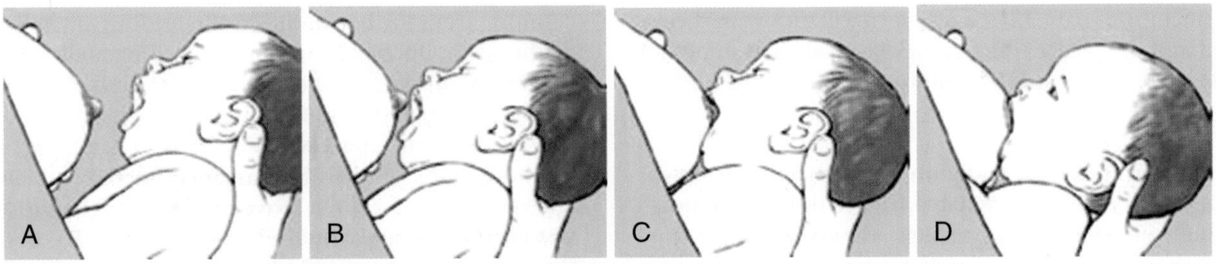

Fig. 26-5 Latching on. **A:** When mouth is wide open, draw baby close. **B:** Nipple should be centred upward in infant's mouth. **C:** As baby latches on, draw infant closer to breast. Chin should be tucked in close to breast. **D:** Baby should be allowed to nurse until he or she stops swallowing. *(Illustrations by Bonnie Ross. Reprinted with written permission from the Province of Nova Scotia.)*

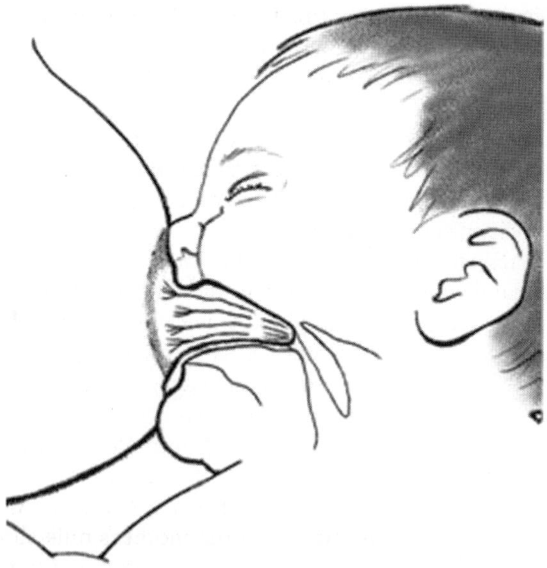

Fig. 26-6 Correct attachment (latch-on) of infant at breast. *(Courtesy Cumberland Health Authority.)*

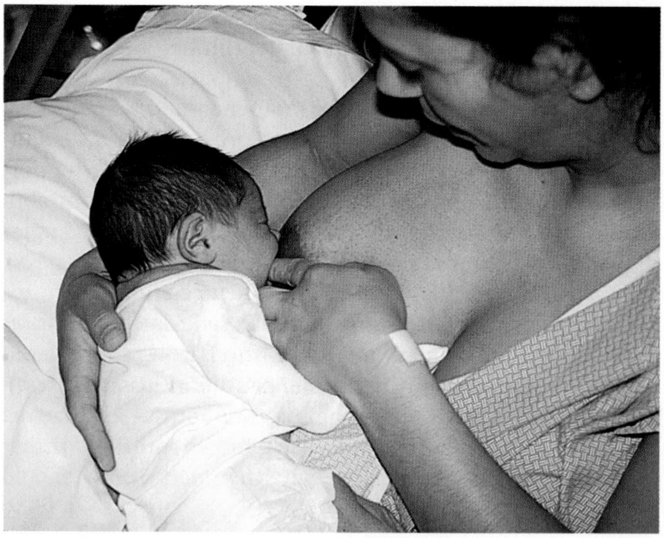

Fig. 26-7 Removing infant from the breast. *(Courtesy Marjorie Pyle, RNC, Lifecircle, Costa Mesa, CA.)*

Sucking creates a vacuum in the intraoral cavity as the breast is compressed between the tongue and the palate. If the mother experiences pinching or pain after the first few sucks or does not feel a firm tugging on the nipple, the latch-on and positioning should be modified.

If each suck is painful, the infant may be having difficulty keeping the tongue out over the lower gum ridge. Clicking or smacking may be audible when this occurs. If repositioning does not alleviate this problem, the nurse or mother can place a finger on the side of the newborn's lower jaw, pulling down gently but firmly as the infant sucks, to help stabilize the jaw so that the tongue stays in place.

Any time the signs of adequate latch-on and sucking are not present, the newborn should be taken off the breast and latch-on attempted again. To prevent nipple trauma as the newborn is taken off the breast, the mother should break the suction by inserting her finger in the side of the infant's mouth between the gums and keeping it there until the nipple is completely out of the newborn's mouth (Fig. 26-7).

When the newborn is latched on correctly and is sucking appropriately, (1) the mother will feel a firm tug on her nipple, but no pinching or pain; (2) the newborn will suck with cheeks rounded, not dimpled; (3) the infant's jaw will glide smoothly with silent sucking; and (4) swallowing will be audible.

Milk Ejection, or Let-Down

As the newborn begins suckling on the nipple, the let-down, or milk ejection reflex, is stimulated. Two to three "let-downs" can occur with each feeding session. The MER can be triggered by thoughts, sights, sounds, or odours that the mother associates with her baby (or other babies), such as hearing the baby cry. Many women report a tingling "pins and needles" sensation in the breasts as let-down occurs, although some mothers can detect milk ejection only by observing the infant's sucking and swallowing. Let-down may also occur during sexual activity because oxytocin is released during orgasm. The following signs indicate that let-down has occurred:

- The mother may feel a tingling sensation in the nipples, although some women do not feel their milk let down.
- The newborn's suck changes from quick, shallow sucks to a slower, deeper, and stronger sucking pattern.
- Swallowing is audible after the newborn sucks.
- The mother feels relaxed, even sleepy, during feedings.
- The mother experiences uterine cramping and increased lochia flow during or after the feeding.
- The opposite breast may leak milk.

Frequency of Feedings

Newborns usually require 8 to 12 feedings in a 24-hour period. During the first 24 to 48 hours after birth, many newborns may not awaken this often to feed. By contrast, some infants may nurse "nonstop" during this period to stimulate milk production. It is important that parents understand that they should awaken the sleepy infant to feed at least every 3 hours during the day and at least every 4 hours at night during the first few weeks of life. Feeding frequency is determined by counting from the beginning of one feeding to the beginning of the next. Once the newborn is feeding well and gaining weight appropriately, he or she can determine the timing of feedings through demand feedings.

Parents should be cautioned about attempting to place newborn infants on strict feeding schedules. Infants should be fed whenever they exhibit feeding cues such as hand-to-mouth movements, rooting, and mouth and tongue movements. Crying is a late sign of hunger, and infants may become frantic when they have to wait too long to feed. Some infants will shut down or go into a deep sleep when their needs are not met. Understanding and responding to an infant's states and cues (see Chapter 24) is essential to the infant feeding interaction.

Frequent skin-to-skin holding helps mothers to notice state changes and early hunger cues and thus provide the frequent feedings required at the breast in the early days (see Evidence-Informed Practice box). One recommendation is that mother and breastfeeding infant sleep in close proximity to promote breastfeeding. The issue of bed-sharing has raised concerns because of the association between a higher incidence of SIDS and bed-sharing with an adult. Health Canada recommends that the safest place for any infant to sleep is in a crib within arm's reach of where the parents sleep. This practice allows for more convenient breastfeeding and at the same time prevents continuous bed-sharing (Health Canada, 2010). Room-sharing is recommended for at least the first 6 months. The back-lying (supine) position for sleep is also recommended for all infants. (See Chapter 25 for more discussion on SIDS).

Duration of Feedings

The duration of breastfeeding sessions is highly variable, as the timing of milk transfer differs for each mother–infant pair. Some infants may complete a feeding in 5 or 10 minutes; others may require 45 minutes or longer. The average time for newborn feeding is 30 to 40 minutes, or approximately 20 minutes per breast, although instructing mothers to feed for a set number of minutes is inappropriate. It is better to teach mothers how to determine when an infant has finished a feeding: The infant's suck-swallow pattern has slowed, and the newborn appears content and may fall asleep or release the nipple. Other, more subtle, satiation cues include extended and relaxed fingers, arms and legs extended, back arching, or pushing away (Spietz et al., 1999).

The amount of intake with each feeding reflects the size of the infant's stomach; approximate increases in stomach capacity for term infants are 5 to 7 mL on day 1; 22 to 27 mL on day 3; and 60 to 81 mL on day 10. Comparing these volumes to a cherry, a walnut, and a hen's egg is one way to help parents visualize the sizes (PHAC, 2009b) (Fig. 26-8).

If a newborn seems to be feeding effectively and is having adequate urine output but not gaining weight well, the mother may be switching to the second breast too soon. The high lactose content in foremilk may cause the newborn to have explosive stools, gas pains, and inconsolable crying. Keeping the infant on the first breast until satiation cues are evident ensures that the infant receives the more calorie-dense, high-fat hindmilk, which usually results in increased weight gain. After repositioning, a newborn will usually restart the feeding on the second breast.

Supplementation

The Canadian Paediatric Society (2005) recommends that, unless a medical indication exists, no supplements be given to breastfeeding infants. Infant conditions that may necessitate supplemental feedings include low birth weight, hypoglycemia, an inborn error of metabolism, or acute water loss. Infants with insufficient weight gain may need supplementation if increased breastfeeding cannot provide sufficient intake. Mothers may be unable to feed because of severe illness, or they may be taking medications incompatible with breastfeeding (Breastfeeding Committee for Canada [BCC], 2011).

Offering a bottle after breastfeeding "just to make sure the baby is getting enough" is unnecessary and should be avoided. Similarly, glucose water feedings are not advised. Blackburn (2007) suggests that early feedings with a carbohydrate source initially increase blood glucose levels; this increase is accompanied by a subsequent increase in plasma insulin levels and the development of cyclic changes in insulin and blood glucose levels in full-term infants. Eidelman (2001) recommends the initiation of breastfeeding within the first 30 to 60 minutes of birth for the healthy term infant and suggests that feedings with water or dextrose water are unnecessary and counterproductive. Supplemental feedings may contribute to nipple confusion (i.e., difficulty knowing how to latch on to the breast) and to low milk supply because the baby becomes overly full and does not breastfeed often enough. Supplementation interferes with the supply-meets-demand cycle of milk production. The parents may interpret the newborn's willingness to take a bottle to mean that the mother's milk supply is inadequate. They need to know that a newborn will automatically suck from a bottle, as the nipple triggers the suck-swallow reflex.

Bottles and Pacifiers

Newborns may become confused going from breast to bottle or bottle to breast when breastfeeding is first initiated. Although there is no research-based evidence to support this idea, there are anecdotal reports of infants who refused the breast once fed from a bottle or even started on a pacifier. Breastfeeding and bottle-feeding require different oral motor skills. The ways newborns use their tongues, jaw, and lips, as well as the swallowing patterns, are very different. Some newborns can transition easily between breast and bottle, whereas others experience considerable difficulty. It is impossible to predict which infants will adapt well and which ones will not. Therefore, many practitioners recommend avoiding bottles until breastfeeding is well established, usually after 3 to 4 weeks. If supplementation is needed, mechanisms such as supplemental nursing systems allow the infant to breastfeed while being supplemented (see Fig. 26-2). Although some parents combine breastfeeding and bottle-feeding, some infants never take a bottle and go directly from the breast to a cup as they grow.

The Canadian Paediatric Society (2003) recommends that health care providers recognize pacifier use as a parental choice determined by the needs of their child and that pacifier use be delayed until breastfeeding is established. Parents should be informed of the relationship between pacifier use and early termination of breastfeeding so they can make an informed decision. Furthermore, pacifier use should not replace actual feeding or suckling. Prohibiting pacifier use will not ensure an increase in the length of breastfeeding. The emphasis should be on allowing the infant to control the pace, frequency, and termination of feeding, instead of allowing the pacifier (or anything else) to become the focus of the interaction.

While dental **malocclusion** has been found in some children using a pacifier, the evidence supporting dental problems is lacking; however, pacifier use should not extend past the age when the permanent teeth erupt (CPS, 2003). The effect of

EVIDENCE-INFORMED PRACTICE Skin-to-Skin Contact for Full-Term Neonates

—Maureen White

Ask the Question

What is the evidence for recommending skin-to-skin contact (STS) for full-term neonates?

Search for Evidence

Search Strategies

Randomized controlled trials, meta-analyses, systematic reviews, experimental research, prospective studies, and guidelines from professional and international health organizations since 2000

Databases Searched

MedLine, PubMed, Ovid CINAHL, Cochrane, and Web sites for the Canadian Paediatric Society (CPS), Association of Women's Health, Obstetric and Neonatal Nurses (AWHONN), Association of Breastfeeding Mothers (ABM), World Health Organization (WHO), Breastfeeding Committee for Canada (BCC), World Alliance for Breastfeeding Action (WABA)

Critically Analyze the Evidence

Health care research concerning STS increased in the 1970s following "kangaroo mother care" (KMC) interventions with premature infants in Bogota, Colombia. Subsequent evidence for clinical, physiological, and psychological advantages of KMC has led to KMC being regarded as safe and superior care for many vulnerable infants worldwide (Kirsten, Bergman, & Hann, 2001). The term *KMC* is now used chiefly to describe a method of intensive care for preterm and very-low-birth-weight infants that involves extended STS, exclusive breastfeeding, and support of the mother–infant dyad. More recently, the research focus includes consideration of the impact of STS on full-term neonates and their parents. STS involves holding the baby naked in a prone position against the skin of the mother's (or father's) chest between the breasts. The baby wears only a diaper and, if needed, a hat. A blanket or shirt can cover baby and parent.

In 2007, a Cochrane Database Systematic Review examined 30 studies involving 1925 mother–infant dyads. The investigators determined that, for full-term infants, STS with their mothers in the first 24 hours of life had a significant positive impact on breastfeeding initiation and duration over the first 4 months. Trends were noted for improved indications of maternal attachment and affection, reduced newborn crying, and improved cardiorespiratory functioning among late preterm infants. No adverse effects were noted (Moore, Anderson, & Bergman, 2007).

Several recent studies have concluded that longer periods of STS lead to increased positive impact on breastfeeding for full-term infants. STS in the first 3 hours of life contributes significantly to rates of exclusive breastfeeding in hospitals (Bramson et al., 2010). In addition to breastfeeding outcomes, recent studies show that STS can be an effective means of maintaining the newborn's temperature, regulating sleep–wake cycles, and minimizing the impact of painful procedures. Parents report high levels of satisfaction with STS, and some evidence is emerging that parent–child interaction is enhanced by STS (Moore et al., 2007; Saloojee, Puig, & Sguassero, 2008). Further research is required to examine more specific implications and best practices in implementing STS for full-term newborns and their families.

Implications for Practice

There is compelling evidence to warrant support of breastfeeding families in initiating STS following birth and encouraging frequent and prolonged skin-to-skin holding in the newborn period. Such support can be achieved through education of health care providers, discussion of STS prenatally with expectant parents, and implementation of supportive policies. In hospitals, policies should include initiating STS as soon as possible after each birth and limiting unnecessary interruptions for care activities—for example, delaying infant weighing and the first newborn bath.

Studies show benefits of STS across cultures and settings; in practice, nurses need to attend to the individual responses of parents related to modesty, culture, and personal feelings (Saloojee et al., 2008). Promoting discreet ways to manage STS and offering practical help in positioning the baby can increase the practice of STS.

Caesarean delivery is a common barrier to initiation of skin-to-skin holding within the first hour following birth because of traditional operating room practices. While it is important to promote early STS and breastfeeding for the postoperative or ill mother, when feasible, encouraging her partner to hold the newborn skin-to-skin can promote stabilization of infant temperature and parental attachment. Most studies focus on breastfeeding outcomes; however, the benefits of STS are not limited to breastfeeding families (Erlandsson, Dsilna, Fagerberg, & Christensson, 2007; Gouchon et al., 2010). Nurses should encourage parents who are formula-feeding to practice frequent skin-to-skin holding so that parents and their infants have more opportunities for attachment and to promote stable infant physiological and behavioural states.

References

Bramson, L., et al. (2010). Effect of early skin-to-skin mother–infant contact during the first 3 hours following birth on exclusive breastfeeding during the maternity hospital stay. *Journal of Human Lactation, 26*(2), 130–137. doi:10.1177/0890334409355779

Erlandsson, K., Dsilna, A., Fagerberg, I., & Christensson, K. (2007). Skin-to-skin care with the father after cesarean birth and its effect on newborn crying and prefeeding behaviour. *Birth, 34*(2), 105–114.

Gouchon, S., Gregori, D., Picotto, A., Patrucco, G., Nangeroni, M., & Di Giulio, P. (2010). Skin-to-skin contact after cesarean delivery: An experimental study. *Nursing Research, 59*(2), 78–84. doi:10.1097/NNR.0b013e3181d1a8bc

Kirsten, G., Bergman, N., & Hann, M. (2001). Kangaroo mother care in the nursery. *Pediatric Clinics of North America, 48*(2), 443–452.

Moore E. R., Anderson G. C., & Bergman N. (2007). Early skin-to-skin contact for mothers and their healthy newborn infants. *Cochrane Database of Systematic Reviews, 3,* Art. No. CD003519. doi:10.1002/14651858.CD003519.pub2

Saloojee, H., Puig, G., & Sguassero, Y. (2008). Early skin-to-skin contact for mothers and their healthy newborn infants: RHL commentary. *WHO Reproductive Health Library*. Geneva: World Health Organization. Retrieved from http://apps.who.int/rhl/newborn/hscom2/en/index.html.

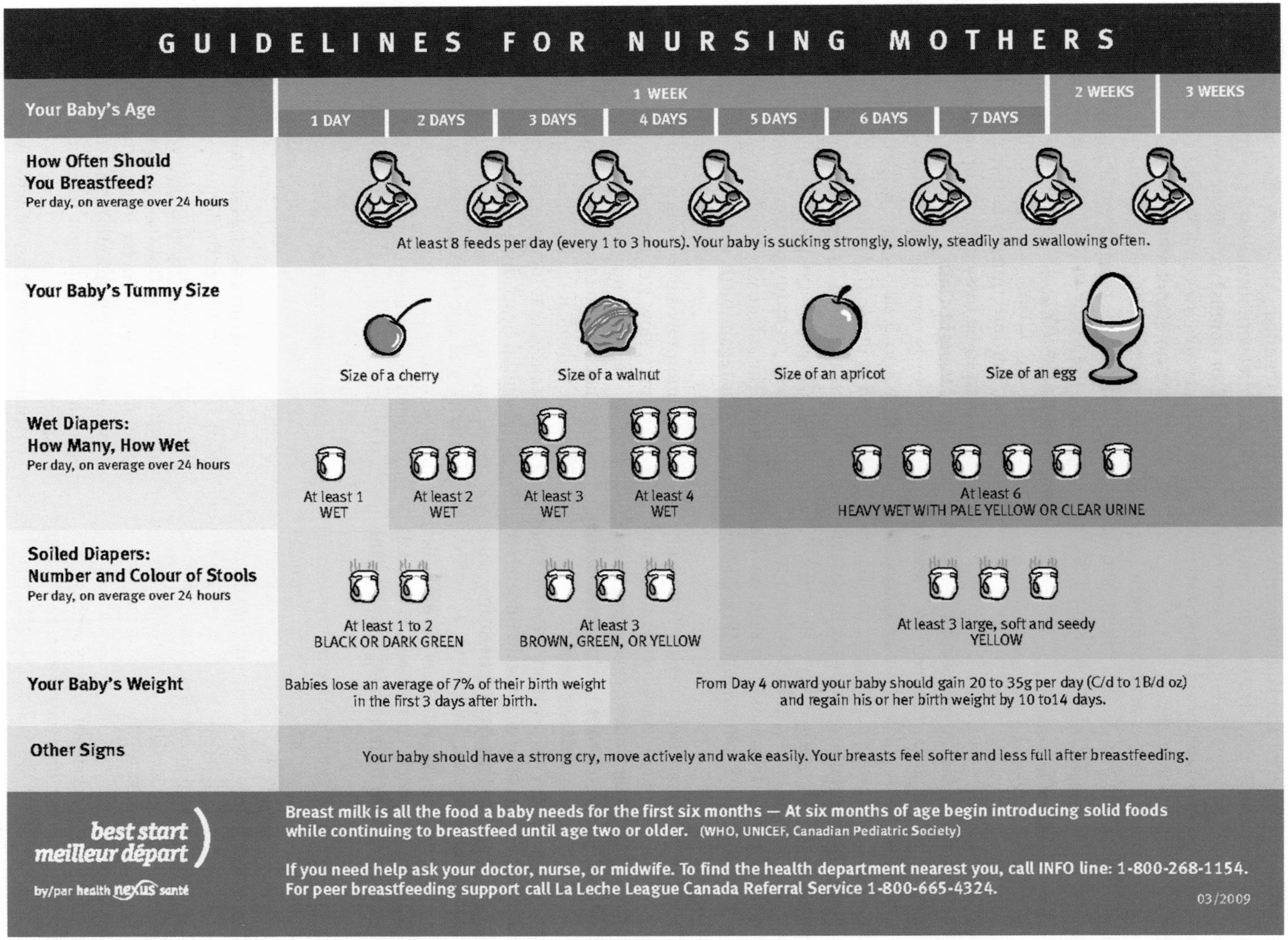
GUIDELINES FOR NURSING MOTHERS
Your Baby's Age
1 WEEK
1 DAY
2 DAYS
3 DAYS
4 DAYS
5 DAYS
6 DAYS
7 DAYS
2 WEEKS
3 WEEKS
How Often Should You Breastfeed?
Per day, on average over 24 hours
At least 8 feeds per day (every 1 to 3 hours). Your baby is sucking strongly, slowly, steadily and swallowing often.
Your Baby's Tummy Size
Size of a cherry
Size of a walnut
Size of an apricot
Size of an egg
Wet Diapers:
How Many, How Wet
Per day, on average over 24 hours
At least 1 WET
At least 2 WET
At least 3 WET
At least 4 WET
At least 6
HEAVY WET WITH PALE YELLOW OR CLEAR URINE
Soiled Diapers:
Number and Colour of Stools
Per day, on average over 24 hours
At least 1 to 2
BLACK OR DARK GREEN
At least 3
BROWN, GREEN, OR YELLOW
At least 3 large, soft and seedy
YELLOW
Your Baby's Weight
Babies lose an average of 7% of their birth weight in the first 3 days after birth.
From Day 4 onward your baby should gain 20 to 35g per day (C/d to 1B/d oz) and regain his or her birth weight by 10 to14 days.
Other Signs
Your baby should have a strong cry, move actively and wake easily. Your breasts feel softer and less full after breastfeeding.
best start
meilleur départ
by/par health nexus santé
Breast milk is all the food a baby needs for the first six months — At six months of age begin introducing solid foods while continuing to breastfeed until age two or older. (WHO, UNICEF, Canadian Pediatric Society)
If you need help ask your doctor, nurse, or midwife. To find the health department nearest you, call INFO line: 1-800-268-1154.
For peer breastfeeding support call La Leche League Canada Referral Service 1-800-665-4324.
03/2009

Fig. 26-8 Guidelines for nursing mothers regarding how often to feed and how to know the baby is getting enough to eat. *(Courtesy Best Start Ontario.)*

continual pacifier use on early speech and language development is unknown, but the pacifier may decrease the infant's desire to imitate sounds and affect intelligibility. Parents need to be alerted that continual dependency on a pacifier may influence social and speech development.

If the infant uses a pacifier, safety considerations in purchasing one must be stressed (see Fig. 25-19). Parents should be cautioned against altering a pacifier, thus, making it more dangerous.

Special Considerations

Sleepy Newborn

During the first few days of life, some newborns need to be awakened for feedings. If the infant is awakened from a sound sleep, attempts at feeding are more likely to be unsuccessful. Unwrapping or undressing the newborn, changing the diaper, sitting the infant upright, talking to the newborn with variable pitch, gently massaging the infant's chest or back, and stroking the arms, legs, palms, or soles may bring the newborn to an alert state. Placing the sleeping infant skin-to-skin on the mother's chest may also stimulate a state change (Fig. 26-9).

Fussy Newborn

Infants sometimes awaken from sleep crying frantically. Although they may be hungry, they cannot focus on feeding until they are calmed. Calming techniques include swaddling, skin-to-skin contact and holding closely, talking soothingly, and allowing the infant to suck on a clean finger.

Some infants cry as soon as they are positioned for feeding. This may be due to a bruised head or previously undetected fractured clavicle. Changing the feeding position may solve the problem.

Fussiness may be related to gastrointestinal distress (i.e., cramping and gas pains); it may occur in response to an occasional feeding of infant formula or be related to something the mother ingested. Although most mothers can consume their normal diet without affecting the infant, foods such as cabbage, broccoli, or onions may irritate some infants' stomachs. Others may react to cow's milk products ingested by the mother. There are no standard foods that all mothers should avoid when breastfeeding; each mother–newborn couple responds individually. One rule of thumb is that if the food causes bloating and gas in the mother, there is a possibility it will do the same for the infant. Persistent crying or refusing to breastfeed can indicate illness, and the health care provider should be notified. Ear infections, sore throat, or oral thrush may cause the infant to be fussy and not breastfeed well.

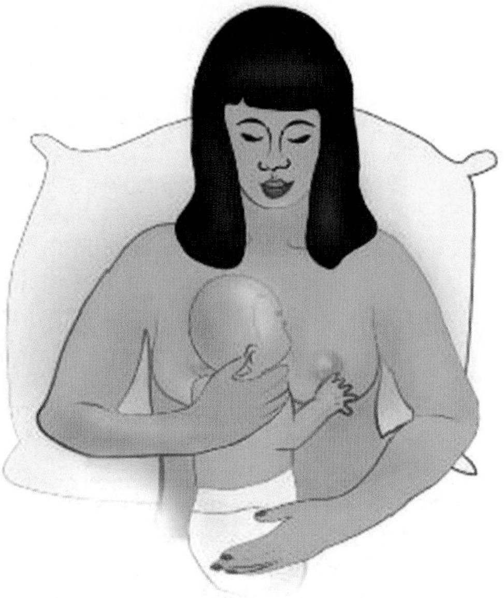

Fig. 26-9 Infant and mother skin-to-skin. Infant is placed between the mother's breasts. *(Courtesy Best Start Ontario.)*

Slow Weight Gain

Newborns may lose up to 10% of their birth weight during the first 3 to 5 days after birth; this is mostly water weight acquired in utero. Thereafter, they should begin to gain weight at the rate of 110 to 200 g/wk, or 20 to 28 g/day. The breastfed infant who loses more than 7% of birth weight requires careful assessment regarding feeding behaviours and maternal milk supply. The infant who continues to lose weight after 5 days, does not regain birth weight by 2 weeks, or whose weight is below the tenth percentile by 1 month should be evaluated and closely monitored by a health care provider.

At times, slow weight gain is related to inadequate breastfeeding. Feedings may be short or infrequent, or the infant may be latching on incorrectly or sucking ineffectively or inefficiently. Other causes are illness; infection; malabsorption; or circumstances that increase the newborn's energy needs, such as congenital heart disease, cystic fibrosis, or being small for gestational age. However, newborns gain weight in differing patterns, and one should not assume that the newborn is ill just because weight gain is not the same as that of another breastfed or bottle-fed infant. Breastfed infants and formula-fed infants have different patterns of growth in the first year. Use of the WHO growth charts is recommended for appropriate growth monitoring. (Dieticians of Canada, Canadian Paediatric Society, Canadian College of Family Physicians, & Public Health Nurses of Canada, 2010).

Maternal factors may also contribute to slow infant weight gain. There may be inadequate emptying of the breasts, pain with feeding, or inappropriate timing of feedings. Inadequate glandular breast tissue or previous breast surgery may affect milk supply. Severe intrapartum or postpartum hemorrhage, illness, or medications may decrease milk supply. Postpartum stress and fatigue may also negatively affect milk production.

Usually the solution to slow weight gain is to improve the feeding technique. Positioning and latch-on should be evaluated and adjustments made. It may help to add a feeding or two in a 24-hour period. Massaging alternate breasts during feedings may help increase the amount of milk going to the infant. With this technique, the mother massages her breast from the chest wall to the nipple whenever the baby has sucking pauses. Some think that this technique may also increase the fat content of the milk, which aids in weight gain.

When newborns are calorie deprived and need supplementation, the extra breast milk or formula can be given with a spoon or cup, a nursing supplemental (see Fig. 26-2), or a bottle. If there are latch-on problems, it is best to avoid bottles and pacifiers. In most cases, supplementation is needed only for a short time until the newborn gains weight and is feeding adequately. Most breastfeeding problems require simple solutions; a lactation consultant can help solve problems by modifying feeding patterns.

Jaundice

Jaundice and **hyperbilirubinemia** in the newborn are discussed in detail in Chapter 25. Colostrum has a natural laxative effect and promotes early passage of meconium. Bilirubin is excreted from the body primarily (98%) through the intestines. Infrequent bowel movements allow bilirubin in the stool to be reabsorbed into the infant's system (enterohepatic shunting), thus promoting hyperbilirubinemia. Infants who receive water or glucose water supplements are more likely to have hyperbilirubinemia because these do not prevent enterohepatic shunting and only 2% of bilirubin is excreted through the kidneys.

Breastfeeding-associated or early breastfeeding jaundice is reported to be related to an increased pattern of enterohepatic shunting, decreased caloric and fluid intake, less frequent stooling, and increased β-glucuronidase in human milk (Blackburn, 2007). This jaundice typically appears around the fourth or fifth day of life and may last as long as 2 weeks. The cause of late-onset breastfeeding jaundice, which may last as long as 12 weeks, is hypothesized to be related to substances in breast milk that interfere with bilirubin conjugation and excretion. These two phases may overlap and be indistinguishable from each other (Blackburn, 2007). Infants with either of these conditions are typically thriving, gaining weight, and stooling normally, and all pathological causes of jaundice have been ruled out. The critical element in breastfeeding-associated jaundice is to encourage early and frequent breastfeeding, often as frequently as every 2 hours in the first week of life, which will enhance stooling and decrease the chance for enterohepatic circulation. Achieving frequent successful latching in the first few days of life and a continuation of this pattern will probably do more to decrease jaundice than other medical therapies. The use of oral supplementation of glucose water or water is strongly discouraged.

The breastfeeding infant who becomes jaundiced should be carefully evaluated for weight loss over 7% of birth weight, decreased milk intake, infrequent bowel movements (less than three or four stools by day 4), decreased urine output (fewer than four to six wet diapers per day), and serum bilirubin levels or transcutaneous monitoring (Blackburn, 2007). The Canadian Paediatric Society recommendations on management of hyperbilirubinemia include professional breastfeeding support and continued exclusive breastfeeding during phototherapy treatment (CPS, 2007b) (see Chapter 25).

Preterm Infants

Human milk is the ideal food for preterm infants, with benefits that are unique to the individual preterm infant in addition to those received by healthy term infants. Initially, preterm human milk contains higher concentrations of energy, fat, sodium, and protein; however, by the second or third week of life, human milk protein content is less than adequate for growth for some preterm or low-birth-weight infants, and supplementation with human milk fortifier is recommended (Askin & Diehl-Jones, 2005). Human milk fortifier contains the protein, minerals (zinc, manganese, calcium, magnesium, phosphorus, sodium, potassium, and copper), and vitamins (folic acid and vitamins B_2, B_6, C, D, E, and K) necessary to support growth and metabolism in the preterm infant (American Academy of Pediatrics, 2009). Human milk fortifiers are available in both liquid and powder form.

Mothers of preterm infants who are unable to breastfeed their infant because of either maternal or neonatal illness should begin pumping their breasts as soon as possible after birth with a hospital-grade electric pump. To establish an optimal milk supply, the mother should use a dual collection kit and pump, beginning slowly and gradually increasing time over the first week. The goal is to pump at least 5 times every 24 hours, aiming to pump for a total of at least 100 minutes per day (Lawrence & Lawrence, 2011). These mothers are taught proper handling and storage of breast milk to minimize bacterial contamination and growth. See the section Breast Milk Storage later in the chapter.

See also Chapter 27 for additional information regarding discharge and nutrition of the preterm infant.

Breastfeeding Twins

Caring for twins takes planning and organization, but breastfeeding means that feedings are always ready instantly, no one has to wash bottles and fix formula, and some mothers can feed both babies at once. The mother with twins will need extra nourishment for herself (200 to 500 kcal/day for each infant).

A typical pattern is that each newborn feeds from one breast per feeding, usually for about 20 to 30 minutes. Some mothers assign each newborn a breast; others switch infants from one breast to the other, either on a schedule or randomly. The mother may find it easiest to use a modified demand feeding schedule; that is, feeding the first infant who wakes up and then waking the second infant for feeding.

During the early weeks, parents may find it helpful to keep a record of feeding times and which breast was used first by which infant. If one twin nurses more vigorously than the other, that infant should be alternated between breasts to equalize breast stimulation.

If the mother wants to feed the newborns simultaneously, she may wish to experiment with positions. For example, one newborn can be held in the football hold and the other in the cradle hold, or the newborns can each be held in the football position. Each infant can be supported on firm pillows while in the football hold. At first, some mothers using this position (Fig. 26-10) may require assistance handling the infants.

Expressing and Storing Breast Milk

In some situations expression of breast milk is necessary or desirable, such as when engorgement occurs, the mother and infant are separated (e.g., preterm or sick infant is in neonatal intensive care), the mother is employed outside the home and wants to maintain her milk supply, the nipples are severely sore or cracked, or the mother leaves the infant with a caregiver and will not be present for feeding.

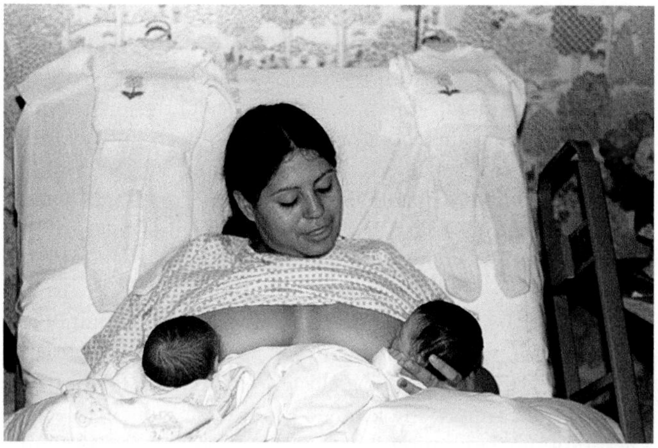

Fig. 26-10 Breastfeeding twins. *(Courtesy Marjorie Pyle, RNC, Lifecircle, Costa Mesa, CA.)*

Because pumping and hand expression are rarely as effective as an infant in removing milk from the breast, the milk supply should never be judged on the basis of volume expressed.

Hand Expression

To manually express milk, after thoroughly washing her hands, the mother places one hand on her breast at the edge of the areola (Fig. 26-11, A). With her thumb above and fingers below, she presses in toward her chest wall and gently compresses the breast while rolling her thumb and fingers forward (Fig. 26-11, B). These motions are repeated rhythmically until the milk begins to flow. While the milk is flowing easily, the mother maintains a steady, light pressure (Fig. 26-11, C). The thumb and fingers should not pinch the breast or slip down to the nipple. The hand should be rotated to reach all sections of each breast. After expressing milk from the second breast, she should return to the first breast and then repeat the procedure until all readily available milk is expressed. This technique was developed by Chele Marmet; more detailed instructions can be found online. All breastfeeding mothers should be given the opportunity to learn and practice the technique for hand expression.

Pumping

There are numerous ways to approach pumping. Some women pump when they first wake up in the morning or when the baby has fed but did not completely empty the breast. Others prefer to pump just before going to sleep. Some pump one breast while the infant is feeding from the other. Double pumping (pumping both breasts at the same time) saves time (Fig. 26-12).

The amount of milk obtained when pumping depends on the type of pump being used, the time of day, how long it has been since the infant breastfed, the mother's milk supply, how practiced she is at pumping, and her comfort level (pumping is uncomfortable for some women). Breast milk may vary in colour and consistency, depending on the time of day, the infant's age, and foods the mother has eaten (e.g., the milk may appear green after the mother has eaten spinach).

Types of Pumps

There are many types of breast pumps (Fig. 26-13). Some are more effective than others, and they vary in price. Manual pumps are the least expensive and may be the most appropriate when portability and quietness of operation are critical, or when a mother is pumping only for an occasional bottle (see Fig. 26-13, B).

Full-service electric pumps, or hospital-grade pumps, are similar to the sucking action and pressure of the breastfeeding infant. These are expensive and are usually rented. When breastfeeding is delayed after birth (e.g., the infant is preterm or ill), or when mother and baby are separated for lengthy periods, these pumps are most appropriate (see Fig. 26-13, A). Electric, self-cycling double pumps are efficient and easy to use. Some of these pumps come with carry bags containing coolers in which to store pumped milk.

Smaller battery-operated or electric pumps are also available. Some have automatic suck-release cycling, and others require use of a finger to regulate strength and speed of suction. These are typically used when pumping is done occasionally, but some models are satisfactory for working mothers or others who pump on a regular basis.

Storage of Breast Milk

Breast milk can be stored safely in any clean glass or plastic container (bisphenol A [BPA] free) (Lawrence & Lawrence, 2011). Plastic bags designed for human milk storage are also available, although not recommended for long-term storage.

Breast milk may be safely kept at room temperature for 6 to 8 hours as long as environmental temperatures do not exceed 25°C and the milk is collected under very clean conditions. Breast milk can be refrigerated safely for 5 days (4°C) after it is expressed. If it is not used within that time, it can be frozen (at 0°C) for up to 2 weeks in a freezer compartment located inside the refrigerator or for up to 6 months in a refrigerator/freezer with a separate freezer door. It should be kept in the middle or toward the back of the freezer to avoid variations in temperature. Milk can be stored for 1 year in a

Fig. 26-11 Hand expression. **A:** One hand is placed on breast with thumb above and fingers below. Press back toward chest. **B:** Gently compress the breast while rolling thumb and fingers forward. Maintain steady, light pressure while milk is flowing. **C:** Relax. Rotate hand to all sections of breast. *(Courtesy of Best Start Ontario.)*

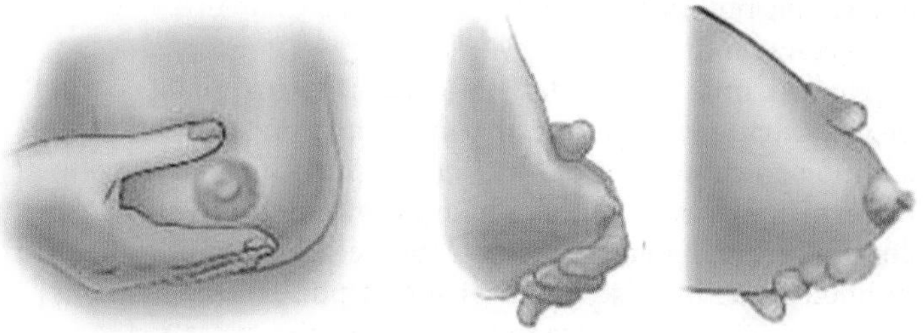

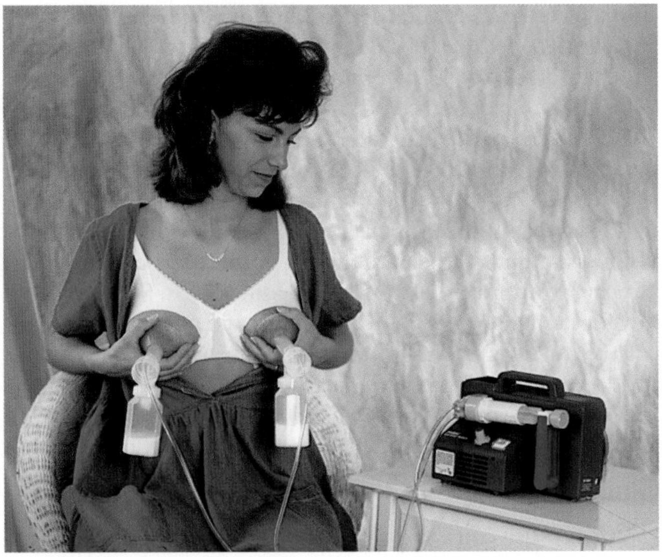

Fig. 26-12 Bilateral breast pumping. *(Courtesy Medela, Inc., McHenry, IL.)*

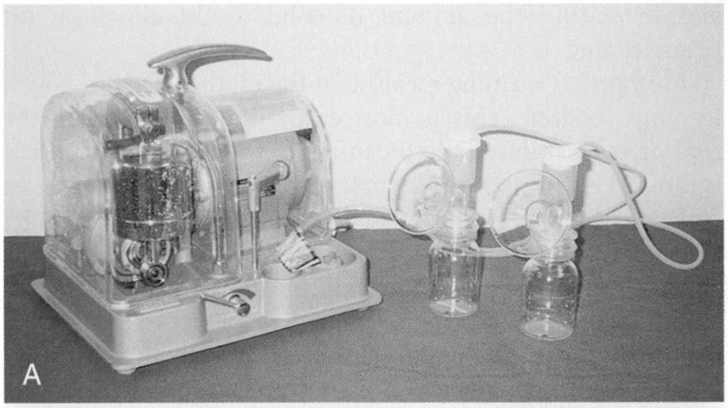

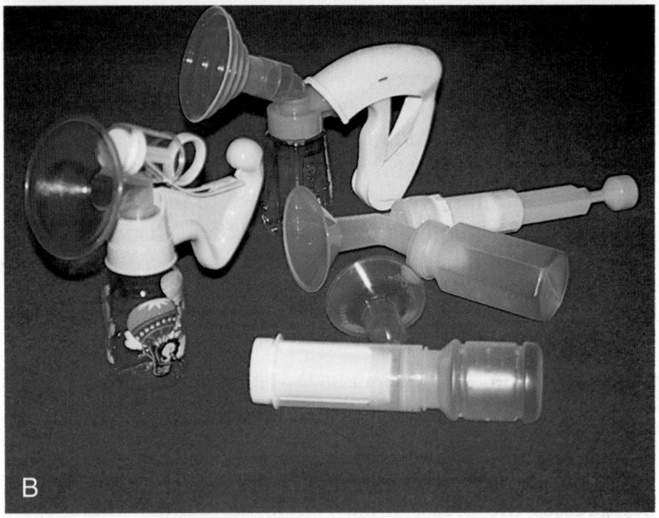

Fig. 26-13 **A:** Hospital-grade electric breast pump. **B:** Manual breast pumps. *(**B**, Courtesy Marjorie Pyle, RNC, Lifecircle, Costa Mesa, CA.)*

freezer at −18°C (Academy of Breastfeeding Medicine, 2010). When breast milk is stored, the container should be dated and the oldest milk used first.

Frozen milk is thawed by placing the container in warm water or in the refrigerator. It should not be refrozen and should be used within 24 hours. After thawing, the container should be shaken gently to mix the layers that have separated. See Nursing Alert.

NURSING ALERT Do not use a microwave to defrost frozen human milk. High-temperature microwaving (72° to 98°C) significantly destroys the anti-infective factors and vitamin C content. The safety of low-temperature microwaving (20° to 53°C) remains questionable. Microwaving does not heat evenly and can cause encapsulated boiling bubbles to form in the center of the liquid. Infants have sustained severe burns to the mouth, throat, and upper gastrointestinal tract as a result of microwaved milk (Lawrence & Lawrence, 2011). One of the best ways to thaw frozen human milk is to place the container under a warm flow of tap water. Another option is to let the frozen milk thaw overnight in the refrigerator to maintain high levels of secretory IgA (Biancuzzo, 2003). Test the temperature of the milk before feeding.

Being Away From the Infant

Many women successfully combine breastfeeding with employment, school, or other commitments. If feedings are missed, the milk supply may be affected. Some women's bodies adjust the milk supply to the times she is with the infant for feedings. Other mothers must pump while away or their supply diminishes rapidly. Employed mothers can continue breastfeeding with guidance and encouragement. Mothers should be encouraged to set realistic goals for employment and breastfeeding, using accurate information regarding the costs, risks, and benefits of available feeding options. Many mothers find that a program of breast pumping when away from home and bottle-feeding the infant the expressed milk with or without formula supplementation is successful. Although feeding the infant at home may occur on a demand basis, pumping milk away from home may be needed every 3 to 4 hours to maintain an adequate supply. Businesses are increasingly making rooms available where mothers can nurse their infants or use breast pumps.

In addition to efficient breast pumping, mothers also need child care by a trusted individual or agency and support and assistance from significant others. As with all breastfeeding mothers, these women must have proper nutrition and rest for adequate lactation. Careful planning, flexibility, and employer support are key to successful breastfeeding by employed mothers (Page, 2008). Canadian maternity benefits permit a new mother who has been employed to have up to 50 weeks of paid leave. Some provinces extend these benefits to self-employed mothers (INFACT Canada, 2005).

Weaning

Typically, weaning is initiated at a time chosen by the mother or the infant. Weaning can be accomplished with little effort and no discomfort when it is done gradually. Abrupt weaning is likely to be distressing for both mother and infant, as well as physically uncomfortable for the mother.

Infant-led weaning means that the infant moves at his or her own pace in omitting feedings. Drinking from a cup and increasing the amount of solid foods substitute for breastfeeding.

Mother-led weaning means that the mother decides which feedings to drop. This is most easily done by omitting the feeding of least interest to the infant or the one that the infant is most likely to sleep through. It can also be the feeding most convenient for the mother to omit. After a week or more, another feeding is dropped, and so on, until the infant is weaned from the breast. Allowing time for the milk supply to adjust before omitting another feeding prevents discomfort for the mother as her supply gradually decreases.

Infants can be weaned directly from the breast to a cup. Bottles are usually offered to infants less than 6 months of age. If the infant is weaned before 1 year of age, formula should be offered instead of whole cow's milk.

If abrupt weaning is necessary, breast **engorgement** often occurs. The mother should be instructed to take mild analgesics, wear a supportive bra, apply ice packs or cabbage leaves to the breasts, and pump milk if needed to increase comfort. The pump should not be used to empty the breasts, since they should remain full enough to promote a decrease in milk production.

Milk Banking

For those infants who cannot be breastfed but who also cannot survive except on human milk, banked donor milk is critically important. Because of the anti-infective and growth-promoting properties of human milk, as well as its superior nutrition, donor milk is used in some neonatal intensive care units for preterm or sick infants when the mother's own milk is not available. Donor milk is also used therapeutically for medical purposes, such as in transplant recipients who are immunocompromised.

The Human Milk Banking Association of North America (HMBANA) (http://www.hmbana.org) has established guidelines for the operation of donor human milk banks (Lawrence & Lawrence, 2011). Donor milk banks collect, screen, process, and distribute milk donated by breastfeeding mothers who are feeding their own infants and pumping a few extra ounces each day for the milk bank. All donors are screened both by interview and serologically for communicable diseases. Donor milk is stored frozen until it is heat processed to kill potential pathogens (bacteria and viruses), and then it is refrozen for storage until it is dispensed for use. The heat processing adds a level of protection for the recipient that is not possible with any other donor tissue or organ. Milk is dispensed only by prescription. A fee is charged by the bank for processing, but the HMBANA guidelines prohibit payment to donors. At the present time, there are three human milk banks in Canada, which are located in Vancouver, Calgary, and Toronto. The Canadian Paediatric Society is advocating for more centres to open across the country, as the health benefits, especially for the very preterm baby, are considerable.

Care of the Mother

Diet

The composition of human milk varies slightly among women, regardless of their diets. The mother's milk automatically contains everything the baby needs, except in rare cases of maternal nutrient deficiencies. For most women, only 200 to 500 extra calories per day need to be added to the diet in order to provide adequate nutrients for the infant while also protecting the mother's body stores. The Institute of Medicine (2005) DRIs provide a guide for energy intake that is adjusted for lactating women. The Estimated Energy Requirement for a lactating woman during the first 6 months is approximately 2700 kcal/day; this amount increases to 2768 kcal/day in the second 6 months. The additional calories can be obtained by eating two to three extra Canada Food Guide Servings from any of the food groups. Additional intake recommendations include micronutrients, vitamins, and minerals. For example, the Institute of Medicine recommends that a 19- to 30-year-old lactating woman consume 3.8 L of water, 210 g of carbohydrate, and 71 g of protein per day. See Chapter 11 for further discussion regarding nutrition during lactation.

There are no specific foods or drinks that all breastfeeding mothers must consume or avoid. Lactating mothers should ideally consume a balanced diet of nutrient-dense foods that includes a wide variety of breads and cereal grains, fruits and vegetables, and three or more servings of milk products daily. Diets or medications that promote rapid weight loss should be avoided, and caffeinated beverages should be consumed in moderation. Adequate amounts of calcium, minerals, and fat-soluble vitamins are important.

If the breastfeeding mother is drinking enough fluids to quench her thirst, she is likely drinking enough to support lactation. Because of her increased need for fluids, the breastfeeding mother may wish to keep a drink within reach while feeding.

Weight Loss

Because it takes energy to produce milk, many mothers experience a gradual weight loss while breastfeeding as fat stores deposited during pregnancy are used. For the mother who is overweight, this fact can present an added incentive for breastfeeding. However, the mother who wants to diet while lactating should avoid losing large amounts of weight quickly because fat-soluble environmental contaminants to which she has been exposed are stored in her body's fat reserves, and these may be released into her milk. In addition, some mothers find that their milk supply decreases when caloric intake is severely restricted. A weight loss of 1 to 2 kg/month will not affect milk production; however, more than that should be carefully evaluated in regard to infant weight gain and feeding pattern (Lawrence & Lawrence, 2011).

Exercise

There is no reason for a breastfeeding woman to restrict her physical activity. Women continue activities such as hiking, jogging, swimming, and aerobics with no detrimental effect on milk supply or composition. Women often find that they are more comfortable if they engage in exercise soon after breastfeeding, when their breasts are as empty as possible. Wearing a well-designed, supportive bra may also help.

Rest

It is important for the breastfeeding mother to rest as much as possible, especially in the first 1 to 2 weeks after birth. Fatigue, stress, and worry may interfere with milk production and let-down. The nurse can encourage the mother to sleep when the baby sleeps. Household chores and care for other children can be done by the partner, grandparents or other relatives, and friends.

Breast Care

The breastfeeding mother's normal bathing routine is all that is required to keep her breasts clean. Soap can have a drying effect on nipples, so she should be instructed to avoid washing the nipples with soap. The small amount of soap that runs down her breasts while washing her face and neck or shampooing her hair is of no concern.

Breast creams should not be used routinely because they may block the natural oil secreted by Montgomery's glands on the areola. Some breast creams contain alcohol, which may dry the nipples. Vitamin E oil or cream is not recommended for use on nipples because it is a fat-soluble vitamin and a breastfeeding infant might consume enough vitamin E from the nipple to reach toxic levels. In addition, some people are allergic to vitamin E oil.

Modified lanolin with reduced allergens can be used safely on dry or sore nipples. Because lanolin is made from sheep's wool, the nurse should ask the mother if she is allergic to wool before applying the ointment. Lanolin is not recommended if it is suspected that nipple soreness may be due to a monilial infection. Antifungal creams are used to treat yeast infections on nipples. Antiseptic sprays and premoistened towelettes containing alcohol are not recommended. A systematic review by Moreland-Schultz and Hill (2005) revealed that no topical agent gave superior results in the prevention or relief of nipple discomfort. Many mothers prefer to use expressed colostrum or milk to soothe sore nipples. Correction of positioning and latch-on problems is the most important factor in avoiding nipple pain.

If a mother needs breast support, she will be more comfortable wearing a bra, since the ligament that supports the breast (Cooper's ligament) will otherwise stretch and be painful. If she is comfortable without a bra, there is no reason for her to wear one. If a woman prefers to wear a bra, it should fit well, offer nonbinding support, and feel comfortable. Underwire bras or improperly fitting bras may contribute to clogged milk ducts. Mothers should be encouraged to breastfeed at least once daily without a bra on so that all milk ducts can empty well.

Leakage of milk between feedings is a problem for some women. Using breast pads (washable or disposable) inside a bra and wearing layered or printed tops can help camouflage the leakage. Plastic-lined pads are not recommended because they trap moisture and may lead to sore nipples. To stop leakage, the mother can be alert to any sensation, such as tingling, that her milk is letting down. If this happens, she can usually stop the let-down by pressing straight back on her nipples. In public, the mother can fold her arms across her chest to apply pressure unobtrusively.

Breast Examination

One to two percent of cases of breast cancer are diagnosed during pregnancy or lactation. If a mother feels a nodule, she should compare breasts, as nodules that match in location in both breasts are almost always breast tissue. Nodules that increase and decrease in size are probably milk glands or ducts. Should a suspicious nodule be discovered, a biopsy can usually be done without interrupting breastfeeding.

Effect of Menstruation

The return of menstrual periods varies among lactating women. Most women will resume menstruation by 6 months postpartum, although for some women this may not occur until lactation has ceased. Menstruation has no effect on breastfeeding. There are no hormonal effects on the infant, although some babies may seem fussy for the first day. The quality of milk is not affected (Lawrence & Lawrence, 2011).

Sexual Sensations

Some women experience rhythmic uterine contractions during breastfeeding. Such sensations are not unusual because uterine contractions and milk ejection are both triggered by oxytocin, but they may be disturbing to some mothers who perceive them to be similar to orgasm.

Breastfeeding and Contraception

Breastfeeding may confer a period of infertility for up to 6 months. Breastfeeding delays the return of ovulation and menstruation; however, ovulation may occur before the first menstrual period after birth. The lactational amenorrhea method of birth control can be a highly effective temporary method of birth control for the first 6 months if the woman is exclusively breastfeeding (see Chapter 7). Hormonal contraceptives, including pills and injectables, may cause a decrease in the milk supply and decreased neonatal growth and are best avoided during the first 6 weeks postpartum. Oral contraceptives have historically not been recommended because of the tendency to decrease milk supply. Lawrence and Lawrence (2011), however, indicate that a number of studies show that low-dose contraceptives containing estrogen can be safely taken by the lactating woman. Progestin-only birth control pills are less likely to interfere with the milk supply. Contraceptives such as the progestin-only injection (Depo-Provera) have not been found to interfere with milk production. Nonhormonal contraceptive methods (e.g., foam, **condom,** nonhormonal intrauterine device, natural family planning, sterilization) are appropriate and have no detrimental effect on breastfeeding.

Recommendation from the World Health Organization is to avoid using combined oral contraceptives from 6 weeks to 6 months postpartum unless appropriate alternative methods are not available (WHO, 2010b). The La Leche League International recommends that breastfeeding women avoid using combined oral contraceptives, and the Society of Obstetricians and Gyneacologists of Canada (SOGC) recommends avoidance of combined oral contraceptives until after 6 weeks postpartum and then only if lactation is well established and the infant's nutritional status is appropriately evaluated (Guthmann, Bang, & Nashelsky, 2005; SOGC, 2004).

Breastfeeding During Pregnancy

It is possible for a breastfeeding woman to conceive and continue breastfeeding throughout the subsequent pregnancy if there are no medical contraindications (e.g., risk of preterm labour). When the second baby is born, colostrum is produced. The practice of breastfeeding a newborn and an older child is called *tandem nursing*. The nurse should remind the mother to always feed the newborn first, to ensure that the newborn is receiving adequate nutrition. The supply-meets-demand principle works just as with breastfeeding multiple babies.

Diabetic Mother

The mother with type 2 diabetes is encouraged to breastfeed. In addition to benefits for the infant and maternal satisfaction, breastfeeding has an antidiabetogenic effect. Blood glucose levels and insulin requirements are lower because of the carbohydrate used in milk production. During lactation, the diabetic woman may be able to eat more food and still take less insulin. However, insulin dosage must be adjusted as the infant is weaned. Some diabetic women are at increased risk for sore nipples caused by monilial infections and may have an increased risk for mastitis (Lawrence & Lawrence, 2011).

Breastfeeding and Medications

Despite much concern about the compatibility of medications and breastfeeding, in fact, few medications are contraindicated during lactation (see Appendix A). Considerations in evaluating the safety of a specific medication during breastfeeding include the pharmacokinetics of the drug in the maternal system and the absorption, metabolism, distribution, storage, and excretion in the infant. The infant's gestational and chronological age, body weight, and breastfeeding pattern are also considered (Lawrence & Lawrence, 2011). Most medications do not cause problems for the infant, but breastfeeding mothers should be cautioned about taking any but essential ones. In certain instances (e.g., radioactive diagnostic agents), the mother should be instructed to pump her breasts and discard the pumped milk until the drug has cleared her body.

Smoking may impair milk production; it also exposes the infant to the risks of secondhand smoke. Mothers who continue to smoke tobacco when lactating should be advised not to smoke within 2 hours before breastfeeding and to never smoke in the same room with the infant. If a mother chooses to consume alcohol, she should be advised to minimize its effects by having only one drink and consuming it immediately after a feeding or waiting for 2 hours after drinking to breastfeed (Koren, 2002). Alcoholic beverages may impair the milk ejection reflex. The mother who is pumping for a preterm or sick infant should avoid alcohol until her baby is healthy.

The caffeine concentration in milk is only about 1% of the level in the mother's plasma. The infant's immature renal system limits the ability to excrete the caffeine; thus, caffeine accumulates in the infant's system and can cause irritability and poor sleeping patterns. Some infants are sensitive to even small amounts of caffeine; mothers of such infants should limit caffeine intake. Caffeine is found in coffee, tea, chocolate, energy drinks, and many soft drinks (Lawrence & Lawrence, 2011).

Herbs and herbal teas are becoming more widely used during lactation. Although some are considered safe, others contain pharmacologically active compounds that may have detrimental effects, particularly on the neonate. A thorough history should include noting the composition of any herbal remedies. Each remedy should then be evaluated for its compatibility with breastfeeding. Herbal teas considered safe during lactation include rose hips, orange spice, chicory, peppermint, raspberry, and red bush tea (Lawrence & Lawrence, 2011). A regional poison control center may provide information on the active properties of herbs.

Mothers using street drugs (e.g., marijuana, cocaine, ecstasy) are usually discouraged from breastfeeding; however, mothers using **methadone** for treatment of opioid dependence can be encouraged to breastfeed, as the benefits of breastfeeding largely outweigh the minimal risks (Glatstein, Garcia-Bournissen, Finkelstein, & Koren, 2008). Consult resources online (e.g., http://www.motherisk.ca) and Appendix A for more information about drugs in breast milk.

Environmental Contaminants

Except under unusual circumstances, breastfeeding is not contraindicated because of exposure to environmental contaminants such as DDT (an insecticide) and tetrachloroethylene (used in dry cleaning) (Lawrence & Lawrence, 2011). It is recommended that breastfeeding mothers not expose their infant to secondhand smoke; this often leads to an increase in the incidence of reactive airway disease, wheezing, and upper respiratory tract infections. Mothers who do not give up smoking should change clothes before breastfeeding because tobacco residue may adhere to clothing. The infant is thus exposed to the effects of nicotine and smoke even in the absence of active smoking.

Special Considerations

The breastfeeding mother may experience some common concerns. In most cases complications are preventable if the mother receives appropriate education about breastfeeding. Early recognition and resolution of problems is important in order to prevent interruption of breastfeeding and promote the mother's comfort and sense of well-being. Emotional support provided by the nurse or lactation consultant is essential to help allay frustration and anxiety and to prevent early cessation of breastfeeding.

Engorgement

Mild engorgement is a common postpartum response of the breasts to the sudden change in hormones and the increased volume of milk. It usually occurs on the second to fifth day postpartum when the mature milk comes in, and it lasts about 24 hours. Painful distention can often be prevented by frequent feedings in the first 48 hours. Intense engorgement can result from accumulation of milk and from the naturally increasing blood supply to the breasts, causing swelling of tissues surrounding the milk ducts. The ducts may be pinched shut, so that the milk does not flow. The breasts become firm, tender, swollen, and hot, and appear shiny and red. The tenderness and swelling may extend into the axilla. The areolae then become firm and the nipples may flatten, making it difficult for the newborn to latch on. Back pressure on full milk glands inhibits milk production if the milk is not removed from the breasts, and the milk supply may diminish.

When engorgement occurs, the nurse should assure the mother that this is a temporary condition that is usually resolved within 24 hours. The mother should be instructed to feed every 2 hours, softening at least one breast, and pumping the other breast to soften. Pumping during engorgement will not cause a problematic increase in milk supply.

Because of the swelling of breast tissue surrounding the milk glands' ducts, ice packs are recommended in a rotation of 15 to 20 minutes on, 45 minutes off between feedings. The ice packs should cover both breasts. Large bags of frozen peas or corn make easy packs and can be refrozen between uses.

Fresh raw cabbage leaves placed over the breasts in between feedings may help reduce the swelling and discomfort (Chapman, 2011; Lawrence & Lawrence, 2011). The cabbage leaves are washed and then placed in the freezer until they are cold; they are then placed over the breasts, leaving just the nipples exposed to air. The leaves are replaced when they begin to wilt. Although the exact mechanism of action of cabbage leaves in treatment of engorgement is not understood, it is thought that continuous application might decrease milk supply. Raw cabbage leaves are often effective for formula-feeding mothers who want their milk to "dry up."

Anti-inflammatory medications such as ibuprofen may help reduce pain and swelling associated with engorgement. Mothers often have an elevated temperature and experience achiness in their breasts; ibuprofen can help remedy this.

Because heat increases blood flow, application of heat to an already congested breast is usually counterproductive. Occasionally, however, standing in a warm shower will start the milk leaking, or the mother may be able to manually express enough milk to soften the areola so that the baby can latch on and feed.

Sore Nipples

Many women expect breastfeeding to be painful, based on stories they have heard from family and friends; however, breastfeeding is not supposed to be painful. While mild nipple discomfort at the beginning of feedings is common, severe soreness and abraded, cracked, or bleeding nipples are not normal and most often result from poor positioning, incorrect latch-on, improper suck, or a monilial infection.

For the first few days after birth, the nursing mother may experience some nipple tenderness with suckling. This should quickly dissipate as the milk begins to flow and acts as a lubricant. To minimize the initial suckling pain, the mother can express a few drops of milk to moisten the nipple and areola before latch-on. The mother should ensure that the newborn is well supported, is in straight body alignment, and has no pressure on the back of her or his head. The newborn's nose, cheeks, and chin should touch the breast, and the mother should support the breast with her hand during the early feedings. The nurse can help to reposition the infant as necessary to resolve the nipple discomfort.

If the mother reports a pinching sensation of the nipple as the infant sucks, it may be helpful to reposition the baby by pulling the baby's buttocks closer to the mother. If the baby cannot open wide enough, it may be appropriate to gently pull down on the side of the newborn's jaw while he or she is sucking to increase the amount of breast tissue in the infant's mouth. If the nipple pain continues, the mother needs to remove the infant from the breast, breaking suction with her finger in the infant's mouth. She can then attempt latch-on again, making certain that the infant's mouth is open wide before the infant is pulled quickly to the breast (see Fig. 26-5).

The infant's suck can be assessed by a lactation consultant or a nurse who is specially trained, by inserting a clean gloved finger in the newborn's mouth and stimulating the newborn to suck. If the newborn is not extruding his or her tongue over the lower gum and the mother reports pain or pinching with sucking, the newborn may have a short frenulum (commonly referred to as being "tongue-tied"). In some cases, ankyloglossia is corrected surgically to free the tongue for less painful, more effective breastfeeding (Dollberg et al., 2006).

The treatment for sore nipples is first to correct the cause. Once the problem is assessed, identified, and corrected, sore nipples should heal within a few days, even though the baby is continuing to breastfeed regularly. A common cause of sore nipples is positioning; the infant's ability to latch effectively should be carefully evaluated (Lawrence & Lawrence, 2011).

When sore nipples occur, it is more comfortable to start the feeding on the least sore nipple. A few drops of milk can be expressed, rubbed into the sore area, and allowed to air dry. Warm water compresses may also be comforting.

If nipples are extremely sore or damaged and the mother cannot tolerate breastfeeding, she may be advised to use an electric breast pump for 24 to 48 hours to allow the nipples to begin healing before resuming breastfeeding. It is important that the mother use a pump that will effectively empty the breasts. Sore nipples should be open to air as much as possible.

Silicone (flexible) nipple shields may be helpful for a mother with flat or inverted nipples and particularly for preterm babies who have trouble latching and maintaining suction and for babies who develop a preference for a bottle nipple and refuse the breast (Riordan & Wambach, 2009). While nipple shields help protect abraded, sore nipples, the cause of the pain must be determined and remedied promptly. The shield should be applied on the nipple areola area just before putting the baby on the breast: flip up the brim of the shield, place the shield directly over the nipple, and gently pat down the brim. Nipple shields should be used for a short time only, or the baby may become so accustomed to them that he or she refuses the breast. In addition, lactation consultants should closely monitor the infant's growth and intake of milk.

Monilial Infections

Sore nipples that occur after the newborn period are often due to a *Candida* or monilial (yeast) infection. The mother usually reports severe nipple pain and tenderness, burning, or stinging, and she may have sharp, shooting, burning pains in the breasts during and after feedings. The nipples appear somewhat pink and shiny or may be scaly or flaky; there may be a visible rash, small blisters, or thrush. Most often, the pain is out of proportion to the appearance of the nipple. Yeast infections of the nipples and breast can be excruciatingly painful and can lead to early cessation of breastfeeding if not recognized and treated promptly.

Infants may or may not exhibit symptoms of monilial infection. Oral thrush and a red, raised diaper rash are common indications of a yeast infection. An affected infant is often fussy and gassy. When feeding, the infant is likely to pull off the breast soon after starting to feed, crying with apparent pain. The infant may be biting or gumming at the breast.

The most common predisposing factors for yeast infections of the breast include previous antibiotic use, vaginal yeast infections, and nipple damage.

Mothers and infants must be treated simultaneously, even if the infant has no visible signs of infection. Treatment for the mother is typically an antifungal cream applied to the nipples after feedings and, in some cases, a systemic antifungal medication such as fluconazole. Most physicians prescribe an oral antifungal medication, such as nystatin or fluconazole, for infants. Treatment should continue for at least 14 days even after symptoms begin to improve in 1 to 2 days (Lawrence & Lawrence, 2011). Good hand hygiene is essential to prevent the spread of yeast.

Plugged Milk Ducts

A milk duct may become plugged or clogged, causing an area of the breast to become swollen and tender. This area typically does not empty or soften with feeding or pumping. There may also be a small white pearl on the tip of the nipple; this is the curd of milk blocking the flow. The mother is afebrile and has no generalized symptoms.

Plugged ducts are most often the result of inadequate emptying of the breast. This may be due to clothing that is too tight, a poorly fitting or underwire bra, or constant use of the same position for feeding. Application of warm compresses to the affected area and to the nipple before feeding helps promote emptying of the breast and release of the plug.

Frequent feeding is recommended, with the infant beginning the feeding on the affected side to foster more complete emptying. The mother should massage the affected area while the infant nurses or while she is pumping. Varying feeding positions and feeding without wearing a bra may be useful in resolving a plugged duct.

If the mother develops fever or flu-like symptoms, she may have developed mastitis and should notify her health care provider. Plugged milk ducts do not necessarily cause mastitis, but milk stasis may increase susceptibility to breast infection.

Mastitis

A breast infection, or **mastitis**, is characterized by the sudden onset of flu-like symptoms, including fever, chills, body aches, and headache. Flu-like symptoms in a breastfeeding mother should be considered indicative of mastitis until proven otherwise. Mastitis is characterized by localized breast pain and tenderness and a hot, reddened area on the breast, often resembling the shape of a pie wedge. Mastitis most commonly occurs in the upper outer quadrant of the breast; it may affect one or both breasts.

Certain factors may predispose a woman to mastitis. Inadequate emptying of the breasts is common, related to engorgement, plugged ducts, a sudden decrease in the number of feedings, abrupt weaning, or underwire bras. Sore, cracked nipples may lead to mastitis by providing a portal of entry for the causative organism (staphylococci, streptococci, and *E. coli* are most common). Maternal stress, fatigue, illness, malnutrition, oversupply of milk, and breast trauma are also predisposing factors for mastitis (Lawrence & Lawrence, 2011).

Breastfeeding mothers should be taught the signs of mastitis before they are discharged from the hospital, and they need to know to call the health care provider promptly if the symptoms occur. Treatment includes antibiotics such as cephalexin or dicloxacillin and analgesic-antipyretic medications such as ibuprofen. Rest is extremely important; the mother should sleep whenever the baby sleeps. The mother should feed the baby or pump frequently, striving to adequately empty the affected side. Warm compresses to the breast before feeding or pumping may be useful; cool compresses may be applied to the breast after feeding. Adequate fluid intake and a balanced diet are important for the mother with mastitis.

Complications of mastitis include breast abscess, chronic mastitis, and fungal infections of the breast. Most complications can be prevented by early recognition and treatment.

Hepatitis B and C

The risk of perinatal transmission of hepatitis C (HCV) is approximately 5 to 6%; transmission is believed to occur primarily at delivery and only in women who are hepatitis C virus ribonucleic acid (HCV RNA) positive at delivery. There is no evidence that HCV is transmitted in breast milk and therefore the Canadian Paediatric Society (2008) maintains there is no increased risk of transmission with breastfeeding as long as the mother is also HIV negative and her nipples are not cracked or bleeding. Breastfeeding by a hepatitis B–positive mother is also reported to pose no additional risk of acquisition to the infant (see Contraindications to Breastfeeding, p. 677).

Role of the Nurse in Promoting Successful Lactation

Nurses play a major role in breastfeeding education and support for new parents. Nurses often work with lactation consultants (LC) in hospitals, physicians' offices, or community settings. Although many lactation consultants are registered nurses, they may come from a variety of educational backgrounds, such as nutrition, physical and occupational therapy, home economics, medicine, psychology, social work, education, or the basic sciences. Lactation consultants have had specialized education, training, and clinical experience working with breastfeeding mothers, and they have passed a certifying examination that requires meeting defined academic and clinical-experience criteria.

Nurses in prenatal settings can educate the mother and her partner about the advantages of breastfeeding and explore reasons why they may prefer bottle-feeding. They can provide expectant parents with current reading materials and information about prenatal classes. At each encounter, the nurse can answer questions and provide additional information as needed.

Assessment of the mother's breasts and nipples during pregnancy is important. Flat or inverted nipples should be identified. The nurse should determine whether the woman has had any breast surgery. Breast reduction or augmentation may interfere with the ability to produce milk and transfer it successfully to the baby. Mothers with a history of breast surgery should be encouraged to seek early lactation support in order to develop realistic goals, and their infants should be continually assessed for appropriate weight gain (West, 2009).

No special nipple preparation is necessary during pregnancy. Efforts to "toughen" the nipples by pulling on them or rubbing them with a rough towel are to be avoided. Such stimulation can cause release of oxytocin and result in preterm labour or damage the outer layer of protective skin cells, which may increase the risk of sore nipples.

In the immediate postpartum period, the nurse is instrumental in helping the mother initiate breastfeeding as soon as possible after birth, preferably within the first 30 to 60 minutes. Encouraging parents to keep the baby in the mother's room (rooming-in) and frequently hold the baby skin-to-skin gives the mother the opportunity to learn feeding cues and to feed the baby when these cues are present. The nurse can provide help with positioning and latch-on until the mother can accomplish this independently. Explanations need to be given early regarding frequency and duration of feedings, how to wake a sleepy baby, and how to determine whether the baby is getting enough milk (see Nursing Care Plan). Information about the transition to mature milk (milk coming in) and how to prevent or deal with engorgement is also needed. The mother should be informed about the prevention and treatment of sore nipples and about signs of mastitis (including the importance of contacting the primary health care provider if these occur). Murray, Ricketts, and Dellaport (2007) found that mothers were more likely to continue breastfeeding when the birth facility supported the following five practices: breastfeeding within the first hour after birth, no pacifiers, infant rooming-in, no supplements given, and a telephone number for consults after discharge.

Parents often expect that because breastfeeding is "natural" it will come naturally for both mother and baby. This misconception needs to be clarified early so that parents may view breastfeeding as a learning process and not have unrealistic expectations. All health care providers who are knowledgeable about breastfeeding can offer needed support and encouragement to parents, to instill a sense of confidence.

In a survey carried out by Arora et al. (2000), breastfeeding mothers indicated that the determining factors for changing to bottle-feeding included the mother's perception of the father's attitude toward breastfeeding and the mother's uncertainty about the amount of milk the infant would receive. These findings have important implications for involving partners in education and discussion about breastfeeding before and during the pregnancy. Partners may express concerns of feeling left out during the newborn period if they have little involvement other than diapering and holding the infant. Encouraging partners regarding their positive role in supporting the mothers' breastfeeding may help decrease feelings of helplessness and isolation and may benefit mother–infant interaction. More recent research reported that fathers of breastfeeding infants considered themselves to be part of the team that supported the mother and the breastfeeding process and wanted to be prepared with strategies and information to perform their unique roles as parents of their newborn (Rempel & Rempel, 2011).

Baby-Friendly Hospital Initiative

The Baby-Friendly Hospital Initiative (BFHI) is a joint effort of the World Health Organization (WHO) and the United Nations Children's Fund (UNICEF) to encourage, promote, and support breastfeeding as the model for optimum infant nutrition. The BFHI developed 10 research-supported practices as a guideline for maternity facilities worldwide to promote breastfeeding (UNICEF, n.d.).

Baby-Friendly Initiative in Canada

The Breastfeeding Committee for Canada (BCC) is the national authority for the BFHI in Canada, which is called the breastfeeding initiative (BFI). The BCC works to protect, promote, and support breastfeeding through the Ten Steps to Successful Breastfeeding, developed by UNICEF and the WHO.

To reflect the continuum of care between hospitals and communities, the BCC describes the international standards within the Canadian context and has developed a set of 10 practice outcome indicators (Box 26-2), which combines the original BFHI Ten Steps to Successful Breastfeeding (UNICEF, n.d.) and the Seven Point Plan for the Promotion, Protection and Support of Breastfeeding in Community Health Care Settings (UNICEF UK BFHI, 2011). These integrated steps are the basis for the process by which hospitals and communities can achieve the Baby-Friendly™ designation, an internationally recognized accomplishment confirming that the 10 BFHI outcomes have been achieved and that there is adherence to

---

NURSING CARE PLAN ● The Newborn With Insufficient Intake of Nutrients

Nursing Diagnosis: Ineffective breastfeeding related to limited knowledge of mother as evidenced by ongoing incorrect latch-on technique

Expected Outcomes

Mother will express increased satisfaction with breastfeeding, and neonate will exhibit satisfaction of hunger and sucking needs.

Nursing Interventions/*Rationales*

Assess the mother's knowledge and motivation for breastfeeding *to acknowledge her desire for an effective outcome and to provide a starting point for teaching.*

Observe a breastfeeding session *to provide a database for positive reinforcement and problem identification.*

Assess the mother's knowledge of hunger cues and satiation cues *to acknowledge her understanding of her baby and provide a basis for teaching on frequency of feedings.*

Describe and demonstrate ways to stimulate the sucking reflex, various positions for breastfeeding, and the use of pillows during a session *to promote maternal and neonatal comfort and effective latch-on.*

Monitor neonatal position of mouth on areola and position of head and body *to give positive reinforcement for the correct latch-on position or to correct a poor latch-on position.*

Teach the mother ways to stimulate the neonate to maintain an awake state by diapering, unwrapping, massaging, or burping the baby *to complete a breastfeeding thoroughly and satisfactorily.*

Give the mother information regarding lactation diet, expression of milk by hand or pump, and storage of expressed breast milk *to provide basic information.*

Make certain the mother has written information on all aspects of breastfeeding *to reinforce verbal instructions and demonstrations.*

Refer to a support group and lactation consultant, if needed, *to provide further information and group support.*

BOX 26-2 Ten Steps to Baby-Friendly Designation

Step 1. Have a written breastfeeding policy that is routinely communicated to all health care providers and volunteers.

Step 2. Ensure that all health care providers have the knowledge and skills necessary to implement the breastfeeding policy.

Step 3. Inform pregnant women and their families about the importance and process of breastfeeding.

Step 4. Place babies in skin-to-skin contact with their mothers immediately following birth for at least an hour or until completion of the first feeding or as long as the mother wishes; encourage mothers to recognize when their babies are ready to feed, offering help as needed.

Step 5. Assist mothers to breastfeed and maintain lactation should they face challenges, including separation from their infants.

Step 6. Infants are not offered food or drink other than human milk for the first 6 months, unless *medically* indicated.

Step 7. Facilitate 24-hour rooming-in for all mothers: Mothers and infants remain together.

Step 8. Encourage baby-led or cue-based breastfeeding. Encourage sustained breastfeeding beyond 6 months with appropriate introduction of complementary foods.

Step 9. Support mothers to feed and care for their breastfeeding babies without the use of artificial teats or pacifiers (dummies or soothers).

Step 10. Provide a seamless transition between the services provided by the hospital, community health services, and peer support programs.

(From Breastfeeding Committee for Canada. [2010]. *Summary: Integrated 10 steps practice outcome indicators for hospitals and community health services*. Retrieved from http://www.breastfeedingcanada.ca/pdf/2010-09_Summary-BCC_Integrated_2010_Steps_Practice_Outcomes_Indicators.pdf.)

the WHO International Code of Marketing of Breastmilk Substitutes (BCC, 2010).

In this initiative, Québec is leading Canada with BFI designation in six hospitals, three birthing centres, and thirteen community facilities. Outside Québec there are three hospitals in Ontario and two in British Columbia and seven community health centres (all in Ontario) that have obtained the BFI designation (BCC, 2010). The BFI requires time and resources to implement and is not without its critics. Some women may not be willing or able to breastfeed and may experience pressure to conform to the new breastfeeding norms. However, the BFI is an important step toward re-establishing a culture that supports breastfeeding in Canada.

Follow-Up After Hospital Discharge

Problems with sore nipples, engorgement, and jaundice may occur after discharge. Thus, it is the hospital nurse's role to educate and prepare the mother for problems she may encounter once she is home. It is critical that the mother be given a list of resources for help with breastfeeding concerns and that she knows when to call for assistance. Community resources for breastfeeding mothers include lactation consultants in hospitals, physicians' offices, or private practice; nurses in pediatric or obstetric offices; public health nurses; support groups such as the La Leche League; and peer counselling programs.

Telephone follow-up by hospital or office nurses within the first day or two after discharge can provide a means of identifying any problems and offering needed advice and support. Infants discharged before 48 hours of age should meet specific criteria for physiological stability and safety (including at least two successful feedings) and have arrangements to be seen by a health care provider within 48 hours (CPS, 2007b; CPS & SOGC, 1996). In some settings and circumstances, home care follow-up is available for mothers after hospital discharge.

Formula-Feeding

Rationale for Formula-Feeding

The decision to feed a baby infant formula may be the result of the mother's or partner's personal preference, the influence of other significant family members, or simply a lack of education and familiarity with breastfeeding. Occasionally, no other option is available: The mother may have extensive breast scarring or may have had a bilateral mastectomy; the mother may be taking medications that preclude breastfeeding; or the baby may be adopted. Breast augmentation or reduction mammoplasty may interfere with the ability to produce an adequate milk supply and successful transfer to the baby. Some mothers are able to induce lactation for an adopted baby by using a supplemental nursing device during breastfeeding. Infants diagnosed with classic galactosemia must be fed a lactose-free formula; this excludes breastfeeding.

Infant formula may be used to supplement breastfeeding if the mother's milk supply is inadequate. It may also be fed to the baby if the mother will be away from home and wishes to leave a bottle of formula instead of expressed breast milk.

Formula-feeding is also recommended for mothers in developed countries who are HIV positive or who are using recreational drugs (e.g., cocaine, methamphetamine, heroin).

Parent Education

Inexperienced mothers and fathers who are formula-feeding their infants usually need instruction, counselling, and support. They may need assistance with the feeding process and with any problems they may experience. Some parents who are formula-feeding may express concern that the baby will suffer as a result of their decision. Emphasis on the beneficial use of feeding times for close contact and socializing with the infant can help relieve some of this concern.

Readiness for Feeding

The first feeding of formula is ideally given after the initial transition to extrauterine life. Feeding readiness cues include stability of vital signs, bowel sounds, an active sucking reflex, an effective breathing pattern, and those feeding cues described for breastfed babies (hands-to-mouth, licking, and sucking).

Feeding Patterns

Typically a newborn initially will take 10 to 15 mL of formula per feeding. Intake gradually increases during the first week of life as the capacity of the stomach increases. Most newborns are drinking 90 to 150 mL per feeding by the end of the second week or sooner. The newborn infant should be fed at least every 3 to 4 hours, even if that requires waking the newborn for the feedings; rigid feeding schedules, however, are not recommended. The infant showing an adequate weight gain can be allowed to sleep at night and be fed only on awakening. Most newborns need six to eight feedings in 24 hours, and the number of feedings decreases as the infant matures. Usually by 3 to 4 weeks after birth a fairly predictable feeding pattern has developed. Scheduling feedings arbitrarily at predetermined intervals may not meet a newborn's needs, but initiating feedings at convenient times often moves the newborn's feedings to times that work for the family.

Mothers will usually notice an increase in the infant's appetite at ages 7 to 10 days, 3 weeks, 6 weeks, 3 months, and 6 months. These appetite spurts correspond to growth spurts. The amount of formula per feeding should be increased by about 30 mL at these times to meet the baby's needs.

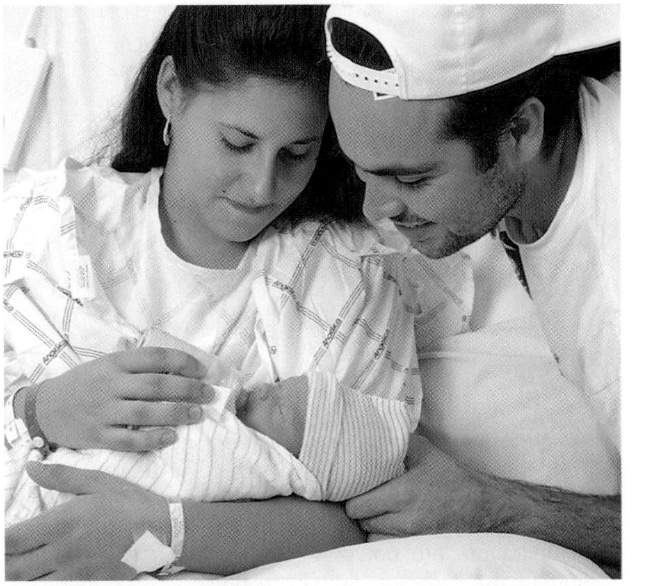

Fig. 26-14 This mother holds her infant close during bottle feeding. The bottle is positioned so that the nipple is filled with milk at all times. The father offers encouragement. *(From Slone-McKenny, E. [2008].* Maternal–child nursing *[3rd ed., p. 577]. St. Louis: Saunders.)*

Feeding Techniques

Parents who choose formula-feeding often need education about feeding techniques. Formula can be fed at room temperature or warmed. Formula should never be heated in a microwave oven. Microwaving does not heat evenly and can cause encapsulated boiling bubbles to form in the center of the liquid. This may not be detected when checking drops of milk for temperature. Babies have sustained severe burns to the mouth, throat, and upper gastrointestinal tract as a result of milk heated in a microwave (Lawrence & Lawrence, 2011). If the formula is warmed, its temperature should be tested before it is given to the infant.

During feedings, parents should be encouraged to sit comfortably, holding the infant closely in a semiupright position. Feedings provide an opportunity to bond with the infant through touching, talking, singing, or reading aloud. Parents should consider feedings, whether breast or bottle, as a time of peaceful relaxation with their newborn (Fig. 26-14).

The bottle should never be propped with a pillow or other inanimate object and left with the infant. Likewise, small children should not be given charge of bottle-feeding the infant unless there is close adult supervision. This practice may result in choking, and it deprives the infant of important interaction during feeding. Moreover, propping the bottle has been implicated in causing nursing-bottle caries, or decay of the first teeth, resulting from continuous bathing of the teeth with carbohydrate-containing fluid as the infant sporadically sucks the nipple.

The bottle should be held so that fluid fills the nipple and none of the air in the bottle is allowed to enter the nipple (see Fig. 26-14). After the newborn period, the infant who falls asleep, turns aside the head, or ceases to suck usually is signaling that enough formula has been taken. Parents should be taught to look for these cues and avoid overfeeding, which could contribute to obesity.

Most infants swallow air when fed from a bottle and should be given a chance to burp several times during a feeding (Fig. 26-15).

Bottles and Nipples

Various brands and styles of bottles and nipples are available. Most babies will feed well with any bottle and nipple. It is important that the bottles and nipples be washed in warm, soapy water using a bottle and nipple brush to facilitate thorough cleansing. Most household dishwashers use hot water and are safe for cleaning bottles and nipples. Boiling of bottles and nipples is not always needed. It is best to check with local Public Health Department regarding recommendations.

Infant Formulas

Commercial Formulas

Because human milk is species specific to meet the needs of the human infant, it is used as the standard for all infant formulas. Commercial infant formulas are designed to resemble human milk as closely as possible, although none has ever duplicated it.

Infants who are not breastfed should be given commercial iron-fortified formulas. If this is too expensive, the family may be eligible for services through income assistance programs.

Commercially prepared formulas are cow's milk–based formulas that have been modified to closely resemble the nutritional content of human milk. These formulas are altered from cow's milk by removing butterfat, decreasing the protein content, and adding vegetable oil and carbohydrate. Some cow's milk–based formulas have demineralized whey added to yield a whey/casein ratio of 60:40. The standard cow's milk–based formulas, regardless of the commercial brand, have essentially the same compositions of vitamins, minerals,

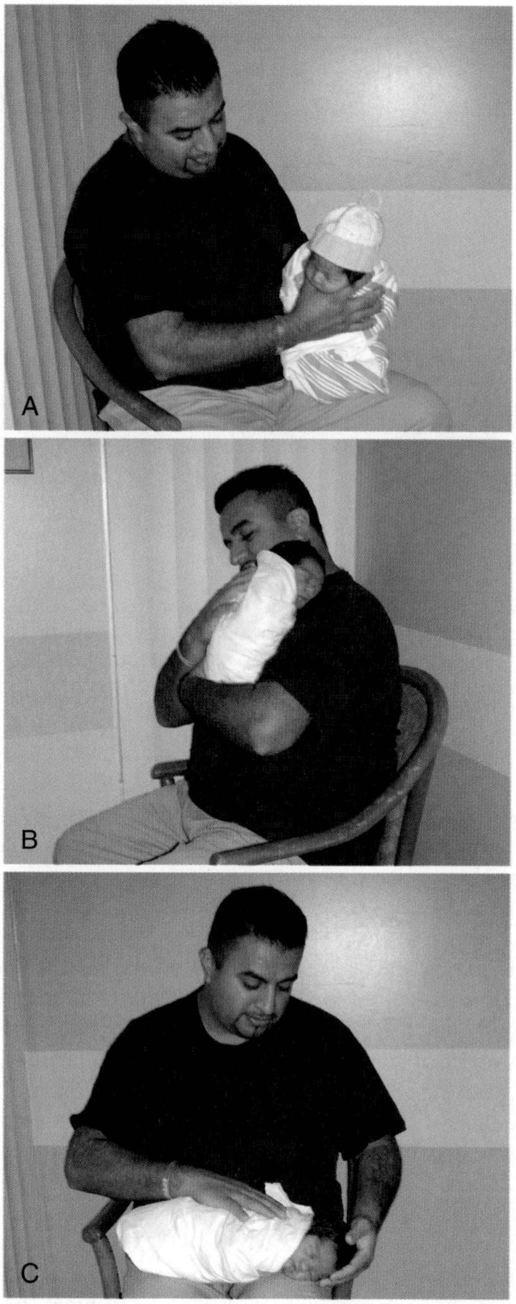

Fig. 26-15 Positions for burping an infant. A: Sitting. B: On the shoulder. C: Across the lap. *(Courtesy Julie Perry Nelson, Loveland, CO.)*

evolve Critical Thinking Exercise—Formula Preparation

protein, carbohydrates, and essential amino acids, with minor variations such as the source of carbohydrate; nucleotides to enhance immune function; and LCPFUA, DHA, and ARA, which are thought to improve central nervous system, visual, and cognitive function (Georgieff, 2001; Gil, Ramirez, & Gil, 2003). The composition, processing, packaging, and labelling of all infant formula is regulated under the Canadian Food and Drug Regulations to ensure product safety and quality (CPS et al., 2005). Iron-fortified cows' milk formulas are designed to meet the nutritional requirements of infants until 9 to 12 months of age. There is no evidence that iron-fortified formula causes constipation in infants (Singhal et al., 2000).

Commercially prepared infant formulas come in four main categories: (1) cow's milk–based formulas, (2) soy-based formulas, commonly used for children who are lactose or cow's milk protein intolerant; (3) casein- or whey-hydrolysate formulas, used primarily for children who cannot tolerate or digest cow's milk or soy-based formulas; and (4) amino acid formulas.

The Canadian Paediatric Society, Dieticians of Canada, and Health Canada Joint Working Groups report that there are few indications for the use of soy protein–based formulas instead of cow's milk–based formulas. Appropriate usage includes infants fed vegan diets and infants with galactosemia (CPS et al., 2005). Infants with documented IgE allergies caused by cow's milk should be fed an extensively hydrolyzed protein formula because about 10 to 14% of infants with cow's milk–based formula intolerance will also have a soy protein allergy. Soy protein–based formulas have not been proved to be effective in colic or in preventing allergy in healthy or high-risk infants.

Commercial formulas are available in three forms: powder, concentrate, and ready-to-feed. All are equivalent in nutritional content (20 kcal/30 mL or 68 kcal/100 mL), but they vary considerably in price. Powdered formulas are least expensive and are convenient because they are lightweight and require no refrigeration before mixing with water and only the amount of formula that is required needs to be made. Concentrated liquid formula is more expensive than powder. It is diluted with water and can be stored in the refrigerator for 24 hours after opening. Ready-to-feed formula is most expensive but easiest to use. The desired amount is poured into the bottle. The opened can is safely refrigerated for 24 hours. This type of formula can also be purchased in individual disposable bottles for the most convenient feeding (Parent Health Information Group, 2008).

Alternate milk sources such as goat's milk; skim or low-fat milk; condensed milk; or raw, unpasteurized milk from any animal source should not be fed to infants, since these are inadequate to support growth and may contain excessive protein or an inadequate calcium/phosphorus ratio, which may cause seizures. Also, the use of honey or corn syrup in infant formula should be avoided as botulism can occur.

Formula Preparation

The commercial infant formula must include label directions for preparation and use of the formula with pictures and symbols for the benefit of individuals who cannot read. Some manufacturers translate the directions into many languages, such as French, Chinese, Punjabi, and Vietnamese, to prevent misunderstanding and errors in formula preparation. It is important to impress on families that the proportions must not be altered—that is, neither diluted to extend the amount of formula nor concentrated to provide more calories.

Although manufacturers of commercial formulas include directions for preparing their products, the nurse should review formula preparation with the mother or primary caretaker. It is especially important that formula be mixed properly. The newborn's kidneys are immature; giving the infant overly concentrated formula may provide protein and minerals in amounts that exceed the kidneys' excretory ability. In contrast, if the formula is diluted too much (sometimes done to save money), the infant does not consume sufficient calories and does not grow appropriately. The water used to mix either powdered or concentrated liquid formula need not contain any fluoride, especially in the first 6 months of life; excess fluoride can permanently stain the teeth once they do appear.

Formula should be prepared with attention to cleanliness. All water used for feeding infants under 4 months of age should be boiled for at least 2 minutes to ensure that it is pathogen free (CPS et al., 2005). When water from a private well is used in formula preparation, parents should be advised to first contact the health department for a chemical and bacteriological analysis of the water. The presence of nitrates, excess fluoride, or bacteria may be harmful to the infant.

If the sanitary conditions in the home appear unsafe, it is better to recommend the use of ready-to-feed formula or to teach the mother to sterilize the formula. The two traditional methods for sterilization are terminal heating and the aseptic method. In the terminal heating method, the prepared formula is placed in the bottles, which are topped with the nipples placed upside down and covered with the caps, and then sealed loosely with the rings. The bottles are then boiled together in a water bath for 25 minutes. In the aseptic method, the bottles, rings, caps, nipples, and any other necessary equipment, such as a funnel, are boiled separately, after which the formula is poured into the bottles. Any formula left in the bottle after the feeding should be discarded because the infant's saliva has mixed with it. (Instructions for formula preparation and feeding are provided in the Home Care box.)

Vitamin and Mineral Supplementation

Commercial iron-fortified formula contains all the nutrients needed by the infant for the first 6 months of life. After

HOME CARE

Formula Preparation and Feeding

Your newborn will be hungry about every 2½ to 3 hours, but sometimes the baby may go 3 to 4 hours between feedings. The newborn should not go longer than 4 hours between feedings until a weight gain pattern is established—usually in about 2 weeks, then newborns should be fed on demand. Your newborn needs to be awake before being fed. If your newborn is sleepy, massage the newborn's back and chest and talk to him or her. Use skin-to-skin holding to increase your sensitivity to the hunger cues.

Your infant's feedings will change a lot in the first week after birth. The first day, most newborns drink only about 15 mL of formula at a feeding. By the time they are 1 week old, most infants drink 30 to 60 mL at a feeding and then gradually increase their intake as they grow. If you do not use all of the formula at a feeding, throw away what is left because it spoils once it has mixed with the infant's saliva.

You may want to write down how many millilitres your infant drinks each day. When you take the infant in for a checkup, the physician or nurse will ask you about how much formula the infant drinks. By 1 to 2 weeks of age, most infants who weigh 3 to 4.0 kg are drinking about 840 mL in 24 hours. Smaller infants may drink a little less because their stomach capacity is less. These figures, however, are approximations only, and infants will consume the amount necessary for growth, provided they are healthy. Do not force-feed an infant if a smaller amount is consumed unless directed by the primary care practitioner.

You will know your baby is drinking enough if the baby is content after feedings and the number of soiled and wet diapers gradually increases from 1 diaper change on the first day to 6 to 10 diaper changes daily after the first week. Formula-fed babies usually return to their birth weight by 2 to 3 weeks and for the first 3 months gain about 1 kg per month.

To feed your newborn, place the nipple in the newborn's mouth on the tongue. It should touch the top of the tongue to stimulate the infant's sucking reflex. Hold the bottle like a pencil. Keep the bottle tipped so that the nipple stays filled with milk and the newborn does not suck in air. With most bottles you will notice air bubbles in the bottle as the infant sucks on the nipple; this means the infant is getting formula from the bottle. The plastic bag bottles will not have as many air bubbles as hard plastic or glass bottles.

Hold your newborn close for feedings. This should be a pleasant time for social interaction and cuddling. Some newborns take longer to feed than others; be patient. It may be necessary to keep the infant awake and encourage continued sucking. Moving the nipple gently in the infant's mouth may stimulate more sucking.

Some newborns swallow air when sucking. Give your infant a chance to burp several times during early feedings. As your infant gets older and you get more experienced, you will know when to stop for burping.

If your infant fusses or cries between feedings, check the diaper to see if he or she needs to be changed and see if the infant needs to be picked up and cuddled. If the child continues to cry and acts hungry, he or she needs to be fed. Infants do not get hungry on a schedule.

Place your baby on his or her back to sleep. Do not use the side-lying position for sleep because the infant may roll forward onto his or her face and stomach. In the event that the infant does not usually sleep after a feeding, he or she may be placed on the tummy provided there is adult supervision.

The stools (bowel movements) of a formula-fed newborn are yellow and soft but formed. The newborn will probably have a stool during or after each feeding in the first 2 weeks, but this will then gradually decrease to one or two stools each day.

Safety Tips

- Infants should be held and never left alone while feeding. Do not prop the bottle: the infant could inhale formula or choke on any that was spit up.
- Know how to use the bulb syringe in case your infant should choke.
- Drinking bottles of formula or juice while falling asleep can cause tooth decay (nursing bottle caries) in young children.
- Juice is not recommended in infants for nutritional purposes.

Continued

HOME CARE

Formula Preparation and Feeding—cont'd

Formula Preparation

- Wash your hands and clean the bottle, nipple, and can opener carefully before preparing formula.
- If new nipples seem too hard, they can be softened by boiling them in water for 5 minutes before use.
- Read the label on the container of formula and mix it exactly according to the directions.
- Use tap water to mix concentrated or powdered formula unless directed otherwise by your infant's physician or nurse. Some manufacturers sell bottles of distilled or fluoridated water for formula preparation; however, neither of these is necessary for preparation of infant formulas unless prescribed by the primary care practitioner.
- Test the size of the nipple hole by holding a prepared bottle upside down. The formula should drip slowly from the nipple. If it runs in a stream, the hole is too big and the nipple should not be used. If it has to be shaken for the formula to come out, the hole is too small. You can either buy a new nipple or enlarge the hole by boiling the nipple for 5 minutes with a sewing needle inserted in the hole.
- If a nipple collapses when your infant sucks, loosen the nipple ring a little to let in air.
- Opened cans of ready-to-feed or concentrated formula should be covered and refrigerated. Any unused portions must be discarded after 48 hours.
- Unopened (sealed) bottles or cans of formula can be stored at room temperature.
- Once a bottle of formula is prepared and fed to the infant, it should be discarded within 1 hour. It is best to prepare only the amount the infant usually takes at each feeding, to prevent discarding large portions of formula.
- If the formula is refrigerated, warm it by placing the bottle in a pan of hot water. Never use a microwave to warm any food to be given to a baby. Test the temperature of the formula by letting a few drops fall on the inside of your wrist. If the formula feels comfortably warm to you, it is the correct temperature.

6 months, fluoride supplementation of 0.25 mg/day is required if the local water supply is not fluoridated. Vitamin D supplementation is discussed earlier in this chapter.

Weaning

The bottle-fed infant will gradually learn to use a cup, and the parents will find that they are preparing fewer bottles. Commonly, the feeding before bedtime is the last one to remain. Infants have a strong need to suck, and the infant who has had the bottle taken away too early or abruptly will compensate with non-nutritive sucking on the fingers or thumb, a pacifier, or even the tongue. Weaning from a bottle should thus be done gradually because the infant has learned to rely on the comfort that sucking provides.

Key Points

- Human milk is species specific and is the recommended form of nutrition for infants. It provides immunological protection against many infections and diseases.
- Breast milk changes in composition with each stage of lactation, during each feeding, and as the infant grows.
- During the prenatal period, parents should be informed of the benefits of breastfeeding for infants, mothers, families, and society.
- Infants should be breastfed as soon as possible after birth and at least 8 to 12 times per day thereafter.
- Nurses play a key role in ensuring that newborns latch onto the breast properly.
- There are objective, measurable indicators that the infant is breastfeeding effectively.
- Breast milk production is based on a supply-meets-demand principle; the more the infant nurses, the greater the milk supply.
- Commercial infant formulas provide satisfactory nutrition for most infants.
- Infants should be held for feedings.
- Parents should be instructed about the types of commercial infant formulas, proper preparation for feeding, and correct feeding technique.
- Unmodified (whole) cow's milk is not appropriate for feeding the infant during the first year of life.

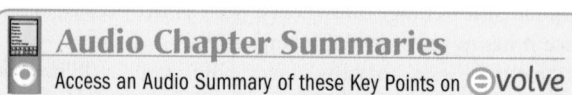

Audio Chapter Summaries

Access an Audio Summary of these Key Points on evolve

References

Academy of Breastfeeding Medicine. (2010). ABM Clinical Protocol #8: Human milk storage information for home use for full-term infants (original protocol March 2004; revision #1 March 2010). *Breastfeeding Medicine, 5*(3), 127–130. doi:10.1089=bfm.2010.9988

Agnew, T., Gilmore, J., & Sullivan, P. (1997). *A multicultural perspective of breastfeeding in Canada.* Ottawa: Health Canada. Retrieved from http://www.phac-aspc.gc.ca/hp-ps/dca-dea/publications/pdf/multicultur-bf-am-eng.pdf.

American Academy of Pediatrics. (2009). *Pediatric nutrition handbook* (6th ed.). Elk Grove Village, IL: Author.

Arora, S., et al. (2000). Major factors influencing breastfeeding rates: Mother's perception of father's attitude and milk supply. *Pediatrics, 106*(5), E67.

Askin, D. F. & Diehl-Jones, W. L. (2005). Improving on perfection: Breast milk and breast-milk additives for preterm neonates. *Newborn and Infant Nursing Reviews, 5*(1), 10–18. doi:10.1053/j.nainr.2005.02.002

Biancuzzo, M. (2003). *Breastfeeding the newborn: Clinical strategies for nurses* (2nd ed.). St. Louis: Mosby.

Blackburn, S. T. (2007). *Maternal, fetal, and neonatal physiology: A clinical perspective* (3rd ed.). St. Louis: Saunders.

Breastfeeding Committee for Canada. (2010). *Summary: Integrated 10 steps practice outcome indicators for hospitals and community health services.*

Retrieved from http://breastfeedingcanada.ca/pdf/2010-09_Summary-BCC_Integrated_2010_Steps_Practice_Outcomes_Indicators.pdf.

Breastfeeding Committee for Canada. (2011). *BFI integrated 10 steps practice outcome indicators for hospitals and community health services*. Retrieved from http://www.breastfeedingcanada.ca/documents/BCC_BFI_20110704_Final_BCC_BFI_Integrated_Indicators_English.pdf.

Canadian Dental Association. (2010). *CDA position on use of fluorides in caries prevention*. Retrieved from http://www.cda-adc.ca/_files/position_statements/Fluorides-English-2010-06-08.pdf.

Canadian Paediatric Society. (2002). The use of fluoride in infants and children. *Paediatrics and Child Health, 7*(8), 569–572. Retrieved from http://www.cps.ca/english/statements/n/n02-01.htm.

Canadian Paediatric Society. (2003). Recommendations for the use of pacifiers. *Paediatrics and Child Health, 8*(8), 515–519. Retrieved from http://www.cps.ca/english/statements/cp/cp03-01.htm.

Canadian Paediatric Society. (2005). Exclusive breastfeeding should continue to six months. *Paediatrics and Child Health, 10*(3), 148. Retrieved from http://www.cps.ca/english/statements/n/breastfeedingmar05.htm.

Canadian Paediatric Society. (2006). Position statement of Infectious Diseases and Immunization Committee—Maternal infectious diseases, antimicrobial therapy or immunizations: Very few contraindications to breastfeeding. *Paediatrics and Child Health, 11*(8), 489–491. Retrieved from http://www.cps.ca/english/statements/ID/PIDnote_Oct2006.htm.

Canadian Paediatric Society. (2007a). *Iron needs of babies and children*. Retrieved from: http://www.caringforkids.cps.ca/pregnancybabies/ironreq.htm.

Canadian Paediatric Society. (2007b). Guidelines for detection, management and prevention of hyperbilirubinemia in term and late preterm newborn infants (35 or more weeks' gestation). *Paediatrics and Child Health, 12*(Suppl B), 1B–12B. Retrieved from http://www.cps.ca/english/statements/FN/FN07-02.pdf.

Canadian Paediatric Society. (2008). Vertical transmission of the hepatitis C virus: Current knowledge and issues. *Paediatrics and Child Health, 13*(6), 529–534. Retrieved from http://www.cps.ca/english/statements/id/id08-05.htm.

Canadian Paediatric Society & College of Family Physicians of Canada. (1997). Routine administration of vitamin K to newborns. *Paediatrics and Child Health, 2*(6), 429–431. Retrieved from http://www.cps.ca/english/statements/FN/fn97-01.htm.

Canadian Paediatric Society, Dieticians of Canada, & Health Canada. (2005). *Nutrition for healthy term infants*. Ottawa: Health Canada. Retrieved from http://www.hc-sc.gc.ca/fn-an/pubs/infant-nourrisson/nut_infant_nourrisson_term-eng.php.

Canadian Paediatric Society & Society of Obstetrician and Gynecologists of Canada. (1996). Facilitating discharge home following a normal term birth. *Paediatrics and Child Health, 1*(2), 165–168. Retrieved from http://www.cps.ca/english/statements/fn/fn96-02.htm.

Carbajal, R., et al. (2003). Analgesic effect of breast feeding in term neonates: Randomized controlled trial. *British Medical Journal, 326*(7379), 13.

Chapman, D. J. (2011). Evaluating the evidence: Is there an effective treatment for breast engorgement? *Journal of Human Lactation, 27*(1), 82–83. doi:10.1177/0890334410396671

Chertok, I. R., Shoham-Vardi, I., & Hallak, M. (2004). Four-month breastfeeding duration in postcesarean women of different cultures in the Israeli Negev. *Journal of Perinatal and Neonatal Nursing, 18*(2), 145–160.

Choudhry, U. K. (1997). Traditional practices of women from India: Pregnancy, childbirth, and newborn care. *Journal of Obstetric, Gynecologic and Neonatal Nursing, 26*(5), 533–539.

Cohen, R., Mrtek, M. B., & Mrtek, R. G. (1995). Comparison of maternal absenteeism and infant illness rates among breast-feeding and formula-feeding women in two corporations. *American Journal of Health Promotion, 10*, 148–153.

Conover, E. & Buehler, B. A. (2004). Use of herbal agents by breastfeeding women may affect infants. *Pediatric Annals, 33*(4), 235–240.

Dieticians of Canada, Canadian Pediatric Society, Canadian College of Family Physicians, & Public Health Nurses of Canada. (2010). *Promoting optimal monitoring of child growth in Canada: Using the new WHO growth charts*. Retrieved from http://www.cps.ca/english/statements/N/growth-charts-statement-FULL.pdf.

Dollberg, S., et al. (2006). Immediate nipple pain relief after frenotomy in breast-fed infants with ankyloglossia: A randomized, prospective study. *Journal of Pediatric Surgery, 41*(9), 1598–1600. doi:10.1016/j.jpedsurg.2006.05.024

Eidelman, A. I. (2001). Hypoglycemia and the breastfed neonate. *Pediatric Clinics of North America, 48*(2), 377–387.

Eisman, J. (1998). Relevance of pregnancy and lactation to osteoporosis. *Clinical Perinatology, 25*(2), 303–326.

Enger, S., et al. (1998). Breastfeeding experience and breast cancer risk among postmenopausal women. *Cancer Epidemiology, Biomarkers and Prevention, 7*(5), 365–369.

Fleith, M. & Clandinin, M. T. (2005). Dietary PUFA for term and preterm infants: Review of clinical studies. *Critical Reviews in Food Science and Nutrition, 45*(3), 205–229. doi:10.1080/10408690590956378

Georgieff, M. K. (2001). Taking a rational approach to the choice of formula. *Contemporary Pediatrics, 18*(8), 112–130.

Gil, A., Ramirez, M., & Gil, M. (2003). Role of long-chain polyunsaturated fatty acids in infant nutrition. *European Journal of Clinical Nutrition, 57*(Suppl 1), S31–S34.

Glatstein, M. M., Garcia-Bournissen, F., Finkelstein, Y., & Koren, G. (2008). Methadone exposure during lactation. *Canadian Family Physician, 54*(12), 1689–1690.

Gray, L., et al. (2002). Breastfeeding is analgesic in healthy newborns. *Pediatrics, 109*(4), 590–593.

Guthmann, R. A., Bang, J., & Nashelsky, J. (2005). FPIN's clinical inquiries: Combined oral contraceptives for mothers who are breastfeeding. *American Family Physician, 72*(7), 1303–1304.

Hale, T. W. (2010). *Medications and mothers' milk* (14th ed.). Amarillo, TX: Hale.

Halken, S. & Host, A. (1996). Prevention of allergic disease: Exposure to food allergens and dietetic intervention. *Pediatric Allergy and Immunology, 7*(9 Suppl), 102–107.

Hartmann, P. E., Cregan, M. D., Ramsey, D. T, Simmer, K., & Kent, J. C. (2003). Physiology of lactation in preterm mothers: Initiation and maintenance. *Pediatric Annals, 32*(5), 351–358.

Health Canada. (2004a). *Exclusive breastfeeding duration—2004 Health Canada recommendations*. Ottawa: Author. Retrieved from http://www.hc-sc.gc.ca/fn-an/nutrition/infant-nourisson/excl_bf_dur-dur_am_excl-eng.php.

Health Canada. (2004b). *Vitamin D supplementation for breastfed infants—2004 Health Canada recommendation*. Retrieved from http://www.hc-sc.gc.ca/fn-an/nutrition/infant-nourisson/vita_d_supp-eng.php.

Health Canada. (2010). *Safe sleep tips*. Ottawa: Author. Retrieved from http://healthycanadians.gc.ca/kids/safe-sleep-tips/?format=pdf.

Heird, W. C. (2007). The feeding of infants and children. In R. M. Kliegman, et al. (Eds.), *Nelson textbook of pediatrics* (18th ed.). Philadelphia: Saunders.

Horta, B. L., Bahl, R., Martines, J. C., & Victora, C. G. (2007). *Evidence on the long-term effects of breastfeeding. WHO Systemic Reviews and Meta-analyses*. Geneva, Switzerland: World Health Organization. Retrieved from http://whqlibdoc.who.int/publications/2007/9789241595230_eng.pdf.

INFACT Canada. (2005). *Maternity benefits and breastfeeding*. Retrieved from http://www.infactcanada.ca/INFACT%20Fall%202005%20NL%20for%20Website.pdf.

Institute of Medicine. (2005). *Dietary reference intakes for energy, carbohydrate, fiber, fatty acids, cholesterol, protein, and amino acids*. Washington, DC: Food and Nutrition Board, Institute of Medicine, National Academies Press.

International Lactation Consultant Association. (2005). *Clinical guidelines for the establishment of exclusive breastfeeding*. Retrieved from http://www.ilca.org/files/resources/ilca_publications/ClinicalGuidelines2005.pdf.

Ip, S., et al. (2007, April). *Breastfeeding and maternal and infant health outcomes in developed countries* (Pub. No. 07-E007). Rockville, MD: Agency for Healthcare Research and Quality.

Johnston, C., et al. (2008). Enhanced kangaroo mother care for heel lance in preterm neonates: A crossover trial. *Journal of Perinatology, 29*(1), 51–56. doi:10.1038/jp.2008.113

Kendall-Tackett, K. (2007). A new paradigm for depression in new mothers: the central role of inflammation and how breastfeeding and anti-inflammatory treatments protect maternal health. *International Breastfeeding Journal, 2*(March 30), 2–6. doi:10.1186/1746-4358-2-2

Koren, G. (2002). Drinking alcohol while breastfeeding: Will it harm my baby? *Canadian Family Physician, 48*, 39–41. Retrieved from http://www.motherisk.org/prof/updatesDetail.jsp?content_id=347.

Kramer, M. S., et al. (2008). Breastfeeding and child cognitive development: New evidence from a large randomized trial. *Archives of General Psychiatry, 65*(5), 578–584.

Kumar, S. P., Mooney, R., Wieser, L. J., & Haystad, S. (2006). The LATCH scoring system and prediction of breastfeeding duration. *Journal of Human Lactation, 22*(4), 391–396. doi:10.1177/0890334406293161

Lawrence, R. A. & Lawrence, R. M. (2011). *Breastfeeding: A guide for the medical profession* (7th ed.). St. Louis: Mosby.

Mannel, R. (2011). Defining lactation acuity to improve patient safety and outcomes. *Journal of Human Lactation, 27*(2), 163–170. doi:10.1177/0890334410397198

McKenna, K. (2009). The practice of prelacteal feeding to newborns among Hindu and Muslim families. *Journal of Midwifery and Women's Health, 54*(1), 78–81. doi:10.1016/j.jmwh.2008.07.012

Millar, W. J. & Maclean, H. (2005). Breastfeeding practices. *Health Reports, 16*(2). Retrieved from http://www.statcan.gc.ca/studies-etudes/82-003/archive/2005/7787-eng.pdf.

Moreland-Schultz, K. & Hill, P. D. (2005). Prevention of and therapies for nipple pain: A systematic review. *Journal of Obstetric, Gynecologic, & Neonatal Nursing, 34*(4), 428–437. doi:10.1177/0884217505276056

Morin, K. H. (2004). Current thoughts on healthy term infant nutrition: The first 12 months. *MCN: American Journal of Maternal Child Nursing, 29*(1), 312–317.

Murray, E. K., Ricketts, S., & Dellaport, J. (2007). Hospital practices that increase breastfeeding duration: Results from a population-based study. *Birth, 34*(3), 202–211.

Page, D. (2008). ILCA's inside track: Breastfeeding and returning to work... working out the details. *Journal of Human Lactation, 24*(1), 85–86. doi:10.1177/08903344073133431

Parent Health Education Resource Working Group. (2008). *How to feed your baby with infant formula*. Halifax: Nova Scotia Department of Health Promotion and Protection.

Pikwer, M., et al. (2009). Breast-feeding, but not oral contraceptives, is associated with a reduced risk of rheumatoid arthritis. *Annals of Rheumatic Disease, 68*(4), 526–530. doi:10.1136/ard.2007.084707

Public Health Agency of Canada. (2008). *The Chief Public Health Officer's report on the state of health in Canada*. Ottawa: Health Canada. Retrieved from http://www.phac-aspc.gc.ca/cphorsphc-respcacsp/2008/fr-rc/cphorsphc-respcacsp07h-eng.php.

Public Health Agency of Canada. (2009a). *What mothers say: The Canadian Maternity Experiences Survey*. Ottawa: Author. Retrieved from http://www.phac-aspc.gc.ca/rhs-ssg/pdf/survey-eng.pdf.

Public Health Agency of Canada. (2009b). *Ten valuable tips for successful breastfeeding* (Cat. HP15-7/2009E-PDF). Retrieved from http://www.phac-aspc.gc.ca/hp-ps/dca-dea/stages-etapes/childhood-enfance_0-2/nutrition/tips-cons-eng.php.

Reading, J. L., Kmetic, A., & Gideon, V. (2007). *Discussion paper for the World Health Organization Commission on Social Determinants of Health*. Retrieved from http://www.afn.ca/cmslib/general/07-05-28_AFN_Paper_to_WHO_Commission_on_Social_Determinants_of_Health.pdf.

Registered Nurses' Association of Ontario. (2003). *Breastfeeding best practice guidelines for nurses*. Toronto: Author. Retrieved from http://rnao.ca/sites/rnao-ca/files/Breastfeeding_Best_Practice_Guidelines_for_Nurses.pdf.

Rempel, L. & Rempel, J. (2011). The breastfeeding team: The role of involved fathers in the breastfeeding family. *Journal of Human Lactation, 27*(2), 115–121. doi:10.1177/0890334410390045

Riordan, J. & Gill-Hopple, K. (2001). Breastfeeding care in multicultural populations. *Journal of Obstetric, Gynecologic and Neonatal Nursing, 30*(2), 216–223.

Riordan, J. & Wambach, K. (2009). *Breastfeeding and human lactation* (4th ed.). Sudbury, MA: Jones & Bartlett Publishers.

Rosenblatt, K. A. & Thomas, D. B. (1995). Prolonged lactation and endometrial cancer: WHO collaborative study of neoplasia and steroid contraceptives. *International Journal of Epidemiology, 24*, 499–503.

Simard, I., et al. (2005). Factors influencing the initiation and duration of breastfeeding among low income women followed by the Perinatal Nutrition Program in four regions of Quebec. *Journal of Human Lactation. 21*(3), 327–337. doi:10.1177/0890334405275831

Simmer, K., Patole, S. K., & Rao, S. C. (2008). Long-chain polyunsaturated fatty acid supplementation in infants born at term. *Cochrane Database of Systematic Reviews, (1)*, CD000376.

Singhal, A., et al. (2000). Clinical safety of iron-fortified formulas. *Pediatrics, 105*(3), e38–e44.

Society of Obstetricians and Gynecologists of Canada. (2004). Canadian contraception consensus. *Journal of Obstetrics and Gynaecology Canada, 26*(4), 347–387. Retrieved from http://www.sogc.org/guidelines/public/143E-CPG3-April2004.pdf.

Spietz, A., Johnson-Crowley, N., Summer, G., & Bernard, K. (1999). *Keys to caregiving: Study guide*. Seattle, WA: NCAST (Nursing Child Assessment Satellite Training), University of Washington School of Nursing.

Statistics Canada. (2009). *Health fact sheet. Breastfeeding, 2009*. Retrieved from http://www.statcan.gc.ca/pub/82-625-x/2010002/article/11269-eng.htm.

UNICEF. (2009). *Canadian supplement to the state of the world's children 2009. Aboriginal children's health: Leaving no child behind*. Retrieved from http://www.unicef.ca/portal/Secure/Community/502/WCM/HELP/take_action/Advocacy/Leaving%20no%20child%20behind%2009.pdf.

UNICEF. (n.d.). *The baby-friendly hospital initiative*. Retrieved from http://www.unicef.org/programme/breastfeeding/baby.htm.

UNICEF UK Baby-Friendly Hospital Initiative. (2011). *Seven point plan*. Retrieved from http://www.unicef.org.uk/BabyFriendly/Health-Professionals/Going-Baby-Friendly/Community/Seven-Point-Plan-for-Sustaining-Breastfeeding-in-the-Community/.

Vallianatos, H., et al. (2006). Beliefs and practices of First Nation women about weight gain during pregnancy and lactation: Implications for women's health. *Canadian Journal of Nursing Research, 38*(1), 102–119.

Vohr, B. R., et al. (2006). Beneficial effects of breast milk in the neonatal intensive care unit on the developmental outcome of extremely low birth weight infants at 18 months of age. *Pediatrics, 118*(1), e115–e123. doi:10.1542/peds.2005-2382

West, D. (2009). *Breastfeeding after breast and nipple surgeries*. Retrieved from http://bfar.org/.

World Health Organization. (2010a). *Exclusive breastfeeding*. Geneva, Switzerland: Author. Retrieved from http://www.who.int/nutrition/topics/exclusive_breastfeeding/en/#.

World Health Organization. (2010b). *Combined hormonal contraceptive use during the postpartum period*. Geneva, Switzerland: Author. Retrieved from http://www.who.int/reproductivehealth/publications/family_planning/rhr_10_15/en/index.htm.

Additional Resources

Beststart: Breastfeeding matters—An important guide to breastfeeding for women and their families: http://www.beststart.org/resources/breastfeeding/pdf/breastfeeding_matters_eng_fnl.pdf

Breastfeeding guidelines for consultants: Desk reference: http://www.beststart.org/resources/breastfeeding/pdf/breastfdeskref09.pdf

Breastfeeding in Peel (Region of Peel Health Department): Multilingual resources for new parents including videos: http://www.peelregion.ca/health/family-health/breastfeeding/

Motherrisk: http://www.motherisk.org

Registered Nurses Association of Ontario—Breastfeeding best practice guideline: http://rnao.ca/bpg/guidelines/breastfeeding-best-practice-guidelines-nurses

Infants With Gestational Age–Related Problems

Learning Objectives

On completion of this chapter, the reader will be able to:

- Compare and contrast the physical characteristics of preterm, term, and postterm neonates.
- Discuss respiratory distress syndrome and the approach to treatment.
- Compare methods of oxygen therapy for the high-risk infant.
- Describe nursing interventions for nutritional care of the preterm infant.
- Discuss the pathophysiology of retinopathy of prematurity and bronchopulmonary dysplasia (chronic lung disease) and identify the predisposing risk factors.
- Describe the treatment of the infant with meconium aspiration.
- Describe risk factors associated with the birth and transition of an infant of a diabetic mother.
- Plan developmentally appropriate care for the high-risk infant.
- Develop a plan to address the unique needs of parents of high-risk infants.

Electronic Resources

Additional information related to the content in Chapter 27 can be found on

evolve the companion Web site at

http://evolve.elsevier.com/Canada/Perry/maternal/

- Animation—Oxygenation Desaturation, Respiratory Failure, in Infant
- Examination Review Questions
- Critical Thinking Exercise—Patent Ductus Arteriosus

Modern technology and expert nursing care have made important contributions to improving the health and survival of high-risk infants. However, infants who are born considerably before term and survive are particularly susceptible to the development of sequelae related to their preterm birth. These conditions include necrotizing enterocolitis (NEC), growth failure, **bronchopulmonary dysplasia** (BPD), intraventricular and periventricular hemorrhage, and **retinopathy of prematurity** (ROP). This chapter focuses on care of the preterm infant; care of other high-risk infants with gestational age–related problems is also discussed. Infants born of mothers with diabetes are included because they may experience problems that place them at risk for improper function and development.

High-risk infants are most often classified according to birth weight, gestational age, and predominant pathophysiological problems (Box 27-1). Intrauterine growth rates are not the same for all infants, and other factors (e.g., heredity, placental insufficiency, and maternal disease) influence intrauterine growth and birth weight.

The Preterm Infant

Preterm infants, those born before 37 completed weeks of gestation, are at risk because their organ systems are immature and they lack adequate physiological reserves to function in an extrauterine environment. The range of birth weight and physiological problems varies widely among preterm infants because of increased survival rates among those who weigh less than 1000 g. However, one general concept is that the lower the birth weight and the gestational age, the lower the chances of survival among infants born preterm. Preterm birth is responsible for 60 to 80% of infant deaths (Joseph, Demissie, & Kramer, 2002; Kramer et al., 2000).

The cause of preterm birth is multifactorial (see Box 19-2). Risk factors for preterm birth include environmental exposures, genetics, infertility, and medical conditions (Public Health Agency of Canada [PHAC], 2008). Specific demographic characteristics related to preterm birth include smoking, infections, the mother being unmarried, younger or older maternal age, low pre-pregnancy weight, low or high

BOX 27-1 Classification of High-Risk Infants

Classification According to Size

Low-birth-weight (LBW)—An infant whose birth weight is less than 2500 g, regardless of gestational age

Very-low-birth-weight (VLBW)—An infant whose birth weight is less than 1500 g

Extremely-low-birth-weight (ELBW)—An infant whose birth weight is less than 1000 g

Appropriate for gestational age (AGA)—An infant whose birth weight falls between the tenth and ninetieth percentiles on intrauterine growth curves

Small for gestational age (SGA)—An infant whose rate of intrauterine growth was restricted and whose birth weight falls below the tenth percentile on intrauterine growth curves

Large for gestational age (LGA)—An infant whose birth weight falls above the ninetieth percentile on intrauterine growth curves

Intrauterine growth restriction (IUGR)—Found in infants whose intrauterine growth does not meet norms for gestational age and sex. Growth may or may not fall before the tenth percentile.

Symmetrical IUGR—Growth restriction in which the weight, length, and head circumference are all affected

Asymmetrical IUGR—Growth restriction in which the head circumference remains within normal parameters as does length, while the birth weight falls below the tenth percentile

Classification According to Gestational Age*

Gestational age is the interval, in completed weeks, between the first day of a woman's last menstrual period and the day of delivery.

Preterm infant—An infant born before 37 completed weeks of gestation, regardless of birth weight

Late preterm infant—An infant born between 34 0/7 and 36 6/7 weeks of gestation, regardless of birth weight*

Term infant—An infant born between 37 through 42 completed weeks of gestation, regardless of birth weight

Postterm infant—An infant born after 42 completed weeks of gestation regardless of birth weight

Classification According to Mortality

Live birth—Birth in which the neonate manifests any heartbeat, breathes, or displays voluntary movement, regardless of gestational age. In Canada, an infant born less than 20 weeks' gestation who dies within the first few minutes after birth may be registered as a live birth and then as an infant death.

Fetal death—Death of the fetus, at any gestational age, before delivery, with absence of any signs of life after birth. Only fetal deaths where the product of conception has a birth weight of 500 g or more or the duration of pregnancy is 20 weeks or longer are registered in Canada.

Neonatal death—Death that occurs in the first 28 days of life; early neonatal death occurs in the first week of life; late neonatal death occurs at 7 to 28 days.

Perinatal mortality—Total number of fetal and early neonatal deaths per 1000 live births

(From Sauve, R. & McCourt, C. [2009]. Infant mortality in Canada. *Journal of Obstetrics and Gynaecology Canada, 31*[4], 351–352; Statistics Canada. [2009]. *Births—2007*. Catalogue no. 84F0210X. Ottawa: Ministry of Industry.)

*Note: Definitions of late preterm vary among experts.

weight gain, previous preterm birth, race and ethnicity, and maternal stress (PHAC, 2008). Other factors associated with preterm birth include gestational hypertension, maternal infection, multifetal pregnancy, HELLP syndrome (hemolysis, elevated liver enzymes, and low platelet count occurring in association with pre-eclampsia), premature dilation of the cervix, and placental or umbilical cord conditions that affect the ability of the fetus to receive nutrients.

According to 2008 data, 7.9% of infants born in Canada were preterm, 7.8% were small for gestational age (SGA) (Public Health Agency of Canada [PHAC], 2012), and approximately 6% were low-birth-weight (LBW) (Statistics Canada, 2009). The incidence of preterm birth is highest among low socioeconomic groups (Canadian Institute for Health Information [CIHI], 2009). This is likely a result of the lack of comprehensive prenatal health care. Although SGA rates have decreased in the past few decades, from 11% in the 1990s, the issue is still a cause for concern.

Opinions vary about the practical and ethical dimensions of resuscitation of extremely-low-birth-weight (ELBW) infants. Ethical issues associated with resuscitation of these infants include whether to resuscitate; who should make that decision; whether the cost of resuscitation is justified; and whether the benefits of technology outweigh the burdens on the infant, family, and society in relation to the infant's quality of life.

Late Preterm Infant

Within the last two decades, several significant changes have occurred in neonatal care. Early postpartum discharge for term and preterm infants gained popularity as health care institutions attempted to cut health care costs. In Canada, early discharge rates increased from 20.1 per 100 hospital live births in 1995–1996 to 27.7 per 100 hospital live births in 2004–2005 (PHAC, 2008). In addition, infants who appeared to be "near" term began to be treated much like term infants; thus, the costs of neonatal intensive care were avoided for infants who appeared to be healthy. Recently, it has been recommended that infants born between 34 0/7 and 36 6/7 weeks of gestation be referred to as *late preterm infants* rather than near-term infants (Engle, 2006; Engle et al., 2007). Late preterm infants may make an effective transition to extrauterine life; however, they remain at risk for problems related to feeding, neurodevelopment, **thermoregulation**, **hypoglycemia**, **hyperbilirubinemia**, sepsis, and respiratory function (Bakewell-Sachs, 2007; Darcy, 2009). In one study, children born at 34 to 36 weeks' gestation were more than three times as likely as children born at term to be diagnosed with cerebral palsy (Petrini et al., 2009). Further, Talge and colleagues (2010) found that late preterm birth was associated with cognitive (lower IQ) and behavioural problems at follow-up in children at 6 years of age.

It is now estimated that late preterm infants represent 70% of the total preterm infant population. The mortality rate for this group is significantly higher than that of term infants (7.9 versus 2.4 per 1000 live births, respectively) (Tomashek, Shapiro-Mendoza, Davidoff, & Petrini, 2007). Because late preterm infants may be cared for in the same manner as healthy term infants, risk factors specific to late preterm infants may be overlooked. Late preterm infants are often discharged early from hospital and have a significantly higher rate of rehospitalization than that of term infants (Escobar, Clark, & Greene, 2006). See Table 27-1 for risk factors and nursing interventions for late preterm infants.

Table 27-1 Late Preterm Infant Assessment and Interventions

RISK FACTORS	ASSESSMENT	INTERVENTIONS*
Respiratory distress	Assess for signs of respiratory distress (nasal flaring, grunting, tachypnea, central cyanosis, retractions) and presence of apnea, especially during feedings. Assess for hypothermia, hypoglycemia.	Perform gestational-age assessment. Observe for signs of respiratory distress; monitor oxygenation by pulse oximetry; provide supplemental oxygen as ordered.
Thermal instability	Monitor axillary temperature every 30 min immediately postpartum until stable; then every 1–4 hr depending on gestational age and ability to maintain thermal stability.	Provide skin-to-skin care in immediate postpartum period for stable infant. Implement measures to avoid excess heat loss (adjust environmental temperature, avoid drafts). Bathe only after thermal stability has been maintained for 1 hr.
Hypoglycemia	Monitor for signs and symptoms of hypoglycemia. Assess feeding ability (latch, nipple feeding). Assess thermal stability and signs and symptoms of respiratory distress. Monitor bedside glucose in infants with additional risk factors (IDM, prolonged labour, respiratory distress, poor feeding).	Initiate early feedings of human milk or, if medically indicated, formula. Avoid dextrose water or water feedings. Provide IV dextrose as necessary for hypoglycemia.
Jaundice	Observe for jaundice in first 24 hr. Evaluate maternal–fetal history for additional risk factors that may cause increased hemolysis and circulating levels of unconjugated bilirubin (Rh, ABO, spherocytosis, bruising). Assess feeding method, voiding and stooling patterns.	Monitor bilirubin [transcutaneous and/or serum] and note risk zone on hour-specific nomogram (see Fig. 25-7).
Feeding problems	Assess ability to coordinate suck-swallow and breathing. Assess for respiratory distress, hypoglycemia, and thermal stability. Assess latch, maternal comfort with feeding method. Determine weight loss (should be ≤10% of birth weight).	Initiate early feedings (human milk or when medically indicated, formula). Ensure maternal knowledge of feeding method and of signs of inadequate feeding (sleepiness, lethargy, colour changes during feeding, apnea during feeding, decreased or absent urine output).
Neurodevelopmental problems	Assess for respiratory distress, neonatal jaundice, hypoglycemia, and thermal instability. Assess neurodevelopmental status. Assess for seizure activity.	Perform newborn screening, including hearing test. Implement individualized developmental care. Encourage parents to keep follow-up appointments with primary care physician for evaluation of growth and development (including cognitive function and achievement of appropriate milestones).
Infection	Evaluate maternal–fetal history for risk factors that may contribute to neonatal septicemia. Assess for signs and symptoms of neonatal infection (see Box 27-2 and Table 28-3).	Use routine practices, especially hand hygiene between infants and after contact with surfaces that may harbour bacteria (e.g., keyboards, telephones). Maintain thermal stability. Administer hepatitis B vaccine if required. Encourage breastfeeding and assist mother and baby with breastfeeding. Encourage parents to decrease infant exposure to respiratory viruses after discharge and to obtain vaccines as appropriate to prevent development of respiratory viruses (e.g., influenza).

(Portions adapted from Askin, D. F., Bakewell-Sachs, S., & Medoff-Cooper, B. [2007]. *Late preterm infant assessment guide*. Washington, DC: Association of Women's Health, Obstetric and Neonatal Nurses [AWHONN].)

IDM, infant of diabetic mother; *IV*, intravenous.

*This is not an exhaustive list of nursing interventions; additional interventions include those discussed under the care of the high-risk infant in this chapter.

Nursing Care Management

Assessment

For the high-risk infant, an accurate assessment of gestational age (see Chapter 25) is critical in helping the nurse identify the potential problems that the newborn is likely to experience. The response of the preterm, late preterm, or **postterm infant** to extrauterine life is different from that of the term infant. By understanding the physiological basis of these differences, the nurse can assess these infants; determine the response of the preterm, late preterm, or postterm infant; and discern which potential problems are most likely to occur.

Respiratory Function

An effective respiratory pattern is usually quickly established in nonstressed newborns and is evidenced by vigorous activity, adequate tissue perfusion, and pink or acrocyanotic colour. However, infants with a potential for respiratory depression at birth because of **asphyxia**, maternal analgesia or illness, pulmonary immaturity, or congenital malformations may exhibit cyanosis, gasping or ineffective respirations, decreased tissue perfusion, retractions, nasal flaring, tachypnea, decreased muscle tone, or a combination of these problems. Clinical tools have been developed to facilitate an objective assessment of the severity of respiratory compromise (Acute Care of at-Risk Newborns [ACoRN], 2010).

The preterm infant is likely to have difficulty making the pulmonary transition from intrauterine to extrauterine life. Numerous problems may affect the respiratory system of preterm infants, including the following:

- Decreased number of functional alveoli
- Deficient surfactant levels
- Smaller airway lumen
- Decreased tracheal cartilage
- Obstruction of respiratory passages
- Insufficient calcification of the bony thorax
- Circulating hormones (prostaglandins) that may affect cardiovascular function
- Immature and fragile pulmonary vasculature
- Greater distance between functional alveoli and capillary bed, especially in ELBW infants

In combination, these deficits severely hinder the infant's respiratory efforts and can produce respiratory distress or respiratory failure. Early signs of respiratory distress include tachypnea, nasal flaring, and expiratory grunting. Depending on the severity of respiratory distress and its cause, retractions may begin as subcostal, intercostal, or suprasternal. Increasing respiratory effort (e.g., paradoxical breathing patterns, retractions, nasal flaring, expiratory grunting, tachypnea, or apnea) indicates increasing distress. As a result of pulmonary immaturity and residual function, very-low-birth-weight (VLBW) and ELBW infants may progress rapidly from respiratory distress to complete respiratory failure. Initially, a compromised infant's colour may be cyanotic centrally or pale. Acrocyanosis is a normal finding in the neonate; however, central cyanosis indicates poor oxygenation.

Periodic breathing is a respiratory pattern commonly seen in preterm infants. Such infants exhibit 5- to 10-second respiratory pauses followed by 10 to 15 seconds of compensatory rapid respirations. Periodic breathing should not be confused with *apnea*: a cessation of respirations for 20 seconds or more associated with hypoxia, bradycardia, or both. The nurse must be prepared to respond to an apneic infant by providing stimulation (e.g., gentle rubbing of back), ventilation, and supplemental oxygen as necessary.

Cardiovascular Function

Evaluation of heart rate and rhythm, skin colour, blood pressure, perfusion, peripheral pulses, oxygen saturation, and acid–base status provides information on cardiovascular status. The nurse must be prepared to intervene if symptoms of **hypovolemia**, shock, or both are found. These symptoms include prolonged capillary refill (longer than 3 seconds); pale colour (pallor); poor muscle tone; lethargy; initial tachycardia then bradycardia; and continued respiratory distress despite the provision of adequate oxygen and ventilation. Hypotension may initially be present or may occur in some infants as a late sign of shock.

Blood pressure is monitored routinely in the sick neonate by either internal or external means. Direct recording with arterial catheters is often used but carries the risks inherent in any procedure in which a catheter is introduced into an artery. An umbilical venous catheter may also be used to monitor the neonate's central venous pressure. Oscillometry is a noninvasive, effective means for detecting alterations in systemic blood pressure (hypotension or hypertension) and implementing appropriate therapy to maintain cardiovascular function.

Body Temperature

Preterm infants are susceptible to temperature instability as a result of numerous factors:

- Large surface area in relation to body weight
- Minimal insulating subcutaneous fat
- Limited stores of brown fat (an internal source for the generation of heat present in normal term infants)
- Decreased or absent reflex control of skin capillaries (vasoconstriction)
- Inadequate muscle mass activity (resulting in inability to produce own heat)
- Poor muscle tone (resulting in more body surface area being exposed to the cooling effects of the environment)
- An immature temperature regulation centre in the brain
- Increased insensible water losses
- Decreased ability to increase oxygen consumption
- Decreased caloric intake

The goal of thermoregulation is a **neutral thermal environment** (NTE), which is the environmental temperature at which oxygen consumption and metabolic rate are minimal but adequate to maintain the body temperature (Blackburn, 2007). The NTE for preterm infants weighing less than 1000 g is very narrow, and the prediction of NTE for each infant is impossible. Extremely immature infants may require environmental temperatures equal to or greater than skin and core temperature to achieve thermoneutrality (Blackburn, 2007). With knowledge of the four mechanisms of heat transfer (i.e., convection, conduction, radiation, and evaporation), the nurse can create an environment for the preterm infant that prevents temperature instability (see Fig. 24-1). Since overheating produces an increase in oxygen and calorie consumption, the infant is also jeopardized if he or she becomes hyperthermic (apnea and flushed colour may indicate hyperthermia). Unlike an older child, the preterm infant is not able to sweat and thus dissipate heat.

Central Nervous System Function

The preterm infant's central nervous system (CNS) is susceptible to injury as a result of the following:

- Birth trauma with damage to immature intracranial structures
- Bleeding from fragile capillaries
- Impaired coagulation process, including prolonged prothrombin time
- Recurrent hypoxic and hyperoxic episodes
- Predisposition to hypoglycemia
- Fluctuating systemic blood pressure with concomitant variation in cerebral blood flow and pressure

In the preterm neonate, neurological function depends on gestational age, illness factors, and predisposing factors (i.e., intrauterine asphyxia). Clinical signs of neurological dysfunction may be subtle, nonspecific, or specific. A neurological assessment should be completed and include an assessment of tone, symmetry and quality of movements, reflexes, and cranial nerves (Blackburn, 2009a; 2009b; Heaberlin, 2009). Preterm infants should be evaluated for seizure activity, hyperirritability, CNS depression, elevated intracranial pressure, and abnormal movements (Blackburn & Ditzenberger, 2007). Primary and tendon reflexes are generally present in preterm infants by 28 weeks of gestation and should be part of the neurological examination. Ongoing assessment and documentation of these neurological signs are needed for their predictive value, discharge teaching, and follow-up recommendations.

Nutritional Status

The initial goal of neonatal nutrition in the preterm infant is to prevent catabolism and excess fluid losses. Once the infant condition has stabilized, the goal of nutrition is to promote optimal growth and development. Maintenance of adequate nutrition in the preterm infant is complicated by problems with intake and metabolism of nutrients adequate to promote physical growth, including brain growth. The preterm infant has the following disadvantages with regard to intake of adequate nutrients: weak or absent suck, swallow, and gag reflexes; small stomach capacity; and immature digestive capacity. The preterm infant's metabolic functions are compromised by a limited store of nutrients, a decreased ability to digest proteins and absorb nutrients, and immature enzyme systems.

The nurse must continually assess the infant's nutritional status. Preterm infants often require parenteral (intravenous [IV]) nutrition or gavage feedings instead of oral feedings, depending on the gestational age, birth weight, and comorbidities, such as respiratory distress.

Renal Function

The preterm infant's immature renal system is unable to (1) adequately excrete metabolites and drugs; (2) concentrate urine; or (3) maintain acid–base, fluid, or electrolyte balance. Therefore, intake and output, as well as specific gravity, must be assessed. Laboratory tests must be performed to assess acid–base and electrolyte balance. Medication levels (e.g., gentamycin) are also monitored in preterm infants because metabolism via renal and hepatic routes is often hindered. Because of great variability in drug metabolism, serum levels are obtained to ensure adequate therapeutic range for treatment and to prevent toxicity.

Hematological Status

The preterm infant is predisposed to hematological problems because of the following conditions:

- Increased capillary fragility
- Increased tendency to bleed (prolonged prothrombin time and partial thromboplastin time)
- Decreased production of red blood cells (RBCs) resulting from physiological rapid decrease in erythropoiesis after birth
- Large amount of fetal hemoglobin (up to 80% of total volume)
- Loss of blood attributable to frequent blood sampling for laboratory tests
- Decreased RBC survival related to the increased size of the RBC and its increased permeability to sodium and potassium
- Decreased levels of circulating albumin

The nurse needs to assess such infants for any evidence of bleeding from puncture sites, the gastrointestinal tract, and pulmonary system. Infants should also be examined for signs of anemia (e.g., decreased hemoglobin and hematocrit levels, pale skin or pallor, apnea, lethargy, tachycardia, and poor weight gain). In high-risk infants, the amount of blood withdrawn for laboratory testing should be monitored.

Infection Prevention

While protection from infection is an integral part of all newborn care, preterm and sick infants are particularly susceptible to infectious organisms. As with all aspects of care, strict hand hygiene is the single most important measure to prevent hospital acquired infections. Personnel with known infectious disorders should be excluded from the unit until they are no longer infectious. Routine practices need to be instituted in all nursery areas as a method of infection control to protect the infants and staff (see Box 6-7).

Neonates are highly susceptible to infection, as a result of diminished nonspecific (inflammatory) and specific (humoral) **immunity**, such as impaired phagocytosis, delayed chemotactic response, decreased complement levels, and minimal or absent immune globulins (Ig) A and M. Because of the infant's poor response to pathogenic agents, there is usually no local inflammatory reaction at the portal of entry to signal an infection, and symptoms tend to be vague and nonspecific. Consequently, diagnosis and treatment may be delayed. Preterm and term infants exhibit various nonspecific signs and symptoms of infection (Box 27-2). Early identification and treatment of sepsis are essential.

Parental Adaptation to the Preterm Infant

Parents who experience the preterm birth of their infant have a much different experience from that of parents giving birth

BOX 27-2 Signs and Symptoms of Neonatal Infection

Signs and symptoms are subtle and nonspecific and include the following:

Temperature instability
- Hypothermia—most common
- Hyperthermia—rarely

Central nervous system changes
- Lethargy
- Irritability
- Altered level of consciousness

Changes in colour
- Cyanosis, pallor
- Mottling
- Jaundice

Cardiovascular instability
- Poor perfusion
- Prolonged capillary refill (>3 seconds)
- Hypotension
- Bradycardia or tachycardia

Respiratory distress
- Tachypnea or bradypnea
- Apnea
- Retractions, nasal flaring, grunting
- Gastrointestinal problems
- Feeding intolerance, increased residuals (when gavage fed)
- Abdominal distension
- Vomiting
- Diarrhea
- Bloody stools (frank or occult positive)
- Metabolic instability
- Glucose instability
- Metabolic acidosis

Other
- Electrolyte imbalance
- Decreased urine output

to a term infant. Thus, parental attachment and adaptation to the parental role may also differ.

Parental Tasks

Parents of preterm infants must accomplish a number of psychological tasks before effective relationships and parenting patterns can evolve. These tasks include the following:

- Experiencing anticipatory grief over the potential loss of the infant. The parents grieve in preparation for the possibility of the infant's death, while clinging to the hope that the infant will survive. This may begin during labour and often lasts until the infant dies or shows evidence of surviving.
- The mother accepting failure to give birth to a healthy, term infant. Grief and depression typify this phase, which persists until the infant is out of danger and is expected to survive.
- Resuming the process of relating to the infant. As the infant's condition improves, the parents can continue the process of developing the attachment to the infant that was interrupted by the infant's critical condition at birth.
- Learning how this infant differs in growth patterns, caregiving needs, and growth and development expectations
- Adapting the home environment to the needs of the new infant (i.e., limiting visitors and exposure to pathogens, adjusting household temperature)

Grandparents and siblings also react to the birth of a preterm infant. Parents may have to deal with grandparents' grief, in addition to bewilderment and anger of the infant's siblings at the amount of parental time spent with the newborn.

Parental Responses

Parents progress through stages as they interact with their infant, from maintaining an **en face** position and stroking and touching their infant (Fig. 27-1) to assuming some child care activities, such as feeding, bathing, and diapering the infant.

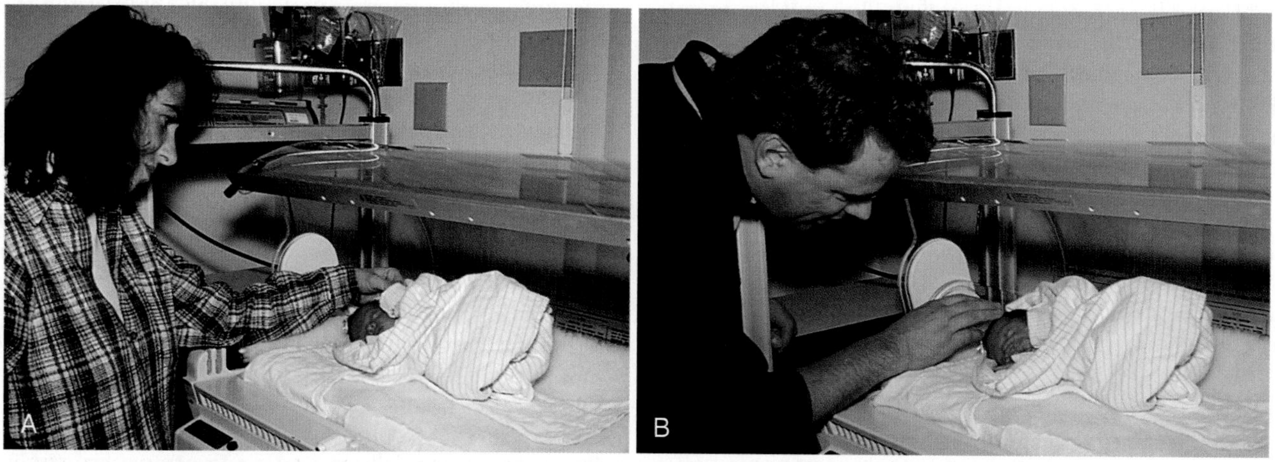

Fig. 27-1 **A:** Mother interacts with her preterm infant by touch. **B:** Father interacts with his newborn by stroking and touching the infant with his fingertips. *(Courtesy Michael S. Clement, MD, Mesa, AZ.)*

Parental Maladaptation

The incidence of physical and emotional abuse is greater among infants who, because of preterm birth or a high-risk condition, are separated from their parents after birth. Physical abuse includes varying degrees of poor nutrition, poor hygiene, and bodily harm. Emotional abuse ranges from subtle lack of interest to outright dislike of the infant. Resources should be made available to assess the parents' feelings about the preterm infant's birth. In addition, proper guidance and counselling should be made available, before and after discharge, to help families adjust to and care for the preterm infant. The ultimate goal is for the family to incorporate the infant as a regular member into their family (see Critical Thinking Exercise).

Factors surrounding the birth may predispose parents to subconsciously or overtly rejecting the infant. These factors might include parental anxiety, unmet personal expectations of the birth experience, financial considerations and extra costs related to the infant's care, or discord in the mother's relationship with her partner. Health care professionals need to identify parents' inadequate coping skills and potentially dysfunctional parenting in order to prevent further problems and enable early intervention.

The nursing process in the care of the preterm and late preterm infant is outlined in the Nursing Process box.

Implementation

The best environment for fetal growth and development is in the uterus of a healthy, well-nourished woman. The goal of care for the preterm infant is to provide an extrauterine environment that approximates a healthy intrauterine environment in order to promote optimal growth and development. Medical and nursing personnel, respiratory therapists, occupational therapists and physiotherapists, dieticians, social workers, case managers, and pharmacists must work as a team to provide the intensive care needed.

The admission of a preterm infant to the intensive care nursery is usually an emergency situation. A rapid initial assessment must be performed to determine the infant's need for lifesaving treatment.

When required, resuscitation is started in the birthing unit and the infant is supported en route to the nursery, where additional resuscitative and stabilization measures are implemented.

Physical Care

The preterm infant's environmental support typically consists of the following equipment and procedures:

- Incubator or radiant warmer to control body temperature and maintain NTE
- Ventilatory support (assisted or mechanical ventilation, oxygen, or both, as necessary)
- Electronic monitoring of respiratory, cardiac, and oxygenation status
- Assistive devices for positioning the infant
- Clustering of care to minimize stimulation and handling

Various metabolic support measures that may be instituted consist of the following:

- Parenteral fluids to support nutrition, hydration, fluid, and electrolyte balance
- IV access for fluids, parenteral nutrition, and medication administration
- Blood work to monitor arterial blood gases (ABGs), glucose, electrolytes, and other diagnostic studies (e.g., complete blood count [CBC]) as indicated

Maintaining Body Temperature

The high-risk infant is susceptible to heat loss and its complications (see Fig. 24-2). In addition, LBW infants may be unable to increase their metabolic rate because of impaired gas exchange, caloric intake restrictions, or poor thermoregulation. Transepidermal water loss (TEWL) is greater in ELBW and VLBW infants and can contribute to temperature instability. The high-risk infant should be transferred from the delivery room in a prewarmed incubator; ELBW infants may be placed in a food-grade polyethylene bag (or wrap) to decrease heat and water loss. Skin-to-skin (kangaroo) contact between the stable preterm infant and parent can help maintain body temperature.

High-risk infants may need an external heat source to achieve an NTE. A probe applied to the infant is attached to the external heat source supplied by a radiant warmer or a servocontrolled incubator. Normal axillary temperatures in the preterm or at-risk newborn may range between 36.3° and 37.2°C (ACoRN, 2010; Brown & Landers, 2011). Guidelines for maintaining NTE in the LBW infant are published; however, further research is needed to define an NTE for the ELBW infant (Brown & Landers, 2011).

CRITICAL THINKING EXERCISE

Late Preterm Infant

A 2010 g male infant is born at an estimated gestational age of 35 weeks. The parents are very excited because they have been trying to become pregnant for 6 years. The baby is placed on the mother's (Patti) abdomen after delivery for skin-to-skin contact but does not breastfeed. The nurse, while assessing the baby, notes that he has some mild grunting, nasal flaring, and intercostal retractions. As a result, the baby is taken to the special care nursery for further evaluation and treatment. Martin, the father, asks when they will be able to hold their son again. Patti is crying and asks to have her baby brought back to her as soon as his condition is stable because she really wants to breastfeed him.

1. Evidence—Is there sufficient evidence to draw conclusions about what to tell Patti and Martin about their infant son?
2. Assumptions—What assumptions can be made about the following?
   a. The mother's and father's reaction to their son's birth
   b. The infant's expected progress
   c. The possibility of Patti breastfeeding the baby
3. What implications and priorities for nursing care can be drawn at this time?
4. Does the evidence objectively support your conclusion?
5. Are there alternative perspectives to your conclusion?

NURSING PROCESS: PRETERM AND LATE PRETERM INFANT CARE

Assessment
The high-risk infant must undergo an initial physical assessment for life-threatening problems. The stable high-risk infant should undergo an initial physical assessment as well as a gestational-age assessment to identify potential risk factors.

Nursing Diagnoses
The following nursing diagnoses may be applicable to high-risk infants and their parents:

Ineffective breathing pattern related to
- decreased number of functional alveoli
- surfactant deficiency
- immature respiratory control
- increased pulmonary vascular resistance

Ineffective thermoregulation related to
- immature central nervous system thermoregulatory control
- increased heat loss to environment and inability to produce heat due to decreased brown fat reserves
- greater body surface exposed to environment

Risk for infection related to
- invasive procedures
- decreased immune response
- ineffective skin barrier

Anxiety (parental) related to
- lack of knowledge about the infant's condition and prognosis (uncertain outcome)
- inability to perform expected caregiving activities
- neonatal intensive care unit (NICU) environment noise and high-tech care

Planning and Implementation
Expected outcomes can apply to either the high-risk infant or the parents and are presented in patient-centred terms. For example, expected outcomes for the infant include that the infant will do the following:
- Maintain adequate physiological functioning (airway, breathing, circulation)
- Receive adequate nutrition for growth
- Maintain stable body temperature
- Remain free of infection
- Experience appropriate parent–infant interactions

Expected outcomes for the parents include that they will do the following:
- Perceive the infant as a family member
- Provide infant care confidently and competently
- Experience pride and satisfaction in the care of the infant
- Organize their time and energies to meet the love, attention, and care needs of the other members of the family as well as their own needs

Numerous nursing implementation strategies are discussed on pp. 710-733.

Evaluation
The nurse can be reasonably assured that care was effective to the extent that expected outcomes for the infant and parents have been achieved.

Care of the Hypothermic Infant
Rapid changes in body temperature may cause apnea and acidosis in the neonate. Therefore, warming a hypothermic infant should occur over a period of hours. Rapid rewarming may cause apnea; too slow rewarming increases metabolic distress and oxygen consumption. Rewarming can proceed at a rate of 1° to 2°C per hour. Rewarming should be individualized for each infant and a servocontrolled environment (radiant warmer or incubator) used. If the infant's condition allows, skin-to-skin contact is an effective method to regulate or increase body temperature.

Transition From the Incubator
To effectively wean the infant from the incubator, the incubator heat is decreased slowly over several hours to days. Infants who are medically stable and gaining weight, tolerate enteral feedings, and weigh 1300 to 1500 g may be transitioned from the incubator. The following guidelines may be followed to wean the infant from the incubator:
- Disconnect the servocontrol probe (if still in use).
- Dress the infant in a diaper, shirt, and cap.
- Lower the incubator temperature no more than 0.5°C every 2 hours.
- Record the temperature of the infant, the air, and the incubator.
- Assess the infant's responses to the changes every hour until four stable readings are obtained.
- Monitor the infant's temperature and other vital signs.

This procedure is repeated until the incubator temperature is the same as the room temperature and the infant's body temperature consistently remains within normal limits. The infant is then placed in an open bassinet (away from any drafts) and reassessed during routine care. If the infant is unable to maintain his or her temperature, the infant is returned to the incubator and the weaning process restarted once the infant is able to regulate his or her temperature. Consistent weight gain and absence of any clinical distress signs (poor feeding, respiratory distress, and temperature instability) are measures of effective weaning to an open bassinet.

Oxygen Therapy
The goals of oxygen therapy are to provide adequate oxygen to the tissues, prevent lactic acid accumulation resulting from **hypoxia**, and avoid the potentially negative effects of hyperoxemia and free radicals. Numerous methods are available to improve oxygenation. All require that the oxygen be warmed and humidified before entering the respiratory tract. If the infant does not require mechanical ventilation, varying concentrations of supplemental oxygen can be supplied by

placement of a plastic hood over the infant's head, by nasal cannula, or by nasal continuous positive airway pressure (CPAP). Because oxygen therapy has inherent risks, each infant must be carefully monitored to prevent hyperoxemia and hypoxemia.

Infants who require oxygen should have frequent assessments of respiratory status and oxygenation; the timing of assessments is based on the infant's status. Oxygenation assessment includes continuous pulse oximetry and ABGs, as ordered. Vital signs should be monitored to ensure adequacy of respiratory function, circulation, and perfusion of tissues.

Preliminary studies of the resuscitation of asphyxiated newborns with 21% oxygen, rather than 100% oxygen, have demonstrated no significant neurological morbidities at 18 to 24 months in newborns resuscitated with 21% oxygen (Saugstad et al., 2003). Proponents of room air resuscitation suggest that fewer complications are associated with oxidative stress and hyperoxemia when room air is administered (Vento et al., 2003). As a result of the International Liaison Committee on Resuscitation (ILCOR) review, the 2010 guidelines for neonatal resuscitation recommend that resuscitation begin with no supplemental oxygen (i.e., 21% oxygen or room air); however, if the infant's condition does not improve within 90 seconds, supplemental oxygen should be available for use. The goal is to minimize oxygen free radicals and avoid both hyperoxia and hypoxia (Perlman et al., 2010). A review of several studies indicates that neonatal mortality is reduced by 30 to 40% when room air is used, instead of 100% oxygen, for neonatal resuscitation; rates of retinopathy of prematurity (ROP) and bronchopulmonary dysplasia (BPD) are lower in infants whose saturation (Sa_{O_2}) is kept between 93 and 95%. Fluctuations in oxygen saturation are also deemed harmful. It is recommended that for ELBW infants, oxygen saturations be maintained at 85 to 93% and not exceed 95% (Saugstad, 2007).

Oxygen Hood

Oxygen in a specified concentration can be administered via hood to infants who do not require positive-pressure mechanical support. The hood is a clear plastic cover sized to fit over the head and neck of the infant (Fig. 27-2, A). Continuous pulse oximetry is used to monitor oxygenation and titrate the amount of oxygen being delivered according to the infant's condition.

Nasal Cannula

Low-flow oxygen can be administered by nasal cannula (see Fig. 27-2, B). A nasal cannula is used for infants who require low concentrations of supplemental oxygen; this is often used for home oxygen administration. The infant receives supplemental oxygen while having optimal vision, positioning, and parental holding. Infants can also breast or bottle feed while receiving oxygen by this method. The nasal prongs must be inspected often to ensure that they are not partially obstructed by milk or secretions.

Continuous Distending Pressure

Infants who are unable to maintain adequate oxygenation (Pa_{O_2}) despite the administration of oxygen by hood or nasal cannula may require the use of continuous distending airway pressure via CPAP. CPAP delivers oxygen at a preset pressure (Fig. 27-3, A) by means of nasal prongs, nasopharyngeal tubes, endotracheal tube, or face mask. Nasal prongs are the most common method of CPAP delivery. CPAP increases the functional residual capacity, improves the diffusion time of pulmonary gases, and can decrease pulmonary vascular resistance (PVR) and intrapulmonary shunting. If implemented early enough, CPAP may preclude the need for mechanical ventilation. CPAP is the preferred mode for infants who require minor distending pressure, as it avoids the trauma associated with endotracheal intubation and its inherent complications (Gardner, Enzman-Hines, & Dickey, 2011). The infant with a nasal CPAP device must be monitored closely for signs of nasal damage and skin breakdown (Squires & Hyndman, 2009). An orogastric tube may be needed to decompress the stomach during the use of CPAP.

Mechanical Ventilation

Mechanical ventilation must be implemented if other methods of therapy cannot correct abnormalities in oxygenation. Its use is indicated whenever blood gas values reveal severe hypoxemia or severe **hypercapnia** (see Fig. 27-3, B). Mechanical ventilation may be required for the infant with apnea, **meconium aspiration syndrome** (MAS), respiratory distress syndrome (RDS), or congenital defects. Ventilator

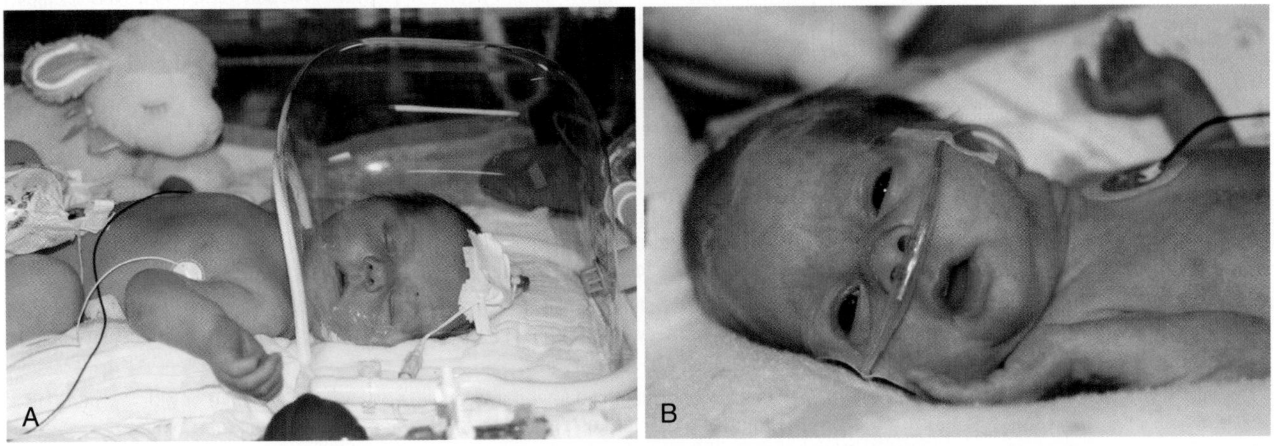

Fig. 27-2 **A:** Infant under hood. **B:** Infant with nasal cannula. *(Courtesy Victoria Langer, RNC, MSN, NNP. From Dickason, E., Silverman, B., & Kaplan, J. [1998].* Maternal–infant nursing care *[3rd ed.]. St. Louis: Mosby.)*

settings are individualized: the ventilator is set to provide a predetermined amount of oxygen during spontaneous respirations and to provide assisted ventilation in the absence of spontaneous respirations. Newer technologies allow oxygen to be delivered at lower pressures and in assist modes. This decreases barotrauma and associated complications such as pneumothorax and pulmonary interstitial emphysema (Greenough & Sharma, 2005, 2007; Wheeler et al., 2010). Table 27-2 outlines the types of mechanical ventilation used in newborns.

Surfactant Replacement Therapy

Surfactant is a surface-active phospholipid secreted by the alveolar epithelium. Surfactant acts much like a detergent and reduces the surface tension of fluids that line the alveoli and

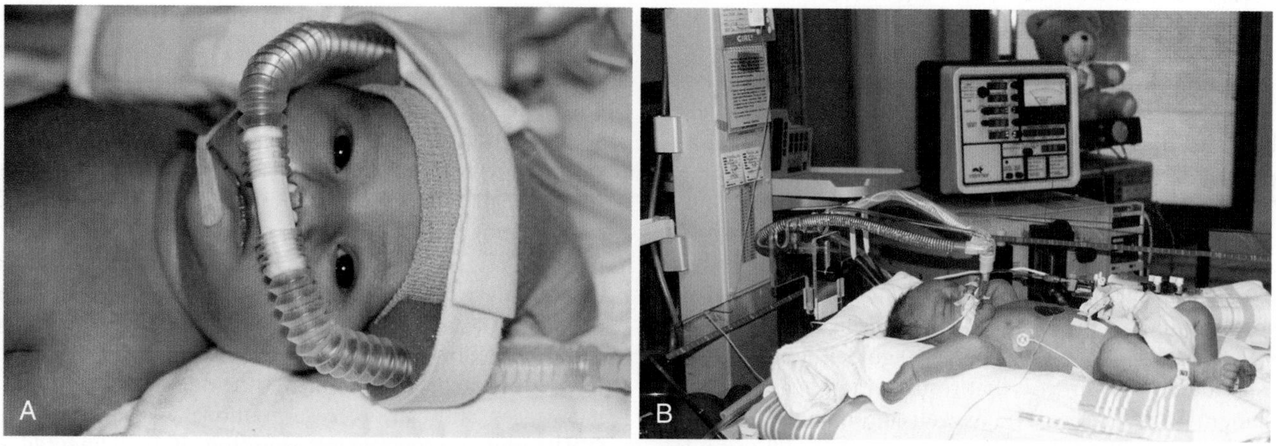

Fig. 27-3 **A:** Infant receiving ventilatory assistance with nasal continuous positive airway pressure (CPAP). **B:** Infant intubated and on ventilator. *(Courtesy Victoria Langer, RNC, MSN, NNP. From Dickason, E., Silverman, B., & Kaplan, J. [1998].* Maternal–infant nursing care *[3rd ed.]. St. Louis: Mosby.)*

Table 27-2 Common Methods for Assisted Ventilation in Neonatal Respiratory Distress*

METHOD	DESCRIPTION	HOW PROVIDED
Continuous positive airway pressure (CPAP)	Provides constant distending pressure to airway in spontaneously breathing infant	Nasal prongs Endotracheal tube Face mask and flow inflating bag Nasal cannula or nasopharyngeal tubes Bubble CPAP using water resistance
Intermittent mandatory ventilation (IMV)	Provides mechanically cycled respirations and pressure at regular preset intervals; infant is able to breathe spontaneously and may have asynchronous ventilation efforts, which diminishes effective gas exchange, air leaks, and air trapping; uses positive end-expiratory pressure (PEEP)	Endotracheal intubation
Synchronized intermittent mandatory ventilation (SIMV)	Mechanically delivered breaths are synchronized to the onset of spontaneous patient breaths Assist/control (A/C) mode facilitates full inspiratory synchrony; involves signal detection of onset of spontaneous respiration from abdominal movement, thoracic impedance, and airway pressure or flow changes Pressure support ventilation provides inspiratory pressure assist when spontaneous breathing is detected to decrease infant's work of breathing	Patient-triggered infant ventilator with signal detector and A/C mode; endotracheal tube SIMV, A/C, and pressure support are also referred to as patient-triggered ventilation
Volume guarantee ventilation	Delivers a predetermined volume of gas using inspiratory pressure that varies according to the infant's lung compliance (often used in conjunction with SIMV)	Volume guarantee ventilator with flow sensor; endotracheal tube
High-frequency oscillation (HFO)	Application of high-frequency, low-volume, sine-wave flow oscillations to airway at rates between 480 and 1200 breaths/min	Variable-speed piston pump (or loudspeaker, fluidic oscillator); endotracheal tube
High-frequency jet ventilation (HFJV)	Uses a separate, parallel, low-compliant circuit and injector port to deliver small pulses or jets of fresh gas deep into airway at rates between 250 and 900 breaths/min	May be used alone or with low-rate IMV; endotracheal tube

*This is not a comprehensive list of available ventilation modes. For more information, consult specific references on mechanical ventilation, such as Donn and Sinha (2003), Gardner, Enzman-Hines, and Dickey (2011), and Wheeler et al. (2010).

respiratory passages. This results in uniform expansion and maintenance of lung expansion at low intra-alveolar pressure. Immature lung development and surfactant deficiency can produce consequences that seriously compromise respiratory efficiency. Deficient surfactant production causes unequal inflation of alveoli on inspiration and the collapse of alveoli on expiration. Without surfactant, infants are unable to keep their lungs inflated and thus exert a great deal of effort to re-expand the alveoli with each breath. As infants tire, they are able to open fewer and fewer alveoli. This inability to maintain lung expansion produces widespread atelectasis.

A lack of alveolar stability (normal functional residual capacity) and progressive atelectasis cause PVR to increase. As a result, there is decreased pulmonary blood flow, and hypoperfusion of the lung tissue occurs. The increase in PVR causes partial reversion to the fetal circulation, with right-to-left shunting of blood through the persisting fetal communications—the ductus arteriosus and foramen ovale. Inadequate pulmonary perfusion and ventilation produce hypoxemia and hypercapnia. Pulmonary arterioles, with their thick muscular layer, are highly reactive to diminished oxygen concentration. Decreased oxygen tension causes vasoconstriction in the pulmonary arterioles; vasoconstriction leads to hypoxemia, which in turn is exacerbated by a decrease in blood pH. Vasoconstriction contributes to a significant increase in PVR. In contrast, during normal transition, with adequate ventilation and increasing oxygen concentration, the ductus arteriosus constricts and the pulmonary vessels dilate to decrease PVR.

Surfactant can be administered as an adjunct to oxygen and ventilation therapy. Generally, infants born before 32 weeks of gestation do not have adequate amounts of pulmonary surfactant. In many centres the use of prophylactic surfactant is reserved for infants at greatest risk for RDS, those between 29 and 32 weeks of gestation (Gardner et al., 2011; Soll & Morley, 2001; Stevens, Blennow, Myers, & Soll, 2007). Exogenous surfactant is manufactured synthetically or extracted from bovine, porcine, or calf lung extract. A course of one or two doses is given through an endotracheal tube. The infant must be monitored for potential adverse effects (apnea, bradycardia, desaturation, plugging of the endotracheal tube, pulmonary hemorrhage). Surfactant has been associated with a significant decrease in duration mechanical ventilation and oxygen therapy. Despite an increased survival rate in preterm infants, surfactant has not significantly decreased the incidence of BPD, intraventricular hemorrhage (IVH), or patent ductus arteriosus (PDA) in extremely immature infants.

When comparing the effects of natural versus synthetic surfactant, studies have shown rapid improvement of respiratory status, less ROP and BPD, lower mortality, and decreased incidence of pneumothorax in infants who received natural surfactant (Gardner et al., 2011; Soll & Blanco, 2001). However, newer synthetic surfactant products may be equally effective. Early administration of surfactant is recommended (Davis et al., 2005; Stevens et al., 2007) for infants with or at risk for RDS, especially ELBW infants and those not exposed to maternal antenatal steroids. The administration of antenatal steroids and surfactant replacement has decreased the incidence of RDS and concomitant morbidities.

Inhaled nitric oxide (INO) and extracorporeal membrane oxygenation (ECMO) are additional therapies used in the treatment of severe respiratory distress and respiratory failure in neonates. INO is used in term and late preterm infants with **persistent pulmonary hypertension** of the newborn (PPHN), MAS, pneumonia, sepsis, and congenital diaphragmatic hernia, to decrease or reverse pulmonary hypertension and vasoconstriction, acidosis, and hypoxemia. Nitric oxide is a colourless, highly diffusible gas that is administered blended with oxygen, through the ventilator circuit. INO therapy may be used in conjunction with surfactant replacement therapy, high-frequency ventilation, or ECMO. INO has been proved to be significantly effective in decreasing RDS and in improving survival rates in preterm infants, although clinical trials are still ongoing (Barrington & Finer, 2007). Clinical trials have demonstrated that the use of INO improved ventilatory status in infants with pulmonary hypertension, decreased requirements for ventilatory support (Sadiq, Mantych, Benawra, Deveskar, & Hocker, 2003), and decreased the need for ECMO (Field et al., 2007).

ECMO may also be used in the management of term infants with acute severe respiratory failure. This therapy involves a modified heart-lung machine, although with ECMO the heart is not stopped and blood does not entirely bypass the lungs. Blood is shunted from a catheter in the right atrium or right internal jugular vein by gravity to a servoregulated roller pump, pumped through a membrane lung where it is oxygenated, through a small heat exchanger where it is warmed, and then returned to the systemic circulation via a major artery (carotid) to the aortic arch. ECMO provides oxygen to the circulation, allowing the lungs to "rest," and decreases pulmonary hypertension and hypoxemia seen with PPHN, congenital diaphragmatic hernia (CDH), sepsis, MAS, and severe pneumonia. ECMO is not used in infants less than 34 weeks' gestation because the anticoagulant therapy required in the pump and circuits may increase the potential for IVH in these infants. In some centres, the success of high-frequency ventilation and INO has greatly decreased the demand for ECMO.

High-Frequency Ventilation

Other modes of ventilator therapy include high-frequency oscillator ventilation and jet ventilation (see Table 27-2). These methods of high-frequency ventilation work by providing smaller volumes of oxygen at a significantly more rapid rate (more than 300 breaths/min) than traditional mechanical ventilators. As a result, the intrathoracic pressure and the risk of barotrauma are decreased.

Weaning From Ventilatory Support

The infant is ready to be weaned from ventilatory support when acid–base balance, ABGs, and oxygen saturation are maintained within normal limits. A spontaneous, adequate respiratory effort must be present, and the infant must show sustained muscle tone during spontaneous respirations. Weaning is done in a stepwise, gradual manner. The infant may be extubated, placed on nasal CPAP, and then weaned to oxygen alone. Throughout the weaning process, the infant's oxygen levels are monitored by pulse oximetry, ABGs, or both.

Some infants are not able to be weaned from oxygen by the time of discharge and may require home oxygen therapy. BPD, congenital anomalies (CDH or tracheal defect), or a neurological insult may prevent weaning.

Parents need to be given consistent information and be reassured about the infant's respiratory progress. Decisions regarding the nature of interventions should be included in an interprofessional care plan, and the therapy should be explained frequently to the family.

Frequent skin care assessments are essential when the infant is receiving supplemental oxygen with any of the methods described here, particularly in infants with poor perfusion and in those requiring equipment that comes in continuous contact with the infant's skin (e.g., nasal CPAP, nasal cannula, pulse oximetry probes).

Nutritional Care

Optimum nutrition is critical in the management of LBW and preterm infants, yet providing for their nutritional needs is difficult. The various mechanisms for ingestion and digestion of foods are not fully developed; the more immature the infant, the greater the challenge. In addition, the nutritional requirements for this group of infants are not known with certainty. It is known that all preterm infants are at risk for nutritional compromise because of poor nutritional stores and physical (immaturity of the gastrointestinal tract) and developmental characteristics (lack of coordinated suck, swallow, and breathe reflexes).

Although some sucking and swallowing activities are demonstrated before birth and in preterm infants, coordination of these mechanisms does not occur until approximately 32 to 34 weeks of gestation, and these activities are not fully synchronized until 36 to 37 weeks. Initial sucking is not accompanied by swallowing, and esophageal contractions are uncoordinated. The gag reflex may not be developed until 36 weeks. Consequently, infants are prone to aspiration and complications thereof. As infants mature, the suck–swallow pattern develops, but it is slow and ineffectual, and these reflexes may also become easily exhausted.

The amount and method of feeding are determined by the infant's size and condition. Nutrition can be provided by either the parenteral or enteral route or by a combination of the two. ELBW, VLBW, or critically ill infants are often initially fed exclusively via the parenteral route because of their inability to digest and absorb enteral nutrition. Organ immaturity and conditions resulting in hypoxia further preclude the use of enteral feeding until the infant's condition has stabilized. **Necrotizing enterocolitis** (NEC) has been associated with enteral feedings in acutely ill or distressed infants (see p. 731). Total parenteral nutrition (TPN) support of acutely ill infants may be accomplished with commercially available IV solutions of protein, amino acids, trace minerals, vitamins, carbohydrates (dextrose), and fat (lipid emulsion). There is evidence to support early (within hours of birth) introduction of parenteral nutrition with the introduction of minimal enteral feedings within the first 5 days of life.

Early introduction of small amounts of enteral feedings in metabolically stable preterm infants is beneficial and has been shown to stimulate the infant's gastrointestinal tract, preventing mucosal atrophy and subsequent enteral feeding difficulties; improve developmental outcome; and prevent growth failure (American Academy of Pediatrics [AAP], 2009; Anderson, Wood, Keller, & Hay, 2011; Ehrenkranz, 2007). Minimal feedings, as little as 0.1 to 4 mL/kg of breast milk or preterm formula, may be given by gavage as early as the first or second postnatal day. Parenteral hydration and nutrition continue until the infant is able to tolerate an amount of enteral feeding sufficient to sustain growth. An increased incidence of NEC in VLBW infants fed with minimal enteral feedings has not been substantiated (Bombell & McGuire, 2008; Henderson, Craig, Brocklehurst, & McGuire, 2009; Mosqueda, Sapiegiene, Glynn, Wilson-Colstello, & Weiss, 2008). Support for initiating minimal enteral feedings includes increased mineral absorption, increased serum calcium and alkaline phosphatase activity, and a substantial decrease in the incidence of bilious gastric residuals and feeding intolerance in preterm infants (Donovan, Puppala, Angst, & Coyle, 2006; Simpson, Schanler, & Lau, 2002).

Type of Nourishment

The types of formulas used, method and volume of feeding, and the infant's feeding schedule are based on assessment of the following variables:

- Weight of the infant
- Pattern of weight gain or loss (Infants <1500 g require more energy for growth and thermoregulation.)
- Presence or absence of suck and swallow reflexes
- Behavioural readiness for oral feedings
- Physical condition (presence or absence of bowel sounds, abdominal distension, bloody stools, respiratory distress, and apnea)
- Residual from previous feeding, if being gavage fed
- Malformations (especially gastrointestinal defects)
- Renal function (urine output) and laboratory values (e.g., electrolyte balance, glucose level)

Human milk is the best source of nutrition for term and preterm infants. Studies indicate that even small preterm infants are able to breastfeed, if they have adequate sucking and swallowing reflexes and no other contraindications (Morton, 2002). Mothers who wish to breastfeed their preterm infants are encouraged to pump their breasts until their infants are stable enough to tolerate breastfeeding. Guidelines for the storage of expressed mother's milk should be followed to decrease the risk of milk contamination and destruction of its beneficial properties (see Chapter 26).

Preterm infants may be able to successfully breastfeed earlier than previously believed (28 to 36 weeks). Breastfed preterm infants have fewer desaturations; warmer skin temperature; and better coordination of breathing, sucking, and swallowing than their bottle-fed counterparts (Gardner & Lawrence, 2011).

Commercially available preterm formulas are cow's milk based and whey predominant and have a higher concentration of protein, calcium, and phosphorus than do term formulas in order to meet the unique needs of the preterm infant (AAP, 2009). Most preterm formulas are either 22 or 24 kcal/30 mL. The preparation of powdered formula for preterm infants should be performed under strict aseptic technique, preferably in a pharmacy, and the formula properly refrigerated to prevent infection (Health Canada, 2010). Preterm infants fed human milk with fortifier (protein, phosphorus, and calcium) have increased weight gain and improved bone mineralization; thus, a human milk fortifier is recommended for LBW preterm infants (Lawrence & Lawrence, 2011). Supplementation with iron, vitamin D, and multivitamins may be considered in exclusively breastfed LBW infants.

NURSING ALERT In the hospital, contamination of powdered infant formula with *Enterobacter sakazakii* has been associated with serious neonatal infections, NEC, and death (Health Canada, 2010; van Acker et al., 2001). When possible, alternatives to powdered formula (i.e., liquid or concentrate) should be chosen; otherwise, such formula should be carefully mixed in a pharmacy or designated formula preparation room using aseptic technique. Continuous infusion of powdered formula should not exceed 4 hours (Centers for Disease Control and Prevention, 2002).

Hydration

High-risk infants often receive supplemental parenteral fluids to supply additional calories, electrolytes, or water. Adequate hydration is particularly important in preterm infants because their extracellular water content is higher (70% in term infants and up to 90% in preterm infants), their body surface is larger, their skin barrier is immature and unable to prevent TEWL losses, and glomerular immaturity decreases the ability to concentrate urine. Therefore, preterm infants are vulnerable to fluid depletion, fluid volume overload, and electrolyte abnormalities.

Infants who are ELBW, tachypneic, receiving phototherapy, or cared for on a radiant warmer have increased insensible water losses that require fluid administration adjustments. Methods to decrease insensible fluid losses include placement of the infant in a highly humidified (60 to 90%) microenvironment (incubator) (Gomella, Cunningham, & Eyal, 2009) and use of plastic wrap, a polyethylene bag, or emollient to decrease TEWL. Concern about the increased incidence of infection associated with the use of emollients has led to a decrease in their use (Darmstadt et al., 2005).

Nurses must monitor fluid status with daily (or more often) weighing of the infant and ensuring accurate intake and output of all fluids, including medications and blood products. Urine specific gravity and dipstick measurements are monitored per unit protocol. Serum electrolytes are obtained as warranted by the infant's condition. ELBW infants often require more frequent monitoring of these parameters because of their inordinate TEWL, immature renal function, and propensity for dehydration or overhydration. Intolerance of even dextrose 5% is not uncommon in the ELBW infant, with subsequent glycosuria and osmotic diuresis. Alterations in behaviour, alertness, or activity level in these infants may signal an electrolyte imbalance, hypoglycemia, or hyperglycemia. The nurse must also assess the VLBW or ELBW infant for tremors or seizures, as these may be a sign of electrolyte imbalance, including hyponatremia or hypernatremia. Weight gain from fluid overload in the sick preterm infant may occur as a result of fluid retention (renal failure), inappropriate fluid administration (parenteral), or congestive heart failure. An increased fluid gain may result in the opening of a previously closed PDA, thus exacerbating associated illness. Growing preterm infants, especially those with BPD and those on oral electrolyte supplements, should be carefully monitored for rapid weight gain that may result in pulmonary congestion, PDA, and electrolyte imbalance. See Box 27-3 for calculation of a weight loss or gain.

Elimination Patterns

Frequency of urination, as well as the amount, colour, pH, and specific gravity of the urine, should be assessed. The assessment of bowel movements includes frequency, character of the stool, and presence of constipation, diarrhea, or loss of fats (steatorrhea). Infants with unexplained abdominal distension are assessed carefully to rule out NEC, ileus, or gastrointestinal tract obstruction.

Oral Feeding

Nourishment by the oral route is preferred for the infant who has adequate strength and gastrointestinal function. Human milk is best and may be provided by breast, bottle, or gavage. Formula, if medically indicated, may be fed by bottle or gavage.

Many high-risk infants cannot suck well enough to breast or bottle-feed until they have recovered from their initial illness or matured physically. Preterm infants may be put to breast to practice non-nutritive suckling as soon as they are medically stable. Mothers should be encouraged to pump their breast milk. Because of the significant breastfeeding attrition rates, these mothers need support and frequent encouragement to continue pumping until their infant is able to nurse.

Gavage Feeding

Gavage feeding is a method of providing breast milk or formula through a nasogastric or orogastric tube (Fig. 27-4). It can be done either intermittently (bolus) or continuously through an indwelling feeding tube. Human milk or formula can be supplied intermittently using a syringe with gravity-controlled flow or can be given continuously using an infusion pump. The type and amount of fluid are recorded with every feed or syringe change. The volume of the continuous feedings is recorded hourly, and gastric aspirates are checked every 2 to 4 hours. When bolus feeding, residuals are measured before each feed. Residuals of less than 25% of a feeding can usually be refed to the infant. It is important to follow unit protocol for specifics and further guidance. Feeding may be stopped if

BOX 27-3 Calculation of a Weight Loss or Gain

Example 1

Day 1 = 1750 g (birth weight)
Day 3 = −1680 g
70 g *loss*

$$\frac{70\text{ g}}{1750\text{ g}} = \frac{x}{100\%}$$

$1750x = 7000\%$

$x = 7000\% \div 1750$
$x = 4.0\%$ weight loss

Example 2

Day 3 = 1680 g
Day 4 = −1720 g
− 40 g = 40 g *gain*

$$\frac{40\text{ g}}{1680\text{ g}} = \frac{x}{100\%}$$

$1680x = 4000\%$

$x = 4000\% \div 1680$
$x = 2.4\%$ weight gain

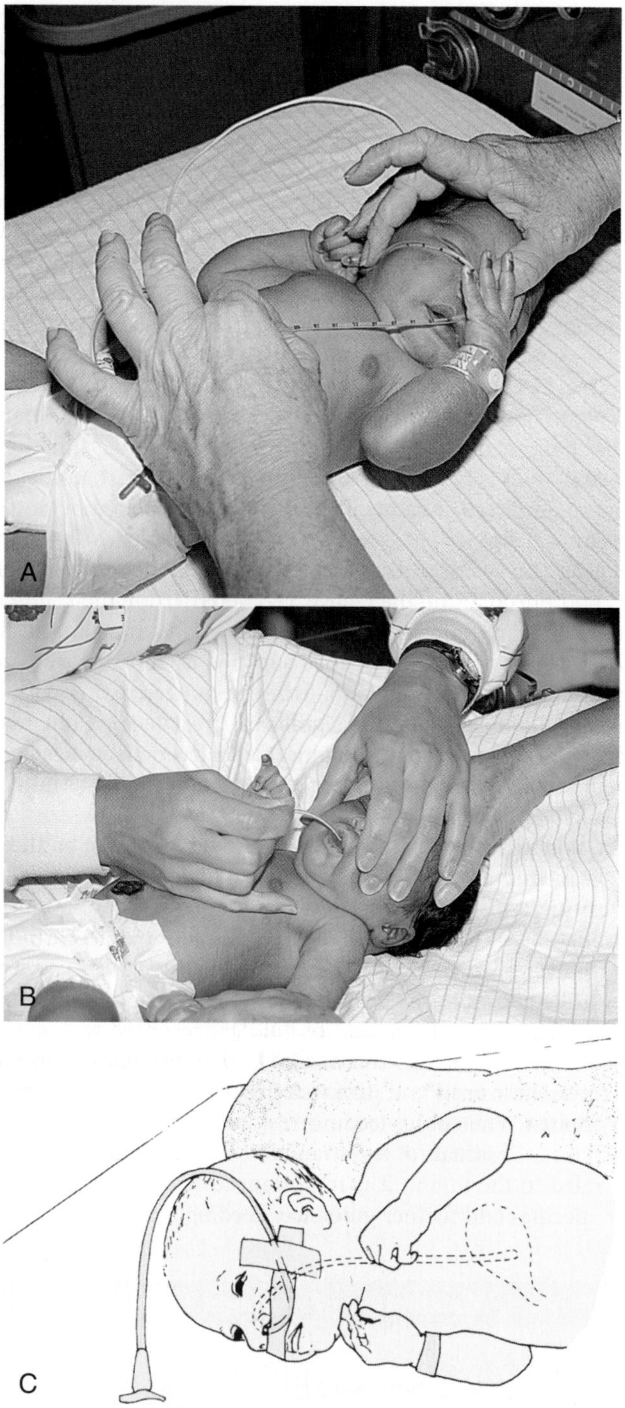

Fig. 27-4 Gavage feeding. **A:** Measurement of gavage feeding tube from tip of nose to earlobe and to midpoint between end of xiphoid process and umbilicus. Tape may be used to mark correct length on tube. **B:** Insertion of gavage tube using orogastric route. **C:** Indwelling gavage tube, nasogastric route. After feeding by orogastric or nasogastric tube, the infant is propped on right side or placed prone (preterm infant) for 1 hour to facilitate emptying of the stomach into the small intestine. Note rolled towel for support. *(**A** and **B**, Courtesy Marjorie Pyle, RNC, Lifecircle, Costa Mesa, CA.)*

the residual is greater than 2 to 4 mL/kg or more than a 1-hour volume of a continuous feed. Feeding is not resumed until the infant can be assessed for a possible feeding intolerance (Anderson et al., 2011).

Theoretically, the orogastric route for gavage feedings may be preferred, as most infants are preferential nose breathers, but this does not seem to be borne out in practice. A recent study in Canada found no consensus on the use of orogastric versus nasogastric tubes. Most of the 28 centres (75%) surveyed used nasogastric tubes the vast majority (more than 90%) of the time (Birnbaum & Limperopoulos, 2009). Smaller flexible feeding tubes (e.g., 5 Fr) may be inserted via the nasal route without interfering with the infant's breathing. The procedure for inserting a gavage feeding tube is described in Box 27-4.

To begin the feeding, the nurse connects the barrel of a syringe to the gavage tube. While clamping (or pinching) the

BOX 27-4 Procedure: Inserting a Gavage Feeding Tube

1. Measure the length of the gavage tube from the tip of the nose to the lobe of the ear to a point midway between the xiphoid process and the umbilicus (see Fig. 27-4, A). Mark the tube with a piece of tape or your finger.
2. Lubricate the tip of the tube with sterile water and insert gently through the nose or mouth (see Fig. 27-4, B) until the predetermined mark is reached. Placement of the tube in the trachea will cause the infant to gag, cough, or become cyanotic.
3. Check correct placement of the tube by doing the following:
   a. Pull back on the plunger to aspirate stomach contents. Lack of stomach aspirate or fluid is not necessarily evidence of improper placement. Aspirate consisting of respiratory secretions may be mistaken for stomach contents; however, the pH of the stomach contents is much lower (more acidic) than the pH of respiratory secretions.
   b. Perform abdominal radiography, which is 100% accurate in determining proper feeding tube placement in infants. In a small pilot study, carbon dioxide measurements of 0 (by capnography) indicated proper feeding tube placement in preterm infants (Ellett, Woodruff, & Stewart, 2007). Proper verification of feeding tube placement in neonates by assessing the pH of the aspirate has yet to be properly established (Ellett, Croffie, Cohen, & Perkins, 2005).
4. Tape the tube in place and also tape it to the cheek to prevent accidental dislodgement and incorrect positioning (see Fig. 27-4, C). Measure and record the length of tube that remains outside the nare.
   a. Assess the infant's skin integrity before taping the tube.
   b. Edematous or very preterm infants should have a pectin barrier placed under the tape to prevent abrasions, or use a hydrocolloid adhesive to prevent epidermal stripping (Lund & Durand, 2011).
5. Tube placement *must* be assessed before each feeding.

feeding tube, the nurse pours the specified amount of breast milk or formula into the syringe. The clamp is then released and the feeding allowed to flow by gravity at a rate that approximates that of an oral feeding (about 1 mL/min). The infant can be held or swaddled to help associate feeding with positive interactions.

Once the prescribed volume has been delivered, the tube is clamped or pinched and the syringe either removed or left in place. If the gavage tube is to be left in situ, it is flushed with sterile water (1–2 mL) or air. If it is to be discontinued, the gavage tube is capped (or the nurse continues to pinch it) and is removed in one steady motion. Capping or pinching the tube prevents breast milk or formula from leaking from the tube and being aspirated during removal of the tube.

Documentation of the procedure includes size of the feeding tube, amount and quality of the residual from the previous feeding, type and quantity of fluid instilled, and the infant's tolerance of the procedure.

Gastrostomy Feeding

Gastrostomy feeding involves the surgical placement of a tube through the skin of the abdomen into the stomach. With percutaneous gastrostomy insertion, feedings are often started within hours of insertion. Feedings by gravity are done slowly over 20 to 30 minutes, depending on the volume. Special care must be taken to avoid a rapid bolus of the fluid because this may lead to respiratory compromise, abdominal distension, reflux into the esophagus, or diarrhea with malabsorption. Meticulous skin care at the tube insertion site is necessary to prevent skin breakdown and infection. Intake and output should be carefully monitored to ensure adequate fluid and calorie intake and adequate renal function. Non-nutritive sucking should be offered with feeds to help the infant associate satiation with suckling.

Advancing Infant Feedings

Feedings are advanced from passive (parenteral and gavage) to active (nipple and breastfeeding) on the basis of the infant's readiness for and ability to tolerate feedings. The infant's sucking patterns and demonstration of a quiet, alert state can also be used to determine readiness to nipple feed.

The infant receiving parenteral nutrition is gradually weaned off this type of nutrition. The nourishment given by gavage feedings is increased as tolerated by the infant, and the parenteral fluids are decreased. Feedings are advanced slowly and cautiously; if feedings are advanced too rapidly, apnea, abdominal distension, vomiting, and diarrhea may result.

Gavage feedings then progress to nipple feedings (breast or bottle). Gavage feedings are decreased as the infant's ability to suckle improves. Often the infant is fed by both nipple and gavage feeding during this transition; this ensures intake of the prescribed volumes of both fluid and nutrients. The parents should be encouraged to interact by holding and talking to the infant and making eye contact with him or her during feedings.

Because preterm infants are often discharged at weights of 1500 g, the need to closely monitor nutritional intake and growth continues after discharge. Often, preterm infants have delayed growth after discharge; it has been recommended that preterm infants receive either fortified human milk or a 22 kcal/30 mL formula until postnatal age of 9 months. A suggested regimen to meet the needs of the growing LBW infant includes breastfeeding with two daily supplemental feedings of a 24 kcal/30 mL preterm formula.

Non-Nutritive Sucking

For the infant who requires gavage or parenteral feedings, non-nutritive sucking on a pacifier during the procedure may improve oxygenation and facilitate earlier transition to nipple feeding (Fig. 27-5). Non-nutritive sucking may lead to decreased energy expenditure and less restlessness. Mothers of preterm infants should be encouraged to let their infant start sucking at the breast during kangaroo care; some infants may have coordinated suck and swallow reflexes as early as 32 weeks of gestation.

Skin Care

The skin of preterm infants is immature relative to that of term infants. Because of its increased sensitivity and fragility, the use of alkaline-based soap should be avoided as it might destroy the acid mantle of the skin. **Vernix caseosa** (when present) has many, previously unrecognized benefits: it acts as an epidermal barrier, decreases bacterial contamination of the skin through its antimicrobial peptides and proteins, and decreases TEWL (Association of Women's Health, Obstetric and Neonatal Nurses [AWHONN], 2007). The increased permeability of the skin allows absorption of components such as cleansers and adhesives that may be toxic. All skin products (e.g., alcohol or povidone-iodine) should be used with caution. The skin is rinsed with sterile water after their use as these substances may cause irritation and chemical burns in LBW infants.

Adhesives used after capillary blood work or to secure IV and monitoring equipment may excoriate the skin or adhere to the surface so firmly that the epidermis is separated from understructures and pulled away with the adhesive. The use of pectin barriers and hydrocolloid adhesives may be useful because these products form well to skin contours and adhere in moist conditions. Recommendations for protecting the integrity of preterm infant skin include using minimal

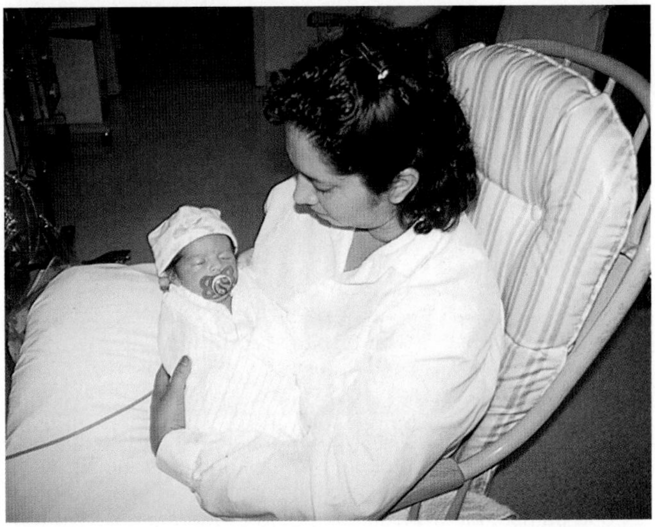

Fig. 27-5 Non-nutritive sucking by infant. *(Courtesy Marjorie Pyle, RNC, Lifecircle, Costa Mesa, CA.)*

adhesive tape, backing the tape with cotton, and delaying adhesive and pectin barrier removal until adherence is reduced (Lund & Kuller, 2007). Solvents used to remove tape are to be avoided because they tend to dry and burn the delicate skin.

An emollient (i.e., Aquaphor) may be used to promote skin integrity and prevent dry, cracking, and peeling skin in infants at risk for skin breakdown. In one small study, emollient application to the skin of infants born at less than 27 weeks' gestation decreased fluid loss during the first 2 weeks of life (Beeram, Olvera, Krauss, Loughran, & Petty, 2006). However, emollient use in infants less than 750 g has been associated with *Staphylococcus epidermidis* infection, and its use must be carefully weighed against the risk of infection (Edwards, Conner, & Soll, 2004).

Guidelines for skin care are listed in the Guidelines box. It is recommended that a validated skin assessment tool such as the Braden Q Scale or Neonatal Skin Condition Score be used once daily to evaluate the high-risk infant's skin condition in order to implement interventions aimed at minimizing skin breakdown (Curley, Razmus, Roberts, & Wypij, 2003; Lund & Osborne, 2004) (see Additional Resources.).

Environmental Concerns

Infants in neonatal intensive care units (NICUs) are exposed to high levels of auditory input from the various machine alarms (Fig. 27-6), which can have adverse effects (Haubrich, 2007). Continuous noise levels of 45 to 85 db are common in the NICU. An incubator produces a constant noise level of approximately 60 db (Thomas & Uran, 2007); each piece of life-support equipment adds to the background noise. The infant's hearing may be damaged if exposed to a constant decibel level of 90 db or frequent decibel levels higher than 110 db.

The noise level from monitoring equipment, alarms, and general unit activity has been correlated with the incidence of intracranial hemorrhage, especially in the ELBW or VLBW infant. Personnel should reduce noise-generating activities, such as slamming doors (including incubator portholes), listening to radios, talking loudly, and handling equipment (e.g., trash containers). Byers, Waugh, and Lowman (2006) suggest monitoring sound levels in the nursery to address problem areas.

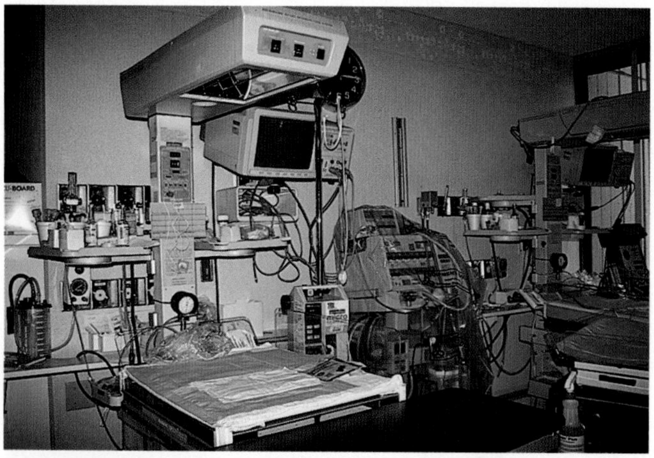

Fig. 27-6 Neonatal intensive care unit (NICU) equipment, although necessary, contributes to environmental noise. Note radiant warmer, gas outlets, suction apparatus, monitor, ventilator, and pumps, all of which contribute to the auditory environment of the NICU. *(Courtesy Marjorie Pyle, RNC, Lifecircle, Costa Mesa, CA.)*

Twenty-four-hour surveillance of sick infants implies maximum visibility and often bright lights. Units should establish a night–day sleep pattern by either darkening the room, covering cribs with blankets, or placing eye patches over the infants' eyes at night. Infants need scheduled rest periods during which the lights are dimmed, the incubators are covered with blankets, and the infants are not disturbed for handling of any kind (Fig. 27-7) (Holditch-Davis & Blackburn, 2007). Sleep periods should be undisturbed for at least 50 minutes to allow complete sleep cycles. Infants' eyes should be shielded from bright lights (e.g., procedure lighting) to prevent potential harm. Many experts suggest that the human face, especially the parent's, is the best visual stimulus and that visual stimuli be kept to a minimum early in development.

Effects of environmental hazards can be potentiated by some medications used for infant therapy. Diuretics (especially furosemide [Lasix]), ototoxic antibiotics such as gentamycin and kanamycin, and antimalarial agents can potentiate noise-induced hearing loss. Routine hearing screening should be performed on all infants before discharge.

Nurses can modify the environment to provide a neurodevelopmentally supportive milieu. In that way, the infant's neurobehavioural and physiological needs can be better met, the infant's developing organization can be supported, and growth and development can be fostered.

Developmental Care

Much attention has been focused on the effects of early developmental intervention on both term and preterm infants. Infants respond to a great variety of stimuli. As stated earlier, the atmosphere and activities of the NICU are overstimulating and can be harmful to infants in the NICU. Nursing care activities, such as taking vital signs, weighing, repositioning, and changing diapers, have been associated with periods of

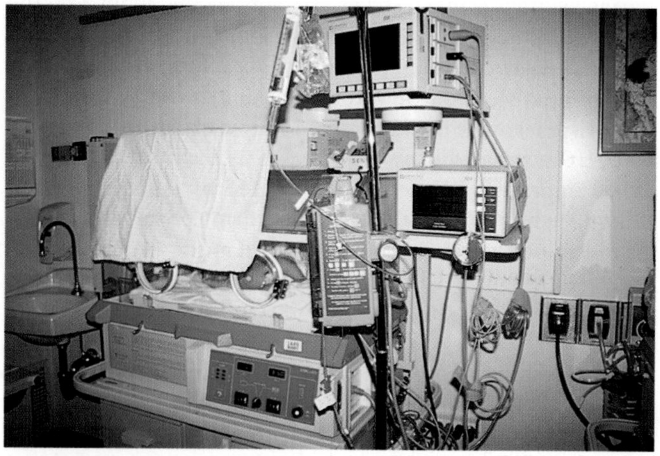

Fig. 27-7 Infant in double-walled incubator with a blanket as a light shield. *(Courtesy Marjorie Pyle, RNC, Lifecircle, Costa Mesa, CA.)*

GUIDELINES Neonatal Skin Care

General Skin Care

Assessment

- Assess skin daily or more often as needed for redness, dryness, flaking, scaling, rashes, lesions, excoriation, or breakdown. An ideal time to assess the skin integrity and condition is during the bath and with diaper changes, but assessment can be performed during vital signs and repositioning.
- Identify risk factors for skin injury: gestational age less than 30 weeks, adhesive use, high-frequency ventilation, nasal CPAP, hypotension requiring vasopressors.
- Use a valid assessment tool to provide reliable and objective measurement of skin condition (e.g., Braden Q Scale or Neonatal Skin Condition Score; see Additional Resources at end of chapter).
- Evaluate and report abnormal skin findings and analyze for possible causes.
- Intervene according to interpretation of findings or physician order.

Bathing

Initial Bath

- Assess for stable temperature a minimum of 2 to 4 hours before the first bath.
- Use cleansing agents with neutral pH and minimal dyes or perfume in water.
- Use routine practices; wear gloves.
- Do not completely remove vernix; allow vernix to wear off with normal care and handling.
- Use warm sterile water to bathe preterm infants (less than 32 weeks gestation) for the first week.

Routine

- Decrease frequency of baths to every second or third day; continue daily cleansing of eyes, oral and diaper areas, and pressure points.
- Use cleanser or soaps no more than two or three times a week.
- Avoid rubbing skin during bathing or drying.
- Immerse stable infants fully (except head) in an appropriate-sized tub.
- Use swaddled immersion bathing technique: slow unwrapping after gently lowering into water for infants needing assistance with motor system reactivity.

Emollients

- Apply sparingly to dry, flaking, fissured areas as needed.
- Choose petrolatum-based products that are free of preservatives, dyes, and perfume.
- Observe neonates who weigh less than 750 g receiving emollient therapy for increased risk of coagulase-negative staphylococcal infections.
- Consider dispensing emollients from the hospital pharmacy in a unit dose or patient-specific container. Follow hospital protocol or consider applying emollient as needed to infants older than 32 weeks for dry, flaking skin.

Adhesives

- Decrease use as much as possible.
- Use semipermeable transparent adhesive dressings to secure intravenous lines (IVs), nasogastric or orogastric tubes, silicone catheters, and central lines.
- Use hydrogel or limb electrodes.
- Consider pectin barriers (e.g., DuoDERM®) beneath adhesives to protect skin.
- Secure pulse oximeter probe or electrodes with elasticized dressing material (carefully to avoid restricting blood flow).
- Do not use adhesive remover, solvents, or bonding agents.
- Avoid removing adhesives for at least 24 hours after application.
- Facilitate adhesive removal using water, mineral oil, or petrolatum.
- Remove adhesives or skin barriers slowly, supporting the skin underneath with one hand and gently peeling away the product from the skin with the other hand.*

Antiseptic Agents

- Apply before invasive procedures.
- Consider the potential for skin breakdown or irritation with disinfectant.
- No specific disinfectant is recommended for all neonates; remove completely with sterile water or saline after use.
- Apply povidone-iodine two times, air dry for 30 seconds in between application; remove completely with sterile water or saline solution immediately after procedure.
- Avoid use of isopropyl alcohol for skin preparation or removal of other disinfectants.

Transepidermal Water Loss

- Minimize TEWL and heat loss in preterm infants less than 30 weeks of gestation by doing the following:
  - Measure ambient humidity during the first weeks of life (incubator).
  - Apply an occlusive food-grade polyethylene bag or wrap at delivery; remove it once the infant is stabilized in the NICU.
  - Maintain the humidity in the microenvironment (incubator) between 60 and 90% for first 7 days and at 50% for the first 28 days (or according to hospital policy).
  - Use supplemental conductive heat and reduce radiant heat source.
  - Apply semipermeable transparent dressings to skin surfaces on the infant's chest, abdomen, and back.

Skin Breakdown

Prevention

- Decrease pressure from externally applied forces using water, air, or gel mattresses; sheepskin; or cotton bedding.
- Provide adequate nutrition, including protein, fat, and zinc.
- Apply transparent adhesive dressings to protect arms, elbows, and knees from friction injury.
- Use tracheostomy and gastrostomy dressings for drainage and relief of pressure from a tracheostomy or gastrostomy tube.
- Use emollient in the diaper area (groin and thighs) to reduce urine irritation.

Treating Skin Breakdown

- Irrigate wound gently every 4 to 8 hours with warm, half-strength normal saline.
- Culture wound and treat if signs of infection are present (excessive redness, swelling, pain on touch, heat, or resistance to healing).
- Use a transparent adhesive dressing for uninfected wounds.
- Apply hydrogel with or without antibacterial or antifungal ointments (as ordered) for infected wounds.
- Use hydrocolloid for deep, uninfected wounds (leave in place for 5 to 7 days) or as an ostomy barrier and to improve

Continued

GUIDELINES Neonatal Skin Care—cont'd

appliance adhesion: warm barrier in your hand for several minutes to soften it before applying it to the skin.
- Avoid use of antiseptic solutions for wound cleansing (use for intact skin only).

Treating Diaper Dermatitis
- Maintain clean, dry skin; use absorbent diapers and change them often.
- If mild irritation occurs, use petrolatum barrier.
- For dermatitis, apply a generous quantity of zinc-oxide barrier; when cleaning, remove only the soiled layer of barrier as excessive friction can cause skin irritation and hinder healing.
- For severe dermatitis, identify the cause and treat (e.g., frequent stooling from spina bifida, severe opiate withdrawal, malabsorption syndrome).
- Treat *Candida albicans* with antifungal ointment or cream.
- Avoid use of powders and antibiotic ointments. (See Chapter 25, Umbilical Cord Care and Care of the Newly Circumcised Infant.)

Other Skin Care Concerns

Use of Substances on Skin
- Evaluate all substances that come in contact with infant's skin. Before using any topical agent, analyze its components and
  - Use sparingly and only when necessary.
  - Confine use to the smallest possible area.
  - Whenever possible and appropriate, wash off with water.
  - Monitor infant carefully for signs of toxicity and systemic effects.

Use of Thermal Devices
- Avoid use of heat lamps because of the increased potential for burns. If needed, measure temperature of the exposed skin every 15 minutes.

  When using heated mattresses,
  - Refer to the manufacturer's instruction manual for proper use.
  - Change the infant's position every 15 minutes initially and then every 1 to 2 hours.
  - Preset temperature of the mattress to less than 40°C.

  When using preheated transcutaneous electrodes,
  - Avoid use on infants.
  - Set at the lowest possible temperature.
  - Use pulse oximetry rather than transcutaneous monitoring whenever possible.
- If prewarming the infant's heels before phlebotomy, avoid temperatures over 40°C.
- Provide warm ambient humidity, directed away from infant; use aerosolized sterile water and maintain ambient temperature so as to not exceed 40°C.
- Document use of all heating devices.

Use of Fluid Therapy and Hemodynamic Monitoring
- Be certain that fingers or toes are visible whenever an extremity is used for peripheral IV or arterial line.
- Secure catheter or needle with transparent dressing and tape for easy visualization of site.
- Assess site hourly for signs of ischemia, infiltration, and inadequate perfusion (check capillary refill, pulses, colour).
- Avoid use of restraints (e.g., arm boards); if used, ensure that they are secured safely and not restricting circulation or movement (check for pressure areas).
- Use commercial IV protector (e.g., I.V. House) with minimal tape.

(Data from Association of Women's Health, Obstetric and Neonatal Nursing. [2007]. *Neonatal skin care: Evidence-based clinical practice guideline* [2nd ed.]. Washington, DC: Author; Taquino, L. T. [2000]. Promoting wound healing in the neonatal setting: Process versus protocol. *Journal of Perinatal and Neonatal Nursing, 14*[1], 108–118.)
*Caution: Scissors should be used with caution for tape or dressing removal because of the hazard of cutting skin or amputating tiny digits.
CPAP, continuous positive airway pressure; *IV*, intravenous; *NICU*, neonatal intensive care unit; *TEWL*, transepidermal water loss.

hypoxia, oxygen desaturation, and elevated intracranial pressure. The more immature the infant, the less able he or she is to habituate to a single procedure without becoming overstimulated. The caregiver needs to use the infant's own behaviour and physiological functioning as the basis for planning care and providing interventions. Through observation, caregivers can identify the infant's strengths, thresholds for disorganization, and areas of vulnerability (Als, 1998).

Developmental care should be tailored to each infant on the basis of a comprehensive behavioural assessment. During the early stages of development (especially before 33 weeks' gestation), external stimulation produces uncoordinated, random activity (jerky limb extension, hyperflexion) and irregular vital signs. At this stage, the infant needs to have minimal environmental stimulation. Using the developmental model of supportive care, the nurse can closely monitor physiological and behavioural signs to foster organization and well-being of the high-risk infant during handling. Softly calling the infant by name and then gently placing a hand on the body signal that care is beginning. The infant should be handled with slow, controlled movements. The infant's random movements should be controlled and limbs held flexed close to the infant's body during turning or other position changes. This containment or facilitated tucking may also be used before doing invasive procedures, such as a heel stick, to alleviate distress. Blanket swaddling and nesting or containment has been shown to decrease physiological and behavioural stress during routine care procedures. A nest constructed by placing blanket rolls underneath the bed sheet helps the infant maintain flexion when prone or side lying.

Skin-to-skin contact (kangaroo care) and short periods of gentle massage can help reduce stress in preterm infants, although such contact must be assessed and implemented individually. Regular skin-to-skin contact between parents and LBW infants has been shown to alleviate stress. The undressed (except for diaper) infant is placed in a vertical position on the parent's bare chest to permit direct eye contact, skin-to-skin sensations, and close proximity. In addition to being a safe and effective method for infant–parent acquaintance, skin-to-skin contact between parent and infant can have a positive healing effect for the mother with a high-risk pregnancy. Mothers may experience psychological healing and regain the mothering role through early skin-to-skin contact with their VLBW infants (Burkhammer, Anderson, & Chiu, 2004). Additional benefits of skin-to-skin care include earlier contact for mechanically ventilated infants, maintenance of neonatal thermal stability and oxygen saturation, increased feeding ability and tolerance, maintenance of organized state, and decreased pain perception during heel sticks (Conde-Agudelo, Belizan, & Diaz-Rossello, 2011; Dodd, 2005). In term and preterm newborns, skin-to-skin contact has a strong analgesic effect during procedures such as heel lance (Johnston et al., 2008; Kostandy et al., 2008). LBW infants receiving skin-to-skin contact maintain higher oxygen saturation and are less likely to have desaturations below 90%. In addition, their mothers are more likely to continue breastfeeding both in the hospital and for 1 month after discharge. Kangaroo care of preterm infants fosters neurobehavioural development by promoting stability of cardiac and respiratory function, minimizing purposeless movements, offering maternal proximity, improving the infant's behavioural state, and permitting self-regulating behaviours (McCain, Ludington-Hoe, Swinth, & Hadeed, 2005) (Fig. 27-8) (see Evidence-Informed Practice box).

Cobedding of twins (or multiples) is another developmental intervention that has been implemented in NICUs and newborn nurseries to provide a better environment for neonatal growth and development (Altimier & Lutes, 2001; Byers, Yovaish, Lowman, & Francis, 2003). Cobedding involves placing twins or other multiples together in the same crib or incubator. Preliminary data from a multicentre study indicate that twins who were cobedded had improved thermoregulation, significantly fewer apnea and bradycardia episodes, more rapid weight gain, and shorter length of stay than their single-bedded counterparts. Parental satisfaction was also significantly greater with cobedded newborns. One major concern with cobedding is cross-transmission of infection between the neonates, but increased infection rates have not occurred with cobedding (LaMar & Dowling, 2006).

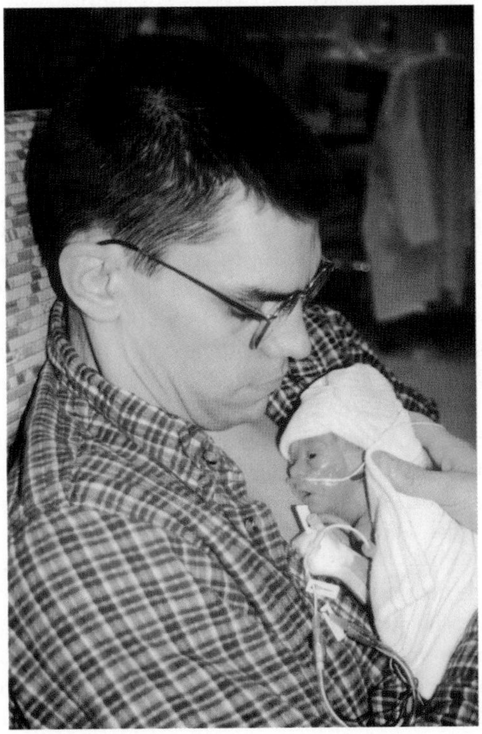

Fig. 27-8 Father providing kangaroo care. *(Courtesy Judy Meyr, St. Louis, MO.)*

Other studies have confirmed the beneficial effects of developmental care with preterm infants. In addition to requiring fewer days of mechanical ventilation, preterm infants who received individualized developmental care had shorter hospital stays; a significant decrease in complications (i.e., IVH and BPD); less need for sedation when critically ill; improved neurodevelopmental scores at 9, 18, and 36 months of life; and a decrease in feeding intolerance (Symington & Pinelli, 2006; Westrup, Sizun, & Lagercrantz, 2007).

Developmental care for preterm infants has expanded to use of a wide variety of interventions, such as infant massage, playing of soothing soft music, recordings of parents reading stories, positioning to enhance self-regulatory abilities, enhancement of hand-to-mouth activities, uninterrupted sleep periods, and minimizing environmental light and noise. These interventions may also lead parents to perceive the NICU environment as less threatening. Active participation in providing a developmentally supportive environment for their infant involves the parents in daily caregiving activities when the newborn is critically ill and cannot be fed or held.

When infants have reached sufficient developmental organization and stability, interventions need to be designed and implemented to support their growing abilities. Nurses and parents must become adept at learning to read the infant's behavioural cues and supplying appropriate interventions. Clues include both approach and avoidance behaviours. Approach behaviours should be encouraged and include tongue extension, hand clasp, hand-to-mouth movements, and sucking. Signs of stress or fatigue that signal the infant's need for time-out include colour changes, tachypnea, periodic breathing, tremors, hiccups, gagging or choking, spitting up, sneezing, yawning, arm or leg extension, arm(s) outstretched with fingers splayed, and oxygen desaturations.

When an infant is medically stable and on room air or minimal amounts of oxygen, ongoing assessment and documentation of his or her behavioural state organization and ability to self-regulate should be continued. Activities need to be individualized according to each infant's cues, temperament, state, behavioural organization, and particular needs. Intervention periods must be short (e.g., 2 to 3 minutes of voices, 5 minutes of quiet music). Auditory and vestibular interventions should be initiated earlier than visual stimulation. Interventions should be introduced one at a time and the infant's tolerance to each assessed and documented. An intervention program for a convalescing infant includes parents and siblings being present early in the infant's hospitalization; teaching parents to be responsive to the infant's individual cues is an important function of the NICU nurse. Parents, siblings, and health care providers should be advised to adhere to the established developmental care plan in order to avoid disruption in the infant's sleep–wake cycles and minimize inappropriate stimuli.

EVIDENCE-INFORMED PRACTICE Skin-to-Skin Contact (Kangaroo Care) for Preterm Infants

—*Pat Gingrich*

Ask the Question

What are the benefits of kangaroo care (skin-to-skin contact)?

Search for Evidence

Search Strategies

Professional organization guidelines, meta-analyses, systematic reviews, randomized controlled trials, nonrandomized prospective studies and retrospective studies since 2006

Databases Searched

CINAHL; Cochrane; Medline; National Guideline Clearinghouse; TRIP Database Plus; and Web sites for the Academy of Breastfeeding Medicine (ABM), Association of Women's Health, Obstetric and Neonatal Nursing (AWHONN), Centers for Disease Control and Prevention (CDC), and Lamaze International

Critically Analyze the Evidence

Kangaroo care (skin-to-skin contact) has proved to be significantly beneficial to the infant and mother (and father) (see Chapter 26). For vulnerable preterm infants, these benefits may be even more protective. A randomized, controlled trial (RCT) comparing kangaroo care with typical care for preterm infants born at 32 to 36 weeks' gestation showed significant exclusive breastfeeding outcomes for as long as 6 months (Hake-Brooks & Anderson, 2008). In addition to breastfeeding and thermoregulation, another RCT concluded that regular skin-to-skin contact helps preterm infants better organize their sleep–awake states into more mature patterns (Ludington-Hoe et al., 2006).

Painful procedures can increase the stress hormones of the already fragile preterm neonate. A single-blind randomized cross-over trial of 61 very preterm infants (gestational ages 28 to 32 weeks) compared the Premature Infant Pain Profile (PIPP) of infants being held in skin-to-skin contact during heel stick with the PIPP of infants swaddled in incubators. The very preterm infants in kangaroo care had significantly lower PIPP scores than those of the controls (Johnston et al., 2008).

Implications for Practice

Skin-to-skin contact between parents and newborns, even preterm infants, is now an accepted way to promote well-being, foster bonding, encourage breastfeeding, and facilitate maturation. The parents feel "needed" and "more comfortable" participating in this highly beneficial intervention (Johnson, 2007). Preterm infants who receive pumped breast milk may not be benefitting from skin-to-skin contact and nurses can advocate for a trial of kangaroo care, as tolerated. Although very preterm infants may not be able to tolerate the stimulation, late preterm infants can benefit very much from a policy of kangaroo care.

Mother–infant pairs should never be left alone during kangaroo care, especially in the first few hours of life, and will need frequent nursing assessment for signs of instability.

References

Hake-Brooks, S. J. & Anderson, G. C. (2008). Kangaroo care and breast-feeding of mother–preterm infant dyads 0–18 months: A randomized, controlled trial. *Neonatal Network, 27*(3), 151–159.

Johnson, A. N. (2007). The maternal experience of kangaroo holding. *Journal of Obstetric, Gynecologic, and Neonatal Nursing, 36*(6), 568–573.

Johnston, C. C., Filion, F., Campbell-Yeo, M., Goulet, C., Bell, L., McNaughton, K., & Walker, C-D. (2008). Kangaroo mother care diminishes pain from heel lance in very preterm neonates: A crossover trial. *BMC Pediatrics, 8*(13), 1–9.

Ludington-Hoe, S. M., Johnson, M. W., Morgan, K., Lewis, T., Gutman, J., Wilson, P. D., & Scher, M. S. (2006). Neurophysiological assessment of neonatal sleep organization: Preliminary results of a randomized, controlled trial of skin contact with preterm infants. *Pediatrics, 117*(5), e909–e923.

Developmental care of the preterm neonate is an ongoing process in the NICU and is incorporated into the daily care given to each infant. The nurse needs to be cognizant of the preterm infant's developmental needs, temperament, and newborn state, as well as environmental conditions that adversely affect the infant. Nursing care should be planned to enhance optimum physical, psychosocial, and neurological development. This task is often difficult to accomplish when invasive treatments or interventions are required to stabilize the critically ill neonate.

Growth and Development Potential

Although it is impossible to predict with complete accuracy the growth and development potential of each preterm newborn, some findings support a favourable outcome in the absence of sequelae that can affect growth, such as BPD, NEC, and CNS problems. The lower the birth weight, the greater the likelihood of negative sequelae.

The age of a preterm newborn is calculated by subtracting the number of weeks born before 40 weeks of gestation from the chronological age. For example, a 6-month-old (chronological age) infant born at 32 weeks of gestation would have a corrected age of 4 months. The infant's responses are evaluated against the norms expected for a 4-month-old infant. For preterm infants, chronological age is not equal to corrected age. Growth and development milestones (e.g., motor milestones, vocalization) are corrected for gestational age until the child is approximately 3 years of age.

An effective discharge plan should include outpatient follow-up visits with a primary care practitioner and a developmental specialist for monitoring growth and achievement of appropriate developmental milestones.

Parental Support

Nurses can help parents interact with their infant and recognize behavioural cues appropriate to his or her development.

If a high-risk birth is anticipated, the family may be given a tour of the NICU or shown a video to prepare them for the sights and activities of the unit. After the birth, the parents may be given a booklet or shown a video about what they will see when they go to the unit to see their infant or have someone describe this. Parents should see and touch their infant as soon as possible so that they can acknowledge the reality of the birth and the infant's appearance and condition (Fig. 27-9). They may need encouragement to accomplish the psychological tasks associated with the preterm birth. A nurse and primary health care provider should be present during the parents' first visit to the infant, for the following reasons:

- To help them "see" the infant rather than focus on the equipment. The nurse and other care providers should explain the significance and function of the apparatus that surrounds the infant.
- To explain the characteristics normal for an infant of their baby's gestational age. In this way, parents do not compare their infant to a healthy term baby.
- To encourage the parents to express feelings about the pregnancy, labour, and birth and the experience of having a preterm infant
- To assess the parents' perceptions of the infant and determine the appropriate time for them to become actively involved in care

Both parents, but especially the mother, should be encouraged to visit the nursery and help with the infant's care. When the family cannot be present physically, staff members can devise appropriate methods to keep the family updated, such as daily phone calls, e-mails, notes written as if from the infant, and video or photographs of the baby (see Family-Centred Teaching box).

Support groups for parents of infants in intensive care nurseries are often a source of comfort and support for parents who may feel isolated from peers because of the birth of the preterm infant. These groups encourage parents experiencing anxiety and grief to share their feelings. A parent with NICU experience often makes contact with a new member and provides additional support. These parents support the new NICU parent through hospital visits, phone contact, and home visits.

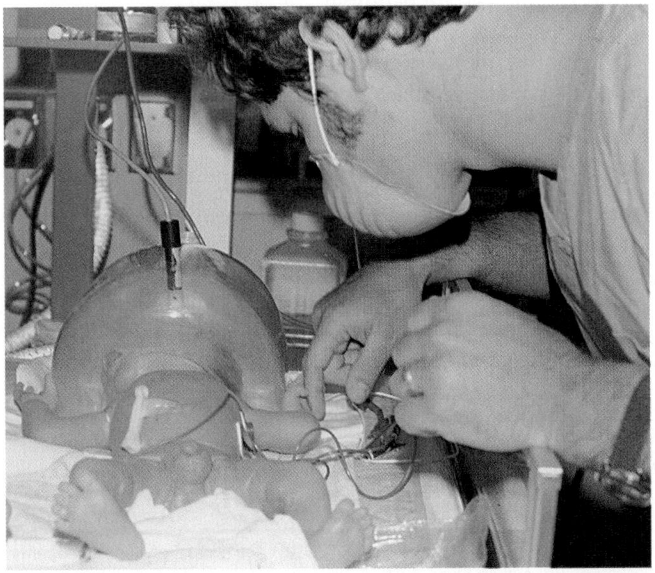

Fig. 27-9 A father caresses his preterm infant receiving oxygen by hood in the NICU. *(Courtesy Marjorie Pyle, RNC, Lifecircle, Costa Mesa, CA.)*

Parents of infants in the NICU have identified the following central themes for NICU staff to consider when caring for the family: (1) nurturing the parents, (2) providing accurate and consistent information, (3) clarifying NICU policies for neonatal treatment and family interaction, and (4) helping parents connect with other parents who have neonates in the NICU and graduates of NICU care (Woodwell, 2002). Ward (2001) developed a 20-item NICU Family Needs Inventory to help identify parents' particular needs. Perceived needs included providing information about the infant's condition and treatment plan, answering parents' questions honestly, actively listening to parents' fears and concerns, assisting parents in understanding the infant's responses, and providing reassurance about the infant's progress.

Some high-risk infants may be discharged earlier than expected. Criteria for early discharge require the infant to be physiologically stable, receive and ingest adequate nutrition, consistently gain weight, and maintain a stable body temperature in an open bassinet. In addition, screening for hyperbilirubinemia, newborn metabolic and hematological conditions, safe transportation (car seat testing), and hearing should occur before the preterm infant's discharge. An evaluation of the home environment, family resources, and arrangements for appropriate medical follow-up are essential. The parents or other caregivers must exhibit physical, emotional, and educational readiness to assume care of the infant. The parents need to show that they know how to take the infant's temperature, recognize signs and symptoms to report, and understand the infant's dietary needs (Whyte et al., 2010).

Parent Education

Cardiopulmonary Resuscitation

Sudden infant death syndrome (SIDS) is more likely to occur in preterm infants than in term infants. Infants discharged from an NICU are almost twice as likely to die unexpectedly during the first year of life as infants in the general population. Instruction in **cardiopulmonary resuscitation** (CPR) is essential for parents of all infants but especially for parents of infants at risk for life-threatening events. Risk factors include preterm birth, apnea or bradycardia spells,

FAMILY-CENTRED TEACHING

Preterm Infant

A multiparous, single woman has a preterm infant born at 28 weeks' gestation and subsequently transported to an NICU in a city 125 kilometres away from her home town. The mother is to be discharged tomorrow. The infant will likely require a stay in the NICU for at least 6 to 8 weeks. What information should the transport team provide the mother? What methods of assistance will this mother need now? Identify resources in the community that have services of potential benefit to the woman. Use your community or town as a guide to such resources.

neurological immaturity, and the tendency to choke. Before taking the infant home, parents must be able to administer infant CPR. All parents should be encouraged to obtain instruction in CPR at the hospital, local Red Cross, or other community agency. It should be emphasized that CPR knowledge does not preclude the need for proper positioning of the infant in the crib (i.e., supine, unless otherwise directed by the primary care physician) when put to sleep. In addition, the bed should have a firm mattress and be free of extra blankets and stuffed animals or toys, which may cause the infant to become entangled and subsequently smothered.

Evaluation

The nurse needs to use the previously stated outcomes of care to evaluate the effectiveness of the physical and psychosocial aspects of care (see Nursing Care Plan).

Complications of Prematurity

Respiratory Distress Syndrome

Respiratory distress syndrome (RDS) is a lung disorder usually affecting preterm infants, although a small percentage of term or late preterm infants may also be affected. The incidence and severity of RDS increase as gestational age decreases. Perinatal asphyxia, hypovolemia, male gender, Caucasian race, maternal diabetes, second-born twin, familial predisposition, Caesarean birth without labour, **hydrops fetalis,** and third-trimester bleeding are factors that place an infant at increased risk for RDS (Gardner et al., 2011). Alternatively, conditions associated with a decrease in the incidence and severity of RDS include female gender; maternal steroid (betamethasone) therapy; **intrauterine growth restriction** (IUGR); and stressors such as maternal hypertension (gestational), maternal drug use, chronic placental abruption, and prolonged rupture of membranes.

RDS is caused by a lack of pulmonary surfactant, which leads to progressive atelectasis, loss of functional residual capacity, and ventilation–perfusion imbalance. Surfactant deficiency may be caused by insufficient surfactant production, abnormal composition and function of surfactant, disruption of surfactant production, or a combination of these factors. Weak respiratory muscles and an overly compliant chest wall, common in preterm infants, exacerbate the condition. Lung capacity is compromised by proteinaceous material and epithelial debris in the airways. The resulting decreased oxygenation, cyanosis, and metabolic or respiratory acidosis can increase PVR. This increased PVR can lead to right-to-left shunting and a reopening of the ductus arteriosus and foramen ovale (Gardner et al., 2011).

Clinical symptoms of RDS include tachypnea, grunting, nasal flaring, intercostal or subcostal retractions, hypercapnia, acidosis, hypotension, and shock. These respiratory symptoms usually appear immediately within 6 hours of birth. Physical examination reveals crackles, poor air exchange, pallor, use of accessory muscles (retractions), and occasionally apnea. Radiographic findings include uniform reticulogranular appearance and air bronchograms. The infant's clinical course is variable. There is usually an increased oxygen requirement and increased respiratory effort as atelectasis, loss of functional residual capacity, and ventilation–perfusion mismatch worsen.

Severe RDS is often associated with a shock-like state, as manifested by diminished cardiac inflow and low arterial blood pressure. The ELBW or VLBW infant, as a result of extreme pulmonary immaturity, decreased glycogen stores, and lack of accessory muscles, may have severe RDS at birth.

RDS is a self-limiting disease with symptoms usually abating after 72 hours; improvement coincides with the production of surfactant in type II cells of the alveoli.

The treatment for RDS is supportive. Adequate ventilation and oxygenation must be established and maintained in an attempt to prevent ventilation–perfusion mismatch and atelectasis. Exogenous surfactant, which alters the typical course of RDS, may be administered at or shortly after birth. Positive-pressure ventilation, CPAP, and oxygen therapy may be needed during the respiratory illness. Prevention of complications associated with mechanical ventilation is critical. These complications include pulmonary interstitial emphysema, pneumothorax, pneumomediastinum, and pneumopericardium.

Acid–base balance is evaluated by monitoring ABG values (Table 27-3). Frequent blood sampling requires arterial access by either umbilical artery catheter or a peripheral arterial line. Pulse oximetry and transcutaneous carbon dioxide and oxygen monitors document trends in ventilation and oxygenation. Capillary blood gas values may be used to evaluate pH and Pco_2 in infants whose condition is more stable.

The maintenance of an NTE continues to be of critical importance in infants with RDS; infants with hypoxemia are unable to increase their metabolic rate when cold stressed.

The clinical and radiographic presentation of neonatal pneumonia may be similar to that of RDS. Therefore, evaluation, including blood culture, CBC with differential, and sometimes a lumbar puncture, is done in infants with RDS to rule out a systemic infection. Laboratory and radiographic tests rarely confirm the diagnosis of neonatal pneumonia; rather, the clinical history and presenting clinical signs provide a basis for the diagnosis and treatment (Stoll, 2007). Broad-spectrum antibiotics should be initiated while the results of cultures are pending.

Fluid and nutrition must be maintained for the infant with RDS. Parenteral nutrition can provide protein and fat to promote a positive nitrogen balance. Daily monitoring of

Table 27-3 Normal Arterial Blood Gas Values for Neonates

VALUE	RANGE
pH	7.35–7.45
Arterial oxygen pressure (Pao_2)	50–80 mm Hg
Carbon dioxide pressure ($Paco_2$)	35–45 mm Hg
Bicarbonate (HCO_3)	18–26 mmol/L
Base excess	(–4) to (+4)
Oxygen saturation	92%–94%

(Adapted from ACoRN Editorial Board. [2010]. *Acute care of at-risk newborns.* Vancouver, BC: Author; Wood, A. M., & Jones Jr., D. [2011]. Acid-base homeostasis and oxygenation. In S. L. Gardner, B. S. Carter, M. Enzman-Hines, & J. A Hernandez. [Eds.], *Merenstein & Gardner's handbook of neonatal intensive care* [7th ed., pp. 153-163]. St. Louis: Mosby.)

NURSING CARE PLAN ● The High-Risk Infant

Nursing Diagnosis: Ineffective breathing pattern related to pulmonary, cardiovascular, and neuromuscular immaturity; decreased energy reserves as evidenced by assessment findings (e.g., nasal flaring, tachypnea, grunting)

Expected Outcome

Infant exhibits adequate oxygenation (i.e., arterial blood gas [ABG] levels and acid-base balance within normal limits [WNL] for age; oxygen saturations 90% or greater; respiratory rate and pattern WNL for age; breath sounds clear; absence of grunting, nasal flaring; minimal retractions, appropriate skin colour).

Nursing Interventions/*Rationales*

Position the neonate prone or supine, avoiding neck hyperextension, *to promote optimum air exchange.* Use a side-lying position to assist in draining excess mucus *to avoid aspiration.* Avoid use of Trendelenburg's position because it can cause increased intracranial pressure (ICP) and reduce lung capacity. **Once the neonate's respiratory status is stable, use supine position.**

Suction nasopharynx, trachea, and endotracheal tube (if intubated) only as necessary *to remove mucus and secretions.* Avoid over-suctioning because it can cause bronchospasm, bradycardia, and hypoxia and can predispose the neonate to intraventricular hemorrhage (IVH).

Administer percussion, vibration, and postural drainage only as necessary *to facilitate drainage of secretions.*

Administer supplemental oxygen as needed *to maintain oxygen saturation WNL* and monitor neonatal response.

Maintain a neutral thermal environment *to conserve oxygen and glucose consumption.*

Monitor ABG levels, acid-base balance, oxygen saturation, respiratory rate and pattern, breath sounds, and airway patency; observe for grunting, nasal flaring, retractions, and cyanosis *to detect signs of respiratory distress.*

Nursing Diagnosis: Ineffective thermoregulation related to immature central nervous system (CNS), decreased brown fat, inability to effectively produce body heat, and minimal subcutaneous fat stores as evidenced by assessment findings (e.g., absent or decreased subcutaneous tissue, body temperature less than 36.3°C)

Expected Outcome

Infant exhibits maintenance of stable body temperature within the normal range for postconceptional age (36.3°C to 37.2°C).

Nursing Interventions/*Rationales*

Place neonate on a prewarmed radiant warmer *to maintain stable temperature.*

Place ELBW infant in a polyethylene bag or wrap immediately after delivery *to decrease heat loss and transepidermal water loss (TEWL).*

Place temperature probe over tissue (not bone) such as the abdomen *to control heat delivered by radiant warmer.*

Take axillary temperature periodically *to monitor temperature and confirm functioning of warmer unit.*

Avoid exposing infant to cool air, drafts, cold equipment (scales, stethoscopes), and prolonged bathing *to avoid heat loss.*

Use microenvironment (polyethylene wrap), double-walled incubator, and/or increased humidity to 60% *to prevent further heat loss from exposure to drafts and air currents and to minimize insensible water loss.*

Monitor temperature probe function (when used) and status frequently *because detachment can cause overheating or warmer-induced hyperthermia.*

Nursing Diagnosis: Risk for infection related to immature immune system and exposure to multiple sources of infection (invasive procedures) as evidenced by assessment findings (e.g., feeding intolerance, apnea, temperature instability)

Expected Outcome

Infant exhibits no evidence of infection.

Nursing Interventions/*Rationales*

Implement hand hygiene before and after handling neonate, ensure that all supplies and equipment are clean before use, and ensure use of strict aseptic technique with invasive procedures *to minimize exposure to infective organisms.*

Prevent contact with persons who have communicable infections and instruct parents in infection-control procedures *to minimize infection risk.*

Administer antibiotics as ordered *to provide coverage for actual or suspected infection.*

Continually monitor vital signs for stability *because instability, hypothermia, or prolonged temperature elevations serve as indicators of infection.*

Nursing Diagnosis: Imbalanced nutrition: less than body requirements related to low birth weight, inability to ingest adequate nutrients for growth secondary to gastrointestinal immaturity, decreased stomach capacity, and associated illness factors as evidenced by inadequate weight gain and feeding intolerance

Expected Outcomes

Infant receives adequate amount of nutrients with sufficient caloric intake to maintain a positive nitrogen balance; demonstrates steady weight gain (as appropriate to acuity).

Nursing Interventions/*Rationales*

Administer parenteral fluid or total parenteral nutrition (TPN) (protein, amino acids, lipids) *to provide adequate nutrition and fluid intake.*

Monitor for signs of intolerance to TPN, *as it can interfere with effective replenishment of nutrients.*

Periodically assess readiness to orally feed (i.e., strong suck, swallow, and gag reflexes) *to provide appropriate transition from gavage to oral feeding as soon as the neonate is ready.*

Advance volume and concentration of formula per unit protocol *to avoid overfeeding and feeding intolerance and to promote growth.*

Provide expressed breast milk (including colostrum) when the infant is stable *to enhance gastrointestinal development, provide natural immunity, and provide other benefits of human milk (digestive enzymes).*

Continued

If the mother wants to breastfeed when the neonate is stable, demonstrate how to express milk *to establish and maintain lactation until the infant can breastfeed.*

Nursing Diagnosis: Risk for imbalanced (specify if deficit or excess) fluid volume related to large extracellular fluid volume, decreased ability to regulate fluid shifts, renal immaturity, permeable skin, and insensible water loss and TEWL as evidenced by excessive weight gain or loss

Expected Outcome

Infant exhibits evidence of fluid homeostasis.

Nursing Interventions/*Rationales*

Administer parenteral fluids as prescribed and regulate carefully *to maintain fluid balance.*

Avoid hypertonic fluids such as undiluted medications and concentrated glucose *to avoid excess solute load on immature kidneys.*

Implement strategies such as use of plastic covers and increasing ambient humidity *to minimize insensible water loss.*

Monitor hydration status (i.e., skin turgor, weight, mucous membranes, fontanels, urine specific gravity, and electrolytes) and intake and output *to evaluate for evidence of dehydration or overhydration.*

Nursing Diagnosis: Risk for impaired skin integrity related to immature skin structure; poor perfusion; immobility; and invasive procedures as evidenced by epidermal stripping with adhesive removal, translucent skin, erythema, and abrasions

Expected Outcome

Infant's skin remains intact without evidence of irritation or injury.

Nursing Interventions/*Rationales*

Cleanse skin as needed with warm water only and apply barrier or emollient to skin (as appropriate) *to prevent dryness and reduce friction across skin surface.*

When performing procedures, minimize use of tape and apply a skin barrier between tape and skin; use transparent elastic film for securing central and peripheral lines; use limb electrodes for monitoring or attach with hydrogel and rotate electrodes often; remove adhesives with water rather than alcohol or acetone-based adhesive removers *to minimize skin damage.*

Promptly remove skin cleansers such as povidone-iodine with water *to decrease absorption and potential toxicity.*

Carefully monitor use of thermal devices such as pulse oximeter probes, biliblankets, or thermal mattresses *to prevent burns.*

Monitor skin closely for evidence of redness, rash, irritation, bruising, breakdown, ischemia, and infiltration *to detect and treat potential complications early.*

Use a validated neonatal skin assessment tool *to objectively monitor the infant's skin status.*

Nursing Diagnosis: Risk for CNS injury related to fluctuating systemic and intracranial pressures; immature CNS vascular bed; immature state regulatory ability; environmental stimuli and episodes of hyperoxia and hypoxia as evidenced by episodes of hypoxia associated with handling, fluctuating blood pressure readings

Expected Outcome

Infant will exhibit normal ICP with no evidence of IVH.

Nursing Interventions/*Rationales*

Institute developmentally supportive care practices (e.g., minimal handling, clustering care, undisturbed sleep periods, light variations to simulate day and night, noise reduction) *to decrease stress responses, which can increase ICP.*

Institute ordered pharmacological and nonpharmacological pain control methods *to manage pain and reduce physical stress.*

Avoid hypertonic solutions and medications *because they increase cerebral blood flow.*

Elevate head of bed 15 to 20 degrees *to decrease ICP.*

Monitor vital signs *for evidence of increased ICP.*

Recognize signs of overstimulation (e.g., flaccidity, yawning, irritability, crying, staring, and active averting) so stimulation can be stopped *to allow rest.*

Nursing Diagnosis: Risk for impaired parenting related to separation and interruption of parent–infant attachment secondary to preterm birth, severity of infant's illness, high-tech NICU environment, and anticipatory grieving over loss of healthy newborn as evidenced by physical separation from parents, verbalization of shock and disbelief at appearance of infant, lack of contact between infant and parent

Expected Outcomes

Parents establish contact with the neonate and demonstrate competent parenting skills and willingness to care for the neonate.

Nursing Interventions/*Rationales*

Before parents' first visit to the NICU, prepare them by explaining what the neonate will look like, what the equipment will look like, and its function *to diminish fear and decrease sense of shock.*

Keep parents informed about the infant's condition (e.g., improvements and setbacks) and important aspects of infant's care; encourage and answer parental questions; actively listen to parental concerns *to establish trust, open communication, and provide a caring atmosphere to aid in coping.*

Encourage parents to contact NICU staff any time, day or night, for concerns regarding the infant's condition *to maintain open channels of communication regarding the infant's status and decrease parents' fear of the unknown.*

Encourage parents to visit the NICU often; to name the infant; to touch, hold, or caress the infant as physical condition permits; to be actively involved in the infant's care; to bring personal items (e.g., clothing, stuffed animals, or pictures of family) *to facilitate formation of emotional bond.*

Reinforce parent involvement and praise care endeavours *to increase self-confidence in their contribution.*

Encourage parents to bring other siblings, as age-appropriate, to visit the preterm infant; explain to siblings what they are seeing; encourage siblings to draw pictures or write letters for the infant and place them in or near the infant's bed *to promote family involvement, help ease sibling fears, and encourage participation in the infant's care.*

Refer parents to social services as needed *to ensure comprehensive care.*

Provide consistent and frequent information regarding the infant's condition through multidisciplinary conferences *to promote parent trust in caregivers and provide consistent information.*

electrolytes, urine output, specific gravity, and weight assists in the evaluation of hydration status.

Respiratory distress, nonpulmonary in origin, may also be caused by sepsis, cardiac defects (structural or functional), exposure to cold, airway obstruction (atresia), IVH, hypoglycemia, metabolic acidosis, acute blood loss, and certain medications. Bacterial or viral pneumonia in the neonatal period may manifest as respiratory distress and may occur alone or as a complication of RDS.

Patent Ductus Arteriosus

The ductus arteriosus is a muscular contractile structure in the fetus connecting the left pulmonary artery and the dorsal aorta. The ductus constricts after birth as oxygenation increases. Other factors that promote ductal closure include catecholamines, low pH, bradykinin, and acetylcholine. When the fetal ductus arteriosus fails to close after birth, a patent ductus arteriosus (PDA) occurs. Ductal closure usually occurs within hours or days in the term infant but may be delayed in preterm infants as a result of oxygenation and circulating **hormones** (prostaglandins).

The clinical presentation of an infant with a PDA includes systolic murmur, active precordium, bounding peripheral pulses, tachycardia, tachypnea, crackles, and hepatomegaly. The systolic murmur is heard best at the second or third intercostal space at the upper left sternal border. An active precordium is caused by an increased left ventricular stroke volume. A widened pulse pressure may result in bounding peripheral pulses.

Radiographic studies of infants with a large shunting PDA typically show cardiac enlargement and pulmonary edema; with a smaller PDA, the radiograph may appear normal for the infant's age (Kenney, Hoover, Williams, & Iskersky, 2011). ABG findings reveal hypercarbia and metabolic acidosis. A colour flow Doppler echocardiograph can demonstrate a PDA and be used to identify the direction of the shunting (left to right, right to left or both) and quantify the amount of blood shunting across the PDA.

A PDA can be managed medically or surgically. Medical management consists of ventilatory support, fluid restriction, diuretics, and nonsteroidal anti-inflammatory drugs (NSAIDs) such as indomethacin or ibuprofen. Indomethacin is a prostaglandin synthetase inhibitor that blocks the effect of the arachidonic acid products on the ductus and causes the PDA to constrict. Ibuprofen administered orally reportedly has fewer adverse effects than indomethacin, yet a recent Cochrane review reports that they are equally effective (Cherif, Jabnoun, & Khrouf, 2010; Ohlsson, Walia, & Shah, 2010).

Ventilatory support is adjusted on the basis of ABG levels. Fluid restriction and diuretic therapy are implemented to decrease cardiovascular volume overload. Surgical ligation is performed when PDA is clinically significant and medical management has failed. Nursing care of the infant with PDA focuses on supportive care. The infant needs an NTE, adequate oxygenation, and meticulous fluid balance. Parental support is imperative.

Periventricular-Intraventricular Hemorrhage

Periventricular-intraventricular hemorrhage (PV-IVH) is one of the more common types of neurological injuries that occurs in neonates and is among the most severe in both short- and long-term outcomes. While the true incidence of PV-IVH is unknown, a general estimate is 15% in infants less than 32 weeks of gestation or under 1501 g (Volpe, 2008). PV-IVH occurs in approximately 3.5 to 5% of term infants, with 50% of those cases caused by asphyxia or trauma. Research has shown that contributing events may occur antenatally and postnatally (Adams-Chapman & Stoll, 2007).

The pathogenesis of PV-IVH includes intravascular factors (e.g., fluctuating or increasing cerebral blood flow, increased cerebral venous pressure, and coagulopathy), vascular factors, extravascular factors (hypoglycemia, acidosis), and routine medical care (rapid volume expansion, blood transfusion). The developing preterm infant's brain has highly vascularized areas with fragile blood vessels that are prone to bleeding when homeostasis is not maintained; the most commonly affected area is in and around the subependymal germinal matrix. PV-IVH events typically occur within the first 72 hours of birth. PV-IVH is classified according to severity, which informs long-term neurodevelopmental outcomes.

Nursing care focuses on recognition of factors that increase the risk of PV-IVH, interventions to decrease the risk of bleeding, and supportive care to infants who have bleeding episodes. The infant should be positioned with his or her head in midline and the head of the bed elevated slightly to prevent or minimize fluctuations in intracranial blood pressure. NTE is maintained, as well as oxygenation. Rapid infusions of fluids should be avoided. Blood pressure should be monitored closely for fluctuations. The infant must be monitored for signs of pneumothorax because it often precedes PV-IVH.

Necrotizing Enterocolitis

Necrotizing enterocolitis (NEC) is an acute inflammatory disease of the gastrointestinal mucosa, commonly complicated by perforation. This often fatal disease occurs in about 1 to 5% of newborns in NICUs. Three factors appear to play an important role in the development of NEC: intestinal ischemia, colonization by pathogenic bacteria, and substrate (formula feeding) in the intestinal lumen. The precise cause of NEC is still uncertain, but it appears to occur in infants whose gastrointestinal tract has suffered vascular compromise. Preterm birth remains the most prominent risk factor in the development of NEC.

The onset of NEC in the term infant, although rare, usually occurs between 4 and 10 days after birth. In the preterm infant the onset may be delayed for up to 30 days. Signs of NEC are nonspecific, a characteristic of many neonatal disease processes. Some general signs include decreased activity, hypotonia, pallor, recurrent apnea and bradycardia, respiratory distress, metabolic acidosis, **oliguria**, hypotension, decreased perfusion, temperature instability, and cyanosis. Gastrointestinal symptoms include abdominal distension, increasing or bile-stained gastric aspirates, vomiting (bile or blood), grossly bloody stools, abdominal tenderness, and erythema of the abdominal wall (Lovvan, Glenn, Pacetti, & Carter, 2011).

Diagnosis of NEC is confirmed by radiographic examination that reveals bowel loop distension, pneumatosis intestinalis, pneumoperitoneum, portal air, or a combination of these findings. The abnormal findings are caused by NEC-associated

evolve Critical Thinking Exercise—Patent Ductus Arteriosus

bacterial colonization of the gastrointestinal tract, resulting in an ileus. Pneumatosis intestinalis, pneumoperitoneum, and portal air are caused by gas produced by the bacteria that invade the wall of the intestines and escape into the peritoneum and portal system when perforation occurs. Laboratory evaluation includes a CBC with differential, blood culture, coagulation studies, ABG analysis, and serum electrolyte levels. The white blood cell count may be either increased or decreased. The platelet count and coagulation studies may be abnormal, with thrombocytopenia and evidence of disseminated intravascular coagulation (DIC). Electrolyte levels may be abnormal, related to leaking capillary beds and fluid shifts seen with the infection.

Treatment of infants with NEC is supportive and preventive for bowel perforation. Feedings should be discontinued to rest the gastrointestinal tract. A nasogastric tube is inserted and placed to low intermittent suction to provide gastric decompression, and parenteral therapy (often TPN) is initiated. NEC is an infectious disease; control of infection is imperative, with an emphasis on careful hand washing before and after infant contact. Systemic antibiotic therapy should be instituted.

With early recognition and treatment, medical management has become increasingly successful. If there is progressive deterioration or evidence of perforation, surgical resection and anastomosis may be performed. Extensive involvement may necessitate surgical intervention and establishment of an ileostomy, jejunostomy, or colostomy. Sequelae include short-bowel syndrome, colonic stricture with obstruction, fat malabsorption, and failure to thrive secondary to intestinal dysfunction. Various surgical interventions for NEC are available and depend on the extent of bowel necrosis, associated illness factors, and infant stability. Intestinal transplantation has been successful in a small number of infants with NEC-associated short-bowel syndrome and life-threatening TPN-related complications. Bowel-lengthening procedures and intestinal transplantation may be lifesaving options for infants who previously faced high morbidity and mortality (Nucci et al., 2008; Vennarecci et al., 2000). Therapy may be prolonged and recovery may be delayed by adhesions, complications of bowel resection, short-bowel syndrome (especially if the ileocecal valve is removed), and intolerance of oral feedings.

NURSING ALERT Observe for early indications of NEC by checking the abdomen for distension (measuring abdominal girth), assessing the infant's feeding tolerance (measuring gastric residuals, assessing bowel sounds), and performing all routine assessments (i.e., vital signs, blood pressure, activity level) for high-risk neonates.

Minimal enteral feedings (trophic feeding, gastrointestinal priming) have gained acceptance. Early findings indicate that such feedings may be protective against NEC in nonasphyxiated preterm infants. An increased incidence of NEC in VLBW infants receiving minimal enteral nutrition has not been substantiated (Reynolds & Thureen, 2007). Human milk may have a protective effect against the development of NEC (Diehl-Jones & Askin, 2004; Sisk, Lovelady, Dillard, Gruber, & O'Shea, 2007). The role of probiotics (*Lactobacillus acidophilus* and *Bifidobacterium infantis*) administered with enteral feedings for the prevention of NEC has yet to be explored fully enough to advocate widespread use in all VLBW infants. In some studies, probiotics decreased the incidence of NEC (Alfaleh & Bassler, 2008; Bin-Nun et al., 2005).

Retinopathy of Prematurity

Retinopathy of prematurity (ROP) is a complex, multicausal disorder that affects the developing retinal vessels of preterm infants. Retinal vessels begin to form in utero at approximately 16 weeks of gestation in response to an unknown stimulus and continue to develop until they reach maturity approximately 42 to 43 weeks after conception. Once the retina is completely vascularized, the retinal vessels are not susceptible to ROP.

The mechanism of injury in ROP is unclear. Elevated oxygen tensions initially result in vasoconstriction. When oxygen therapy is discontinued, neovascularization occurs in the retina and vitreous, with resulting capillary hemorrhages, fibrotic resolution, and possible retinal detachment. Scar tissue formation and consequent visual impairment may be mild or severe. The entire disease process in severe cases may take as long as 5 months to evolve. Examination by an ophthalmologist before discharge and a schedule for repeat examinations thereafter are recommended.

Studies have demonstrated an association between the development of ROP and high arterial oxygen saturations in ELBW and VLBW infants. Fluctuations in arterial oxygen saturation in the first few weeks of life have also been implicated in the development of ROP. Although there is no consensus on what the ideal arterial oxygen saturation is in preterm infants, there is irrefutable evidence that oxygen saturations of 100% are undesirable and may have a significant role in the development of ROP in preterm infants. Further studies are needed to clarify optimal arterial oxygen saturation (Pollan, 2009). The Canadian Oxygen Trial (COT) is attempting to answer that very question for preterm infants born between 23^0 and 27^6 weeks of gestation (Schmidt, & Canadian Oxygen Trial Collaborators, 2005).

All caregivers should use supplemental oxygen judiciously, monitor oxygen blood levels carefully, promptly attend to saturation monitor alarms, and prevent wide fluctuations in oxygen blood levels (hyperoxemia and hypoxemia).

Circumferential cryopexy, laser photocoagulation, vitamin E therapy, and decreased intensity of ambient light are used in the treatment of ROP, with varying results. Early screening and detection should be provided in infants who are born at less than 32 weeks' gestation and who weigh less than 1500 g, and in infants believed to be at high risk for development of ROP (Ells & Hindle, 2000; Jefferies et al., 2010). The Early Treatment for Retinopathy of Prematurity study found that early treatment of prethreshold ROP improved retinal and visual outcomes at 9 months corrected age (Jones et al., 2005).

Bronchopulmonary Dysplasia

Bronchopulmonary dysplasia (BPD), or chronic lung disease, is a result of lung injury in infants who require mechanical ventilation and supplemental oxygen (Dudell & Stoll, 2007). The etiology of BPD is multifactorial and includes pulmonary immaturity, surfactant deficiency, barotrauma, inflammation caused by oxygen exposure, fluid overload, ligation of a PDA, and genetic predisposition (Gardner et al., 2011). The type of BPD observed over the past decade has changed, with the "classic" form observed less frequently; these changes are primarily morphological rather than etiological. The "new" BPD is characterized by impeded lung development and remains a disease seen primarily in infants weighing less than 1000 g who are born at less than 28 weeks' gestation (Dudell & Stoll, 2007; Sahni et al., 2005). The incidence of BPD in infants weighing less than 1500 g who require mechanical ventilation for RDS ranges from 23 to 80% (Berger, Bachmann, Adams, & Schubiger, 2004; Gracey, Talbot, Lankford, & Dodge, 2002).

Clinical symptoms of BPD include tachypnea, retractions, nasal flaring, increased work of breathing, exercise intolerance (to handling and feeding), and tachycardia (Gardner et al., 2011). Auscultation of lung fields in affected infants reveals crackles, decreased air movement, and occasionally expiratory wheezing.

Treatment for BPD includes oxygen therapy, nutrition, fluid restriction, and medications (e.g., diuretics, corticosteroids, and bronchodilators). The use of corticosteroids to prevent or treat BPD is controversial because of the adverse effects and varied results in clinical trials; however, corticosteroids are used in many centres to treat or prevent BPD (Van Aerde, Shah, Stark, & Ohlsson, 2002). The key to management of BPD is prevention, by reducing the incidence of preterm births and RDS and by using surfactant, giving antenatal steroids, and minimizing lung trauma from mechanical ventilation and high oxygen concentrations.

The prognosis for infants with BPD depends on the degree of pulmonary dysfunction. Most deaths occur within the first year of life as a result of cardiorespiratory failure, sepsis, or respiratory tract infection; in some infants death is sudden and unexplained.

The Postterm Infant

Postterm (or postmature) infants are those whose gestation is prolonged beyond 42 weeks, regardless of birth weight. These infants may be LGA or SGA, but most often their weight is appropriate for gestational age. The rate of infants born postterm has been declining, and in 2008 it was 0.62% down from 1.46% in 1999 (PHAC, 2012). The cause of prolonged pregnancy is unknown. **Postmaturity** can be associated with placental insufficiency, resulting in a newborn that has a thin, emaciated appearance *(dysmature)* at birth because of loss of subcutaneous fat and muscle mass. Not all postterm infants show signs of dysmaturity. There may be meconium staining of the fingernails, the hair and nails may be long, and vernix may be absent. The skin may also peel off.

Perinatal mortality is significantly higher in the postterm infant. During labour and birth, increased oxygen demands of the postterm fetus may not be met. Insufficient gas exchange in the postterm placenta increases the likelihood of intrauterine hypoxia. This may result in the passage of meconium in utero and the risk for meconium aspiration syndrome (MAS). In one study, postterm infants were found to have a mortality rate almost three times higher than that of a control group of term infants (Stoll & Adams-Chapman, 2007).

Meconium Aspiration Syndrome

Meconium-staining of the amniotic fluid can be indicative of atypical or abnormal fetal heart rate status. It appears in 10 to 15% of all births, primarily in term and postterm births. Many infants with meconium-staining exhibit no signs of depression at birth; however, the presence of meconium in the amniotic fluid necessitates careful supervision of labour and close monitoring of fetal well-being. The presence of a team skilled in neonatal resuscitation is required at the birth of any infant with meconium-stained amniotic fluid (Fig. 27-10). The infant's mouth and nares are no longer routinely suctioned on the perineum before the infant's first breath. In a multicentred, randomized, controlled trial, Vain and colleagues (2005) found no difference in outcomes between those infants who were suctioned and those who were not. Current resuscitation guidelines (Perlman et al., 2010) assert that there is not enough evidence at this time to change the current practice of intubation and suctioning below the cords for nonvigorous infants. More research is recommended.

If meconium is not removed from the airway at birth, it can migrate down to the terminal airways, causing mechanical obstruction and leading to MAS. The fetus may aspirate meconium in utero, causing a chemical pneumonitis. These infants may develop persistent pulmonary hypertension of the newborn, further complicating their management. Surfactant administration in infants with MAS decreased the severity of respiratory failure and the need for ECMO and improved oxygenation (Davis et al., 2005).

Persistent Pulmonary Hypertension of the Newborn

Persistent pulmonary hypertension of the newborn (PPHN) is a term applied to the combined findings of pulmonary hypertension, right-to-left shunting, and a structurally normal heart. PPHN may manifest either as a single entity or a sequela

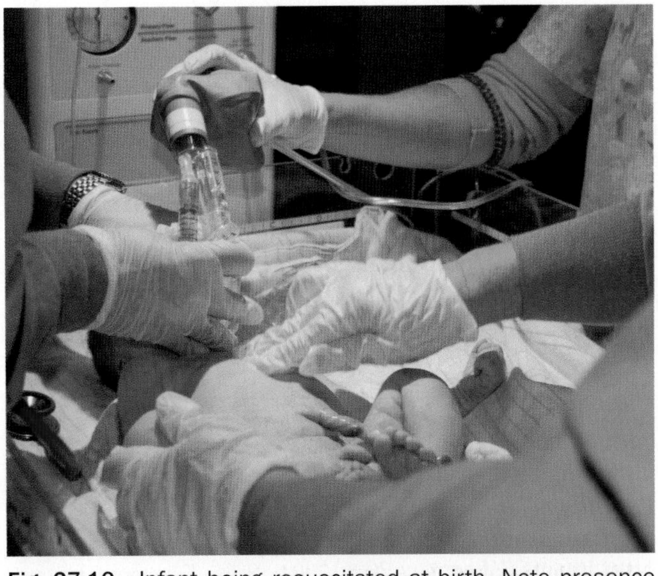

Fig. 27-10 Infant being resuscitated at birth. Note presence of meconium on abdomen, umbilical cord, and overbed warmer. *(Courtesy Shannon Perry, Phoenix, AZ.)*

of MAS, CDH, RDS, hyperviscosity syndrome, neonatal pneumonia, or sepsis. PPHN is also called *persistent fetal circulation* because the syndrome involves reversion to fetal pathways of blood flow.

A brief review of fetal blood flow can help in visualization of the problems with PPHN (see Fig. 8-12). In utero, oxygen-rich blood leaves the placenta via the umbilical vein, goes through the ductus venosus, and enters the inferior vena cava. From there it empties into the right atrium and is mostly shunted across the foramen ovale to the left atrium, effectively bypassing the lungs. This blood enters the left ventricle, leaves through the aorta, and preferentially perfuses the carotid and coronary arteries: the heart and brain receive the most oxygenated blood. Blood drains from the brain into the superior vena cava, re-enters the right atrium, proceeds to the right ventricle, and exits through the main pulmonary artery. The lungs, a high-pressure circuit, need only enough perfusion for growth and nutrition. The ductus arteriosus (connecting the main pulmonary artery and the aorta) is the path of least resistance for the blood leaving the right side of the fetal heart and shunts most of the cardiac output away from the lungs and toward the systemic system. This right-to-left shunting is the key to fetal circulation.

After birth, both the foramen ovale and the ductus arteriosus close in response to biochemical processes, pressure changes within the heart, and dilation of the pulmonary vessels. This dilation allows virtually all of the cardiac output to enter the lungs, become oxygenated, and provide oxygen-rich blood to the tissues. Any process that interferes with this transition from fetal to neonatal circulation may precipitate PPHN. PPHN characteristically proceeds into a downward spiral of increasing hypoxia and pulmonary vasoconstriction. Prompt recognition and aggressive intervention are required to reverse this process.

The infant with PPHN is typically born at term or postterm and exhibits tachycardia and cyanosis that, within minutes or hours, progresses to severe respiratory compromise with concomitant acidosis, further compromising pulmonary perfusion and oxygenation. Management depends on the underlying cause of the persistent pulmonary hypertension. The use of INO and ECMO has improved survival in some of these infants.

Another mode of treatment for PPHN and other respiratory disorders is high-frequency ventilation, an assisted-ventilation method that delivers small volumes of gas at high frequencies and limits the development of high airway pressure, thus theoretically reducing barotrauma.

Other Problems Related to Gestation

Small-for-Gestational-Age Infants and Intrauterine Growth Restriction

Infants who are SGA or IUGR are considered high risk, with a perimortality rate 5 to 20 times greater than that for normal term infants (Kliegman, 2006).

Conditions occurring in the first trimester (e.g., infections, **teratogens**, chromosomal abnormalities) can affect all aspects of fetal growth. Extrinsic conditions early in pregnancy can also result in symmetrical IUGR (i.e., head circumference, length, and weight are all less than the tenth percentile). Infants with symmetrical growth restriction have a smaller head circumference and concomitant reduced brain growth. Growth restriction during later stages of pregnancy, due to maternal or placental factors, results in asymmetrical growth restriction—weight will be less than the tenth percentile, whereas length and head circumference will be greater than the tenth percentile, possibly within normal limits. Infants with asymmetrical IUGR have the potential for normal growth and development.

Care of the SGA infant is guided by the accompanying clinical problems and is comparable to the care provided to preterm infants with similar problems. Gas exchange is supported by maintaining a clear airway and preventing cold stress. Hypoglycemia is treated with oral feedings (e.g., breast, formula) or IV dextrose as the infant's condition warrants. An external heat source (radiant warmer or incubator) should be used until the infant is able to maintain an adequate body temperature. Nursing support of parents is the same as that given to parents of preterm infants.

Common problems that affect SGA or IUGR infants are perinatal asphyxia, meconium aspiration (discussed previously), immunodeficiency, hypoglycemia, **polycythemia**, and temperature instability.

Perinatal Asphyxia

Commonly, IUGR infants have been exposed to chronic hypoxia for varying periods before labour and birth. Labour is a stressor to the normal fetus; it is an even greater stressor for the growth-restricted fetus. The chronically hypoxic infant is severely compromised by a normal labour and has difficulty compensating after birth. The alert, wide-eyed appearance of the newborn is attributed to prolonged fetal hypoxia. Appropriate management and resuscitation are essential for the depressed infant.

The birth of the SGA newborn with perinatal asphyxia may be associated with a maternal history of heavy cigarette smoking; gestational hypertension; low socioeconomic status; multifetal gestation; congenital infections such as rubella, cytomegalovirus, and toxoplasmosis; advanced diabetes mellitus; and cardiac problems. Sequelae of perinatal asphyxia include MAS and hypoglycemia.

Hypoglycemia and Hyperglycemia

All high-risk infants are at risk for hypoglycemia. Infants who experience physiological stress may experience hypoglycemia as a result of a decreased glycogen supply, inadequate gluconeogenesis, or overutilization of glycogen stored during fetal and postnatal life. Preterm infants may also become hypoglycemic as a result of inadequate intake and increased metabolic demands due to illness (Blackburn, 2007). There is insufficient evidence to support the concept that the preterm or high-risk infant can tolerate lower levels of serum glucose any better than healthy term infants (Blackburn, 2007) (see Chapter 25, p. 654, for discussion of hypoglycemia). The SGA infant, not unlike the preterm infant, is at higher risk for hypoglycemia as a result of decreased fetal stores and decreased rate of gluconeogenesis.

Hyperglycemia is defined as a blood glucose level greater than 6.9 mmol/L (whole blood) or plasma glucose of 8.0 to

8.3 mmol/L (Blackburn, 2007). This condition is seen primarily in ELBW and VLBW infants receiving parenteral nutrition with dextrose concentrations of 5% or higher. Hyperglycemia may be just as harmful to the preterm infant as hypoglycemia. Increased circulating levels of glucose may lead to osmotic changes, increased urine output, and fluid shifts in the already compromised CNS of the preterm infant. The net result of hyperglycemia may be cellular dehydration and IVH. Preterm infants undergoing stress (i.e., surgery) may also become hyperglycemic with increased catecholamine release, which inhibits insulin release and glucose utilization (Blackburn, 2007). In summary, ELBW and VLBW infants should be monitored closely for both hypoglycemia and hyperglycemia while receiving parenteral nutrition, both during the acute phase of illness and perioperatively.

Heat Loss

SGA infants are particularly susceptible to temperature instability as a result of decreased **brown fat** deposit; decreased adipose tissue; large body surface exposure; inability to accomplish flexed position due to poor muscle tone; and decreased glycogen storage in major organs such as the liver and heart. Close attention must be given to maintenance of a neutral thermal environment.

Large-for-Gestational-Age Infants

An infant is considered large for gestational age (LGA) despite gestational age when the weight is above the ninetieth percentile on growth charts or 2 standard deviations above the mean weight for gestational age. The LGA infant is at greater risk for morbidity than the SGA and preterm infant; such infants have a higher incidence of birth injuries, asphyxia, and congenital anomalies such as heart defects (Stoll & Adams-Chapman, 2007). In Canada the rate of infants born who were LGA was 11.1% in 2008 (PHAC, 2012).

All pregnancies of longer than 42 weeks of gestation must be carefully evaluated. LGA newborns may be preterm, term, or postterm; they may be infants of diabetic mothers (IDMs). Each of these problems carries special concerns. Regardless of coexisting potential problems, the LGA infant is at risk by virtue of size alone.

The nurse needs to assess the LGA infant for hypoglycemia and trauma resulting from vaginal or Caesarean birth. Any specific birth injuries should be identified and treated appropriately.

Infants of Diabetic Mothers

All infants born to mothers with diabetes are at some risk for complications. The degree of risk is influenced by the severity and duration of maternal disease. Problems seen in IDMs include congenital anomalies (especially cardiac), macrosomia, birth trauma and perinatal asphyxia, RDS, hypoglycemia, cardiomyopathy, hyperbilirubinemia, and polycythemia (see Chapter 14). Because some of these problems are also seen in infants with gestational age–related problems, discussion of IDMs is included here.

Pathophysiology

The mechanisms responsible for the problems seen in IDMs are not fully understood. Congenital anomalies are believed to be caused by fluctuations in blood glucose levels and episodes of ketoacidosis in early pregnancy. Later in pregnancy, when the mother's pancreas cannot release sufficient insulin to meet increased demands, maternal hyperglycemia results. The high levels of glucose cross the placenta and stimulate the fetal pancreas to release insulin. The combination of the increased supply of maternal glucose and other nutrients, the inability of maternal insulin to cross the placenta, and increased fetal insulin result in excessive fetal growth called *macrosomia.*

Hyperinsulinemia accounts for many of the problems that the fetus or infant develops. In addition to fluctuating glucose levels, maternal vascular involvement or superimposed maternal infection adversely affects the fetus. Normally, maternal blood has a more alkaline pH than does carbon dioxide–rich fetal blood. This phenomenon encourages the exchange of oxygen and carbon dioxide across the placental membrane. When maternal blood is more acidotic than the fetal blood (i.e., during ketoacidosis), minimal exchange of carbon dioxide or oxygen occurs at the level of the placenta. The mortality for the unborn infant resulting from an episode of maternal ketoacidosis may be as high as 50% or more (Kalhan & Parimi, 2006).

The single most important factor influencing fetal well-being is the mother's glycemic status. There are indications that some neonatal conditions (e.g., macrosomia, hypoglycemia, preterm birth) may be eliminated, or the incidence decreased, by maintaining control over maternal glucose levels within narrow limits (Berger et al., 2002). Tight glucose control is defined as maintenance of 1-hour postprandial maternal blood glucose levels between 5.5 and 7.7 mmol/L or a **glycosylated hemoglobin** (A_{1c}) between 6 and 7% (see Box 14-1) (Brophy, Scarlett-Fergusson, & Webber, 2010; Canadian Diabetes Association, 2008).

Congenital Anomalies

Congenital anomalies occur in about 7 to 10% of IDMs—an incidence two to four times that of infants born to mothers without diabetes. The incidence is greatest among SGA newborns. Growth restriction and SGA infants result when severe maternal vascular disease is present. The most commonly occurring anomalies involve the cardiac, musculoskeletal, and central nervous systems. Most anomalies associated with diabetic pregnancies occur before the eighth week of gestation, thus reinforcing the importance of glycemic control both antenatally and in the early stages of pregnancy.

The incidence of congenital heart lesions in IDMs is five times higher than the general population. Coarctation of the aorta, transposition of the great vessels, and septal defects are the most common lesions. Maternal glycemic control is correlated with the incidence of defects; the better the control, the lower the risk of defects.

CNS anomalies include anencephaly, encephalocele, meningomyelocele, and hydrocephalus. The musculoskeletal system may be affected by caudal regression syndrome (i.e., sacral agenesis, deformities of the lower extremities, shortening or deformity of the femurs). Hypertrichosis on the pinnae (excessive hair growth on the external ear) is common. Other defects may include gastrointestinal atresia and urinary tract malformations.

Macrosomia

Despite improvements in maintaining maternal glycemic control, the incidence of macrosomia in infants of insulin-dependent diabetics is higher than in infants born of mothers who are not diabetic. At birth, the typical LGA infant has a round, cherubic ("tomato" or cushingoid) face, chubby body, and a plethoric or flushed complexion (Fig. 27-11). The infant has enlarged internal organs (i.e., hepatosplenomegaly, cardiomegaly) and increased body fat, especially around the shoulders. The placenta and umbilical cord are larger than average. The brain is the only organ that is not enlarged. IDMs may be LGA but physiologically immature.

The macrosomic infant is at risk for hypoglycemia, hypocalcemia, hyperviscosity, and hyperbilirubinemia. The excessive shoulder size in these infants often leads to dystocia, particularly because the head may be smaller in proportion to the shoulders than in a nonmacrosomic infant. Macrosomic infants may incur birth trauma.

Birth Trauma and Perinatal Asphyxia

Birth injury (resulting from macrosomia or method of birth) and perinatal asphyxia occur in 20% of infants of gestational diabetic mothers and 35% of IDMs. Examples of birth trauma include cephalohematoma; paralysis of the facial nerve (see Fig. 28-3); fractured clavicle or humerus; brachial plexus paralysis, usually Erb-Duchenne palsy (see Figs. 28-1 and 28-2); and phrenic nerve paralysis, invariably associated with diaphragmatic paralysis.

Respiratory Distress Syndrome

IDMs are four to six times more likely than infants of nondiabetic mothers to develop RDS. With improved maternal glycemic control, this risk has been substantially reduced.

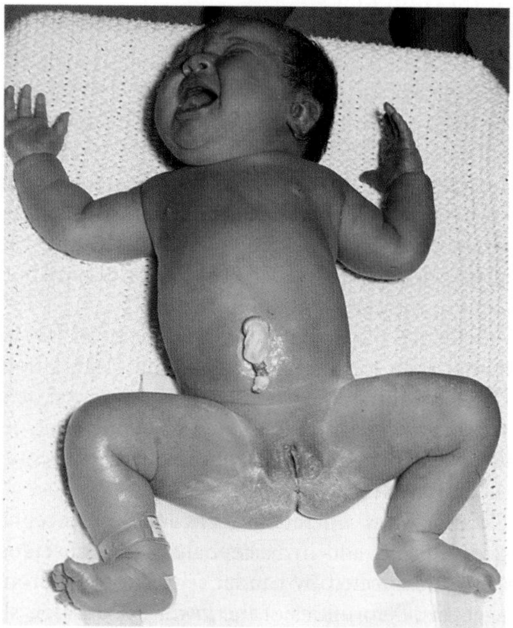

Fig. 27-11 Macrosomic newborn. *(From O'Doherty, N. [1986].* Neonatology: Micro atlas of the newborn. *Nutley, NJ: Hoffmann-La Roche.)*

Synthesis of surfactant may be delayed because of the high fetal serum level of insulin. Before delivery, fetal lung maturation tests via amniocentesis may be done, including lecithin/sphingomyelin ratio, phosphatidylglycerol, and disaturated phosphatidylcholine measurements. In the IDM, the presence of phosphatidylglycerol in the amniotic fluid is the best predictor of normal neonatal respiratory function.

Hypoglycemia

Hypoglycemia affects many IDMs. After constant exposure to high circulating levels of glucose, the fetal pancreas undergoes hyperplasia, resulting in hyperinsulinemia. Disruption of the fetal glucose supply occurs with the clamping of the umbilical cord, and the neonate's blood glucose level falls rapidly because of fetal hyperinsulinism. Hypoglycemia is most common in the macrosomic or SGA infant, but blood glucose levels should be monitored in all infants of known or suspected diabetic mothers.

Asymptomatic or symptomatic hypoglycemia most commonly manifests within the first 1 to 3 hours after birth. Signs of hypoglycemia include jitteriness, apnea, tachypnea, and cyanosis. Significant hypoglycemia may result in seizures. Hypoglycemia is worsened by the presence of hypothermia or respiratory distress.

Studies confirm the importance of maintaining serum glucose levels above 2.8 mmol/L in hyperinsulinemic infants with hypoglycemia to prevent serious neurological sequelae (Aziz et al., 2004; Cowett & Loughead, 2002).

Hypocalcemia and Hypomagnesemia

Hypocalcemia occurs in as many as 50% of IDMs. A number of these cases are related to hypoxia or prematurity; however, the overall incidence of hypocalcemia is higher than in nondiabetic pregnancies. Hypomagnesemia is believed to develop because of maternal renal losses that occur in diabetes. Hypocalcemia is associated with preterm birth, birth trauma, and perinatal asphyxia. Signs of hypocalcemia are similar to those of hypoglycemia, but they occur within the first 24 hours of age.

Cardiomyopathy

All IDMs need careful observation for cardiomegaly and heart failure, common findings among these infants. Two types of cardiomyopathy can occur—hypertrophic (HCM) and nonhypertrophic (non-HCM). Clinicians must be alert to identify correctly the type of lesion so that appropriate therapy is instituted. Both types of lesions are associated with respiratory symptoms and congestive heart failure.

HCM is characterized by a hypercontractile and thickened myocardium. The ventricular walls are thickened, as is the septum, which, in severe cases, results in outflow tract obstructions. The mitral valve functions poorly. In non-HCM, the myocardium is poorly contractile and overstretched. The ventricles are increased in size, but there is no outflow obstruction. Most infants are asymptomatic, but severe outflow obstruction may cause left ventricular heart failure. HCM may be treated with a β-adrenergic blocker (i.e., propranolol) to decrease contractility and heart rate. A cardiotonic agent is used to treat non-HCM (i.e., digoxin) to increase contractility and decrease heart rate. The abnormality usually resolves in 3 to 12 months.

Hyperbilirubinemia and Polycythemia

IDMs are at increased risk of developing hyperbilirubinemia. Many IDMs are polycythemic. Polycythemia increases blood viscosity, thereby impairing circulation. In addition, an increased number of RBCs and accompanying hemolysis increases the potential bilirubin load that the neonate must clear. The additional RBCs are produced in extramedullary foci (liver and spleen) in addition to the usual sites (bone marrow). Therefore, both liver function and bilirubin clearance may be adversely affected. Bruising associated with the birth of a macrosomic infant will contribute further to high bilirubin levels.

Nursing Care

Ideally, planning for the IDM begins during the antenatal period. It is beneficial if members of the neonatal team are present at the birth. Implementation of care depends on the neonate's particular problems. If the maternal blood glucose level was well controlled throughout the pregnancy, the infant may require only monitoring. Because **euglycemia** is not always possible, the nurse must promptly recognize and treat any consequences of maternal diabetes that arise (see Nursing Care Plan).

Discharge Planning and Transport

Discharge Planning

Discharge planning for the high-risk newborn begins early in the hospitalization. Throughout the infant's hospitalization, the nurse must gather information from the health care team members and the family. This information is used to determine the infant's and family's readiness for discharge.

As the nurse assesses the discharge needs of the infant's parents, he or she needs to take steps to eliminate any knowledge deficits. Discharge teaching for the high-risk newborn's family is extensive, requires time and planning, and cannot be accomplished on the day of discharge alone. Information should be provided about infant care, especially as it pertains to the particular infant's needs (e.g., supplemental oxygen, gastrostomy feedings, follow-up medical visits). Parent education includes having them give return demonstrations of their infant care skills to show whether they are becoming increasingly independent in providing care for their infant. Parents of a preterm infant or one with special needs should be given

NURSING CARE PLAN ● The Infant of Mother With Diabetes Mellitus

Nursing Diagnosis: Risk for unstable blood glucose related to hypoglycemia secondary to hyperinsulinemia and maternal diabetes

Expected Outcome

Infant will exhibit serum blood glucose levels that are within normal limits.

Nursing Interventions/*Rationales*

Monitor blood glucose levels in infants at known risk for hypoglycemia (e.g., SGA, preterm [ELBW, VLBW], IDM) *to assess and detect early onset to prevent complications.*

Observe for signs of hypoglycemia (e.g., jitteriness, lethargy, poor feeding, seizures, cyanosis, diaphoresis) *to assess and respond appropriately to prevent complications.*

Institute early feeding of breast milk or infant formula *to prevent or treat early hypoglycemia.*

Reduce adverse environmental factors (e.g., cold stress, hypoxia, respiratory distress) *that can predispose infant to hypoglycemia.*

Nursing Diagnosis: Ineffective breathing pattern related to lung immaturity secondary to maternal diabetes (gestational or pre-existing)

Expected Outcome

Infant will exhibit breathing pattern adequate to maintain oxygenation (i.e., respiratory rate, rhythm, and characteristics within normal limits).

Nursing Interventions/*Rationales*

Monitor infant's vital signs and patency of airway *to evaluate pulmonary and circulatory status.*

Avoid activities that may lower body temperature and lead to cold stress, *which can induce or worsen respiratory distress.*

Suction as needed *to keep airway patent and prevent aspiration.*

Position infant on side initially *to facilitate mucus drainage.*

Have resuscitation equipment and oxygen available *for quick treatment of respiratory distress.*

Nursing Diagnosis: Risk for temperature instability related to physiological immaturity

See Body Temperature Maintenance on p. 646 in Chapter 25.

Nursing Diagnosis: Anxiety (parental—risk for powerlessness, situational low self-esteem, ineffective coping) related to neonate's condition, management, and prognosis

Expected Outcome

Parents demonstrate understanding of prognosis and therapy for infant.

Nursing Interventions/*Rationales*

Explain potential effects of maternal diabetic condition on newborn *to relieve fear of unknown and support ability to cope.*

Encourage open communication (e.g., inform parents of ongoing condition, procedures, and treatment; answer questions; correct misperceptions; actively listen to parental concerns) *to provide support and help provide a sense of control.*

Encourage parents to interact with the infant and become involved in care routines *to foster emotional connection.*

Arrange for return demonstration of care by parents *to assess competence, provide positive reinforcement, and decrease their anxiety.*

the opportunity to room-in and spend a night or two providing care for their infant away from the NICU. This affords them the opportunity to become more aware of the necessary care and to have transition time in which to ask questions regarding home care. Additional parent teaching should include bathing and skin care; requirements for meeting nutritional needs after discharge; safety in the home, including supine sleep position and prevention of infection (e.g., respiratory syncytial virus); and medication administration.

Medical equipment and supplies required for the care of the infant in the home should be delivered to the home before discharge; parents and care providers should have education and ample practice in its use. Parents of an infant being discharged with special needs (i.e., gavage or gastrostomy feedings, oxygen, tracheostomy, or colostomy) should receive several days of carefully planned education in the various procedures before discharge.

Parents should obtain an age-appropriate car seat before discharge and demonstrate its use with the infant. Car seat safety is an essential aspect of discharge planning, and infants at less than 37 weeks of gestation should have a period of observation in an appropriate car seat to monitor for possible apnea, bradycardia, and desaturations (see Chapter 25, p. 669) (see Community Focus box).

Preterm infants have a high rate of readmission to hospital and emergency department visits. It is imperative that the family have a health care professional they can contact for questions regarding infant care and behaviour once they are home.

Before discharge, all high-risk or preterm infants should receive the appropriate immunizations, metabolic screening, hematology assessment (bilirubin risk as appropriate), and evaluation of hearing. Successful discharge of a high-risk infant requires an interprofessional approach. Medical, nursing, social services, and other professionals (physiotherapy, occupational therapy, developmental follow-up specialist) are crucial to the smooth transition of these infants and their families to the community and home. If the infant is retro-transferred to the community hospital that referred either the mother before the infant's birth or the infant after birth, inter-facility communication is essential to continuity of care.

Discharge to home for high-risk infants does not mean they can be treated like healthy term newborns. Follow-up by a practitioner familiar with the issues common to the high-risk newborn is essential. Further follow-up of specific complications by qualified specialists and referral to centres for developmental interventions can help ensure the best outcome possible for these infants.

Referrals for appropriate community resources also need to be made for infants with developmental disabilities or those at risk for further problems (e.g., preterm infants). Social-service involvement is especially important for young or psychosocially high-risk parents (e.g., parents with a history of substance use or child maltreatment).

For the family of the child who is technology dependent, special education needs should be discussed before discharge. For further discussion of home care, see Chapter 43.

Transport to a Regional Centre

If a hospital is not equipped to care for a high-risk mother and fetus or a high-risk infant, transfer to a specialized perinatal or regional tertiary care centre is arranged. Maternal transport occurs with the fetus in utero and this has two distinct advantages: (1) neonatal morbidity and mortality are decreased, and (2) the mother and infant are not separated at birth.

COMMUNITY FOCUS

Preterm and Late-Term Infant Car Seat Evaluation

The Canadian Paediatric Society (2010) recommends that late preterm infants be evaluated for apnea, hyperbilirubinemia, temperature stability, and feeding ability before hospital discharge. Based on the available literature, suggestions for providing a car seat evaluation of infants born before 37 weeks of gestation to assess for apnea, bradycardia, and oxygen desaturation episodes, include the following:

- Use the parents' car seat for the evaluation.
- Perform the evaluation 1 to 7 days before the infant's anticipated discharge.
- Secure the infant in the car seat per guidelines, using blanket rolls on sides, if necessary.
- Set pulse oximeter low alarm at 88% (arbitrary).
- Set heart rate low alarm limit at 80 beats/min and apnea alarm at 20 seconds (cardiorespiratory monitor).
- Leave the infant undisturbed in the car seat for 90 to 120 minutes or for the time it will take to drive home (if more than 90 minutes).
- Document the infant's tolerance to car seat evaluation.
- An episode of desaturation, bradycardia, or apnea (20 seconds or more) constitutes a failure, and evaluation by the practitioner must occur before discharge.
- Repeat the test once modifications are made to the car seat, car bed, or infant's position in either restraint system (supplemental oxygen may be required).
- A certified car seat technician may be consulted to assist with proper placement of (1) the infant in the car seat (or bed) and (2) the car seat (or bed) in the vehicle.
- The technician will demonstrate to the parents the appropriate positioning of the infant in the restraint device and have the parents do a return demonstration.
- Document the interventions, the infant's tolerance, and the parents' return demonstration.

(Information from American Academy of Pediatrics. [2009]. Safe transportation of preterm and low birth weight infants at hospital discharge. *Pediatrics, 123*[5], 1424–1429; Canadian Paediatric Society. [2010]. Safe discharge of the late preterm infant. *Paediatrics and Child Health, 15*[10], 655–660; Transport Canada. [2008]. *Transporting infants and children with special needs in personal vehicles: A best practices guide for healthcare practitioners.* Ottawa, ON: Author; van Schaik, C., & Canadian Paediatric Society, Injury Prevention Committee. [2008]. Transportation of infants and children in motor vehicles. *Paediatrics and Child Health, 13*[4], 313–318.)

For a variety of reasons, it is not always possible to transport the mother before the birth. Therefore, physicians and nurses in all facilities must have the skills and equipment necessary for making an accurate diagnosis and implementing emergency interventions to stabilize the infant's condition until transport can occur (Rojas, Shirley, & Rush, 2011). The goal of these interventions is to maintain the infant's condition within the normal physiological range. Specific attention should be given to vital signs, oxygenation and ventilation, thermoregulation, acid–base balance, fluid and electrolyte status, blood glucose, and developmental interventions.

Arrangements for transport to a tertiary centre should be made as soon as the high-risk infant is identified (see Community Focus box). The infant must be kept warm and adequately oxygenated (including intubation and surfactant replacement as indicated); have vital signs and oxygen saturation monitored; and, when indicated, receive an IV infusion. The infant must be transported in a specially designed incubator unit containing a complete life support system and other emergency equipment that can be carried by ambulance, helicopter, or a fixed-wing aircraft (Fig. 27-12).

The transport team may consist of physicians, nurse practitioners, nurses, and respiratory therapists. The team must have experience in resuscitation, stabilization, and provision of critical care during the transport. Teams can provide information for the parents about the tertiary centre as well as allow the parents to see the newborn prior to transfer (Box 27-5).

The birth of any high-risk infant can cause profound parental stress. Parents often grieve the loss of the ideal infant and fear the possible eventual outcomes. They must also deal with the technological world surrounding their infant. Amid all the equipment, it is sometimes difficult for them to perceive the infant and respond to his or her needs. Parents of high-risk infants who have been transported to a regional centre often need additional support.

Transport From a Regional Centre

Infants may need to be transferred back (retrotransport or retrotransfer) to the referring facility. Preterm infants who require thermoregulation and gavage feedings may be cared for in community hospitals closer to the parents' home. This allows parents to visit their infant more easily and to work with their personal health care provider on the long-range expected outcomes for the infant. Specialized incubators make these trips possible (see Fig. 27-12). However, parents may express mixed feelings about such return transports and may be reluctant to adapt to a different facility and group of caregivers. To minimize some of these concerns, it is important to give the parents clear information about return transports during the initial discharge planning.

Although at the time of discharge parents may not recognize the need for information on the various resources available to help them in the care of their infant, they can be given lists of agencies and telephone numbers for later use. Providing them with a patient-specific directory of special programs, community and social support, as well as funding resources can help them make the transition to home. As the nurse continually reinforces the idea that the infant will go home, the parents are prompted to plan for the days ahead and be more prepared to take their infant home when the time comes.

COMMUNITY FOCUS

Neonatal Transport

During a scheduled clinical experience in the NICU, observe a transport team leaving to pick up an infant from a referring hospital. Who are the transport team members? What are their job responsibilities when not transporting patients? What equipment are they taking on the transport? How was the referral made? What communication links exist between the NICU and the community hospitals in the surrounding area? What communication links exist between the NICU and the transport team when they are transporting the sick infant? How are the parents kept informed of the infant's condition?

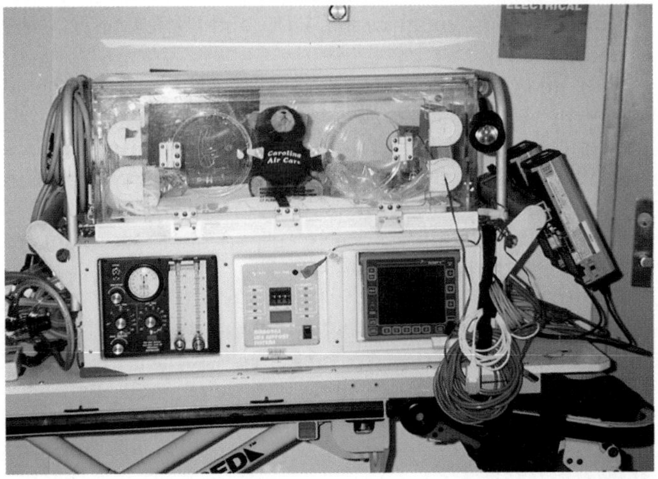

Fig. 27-12 Total life support system for transport of high-risk newborns. *(Courtesy UNC Hospitals, Carolina Air Care, Chapel Hill, NC.)*

BOX 27-5 Information for Parents About the Tertiary Centre

- Exact location of the unit—address, map, waiting area for relatives and friends
- Visiting hours and hospital rules
- Telephone numbers
- Names of individuals likely to be involved with the newborn's care (e.g., primary nurse, neonatologist, clinical manager)
- Information about the neonatal intensive care unity (NICU) or special care unit
- Location of parking facilities, nearby lodging, and guidelines regarding visitation by siblings
- Any particular rules or regulations regarding the special care unit

(From Rojas, M. A., Shirley, K., & Rush, M. G. [2011]. Perinatal transport and levels of care. In S. L. Gardner, B. S. Carter, M. Enzman-Hines, & J. A Hernandez [Eds.], *Merenstein & Gardner's handbook of neonatal intensive care* [7th ed., pp. 39–51]. St. Louis: Mosby.)

Key Points

- Preterm infants are at risk for problems related to the immaturity of their organ systems.
- Late preterm infants are at higher risk for feeding problems, respiratory distress, jaundice, poor neurodevelopment, hypoglycemia, infection, and thermoregulation than their term counterparts.
- RDS, ROP, and chronic lung disease (BPD) are associated with preterm birth.
- High-risk infants must be observed for respiratory distress and other early signs of physiological distress.
- The adaptation of parents to preterm or high-risk infants differs from that of parents of term infants.
- Parents need special instruction (e.g., CPR, oxygen therapy, suctioning, developmental care) before they take a high-risk infant home.
- Infants born to diabetic mothers (gestational or otherwise) are at risk for hypoglycemia, RDS, and birth asphyxia and trauma.
- SGA infants are considered to be at risk because of fetal growth restriction.
- Atypical or abnormal fetal status among postterm infants is related to the progressive placental insufficiency that can occur in a postterm pregnancy.
- Specially trained nurses may transport high-risk infants to and from special care units.

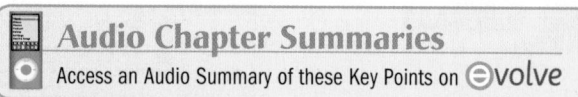

Audio Chapter Summaries

Access an Audio Summary of these Key Points on evolve

References

ACoRN Editorial Board. (2010). *Acute care of at-risk newborns*. Vancouver, BC: Author.

Adams-Chapman, I., & Stoll, B. (2007). Nervous system disorders. In R. M. Kliegman, R. E. Behrman, H. B. Jenson, & B. F. Stanton (Eds.), *Nelson textbook of pediatrics* (18th ed.). Philadelphia: Saunders.

Alfaleh, K., & Bassler, D. (2008). Probiotics for prevention of necrotizing enterocolitis in preterm infants. *Cochrane Database of Systematic Reviews*, Issue 1. Art. No. CD005496. doi:10.1002/14651858.CD005496.pub2

Als, H. (1998). Developmental care in the newborn intensive care unit. *Current Opinion in Pediatrics, 10*(2), 138–142.

Altimier, L., & Lutes, L. (2001). Cobedding multiples. *Newborn and Infant Nursing Reviews, 1*(4), 205–206.

American Academy of Pediatrics. (2009). *Pediatric nutrition handbook* (6th ed.). Elk Grove Village, IL: Author.

Anderson, M. S., Wood, L. L., Keller, J. A., & Hay, Jr., W. W. (2011). Enteral nutrition. In S. L. Gardner, B. S. Carter, M. Enzman-Hines, & J. A. Hernandez (Eds.), *Merenstein & Gardner's handbook of neonatal intensive care* (7th ed., pp. 398–433). St. Louis: Mosby.

Association of Women's Health, Obstetric and Neonatal Nurses. (2007). *Neonatal skin care: Evidence-based clinical practice guideline* (2nd ed.). Washington, DC: Author.

Aziz, K., Dancy, P., & Canadian Paediatric Society, Fetus and Newborn Committee. (2004). Screening guidelines for newborns at risk for low blood glucose. *Paediatrics and Child Health, 9*(10), 723–729.

Bakewell-Sachs, S. (2007). Near-term/late preterm infants. *Newborn and Infant Nursing Reviews, 7*(2), 67–71. doi:10.1053/j.nainr.2007.05.001

Barrington, K. J. & Finer, N. N. (2007). Inhaled nitric oxide for respiratory failure in preterm infants: A systematic review. *Pediatrics, 120*(5), 1088–1099. doi:10.1542/peds.2007-0726

Beeram, M., Olvera, R., Krauss, D., Loughran, C., & Petty, M. (2006). Effects of topical emollient therapy on infants at or less than 27 weeks' gestation. *Journal of the National Medical Association, 98*(2), 261–264.

Berger, H., et al (2002). SOGC clinical practice guideline: Screening for gestational diabetes mellitus. *Journal of Obstetrics and Gynaecology Canada, 24*(11), 894–903.

Berger, T. M., Bachmann, I. I., Adams, M., & Schubiger, G. (2004). Impact of improved survival of very low–birth-weight infants on incidence and severity of bronchopulmonary dysplasia. *Biology of the Neonate, 86*(2), 124–130.

Bin-Nun, A., Bromiker, R., Wilschanski, M., Kaplan, M., Rudensky, B., Caplan, M., & Hammerman, C. (2005). Oral probiotics prevent necrotizing enterocolitis in very low birth weight neonates. *Journal of Pediatrics, 147*(2), 143–146. doi:10.1016/j.jpeds.2005.03.054

Birnbaum, R., & Limperopoulos, C. (2009). Nonoral feeding practices for infants in the neonatal intensive care unit. *Advances in Neonatal Care, 9*(4), 180–184. doi:10.1097/ANC.0b013e3181aa9c65

Blackburn, S. T. (2007). *Maternal, fetal, and neonatal physiology: A clinical perspective* (3rd ed.). St. Louis: Saunders.

Blackburn, S. T. (2009a). Central nervous system vulnerabilities in preterm infants, part I. *Journal of Perinatal and Neonatal Nursing, 23*(1), 12–14. doi:10.1097/JPN.0b013e31819685cc

Blackburn, S. T. (2009b). Central nervous system vulnerabilities in preterm infants, part II. *Journal of Perinatal and Neonatal Nursing, 23*(2), 108–110. doi:10.1097/JPN.0b013e3181a3924b

Blackburn, S. T., & Ditzenberger, G. R. (2007). Neurologic system. In C. Kenner & J. W. Lott (Eds.), *Comprehensive neonatal care: An interdisciplinary approach* (4th ed., pp. 267–299). St. Louis: Saunders.

Bombell, S. & McGuire, W. (2008). Delayed introduction of progressive enteral feeds to prevent necrotising enterocolitis in very low birth weight infants. *Cochrane Database of Systematic Reviews*, Issue 2. Art. No. CD001970. doi:10.1002/14651858.CD001970.pub2

Brophy, K. M., Scarlett-Fergusson, H., & Webber, K. S. (2010). Drug use in pregnancy and lactation. In K. M. Brophy, H. Scarlett-Fergusson, K. S. Webber, A. D. Abrans, S. S. Pennington, & C. B. Lammon (Eds.), *Clinical drug therapy for Canadian practice* (2nd ed.). Toronto: Lippincott.

Brown, W. D. & Landers, S. (2011). Heat balance. In S. L. Gardner, B. S. Carter, M. Enzman-Hines, & J. A Hernandez (Eds.), *Merenstein & Gardner's handbook of neonatal intensive care* (7th ed., pp. 113–133). St. Louis: Mosby.

Burkhammer, M. D., Anderson, G. C., & Chiu, S-H. (2004). Grief, anxiety, perinatal problems: Healing with kangaroo care. *Journal of Obstetric, Gynecologic, and Neonatal Nursing, 33*(6), 774–782.

Byers, J. F., Waugh, W. R., & Lowman, L. B. (2006). Sound level exposure of high-risk infants in different environmental conditions. *Neonatal Network, 25*(1), 25–32.

Byers, J. F., Yovaish, W., Lowman, L. B., & Francis, J. D. (2003). Co-bedding versus single-bedding of premature multiple-gestation infants in incubators. *Journal of Obstetric, Gynecologic, and Neonatal Nursing, 32*(3), 340–347.

Canadian Diabetes Association. (2008). Clinical practice guidelines for the prevention and management of diabetes in Canada. *Canadian Journal of Diabetes, 32*(Suppl 1), S1–S201. Retrieved from http://www.diabetes.ca/for-professionals/resources/2008-cpg/.

Canadian Institute for Health Information (CIHI). (2009). *Too early, too small: A profile of small babies across Canada*. Ottawa: Author.

Centers for Disease Control and Prevention. (2002). *Enterobacter sakazakii* infections associated with the use of powdered infant formula—Tennessee, 2001. *MMWR: Morbidity and Mortality Weekly Report, 51*(14), 297–300.

Cherif, A., Jabnoun, S., & Khrouf, N. (2007). Oral ibuprofen in early curative closure of patent ductus arteriosus in very premature infants. *American Journal of Perinatology, 24*(6), 339–345. doi:10.1055/s-2007-981853

Conde-Agudelo, A., Belizan, J. M., & Diaz-Rossello, J. (2011). Kangaroo mother care to reduce morbidity and mortality in low birthweight infants. *Cochrane Database of Systematic Reviews*, Issue 3. Art. No. CD002771. doi:10.1002/14651858.CD002771.pub2

Cowett, R. M., & Loughead, J. L. (2002). Neonatal glucose metabolism: Differential diagnoses, evaluation, and treatment of hypoglycemia. *Neonatal Network, 21*(4), 9–19.

Curley, M. A., Razmus, I. S., Roberts, K. E., & Wypij, D. (2003). Predicting pressure ulcer risk in pediatric patients: The Braden Q scale. *Nursing Research, 52*(1), 22–33.

Darcy, A. E. (2009). Complications of the late preterm infant. *Journal of Perinatal and Neonatal Nursing, 23*(1), 78–86. doi:10.1097/JPN.0b013e31819685b6

Darmstadt, G. L., et al. (2005). Effect of topical treatment with skin barrier–enhancing emollients on nosocomial infections in preterm infants in

Bangladesh: A randomised controlled trial. *Lancet, 365*(9464), 1039–1045. doi:10.1016/S0140-6736(05)71140-5

Davis, D. J., Barrington, K. J., & Canadian Paediatric Society, Fetus and Newborn Committee. (2005). Recommendations for neonatal surfactant therapy. *Paediatrics and Child Health, 10*(2), 109–116.

Diehl-Jones, W. L., & Askin, D. F. (2004). Nutritional modulation of neonatal outcomes. *AACN Clinical Issues, 15*(1), 83–96.

Dodd, V. L. (2005). Implications of kangaroo care for growth and development in preterm infants. *Journal of Obstetric, Gynecologic, and Neonatal Nursing, 34*(2), 218–232. doi:10.1177/0884217505274698

Donn, S. M., & Sinha, S. K. (2003). Invasive and noninvasive neonatal mechanical ventilation. *Respiratory Care, 48*(4), 426–441.

Donovan, R., Puppala, B., Angst, D., & Coyle, B. W. (2006). Outcomes of early nutrition support in extremely low-birth-weight infants. *Nutrition in Clinical Practice, 21*, 395–400. doi:10.1177/0115426506021004395

Dudell, G. G., & Stoll, B. J. (2007). Respiratory tract disorders. In R. M. Kliegman, R. E. Behrman, H. B. Jenson, & B. F. Stanton (Eds.), *Nelson textbook of pediatrics* (18th ed., pp. 728–752). Philadelphia: Saunders.

Edwards, W., Conner, J., & Soll, R. (2004). The effect of prophylactic ointment therapy on nosocomial sepsis rates and skin integrity in infants with birth weights of 501–1000g. *Pediatrics, 113*(5), 1195–1203.

Ehrenkranz, R. A. (2007). Early, aggressive nutritional management for very low birth weight infants: What is the evidence? *Seminars in Perinatology, 31*(2), 48–55. doi:10.1053/j.semperi.2007.02.001

Ellett, M. L., Croffie, J. M., Cohen, M. D., & Perkins, S. M. (2005). Gastric tube placement in young children. *Clinical Nursing Research, 14*(3), 238–252. doi:10.1177/1054773805275121

Ellett, M. L., Woodruff, K., & Stewart, D. (2007). The use of carbon dioxide monitoring to determine orogastric tube placement in premature infants: A pilot study. *Gastroenterology Nursing, 30*(6), 414–417. doi:10.1097/01.SGA.0000305222.16522.a4

Ells, A. & Hindle, W. (2000). Commentary on guidelines for screening for retinopathy of prematurity. *Canadian Journal of Ophthalmology, 35*(5), 253–254.

Engle, W. A. (2006). A recommendation for the definition of "late preterm" (near-term) and the birth weight–gestational age classification system. *Seminars in Perinatology, 30*(1), 2–7. doi:10.1053/j.semperi.2006.01.007

Engle, W. A., Tomashek, K. M., Wallman, C., & American Academy of Pediatrics, Committee on Fetus and Newborn. (2007). Late-preterm infants: A population at risk. *Pediatrics, 120*(6), 1390–1401. doi:10.1542/peds.2007-2952

Escobar, G. J., Clark, R. H., & Greene, J. D. (2006). Short-term outcomes of infants born at 35 and 36 weeks gestation: We need to ask more questions. *Seminars in Perinatology, 30*(1), 28–33. doi:10.1053/j.semperi.2006.01.005

Field, D., Elbourne, D., Hardy, P., Fenton, A. C., Ahluwalia, H. L., Halliday, N., on behalf of the INNOVO Trial Collaborating Group. (2007). Neonatal ventilation with inhaled nitric oxide vs. ventilatory support without inhaled nitric oxide for infants with severe respiratory failure born at or near term: The INNOVO multicenter randomised controlled trial. *Neonatology, 91*(2), 73–82. doi:10.1542/peds.2004-1209

Gardner, S., Enzman-Hines, M., & Dickey, L. A. (2011). Respiratory diseases. In S. L. Gardner, B. S. Carter, M. Enzman-Hines, & J. A Hernandez. (Eds.), *Merenstein & Gardner's handbook of neonatal intensive care* (7th ed., pp. 581–677). St. Louis: Mosby.

Gardner, S. L. & Lawrence, R. A. (2011). Breastfeeding the neonate with special needs. In S. L. Gardner, B. S. Carter, M. Enzman-Hines, & J. A Hernandez. (Eds.), *Merenstein & Gardner's handbook of neonatal intensive care* (7th ed., pp. 434–481). St. Louis: Mosby.

Gomella, T. L., Cunningham, M. D., & Eyal, F. G. (2009). *Neonatology: Management, procedures, on-call problems, diseases, and drugs* (6th ed.). Toronto: McGraw-Hill.

Gracey, K., Talbot, D., Lankford, R., & Dodge, P. (2002). The changing face of bronchopulmonary dysplasia. Part 1. *Advances in Neonatal Care, 2*(6), 327–338.

Greenough, A., & Sharma, A. (2005). Optimal strategies for newborn ventilation—A synthesis of the evidence. *Early Human Development, 81*, 957–964. doi:10.1016/j.earlhumdev.2005.10.002

Greenough, A., & Sharma, A. (2007). What is new in ventilation strategies for the neonate? *European Journal of Pediatrics, 166*, 991–996. doi:10.1007/s00431-007-0513-0

Haubrich, K. (2007). Auditory system. In C. Kenner & J. W. Lott (Eds.), *Comprehensive neonatal nursing: A physiologic perspective* (4th ed., pp. 300–312). Philadelphia: Saunders.

Heaberlin, P. D. (2009). Neurologic assessment. In E. P. Tappero & M. E. Honeyfield (Eds.), *Physical assessment of the newborn: A comprehensive approach to the art of physical examination* (4th ed., pp. 159–183.). Santa Rosa, CA: NICU Ink.

Health Canada. (2010). *Recommendations for the preparation and handling of powdered infant formula (PIF)*. Retrieved from http://www.hc-sc.gc.ca/fn-an/nutrition/infant-nourisson/pif-ppn-recommandations-eng.php.

Henderson, G., Craig, S., Brocklehurst, P., & McGuire, W. (2009). Enteral feeding regimens and necrotising enterocolitis in preterm infants: A multicentre case-control study. *Archives of Diseases in Childhood, Fetal-Neonatal Edition, 94*, F120–F123. doi:10.1136/adc.2007.119560

Holditch-Davis, D. & Blackburn, S. T. (2007). Neurobehavioral development. In C. Kenner & W. J. Lott (Eds.), *Comprehensive neonatal care: An interdisciplinary approach* (4th ed., pp. 448–479). St. Louis: Saunders.

Jefferies, A. L. & Canadian Paediatric Society, Fetus and Newborn Committee. (2010). Retinopathy of prematurity: Recommendations for screening. *Paediatrics and Child Health, 15*(10), 667–670.

Johnston, C. C., Filion, F., Campbell-Yeo, M., Goulet, C., Bell, L., McNaughton, K., et al. (2008). Kangaroo mother care diminishes pain from heel lance in very preterm neonates: A crossover trial. *BMC Pediatrics, 8*(13), 1–9. doi:10.1186/1471-2431-8-13

Jones J. G., et al. (2005). The Early Treatment for ROP (ETROP) randomized trial: Study results and nursing care adaptations. *Insight, 30*(2), 7–13.

Joseph, K. S., Demissie, K., & Kramer, M. S. (2002). Obstetric intervention, stillbirth, and preterm birth. *Seminars in Perinatology, 26*(4), 250–259.

Kalhan, S. C. & Parimi, P. S. (2006). Disorders of carbohydrate metabolism. In R. J. Martin, A. A. Fanaroff, & M. C. Walsh (Eds.), *Fanaroff & Martin's neonatal–perinatal medicine: Diseases of the fetus and infant* (8th ed.). Philadelphia: Mosby.

Kenney, P. M., Hoover, D., Williams, L. C., & Iskersky, V. (2011). Cardiovascular diseases and surgical interventions. In S. L. Gardner, B. S. Carter, M. Enzman-Hines, & J. A Hernandez (Eds.), *Merenstein & Gardner's handbook of neonatal intensive care* (7th ed., pp. 678–716). St. Louis: Mosby.

Kliegman, R. M. (2006). Intrauterine growth restriction. In R. J. Martin, A. A. Fanaroff, & M. C. Walsh (Eds.), *Fanaroff & Martin's neonatal–perinatal medicine: Diseases of the fetus and infant* (8th ed.). Philadelphia: Mosby.

Kostandy, R. R., Ludington-Hoe, S. M., Cong, X., Abouelfettoh, A., Bronson, C., Stankus, A., & Jarrell, J. R. (2008). Kangaroo care (skin contact) reduces crying response to pain in preterm neonates: Pilot results. *Pain Management Nursing, 9*(2), 55–65. doi:10.1016/j.pmn.2007.11.004

Kramer, M. S., Demissie, K., Hong, Y., Platt, R. W., Sauve, R., & Liston, R. (2000). The contribution of mild and moderate preterm birth to infant mortality. *Journal of the American Medical Association, 284*(7), 843–849.

LaMar, K., & Dowling, D. A. (2006). Incidence of infection for preterm twins cared for in cobedding in the neonatal intensive-care unit. *Journal of Obstetric, Gynecologic, and Neonatal Nursing, 35*(2), 193–198. doi:10.1111/j.1552-6909.2006.00025.x

Lawrence, R. A., & Lawrence, R. M. (2011). *Breastfeeding: A guide for the medical profession* (7th ed.). Philadelphia: Mosby.

Lovvan III, H. N., Glenn, J. B., Pacetti, A. S., & Carter, B. S. (2011). Neonatal surgery. In S. L. Gardner, B. S. Carter, M. Enzman-Hines, & J. A Hernandez (Eds.), *Merenstein & Gardner's handbook of neonatal intensive care* (7th ed., pp. 812–848). St. Louis: Mosby.

Lund, C. H., & Durand, D. J. (2011). Skin and skin care. In S. L. Gardner, B. S. Carter, M. Enzman-Hines, & J. A Hernandez (Eds.), *Merenstein & Gardner's handbook of neonatal intensive care* (7th ed., pp. 482–501). St. Louis: Mosby.

Lund, C. H., & Kuller, J. M. (2007). Assessment and management of the integumentary system. In C. Kenner & J. W. Lott (Eds.), *Comprehensive neonatal care: An interdisciplinary approach* (4th ed., pp. 65–91). St. Louis: Saunders.

Lund, C. H., & Osborne, J. W. (2004). Validity and reliability of the Neonatal Skin Condition Score. *Journal of Obstetric, Gynecologic, and Neonatal Nursing, 33*(3), 320–327.

McCain, G. C., Ludington-Hoe, S. M., Swinth, J. Y., & Hadeed, A. J. (2005). Heart rate variability responses of a preterm infant to kangaroo care. *Journal of Obstetric, Gynecologic, and Neonatal Nursing, 34*(6), 689–694. doi:10.1177/0884217505281857

Morton, J. A. (2002). Strategies to support extended breastfeeding of the premature infant. *Advances in Neonatal Care, 2*(5), 267–282.

Mosqueda, E., Sapiegiene, L., Glynn, L., Wilson-Colstello, D., & Weiss, M. (2008). The early use of minimal enteral nutrition in extremely low birth weight newborns. *Journal of Perinatology, 28*(4), 264–269. doi:10.1038/sj.jp.7211926

Nucci, A., Burns, R. C., Armah, T., Lowery, K., Yaworski, J. A., Strohm, S., & Squires, R. (2008). Interdisciplinary management of pediatric intestinal failure: A 10-year review of rehabilitation and transplantation. *Journal of Gastrointestinal Surgery, 12*(3), 429–435. doi:10.1007/s11605-007-0444-0

Ohlsson, A., Walia, R., & Shah, S. S. (2010). Ibuprofen for the treatment of patent ductus arteriosus in preterm and/or low birth weight infants. *Cochrane Database of Systematic Reviews* Issue 4. Art. No. CD003481. doi:10.1002/14651858.CD003481.pub4

Perlman, J. M., Wyllie, J., Kattwinkel, J., Atkins, D. L., Chameides, L., Goldsmith, J. P., & Velaphi, S. on behalf of the Neonatal Resuscitation Chapter Collaborators. (2010). Part 11: Neonatal resuscitation: 2010 international consensus on cardiopulmonary resuscitation and emergency cardiovascular care science with treatment recommendations. *Circulation, 122*(Suppl 2), S516–S538. doi:10.1161/CIR.0b013e3181fdf77e

Petrini, J. R., Dias, T., McCormick, M. C., Massolo, M. L., Green, N. S., & Escobar, G. J. (2009). Increased risk of adverse neurological development for late preterm infants. *Journal of Pediatrics, 154*(2), 169–176. doi:10.1016/j.jpeds.2008.08.020

Pollan, C. (2009). Retinopathy of prematurity: An eye toward better outcomes. *Neonatal Network, 28*(2), 93–101.

Public Health Agency of Canada. (2008). *Canadian perinatal health report: 2008 edition*. Ottawa: Author.

Public Health Agency of Canada. (2012). *Perinatal Health Indicators for Canada 2011*. Cat. No. HP7-1/2011 Ottawa: Author.

Reynolds, R. M., & Thureen, P. J. (2007). Special circumstances: Trophic feeds, necrotizing enterocolitis and bronchopulmonary dysplasia. *Seminars in Fetal and Neonatal Medicine, 12*(1), 64–70. doi:10.1016/j.siny.2006.11.002

Rojas, M. A., Shirley, K., & Rush, M. G. (2011). Perinatal transport and levels of care. In S. L. Gardner, B. S. Carter, M. Enzman-Hines, & J. A Hernandez. (Eds.), *Merenstein & Gardner's handbook of neonatal intensive care* (7th ed., pp. 39–51). St. Louis: Mosby.

Sadiq, H. F., Mantych, G., Benawra, R, Deveskar, U. P., & Hocker, J. (2003). Inhaled nitric oxide in the treatment of moderate persistent pulmonary hypertension of the newborn: A randomized controlled, multicenter trial. *Journal of Perinatology, 23*(2), 98–103.

Sahni, R., Ammari, A., Suri, M. S., Milisavljevic, V., Ohira-Kist, K., Wung, J. T., & Polin, R. A. (2005). Is the new definition of bronchopulmonary dysplasia more useful? *Journal of Perinatology, 25*, 41–46. doi:10.1038/sj.jp.7211210

Saugstad, O. D. (2007). Optimal oxygenation at birth and in the neonatal period. *Neonatology, 91*(4), 319–322. doi:10.1159/000101349

Saugstad, O. D., et al. (2003). Resuscitation of newborn infants with 21% or 100% oxygen: Follow-up at 18 and 24 months. *Pediatrics, 112*(2), 296–300.

Schmidt, B. K., & Canadian Oxygen Trial Collaborators. (2005). Efficacy and safety of targeting lower arterial oxygen saturations to reduce oxygen toxicity and oxidative stress in very preterm infants: The Canadian oxygen trial (COT). *Canadian Institutes of Health Research*. Retrieved from http://clinicaltrials.gov/ct2/show/NCT00637169.

Simpson, C., Schanler, R. J., & Lau, C. (2002). Early introduction of oral feeding in preterm infants. *Pediatrics, 110*(3), 517–522.

Sisk, P. M., Lovelady, C. A., Dillard, R. G., Gruber, K. J., & O'Shea, T. M. (2007). Early human milk feeding is associated with a lower risk of necrotizing enterocolitis in very low birth weight infants. *Journal of Perinatology, 27*(7), 428–433. doi:10.1038/sj.jp.7211758

Soll, R., & Blanco, F. (2001). Natural surfactant extract versus synthetic surfactant for neonatal respiratory distress syndrome. *Cochrane Database of Systematic Reviews*, Issue 2. Art. No. CD000144. doi:10.1002/14651858.CD000144

Soll, R., & Morley, C. J. (2001). Prophylactic versus selective use of surfactant in preventing morbidity and mortality in preterm infants. *Cochrane Database of Systematic Reviews*, Issue 2. Art. No. CD000510. doi:10.1002/14651858.CD000510

Squires, A. J., & Hyndman, M. (2009). Prevention of nasal injuries secondary to NCPAP application in the ELBW infant. *Neonatal Network, 28*(1), 13–27.

Statistics Canada. (2009). *Births 2007* (Cat. No. 84F0210X). Ottawa: Author. Retrieved from http://www.statcan.gc.ca/pub/84f0210x/84f0210x2007000-eng.pdf.

Stevens, T. P., Blennow, M., Myers, E. H., & Soll, R. (2007). Early surfactant administration with brief ventilation vs. selective surfactant and continued mechanical ventilation for preterm infants with or at risk for respiratory distress syndrome. *Cochrane Database of Systematic Reviews*, Issue 4. Art. No. CD003063. doi:10.1002/14651858.CD003063.pub3

Stoll, B. J. (2007). Infections in the neonatal infant. In R. M. Kliegman, R. E. Behrman, H. B. Jenson, & B. F. Stanton (Eds.), *Nelson textbook of pediatrics* (18th ed. pp. 794–812). Philadelphia: Saunders.

Stoll, B. J., & Adams-Chapman, I. (2007). The high-risk infant. In R. M. Kliegman, R. E. Behrman, H. B. Jenson, & B. F. Stanton (Eds.), *Nelson textbook of pediatrics* (18th ed., pp. 698–710). Philadelphia: Saunders.

Symington, A., & Pinelli, J. (2006). Developmental care for promoting development and preventing morbidity in preterm infants. *Cochrane Database Systematic of Reviews*, Issue 2. Art. No. CD001814. doi:10.1002/14651858.CD001814.pub2

Talge, N. M., Holzman, C., Wang, J., Lucia, V., Gardiner, J., & Breslau, N. (2010). Late-preterm birth and its association with cognitive and socioemotional outcomes at 6 years of age. *Pediatrics, 126*, 1124–1131. doi:10.1542/peds.2010-1536

Thomas, K. A., & Uran, A. (2007). How the NICU environment sounds to a preterm infant. *MCN: American Journal of Maternal/Child Nursing, 32*(4), 250–253. doi:10.1097/01.NMC.0000281966.23034.e9

Tomashek, K. M., Shapiro-Mendoza, C. K., Davidoff, M. J., & Petrini, J. R. (2007). Differences in mortality between late-preterm and term singleton infants in the United States, 1995–2002. *Journal of Pediatrics, 151*(5), 450–456. doi:10.1016/j.jpeds.2007.05.002

Vain, N. E., Szyld, E. G., Prudent, L. M., Wiswell, T. E., Aquilar, A. M., & Vivas, N. I. (2005). Oropharyngeal and nasopharyngeal suctioning of meconium-stained neonates before delivery of their shoulders: Multicenter, randomized, controlled trial. *Lancet, 364*, 597–602. doi:10.1016/S0140-6736(04)16852-9

van Acker, J., de Smet, F., Muyldermans, G., Bouqatef, A., Naessens, A., & Lauwers, S. (2001). Outbreak of necrotizing enterocolitis associated with *Enterobacter sakazakii* in powdered milk formula. *Journal of Clinical Microbiology, 39*(1), 293–297.

Van Aerde, J., Shah, V., Stark, A. R., & Ohlsson, A. (2002). Postnatal corticosteroids to treat of prevent chronic lung disease in preterm infants: A joint statement with the American Academy of Pediatrics and Canadian Paediatric Society. *Paediatrics and Child Health, 7*(1), 20–28.

Vennarecci, G., et al. (2000). Intestinal transplantation for short gut syndrome attributable to necrotizing enterocolitis. *Pediatrics, 105*(2), 1–5.

Vento, M., Aseni, M., Sastre, J., Lloret, A., Garcia-Sala, F., & Vina, J. (2003). Oxidative stress in asphyxiated term infants resuscitated with 100% oxygen. *Journal of Pediatrics, 142*(3), 240–246.

Volpe, J. J. (2008). *Neurology of the newborn* (5th ed.). Philadelphia: Saunders.

Ward, K. (2001). Perceived needs of parents of critically ill infants in a neonatal intensive care unit (NICU). *Pediatric Nursing, 27*(3), 281–286.

Westrup, B., Sizun, J., & Lagercrantz, H. (2007). Family-centered developmental supportive care: A holistic and humane approach to reduce stress and pain in neonates. *Journal of Perinatology, 27*(Suppl 1), S12–S18. doi:10.1038/sj.jp.7211724

Wheeler, K., Klingenberg, C., McCallion, N., Morley, C. J., & Davis, P. G. (2010). Volume-targeted versus pressure-limited ventilation in the neonate. *Cochrane Database of Systematic Reviews*, Issue 11. Art. No. CD003666. doi:10.1002/14651858.CD003666.pub3

Whyte, R. K., & Canadian Paediatric Society, Fetus and Newborn Committee. (2010). Safe discharge of the late preterm infant. *Paediatrics and Child Health, 15*(10), 655–660.

Woodwell, W. H. (2002). The long road home: Perspectives on parenting in the NICU. *Advances in Neonatal Care, 2*(3), 161–169.

Additional Resources

AWHONN Neonatal Skin Condition Score: http://www.awhonn.org/awhonn/content.do?name=03_JournalsPubsResearch%2F3G4_NeonatalSkinCare.htm

Therapy BC: Modified Braden Q Scale: http://www.therapybc.ca/eLibrary/docs/Resources/Braden%20Q%20scale%20for%20paeds.pdf

The Newborn at Risk: Acquired and Congenital Problems

28

Learning Objectives

On completion of this chapter, the reader will be able to:

- Summarize assessment and care of the newborn who has soft tissue, skeletal, and nervous system injuries due to birth trauma.
- Identify maternal conditions that place the newborn at risk for infection.
- Describe methods used to identify infection in the newborn.
- Identify the effects of maternal use of alcohol, heroin, methadone, marijuana, methamphetamine, cocaine, and tobacco on the fetus and newborn.
- Describe the assessment of a newborn exposed to recreational drugs in utero.
- Identify clinical signs of infection in the newborn.
- Describe the nurse's role in the diagnosis of neonatal sepsis.
- Compare characteristics of neonatal Rh and ABO incompatibility.
- Describe preoperative and postoperative nursing care of the newborn.
- Describe congenital disorders presented in this chapter and identify the priority of nursing care for each.

Electronic Resources

Additional information related to the content in Chapter 28 can be found on

evolve **the companion Web site at**

http://evolve.elsevier.com/Canada/Perry/maternal/

- Examination Review Questions
- Critical Thinking Exercise—Fetal Alcohol Syndrome

The birth of an at-risk or high-risk infant is a challenge for health care providers as transition to extrauterine life is complicated by additional conditions or circumstances. The infant may be considered high risk because of antenatal, intrapartum, or neonatal conditions such as maternal substance use, birth trauma, infection, or congenital anomalies. Birth trauma includes physical injuries a neonate sustains during labour and birth. Congenital anomalies include such conditions as gastrointestinal malformations, neural tube defects, abdominal wall defects, and cardiac defects.

At times, the nurse can anticipate problems, such as when a woman is admitted in preterm labour or a congenital anomaly is diagnosed in the antenatal period. At other times, the birth of a high-risk infant is unanticipated. In either case, the personnel and equipment necessary for immediate care of the infant must be available.

Birth Trauma

Birth trauma (injury) is physical injury sustained by a neonate during labour and birth. It remains an important source of neonatal morbidity. Most birth injuries are avoidable, especially with careful assessment of risk factors and appropriate planning of the birth. The use of fetal ultrasonography allows antepartum diagnosis of certain fetal conditions that may be treated in utero or shortly after birth. Elective Caesarean birth can be chosen for some pregnancies to prevent significant birth injury. A small percentage of significant birth injuries, such as prolonged labour or an abnormal fetal presentation, are unavoidable despite skilled and competent obstetrical care. Emergency Caesarean birth may improve outcome in some circumstances, but in others the injury may be unavoidable. The same injury might be caused in several ways; for example, a cephalohematoma could result from an instrumented birth (forceps or vacuum extraction) or from pressure of the fetal skull against the pelvis.

Many injuries are minor and resolve without treatment in the neonatal period. Others require some degree of intervention; few are serious enough to be fatal. The nurse's contributions to the newborn's welfare begin with early observation of his or her transition. Prompt recognition and reporting of signs that indicate deviations from normal transition facilitates early initiation of appropriate therapy. Table 28-1 provides an overview of birth injuries and the sites in which they occur.

Nursing Care Management

When the infant is born, the nurse performs a rapid inspection and physical assessment to determine whether there are any life-threatening conditions requiring immediate medical or surgical attention. A comprehensive physical assessment of the newborn is performed after the parents have had the opportunity to interact with their new baby. Because evidence of some birth injuries may not be immediately apparent, ongoing assessment is necessary and should occur during each contact with the infant.

Soft-tissue injuries that commonly occur at birth are discussed at length in Chapter 25. Caput succedaneum and cephalohematoma are considered normal findings in the newborn and are discussed in Chapter 24.

Table 28-1 Types of Birth Injuries

SITE OF INJURY	TYPE OF INJURY
Scalp	Subgaleal hemorrhage
Skull	Linear fracture Depressed fracture Occipital osteodiastasis (abnormal separation of adjacent bones)
Intracranial	Epidural hematoma Subdural hematoma (laceration of falx, tentorium, or superficial veins) Subarachnoid hemorrhage Cerebral contusion Cerebellar contusion Intracerebellar hematoma
Spinal cord (cervical)	Vertebral artery injury Intraspinal hemorrhage Spinal cord transection or injury
Plexus	Erb's palsy Klumpke's paralysis Total (mixed) brachial plexus injury Horner's syndrome Diaphragmatic paralysis Lumbosacral plexus injury
Cranial and peripheral nerve	Radial nerve palsy Medial nerve palsy Sciatic nerve palsy Laryngeal nerve palsy Diaphragmatic paralysis Facial nerve palsy

(From Verklan, M. T., & Lopez, S. M. [2011]. Neurologic disorders. In S. L. Gardner, B. S. Carter, M. Enzman-Hines, & J. A Hernandez [Eds.], *Merenstein & Gardner's handbook of neonatal intensive care* [7th ed., pp. 748–786]. St. Louis: Mosby.)

Skeletal Injuries

The newborn's immature, flexible skull can withstand a great degree of deformation (moulding) before fracture results. Considerable force is required to fracture the newborn's skull. Two types of skull fractures typically occur: linear fractures and depressed fractures. The location of the fracture and involvement of underlying structures determine its significance.

If an artery lying in a groove on the undersurface of the skull is torn as a result of the fracture, increased intracranial pressure (ICP) will result. Unless a blood vessel is involved, linear fractures, which account for 70% of all fractures in this age group, heal without special treatment. The infant's skull may become indented without laceration of either the skin or the dural membrane. These depressed fractures, or ping-pong ball indentations, may occur during difficult births from pressure of the head on the bony pelvis. They also can occur as a result of injudicious application of forceps.

The clavicle is the bone most often fractured during birth as a result of shoulder dystocia. Generally, the break is in the middle third of the bone (Fig. 28-1). Common findings associated with a fractured clavicle include decreased movement of the arm on the affected side; crepitus over the bone; and absence of the Moro reflex, again, on the affected side. Treatment for a fractured clavicle includes gentle handling, containment of the limb against the chest, and pain management. Generally, the prognosis is good. The humerus and femur are other bones that may be fractured during a difficult birth. Fractures in newborns generally heal rapidly. Immobilization is accomplished with slings, splints, swaddling, and other immobilization devices.

The parents need support when handling their infant with a skeletal injury because they often are fearful of hurting the baby. Nurses can encourage and offer support to parents as they handle, change, and feed their infant. This increases parental knowledge and confidence and facilitates attachment.

Peripheral Nervous System Injuries

Plexus injury results from forces that alter the normal position and relationship of the arm, shoulder, and neck. Erb palsy

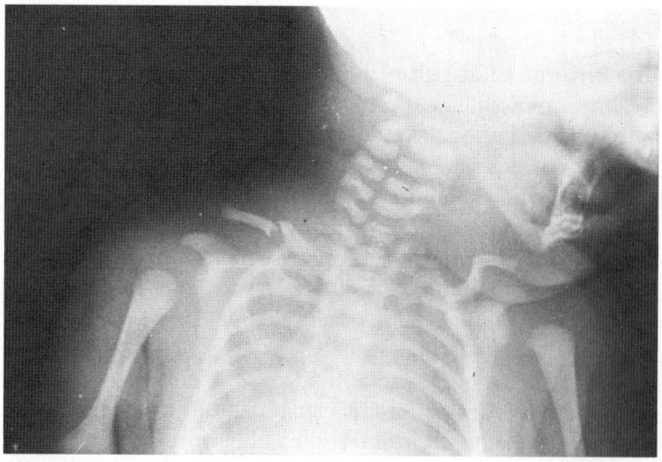

Fig. 28-1 Fractured clavicle after shoulder dystocia. *(From O'Doherty, N. [1986].* Neonatology: Micro atlas of the newborn. *Nutley, NJ: Hoffmann–La Roche.)*

(Erb-Duchenne paralysis) is caused by damage to the upper plexus and usually results from a stretching or pulling away of the shoulder from the head. Erb palsy may occur with shoulder dystocia or with a difficult vertex or breech delivery. The less common lower plexus palsy, or Klumpke palsy, results from severe stretching of the upper extremity while the trunk is relatively less mobile.

The clinical manifestations of Erb palsy are related to the paralysis of the affected extremity and muscles. The arm hangs limply alongside the body. The shoulder and arm are adducted and internally rotated; the elbow is extended, and the forearm is pronated, with the wrist and fingers flexed. Despite this paralysis, a grasp reflex may be present because finger and wrist movement remains normal (Adams-Chapman & Stoll, 2007) (Fig. 28-2). In lower plexus palsy, the muscles of the hand are paralyzed, with resultant wrist drop and relaxed fingers. In a third and more severe form of brachial palsy, the entire arm is paralyzed and hangs limply and motionless at the infant's side. The Moro reflex is absent on the affected side in all forms of brachial palsy.

The goal of treatment for any of the palsies described above is twofold: prevention of contractures and maintenance of correct placement of the humeral head within the glenoid fossa of the scapula. Complete recovery from stretched nerves usually takes 3 to 6 months. However, avulsion (disconnection) of the nerves of the ganglia from the spinal cord results in permanent damage. For those injuries that do not improve by 3 to 6 months, surgical intervention may be needed to relieve pressure on the nerves or to repair the nerves with grafting (Adams-Chapman & Stoll, 2007).

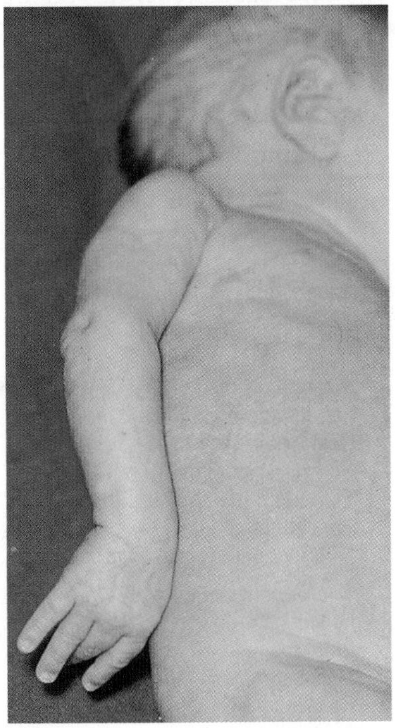

Fig. 28-2 Erb-Duchenne paralysis in newborn infant. Moro reflex is absent in right upper extremity. Recovery was complete. *(From O'Doherty, N. [1986].* Neonatology: Micro atlas of the newborn. *Nutley, NJ: Hoffmann–La Roche.)*

Nursing care of the newborn with brachial palsy is concerned primarily with proper positioning of the affected arm: it should be abducted 90 degrees with external shoulder rotation, forearm supination, and extension at the wrist with the palm facing the infant's face (Adams-Chapman & Stoll, 2007). Passive range-of-motion exercises of the shoulder, wrist, elbow, and fingers are initiated in the latter part of the first week. Wrist flexion contractures may be prevented with the use of a wrist splint. In dressing the infant, preference is given to the affected arm to prevent unnecessary manipulation and stress on the paralyzed muscles; undressing begins with the unaffected arm. Parents need to be taught to use the football position when holding the infant and to avoid picking the child up from under the axillae or by pulling on the arms.

Pressure on the facial nerve (cranial nerve VII) during delivery may result in injury to it. The primary clinical manifestations are loss of movement on the affected side, such as an inability to completely close the eye, drooping of the mouth, and absence of wrinkling of the forehead and nasolabial fold (Fig. 28-3). Facial palsy or paralysis is most noticeable when the infant cries. The mouth is drawn to the unaffected side, wrinkles are deeper on the normal side, and the eye on the involved side remains open. Often the condition is temporary, resolving within hours or days of birth. Permanent paralysis is rare unless the nerve fibres were torn, in which case surgical intervention may be necessary.

Nursing care of the infant with facial nerve paralysis involves assisting the infant to suck and helping the mother with feeding techniques. The infant may require gavage feeding to prevent aspiration. While breastfeeding is not contraindicated, the mother may need additional assistance to help the infant latch onto the breast.

If the eyelid on the affected side does not close completely, artificial tears can be instilled daily to prevent drying of the

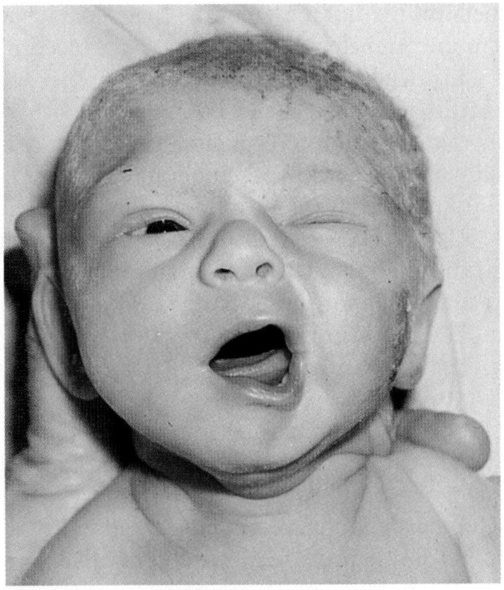

Fig. 28-3 Facial paralysis 15 minutes after forceps birth. Absence of movement on the affected side is especially noticeable when the infant cries. *(From O'Doherty, N. [1986].* Neonatology: Micro atlas of the newborn. *Nutley, NJ: Hoffmann–La Roche.)*

conjunctiva, sclera, and cornea. The lid is often taped shut to prevent accidental injury. If eye care is needed at home, the parents should be taught to administer eye drops prior to discharge.

Phrenic nerve paralysis results in diaphragmatic paralysis as demonstrated by ultrasonography, which shows paradoxical chest movement and an elevated diaphragm. An elevated diaphragm may not be obvious if the neonate is receiving positive-pressure ventilation (Volpe, 2008). This injury sometimes occurs in conjunction with brachial palsy. Respiratory distress is the most common and important sign of injury. Because injury to the phrenic nerve is usually unilateral, the lung on the affected side does not expand and respiratory efforts are ineffective. The infant needs to be positioned on the affected side to facilitate maximum expansion of the uninvolved lung. Breathing is primarily thoracic, and cyanosis, tachypnea, or complete respiratory failure may be seen. Pneumonia and atelectasis on the affected side may also occur.

The infant with phrenic nerve paralysis requires the same nursing care as that for any infant with respiratory distress. As with other birth injuries, the family's emotional needs are similar to those discussed for soft-tissue injury (see Chapter 25). Follow-up is essential because of the extended length of recovery.

Central Nervous System Injuries

Many types of intracranial hemorrhage (ICH) occur in newborns. ICH as a result of birth trauma is more likely to occur in the full-term macrosomic infant. The frequency and degree of severity of ICH is different in the newborn than in older children or adults. In the newborn, more than one type of hemorrhage can and does commonly occur.

A subdural **hematoma**, a life-threatening collection of blood in the subdural space, is most often caused by the stretching and tearing of the large veins in the tentorium of the cerebellum, the dural membrane that separates the cerebrum from the cerebellum. When this type of bleeding occurs, the typical history includes a primiparous mother with a precipitous birth (total labour and birth occurring in less than 3 hours); mid- or high-forceps application; or a large-for-gestational-age (LGA) infant. Subdural hematoma occurs infrequently related to improvements in obstetrical care. However, it is especially serious because of the associated risk of treatment: bleeding related to aspiration or subdural tap.

Subarachnoid hemorrhage occurs rarely and often without clinical manifestations. Small hemorrhages are most common. Bleeding is of venous origin and underlying contusion may occur.

The clinical presentation of hemorrhage in the full-term infant can vary considerably. In many infants, signs are absent. Hemorrhage may be diagnosed as a result of abnormal findings on lumbar puncture (red blood cells [RBCs] in the cerebrospinal fluid) or as seen on a computed tomography (CT) scan. The initial clinical manifestations of neonatal subarachnoid hemorrhage may be evidenced by alternating central nervous system (CNS) depression and irritability, with refractory seizures. Poor feeding, apnea, and unequal pupils may suggest an intracranial insult. The nursing care of an infant with ICH is supportive and includes monitoring of neurological signs, observation and management of seizures, prevention of increased ICP, and intravenous (IV) therapy.

Spinal cord injuries almost always result from complicated breech births, especially difficult ones in which version and extraction are used. Clinical manifestations include respiratory failure and flaccid extremities; stillbirth is not uncommon.

Neonatal Infections

Sepsis

Sepsis continues to be one of the most significant causes of neonatal morbidity and mortality. Maternal immune globulin M (IgM) does not cross the placenta. IgG is the most abundant and active immunoglobulin in humans and accounts for 70 to 75% of all antibody activity and does cross the placenta (Askin, 2004). IgG levels in term infants are equal to maternal levels; however, in preterm infants the amount of IgG is directly proportional to gestational age (Stoll, 2007). Neonatal neutrophils are present in term infants but have decreased functional capabilities; response to infections is sluggish. Phagocytosis is less efficient. Serum complement levels are low in term infants and even lower in preterm infants; serum complement is involved in immunological reactions, some of which kill or lyse bacteria and enhance phagocytosis.

Table 28-2 outlines risk factors for neonatal sepsis. Special precautions for preventing infection, as well as prompt recognition when it occurs, are necessary for optimum newborn care. Neonatal infections may be acquired in utero, at birth, or shortly thereafter and may be hospital acquired.

Neonatal bacterial infection is classified into two categories according to the time of presentation—early onset and late onset. Early-onset (congenital) sepsis usually manifests within

Table 28-2 Risk Factors for Neonatal Sepsis

SOURCE	RISK FACTORS
Maternal	Low socioeconomic status Poor prenatal care Poor nutrition Substance use Sexually transmitted infections
Intrapartum	Premature rupture of fetal membranes Maternal fever Chorioamnionitis Prolonged labour Rupture of membranes >18 hr Premature labour Maternal urinary tract infection
Neonatal	Twin or multiple gestation Male Birth asphyxia Meconium aspiration Congenital anomalies of skin or mucous membranes Galactosemia Absence of spleen Low birth weight or prematurity Malnourishment Prolonged hospitalization

24 to 48 hours of birth, progresses more rapidly than later-onset infection, and carries a mortality rate as high as 50%. Early-onset sepsis is acquired in the perinatal period; infection can occur from direct contact with organisms from the maternal gastrointestinal and genitourinary tracts. The most common organism is *Escherichia coli*, whereas group B streptococci (GBS) rates remain low (Stoll et al., 2005). *E. coli*, which may be present in the vagina, accounts for approximately half of all cases of sepsis caused by gram-negative organisms. GBS is an extremely virulent organism in neonates, with a high (50%) mortality rate in affected infants (see discussion on p. 755). Other bacteria noted to cause early-onset infection include *Haemophilus influenzae*, *Citrobacter* and *Enterobacter* organisms, coagulase-negative staphylococci, and *Streptococcus viridans* (Stoll et al., 2005). Other pathogens that are harboured in the vagina and may infect the infant include gonococci, *Candida albicans*, herpes simplex virus (HSV type 2), and chlamydia. Early-onset sepsis is associated with a history of obstetrical events such as preterm labour, prolonged rupture of membranes (more than 18 hours), maternal fever during labour, and chorioamnionitis (Venkatesh, Adams, & Weisman, 2011).

Late-onset sepsis, occurring approximately at 7 to 30 days of age, may include maternally derived infection or hospital acquired infection; the offending organisms are usually staphylococci, *Klebsiella* organisms, enterococci, *E. coli*, and *Pseudomonas* or *Candida* species (Stoll, 2007). Coagulase-negative staphylococci, considered to be primarily a contaminant in older children and adults, are commonly found to be the cause of septicemia in extremely-low-birth-weight (ELBW) and very-low-birth-weight (VLBW) infants. Additional infections of concern include methicillin-resistant *Staphylococcus aureus* (MRSA), vancomycin-resistant enterococci (VRE), and multidrug-resistant gram-negative pathogens (Stoll, 2007). Bacterial invasion can occur through the umbilical stump; the skin; mucous membranes of the eye, nose, pharynx, and ear; and respiratory, nervous, urinary, and gastrointestinal systems.

Perinatally acquired infections may cause miscarriage, stillbirth, intrauterine infection, congenital malformations, and acute neonatal disease. Other viral infections such as respiratory syncytial virus (RSV), rotavirus, herpes, influenza, and varicella may occur in the neonatal intensive care unit (NICU). These pathogens also may cause chronic infection, with subtle manifestations that may be recognized only after a prolonged period. It is important to recognize the manifestations of infections in the neonatal period in order to be able to treat the acute infection, prevent hospital-acquired infections, and anticipate effects on the infant's subsequent growth and development.

Fungal infections are of greatest concern in the immunocompromised or preterm infant. Occasionally, fungal infections, such as thrush, are found in otherwise healthy term infants.

Pneumonia, the most common form of neonatal infection, is one of the leading causes of perinatal death. Bacterial meningitis occurs in approximately 0.2 to 0.4 cases per 1000 live births, with a higher rate in preterm infants. Gastroenteritis is sporadic, depending on epidemic outbreaks. Infection continues to be a significant factor in fetal and neonatal morbidity and mortality in Canada.

Nursing Care Management

Assessment

The prenatal record should be reviewed for risk factors associated with infection and the signs and symptoms suggestive of infection. Maternal vaginal or perineal infection may be transmitted directly to the infant during passage through the birth canal. Psychosocial history and history of sexually transmitted infections (STIs) may indicate possible human immunodeficiency virus (HIV), hepatitis B virus (HBV), herpes (type 2), or cytomegalovirus (CMV) infection.

Perinatal events should also be reviewed. Premature rupture of membranes (PROM) may be caused by maternal or intrauterine infection. Ascending infection may occur after prolonged PROM, prolonged labour, or intrauterine fetal monitoring. In some cases infection may occur with intact membranes or contribute to early rupture. A maternal history of fever during labour or the presence of foul-smelling amniotic fluid may also indicate infection. Antibiotic therapy initiated during labour should be noted. The neonate's gestational age, birth weight, and gender all affect the incidence of infection. Sepsis occurs about twice as often and results in a higher mortality in male infants than in female infants.

During the postnatal period, the time of onset of suspicious signs needs to be noted. Onset within the first 48 hours of life is more often associated with prenatal or perinatal predisposing factors; onset after 2 or 3 days more often reflects a hospital-acquired infection.

The earliest clinical signs of neonatal sepsis are characterized by a lack of specificity. The nonspecific signs include lethargy, poor feeding, poor weight gain, and irritability. The nurse or parent may simply note that the infant is not doing as well as before. Differential diagnosis may be difficult because signs of sepsis are similar to signs of noninfectious neonatal problems such as hypoglycemia and respiratory distress. Additional clinical and laboratory information, including cultures, will substantiate the findings described. Table 28-3 outlines the clinical signs associated with neonatal sepsis.

Laboratory studies are important in assessing for neonatal infection. Specimens for cultures include blood, cerebrospinal fluid (CSF), stool, and urine. Fluids such as urine and CSF may be evaluated by counterimmune electrophoresis or latex agglutination to assist in the identification of the bacteria. A complete blood cell count (CBC) with differential should be performed to determine the presence of bacterial infection or increased or decreased white blood cell count (the latter is an ominous sign). The total neutrophil count, immature to total neutrophil (I/T) ratio, absolute neutrophil count (ANC), and C-reactive protein may be used to determine the presence of sepsis. Detection of viral deoxyribonucleic acid (DNA) or antibodies by polymerase chain reaction (PCR) amplification in fluids is also an important diagnostic tool (Frenkel, 2005). Treatment with antibiotics should be initiated after blood cultures are obtained. Once the pathogen is identified, antibiotic, antiviral, or antifungal therapy may be modified. Vigilant assessment needs to continue during and after treatment.

The newborn should undergo ongoing assessment for sequelae to septicemia, which include meningitis, disseminated intravascular coagulation (DIC), necrotizing enterocolitis (NEC), pneumonia, and septic shock. Septic shock results

Table 28-3 Signs of Sepsis*

SYSTEM	SIGNS
Respiratory	Apnea, bradycardia Tachypnea Grunting, nasal flaring Retractions Decreased oxygen saturation Metabolic acidosis
Cardiovascular	Decreased cardiac output Tachycardia Hypotension Decreased perfusion
Central nervous	Temperature instability Lethargy Hypotonia Irritability, seizures
Gastrointestinal	Feeding intolerance (increasing residuals) Abdominal distension Vomiting, diarrhea
Integumentary	Jaundice Pallor Petechiae Mottling

(Modified from Askin, D. F. [1995]. Bacterial and fungal sepsis in the neonate. *Journal of Obstetric, Gynecologic, and Neonatal Nursing, 24*[7], 635–643.)
*Laboratory findings include neutropenia, increased bands, hypoglycemia or hyperglycemia, metabolic acidosis, and thrombocytopenia.

from the toxins released into the bloodstream. The most common signs include decreasing oxygen saturation, poor perfusion (prolonged capillary refill, cool extremities, mottling), tachycardia, respiratory distress, and hypotension.

The nursing process in the care of the infant with suspected or confirmed infection (sepsis), or with risk factors that predispose to sepsis, is outlined in the Nursing Process box.

Plan of Care and Implementation

Prevention

Virtually all controlled clinical trials have demonstrated that effective hand washing is responsible for the prevention of hospital-acquired infection in nursery units. Nurses are responsible for minimizing or eliminating environmental sources of infectious agents in the nursery. Measures to be taken include routine practices, careful and thorough cleaning of contaminated equipment, frequent replacement of used equipment (e.g., changing IV and nasogastric tubing per hospital protocol; cleaning resuscitation and ventilation equipment, IV pumps, and incubators), and appropriate disposal of contaminated linens and diapers. Overcrowding must be avoided in nurseries. Guidelines regarding infection control, space, and visitation in areas where newborns receive care have been established and should be followed (Health Canada, 2000; Public Health Agency of Canada [PHAC], 2010a).

NURSING PROCESS: NEWBORN WITH SUSPECTED SEPSIS

Assessment

The prenatal and birth histories, the newborn's physical, and gestational age assessment are reviewed for risk factors. Individual assessment findings are used to plan care for each newborn.

Nursing Diagnoses

Various nursing diagnoses are possible, depending on the type of infection, the newborn's gestational age, birth weight, and clinical manifestations. Examples of nursing diagnoses related to neonatal infections include the following:

Neonate

Risk for infection related to
- maternal infection (suspected or confirmed; e.g., chorioamnionitis)
- invasive procedures (indwelling umbilical catheters)
- intrauterine electronic fetal monitoring
- fetal dysmaturity, intrauterine growth restriction, preterm birth

Ineffective thermoregulation related to
- systemic infection

Impaired skin integrity related to
- use of multiple supportive invasives (i.e., intubation, venipuncture, IV insertion)

Pain (acute) related to
- multiple supportive invasive measures

Parents and Family

Anxiety, fear, or anticipatory grieving related to
- uncertainty about infant's prognosis
- therapy (invasive)

Risk for impaired parent–infant attachment related to
- separation of parent and newborn
- feelings of inadequacy in caring for infant

Powerlessness or spiritual distress related to
- perinatal events or newborn's condition beyond parents' control

Planning and Implementation

Parents and family are encouraged to participate in planning. Expected outcomes include the following:

- The newborn will remain free of infection.
- The newborn's clinical manifestations or suspicion of sepsis will be recognized and reported; appropriate diagnosis and therapy will be instituted.
- If therapy is necessary, the newborn will suffer no harmful sequelae.
- Parents will interact and care for the newborn and be involved in his or her care.
- Parents will maintain self-esteem by understanding that their role as parents is important to the newborn's well-being.

A number of implementation strategies are discussed on pp. 747–749.

Evaluation

The nurse can be reasonably assured that care was effective if the outcomes established for care are met.

Infants cared for in NICUs are at high risk for infection. In a study of infants admitted at less than 4 days of age to 1 of 17 NICUs in the Canadian Neonatal Network, 23.5% of infants with a birth weight less than 1500 g developed a hospital-acquired infection, as did 2.5% of infants with a birth weight greater than 1500 g. Infection rates varied considerably between facilities, with 6.7 to 74.5% of infants having one episode of confirmed infection (Aziz et al., 2005). While hand washing is the single most effective measure to reduce infection, the rate of compliance with standards for hand hygiene is only 22%. The combined use of alcohol, hand hygiene, and gloves is even more effective in reducing the incidence of systemic infection (Buus-Frank, 2004). It is incumbent on caregivers to strictly adhere to recommended guidelines for hand hygiene.

The skin, its secretions, and normal flora are natural defenses that protect against invading pathogens, thus care practices that preserve this protection should be used. Warm water may be used to remove blood and meconium from the neonate's face, head, and body. A mild nonmedicated soap (in single-use container) can be used with careful water rinsing. Vernix caseosa should not be scrubbed vigorously for removal, since this further disrupts the skin barrier properties. No single method of cord care has been shown to be more effective in the promotion of drying, separation, and prevention of colonization. Nurses must follow agency protocols for cord care and can advocate for revision of protocols based on research (see also Chapter 25, Umbilical Cord Care, p. 671).

NURSING ALERT Artificial and long natural fingernails worn by nurses have been associated with serious neonatal infection and morbidity from *Pseudomonas aeruginosa* (Moolenaar et al., 2000) and *Klebsiella* organisms in the NICU (Gupta et al., 2004). Thus, nurses caring for neonates should aim to keep their fingernails short.

Care Management

Breastfeeding or feeding the newborn breast milk from the mother is encouraged. Breast milk provides the infant with protective mechanisms against infection. Colostrum contains IgA, which offers protection against infection in the gastrointestinal tract. Human milk contains iron-binding protein that exerts a bacteriostatic effect on *E. coli*. Human milk also contains macrophages and lymphocytes. The vulnerability of infants to common mucosal pathogens such as RSV may be reduced by passive transfer of maternal immunity in the colostrum and breast milk. Some evidence indicates that early enteral feedings with human milk (trophic or minimal enteral feedings) may be beneficial in establishing a natural barrier to infection in ELBW and VLBW infants (Anderson et al., 2011). Human milk is thought to provide some degree of protection from necrotizing enterocolitis (Diehl-Jones & Askin, 2004).

Administering medications, taking precautions when performing treatments, and following isolation procedures are nursing interventions that can help prevent and treat neonatal sepsis.

Monitoring the IV infusion rate and administering antibiotics are nursing responsibilities. It is important to administer the prescribed dose of antibiotic within 1 hour after it is prepared, to avoid loss of drug stability. If the IV fluid that the infant is receiving contains electrolytes, vitamins, or other medications, the nurse should check with the hospital pharmacy before adding antibiotics. The antibiotic (or other medication) may be deactivated or may form a precipitate when combined with other medications.

Care must be taken in suctioning secretions from any newborn's oropharynx or trachea. Routine suctioning is not recommended and may further compromise the infant's immune status, cause hypoxia, and increase ICP. Isolation procedures should be implemented as indicated according to hospital policy. Isolation protocols change rapidly, so the nurse needs to participate in continuing education and in-service programs in order to remain up to date.

Perinatally Acquired Infections

The occurrence of certain maternal infections during early pregnancy is known to be associated with various congenital malformations and disorders. An acronym that is often used in clinical practice is TORCH, which stands for *t*oxoplasmosis, *o*ther (gonorrhea, hepatitis B, syphilis, varicella-zoster virus, parvovirus B19 and HIV), *r*ubella, *c*ytomegalovirus, and *h*erpes simplex virus (HSV) (Box 28-1). Additional diagnostic studies specific to perinatal infectious agents also need to be considered. One of the problems with these viral infections is the lack of maternal symptomatology, resulting in lack of treatment and an affected newborn at birth. With the advent of newer diagnostic methods, however, viral infections may be diagnosed in utero and interventions initiated based on the availability of intrauterine treatments.

HSV may result in a severe, often fatal systemic illness in neonates. Survivors of herpetic infection may have residual CNS damage (encephalitis) and chorioretinitis. The other congenital infections also may result in encephalopathy with various anomalies, including microcephaly, chorioretinitis, intracranial calcifications, microphthalmos, and cataracts. To a certain extent, the varied clinical manifestations of these infections overlap; a specific diagnosis can be made by the clustering of clinical findings and specific antibody studies.

Toxoplasmosis

Toxoplasmosis is a multisystem disease caused by the protozoan *Toxoplasma gondii*. Cats that hunt infected birds and mice harbour the parasite and excrete the infective oocysts in their feces. Human infection follows hand-to-mouth contact, such as after disposing of cat litter or after handling

BOX 28-1 TORCH Infections Affecting Newborns

T—Toxoplasmosis
O—Other: gonorrhea, syphilis, varicella, hepatitis B virus, human parvovirus B19, human immunodeficiency virus (HIV)
R—Rubella
C—Cytomegalovirus (CMV)
H—Herpes simplex virus (HSV)

or ingesting raw meat from cattle or sheep that grazed in contaminated fields or from eating unwashed or unpeeled fruits or vegetables. In Canada, up to 25% of individuals are IgG positive related to past exposure to the pathogen (Many & Koren, 2006). First-trimester exposure to the protozoan is more serious for the fetus than third-trimester or perinatal transmission. Intrauterine detection of the condition may occur as early as 18 weeks using PCR of the gene (B1) of the protozoa in amniotic fluid. The detection of intrauterine infection and subsequent maternal treatment with spiramycin may prevent fetal infection (Boyer & Boyer, 2004).

More than 70% of affected infants are free of symptoms. The clinical features of toxoplasmosis resemble those of cytomegalic inclusion disease in the infant. Both diseases are responsible for serious perinatal mortality and morbidity: 10 to 15% die, 85% have severe psychomotor problems or cognitive impairment by age 2 to 4 years, and 50% have visual problems by age 1 year.

Severe toxoplasmosis is associated with preterm birth, growth restriction, microcephaly or hydrocephaly, microphthalmos, chorioretinitis, CNS calcification, thrombocytopenia, jaundice, and fever. Petechiae or a maculopapular rash may also be evident. Some clinical manifestations do not develop until later in life. The affected infant may be treated with pyrimethamine and oral sulfadiazine. Folic acid supplement will be required to prevent anemia.

Gonorrhea

The incidence of gonococcal infection in pregnant women ranges from 2.5 to 7.3%. In Canada, between 1997 and 2006, the number of reported cases of gonococcal infections doubled (PHAC, 2008b). Many women with gonorrhea often have a concurrent *Chlamydia trachomatis* infection (PHAC, 2008b). After rupture of membranes, ascending *Neisseria gonorrhoeae* infection can be transmitted to the fetus. The organism may invade mucosal surfaces such as the conjunctiva (ophthalmia neonatorum), rectal mucosa, and pharynx. Approximately one-third of infants born vaginally to women with gonococcal infection will develop ophthalmia neonatorium (Askin, 2004). Contamination may occur postnatally from an infected adult. Neonatal conjunctivitis usually appears 2 to 5 days after delivery. Neonatal gonococcal arthritis, septicemia, meningitis, vaginitis, and scalp abscesses can also develop.

Eye prophylaxis with erythromycin ointment is administered within the first 2 hours after birth to prevent ophthalmia neonatorum (Embree et al., 2002). The infant with a mild infection often recovers completely with appropriate treatment (e.g., single dose of intramuscular [IM] or IV ceftriaxone). Occasionally, permanent visual damage may result (Embree et al., 2002), or death may occur as a result of overwhelming infection in the early neonatal period. The newborn with clinical disease should be admitted to a hospital for treatment (PHAC, 2008b).

Syphilis

Congenital and neonatal syphilis have re-emerged in recent years as significant health problems (PHAC, 2008a; Robinson et al., 2009). It is estimated that for every 100 women diagnosed with primary or secondary disease, 2 to 5 infants will contract congenital syphilis. If syphilis (primary or secondary) during pregnancy is left untreated, 70 to 100% of neonates born to these women will have symptomatic congenital syphilis. In approximately 40% of pregnancies, fetal demise may occur (Robinson et al., 2009). Because the incidence of syphilis has increased in recent years, universal screening of all pregnant women, ideally in the first trimester, is recommended (PHAC, 2008b). Treatment failure can occur, particularly when treatment is given in the third trimester; therefore, infants born to women treated after 20 weeks of gestation should be investigated for congenital syphilis.

Fetal infestation with the spirochete *Treponema pallidum* is blocked by Langhans' layer in the chorion until this layer begins to atrophy between 16 and 18 weeks of gestation. If spirochetemia is left untreated, it will result in fetal death by midtrimester, miscarriage, or stillbirth (in 1 in 4 cases). All neonates in whom the infection occurs before 7 months of gestation are affected. Only 60% are affected if the infection occurs late in pregnancy. If maternal infection is treated adequately before the eighteenth week, neonates seldom demonstrate signs of the disease. Although treatment after the eighteenth week may cure fetal spirochetemia, pathological changes may not be prevented completely.

Because the fetus becomes infected after the period of organogenesis (first trimester), organs develop normally. Congenital syphilis may stimulate preterm labour, but no evidence indicates that it causes IUGR. Organs affected later by congenital syphilis may include the liver, spleen, kidneys, adrenal glands, and bone covering and marrow. Disorders of the CNS, teeth, and cornea may not become evident until several months after birth.

The most severely affected infants are born to untreated mothers. The newborn may be hydropic (edematous) and anemic, with enlarged liver and spleen. Hepatosplenomegaly likely results from extramedullary hematopoietic activity stimulated by the severe anemia. In some infants, signs of congenital syphilis do not appear until late in the neonatal period. In these newborns, early nonspecific signs such as poor feeding, slight hyperthermia, and "snuffles" may be present. The term *snuffles* refers to the copious, clear, serosanguineous mucous discharge from the neonate's nose. A mucopurulent discharge indicates secondary infection, usually by streptococci or staphylococci organisms. Infants who display any signs or symptoms associated with congenital syphilis should be tested, even if the mother was seronegative at delivery, as she may have been infected more recently (PHAC, 2008b).

By the end of the first week of life, a copper-coloured maculopapular dermal rash appears in untreated newborns. The rash is first noticeable on the palms of the hands, on the soles of the feet (Fig. 28-4), in the diaper area, and around the mouth and anus. The maculopapular lesions may become vesicular and confluent and extend over the trunk and extremities. **Condylomata** (elevated, wartlike lesions) may be seen around the anus. Rough, cracked, mucocutaneous lesions of the lips heal to form circumoral radiating scars known as *rhagades*.

If the mother was adequately treated before giving birth and serological testing of the infant does not reveal syphilis,

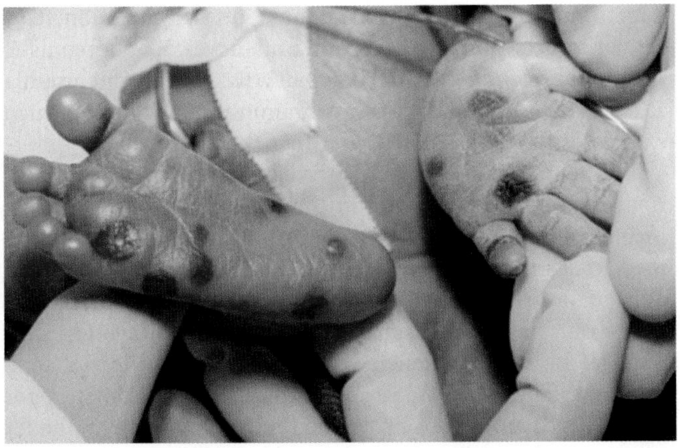

Fig. 28-4 Neonatal syphilis lesions on hands and feet. *(Courtesy Mahesh Kotwal, MD, Phoenix, AZ.)*

generally the infant is not treated with antibiotics. Follow-up surveillance is usually recommended and may include monthly assessments for signs and symptoms of congenital syphilis, as well as periodic evaluation of serology, often every 3 months (PHAC, 2008b). Some physicians recommend antibiotic therapy for asymptomatic or inconclusive cases.

A 10-day course of crystalline penicillin G (consult drug references for dosage and administration route for each) is the usual treatment for congenital syphilis (Robinson et al., 2009). Erythromycin is the substitute antibiotic of choice for infants sensitive to penicillin.

NURSING ALERT The infant with congenital syphilis may be entirely asymptomatic until after discharge from the birth hospital. It is therefore imperative that caregivers use routine precautions with all newborns.

In general, treatment of syphilis is more effective if it is begun early rather than later in the course of the disease. Regardless, a recurrence rate of 5% can be expected, and adequate treatment of congenital syphilis after birth does not always prevent late complication (e.g., 5 to 15 years after initial infection). Potential complications include neurosyphilis, deafness, Hutchinson's teeth (notched incisors), saber shins, joint involvement, saddle nose (depressed bridge), gummas (soft, gummy tumours) over the skin and other organs, and interstitial keratitis (inflammation of the cornea).

Varicella Zoster

The varicella zoster virus responsible for chickenpox and shingles is a member of the herpes family. About 90% of women in their childbearing years are immune; therefore, the risk of infection in pregnancy is low (Society of Obstetricians and Gynaecologists of Canada [SOGC], 2008).

Varicella transmission to the fetus may occur when the disease is contracted in the first half of pregnancy, but this is relatively infrequent. When transmission to the fetus does occur, the effects on the fetus include limb atrophy, neurological abnormalities, eye abnormalities, and IUGR.

When maternal infection occurs in the last few days of pregnancy, 20% of infants will develop clinical varicella (Boyer & Boyer, 2004). The severity of the infant's illness increases greatly if maternal infection occurred within 5 days before or 2 days after birth (Askin, 2004). The neonatal mortality in severe illness is 30% (Sauerbrei & Wutzler, 2007).

Infants born to mothers who develop chickenpox between 5 days before birth and 2 days after birth should be given varicella zoster immune globulin (VariZIG) at birth because of the risk of severe disease. Acyclovir can be used to treat infants with generalized involvement and pneumonia (Myers, Seward, & LaRussa, 2007).

Term infants exposed to chickenpox after birth will have either a mild infection or no infection if they are born to immune mothers. Those born to nonimmune mothers may develop chickenpox, but the course is not usually severe. All hospitalized preterm infants (28 or more weeks of gestation) whose mother lacks a reliable history of varicella or no evidence of protection, and hospitalized preterm infants less than 28 weeks of gestation or less than 1000 g at birth, are at risk regardless of their mother's status and should receive either acyclovir or VariZIG if exposed to chickenpox (Langley et al., 2005).

Hepatitis B Virus

Hepatitis B virus (HBV) infection during pregnancy is not associated with an increase in malformations, stillbirths, or IUGR; however, the risk for preterm birth increases by about 32%. The transmission rate of HBV to the newborn ranges from 70 to 90% when the mother is seropositive for both hepatitis B surface antigen (HBsAg) and hepatitis B e antigen (HBeAg) (American Academy of Pediatrics [AAP], 2006). More than 90% of infants infected in the perinatal period will develop chronic HBV infection. Transmission occurs infrequently (less than 2%) and occurs transplacentally; serum to serum; and by contact with contaminated blood, urine, feces, saliva, semen, or vaginal secretions during birth. Infants are most commonly infected during birth or in the first few days of life. The rate of transmission is highest when the mother contracts the virus immediately before birth. These mothers will be positive for HBsAg. Transmission may occur through breast milk, but antigens also develop in formula-fed infants at the same or higher rate. Diagnosis is made by viral culture of amniotic fluid and by the presence of HBsAg and IgM in the cord blood or newborn's serum.

Neonatal and fetal effects are serious. Infants may be symptom free at birth or show evidence of acute hepatitis with changes in liver function. The mortality rate for severe cases of hepatitis is 75%. Infants who become carriers are at high risk for chronic hepatitis, cirrhosis of the liver, or liver cancer even years later (Yudin & Gonik, 2006). As a result, routine screening for HBsAg is recommended for all pregnant women (PHAC, 2006).

Infants whose mothers have antibodies for HBsAg or who have developed hepatitis during pregnancy or the postpartum period should be treated with hepatitis B immune globulin (0.5 mL IM) as soon as possible after birth or within the first 12 hours of life (see Chapter 25, Medication Guide, p. 661). The hepatitis B vaccine should be given concurrently, but at a different site (PHAC, 2006). The second dose of vaccine is given at 1 month and the third dose at 6 months (PHAC, 2006). Response to the hepatitis B vaccine may be less than optimal in infants that weigh less than 2000 g at birth. As a result, immunization of these infants (born to mothers who are negative for HBsAG) should be delayed until the weight reaches 2000 g or 1 month of age. If the mother was positive for HBsAg, the infant should receive immunoglobulin and the vaccine within 12 hours of birth and will also require a fourth does of the vaccine (PHAC, 2006). The vaccine should protect the child for up to 9 years. Breastfeeding may be initiated prior to receiving the vaccine. Vaccination for infants not exposed to maternal HBV is provided in some provinces before discharge from the hospital.

Human Immunodeficiency Virus (Type 1)

It is estimated that, at the end of 2004, 2.2 million children under the age of 15 years were infected with HIV; more than 90% of those children lived in developing countries. The number of infants perinatally exposed to the virus has decreased significantly in Canada. The decline is reportedly due to decreased perinatal transmission of the virus as a result of decreased maternal-to-infant transmission and potent antiretroviral medication therapy (AAP, 2006). In 2009, there were 180 infants perinatally exposed to HIV; of those, only 1 infant had confirmed infection (PHAC, 2010b). The majority of cases of pediatric acquired immunodeficiency syndrome (AIDS) (90% or more) result from maternal-to-fetal transmission. Universal counselling and screening of pregnant women is recommended in Canada.

Transmission of HIV from mother to infant may occur transplacentally at various gestational ages. The risk of infection in an infant born to an HIV-positive mother (not treated) is approximately 13 to 39% (AAP, 2006). Globally the rate of maternal transmission of the virus is estimated to be 25%. With antepartum, intrapartum, and neonatal zidovudine treatment, the incidence of neonatal HIV infection is decreased to 5 to 8%, and compliance with antiretroviral therapy (ART) is said to further reduce newborn infection rates to 1 to 2% (AAP, 2008; Cooper et al., 2002; Kriebs, 2002; PHAC, 2010b). An elective Caesarean section is said to further decrease perinatal transmission by 87% when zidovudine therapy is administered to both the mother and newborn. Women receiving appropriate retroviral therapy and with complete suppression of the viral load may deliver vaginally without significant risk of vertical transmission (Burdge et al., 2003). A critical factor in perinatal transmission is the maternal viral load; a high viral load (especially more than 100,000 copies/mL) creates a greater chance (up to 40%) for perinatal transmission of the virus. Postpartum transmission may also occur, with an additional risk of 14% attributed to breast milk contact (AAP, 2006; Burdge et al., 2003).

Diagnosis of HIV infection in the neonate is complicated by the presence of maternal IgG antibodies, which cross the placenta after 32 weeks of gestation. The most accurate test for newborns and infants younger than 18 months is the HIV-1 DNA PCR assay, which is performed on neonatal blood, not cord blood (AAP, 2006). Follow-up testing for infants born to HIV-positive mothers is recommended at several intervals within the first year of life.

Typically, the HIV-infected neonate is asymptomatic at birth. Early-onset illness (i.e., virus detected within 48 hours of birth) is attributed to prenatal infection and occurs in 10 to 15% of infected infants. These infants develop opportunistic infections (*Candida* and *pneumocystis carinii* pneumonia [PCP]) and rapid progression of immunodeficiency, which progresses to death in the first 1 to 2 years of life.

The remainder of infants seroconvert over a period of months to years. By 1 year of life, 80 to 90% of perinatally infected infants show signs of infection. Some children infected at birth show no signs of disease 8 to 10 years later. The age of onset of symptoms predicts the length of survival.

The presenting signs and symptoms of HIV infection vary from severe immunodeficiency to nonspecific findings such as growth failure, parotitis, and recurrent or persistent upper respiratory tract infections. In the first year of life, lymphadenopathy and hepatosplenomegaly are common. The infant may have fever, chronic diarrhea, chronic dermatitis, interstitial pneumonitis, persistent thrush, and AIDS-defining opportunistic infections. Common secondary opportunistic infections include PCP, candidiasis, CMV, cryptosporidiosis, herpes simplex or herpes zoster virus, and disseminated varicella.

Nursing Care Management

Although it is rare for an infant to be born with symptoms of HIV infection, all infants born to seropositive mothers should be presumed to be HIV positive until proven otherwise. Management begins by implementing routine practices. Measures should also be taken to protect the infant from further exposure to maternal blood and body fluids. In developed countries, breastfeeding should be avoided completely if the mother is HIV positive. Regimens for the prevention of HIV transmission include antepartum, intrapartum, and neonatal treatment with ART. Children who are HIV positive may be treated with a combination of three antiretroviral medications: two nucleoside reverse transcriptase inhibitors, such as zidovudine and stavudine, plus either a protease inhibitor such as nelfinavir, lopinavir, or saquinavir, or a non-nucleoside reverse transcriptase such as nevirapine (AAP, 2006; Yogev & Chadwick, 2007). Some children may not require treatment if the viral load is low and risk for disease progression is minimal. In either case, a consultation with a pediatric HIV specialist is recommended. If the infant is diagnosed with HIV infection, the family should be counselled about conventional and investigational treatment options.

The goal in the administration of antivirals is the suppression of the virus to undetectable concentrations; the available antiviral medications do not, however, cure the child's disease (AAP, 2006). HIV diagnosis in the neonatal period, combined with aggressive antibiotic treatment of opportunistic infections such as PCP, has the potential to prolong survival in children (AAP, 2006). Studies of HIV symptoms in children treated in the era of ART show a significant decrease in the incidence of secondary opportunistic infections (Nesheim et al., 2007). Long-term outcomes (18 and 36 months) in children treated with ART show that children exposed to therapy had lower developmental scores and adaptive behaviour scores than those of children who had not been exposed to ART; however, the researchers attributed the lower scores to a high incidence and subsequent effect of maternal substance use (Alimenti et al., 2006).

Counselling regarding the care of the mothers themselves, the family's care of the infant, and future pregnancies should be provided. The risk for transmission among members of the same household is minimal. Social services are required in these cases.

In North America, breastfeeding by the HIV-positive mother is contraindicated; however, in developing countries, the risks versus benefits in relation to number of infant deaths attributed to poor sanitary conditions and availability of an appropriate food supply for infants are considered. The World Health Organization (2010) recommends exclusive breastfeeding for 12 months in infants with HIV-positive mothers in developing countries where the infant food supply is not readily available or has a greater chance of contamination (poor sanitary conditions, water supply). Studies in developing countries show that interrupting breastfeeding at 3 to 4 months, even if the mother is HIV positive, increases infant mortality rates from diarrhea and other illnesses (Ogundele & Coulter, 2003).

The family must be counselled about vaccinations. Children with symptomatic or asymptomatic HIV infection should receive all routine vaccines. Although data on children with HIV and varicella vaccine are limited, the Public Health Agency of Canada (2006) and the American Academy of Pediatrics (2006) both recommend that children with no or mild symptoms be immunized for varicella.

Rubella Infection

Since rubella vaccination was begun in 1983, cases of congenital rubella have been reduced from 5300 (1971–1982) to 30 cases (1998–2004) (PHAC, 2006); however, it is still seen occasionally in the newborn. Vaccination failures, failure to complete recommended vaccination schedule, and the immigration of unimmunized persons result in periodic outbreaks of rubella, also known as German, or 3-day, measles.

The risk for congenital anomalies varies with the fetus's gestational age at the time maternal infection occurs. Abnormalities are most severe if the mother contracts the virus during the first trimester, with occurrence of congenital defects as high as 85% in the first 12 weeks of gestation; infection during this time may also result in miscarriage or stillbirth (PHAC, 2006).

More than two-thirds of infected infants have no symptoms apparent at birth, but sequelae may develop years later, such as diabetes mellitus. Hearing loss, a common finding, appears to be progressive after birth. Initially, the newborn may be seen with hepatosplenomegaly, lymphedema, IUGR, jaundice, hepatitis, thrombocytopenic purpura with petechiae, and the characteristic blueberry muffin lesions (dermal erythropoiesis). Congenital rubella syndrome often includes chronic problems such as cataracts or glaucoma, sensorineural hearing impairment, hypogammaglobulinemia, peripheral pulmonary stenosis, congenital heart defects, and subnormal mental development (Boyer & Boyer, 2004; PHAC, 2006; Robinson et al., 2007). The rubella virus has been cultured in infants for up to 18 months after their birth. These infants are a serious source of infection to susceptible individuals, particularly women in the childbearing years. Extended pediatric isolation is mandatory until the noncontagious stage of rubella has been reached (i.e., the infant should be isolated until pharyngeal mucus and the urine are free of virus).

Cytomegalovirus Infection

CMV infection during pregnancy may result in miscarriage, stillbirth, or congenital illness. It is the most common cause of congenital viral infections in North America (Boyer & Boyer, 2004; Michaels, 2007; Yinon, Farine, & Yudin, 2010). Most (90 to 95%) of the infected infants are asymptomatic at birth; however, sensorineural hearing impairment and learning disabilities have been reported in previously asymptomatic infants.

Only approximately 10% of infants with congenital CMV will display severe involvement and may have IUGR and microcephaly. The neonate may also have a rash, jaundice, and hepatosplenomegaly (Fig. 28-5). Anemia, thrombocytopenia, and hyperbilirubinemia are common in the early stages of the illness. Intracranial, periventricular calcification often is noted on radiography. Inclusion bodies ("owl's eye" figures) in cells sedimented from freshly voided urine or in liver biopsy specimens are typical.

The virus may be isolated from urine or saliva of the newborn using the PCR assay. Differential diagnosis includes other causes of jaundice, syphilis (positive Venereal Disease Research Laboratories [VDRL] findings), toxoplasmosis (positive Sabin-Feldman dye test result), hemolytic disease of the newborn (positive Coombs' test reaction), or coxsackievirus infection (positive culture).

Milder forms of the disease often result when the fetus is infected late in pregnancy. CMV can be transmitted through breast milk while the mother is experiencing acute CMV syndrome. CMV infections acquired after birth are often asymptomatic and have no sequelae. Exceptions to this occur in preterm infants, in whom postnatal acquisition of CMV can result in pneumonia, hepatitis, thrombocytopenia, and long-term neurological sequelae.

Antenatally infected infants who are asymptomatic at birth are at risk for late sequelae. Hearing loss may not be apparent

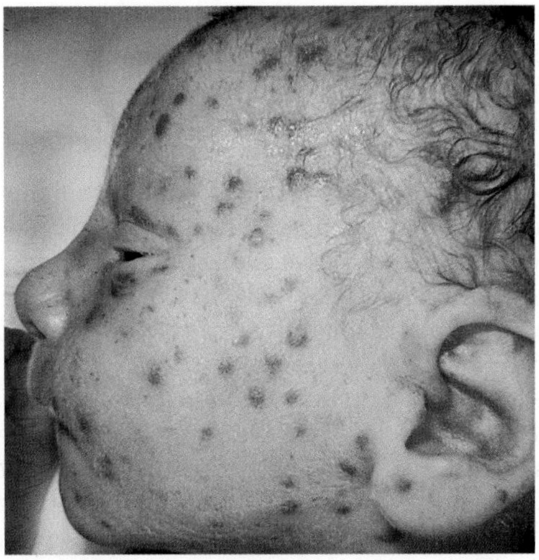

Fig. 28-5 Neonatal cytomegalovirus infection. Shown here is a typical rash in a severely affected infant. *(Courtesy David A. Clarke, Philadelphia, PA.)*

until after the first year of life. Chorioretinitis, microcephaly, cognitive impairment, and neuromuscular deficits may occur by 2 years of age. Some children are at risk for a defect in tooth enamel, resulting in severe caries.

Treatment of the infected newborn with ganciclovir has proved effective in decreasing neurological sequelae, particularly sensorineural hearing loss (Schleiss, 2008).

Herpes Simplex Virus

HSV infections among newborns are being diagnosed more frequently and are estimated to occur in as many as 1 in 3000 to 1 in 20,000 births. HSV type 2 is the most common cause of HSV illness in neonates (70 to 75%) (Allen et al., 2006).

The neonate may acquire the virus by any of four modes of transmission:

1. Transplacental infection
2. Ascending infection by way of the birth canal
3. Direct contamination during passage through an infected birth canal
4. Direct transmission from infected personnel or family

Congenital infection is rare and characterized by in utero destruction of normally formed organs. Affected infants are growth restricted and are more likely to be born preterm. They have severe psychomotor restriction, with intracranial calcifications, microcephaly, hypertonicity, and seizures. They suffer eye involvement, including microphthalmos, cataracts, chorioretinitis, blindness, and retinal dysplasia. Some infants have patent ductus arteriosus, limb anomalies, and recurrent skin vesicles, with a short life expectancy.

Most infants are infected directly during passage through the birth canal. The risk of infection during vaginal birth in the presence of genital herpes is estimated to be 33 to 50%, with active primary infection at term. The transmission rate of chronic vaginal herpes from the pregnant woman to her newborn is low. Passive intrauterine immunity to herpes may be responsible (Money et al., 2008). In a recent study, clinical and laboratory features associated with neonatal herpes included maternal primary HSV infection, vaginal delivery, preterm birth, neonatal seizures, elevated liver enzymes, vesicular rash, and elevated CSF counts (Caviness, Demmler, & Selwyn, 2008).

Postnatal acquisition of the virus and spread within the nursery has been documented by DNA analysis. Both mother (including maternal breast lesions) and father have been implicated in neonatal infections. There also is concern regarding symptomatic and asymptomatic shedding among hospital personnel. Nursery personnel with cold sores should practice strict hand hygiene and wear a mask, although no evidence indicates that they should be removed from the nursery unless they have a herpetic whitlow (primary HSV infection of the terminal segment of a finger).

Clinically, neonatal HSV infections are classified as disseminated infection; localized CNS disease; or localized infection of the skin, eye, or mouth. Disseminated infections may involve virtually every organ system, but those primarily involved are the liver, adrenal glands, and lungs. Affected infants exhibit initial symptoms usually in the first week of life but sometimes in the second week, with signs of bacterial sepsis or shock. Clinical manifestations include skin vesicles in about 33% of infants. Death results from progression of CNS involvement, respiratory distress and pneumonitis, shock, DIC, and bleeding; the mortality rate without antiviral therapy is approximately 25% (Allen et al., 2006).

Nursing Care Management

Routine practices should be observed when caregivers have contact with infants infected with HSV. The neonate's eyes, oral cavity, and skin should be inspected carefully for the presence of any lesions (Fig. 28-6). Cultures need to be obtained from the mouth, eyes, and any lesions. Circumcision, if performed, should be delayed until the infant is ready to be discharged. The infant may be discharged with the mother if the infant's cultures are negative for the virus. As long as no suspicious lesions are on the mother's breasts, breastfeeding is allowed. For the infant at risk, a prophylactic topical eye ointment (vidarabine, iododeoxyuridine, or trifluridine) is administered for 5 days to prevent keratoconjunctivitis. Parenteral acyclovir is recommended as standard therapy for neonatal herpes; neonates with ocular manifestations should receive acyclovir as well as the eye ointment. Blood, urine, and CSF specimens should be cultured when indicated clinically. If herpetic lesions first occur after 6 weeks of life, the risk of dissemination and severe illness is very low (Baley & Toltzis, 2006).

Parvovirus B19

Parvovirus B19 is well known in older children as fifth disease or "slapped cheek illness" because of the characteristic facial appearance of the affected child. During pregnancy, infection may result in fetal miscarriage or the development of fetal hydrops and IUGR (Crane et al., 2002). The estimated risk of transplacental transmission is approximately 30%, and fetal death may occur in about 9% of those affected (Boyer & Boyer, 2004). Protocols for intrauterine management have not been well developed; intrauterine transfusion to treat anemia is the only currently accepted therapy (de Jong et al., 2006). Serial ultrasounds to detect fetal hydrops are possible. The virus may

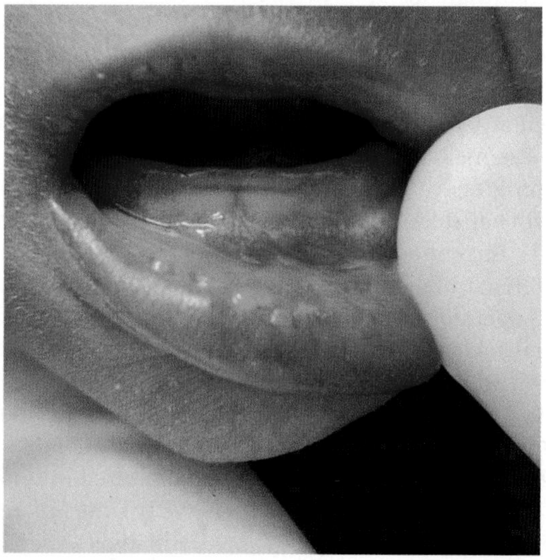

Fig. 28-6 Herpes simplex virus oral lesions. *(Courtesy David A. Clarke, Philadelphia, PA.)*

be isolated from amniotic fluid, fetal blood, or tissues using DNA PCR assay (Boyer & Boyer, 2004). Pericardial, pleural, and peritoneal effusions are common and are fatal if not treated immediately, with cardiac failure from anemia being the most common cause of death.

Bacterial Infections

Group B Streptococcus

Historically, GBS was one of the more common causes of neonatal sepsis and meningitis in North America; however, antepartum maternal screening and administration of penicillin have significantly decreased the incidence of GBS. As a result of screening and treatment of maternal GBS in the 1990s, the incidence of neonatal GBS decreased by 70% to a low of 0.5 cases per 1000 live births in 1999 (Centers for Disease Control and Prevention [CDC], 2010; Money et al., 2004). Early-onset GBS rates have decreased in both Canada and the United States to approximately 0.3 cases per 1000 live births (CDC, 2009; Davies et al., 2001). Early-onset GBS infection in the neonate occurs in the first 7 days of life but most commonly manifests in the first 24 hours after birth. Risk factors for the development of early-onset GBS include low birth weight, preterm birth, rupture of membranes of more than 18 hours, maternal fever, previous GBS infant, maternal GBS bacteriuria, and multiple gestation. Usually a result of vertical transmission from the birth canal, early-onset disease results in a respiratory illness that mimics the symptoms of severe respiratory distress syndrome. The infant may rapidly develop septic shock, which has a significant mortality rate.

Late-onset GBS infection manifests between 1 week and 3 months of age with an average age of onset of 24 days. Eighty-five percent of infants with late-onset GBS have meningitis; this population has a mortality rate of 5%. Fifty percent of the survivors develop neurological damage.

In the newborn with presumptive or confirmed GBS infection, ampillicin or penicillin and an aminoglycoside are the therapy of choice (AAP, 2006; Barrington et al., 2007). The newborn born to a mother who did not receive complete intrapartum prophylaxis is observed for 24 to 48 hours before discharge (Barrington et al., 2007; CDC, 2010).

Escherichia coli

E. coli is a common cause of neonatal sepsis and meningitis in North America. It is postulated that the incidence of this organism has increased in the VLBW and term infant as a result of maternal prophylaxis for GBS (Stoll, 2007). *E. coli* is found in the gastrointestinal tract soon after birth and makes up the bulk of human fecal flora. In addition to meningitis, *E. coli* can also cause infections in other body systems, including the urinary tract.

Tuberculosis

The incidence of tuberculosis (TB), which is caused by *Mycobacterium tuberculosis*, is increasing in Canada; most cases observed in children under 14 are in international adoptees, foreign-born immigrants, and First Nations, Métis, and Inuit children (AAP, 2006; Health Canada, 2012). Congenitally acquired TB, although rare, can cause otitis media, pneumonia, hepatosplenomegaly, enlarged lymph glands, or disseminated disease. After birth, exposed infants contract TB through droplets expelled by infected individuals, which results in pneumonia and necrosis of lung tissue. Untreated neonatal tuberculosis is almost always fatal.

Chlamydia Infection

Chlamydia trachomatis is an intracellular bacterium that causes neonatal conjunctivitis and pneumonia. Chlamydia infection is the most common reportable disease in Canada; the rate of this STI is increasing (PHAC, 2009). Pregnant women should be screened for chlamydia early in pregnancy; women who are positive or high risk for reinfection should be rescreened during the third trimester (PHAC, 2008b). Conjunctivitis, with minimal watery discharge, develops 5 days to 2 weeks after birth (see Critical Thinking Exercise). Inclusion conjunctivitis is usually self-limiting, but if it is left untreated, chronic follicular conjunctivitis (trachoma) with conjunctival scarring and corneal microgranulations may occur. The organism may spread to the lungs from nasal secretions if left untreated, causing chlamydia pneumonia in about 33% of infected infants, with symptoms of a repetitive staccato cough, tachypnea, rales, hyperinflation, and bilateral diffuse infiltrates on radiographic examination (Popovich & McAlhany, 2004).

Ophthalmic 0.5% erythromycin and 1% tetracycline are not effective against *C. trachomatis*; therefore, it is recommended that infants born to mothers who are positive for chlamydia be monitored closely for the development of symptoms. The neonate with positive cultures should be treated with oral erythromycin (PHAC, 2008b) or oral sulfonamide

CRITICAL THINKING EXERCISE

Neonate With Chlamydia

An 8-day-old male infant is brought to the pediatric urgent care centre on a Sunday morning by Maggie, an 18-year-old single mother, because of eye drainage for 2 days. Maggie is breastfeeding and states that she was diagnosed and partially treated for a couple of sexually transmitted infections late in pregnancy; she does not remember the names but says one started with a "C." The medications made her sick to her stomach so she quit taking them after 2 days. The practitioner examines the infant, who has a purulent yellowish discharge from both eyes but otherwise appears healthy; she suspects chlamydial conjunctivitis and orders cultures of the eye drainage. The retrieved medical record from the infant's birth indicates that eye prophylaxis with erythromycin ophthalmic ointment was administered.

1. Evidence—Is there sufficient evidence to draw conclusions about the cause of the infant's eye drainage?
2. Assumptions—What assumptions can be made about the following factors:
   a. Treatment for neonatal chlamydia infection
   b. Neonatal sequelae of inadequate chlamydia treatment in newborn
   c. The mother's health status and possible treatment (she is not allergic to penicillin)
3. What implications and priorities for nursing care can be drawn at this time?
4. Does the evidence objectively support your conclusion?
5. Are there alternative perspectives to your conclusion?

for 2 to 3 weeks. Erythromycin administration in infants younger than 6 weeks has been associated with an increased risk of infantile hypertrophic pyloric stenosis; therefore, parents should be educated regarding the symptoms of the condition (feeding intolerance, projectile vomiting, and abdominal distension).

Fungal Infections

Candidiasis

Candida infections, formerly known as moniliasis, may occur in the newborn. *C. albicans*, the organism usually responsible, may cause disease in any organ system. It is a yeastlike fungus (producing yeast cells and spores) that can be acquired from a maternal vaginal infection during birth; by person-to-person transmission; or from contaminated hands, bottles, nipples, or other articles. It usually is a benign disorder in the neonate, often confined to the oral and diaper regions. Diaper dermatitis caused by *Candida* organisms manifests as a moist, erythematous eruption with small white or yellow pebbly pustules. Small areas of skin erosion may also be seen.

Candidal diaper dermatitis appears on the perianal area, inguinal folds, and lower portion of the abdomen. The affected area is intensely erythematous, with a sharply demarcated, scalloped edge, often with numerous satellite lesions that extend beyond the larger lesion. The source of the infection can be through the gastrointestinal tract or caretakers' hands.

Topical application of 1 mL nystatin (Mycostatin) over the surfaces of the oral cavity four times a day (every 6 hours) is usually sufficient to prevent spread of the disease or prolongation of its course. Several other medications may be used, including amphotericin B, clotrimazole (Canesten), fluconazole (Diflucan), or miconazole (Monistat, Micatin) given intravenously, orally, or topically. To prevent relapse, therapy should be continued for at least 2 days after the lesions disappear (Lawrence & Lawrence, 2011). Gentian violet solution may be used in addition to one of the antifungal medications in chronic cases of oral thrush; however, the former does not treat gastrointestinal candida and may irritate the oral mucosa.

NURSING ALERT Nystatin is best absorbed when given either 1 hour before feeding or after a feeding. Using a needleless syringe or medicine dropper, apply the medication to each side of the infant's mouth for optimal absorption.

Oral candidiasis (thrush or mycotic stomatitis) is characterized by white plaques on the oral mucosa, gums, and tongue. The white patches are easily differentiated from milk curds; the patches cannot be removed and tend to bleed when touched. In most cases the infant does not seem to be in discomfort from the infection; however, some will pull away from the breast or bottle and cry. The child may be brought to the primary care provider with a complaint of poor oral intake.

Infants who are sick, debilitated, or receiving prolonged antibiotic therapy are more susceptible to thrush. Those with conditions such as cleft lip or palate, neoplasms, and hyperparathyroidism seem to be more vulnerable to mycotic infection.

Nursing Care Management

The objectives of management are to eradicate the causative organism and to control exposure to *C. albicans*. Interventions include maintenance of scrupulous cleanliness (by nursing personnel, parents, and others) to prevent reinfection. Good hand hygiene is always essential. Clean surfaces should be provided for changing neonates' diapers. Diaper dermatitis is treated with a topical fungicide at each diaper change. For the infant who is prone to diaper dermatitis, a barrier cream such as zinc oxide may be helpful, provided there is not already an infection. Diaper dermatitis that is not caused by *Candida* organisms may require treatment with a mild topical hydrocortisone ointment. When possible, exposing the perineal area to dry air is recommended because yeast prefers a moist environment. Other measures to control thrush include rinsing the infant's mouth with plain water after each feeding before applying the medication, and boiling reusable nipples and bottles for at least 20 minutes after a thorough washing (spores are heat resistant). Pacifiers should be boiled for at least 20 minutes once daily, and the nipples of breastfeeding mothers should be treated with an antifungal to prevent reinfection.

Infants who are breastfed may acquire thrush from the mother. If the mother is colonized, treatment for mother and infant is recommended. There is no need to stop breastfeeding even if the mother is receiving systemic antifungal medications (Lawrence & Lawrence, 2011).

Substance Use

Certain maternal behaviours can result in perinatal risk. Maternal habits hazardous to the fetus and neonate include recreational drug use, tobacco smoking, and alcohol consumption. Other than alcohol and tobacco use, cocaine and marijuana are the most commonly used substances by pregnant women.

Physiological signs of withdrawal have been reported in neonates whose mothers used, to excess, barbiturates, alcohol, opioids, or amphetamines. Prescription opioids such as oxycodone have been identified as increasingly popular drugs of use, which may cause withdrawal symptoms in neonates (Rao & Desai, 2002; Sander & Hays, 2005). Serious withdrawal reactions may be seen in neonates whose mothers use psychoactive drugs. Infants of women receiving methadone as part of a substance use treatment program may exhibit withdrawal symptoms requiring treatment. Almost 50% of pregnancies of women addicted to opioids result in low-birth-weight (LBW) infants who are not necessarily preterm.

Alcohol is a teratogen that produces CNS effects that may not be evident for years. Maternal ethanol use during pregnancy can lead to a range of effects known as **fetal alcohol spectrum disorder** (FASD) and may include fetal alcohol syndrome (FAS), alcohol-related birth defects (ARBD), or neurobehavioural and cognitive problems that may be identified only by maternal history and behavioural characteristics (PHAC, 2008d).

Historically, the focus of maternal substance use has been on identifying the affected neonate and treating the withdrawal. However, these infants are often not easily identifiable in the perinatal period as withdrawal may or may not occur. Low birth weight is a common result of maternal substance use. LBW infants, a population with considerable morbidity and mortality, have increased risk of long-term behavioural and neurodevelopmental effects that result from the effects of substance use.

In this context of substance use, the term *addiction* is often associated with behaviours in which an individual seeks drug(s) to experience a high, achieve euphoria, escape from reality, or satisfy a personal need. Newborns who have been exposed to drugs in utero are not addicted in a behavioural sense, yet they may experience mild to strong physiological signs of addiction as a result of the exposure. Thus, to say that an infant born to a mother who uses substances is addicted is incorrect; *drug-exposed newborn*, which implies intrauterine drug exposure, is a better term.

The adverse effects of fetal exposure to drugs are varied and include transient changes, such as differences in fetal breathing movements to irreversible effects such as IUGR, structural malformations, and fetal death. Some effects may not be identified until after the neonatal period, possibly not until school entry, and include cognitive and motor delay as well as behavioural problems. Critical determinants of the drug's effect on the fetus depend on the specific drug, the dosage, the route of administration, the genotype of the mother or fetus, and the timing of the drug exposure. Fig. 28-7 shows critical periods in human embryogenesis and the teratogenic effects of drugs. Table 28-4 summarizes the effects of commonly used substances on the fetus and neonate.

Alcohol

The incidence of FASD in Canada has been estimated at approximately 9 per 1000 live births (Schröter et al., 2010). The term *fetal alcohol spectrum disorder* includes children with ARBD, FAS, or alcohol-related neurodevelopment disorder (ARND), all of which occur as a result of fetal exposure to alcohol. FAS is diagnosed in the presence of the following

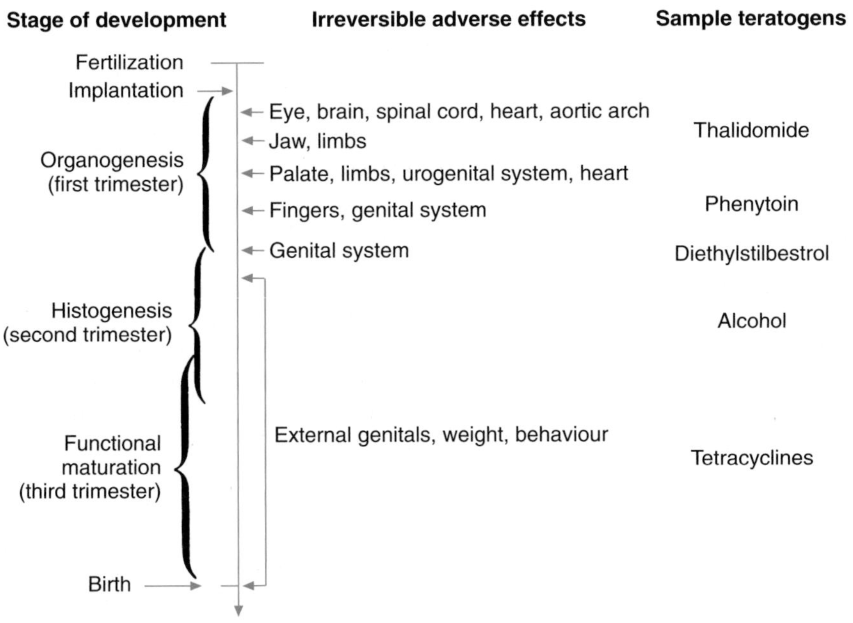

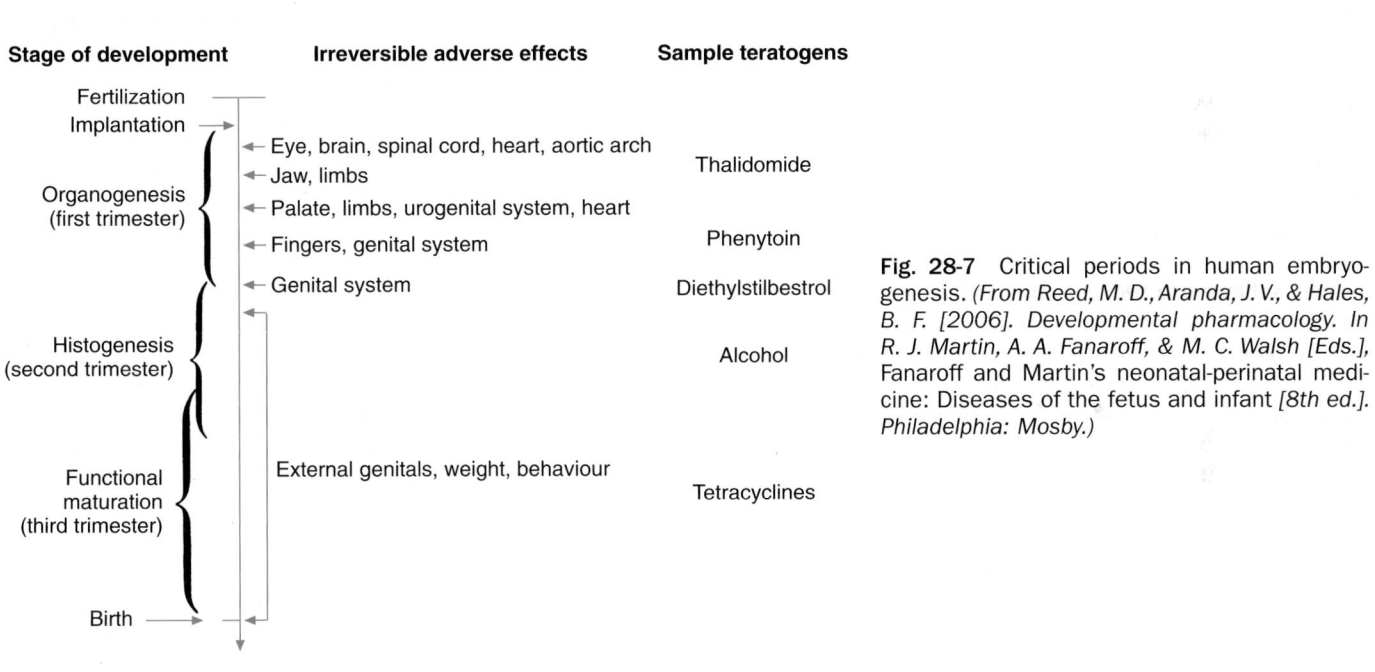

Fig. 28-7 Critical periods in human embryogenesis. *(From Reed, M. D., Aranda, J. V., & Hales, B. F. [2006]. Developmental pharmacology. In R. J. Martin, A. A. Fanaroff, & M. C. Walsh [Eds.],* Fanaroff and Martin's neonatal-perinatal medicine: Diseases of the fetus and infant *[8th ed.]. Philadelphia: Mosby.)*

Table 28-4 Summary of Neonatal Effects of Commonly Used Substances

SUBSTANCE	NEONATAL EFFECTS
Alcohol	*Fetal alcohol syndrome (FAS)*—Craniofacial features varied and may include short eyelid opening, flat midface, flat upper lip groove, thin upper lip; also may involve microcephaly, hyperactivity, developmental delays, attention deficits *Alcohol-related neurodevelopmental disorder (ARND)*—Varying forms of FAS; cognitive, behavioural, and psychosocial problems without typical physical features
Cocaine	Preterm birth, small for gestational age, microcephaly, poor feeding, irregular sleep patterns, diarrhea, visual attention problems, hyperactivity, difficulty being consoled, hypersensitivity to noise and external stimuli, irritability, developmental delays, congenital anomalies such as prune belly syndrome (i.e., distended, flabby, wrinkled abdomen caused by lack of abdominal muscles)
Heroin	Low birth weight, small for gestational age, irritability, tachypnea, feeding difficulties, vomiting, high-pitched cry, seizures
Methamphetamine	Small for gestational age, preterm birth, poor weight gain, lethargy, behavioural problems later in childhood
Tobacco	Preterm birth; low birth weight; increased risk for sudden infant death syndrome; increased risk for bronchitis, pneumonia, developmental delays, orofacial clefts
Marijuana	Possible neonatal tremors, low birth weight, growth restriction

features: (1) midfacial dysmorphisms, (2) growth restriction, and (3) evidence of neurological impairment (CDC, 2005; Chudley et al., 2005; Schröter et al., 2010).

Any single or multiple combinations of these may be present in addition to confirmed or unknown history of maternal alcohol consumption. The diagnosis of FAS is complicated by the absence of a specific single biological marker and by manifestations that are often seen in other childhood conditions.

FAS is recognized as the leading cause of cognitive impairment (AAP, 2000; Schröter et al., 2010). Alcohol (ethanol and ethyl alcohol) interferes with normal fetal development; the effects on the fetal brain are permanent, and even moderate use of alcohol during pregnancy may cause long-term postnatal difficulties, including impaired maternal–infant attachment. Because there is no known safe level of alcohol consumption in pregnancy, women should stop consuming alcohol at least 3 months before they plan to conceive.

Fetal abnormalities are not related to the amount of the mother's alcohol intake per se, but to the amount consumed in excess of the liver's ability to detoxify it. The liver's capacity to detoxify alcohol is limited and inflexible; when the liver receives more alcohol than it is able to handle, the excess is continually recirculated until the organ is able to reduce it to carbon dioxide and water. This circulating alcohol has a special affinity for brain tissue. Other factors that contribute to the teratogenic effects include toxic acetyl aldehyde (a degradation by-product of ethanol) and other substances that may be added to the alcohol. Poor nutritional state, smoking, polydrug intake, and infrequent or lack of prenatal care may compound the problem of alcohol use during pregnancy (Jones & Bass, 2003).

The effects on the fetal brain are reflected in CNS manifestations of FAS (Box 28-2). Cognitive and motor delays, hearing disorders, and a variety of defects in craniofacial development are prominent features (Fig. 28-8). Magnetic resonance imaging (MRI) studies of children with diagnosed FAS have revealed structural anomalies, including alteration in the midbrain anomalies, particularly micrencephaly (Guerri, Bazinet, & Riley, 2009; Swayze et al., 1997). Some affected infants display physical features of the syndrome; behaviours, however, are nonspecific in newborns and may

BOX 28-2 Characteristics for Diagnosing Fetal Alcohol Syndrome (FAS)

Facial Dysmorphia

Despite consideration of racial norms (i.e., those appropriate for a person's race), the person exhibits all three of the following characteristic facial features:

1. Smooth philtrum (University of Washington Lip-Philtrum Guide* rank 4 or 5*)
2. Thin vermillion border (University of Washington Lip-Philtrum Guide rank 4 or 5)
3. Small palpebral fissures (≤10th percentile)

Growth Problems

Confirmed, documented prenatal or postnatal height, weight, or both below the tenth percentile, adjusted for age, sex, gestational age, and race or ethnicity

Central Nervous System Abnormalities

Structural

Head circumference ≤10th percentile, adjusted for age and sex

Clinically meaningful brain abnormalities observable through imaging (e.g., reduction in size or change in shape of the corpus callosum, cerebellum, or basal ganglia)

Neurological

Neurological problems (e.g., motor problems or seizures) not resulting from sepsis, metabolic disturbances, postnatal insult, or other soft neurological signs outside normal limits

Functional

Test performance substantially below that expected for a person's age, schooling, or circumstances as evidenced by either:

1. Global cognitive or intellectual deficits representing multiple domains of deficit (or substantial developmental delay in younger children) with performance below the third percentile (i.e., 2 standard deviations below the mean for standardized testing); or
2. Functional deficits below the sixteenth percentile (i.e., 1 standard deviation below the mean for standardized testing) in at least three of the following domains:
   - Cognitive or developmental deficits or discrepancies
   - Executive functioning deficits
   - Motor functioning delays
   - Problems with attention or hyperactivity
   - Social skills
   - Other (e.g., sensory problems, pragmatic language problems or memory deficits)

Maternal Alcohol Exposure

Confirmed prenatal exposure to alcohol

Unknown prenatal exposure to alcohol

Criteria for FAS Diagnosis

Diagnosis requires all three of the following findings:

1. Documentation of all three facial abnormalities listed above
2. Documentation of growth problems
3. Documentation of central nervous system abnormality

(Adapted from Bertrand, J., Floyd, R. L., Weber, M. K., O'Connor, M., Riley, E. P., Johnson, K. A., National Task Force on FAS/FAE. [2004]. *Fetal alcohol syndrome: Guidelines for referral and diagnosis.* Atlanta, GA: Centers for Disease Control and Prevention; Chudley, A. E., Conry, J., Cook, J. L., Loock, C., Rosales, T., & LeBlanc, N. [2005]. Fetal alcohol spectrum disorder: Canadian guidelines for diagnosis. *Canadian Medical Association Journal 172* [5 Suppl], S1–S21. doi:10.1503/cmaj.1040302.)

*Astley, S. J. (2004). *Diagnostic guide for fetal alcohol spectrum disorders: The four-digit diagnostic code* (3rd ed.). Seattle: University of Washington.

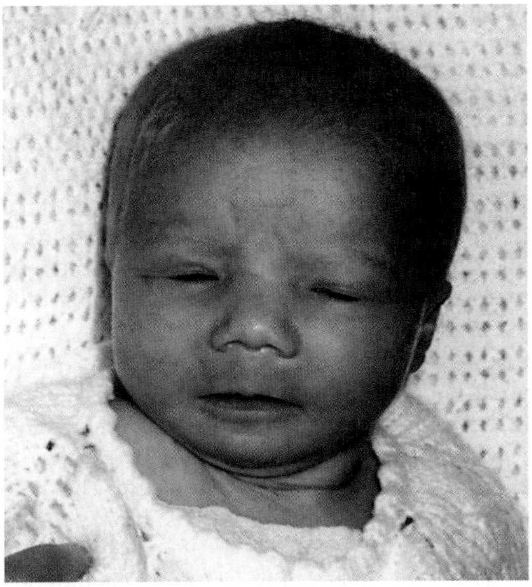

Fig. 28-8 Infant with fetal alcohol syndrome. *(From Markiewicz, M., & Abrahamson, E. [1999].* Diagnosis in color: Neonatology. *St. Louis: Mosby.)*

thus pass undetected. These features include difficulty in establishing respiration, irritability, lethargy, poor suck reflex, and abdominal distension.

The effects of FAS have been identified in adolescents and young adults, primarily in relation to growth deficiencies, delayed motor development, and cognitive impairment. In one study, children who were exposed to only small amounts of alcohol prenatally showed more aggressiveness, delinquent behaviour, and attention problems at 6 to 7 years of age compared with unexposed controls (Sood et al., 2001). Another study found that young-adult offspring prenatally exposed to alcohol had significant alcohol-related problems by age 21 (Baer et al., 2003). Facial characteristics in adults tend to be more subtle than in infants and children.

Nursing care of affected infants involves the same assessment and observations employed for any high-risk infant. Poor feeding is characteristic of infants with FAS and can be a significant problem throughout infancy. The provision of individualized developmental care is paramount and includes reduction of noxious environmental stimuli and helping the infant achieve self-regulation. Special emphasis is placed on monitoring weight gain, assessing feeding behaviours, and devising strategies to promote nutritional intake (LaGasse et al., 2003).

Early diagnosis and intervention are reported to be beneficial for reducing the effects of alcohol exposure on the growing child (Stoler & Holmes, 2004). Therefore, nurses should be actively involved in identifying and referring children exposed to alcohol prenatally.

When possible, long-term disabilities may be mitigated through early evaluation and implementation of therapy. The family should be taught any special techniques needed for the care of their infant and the signs of complications or possible sequelae. When sequelae are inevitable, the family will need assistance in determining how to best cope, such as with home care assistance or referral to appropriate agencies.

The dangers of heavy drinking are well known, and all women should be counselled about the risks to the fetus. The major goal of nursing care is prevention of these disorders through provision of adequate prenatal care for the expectant mother and precautions regarding exposure to potentially harmful infections. The nurse should emphasize to all women of childbearing age that there is no known "safe" amount of alcohol intake during pregnancy and recommend abstinence in order to preclude FAS, ARBD, ARND, and fetal alcohol effects (SOGC, 2010). Furthermore, FAS is a totally preventable birth defect. A change in drinking habits even as late as the third trimester (when brain growth in the fetus is greatest) is associated with improved fetal outcome.

Tobacco

Cigarette smoking during pregnancy is associated with birth weight deficits of up to 250 g for a full-term neonate (Reed, Aranda, & Hales, 2006). Maternal cigarette smoking is implicated in 21 to 39% of LBW infants. Passive exposure to secondhand smoke by a pregnant woman may also result in the birth of an LBW infant. The rate of miscarriage and preterm birth is increased in women who smoke. Nicotine and cotinine, the two pharmacologically active substances in tobacco, are found in higher concentrations in infants whose mothers smoke. These substances can be secreted in breast milk for up to 2 hours after the mother has smoked. Further, cigarette smoke contains more than 2000 compounds, including carbon monoxide, dioxin, cyanide, and cadmium. Deficits in growth, intellectual and emotional development, poor auditory responsiveness, increased fine motor tremors, hypertonicity, and decreased verbal comprehension have been observed in infants exposed to smoke. There is also a positive dose-response relationship between the amount of tobacco exposure and newborn neurobehaviour; increased tobacco exposure in utero is related to more negative neurobehavioural effects (Law et al., 2003). In addition, it is now recognized that neonates may experience withdrawal symptoms following exposure to nicotine.

Pregnant women must be informed about the harmful effects of smoking on their unborn baby's health. These include IUGR, miscarriage, preterm rupture of membranes (PROM), placenta previa, perinatal death, LBW, deficits in learning and behaviour, and sudden infant death syndrome (SIDS). The association between maternal smoking and SIDS (Fleming & Blair, 2007; Sawnani, Olsen, & Simakajornboon, 2010) reflects both in utero exposure and passive exposure postnatally. Other congenital defects or childhood problems associated with maternal tobacco use include heart defects, in particular septal defects (Malik et al., 2008), orofacial clefts (cleft lip, cleft palate) (Honein et al., 2007), and increased incidence of childhood otitis media. Smoking cessation during pregnancy greatly decreases the chance of fetal complications; thus, women should be counselled regarding smoking cessation programs (see Family-Centred Teaching box). All individuals should refrain from smoking near an infant; the house and car should be smoke-free zones for infants and children. Some Canadian provinces have laws that make it illegal for anyone to smoke in a vehicle with children under the age of 18.

FAMILY-CENTRED TEACHING

Smoking Cessation

You are the nurse working in a family health team clinic; you observe that many of the young mothers with newborns seen in the clinic smoke cigarettes. One young mother said, "I know it's bad for me but I can't quit. At least I don't smoke around the baby." What advice could you provide for the young mothers about the effect of tobacco smoke on young infants, especially those under 6 months of age? Prepare a short presentation that can be shared with the young mothers about the effects of tobacco on an infant's long-term health. Discuss options and resources for smoking cessation that are available from local community agencies.

Marijuana

Marijuana use in Canada has been decreasing since 2004, although the rates are high compared to the rest of the world at 12.6% in the adult population in 2009 (United Nations Office on Drugs and Crime, 2011). While marijuana has not been classified as a teratogen, it does cross the placenta and subtle negative neurobehavioural effects have been identified, including sleep disturbances, hyperactivity, inattention, and an increased risk for delinquency (Kozer, & Koren, 2001). An association has been reported between the use of marijuana and a decrease in fetal growth and infant birth weight and length (Hurd et al., 2005). Other investigators have found a higher incidence of meconium staining (Bandstra & Accornero, 2006). It is difficult to isolate the specific effects of marijuana as in many instances it is only one of many substances used. Long-term follow-up studies on exposed infants are needed.

Cocaine

Cocaine, a common illicit drug used in North America, has multiple modes of use. However, use of the relatively inexpensive and easily administered "crack" form is increasingly common, especially among women of childbearing age (Campbell, 2003). Because crack vaporizes at low temperatures, it is smoked and absorbed in large quantities through pulmonary vasculature. The drug readily crosses the placenta, placing the fetus at risk.

Cocaine is a CNS stimulant and peripheral sympathomimetic. Legally it is classified as a narcotic, but it is not an opioid. The effects on the fetus are secondary to maternal effects of increased blood pressure, decreased uterine blood flow, and increased vascular resistance. Consequently, the fetus suffers decreased blood flow and oxygenation as a result of placental and fetal vasoconstriction. The difficulties encountered by cocaine-exposed infants are compounded when the mother is taking the drug in conjunction with other illicit drugs (Askin & Diehl-Jones, 2001). Researchers have concluded that variables such as the mother's lack of prenatal care; poor nutrition; and use of tobacco, alcohol, and other drugs during pregnancy add to the effects of cocaine exposure in the infant (Askin & Diehl-Jones, 2001).

Infants may appear normal at birth or they may show neurological problems that may continue during the neonatal period. Fortunately, these findings are transient and there has been little evidence of permanent sequelae. One of two types of behaviour may emerge as a result of cocaine effects on fetal development: neurobehavioural depression or excitability. The behaviours of the depressed infant include lethargy, poor suck, hypotonia, weak cry, and difficulty in arousing. The behaviours of the excitable neonate may include a high-pitched cry, hypertonicity, rigidity, irritability, inability to be consoled, and intolerance to a change in routine Other possible behaviours are frequent startling, poor awake state, sleeping difficulties, and persistent primitive reflexes. Some infants develop late onset of symptoms (2 to 8 weeks). They may become irritable and hypertonic, experience sleep–awake disruptions, and demonstrate an inability to tolerate change; they may also be slightly febrile. The adverse effects on the cocaine-exposed neonate have a dose-response relationship: the higher the dose, the more effects, such as IUGR, hypertonia, and decreased fetal head growth.

Sequelae of prenatal cocaine exposure include a smaller head circumference, decreased birth length, and decreased weight. Head growth may be one of the best predictors of long-term development (Bateman & Chiriboga, 2000). Other neonatal effects of cocaine exposure include increased incidence of gastroschisis, genitourinary anomalies, and periventricular and intraventricular hemorrhage. Some studies have found that long-term sequelae for newborns exposed to cocaine include lower language, motor, and cognitive scores as well as an increased risk for learning disabilities (Singer et al., 2002; Morrow et al., 2006); however, one study showed no significant differences in the total or verbal IQ scores but did note an increased risk of specific cognitive impairments (Singer et al., 2004). In a large controlled study of children exposed to cocaine and opiates in utero, only subtle deficiencies in mental and psychomotor functioning were noted at 3 years of age (Messinger et al., 2004). Others have suggested that the effects of cocaine in the newborn period are transient; in one study, cognitive function was only affected in relation to restriction of head growth (Chiriboga, 2003). No significant differences were noted in mental, psychomotor, or behavioural functioning. The environmental factors to which these children were exposed were perceived as an important factor in their development. Further long-term studies of exposed infants have been recommended (Messinger et al., 2004).

Scores on the Brazelton Neonatal Behavioural Assessment Scale have shown cocaine-affected infants to be low in responding appropriately to arousal, auditory, and visual stimuli (Eyler et al., 1998).

Nursing care of cocaine-exposed infants is the same as that for other drug-exposed infants. Because they have increased flexor tone, these infants respond to swaddling in a semiflexed position (Askin & Diehl-Jones, 2001). Positioning, infant massage, and limited tactile stimulation have been shown to be effective interventions. Traces of the drug have been detected in breast milk (Moretti, Lee, & Ito, 2000); mothers should be cautioned about this hazard to their infants.

Because cocaine-exposed children often live in an impoverished environment, they are at high risk for cognitive delays, lack of health care, and inadequate nutrition. Referral to early-intervention programs, including child health care, parental drug treatment, individualized developmental care, and parenting education, is essential in promoting the optimum outcome for these children.

Phencyclidine ("Angel Dust")

Phencyclidine (PCP) increases the risk of injury to the pregnant woman and thus also to her fetus. The user may be unaware that she is ingesting PCP because it often is misrepresented as another drug of use or is mixed with other drugs.

PCP crosses the placenta and is found in breast milk. Literature about the effects on infants is limited. Infants exposed to PCP may exhibit abnormal motor behaviour such as irritability, jitteriness, and hypertonicity.

Heroin

Heroin crosses the placenta and often results in IUGR. Heroin may have a direct growth-inhibiting effect on the fetus, but the exact mechanisms of growth inhibition are not clear. Among mothers who use heroin there is an increased rate of stillbirths but not of congenital anomalies in their infants. Additional neonatal effects include meconium aspiration, increased neonatal death, microcephaly, neurobehavioural problems, and a 74-fold increase in SIDS (Minozzi, Amato, Vecchi, & Davoli, 2008).

Many of the medical complications attributed to heroin ingestion result from preterm birth. Other risks include physical dependence in the fetus and the increased risk of exposure to infections, including hepatitis B and C virus and HIV.

Drug withdrawal in the expectant mother is accompanied by fetal withdrawal. Heroin withdrawal occurs in infants born to addicted mothers, usually within the first 24 to 72 hours of life (Finnegan, Pacini, & Maremmani, 2010). The signs depend on the length of maternal addiction, the amount of drug taken, and the time of injection before birth. The infant whose mother is taking methadone may not demonstrate signs of withdrawal until a week or so after birth. The symptoms of infants whose mothers used heroin or methadone are similar. Initially the infant may be depressed. The withdrawal syndrome may manifest as a combination of any of the following signs:

- The infant may be jittery and hyperactive.
- Cry is shrill and persistent.
- The infant may yawn or sneeze frequently.
- Tendon reflexes are increased; Moro reflex is decreased.
- The infant may exhibit poor feeding and sucking, tachypnea, vomiting, diarrhea, hypothermia, or hyperthermia and sweating.
- The infant may exhibit an abnormal sleep cycle, with absence of quiet sleep and disturbance of active sleep.

The risk of SIDS is higher for infants with significant withdrawal problems than for infants in the general population. If withdrawal is not treated, vomiting, diarrhea, dehydration, apnea, and seizures may develop. Death may follow.

Therapy needs to be individualized. Dehydration and electrolyte imbalance should be prevented or treated. Usually the following drugs are given, singly or in combination: phenobarbital, diluted tincture of opium (paregoric), methadone, and morphine.

NURSING ALERT The use of naloxone (Narcan) is contraindicated in infants born to narcotic addicts because it may exacerbate neonatal abstinence syndrome (NAS) and cause seizures.

Methadone

Methadone, a synthetic opiate, has been the therapy of choice for heroin addiction since 1965. Methadone crosses the placenta. An increasing number of infants have been born to methadone-maintained mothers, women who seem to have better prenatal care and a somewhat better lifestyle than those taking heroin.

Some question exists concerning the benefits of methadone therapy during pregnancy because of its effect on the fetus. Methadone withdrawal in infants resembles heroin withdrawal but tends to be more severe and prolonged. Signs of methadone withdrawal include tremors, irritability, state lability, hypertonicity, hypersensitivity, vomiting, mottling, and nasal stuffiness (Jansson, Velez, & Harrow, 2004). These infants exhibit a disturbed sleep pattern similar to that seen in heroin withdrawal. They have a higher birth weight than those infants in heroin withdrawal and usually are appropriate for gestational age. No increased incidence of congenital anomalies is seen. Women in a methadone treatment program are encouraged to breastfeed, regardless of the methadone treatment dosage (Finnegan et al., 2010). Follow-up counselling and monitoring of the mother and infant are recommended. The few available follow-up studies of these infants indicate a high incidence of hyperactivity, learning and behaviour disorders, and poor social adjustment.

Late-onset withdrawal occurs at age 2 to 4 weeks and may continue for weeks or months. A higher incidence of SIDS also has been reported in these infants (Burns, Conroy, & Mattick, 2010). This risk factor is important for perinatal nurses to recognize as they coordinate the follow-up care for the infant and provide education for the mother or other caregivers. Community health nurses must know about the potential for withdrawal symptoms.

Therapy for methadone withdrawal is similar to that for heroin withdrawal. Buprenorphine, an opioid analgesic, has gained acceptance in the treatment of opioid addiction. Preliminary studies indicate that this medication may have advantages over methadone in relation to neonatal outcomes. Offspring of mothers treated with buprenorphine had higher birth weights than those exposed to methadone, had shorter hospital stays, and had lower NAS scores (Jones et al., 2005; Kakko, Heilig, & Sarman, 2008).

Methamphetamine

The fetal and neonatal effects of maternal use of methamphetamines in pregnancy are not well known but appear to be dose related (Smith et al., 2003). LBW, preterm birth, and perinatal mortality may be consequences of higher doses used throughout pregnancy. In addition, a higher incidence of cleft lip and palate and cardiac defects has been reported in infants exposed to methamphetamines in utero.

Methamphetamine use has increased considerably in recent years; 63% of pregnant women who reported methamphetamine use reported using it throughout the pregnancy

(Smith et al., 2003). A higher incidence of preterm delivery and placental abruption was associated with methamphetamine use. In addition, fetal growth restriction (being small for gestational age) was slightly higher in methamphetamine-exposed offspring; however, 80% of these neonates' mothers also had significant intake of alcohol and tobacco use (Smith et al., 2003, 2006).

Reports vary in the time of clinical manifestations of withdrawal from this drug; one study did not identify any signs of withdrawal in the first 3 days after birth, but long-term data were not collected (Smith et al., 2003). After birth, infants may experience bradycardia or tachycardia that resolves as the drug is cleared from the infant's system. Lethargy may continue for several months, along with frequent infections and poor weight gain. Emotional disturbances and delays in gross and fine motor coordination may be seen during early childhood.

One study found that prenatal methamphetamine users were also likely to smoke tobacco (25%), drink alcohol (22.8%), use marijuana (6%), and take barbiturates (1.3%) prenatally (Arria et al., 2006). Prenatal methamphetamine use was strongly associated with greater incidence of substance use among family and friends, lower maternal perception of quality of life, increased risk of legal difficulties, and increased likelihood of developing a substance use disorder (Derauf et al., 2007).

The long-term effects of methamphetamine exposure on children living in households where the product is manufactured are not known, but there are early reports of burns in exposed children and concerns regarding the effects of the toxic by-products of methamphetamine production on small children. Skin rashes and respiratory illnesses are common problems seen in methamphetamine-exposed children; physical neglect and speech and language developmental delays are of significant concern as well (Crocker, 2005).

Phenobarbital

Phenobarbital crosses the placenta readily and is subsequently found in high levels in the fetal liver and brain. Because of its slow metabolic rate, withdrawal onset is generally 2 to 14 days after birth and can last between 2 to 4 months. Irritability, crying, hiccups, and sleepiness mark the initial response. As withdrawal continues, the infant is extremely hungry, regurgitates and gags frequently, and demonstrates episodic irritability, sweating, and disturbed sleep patterns.

Caffeine

Although caffeine has not been implicated as a teratogen in humans, limiting intake to 300 mg/day during pregnancy is recommended; that is the equivalent of two cups of coffee a day (PHAC, 2008a). A meta-analysis suggested that the risk for miscarriage and fetal growth restriction were increased when amounts greater than the above were consumed; however, prenatal smoking may have been a confounding factor (Koren, 2000). Bracken and colleagues (2003) reported a slight decrease in birth weight in offspring of women consuming coffee during pregnancy; these authors indicated that caffeine intake of less than 600 mg/day is unlikely to have a significant impact on fetal growth. Caffeine is found in chocolate and many beverages, including colas, tea, and diet drinks. High quantities of caffeine are also found in energy drinks.

Nursing Care Management

Assessment

Assessment of the newborn of a substance-using mother requires a review of the mother's prenatal record. A medical and social history of substance use, methadone treatment, and STIs should be noted. The infant may have IUGR or be preterm and LBW. The woman who is using chemical substances may have infections that compound the risk to the infant, such as hepatitis B, STIs, or HIV.

The nurse often is the first one to observe the signs of drug withdrawal in the infant; however, in many cases the newborn may be discharged before the appearance of any manifestations of withdrawal. The infant should be assessed according to the guidelines discussed in Chapter 25. The infant's gestational age and maturity need to be noted. In utero exposure to some teratogens results in observable malformations or dysmorphism. Neonatal behaviour may arouse suspicion. **Neonatal abstinence syndrome** (NAS) is the term used to describe the set of behaviours exhibited by an infant exposed to chemical substances in utero (Table 28-5). Fig. 28-9 provides an example of an NAS scoring system for assessing withdrawal symptoms. Because many women are multidrug users, the newborn initially may exhibit a variety of withdrawal manifestations.

Another scoring tool, developed to measure neurological behaviour and resultant effects on the neonate exposed to substances during pregnancy, is the NICU Network Neurobehavioral Scale (NNNS). The NNNS was developed by the U.S. National Institutes of Health and provides an assessment of neurological, behavioural, and stress-abstinence function in the neonate. The test combines items from other tests such as the Neonatal Behavioral Assessment Scale; stress-abstinence items developed by Finnegan (see Fig. 28-9); and a complete neurological examination, which includes primitive reflexes and active and passive tone (Law et al., 2003; Lester & Tronick, 2004; Tronick, 2007).

Newborn urine, hair, or meconium sampling may be required to identify drug exposure and to implement appropriate early interventional therapies aimed at minimizing the consequences of intrauterine drug exposure (Koren, Hutson, & Gareri, 2008). Methamphetamine may be found in fetal hair samples when intrauterine exposure occurs. Meconium

Table 28-5 Signs of Neonatal Abstinence Syndrome

SYSTEM	SIGNS
Gastrointestinal	Poor feeding, vomiting, regurgitation, diarrhea, excessive sucking
Central nervous	Irritability, tremors, shrill cry, incessant crying, hyperactivity, little sleep, excoriations on face, convulsions
Metabolic, vasomotor, respiratory	Nasal congestion, tachypnea (>60 breaths/min), sweating, frequent yawning, temperature >37.2°C

NEONATAL ABSTINENCE SCORING SYSTEM

System	Signs and Symptoms	Score	AM	PM	Comments
Central Nervous System Disturbances	Excessive high-pitched (or other) cry Continuous high-pitched (or other) cry	2 3			Daily weight:
	Sleeps <1 hour after feeding Sleeps <2 hours after feeding Sleeps <3 hours after feeding	3 2 1			
	Hyperactive Moro reflex Markedly hyperactive Moro reflex	2 3			
	Mild tremors disturbed Moderate-severe tremors disturbed	1 2			
	Mild tremors undisturbed Moderate-severe tremors undisturbed	3 4			
	Increased muscle tone	2			
	Excoriation (specific area)	1			
	Myoclonic jerks	3			
	Generalized convulsions	5			
Metabolic/Vasomotor/Respiratory Disturbances	Sweating	1			
	Fever 37.2–38.2°C Fever > 38.4°C	1 2			
	Frequent yawning (>3 or 4 times/interval)	1			
	Mottling	1			
	Nasal stuffiness	1			
	Sneezing (>3 or 4 times/interval)	1			
	Nasal flaring	2			
	Respiratory rate >60/min Respiratory rate >60/min with retractions	1 2			
Gastrointestinal Disturbances	Excessive sucking	1			
	Poor feeding	2			
	Regurgitation Projectile vomiting	2 3			
	Loose stools Watery stools	2 3			
	Total Score				
	Initials of Scorer				

Fig. 28-9 Neonatal Abstinence Scoring (NAS) system: developed by L. Finnegan. *(From Nelson, N. [1990].* Current therapy in neonatal-perinatal medicine *[2nd ed.]. St. Louis: Mosby.)*

sampling for fetal drug exposure is reported to provide more screening accuracy than urine, since drug metabolites accumulate in meconium (Ostrea, 2001). Urine toxicology screening has less accuracy because it reflects only recent substance intake by the mother (Huestis & Choo, 2002). Meconium testing for drug metabolites has the advantage of being easy to collect, noninvasive, and more accurate.

The nursing process in the care of the drug-exposed neonate is outlined in the Nursing Process box.

Plan of Care and Implementation

Caring for the infant born to a substance-using mother presents a challenge to the health care team. The mother, often single, needs to be included in planning for the newborn's care and encouraged to plan for her own care. An interprofessional approach is needed that includes community resource personnel (e.g., regulatory agencies such as child protective services). Education and social support to prevent use of drugs is the ideal approach. However, given the scope of the drug use problem, total prevention may be unrealistic.

D'Apolito and Hepworth (2001) studied a small group (14) of infants exposed to multiple drugs in utero; these included opioids, stimulants, depressants, and sedatives. The most common symptoms observed were increased tone, increased respiratory rate, disturbed sleep, fever, frantic and increased sucking, and loose or watery stools. For nurses working in neonatal and obstetrical areas, the presence of these symptoms should alert the nurse to the possibility of withdrawal. In response, reporting and documentation of the events (per the NAS scoring tool or another objective measure) should occur so that appropriate therapy is implemented. Initial nursing interventions such as providing a quiet environment and offering a pacifier for characteristic frantic, excessive sucking may be implemented independently. It is important not to overfeed infants who demand frequent sucking as part of the withdrawal process. Specific suggestions for providing care to

NURSING PROCESS: DRUG-EXPOSED NEWBORN

Assessment

A comprehensive review of the maternal history and assessment of the neonate, including gestational age assessment, are performed on admission.

Nursing Diagnoses

Nursing diagnoses that may be derived from the neonatal assessment findings include the following:

Neonate

Risk for infection related to
- maternal risk behaviours for sexually transmitted infections
- prolonged rupture of membranes
- intrauterine growth restriction, preterm birth

Risk for disorganized infant behaviour related to
- chemical effects of maternal substance use
- caregiver cue misreading
- caregiver cue knowledge deficit
- sensory overstimulation

Disturbed sleep pattern related to
- drug, chemical withdrawal

Risk for injury related to
- effects of drug exposure on growing fetal tissues

Parents

Risk for impaired parenting related to
- continuation of substance use or detoxification program
- guilt about infant's condition
- inability to cope with care needs of a drug-exposed infant

Anxiety related to lack of knowledge regarding
- care needs of a drug-exposed infant

Violence: self-directed or directed toward infant related to
- drug-dependent lifestyle

Planning and Implementation

Examples of expected outcomes for neonates and parents are as follows:

Neonate

- The neonate will remain free of infection.
- Early manifestations of infection (viral or bacterial) will be recognized and appropriate therapy to minimize effects of disease will be implemented.
- Newborn manifestation of withdrawal (neonatal abstinence syndrome) will be recognized and appropriate therapy implemented to provide newborn state regulation.
- The newborn will receive appropriate physical and emotional care to minimize effects of maternal chemical substance use.
- The neonate will have regular periods of uninterrupted sleep throughout the day.
- The neonate will demonstrate appropriate growth and development.

Parents

- Parent(s) will demonstrate the ability to consistently meet basic caregiving needs of the neonate.
- Parent(s) will continue to participate in a substance use program to enhance their ability to cope with life and effectively parent the newborn.
- Parent(s) will receive counselling and information from health care staff regarding newborn behaviour, cues requiring comfort and feeding, signs of withdrawal, and general infant care.
- Parent(s) will recognize patterns of self-destructive behaviour (substance use) and seek intervention.

A number of nursing interventions for the drug-exposed neonate are discussed on pp. 762–765.

Evaluation

Evaluation is based on the expected outcomes of care. The plan is revised as needed on the basis of evaluation findings.

infants experiencing withdrawal are listed in the Patient Teaching box.

Pharmacological treatment is based on the severity of withdrawal symptoms, as determined by an assessment tool (see Fig. 28-9). An evaluation of NAS is recommended within 2 hours of the newborn's admission to the nursery and every 4 hours thereafter. A score of 8 or higher requires more frequent assessment. With three consecutive scores of 8 or more, pharmacological interventions are recommended (Weiner & Finnegan, 2011). Medication therapies to decrease the adverse effects of withdrawal include administration of phenobarbital, morphine, diluted tincture of opium (paregoric), or methadone (Coyle, Fergusson, Lagasse, Oh, & Lester, 2002; Johnson, Gerada, & Greenough, 2003). A combination of these drugs may be necessary to treat infants exposed to multiple drugs in utero, and careful attention should be given to possible adverse effects of the treatment medications (Johnson et al., 2003).

When NAS is identified in an infant, nursing care is directed toward treating the presenting signs, decreasing stimuli that may precipitate hyperactivity and irritability (e.g., dimming the lights, decreasing noise levels), providing adequate nutrition and hydration, and promoting positive maternal–infant relationships (promoting skin-to-skin contact) (see Nursing Care Plan). Appropriate individualized developmental care should be implemented to facilitate self-consoling and self-regulating behaviours. Irritable and hyperactive infants have been found to respond to physical comforting, movement, and close contact. Wrapping infants snugly and rocking and holding them tightly limit their ability to self-stimulate. The infant's arms should remain flexed with hands in close proximity of the mouth for sucking, as sucking on fingers or hands is a form of self-control and comfort. Organizing of nursing activities and clustering of care reduce the amount of handling and help decrease exogenous stimulation.

Loose stools, poor intake, and regurgitation after feeding predispose these infants to malnutrition, dehydration, and electrolyte imbalance. Careful monitoring of intake and output as well as of electrolytes, additional caloric supplementation, and daily weighing may be necessary. These infants have a tendency to burn up additional energy as a result of continuous activity and have increased oxygen consumption at the cellular level. It takes considerable time and patience to ensure that they receive a sufficient caloric and fluid intake.

In addition, these infants must be protected from skin abrasions on the knees, toes, and cheeks caused by rubbing on bed linens while in a prone position. The incidence of SIDS is high, and parents should be reminded that the supine position for sleep is preferred. Monitoring and recording the infant's tolerance for routine activities (feeding, diaper changes) and preventing complications are important nursing functions.

Breastfeeding is encouraged for mothers who are not using illicit substances, are negative for HIV infection, and are compliant with a methadone program. Breastfeeding promotes maternal–infant bonding, and the small amount of methadone passed through breast milk has not proved to be harmful to the neonate (Berghella et al., 2003; Hale, 2002; Philipp, Merewood, & O'Brien, 2003). Lawrence and Lawrence (2011) suggest, however, that maternal methadone regimens of 100 mg/day or more may cause increased withdrawal in infants, requiring paregoric for 6 to 8 weeks. Because many new medications are being manufactured, the reader is advised to consult with updated references regarding the safety of medications for breastfeeding. It is important to teach pregnant women the effects of the recreational drugs discussed earlier.

PATIENT TEACHING Care of the Infant Experiencing Withdrawal

- Place the awake infant in a side-lying position with the spine and legs flexed.
- Position the infant's hands in midline with the arms at the side.
- Carry the infant in a flexed position.
- When interacting with the infant, introduce one stimulus at a time when the infant is in a quiet, alert state. Watch for time-out or distress signals (e.g., gaze aversion, yawning, sneezing, hiccups, arching, mottled colour).
- When the infant is distressed, swaddle in a flexed position and rock in a slow, rhythmic fashion.
- Put the infant in a sitting position with chin tucked down for feeding.

Hemolytic Disorders

Hyperbilirubinemia, physiological jaundice, and pathological jaundice are discussed in Chapter 25.

Hemolytic Disease of the Newborn

Hemolytic disease occurs when the blood groups of the mother and newborn are different; the most common of these are RhD factor and ABO incompatibilities. Hemolytic disorders occur when maternal antibodies are present naturally or form in response to an antigen from the fetal blood crossing the placenta and entering the maternal circulation. Maternal IgG antibodies cross the placenta and cause hemolysis of the fetal RBCs, resulting in fetal anemia, neonatal jaundice, and hyperbilirubinemia.

Rh Incompatibility

Rh incompatibility, or isoimmunization, occurs when an RhD-negative mother has an RhD-positive fetus who inherits the dominant Rh-positive gene from the father. The Rh blood group consists of several antigens (since D is the most prevalent Rh antigen, the following discussion focuses on RhD isoimmunization). When the mother is Rh negative and the father is Rh positive (and homozygous for the Rh factor), all of the offspring will be Rh positive. When the father is heterozygous for the factor, there is a 50% chance that each infant will be Rh positive and a 50% chance that each will be Rh negative. An Rh-negative fetus is in no danger because he or she has the same Rh factor as the mother. An Rh-negative fetus with an Rh-positive mother is also in no danger. Only the Rh-positive offspring of an Rh-negative mother is at risk. From 10 to 15% of all White couples and about 5% of Black couples have Rh incompatibility. Incompatibility is rare in

NURSING CARE PLAN ● The Drug-Exposed Newborn

Nursing Diagnosis: Risk for injury related to hyperactivity, irritability, and disorganized state

Expected Outcome

Infant exhibits age-appropriate state modulation regulation and stability (i.e., quiet alert, deep sleep, and drowsy states) with minimal irritability and inability to modulate state.

Nursing Interventions/*Rationales*

Use an objective measure or tool such as the Neonatal Abstinence Scoring system *to verify and document behaviours associated with withdrawal.**

Perform a comprehensive neurobehavioural assessment of the infant *to assist in planning individualized care appropriate for the infant experiencing withdrawal as a result of intrauterine drug exposure.**

Administer medications as ordered *to decrease CNS irritability.*

Decrease environmental stimuli *that may trigger irritability and hyperactive behaviours.*

Plan care activities carefully *to allow for appropriate interaction as per infant's behavioural clues.*

Wrap infant snugly and hold infant tightly *to reduce self-stimulating behaviours.*

Monitor activity level, noting the relationship between activity level and external stimulation, and stop external stimulation *if it causes activity increase.*

Provide scheduled periods of rest, decreased overhead lighting, and no physical *care to allow time for recovery of quiet state after periods of care.*

Help mother understand that infant behavioural cues are not a sign of rejection of her caregiving abilities, *to facilitate long-lasting maternal–infant interaction, decrease maternal guilt, and enhance environment conducive to infant growth (promote infant's sense of trust).*

Nursing Diagnosis: Imbalanced nutrition: less than body requirements related to central nervous system irritability; disorganized sucking pattern; vomiting; and loose, watery stools

Expected Outcome

Infant exhibits appropriate weight gain.

Nursing Interventions/*Rationales*

Observe for feeding cues indicating readiness for interaction (quiet alert, rooting) and feed frequent small amounts and burp well *to diminish vomiting and aspiration.*

Monitor weight daily and maintain strict intake and output *to evaluate success of feeding.*

If intake is insufficient, feed by gavage *to ensure ingestion of needed nutrients.*

Modify environment of feeding area as necessary *to decrease stimuli that detract from feeding process and interaction with caregiver.*

Nursing Diagnosis: Risk for impaired skin integrity related to hyperactivity; elbows and ankles rubbing against linen; and loose, watery stools

Expected Outcome

Infant exhibits evidence of intact skin.

Nursing Interventions/*Rationales*

Position infant supine with knees and arms flexed and place a blanket roll at front and back *to promote containment and comfort and minimize frantic, irritable activity.*

Monitor hydration and nutritional status (i.e., skin turgor, weight, mucous membranes, fontanels, urine specific gravity, electrolytes) *to decrease risk for skin breakdown.*

Administer medications intended to decrease hyperactivity, irritability, and frantic posturing *to decrease exposure of skin to surfaces that may cause skin breakdown.*

Cleanse face and diaper area promptly after regurgitation or stooling *to prevent skin breakdown.*

Wrap infant snugly in blanket and place hands in midline next to face *to promote self-comforting and decrease frantic activity.*

Cuddle infant *to promote quiet and relaxation.*

Nursing Diagnosis: Ineffective maternal coping, anxiety, and powerlessness related to drug dependence, infant distress during withdrawal, and poor social support

Expected Outcome

Mother will accept newborn's condition and participate in care activities, showing evidence of maternal–infant bonding process.

Nursing Interventions/*Rationales*

Explain effects of maternal drug use on newborn and the withdrawal process *to provide understanding and information concerning effects of drug use.*

Encourage open communication (e.g., inform mother of ongoing condition, procedures, and treatment; answer questions; correct misperceptions; actively listen to her concerns) *to provide a sense of respect, provide support, and encourage a sense of control.*

Encourage mother to interact with the infant and to become involved in care routines *to foster emotional connection.*

Explain how to do care procedures, how to avoid excess stimulation, and how to hold and comfort the infant *to enhance mother's care abilities and her sense of confidence and control.*

Encourage skin-to-skin contact, whenever possible *to enhance bonding.*

If the infant demonstrates signs of withdrawal, explain to mother the infant's inability to interact, gaze aversion, arching back, and lack of response to cuddling, *to enhance understanding of infant behaviours and maintenance of maternal–infant attachment.*

Make appropriate referrals to community and social agencies for treatment of maternal substance use, for infant development programs, and for other needed support services *to ensure adequate resources for care of self and infant.*

Encourage maternal participation in a substance use counselling (and methadone maintenance, as appropriate) program *to enhance maternal coping skills for effective caretaking of drug-exposed newborn.*

*Note: These first two interventions take precedence over all others because manifestations of withdrawal may vary from one infant to another.

Asian couples. The incidence of Rh sensitization and resulting hemolytic disease of the newborn have decreased dramatically since the development of $Rh_o(D)$ immune globulin in 1968.

The pathogenesis of Rh incompatibility is as follows: hematopoiesis in the fetus, or the formation of blood cells, begins as early as the eighth week of gestation; in up to 40% of pregnancies, these cells pass through the placenta into the maternal circulation. When the fetus is Rh positive and the mother Rh negative, the mother forms antibodies against the fetal blood cells: first IgM antibodies that are too large to pass through the placenta and then IgG antibodies that can cross the placenta. The process of antibody formation is called *maternal sensitization*. Sensitization may occur during pregnancy, birth, induced abortion or miscarriage, or amniocentesis. Usually women become sensitized in their first pregnancy with an Rh-positive fetus but do not produce enough antibodies to cause lysis (destruction) of the fetal blood cells. In subsequent pregnancies, antibodies form in response to repeated contact with the antigen from the fetal blood and lysis results. In approximately 10 to 15% of sensitized mothers, there is no hemolytic reaction in the newborn. In addition, some Rh-negative women, even though exposed to Rh-positive fetal blood, are immunologically unable to produce antibodies to the foreign antigen (Neal, 2001). Multiple gestations, abruptio placentae, placenta previa, manual removal of the placenta, and Caesarean delivery increase the incidence of transplacental hemorrhage and subsequent isoimmunization (Moise, 2002).

Severe Rh incompatibility results in marked fetal hemolytic anemia because the fetal erythrocytes are destroyed by maternal Rh-positive antibodies. Although the placenta usually clears the bilirubin generated by the RBC breakdown, in extreme cases fetal bilirubin levels increase. The fetus compensates for the anemia by producing large numbers of immature erythrocytes to replace those hemolyzed—thus the name for this condition: *erythroblastosis fetalis*. In hydrops fetalis, the most severe form of this disease, the fetus has marked anemia, cardiac decompensation, cardiomegaly, and hepatosplenomegaly. Hypoxia results from the severe anemia. In addition, because of the decreased intravascular oncotic pressure involved, fluid leaks out of the intravascular space, resulting in generalized edema and effusions into the peritoneal (ascites), pericardial, and pleural (hydrothorax) spaces. The placenta is often edematous, which, along with the edematous fetus, can cause the uterus to rupture.

Intrauterine or early neonatal death may occur as a result of hydrops fetalis, although intrauterine transfusions and early delivery of the fetus may avert this. Intrauterine transfusion involves the infusion of Rh-negative, type O blood into the umbilical vein. The frequency of intrauterine transfusions may vary according to institution and fetal hydropic status, but it may be as often as every 2 weeks until the fetus reaches pulmonary maturity at approximately 37 to 38 weeks of gestation (Moise, 2002).

ABO Incompatibility

ABO incompatibility is more common than Rh incompatibility, but it causes less severe problems in the affected infant. It occurs if the fetal blood type is A, B, or AB and the maternal type is O. It occurs rarely in infants with type B blood born to mothers with type A blood. The incompatibility arises because naturally occurring anti-A and anti-B antibodies are transferred across the placenta to the fetus. Unlike the situation that pertains to Rh incompatibility, first-born infants may be affected because mothers with type O blood already have anti-A and anti-B antibodies in their blood. Such a newborn may have a weakly positive direct Coombs' test (also referred to as a *direct antiglobulin test*). The cord bilirubin level usually is less than 68 mmol/L, and any resulting hyperbilirubinemia usually can be treated with phototherapy. Exchange transfusions are required only occasionally. Although ABO incompatibility is a common cause of hyperbilirubinemia, it rarely precipitates significant anemia resulting from the hemolysis of RBCs.

Other Hemolytic Disorders

It is not within the scope of this text to discuss the many potential causes of hemolytic jaundice in childhood. However, in some populations there is a high incidence of glucose-6-phosphate dehydrogenase deficiency (G6PD), which may cause an exaggerated jaundice in a newborn within 24 to 48 hours of birth. G6PD red cells hemolyze at a greater rate than healthy red cells, thus overwhelming the immature neonatal liver's ability to conjugate the indirect bilirubin. Some of the triggers that potentiate hemolysis include vitamin K, acetaminophen, aspirin, sepsis, and exposure to certain chemicals (Reiser, 2004). Hereditary spherocytosis may also cause serious neonatal hemolytic anemia as a result of high quantities of fetal hemoglobin; jaundice may develop rapidly and require phototherapy (Segel, 2007). Treatment is the same as for any newborn with rapidly rising serum bilirubin levels.

Other metabolic and inherited conditions that increase hemolysis and may cause jaundice in the infant include galactosemia, Crigler-Najjar disease, and hypothyroidism.

Nursing Care Management

At the first prenatal visit of an Rh-negative woman with a fetus who may be Rh positive, an indirect Coombs' test should be done to determine whether she has antibodies to the Rh antigen. In this test, the maternal blood serum is mixed with Rh-positive RBCs. If the Rh-positive RBCs agglutinate or clump, this indicates that maternal antibodies are present or that the mother has been sensitized. The dilution of the specimen of blood at which clumping occurs determines the titre, or level, of maternal antibodies. This titre indicates the degree of maternal sensitization. A level of 1:8 rarely results in fetal jeopardy. If the titre reaches 1:16, amniocentesis is performed to determine the delta optical density (ΔOD) of the amniotic fluid to estimate fetal hemolytic process (see Table 12-1). Rising bilirubin levels may indicate the need for an intrauterine transfusion. Genetic testing allows early identification of paternal zygosity at the RhD gene locus, thus allowing earlier detection of the potential for isoimmunization and precluding further maternal or fetal testing (Moise, 2002).

The indirect Coombs' test is repeated at 28 weeks. If the result remains negative, indicating that sensitization has not occurred, the woman is given an IM injection of $Rh_o(D)$ immune globulin. If the test result is positive, showing that sensitization has occurred, the test is repeated at 4- to 6-week intervals to monitor the maternal antibody titre as just described.

At birth, the neonate's cord blood is sent to the laboratory to determine the infant's blood type and Rh status. A direct Coombs' test is performed on cord blood to determine whether maternal antibodies are present in the fetal blood. If antibodies are present, the titre, which indicates the degree of maternal sensitization, is measured. The prevention of or prompt therapy for perinatal asphyxia, acidosis, cold stress, sepsis, and hypoglycemia will decrease the newborn's risk for severe hemolytic disease and his or her susceptibility to kernicterus. In the stable newborn, early feeding is initiated to stimulate stooling and thus facilitate the removal of bilirubin.

If jaundice is present, the cause is determined and therapeutic management is begun. Phototherapy is used to reduce rapidly increasing serum bilirubin levels. See Chapter 25 for a discussion of phototherapy.

Exchange transfusions are needed infrequently because of the decrease in the incidence of severe hemolytic disease in newborns resulting from isoimmunization. Other factors must be considered, particularly the infant's clinical condition, because it is a procedure with potential complications. Guidelines for the initiation of exchange transfusion for infants 35 weeks of gestation or greater have been developed by the Canadian Paediatric Society (Barrington, Sankaran et al., 2007).

Exchange transfusion is accomplished by alternately removing a small amount of the infant's blood and replacing it with an equal amount of donor blood. If the infant has Rh incompatibility, type O Rh-negative blood is used for transfusion, so the maternal antibodies still present in the infant do not hemolyze the transfused blood. Depending on the infant's size, gestational age, and condition, 5 to 20 mL of the infant's blood are removed at one time and replaced with an equal amount of warmed donor blood. Preservatives in donor blood lower the infant's serum calcium level; therefore, calcium gluconate is often given during the exchange transfusion. The neonate is monitored closely for signs of a blood transfusion reaction as well as hypotension, temperature instability, and cardiorespiratory compromise.

Congenital Anomalies

Congenital defects are reported to occur in 2 to 3% of all live births (Bay, Steele, & Davis, 2007; Health Canada, 2002), but this number increases to about 6% by 5 years of age, when more anomalies are diagnosed. If one considers the total number of births (i.e., live births and stillbirths), the prevalence of congenital anomalies in Canada was 4.1% in 2007 (PHAC, 2012). Major congenital defects are a leading cause of death in infants younger than 1 year of age in Canada and account for almost 24% of neonatal deaths (PHAC, 2008c). Although the incidences of other causes of neonatal mortality have decreased, the death rate associated with most congenital anomalies has essentially remained stable.

The most common major congenital anomalies that cause serious problems in the neonate are congenital heart disease, abdominal wall defects, imperforate anus, neural tube defects (NTDs), cleft lip or palate, clubfoot, and developmental dysplasia of the hip. These are thought to result from the interaction of multiple genetic and environmental factors.

Ways of detecting and preventing some of these anomalies are being improved continuously, as are some surgical techniques for the care of the fetus with certain anomalies. Promoting the availability of these services to populations at risk can challenge community health care systems. An interdisciplinary team approach is vital for providing holistic care: the surgical treatment, rehabilitation, and education of the child, as well as psychosocial and financial assistance for the parents. Parental disappointment and disillusion add to the complexity of the nursing care needed for these infants.

Central Nervous System Anomalies

Most congenital anomalies of the CNS result from defects in the closure of the neural tube during fetal development. Although the cause of NTDs is unknown, they are thought to stem from the interaction of many genes that may be influenced by factors in the fetal environment. Environmental influences such as treatment with valproic acid (an anticonvulsant), treatment with methotrexate (a chemotherapeutic agent), and alcohol and tobacco consumption have been implicated. Maternal folic acid deficit has a direct bearing on failure of the neural tube to close; therefore, folic acid supplementation is recommended for women of childbearing age. In Canada, the rate of NTDs decreased from 11.1 to 5.6 per 10,000 total births between 1989 and 1999 (Health Canada, 2002) and to 4.0 per 10,000 total births in 2004 (PHAC, 2008c). This decline has been attributed to increases in vitamin supplementation, prenatal diagnosis, and termination of affected pregnancies (Health Canada, 2002). Further, the decrease in prevalence has been attributed to the addition of folic acid to cereal grain products (Honein, 2001; PHAC, 2008c).

Although an NTD is usually an isolated defect, it can occur with some chromosomal abnormalities and syndromes and also with other defects, such as cleft palate, ventricular septal defect, tracheoesophageal fistula (TEF), congenital diaphragmatic hernia (CDH), imperforate anus, and renal anomalies.

Encephalocele and Anencephaly

Encephalocele and anencephaly are abnormalities resulting from failure of the anterior end of the neural tube to close. An encephalocele is a herniation of the brain and meninges through a skull defect, usually at the base of the neck. The defect may be associated with hydrocephalus; the resulting sequelae depend on the amount of neural tissue within the protruding sac and associated neurological defects. Treatment consists of surgical repair and shunting to relieve hydrocephalus, unless a major brain malformation is present. Anencephaly is the absence of both cerebral hemispheres and of the overlying skull. It is a condition that is incompatible with life; many of the infants are stillborn or die within a few days of birth. Comfort measures are provided until the infant eventually dies of temperature instability and respiratory failure.

Spina Bifida

Spina bifida, the most common defect of the CNS, results from failure of the neural tube to close at some point. There are two categories of spina bifida: spina bifida occulta and spina bifida cystica. Spina bifida occulta is a malformation in which the posterior portion of the laminae fails to close but the spinal cord or meninges do not herniate or protrude through the defect. It is usually asymptomatic and may not be diagnosed unless there are associated problems. Spina bifida cystica includes meningocele and myelomeningocele. A *meningocele* is an external sac that contains meninges and CSF and that protrudes through a defect in the vertebral column. A *myelomeningocele* is similar, except that it also contains nerves; thus, the infant has motor and sensory deficits below the lesion. A myelomeningocele is visible at birth, most often in the lumbosacral area. It is usually covered by a fragile, thin membrane (Fig. 28-10). The sac can tear easily, allowing CSF to leak out and providing an entry for infectious agents into the CNS (see Fig. 28-10, B). Myelomeningocele may be associated with an Arnold-Chiari malformation (70%), which results from the improper development and downward displacement of part of the brain into the cervical spinal canal. This in turn results in the development of hydrocephalus, which affects about 90% of children with myelomeningocele, although it is usually not present at birth.

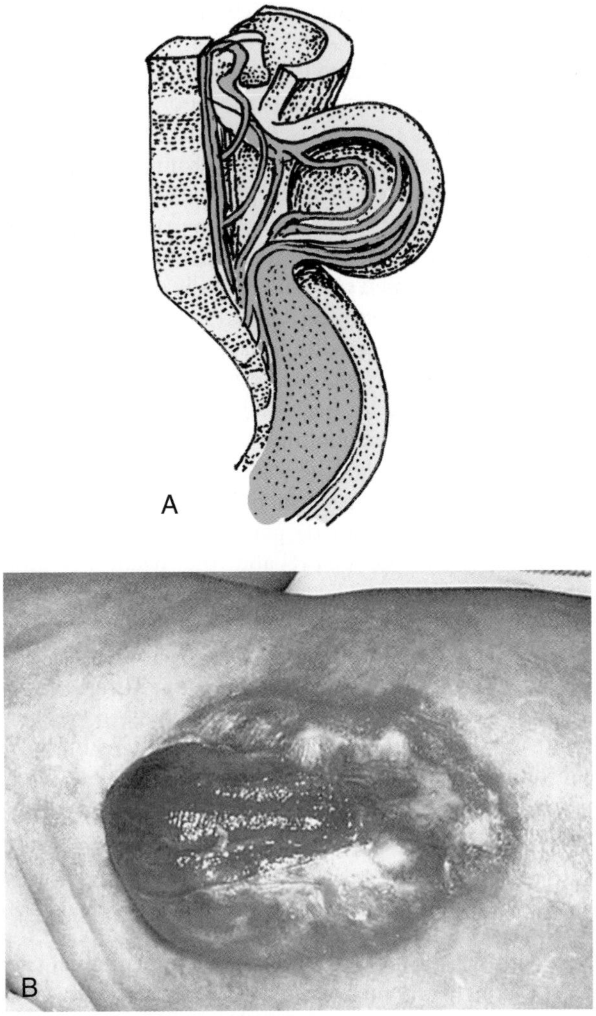

Fig. 28-10 **A:** Myelomeningocele. Note absence of vertebral arches. **B:** Myelomeningocele (ruptured sac exposing defect). *(From Zitelli, B. J., & Davis, H. W. [2007].* Atlas of pediatric physical diagnosis *[5th ed., p. 8]. St. Louis: Mosby.)*

The long-term prognosis of an affected infant can be determined, to a large extent, at birth, with the degree of neurological dysfunction related to the level of the lesion and the nerves involved. Most neurosurgeons recommend that treatment be instituted regardless of the level of the lesion unless there is a severe CNS anomaly, advanced hydrocephalus at birth, severe anoxic brain damage, active CNS infection, or a malformation or syndrome incompatible with long-term survival. Prenatal diagnosis makes possible a scheduled Caesarean birth, allowing for more careful delivery of the infant's back to prevent rupture of the meningeal sac.

Preoperatively, an important nursing intervention for a neonate with a myelomeningocele is to protect the protruding sac from injury, rupture, and risk of CNS infection. Infants should be positioned in a side-lying or prone position to prevent pressure on the sac until surgical repair is done. If the infant is able to be held, the nurse or parent must be careful to keep the defect from injury. The sac should be covered with a sterile, moist, nonadherent dressing and cared for using sterile technique. The skin around the defect must be cleansed and dried carefully to prevent breakdown, which would establish a portal of entry for infectious agents. An important nursing intervention is providing support and information to parents as they learn to cope with an infant who has immediate intensive care needs and who will have long-term needs as well. Surgical repair is performed in the neonatal period, often within the first 24 to 48 hours. Early closure can prevent CNS infection and trauma to the exposed nerves. It can also prevent stretching of other nerve roots, which can occur as the sac continues to enlarge after birth. Surgical interventions to prevent hydrocephalus, such as shunt insertion, may be needed. Complications, including infection, are treated as they occur.

Hydrocephalus

Hydrocephalus is a condition in which the ventricles of the brain are enlarged as a result of an imbalance between the production and absorption of the CSF. Congenital hydrocephalus usually arises as a result of a malformation in the brain or an intrauterine infection. About one third of all cases of congenital hydrocephalus result from stenosis of the aqueduct of Sylvius in the brain. Hydrocephalus often occurs in conjunction with a myelomeningocele, which blocks the flow of CSF.

An infant with congenital hydrocephalus initially has a bulging anterior fontanel and a head circumference that increases at an abnormal rate, as a result of increasing CSF pressure. Depressed eyes that are rotated downward, causing a "setting sun" sign, occurs as the condition worsens. If surgical shunting of excess CSF from the brain is not done soon after birth, the ensuing increase in ICP will lead to irreversible neurological damage, as evidenced by palpably widening sutures and fontanels; distended scalp veins; lethargy; poor feeding; vomiting; irritability; opisthotonic positioning; and a high-pitched, shrill cry. Fetal ultrasound is helpful in the detection of hydrocephalus.

Nursing actions for the newborn with hydrocephalus include care similar to that for any high-risk newborn. Measurement of the head circumference and neurological assessments should be done frequently. If the infant's head is large, a special pressure-sensitive mattress and frequent position changes are necessary to prevent skin breakdown. Chapter 51 contains a more detailed description of the evaluation and management of the child with hydrocephalus.

Microcephaly

Microcephaly refers to a head circumference that measures more than 3 standard deviations below the mean for age and sex. Brain growth is usually restricted and thus cognitive impairment is common. Microcephaly can be the result of an autosomal-dominant disorder; a chromosomal abnormality; fetal exposure to teratogens such as radiation; maternal substance use; and congenital infections such as rubella, toxoplasmosis, or CMV. Infants with microcephaly require supportive nursing care and medical observation to determine the extent of the psychomotor delay that almost always accompanies this abnormality. There is no treatment. Parents need support to learn to care for a child with cognitive impairment.

Cardiovascular System Anomalies

Congenital heart defects (CHDs) are anatomical abnormalities of the heart that are present at birth, although they may not be diagnosed immediately. Some type of congenital heart disease occurs in approximately 0.5 to 0.8% of live births, and about 2 to 3 in 1000 newborns will be symptomatic with heart disease in the first year of life (Bernstein, 2007). Ventricular septal defects, constituting more than 20 to 25% of all CHDs, are the most common type of acyanotic lesion. Tetralogy of Fallot constitutes 5 to 7% of all CHDs and is the most common lesion resulting in cyanosis. CHDs, often in association with other congenital anomalies, are the second major cause of death in the first year of life (the first being preterm birth).

In many cases the cause of CHDs is unknown. Approximately 8% have a clear genetic cause, and most are associated with a chromosomal anomaly, such as Down syndrome (40%) (Blackburn, 2007). Maternal factors associated with a higher incidence of CHD include diabetes mellitus, rubella, alcohol intake, systemic lupus erythematosus, phenylketonuria (PKU), poor nutrition, or antiepileptic medication use.

As a rule, CHDs are thought to be multifactorial in origin, involving both genetic and environmental influences; however, a familial occurrence of virtually all forms of CHD has been noted. See Chapter 48 for a discussion of classifications of CHDs.

Some CHDs are evident immediately after birth, especially those defects that cause central cyanosis (e.g., transposition of the great vessels) despite 100% oxygen administration. Infants with these anomalies are transferred directly to a tertiary centre with a neonatal or pediatric intensive care unit.

Affected newborns may have cyanosis that is unrelieved by oxygen treatment, with the cyanosis increasing whenever the child cries. Pulse oximetry readings that remain low (below 89%) despite oxygen administration are not unusual; respiratory distress may or may not be present. In many cases the infant's colour is unrelated to the severity of the defect. Infants may be acyanotic and pale, with or without mottling on exertion, such as crying, feeding, or stooling.

The affected newborn's activity level varies from restlessness to lethargy and possible unresponsiveness, except in response to pain. Persistent bradycardia (i.e., resting heart rate of less than 80 to 100 beats/min) or tachycardia (i.e., rate exceeding 160 to 180 beats/min) may be noted. The infant born to a mother with systemic lupus may exhibit bradycardia with normal sinus rhythm and good perfusion; eventually, cardioversion may be required if the rhythm persists. The cardiac rhythm may be abnormal, and a murmur may or may not be heard. In many cases, however, ductal (ductus arteriosus) dependent defects or large shunts will not be seen with a murmur. Signs of congestive heart failure, diminished cardiac output, and poor tissue perfusion may occur within several days of birth.

Because the cardiac and respiratory systems function together, cardiac disease may also be manifested by respiratory signs and symptoms. The respiratory rate should be determined when the newborn is in a resting state. Abnormal findings may include tachypnea (60 breaths/min or more); retractions with nasal flaring; grunting occurring with or without exertion; and dyspnea, which may worsen with crying and activity.

A major role of the nurse is to assess infants for abnormal findings such as central cyanosis and poor perfusion, which may be indications of decreased cardiac output. Newborns exhibiting these symptoms require prompt attention and appropriate therapy in a neonatal or pediatric intensive care unit. Interventions initiated when a nursing diagnosis of decreased cardiac output is made include administering oxygen, although oxygen content is usually decreased once the defect is identified; administering cardiotonic medications to increase cardiac output, medications (prostaglandin) designed to prevent closure of the ductus arteriosus, and diuretic agents, as needed, for congestive heart failure; decreasing the work load of the heart by maintaining a thermoneutral environment; and feeding through the least strenuous method necessary. Various diagnostic tests such as echocardiography and cardiac catheterization can be performed to obtain specific information about the defect and the need for surgical intervention.

Respiratory System Anomalies

Screening for congenital anomalies of the respiratory system is necessary even in infants who are apparently normal at birth. Respiratory distress at birth or shortly thereafter may be the result of lung immaturity or anomalous development. Respiratory distress caused by CDH and TEF may appear immediately or be delayed, depending on the severity of the defect.

Choanal Atresia

Choanal atresia, the most common congenital anomaly of the nose, is a bony or membranous septum located between the nose and the pharynx (Fig. 28-11). The atresia may be unilateral or bilateral. Because most infants are preferential nose breathers, bilateral choanal atresia may be associated with apnea and cyanosis when the infant is at rest. When the infant

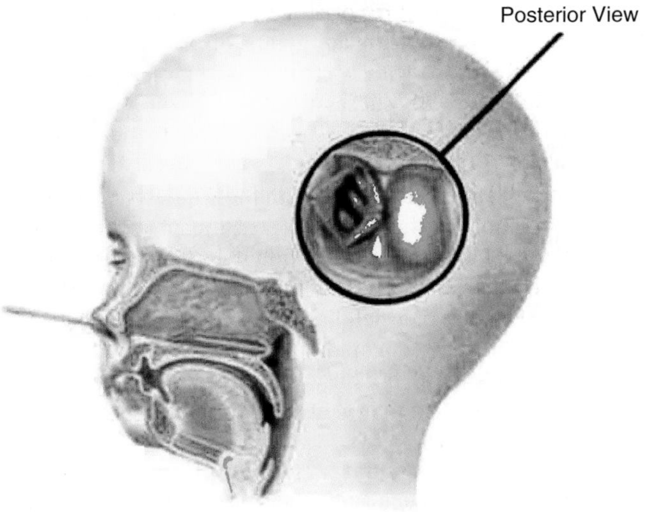

Fig. 28-11 Choanal atresia. Posterior nares are obstructed by membrane or bone, either bilaterally or unilaterally. Infant becomes cyanotic at rest. With crying, the newborn's colour improves. Nasal discharge is present. Snorting respirations often are observed with increased respiratory effort. The newborn may be unable to breathe and eat at the same time. Diagnosis is made by noting inability to pass a small feeding tube through one or both nares. *(Used with permission of Ross Products Division, Abbott Laboratories, Inc., Columbus, OH. From Clinical Education Aid No. 6, Copyright © 1963, Ross Products Division, Abbott Laboratories, Inc.)*

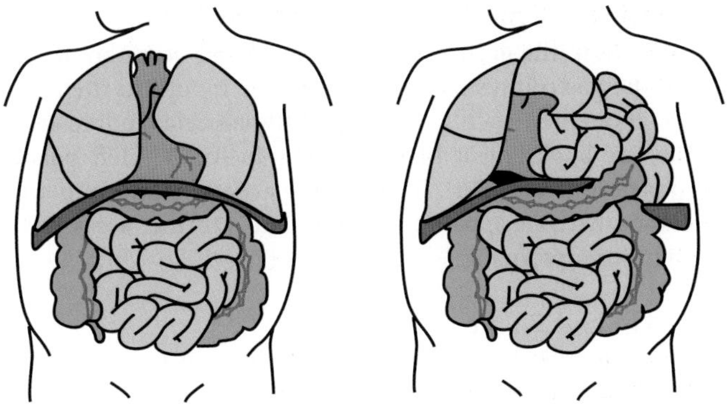

Fig. 28-12 A: Normal diaphragm separating the abdominal and thoracic cavities. B: Diaphragmatic hernia with a small lung and abdominal contents in the thoracic cavity. *(From Ehrlich, P. F., & Coran, A. G. [2007]. Diaphragmatic hernia. In R. M. Kliegman, R. E. Behrman, H. B. Jenson, & B. F. Stanton [Eds.],* Nelson textbook of pediatrics *[18th ed., pp. 746–748]. Philadelphia: Saunders.)*

cries, he or she breathes in through the mouth and pinks up. Unilateral choanal atresia may not be associated with apnea. Inability to pass a suction catheter through the nose into the pharynx or cyanosis without obvious respiratory distress usually leads to detection of choanal atresia. Nearly half of the infants with choanal atresia have other anomalies.

Congenital Diaphragmatic Hernia

CDH results from a defect in the formation of the diaphragm, allowing the abdominal organs to be displaced into the thoracic cavity. It occurs in approximately 1 in 2000 to 1 in 5000 live births (Ehrlich & Coran, 2007). Herniation of the abdominal viscera into the thoracic cavity may cause severe respiratory distress and represent a neonatal emergency (Fig. 28-12). The defect and herniation may be minimal and easily repaired, or the defect may be so extensive that the viscera present in the thoracic cavity during embryonic life have prevented the normal development of pulmonary tissue. The defect is usually on the left (85%) because that is the side of the diaphragm that fuses last.

Most CDHs are discovered prenatally on ultrasound. Hernias may be repaired by fetal surgery in some research institutions. Intrauterine surgical correction of CDH has met with poor neonatal outcomes in many cases, primarily as a result of tocolysis failure and early delivery. At birth, most affected infants have severe respiratory distress, and respiratory assessment reveals worsening distress as the bowel fills with air. Typically, breath sounds are diminished and bowel sounds are heard in the chest. Heart sounds may be shifted to the right side of the chest because the heart has been displaced by the abdominal contents. Physical examination reveals a flat or scaphoid abdomen and a prominent ipsilateral chest. Diagnosis can be made on the basis of the x-ray finding of loops of intestine in the thoracic cavity and the absence of intestine in the abdominal cavity.

Preoperatively, nursing interventions include assessment and stabilization of the infant's condition until surgical repair can be performed. Conventional mechanical ventilation, high-frequency oscillatory ventilation, and extracorporeal membrane oxygenation (ECMO) may be used as respiratory support. Permissive hypercapnia may be allowed as long as the pH is maintained above or equal to 7.30 (Ehrlich & Coran, 2007). Inhaled nitric oxide to relieve pulmonary hypertension of CDH has also been used in some cases, with mixed results. Gastric contents are aspirated and suction applied to decompress the gastrointestinal tract and prevent further cardiothoracic compromise. Oxygen therapy, mechanical ventilation, and the correction of acidosis are necessary in infants with early clinical respiratory distress from CDH. ECMO may be used in infants with severe circulatory and respiratory complications. Traditional management has been early surgical repair of the defect. However, increased survival rates have been reported with surgery after a period of preoperative stabilization and resolution of pulmonary hypertension.

The prognosis depends largely on the degree of fetal pulmonary development, but the prognosis in severe cases is often poor. The overall survival rate for live-born infants is 67% (Ehrlich & Coran, 2007). The incidence of gastroesophageal reflux (GER) disease in survivors is approximately 50%, and a significant number will have neurocognitive deficits.

Gastrointestinal System Anomalies

Anomalies in the gastrointestinal system can occur anywhere along the gastrointestinal tract, from the mouth to the anus. Some anomalies, such as cleft lip, omphalocele, and gastroschisis, are apparent at birth. Others, including cleft palate, esophageal atresia (EA), intestinal obstruction, and imperforate anus, become apparent as the infant is further assessed or becomes symptomatic.

Cleft Lip and Palate

Cleft lip or palate is a commonly occurring congenital midline fissure, or opening, in the lip or palate resulting from failure of the primary palate to fuse (Fig. 28-13). One or both deformities may occur and affect 400 to 500 infants each year in Canada (Health Canada, 2002). The rate of cleft lip with or without cleft palate declined between 1998 and 2007 with no further trend noted recently (PHAC, 2012). Multiple genetic and, to a lesser extent, environmental factors (e.g., maternal infection; tobacco exposure; radiation exposure; alcohol ingestion; and medications such as corticosteroids, some tranquilizers, and antiepileptics) appear to be involved in their development. Pathophysiology, evaluation, and treatment are addressed in Chapter 47.

Feeding is difficult because the cleft lip renders the newborn unable to maintain a seal around a nipple; the cleft palate renders the infant unable to form a vacuum to maintain suction when feeding. The inability to suck and swallow normally allows milk to pool in the nasopharynx, which increases the likelihood of aspiration. In addition, as the infant attempts to suck, milk often comes out through the cleft and out of the nares. Although the degree of difficulty depends on the size of the cleft, feeding problems are greater in infants with a cleft palate than in those with a cleft lip alone (see Fig. 28-13). Breastfeeding can be successful in some infants. Special nipples, bottles, and appliances are available to aid in feeding (Fig. 28-14).

In general, parents of infants with these defects need education and support as they learn to feed their baby, to prevent what should be a normal part of infant care from becoming a frustrating experience. Parents may also need support, particularly in the case of a cleft lip, as this is both a cosmetic and functional defect. Recognizing that it may interfere with normal parent–infant bonding in the neonatal period, the nurse must assess and intervene appropriately.

Esophageal Atresia and Tracheoesophageal Fistula

EA and TEF often occur together, although they can also occur separately. EA is a congenital anomaly in which the esophagus ends in a blind pouch or narrows into a thin cord, thus failing to form a continuous passageway to the stomach (Fig. 28-15, A). TEF is an abnormal connection between the esophagus and trachea (Fig. 28-15, B–E).

Polyhydramnios is a common antenatal finding, particularly if the fetus has an EA without TEF. The infant with EA or TEF may also show some fetal growth restriction and as a result will be SGA. The presence of EA or TEF, a midline defect, is often accompanied by another significant embryonic defect such as a cardiac anomaly; cleft lip, cleft palate, or both; or vertebral, genitourinary, or abdominal wall defect (Lovvan, Glenn, Pacetti, & Carter, 2011). Variations of the anomalies

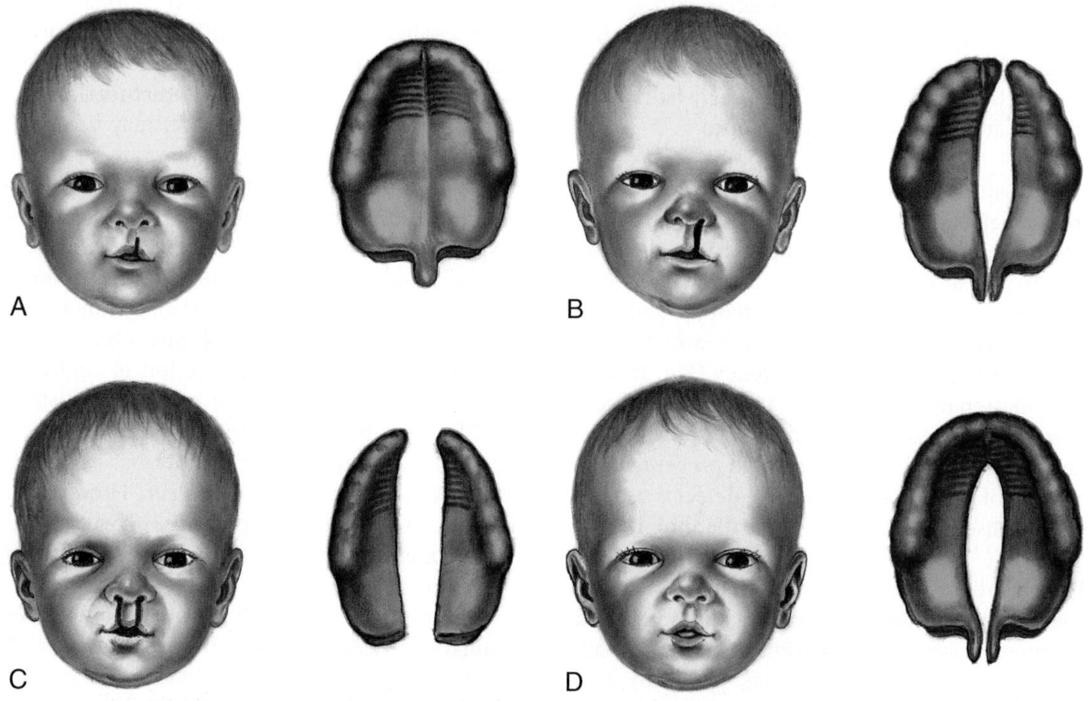

Fig. 28-13 Variations in clefts of lip and palate at birth. **A:** Notch in vermilion border. **B:** Unilateral cleft lip and cleft palate. **C:** Bilateral cleft lip and cleft palate. **D:** Cleft palate. *(From Hockenberry, M. J., & Wilson, D. [2011].* Wong's essentials of pediatric nursing *[9th ed., p. 429]. St. Louis: Mosby.)*

are possible, depending on the presence or absence of a TEF, the site of the fistula, and the location and degree of esophageal obstruction (see Fig. 28-15).

Infants with EA and TEF may demonstrate limited respiratory difficulty immediately after birth. EA with or without TEF results in excessive oral secretions, choking, and spitting up. When fed, the infant may swallow, but then cough, gag, and have the fluid return through the nose and mouth. Respiratory distress can result from aspiration or from the acute gastric distension produced by the TEF. Choking, coughing, and cyanosis occur after even a small amount of fluid is taken by mouth.

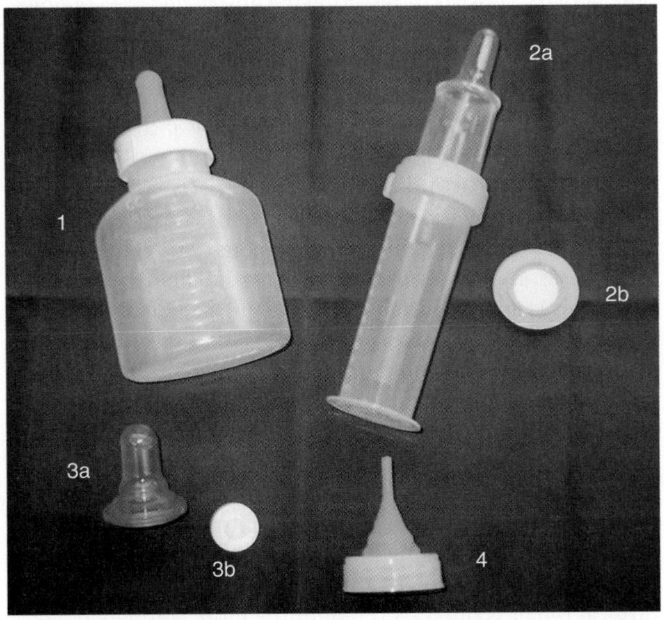

Fig. 28-14 Mead Johnson bottle and nipple for cleft palate (1). Cleft palate nipple system (2a) with valve (2b) to regulate flow. Haberman feeder (3a) with disc (3b) to control flow of milk. Ross cleft palate assembly (4). Nipple can be trimmed to accommodate palate size. *(Courtesy Shannon Perry, Phoenix, AZ.)*

Nursing interventions are supportive until surgery is performed. Any infant with excessive oral secretions and respiratory distress should not be fed orally until further evaluation is carried out. The head of the bed should be raised approximately 30 degrees and the infant placed supine to minimize the risk of aspiration of secretions. Further, a double-lumen catheter should be placed in the proximal esophageal pouch and set on low continuous suction to allow drainage of swallowed secretions. Other supportive measures include thermoregulation, fluid and electrolyte balance, acid–base balance, and prevention of complications as a result of an associated defect. Surgical correction of a TEF, often performed in one stage, consists of ligating the fistula and anastomosing the two segments of the esophagus. With EA, a staged repair may be necessary, especially when there is a significant gap between the proximal pouch and the distal esophagus (Fig. 28-15, A). The chances for survival in those infants in a good-risk category exceed 95, depending on the presence of associated defects and the infant's birth weight. Many infants with EA and TEF will have postoperative issues related to feeding difficulties such as GER and esophageal strictures requiring periodic dilation. (See Chapter 47 for further discussion of surgical treatment and nursing care.)

Omphalocele and Gastroschisis

Omphalocele and gastroschisis are two of the more common congenital defects that occur in the abdominal wall. They are rare, however, with omphalocele occurring in approximately 1 in 3000 to 10,000 live births, whereas the incidence of gastroschisis is 1 in 6000 live births (Blackburn, 2007).

An *omphalocele* is a covered defect of the umbilical ring into which varying amounts of the abdominal organs may herniate (Fig. 28-16). Although it is covered with a thin, often translucent peritoneal sac, the sac may rupture during or after birth. Many infants born with an omphalocele are preterm, and more than half have other defects involving the gastrointestinal, cardiac, genitourinary, musculoskeletal, and nervous systems.

Gastroschisis is the herniation of the bowel through a defect in the abdominal wall to the right of the umbilical cord. Unlike

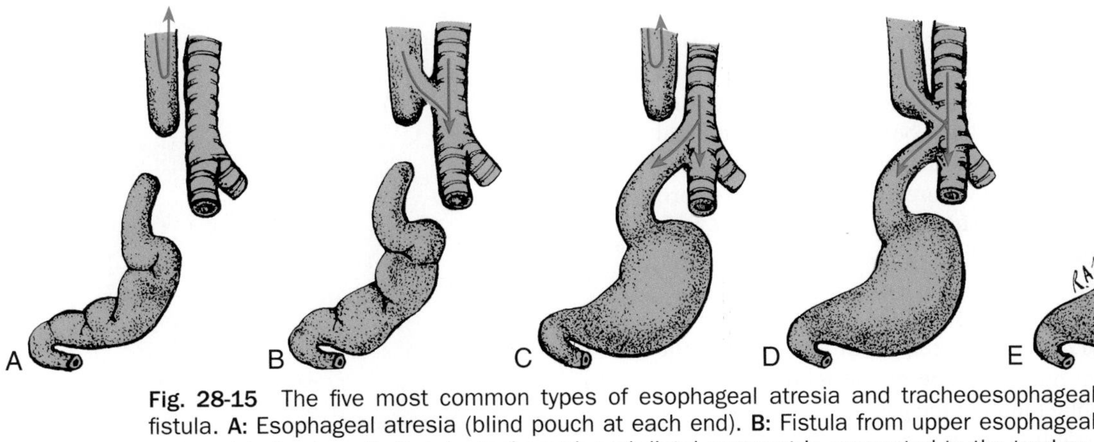

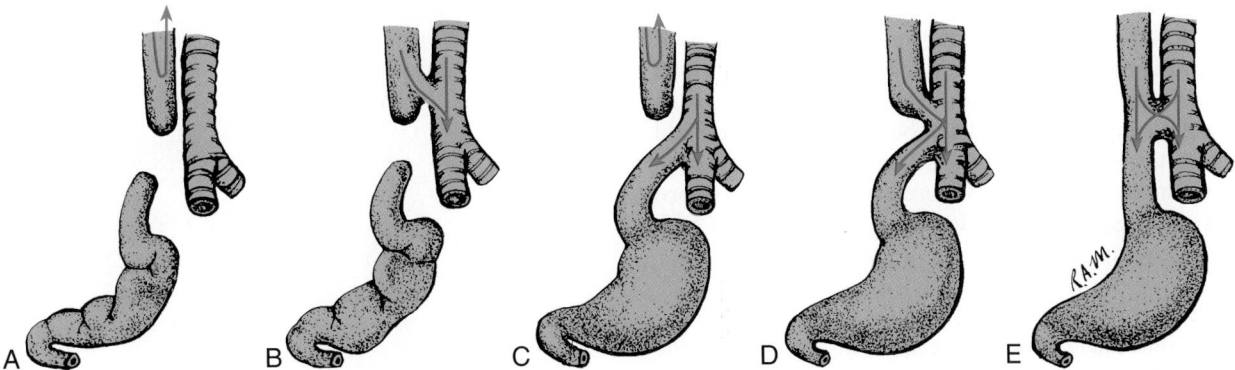

Fig. 28-15 The five most common types of esophageal atresia and tracheoesophageal fistula. **A:** Esophageal atresia (blind pouch at each end). **B:** Fistula from upper esophageal segment to trachea. **C:** Esophageal pouch and distal segment is connected to the trachea. **D:** Fistula to upper and lower segment of esophagus from trachea. **E:** Normal esophagus and trachea connected by a fistula.

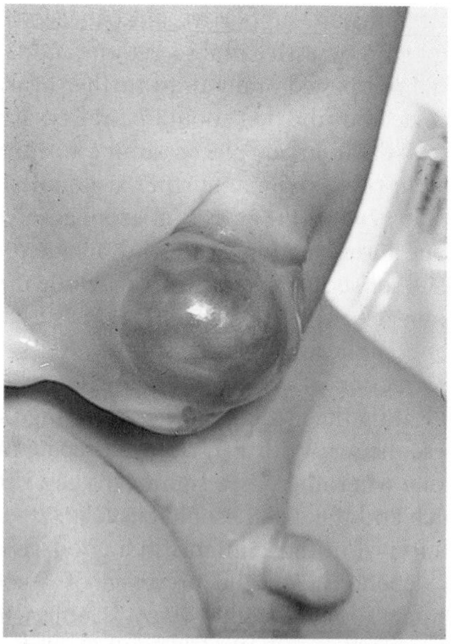

Fig. 28-16 Omphalocele. *(From O'Doherty, N. [1986].* Neonatology: Micro atlas of the newborn. *Nutley, NJ: Hoffmann–La Roche.)*

an omphalocele, there is no membrane covering the organs. In contrast to infants with omphalocele, there is less than 10 to 15% likelihood of associated anomalies, including intestinal atresia and cardiac anomalies.

The preoperative nursing care is similar for infants with either defect. Exposure of the viscera causes problems with thermoregulation and fluid and electrolyte balance. Before closure is performed, the exposed viscera are covered with moistened saline gauze and plastic wrap. In some cases the infant may be placed in an impermeable, clear plastic bowel bag to decrease insensible water losses, maintain thermoregulation, and prevent contamination of the exposed viscera (Lovvan et al., 2011). Antibiotics, fluid and electrolyte replacement, gastric decompression, and thermoregulation are needed for physiological support. If complete closure is impossible because of the small size of the abdominal cavity and the large amount of viscera to be replaced, a Silastic silo pouch is created and sewn to the fascia of the abdominal defect. The defect is closed surgically after the reduction of contents is complete, which usually takes 7 to 10 days. With surgical treatment, nutritional support, and medical management, the prognosis has improved for infants born with an abdominal wall defect. It is estimated that more than 80% of infants born with omphalocele survive, as do more than 90% of those born with gastroschisis, although residual feeding difficulties such as GER are not uncommon.

Intestinal Obstruction

Congenital intestinal obstruction can occur anywhere in the gastrointestinal tract and takes one of the following forms: atresia, a complete obliteration of the passage; partial obstruction, in which the symptoms may vary in severity and sometimes not be detected in the neonatal period; or malrotation of the intestine, which leads to twisting of the intestine (volvulus) and obstruction. EA, discussed previously, is a type of gastrointestinal obstruction. Meconium ileus is an obstruction caused by impacted meconium and is the earliest symptom of cystic fibrosis, a life-threatening chronic illness. Infants with this type of obstruction should be tested for cystic fibrosis because 95% of infants with meconium ileus have the disease. In addition to a history of polyhydramnios, the infant with an ileus shows the following cardinal signs and symptoms: bilious vomiting, abdominal distension, and failure to pass normal amounts of meconium in the first 24 hours.

Nursing care is aimed at supporting the infant until surgical intervention can be carried out to eliminate the obstruction. Oral feedings are held, a nasogastric tube is inserted for decompression and IV therapy is initiated to provide needed fluids and electrolytes. In infants with an intestinal obstruction, surgery consists of resecting the obstructed area of bowel and anastomosing the unaffected bowel. In recent years, the survival rate for these infants has risen to 90 to 95% as a result of better treatments, improved neonatal intensive care, and an increased understanding of the problem.

Anorectal Malformation

Anorectal malformation is a term used to describe a wide range of congenital disorders involving the anus and rectum and, in many cases, the genitourinary system. The incidence of these anomalies is approximately 1 in 5000 to 1 in 15,000 live births (Blackburn, 2007). Occurring more often in male than female infants, they result from the failure of anorectal development in weeks 7 and 8 of fetal life. Infants have no anal opening (Fig. 28-17) and often have a fistula from the rectum to the perineum or genitourinary system. Types of anorectal malformations include the typical cloaca in females, in which the vagina, colon, and urethra form a single common passage in the perineum. Others include the low rectovaginal fistula (female) and rectourethral bulbar fistula (male). Extensive and staged surgical repair is often required for the more complex types of anorectal malformations. In some cases, the anomaly may involve stenotic areas, or there may be a thin translucent membrane covering the anal opening. Treatment for such a

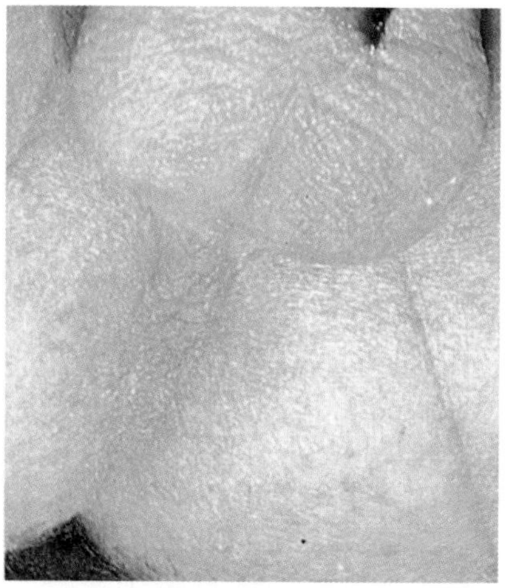

Fig. 28-17 Anorectal malformation (imperforate anus). *(From Chessell, G., Jamieson, M. J., & Morton, M. [1984].* Diagnostic picture tests in clinical medicine: Vol. 2. *St. Louis: Mosby-Wolfe.)*

membrane is excision followed by daily dilation, which parents are taught to do. (See Chapter 47 for further discussion of surgical treatment.)

Musculoskeletal System Anomalies

Developmental Dysplasia of the Hip

The broad term *developmental dysplasia of the hip* (DDH) describes a spectrum of disorders related to abnormal development of the hip that may appear at any time during fetal life, infancy, or childhood. A change in terminology from congenital hip dysplasia and congenital dislocation of the hip to DDH more properly reflects a variety of hip abnormalities in which there is a shallow acetabulum, subluxation, or dislocation.

The incidence of hip instability of some kind is approximately 10 per 1000 live births. The incidence of frank dislocation or a dislocatable hip is 1 to 1.5 per 1000 live births (Hosalkar, Horn, Friedman, & Dormans, 2007).

The cause of DDH is unknown, but certain factors such as sex, birth order, family history, intrauterine position, birth type, joint laxity, and postnatal positioning are believed to affect the risk of DDH. Predisposing factors associated with DDH may be divided into three broad categories: (1) physiological factors, which include maternal hormone secretion and intrauterine positioning; (2) mechanical factors, which involve breech presentation, multiple fetuses, oligohydramnios, and large infant size; other mechanical factors may include continued maintenance of the hips in adduction and extension that will in time cause a dislocation; and (3) genetic factors, which entail a higher incidence (6%) of DDH in siblings of affected infants and an even greater incidence (36%) of occurrence if a sibling and one parent were affected.

Three degrees of DDH are as follows (Fig. 28-18):

1. *Acetabular dysplasia (or preluxation)*: This is the mildest form of DDH; there is neither subluxation nor dislocation. There is a delay in acetabular development evidenced by osseous hypoplasia of the acetabular roof that is oblique and shallow, although the cartilaginous roof is comparatively intact. The femoral head remains in the acetabulum.
2. *Subluxation*: The largest percentage of DDH, subluxation implies incomplete dislocation of the hip and is sometimes regarded as an intermediate stage in the development from primary dysplasia to complete dislocation. The femoral head remains in contact with the acetabulum, but a stretched capsule and ligamentum teres cause the head of the femur to be partially displaced. Pressure on the cartilaginous roof inhibits ossification and produces a flattening of the socket.
3. *Dislocation*: The femoral head loses contact with the acetabulum and is displaced posteriorly and superiorly over the fibrocartilaginous rim. The ligamentum teres is elongated and taut.

DDH is often not detected at the initial examination after birth; thus, all infants should be carefully monitored for hip dysplasia at follow-up visits throughout the first year of life. In the newborn period, dysplasia usually appears as hip joint laxity rather than as outright dislocation. Subluxation and the tendency to dislocate can be demonstrated by the Ortolani (see Fig. 24-10) or Barlow tests. The Ortolani and Barlow tests are most reliable from birth to 2 or 3 months of age. Other signs of DDH are shortening of the limb on the affected side (Galeazzi sign, Allis sign), asymmetrical thigh and gluteal folds, and broadening of the perineum (in bilateral dislocation) (see Fig. 24-8).

NURSING ALERT The Ortolani and Barlow tests must be performed by an experienced clinician to prevent fracture or further damage to the hip. If these tests are performed too vigorously in the first 2 days of life, when the hip subluxates freely, persistent dislocation may occur.

Treatment should be initiated as soon as the condition is recognized, since early intervention is more likely to restore normal bony architecture and function. The longer treatment is delayed, the more severe the deformity, the more difficult the treatment, and the less favourable the prognosis. The treatment varies with the child's age and the extent of the dysplasia. The goal of treatment is to obtain and maintain a safe, congruent position of the hip joint in order to promote normal hip joint development and ambulation.

The hip joint needs to be maintained in a safe position with the proximal femur centred in the acetabulum in an attitude of flexion by dynamic splinting. Of the numerous devices available, the Pavlik harness is the most widely used, and with

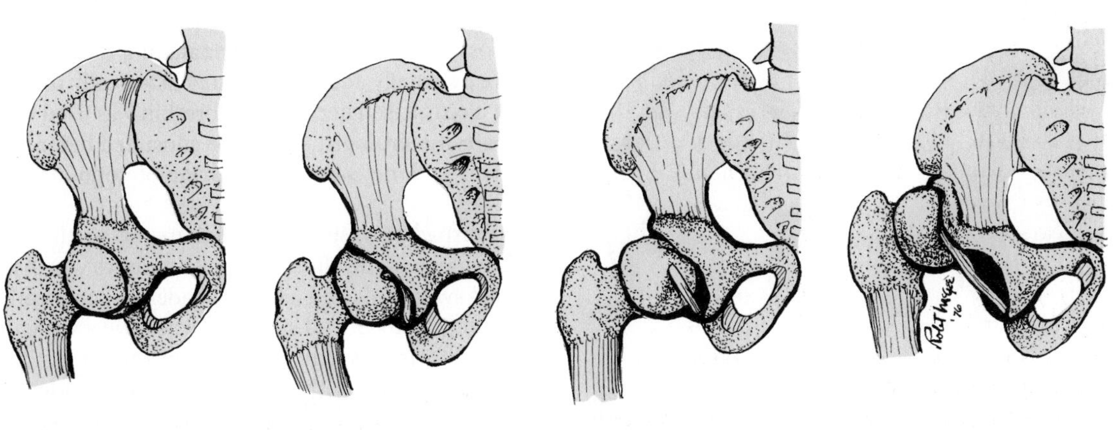

Fig. 28-18 Configuration and relationship of structures in developmental dysplasia of the hip.

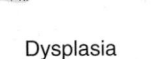

time, motion, and gravity, the hip works into a more abducted, reduced position (Fig. 28-19). The harness is worn continuously until the hip is proved stable on clinical and radiographic examination, usually about 3 to 5 months.

NURSING ALERT The practice of double- or triple-diapering for DDH is not recommended because it promotes hip extension, thus worsening proper hip alignment.

See Chapter 54 for more detailed discussion of DDH.

Clubfoot

Congenital clubfoot is a complex deformity of the ankle and foot that includes forefoot adduction, midfoot supination, hindfoot varus, and ankle equinus. Deformities of the foot and ankle are described according to the position of the ankle and foot. The more common positions involve the following variations:

Talipes varus: An inversion, or a bending inward
Talipes valgus: An eversion, or bending outward
Talipes equinus: Plantar flexion, in which the toes are lower than the heel
Talipes calcaneus: Dorsiflexion, in which the toes are higher than the heel

Most cases of clubfoot are a combination of these positions. The most common type of clubfoot (approximately 95%) is the composite deformity talipes equinovarus, in which the foot is pointed downward and inward in varying degrees of severity (see Fig. 54-9, p. 1702). Unilateral clubfoot is somewhat more common than bilateral clubfoot and may occur as an isolated defect or in association with other disorders or syndromes, such as chromosomal anomalies, arthrogryposis (a generalized immobility of the joints), cerebral palsy, or spina bifida.

The goal of treatment for clubfoot is to achieve a painless, plantigrade (ability to walk on the sole of the foot with the heel on the ground), and stable foot. Treatment of clubfoot involves three stages: (1) correction of the deformity, (2) maintenance of the correction until normal muscle balance is regained, and (3) follow-up observation to avert possible recurrence of the deformity. Some feet respond to treatment readily; some respond only to prolonged, vigorous, and sustained efforts; and improvement in others remains disappointing even with maximum effort on the part of all concerned.

Serial casting is begun shortly after birth, often before discharge from the nursery. Successive casts allow for gradual stretching of skin and tight structures on the medial side of the foot. Manipulation and casting need to be repeated frequently (every week) to accommodate the rapid growth of early infancy. In some cases, daily manipulation and stretching of tissues are accomplished with taping and splinting of the affected extremity. A continuous passive motion machine may be used several hours daily to stretch and strengthen muscle groups involved (Faulks & Luther, 2005). The extremity or extremities are often casted or splinted until maximum correction is achieved, usually within 8 to 12 weeks. An apparatus with foot splints attached to a cross bar (Denis Browne splint) may be used to manage feet that correct with casting and manipulation.

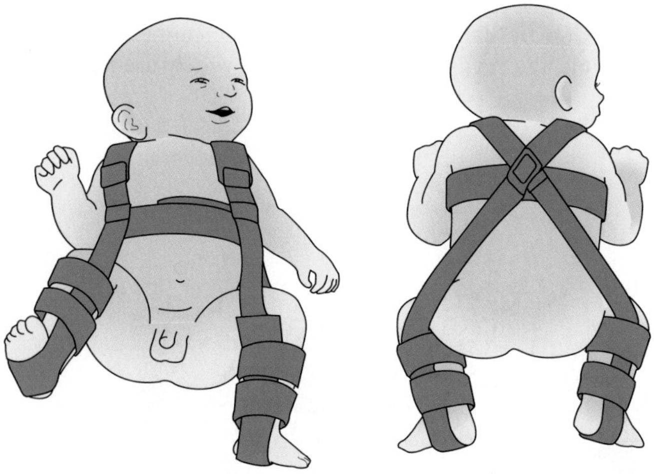

Fig. 28-19 Treatment for developmental hip dysplasia with Pavlik harness. *(From Ball, J. [1998].* Mosby's pediatric patient teaching guides. *St. Louis: Mosby.)*

Polydactyly

Occasionally, hands or feet are seen with extra digits. In some instances, polydactyly is hereditary. If there is little or no bone involvement, the extra digit is tied with silk suture soon after birth. The digit falls off within a few days, leaving a small scar. When there is bone involvement, surgical repair is indicated.

Genitourinary System Anomalies

Hypospadias and Epispadias

Hypospadias constitutes a range of penile anomalies associated with an abnormally located urinary meatus. The meatus can open below the glans penis or anywhere along the ventral surface of the penis, the scrotum, or the perineum. It is the most common anomaly of the penis, occurring in approximately 1 in 250 to 300 live births (Gray & Moore, 2009). It is classified according to the location of the meatus and the presence or absence of chordee, which is a ventral curvature of the penis.

Mild cases of hypospadias (Fig. 28-20) are often repaired for cosmetic reasons and involve a single surgical procedure. The goals are to improve the appearance of the genitalia, make it possible for the child to urinate in a standing position, and have a sexually adequate organ. Historically these infants were not circumcised because the foreskin was used during surgical repair; the urologist should be consulted before circumcision. Repair is done early, often during or soon after the first year of life.

Epispadias results from failure of urethral canalization. About 55% of the affected infants are boys who have a widened pubic symphysis and a broad spadelike penis with the urethra opening on its dorsal surface. Girls have a wide urethra and a bifid clitoris. Severity ranges from mild anomaly to a severe form associated with exstrophy of the bladder. Surgical correction is necessary, and affected male infants should not be circumcised.

Exstrophy of the Bladder

The most common bladder anomaly is exstrophy (Fig. 28-21), which often occurs in conjunction with epispadias. It is rare, occurring only in about 1 in 35,000 to 40,000 live births (Elder, 2007). It results from abnormal development of the bladder, abdominal wall, and symphysis pubis that causes the bladder, urethra, and ureteral orifices to all be exposed. The bladder is visible in the suprapubic area as a red mass with numerous folds, with urine draining from it onto the infant's skin.

Immediately after birth, the exposed bladder is covered with a sterile, nonadherent dressing to protect it until closure can be performed. It is recommended that reconstructive surgery be started in the neonatal period, preferably with the bladder being closed during the first or second day of life.

Disorders of Sex Development

A disorder of sex development (DSD) in the newborn (Fig. 28-22) often is discovered by the nurse during a physical assessment. Erroneous or abnormal sexual differentiation may be a genetic defect, such as congenital adrenal hypoplasia, which can be life threatening because it involves deficiency of all adrenocortical hormones. Other possible causes of DSD include chromosomal abnormalities, defective sex hormone synthesis in males, and the placental transfer of masculinizing agents to female fetuses. Gender assignment should be based on data gathered from the following sources: maternal and family history, including the ingestion of steroids during pregnancy and relatives who had DSD or who died during the neonatal period; physical examination; chromosomal analysis (results are available in 2 or 3 days); endoscopy, ultrasonography and radiographic contrast studies; biochemical tests, such as analysis of urinary steroid excretion, which helps detect several of the adrenocortical syndromes; and, in some instances, laparotomy or gonad biopsy.

Therapeutic intervention, including any counselling and surgery, should be started as soon as possible. Any child born with DSD should not receive gender assignment until a proper assessment has been done. Gender assignment should be based on age at presentation, potential for mature sexual function, potential fertility, and the long-term psychological and emotional impact on the child and family. Parents need much support as they learn to deal with this challenging situation.

Teratoma

A *teratoma* is an embryonal tumour that may be solid, cystic, or mixed. It is composed of at least two and usually three types of embryonal tissue: ectoderm, mesoderm, and endoderm. A teratoma in the newborn may occur in the skull, mediastinum, abdomen, or sacral area; more than half are located in the sacrococcygeal area. The treatment of choice is complete surgical resection of the teratoma. Approximately 80% of all teratomas are benign and no additional therapy is needed after

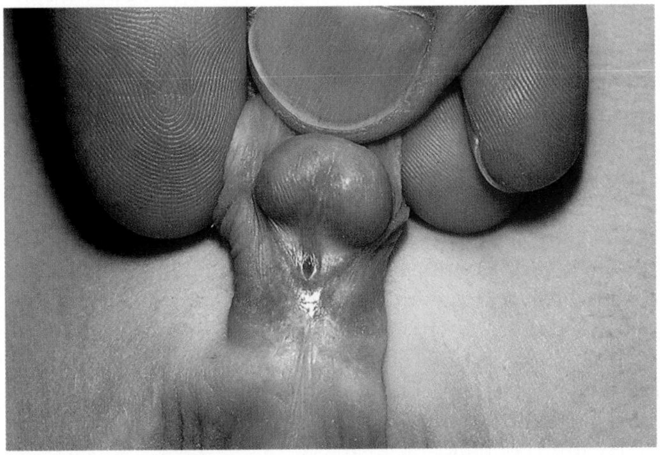

Fig. 28-20 Hypospadias. *(Courtesy H. Gil Rushton, MD, Children's National Medical Center, Washington, DC.)*

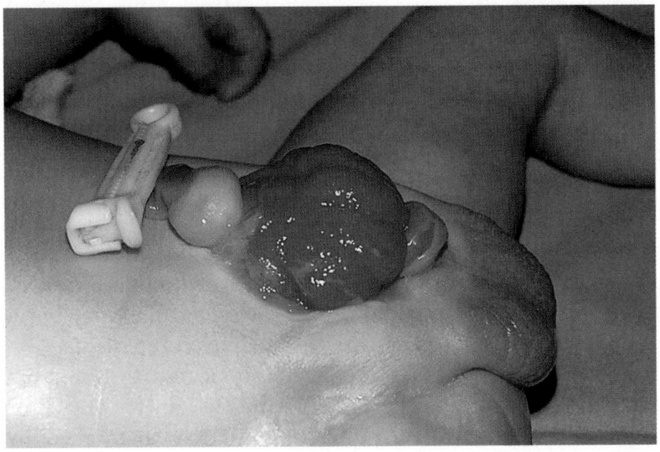

Fig. 28-21 Exstrophy of bladder. *(Courtesy H. Gil Rushton, MD, Children's National Medical Center, Washington, DC.)*

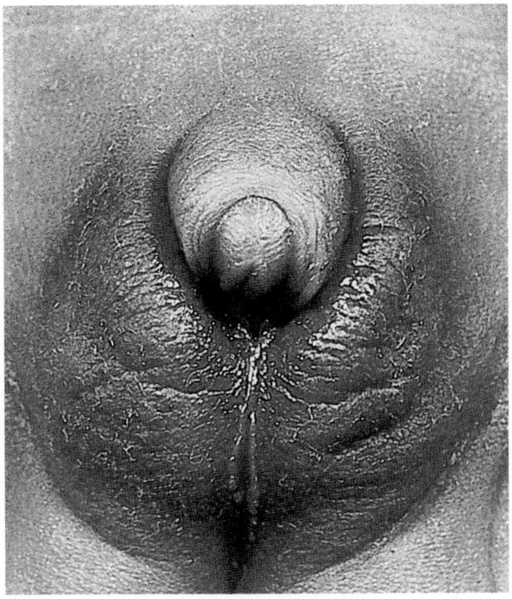

Fig. 28-22 Ambiguous external genitalia (i.e., structure may be enlarged clitoral hood and clitoris or micropenis and bifid scrotum). *(Courtesy Edward S. Tank, MD, Division of Urology, Oregon Health Sciences University, Portland, OR.)*

complete resection. If the tumour is not surgically resected before the infant is 1 to 2 months old, the likelihood of the teratoma becoming malignant increases rapidly.

Nursing Care Management

Any deviations from normal should be reported to the primary health care provider immediately. A thorough assessment of all body systems needs to be completed, with identification of both visible anomalies and those that might not be visible.

Some infants have multiple congenital anomalies. A recognized pattern of malformations is referred to as a *syndrome*. The most common one is Down syndrome, with the diagnosis confirmed early in the neonatal period.

Genetic Diagnosis

Diagnostic procedures for the detection of genetic disorders are performed after birth, any time from the postnatal period through adulthood. Many tests are available for various disorders; only the most commonly used ones are discussed here.

Newborn Screening

The most widespread use of postnatal testing for genetic disease is the routine screening of newborns for inborn errors of metabolism (IEMs) such as PKU and hypothyroidism (see Table 25-3).

An IEM is the term applied to a large group of disorders caused by a metabolic defect that results from the absence of or change in a protein, usually an enzyme, and mediated by the action of a certain gene. These defects can involve any substrate produced from protein, carbohydrate, or fat metabolism. IEMs are recessive disorders and an individual must receive a defective gene from each parent for them to occur. The parents usually are unaffected because their dominant gene directs the synthesis of sufficient protein to meet their metabolic needs under normal circumstances.

With the advent of new biochemical techniques, it is now possible to detect the gene responsible for causing an increasing number of these disorders early in the neonatal period so that appropriate therapies to prevent further morbidity may be implemented. Tandem mass spectrometry has the potential for identifying up to as many as 40 IEMs. With tandem mass spectrometry, earlier identification of IEMs may prevent further developmental delays and morbidities in affected children.

Phenylketonuria

PKU results from a deficiency of the enzyme phenylalanine dehydrogenase. The test for PKU is not reliable until the newborn has ingested an ample amount of the amino acid phenylalanine, a constituent of both human and cow's milk. The nurse must document the initial ingestion of milk and perform the test at least 24 hours after that time. The current trend toward early infant discharge from the hospital has the potential to cause neonates with a disorder such as PKU not to be adequately screened. A number of agencies have developed guidelines to minimize the risk of this happening and recommend the following:

- Obtain a subsequent sample by 2 weeks of age if the initial specimen is collected before the newborn is 24 hours old.
- Designate a primary care provider for all newborns before discharge for adequate newborn screening follow-up.
- Collect the initial specimen as close as possible to discharge and no later than 7 days after birth (Newborn Screening Ontario, n.d.; Perinatal Services BC, 2010).

If the infant is found to have PKU, a diet low in phenylalanine is begun soon after birth. A new medication, sapropterin dihydrochloride, has been approved for use in persons with PKU; the drug acts to decrease blood phenylalanine levels in persons with hyperphenylalaninemia (Stokowski, 2008). Breastfeeding or partial breastfeeding may be possible for some infants if the phenylalanine levels are monitored carefully and remain within acceptable limits (Lawrence & Lawrence, 2011). Many affected children have some intellectual impairment. Successful management and outcome are largely dependent on early identification of the condition, modification of the diet, and compliance with the treatment regimen throughout the entire life.

Galactosemia

Galactosemia, a deficiency of the enzyme galactose-1-phosphate uridyltransferase, results in the inability to convert galactose to glucose. Galactosemia can be detected by measuring the serum galactose in newborns suspected of having the disease after they have ingested human milk (which contains galactose) or formula containing galactose. Infants with galactosemia appear well at birth, but after ingestion of milk (which has a high lactose content), they begin to show progressive symptoms, including vomiting, diarrhea, and weight loss (Askin & Diehl-Jones, 2003). *E. coli* sepsis is another common initial clinical sign. If the disorder goes untreated, the galactose levels will continue to increase and the infant will show growth failure, cognitive impairment, cataracts, jaundice, hepatomegaly, and cirrhosis of the liver, with death possible within the first month of life. Therapy consists of eliminating lactose from the diet. This condition precludes breastfeeding, since lactose is present in breast milk.

Hypothyroidism

Congenital hypothyroidism results from a deficiency of thyroid hormones; it affects approximately 1 of every 3000 to 4000 newborns (Kaye & AAP, Committee on Genetics, 2006; Ontario Newborn Screening Program, 2006). All provinces in Canada routinely screen for hypothyroidism. Although a heel stick blood sample for the test is best obtained between 2 and 6 days of age, specimens are usually taken within the first 24 to 48 hours or before discharge as part of a concurrent screening for other metabolic defects. At this time, the normally expected increase in thyroxine (T_4) would be lacking in newborns with hypothyroidism.

Neonatal screening consists of an initial filter paper blood spot T_4 measurement followed by measurement of thyroid-stimulating hormone (TSH) in specimens with low T_4 values. Early screening may have false-positive results. In the newborn, thyroid function studies are elevated in comparison with values in older children; therefore, it is important to document the timing of the tests. In preterm and sick full-term infants thyroid function tests are usually lower than in the healthy full-term infant. A repeat T_4 and TSH may be evaluated after 30 weeks (corrected age) in newborns born before that time and after resolution of the acute illness in the sick full-term infant.

Treatment involves lifelong thyroid hormone replacement therapy that begins as soon as possible after diagnosis to alleviate signs of hypothyroidism and to reestablish normal physical and mental development. The medication of choice is synthetic levothyroxine sodium (Synthroid, Levothroid).

Genetic Evaluation and Counselling

Genetic counselling addresses the problems associated with the occurrence or risk of occurrence of a genetic disorder in a family. It involves the relaying of information about the diagnosis, treatment options, recurrence risk, and availability of prenatal diagnosis. With the completion of the Human Genome Project, the international project to determine the total genetic information in humans, a new era of human genetics is unfolding (International Human Genome Sequencing Consortium, 2004), and advances will lead to a better understanding of how genetic variation contributes to health and disease. It is essential that nurses understand basic principles of heredity, understand how heredity contributes to disorders, and be aware of the types of genetic testing available.

Nurses frequently encounter children with a genetic disorder, including an IEM, as well as families in which there is a risk that a disorder may be transmitted to, or occur in, an offspring. It is the nurse's responsibility to be alert to situations in which persons could benefit from genetic evaluation and counselling. Nurses also need to be aware of the local genetic resources, aid the family in finding related services, and offer support and care for children and families affected by genetic conditions.

Nursing Care

Newborn

A collaborative health team approach that includes specialists and community service representatives is needed in the care of the infant with a congenital anomaly. Surgical intervention in the neonatal period may be necessary for the infant requiring either immediate correction or a palliative procedure to relieve the symptoms of the anomaly until definitive correction can be done. There is higher morbidity and mortality in neonates than in older children or adults undergoing similar procedures. However, despite the problems unique to neonates, advances in surgical techniques, fluid and electrolyte management, anaesthesia, pain management, and the nursing care given in intensive care nurseries have together been responsible for decreasing the risk of surgery in neonates.

The health care team must be highly skilled to meet the infant's needs. These needs are similar to those of other high-risk infants. In addition to stabilization of the infant's condition (oxygenation and perfusion of tissues), other preoperative interventions, such as nasogastric tube placement for abdominal decompression, pain management, and the maintenance of fluid and electrolyte balance, are implemented to manage specific problems.

Postoperatively, the infant is often returned to the intensive care nursery, where he or she needs to be closely monitored. The infant's respiratory efforts need to be supported; this often requires mechanical ventilation. Constant surveillance is necessary to detect any respiratory complications resulting from the anaesthesia. A pulse oximeter is attached to measure the oxygen saturation and oxygen is provided as needed. An indwelling gastric catheter may be placed to remove gastric secretions, thereby preventing aspiration and abdominal distension. The infant's fluid, electrolyte, and acid–base balance should be monitored and adjusted as needed. Urine output is also monitored and should equal 1 to 2 mL/kg/hr. Other nursing interventions include assessment and care of the surgical site, thermoregulation, pain management, and promoting comfort.

Parents and Family

While the infant is receiving care, the parents also have needs that must be met as they deal with the crisis of having an infant with an abnormal condition. Their reactions should be carefully assessed and are likely to be those typical of a grief response. Facilitating their understanding of the information given them about their infant's condition is a vital nursing intervention. A newly diagnosed disorder often implies the need for the implementation of a therapeutic regimen. For example, the disorder may be an IEM, such as PKU, which requires consistent and rigid adherence to a diet. The family may need help securing the required formula and may require counselling from a clinical dietician. The importance of maintaining the diet, keeping an adequate supply of special preparations, and avoiding the use of unauthorized substitutions must be impressed upon the family. These conditions often require a drastic change in family lifestyle and functioning; families often depend on others for assistance. Family coping skills and resources may be stretched thin with a diagnosis such as PKU or galactosemia.

Referral to appropriate agencies is another essential component of the follow-up management, and the nurse should make the parents aware of all possible sources of aid, including pertinent literature, parent groups, and national organizations. Many organizations and foundations (e.g., Canadian Organization of Rare Disorders) provide services and counselling for families of affected children. Numerous parent support groups are also available, where they can share experiences and derive mutual support in coping with problems similar to those of other group members. Nurses must be familiar with the services available in their community that provide assistance and education to families with these particular needs.

A major nursing role is the provision of emotional support during all phases of care to the family of an infant with an anomaly or disorder. The feelings that stem from the real or imagined threat posed by a congenital anomaly are as varied as the people being counselled. Responses may include apathy, denial, anger, hostility, fear, embarrassment, grief, and loss of self-esteem.

Parents may benefit from seeing before-and-after pictures of other babies born with the same defect. In addition to verbal and nonverbal supportive care, this visual reassurance may be effective in allaying their concerns.

Families need much information, guidance, and support as they make decisions regarding their infant's care. Once parents have been given the facts, possible consequences, and any assistance they need in problem solving, the final decision regarding a course of action must be their own. It is then incumbent on health care providers to support the family's decision.

Key Points

- The identification of maternal and fetal risk factors in the antepartum and intrapartum periods is vital for planning adequate care of high-risk infants.
- A small percentage of significant birth injuries may occur despite skilled and competent obstetrical care.
- Metabolic abnormalities of diabetes mellitus in pregnancy adversely affect embryonic and fetal development.
- Infection in the newborn may be acquired in utero, at birth, in breast milk, or from within the nursery.
- The most common maternal infections during early pregnancy that are associated with various congenital malformations include toxoplasmosis, herpes, CMV, rubella, parvovirus B19, and varicella.
- HIV transmission from mother to infant occurs transplacentally at various gestational ages, perinatally by maternal blood and secretions, and postnatally through breast milk.
- Preterm infants are at risk for problems related to the immaturity of organ systems.
- Maternal–fetal Rh and ABO incompatibility may cause significant hemolysis and jaundice in the neonatal period.
- The injection of Rho(D) immune globulin in Rh-negative and Coombs' test–negative women minimizes the possibility of isoimmunization.
- The nurse often is the first person to observe signs of newborn drug withdrawal (NAS) and then acquires additional information from the maternal history.
- Congenital defects are now the leading cause of death in the first year of life.
- The curative and rehabilitative problems of a child with a congenital disorder are often complex, requiring an interprofessional approach to care.
- Parents often need special instruction (e.g., cardiopulmonary resuscitation, oxygen therapy, or nutrition requirements) before they take a high-risk infant home.
- The supportive care given to the parents of infants with a congenital anomaly or inborn error of metabolism must begin at birth or at the time of diagnosis and continue for years.

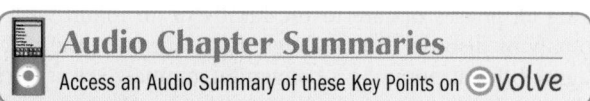

Audio Chapter Summaries

Access an Audio Summary of these Key Points on Evolve

References

Adams-Chapman, I., & Stoll, B. (2007). Nervous system disorders. In R. M. Kliegman, R. E. Behrman, H. B. Jenson, & B. F. Stanton (Eds.), *Nelson textbook of pediatrics* (18th ed., pp. 713–722). Philadelphia: Saunders.

Alimenti, A., et al. (2006). A prospective controlled study of neurodevelopment in HIV-uninfected children exposed to combination retroviral drugs in pregnancy. *Pediatrics, 118*(4), e1139–e1145. doi:10.1542/peds.2006-0525

Allen, U., & Canadian Paediatric Society, Infectious Diseases and Immunization Committee. (2006). Current management of herpes simplex virus infection in pregnant women and their newborn infants. *Paediatrics and Child Health, 11*, 363–365.

American Academy of Pediatrics. (2000). Fetal alcohol syndrome and alcohol-related neurodevelopmental disorders. *Pediatrics, 106*(2), 358–361.

American Academy of Pediatrics, Committee on Infectious Diseases. (2006). *Red book: 2006 report of the committee on infectious diseases* (27th ed.). Elk Grove Village, IL: Author.

American Academy of Pediatrics, Committee on Pediatric AIDS. (2008). HIV testing and prophylaxis to prevent mother-to-child transmission in the United States. *Pediatrics, 122*(5), 1127–1134. doi:10.1542/peds.2008-2175

Anderson, M. S., Wood, L. L., Keller, J. A., & Hay, W. W., Jr. (2011). Enteral nutrition. In S. L. Gardner, B. S. Carter, M. Enzman-Hines, & J. A Hernandez. (Eds.), *Merenstein & Gardner's handbook of neonatal intensive care* (7th ed., pp. 398–433). St. Louis: Mosby.

Arria, A. M., et al. (2006). Methamphetamine and other substance use during pregnancy: Preliminary estimates from the Infant Development, Environment, and Lifestyle (IDEAL) study. *Maternal and Child Health, 10*(3), 293–302. doi:10.1007/s10995-005-0052-0

Askin, D. F. (2004). *Infection in the neonate: A comprehensive guide to assessment, management, and nursing care.* Santa Rosa, CA: NICU Ink.

Askin, D. F., & Diehl-Jones, B. (2001). Cocaine: Effects of in utero exposure on the fetus and newborn. *Journal of Perinatal and Neonatal Nursing, 14*(4), 83–102.

Askin, D. F., & Diehl-Jones, B. (2003). Liver. Part 3: Pathophysiology of liver dysfunction. *Neonatal Network, 22*(3), 5–15.

Aziz, K., et al. (2005). Variations in rates of nosocomial infection among Canadian neonatal intensive care units may be practice-related. *BMC Pediatrics, 5*(22). doi:10.1186/1471-2431-5-22

Baer, J. S., Sampson, P. D., Barr, H. M., Connor, P. D., & Streissguth, A. P. (2003). A 21-year longitudinal analysis of the effects of prenatal alcohol exposure on young adult drinking. *Archives of General Psychiatry, 60*(4), 377–385.

Baley, J. E., & Toltzis, P. (2006). Viral infections. In R. J. Martin, A. A. Fanaroff, & M. C. Walsh (Eds.), *Fanaroff and Martin's neonatal-perinatal medicine: Diseases of the fetus and infant* (8th ed.). Philadelphia: Mosby.

Bandstra, E. S., & Accornero, V. H. (2006). Infants of substance abusing mothers. In R. J. Martin, A. A. Fanaroff, & M. C. Walsh (Eds.), *Fanaroff and Martin's neonatal-perinatal medicine: Diseases of the fetus and infant* (8th ed.). Philadelphia: Mosby.

Barrington, K. J., & Canadian Paediatric Society, Fetus and Newborn Committee. (2007). Management of the infant at increased risk for sepsis. *Paediatrics and Child Health, 12*(10), 893–898.

Barrington, K., Sankaran, K., & Canadian Paediatric Society, Fetus and Newborn Committee. (2007). Guidelines for detection, management and prevention of hyperbilirubinemia in term and late preterm newborn infants (35 or more weeks' gestation). *Paediatrics and Child Health 12*(5), 1B–12B.

Bateman, D. A., & Chiriboga, C. A. (2000). Dose-response effect of cocaine on newborn head circumference. *Pediatrics, 106*(3), e33.

Bay, C. A., Steele, M. W., & Davis, H. (2007). Genetic disorders and dysmorphic conditions. In B. Zitelli, & H. Davis (Eds.), *Atlas of pediatric physical diagnosis* (5th ed.). St. Louis: Mosby.

Berghella, V., et al. (2003). Maternal methadone dose and neonatal withdrawal. *American Journal of Obstetrics and Gynecology, 189*(2), 312–317.

Bernstein, D. (2007). Congenital heart disease. In R. M. Kliegman, R. E. Behrman, H. B. Jenson, & B. F. Stanton (Eds.), *Nelson textbook of pediatrics* (18th ed., pp. 1878–1941). Philadelphia: Saunders.

Blackburn, S. (2007). *Maternal, fetal, and neonatal physiology: A clinical perspective* (3rd ed.). St. Louis: Saunders.

Boyer, S. G., & Boyer, K. M. (2004). Update on TORCH infections in the newborn infant. *Newborn and Infant Nursing Reviews, 4*(1), 70–80.

Bracken, M. B., Triche, E. W., Belanger, K., Hellenbrand, K., & Leaderer, B. P. (2003). Association of maternal caffeine consumption with decrements in fetal growth. *American Journal of Epidemiology, 157*(5), 456–466.

Burdge, D. R., et al. (2003). Canadian consensus guidelines for the management of pregnant HIV-positive women and their offspring. *Canadian Medical Association Journal, 168*(14), 1683–1688.

Burns, L., Conroy, E., & Mattick, R. P. (2010). Infant mortality among women on a methadone program during pregnancy. *Drug and Alcohol Review, 29*(5), 551–556. doi:10.1111/j.1465-3362.2010.00176.x

Buus-Frank, M. (2004). Hands that heal—hands that harm. *Advances in Neonatal Care, 4*(5), 251–255.

Campbell, S. (2003). Prenatal cocaine exposure and neonatal/infant outcomes. *Neonatal Network, 22*(1), 19–21.

Caviness, A. C., Demmler, G. J., & Selwyn, B. J. (2008). Clinical and laboratory features of neonatal herpes simplex infection: A case-control study. *Pediatric Infectious Disease Journal, 27*(5), 425–430. doi:10.1097/INF.0b013e3181646d95

Centers for Disease Control and Prevention. (2005). Guidelines for identifying and referring persons with fetal alcohol syndrome. *MMWR: Morbidity and Mortality Weekly Report, 54*(RR-11), 1–15. Retrieved from http://www.cdc.gov/mmwr/preview/mmwrhtml/rr5411a1.htm.

Centers for Disease Control and Prevention. (2009). Trends in perinatal group B streptococcal disease—United States, 2000–2006. *MMWR: Morbidity and Mortality Weekly Report, 58*(5), 109–112. Retrieved from http://www.cdc.gov/mmwr/preview/mmwrhtml/mm5805a2.htm.

Centers for Disease Control and Prevention. (2010). Prevention of perinatal group B streptococcal disease. *MMWR: Morbidity and Mortality Weekly Report, 59*(RR10), 1–32. Retrieved from http://www.cdc.gov/mmwr/preview/mmwrhtml/rr5910a1.htm.

Chiriboga, C. A. (2003). Fetal alcohol and drug effects. *Neurologist, 9*(6), 267–279.

Chudley, A. E., et al. (2005). Fetal alcohol spectrum disorder: Canadian guidelines for diagnosis. *Canadian Medical Association Journal, 172*(Suppl. 5), S1–S21. doi:10.1503/cmaj.1040302

Cooper, E. R., et al. (2002). Combination antiretroviral strategies for the treatment of pregnant HIV-1 infected women and prevention of perinatal HIV-1 transmission. *Journal of AIDS, 29*, 484–494.

Coyle, M. G., Fergusson, A., Lagasse, L., Oh, W., & Lester, B. (2002). Diluted tincture of opium (DTO) and phenobarbital versus DTO alone for neonatal opiate withdrawal in term infants. *Journal of Pediatrics, 140*(5), 561–564.

Crane, J., & Society of Obstetricians and Gynaecologists of Canada, Maternal Fetal Medicine and Infectious Diseases Committees. (2002). Parvovirus B19 infection in pregnancy. *Journal of Obstetrics and Gynaecology Canada, 24*(9), 727–734.

Crocker, E. (2005). Meth's burning issues. *Nurse Week, Heartland Edition, 6*(8), 22–23.

D'Apolito, K., & Hepworth, J. T. (2001). Prominence of withdrawal symptoms in polydrug-exposed infants. *Journal of Perinatal and Neonatal Nursing, 14*(4), 46–60.

Davies, H. D., et al. (2001). Population-based active surveillance for neonatal group B streptococcal infections in Alberta, Canada: Implications for vaccine formulation. *Pediatric Infectious Disease Journal, 20*(9), 879–894.

de Jong, E. P., et al. (2006). Parvovirus B19 infection in pregnancy. *Journal of Clinical Virology, 36*(1), 1–7. doi:10.1016/j.jcv.2006.01.004

Derauf, C., et al. (2007). Demographic and psychosocial characteristics of mothers using methamphetamine during pregnancy: Preliminary results of the Infant Development, Environment and Lifestyle (IDEAL) study. *American Journal of Drug and Alcohol Abuse, 33*(2), 281–289. doi:10.1080/00952990601175029

Diehl-Jones, W., & Askin, D. F. (2004). Nutritional modulation of neonatal outcomes. *AACN Clinical Issues, 15*(1), 83–96.

Ehrlich, P. J., & Coran, A. G. (2007). Diaphragmatic hernia. In R. M. Kliegman, R. E. Behrman, H. B. Jenson, & B. F. Stanton (Eds.), *Nelson textbook of pediatrics* (18th ed., pp. 746–748). Philadelphia: Saunders.

Elder, J. S. (2007). Urologic disorders in infants and children: Anomalies of the bladder. In R. M. Kliegman, R. E. Behrman, H. B. Jenson, & B. F. Stanton (Eds.), *Nelson textbook of pediatrics* (18th ed., pp. 2221–2272). Philadelphia: Saunders.

Embree, J., & Canadian Paediatric Society, Infectious Diseases and Immunization Committee. (2002). Recommendations for the prevention of neonatal ophthalmia. *Paediatrics and Child Health, 7*(7), 480–483.

Eyler, F. D., Behnke, M., Conlon, M., & Woods, N. S. (1998). Birth outcome from a prospective, matched study of prenatal crack/cocaine use: II. Interactive and dose effects on neurobehavioral assessment. *Pediatrics, 101*(2), 237–241.

Faulks, S., & Luther, B. (2005). Changing paradigm for the treatment of clubfeet. *Orthopedic Nursing, 24*(1), 25–30.

Finnegan, L., Pacini, M., & Maremmani, I. (2010). Methadone treatment for pregnant heroin addicted women. *Heroin Addiction and Related Clinical Problems, 12*(2), 29–36.

Fleming, P., & Blair, P. S. (2007). Sudden infant death syndrome and parental smoking. *Early Human Development, 83*(11), 721–725. doi:10.1016/j.earlhumdev.2007.07.011

Frenkel, L. (2005). Challenges in the diagnosis and management of neonatal herpes simplex virus encephalitis. *Pediatrics, 115*(3), 795–797. doi:10.1542/peds.2004-1941

Gray, M., & Moore, K. N. (2009). *Urologic disorders: Adult and pediatric care.* St. Louis: Mosby.

Guerri, C., Bazinet, A., & Riley, E. P. (2009). Fetal alcohol spectrum disorders and alterations in brain and behaviour. *Alcohol and Alcoholism, 44*(2), 108–114. doi:10.1093/alcalc/agn105

Gupta, A., et al. (2004). Outbreak of extended-spectrum beta-lactamase-producing *Klebsiella pneumoniae* in a neonatal intensive care unit linked to artificial nails. *Infection Control and Hospital Epidemiology, 25*(3), 210–215.

Hale, T. W. (2002). *Medications and mothers' milk.* Amarillo, TX: Pharmasoft Medical.

Health Canada. (2000). *Family-centred maternity and newborn care—National guidelines.* Ottawa: Author.

Health Canada. (2002). *Congenital anomalies in Canada—A perinatal health report.* Ottawa: Minister of Public Works and Government Services Canada.

Health Canada. (2012). *First Nations, Inuit and Aboriginal health. Tuberculosis.* Retrieved from http://www.hc-sc.gc.ca/fniah-spnia/diseases-maladies/tuberculos/index-eng.php.

Honein, M. A. (2001). Impact of folic acid fortification of the U.S. food supply and occurrence of neural tube defects. *Journal of the American Medical Association, 285*(23), 2981–2986.

Honein, M. A., et al. (2007). Maternal smoking and environmental tobacco smoke exposure and the risk of orofacial clefts. *Epidemiology, 18*(2), 226–233. doi:10.1097/01.ede.0000254430.61294.c0

Hosalkar, H. S., Horn, B. D., Friedman, J. E., & Dormans, J. P. (2007). The hip. In R. M. Kliegman, R. E. Behrman, H. B. Jenson, & B. F. Stanton (Eds.), *Nelson textbook of pediatrics* (18th ed., pp. 2800–2810). Philadelphia: Saunders.

Huestis, M. A., & Choo, R. E. (2002). Drug abuse's smallest victims: In utero drug exposure. *Forensic Science International, 128*(1–2), 20–30.

Hurd, Y. L., Wang, X., Anderson,V., Beck, O., Minkoff, H., & Dow-Edwards, D. (2005). Marijuana impairs growth in mid-gestation fetuses. *Neurotoxicology and Teratology, 27*(2), 221–229. doi:10.1016/j.ntt.2004.11.002

International Human Genome Sequencing Consortium. (2004). Finishing the euchromatic sequence of the human genome. *Nature, 431*, 931–945.

Jansson, L. M., Velez, M., & Harrow, C. (2004). Methadone maintenance and lactation: A review of the literature and current management guidelines. *Journal of Human Lactation, 20*(1), 62–71.

Johnson, K., Gerada, C., & Greenough, A. (2003). Treatment of neonatal abstinence syndrome. *Archives of Disease in Childhood: Fetal Neonatal Edition, 88*(1), F2–F5.

Jones, H. E., et al. (2005). Buprenorphine versus methadone in the treatment of pregnant opioid-dependent patients: Effects on the neonatal abstinence syndrome. *Drug and Alcohol Dependence, 79*(1), 1–10. doi:10.1016/j.drugalcdep.2004.11.013

Jones, M. W., & Bass, W. T. (2003). Fetal alcohol syndrome. *Neonatal Network, 22*(3), 63–70.

Kakko, J., Heilig, M., & Sarman, I. (2008). Buprenorphine and methadone treatment of opiate dependence during pregnancy: Comparison of fetal growth and neonatal outcomes in two consecutive case series. *Drug and Alcohol Dependence, 96*(1–2), 69–78. doi:10.1016/j.drugalcdep.2008.01.025

Kaye, C. I., & American Association of Pediatrics, Committee on Genetics. (2006). Newborn screening fact sheets. *Pediatrics, 118*(3), e934–e963. doi:10.1542/peds.2006-1783

Koren, G. (2000). Caffeine during pregnancy? In moderation. *Canadian Family Physician, 46*, 801–803.

Koren, G., Hutson, J., & Gareri, J. (2008). Novel methods for the detection of drug and alcohol exposure during pregnancy: Implications for maternal and child health. *Clinical Pharmacology and Therapeutics, 83*, 631–634. doi:10.1038/sj.clpt.6100506

Kozer, E., & Koren, G. (2001). Effects of prenatal exposure to marijuana. *Canadian Family Physician, 47*, 263–264.

Kriebs, J. M. (2002). The global reach of HIV: Preventing mother-to-child transmission. *Journal of Perinatal and Neonatal Nursing, 16*(3), 1–10.

LaGasse, L. L., et al. (2003). Prenatal drug exposure and maternal and infant feeding behaviour. *Archives of Diseases in Childhood, Fetal and Neonatal Edition, 88*(5), F391–F399.

Langley, J., & Canadian Paediatric Society, Infectious Diseases and Immunization Committee. (2005). Prevention of varicella in children and adolescents. *Paediatrics and Child Health, 10*(7), 409–412.

Law, K. L., et al. (2003). Smoking during pregnancy and newborn neurobehavior. *Pediatrics, 111*(6), 1318–1323.

Lawrence, R. A., & Lawrence, R. M. (2011). *Breastfeeding: A guide for the medical profession* (7th ed.). St. Louis: Mosby.

Lester, B. M., & Tronick, E. Z. (2004). History and description of the Neonatal Intensive Care Unit Network Neurobehavioral Scale. *Pediatrics, 113*(3 Pt 2), 634–640.

Lovvan, H. N., III, Glenn, J. B., Pacetti, A. S., & Carter, B. S. (2011). Neonatal surgery. In S. L. Gardner, B. S. Carter, M. Enzman-Hines, & J. A Hernandez.

(Eds.), *Merenstein & Gardner's handbook of neonatal intensive care* (7th ed., pp. 398–433). St. Louis: Mosby.

Malik, S., et al. (2008). Maternal smoking and congenital heart defects. *Pediatrics, 121*(4), e810–e816. doi:10.1542/peds.2007-1519

Many, A., & Koren, G. (2006). *Toxoplasmosis during pregnancy*. Retrieved from http://www.motherisk.org/prof/updatesDetail.jsp?content_id=826.

Messinger, D. S., et al. (2004). The maternal lifestyle study: Cognitive, motor, and behavioral outcomes of cocaine-exposed and opiate-exposed infants through 3 years of age. *Pediatrics, 113*(6), 1677–1685.

Michaels, M. G. (2007). Treatment of congenital cytomegalovirus: Where are we now? *Expert Review of Anti-Infective Therapy, 5*(3), 441–448. doi:10.1586/14787210.5.3.441

Minozzi, S., Amato, L., Vecchi, S., & Davoli, M. (2008). Maintenance agonist treatments for opiate dependent pregnant women. *Cochrane Database of Systematic Reviews, Issue 2*. Art. No. CD006318. doi:10.1002/14651858.CD006318.pub2

Moise, K. J. (2002). Management of rhesus alloimmunization in pregnancy. *Obstetrics and Gynecology, 100*(3), 600–611.

Money, D., Dobson, S., & Society of Obstetricians and Gynaecologists of Canada Infectious Disease Committee. (2004). SOGC clinical practice guideline: The prevention of early-onset neonatal group B streptococcal disease. *Journal of Obstetrics and Gynaecology Canada, 26*(9), 826–832. Retrieved from http://www.sogc.org/guidelines/public/149E-CPG-September2004.pdf.

Money, D., Steben, M., & Society of Obstetricians and Gynaecologists of Canada Infectious Disease Committee. (2008). Guidelines for the management of herpes simplex virus in pregnancy. *Journal of Obstetrics and Gynaecology Canada, 30*(6), 514–519. Retrieved from http://www.sogc.org/guidelines/documents/gui208CPg0806.pdf.

Moolenaar, R. L., et al. (2000). A prolonged outbreak of *Pseudomonas aeruginosa* in a neonatal intensive care unit: Did staff fingernails play a role in disease transmission? *Infection Control and Hospital Epidemiology, 21*(2), 80–85.

Moretti, M. E., Lee, A., & Ito, S. (2000). Which drugs are contraindicated during breastfeeding? Practice guidelines. *Canadian Family Physician, 46*, 1754–1757.

Morrow, C. E., et al. (2006). Learning disabilities and intellectual functioning in school-aged children with prenatal cocaine exposure. *Developmental Neuropsychology, 30*(3), 905–931. doi:10.1207/s15326942dn3003_8

Myers, M. G., Seward, J. F., & LaRussa, P. S. (2007). Varicella-zoster virus. In R. M. Kliegman, R. E. Behrman, H. B. Jenson, & B. F. Stanton (Eds.), *Nelson textbook of pediatrics* (18th ed., pp. 1366–1371). Philadelphia: Saunders.

Neal, J. L. (2001). RhD isoimmunization and current management modalities. *Journal of Obstetrics, Gynecology and Neonatal Nursing, 30*(6), 589–607.

Nesheim, S. R., et al. (2007). Trends in opportunistic infections in the pre- and post-highly active antiretroviral therapy eras among HIV-infected children in the Perinatal AIDS Collaborative Transmission Study, 1986–2004. *Pediatrics, 120*(1), 100–109. doi:10.1542/peds.2006-2052

Newborn Screening Ontario. (n.d.). *Information for health care providers*. Retrieved from http://www.newbornscreening.on.ca/bins/content_page.asp?cid=7-272.

Ogundele, M. O., & Coulter, J. B. (2003). HIV transmission through breastfeeding: Problems and prevention. *Annals of Tropical Paediatrics, 23*(2), 91–106.

Ontario Newborn Screening Program. (2006). *Congenital hypothyroidism (CH)*. Ottawa: Author. Retrieved from http://www.health.gov.on.ca/english/providers/program/child/screening/pdf/fs_ch.pdf.

Ostrea, E. (2001). Understanding drug testing in the neonate and the role of meconium analysis. *Journal of Perinatal and Neonatal Nursing, 14*(4), 61–82.

Perinatal Services BC. (2010). *Neonatal guideline 9: Newborn screening*. Retrieved from http://www.perinatalservicesbc.ca/NR/rdonlyres/5DF1127B-9015-4714-9B31-01E52BC3747D/0/NBGuidelinesScreening9.pdf.

Philipp, B. L., Merewood, A., & O'Brien, S. (2003). Commentary: Methadone and breastfeeding: new horizons. *Pediatrics, 111*(6 Pt 1), 1429–1430.

Popovich, D. M., & McAlhany, A. (2004). Practitioner care and screening guidelines for infants born to Chlamydia-positive mothers. *Newborn Infant Nursing Review, 4*(1), 51–55.

Public Health Agency of Canada. (2006). *Canadian immunization guide* (7th ed.). Ottawa: Author. Retrieved from http://www.phac-aspc.gc.ca/publicat/cig-gci/index-eng.php.

Public Health Agency of Canada. (2008a). *Caffeine in pregnancy*. Ottawa: Author. Retrieved from http://www.phac-aspc.gc.ca/hp-gs/know-savoir/caffeine-eng.php.

Public Health Agency of Canada. (2008b). *Canadian guidelines on sexually transmitted infections*. Ottawa: Author. Retrieved from http://www.phac-aspc.gc.ca/std-mts/sti-its/guide-lignesdir-eng.php.

Public Health Agency of Canada. (2008c). *Canadian perinatal health report—2008 edition*. Ottawa: Author. Retrieved from http://www.phac-aspc.gc.ca/publicat/2008/cphr-rspc/index-eng.php.

Public Health Agency of Canada. (2008d). *Fetal alcohol spectrum disorder (FASD) prevention: Canadian perspectives: Multiple approaches to FASD prevention*. Ottawa: Author. Retrieved from: http://www.phac-aspc.gc.ca/hp-ps/dca-dea/prog-ini/fasd-etcaf/publications/cp-pc/index-eng.php.

Public Health Agency of Canada. (2009). *Brief report on sexually transmitted infections in Canada: 2007* (Cat. No. HP37-10/2007E-PDF). Ottawa: Author. Retrieved from http://www.phac-aspc.gc.ca/publicat/2009/sti-its/pdf/sti_brief-its_bref_2009-eng.pdf.

Public Health Agency of Canada. (2010a). *Essential resources for effective infection prevention and control programs: A matter of patient safety—A discussion paper*. Ottawa: Author. Retrieved from http://www.phac-aspc.gc.ca/nois-sinp/guide/ps-sp/partII-eng.php#b61.

Public Health Agency of Canada. (2010b). *HIV and AIDS in Canada. Surveillance report to December 31, 2009*. Ottawa: Author.

Public Health Agency of Canada. (2012). *Perinatal health indicators for Canada, 2011*. Ottawa: Author.

Rao, R., & Desai, N. S. (2002). OxyContin and neonatal abstinence syndrome. *Journal of Perinatology, 22*(4), 324–325.

Reed, M. D., Aranda, J. V., & Hales, B. F. (2006). Developmental pharmacology. In R. J. Martin, A. A. Fanaroff, & M. C. Walsh (Eds.), *Fanaroff and Martin's neonatal-perinatal medicine: Diseases of the fetus and infant* (8th ed.). St. Louis: Mosby.

Reiser, D. J. (2004). Neonatal jaundice: Physiologic variation or pathologic process. *Critical Care Nursing Clinics of North America, 16*, 257–269.

Robinson, J. L., & Canadian Paediatric Society, Infectious Diseases and Immunization Committee. (2007). Prevention of congenital rubella syndrome. *Paediatrics and Child Health, 12*(9), 795–797.

Robinson, J. L., & Canadian Paediatric Society, Infectious Diseases and Immunization Committee. (2009). Congenital syphilis: No longer just of historical interest. *Paediatrics and Child Health, 14*(5), 337.

Sander, S. C., & Hays, L. R. (2005). Prescription opioid dependence and treatment with methadone in pregnancy. *Journal of Opioid Management, 1*(2), 91–97.

Sauerbrei, A., & Wutzler, P. (2007). Herpes simplex and varicella-zoster virus infections during pregnancy: Current concepts of prevention, diagnosis and therapy. Part 2: Varicella-zoster virus. *Medical Microbiology and Immunology, 196*(2), 95–102. doi:10.1007/s00430-006-0032-z

Sawnani, H., Olsen, E., & Simakajornboon, N. (2010). The effect of in utero cigarette smoke exposure on development of respiratory control: A review. *Pediatric Allergy, Immunology, and Pulmonology, 23*(3), 161–167. doi:10.1089/ped.2010.0036

Schleiss, M. R. (2008). Congenital cytomegalovirus infection: Update on management strategies. *Current Treatment Options in Neurology, 10*(3), 186–192. doi:10.1007/s11940-008-0020-2

Schröter, H., & Canadian Paediatric Society, First Nations, Inuit and Métis Health Committee. (2010). *Fetal alcohol spectrum disorder: Diagnostic update*. Retrieved from http://www.cps.ca/english/statements/II/ii02-01.htm#ADDENDUM.

Segel, G. B. (2007). Hereditary spherocytosis. In R. M. Kliegman, R. E. Behrman, H. B. Jenson, & B. F. Stanton (Eds.), *Nelson textbook of pediatrics* (18th ed., pp. 2020–2023). Philadelphia: Saunders.

Singer, L. T., et al. (2002). Cognitive and motor outcomes of cocaine-exposed infants. *Journal of the American Medical Association, 287*(15), 1952–1960.

Singer, L. T., et al. (2004). Cognitive outcomes of preschool children with prenatal cocaine exposure. *Journal of the American Medical Association, 291*(20), 2448–2456.

Smith, L., et al. (2003). Effects of prenatal methamphetamine exposure on fetal growth and drug withdrawal symptoms in infants born at term. *Journal of Development and Behavior in Pediatrics, 24*(1), 17–23.

Smith, L. M., et al. (2006). The infant development, environment, and lifestyle study: Effects of prenatal methamphetamine exposure, polydrug exposure, and poverty on intrauterine growth. *Pediatrics, 118*(3), 1149–1156. doi:10.1542/peds.2005-2564

Society of Obstetricians and Gynecologists of Canada. (2008). SOGC clinical practice guideline: Immunization in pregnancy. *Journal of Obstetrics and Gynaecology Canada, 30*(12), 1149–1154. Retrieved from http://www.sogc.org/guidelines/documents/gui220CPG0812.pdf.

Society of Obstetricians and Gynecologists of Canada. (2010). SOGC clinical practice guideline: Alcohol use and pregnancy consensus clinical guidelines. *Journal of Obstetrics and Gynaecology Canada, 32*(8) (Suppl. 3), S1–S33. Retrieved from http://www.sogc.org/guidelines/documents/gui245CPG1008E.pdf.

Sood, B., et al. (2001). Prenatal alcohol exposure and childhood behavior at age 6 to 7 years: I. Dose-response effect. *Pediatrics, 108*(2), e34.

Stokowski, I. A. (2008). *Noteworthy professional news: Drug to treat phenylketonuria approved.* Advances in Neonatal Care, *8*(3), 139–140. doi:10.1097/01.ANC.0000324334.56228.14

Stoler, J. M., & Holmes, L. B. (2004). Recognition of facial features of fetal alcohol syndrome in the newborn. *American Journal of Medical Genetics: Part C: Seminars in Medical Genetics, 127*(1), 21–27.

Stoll, B. J. (2007). Infections in the neonatal infant. In R. M. Kliegman, R. E. Behrman, H. B. Jenson, & B. F. Stanton (Eds.), *Nelson textbook of pediatrics* (18th ed., pp. 794–812). Philadelphia: Saunders.

Stoll, B. J., et al. (2005). Very low birth weight preterm infants with early onset neonatal sepsis: The predominance of gram-negative infections continues in the National Institute of Child Health and Human Development Neonatal Research Network, 2002–2003. *Pediatric Infectious Diseases Journal, 24*(7), 635–639. doi:10.1097/01.inf.0000168749.82105.64

Swayze, V. W., et al. (1997). Magnetic resonance imaging of brain anomalies in fetal alcohol syndrome. *Pediatrics, 99*(2), 232–240.

Tronick, E. Z. (Ed.). (2007). *The neurobehavioral and social-emotional development of infants and children.* New York: W.W. Norton.

United Nations Office on Drugs and Crime. (2011). *World drug report: 2011.* Vienna: United Nations. Retrieved from http://www.unodc.org/documents/data-and-analysis/WDR2011/World_Drug_Report_2011_ebook.pdf.

Venkatesh, M., Adams, K. M., & Weisman, L. E. (2011). Infection in the neonate. In S. L. Gardner, B. S. Carter, M. Enzman-Hines, & J. A Hernandez (Eds.), *Merenstein & Gardner's handbook of neonatal intensive care* (7th ed., pp. 553–580). St. Louis: Mosby.

Volpe, J. J. (2008). *Neurology of the newborn* (5th ed.). Philadelphia: Saunders.

Weiner, S. M., & Finnegan, L. P. (2011). Drug withdrawal in the neonate. In S. L. Gardner, B. S. Carter, M. Enzman-Hines, & J. A Hernandez (Eds.), *Merenstein & Gardner's handbook of neonatal intensive care* (7th ed., pp. 201–222). St. Louis: Mosby.

World Health Organization. (2010). *Principles and recommendations for infant feeding in the context of HIV and a summary of evidence.* Geneva, Switzerland: Author. Retrieved from http://whqlibdoc.who.int/publications/2010/9789241599535_eng.pdf.

Yinon, Y., Farine, D., & Yudin, M. H. (2010). SOGC clinical practice guideline: Cytomegalovirus infection in pregnancy. *Journal of Obstetrics and Gynaecology Canada, 32*(4), 348–354. Retrieved from http://www.sogc.org/guidelines/documents/gui240CPG1004E.pdf.

Yogev, R., & Chadwick, E. G. (2007). Acquired immunodeficiency syndrome (human immmunodeficiency virus). In R. M. Kliegman, R. E. Behrman, H. B. Jenson, & B. F. Stanton (Eds.), *Nelson textbook of pediatrics* (18th ed., pp. 1427–1442). Philadelphia: Saunders.

Yudin, M. H., & Gonik, B. (2006). Perinatal infections. In R. J. Martin, A. A. Fanaroff, & M. C. Walsh (Eds.), *Fanaroff and Martin's neonatal-perinatal medicine: Diseases of the fetus and infant* (8th ed.). Philadelphia: Mosby.

Part 2

Pediatric Nursing

Unit 7 Children, Their Families, and the Nurse

Unit 8 Assessment of the Child and Family

Unit 9 Health Promotion and Special Health Problems

Unit 10 Special Needs, Illness, and Hospitalization

Unit 11 Health Problems of Children

Unit 7

29 Contemporary Pediatric Nursing in Canada

Learning Objectives

On completion of this chapter, the reader will be able to:

- Define the terms *mortality* and *morbidity*.
- Identify two ways in which knowledge of mortality and morbidity can improve child health.
- List three major causes of death during infancy, early childhood, later childhood, and adolescence.
- List two major causes of illness during childhood.
- Describe five broad functions of the pediatric nurse in promoting the health of children.
- Define the term *critical thinking*.
- Identify the five steps of the nursing process.
- Define the term *nursing diagnosis*.
- Define *evidence-informed practice*.

Electronic Resources

Additional information related to the content in Chapter 29 can be found on

evolve the companion Web site at

http://evolve.elsevier.com/Canada/Perry/maternal/

- Examination Review Questions

Health Care for Children

The pediatric nurse has a very important role in helping children and their families achieve optimum health. The major goal of pediatric nursing is to improve the quality of health care for children. When providing nursing care to children, it is essential that the pediatric nurse do so in the context of the family. To provide effective care, the pediatric nurse must develop a trusting and collaborative relationship with the child and family. Respect for social and cultural differences and beliefs is the cornerstone of high-quality pediatric care.

There were approximately 5,607,345 children under age 14 living in Canada in 2011 (Statistics Canada, 2012). The health of Canadian children has steadily improved over time. Many factors, discussed in this and subsequent chapters, have played a role in this improvement and explain why more Canadian children are healthier.

Children's health is influenced by a multitude of agents, technology being a leading force. In today's world, there are myriad technological advances that have helped to improve the health of children and their families. For example, researchers have significantly decreased mortality rates of childhood cancer and have significantly increased rates of infant heart transplants. At the same time, this new technological world has also created many challenges that can have a negative impact on the health of children and their families. Global warming from increased industrialization has thinned the ozone layer, leading to a significant increase in the rate of skin cancer. Another example is increasing sedentary activity levels related to greater use of electronic devices (e.g., watching television, playing computer games); this lifestyle has contributed to the higher rates of obesity and type 2 diabetes among children.

Another factor that affects children's health is family income level. The Canadian government has identified income level and socioeconomic status as having the greatest impact on health, with poverty having a detrimental effect on children's health. Poverty levels are highest in the First Nations, Métis, and Inuit, new immigrant, and child services' populations of Canada.

In Canada, the Medicare system provides health care for all of its legal residents (see Chapter 1). The government is gradually shifting the emphasis in health care from treatment of illnesses to health promotion and prevention. In order to promote good health, the many, complex influences on health need to be investigated and understood. To this end, the federal government has outlined the *determinants of health* (see Box 1-3 and Table 29-1). These determinants provide a blueprint for health care policies and help direct population health research with the goal of improving health for its citizens (Public Health Agency of Canada [PHAC], 2010). Understanding of these health determinants is continuing to evolve as researchers discover more evidence to add to the Canadian health database. Please refer to Table 29-1 for further details.

In this second part of the textbook, we focus on the complex factors that influence health in the Canadian pediatric

Table 29-1 Determinants of Health

HEALTH DETERMINANTS	DESCRIPTION
1. Income and social status	Greatest influence on health status and behaviours and use of health care services. Lower-income Canadians have poorer health, with more chronic illness and earlier death, than that of higher-income Canadians, regardless of age, gender, culture, race, or residence. Only 46% of Canadians with the least income rate their health as very good or excellent, compared with 73% for those in the highest income group (PHAC, 2010). Higher social status, with its associated health behaviours and access to health care, may protect individuals from cardiovascular disease.
2. Social support networks	Social contacts and support networks are linked with better health by providing emotional support, care giving, and improved management of adversity.
3. Education and literacy	Higher education improves a person's state of health. Education increases opportunities for earning higher incomes, improves problem-solving capacity, and access to health information.
4. Employment/working conditions	Unemployment or employment that is stressful or unsafe is linked to poorer health. Income, social contacts, and emotional health are all affected by the workplace.
5. Social environments	The community, region, province, and country provide resource sharing and social networks that create safety nets and improve overall health for community members.
6. Physical environments	Environmental contaminants in the air, soil, water, and food can cause poor health, such as respiratory conditions or other serious illnesses. Environments in the built community can affect health in many ways, such as through poor air quality and unsafe building codes.
7. Personal health practices and coping skills	There are measures that individuals can carry out themselves to promote their own health and manage challenges. Self-sufficiency and making healthy choices will optimize their level of health.
8. Healthy child development	What happens to a child during the growing years will have an impact on the child's long-term health and may lead to the development of chronic illness—e.g., low-birth-weight infants have almost twice the incidence of lifelong diseases.
9. Biology and genetic endowment	Genetics play an important role in individuals' health status. Genetic predisposition to certain conditions, as well as environmental interrelationships, puts certain individuals at risk for specific diseases.
10. Health services	Availability of health services has a direct impact on individuals', families', groups', and communities' ability to prevent disease and adequately treat secondary conditions. There are still inequities in accessibility to these essential services—e.g., urban populations with increased access to health services have better morbidity and mortality rates than those of rural populations with less access to health care.
11. Gender	*Gender* refers to differences in biologics, roles in society, personalities, attitudes, values, and socioeconomic position. These differences have a direct bearing on health. There are also gender-specific predispositions toward certain disease states and treatments programs.
12. Culture	Health risks related to cultural and ethnic backgrounds can affect an individual and the family. A person's culture may influence his or her health choices. For example, access to health care may be difficult for new immigrants who do not know the language or how to enter and manoeuvre the health care system. It is essential that culturally appropriate care be available to everyone.

(Adapted from Public Health Agency of Canada [2010]. *What makes Canadians healthy or unhealthy?* Retrieved from http://www.phac-aspc.gc.ca/ph-sp/determinants/index-eng.php.)

population, from the infant to the adolescent. The chapters in Part 2 provide foundational knowledge on how the determinants of health affect each age group. Topics addressed include children, their families, and the nurse; assessment of the family and the child; health promotion and special health problems; special needs, illness, and hospitalization; and health problems of children. All of these topics are discussed in the context of pediatric nursing.

Health Promotion

Many of the leading causes of death, disease, and disability—including cardiovascular disease, cancer, chronic lung diseases, depression, **violence**, **substance use**, injuries, nutritional deficiencies, and human **immunodeficiency** virus/acquired immunodeficiency syndrome (HIV/AIDS)—can be significantly reduced in children and adolescents through the prevention of six categories of behaviour (World Health Organization, 2007):

1. Tobacco use
2. Behaviour that results in injury and violence
3. Alcohol and substance use
4. Dietary and hygienic practices that cause disease
5. Sedentary lifestyle
6. Sexual behaviour that causes unintended pregnancy and disease

Child health promotion opens up opportunities to reduce differences in health status among members of various groups and helps ensure that all children have equal opportunities and resources to achieve their fullest health potential.

Nutrition

Nutrition is an essential component for healthy growth and **development**, and its promotion begins at birth. Human milk is the preferred form of nutrition for all infants up to 6 months of age; at that time other foods can be introduced, although breastfeeding can continue for 2 years or longer. Breastfeeding provides the infant with micronutrients, immunological properties, and several enzymes that enhance digestion and absorption of these **nutrients** (see Chapter 26). Many working mothers tend to wean their infants early to avoid breast pumping during the workday. However, there has been a resurgence in breastfeeding due to the education of mothers and fathers regarding its benefits.

Young children tend to establish eating habits during the first 2 to 3 years of life. The nurse can be instrumental in guiding parents in the selection of nutritious foods. During childhood, the eating preferences and attitudes related to food habits are established by family influences and **culture**. During **adolescence**, parental influence diminishes as the adolescent makes food choices related to peer acceptability and sociability; these choices may be detrimental to the health of the chronically ill child with diabetes, hypertension, or heart or renal disease.

Unhealthy diets are common among lower income families, often because of the lack of nutritious fresh fruits and vegetables and adequate milk and protein intake. In addition, the lifestyles of homeless and migrant children place these populations at risk for inadequate food, causing nutrient deficiencies, developmental and growth delays, depression, hunger, and behavioural problems.

Dental Care

Dental **caries** is the single most common chronic disease of childhood (Heuer, 2007). The most common form of early dental disease is early childhood caries, which may begin at the first birthday and progress to **pain** and **infection** within the first 2 years of life (Edelstein, 2005). Preschoolers of low-income families are twice as likely to develop tooth decay and only half as likely to visit the dentist as other children (Edelstein, 2005). Since this is a preventable disease, nursing plays an essential role in the promotion of early tooth care. Nurses can instruct children and their parents in dental hygiene, prior to the first tooth eruption; encourage them to drink fluoridated water, including bottled water; and promote early dental preventive care.

Dental care is not covered under the Canadian Medicare program. Individual provinces and territories have variable plans to cover dental care for families with low incomes. The Aboriginal peoples have government coverage for dental care (PHAC, 2009).

Immunizations

The two public health interventions that have had the greatest impact on world health are clean drinking water and vaccines. The Canadian Institutes of Health Research (2003) has identified vaccination as one of the most important public health interventions provided to Canadians. A child's immunization record should be reviewed at each clinic visit, and parents should be instructed to keep immunizations current. Children's vaccines are generally paid for by the Canadian provincial and territorial governments (PHAC, 2008c).

Childhood Health Problems

The health of Canada's children continues to improve in many areas, such as lower pregnancy rates for adolescents and expanded vaccine coverage. However, changes in modern society, including disruptive influences on the family, and the greater use of technology, such as watching video games for long periods of time, are contributing to significant medical problems that affect the health of children (Lichter, 2005). Recent concern has focused on specific groups of children who have increased **morbidity**: homeless and immigrant children; children living in poverty; First Nations, Métis, and Inuit peoples; children in child services; low-birth-weight (LBW) children; children with **chronic illnesses**; immigrant adopted children; and children in day care centres. A number of factors identified in the determinants of health (PHAC, 2010), such as lower income and socioeconomic status, lack of social support networks, lack of education, environmental contaminants, and decreased access to health care (see Table 29-1), place these groups at risk for poor health. Also, while infants of very low birth weight (VLBW) have improved survival over that of previous decades, these children are twice as prone to having chronic lifelong health problems (PHAC, 2010).

In addition to disease and injury, children face behavioural, social (family), and educational problems that are referred to as the *new morbidity* or *pediatric social illness*. These problems (e.g., poverty, violence, aggression, noncompliance, school failure, and adjustment to divorce or bereavement) interfere with children's social and academic development. Mental health issues also affect the well-being of children and adolescents. Examples of increasing pediatric problems include obesity, type 2 diabetes, injuries, violence, substance use, and emotional and mental health problems during adolescence.

Obesity and Type 2 Diabetes

Childhood obesity is the most common nutritional problem among Canadian children and is increasing at epidemic proportions, as is type 2 diabetes. The childhood obesity rate in Canada has tripled since 1975 (Ontario Ministry of Health Promotion and Sport, 2010). *Obesity* in children and adolescents is defined as a body mass index (BMI) at or greater than the 95th percentile for youth of the same age and gender (Dietz, 2005).

Advancements in entertainment and technology, such as television, computers, and video games, have made these devices more appealing, resulting in greater time spent at sedentary activity. This pattern has contributed to the growing childhood obesity problem in Canada. Canadian children watch television, talk online, or play virtual games for about 6 hours every weekday and 7 hours on the weekend (Ontario Ministry of Health Promotion and Sport, 2010).

Lack of outside physical activity because of unsafe environments and inconvenient facilities for physical activities, combined with easy access to video games and television within the home, tends to result in obesity among low-income children. The levels of obesity vary across the different **ethnic** groups. Research has shown that the First Nations, Métis, and Inuit population has the highest level of obesity among all ethnic backgrounds in Canada for the child and adult age groups (Katzmarzyk, 2008). Obesity is an important focus for Health Canada and its Healthy Canadians program (Fig. 29-1). Nurses play an important role in prevention of obesity; teaching health promotion strategies can assist in the number of overweight children. For more information on childhood obesity in Canada, visit http://www.healthycanadians.gc.ca/init/kids-enfants/obesit/index-eng.php..

Childhood Injuries

Injuries are the most common cause of death and disability among children in Canada. Unintentional injuries are the leading cause of death for Canadian children ages 1 to 14. Injury accounts for more deaths than all of the other causes combined. The major causes of injury-related deaths in children aged 0 to 14 years are mostly preventable. See Table 29-2 for the rates and causes of injuries and hospitalizations among Canadian children. The rates of childhood injuries have decreased from approximately 0.8 per 10,000 in 1994 to 0.5 per 10,000 in 2003, but they are still high. First Nations, Métis, and Inuit people have a 26% injury mortality rate for all age groups compared to 6% for the rest of the country (Health Canada, 2008). Canada and the United States still do not have a national injury prevention strategy for children and youth, which could help reduce childhood injuries (Health Canada, 2009).

The type of injury and the circumstances surrounding it are closely related to normal growth and developmental behaviour. As children develop, their innate curiosity impels them to investigate activities and to mimic the behaviour of others. While it is essential to acquire competency in this trait as an adult, it predisposes children to numerous hazards.

The pattern of deaths caused by unintentional injuries, especially from motor vehicles, drowning, and burns, is remarkably consistent in most Western societies. Fortunately, prevention strategies such as the use of car restraints, bicycle helmets, and smoke detectors have resulted in a significant decrease in fatalities among children. The Government of Canada has enacted new safety regulations for motor vehicles and booster seat safety that require manufacturers to modify car seats and booster seats to improve the safety level by December 31, 2011. The Ministry of Transport reported that the improved use and design of child restraints reduced the child passenger mortality rates by 50% between 1993 and 2006 (Safe Kids Canada, 2010) (Fig. 29-2). Safe Kids Canada has information on the Ministry regulations and motor vehicle safety tips, at http://www.safekidscanada.ca/Professionals/Safety-Information/Child-Passenger-Safety/Index.aspx.

Pedestrian injuries in children account for significant numbers of motor vehicle–related deaths. Most pedestrian injuries occur at midblock, at intersections, in driveways, and in parking lots. Driveway injuries typically involve small children, and large vehicles backing up. Parents may not be alert to the dangers leading to such injuries and consequently fail to protect their children.

Bicycle injuries are another significant cause of childhood deaths. Children ages 5 to 9 years are at greatest risk of bicycling fatalities. Most bicycling deaths are from head injuries. Helmet use reduces the risk of head injury by 85%

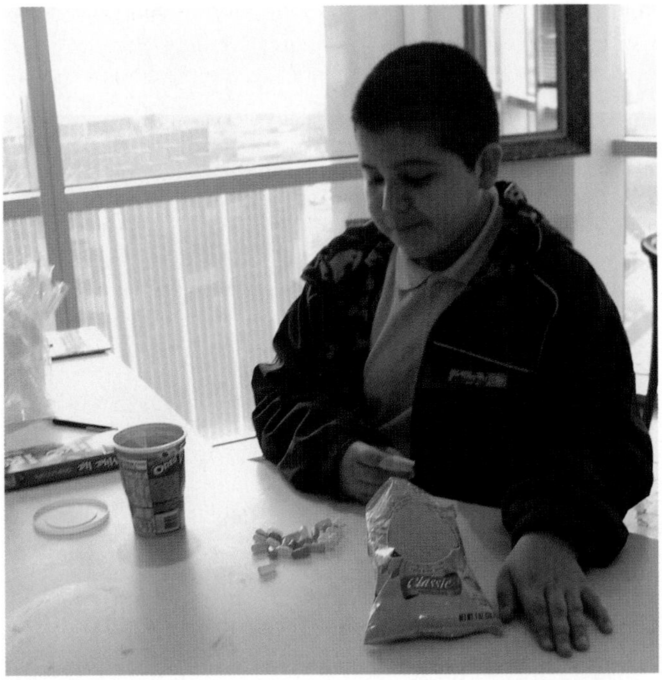

Fig. 29-1 The Canadian cultural tendency toward excessive intake of high-caloric, fatty foods contributes to obesity in children.

Table 29-2 Major Causes of Unintentional Injury Deaths and Hospitalization Among Canadian Children Ages 0–14 Years, 2000–2005

Major causes of unintentional injury deaths among Canadian children aged 0–14 years, 2000-2005	Drowning 15% Motor vehicle accident (passenger) 14% Suffocation 13% Pedestrian 12% Fire/burns 8% Cyclist 4% Fall 3% Struck by/against 2% Poisoning 1% Firearms 1% Other causes 26%
Major causes of unintentional injury hospitalizations among Canadian children aged 0-14, 2000-2005	Falls 37% Playground 8% Struck by/against 9% Cycling 9% Poisoning 6% Motor vehicle accident (passenger) 3% Fire/burns 3% Pedestrian 2% Cut or pierce 2% Suffocation 1% Drowning 1% Other causes 21%

(Adapted from Safe Kids Canada. [2010]. *About injuries*. Retrieved from http://www.safekidscanada.ca/Professionals/Safety-Information/About-Injuries/Index.aspx.)

(Thompson, Rivara, & Thompson, 2009). Community-wide bicycle helmet use campaigns and mandatory-use laws have resulted in significant increases in helmet use. Still, issues such as stylishness, comfort, and social acceptability remain important factors in whether children will actually wear a helmet. Children ages 10 to 14 are those most likely not to wear helmets (Safe Kids Canada, 2010).

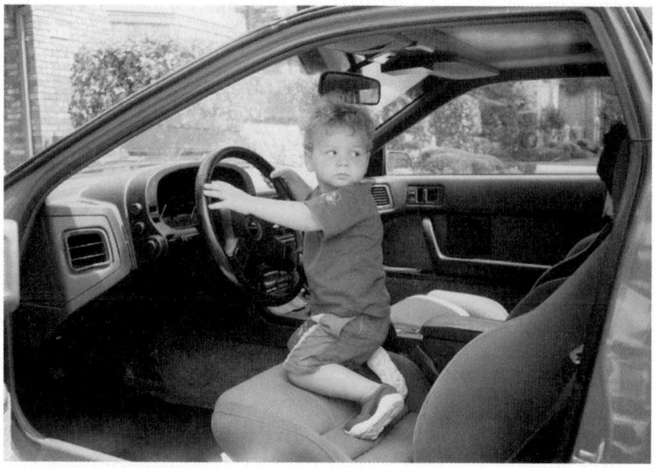

Fig. 29-2 Motor vehicle injuries are the leading cause of death in children older than 1 year of age. Despite mandatory-seatbelt legislation, some children still remain unrestrained and are at higher risk of injuries.

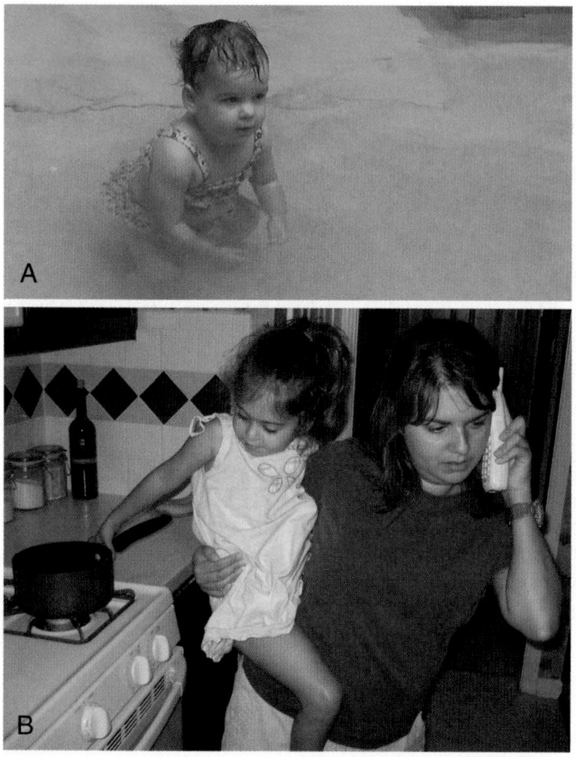

Fig. 29-3 **A:** Drowning is one of the leading causes of death among children. Children left unattended are unsafe even in shallow water. **B:** Burns are among the top three leading cause of death from injury in children ages 1 to 14 years.

Nurses can educate children and their families about pedestrian and bicycle safety. In particular, school nurses can promote helmet wearing and encourage peer leaders to act as role models. When parents wear helmets, their children are more likely to wear them (Safe Kids Canada, 2010).

Drowning, suffocation, and burns are also leading causes of death throughout childhood (Fig. 29-3). During infancy, more males succumb to death from aspiration or suffocation than do females (Fig. 29-4). The leading cause of unintentional poisoning in children under 5 years of age is medication **ingestion,** although household cleaners and personal care products are also ingested (Health Canada, 2010) (Fig. 29-5). The Canadian Association of Poison Control Centres reports that their centres receive thousands of calls regarding unintentional poisonings every year. Contact information for individual provincial and territorial poison control centres can be found at the Association's Web site: http://www.capcc.ca/provcentres/centres.html.

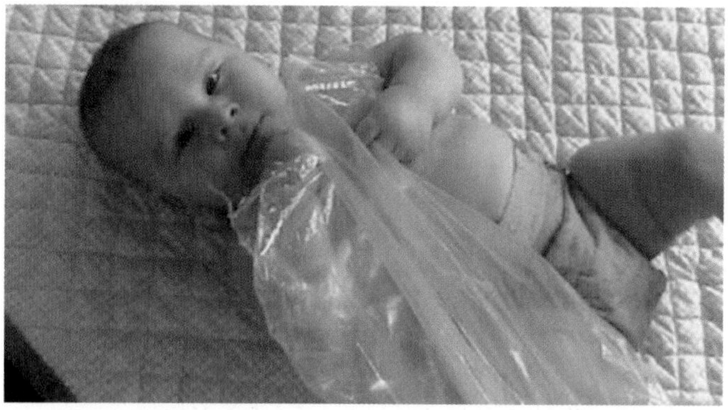

Fig. 29-4 Suffocation is the leading cause of death from injury in infants.

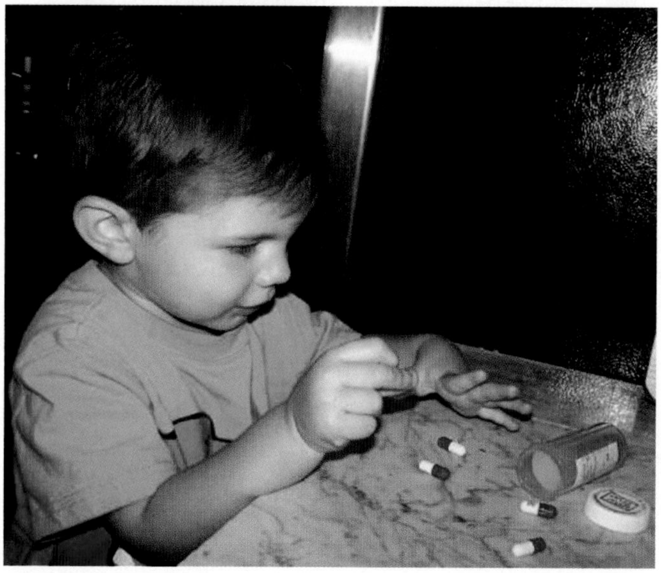

Fig. 29-5 Poisoning causes a considerable number of injuries in children under 4 years of age. Prescription medications should never be left where young children can reach them.

Violence

Children are one of the more vulnerable populations in the context of violence. Violence against children most commonly occurs within the family. In 2008, there were 236,842 child maltreatment and neglect investigations carried out by children's services in Canada. From 1998 to 2003, there was an increase of 100,000 investigations; this rate then levelled off, without a further increase between 2003 and 2008. The major reasons for these investigations were neglect (34%) and exposure to domestic violence (34%) (PHAC, 2008a). First Nations, Métis, and Inuit children continue to be overrepresented in Canadian child welfare organizations, as found in a comparison study of Aboriginal and non-Aboriginal children investigated for child maltreatment in 2003 (MacLaurin et al., 2011). More information on family violence and child maltreatment in Canada is available from the Canadian Family Violence Initiative under the Department of Justice (http://canada.justice.gc.ca/eng/pi/fv-vf/facts-info/child-enf.html#widespread). A national Kids' Help Line (1-800-668-6868) gives children a way to seek help when experiencing violence.

In Canada, child homicides rates are on the decline. In 2007, 56 homicides were committed against children and youth under 18 years of age. The largest number, 41%, were committed by family members (86% by a parent); 27% were committed by nonfamily members; and 27% were committed by strangers. In 2005 and 2007, the family rate was below the nonfamily rate, to just over 3 homicides per million children—the lowest rate in over 30 years. Of the children killed by a parent between 1978 and 2007, 54% were killed by the father. During this time period, 30% of the child homicides were infants under 1 year of age who were killed by their mother (51%) or their father (47%). Infant boys were at a higher risk of death, at 35 per million for boys and 27 per million for girls. The next largest child homicide age group is children 1 to 3 years of age. The methods used in child homicides were different or individual age groups. Usually, physical force (e.g., strangulation, beating, or shaken baby syndrome) was used against children under 6 years of age. Homicide victims in the older age group of 7 to 17 years of age were most frequently killed by a weapon (e.g., knife or firearm) (Statistics Canada, 2009a).

Violence permeates North American households through the violent images portrayed in television programs, commercials, video games, and movies, which tend to desensitize children toward violence. The average Canadian child sees 12,000 violent acts on television annually, including many scenes of murder and rape (Canadian Paediatric Society [CPS], 2011). Canada was one of the first countries to research this issue; Canadian researchers identified that children's exposure to media violence early in the school year predicted higher verbally aggressive behaviour, higher relationally aggressive behaviour, higher physically aggressive behaviour, and less prosocial behaviour later in the school year (Gentile, Coyne, & Walsh, 2011). Debate is still ongoing over the degree to which violence in the media translates into aggressive behaviour in the child viewer. Violence also permeates the schools, with the availability of guns and illicit drugs and the presence of gangs (Fisher & Kettl, 2003).

The number of Canadian children as offenders (ages 12 to 17) has declined by 23% since 2002/2003. Youth courts in Canada processed 58,379 cases in 2008/2009. This decrease has taken place since the enactment of the *Youth Criminal Justice Act*, which diverts minor crimes away from the criminal court system and usually involves community service for the young offender found guilty (Statistics Canada, 2010). Despite this decrease in the youth crime rate, however, assessment of high-risk behaviours in youth must continue to be a major focus of health promotion.

The causes of violence against children and self-inflicted violence are not fully understood. In all cases, the problem of child homicide is extremely complex and involves numerous social, economic, and other influences. Prevention lies in better understanding of the social and psychological factors that lead to the high rates of homicide and suicide. Nurses need to be especially aware of young people who are depressed, are repeatedly in trouble with the criminal justice system, or are associated with groups known to be violent. Prevention requires identification of these young people and therapeutic intervention by qualified professionals.

Pediatric nurses can assess children and adolescents for risk related to violence. For instance, families that own firearms must be educated about their safe use and storage. A home with a gun is five times more likely to be a scene of a suicide than a home without a gun and increases the risk of homicide (Canadian Safety Council, 2009). The suicide risk is higher in the First Nations, Métis, and Inuit communities, where there are more firearms in homes (Health Canada, 2006). In Canada, suicide prevention experts have emphasized the importance of stronger gun laws, which have successfully reduced suicide rates overall, particularly those for youth (Gagné, 2008). Canadian gun law efforts have focused on preventing specific groups, such as felons and children, from having access to firearms (Canadian Safety Council, 2009). Technological changes such as childproof safety devices, safer storage, and loading indicators could improve the safety of firearms.

Substance Use

Risk-taking behaviours, particularly among males, tend to begin in the first decade of life and continue into adolescence with drinking alcohol while driving, speeding, carrying a weapon, or using illicit drugs. In children and young adults, alcohol and illicit drug use occurs most commonly between ages 12 and 24 and is associated with violence and injury (Canadian Centre on Substance Abuse, 2007).

Substance use is a major health care problem in Canada. Early substance use and hazardous drug ingestion during adolescence can lead to the development of serious long-term problems in adulthood, such as **addiction**. Evolving research in this age group suggests that some adolescents use substances to help cope with toxic environments, untreated trauma, and underlying psychological conditions. Alcohol, tobacco, and cannabis are most commonly used. Hallucinogenic drugs such as psilocybin and mescaline are next in line, with 10% of middle and high school students reporting use. Among Western nations, Canada has the highest rates of alcohol and cannabis use in the 12- to 24-year-old age groups (United Nations Office on Drugs and Crime, 2011). Alcohol is the most commonly used substance and is a major factor in causing injury and death, such as in motor vehicle accidents. In Canada, recent surveys indicate that over one third of students in grades 7 to 9 students had binged on alcohol. Over 40% of 15- to 19-year-olds had binged on alcohol at least once in the past year and had binged 12 or more times in the past year. While tobacco smoking rates among adolescents have decreased, cannabis rates still remain high. In grades 5 to 9, 19% of students had tried smoking a cigarette, and 2% smoked daily. Surveys also identified that 18% of adolescents from 15 to 19 years of age were current smokers (Canadian Centre on Substance Abuse, 2007).

Mental Health Problems

There are many children and youth in Canada who have mental health problems; as many as 15%, or 1.2 million, Canadian children are affected by anxiety, attention deficit, depression, addiction, and other mental health issues. In 2006, a Senate committee report on mental health and mental illness identified that Canadian children and youth are at significant risk compared to other groups affected by mental illness and that the mental health system fails them more severely (Standing Senate Committee on Social Affairs, Science and Technology, 2006). Mental illness in this age group is often the beginning of an adult mental illness. The Offord Centre for Child Studies reported that 20% of children and adolescents have developmental, emotional, and behavioural problems and that 1 in 10 children have an aggressive behavioural problem. Such mental health issues have a direct and significant impact on family caregivers as well. Unfortunately, there are many gaps in service and long waits for services for this population (Canadian Paediatric Society, 2009). Canada needs a national program to coordinate the various mental health services.

Suicide among children and youth remains a serious issue in Canada. Suicide is the second leading cause of death among youth in Canada and one of the top three causes of death among youth worldwide. Each year, 2 out of every 100,000 children aged 10 to 14 years commit suicide. For adolescents aged 15 to 19 years, the rate increases to 10 of every 100,000 children, with substantial variation across provinces and territories (Kutcher & Szumilas, 2008). These statistics mean that 256 young Canadians die every year from suicide. In addition to these children, there are many more individuals in these age groups who contemplate or attempt suicide (Statistics Canada, 2009b). Untreated mental disorder, the most important risk factor for suicide, is present in as many as 90% of adolescent suicide victims (Kutcher & Szumilas, 2008). Depression is one of the more common factors and occurs in 60% of suicides and in 40 to 80% of adolescents who have suicidal ideation or have attempted suicide (Barbe, Bridge, Birmaher, Kolko, & Brent, 2004). Substance use and conduct disorder are often present in youth suicides, particularly among boys (Kutcher & Szumilas, 2008). In order to reduce the suicide rate in this young population, it is important to treat and prevent mental health disorders. Another cause of adolescent suicide is bullying. Health Canada provides bullying prevention programs (see Additional Resources).

In British Columbia, the Aboriginal suicide rate varies from 5 to 20 times higher than that of the general population. Researchers found that some of the First Nations, Métis, and Inuit bands had rates as high as 800 times the national average, but more than half had no youth suicides between 1987 and 2000. The research showed that strong cultural continuity of the band, including women leaders; pursuit of land claims; culture-designated buildings; and community control of child services, lower of fostering rates, band school, band health, and fire and police services, protected the band from youth suicide (Chandler & Lalonde, 2009).

Suicide is a preventable occurrence, placing a heavy burden on nurses to identify the at-risk child or adolescent who may display mental health and emotional problems. More completely integrated medical and mental health services for children and adolescents are needed (Coury, 2006).

Mortality

Figures describing rates of occurrence of events such as death among children are referred to as *vital statistics*. *Mortality statistics* describe the incidence, or number of individuals who have died over a specific period. These statistics are usually presented as rates per 1,000 and are calculated from a sample of death certificates. Statistics Canada, under the auspices of the federal government, is responsible for the collection, analysis, and dissemination of data on the health of the Canadian people.

Infant Mortality

Over the past 50 years, the mortality rate for newborns that die before reaching the age of 5 has significantly decreased. In 1960, the mortality rate for this group had the probability factor of 32.6 per 1000, and in 2009 it dropped to 6.1 per 1000 (World Bank, 2010a). In 2010, the mortality rate for infants under 1 year of age in Canada was 4.99 per 1000 live births.

From a worldwide perspective, however, Canada lags behind other nations in reducing infant mortality. In 2010, Canada ranked 186th among 221 nations that have equal to or lower **infant mortality rates** than that of Canada. The top three ranked countries with the three lowest rates are Singapore, Bermuda, and Sweden (World Bank, 2010b). Researchers suggest that Canada has had an increase in higher risk births because of success in delivery of early **preterm infants** and more multiple births occurring from fertility programs. There is also variation in how countries define the parameters of low birth weight and in registration of births and deaths (Conference Board of Canada, 2011).

Birth weight is considered the major determinant of neonatal death in technologically developed countries; there is a definite relationship between birth weight and infant morbidity and mortality (Martin et al., 2005). Access to and use of high-quality prenatal care is the single most important preventive strategy to decrease early delivery and infant mortality rates (Martin et al., 2005).

Many of the leading causes of death during infancy continue to occur during the perinatal period. From 2000 to 2004, the first two causes of infant deaths were **congenital** anomalies and preterm birth, which led to over one third of infant deaths in Canada. The infant mortality rate for preterm birth increased by one third from 2000 until 2004, whereas congenital anomalies decreased (PHAC, 2008b).

Researchers compared rates of infant mortality among indigenous children in Canada, the United States, Australia, and New Zealand. In all four countries, the infant mortality rates were 1.7 to 4 times higher for indigenous infants than for nonindigenous infants (Kermode-Scott, 2009).

Morbidity

Measurements of the prevalence of specific illnesses in the population at a particular time are known as *morbidity statistics*, generally presented as rates per 1000 population because of their **frequency** of occurrence. Unlike mortality, morbidity is difficult to define and may denote acute illness, chronic disease, or disability. Sources of data for morbidity statistics include reasons for visits to physicians, diagnoses qualifying for hospital admission, and household interviews. Unlike death rates, which are updated annually, morbidity statistics are revised less frequently and may not represent the general population.

Childhood Morbidity

Acute illness is defined as symptoms severe enough to limit activity or require medical attention. Respiratory illness accounts for about 50% of all acute conditions; infections and parasitic disease cause 11%, and injuries cause 15%. The common cold is the illness that occurs most frequently.

The types of diseases that children contract during childhood vary according to age. For example, upper respiratory tract infections and diarrhea decrease with age, but other disorders such as acne and headaches increase in occurrence. Children who have had a particular type of problem are more likely to have that problem again. Morbidity is not distributed randomly in children.

The Art of Pediatric Nursing

Philosophy of Care

Pediatric nursing in Canada follows the practice guidelines and standards set by the Canadian Nurses Association (CNA) and the individual provincial and territorial regulatory bodies.

The Hospital for Sick Children (HSC) (2011) in Toronto is an example of a tertiary pediatric centre that has developed a pediatric nursing philosophy that integrates Canadian nursing practice standards, as follows:

1. Staff are committed to achieving the highest level of nursing care for children and their families.
2. The diversity of the community and uniqueness of each individual child and family are recognized and respected.
3. Through partnerships and collaboration, nurses strive to promote and restore optimal health and to assist children and families to effectively adjust to health challenges.
4. A work environment is fostered in which excellence and innovation in practice, education, and research are valued.
5. Nursing knowledge, skills, and judgement are used to provide safe, competent, and high-quality care.

Family-Centred Care

The philosophy of family-centred care recognizes the family as the one constant in a child's life. Health care providers must support, respect, encourage, and enhance the family's strength and competence by developing a partnership with parents (Newton, 2000). Nurses support families in their natural caregiving and decision-making roles by building on families' unique strengths and acknowledging their expertise in caring for their child both within and outside the hospital setting (Newton, 2000). The needs of all family members, not just the child's, are considered (Box 29-1). Family-centred

BOX 29-1 Key Elements of Family-Centred Care

Incorporating into policy and practice the recognition that the family is the constant in a child's life while the service systems and support personnel within those systems fluctuate

Facilitating family–professional collaboration at all levels of hospital, home, and community care:
- Care of an individual child
- Program development, implementation, and evaluation
- Policy formation

Exchanging complete and unbiased information between family members and professionals in a supportive manner at all times

Incorporating into policy and practice the recognition and honouring of cultural diversity, strengths, and individuality within and across all families, including ethnic, racial, spiritual, social, economic, educational, and geographical diversity

Recognizing and respecting different methods of coping and implementing comprehensive policies and programs that provide developmental, educational, emotional, environmental, and financial support to meet the diverse needs of families

Encouraging and facilitating family-to-family support and networking

Ensuring that home, hospital, and community service and support systems for children needing specialized health and developmental care and their families are flexible, accessible, and comprehensive in responding to diverse family-identified needs

Appreciating families as families and children as children, recognizing that they possess a wide range of strengths, concerns, emotions, and aspirations beyond their need for specialized health and developmental services and support

(From Shelton, T. L., & Stepanek, J. S. [1994]. *Family-centred care for children needing specialized health and developmental services.* Bethesda, MD: Association for the Care of Children's Health.)

care addresses the diversity among family structures and backgrounds; family goals, dreams, strategies, and actions; and family support, service, and information needs. It is essential that the pediatric nurse work within the framework of family-centred care. For additional resources on family-centred care, visit the Web site of the Institute for Family-Centred Care (http://www.ipfcc.org/pdf/getting_started.pdf).

Two basic concepts in family-centred care are enabling and empowerment. Professionals enable families by creating opportunities for all family members to display their current abilities and competencies and to acquire new ones that are necessary for meeting the needs of the child and family. **Empowerment** is interaction of professionals with families in a way that assists families to maintain or acquire a sense of control over their lives and make positive changes through the fostering of their own strengths, abilities, and actions.

Atraumatic Care

Although tremendous advances have been made in pediatric care, many changes that have cured illnesses and prolonged life are also traumatic, painful, upsetting, and frightening. Unfortunately, minimizing the trauma of medical interventions has not kept pace with technological advances. With knowledge of the treatment-related stressors imposed on ill children and their families and equipped with interventions that are safe and effective in eliminating or reducing these stressors, health care professionals can direct their attention to providing atraumatic care.

Atraumatic care is the provision of therapeutic care in settings, by personnel, and through the use of appropriate interventions that eliminates or minimizes the psychological and physical distress experienced by children and their families in the health care system. *Therapeutic care* encompasses the prevention, diagnosis, treatment, and palliation of chronic or acute conditions. *Setting* refers to whatever place in which care is given—the home, the hospital, or any other health care setting. *Personnel* include anyone directly involved in providing therapeutic care. *Interventions* range from psychological approaches, such as preparing children for procedures, to physical interventions, such as providing space for a parent to room in with a child. *Psychological distress* may include anxiety, fear, anger, disappointment, sadness, shame, or guilt. *Physical distress* may range from sleeplessness and immobilization to disturbing sensory stimuli such as pain, temperature extremes, loud noises, bright lights, or darkness. In short, atraumatic care is concerned with the who, what, when, where, why, and how of any procedure performed on a child, for the purpose of preventing or minimizing psychological and physical stress (Wong, 1989).

The overriding goal in providing atraumatic care is first, *do no harm*. Three principles constitute the framework for achieving this goal: (1) prevent or minimize the child's separation from the family; (2) promote a sense of control; and (3) prevent or minimize bodily injury and pain. Examples of atraumatic care include fostering the parent–child relationship during hospitalization, preparing the child before any unfamiliar treatment or procedure, controlling pain, allowing the child privacy, providing play activities for expression of fear and aggression, offering choices to children, and respecting cultural differences.

Role of the Pediatric Nurse

Pediatric nurses are involved in every aspect of a child's and family's growth and development. Nursing functions vary according to regional job structures, individual education and experience, and personal career goals. Just as patients (children and their families) have unique backgrounds, each nurse brings an individual set of variables that affect the nurse–patient relationship. No matter where pediatric nurses practice, their primary concern is the welfare of the child and family.

Therapeutic Relationship

The establishment of a **therapeutic relationship** is the essential foundation for providing high-quality nursing care. Pediatric nurses need to have meaningful relationships with the children and families they encounter and yet remain separate enough to distinguish their own feelings and needs. In a therapeutic relationship, caring, well-defined boundaries separate the nurse from the child and family. These boundaries are positive and professional and promote the family's control over the child's health care. For effective family advocacy to occur, these boundaries need to be established and therapeutic relationships promoted. Both the nurse and the family are empowered, and open communication is maintained. In a nontherapeutic relationship, these boundaries are blurred, and many of the nurse's actions may serve personal needs, such as a need to feel wanted and involved, rather than the family's needs.

Exploring whether relationships with patients are therapeutic or nontherapeutic can help nurses identify problem areas early in their interactions with children and families. Although questions for exploring types of involvement can be labelled negative or positive, no one action makes a relationship therapeutic or nontherapeutic. For example, nurses may spend additional time with the family but still recognize their own needs and maintain professional separateness.

Family Advocacy and Caring

Although nurses are responsible to themselves, the profession, and the institution of employment, their primary responsibility is to the consumer of nursing services—the child and the family. The nurse must work with family members, identify their goals and needs, and plan interventions that meet the defined problems. As an advocate, the nurse assists children and their families in making informed choices and acting in the child's best interest. **Advocacy** involves ensuring that families are aware of all available health services, informed of treatments and procedures, involved in the child's care, and encouraged to change or support existing health care practices. The United Nations Declaration of the Rights of the Child (Box 29-2) provides guidelines for nursing practice that can be used to ensure that every child receives optimum care. The nurse can use this knowledge to adapt care for the child's physical and emotional well-being.

BOX 29-2 United Nations Declaration of the Rights of the Child

All children need:

- To be free from discrimination
- To develop physically and mentally in freedom and dignity
- To have a name and nationality
- To have adequate nutrition, housing, recreation, and medical services
- To receive special treatment, if handicapped
- To receive love, understanding, and material security
- To receive an education and to develop their abilities
- To be the first to receive protection in disaster
- To be protected from neglect, cruelty, and exploitation
- To be brought up in a spirit of friendship among people

(From United Nations. [1995]. *Children's rights*. Retrieved from http://www.un.org/rights/dpi1765e.htm.)

As nurses care for children and families, they must demonstrate caring, compassion, and **empathy** for others. Aspects of caring embody the concepts of atraumatic care and the development of a therapeutic relationship with patients. Parents perceive caring as a sign of high-quality nursing care, which is often focused on the nontechnical needs of the child and family. Parents describe "personable" care as actions by the nurse that include acknowledging the parents' presence, listening, making the parents feel comfortable, involving both the parents and the child in care, showing interest and concern for their welfare, showing affection and sensitivity to the parent and child, communicating with them, and individualizing the nursing care. Parents perceive personable nursing care as an integral part of a positive relationship.

Disease Prevention and Health Promotion

Every nurse involved with child care must practice preventive health care. Regardless of the identified problem, the nurse's role is to plan care that fosters every aspect of growth and development. On the basis of a thorough assessment process, problems related to nutrition, immunizations, safety, dental care, development, socialization, **discipline**, or schooling often become obvious. Once the problem is identified, the nurse can intervene directly or refer the family to other health care providers or agencies.

The best approach to prevention is education and **anticipatory guidance**. An appreciation of the hazards or conflicts of each developmental period enables the nurse to guide parents regarding childrearing practices aimed at preventing potential problems. One of the most significant examples is safety. Because each age group is at risk for special types of injuries, preventive teaching can significantly reduce the rate of injuries, in turn lowering permanent disability and mortality rates.

Prevention also involves less obvious aspects of care. In addition to preventing physical disease or injury, the nurse should also promote mental health. For example, it is not sufficient to administer immunizations without regard to the psychological trauma associated with the procedure. The nurse and all other health care providers must ensure that humane care is provided.

Health Teaching

Health teaching is inseparable from family advocacy and prevention. Health teaching may be direct, as during parenting classes, or indirect, as when nurses help parents and children understand a diagnosis or treatment, encourage children to ask questions about their bodies, refer families to health-related professional or lay groups, supply appropriate literature, and provide anticipatory guidance. Health teaching is one area in which nurses often need preparation and practice with competent role models as it involves the transmission of information at the child's and family's levels of understanding and desire for information. As an effective educator, the nurse focuses on providing the appropriate health teaching along with generous feedback and evaluation to promote learning.

Support and Counselling

Attention to emotional needs requires support and sometimes counselling. The role of child advocate or health teacher requires an individualized approach. Support can be offered by listening, by touching, and through physical presence. Touching and physical presence are helpful to use with children because these interventions facilitate nonverbal communication.

Counselling involves a mutual exchange of ideas and opinions that provides the basis for mutual problem solving. It involves supporting, teaching, fostering expression of feelings or thoughts, and helping families cope with stress. Optimally, counselling not only helps resolve a crisis or problem but also enables the family to attain a higher level of functioning, greater **self-esteem**, and closer relationships. Counselling techniques are discussed in this text (see Chapters 2 and 34) to help students and nurses cope with immediate crises and refer families for additional professional assistance.

Coordination and Collaboration

As a member of the health care team, the nurse collaborates and coordinates nursing services with the activities of other professionals. Working in isolation does not serve the child's best interest. The concept of holistic care can only be realized through a unified interdisciplinary approach. Being aware of individual contributions and limitations to the child's care, the nurse collaborates with other specialists to provide high-quality health services. Failure to recognize one's limitations can be nontherapeutic and perhaps destructive. For example, the nurse who feels competent in counselling but who is really inadequate in this area may not only not prevent the child from dealing with a crisis but may also impede future success with a qualified professional.

Even nurses who practice in isolated geographic areas separated from other health care professionals cannot be considered independent. Every nurse works interdependently with the child and family, collaborating on needs and interventions so that the final care plan is one that truly meets the child's needs. Unfortunately, collaboration and coordination with the child and the family are sometimes not included in health care planning. Staff from numerous disciplines often work together to formulate a comprehensive approach without consulting the child and the family about their preferences. The nurse is in a vital position to include the child and family members in their care, either directly or indirectly, by communicating their thoughts to the health care team.

Ethical Decision Making

Ethical dilemmas arise when competing moral considerations underlie various alternatives. Parents, nurses, physicians, and other health care team members may reach different but morally defensible decisions by assigning different weight to the competing moral values. These competing moral values may include *autonomy*, the patient's right to be self-governing; *nonmaleficence*, the obligation to minimize or prevent harm; *beneficence*, the obligation to promote the patient's well-being; and *justice*, the concept of fairness. Nurses are important role models for demonstrating how to create an environment of mutual respect and understanding for patients and their families. Respect for the individuals they care for is the affirmation that other persons matter in the same way as the nurses themselves (Milton, 2005).

Nurses must prepare themselves systematically for collaborative ethical decision making. This can be accomplished through taking formal coursework and continuing education, reading contemporary literature, and working to establish an environment conducive to ethical discourse. Moreover, nurses need to be educated in the mechanisms for dispute resolution, case review by **ethics** committees, procedural safeguards, Canadian legislation, and case law (Woods, 2005).

The nurse can also use the professional code of ethics for guidance and as a means for professional self-regulation. The *Code of Ethics for Registered and Registered Practical or Licensed Nurses*, by the Canadian Nurses Association (CNA), provides the framework and core responsibilities for nursing practice. The *Code of Ethics* focuses on the nurse's accountability and responsibility to the patient (CNA, 2008a) and emphasizes the nursing role as an independent professional, one that upholds its own legal liability (Box 29-3).

BOX 29-3 Canadian Nurses Association Code of Ethics for Registered Nurses

The registered nurse integrates ethical provisions in all areas of practice.

The registered nurse will:

1. Provide safe, compassionate, and competent care
2. Promote health and well-being
3. Promote and respect informed decision making
4. Preserve dignity
5. Maintain privacy and confidentiality
6. Promote justice
7. Be accountable

(From Canadian Nurses Association. [2008]. *Code of ethics for registered nurses*. Retrieved from http://www.cna-nurses.ca/CNA/documents/pdf/publications/Code_of_Ethics_2008_e.pdf. © Canadian Nurses Association. Reprinted with permission. Further reproduction prohibited.)

Nurses may face ethical issues regarding patient care, such as the use of lifesaving measures for VLBW newborns or the terminally ill child's right to refuse treatment. They may struggle with questions involving truthfulness, balancing their rights and responsibilities in caring for children with AIDS, whistle-blowing, or allocating resources.

Research

Practicing nurses should contribute to research because they are the individuals observing human responses to health and illness. The current emphasis on measurable outcomes to determine the efficacy of interventions (often in relation to the cost) demands that nurses know whether clinical interventions result in positive outcomes for their patients. This demand has influenced the current trend toward evidence-informed practice (EIP), which involves questioning why something is effective and whether a better approach exists. The concept of EIP also involves analyzing published clinical research and translating it into the everyday practice of nursing. When nurses base their clinical practice on science and research and document their clinical outcomes, they are better able to validate their contributions to health, wellness, and cure, not only to their patients and institutions, but also to the nursing profession. Evaluation is essential to the nursing process, and research is one of the best ways to accomplish this.

Critical Thinking and the Process of Nursing Children and Families

Critical Thinking

A systematic thought process is essential to the nursing profession. It assists the professional in meeting the patient's needs. *Critical thinking* is purposeful, goal-directed thinking that assists individuals in making judgements based on evidence rather than on guesswork (Alfaro-LeFevre, 2005). It is based on the scientific method of inquiry, which is also the root of the nursing process. Critical thinking and the nursing process are considered crucial to professional nursing in that they constitute a holistic approach to problem solving.

Critical thinking is a complex developmental process based on rational and deliberate thought. In becoming a critical thinker one has a common denominator for knowledge that exemplifies disciplined and self-directed thinking. The knowledge is acquired, assessed, and organized by thinking through the clinical situation and developing an outcome focused on optimum patient care. The cognitive skills used in high-quality thinking include intellectual discipline, self-evaluation, creativity, persistence, risk taking, and intuition (Ignatavicius, 2001). Critical thinking transforms the way in which individuals view themselves, understand the world, and make decisions.

Evidence-Informed Practice

Evidence-informed practice is the collection, interpretation, and integration of valid, important, and applicable patient-reported, nurse-observed, and research-derived information (Simpson, 2004). Evidence-informed nursing practice combines knowledge with clinical experience and intuition. It provides a rational approach to decision making that facilitates best practice (Newhouse et al., 2005). EIP is an important tool that complements the nursing process by using critical thinking skills to make decisions based on existing knowledge. The traditional nursing process approach to patient care (discussed further in the next section) can be used to conceptualize the essential components of evidence-informed nursing.

During the assessment and diagnostic (first and second) phases of the nursing process, the nurse establishes important clinical questions and completes a critical review of existing knowledge. EIP also begins with identification of the problem. The nurse asks clinical questions in a concise, organized way that elicits clear answers. Once the specific questions are identified, extensive searching for the best information to answer the question begins. The nurse evaluates clinically relevant research, analyzes findings from the **history** and physical examinations, and reviews the specific pathophysiology of the defined problem. The third step in the nursing process is to develop a care plan. In evidence-informed nursing practice, the care plan is established after a critical appraisal of what is known and not known about the defined problem. Next, in the traditional nursing process, the nurse implements the care plan. By integrating evidence with clinical expertise, the nurse focuses care on the patient's unique needs. The final step in EIP is consistent with the final phase of the nursing process: to evaluate the effectiveness of the care plan.

Searching for evidence in this modern era of technology can be overwhelming. Appropriate resources must be available for nurses to implement EIP. Resources include online search engines and journal access to the most recent information. In many institutions, computer terminals are available on patient care units, with the Internet and online journals easily accessible. Another important resource for the implementation of EIP is time. The nursing shortage and ongoing changes that many institutions face have compounded the issue of nursing time allocation for patient care, education, and training. In some institutions, nurses are given paid time away from performing patient care to participate in activities that promote EIP. This requires an organizational environment that values EIP and its potential impact on patient care. As knowledge is generated regarding the significant impact of EIP on patient care outcomes, it is hoped that the organizational culture will change to support the staff nurse's participation in EIP. As the amount of available evidence increases, so does the need to critically evaluate the evidence.

Nursing Process

The *nursing process* is a method of problem identification and problem solving that describes what the nurse actually does (Alfaro-LeFevre, 2005). The five-step model accepted as the nursing process is assessment, diagnosis (problem identification), planning (with outcome development), implementation, and evaluation.

The first step of the nursing process is assessment. The second step, **nursing diagnosis**, involves naming of the child's or family's problem in standardized nursing language; cue clusters are obtained during the assessment phase. According to NANDA International (formerly the North American Nursing Diagnosis Association), the currently accepted definition of the term *nursing diagnosis* is that it is a clinical judgement about individual, family, or community responses to actual and potential health problems and life processes. Nursing diagnoses provide the basis for selecting nursing interventions aimed at achieving the best possible patient outcomes and for which the nurse is accountable (Johnson et al., 2006). The Nursing Interventions Classification (NIC) consists of a standardized list of more than 400 examples of care provided by nurses in clinical practice. The Nursing Outcomes Classification (NOC) is a comprehensive, standardized system of patient outcomes that can be used to evaluate the results of specific nursing interventions.

Not all children have actual health problems; some have a potential health problem, which is a risk state that requires nursing intervention to prevent the development of an actual problem. Potential health problems may be indicated by the presence of *risk factors*, or signs, that predispose a child and family to a dysfunctional health pattern and are limited to individuals at greater risk than the population as a whole. Nursing interventions are directed toward reducing risk factors. To differentiate actual from potential health problems, the word *risk* is included in the nursing diagnosis statement (e.g., risk for infection).

Signs and symptoms refer to a cluster of cues and defining characteristics that are derived from patient assessment and indicate actual health problems. When a defining characteristic is essential for the diagnosis to be made, it is considered critical. These critical defining characteristics help differentiate between diagnostic categories. For example, in deciding between the diagnostic categories related to family function and coping, the defining characteristics are critical in choosing the most appropriate nursing diagnosis.

Documentation

Although documentation is not one of the five steps of the nursing process, it is essential for evaluation. The nurse can assess, diagnose, and identify problems; plan care; and implement and evaluate treatment interventions. There should be written evidence of progress toward outcomes.

Currently, along with health promotion, attention in health care is focused on patient outcomes. The patient's care is evaluated not only at discharge but also thereafter, to ensure that outcomes are met and that there is adequate care for assisting the patient in resolving existing or potential health problems.

Health Care Planning

The nurse's role has expanded beyond the nucleus of the family to include the community-based, health-driven system. Traditionally, nurses were involved in public health either on a continuous or an episodic basis. Nurses were less frequently involved in health care planning on a political or legislative level. Future nurses will need to incorporate a political component into their professional identity and attempt to influence the decision-making arm of government. Some Canadian professional nursing organizations provide organizational mechanisms to respond to political issues.

As the largest health care profession, nursing has a valuable voice, especially as a family and consumer advocate. Nurses must become aware of community needs, be interested in the formulation of bills, and be supportive of politicians to ensure passage (or rejection) of significant legislation. Nurses also need to become actively involved with groups dedicated to the welfare of children (e.g., professional nursing societies, parent–teacher organizations, parent support groups, and volunteer organizations).

Health care planning involves not only providing new services to children and their families but also promoting the highest quality in existing services. In addition to following the Canadian Code of Ethics for Registered Nurses, nurses can ensure excellence in their profession by following standards of practice and required competency levels set by the CNA and provincial and territorial regulatory bodies. In the past, pediatric nursing had no national or international standards of care or education. Most pediatric nurses merged pediatrics with other specialties within nursing and followed the Standards of Maternal-Child Health Nursing or the standards of several of the pediatric specialties, such as pediatric oncology nursing or school nursing. However, pediatric nursing is increasing in momentum in Canada. For example, the CNA offers a Critical Care Pediatric Certificate, and the British Columbia Institute of Technology offers a Pediatric Nursing Specialty Option.

The highest standards of nursing practice are reflected in the emphasis on thorough assessment, the focus on scientific rationale as the basis for care, the summary of nursing care goals and responsibilities, and the comprehensive discussion of growth and development.

Future Trends

The current shift from treatment of disease to promotion of health has expanded nurses' roles in ambulatory care and highlighted the prevention and health teaching aspects of nursing practice. The need for home care and community health services require nurses to be more independent and to acquire skills useful in settings beyond the hospital. As changing social policy shapes the expanding health care arena, the focus of nursing care has shifted from what we do *for* families to what we do *in partnership with* them. The philosophy of family-centred care is no longer an option but a mandate.

Today, technological advances and the demand for computer knowledge in the work setting are obvious. The current shortage of nurses will persist into the future, and the pressure to create positions in the health care system that do not require a nursing background will intensify. As new categories of workers enter the health care field, nurses will need to continue to update their knowledge of technology and prove their unique contribution to health care. Nurses must use technology and learn to work collaboratively with unregulated health workers—a variety of health care providers not licensed or regulated by any professional, governmental, or regulatory body (CNA, 2008b).

Changing demographics will also influence pediatric nursing. The adult population is growing faster than the pediatric population; consequently, the number of pediatric hospital beds is decreasing, particularly in rural areas. Pediatric units may amalgamate with obstetrical units, creating maternal child nursing units. Because older adults make up a larger percentage of the population, health care dollars will be split between the youngest and oldest groups, with shrinking resources available to meet the needs of both. Nurses will need to be aware of developments in pediatric medicine and continually adapt their care to the cultural milieu in which they practice.

Finally, cost containment will present an ever-present challenge to providing high-quality care.

Key Points

- The *Healthy Canadians* government program broadened the health care objectives of the past and shifted the focus to prevention as the method to accomplish health goals.
- The determinants of health provide a blueprint for health care policies and help direct public health research focused on improving the health of Canadian citizens.
- While the infant mortality rate in Canada is at an all-time low, it continues to be higher than that in other major countries.
- LBW, which is closely related to early gestational age, is a leading cause of neonatal death in Canada.
- Injuries are the leading cause of death in children over age 1 year, with the majority being motor vehicle injuries.
- Childhood morbidity encompasses acute illness, chronic disease, and disability.
- The *new morbidity* refers to behavioural, social, and educational problems that can significantly alter a child's health.
- Developmental stage and environment are important factors in the prevalence of injuries at every age and should guide injury prevention measures.
- The philosophy of family-centred care recognizes the family as the constant in a child's life and that service systems and personnel must support, respect, encourage, and enhance the family's strength and competence.
- Atraumatic care is the provision of therapeutic care in settings, by personnel, and through the use of interventions that eliminate or minimize the psychological and physical distress experienced by children and their families in the health care system.
- Roles of the pediatric nurse include establishing a therapeutic relationship, advocating for families, preventing disease and promoting health, providing health teaching, providing support and counselling, coordinating and collaborating on care, making ethical decisions, and doing research.
- With the shift in focus from treatment of disease to promotion of health, nurses' roles have expanded beyond working in traditional health care facilities to providing care in ambulatory care centres, schools, the family's home, and the community.
- Evidence-informed practice is the collection, interpretation, and integration of valid, important, and applicable patient-reported, nurse-observed, and research-derived information.

- The process of nursing for children and families includes accurate and complete assessment, analysis of assessment data to arrive at a nursing diagnosis, planning of care, implementation of the plan, evaluation of interventions, and documentation.

Audio Chapter Summaries
Access an Audio Summary of these Key Points on evolve

References

Alfaro-LeFevre, R. (2005). *Applying nursing process: A tool for critical thinking* (6th ed.). Philadelphia: Lippincott.

Barbe, R. P., Bridge, J., Birmaher, B., Kolko, D., & Brent, D. A. (2004). Suicidality and its relationship to treatment outcome in depressed adolescents. *Suicide and Life-Threatening Behavior, 34*, 44–55.

Canadian Centre on Substance Abuse. (2007). *Substance abuse in Canada: Youth in focus*. Retrieved from http://www.ccsa.ca/2007%20CCSA%20Documents/ccsa-011521-2007-e.pdf.

Canadian Institutes of Health Research. (2003). *Research in infection and immunity*. Retrieved from http://www.cihr-irsc.gc.ca.

Canadian Nurses Association. (2008a). *Code of ethics for Canadian registered nurses*. Retrieved from http://www.cna-aiic.ca/CNA/practice/ethics/code/default_e.aspx.

Canadian Nurses Association. (2008b). *Maximizing human resources: Valuing unregulated health care workers*. Retrieved from http://www.cna-aiic.ca/cna/documents/pdf/publications/UHW_Final_Report_e.pdf.

Canadian Paediatric Society. (2009). *Child and youth mental health abandoned by health care system: Hon. Michael Kirby*. Retrieved from http://www.cps.ca/english/publications/CPSNews/SepOct09.pdf.

Canadian Paediatric Society. (2011). *Impact of media use on children and youth*. Retrieved from http://www.cps.ca/english/statements/CP/pp03-01.

Canada Safety Council. (2009). *Unload and lock your firearms, store them safely!* Retrieved from http://canadasafetycouncil.org/news/unload-and-lock-your-firearms-store-them-safely.

Chandler, M. J., & Lalonde, C. E. (2009). Cultural continuity as a moderator of suicide risk among Canada's First Nations. In L. J. Kirmayer & G. Valaskakis (Eds.), *Healing traditions: The mental health of Aboriginal peoples in Canada* (pp. 221–248). Vancouver, BC: UBC Press.

Conference Board of Canada. (2011). *Health infant mortality*. Retrieved from http://www.conferenceboard.ca/hcp/details/health/infant-mortality-rate.aspx.

Coury, D. L. (2006). Over the rainbow: Advancing child health in the new millennium. *Ambulatory Pediatrics, 6*(3), 134–137. doi:10.1016/j.ambp.2005.12.001

Dietz, W. H. (2005). Overweight: An epidemic. In A. G. Cosby, et al. (Eds.), *About children: An authoritative resource on the state of childhood today*. Elk Grove Village, IL: American Academy of Pediatrics.

Edelstein, B. L. (2005). Tooth decay: The best of times, the worst of times. In A. G. Cosby, et al. (Eds.), *About children: An authoritative resource on the state of childhood today*. Elk Grove Village, IL: American Academy of Pediatrics.

Fisher, K., & Kettl, P. (2003). Teachers' perceptions of school violence. *Journal of Pediatric Health Care, 17*, 79–83.

Gagné, M-P. (2008). *L'effet des législations canadiennes entourant le contrôle des armes à feu sur les homicides et les suicides*. M.Sc. Thesis, Université de Montréal.

Gentile, D. A., Coyne, S., & Walsh, D. A. (2011). Media violence, physical aggression, and relational aggression in school age children: A short-term longitudinal study. *Aggressive Behavior, 37*(2), 193–206. doi:10.1002/ab.20380

Health Canada. (2006). *Suicide prevention*. Retrieved from http://www.hc-sc.gc.ca/fniah-spnia/pubs/promotion/_suicide/prev_youth-jeunes/index-eng.php#s21.

Health Canada. (2008). *Keeping safe—Injury prevention*. Retrieved from http://www.hc-sc.gc.ca/fniah-spnia/promotion/injury-bless/index-eng.php.

Health Canada. (2009). *Reaching for the top: A report by the Advisor on Healthy Children and Youth*. Retrieved from http://www.hc-sc.gc.ca/hl-vs/pubs/child-enfant/advisor-conseillere/prevention-eng.

Health Canada. (2010). *Health Canada reminds parents and caregivers to take steps to prevent unintentional poisoning*. Retrieved from http://www.hc-sc.gc.ca/ahc-asc/media/nr-cp/_2010/2010_38-eng.php.

Heuer, S. (2007). Family-centred care. *Journal for Specialists in Pediatric Nursing, 12*(1), 61–65. doi: 10.1111/j.1744-6155.2007.00091.x

Hospital for Sick Children. (2011). *Nursing*. Retrieved from http://www.sickkids.ca/Nursing/index.html.

Ignatavicius, D. (2001). Critical thinking skills for at the bedside success. *Nursing Management, 32*(1), 37–39.

Johnson, M., et al. (2006). *NANDA, NOC, and NIC linkages: Nursing diagnoses, outcomes and interventions* (2nd ed.). St. Louis: Mosby.

Katzmarzyk, P. (2008). Obesity and physical activity among Aboriginal Canadians. *Obesity, 16*, 184–190. doi:10.1038/oby.2007.51

Kermode-Scott, B. (2009). Rates of infant mortality higher among indigenous children in Canada, the US, Australia, and New Zealand. *British Medical Journal, 338*(1379). doi: 10.1136/bmj.b1379

Kutcher, R., & Szumilas, M. (2008). Youth suicide prevention. *Canadian Medical Association Journal, 178*(3), 282–285. doi: 10.1503/cmaj.071315

Lichter, D. T. (2005). Families: Diversity and change. In A. G. Cosby, et al. (Eds.), *About children: An authoritative resource on the state of childhood today*. Elk Grove Village, IL: American Academy of Pediatrics.

MacLaurin, B., Trocmé, N., Fallon, B., Blackstock, C., Pitman, L., & McCormack, M. (2011). *A comparison of First Nations and non-Aboriginal children investigated for maltreatment in Canada in 2003*. Retrieved from http://www.cecw-cepb.ca/publications/537.

Martin, J. A., et al. (2005). Annual summary of vital statistics: 2003. *Pediatrics, 115*(3), 619–634. doi: 10.1542/peds.2004-2695

Milton, C. L. (2005). The ethics of respect in nursing. *Nursing Science Quarterly, 18*(1), 20–23. doi: 10.1177/0894318404272103

Newhouse, R., et al. (2005). Evidence-based practice: A practical approach to implementation. *Journal of Nursing Administration, 35*(1), 35–40.

Newton, M. S. (2000). Family-centred care: Current realities in parent participation. *Pediatric Nursing, 26*(2), 164–168.

Ontario Ministry of Health Promotion and Sport. (2010). *Active living: Help your kids get active*. Retrieved from http://www.mhp.gov.on.ca/en/healthy-ontario.asp?utm_campaign=jan2011.

Public Health Agency of Canada. (2008a). *Canadian incidence study of reported child abuse and neglect 2008 (CIS-2008): Major findings*. Retrieved from http://www.cecw-cepb.ca/publications/2117.

Public Health Agency of Canada. (2008b). *Canadian perinatal health report*. Ottawa: Author. Retrieved from http://www.phac-aspc.gc.ca/publicat/2008/cphr-rspc/pdf/cphr-rspc08-eng.pdf.

Public Health Agency of Canada. (2008c). *Vaccine safety*. Retrieved from http://www.phac-aspc.gc.ca/im/vs-sv/vs-faq17-eng.php.

Public Health Agency of Canada. (2009). *Oral diseases*. Retrieved from http://www.hc-sc.gc.ca/hl-vs/oral-bucco/disease-maladie/index-eng.php.

Public Health Agency of Canada. (2010). *What determines health*? Retrieved from http://www.phac-aspc.gc.ca/ph-sp/determinants/index-eng.php.

Safe Kids Canada. (2010). *Safe cycling*. Retrieved from http://www.safekidscanada.ca/Professionals/Safety-Information/Wheeled-Activities/Cycling/Safe-Cycling.aspx.

Simpson, R. (2004). Evidence-based nursing offers certainty in the uncertain world of healthcare. *Nursing Management, 35*(10), 10–12.

Standing Senate Committee on Social Affairs, Science and Technology. (2006). *Out of the shadows at last: Transforming mental health, mental illness and addiction services in Canada*. Retrieved from http://www.parl.gc.ca/Content/SEN/Committee/391/soci/rep/rep02may06-e.htm.

Statistics Canada. (2009a). *Family homicides*. Retrieved from http://www.statcan.gc.ca/pub/85-224-x/2009000/part-partie5-eng.htm.

Statistics Canada. (2009b). *Table 102-0551: Suicides and suicide rate, by sex and by age group (both sexes)*. Retrieved from http://www40.statcan.gc.ca/cbin/sf01.cgi?se=suicide&searchbut01=Go&mod=cst&lan=eng.

Statistics Canada. (2010). *Youth court statistics, 2008/2009*. Retrieved from http://www.statcan.gc.ca/pub/85-002-x/2010002/article/11294-eng.htm.

Statistics Canada (2012). *2011 Census of population*. Ottawa: Author. Retrieved from http://www12.statcan.gc.ca/census-recensement/index-eng.cfm

Thompson, D. C., Rivara, F., & Thompson, R. (2009). Helmets for preventing head and facial injuries in bicyclists. *Cochrane Database of Systematic Reviews*, (1).

United Nations Office on Drugs and Crime. (2011). *World drug report: 2011*. Vienna: United Nations. Retrieved from http://www.unodc.org/documents/data-and-analysis/WDR2011/World_Drug_Report_2011_ebook.pdf.

Wong, D. (1989). Principles of atraumatic care. In V. Feeg (Ed.), *Pediatric nursing: Forum on the future: Looking toward the 21st century*. Pitman, NJ: Anthony J. Jannetti.

Woods, M. (2005). Nursing ethics education: Are we really delivering the good(s)? *Nursing Ethics, 12*(1), 5–18. doi:10.1191/0969733005ne754oa
World Bank. (2010a). *Mortality rate under 5*. Retrieved from http://www.google.com/publicdata?ds=wb-wdi&met=sh_dyn_mort&idim=country:CAN&dl=en&hl=en&q=child+mortality+rates+in+canada#met=sh_dyn_mort&idim=country:CAN:BLZ:USA.
World Bank. (2010b). *Canada infant mortality rate*. Retrieved from http://www.indexmundi.com/canada/infant_mortality_rate.html.
World Health Organization. (2007). *School health and youth health promotion*. Retrieved from http://www.who.int/topics/school_health_promotion/en/.

Additional Resources

About Kids Health: http://www.aboutkidshealth.ca/Default.aspx
Canadian Paediatric Society: http://www.cps.ca/english/index.html
Caring for Kids: http://www.caringforkids.cps.ca/
Health Canada Bullying Prevention Programs: http://www.healthycanadians.gc.ca/init/kids-enfants/intimidation/prevention/index-eng.php.
Institute for Family-Centred Care: http://www.ipfcc.org
Safe Kids Canada: http://www.sickkids.ca

Unit 7

Community-Based Nursing Care of the Child and Family

30

Learning Objectives

On completion of this chapter, the reader will be able to:

- Describe community health nursing.
- Identify the roles and functions of the community health nurse.
- Discuss selected aspects of the epidemiological process.
- Explain the purpose of an economic evaluation.
- Discuss the components of the community nursing process.

Electronic Resources

Additional information related to the content in Chapter 30 can be found on

evolve the companion Web site at

http://evolve.elsevier.com/Canada/Perry/maternal/

Nursing in the Community

The health of children and their families is greatly influenced by their community, and nurses can make a significant contribution by working with the community to promote children's health. Nurses working with pediatric populations in the community need an understanding of the concepts and processes critical to addressing pediatric concerns from a community health perspective. Healthy communities not only provide excellent medical care; they also provide children a nurturing, safe place in which to live and grow. Healthy communities address concerns through collaboration between and among citizens, health care providers, businesses, and governmental and private agencies (Flynn & Ivanov, 2004).

This chapter discusses community health nursing as it relates to children. First it identifies and defines the concepts and principles that serve as the basis of community health nursing. Then it describes the community health nursing process, step by step. It includes a demonstration of the process used to address a very real child health concern: obesity.

Community health nurses work in the community to partner with people where they live, work, learn, meet, and play in order to promote health. As nurses work in the community with families and individuals, the goal is to promote health, build individual and community capacity, connect with and care for patients, facilitate access and equity, and demonstrate professional responsibility and accountability (Community Health Nurses of Canada, 2009). The essential functions of public health and community health nurses are as follows: public health, health promotion, disease and injury prevention, health protection, health surveillance, population health assessment, and emergency preparedness and response (Canadian Public Health Association, 2010).

There are several ways to define a community. A *community* is a group of individuals with shared characteristics or interests who interact with each other (Allender & Spradley, 2005). A community is a system that includes children and families, the physical environment, educational facilities, safety and transportation resources, political and governmental agencies, health and social services, communication resources, economic resources, and recreational facilities. The community is also the patient of the community health nurse (Anderson, 2008). The core of the community is the people, characterized by their age, sex, socioeconomic status, educational level, occupation, **ethnicity**, and religion. The community is often defined by the geography or geopolitical boundaries, which can be used to determine the location of service delivery (Anderson, & McFarlane, 2008). Community health initiatives are directed at either the general health of the community as a whole or specific populations within the community that have unique needs. In this context, *populations* can be described as groups of people who live in a community, for example, school-age children. *Target populations* or *subpopulations* are more narrowly defined groups (e.g., unimmunized preschoolers, or obese middle school children) toward whom nurses direct activities to improve the health status of individuals in the group. Common values often guide behaviours of populations and subpopulations in relation to health promotion and disease prevention (McEwen & Nies, 2007; Williams, 2011).

The Public Health Agency of Canada's (PHAC's) primary goal is to strengthen Canada's capacity to protect and improve the health of Canadians (PHAC, 2010e). This is done by promoting health; preventing and controlling chronic diseases, injuries, and infectious diseases; preparing and responding to public health emergencies; and strengthening public health capacity, through greater understanding of determinants of health and common factors that maintain health or lead to disease and injury. The government of Canada has recognized the importance of health promotion by creating programs that address child health, healthy pregnancy and infancy, healthy living, injury prevention, mental health, family violence, obesity, physical activity, population health, rural health, and older adult health (PHAC, 2010a). Capacity building involves the implementation of health promotion initiatives and sustaining of positive health outcomes over time through the development and strengthening of capabilities of an individual, organization, community, or health system (Joffres et al., 2004). The PHAC (2007) recognizes the following as tools for capacity building: participation; leadership; community structures; role of external support (e.g., a funding agency); asking why; skills, knowledge, and **learning**; linking with others; sense of community; and ability to obtain resources.

Although community health concepts can be used to address health concerns in any setting, traditional community health settings include the following: home health agencies, schools, physicians' offices, ambulatory health clinics, emergency rooms, **triage** call centres, insurance agencies, health departments, international relief agencies, health education agencies, juvenile detention facilities, camps, day care centres, foster care facilities, and rehabilitation agencies.

Roles and Functions

The roles and functions of the community health nurse continue to evolve. In the future, many pediatric nurses will be working in community settings. In 2007, 16% of the nursing workforce worked in community health (Underwood et al., 2009).

Traditionally, the roles and functions of community health nurses included caregiver, advocate, case manager, case finder, counselor, educator, epidemiologist, group process leader, health planner, and manager. The nurse provides **case management** by coordinating care between the disciplines, provides counselling by supporting the child and family through developmental crises, and acts as a case finder by identifying risk factors in the child's siblings.

The PHAC (2007) developed core competencies for all public health care professionals, including community nurses, to improve the health of the public and guide their work. The eight competencies are public health and nursing sciences; assessment and analysis; policy and program planning, implementation, and evaluation; partnership or collaboration and **advocacy**; diversity and inclusiveness; communication; leadership; and professional responsibility and accountability. These competencies are designed to evolve and change over time, reflecting the changes in nursing and public health practices. The competencies were identified as a priority by both the Community Health Nurses Association of Canada (2009) and the PHAC (2007), and they surpass discipline boundaries, independent of program and topic.

The community health standards of care, developed to ensure high-quality nursing care, apply to all public health nurses, whether working in schools, promoting community **development**, or running immunization clinics (Canadian Community Health Nursing, 2003). Such care includes using knowledge and critical thinking skills related to population health, as the Canadian population is diverse and rich in **culture**. The community health nurse practices these standards of care by being culturally sensitive and professional and by providing safe care, as when responding to an influenza pandemic in an immunization clinic focused on the pediatric population or in schools. The nurse may have to evaluate the number of eligible participants for the flu clinic, the cost of the clinic, and the subsequent cost on the system if the immunizations are not available. This may also include educating the child and family about determinants of health and steps to take in order to prevent the spread of influenza.

NURSING ALERT Nurses must be able to communicate and work with professionals from other disciplines. This includes being able to understand the terms used by demographers, epidemiologists, and economists.

Demography

Demography is the study of population characteristics. Demographic characteristics include age, gender, race and **ethnicity**, socioeconomic status, and education. Individuals, families, and communities may have demographic characteristics that affect their health risks (Cashaw, 2008). *Risk* is an increased probability of developing a disease, injury, or illness. Age is one of the most important risk factors for disease prevention and certain health conditions. For example, infants are more likely to die as a result of **congenital** malformations; children and adolescents, as a result of accidents; and middle-age adults, as a result of cancer (Statistics Canada, 2008). Gender also plays an important role. Males are at greater risk of having hemophilia A and B than females. Race and ethnicity have long been associated with increased risk for disease and disability, but it is now thought that, aside from **genetic** predisposition, there is a complicated relationship between minority status and socioeconomic status that increases the risk for disease and disability (PHAC, 2010b). Low socioeconomic status, an important determinant of health, predisposes children to a variety of problems. Poor children are more likely to be obese and to have untreated dental problems. They are more likely to have no regular site for medical care and to be treated in emergency departments (PHAC, 2010b).

Epidemiology

Epidemiology is the science of population health applied to the detection of **morbidity** and mortality in a population. Through the epidemiological process, the distribution and causes of disease or injury across a population are identified (Cashaw, 2008). It also serves as an important component in developing health programs. For example, the Community Action Program for Children incorporated the process to develop programs that promote the healthy development of young children ages 0 to 6 years (PHAC, 2010c). Health care professionals in community, provincial, and national health care organizations use the epidemiological process as a guide to develop programs that have the greatest impact on children's health.

Distribution of Disease, Injury, or Illness

Morbidity rates are used to measure disease and injury and, along with natality and mortality rates, present an objective picture of a community's health status. There are two types of morbidity rates: incidence and prevalence. *Incidence* measures the occurrence of new events in a population during a period of time. *Prevalence* measures existing events in a population during a period of time (Hennekens & Buring, 1987). For example, the incidence of type 1 diabetes in a community is estimated by counting the new cases of type 1 diabetes in a population and dividing that figure by the size of the population at risk. The prevalence of type 1 diabetes is estimated by counting the existing cases of type 1 diabetes in a population and dividing that figure by the size of the population at risk. Both incidence and prevalence are usually given as rates per 1000, 10,000, or 100,000 population, depending on their frequency. Box 30-1 presents frequently used mortality and morbidity rates.

BOX 30-1 Frequently Used Mortality and Morbidity Rates

Crude Birth Rate

$$\frac{\text{Number of births in a population}}{\text{Total population}} \text{ within a time period} \times 1000$$

Crude Death Rate

$$\frac{\text{Number of deaths in a population}}{\text{Total population}} \text{ within a time period} \times 1000$$

Cause-Specific Death Rate

$$\frac{\text{Number of deaths in a population due to a certain disease}}{\text{Total population}} \text{ within a time period} \times 1000$$

Age-Specific Death Rate

$$\frac{\text{Number of deaths in a population in a certain age-group}}{\text{Total population in that age-group}} \text{ within a time period} \times 1000$$

Incidence of Disease

$$\frac{\text{Number of new events in a population}}{\text{Total at-risk population}} \text{ within a time period} \times 1000$$

Prevalence of Disease

$$\frac{\text{Number of existing events in a population}}{\text{Total at-risk population}} \text{ within a time period} \times 1000$$

Epidemiological Triangle

Three factors form the epidemiological triangle, and their interrelationship alters the risk of acquiring a disease or condition (McKeown & Hilfinger, 2004). These factors are agent, **host**, and environment (Fig. 30-1).

An *agent* is responsible for causing a disease and may be an infectious agent, such as *Mycobacterium tuberculosis*; a chemical agent, such as lead in paint; or a physical agent, such as fire. *Host factors* are those that are specific to an individual or group. These may be genetic factors, which cannot be controlled, or they may be lifestyle factors, such as food selections or exercise patterns. *Environmental factors* provide a setting for the host and include the climatic conditions in which the host lives and factors related to the home, neighborhood, and school.

Levels of Prevention

Community health programs are based on three classic levels of prevention (Leavell & Clark, 1965). *Primary prevention* focuses on health promotion and prevention of disease or injury. Examples of primary prevention activities include well-child care clinics, immunization programs, safety programs (bike helmets, car seats, seat belts, child-proof containers), nutrition programs, environmental efforts (clean air programs), sanitation measures (chlorinated water, garbage removal, sewage treatment), and community parenting classes. *Secondary prevention* focuses on screening and early diagnosis of disease. Examples of secondary interventions include tuberculosis and lead screening programs, and mental health counselling for stressful events such as separation, divorce, death, or community natural disasters (e.g., earthquakes, floods, and hurricanes). *Tertiary prevention* focuses on optimizing function for children with a disability or chronic disease. Tertiary interventions include rehabilitation and disease management programs for asthma, sickle cell disease, cancer, and anorexia and special education programs for children.

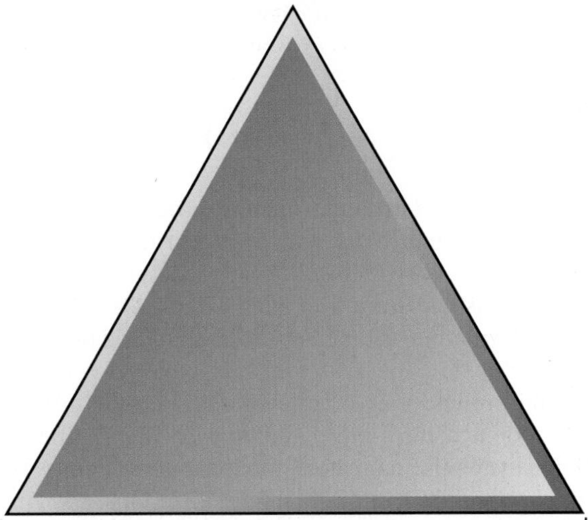

Fig. 30-1 The epidemiological triangle.

Screening

Community health nurses are frequently involved in *screening*, a secondary prevention activity. The purpose of screening is to detect and treat disease early in the period of pathogenesis in order to prevent the spread and progression of the disease (Wilson & Jungner, 1968). However, screening is not appropriate for every condition. Although screening may bring benefits, a certain amount of risk is associated with any intervention. It is essential to determine the evidence for a proposed screening program before beginning it so that the benefits of screening exceed the risks and cost. For example, acanthosis nigricans (AN) is a thickening and darkening of the skin that is commonly found on the neck and is associated with insulin resistance (Centers for Disease Control and Prevention, 2005). Some school health officials have recommended screening for AN as a way to identify early type 2 diabetes in children, but others have argued that screening may not be effective. Because of this controversy, AN is a good example of the need to determine the evidence before establishing a screening program.

Economics

A basic understanding of the economics of health care enables the nurse to participate in decision making about the worth of children's health programs. Economists theorize that individuals and societies view health as a basic utility, that is, something that is perceived as valuable (Gold et al., 1996). Other basic utilities are food, shelter, and clothing. People are willing to trade resources, such as money and time, for a program or intervention that will improve their health. Economists measure the amount of resources that individuals and communities are willing to pay for good health. Methods for defining and estimating cost have been well described, as has the need for a standardized approach to the measurement of cost and effects (Brosnan & Swint, 2001; Drummond et al., 2005).

Economic evaluation provides objective information to establish a program's value to the community. An example is the evaluation of a school-based hepatitis B vaccination program (Dobson, Scheifele, & Bell, 1995). The higher vaccination student rate of 95.4% potentially saved money that might have eventually been spent to treat these children for hepatitis, cirrhosis, or cancer.

Community Nursing Process

In community nursing, the nursing process shifts its focus from the individual child and family to the community or target population (Box 30-2). The stages of the process (assessment, diagnosis, planning, implementation, and evaluation) are similar, whether the patient is one child or a population of children.

Community nursing is collaborative, and the nurse is one member of a community team that includes other health care professionals, educators, politicians, religious leaders, members of public and voluntary organizations, and consumers. The nurse's role depends on the project's scope, the target population, and the expertise of team members.

The community partnership model is an example of a model that enables nursing students to become part of a collaborative team and to directly contribute to a community's well-being. In this model, the missions of nursing education, research, and practice are linked through three processes: evidence-informed practice, service learning, and scholarly teaching (Brosnan et al., 2005).

Community Needs Assessment and Diagnosis

The assessment phase of the community nursing process is called a *community needs assessment* (see Chapter 3, p. 30). Assessment involves the collection of subjective and objective information about a community. Subjective information indicates what community members say are their most important needs and can be determined in a number of ways. Objective information is data that the nurse collects either by direct observation or through written sources. A community walk-through is one method of direct observation. Nurses walk or drive through a neighbourhood and take notes about the environment, such as the number of public areas (see Community Focus box, p. 32). Objective information about the community's health status can also be obtained from such sources as the local chamber of commerce, Statistics Canada, libraries, provincial health departments, and the Internet sites of voluntary health organizations or government agencies. Information about service agencies can be found in resource directories, including the local telephone book, and population-specific books provided by public and voluntary agencies.

One way to organize an assessment is to use a guide that lists community systems that need to be examined. This process is similar to using a physical assessment guide to examine the different body systems in an individual patient. Anderson and McFarlane (2008) have described eight community systems that the nurse should examine: health and social services, communication, recreation, physical environment, education, safety and transportation, politics and government, and economics. During the assessment, the nurse studies how well each component in the community functions and interacts to meet children's health needs, identifies the community's strengths, and determines whether any barriers disrupt the components and prevent access to care for children and their families.

After the assessment is completed, the community nurse can collaborate with team members to analyze the results of surveys

BOX 30-2 The Community Nursing Process

Assessment and diagnosis—The nurse collects subjective and objective information about a community and develops a diagnosis based on community needs and problems.

Planning—The nurse develops community-centred goals to address the identified needs and problems.

Intervention—The nurse implements a program that enables community members to reach their goals.

Evaluation—The nurse conducts a systematic evaluation to determine that goals and program objectives were met.

and questionnaires and determine whether the needs described by community members can be met by existing community agencies. During the analysis, the community's demographic characteristics, morbidity rates, and mortality rates are compared with a standard. In time comparisons, the nurse contrasts the rates in the current year with the rates during an earlier period. In comparisons of place, the nurse contrasts the rates in the community with those of a standard population. Standard rates may come from another community or from city, province/territory, or national data. For example, the rate of tuberculosis in a group of preschool children in the community in 2011 could be compared with the rate of tuberculosis in preschool children in the province in 2011.

A *community health diagnosis* is the reflection of health status, risks, or needs as determined by a causative agent. A community diagnosis is similar to that of an individual **nursing diagnosis** with a problem (need) and an etiology related to that problem (causative agent). An example of a community nursing diagnosis is childhood obesity related to poor socioeconomic environment.

Community Planning

The nurse can collaborate with community members in developing a plan that addresses the target population's needs and problems utilizing population health. To maximize the use of community resources, problems should first be prioritized on the basis of their severity, the community's felt needs, and the community nurse's ability to bring about change. The nurse works with community members to develop at least one goal for each problem. *Goals* are outcomes that give direction to interventions and provide a measure of the change the interventions produced. Community interventions frequently take the form of health programs for improving the target population's health status. Community health programs are based on the three levels of prevention: primary, secondary, and tertiary. For example, a goal for preventing bicycle injuries is, "Within 1 year all students in the first grade will wear bicycle helmets." The nurse and community members can then plan a program that includes health education about bicycle safety for students and their parents (primary prevention).

The planning group will consider the resources that are already available in the community and resources that will be needed for implementing a health program, including personnel, supplies, and equipment. Decisions are made about the program's timeline, the budget, and strategies to obtain funding. Program descriptions are found through professional contacts, online resources, and a review of the literature. An example of a community assessment and planning project is presented in Box 30-3.

BOX 30-3 An Example of Community Assessment and Planning

Rivers is an elementary school with 500 pre-kindergarten to sixth-grade children. The school nurse has been asked to conduct an assessment of the school community and to develop a care plan. The schoolchildren and their families are the target population.

Community Needs Assessment and Diagnosis

The school nurse formed a team of community members that included parents of students who attend Rivers Elementary School, faculty and staff, health care providers, local religious leaders, and politicians. Their first task was to complete the community assessment. Team members mailed questionnaires to a random sample of families who had children attending Rivers. They held focus groups with community members to obtain subjective information about the needs of the school community. Team members obtained objective data from the local health department, school records, and Statistics Canada. The nurse also conducted a community walk-through of the neighborhood surrounding the school. The following information was collected:

People—Rivers is located in an ethnically diverse area composed of 30% First Nations, Métis, and Inuit; 30% White; 30% Asian; and 10% Black. The ethnicity of students in the school is representative of the surrounding area. Rivers is located in a large prairie city.

Safety and transportation—School bus service was rated very good to excellent by a majority of those surveyed. Transportation records indicated that the last school bus accident occurred 1 year ago. There were no fatalities, but a number of children were injured. Other accidents occurred 2 years and 10 years before the most recent accident.

Economics—Although 94% of families had at least one fully employed member, 20% of the families lived below the poverty level. The number below poverty level had not changed in 10 years.

Education—Seventy-five percent of the adult population had a high school diploma, and 15% of this group had completed at least 1 year of college. School attendance at Rivers was higher than overall provincial attendance rates.

Communication—Ninety-five percent of homes had telephones, compared with 85% 10 years ago. An estimated 10% of the target population did not speak English, as Asian, African, or Cree dialects were the primary language spoken in this group.

Recreation—Few places were available for small children to play. The focus groups recommended more parks and playgrounds.

Politics and government—The school system was strongly centralized and headed by a school superintendent. The city had a mayor and city council.

Social—Of those families living below the poverty level, 60% received some type of welfare assistance, including food stamps. The school breakfast and lunch program served 80% of the children attending the school.

Health—The childhood immunization rate for all diseases among children in the community who were less than 2 years of age was 85%, which compared favourably with the national level of 61% of children being up to date on

Continued

BOX 30-3 An Example of Community Assessment and Planning—cont'd

immunizations (PHAC, 2010d). The immunization rate for children attending Rivers Elementary School was 91%. Vision and hearing screening programs at Rivers resulted in the referral of 5% of the students for vision problems and 2% of the students for hearing problems. Review of student records indicated that all those children referred received diagnostic follow-up and treatment when indicated. Heights and weights were obtained on all students annually. Results indicated that 34% of students were above the 95th percentile for age and sex (PHAC, 2010d). In focus groups, students and teachers noted that school breakfasts and lunches were high in carbohydrates and fats. They also observed that decreased recess time resulted in decreased student activity during school hours. Adverse weather, especially during the winter months, also decreased activity during recess.

On the basis of these assessments, the following community diagnoses were made:

1. Increase in injuries related to school bus accidents
2. Increase in obesity among students compared with the national standard related to high intake of calories and sedentary lifestyle

Planning

Team members agreed that the number of school bus accidents should be closely monitored over the next 5 years. However, there was a consensus that increased obesity among students was the priority problem, and the team developed the following two goals:

1. Within 2 years, the percentage of students with BMIs above the 95th percentile for age and sex will be 25% (World Health Organization, 2010).
2. Within 5 years, that percentage will be 15%.

Team members reviewed the literature for examples of communities that had experienced similar problems, contacted school and health department officials in other areas of the country, examined the results of successful programs, and planned a health program that addressed the unique needs of the target population. The program was titled "Rivers Excels in Health." Program activities were as follows:

- Each September, the nurse will address the school's parent association about the program and will discuss the importance of a healthy diet and exercise for all family members.
- Every month, teachers will set aside 1 hour to talk with their students about healthy food choices and about the importance of limiting television viewing time.
- Within 6 months, school administrators and community members will petition the city to provide a neighbourhood park.
- Within 1 year, the school dietitian will assess the nutritional value of the current school meals and, if indicated, revise the meal plan to ensure a healthy diet.
- Within 1 year, the school will develop a plan to allow a minimum of 30 minutes of unrestricted play during the school day.

Team members determined the resources needed to implement the program, including personnel, supplies, and equipment. They estimated the total cost of setting up the program and maintaining it for 5 years and applied for funding to the school district and to the city and provincial health departments.

Implementation and Evaluation

The school nurse and other team members assumed responsibility for the timely implementation and evaluation of the Rivers Excels in Health program.

Community Intervention

During program implementation, the nurse and community members carry out the intervention. Whether the program is simple or complex, oversight is needed to ensure that everyone involved is communicating with one another, following the plan's guidelines, keeping within the timeline, and documenting daily activities and expenses. The documentation will prove invaluable during the evaluation phase of the process.

Community Evaluation

Evaluation is used to identify whether the goals and program objectives were met. There are various models of program evaluation. Health care organizations commonly use the structure, process, and outcomes method. Donabedian (1980) have described this approach, which focuses on the following:

Structure—the qualifications of personnel; the adequacy of buildings and offices, supplies, and equipment; and the target population's characteristics

Process—the number of people who attended a health education program, the number of pamphlets distributed, and the program's efficiency

Outcomes—whether program objectives and community goals were met. Program evaluation should be ongoing so that an improvement in the way health care is delivered will affect the target population's health status.

Key Points

- Caring for children within a community requires a multidisciplinary approach.
- Healthy communities provide children with high-quality medical care and a nurturing, safe place to live and grow.
- Community health nursing focuses on promoting and maintaining the health of individuals, families, and groups in the community setting.
- Individual families and communities may have demographic characteristics that affect their risk for disease or injury.
- Epidemiology is the science of population health applied to the detection of morbidity and mortality in a population.
- Community health programs are based on three levels of intervention: primary, secondary, and tertiary.

- Economic evaluations provide objective information to establish a program's value to society.
- A community needs assessment involves collection of subjective and objective information about the community.
- A community health diagnosis is a problem with a defined cause related to a community problem.
- Program planning and implementation in the community require collaboration between the nurse and community members who are in positions to promote change.
- Evaluation of effective community programs includes consideration of the structure, process, and outcomes related to the program.

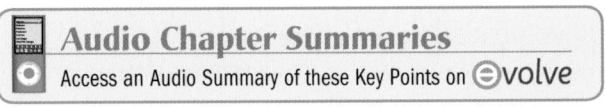

Audio Chapter Summaries

Access an Audio Summary of these Key Points on evolve

References

Allender, J. A., & Spradley, B. W. (2005). Opportunities and challenges of community health nursing. In J. A. Allender & B. W. Spradley (Eds.), *Community health nursing: Promoting and protecting the public's health*. Philadelphia: Lippincott Williams & Wilkins.

Anderson, E. T. (2008). A model to guide practice. In E. T. Anderson & J. McFarlane (Eds.), *Community as partner: Theory and practice in nursing* (5th ed.). Philadelphia: Lippincott Williams & Wilkins.

Anderson, E. T., & McFarlane, J. (2008). Community assessment. In E. T. Anderson & J. McFarlane (Eds.), *Community as partner: Theory and practice in nursing* (5th ed.). Philadelphia: Lippincott Williams & Wilkins.

Brosnan, C. A., & Swint, J. M. (2001). Cost analysis: Concepts and application. *Public Health Nursing, 18*(1), 13–18. doi: 10.1111/j.1525-1446.2001.00013.x

Brosnan, C. A., et al. (2005). Student nurses participate in public health research and practice through a school-based screening program. *Public Health Nursing, 22*(3), 260–266. doi: 10.1111/j.0737-1209.2005.220310.x

Canadian Community Health Nursing. (2003). Canadian community health nursing: Standards of practice. Retrieved from http://www.chnc.ca/documents/chn_standards_of_practice_mar08_english.pdf.

Canadian Public Health Association. (2010). *Public health ~ Community health nursing practice in Canada: Roles and activities* (4th ed.). Retrieved from http://www.chnc.ca/documents/PublicHealth-CommunityHealthNursinginCanadaRolesandActivities2010.pdf.

Cashaw, S. A. (2008). Epidemiology, demography and community health. In E. T. Anderson & J. McFarlane (Eds.), *Community as partner: Theory and practice in nursing* (5th ed.). Philadelphia: Lippincott Williams & Wilkins.

Centers for Disease Control and Prevention. (2005). *CDC statement on screening children for Acanthosis nigricans in schools and communities*. Retrieved from http://www.cdc.gov/diabetes/news/docs/an.htm.

Community Health Nurses of Canada. (2009). *Public health nursing discipline specific competencies version 1.0*. Retrieved from http://www.chnc.ca/documents/competencies_june_2009_english.pdf.

Dobson, S., Scheifele, D., & Bell, A. (1995). Assessment of a universal, school-based hepatitis B vaccination program. *Journal of the American Medical Association, 274*(15), 1209–1213. doi: 10.1001/jama.1995.03530150033030

Donabedian, A. (1980). *The definition of quality and approaches to its assessment*. Ann Arbor, MI: Health Administration Press.

Drummond, M. F., et al. (2005). *Methods for the economic evaluation of health care programmes* (3rd ed.). New York: Oxford University Press.

Flynn, B. C., & Ivanov, L. L. (2004). Health promotion through healthy communities and cities. In M. Stanhope & J. Lancaster (Eds.), *Community and public health nursing* (6th ed.). St. Louis: Mosby.

Gold, M. R., et al. (1996). Identifying and valuing outcomes. In M. R. Gold, et al. (Eds.), *Cost-effectiveness in health and medicine*. New York: Oxford University Press.

Hennekens, C. H., & Buring, J. E. (1987). *Epidemiology in medicine*. Boston: Little, Brown.

Joffres, C., Heath, S., Farquharson, J., Barkhouse, K., Latter, C., & MacLean, D. (2004). Facilitators and challenges to organizational capacity building in heart health promotion. *Quality Health Research, 14*(1), 39–60. doi: 10.1177/1049732303259802

Leavell, H. R., & Clark, E. G. (1965). *Preventive medicine for the doctor in his community: An epidemiologic approach*. New York: McGraw-Hill.

McEwen, M., & Nies, M. A. (2007). Health: a community view. In M. A. Nies & M. McEwen (Eds.), *Community/public health: Promoting the health of populations*. Philadelphia: Saunders.

McKeown, R. E., & Hilfinger, D. K. (2004). Epidemiology. In M. Stanhope & J. Lancaster (Eds.), *Community and public health nursing* (6th ed.) St. Louis: Mosby.

Public Health Agency of Canada. (2007). *Community capacity building tool: A tool for planning, building and reflecting on community capacity in community based health projects*. Retrieved from http://www.phac-aspc.gc.ca/canada/regions/ab-nwt-tno/documents/CCBT_English_web_000.pdf.

Public Health Agency of Canada. (2010a). *Centre for health promotion*. Retrieved from http://www.phac-aspc.gc.ca/chhd-sdsh/index-eng.php.

Public Health Agency of Canada. (2010b). *What determines health?* Retrieved from http://www.phac-aspc.gc.ca/ph-sp/determinants/index-eng.php.

Public Health Agency of Canada. (2010c). *Community action program for children*. Retrieved from http://www.phac-aspc.gc.ca/hp-ps/dca-dea/prog-ini/capc-pace/index-eng.php.

Public Health Agency of Canada. (2010d). *Curbing childhood obesity: A federal, provincial and territorial framework for action to promote healthy weights*. Retrieved from http://www.phac-aspc.gc.ca/hp-ps/hl-mvs/framework-cadre/index-eng.php.

Public Health Agency of Canada. (2010e). *Health promotion*. Retrieved from http://www.phac-aspc.gc.ca/hp-ps/index-eng.php.

Statistics Canada. (2008). *Leading causes of death in Canada, 2008*. Retrieved from http://www.statcan.gc.ca/pub/84-215-x/84-215-x2011001-eng.htm.

Underwood, J. M., et al. (2009). Building community and public health nursing capacity: A synthesis report of the National Community Health Nursing Study. *Canadian Journal of Public Health, 100*(5), 1–11.

Williams, C. A. (2011). Populations-focused practice: The foundation of specialization in public health practice. In M. Stanhope & J. Lancaster (Eds.), *Community and public health nursing* (7th ed.). St. Louis: Mosby.

Wilson, J. M., & Jungner, G. (1968). *Principles and practice of screening for disease. Public Health Papers*, No. 34. Geneva: World Health Organization.

World Health Organization. (2010). *Immunization surveillance, assessment and monitoring*. Retrieved from http://www.who.int/immunization_monitoring/data/en/index.html.

Additional Resources

Canadian Public Health Association: http://www.cpha.ca/en/default.aspx
Community Health Nurses of Canada: http://www.chnc.ca/default.cfm

Unit 7

31 Family Influences on Child Health Promotion

Learning Objectives

On completion of this chapter, the reader will be able to:

- Discuss definitions of family.
- Describe three major family theories.
- Identify different family structures found in Canada.
- Discuss the effect of family size and configuration on personality development.
- Discuss role transition experienced by new parents.
- Explain various parenting behaviours, such as parenting styles, disciplinary patterns, and communication skills.
- Demonstrate an understanding of special parenting situations, such as adoption, divorce, lone parenting, parenting in reconstituted families, and dual-earner families.

Electronic Resources

Additional information related to the content in Chapter 31 can be found on

evolve the companion Web site at

http://evolve.elsevier.com/Canada/Perry/maternal/

- Examination Review Questions
- Case Study—Family Functioning

General Concepts

Definition of Family

The term **family** has been defined in many different ways according to the individual's own frame of reference, value judgement, or **discipline**. There is no universal definition of family; a family is what an individual considers it to be. Biologists describe the family as fulfilling the biological function of perpetuation of the species. Psychologists emphasize interpersonal aspects of family and its responsibility for personality development. Economists view the family as a productive unit providing for material needs. In sociology, the family is depicted as a social unit interacting with the larger society, creating contexts within which cultural values and identity are formed. Others define family in terms of the relationships of the persons who make up the family units. The most common types of relationships are *consanguineous* (blood relationships), *affinal* (marital relationships), and *family of origin* (family unit a person is born into).

Earlier definitions of family emphasized that family members were related by legal ties or genetic relationships and lived in the same household with specific roles. Later definitions have been broadened to reflect structural and functional changes. A family can be defined as an institution in which individuals, related through biology or enduring commitments and representing similar or different generations and genders, participate in roles involving mutual socialization, nurturance, and emotional commitment (Lerner, Sparks, & McCubbin, 1999).

Considerable controversy has been generated about the newer concepts of family, such as communal families, lone-parent families, and gay and lesbian families. To accommodate these and other varieties of family styles, the descriptive term *household* is frequently used (see Chapter 2, p. 17, for discussion of various family formations).

Nursing of infants and children is intimately involved with care of the child *and* the family. Consequently, nurses must be aware of the functions of the family, various types of family structures, and theories that provide a foundation for understanding the changes within a family and for directing family-oriented interventions.

Family Nursing Interventions

In working with children, nurses must include family members in their care plan. To discover family dynamics, strengths, and weaknesses, a thorough family assessment is necessary (see Chapter 34). When working with families, the nurse's choice of interventions depends on the theoretic family model that is used (Box 31-1) (for a brief synopsis of family theories, see Table 2-1). For example, in family systems theory, the focus is on the interaction of family members within larger environments. In this case, using group dynamics to involve all

BOX 31-1 Family Nursing Interventions

- Behaviour modification
- Case management and coordination
- Collaborative strategies
- Contracting
- Counselling, including support, cognitive reappraisal, and reframing
- Empowering families through active participation
- Environmental modification
- Family advocacy
- Family crisis intervention
- Networking, including use of self-help groups and social support
- Providing information and technical expertise
- Role modelling
- Role supplementation
- Teaching strategies, including stress management, lifestyle modifications, and anticipatory guidance

(From Friedman, M. M., Bowden, V. R., & Jones, E. G. [2003]. *Family nursing: Research theory and practice* [5th ed.]. Upper Saddle River, NJ: Pearson Education.)

members in the intervention process and being a skilful communicator are essential. Systems theory also presents excellent opportunities for **anticipatory guidance**. Because each family member reacts to every **stress** experienced by that system, nurses can intervene to help the family prepare for and cope with changes. Each stress point represents an opportunity for change and **learning** because families are more open to interventions at this time (Brazelton, 1995). In the family stress theory, crisis intervention strategies are employed to help family members cope with the challenging event. In developmental theory, the nurse provides anticipatory guidance to prepare members for transition to the next family stage.

Family Roles, Relationships, and Strengths

Each individual has a position, or status, in the family structure and plays culturally and socially defined roles in interactions within the family. Each family also has its own traditions and values and sets its own standards for interaction within and outside the group. Each determines the experiences the children should have, those they are to be shielded from, and how each of these experiences meets the needs of family members. When family ties are strong, social control is highly effective, and most members conform to their roles willingly and with commitment. Conflicts arise when people do not fulfill their roles in ways that meet other family members' expectations, either because they are unaware of the expectations, they choose not to meet them, or they are incapable of meeting them.

Parental Roles

In all family groups the socially recognized status of father and mother exists with socially sanctioned roles that prescribe appropriate sexual behaviour and childrearing responsibilities. Guides for behaviour in these roles serve to control sexual conflict in society and provide for prolonged care of children. The degree to which parents are committed and the ways in which they play their roles are influenced by a number of variables and by the parents' unique socialization experience.

Parental role definitions are changing as a result of the changing economy and increased opportunities for women. Women are achieving equality with men in education, more women have entered the workforce, and the number of women who choose to have fewer children or none at all is increasing. As the role of women has changed, the complementary role of men has also changed. Many fathers are taking a more active role in childrearing and household tasks. As the redefinition of gender roles continues in Canadian families, there may be role conflicts in many families because of a cultural lag of persisting traditional role definitions.

Role Learning

Roles are learned through the socialization process. During all stages of **development**, children learn and practise, through interaction with others and in their play, a set of social roles and characteristics of other roles. They behave in patterned and more or less predictable ways because they learn roles that define mutual expectations in typical social relationships. Although role definitions are changing, the basic determinants of parenting remain the same. Several determinants of parenting infants and young children are parental personality and mental well-being, systems of support, and child characteristics. These determinants have been used as consistent measurements to determine a person's success in fulfilling the parental role.

Parents, peers, authority figures, and other socializing agents who use positive and negative sanctions to ensure conformity to their norms transmit role conceptions. Role behaviours positively reinforced by rewards such as love, affection, friendship, and honours are strengthened. Negative reinforcement takes the form of ridicule, withdrawal of love, expressions of disapproval, or banishment.

In some **cultures**, the role behaviour expected of children conflicts with desirable adult behaviour. For example, in some North American families, children are expected to be submissive in childhood but dominant as adults. This conflict of expectations is known as *role discontinuity*. Other cultures value the same behaviours, such as courage and aggression, in both children and adults; this provides *role continuity*.

One responsibility of the family is to develop culturally appropriate role behaviour in children. Children learn to perform in expected ways that are consistent with their position in the family and culture. The observed behaviour of each child is a single manifestation—a combination of social influences and individual psychological processes. In this way, the uniting of the children's intrapersonal system (the self) with the family's interpersonal system is simultaneously understood as the child's conduct.

Role structuring initially takes place within family units, in which children fulfill a set of roles and respond to the roles of their parents and other family members. The children's roles are shaped primarily by the parents, who apply direct or evolve Case Study—Family Functioning

indirect pressures to induce or force children into the desired patterns of behaviour or direct their efforts toward modification of the child's role responses on a mutually acceptable basis. Children respond to life situations according to behaviours learned in reciprocal transactions. As they acquire important role-taking skills, their relationships with others change. For instance, when a teenager is also a mother but lives in a household with her grandmother, the teenager may be viewed more as an adolescent than as a mother. Children become proficient at understanding others as they acquire the ability to discriminate their own perspectives from those of others. Children who get along well with others and attain status in the peer group have well-developed role-taking skills.

Family Size and Configuration

Parenting practices differ between small and large families. In small families, more emphasis is placed on the individual development of the children. Parenting is intensive rather than extensive, and there is constant pressure to measure up to family expectations. Children's development and achievement are measured against those of other children in the neighbourhood and social class. In small families, there tends to be more democratic participation by the children than in larger families. Adolescents in small families often identify more strongly with their parents and rely more on parental advice. They have well-developed, autonomous inner controls as contrasted with adolescents from larger families, who may rely more on adult authority.

Children in a large family are generally able to adjust to a variety of changes and crises. There is often more emphasis on the group and less on the individual (Fig. 31-1). Cooperation is essential, often because of economic necessity. The large number of people sharing a limited amount of space requires a greater degree of organization, administration, and authoritarian control. A dominant family member (a parent or older child) wields control and discipline. The number of children can reduce the intimate, one-to-one contact between the parent and any individual child. Consequently, children turn to each other for what they cannot get from their parents. The reduced parent–child contact encourages individual children to adopt specialized roles to gain recognition in the family. Siblings are usually attuned to what constitutes misbehaviour. Sibling disapproval or ostracism is frequently a more meaningful disciplinary measure than parental interventions. In situations such as death or illness of a parent, an older sibling often assumes responsibility for the family at considerable personal sacrifice. Large families generate a sense of security in the children that is fostered by sibling support and cooperation. Adolescents from a large family tend to be more peer- than family-oriented.

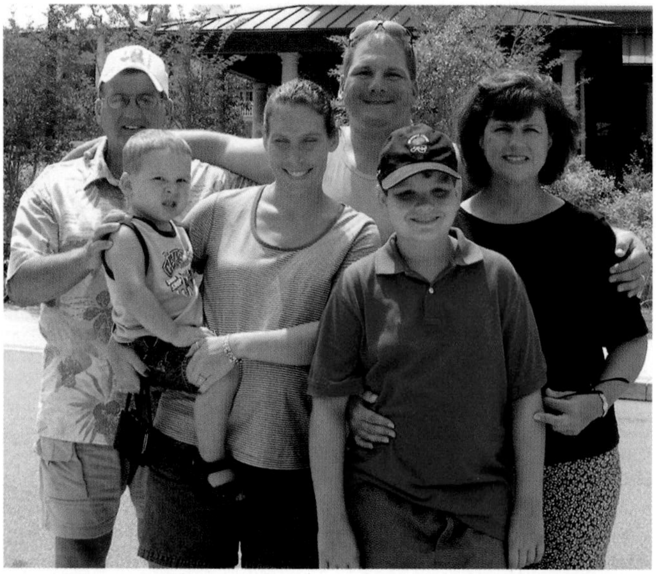

Fig. 31-1 Family structure promotes strong relationships among its members.

Sibling Interactions

Spacing of Children

Age differences between siblings affect the childhood environment, but to a lesser extent than does the sex of the sibling. The arrival of a sibling is often difficult for toddlers and preschool children, especially between the ages of 2 and 3 years old. At this age, they are still attached to their parents and do not understand the concept of sharing. An older child is able to understand the situation and is less likely to see the newcomer as a threat, although the child does feel the loss of the only-child status. In general, the narrower the spacing between siblings, the more the children influence one another, especially in emotional characteristics. The wider the spacing, the greater the influence of the parents.

Traditionally, sibling relationships were viewed from a Freudian perspective that emphasized the concept of **sibling rivalry**. Recently, researchers have viewed siblings through developmental or ecological frameworks that focus on interactions within family systems (Friedman, Bowden, & Jones, 2003). The results of these broader perspectives provide a picture of rich and varied sibling interactions (Fig. 31-2).

Sibling Functions

The sibling relationship's most unique feature is its duration. The longest relationship one will share with another human being is usually the sibling relationship, which lasts

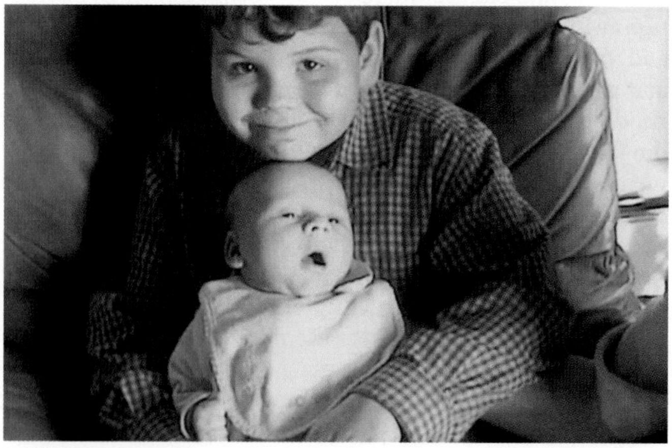

Fig. 31-2 Older school-age children often enjoy taking responsibility for the care of a younger sibling.

through a lifetime (often 50 to 80 years), compared to a parent relationship of approximately 30 to 50 years.

Siblings exert power, exchange services, and express feelings in reciprocal ways that are often not revealed in the presence of the parents. They see themselves in their brother or sister, experience life vicariously through their sibling's behaviour, and begin to expand on their own possibilities. Siblings can also be touchstones for what the other would not like to be, and they use each other as yardsticks for comparison. They provide a sounding board for each other and offer a safe forum for experimenting with new behaviours and roles. Brothers and sisters provide each other with tangible services (e.g., lending money, clothing, toys, or sports equipment; teaching a skill), help each other with childhood problems, provide support in dealing with parents or others outside the family, and provide introductions to new friendship groups. Children learn to negotiate and bargain, and sometimes to manipulate, from their siblings. Their interactions with each other provide opportunities for conflict and conflict resolution. They protect one another from parental-executive abuse of power and can form a coalition to deal with issues of authority, power, and emotional support. Negotiating with parents is stronger when siblings act together rather than singly.

Siblings interpret the outside world for each other and perform educative functions for the parents. A related function is *pioneering*, in which one sibling initiates a process, thereby giving the others permission to follow, such as breaking explicit family rules, taking new pathways, or adopting different moral or political codes and lifestyles.

Tattling can be an important lever in sibling interactions. On the other hand, there is often a conspiracy of silence among siblings, leaving the parents feeling isolated and excluded. A willingness to maintain each other's privacy often serves as a powerful bond of loyalty that distinguishes the relationship between siblings from that between friends.

More Active Sibling Relationships

Sibling relationships vary among cultures. Also, some social factors are giving the sibling relationship greater significance in North American families than in the past. Shrinking family size, longer lifespans, divorce and remarriage, geographic mobility, maternal employment, alternative sources of child care, competitive pressures, stress, and parental insufficiency may be propelling siblings into greater contact with each other and emotional interdependence than ever before. Siblings often join forces to confront the trauma of divorce, and they frequently rely on each other for support when parents remarry. With larger numbers of mothers now working outside the home, young siblings can have significant amounts of time when a personally committed adult does not monitor their relationship, resulting in more unsupervised children. In a worried, mobile, small-family, high-stress, fast-paced, parent-absent society, children often turn to a brother or sister to meet their needs for contact, constancy, and permanency.

Ordinal Position

Researchers have observed that the birth position of children affects their personalities. Parents treat children differently, and sibling interactions are different, depending on the child's position within the family. Power is unequally distributed among siblings. Older siblings attempt to dominate younger ones; younger siblings develop interpersonal skills, learn the ability to negotiate, and accept unfavourable outcomes to a greater extent than older siblings. Later-born children are obliged to interact with other siblings from birth and seem to be more outgoing and make friends more easily than firstborns. General characteristics of children in the ordinal positions are presented in Box 31-2. It is important to bear in mind, however, that children vary tremendously, and such generalizations do not always apply to individuals.

The Only Child

Being the only child in a family has traditionally been considered a disadvantage. Only children have been described as selfish, spoiled, dependent, and lonely. However, they do not demonstrate more evidence of maladjustment or self-centredness than other children, and they tend to strongly

BOX 31-2 Influence of Ordinal Position on Children

Firstborn Children

- Are more achievement oriented
- Are more dominant
- Receive more physical punishment
- Have stronger consciences; are more self-disciplined and inner directed
- Are more socially anxious
- Are prone to feelings of guilt
- Identify more with parents than with peers
- Are more conservative
- Are subject to greater parental expectations
- Begin to speak earlier in life
- Demonstrate higher intellectual achievement
- Plan better and experience fewer frustrations

Middle Children

- Have more demands made on them for household help
- Are praised less often
- Receive less of the parents' time
- Learn to compromise and be adaptable
- Are less stimulated toward achievement
- Are more difficult to characterize because of a variety of positions in the family

Youngest Children

- Are less dependent than firstborn children
- Are less tense, more affectionate, and more good-natured
- Tend to identify more with a peer group than with parents
- Are more flexible in their thinking
- Have fewer demands placed on them for household help

Only Children

- Resemble firstborn children
- Are more mature and cultivated
- Experience greater parental pressure for mature behaviour and achievement
- Demonstrate superiority in language facility
- Rarely develop into the stereotype of a spoiled, selfish child
- Often enjoy a rich fantasy life as a result of isolation

resemble firstborn children in respects such as higher educational goals. Only children perform better on cognitive tests, are more mature and socially sensitive, and demonstrate superiority in language facility.

Only children enjoy the advantage of having parents who can devote more time to them, talk to them, and stimulate them in intellectual activities. Parents also exert greater pressure for mature behaviour at an early age and for achievement. Relative isolation from peers contributes to intellectual pursuits and encourages a rich fantasy life, independence, and originality.

Multiple Births

Multiple births occur with variable frequency. While twins are not uncommon in the population, triplets are rare, and quadruplets or quintuplets are extremely unusual. In 2004, Statistics Canada reported the incidence of multiple births without assistance of fertility treatment to be as follows: 1 in 90 births for twins; 1 in 8100 births for triplets; 1 in 729,000 births for quadruplets; and 1 in 65,610,000 for quintuplets. In any of these situations, the offspring can be of the like or unlike sex (i.e., derived from a single ovum; from multiple ova; or from a combination of the two, which can involve one or more cell divisions). The cause of twinning is unknown, but the increase in the number of larger multiples (quintuplets, sextuplets) during recent years has been associated with reproductive technologies (see Chapter 7, section on assisted reproductive technologies, p. 133), which has contributed to 35% of all Canadian multiple births (PHAC, 2004). Even though there has been a 19% drop in the overall Canadian birth rate between the years 1993 and 2002, the rate of multiple births has increased by 18%; it has risen from 2.2% in 1995 to 3.0% in 2008 (PHAC, 2004, 2012; Statistics Canada, 2004). Because women in their 30s are almost 2.5 times as likely as women in their 20s to have higher-order plural births, the rise in the multiple-birth ratio has been associated with increased childbearing among older women and the expanded use of fertility drugs (Hamilton et al., 2007).

Twins are of two distinct types: *identical*, or *monozygotic* (MZ), and *fraternal*, or *dizygotic* (DZ) (Box 31-3). Statistics Canada (2004) reported that approximately 3% of Canadian babies are born in sets of two and three and about 95% of these births were twins. On average, there are 26 multiple births every day in Canada; as of 2004, approximately 41% of these children were born in Ontario (Statistics Canada, 2004).

A special kind of sibling relationship is observed in twins, although getting along with each other and quarrelling are not much different from these behaviours in any other two siblings, especially if they are different-sex fraternal twins. Twins tend to work out a relationship that is reasonably satisfactory to both and demonstrate early independence from parental attention. They develop a remarkable capacity for **cooperative play** and considerable loyalty and generosity toward each other. It is not uncommon for a private language to evolve between the twins that may interfere with the development of the family language.

In a twinship, one member of the pair, to a greater or lesser extent, is more dominant, outgoing, and assertive than the other, often to the parents' consternation. The seemingly more passive twin is nonetheless able to accomplish as much and get his or her way as frequently as the more assertive twin.

BOX 31-3 Characteristics of Twins

Monozygotic (Identical) Twins	Dizygotic (Fraternal) Twins
Result of one fertilized ovum that became separated early in development	Result of fertilization of two ova
Alike physically and genetically	Differ physically and genetically
Same sex	May be same or opposite sex
Frequency—Occurs uniformly in all populations	Frequency—Varies among races (highest in Blacks; lowest in Asians; intermediate in Whites)
Unaffected by maternal age	More common with advancing maternal age (maximum at age 35 to 39 years, then decreases rapidly)
Tendency unaffected by heredity	Marked familial tendency Expressed only in the female Fathers appear to transmit disposition toward double ovulation to daughters
Similar behaviour	Dissimilar behaviour; more sibling rivalry

Researchers have also observed a difference in behaviour between identical and fraternal twins. There is near-unison in the actions of identical twins (although they alternate in assuming the leadership), but fraternal twins, even of the same sex, do not display this quality. Sibling rivalry can be pronounced in fraternal twins, especially in different-sex twins.

Identical twins also differ in their response to the tendency of some parents to treat twins exactly alike. The present philosophy is to determine the degree to which the children demonstrate an inclination toward togetherness. Some twins thrive best when they are constantly in each other's company; others prefer more individuality and separateness. The conservative approach is to allow the children to follow their natural inclinations. Early years of togetherness are often the basis of the children's security, and separating them too early may produce unnecessary stress. Fostering individual differences as they become evident could ease the process of separation, when it becomes advisable.

Parental Adjustment

The entrance of any new member into a household creates stress, but with multiple births, two or more new members must be incorporated into the family at the same time. The problems are obvious. Two infants must be provided with physical care, including feeding and diapering, and all of the purchasing and preparation that accompanies the care of any infant is multiplied. Scheduling becomes crucial, and advancement in development brings new problems and adjustments (e.g., space and sleeping arrangements, selection of a stroller and other equipment). Toys must be selected carefully. As play becomes a serious business, some toys that would be safe and appropriate for a single child can become weapons when two infants share a playpen. It is a good idea to select different toys for each child as they grow older and to encourage sharing.

Parenting

Motivation for Parenthood

A dominant characteristic in all societies is that adults are expected to become parents and to be gratified by the experience. Pressures of tradition, sentiment regarding the state of parenthood, and religious beliefs influence decision making related to becoming a parent because conformity to social-role expectations is a strong influence in family planning.

Factors that influence family size are social class, religion, race, financial stability, type of conjugal-role relationships, and the social–psychological aspects of sexual relations. With divorce and remarriage, an individual may decide to have more children with the new spouse.

Preparation for Parenthood

The basic goals of parenting are to promote children's physical survival and health, foster the skills and abilities that are necessary to be a self-sustaining adult, and foster behavioural capabilities for optimizing cultural values and beliefs. New parents often approach parenthood with limited experience and knowledge. Parents learn by trial and error, committing the same mistakes that have been committed by countless other parents, but they somehow manage to accomplish the task, becoming more skilled with each additional child. Tradition, rather than rational planning, furnishes the chief norms for childrearing. Experience in having been nurtured as a child is an essential component of successful parenting.

Their own parents are probably the only persons whom parents observe intimately in the parental role. This results in *generational continuity*—parents often rear their own children in much the same way as they themselves were reared. Other essential skills that parents need in order to feel comfortable in the parenting role include a basic understanding of childhood growth and development, bathing, feeding, use of play, and interpersonal communication skills.

Transition to Parenthood

The birth of a child is a major transition within a family; the early weeks of an infant's life require parents to make drastic adjustments. Even though the parents have anticipated and prepared for the child's arrival, the birth presents challenges of providing total care 24 hours a day for a new member of the family. A crisis may occur if the event is perceived as disturbing old habits and relationships and eliciting new responses. The birth requires role changes or significantly modifies former relationships. In addition to the roles of husband and wife, the couple must assume the roles of father and mother (or in the case of same-sex couples, of becoming parents).

The advent of a new family member requires that the family cope with greater financial responsibilities, a possible loss of income, changes in sleeping habits, and less time for parents to spend with each other (especially if it is a firstborn) and with other children. If these events are perceived as adverse, the couple's bond may be disrupted and the couple's intimacy and affection reduced.

Other factors influencing the transition to the parental role include the following:

- Parents with previous experience, such as having another child, appear to be more relaxed, have less conflict in disciplinary relationships, and are more aware of normal growth and development.
- The amount of stress experienced by one or both parents may interfere with their ability to exhibit patience and understanding and to cope with their children's behaviour.
- Special characteristics of the infant, such as being temperamentally difficult, can cause the parents to lose confidence and doubt their abilities. Infants with special care needs (such as those associated with a disability) can be a significant source of added stress.
- Fathers who are highly involved with their child often feel more comfortable in the parenting role (Fig. 31-3).
- Stressed marital relationships can have a negative effect on parental transition because marital tension can alter caregiving routines and interfere with enjoyment of the infant. Conversely, parents' support and encouragement of one another serve as positive influences on the establishment of a satisfying parental role.

Support Systems

Successful adaptation to the stress of transition to parenthood involves at least two types of family resources (McCubbin & McCubbin, 1994). *Internal resources* such as adaptability and integration are the first type. Changing from an orderly, predictable life to a relatively disordered, unpredictable one is a universal adaptation that families must make. Rigid schedules are impossible to maintain, and former activities must be curtailed or abandoned. Spending quality time with a child can promote health and a successful transition (Fig. 31-4). *Adaptation* is reflected in learning to be patient, becoming better organized, and becoming more flexible. *Integration* refers to the couple's attempt to continue some activities they engaged in before they became parents. In this way, couples are able to

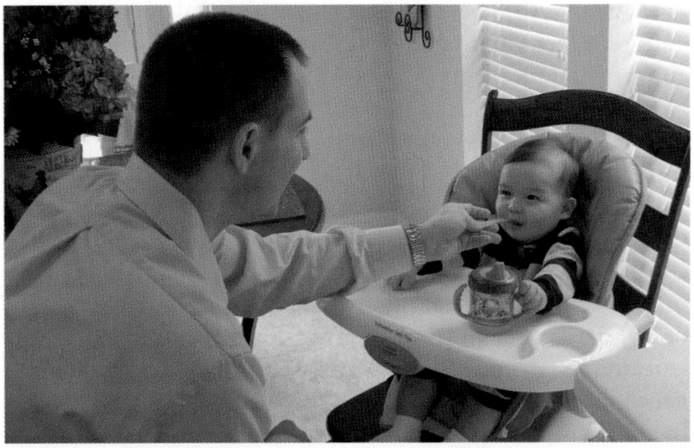

Fig. 31-3 Fathers who assume care of their children may feel more comfortable and successful in their parenting role.

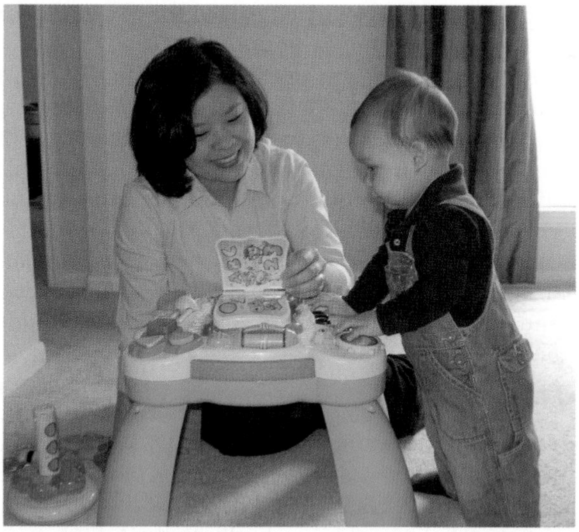

Fig. 31-4 Quality time spent with a child is essential to a family's health and well-being.

maintain a sense of continuity and appreciate the importance of the husband–wife or partner–spouse relationship.

The second resource for dealing with stress is the use of *coping strategies* that strengthen the family's organization and functioning. These include the use of social support systems and community resources and the adoption of a future orientation. Interpersonal supports that provide information, advice, and caretaking can be derived from friends, relatives, and neighbours. Relationships with family, friends, and community are essential. For parents, positive, supportive work relationships are important. Equally important is time spent with friends. Arranging for time away from the child is also beneficial. One parent can assume care of the family to allow the other parent some time to himself or herself. Adoption of a future orientation reassures parents that things will get better, that they will cope, and that it is realistic to plan for the time when they will be able to engage in self-fulfilling activities.

It is also reassuring to know that others experience ambivalent feelings toward parenthood and share the same difficulties and frustrations. Exchanging ideas and experiences with other parents and with one's partner provides an opportunity to voice concerns and to learn new ways to cope with multiple childrearing problems.

Parenting Behaviours

Parental Styles of Control

Parenting styles can be described as authoritarian, permissive, or authoritative. *Authoritarian* or *dictatorial* parents try to control their children's behaviour and attitudes through unquestioned mandates. They establish rules and regulations or standards of conduct that they expect to be followed rigidly and unquestioningly. They value and reward absolute obedience, mute acceptance of their word, and unfailing respect for the family's principles and beliefs. They forcefully punish any behaviour that is contrary to parental standards. Parental authority is exercised with little explanation and little involvement of the child in decision making. The message is: "Do it because I say so." Punishment may not be corporal but may involve stern withdrawal of love and approval.

Careful training often results in rigidly conforming behaviour in children, who tend to be sensitive, shy, self-conscious, retiring, and submissive. They are more apt to be courteous, loyal, honest, and dependable but docile. These behaviours are more typically observed when close supervision and affection accompany parental authority. If not, this style of parenting may be associated with defiant and antisocial behaviour.

Permissive or *laissez-faire* parents exert little or no control over their children's actions. They avoid imposing their own standards of conduct and allow their children to regulate their own activity as much as possible. These parents consider themselves to be resources for the children, not role models. If rules do exist, the parents explain the underlying reason, elicit the children's opinions, and consult them in decision-making processes. They employ lax, inconsistent discipline; do not set sensible limits; and do not prevent the children from upsetting the home routine. These parents rarely punish the children. Consequently, the children control the parents and are often disobedient, disrespectful, and generally defiant of authority.

Authoritative or *democratic* parents combine practices from both of the previously described parenting styles. They direct their children's behaviour and attitudes by emphasizing the reason for rules and negatively reinforcing deviations. They respect each child's individuality and allow him or her to voice objections to family standards or regulations. Parental control is firm and consistent but tempered with encouragement, understanding, and security. Control is focused on the issue, not on withdrawal of love or fear of punishment. These parents foster "inner-directedness," a conscience that regulates behaviour based on feelings of guilt or shame for wrongdoing, not on fear of being caught or punished. Parents' realistic standards and reasonable expectations produce children with high self-esteem who are self-reliant, assertive, inquisitive, content, and highly interactive with other children.

Limit Setting and Discipline

In its broadest sense, *discipline* means to *teach* or refers to a set of rules governing conduct. In a narrower sense, it refers to the action taken to enforce the rules after noncompliance. *Limit setting* refers to establishing the rules or guidelines for behaviour. For example, parents can place limits on the amount of time children spend watching television or chatting online. The clearer the limits that are set and the more consistently they are enforced, the less need there is for disciplinary action.

Nurses can help parents establish realistic and concrete "rules." Limit setting and discipline are positive, necessary components of childrearing and serve several useful functions as they help children do the following:

- Test their limits of control
- Achieve in areas appropriate for mastery at their level
- Channel undesirable feelings into constructive activity
- Protect themselves from danger
- Learn socially acceptable behaviour

Children want and need limits. Unrestricted freedom is a threat to their security and safety. Through testing the limits imposed on them, children learn the extent to which they can manipulate their environment and gain reassurance from knowing that others are there to protect them from potential harm.

Minimizing Misbehaviour

The reasons for misbehaviour may include attention, power, defiance, and a display of inadequacy (e.g., the child misses classes because of a fear that he or she is unable to do the work). Children may also misbehave because the rules are not clear or consistently applied. Acting-out behaviour, such as a temper tantrum, may represent uncontrolled frustration, anger, depression, or pain. The best approach is to structure interactions with children so that unacceptable behaviour is prevented or minimized (see Family-Centred Teaching box).

General Guidelines for Implementing Discipline

Regardless of the type of discipline used, certain principles are essential to ensure efficacy of the approach (see Family-Centred Teaching box). Many strategies, such as behaviour modification, can only be implemented effectively when principles of consistency and timing are followed. A pattern of intermittent or occasional enforcement of limits actually prolongs the undesired behaviour because children learn that if they are persistent, the behaviour is permitted eventually. Delaying punishment weakens its intent, and practices such as telling the child, "Wait until your father comes home," are not only ineffectual but also convey negative messages about the other parent.

FAMILY-CENTRED TEACHING

Minimizing Misbehaviour

- Set realistic goals for acceptable behaviour and expected achievements.
- Structure opportunities for small successes to lessen feelings of inadequacy.
- Praise children for desirable behaviour with attention and verbal approval.
- Structure the environment to prevent unnecessary difficulties (e.g., place fragile objects in inaccessible areas).
- Set clear and reasonable rules; expect the same behaviour regardless of the circumstances; if exceptions are made, clarify that the change is for one time only.
- Teach desirable behaviour through your own example, such as using a quiet, calm voice rather than screaming.
- Review expected behaviour before special or unusual events, such as visiting a relative or having dinner in a restaurant.
- Phrase requests for appropriate behaviour positively, such as "Put the book down," rather than "Don't touch the book."
- Call attention to unacceptable behaviour as soon as it begins; use distraction to change the behaviour or offer alternatives to annoying actions, such as a quiet toy for one that is excessively noisy.
- Give advance notice or "friendly reminders," such as "When the TV program is over, it is time for dinner" or "I'll give you to the count of three and then we have to go."
- Be attentive to situations that increase the likelihood of misbehaving, such as overexcitement or fatigue, or to decreased personal tolerance to minor infractions.
- Offer sympathetic explanations for not granting a request, such as "I am sorry I can't read you a story now, but I have to finish dinner. Then we can spend time together."
- Keep any promises made to children.
- Avoid outright conflicts; temper discussions with statements such as "Let's talk about it and see what we can decide together" or "I have to think about it first."
- Provide children with opportunities for power and control.

FAMILY-CENTRED TEACHING

Implementing Discipline

Consistency—Implement disciplinary action exactly as agreed on and for each infraction.

Timing—Initiate discipline as soon as the child misbehaves; if delays are necessary, such as to avoid embarrassment, verbally disapprove of the behaviour and state that disciplinary action will be implemented.

Commitment—Follow through with the details of the discipline, such as timing of minutes; avoid distractions that may interfere with the plan, such as telephone calls.

Unity—Make certain that all caregivers agree on the plan and are familiar with the details to prevent confusion and alliances between the child and one parent.

Flexibility—Choose disciplinary strategies that are appropriate to the child's age and temperament and the severity of the misbehaviour.

Planning—Plan disciplinary strategies in advance and prepare the child, if feasible (e.g., explain use of time-out); for unexpected misbehaviour, try to discipline when you are calm.

Behaviour orientation—Always disapprove of the behaviour, not the child, with such statements as "That was a wrong thing to do. I am unhappy when I see behaviour like that."

Privacy—Administer discipline in private, especially with older children, who may feel ashamed in front of others.

Termination—After the discipline is administered, consider the child as having a "clean slate," and avoid bringing up the incident or lecturing.

Most important is the rewarding of good behaviour. Children need to know that you recognize their good behaviour. Praise and affection go a long way. Be specific, for example by stating "Thank you for picking up your toys when I asked you." Avoid general statements, such as "You were a good boy today."

Types of Discipline

In order to deal with misbehaviour, parents need to implement appropriate disciplinary action. Many approaches are available. *Reasoning* involves explaining why an act is wrong and is usually appropriate for older children, especially when moral issues are involved. Young children cannot be expected to "see the other side" because of their egocentrism. Children in the preoperative stage of cognitive development (toddlers and preschoolers) have a limited ability to distinguish between their point of view and those of others. Sometimes children use "reasoning" as a way of gaining attention. For example, they may misbehave thinking parents will give them a lengthy explanation of the wrongdoing and knowing that negative attention is better than no attention. When children use this technique, parents should end the explanation by stating, "This is the rule, and this is how I expect you to behave. I won't explain it any further."

Unfortunately, reasoning is often combined with *scolding*, which sometimes takes the form of shame or criticism. For example, the parent may state, "You are a bad boy for hitting your brother." Children take such remarks seriously and personally, believing that they *are* bad.

NURSING ALERT When reprimanding children, focus only on the misbehaviour, not on the child. Use of "I" messages rather than "you" messages expresses personal feelings without accusation or ridicule. For example, an "I" message attacks the behaviour—"I am upset when Johnny is punched; I don't like to see him hurt"—not the child.

Positive and negative reinforcement is the basis of *behaviour modification* theory—behaviour that is rewarded will be repeated; behaviour that is not rewarded will stop. Using rewards is a positive approach. By encouraging children to behave in specified ways, the parents can decrease tendencies to misbehave. With young children, using star stickers is an effective method. For older children, the "token system" is appropriate, especially if a certain number of tokens yields a special reward, such as a trip to the movies or a new book. In planning a *reward* system, parents must explain expected behaviours to children and establish rewards that are reinforcing. A chart should be used to record the stars or tokens, and an earned reward should be given promptly. Verbal approval should always accompany extrinsic rewards.

Consistently *ignoring* behaviour will eventually stop or minimize the act. Although this approach sounds simple, it is often difficult to implement consistently. Parents frequently give in and resort to previous patterns of discipline. Consequently, the behaviour is actually reinforced because the child learns that persistence gains parental attention. For ignoring to be effective, parents should (1) understand the process, (2) record the undesired behaviour before using ignoring to determine whether a problem exists and to compare results after ignoring is begun, (3) determine whether parental attention acts as a reinforcer, and (4) be aware of "response burst." *Response burst* occurs when the undesired behaviour increases after ignoring is initiated because children are testing the parents to see if they are serious about the plan.

The strategy of *consequences* involves allowing children to experience the results of their misbehaviour. It includes three types:

Natural—Those that occur without any intervention, such as being late and missing dinner

Logical—Those that are directly related to the rule, such as not being allowed to play with another toy until the used ones are put away

Unrelated—Those that are imposed deliberately, such as no playing until homework is completed or the use of time-out

Natural or logical consequences are preferred and effective if they are meaningful to children. For example, the natural consequence of living in a messy room may do little to encourage cleaning up, but allowing no friends over until the room is neat can be motivating! Withdrawing privileges is often an unrelated consequence. After the child experiences consequences, the parent should refrain from any comment, since the usual tendency is for the child to try to place blame for imposing the rule.

Time-out is actually a refinement of the common practice of sending children to their room and is a type of unrelated consequence. It is based on the premise of removing the reinforcer (i.e., the satisfaction or attention the child is receiving from the activity). When placed in an unstimulating and isolated place, children become bored and consequently agree to behave in order to re-enter the family group. Time-out avoids many of the problems of other disciplinary approaches. No physical punishment is involved; no reasoning or scolding is given; and parents do not need to be present for all of the time-out, thus facilitating their ability to consistently apply this type of discipline. Time-out offers children and parents a "cooling off" time. To be effective, the time-out must be planned in advance (see Family-Centred Teaching box).

Corporal or *physical punishment* most often takes the form of spanking. Based on the principles of aversive therapy, inflicting pain through spanking causes a dramatic short-term decrease in the behaviour. This approach has serious flaws: (1) it teaches children that violence is acceptable; (2) it may physically harm the child if it is the result of parental rage; and (3) children become accustomed to spanking, requiring more severe corporal punishment each time. Spanking can result in severe physical and psychological injury, and it interferes with effective parent–child interaction. In addition, when the parent is not around, the misbehaviour is likely to occur, since children have not learned to behave well for their own sake. Parental use of corporal punishment may also interfere with the child's development of moral reasoning.

In Canada, corporal punishment is allowed in only a mild form as a means to discipline children. The difference between child abuse and a mild form of discipline is outlined in Section 43 of the Criminal Law: "Every schoolteacher, parent or person standing in the place of a parent is justified in using force by way of correction toward a pupil or child, as the case may be, who is under his care, if the force does not exceed what is reasonable under the circumstances" (R.S.C. 1985, c. C-46, s.43) (Canadian Legal Information Institute, 2012). The vagueness noted in the wording of this law leads to possible misinterpretation and use of child abuse instead of discipline.

FAMILY-CENTRED TEACHING

Using Time-Out

Select an area for time-out that is safe, convenient, and unstimulating, but where the child can be monitored, such as the hallway, sitting on the first step of the stairs, or the couch or chair.

Determine what behaviours warrant a time-out.

Make certain children understand the "rules" and how they are expected to behave.

Explain to children the process of time-out:

- When they misbehave, they will be given one warning.
- If they do not obey, they will be sent to the place designated for time-out.
- They are to sit there for a specified period.
- If they cry, refuse, or display any disruptive behaviour, the time-out period will begin *after* they quiet down.
- When they are quiet for the duration of the time, they can then leave the room or place where they have been sent.
- A rule for the length of time-out is *1 minute per year of age*; use a kitchen timer with an audible bell to record the time rather than a watch.
- Implement time-out in a public place by selecting a suitable area, or explain to children that time-out will be spent immediately on returning home.

In 2009, two thirds of the 15,000 Canadian child and youth victims were physically assaulted by family-related members. Some of these assaults involved inappropriate use of discipline (Statistics Canada, 2009).

Special Parenting Situations

Parenting is a demanding task under ideal circumstances, but when parents and children are faced with additional challenging situations, the potential for family disruption is increased. Situations that can prove stressful for families are divorce, lone parenthood, blended families, adoption, and balancing of career and parenting. In addition, as cultural diversity increases in our communities, many immigrants are having to make the transitions to parenthood and to a new country, culture, and language simultaneously. Other situations that create unique parenting challenges are parental alcoholism, homelessness, and incarceration. Although these topics are not addressed here, the reader may wish to investigate them further.

Parenting the Adopted Child

While adoption laws in Canada vary from province to province and territories, in general they follow similar requirements and guidelines from child protection legislation, defining *parent* as anyone who has decision-making authority over a child and assumes all the rights, duties, obligations and responsibilities of the child. Certain adoption agencies may have specific requirements for adoptive parents, but in general anyone who is over 18 years and is a Canadian citizen without a criminal record is eligible to adopt a child (Department of Justice Canada, 2011).

Adoption establishes a legal relationship between a child and parents who are not related by birth but who have the same rights and obligations that exist between children and their biological parents. In the past, the biological mother alone made the decision to relinquish the rights to her child. In recent years, the courts have acknowledged the legal rights of the biological father regarding this decision. Concerned child advocates have questioned whether decisions that honour the father's rights are in the child's best interests. As the rights of the child have become recognized, older children have successfully dissolved their legal bond with their biological parents to pursue adoption by adults of their choice. Furthermore, there is a growing demand within the gay and lesbian community to adopt.

Unlike biological parents, who prepare for their child's birth with prenatal classes and the support of friends and relatives, adoptive parents have few sources of support and preparation for the new addition to their family. Nurses can provide the information, support, and reassurance needed to reduce parental anxiety regarding the adoptive process and can refer adoptive parents to parental support groups. Such resources can be contacted through a department of health or provincial or territorial social services office.

Most problems faced by adoptive parents are not different from those encountered by natural parents, but the desire to be a good parent is often intensified in adoptive parents. Adoptive parents have been portrayed as more apprehensive, insecure, and in need of assistance than biological parents. Some adoptive parents may actually need less assistance than biological parents. This situation may be related to adoptive parents' completely voluntary decision to become parents, the relatively long period of time they have to prepare for parenting, and maturity associated with adoption.

The sooner infants enter their adoptive home, the better the chances of **parent–infant attachment**. The more caregivers the infant had before adoption, the greater the risk for attachment problems. The infant must break the bond with the previous caregiver and form a new bond with the adoptive parents. Difficulties in forming an attachment depend on the amount of time infants have spent with earlier caregivers (e.g., birth mother, nurse, adoption agency personnel).

Siblings, adopted or biological, who are old enough to understand should be included in decisions regarding the commitment to adopt, with reassurance that they are not being replaced. Ways in which the siblings can interact with the adopted child should be stressed (Fig. 31-5).

Issues of Origin

The task of telling children that they are adopted can be a cause of deep concern and anxiety. There are no clear-cut guidelines for parents to follow in determining when and at what age children are ready for the information. Parents are naturally reluctant to present children with such potentially unsettling news. It is important that parents not withhold knowledge of the adoption from the child, since it is an essential component of the child's identity.

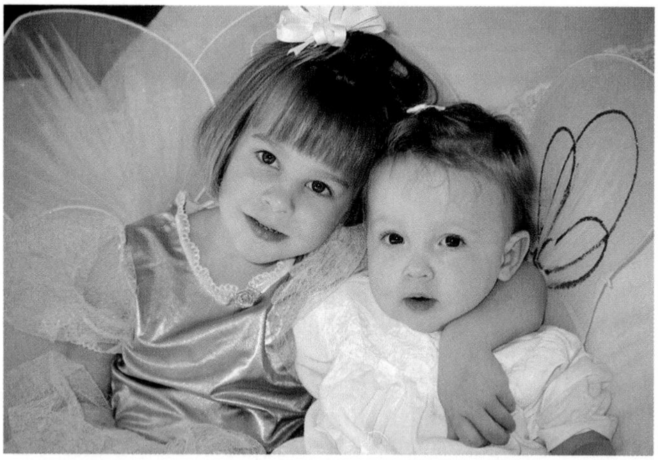

Fig. 31-5 An older sister lovingly embraces her adopted sister.

The timing arises naturally, as parents become aware of the child's readiness. Most authorities believe that children should be informed at an age young enough so that, as they grow older, they do not remember a time when they did not know they were adopted. The time is highly individual but must be right for parents and the child. It may be when children ask where babies come from, at which time children can also be told the facts of their adoption. If they are told in a way that conveys the idea that they were active participants in the selection process, they will be less likely to feel that they were abandoned, helpless victims. For example, parents can tell children that their personal qualities drew the parents to them. It is wise for parents to tell children that they are adopted before the children enter school, to avoid having them hear it from third parties. Complete honesty between parents and children strengthens the relationship.

Parents should anticipate behaviour changes after disclosure, especially in older children. Children who are struggling with the revelation that they are adopted may benefit from individual and family counselling. Children may use the fact of their adoption as a weapon to manipulate and threaten parents. Statements such as "My real mother would not treat me like this" or "You don't love me as much because I'm adopted" can hurt parents and increase their feelings of insecurity. Such statements may also cause parents to become overpermissive. Adopted children need the same undemanding love, combined with firm discipline and limit setting, as any other child.

Adolescence

Adolescence may be an especially trying time for parents. Whether adopted children have more adjustment issues than nonadopted children is debatable; more evidence-informed research on this area needs to be done in Canada. The normal confrontations of adolescents and parents can assume more painful aspects in adoptive families. Adolescents may use their adoption to defy parental authority or as a justification for aberrant behaviour. As they attempt to master the task of **identity formation**, the feeling of abandonment by their biological parents can come into awareness and may be intensified.

Adopted children fantasize about their biological parents and may feel the need to discover their parents' identity to define themselves and their own identity. It is important for parents to keep the lines of communication open and to reassure their child that they understand the need to search for their identity. In some provinces and territories, birth certificates are made legally available to adopted children when they come of age. It is important for parents to be honest with questioning adolescents and to tell them of this possibility (the parents themselves are unable to obtain the birth certificate; it is the responsibility of the adopted children, if they desire it).

Cross-Racial and International Adoption

Since 1993, Canadian parents considering international adoption must follow the laws of the adopting countries, which are governed by the Hague Convention. The Hague Convention on Protection of Children and Co-operation in Respect of Intercountry Adoption's main goals are to (1) protect the best interests of adopted children; (2) standardize the process between countries; and (3) prevent child abuse and child trafficking.

In 2009, 2122 international adoptions were reported in Canada, with the majority of children being welcomed from China, Haiti, the United States, and Vietnam. Canadian law offers parents seeking international adoptions two avenues: (1) The citizenship process, which makes the child a Canadian citizen, or (2) the immigration process, which makes the child a permanent resident (Citizenship and Immigration, 2010; Statistics Canada, 2011).

Adoption of children from racial backgrounds different from that of the family is commonplace. In addition to the problems faced by adopted children in general, children of a cross-racial adoption must deal with physical and sometimes cultural differences. It is advised that parents who adopt such children do everything possible to preserve the adopted children's racial heritage.

NURSING ALERT As a health care provider, it is important not to ask the wrong questions, such as "Is she yours, or is she adopted?" "What do you know about the 'real' mother?" "Do they have the same father?" or "How much did it cost to adopt him?"

Although the children are full-fledged members of an adopting family and citizens of the adopted country, if they have a strikingly different appearance from other family members or exhibit distinct racial or ethnic characteristics, challenges may be encountered outside the family. Bigotry may appear among relatives and friends. Strangers may make thoughtless comments and talk about the children as though they were not members of the family. It is vital that family members declare to others that this is their child and a cherished member of the family.

In international adoptions the medical information that parents receive may be incomplete or sketchy; weight, height, and head circumference are often the only objective information present in the child's medical record. Many internationally adopted children were born prematurely, and common health problems such as infant diarrhea and malnutrition delay growth and development. Some children have serious or multiple health problems that can be stressful for the parents.

Parenting and Divorce

Since the introduction of the divorce laws in 1968, there has been a steady increase in the Canadian divorce rate. However, since the 1990s, the divorce rate has remained relatively stable, with a less than 2% increase per year. The divorce rate is approximately 220.7 per 100,000 population (Statistics Canada, 2005). The process of divorce begins with a period of marital conflict of varying length and intensity, followed by a separation, the actual legal divorce, and re-establishment of different living arrangements. Because a function of parenthood is to provide for the security and emotional welfare of children, disruption of the family structure often engenders strong feelings of guilt in the divorcing parents.

During a divorce, parents' coping abilities may be compromised. The parents may be preoccupied with their own feelings, needs, and life changes and unable to be available and supportive to their children. Newly employed parents, usually mothers, are likely to leave children with new caregivers, in strange settings, or alone after school. The parent may also spend more time away from home, searching for or establishing new relationships. Sometimes, the adults feel frightened and alone and begin to depend on children as a substitute for the absent parent, which places an enormous burden on the child.

Common characteristics in the custodial household after separation and divorce include disorder, coercive types of control, inflammable tempers in parents and children, reduced parental competence, a greater sense of parental helplessness, poorly enforced discipline, and diminished regularity in enforcing household routines. Noncustodial parents are seldom prepared for the role of visitor, may assume the role of recreational and "fun" parent, and may not have a residence suitable for children's visits. They may also be concerned about maintaining the arrangement over the years to follow.

Impact of Divorce on Children

Numerous studies indicate that divorce has a profound effect on children. Many youngsters suffer for years from psychological and social difficulties associated with continuing or new stresses in the post-divorce family. Even when a divorce is amicable and open, children recall parental separation with the same emotions felt by victims of a natural disaster: loss, grief, and vulnerability to forces beyond their control.

The impact of divorce on children depends on several factors, including children's age and sex, parental interaction or conflict, and the quality of the parent–child relationship and parental care during the years following the divorce. Family characteristics are more crucial to the child's well-being than specific child characteristics, such as age or sex. High levels of ongoing family conflict are related to problems of social development, emotional stability, and cognitive skills for the child.

Complications associated with divorce include efforts on the part of one parent to subvert the child's loyalties to the other, abandonment to other caregivers, and adjustment to a step-parent. A major problem occurs when children are "caught in the middle" between divorced parents. They become message bearers between parents, are often quizzed about activities of the other parent, and have to listen to one parent criticize the other. A nurse may be able to intercede by helping the child get out of the middle by using "I messages" based on the formula of "I feel … (state the feeling) when you … (state the source). I would like it if you. …" This approach enables children to feel in control. An example of an "I message" is as follows: "I do not feel comfortable when you ask me questions about Mom; maybe you could ask her yourself."

Feelings of children toward divorce vary with age (Box 31-4). Some children feel a sense of shame and embarrassment about the family situation. Some feelings cause children to see themselves as different, inferior, or unworthy of love, especially if they feel responsible for the family dissolution. Although the social stigma attached to divorce no longer produces the emotions it did in the past, such feelings may still exist in small towns or in some cultural groups and can reinforce children's negative self-image. Lasting effects of divorce depend on the children's and parents' adjustment to the transition from an intact family to a lone-parent family and, often, to a reconstituted family.

Although most studies have concentrated on the negative effects of divorce on youngsters, some positive outcomes of divorce have been reported. A successful post-divorce family, either a lone-parent or a reconstituted family, can improve the quality of life for adults and children. If conflict is resolved, a better relationship with one or both parents may result, and some children may have less contact with a disturbed parent. Greater stability in home settings and the removal of arguments between parents at home can be a positive outcome for children's long-term well-being.

Age- and Gender-Related Responses to Divorce

Previously, it was believed that divorce had a greater impact on younger children, but recent observations indicate that divorce constitutes a major disruption for children of all ages. While feelings and behaviours of children may be different for various ages and genders, all children suffer stress second only to the stress produced by the death of a parent. Although considerable research has looked at gender differences in children's adjustments to divorce, the findings are not conclusive.

Telling the Children

Parents are understandably hesitant to tell children about their decision to divorce. Most parents neglect to discuss either the divorce or its inevitable changes with their preschool child. Without preparation, even children who remain in the family home are confused by parental separations. Frequently, children are already experiencing vague, uneasy feelings that are more difficult to cope with than being told the truth about the situation. If possible, the initial disclosure should include both parents and siblings, followed by individual discussions with each child. Sufficient time should be set aside for these discussions in a period of calm, not after an argument, and include reasons for the divorce (if age appropriate) and reassurance that the divorce is not the children's fault.

BOX 31-4 Children's Feelings and Behaviours Related to Divorce

Infants
- Effects of reduced mothering or lack of mothering
- Increased irritability
- Disturbance in eating, sleeping, and elimination
- Interference with attachment process

Early Preschool Children (Ages 2 to 3 Years)
- Frightened and confused
- Blame themselves for the divorce
- Fear of abandonment
- Increased irritability, whining, tantrums
- Regressive behaviours (e.g., thumb sucking, loss of elimination control)
- Separation anxiety

Later Preschool Children (Ages 3 to 5 Years)
- Fear of abandonment
- Blame themselves for the divorce; decreased self-esteem
- Bewilderment regarding all human relationships
- Become more aggressive in relationships with others (e.g., siblings, peers)
- Engage in fantasy to seek understanding of the divorce

Early School-Age Children (Ages 5 to 6 Years)
- Depression and immature behaviour
- Loss of appetite and sleep disorders
- May be able to verbalize some feelings and understand some divorce-related changes
- Increased anxiety and aggression
- Feelings of abandonment by departing parent

Middle School-Age Children (Ages 6 to 8 Years)
- Panic reactions
- Feelings of deprivation—loss of parent, attention, money, and secure future
- Profound sadness, depression, fear, and insecurity
- Feelings of abandonment and rejection
- Fear about the future
- Difficulty expressing anger at parents
- Intense desire for reconciliation of parents
- Impaired capacity to play and enjoy outside activities
- Decline in school performance
- Altered peer relationships—become bossy, irritable, demanding, and manipulative
- Frequent crying, loss of appetite, sleep disorders
- Disturbed routine, forgetfulness

Later School-Age Children (Ages 9 to 12 Years)
- More realistic understanding of divorce
- Intense anger directed at one or both parents
- Divided loyalties
- Ability to express feelings of anger
- Ashamed of parental behaviour
- Desire for revenge; may wish to punish the parent they hold responsible
- Feelings of loneliness, rejection, and abandonment
- Altered peer relationships
- Decline in school performance
- May develop somatic complaints
- May engage in aberrant behaviour such as lying, stealing
- Temper tantrums
- Dictatorial attitude

Adolescents (Ages 12 to 18 Years)
- Able to disengage themselves from parental conflict
- Feelings of a profound sense of loss—of family, childhood
- Feelings of anxiety
- Worry about themselves, parents, siblings
- Expression of anger, sadness, shame, embarrassment
- May withdraw from family and friends
- Disturbed concept of sexuality
- May engage in acting-out behaviours

Parents should not fear crying in front of the children because their crying gives the children permission to cry also. Children may feel guilt, a sense of failure, or that they are being punished for misbehaviour. They normally feel anger and resentment and should be allowed to communicate these feelings without punishment. They need consistency and order in their lives. They want to know where they will live, who will take care of them, if they will be with their siblings, and if there will be enough money to live on. Children fear that if their parents stopped loving each other, they could stop loving them. Their need for love and reassurance is tremendous at this time. Children may also wonder what will happen on special days such as birthdays and holidays, whether both parents will come to school events, and whether they will still have the same friends.

Custody and Parenting Partnerships

In the past, when parents separated, mothers were given custody of the children, with visitation agreements for fathers. Now both parents and the courts are seeking alternatives. Current belief is that neither fathers nor mothers should be awarded custody automatically. Custody should be awarded to parents who are best able to provide for the children's welfare. In some cases, children experience severe stress when living or spending time with a parent.

Two other types of custody arrangements are divided custody and joint custody. *Divided*, or *split, custody* means that each parent is awarded custody of one or more of the children, thereby separating siblings. For example, sons might live with the father and daughters with the mother.

Joint custody takes one of two forms. In *joint physical custody*, the parents alternate the physical care and control of the children on an equitable basis while maintaining shared parenting responsibilities legally. This custody arrangement works well for families who live close to each other and whose occupations permit an active role in the care and rearing of the children. In *joint legal custody*, children reside with one parent but both parents are the children's legal guardians and participate in childrearing. In Canada in 2005, joint custody was awarded to both parents in 37% of the custody cases (Juby, Marcil-Gratton, & Le Bourdais, 2005). The number of fathers awarded sole custody has decreased to under 10% of cases, and sole custody was awarded to mothers in slightly more than 50% of custody cases (Juby et al., 2005).

Coparenting offers substantial benefits for the family: children can be close to both parents, and life with each parent can be more normal (as opposed to having a disciplinarian mother and a recreational father). To be successful, parents in these arrangements must place high value on the commitment to provide normal parenting and to separate their marital conflicts from their parenting roles. The primary consideration is the welfare of the children.

Lone Parenting

An individual may become a lone parent as a result of divorce, separation, death of a spouse, or birth or adoption of a child. Although divorce rates have stabilized, the number of lone-parent households continues to rise. In 2004, these families accounted for 25% of all Canadian families, with 81% being headed by women (Canadian Council on Social Development, 2006). It is estimated that at least half of the children born during the 2000s will spend part of their life in a family headed by a divorced, separated, widowed, or never-married mother. Although some women are lone parents by choice, most never planned on being parents on their own, and many feel pressure to marry or remarry.

Managing shortages of money, time, and energy is a major concern for lone parents. Studies repeatedly confirm the financial difficulties of lone-parent families, particularly single mothers, (Gucciardi, Celasun, & Stewart, 2004). The stigma of poverty may be more keenly felt than the discrimination associated with being a lone parent. These families are often forced by their financial status to live in communities with inadequate housing and personal safety concerns. Lone parents often feel guilty about the time spent away from their children.

Over the last 25 years, the number of teenage pregnancies has declined in Canada; the rate dropped almost 37% between 1996 and 2006 (McKay & Barrett, 2010). In 2006, the Canadian adolescent birth and abortion rate was 27.9 per 1000 women aged 15 to 19 (McKay & Barrett, 2010). Being a teenage parent adds to the financial burden of being a lone parent and can have long-term consequences for the mother and her child. Poverty is a well-known determinant of health that can have adverse effects on a child's health and well-being.

Single Fathers

Fathers who have custody of their children have many of the same problems that divorced mothers have. They feel overburdened by the responsibility, depressed, and concerned about their ability to cope with the emotional needs of the children, especially girls. Some fathers find it difficult at first to coordinate household tasks, school visits, and other activities. Fathers often demand more assistance with household tasks and more independence from their children than custodial mothers do, and are likely to make use of alternative care giving and support systems.

Same-Sex Marriages and Parenting

In Canada, same-sex marriage became legal in 2005. The 2006 Census indicated 15,000 persons living as same-sex married couples, which is about 0.1% of all married couples. Statistics Canada (2006) reported an increase in 2001 from 34,200 same-sex common-law couples to 37,885 in 2006. Among married same-sex men, 9% had children in their home; less than 2% of male common-law partners had children. Of married same-sex women, 24% had children in their home, and less than 15% of common-law partners had children (Statistics Canada, 2006). There is a lack of research on the effect of same-sex parenting on children, particularly when there are two male partners. In 2006, the Department of Justice Canada released a report completed in 2003 that studied the available research. The researchers concluded that there was very little difference in socialization and social competence of children raised by heterosexual parents compared to that of children raised by gay or lesbian parents (Hastings et al., 2006).

Parenting in Reconstituted Families

In North America, many of the children living in homes where parents have divorced will experience another major change in their lives, such as the addition of a step-parent or new siblings. In Canada, 12% of coupled families are made up of stepfamilies (Bechard, 2006). The entry of a step-parent into an existing family requires adjustments for all family members. Some obstacles to the role adjustments and family problem solving include disruption of previous lifestyles and interaction patterns, complexity in the formation of new ones, and lack of social supports. Most children from divorced families still want to live in a two-parent home.

Cooperative parenting relationships can allow more time for each set of parents to be alone to establish their own relationship with the children. Under ideal circumstances, power conflicts between the two households can be reduced, and tension and anxiety can be lessened for all family members. In addition, the children's self-esteem can be increased, and there is a greater likelihood of continued contact with grandparents. Flexibility, mutual support, and open communication are critical to forming successful relationships in stepfamilies. Unfortunately, stepfamilies usually do not seek help to prevent problems. Typically, information and counselling are sought only when problems have surfaced and can no longer be ignored.

Parenting in Dual-Earner Families

No change in family lifestyle has had a greater impact than the trend of larger numbers of women entering the workplace and moving away from the traditional homemaker role. As a result, the family is subjected to considerable stress as members attempt to meet the often competing demands of occupational needs and those regarded as necessary for a rich family life.

Role definitions are frequently altered to arrange an equitable division of time and labour, as well as to resolve conflict, especially conflict related to the traditional norms of the culture. Overload is a common source of stress in a dual-earner family, and social activities are often significantly curtailed. Time demands and scheduling for working parents are intense. Dual-earner couples may increase the strain on themselves to avoid creating stress for their children. Although there is no evidence to indicate that the dual-earner lifestyle is stressful to children, the stress experienced by the parents may affect the children indirectly.

Working Mothers

Working mothers have become the norm in North America. Child care is critical to the working mother's sense of well-being. The quality of child care is a persistent concern for all working parents. Determinants of child care quality are based on health and safety requirements, responsive and warm interaction between staff and children, developmentally appropriate activities, trained staff, limited group size, age-appropriate caregivers, adequate staff-to-child ratios, and adequate indoor and outdoor space. Nurses play an important role in helping families find suitable sources of child care and preparing children for this experience.

Foster Parenting

Foster care is defined as placement in an approved living situation away from the family of origin. The living situation may be an approved foster home, possibly with other children, or a preadoptive home. The child welfare services from each province and territory offers training and ongoing education for foster parents. Each province and territory has guidelines regarding the relative health of the prospective foster parents and their families, background checks regarding legal issues for the adults, personal interviews, and a safety inspection of the residence and surroundings.

In 2007, it was estimated that nearly 76,000 children were living in foster care, with many children facing developmental concerns (Mulcahy & Trocme, 2007). From 2000 to 2006, the children requiring foster care increased by 24% (Ontario Association of Children's Aid Societies, 2007). Children in foster care tend to have a higher than normal incidence of acute and chronic health problems and may experience feelings of isolation or confusion. Nurses should strive to implement strategies that will improve the health care for this group of children.

Accommodating Contemporary Parenting Situations

During recent years, private and government sectors have identified specific problems of contemporary families. Many of these issues involve working parents. One significant stressor for the working lone parent or for dual-earner families is when a child becomes ill. The frequency of childhood illness, exclusion practices of most licensed child care programs, and employers' limited sick-leave policies are other contributing factors. Some employers have become more family focused and provide time off for parents to be with sick children. Flexible work schedules and family-oriented legislation can ease the burden of managing family and work responsibilities. The *Family Medical Leave Act* allows eligible employees to take up to 12 weeks of unpaid leave each year to care for newborn or newly adopted children, to care for parents or spouses who have serious health conditions, or to recover from their own serious health condition.

Key Points

- Because there is no agreement on the definition of family, a family is what an individual considers it to be.
- Three theories that have significant relevance and application to pediatric nursing are family systems theory, family stress theory, and developmental theory.
- Although the traditional family structure was nuclear or extended, in recent years other forms, such as the lone-parent family, have emerged.
- Family size and position within the family structure have a strong impact on a child's development.
- Interpersonal skills and a basic understanding of childhood growth and development are essential areas of focus for parents.
- Parental control tends to be predominantly one of three types: authoritarian, permissive, or authoritative.
- Three areas of special concern to adoptive families include the initial attachment process, the task of telling children that they are adopted, and identity formation during adolescence.
- Marital factors within the home significantly influence a child's development. The impact of divorce on a child depends on the child's age, the outcome, and the quality of the parent–child relationship and parental care following the divorce.
- Lone parenting and step-parenting create adjustment difficulties and add stress to the already demanding parental role. Significant numbers of children will live in a lone-parent or reconstituted family at some point.

Audio Chapter Summaries
Access an Audio Summary of these Key Points on evolve

References

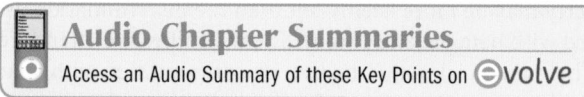

Bechard, M. (2006). *General social survey, cycle 20: Family transition survey, family structure by region, Statistics Canada, Social and Aboriginal Statistic Division.* Retrieved from http://dsp-psd.pwgsc.gc.ca/collection_2007/statcan/89-625-X/89-625-XIE2007001.pdf.

Brazelton, T. B. (1995). Working with families: Opportunities for early intervention. *Pediatric Clinics of North America, 42*(1), 1–10.

Canadian Council on Social Development. (2006). *The progress of Canada's children and youth, 2006.* Retrieved from http://www.ccsd.ca/pccy/2006/pdf/pccy_2006.pdf.

Canadian Legal Information Institute. (2012). *Criminal Code, R.S.C. 1985, c. C-46.* Retrieved from http://canlii.ca/en/ca/laws/stat/rsc-1985-c-c-46/97962/rsc-1985-c-c-46.html.

Citizenship and Immigration. (2011). *Intercountry adoption.* Retrieved from http://www.cic.gc.ca/english/immigrate/adoption/index.asp.

Department of Justice Canada. (2011). *An analysis of options for changes in the legal regulation of child custody and access: Adoption.* Retrieved from http://www.justice.gc.ca/eng/pi/fcy-fea/lib-bib/rep-rap/2001/2001_2b/option1a.html.

Friedman, M. M., Bowden, V. R., & Jones, E. G. (2003). *Family nursing: Research theory and practice* (5th ed.). Upper Saddle River, NJ: Prentice Hall.

Gucciardi, E., Celasun, N., & Stewart, D. (2004). Single-mother families in Canada. *Canadian Journal of Public Health, 95*(1), 70–73.

Hamilton, B. E., et al. (2007). Annual summary of vital statistics: 2005. *Pediatrics, 119*(2), 345–360. doi:10.1542/peds.2006-3226

Hastings, P. D., et al. (2006). *Children's development of social competence across family types*. Ottawa, ON: Department of Justice. Retrieved from http://www.samesexmarriage.ca/docs/Justice_Child_Development.pdf.

Juby, H., Marcil-Gratton, N., & Le Bourdais, C. (2005). *When parents separate: Further findings from the national longitudinal survey of children and youth*. Ottawa: Department of Justice. Retrieved from http://dsp-psd.pwgsc.gc.ca/Collection/J3-2-2004-6E.pdf.

Lerner, R. M., Sparks, E. E., & McCubbin, L. D. (1999). *Family diversity and family policy: Strengthening families for America's children*. Boston: Kluwer.

McCubbin, M. A., & McCubbin, H. I. (1994). Families coping with illness: Resiliency model of family stress, adjustment, and adaptation. In C. B. Danielson, B. H. Bissel, & P. Winstead-Fry (Eds.), *Families, health, and illness*. St. Louis: Mosby.

McKay, A., & Barrett, M. (2010). Trends in teen pregnancy rates from 1996 to 2006: A comparison of Canada, Sweden, U.S.A., and England/Wales. *Canadian Journal of Human Sexuality, 19*(1/2), 43–52.

Mulcahy, M., & Trocme, N. (2007). *Children and youth in out-of-home care in Canada*. Retrieved from http://www.cecw-cepb.ca/sites/default/files/publications/en/ChildrenInCare78E.pdf.

Ontario Association of Children's Aid Societies. (2007). *More foster families needed in Ontario*. Retrieved from http://www.oacas.org/newsroom/releases/newsreleasefosterfamily07oct21.pdf.

Public Health Agency of Canada. (2004). *Canadian perinatal health report 2003*. Ottawa: Minister of Public Works and Government Services Canada. Retrieved from http://www.phac-aspc.gc.ca/publicat/cphr-rspc03/index-eng.php.

Public Health Agency of Canada. (2012). *Perinatal health indicators for Canada 2011*. (Cat. No. HP7-1/2011). Ottawa: Author.

Statistics Canada. (2004). *Birth*. Ottawa: Ministry of Industry. Retrieved from http://www.statcan.ca/english/freepub/84F0210XIE/84F0210XIE2002000.htm.

Statistics Canada. (2005). *The daily: Divorces, 2003*. Retrieved from http://www.statcan.gc.ca/daily-quotidien/050309/dq050309b-eng.htm.

Statistics Canada. (2006). *2006 census information on same-sex, common-law and married couples*. Retrieved from http://www12.statcan.ca/census-recensement/2006/ref/info/same_sex-meme_sexe-eng.cfm.

Statistics Canada. (2009). *Family violence in Canada: A statistical profile*. Retrieved from http://www.statcan.gc.ca/pub/85-224-x/85-224-x2010000-eng.pdf.

Statistics Canada. (2011). *Migration International: 2009*. Ottawa: Ministry of Industry. Retrieved from http://www.statcan.gc.ca/pub/91-209-x/2011001/article/11526-eng.pdf.

Additional Resources

Canadian Institute of Child Health: http://www.cich.ca/about.html

Service Canada for Families and Children: http://www.servicecanada.gc.ca/eng/audiences/families/index.shtml

Unit 7

32 Social, Cultural, and Religious Influences on Child Health Promotion

Learning Objectives

On completion of this chapter, the reader will be able to:

- Define culture, cultural competence, ethnocentrism, and cultural relativism.
- Describe the subcultural influences of socioeconomic status, poverty, religion, and schools on child development.
- Discuss the population shifts in numbers of minority children in Canada.
- Identify four common diseases or disorders that affect certain ethnic or cultural groups.
- Identify potential conflicts of values and customs for a nurse interacting with a family with a cultural or ethnic background different from that of the nurse.
- Describe three religious groups whose beliefs significantly affect their health practices.

Electronic Resources

Additional information related to the content in Chapter 32 can be found on

evolve the companion Web site at

http://evolve.elsevier.com/Canada/Perry/maternal/

- Examination Review Questions
- Case Study—Cultural Considerations
- Skill—Providing Culturally Sensitive Care

Social Determinants of Health

Social determinants of health exist at an individual as well as a population level, and they affect the degree to which each person has the necessary resources to meet their daily needs and achieve their goals. While early research focused largely on family income and social status as primary influences on health, more recently the boundaries of these factors have been broadened (Halfon, Larson, & Russ, 2010). The following are now more widely accepted as key determinants of health: family wealth and assets, social status, employment, working conditions, education, literacy, quality and nature of housing, race, ethnicity, gender, biology and genetic endowment, family structure, culture, social relationships and support networks, quality of parenting and caregiving, child development, exposure to domestic violence, neighbourhood safety, natural environment (air, water, soil, climate changes), built environment (land use, community design), living conditions (transportation, nutritious foods), media use, personal health literacy and practices, coping skills, and available health care services (see Table 29-1) (Halfon et al., 2010; Postl, Cook, & Moffatt, 2010; Public Health Agency of Canada, 2011).

Key Social-Determinant Influences

Although there is no general agreement on the categorization of social determinants, there is strong evidence that social factors are interconnected and complex and that they have a significant influence on health. Health is a developmental process, a product of interactions among personal, physical, and environmental factors. Children are particularly sensitive to social determinants, especially in their younger years; the first 3 years of life present a crucial period during which they are susceptible to both negative and positive influences. If the exposure to negative influences outweighs that to positive ones, their adaptation can be compromised, setting the stage for greater problems later in life. While very young children are dependent on supportive caregiving for healthy development, older children are more dependent on relationships with peers and on school and neighbourhood environments (Halfon et al., 2010).

Culture

The future of any society depends on its children; therefore, society must provide for their care, nurturing, and socialization. Culture plays a critical role in shaping parenting behaviours that facilitate children's development (Meléndez, 2005). The culture's customs and values help to organize a society's childrearing system and are transmitted from one generation to the next through the family. A holistic view of any child requires that nurses develop some understanding of the ways in which culture contributes to the development of social and emotional relationships and influences childrearing practices and attitudes toward health.

Culture is a pattern of learned beliefs, values, and practices that are shared within a group; it includes practices; customs; views on roles and relationships, including parenting; and communication patterns and language (Betancourt, 2004). Culture differs from both race and ethnicity. *Race* is defined as a classification of humans on the basis of traits that are not only transmissible by descent but also socially constructed. **Ethnicity** is the affiliation of a set of persons who share a unique cultural, social, and linguistic heritage (Fig. 32-1). *Socialization* is the process by which society imparts its competencies, values, and expectations to children (Trawick-Smith, 2006).

Culture is a complex whole in which each component is interrelated. It provides the lens through which all facets of human behaviour can be interpreted (Spector, 2004). Culture is not a surface veneer that covers a basic outlook shared by all human beings; rather, it is an ingrained orientation toward life that serves as a frame of reference for individual perception and judgement. People from one culture differ from those in other cultures in the ways that they think, solve problems, and perceive and structure the world. Culture is, essentially, the way of life of a group of people that incorporates experiences of the past, influences thought and action in the present, and transmits these traditions to future group members. Adaptation is necessary, however, for the culture to survive in an ever-changing world. Consciously and unconsciously, the members abandon, modify, or assume new patterns to meet the group's needs.

The cultural setting in which children are raised can influence many aspects of their life—from the food they eat to the way they behave in a social setting. To be acceptable members of the culture, children must learn how the culture expects them to behave toward others in the group. In turn, they learn how they can expect others to behave toward them.

Cultures and subcultures contribute to the uniqueness of child members in such a subtle way and at such an early age that children grow up to think that their beliefs, attitudes, values, and practices are the "correct" or "normal" ones. By age 5, children can identify persons who belong to their own race or cultural background. During later primary years, children are able to identify people from different cultures (Trawick-Smith, 2006). A set of values learned in childhood is likely to characterize children's attitudes and behaviour for life, guiding their long-range strivings and informing their short-range, impulsive inclinations. Thus every ongoing society socializes each succeeding generation to its cultural heritage.

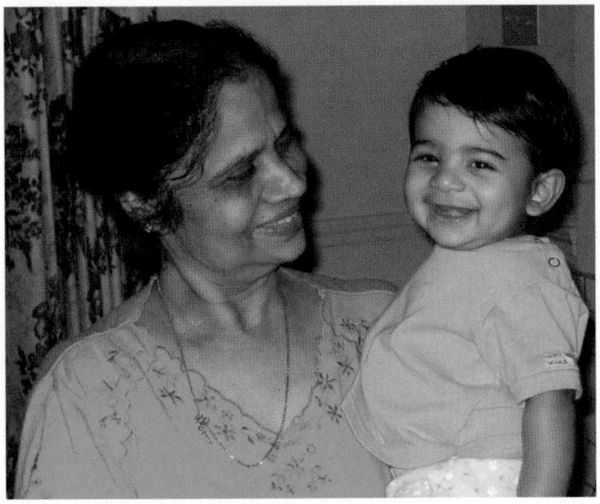

Fig. 32-1 Ethnicity is an individual's association with a shared cultural, social, and linguistic heritage.

The manner and sequence of growth and development are universal and fundamental features of all children; however, the variations in behavioural responses that children display to similar events are believed to be determined by their culture. Children acquire the skills, knowledge, beliefs, and values important to their own family and culture. The pace of acquisition of cognitive and motor skills can differ by cultural background, as can the child's social and emotional development (Trawick-Smith, 2006).

Cultures may also differ in whether status in the group is based on age or on skill. Even children's play and their types of games are culturally determined. In some cultures, children play in groups composed of members of the same sex; in others, they play in mixed-sex groups. In some cultures, team games predominate; in others, most play is limited to individual games.

Standards and norms vary from culture to culture and from location to location; a practice that is accepted in one area may meet with disapproval or create tension in another. The extent to which cultures tolerate divergence from the established norm also varies among cultures and subcultural groups. Although conformity provides a degree of security, it is often a deterrent to change.

Except in rare situations, children grow and develop in a blend of cultures and subcultures. In a large, complex society such as that of Canada, different groups have their own sets of standards, values, and expectations within the collective ways of the larger culture. Although many cultural differences are related to geographic boundaries, subcultures are not always restricted by location.

Children's membership in a cultural subgroup is, for the most part, involuntary. They are born into a family with a specific **ethnic** or racial heritage, socioeconomic level, and set of religious beliefs. Although in North American society there are countless subcultures and considerable variations in the way of life, those subcultures that seem to exert the greatest influence on childrearing are ethnicity, social status, and occupational role. In addition, schools and peer-group subcultures are strong influences in the socialization of the child.

Social Roles

Much of children's self-concept is derived from their ideas about their social roles. Roles are cultural creations; therefore, the culture prescribes patterns of behaviour for persons in a variety of social positions. All persons who hold similar social positions have an obligation to behave in a particular manner. A role prohibits some behaviours and allows others. Because it delineates and clarifies roles, the culture is a significant influence on the development of children's self-concept (i.e., attitudes and beliefs they have about themselves).

A social group consists of a system of roles carried out in primary and secondary groups. A *primary group* is characterized by intimate, continued, face-to-face contact; mutual support of members; and the ability to order or constrain a considerable proportion of individual members' behaviour. Two such groups are the family and the peer group, both of which exert a great deal of influence on the child.

Secondary groups are groups that have limited, intermittent contact and in which there is generally less concern about members' behaviour. These groups offer little in terms of support or pressure toward conformity except in rigidly limited areas. Examples of secondary groups are professional associations and church organizations (also considered in relation to subgroups). The childrearing orientation in a secondary group environment, such as urban communities, differs considerably from that of a primary group community. An urban community is dynamic and rapidly changing; thus many of the traditional behaviours and values do not meet its needs. Consequently, parents are often uncertain about what to teach their children. They may wish to rear their children with values consistent with their own, but the differences in experience between the generations are too great. As a result, they often grant their children autonomy in some areas of decision making early in the developmental process, and other secondary groups assume a greater influence. The children are exposed to an assortment of social groups with diverse sets of values and expectations. None of the groups is highly dominant in its influence; children are exposed to an eclectic set of values, some in agreement and some in conflict with the others. From these they must ultimately select those values that they determine to be best for them and adopt them to form a consistent set of roles and behaviours to be incorporated into their self-concept.

Self-Esteem

A child's **self-esteem** is influenced by his or her culture. Some cultures are more collective in thought and action. A child from a collective culture will hold an inclusive view of self. Self-evaluation is related to the accomplishments or competencies of the entire family or community. School experiences that focus on personal achievement may promote positive self-esteem in some children but not in others, who are more dependent on the success of a whole family or peer group. A child's sense of control may not come from individual self-reliance but rather from a feeling of worthiness in his or her family or community (Trawick-Smith, 2006).

evolve Case Study-Cultural Considerations

Families and culture also influence the criteria that children use to evaluate their own abilities. Additionally, cultures vary in the degree to which they instill an internal locus of control (a belief in the ability to regulate one's own life). Effects on self-esteem are minimal if these beliefs are directed by parents and are in accordance with cultural customs. What is damaging to emotional health is the helplessness that can stem from prejudice. Ethnic pride has helped individuals maintain a positive self-image and protect against the damage that prejudice can cause (Trawick-Smith, 2006).

Ethnicity

As stated earlier, *ethnicity* is the classification of or affiliation with any of the basic groups or divisions of humans or any heterogeneous population differentiated by customs, characteristics, language, or similar distinguishing factors. Ethnic differences extend to many areas and include such manifestations as family structure, language, food preferences, moral codes, and expression of emotion. Some standards of behaviour result from the cultural heritage of the specific ethnic group. The term *ethnic* has aroused strong negative feelings and is often rejected by the general population (Spector, 2004).

To establish their place in the group, children learn how to adhere to a mode of behaviour that is in accordance with standards distinctive to the group and learn how they can expect others to behave toward them. They take their cues by observing and imitating those to whom they are exposed. For example, children of a racial minority form a perception of their role as a group member by observing the manner in which role models within the subgroup respond to treatment by people outside the subgroup. If they see group members display an attitude of inferiority, they may assume this to be appropriate behaviour and incorporate these perceptions into their own self-concept. Children observing the rejection of bigotry may develop a more positive self-concept.

While Canada embraces diversity, the cross-cultural lines may become blurred as subcultures live within the larger culture (Fig. 32-2). It may be particularly difficult for persons to attempt to maintain an identity with a subculture while living and conforming to the requirements of the dominant culture. Universal customs and language used in commercial and educational systems are different from those of the minority culture. Consequently, children reared in this environment can be confused about roles and values and may adopt those of the more influential or higher-status culture. Youths, in particular, are influenced by the locally dominant group.

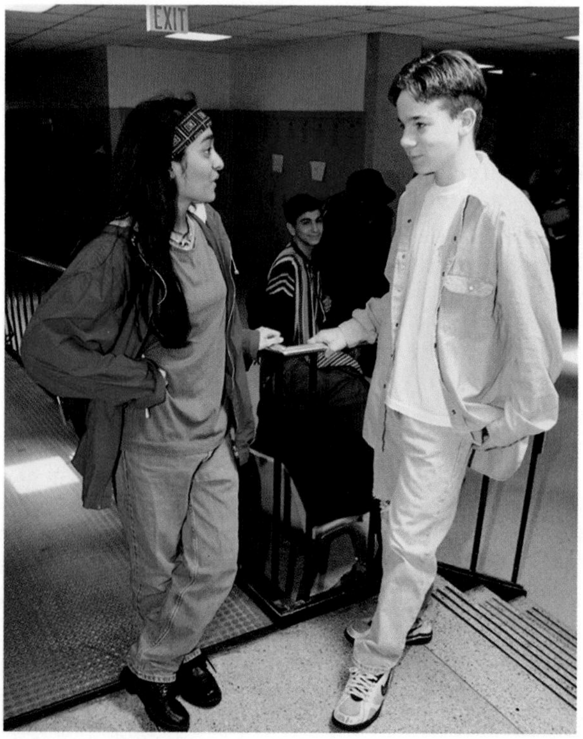

Fig. 32-2 Teenagers from different cultural backgrounds interact within the larger culture.

Ethnocentrism is the concept that one's own culture is the right and natural way to do things while all other ways are unnatural and inferior (Galanti, 2004). *Ethnic stereotyping* or labelling stems from ethnocentric views of people. Ethnocentrism implies that all other groups are inferior and that their ways are not in the best interests of the group. It is a common attitude among a dominant ethnic group and strongly influences the ability of one person to objectively evaluate the beliefs and behaviours of others. This inherent viewpoint of individuals tends to bias their interpretation and understanding of the behaviour of others. The culturally competent nurse should be empathetic and aware of his or her own views and that they may differ from another's, based on culture or ethnicity. The nurse should be willing to ask questions that will provide a better understanding of patient or family views, when appropriate.

Socioeconomic Status

Socioeconomic status relates to a family's economic and education levels. As a determinant of health, the influence of socioeconomic class cannot be overlooked; the most overwhelming adverse influence on health is low socioeconomic status. At any one time, a higher percentage of low-income individuals suffers from some health problem than any other group.

The sum of all aspects of a low-income family's living situation contributes to and compounds health problems; this includes crowded living conditions and poor sanitation, which facilitate transfer of disease (e.g., tuberculosis). Lack of funds or inaccessibility of health services can inhibit treatment for any but severe illness or injury. Sometimes health care is inadequate because of lack of information. In some areas, a disorder is so commonplace that it is looked on as unavoidable; it is not recognized as something that requires (or is amenable to) treatment. The parents may not have information regarding causes, treatment, outcome of the illness, or preventive measures. The nurse can use the few opportunities when the family does use the health care system to inquire about immunizations, screen for vision problems, provide nutritional information, and offer additional prevention and health promotion resources.

Strong family relationships may exist among those with low income or education level, as these individuals have few resources and must rely on the support of a family network to meet their physical needs. Middle- and upper-class people often have resources that reach beyond the extended family, enabling them to access physical and emotional support in the community (Giger & Davidhizar, 2008). It is also important to recognize that family relationships may be stronger among some ethnic or cultural groups than others. The term *socioeconomic status* should not be confused, however, with cultural or ethnic diversity. Children of a specific race are not necessarily of low socioeconomic status (Trawick-Smith, 2006).

Poverty

Recognized as one of the more influential determinants of health, the term *poverty* implies both visible and invisible impoverishment. It is a condition in which families live without adequate resources (Denburg & Daneman, 2010; Trawick-Smith, 2006). *Visible poverty* refers to lack of money or material resources, which includes insufficient clothing, poor sanitation, and deteriorating housing. *Invisible poverty* refers to social and cultural deprivation, such as limited employment opportunities, inferior educational opportunities, lack of or inferior medical services and health care facilities, and an absence of public services.

Although Canada has no official definition of poverty, it is typically measured using the Low Income Cut-Offs (LICO)—before and after tax, the Low Income Measures (LIM)—before and after tax, and the Market Basket Measures (MBM) (Statistics Canada, 2008). The LICO is meant to express the income level at which a family faces constraints because it has to spend a higher percentage of its income on basic resources—e.g. shelter, clothes, food—than the average similar size family.

The number of children living in poverty has continued to increase during the twenty-first century. The child poverty rate in Canada is among the highest in the developed world. In 2004, an average of 13% of children were living in poverty, virtually the same rates that existed in 1989, despite the economic growth in Canada (Fleury, 2008). Large urban centres have child poverty rates as high as 29% (McNeill, 2010). Persistent poverty puts children at risk for suffering health problems, including infant mortality, asthma, obesity, poor literacy, developmental delays, and behavioural and mental health difficulties. These children also tend to attain lower levels of education and are more likely to live in poverty as adults (Canadian Paediatric Society [CPS], 2007; Fleury, 2008).

Families living in poverty struggle to provide health care for themselves and for their children. Travel to health care facilities often requires finding money for public transit or a taxi, borrowing a car, or seeking other means of transportation. They must find care for dependents, such as other infants and small children, or have them accompany them when taking the child for care. Families tend to delay preventive care indefinitely unless health services are relatively accessible. They are more likely to consult traditional practitioners or other persons within their community. Day-to-day needs of food, clothing, and lodging take precedence over health care as long as the ailing person feels able to perform activities of daily living.

Homelessness

One of the more pressing problems in Canada is the growing number of homeless families. Homeless individuals are those who lack resources and community ties necessary to provide for their own adequate shelter. It is estimated that there are 150,000 to 300,000 homeless people in Canada, living either in shelters or on the streets. Most nights, shelters accommodate approximately 40,000 people. Although single men are the highest portion of homeless people in Canada, families with children living in poverty; street youth; First Nations, Métis, and Inuit persons with mental illness; and new immigrants are disproportionately reflected in the homeless population (Human Resources and Skills Development Canada, 2012).

There are a variety of causes of homelessness in Canada, including a lack of affordable housing, low income, job layoffs, the gap between incomes and affordability of resources, parental mental illness, substance use, intimate partner conflict and violence, unexpected family crises, and inadequate discharge coordination between mental health services, justice facilities, and the social services system. Homeless children experience all of the health problems associated with poverty, as well as other types of disorders. Most of these children experience poor health. They may not have a regular source of health care, and the focus of their care may not be preventive. Their care is likely fragmented, crisis oriented, and often sought in emergency departments of hospitals. Another group of homeless children are the "runaway" and "throwaway" adolescents, who are at risk for violence, victimization, sexually transmitted infections, and substance use (Human Resources and Skills Development Canada, 2012; Tropello, 2000).

Religion

Many immigrants came to Canada for religious freedom and established a religious and moral atmosphere that persists today. At the same time, individual differences are also part of the general culture. Many religions are practised in Canada, such as Judaism, Christianity, and Islam. Because of recent immigration patterns, there has been an increase in religious diversity in Canada.

The family's religious orientation can dictate a code of morality and influence the family's attitudes toward education, male and female role identity, and beliefs regarding their ultimate destiny (Fig. 32-3). Religion may also be a factor in determining the school that children attend, the companions with whom they associate, and, often, their mate selection. In a few instances, such as in Mennonite and Amish communities, religion is the basis for a common way of life that determines both where children are reared and their lifestyle (see also Religious Beliefs, p. 837).

School

Next to family, schools are a major force in providing continuity between generations, by conveying a vast amount of culture from older members of society to the young. In this way, children are prepared to carry out the traditional social roles

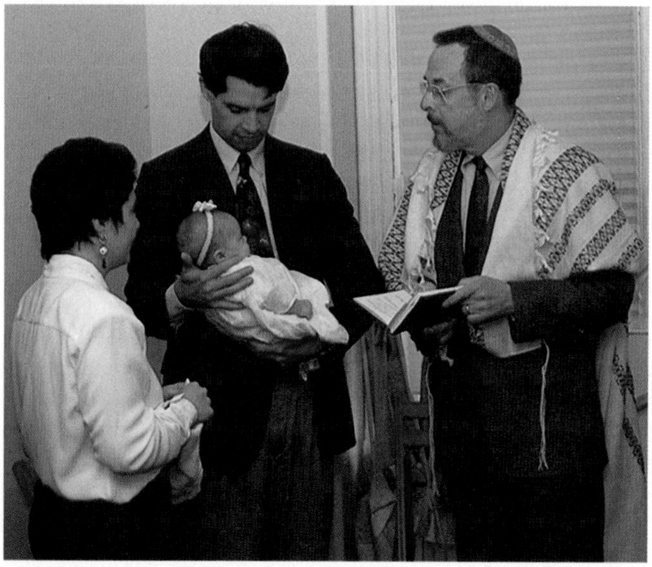

Fig. 32-3 Many families have a special religious ceremony soon after an infant is born.

expected of them as adults in society. School rules and regulations regarding attendance, authority relationships, and the system of sanctions and rewards based on achievement transmit to the child the behavioural expectations of the adult world of employment and relationships. School is often the only institution in which children systematically learn about the negative consequences of behaviours that deviate from societal expectations. Teachers are expected to stimulate and guide the intellectual development of children and their sense of aesthetics and to foster their capacity for creative problem solving. Through education, individuals of lower socioeconomic status are offered the opportunity and capacity to move up in the social strata.

Traditionally, the socialization process of school began when the child entered kindergarten or first grade. Today, with almost 70% of mothers of preschool children working outside the home, this socialization process begins much earlier for a significant number of children in a variety of child care settings (Statistics Canada, 2007).

Community

The child's or adolescent's community is made up of the family, school, neighbourhood, youth organizations, and other members. These all contribute to the young person's experience within any culture (Search Institute, 2011). Studies of students in grades 6 through 12 have shown that those who experience a higher number of relationships, opportunities, and personal qualities, or assets, that they need to thrive in their lives are more likely to make healthy choices and avoid high-risk behaviours. These assets offer a framework for positive child and adolescent development.

Four categories of external assets that youth receive from the community are as follows (Search Institute, 2011):

1. **Support**—Young people need to feel support, care, and love from their families, neighbours, and others. They also need organizations and institutions that offer positive, supportive environments.
2. **Empowerment**—Young people need to feel valued by their community and be able to contribute to others. They need to feel safe and secure.
3. **Boundaries and expectations**—Young people need to know what is expected of them and what actions and behaviours are within the community boundaries and what are outside of them.
4. **Constructive use of time**—Young people need opportunities for growth through constructive, enriching opportunities and quality time at home.

Internal assets must also be nurtured in the community's younger members. These internal qualities guide choices and create a sense of centredness, purpose, and focus. The four categories of internal assets are as follows (Search Institute, 2011):

1. **Commitment to learning**—Young people need to develop a commitment to education and life-long **learning.**
2. **Positive values**—Youth need to have a strong sense of values that direct their choices.
3. **Social competencies**—Young people need competencies that help them make positive choices and build relationships.

4. **Positive identity**—Young people need a sense of their own power, purpose, worth, and promise.

Peer Culture

Peer groups also have an impact on the socialization of children. Peer relationships become increasingly important and influential as children proceed through school. Children have what can be regarded as a culture of their own, which is most apparent in school and in the unsupervised play group. The play group presents this culture in a much purer form than does the school, in which culture is partly produced by adults.

Throughout their lives, children are exposed to value systems, such as those of the family, ethnic group, and social class. In peer-group interaction, they are confronted with a variety of these sets of values. The values imposed by the peer group are especially compelling because children must accept and conform to them in order to be accepted as members of the group. When peer values are not too different from those of family and teachers, the mild conflict created by these small differences serves to separate children from the adults in their lives and to strengthen the feeling of belonging to the peer group. The relationships in a peer group change over time, and leadership may shift (Trawick-Smith, 2006).

The kind of socialization provided by the peer group depends on the special subculture that develops from the background, interests, and capabilities of its members. Some groups support school achievement, others focus on athletic prowess, and still others are decidedly antithetical to educative goals. Scholastic achievement is strongly related to the value system of the peer groups. Many conflicts between teachers and students and between parents and students can be attributed to fear of rejection by peers. A conflict between what is expected from parents regarding academic achievement and what is expected from the peer culture can be especially pronounced in high school.

Although the peer group has neither the traditional authority of the parents nor the legal authority of the schools for teaching information, it manages to convey a substantial amount of information to its members. Peer relationships also provide an important social context for the development of body image among adolescent girls and boys. Although other subcultural forces such as the family and media influence the development of body image, adolescents' perception of what is a desirable appearance is created by norms and expectations that are modelled and reinforced within the peer group (Jones & Crawford, 2006). It is through peer relationships that children learn ways to deal with dominance and hostility and to relate with persons in positions of leadership and authority. The peer subculture relieves boredom and provides the recognition that individual members may not receive from teachers and other authority figures.

The Child and Family in North America

The frontier background of North American culture has contributed to the overall orientation toward life and childrearing. There has always been a basic optimistic view of the world, a belief that things can be better and that the children can and will be better off than their parents. This hopeful outlook and a general future orientation, together with the possibility of upward social mobility, have created a pervasive attitude of optimism. Increasing development of self-confidence and autonomy in children is fostered and encouraged. Children in North America are generally permitted a greater degree of freedom than in some more tradition-oriented cultures, where individuals remain in one class for life.

Family life in North America is characterized by increasing geographic and economic mobility. There is less reliance on tradition, families are fragmented, and there are fewer opportunities to transmit and acquire traditional and accepted customs of a culture. Consequently, young adults rely to a greater extent on professed experts, peers, and mass media for acquisition of acceptable patterns of behaviour, including childrearing practices. Conflicting information can be a source of confusion and frustration as parents attempt to determine the comparatively stable, essential components of the culture and transmit these to their children.

Children in North America grow up with a number of adults who differ from one another but who all provide input as role models, teachers, and standards for behaviour. Most children live in some form of nuclear family located in differentiated neighbourhoods determined by income and ethnic status, within a highly technological, largely urban society. Far fewer children and families live in rural communities.

Unlike the the rest of Canada's population, Aboriginal youth under 25 years of age make up over 50% of the First Nations, Métis, and Inuit populations. This population is growing twice as fast as the general Canadian population, with the largest increase occurring in families living on the reserves (Aboriginal Affairs and Northern Development Canada, 2012).

Visible Minority Groups

The *Employment Equity Act* defines visible minorities as persons, other than Aboriginal peoples, who are non-White in race or colour. The 2006 census estimated that 16.2% of Canada's total population (5.1 million) belongs to a visible minority group, up from 4.7% in 1981. South Asians represent 25% of all visible minorities; Chinese represent 24%; and Blacks represent almost 16% (the majority indicating Caribbean descent, and a smaller proportion, African descent). Approximately one third of visible minorities are Filipinos (8%), Latin Americans (6%), Arabs (5%), Southeast Asians (4.7%), West Asians (3%), Koreans (3%), and Japanese (1.6%). The remaining 4% indicated that they are either Pacific Islanders or belong to more than one visible minority group (Natural Resources Canada, 2009) (see Cultural Awareness box).

When minority groups emigrate to another country, a certain degree of cultural and ethnic blending occurs through the involuntary process of *acculturation*, those gradual changes produced in a culture by the influence of another culture that cause one or both cultures to be more similar to the other. This process is involuntary; the minority group member is forced to learn the new culture to survive (Spector, 2004). However, the changes occur to various degrees in different families and groups. Many groups continue to identify with their traditional heritage while adapting to the ill-defined concept of "a better life" (Spector, 2004).

CULTURAL AWARENESS

Overview of Visible Minority Status in 2006 Canada Census

The definitions of visible minority groups included the following (Statistics Canada. 2008):

- South Asians include people whose origins are in East India, Pakistan, Sri Lanka, etc.
- Southeast Asians are defined as people whose origins include Vietnam, Cambodia, Malaysia, Laos, etc.
- West Asians are defined as those who have origins in Iran, Afghanistan, etc.
- Black Canadians typically are referred to by their origin—either Canadian of African origins or Canadian with origins in the Caribbean.
- Latin Americans are defined as people having origins in areas in the Americas where primarily Spanish and Portuguese are spoken.
- Pacific Islanders are people whose origins trace from any of the original peoples of Guam, Samoa, or other Pacific Islands.

Evidence indicates that changes in attitudes are slowly taking place in some groups and in some places. An attitude of cultural relativism assists in understanding behaviours in their cultural context and seeing other ways of doing things as different but equally valid (Galanti, 2004). In Canada, diversity is embraced and valued, and minority-group children are encouraged to feel secure and confident in their racial or ethnic identity. As with all children, the most important influences on development of a positive self-image are warm, understanding parents who take an active interest in fostering their children's growth. Parents who accept their children and react positively and constructively rather than in a negative and demeaning manner will help their children develop feelings of self-worth, self-esteem, and self-acceptance. The more adequate children feel, the more positive their attitudes will be toward majority and minority children will be reduced.

Aboriginal Peoples

Aboriginal peoples is the name given for the original peoples of North America. In Canada, the Constitution recognizes three groups of Aboriginal people: First Nations (made up of more than 615 bands across the country), Métis (European–First Nation ancestry), and Inuit (Arctic-situated Aboriginal peoples). These three peoples have distinct histories, languages, cultural practices, and spiritual beliefs. According to the 2006 census, there are greater than one million people in Canada who identify themselves as Aboriginal persons (Aboriginal Affairs and Northern Development Canada, 2010a).

Aboriginal Affairs and Northern Development Canada is one of the federal government departments responsible for fulfilling the government's constitutional responsibilities, obligations, and commitments to First Nations, Inuit, and Métis peoples and to Northerners. The aim is to improve their social well-being and economic prosperity, develop healthier communities, and promote more participation in Canada's political, social, and economic development (Aboriginal Affairs and Northern Development Canada, 2010b). Aboriginal communities are trying to pass on to their children the many traditions that are part of their Canadian heritage, so that these traditions can be preserved.

First Nations, Métis, and Inuit peoples tend to experience health problems that are common to people living in poverty, related largely to the position they have historically held in Canadian society (Waldram, Herring, & Kue Young, 2006). Children under 16 years of age make up 40% of the total Aboriginal population, and their health lags behind that of other Canadian children. Infant mortality rates are three times higher, immunization rates are lower, and infectious diseases continue to be a key factor of morbidity for Aboriginal children. The rates of diabetes in adolescents are higher, and the number of deaths related to injuries (motor vehicle accidents, fires, self-harm, and harm to others) is four times higher than that of the overall Canadian population. In addition, the suicide rate is almost four times higher than the national average, and suicide frequently occurs in clusters. The most common reasons for poorer health status among First Nations, Métis, and Inuit peoples are lower incomes, a higher jobless rate, poor shelter, lower education level, and inadequate water and sewage systems (CPS, 2010; Lemchuk-Favel & Jock, 2004; Postl et al., 2010).

Immigrant Families

Immigration to Canada has been on the rise over the past two decades. In the 2006 census, immigrants made up 19.8% of the population, up from 17.4% in 1996 (Barozzino, 2010). In 2009, more than 250,000 people immigrated to Canada, with just over 50,000, or 20%, being children under the age of 15 years (Citizenship and Immigration Canada, 2010).

Canada's national health insurance program—usually referred to as "Medicare"—is designed to ensure that residents have reasonable access to medically necessary hospital and physician services. The national program, with common features and coverage standards, is administered by the provinces and territories (Health Canada, 2010). Immigrants to Canada who are classified as permanent residents, whether approved applicants or refugees, typically are able to receive health care benefits after 3 months in the country. Temporary residents who enter Canada for a variety of reasons (as students, contract employees, or if not admissible under the Immigration and Refugee Protection Act) do not consistently have health insurance coverage, depending on the province or territory of residence and reason for entry (Elgersma, 2008).

For decades it was generally accepted that immigrants to Canada arrived with a variety of health issues and were in need of health care that was absent in their countries of origin. More recent research and observations have revealed that new immigrants arrive with relatively better overall health (lower chronic disease and mortality rates) than that of their Canadian-born counterparts (with the exception of HIV/AIDS and tuberculosis) and maintain this health for 5 to 10 years—this is termed the *healthy migrant effect* (Barozzino, 2010).

Social determinants of health are thought to affect immigrants to Canada more significantly than native-born

Canadians, leading to a phenomenon known as *immigrant overshoot*, where immigrants' health not only deteriorates to the Canadian average but also may get worse as a result of the impact of the social determinants of health that affect immigrants more powerfully (Barozzino, 2010). Immigrant families face unique challenges, including language barriers, lack of recognition of their skills and credentials, lack of access to affordable housing and to appropriate community and settlement supports, limited health care coverage until provincial or territorial health insurance is arranged, limited access to and navigation of the health care system, and health care providers who lack any significant knowledge of and sensitivity to their diverse health care needs.

NURSING ALERT Because Canadian cultures and subcultures can be so diverse, it is essential that nurses be aware of and knowledgeable about the predominant groups in their work community and apply the knowledge in their practice.

NURSING ALERT Generalizations made about an **ethnic** group may not apply to certain groups and individuals.

Cultural, Ethnic, and Religious Influences on Health Care

Susceptibility to Health Problems

Some groups of people are more susceptible than others to certain illnesses. An innate susceptibility is acquired through generations of evolutionary changes that take place within constrained or segregated populations. The proximity to disease, environmental factors, and general physical status are significant factors associated with health problems.

Hereditary Factors

Heredity is one of the determinants of health, and many diseases have a genetic basis. Access to screening for these diseases will challenge the effectiveness of genetic testing and counselling. Such screening can present complex moral dilemmas for individual patients and their family, as well as for society.

A number of conditions show ethnic or racial differences based on genetics. For example, Tay-Sachs disease, characterized by early neurological deterioration and cognitive impairment, affects primarily Ashkenazi Jewish families, particularly those of Northeastern European origin, whereas Sephardic Jewish families appear to be no more at risk for the disease than other populations. The incidence of cystic fibrosis is highest in Whites but almost nonexistent in Asians, and the rare affected Canadian of African or Caribbean origin is usually in a person who is likely to be of mixed ancestry. A classic disorder of African- or Caribbean-origin Canadians is sickle cell disease. First Nations, Métis, and Inuit are at risk for type 2 diabetes and cardiovascular disease. Such racial and ethnic differences are further considered in relation to diseases and defects as they are discussed individually throughout the book.

Common food items and medications may cause health problems in certain ethnic groups. For example, persons of Mediterranean, African, Near Eastern, and Asian origin frequently have glucose-6-phosphate dehydrogenase deficiency. They may develop acute hemolytic anemia after they ingest fava beans or certain medications such as aspirin preparations, sulphonamides, or primaquine (the medication used to treat malaria). Other groups, especially Southern Europeans, Jews, Arabs, African- or Caribbean-origin Canadians, and Asians, are more likely to have a deficiency of lactase, the enzyme needed to metabolize lactose. Ingestion of lactose can cause abdominal distension, flatus, and diarrhea (Purnell & Paulanka, 2003). Unknowing but well-meaning health care workers may be responsible for these symptoms in their patients when they prescribe or provide foods or food supplements containing lactose as sources of nutrients.

Physical Characteristics

Among racial groups there are observable differences in physical appearance. The most obvious are skin and hair colouring and texture. Skin colour is determined by the amount of melanin pigment present in the skin. Persons from countries located near the equator have darkly pigmented skin, which serves to protect the skin from year-round exposure to the sun's rays. Persons from northern countries have very light skin, which provides for maximum exposure to the sun's rays (necessary for vitamin D metabolism) during the short daylight hours. There can be wide variations in skin colour between these two extremes as a result of geographic origin or intermixing of persons with dark and light skin colour. In patients with dark pigmentation, the detection of skin colour changes (e.g., vasomotor alterations, cyanosis, jaundice) can be difficult and requires modified assessment techniques.

Variations in the newborn are often related to racial or ethnic origin. For example, newborn infants of parents of Asian and African or Caribbean origin are smaller than infants of White parents, and bluish pigmented areas (Mongolian spots) on the sacral region are a common observation in infants with darker skin colouring. It is important that health care providers be familiar with these birthmarks. They should be documented at newborn examinations and subsequent visits so that they are not suddenly interpreted as bruises (Garwick & Auger, 2000).

Evaluation of stature and body build reveals some racial tendencies. "Typical" growth descriptions are often based on observations of middle-class White Canadian children. Children from Asian countries are commonly smaller, falling below the tenth percentile on weight and height charts used for North American–born children (Trawick-Smith, 2006). This difference in stature can lead to misinterpretation of health status and capabilities.

Cultural Customs

Nurses must be aware of the need to consider cultural differences among patients when providing health care. An understanding of the various beliefs regarding the causation of illness and disease, as well as traditional health practices, is essential to successful intervention. The more nurses know about the values, beliefs, and customs of various ethnic groups, the better they will be able to meet the needs of families and work together to plan care.

NURSING ALERT Cultural resources that include a brief description of the culture and views on health, illness, diet, and other matters are available on the Internet; some institutions develop their own quick references. A newer approach to cultural competence focuses on educating providers to be aware of certain cross-cutting cultural and social issues and health beliefs that are present in all cultures (Betancourt et al., 2003).

Cultural Relativism

Although clinical characteristics of a disease or condition are essentially the same across cultures, the way in which a child or family interprets or experiences it varies. Culture as an influence is one obvious explanation for variance. *Cultural relativism* is the concept that any behaviour must be assessed first in the context of the culture in which it occurs (Purnell & Paulanka, 2003). Nurses must first relate to the family's perceptions and interpretations of experiences from the family's background and cultural belief system before they can effectively intervene.

For example, some cultures may view a chronic illness or disability as affecting only particular aspects of a child's life, and the child as a whole is viewed as normal. In contrast, Chinese families frequently describe the illness as having global effects on many aspects of the child's present and future life (Martinson, Armstrong, & Qiao, 1997). These contrasting views may result in parents having different goals and expectations for their children.

In some cultures, the child's gender may influence a family's perception of the implications of an illness or disability. For example, in Arabic and Asian cultures, boys are held in higher esteem than girls. This also holds true for some families of Jewish, Italian, Greek, and East Indian origin. Boys may receive better health care and more food because they are expected to take care of their parents in old age (Galanti, 2004).

Perceptions of disease or signs and symptoms of illness are also influenced by culture. Some cultures, for example, see diarrhea as a cleansing of the body that is essential for health maintenance and prevention or cure of illness. Furthermore, signs or symptoms resulting from diarrhea and ensuing dehydration, such as malaise, fever, anorexia, and irritability, may be viewed as separate illness entities.

Nurses can often recognize a family's health-related cultural perceptions and interpretations through discussion and observation. Implications of these perceptions should be explored with the family and considered when planning culturally appropriate interventions.

Cultural Shock

The term *cultural shock* describes the "feelings of helplessness and discomfort and a state of disorientation experienced by an outsider attempting to comprehend or effectively adapt to a different cultural group because of differences in cultural practices, values, and beliefs" (Leininger, 1978). This state occurs with both patients and health care providers who move from one cultural setting to another. It can happen to persons who immigrate to a new country (such as refugees) or to those from a subcultural group who must adjust to the ways of an unfamiliar subgroup (such as children entering the school subculture or consumers entering the hospital subculture). Cultural shock is characterized by the inability to respond to or function in a new or strange situation (see Critical Thinking Exercise).

Numerous factors influence reactions to a new environment. Language barriers, including dialects and jargon (such as medical language) specific to a subcultural group, inhibit effective communication. Unfamiliar habits and customs (such as different role behaviours or etiquette) and differences in attitudes and beliefs can be puzzling to the stranger in a new environment. The outsider can experience intense feelings of isolation, loneliness, and nonrelatedness.

Nurses are challenged to overcome cultural shock and to develop the dynamics of cultural sensitivity, an awareness of cultural similarities and differences. In doing so, the nurse is enabled to practise culturally competent care.

Relationships With Health Care Providers

Communication in the health care setting can be challenging when both parties speak the same language. It becomes even more complex when the patient and health care provider speak different languages. The same word can have different meanings in different cultures. Patients may say "yes" to a question they do not understand when they mean "no." Communication styles can differ by style and demeanour, use of silence, eye contact, gestures, and body language (Galanti, 2004).

In relation to time, some cultures are oriented toward the clock, whereas others are more focused on activities. Conflicts can arise during an interaction involving these two orientations. For example, some cultures tend to be flexible in their time orientation; they may be late for or miss appointments because other issues take precedence, and the family may not communicate this to the health agency. Japanese individuals, by contrast, consider time to be valuable and to be used wisely.

Family roles differ by culture as well. Decision making may involve the extended family. Authority figures in a family may be a mother, father, or grandparent. Kinship structure is also determined by culture. Many cultures are unilateral in that

CRITICAL THINKING EXERCISE

Reducing Cultural Shock

A woman from an Arab country in the Middle East is visiting her child, who is being hospitalized for a serious illness. Her husband left for home a short time ago to wash and change clothes. She speaks little English. You need to obtain consent from her for an emergency procedure. She is hesitant and refuses to sign the consent form. What should you do?

1. Evidence—Is there sufficient information to draw any conclusions about this woman's actions?
2. Assumptions—Describe some underlying assumptions about each of the following:
   a. Arab culture
   b. Need for interpreter
   c. Consent process for obtaining approval for emergency procedures
3. What priorities for nursing care should be established at this time?
4. Does the evidence support your nursing intervention(s)?
5. What alternative perspectives might you have?

they trace their descent from either a male or a female ancestor (Galanti, 2004).

NURSING ALERT In working with families, it is essential for nurses to identify key members. Failure to include these significant individuals in communication or teaching can seriously hinder working together to achieve the care plan.

Nurses should inform themselves of any specific attitudes regarding the manner of approach to a child in a given culture. Some cultures may view their children as being able to make decisions for themselves, even those that are typically regarded as too young to do so in Canada. They may allow a child to decide whether to take a medicine or not, whereas in other cultures this view might be viewed as irresponsible (Purnell & Paulanka, 2003). Some ethnic groups, such as the Amish, consider a child's admission to the hospital to be a family affair, with all members gathering to support and console the child and parents. In other groups, such as the Samoan family, the family is willing to relinquish the care of the child to the hospital authority without interference. Their visits with the child are short, although intense; this behaviour may be misinterpreted by the hospital staff as indifference or abandonment.

All ethnic groups are entitled to be treated with dignity and respect. Stereotyping is to be condemned. People are individuals who are evaluated in relation to their cultural standards, needs, and preferences. For example, believing that fathers are never involved in the direct care of their child can result in wrong assumptions about a culture (Fig. 32-4).

Nurses who are members of a majority culture may encounter tension and distrust in a child from a minority culture as a result of the child's learned perception of or relationships with other persons in the majority group. On the basis of these biases, minority children may suspect that nurses have hostile feelings toward them and may fear ill treatment. When such children are hospitalized, this feeling compounds the feelings of loneliness and helplessness, which accompany frightening experiences and separation from families. The reverse situation may be encountered by a nurse from a minority culture attempting to meet the needs of a child who has been conditioned to view the nurse's culture, ethnic group, or gender as inferior.

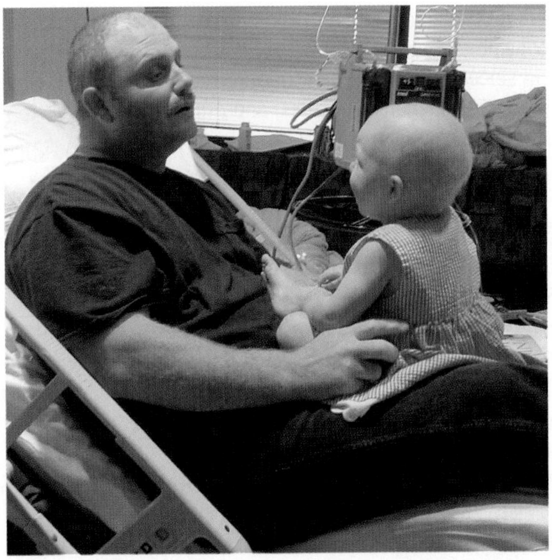

Fig. 32-4 A father with his hospitalized child. *(Courtesy E. Jacob, Texas Children's Hospital, Houston.)*

Communication

Communication may be a source of distress and misunderstanding between persons from different ethnic groups, especially if the languages are different. Lack of interpreter services and linguistically appropriate health education materials is associated with patient dissatisfaction, poor understanding and compliance, and lower-quality health care (Betancourt et al., 2003). Health care organizations must ensure the competence of language assistance provided to persons with limited English proficiency by interpreters and bilingual staff. Family and friends should not be used for interpretation services, except on request by the patient if no other trained professional medical interpreters are available (Shaw-Taylor, 2002).

Some persons with poor or limited language comprehension may simply smile and nod in agreement if they do not understand the questions or directives. It is vital that the family fully understand all implications of a child's care and management before they sign permissions for special procedures or assume responsibility for the child's care. It is not uncommon for a Vietnamese or a Japanese family to indicate "yes" in order to avoid social disharmony, when in fact they mean "no". They tend to use indirectness rather than confrontation and may become evasive when direct questioning makes them uncomfortable.

NURSING ALERT Helpful communication tools include the following:

- Have a series of audio and audiovisual recordings in several languages designed to greet the family and familiarize them with the hospital.
- If an interpreter is not available on site, attempts should be made to access an interpreter via telephone. Many communities have interpreters available as a back-up system.
- Have legal consent forms and explanations of common diagnostic tests available in several languages.
- Keep cards with common greetings, phrases, and names of body parts and pictures in the family's language with the patient's chart.

Many First Nations, Métis, and Inuit people practise nonverbal communication and are highly sensitive to body language. They use periods of silence to formulate thoughts in preparation for speech and often remain silent after listening to statements by others in order to properly assimilate what has been said. Interruption, interjection, or haste in arriving at conclusions is perceived as immature behaviour.

The level of comfort with body space or distance from others varies among cultures. For example, Latin Americans tend to get closer whereas Asians prefer a greater distance between people. Eye contact is also viewed differently in cultures. Although Anglo-Canadians are advised to look people straight in the eye, it is not uncommon for persons in some ethnic groups to avoid eye contact and become uncomfortable when conversing with health workers. A Vietnamese patient may not look directly into the nurse's eyes as a sign of respect.

Some Aboriginal people will make eye contact during the initial greeting, but continued, unwavering eye contact is considered insulting and disrespectful. Some Asians may consider eye contact a sign of hostility or impoliteness.

Families may be reluctant to question or otherwise initiate contact with health care providers. In Asian cultures, for example, it is considered a sign of disrespect to question those who are viewed as persons of authority. A Japanese family may wait silently rather than ask questions or question decisions being made. They believe that health care providers know best and will meet their needs without their being asked. It is also important to avoid criticism. Criticism can cause some Asians to "lose face," or feel ashamed, which is highly undesirable.

Lack of fluency in the dominant language has been considered a significant barrier to the use of health care services by many families (Betancourt et al., 2003; Bowen, 2001). Often families may have poor comprehension of the health care providers' language, so it is necessary to speak slowly and carefully, not loudly, when conversing with them. Many persons are able to read and write English or French better than they can speak or understand it. Also, the dominant language usually takes over in anxiety-provoking situations, even among those who are able to communicate satisfactorily under ordinary circumstances.

Terms of address and the use of first and last names also vary among cultures and can create confusion. For example, in traditional Asian cultures, the family name is given first, out of respect for the family, and the given name follows. Therefore, all siblings in a family have the same first name. Ethiopians have a complex system whereby women retain their last names after marriage and the paternal grandfather's name becomes the child's last name.

The expression of emotion also varies by culture. In some cultures (e.g., Latin American), emotions tend to be expressed openly and members are accustomed to sharing their sorrows and joys with family and friends. Conversely, Nordic and Asian groups are more restrained.

Health care providers generally ask questions and use handouts, booklets, and—particularly with children—dolls and pictures as communication aids. This practice is uncommon in some cultures. For example, Aboriginal healers ask few questions and do not use forms. Nurses need to consider both verbal and nonverbal communication techniques to interact effectively with children and their families from different cultures (see Guidelines box).

GUIDELINES Culturally Sensitive Interactions

Nonverbal Strategies

- Invite family members to choose where they would like to sit or stand, allowing them to select a comfortable distance for personal space.
- Observe interactions with others to determine which body gestures (e.g., shaking hands) are acceptable and appropriate. Ask when in doubt.
- Avoid appearing rushed.
- Be an active listener.
- Observe for cues regarding appropriate eye contact.
- Learn appropriate use of pauses or interruptions for different cultures.
- Ask for clarification if nonverbal meaning is unclear.

Verbal Strategies

- Learn the proper terms of address.
- Use a positive tone of voice to convey interest.
- Speak slowly and carefully, not loudly, when families have poor language comprehension.
- Encourage questions.
- Learn basic words and sentences of the family's language, if possible.
- Avoid medical jargon and use more basic words when asking questions or describing treatments or other aspects of care.
- When asking questions, tell the family why the questions are being asked, the way in which the information they provide will be used, and how it might benefit their child.
- Repeat important information more than once.
- Always give the reason or purpose for a treatment or prescription.
- Use information written in the family's language.
- Obtain the services of an interpreter whenever the child or family are not fluent in English or French. Some families may be reluctant to use the services as they may be concerned there will be a charge—explain that many families use and benefit from this free service.
- Learn from families and representatives of their culture some methods of communicating information without creating discomfort.
- Address intergenerational needs (e.g., family's need to consult with others).
- Be sincere, open, and honest and, when appropriate, share personal experiences, beliefs, and practices to establish rapport and trust.

Food Customs

Food customs and symbolism are an integral part of various cultural, ethnic, and religious groups. Although in a large country such as Canada many persons have adopted the eclectic food habits that have evolved over countless generations, many ethnic and geographic food traditions and preferences have been retained. Special holidays, ceremonies, and life experiences such as births, birthdays, weddings, and death are often marked by special food items or feasts. In many cultures, specific food practices are followed during pregnancy in the belief that certain foods damage the developing fetus.

The distinctive food customs of ethnic groups are a product of their native environment and were determined by availability. Fish is a staple food of persons living near the ocean, such as people from Japan, Polynesia, Southern Europe, and Scandinavia. Fruit and vegetable preferences are directly related to the climate in which the foods grow naturally or can be cultivated. The types of grain that are ethnically associated are also those that grow best in immigrants' native lands. In some cultures, food is highly spiced; in others, foods tend to be bland.

Children may have a number of food restrictions. Some have a physiological origin, such as lack of dairy foods in the diets of some persons of African or Asian ancestry, in whom a hereditary lactase deficiency prevents digestion of foods containing lactose. Others have religious restrictions, such as kosher foods and restrictions on food preparation according to the Orthodox Jewish faith; avoidance of pork by persons of Islamic faith; and the vegetarian diet of Seventh-Day Adventists.

Children in a strange environment, such as the hospital, feel much more comfortable when they are served familiar foods (Fig. 32-5). Hospital food often tastes strange and bland. The family may be concerned that their child is not receiving foods appropriate to their culture and beliefs. When possible, it is advisable to provide children foods that are familiar to them or allow families to bring favourite foods. Concern for differences in food habits and patterns conveys an attitude of respect for the family's ethnic or religious heritage.

Health Beliefs and Practices

Health Beliefs

Beliefs related to the cause of illness and maintenance of health are an integral part of the cultural heritage of families. Often inseparable from religious beliefs, health beliefs influence the ways in which families cope with health problems and respond to health care providers. Predominant among most cultures are beliefs related to natural forces, supernatural forces, and imbalance between forces.

Natural Forces

The most common natural forces held responsible for ill health are cold air entering the body and impurities in the air; if the body is not adequately protected, illness can ensue. For example, a Chinese mother may overdress her infant in an effort to keep cold wind from entering the child's body. The Chinese believe that cold weather, rain, and wind are responsible for "cold" conditions. Among Canadians of African origin, natural phenomena such as phases of the moon, seasons of the year, and planet positions are believed to affect the body and its processes; thus health maintenance is strongly associated with the ability to read "the signs." Most First Nations, Métis, and Inuit people consider health to be a state of harmony with nature and the universe.

Supernatural Forces

High on the list of causes of illness are forces beyond comprehension and logical explanation. Evil influences such as voodoo, witchcraft, or evil spirits are viewed in some cultures as causes of adverse health, especially those illnesses that cannot be explained by other means.

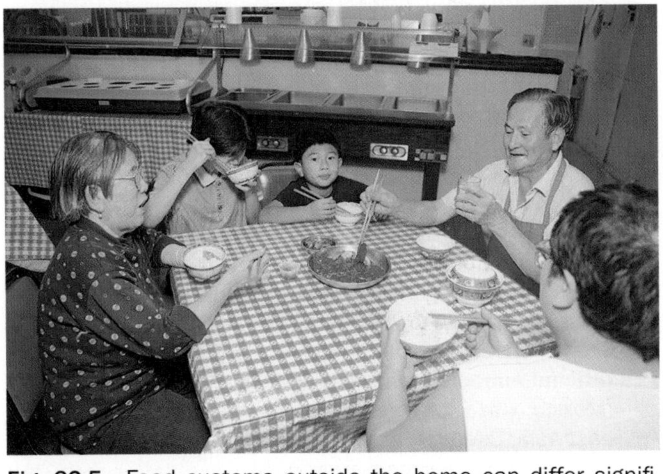

Fig. 32-5 Food customs outside the home can differ significantly from traditional cultural practices.

A health belief common among people from Central America, the Middle East, the Mediterranean, and some Asian and African societies is the concept of the evil eye (Galanti, 2004). The general belief is that one person inflicts evil on another and causes the victim to fall ill. The motive is usually envy. Each culture that believes in the evil eye also has ways to neutralize it. This is part of the concept of health as a state of balance, and illness as a state of imbalance (see Imbalance of Forces, below). Infants and small children, because of immature development of their internal strength–weakness states, are especially vulnerable to the gaze of the evil eye. Consequently, the evil-eye concept serves to rationalize an inexplicable onset of illness in children who display such symptoms as restlessness, crying, diarrhea, vomiting, and fever.

The belief that a witch can cast a spell over others at the request of someone who wishes them ill is found in Caribbean, African, and Australian aboriginal cultures. The victim is often tortured in effigy by pins driven into a doll at the location where the intended victim is to be hurt. "Voodoo deaths" have occurred from the victim's belief in the curse and may result from dehydration as the victim gives up the will to live and refuses to drink (Chidester, 2001). Because this belief is seldom expressed to health care providers, they may not be aware of its influence on patients.

Imbalance of Forces

The concept of balance or equilibrium is widespread throughout the world. One of the most common imbalances supported by Latin American, Filipino, Chinese, and Arab cultures is that which exists between "hot" and "cold." This belief is reputedly derived from the Hippocratic theory of humoral pathology, which states that illness is caused by an imbalance of the four humours: phlegm, blood, black bile, and yellow bile. "Hot" and "cold" describe certain properties and conditions completely unrelated to temperature. Diseases, areas of the body, foods, and illnesses are classified as either "hot" or "cold." In Chinese health belief, the forces are termed *yin* (cold) and *yang* (hot). To maintain health, these "hot" and "cold" forces must be kept in balance.

Illness is treated by restoring normal balance through the application of appropriate "hot" or "cold" remedies. A "cold" condition such as a respiratory tract disease is believed to be caused by exposure to cold weather, rain, or cold wind entering the body; it is treated by administering "hot" foods, herbs, or medications. Menstruation is considered to be a "hot" condition; therefore women are cautioned against ingesting "hot" foods, which might increase menstrual flow or produce cramping. Ingesting too much of either "hot" or "cold" foods can also be interpreted as a cause of illness.

Health care workers who are aware of this belief are better able to understand why some persons refuse to eat certain foods. It is possible to help families devise a diet that contains the necessary balance of basic food groups prescribed by the medical subculture while still following the beliefs of the ethnic subculture.

The hot–cold food classification may have adverse effects. For example, newborn infants are often started on milk formulas. Milk formula is considered to be a "hot" food, whereas whole milk is viewed as a "cold" food. Infants tend to develop rashes, which are believed to be caused by "hot" foods; in such cases, parents may decide to switch to whole milk. However, parents fear that it is dangerous to change too rapidly, so they often feed the child some type of neutralizing substance, which may create additional health problems. Such a problem might be averted if the family's preference is determined before discharge from the hospital, with a formula recommended that is agreeable to both the family and the practitioner.

Health Practices

There are numerous similarities among cultures regarding prevention and treatment of illness. All cultures have some types of home remedies that they apply before seeking help from other persons. Within some ethnic communities, traditional healers who are endowed with the ability to "cure" maladies are sought for special situations and when home remedies are unsuccessful. Some Asians will consult an herbalist, knowledgeable in medicines, or an ethnic practitioner practiced in Asian therapies, including acupuncture (insertion of needles), acupressure (application of pressure), and moxibustion (application of heat). First Nations, Métis, and Inuit people may consult a variety of traditional healers with specific skills and knowledge. Specialized healers diagnose illness, provide nonsacred treatments (usually by way of massage and herbs), and care for souls. Other specialists perform services or affect cures through spiritual means.

Traditional healers are powerful persons in their community. They "speak the language" of the family who seeks help and often combine their rituals and potions with prayer and entreaties to God. They also are able to create an atmosphere conducive to successful management. Furthermore, they exhibit a sincere interest in the family and their problem.

Some traditional remedies are compatible with the medical regimen and can be used to reinforce the treatment plan. For example, most of the foods contraindicated for persons with peptic ulcers are "hot" foods and would be avoided because of their belief systems. Also, aspirin (a "hot" medication) is an appropriate therapy for "cold" diseases such as the common cold and arthritis. It is not uncommon to discover that a traditional prescription has a scientific basis. However, no scientific basis has been found for numerous health remedies or preventive practices, such as the use of garlic or asafetida (a bad-smelling gum resin, obtained from various Asiatic plants, that looks like a dried sponge), which is worn around the neck to prevent contagious diseases. Also, wearing copper or silver bracelets to protect the wearer as he or she grows has no scientific basis.

Practices that do no harm should be respected. Overcoming the effect of the evil eye usually requires specialized rituals conducted by the appropriate practitioner. Sometimes the faith in the traditional practitioner results in a delay in obtaining needed medical treatment, although the practitioner will usually suggest medical care if his or her ministrations are unsuccessful.

Health practices of different cultures may also present problems in assessment and interpretation. For example, certain cultural practices or remedies can be misdiagnosed as evidence of child abuse by uninformed professionals (Box 32-1). It is important to explain why these and other familiar remedies may now be considered harmful. Health care providers need to be aware of the practices so they do not misinterpret symptoms, such as red welts from coining. Families need to understand how such practices can place them in jeopardy with child protective services (Galanti, 2004). Cultural health remedies that are detrimental to health include eating clay, excessive amounts of salt, or compounds that contain lead. While a careful history can reveal these remedies, it may require the collaboration of a traditional healer to convince a user to stop the practice.

Faith healing and religious rituals are closely allied with many traditional healing practices. The wearing of amulets, medals, and other religious relics believed by the culture to protect the individual and facilitate healing is a common practice. It is important for health workers to recognize the value of this practice and keep the items where the family has placed them or nearby. It offers comfort and support and rarely impedes medical and nursing care. If an item must be removed during a procedure, it should be replaced, if possible, when the procedure is completed. The reason for its temporary removal should be explained to the family, and they should be reassured that their wishes will be respected.

Nurses can be most effective by operating from a multicultural perspective. This means using appropriate aspects of

BOX 32-1 Cultural Practices Possibly Considered Abusive by the Dominant Culture

Coining—An Asian practice that may produce weltlike lesions on the child's back when a coin, held on edge, is repeatedly rubbed lengthwise on the oiled skin to rid the body of a disease (Galanti, 2004)

Cupping—A practice in many parts of the world (Asia, Latin America, parts of Europe) of placing a container (e.g., tumbler, bottle, jar) containing steam against the skin surface to "draw out the poison" or other evil element. When the heated air within the container cools, a vacuum is created that produces a bruiselike blemish on the skin directly beneath the mouth of the container (Galanti, 2004).

Burning—A practice of some Southeast Asian groups whereby small areas of skin are burned to treat enuresis and temper tantrums

Female genital mutilation (female circumcision)—Removal of or injury to any part of the female genital organ; practised in some parts of Africa (Galanti, 2004)

Forced kneeling—A discipline measure of some Caribbean groups in which a child is forced to kneel for a long time

Topical garlic application—A practice of Yemenite Jews in which crushed garlic cloves or garlic–petroleum jelly plaster is applied to the wrists to treat infectious disease. The practice can result in blisters or garlic burns.

Traditional remedies that contain lead—Greta and azarcon (Mexico; used for digestive problems), paylooah (Southeast Asia; used for rash or fever), and surma (India; used as a cosmetic to improve eyesight)

each culture's orientation toward health in developing culturally acceptable health care interventions.

NURSING ALERT Avoid directly criticizing traditional cultural health beliefs and practices as wrong or harmful or implying that biomedical measures are uniformly correct and effective and the only way to prevent illness or treat sickness. Such criticisms usually result in rejection of both biomedical health care practitioners and their health teaching. When traditional practices do not interfere with the patient's welfare, they need not be discouraged. Often a compromise can be reached that accomplishes the nurse's goal while maintaining the dignity and self-esteem of the child and family.

Religious Beliefs

Religious and spiritual dimensions are among the most important influences in many people's lives. The term *spirituality* relates to an individual's personal beliefs, transcendent experiences, and principles; *religion* refers to an organized system of beliefs or a place of worship. The pediatric nurse who learns how the patient and family view their traditions, values, and beliefs can then understand how these dimensions may affect the patient's health (McEvoy, 2003). Three areas to explore for information about the family's culture, religion, or spirituality are beliefs and values, daily practices, and community involvement. An assessment tool can be easily used for integrating culture and spirituality into the nursing assessment (Box 32-2).

BOX 32-2 Belief Framework for Integrating Culture and Spirituality Into the Nursing Assessment

Belief system—A spiritual belief system is one that gives structure and meaning, often in relation to a higher power, to everyday lives.

Ethics or values—Ethical or personal belief system that guides the family's everyday life. The family may not follow a formal religion but still adhere to core values.

Lifestyle—Diet, nutrition, use of caffeine and alcohol, prayer and meditation, clothing, and medicinal practices all are examples in which culture, religion, and spirituality may be closely connected.

Involvement in a spiritual community—The community can provide the family the benefits of identity, socialization, and support, while keeping children and adolescents involved in safe and healthy social activities.

Education—Religious education affects the cultural, moral, and ethical development of children. The children's belief system influences their coping mechanisms, especially during chronic illness.

Future events—Knowledge of the patient and family's belief system allows the nurse to provide individualized and sensitive anticipatory guidance for future health events.

(From McEvoy, M. [2003]. Culture and spirituality as an integrated concept in pediatric care. *MCN: American Journal of Maternal Child Nursing, 28*[1], 39–43.)

Religion affects the way in which people interpret and respond to illness (Spector, 2004). Among many groups, illness, injury, or death is believed to be sent by God as a punishment for sin. Some may believe that health workers will be unable to help a person whom God is punishing and may express a fatalistic attitude toward treatment, stating it is "the will of God." Others view it as a test of strength, like the testing of Job in the Bible, and strive to remain faithful and overcome the conflicts.

Religious affiliation has implications for many health-related functions and procedures. It is comforting for the family of an ill child to have this need recognized and respected. Nurses need to determine whether there are any special considerations, including dietary restrictions, related to spiritual practices that are important to the family. Family members should be asked whether they want a clergy member present and whether they prefer hospital staff to call the clergy person or prefer to do this on their own.

It is also important to determine the wishes of the family regarding baptism, rites or practices related to death, and other religious rituals (such as circumcision, communion, or use of amulets or icons). Religion, which offers families understanding and spiritual support, is a valuable asset to health care. Characteristics of selected religions with beliefs that affect health care are outlined in Table 32-1.

Importance of Culture and Religion to Nursing

A general agreement exists among nurses to raise the cultural competence of professional nursing practice. The nurse who seeks to gain cultural competence learns about other cultures, is able to assess the perspectives of others, and shares his or her own culture with others (Dunn, 2002). Cultural competence is an ongoing, interactive process (Dunn, 2002). It has been described as a set of congruent behaviours, attitudes, and policies that come together to enable a system, organization, or professionals to work effectively in cross-cultural situations (Cross, 1988). More recently it has been defined as cultural awareness that includes curiosity, perceptiveness, respect, and a desire to connect with the patient and family in order to determine the most appropriate goals and the interventions most likely to achieve those goals (Srivastava, 2008). Six elements of fostering cultural competence are as follows (Canadian Nurses Association, 2010; Dunn, 2002) (see Chapter 2):

1. Working on changing one's world view by examining one's own values and behaviours and striving to reject racism and institutions that support it
2. Becoming familiar with core cultural issues by recognizing these issues and exploring them with patients
3. Becoming knowledgeable about the cultural groups one works with while learning about each individual patient's unique history
4. Becoming familiar with core cultural issues related to health and illness and communicating in a way that encourages patients to explain what an illness means to them
5. Developing a relationship of trust with patients and creating a welcoming atmosphere in the health care setting
6. Negotiating for mutually acceptable and understandable interventions of care

evolve Skill—Providing Culturally Sensitive Care

Table 32-1 Religious Beliefs That May Affect Nursing Care

BIRTH AND DEATH	DIET AND FOOD PRACTICES	MEDICAL CARE
Buddhist		
Birth—No baptism Infant presentation **Death**—Last rite chanting is often practised at bedside soon after death; the deceased's family or Buddhist priest should be contacted. **Organ donation/transplantation**—Organ donation is a matter of individual conscience.	Restrictions on some food combinations; extremes must be avoided. Some sects are strictly vegetarian. Discourage use of alcohol and drugs	Illness is believed to be a trial to aid development of soul; illness results from Karmic causes. Surgery is permitted, but extremes must be avoided. Cleanliness is of great importance. Family, community, and a Buddhist priest are supportive visitors.
Church of Christ, Scientist (Christian Science)		
Birth—No baptism **Death**—No last rites; autopsy is not permitted except in cases of sudden death; individuals can choose burial or cremation. **Organ donation/transplantation**—Church takes no specific position on transplantation as distinct from other medical or surgical procedures. Individuals decide on organ donation.	Abstain from alcohol and some forms of tea and coffee	Oppose human intervention with medications or other therapies; however, may accept legally required immunizations Accept physical and moral healing Family, friends, and members of the spiritual community may visit.
Church of Jesus Christ of Latter-Day Saints (Mormon)		
Birth—No baptism Infant is blessed by a church official at first opportunity after birth (in church). Baptism is by immersion at 8 years. **Death**—Believe that it is proper to bury the dead in the ground; cremation is discouraged. **Organ donation/transplantation**—Individuals can choose whether to will organs to be used in transplants.	Prohibit tea (except herbal), coffee, and alcohol Some individuals avoid chocolate and other products that contain caffeine. Fasting for 24 hours each month	Devout adherents believe in divine healing. Medical therapy is not prohibited. **Spiritual items**—A "garment" (type of underwear) that is considered sacred; the person may not want to remove it. Family, friends, and church members are supportive visitors.
Hindu		
Birth—No baptism **Death**—Certain prescribed rites are followed after death; a priest may tie a thread around the neck or wrist to signify blessing; the family will wash the body and are particular about who touches the dead; bodies are to be cremated. **Organ donation/transplantation**—No religious laws prohibiting donation; this is an individual decision.	Many dietary restrictions Eating meat is forbidden.	With an amputation, loss of a limb is believed to represent sins committed in a previous life. Accept most modern medical practices; some belief in faith healing **Spiritual items**—Person may wear a thread around the wrist or body; do not remove it. Family, community members, and the priest are supportive visitors.
Islam (Muslim)		
Birth—At birth, the first words said to the infant in his or her right ear are *Allah-o-Akbar* (Allah is great), and the remainder of the Call for Prayer is recited. An *Aqeeqa* (party) to celebrate the birth of the child is arranged by the parents. Male children are circumcised. **Death**—At the time of death, specific rituals (e.g., bathing, wrapping the body in cloth) must be done by a same-sex Muslim. Before moving and handling the body, it is preferable to contact someone from the person's mosque or the local Islamic Society to perform these rituals. **Organ donation/transplantation**—Individual decides on organ donation/transplantation.	All pork products and alcohol are prohibited. Fasting is practised during the ninth month of the Islamic year (Ramadan).	Believers are encouraged in the Qu'ran to seek treatment. It is taught that only Allah cures; however, Muslims are taught not to refuse treatment in the belief that Allah will take care of them because he also chooses at times to work through the efforts of humans. **Other practices**—Right hand is used for eating; left hand is for hygiene. Family and friends are supportive visitors.
Jehovah's Witnesses		
Birth—No baptism **Death**—No official last rites are practised when death occurs. **Organ donation/transplantation**—Organ donation is forbidden.	No tobacco; moderate alcohol is permissible.	Blood or blood products are not allowed; volume expanders are permissible if not derived from blood.

Table 32-1 Religious Beliefs That May Affect Nursing Care—cont'd

BIRTH AND DEATH	DIET AND FOOD PRACTICES	MEDICAL CARE
Judaism (Orthodox and Conservative)		
Birth—No baptism Ritual circumcision of male infants occurs on the eighth day; performed by a mohel (ritual circumciser familiar with Jewish law and aseptic technique). **Death**—According to tradition, during last moments of life, relatives and close friends remain with the deceased. Amputated limbs or surgically removed tissues should be made available to the family for burial. Cremation is not allowed. Burial usually occurs quickly. **Organ donation/transplantation**—Organ transplantation/donation is complex issue; sometimes they are practised.	Numerous dietary kosher laws exist; followers are allowed only meat from animals that are vegetable eaters and are ritually slaughtered; predatory fowl, shellfish, and pork are prohibited. Milk products served first can be followed by meat in a few minutes, but milk may not be consumed for several hours after eating meat. Fasting is part of Yom Kippur observance. Matzo replaces leavened bread during Passover week.	May resist surgical procedures during Sabbath, which extends from sundown Friday until sundown Saturday. Illness is grounds for violating dietary laws. **Spiritual items**—Men may wear a prayer shawl, yarmulka (cap), or both while praying. Family, friends, and the rabbi are supportive visitors.
Roman Catholicism		
Birth—Infant baptism; this is especially urgent if there is a poor prognosis, when it may be performed by anyone. **Death**—Sacrament of the Sick is performed if prognosis is poor while patient is alive. **Organ donation/transplantation**—Transplantation of organs is ethically and morally acceptable to the Vatican; organ donation is viewed as an act of charity.	Abstaining from meat is practised on Ash Wednesday, Good Friday, and Fridays during Lent (as a rule).	Encourage anointing of the sick **Spiritual items**—Rosary beads, crucifix Traditional church teaching does not approve of contraceptives or abortion.
First Nations, Métis, and Inuit		
Most Aboriginal peoples practise some form of Christian religion, along with the traditional spiritual beliefs and practices that are primarily passed from generation to generation orally. **Birth**—Viewed as a sacred event experienced by the whole family **Death**—Typically, practices of the Christian religion are followed, but may include traditional rituals, such as family members cutting their hair, lighting ceremonial fires	Fasting is common in order to participate in certain spiritual experiences. Specific foods may be used as symbols during ceremonies or rituals—these foods differ from area to area.	Follow the practices of the Christian religion Individuals may burn sweetgrass, tobacco or other sacred herb to aid in healing.

(Data from Galanti, G. [2004]. *Caring for patients from different cultures* [3rd ed.]. Philadelphia: University of Pennsylvania Press; Lipson, J. G., Dibble, S. L., & Minarik, P. A. [2005]. *Culture and clinical care: A pocket guide*. San Francisco: UCSF Nursing Press; Purnell, L. D., & Paulanka, B. J. [2003]. *Transcultural health care: A culturally competent approach*. Philadelphia: Davis; Spector, R. E. [2004]. *Cultural diversity in health and illness* [6th ed.]. Upper Saddle River, NJ: Prentice Hall; National Defence and the Canadian Forces. [2009]. *Religions in Canada: Native spirituality.*)

NURSING ALERT Cultural knowledge helps nurses better understand the behaviour of their patients and families so that they do not consider it pathological. This knowledge helps to ensure that nurses are not making assumptions about patients' behaviour in a clinical context. By performing a cultural assessment, the nurse can elicit the patient's and family's understanding of their illness and individualize the patient's care plan. Cultural competence is nursing competence (Dreher & MacNaugton, 2002).

With globalization increasing the ethnic, racial, and cultural diversity of our society, it is important that nurses become competent in transcultural nursing knowledge so that they can provide safe and meaningful care to people from all corners of the globe (Leininger & McFarland, 2002). To begin to understand and deal effectively with families in a multicultural community, nurses need to recognize the barriers to transcultural communication and work toward removing these barriers (Muñoz & Luckmann, 2005). Nurses, too, are a product of their own cultural background. They need to recognize that they are part of the "nursing culture." Nurses function within the framework of a professional culture with its own values and traditions and, as such, become socialized into their professional culture in their educational program and later in their work environments and professional associations.

Frequently, nurses and other health care workers are not aware of their own cultural values and how those values influence their thoughts and actions. A model for self-examination on cultural competence is the ASKED model (Box 32-3).

Recognizing that a behaviour may be characteristic of a culture rather than an "abnormal" behaviour places nurses at an advantage in their relationships with families. When nurses respect a family's cultural differences, they are better able to determine whether the behaviour is distinctive to the individual or a characteristic of the culture.

BOX 32-3 Exploring Your Cultural Competence: ASKED Model of Cultural Competence

Awareness—Am I aware of my personal biases and prejudices toward cultural groups different from mine? Have I examined my own values, beliefs, and assumptions?
Skill—Do I have the skill to conduct a cultural assessment and perform a culturally based physical assessment in a sensitive manner?
Knowledge—Do I have knowledge of the patient's world view and the field of biocultural ecology?
Encounters—How many face-to-face encounters have I had with patients from diverse cultural backgrounds?
Desire—What is my genuine desire to want to be culturally competent?

(Data from Campinha-Bacote, J. [2003]. Many faces: Addressing diversity in health care. *Online Journal of Issues in Nursing, 8*[1]. Retrieved from http://www.nursingworld.org/MainMenuCategories/ANAMarketplace/ANAPeriodicals/OJIN/TableofContents/Volume82003/No1Jan2003/AddressingDiversityinHealthCare.html.)

Cultural standards and values, family structure and function, and experience with health care influence a family's feelings and attitudes toward health, their children, and health care delivery systems. It is often difficult for nurses to be nonjudgemental and objective in working with families whose behaviours and attitudes differ from or conflict with their own. Nurses need to understand how their own cultural background influences the way in which they deliver care, and they need to be responsible and accountable for incorporating culturally competent care into their practice, regardless of domain (Canadian Nurses Association, 2010). Relying on one's own values and experiences for guidance can result in frustration and disappointment. It is one thing to know what is needed to deal with a health problem; it is often quite another to implement a fruitful course of action within the cultural and socioeconomic framework of the family.

Rather than attempting to change longstanding beliefs, it is beneficial to adapt a family's ethnic practices to their health needs. In the effort to understand and respect the cultural beliefs of families, nurses need to develop knowledge of how cultural groups understand life processes, define health and illness, and view the causes of illness. Nurses need to combine their cross-cultural knowledge with excellent communication skills to learn from the individual patient and family about issues important to their care (Betancourt et al., 2003).

Some broad health care–related characteristics of selected cultures are outlined in Table 32-2. Tables 32-1 and 32-2 are

Table 32-2 Broad Cultural Characteristics Related to Health Care of Children and Families

HEALTH BELIEFS	HEALTH PRACTICES	FAMILY RELATIONSHIPS	COMMUNICATION
African			
Illness classified as: **Natural**–Affected by forces of nature without adequate protection (e.g., cold air, pollution, food and water) **Unnatural**–God's punishment for improper behaviour May see illness as the "will of God"	Self-care and traditional medicine are prevalent. Traditional therapies are usually religious in origin. Traditional therapies often are not shared with the medical provider. Prayer is a common means for prevention and treatment.	Strong kinship bonds in extended family; members come to aid of others in crisis Less likely to view illness as a burden Place strong emphasis on work and ambition Elders are cared for and respected.	Alert to any evidence of discrimination Place importance on nonverbal behaviour Affection is shown by touching and hugging. Silence may indicate lack of trust. Initial eye contact is made to show respect; maintaining eye contact can be viewed as aggressive. It is best to use a direct but caring approach.
Chinese			
A healthy body is viewed as a gift from parents and ancestors and must be cared for. Health is seen as one of the results of balance between the forces of *yin* (cold) and *yang* (hot)–energy forces that rule the world. Illness is caused by imbalance. Blood is believed to be the source of life and is not regenerated. *Chi* is innate energy.	Goal of therapy–To restore balance of yin and yang Acupuncture needles are applied to appropriate meridians identified in terms of yin and yang. Acupressure and tai chi are replacing acupuncture in some areas. Use of *moxibustion*–application of heat to skin over specific meridians There is wide use of medicinal herbs procured and applied in prescribed ways. Meals may or may not be planned to balance hot and cold.	Extended family pattern common Strong concept of loyalty of young to old Respect for elders is taught at an early age–acceptance without questioning or talking back Children's behaviour is a reflection on the family. Family and individual honour and "face" are important. Self-reliance and self-esteem are highly valued; self-expression is repressed.	Open expression of emotions is unacceptable. Often they smile when they do not comprehend. Eye contact is avoided as sign of respect.

Table 32-2 Broad Cultural Characteristics Related to Health Care of Children and Families—cont'd

HEALTH BELIEFS	HEALTH PRACTICES	FAMILY RELATIONSHIPS	COMMUNICATION
Haitian			
Illness is seen as a punishment. **Natural** (*maladi bone die*—disease of the Lord) caused by environmental factors, movement of blood within the body, changes between hot and cold, and bone displacement **Supernatural** (*loa*—spirits' anger) Good health seen as maintenance of equilibrium Prayer and good spiritual habits are important.	Health a personal responsibility. Foods have properties of "hot" or "cold" and "light" or "heavy" and must be in harmony with one's life cycle and bodily states. Natural illnesses are treated by home and traditional remedies first. May use religious medallions, rosary beads, or figure of saint to pray with	Maintenance of family reputation is paramount. Lineal authority is supreme; children are in a subordinate position in the family hierarchy. Children are valued for parental security in old age and are expected to contribute to family welfare at an early age.	Often they smile and nod in agreement when they do not understand. Quiet and gentle communication style and lack of assertiveness lead health care providers to falsely believe that they comprehend health teaching and are compliant. They may not ask questions if the health care provider is busy or rushed.
Japanese			
Shinto religious influence Humans are inherently good. Evil is caused by outside spirits. Illness is caused by contact with polluting agents (e.g., blood, corpses, skin diseases) Health is achieved through harmony and balance between self and society. Disease is caused by disharmony with society and not caring for the body.	Energy is restored by means of acupuncture, acupressure, massage, and moxibustion along affected meridians. *Kampō medicine*—use of natural herbs Believe in removal of diseased parts The trend is to use both Western and Asian healing methods. Care for disabled is viewed as the family's responsibility. Take pride in child's good health Seek preventive care, medical care for illness	Close intergenerational relationships Generational categories: *Issei*—first generation to live outside Japan *Nisei*—second generation *Sansei*—third generation *Yonsei*—fourth generation Family tends to keep problems to themselves. Value self-control and self-sufficiency Concept of *haji* (shame) imposes strong control; unacceptable behaviour of children reflects on the family.	Individuals make significant use of nonverbal communication with subtle gestures and facial expression. They tend to suppress emotions. They will often wait silently.
First Nations, Métis, and Inuit			
Believe health is state of harmony with nature and universe Believe that disease can be caused by natural forces or by a loss of spirit Respect bodies through proper management Depend on individual belief in traditional culture Traditional health beliefs are holistic and wellness oriented.	Distinction is made between an indigenous health problem requiring a native healer or practice and Western disease requiring other medical care. Health practices include self-sufficiency and harmonious living. Participation in religious ceremonies, prayer, and traditional healing ceremonies (e.g., sweat lodges) promote health.	Cultures vary in kinship structure. Extended family structure—usually includes relatives from both sides of the family. Elder members assume leadership roles.	Individuals use anecdotes or metaphors to discuss a situation. Long pauses indicate careful consideration. Nonverbal communication is used. Respect is indicated by avoiding eye contact. Individuals usually speak for themselves.
Vietnamese			
Good health is considered to be a balance between yin and yang. Concept of health is based on harmony and balance. Rituals are used to prevent illness.	Family uses all means possible before using outside agencies for health care. They regard health as a family responsibility; outside aid is sought when resources run out. Herbal medicine, spiritual practices, and acupuncture are used. Individuals may consider the head sacred and feet profane; avoid touching the head after touching feet. They may use cupping, coin rubbing, or pinching skin. They may inhale aromatic oils, take herbal teas, or wear strings tied on the body.	Family is a revered institution. Multigenerational families Family is the chief social network. Children are highly valued. Individual needs and interests are subordinate to those of a family group. Father is the main decision maker. Women are taught submission to men. Parents expect respect and obedience from their children.	Individuals may hesitate to ask questions. Questioning authority is a sign of disrespect; asking questions is considered impolite. They may avoid eye contact with health care providers as a sign of respect.

(From Galanti, G. [2004]. *Caring for patients from different cultures* [3rd ed.]. Philadelphia: University of Pennsylvania Press; Lipson, J. G., Dibble, S. L., & Minarik, P. A. [2005]. *Culture and clinical care: A pocket guide*. San Francisco: UCSF Nursing Press; Purnell, L. D., & Paulanka, B. J. [2003]. *Transcultural health care: A culturally competent approach*. Philadelphia: Davis; Spector, R. E. [2004]. *Cultural diversity in health and illness* [6th ed.]. Upper Saddle River, NJ: Prentice Hall; The Canadian Encyclopedia. [2010]. *Native people, Religion*. Retrieved from http://www.thecanadianencyclopedia.com/articles/indian-reserve.)

presented as beginning frameworks for practising transcultural nursing. Nurses must assess the cultural and religious practices of families to identify how these practices are similar to and different from those of their own cultural and religious backgrounds. At the same time, they must remember to treat each patient as an individual, not simply a member of a particular group.

NURSING ALERT These generalizations are presented to help nurses learn the unique beliefs and practices of various groups and are not meant to be used as stereotypes of any group. A stereotype is an end point; the nurse does not attempt to learn where the individual fits the statement. A generalization provides a beginning point from which the nurse can inquire further, to obtain more information and individualize the patient's care (Galanti, 2004).

Key Points

- Culture is the sum total of mores, traditions, and beliefs about how people function and encompasses other products of human works and thoughts specific to members of an intergenerational group, community, or population.
- Nurses have a responsibility to continually develop cultural competence. This includes understanding and respecting the influence of culture, race, and ethnicity on the development of social and emotional relationships, childrearing practices, and attitudes toward health.
- A child's self-concept evolves from ideas about his or her social roles.
- Key social determinants of health that influence children include culture, ethnicity, socioeconomic status, poverty, homelessness, immigration, religion, schools, community, and peer groups.
- Membership in a minority group may present special challenges for children.
- A child's physical characteristics and susceptibility to health problems can be related to ethnic and cultural variations of hereditary and socioeconomic forces.
- Groups of children suffering from greater physical and mental health problems are those living in poverty; those who are homeless; First Nations, Métis, and Inuit peoples; and those who are recent immigrants to Canada.
- Because verbal and nonverbal communication is an important cultural consideration, nurses need to acknowledge and respect their patients' communication practices for productive interaction to occur.
- Cultural and religious beliefs related to the cause of illness and maintenance of health may focus on natural forces, supernatural forces, or imbalance of forces.
- In planning and implementing patient care, nurses need to strive to adapt ethnic practices to the family's health needs rather than attempt to change longstanding beliefs.
- No cultural group is homogeneous; every racial and ethnic group contains great diversity.
- Culturally competent care is family-centred care, as it focuses on exploring the child's and family's meaning of illness, preferences, and needs.

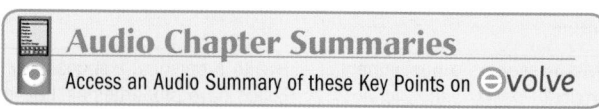

Audio Chapter Summaries

Access an Audio Summary of these Key Points on Evolve

References

Aboriginal Affairs and Northern Development Canada. (2010a). *Aboriginal peoples and communities.* Retrieved from http://www.ainc-inac.gc.ca/ap/index-eng.asp.

Aboriginal Affairs and Northern Development Canada. (2010b). *About AANDC.* Retrieved from http://www.ainc-inac.gc.ca/ai/index-eng.asp.

Aboriginal Affairs and Northern Development Canada. (2012). *Aboriginal demography—Population, household and family projections, 2001-2026.* Retrieved from http://www.aadnc-aandc.gc.ca/eng/1309463897584.

Barozzino, T. (2010). Immigrant health and the children and youth of Canada: Are we doing enough? *Healthcare Quarterly, 14,* 52–59.

Betancourt, J. R. (2004). Cultural competence—marginal or mainstream movement. *New England Journal of Medicine, 351*(10), 953–954.

Betancourt, J. R., et al. (2003). Defining cultural competence: A practical framework for addressing racial/ethnic disparities in health and healthcare. *Public Health Reports, 118,* 292–302.

Bowen, S. (2001). *Language barriers in access to health care.* Cat. No. H39-578/2001E. Ottawa: Health Canada. Retrieved from http://www.hc-sc.gc.ca/hcs-sss/alt_formats/hpb-dgps/pdf/pubs/2001-lang-acces/2001-.lang-acces-eng.pdf.

Canadian Nurses Association. (2010). *Position statement: Promoting cultural competence in nursing.* Retrieved from http://www2.cna-aiic.ca/CNA/documents/pdf/publications/PS114_Cultural_Competence_2010_e.pdf.

Canadian Paediatric Society. (2007). *Canadian paediatricians join international efforts to eradicate poverty.* Retrieved from http://www.cps.ca/english/media/newsreleases/2007/Poverty.htm.

Canadian Paediatric Society. (2010). *Aboriginal children and youth.* Retrieved from http://www.cps.ca/English/Advocacy/Aboriginal.htm.

Chidester, D. (2001). *Patterns of transcendence: Religion, death, and dying* (2nd ed.). Belmont, CA: Wadsworth.

Citizenship and Immigration Canada. (2010). *Research and statistics: Facts and figures.* (Modified February 16, 2012). Retrieved from http://www.cic.gc.ca/english/resources/statistics/menu-fact.asp.

Cross, T. (1988). Service to minority populations. *Focal Point, 3,* 1–4.

Denburg, A., & Daneman, D. (2010). The link between social inequality and child health outcomes. *Healthcare Quarterly, 14,* 21–31.

Dreher, M., & Macnaughton, N. (2002). Cultural competence in nursing: Foundation or fallacy? *Nursing Outlook, 50,* 181–186.

Dunn, A. M. (2002). Culture competence and the primary care provider. *Journal of Pediatric Health Care, 16,* 105–111.

Elgersma, S. (2008). *Immigration status and legal entitlement to insured health services.* Ottawa: Library of Parliament.

Fleury, D. (May 2008). Low-income children. *Perspectives* (Cat. No. 75-001-X). Statistics Canada. Retrieved from http://www.statcan.gc.ca/pub/75-001-x/2008105/pdf/10578-eng.pdf.

Galanti, G. (2004). *Caring for patients from different cultures* (3rd ed.). Philadelphia: University of Pennsylvania Press.

Garwick, A., & Auger, S. (2000). What do providers need to know about American Indian culture? Recommendations from urban Indian family caregivers. *Family, Systems and Health, 18,* 177–189.

Giger, J. N., & Davidhizar, R. E. (2008). *Transcultural nursing: Assessment and intervention* (5th ed.). St. Louis: Mosby.

Halfon, N., Larson, K., & Russ, S. (2010). Why social determinants? *Healthcare Quarterly, 14,* 9–20.

Health Canada. (2010). *Canada's health care system: Medicare.* Retrieved from http://www.hc-sc.gc.ca/hcs-sss/medi-assur/index-eng.php.

Human Resources and Skills Development Canada. (2012). *Homeless partnering strategy.* Retrieved from http://www.hrsdc.gc.ca/eng/homelessness/index.shtml.

Jones, D. C., & Crawford, J. K. (2006). The peer appearance culture during adolescence: Gender and body mass variations. *Journal of Youth and Adolescence, 2,* 257–269.

Leininger, M. (1978). *Transcultural nursing.* New York: John Wiley & Sons.

Leininger, M., & McFarland, M. (2002). *Transcultural nursing: Concepts, theories, research and practice* (3rd ed.). New York, Chicago, Toronto: McGraw-Hill.

Lemchuk-Favel, L., & Jock, R. (2004). Aboriginal health systems in Canada: Nine case studies. *Journal of Aboriginal Health, 1*(1), 28–51.

Martinson, I. M., Armstrong, V., & Qiao, J. (1997). The experience of the family of children with chronic illness at home in China. *Pediatric Nursing, 23*(4), 371–375.

McEvoy, M. (2003). Culture and spirituality as an integrated concept in pediatric care. *MCN: American Journal of Maternal Child Nursing, 28*(1), 39–43.

McNeill, T. (2010). Family as a social determinant of health. *Healthcare Quarterly, 14*, 60–67.

Meléndez, L. (2005). Parental beliefs and practices around early self-regulation: The impact of culture and immigration. *Infants and Young Children, 18*(2), 136–146.

Muñoz, C., & Luckmann, J. (2005). *Transcultural communication in nursing* (2nd ed.). Clifton Park, NY: Thomson Delmar Learning.

Natural Resources Canada. (2009). *The atlas of Canada—Visible minority population.* Retrieved from http://atlas.nrcan.gc.ca/site/english/maps/peopleandsociety/population/visible_minority.

Postl, B., Cook, C., & Moffatt, M. (2010). Aboriginal child health and the social determinants: Why are these children so disadvantaged? *Healthcare Quarterly, 14*, 42–51.

Public Health Agency of Canada. (2011). *Determinants of health: What makes Canadians healthy or unhealthy?* Retrieved from http://www.phac-aspc.gc.ca/ph-sp/determinants/index-eng.php#determinants.

Purnell, L. D., & Paulanka, B. J. (2003). *Transcultural health care: A culturally competent approach* (2nd ed.). Philadelphia: Davis.

Search Institute. (2011). *What kids need: Developmental assets tools.* Retrieved from http://www.search-institute.org/assets/forty.htm.

Shaw-Taylor, Y. (2002). Culturally and linguistically appropriate health care for racial or ethnic minorities: Analysis of the US Office of Minority Health's recommended standards. *Health Policy, 62*, 211–221.

Spector, R. E. (2004). *Cultural diversity in health and illness* (6th ed.). Upper Saddle River, NJ: Prentice-Hall.

Srivastava, R. (2008). The ABC (and DE) or cultural competence in clinical care. *Ethnicity and Inequalities in Health and Social Care, 1*(1), 27–33.

Statistics Canada. (2007). *Women in Canada: Work chapter updates.* Retrieved from http://www.statcan.gc.ca/pub/89f0133x/89f0133x2006000-eng.htm.

Statistics Canada. (2008). *2006 census data products* (modified March 15, 2012). Retrieved from http://www12.statcan.gc.ca/census-recensement/2006/dp-pd/index-eng.cfm.

Trawick-Smith, J. (2006). *Early childhood development: A multicultural perspective* (4th ed.). Upper Saddle River, NJ: Pearson Education.

Tropello, P.D. (2000). The many faces of homelessness. In M. L. Kelley & V. M. Fitzsimons (Eds.), *Understanding cultural diversity.* Sudbury, MA: Jones & Bartlett.

Waldram, J. B., Herring, D. A., and Kue Young, T. (2006). *Aboriginal health in Canada: Historical, cultural and epidemiological perspectives* (2nd ed.). Toronto, Buffalo, London: University of Toronto Press.

Unit 7

33 Developmental Influences on Child Health Promotion

Learning Objectives

On completion of this chapter, the reader will be able to:

- Describe major trends in growth and development.
- Explain the alterations in the major body systems that take place during the process of growth and development.
- Discuss the development of personality, cognition, language, morality, spirituality, and self-concept and how they are related to each other.
- Describe the role of play in the growth and development of children.
- Demonstrate an understanding of the role of innate and environmental factors in the physical and emotional development of children.

Electronic Resources

Additional information related to the content in Chapter 33 can be found on

evolve the companion Web site at

http://evolve.elsevier.com/Canada/Perry/maternal/

- Examination Review Questions
- Critical Thinking Exercise—Growth Trends During Infancy

Growth and Development

Foundations of Growth and Development

Growth and **development**, usually referred to as a unit, express the sum of the numerous changes that take place during the lifetime of an individual. The entire course is a dynamic process that encompasses several interrelated dimensions:

Growth—An increase in the number and size of cells as they divide and synthesize new proteins; results in increased size and weight of the whole or any of its parts

Development—A gradual change and expansion; advancement from lower to more advanced stages of complexity; the emerging and expanding of the individual's capacities through growth, maturation, and learning

Maturation—An increase in competence and adaptability; aging; usually used to describe a qualitative change; a change in the complexity of a structure that makes it possible for that structure to begin functioning; to function at a higher level

Differentiation—Processes by which early cells and structures are systematically modified and altered to achieve specific and characteristic physical and chemical properties; sometimes used to describe the trend of mass to specific; development from simple to more complex activities and functions

All of these processes are interrelated, simultaneous, and ongoing; none occurs apart from the others. The processes depend on a sequence of endocrine, genetic, constitutional, environmental, and nutritional influences (Seidel et al., 2006). The child's body becomes larger and more complex; the personality simultaneously expands in scope and complexity. Very simply, *growth* can be viewed as a quantitative change, and *development* as a qualitative change.

Stages of Development

Most authorities in the field of child development conveniently categorize child growth and behaviour into approximate age stages or in terms that describe the features of an age group. The age ranges of these stages are admittedly arbitrary and, because they do not take into account individual differences, cannot be applied to all children with any degree of precision. However, categorization affords a convenient means to describe the characteristics associated with the majority of children at periods when distinctive developmental changes appear and specific developmental tasks must be accomplished. (A *developmental task* is a set of skills and competencies peculiar to each developmental stage that children must accomplish or master in order to deal effectively with their environment.) It is also significant for nurses to know that there are characteristic health problems peculiar to each major phase of development. The sequence of descriptive age periods and subperiods that are used here and elaborated on in subsequent chapters is listed in Box 33-1.

Patterns of Growth and Development

There are definite and predictable patterns in growth and development that are continuous, orderly, and progressive. While these patterns, or trends, are universal and basic to all human beings, each person accomplishes these in a manner and time unique to that individual.

Directional Trends

Growth and development proceed in regular, related directions, or gradients, and reflect the physical development and maturation of neuromuscular functions (Fig. 33-1). The first pattern is the *cephalocaudal*, or head-to-tail, direction. The head end of the organism develops first and is large and complex, whereas the lower end is small and simple and takes shape at a later period. While the physical evidence of this trend is most apparent during the period before birth, it also applies to postnatal behaviour development. Infants achieve structural control of the head before they have control of the trunk and extremities, hold their back erect before they stand, use their eyes before their hands, and gain control of their hands before they have control of their feet.

The second pattern, the **proximodistal**, or near-to-far, trend, applies to midline-to-peripheral development. A conspicuous illustration is the early embryonic development of limb buds, which is followed by rudimentary fingers and toes. In the infant, shoulder control precedes mastery of the hands, the whole hand is used as a unit before the fingers can be manipulated, and the central nervous system develops more rapidly than the peripheral nervous system.

These patterns are bilateral and appear symmetrical—each side develops in the same direction and at the same rate as the other. For some of the neurological functions, this symmetry

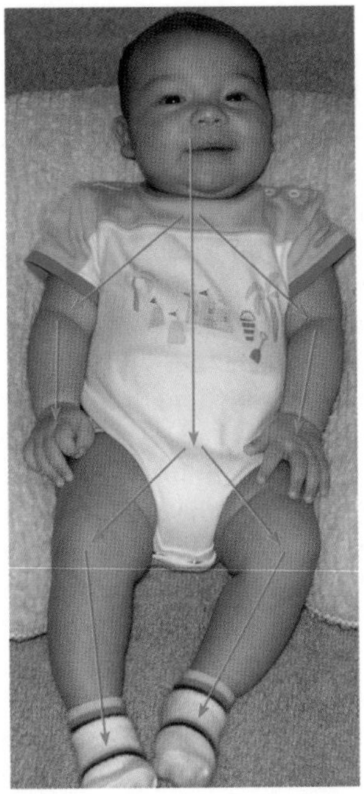

Fig. 33-1 Directional trends in growth.

BOX 33-1 Developmental Age Periods

Prenatal Period—Conception to Birth

Germinal—Conception to approximately 2 weeks
Embryonic—2 to 8 weeks
Fetal—8 to 40 weeks (birth)

A rapid growth rate and total dependency make this one of the most crucial periods in the developmental process. The relationship between maternal health and certain manifestations in the newborn emphasizes the importance of adequate prenatal care to the infant's health and well-being.

Infancy Period—Birth to 12 Months

Neonatal—Birth to 27 or 28 days
Infancy—1 month to approximately 12 months

The infancy period is one of rapid motor, cognitive, and social development. Through mutuality with the caregiver (parent), the infant establishes a basic trust in the world and the foundation for future interpersonal relationships. The critical first month of life, although part of the infancy period, is often differentiated from the remainder because of the infant's major physical adjustments to extrauterine existence and the parent's psychological adjustment.

Early Childhood—1 to 6 Years

Toddler—1 to 3 years
Preschool—3 to 6 years

This period, which extends from the time children attain upright locomotion until they enter school, is characterized by intense activity and discovery. It is a time of marked physical and personality development. Motor development advances steadily. Children at this age acquire language and wider social relationships, learn role standards, gain self-control and mastery, develop increasing awareness of dependence and independence, and begin to develop a self-concept.

Middle Childhood—6 to 10 Years

Frequently referred to as the school age, this period of development is one in which the child is directed away from the family group and centred around the wider world of peer relationships. There is steady advancement in physical, mental, and social development, with emphasis on developing skill competencies. Social cooperation and early moral development take on more importance with relevance for later life stages. This is a critical period in the development of a self-concept.

Later Childhood—11 to 19 Years

Prepubertal—10 to 13 years
Adolescence—13 to approximately 18 years

The tumultuous period of rapid maturation and change known as adolescence is considered to be a transitional period that begins at the onset of puberty and extends to the point of entry into the adult world—usually high school graduation. Biological and personality maturation are accompanied by physical and emotional turmoil, and there is redefining of the self-concept. In the late adolescent period, the young person begins to internalize all previously learned values and to focus on an individual, rather than a group, identity.

evolve Critical Thinking Exercise—Growth Trends During Infancy is only external because of unilateral differentiation of function at an early stage of postnatal development. For example, by the age of approximately 5 years, the child has demonstrated a decided preference for the use of one hand over the other, even though previously either one had been used.

The third trend, *differentiation*, describes development from simple operations to more complex activities and functions. From broad, global patterns of behaviour, more specific, refined patterns emerge. All areas of development (physical, mental, social, and emotional) proceed in this direction. Through the process of development and differentiation, early embryonal cells with vague, undifferentiated functions progress to an immensely complex organism composed of highly specialized and diversified cells, tissues, and organs. Generalized development precedes specific or specialized development; gross, random muscle movements take place before fine muscle control.

Sequential Trends

In all dimensions of growth and development there is a definite, predictable sequence, with each child normally passing through every stage. Children crawl before they creep, creep before they stand, and stand before they walk. Later facets of the personality are built on the early foundation of **trust**. The child babbles, then forms words and, finally, sentences; writing emerges from scribbling.

Developmental Pace

Although development has a fixed, precise order, it does not progress at the same rate or pace in each child. There are periods of accelerated growth and periods of decelerated growth in both total body growth and the growth of subsystems. Not all areas develop at the same pace. When a spurt occurs in one area such as gross motor, minimal advances may take place in language, fine motor, or social skills. Once the gross motor skill has been achieved, then development will shift to another area. The rapid growth before and after birth gradually levels off throughout early childhood. Growth is relatively slow during middle childhood, markedly increases at the beginning of adolescence, and levels off in early adulthood. Each child grows at his or her own pace. Distinct differences are observed between children as they reach developmental milestones.

Sensitive Periods

There are limited times during the process of growth when the organism will interact with a particular environment in a specific manner. Periods termed *critical*, *sensitive*, *vulnerable*, and *optimal* are those times in the life of an organism when it is more susceptible to positive or negative influences.

The quality of interactions during these sensitive periods determines whether the effects on the organism will be beneficial or harmful. For example, physiological maturation of the central nervous system is influenced by adequacy and timing of contributions from the environment such as stimulation and nutrition. The first 3 months of prenatal life are sensitive periods for physical growth of the fetus.

Psychological development also appears to have sensitive periods, when an environmental event has maximal influence on the developing personality. For example, primary socialization occurs during the first year when the infant makes the initial social attachments and establishes a basic trust in the world. A warm relationship with a parent figure is fundamental to a healthy personality. The same concept might be applied to readiness for learning skills such as toilet training or reading. In these instances, there appears to be an opportune time when the skill is best learned.

Individual Differences

Each child grows in his or her own unique and personal way. Great individual variation exists in the age at which developmental milestones are reached. The sequence is predictable; the exact timing is not. Rates of growth vary, and measurements are defined in terms of ranges, to allow for individual differences. Some children are fast growers, others are moderate, and some are slower to reach maturity. Periods of fast growth, such as the pubescent growth spurt, may begin earlier or later in some children than in others. Children may grow fast or slowly during the spurt and may finish sooner or later than other children. Gender is an influential factor; girls seem to be more advanced in physiological growth at all ages.

Biological Growth and Physical Development

As children grow, their external dimensions change. These changes are accompanied by corresponding alterations in structure and function of internal organs and tissues that reflect the gradual acquisition of physiological competence. Each part has its own rate of growth, which may be directly related to alterations in the child's size (e.g., the heart rate). Skeletal muscle growth approximates whole-body growth; brain, lymphoid, adrenal, and reproductive tissues follow distinct and individual patterns (Fig. 33-2). When growth deficiency has a secondary cause, such as severe illness or acute malnutrition, recovery from the illness or establishment of an adequate diet will produce a dramatic acceleration of the growth rate that usually continues until the child's individual growth pattern is resumed.

External Proportions

Variations in the growth rate of different tissues and organ systems produce significant changes in body proportions during childhood. The cephalocaudal trend of development is most evident in total body growth as indicated by these changes. During fetal development, the head is the fastest growing body part, and at 2 months of gestation the head constitutes 50% of total body length. During infancy, growth of the trunk predominates; the legs are the most rapidly growing part during childhood; in adolescence, the trunk once again elongates. In the newborn infant, the lower limbs are one-third the total body length but only 15% of the total body weight; in the adult, the lower limbs constitute one half of the total body height and 30% or more of the total body weight. As growth proceeds, the midpoint in head-to-toe measurements gradually descends from a level even with the umbilicus at birth to the level of the symphysis pubis at maturity.

Biological Determinants of Growth and Development

The most prominent feature of childhood and adolescence is physical growth (Fig. 33-3). Throughout development various tissues in the body undergo changes in size, composition, and

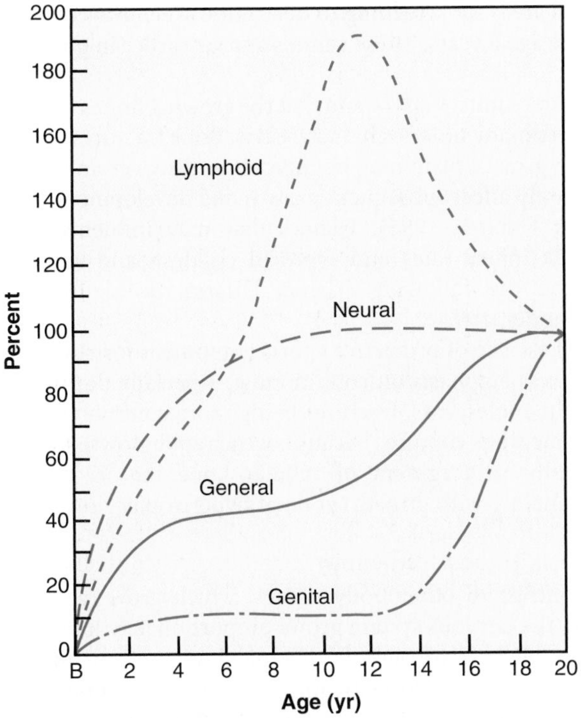

Fig. 33-2 Growth rates for the body as a whole and three types of tissues. Lymphoid: thymus, lymph nodes, and intestinal lymph masses. Neural: brain, dura, spinal cord, optic apparatus, and head dimensions. General: body as a whole; external dimension; and respiratory, digestive, renal, circulatory, and musculoskeletal systems. *B,* Birth. *(From Jackson, J. A., Patterson, D. G., & Harris, R. E. [1930].* The measurement of man. *Minneapolis: University of Minnesota Press.)*

structure. In some tissues the changes are continuous (e.g., bone growth and dentition); in others, significant alterations occur at specific stages (e.g., appearance of secondary sex characteristics). When these measurements are compared with standardized norms, a child's developmental progress can be determined with a high degree of confidence (Table 33-1). Some pediatric illnesses will lead to slower growth patterns. For example, children with Down syndrome have a lower growth velocity, which can be monitored more accurately using an adapted Down syndrome growth chart (Cronk et al., 1988; Myrelid et al., 2002).

Linear growth, or height, occurs almost entirely as a result of skeletal growth and is considered a stable measurement of

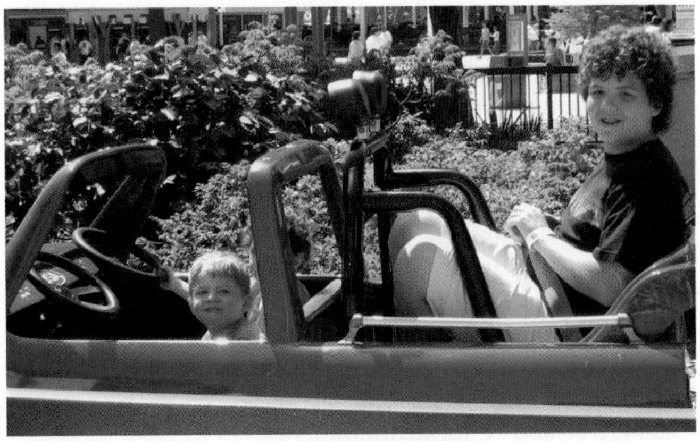

Fig. 33-3 Changes in body proportions occur dramatically during childhood.

Table 33-1 General Trends in Height and Weight Gain During Childhood

AGE GROUP	WEIGHT*	HEIGHT*
Infants		
Birth-6 mo	Weekly gain—140-200 g Birth weight doubles by end of first 4-7 mo†	Monthly gain—2.5 cm
6-12 mo	Weekly weight gain—85-140 g Birth weight triples by end of first year	Monthly gain—1.25 cm Birth length increases by approximately 50% by end of first year
Toddlers	Birth weight quadruples by age 2½	Height at age 2 yr is approximately 50% of eventual adult height Gain during second year—about 12 cm Gain during third year—about 6-8 cm
Preschoolers	Yearly gain—2-3 kg	Birth length doubles by age 4 yr Yearly gain—5-7.5 cm
School-age children	Yearly gain—2-3 kg	Yearly gain after age 7 yr—5 cm Birth length triples by about age 13
Pubertal Growth Spurt		
Females—10-14 yr	Weight gain—7-25 kg Mean—17.5 kg	Height gain—5-25 cm; approximately 95% of mature height achieved by onset of menarche or skeletal age of 13 yr Mean—20.5 cm
Males—11-16 yr	Weight gain—7-30 kg Mean—23.7 kg	Height gain—10-30 cm; approximately 95% of mature height achieved by skeletal age of 15 yr Mean—27.5 cm

*Yearly height and weight gains for each age group represent averaged estimates from a variety of sources.
†Jung, F. E., & Czajka-Narins, D. M. (1985). Birth weight doubling and tripling times: An updated look at the effects of birth weight, sex, race, and type of feeding. *American Journal of Clinical Nutrition, 42,* 182-189.

general growth. Growth in height is not uniform throughout life but ceases when maturation of the skeleton is complete. The maximum rate of growth in length occurs before birth, but the newborn continues to grow at a rapid, though slower, rate.

NURSING ALERT A common method for predicting an adult height is to double the child's height at the age of 2 years to estimate how tall he or she may be as an adult. However, it is very difficult to predict height because of differences in individual growth velocities. A kinesiology research group from Saskatchewan has developed a more accurate method to predict children's adult heights (Sherar, Mirwald, Baxter-Jones, & Tomis, 2005). This formula can be found at http://taurus.usask.ca/growthutility.

At birth, weight is more variable than height and is, to a greater extent, a reflection of the intrauterine environment. The average newborn weighs from 3175 to 3400 g. In general, the birth weight doubles by 4 to 7 months of age and triples by the end of the first year. By the age of 2 to 2½ years the birth weight usually quadruples. After this point the "normal" rate of weight gain, just as the growth in height, assumes a steady annual increase of approximately 2 to 2.75 kg per year until the adolescent growth spurt.

Both bone age determinants and state of dentition are used as indicators of development. These indicators are discussed elsewhere in the text (see next section for bone age; see also Chapters 36 and 38 for dentition).

Skeletal Growth and Maturation

The most accurate measure of general development is skeletal or bone age, the radiological determination of osseous maturation. Skeletal age appears to correlate more closely with other measures of physiological maturity (such as onset of menarche) than with chronological age or height. Bone age is determined by comparing the mineralization of ossification centres and advancing bony form to age-related standards.

Bone formation begins during the second month of fetal life when calcium salts are deposited in the intercellular substance (matrix) to form calcified cartilage first and then true bone. In small bones, the bone continues to form in the centre and cartilage continues to be laid down on the surfaces. In long bones, the ossification begins in the *diaphysis* (the long central portion of the bone) and continues in the *epiphysis* (the end portions of the bone). Between the diaphysis and the epiphysis an epiphyseal cartilage plate (or growth plate) unites with the diaphysis by columns of spongy tissue, the *metaphysis*. Active growth in length takes place in the epiphyseal growth plate. Interference with this growth site by trauma or infection can result in deformity.

The first centres of ossification appear in the 2-month-old embryo, and at birth the number is approximately 400, about half the number at maturity. New centres appear at regular intervals during the growth period and represent bone age. Postnatally the earliest centres to appear (at 5 to 6 months of age) are those of the capitate and hamate bones in the wrist. Therefore, radiographs of the hand and wrist provide the most useful areas for screening to determine skeletal age, especially before age 6 years. These centres appear earlier in girls than in boys.

Nurses must understand that the growing bones of children possess many unique characteristics. Bone fractures occurring at the growth plate may be difficult to discover and may significantly affect subsequent growth and development (Urbanski & Hanlon, 1996). Factors that may influence skeletal muscle injury rates and types in children and adolescents include the following (Caine, DiFiori, & Maffulli, 2006; Kaczander, 1997):

- Less use of protective sports equipment for children
- Less emphasis on conditioning, especially flexibility
- In adolescents, fractures being more common than ligamentous ruptures because of the rapid growth rate of the physeal (segment of tubular bone that is concerned mainly with growth) zone of hypertrophy

Neurological Maturation

In contrast to other body tissues, which grow rapidly after birth, the nervous system grows proportionately more rapidly before birth. Two periods of rapid brain cell growth occur during fetal life: a dramatic increase in the number of neurons between 15 and 20 weeks of gestation and another increase at 30 weeks, which extends to 1 year of age. The rapid growth of infancy continues during early childhood and then slows to a more gradual rate during later childhood and adolescence.

Postnatal growth consists of increasing the amount of cytoplasm around the nuclei of existing cells, increasing the number and intricacy of communications with other cells, and advancing their peripheral axons to keep pace with expanding body dimensions. This allows for increasingly complex movement and behaviour. Neurophysiological changes also provide the foundation for language, learning, and behaviour development. Neurological or electroencephalographic development is sometimes used as an indicator of maturational age in the early weeks of life.

Lymphoid Tissues

Lymphoid tissues contained in the lymph nodes, thymus, spleen, tonsils, adenoids, and blood lymphocytes follow a growth pattern unlike that of other body tissues. These tissues are small in relation to total body size, but they are well developed at birth. They increase rapidly to reach adult dimensions by 6 years of age and continue to grow. At about age 10 to 12 years, they reach a maximum development that is approximately twice their adult size. This is followed by a rapid decline to stable adult dimensions by the end of adolescence.

Development of Organ Systems

All tissues and organ systems undergo changes during development. Some are striking; others are subtle. Many have implications for assessment and care. Because the major importance of these changes relates to their dysfunction, the developmental characteristics of various systems and organs are discussed throughout the book as they relate to these areas. Physical characteristics and physiological changes that vary with age are included in age group descriptions (see Unit 9).

Physiological Changes

Physiological changes that take place in all organs and systems are discussed as they relate to dysfunction (see Unit 11). Other changes such as pulse and respiratory rates and blood pressure are an integral part of physical assessment (see Chapter 34). In addition, changes occur in basic functions, including metabolism, temperature, and patterns of sleep and rest.

Metabolism

The rate of metabolism when the body is at rest (basal metabolic rate [BMR]) demonstrates a distinctive change throughout childhood. Highest in the newborn infant, the BMR closely relates to the proportion of surface area to body mass, which changes as the body increases in size. In both sexes the proportion decreases progressively to maturity. The BMR is slightly higher in boys at all ages and further increases during pubescence over that in girls.

The rate of metabolism determines the child's caloric requirements. The basal energy requirement is about 108 kcal/kg of body weight in infancy and decreases to 40 to 45 kcal/kg at maturity. Water requirements throughout life remain at approximately 1.5 mL/calorie of energy expended. Children's energy needs vary considerably at different ages and with changing circumstances. The energy requirement to build tissue steadily decreases with age, following the general growth curve; however, energy needs vary with the individual child and may be considerably higher. For short periods (e.g., during strenuous exercise) and more prolonged periods (e.g., illness), the needs can be very high.

Temperature

Body temperature, reflecting metabolism, decreases over the course of development. Thermoregulation is one of the most important adaptation responses of the infant during the transition from intrauterine to extrauterine life. In the healthy neonate, hypothermia can result in several negative metabolic consequences, such as hypoglycemia, elevated bilirubin levels, and metabolic acidosis. Skin-to-skin care, also referred to as kangaroo care, is an effective way to prevent neonatal hypothermia in infants (see Chapter 26, Evidence-Informed Practice box). Unclothed, diapered infants are placed on the parent's bare chest after birth, promoting thermoregulation and attachment (Galligan, 2006). After the unstable regulatory ability in the neonatal period, heat production steadily declines as the infant grows into childhood. Individual differences of −8.6° to −17.2°C are normal, and occasionally a child will normally display an unusually high or low temperature. Beginning at approximately 12 years of age, girls' temperature remains relatively stable, whereas the temperature in boys continues to fall for a few more years. Females maintain a temperature slightly above that of males throughout life.

Even with improved temperature regulation, infants and young children are highly susceptible to temperature fluctuations. Body temperature responds to changes in environmental temperature and is increased with active exercise, crying, and emotional stress. Infections can cause a higher and more rapid temperature increase in infants and young children than in older children. In relation to body weight, an infant produces more heat per unit than adolescents. Consequently, during active play or when heavily clothed, an infant or small child is likely to become overheated.

Sleep and Rest

Sleep, a protective function in all organisms, allows for repair and recovery of tissues after activity. As in most aspects of development, there is wide variation among individual children in the amount and distribution of sleep at various ages. As children mature, the total time they spend in sleep and the amount of time they spend in deep sleep change.

Newborn infants sleep much of the time. As infants grow older, the total sleep time gradually decreases, they remain awake for longer periods, and they sleep longer at night. For example, the length of a sleep cycle increases from approximately 50 to 60 minutes for the newborn infant to approximately 90 minutes in adolescence (Anders, Sadeh, & Appareddy, 2005). During the latter part of the first year, most children sleep through the night and take one or two naps during the day. By the time they are 12 to 18 months old, most children have eliminated the second nap. After age 3 years, the child has usually given up daytime naps, except in cultures in which an afternoon nap or siesta is customary. Sleep time declines slightly from ages 4 to 10 and then increases somewhat during the pubertal growth spurt.

The quality of sleep changes as children mature. As children develop through adolescence, their need for sleep does not decline, but their opportunity for sleep may be affected by social activity and academic schedules. The time spent in deep, restful sleep increases from 50% in infancy to 80% in the older child.

Temperament

Temperament is defined as "the manner of thinking, behaving, or reacting characteristic of an individual" (Chess & Thomas, 1999) and refers to the way in which a person deals with life. From the time of birth, children exhibit marked individual differences in the way they respond to their environment and the way that others, particularly the parents, respond to them and their needs. A genetic basis has been suggested for some differences in temperament. Nine characteristics of temperament have been identified through interviews with parents (Box 33-2). Temperament refers to behavioural tendencies, not to discrete behavioural acts; there are no implications of good or bad. Most children can be placed into one of three common categories based on their overall pattern of temperamental attributes:

1. **The easy child**—Easy-going children are even tempered, are regular and predictable in their habits, and have a positive approach to new stimuli. They are open and adaptable to change and display a mild to moderately intense mood that is typically positive. Approximately 40% of children fall into this category.
2. **The difficult child**—Difficult children are highly active, irritable, and irregular in their habits. Negative withdrawal responses are typical, and they require a more structured environment. These children adapt slowly to new routines, people, or situations. Mood expressions are usually intense

and primarily negative. They exhibit frequent periods of crying, and frustration often produces violent tantrums. This group represents about 10% of children.

3. **The slow-to-warm-up child**—Slow-to-warm-up children typically react negatively and with mild intensity to new stimuli and, unless pressured, adapt slowly with repeated contact. They respond with only mild but passive resistance to novelty or changes in routine. They are inactive and moody but show only moderate irregularity in functions. Approximately 15% of children demonstrate this temperament pattern.

Roughly 35% of children either have some, but not all, of the characteristics of one of the categories or are inconsistent in their behavioural responses. Many normal children demonstrate this wide range of behavioural patterns.

Significance of Temperament

Observations indicate that children who display the difficult or slow-to-warm-up patterns of behaviour are more vulnerable to the development of behavioural problems in early and middle childhood. Any child can develop behavioural problems if there is dissonance between the child's temperament and the environment. Demands for change and adaptation that are in conflict with the child's capacities can become excessively stressful. However, authorities emphasize that it is not the children's temperament patterns that place them at risk; it is the degree of fit between children and their environment, specifically their parents, that determines the degree of vulnerability. The potential for optimum development exists when environmental expectations and demands fit with the individual's style of behaviour and the parents' ability to navigate this period (Chess & Thomas, 1999) (see Chapter 36, Growth Failure [Failure to Thrive]).

Early identification of temperament provides a useful tool for caregivers in anticipating probable areas of difficulty or risk associated with development. For example, "difficult" children may be prone to colic in infancy, active children require more vigilance to prevent injury, and school entry requires different approaches for children with different temperaments.

Research indicates that irritable and inadaptable infants can raise doubts in mothers about their competence (Beck, 1996). Additional research indicates that a child's temperament can affect parent–child interactions and influence the parents' self-esteem, marital harmony, mood, and overall satisfaction as parents (Carey, 1998). Studies on the relationship between temperament and the ability to perform a task successfully (mastery motivation) have found that infants with high mastery are more cooperative and less difficult (Morrow & Camp, 1996). Principles that nurses can use in direct patient care and anticipatory guidance to promote mastery of performing tasks are listed in Box 33-3.

BOX 33-2 Attributes of Temperament

Activity—Level of physical motion during activity such as sleep, eating, play, dressing, and bathing

Rhythmicity—Regularity in the timing of physiological functions such as hunger, sleep, and elimination

Approach–withdrawal—Nature of initial responses to new stimuli such as people, situations, places, foods, toys, and procedures (Approach responses are positive and are displayed by activity or expression; withdrawal responses are negative expressions or behaviours.)

Adaptability—Ease or difficulty with which the child adapts or adjusts to new or altered situations

Threshold of responsiveness (sensory threshold)—Amount of stimulation, such as sounds or light, required to evoke a response in the child

Intensity of reaction—Energy level of the child's reactions, regardless of quality or direction

Mood—Amount of pleasant, happy, friendly behaviour compared with unpleasant, unhappy, crying, unfriendly behaviour exhibited by the child in various situations

Distractibility—Ease with which a child's attention or direction of behaviour can be diverted by external stimuli

Attention span and persistence—Length of time a child pursues a given activity (attention) and the continuation of an activity in spite of obstacles (persistence)

Development of Personality and Mental Function

Personality and cognitive skills develop in much the same manner as biological growth—new accomplishments build on previously mastered skills. Many aspects depend on physical growth and maturation. The following discussion acts as an introduction to the multiple facets of personality and behaviour development; many aspects of this development are also integrated with the later discussion of children's emotional and social development at various ages (see Unit 9). Table 33-2 summarizes some of the developmental theories.

Theoretical Foundations of Personality Development

Psychosexual Development (Freud)

According to Freud, all human behaviour is energized by psychodynamic forces, and this psychic energy is divided among three components of personality: the id, the ego, and the superego. The *id*, the *unconscious mind*, is the inborn component that is driven by instincts. The id obeys the pleasure

BOX 33-3 Activities to Promote Mastery Motivation

- Provide inconspicuous assistance during play.
- Share pleasure with infant in accomplishments.
- Do not give immediate assistance during tasks.
- Do not interrupt infant during tasks.
- Let infant initiate activities.
- Limit controlling feedback during play.
- Provide audio and visually responsive toys.
- Provide early kinesthetic stimulation (picking up, rocking).

(From Morrow, J. D., & Camp, B. W. [1996]. Mastery motivation and temperament of 7-month-old infants. *Pediatric Nursing, 22*[3], 211–217.)

Table 33-2 Summary of Personality, Cognitive, and Moral Development Theories

PSYCHOSEXUAL (FREUD)	PSYCHOSOCIAL (ERIKSON)	COGNITIVE (PIAGET)	MORAL JUDGEMENT (KOHLBERG)	SPIRITUAL (FOWLER)
I. Infancy—Birth to 1 Yr				
Oral-sensory	Trust vs. mistrust	Sensorimotor (birth–2 yr)		Undifferentiated
II. Toddlerhood—1 to 3 Yr				
Anal-urethral	Autonomy vs. shame and doubt	Preoperational thought, preconceptual phase (transductive reasoning [e.g., specific to specific] (2–4 yr)	Preconventional (premoral) level Punishment and obedience orientation	Intuitive-projective
III. Early Childhood—3 to 6 Yr				
Phallic-locomotion	Initiative vs. guilt	Preoperational thought, intuitive phase (transductive reasoning) (4–7 yr)	Preconventional (premoral) level Naive instrumental orientation	Mythical-literal
IV. Middle Childhood—6 to 12 Yr				
Latency	Industry vs. inferiority	Concrete operations (inductive reasoning and beginning logic) (7–11 yr)	Conventional level Good-boy, nice-girl orientation Law-and-order orientation	Synthetic-convention
V. Adolescence—12 to 18 Yr				
Genitality	Identity vs. role confusion	Formal operations (deductive and abstract reasoning) (11–15 yr)	Postconventional or principled level Social-contract orientation Universal ethical principle orientation	Individuating-reflexive

principle of immediate gratification of needs, regardless of whether the object or action can actually do so. The *ego*, the *conscious mind*, serves the reality principle. It functions as the conscious or controlling self that is able to find realistic means for gratifying the instincts while blocking the irrational thinking of the id. The *superego*, the *conscience*, functions as the moral arbitrator and represents the ideal. It is the mechanism that prevents individuals from expressing undesirable instincts that might threaten the social order.

Freud considered the sexual instincts to be significant in the development of the personality. However, he used the term *psychosexual* to describe any sensual pleasure. During childhood, certain regions of the body assume a prominent psychological significance as the source of new pleasures and new conflicts gradually shifts from one part of the body to another at particular stages of development:

Oral stage (birth to 1 year)—During infancy, the major source of pleasure seeking is centred on oral activities such as sucking, biting, chewing, and vocalizing. Children may prefer one of these over the others, and the preferred method of oral gratification can provide some indication of the personality they develop.

Anal stage (1 to 3 years)—Interest during the second year of life centres on the anal region as sphincter muscles develop and children are able to withhold or expel fecal material at will. At this stage, the climate surrounding toilet training can have lasting effects on children's personalities.

Phallic stage (3 to 6 years)—During the phallic stage, the genitalia become an interesting and sensitive area of the body. Children recognize differences between the sexes and become curious about the dissimilarities. This is the period around which the controversial issues of the Oedipus and Electra complexes, penis envy, and castration anxiety are centred.

Latency period (6 to 12 years)—During the latency period, children elaborate on previously acquired traits and skills. Physical and psychic energy are channelled into acquisition of knowledge and into vigorous play.

Genital stage (age 12 and older)—The last significant stage begins at puberty with maturation of the reproductive system and production of sex hormones. The genital organs become the major source of sexual tensions and pleasures, but energies are also invested in forming friendships and preparing for marriage.

Psychosocial Development (Erikson)

The most widely accepted theory of personality development is that advanced by Erikson (1963). Although built on Freudian theory, it is known as *psychosocial* development and emphasizes a healthy personality as opposed to a pathological approach. Erikson also uses the biological concepts of critical periods and epigenesis, describing key conflicts or core problems that the individual strives to master during critical periods in personality development. Successful completion or mastery of each of these core conflicts is built on the satisfactory completion or mastery of the previous stage.

Each psychosocial stage has two components—the favourable and the unfavourable aspects of the core conflict—and progress to the next stage depends on resolution of this conflict. No core conflict is ever mastered completely but remains a recurrent problem throughout life. No life situation is ever secure. Each new situation presents the conflict in a new form. For example, when children who have satisfactorily achieved a sense of trust encounter a new experience (e.g., hospitalization), they must again develop a sense of trust in those responsible for their care in order to master the situation. Erikson's lifespan approach to personality development consists of eight stages; however, only the first five relating to childhood are included here:

1. **Trust versus mistrust (birth to 1 year)**—The first and most important attribute to develop for a healthy personality is basic *trust*. Establishment of basic trust dominates the first year of life and describes all of the child's satisfying experiences at this age. Corresponding to Freud's oral stage, it is a time of "getting" and "taking in" through all the senses. It exists only in relation to something or someone; therefore, consistent, loving care by a mothering person is essential for development of trust. *Mistrust* develops when trust-promoting experiences are deficient or lacking or when basic needs are inconsistently or inadequately met. Although shreds of mistrust are sprinkled throughout the personality, from a basic trust in parents stems trust in the world, other people, and oneself. The result is faith and optimism.
2. **Autonomy versus shame and doubt (1 to 3 years)**—Corresponding to Freud's anal stage, the problem of *autonomy* can be symbolized by the holding on and letting go of the sphincter muscles. The development of autonomy during the toddler period is centred on children's increasing ability to control their bodies, themselves, and their environment. They want to do things for themselves, using their newly acquired motor skills of walking, climbing, and manipulating and their mental powers of selecting and decision making. Much of their learning is acquired by imitating the activities and behaviour of others. Negative feelings of *doubt* and *shame* arise when children are made to feel small and self-conscious, when their choices are disastrous, when others shame them, or when they are forced to be dependent in areas in which they are capable of assuming control. The favourable outcomes are *self-control* and *willpower*.
3. **Initiative versus guilt (3 to 6 years)**—The stage of *initiative* corresponds to Freud's phallic stage and is characterized by vigorous, intrusive behaviour; enterprise; and a strong imagination. Children explore the physical world with all their senses and powers (Fig. 33-4). They develop a conscience. No longer guided only by outsiders, they have an inner voice that warns and threatens. Children sometimes undertake goals or activities that are in conflict with those of parents or others, and being made to feel that their activities or imaginings are bad produces a sense of guilt. Children must learn to retain a sense of initiative without impinging on the rights and privileges of others. The lasting outcomes are *direction* and *purpose*.
4. **Industry versus inferiority (6 to 12 years)**—The stage of *industry* is the latency period of Freud. Having achieved the more crucial stages in personality development, children are ready to be workers and producers. They want to engage in tasks and activities that they can carry through to completion; they need and want real achievement. Children learn to compete and cooperate with others, and they learn the rules. It is a decisive period in their social relationships with others. Feelings of *inadequacy* and *inferiority* may develop if too much is expected of them or if they believe that they cannot measure up to the standards set for them by others. The ego quality developed from a sense of industry is competence.
5. **Identity versus role confusion (12 to 18 years)**—Corresponding to Freud's genital period, the development of *identity* is characterized by rapid and marked physical changes. Previous trust in their bodies is shaken, and children become overly preoccupied with the way they appear in the eyes of others as compared with their own self-concept. Adolescents struggle to fit the roles they have played and those they hope to play with the current roles and fashions adopted by their peers, to integrate their concepts and values with those of society, and to come to a decision regarding an occupation. Inability to solve the core conflict results in *role confusion*. The outcome of successful mastery is *devotion* and *fidelity* to others and to values and ideologies.

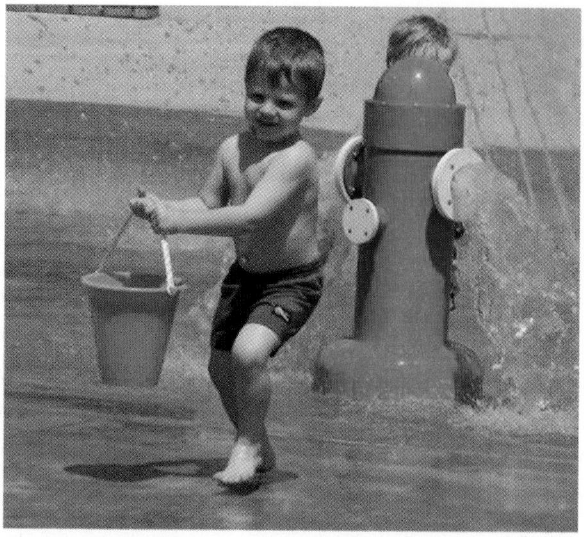

Fig. 33-4 The stage of initiative is characterized by physical activity and imagination while children explore the physical world around them.

Theoretical Foundations of Mental Development

The term *cognition* refers to the process by which developing individuals become acquainted with the world and the objects it contains. Children are born with inherited potentials for intellectual growth, but they must develop that potential through interaction with the environment. By assimilating information through the senses, processing it, and acting on it, they come to understand relationships between objects and between themselves and their world. With cognitive development, children acquire the ability to reason abstractly, to think in a logical manner, and to organize intellectual functions or performances into higher-order structures. Language, morals, and spiritual development emerge as cognitive abilities advance.

Cognitive Development (Piaget)

Cognitive development consists of age-related changes that occur in mental activities. The best-known theory regarding children's thinking, and a more comprehensive developmental theory than those already described, was developed by the Swiss psychologist Jean Piaget (1969). According to Piaget, intelligence enables individuals to make adaptations to the environment that increase the probability of survival, and through their behaviour individuals establish and maintain equilibrium with the environment.

Piaget (1969) proposed three stages of reasoning: (1) intuitive, (2) concrete operational, and (3) formal operational. When children enter the stage of concrete logical thought at about age 7 years, they are able to make logical **inferences,** classify, and deal with quantitative relationships about concrete things. Not until adolescence are they able to reason abstractly with any degree of competence. Each stage is derived from and builds on the accomplishments of the previous stage in a continuous, orderly process. The course of intellectual development is both maturational and invariant and is divided into the following stages (ages are approximate):

Sensorimotor (birth to 2 years)—The sensorimotor stage of intellectual development consists of six substages (see pp. 964 and 1024 for more in-depth discussion) that are governed by sensations in which simple learning takes place. Children progress from reflex activity through simple repetitive behaviours to imitative behaviour. They develop a sense of cause and effect as they direct behaviour toward objects. Problem solving is primarily by trial and error. They display a high level of curiosity, experimentation, and enjoyment of novelty and begin to develop a sense of self as they are able to differentiate themselves from their environment. They become aware that objects have permanence—that an object exists even though it is no longer visible. Toward the end of the sensorimotor period, children begin to use language and representational thought.

Preoperational (2 to 7 years)—The predominant characteristic of the preoperational stage of intellectual development is egocentrism, which in this sense does not mean selfishness or self-centredness but the inability to put oneself in the place of another. Children interpret objects and events not in terms of general properties, but in terms of their relationships or their use to them. They are unable to see things from any perspective other than their own; they cannot see another's point of view, nor can they see any reason to do so (see Chapter 38, Cognitive Development). Preoperational thinking is concrete and tangible. Children cannot reason beyond the observable, and they lack the ability to make deductions or generalizations. Thought is dominated by what they see, hear, or otherwise experience. However, they are increasingly able to use language and symbols to represent objects in their environment. Through imaginative play, questioning, and other interactions, they begin to elaborate concepts and to make simple associations between ideas. In the latter stage of this period, their reasoning is intuitive (e.g., the stars have to go to bed just as children do), and they are only beginning to deal with problems of weight, length, size, and time. Reasoning is also transductive—because two events occur together, they cause each other, or knowledge of one characteristic is transferred to another (e.g., all women with big bellies have babies).

Concrete operations (7 to 11 years)—At this age, thought becomes increasingly logical and coherent. Children are able to classify, sort, order, and otherwise organize facts about the world to use in problem solving. They develop a new concept of permanence—conservation (see Chapter 39, Cognitive Development [Piaget]); that is, they realize that physical factors such as volume, weight, and number remain the same even though outward appearances are changed. They are able to deal with a number of different aspects of a situation simultaneously. They do not have the capacity to deal in abstraction; they solve problems in a concrete, systematic fashion based on what they can perceive. Reasoning is inductive. Through progressive changes in thought processes and relationships with others, thought becomes less self-centred. They can consider points of view other than their own. Thinking has become socialized.

Formal operations (11 to 15 years)—Formal operational thought is characterized by adaptability and flexibility. Adolescents can think in abstract terms, use abstract symbols, and draw logical conclusions from a set of observations. For example, they can solve the following question: If A is larger than B, and B is larger than C, which symbol is the largest? (The answer is A.) They can make hypotheses and test them; they can consider abstract, theoretical, and philosophical matters. Although they may confuse the ideal with the practical, most contradictions in the world can be dealt with and resolved.

Language Development

Children are born with the mechanism and capacity to develop speech and language skills. However, they do not speak spontaneously. The environment must provide a means for them to acquire these skills. Speech requires intact physiological structure and function (including respiratory, auditory, and cerebral) plus intelligence, a need to communicate, and stimulation.

The rate of speech development varies from child to child and is directly related to neurological competence and cognitive development. Gesture precedes speech, and in this way a small child communicates satisfactorily. As speech develops, gesture recedes but never disappears entirely. Research suggests that infants can learn sign language before vocal language and that it may enhance the development of vocal language (Thompson et al., 2007). At all stages of language development, children's comprehension vocabulary (what they understand) is greater than their expressed vocabulary (what they can say), and this development reflects a continuing process of modification that involves both the acquisition of new words and the expansion and refinement of word meanings previously learned. By the time they begin to walk, children are able to attach a name to objects and persons.

The first parts of speech used are nouns, sometimes verbs (e.g., "go"), and combination words (such as "bye-bye"). Responses are usually structurally incomplete during the toddler period, although the meaning is clear. Next they begin to use adjectives and adverbs to qualify nouns, followed by adverbs to qualify nouns and verbs. Later, pronouns and gender words are added (such as "he" and "she"). By the time children enter school, they are able to use simple, structurally complete sentences that average five to seven words.

Moral Development (Kohlberg)

Children also acquire moral reasoning in a developmental sequence. Moral development, as described by Kohlberg (1968), is based on cognitive developmental theory and consists of the following three major levels, each of which has two stages:

1. **Preconventional level**—The preconventional level of moral development parallels the preoperational level of cognitive development and intuitive thought. Culturally oriented to the labels of good/bad and right/wrong, children integrate these in terms of the physical or pleasurable consequences of their actions. At first, children determine the goodness or badness of an action in terms of its consequences. They avoid punishment and obey without question those who have the power to determine and enforce the rules and labels. They have no concept of the basic moral order that supports these consequences. Later, children determine that the right behaviour consists of that which satisfies their own needs (and sometimes the needs of others). Although elements of fairness, give and take, and equal sharing are evident, they are interpreted in a practical, concrete manner without loyalty, gratitude, or justice.
2. **Conventional level**—At the conventional stage, children are concerned with conformity and loyalty. They value the maintenance of family, group, or community expectations regardless of consequences. Behaviour that meets with approval and pleases or helps others is considered good. One earns approval by being "nice." Obeying the rules, doing one's duty, showing respect for authority, and maintaining the social order are the correct behaviours. This level is correlated with the stage of concrete operations in cognitive development.
3. **Postconventional, autonomous, or principled level**—At the postconventional level, the individual has reached the cognitive stage of formal operations. Correct behaviour tends to be defined in terms of general individual rights and standards that have been examined and agreed on by the entire society. Although procedural rules for reaching consensus become important, with emphasis on the legal point of view, there is also emphasis on the possibility for changing law in terms of societal needs and rational considerations.

The most advanced level of moral development is one in which self-chosen ethical principles guide decisions of conscience. These are abstract and ethical but universal principles of justice and human rights with respect for the dignity of persons as individuals. Kohlberg believed that few persons reach this stage of moral reasoning.

Spiritual Development (Fowler)

Spiritual beliefs are closely related to the moral and ethical portion of the child's self-concept and, as such, must be considered as part of the child's basic needs assessment. Children need to have meaning, purpose, and hope in their lives. Also, the need for confession and forgiveness is present, even in very young children. Extending beyond religion (an organized set of beliefs and practices), spirituality affects the whole person: mind, body, and spirit. Fowler (1981) has identified six stages in the development of faith, four of which are closely associated with and parallel cognitive and psychosocial development in childhood:

Stage 0: Undifferentiated—This stage of development encompasses the period of infancy, during which children have no concept of right or wrong, no beliefs, and no convictions to guide their behaviour. However, the beginnings of a faith are established with the development of basic trust through their relationships with the primary caregiver.

Stage 1: Intuitive-projective—Toddlerhood is primarily a time of imitating the behaviour of others. Children imitate the religious gestures and behaviours of others without comprehending any meaning of or significance to the activities. During the preschool years, children assimilate some of their parents' values and beliefs. Parental attitudes toward moral codes and religious beliefs convey to children what they consider to be good and bad. Children still imitate behaviour at this age and follow parental beliefs as part of their daily lives rather than through an understanding of their basic concepts.

Stage 2: Mythic-literal—Through the school-age years, spiritual development parallels cognitive development and is closely related to children's experiences and social interaction. Most have a strong interest in religion during the school-age years. They accept the existence of a deity, and petitions to an omnipotent being are important and expected to be answered; good behaviour is rewarded, and bad behaviour is punished. Their developing conscience bothers them when they disobey. They have a reverence for thoughts about spiritual matters and are able to articulate their faith. They may even question its validity.

Stage 3: Synthetic-conventional—As children approach adolescence, however, they become increasingly aware of spiritual disappointments. They recognize that prayers are not always answered (at least on their own terms), and they may begin to abandon or modify some religious practices. They begin to reason, to question some of the established parental religious standards, and to drop or modify some religious practices.

Stage 4: Individuative-reflective—Adolescents become more skeptical and begin to compare their parents' religious standards with those of others. They attempt to determine which to adopt and incorporate into their own set of values. They also begin to compare religious standards with the scientific viewpoint. It is a time of searching rather than reaching conclusions. Adolescents are uncertain about many religious ideas but will not achieve profound insights until late adolescence or early adulthood.

Stage 5: Conjunctive—In this stage, which occurs during mid-life adulthood, individuals recognize paradoxes in their faith and can transcend the reality of the religious symbols.

Stage 6: Universalizing—Adults become enlightened about their faith and what religious symbolism means.

Development of Self-Concept

Self-concept is how an individual describes himself or herself. The term *self-concept* includes all the beliefs and convictions that constitute an individual's self-knowledge and that influence relationships with others. It develops gradually as a result of unique experiences within the self, with significant others, and with the realities of the world. However, an individual's self-concept may or may not reflect reality.

In infancy the self-concept is primarily an awareness of one's independent existence learned in part as a result of social contacts and experiences with others. The process becomes more active during toddlerhood as children explore the limits of their capacities and the nature of their impact on others. School-age children are more aware of differences among people, are more sensitive to social pressures, and become more preoccupied with issues of self-criticism and self-evaluation. During early adolescence, children focus more on physical and emotional changes taking place and on peer acceptance. Self-concept is crystallized during later adolescence as young people organize their self-concept around a set of values, goals, and competencies acquired throughout childhood.

Body Image

A vital component of self-concept, *body image* refers to the subjective concepts and attitudes that individuals have toward their own bodies. It consists of the physiological (the perception of one's physical characteristics), psychological (values and attitudes toward the body, abilities, and ideals), and social nature of one's image of self (the self in relation to others). All three components interrelate with one another. Body image is a complex phenomenon that evolves and changes during the process of growth and development. Any actual or perceived deviation from the "norm" (no matter how this is interpreted) is cause for concern and is influenced by the attitudes and behaviour of those around them.

The significant others in children's lives exert the most important and meaningful impact on children's body image. Labels that are attached to them (such as "skinny," "pretty," or "fat") or body parts (such as "ugly mole," "bug eyes," or "yucky skin") are incorporated into the body image. Because they lack the understanding of deviations from the physical standard or norm, children notice prominent differences in others and unwittingly make rude or cruel remarks about such minor deviations as large or widely spaced front teeth, large or small eyes, moles, or extreme variations in height.

Infants receive input about their bodies through self-exploration and sensory stimulation from others. As they begin to manipulate their environment, they become aware of their bodies as separate from others. Toddlers learn to identify the various body parts and are able to use symbols to represent objects. Preschoolers become aware of the wholeness of their bodies and discover the genitalia. Exploration of the genitalia and the discovery of differences between the sexes become important. They have only a vague concept of internal organs and function (Stuart & Laraia, 2000).

School-age children begin to learn about internal body structure and function and become aware of differences in body size and configuration. They are highly influenced by the cultural norms of society and current fads. Children whose bodies deviate from the norm are often criticized or ridiculed. Adolescence is the age when children become most concerned about the physical self. The unfamiliar body changes, and the new physical self must be integrated into the self-concept. Adolescents face conflicts over what they see and what they visualize as the ideal body structure. Body image formation during adolescence is a crucial element in the shaping of identity, the psychosocial crisis of adolescence.

Self-Esteem

Self-esteem is the value that an individual places on himself or herself and refers to an overall evaluation of oneself (Willoughby, King, & Polatajko, 1996). *Self-esteem* is described as the affective component of the self, whereas *self-concept* is the cognitive component; however, the two terms are almost indistinguishable and are often used interchangeably.

The term *self-esteem* refers to a personal, subjective judgement of one's worthiness derived from and influenced by the social groups in the immediate environment and individuals' perceptions of how they are valued by others. Self-esteem changes with development. Highly egocentric toddlers are unaware of any difference between competence and social approval. By contrast, preschool and early school-age children are increasingly aware of the discrepancy between their competencies and the abilities of more advanced children. Being accepted by adults and peers outside the family group becomes more important to them. Positive feedback enhances their self-esteem; they are vulnerable to feelings of worthlessness and are anxious about failure.

As children's competencies increase and they develop meaningful relationships, their self-esteem rises. Their self-esteem is again at risk during early adolescence when they are defining an identity and sense of self in the context of their peer group. Unless children are continually made to feel incompetent and of little worth, a decrease in self-esteem during vulnerable times is only temporary. Children assess the following aspects of themselves in forming an overall evaluation of their self-esteem (Sieving & Zirbel-Donisch, 1990):

Competence—How adequate are my cognitive, physical, and social skills?

Sense of control—How well can I complete tasks needed to produce desired actions? Are my successes or failures due to someone or something specific or is it due to luck?

Moral worth—How well do my actions and behaviours meet moral standards that have been set?

Worthiness of love and acceptance—How worthy am I of love and acceptance from parents, other significant adults, siblings, and peers?

Factors that influence the formation of a child's self-esteem include (1) the child's temperament and personality, (2) abilities and opportunities available to accomplish age-appropriate developmental tasks, (3) how significant others interact with the child, and (4) social roles assumed and the expectations surrounding these roles (see also Chapter 34, Psychosocial History).

Role of Play in Development

Through the universal medium of play, children learn what no one can teach them. They learn about their world and how to deal with this environment of objects, time, space, structure, and people. They learn about themselves operating within that environment—what they can do, how to relate to things and situations, and how to adapt themselves to the demands society makes on them. Play is the work of the child. In play, children continually practise the complicated, stressful processes of living, communicating, and achieving satisfactory relationships with other people.

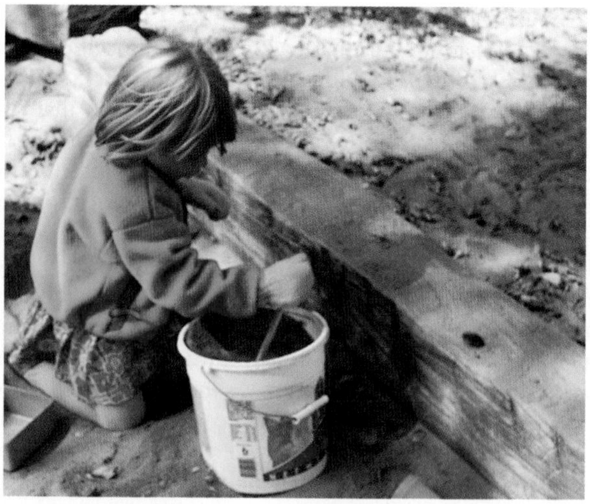

Fig. 33-5 Children derive pleasure from handling raw materials.

Classification of Play

From a developmental point of view, patterns of children's play can be categorized according to content and social character. In both there is an additive effect; each builds on past accomplishments, and some element of each is maintained throughout life. At each stage in development the new predominates.

Content of Play

The content of play involves primarily the physical aspects of play, although social relationships cannot be ignored. Play follows the simple to the complex:

Social-affective play—Play begins with social-affective play, in which infants take pleasure in relationships with people. As adults talk to, touch, and nuzzle an infant and in various ways elicit a response from an infant, the infant soon learns to provoke parental emotions and responses with such behaviours as smiling, cooing, or initiating games and activities. The type and intensity of the adult behaviour with children vary among cultures.

Sense-pleasure play—Sense-pleasure play is a nonsocial stimulating experience that originates from without. Objects in the environment—light and colour, tastes and odours, textures and consistencies—attract children's attention, stimulate their senses, and give them pleasure. Pleasurable experiences are derived from handling raw materials (water, sand, food), from body motion (swinging, bouncing, rocking), and from other uses of senses and abilities (smelling, humming) (Fig. 33-5).

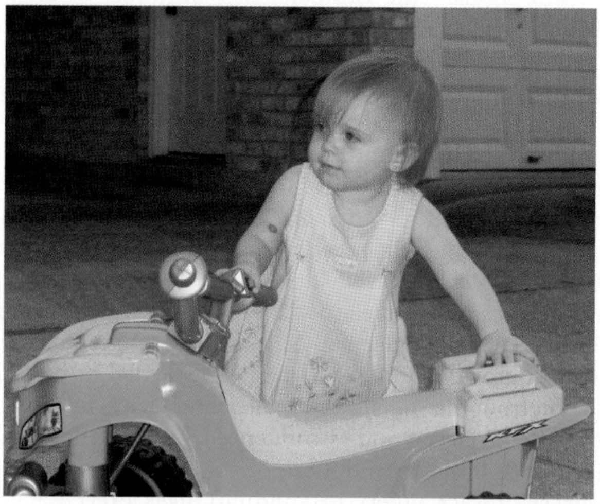

Fig. 33-6 After infants develop new skills to grasp and manipulate, they begin to conquer new abilities such as getting on a play motorcycle.

Skill play—After infants have developed the ability to grasp and manipulate, they persistently demonstrate and exercise their newly acquired abilities through skill play, repeating an action over and over. The element of sense-pleasure play is often evident in practicing a new ability, but frequently the determination to conquer the elusive skill produces pain and frustration (e.g., learning to get into a play car) (Fig. 33-6).

Unoccupied behaviour—In unoccupied behaviour, children are not playful but focusing their attention momentarily on anything that strikes their interest. Children daydream, fiddle with clothes or other objects, or walk aimlessly. This role differs from that of onlookers, who actively observe the activity of others.

Dramatic, or pretend, play—One of the vital elements in children's process of identification is dramatic play, also known as **symbolic** or **pretend** play. It begins in late infancy (11 to 13 months) and is the predominant form of play in the preschool child. After children begin to invest situations and people with meanings and to attribute affective significance to the world, they can pretend and fantasize almost anything. By acting out events of daily life, children learn and practise the roles and identities modelled by the members of their family and society. Children's toys, replicas of the tools and pastimes of society, provide a medium for learning about adult roles and activities that may be puzzling and frustrating to them. Interacting with the world is one way children get to know it. The simple, imitative, dramatic play of the toddler, such as using the telephone or computer, driving a car, or rocking a doll, evolves into more complex, sustained dramas of the preschooler, which extend beyond common domestic matters to the wider aspects of the world and the society, such as playing police officer, storekeeper, teacher, or nurse. Older children work out elaborate themes, act out stories, and compose plays.

Games—Children in all cultures engage in games alone and with others. Solitary activity involving games begins as very small children participate in repetitive activities and progress to more complicated games that challenge their independent skills, such as puzzles, solitaire, and computer or video games. Very young children participate in simple, imitative games such as pat-a-cake and peek-a-boo. Preschool children learn and enjoy formal games, beginning with ritualistic, self-sustaining games such as ring-around-a-rosy and London Bridge. With the exception of some simple board games, preschool children do not engage in competitive games. Preschoolers hate to lose and will try to cheat, want to change rules, or demand exceptions and opportunities to change their moves. School-age children and adolescents enjoy competitive games, including computer or smartphone video games, cards, chess, and physically active games such as baseball.

Social Character of Play

The play interactions of infancy are between the child and an adult. Children continue to enjoy the company of adults but are increasingly able to play alone. As children grow, interaction with age-mates increases in importance and becomes an essential part of the socialization process. Through interaction, highly egocentric infants, unable to tolerate delay or interference, ultimately acquire concern for others and the ability to delay gratification or even to reject gratification at the expense of another. A pair of toddlers will engage in considerable combat because their personal needs cannot tolerate delay or compromise. By the time they reach age 5 or 6 years, children are able to arrive at a compromise or make use of arbitration, usually after they have attempted but failed to gain their own way. Through continued interaction with peers and the growth of conceptual abilities and social skills, children are able to increase participation with others in the following types of play:

Onlooker play—During onlooker play, children watch what other children are doing but make no attempt to enter into the play activity. Watching an older sibling bounce a ball is a common example of the onlooker role.

Solitary play—During solitary play, children play alone with toys different from those used by other children in the same area. They enjoy other children but make no effort to get close to or speak to them. Their interest is centred on their own activity, which they pursue with no reference to the activities of the others.

Parallel play—During parallel activities, children play independently beside but not with other children. They play with toys like those the children around them are using, but as each child sees fit, neither influencing nor being influenced by the other children (Fig. 33-7). There is no group association. Parallel play is the characteristic of toddlers, but it may occur at other ages. Individuals who are involved in a creative craft with each person separately working on an individual project are engaged in parallel play.

Associative play—Children play together and are engaged in a similar or even identical activity, but there is no organization, division of labour, leadership assignment, or mutual group goal. Children borrow and lend play materials, follow each other with wagons and tricycles, and sometimes attempt to control who may or may not play in the group (Fig. 33-8). For example, two children play with dolls, borrowing articles of clothing from each other and engaging in similar conversation, but neither directs the other's actions or establishes rules regarding the limits of the play session. When one child initiates an activity, often, the entire group follows the example.

Cooperative play—Children play in a organized group *with* other children (Fig. 33-9). They discuss and plan activities for the purposes of accomplishing an end—to make something, to attain a competitive goal, to dramatize situations of adult or group life, or to play formal games. The group is loosely formed, but there is a marked sense of belonging or not belonging. The goal and its attainment require

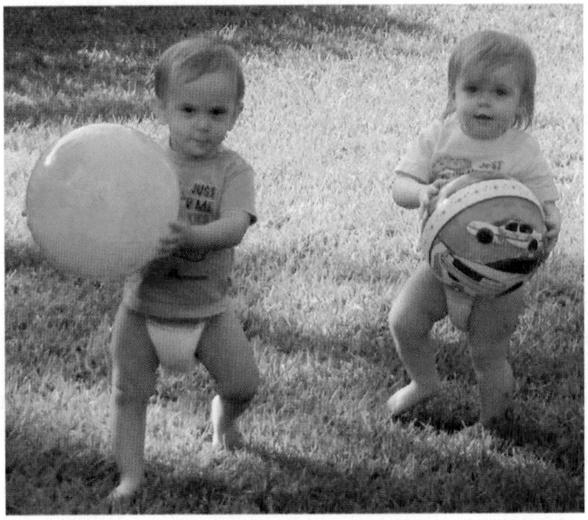

Fig. 33-7 Parallel play.

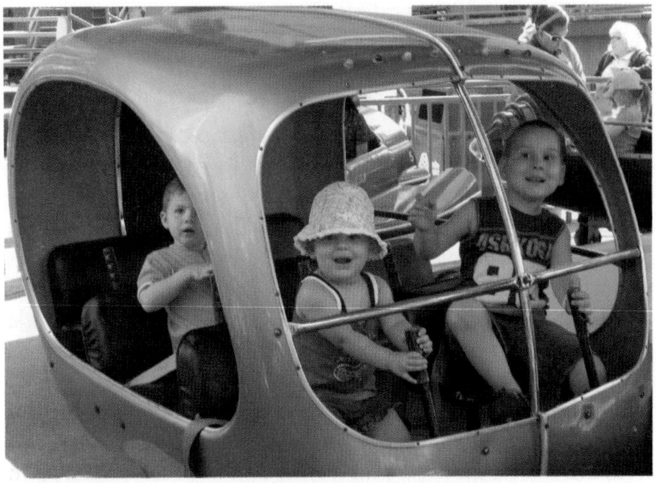

Fig. 33-8 Associative play.

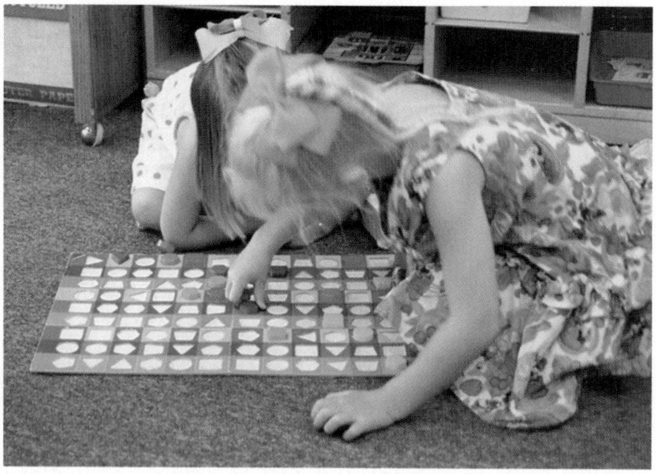

Fig. 33-9 Cooperative play.

organization of activities, division of labour, and role playing. The leader–follower relationship is definitely established, and the activity is controlled by one or two members who assign roles and direct the activity of the others. The activity is organized to allow one child to supplement another's function to complete the goal.

Functions of Play

Sensorimotor Development

Sensorimotor activity is a major component of play at all ages and is the predominant form of play in infancy. Active play is essential for muscle development and serves a useful purpose as a release for surplus energy. Through sensorimotor play, children explore the nature of the physical world. Infants gain impressions of themselves and their world through tactile, auditory, visual, and kinesthetic stimulation. Toddlers and preschoolers revel in body movement and exploration of objects in space. With increasing maturity, sensorimotor play becomes more differentiated and involved. Whereas very young children run for the sheer joy of body movement, older children incorporate or modify the motions into increasingly complex and coordinated activities such as racing, playing games, skateboarding, and bicycle riding.

Intellectual Development

Through exploration and manipulation children learn colours, shapes, sizes, textures, and the significance of objects. They learn the significance of numbers and how to use them; they learn to associate words with objects; and they develop an understanding of abstract concepts and spatial relationships, such as *up*, *down*, *under*, and *over*. Activities such as puzzles and games help them develop problem-solving skills. Books, stories, films, and collections expand knowledge and provide enjoyment as well. Play provides a means to practise and expand language skills. Through play, children continually rehearse past experiences to assimilate them into new perceptions and relationships. Play helps children comprehend the world in which they live and distinguish between fantasy and reality.

Creativity

Children can experiment and try out their creative ideas in play through every medium at their disposal, including raw materials, fantasy, and exploration. Creativity is stifled by pressure toward conformity; therefore, striving for peer approval may inhibit creative endeavours in the school-age or adolescent child. Creativity is primarily a product of solitary activity, yet creative thinking is often enhanced in group settings where listening to others' ideas stimulates further exploration of one's own ideas. After children feel the satisfaction of creating something new and different, they transfer this creative interest to situations outside the world of play.

Self-Awareness

Beginning with active explorations of their bodies and awareness of themselves as separate from the mother, the process of developing a self-identity is facilitated through play activities. Children learn who they are and their place in the world. They become increasingly able to regulate their own behaviour, to learn what their abilities are, and to compare their abilities with those of others. Through play, children are able to test their abilities, to assume and try out various roles, and to learn the effect their behaviour has on others. They learn the gender role that society expects them to fulfill, as well as approved patterns of behaviour and deportment.

Therapeutic Value

Play is therapeutic at any age (Fig. 33-10). In play, children can express emotions and release unacceptable impulses in a socially acceptable fashion. Children are able to experiment and test fearful situations and can assume and vicariously master the roles and positions that they are unable to perform in the world of reality. Children reveal much about themselves in play. Through play, children are able to communicate to the alert observer the needs, fears, and desires that they are unable to express with their limited language skills. Throughout their play, children need the acceptance of adults and their presence to help them control aggression and channel their destructive tendencies.

Moral Value

Although children learn at home and at school those behaviours considered right and wrong in the culture, the interaction with peers during play contributes significantly to their moral training. Nowhere is the enforcement of moral standards as rigid as in the play situation. If they are to be members of the group, children must adhere to the accepted codes of behaviour of the culture (e.g., fairness, honesty, self-control, consideration for others). Children soon learn that their peers are less tolerant of violations than are adults and that to maintain a place in the play group, they must conform to the group's standards.

Toys

The type of toys chosen by or provided for children can support and enhance the child's development in the areas just described. Although no scientific evidence shows that any toy is necessary for optimal learning, toys offer an opportunity to bring the child and parent together. Toys that are small

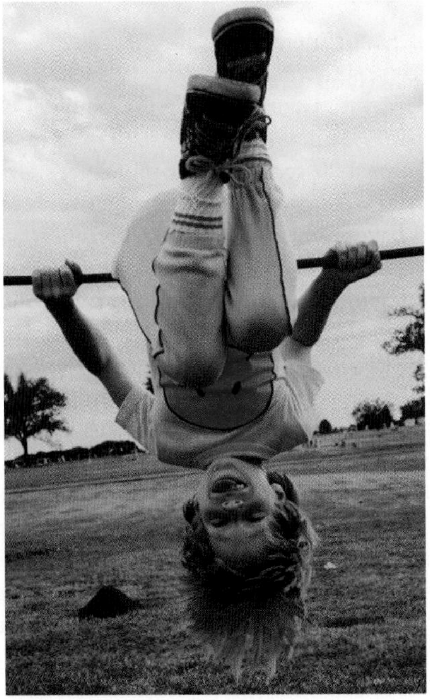

Fig. 33-10 Play is therapeutic at any age and provides a means for release of tension and stress.

replicas of the culture and its tools help children assimilate into their culture. Toys that require pushing, pulling, rolling, and manipulating teach them about physical properties of the items and help develop muscles and coordination. Rules and the basic elements of cooperation and organization are learned through board and some video games.

Raw materials with which children can exercise their own creativity and imaginations are sometimes superior to ready-made items. For example, building blocks can be used to construct a variety of structures, to count, and to learn shapes and sizes.

Toy Safety

Selection of toys and play equipment is a joint effort between parents and children, but evaluation of their safety is the adult's responsibility. Government agencies do not inspect and police all toys on the market. Thus adults who purchase toys, supervise purchases, or allow children to use play equipment need to evaluate such equipment for its safety and age appropriateness. This includes toys that are gifts or those that are purchased by the children themselves (see Family-Centred Teaching box).

A choke tube tester such as a cardboard toilet paper roll (diameter 3 cm) can be used to see if a toy fits inside the tube and will be a choking hazard for children under 3 years (Safe Kids Canada, 2010). Parents should also be alert to notices of toys determined to be defective and recalled by the manufacturers. Parents and health care workers can obtain information on a variety of recalled products and can report potentially dangerous toys and child products to the Canadian Toy Testing Council (see Additional Resources section). The Council has links to various government and consumer Web sites that contain warnings about the safety of specific toys. The Canadian federal government has passed a new toy safety *Consumer Product Safety Act* that is intended to deal quickly with any toy safety issues. For example, Canada is the only country to ban the importation, advertisement, and sale of wheeled baby walkers (Safe Kids Canada, 2010).

Selected Factors That Influence Development

Heredity

Inherited characteristics have a profound influence on development. The child's sex, determined by random selection at the time of conception, directs both the pattern of growth and the behaviour of others toward the child. In all cultures, attitudes and expectations are shaped by the child's sex. Sex and other hereditary determinants strongly affect the progress and end result of growth. There is a high correlation between parent and child with regard to traits such as height, weight, and rate of growth. Most physical characteristics, including shape and form of features, body build, and physical peculiarities, are inherited and can influence the way in which children grow and interact with their environment. Many dimensions of personality, such as temperament, activity level, responsiveness, and a tendency toward shyness, are believed to be inherited.

Differences in children's health and vigour may be attributed to hereditary traits. An inherited physical or mental disorder will alter or modify a child's physical or emotional growth and interactions.

Neuroendocrine Factors

The hypothalamic–pituitary axis produces a number of releasing and inhibitory hormones that influence growth. Probably all hormones affect growth in some fashion. Three hormones—growth hormone, thyroid hormone, and androgens—when given to persons deficient in these hormones, stimulate protein anabolism and thereby produce retention of elements essential for building protoplasm and bony tissue. It appears that each of the hormones that has a significant influence on growth manifests its major effect at a different period of growth (see Chapter 52).

Nutrition

Nutrition is probably the single most important influence on growth. Dietary factors regulate growth at all stages of development, and their effects are exerted in numerous and complex ways. During the rapid prenatal growth period, poor nutrition may influence development from the time of implantation of the ovum until birth (see Chapter 11). During infancy and childhood, the demand for calories is relatively great, as evidenced by the rapid increase in both height and weight (see Table 33-1). At this time, protein and caloric requirements are higher than at almost any period of postnatal development. As the growth rate slows, with its concomitant decrease in metabolism, there is a corresponding reduction in caloric and protein requirements.

FAMILY-CENTRED TEACHING

Toy Safety

Selection

Select toys that suit the skills, abilities, and interests of children.

Select toys that are safe for the specific child; look for a label that indicates the intended age group. Toys that are safe for one age may not be safe for another.

For infants, toddlers, and all children who still mouth objects, avoid toys with small parts that may pose a fatal choking or aspiration hazard. Toys in this category are usually labelled "Not recommended for children under 3 years."

For infants, avoid toys with strings or cords that are 18 cm or longer because they may cause strangulation. Remove all crib toys strung across the crib as soon as the infant starts to push up on hands or knees or is 5 months old (whichever comes first).

For all children younger than 8 years, avoid electric toys with heating elements.

For children younger than 5 years, avoid arrows or darts.

Check for clear safety labels such as "flame retardant" or "flame resistant" and that toys are nontoxic.

Select toys durable enough to survive rough play; look for sturdy construction such as tightly secured eyes, nose, or any small parts.

Select toys light enough that they will not cause harm if one falls on a child.

Look for toys with smooth, rounded edges. Avoid toys with sharp edges that can cut or that have sharp points. Points on the inside of the toy can puncture the skin if the toy is broken.

Avoid toys with any shooting or throwing objects that can injure eyes. This includes toys with which other missiles such as sticks or pebbles might be used as substitutes for the intended projectiles.

Arrows and darts used by children should have blunt tips and be manufactured from resilient materials; make certain the tips are securely attached.

Avoid toys that make loud noises that might damage a child's hearing. Even some squeaking toys are too loud when held close to the ear.

If selecting caps for cap guns, look for the label on boxes or packages of caps which states: "Warning—Do not fire closer than 30 cm to the ear. Do not use indoors."

If selecting a toy gun, be certain that the barrel or the entire gun is brightly coloured, to avoid being mistaken for a real gun.

BB guns or pellet rifles should not be given to children under the age of 16.

Toys with magnets are a significant swallowing risk for the under-6 age group, which can lead to serious gastrointestinal complications. The magnet toy must contain a warning label on it with an alert symbol (/!\) and "WARNING!".

Battery-operated toys must be in good condition and the batteries not in reach of children. Button-type batteries, when swallowed, can cause internal poisoning or chemical burns.

Supervise children who are playing with balloons. Throw away immediately any pieces of the balloon that are broken. Use Mylar (foil) balloons because latex balloons pose a choking hazard.

Do not let children chew on metal jewellery. Some jewellery can contain large levels of lead, which can lead to serious illness in children.

Do not use baby walkers that allow young babies to move quickly, as babies may then fall down stairs or get burned from pulling hot objects or liquid onto themselves.

Never use baby rings or bath seats as they can tip over and cause young children to drown or nearly drown.

Do not put stuffed toys in an infant's crib, as they can pose a suffocation hazard. Secure televisions with brackets or straps to prevent them from toppling onto children; this can cause serious injuries.

Supervision

Maintain a safe play environment.

Remove and discard plastic wrappings on toys immediately; they could suffocate a child.

Remove large toys, bumper pads, and boxes from playpens; an adventuresome child can use such items as a means of climbing or falling out.

Set ground rules for play.

Supervise young children closely during play.

Teach children how to use toys properly and safely.

Instruct older children to keep their toys away from younger brothers, sisters, and friends.

Keep children who are playing with riding toys away from stairs, hills, traffic, and swimming pools.

Establish and enforce rules regarding protective gear.

- Insist that children wear helmets when using bicycles, skateboards, skis, or in-line skates.
- Insist that children wear gloves and wrist, elbow, and knee pads when using skateboards or in-line skates.

Instruct children on electrical safety and how to properly unplug an electric toy—pull on the plug.

- Teach children to beware of electric appliances and even electrically operated playthings; often children are unfamiliar with the hazards of electricity in association with water.
- Teach children the safe use of utensils or other items that under certain circumstances can cause injury—scissors, knives, needles, heating elements, loops, long string, or cord.

Maintenance

Inspect old and new toys regularly for breakage, loose parts, and other potential hazards.

Look for jagged or sharp edges or broken parts that might constitute a choking hazard.

Check movable parts to make certain they are attached securely to the toys; sometimes pieces that are safe when attached to the toy become a danger when detached.

FAMILY-CENTRED TEACHING

Toy Safety—cont'd

Examine all outdoor toys regularly for rust and weak or sharp parts that could become a danger to a child.

Check electrical cords and plugs for cracked or fraying parts.

Maintain toys in good repair, without signs of possible hazards such as sharp edges, splinters, weak seams, or rust.

Make repairs immediately, or discard out of reach of children.

Sand sharp wooden toys or splintered surfaces so they are smooth.

Use only paint labelled "nontoxic" to repaint toys, toy boxes, or children's furniture.

Storage

Provide a safe place for children to store toys safely to prevent accidental injury from stepping, tripping, or falling on a toy.

Select a toy chest or toy box that is ventilated and is free of self-locking devices that could entrap or suffocate a child inside. It must have a spring-loaded lid support, designed not to pinch a child's fingers or fall on a child's head.

Playthings meant for older children and adults should be safely stowed away in areas unavailable to younger children.

(Adapted from Safe Kids Canada. [2010]. *Toy safety.* Retrieved from http://www.safekidscanada.ca/parents/safety-information/product-safety/toy-safety/toy-safety.aspx.)

Growth is uneven during the periods of childhood between infancy and adolescence, when there are plateaus and small growth spurts. The child's appetite fluctuates in response to these variations until the turbulent growth spurt of adolescence, when adequate nutrition is extremely important but may be subject to numerous emotional influences. Adequate nutrition is closely related to good health throughout life, and an overall improvement in nourishment is evidenced by the gradual increase in size and early maturation of children in this century (see Community Focus box).

COMMUNITY FOCUS

Healthy Food Choices

Current research indicates that new lower-fat recipes in school lunch programs are well accepted by children (Matvienko, 2007). However, less-healthy foods are still more available than more-healthy foods in our nation's schools. Because students consume about 30% of their daily food at school, this situation can contribute to a higher rate of obesity. Indeed, obesity is on the increase in the pediatric population in Canada, which can have a long-term negative impact on health. The Dietitians of Canada (2010) support healthy nutrition programs in day care centres and schools across Canada with the goal of children developing lifelong healthy eating habits. This group has been involved with school policies regarding the provision of healthier food choices. Many provinces and territories such as Manitoba, British Columbia, and Ontario, along with multiple school districts, have tried to improve food options in cafeterias and vending machines. One unexpected outcome, however, is that some students go outside the school to buy unhealthy food at fast-food outlets. This pattern can decrease the income of food delivery companies as well as the income of schools, which share in the food profits (Finkelstein, 2009). The provision of healthier choices in food delivery in schools remains a challenge.

Interpersonal Relationships

Relationships with significant others play a critical role in development, particularly in emotional, intellectual, and personality development. Not only do the quality and quantity of contacts with other persons exert an influence on the growing child, but the widening range of contacts is essential to learning and developing a healthy personality.

The mothering person is unquestionably the single most influential person during early infancy who meets the infant's basic needs of food, warmth, comfort, and love. He or she stimulates the child's senses and facilitates his or her expanding capacities. Through this person the child learns to trust the world and feel secure to venture in increasingly wider relationships.

Generally, the parents are most influential in helping the child to assume sex-role identification. Parents define and reinforce acceptable sex-role behaviour and provide sex-appropriate role models for the child. In the absence of a sex-role model in the family setting, the child may adopt some characteristics of the opposite-sex parent or sibling. Frequently, the child identifies with a teacher or other significant person of the same sex.

Siblings are children's first peers, and the way in which they learn to relate to each other affects later interactions with peers outside the family group. The sphere of persons from whom children seek approval widens to include other members of their family, their peers, and, to a lesser extent, other authority figures (e.g., teachers). The increasing importance of the peer group in determining the behaviour of school-age children and adolescents is well documented (Fig. 33-11).

When children fail to have high-quality interpersonal relationships with mothering persons, they experience *emotional deprivation.* The most prominent feature of emotional deprivation, particularly during the first year, is developmental delays. Much of the information regarding the adverse effects of interpersonal influences on development has been acquired through retrospective studies of gross deprivation and trauma. The most notable instances involved homeless infants who were placed in institutions for care (Bowlby, 1951). Those

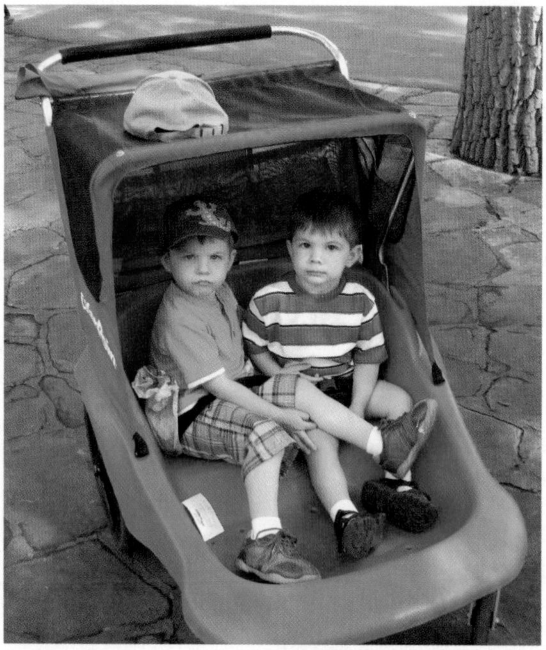

Fig. 33-11 Peers become increasingly important as children develop friendships outside the family group.

infants who did not receive consistent mothering care failed to gain weight even with an adequate diet; were pale, listless, and immobile; and were unresponsive to stimuli such as smiling or cooing that usually elicit a response from the normal infant. If emotional deprivation continues for a sufficient length of time, the child may not survive infancy. The term *masked deprivation* has been used to describe children reared in homes in which there is a distorted parent–child relationship or otherwise disordered home environment. Infants do not thrive if the caregiving person is hostile, fearful of handling them, or indifferent to them and their needs. Such children exhibit poor growth even though they are apparently free of physical disease. Growth delays in these children are believed to be caused by a psychologically induced endocrine imbalance that interferes with growth. These same infants and children display "catch-up" growth in a changed environment, however (see Chapter 36, Growth Failure [Failure to Thrive]). Le Mare and Audet (2006) studied adoptees from Romanian orphanages who were adopted by Canadians. These researchers discovered that all of the adoptees had growth delays when they first arrived in Canada but then thrived and achieved normal growth patterns after 10.5 years.

Socioeconomic Level

Evidence indicates that the families' socioeconomic level has a significant impact on children's growth and development (see Table 29-1). At all ages, children from upper- and middle-class families are taller than comparative children of families in the lower socioeconomic strata. The cause of these differences is less definite, although the poorer health and nutrition of children in lower socioeconomic levels are probably significant factors. Nutritious food sources (especially proteins) are scarce, and other factors (e.g., larger family size and irregularity in eating, sleeping, and exercise) may play a role.

Families from lower socioeconomic groups may lack the knowledge or resources needed to provide the safe, stimulating, and enriched environment that fosters optimum development for children. They may be unable to move from unsafe neighbourhoods where drug traffic and drive-by shootings are common. The effects on the emotional development of children living under these conditions have been compared with those experienced by children living in war zones (Garbarino, 2001).

Canadian researchers studied the impact of living in poor neighbourhoods on families' health. Some of the parents in these neighbourhoods had poorer mental health and more strained family relations compared with parents in higher-income neighbourhoods and used more punitive parenting (Kohen, Leventhal, Dahinten, & McIntosh, 2008), which can put children at risk for behavioural and emotional problems.

Disease

Altered growth and development are one of the clinical manifestations in a number of hereditary disorders. Growth impairment is particularly marked in skeletal disorders, such as the various forms of dwarfism and at least one of the chromosomal anomalies (Turner's syndrome). Many of the disorders of metabolism, such as vitamin D–resistant rickets, the mucopolysaccharidoses, and the numerous endocrine disorders, interfere with the normal growth pattern. In other disorders (e.g., Klinefelter's and Marfan syndromes) the tendency is toward the upper percentile of height.

Many chronic illnesses associated with varying degrees of growth failure are congenital cardiac anomalies, chronic renal disease, and respiratory disorders such as cystic fibrosis. Any disorder characterized by the inability to digest and absorb body nutrients will have an adverse effect on growth and development.

Environmental Hazards

Hazards in the environment, another determinant of health, are a source of concern to health care providers and others interested in health and safety. Physical injuries are the most prevalent consequences of environmental dangers; these are discussed extensively throughout the Pediatric Nursing section (Part 2) of this book in relation to age, specific hazards, and selected physical disabilities.

Children are at a high risk for harm resulting from the chemical residues present in the environment. The hazards of these chemical residues relate to their potential carcinogenicity, enzymatic effects, and accumulation (Baum & Shannon, 1995). The harmful agents most often associated with health risks are chemicals and radiation, including sun exposure (see Community Focus box). Water, air, and food contamination from a variety of sources are well documented. Significant means of exposure are the presence of substances, such as asbestos and lead, in the immediate environment; secretion of chemicals in breast milk (especially prescribed drugs and nicotine); and contamination within well-insulated homes (especially from disinfectants or burning of substances that produce toxic fumes) (Newman, 2009). Passive inhalation of tobacco smoke by infants and children is a hazard at all stages of development. The harmful effects of large doses of radiation

COMMUNITY FOCUS

Sun Protection Basics

The incidence of skin cancer is increasing in children, accounting for about 4% of pediatric malignancies. A resource to use for protecting children from harmful sun exposure is the Environment Canada UV (ultraviolet) Index level, with a scale from 1 to 11, which has associated precautions, including sunglasses, sunscreens, sun-protective clothing, and sun avoidance. Environment Canada predicts the maximum daily UV index levels, which measure the sun's burning UV rays on a daily basis, country wide. This information is available on the Health Canada Web site at http://www.weatheroffice.gc.ca/forecast/textforecast_e.html?Bulletin=fpcn48.cwao. Following are some practices to protect children from harmful UV exposure:

- Children's sunglasses must absorb at least 99% of UV radiation. Choose sunglasses with the label "Blocks 99% of UV rays." The glasses must have unbreakable plastic lenses with a wrap-around style that closely fits, to maximize UV and light protection. The glasses should be worn on cloudy as well as sunny days.
- Allow children to choose their sunglasses. A child who wears prescription glasses should also wear prescription sunglasses.
- Avoid sun exposure between 10 A.M. and 2 P.M. High altitude, sand, concrete, snow, and water increase UV exposure.
- Wear wide-brim hats and sun-protective clothing.
- Apply an adequate layer of sunscreen, preferably waterproof or water resistant, and reapply at regular intervals.

(Sources: Maguire-Eisen, M., Rothman, K., & Demierre, M. [2005]. The ABC's of sun protection. *Dermatology Nursing, 17*[6], 419–433; Health Canada. [2007]. *Babies, children and sun safety*. Retrieved from http://www.hc-sc.gc.ca/hl-vs/pubs/sun-sol/babies_child-bebes_enfant-eng.php.)

are unquestioned, although the effects of low-dose or short-term radiation are debatable, as are the dosage levels considered safe or harmful.

Stress in Childhood

Defined from both a physiological and an emotional point of view, *stress* is "an imbalance between environmental demands and a person's coping resources that . . . disrupts the equilibrium of the person" (Masten et al., 1988).

Although all children experience stress, some youngsters appear to be more vulnerable than others and are affected by age, temperament, life situation, and state of health in their reactions and ability to handle stress. Also, the responses to a stressor can be behavioural, psychological, or physiological. It is impossible and undesirable to protect children from stress, but providing them with interpersonal security helps them develop coping strategies for dealing with stress. The concept of an *emotional bank*, in which deposits and withdrawals can be made, can help parents and caregivers maintain a proper perspective on the effects of stress and coping. Children with a good, positive balance in the account can tolerate significant withdrawal experiences. For children with a low balance, even a minor withdrawal may bankrupt the account, causing it to be overdrawn.

Parents and other caregivers can try to recognize signs of stress to help children deal with stressors before they become overwhelming. Signs of stress take many forms but are typically the same ones seen in children who are abused (see Chapter 38) or depressed (see Chapter 40). If a number of stressors are imposed on children at the same time, the children are more vulnerable. When a succession of stressors produces an excessive stress load, children may experience a serious change in health or behaviour.

It is important that parents and persons working with children understand the nature of childhood stress and ways in which it can be recognized or anticipated. Caregivers must listen to children so that they are aware of children's fears and concerns. They must let children know that they are important and that what they say matters. Physical contact is usually comforting and reassuring to children. Simply holding, touching, or hugging children can be both relaxing and comforting and facilitate communication. Spending unhurried time with children, taking family outings or vacations, and exposing children to positive influences can help build children's strength and security. Supportive interpersonal relationships are essential to children's psychological well-being.

Coping

Coping refers to a special class of individual reactions to stressors—specifically, a reaction to a stressor that resolves, reduces, or replaces the affective state classified as stressful. *Coping strategies* are the specific ways in which children cope with stressors, as distinguished from *coping styles*, which are relatively unchanging personality characteristics or outcomes of coping (Wachs, 2006). Research indicates that, as children age, they tend toward a more internal locus of control and use more vigilant modes of coping (LaMontagne et al., 1996). Children, like adults, respond to everyday stress by trying to change the circumstances or trying to adjust to circumstances the way they are. Any strategy that provides relaxation is effective in reducing stress, and most children have their own natural methods of dealing with stress, such as withdrawing, engaging in physical activity, reading, listening to music, working on a project, or taking a nap. Some turn to parents to solve their problems, or they may develop socially unacceptable strategies, such as cheating, stealing, or lying.

Children can be taught stress-reduction techniques to use in coping. First, they must be helped to recognize signs of tension in themselves. Then they can be taught any of a variety of appropriate strategies—special exercises, relaxation and breathing, mental imagery, and numerous other simple activities. Also, parents and other caregivers can anticipate possible stress-provoking events and prepare children for coping by role playing a scenario or "talking it through" so that they can learn how to solve problems. When children can view any new situation as a problem to be solved and an opportunity to learn, they are not vulnerable to the control of others. It provides them with a sense of mastery over their own lives and reinforces the fact that they have within themselves the ability and information to handle whatever comes their way. Problem-solving skill gives them the confidence to know where and how to seek help when they need it.

Influence of Mass Media

The media can have an enormous influence on the developing child. There is no doubt that the media provide children with a means of extending their knowledge about the world in which they live and have helped narrow the differences between classes. However, there is growing concern about the enormous influence that the media can have on the developing child because of the large number of hours children spend watching television. For instance, the images of risky behaviour presented in the media may establish or reinforce teenagers' perceptions of their social environment.

Children may identify closely with and be influenced by people or characters portrayed in reading materials, movies, video games, and television programs and commercials. The role of each of these genres in children's development is discussed in the next sections.

Reading Materials

Books, newspapers, and magazines are the oldest form of mass media. They contribute to children's competence in almost every respect and also provide enjoyment. Recognition of the impact that reading matter used in the schools has on the value system and socialization processes has prompted re-evaluation of the content of textbooks in terms of the biased presentation of male and female role models, the sugar-coated view of life situations, and the biased history of minority groups.

Fairy tales, for generations the mainstay of young children's literature, were condemned for a time for being sexist; violent; and riddled with unfavourable stereotypes, such as the wicked stepmother, dwarves, and physical unattractiveness associated with evil. They are now believed to provide an excellent medium for explaining puzzling and important topics such as death, step-parents, and inner feelings and turmoil. Although they do not provide solutions, fairy tales confront children with emotional predicaments and offer suggestions for dealing with them.

Comic books and other reading materials have been popular in every generation, usually at the expense of literature provided by schools, libraries, and parents. Many children have nothing else to read. The easy reading, quick action, and adventure in brief episodes seem to fulfill a need for children who are striving to understand both aggression in others and their own impulses. Reading ability, intelligence, and school adjustment apparently have no relationship to the number and type of comic books read. Most comic books appear to be relatively harmless to the majority of children and may be beneficial. Comic books seem to have only a minor influence on acquisition of beliefs, values, and behaviours. The popularity of this medium has prompted some educators to encourage translations of literature into comic book form to stimulate students' interest in the classics.

Movies

Movies that are not closely bound to reality and portray an assortment of socially approved behaviours may contribute to children's value systems and provide opportunities for desirable social learning. On the other hand, children, especially adolescents, flock to the "macho" movies and those whose heroes resort to violent resolution of problems, such as karate and wild automobile chases.

Another concern is the plethora of "slasher" and R-rated movies available to children and teenagers in theatres and through cable television and DVDs. The content of movies has changed markedly during the past few decades, with violence and mutilation being major themes. To children who are unable to distinguish between reality and fantasy, these films play on their deepest fears and result in bedtime fears, nightmares, and a fearful view of the world.

Young children can be frightened by some of the movies considered safe for family viewing. For example, Bambi can frighten young children, and the villainous witches in *Snow White* and *The Wizard of Oz* are terrifying figures. Also, certain classic children's movies, such as *Snow White* and *Cinderella*, depict stepmothers as evil, destructive persons; such portrayals can have a deleterious effect on child–stepmother relationships or can be confusing to children who have developed a positive relationship with a stepmother.

Television

The medium with the most impact on children in North America today is television, which has become one of the most significant socializing agents in the lives of young children. The content of programs and commercials provides multiple sources for acquiring information, modelling behaviours, and observing value orientations. Besides producing a levelling effect on class differences, television exposes children to a wider variety of topics and events than they encounter in day-to-day life. Television always has time to "talk" to children and is a form of access to the adult world.

Television viewing has a direct impact on child development and behaviour. Several studies have found that violence on television and the mass media in general can contribute to the development of unhealthy behaviours and violence in children (Brown & Witherspoon, 2002; Earles et al., 2002; Monsen, 2002). Several factors encourage the learning or performing of television-influenced behaviours (Box 33-4). The Canadian Paediatric Society (2003) has developed a position statement that supports this view on the impact of media use on children and youth.

Most researchers have concluded that protracted television viewing can have detrimental effects on children. For example, in one study, television viewing was implicated as contributing to irregular sleep schedules in children under 3 years of age (Thompson & Christakis, 2005). Recognizing the negative effects of television viewing, the Canadian Paediatric Society (2003) has recommended that children watch no more than 1 to 2 hours of high-quality television a day. However, this warning has not been heeded, with approximately 40% of infants already watching television by 3 months of age and the number increasing to 90% by age 24 months. Parents reported the three primary reasons they allowed their infants to watch television was because they thought it was educational for them, they thought it was entertaining, and they needed time to get other things done. Parents did watch television with

BOX 33-4 Factors That Encourage Learning or Performing of Television-Influenced Behaviours

Age—Younger children focus on behaviours rather than on motives or consequences. They view alternatives in a concrete manner, and they are unable to differentiate between central and peripheral plot information.

Identification with characters or situations—Children often imitate behaviours of persons in situations similar to those in their own lives.

Reward and punishment syndrome—Children imitate behaviours they see rewarded or not punished when it is expected. They are less likely to repeat an act they see punished; their attention is immediately attracted when they see an act committed that they know should be punished but is not.

Opportunity to reproduce behaviours—Children imitate behaviours when given the right environment or when violence seems an accepted solution. When children see a situation on television, they use this information when they encounter a similar situation that requires a solution.

Motivation to reproduce behaviours—Children imitate behaviour when given the appropriate incentives: expectation of reward or lack of punishment. Some children have self-control; others do not.

their infants more than half the time (Zimmerman, Christakis, & Meltzoff, 2007).

The passive activity of television viewing is frequently accompanied by eating—in many cases, high-calorie snacks. Furthermore, children may expend tremendous mental energy processing the audiovisual messages from television, which may be exhausting and make them less likely to engage in physical activity later. Tremblay and Willms (2003) found that the incidence of body fat increased in direct proportion to the number of hours of television watched by children in Canada; as viewing increased, children were less likely to participate in vigorous physical activities.

In a study to identify children at risk for heart disease, researchers found that more than half of the children with high cholesterol levels watched at least 2 hours of television each day. Using a family history of heart disease or high cholesterol as the screening indicator, researchers identified three out of four children with high cholesterol levels. When these families were also questioned about the time their children spent watching television, investigators were able to identify 90% of the children with high cholesterol levels by using 2 or more viewing hours as the risk factor (Goldsmith, 1990).

It is especially important to identify at-risk children and control their viewing. The more at-risk groups may include children left without adult supervision, emotionally disturbed children, children with learning disabilities, children who are abused by their parents, and children in families in distress (Canadian Paediatric Society, 2003). For all children, house rules that specify the type and amount of television help children understand limits, and recorded selections of appropriate programs can be substituted for less desirable offerings. Parents need to carefully monitor cable and other pay-television programming. Lockboxes, V-chips, and blocking devices are available for cable receivers to prevent children from viewing uncensored programs when unsupervised.

Like movies, some television programs and commercials contain many implicit and explicit messages that promote alcohol consumption, smoking, violence, and promiscuous or unsafe sexual activity. There is evidence documenting a relationship between viewing these activities on television and the actual use of alcohol or tobacco, violence, and aggressive behaviour. Canadian researcher Paquette (2004) studied Canadian television and found that between 1993 and 2001, televised incidents of physical violence increased by 378%. In 2001, television shows averaged 40 acts of violence per hour. Franchophone viewers experienced an increase of 540%. Paquette also identified a 325% increase in psychological violence on television from 1999 to 2001; this type of violence is now shown more frequently than physical violence on all Canadian stations.

Parents can help children evaluate violence on television by pointing out the subtleties that children miss, such as the aggressor's motives and intentions and the unpleasant consequences that the perpetrators suffer as a result of their aggressive acts. Often the consequence is separated from the act by a commercial, thus children cannot make the correlation. Parents need to point out that conflicts can be resolved without resorting to violent behaviour. They can also stress the program's purpose—primarily entertainment—and explain why they like or dislike something on television (e.g., "This show is trying to tell you that crime does not pay and that if one does wrong, one will go to jail"). Explanations and discussions can take place between shows (with the volume turned down), and young children can learn from both older children and adults. These discussions can be effective when begun early and carried out consistently.

Television is the medium by which most children learn of a natural disaster or act of terrorism. For example, there was extensive media coverage in Canada of the September 11, 2011 terrorist attacks. Research on the effects of these terrorist attacks suggests that post-traumatic stress reactions increase with greater exposure to media coverage. Reading, rather than watching the event on television, may lead to better retention of the experience (Pfefferbaum et al., 2003). After the events of September 11, 85% of children in one study reported concerns for their safety and security (Phillips, Prince, & Schiebelhut, 2004). More than half of the children in this study coped by volunteering their time or donating materials for relief teams. In addition, parents should limit the exposure to media coverage of traumatic events, talk to their child about the event, and maintain routines as much as possible.

While there are not any Canadian statistics available on this topic, the Canadian Media Awareness group has expressed concern about television news programs having increased crime coverage, which can frighten children and exaggerate the actual risk. Statistics Canada found that 46% of those polled feared more for their safety at the time of the polling than they did 5 years previously, even though the actual risk of violence had not increased (Brandao, 1995).

On the plus side, television has been shown to have a positive influence on children's abilities to deal with a variety of social issues, such as divorce, the arrival of a new baby, discrimination, honesty, and helpfulness. Children who view educational programming for an extended period become more affectionate, considerate, cooperative, and helpful toward their playmates. A systematic review of preschoolers and television found that educational viewing can increase their knowledge, affect their racial attitudes, and increase their imaginative behaviour (Thakkar, Garrison, & Christakis, 2006). The ways in which minority and ethnic characters are portrayed on television can have an impact on the ways in which the majority culture views minority persons and on the self-image of minority children. The impact can be positive or negative, depending on whether the characters are treated with respect or discrimination.

In short, parents need to supervise the amount and type of television programs their children watch and to teach their children how to watch television (Box 33-5 and Family-Centred Care box). As the Canadian Paediatric Society (2003) recommends, parental role modelling may have a more positive influence on the child's behaviour than television programming. They recommend that parents watch television with children and help children understand the difference between their life and habits and those of persons represented on television.

Nurses and parents can be powerful forces in influencing the media. They can watch closely for an increase in violence and other undesirable programming and complain to sponsors and television stations if they believe it is not appropriate. Good programming can be both educational and entertaining.

Video Games

With the popularity of home gaming systems, children are spending more hours playing video games. Unfortunately, many of the video games available are violent, portraying virtual crimes and violence against others, particularly women. Video games allow the player to be the aggressor, making an ideal environment for a child to learn violent behaviour (American Academy of Pediatrics, Committee on Public Education, 2001). Although video games come with violence and age ratings, many parents are not aware of or choose to ignore the rating appropriate for their child. The Canadian Paediatric Society (2003) recommends restricted time limits to avoid the violence overexposure and to prevent the other issues of inactivity, undeveloped social skills, and a form of addictive behaviour.

BOX 33-5 Five Important Ideas to Teach Children and Adolescents About Television

1. You are smarter than what you see on your television.
2. The television world is not real.
3. Television teaches that some people are more important than others.
4. Television keeps showing the same things over and over again.
5. Somebody is always trying to make money with television.

(Modified from Davis, J. [1992]. Five important ideas to teach your children about TV. *Media Values, 59/60*, 10–14.)

Internet

The use of computers and personal tablets in both the classroom and household has affected childhood learning and development. Many schools offer computer programs and use digital devices that enable children of all ages to research a range of topics and broaden their world view. These technologies can be used for interactive learning, and their use can improve hand–eye coordination. Parents have a wide variety of computer software choices for their children's learning and gaming.

The Internet and e-mail have made correspondence and information available to children from around the world in minutes. Social networking sites (e.g., Twitter, Facebook) provide opportunities for children and adolescents to express themselves through blogs, music, pictures, and videos, and the overwhelming majority of adolescents use these sites responsibly (Hinduja & Patchin, 2008; Ybarra & Mitchell, 2008).

Although computer and digital technology has enhanced many forms of learning and recreation, there are potential dangers to children. The negative aspects of television and video games also apply to the Internet. It is important for parents to be aware of the Web sites that their children access as they are vulnerable to exposure to pornographic sites. Children can also be lured into interactions with pedophiles. Locks that block certain Web sites should be considered. Children can also spend too much time sitting in front of a computer screen. With excessive use of digital devices such as smartphones they can also develop repetitive-use injuries.

FAMILY-CENTRED TEACHING

Television Viewing

Provide a positive role model by developing television substitutes such as reading, athletics, physical conditioning, and hobbies.

Together with your child, construct a time chart of activities (homework, television viewing, scheduled and other outside activities, playing with a friend).

Require that the child choose to do something from this list before watching television.

Limit the child's viewing to 2 hours or less per day.

Rule out television at specific times (e.g., mealtimes, before breakfast, or on school nights).

Discuss the purpose of a program and of commercial content with the child:

- Distinguish between the real and the unreal.
- Correlate consequences with actions.
- Point out subtle messages.
- Explore alternatives to aggressive conflict resolution.

Remove televisions from children's bedrooms.

Limit use of television as a safe distraction to potentially stressful times (e.g., keeping the children occupied while the parent gets organized after a difficult day).

Nurses must be involved in encouraging parents to be knowledgeable of their children's Internet activities while providing appropriate learning activities unique to computers and digital devices. One helpful strategy is to locate the computer in a public area of the home, such as the kitchen or family room, to enable parents to easily monitor its use.

Key Points

- Growth describes a change in quantity and occurs when cells divide and synthesize new proteins.
- Maturation, a qualitative change, describes the aging process or an increase in competence and adaptability.
- Differentiation refers to biological processes by which early cells and structures are modified and altered to achieve specific and characteristic physical and chemical properties.
- Development involves change from a lower to a more advanced stage of complexity.
- The five major developmental periods are prenatal, infancy, early childhood, middle childhood, and later childhood (pubescence and adolescence).
- Growth and development proceed in predictable patterns of direction, sequence, and pace.
- The directional trends in growth and development are cephalocaudal, proximodistal, and mass to specific.
- Physical development includes increase in height and weight and changes in body proportion, dentition, and some body tissues.
- The three broad classifications of child temperament are the easy child, the difficult child, and the slow-to-warm-up child.
- The developmental theories most widely used in explaining child growth and development are Freud's psychosexual stages, Erikson's stages of psychosocial development, Piaget's stages of cognitive development, Kohlberg's stages of moral development, and Fowler's stages of spiritual development.
- To develop a positive self-concept, children need recognition for their achievements and the approval of others.
- Through play, children learn about their world and how to relate to objects, people, and situations.
- Play provides a means of development in the areas of sensorimotor and intellectual progress, socialization, creativity, self-awareness, and moral behaviour; it serves as a means for the release of tension and expression of emotions.
- Growth and development are affected by a variety of conditions and circumstances, including heredity, physiological function, gender, disease, physical environment, nutrition, and interpersonal relationships.
- Children's vulnerability and reaction to stress depend to a large extent on their age, coping behaviours, and support systems.
- Mass media can be influential in children's learning and behaviour.

References

American Academy of Pediatrics, Committee on Public Education. (2001). Media violence. *Pediatrics, 108*(5), 1222–1226.

Anders, T. F., Sadeh, A., & Appareddy, V. (2005). Normal sleep in neonates and children. In S. Sheldon, R. Ferber, & M. Kryger (Eds.), *Principles and practice of sleep medicine in the child*. Philadelphia: Saunders.

Baum, C., & Shannon, M. (1995). Environmental toxins: cutting the risks. *Contemporary Pediatrics, 12*(7), 20–43.

Beck, C. T. (1996). A meta-analysis of the relationship between postpartum depression and infant temperament. *Nursing Research, 45*(4), 225–230.

Bowlby, J. (1951). *Maternal care and mental health*. Geneva, Switzerland: World Health Organization.

Brandao, C. (1995). *Crime-time news: How Toronto's TV stations distort the picture of what's really happening on the streets*. Media Awareness Network. Retrieved from http://209.29.148.33/english/resources/educational/teaching_backgrounders/crime/crime_time_news.cfm.

Brown, J. D., & Witherspoon, E. M. (2002). The mass media and American adolescents' health. *Journal of Adolescent Health, 31*(6S), 153–170.

Caine, D., DiFiori, J., & Maffulli, N. (2006). Physeal injuries in children's and youth sports: Reasons for concern? *British Journal of Sports Medicine, 40*(9), 749–760. doi:10.1136/bjsm.2005.017822

Canadian Paediatric Society, Psychosocial Paediatrics Committee. (2003). Canadian Paediatric Society position statement: Impact of media use on children and youth. *Paediatrics and Child Health, 8*(5), 301–306. (Reaffirmed February 2011.)

Carey, W. B. (1998). Teaching parents about infant temperament. *Pediatrics, 102*(5 Suppl E), 1311–1316.

Chess, S., & Thomas, A. (1999). *Goodness of fit: Clinical applications from infancy through adult life*. London: Routledge.

Cronk, C., et al. (1988). Growth charts for children with Down syndrome: 1 month to 18 years of age. *Pediatrics, 81*(1), 102–110.

Dietitians of Canada. (2010). *School nutrition policy*. Retrieved from http://www.dietitians.ca/Dietitians-Views/School-Nutrition-Policy.aspx.

Earles, K. A., et al. (2002). Media influences on children and adolescents: Violence and sex. *Journal of the National Medical Association, 94*(9), 797–801.

Erikson, E. H. (1963). *Childhood and society* (2nd ed.). New York: Norton.

Finkelstein, P. (2009). School nutrition: Are we failing Canadian kids? *Best Health Magazine*, March/April. Retrieved from http://www.besthealthmag.ca/eat-well/nutrition/school-nutrition-are-we-failing-canadas-kids.

Fowler, J. (1981). *Stages of faith: The psychology of human development and the quest for meaning*. New York: HarperCollins.

Galligan, M. (2006). Proposed guidelines for skin to skin treatment of neonatal hypothermia. *MCN: American Journal of Maternal Child Nursing, 31*(5), 298–304.

Garbarino, J. (2001). An ecological perspective on the effects of violence on children. *Journal of Community Psychology, 29*(3), 361–378.

Goldsmith, M. (1990). Youngsters dialing up cholesterol levels? *Journal of the American Medical Association, 264*(23), 2976.

Hinduja, S., & Patchin, J. W. (2008). Personal information of adolescents on the Internet: A quantitative content analysis of MySpace. *Journal of Adolescence, 31*(1), 125–146. doi:10.1016/j.adolescence.2007.05.004

Kaczander, B. I. (1997). Pediatric sports medicine: A unique perspective. *Podiatry Management, 16*(2), 53–60.

Kohen, D. E., Leventhal, T., Dahinten, V. S., & McIntosh, C. N. (2008). Neighborhood disadvantage: Pathways of effects for young children. *Child Development, 79*(1), 156–169. doi:10.1111/j.1467-8624.2007.01117.x

Kohlberg, L. (1968). Moral development. In D. L. Sills (Ed.), *International encyclopedia of the social sciences*. New York: Macmillan.

LaMontagne, L. L., et al. (1996). Children's preoperative coping and its effects on postoperative anxiety and return to normal activity. *Nursing Research, 45*(3), 141–147.

Le Mare, L., & Audet, K. (2006). A longitudinal study of the physical growth and health of postinstitutionalized Romanian adoptees. *Paediatrics and Child Health, 11*(2), 85–91.

Masten, A. S., et al. (1988). Competence and stress in school children: Moderating effects of individual and family qualities. *Journal of Child Psychology and Psychiatry, 29*, 747–764.

Matvienko, O. (2007). Impact of a nutrition education curriculum on snack choices of children ages six and seven years. *Journal of Nutrition Education & Behavior, 39*(5), 281–285. doi:10.1016/j.jneb.2007.01.004

Monsen, R. B. (2002). Children and the media. *Journal of Pediatric Nursing, 17*(4), 309–310.

Morrow, J. D., & Camp, B. W. (1996). Mastery motivation and temperament of 7-month-old infants. *Pediatric Nursing, 22*(3), 211–217.

Myrelid, A., et al. (2002). Growth charts for Down's syndrome from birth to 18 years of age. *Archives of Disease in Childhood, 87*(2), 97–103.

Newman, J. (2009). *Canadian Breast Feeding Foundation: Toxins and infant feeding*. Retrieved from http://www.canadianbreastfeedingfoundation.org/basics/toxins.shtml.

Paquette, G. (2004). Violence on Canadian television networks. *Canadian Child Adolescent Psychiatry, 13*(1), 13–15.

Pfefferbaum, B., et al. (2003). Media exposure in children 100 miles from a terrorist bombing. *Annals of Clinical Psychiatry, 15*(1), 1–8.

Phillips, D., Prince, S., & Schiebelhut, L. (2004). Elementary school children's responses 3 months after the September 11 terrorist attacks: A study in Washington, DC. *American Journal of Orthopsychiatry, 75*(4), 509–528.

Piaget, J. (1969). *The theory of stages in cognitive development*. New York: McGraw-Hill.

Safe Kids Canada. (2010). *Toy safety*. Retrieved from http://www.safekidscanada.ca/Parents/Safety-Information/Product-Safety/Toy-Safety-Prod/Toy-Safety.aspx.

Seidel, H. M., et al. (2006). *Mosby's guide to physical examination* (6th ed.). St. Louis: Mosby.

Sherar, L. B., Mirwald, R. L., Baxter-Jones, A., & Tomis, M. (2005). Prediction of adult height using maturity-based cumulative height velocity curves. *Journal of Pediatrics, 147*(4), 508–514.

Sieving, R. E., & Zirbel-Donisch, S. T. (1990). Development and enhanceiment of self-esteem in children. *Journal of Pediatric Health Care, 4*(6), 290–296.

Stuart, G. W., & Laraia, M. T. (2000). *Principles and practice of psychiatric nursing* (7th ed.). St. Louis: Mosby.

Thakkar, R., Garrison, M., & Christakis, D. (2006). A systematic review for the effects of television viewing by infants and preschoolers. *Pediatrics, 118*(5), 2025–2031. doi:10.1542/peds.2006-1307.

Thompson, D. A., & Christakis, D. A. (2005). The association between television viewing and irregular sleep schedules among children less than 3 years of age. *Pediatrics, 116*(4), 851–856. doi:10.1542/peds.2004-2788

Thompson, R., et al. (2007). Enhancing early communication through infant sign training. *Journal of Applied Behavior Analysis, 40*(1), 15–23. doi:10.1901/jaba.2007.23-06

Tremblay, M. S., & Willlms, J. D. (2003). Is the Canadian childhood obesity epidemic related to physical inactivity? *International Journal of Obesity, 27*, 1100–1105. doi:10.1038/sj.ijo.0802376

Urbanski, L. F., & Hanlon, D. P. (1996). Pediatric orthopedics. *Topics in Emergency Medicine, 18*(2), 73–90.

Wachs, T. (2006). Contributions of temperament to buffering and sensitization processes in children's development. *Annals of the New York Academy of Science, 1094*, 28–30.

Willoughby, C., King, G., & Polatajko, H. (1996). A therapist's guide to children's self-esteem. *American Journal of Occupational Therapy, 50*(2), 124–132.

Ybarra, M. L., & Mitchell, K. J. (2008). How risky are social networking sites? A comparison of places online where youth sexual solicitation and harassment occurs. *Pediatrics, 121*(2), e350–357. doi:10.1542/peds.2007-0693.

Zimmerman, F., Christakis, D., & Meltzoff, A. (2007). Television and DVD/video viewing in children younger than 2 years. *Archives of Pediatric and Adolescent Medicine, 161*, 473–479.

Additional Resources

Canadian Toy Testing Council: http://www.toy-testing.org.

Dietitians of Canada—A comprehensive resource for healthy nutrition programs and safe food supplies; a tracking system is available that can help individuals make healthy choices: http://www.dietitians.ca

MediaSmarts: Canada's Centre for Digital and Media Awareness (formerly Media Awareness Network) http://www.mediasmarts.ca/

Motion Picture Association—Movie rating categories: http://www.mpaa.org

Unit 8

34 Communication, History, Physical, and Developmental Assessment

Learning Objectives

On completion of this chapter, the reader will be able to:

- Identify communication strategies for interviewing parents.
- Formulate guidelines for using an interpreter.
- Identify communication strategies for communicating with children of different age groups.
- Describe four communication techniques that are useful with children.
- State the components of a complete health history.
- List three areas that are evaluated as part of a nutritional assessment.
- Prepare a child for a physical examination based on his or her developmental needs.
- Perform a comprehensive physical examination in a sequence appropriate to the child's age.
- Recognize expected normal findings for children at various ages.
- Record the physical examination according to the head-to-toe format.

Electronic Resources

Additional information related to the content in Chapter 34 can be found on

evolve the companion Web site at

http://evolve.elsevier.com/Canada/Perry/maternal/

- Examination Review Questions
- Anatomy Reviews
- Animation—Abdominal Anatomy
- Animation—Cranial Nerves
- Animation—Organ Systems 3-D Tour
- Assessment Video Clips
- Case Study—Communicating With Adolescents
- Case Study—Immunizations
- Case Study—Pediatric Assessment
- Critical Thinking Exercise—Cardiovascular Assessment
- Critical Thinking Exercise—The Interview
- Skill—Communicating With Children
- Skill—Measuring Body Temperature
- Skill—Measuring Physical Growth

Guidelines for Communication and Interviewing

The most widely used method of communicating with parents and children on a professional basis is the interview process. Unlike social conversation, interviewing is a specific form of goal-directed communication. As nurses converse with children and adults, they focus on the individuals to determine the kind of persons they are, their usual mode of handling problems, whether help is needed, and the way they react to counselling. Developing interviewing skills requires time and practice, but following some guiding principles can facilitate this process. An organized approach is most effective when using interviewing skills in patient teaching.

Establishing a Setting for Communication

Appropriate Introduction

When first meeting a patient and his or her **family**, the nurse needs to introduce herself or himself to, and ask the name of, each family member who is present. Parents or other adults should be addressed by their appropriate titles, such as "Mr." and "Mrs.," unless they specify a preferred name. The nurse should record the preferred name on the medical record. Using formal address or their preferred names, rather than using first names or "mother" or "father," conveys respect and regard for the parents or other caregivers (Seidel et al., 2006).

At the beginning of the visit, children should be included in the interaction by asking them their name, age, and other information. Nurses often direct all questions to adults, even when children are old enough to speak for themselves. This practice serves to terminate one extremely valuable source of information: the patient. When the child is included in the interview, one can use the general rules for communication that are given in the Guidelines box on communicating with children (p. 874).

evolve Critical Thinking Exercise—The Interview

Assurance of Privacy and Confidentiality

The place where the interview is conducted is almost as important as the interview itself. The physical environment should allow for as much privacy as possible, with distractions, such as interruptions, noise, or other visible activity, kept to a minimum. At times it is necessary to turn off a television or radio. The environment should also have some toys for young children to keep them occupied during the parent–nurse interview (Fig. 34-1). Parents who are constantly interrupted by their children are unable to concentrate fully and tend to give brief answers in order to finish the interview as quickly as possible.

Confidentiality is another essential component of the initial phase of the interview. One of the primary nursing values of the Canadian Nurses Association (2010) is to recognize the importance of privacy and confidentiality and to *protect personal, family, and community information obtained within the framework of a professional relationship.* Since the interview is usually shared with other members of the health team care or with a teacher (in the case of students), it is imperative to inform the family of the limits regarding confidentiality. If confidentiality is a concern in a particular situation, such as when talking to a parent suspected of child abuse or a teenager contemplating suicide, this should be dealt with directly and the person informed that in such instances confidentiality cannot be ensured. However, the nurse needs to judiciously protect information of a confidential nature.

NURSING ALERT In Canada, the *Privacy Act of 1985* is the law that protects the privacy of individuals with respect to personal information about themselves held by a government institution and that provides individuals with a right of access to that information. The *Personal Information Protection and Electronic Documents Act (PIPEDA)* protects the privacy and confidentiality of an individual's personal information within the private and health care sectors and applies in jurisdictions that have not adopted similar legislation (eg. Québec, Alberta, Ontario) (Office of the Privacy Commissioner of Canada, 2009) (see Additional Resources).

Computer Privacy and Applications in Nursing

The use of computer technology to store and retrieve health information has become widespread. Throughout the health

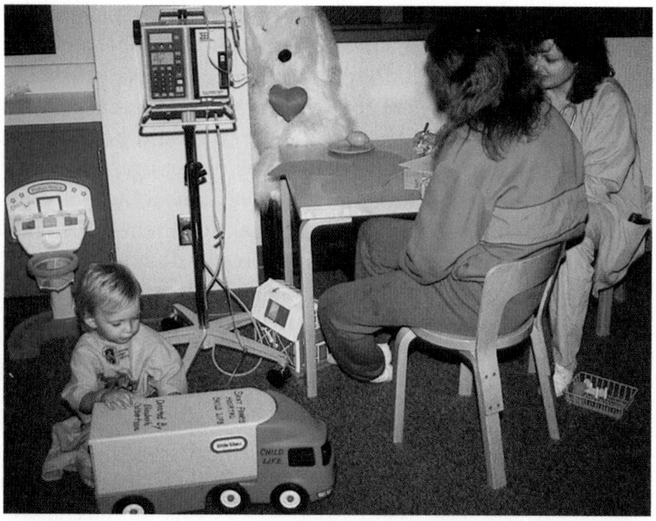

Fig. 34-1 A child plays while the nurse interviews the parent.

care community, the privacy and security of this health information has become a growing concern. Any person accessing confidential health information is charged with managing safeguards for disclosure, since violations might incur civil damages.

In 2005, a Pan-Canadian Health Information Privacy and Confidentiality Framework was developed by Deputy Ministers of Health to inform and influence any private legislative process regarding health information and to provide more consistent privacy protocols among health care jurisdictions. This framework includes the development of electronic health record systems and primary health care reform (Health Canada, 2005).

Many institutions use computer and information applications in nursing (nursing informatics), such as electronic medical records, to record care and access information. Two health care applications are record transmission, via facsimile (fax) or electronic mail (e-mail), and telemedicine. The telemedicine application is capable of two-way video conferencing, transmission of radiographs, and clinical consultation between remote sites and centralized resources.

Telephone Triage and Counselling

Nurses are increasingly responsible for assessing children's symptoms and providing clinical judgement regarding further medical care (triage) by means of telephone report. Most often, health problems are assessed and prioritized according to urgency, and treatment is judiciously provided via telephone services. The goal of telephone triage care management is to increase access to high-quality health care services and to significantly increase patient satisfaction. Successful outcomes are based on the consistency and accuracy of the information provided, and parents are empowered to participate in their child's medical care. While more research is needed to investigate actual outcomes of this type of care, Canadian researchers have audited the appropriateness of advice given by telephone triage nurses and found that 90% of the advice was appropriate. Theses nurses erred on the side of caution, with no adverse effects (Goodwin 2007; Stacey, Hussein, Fisher, Robinson, & Pong, 2003). With the use of telephone triage, unnecessary physician office visits have decreased, saving medical costs and time (along with less absence from work) for families in need of health care. The most common telephone triage call is for a fever.

A well-designed telephone triage program is essential for safe, prompt, and consistent-quality health care (Rutenberg, 2000). Typically, guidelines for telephone triage include asking screening questions; determining when to immediately refer to emergency medical services (dial 911); and determining when to refer to same-day appointments, appointments in 24 to 72 hours, appointments in 4 days or more, or home care (Box 34-1).

Many provinces and territories have telephone health advice services. For example, Telehealth Ontario (http://www.health.gov.on.ca/en/public/programs/telehealth/) has registered nurses available 24 hours a day providing free, confidential telephone service that the public can call to get health advice or general health information.

BOX 34-1 Telephone Triage Guidelines

Date and time
Background
- Name, age, sex
- Chronic illness
- Allergies, current medications, treatments, or recent immunizations

Chief health concern
General symptoms
- Severity
- Duration
- Other symptoms
- Pain

Systems review
Steps taken
- Advised to call emergency medical services (911)
- Advised to see practitioner
- Advice given for home care
- Call back if symptoms worsen or fail to improve

Resources for Telephone Triage Protocols

Briggs, J. K. (2011). *Telephone triage protocols for nurses* (4th ed.). Philadelphia: Lippincott Williams & Wilkins.

Schmitt, B. D. (2009). *Pediatric telephone protocols: Office version* (12th ed.). Elk Grove Village, IL: American Academy of Pediatrics.

The Canada Health Infoway's telehealth program also provides improved access to health care services using electronic solutions. This program focuses on Aboriginal, official-language minority, northern, and remote communities. Nurses play many different roles in this system, particularly in the area of health education. For example, Infoway is aiming toward having 40% of First Nations, Métis, and Inuit communities telehealth enabled, with a focus on mental health and drug addiction services (Canada Health Infoway, 2011).

Communicating With Families

Communicating With Parents

Although the parent and child are separate and distinct individuals, the nurse's relationship with the child is frequently mediated by the parent, particularly for younger children. For the most part, information about the child is acquired by direct observation or is communicated to the nurse by the parents. Usually it can be assumed that because of the close contact with the child, the parent gives reliable information. Making an assessment of the child requires input from the child (verbal and nonverbal), information from the parent, and the nurse's own observations of the child and interpretation of the relationship between the child and the parent. Counselling and guidance must be directed to the caregiver of infants and small children; when children are old enough to be active participants in their own health maintenance, the parent becomes a collaborator in health care.

Encouraging the Parent to Talk

Interviewing parents provides the opportunity to not only determine the child's health and developmental status but also to obtain information about factors that influence the child's life. Whatever the parent sees as a problem should be a concern of the nurse. These problems are not always easy to identify. Nurses need to be alert for clues and signals by which a parent communicates worries and anxieties. Careful phrasing with broad, open-ended questions, such as "What is Jimmy eating now?" provides more information than several single-answer questions, such as "Is Jimmy eating what the rest of the family eats?"

Sometimes the parent will take the lead without prompting. At other times, it may be necessary to direct another question on the basis of an observation, such as "Consuela seems unhappy today" or "How do you feel when Jamil cries?" If the parent appears to be tired or distraught, consider asking, "What do you do to relax?" or "What help do you have with the children?" A comment such as "You handle the baby very well. What kinds of experience have you had with babies?" to new parents who appear comfortable with their first child gives positive reinforcement and provides an opening for any questions they might have regarding the infant's care. Often all that is required to keep parents talking is a nod or saying "yes" or "uh-huh."

When attempting to elicit feelings and covert problem areas, avoid closed-ended questions that begin with "Does ... ," "Did ... ," or "Is ... ," which usually require only a single response. In addition, asking questions such as "Does your son have any problems at school?" subtly implies a lack of parental skills and evokes defensiveness. Instead, say, "What ... ," "How ... ," or "Tell me about ... ," and encourage elaboration with "You were saying ..." or "You say that ... ," or by reflecting back a key word. Open-ended questions are nonthreatening and encourage description.

Directing the Focus

The ability to direct the focus of the interview while allowing for maximum freedom of expression is one of the most difficult goals in effective communication. One approach is the use of open-ended or broad questions, followed by guiding statements. For example, if the parent proceeds to list the other children by name, say, "Tell me their ages, too." If the parent continues to describe each child in depth, which is not the purpose of the interview, redirect the focus by stating, "Let's talk about the other children later. You were beginning to tell me about Paul's activities at school." This approach conveys interest in the other children but focuses the assessment on the patient.

Listening and Cultural Awareness

Listening is the most important component of effective communication. When listening is truly aimed at understanding the patient, it is an active process that requires concentration and attention to all aspects of the conversation—verbal, nonverbal, and abstract. Major blocks to listening are environmental distraction and premature judgement.

The nurse's attitudes and feelings are easily injected into an interview. Often nurses' perceptions of a parent's behaviour are influenced by their own perceptions, prejudices, and **assumptions,** which may include racial, religious, and cultural stereotypes. What may be interpreted as a parent's passive hostility or lack of interest may be shyness or an expression of anxiety. For example, in Western cultures, eye contact and directness are signs of paying attention. However, in many non-Western cultures, including some First Nations, Métis, and Inuit cultures, directness, such as looking someone in the eye, is considered rude. Children are taught to avert their gaze and to look down when being addressed by an adult, especially one with authority (Seidel et al., 2006). Therefore, judgements about listening and verbal interactions need to be made with an appreciation of cultural differences (see Guidelines box, p. 834, and Chapter 32).

Although it is necessary for the nurse to make some preliminary judgements, it is important to listen with as much objectivity as possible by clarifying meanings and attempting to see the situation from the parent's point of view. Effective interviewers control their reactions, responses, and the techniques that they use.

Minimal speaking along with active listening can facilitate parents' involvement. While it is tempting to spend time explaining, describing, and interpreting health information when the opportunity presents itself, it is possible to provide effective health education by timing the information properly and presenting only as much as is necessary at the moment.

The nurse who practises careful listening will use cues, verbal leads, or signals from the interviewee to move the interview along. Frequent references to an area of concern, repetition of certain key words, or special emphasis on something or someone can serve as cues to the interviewer for directing the inquiry. Parents' concerns and anxieties are often mentioned in a casual, offhand manner; however, they are nonetheless important and deserve careful scrutiny to identify problem areas. For example, a parent who is concerned about a child's habit of bed-wetting may mention that the child's bed was "wet this morning."

Using Silence

Responding with silence is often one of the most difficult interviewing techniques to learn. It requires a sense of confidence and comfort on the part of the interviewer to allow the interviewee space in which to think without interruptions. Silence permits the interviewee to sort out thoughts and feelings and search for responses to questions. Silence can also be a cue for the interviewer to go more slowly, re-examine the approach, and not push too hard (Seidel et al., 2006).

Sometimes it is necessary to break the silence and reopen communication. This should be done in a way that encourages the person to continue talking about what is considered important. Breaking a silence by introducing a new topic or with prolonged talking essentially terminates the interviewee's opportunity to use the silence. Suggestions for breaking the silence include statements such as the following: "Is there anything else you wish to say?" "I see you find it difficult to continue; how may I help?" or "I don't know what this silence means. Perhaps there is something you would like to put into words but find difficult to say."

Being Empathic

Empathy is the capacity to understand what another person is experiencing from within that person's frame of reference; it is often described as the ability to put oneself in another's shoes. The essence of empathic interaction is accurate understanding of another's feelings (Price & Archbold, 1997; Reynolds, Scott, & Jessiman, 1999; White, 1997). Empathy differs from sympathy, which is *having* feelings or emotions in common with another person, rather than *understanding* those feelings. Sympathy is not therapeutic in the helping relationship because it leads to overinvolvement emotionally and potentially to professional burnout (Yegdich, 1999).

Providing Anticipatory Guidance

The ideal way to handle a situation is to deal with it *before* it becomes a problem. The best preventive measure is anticipatory guidance. Traditionally, anticipatory guidance has focused on providing families with information on normal growth and development, as well as nurturing childrearing practices. For example, one of the most significant areas in pediatrics is injury prevention. Beginning prenatally, parents need specific instructions on home safety. Because of the child's maturing developmental skills, home safety changes must be implemented early to minimize risks to the child.

Many normal developmental changes can disturb unprepared parents, such as a toddler's diminished appetite, negativism, altered sleeping patterns, and anxiety toward strangers. The nurse can allay parents' fear by providing relevant information about such behaviours. Topics like these are discussed in the chapters on health promotion (Unit 9) to provide the nurse with information for counselling parents.

Anticipatory guidance should extend beyond merely providing information to empowering families to use the information as a means of building confidence in their parenting abilities. In order to achieve this level of anticipatory guidance, the nurse should do the following:

- Base interventions on needs identified by the family, not by the professional.
- View the family as competent or as having the ability to be competent.
- Provide opportunities for the family to achieve competence.

Avoiding Blocks to Communication

A number of blocks to communication can adversely affect the quality of the helping relationship. Many of these barriers are initiated by the interviewer, such as giving unrestricted advice or forming prejudged conclusions. Sometimes the interviewees reach information overload. When individuals are presented with too much information or information that is overwhelming, they will often demonstrate signs of increasing anxiety or decreasing attention. Such signals should alert the interviewer to give less information or to clarify what has been said. Some of the more common blocks to communication, including signs of information overload, are listed in Box 34-2.

BOX 34-2 Blocks to Communication

Communication Barriers (Nurse)

- Socializing
- Giving unrestricted and sometimes unasked-for advice
- Offering premature or inappropriate reassurance
- Giving over-ready encouragement
- Defending a situation or opinion
- Using stereotyped comments or clichés
- Limiting expression of emotion by asking directed, closed-ended questions
- Interrupting and finishing the person's sentence
- Talking more than the interviewee
- Forming prejudged conclusions
- Deliberately changing the focus

Signs of Information Overload (Patient)

- Long periods of silence
- Wide eyes and fixed facial expression
- Constant fidgeting or attempting to move away
- Nervous habits (e.g., tapping, playing with hair)
- Sudden disruptions (e.g., asking to go to the bathroom)
- Looking around
- Yawning, eyes drooping
- Frequently looking at a watch or clock
- Attempting to change the topic of discussion

Communicating With Families Through an Interpreter

Sometimes communication is impossible because the health care provider and the patient speak different languages. In this case, it is necessary to obtain information through a third party, the interpreter. When an interpreter is used, the same interviewing guidelines as those used without an interpreter apply. Specific guidelines for using an adult interpreter are presented in the Guidelines box.

Communicating with families through an interpreter requires sensitivity to cultural, legal, and ethical considerations. For example, in some cultures using a child as an interpreter is considered an insult to an adult because children are expected to show respect by not questioning their elders. In some cultures, class differences between the interpreter and the family may cause the family to feel intimidated and less inclined to offer information. Thus it is important to choose the translator carefully and provide time for the interpreter and family to establish rapport. If possible, family members should not be used as interpreters.

Issues of legal and ethical concerns may also arise. For example, in obtaining informed consent through an interpreter, it is important that the family be fully informed of all aspects of the particular procedure to which they are consenting. Issues of confidentiality may arise when family members related to another patient are asked to interpret for the family, thus revealing sensitive information that may be shared with other families on the unit. Because of increased sensitivity toward patient rights and confidentiality, many institutions now require consent forms to be produced in the patient's primary language.

GUIDELINES Using an Interpreter

- Explain to the interpreter the reason for the interview and the type of questions that will be asked.
- Clarify whether a detailed or brief answer is required and whether the translated response can be general or literal.
- Introduce the interpreter to the family and allow some time before the interview for them to become acquainted.
- Communicate directly with family members when asking questions in order to reinforce interest in them and to observe nonverbal expressions, but do not ignore the interpreter.
- Pose questions to elicit only one answer at a time, such as "Do you have pain?" rather than "Do you have any pain, tiredness, or loss of appetite?"
- Refrain from interrupting the family member and interpreter while they are conversing.
- Avoid commenting to the interpreter about family members, since they may understand some English.
- Be aware that some medical words, such as *allergy*, may have no similar word in another language; avoid medical jargon whenever possible.
- Be aware that cultural differences may exist regarding views on sex, marriage, or pregnancy.
- Allow time after the interview for the interpreter to share something that he or she thought could not be said earlier; ask about the interpreter's impression of nonverbal clues to communication and family members' ease in revealing information.
- Arrange for the family to speak with the same interpreter on subsequent visits whenever possible.

When no one else is available to translate, children within the family may be asked to assume this role. In this situation, it is important to stress literal translation of parent responses. To ensure correct translations, it may be necessary to interrupt the parent and ask the child to translate every few sentences. When using children as interpreters, questions should be directed at specific answers and the interpreted translation assessed along with nonverbal expressions of communication. Some institutions prohibit or discourage the use of children as interpreter; check institutional policy to ensure compliance with procedure.

evolve Skill—Communicating With Children

Communicating With Children

Although the greatest amount of verbal communication is usually carried out with the parent, the child should not be excluded during the interview. Infants and younger children can be observed through play; occasionally younger children can answer questions or respond to remarks. Older children should be included as active participants in the interview.

In communication with children of all ages, the nonverbal components of the communication process convey the most significant messages (Fig. 34-2). It is difficult to disguise feelings, attitudes, and anxiety when relating to children. They are alert to surroundings and attach meaning to every gesture and move that is made; this is particularly true of very young children.

Active attempts to make friends with children before they have had an opportunity to evaluate an unfamiliar person tend to increase their anxiety. It is helpful to continue to talk to the child and parent but go about activities that do not involve the child directly, thus allowing the child to observe from a safe position. If the child has a special toy or doll, the nurse can "talk" to the doll first. Simple questions such as "Does your teddy bear have a name?" can be asked to ease the child into conversation. Other guidelines for communicating with children are presented in the Guidelines box.

Communication Related to Development of Thought Processes

The normal development of language and thought in children offers a frame of reference for communicating with children.

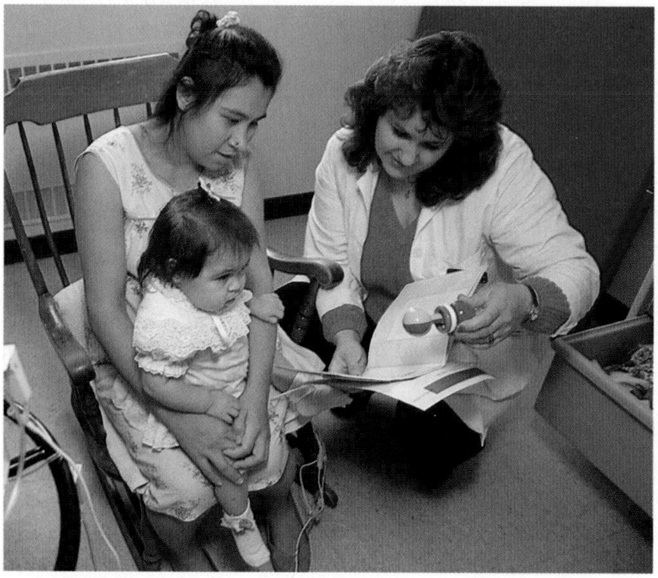

Fig. 34-2 Nurse assumes position at child's level.

GUIDELINES Communicating With Children

- Allow children time to feel comfortable.
- Avoid sudden or rapid advances, broad smiles, extended eye contact, or other gestures that may be seen as threatening.
- Talk to the parent if the child is initially shy.
- Communicate through transition objects such as dolls, puppets, and stuffed animals before questioning a young child directly.
- Give older children the opportunity to talk without the parents present.
- Assume a position that is at eye level with the child (see Fig. 34-2).
- Speak in a quiet, unhurried, and confident voice.
- Speak clearly, be specific, and use simple words and short sentences.
- State directions and suggestions positively.
- Offer a choice only when one exists.
- Be honest with children.
- Allow them to express their concerns and fears.
- Use a variety of communication techniques.

Thought processes progress from sensorimotor to perceptual to concrete and, finally, to abstract, formal operations. The early social communicative development of children has been divided into three stages: (1) *perlocutionary stage*—unintentional communication behaviour; (2) *illocutionary stage*—true intent in communication efforts; and (3) *locutionary stage*—intentional communication behaviours and use of symbols (Hoge & Parette, 1995). An understanding of the typical characteristics of these stages provides the nurse with a framework to facilitate social communication (Box 34-3).

Infancy

Because infants are unable to use words, they primarily use and understand nonverbal communication. Infants communicate their needs and feelings through nonverbal behaviours and vocalizations that can be interpreted by someone who is around them for a sufficient time. Infants smile and coo when content and cry when distressed. Crying is provoked by unpleasant stimuli from inside or outside, such as hunger, pain, body restraint, or loneliness. Adults interpret this to mean that an infant needs something and consequently try to alleviate the discomfort and reduce tension. Crying (or the desire to cry) persists as a part of everyone's communication repertoire.

Infants respond to adults' nonverbal behaviours. They become quiet when they are cuddled, are patted, or receive other forms of gentle physical contact. They derive comfort from the sound of a voice, even though they do not understand the words that are spoken. Until infants reach the age at which they experience stranger anxiety, they readily respond to any firm, gentle handling and quiet, calm speech. Loud, harsh sounds and sudden movements are frightening to infants.

Older infants' attention is centred on themselves and their parents; therefore, any stranger is a potential threat until proved otherwise. Holding out one's hands and asking the child to come is seldom successful, especially if the infant is with the parent. If infants must be handled, they should simply be picked up firmly, without gestures. The nurse should

BOX 34-3 Characteristics of Communicative Development in Young Children

Perlocutionary Stage (0 to 8–9 Months)

Child is reflexive to stimuli.

Child shows increasing purpose in action.

Emerging Illocutionary Stage (8–9 to 12–15 Months)

Child communicates intentionally with signals and gestures.

Conventional Illocutionary—Emerging Locutionary Stage (12–15 to 18–24 Months)

Child communicates intentionally with gestures, vocalizations, and verbalizations.

(Modified from Hoge, D. R., & Parette, H. P. [1995]. Facilitating communicative development in young children with disabilities. *Transdisciplinary Journal, 5*[2], 113–130.)

observe the position in which the parent holds the infant. Most infants learn to prefer a particular position and manner of handling. In general, infants are more at ease upright than horizontal. Also, infants should be held in such a way that they can see their parents. Until they develop the understanding that an object (in this case the parent) removed from sight can still be present, they have no way of knowing the object is still there.

Early Childhood

Children younger than 5 years of age are egocentric. They see things only in relation to themselves and from their point of view. Therefore, communication needs to be focused on them. They should be told what they can do or how they will feel. Experiences of others are of no interest to them. It is futile to use another child's experience in an attempt to gain the cooperation of small children. They should be allowed to touch and examine articles that will come in contact with them. A stethoscope bell will feel cold; palpating a neck might tickle. Although they have not yet acquired sufficient language skills to express their feelings and wants, toddlers are able to communicate effectively with their hands to transmit ideas without words. They will push an unwanted object away, pull another person to show them something, point, and cover the mouth that is saying something they do not wish to hear.

Everything is direct and concrete to small children. They are unable to work with abstractions and interpret words literally. Analogies escape them because they are unable to separate fact from fantasy. For example, they attach literal meaning to such common phrases as "two-faced," "sticky fingers," or "coughing your head off." Children who are told they will get "a little stick in the arm" may not be able to envision an injection (Fig. 34-3). Therefore, avoid using a phrase that might be misinterpreted by a small child.

Young children assign human attributes to inanimate objects. Consequently, they fear that objects may jump, bite, cut, or pinch all by themselves. Children do not know that these devices are unable to perform without human direction. To minimize their fear, unfamiliar equipment should be kept out of view until it is needed.

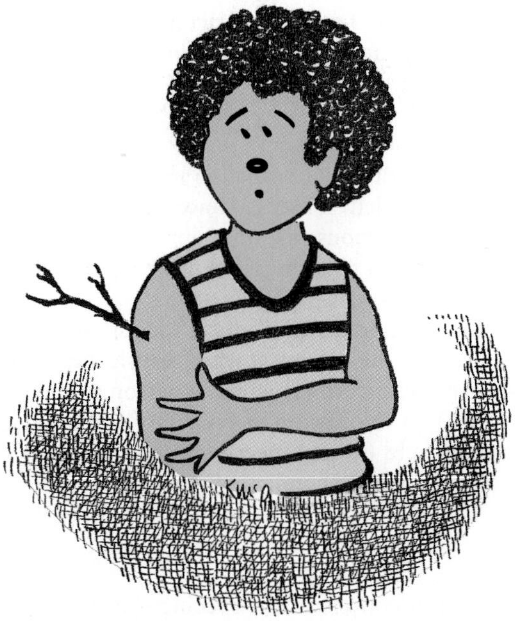

Fig. 34-3 A young child may take the expression "a little stick in the arm" literally.

School-Age Years

Younger school-age children rely less on what they see and more on what they know, when faced with new problems. They want explanations and reasons for everything but require no verification beyond that. They are interested in the functional aspect of all procedures, objects, and activities. They want to know why an object exists, why it is used, how it works, and the intent and purpose of its user. They need to know what is going to take place and why it is being done to them specifically. For example, to explain a procedure such as taking blood pressure (BP), show the child how squeezing the bulb pushes air into the cuff and makes the "silver" in the tube go up. Let the child operate the bulb. An explanation for the procedure might be as simple as, "I want to see how far the silver goes up when the cuff squeezes your arm." The child then becomes an enthusiastic participant.

School-age children have a heightened concern about body integrity. Because of the special importance they place on their body, they are sensitive to anything that constitutes a threat or suggestion of injury to it. This concern extends to their possessions, so that they may appear to overreact to loss or threatened loss of treasured objects. Helping children voice their concerns enables the nurse to provide reassurance and to implement activities that reduce their anxiety. For example, if a shy child dislikes being the centre of attention, the child should be ignored by talking and relating to other children in the family or group. When children feel more comfortable, they will usually interject personal ideas, feelings, and interpretations of events.

evolve Case Study—Communicating With Adolescents

Older children have an adequate and satisfactory use of language. They still require relatively simple explanations, but their ability to think concretely can facilitate communication and explanation. Commonly, they have sufficient experience with health and health care workers to understand what is transpiring and what is generally expected of them.

Adolescence

As children move into adolescence, they fluctuate between child and adult thinking and behaviour. They are riding a current that is moving them rapidly toward a maturity that may be beyond their coping ability. Thus when tensions rise, they may seek the security of the more familiar and comfortable expectations of childhood. Anticipating these shifts in identity allows the nurse to adjust the course of interaction to meet the needs of the moment. No single approach can be relied on consistently; one can expect to encounter cooperation, hostility, anger, bravado, and a variety of other behaviours and attitudes. It is as much a mistake to regard the adolescent as an adult with an adult's wisdom and control as it is to assume that the teenager has the concerns and expectations of a child.

Frequently adolescents are more willing to discuss their concerns with an adult outside the family, and they often welcome the opportunity to interact with a nurse outside the presence of their parents. They are usually accepting of anyone who displays a genuine interest in them. However, adolescents are quick to reject persons who attempt to impose their values on them, whose interest is feigned, or who appear to have little respect for who they are and what they think or say.

Interviewing the adolescent presents some special issues. The first may be whether to talk with the adolescent alone or with the adolescent and parents together. Of course, if the parent is not there, the only question is whether to suggest to the teenager that the parents be interviewed at another time. If the parents and teenager are together, talking with the adolescent first has the advantage of immediately identifying with the young person, thus fostering the interpersonal relationship. However, talking with the parents initially may provide insight into the family relationship. In either case, both parties should be given an opportunity to be included in the interview. If time constraints are important, such as during history taking, clarify this at the outset to avoid appearing to "take sides" by talking more with one person than with the other.

Confidentiality is of great importance when interviewing adolescents. Parents and teenagers need to have the limits of confidentiality explained to them, specifically that young persons' disclosures will not be shared unless they indicate a need for intervention, as in the case of suicidal behaviour.

Another dilemma in interviewing adolescents is that two views of a problem frequently exist—the teenager's and the parents'. Clarification of the problem is a major task. However, providing both parties an opportunity to discuss their perceptions in an open and unbiased atmosphere can, by itself, be therapeutic. The demonstration of positive communication skills can help families communicate more effectively (see Guidelines box).

evolve Case Study—Pediatric Assessment

Communication Techniques

In addition to such conventional interviewing methods as reflection and open-ended questions, a number of techniques encourage family members to express their thoughts and feelings in a less directive and confrontational manner. Several approaches are *projective*—they present nonspecific material that enables individuals to externalize or project inner aspects of themselves to others.

A variety of verbal techniques can be used to encourage communication. Some of these techniques can be used to pose questions or to explore concerns in a less threatening manner. Others can be presented as "word games," which are often well received by children. However, for many children and adults, talking about feelings is difficult, and verbal communication may be more stressful than supportive. In such instances, several nonverbal techniques can be used to encourage communication.

Both verbal and nonverbal techniques of communicating with children are described in Box 34-4. Play is an important part of this process and is discussed more extensively in Chapter 33. Any of the verbal or nonverbal techniques can give rise to strong feelings that surface unexpectedly. Be prepared to handle them or to recognize when issues go beyond your ability to deal with them. At that point, consider an appropriate referral.

GUIDELINES Communicating With Adolescents

Build a Foundation
- Spend time together.
- Encourage expression of ideas and feelings.
- Respect their views.
- Tolerate differences.
- Praise good points.
- Respect their privacy.
- Set a good example.

Communicate Effectively
- Give undivided attention.
- Listen, listen, listen.
- Be courteous, calm, and open minded.
- Try not to overreact. If you do, take a break.
- Avoid judging or criticizing.
- Avoid the "third degree" of continuous questioning.
- Choose important issues when taking a stand.
  After taking a stand:
  - Think through all options.
  - Make expectations clear.

History Taking

Performing a Health History

The format used for history taking may be (1) *direct*, where the nurse asks for information via direct interview with the informant; or (2) *indirect*, where the informant supplies the information by completing some type of questionnaire. The direct method is superior to the indirect approach or a combination of both. However, in view of time constraints, the direct approach is not always practical. If the direct approach cannot be used, the parents' written responses should be reviewed and the parents questioned regarding any unusual answers. The nurse taking a pediatric history can use the categories listed in Box 34-5, which encompass children's current and past health status and information about their psychosocial environment.

Identifying Information

Much of the identifying information may already be available from other recorded sources. However, if the parent and youngster seem anxious, use this opportunity to ask about such information to help them feel more comfortable.

Informant

One of the important elements of identifying information is the informant, the person(s) who furnish the information. The nurse should record (1) who the person is (child, parent, or other), (2) an impression of reliability and willingness to communicate, and (3) any special circumstances, such as the use of an interpreter or conflicting answers by more than one person.

Health Issue or Concern

The chief health concern is the specific reason for the child's visit to the clinic, office, or hospital. It may be viewed as the theme, with the present illness viewed as the description of the

BOX 34-4 Creative Communication Techniques With Children

Verbal Techniques

"I" Messages

Relate a feeling about a behaviour in terms of "I."

Describe the effect that the behaviour had on the person.

Avoid use of "you;" "you" messages are judgemental and provoke defensiveness.

Example—"You" message: "You are being uncooperative about doing your treatments."

Example—"I" message: "I am concerned about how the treatments are going because I want to see you get better."

Third-Person Technique

Express a feeling in terms of a third person ("he," "she," "they"). This is less threatening than directly asking children how they feel because it gives them an opportunity to agree or disagree without being defensive.

Example—"Sometimes when a person is sick a lot, he feels angry and sad because he cannot do what others can." Either wait silently for a response or encourage a reply with a statement such as "Did you ever feel that way?"

This approach allows children three choices: (1) to agree and possibly express how they feel; (2) to disagree; or (3) to remain silent, which means they probably have such feelings but are unable to express them at this time.

Facilitative Response

Listen carefully and reflect back to patients the feelings and content of their statements.

Responses are empathic and nonjudgemental and legitimize the person's feelings.

Formula for facilitative responses: "You feel ________ because ________."

Example—If the child states, "I hate coming to the hospital and getting needles," a facilitative response is, "You feel unhappy because of all the things that are done to you."

Storytelling

Use the language of children to probe into areas of their thinking while bypassing conscious inhibitions or fears.

The simplest technique is asking the child to relate a story about an event, such as "being in the hospital."

Other approaches:

- Show the child a picture of a particular event, such as a child in a hospital with other people in the room, and ask the child to describe the scene.
- Cut out comic strips, remove words, and have the child add statements for scenes.

Mutual Storytelling

Reveal the child's thinking and attempt to change the child's perceptions or fears by retelling a somewhat different story (more therapeutic approach than storytelling).

Begin by asking the child to tell a story about something, then tell another story that is similar to the child's tale but with differences that help the child in problem areas.

Example—The child's story is about going to the hospital and never seeing his or her parents again. The nurse's story is also about a child (using different names but similar circumstances) in a hospital, but whose parents visit every day, in the evening after work, until the child is better and goes home with them.

Bibliotherapy

Use books in a therapeutic and supportive process.

Provide children with an opportunity to explore an event that is similar to their own but sufficiently different to allow them to distance themselves from it and remain in control.

General guidelines for using bibliotherapy are as follows:

1. Assess the child's emotional and cognitive development in terms of readiness to understand the book's message.
2. Be familiar with the book's content (intended message or purpose) and the age for which it is written.
3. Read the book to the child if he or she is unable to read.
4. Explore the meaning of the book with the child by having child do the following:
   - Retell the story
   - Read a special section with the nurse or parent
   - Draw a picture related to the story and discuss the drawing
   - Talk about the characters
   - Summarize the moral or meaning of the story

Dreams

Dreams often reveal unconscious and repressed thoughts and feelings.

Ask the child to talk about a dream or nightmare.

Explore with the child what meaning the dream could have.

"What If" Questions

Encourage the child to explore potential situations and to consider different problem-solving options.

Example—"What if you got sick and had to go the hospital?" Children's responses reveal what they know already and what they are curious about, providing an opportunity for them to learn coping skills, especially in potentially dangerous situations.

Three Wishes

Ask, "If you could have any three things in the world, what would they be?"

If child answers, "That all my wishes come true," ask child for specific wishes.

Rating Game

Use some type of rating scale (numbers, sad to happy faces) to have the child rate an event or feeling.

Example—Instead of asking youngsters how they feel, ask how their day has been "on a scale of 1 to 10, with 10 being the best."

Word Association Game

State key words and ask children to say the first word they think of when they hear the word.

Start with neutral words and then introduce more anxiety-producing words, such as "illness," "needles," "hospitals," and "operation."

Select key words that relate to some relevant event in the child's life.

Continued

BOX 34-4 Creative Communication Techniques With Children—cont'd

Sentence Completion

Present a partial statement and have the child complete it. Some sample statements are as follows:

- The thing I like best (least) about school is ________.
- The best (worst) age to be is ________.
- The most (least) fun thing I ever did was ________.
- The thing I like most (least) about my parents is ________.
- The one thing I would change about my family is ________.
- If I could be anything I wanted, I would be ________.
- The thing I like most (least) about myself is ________.

Pros and Cons

Select a topic, such as "being in the hospital," and have the child list "five good things and five bad things" about it.

This is an exceptionally valuable technique when applied to relationships, such as things family members like and dislike about each other.

Nonverbal Techniques

Writing

Writing is an alternative communication approach for older children and adults. Specific suggestions include the following:

- Keep a journal or diary.
- Write down feelings or thoughts that are difficult to express.
- Write "letters" that are never mailed (a variation is making up a pen pal to write to).
- Keep an account of the child's progress from both a physical and an emotional viewpoint.

Drawing

Drawing is one of the most valuable forms of communication—both nonverbal (from looking at the drawing) and verbal (from the child's story of the picture).

Children's drawings tell a great deal about them because they are projections of their inner selves.

Spontaneous drawing involves giving child a variety of art supplies and providing the opportunity to draw.

Directed drawing involves a more specific direction, such as "draw a person" or the "three themes" approach (state three things about the child and ask the child to choose one and draw a picture).

Guidelines for Evaluating Drawings

Use spontaneous drawings and evaluate more than one drawing whenever possible.

Interpret drawings in light of other available information about the child and family, including the child's age and stage of development.

Interpret drawings as a whole rather than focusing on specific details of the drawing.

Consider individual elements of the drawing that may be significant:

Gender of figure drawn first—Usually relates to child's perception of his or her own gender role

Size of individual figures—Expresses importance, power, or authority

Order in which figures are drawn—Expresses priority in terms of importance

Child's position in relation to other family members—Expresses feelings of status or alliance

Exclusion of a member—May denote feeling of not belonging or desire to eliminate a family member

Accentuated parts—Usually express concern for areas of special importance (e.g., large hands may be a sign of aggression)

Absence of or rudimentary arms and hands—Suggest timidity, passivity, or intellectual immaturity; tiny, unstable feet may express insecurity, and hidden hands may mean guilt feelings

Placement of drawing on the page and type of stroke—Free use of paper and firm, continuous strokes express security, whereas drawings restricted to a small area and lightly drawn in broken or wavering lines may be a sign of insecurity

Erasures, shading, or cross-hatching—Expresses ambivalence, concern, or anxiety with a particular area

Magic

Use simple magic tricks to help establish rapport with the child, encourage cooperation with health interventions, and provide effective distraction during painful procedures.

Although the magician talks, no verbal response from the child is required.

Play

Play is the universal language and "work" of children.

It tells a great deal about children because they project their inner selves through the activity.

Spontaneous play involves giving the child a variety of play materials and providing the opportunity to play.

Directed play involves a more specific direction, such as providing medical equipment or a dollhouse for focused reasons, such as exploring the child's fear of injections or exploring family relationships.

problem. The health issue is elicited by asking open-ended, neutral questions, such as "What seems to be the matter?" "How may I help you?" or "Why did you come here today?" Labelling-type questions, such as "How are you sick?" or "What is the problem?", should be avoided; it is possible that the reason for the visit is not an illness or problem.

Occasionally, it is difficult to isolate one symptom or problem as the health issue because the parent may identify many. In this situation, the nurse should be as specific as possible when asking questions. For example, asking informants to state which one problem or symptom prompted them to seek help now may help them focus on the most immediate concern.

BOX 34-5 Outline of a Pediatric Health History

Identifying information
1. Name
2. Address
3. Telephone
4. Birth date and place
5. Race/ethnic group
6. Sex
7. Religion
8. Date of interview
9. Informant

Presenting health issue—To establish the major specific reason for the child's and parents' seeking professional health attention

Present illness (PI)—To obtain all details related to the chief health concern

Past history (PH)—To elicit a profile of the child's previous illnesses, injuries, or operations
1. Birth history (pregnancy, labour and delivery, perinatal history)
2. Previous illnesses, injuries, or operations
3. Allergies
4. Current medications
5. Immunizations
6. Growth and development
7. Habits

Sexual history—To elicit information about the child's sexual concerns or activities and any pertinent data regarding adults' sexual activity that influences the child

Family medical history—To identify genetic traits or diseases that have familial tendencies and to assess exposure to a communicable disease in a family member and family habits that may affect the child's health, such as smoking and chemical use

Family structure—To develop an understanding of the child as an individual and as a member of a family and a community
1. Family composition
2. Home and community environment
3. Occupation and education of family members
4. Cultural and religious traditions
5. Family function and relationships

Psychosocial history—To elicit information about the child's self-concept

Nutritional assessment—To elicit information on the adequacy of the child's nutritional intake and needs
1. Dietary intake
2. Clinical examination

Review of systems (ROS)—To elicit information concerning any potential health problem
1. General
2. Integument
3. Head
4. Eyes
5. Ears
6. Nose
7. Mouth
8. Throat
9. Neck
10. Chest
11. Respiratory
12. Cardiovascular
13. Gastrointestinal
14. Genitourinary
15. Gynecological
16. Musculoskeletal
17. Neurological
18. Endocrine

Present Illness

The history of the present illness* is a narrative of the health issue from its earliest onset through its progression to the present. Its four major components are (1) the details of onset, (2) a complete interval history, (3) the present status, and (4) the reason for seeking help now. The focus of the present illness is on all factors relevant to the main problem, even if they have disappeared or changed during the onset, interval, and present.

Analyzing a Symptom

Because **pain** is often the most characteristic symptom denoting the onset of a physical problem, it is used as an example for analysis of a symptom. Assessment includes (1) type, (2) location, (3) severity, (4) duration, and (5) influencing factors (see Guidelines box; see also Pain Assessment, Chapter 35).

*The term *illness* is used in its broadest sense to denote any problem of a physical, emotional, or psychosocial nature. It is actually a history of the health issue.

History

The **history** contains information relating to all previous aspects of the child's health status and concentrates on several areas that are ordinarily passed over in the history of an adult, such as birth history, detailed feeding history, immunizations, and growth and development. Since a great deal of information is included in this section, a combination of open-ended and fact-finding questions should be used. For example, interviewing for each section can start with an open-ended statement, such as "Tell me about your child's birth," to provide the informants with the opportunity to relate what they think is most important. Fact-finding questions related to specific details can be asked whenever necessary to focus the interview on certain topics.

Birth History

The birth history includes all data concerning (1) the mother's health during pregnancy, (2) the labour and delivery, and (3) the infant's condition immediately after birth. Since prenatal influences have significant effects on a child's physical and emotional development, a thorough investigation of the birth history is essential. Because parents may question what relevance pregnancy and birth have on the child's present condition, particularly if the child is past infancy, the nurse needs to explain why such questions are included. An appropriate statement may be, "I will be asking you some questions about your pregnancy and ____'s [refer to child by name] birth. Your answers will give me a more complete picture of your child's overall health."

Because emotional factors also affect the outcome of pregnancy and the subsequent parent–child relationship, it is important to investigate (1) concurrent crises during pregnancy and (2) prenatal attitudes toward the fetus. It is best to approach the topic of parental acceptance of pregnancy through indirect questioning. Asking parents if the pregnancy was planned is a leading statement because they may respond affirmatively for fear of criticism if the pregnancy was unexpected. Rather, parents should be encouraged to disclose their true reactions by referring to specific facts relating to the pregnancy, such as the spacing between offspring, an extended or short interval between marriage and conception, or the concurrent experience of pregnancy and adolescence. Parents can choose to explore such statements with further explanations or, for the moment, may not be able to reveal related feelings. If the parents or parent remains silent, this topic can be revisited later in the interview.

Previous Illnesses, Injuries, and Operations

When inquiring about past illnesses, the nurse should begin with a general statement such as "What other illnesses has your child had?" Since parents are most likely to recall serious health problems, they should be asked specifically about colds; earaches; and childhood diseases such as measles, rubella (German measles), chicken pox, mumps, pertussis (whooping cough), diphtheria, tuberculosis, scarlet fever, strep throat, tonsillitis, or allergic manifestations.

In addition to illnesses, the nurse needs to ask about injuries that required medical intervention, operations, and any other reason for hospitalization, including the dates of each incident. It is important to focus on injuries such as accidental falls, poisoning, choking, or burns, since these may be potential areas for parental guidance.

Allergies

It is important to ask about commonly known allergic disorders such as hay fever and asthma; unusual reactions to medications, food, or latex products; and reactions to other contact agents such as poisonous plants, animals, household products, or fabrics. If asked appropriate questions, most people can give reliable information about medication reactions (see Guidelines box).

NURSING ALERT Information about allergic reactions to medications or other products is essential. Failure to document a serious reaction places the child at risk if the medication is given.

GUIDELINES Analyzing the Symptom: Pain

Type

Be as specific as possible. With young children, asking the parents how they know the child is in pain may help describe its type, location, and severity. For example, a parent may state, "My child must have a severe earache because she pulls at her ears, rolls her head on the floor, and screams. Nothing seems to help." Help older children describe the "hurt" by asking them if it is sharp, throbbing, dull, or stabbing. Record whatever words they use in quotes.

Location

Be specific. "Stomach pains" is too general a description. Children can better localize the pain if they are asked to "point with one finger to where it hurts" or to "point to where Mommy or Daddy would put a Band-Aid." Determine if the pain radiates, by asking, "Does the pain stay there or move? Show me with your finger where the pain goes."

Severity

Severity is best determined by finding out how it affects the child's usual behaviour. Pain that prevents a child from playing, interacting with others, sleeping, and eating is most often severe. Assess pain intensity using a rating scale, such as a numeric or FACES scale (see Chapter 35).

Duration

Include the duration, onset, and frequency of the pain. Describe this in terms of activity and behaviour, such as "pain reported to last all night, child refused to sleep and cried intermittently."

Influencing Factors

Include anything that causes a change in the type, location, severity, or duration of the pain: (1) precipitating events (those that cause or increase the pain), (2) relieving events (those that lessen the pain, such as medications), (3) temporal events (times when the pain is relieved or increased), (4) positional events (standing, sitting, lying down), and (5) associated events (meals, stress, coughing).

GUIDELINES Taking an Allergy History

- Has your child ever taken any medications or tablets that have disagreed with him or her or caused an allergic response? If yes, can you remember the name(s) of these medications?
- Can you describe the reaction?
- Was the medication taken by mouth (as a tablet or syrup), or was it an injection?
- How soon after starting the medication did the reaction happen?
- How long ago did this happen?
- Did anyone tell you it was an allergic reaction, or did you decide for yourself?
- Has your child ever taken this medication, or a similar one, again? If yes, did your child experience the same problems?
- Have you told the doctors or nurses about your child's reaction or allergy?

(Modified from Cantrill, J. A., & Cottrell, W. N. [1997]. Accuracy of drug allergy documentation. *American Journal of Health-System Pharmacy, 54*, 1627–1629.)

Current Medications

The nurse should inquire about current medication regimens, including vitamins, antipyretics (especially aspirin), antibiotics, antihistamines, decongestants, or antitussives. All medications need to be listed, including name, dose, schedule, duration, and reason for administration. Often parents are unaware of the medication's actual name. Whenever possible, parents should bring the containers with them to the next visit, or the nurse can ask for the name of the pharmacy and call for a list of all the child's recent prescription medications. However, this list will not include over-the-counter medications or herbal remedies, which are important to know.

Immunizations

A record of all immunizations is essential. Since many parents are unaware of the exact name and date of each immunization, the most reliable source of information is a hospital, clinic, or private practitioner's record. All immunizations and "boosters" will be listed, stating (1) the name of the specific disease, (2) the number of injections, (3) the dosage (sometimes lesser amounts are given if a reaction is anticipated), (4) the ages when administered, and (5) the occurrence of any reaction following the immunization.

Growth and Development

The most important previous growth patterns to record are the following:

- Approximate weight at 1 week, 2 months, 4 months, 6 months, 12 to 13 months, and 18 months, then yearly (Canadian Paediatric Society [CPS], 2010a)
- Approximate length at 1 week, 2 months, 4 months, 6 months, 12 to 13 months, and 18 months, then yearly (CPS, 2010a)
- Dentition, including age of onset, number of teeth, and symptoms during teething

Developmental milestones include the following:

- Age of holding up head steadily
- Age of sitting alone without support
- Age of walking without assistance
- Age of saying first words with meaning
- Present grade in school
- Scholastic grades
- Interactions with other children, peers, and adults

The nurse should use specific and detailed questions when inquiring about each developmental milestone. For example, "sitting up" can mean many different activities, such as sitting propped up, sitting in someone's lap, sitting with support, sitting up alone but in a hyperflexed position for assisted balance, or sitting up unsupported with the back slightly rounded. A clue to misunderstanding of the requested activity may be an unusually early age of achievement (see Developmental Assessment, p. 928).

Habits

Habits are an important area to explore during the interview (Box 34-6). Parents frequently express concerns during this part of the history. The nurse needs to encourage their input, by saying, "Please tell me any concerns you have about your child's habits, activities, or development." Any concerns expressed should be investigated further.

One of the most common concerns relates to sleep. Many children develop a normal sleep pattern, and all that is required during the assessment is a general overview of nighttime sleep and nap schedules. However, a number of children also develop sleep problems (see Sleep Problems, Chapters 36 and 38). When sleep problems do occur, a more detailed sleep history is required to guide appropriate interventions.

Habits related to use of chemicals apply primarily to older children and adolescents. If a youngster admits to smoking, drinking, or drug use, he or she should be asked about the quantity and frequency. Questions such as "Have you ever had a drinking or drug problem?" or "When was the last time you had a drink or took drugs?" may yield more reliable data than questions such as "How much do you drink?" or "How often do you drink or take drugs?" The nurse needs to clarify that "drinking" includes all types of alcohol, such as beer and wine. When quantities such as a "glass" of wine or a "can" of beer are given, the size of the container needs to be determined.

If older children deny use of chemical substances, they should be asked about past experimentation. Asking, "You mean you never tried to smoke or drink?" implies that the nurse expects some such activity, and the youngster may be more inclined to answer truthfully. It is important to be aware of the confidential nature of such questioning, the adverse effect that the parents' presence may have on the adolescent's willingness to answer, and the fact that self-reporting may not be an accurate account of chemical abuse.

BOX 34-6 Habits to Explore During a Health Interview

- Behaviour patterns such as nail biting, thumb sucking, pica (habitual ingestion of nonfood substances), rituals ("security" blanket or toy), and unusual movements (head banging, rocking, overt masturbation, walking on toes)
- Activities of daily living, such as the hour of going to sleep and arising, duration of nighttime sleep and naps, type and duration of exercise, regularity of stools and urination, age of toilet training, and daytime or nighttime bed-wetting
- Unusual disposition; response to frustration
- Use of alcohol, drugs, coffee, or tobacco

Sexual History

The sexual history is an essential component of adolescents' health assessment. The history uncovers areas of concern related to sexual activity; alerts the nurse to circumstances that may indicate screening for sexually transmitted infections (STIs) or testing for pregnancy; and provides information related to the need for sexual counselling, such as safer sex practices. Guidelines for anticipatory guidance topics for parents and adolescents are found in Box 34-7.

One approach to initiating a conversation about sexual concerns is to begin with a history of peer interactions. Open-ended statements such as "Tell me about your social life" or "Who are your closest friends?" generally lead into a discussion of dating and sexual issues. To probe further, the nurse can include questions about the adolescent's attitudes on such topics as sex education, going steady, living together, and premarital sex. Such questions should be phrased to

BOX 34-7 Anticipatory Guidance—Sexuality

Ages 12 to 14 Years

Have the adolescent identify a supportive adult to discuss sexuality issues and concerns with.
Discuss advantages of delaying sexual activity.
Discuss making responsible decisions regarding normal sexual feelings.
Discuss roles of gender, peer pressure, and the media in sexual decision making.
Discuss contraceptive options (advantages and disadvantages).
Provide education regarding sexually transmitted infections (STIs) and human immunodeficiency virus (HIV) infection; clarify risks and discuss the use of condoms.
Discuss abuse prevention: avoiding dangerous situations, the role of drugs and alcohol, and the use of self-defence.
Have the adolescent clarify values, needs, and the ability to be assertive.
If the adolescent is sexually active, discuss the use of condoms, limiting the number of partners, and contraceptive options.
Have a confidential interview with the adolescent (including a sexual history).
Discuss the evolution of sexual identity and expression.
Discuss breast examination or testicular examination.

Ages 15 to 18 Years

Clarify values; encourage responsible decision making.
Discuss alternatives to intercourse.
Discuss "When are you ready for sex?"
Discuss consequences of unprotected sex: early pregnancy; STIs, including HIV infection.
Discuss negotiating with the partner and barriers to safer sex.
If the adolescent is sexually active, discuss the use of condoms, limiting the number of partners, and contraceptive options.
Emphasize that sex should be safe and pleasurable for both partners.
Have a confidential interview with the adolescent.
Discuss concerns about sexual identity and expression.

(Modified from Wright, K. [1997]. Anticipatory guidance: developing a healthy sexuality. *Pediatric Annals, 26*[2 Suppl], S142–S144, C3.)

reflect concern rather than judgement or criticism of sexual practices.

In any conversation regarding sexual history, it is important be aware of the language used in either eliciting or conveying sexual information. For example, the nurse should avoid asking whether the adolescent is "sexually active," because this term is broadly defined. "Are you having sex with anyone?" is probably the most direct and best understood question. Since same-sex experimentation may occur, all sexual contacts should be referred to in nongender terms, such as "anyone" or "partners," rather than "girlfriends" or "boyfriends."

A detailed account of sexual partners is needed if the patient has a history of, displays any symptoms of, or asks for treatment of an STI. A difficult but necessary part of the interview is to determine the sites of possible infection. Since sexual diseases can be contracted in any of the body orifices, the adolescent should be informed that an STI can be acquired without visible signs of disease at nongenital sites.

Family Medical History

The family medical history is used primarily for discovering the potential existence of hereditary or familial diseases in the parents and child. In general, it is confined to first-degree relatives (parents, siblings, grandparents, and immediate aunts and uncles). Information for each family member includes age, marital status, state of health if living, cause of death if deceased, and any evidence of the following conditions: heart disease, hypertension, cancer, diabetes mellitus, obesity, congenital anomalies, allergy, asthma, seizures, tuberculosis, sickle cell disease, cognitive impairment, mental disorders such as depression or psychosis, emotional problems, syphilis, or rheumatic fever. The nurse needs to confirm the accuracy of the reported disorders by inquiring about the symptoms, course, treatment, and sequelae of each diagnosis.

Geographic Location

One of the important areas to explore when assessing the family health history is geographic location, including the birthplace and travel to different areas in or outside of the country, for identification of possible exposure to endemic diseases. Although the primary interest focuses on the child's temporary residence in various localities, the nurse should also inquire about close family members' travel, especially travel during tours of military service or business trips. Children are particularly susceptible to parasitic infestation in areas of poor sanitary conditions and to vector-borne diseases, such as those from mosquitoes or ticks in warm and humid or heavily wooded regions.

Family Structure

Assessment of the family, both its structure and function, is an important component of the history-taking process. Because the quality of the functional relationship between the child and family members is a major factor in emotional and physical health, family assessment is discussed separately and in greater detail apart from the more traditional health history.

Family assessment is the collection of data about the family's composition and the relationships among its members. In its broadest sense, *family* refers to all those individuals who are considered by the patient to be significant to the nuclear unit, including relatives, friends, and social groups such as the school and church. Although family assessment is not family therapy, it can and frequently is therapeutic. Involving family members in the discussion of family characteristics and activities can provide insight into family dynamics and relationships.

Because of the time involved in performing an in-depth family assessment as presented here, the nurse needs to be selective in deciding when knowledge of family function may facilitate nursing care (see Guidelines box). During brief contacts with families, a full assessment is not appropriate, and screening with one or two questions from each category may reflect the health of the family system or the need for additional assessment.

GUIDELINES Initiating a Comprehensive Family Assessment

Perform a comprehensive assessment on the following:
- Children receiving comprehensive well-child care
- Children experiencing major stressful life events (e.g., chronic illness, disability, parental divorce, death of a family member)
- Children requiring extensive home care
- Children with developmental delays
- Children with repeated accidental injuries and those with suspected child abuse
- Children with behavioural or physical problems that could be caused by family dysfunction

Family structure refers to the family's composition—who lives in the home and those social, cultural, religious, and economic characteristics that influence the child's and family's overall psychobiological health (see also Chapters 31 and 32). Since the information elicited in this part of the history is often the most personal and confidential, it should be included toward the end of the interview, when rapport is well established.

The most common method of eliciting information on the family structure is to interview family members. The principal areas of concern (Box 34-8) are (1) family composition, (2) home and community environment, (3) occupation and education of family members, and (4) cultural and religious traditions.

BOX 34-8 Family Assessment Interview

General Guidelines

Schedule the interview with the family at a time that is most convenient for all parties; include as many family members as possible; clearly state the purpose of the interview.
Begin the interview by asking each person's name and their relationship to one another.
Restate the purpose of the interview and the objective.
Keep the initial conversation general to put members at ease and to learn the "big picture" of the family.
Identify major concerns and reflect these back to the family to be certain that all parties receive the same message.
Terminate the interview with a summary of what was discussed and a plan for additional sessions, if needed.

Structural Assessment Areas

Family Composition

Immediate members of the household (names, ages, and relationships)
Significant extended family members
Previous marriages, separations, death of spouses, or divorces

Home and Community Environment

Type of dwelling, number of rooms, occupants
Sleeping arrangements
Number of floors, accessibility of stairs and elevators
Adequacy of utilities
Safety features (fire escape, smoke and carbon monoxide detectors, guardrails on windows, use of car restraint)
Environmental hazards (e.g., chipped paint, poor sanitation, pollution, heavy street traffic)
Availability and location of health care facilities, schools, play areas
Relationship with neighbours
Recent crises or changes in home
Child's reaction and adjustment to recent stresses

Occupation and Education of Family Members

Types of employment
Work schedules
Work satisfaction
Exposure to environmental or industrial hazards
Sources of income and adequacy
Effect of illness on financial status
Highest degree or grade level attained

Cultural and Religious Traditions

Religious beliefs and practices
Cultural and ethnic beliefs and practices
Language spoken in home
Assessment questions include the following:
- Does the family identify with a particular religious or ethnic group? Are both parents from that group?
- How is religious or ethnic background part of family life?
- What special religious or cultural traditions are practised in the home (e.g., food choices and preparation)?
- Where were family members born, and how long have they lived in this country?
- What language does the family speak most often?
- Do they speak and understand English?
- What do they believe causes health or illness?
- What religious or ethnic beliefs influence the family's perception of illness and its treatment?
- What methods are used to prevent or treat illness?
- How does the family know when a health problem needs medical attention?
- Whom does the family contact when a member is ill?
- Does the family rely on cultural or religious healers or remedies? If so, ask them to describe the type of healer or remedy.
- Whom does the family go to for support (clergy, medical healer, relatives)?
- Does the family experience discrimination because of their race, beliefs, or practices? Ask them to describe.

Functional Assessment Areas

Family Interactions and Roles

Interactions refer to ways in which family members relate to each other.

Continued

BOX 34-8 Family Assessment Interview—cont'd

The chief concern is the amount of intimacy and closeness among the members, especially spouses.

Roles refer to behaviours of people as they assume a different status or position.

Observations include the following:

- Family members' responses to each other (cordial, hostile, cool, loving, patient, short tempered)
- Obvious roles of leadership versus submission
- Support and attention shown to various members

Assessment questions include the following:

- What activities does the family perform together?
- Whom do family members talk to when something is bothering them?
- What are members' household chores?
- Who usually oversees what is happening with the children, such as at school or for health care?
- How easy or difficult is it for the family to change or accept new responsibilities for household tasks?

Power, Decision Making, and Problem Solving

Power refers to individual member's control over others in the family; it is manifested through family decision making and problem solving.

The chief concern is clarity of boundaries of power between parents and children.

One method of assessment involves offering a hypothetical conflict or problem, such as a child failing school, and asking the family how they would handle this situation.

Assessment questions include the following:

- Who usually makes the decisions in the family?
- If one parent makes a decision, can the child appeal to the other parent to change it?
- What input do children have in making decisions or discussing rules?
- Who makes and enforces the rules?
- What happens when a rule is broken?

Communication

Communication is concerned with clarity and directness of communication patterns.

Further assessment includes periodically asking family members if they understood what was just said and to repeat the message.

Observations include the following:

- Who speaks to whom?
- If one person speaks for another or interrupts
- If members appear uninterested when certain individuals speak
- If there is agreement between verbal and nonverbal messages

Assessment questions include the following:

- How often do family members wait until others are through talking before "having their say"?
- Do parents or older siblings tend to lecture and preach?
- Do parents tend to "talk down" to the children?

Expression of Feelings and Individuality

Expressions are concerned with personal space and freedom to grow with limits and structure needed for guidance.

Observing patterns of communication offers clues to how freely feelings are expressed.

Assessment questions include the following:

- Is it OK for family members to get angry or sad?
- Who gets angry most of the time? What do they do?
- If someone is upset, how do other family members try to comfort this person?
- Who comforts specific family members?
- When someone wants to do something, such as try out for a new sport or get a job, what is the family's response (offer assistance, discouragement, or no advice)?

NURSING ALERT In assessing family composition, it is sometimes difficult to ascertain the status of the adult relationships. If the parent fails to mention the other parent, ask, "Where is the child's father [or mother]?" Avoid saying "husband" or "wife" because this assumes that only marital relationships exist.

Psychosocial History

The traditional medical history includes a personal and social section that concentrates on children's personal status, such as school adjustment and any unusual habits, and the family and home environment. Since several personal aspects are covered under development and habits, only those issues related to children's ability to cope and their self-concept are presented here.

Through observation, the nurse can obtain a general idea of how confident children are in dealing with others, answering questions, and coping with new situations. It is important to observe the parent–child relationship for the types of messages sent to children about their coping skills and self-worth. Do the parents treat the child with respect, focusing on strengths, or is the interaction one of constant reprimands, with emphasis on weaknesses and faults? Do the parents help the child learn new coping strategies or support the ones the child uses?

Messages about body image are also conveyed through the parent–child interaction. Do the parents label the child and body parts, such as "bad boy," "skinny legs," or "ugly scar"? Do the parents handle the child gently, using soothing touch to calm an anxious child, or do they treat the child roughly, using slaps or restraint to force compliance? If the child touches certain parts of the body, such as the genitalia, do the parents make negative comments?

With older children many of the communication strategies discussed earlier in the chapter are useful in eliciting more definitive information about their coping and self-concept. Children can write down five things they like and dislike about themselves. The nurse can use sentence completion statements, such as "The thing I like best (or worst) about myself is ____________," "If I could change one thing about myself, it would be ____________," or "When I am scared, I ____________."

Review of Systems

The *review of systems* is a specific review of each body system, following an order similar to that of the physical examination (see Guidelines box). Often the history of the present illness provides a complete review of the system involved in the chief health concern. Since asking questions about other body systems may appear unrelated and irrelevant to the parents or child, the questioning should be preceded by an explanation of why the data are needed (similar to the explanation concerning the relevance of the birth history) and the parents reassured that the child's main problem has not been forgotten.

The review of a specific system begins with a broad statement such as "How has your child's general health been?" or "Has your child had any problems with his eyes?" If the parent states that the child has had problems with some body function, this should be pursued with an encouraging statement, such as "Tell me more about that." If the parent denies any problems, the nurse can query for specific symptoms (e.g., "No headaches, bumping into objects, or squinting?"). If the parent reconfirms the absence of such symptoms, the nurse should record positive statements in the history, such as "Mother denies headaches, bumping into objects, or squinting." In this way, anyone who reviews the health history is aware of exactly what symptoms were investigated.

GUIDELINES Review of Systems

General—Overall state of health, fatigue, recent or unexplained weight gain or loss (period of time for either), contributing factors (change of diet, illness, altered appetite), exercise tolerance, fevers (time of day), chills, night sweats (unrelated to climatic conditions), frequent infections, general ability to carry out activities of daily living

Integument—Pruritus, pigment or other colour changes, acne, eruptions, rashes (location), tendency for bruising, petechiae, excessive dryness, general texture, disorders or deformities of nails, hair growth or loss, hair colour change (for adolescents, use of hair dyes or other potentially toxic substances, such as hair straighteners)

Head—Headaches, dizziness, injury (specific details)

Eyes—Visual problems (behaviours indicative of blurred vision, such as bumping into objects, clumsiness, sitting close to television, holding a book close to the face, writing with head near the desk, squinting, rubbing the eyes, bending head in an awkward position), cross-eyes (strabismus), eye infections, edema of lids, excessive tearing, use of glasses or contact lenses, date of last optic examination

Ears—Earaches, discharge, evidence of hearing loss (ask about behaviours, such as need to repeat requests, loud speech, inattentive behaviour), results of any previous auditory testing

Nose—Nosebleeds (epistaxis), constant or frequent runny or stuffy nose, nasal obstruction (difficulty breathing), alteration or loss of sense of smell

Mouth—Mouth breathing, gum bleeding, toothaches, tooth brushing, use of fluoride, difficulty with teething (symptoms), last visit to dentist (especially if temporary dentition is complete), response to dentist

Throat—Sore throat, difficulty swallowing, choking (especially when chewing food—may be from poor chewing habits), hoarseness or other voice irregularities

Neck—Pain, limitation of movement, stiffness, difficulty holding head straight (torticollis), thyroid enlargement, enlarged nodes or other masses

Chest—Breast enlargement, discharge, masses, enlarged axillary nodes

Respiratory—Chronic cough, frequent colds (number per year), wheezing, shortness of breath at rest or on exertion, difficulty breathing, sputum production, infections (pneumonia, tuberculosis), date of last chest x-ray examination, skin reaction from tuberculin testing

Cardiovascular—Cyanosis or fatigue on exertion, history of heart murmur or rheumatic fever, anemia, date of last blood count, blood type, recent transfusion

Gastrointestinal (questions in regard to appetite, food tolerance, and elimination habits are asked elsewhere)—Nausea, vomiting (not associated with eating, may be indicative of brain tumour or increased intracranial pressure), jaundice or yellowing skin or sclera, belching, flatulence, recent change in bowel habits (blood in stools, change of colour, diarrhea, or constipation)

Genitourinary—Pain on urination, frequency, hesitancy, urgency, hematuria, nocturia, polyuria, unpleasant odour to urine, force of stream, discharge, change in size of scrotum, date of last urinalysis (for adolescents, sexually transmitted infection, type of treatment)

Gynecological—Menarche, date of last menstrual period, regularity or problems with menstruation, vaginal discharge, pruritus, date and result of last Papanicolaou (Pap) smear (include obstetric history, as discussed under birth history, when applicable); if sexually active, type of contraception, sexually transmitted disease and type of treatment

Musculoskeletal—Weakness, clumsiness, lack of coordination, unusual movements, back or joint stiffness, muscle pains or cramps, abnormal gait, deformity, fractures, serious sprains, activity level

Neurological—Seizures, tremors, dizziness, loss of memory, general affect, fears, nightmares, speech problems, any unusual habits

Endocrine—Intolerance to weather changes, excessive thirst or urination, excessive sweating, salty taste to skin, signs of early puberty

Nutritional Assessment

Dietary Intake

Food consumption patterns of children have changed over the past 30 years (Nicklas et al., 2004). The prevalence of overweight and obesity among children and adolescents has significantly increased (Hedley et al., 2004). Thus knowledge of the child's dietary intake is an essential component of a nutritional assessment. However, it is also one of the most difficult factors to assess. Individuals' recall of food consumption, especially amounts eaten, is frequently unreliable. The food intake history of children and adolescents is prone to reporting error, mostly in the form of underreporting (Livingstone, Robson, & Wallace, 2004). Also, people from different cultures may have difficulty adequately describing the types of food they eat. Despite these obstacles, a dietary evaluation is an important component of the child's assessment.

Specific questions used to conduct a nutritional assessment are included in Box 34-9. Every nutritional assessment should begin with a dietary history. The exact questions used to elicit a dietary history vary with the child's age. In general, the younger the child, the more specific and detailed the history should be.

The overview elicited from the dietary history can be helpful in evaluating frequency of food intake. The history should also be concerned with financial and cultural factors that influence food selection and preparation (see Cultural Awareness box).

The most common and probably easiest method of assessing daily intake is the 24-hour recall. The child or parent recalls every item eaten in the past 24 hours and the approximate amounts. The 24-hour recall is most beneficial when it represents a typical day's intake. Some of the difficulties with a daily recall are the family's inability to remember exactly what was eaten and inaccurate estimation of portion size. To increase accuracy of reporting portion sizes, the use of food models and additional questioning are recommended. In general, this method is most useful in providing qualitative information about the child's diet.

BOX 34-9 Dietary Assessment for an Individual

Dietary History

What are the family's usual mealtimes?
Do family members eat together or at separate times?
Who does the family grocery shopping and meal preparation?
How much money is spent to buy food each week?
How are most foods prepared—baked, broiled, fried, other?
How often does the family or your child eat out?
- What kinds of restaurants do you go to?
- What kinds of food does your child typically eat at restaurants?

Does your child eat breakfast regularly?
Where does your child eat lunch?
What are your child's favourite foods, beverages, and snacks?
- What are the average amounts eaten per day?
- What foods are artificially sweetened?
- What are your child's snacking habits?
- When are sweet foods usually eaten?
- What are your child's tooth-brushing habits?

What special cultural practices are followed? What ethnic foods are eaten?
What foods and beverages does your child dislike?
How would you describe your child's usual appetite (hearty eater, picky eater)?
What are your child's feeding habits (breast, bottle, cup, spoon, eats by self, needs assistance, any special devices)?
Does your child take vitamins or other supplements? Do they contain iron or fluoride?
Does your child have any known or suspected food allergies? Is your child on a special diet?
Has your child lost or gained weight recently?
Are there any feeding problems (excessive fussiness, spitting up, colic, difficulty sucking or swallowing)? Are there any dental problems or appliances, such as braces, that affect eating?
What types of exercise does your child do regularly?
Is there a family history of cancer, diabetes, heart disease, high blood pressure, or obesity?

Additional Questions Regarding Infants

What was the infant's birth weight? When did it double? Triple?
Was the infant preterm?
Are you breastfeeding or have you breastfed your infant? For how long?
If you use a formula, what is the brand?
- How long has the infant been taking it?
- How many millilitres does the infant drink a day?

Are you giving the infant cow's milk (whole, low fat, skim)?
- When did you start?
- How many millilitres does the infant drink a day?

Do you give your infant extra fluids (water, juice)?
If the infant takes a bottle to bed at nap time or nighttime, what is in the bottle?
At what age did the child start on cereal, vegetables, meat or other protein sources, fruit or juice, finger food, table food?
Do you make your own baby food or use commercial foods, such as infant cereal?
Does the infant take a vitamin or mineral supplement? If so, what type?
Has the infant had an allergic reaction to any food(s)? If so, list the foods and describe the reaction.
Does the infant spit up frequently; have unusually loose stools; or have hard, dry stools? If so, how often?
How often do you feed your infant?
How would you describe your infant's appetite?

(Modified from Murphy, S. P., & Poos, M. I. [2002]. Dietary reference intakes: Summary of applications in dietary assessment. *Public Health Nutrition*, 5[6A], 843–849.)

CULTURAL AWARENESS

Food Practices

Because cultural practices are prevalent in food preparation, consider carefully the kinds of questions that are asked and the judgements made during counselling (see Food Customs, Chapter 32). For example, some First Nations, Métis, and Inuit people eat food that is different from food listed in *Eating Well With Canada's Food Guide*. The Canadian Dietetic Association has adapted the *Guide* to include foods such as moose stew, char, and bannock. There has never been a national food guide that has reflected the values, traditions, and food choices of First Nations, Métis, and Inuit cultures. The *Guide* includes traditional as well as store-bought foods that are usually affordable, available, and accessible across Canada. This guide is also available in Inuktitut, Ojibwe, Plains Cree, and Woods Cree languages. For more information, visit the *Food Guide* Web site: http://www.hc-sc.gc.ca/fn-an/food-guide-aliment/fnim-pnim/index-eng.php.

To improve the reliability of the daily recall, the family can complete a food diary by recording every food and liquid consumed for a certain number of days. A 3-day record consisting of 2 weekdays and 1 weekend day is representative for most people. Providing specific charts to record intake can improve compliance. The family should record items immediately after eating.

A food frequency questionnaire or record provides information about the number of times in a day, week, or month a child consumes items from the different food groups. In general, it provides a qualitative overview but has the advantage of avoiding recall based on a "typical" day. It can be especially useful when verifying a food history or diary.

Clinical Examination

A significant amount of information regarding nutritional deficiencies can be elicited from a clinical examination, especially from assessing the skin, hair, teeth, gums, lips, tongue, and eyes. The hair, skin, and mouth are vulnerable because of the rapid turnover of epithelial and mucosal tissue. Table 34-1 summarizes clinical signs of possible nutritional deficiency or excess (see also Table 11-6). Few are diagnostic for a specific nutrient, and if suspicious signs are found, they must be

Table 34-1 Clinical Assessment of Nutritional Status

EVIDENCE OF ADEQUATE NUTRITION	EVIDENCE OF DEFICIENT OR EXCESS NUTRITION	DEFICIENCY OR EXCESS*
General Growth		
Between 5th and 95th percentiles for height, weight, and head circumference	Below 5th or above 95th percentile for growth	Protein, calories, fats, and other essential nutrients, especially vitamin A, pyridoxine, niacin, calcium, iodine, manganese, zinc
Steady gain with expected growth spurts during infancy and adolescence	Absence of or delayed growth spurts; poor weight gain	
Sexual development appropriate for age	Delayed sexual development	Excess vitamins A, D
Skin		
Smooth, slightly dry to touch Elastic and firm Absence of lesions Colour appropriate to genetic background	Hardening and scaling	Vitamin A
	Seborrheic dermatitis	Excess niacin
	Dry, rough, petechiae	Riboflavin
	Delayed wound healing	Vitamin C
	Scaly dermatitis on exposed surfaces	Riboflavin, vitamin C, zinc
	Wrinkled, flabby	Niacin
	Crusted lesions around orifices, especially nares	Protein, calories, zinc
	Pruritus	Excess vitamin A, riboflavin, niacin
	Poor turgor	Water, sodium
	Edema	Protein, thiamine
		Excess sodium
	Yellow tinge (jaundice)	Vitamin B_{12}
		Excess vitamin A, niacin
	Depigmentation	Protein, calories
	Pallor (anemia)	Pyridoxine; folic acid; vitamins B_{12}, C, E (in preterm infants); iron
		Excess vitamin C, zinc
	Paresthesia	Excess riboflavin

*Nutrients listed are deficient unless specified as excess.

Continued

Table 34-1 Clinical Assessment of Nutritional Status—cont'd

EVIDENCE OF ADEQUATE NUTRITION	EVIDENCE OF DEFICIENT OR EXCESS NUTRITION	DEFICIENCY OR EXCESS*
Hair		
Lustrous, silky, strong, elastic	Stringy, friable, dull, dry, thin	Protein, calories
	Alopecia	Protein, calories, zinc
	Depigmentation	Protein, calories, copper
	Raised areas around hair follicles	Vitamin C
Head		
Even moulding, occipital prominence, symmetrical facial features	Softening of cranial bones, prominence of frontal bones, skull flat and depressed toward middle	Vitamin D
Fused sutures after 18 mo	Delayed fusion of sutures	Vitamin D
	Hard, tender lumps in occiput	Excess vitamin A
	Headache	Excess thiamine
Neck		
Thyroid not visible, palpable in midline	Thyroid enlarged, may be grossly visible	Iodine
Eyes		
Clear, bright	Hardening and scaling of cornea and conjunctiva	Vitamin A
Good night vision	Night blindness	Vitamin A
Conjunctiva—Pink, glossy	Burning, itching, photophobia, cataracts, corneal vascularization	Riboflavin
Ears		
Tympanic membrane—Pliable	Calcified (hearing loss)	Excess vitamin D
Nose		
Smooth, intact nasal angle	Irritation and cracks at nasal angle	Riboflavin
		Excess vitamin A
Mouth		
Lips—Smooth, moist, darker colour than skin	Fissures and inflammation at corners	Riboflavin
		Excess vitamin A
Gums—Firm, coral pink, stippled	Spongy, friable, swollen, bluish red or black, bleed easily	Vitamin C
Mucous membranes—Bright pink, smooth, moist	Stomatitis	Niacin
Tongue—Rough texture, no lesions, taste sensation	Glossitis	Niacin, riboflavin, folic acid
	Diminished taste sensation	Zinc
Teeth—Uniform white colour, smooth, intact	Brown mottling, pits, fissures	Excess fluoride
	Defective enamel	Vitamins A, C, D; calcium; phosphorus
	Caries	Excess carbohydrates
Chest		
In infants, shape almost circular	Depressed lower portion of rib cage	Vitamin D
In children, lateral diameter increased in proportion to anteroposterior diameter	Sharp protrusion of sternum	Vitamin D
Smooth costochondral junctions	Enlarged costochondral junctions	Vitamins C, D
Breast development—Normal for age	Delayed development	See under General Growth; especially zinc

Table 34-1 Clinical Assessment of Nutritional Status—cont'd

EVIDENCE OF ADEQUATE NUTRITION	EVIDENCE OF DEFICIENT OR EXCESS NUTRITION	DEFICIENCY OR EXCESS*
Cardiovascular System		
Pulse and blood pressure (BP) within normal limits	Palpitations	Thiamine
	Rapid pulse	Potassium
		Excess thiamine
	Arrhythmias	Magnesium, potassium
		Excess niacin, potassium
	Increased BP	Excess sodium
	Decreased BP	Thiamine
		Excess niacin
Abdomen		
In young children, cylindrical and prominent	Distended, flabby, poor musculature	Protein, calories
	Prominent, large	Excess calories
In older children, flat	Potbelly, constipation	Vitamin D
Normal bowel habits	Diarrhea	Niacin
		Excess vitamin C
	Constipation	Excess calcium, potassium
Musculoskeletal System		
Muscles—Firm, well developed, equal strength bilaterally	Flabby, weak, generalized wasting	Protein, calories
	Weakness, pain, cramps	Thiamine, sodium, chloride, potassium, phosphorus, magnesium
		Excess thiamine
	Muscle twitching, tremors	Magnesium
	Muscular paralysis	Excess potassium
Spine—Cervical and lumbar curves (double S curve)	Kyphosis, lordosis, scoliosis	Vitamin D
Extremities—Symmetrical; legs straight with minimum bowing	Bowing of extremities, knock-knees	Vitamin D, calcium, phosphorus
	Epiphyseal enlargement	Vitamins A, D
	Bleeding into joints and muscles, joint swelling, pain	Vitamin C
Joints—Flexible, full range of motion, no pain or stiffness	Thickening of cortex of long bones with pain and fragility, hard tender lumps in extremities	Excess vitamin A
	Osteoporosis of long bones	Calcium
		Excess vitamin D
Neurological System		
Behaviour—Alert, responsive, emotionally stable	Listless, irritable, lethargic, apathetic (sometimes apprehensive, anxious, drowsy, mentally slow, confused)	Thiamine, niacin, pyridoxine, vitamin C, potassium, magnesium, iron, protein, calories
		Excess vitamins A, D; thiamine; folic acid; calcium
Absence of tetany, convulsions	Masklike facial expression, blurred speech, involuntary laughing	Excess manganese
	Convulsions	Thiamine, pyridoxine, vitamin D, calcium, magnesium
		Excess phosphorus (in relation to calcium)
Intact peripheral nervous system	Peripheral nervous system toxicity (unsteady gait, numb feet and hands, fine motor clumsiness)	Excess pyridoxine
Intact reflexes	Diminished or absent tendon reflexes	Thiamine, vitamin E

confirmed with dietary and biochemical data. Generally, the clinical examination does not reveal children's risk for a deficiency or excess.

Anthropometry, an essential parameter of nutritional status, is the measurement of height, weight, head circumference, proportions, skin fold thickness, and arm circumference in young children. Height and head circumference reflect past nutrition, whereas weight, skin fold thickness, and arm circumference reflect present nutritional status, especially of protein and fat reserves. Skin fold thickness is a measurement of the body's fat content; approximately half the body's total fat stores are directly beneath the skin. The upper arm muscle circumference is correlated with measurements of total muscle mass. Since muscle serves as the body's major protein reserve, this measurement is considered an index of the body's protein stores. Ideally, growth measurements are recorded over time, and comparisons are made regarding the velocity of growth based on previous and present values. Numerous biochemical tests available for assessing nutritional status include analysis of plasma; blood cells; urine; and tissues from liver, bone, hair, and fingernails. Many of these tests are complicated and are not performed routinely. Common laboratory procedures for nutritional status include measurement of hemoglobin, hematocrit, transferrin, albumin, creatinine, and nitrogen. Laboratory values for these tests and more specific nutrient measurements are given in Appendix D.

Evaluation of Nutritional Assessment

After collecting the data needed for a thorough nutritional assessment, the nurse needs to evaluate the findings to plan appropriate counselling. From the data, assessment can be made as to whether the child is (1) malnourished, (2) at risk for becoming malnourished, or (3) well nourished with adequate reserves.

The **Dietary Reference Intakes** (DRIs) are a set of four nutrient-based reference values that provide quantitative estimates of nutrient intake for use in assessing and planning dietary intake (American Academy of Pediatrics [AAP], 2004; Murphy & Poos, 2002). The specific DRIs include the following:

Estimated average requirement (EAR)—Nutrient intake estimated to meet the requirement of half the healthy individuals (50%) for a specific age and gender group. The EAR is used to examine the possibility of inadequacy.

Recommended dietary allowance (RDA)—Average daily dietary intake sufficient to meet the nutrient requirement of nearly all (97 to 98%) of healthy individuals for a specific age and gender group. Dietary intake at or above this level usually has a low probability of inadequacy.

Adequate intake (AI)—Recommended intake level based on estimates of nutrient intake by healthy groups of individuals. Dietary intake at or above this level usually has a low probability of inadequacy.

Tolerable upper intake level (UL)—Highest average daily nutrient intake level likely to pose no risk of adverse health effects. As intake increases above the UL, risk of adverse effects increases. Dietary intake above this level usually places an individual at risk of adverse effects from excessive nutrient intake.

Another resource for assessing nutrition is Health Canada's (2007) *Eating Well With Canada's Food Guide*. The *Food Guide* is based on current nutritional science and is intended to help individuals make good food choices that promote health and prevent nutrition-related illnesses. It is not prescriptive but promotes desirable ways of eating (Katamay et al., 2007). The Canada *Food Guide* provides special recommendations for children, women of childbearing age, and adults over age 50. There are also different adaptations of the *Food Guide*, including one for First Nations, Métis, and Inuit populations. In addition to the English and French versions, the *Food Guide* has been translated into Arabic, Chinese (traditional or simplified), Farsi, Korean, Russian, Punjabi, Spanish, Tagalog, Tamil, and Urduhas (Health Canada, 2007). The Web site for the *Food Guide* contains interactive guides for tracking food choices, at http://www.hc-sc.gc.ca/fn-an/food-guide-aliment/myguide-monguide/index-eng.php.

It is important to analyze the daily food diary for the variety and amounts of foods suggested in *Eating Well With Canada's Food Guide*. For example, if the list includes no vegetables, the nurse can inquire about this rather than assuming that the child dislikes vegetables, since it could be that none were served that day. Also, information should be evaluated in terms of the family's ethnic practices and financial resources. Encouraging increased protein intake with additional meat may be unfeasible for families on a limited budget or in conflict with food practices that use meat sparingly.

General Approaches Toward Examining the Child

Sequence of the Examination

Ordinarily, the sequence for examining patients follows a head-to-toe direction. The main function of such a systematic approach is to avoid omitting segments of the examination. The standard recording of data also facilitates exchange of information among different health care providers. This orderly sequence is frequently altered to accommodate the child's developmental needs, although the examination is recorded following the head-to-toe model. Using developmental and chronological age as the main criteria for assessing each body system accomplishes several goals:

- Minimizes stress and anxiety associated with assessment of various body parts
- Fosters a trusting nurse–child–parent relationship
- Allows for maximum **preparation** of the child
- Preserves the essential security of the parent–child relationship, especially with young children
- Maximizes the accuracy and reliability of assessment findings

Preparation of the Child

Although the physical examination consists of painless procedures, to a child the use of a tight arm cuff, probes in the ears and mouth, pressure on the abdomen, and a cold piece of metal to listen to the chest can be stressful. Therefore, the same considerations discussed in Chapter 45 for preparing children for procedures are followed here. In addition to that discussion, general guidelines related to the examining process are presented in the Guidelines box.

The physical examination should be as pleasant as possible and educational. For example, the nurse can use a detailed drawing or anatomically correct doll to help preschoolers and older children learn about their bodies (Vessey, 1995). The paper-doll technique is a useful approach to teaching children about the body part that is being examined (Fig. 34-4). At the conclusion of the visit, the child can bring home the paper doll as a memento of the experience.

Table 34-2 summarizes guidelines for positioning, preparing, and examining children at various ages. Because no child fits precisely into one age category, it may be necessary to vary the approach after a preliminary assessment of the child's developmental achievements and needs. Even with the best approach, many toddlers find the procedure difficult and are inconsolable for much of the physical examination. However, some seem intrigued by the new surroundings and unusual equipment and respond more like preschoolers than toddlers. Likewise, some early preschoolers may require more of the "security measures" employed with younger children, such as continued parent–child contact, and less of the preparatory measures used with preschoolers, such as playing with the equipment before and during the actual examination (Fig. 34-5).

Although the variations in the general approaches are numerous, some common ones are elaborated on here. For example, the suggested sequence may change considerably when the child is in pain or when obvious physical defects are present. In either situation, the affected area needs to be

GUIDELINES Performing a Pediatric Physical Examination

Perform the examination in an appropriate, nonthreatening area.
- Have the room well lit and decorated with neutral colours.
- Have room temperature comfortably warm.
- Place all strange and potentially frightening equipment out of sight.
- Have some toys, dolls, stuffed animals, and games available for the child.
- If possible, have rooms decorated and equipped for different-age children.
- Provide privacy, especially for school-age children and adolescents.

Provide time for play and becoming acquainted.

Observe behaviours that signal the child's readiness to collaborate:
- Talking to the nurse
- Making eye contact
- Accepting the offered equipment
- Allowing physical touching
- Choosing to sit on the examining table rather than the parent's lap

If signs of readiness are not observed, use the following techniques:
- Talk to the parent while essentially "ignoring" the child; gradually focus on the child or a favourite object, such as a doll.
- Make complimentary remarks about the child, such as appearance, dress, or a favourite object.
- Tell a funny story or play a simple magic trick.
- Have a nonthreatening "friend" available, such as a hand puppet to "talk" to the child for the nurse (see Fig. 34-25, A).

If the child refuses to collaborate, use the following techniques:
- Assess reason for behaviour; consider that a child who is unduly afraid may have had a traumatic experience.
- Try to involve the child and parent in the process.
- Avoid prolonged explanations about the examining procedure.
- Use a firm, direct approach regarding expected behaviour.
- Perform the examination as quickly as possible.
- Have an attendant gently restrain the child.
- Minimize any disruptions or stimulation.
- Limit the number of people in the room.
- Use an isolated room.
- Use a quiet, calm, confident voice.

Begin the examination in a nonthreatening manner for young children or children who are fearful:
- Use activities that can be presented as games, such as the test for cranial nerves (see Table 34-13) or parts of developmental screening tests (pp. 928–929).
- Use approaches such as "Simon Says" to encourage the child to make a face, squeeze a hand, stand on one foot, and so on.
- Use the paper-doll technique:
  1. Lay the child supine on an examining table or floor that is covered with a large sheet of paper.
  2. Trace around the child's body outline.
  3. Use body outline to demonstrate what will be examined, such as drawing a heart and listening with a stethoscope, before performing the activity on the child.

If several children in the family will be examined, begin with the child who is most willing to be examined to model desired behaviour.

Involve the child in the examination process:
- Provide choices, such as sitting on the table or in the parent's lap.
- Allow the child to handle or hold equipment.
- Encourage the child to use equipment on a doll, family member, or examiner.
- Explain each step of the procedure in simple language.

Examine the child in a comfortable and secure position:
- Sitting in parent's lap
- Sitting upright if in respiratory distress

Proceed to examine the body in an organized sequence (usually head to toe) with the following exceptions:
- Alter sequence to accommodate needs of different-age children (see Table 34-2).
- Examine painful areas last.
- In an emergency situation, examine vital functions (airway, breathing, and circulation) and injured area first.

Reassure the child throughout examination, especially about bodily concerns that arise during puberty.

Discuss findings with the family (if appropriate) at the end of the examination.

Praise the child for their assistance during the examination; give a reward such as a small toy or sticker.

Table 34-2 Age-Specific Approaches to Physical Examination During Childhood

POSITION	SEQUENCE	PREPARATION
Infant		
Before able to sit alone—Supine or prone, preferably in parent's lap; before 4–6 mo, can place on examining table **After able to sit alone**—Sitting in parent's lap whenever possible; if on table, place with parent in full view	If quiet, auscultate heart, lungs, abdomen. Record heart and respiratory rates. Palpate and percuss same areas. Proceed in usual head-to-toe direction. Perform traumatic procedures last (eyes, ears, mouth [while crying]). Elicit reflexes as body part is examined. Elicit Moro reflex last.	Completely undress if room temperature permits. Leave diaper on male infant. Gain cooperation with distraction, bright objects, rattles, talking. Smile at infant; use soft, gentle voice. Use pacifier or feeding if necessary. Enlist parent's aid for restraining to examine ears, mouth. Avoid abrupt, jerky movements.
Toddler		
Sitting or standing on or by parent Prone or supine in parent's lap	Inspect body area through play: "count fingers," "tickle toes." Use minimum physical contact initially. Introduce equipment slowly. Auscultate, percuss, palpate whenever quiet. Perform traumatic procedures last (same as for infant).	Have parent remove outer clothing. Remove underwear as body part is examined. Allow child to inspect equipment; demonstrating use of equipment is usually ineffective. If uncooperative, perform procedures quickly. Use restraint when appropriate; request parent's assistance. Talk about examination; use short phrases. Praise for assisting.
Preschool Child		
Prefer standing or sitting Usually most helpful prone or supine Prefer parent's closeness	If cooperative, proceed in head-to-toe direction. If having difficuly, proceed as with toddler.	Request self-undressing. Allow to wear underpants if shy. Offer equipment for inspection; briefly demonstrate use. Make up story about procedure (e.g., "I'm seeing how strong your muscles are" [blood pressure]). Use paper-doll technique. Give choices when possible. Use positive statements (e.g., "Open your mouth").
School-Age Child		
Prefer sitting Helpful in most positions Younger child prefers parent's presence Older child may prefer privacy	Proceed in head-to-toe direction. May examine genitalia last in older child	Respect need for privacy. Request self-undressing. Allow to wear underpants. Give gown to wear. Explain purpose of equipment and significance of procedure, such as otoscope to see eardrum, which is necessary for hearing. Teach about body function and care.
Adolescent		
Same as for school-age child Offer option of parent's presence	Same as older school-age child May examine genitalia last	Allow to undress in private. Give gown. Expose only area to be examined. Respect need for privacy. Explain findings during examination: "Your muscles are firm and strong." Matter-of-factly comment about sexual development: "Your breasts are developing as they should be." Emphasize normalcy of development. Examine genitalia as any other body part; may leave to end.

examined last, to minimize distress early in the examination and to focus on normal, healthy, functioning body parts.

Physical Examination

Although the approach to and sequence of the physical examination differ according to the child's age, the following discussion outlines the traditional model for physical assessment. The focus includes all pediatric age groups; the reader is referred to Chapter 25 for a detailed discussion of a newborn assessment.

Along with physical examination, another vital part of preventive pediatric care is assessment of immunization status. A schedule for the Canadian periodic health visits is given in Figure 34-6.

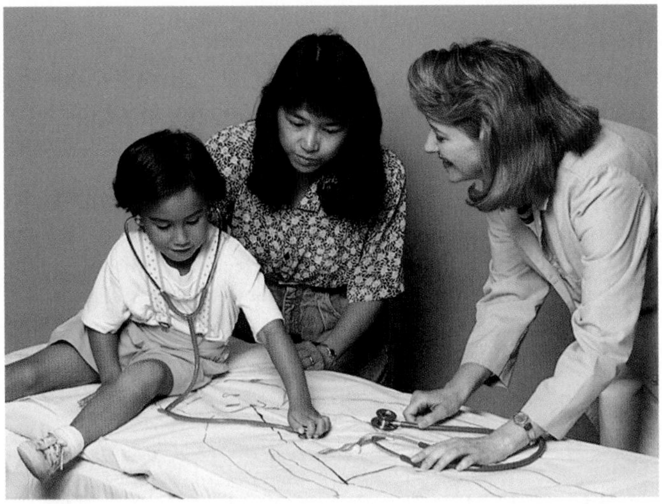

Fig. 34-4 Using paper-doll technique to prepare child for physical examination.

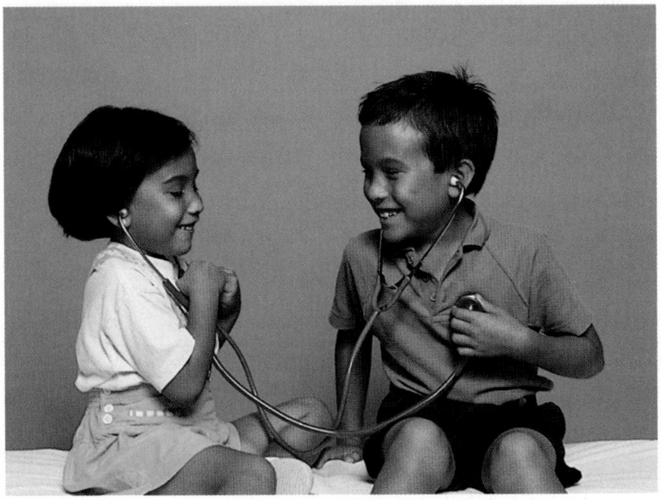

Fig. 34-5 Preparing children for physical examination.

Growth Measurements

Measurement of physical growth in children is a key element in evaluating their health status. Physical growth parameters include weight, height (length), skin fold thickness, arm circumference, and head circumference. Values for these growth parameters are plotted on percentile charts, and the child's measurements in percentiles are compared with those of the general population.

Growth Charts

The growth charts used in Canada have been adapted from the 2006 and 2007 World Health Organization (WHO) Growth Standards and Growth References. The Canadian Paediatric Society (2010b) adapted the WHO growth charts in collaboration with Dietitians of Canada, the College of Family Physicians of Canada, and Community Health Nurses of Canada. The charts were adapted in order to provide health care providers with consistent practices in monitoring growth and assessing patterns of linear growth and weight gain to support healthy children. These new charts reflect the 0 to 5 years of age population with optimal health conditions. It also reflects an increase in the multi-ethnic international population and an improvement in the tool to identify children at risk for obesity. The Canadian Paediatric Society Web site contains the charts, professional health guidelines, and a parent handout at http://www.cps.ca/english/Publications/CPS10-01.htm.

NURSING ALERT The definition of body mass index for age (BMI) is weight in kilograms divided by height in metres squared: BMI = Weight (kg) ÷ Height (m^2). BMI correlates with the amount of body fat. BMI in children has been linked to future obesity and resultant negative impact on health. A BMI of 28 begins to decrease in later infancy and reaches a low at around 4 to 6 years of age. There is then an increase throughout childhood and adolescence (CPS, 2010c).

Breastfed and Formula-Fed Infants

For assessment of growth in these infants the Canadian WHO growth charts for the 0 to 5 age group are used. The charts include a recommendation of a minimum of 4 to 6 months of breastfeeding to help maximize nutritional levels and optimize growth (CPS, 2010b).

Special Groups

The WHO growth charts do not include premature infants or very low-birth-weight infants who weigh less than 1500 g. These infants do not grow in the same manner as full-term infants. Once these preterm infants are discharged from the neonatal intensive care unit, the WHO charts can then be used for them. Measurements should be plotted with the corrected postnatal age for prematurity (40 weeks—gestational age in weeks) until the child is 24 to 36 months of age. As an alternative, Fenton's growth chart, which updated the Babson and Benda charts, can be used for plotting growth from 22 gestational weeks to 10 weeks postterm. (CPS, 2010c; Fenton, 2003). Children with specific intellectual, developmental, genetic, or other conditions often have growth patterns that are different from those of healthy children. Their growth can also be plotted on the WHO growth charts alone, or in conjunction with specific growth curves that exist for some of these disorders (CPS, 2010c; Cronk et al., 1988).

NURSING ALERT The 2007 WHO Growth Reference Charts include data that reflect healthy growth and can be used to identify children who are at risk for obesity. The BMI-for-age values that suggest overweight (BMI of 25 kg/m^2) and obesity (BMI of 30 kg/m^2) match the adult cut-offs for overweight and obesity at 19 years (CPS, 2010b).

Children whose growth may be questionable include the following:

- Children whose height and weight percentiles are widely disparate (e.g., height in the tenth percentile and weight in the ninetieth percentile, especially with above-average skin fold thickness)
- Children who fail to show the expected growth rates in height and weight, especially during the rapid growth periods of infancy and adolescence
- Children who show a sudden increase (except during puberty) or decrease in a previously steady growth pattern

Because growth is a continuous but uneven process, the most reliable evaluation lies in comparing growth measurements over time. It is important to remember that normal growth patterns vary among children of the same age (Fig. 34-7).

Length

The term *length* refers to measurements taken when children are supine (also referred to as recumbent length). Until children are 24 months old (or 36 months if using the chart for birth to 36 months), recumbent length is measured. Because of the normally flexed position during infancy, the body should be fully extended by (1) holding the head in midline, (2) grasping the knees together gently, and (3) gently pushing down on the knees until the legs are fully extended and flat against the table. If using a measuring board, place the head firmly at the top of the board and the heels of the feet firmly against the footboard.

If such a measuring device is not available, length can be measured by placing the child on a paper-covered surface, marking the end points of the top of the head and the heels of the feet, and measuring between these two points (Fig. 34-8). For accurate measurement, the nurse should hold the writing utensil at a right angle to the table when marking the cephalic

Routine Immunizations for Infants and Children

Age at vaccination	DTaP-IPV	Hib	MMR	Var	HB	Pneu-C-7	Men-C	Tdap	Inf
Birth					Infancy 3 doses ★				
2 months	○	✦				⧗	◉		
4 months	○	✦				⧗	(◉)		
6 months	○	✦				⧗	◉ or		6–23 months ⊕ 1–2 doses
12 months			■	●	or	⧗ 12–15 months	◉ if not yet given		
18 months	○	✦	■						
4–6 years	○		or ■						
14–16 years					Pre-teen/ teen 2–3 doses		◉ if not yet given	▲	

Routine Immunization Schedule for Children <7 Years of Age Not Immunized in Early Infancy

Timing	DTaP-IPV	Hib	MMR	Var	HB	Pneu-C-7	Men-C	Tdap
First visit	○	✦	■	●	★	⧗	◉	
2 months later	○	(✦)	■		★	(⧗)	(◉)	
4 months later	○					(⧗)		
6–12 months later	○	(✦)			★			
4–6 years of age	(○)							
14–16 years of age								▲

Routine Immunizations for Children ≥ 7 Years of Age Up to 17 Years of Age Not Immunized in Early Infancy

Timing	Tdap	IPV	MMR	Var	HB	Men-C
First visit	▲	⬟	■	●	★	◉
2 months later	▲	⬟	■	(●)	(★)	
6–12 months later	▲	⬟			★	
10 years later	▲					

Fig. 34-6 Recommended Immunization Schedules from Public Health Agency of Canada (2006). *(From the Public Health Agency of Canada. [2006].* Canadian immunization guide, *7th ed. Retrieved from http://www.phac-aspc.gc.ca/publicat/cig-gci/pdf/cig-gci-2006_e.pdf [pp. 93–94].)*

Notes

() Symbols with brackets around them imply that these doses may not be required, depending upon the age of the child or adult.

Diphtheria, tetanus, acellular pertussis, and inactivated polio virus vaccine (DTaP-IPV): DTap-IPV(±Hib) vaccine is the preferred vaccine for all doses in the vaccination series, including completion of the series in children who have received one or more doses of DPT (whole cell) vaccine (e.g., recent immigrants). In the top and middle tables, the 4–6 year dose can be omitted if the fourth dose was given after the fourth birthday.

***Haemophilus influenzae* type b conjugate vaccine (Hib):** The Hib schedule shown is for the *Haemophilus* b capsular polysaccharide – polyribosylribitol phosphate (PRP) conjugated to tetanus toxoid (PRP-T). For catch-up, the number of doses depends on the age at which the schedule is begun. This vaccine is not usually required past age 5 years.

Measles, mumps, and rubella vaccine (MMR): A second dose of MMR is recommended for children at least 1 month after the first dose for the purpose of better measles protection. For convenience, options include giving it with the next scheduled vaccination at 18 months of age or at school entry (4–6 years) (depending on the provincial/territorial policy) or at any intervening age that is practical. In the catch-up schedule (see middle table), the first dose should not be given until the child is ≥12 months old. MMR should be given to all susceptible adolescents and adults.

Varicella vaccine (Var): Children aged 12 months to 12 years should receive one dose of varicella vaccine. Susceptible individuals ≥13 years of age should receive two doses at least 28 days apart.

Hepatitis B vaccine (HB): Hepatitis B vaccine can be routinely given to infants or pre-adolescents, depending on the provincial/territorial policy. For infants born to chronic carrier mothers, the first dose should be given at birth (with hepatitis B immunoglobulin), otherwise the first dose can be given at 2 months of age to fit more conveniently with other routine infant immunization visits. The second dose should be administered at least 1 month after the first dose, and the third at least 2 months after the second dose, but these may fit more conveniently into the 4- and 6-month immunization visits. A two-dose schedule for adolescents is an option.

Pneumococcal conjugate vaccine – 7-valent (Pneu-C-7): Recommended for all children under 2 years of age. The recommended schedule depends on the age of the child when vaccination is begun.

Pneumococcal polysaccharide – 23-valent (Pneu-P-23): This is recommended for all adults ≥65 years of age.

Meningococcal C conjugate vaccine (Men-C): Recommended for children under 5 years of age, adolescents, and young adults. The recommended schedule depends on the age of the individual and the conjugate vaccine used. At least one dose in the primary infant series should be given after 5 months of age. If the provincial/territorial policy is to give Men-C to persons ≥12 months of age, one dose is sufficient.

Diphtheria, tetanus, acellular pertussis vaccine – adult/adolescent formulation (Tdap): A combined adsorbed "adult-type" preparation for use in people ≥7 years of age. It contains less diphtheria toxoid and fewer pertussis antigens than preparations given to younger children and is less likely to cause reactions in older people.

Diphtheria, tetanus vaccine (Td): A combined adsorbed "adult-type" preparation for use in people ≥7 years of age. It contains less diphtheria toxoid antigen than preparations given to younger children and is less likely to cause reactions in older people. It is given to adults not immunized in childhood as the second and third doses of their primary series and subsequent booster doses; Tdap is given only once under these circumstances as it is assumed that previously unimmunized adults will have encountered *Bordetella pertussis* and have some pre-existing immunity.

Influenza vaccine (Inf): Recommended for all children 6–23 months of age and all persons ≥65 years of age. Previously unvaccinated children <9 years of age require two doses of the current season's vaccine with an interval of at least 4 weeks. The second dose within the same season is not required if the child received one or more doses of influenza vaccine during the previous influenza season.

IPV Inactivated polio virus

Fig. 34-6, cont'd

point; the feet are positioned with the toes pointing directly to the ceiling when marking the heel point. Regardless of the method used, someone needs to assist the nurse in holding the child's head in midline while extending the legs and taking the measurements.

Height

The term *height* (or stature) refers to the measurement taken when children are standing upright. Height is measured by having the child, with shoes removed, stand as tall and straight as possible, with the head in midline and the line of vision parallel to the ceiling and floor. The child's back needs to be against the wall or other vertical flat surface, with the heels, buttocks, and back of the shoulders touching the wall and the medial malleoli touching, if possible (Fig. 34-9). The nurse should check for and correct bending of the knees, slumping of the shoulders, or raising of the heels.

For the most accurate measurement, a wall-mounted unit (stadiometer; see Fig. 34-9) can be used. The movable measuring rod of platform scales is accurate only if it maintains a parallel position to the floor and rests securely on the topmost part of the head. To improvise a flat surface for measuring

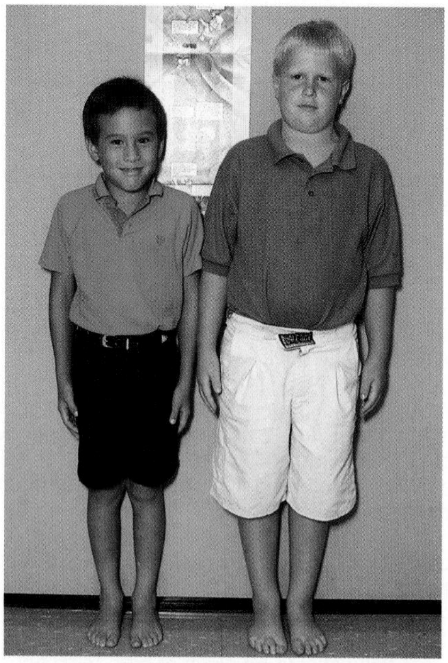

Fig. 34-7 These children of identical age (8 years) are markedly different in size. The child on the left, of Asian descent, is at the fifth percentile for height and weight. The child on the right is above the ninety-fifth percentile for height and weight. However, both children demonstrate normal growth patterns.

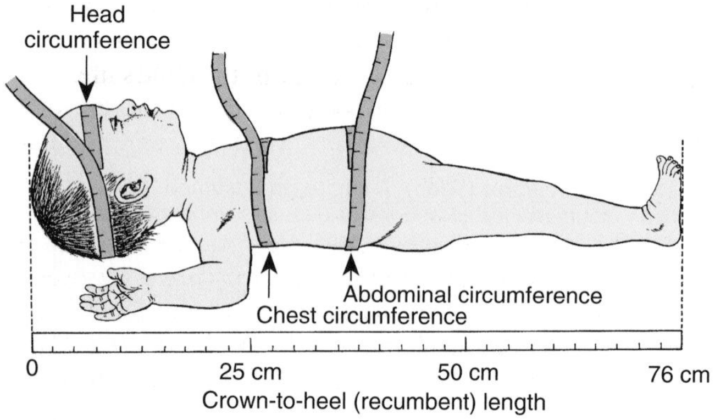

Fig. 34-8 Measurement of head, chest, and abdominal circumference and crown-to-heel (recumbent) length.

length, attach a paper or metal tape or yardstick to the wall, position the child adjacent to the tape, and place a three-dimensional object, such as a thick book or box, on top of the head. Rest the side of the object firmly against the wall to form a right angle. Measure length or stature to the nearest 1 mm.

Weight

Weight is measured with an appropriately sized beam balance scale, which measures weight to the nearest 10 g for infants and 100 g for children. Before the child is weighed, the nurse needs to balance the scale by setting it at 0 and noting if the balance registers exactly in the middle of the mark. If the end of the balance beam rises to the top or bottom of the mark, more or less weight, respectively, is needed. Some scales are designed to allow for self-correction, but others need to be

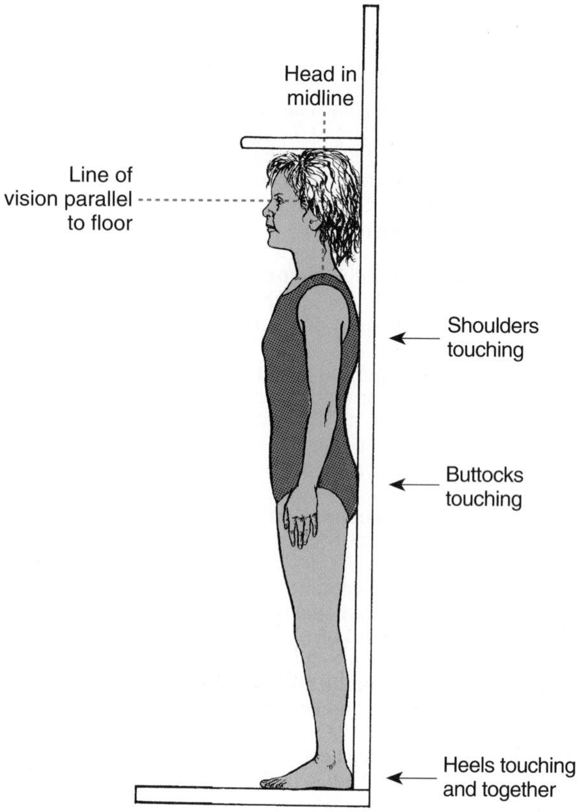

Fig. 34-9 Measurement of height. *(Redrawn from* Human growth and growth disorders: An update. *San Francisco: Genentech. 1989.)*

recalibrated by the manufacturer. Scales vary in their accuracy; infant scales tend to be more accurate than adult platform scales, and newer scales tend to be more accurate than older ones, especially at the upper levels of weight measurement. When precise measurements are needed, two nurses should take the weight independently; if there is a discrepancy, a third reading should be taken.

Measurements should be taken in a comfortably warm room. From birth to 36 months, children should be weighed nude. Older children are usually weighed while wearing their underpants or a light gown. However, always respect the privacy of all children. If the child must be weighed wearing some article of clothing or some type of special device, such as a prosthesis or an armboard for an intravenous device, note this when recording the weight. Children who are measured for recumbent length are usually weighed on an infant platform scale and placed in a lying or sitting position. When weighing children, the nurse should place a hand lightly above the infant's body to prevent the child from accidentally falling off the scale (Fig. 34-10, A) or stand close to the toddler, ready to prevent a fall (see Fig. 34-10, B). For maximum asepsis, the scale should be covered with a clean sheet of paper and cleaned between each child's measurement.

Skin Fold Thickness and Arm Circumference

Measures of relative weight and stature cannot distinguish between adipose (fat) tissue and muscle. One convenient

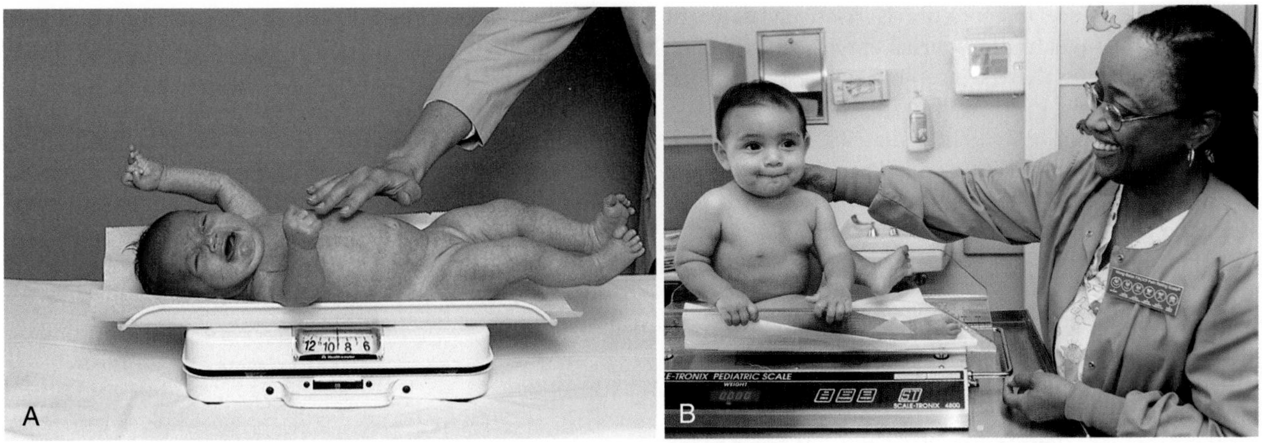

Fig. 34-10 A: Infant on scale. B: Toddler on scale. Note presence of nurse to prevent falls. *(B, Courtesy Paul Vincent Kuntz, Texas Children's Hospital, Houston.)*

measure of body fat is skin fold thickness, which is increasingly recommended as a routine measurement. Skin fold thickness is measured with special calipers, such as the Lange calipers. The most common sites for measuring skin fold thickness are the triceps (most practical for routine clinical use), subscapula, suprailiac, abdomen, and upper thigh. For greatest reliability the exact procedure for measurement must be followed and the average of at least two measurements of one site recorded.

Arm circumference is an indirect measure of muscle mass. Measurement of arm circumference follows the same procedure as that for skin fold thickness except the midpoint is measured with a paper or steel tape. The tape is placed vertically, along the posterior aspect of the upper arm from the acromial process to the olecranon process; half the measured length is the midpoint. Percentiles for triceps skin fold and arm circumference in children are listed on the Evolve site and may be used as reference data. However, the percentiles are not standards or norms, since values between the fifth and ninety-fifth percentiles are not ranges of normal.

Head Circumference

Head circumference in children is measured up to 36 months of age and in any child whose head size is questionable. The head is measured at its greatest circumference, usually slightly above the eyebrows and pinna of the ears and around the occipital prominence at the back of the skull (see Fig. 34-8). Because head shape can affect the location of the maximum circumference, more than one measurement at points above the eyebrows may be needed to obtain the most accurate measure. A paper or metal tape should be used, since a cloth tape can stretch and give a falsely small measurement. For greatest accuracy, devices with tenths of a centimeter are best, since the percentile charts have only 0.5-cm increments.

The nurse can plot the head size on the appropriate growth chart under head circumference. Generally, head and chest circumferences are equal at about 1 to 2 years of age. During childhood, chest circumference exceeds head size by about 5 to 7 cm. (For newborns, see Chapter 24, Table 24-2.)

Physiological Measurements

Physiological measurements, key elements in evaluating physical status of vital functions, include temperature, pulse, respiration, and BP. Each physiological recording should be compared with normal values for that age group. In addition, the values taken on preceding health visits need to be compared with present recordings. For example, a falsely elevated BP reading may not indicate hypertension if previous recent readings have been within normal limits. The isolated recording may indicate some stressful event in the child's life.

As in most procedures carried out with children, older children and adolescents are treated much the same as adults. However, special consideration must be given to preschool children (see Atraumatic Care box).

For best results in taking vital signs of infants, the nurse should count respirations first (before the infant is disturbed), take the pulse next, and measure temperature last. If vital signs cannot be taken without disturbing the child, the nurse should record the child's behaviour (e.g., crying) along with the measurement.

Temperature

Temperature is the measure of heat content within an individual's body. The core temperature most closely reflects the temperature of the blood flow through the carotid arteries to

evolve Skill—Measuring Body Temperature

> **ATRAUMATIC CARE**
>
> *Reducing Young Children's Fears*
>
> Young children, especially preschoolers, fear intrusive procedures because of their poorly defined body boundaries. Therefore, avoid invasive procedures, such as measuring rectal temperature, whenever possible. Also, avoid using the word "take" when measuring vital signs, since young children interpret words literally and may think that their temperature or other function will be taken away. Instead, say, "I want to know how warm you are."

the hypothalamus. Core temperature is relatively constant despite wide fluctuations in the external environment. When a child's temperature is altered, receptors in the skin, spinal cord, and brain respond in an attempt to achieve *normothermia*, a normal temperature state. In pediatrics, there is a lack of consensus on what temperature constitutes normothermia for every child. For rectal temperatures in children, 36.6°C to 38°C is an acceptable range, where heat loss and heat production are balanced (CPS, 2003). For neonates, an axillary temperature between 36.5° and 37.2°C is a desirable range (see Chapter 24). In the neonate, temperature measurements are obtained for monitoring adequacy of thermoregulation, not fever; therefore, temperature measurements in each infant should be carefully considered in the context of the purpose and the environment. Temperature definitions of fever based on age are found in Box 34-10.

Temperature in healthy children can be measured at several body sites via the oral, rectal, axillary, ear canal, tympanic membrane, temporal artery, or skin route (Box 34-11). For the ill child, other sites for temperature measurement that have been investigated include the urinary bladder, pulmonary artery, and esophageal and nasopharyngeal sites (Martin & Kline, 2004) (Box 34-12). One of the most important influences on the accuracy of temperature is improper temperature-taking technique. Detailed discussion of temperature-taking methods and visual examples of proper techniques are shown in Table 34-3. For a critical review of the evidence on temperature-taking methods, see the Evidence-Informed Practice box.

BOX 34-10 Fever in Infants and Children

Measurement Method	Normal Temperature Range
Rectal	36.6°C to 38°C (97.9°F to 100.4°F)
Tympanic membrane	35.8°C to 38°C (96.4°F to 100.4°F)
Oral	35.5°C to 37.5°C (95.9°F to 99.5°F)
Axillary	34.7°C to 37.3°C (94.5°F to 99.2°F)

Temperature depends on the time of day, age, and physical activity. In general, fever is defined as a temperature of 38°C or greater (100.4°F) rectally.

Please note that in newborns, the normal axillary temperature is 36.5°C (97.9°F) to 37.2°C (99.0°F).

(Adapted from Canadian Paediatric Society [2003]. *Temperature measurement in paediatrics.* [Reaffirmed February 2011] Retrieved from http://www.cps.ca/english/statements/CP/cp00-01.htm.)

BOX 34-11 Recommended Temperature Screening Routes in Infants and Children

Birth to 2 Years

Rectal—if definitive temperature reading is needed for infants over 1 month of age

Axillary—screening low-risk children

2 to 5 Years

Axillary

Tympanic or temporal artery—if in hospital for screening

Rectal—if definitive temperature reading is needed

Over 5 Years

Oral—definitive

Axillary, tympanic or temporal artery—if in hospital for screening

(Adapted from Canadian Paediatric Society. [2003]. *Temperature measurement in paediatrics.* [Reaffirmed February 2011] Retrieved from http://www.cps.ca/english/statements/CP/cp00-01.htm.)

BOX 34-12 Alternative Temperature Measurement Sites for the Ill Child

Skin

Probe is placed on the skin to determine heat output in response to changes in the patient's skin temperature.

Skin temperature sensors are most often used for neonates and infants placed in radiant heat warmers or isolettes (using servocontrol feature of the apparatus). In turn, the heater unit warms to a set point to maintain the infant's temperature within a specified range.

Urinary Bladder

A thermistor or thermocouple is placed within the indwelling bladder catheter. The catheter tip immersed in the bladder provides a continuous temperature read-out on the bedside monitor.

This is not a true measure of core temperature but responds better than rectal and skin temperatures to core body changes.

Because of thermistor sizes, this method is unusable in neonates and small infants.

Pulmonary Artery

A catheter is placed into the heart to obtain a reading in the pulmonary artery.

It is used in critical care settings or operating rooms only in patients requiring aggressive monitoring.

The catheter is not available in sizes for neonates or small infants.

Esophageal Site

Probe is inserted into the lower third of the esophagus at the level of the heart.

This is used in critical care settings or operating rooms.

Several companies have esophageal stethoscopes with temperature probe monitors that show a continuous temperature reading for patients in the operating room.

Nasopharyngeal Site

Probe is inserted into the nasopharynx, posterior to the soft palate, and provides an estimate of hypothalamic temperature.

This is used in critical care settings or operating rooms.

(Data from Kumar, P. R., Nisarga, R., & Gowda, B. [2004]. Temperature monitoring in newborns using ThermoSpot. *Indian Journal of Pediatrics, 71*[9], 795–796; Martin, S. A., & Kline, A. M. [2004]. Can there be a standard for temperature measurement in the pediatric intensive care unit? *AACN Clinical Issues, 15*[2], 254–266; Maxton, F. J., Justin, L., & Gilles, D. [2004]. Estimating core temperature in infants and children after cardiac surgery: A comparison of six methods. *Journal of Advanced Nursing, 45*[2], 214–222.)

Table 34-3 Temperature Measurement Locations for Infants and Children

TEMPERATURE SITE

Oral

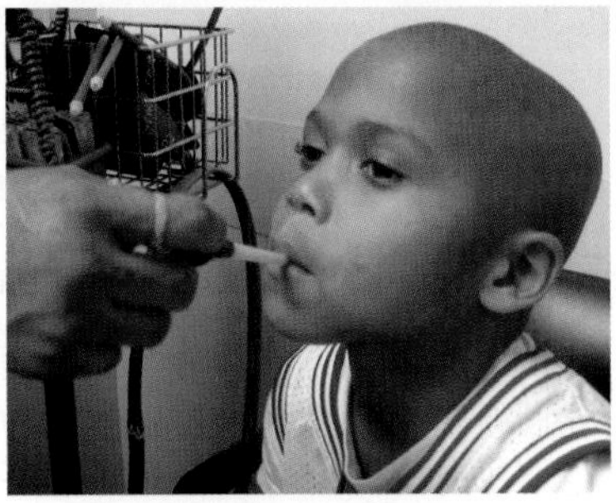

Place tip under tongue in right or left posterior sublingual pocket, not in front of tongue. Have child keep the mouth sealed, with the tongue depressed for 3 to 4 min, which is hard for young children.

Oral measurement cannot be used with young children or in uncooperative or unconscious children. The accuracy is somewhere between that of axillary and rectal thermometry. Accuracy will be better in older children, mostly because they can use the proper technique.

Digital thermometers are recommended by the Canadian Paediatric Society and have replaced mercury ones.

Pacifier thermometers measure intraoral or supralingual temperature and are available but lack support in the literature.

Several factors affect mouth temperature: eating and mastication, hot or cold beverages, open-mouth breathing, and ambient temperature.

Axillary

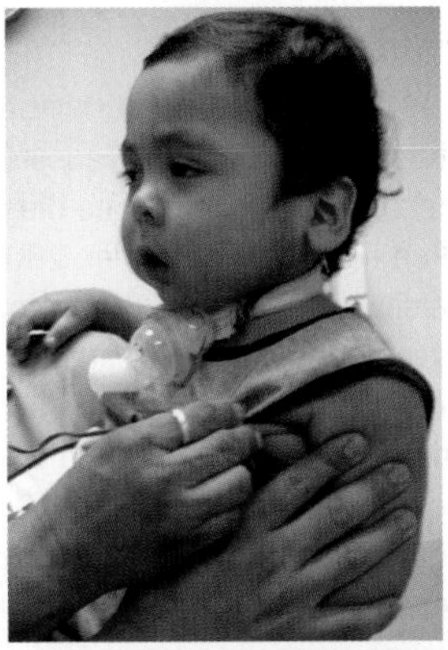

Place tip under the arm in centre of axilla and keep close to the skin, not clothing. Hold child's arm firmly against side. Temperature may be affected by poor peripheral perfusion (results in lower value), clothing or swaddling, use of radiant warmer, or amount of brown fat in cold-stressed neonate (results in higher value).

The advantage is that use of this site avoids an intrusive procedure and eliminates the risk of rectal perforation.

Ear Based (Aural)

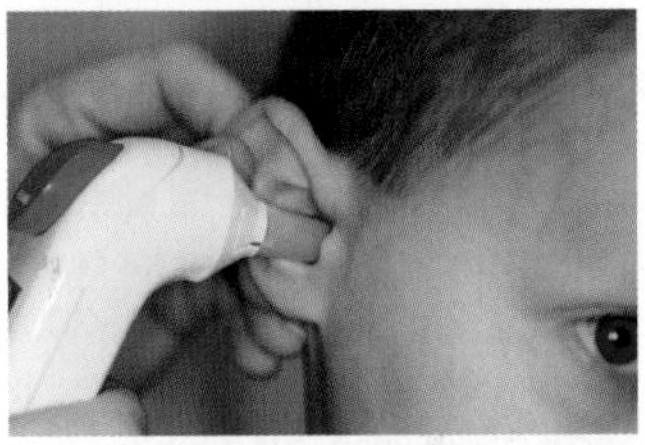

Insert small infrared probe deeply into canal to allow sensor to obtain measurement. The size of probe (most are 8 mm) may influence accuracy of the result. In young children this may be a problem because of the small diameter of the canal. For proper placement of the ear, it is debated as to whether the pinna should be pulled in a manner similar to that used during otoscopy (see Fig. 34-23).

Rectal

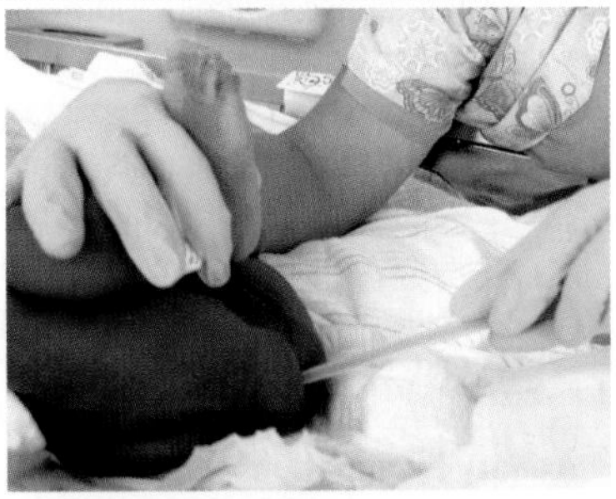

Place well-lubricated tip at maximum 2.5 cm into rectum for children and 1.5 cm for infants; securely hold thermometer close to anus.

Child may be placed in side-lying, supine, or prone position (i.e., supine with knees flexed toward abdomen); cover the penis, since the procedure may stimulate urination. A small child may be placed prone across the parent's lap.

Rectal temperatures are slow to change in relation to changing core temperature and can stay elevated well after the patient's core temperature has begun to fall, and vice versa. Rectal readings are affected by the depth of a measurement, conditions affecting local blood flow, and the presence of stool. Rectal perforation has occurred; the thermometer can spread contaminants if not sterilized.

Temporal Artery

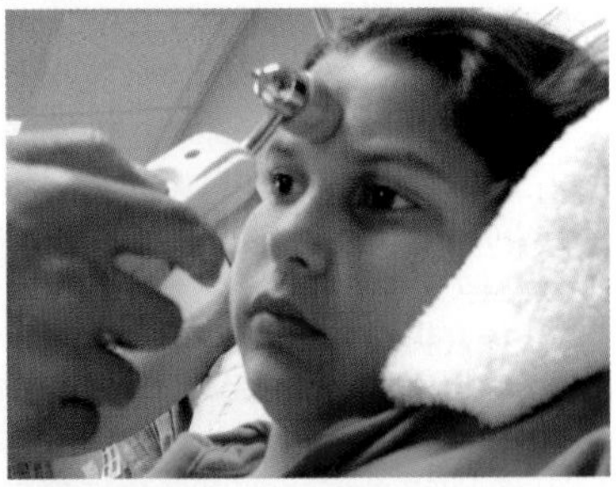

An infrared sensor probe scans across the forehead, capturing heat from arterial blood flow. The temporal artery is the only artery close enough to the skin's surface to provide access for accurate temperature measurement.

These probes have been shown to be more accurate than tympanic thermometry and are better tolerated than rectal thermometry.

(Data from Canadian Paediatric Society. [2003]. *Temperature measurement in paediatrics.* [Reaffirmed February 2011] Retrieved from http://www.cps.ca/english/statements/CP/cp00-01.htm#Rectal; Falzon, A., et al. [2003]. How reliable is axillary temperature measurement? *Acta Paediatrica, 92*[3], 309–313; Martin, S. A., & Kline, A. M. [2004]. Can there be a standard for temperature measurement in the pediatric intensive care unit? *AACN Clinical Issues, 15*[2], 254–266.)

Oral, axillary, rectal, and temporal artery images courtesy Paul Vincent Kuntz, Texas Children's Hospital, Houston.

EVIDENCE-INFORMED PRACTICE Temperature Measurement in Pediatrics

Ask the Question

In infants and children, what is the most accurate method for measuring temperature?

Search for Evidence

Search Strategies

English publications, published within past 10 years, research-based articles (level 3 or lower), infant and child populations, comparisons to gold standard: rectal thermometry

Databases Searched

PubMed, Cochrane Collaboration, MD Consult, Joanna Briggs Institute, National Guideline Clearinghouse (AHRQ), TRIP Database Plus, PedsCCM, BestBETs

Critically Analyze the Evidence

Rectal temperature–Rectal measurement remains the clinical gold standard for the precise diagnosis of fever in infants and children (Greenes & Fleisher, 2004; Riddell & Eppich, 2003; University of Michigan, 2003). However, this procedure is more invasive and is contraindicated for infants less than 1 month old, children with recent rectal surgery, children with diarrhea or anorectal lesions, and children receiving chemotherapy (cancer treatment usually affects mucosa and causes neutropenia). Findings are affected by depth of insertion and presence of stool. Rectal temperatures are slow to change in relation to changing core temperature. Many parents are uncomfortable with this method, and children may resent it. It has the capacity to spread contaminants found in stool.

Oral temperature (OT)–OT indicates rapid changes in core body temperature, but accuracy may be an issue when compared with that using the rectal site (Jensen et al., 2000). OT is considered the standard for temperature measurement (Gilbert, Barton, & Counsell, 2002) but is contraindicated in children who have an altered level of consciousness, are receiving oxygen, are mouth breathing, are experiencing mucositis, had recent oral surgery or trauma, or are under 5 years of age (Carroll, 2000; El-Radhi & Barry, 2006). Limitations of OT include the effect of ambient room temperature and recent oral intake (Carroll, 2000; Martin & Kline, 2004). Even patients with no obvious mouth breathing were found to have OTs in the normal range despite the presence of clinical fever (Tandberg & Sklar, 1983). O'Brien and colleagues (2000) found OT-predictive thermometers to read significantly lower than other core temperature measurements and to miss one out of seven fevers.

Axillary temperature–This method is inconsistent and insensitive in infants and children over 1 month old (Falzon et al., 2003; Jean-Mary et al., 2002). In neonates with fever, the axillary temperature cannot be used interchangeably with rectal measurement (Muller, Van Berkel, & de Beaufort, 2008). Despite its low sensitivity and specificity in detecting fever, the axillary site is recommended by the Canadian Paediatric Society (2003) as a screening test for fever in infants less than 1 month of age.

Ear (aural) temperature–This is not a precise measurement of body temperature. Meta-analysis of 101 studies comparing tympanic membrane temperatures with rectal temperatures in children concluded that the tympanic method demonstrated a wide range of variability, limiting its application in a pediatric setting (Craig et al., 2002). More recently published reviews continue to find poor sensitivity using infrared ear thermometry (Dodd et al., 2006). Diagnosis of fever without a focus should not be made on the basis of tympanic thermometry, since it is not an accurate measure of core temperature (Craig et al., 2002; Dodd, et al., 2006; Riddell & Eppich, 2003).

Temporal artery temperature (TAT)–TAT was not predictable in the assessment of fever in children under 3 months of age but could be used as a screening tool for detecting fever less than 38°C in children 3 to 24 months old (Schuh et al., 2004). Temporal temperature can be used as a rapid assessment screening tool to identify fever over 39°C in children 3 to 24 months old, but is unreliable as a screening tool for infants under 3 months (Siberry et al., 2002). These published studies examining the accuracy and precision of TATs in infants and children are limited by small sample sizes. Previous samples included subjects primarily under the age of 36 months, although one abstract was found of a study that examined 75 TATs in children 6 to 12 years old (Pidwell et al., 2000). Settings used to study TATs in pediatric patients include the emergency department (Greenes & Fleisher, 2001; Pidwell et al., 2000; Schuh et al., 2004; Siberry et al., 2002), physician's office (Callanan, 2003), pediatric intensive care unit (Hebbar et al., 2005), and operating room (Al-Mukhaizeem et al., 2004).

Apply the Evidence: Nursing Implications

No single site used for temperature assessment provides unequivocal estimates of core body temperature. Studies show that the axillary and tympanic measures demonstrate poor agreement when these modes are compared with more accurate core temperature methods. The differences are more evident as temperature increases, regardless of age. When an accurate method for obtaining a correct reflection of core temperature is needed, the rectal temperature is recommended in younger children and the oral route in older children. For infants less than 1 month of age, the Canadian Paediatric Society (2003) recommends axillary temperatures.

References

Al-Mukhaizeem, F., et al. (2004). Comparison of temporal artery, rectal and esophageal core temperatures in children: Results of a pilot study. *Paediatrics and Child Health, 9*(7), 461–465.

Callanan, D. (2003). Detecting fever in young infants: reliability of perceived, pacifier, and temporal artery temperatures in infants younger than 3 months of age. *Pediatric Emergency Care, 19*(4), 240–243.

Canadian Paediatric Society. (2003). *Temperature measurement in paediatrics.* (Reaffirmed February 2011) Retrieved from http://www.cps.ca/english/statements/CP/cp00-01.htm#Rectal.

Carroll, M. (2000). An evaluation of temperature measurement. *Nursing Standard, 14*(44), 39–43.

Craig, J. V., et al. (2002). Infrared ear thermometry compared with rectal thermometry in children: A systemic review. *Lancet, 360*, 603–609.

Dodd, S. R., et al. (2006). In a systematic review, infrared ear thermometry for fever diagnosis in children finds poor sensitivity. *Journal of Clinical Epidemiology, 59*, 354–357.

El-Radhi, A. S., & Barry, W. (2006). Thermometry in paediatric practice. *Archives of Diseases in Childhood, 91*(4), 351–356.

Falzon, A., et al. (2003). How reliable is axillary temperature measurement? *Acta Paediatrica, 92*(3), 309–313.

Gilbert, M., Barton, A. J., & Counsell, C. M. (2002). Comparison of oral and tympanic temperatures in adult surgical patients. *Applied Nursing Research, 15*(1), 42–47.

EVIDENCE-INFORMED PRACTICE Temperature Measurement in Pediatrics—cont'd

Greenes, D. S., & Fleisher, G. R. (2001). Accuracy of a noninvasive temporal artery thermometer for use in infants. *Archives of Pediatrics and Adolescent Medicine, 155*(3), 376–381.

Greenes, D. S., & Fleisher, G. R. (2004). When body temperature changes, does rectal temperature lag? *Journal of Pediatrics, 144*(6), 824–826.

Hebbar, K., et al. (2005). Comparison of temporal artery thermometer to standard temperature measurement in pediatric intensive care unit patients. *Pediatric Critical Care Medicine, 6*(5), 557–561.

Jean-Mary, M. B., et al. (2002). Limited accuracy and reliability of infrared axillary and aural thermometers in a pediatric outpatient population. *Journal of Pediatrics, 141*(5), 671–676.

Jensen, B. N., et al. (2000). Accuracy of digital tympanic, oral, axillary, and rectal thermometers compared with standard rectal mercury thermometers. *European Journal of Surgery, 166*(11), 848–851.

Martin, S. A., & Kline, A. M. (2004). Can there be a standard for temperature measurement in the pediatric intensive care unit? *AACN Clinical Issues, 15*(2), 254–266.

Muller, P. C. E., Van Berkel, L. H., & de Beaufort, A. J. (2008). Axillary and rectal temperature measurements poorly agree in newborn infants. *Neonatology, 94*, 31–34.

O'Brien, D. L., et al. (2000). The accuracy of oral predictive and infrared emission detection tympanic thermometers in an emergency department setting. *Academy of Emergency Medicine, 7*(9), 1061–1064.

Pidwell, W. B., et al. (2000). Accuracy of temporal artery thermometer (abstract). *Annals of Emergency Medicine, 36*(4), S5.

Riddell, A., & Eppich, W. (2003). *Should tympanic temperature measurement be trusted? BestBETs*. Retrieved from http://www.bestbets.org/cgi-bin/bets.pl?record=00340.

Schuh, S., et al. (2004). Comparison of the temporal artery and rectal thermometry in children in the emergency department. *Pediatric Emergency Care, 20*(11), 736–741.

Siberry, G. K., et al. (2002). Comparison of temple temperatures with rectal temperatures in children under 2 years of age. *Clinical Pediatrics, 41*(6), 405–414.

Tandberg, D., & Sklar, D. (1983). Effect of tachypnea on the estimation of body temperature by an oral thermometer. *New England Journal of Medicine, 308*(16), 945–946.

University of Michigan. (2003). *Rectal temperature is still the gold standard for determining the presence or absence of fever*. Evidence-Based Pediatrics Web site. Retrieved from www.med.umich.edu/pediatrics/ebm/cats/fever.htm.

NURSING ALERT Glass mercury thermometers used in many studies as the "gold standard" are no longer recommended for use (Goldman & Shannon, 2001).

The following thermometers can be used for measuring temperature in infants and children:

Electronic intermittent thermometers—Measure the patient's temperature at oral, rectal, and axillary sites and are used as primary diagnostic indicators.

Infrared thermometers—Measure the patient's temperature by collecting emitted thermal radiation from a particular site (e.g., ear canal)

Electronic continuous thermometers—Measure the patient's temperature during the administration of general anaesthesia, treatment of hypothermia or hyperthermia, and other situations that require continuous monitoring

A detailed description of these devices is found in Box 34-13.

NURSING ALERT The belief that core temperature can be estimated by adding 1°C to the temperature taken in the axilla is incorrect. Do not add a degree to the finding obtained by taking a temperature by the axillary route (Craig et al., 2000).

Pulse

A satisfactory pulse can be taken radially in children older than 2 years of age. However, in infants and young children, the apical impulse (heard through a stethoscope held to the chest at the apex of the heart) is more reliable (see Fig. 34-32 for location of pulses). The pulse is counted for 1 full minute in infants and young children because of possible irregularities in rhythm. However, when frequent apical rates are needed, shorter counting times (e.g., 15- or 30-second intervals) can be used. For greater accuracy, the apical rate is measured while the child is asleep; the nurse should record the child's behaviour along with the rate. Pulses may be graded according to the criteria in Table 34-4. Radial and femoral pulses need to be compared at least once during infancy to detect the presence of circulatory impairment, such as coarctation of the aorta.

Respiration

The respiratory rate in children is measured in the same manner as for the adult patient. However, in newborns and infants, respirations are **auscultated** at the same time as observing the abdomen for movement, since respirations are primarily diaphragmatic. Because the movements are irregular, they should be counted for 1 full minute for accuracy (see also Appendix E).

Blood Pressure

BP measurement by noninvasive methods is part of a routine vital sign determination. BP should be measured annually in children 3 years of age through adolescence and in children with symptoms of hypertension, children in emergency departments and critical care units, and high-risk infants (National High Blood Pressure Education Program Working Group on High Blood Pressure in Children and Adolescents, 2004). Ambulatory BP monitoring in children and adolescents is a valuable method for assessing and managing suspected hypertension (Bald, 2002).

Measurement Devices

BP can also be measured using electronic devices that employ oscillometric or Doppler techniques. In oscillometry, pressure changes are transmitted through the arterial wall to the pressure cuff, and the oscillations are detected by a pressure-sensitive indicator. Oscillometers have digital readouts for systolic, diastolic, and mean arterial pressures (MAP) and for pulse. The MAP is not the same as the mean BP (arithmetic average of systolic and diastolic pressures). Rather, it is a value somewhat lower than the arithmetic mean. BP readings using oscillometry, such as Dinamap, are generally higher (10 mm Hg higher) than measurements using auscultation (Park, Menard, & Schoolfield, 2005) (Table 34-5). Differences between Dinamap and auscultatory readings prevent the interchange of the readings by the two methods. The oscillometric BP monitoring method is a reliable screening tool used in a variety of age groups (Mattu, Heran, & Wright, 2004a, 2004b).

BOX 34-13 Types of Thermometers Used to Measure Temperature in Infants and Children

Electronic Thermometer

Temperature is sensed with an electronic component called a thermistor, which is mounted at the tip of a plastic and stainless steel probe and is connected to an electronic recorder. A disposable plastic cover is used for infection control.

Temperature measurement appears on a digital display within 60 seconds.

Probe can be placed in the mouth, axilla, or rectum.

Infrared Thermometer

Thermal radiation is measured from the axilla, ear canal, or tympanic membrane.

Temperature measurement appears on a digital display in approximately 1 second.

Three types are available for ear-based use: tympanic, ear canal, and arterial heat balance via the ear canal (AHBE).

Often these devices are all inappropriately referred to as tympanic thermometers.

Temperatures measured in this way reflect arterial (bloodstream) temperature.

Ear-Based Temperature Sensor

Although this is frequently used in pediatric settings (especially ambulatory clinics), debate still continues on the reliability of ear-based thermometry in screening febrile children.

Most models use "offsets" for internal calculations that transform ear temperature into supposedly equivalent oral or rectal temperatures.

Ear Sensor (LighTouch LTX)

This measures the infrared heat energy radiating from the canal opening, scans the canal for the highest temperature reading, and then calculates the arterial temperature (which correlates highly with core or internal body temperature).

It is available in two sizes; the smaller size of LighTouch Pedi-Q is for infants and toddlers.

Axillary Sensor (LighTouch LTN)

This measures the infrared heat energy radiating from the axilla.

It can be used on wet skin; in incubators; or under radiant heaters, warming pads, or other heat sources.

Digital Thermometer

Probe is connected to a microprocessor chip, which translates signals into degrees and sends temperature measurement to a digital display.

It is used like an oral electronic thermometer and can be used for measuring oral, rectal, and axillary temperature.

It is more accurate and easier to read, but somewhat more expensive than a plastic strip thermometer.

Liquid Crystal Skin Contact Thermometer (Chemical Dot Thermometer)

This single-use, disposable, flexible thermometer has a specific chemical mixture in each circle that changes colour to measure temperature increments of 2/10 of a degree.

There are two types:

1. Kept in mouth (1 minute), axilla (3 minutes), or rectum (3 minutes); colour change is read 10 to 15 seconds after removing thermometer
2. Wearable, continuous-use thermometer, which is placed in the axilla; may be read within 2 to 3 minutes after placement and continuously thereafter; discard and replace every 48 hours

Table 34-4 Grading of Pulses

GRADE	DESCRIPTION
0	Not palpable
+1	Difficult to palpate, thready, weak, easily obliterated with pressure
+2	Difficult to palpate, may be obliterated with pressure
+3	Easy to palpate, not easily obliterated with pressure (normal)
+4	Strong, bounding, not obliterated with pressure

Table 34-5 Normative Dinamap Blood Pressure Values

	Systolic/Diastolic (Mean Arterial Pressure)		
AGE GROUP	MEAN	90TH PERCENTILE	95TH PERCENTILE
Newborn (1-3 days)	65/41 (50)	75/49 (59)	78/52 (62)
1 mo–2 yr	95/58 (72)	106/68 (83)	110/71 (86)
2–5 yr	101/57 (74)	112/66 (82)	115/68 (85)

(From Park, M., & Menard, S. [1989]. Normative oscillometric blood pressure values in the first 5 years in an office setting. *American Journal of Diseases in Childhood, 143*[7], 860–864.)

Doppler ultrasound translates changes in ultrasound frequency caused by blood movement within the artery to audible sound by means of a transducer in the cuff. This technique is useful for systolic pressure measurement but is unreliable for diastolic pressure measurement. Oscillometric and Doppler instruments are useful in measuring BP in infants and have largely replaced the flush method, which reflects only the mean BP, and the auscultatory method.

Selection of Cuff

No matter what type of noninvasive technique is used, the most important factor in accurately measuring BP is the use of an appropriately sized cuff (cuff size refers only to the inner inflatable bladder, not the cloth covering). A technique to establish an appropriate cuff size is to choose a cuff having a bladder width that is approximately 40% of the arm circumference midway between the olecranon and the acromion. This will usually be a cuff bladder that covers 80 to 100% of the circumference of the arm (Fig. 34-11) (Beevers, Lip, & O'Brien, 2001; National Institutes of Health & National Heart, Lung, and Blood Institute, 1996). Researchers have found that selection of a cuff with a bladder width equal to 40% of the upper arm circumference most accurately reflects

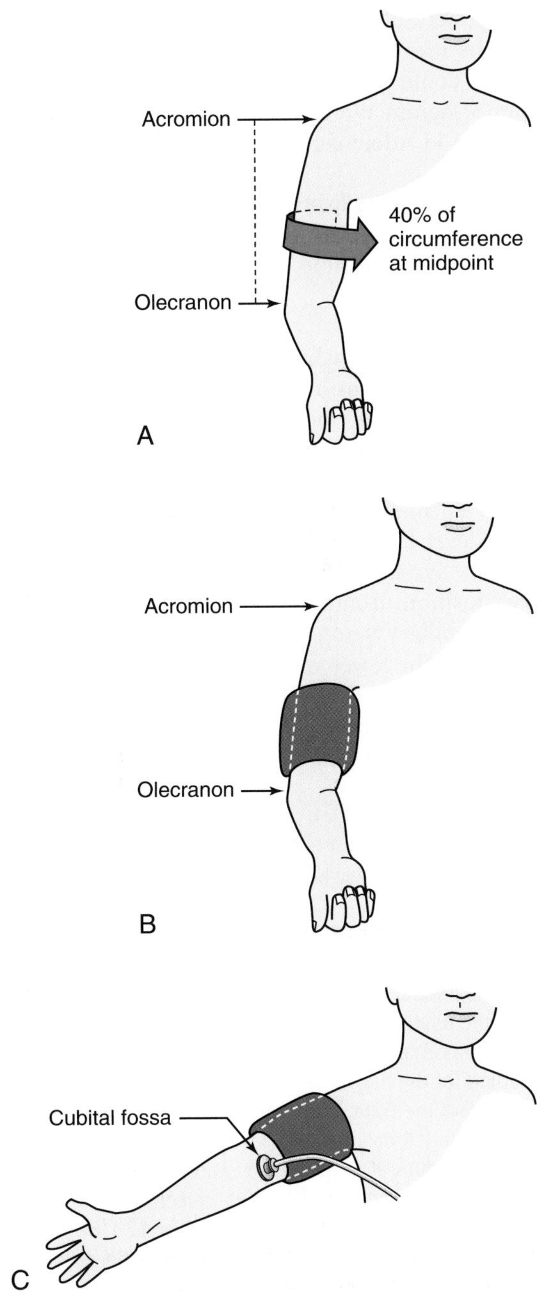

Fig. 34-11 Determination of proper cuff size. **A:** Cuff bladder width should be approximately 40% of circumference of arm measured at a point midway between olecranon and acromion. **B:** Cuff bladder length should cover 80 to 100% of circumference of arm. **C:** Blood pressure should be measured with cubital fossa at heart level. The arm should be supported. The stethoscope bell is placed over brachial artery pulse, proximal and medial to cubital fossa and below bottom edge of cuff. *(From National Institutes of Health, National Heart, Lung, and Blood Institute. [1996, September].* Update on the Task Force Report [1987] on high blood pressure in children and adolescents: A working group report from the National High Blood Pressure Education Program *[NIH Pub No 96-3790]. Bethesda, MD: Author.)*

directly measured radial arterial pressure (Clark et al., 2002) (Table 34-6).

Using limb circumference for selecting cuff width more accurately reflects direct arterial BP than using limb length, since this method takes into account variations in arm thickness and the amount of pressure required to compress the artery (Gillman & Cook, 1995). For measurement sites other than the upper arms, the limb circumference guidelines can be used, although the shape of the limb (e.g., conical shape of the thigh) may prevent appropriate placement of the cuff and inaccurately reflect intra-arterial BP.

Cuffs that are either too narrow or too wide affect the accuracy of BP measurements. If the cuff size is too small, the reading on the device is falsely high. If the cuff size is too large, the reading is falsely low (Clark et al., 2002).

When another site is used, BP measurements using noninvasive techniques may differ. Generally, systolic pressure in the lower extremities (thigh or calf) is greater than pressure in the upper extremities, and systolic BP in the calf is higher than that in the thigh, although diastolic pressure should be similar (Fig. 34-12). These differences are listed in Table 34-7 and apply to oscillometric measurements taken on the right extremities with the child supine and the cuff size, based on the circumference method (Park, Lee, & Johnson, 1993).

Table 34-6 Recommended Dimensions for Blood Pressure Cuff Bladders

AGE RANGE	WIDTH (CM)	LENGTH (CM)	MAXIMUM ARM CIRCUMFERENCE (CM)*
Newborn	4	8	10
Infant	6	12	15
Child	9	18	22
Small adult	10	24	26
Adult	13	30	34
Large adult	16	38	44
Thigh	20	42	52

(From National High Blood Pressure Education Program Working Group on High Blood Pressure in Children and Adolescents. [2004]. The fourth report on the diagnosis, evaluation, and treatment of high blood pressure in children and adolescents. *Pediatrics, 114*[2 Suppl 4th Rep], 555–576.)

*Calculated so that largest arm would still allow bladder to encircle arm by at least 80%.

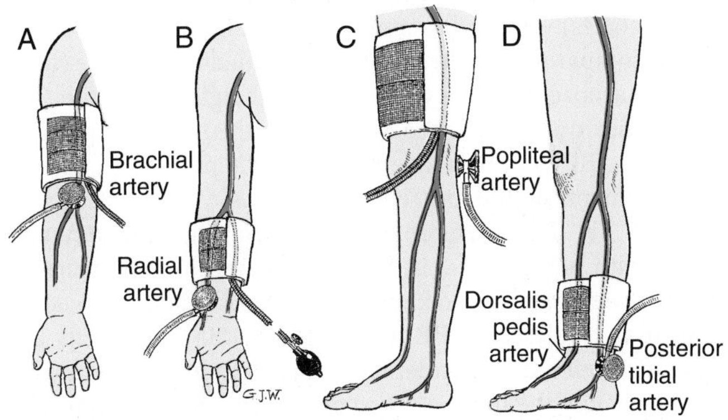

Fig. 34-12 Sites for measuring blood pressure. **A:** Upper arm. **B:** Lower arm or forearm. **C:** Thigh. **D:** Calf or ankle.

Table 34-7 Differences in Oscillometric Systolic Blood Pressure Between Arm and Lower-Extremity Sites in Normal Children

	Systolic Blood Pressure × (Mean ± SD)	
AGE GROUP (YR)	ARM–THIGH	ARM–CALF
4–8	−7.1 ± 6.8	−9.3 ± 7.4
9–16	−2.4 ± 7.7	−5.0 ± 26.9

(From Park, M., Lee, D., & Johnson, G. A. [1993]. Oscillometric blood pressures in the arm, thigh, and calf in healthy children and those with aortic coarctation. *Pediatrics, 91*[4], 761–765.)

NURSING ALERT When taking BP, use an appropriately sized cuff. When the correct size is not available, use an oversized cuff rather than an undersized one or use another site that more appropriately fits the cuff size. Do not choose a cuff based on the name of the cuff (e.g., an "infant" cuff may be too small for some infants). When taking an extremity blood pressure, ensure that the cuff is specific for taking extremity blood pressure measurements.

NURSING ALERT Compare BP in the upper and lower extremities will help detect abnormalities, such as coarctation of the aorta, in which the lower extremity pressure is less than the upper extremity pressure.

Measurement and Interpretation

Measuring and interpreting BP in infants and children requires additional attention to correct procedure because (1) limb sizes vary and cuff selection must accommodate the circumference; (2) excessive pressure on the antecubital fossa affects the Korotkoff sounds; (3) children easily become anxious, which can elevate BP; and (4) BP values change with age and growth. In children and adolescents, the normal range of BP is determined by body size and age. BP standards that are based on gender, age, and height provide a more precise classification of BP according to body size. This approach avoids misclassifying children who are very tall or very short. The revised BP tables now include the fiftieth, ninetieth, ninety-fifth, and ninety-ninth percentiles (with standard deviations) by gender, age, and height (see Appendix E).

To use the tables in a clinical setting, the height percentile is determined by using the newly revised Centers for Disease Control and Prevention growth charts (http://www.cdc.gov/growthcharts). The child's measured systolic BP and diastolic BP are compared with the numbers provided in the table (boys or girls) according to the child's age and height percentile. The child is normotensive if the BP is below the ninetieth percentile. If the BP is at or above the ninetieth percentile, the BP measurement should be repeated at that visit to verify an elevated BP. BP measurements between the ninetieth and ninety-fifth percentiles indicate prehypertension and warrant reassessment and consideration of other risk factors. In addition, if an adolescent's BP is more than 120/80 mm Hg, the patient should be considered prehypertensive even if this value is below the ninetieth percentile. This BP level typically occurs for systolic BP at 12 years old and for diastolic BP at 16 years old. If the child's BP (systolic or diastolic) is at or above the ninety-fifth percentile, the child may be hypertensive, and the measurement must be repeated on at least two occasions to confirm diagnosis (National High Blood Pressure Education Program Working Group on High Blood Pressure in Children and Adolescents, 2004) (see Guidelines box).

NURSING ALERT Published norms for BP, such as those located in Appendix E, are valid only if the same method of measurement (auscultation and cuff size determination) is used in clinical practice.

Orthostatic Hypotension

Orthostatic hypotension (OH), also called *postural hypotension* or *orthostatic intolerance*, is often manifested as syncope (fainting), vertigo (dizziness), or lightheadedness and is caused by decreased blood flow to the brain (cerebral hypoperfusion). Normally, blood flow to the brain is maintained at a constant level by a number of compensating mechanisms that regulate systemic BP. When one assumes a sitting or standing position from a supine or recumbent position, peripheral capillary vasoconstriction occurs, and blood that was pooling in the lower vasculature is returned to the heart for redistribution to the head and remainder of the body. When this mechanism fails or is slow to respond, the person

GUIDELINES Using the Blood Pressure Tables

1. Use the standard height charts to determine the height percentile.
2. Measure and record the child's systolic blood pressure (SBP) and diastolic blood pressure (DBP).
3. Use the correct gender table for SBP and DBP.
4. Find the child's age on the left side of the table. Follow the age row horizontally across the table to the intersection of the line for the height percentile (vertical column).
5. There, find the 50th, 90th, 95th, and 99th percentiles for SBP in the left columns and for DBP in the right columns.
   - BP less than 90th percentile is normal.
   - BP between the 90th and 95th percentile is prehypertension. In adolescents, BP of 120/80 mm Hg or greater is prehypertension, even if this figure is less than the 90th percentile.
   - BP over 95th percentile may be hypertension.
6. If the BP is over the 90th percentile, the BP should be repeated twice at the same office visit, and an average SBP and DBP should be used.
7. If the BP is over the 95th percentile, BP should be staged. If BP is stage 1 (95th to 99th percentile plus 5 mm Hg), BP measurements should be repeated on two more occasions. If hypertension is confirmed, evaluation should proceed. If BP is stage 2 (greater than 99th percentile plus 5 mm Hg), prompt referral should be made for evaluation and therapy. If the patient is symptomatic, immediate referral and treatment are indicated.

(From National High Blood Pressure Education Program Working Group on High Blood Pressure in Children and Adolescents. [2004]. The fourth report on the diagnosis, evaluation, and treatment of high blood pressure in children and adolescents. *Pediatrics, 114*[2 Suppl 4th Rep], 555–576.)

may experience vertigo or syncope. One of the most common causes of OH is hypovolemia, which may be induced by medications such as diuretics, vasodilators, and prolonged immobility or bed rest. Other causes of OH include dehydration, diarrhea, emesis, fluid loss from sweating and exertion, alcohol intake, dysrhythmias, diabetes mellitus, sepsis, and hemorrhage.

BP measurements taken with the child supine then standing (at least 2 minutes in each position) may demonstrate variability and assist in the diagnosis of OH. The child with a sustained drop in systolic pressure of more than 20 mm Hg or in diastolic pressure of more than 10 mm Hg after standing for 2 minutes without an increase in heart rate of more than 15 beats/min most likely has an autonomic deficit. Non-neurogenic causes of OH have a compensatory increase in pulse of more than 15 beats/min as well as a drop in BP, as noted previously. For the child or adolescent who is seen with vertigo, lightheadedness, nausea, syncope, diaphoresis, and pallor, it is important to monitor BP and heart rate to determine the original cause. BP is an important diagnostic measurement in children and adolescents and must be a part of the routine monitoring of vital signs.

General Appearance

The child's general appearance is a cumulative, subjective impression of the child's physical appearance, state of nutrition, behaviour, personality, interactions with parents and nurse (also siblings if present), posture, development, and speech. Although general appearance is recorded at the beginning of the physical examination, it encompasses all the observations of the child during the interview and physical assessment.

The nurse should note the facies (the child's facial expression and appearance). For example, the facies may give clues to children who are in pain; have difficulty breathing; feel frightened, discontented, or unhappy; are mentally deficient; or are acutely ill.

The posture, position, and types of body movement should also be observed. The child with hearing or vision loss may characteristically tilt the head in an awkward position to hear or see better. The child in pain may favour a body part. The child with low self-esteem or a feeling of rejection may assume a slumped, careless, and apathetic pose. Likewise, a child with confidence, a feeling of self-worth, and a sense of security usually demonstrates a tall, straight, well-balanced posture. While observing such body language, the nurse should not interpret too freely but rather record objectively.

The child's hygiene is noted in terms of cleanliness; unusual body odour; the condition of the hair, neck, nails, teeth, and feet; and the condition of the clothing. Such observations are excellent clues to possible instances of neglect, inadequate financial resources, housing difficulties (e.g., no running water), or lack of knowledge concerning children's needs.

Behaviour includes the child's personality, activity level, reaction to stress, requests, frustration, interactions with others (primarily the parent and nurse), degree of alertness, and response to stimuli. Some questions that serve as reminders for observing behaviour include the following: What is the child's overall personality? Does the child have a long attention span, or is he or she easily distracted? Can the child follow two or three commands in succession without the need for repetition? What is the youngster's response to delayed gratification or frustration? Is eye contact used during conversation? What is the child's reaction to the nurse and family members? Is the child quick or slow to grasp explanations?

Development can be assessed by carefully observing the child, but the nurse needs to verify impressions with screening tests. Various tests for assessing development, speech, vision, and hearing are discussed later in this chapter and in Chapter 42.

Under general appearance, the nurse should record an overall estimate of the child's speech development, motor skills, coordination, and recent area of achievement. For example, the following statement may apply to an 18-month-old child: "Motor development advanced for age; climbs, runs, jumps (most recent motor skill), manipulates small objects with ease; excellent coordination and balance; beginning to name many objects; uses two-word phrases; and enjoys 'talking' to self and others."

Skin

Skin is assessed for colour, texture, temperature, moisture, and turgor. Examination of the skin and its accessory organs primarily involves inspection and palpation. Touch allows the nurse to assess the texture, turgor, and temperature of the skin (Turnbull, 2000). The normal colour in light-skinned children varies from a milky white and rose to a deeply hued pink. Dark-skinned children, such as those of Aboriginal, Latin American, or African descent, have inherited various brown, red, yellow, olive green, and bluish tones in their skin. Asian persons have skin that is normally of a yellow tone. Several variations in skin colour can occur, some of which warrant further investigation. The types of colour change and their appearance in children with light or dark skin are summarized in Table 34-8.

Normally the skin texture of young children is smooth, slightly dry, and not oily or clammy. Skin temperature is evaluated by symmetrically feeling each part of the body and comparing upper areas with lower ones. Note any difference in temperature.

Tissue turgor, or elasticity in the skin, can be determined by grasping the skin on the abdomen between the thumb and index finger, pulling it taut, and quickly releasing it. Elastic tissue immediately assumes its normal position without residual marks or creases. In children with poor skin turgor, the skin remains suspended or tented for a few seconds before slowly falling back on the abdomen. Skin turgor is one of the best estimates of adequate hydration and nutrition.

Accessory Structures

Inspection of the accessory structures of the skin may be performed while the skin is being examined or when the scalp and extremities are being assessed.

The hair is inspected for colour, texture, quality, distribution, and elasticity. Children's scalp hair is usually lustrous, silky, strong, and elastic. Genetic factors affect the appearance of hair. For example, the hair of Black children is usually

Table 34-8 Differences in Colour Changes of Racial Groups

DESCRIPTION	APPEARANCE IN LIGHT SKIN	APPEARANCE IN DARK SKIN
Cyanosis—Bluish tone through skin; reflects reduced (deoxygenated) hemoglobin	Bluish tinge, especially in palpebral conjunctiva (lower eyelid), nail beds, earlobes, lips, oral membranes, soles, and palms	Ashen grey lips and tongue
Pallor—Paleness; may be sign of anemia, chronic disease, edema, or shock	Loss of rosy glow in skin, especially face	Ashen grey appearance in black skin More yellowish brown colour in brown skin
Erythema—Redness; may be result of increased blood flow from climatic conditions, local inflammation, infection, skin irritation, allergy, or other dermatoses, or may be caused by increased numbers of red blood cells as compensatory response to chronic hypoxia	Redness easily seen anywhere on body	Much more difficult to assess; rely on palpation for warmth or edema
Ecchymosis—Large, diffuse areas, usually black and blue, caused by hemorrhage of blood into skin; typically result of injuries	Purplish to yellow-green areas; may be seen anywhere on skin	Very difficult to see unless in mouth or conjunctiva
Petechiae—Same as ecchymosis except for size: small, distinct, pinpoint hemorrhages ≤2 mm in size; can denote some type of blood disorder, such as leukemia	Purplish pinpoints most easily seen on buttocks, abdomen, and inner surfaces of arms or legs	Usually invisible except in oral mucosa, conjunctiva of eyelids, and conjunctiva covering eyeball
Jaundice—Yellow staining of skin usually caused by bile pigments	Yellow staining seen in sclerae of eyes, skin, fingernails, soles, palms, and oral mucosa	Most reliably assessed in sclerae, hard palate, palms, and soles

curlier and coarser than that of White children. Hair that is stringy, dull, brittle, dry, friable, and depigmented may suggest poor nutrition. The nurse should record any bald or thinning spots. Loss of hair in infants may indicate lying in the same position and may be a clue for counselling parents concerning the child's stimulation needs.

The hair and scalp are inspected for general cleanliness. Persons in various ethnic groups condition their hair with oils or lubricants that, if not thoroughly washed from the scalp, can clog the sebaceous glands, causing scalp infections. The area should also be examined for lesions; scaliness; evidence of infestation, such as lice or ticks; and signs of trauma, such as ecchymosis, masses, or scars.

In children who are approaching puberty, the nurse should look for growth of secondary hair as a sign of normally progressing pubertal changes. Precocious or delayed appearance of hair growth should be noted because, although not always suggestive of hormonal dysfunction, it may be of great concern to the early- or late-maturing adolescent.

The nails are inspected for colour, shape, texture, and quality. Normally the nails are pink, convex, smooth, and hard but flexible (not brittle). The edges, which are usually white, should extend over the fingers. Dark-skinned individuals may have more deeply pigmented nail beds. Short, ragged nails are typical of habitual biting. Uncut, dirty nails are a sign of poor hygiene.

The palm normally shows three flexion creases (Fig. 34-13, A). In some situations, such as Down syndrome, the two distal horizontal creases are fused to form a single horizontal crease (the single palmar crease, or transpalmar crease, called a *Simian crease*) (see Fig. 34-13, B). If grossly abnormal lines or folds are observed, the nurse should sketch a picture to

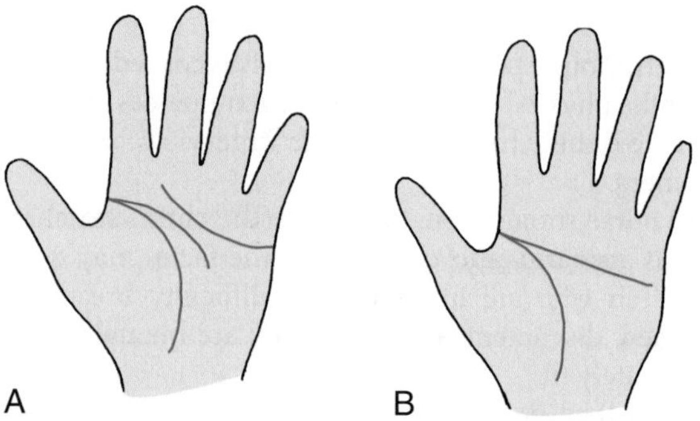

Fig. 34-13 Examples of flexion creases on palm. **A:** Normal. **B:** Transpalmar crease.

describe them and refer the finding to a specialist for further investigation.

Lymph Nodes

Lymph nodes are usually assessed when the part of the body in which they are located is examined. The body's lymphatic drainage system is extensive; the usual sites for palpating accessible lymph nodes are shown in Figure 34-14.

Nodes are palpated using the distal portion of the fingers and gently but firmly pressing in a circular motion along the regions where nodes are normally present. During assessment of the nodes in the head and neck, the child's head is tilted upward slightly but without tensing the sternocleidomastoid or trapezius muscles. This position facilitates palpation of the submental, submandibular, tonsillar, and cervical nodes. The nurse should palpate the axillary nodes with the child's arms relaxed at the sides but slightly abducted. The inguinal nodes

evolve Anatomy Review—Superficial Lymph Nodes

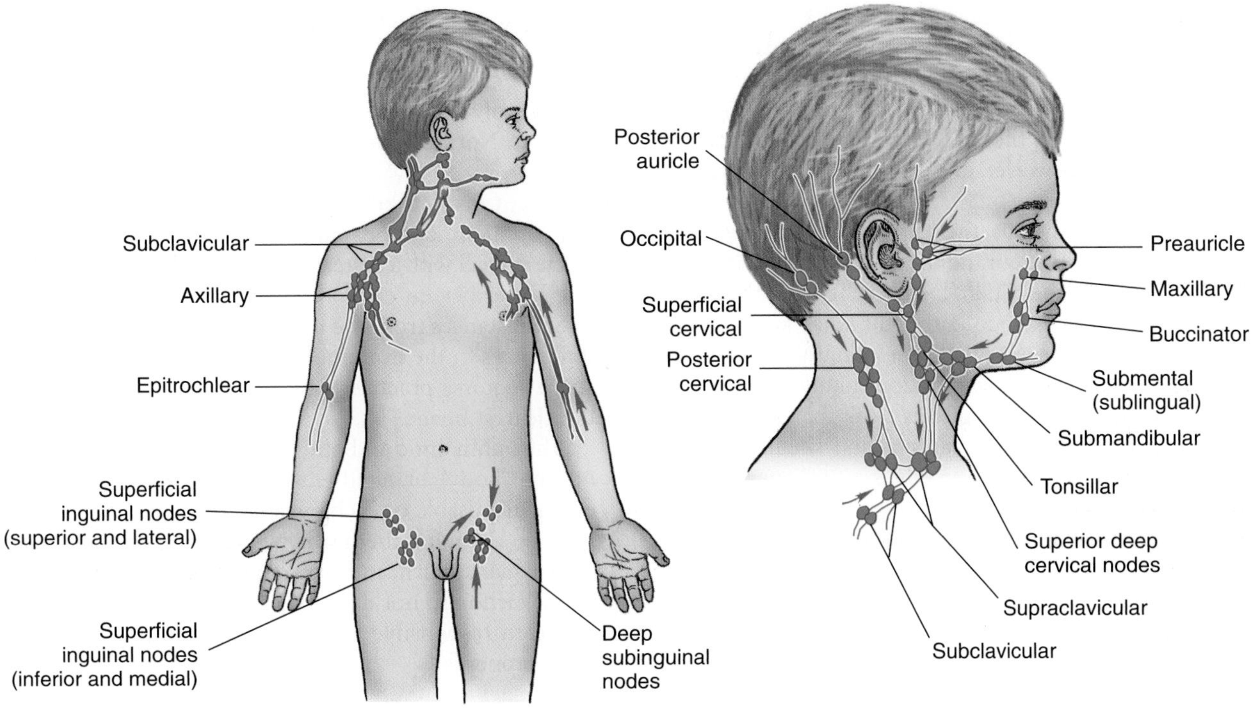

Fig. 34-14 Location of superficial lymph nodes. *Arrows* indicate directional flow of lymph.

are assessed with the child in the supine position. The nurse needs to note size, mobility, temperature, and tenderness, as well as reports by the parents regarding any visible change of enlarged nodes. In children, small, nontender, movable nodes are usually normal. Tender, enlarged, warm lymph nodes generally indicate infection or inflammation close to their location. Such findings need to be reported for further investigation.

Head and Neck

The head is observed for general shape and symmetry. A flattening of one part of the head, such as the occiput, may indicate that the child continually lies in this position. Marked asymmetry is usually abnormal and may indicate premature closure of the sutures (craniosynostosis).

NURSING ALERT Significant head lag after 6 months of age strongly indicates cerebral injury and is referred for further evaluation.

The nurse should note head control in infants and head posture in older children. Most infants by 4 months of age should be able to hold the head erect and in midline when in a vertical position.

Range of motion is evaluated by asking the older child to look in each direction (to either side, up, and down) or by manually putting the younger child through each position. Limited range of motion may indicate wryneck, or torticollis, in which the child holds the head to one side with the chin pointing toward the opposite side as a result of injury to the sternocleidomastoid muscle.

NURSING ALERT Hyperextension of the head (opisthotonos) with pain on flexion is a serious indication of meningeal irritation and needs to be referred for immediate medical evaluation.

The skull is palpated for patent sutures, fontanels, fractures, and swellings. Normally the posterior fontanel closes by the second month of life, and the anterior fontanel fuses between 12 and 18 months of age. Early or late closure should be noted, since either may be a sign of a pathological condition.

While examining the head, the nurse should observe the face for symmetry, movement, and general appearance. Ask the child to "make a face," to assess symmetrical movement and disclose any degree of paralysis. Any unusual facial proportion, such as an unusually high or low forehead; wide- or close-set eyes; or a small, receding chin needs to be noted.

In addition to assessment of the head and neck for movement, the neck is inspected for size and its associated structures palpated. The neck is normally short, with skin folds between the head and shoulders during infancy; however, it lengthens during the next 3 to 4 years.

NURSING ALERT If any masses are detected in the neck, report them for further investigation. Large masses can block the airway.

Eyes

Inspection of External Structures

The lids should be inspected for proper placement on the eye. When the eye is open, the upper lid should fall near the upper evolve Anatomy Review—Structures of the Eye

iris (Fig. 34-15). When the eyes are closed, the lids should completely cover the cornea and sclera.

The general slant of the palpebral fissures or lids is determined by drawing an imaginary line through the two points of the medial canthus and across the outer orbit of the eyes and aligning each eye on the line. Usually the palpebral fissures lie horizontally. However, in Asians the slant is normally upward.

The inside lining of the lids, the palpebral conjunctiva, also needs to be inspected To examine the lower conjunctival sac, pull the lid down while the patient looks up. To evert the upper lid, hold the upper lashes and gently pull *down* and *forward* as the child looks down. Normally the conjunctiva appears pink and glossy. Vertical yellow striations along the edge are the meibomian, or sebaceous, glands near the hair follicle. Located in the inner or medial canthus and situated on the inner edge of the upper and lower lids is a tiny opening, the lacrimal punctum. Any excessive tearing, discharge, or inflammation of the lacrimal apparatus should be noted.

The bulbar conjunctiva, which covers the eye up to the limbus, or junction of the cornea and sclera, should be transparent. The sclera, or white covering of the eyeball, should be clear. Tiny black marks in the sclera of heavily pigmented individuals are normal.

The cornea, or covering of the iris and pupil, should be clear and transparent. The nurse needs to record opacities because they can be signs of scarring or ulceration, which can interfere with vision. The best way to test for opacities is to illuminate the eyeball by shining a light at an angle (obliquely) toward the cornea.

The pupils are compared for size, shape, and movement. They should be round, clear, and equal. Their reaction to light is tested by quickly shining a light toward the eye and removing it. As the light approaches, the pupils should constrict; as the light fades, the pupils should dilate. The pupil is tested for any response of accommodation by having the child look at a bright, shiny object at a distance and quickly moving the object toward the face. The pupils should constrict as the object is brought near the eye. Normal findings on examination of the pupils may be recorded as *PERRLA*, which stands for "*P*upils *E*qual, *R*ound, *R*eact to *L*ight, and *A*ccommodation."

The iris and pupil are inspected for colour, size, shape, and clarity. Permanent eye colour is usually established by 6 to 12 months of age. While inspecting the iris and pupil, look for the lens. Normally the lens is not visible through the pupil.

Inspection of Internal Structures

The ophthalmoscope enables visualization of the interior of the eyeball with a system of lenses and a high-intensity light. The lenses permit clear visualization of eye structures at different distances from the nurse's eye and correct **visual acuity** differences in the examiner and child. Use of the ophthalmoscope requires practice to know which lens setting produces the clearest image.

The ophthalmic and otic heads are usually interchangeable on one "body" or handle, which encloses the power source, either disposable or rechargeable batteries. The nurse should practise changing the heads, which snap on and are secured with a quarter turn, and replacing the batteries and light bulbs. Nurses who are not directly involved in physical assessment are often responsible for ensuring that the equipment functions properly.

Preparing the Child

The nurse can prepare the child for the ophthalmoscopic examination by showing the child the instrument, demonstrating the light source and how it shines in the eye, and explaining the reason for darkening the room. For infants and young children who do not respond to such explanations, it is best to use distraction to encourage them to keep their eyes open. Forcibly parting the lids results in an uncooperative, watery-eyed child and a frustrated nurse. Usually, with some practice, the nurse can elicit a red reflex almost instantly while approaching the child and may also gain a momentary inspection of the blood vessels, macula, or optic disc.

Funduscopic Examination

Figure 34-16 shows the structures of the back of the eyeball, or the *fundus*. The fundus is immediately apparent as the red reflex. The intensity of the colour increases in darkly pigmented individuals.

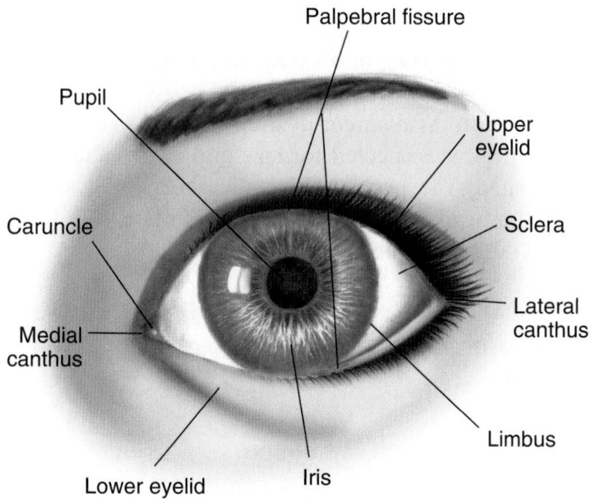

Fig. 34-15 External structures of the eye.

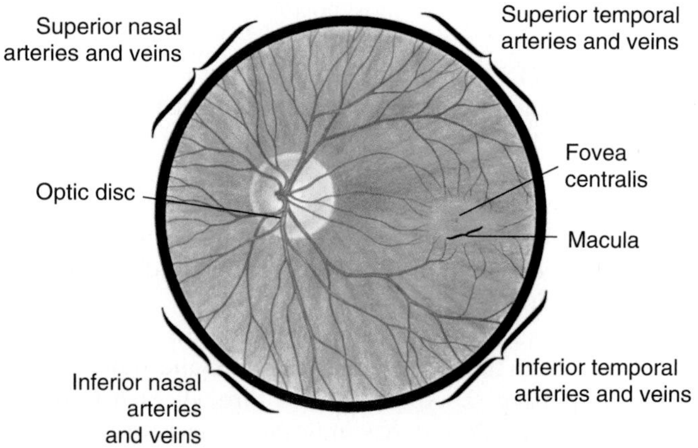

Fig. 34-16 Structures of the fundus. *(Seidel, H. M., et al. [2006].* Mosby's guide to physical examination *[6th ed., p. 296]. St. Louis: Mosby [Fig 11-24].)*

NURSING ALERT A brilliant, uniform red reflex is an important sign because it rules out many serious defects of the cornea, aqueous chamber, lens, and vitreous chamber. Any dark shadows or opacities should be recorded because they indicate some abnormality in any of these structures.

As the ophthalmoscope is brought closer to the eye, the most conspicuous feature of the fundus is the optic disc, the area where the blood vessels and optic nerve fibres enter and exit from the eye. The colour of the disc is creamy pink; it is lighter in colour than the surrounding fundus. Normally it is round or vertically oval.

After the optic disc is located, the area is inspected for blood vessels. The central retinal artery and vein appear in the depths of the disc and emanate outward with visible branching. The veins are darker and about one-fourth larger than the arteries. Normally the branches of the arteries and veins cross one another.

Other structures that may be seen are the macula, the area of the fundus with the greatest concentration of visual receptors; and, in the centre of the macula, a minute glistening spot of reflected light called the fovea centralis, which is the area of most perfect vision.

Vision Testing

Several tests are available for assessing vision. This discussion focuses on four areas: (1) ocular alignment, (2) visual acuity, (3) peripheral vision, and (4) colour vision. Vision screening should be performed at the earliest possible age and at regular intervals. A new survey in Canada has identified that most children under the age of 4 years have yet to visit an optometrist. A common myth is that parents think that children need to be able to read in order to have their eyes examined. Guidelines recommend routine eye examinations starting at the age of 6 months (Canadian Association of Optometrists, 2010; Wall et al., 2002). Behavioural and physical signs of visual impairment are discussed in Chapter 42.

Ocular Alignment

Normally, by the age of 3 to 4 months, children are able to fixate on one visual field with both eyes simultaneously (binocularity). One of the most important tests for binocularity is alignment of the eyes to detect nonbinocular vision, or strabismus (Halle, 2002). In **strabismus**, or cross-eye, one eye deviates from the point of fixation. If the misalignment is constant, the weak eye becomes "lazy," and the brain eventually suppresses the image produced by that eye. If strabismus is not detected and corrected by ages 4 to 6 years, blindness from disuse, known as **amblyopia**, may result.

Tests commonly used to detect misalignment are the corneal light reflex and the cover tests. To perform the corneal light reflex test, or Hirschberg test, shine a flashlight or the light of the ophthalmoscope directly into the patient's eyes from a distance of about 40.5 cm. If the eyes are orthophoric, or normal, the light falls symmetrically within each pupil (Fig. 34-17, A). If the light falls off centre in one eye, the eyes are misaligned. Epicanthal folds, excess folds of skin that extend from the roof of the nose to the inner termination of the eyebrow and that partially or completely overlap the inner canthus of the eye, may give a false impression of misalignment (pseudostrabismus) (see Fig. 34-17, B). Epicanthal folds are often found in Asian children.

In the cover test, one eye is covered, and the movement of the *uncovered* eye is observed while the child looks at a near (33 cm) or distant (6 m) object. If the uncovered eye does not move, it is aligned. If the uncovered eye moves, a misalignment is present because, when the stronger eye is temporarily covered, the misaligned eye attempts to fixate on the object.

In the alternate-cover test, occlusion shifts back and forth from one eye to the other, and movement of the eye that was covered is observed as soon as the occluder is removed while the child focuses on a point in front of him or her (Fig. 34-18). If normal alignment is present, shifting the cover from one eye to the other will not cause the eye to move. If misalignment is present, eye movement will occur when the cover is moved. This test takes more practice to perform than the other cover test because the occluder must be moved back and forth quickly and accurately to see the eye move. Because deviations can occur at different ranges, it is important to perform the cover tests at both close and far distances.

NURSING ALERT The cover test is usually easier to perform if the examiner uses his or her own hand rather than

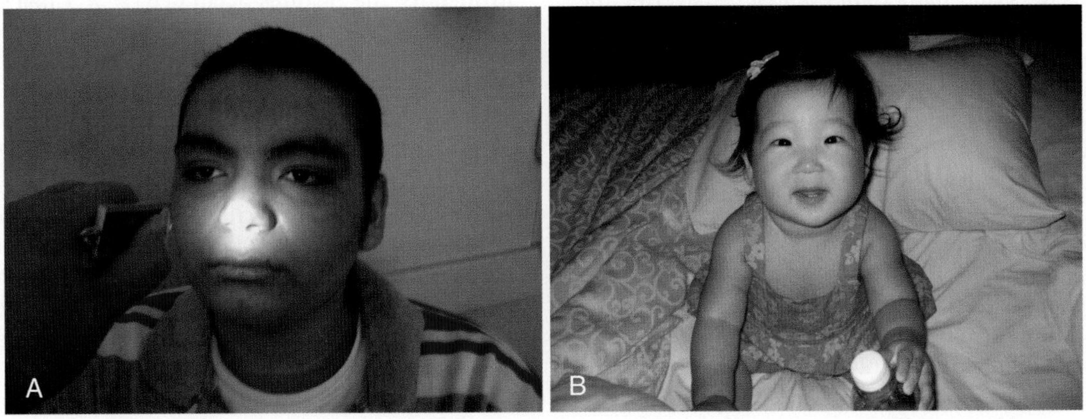

Fig. 34-17 **A:** Corneal light reflex test demonstrating orthophoric eyes. **B:** Pseudostrabismus. Inner epicanthal folds cause eyes to appear misaligned; however, corneal light reflexes fall perfectly symmetrically.

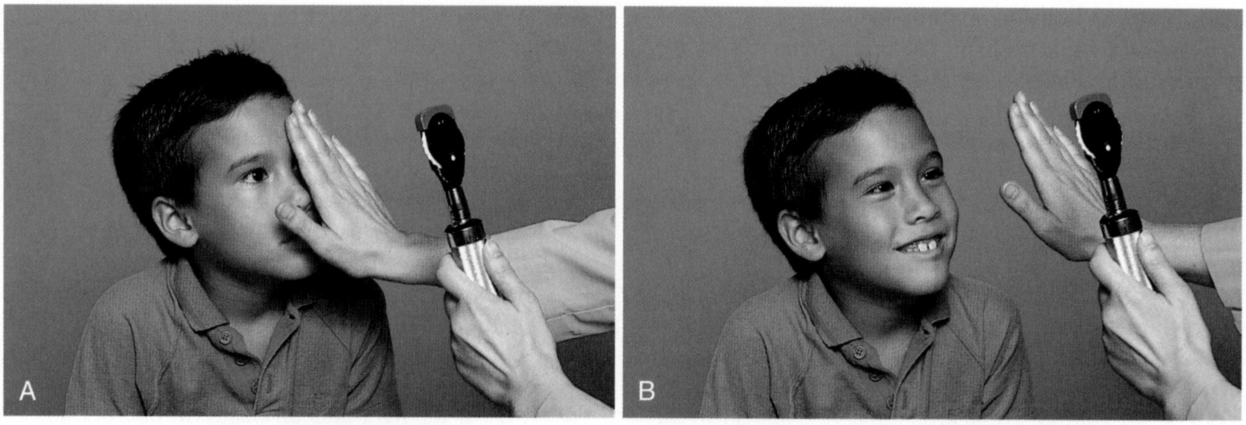

Fig. 34-18 Alternate-cover test to detect amblyopia in patient with strabismus. **A:** Eye is occluded, and child is fixating on light source. **B:** If eye does not move when uncovered, eyes are aligned.

a card-type occluder (see Fig. 34-18). Attractive occluders fashioned like an ice cream cone or happy-face lollipop cut from cardboard are also well received by young children.

Photoscreening is a technique used to screen for amblyopia, refractive disorders, and media opacities (AAP, Committee on Practice and Ambulatory Medicine, Section on Ophthalmology, 2003; Berry et al., 2001). Using a camera, the nurse obtains images of the pupillary reflexes (reflections) and red reflexes (Bruckner test) (AAP, Committee on Practice and Ambulatory Medicine, Section on Ophthalmology, 2003). Photoscreening offers an effective way to screen infants, preverbal children, and those with developmental delays who are difficult to screen.

Visual Acuity Testing in Children Beyond Infancy

The most common test for measuring visual acuity is the Snellen letter chart, which consists of lines of letters of decreasing size (see the Evolve site). The American Academy of Pediatrics, Committee on Practice and Ambulatory Medicine, Section on Ophthalmology (2003) recommends that during testing, children stand 3 metres from the chart with their heels at the 3-metre line. When screening for visual acuity in children, the nurse tests the child's right eye first by covering the left. Children who wear glasses should be screened with them on. Tell the child to keep both eyes open during the examination. If the child fails to read the current line, move up the chart to the next larger line. Continue up the chart until a line is found that the child can pass. Then begin moving down the chart again until the child fails to read the line. To pass each line, the child must correctly identify four of six symbols on the line. Repeat the procedure, covering the right eye. Table 34-9 provides a list of visual screening tests for children and guidelines for referral recommended by the American Academy of Pediatrics, Committee on Practice and Ambulatory Medicine, Section on Ophthalmology (2003). The Canadian Paediatric Society (2009) recommends using the same guidelines.

For children unable to read letters and numbers, the tumbling E or HOTV test is useful (Coats & Jenkins, 1997). The tumbling E test uses the capital letter E pointing in four different directions. The child is asked to point in the direction that the E is facing. The HOTV test consists of a wall chart composed of the letters H, O, T, and V. The child is given a board containing a large H, O, T, and V. The examiner points to a letter on the wall chart, and the child matches the correct letter on the board held in his or her hand. The tumbling E and HOTV tests are excellent tests for preschool-age children.

When a child is unable to perform the tumbling E or HOTV test, the LEA symbol or Allen card test may be used. The Allen card test uses common figures to test the child's vision. It is important to assess whether the child is able to identify the pictures before actual vision testing. The examiner walks backward slowly, flipping through the cards and presenting different pictures to the child. The examiner continues to move backward as the child correctly calls out the figures. When the child begins to miss the figure on the cards, the examiner moves forward to confirm that the child is able to identify the figures at that point. All Allen card figures are 20/30 in size. The farthest distance at which the child is able to accurately identify the pictures becomes the numerator, and 30 becomes the denominator. For example, if the child is able to identify the pictures accurately at 4.5 metres, the visual acuity is recorded as 15/30. This is equivalent to 20/40 or 10/20 visual acuity.

Visual Acuity Testing in Infants and Difficult-to-Test Children

In newborns, vision is tested mainly by checking for light perception by shining a light into the eyes and noting responses such as pupillary constriction, blinking, following the light to midline, increased alertness, or refusal to open the eyes after exposure to the light. Although the simple manoeuvre of checking light perception and eliciting the pupillary light reflex indicates that the anterior half of the visual apparatus is intact, it does not confirm that the infant can see. In other words, this test does not assess whether the brain receives the visual message and interprets the signals.

Another test of visual acuity is the infant's ability to fix on and follow a target. Although any brightly coloured or

Table 34-9 Eye Examination Guidelines*

FUNCTION	RECOMMENDED TESTS	REFERRAL CRITERIA	COMMENTS
Ages 3–5 Yr			
Distance visual acuity	Snellen letters Snellen numbers Tumbling E HOTV test Picture test • Allen figures • LEA symbols	1. Fewer than 4 of 6 correct on 6-m line with either eye tested at 3 m monocularly (i.e., <10/20 or 20/40) or 2. Two-line difference between eyes, even within passing range (i.e., 10/12.5 and 10/20 or 20/25 and 20/40)	1. Tests are listed in decreasing order of cognitive difficulty; highest test that child is capable of performing should be used; in general, tumbling E or HOTV test should be used for children 3–5 yr of age and Snellen letters or numbers for children 6 yr and older. 2. Testing distance of 3 m is recommended for all visual acuity tests. 3. Line of figures is preferred over single figures. 4. Nontested eye should be covered by occluder held by examiner or by adhesive occluder patch applied to eye; examiner must ensure that it is not possible to peek with nontested eye.
Ocular alignment	Cross cover test at 3 m Random dot E stereo test at 40 cm Simultaneous red reflex test (Bruckner test)	Any eye movement Fewer than 4 of 6 correct Any asymmetry of pupil colour, size, brightness	Child must be fixing on a target while cross cover test is performed. Use direct ophthalmoscope to view both red reflexes simultaneously in a darkened room from 60–90 cm away; detects asymmetrical refractive errors as well.
Ocular media clarity (cataracts, tumours, etc.)	Red reflex	White pupil, dark spots, absent reflex	Use direct ophthalmoscope in a darkened room. View eyes separately at 30–45 cm; white reflex indicates possible retinoblastoma.
6 Yr and Older			
Distance visual acuity	Snellen letters Snellen numbers Tumbling E HOTV test Picture test • Allen figures • LEA symbols	1. Fewer than 4 of 6 correct on 4.5-m line with either eye tested at 3 m monocularly (i.e., <10/15 or 20/30) or 2. Two-line difference between eyes, even within the passing range (i.e., 10/10 and 10/15 or 20/20 and 20/30)	1. Tests are listed in decreasing order of cognitive difficulty; highest test that child is capable of performing should be used; in general, tumbling E or HOTV test should be used for children 3–5 yr of age and Snellen letters or numbers for children 6 yr and older. 2. Testing distance of 3 m is recommended for all visual acuity tests. 3. Line of figures is preferred over single figures. 4. Nontested eye should be covered by occluder held by examiner or by adhesive occluder patch applied to eye; examiner must ensure that it is not possible to peek with nontested eye.
Ocular alignment	Cross cover test at 3 m Random dot E stereo test at 40 cm Simultaneous red reflex test (Bruckner test)	Any eye movement Fewer than 4 of 6 correct Any asymmetry of pupil colour, size, brightness	Child must be fixing on target while cross cover test is performed. Use direct ophthalmoscope to view both red reflexes simultaneously in a darkened room from 60–90 cm away; detects asymmetrical refractive errors as well.
Ocular media clarity (cataracts, tumours, etc.)	Red reflex	White pupil, dark spots, absent reflex	Use direct ophthalmoscope in a darkened room. View eyes separately at 30–45 cm; white reflex indicates possible retinoblastoma.

(From American Academy of Pediatrics, Committee on Practice and Ambulatory Medicine, Section on Ophthalmology. [1996]. Eye examination in infants, children, and young adults. *Pediatrics 98:* 1, 153–157.)

*The Canadian Paediatric Society has adapted these guidelines to be used by physicians, nurses, educational institutions, public health departments, and other health care providers who perform vision evaluation services.

patterned object can be used, the human face is excellent. Hold the infant upright while moving your face slowly from side to side.

NURSING ALERT If visual fixation and following are not present by 3 to 4 months of age, further ophthalmological evaluation is needed.

Other signs that may indicate visual loss or other serious eye problems include fixed pupils, strabismus, constant nystagmus, the setting-sun sign, and slow lateral movements. Unfortunately, it is difficult to test each eye separately; the presence of such signs in one eye could indicate unilateral blindness.

Special tests are available for testing infants and other difficult-to-test children to assess acuity or confirm blindness. For example, in visually evoked potentials, the eyes are stimulated with a bright light or pattern, and electrical activity to the visual cortex is recorded through scalp electrodes. Acuity is assessed by using progressively smaller patterns.

evolve Anatomy Review—Landmarks of the Pinna

Peripheral Vision

In children who are old enough to cooperate, peripheral vision, or the visual field of each eye, can be estimated by having the children fixate on a specific point directly in front of them as an object, such as a finger or a pencil, is moved from beyond the field of vision into the range of peripheral vision. Each eye is checked separately and for each quadrant of vision. As soon as children see the object, they should say "stop." At that point, the examiner measures the angle from the anteroposterior axis of the eye (straight line of vision) to the peripheral axis (point at which the object is first seen). Normally, children see about 50 degrees upward, 70 degrees downward, 60 degrees nasalward, and 90 degrees temporally. Limitations in peripheral vision may indicate blindness from damage to structures within the eye or to any of the visual pathways.

Colour Vision

Another important test is for colour vision. It is estimated that 8 to 10% of White males and less than half that percentage of Black males inherit the X-linked disorder known as *colour vision deficit* (also known as *colour blindness*, a less acceptable term). From 0.5 to 1% of White females are affected. Although the severity of impaired perception of colour varies considerably, the two most common types are *protanomaly*, in which the child confuses grey with pink or pale blue with green, and *deuteranomaly*, in which the child confuses grey with pale purple or green. In most of these individuals the colour vision deficit causes no major problems. However, some individuals with more severe deficits may be unable to distinguish amber or red traffic lights, fail to see a red brake light on the rear of a car, have difficulty distinguishing green traffic lights from certain types of incandescent street lamps, and have a poor sense of colour coordination of clothing. For school-age children, the greatest difficulty lies in performance of academic skills that use colour as a visual aid. Adolescents may be ineligible for certain vocational opportunities, such as electronics, photography, printing, interior decorating, pharmaceuticals, textiles, police work, and several types of military service.

The tests available for colour vision include the Ishihara test and the Hardy-Rand-Rittler test. Each consists of a series of cards (pseudoisochromatic) on which is printed a colour field composed of spots of a certain "confusion" colour. Against the field is a number or symbol similarly printed in dots but of a colour likely to be confused with the field colour by the person with a colour vision deficit. As a result, the figure or letter is invisible to an affected individual but is clearly seen by a person with normal vision.

Ears

Inspection of External Structures

The entire external earlobe is called the *pinna*, or *auricle*; one is located on each side of the head. The height alignment of the pinna is measured by drawing an imaginary line from the outer orbit of the eye to the occiput, or most prominent protuberance of the skull. The top of the pinna should meet or cross this line. Low-set ears are commonly associated with renal anomalies or cognitive impairment. The angle of the pinna is measured by drawing a perpendicular line from the imaginary horizontal line and aligning the pinna next to this mark. Normally, the pinna lies within a 10-degree angle of the vertical line (Fig. 34-19) (see also Table 24-2, p. 631). If it falls outside this area, the nurse should record the deviation and look for other anomalies.

Normally the pinnae extend slightly outward from the skull. Except in newborn infants, ears that are flat against the head or protruding away from the scalp may indicate problems. Flattened ears in an infant may suggest a frequent side-lying position and, just as with isolated areas of hair loss, may indicate a need to investigate parents' understanding of the child's stimulation needs.

The skin surface around the ear should be inspected for small openings, extra tags of skin, or sinuses. If a sinus is found, the nurse should note this because it may represent a fistula that drains into some area of the neck or ear. Cutaneous tags represent no pathological process but may cause parents concern in terms of the child's appearance.

The ear should also be assessed for hygiene. An otoscope is not necessary for looking into the external canal to note

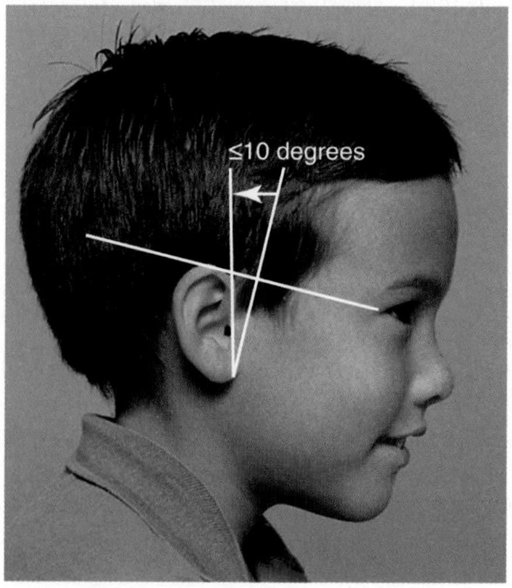

Fig. 34-19 Ear alignment.

the presence of cerumen, a waxy substance produced by the ceruminous glands in the outer portion of the canal. Cerumen is usually yellow-brown and soft. If an otoscope is used and any discharge is seen, its colour and odour are noted. Avoid transmitting potentially infectious material to the other ear or to another child through hand washing and using disposable specula or sterilizing reusable specula between each examination.

Inspection of Internal Structures

The head of the otoscope enables visualization of the tympanic membrane by use of a bright light, a magnifying glass, and a speculum. Some otoscopes have an attachment for a pneumonic device to insert air into the canal to determine membrane compliance (movement). The speculum, which is inserted into the external canal, comes in a variety of sizes to accommodate different canal widths. The largest speculum that fits comfortably into the ear is used to achieve the greatest area of visualization. The lens, or magnifying glass, is movable, allowing the examiner to insert an object, such as a curette, into the ear canal through the speculum while still viewing the structures through the lens.

Positioning the Child

Before the start of the otoscopic examination, the child should be positioned properly and restrained, if necessary. Older children are usually able to assist. However, the nurse should prepare them for the procedure by allowing them to play with the instrument, demonstrating how it works, and stressing the importance of remaining still. It may be helpful to have them observe the nurse examining the parent's ear. Restraint is needed for younger children because the ear examination upsets them (see Atraumatic Care box).

As the speculum is inserted into the meatus, move it around the outer rim to accustom the child to the feel of something entering the ear. If examining a painful ear, touch a nonpainful part of the affected ear, then examine the unaffected ear, and finally return to the painful ear. By this time the child is usually less fearful of anything causing discomfort to the ear and will cooperate more.

For their protection and safety, infants and toddlers must be restrained for the otoscopic examination. There are two general positions of restraint. In one, the child is seated sideways in the parent's lap with one arm hugging the parent and the other arm at the side. The ear to be examined is toward the nurse. With one arm, the parent holds the child's head firmly against his or her chest, and with the other arm hugs the child, thereby securing the child's free arm (Fig. 34-20, A). The ear is examined using the same procedure for holding the otoscope as described in the discussion that follows.

The other position involves placing the child on the side, back, or abdomen with the arms at the side and the head turned so that the ear to be examined points toward the ceiling. The examiner leans over the child, uses the upper part of the body to restrain the arms and upper trunk movements, and uses the examining hand to stabilize the head. This position is practical for young infants or for older children who need minimum restraint, but it may not be feasible for other children who protest vigorously. For safety, enlist the parent's or an assistant's help in immobilizing the head by firmly placing one hand above the ear and the other on the child's side, abdomen, or back (see Fig. 34-20, B).

With children who are able to help, the ear is examined with the child in a side-lying, sitting, or standing position. One disadvantage to standing is that the child may "walk away" as the otoscope enters the canal. If the child is standing or sitting, tilt the head slightly toward the child's opposite shoulder to achieve a better view of the drum (Fig. 34-21).

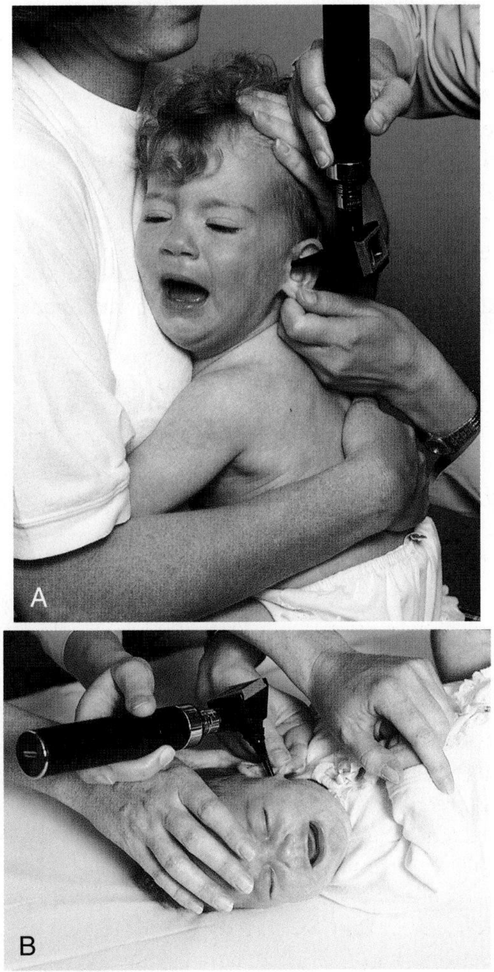

Fig. 34-20 Position for restraining child (A) and infant (B) during otoscopic examination.

ATRAUMATIC CARE

Reducing Distress from Otoscopy in Young Children

Make examining the ear a game by explaining that you are looking for a "big elephant" in the ear. This kind of make-believe is an absorbing distraction and usually elicits cooperation. After examining the ear, clarify that "looking for elephants" was only pretend and thank the child for letting you look in his or her ear. Another great distraction technique is asking the child to put a finger on the opposite ear to keep the light from getting out.

evolve Anatomy Review—External, Middle, and Inner Ear

With the thumb and forefinger of the free (usually non-dominant) hand, grasp the auricle. For the two positions of restraint, hold the otoscope upside down at the junction of its head and handle with the thumb and index finger. Place the other fingers against the skull to allow the otoscope to move with the child in case of sudden movement. In examining a child who is helpful, hold the handle with the otic head upright or upside down. Use the dominant hand to examine both ears or reverse hands for each ear, whichever is more comfortable.

Before using the otoscope, visualize the external ear and the tympanic membrane as being superimposed on a clock (Fig. 34-22). The numbers become important geographic landmarks. Introduce the speculum into the meatus between the 3 and 9 o'clock positions in a *downward* and *forward* position. Because the canal is curved, the speculum does not permit a panoramic view of the tympanic membrane unless the canal is straightened. In infants the canal curves upward. Therefore, pull the pinna *down* and *back* to the 6 to 9 o'clock range to straighten the canal (Fig. 34-23, A).

With older children, usually those older than 3 years of age, the canal curves downward and forward. Therefore, pull the pinna *up* and *back* toward a 10 o'clock position (see Fig. 34-23, B). If you have difficulty visualizing the membrane, try repositioning the head, introducing the speculum at a different angle, and pulling the pinna in a slightly different direction. Do not insert the speculum past the cartilaginous (outermost) portion of the canal, usually a distance of 0.60 to 1.25 cm in older children. Insertion of the speculum into the posterior or bony portion of the canal causes pain.

In neonates and young infants, the walls of the canal are pliable and floppy because of the underdeveloped cartilaginous and bony structures. Therefore, the very small 2-mm speculum usually needs to be inserted deeper into the canal

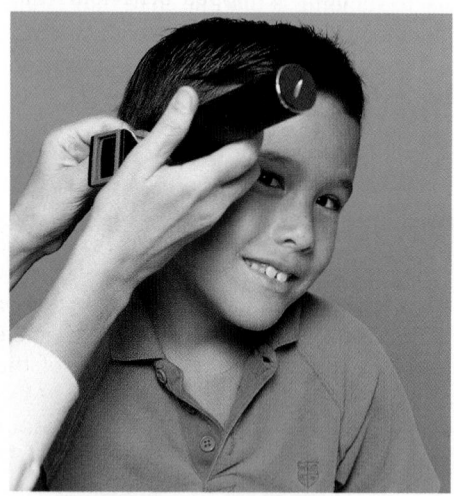

Fig. 34-21 Positioning head by tilting it toward opposite shoulder for full view of tympanic membrane.

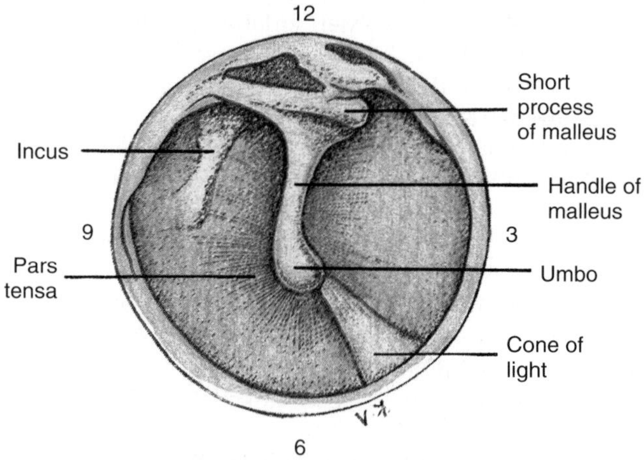

Fig. 34-22 Landmarks of tympanic membrane with "clock" superimposed. *(Adapted from Potter, P. A. & Perry, A. G. [2006]. Basic nursing: Essentials for practice [6th ed.]. St. Louis: Mosby.)*

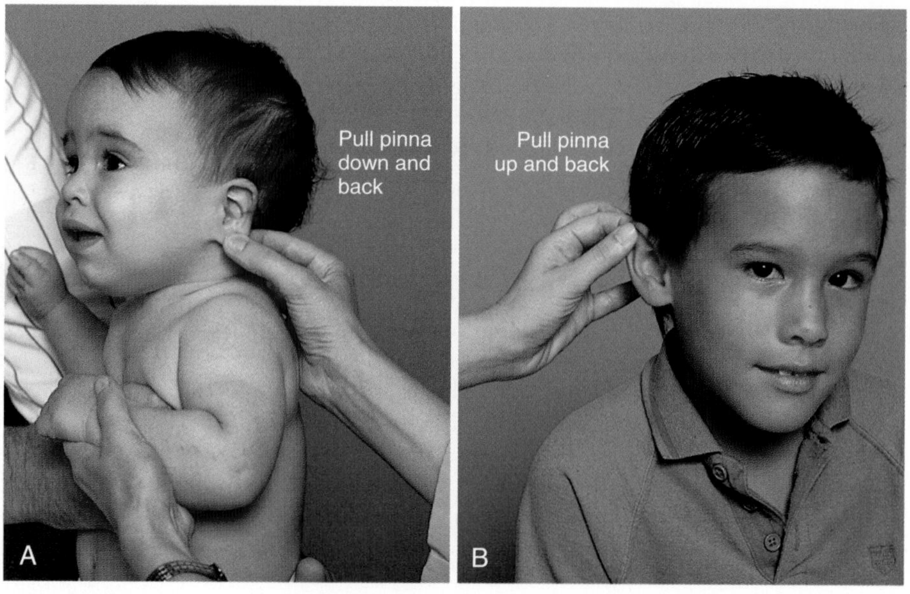

Fig. 34-23 Positioning for visualizing eardrum in infant **(A)** and in child older than 3 years of age **(B)**.

than in older children. Great care must be exercised not to damage the walls or drum. For this reason, only an experienced examiner should insert an otoscope into the ears of very young infants.

Otoscopic Examination

As the speculum is introduced into the external canal, the examiner inspects the walls of the canal, the colour of the tympanic membrane, the light reflex, and the usual landmarks of the bony prominences of the middle ear. The walls of the external auditory canal are pink, although they are more pigmented in dark-skinned children. Minute hairs are evident in the outermost portion, where cerumen is produced. Note signs of irritation, foreign bodies, or infection.

Foreign bodies in the ear are not uncommon in children and range from erasers to beans. Symptoms may include pain, discharge, and affected hearing. Soft objects, such as paper or insects, can be removed with forceps. Small, hard objects, such as pebbles, can be removed with a suction tip, a hook, or irrigation. However, irrigation is contraindicated if the object is vegetative matter, such as beans or pasta, which swells when in contact with fluid.

The tympanic membrane is a translucent, light pearly pink or grey. Marked erythema (which may indicate suppurative otitis media), a dull nontransparent greyish colour (sometimes suggestive of serous otitis media), or ashen grey areas (signs of scarring from a previous perforation) should be noted. A black area usually suggests a perforation of the membrane that has not healed.

The characteristic tenseness and slope of the tympanic membrane cause the light of the otoscope to reflect at about the 5 or 7 o'clock position. The light reflex is a fairly well-defined, cone-shaped reflection, which normally points away from the face.

The bony landmarks of the drum are formed by the umbo, or tip of the malleus. It appears as a small, round, opaque, concave spot near the centre of the drum. The manubrium (long process or handle) of the malleus appears to be a whitish line extending from the umbo upward to the margin of the membrane. At the upper end of the long process near the 1 o'clock position (in the right ear) is a sharp, knoblike protuberance, representing the short process of the malleus. Note the absence of the light reflex or loss or abnormal prominence of any of these landmarks.

Auditory Testing

Several types of hearing tests are available and recommended for screening in infants and children (AAP, Committee on Practice and Ambulatory Medicine, Section on Otolaryngology and Bronchoesophagology, 2003; CPS, 2008) (Table 34-10). Many provinces have mandatory hearing screening for newborns prior to discharge in order to detect hearing loss. The nurse must have a high index of suspicion for those children who appear to have conditions associated with hearing loss and who may have developed behaviours that indicate auditory impairment (Cunningham & Cox, 2003).

Nose

Inspection of External Structures

The nose is located in the middle of the face just below the eyes and above the lips. Its placement and alignment are compared by drawing an imaginary vertical line from the centre point between the eyes down to the notch of the upper lip. The nose should be directly centred on this line, with each side exactly symmetrical. Its location, any deviation to one side, and asymmetry in overall size and in diameter of the nares (nostrils) should be noted. The bridge of the nose is sometimes flat in Asian and Black children. Observe the alae nasi for any sign of flaring, which indicates respiratory difficulty. The nurse should always report any flaring of the alae nasi.

evolve Anatomy Review—External and Internal Structures of the Nose

Table 34-10 Audiological Tests for Infants and Children

AGE	AUDITORY TEST AND AVERAGE TIME	TYPE OF MEASUREMENT	PROCEDURE
All ages	Evoked otoacoustic emissions, 10-min test	Physiological test specifically measuring cochlear (outer hair cell) response to presentation of stimulus	Small probe containing sensitive microphone is placed in ear canal for stimulus delivery and response detection
Birth–9 mo	Auditory brainstem response, 15-min test	Electrophysiological measurement of activity in auditory nerve and brainstem pathways	Placement of electrodes on child's head detects auditory stimuli presented though earphones one ear at a time
9 mo–2½ yr	Conditioned oriented responses or visual reinforced audiometry, 30-min test	Behavioural tests measuring child's responses to speech and frequency-specific stimuli presented through speakers	Both techniques condition child to associate speech or frequency-specific sound with reinforcement stimulus, such as a lighted toy
2½–4 yr	Play audiometry, 30-min test	Behavioural test measuring auditory thresholds in response to speech and frequency-specific stimuli presented through earphones and/or bone vibrator	Child is conditioned to put peg in peg board or drop block in a box when stimulus tone is heard
4 yr–adolescence	Conventional audiometry, 30-min test	Behavioural test measuring auditory thresholds in response to speech and frequency-specific stimuli presented through earphone and/or bone vibrator	Patient is instructed to raise hand when stimulus is heard

(Modified with permission from Bachmann, K. R., & Arvedson, J. C. [1998]. Early identification and intervention for children who are hearing impaired. *Pediatrics in Review, 19*[5], 155–165.)

Figure 34-24 illustrates the landmarks used in describing the external structures of the nose.

Inspection of Internal Structures

The anterior vestibule of the nose is inspected by pushing the tip upward, tilting the head backward, and illuminating the cavity with a flashlight or otoscope without the attached ear speculum. The colour of the mucosal lining should be noted, which is normally redder than the oral membranes, as well as any swelling, discharge, dryness, or bleeding. There should be no discharge from the nose.

On looking deeper into the nose, the nurse should inspect the turbinates, or concha, plates of bone that jut into the nasal cavity and are enveloped by mucous membrane. The turbinates greatly increase the surface area of the nasal cavity as air is inhaled. The spaces or channels between the turbinates are called the *meatus* and correspond to each of the three turbinates. Normally the front end of the inferior and middle turbinate and the middle meatus are seen. They should be the same colour as the lining of the vestibule.

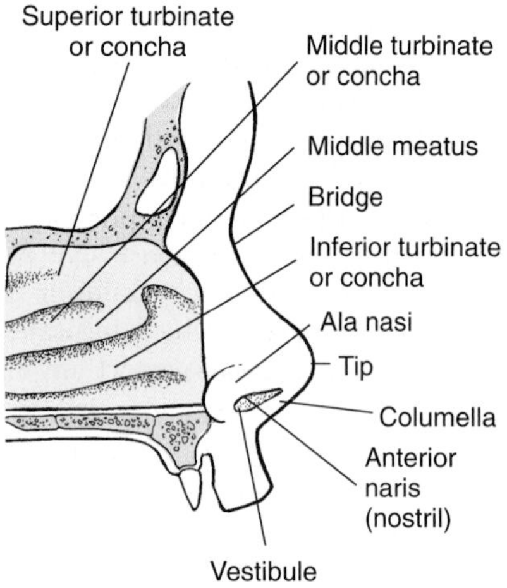

Fig. 34-24 External landmarks and internal structures of the nose.

evolve Anatomy Review—Interior Structures of the Mouth

The septum is also inspected, which should divide the vestibules equally. Any deviation should be noted, especially if it causes an occlusion of one side of the nose. A perforation may be evident within the septum. If this is suspected, shine the light of the otoscope into one naris and look for admittance of light to the other. Because olfaction is an important function of the nose, testing for smell may be done at this point or as part of the cranial nerve assessment (see Table 34-13).

Mouth and Throat

With a child who is helpful, almost the entire examination of the mouth and throat can be accomplished without the use of a tongue blade. Ask the child to open the mouth wide; to move the tongue in different directions for full visualization; and to say "ahh," which depresses the tongue for full view of the back of the mouth (tonsils, uvula, and oropharynx) (Fig. 34-25, B). For a closer look at the buccal mucosa, or lining of the cheeks, ask children to use their fingers to move the outer lip and cheek to one side (see Atraumatic Care box).

Infants and toddlers usually resist attempts to keep the mouth open. Because inspection of the mouth is upsetting, it should be left for the end of the physical examination (along with examination of the ears) or done during episodes of crying. However, the use of a tongue blade (preferably

> **ATRAUMATIC CARE**
>
> ***Encouraging Opening the Mouth for Examination***
>
> - Perform the examination in front of a mirror.
> - Let the child first examine someone else's mouth, such as in the parent, the nurse, or a puppet (see Fig. 34-25, A), and then examine the child's mouth.
> - Instruct the child to tilt the head back slightly, breathe deeply through the mouth, and hold the breath; this action lowers the tongue to the floor of the mouth without the use of a tongue blade.
> - Lightly brushing the palate with a cotton swab also may open the mouth for assessment.

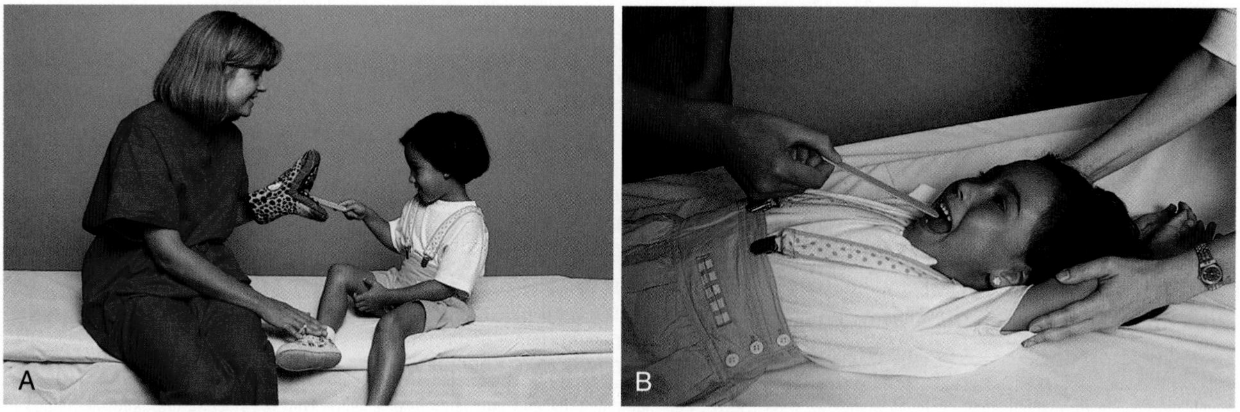

Fig. 34-25 **A:** Encouraging child to cooperate. **B:** Positioning child for examination of the mouth.

flavoured) to depress the tongue is necessary. The tongue blade is placed along the *side* of the tongue, not in the centre back area where the gag reflex is elicited. Figure 34-25, B illustrates proper positioning of the child for the oral examination.

The major structure of the exterior of the mouth is the lips. The lips should be moist, soft, smooth, and pink, or a deeper hue than the surrounding skin. The lips should be symmetrical when relaxed or tensed. The nurse can assess symmetry when the child talks or cries.

Inspection of Internal Structures

The major structures visible within the oral cavity and oropharynx are the mucosal lining of the lips and cheeks, gums (or gingiva), teeth, tongue, palate, uvula, tonsils, and posterior oropharynx (Fig. 34-26). The nurse needs to inspect all areas lined with mucous membranes (inside the lips and cheeks, gingiva, underside of the tongue, palate, and back of the pharynx) for colour, any areas of white patches or ulceration, bleeding, sensitivity, and moisture. The membranes should be bright pink, smooth, glistening, uniform, and moist.

The teeth are inspected for number in each dental arch, for hygiene, and for occlusion or bite. Discolouration of tooth enamel with obvious plaque (whitish coating on the surface of the teeth) is a sign of poor dental hygiene and indicates a need for counselling. Brown spots in the crevices of the crown of the tooth or between the teeth may be **caries** (cavities). Chalky white to yellow or brown areas on the enamel may indicate fluorosis (excessive fluoride ingestion). Teeth that appear greenish black may be stained temporarily from ingestion of supplemental iron.

The gums (gingiva) surrounding the teeth should also be examined. The colour is normally coral pink, and the surface texture is stippled, similar to the appearance of an orange peel. In dark-skinned children the gums are more deeply coloured, and a brownish area is often observed along the gum line.

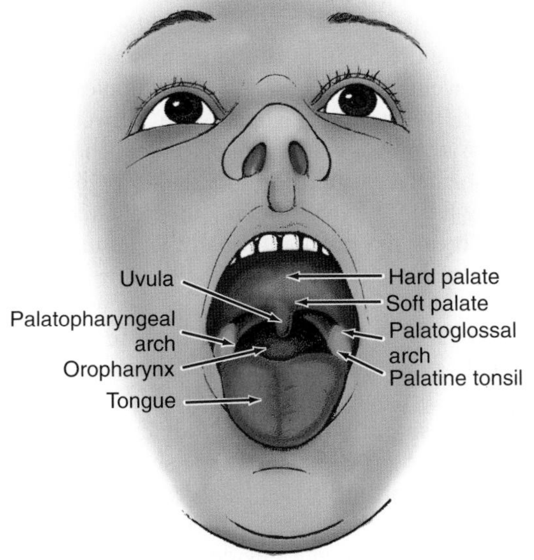

Fig. 34-26 Interior structures of the mouth.

The tongue is inspected for papillae, small projections that contain several taste buds and give the tongue its characteristic rough appearance. The size and mobility of the tongue should be noted. Normally the tip of the tongue should extend to the lips or beyond.

The roof of the mouth consists of the hard palate, which is located near the front of the oral cavity, and the soft palate, which is located toward the back of the pharynx and has a small midline protrusion called the *uvula*. The nurse should carefully inspect the palates to ensure that they are intact. The arch of the palate should be dome shaped. A narrow, flat roof or a high, arched palate affects the placement of the tongue and can cause feeding and speech problems. Movement of the uvula is tested by eliciting a gag reflex. The uvula should move upward to close off the nasopharynx from the oropharynx.

The nurse should examine the oropharynx and note the size and colour of the palatine tonsils. They are normally the same colour as the surrounding mucosa; glandular, rather than smooth in appearance; and barely visible over the edge of the palatoglossal arches. The size of the tonsils varies considerably during childhood. However, any swelling, redness, or white areas on the tonsils should be reported.

Chest

The chest is inspected for size, shape, symmetry, movement, breast development, and the bony landmarks formed by the ribs and sternum. The rib cage consists of 12 ribs on each side and the sternum, or breast bone, located in the midline of the trunk (Fig. 34-27). The sternum is composed of three main parts. The manubrium, the uppermost portion, can be felt at the base of the neck at the suprasternal notch. The largest segment of the sternum is the body, which forms the sternal angle (angle of Louis) as it articulates with the manubrium. At the end of the body is a small, movable process called the *xiphoid*. The angle of the costal margin as it attaches to the sternum is called the *costal angle* and is normally about 45 to 50 degrees. These bony structures are important landmarks in the location of ribs and intercostal spaces (ICSs), which are the spaces between the ribs. They are numbered according to the rib directly above the space. For example, the space immediately below the second rib is the second ICS.

The thoracic cavity is also divided into segments by drawing imaginary lines on the chest and back. Figure 34-28 illustrates the anterior, right lateral, and posterior divisions.

The size of the chest is measured by placing the measuring tape around the rib cage at the nipple line (see Fig. 34-8). For greatest accuracy, two measurements are needed—one during inspiration and the other during expiration—and the average recorded. Chest size is important mainly in relation to head circumference, which is discussed on p. 897. The nurse should always report marked disproportions because most are caused by abnormal head growth, although some may be a result of altered chest shape, such as barrel chest (chest is round) or pigeon chest (sternum protrudes outward).

During infancy, the chest's shape is almost circular, with the anteroposterior (front-to-back) diameter equalling the transverse, or lateral (side-to-side), diameter. As the child grows, the chest normally increases in the transverse direction, causing the anteroposterior diameter to be less than the lateral

evolve Anatomy Review—Rib Cage
evolve Anatomy Review—Imaginary Landmarks of the Chest

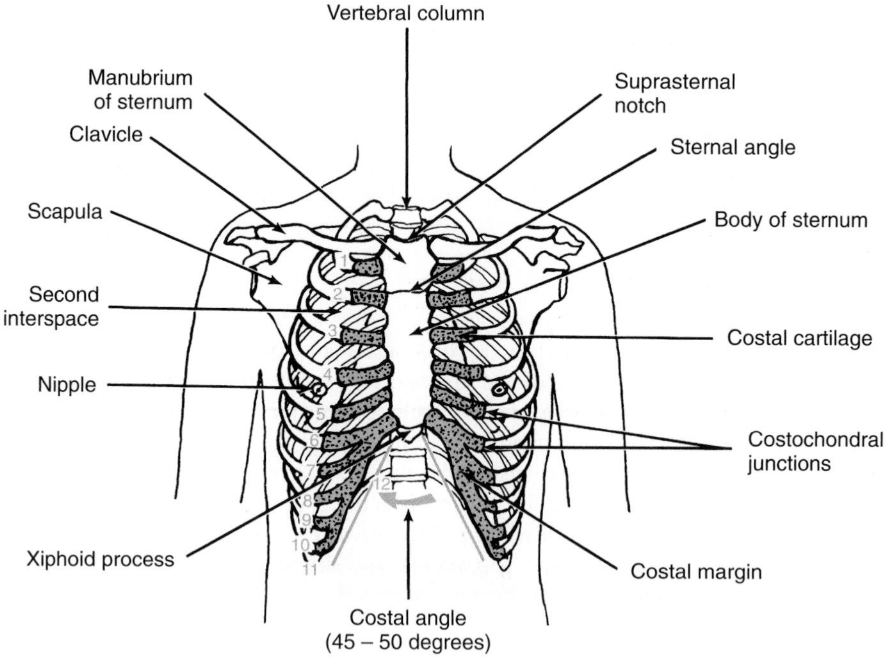

Fig. 34-27 Rib cage.

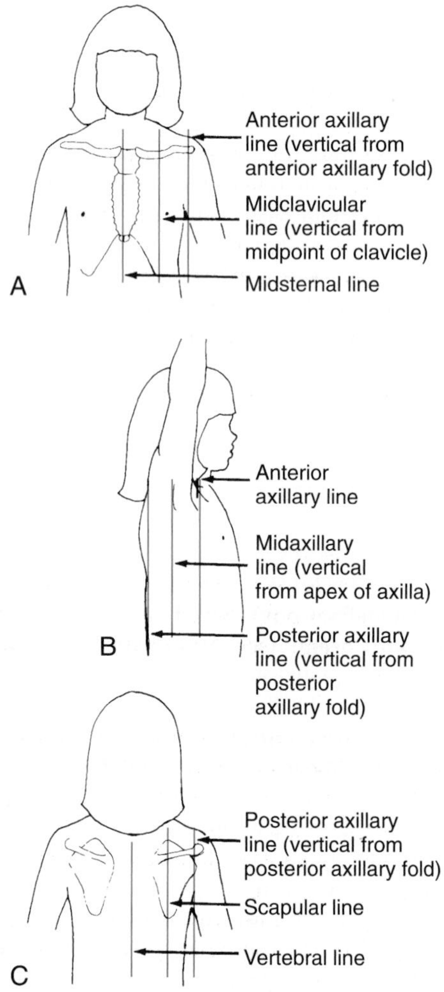

Fig. 34-28 Imaginary landmarks of the chest. **A:** Anterior. **B:** Right lateral. **C:** Posterior.

diameter. The nurse should note the angle made by the lower costal margin and the sternum, and palpate the junction of the ribs with the costal cartilage (costochondral junction) and sternum, which should be fairly smooth.

Movement of the chest wall should be symmetrical bilaterally and coordinated with breathing. During inspiration, the chest rises and expands, the diaphragm descends, and the costal angle increases. During expiration, the chest falls and decreases in size, the diaphragm rises, and the costal angle narrows (Fig. 34-29). In children younger than 6 or 7 years of age, respiratory movement is principally abdominal or diaphragmatic. In older children, particularly girls, respirations are chiefly thoracic. In either type the chest and abdomen should rise and fall together. Any asymmetry of movement must be reported.

While inspecting the skin surface of the chest, the nurse should observe the position of the nipples and any evidence of breast development. Normally the nipples are located slightly lateral to the midclavicular line, between the fourth and fifth ribs. Symmetry of nipple placement should be noted as well as normal configuration of a darker pigmented areola surrounding a flat nipple in the prepubertal child.

Pubertal breast development usually begins in girls between 10 and 14 years of age. Early (precocious) or delayed breast development should be recorded, as well as evidence of any other secondary sexual characteristics. In males, breast enlargement (gynecomastia) may be caused by hormonal or systemic disorders, but more commonly it is a result of adipose tissue from obesity or a transitory body change during early puberty. In either situation, the nurse should investigate the child's feelings regarding breast enlargement.

In adolescent girls who have achieved sexual maturity, the breasts need to be palpated for evidence of any masses or hard nodules. The nurse can use this opportunity to discuss how to

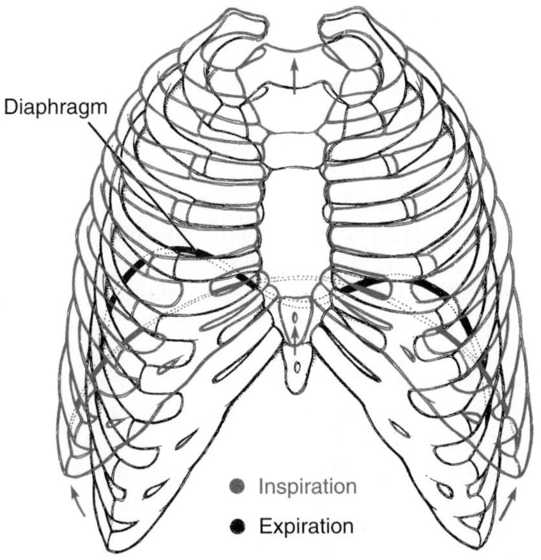

Fig. 34-29 Movement of chest during respiration.

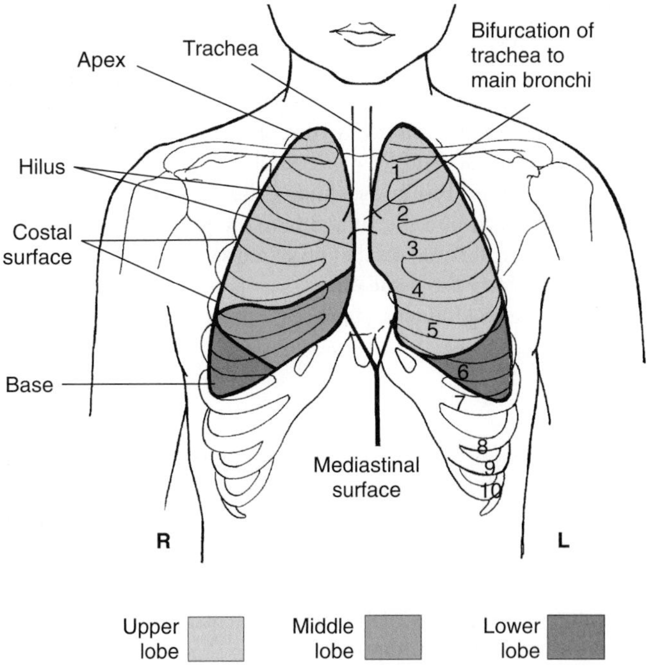

Fig. 34-30 Location of lobes of lungs within thoracic cavity.

evolve Anatomy Review—Percussion Sounds in the Thorax

do a breast examination. Most palpable masses are benign, thus it is important to convey this tendency, to decrease any fear or concern that results when a mass is felt.

Lungs

The lungs are situated inside the thoracic cavity, with one lung on each side of the sternum. Each lung is divided into an apex, which is slightly pointed and rises above the first rib; a base, which is wide and concave and rides on the dome-shaped diaphragm; and a body, which is divided into lobes. The right lung has three lobes: the upper, middle, and lower. The left lung has only two lobes, the upper and lower, because of the space occupied by the heart (Fig. 34-30).

Inspection of the lungs primarily involves observation of respiratory movements, which were discussed previously. Respirations are evaluated for rate (number per minute), rhythm (regular, irregular, or periodic), depth (deep or shallow), and quality (effortless, automatic, difficult, or laboured). The nurse should note the character of breath sounds, such as noisy, grunting, snoring, or heavy.

Respiratory movements are evaluated by placing each hand flat against the back or chest with the thumbs in midline along the lower costal margin of the lungs. The child should be sitting during this procedure and should take several deep breaths. During respiration, the examiner's hands will move with the chest wall. The amount and speed of respiratory excursion should be assessed and any asymmetry of movement noted.

Experienced examiners may **percuss** the lungs. The anterior lung is percussed from apex to base, usually with the child in the supine or sitting position. Each side of the chest is percussed in sequence to compare the sounds. When the posterior lung is percussed, the procedure and sequence are the same, although the child should be sitting. Resonance is heard over all the lobes of the lungs that are not adjacent to other organs. Any deviation from the expected sound should be recorded and reported.

GUIDELINES Effective Auscultation

- Make certain the child is relaxed and not crying, talking, or laughing. Record if the child is crying.
- Check that the room is comfortable and quiet.
- Warm the stethoscope before placing it against the skin.
- Apply firm pressure on chest piece but not enough to prevent vibrations and transmission of sound.
- Avoid placing the stethoscope over hair or clothing, moving it against skin, breathing on tubing, or sliding fingers over chest piece, which may cause sounds that falsely resemble pathological findings.
- Use a symmetrical and orderly approach for comparing sounds.

Auscultation

Auscultation involves using the stethoscope to evaluate breath sounds (see Guidelines box). Breath sounds are best heard if the child inspires deeply (see Atraumatic Care box). In the lungs, breath sounds are classified as vesicular, bronchovesicular, or bronchial (Box 34-14).

Absent or diminished breath sounds are always an abnormal finding warranting investigation. Fluid, air, or solid masses in the pleural space all interfere with the conduction of breath sounds. Diminished breath sounds in certain segments of the lung can alert the nurse to pulmonary areas that may benefit from chest physiotherapy. Increased breath sounds after pulmonary therapy indicate improved passage of air through the respiratory tract. Terms used to describe various respiration patterns are found in Box 34-15.

Various pulmonary abnormalities produce adventitious sounds that are not normally heard over the chest. These

ATRAUMATIC CARE
Encouraging Deep Breaths

- Ask the child to "blow out" the light on an otoscope or pocket flashlight; discreetly turn off the light on the last try so that the child feels successful.
- Place a cotton ball in the child's palm; ask the child to blow the ball into the air and have the parent catch it.
- Place a small tissue on the top of a pencil and ask the child to blow the tissue off.
- Have the child blow a pinwheel, a party horn, or bubbles.

BOX 34-14 Classification of Normal Breath Sounds

Vesicular Breath Sounds

These sounds are heard over the entire surface of the lungs, with the exception of the upper intrascapular area and area beneath the manubrium.

Inspiration is louder, longer, and higher pitched than expiration.

Sound is a soft, swishing noise.

Bronchovesicular Breath Sounds

These sounds are heard over the manubrium and in the upper intrascapular regions where the trachea and bronchi bifurcate.

Inspiration is louder and higher pitched than in vesicular breathing.

Bronchial Breath Sounds

These sounds are heard only over the trachea near the suprasternal notch.

The inspiratory phase is short, and expiratory phase is long.

sounds occur in addition to normal or abnormal breath sounds. They are classified into two main groups: crackles, which result from the passage of air through fluid or moisture; and wheezes, which are produced as air passes through narrowed passageways, regardless of the cause, such as exudate, inflammation, spasm, or tumour. Considerable practice with an experienced tutor is necessary to differentiate the various types of lung sounds. Often it is best to describe the type of sound heard in the lungs rather than trying to label it. The nurse should always report any abnormal sounds for further medical evaluation.

Heart

The heart is situated in the thoracic cavity between the lungs in the mediastinum and above the diaphragm (Fig. 34-31). About two thirds of the heart lies within the left side of the rib cage, with the other third on the right side as it crosses the sternum. The heart is positioned in the thorax like a trapezoid:

- *Vertically* along the right sternal border (RSB) from the second to the fifth rib

evolve Critical Thinking Exercise—Cardiovascular Assessment

evolve Anatomy Review—Location of Pulses

BOX 34-15 Various Patterns of Respiration

Tachypnea—Increased rate
Bradypnea—Decreased rate
Dyspnea—Distress during breathing
Apnea—Cessation of breathing
Hyperpnea—Increased depth
Hypoventilation—Decreased depth (shallow) and irregular rhythm
Hyperventilation—Increased rate and depth
Kussmaul respiration—Hyperventilation, gasping and laboured respiration; usually seen in diabetic coma or other states of respiratory acidosis
Cheyne-Stokes respiration—Gradually increasing rate and depth with periods of apnea
Biot respiration—Periods of hyperpnea alternating with apnea (similar to Cheyne-Stokes except that depth remains constant)
Seesaw (paradoxical) respirations—Chest falls on inspiration and rises on expiration
Agonal—Last gasping breaths before death

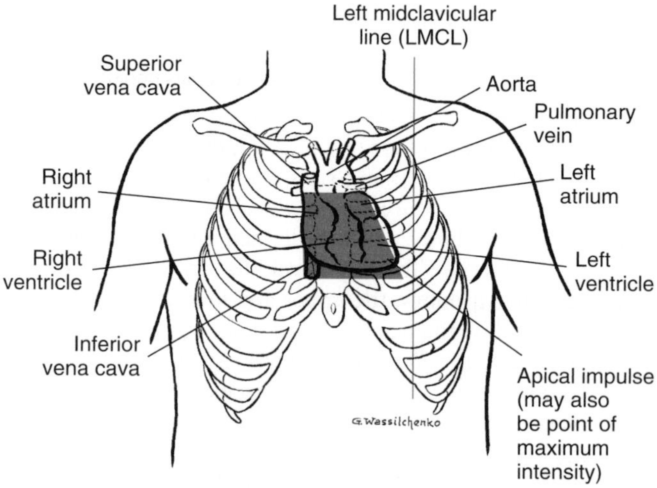

Fig. 34-31 Position of heart within the thorax.

- *Horizontally* (long side) from the lower right sternum to the fifth rib at the left midclavicular line (LMCL)
- *Diagonally* from the left sternal border (LSB) at the second rib to the LMCL at the fifth rib
- *Horizontally* (short side) from the RSB and LSB at the second ICS—base of the heart

Inspection is best done with the child sitting in a semi-Fowler position. Look at the anterior chest wall from an angle, comparing both sides of the rib cage with each other. Normally they should be symmetrical. In children with thin chest walls, a pulsation may be visible. Because comprehensive evaluation of cardiac function is not limited to the heart, also consider other findings such as the presence of all pulses (especially the femoral pulses) (Fig. 34-32), distended neck veins, clubbing of the fingers, peripheral cyanosis, edema, BP, and respiratory status.

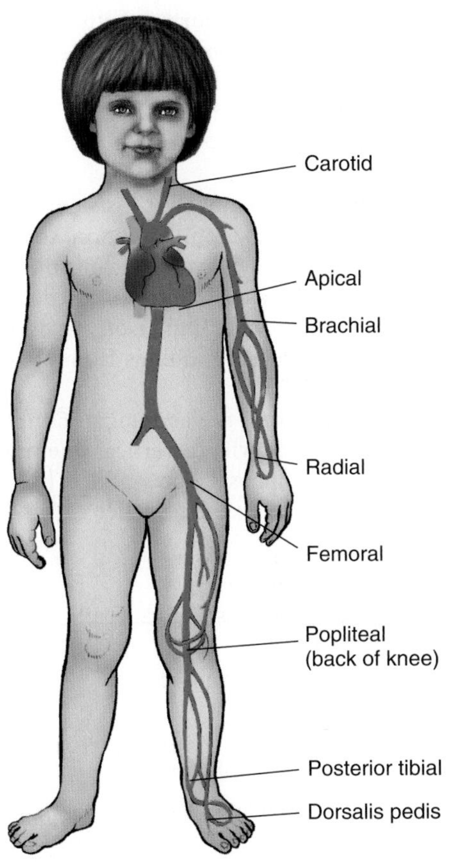

Fig. 34-32 Location of pulses.

Palpation is used to determine the location of the apical impulse (AI), the most lateral cardiac impulse that may correspond to the apex. The AI is found:

Just lateral to the LMCL and fourth ICS in children over 7 years of age.

At the LMCL and fifth ICS in children less than 7 years of age.

Although the AI gives a general idea of the size of the heart (with enlargement, the apex is lower and more lateral), its normal location is variable, making it an unreliable indicator of heart size.

The **point of maximum impulse** (PMI), as the name implies, is the area of most intense pulsation. Usually the PMI is located at the same site as the AI, but it can occur elsewhere. For this reason, the two terms should not be used synonymously.

Capillary refill time, an important test for peripheral circulation, is assessed by pressing the skin lightly on a central site, such as the forehead, or a peripheral site, such as the top of the hand, to produce a slight blanching. The time it takes for the blanched area to return to its original colour is the capillary refill time.

NURSING ALERT Capillary refill should be brisk—less than 2 seconds; prolonged refill may be associated with poor systemic perfusion or a cool ambient temperature.

Auscultation

Origin of Heart Sounds

The heart sounds are produced by the opening and closing of the valves and the vibration of blood against the walls of the heart and vessels. Normally two sounds—S_1 and S_2—are heard, which correspond, respectively, to the familiar "lub dub" often used to describe the sounds. S_1 is caused by closure of the tricuspid and mitral valves (sometimes called the *atrioventricular valves*). S_2 is the result of closure of the pulmonic and aortic valves (sometimes called *semilunar valves*). Normally the split of the two sounds in S_2 is distinguishable and widens during inspiration. Physiological splitting is a significant normal finding.

NURSING ALERT Fixed splitting, in which the split in S_2 does not change during inspiration, is an important diagnostic sign of atrial septal defect.

Two other heart sounds—S_3 and S_4—may be produced. S_3 is normally heard in some children; S_4 is rarely heard as a normal heart sound; it usually indicates the need for further cardiac evaluation.

Differentiating Normal Heart Sounds

Figure 34-33 illustrates the approximate anatomical position of the valves within the heart chambers. Note that the anatomical location of valves does not correspond to the area where the sounds are heard best. The auscultatory sites are located in the direction of the blood flow through the valves. Normally, S_1 is louder at the apex of the heart in the mitral and tricuspid area, and S_2 is louder near the base of the heart in the pulmonic and aortic area (Table 34-11). Listen to each sound by inching down the chest. The following areas should also be auscultated for sounds, such as murmurs, which may radiate to these sites: sternoclavicular area above the clavicles and manubrium, area along the sternal border, area along the left midaxillary line, and area below the scapulae.

NURSING ALERT To distinguish between S_1 and S_2 heart sounds, simultaneously palpate the carotid pulse with the index and middle fingers and listen to the heart sounds; S_1 is synchronous with the carotid pulse.

The nurse should auscultate the heart with the child in at least two positions: sitting and reclining. If adventitious sounds are detected, they should be further evaluated with the child standing, sitting and leaning forward, and lying on the left side. For example, atrial sounds such as S_4 are heard best with the person in a recumbent position and usually fade if the person sits or stands.

Heart sounds are evaluated for (1) quality (they should be clear and distinct, not muffled, diffuse, or distant); (2) intensity, especially in relation to the location or auscultatory site (they should not be weak or pounding); (3) rate (they should have the same rate as the radial pulse); and (4) rhythm (they should be regular and even). A particular arrhythmia that occurs normally in many children is *sinus arrhythmia*, in which the heart rate increases with inspiration and decreases with expiration. This rhythm is differentiated from a truly abnormal arrhythmia by having children hold their breath. In

evolve Anatomy Review—Direction of Heart Sounds

sinus arrhythmia, cessation of breathing causes the heart rate to remain steady.

Heart Murmurs

Another important category of the heart sounds is murmurs, which are produced by vibrations within the heart chambers or in the major arteries from the back-and-forth flow of blood. Murmurs are classified as follows:

Innocent—No anatomical or physiological abnormality exists.

Functional—No automatic cardiac defect exists, but a physiological abnormality such as anemia is present.

Organic—A cardiac defect with or without a physiological abnormality exists.

The description and classification of murmurs are skills that require considerable practice and training. In general, recognize murmurs as distinct swishing sounds that occur in addition to the normal heart sounds and record the (1) location, or the area of the heart in which the murmur is heard best; (2) time of the occurrence of the murmur within the S_1–S_2 cycle; (3) intensity (evaluate in relationship to the child's position); and (4) loudness. The usual subjective method of grading the loudness or intensity of a murmur is listed in Table 34-12.

Abdomen

Examination of the abdomen involves inspection, followed by auscultation and then palpation. Palpation should be performed last because it may distort the normal abdominal sounds, assessed during auscultation. Knowledge of the anatomical placement of the abdominal organs is essential to differentiate normal, expected findings from abnormal ones (Fig. 34-34).

For descriptive purposes, the abdominal cavity is divided into four quadrants by drawing a vertical line midway from the sternum to the symphysis pubis and a horizontal line across the abdomen through the umbilicus. The sections are named as follows:

Table 34-11 Sequence of Auscultating Heart Sounds*

AUSCULTATORY SITE	CHEST LOCATION	CHARACTERISTICS OF HEART SOUNDS
Aortic area	Second right intercostal space close to sternum	S_2 heard louder than S_1; aortic closure heard loudest
Pulmonic area	Second left intercostal space close to sternum	Splitting of S_2 heard best, normally widens on inspiration; pulmonic closure heard best
Erb's point	Second and third left intercostal spaces close to sternum	Frequent site of innocent murmurs and those of aortic or pulmonic origin
Tricuspid area	Fifth right and left intercostal spaces close to sternum	S_1 heard as louder sound preceding S_2 (S_1 synchronous with carotid pulse)
Mitral or apical area	Fifth intercostal space, left midclavicular line (third to fourth intercostal space and lateral to left midclavicular line in infants)	S_1 heard loudest; splitting of S_1 may be audible because mitral closure is louder than tricuspid closure
		S_1 heard best at beginning of expiration with child in recumbent or left side-lying position; occurs immediately after S_2; sounds like word S_1 S_2 S_3: "Ken-tuc-ky"
		S_4 heard best during expiration with child in recumbent position (left side-lying position decreases sound); occurs immediately before S_1; sounds like word S_4 S_1 S_2: "Ten-nes-see"

*Use both diaphragm and bell chest pieces when auscultating heart sounds. Bell chest piece is necessary for low-pitched sounds of murmurs, S_3, and S_4. See Fig. 34-33 for sites.

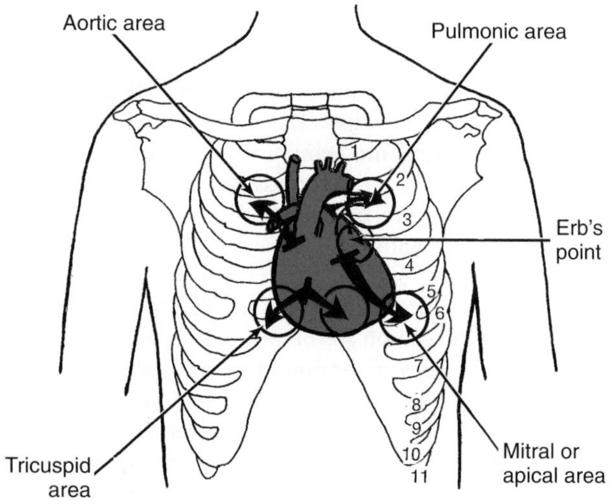

Fig. 34-33 Direction of heart sounds for anatomical valve sites and areas (*circled*) for auscultation.

Table 34-12 Grading of the Intensity of Heart Murmurs

GRADE	DESCRIPTION
I	Very faint; often not heard if child sits up
II	Usually readily heard; slightly louder than grade I; audible in all positions
III	Loud, but not accompanied by a thrill
IV	Loud, accompanied by a thrill
V	Loud enough to be heard with a stethoscope barely touching the chest; accompanied by a thrill
VI	Loud enough to be heard with the stethoscope not touching the chest; often heard with the human ear close to the chest; accompanied by a thrill

- Left upper quadrant
- Left lower quadrant
- Right upper quadrant
- Right lower quadrant

Inspection

The contour of the abdomen is inspected with the child erect and supine. Normally the abdomen of infants and young children is cylindrical and, in the erect position, fairly prominent because of the physiological lordosis of the spine. In the supine position, the abdomen appears flat. A midline protrusion from the xiphoid to the umbilicus or symphysis pubis is usually diastasis recti, or failure of the rectus abdominis muscles to join in utero. In a healthy child, a midline protrusion is usually a variation of normal muscular development.

NURSING ALERT A tense, boardlike abdomen is a serious sign of paralytic ileus and intestinal obstruction.

The skin covering the abdomen should be uniformly taut, without wrinkles or creases. Sometimes silvery, whitish striae ("stretch marks") are seen, especially if the skin has been stretched, as in obesity. Superficial veins are usually visible in light-skinned, thin infants, but distended veins are an abnormal finding.

The nurse should observe movement of the abdomen. Normally, chest and abdominal movements are synchronous. In infants and thin children, peristaltic waves may be visible through the abdominal wall; they are best observed by standing at eye level to and across from the abdomen. This finding should always be reported.

The umbilicus is examined for size, hygiene, and evidence of any abnormalities, such as hernias. The umbilicus should be flat or only slightly protruding. If a herniation is present, the nurse should palpate the sac for abdominal contents and estimate the approximate size of the opening. Umbilical hernias are common in infants, especially in Black children.

Hernias may exist elsewhere on the abdominal wall (Fig. 34-35). An *inguinal hernia* is a protrusion of peritoneum through the abdominal wall in the inguinal canal. It occurs mostly in males, is frequently bilateral, and may be visible as a mass in the scrotum. To locate a hernia, slide the little finger into the external inguinal ring at the base of the scrotum and ask the child to cough. If a hernia is present, it will hit the tip of the finger.

A *femoral hernia*, which occurs more frequently in girls, is felt or seen as a small mass on the anterior surface of the thigh just below the inguinal ligament in the femoral canal (a potential space medial to the femoral artery). Feel for a hernia by placing the index finger of your right hand on the child's right femoral pulse (left hand for left pulse) and the middle finger flat against the skin toward the midline. The ring finger lies over the femoral canal, where the herniation occurs. Palpation of hernias in the pelvic region is often part of the genital examination.

Auscultation

The most important finding to listen for is *peristalsis*, or bowel sounds, which sound like short metallic clicks and gurgles. Their frequency per minute should be recorded (e.g., 5 sounds/min). Bowel sounds may be stimulated by stroking the abdominal surface with a fingernail. Absence of bowel sounds or hyperperistalsis should be reported, since either usually denotes an abdominal disorder.

Palpation

Two types of palpation are performed: superficial and deep. For superficial palpation, the examiner should lightly place the hand against the skin and feel each quadrant, noting any areas

evolve Anatomy Review—Location of Hernias

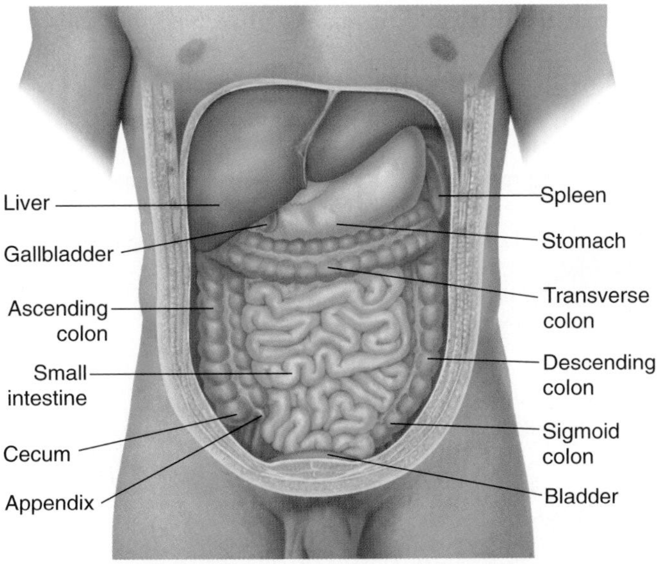

Fig. 34-34 Location of structures in the abdomen. *(From Seidel, H. M., et al. [2006]. Mosby's guide to physical examination [6th ed.]. St. Louis: Mosby.)*

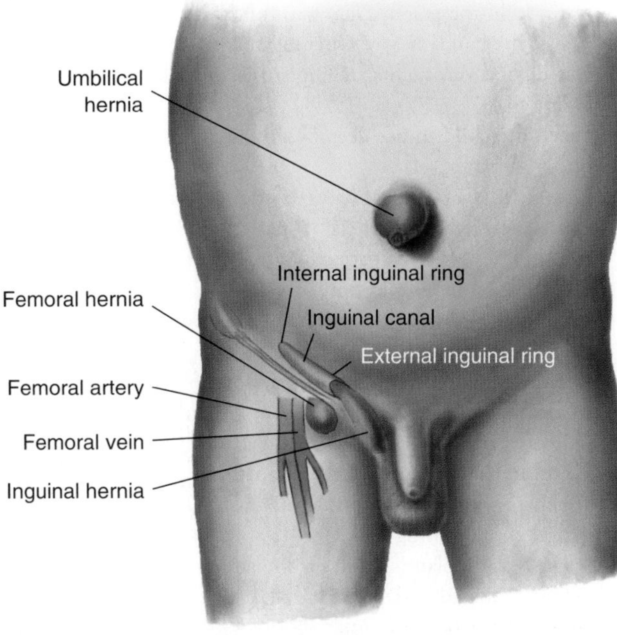

Fig. 34-35 Location of hernias.

of tenderness, muscle tone, and superficial lesions such as cysts. Because superficial palpation is often perceived as tickling, several techniques can be used to minimize this sensation and relax the child (see Atraumatic Care box). Admonishing the child to stop laughing only draws attention to the sensation and may make it more difficult to complete the assessment.

Deep palpation is used for palpating organs and large blood vessels and for detecting masses and tenderness that were not discovered during superficial palpation. Palpation usually begins in the lower quadrants and proceeds upward to avoid missing the edge of an enlarged liver or spleen. Except for palpating the liver, successful identification of other organs, such as the spleen, kidney, and part of the colon, requires considerable practice with tutored supervision. Any questionable mass should be reported. The lower edge of the liver is sometimes felt in infants and young children as a superficial mass 1 to 2 cm below the right costal margin (the distance is sometimes measured in fingerbreadths). Normally, the liver descends during inspiration as the diaphragm moves downward. This downward displacement should not be mistaken as a sign of liver enlargement.

NURSING ALERT If the liver is palpable 3 cm below the right costal margin or the spleen is palpable more than 2 cm below the left costal margin, these organs are enlarged—a finding that is always reported for further medical investigation.

The femoral pulses are palpated by placing the tips of two or three fingers (index, middle, or ring) along the inguinal ligament about midway between the iliac crest and symphysis pubis. Both pulses should be felt simultaneously to make certain that they are equal and strong (Fig. 34-36).

NURSING ALERT Absence of femoral pulses is a significant sign of coarctation of the aorta and needs to be referred for medical evaluation.

ATRAUMATIC CARE

Promoting Relaxation During Abdominal Palpation

- Position the child comfortably, such as in a semireclining position in the parent's lap, with knees flexed.
- Warm the hands before touching the skin.
- Use distraction, such as telling stories or talking to the child.
- Teach the child to use deep breathing and to concentrate on an object.
- Give infants a bottle (if being bottle-fed) or pacifier.
- Begin with light, superficial palpation and gradually progress to deeper palpation.
- Palpate any tender or painful areas last.
- Have the child hold the parent's hand and squeeze it if palpation is uncomfortable.
- Use the nonpalpating hand to comfort the child, such as placing the free hand on the child's shoulder while palpating the abdomen.
- To minimize sensation of tickling during palpation:
  - Have children "help" with palpation by placing a hand over the palpating hand.
  - Have them place a hand on the abdomen with the fingers spread wide apart, and palpate between their fingers.

Genitalia

Examination of genitalia conveniently follows assessment of the abdomen while the child is still supine. In adolescents, inspection of the genitalia may be left to the end of the examination. The best approach is to examine the genitalia matter-of-factly, placing no more emphasis on this part of the assessment than on any other segment. It helps to relieve children's and parents' anxiety by telling them the results of the findings; for example, the nurse might say, "Everything looks fine here."

If it is necessary to ask questions, such as about discharge or difficulty urinating, respect the child's privacy by covering the lower abdomen with the gown or underpants. To prevent embarrassing interruptions, keep the door or curtain closed and post a "do not disturb" sign. Have a drape ready to cover the genitalia if someone enters the room.

In examining the genitalia, gloves should be worn when touching body substances. It might be helpful for the adolescent to know that wearing gloves also prevents skin-to-skin contact.

The genital examination is an excellent time for eliciting questions or concerns about body function or sexual activity. The nurse can also use this opportunity to increase or reinforce the child's knowledge of reproductive anatomy by naming each body part and explaining its function. This is a good time to discuss testicular cancer, although testicular self-examination is not recommended.

Male Genitalia

In examining the male genitalia, the nurse should note the external appearance of the glans and shaft of the penis, the

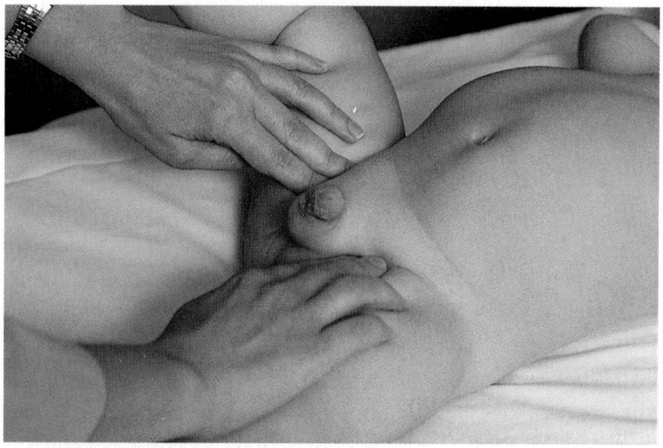

Fig. 34-36 Palpating femoral pulses.

prepuce, the urethral meatus, and the scrotum (Fig. 34-37). The penis is generally small in infants and young boys until puberty, when it begins to increase in both length and width. In an obese child, the penis often looks abnormally small because of the folds of skin partially covering it at the base. It is important to be familiar with normal pubertal growth of the external male genitalia in order to compare the findings with the expected sequence of maturation.

The glans (head of the penis) and shaft (portion between the perineum and prepuce) are examined for signs of swelling, skin lesions, inflammation, or other irregularities. Any of these signs may indicate underlying disorders, especially STIs.

The urethral meatus is carefully inspected for location and evidence of discharge. Normally it is centred at the tip of the glans.

Hair distribution should also be noted. Normally, before puberty, no pubic hair is present. Soft, downy hair at the base of the penis is an early sign of pubertal maturation. In older adolescents, hair distribution is diamond shaped from the umbilicus to the anus.

The location and size of the scrotum should be noted. The scrota hang freely from the perineum behind the penis, and the left scrotum normally hangs lower than the right. In infants, the scrota appear large in relation to the rest of the genitalia. The skin of the scrotum is loose and highly rugated (wrinkled). During early adolescence, the skin normally becomes redder and coarser. In dark-skinned children, the scrota are usually more deeply pigmented.

Palpation of the scrotum includes identification of the testes, epididymis, and, if present, inguinal hernias. The two testes are felt as small, ovoid bodies about 1.5 to 2 cm long—one in each scrotal sac. They do not enlarge until puberty, when they approximately double in size.

When palpating for the presence of the testes, the nurse should avoid stimulating the cremasteric reflex, which is stimulated by cold, touch, emotional excitement, or exercise. This reflex pulls the testes higher into the pelvic cavity. Several measures are useful in preventing the cremasteric reflex during palpation of the scrotum. First, warm the hands. Second, if the child is old enough, he should be examined in a "tailor" position, which stretches the muscle, preventing its contraction (Fig. 34-38, A). Third, block the normal pathway of ascent of the testes by placing the thumb and index finger over the upper part of the scrotal sac along the inguinal canal (see Fig. 34-38, B). If there is any question concerning the existence of two testes, place the index and middle fingers in a scissors fashion to separate the right and left scrota. If, after using these techniques, the testes have not been palpated, feel along the inguinal canal and perineum to locate masses that may be undescended testes. Although undescended testes may descend at any time during childhood and are checked at each visit, failure to palpate testes should be reported.

Female Genitalia

The examination of female genitalia is limited to inspection and palpation of external structures. If a vaginal examination is required, an appropriate referral is made unless the nurse is qualified to perform the procedure. A convenient position for examination of the genitalia involves placing the young child supine on the examining table or in a semireclining position on the parent's lap with the feet supported on the nurse's knees as the nurse sits facing the child. The child's attention can be diverted from the examination by instructing her to try to keep the soles of her feet pressed against each other. Separate the labia majora with the thumb and index finger and retract

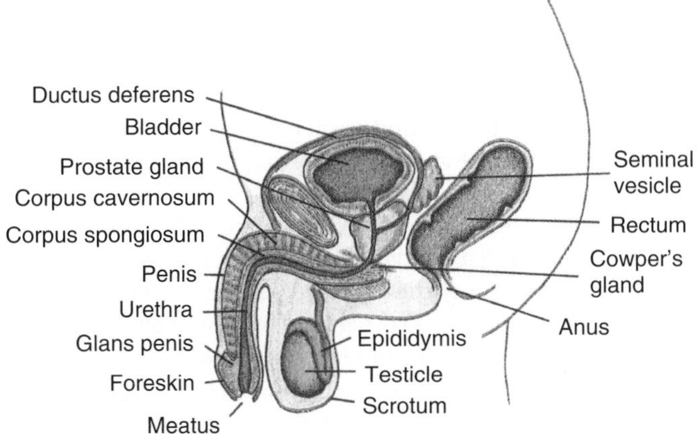

Fig. 34-37 Major structures of genitalia in uncircumcised postpubertal male. *(Potter, P. A. & Perry, A. G. [2009]. Fundamentals of nursing [7th ed., p. 621]. St. Louis: Mosby [Fig. 33-69].)*

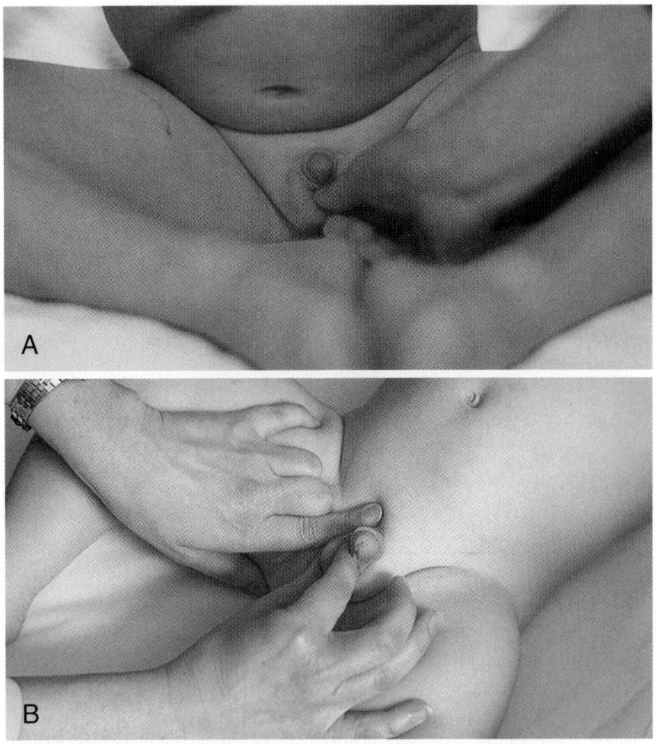

Fig. 34-38 **A:** Preventing cremasteric reflex by having child sit in "tailor" position. **B:** Blocking inguinal canal during palpation of scrotum for descended testes.

outward to expose the labia minora, urethral meatus, and vaginal orifice.

The female genitalia are examined for size and location of the structures of the vulva, or pudendum (Fig. 34-39). The *mons pubis* is a pad of adipose tissue over the symphysis pubis. At puberty, the mons is covered with hair, which extends along the labia. The usual pattern of female hair distribution is an inverted triangle. The appearance of soft, downy hair along the labia majora is an early sign of sexual maturation. The nurse should note the size and location of the *clitoris*, a small, erectile organ located at the anterior end of the labia minora. It is covered by a small flap of skin, the *prepuce*.

The *labia majora* are two thick folds of skin running posteriorly from the mons to the posterior commissure of the vagina. Internal to the labia majora are two folds of skin called the *labia minora*. Although the labia minora are usually prominent in the newborn, they gradually atrophy, which makes them almost invisible until their enlargement during puberty. The inner surface of the labia should be pink and moist. The size of the labia should be noted as well as any evidence of fusion, which may suggest male scrota. Normally, no masses are palpable within the labia.

The urethral meatus is located posterior to the clitoris and is surrounded by Skene's glands and ducts. Although not a prominent structure, the meatus appears as a small V-shaped slit. Its location should be noted, especially if it opens from the clitoris or inside the vagina. Gently palpate the glands, which are common sites of cysts and sexually transmitted lesions.

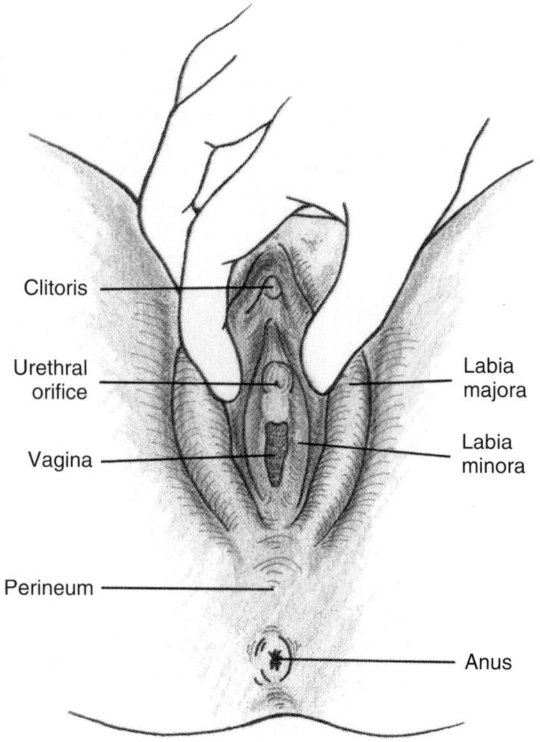

Fig. 34-39 External structures of genitalia in postpubertal female. Labia are spread to reveal deeper structures. *(Potter, P. A. & Perry, A. G. [2009]. Fundamentals of nursing [7th ed., p. 620]. St. Louis: Mosby [Fig 33-68].)*

The vaginal orifice is located posterior to the urethral meatus. Its appearance varies depending on individual anatomy and sexual activity. Ordinarily, examination of the vagina is limited to inspection. In virgins, a thin crescent-shaped or circular membrane, called the *hymen*, may cover part of the vaginal opening. In some instances it completely occludes the orifice. After rupture, small rounded pieces of tissue called *caruncles* remain. Although an imperforate hymen denotes lack of penile intercourse, a perforate one does not necessarily indicate sexual activity.

NURSING ALERT In girls who have undergone female genital mutilation the genitalia will appear different. Do not show surprise or disgust, but note the appearance and discuss the procedure with the young woman (see Chapter 4, Cultural Awareness box, p. 54).

Surrounding the vaginal opening are Bartholin's glands, which secrete a clear, mucoid fluid into the vagina for lubrication during intercourse. The ducts should be palpated for cysts. The nurse should also note the discharge from the vagina, which is usually clear or white.

Anus

After examination of the genitalia, the anal area is easily examined, although the child should be placed on the abdomen. Note the general firmness of the buttocks and symmetry of the gluteal folds. The tone of the anal sphincter can be assessed by eliciting the anal reflex. Gently scratching the anal area results in an obvious quick contraction of the external anal sphincter.

Back and Extremities

Spine

The general curvature of the spine is noted. Normally, the back of a newborn is rounded or C-shaped from the thoracic and pelvic curves. The development of the cervical and lumbar curves approximates development of various motor skills, such as cervical curvature with head control, and gives the older child the typical double S curve.

Marked curvatures in posture are abnormal. *Scoliosis*, lateral curvature of the spine, is an important childhood problem, especially in girls. Although scoliosis may be identified by observing and palpating the spine and noting a sideways displacement, more objective tests include the following:

- With the child standing erect, clothed only in underpants (and bra if older girl), observe from behind, noting asymmetry of the shoulders and hips.
- With the child bending forward so that the back is parallel to the floor, observe from the side, noting asymmetry or prominence of the rib cage (see Fig. 54-11).

A slight limp, a crooked hemline, or complaints of a sore back are other signs and symptoms of scoliosis.

The back should be inspected, especially along the spine, for any tufts of hair, dimples, or discolouration. Mobility of the vertebral column is easily assessed in most children because of their propensity for constant motion during the examination. However, mobility can be tested by asking the child to sit up from a prone position or to do a modified sit-up exercise.

Movement of the cervical spine is an important diagnostic sign of neurological problems, such as meningitis. Normally, movement of the head in all directions is effortless.

NURSING ALERT Hyperextension of the neck and spine, or *opisthotonos,* which is accompanied by pain when the head is flexed, is always referred for immediate medical evaluation.

Extremities

Each extremity needs to be inspected for symmetry of length and size; any deviation should be referred for orthopaedic evaluation. The nurse should count the fingers and toes to be certain of the normal number. This is so often taken for granted that an extra digit (*polydactyly*) or fusion of digits (*syndactyly*) may go unnoticed.

The arms and legs are inspected for temperature and colour, which should be equal in each extremity, although the feet may normally be colder than the hands.

The shape of bones should also be assessed. Several variations of bone shape may be observed in children. Although many of them cause parents concern, most are benign and require no treatment. *Bowleg,* or genu varum, is lateral bowing of the tibia. It is clinically present when the child stands with the medial malleoli (rounded prominence on either side of the ankle) opposite each other and the space between the knees is greater than approximately 5 cm (Fig. 34-40). Toddlers are usually bowlegged after beginning to walk until all their lower back and leg muscles are well developed. Unilateral or asymmetrical bowlegs that are present beyond the age of 2 to 3 years, particularly in Black children, may represent pathological conditions requiring further investigation.

Knock-knee, or genu valgum, appears as the opposite of bowleg, in that the knees are close together but the feet are spread apart. It is determined clinically by using the same method as for genu varum but by measuring the distance between the malleoli, which normally should be less than 7.5 cm (Fig. 34-41). Knock-knee is normally present in children from about 2 to 7 years of age. Knock-knee that is excessive, asymmetrical, accompanied by short stature, or evident in a child nearing puberty requires further evaluation.

Next, the feet are inspected. Infants' and toddlers' feet appear flat because the foot is normally wide and the arch is covered by a fat pad. Development of the arch occurs naturally from the action of walking. Normally, at birth the feet are held in a valgus (outward) or varus (inward) position. To determine whether a foot deformity at birth is a result of intrauterine position or development, scratch the outer, then inner, side of the sole. (See Chapter 28 for a discussion of clubfoot and Fig. 54-9.) If the foot position is self-correctable, it will assume a right angle to the leg. As the child begins to walk, the feet turn outward less than 30 degrees and inward less than 10 degrees.

Toddlers have a "toddling" or broad-based gait, which facilitates walking by lowering the centre of gravity. As the child reaches preschool age, the legs are brought closer together. By school age the walking posture is much more graceful and balanced.

The most common gait problem in young children is *pigeon toe,* or toeing in, which usually results from torsional deformities, such as internal tibial torsion (abnormal rotation or bowing of the tibia). Tests for tibial torsion include measuring the thigh–foot angle, which requires considerable practice for accuracy.

The plantar or grasp reflex can be elicited by exerting firm but gentle pressure with the tip of the thumb against the lateral sole of the foot from the heel upward to the little toe and then across to the big toe. The normal response in children who are walking is flexion of the toes. *Babinski sign,* dorsiflexion of the big toe and fanning of the other toes, is normal during infancy but abnormal after about 1 year of age or when locomotion begins (see Fig. 36-6).

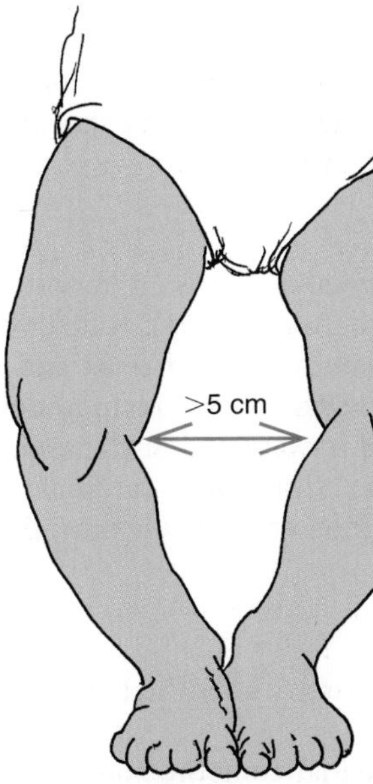

Fig. 34-40 Bowleg.

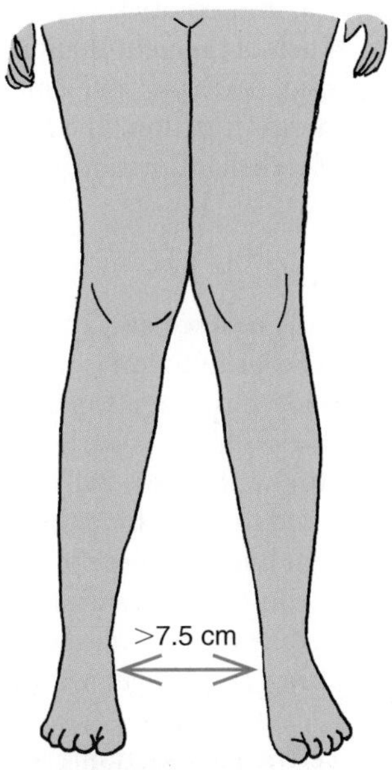

Fig. 34-41 Knock-knee.

Joints

The joints are evaluated for range of motion. Normally this requires no specific testing if the nurse has observed the child's movements during the examination. However, the hips should be routinely investigated in infants for congenital dislocation by a qualified health care provider (see Chapter 54). Any evidence of joint immobility or hyperflexibility needs to be reported.

The joints are palpated for heat, tenderness, and swelling. These signs, as well as redness over the joint, warrant further investigation.

Muscles

The symmetry and quality of muscle development, tone, and strength should be noted. Development is observed by looking at the shape and contour of the body in both a relaxed and a tensed state. Tone is estimated by grasping the muscle and feeling its firmness when it is relaxed and contracted. A common site for testing tone is the biceps muscle of the arm. Children are usually willing to "make a muscle" by clenching their fist.

Estimate strength by having the child use an extremity to push or pull against resistance, as in the following examples:

Arm strength—Child holds the arms outstretched in front of the body and tries to raise the arms while downward pressure is applied.

Hand strength—Child shakes hands with nurse and squeezes one or two fingers of the nurse's hand.

Leg strength—Child sits on a table or chair with the legs dangling and tries to raise the legs while downward pressure is applied.

Symmetry of strength in the extremities, hands, and fingers should be noted and evidence of paresis, or weakness, needs to be reported.

Neurological Assessment

The assessment of the nervous system is the broadest and most diverse part of the examination process, since every human function, both physical and emotional, is controlled by neurological impulses. Much of the neurological examination has already been discussed, such as assessment of behaviour, sensory testing, and motor function. The following focuses on a general appraisal of cerebellar function, deep tendon reflexes, and the cranial nerves.

Cerebellar Function

The cerebellum controls balance and coordination. Much of the assessment of cerebellar function is included in observing the child's posture, body movements, gait, and development of fine and gross motor skills. Tests such as balancing on one foot and the heel-to-toe walk assess balance. Coordination is tested by asking the child to reach for a toy, button clothes, tie shoes, or draw a straight line on a piece of paper (provided the child is old enough to do these activities). Coordination can also be tested by any sequence of rapid, successive movements, such as quickly touching each finger with the thumb of the same hand.

Several tests for cerebellar function can be performed as games (Box 34-16). When a Romberg test is done, stay beside the child if there is a possibility that the child may fall. School-age children should be able to perform these tests, although in the finger-to-nose test, preschoolers normally can only bring the finger within 5 to 7.5 cm of the nose. Difficulty in performing these exercises indicates poor sense of position (especially with the eyes closed) and incoordination (especially with the eyes opened).

evolve Animation—Cranial Nerves

BOX 34-16 Tests for Cerebellar Function

Finger-to-nose test—With the child's arm extended, ask the child to touch the nose with the index finger with eyes open and then closed.

Heel-to-shin test—Have the child stand and run the heel of one foot down the shin or anterior aspect of the tibia of the other leg, both with eyes opened and then closed.

Romberg test—Have the child stand with eyes closed and heels together; falling or leaning to one side is abnormal and is called the Romberg sign.

Reflexes

Testing reflexes is an important part of the neurological examination. Persistence of primitive reflexes, loss of reflexes, or hyperactivity of deep tendon reflexes is usually a result of a cerebral insult.

Reflexes can be elicited by using the rubber head of the reflex hammer, flat of the finger, or side of the hand. If the child is easily frightened by equipment, use your hand or finger. Although testing reflexes is a simple procedure, the child may inhibit the reflex by unconsciously tensing the muscle. To avoid tensing, distract younger children with toys or talk to them. Older children can concentrate on the exercise of grasping their two hands in front of them and trying to pull them apart. This diverts their attention from the testing and causes involuntary relaxation of the muscles.

Deep tendon reflexes are stretch reflexes of a muscle. The most common deep tendon reflex is the knee jerk, or patellar reflex (sometimes called the quadriceps reflex). The reflexes normally elicited are described in Figures 34-42 to 34-45. Any diminished or hyper-reflexive response should be reported for further evaluation.

Cranial Nerves

Assessment of the cranial nerves is an important area of neurological assessment (Table 34-13). With young children, present the tests as games to foster **trust** and security at the beginning of the examination. Or include the cranial nerve test when each system is examined, such as tongue movement and strength, gag reflex, swallowing, cardinal positions of gaze (Fig. 34-46), and position of the uvula during examination of the mouth.

Developmental Assessment

One of the most essential components of a complete health appraisal is assessment of developmental function. Screening

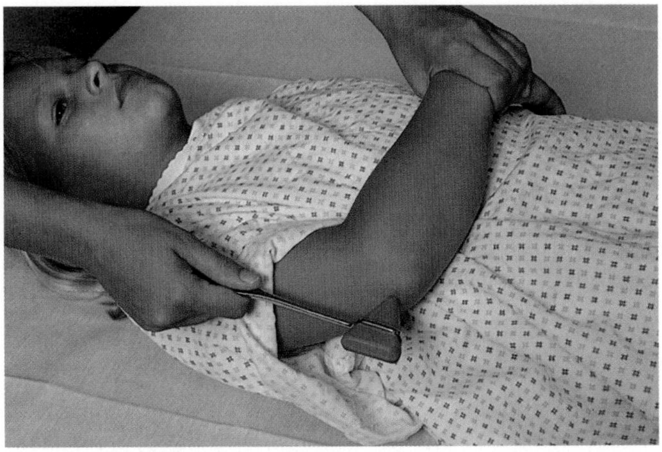

Fig. 34-42 Testing for triceps reflex. The child is placed supine, with forearm resting over chest, and triceps tendon is struck. Alternate procedure: child's arm is abducted, with upper arm supported and forearm allowed to hang freely. Triceps tendon is struck. Normal response is partial extension of the forearm.

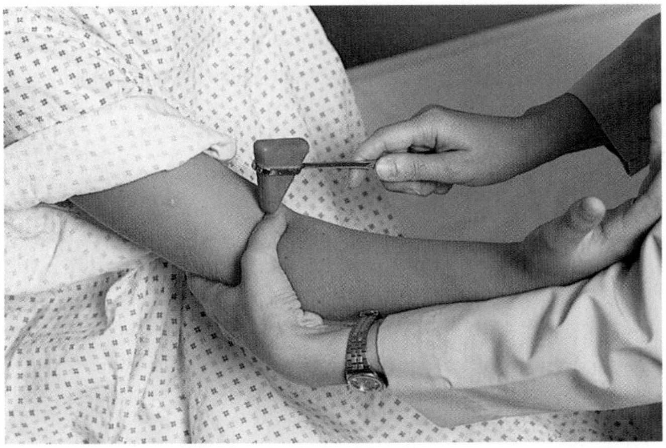

Fig. 34-43 Testing for biceps reflex. The child's arm is held by placing the partially flexed elbow in the examiner's hand with thumb over antecubital space. The examiner's thumbnail is struck with a hammer. Normal response is partial flexion of the forearm.

procedures are designed to identify quickly and reliably those children whose developmental level is below normal for their age and who thus require further investigation. They also provide a means of recording objective measurements of present developmental function for future reference. Nurses play a vital role in providing a developmental assessment of children with disabilities. The procedures discussed in this section can be administered in a variety of settings: home, school, day care centre, hospital, practitioner's office, or clinic.

Nipissing District Developmental Screen

In Canada, much of the pediatric primary care is provided by family practitioners. Most physicians perform a developmental assessment of some kind, during the well-child visits, but it is unknown how many use a consistent standardized assessment. It is very important that all children be assessed for

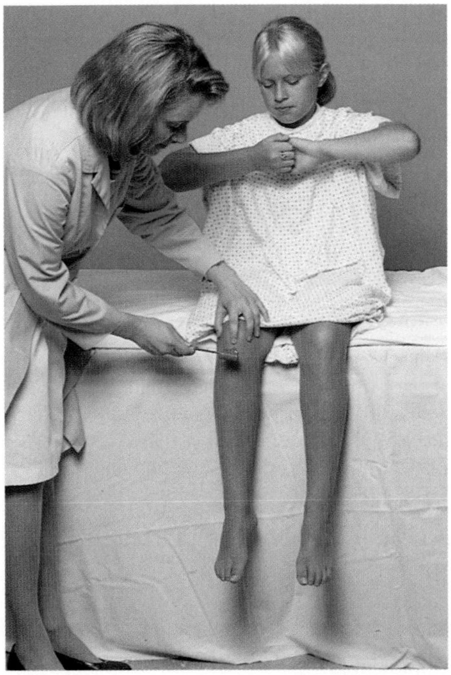

Fig. 34-44 Testing for patellar, or knee jerk, reflex, using distraction. The child sits on edge of the examining table (or on parent's lap) with lower legs flexed at the knee and dangling freely. The patellar tendon is tapped just below the kneecap. Normal response is partial extension of the lower leg.

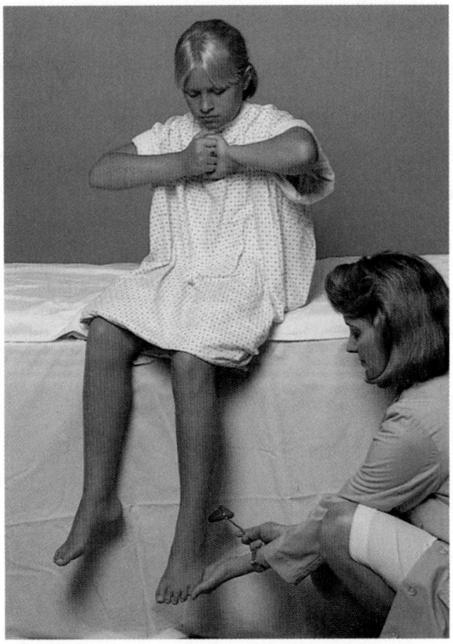

Fig. 34-45 Testing for Achilles reflex. The child should be in the same position as for knee jerk reflex. The foot is supported lightly in the examiner's hand, and the Achilles tendon is struck. Normal response is plantar flexion of the foot (foot pointing downward).

developmental disabilities. Developmental delay affects between 4 and 16% of children and is the leading cause of disability among children younger than 4 years of age in Canada. Early diagnosis and intervention is critical to improve long-term outcomes. However, only 30% of children with

Table 34-13 Assessment of Cranial Nerves

DESCRIPTION AND FUNCTION	TESTS
I—Olfactory Nerve	
Olfactory mucosa of nasal cavity Smell	With eyes closed, have child identify odours such as coffee, alcohol from a swab, or other smells; test each nostril separately.
II—Optic Nerve	
Rods and cones of retina, optic nerve Vision	Check for perception of light, visual acuity, peripheral vision, colour vision, and normal optic disc.
III—Oculomotor Nerve	
Extraocular muscles of the eye: Superior rectus (SR)—moves eyeball up and in Inferior rectus (IR)—moves eyeball down and in Medial rectus (MR)—moves eyeball nasally Inferior oblique (IO)—moves eyeball up and out	Have child follow an object (toy) or light in six cardinal positions of gaze (see Fig. 34-46).
Pupil constriction and accommodation	Perform PERRLA (*P*upils *E*qual, *R*ound, *R*eact to *L*ight, and *A*ccommodation).
Eyelid closing	Check for proper placement of lid.
IV—Trochlear Nerve	
Superior oblique muscle (SO)—moves eye down and out	Have child look down and in (see Fig. 34-46).
V—Trigeminal Nerve	
Muscles of mastication	Have child bite down hard and open jaw; test symmetry and strength.
Sensory—face, scalp, nasal and buccal mucosa	With child's eyes closed, see if child can detect light touch in mandibular and maxillary regions. Test corneal and blink reflex by touching cornea lightly (approach from the side so that child does not blink before cornea is touched).
VI—Abducens Nerve	
Lateral rectus (LR) muscle—moves eye temporally	Have child look toward temporal side (see Fig. 34-46)
VII—Facial Nerve	
Muscles for facial expression	Have child smile, make funny face, or show teeth to see symmetry of expression.
Anterior two thirds of tongue (sensory)	Have child identify sweet or salty solution; place each taste on anterior section and sides of protruding tongue; if child retracts tongue, solution will dissolve toward posterior part of tongue.
VIII—Auditory, Acoustic, or Vestibulocochlear Nerve	
Internal ear Hearing and balance	Test hearing; note any loss of equilibrium or presence of vertigo.
IX—Glossopharyngeal Nerve	
Pharynx, tongue	Stimulate posterior pharynx with a tongue blade; child should gag.
Posterior third of tongue Sensory	Test sense of sour or bitter taste on posterior segment of tongue.
X—Vagus Nerve	
Muscles of the larynx, pharynx, some organs of gastrointestinal system, sensory fibres of root of tongue, heart, and lung	Note hoarseness of voice, gag reflex, and ability to swallow. Check that uvula is in midline; when stimulated with tongue blade, it should deviate upward and to stimulated side.
XI—Accessory Nerve	
Sternocleidomastoid and trapezius muscles of the shoulder	Have child shrug shoulders while applying mild pressure; with examiner's hands placed on shoulders, have child turn head against opposing pressure on either side; note symmetry and strength.
XII—Hypoglossal Nerve	
Muscles of the tongue	Have child move tongue in all directions; have child protrude tongue as far as possible; note any midline deviation. Test strength by placing tongue blade on one side of tongue and having child move it away.

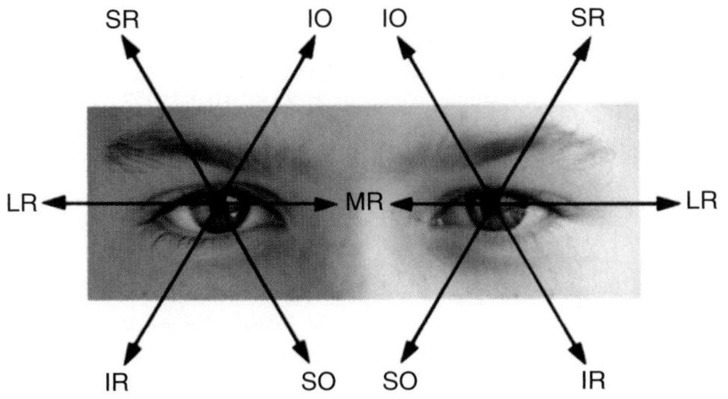

Fig. 34-46 Testing cardinal positions of gaze. Muscles responsible for movement: *SR*, superior rectus; *IR*, inferior rectus; *MR*, medial rectus; *IO*, inferior oblique; *SO*, superior oblique; *LR*, lateral rectus.

BOX 34-17 Nipissing Developmental Assessment Screening

The Nipissing District Developmental Screen™* was compiled by a multidisciplinary team and is free of charge. This straightforward, easy tool tests 13 critical developmental stages at ages 1 and 2 months, 4 months, 6 months, 9 months, 12 months, 15 months, 18 months, 2 years, 30 months, 3 years, 4 years, 5 years, and 6 years. The Screen is available in English, French, Spanish, Chinese, and Vietnamese. Age-appropriate activities that promote overall development are included in the Screens.

The Screen examines a child's skills in the following areas:

- Vision
- Hearing
- Speech and language
- Communication
- Gross motor and fine motor
- Cognitive
- Social/emotional
- Self-help

*The NDDS is available from http://www.ndds.ca/canada/.

disabilities are identified before starting school, and up to one quarter of the first grade children will have learning, health, and behavioural problems that will interfere with their academic and social performance. Nurses provide a valuable service by doing developmental assessments (Limbos, Joyce, & Roberts, 2010).

The Nipissing District Developmental Screen (NDDS) is an accurate, brief screening tool for children aged 1 to 72 months that health care providers can use (Department of Health and Social Services of Yellowknife, 2001). The assessment includes vision, hearing, speech, language, and communication, gross and fine motor function, self-help, and cognitive, social, and emotional function (Box 34-17). The NDDS forms and complete instructions, as well as a computer software program, are provided at the following website: http://www.ndds.ca/canada/. People in some provinces may pay for this service, and in some provinces it is free.

Key Points

- In order to effectively establish a setting for communication, nurses must make an appropriate introduction and ensure privacy and confidentiality.
- When communicating with parents, nurses need to encourage parental involvement, listen carefully, use silence, and be empathic.
- Communication with children needs to reflect their developmental stage.
- Nonverbal communication with children may take the form of writing, drawing, and play.
- The objectives of performing a health history are to identify pertinent information, determine the chief health concern, analyze the present illness, secure the patient's health history, review biological systems, and record a family medical history and child psychosocial and sexual history.
- Family assessment is the collection of data about family composition and relationships among its members; it also focuses on home and community environment, parents' occupation and education, and cultural and religious traditions.
- Nutritional assessment is performed by determination of dietary intake, clinical examination, and biochemical analysis.
- Growth measurements during the physical examination focus on length or height, weight, skin fold thickness, and arm and head circumference. Assessment of growth is measured against standard growth charts to determine a child's status in comparison with that of other children the same age.
- Measurements of temperature, pulse, respiration, and BP constitute the physiological approach to assessment.
- The general appearance of a child is a cumulative, subjective impression of physical appearance, state of nutrition, behaviour, personality, interactions with parents and nurse, posture, development, and speech.
- Assessment of the skin, which primarily involves inspection and palpation, focuses on colour, texture, temperature, moisture, and turgor. The nurse needs to be aware of both physiological and ethnic factors that may affect these areas.
- In assessment of the lymph nodes, the nurse examines, by palpation, the part of the body in which the glands are located.
- The head is inspected for shape, symmetry, mobility, and muscle control.
- Examination of the eyes includes placement and alignment, inspection of external and internal structures, and vision testing.
- The ear examination encompasses placement and alignment, external and internal structures, and auditory testing.
- The lungs are examined by inspection, palpation, percussion, and auscultation.
- Auscultation is the most important procedure for examining the heart.
- Abdominal assessment follows an orderly sequence of inspection, auscultation, percussion, and, finally, palpation, since palpation may distort normal abdominal sounds assessed during auscultation.

- Examination of the genitalia may provoke anxiety in the child, and the nurse must avoid any transference of anxiety.
- Neurological assessment addresses behaviour; motor, sensory, and cerebellar function; reflexes; and cranial nerves.
- The Nipissing District Developmental Screen™ is an accurate, brief developmental assessment tool for children ages 1 to 72 months.

References

American Academy of Pediatrics. (2004). *Pediatric nutrition handbook* (5th ed.). Elk Grove Village, IL: Author.

American Academy of Pediatrics, Committee on Practice and Ambulatory Medicine, Section on Ophthalmology. (2003). Eye examination in infants, children, and young adults by pediatricians. *Pediatrics, 111*(4), 902–907.

American Academy of Pediatrics, Committee on Practice and Ambulatory Medicine, Section on Otolaryngology and Bronchoesophagology. (2003). Hearing assessment in infants and children: Recommendations beyond neonatal screening. *Pediatrics, 111*(2), 436–440.

Bald, M. (2002). Ambulatory blood pressure monitoring in children and adolescents. *Minerva Pediatrica, 54*(1), 13–24.

Beevers, G., Lip, G. Y., & O'Brien, E. (2001). ABC of hypertension blood pressure measurement, part I, sphygmomanometry: Factors common to all techniques. *British Medical Journal, 322*(7292), 981–985.

Berry, B. E., et al. (2001). Preschool vision screening using the MTI-Photoscreener. *Pediatric Nursing 27*(1), 27–34.

Canada Health Infoway. (2011). *Infoway vision.* Retrieved from https://www.infoway-inforoute.ca/lang-en/about-infoway/vision.

Canadian Association of Optometrists. (2010). *Life view: Children's vision is overlooked by Canadian parents.* Retrieved from http://www.northumberlandview.ca/index.php?module=news&func=display&sid=4555.

Canadian Nurses Association. (2010). *Nursing ethics. Code of ethics for registered nurses (2008 centennial edition).* Retrieved from http://www.cna-aiic.ca/CNA/practice/ethics/code/default_e.aspx.

Canadian Paediatric Society. (2003). *Temperature measurement in paediatrics.* (Reaffirmed February 2011) Retrieved from http://www.cps.ca/english/statements/CP/cp00-01.htm.

Canadian Paediatric Society. (2008). *Your baby's hearing.* Retrieved from http://www.caringforkids.cps.ca/pregnancybabies/BabyHearing.htm.

Canadian Paediatric Society. (2009). Vision screening in infants, children, and youths. *Paediatrics and Child Health, 14*(4), 246–248.

Canadian Paediatric Society. (2010a). The Greig health record. *Paediatrics and Child Health, 15*(3), 157–159.

Canadian Paediatric Society. (2010b). *Promoting optimal monitoring of child growth in Canada: Using the new WHO growth charts.* Retrieved from http://www.cps.ca/english/Publications/CPS10-01.htm.

Canadian Paediatric Society. (2010c). *A health professional's guide to using the new WHO growth charts.* Retrieved from http://www.cps.ca/ENGLISH/statements/N/DC_HealthProGrowthGuide_BW.pdf.

Clark, J. A., et al. (2002). Discrepancies between direct and indirect blood pressure measurements using various recommendations for arm cuff selection. *Pediatrics, 110*(5), 920–923.

Coats, D. K., & Jenkins, R. H. (1997). Vision assessment of the pediatric patient: Refinements. *American Academy of Ophthalmology, 1*(1), 1–12.

Craig, J. V., et al. (2000). Temperature measured at the axilla compared with rectum in children and young people: Systematic review. *British Medical Journal, 320*(7243), 1174–1178.

Cronk, C., Crocker, A. C., Pueschel, S. M., et al. (1988). Growth charts for children with Down syndrome: 1 month to 18 years of age. *Pediatrics 81*, 102–110. Retrieved from http://pediatrics.aappublications.org/cgi/content/abstract/81/1/102.

Cunningham, M., & Cox, E. O. (2003). Hearing assessment in infants and children: Recommendations beyond neonatal screening. *Pediatrics, 111*(2), 436–440.

Department of Health and Social Services of Yellowknife. (2001). *Evaluation. Field test of the Nipissing developmental assessment screening.* Retrieved from http://www.ndds.ca/pdf2/Evaluation%20-%20Field%20Test%20of%20NDDS%20Screen%20in%20NWT.pdf.

Fenton, T. R. (2003). A new growth chart for preterm babies: Babson and Benda's chart updated with recent data and a new format. *BMC Pediatrics, 3*, 13. Retrieved from http://www.biomedcentral.com/1471-2431/3/13. doi:10.1186/1471-2431-3-13.

Gillman, M. W., & Cook, N. R. (1995). Blood pressure measurement in childhood epidemiological studies. *Circulation, 92*(4), 1049–1057.

Goldman, L. R., & Shannon, M. W. (2001). Technical report: Mercury in the environment: Implications for pediatricians. *Pediatrics, 108*(1), 197–205.

Goodwin, S. (2007). Telephone nursing: An emerging area. *Nursing Leadership, 20*(4), 37–45.

Halle, C. (2002). Achieve new vision screening objectives. *The Nurse Practitioner, 27*(3), 15–35.

Health Canada. (2005). *Pan-Canadian health information privacy and confidentiality framework.* Ottawa: Author. Retrieved from http://www.hc-sc.gc.ca/hcs-sss/pubs/ehealth-esante/2005-pancanad-priv/index-eng.php.

Health Canada. (2007). *Eating well with Canada's food guide.* Ottawa: Author. Retrieved from http://www.hc-sc.gc.ca/fn-an/food-guide-aliment/myguide-monguide/index-eng.php.

Hedley, A. A., et al. (2004). Prevalence of overweight and obesity among U.S. children, adolescents, and adults, 1999–2002. *Journal of the American Medical Association, 291*(23), 2847–2850.

Hoge, D. R., & Parette, H. P. (1995). Facilitating communicative development in young children with disabilities. *Transdisciplinary Journal, 5*(2), 113–130.

Katamay, S., et al. (2007). Eating well with Canada's food guide: Development of the food intake pattern. *Nutrition Reviews, 65*(4), 155–156. doi:10.1111/j.1753-4887.2007.tb00295.x

Limbos, M. M., Joyce, D. P., & Roberts, G. J. (2010). Nipissing District Developmental Screen. Patterns of use by physicians in Ontario, *Canadian Family Physician, 56*(2), e66–e72.

Livingstone, M. B., Robson, P. J., & Wallace, M. W. (2004). Issues in dietary intake assessment of children and adolescents. *British Journal of Nutrition, 92*(Suppl 2), S213–S222.

Martin, S. A., & Kline, A. M. (2004). Can there be a standard for temperature measurement in the pediatric intensive care unit? *AACN Clinical Issues, 15*(2), 254–266.

Mattu, G. S., Heran, B. S., & Wright, J. M. (2004a). Comparison of the automated non-invasive oscillometric blood pressure monitor (BpTRU™) with the auscultatory mercury sphygmomanometer in a paediatric population. *Blood Pressure Monitoring, 9*(1), 39–45.

Mattu, G. S., Heran, B. S., & Wright, J. M. (2004b). Overall accuracy of the BpTRU™—an automated electronic blood pressure device. *Blood Pressure Monitoring, 9*(1), 47–52.

Murphy, S. P., & Poos, M. I. (2002). Dietary reference intakes: Summary of applications in dietary assessment. *Public Health and Nutrition, 5*(6A), 843–849.

National High Blood Pressure Education Program Working Group on High Blood Pressure in Children and Adolescents. (2004). The fourth report on the diagnosis, evaluation, and treatment of high blood pressure in children and adolescents. *Pediatrics, 114*(2 Suppl 4th Rep), 555–576.

National Institutes of Health, National Heart, Lung, and Blood Institute. (1996, September). *Update on the Task Force Report (1987) on high blood pressure in children and adolescents: A working group report from the National High Blood Pressure Education Program* [NIH Pub No 96-3790]. Bethesda, MD: Author.

Nicklas, T. A., et al. (2004). Children's food consumption patterns have changed over 2 decades (1973–1994): The Bogalusa heart study. *Journal of the American Dietetic Association, 104*(7), 1127–1140.

Office of the Privacy Commissioner of Canada. (2009). *A guide for individuals. Your guide to PIPEDA.* Ottawa: Author. Retrieved from http://www.priv.gc.ca/information/02_05_d_08_e.cfm.

Park, M., Lee, D., & Johnson, G. A. (1993). Oscillometric blood pressures in the arm, thigh, and calf in healthy children and those with aortic coarctation. *Pediatrics, 91*(4), 761–765.

Park, M. K., Menard, S. W., & Schoolfield, J. (2005). Oscillometric blood pressure standards for children. *Pediatric Cardiology, 26*(5), 601–607.

Price, V., & Archbold, J. (1997). What's it all about, empathy? *Nursing Education Today, 17*(2), 106–110.

Reynolds, W. H., Scott, B., & Jessiman, W. C. (1999). Empathy has not been measured in clients' terms or effectively taught: A review of the literature. *Journal of Advanced Nursing, 30*(5), 1177–1185.

Rutenberg, C. D. (2000). Telephone triage. *American Journal of Nursing, 100*(3), 77–78, 80–81.

Seidel, H. M., et al. (2006). *Mosby's guide to physical examination* (6th ed.). St. Louis: Mosby.

Stacey, D. Z., Hussein, A., Fisher, D., Robinson, J., & Pong, R. (2003). *Telephone triage services: Systematic review and a survey of Canadian call service programs*. Ottawa: Canadian Coordinating Office for Health Technology Assessment.

Turnbull, R. (2000). Skin assessment in children: A methodical approach. *Nursing Times, 96*(41), 33–34.

Vessey, J. A. (1995). Developmental approaches to examining young children. *Pediatric Nursing, 21*(1), 53–56.

Wall, T. C., et al. (2002). Compliance with vision-screening guidelines among a national sample of pediatricians. *Ambulatory Pediatrics, 2*(6), 449–455.

White, S. J. (1997). Empathy: A literature review and concept analysis. *Journal of Clinical Nursing, 6*(4), 253–257.

Yegdich, T. (1999). On the phenomenology of empathy in nursing: Empathy or sympathy? *Journal of Advanced Nursing, 30*(1), 83–93.

Additional Resources

Canadian Nursing Informatics Association: http://www.cnia.ca/about.htm

Hockenberry, M. (2008). Communication and physical assessment of the child. In D. Wilson & M. Hockenberry (Eds.), *Wong's clinical manual of pediatric nursing* (7th ed.). St. Louis: Mosby.

Office of Privacy Commissioner of Canada (Information on the *Privacy Act and PIPEDA*): http://www.priv.gc.ca/information/02_05_d_08_e.cfm

Unit 8

35 Pain Assessment and Management

Learning Objectives

On completion of this chapter, the reader will be able to:

- Identify measures to assess pain in children.
- List various types of pain assessment tools that are used with children.
- Outline essential pain management strategies of reducing pain in children.
- Review common types of pain experienced by children.
- Discuss evidence supporting specific pain management strategies.

Electronic Resources

Additional information related to the content in Chapter 35 can be found on

evolve the companion Web site at

http://evolve.elsevier.com/Canada/Perry/maternal/

- Examination Review Questions
- Skill—Calculating Safe Dosages for Children
- Skill—Managing Pain

Pain Assessment

Although the ability to measure **pain** in children has improved dramatically in recent years, assessment of pain in children continues to be complex and challenging. Children's ability to describe pain changes as they grow older and as they cognitively and linguistically mature (Box 35-1). Three types of measures—behavioural, physiological, and self-report—have been developed to measure children's pain, and their applicability depends on the child's cognitive and linguistic abilities.

Behavioural Measures

Distress behaviours, such as vocalization, facial expression, and body movement, have been associated with pain (Figs. 35-1 and 35-2). These behaviours are helpful in evaluating pain in infants and children with limited communication skills. However, discriminating between pain behaviours and reactions from other sources of distress, such as hunger, anxiety, or other types of discomfort, is not always easy, thus the specificity and sensitivity of behavioural measures may be decreased (Table 35-1).

Behavioural assessment is useful for measuring pain in infants and preverbal children who do not have the language skills to communicate that they are in pain, or in children with mental clouding and confusion that limit their ability to communicate meaningfully (McGrath, 1998). Behaviour provides important information that cannot be obtained from self-report. Behavioural assessment may give a more complete picture of the total pain experience when done in conjunction with a subjective self-report measure. However, behavioural pain scales may be more time consuming to conduct than obtaining self-reports. These measures depend on a trained observer to watch and record children's behaviours, such as vocalization, facial expression, and body movements, that suggest discomfort.

Behavioural measures are most reliable when measuring short, sharp procedural pain, such as during injections or lumbar punctures. They are less reliable when measuring longer-lasting pain. In older children, pain scores on behavioural measures do not always correlate with the children's own reports of pain intensity.

The four most commonly used behavioural pain measures are FLACC, CHEOPS (Children's Hospital of Eastern Ontario Pain Scale), TPPPS (Toddler-Preschooler Postoperative Pain Scale), and PPPRS (Parent's Postoperative Pain Rating Scale). The FLACC Pain Assessment Tool is an interval scale that includes five categories of behaviour: *F*acial expression, *L*eg movement, *A*ctivity, *C*ry, and *C*onsolability (Manworren & Hynan, 2003) (Table 35-2). It measures pain by quantifying pain behaviours with scores ranging from 0 (no pain behaviours) to 10 (most possible pain behaviours). The FLACC observational pain tool has been revised and validated to include behaviours specific to individuals with cognitive impairment (Malviya et al., 2006).

Physiological Measures

Physiological measures are not able to distinguish between physical responses to pain and other forms of stress to the body (Sweet & McGrath, 1998). Profound physiological changes often accompany the experience of pain. Physiological parameters such as heart rate, respiratory rate, blood pressure, palmar sweating, cortisone levels, transcutaneous oxygen, vagal tone, and endorphin concentrations reflect a generalized and complex response to stress. They are not localized responses to pain, but they provide useful information about general distress levels of children experiencing pain. Like

BOX 35-1 Developmental Characteristics of Children's Responses to Pain

Young Infant

Generalized body response of rigidity or thrashing, possibly with local reflex withdrawal of stimulated area
Loud crying
Facial expression of pain (brows lowered and drawn together, eyes tightly closed, mouth open and squarish)
No association demonstrated between approaching stimulus and subsequent pain

Older Infant

Localized body response with deliberate withdrawal of stimulated area
Loud crying
Facial expression of pain or anger
Physical resistance, especially pushing the stimulus away after it is applied

Young Child

Loud crying, screaming
Verbal expressions such as "Ow," "Ouch," "It hurts"
Thrashing of arms and legs
Attempts to push stimulus away before it is applied
Lack of cooperation; need for physical restraint
Requests for termination of procedure
Clinging to parent, nurse, or other significant person
Requests for emotional support, such as hugs or other forms of physical comfort
Becoming restless and irritable with continuing pain
Behaviours occurring in anticipation of actual painful procedure

School-Age Child

May see all behaviours of young child, especially during actual painful procedure, but less in anticipatory period
Stalling behaviour, such as "Wait a minute" or "I'm not ready"
Muscular rigidity, such as clenched fists, white knuckles, gritted teeth, contracted limbs, body stiffness, closed eyes, wrinkled forehead

Adolescent

Less vocal protest
Less motor activity
More verbal expressions, such as "It hurts" or "You're hurting me"
Increased muscle tension and body control

(Data from Craig, K. D., et al. [1984]. Developmental changes in infant pain expression during immunization injections. *Social Science and Medicine, 19*[12], 1331–1337; Katz, E. R., Kellerman, J., & Siegel, S. E. [1980]. Behavioral distress in children with cancer undergoing medical procedures: Developmental considerations. *Journal of Consulting and Clinical Psychology, 48*[3], 356–365.)

behavioural scales, physiological measures may be useful for infants and children who are not able to communicate verbally. The physiological parameters provide indirect estimates of pain, and the presence and strength of pain can only be inferred from the changes in these parameters. Most of the

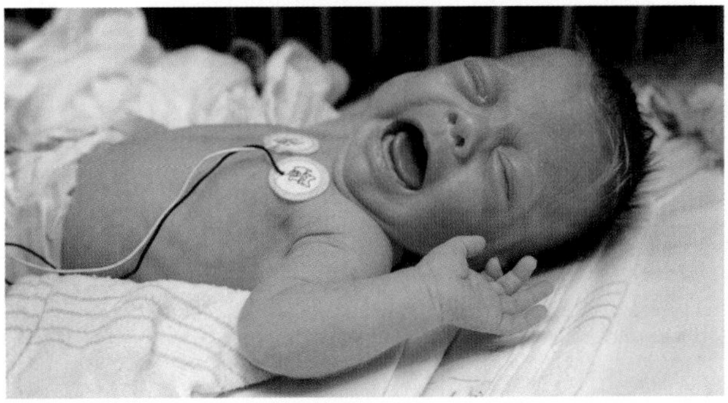

Fig. 35-1 Full, robust crying of preterm infant after heel stick. *(Courtesy Halbouty Premature Nursery, Texas Children's Hospital, Houston; photo by Paul Vincent Kuntz.)*

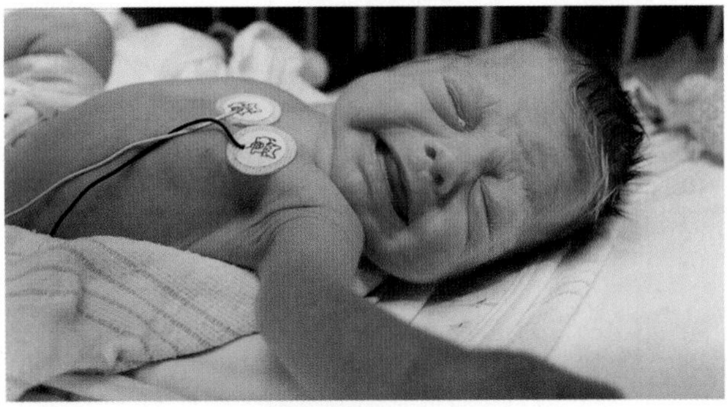

Fig. 35-2 The face of pain after heel stick. Note eye squeeze, brow bulge, nasolabial furrow, and widespread mouth. *(Courtesy Halbouty Premature Nursery, Texas Children's Hospital, Houston; photo by Paul Vincent Kuntz.)*

studies on physiological parameters involved predominantly infants.

Self-Report Measures

Although children who are 4 or 5 years old are able to use self-report measures (Table 35-3), their ability to use them may be influenced by the cognitive characteristics of the preoperational stage (Stanford, Chambers, & Craig, 2006). The child's thinking tends to be egocentric, concrete, and perceptually dominated. Simple, concrete anchor words, such as "no hurt" to "biggest hurt," are more appropriate than "least pain sensation to worst intense pain imaginable."

The ability to discriminate degrees of pain in facial expressions appears to be reasonably established by 3 years of age (Stanford et al., 2006). *Faces pain scales* developed for young children may be a measure of pain intensity, pain affect, or both, particularly when the faces are anchored by a smiling face on one end and a face with tears on the other end (Chambers et al., 1999, 2005). Although clinicians may think that the smiling-face anchor confounds the emotion of "feeling happy" with being "pain free," there is no evidence to support this notion. Researchers compared the effects of the smiling face (e.g., the Wong-Baker [WB] FACES Pain Scale) with those of the neutral-anchor faces (e.g., Bieri Faces Pain Scale—Revised) on measurement of pain. Chambers and colleagues (2005) demonstrated a high correlation between the two forms of

Table 35-1 Selected Behavioural Pain Assessment Scales for Infants and Young Children

AGES OF USE	INSTRUMENT
4 mo–18 yr	Objective Pain Score (OPS) (Hannallah et al., 1987)
1–5 yr	Children's Hospital of Eastern Ontario Pain Scale (CHEOPS) (McGrath et al., 1985)
Newborn–16 yr	Nurses Assessment of Pain Inventory (NAPI) (Stevens, 1990)
3–36 mo	Behavioural Pain Score (BPS) (Robieux et al., 1991)
4–6 mo	Modified Behavioural Pain Scale (MBPS) (Taddio et al., 1995)
<36 mo and children with cerebral palsy	Riley Infant Pain Scale (RIPS) (Schade et al., 1996)
2 mo–7 yr	FLACC Postoperative Pain Tool (Merkel et al., 1997)
1–7 mo	Postoperative Pain Score (POPS) (Barrier et al., 1987)
Average gestational age 33.5 wk	Neonatal Infant Pain Scale (NIPS) (Lawrence et al., 1993)
27 wk gestational age to full term	Pain Assessment Tool (PAT) (Hodgkinson et al., 1994)
1–36 mo	Pain Rating Scale (PRS) (Joyce et al., 1994)
32–60 wk gestational age	CRIES (Krechel & Bildner, 1995)
28–40 wk gestational age	Premature Infant Pain Profile (PIPP) (Stevens et al., 1996)
0–28 days	Scale for Use in Newborns (SUN) (Blauer & Gerstmann, 1998)
Birth (23 wk gestational age) and full-term newborns up to 100 days	Neonatal Pain, Agitation, and Sedation Scale (NPASS) (Puchalski & Hummel, 2002)

Table 35-2 FLACC Scale

	0	1	2
Face	No particular expression or smile	Occasional grimace or frown, withdrawn, disinterested	Frequent to constant frown, clenched jaw, quivering chin
Legs	Normal position or relaxed	Uneasy, restless, tense	Kicking, or legs drawn up
Activity	Lying quietly, normal position, moves easily	Squirming, shifting back and forth, tense	Arched, rigid, or jerking
Cry	No cry (awake or asleep)	Moans or whimpers, occasional complaint	Crying steadily, screams or sobs, frequent complaints
Consolability	Content, relaxed	Reassured by occasional touching, hugging, or talking to; distractible	Difficult to console or comfort

(From Merkel, S., et al. [1997]. The FLACC: A behavioral scale for scoring postoperative pain in young children. *Pediatric Nursing, 23*[3], 293–297. Used with permission of Jannetti Publications, Inc., and the University of Michigan Health System. Can be reproduced for clinical and research use.)

faces scales, with $r = 0.91$ between the Bieri Faces Pain Scale (neutral anchor) and WB-FACES Pain Scale (smiling anchor). These data suggest that children are able to use either scale for communicating the amount of pain they experience.

Multidimensional Measures

Several cognitive skills, such as measurement, classification, and seriation (the ability to accurately place in ascending or descending order), become explicit between approximately 7 and 10 years of age. Older children are able to use the 0-to-10 numeric rating scale currently used with adolescents and adults. However, use of this scale is only an assessment of pain intensity, which may not change in some pain states (Jacob et al., 2003a; Jacob, 2003b). Other dimensions such as pain quality, pain location, and spatial distribution of pain may change without a change in pain intensity.

Two multidimensional assessment tools that have been well validated in children 8 years of age and older assess not only pain intensity but also pain location and pain quality. Modelled after the McGill Pain Questionnaire (Melzack, 1975), the *Adolescent Pediatric Pain Tool (APPT)* is a multidimensional pain instrument for children and adolescents that is used to assess three dimensions of pain: location, intensity, and quality. The *Pediatric Pain Questionnaire (PPQ)* is a multidimensional pain instrument to assess patient and parental perceptions of the pain experience in a manner appropriate for the cognitive-developmental level of children and adolescents. The PPQ represents an attempt to assess the complexities of pediatric chronic, recurrent pain and targeted chronic musculoskeletal pain in children with juvenile rheumatoid arthritis. It consists of eight questions about the following: (1) the pain history, (2) pain language, (3) the colours that children associate with pain, (4) the emotions they experience, (5) their worst pain experiences, (6) the ways in which they cope with pain, (7) the positive aspects of pain, and (8) the location of their current pain.

Table 35-3 Pain Rating Scales for Children

PAIN SCALE, DESCRIPTION	RECOMMENDED AGE, COMMENTS
FACES Pain Rating Scale (Wong & Baker, 1988) Uses six cartoon faces ranging from smiling face for "no pain" to tearful face for "worst pain"	Children as young as 3 yr Using original instructions without affect words, such as *happy* or *sad*, or brief words resulted in same range of pain rating, probably reflecting child's rating of pain intensity. For coding purposes, numbers 0, 2, 4, 6, 8, 10 can be substituted for 0–5 system to accommodate 0–10 system. Provides three scales in one: facial expressions, numbers, and words. Research supports cultural sensitivity of FACES for White, Black, Latin American, Thai, Chinese, and Japanese children.

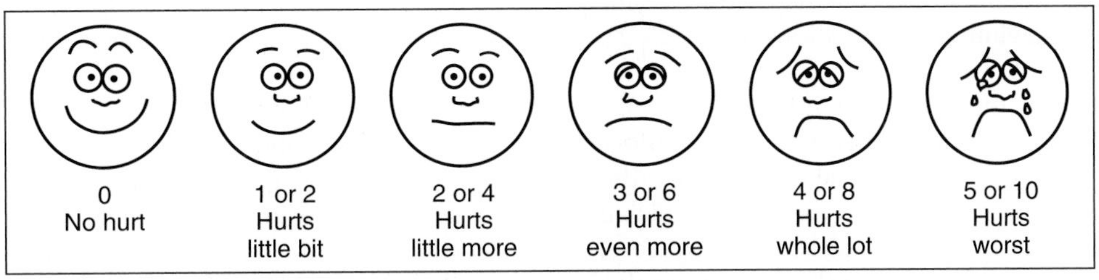

(From Hockenberry, M. J., et al. [2005]. Wong's essentials of pediatric nursing, ed 7, St. Louis: Mosby, p. 1259. Used with permission. Copyright, Mosby.)

PAIN SCALE, DESCRIPTION	RECOMMENDED AGE, COMMENTS
Oucher (Beyer, Denyes, & Villarruel, 1992) Uses six photographs of White child's face representing "no hurt" to "biggest hurt you could ever have"; also includes vertical scale with numbers from 0 to 100; scales for Black and Latin American children have been developed (Villarruel & Denyes, 1991)	Children 3–13 yr Use numeric scale if child can count to 100 by ones and identify the larger of any two numbers, or by tens (Jordan-Marsh et al., 1994). Determine whether child has cognitive ability to use photographic scale; child should be able to rate six geometric shapes from largest to smallest. Determine which ethnic version of Oucher to use. Allow child to select version of Oucher, or use version that most closely matches child's physical characteristics. Note: Child may not prefer ethnically similar scale when given choice of ethnically neutral cartoon scale (Luffy & Grove, 2003).
Poker Chip Tool (Hester et al., 1998) Uses four red poker chips placed horizontally in front of child to denote varying intensities of pain	Children as young as 4 yr Determine whether child has cognitive ability to use numbers by identifying larger of any two numbers.
Word-Graphic Rating Scale (Tesler et al., 1991) Uses descriptive words (may vary in other scales) to denote varying intensities of pain	Children 4–17 yr

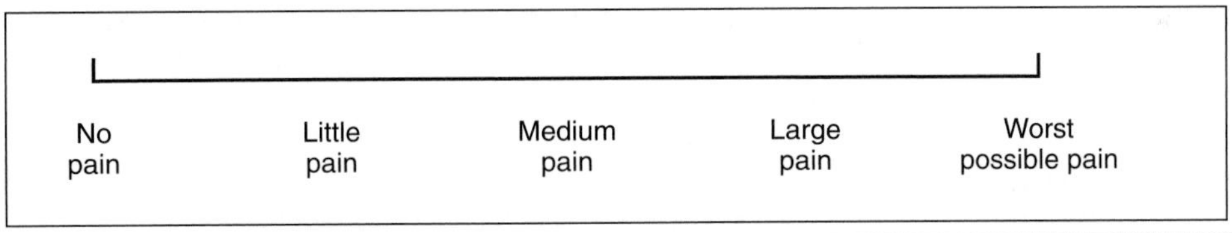

PAIN SCALE, DESCRIPTION	RECOMMENDED AGE, COMMENTS
Numeric Scale Uses straight line with end points identified as "no pain" and "worst pain" and sometimes "medium pain" in the middle; divisions along line marked in units from 0 to 10 (high number may vary)	Children as young as 5 yr, as long as they can count and have some concept of numbers and their values in relation to other numbers. Scale may be used horizontally or vertically. Number coding should be the same as in other scales used in facility.

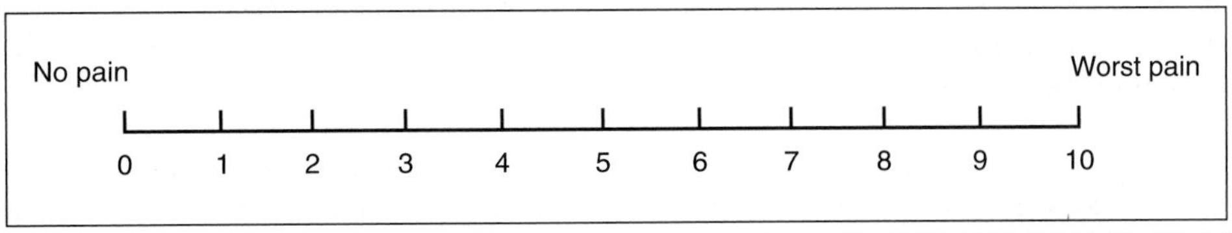

PAIN SCALE, DESCRIPTION	RECOMMENDED AGE, COMMENTS
Visual Analogue Scale (VAS) (Cline et al., 1992) A vertical or horizontal line is drawn to a certain length, such as 10 cm, and anchored by items that represent extremes of the subjective phenomenon, such as pain, that is measured	Children as young as $4\frac{1}{2}$ yr, preferably 7 yr Vertical or horizontal scale may be used. Research shows that children ages 3–18 yr prefer VAS less than other scales (Luffy & Grove, 2003; Wong & Baker, 1988).

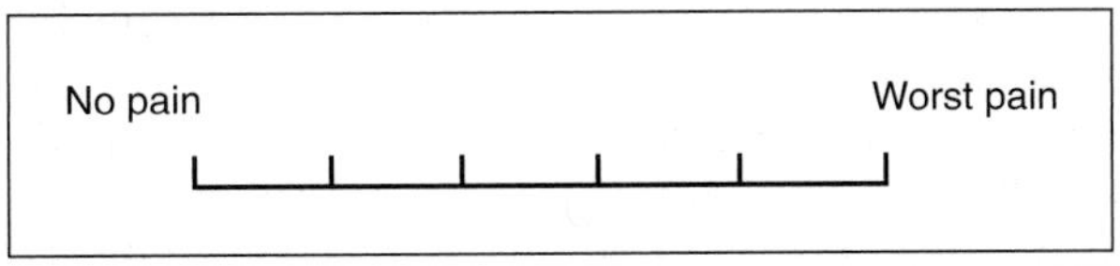

PAIN SCALE, DESCRIPTION	RECOMMENDED AGE, COMMENTS
Colour Tool (Eland & Banner, 1999) Uses markers for child to construct own scale that is used with body outline; different-coloured markers denote different levels of pain in different body areas	Children as young as 4 yr, provided they know their colours, are not colour blind, and are able to construct the scale if in pain

Pain Assessment in Specific Populations

Pain in Neonates

Assessment of pain is difficult in the preverbal child, especially the neonate, since the most reliable indicator of pain, self-report, is not possible. Evaluation must be based on physiological changes and behavioural observations (Box 35-2). Although behaviours such as vocalizations, facial expressions, and body movements are common to all infants, they vary with different situations. Crying associated with pain is more intense and sustained (see Fig. 35-1). Facial expression is the most consistent and specific characteristic; scales are available to systematically evaluate facial features, such as eye squeeze, brow bulge, open mouth, and taut tongue (Hadjistavropoulos et al., 1997). Most infants respond with increased body movements, but the infant may be experiencing pain even when lying quietly with eyes closed. The preterm infant's response to pain may be behaviourally blunted or absent; however, there is ample evidence that such infants are neurologically capable of feeling pain. In addition, infants in awake or alert states demonstrate a more robust reaction to painful stimuli than do infants in sleep states. Also, an infant receiving a muscle-paralyzing agent such as vecuronium will be incapable of a behavioural or visible pain response.

Although regular use of pain assessment tools can assist caregivers in determining whether the infant is in pain, caregivers must consider the infant's maturity, behavioural state, energy resources available to respond, and risk factors for pain. In infants with diminished ability to respond robustly to pain, it is imperative to presume that pain exists in all situations that are usually considered painful for adults and children, even in the absence of behavioural or physiological signs (Sweet & McGrath, 1998).

Several pain assessment tools have been developed for the assessment of pain in the neonate. One such tool used by nurses who work with preterm and full-term infants in the neonatal intensive care setting is called *CRIES*, which is an acronym for the tool's physiological and behavioural indicators of pain: *C*rying, *R*equires increased oxygen, *I*ncreased vital signs, *E*xpression, and *S*leeplessness (Table 35-4). Each indicator is scored from 0 to 2—similar to the Apgar score for neonates. The total possible pain score, representing the worst pain, is 10. A pain score greater than 4 should be considered significant. This tool has been tested for reliability and validity for postoperative pain in infants between the ages of 32 weeks of gestation up to 20 weeks postterm (60 weeks) (Sweet & McGrath, 1998).

The *Premature Infant Pain Profile (PIPP)* is unique because it has been developed specifically for preterm infants (Sweet & McGrath, 1998). The category "gestational age at time of observation" gives a higher pain score to infants with lower gestational age. Infants who are asleep 15 seconds before the painful procedure also receive additional points for their blunted behavioural responses to painful stimuli.

BOX 35-2 Manifestations of Acute Pain in the Neonate

Physiological Responses

Vital signs—Observe for variations.
- Increased heart rate
- Increased blood pressure
- Rapid, shallow respirations

Oxygenation
- Decreased transcutaneous oxygen saturation ($tcPo_2$)
- Decreased arterial oxygen saturation (Sao_2)

Skin—Observe colour and character.
- Pallor or flushing
- Diaphoresis
- Palmar sweating

Laboratory evidence of metabolic or endocrine changes
- Hyperglycemia
- Lowered pH
- Elevated corticosteroids
- Other observations
- Increased muscle tone
- Dilated pupils
- Decreased vagal nerve tone
- Increased intracranial pressure

Behavioural Responses

Vocalizations—Observe quality, timing, and duration.
- Crying
- Whimpering
- Groaning

Facial expression—Observe characteristics, timing, and orientation of eyes and mouth.
- Grimaces
- Brow furrowed
- Chin quivering
- Eyes tightly closed
- Mouth open and squarish

Body movements and posture—Observe type, quality, and amount of movement or lack of movement; consider in relationship to other factors.
- Limb withdrawal
- Thrashing
- Rigidity
- Flaccidity
- Fist clenching

Changes in state—Observe sleep, appetite, and activity level.
- Changes in sleep–wake cycles
- Changes in feeding behaviour
- Changes in activity level
- Fussiness, irritability
- Listlessness

Table 35-4 CRIES Neonatal Postoperative Pain Scale

	0	1	2
Crying	No	High pitched	Inconsolable
Requires oxygen for saturation >95%	No	<30%	>30%
Increased vital signs	Heart rate and blood pressure ≤ preoperative state	Heart rate and blood pressure increase <20% of preoperative state	Heart rate and blood pressure increase >20% of preoperative state
Expression	None	Grimace	Grimace, grunt
Sleepless	No	Wakes at frequent intervals	Constantly awake

Children With Communication and Cognitive Impairment

The assessment of pain in children with communication and cognitive impairment can be challenging. Children who have significant difficulties communicating with others about their pain include those with significant neurological impairments (e.g., cerebral palsy), cognitive impairment, metabolic disorders, autism, severe brain injury, or communication barriers (e.g., critically ill children who are on ventilators or heavily sedated or have neuromuscular disorders, loss of hearing, or loss of vision). These children are at greater risk than other children for undertreatment of pain because they have medical problems that may cause pain and they undergo painful procedures. Their behaviours include moaning, inconsistent patterns of play and sleep, changes in facial expression, and other physical problems that may mask expression of pain and be difficult to interpret (Hadden & von Baeyer, 2002). These children may experience spasticity, contractures, and orthopaedic surgical treatment that may be painful.

The mother or primary caregiver is an important source of information during assessment (Breau et al., 2003). Up to 60% of parents of children with severe cognitive impairment reported that their child experienced pain or severe discomfort that was not being effectively managed (Lenton et al., 2001; Stallard et al., 2002a). The most frequently reported pain behaviours are crying; being less active; seeking comfort; moaning; not cooperating; being irritable; being stiff, spastic, tense, or rigid; sleeping less; being difficult to satisfy or pacify; flinching or moving a body part away; and being agitated or fidgety (Hadden & von Baeyer, 2002). Parents also reported pain during some daily living activities such as assisted stretching and walking; independent standing; toileting; putting on splints; and doing occupational therapy, range-of-motion exercises, or physical therapy.

The *Non-Communicating Children's Pain Checklist* is a pain measurement tool specifically designed for children with cognitive impairments (Breau et al., 2002). The scale discriminates between periods of pain and those of calm and can predict behaviour during subsequent episodes of pain. The scale consists of six subscales (vocal, social, facial, activity, body and limbs, physiological), which are scored on the basis of number of times the items are observed over a 10-minute period (0 = not at all; 1 = just a little; 2 = fairly often; 3 = very often).

Another tool, the *Pain Indicator for Communicatively Impaired Children (PICIC)*, is used to distinguish between pain and nonpain in communicatively impaired children with life-threatening illness (Stallard et al., 2002a, 2002b). The PICIC has six core pain cues: (1) crying with or without tears; (2) screaming, yelling, groaning, or moaning; (3) screwed-up or distressed-looking face; (4) body appearing stiff or tense; (5) difficulty in being comforted or consoled; and (6) flinching or moving away if touched. The items are rated using a 4-point Likert scale (1 = not at all, 2 = a little, 3 = often, 4 = all the time).

Cultural Issues in Pain Assessment

A major challenge in the assessment and management of pain in children is the cultural appropriateness of pain assessment tools that have been validated only in White and English-speaking children. Observational scales and interview questionnaires for pain may not be as reliable for pain assessment as self-report scales in non-White and non-English-speaking children. In Chinese children who learned to read Chinese characters vertically downward and from right to left, the use of vertically oriented visual analogue scales resulted in less error than horizontally oriented scales. Cultural background may thus influence the reliability of pain assessment tools developed in a single-cultural context (Bernstein & Pachter, 2003).

The *Oucher Pain Scale* (see Table 35-3), originally developed and validated as a self-report of pain intensity for White children 3 to 12 years old, now features culturally specific photographs of children who better represent the physical characteristics of Black and Latin American children (Beyer & Knott, 1998). The Oucher Pain Scale consists of six photographs on the right side and a 0-to-100 scale marked off in tens on the left side. The photographs show the face of one child with the pictures arranged to show increasing levels of discomfort. Each version has been tested primarily with children of the ethnic group (White, Black, Latin American) depicted in the photographs. Children ages 3 to 12 years old use the Oucher by selecting a photograph or number that most closely represents the level of pain intensity that they are experiencing (Beyer & Knott, 1998). This tool is designed to promote cultural sensitivity during pain assessment for non-White children.

evolve Skill—Managing Pain

Children With Chronic Illness and Complex Pain

Questionnaires and pain assessment scales do not always provide the most meaningful means of assessing pain in children, particularly for those with complex pain. Some children cannot relate to a face or a number that describes their pain and may not be able to isolate pain from other symptoms they are experiencing. Children with cancer experience multiple symptoms, making it difficult to isolate the pain symptom from other symptoms. Rating the pain does not always accurately convey to others how they really feel (Woodgate & Yanofsky, 2004).

In children with chronic illness, particularly those with complex pain, the most important aspect of assessment is to develop a trusting relationship with the child and the family so that a deeper understanding of the pain experience may be obtained. The pain experience may be complicated by pain processes that occur in the central nervous system (such as hyperalgesia, central sensitization, windup), by other symptoms (such as fatigue, nausea, vomiting, diarrhea, constipation) that accompany medical treatments, and by complications (such as infections, unexpected development of fistulas, typhlitis) from disease or treatments (Turner, 2005). The pain experience may interfere with the child's ability to eat, sleep, and perform daily activities and routines (Miaskowski & Lee, 1999; Morin, Gibson, & Wade, 1998).

Other important components of assessment include the onset of pain; pain duration or pattern; the effectiveness of the current treatment; factors that aggravate or relieve the pain; other symptoms and complications concurrently felt; and interference with the child's **mood**, function, and interactions with family (Turner, 2005). In addition to asking the child or parent when the pain started and how long the pain lasts, the nurse can assess variations and rhythms by asking if the pain is better or worse at certain times during the day or night. If the child has had pain for a while, the child or parent may know which medications and doses are helpful. They may also have found some nonpharmacological methods that have helped. The nurse may ask the child or parent if there are activities, positions, and other events that may increase the pain. Pain may be accompanied by other symptoms such as nausea and poor appetite.

Other factors warranting careful assessment that may pose barriers to effective management include family issues and relationships, fears and concerns about addiction (see Family-Centred Teaching box), the clinician's and family's lack of knowledge about pain, inappropriate use of pain medications, ineffective management of adverse effects from medications, and the use of different pain interventions (Turner, 2005).

FAMILY-CENTRED TEACHING

Fear of Opioid Addiction

One of the reasons for the unfounded but prevalent fear of addiction from opioids used to relieve pain is a misunderstanding of the differences between physical dependence, tolerance, and addiction. Health care providers and the community often confuse addiction with the physiological effects of opioids, when in reality physical dependence, tolerance, and addiction are unrelated. The Canadian Pain Society defines these terms as follows:

Physical dependence is a state of adaptation that often includes tolerance and is manifested by a drug class–specific withdrawal syndrome that can be produced by abrupt cessation, rapid dose reduction, decreasing blood level of the drug, or administration of an antagonist. It is not the same thing as addiction. The symptoms of withdrawal include hypertension, nausea, vomiting, fever, shivering, diarrhea, and muscle aches. These symptoms can be minimized by slowly decreasing the dose of opioids. Weaning should be planned for any patient who has been taking opioids for more than 1 week.

Tolerance is a state of adaptation in which exposure to a drug induces changes that result in a diminution of one or more of the drug's effects over time. This is also not the same as addiction.

Addiction is a primary, chronic, neurobiological disease, with genetic, psychosocial, and environmental factors influencing its development and manifestations. Addiction is characterized by behaviours that include one or more of the following (4 C's):

- Impaired Control over drug use
- Compulsive use
- Craving
- Continued use despite harm (Consequences)

Unfortunately, individuals who have severe, unrelieved pain may become intensely focused on finding relief. Sometimes behaviours such as "clock watching" make patients appear to others to be preoccupied with obtaining opioids. However, this preoccupation centres on finding relief of pain, not on using opioids for reasons other than pain control. This phenomenon has been termed *pseudoaddiction* and must not be confused with real addiction.

Nurses must educate older children, parents, and other health care providers about the extremely low risk of real addiction (less than 0.1%) from the use of opioids to treat pain. Infants, young children, and comatose or terminally ill children simply cannot become addicted because they are incapable of a consistent pattern of drug-seeking behaviour, such as stealing, drug dealing, prostitution, or use of family income, to obtain opioids for nonanalgesic reasons.

(Data from The Canadian Pain Society. [2005, November]. *Accreditation pain standard: Making it happen!* Retrieved from http://www.canadianpainsociety.ca/pdf/accreditation_manual.pdf.)

Pain Management

Unrelieved pain may lead to potential long-term physiological, psychosocial, and behavioural consequences (Goldschneider & Anand, 2003; Weisman, Bernstein, & Schechter, 1998). Management of pain should be a priority for all clinicians.

Nonpharmacological Management

Pain is often associated with fear, anxiety, and stress (Kain et al., 2006). A number of nonpharmacological techniques (see Guidelines box), such as distraction, relaxation, guided imagery, and cutaneous stimulation, provide **coping** strategies that may help reduce **pain perception**, make pain more tolerable, decrease anxiety, and enhance the effectiveness of **analgesics** or reduce the dosage required (Rusy & Weisman, 2000). In addition, these techniques decrease the perceived threat of pain, provide a sense of control, enhance comfort, and promote rest and sleep (Greco & Berde, 2005). Although there is little research on the effectiveness of many of these interventions, the strategies are safe, noninvasive, and inexpensive.

GUIDELINES Nonpharmacological Strategies for Pain Management

General Strategies

Use nonpharmacological interventions to supplement, not replace, pharmacological interventions, and use them for mild pain and pain that is reasonably well controlled with analgesics.

Form a trusting relationship with the child and family.

Express concern regarding their reports of pain and intervene appropriately.

Take an active role in seeking effective pain management strategies.

Use general guidelines to prepare the child for a procedure.

Prepare the child before potentially painful procedures, but avoid "planting" the idea of pain.

- For example, instead of saying, "This is going to (or may) hurt," say, "Sometimes this feels like pushing, sticking, or pinching, and sometimes it doesn't bother people. Tell me what it feels like to you."
- Use "nonpain" descriptors when possible (e.g., "It feels like heat" rather than "It's a burning pain"). This allows for variation in sensory perception, avoids suggesting pain, and gives the child control in describing reactions.
- Avoid evaluative statements or descriptions (e.g., "This is a terrible procedure" or "It really will hurt a lot").

Stay with child during a painful procedure.

- Allow parents to stay with the child if the child and parent desire; encourage the parent to talk softly to the child and to remain near the child's head.
- Involve parents in learning specific nonpharmacological strategies and in assisting the child with their use.

Educate the child about the pain, especially when explanation may lessen anxiety (e.g., that pain may occur after surgery and does not indicate something is wrong); reassure the child that he or she is not responsible for the pain.

For long-term pain control, give the child a doll, which represents "the patient," and allow the child to do everything to the doll that is done to the child; pain control can be emphasized through the doll by stating, "Dolly feels better after the medicine."

Teach procedures to the child and family for later use.

Specific Strategies

Distraction

Involve the parent and child in identifying strong distracters.

Involve the child in play; use a radio, CD player, MP3 player, or computer game; have the child sing or use rhythmic breathing.

Have the child take a deep breath and blow it out until told to stop.

Have the child blow bubbles to "blow the hurt away."

Have the child concentrate on yelling or saying "ouch," with instructions to "yell as loud or soft as you feel it hurt; that way I know what's happening."

Have the child look through a kaleidoscope (one with glitter suspended in fluid-filled tube) and encourage him or her to concentrate, by asking, "Do you see the different designs?"

Use humour, such as watching cartoons, telling jokes or funny stories, or acting silly with the child.

Have the child read, play games, or visit with friends.

Relaxation

With an infant or a young child:

- Hold the child in a comfortable, well-supported position, such as vertically against the chest and shoulder.
- Rock the child in a wide, rhythmic arc in a rocking chair or sway back and forth, rather than bouncing the child.
- Repeat one or two words softly, such as "Mommy's here."

With a slightly older child:

- Ask the child to take a deep breath and "go limp as a rag doll" while exhaling slowly; then ask the child to yawn (demonstrate if needed).
- Help the child assume a comfortable position (e.g., pillow under neck and knees).
- Begin progressive relaxation: starting with the toes, systematically instruct the child to let each body part "go limp" or "feel heavy"; if the child has difficulty relaxing, instruct the child to tense or tighten each body part and then relax it.
- Allow the child to keep eyes open, since children may respond better if eyes are open rather than closed during relaxation.

Guided Imagery

Have the child identify some highly pleasurable real or imaginary experience.

Have the child describe details of the event, including as many senses as possible (e.g., "feel the cool breezes," "see the beautiful colours," "hear the pleasant music").

Have the child write down or record the script.

Encourage the child to concentrate only on the pleasurable event during the painful time; enhance the image by recalling specific details through reading the script or playing the recording.

Combine with relaxation and rhythmic breathing.

Positive Self-Talk

Teach the child positive statements to say when in pain (e.g., "I will be feeling better soon," "When I go home, I will feel better, and we will eat ice cream").

Thought Stopping

Identify positive facts about the painful event (e.g., "It does not last long").

Identify reassuring information (e.g., "If I think about something else, it does not hurt as much").

Condense positive and reassuring facts into a set of brief statements and have child memorize them (e.g., "short procedure, good veins, little hurt, nice nurse, go home").

Have child repeat the memorized statements whenever thinking about or experiencing the painful event.

Behavioural Contracting

Informal—May be used with children as young as 4 or 5 years of age:

- Use stars, tokens, or cartoon character stickers as rewards.
- Give a child who is uncooperative or procrastinating during a procedure a limited time (measured by a visible timer) to complete the procedure.
- Proceed as needed if the child is unable to comply.
- Reinforce cooperation with a reward if the procedure is accomplished within a specified time.

Formal—Use a written contract, which includes the following:

- Realistic (seems possible) goal or desired behaviour
- Measurable behaviour (e.g., agreeing not to hit anyone during procedures)
- Date and signature of all persons involved in any of the agreements
- Identified rewards or consequences that are reinforcing
- Goals that can be evaluated
- Commitment and compromise requirements for both parties (e.g., while timer is used, the nurse will not nag or prod the child to complete the procedure)

Environmental and psychological factors may play a large role in children's pain perceptions and may be modified by using psychosocial strategies, education, parental support, and cognitive-behavioural interventions. For children undergoing repeated painful procedures, cognitive-behavioural interventions are effective for decreasing anxiety and distress (McGrath & Hillier, 2003).

If the child cannot identify a familiar coping technique, the nurse can describe several strategies and let the child select the most appealing one. Experimentation with several strategies that are suitable to the child's age, pain intensity, and abilities is often necessary to determine the most effective approach. Parents should be involved in the selection process; they may be familiar with the child's usual coping skills and can help identify potentially successful coping strategies. Involving parents also encourages their participation in learning the relevant skill with the child and acting as coach. If the parent cannot assist the child, other appropriate persons may include a grandparent, older sibling, nurse, or child life specialist (McGrath & Hillier, 2003).

Children should learn to use a specific strategy before pain occurs or before it becomes severe. Children are responsive to pain-controlling strategies that involve their imagination and sense of play (Gerik, 2005). To reduce the child's effort, instructions for a strategy, such as distraction or relaxation, can be recorded and played during a period of comfort. However, even after they have learned an intervention, children often need help using it during a painful procedure. The intervention can also be used after the procedure. This gives the child a chance to recover, feel mastery, and cope more effectively (McGrath & Hillier, 2003).

Virtual reality has been identified as a potentially effective tool for pain distraction (Gold et al., 2006). The participant's attention is drawn away from the "real world" and into the "virtual world" with the incorporation of visual, auditory, and tactile stimuli.

Several studies have documented the effectiveness of non-pharmacological analgesia, such as containment, positioning, non-nutritive sucking (Fig. 35-3), and kangaroo holding, during painful procedures in neonates. Containment is achieved through positioning the child and wrapping him or her in blanket rolls (Cole & Jorgensen, 1997). It provides a "nest" that enhances the infant's feelings of security and decreases stress. Comforting measures and swaddling have been demonstrated to reduce crying and heart rate after procedures such as heel punctures and injections. In infants between 27 and 34 weeks of gestational age, those infants who were swaddled after a routine heel stick procedure were able to calm their crying immediately, decrease their heart rate, and return to a sleep state; in comparison, infants who were not swaddled took a minimum of 10 minutes to return to baseline physiological and behavioural levels (Fearon et al., 1997). Proper positioning with the infant held in a midline orientation, hand-to-mouth activity, and proper flexion can promote self-soothing behaviours. *Facilitated tucking*, which is holding the infant's extremities flexed and contained close to the trunk during heel lance procedures has been demonstrated to decrease heart rate, decrease crying time, and promote stability in the sleep–wake cycles after the lance (Cignacco et al., 2012)

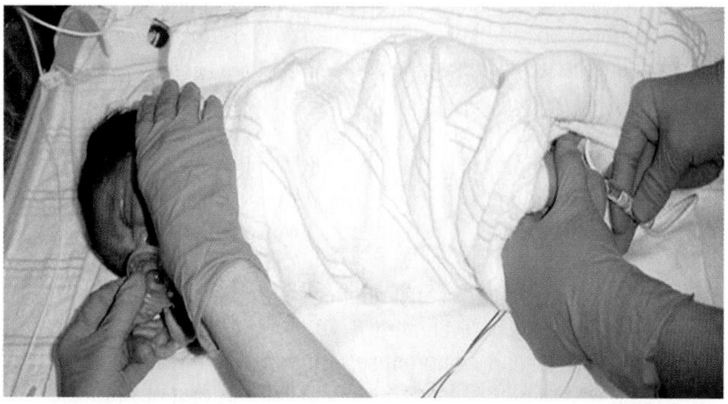

Fig. 35-3 Sucking following oral sucrose can enhance analgesia before a heel stick in a preterm infant.

Non-nutritive sucking (pacifier) attenuates behavioural, physiological, and hormonal responses to pain from procedures such as heel punctures, venipuncture, and immunization injections. The administration of concentrated sucrose with or without non-nutritive sucking has been shown to have calming and pain-relieving effects for invasive procedures in neonates. The amount of crying time was decreased with the oral administration of 2 mL of a 12 to 24% sucrose solution, 2 minutes before a heel lance or venipuncture (Stevens, Yamada, & Ohlsson, 2005).

Kangaroo care is skin-to-skin holding of infants dressed only in diapers against their mother's or father's chest (Gray, Watt, & Blass, 2000; Johnston et al., 2003) (see Chapter 26, Evidence-Informed Practice box). Infants who spent 1 to 3 hours in kangaroo care experienced quiet sleep more often, had a longer duration of quiet sleep, and cried less when returned to the neonatal intensive care unit. They also cried less at age 6 months than neonates who did not receive skin-to-skin contact. Significant differences were found in pain responses during heel lancing between infants who were kangaroo held and those who were not. In the study by Gray and colleagues (2000), heart rate increased by 8 to 10 beats/min in the kangaroo care group in contrast to an increase by 36 to 38 beats/min in the control group of neonates who were swaddled in bassinets. Grimacing was 64% less, and crying was 82% less frequent.

In another study, infant responses to pain during heel lance procedures were compared using kangaroo holding (Fig. 35-4), with the neonate held upright at a 60-degree angle between the mother's breasts for maximal skin-to-skin contact (Johnston et al., 2003). A blanket was placed over the neonate's back, and the mother's clothes were wrapped around the neonate for 30 minutes before the lancing procedure, during, and at least 30 minutes after the heel stick. Another group remained in the isolette in a prone position, swaddled with a blanket and the heel accessible, for 30 minutes before the heel-lancing procedure. Pain scores were significantly lower for kangaroo-held infants.

Complementary Pain Medicine

Many terms are used to describe approaches to health care that are outside the realm of conventional medicine as

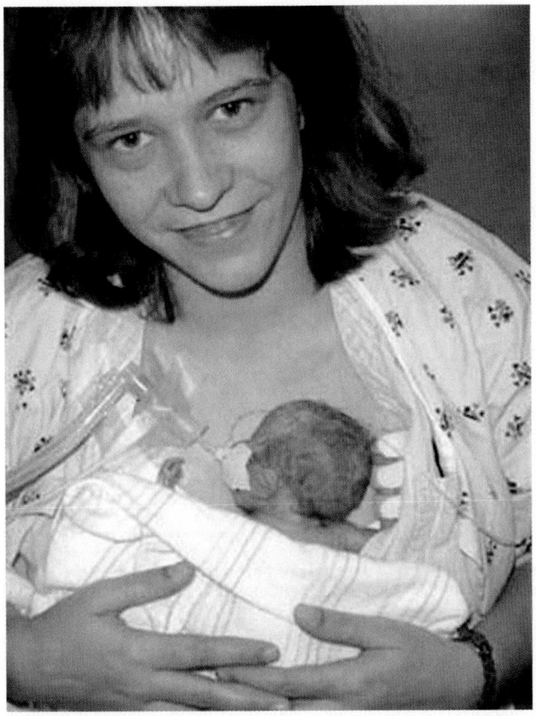

Fig. 35-4 Mother using kangaroo hold with her newborn infant. Note placement of the infant directly on the mother's skin.

practised in Canada. *Complementary and alternative medicine (CAM)*, as defined by the Canadian Interdisciplinary Network for Complementary and Alternative Medicine Research (INCAM), is a group of diverse medical and health care systems, practices, and products that are not currently considered part of conventional medicine. Although some scientific evidence exists regarding the efficacy of some CAM therapies, questions remain to be answered through well-designed scientific studies, such as whether these therapies are safe and whether they work for the diseases or medical conditions for which they are used.

CAM therapies may be grouped into five classes:

1. **Biologically based**—Foods, special diets, herbal or plant preparations, vitamins, other supplements
2. **Manipulative treatments**—Chiropractic, osteopathy, massage
3. **Energy based**—Reiki, bioelectric or magnetic treatments, pulsed fields, alternating and direct currents
4. **Mind-body techniques**—Mental healing, expressive treatments, spiritual healing, hypnosis, relaxation
5. **Alternative medical systems**—Homeopathy; naturopathy; ayurvedic; and traditional Chinese medicine, including acupuncture and moxibustion

Current estimates of pediatric CAM use range from 10 to 15%, derived from children sampled at health care facilities, with chronic conditions, and from countries other than the United States. For the Canadian population, pediatric CAM use was estimated to be 11%. Homeopathy is one of the more popular alternative therapies used in children for dermatological; ear, nose and throat; respiratory; and emotional disorders (Canadian Paediatric Society, Community Paediatrics Committee, 2005). Other therapies that are increasingly used include herbal medicine, massage, megavitamins, self-help groups, traditional remedies, and energy healing (Myers et al., 2005; Rusy & Weisman, 2000).

Pharmacological Management

Nonopioids, including acetaminophen (Tylenol, Tempra) and nonsteroidal anti-inflammatory drugs (NSAIDs), are suitable for mild to moderate pain (Table 35-5); *opioids* are needed for moderate to severe pain (Table 35-6). A combination of the two analgesics acts on the pain system on two levels: nonopioids act primarily at the peripheral nervous system, and opioids act primarily at the central nervous system. The combination of NSAIDs and opioids provides increased analgesia without increased adverse effects. Several combinations, such as acetaminophen with codeine, may have increasing doses of the opioid but a constant dose of the nonopioid. Before increasing the opioid, it may be preferable to increase the nonopioid component, for example, by adding one regular-strength acetaminophen tablet (325 mg) to acetaminophen 300 mg with codeine 15 mg (Tylenol No. 2) before advancing to acetaminophen 300 mg with codeine 30 mg (Tylenol No. 3) or codeine 60 mg (Tylenol No. 4). However, if this approach is not successful, pain management will require a stronger opioid (see Table 35-6). Oxycodone is available without a nonopioid in an immediate-release and controlled-release preparation. The oxycodone dose can be safely increased without the risk of toxicity from excessive acetaminophen use.

Actions of various opioids differ. Morphine is considered the gold standard for the management of severe pain. When morphine is not a suitable opioid, drugs such as hydromorphone (Dilaudid) and fentanyl (Sublimaze) are effective substitutes. Although fentanyl is used as an anaesthetic in the operating room, it is classified as an analgesic. It can be safely administered by nurses by the intravenous (IV), intramuscular (IM), transmucosal, and transdermal routes (Algren et al., 1998).

Several drugs known as *coanalgesics* or **adjuvant** *analgesics* may be used alone or with opioids to control pain symptoms and opioid adverse effects. Drugs frequently used to relieve anxiety, cause sedation, and provide amnesia are diazepam (Valium) and midazolam (Versed); however, these drugs are not analgesics and should be used to enhance the effects of analgesics, not as a substitute for analgesics. Other adjuvants include tricyclic antidepressants (e.g., amitriptyline, imipramine) and anti-epileptics (e.g., gabapentin, carbamazepine, clonazepam) for neuropathic pain (Table 35-7), stool softeners and laxatives for constipation, anti-emetics for nausea and vomiting, diphenhydramine for itching, steroids for inflammation and bone pain, and dextroamphetamine and caffeine for possible increased analgesia and decreased sedation (Greco & Berde, 2005).

The use of placebos to determine whether the patient is having pain is unjustified and unethical. A positive response to a placebo, such as a saline injection, is common in patients who have a documented organic basis for pain. Therefore, the deceptive use of placebos does not provide useful information about the presence or severity of pain. The use of placebos can cause adverse effects similar to those of opioids, can destroy

evolve Skill—Calculating Safe Dosages for Children

Table 35-5 Nonopioid and Nonsteroidal Anti-inflammatory Drugs (NSAIDs) Approved for Use in Children*

DRUG	DOSAGE	COMMENTS
Nonopioids		
Acetaminophen (Tylenol)	Oral: 10-15 mg/kg/dose q4-6h	Available in numerous preparations
	Rectal: 10-20 mg/kg/dose q4-6h	Nonprescription
	Not to exceed 5 doses in 24 hr or 75 mg/kg/day	Higher dosage range may provide increased analgesia
Nonsteroidal Anti-inflammatory Drugs (NSAIDS)		
Ibuprofen (children's Motrin, children's Advil)	Children 6 mo to 12 yr: 5-10 mg/kg/dose q6-8h; maximum: 40 mg/kg/day >12 yr: 200-400 mg po q4-6h	Available in numerous preparations Available in suspension (100 mg/5 mL) and drops (100 mg/2.5 mL) Nonprescription
Naproxen (Naprosyn)	10-20 mg/kg/day po divided into 2 doses	Available in suspension (25 mg/mL) and several different dosages for tablets
	25-49 kg: 250 mg/dose pr	Suppository 500 mg
	>49 kg: 500 mg/dose pr	Nonprescription
Ketorolac (Toradol)	I mg/kg/dose IM, single dose only	

(Data from *Drug facts and comparisons*. Philadelphia: Lippincott Williams & Wilkins, 2008. Dosages from The Sick Kids Drug Handbook and Formulary, Toronto: The Hospital for Sick Children, 2012.)
Acetylsalicylic acid (aspirin) is also an NSAID but is not recommended for children because of its possible association with Reye's syndrome. The NSAIDs in this table have no known association with Reye's syndrome. However, caution should be exercised in prescribing any salicylate-containing drug for children with known or suspected viral infection.
*All NSAIDs in this table have significant anti-inflammatory, antipyretic, and analgesic actions. Acetaminophen has a weak anti-inflammatory action. Patients respond differently to various NSAIDs; thus changing from one drug to another may be necessary for maximum benefit.
Adverse effects of ibuprofen and naproxen include nausea, vomiting, diarrhea, constipation, gastric ulceration, bleeding nephritis, and fluid retention.
Acetaminophen is well tolerated in the gastrointestinal tract and does not interfere with platelet function. NSAIDs should not be given to patients with allergic reactions to salicylates. All the NSAIDs should be used cautiously in patients with renal impairment.
IM, intramuscularly; *po*, orally; *pr*, rectally; *q*, every.

the patient's trust in the health care staff, and raises serious ethical and legal questions (McCaffery & Pasero, 1999).

NURSING ALERT The optimum dosage of an analgesic is one that controls pain without causing severe adverse effects. This usually requires *titration*, the gradual adjustment of drug dosage (usually by increasing the dose), until optimum pain relief without excessive sedation is achieved. Dosage recommendations are only safe initial dosages (see Tables 35-5 and 35-6), not optimum dosages.

Children (except infants younger than about 3 to 6 months) metabolize drugs more rapidly than adults; younger children may require higher doses of opioids to achieve the same analgesic effect. Therefore, the therapeutic effect and duration of analgesia vary. Children's dosages are usually calculated according to body weight, except in children with a weight greater than 50 kg, where the weight formula may exceed the average adult dosage. In this case, the adult dosage is used.

A reasonable starting dose of opioid for infants under 6 months who are not mechanically ventilated is one fourth to one third of the recommended starting dose for older children. The infant needs to be monitored closely for signs of pain relief and respiratory depression. The dose should be titrated to effect. Because tolerance can develop rapidly, large doses may be needed for continued severe pain (Greco & Berde, 2005). If pain relief is inadequate, the initial dose is increased (usually by 25 to 50% if pain is moderate, or by 50 to 100% if pain is severe) to provide greater analgesic effectiveness. Decreasing the interval between doses may also provide more continuous pain relief. A major difference between opioids and nonopioids is that nonopioids have a *ceiling effect*, which means that dosages higher than the recommended dosage will not produce greater pain relief. Opioids do not have a ceiling effect other than that imposed by adverse effects; therefore, larger dosages can be safely given for increasing severity of pain.

Parenteral and oral dosages of opioids are not the same. Because of the *first-pass effect*, an oral opioid is rapidly absorbed from the gastrointestinal tract and is partially metabolized in the liver before reaching the central circulation. Thus oral dosages must be larger to compensate for the partial loss of analgesic potency to achieve *equianalgesia* (equal analgesic effect). Conversion factors (Table 35-8) for selected opioids must be used when a change is made from IV (preferred) or IM to oral administration. Immediate conversion from IM or IV to the suggested equianalgesic oral dose may result in a substantial error. For example, the dose may be significantly more or less than what the child requires. Small changes ensure small errors. Several routes of analgesic administration can be used (Box 35-3); the most effective and least traumatic one should be selected.

Patient-Controlled Analgesia

A significant advance in the administration of IV, **epidural**, or subcutaneous analgesics is the use of patient-controlled analgesia (PCA). As the name implies, the patient controls the amount and frequency of the analgesic, which is typically delivered through a special infusion device. Children who are physically able to "push a button" (i.e., 5 to 6 years of age) and

Table 35-6 Dosage of Selected Opioids for Children

DRUG	APPROPRIATE EQUIANALGESIC	APPROXIMATE EQUIANALGESIC PARENTERAL DOSE	*Recommended Starting Dosage (Children <50 kg Body Weight)** ORAL	PARENTERAL*
Morphine	30 mg q3–4h	10 mg q3–4h	0.2–0.4 mg/kg q3–4h 0.3–0.6 mg/kg time released q12h	0.1–0.2 mg/kg IM q3–4h 0.02–0.1 mg/kg IV bolus q2h 0.015 mg/kg q8min PCA 0.01–0.02 mg/kg/hr IV infusion (neonates) 0.01–0.06 mg/kg/hr IV infusion (child)
Fentanyl (Sublimaze) (oral mucosal form [Actiq])†	Not available	0.1 mg IV	5–15 mcg/kg; maximum dose: 400 mcg	0.5–1.5 mcg/kg IV bolus q30min 1–2 mcg/hr IV infusion
Codeine‡	200 mg q3–4h	130 mg q3–4h	Not recommended	Not recommended
Hydromorphone (Dilaudid)§	7.5 mg q3–4h	1.5 mg q3–4h	0.04–0.1 mg/kg q3–4h	0.02–0.1 mg/kg q3–4h 0.005–0.2 mg/kg IV bolus q2h
Hydrocodone and acetaminophen (Lorcet, Lortab, Vicodin)	30 mg q3–4h	Not available	0.2 mg/kg q3–4h	Not available
Levorphanol (Levo-Dromoran)	4 mg q6–8h	2 mg q6–8h	0.04 mg/kg q6–8h	0.02 mg/kg q6–8h
Methadone (Dolophine)**	20 mg q6–8h	10 mg q6–8h	0.2 mg/kg q6–8h	0.1 mg/kg q6–8h
Oxycodone (Roxicodone; also in Percocet, Percodan, Tylox)	20 mg q3–4h	Not available	2 mg/kg q3–4h††	Not available

(Data from Acute Pain Management Guideline Panel. [1992]. *Acute pain management: Operative or medical procedures and trauma: Clinical practice guideline* [AHCPR Pub No 92-0032]. Rockville, MD: Agency for Health Care Policy and Research, Public Health Service, U.S. Department of Health and Human Services; Berde, C., et al. [1990]. American Academy of Pediatrics Report of the Subcommittee on Disease-Related Pain in Childhood Cancer. *Pediatrics, 86*[5 Pt 2], 818-825. Codeine dosages from McCaffery, M., & Pasero, C. [1999]. *Pain: A clinical manual* [2nd ed.]. St. Louis: Mosby.)

**Caution:* Dosages listed for patients with body weight <50 kg cannot be used as initial starting doses in infants <6 months of age. For nonventilated infants younger than 6 months, the initial opioid dose should be about one fourth to one third of the dose recommended for older infants and children. For example, morphine could be used at a dose of 0.03 mg/kg instead of the traditional 0.1 mg/kg.

†Actiq is indicated only for management of breakthrough cancer pain in patients with malignancies who are already receiving and are tolerant of opioid therapy, but it can be used for preoperative or preprocedural sedation and analgesia.

‡*Caution:* Codeine doses above 65 mg often are not appropriate because of diminishing incremental analgesia with increasing doses along with continually increasing constipation and other adverse effects.

§For morphine, hydromorphone, and oxymorphone, rectal administration is an alternate route for patients unable to take oral medications, but equianalgesic doses may differ from oral and parenteral doses because of pharmacokinetic differences.

**Restricted to physicians who have methadone prescribing privileges per Health Canada, 2002, http://www.hc-sc.gc.ca/hc-ps/pubs/adp-apd/methadone-bp-mp/background-contexte-eng.php.

††*Caution:* Doses of aspirin and acetaminophen in combination with opioid or nonsteroidal anti-inflammatory drug preparations must also be adjusted to patient's body weight. Daily dose of acetaminophen should not exceed 75 mg/kg or 4000 mg.

Note: Published tables vary in suggested doses that are equianalgesic to morphine. Clinical response is the criterion that must be applied for each patient; titration to clinical response is necessary. Because there is not complete cross-tolerance among these drugs, it is usually necessary to use a lower than equianalgesic dose when changing drugs and to retitrate to response.

Caution: Recommended dosages do not apply to patients with renal or hepatic insufficiency or other conditions affecting drug metabolism and kinetics.

IM, intramuscular; *IV,* intravenous; *PCA,* patient-controlled analgesia; *q,* every.

who can understand the concept of pushing a button to obtain pain relief can use PCA (Maxwell & Yaster, 2000). Although controversial, the IV PCA system for children has been used by parents and nurses. Children can use the IV PCA system if they are old enough and capable of effectively managing their own pain. Nurses can efficiently use the infusion device on a child of any age to administer analgesics to avoid signing for and preparing opioid injections every time one is needed (Fig. 35-5). When PCA is used as "nurse- or parent-controlled" analgesia, the concept of patient control is negated, and the inherent safety of PCA needs to be monitored. Researchers have reported safe and effective analgesia in children when the PCA was controlled by the patient, parent, or nurse (Algren et al., 1998; Maxwell & Yaster, 2000).

PCA infusion devices typically allow for three methods or modes of drug administration to be used alone or in combination:

1. Patient-administered boluses that can only be infused according to the preset amount and *lockout interval* (time between doses). More frequent attempts at self-administration usually mean that the patient may need the dose and time adjusted for better pain control.
2. Nurse-administered boluses that are typically used to give an initial loading dose to increase blood levels rapidly and to relieve *breakthrough pain* (pain not relieved with the usual programmed dose)
3. Continuous basal rate infusion that delivers a constant amount of analgesic and prevents pain from returning during those times, such as sleep, when the patient cannot control the infusion

As with any type of analgesic management plan, continued assessment of the child's pain relief is essential for the greatest benefit from PCA. Typical uses of PCA are for controlling pain from surgery, sickle cell crisis, trauma, and cancer. Morphine is the drug of choice for PCA and is usually prepared in a concentration of 10 mcg/mL (Table 35-9). Other options are hydromorphone (2 mcg/mL) and fentanyl (0.1 mcg/mL). Hydromorphone is often used when patients are not able to

Table 35-7 Coanalgesic Adjuvant Drugs

DRUG	DOSAGE	INDICATIONS	COMMENTS
Antidepressants			
Amitriptyline	0.2–0.5 mg/kg po hs Titrate upward by 0.25 mg/kg q5–7 days prn Available in 10- and 25-mg tablets Usual starting dose: 10–25 mg	Continuous neuropathic pain with burning, aching, dysthesia with insomnia	Provides analgesia by blocking reuptake of serotonin and norepinephrine, possibly slowing transmission of pain signals Helps with pain related to insomnia and depression (use nortriptyline if patient is oversedated) Analgesic effects seen earlier than antidepressant effects Adverse effects include dry mouth, constipation, urinary retention
Nortriptyline	0.2–1.0 mg/kg po A.M. or bid Titrate up by 0.5 mg q5–7 days Maximum: 25 mg/dose	Neuropathic pain as above without insomnia	
Anticonvulsants			
Gabapentin	5 mg/kg po hs Increase to bid on day 2, tid on day 3 Maximum: 300 mg/day	Neuropathic pain	Mechanism of action unknown Adverse effects include sedation, ataxia, nystagmus, dizziness
Carbamazepine	*<6 years:* 2.5–5 mg/kg po bid initially Increase 20 mg/kg/24 hr, divide bid every week prn Maximum: 100 mg bid ***6–12 years:*** 5 mg/kg po bid initially Increase 10 mg/kg/24 hr, divide bid every week prn to usual maximum: 100 mg bid *>12 years:* 200 mg po bid initially Increase 200 mg/24 hr, divide bid every week prn to maximum: 1.6–2.4 g/24 hr	Sharp, lancinating neuropathic pain Peripheral neuropathies Phantom limb pain	Similar analgesic effect to that of amitriptyline Monitor blood levels for toxicity only Adverse effects include decreased blood counts, ataxia, gastrointestinal irritation
Anxiolytics			
Lorazepam	0.03–0.1 mg/kg q4–6h po or IV Maximum: 2 mg/dose	Muscle spasm Anxiety	May increase sedation in combination with opioids Can cause depression with prolonged use
Diazepam	0.1–0.3 mg/kg q4–6h po or IV Maximum: 10 mg/dose		
Corticosteroids			
Dexamethasone	Dose depends on clinical situation; higher bolus doses in cord compression, then lower daily dose Try to wean to NSAIDs if pain allows Cerebral edema: 1–2 mg/kg load then 1–1.5 mg/kg/day divided q6h Maximum: 4 mg/dose Anti-inflammatory: 0.08–0.3 mg/kg/day divided q6–12h	Pain from increased intracranial pressure Bony metastasis Spinal or nerve compression	Adverse effects include edema, gastrointestinal irritation, increased weight, acne Use gastroprotectants such as H_2 blockers (ranitidine) or proton pump inhibitors such as omeprazole for long-term administration of steroids or NSAIDs in end-stage cancer with bony pain
Others			
Clonidine	2–4 mcg/kg po q4–6h May also use a 100-mcg transdermal patch q7 days for patients >40 kg	Neuropathic pain Lancinating, sharp, electrical, shooting pain Phantom limb pain	α_2-Adenoreceptor agonist modulates ascending pain sensations Routes of administration: oral, transdermal, and spinal Management of withdrawal symptoms Monitor for orthostatic hypertension, decreased heart rate Sedation is common
Mexiletine	2-3 mg/kg/dose po tid, may titrate 0.5 mg/kg q2–3 wk prn Maximum: 300 mg/dose		Similar to lidocaine, longer acting Stabilizes sodium conduction in nerve cells, reduces neuronal firing Can enhance action of opioids, antidepressants, anticonvulsants Adverse effects include dizziness, ataxia, nausea, vomiting May measure blood levels for toxicity

bid, twice a day; *hs,* at bedtime; *IV,* intravenous; *NSAIDs,* nonsteroidal anti-inflammatory drugs; *po,* by mouth; *prn,* as needed; *q,* every; *tid,* three times a day.

Table 35-8 Equianalgesia of Selected Analgesics

DRUG*	EQUAL TO ORAL MORPHINE (MG)	EQUAL TO IM OR IV MORPHINE (MG)
Hydromorphone (Dilaudid) 1 mg	4	1.3
Codeine 30 mg	4.5	1.5
Meperidine (Demerol) 50 mg	4.8	1.6
Codeine 30 mg, acetaminophen 300 mg (Tylenol No. 3)	7.2	2.4
Oxycodone 5 mg, acetaminophen 325 mg (Percocet)	7.2	2.4
Oxycodone 5 mg, aspirin 325 mg (Percodan)	7.2	2.4
Hydrocodone 5 mg, acetaminophen 500 mg (Vicodin, Lortab)	9	3
Oxycodone 5 mg, acetaminophen 500 mg (Tylox)	9	3
Methadone (Dolophine) 10 mg	15	7.5
Acetaminophen 325 mg (Tylenol)	2.7	0.9
Aspirin 325 mg	2.7	0.9
Acetaminophen 500 mg (Tylenol Extra Strength)	4	1.3
Codeine 60 mg, acetaminophen 300 mg (Tylenol No. 4)	11.7	3.9
Fentanyl transdermal patch (Duragesic) (based on 25 mcg/hr patch applied q3 days = 50 mg oral morphine q24h or divided into 6 doses = 8.3 mg) or use:	8.3	2.77

Recommended Initial Duragesic Dose Based on Daily Oral Morphine Dose†

ORAL 24-HR MORPHINE (MG/DAY)	DURAGESIC DOSE (MG/HR)
45–134	25
135–224	50
225–314	75
315–404	100
405–494	125
495–584	150
585–674	175
675–764	200
765–854	225
855–944	250
945–1034	275
1035–1124	300

(Courtesy Betty R. Ferrell, PhD, FAAN, 1999. Used with permission.)
*Oral medication with exception of fentanyl.
†Data from Duragesic package insert, Janssen Pharmaceutical Products, Titusville, NJ, 2001, USA.
Note: When converting to oral oxycodone from oral morphine, an appropriate conservative estimate is 15–20 mg oxycodone per 30 mg morphine; however, when converting to oral morphine from oral oxycodone, an appropriate conservative estimate is 30 mg morphine per 30 mg oxycodone (McCaffery, M., & Pasero, C. [1999]. *Pain: A clinical manual* [2nd ed.]. St. Louis: Mosby).
IM, intramuscular; *IV*, intravenous; *q*, every.

tolerate the adverse effects, such as pruritus and nausea, from the morphine PCA (Algren et al., 1998; Maxwell & Yaster, 2000).

Some physicians may still prescribe meperidine. However, meperidine is the least potent and shortest acting of the synthetic opioids and the least effective in providing analgesia for severe pain. More important, it may increase the risk of seizures when administered chronically because of the excitatory effects on the nervous system of its metabolite, normeperidine.

Epidural Analgesia

Epidural analgesia may also be used to manage pain, in selected cases. Although an epidural catheter may be inserted at any vertebral level, it is usually placed into the **epidural space** of the spinal column at the lumbar or caudal level (Fig. 35-6). The thoracic level is usually reserved for older children or adolescents who have had an upper abdominal or thoracic procedure, such as a lung transplant. An opioid (usually fentanyl, hydromorphone, or preservative-free morphine, which is often combined with a long-acting local anaesthetic such as bupivacaine or ropivacaine) is instilled via single or intermittent bolus, continuous infusion, or patient-controlled epidural analgesia. Analgesia results from the drug's effect on opiate receptors in the dorsal horn of the spinal cord, rather than the brain. As a result, respiratory depression is rare, but if it occurs, it develops slowly, typically 6 to 8 hours after administration

BOX 35-3 Routes and Methods of Analgesic Drug Administration

Oral

Oral route preferred because of convenience, cost, and relatively steady blood levels

Higher dosages of oral form of opioids required for equivalent parenteral analgesia

Peak drug effect after 1 to 2 hours for most analgesics

Delay in onset is a disadvantage when rapid control of severe pain or of fluctuating pain is desired

Sublingual, Buccal, or Transmucosal

Tablet or liquid placed under tongue (sublingual), between cheek and gum (buccal), or through the mucous membrane (transmucosal)

Highly desirable because more rapid onset than with oral route

- Produces less first-pass effect through liver than with oral route, which normally reduces analgesia from oral opioids (unless sublingual or buccal form is swallowed, which occurs often in children)

Few drugs are commercially available in this form

Many drugs can be compounded into sublingual troche or lozenge.

- Actiq—Oral transmucosal fentanyl citrate in hard confection base on a plastic holder; indicated only for management of breakthrough cancer pain in patients with malignancies who are already receiving and are tolerant of opioid therapy, but can be used for preoperative or preprocedural sedation and analgesia

Intravenous (Bolus)

Preferred for rapid control of severe pain

Provides most rapid onset of effect, usually in about 5 minutes

Advantage for acute pain, procedural pain, and breakthrough pain

Needs to be repeated hourly for continuous pain control

Preferable for drugs with short half-life (morphine, fentanyl, hydromorphone) to avoid toxic accumulation of drug

Intravenous (Continuous)

Preferred over bolus and intramuscular injection for maintaining control of pain

Provides steady blood levels

Easy to titrate dosage

Subcutaneous (Continuous)

Used when oral and intravenous (IV) routes not available

Provides equivalent blood levels to continuous IV infusion

Suggested initial bolus dose to equal 2-hour IV dose; total 24-hour dose usually requires concentrated opioid solution to minimize infused volume; use smallest gauge needle that accommodates infusion rate

Patient-Controlled Analgesia

Generally refers to self-administration of drugs, regardless of route

Typically involves programmable infusion pump (IV, epidural, subcutaneous [SC]) that permits self-administration of boluses of medication at preset dose and time interval (*lockout interval* is time between doses)

Patient-controlled analgesia (PCA) bolus administration is often combined with initial bolus and continuous (basal or background) infusion of opioid

Optimum lockout interval is not known but must be at least as long as time needed for onset of drug

- Should effectively control pain during movement or procedures
- Longer lockout requires larger dose

Family-Controlled Analgesia

One family member (usually a parent) or other caregiver is designated as child's primary pain manager with responsibility for pressing PCA button

Guidelines for selecting a primary pain manager for family-controlled analgesia:

- Spends a significant amount of time with the patient
- Is willing to assume responsibility of being primary pain manager
- Is willing to accept and respect patient's reports of pain (if able to provide) as best indicator of how much pain the patient is experiencing; knows how to use and interpret a pain rating scale
- Understands the purpose and goals of patient's pain management plan
- Understands concept of maintaining a steady analgesic blood level
- Recognizes signs of pain and adverse reactions to opioid

Nurse-Activated Analgesia

Child's primary nurse is designated as primary pain manager and is only person who presses PCA button during that nurse's shift

Guidelines for selecting primary pain manager for family-controlled analgesia are also applicable to nurse-activated analgesia

May be used in addition to a basal rate to treat breakthrough pain with bolus doses; patients assessed every 30 minutes for the need for a bolus dose

May be used without a basal rate as a means of maintaining analgesia with around-the-clock bolus doses

Intramuscular

Not recommended for pain control; not current standard of care

Painful administration (hated by children)

Tissue and nerve damage possible with some drugs

Wide fluctuation in absorption of drug from muscle

Faster absorption from deltoid than from gluteal sites

Shorter duration and more expensive than oral drugs

Time consuming for staff and unnecessary delay for child

Intranasal

Available commercially as butorphanol (Stadol NS); approved for those older than 18 years of age

Should not be used in patient receiving morphinelike drugs because butorphanol is partial antagonist that will reduce analgesia and may cause withdrawal

BOX 35-3 Routes and Methods of Analgesic Drug Administration—cont'd

Intradermal

Used primarily for skin anaesthesia (e.g., before lumbar puncture, bone marrow aspiration, arterial puncture, skin biopsy)

Local anaesthetics (e.g., lidocaine) cause stinging, burning sensation

Duration of stinging dependent on type of "caine" used

To avoid stinging sensation associated with lidocaine:

- Buffer the solution by adding 1 part sodium bicarbonate (1 mmol/mL) to 9 or 10 parts 1% or 2% lidocaine with or without epinephrine

Normal saline with preservative, benzyl alcohol, used to anaesthetize venipuncture site

Use same dose as for buffered lidocaine

Topical or Transdermal

EMLA (eutectic mixture of local anaesthetics [lidocaine and prilocaine]) cream and anaesthetic disk or LMX4 (4% lidocaine cream)

- Eliminates or reduces pain from most procedures involving skin puncture
- Must be placed on intact skin over puncture site and covered by occlusive dressing or applied as anaesthetic disk for 1 hour or more before procedure

LAT (lidocaine-adrenaline-tetracaine) or tetracaine-phenylephrine (tetraphen)

- Provides skin anaesthesia about 15 minutes after application on nonintact skin
- Gel (preferable) or liquid placed on wounds for suturing
- Adrenaline not for use on end arterioles (fingers, toes, tip of nose, penis, earlobes) because of vasoconstriction

Numby Stuff system

- Uses iontophoresis to transport lidocaine 2% and epinephrine 1:100,000 (Iontocaine) into the skin
- Current delivered by small battery-powered device that has an electrode with Iontocaine and a ground electrode
- Produces local dermal anaesthesia in about 10 minutes to a depth of approximately 10 mm at maximum setting
- May be frightening to young children when they see the device and feel the current
- Observe child during iontophoresis and remove all metal, such as jewellery, from application site to prevent burns

Transdermal fentanyl (Duragesic)

- Available as patch for continuous pain control
- Safety and efficacy not established in children younger than 12 years of age
- Not appropriate for initial relief of acute pain because of long interval to peak effect (12 to 24 hours); for rapid onset of pain relief, give an immediate-release opioid
- Orders for "rescue doses" of an immediate-release opioid recommended for breakthrough pain (a flare of severe pain that breaks through the medication being administered at regular intervals for persistent pain)
- Has duration of up to 72 hours for prolonged pain relief
- If respiratory depression occurs, possible need for several doses of naloxone

Vapocoolant

- Use of prescription spray coolant, such as fluorimethane (Spray and Stretch) or ethyl chloride (Pain Ease)
- Applied to the skin for 10 to 15 seconds immediately before the needle puncture; anaesthesia lasts about 15 seconds
- Cold disliked by some children; may be more comfortable for child to spray coolant on a cotton ball and then apply this to the skin
- Application of ice to the skin for 30 seconds found to be ineffective

Rectal*

Alternative to oral or parenteral routes

Variable absorption rate

Generally disliked by children

Regional Nerve Block

Use of long-acting local anaesthetic (bupivacaine or ropivacaine) injected into nerves to block pain at site

Provides prolonged analgesia postoperatively, such as after inguinal herniorrhaphy

May be used to provide local anaesthesia for surgery, such as dorsal penile nerve block for circumcision or for reduction of fractures

Inhalation

Use of anaesthetics, such as nitrous oxide, to produce partial or complete analgesia for painful procedures

Adverse effects (e.g., headache) possible from occupational exposure to high levels of nitrous oxide

Epidural or Intrathecal

Involves catheter placed into epidural, caudal, or intrathecal space for continuous infusion or single or intermittent administration of opioid with or without a long-acting local anaesthetic (e.g., bupivacaine, ropivacaine)

Analgesia primarily from drug's direct effect on opioid receptors in spinal cord

Respiratory depression is rare but may have slow and delayed onset; can be prevented by checking level of sedation and respiratory rate and depth hourly for initial 24 hours and decreasing dose when excessive sedation is detected

Nausea, itching, and urinary retention are common dose-related adverse effects from the epidural opioid

Mild hypotension, urinary retention, and temporary motor or sensory deficits are common unwanted effects of epidural local anaesthetic

Catheter for urinary retention is inserted during surgery to decrease trauma to child; if inserted when child is awake, anaesthetize urethra with lidocaine

(Data from American Pain Society. [1999]. *Principles of analgesic use in the treatment of acute pain and chronic cancer pain* [4th ed.]. Skokie, IL: Author; McCaffery, M., & Pasero, C. [1999]. *Pain: A clinical manual* [2nd ed.]. St. Louis: Mosby.)

*Many drugs can be compounded into rectal suppositories. For further information about compounding drugs in troche or suppository form, contact Professional Compounding Centers of America (PCCA), Canada, 744 Third Street, London, ON, N5V 5J2, 800.668.9453, http://www.pccarx.ca/.

(Golianu et al., 2000). Proper securing of the epidural catheter with an occlusive dressing decreases the possibility of soiling or inadvertently displacing the catheter. Careful monitoring of sedation level and respiratory status is critical to prevent opioid-induced respiratory depression. Assessment of pain and of the skin condition around the catheter site is an important aspect of related nursing care.

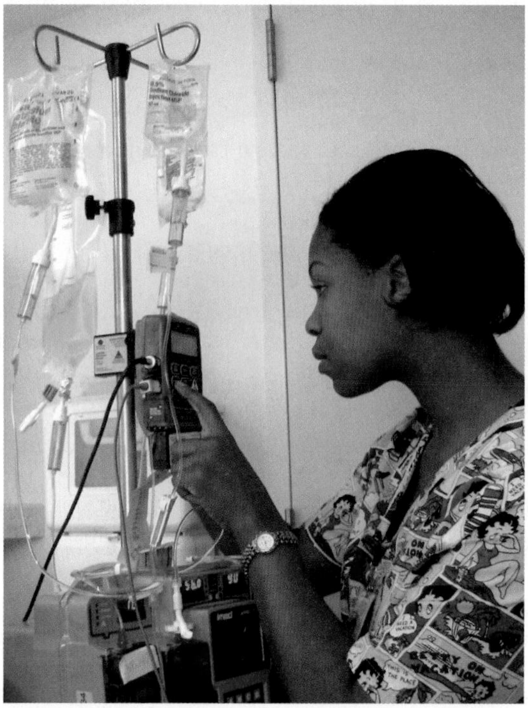

Fig. 35-5 Nurse programming a patient-controlled analgesia pump to administer analgesic.

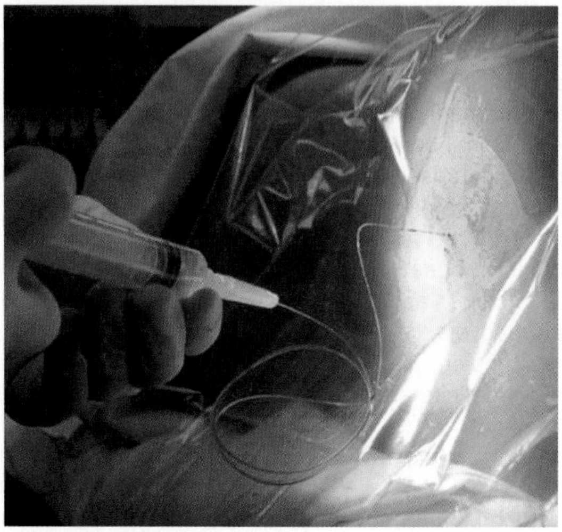

Fig. 35-6 Epidural analgesia catheter placement.

Transmucosal and Transdermal Analgesia

Fentanyl is also available as a transdermal patch (Duragesic). Although contraindicated for acute pain management, it may be used for older children and adolescents who have cancer pain or sickle cell pain or for patients who are opioid tolerant.

One of the most significant improvements in the ability to provide atraumatic care to children is the anaesthetic cream LMX (a 4% liposomal lidocaine cream) or EMLA (a eutectic mixture of local anaesthetics) (Abdelkefi et al., 2004; Gad et al., 2005; Rogers & Ostrow, 2004). The eutectic mixture (lidocaine 2.5% and prilocaine 2.5%), whose melting point is lower than that of the two anaesthetics alone, permits effective concentrations of the drug to penetrate intact skin (Fig. 35-7).

A needle-free system containing 0.5 mg of sterile lidocaine powder (Zingo) is now available and provides a rapid onset of action to reduce pain associated with peripheral IV insertions or blood draws. Two randomized, double-blind, placebo-controlled studies conducted at 15 centres across the United States found significant reduction in procedural pain compared with placebo in children 3 to 18 years of age (Migdal et al., 2006; Zempsky et al., 2008).

In some situations, refrigerant sprays such as ethyl chloride and fluorimethane can be used (Reis & Holubkov, 1997).

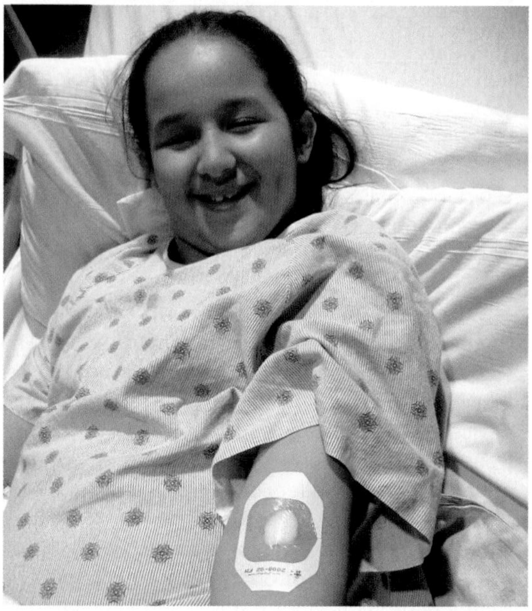

Fig. 35-7 LMX is an effective analgesic before intravenous insertion or blood draw.

Table 35-9 Suggested Intravenous Patient-Controlled Analgesia Opioid Infusion Orders

DRUG	BASAL RATE (MCG/KG/HR)	BOLUS RATE (MCG/KG/DOSE)	LOCKOUT PERIOD (MIN)	MAXIMUM DOSE/HR (MG/KG)
Morphine	10–30	10–30	6–10	0.1–0.15
Hydromorphone	3–5	6–10	0.015–0.02	3–5
Fentanyl	0.5–1.0	0.5–1.0	6–10	0.002–0.004

(From Yaster, M., et al. [1997]. *Pediatric pain management and sedation handbook.* St. Louis: Mosby.)

When sprayed on the skin, these sprays vaporize, rapidly cooling the area and providing superficial **anaesthesia**. Hospital formularies may have other products with lidocaine, prilocaine, or amethocaine topical preparations that require less time for application.

The LidoSite Topical System is another method used to help reduce needlestick pain associated with procedures such as IV cannulation, venipuncture, or laser ablation of superficial skin lesions for patients ages 5 years and older. The LidoSite system delivers numbing medication to the procedure site quickly and effectively after a 10-minute application. The system consists of a single-use, prefilled LidoSite patch, filled with lidocaine hydrochloride 10% and epinephrine 0.1%, and the LidoSite controller, an easy-to-use preprogrammed device that activates the patch. It provides pain reduction equivalent to that of a lidocaine (Xylocaine) injection, without the needlestick. Through iontophoresis, a mild current from the controller activates the patch to accelerate delivery of lidocaine—the anaesthetic medication—to the injection site. Epinephrine contained in the LidoSite patch helps focus the anaesthetic effect directly under the patch and extends the duration of the effect for an hour.

The intradermal route is sometimes used to inject a local anaesthetic, typically lidocaine, into the skin to reduce the pain from a lumbar puncture, bone marrow aspiration, or venous or arterial access. One problem with the use of lidocaine is the stinging and burning that initially occur. However, the use of buffered lidocaine with sodium bicarbonate (see Evidence-Informed Practice box) reduces the stinging sensation (Wong & Pasero, 1997a, 1997b). Warming the lidocaine to 37°C may accomplish the same effect.

Timing of Analgesia

The right timing for administering analgesics depends on the type of pain. For continuous pain control, such as for postoperative or cancer pain, a preventive schedule of medication around the clock (ATC) is effective. The ATC schedule avoids the low concentrations of medications in plasma that permit breakthrough pain. If analgesics are administered only when pain returns (a typical use of the prn, or "as needed," order), pain relief may take several hours. The patient may then require higher doses, leading to a cycle of undermedication of pain, alternating with periods of overmedication and drug toxicity. This cycle of erratic pain control also promotes "clock watching," which may be erroneously equated with addiction. Nurses can effectively use prn orders by giving the drug at regular intervals, since "as needed" should be interpreted as "as needed to prevent pain," not "as little as possible."

Preventive pain control is best provided through continuous IV infusion rather than intermittent boluses. If intermittent boluses are given, the intervals between doses should not exceed the drug's expected duration of effectiveness. For extended pain control with fewer administration times, drugs that provide longer duration of action (e.g., some NSAIDs, time-released morphine or oxycodone, methadone, levorphanol) can be used.

Continuous analgesia is not always appropriate, since not all pain is continuous. Frequently, temporary pain control or conscious sedation is needed to provide analgesia before a scheduled procedure. When pain can be predicted, the drug's peak effect should be timed to coincide with the painful event. For example, with opioids the peak effect is approximately a half-hour for the IV route; with nonopioids the peak effect occurs about 2 hours after oral administration. For rapid onset and peak of action, opioids that quickly penetrate the blood–brain barrier (e.g., IV fentanyl) provide excellent pain control.

Monitoring Adverse Effects

Both NSAIDs and opioids have adverse effects, although the major concern is with those from opioids (Box 35-4). Respiratory depression is the most serious complication and is most likely to occur in sedated patients. The respiratory rate may decrease gradually, or respirations may cease abruptly, and thus must be monitored closely. Lower limits of normal are not established for children, but any significant change from a previous rate calls for increased vigilance. A slower respiratory rate does not necessarily reflect decreased arterial oxygenation; an increased depth of ventilation may compensate for the altered rate. If respiratory depression or arrest occurs,

BOX 35-4 Adverse Effects of Opioids

General

Constipation (possibly severe)
Respiratory depression
Sedation
Nausea and vomiting
Agitation, euphoria
Mental clouding
Hallucinations
Orthostatic hypotension
Pruritus
Urticaria
Sweating
Miosis (may be sign of toxicity)
Anaphylaxis (rare)

Signs of Tolerance

Decreasing pain relief
Decreasing duration of pain relief

Signs of Withdrawal Syndrome in Patients With Physical Dependence

Initial Signs of Withdrawal

Lacrimation
Rhinorrhea
Yawning
Sweating

Later Signs of Withdrawal

Restlessness
Irritability
Tremors
Anorexia
Dilated pupils
Gooseflesh
Nausea, vomiting

EVIDENCE-INFORMED PRACTICE Buffered Lidocaine for Pain Reduction During Peripheral Intravenous Access in Children

—Angela C. Morgan

Ask the Question

In children, is buffered lidocaine an appropriate anaesthetic for reducing pain during peripheral intravenous (PIV) access?

Search for Evidence

Search Strategies

English publications within the past 5 years, research-based articles (level 3 or lower) on children undergoing PIV access; two articles more than 5 years old included on the basis of limited literature in this area

Databases Searched

PubMed, Cochrane Collaboration, MD Consult, Joanna Briggs Institute, National Guideline Clearinghouse (AHQR), TRIP Database, PedsCCM, Best BETs

Critically Analyze the Evidence

A review of the literature revealed 10 studies evaluating buffered lidocaine given before PIV access from 1991 through 2012 (Murphy & Carley, 2000). Four of the studies were specific to pediatrics. Findings from the pediatric studies support buffered lidocaine as a pain reduction measure in children before PIV access.

- A randomized trial consisting of 69 subjects ranging from 4 to 17 years of age (61% female) evaluated buffered lidocaine versus LMX (liposomal lidocaine cream) before PIV access. Results showed that both interventions decreased pain and resulted in no significant differences in pain levels. The LMX group stated that the pain came with the removal of the occlusive dressing from the site (Luhmann et al., 2004).
- Fein and colleagues (1998) evaluated buffered lidocaine versus no pain-control measures in a group of 99 children requiring PIV access in the emergency department (ED). PIV access without buffered lidocaine was significantly more painful than PIV access with buffered lidocaine.
- Sacchetti and Carraccio (1996) evaluated subcutaneous lidocaine versus no pain-control measures in 110 children less than 2 years of age before PIV access in the ED. No significant differences in pain levels were found between the groups. A weakness to this trial was that it was not blinded or randomized.
- A randomized clinical trial of 59 children requiring PIV access in the ED evaluated the use and nonuse of subcutaneous lidocaine before PIV access. PIV access without lidocaine was significantly more painful than PIV access with lidocaine regardless of catheter size. Trial weaknesses included a small sample size with wide confidence levels and no randomization (Klein et al., 1995).
- In 2011, a nursing group compared use of intradermal buffered lidocaine with that of intradermal bacteriostatic normal saline in a group of adults for producing an anaesthetic result before insertion of an intravenous catheter. Previously, it had been suggested that normal saline might be as effective as lidocaine. The study results showed that lidocaine was superior in managing procedural pain (Burke, Vercler, Bye, Desmond, & Rees, 2011).

Apply the Evidence: Nursing Implications

Age—More than 2 years
Time of onset—Immediate
Duration—1 hour
Multiple sites—Yes
Use with abraded skin—No
Impact on PIV access difficulty—Possibility of some vasoconstriction
Timing—Do not use within 2 hours before vesicants
Dose—0.1 to 0.5 mL buffered 1% lidocaine, to a maximum of 0.45 mL/kg/dose; can repeat dose after 2 hours
Considerations—An "extra stick" and ineffective buffered lidocaine administration may result in pain during both local administration and PIV access. Expertise in administering buffered lidocaine is an important factor related to its effectiveness.

References

Burke, S. D., Vercler, S. J., Bye, O. R., Desmond, P. C., & Rees, Y. W. (2011). Local anesthesia before IV catheterization. *American Journal of Nursing, 111*(2), 40–45.

Fein, J. A., et al. (1998). Saline with benzyl alcohol as intradermal anesthesia for intravenous line placement in children. *Pediatric Emergency Care, 14*(2), 119–122.

Klein, E. J., et al. (1995). Buffered lidocaine: Analgesia for intravenous line placement in children. *Pediatrics, 95*(5), 709–712.

Luhmann, J., et al. (2004). A comparison of buffered lidocaine versus ELA-Max before peripheral intravenous catheter insertions in children. *Pediatrics, 113*(3 Pt 1), 217–220.

Murphy, R., & Carley, S. (2000). Prior injection of local anaesthetic and the pain and success of intravenous cannulation. *Journal of Accident and Emergency Medicine, 17*(6), 406–408. doi:10.1136/emj.17.6.406

Sacchetti, A. D., & Carraccio, C. (1996). Subcutaneous lidocaine does not affect the success rate of intravenous access in children less than 24 months of age. *Academic Emergency Medicine, 3*(11), 1016–1019.

the nurse must be prepared to intervene quickly (see Guidelines box).

Although respiratory depression is the most feared adverse effect, constipation is a common, and sometimes serious, adverse effect of opioids, which decrease peristalsis and increase anal sphincter tone. Prevention with stool softeners and laxatives is more effective than treatment once constipation occurs. Dietary treatment, such as increased fibre, is usually not sufficient to promote regular bowel evacuation. However, dietary measures, such as greater fluid and fruit intake, and physical activity are encouraged. Pruritus from epidural or IV infusion can be treated with low doses of IV naloxone, nalbuphine, or diphenhydramine. Nausea, vomiting, and sedation usually subside after 2 days of opioid administration; however, oral or rectal antiemetics may be necessary.

Both tolerance and physical dependence can occur with prolonged use of opioids (see Family-Centred Teaching box, p. 940). *Physical dependence* is a normal, natural, physiological state of neuroadaptation. When opioids are abruptly

GUIDELINES Managing Opioid-Induced Respiratory Depression

If Respirations Are Depressed
- Assess sedation level.
- Reduce infusion by 25% when possible.
- Stimulate patient (shake shoulder gently, call by name, ask to breathe).

If Patient Cannot Be Aroused or Is Apneic
Administer naloxone (Narcan).
- For children weighing less than 40 kg, dilute 0.1 mg naloxone in 10 mL sterile saline to make 10 mcg/mL solution, and give 0.5 mcg/kg.
- For children weighing more than 40 kg, dilute 0.4-mg ampule in 10 mL sterile saline, and give 0.5 mL.

Administer bolus by slow intravenous push every 2 minutes until effect is obtained.
Closely monitor patient. Naloxone's duration of antagonist action may be shorter than that of opioid, requiring repeated doses of naloxone.

Note: Respiratory depression caused by benzodiazepines (e.g., diazepam [Valium] or midazolam [Versed]) can be reversed with flumazenil (Romazicon). Pediatric dosing experience suggests 0.01 mg/kg (0.1 mL/kg); if there is no (or inadequate) response after 1 to 2 minutes, administer the same dose and repeat as needed at 60-second intervals for a maximum dose of 1 mg (10 mL).

(Adapted from Yaster, M., et al. [1997]. *Pediatric pain management and sedation handbook*. St. Louis: Mosby.)

discontinued without weaning, withdrawal symptoms occur. Symptoms of withdrawal occur at 24 hours after abrupt discontinuation and reach a peak within 72 hours. Symptoms of withdrawal include signs of neurological excitability (irritability, tremors, seizures, increased motor tone, insomnia), gastrointestinal dysfunction (nausea, vomiting, diarrhea, abdominal cramps), and autonomic dysfunction (sweating, fever, chills, tachypnea, nasal congestion, rhinitis). Withdrawal symptoms can be anticipated and prevented by weaning patients from opioids that were administered for more than 5 to 10 days. Adherence to a weaning protocol to prevent or minimize withdrawal symptoms from opioids will be required. A weaning flow sheet may be used to assess the efficacy of opioid weaning in neonates (Franck & Vilardi, 1995; Franck et al., 1998) (Fig. 35-8).

Tolerance occurs when the dose of an opioid needs to be increased to achieve the same analgesic effect that was previously achieved at a lower dose. Tolerance may develop after 10 to 21 days of morphine administration. Treatment of tolerance involves increasing the dose or decreasing the duration between doses. Treatment of physical dependence involves gradually reducing the dose over several days to prevent withdrawal symptoms. The following are guidelines for treating physical dependence from morphine:

- Gradually reduce the dose (similar to tapering of steroids).
- Give one half of the previous daily dose every 6 hours for the first 2 days.
- Then reduce the dose by 25% every 2 days. Continue this schedule until total daily dosage of 0.6 mg/kg/day of morphine (or equivalent) is reached. After 2 days on this dose, discontinue opioid.
- A switch to oral methadone may also be made, using one fourth of an equianalgesic dose as the initial weaning dose and proceeding as described above.

Parents and older children may fear addiction when opioids are prescribed. The nurse should address these concerns with assurance that any such risk is extremely low. It may be helpful to ask the question, "If you did not have this pain, would you want to take this medicine?" The answer is invariably no, which reinforces the solely therapeutic nature of the drug. It is also important to avoid making statements to the family such as "We don't want you to get used to this medicine," or "By now you shouldn't need this medicine," which may reinforce the fear of becoming addicted. Whereas both physical dependence and tolerance are physiological states, *addiction* or *psychological dependence* is a psychological state and implies a "cause–effect" mode of thinking, such as "I need the drug because it makes me feel better." Infants and children do not have the cognitive ability to make the cause-effect association and therefore cannot become addicted. The use of opioid analgesics early in life has not been demonstrated to increase the risk for addiction later in life. Nurses need to explain to parents the differences between physical dependence, tolerance, and addiction and allow parents to express concerns about the use and duration of use of opioids. Infants and children, when treated appropriately with opioids, may be at risk for physical tolerance and physical dependence, but not psychological dependence or addiction (Greco & Berde, 2005; Turner, 2005).

Evaluation of Effectiveness of Pain Regimen

The effectiveness of analgesics can be enhanced by a supportive attitude toward the child. By reinforcing the cause and effect of the medication and analgesia, the nurse can condition the child to expect pain relief, provided the regimen is likely to be effective. A pain relief scale or periodic ratings of pain intensity should be used for evaluation of effectiveness of pain regimens.

The response to therapy should be evaluated 15 to 30 minutes after each parenteral drug dose, 1 hour after immediate-release analgesic, 4 hours after sustained-release analgesic or transdermal patch, or 30 minutes after a nonpharmacological intervention. Titration should continue to the point of highest achievable amount of relief (Registered Nurses' Association of Ontario, 2002). The Joint Commission on Accreditation of Healthcare Organizations (Colleau, 2001) advocates assessment of pain as the fifth vital sign (Lynch, 2001; Merboth & Barnason, 2000).

Pediatric pain interventions are still a concern; many children undergo painful procedures and lack effective pain management. A pain study done for the Canadian Institute of Health Research investigated 2987 children who had undergone at least one painful procedure in the previous 24 hours. The results showed that only 28.3% of the children received one or more pain interventions, and there was documentation specifically for a painful procedure. The highest number of

Children's Hospital Oakland Opioid Weaning Flowsheet and Guidelines for Use of the Form

Analgesia/sedation orders (drug/dose/frequency)

Date		
Drug		
Administration time		
Dose ↑ or ↓ or freq change		

	Time:		
Choose one: Crying/agitated 25%–50% of interval Crying/agitated >50% of interval	 2 3		
Choose one: Sleeps ≤25% of interval Sleeps 26%–75% of interval Sleeps >75% of interval	 3 2 1		
Choose one: Hyperactive Moro Markedly hyperactive Moro	 2 3		
Choose one: Mild tremors, disturbed Moderate/severe tremors, disturbed	 1 2		
Increased muscle tone	2		
Temperature 37.2°-38.4°C	1		
Temperature >38.4°C	2		
Respiratory rate >60 (extubated)	2		
Suction >twice/interval (intubated)	2		
Sweating	1		
Frequent yawning (>3–4/interval)	1		
Sneezing (>3–4/interval)	1		
Nasal stuffiness	1		
Emesis	2		
Projectile vomiting	3		
Loose stools	2		
Watery stools	3		
TOTAL SCORE			
ADJUSTED SCORE			
INITIALS OF PERSON SCORING			

Directions: Score every 2–4 hours per guideline
Score greater than 8–12 may indicate withdrawal

Guidelines for use of the flow sheet

Use of form

Use the flowsheet for all infants who have received continuous or around-the-clock opioid medication for 3 days or more, or more than 3 doses per day for more than 5 days. This patient population will most often include postoperative patients, agitated intubated infants, and all post-ECMO patients.

Instructions

1. Write drug, dose, and frequency of analgesics and sedatives ordered
2. Enter date, name of drug (abbreviated MS=morphine sulfate or FENT=fentanyl), and administration time of drugs given in the appropriate boxes; indicate if dose frequency given is an increase or decrease from the ordered dose
3. Scoring must be performed every 4 hours during weaning of opioids, every 2 hours if score is 8 or greater. The score for each item indicates the presence of the sign during the previous 2–4 hours (depending on the scoring interval). Every 4–hour scoring should continue until the patient is off all opioids for 48-72 hours. Place a "0" in the column after the sign if it is not seen during the scoring period.

Central nervous system

Crying behavior: Score 2 points if patient exhibits crying or cry behavior for a duration of ≤50% of the scoring interval. Score 3 points if cumulative crying behavior totals >50% of the scoring interval.
NOTE: Crying behavior is accompanied by the facial expressions associated with crying, but without audible sounds because of endotracheal intubation.
Sleeping: Score 3 points if patient sleeps for ≤25% of the scoring interval. Score 2 points if patient sleeps for 26%–75% of the scoring interval. Score 1 point if patient sleeps for >75% of the scoring interval.
Moro (startle) reflex: Score 2 points if patient has some arm and/or leg extension when touched or when disturbed by loud noises. Score 3 points if patient has marked arm and/or leg extension that is accompanied by crying behavior, hyperalert state, or continued arm and/or leg tremors after being startled.
Tremors—disturbed: Score 1 point if patient has mild tremors when disturbed. Score 2 points if patient has moderate to severe tremors when disturbed. NOTE: Tremors are alternating movements that are rhythmic, of equal rate and amplitude, and can usually be stopped by flexion of the limb.
Increased muscle tone: Score 2 points if patient exhibits fisting or tight flexion of extremities that are difficult to extend.

Metabolic

Temperature: Score 1 point if patient's temperature is 37.2°–38.4°C. Score 2 points if patient's temperature is >38.4°C.
Respiratory rate: Score 1 point if patient's spontaneous respiratory rate is >60/minute. Score 2 points if patient's spontaneous respiratory rate is >60/minute and accompanied by retractions.
Suction: Score 2 points if patient is suctioned more than twice during a 4-hour period.
Sweating: Score 1 point if patient exhibits any type of sweating, including beads of sweat, or if skin is moist to touch.
Yawning: Score 1 point if patient yawns >3–4 times in succession or yawns 1–2 times often during a 4-hour period.
Sneezing: Score 1 point if patient sneezes >3–4 times in succession or sneezes 1–2 times during a 4-hour period.
Nasal stuffiness: Score 1 point for nasal stuffiness.

Gastrointestinal

Emesis of formula/stomach contents: Score 2 points if patient has 1 or more episodes of emesis during a 4-hour period.
Projectile vomiting: Score 3 points if patient has 1 or more episodes of projectile vomiting.
Loose stools: Score 2 points if patient has loose stools characterized by a water ring around some solid stool. The stools will often be frequent. NOTE: Do not score for "breast milk" stools: frequent, small, seedy, yellow stools.
Watery stools: Score 3 points if patient has stools that consist of only liquid. The stools will often be frequent.

Total score: Add up all the scores in the column and place the total score in this box. Clinical signs that appear continuously, such as respiratory rate >60 or regular poor feeding, should be included in the total score.
Adjusted score: The adjusted score is used when a sign is detected that is expected to occur independently of withdrawal, due to a preexisting condition (high respiratory rate in infant with bronchopulmonary dysplasia). The decision to adjust the score should be made after discussion with the healthcare team during rounds, and the rationale should be recorded in a problem-oriented note. Circle the signs to be excluded and deduct the points from the total score to obtain the adjusted score.
Initials of person scoring: The person scoring should write his/her initials in this space.

Fig. 35-8 Weaning flow sheet to monitor weaning in neonates.

pain procedures and analgesics that were administered were reported by pediatric intensive care units (Stevens et al., 2011).

Several harmful effects occur with unrelieved pain, particularly when pain is prolonged. A number of physiological stress responses in the body are triggered during pain, and they lead to negative consequences that involve multiple systems. Unrelieved pain may prolong the stress response and adversely affect an infant or child's recovery, whether it is from trauma, surgery, or disease. In a landmark study by Anand and Hickey (1992), 30 neonates received deep intraoperative anaesthesia with high doses of the opioid sufentanil, followed postoperatively by an infusion of opioids for 24 hours, and 15 neonates received lighter anaesthesia with halothane and morphine, followed postoperatively by intermittent morphine and diazepam. The 15 neonates who received the lighter anaesthesia and intermittent postoperative opioids had more severe hyperglycemia and lactic acidemia, and four postoperative deaths occurred in the group. The 30 neonates who received deep anaesthesia had a lower incidence of complications (sepsis, metabolic acidosis, disseminated intravascular coagulation) and no deaths.

Poorly controlled acute pain can predispose patients to *chronic pain syndromes*. A guiding principle in pain management is that prevention of pain is always better than treatment (Benjamin, Swinson, & Nagel, 2000). Pain that is established and severe is often more difficult to control. When pain is unrelieved, sensory input from injured tissues reaches spinal cord neurons and may enhance subsequent responses. Long-lasting changes in cells within spinal cord pain pathways may occur after a brief painful stimulus and may lead to the development of chronic pain conditions. Basbaum (1999a, 1999b) reported a series of studies emphasizing a distinct neurochemistry of acute and persistent pain, and they concluded that persistent pain is not merely a prolonged acute pain symptom of some other disease. Underlying physiological mechanisms lead to the persistence of pain (Marx, 2004; Woolf & Salter, 2000).

In a study of nursing practice related to pain assessment and management in different pediatric specialty units, Jacob and Puntillo (2000) noted that nurses were aware of patients' indications of pain but seldom documented patient-specific pain scores or notations about responses to analgesics after administration. Pain scores were not available before and after giving analgesics, and it was thus not possible to conclude whether analgesics were effective. Nurses need to evaluate and monitor pain in a timely fashion after administration of analgesics; titrate dosage to effect; or make recommendations for an alternate analgesic, for addition of another analgesic, or for a combination of analgesics, adjuvants, and nonpharmacological strategies.

Key Points

- Although the ability to measure pain in children has improved dramatically in recent years, assessment of pain in children continues to be complex and challenging.
- Behavioural assessment is useful for measuring pain in infants and preverbal children who do not have the language skills to communicate that they are in pain, or when mental clouding and confusion limit a child's ability to communicate.
- Physiological measures do not distinguish between physical responses to pain and other forms of stress to the body.
- The number of pain measures available for use in infants and young children has increased dramatically and adds a layer of complexity to the assessment of pain in children.
- Important components of assessment include the onset of pain; pain duration or pattern; effectiveness of the current treatment; factors that aggravate or relieve the pain; other symptoms and complications concurrently felt; and interference with the child's mood, function, and interactions with family.
- The administration of sucrose with or without non-nutritive sucking and use of kangaroo care have been demonstrated to have calming and pain-relieving effects in neonates undergoing invasive procedures.
- One of the most significant improvements in the ability to provide atraumatic care to children is use of the anaesthetic creams LMX and EMLA.
- Nonopioids, including acetaminophen and NSAIDs, are suitable for mild to moderate pain; opioids are needed for moderate to severe pain.
- Several drugs—coanalgesics or adjuvant analgesics—may be used alone or with opioids to control pain symptoms and opioid adverse effects.
- A significant advance in the administration of IV, epidural, or subcutaneous analgesics is the use of PCA.
- Although respiratory depression is the most feared adverse effect of opioids, they also decrease peristalsis and increase anal sphincter tone, which can result in constipation, a common and sometimes serious adverse effect.
- Several harmful effects occur with unrelieved pain, particularly when pain is prolonged.
- Surgery and traumatic injuries generate a catabolic state as a result of increased secretion of catabolic hormones and lead to alterations in blood flow, coagulation, fibrinolysis, substrate metabolism, and water and electrolyte balance, and increase the demands on the cardiovascular and respiratory systems.

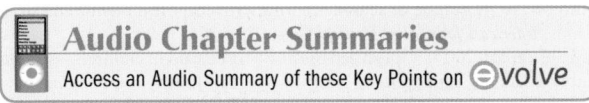

Audio Chapter Summaries
Access an Audio Summary of these Key Points on evolve

References

Abdelkefi, A., et al. (2004). Effectiveness of fixed 50% nitrous oxide oxygen mixture and EMLA cream for insertion of central venous catheters in children. *Pediatric Blood and Cancer, 43*(7), 777–779.

Algren, J. T., et al. (1998). The effect of nitrous oxide diffusion on laryngeal mask airway cuff inflation in children. *Paediatrica Anaesthesia, 8*(1), 31–36.

Anand, K. J., & Hickey, P. R. (1992). Halothane-morphine compared with high-dose sufentanil for anaesthesia and postoperative analgesia in neonatal cardiac surgery. *New England Journal of Medicine, 326*(1), 1–9.

Barrier, G., et al. (1987). Measurement of postoperative pain and narcotic administration in infants using a new clinical scoring system. *Anesthesiology, 67*(3A), A532.

Basbaum, A. I. (1999a). Distinct neurochemical features of acute and persistent pain. *Proceedings of the National Academy of Sciences U S A, 96*(14), 7739–7743.

Basbaum, A. I. (1999b). Spinal mechanisms of acute and persistent pain. *Regional Anesthesia and Pain Medicine, 24*(1), 59–67.

Benjamin, L., Swinson, G., & Nagel, R. (2000). Sickle cell anemia day hospital: An approach for the management of uncomplicated painful crises. *Blood, 95,* 1130–1137.

Bernstein, B., & Pachter, L. (2003). Cultural considerations in children's pain. In N. Schechter, C. Berde, & M. Yaster (Eds.), *Pain in infants, children, and adolescents.* Philadelphia: Lippincott Williams & Wilkins.

Beyer, J. E., Denyes, M. J., & Villarruel, A. M. (1992). The creation and development of the Oucher: A measure of pain intensity in children. *Journal of Pediatric Nursing, 7*(5), 335–346.

Beyer, J. E., & Knott, C. B. (1998). Construct validity estimation for the African-American and Hispanic versions of the Oucher scale. *Journal of Pediatric Nursing, 13*(1), 20–31.

Blauer, T., & Gerstmann, D. (1998). A simultaneous comparison of three neonatal pain scales during common NICU procedures. *Clinical Journal of Pain, 14*(1), 39–47.

Breau, L. M., et al. (2003). Caregivers' beliefs regarding pain in children with cognitive impairment: Relation between pain sensation and reaction increases with severity of impairment. *Clinical Journal of Pain, 19*(6), 335–344.

Breau, L. M., et al. (2002). Psychometric properties of the Non-communicating Children's Pain Checklist—Revised. *Pain, 99,* 349–357.

Canadian Paediatric Society, Community Paediatrics Committee. (2005). Canadian Paediatric Society position statement: Homeopathy in the paediatric population. *Paediatrics and Child Health, 10*(3), 173–177. (Reaffirmed February 2011) Retrieved from http://www.cps.ca/english/statements/cp/cp05-01.htm.

Chambers, C. T., et al. (1999). A comparison of faces scales for the measurement of pediatric pain: Children's and parents' ratings. *Pain, 83,* 25–35.

Chambers, C. T., et al. (2005). Faces scales for the measurement of postoperative pain intensity in children following minor surgery. *Clinical Journal of Pain, 21*(3), 277–285.

Cignacco, E. L., et al. (2012). Oral sucrose and "facilitated tucking" for repeated pain relief in preterms: A randomized controlled trial. *Pediatrics, 129*(2), 299–308. doi:10.1542/peds.2011-1879

Cline, M. E., et al. (1992). Standardization of the visual analogue scale. *Nursing Research, 41*(6), 378–380.

Cole, J., & Jorgensen, K. (1997). Medical, developmental, and pharmacologic intervention: The essence of collaboration. *Neonatal Network, 16,* 56–58.

Colleau, S. (2001). New pain standards: A giant opportunity to change patterns of care in the US. *WHO Pain & Palliative Care Communications Program, 4*(2). Retrieved from http://www.whocancerpain.wisc.edu/?q=node/186.

Eland, J. A., & Banner, W. (1999). Analgesia, sedation, and neuromuscular blockage in pediatric critical care. In M. E. Hazinski (Ed.), *Manual of pediatric critical care.* St. Louis: Mosby.

Fearon, I., et al. (1997). Swaddling after heel lance: Age-specific effects on behavioral recovery in preterm infants. *Developmental and Behavioral Pediatrics, 18,* 222–232.

Franck, L., & Vilardi, J. (1995). Assessment and management of opioid withdrawal in ill neonates. *Neonatal Network, 14*(2), 39–48.

Franck, L. S., et al. (1998). Opioid withdrawal in neonates after continuous infusions of morphine or fentanyl during extracorporeal membrane oxygenation. *American Journal of Critical Care, 7*(5), 364–369.

Gad, L. N., et al. (2005). Optimized use of EMLA cream in children—secondary publication: A randomized, prospective, controlled comparison of two application regimes. *Ugeskrift for Laeger, 167*(4), 404–407.

Gerik, S. M. (2005). Pain management in children: Developmental considerations and mind-body therapies. *Southern Medical Journal, 98*(3), 295–302.

Gold, J. I., et al. (2006). Effectiveness of virtual reality for pediatric pain distraction during IV placement. *Cyberpsychological Behavior, 9*(2), 207–212. doi:10.1089/cpb.2006.9.207.

Goldschneider, K., & Anand, K. (2003). Long-term consequences of pain in neonates. In N. Schechter, C., Berde, & M. Yaster (Eds.), *Pain in infants, children, and adolescents.* Philadelphia: Lippincott Williams & Wilkins.

Golianu, B., et al. (2000). Pediatric acute pain management. *Pediatric Clinics of North America, 47*(3), 559–587.

Gray, L., Watt, L., & Blass, E. (2000). Skin-to-skin contact is analgesic in healthy newborns. *Pediatrics, 105*(1), 110–111.

Greco, C., & Berde, C. (2005). Pain management for the hospitalized pediatric patient. *Pediatric Clinics of North America, 52*(4), 995–1027. doi:10.1016/j.pcl.2005.04.005.

Hadden, K. L., & von Baeyer, C. L. (2002). Pain in children with cerebral palsy: Common triggers and expressive behaviors. *Pain, 99*(1-2), 281–288.

Hadjistavropoulos, H. D., et al. (1997). Judging pain in infants: Behavioural, contextual, and developmental determinants. *Pain, 73*(3), 319–324.

Hannallah, R. S., et al. (1987). Comparison of caudal and ilioinguinal/iliohypogastric nerve blocks for control of post-orchiopexy pain in pediatric ambulatory surgery. *Anesthesiology, 66,* 832–834.

Hester, N. O., et al. (1998). Putting pain measurement into clinical practice. In G. A. Finley & P. J. McGrath (Eds.), *Measurement of pain in infants and children, Vol. 10.* Seattle: IASP Press.

Hodgkinson, K., et al. (1994). Measuring pain in neonates: Evaluating an instrument and developing a common language. *Australian Journal of Advanced Nursing, 12*(1), 17–22.

Jacob, E., & Puntillo, K. A. (2000). Variability of analgesic practices for hospitalized children on different pediatric specialty units. *Journal of Pain Symptom Management, 20*(1), 59–67.

Jacob, E., et al. (2003a). Changes in intensity, location, and quality of vaso-occlusive pain in children with sickle cell disease. *Pain, 102*(1-2), 187–193.

Jacob, E., et al. (2003b). Management of vaso-occlusive pain in hospitalized children with sickle cell disease. *Journal of Pediatric Hematology/Oncology, 25*(4), 307–311.

Johnston, C. C., et al. (2003). Kangaroo care is effective in diminishing pain response in preterm neonates. *Archives of Pediatrics and Adolescent Medicine, 157*(11), 1084–1088.

Jordan-Marsh, M., et al. (1994). Alternate Oucher form testing: Gender, ethnicity, and age variations. *Research in Nursing and Health, 17,* 111–118.

Joyce, B. A., et al. (1994). Reliability and validity of preverbal pain assessment tools. *Issues in Comprehensive Pediatric Nursing, 17,* 121–135.

Kain, Z. N., et al. (2006). Preoperative anxiety, postoperative pain, and behavioral recovery in young children undergoing surgery. *Pediatrics, 118*(2), 651–658. doi:10.1542/peds.2005-2920

Krechel, S. W., & Bildner, J. (1995). CRIES: A new neonatal postoperative pain measurement score: Initial testing of validity and reliability. *Paediatric Anaesthesia, 5,* 53–61.

Lawrence, J., et al. (1993). The development of a tool to assess neonatal pain. *Neonatal Network, 12*(6), 59–66.

Lenton, S., et al. (2001). Prevalence and morbidity associated with non-malignant, life-threatening conditions in childhood. *Child Care and Health Development, 27*(5), 389–398.

Luffy, R., & Grove, S. K. (2003). Examining the validity, reliability, and preference of three pediatric pain measurement tools in African-American children. *Pediatric Nursing, 29*(1), 54–60.

Lynch, M. (2001). Pain: The fifth vital sign. Comprehensive assessment leads to proper treatment. *Advance for Nurse Practitioners, 9*(11), 28–36.

Malviya, S., et al. (2006). The revised FLACC observational pain tool: Improved reliability and validity for pain assessment in children with cognitive impairment. *Paediatric Anaesthesia, 16*(3), 258–265. doi:10.1542/peds.2005-2920.

Manworren, R., & Hynan, L. (2003). Clinical validation of FLACC: Preverbal patient pain scale. *Pediatric Nursing, 29*(2), 140–146.

Marx, J. (2004). Pain research: Prolonging the agony. *Science, 305*(5682), 326–329.

Maxwell, L., & Yaster, M. (2000). Perioperative management issues in pediatric patients. *Anesthesiology Clinics of North America, 18*(3), 601–632.

McCaffery, M., & Pasero, C. (1999). *Pain clinical manual* (2nd ed.). St. Louis: Mosby.

McGrath, P. (1998). Behavioral measures of pain. In G. Finley & P. McGrath (Eds.), *Measurement of pain in infants and children.* Seattle: IASP Press.

McGrath, P. & Hillier, L. (Eds.). (2003). *Modifying the psychologic factors that intensify children's pain and prolong disability.* Philadelphia: Lippincott Williams & Wilkins.

McGrath, P. J., et al. (1985). The CHEOPS: A behavioral scale to measure postoperative pain in children. In H. Fields, R. Dubner, & F. Cervero (Eds.), *Advances in pain research and therapy.* New York: Raven Press.

Melzack, R. (1975). The McGill pain questionnaire: Major properties and scoring methods. *Pain, 1,* 277–299.

Merboth, M. K., & Barnason, S. (2000). Managing pain: The fifth vital sign. *Nursing Clinics of North America, 35*(2), 375–383.

Merkel, S. I., et al. (1997). The FLACC: A behavioral scale for scoring postoperative pain in young children. *Pediatric Nursing, 23*(3), 293–297.

Miaskowski, C., & Lee, K. (1999). Pain, fatigue, and sleep disturbances in oncology outpatients receiving radiation therapy for bone metastasis: A pilot study. *Journal of Pain Symptom Management, 17*(5), 320–332.

Migdal, M., et al. (2006). Rapid, needle-free delivery of lidocaine for reducing the pain of venipuncture among pediatric subjects. *Pediatrics, 115*(4), e393–e398. doi:10.1016/j.jpeds.2007.07.018

Morin, C., Gibson, D., & Wade, J. (1998). Self-reported sleep and mood disturbance in chronic pain patients. *Clinical Journal of Pain, 14*(4), 311–314.

Myers, C., et al. (2005). Complementary therapies and childhood cancer. *Cancer Control, 12*(3), 172–180.

Puchalski, M., & Hummel, P. (2002). The reality of neonatal pain. *Advances in Neonatal Care, 2*(5), 233–244.

Registered Nurses' Association of Ontario. (2002). *Best practice guidelines: Assessment and management of pain*. (Supplement, 2007) Retrieved from http://www.rnao.org/Storage/29/2351_BPG_Pain_and_Supp.pdf.

Reis, E., & Holubkov, R. (1997). Vapocoolant spray is equally effective as EMLA cream in reducing immunization pain in school-aged children. *Pediatrics, 100*(6), E5.

Robieux, I., et al. (1991). Assessing pain and analgesia with a lidocaine-prilocaine emulsion in infants and toddlers during venipuncture. *Journal of Pediatrics, 118*(6), 971–973.

Rogers, T. L., & Ostrow, C. L. (2004). The use of EMLA cream to decrease venipuncture pain in children. *Journal of Pediatric Nursing, 19*(1), 33–39.

Rusy, L., & Weisman, S. (2000). Complementary therapies for acute pediatric pain management. *Pediatric Clinics of North America, 47*(3), 589–599.

Schade, J. G., et al. (1996). Comparison of three preverbal scales for postoperative pain assessment in a diverse pediatric sample. *Journal of Pain Symptom Management, 12*(6), 348–359.

Stallard, P., et al. (2002a). The development and evaluation of the Pain Indicator for Communicatively Impaired Children (PICIC). *Pain, 98*(1-2), 145–149.

Stallard, P., et al. (2002b). Intervening factors in caregivers' assessments of pain in non-communicating children. *Developmental Medicine and Child Neurology, 44*(3), 213–214.

Stanford, E. A., Chambers, C. T., & Craig, K. D. (2006). The role of developmental factors in predicting young children's use of a self-report scale for pain. *Pain, 120*(1-2), 16–23. doi:10.1016/j.pain.2005.10.004

Stevens, B. (1990). Development and testing of a pediatric pain management sheet. *Pediatric Nursing, 16*(6), 543–548.

Stevens, B., et al. (2011). Epidemiology and management of painful procedures in children in Canadian hospitals. *Canadian Medical Association Journal, 183*(7), E403–E410. doi:10.1503/cmaj.101341

Stevens, B., et al. (1996). Premature Infant Pain Profile: Development and initial validation. *Clinical Journal of Pain, 12*, 13–22.

Sweet, S., &, McGrath, P. (1998). Physiological measures of pain. In G. Finley & P. McGrath (Eds.), *Measurement of pain in infants and children*. Seattle: IASP Press.

Stevens, B., Yamada, J., & Ohlsson, A. (2005). Sucrose for analgesia in newborn infants undergoing painful procedures (review). In *Cochrane Neonatal Collaboration*. Retrieved from http://discuss.pediatricpainresearch.ca/resources/Sucrose%20review%202010.pdf.

Taddio, A., et al. (1995). A revised measure of acute pain in infants. *Journal of Pain Symptom Management, 10*(6), 456–463.

Tesler, M. D., et al. (1991). The Word-Graphic Rating Scale as a measure of children's and adolescents' pain intensity. *Research in Nursing and Health, 14*, 361–371.

Turner, H. N. (2005). Complex pain consultations in the pediatric intensive care unit. *AACN Clinical Issues, 16*(3), 388–395.

Villarruel, A. M., & Denyes, M. J. (1991). Pain assessment in children: Theoretical and empirical validity *ANS Advances in Nursing Science, 14*(2), 32–41.

Weisman, S., Bernstein, B., & Schechter, N. (1998). Consequences of inadequate analgesia during painful procedures in children. *Archives of Pediatric and Adolescent Medicine, 152*, 147–149.

Wong, D. L., & Baker, C. M. (1988). Pain in children: Comparison of assessment scales. *Pediatric Nursing, 14*(1), 9–17.

Wong, D., & Pasero, C. L. (1997a). Reducing the pain of lidocaine. *American Journal of Nursing, 97*(1), 17–18.

Wong, D., & Pasero, C. L. (1997b). Using local anesthetics to control procedural pain. *American Journal of Nursing, 97*(1), 17.

Woodgate, R., & Yanofsky, R. (2004). A different perspective to approaching cancer symptoms in children. *Journal of Pain Symptom Management, 26*(3), 800–817.

Woolf, C. J., & Salter, M. W. (2000). Neuronal plasticity: Increasing the gain in pain. *Science, 288*(5472), 1765–1769.

Zempsky, W. T., et al. (2008). Needle-free powder lidocaine delivery system provides rapid effective analgesic for venipuncture or cannulation pain in children: Randomized, double-blind comparison of venipuncture and venous cannulation pain after fast-onset needle-free powder lidocaine or placebo treatment trial. *Pediatrics, 121*(5), 978–987.

Additional Resources

The four most commonly used behavioural pain measures are FLACC, CHEOPS, TPPPS, and PPPRS. More information on these pain scales can be found at the following Web sites:

- FLACC scale assessment from the Canadian Agency for Drugs & Technologies in Health (CADTH): Ens, B. (2010). *Pain scales: Reliability and accuracy to measure 5th vital sign*. http://www.usask.ca/nursing/cne/docs/Pain%202010/Presentations/Pain%20Scales%20-%20Moose%20Jaw%20CNE%20Conference%20Nov%202010.pdf
- General pain research information as well as CHEOPS and PPPRS scale information is available from the Centre for Pediatric Research. http://pediatric-pain.ca/content
- TPPPS scale information: Chambers, C. T., Finley, A. G., McGrath, P. J., & Walsh, T. M. (2003). *The parents' postoperative pain measure: Replication and extension to 2- to 6-year-old children. Pain, 105*, 437–443. http://www.pediatric-pain.ca/files/01/23/Pain2003.pdf

Other guidelines for pain management:

- Canadian Interdisciplinary Network for Complementary and Alternative Medicine Research (INCAM). http://www.incamresearch.ca/index.php?id=11,0,0,1,0,0&menu=14
- Registered Nurses' Association of Ontario. (2002). *Nursing Best Practice Guideline: Assessment and management of pain* (supplement 2007) (includes resources on how to develop an organizational program for pain and provides E-learning nursing interventions). http://www.rnao.org/Storage/29/2351_BPG_Pain_and_Supp.pdf

Unit 9

36 The Infant and Family

Learning Objectives

On completion of this chapter, the reader will be able to:

- Identify the major biological, psychosocial, cognitive, and social developments that occur during the first year of life.
- Relate parent–child attachment, separation anxiety, and stranger fear to developmental achievements during infancy.
- Provide anticipatory guidance to parents regarding common parental concerns during infancy.
- Provide anticipatory guidance to parents regarding recommendations for feeding infants.
- Outline immunization requirements during infancy, early childhood, and adolescence.
- List general contraindications, precautions, and administration routes for immunizations.
- Provide anticipatory guidance to parents regarding injury prevention based on the infant's developmental achievements.
- Provide anticipatory guidance in the care of the family with an infant who is experiencing colic.
- Plan nursing care that can meet the physical and emotional needs of the child with growth failure as well as needs of the family.
- Provide anticipatory guidance for the prevention of sudden infant death syndrome.
- Provide nursing care that aims to meet the immediate and long-term needs of the family that has lost a child from sudden infant death syndrome.
- Identify needs of the family whose child is home monitored for apnea.

Electronic Resources

Additional information related to the content in Chapter 36 can be found on

evolve the companion Web site at

http://evolve.elsevier.com/Canada/Perry/maternal/

- Examination Review Questions
- Assessment Video Clips
- Case Study—Child Abuse
- Case Study—Health Problems of Infants
- Case Study—Infant Growth and Development
- Critical Thinking Exercise—Infant Safety
- Skill—Fostering Healthy Sleep Patterns in Children

Promoting Optimum Growth and Development

Biological Development

At no other time in life are physical changes and developmental achievements as dramatic as during infancy. All major body systems undergo progressive maturation, and there is concurrent development of skills that increasingly allow infants to respond to and cope with the environment. Acquisition of these fine and gross motor skills occurs in an orderly head-to-toe and centre-to-periphery (**cephalocaudal** and **proximodistal**) sequence.

Proportional Changes

Growth is very rapid during the first year, especially during the initial 6 months. Infants gain 150 to 200 g weekly until approximately age 5 to 6 months, when the birth weight has at least doubled. An average weight for a 6-month-old child is 7.0 kg. Weight gain slows during the second 6 months. By 1 year of age the infant's birth weight has tripled, for an average weight of 9.75 kg. Height increases by 2.5 cm a month during the first 6 months and also slows during the second 6 months. Increases in length occur in sudden spurts, rather than in a slow, gradual pattern. Average height is 65 cm at 6 months and 74 cm at 12 months. By age 1 year, the birth length has increased by almost 50%. This increase occurs mainly in the trunk, rather than in the legs, and contributes to the infant's characteristic physique. It is important for individual children to have specific measurements taken to accurately track their growth patterns. These measurements need to be done on a regular basis with a growth chart that compares them with the average measurements of other children. The Dietitians of Canada, Canadian Paediatric Society (CPS), the College of Family Physicians, and the Community Health Nurses of Canada (2010) have put forth a joint recommendation to use the World Health Organization (WHO) 2006 Child Growth Standards and the 2007 WHO Growth Reference growth charts for Canadian children (see Appendix C).

Head growth is also rapid. During the first 6 months, head circumference increases approximately 1.5 cm a month, but the rate of increase falls to only 0.5 cm monthly during the second 6 months. The average size is 43 cm at 6 months and 46 cm at 12 months. By 1 year of age, head size has increased by almost 33%. Closure of the cranial sutures occurs, with the posterior fontanel closing by 6 to 8 weeks of age and the anterior fontanel closing by 12 to 18 months of age (the average age being 14 months).

Expanding head size reflects the growth and differentiation of the nervous system. By the end of the first year, the brain has increased in weight about 2½ times. Maturation of the brain is exhibited in the dramatic developmental achievements of infancy (see Table 36-2, p. 971). Primitive reflexes are replaced by voluntary, purposeful movement, and new reflexes that influence motor development appear.

The chest assumes a more adult contour, with the lateral diameter becoming larger than the anteroposterior diameter. The chest circumference approximately equals the head circumference by the end of the first year. The heart grows less rapidly than the rest of the body. Its weight is usually doubled by 1 year of age; in comparison, body weight triples during the same period. The size of the heart is still large in relation to the chest cavity; its width is approximately 55% of the chest width.

Maturation of Systems

Other organ systems also change and grow during infancy. The respiratory rate slows somewhat (see Appendix E) and is relatively stable. Respiratory movements continue to be abdominal. Several factors predispose the infant to more severe and acute respiratory problems. Because of the close proximity of the trachea to the bronchi and its branching structures, infectious agents can be rapidly transmitted from one anatomical location to another. The short, straight eustachian tube closely communicates with the ear, allowing **infection** to ascend from the pharynx to the middle ear. In addition, because the infant's immune system is unable to produce sufficient immune globulin A (IgA) in the mucosal lining, there is less protection against infection in infancy than during later childhood.

The heart rate slows (see Appendix E), and the rhythm is often sinus arrhythmia (i.e., rate increases with inspiration and decreases with expiration). Blood pressure also changes during infancy (see Appendix E). Systolic pressure rises during the first 2 months as a result of the increasing ability of the left ventricle to pump blood into the systemic circulation. Diastolic pressure decreases during the first 3 months then gradually rises to values close to those at birth. Fluctuations in blood pressure occur during varying states of activity and emotion.

Significant hematopoietic changes occur during the infant's first year (see Appendix D). Fetal hemoglobin (HgbF) is present in large quantities for the first 5 months, with adult hemoglobin steadily increasing through the first half of infancy. Fetal hemoglobin has a shorter lifespan than that of adult hemoglobin; thus there is an increased turnover of these cells and a gradual decrease in hemoglobin. This process results in a physiological anemia around 3 to 6 months of age. High levels of HgbF depress the production of erythropoietin, a hormone released by the kidney that stimulates red blood cell production. Hemoglobin levels decrease to a point at which tissue oxygenation needs stimulate erythropoietin, and erythropoiesis resumes, forming new red blood cells (Blackburn, 2007). This anemia can be decreased if there is a delay in clamping the cord at birth (Hutton and Hassan, 2007).

Maternal iron stores are present for the infant's first 5 to 6 months and then gradually diminish, which also accounts for lowered hemoglobin levels toward the end of the first 6 months. The occurrence of physiological anemia is not affected by an adequate supply of iron. However, when erythropoiesis is stimulated, iron supplies are necessary for the formation of hemoglobin.

The digestive processes are immature at birth. Saliva is secreted in small amounts, but most of the digestive processes do not begin functioning until age 3 months, when drooling is common because of the poorly coordinated swallowing reflex. The enzyme amylase is present in small amounts but usually has little effect on the foodstuffs because of the small amount of time the food stays in the mouth. Gastric digestion in the stomach consists primarily of the action of hydrochloric acid and rennin, an enzyme that acts specifically on the casein in milk to cause the formation of curds (i.e., coagulated semi-solid particles of milk). The curds cause the milk to be retained in the stomach long enough for digestion to occur.

Digestion also takes place in the duodenum, where pancreatic enzymes and bile begin to break down protein and fat. Secretion of the amylase, which is needed for digestion of complex carbohydrates, is deficient until about the fourth to sixth month of life. Lipase is also limited, and infants do not achieve adult levels of fat absorption until 4 to 5 months of age. Trypsin is secreted in sufficient quantities to catabolize protein into polypeptides and some amino acids.

The immaturity of the digestive processes is evident in the appearance of stools. During infancy, solid foods (e.g., peas, carrots, corn, and raisins) are passed incompletely broken down in the feces. An excess quantity of fibre easily disposes the child to loose, bulky stools. During infancy, the stomach enlarges to accommodate a greater volume of food. By the end of the first year, the infant is able to tolerate three meals a day and an evening bottle and may have one or two bowel movements daily. With any type of gastric irritation, however, the infant is vulnerable to diarrhea, vomiting, and dehydration (see Chapter 47).

The liver is the most immature of all the gastrointestinal organs throughout infancy. The ability to conjugate bilirubin and secrete bile is achieved after the first couple of weeks of life. However, the capacities for gluconeogenesis, formation of plasma protein and ketones, storage of vitamins, and deamination of amino acids remain relatively immature for the first year of life.

Maturation of the suckling, sucking, and swallowing reflexes and the eruption of teeth (see Teething, p. 977) parallel the changes in the gastrointestinal tract and prepare the infant for the introduction of solid foods.

The immunological system undergoes numerous changes during the first year. IgA is present in large amounts in colostrum; this is believed to have a protective role in the gastrointestinal tract against many bacteria, such as *Escherichia coli*, and viruses such as poliovirus. The function and quantity of T-lymphocytes, lymphokines, and complement are reduced in early infancy, thus preventing optimal response to certain bacteria and viruses.

The full-term newborn receives significant amounts of maternal IgG, which for approximately 3 months confers immunity against **antigens** to which the mother was exposed. During this time, the infant begins to synthesize IgG; approximately 40% of adult levels are reached by 1 year of age. Significant amounts of IgM are produced at birth, and adult levels are reached by 9 months of age. The production of IgA, IgD, and IgE is much more gradual. Please see Appendix D for serum values.

During infancy, thermoregulation becomes more efficient; the ability of the skin to contract and of muscles to shiver in response to cold increases. The peripheral capillaries respond to changes in ambient temperature to regulate heat loss. The capillaries constrict in response to cold, conserving core body temperature and decreasing potential evaporative heat loss from the skin surface. The capillaries dilate in response to heat, decreasing internal body temperature through evaporation, conduction, and convection. Shivering (**thermogenesis**) causes the muscles and muscle fibres to contract, generating metabolic heat that is distributed throughout the body. Increased adipose tissue during the first 6 months insulates the body against heat loss.

A shift in the total body fluid also occurs. At birth, 75% of the term infant's body weight is water, and there is an excess of **extracellular fluid** (ECF). As the percentage of body water decreases, so does the amount of ECF—from 40% at term to 20% in adulthood. The high proportion of ECF, which is composed of blood plasma, **interstitial fluid**, and lymph, predisposes the infant to a more rapid loss of total body fluid and, consequently, dehydration.

The immaturity of the renal structures also predisposes the infant to dehydration. Complete maturity of the kidney occurs during the latter half of the second year, when the cuboidal epithelium of the glomeruli becomes flattened. Before this time the glomeruli's filtration capacity is reduced. Urine is voided frequently and has a low specific gravity (i.e., 1.000 to 1.010).

Auditory acuity is at adult levels during infancy. Visual acuity begins to improve, and binocular fixation is established. Binocularity, or the fixation of two ocular images into one cerebral picture (fusion), begins to develop by 6 weeks of age and should be well established by age 4 months. Depth perception (**stereopsis**) begins to develop by age 7 to 9 months but may exist earlier as an innate safety mechanism against accidental falling.

Fine Motor Development

Fine motor behaviour includes the use of the hands and fingers in the prehension (grasp) of an object. Grasping occurs during the first 2 to 3 months as a reflex and gradually becomes voluntary. At 1 month of age the hands are predominantly closed, and by 3 months they are mostly open. By this time, infants demonstrate a desire to grasp an object, but they "grasp" it more with the eyes than with the hands. If a rattle is placed in the hand, the infant will actively hold onto it. By 4 months of age, the infant regards both a small pellet and the hands and then looks from the object to the hands and back again. By 5 months the infant is able to voluntarily grasp an object.

Gradually the palmar grasp (using the whole hand) is replaced with a **pincer grasp** (using the thumb and index finger). The infant uses a crude pincer grasp by 8 to 9 months of age and has progressed to a neat pincer grasp by 11 months (Fig. 36-1).

By 6 months of age, infants have increased manipulative skill: they hold their bottle, grasp their feet and pull them to their mouth, and feed themselves a cracker. By 7 months they transfer objects from one hand to the other, use one hand for grasping, and hold a cube in each hand simultaneously. They enjoy banging objects and will explore the movable parts of a toy.

By 10 months of age, the pincer grasp is sufficiently established to enable infants to pick up a raisin and other finger foods. They can deliberately let go of an object and will offer it to someone. By 11 months they can put objects into a container and like to remove them. By age 1 year, infants try, but may fail, to build a tower of two blocks.

Gross Motor Development

Head Control

The full-term newborn can momentarily hold the head in midline and parallel when the body is suspended ventrally and can lift and turn the head from side to side when prone. This is not the case when the infant is lying prone on a pillow

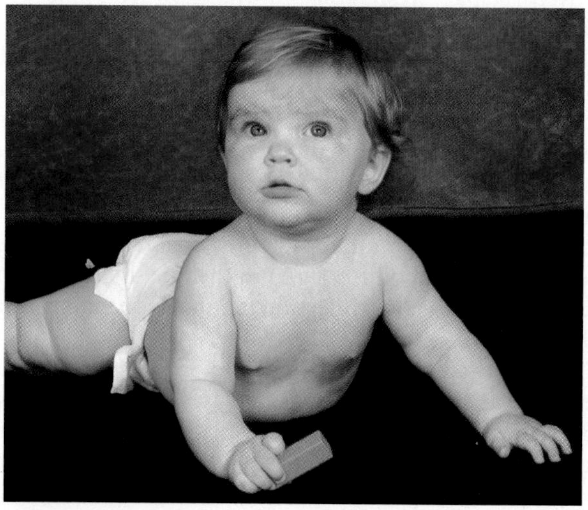

Fig. 36-1 Crude pincer grasp at 8 to 10 months. *(Photo by Paul Vincent Kuntz, Texas Children's Hospital, Houston.)*

or soft surface; infants do not have the head control to lift their head out of the depression of the object and thus risk possible suffocation in the prone position early in infancy (see Sudden Infant Death Syndrome, p. 1008, and Chapter 25, p. 667). Marked head lag is evident when the infant is pulled from a lying to a sitting position. By 3 months of age, infants can hold their head well beyond the plane of the body. By 4 months infants can lift the head and front portion of the chest approximately 90 degrees above the table, bearing their weight on the forearms. Only slight head lag is evident when the infant is pulled from a lying to a sitting position, and by 4 to 6 months head control is well established (Figs. 36-2 and 36-3).

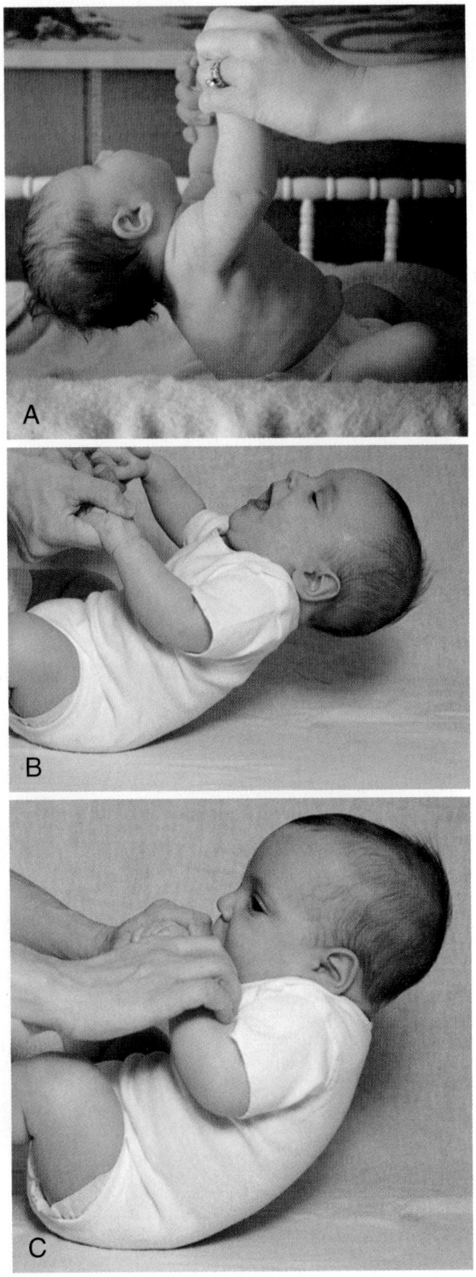

Fig. 36-2 Head control while pulled to sitting position. **A:** Complete head lag at 1 month. **B:** Partial head lag at 2 months. **C:** Almost no head lag at 4 months.

NURSING ALERT An infant who displays head lag at 6 months of age should have a developmental and neurological evaluation.

Rolling Over

Newborns may roll over accidentally because of their rounded back. The ability to willfully turn from the abdomen to the back generally occurs at 5 months, and the ability to turn from the back to the abdomen occurs at 6 months. Infants put to sleep on their sides may easily roll over to a prone (face-down) position, thus placing them at higher risk for sudden infant death syndrome (SIDS). It is therefore important to place infants in a supine position for sleep. While the infant is awake and being observed, a prone position is acceptable to

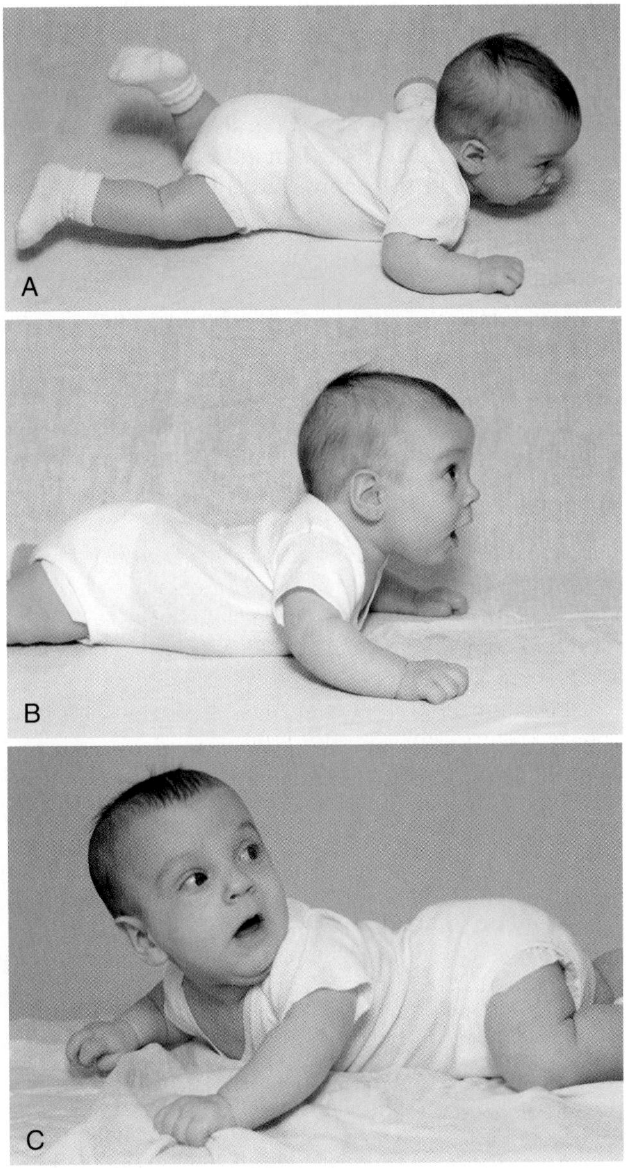

Fig. 36-3 Head control while prone. **A:** Infant momentarily lifts head at 1 month. **B:** Infant lifts head and chest 90 degrees and bears weight on forearms at 4 months. **C:** Infant lifts head, chest, and upper abdomen and can bear weight on hands at 6 months. Note how this position facilitates turning from abdomen to back.

enhance achievement of milestones such as head control, crawling, creeping, and turning over. The parachute reflex (Fig. 36-4), a protective response to falling, appears at 7 months.

Sitting

The ability to sit follows progressive head control and straightening of the back (Fig. 36-5). For the first 2 to 3 months the back is uniformly rounded. The convex cervical curve forms at approximately 3 to 4 months of age, when head control is established. The convex lumbar curve appears when the child begins to sit, at about age 4 months. As the spinal column straightens, the infant can be propped in a sitting position. By age 7 months infants can sit alone, leaning forward on their hands for support. By age 8 months they can sit well while unsupported and begin to explore their surroundings in this position rather than in a lying position. By 10 months they can manoeuvre from a prone to a sitting position.

Locomotion

Locomotion involves acquiring the ability to bear weight, propel forward on all four extremities, stand upright with support, and, finally, walk alone (Fig. 36-6). Following a cephalocaudal pattern, infants 4 to 6 months old develop increasing coordination in their arms. Initial locomotion results in

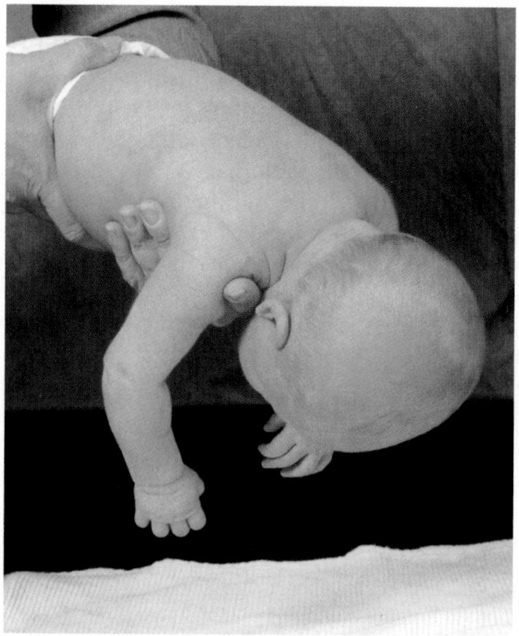

Fig. 36-4 Parachute reflex. *(Photo by Paul Vincent Kuntz, Texas Children's Hospital, Houston.)*

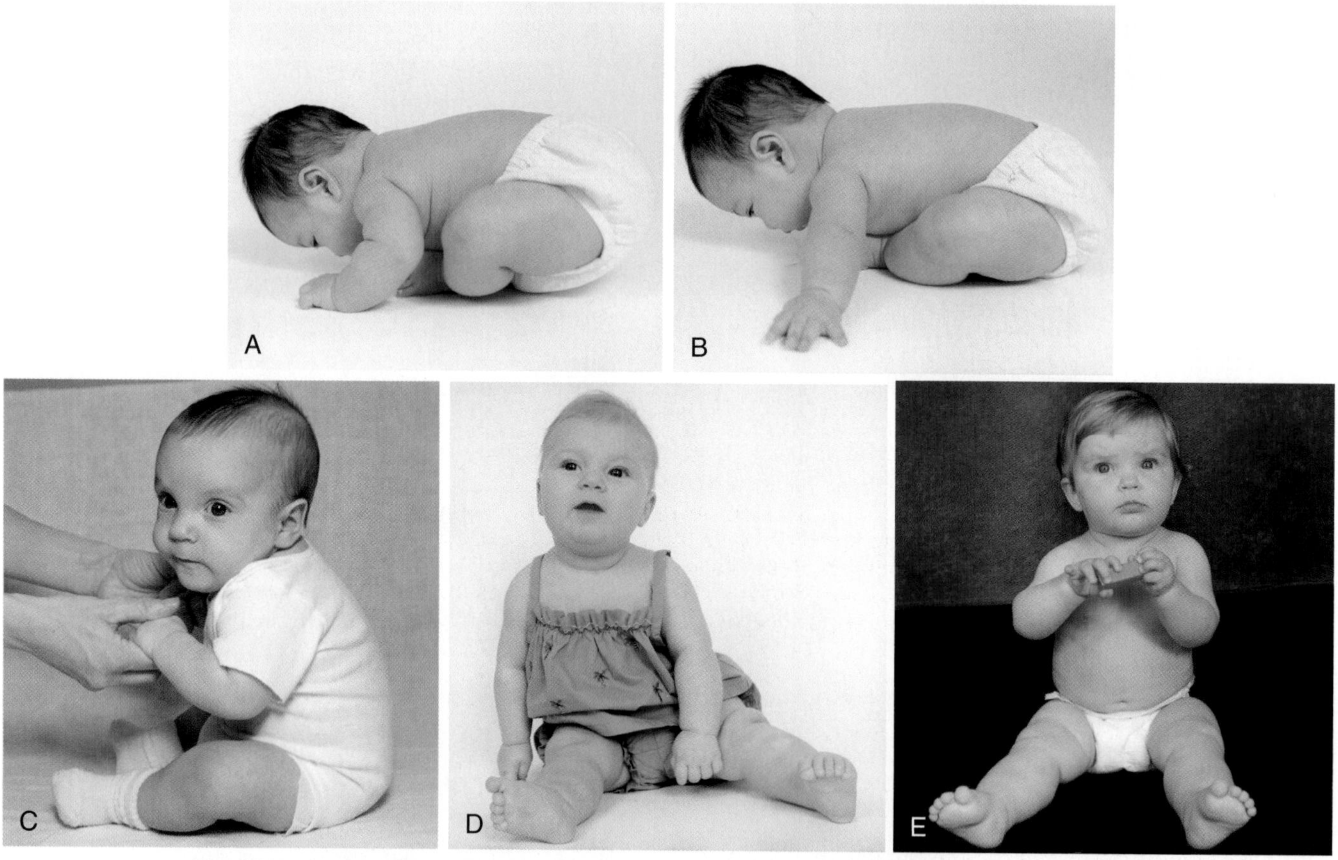

Fig. 36-5 Development of sitting. **A:** Back is completely rounded, and infant has no ability to sit upright at 1 month. **B:** At 2 months, infant exhibits more control; back is still rounded, but infant can sit up momentarily with some head control. **C:** Back is rounded only in lumbar area, and infant is able to sit erect with good head control at 4 months. **D:** Infant can sit alone, leaning on hands for support, at 7 months. **E:** Infant sits without support at 8 months. Note the transferring of objects that occurs, beginning at 7 months. *(Photos by Paul Vincent Kuntz, Texas Children's Hospital, Houston.)*

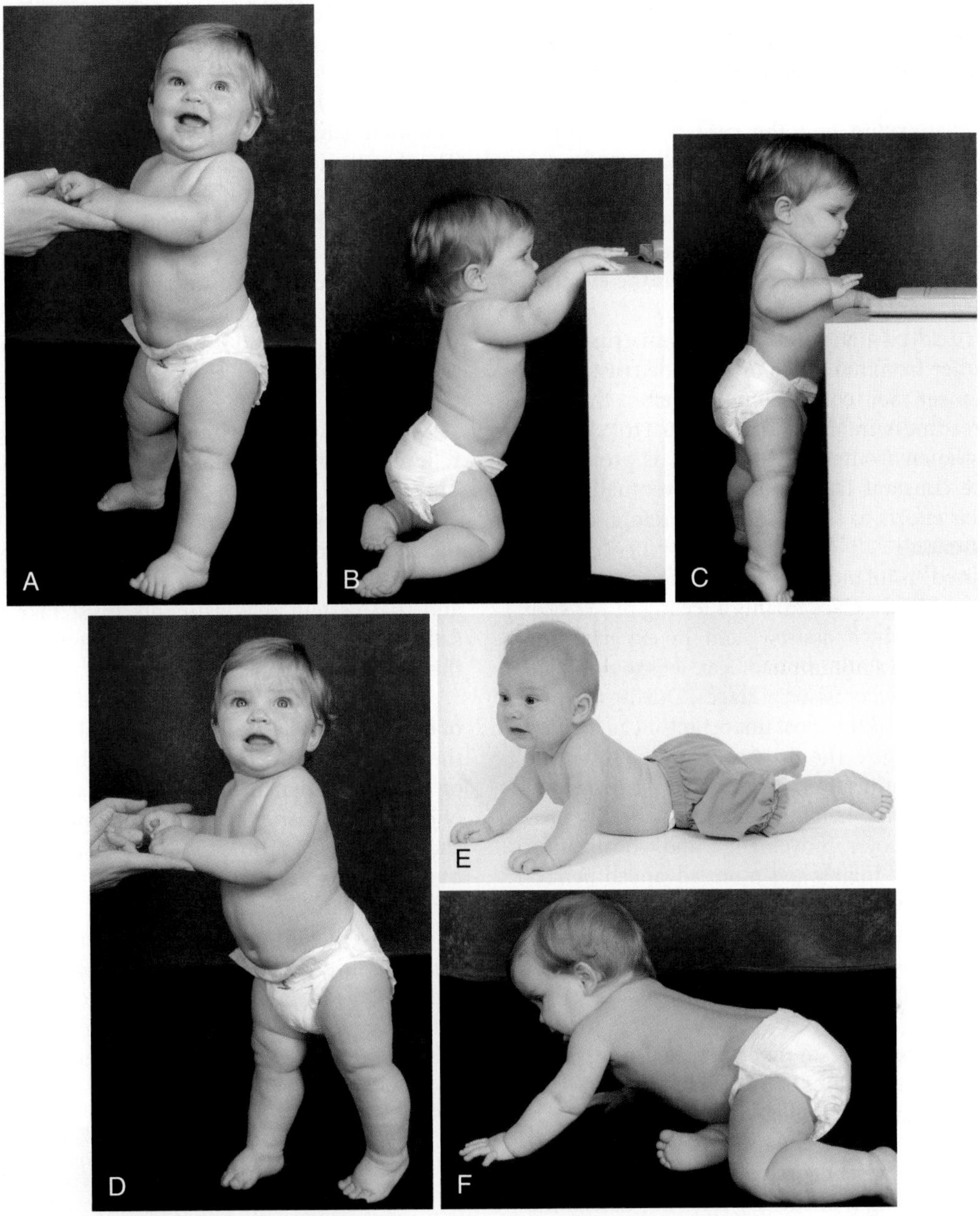

Fig. 36-6 Development of locomotion. **A:** Infant bears full weight on feet by 7 months. **B:** Infant can manoeuvre from sitting to kneeling position. **C:** Infant can stand holding onto furniture at 9 months. **D:** While standing, infant takes deliberate step at 10 months. **E:** Infant crawls with abdomen on floor and pulls self forward, and then **(F)** creeps on hands and knees at 9 months. *(Photos by Paul Vincent Kuntz, Texas Children's Hospital, Houston.)*

infants propelling themselves backward by pushing with the arms. By 6 to 7 months of age, they are able to bear all their weight on their legs with assistance. Crawling (propelling forward with belly on floor) progresses to creeping (on hands and knees with belly off floor) by 9 months. At this time, they stand while holding onto furniture and can pull themselves to the standing position, but they are unable to manoeuvre back down except by falling. By 11 months they can usually walk while holding onto furniture or with both hands held, and by age 1 year they may be able to walk with one hand held. A number of infants attempt their first independent steps by their first birthday.

NURSING ALERT An infant who does not pull to a standing position by 11 to 12 months of age should be further evaluated for possible developmental **dysplasia** of the hip (see Fig. 24-10). Although there is considerable variation among infants for the achievement of these milestones, they provide guidelines for early intervention.

Psychosocial Development

Developing a Sense of Trust (Erikson)

Erikson's (1963) phase I (birth to 1 year) is concerned with acquiring a sense of **trust** while overcoming a sense of **mistrust** (termed "Trust versus Mistrust") (see Chapter 33). The trust that develops is a trust of self, of others, and of the world. Infants "trust" that their feeding, comfort, stimulation, and caring needs will be met. The crucial element for the achievement of this task is the quality of both the parent–child (or caregiver–child) relationship and the care that the infant receives. The provision of food, warmth, and shelter alone is inadequate for the development of a strong sense of self. The infant and parent must jointly learn to satisfactorily meet their needs in order for mutual regulation of frustration to occur. When this synchrony fails to develop, mistrust is the eventual outcome.

Failure to learn delayed gratification leads to mistrust. Mistrust can result either from too much or too little frustration. If parents always meet their children's needs before the children signal their readiness, infants will never learn to test their ability to control the environment. If the delay is prolonged, infants experience constant frustration and eventually mistrust others in their efforts to satisfy them. Therefore, consistency of care is essential.

The trust acquired in infancy provides the foundation for all succeeding phases. Trust gives infants a feeling of physical comfort and security, which assists them in experiencing unfamiliar situations with a minimum of fear. Erikson divided the first year of life into two oral/social stages. During the first 3 to 4 months, food intake is the most important social activity in which the infant engages. The newborn can tolerate little frustration or delay of gratification. Primary **narcissism** (total concern for oneself) is at its height. However, as bodily processes such as vision, motor movements, and vocalization become better controlled, infants use more advanced behaviours to interact with others. For example, rather than cry, infants may put their arms up to signify a desire to be held.

The next social modality involves a mode of reaching out to others through grasping. *Grasping* is initially reflexive, but even as a reflex it has a powerful social meaning for the parents. The reciprocal response to the infant's grasping is the parents' holding on and touching. Both the child and parents experience pleasurable tactile stimulation.

Tactile stimulation is extremely important in the total process of acquiring trust. The degree of mothering skill, the quantity of food, or the length of sucking does not determine the quality of the experience. Rather, it is the overall quality of the interpersonal relationship that influences the infant's formulation of trust.

During the second stage, the more active and aggressive modality of biting occurs. Infants learn that they can hold onto what is their own and can more fully control their environment. During this stage, infants may be confronted with one of their first conflicts. If they are breastfeeding, they quickly learn that biting causes the mother to become upset and withdraw the breast. Yet biting also brings internal relief from teething discomfort and a sense of power or control.

This conflict may be solved in a variety of ways. The infant can be taught not to bite by the mother saying "no" and withdrawing the nipple from the baby's mouth. The mother may wean the infant from the breast and begin bottle-feeding, or the infant may learn to bite substitute "nipples," such as a pacifier, and retain pleasurable breastfeeding. The successful resolution of this conflict strengthens the mother–child relationship because it occurs at a time when infants are recognizing the mother as the most significant person in their life.

Cognitive Development

Sensorimotor Phase (Piaget)

The theory most commonly used to explain cognition, or the ability to know, is that of Piaget (1952) (see Chapter 33). The period from birth to 24 months is termed the **sensorimotor phase** and is composed of six stages; however, because this discussion is concerned with ages birth to 12 months, only the first four stages are discussed here. The last two stages (tertiary circular reactions and invention of new means) occur during the toddler period of 12 to 24 months and are discussed in Chapter 37.

During the sensorimotor phase, infants progress from reflex behaviours to simple repetitive acts to imitative activity. Three crucial events take place during this phase. The first event involves *separation*, in which infants learn to separate themselves from other objects in the environment. They realize that others besides themselves control the environment and that certain readjustments must take place for mutual satisfaction to occur. This coincides with Erikson's concept of the formation of trust.

The second major accomplishment is achieving the concept of **object permanence**, or the realization that objects that leave the visual field still exist. A typical example of the development of object permanence is when infants are able to pursue objects they observe being hidden under a pillow or behind a chair (Fig. 36-7). This skill develops at approximately 9 to 10 months of age, which corresponds to the time of increased locomotion skills.

The last major intellectual achievement of this period is the ability to use *symbols*, or *mental representation*. The use of symbols allows the infant to think of an object or situation without actually experiencing it. The recognition of symbols is the beginning of the understanding of time and space.

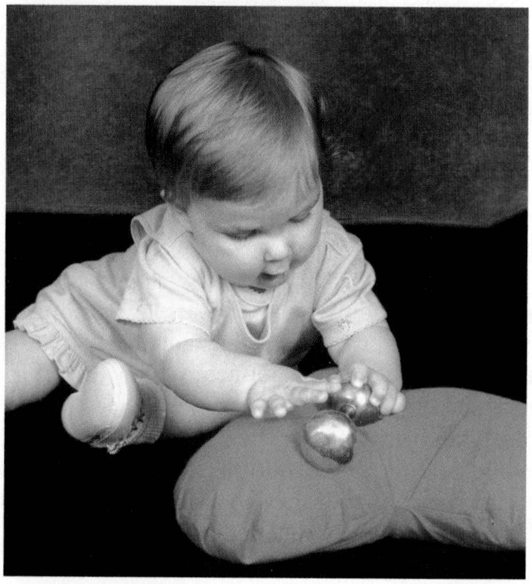

Fig. 36-7 Nine-month-old infant actively searches for object hidden behind pillow. *(Photo by Paul Vincent Kuntz, Texas Children's Hospital, Houston.)*

Piaget's first stage, from birth to 1 month, is identified by the infant's *use of reflexes*. At birth, the infant's individuality and temperament are expressed through the physiological reflexes of sucking, rooting, grasping, and crying. The repetitious nature of the reflexes is the beginning of associations between an act and a sequential response. When infants cry because they are hungry, a nipple is put in the mouth, and they suck, feel satisfaction, and sleep. They are assimilating this experience while perceiving auditory, tactile, and visual cues. This experience of perceiving certain patterns, or "ordering," provides a foundation for the subsequent stages.

The second stage, *primary circular reactions*, marks the beginning of the replacement of reflexive behaviour with voluntary acts. During the period from 1 to 4 months, activities such as sucking or grasping become deliberate acts that elicit certain responses. The beginning of accommodation is evident. Infants incorporate and adapt their reactions to the environment and recognize the stimulus that produced a response. Previously they would cry until the nipple was brought to the mouth. Now they associate the nipple with the sound of the parent's voice. They accommodate this new piece of information and adapt by ceasing to cry when they hear the voice—before receiving the nipple. What is taking place is a realization of causality and a recognition of an orderly sequence of events. The environment is taken in with all of the senses and with whatever motor ability is present.

The *secondary circular reactions* stage is a continuation of primary circular reactions and lasts until 8 months of age. In this stage, the primary circular reactions are repeated and prolonged for the response that results. Grasping and holding now become shaking, banging, and pulling. Shaking is performed to hear a noise, not solely for the pleasure of shaking. The quality and quantity of an act become evident. More or less shaking produces different responses. Understanding of causality, time, deliberate intention, and separateness from the environment begins to develop.

Three new processes of human behaviour occur. *Imitation* requires the differentiation of selected acts from several events. By the second half of the first year, infants can imitate sounds and simple gestures. *Play* becomes evident as they take pleasure in performing an act after they have mastered it. Many of the infant's waking hours are absorbed in sensorimotor play. *Affect* (the outward manifestation of emotion and feeling) is seen as infants begin to develop a sense of permanency. During the first 6 months, infants believe that an object exists only for as long as they can visually perceive it—in other words, out of sight, out of mind. Affect in relation to external objects is evident when the object continues to be present or remembered even though it is beyond the range of perception. Object permanence is a critical component of parent–child attachment and is seen in the development of **separation anxiety** at 6 to 8 months of age (see p. 966).

During the fourth sensorimotor stage, *coordination of secondary schematas and their application to new situations*, infants use previous behavioural achievements primarily as the foundation for adding new intellectual skills to their expanding repertoire. This stage is largely transitional. Increasing motor skills allow for greater exploration of the environment. They begin to discover that hiding an object does not mean that it is gone but that removing an obstacle will reveal the object. This marks the beginning of intellectual reasoning. Furthermore, they can experience an event by observing it, and they begin to associate symbols with events (e.g., "bye-bye" with "Daddy goes to work"), but the classification is purely their own. In this stage, they learn from the object itself; this is in contrast to the second stage, in which infants learn from the type of interaction between objects or individuals. Intentionality is further developed, in that infants now actively attempt to remove a barrier to the desired (or undesired) action (see Fig. 36-7). If something is in their way, they attempt to climb over it or push it away. Previously, an obstacle would have caused them to give up any further attempt to achieve the desired goal.

Development of Body Image

The development of body image parallels sensorimotor development. Infants' kinesthetic and tactile experiences are the first perceptions of their body, and the mouth is the principal area of pleasurable sensations. Other parts of the body are primarily objects of pleasure—the hands and fingers to suck and the feet to play with. As physical needs are met, they feel comfort and satisfaction with their body. Messages conveyed by the caregivers reinforce these feelings. For example, when infants smile, they receive emotional satisfaction from others who smile back.

Achieving the concept of object permanence is basic to the development of self-image. By the end of the first year, infants recognize that they are distinct from their parents. At the same time, they have increasing interest in their own image, especially in the mirror (Fig. 36-8). As motor skills develop, they learn that parts of the body are useful; for example, the hands bring objects to the mouth, and the legs help them move to different locations. All of these achievements transmit messages to them about themselves. Therefore, it is important to transmit positive messages to infants about their bodies.

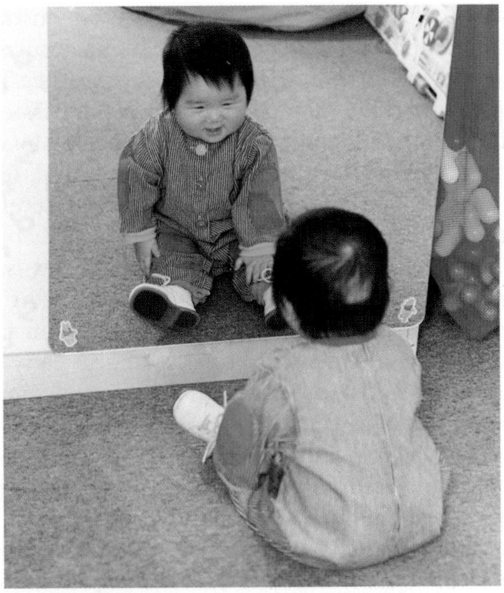

Fig. 36-8 Nine-month-old infant enjoying own image in mirror.

Social Development

Infants' social development is initially influenced by their reflexive behaviour, such as the grasp, and eventually depends primarily on the interaction between them and the principal caregivers. Attachment to the parent is increasingly evident during the second half of the first year, and tremendous strides are made in communication and personal–social behaviour. Whereas crying and reflexive behaviour are initial ways in which neonates meet their needs, the social smile is an early step in social communication. This has a profound effect on family members and is stimulus for evoking continued responses from others. By 4 months of age, infants can laugh out loud.

Play is a major socializing agent and provides stimulation needed to learn from and interact with the environment. By age 6 months infants are personable. They can play games such as peek-a-boo when their head is hidden in a towel, signal their desire to be picked up by extending their arms, and show displeasure when a toy is removed or their face is being washed.

Attachment

The importance to infants of human physical contact cannot be overemphasized. Parenting is not an instinctual ability but a learned, acquired process. The attachment of parent and child, which begins before birth, assumes even greater importance at birth and during the first year (see Chapter 22, Parental Attachment, Bonding, and Acquaintance). In the following discussion of attachment, the term *mother* is used in the broad context of the consistent caregiver with whom the child relates more than anyone else. However, in society's changing social climate and sex-role stereotypes, this person may very well be the father or a grandparent. Having two mothers or two fathers is not unusual. According to the 2006 Census, the second in Canadian history to collect data on same-sex families, 0.6% of all couples in Canada were of the same sex. Out of that number, approximately 9% of lesbian couples and 3% of gay male couples were caring for children in their home (Statistics Canada, 2007).

evolve Case Study—Child Abuse

Studies on paternal–infant attachment demonstrate that stages similar to those in maternal attachment occur and that fathers are often more involved in child care when mothers are employed outside the home (although mothers continue to do the majority of infant care) (McConnell & Moss, 2011). Additional research has shown that inexperienced, first-time fathers are as capable as experienced fathers of developing a close attachment with their infants (Yu, Hung, Chan, Yeh, & Lai, 2012). The father's attachment with the infant is also an important factor in the mother's emotional well-being. Breastfeeding mothers reported that the most important factor in establishing and maintaining breastfeeding in early infancy was the father's acceptance of breastfeeding and support for the mother (Arora et al., 2000).

Attachment progresses during infancy, with the child assuming an increasingly significant role. Two components of cognitive development are required for attachment: (1) the ability to discriminate the mother from other individuals, and (2) the achievement of object permanence. Both of these processes prepare the infant for an equally important aspect of attachment: separation from the parent. Separation–individuation should occur as a harmonious, parallel process with emotional attachment.

During the formation of attachment to the parent, the infant progresses through four distinct but overlapping stages. For the first few weeks, infants respond indiscriminately to anyone. Beginning at approximately 8 to 12 weeks of age, they cry, smile, and vocalize more to the mother than to anyone else but continue to respond to others, whether familiar or not. At approximately 6 months of age, infants show a distinct preference for the mother. They follow her more, cry when she leaves, enjoy playing with her more, and feel most secure in her arms. About 1 month after showing attachment to the mother, many infants begin attaching to other members of the family, most often the other parent.

Infants acquire other developmental behaviours that influence the attachment process. These include (1) differential crying, smiling, and vocalization (more to the mother than to anyone else); (2) visual-motor orientation (looking more at the mother, even if she is not close); (3) crying when the mother leaves the room; (4) approaching through locomotion (crawling, creeping, or walking); (5) clinging (especially in the presence of a stranger); and (6) exploring away from the mother while using her as a secure base.

Reactive attachment disorder (RAD) is a psychological and developmental problem that stems from maladaptive or absent attachment between the infant and parent (or primary caregiver) and may persist into childhood and even adulthood (Wilson, 2001; Zeanah & Fox, 2004). Infants at risk for RAD include those who have been victims of physical abuse, sexual abuse, or neglect; infants exposed to parental alcoholism, mental illness, and substance use; and infants who have experienced the absence of a consistent primary caregiver as a result of foster care, institutionalization, parental abandonment, and parental incarceration. Two different patterns of RAD have emerged: the emotionally withdrawn–inhibited pattern and an indiscriminate-disinhibited pattern (Hornor, 2008; Zeanah & Fox, 2004). Signs of RAD are usually seen before the age of 5 years in infants who had insecure attachments to the mother or other primary caretaker (American Psychiatric Association, 2000). The child may manifest behaviours such as not being cuddly with parents, failing to make eye contact with significant others, having poor impulse control, and being destructive to self and others. Without early intervention, some of these children fail to develop a conscience and suffer from an antisocial personality disorder that may lead to criminal acts. The American Academy of Pediatrics (2012) position statement on RAD strongly recommends against the use of coercive holding therapies or rebirthing techniques for the treatment of RAD. It is not within the scope of this text to discuss the full array of attachment disorders and associated therapies.

Separation Anxiety

Between ages 4 and 8 months, the infant progresses through the first stage of separation–individuation and begins to have some awareness of self and mother as separate beings. At the same time, the sense of object permanence is developing, and the infant is aware that the parent can be absent. Thus, separation anxiety develops and is manifested through a predictable sequence of behaviours.

During the early second half of the first year, infants usually protest when placed in their crib, and a short time later they will object when the mother leaves the room. Infants may not notice the mother's absence if they are absorbed in an activity. However, when they realize her absence, they may protest. From this point on, they become very alert to her activities and whereabouts. By 11 to 12 months of age, they are able to anticipate her imminent departure by watching her behaviours, and they may begin to protest before she leaves. At this point, many parents learn to postpone alerting the child to their departure until just before leaving.

Fear of Strangers

As infants demonstrate attachment to one person, they correspondingly exhibit less friendliness to others. Between 6 and 8 months of age, fear of strangers and **stranger anxiety** become prominent and are related to infants' ability to discriminate between familiar and unfamiliar people. Behaviours such as clinging to the parent, crying, and turning away from the stranger are common (Fig. 36-9).

Language Development

The infant's first means of verbal communication is crying. Crying as a biological sign conveys a message of urgency and signals displeasure, such as hunger. However, crying is also a social event that affects the development of the parent–infant relationship—either by its absence, which usually has a positive effect on parents, or its presence, which may involve a negative response or persuade parents to minister to the child's physical or emotional needs.

In the first few weeks of life, crying has a reflexive quality and is mostly related to physiological needs. Infants cry for 1 to 1½ hours a day up to 3 weeks of age, then build up to 2 and even 4 hours a day by 6 weeks. Crying tends to decrease by 12 weeks of age. It is thought that the increase in crying for no apparent reason during the first few months may be related to the discharge of energy and the maturational changes in the central nervous system. During the end of the first year, infants cry for attention; from fear (especially stranger fear); and from frustration, usually in response to their developing but inadequate motor skills.

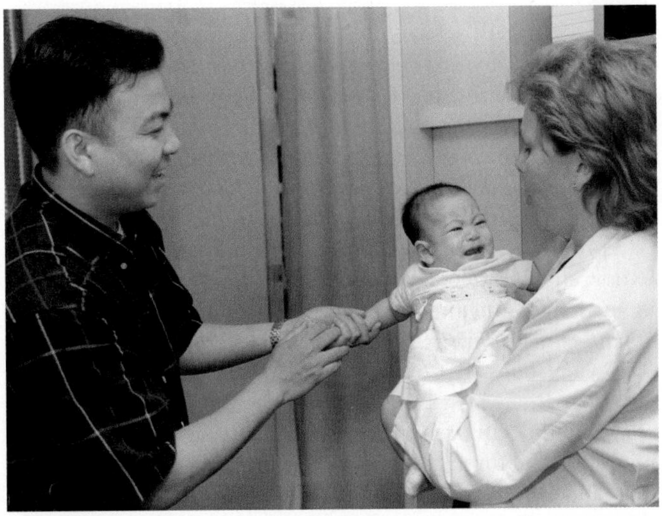

Fig. 36-9 Behaviours related to fear of strangers include clinging to the parent and turning away from the stranger. *(Photo by Paul Vincent Kuntz, Texas Children's Hospital, Houston.)*

NURSING ALERT Be alert to parents' reports about maternal postpartum depression and infant crying, since these concerns may indicate a stressed mother–infant relationship. Depression is a serious issue that may have started earlier in the pregnancy. Please see Chapter 23 (Postpartum Complications) for further information.

Depression is diagnosed if a woman is experiencing signs, almost every day for 2 weeks, that significantly affect her ability to care for herself, her children, and home, as well as her ability to work (Public Health Agency of Canada [PHAC], 2012b):

- Depressed mood or extreme sadness
- Crying spells for no apparent reason
- Guilty thoughts; feelings of worthlessness or hopelessness
- Restlessness, lack of control, or lack of energy
- Difficulty concentrating; disorganized thoughts
- Feelings of guilt or inadequacy as a mother
- Changes in sleep or appetite; for example, sleeping or eating too little or too much
- Withdrawing from her partner, family, friends, and coworkers
- Having thoughts of suicide or other frightening thoughts of hurting others

Vocalizations heard during crying eventually become syllables and words (e.g., the "mama" heard during vigorous crying). Infants vocalize as early as 5 to 6 weeks of age by making small throaty sounds. By 2 months they can make single-vowel sounds such as *ah*, *eh*, and *uh*. By 3 to 4 months of age, the consonants *n*, *k*, *g*, *p*, and *b* are added, and infants coo, gurgle, and laugh out loud. By 8 months they can imitate sounds; add the consonants *t*, *d*, and *w*; and combine syllables (e.g., "dada"), but they do not ascribe meaning to the word until 10 to 11 months of age (see Family-Centred Teaching box). By 9 to 10 months of age, they comprehend the meaning of the word "no" and obey simple commands. By age 1 year they can say three to five words with meaning.

FAMILY-CENTRED TEACHING

Child's Developing Language Skills

During the acquisition of new language skills the child temporarily may stop using other recently learned sounds or words. This is often distressing for parents, who have waited in anticipation for the words "dada" or "mama," because these sounds are commonly replaced by other vocalizations and may not be repeated for several weeks. Nurses can reassure parents that the child will again say these special words, and with increased meaning.

Play

Play during infancy represents the various social modalities observed during cognitive development (see Chapter 33, Role of Play in Development). Infants' activity is primarily narcissistic and revolves around their own body. As discussed under Development of Body Image (p. 965), body parts are primarily objects of play and pleasure.

During the first year, play becomes more sophisticated and interdependent. From birth to 3 months of age, infants' responses to the environment are global and largely undifferentiated. Play is dependent; pleasure is demonstrated by a quieting attitude (1 month), a smile (2 months), or a squeal (3 months). From 3 to 6 months, infants show more discriminate interest in stimuli and begin to play alone with a rattle or a soft stuffed toy or with someone else. There is much more interaction during play. By 4 months of age, they laugh out loud, show a preference for certain toys, and become excited when food or a favourite object is brought to them. They recognize an image in a mirror, smile at it, and vocalize to it.

By age 6 months to 1 year, play involves sensorimotor skills. Actual games such as peekaboo and pat-a-cake are played. Verbal repetition and imitation of simple gestures occur in response to demonstration. Play is much more selective, not only in terms of specific toys but also in terms of "playmates." Although play is solitary or one-sided, infants choose with whom they will interact. At 6 to 8 months of age they usually refuse to play with strangers. Parents are definite favourites, and infants know how to attract their attention. At 6 months they will extend the arms to be picked up, at 7 months cough or squeal to make their presence known, at 10 months pull the parent's clothing, and at 12 months call them by name. This represents a tremendous advance from the newborn who signaled biological needs by merely crying to express displeasure.

Stimulation is as important for psychosocial growth as food is for physical growth. Knowledge of **developmental milestones** allows nurses to guide parents regarding proper play for infants. For instance, it is not sufficient to place a mobile over a crib and toys in a playpen for a child's optimum social, emotional, and intellectual development. Play must provide interpersonal contact and recreational and educational stimulation. Infants need to be *played with*, not merely *allowed to play*. Although the type of play infants engage in is called *solitary*, this is a figurative, not literal, term to denote one-sided play. The type of toys given to the child is much less important than the quality of personal interaction that occurs.

Table 36-1 lists play activities appropriate for the developmental level of the infant in view of their motor, language, and personal–social achievements. Although the activities are grouped according to the major mode of stimulation provided, there is overlap in many instances. In addition, play activities suggested for one age group may be appropriate for older infants but inappropriate for younger infants.

Temperament

The infant's temperament or behavioural style influences the type of interaction that occurs between the child and parents, especially the mother, and other family members (see general discussion of temperament in Chapter 33). In assessments of a child's temperament, it is the parents' perception of the child and the degree of fit between their expectations and the child's actual temperament that are important. The more dissonance, or lack of harmony, between the child's temperament and the parent's ability to accept and deal with the behaviour, the more risk there is for subsequent parent–child conflicts.

Although most behavioural researchers agree that there is a strong biological component to temperament, researchers also suggest that temperament may be modified by the environment, particularly the family (Wilson et al., 2000). Family interaction with the infant is perceived as a circular process in which family members affect each other and the family as a unit. With these concepts in mind, the nurse has an important role in helping the family understand the infant's temperament as it relates to family dynamics and the eventual well-being of the child and family unit (Wilson et al., 2000).

The Revised Infant Temperament Questionnaire (RITQ) (Carey & McDevitt, 1978) can be used as a screening tool with parents. The questionnaire focuses on nine temperament variables, and the 95 questions relate specifically to activities such as sleeping, feeding, playing, diapering, and dressing. The scores from the RITQ help identify the child's temperamental style. Use of the RITQ is well accepted by parents and should be accompanied by an adequate explanation of the results. In discussing the results, the nurse should avoid descriptors such as *difficult* and instead describe such infants using terms such as *intense* or *less predictable.*

The Early Infancy Temperament Questionnaire, a 76-item parent questionnaire, was adapted from the RITQ to specifically evaluate temperament characteristics of infants 1 to 4 months old. The RITQ is best suited for infants 4 months old and older (Medoff-Cooper, Carey, & McDevitt, 1993).

With knowledge of the infant's temperament, nurses are better able to (1) provide parents with background information that will help them see their child in a better perspective, (2) offer a more organized picture of their child's behaviour and possibly reveal distortions in their perceptions of the behaviour, and (3) guide parents in choosing appropriate childrearing techniques.

Childrearing Practices Related to Temperament

Most parents realize that their infant is born with unique characteristics, and few parents of difficult infants need to be told of the challenge of caring for them. However, few parents are aware of the significance of the temperamental characteristics and of constructive approaches to dealing with them. The following discussion includes examples of interventions that promote more positive parenting of infants with different temperament styles. Recommended resources for parents include the *Canadian Paediatric Society Guide to Caring for Your Child From Birth to Age 5* (Sacks, 2009) and *Canada's Baby Care Book: A Complete Guide From Birth to 12 Months Old* (Friedman & Saunders, 2007).

"Difficult" children may respond better to scheduled feedings and structured caregiving routines than to demand feedings and frequent changes in daily routines. These children sleep less and may need more structured approaches to bedtime to prevent bedtime problems. "Highly distractible" children may require additional soothing measures such as

Table 36-1 Play During Infancy

AGE (MO)	VISUAL STIMULATION	AUDITORY STIMULATION	TACTILE STIMULATION	KINETIC STIMULATION
Suggested Activities				
Birth–1	Look at infant at close range. Hang bright, shiny object within 20–25 cm of infant's face and in midline. Hang mobiles with black-and-white designs.	Talk to infant; sing in soft voice. Play music box, CD, or MP3 player. Have ticking clock or metronome nearby.	Hold, caress, and cuddle infant. Hold infant skin-to-skin. Keep infant warm. Infant may like to be swaddled.	Rock infant; place in cradle. Use stroller for walks.
2–3	Provide bright objects. Make room bright with pictures or mirrors. Take infant to various rooms while doing chores. Place infant in infant seat for vertical view of environment.	Talk to infant. Include infant in family gatherings. Expose infant to various environmental noises other than those of home. Use rattles, wind chimes.	Caress infant while bathing, at diaper change. Comb hair with a soft brush. Give massage.	Use infant swing. Take infant in car for rides. Exercise body by moving extremities in swimming motion. Use cradle gym.
4–6	Place infant in front of unbreakable mirror. Give brightly coloured toys to hold (small enough to grasp).	Talk to infant; repeat sounds infant makes. Laugh when infant laughs. Call infant by name. Crinkle different papers by infant's ear. Place rattle or ball in infant's hand.	Give infant soft squeeze toys of various textures. Allow to splash in bath. Place infant nude on soft, furry rug and move extremities.	Use swing or stroller. Bounce infant in lap while holding in standing position. Support infant in sitting position; let infant lean forward to balance self. Place infant on floor to crawl, roll over, sit.
6–9	Give infant large toys with bright colours, movable parts, and noisemakers. Place unbreakable mirror where infant can see self. Play peek-a-boo, especially hiding face in a towel. Make funny faces to encourage imitation. Give ball of yarn or string to pull apart.	Call infant by name. Repeat simple words such as "dada," "mama," "bye-bye." Speak clearly. Name parts of body, people, and foods. Tell infant what you are doing. Use "no" only when necessary. Give simple commands. Show how to clap hands, bang a drum.	Let infant play with fabrics of various textures. Have bowl with foods of different sizes and textures to feel. Let infant "catch" running water. Encourage "swimming" in large bathtub or shallow pool. Give infant wad of sticky tape to manipulate.	Hold infant upright to bear weight and bounce. Pick up infant, say "up." Put down infant, say "down." Place toys out of reach; encourage infant to get them. Play pat-a-cake.
9–12	Show infant large pictures in books. Take infant to places where there are animals, many people, different objects (e.g., shopping centre). Play ball by rolling it to child, demonstrate "throwing" it back. Demonstrate building a two-block tower.	Read infant simple nursery rhymes. Point to body parts and name each one. Imitate sounds of animals.	Give infant finger foods of different textures. Let infant mess and squash food. Let infant feel cold (ice cube) or warm objects; say what temperature each one is. Let infant feel a breeze (fan blowing).	Give large push-pull toys. Place furniture in a circle to encourage cruising. Turn infant in different positions.
Suggested Toys				
Birth–6	Nursery mobiles Unbreakable mirrors Contrasting coloured sheets	Music boxes Musical mobiles Crib dangle bells Small-handled, clear rattle	Stuffed animals Soft clothes Soft or furry quilt Soft mobiles	Rocking crib or cradle Weighted or suction toy Infant swing
6–12	Various coloured blocks Nested boxes or cups Books with rhymes and bright pictures Strings of big beads Simple take-apart toys Large ball Cup and spoon Large puzzles Jack-in-the-box	Rattles of different sizes, shapes, tones, and bright colours Squeaky animals and dolls Light, rhythmic music	Soft, different-textured animals and dolls Sponge toys, floating toys Squeeze toys Teething toys Books with various textures or objects, such as fur and zipper	Activity box for crib Push-pull toys Wind-up swing

swinging, rocking, or being carried in a pack worn across the parent's chest or back. Children with "high activity" levels require vigilant watching, and parents need to take extra precautions to make the home safe for the child. These children benefit from increased opportunities for gross motor activity to constructively channel their energy.

The child who is "slow to warm up" may demonstrate a higher level of fear of strangers than that of other children and may require gradual and frequent preparation for new situations, such as substitute child care. Even the "easy child" can present problems: the parents may need reminders to feed the infant who sleeps for prolonged intervals and rarely cries. Appropriate counselling based on awareness of the child's temperament can greatly enhance the quality of interaction between parents and infant. Even just letting parents know that "difficult" traits are innate can relieve feelings of guilt and incompetence.

Because of the complexity of the developmental process during the first 12 months, Table 36-2 is provided to help organize and clarify the data already discussed. Although all milestones are important, some (designated by an asterisk in the table) represent essential integrative aspects of development that lay the foundation for achievement of more advanced skills. The table presents the average monthly age at which various skills are attained. It must be remembered that although the sequence of milestones is the same, the rate will vary among children.

evolve Case Study—Infant Growth and Development

Coping With Concerns Related to Normal Growth and Development

Separation and Fear of Strangers

Parents can have a number of fears regarding their child during infancy. However, the fear that causes parents the most concern is fear related to strangers and separation. Although erroneously interpreted by some as a sign of undesirable, antisocial behaviour, fear of strangers and separation anxiety are important components of a strong, healthy, parent–child attachment. Nevertheless, this period can present difficulties for the parent and child. Parents may experience guilt at having to leave the infant because he or she violently protests having a baby-sitter. To accustom the infant to new people, parents can have close friends or relatives visit often. This gives the child the opportunity to become comfortable with other persons and can give parents time for themselves.

Infants also need opportunities to safely experience strangers. Usually toward the end of the first year, infants begin to venture away from the parent and demonstrate curiosity about strangers. If allowed to explore at their own rate, many infants eventually "warm up" to strangers. If parents hold the child away from their face, the infant can observe while maintaining close physical contact.

The best approach for the stranger (who may be the nurse) is to talk softly; meet the child at eye level (to appear smaller); maintain a safe distance from the infant; and avoid sudden, intrusive gestures, such as holding the arms out and smiling broadly.

Parents also may wonder whether they should encourage the child's clinging, dependent behaviour, especially if there is pressure from others who view this as "spoiling" (see the following discussion). Parents need to be reassured that such behaviour is healthy, desirable, and necessary for the child's optimum emotional development. If parents can reassure the infant of their presence, the infant will learn to realize that they are still there even if not physically present. Talking to infants when leaving the room, allowing them to hear one's voice on the telephone, and using transitional objects (e.g., a favourite blanket or toy) reassures them of the parent's continued presence.

Alternative Child Care Arrangements

For many parents, especially working parents, locating safe and competent child care facilities for the infant is an increasingly difficult problem—one that is compounded by the number of families with both parents working outside the home. Over the years, there has been a marked shift in child care arrangements; whereas most children are cared for in group centres or other settings, an increasing number of children are being cared for in home settings.

The basic types of care are in-home care, either in the parents' or caregivers' home, and centre-based care, usually in a day care centre. In-home care may consist of a full-time baby-sitter who lives in the home, a full-time baby-sitter who comes to the home, cooperative arrangements such as exchange baby-sitting, and family day care. A licenced in-home day care typically provides care and protection for up to five children for part of a day and does not include informal arrangements such as exchange baby-sitting or caregivers in the child's own home. The five children include the day care provider's own children younger than 6 years of age living in the home. Unfortunately, many day care homes operate without a licence and may care for large numbers of infants without adequate staff and facilities.

Child centre–based care usually refers to a licensed day care facility that provides care for six or more children, for 6 or more hours a day. Work-based group care is another option that is becoming increasingly popular as employers recognize the benefit of providing high-quality and convenient child care to their employees. Sick-child care may also be available for times when the youngster is ill. A major nursing responsibility is guiding parents in locating suitable facilities that have a well-qualified staff.

Provincial licensing regulations exist in most provinces and territories to ensure that facilities meet minimum standards for such things as staff qualifications, the ratio of staff to children, the safety and cleanliness of the care environment, and behaviour management. These regulations help ensure that any potential risks to the child's well-being are kept to a minimum. Community agencies can assist parents in identifying day care centres that accept children of specific age groups and that are convenient to home and work. Their records should be available to the public and provide reports from the health, safety, and fire departments; periodic evaluations from the licensing agency; complaints filed against the centre; and qualifications of the centre's employees. Early-childhood programs may also belong to a voluntary accreditation system, for example, the Association of Day Care Operators of Ontario, which serves as a model for optimum care. References from other parents are helpful, provided that they have investigated

Table 36-2 Growth and Development During Infancy

AGE (MO)	PHYSICAL	GROSS MOTOR	FINE MOTOR	SENSORY	VOCALIZATION	SOCIALIZATION/COGNITION
1	Weight gain of 150–200 g weekly for first 6 mo Height gain of 2.5 cm monthly for first 6 mo Head circumference increases by 1.5 cm monthly for first 6 mo Primitive reflexes present and strong Doll's eye reflexes and dance reflex fading Obligatory nose breathing (most infants)	Assumes flexed position with pelvis high but knees not under abdomen when prone (at birth, knees flexed under abdomen)* Can turn head from side to side when prone; lifts head momentarily from bed (see Fig. 36-3, A)* Has marked head lag, especially when pulled from lying to sitting position (see Fig. 36-2, A) Holds head momentarily parallel and in midline when suspended in prone position Assumes asymmetrical tonic neck reflex position when supine When held in standing position, body is limp at knees and hips In sitting position, back is uniformly rounded, absence of head control	Hands predominantly closed Grasp reflex strong Hand clenches on contact with rattle	Able to fixate on moving object in range of 45 degrees when held at a distance of 20–25 cm Visual acuity approaches 20/100† Follows light to midline Quiets when hears a voice	Cries to express displeasure Makes small, throaty sounds Makes comfort sounds during feeding	Is in sensorimotor phase—stage I, use of reflexes (birth–1 mo), and stage II, primary circular reactions (1–4 mo) Watches parent's face intently as parent talks to infant
2	Posterior fontanel closed Crawling reflex disappears	Assumes less flexed position when prone—hips flat, legs extended, arms flexed, head to side* Less head lag when pulled to sitting position (see Fig. 36-2, B) Can maintain head in same plane as rest of body when held in ventral suspension When prone, can lift head almost 45 degrees off table When moved to sitting position, head is held up but bends forward (see Fig. 36-5, B) Assumes asymmetrical tonic neck reflex position intermittently	Hands often open Grasp reflex fading	Binocular fixation and convergence to near objects beginning When supine, follows dangling toy from side to point beyond midline Visually searches to locate sounds Turns head to side when sound is made at level of ear	Vocalizes, distinct from crying* Crying becomes differentiated Coos Vocalizes to familiar voice	Demonstrates social smile in response to various stimuli*

*Milestones that represent essential integrative aspects of development that lay the foundation for the achievement of more advanced skills.
†Degree of visual acuity varies according to vision measurement procedure used.

Continued

Table 36-2 Growth and Development During Infancy—cont'd

AGE (MO)	PHYSICAL	GROSS MOTOR	FINE MOTOR	SENSORY	VOCALIZATION	SOCIALIZATION/COGNITION
3	Primitive reflexes fading	Able to hold head more erect when sitting, but still bobs forward Has only slight head lag when pulled to sitting position Assumes symmetrical body positioning Able to raise head and shoulders from prone position to a 45- to 90-degree angle from table; bears weight on forearms When held in standing position, able to bear slight fraction of weight on legs Regards own hand	Actively holds rattle but will not reach for it* Grasp reflex absent Hands kept loosely open Clutches own hand; pulls at blankets and clothes	Follows object to periphery (180 degrees)* Locates sound by turning head to side and looking in same direction* Begins to have ability to coordinate stimuli from various sense organs	Squeals aloud to show pleasure* Coos, babbles, chuckles Vocalizes when smiling "Talks" a great deal when spoken to Less crying during periods of wakefulness	Displays considerable interest in surroundings Ceases crying when parent enters room Can recognize familiar faces and objects, such as feeding bottle Shows awareness of strange situations
4	Drooling begins Moro, tonic neck, and rooting reflexes have disappeared*	Has almost no head lag when pulled to sitting position (see Fig. 36-2, C)* Balances head well in sitting position (see Fig. 36-5, C)* Back less rounded, curved only in lumbar area Able to sit erect if propped up Able to raise head and chest off surface to angle of 90 degrees (see Fig. 36-3, B) Assumes predominant symmetrical position Rolls from back to side*	Inspects and plays with hands; pulls clothing or blanket over face in play* Tries to reach objects with hand but overshoots Grasps object with both hands Plays with rattle placed in hand, shakes it, but cannot pick it up if dropped Can carry objects to mouth	Able to accommodate to near objects Binocular vision fairly well established Can focus on a 1.25 cm block Beginning eye–hand coordination	Makes consonant sounds *n, k, g, p, b* Laughs out loud* Vocalization changes according to mood	Is in stage III, secondary circular reactions Demands attention by fussing; becomes bored if left alone Enjoys social interaction with people Anticipates feeding when sees bottle or mother if breastfeeding Shows excitement with whole body, squeals, breathes heavily Shows interest in strange stimuli Begins to show memory
5	Beginning signs of tooth eruption Birth weight doubles	No head lag when pulled to sitting position When sitting, able to hold head erect and steady Able to sit for longer periods when back is well supported Back straight When prone, assumes symmetrical positioning with arms extended Can turn over from abdomen to back* When supine, puts feet to mouth	Able to grasp objects voluntarily* Uses palmar grasp, bidextrous approach Plays with toes Takes objects directly to mouth Holds one cube while regarding a second one	Visually pursues a dropped object Is able to sustain visual inspection of an object Can localize sounds made below ear	Squeals Makes cooing vowel sounds interspersed with consonant sounds (e.g., *ah-goo*)	Smiles at mirror image Pats breast or bottles with both hands More enthusiastically playful, but may have rapid mood swings Is able to discriminate strangers from family Vocalizes displeasure when object is taken away Discovers parts of body

6	Growth rate may begin to decline Weight gain of 90–150 g weekly for next 6 mo Height gain of 1.25 cm monthly for next 6 mo Teething may begin with eruption of two lower central incisors* Chewing and biting occur*	When prone, can lift chest and upper abdomen off surface, bearing weight on hands (see Fig. 36-3, C) When about to be pulled to a sitting position, lifts head Sits in high chair with back straight Rolls from back to abdomen When held in standing position, bears almost all of weight Hand regard absent	Resecures a dropped object Drops one cube when another is given Grasps and manipulates small objects Holds bottle Grasps feet and pulls to mouth	Adjusts posture to see an object Prefers more complex visual stimuli Can localize sounds made above ear Will turn head to the side, then look up or down	Begins to imitate sounds* Babbling resembles one-syllable utterances—*ma, mu, da, di, hi** Vocalizes to toys, mirror image Takes pleasure in hearing own sounds (self-reinforcement)	Recognizes parents; begins to fear strangers Holds arms out to be picked up Has definite likes and dislikes Begins to imitate (cough, protrusion of tongue) Excites on hearing footsteps Laughs when head is hidden in a towel Briefly searches for a dropped object (object permanence beginning)* Frequent mood swings—from crying to laughing with little or no provocation
7	Eruption of upper central incisors	When supine, spontaneously lifts head off surface Sits, leaning forward on hands (see Fig. 36-5, D)* When prone, bears weight on one hand Sits erect momentarily Bears full weight on feet (see Fig. 36-6, A) When held in standing position, bounces actively	Transfers objects from one hand to the other (see Fig. 36-5, E)* Has unidextrous approach and grasp Holds two cubes more than momentarily Bangs cube on table Rakes at a small object	Can fixate on very small objects* Responds to own name Localizes sound by turning head in a curving arch Beginning awareness of depth and space Has taste preferences	Produces vowel sounds and chained syllables—*baba, dada, kaka** Vocalizes four distinct vowel sounds "Talks" when others are talking	Increasing fear of strangers; shows signs of fretfulness when parent disappears* Imitates simple acts and noises Tries to attract attention by coughing or snorting Plays peekaboo Demonstrates dislike of food by keeping lips closed Exhibits oral aggressiveness in biting and mouthing Demonstrates expectation in response to repetition of stimuli
8	Begins to show regular patterns in bladder and bowel elimination Parachute reflex appears (see Fig. 36-4)	Sits steadily unsupported (see Fig. 36-5, E)* Readily bears weight on legs when supported; may stand holding onto furniture Adjusts posture to reach an object	Has beginning pincer grasp using index, fourth, and fifth fingers against lower part of thumb Releases objects at will Rings bell purposely Retains two cubes while regarding third cube Secures an object by pulling on a string Reaches persistently for toys out of reach		Makes consonant sounds *t, d, w* Listens selectively to familiar words Utterances signal emphasis and emotion Combines syllables, such as *dada*, but does not ascribe meaning to them	Increasing anxiety over loss of parent, particularly mother, and fear of strangers Responds to word "no" Dislikes dressing, diaper change

*Milestones that represent essential integrative aspects of development that lay the foundation for the achievement of more advanced skills.

Continued

Table 36-2 Growth and Development During Infancy—cont'd

AGE (MO)	PHYSICAL	GROSS MOTOR	FINE MOTOR	SENSORY	VOCALIZATION	SOCIALIZATION/COGNITION
9	Eruption of upper lateral incisor may begin	Creeps on hands and knees Sits steadily on floor for prolonged time (10 min) Recovers balance when leaning forward but cannot do so when leaning sideways Pulls self to standing position and stands holding onto furniture (see Fig. 36-6, B and C)*	Uses thumb and index fingers in crude pincer grasp (see Fig. 36-1)* Preference for use of dominant hand now evident Grasps third cube Compares two cubes by bringing them together	Localizes sounds by turning head diagonally and directly toward sound Depth perception increasing	Responds to simple verbal commands Comprehends "no-no"	Parent (mother) is increasingly important for own sake Shows increasing interest in pleasing parent Begins to show fears of going to bed and being left alone Puts arms in front of face to avoid having it washed
10	Labyrinth-righting reflex is strongest–when infant is in prone or supine position, is able to raise head	Can change from prone to sitting position Stands while holding onto furniture, sits by falling down Recovers balance easily while sitting While standing, lifts one foot to take a step (see Fig. 36-6, D)	Crude release of an object beginning Grasps bell by handle		Says "dada," "mama" with meaning* Comprehends "bye-bye" May say one word (e.g., "hi," "bye," "no")	Inhibits behaviour to verbal command of "no-no" or own name Imitates facial expressions; waves bye-bye Extends toy to another person but will not release it Develops object permanence* Repeats actions that attract attention and cause laughter Pulls clothes of another to attract attention Plays interactive game such as pat-a-cake Reacts to adult anger; cries when scolded Demonstrates independence in dressing, feeding, locomotive skills, and testing of parents Looks at and follows pictures in a book

11	Eruption of lower lateral incisor may begin	When sitting, pivots to reach toward back to pick up an object Cruises or walks holding onto furniture or with both hands held*	Explores objects more thoroughly (e.g., clapper inside bell) Has neat pincer grasp Drops object deliberately for it to be picked up Puts one object after another into a container (sequential play) Able to manipulate an object to remove it from tight-fitting enclosure		Imitates definite speech sounds	Experiences joy and satisfaction when a task is mastered Reacts to restrictions with frustration Rolls ball to another on request Anticipates body gestures when a familiar nursery rhyme or story is being told (e.g., holds toes and feet in response to "This little piggy went to market") Plays game up-down, "so big," or peek-a-boo Shakes head for "no"
12	Birth weight tripled* Birth length increased by 50%* Head and chest circumference equal (head circumference 46 cm) Has total of six to eight deciduous teeth Anterior fontanel almost closed Landau reflex fading Babinski reflex disappears Lumbar curve develops; lordosis evident during walking	Walks with one hand held* Cruises well May attempt to stand alone momentarily; may attempt first step alone* Can sit down from standing position without help	Releases cube in cup Attempts to build two-block tower but fails Tries to insert a pellet into a narrow-necked bottle but fails Can turn pages in a book, many at a time	Discriminates simple geometric forms (e.g., circle) Amblyopia may develop with lack of binocularity Can follow rapidly moving object Controls and adjusts response to sound; listens for sound to recur	Says three to five words besides "dada," "mama"* Comprehends meaning of several words (comprehension always precedes verbalization) Recognizes objects by name Imitates animal sounds Understands simple verbal commands (e.g., "Give it to me," "Show me your eyes")	Shows emotions such as jealousy, affection (may give hug or kiss on request), anger, fear Enjoys familiar surroundings and explores away from parent Is fearful in strange situation; clings to parent May develop habit of "security blanket" or favourite toy Has increasing determination to practise locomotor skills Searches for an object even if it has not been hidden, but searches only where object was last seen*

*Milestones that represent essential integrative aspects of development that lay the foundation for the achievement of more advanced skills.

the centre carefully and have remained involved with the centre's activities. Information for parents on what to consider when selecting a child care facility can be found in the Additional Resources section at the end of the chapter.

The same attention should be applied to locating competent baby-sitters. References from other parents are essential, and there is no substitute for observing the interaction between the individual and the child. Although very young infants need little if any preparation for the introduction of a new caregiver, older infants may benefit from a gradual placement to reduce stranger anxiety. At all times, the parent should have the right to visit the child, and regular conferences should be established to review the child's progress. Some child care centres provide a service whereby the parent may log on to the Internet from work and view the child's activity at the centre for reassurance that the child is well.

One of the areas that is increasingly important in selecting child care is the centre's health practices; however, parents often do not check the centre for health and safety features. The Canadian Paediatric Society (2008) has described the factors that promote high-quality child care centres and provided evidence for the developmental and behavioural outcomes of children in these centres.

Children in day care centres, especially those under 3 years of age, tend to have more illnesses—especially diarrhea, otitis media, respiratory tract infections (especially if the caregiver smokes), hepatitis A, meningitis, and cytomegalovirus—than children cared for in their home (Canadian Paediatric Society [CPS], 2009). The strongest predictor of risk of illness is the number of unrelated children in the room. Proactive infection control measures and education of staff have been effective in reducing the incidence of upper respiratory tract infections, diarrhea, and rotavirus in day care centres (Kotch et al., 2007). It has been reported that families who have children in out-of-home child care lose an estimated 13 days of work per year as a result of childhood infections (Brady, 2005). Parents should inquire about the centre's policy regarding the attendance and care of sick children.

Limit-Setting and Discipline

As infants' motor skills advance and mobility increases, parents face the need to set safe limits to protect the child and establish a positive and supportive parent–child relationship (see Nurse's Role in Injury Prevention, p. 1001). Although there are numerous disciplinary techniques, some are more appropriate for this age than others. An effective approach used in disciplining a child is the use of "time-out." The basic principles are the same as those discussed in Chapter 31, except that the place for time-out needs to be commensurate with the child's abilities. For example, the playpen is better for most infants than a chair. Although parents may be concerned with instituting discipline during infancy, it is important to stress that the earlier effective disciplinary methods are employed, the easier it is to continue these approaches.

Parents must recognize the child's cognitive and behavioural limitations; adequate protection from hazards must be implemented because infants and toddlers do not understand a cause–effect relationship between dangerous objects and physical harm. Children will innately test limits and explore during the exploratory phase of growth; instead of discouraging exploration, parents should provide safe alternatives, put away dangerous household items, and provide consistent discipline and nurturing.

Thumb-Sucking and Use of a Pacifier

As discussed in Chapter 25, sucking is the infant's chief pleasure and may not be satisfied entirely by breastfeeding or bottle-feeding. To address this natural urge, infants may need to engage in **non-nutritive sucking** by sucking on their thumb or fingers, or parents may introduce use of a pacifier. Some parents may have concerns about infant thumb-sucking and pacifier use; for discussion of these concerns, as well as counselling of parents regarding pacifier use, see Chapter 25 (Non-Nutritive Sucking, p. 670).

Non-nutritive sucking, particularly in preterm infants, can result in increased weight gain, decreased length of hospital stay, and improved pain management (Pinelli & Symington, 2000; Pinelli, Symington, & Ciliska, 2002). Thus non-nutritive sucking should not be withheld from preterm infants as there is no evidence that pacifier use has any effect on the initiation and length of breastfeeding, specifically in preterm infants. Non-nutritive sucking should also be offered in conjunction with the use of concentrated sucrose for pain management (see Atraumatic Care, p. 658).

Pacifier use, particularly in the early days after birth and in the birth hospital, has gained considerable attention in the scientific literature. Lawrence and Lawrence (2011), as well as other experts in breastfeeding, recommend that health care workers not introduce pacifiers to breast-fed infants unless at the request of the parent. Pacifier use is not recommended as part of the Baby-Friendly Hospital Initiative (see Box 26-2, p. 700). A review of studies by the Joanna Briggs Institute (2005) found an association between pacifier use in infancy and a reduction in breastfeeding and exclusive breastfeeding. However, the authors concluded that pacifier use did not cause a reduction in breastfeeding; rather it was a "marker for socioeconomic, demographic, psychosocial, and cultural factors that determine pacifier use and breastfeeding." (For further discussion of the relation between breastfeeding and pacifier use, see Chapter 26, Bottles and Pacifiers, pp. 687–690.) In addition, the researchers found that infants put to sleep with a pacifier had a reduced risk of SIDS (see Sudden Infant Death Syndrome: Etiology, p. 1008). Regarding other possible correlations with pacifier use, such as increased risk of infections or dental **malocclusion**, the authors were unable to make any recommendations for or against pacifier use, because of the limited number of studies (Hanzer et al., 2010; Jenik, Vain, Gorestein, & Jocobi, 2009; Joanna Briggs Institute, 2005).

Infants' use of a pacifier has also been suggested as a causative factor in the increase in episodes of acute otitis media (Niemela, Uhari, & Mottonen, 1995). However, a later study showed a significant decrease in the incidence of acute otitis media when a pacifier was used only at bedtime (Niemela et al., 2000).

The Canadian Paediatric Society (2003) position paper on the use of pacifiers also states that such use may decrease the risk of SIDS, but given the lack of definitive research on pacifiers the decision on their use is left to the parents. If pacifiers are used, they should not be given to the child until breastfeeding is well established and should be restricted if infants and children experience frequent or recurrent otitis media (CPS, 2003). Families need to receive instruction on the safe and appropriate use of pacifiers (CPS, Community Paediatrics Committee, 2012), and safety considerations in purchasing one must be stressed (see Fig. 25-19). Parents should be cautioned against altering a pacifier, thus making it more dangerous (see Aspiration of Foreign Objects, p. 993).

To decrease dependence on non-nutritive sucking in young infants, sucking pleasure can be increased by prolonging feeding time. Also, if a parent is overusing a pacifier, the parent's excessive use of the pacifier to calm the child should be explored. It is not unusual for parents to place a pacifier in the infant's mouth as soon as crying begins, thus reinforcing a pattern of distress–relief.

See Additional Resources at the end of this chapter for further information from Health Canada on the safety of baby equipment, including pacifiers.

During infancy and early childhood there is no need to restrain non-nutritive sucking of the fingers. Malocclusion may occur if thumb-sucking persists past 4 to 6 years of age, or when the permanent teeth erupt. Pacifiers may be perceived by some parents as less damaging because they are discarded by 2 to 3 years of age, whereas thumb-sucking may persist well into school-age years. Both pacifier use and thumb-sucking may also have significant cultural variations. Thumb-sucking reaches its peak at age 18 to 20 months and is most prevalent when the child is hungry, tired, or feeling insecure. Persistent thumb-sucking in a listless, apathetic child always warrants investigation. It may be a sign of an emotional problem between parent and child or of boredom, isolation, and lack of stimulation.

Teething

One of the more difficult periods in the infant's (and parents') life is the eruption of the deciduous (primary) teeth, often referred to as *teething*. The age of tooth eruption varies considerably among children, but the order of their appearance is fairly regular and predictable (Fig. 36-10). The first primary teeth to erupt are the lower central incisors, which appear at approximately 6 to 10 months of age (average 8 months). These are followed closely by the upper central incisors. The following is a quick guide to assessment of deciduous teeth during the first 2 years:

Age of the child in months − 6 = Number of teeth

For example: 8 months of age − 6 = 2 teeth

Teething is a physiological process; some discomfort is common as the crown of the tooth breaks through the periodontal membrane. Some children show minimum evidence of teething, such as drooling, increased finger sucking, or biting on hard objects. Others are very irritable, have difficulty sleeping, and refuse to eat. Generally, signs of illness such as fever, vomiting, or diarrhea are not symptoms of teething but of illness and may warrant further investigation. Anderson (2004) suggests that frequent waking periods are related to environmental, behavioural, or developmental changes rather than to teething. The author also cautions parents (and health care workers) to not overdiagnose teething; the ill-appearing child or child with a temperature over 38°C should be evaluated by the practitioner.

Because teething pain is a result of **inflammation**, cold is soothing. Giving the child a frozen teething ring or a clean wet washcloth placed in the freezer for about 30 minutes can help relieve the inflammation. Several nonprescription topical anaesthetic ointments are available, such as Baby Orajel, although parents and health care workers should be aware of the risks of using topical anaesthetic products (absorption rates vary in infants) (Anderson, 2004). The active ingredient in most of these is benzocaine. If such products are used, parents are advised to apply them correctly. In the event of persistent irritability that affects sleeping and feeding, systemic analgesics such as acetaminophen or ibuprofen (age-appropriate dose) can be given for no more than 3 days. However, parents should know that this is a temporary measure and should contact the health care practitioner if symptoms persist or if the child's condition changes.

NURSING ALERT The use of teething powders or procedures, such as cutting the gums or rubbing them with aspirin, is discouraged because ingestion of the powder, infection or irritation of the tissue, or aspiration of the aspirin can occur. Hard candy may cause accidental choking or aspiration and should be avoided at this age.

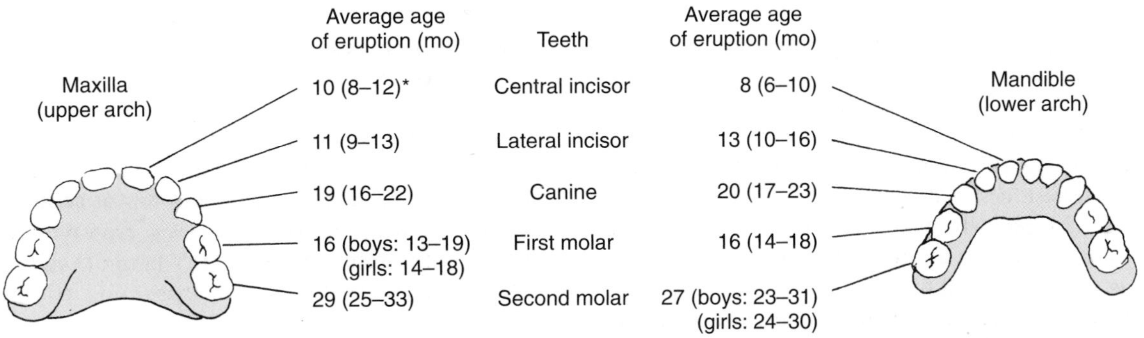

Fig. 36-10 Sequence of eruption of primary teeth. *Range represents ±1 standard deviation, or 67% of subjects studied. *(Data from McDonald, R. E., & Avery, D. R. [1994].* Dentistry for the child and adolescent *[6th ed.] St. Louis: Mosby.)*

Infant Shoes

Many parents are unaware of the type of shoes that are appropriate for the older infant and buy expensive infant shoes because of misleading advertising claims. Inflexible shoes that have hard soles can be detrimental. They can delay walking, aggravate intoeing or outtoeing, and impede the development of supportive foot muscles. Therefore, the counselling of parents regarding footwear should begin when infants are 6 months old—well before they are walking.

It is helpful to begin by explaining to parents that changes in the feet occur during infancy and early childhood as locomotion and weight bearing progress. At birth, the feet are flat because the arches are protected by fat pads on the soles. As the bones in the arches develop, the pads disappear and the feet begin to assume a mature shape. A normal arch is determined by proper alignment of all the bones and development of the surrounding musculature, not by the height of the arch.

When children begin walking, the main reason for shoes is protection. To provide protection, the shoe should retain its fit; be made of durable material with a smooth interior and few construction seams to irritate the skin; and be soft and flexible, especially in the toe area. A high-top shoe is not necessary for support but may be helpful in keeping the foot in the shoe.

A good shoe conforms to the anatomical shape of the foot, with a rounded toe and sufficient toe room. During weight bearing there should be at least the space of half the width of the thumbnail, or 1.25 cm, between the end of the longest toe and the shoe. Roomy and square-toed socks allow for proper growth and alignment. Inexpensive but well-constructed sneakers or soft-leather moccasin-type shoes are suggested as adequate footgear for walking infants. Even if the shoes are fitted properly, frequent changes are needed to accommodate the infant's rapidly growing feet. Shoe size changes at approximately 3-month intervals between 12 and 36 months; during this time the child's foot should be measured every 3 months. Curled toes when shoes are removed, and redness and irritation of the skin on the bottom of the toes indicate the need for a larger shoe size.

Promoting Optimum Health During Infancy

Nutrition

Ideally, discussion of optimum nutrition should begin prenatally with the decision to breastfeed or bottle-feed the infant. The choice for either is highly individual and is discussed in Chapter 26. This section is primarily concerned with infant nutrition up to the age of 12 months, when growth needs and developmental milestones ready the child for the introduction of solid foods. Table 36-3 shows the Dietary Reference Intake Adequate Intakes for infants for carbohydrate, fat, and protein intake during the first year of life.

Among health care providers there is concern that, despite adequate availability of optimum nutrient sources, infants are not being fed appropriately. These practices may have far-reaching, long-term health consequences for infants. It has been shown that infant health practices have an impact on the child's life. Certain chronic health conditions have been linked to feeding practices in infancy. Nurses must thus be proactive in teaching parents about what constitutes appropriate infant nutrition and nutritional habits, which can provide the opportunity to grow and develop into a healthy child and adult.

Table 36-3 Dietary Reference Intake: Adequate Intake (AI)* for Infants

AGE	AI	COMMENTS
Carbohydrate		
0–6 mo	60 g/day	Human milk; predominant source is lactose
7–12 mo	95 g/day	Human milk and complementary foods
Fat (n-6 Polyunsaturated Fatty Acids)		
0–6 mo	4.4 g/day	Human milk
7–12 mo	4.6 g/day	Human milk and complementary foods
Protein		
0–6 mo	1.52 g/kg/day	Human milk
7–12 mo	1.6 g/kg/day	Human milk and complementary foods

(Data from Institute of Medicine. [2005]. *Dietary reference intakes for energy, carbohydrate, fiber, fatty acids, cholesterol, protein, and amino acids*. Washington, DC: Food and Nutrition Board, Institute of Medicine, National Academies Press.)
*AI—The recommended average daily intake level based on observed or experimentally determined approximations or estimates of nutrient intake by a group (or groups) of apparently healthy individuals that are assumed to be adequate; used when a recommended dietary allowance cannot be determined.

Health care providers have become more aware of the use of complementary and alternative medical therapies in children that may not be as beneficial as indicated in various media sources. One concern is children's intake of megavitamins and herbs; parents may assume that the word *natural* in reference to ingredients means the product is safe, when this may not be the case. One report cited the home administration of star anise tea to treat colic as the cause of adverse neurological reactions in seven infants (Ize-Ludlow et al., 2004). It is important for nurses to be aware of the effects, availability, and practice of complementary therapies and to be able to cogently discuss their use with parents.

The First 6 Months

Human milk is the most desirable complete diet for the infant during the first 6 months. The healthy term infant receiving breast milk usually requires no vitamin and mineral supplements, with a few exceptions. Daily supplementation of vitamin D is indicated because many Canadian mothers and babies, especially those in northern communities, do not get enough vitamin D. The Canadian Paediatric Society has issued a recommendation that all breastfed infants receive a daily supplement of 400 International Units (IU) (10 mcg) of vitamin D beginning in the first few days of life. to prevent rickets and vitamin D deficiency. Vitamin D supplementation should occur until the infant is consuming at least 1 L/day of vitamin D–fortified formula (CPS, First Nations, Inuit and Métis Health Committee, 2007).

Nonbreastfed infants who are taking less than 1 L/day of vitamin D–fortified formula should also receive a daily vitamin

D supplement of 400 IU (10 mcg) and should receive more if living in a northern community. If the infant is exclusively breastfed after 4 to 6 months (when fetal iron stores are depleted), iron supplementation, which may be accomplished with iron-fortified cereal, is recommended to offset the decrease in iron available in human milk at this time and to enhance erythropoiesis. Whether breastfed or bottle-fed, infants do not require additional fluids, especially water or juice, during the first 6 months of life. Excessive intake of water in infants may result in water intoxication and hyponatremia.

Mothers working outside the home can continue breastfeeding with guidance and encouragement. Mothers should be encouraged to set realistic goals for employment and breastfeeding, with accurate information regarding the costs, risks, and benefits of available feeding options (see Chapter 26, Being Away From the Infant, p. 693).

Expressed breast milk may be stored in the refrigerator (4°C) without danger of bacterial contamination for up to 5 days (Lawrence & Lawrence, 2011). To thaw frozen milk, the container should be placed under a lukewarm water bath (less than 40.5°C) or placed in the refrigerator overnight. Although microwaving bottles and baby food is not recommended, it remains a common practice. Parents should be taught that microwaving does not heat evenly and can cause encapsulated boiling bubbles to form in the center of the liquid. Infants have sustained severe burns to the mouth, throat, and upper gastrointestinal tract as a result of microwaved milk (Lawrence & Lawrence, 2011). For more detailed information on the expression, pumping, and storage of breast milk, see Chapter 26, Hand Expression and Storage of Breast Milk, pp. 692–693.

In addition to efficient breast pumping, mothers need child care by a trusted individual or agency and support and assistance from significant others. As with all breastfeeding mothers, these women must have proper nutrition and rest for adequate lactation. Maternal fatigue is considered the biggest threat to successful breastfeeding in employed mothers (Corbett-Dick & Bezek, 1997).

An alternative to breastfeeding is commercial iron-fortified formula. It supplies the **nutrients** needed by the infant for the first 6 months.

Unmodified whole cow's milk, low-fat cow's milk, skim milk, other animal milks, and imitation milks are not acceptable as a major source of nutrition for infants because of infants' limited ability to digest these foods, the increased risk of contamination, and the lack of nutritional components in animal milk that are needed for appropriate growth. Pasteurized whole cow's milk is deficient in iron, zinc, and vitamin C and has a high renal solute load, which makes it undesirable for infants less than 12 months of age (American Academy of Pediatrics [AAP], 2009).

Dietary fat should not be restricted in infancy unless such restriction is under medical supervision. Substituting skim or low-fat milk is unacceptable because the essential fatty acids are inadequate and the solute concentration of protein and electrolytes, such as sodium, is too high.

The amount of formula per feeding and the number of feedings per day vary among infants. Infants on demand feeding usually determine their own feeding schedule, but some infants may need a more planned schedule based on average feeding patterns to ensure their receiving sufficient nutrients. In general, the number of feedings per day decreases from six at 1 month of age to four or five at 6 months. Regardless of the number of feedings, the total amount of formula ingested will usually level off at about 960 mL/day. (See discussion of formula-feeding in Chapter 26, p. 700.)

Bottled water for mixing powdered or concentrated formula is a relatively safe alternative to tap water if available tap water has a high content of contaminants such as lead. Bottled water, however, should not be assumed to be sterile unless specifically stated on the container. Fluoridated bottled water is not necessary for mixing powdered formula unless the local water source is low in fluoride, in which case fluoride supplementation is recommended after age 6 months (see Dental Health, p. 983). If powdered formula is being used, parents should be instructed in its safe preparation (see Chapter 26, Home Care box). Powdered formula has a greater risk of contamination by microorganisms than concentrated formula. Recommendations for preparation of powdered infant formula in the home or in a professional setting (i.e., hospitals and day-care centres) are provided by Health Canada at http://www.hc-sc.gc.ca/fn-an/nutrition/infant-nourisson/pif-ppn-recommandations-eng.php.

Parents should be cautioned to not feed their infant juices and non-nutritive drinks such as fruit-flavoured drinks or carbonated beverages (soft drinks). Many of these drinks do not provide sufficient caloric intake for infants less than 12 months of age. Such drinks do not replace the nutrients in milk (formula), and their use may lead to growth or health problems.

The addition of solid foods before 6 months of age is also not recommended (CPS, 2006). During the first months of an infant's life, solid foods are not compatible with the ability of the gastrointestinal tract and the infant's nutritional needs. Developmentally, infants are not ready for solid food. The extrusion (protrusion) reflex is strong and causes food to be pushed out of the mouth. Early introduction of solid foods is a type of forced feeding that may lead to excessive weight gain and increased predisposition to allergies and iron deficiency anemia. Despite these recommendations, and lacking evidence-based information to support such practices, many parents introduce solids as early as 2 weeks of age. In such cases, rice cereal is often added to the formula to help the infant sleep better at night or to enhance weight gain; however, this practice is not substantiated by any scientific evidence (Morin, 2004).

The Second 6 Months

During the second half of the infant's first year, human milk or formula continues to be the primary source of nutrition. Fluoride supplementation should begin, depending on the infant's intake of fluoridated tap water (see Dental Health, p. 983). If breastfeeding is discontinued, a commercial iron-fortified formula should be substituted. Follow-up or transition formulas specially marketed for older infants offer no special advantages over other infant formulas (AAP, 2009).

The major change in feeding habits is the addition of solid foods to the infant's diet. Physiologically and developmentally, the infant at 6 months of age is in a transition period. By this time, the gastrointestinal tract has matured sufficiently to handle more complex nutrients and is less sensitive to potentially allergenic foods. Tooth eruption is beginning and facilitates biting and chewing. The extrusion reflex has disappeared, and swallowing is more coordinated to allow the infant to accept solids easily. Head control is well developed, which permits infants to sit with support and purposely turn the head away to communicate disinterest in food. Voluntary grasping and improved eye–hand coordination gradually allow infants to pick up finger foods and feed themselves. Their increasing sense of independence is evident in their desire to hold the bottle and try to "help" during feeding.

Selection and Preparation of Solid Foods

The choice of solid foods to introduce first is variable but should meet the criteria for feeding solids, such as supplying nutrients not found in formula or breast milk. Iron-fortified infant cereal is generally introduced first because of its high iron content (7 mg prepared dry cereal). Commercially prepared ready-to-serve dry cereals for infants include rice, barley, oatmeal, and high-protein cereals; rice is usually suggested as an initial food because of its easy digestibility and low allergenic potential. Cereals such as cream of farina should not be used because infant commercial cereals are a better source of iron. Some of the commercial baby cereals are combined with fruit. There is little nutritional benefit from these preparations, they are more expensive, and some may contain additional, unneeded calories. New foods should be added one at a time; thus parents should avoid cereal combinations when beginning a new grain.

Infant cereal (iron fortified) should be mixed with formula until whole milk is given. If the infant is being breastfed, the cereal should be mixed with expressed breast milk or water. The addition of solid foods to the exclusively breastfed infant's diet does not significantly increase overall caloric intake or weight gain (Dewey, 2001). After 6 months of age, small amounts of fruit juices can be mixed with the dry cereal; the vitamin C content of the juice enhances the absorption of iron in the cereal. Because of their benefit as a source of iron, infant cereals should be continued until the child is 18 months of age.

When infants are 6 months of age or older, fruit juice can be offered from a cup for its rich source of vitamin C, although it should not be offered as a milk replacement. Large quantities of certain juices (e.g., apple, pear, prune, sweet cherry, peach, grape) should be avoided because they may cause abdominal pain, diarrhea, or bloating in some children. White grape juice is better absorbed and safe for infants this age (less than 180 mL/day) without causing gastrointestinal distress. Fruit-flavoured drinks, which may be marketed as juices but contain high concentrations of complex sugars, should be avoided. The Canadian Paediatric Society (2006) recommends that fruit juice intake not exceed 120 to 180 mL per day and that juices not be given to infants less than 6 months old; only 100% fruit juice should be given. Because vitamin C is naturally destroyed by heat, juice should not be not warmed. Juice containers should always be kept covered and refrigerated to prevent further vitamin loss. Fruit juice should be offered from a cup, not a bottle, to prevent the development of nursing **caries** (see Chapter 37, Low-Cariogenic Diet).

Following is a recommended sequence for introducing foods (CPS, 2006; Health Canada, 2012):

- **Grain products**—At 6 to 9 months, offer up to 30 to 60 mL of iron-fortified infant cereal, twice a day. Then try other grain products such as small pieces of dry toast or unsalted crackers. At 9 to 12 months, offer other plain cereals, whole grain bread, rice, and pasta.
- **Vegetables**—At 6 to 9 months, offer puréed cooked vegetables—yellow, green, or orange. At 9 to 12 months, progress to soft, mashed cooked vegetables.
- **Fruits**—At 6 to 9 months, offer puréed cooked fruits, very ripe mashed fruits (such as bananas). At 9 to 12 months, try soft fresh fruits, peeled, seeded, and diced or canned fruit, packed in water or juice (not syrup). Avoid whole grapes as they are a choking hazard.
- **Meat and alternatives**—At 6 to 9 months, offer puréed cooked meat, fish, chicken, tofu, mashed beans, and egg yolk. At 9 to 12 months, mince or dice these foods.
- **Milk and milk products**—At 9 months, offer dairy foods like yogourt (3.25% or higher), cottage cheese, or grated hard cheese. Wait until the infant is 9 to 12 months old before introducing whole cow's milk (3.25%). After 12 months of age, the infant should not take more than 720 mL of milk products per day. Too much milk can lead to iron deficiency anemia.

Commercially prepared baby foods are the most commonly used types of food served to infants in Canada. They are convenient and usually contain no added salt or sugar, but they are relatively expensive. An alternative is to prepare baby foods at home, which is a simple and inexpensive process. Fruits and vegetables can be steamed in a small amount of water and puréed in a blender or food processor. Many of them, such as ripe banana, can be mashed fine with a fork. Fruits such as apples or pears require little or no water in the cooking process. Vegetables such as carrots, potatoes, or string beans require additional water in the cooking and blending process.

Preferably, infant foods prepared at home should start with fresh or frozen foods, since canned foods, other than those prepared for infants, may contain excessive sodium or sugar or be a source of lead from the container. If sweetening is needed, refined sugar can be used, but honey and corn syrup should be avoided because of the risk of infant botulism. There is no evidence that the addition of salt to foods such as vegetables increases the infant's acceptance of the new food. Additional guidelines for the home preparation of baby foods are provided by Morin (2005).

Parents should be cautioned to avoid reliance on foods and supplements marketed as iron- or vitamin-fortified as primary sources of minerals. Instead, they should be encouraged to offer the child a variety of fruits, vegetables, whole grains, and those known to naturally be rich in iron.

Infants and toddlers should not be given low-calorie foods unless a strict, medically prescribed diet is required. The infant's growth during this phase is crucial to future development, and curtailing dietary fat should be done with great caution. Many parents may be concerned that their child is getting too much dietary fat; in such cases, the primary practitioner should be consulted before dietary substitutions are made. On the other hand, making an infant or toddler finish a bottle or "clean up the plate" may lead to unhealthy eating habits (see Chapter 40, Obesity).

Introduction of Solid Foods

When the spoon is first introduced, infants often push it away and appear dissatisfied. Patience and skill are required to overcome this initial response. As infants become accustomed to the spoon, they more eagerly accept the food and eventually will open the mouth in anticipation (or keep it closed in dislike). Because the first introduction of food is a new experience, spoon feeding should be attempted after ingestion of some breast milk or formula to associate this activity with a pleasurable and satisfying experience. After several spoon feedings, food can be introduced at the beginning of a meal. It is best to introduce many foods, one at a time, during the first year, when the infant is more likely to eat them; the infant will have a hearty appetite because of a rapid growth rate. During the toddler years, eating becomes less of an adventure, and strong food preferences become evident.

Because feeding is a learning process, as well as a means of nutrition, new foods should be given alone, not mixed with others, to allow the child to learn new tastes and textures. Food should not be mixed in the bottle and fed through a nipple with a large hole; this deprives the child of the pleasure of learning new tastes and of developing a discriminating palate. It can also cause problems with poor chewing of food later in life because of lack of experience. Guidelines for the introduction of new foods are given in the Patient Teaching box.

The infant's first, second, and often twentieth try at self-feeding or cup feeding is a sloppy experience. Finger foods such as soft fruits or vegetables are just as good as playthings as they are food. However, all of this is part of learning, and mastery follows many accidents.

Parents need to be encouraged to interpret their infant's signals of discomfort and intervene in ways other than through feeding. Crying, fussiness, and sucking do not necessarily indicate hunger. Rocking, stroking, holding, and offering a toy or a pacifier may be more appropriate than automatically responding with food.

PATIENT TEACHING Introducing Solid Foods to Infants

- Introduce solid foods when the infant is hungry.
- Begin spoon feeding by pushing food to the back of the tongue because of the infant's natural tendency to thrust the tongue forward.
- Use a small spoon with a straight handle; begin with 5 or 10 mL of food; gradually increase to a couple of tablespoons per feeding.
- Introduce one food at a time, usually at intervals of 4 to 7 days, to allow for identification of food allergies.
- Feed new foods in small amounts, from 5 to 30 mL. As the amount of solid food increases, the quantity of milk is decreased to less than 1 L daily to prevent overfeeding.
- Do not introduce foods by mixing them with formula in the bottle.

Weaning

Defined as the process of giving up one method of feeding for another, *weaning* usually refers to relinquishing the breast or bottle for a cup (see Chapter 26). In Western societies this is generally regarded as a major task for infants and is often seen as a potentially traumatic experience. It is psychologically significant because the infant is required to give up a major source of oral pleasure and gratification.

While there is no one time for weaning that is best for every child, most infants show signs of readiness during the second half of the first year. They have learned that good things come from a spoon. Their increasing desire for freedom of movement may lessen their desire to be held close for feedings. They are acquiring more control over their actions and can easily manipulate a cup to their lips. Imitation becomes a powerful motivator by age 8 or 9 months, and they enjoy using a cup or glass like others do (Lawrence & Lawrence, 2011).

Weaning should be individualized and gradual, replacing one bottle-feeding or breastfeeding at a time. The nighttime feeding is usually the last feeding to be discontinued. A child should not be allowed to take a bottle of milk to bed, as this is a major cause of caries. If breastfeeding is terminated before 5 or 6 months of age, weaning should be to a bottle to provide for the sucking needs. If breastfeeding is discontinued later, weaning can be directly to a cup, especially by age 12 to 14 months.

Sleep and Activity

Sleep patterns vary among infants, with active infants typically sleeping less than placid children. Infants in the age group newborn to 6 months sleep approximately 16 hours per day, 3 to 4 hours at a time, with about three naps a day. Infants aged 6 months to 1 year sleep approximately 14 hours per day and gradually will require only two naps (CPS, 2007). Breastfed infants usually sleep for less prolonged periods, with more frequent waking, especially during the night, than do bottle-fed infants.

Most infants are naturally active and need no encouragement to be mobile. If devices such as playpens, strollers, commercial swings, and walkers are used excessively, they can restrict movement and prevent infants from exploring and developing gross motor skills. Walkers do not enhance coordination and are dangerous if tipped over or placed near stairs. Health Canada (2005) has recommended a ban on the sale of infant walkers because of the large number of associated injuries. Newer models of infant walkers have been designed without wheels to decrease infant injuries (see Falls, p. 997).

evolve Skill—Fostering Healthy Sleep Patterns in Children

Sleep Problems

A number of sleep problems have been identified in small children. One of the two major categories is *dyssomnia*: the child has trouble either falling or staying asleep at night, or has difficulty staying awake during the day. The second category, *parasomnias*, are characterized as confusional arousals, sleep-walking, sleep terrors, nightmares, and rhythmic movement disorders; these typically occur in children 3 to 8 years old (Dahl, 1998) and decline in incidence as the child matures

(Davis, Parker, & Montgomery, 2004). The discussion here focuses on minor sleep issues in infants, such as refusal to go to sleep or frequent waking during the night (Table 36-4). Other sleep disturbances include obstructive sleep apnea (see Chapter 46) and sleep terrors (see Chapters 37 and 38).

Concerns regarding sleep are common during infancy. Sometimes these concerns are as basic as parents' questioning whether the infant needs additional sleep. In this case, it is best to investigate the reason for their concern, stressing each child's individual needs. Infants who are active during wakeful periods and growing normally are sleeping a sufficient amount of time.

Sleep problems in early infancy have also been positively correlated with higher maternal depression scores (Hawkins-Walsh, 2003; Hiscock & Wake, 2001) and poorer general and mental health in both mothers and fathers (Martin et al., 2007). Therefore, nurses must discuss infant sleep problems with the mother (and family) in addition to other developmental aspects of newborn care.

When a sleeping problem exists, a careful assessment is essential. Charting sleep habits both before and after interventions is also an important strategy. Questions regarding the frequency and duration of waking, the usual bedtime routine, the number of nighttime feedings, the perceived problem (e.g., how much disruption the behaviour generates), and the attempted interventions are important in planning effective approaches designed for the specific sleep problem. A common suggestion given for any type of sleep problem—"Let the child cry until he or she falls asleep"—is very difficult to implement and is inappropriate for certain conditions. Once the parents relent and console the child, they have only reinforced the crying.

An equally effective and more atraumatic approach to night crying, known as *graduated extinction*, is to let the child cry for progressively longer times between brief parental interventions that consist only of reassurance—not rocking, holding, or using a bottle or pacifier. For example, the parents may check on the child every 5 minutes during the first night

Table 36-4 Selected Sleep Disturbances During Infancy and Early Childhood

DISORDER/DESCRIPTION	MANAGEMENT
Nighttime Feeding	
Child has a prolonged need for middle-of-night breastfeeding or bottle-feeding. Child goes to sleep at breast or with a bottle. Awakenings are frequent (may be hourly). Child returns to sleep after feeding; other comfort measures (e.g., rocking or holding) are usually ineffective.	Increase daytime feeding intervals to 4 hr or more (may need to be done gradually). Offer last feeding as late as possible at night; may need to gradually reduce amount of formula or length of breastfeeding. Offer no bottles in bed. Put child to bed *awake*. When child is crying, check at progressively longer intervals each night; reassure child but do not hold, rock, take to parent's bed, or give bottle or pacifier.
Developmental Night Crying	
Child age 6–12 mo with undisturbed nighttime sleep now wakens abruptly; may be accompanied by nightmares.	Parents should be reassured that this phase is temporary. Enter room immediately to check on child but keep reassurances *brief*. Avoid feeding, rocking, taking to child parent's bed, or any other routine that may initiate trained night crying.
Trained Night Crying (Inappropriate Sleep Associations)	
Child typically falls asleep in place other than own bed (e.g., rocking chair or parent's bed) and is taken to own bed while asleep; on awakening, cries until usual routine is instituted (e.g., rocking).	Put child in own bed when awake. If possible, arrange sleeping area separate from other family members. When child is crying, check at progressively longer intervals each night; reassure child but do not resume usual routine.
Refusal to Go to Sleep	
Child resists bedtime and comes out of room repeatedly. Nighttime sleep may be continuous, but frequent awakenings and refusal to return to sleep may occur and become a problem if parent allows child to deviate from usual sleep pattern.	Evaluate whether hour of sleep is too early (child may resist sleep if not tired). Parents should be assisted in establishing consistent before-bedtime routine and enforcing consistent limits regarding child's bedtime behaviour. If child persists in leaving bedroom, close door for progressively longer periods. Use reward system with child to provide motivation.
Nighttime Fears	
Child resists going to bed or wakens during the night because of fears. Child seeks parent's physical presence and falls asleep easily with parent nearby, unless fear is overwhelming.	Evaluate whether hour of sleep is too early (child may fantasize when there is nothing to do but think in dark room). Calmly reassure the frightened child; keeping a night light on may help. Use reward system with child to provide motivation to deal with fears. Avoid patterns that can lead to additional problems (e.g., sleeping with child or taking child to parent's room). If child's fear is overwhelming, consider desensitization (e.g., progressively spending longer periods of time alone; consult professional help for protracted fears). Distinguish between nightmares and sleep terrors (confused partial arousals).

(Modified from Ferber, R. [1987]. Behavioural "insomnia" in the child. *Psychiatric Clinics of North America, 10*[4], 641–653.)

and progressively extend this interval by 5 minutes on successive nights.

Families who cannot tolerate unexpected crying spells while everyone else is asleep can try the two-step approach. Graduated extinction is used during naps and at bedtime until the parents go to bed. If the child cries during the night, the parents use comforting measures. However, once the child is partially trained, step 2 is initiated—the use of graduated extinction at all times.

Children who learn to fall asleep on their own at bedtime have longer sustained sleep periods than those who fall asleep with a parent present (Davis et al., 2004). In addition, comforting children outside their own bed at night once they awaken has been associated with poor sleep consolidation. For example, feeding 5-month-old children after awakening at night resulted in fewer consecutive sleep hours (Touchette et al., 2005). The authors of this study recommend parental presence at bedtime until the child is drowsy, then placing the child in his or her own bed for a night's sleep.

The best way to prevent sleep problems is to encourage parents to establish bedtime rituals that do not foster problematic patterns. One of the most constructive habits parents can form is to place the infant awake in his or her own crib. When infants are accustomed to falling asleep somewhere else, such as in their parent's arms, and then being transferred to their crib, they awaken in unfamiliar surroundings and are unable to fall asleep until the routine is repeated. In addition, the bed should be used for sleeping only—not as a playpen. It is advisable to not hang playthings over or on the bed; in this way the child associates the bed with sleep, not with activity. Although the interventions described previously and in Table 36-4 are usually successful, it is much easier to prevent the problem with appropriate counselling during the early months of the infant's life.

Dental Health

Good dental hygiene begins with appropriate maternal dental health and with counselling during early infancy regarding dietary intake for the promotion of optimal oral hygiene (Douglass, Douglass, & Silk, 2004). Parents also need to be counselled on the risk of feeding practices that increase the risk of poor dental health. Some of these, discussed previously, include not propping the milk bottle or giving the milk bottle in the bed, and not giving fruit juices in a bottle, especially before 6 months of age.

Cleaning can commence right after birth: parents should be taught to clean the infant's gums with a piece of gauze or cloth so that children become accustomed to cleaning of the mouth. Once the primary teeth erupt, the teeth and gums are initially cleaned by wiping with a damp cloth; toothbrushing is too harsh for the tender gingiva. The caregiver can stabilize the infant by cradling the child with one arm and using the free hand to cleanse the teeth. Oral hygiene can be made pleasant by singing or talking to the infant.

The Canadian Dental Association (2010) recommends that all children have their first visit to a dentist in their first year of life. It is generally recommended that a small, soft-bristled toothbrush be used as more teeth erupt and the infant adjusts to the routine of cleaning. Water is preferred to toothpaste, which the infant will swallow (and if the toothpaste is fluoridated, the infant will ingest excessive amounts of fluoride).

Fluoride, an essential mineral for building caries-resistant teeth, needs to be supplemented beginning at 6 months of age if the infant does not already receive water with adequate fluoride content. The Canadian Dental Association (2010) recommends that parents discuss their infant's fluoride needs with a dentist. Many communities fluoridate public drinking water. Thus if bottled water is used to reconstitute powdered or concentrated formula, it should either be fluoride free or contain low levels of fluoride (American Dental Association, 2007).

Dietary considerations are also important to dental health because habits begun during infancy tend to continue into later years. Foods with added concentrated sugar should be used sparingly (if at all) in the infant's diet. The practice of coating pacifiers with honey or using commercially available hard-candy pacifiers is discouraged. Besides being cariogenic, honey also may cause infant botulism, and parts of the candy pacifier can be aspirated (see Aspiration of Foreign Objects, p. 993). Parents need to be counselled regarding the detrimental effects of frequent and prolonged bottle-feeding or breastfeeding during sleep, when the sweet milk or other fluid, such as juice, bathes the teeth, producing caries. In addition, carbonated beverages should be avoided in infancy. (See Chapter 37 for a more extensive discussion of dental care, including nursing caries.)

Immunizations

Perhaps one of the most dramatic advances in pediatrics has been the decline of infectious diseases during the twentieth century because of the widespread use of immunization for preventable diseases. In recent years, however, childhood vaccines have been widely criticized, and fear related to vaccine components has prompted some families to avoid childhood vaccines. In addition, many of the diseases for which children are vaccinated are rarely seen on a large-scale basis, leading some parents to believe that such vaccines are no longer necessary in the twenty-first century. A variety of information is available suggesting that parents avoid childhood vaccines altogether; a number of "vaccine myths" exist, which are based on erroneous information. Several URL links to objective and scientifically accurate information regarding childhood vaccination are provided in the Resources section on the Evolve site for this text. It is the nurse's responsibility to provide parents with accurate information about childhood illnesses and available vaccines; the parents must then make an informed decision about the child's vaccinations. Nurses should address parents' concerns about childhood vaccines and avoid judgemental attitudes regarding the parents' decision to not vaccinate their children.

Although many of the immunizations can be given to individuals of any age, the recommended primary schedule begins during infancy and, with the exception of boosters, is completed during early childhood. Therefore, the discussion of childhood immunizations for diphtheria, tetanus, pertussis (DTaP); polio; measles, mumps, rubella (MMR); *Haemophilus influenzae* type b (Hib); hepatitis A virus (HAV), hepatitis B virus (HBV); pneumococcus; influenza; meningococcus; and chickenpox is included under health promotion during infancy. Selected vaccines generally reserved for children considered at high risk for the respective disease are also discussed here and as appropriate throughout the text. (See also Chapter 38, Communicable Diseases, for a discussion of several of the diseases for which vaccines are available.)

Schedule for Immunizations

In Canada, recommendations for immunization are from the National Advisory Committee on Immunization, under the authority of the Minister of Health and Public Health Agency of Canada. The policies of each committee are recommendations, not rules, and they change as a result of advances in the field of immunology. Most countries have different immunization recommendations. Thus, with the increasing number of children in Canada who come from other countries, it is important that nurses obtain all immunization information from the family.

Nurses need to keep informed of the latest advances and changes in immunization policies and guidelines (PHAC, 2011a). Please see Figure 34-6 for the 2006 Canadian immunization schedule (in revision as of this writing).

Children who began primary immunization at the recommended age but then failed to receive all of the doses do not need to begin the series again but instead should receive only the missed doses. When there is doubt that the child will return for immunization according to the optimum schedule, any of the recommended vaccines can be administered simultaneously. Parenteral vaccines are given in separate syringes in different injection sites.

Recommendations for Routine Immunizations

Because of constant changes in the pharmaceutical industry, trade names of some single and combination vaccines in this section may differ from those currently available. The reader is encouraged to access the Canadian Immunization Guide, which is updated periodically, at http://www.phac-aspc.gc.ca/publicat/cig-gci/pdf/avtables_revised0803-eng.pdf.

Hepatitis B Virus (HBV)

HBV is a significant pediatric disease because HBV infections that occur during childhood and adolescence can lead to fatal consequences from cirrhosis or liver cancer during adulthood. Up to 90% of infants infected perinatally and 25 to 50% of children infected before age 5 years become HBV carriers. In addition, the incidence of HBV infection increases rapidly during adolescence (AAP, Committee on Infectious Diseases & Pickering 2009).

It is recommended that newborns receive the hepatitis B vaccine (HepB) within 12 hours of birth if the mother is infected with hepatitis B, because of the high risk of long-term complications if infection occurs (see Chapter 25, Medication Guide: Hepatitis B Vaccine, p. 661) (PHAC, 2006). Both full-term and preterm infants born to mothers whose HBsAg status is positive should also receive hepatitis B immune globulin (HBIG), 0.5 mL (see Chapter 25, Medication Guide: Hepatitis B Immune Globulin). The HepB vaccine and the HBIG should be given at two different injection sites. Parental consent must be obtained prior to administering the medication. If the mother's status is unknown, testing should be done at the time of delivery. If maternal HBV status is not available within 12 hours of delivery, serious consideration should be given to administering HepB vaccine and HBIG while the results are pending, taking into account the mother's risk factors and erring on the side of providing vaccine and HBIG if there is any suspicion that the mother could be infected (PHAC, 2006). Because the immune response to HepB is not optimum in newborns weighing less than 2000 g, the first HepB dose should be given to such infants at 1 month, as long as the mother's HBsAg status is negative (PHAC, 2006). In the event that the preterm infant is given a dose at birth, the current recommendation is that the infant be given the full series (three additional doses) at 1, 2, and 6 months of age. In the late 1990s, HepB contained small amounts of mercury (thimerosal) as a preservative, which generated concern regarding possible mercury poisoning in infants and led to a subsequent decrease in HepB immunization rates in newborns. To date, studies have not found any association between thimerosal in vaccines and neurological **developmental disorders** such as autism spectrum disorder (de Los Reyes, 2010; Mrozek-Budzn, Kieltyka, & Majewska, 2010). The Public Health Agency of Canada (2011a) encourages immunization of all children before or in early adolescence. Since the early 1990s, all provinces and territories have had either a universal school-based hepatitis B vaccination program aimed at children aged 9 to 13 or an infant vaccination program (PHAC, 2006).

The vaccine is given intramuscularly in the vastus lateralis in newborns (see Fig. 25-11) or in the deltoid for older infants and children. Regardless of age, the dorsogluteal site should never be used for intramuscular injections, because it has been associated with low antibody **seroconversion** rates, indicating a reduced immune response (Zuckerman, Cockcroft, & Zuckerman, 1992). No data exist regarding the seroconversion when the ventrogluteal site is used. The vaccine can be safely administered simultaneously at a separate site with DTaP, MMR, and Hib vaccines.

Hepatitis A Virus (HAV)

HAV has been recognized as a significant child health problem, particularly in communities where widespread childhood HepA immunization has not been historically recommended. HAV is spread by the fecal–oral route and from person-to-person contact, by ingestion of contaminated food or water, and rarely by blood transfusion. The illness has an abrupt onset, with fever, malaise, anorexia, nausea, abdominal discomfort, dark urine, and jaundice being the most common clinical signs of infection. In children under 6 years of age the disease may be asymptomatic, and jaundice is rarely evident.

In Canada, universal HepA vaccination is not recommended. Individuals at risk, such as those travelling to countries where hepatitis A is endemic, should be immunized (PHAC, 2006). If HepA vaccine is given, it is given in a two dose series with the second dose administered no sooner than 6 months after the first dose.

Diphtheria

Although cases of diphtheria are rarely seen in Canada, the disease can result in significant morbidity. Respiratory manifestations include respiratory nasopharyngitis or obstructive laryngotracheitis with upper airway obstruction. The cutaneous manifestations of the disease include vaginal, otic, conjunctival, or cutaneous lesions, which are primarily seen in the tropics (PHAC, 2006). Diphtheria vaccine is commonly administered (1) in combination with tetanus and acellular pertussis vaccines (DTaP) or DTaP and Hib vaccines for children younger than 7 years of age, (2) in combination with a conjugate Hib vaccine (see Fig. 34-6), (3) in a combined vaccine with tetanus (DT) for children younger than 7 years of age who have some contraindication to receiving pertussis vaccine, or (4) as a single antigen when combined antigen preparations are not indicated. Although the diphtheria vaccine does not produce absolute immunity, protective antitoxin persists for 10 years or more when given according to the recommended schedule, and boosters are given every 10 years for life (see discussion below for adolescent diphtheria and acellular pertussis and tetanus toxoid recommendation). Several vaccines contain diphtheria toxoid (Hib, meningococcal, pneumococcal), but this does not confer immunity to the disease.

Tetanus

Two forms of tetanus vaccine—tetanus toxoid and tetanus immune globulin (TIG) (human)—are available. Tetanus toxoid is used for routine primary immunization, usually in one of the combinations listed for diphtheria, and provides protective antitoxin levels for approximately 10 years.

Tetanus and diphtheria toxoids as well as acellular pertussis vaccine (Tdap–adolescent formulation) are now recommended for children 11 to 12 years of age who have completed the recommended DTaP/DTP vaccine series yet have not received the tetanus (Td) booster dose. Adolescents who are 13 to 18 years of age and have not received the Td/Tdap booster should receive a single Tdap booster, provided the routine DTaP/DTP childhood immunization series has been previously received (see Fig. 34-6). Boostrix (Tdap) is currently licensed for children 10 to 18 years of age, whereas Adacel (Tdap) is licensed for individuals 11 to 64 years of age.

For wound management, **passive immunity** is available with TIG. This is recommended for children who have immune deficiency, in addition to the vaccine. In persons with a history of two previous doses of tetanus toxoid, a booster dose of the toxoid can be given. Separate syringes and different sites are used when tetanus toxoid and TIG are given concurrently. For children over age 7 years who require wound prophylaxis, tetanus immunization may be accomplished by administering Td (adult-type diphtheria and tetanus toxoids).

Pertussis

Pertussis vaccine is recommended for all children 6 weeks through 6 years of age (up to the seventh birthday) who have no neurological contraindications to its use. Concerns over outbreaks of the disease in the past decade have prompted discussion about vaccinating infants and adults; many cases of pertussis have been seen in children less than 6 months or persons over 7 years of age, both groups falling in the category for which there was inadequate vaccine protection from pertussis infection (PHAC, 2006). The tetanus and diphtheria toxoids and acellular pertussis vaccine (Tdap) is now recommended at ages 11 to 12 years for children who have completed the DTaP/DTP childhood series; the Tdap is also recommended for adolescents 13 to 18 years old who have not received a tetanus booster (Td) or Tdap dose and have completed the childhood DTaP/DTP series. When the Tdap is used as a booster dose, it may be administered 5 years from the last Td dose or earlier if pertussis immunity is necessary (PHAC, 2006).

Only acellular vaccines made from purified antigens of *B. pertussis* are now available in Canada; whole-cell preparations are no longer in use. Acellular vaccines have decreased the frequency and severity of both local and systemic adverse reactions compared with those from whole-cell pertussis vaccines. In Canada, there is no monovalent acellular pertussis vaccine. Pertussis vaccine is only available in combined form with other agents such as diphtheria (D) and tetanus (T) toxoids with or without inactivated polio vaccine (IPV) and/or Hib conjugate vaccine (Hib).

The acellular pertussis vaccine contains one or more immunogens derived from the *B. pertussis* organism. Health care workers who may be susceptible to pertussis as a result of waning immunity and who have potential exposure to children or adults with pertussis should take the necessary protective precautions against droplet contamination (wear procedural or surgical masks and practise hand hygiene). The diagnosis of pertussis may be missed or delayed in unvaccinated infants, who often are seen with respiratory distress and apnea without the typical cough. Additional guidelines for prevention and treatment of pertussis among health care workers and close contacts are found in the Canadian Immunization Guide (PHAC, 2006) and the *2009 Red Book: Report of the Committee on Infectious Diseases* (AAP, Committee on Infectious Diseases & Pickering, 2009).

Polio

An all-inactivated polio virus (IPV) schedule for routine childhood polio vaccination is now recommended; oral poliovirus (OPV) is no longer used in Canada. For routine immunization beginning in infancy, four doses of IPV are recommended, in combination with other routinely administered vaccines (DTaP and Hib) at 2 months, 4 months, 18 months, and 4 to 6 years of age (preschool booster). The fourth dose is not needed if the third dose is given on or after the fourth birthday. It is acceptable to give an additional dose of IPV at 6 months of age for convenience of administration in combination with DTaP and Hib (PHAC, 2006).

Poliomyelitis is a disease that may cause irreversible paralysis in less than 1% of infected individuals. It is a highly infectious disease that is spread from person to person, principally through the fecal-oral route (PHAC, 2006). Canada was certified polio-free in 1994. The last major Canadian epidemic of wild poliovirus occurred in 1959, with 1887 paralytic cases reported. Smaller clusters occurred after that time. In 1978–79, there were 11 paralytic cases among unimmunized individuals in religious groups in Ontario, Alberta, and British Columbia, who had had contact with imported cases. In 1993, 22 asymptomatic persons with imported wild polio infection were found in the same religious group in Alberta, and in 1996 an asymptomatic person was reported in Ontario. In none of these instances was spread of the virus seen outside the unimmunized groups, presumably because of high levels of immunization in the rest of the population, nor did cases of clinical illness occur in the affected communities in Canada.

The change from the exclusive use of OPV to the exclusive use of IPV is related to the rare risk of vaccine-associated polio paralysis (VAPP) from OPV. Vaccine programs in Canada switched from OPV to IPV in 1995/1996; the last VAPP case occurred in 1995 (PHAC, 2006).

Measles

For routine immunization of all children, two doses of measles vaccine should be given. Infants should receive a first dose combined with mumps and rubella vaccines (MMR) on or shortly after their first birthday; the second dose should be given after 15 months of age but before school entry. It is convenient to link this dose with other routinely scheduled immunizations. Options include giving it with the scheduled immunization at 15 or 18 months of age, with school entry immunization at 4 to 6 years, or at any intervening age that is practicable (such as entry to day care).

Two doses of vaccine given at least 4 weeks apart are recommended for children who

- Have missed MMR immunization on the routine schedule
- Are without an immunization record
- Are without reliable records of measles immunization (e.g., immigrants)
- Were given live measles vaccine and immune globulin (Ig) separated by an inappropriate interval (PHAC, 2006).

Vaccine may be recommended for children less than 12 months of age during outbreaks or international travel to an area where measles is common. MMR may be given as early as 6 months of age. Under these circumstances, or if vaccine was inappropriately given before the child's first birthday, two doses of MMR should still be given after the first birthday.

Individuals born before 1970 are thought to be immune from exposure to natural measles virus. Because of the continuing occurrence of measles in older children and young adults, potentially susceptible adolescents and young adults should be identified and immunized if two doses of measles vaccine have not been administered previously or the person had a confirmed case of the illness (PHAC, 2006).

Mumps

One dose of MMR vaccine should be administered for mumps protection, with the second dose given for measles protection. The first dose should be given on or after the first birthday and the second dose given at least 1 month after the first dose and before school entry. The standard dose is 0.5 mL.

In Canada, the number of reported mumps cases has decreased from approximately 34,000 cases in the 1950s to less than 400 cases yearly in the 1990s (Canada Communicable Disease Report, 2010). Large Canadian outbreaks have been rare in recent years, but three localized outbreaks did occur between 2001 and 2005. The first outbreak, of 193 cases, occurred between September 2001 and March 2002 and involved an undervaccinated community in northern Alberta following importation of the disease from Bolivia (Canada Communicable Disease Report, 2010). Most members of the community were philosophically opposed to vaccination. Immunization rates in the affected community were greatly below the provincial average. The majority of cases (80%) were in unimmunized individuals, spreading through area schools and, to a lesser extent, the surrounding community. Two small outbreaks involving 13 and 19 patients occurred in Nova Scotia in the spring and fall of 2005, respectively. The patients ranged in age from 13 to 19 years (average age 14) in the spring outbreak and 20 to 27 years in a university community (average age 23 years) in the fall outbreak. Four of the 13 cases in the first Nova Scotia outbreak and all of the cases in the second outbreak reported receiving only one dose of MMR. The latter outbreak resulted in three secondary cases in other provinces (Canada Communicable Disease Report, 2010). In 2007, 1284 confirmed cases of mumps were reported from 10 out of 13 Canadian provinces and territories (PHAC, 2009).

Rubella

Rubella is a relatively mild infection in children. The main goal of immunization is the prevention of rubella infection in pregnancy, which may give rise to congenital rubella syndrome (CRS). This syndrome can result in miscarriage, stillbirth, and fetal malformations, including congenital heart disease, cataracts, deafness, and mental disabilities. Fetal infection can occur at any stage of pregnancy, but the risk of fetal damage following maternal infection is particularly high in the earliest months after conception (85% in the first trimester). One dose of rubella-containing vaccine (MMR) is recommended routinely for all children on or as soon as practical after their first birthday. The second dose, given for measles protection, should be given after 15 months of age and before school entry. The acceptable minimum interval between the first and second dose is at least 1 month. All unimmunized prepubertal children, susceptible adolescents, and adult women in the childbearing age group should be vaccinated, particularly those who have emigrated from countries that do not routinely vaccinate for rubella. Because the live attenuated virus may cross the placenta and theoretically present a risk to the developing fetus, rubella vaccine is not given to any pregnant woman (PHAC, 2006).

Pneumococcus

A pneumococcal conjugate vaccine (Prevnar®) is approved for use in Canada for children from 6 weeks to 9 years of age and is composed of the purified polysaccharides of the capsular antigens of seven *Streptococcus pneumoniae* serotypes, individually conjugated to CRM197 (cross-reacting material 197), a purified nontoxic variant of diphtheria **toxin** (PHAC, 2006). Streptococcal pneumococci are responsible for a number of bacterial infections in children under 2 years of age, which may cause serious morbidity and mortality. Among these are generalized infections such as septicemia and meningitis or localized infections such as otitis media, sinusitis, and pneumonia. These illnesses are particularly problematic in children who attend day care facilities (the incidence among children in day care centres is two to three times higher than in children not attending out-of-home day care) and in those who are immunocompromised.

The recommended optimal schedule for infants is four doses of the conjugate vaccine administered at 2, 4, 6, and 12 to 15 months of age. Infants of very low birth weight (<1500 grams) should be given their first dose according to their chronological age and not their calculated gestational age. Children 7 to 11 months old who have not been previously immunized against invasive pneumococcal disease (IPD) should receive two doses at least 4 weeks apart, followed by a third dose after 12 months of age and at least 2 months after the second dose. Children 12 to 23 months of age not previously immunized should receive two doses at least 2 months apart. For children 2 to 5 years old, one dose is sufficient for healthy children, but two doses given 2 months apart is recommended for children with chronic conditions that place them at higher risk of IPD (PHAC, 2006). The long-term efficacy of the conjugate pneumococcal vaccines is not known, but immunological memory has been demonstrated 18 months after two to three doses in infancy and up to 20 months after one dose in children 2 to 3 years of age.

Conjugate pneumococcal vaccine is recommended for routine administration to all children 23 months of age or younger. It is also recommended for children 24 to 59 months of age at higher risk of IPD: those who attend child care centres; Aboriginal children; those who have sickle cell disease and other sickle cell hemoglobinopathies or who have other types of functional or anatomical asplenia, HIV infection, immunocompromising conditions (e.g., primary immunodeficiencies; malignancies; conditions resulting from immunosuppressive therapy, solid organ transplantation, or the use of long-term systemic corticosteroids; nephrotic syndrome), or chronic medical conditions (e.g., chronic cardiac and pulmonary disease such as bronchopulmonary dysplasia, diabetes mellitus, chronic renal disease, or cerebrospinal fluid leak); and children with cochlear implants or those receiving cochlear implants (PHAC, 2006).

The polysaccharide vaccine (PPV) is not recommended for children <2 years of age, as it is relatively ineffective and the conjugate vaccine is superior. Children aged 2 years to <5 years of age who are at increased risk of IPD should receive the conjugate vaccine with the polysaccharide vaccine being used as a booster dose in this age group to increase the serotype coverage.

The polysaccharide vaccine should be given to all individuals older than 5 years of age who have not received the vaccine previously and who are at higher risk of IPD (PHAC, 2006).

Haemophilus influenzae Type B (Hib)

Hib conjugate vaccines protect against a number of serious infections caused by Hib, especially bacterial meningitis, **epiglottitis**, bacterial pneumonia, septic arthritis, and sepsis (Hib is not associated with the viruses that cause influenza, or "flu"). Hib vaccines that are currently available in Canada include PedvaxHIB, Pentacel, and ActHIB. These conjugate vaccines connect Hib to a nontoxic form of another organism, such as meningococcal protein or diphtheria protein. While there is no **antibody** response to these nontoxic proteins, they significantly improve the antibody response to Hib, especially in infants. The use of combination vaccines provides equivalent immunogenicity and decreases the number of injections an infant receives; however, it is important that they be given to the appropriate-age child.

All Canadian provinces and territories include Hib conjugate vaccine in their immunization program for children. Hib polysaccharide–protein conjugate vaccines are the second generation of vaccines against Hib disease, having replaced an earlier polysaccharide product. Polysaccharide–protein conjugate antigens have the advantage of producing greater immune response in infants and young children than that with purified polysaccharide vaccine. The latter stimulates only B cells, whereas the former activates macrophages, T-helper cells, and B cells, resulting in greatly enhanced antibody responses and establishment of immunological memory (PHAC, 2006).

The 2009 Centers for Disease Control and Prevention immunization guidelines indicate limited data for administering the Hib vaccine to persons 5 years and older. However, children with sickle cell disease, leukemia, or HIV infection or children who have had a splenectomy may benefit from one dose of the Hib vaccine (PHAC, 2006).

When possible, the Hib conjugate vaccine used at the first vaccination should be used for all subsequent vaccinations in the primary series. All Hib vaccines are administered by intramuscular injection using a separate syringe and at a site separate from any concurrent vaccinations.

Varicella

Unlike the United States, Canada does not have as a goal the elimination of varicella, and the National Advisory Committee on Immunization (NACI) continues to recommend a single-dose vaccine strategy for children (two doses for adults and adolescents at least 13 years of age). Administration of the cell-free live-attenuated varicella vaccine (Varivax) is recommended for any susceptible child (one who lacks proof of varicella vaccination or has a reliable history of varicella infection). A single dose of varicella vaccine is recommended for children ages 12 to 15 months. The NACI does not recommend booster doses (PHAC, 2006). A single dose of 0.5 mL should be given by subcutaneous injection. Children 13 years of age or older who are susceptible should receive two doses administered at least 4 weeks apart. The vaccine should be kept frozen in the lyophilic form (stable particles that readily go into solution) and used within 30 minutes of being reconstituted to ensure viral potency.

Varicella vaccine may be administered simultaneously with MMR. However, separate syringes and injection sites should be used. If they are not administered simultaneously, the interval between administration of varicella vaccine and MMR should be at least 1 month. Varicella vaccine may also be given simultaneously with DTaP, IPV, HBV, or Hib (PHAC, 2006).

Influenza

Influenza vaccine may be administered to any healthy individual for whom contraindications are not present. To reduce the morbidity and mortality associated with influenza and the impact of illness in our communities, immunization programs should focus on those at high risk of influenza-related complications, those capable of transmitting influenza to individuals at high risk of complications, and those who provide essential community services. However, significant morbidity and societal costs are also associated with seasonal interpandemic influenza illness and its complications occurring in healthy children and adults. For this reason, healthy children and adults should be encouraged to receive the vaccine annually, particularly children 6 months to 18 years (PHAC, 2006). Children who have a reported anaphylactic hypersensitivity to eggs should not receive the vaccine.

The vaccine is administered in early fall before the flu season begins and is repeated yearly for ongoing protection. The intramuscular vaccine is administered as two separate doses 4 weeks apart in first-time recipients under the age of 9 years (PHAC, 2006). The dose is 0.25 mL for children ages 6 to 35 months and 0.5 mL for children 3 years and above. The vaccine may be given simultaneously with other vaccines but at a separate site. The vaccine is administered yearly because different strains of influenza are used each year in the manufacture of the vaccine.

Meningococcus

Invasive meningococcal disease (IMD) is endemic in Canada, showing periods of increased activity roughly every 10 to 15 years with no consistent pattern. The incidence rate varies considerably with different serogroups of *Neisseria meningitidis,* age groups, geographic locations, and time. Implementation of universal meningococcal C immunization programs will also affect disease epidemiology (PHAC, 2006).

Since 1985, the overall incidence of IMD has remained at or below 2 per 100,000 per year. Overall, the incidence rate has been highest among children less than 1 year of age and then declines as age increases, except for a smaller peak in the 15- to 19-year age group. An average of 298 cases of meningococcal disease have been reported annually. Disease occurs year round, but there is seasonal variation, with most cases occurring in the winter months (PHAC, 2006).

Meningococcal C conjugate vaccines are recommended for routine immunization of infants. The recommended schedule differs depending on the vaccine used. Three doses of either Meningitec™ or Menjugate™ are recommended to be given to infants beginning no earlier than 2 months of age and separated by at least 1 month. Two doses of NeisVac-C™ should be administered at least 2 months apart, with the first dose not to be administered before 2 months of age. At least one dose of the primary immunization series should be given after 5 months of age. Infants 4 to 11 months of age who have not previously received the vaccine should be immunized with two doses given at least 4 weeks apart. Infants born prematurely should receive the vaccine at the same **chronological age** as term infants. Polysaccharide vaccine is not recommended for routine infant immunization.

There have been recent concerns regarding reports of an association between quadrivalent meningococcal conjugate vaccine (Menactra) and cases of Guillain-Barré syndrome in vaccinated persons 11 to 19 years of age; onset of symptoms occurred within 2 to 23 days of vaccination. A preliminary survey by the Centers for Disease Control and Prevention (2006) indicates insufficient data to change the 2005 recommendation for adolescents, college freshmen residing in dormitories, and other high-risk populations.

Recommendations for Selected Immunizations

Two additional vaccines are recommended for children and adolescents at high risk for particular diseases: RotaTeq and Rotarix, two rotavirus vaccines, are available for distribution in Canada. Rotavirus is one of the leading causes of severe diarrhea in infants and young children. RotaTeq is licensed for administration to infants 6 to 12 weeks of age, with two additional doses administered at 4- to 10-week intervals but not after 32 weeks of age. The dose is 2 mL, and the product must be protected from light until administration. Rotarix (1 mL) may be administered beginning at 6 weeks of age with a second dose at least 4 weeks after the first dose but before 24 weeks of age. Both vaccines are administered orally. At the time of publication, neither vaccine was covered by provincial or territorial health care plans, thus parents will need to pay for it (CPS, Infectious Diseases and Immunization Committee, 2010).

A quadrivalent human papillomavirus (HPV) vaccine, Gardasil®, has been approved and is recommended for female children and adolescents to prevent HPV-related cervical cancer (see Chapter 6, p. 103). HPV is described as the most common sexually transmitted infection (STI). The overall prevalence of HPV infection in Canada ranges between 11 and 29%, with peak prevalence in adolescents and young adults (younger than 25 years of age). The highest rates of HPV acquisition occur in the first 5 years following the onset of sexual activity, with most cases being unrecognized and self-limited. The vaccine is administered intramuscularly in three separate doses; the first dose in the series may be given at 11 to 12 years of age (minimum age 9 years), the second dose is administered 2 months after the first, and the third dose is given 6 months after the first dose. The vaccine is covered by all provincial and territorial health plans (PHAC, 2011a).

Immunizations that may be used in older children and adolescents in the future and that are being evaluated include vaccines for preventing diseases such as herpes simplex virus, human cytomegalovirus, and Epstein-Barr virus.

Reactions

Vaccines used for routine immunizations are among the safest and most reliable medications available. However, minor adverse effects do occur after many of the immunizations, and, rarely, a serious reaction may result from the vaccine (PHAC, 2006, 2012a).

With inactivated antigens, such as DTaP, adverse effects are most likely to occur within a few hours or days of administration and are usually limited to local tenderness, **erythema**, and swelling at the injection site; low-grade fever; and behavioural changes (e.g., drowsiness, fretfulness, eating less, and prolonged or unusual cry). Local reactions tend to be less severe when the deltoid (except in small infants) rather than the vastus lateralis site is used and when a needle of sufficient length to deposit the vaccine in the muscle is used (see Atraumatic Care box). Rarely, more severe reactions may occur, especially with pertussis (Table 36-5). Reactions to DTaP tend to be more severe if they occurred with a previous immunization.

Hib vaccine is one of the safest vaccines available but may be associated with low-grade fever and mild local reactions at the site of injection, which resolve rapidly. Fever (temperature higher than 38.5°C) may rarely occur.

A number of inactive components are incorporated in vaccines to enhance their effectiveness and safety. Some of these components include preservatives, stabilizers, adjuvants, antibiotics, and purified culture medium proteins to enhance effectiveness. A child may react to the preservative in the vaccine rather than the vaccine component; an example of this is the HepB vaccine, which is prepared from yeast cultures. Yeast hypersensitivity would preclude one from receiving that particular vaccine (Schuval, 2003). Trace amounts of neomycin are used to decrease bacterial growth within certain vaccine preparations, and persons with documented anaphylactic reactions to neomycin should avoid those vaccines. Most vaccine preparations now contain vial stoppers with a synthetic rubber to prevent latex **allergy** reactions. In the event that an individual has a severe reaction to a vaccine and

Table 36-5 Contraindications and Precautions to Vaccinations*

TRUE CONTRAINDICATIONS	PRECAUTIONS†	NOT CONTRAINDICATIONS (VACCINES MAY BE ADMINISTERED)
General for All Vaccines (DTaP, IPV, MMR, Hib, HepB, Varicella, PCV, HepA, Influenza, Meningococcal)		
Anaphylactic reaction to vaccine is contraindication to further doses of that vaccine or to use of vaccines containing that substance. Moderate or severe illnesses with or without fever		Mild to moderate local reaction (soreness, redness, swelling) after a dose of injectable antigen Mild acute illness with or without low-grade fever Current antimicrobial therapy Convalescent phase of illnesses Prematurity (same dosage and indications as for normal, full-term infants) Recent exposure to infectious disease History of penicillin or other nonspecific allergies or family history of such allergies
Diphtheria, Tetanus, and Pertussis or Acellular Pertussis Vaccine (DTP or DTaP)		
Encephalopathy within 7 days of administration of previous dose of DTaP	Fever of ≥40.5°C within 48 hr after vaccination with prior dose of DTaP Collapse or shock-like state (hypotonic-hyporesponsive episode) within 48 hr of receiving prior dose of DTaP Seizures within 3 days of receiving prior dose of DTaP‡ Persistent, inconsolable crying lasting ≥3 hr within 48 hr of receiving prior dose of DTaP	Temperature of <40.5°C after previous dose of DTaP Family history of seizures‡ Family history of sudden infant death syndrome Family history of adverse event after DTaP administration
Diphtheria, Tetanus (DT, Td)		
Severe allergic reaction after a previous dose or to a vaccine component	GBS ≤6 wk after previous dose of tetanus toxoid–containing vaccine Moderate or severe acute illness with or without fever	Same as DTaP or DTP
Inactivated Poliovirus Vaccine (IPV)		
Anaphylactic reaction to neomycin or streptomycin	Pregnancy	Breastfeeding Diarrhea
Measles, Mumps, Rubella Vaccine (MMR)		
Pregnancy Known altered immunodeficiency (hematological and solid tumours, congenital immunodeficiency, long-term immunosuppressive therapy)	Recent immune globulin administration Immune globulin products and MMR should not be given simultaneously; if unavoidable, give at different sites and revaccinate or test for seroconversion in 3 mo; if immune globulin is given first, MMR should not be given for at least 3-6 mo, depending on dose; if MMR is given first, immune globulin should not be given for 2 wk. Thrombocytopenia or thrombocytopenic purpura	Tuberculosis or positive tuberculin skin test Simultaneous tuberculosis skin testing§ Breastfeeding Pregnancy of mother of recipient Immunodeficient family member or household contact Infection with HIV Nonanaphylactic reactions to eggs or neomycin Consider MMR for mildly symptomatic HIV-infected children (PHAC, 2006)
***Haemophilus influenzae* Type b Vaccine (Hib)**		
None identified		History of Hib disease
Hepatitis B Virus Vaccine (HepB)		
Anaphylactic reaction to common baker's yeast	Preterm birth	Pregnancy‖
Pneumococcal Vaccine (PCV)		
Severe allergic reaction after a previous dose or to a vaccine component	Moderate or severe acute illness with or without fever A child who has received pneumococcal polysaccharide vaccine (PPV) previously should wait at least 2 mo before receiving PCV.	Minor illnesses with or without fever Mild upper respiratory tract infection Allergic rhinitis

Continued

Table 36-5 Contraindications and Precautions to Vaccinations—cont'd

TRUE CONTRAINDICATIONS	PRECAUTIONS†	NOT CONTRAINDICATIONS (VACCINES MAY BE ADMINISTERED)
Varicella Vaccine		
Severe allergic reaction after a previous dose or to a vaccine component (e.g., neomycin or gelatin) Infection with HIV Known altered immunodeficiency (hematological and solid tumours, congenital immunodeficiency, and long-term immunosuppressive therapy) Pregnancy Children receiving corticosteroids	Recent immune globulin administration (see MMR, above) (PHAC, 2006). Family history of immunodeficiency	Breastfeeding
Rotavirus Vaccine		
Severe allergic reaction after a previous dose or to a vaccine component Infants born to HIV-positive mother Known or suspected weakened immune system caused by radiation; medications; or conditions such as leukemia, blood disorders, cancer	Altered immunocompetence Moderate to severe acute gastroenteritis Moderate to severe febrile illness Chronic gastrointestinal diseases Intussusception	Pregnancy Previous history of rotavirus infection; history of intussusception; temperature ≥38°C; close contact with immunocompromised person(s); blood transfusion or immune globulins within previous 42 days
Influenza Vaccine (Inactivated/Live-Attenuated)¶		
Severe allergic reaction after a previous dose or to a vaccine component, including eggs Egg hypersensitivity LAIV should not be administered to persons taking salicylates, with known or suspected immunodeficiency, with a history of GBS, or with a reactive airway disease or other chronic disorder considered high risk for severe influenza.	GBS within 6 wk after previous influenza immunization	Pregnancy
Meningococcal Vaccine		
MCV4—Allergy to vaccine components, including diphtheria toxoid, and possible reaction to latex stopper; history of GBS		Pregnancy
MPSV4—Allergy to vaccine components		Pregnancy
Tetanus (Booster Toxoid), Reduced Diphtheria Toxoid, Acellular Pertussis Adsorbed (Tdap)		
Serious reaction to any vaccine component History of encephalopathy (e.g., coma, prolonged seizures) within 7 days of administration of a pertussis vaccine that is not attributable to another identifiable cause	GBS ≤6 wk after previous dose of a tetanus toxoid vaccine Progressive neurological disorder, uncontrolled epilepsy, or progressive encephalopathy until the condition has stabilized	Temperature ≥40.5°C within 48 hr after DTP/DTaP immunization not attributable to another cause Collapse or shocklike state within 48 hr after DTP/DTaP immunization Persistent crying lasting ≥3 hr, occurring within 48 hr after DTP/DTaP immunization Seizures with or without fever, occurring within 3 days after DTaP/DTP immunization History of entire limb swelling reaction after pediatric DTaP/DTP or Td immunization that was not an Arthus hypersensitivity reaction Stable neurological disorder, including well-controlled seizures, history of seizure disorder, and CP Brachial neuritis Latex allergy other than anaphylactic allergies (e.g., history of contact to latex gloves) Immunosuppression, including persons with HIV Antibiotic use Intercurrent minor illness

Table 36-5 Contraindications and Precautions to Vaccinations—cont'd

TRUE CONTRAINDICATIONS	PRECAUTIONS†	NOT CONTRAINDICATIONS (VACCINES MAY BE ADMINISTERED)
Human Papillomavirus Vaccine		
Pregnancy Hypersensitivity to yeast or any vaccine component		Immunosuppressed female Minor acute illness Lactation

(Modified from American Academy of Pediatrics, Committee on Infectious Diseases & Pickering, L. [Ed.], [2009]. *2009 Red book: Report of the Committee on Infectious Diseases* [28th ed.]. Elk Grove Village, IL: Author.)
See also the National Advisory Committee on Immunizations (Public Health Agency of Canada) at: http://www.phac-aspc.gc.ca/naci-ccni/.
*This information is based on the recommendations of the Advisory Committee on Immunization Practices (ACIP) and those of the Committee on Infectious Diseases (Red Book Committee) of the American Academy of Pediatrics. Sometimes these recommendations vary from those contained in manufacturer's package inserts. For more detailed information, consult published recommendations of the ACIP and American Academy of Pediatrics and manufacturer's package inserts.
†Events or conditions listed as precautions, although not contraindications, should be carefully reviewed. Benefits and risks of administering a specific vaccine to an individual under the circumstances should be considered. If risks are believed to outweigh benefits, vaccination should be withheld; if benefits are believed to outweigh risks (e.g., during an outbreak or foreign travel), vaccination should be administered. Whether and when to administer DTaP to children with proven or suspected underlying neurological disorders should be decided on an individual basis. It is prudent on theoretical grounds to avoid vaccinating pregnant women.
‡Acetaminophen given before administering DTaP and thereafter every 4 hr for 24 hr should be considered for children with a personal history of seizures or family history of seizures in siblings or parents.
§Measles vaccination may temporarily suppress tuberculin reactivity. If testing cannot be done the day of MMR vaccination, the test should be postponed for 4 to 6 wk.
||Birth weight <2000 g and unknown or hepatitis B surface antigen–positive mother is not a contraindication for vaccination.
¶See James, J. M., et al. (1998). Safe administration of influenza vaccine to patients with egg allergies. *Journal of Pediatrics, 133*(5), 624-628.
CP, cerebral palsy; *GBS,* Guillain-Barré syndrome; *HIV,* human immunodeficiency virus; *LAIV,* live-attenuated influenza vaccine; *PPD,* purified protein derivative.

ATRAUMATIC CARE

Immunizations

Needle length is an important factor and must be considered for each individual child; fewer reactions to immunizations are observed when the vaccine is given deep into the muscle rather than into subcutaneous tissue. Contrary to previous belief, deep intramuscular tissue has a better blood supply and fewer pain receptors than adipose tissue, thus providing an optimum site for immunizations with fewer adverse effects (Zuckerman, 2000).

To minimize local reactions from vaccines:

- Recommended needle length for newborn to 2 months is 16 mm
- Select a needle of adequate length (2 mm in infants) to deposit the antigen deep in the muscle mass.
- Toddlers and older children require a needle length of 16 to 25 mm for deltoid, or 25 to 32 mm for vastus lateralis (Schechter et al., 2007).
- Adolescents require a needle length of 25 to 51 mm in deltoid or vastus lateralis (Schechter et al., 2007).
- Inject into the vastus lateralis or ventrogluteal muscle; the deltoid may be used in children 18 months of age or older.
- Do not withdraw plunger in syringe after injecting needle.

To minimize pain:

- Apply a topical anaesthetic such as EMLA® (lidocaine-prilocaine) or Maxalene® to the injection site and cover with an occlusive dressing for at least 1 hour.*

*The use of the EMLA patch before administration of diphtheria-tetanus–acellular pertussis–inactivated poliovirus–*Haemophilus influenzae* type b (DTaP-IPV-Hib) and hepatitis B vaccines did not decrease antibody titres in immunized infants and was effective in reducing pain in 6-month-old children (Halperin et al., 2002).

OR

- Apply the topical anaesthetic LMX4 (4% lidocaine) to the injection site 30 minutes before the injection; there is no evidence that an occlusive dressing is required except to prevent ingestion or accidental application to the eyes in infants (Wong, 2003). To date, the studies for LMX4 have only discussed pain from procedures such as venipuncture, not injections.
- Apply a vapocoolant spray (e.g., ethyl chloride or FluoriMethane) directly to the skin or to a cotton ball, which is placed on the skin for 15 seconds immediately before the injection (Reis & Holubkov, 1997).
- There is increasing evidence that a concentrated oral sucrose solution (24%) and non-nutritive sucking (pacifier) decrease the pain related to minor invasive procedures in neonates and infants (Harrison, Yamada, & Stevens, 2010; Stevens et al., 1999; Stevens, Yamada, & Ohlsson, 2001) (see Chapter 25, Atraumatic Care box: Heel Punctures, p. 658). Most studies have focused on heel lance, venipuncture, and circumcision (neonatal period), but one institution has incorporated a neonatal oral sucrose pain protocol for painful procedures, including injections (Thompson, 2005). Hatfield (2008) found that 2- and 4-month-old infants who received a 0.6 mL/kg dose of 24% sucrose and non-nutritive sucking 2 minutes before immunization administration had decreased pain behavioural responses in comparison to a control group of infants who received only sterile water and non-nutritive sucking 2 minutes before the injection. Therefore, it is recommended that a concentrated oral sucrose solution (1 to 2 mL) be administered orally 2 minutes before the injection,

Continued

ATRAUMATIC CARE

Immunizations—cont'd

during the injection, and up to 3 minutes after the procedure to decrease neonatal pain with immunizations.
- In preschool children, use distraction, such as telling the child to "take a deep breath and blow and blow and blow until I tell you to stop."
- Two studies in adult patients receiving intramuscular injections documented a decrease in pain sensation at the time of the injection when manual pressure was applied to the site before the injection; pressure was applied for 10 seconds in both studies (Barnhill et al., 1996; Chung, Ng, & Wong, 2002). To date, there are no published studies involving the use of this technique in children.
- The use of a needleless system to deliver lidocaine to the skin has been used in older children for venipuncture; the J-Tip delivers 1% buffered lidocaine, which numbs the skin within 1 to 3 minutes (Jimenez et al., 2006; Spanos et al., 2008; Zempsky, 2008). However, at time of this writing, this product is not approved for use in Canada.
- NOTE: Changing the needle on the syringe after drawing up the vaccine and before injecting it has not been shown to decrease local reactions. In children 4 to 6 years of age, the administration of sequential injections or simultaneous injections of vaccines did not alter their perceptions of distress, but parents preferred the simultaneous method (Horn & McCarthy, 1999).

subsequent immunizations are required, an allergist may be consulted to determine the best course of action (Schuval, 2003).

Unlike the inactivated antigens, live attenuated virus vaccines such as MMR multiply for days or weeks, and unfavourable reactions and vaccine-associated disorders can occur for 30 to 60 days. These reactions are usually mild, although reactions to rubella tend to be more troublesome in older children and adults.

Studies in the United States and in various European countries (Denmark, Finland) have found no association between the MMR vaccine and the incidence of autism (Campion, 2002; Dales, Hammer, & Smith, 2001; de Los Reyes, 2010; DeStefano, 2007; Hviid et al., 2003; Institute of Medicine, 2004, Mrozek-Budzn et al., 2010).

Contraindications and Compliance

Nurses need to be aware of the reasons for withholding immunizations—both for the child's safety in terms of avoiding reactions and for the child's maximum benefit from receiving the vaccine. Unfounded fears and lack of knowledge of contraindications can needlessly prevent a child from having protection from life-threatening diseases. Issues that have surfaced regarding vaccines include the misconception that administering combination vaccines may overload the child's immune system; the combined vaccines have undergone rigorous study in relation to adverse effects and immunogenicity rates following administration. Parents must be given appropriate information about vaccine safety, benefits, and risks so that they can make informed decisions regarding vaccinations for their children (Koslap-Petraco & Parsons, 2003). The advantage of widespread media via television and the Internet is that information is readily available at any given moment; the disadvantage is that some of this information may be incorrect, incomplete, or misleading and may influence parents to make decisions that may have deleterious consequences on their children's health. In one survey of parents, fear of adverse effects was the most commonly expressed reason (52%) for vaccination refusal; other common reasons included the belief that the particular disease was not harmful (26%), religious beliefs that prohibit immunization (28%), and philosophical reasons (26%) (Fredrickson et al., 2004). To help parents make informed decisions about immunizations for their children, parents may be directed to resources such as the Canadian Paediatric Society's *A Parent's Guide to Immunization Information on the Internet* (http://www.cps.ca/caringforkids/immunization/ImmunizationInfo.htm).

Strategies that may ensure parents follow immunization guidelines include giving parents vaccine information at the time of the newborn's discharge, mailing reminder cards, making immunization services readily available, removing barriers to vaccination (such as long waiting times and appointment-only systems), and taking every opportunity to immunize children when they enter a health care facility (such as emergency departments, clinics, private offices, and hospitals).

For contraindications to the usual childhood vaccines, see Table 36-5.

Administration

The principal precautions in administering immunizations include proper storage of the vaccine to protect its potency and the institution of recommended procedures for injection. The nurse must be familiar with the manufacturer's directions for storage and reconstitution of the vaccine. For example, if the vaccine is to be refrigerated, it should be stored on a centre shelf and not in the door, where frequent temperature increases from opening the refrigerator can alter the vaccine's potency. For protection against light, the vial can be wrapped in aluminum foil. Periodic checks should be scheduled to ensure that no vaccine is used after its expiration date.

The DTaP vaccines contain the adjuvant alum to retain the antigen at the injection site and to prolong the stimulatory effect. One of the most important features of injecting vaccines is adequate penetration of the muscle for deposition of the medication intramuscularly and not subcutaneously. The use of appropriate needle length is an essential component of administering vaccines. In two studies, the use of longer needles significantly decreased the incidence of localized edema and tenderness when vaccines were administered to a group of infants (Diggle & Deeks, 2000; Diggle, Deeks, & Pollard, 2006). Because subcutaneous or intracutaneous injection of the adjuvant can cause local irritation, inflammation, or abscess formation, attention to excellent intramuscular injection technique must be used (see Atraumatic Care box on immunization).

The total series requires several injections, and every attempt should be made to rotate the sites and administer the injections as painlessly as possible (see discussion on intramuscular injections in Chapter 45). When two or more injections are given at separate sites, the order of injections is arbitrary. Some practitioners suggest injecting the less painful one first. Some believe this is DTaP, whereas others suggest the MMR or Hib vaccine is less painful. Still others advocate injecting at two sites simultaneously (which requires two operators).

One study found that children ages 4 to 6 years rated sequential injections for immunizations versus simultaneous injections as being equally successful (Horn & McCarthy, 1999). Parents in the study preferred simultaneous immunization injections.

Because allergic reactions can occur after injection of vaccines, appropriate precautions need to be taken (see Chapter 48, Anaphylaxis).

Because nurses often administer vaccines, they have the responsibility of adequately informing parents of the nature, prevalence, and risks of the disease; the type of immunization product to be used; the expected benefits, and the risk of adverse effects of the vaccine; and the need for accurate immunization records. Referring to immunizations as "baby shots" and limiting the discussion to vague statements about the vaccines are unacceptable practices.

Another important nursing responsibility is accurate documentation. Each child should have an immunization record for parents to keep, especially for families who move often. Although immunization rates have increased significantly, health care providers should use every opportunity to encourage complete immunization of all children. Blank immunization records may be downloaded from a number of Web sites, including Immunize Canada (http://immunize.ca/en/learn/records.aspx), which has vaccine information and records.

The following information is documented on the medical record: day, month, and year of administration; manufacturer and lot number of vaccine; expiration date of vaccine; and the name, work address, and title of the person administering the vaccine. Additional data to record are the site and route of administration and evidence that the parent or legal guardian gave informed consent before the immunization was administered.

Practitioners are required to fully inform families of the risks and benefits of the vaccines. Any adverse reactions after the administration of any vaccine should be reported to the Canadian Adverse Events Following Immunization Surveillance System (CAEFISS) (PHAC, 2012a). See the Additional Resources section at the end of this chapter for additional information on immunization.

Injury Prevention

Injuries are a major cause of death during infancy, especially for children 6 to 12 months old. The main causes of death in children under 1 year of age are threats to breathing (41%), being a passenger in a motor vehicle accident (14%), and drowning (8%) (Safe Kids Canada, 2006). The main reason for hospitalization of children under age 1 year is falls (50%) (Safe Kids Canada, 2006).

Constant vigilance, awareness, and supervision are essential as the child gains increased locomotor and manipulative skills that are coupled with an insatiable curiosity about the environment. Box 36-1 lists the major developmental achievements of each period during infancy and the appropriate corresponding injury prevention plan.

Aspiration of Foreign Objects

Asphyxiation by foreign material in the respiratory tract, combined with mechanical suffocation, is one of the leading causes of fatal injury in children younger than 1 year of age. The most common foreign bodies ingested and found in the gastrointestinal tract include both food and nonfood items. The size, shape, and consistency of foods or objects are important determinants of fatal obstruction. For example, small spherical or cylindrical and pliable objects (less than 3.2 cm) are more likely to completely obstruct the airway. Unfortunately, many common household items can be deadly to infants.

As soon as infants have the ability to find their mouth, they are vulnerable to aspiration of small objects, such as those left within reach or removable parts of objects that may on initial inspection appear safe. All toys must be carefully inspected for potential danger. Rattles, for example, have small beads in them to produce noise. A broken or cracked rattle can be dangerous because the beads can easily be aspirated while the infant has the toy in the mouth. Stuffed animals are another potentially dangerous toy if any of the parts, such as the eyes or nose, are removable buttons or plastic pieces. An active infant can grab a low-hanging mobile and quickly chew off a small piece. As soon as the infant crawls or plays on the floor, the floor must be kept free of any small articles that can be picked up and swallowed, such as coins, buttons, or small round batteries.

When infant clothes are purchased, the type of closure is important. A front button can easily be pulled off and swallowed. Safety pins for diapers should be kept closed and away from the dressing table. Even though a young infant may not search for them, practising this good habit from the beginning prevents future injuries.

Food items are a common cause of aspiration; the most common offenders are hot dogs, candy, nuts, and grapes. When new foods are given to the child, nuts, hard candies, marshmallows, large amounts of peanut butter, and fruits with pits or seeds should be avoided. When travelling or entertaining, parents must keep snack foods such as peanuts and popcorn away from young children. If given to young children, hot dogs must be cut into small, irregular pieces rather than served whole or in slices, since their size (diameter), round shape, and consistency allow for complete occlusion of the airway. Perhaps the most dangerous foods are dried beans,

evolve Critical Thinking Exercises—Infant Safety

BOX 36-1 Injury Prevention During Infancy

Birth to 4 Months

Major Developmental Accomplishments

Exhibits involuntary reflexes (e.g., crawling reflex may propel infant forward or backward; startle reflex may cause the body to jerk)
May roll over
Has increasing eye–hand coordination and voluntary grasp reflex

Injury Prevention

Aspiration

Aspiration is not as great a danger to this age group as in older infants, but parents should begin practising safeguarding early (see under Age 4 to 7 Months).
Baby powder should never be shaken directly on the infant; place powder in the hand and then on the infant's skin; store container closed and out of infant's reach.
Hold the infant for feeding; do not prop bottle.
Know emergency procedures for choking.
Use a pacifier with one-piece construction and loop handle.

Burns

Install smoke detectors in the home.
Use caution when warming formula in a microwave oven; always check temperature of liquid before feeding.
Check bathwater.
Do not pour or drink hot liquids when the infant is close by, such as when sitting on your lap.
Beware of cigarette ashes that may fall on the infant.
Do not leave infant in the sun for more than a few minutes; keep skin covered.
Wash flame-retardant clothes according to label directions.
Use cool-mist vaporizers.
Do not leave the child in a parked car.
Check surface heat of the car restraint before placing child in the seat.

Suffocation and Drowning

Keep all plastic bags stored out of the infant's reach; discard large plastic garment bags after tying in a knot.
Do not cover mattress with plastic.
Use firm mattress and loose blankets, with no pillows.
Make certain the crib design follows government regulations and the mattress fits snugly. No crib manufactured before September 1986 should be used for infants (Health Canada, 2010a). Position the crib away from other furniture and away from radiators.
Keep all cords and strings out of reach and do not tie pacifier on a string around infant's neck.
Remove bibs at bedtime.
Never leave an infant alone in the bath.
Do not leave an infant under age 1 year alone on an adult or youth mattress or "beanbag"-type seats.

Motor Vehicles

Transport infant in a Transport Canada–approved, rear-facing car seat, preferably in the back seat.
Do not place infant on the seat (of car) or in your lap.
Do not place child in a carriage or stroller behind a parked car.
Do not place infant or child in the front passenger seat with an activated air bag.

Falls

Always raise crib rails.
Never leave an infant alone on a raised, unguarded surface.
When in doubt as to where to place the child, use the floor.
Restrain child in an infant seat or stroller, and never leave child unattended while the seat is resting on a raised surface.
Avoid using a high chair until the child can sit well with support.

Poisoning

Poisoning is not as great a danger in this age group as in older infants, but parents should begin practising safeguards early (see under Age 4 to 7 Months)

Bodily Damage

Keep sharp or jagged objects such as knives and broken glass out of child's reach.
Keep diaper pins closed and away from the infant.

Age 4 to 7 Months

Major Developmental Accomplishments

Rolls over
Sits momentarily
Grasps and manipulates small objects
Resecures a dropped object
Has well-developed eye–hand coordination
Can focus on and locate small objects
Places objects in mouth (hand-to-mouth)
Can push up on hands and knees
Crawls backward

Injury Prevention

Aspiration

Keep buttons, beads, syringe caps, and other small objects out of infant's reach.
Keep floor free of any small objects.
Do not feed infant hard candy, nuts, food with pits or seeds, or whole or circular pieces of hot dog or grapes.
Exercise caution when giving teething biscuits, since large chunks may be broken off and aspirated.
Do not feed the infant while he or she is lying down.
Inspect toys for removable parts. Use only toys approved for the age of your child.
Use only cornstarch baby powder, if powder is needed, and keep out of reach.

Suffocation

Keep all latex balloons out of reach.
Remove all crib toys that are strung across the crib or playpen when the child begins to push up on hands or knees or is 5 months old.

Burns

Keep water faucets out of reach.
Place hot objects (cigarettes, candles, incense) on a high surface out of the child's reach.
Limit the child's exposure to sun; apply sunscreen.

Falls

Restrain the child in a high chair.
Keep crib rails raised to full height.

Motor Vehicles

See under Birth to 4 Months.

Poisoning

Make certain that paint for furniture or toys does not contain lead.
Place toxic substances on a high shelf or in locked cabinet.
Keep medication vials and bottles locked in a secure place.

BOX 36-1 Injury Prevention During Infancy—cont'd

Hang plants or place them on a high surface rather than on the floor.
Avoid storing large quantities of cleaning fluid, paints, pesticides, and other toxic substances.
Discard used containers of poisonous substances.
Do not store toxic substances in food or drink containers.
Discard used button-size batteries; store new batteries in a safe area.
Know the telephone number of the provincial or territory poison control centre (usually listed in front of telephone directory).

Bodily Damage
Give the child toys that are smooth and rounded, preferably made of wood or plastic.
Avoid long, pointed objects as toys.
Avoid toys that are excessively loud.
Keep sharp objects out of infant's reach.

Age 8 to 12 Months

Major Developmental Accomplishments
Crawls or creeps
Stands, holding onto furniture
Stands alone
Cruises around furniture
Walks
Climbs
Pulls on objects
Throws objects
Is able to pick up small objects; has pincer grasp
Explores by putting objects in mouth
Dislikes being restrained
Explores away from parent
Increasingly understands simple commands and phrases

Injury Prevention

Aspiration
Keep small objects off the floor, off furniture, and out of reach of children.
When feeding the child solid table food, give it in very small pieces.
Do not use beanbag toys or allow the child to play with dried beans.
See also under Age 4 to 7 Months.

Bodily Damage
See under Age 4 to 7 Months.
Avoid placing televisions or other large objects on top of furniture, which may be overturned when the infant pulls self to standing position.

Falls
Avoid walkers, especially near stairs.†
Ensure that furniture is sturdy enough for the child to pull self to standing position and cruise.
Fence stairways at the top and bottom if the child has access to either end.†
Dress infant in safe shoes and clothing (soles that do not "catch" on floor, tied shoelaces, pant legs that do not touch floor).

Suffocation and Drowning
Keep doors of the oven, dishwasher, refrigerator, cooler, and front-loading clothes washer and dryer closed at all times.
If storing an unused large appliance, such as a refrigerator, lock or remove the door.
Supervise contact with inflated balloons; immediately discard popped balloons, and keep uninflated balloons out of reach.
Fence swimming pools and other bodies of standing water such as decorative fountains; lock gates to swimming pools so only adult can gain access.
Always supervise the child when near any source of water, such as cleaning buckets, drainage areas, and toilets.
Keep bathroom doors closed.
Eliminate unnecessary pools of water.
Keep one hand on the child at all times when in the tub.

Poisoning
Administer medications as a drug, not as a candy.
Do not administer medications unless prescribed by a practitioner.
Return medications and poisons to a safe storage area immediately after use; replace caps properly if a child-protector cap is used.
Have the provincial or territory poison control centre number on the telephone and refrigerator.

Burns
Place guards in front of or around any heating appliance, fireplace, or furnace.
Keep electrical wires hidden or out of reach.
Place plastic guards over electrical outlets; place furniture in front of outlets.
Keep hanging tablecloths out of reach (the child may pull down hot liquids or heavy or sharp objects).

†Information on many items such as cribs or walkers is available from Health Canada, at http://www.hc-sc.gc.ca/index-eng.php.

which, if aspirated, enlarge when they come in contact with the wet mucosa and can block the airway.

Pacifiers can also be dangerous because the entire object may be aspirated if it is small, or the nipple and shield may become detached from the handle and become lodged in the pharynx. Improvised pacifiers also present dangers. To eliminate the hazards of improvised pacifiers, hospitals should use only safe, commercial types (see Fig. 25-19). Pacifiers should not be altered from their original shape to encourage or discourage usage. Candy pacifiers pose dangers because the candy portion can dislodge from the circular base and be aspirated. To be safe, pacifiers should have the following features:

- Sturdy, one-piece construction with material that is nontoxic, flexible, and firm but not brittle
- An easily grasped handle
- A mouthguard that cannot be separated from the nipple, that has two ventilating holes, and that is too large to be aspirated

- No detachable ribbon or string
- A label warning against tying the pacifier around the infant's neck

Using a syringe to accurately measure and dispense oral liquid medications to young children has become common practice. However, the syringe cap is a potential aspiration hazard. As a precaution, parts of medication devices should be kept out of the reach of children and the cap removed before dispensing medication. Medication administration syringes without caps are now available; syringes with caps should not be used for medication administration.

Another hazardous substance if aspirated is baby powder, which is usually a mixture of talc (hydrous magnesium silicate) and other silicates. Although the use of talc has been discouraged, it is a common baby care product and can cause severe and often fatal aspiration pneumonia. One of the factors involved in talc aspiration is the similar appearance of baby powder containers and nursing bottles. Talc containers often become favourite playthings and are placed in the mouth. Improperly using powder by sprinkling it directly on the skin creates a cloud of talc dust that is easily inhaled. Parents need to be advised of the danger of baby powder and discouraged from using it. If they prefer to use a powder, a cornstarch preparation can be substituted (see Chapter 53, Diaper Dermatitis).

Suffocation

Mechanical suffocation includes suffocation by covering of the airway (i.e., mouth and nose); by pressure on the throat and chest; and by exclusion of air, such as by refrigerator entrapment. Nonfood items cause the majority of deaths in young children.

Latex balloons, whether partially inflated, uninflated, or popped, are a leading cause of pediatric choking deaths from children's products. They should be kept away from infants and young children. Even the practice of inflating latex gloves to amuse children in health care settings may pose a danger, especially if the child is latex sensitive. Adults should be encouraged to blow up balloons for children, supervise children's balloon play, pick up and dispose of broken balloon pieces, warn older children of dangers of chewing or sucking on balloons, and substitute Mylar or paper balloons for latex balloons.

Another hazard is the accessibility of the plastic linings of diapers used on the infant or on dolls, which is especially dangerous to young children.

The bed or crib poses a number of hazards. An infant who is placed in a bed under tucked-in blankets and sheets can be caught under them and become unable to wriggle free. Baby pillows filled with plastic foam beads, resembling small beanbags, are dangerous; very young infants are suffocated when the pillow contours to the face and blocks the airway. When adults sleep with a small infant there is the possibility of an adult rolling over and smothering the child (overlaying). The most common causes of infant suffocation are wedging between a bed or mattress and a wall and oronasal obstruction by a plastic bag. For the crib itself, there should be no more than 6 cm between the crib and cradle bars to prevent the infant's head from becoming trapped between the bars and mattresses or other items in the crib. The bed must meet Canadian standards: the mattress should be firm, not worn, and should fit tight all around the crib or cradle. In addition, no crib or cradle with decorative cut-outs, lead paint, loose screws, missing pieces, splinters, or corner posts more than 3 mm in height should be used, nor if it was manufactured before September 1986 (Health Canada, 2010a). See Additional Resources at the end of this chapter for parent education regarding safe sleep environments for infants.

Mesh-sided playpens and cribs can result in death if the sides are left in the lowered position. Infants have suffocated when they fell off the edge of the mattress and the head or chest was compressed between the floorboard and mesh side. Parents should be advised of this danger and encouraged to always keep the sides locked securely in the up position whenever the child is in the playpen or crib. The crib should be positioned away from large furniture, since children who crawl out of the crib may become caught between the two objects. Cribs should also be located away from windows, where drape or blind cords can become wrapped around the infant's neck.

Plastic bags, another source of suffocation, are very lightweight and can easily and quickly be wrapped around the head of an active infant or pressed against the face. For this reason, pillows and mattresses should not be covered with plastic. Older infants may play with a plastic bag and accidentally pull it over their heads. Because plastic is nonporous, suffocation occurs in a matter of minutes.

Cords (e.g., drapery or window blinds) located near the infant are a potential cause of strangulation. Bibs should be removed at bedtime, and objects such as pacifiers should never be hung on a string around the infant's neck. This is a common practice in some cultures that can be remedied by tying a short string to a pacifier and clipping the string to the child's shirt.

Toys that have strings attached (e.g., a telephone) or toys that are tied to cribs or playpens can be hazards because the string can become wrapped around the child's neck or the child can become entrapped in the toy. As a precaution, all cords should be less than 30 cm long. Crib toys should be hung high enough that the infant cannot become entangled in them and should no longer be used once the child is able to reach them.

If applied too loosely or left unfastened, restraining straps can be a hazard. For example, a child may slide off a high chair beneath the tray and become strangled on the loose strap. All straps should be fastened securely.

Motor Vehicle Injuries

Automobile injuries are the leading cause of accidental death in children in Canada between the ages of 1 and 9 years (Safe Kids Canada, 2012). A significant number of nonfatal vehicle-related injuries in children between 1 and 4 years of age occur as a result of a car backing out while children are playing in a driveway (Centers for Disease Control and Prevention, 2005). In addition, a significant number of infants are injured or die from improper restraint within the vehicle, most often from riding on the lap of another occupant or from riding unrestrained in the back seat of the vehicle. Reports indicate that child-restraint use decreases with increasing age of children and increasing number of occupants in the vehicle. Lack of proper child restraint continues to be a major factor in fatal accidents involving children. All infants must be secured in a Transport Canada–approved restraint rather than being held or placed on the seat of the car (see Additional Resources section). There is no safe alternative.

Infant restraints are designed either as an infant-only model or as a convertible infant-toddler model (Fig. 36-11). Either restraint is a semireclined seat that faces the rear of the car. A rear-facing car seat provides the best protection for the disproportionately heavy head and weak neck of a young child. This position minimizes the stress on the neck by spreading the forces of a frontal crash over the entire back, neck, and head; the spine is supported by the back of the car seat. If the seat were faced forward, the head would whip forward because of the force of the crash, creating enormous stress on the neck.

A recent study indicated that children 0 to 3 years of age riding properly restrained in the middle of the back seat had a 43% lower risk of injury than that of children riding in the outboard (window) seat during a crash (Kallan et al., 2008). Another study has shown that children 0 to 23 months riding in a rear-facing restraint were less likely to be injured than those riding in a forward-facing restraint (Henary et al., 2007).

The restraint is anchored to the vehicle with the vehicle's seat belt, and the restraint has a harness system for securing the infant. The five-point harness system provides the most effective support for an infant restraint. Many infant seats have a plastic base that can be left in the car; the seat latches or clicks into the base so that the base does not have to be installed each time the car seat is removed. The universal anchorage system (UAS) provides car seat anchors between the front cushion and backrest so that the seat belt does not have to be used. Some automobiles have tether anchors for rear-facing infant-only seats as well (see Chapter 37). Although many infant restraints can be recliners, they are used in the car only in the position specified by the manufacturer.

NURSING ALERT Infants should ride in a rear-facing car seat from birth to a weight of 10 kg and until at least 1 year of age. If the child weighs 10 kg but is not 1 year old, the rear-facing position is still recommended. Infants and children must be in a car seat or booster seat until age 8 years. All children's car seats and booster seats sold in Canada must have a Transport Canada sticker on them and will have an expiration or useful life date on them. Manufacturers place expiratory or useful-life dates to inform current owners and prospective buyers of the potential risks of using car seats and booster seats that may be missing important parts, labels, or instructions or that may have an unknown history that could lead to inadequate performance when needed. People should not use children's car seats and booster seats past their expiration or useful-life date (Safe Kids Canada, 2010a).

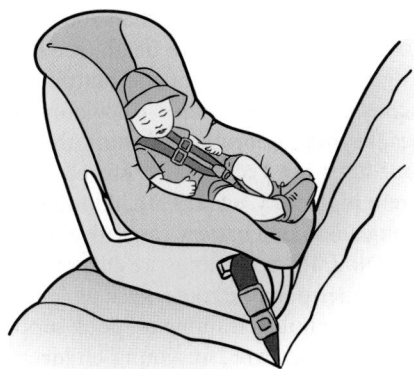

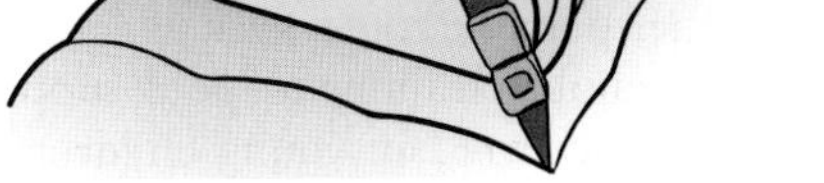

Fig. 36-11 A rear-facing infant car restraint that is approved by Transport Canada and placed in the back seat provides the best protection.

Severe injuries and deaths in children have occurred from air bags deploying on impact in the front passenger seat; thus the back seat is the safest area of the car. If this is not an option, an infant restraint may be positioned in the front seat provided that the seat belt can be locked into position and there is no passenger-side air bag. If there is a passenger-side air bag and the child has special health care needs or requires constant observation and no other adult is available to ride in the back seat with the child, an on/off switch may be installed to prevent the air bag from deploying and injuring the child. For vehicles without a back seat it is best that the front passenger seat be placed as far back as possible and appropriate child safety restraint be used. With advanced technology, new, "smart" air bags include features that make them a safer alternative for children. See Additional Resources for more information on motor vehicle restraints.

For restraints to be effective, they must be used properly. Dressing the infant in a light-weight outfit with sleeves and legs allows the harness to hold the child securely in the seat. A small blanket or towel rolled tightly can be placed on either side of the head to minimize movement and keep the infant's hips against the back of the seat. Padding between the infant's legs and crotch can be added to prevent slouching. Thick, soft padding should not be placed under the infant or behind the back, and if possible, the infant should not be wearing a snowsuit or heavy coat because during the impact the padding will compress, leaving the harness straps loose. Only padding that came with the car seat should be used. Preterm infants being discharged home should be placed in an appropriate car seat restraint before it is placed in the car, and the infant's oxygen saturations should be monitored for a determined period to detect any potential problems with airway occlusion. (For further discussion of car seat restraints, see Chapter 37; for preterm infant car restraint test guidelines, see Chapter 27, Community Focus box: Preterm and Late-Term Infant Car Seat Evaluation, p. 738.)

Another automobile-related hazard for infants is overheating (hyperthermia) and subsequent death when left in a vehicle in hot weather (over 26°C). Infants dissipate heat poorly, and an increase in body temperature may cause death in a few hours. Parents should be cautioned against leaving infants in a vehicle alone *for any reason*. A small sign or placard has been designed to hang in the rear-view mirror to remind the parent that there is a child in the back seat. Busy parents may forget that the child is in the back.

Falls

Residential injuries, especially falls, accounted for the highest incidence of unintentional injuries to children seen in emergency departments in Canada. Young children are at risk for falls from furniture, down stairs, or from windows. For example, Safe Kids Canada (2009) reported that between 1990 and 2007, more than 5403 injuries from bunk beds were reported; children who fell from the top bunk were twice as likely to be hospitalized. Falls are most common after 4 months of age, when the infant has learned to roll over, but they can occur at any age.

The best advice for prevention of falls is to never place a child of any age unattended on a raised surface that is not designed to protect the child from accidentally falling. When in doubt, the safest place is the floor. Even though young infants cannot climb over a partially raised crib rail, it is best to form a habit of raising the rail all the way, since some day that infant will be able to climb out. Crib sides should have a latching device that cannot be easily released. The welds attaching the crib corner locks to the corner posts should not be cracked or broken. If the welds are damaged, the bedspring could fall to the floor. Ideally, cribs should be placed on carpeted, not hard, floors.

Another danger area for falling is the changing table, which is usually high and narrow. Although these tables have a restraining belt, restrained children should never be left unattended. The area should be arranged with all necessary articles within easy reach so that the child is always in full sight. It takes only a fraction of a second for an infant to fall off. During the latter half of the first year, infants usually resist dressing and diapering and may be difficult to manage. If there is danger that the child is strong enough to resist restraining, the infant should be changed on a safer surface, such as a clean floor.

Infant seats, high chairs, walkers, and swings present additional opportunities for falls. If the infant seat is placed on a table, the child should never be left unrestrained or unattended. The same rule is essential for other baby equipment, particularly when the child has learned to crawl and to stand up. High chairs are designed for older infants who can sit well and who are tall enough to have the tray at the level of their chest or abdomen. Small infants can slip through a high chair if a protective harness is not used. Infant walkers are responsible for a number of different types of injuries that occur because the walker tipped over or fell down stairs. Parents need to be warned of these dangers and know that infant walkers have been prohibited in Canada since 2004 (Health Canada, 2005). One alternative is to use a stationary play station with a seat similar to that in a walker. There is no evidence that use of infant walkers helps infants walk sooner.

Once infants are mobile, they should not be allowed to crawl unsupervised on any raised surface, near stairs, or near any water reservoir. Gates should be used at the bottom *and* top of stairs, since both present dangers to the crawling and climbing infant. However, certain types of gates can present hazards. Freestanding enclosures constructed of crisscrossed wood slats that expand and contract can trap the head or neck when children attempt to climb over them. If these types of gates are used, they must be securely fastened to prevent mobility of the slats.

As children begin to pull themselves to a standing position, heavy objects, such as unsturdy furniture or any freestanding item (e.g., wrought iron fish tank stands or televisions), can be extremely dangerous if pulled down on top of the child. Televisions should be placed on lower furniture, as far back as possible, and angle anchors can be used to secure furniture to walls.

Even when the environment is made safe, infants may sometimes literally trip over their own feet from clothing. Slippery socks; hard, slick soles on shoes or rubber soles that can catch, especially on a carpet; and long pants or pajama bottoms can easily upset a child's balance. Such dangers need to be pointed out to parents, especially when infants are taking their first steps.

An alarming number of small children fall out of windows and are hurt; this is especially common with window ledges such as bay windows that have wide ledges for children to sit on. Window screens are not fall-prevention devices; rather, window guards should be installed to prevent falls from any window, regardless of the height. Furniture should be kept away from windows so that children cannot climb onto the furniture and access the window.

Poisoning

Poisoning is one of the major causes of death in children younger than 5 years of age. The highest incidence occurs in the 2-year-old group, with the second highest incidence occurring in 1-year-old children. Infants who do not crawl are relatively free from the danger of poisonous agents. With locomotion, danger from poisoning is present almost everywhere. The average home contains more than 500 toxic substances, and approximately one third of all poisonings occur in the kitchen.

The major reason for ingestion of poisons is improper storage. To protect the infant, toxic agents should not be placed on a low shelf, a low table, or the floor. Medications that are kept in a purse pose additional dangers if infants play with it; they may open it and ingest the medication. Another unrecognized hazard occurs during diaper changes, when infants are near many toxic substances such as ointments, creams, oils, and talc. Common household over-the-counter medications such as acetaminophen and cold and cough preparations, cosmetics and personal care products, and cleaning products are also sources of childhood poisoning (Wilkerson, Northington, & Fisher, 2005). Toys need to be at hand to avoid an infant playing with a toxic substance.

Plants are another source of poisoning for infants. Plants are commonly placed on the floor, and the leaves or flowers are attractive and easy to pull off. More than 700 species of plants are known to have caused illness or death (see Box 47-22).

Another danger is ingestion of the button-sized batteries used in devices such as hearing aids, calculators, watches, and cameras. Because they are bright and shiny, they are attractive to children and thus need to be safely stored. If ingested they can cause severe morbidity, even death, if lodged in the esophagus. The strong alkali in a battery can leak and cause a severe caustic burn. Not all poisonings result from ingestion—inhalation is another possible route, such as inhaling chlorine vapours from household cleaning or pool supplies. Passive cocaine toxicity has occurred in young children exposed to freebase cocaine ("crack") smoking by adults. Children should be protected from environments in which airborne toxins exist. (For a discussion of passive secondhand tobacco smoke, see Chapter 46.)

The production of methamphetamines, a common central nervous system stimulant also known as ice, speed, or crystal, involves the use of a number of chemicals that may be toxic alone (via contact or ingestion) or during the production (cooking) of the drug itself. Methamphetamine laboratories are commonly in household areas where children may be exposed to harmful inhalants as well as open fires where meth is "cooked." Methamphetamine use and exposure can cause developmental problems and short- and long-term brain damage, particularly in children. Reports of the number of children exposed daily to methamphetamine laboratories in North America are alarming; such children are also at high risk for abuse and neglect because their caretakers are preoccupied with the production, sale, and use of the drug (Bellemare, 2008; Matteucci et al., 2007; Mecham & Melini, 2002). Children should be protected from environments in which inhaled toxins exist (see Chapter 28 for a discussion of the effects of chemical substances on the fetus and neonate).

The only sure way to prevent poisoning is to remove toxic agents from the proximity of children; this means placing containers out of the infant's reach or contact. It is best to keep all toxic agents, especially medications, in a locked cabinet. Special plastic hooks can be attached to the inside of cabinet doors to keep them securely closed (Fig. 36-12). Firm thumb pressure is required to unlatch the hook, and small children are usually unable to manipulate them.

With several hundred toxic substances in each house, locking up all potentially toxic substances can present a problem; however, careful planning can help. A large surplus of cleaning agents, furniture polishes, laundry additives, paints, insecticides, and solvents should be avoided. Used poison containers should be promptly discarded and not used to store another poison without adequately marking the package. Potentially hazardous substances should not be stored in any type of food container. A popular container used to store toxic liquids is a soft drink bottle; this can entice a child to drink from it.

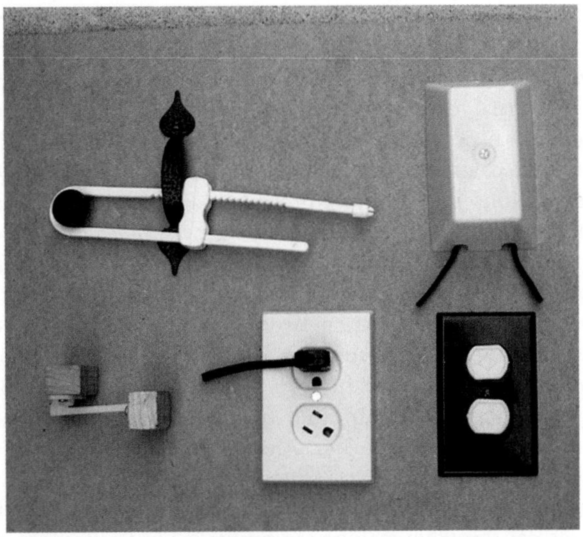

Fig. 36-12 Safety demonstration board. Clockwise from lower left: Two types of cabinet latches, a shock guard for an electrical outlet in use, and two types of outlet covers (the one with the white cover has passive devices that automatically cover the outlet when a plug is removed).

NURSING ALERT Parents should know the telephone number of the local poison centre, and call this number in the event of a suspected poisoning. Ipecac, used to induce vomiting, is no longer a standard recommendation. If the child is not breathing, the parent should call 911 immediately.

Emergency measures for poisoning are discussed in Chapter 47.

Burns

Scalding from water that is too hot; excessive sunburn; and burns from house fires, electrical wires, sockets, and heating elements such as radiators, registers, and electric floor heaters cause a significant number of deaths and many more injuries in infants. The infant's skin is particularly sensitive to irritation, and the mechanisms for temperature perception are not completely developed. As a general precaution, all homes should have smoke alarms installed near the bedroom areas and on each level of the building.

Scald burns from hot tap water can be prevented by lowering the water heater temperature to a safe temperature of 49°C. Bathwater should be checked before the infant is immersed. The most common type of scald injury is from infants pulling hot pans of water off a stove or an elevated surface onto themselves (Drago, 2005). Scalds can also occur from bathing infants in the kitchen sink when the garbage disposal, occluded with debris, causes the draining dishwasher effluent to back up into the sink. Caregivers should not bathe small children in the sink when the dishwasher is running.

If food is warmed in a microwave oven, it must be checked before feeding because the container may remain cool while the contents are hot. Another danger is explosion of the container from the buildup of steam. Because of these dangers, Health Canada (2010b) does not recommend microwaving infant formula or food but rather using conventional warming, for example, with baby-bottle warmers. If a microwave oven is used, it is important to stop halfway through warming of the food and stir the fluid or food, use only containers that are labelled microwave safe, use oven mitts to remove containers from the oven, and shake the contents and test the food's temperature before feeding it to the child. The handles of cooking utensils should be turned toward the back of the stove. When the infant is underfoot, pouring hot liquids and cooking with hot oil should be avoided. Hanging tablecloths should also be placed out of the infant's reach to prevent the infant from pulling hot items off the table.

Sunburn can be a source of a first- or second-degree burn. Exposure to direct sunlight should be avoided for the infant's first 6 months. When infants are in the sun, the body, especially the face and head, should be covered. Sunscreen can be used on older infants but should be used on small areas of the body and only sparingly in infants under 6 months (see Chapter 53, Sunburn). Although infants burn less readily, their thin skin can become sunburned and needs protection.

Electrical outlets should be covered with protective plastic caps that prevent the child from putting objects such as hairpins into the outlet (see Fig. 36-12). Extension cords should be placed out of reach so that curious infants cannot chew on them and break the rubber coating (Fig. 36-13). Infants should not be allowed to play near television sets, stereo units, or other appliances.

Any heat-producing element should have a guard placed in front of it. Fireplaces should be well screened because they are appealing and within easy access. Small, portable heaters should be placed on a high surface. Floor furnaces should have barrier gates to prevent children from crawling or walking over them. Burning cigarettes, candles, and incense should be kept out of reach, and infants should not be held by a smoking adult because falling ashes are a hazard, especially to the eyes. Heated-mist vaporizers are a source of burns; only cool-mist vaporizers are safe. Handheld curling irons are also a common source of hand burns in small children.

By law, all infant sleepwear must be flame retardant. Unfortunately, this does not apply to all infant clothing. Flame-retardant fabric must never be viewed as the ultimate protection against burns. Repeated washing with soap or bleach destroys the protection. Home-sewn sleepwear should be made of specially treated, flame-retardant fabric.

Children can also be burned by overheated metal hardware and vinyl seats in cars parked in the sun. As a precaution, the surface heat of car restraints should be determined before placing children in them. Covering the restraints and hardware (such as metal latches on seat belts) may be necessary to prevent skin burns. An additional safeguard is buying a light-coloured restraint, which absorbs less heat.

Drowning

Drowning in this age group can occur in just a few centimetres of water. Consequently, infants should always be supervised in a bathtub and when they are near a source of water such as a swimming pool, hot tub, lake, toilet, or bucket. Most unintentional infant drownings occur in the home setting; of infants younger than 1 year who drowned, most drowned in a toilet, bathtub, or bucket (Brenner & AAP, Committee on Injury, Violence, and Poison Prevention, 2003; Lassman, 2002); 20-litre buckets are particularly dangerous because the child may inadvertently fall in head first and, because of the weight of the upper body at this age, cannot withdraw from the bucket. Inadequate supervision is often associated with childhood drowning.

Safe Kids Canada (2010b) does not recommend swimming lessons for children under 5 years of age because of their lack of physical ability. Toddler lessons should focus on an introduction to water and on teaching parents the importance of water safety. No infant can be expected to learn the elements of water safety or to react appropriately in an emergency. Therefore, all young children need to be considered at risk when near water. Infants and toddlers are also at increased risk of infection and seizures from swallowing large amounts of water.

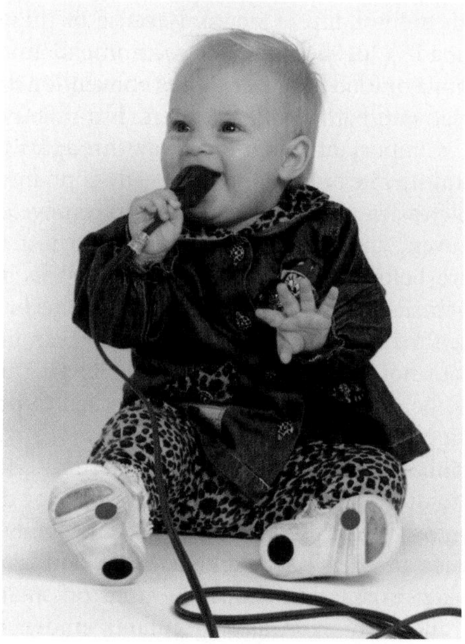

Fig. 36-13 Infants can find hazardous electrical wires. *(Photo by Paul Vincent Kuntz, Texas Children's Hospital, Houston.)*

Bodily Damage

Injuries in children may occur in numerous ways. Sharp, jagged-edged objects can cause wounds in the skin. Long, pointed articles, such as the common toothpick or fork, can be poked into the eye or ear, causing serious damage. Such articles should be safely stored away from the infant's reach; forks are best avoided for self-feeding until the child has mastered the spoon, usually by age 18 months.

In addition to hazards such as aspiration, small articles can be placed in the ear or nose, and excessive noise from toys can result in sensorineural hearing loss. Although toys with the highest noise levels are model airplanes, air guns, and toy cap guns, even common squeaking toys used by young children may be harmful if placed close to the ear.

Another cause of injuries in children is child maltreatment, which remains a serious issue in Canada. In 2008, the Canadian Incidence Study of Reported Child Abuse and Neglect was conducted for the Public Agency of Canada (2010). It was the third study of its kind, all of them done 5 years apart. From 1998 to 2003 there was a significant increase in the number of maltreatment cases reported; in 2008 the level remained steady. An estimated 235,842 maltreatment-related investigations were carried out in Canada, representing a rate of 39.16 investigations per 1000 children. Children of First Nations, Métis, and Inuit heritage had a four times higher rate of confirmed child maltreatment than that of non-Aboriginal children. Of all child maltreatment cases, 7% were infants under 1 year of age and 19% were between 1 and 3 years of age. Social determinants of health such as poverty played a role in some families in which maltreatment was present. For example, 33% of the families in which child maltreatment occurred were receiving social assistance or other benefits.

Another common and often unrecognized danger to infants is animal attacks. As newcomers to the home, helpless infants can provoke jealousy in animals, especially dogs and cats. Parents must be constantly vigilant to protect the child from household pets and farm animals (see Chapter 53, Animal Bites).

Shaken Baby Syndrome

Shaken baby syndrome (SBS) is a serious form of child abuse caused by violent shaking of infants and young children. This shaking can be easily recognized by others as dangerous (CPS, 2001, PHAC, 2011c) and is most often a result of the caregiver's frustration with an infant's crying. Shaken babies can have serious neurological injuries with significant morbidity and mortality. The Canadian Paediatric Society (2010) surveillance program found in 2006 that the annual incident rate per 100,000 is 14.1 in those under 1 year old, 3.2 for 1- to 2-year-olds, 0.8 for 2- to 4-year-olds, and 0.8 for children over 4 years old. Thirty percent of children had previously been reported to Child Welfare Services. Over 50% of the children died or had neurological sequelae.

It is important to understand what happens in SBS. Infants have a large head-to-body ratio, weak neck muscles, and a large amount of water in the brain. Violent shaking causes the brain to rotate within the skull, resulting in shearing forces that tear blood vessels and neurons. The characteristic injuries that occur are intracranial bleeding (subdural and subarachnoid hematomas) and retinal hemorrhages, but they may also include fractures of the ribs and long bones. Most often there are no external signs of injury. SBS is often not an isolated event; in one study, 45% of the children with inflicted traumatic brain injury caused by shaking showed some evidence of prior injury (CPS, 2001).

Victims of SBS can manifest a variety of symptoms, from generalized flulike symptoms to unresponsiveness with impending death (CPS, 2001). Many of the presenting symptoms, such as vomiting, irritability, poor feeding, and listlessness, are often mistaken for common infant and childhood ailments. In more severe forms, presenting symptoms may include seizures, posturing, alterations in level of consciousness, apnea, bradycardia, or death. The long-term outcomes of SBS include seizure disorder; visual impairments, including blindness; developmental delays; hearing loss; cerebral palsy; and mild to profound mental, cognitive, and motor impairments (CPS, 2001). Nurses can take an active role in prevention of SBS by teaching all caregivers about crying and techniques to cope with inconsolable crying.

NURSING ALERT Nurses should emphasize to parents the danger of shaking an infant (shaking can cause SBS). Education must include coping mechanisms for caring for children with inconsolable crying.

Nurse's Role in Prevention of Injury

The task of injury prevention can be appreciated only when the potential environmental dangers to which infants are vulnerable are considered. Injury prevention and parent education should be handled on a growth and developmental basis. It is simply impossible to completely protect infants and small children from all potential dangers without placing them in a sterile, impractical environment. However, a large percentage of childhood deaths that are the result of preventable injuries continue to occur. Nurses must be aware of the possible causes of injury in each age group in order to carry out anticipatory preventive teaching. For example, the guidelines for injury prevention during infancy presented in Box 36-1 should be discussed before the child reaches the susceptible age group. Preventive teaching ideally occurs during pregnancy.

Two thirds of all injuries to children occur in the home, thus the importance of safety cannot be overemphasized. The Patient Teaching box contains a home safety checklist that can be presented to parents to increase their awareness of danger areas in the home and assist them in implementing safety devices and practices before their absence leads to injury in infants. In addition, displays such as a safety demonstration board can be helpful in familiarizing parents with inexpensive commercial devices that can be used in the home to prevent injuries (Fig. 36-15). To help parents appreciate the dangers to young children that are present in their home, the nurse can suggest that they get down on the floor at the child's eye level to survey the environment from a child's viewpoint.

Injury prevention requires protection of the child and education of the caregiver. Nurses in ambulatory care settings, health maintenance centres, or visiting nurse agencies are in a favourable position to provide injury education. Nurses in inpatient facilities could use visiting times as an opportunity for discussing this topic.

One approach to teaching prevention of injury is to relate why children in various age groups are prone to specific types of injuries. Stressing prevention is just as important as emphasizing the "why" of the injury. However, injury prevention must also be practical. Asking parents for their ideas can lead to realistic suggestions to be followed.

If an injury has occurred, the nurse should not be too quick to admonish the parent; injuries do not always indicate neglect. It is a difficult task to watch children carefully without overprotecting or unnecessarily confining them. Allowing children to explore while maintaining consistent, age-appropriate limits is sound advice.

Parents need to remember that infants and young children cannot anticipate danger or understand when it is or is not present. A dead electrical wire may present no actual harm; but if the child is allowed to play with it, a poor behaviour develops and may be practised when the child encounters a live wire. Although it is always wise to explain why something is dangerous, it must be remembered that small children need to be physically removed from the situation.

It is not easy to teach safety, supervise closely, and refrain from saying "no" a hundred times a day. Parents become acutely aware of this dilemma as soon as the infant learns to crawl. Preventing injuries to children is usually the first reason for limit-setting and discipline, but limits are also set to prevent danger to valuable household objects. When small children are in the home, dangerous objects must be removed or guarded and valuable articles placed out of reach.

When children are taught the meaning of "no," they should also be taught what "yes" means. Children should be praised for playing with suitable toys, their efforts at behaving or listening should be reinforced, and innovative and creative recreational toys should be provided for them. Infants love to tear paper and avidly pursue books, magazines, or newspapers left on the floor. Instead of always scolding them for destroying a valued book, child-safe books (such as those constructed of

PATIENT TEACHING Child Safety Home Checklist

Safety: Fire, Electrical, Burns

__ Guards in front of or around any heating appliance, fireplace, or furnace (including electric heaters)*
__ Electrical wires are hidden or out of reach*
__ No frayed or broken wires; no overloaded sockets
__ Plastic guards or caps over electrical outlets, furniture in front of outlets*
__ Hanging tablecloths are out of reach, away from open fires*
__ Smoke detectors tested and operating properly
__ Kitchen matches stored out of child's reach*
__ Large, deep ashtrays throughout house (if used)
__ Small stoves, heaters, and other hot objects (cigarettes, candles, coffee pots, slow-cookers) are placed where they cannot be tipped over or reached by children
__ Hot water heater is set at 49°C or lower
__ Pot handles are turned toward back of stove, centre of table
__ No loose clothing is worn near stove
__ No cooking or eating of hot foods or liquids with the child standing nearby or sitting in lap
__ All small appliances, such as irons, are turned off, disconnected, and placed out of reach when not in use
__ A cool, not hot, mist vaporizer is used
__ Fire extinguisher is available on each floor and checked periodically
__ Electrical fuse box and gas shutoff accessible
__ Family escape plan in case of a fire is practised periodically; fire escape ladder is available on upper-level floors
__ Telephone number of fire or rescue squad and address of home with nearest cross street posted near phone

Safety: Suffocation and Aspiration

__ Small objects are stored out of reach*
__ Toys inspected for small removable parts or long strings*
__ Hanging crib toys and mobiles placed out of reach
__ Plastic bags are stored away from young child's reach, large plastic garment bags discarded after tying in knots*
__ Mattress or pillow is not covered with plastic or in manner accessible to child*
__ Crib design is according to government regulations (crib slats less than 6 cm apart) with snug-fitting mattress*†
__ Crib is positioned away from other furniture or windows*
__ Portable playpen gates are up at all times while in use*
__ Accordion-style gates are not used*
__ Bathroom doors are kept closed and toilet seats down*
__ Faucets are turned off firmly*
__ Pool is fenced with locked gate
__ Proper safety equipment is at poolside
__ Electric garage door openers are stored safely and garage door adjusted to rise when door strikes object
__ Doors of oven, trunks, dishwasher, refrigerator, and front-loading clothes washer and dryer are kept closed*
__ Unused appliance, such as a refrigerator, is securely locked or doors are removed*
__ Food is served in small, noncylindrical pieces*
__ Toy chests are without lids or with lids that securely lock in open position*
__ Buckets and wading pools are kept empty when not in use*
__ Clothesline is above head level
__ At least one member of household is trained in basic life support (cardiopulmonary resuscitation), including first aid for choking

Safety: Poisoning

__ Toxic substances, including batteries, are placed on a high shelf, preferably in locked cabinet
__ Toxic plants are hung or placed out of reach*
__ Excess quantities of cleaning fluids, paints, pesticides, medications, and other toxic substances are not stored in home
__ Used containers of poisonous substances discarded where child cannot obtain access
__ Telephone number of local poison control centre and address of home with nearest cross street posted near phones
__ Medicines are clearly labelled in childproof containers and stored out of reach
__ Household cleaners, disinfectants, and insecticides are kept in their original containers, separate from food, and out of reach
__ Smoking takes place in areas away from children, with no smoking in child's room or bed

Safety: Falls

__ Nonskid mats, strips, or surfaces in tubs and showers
__ Exits, halls, and passageways in rooms are kept clear of toys, furniture, boxes, or other items that could be obstructive
__ Stairs and halls are well lighted, with switches at both top and bottom
__ Sturdy handrails for all steps and stairways
__ Nothing stored on stairways
__ Treads, risers, and carpeting in good repair
__ Glass doors and walls are marked with decals
__ Safety glass is used in doors, windows, and walls
__ Gates are on top and bottom of staircases and elevated areas, such as porch, fire escape*
__ Guardrails are on upstairs windows with locks that limit height of window opening and access to areas such as fire escape*
__ Crib side rails are raised to full height; mattress lowered as child grows*
__ Restraints are used in high chairs or other baby furniture; preferably, walkers with wheels are not used*
__ Scatter rugs are secured in place or used with nonskid backing
__ Walks, patios, and driveways are in good repair

Safety: Bodily Injury

__ Knives, power tools, and unloaded firearms are stored safely or placed in locked cabinet
__ Garden tools are returned to storage racks after use
__ Pets are properly restrained and immunized for rabies
__ Swings, slides, and other outdoor play equipment are kept in safe condition
__ Yard is free of broken glass, nail-studded boards, other litter
__ Cement birdbaths are placed where young child cannot tip them over*

*Safety measures are specific for homes with young children. All safety measures should be implemented in homes where children reside and visit frequently, such as those of grandparents or baby-sitters. Information about home safety can be obtained at http://www.safekidscanada.ca.
†Government regulations are available at Health Canada: http://www.hc-sc.gc.ca/index-eng.php.

fabric) can be kept available for them to play with. If they enjoy pots and pans, a cabinet can be arranged with safe utensils for them to explore.

One additional factor must be stressed concerning injury prevention and education: Children are imitators; they copy what they see and hear. *Practising safety teaches safety.* This applies to parents and their children and to nurses and their patients. Saying one thing but doing another confuses children and can lead to difficulties as the child grows older.

Anticipatory Guidance—Care of Families

Childrearing is no easy task; it presents challenges to both new and "seasoned" parents. Society's changing roles and mores, combined with a highly mobile population, leave little stability for traditional role models and time-honoured methods of raising children. As a result, parents look to professionals for guidance. Nurses are in an advantageous position to render assistance and offer suggestions. Every phase of a child's life has its particular traumas—toilet training for toddlers, unexplained fears for preschoolers, and identity crises for adolescents. For parents of an infant, some challenges centre around dependency, discipline, increased mobility, and safety. Major areas for parental guidance during the first year are listed in the Patient Teaching box.

PATIENT TEACHING Guidance During Infant's First Year

First 6 Months

- Teach car safety with use of a government-approved restraint, facing toward the rear, in the middle of the back seat—not in a front seat with an air bag.
- Understand each parent's adjustment to the newborn, especially the mother's postpartum emotional needs.
- Teach care of the infant and help parents understand the infant's individual needs and temperament and that the infant expresses wants through crying.
- Reassure parents that the infant cannot be spoiled by too much attention during the first 4 to 6 months.
- Encourage parents to establish a schedule that meets the needs of the child and themselves.
- Help parents understand the infant's need for stimulation in the environment.
- Support parents' pleasure in seeing the child's growing friendliness and social response, especially smiling.
- Plan anticipatory guidance for safety.
- Stress the need for immunizations.
- Prepare parents for the introduction of solid foods.

Second 6 Months

- Prepare parents for the child's "stranger anxiety."
- Encourage parents to allow the child to cling to them and avoid long separation from either parent.
- Guide parents in disciplining their child because of the infant's increasing mobility.
- Encourage use of negative voice and eye contact rather than physical punishment as a means of discipline.
- Encourage showing the most attention when the infant is behaving well, rather than when the infant is crying.
- Teach injury prevention, because of the child's advancing motor skills and curiosity.
- Encourage parents to leave the child with a suitable caregiver to allow them some free time.
- Discuss readiness for weaning (as desired).
- Explore parents' feelings about their infant's sleep patterns.

SPECIAL HEALTH PROBLEMS

Feeding Difficulties

Regurgitation and "Spitting Up"

The return of small amounts of food after a feeding is a common occurrence during infancy. It should not be confused with actual vomiting, which can be associated with a number of disturbances that may be insignificant or serious. Regurgitation is usually benign, although persistent regurgitation necessitates medical evaluation to rule out gastroesophageal reflux. For clarification, the following terms are defined:

Regurgitation—Return of undigested food from the stomach, usually accompanied by burping

Spitting up—Dribbling of unswallowed formula from the infant's mouth immediately after a feeding

The normal occurrence of regurgitation or spitting up should be explained to parents, especially to those who are unduly concerned about it. Regurgitation can be reduced by some simple measures such as frequent burping during and after feeding, minimum handling during and after feeding, and positioning the child on the right side with the head slightly elevated after feeding. The inconvenience of spitting up can be managed with the use of absorbent bibs on the infant and protective cloths on the parent.

Sometimes frequent dribbling of formula causes **excoriation** of the chin, neck, and corners of the mouth. Keeping the area dry promotes healing but can be difficult to maintain. Helpful suggestions include applying a thin film of a moisture barrier cream such as A&D emollient ointment to the affected areas after cleansing and using absorbent, nonplastic-lined terry cloth bibs.

Colic (Paroxysmal Abdominal Pain)

Colic is reported to occur in 5 to 30% of all infants (Neu & Robinson, 2003) and has no particular affinity with regard to the gender, race, or socioeconomic status of the infant and family (Cirgin Ellett, 2003). The condition is generally described as paroxysmal abdominal pain or cramping that is manifested by loud crying and drawing the legs up to the abdomen. Other definitions include variables such as duration of cry greater than 3 hours a day, occurring more than 3 days per week, and parental dissatisfaction with the child's behaviour. Some studies report an increase in symptoms (fussiness and crying) in the late afternoon or evening; however, in some infants the onset of symptoms occurs at another time. Colic is more common in infants under 3 months of age than in older infants, and infants with so-called difficult temperaments are more likely to be colicky. Despite the obvious behavioural indications of pain, the child tolerates breast milk or some type of infant formula well, gains weight, and usually thrives. There is no evidence of a residual effect of colic on older children, except perhaps a strained parent–child relationship in some cases; in other words, infants who are colicky grow up to be normal children and adults.

Among the theories that have been investigated as potential causes are too-rapid feeding, overeating, swallowing excessive air, improper feeding technique (especially in positioning and burping), and emotional stress or tension between parent and child. Although all of these may occur, there is no evidence that one factor is consistently present. In some infants, colic may be a sign of cow's milk allergy (CMA) or intolerance, and eliminating cow's milk products from the diets of infants and lactating mothers can reduce the symptoms; in some infants, soy milk may cause the same discomfort as cow's milk. Parental smoking, strained parent–infant interaction, lactase deficiency, difficult infant temperament, difficulty regulating emotions, central nervous system immaturity, and neurochemical dysregulation in the brain have also been proposed as potential causes of colic (Cirgin Ellett, 2003; Neu & Robinson, 2003). A positive association between the consumption of fruit juices (carbohydrate malabsorption) and colic has been demonstrated in some cases (Duro et al., 2002). The consensus of most experts who study colic is that it is multifactorial in nature and no single treatment for every colicky infant will be effective in alleviating the symptoms.

Therapeutic Management

Management of colic should begin with an investigation of possible organic causes, such as CMA, intussusception, or other gastrointestinal problem. If a sensitivity to cow's milk is strongly suspected, a trial substitution of another formula such as an extensively hydrolyzed (Nutramigen, Alimentum, Pregestimil), whey hydrolysate, or amino acid (Neocate, EleCare) formula is warranted. Soy formulas are usually avoided because of the possibility of sensitivity to soy protein as well. Oral administration of *Lactobacillus reuteri* to colicky breastfed infants decreased symptoms within 1 week of initiation in one small study (Savino et al., 2007).

The use of medications, including sedatives, antispasmodics, antihistamines, and antiflatulents, is sometimes recommended. The most commonly used sedatives are phenobarbital, hydroxyzine hydrochloride (Atarax), and chloral hydrate. Simethicone (Mylicon) may also help allay the symptoms of colic. However, in most controlled studies, none of these medications completely eliminated the symptoms of colic. Chamomile tea offered at the onset of crying and up to three times daily has proved effective in relieving the symptoms of colic in some infants (Weizman et al., 1993); however, parents are to be cautioned regarding the unknown safety of this treatment (Crotteau, Wright, & Eglash, 2006). Behavioural interventions have not proved effective at reducing symptoms of colic but have helped parents deal with the crying infant in a more positive manner. The addition of lactase to infant formula has produced mixed results in the abatement of overall symptoms.

One study found that a combination of interventions—massage, herbal tea, sucrose solution, and hydrolyzed formula—decreased crying in reported colicky infants; the administration of the hydrolyzed formula achieved best results, whereas massage was least effective at reducing crying (Arikan et al., 2008).

An extensive review of a wide variety of interventions for colic indicates that there are no specific safe remedies to alleviate symptoms of colic in every infant; dietary changes such as eliminating cow's milk protein from the lactating mother's diet and behavioural interventions were shown to be effective in helping parents reduce stimulation and respond to the infant's crying, yet these interventions are perceived only as moderately effective (Joanna Briggs Institute, 2004).

Nursing Care Management

The initial step in managing colic is to take a thorough, detailed history of the usual daily events. Areas that should be stressed include (1) the infant's diet; (2) the diet of the breastfeeding mother; (3) the time of day when crying occurs; (4) the relationship of the crying to feeding time; (5) the presence of specific family members during the crying and habits of family members, such as smoking; (6) activity of the mother or usual caregiver before, during, and after the crying; (7) characteristics of the cry (e.g., duration, intensity); (8) measures used to relieve the crying and their effectiveness; and (9) the infant's stooling, voiding, and sleeping patterns. Of special emphasis is a careful assessment of the feeding process via demonstration by the parent.

If cow's milk sensitivity is suspected, breastfeeding mothers should follow a milk-free diet for a minimum of 3 to 5 days in an attempt to reduce the infant's symptoms. Mothers need to be cautioned that some nondairy creamers may contain calcium caseinate, a cow's milk protein. If a milk-free diet is helpful, lactating mothers may need calcium supplements to meet the body's requirement. Bottle-fed infants may improve with the same dietary modifications as for the child with CMA (CPS, Nutrition and Gastroenterology Committee, 2011).

Perhaps the most important nursing intervention (once the diagnosis of colic is established) is reassurance of both parents that they are not doing anything wrong and that the infant is not experiencing any physical or emotional harm. Parents, especially mothers, become easily frustrated with the infant's crying and perceive this as a sign that there is something horribly wrong. An empathetic, gentle, and reassuring attitude, in addition to suggestions about remedies for treatment, will help allay parents' anxieties, which are usually exacerbated by loss of sleep and preoccupation over the infant's welfare. Other support persons and extended family members may be enlisted to help support the parents during this difficult time.

When no cause can be identified, helping parents understand the infant's crying behaviour and modifying parent interventions to promptly attend to the infant's needs can decrease the length of fussiness and crying. Other approaches for managing colic are listed in the Patient Teaching box. Parents should be encouraged to try as many of these approaches as possible, since not all are effective for every infant.

One author suggests that a problem-solving discussion with the parents, in addition to acknowledgment that the infant has colic, is an optimal strategy for helping parents manage the infant with colic until a cure is found (Cirgin Ellett, 2003). Nurses must also be aware that once colic symptoms are resolved, family function may be negatively affected by residual feelings and emotions experienced during the acute phase of the colic (Ellett, Schuff, & Davis, 2005).

PATIENT TEACHING Managing the Colicky Infant

- Place the awake infant prone over a covered hot-water bottle, heated towel, or covered heating pad.
- Massage the infant's abdomen.
- Respond immediately to the crying.
- Change the infant's position frequently; walk with the child's face down and body across the parent's arm, with the parent's hand under the infant's abdomen, applying gentle pressure (Fig. 36-14).
- Use a front carrier for transporting the infant.
- Swaddle the infant tightly with a soft, stretchy blanket.
- Place the infant in a wind-up swing.
- Take the infant for car rides or outside for a change in environment.
- Use bottles that minimize air swallowing (curved bottle or inner collapsible bag).
- Play soothing "white noise," in utero sounds, or music.*
- Provide smaller, frequent feedings; burp the infant during and after feedings using the shoulder position or sitting upright, and place the infant in an upright seat after feedings.
- Introduce a pacifier for added sucking.
- For breastfed infants, the mother could try avoiding all milk products for a trial period.
- If household members smoke they should avoid smoking near the infant; smoking must be done outside the home.
- Give an appropriate dose of acetaminophen elixir or suppository if suggested by the health care provider; this is not recommended for daily use.
- If nothing reduces the crying, place the infant in the crib and allow to cry; periodically hold and comfort the child and put down again.

*Suggested infant relaxation music: Heartbeat Lullabies, by Terry Woodford. Available from Baby-Go-To-Sleep Center, Audio Therapy Innovations, Inc., PO Box 550, Colorado Springs, CO 80901; 800-537-7748; http://www.babygotosleep.com.

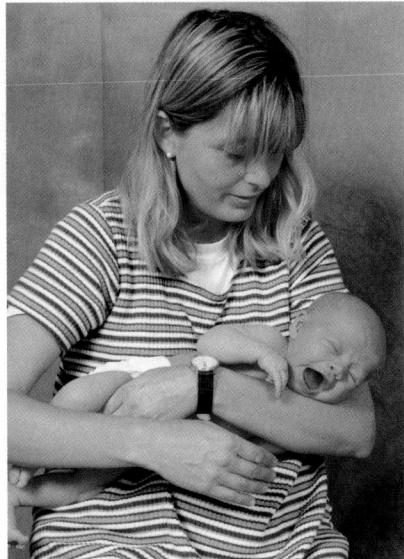

Fig. 36-14 The "colic carry" may be comforting to an infant with colic. *(Photo by Paul Vincent Kuntz, Texas Children's Hospital, Houston.)*

Practical parental support interventions include the provision of a colic hotline (mother-to-nurse practitioner or nurse) and nurse-managed colic support groups (Ellett et al., 2005).

Growth Failure (Failure to Thrive)

Growth failure, or *failure to thrive* (FTT), is a sign of inadequate growth resulting from an inability to obtain or use calories required for growth. FTT has no universal definition, although one of the more common parameters is a weight (and sometimes height) that falls below the fifth percentile for the child's age. Another definition of FTT includes a weight for age (height) z-value of less than −2.0 (a z-value is a standard deviation value that represents anthropometric data normalizing for sex and age with greater precision than growth percentile curves) (Markowitz & Duggan, 2003). The new Canadian growth charts, developed by the Dietitians of Canada, Canadian Paediatric Society, the College of Family Physicians of Canada, and the Community Health Nurses of Canada (2010), should be used to measure growth. Growth measurements alone, however, are not used to diagnose children with FTT. Rather, the finding of a pattern of persistent deviation from established growth parameters is cause for concern. In addition to lack of consensus on the precise definition of FTT, there are those who advocate for a change in terminology; thus terms such as *growth failure* and *pediatric undernutrition* are used in the literature for FTT (Locklin, 2005).

Some experts, however, suggest that the previously used classifications of organic FTT and nonorganic FTT are too simplistic because most cases of growth failure have mixed causes. They suggest that FTT be classified according to pathophysiology in the following categories: (1) inadequate caloric intake—incorrect formula preparation, neglect, food fads, excessive juice consumption, poverty, behavioural problems affecting eating, or central nervous system problems affecting intake; (2) inadequate absorption—cystic fibrosis, celiac disease, vitamin or mineral deficiencies, biliary atresia, or hepatic disease; (3) increased metabolism—hyperthyroidism, congenital heart defects, or chronic immunodeficiency; and (4) defective utilization—genetic anomaly such as trisomy 21 or 18, congenital infection, or metabolic storage diseases (Krugman & Dubowitz, 2003). The cause of growth failure is often multifactorial and involves a combination of infant organic disease, dysfunctional parenting behaviours, subtle neurological or behavioural problems, and disturbed parent–child interactions (Block, Krebs, & AAP, Committee on Child Abuse and Neglect and Committee on Nutrition, 2005).

Other factors that can contribute to inadequate caloric intake in infancy include poverty, health or childrearing beliefs such as fad diets, inadequate nutritional knowledge, family stress, feeding resistance, and insufficient breast milk.

Diagnostic Evaluation

Diagnosis is initially made from evidence of growth failure. If FTT is recent, the weight, but not the height, is below accepted standards (usually the fifth percentile); if FTT is longstanding, both weight and height are low, indicating chronic malnutrition. Perhaps as important as anthropometric measurements are a complete health and dietary history (including perinatal history), physical examination for evidence of organic causes, developmental assessment, and family assessment. A dietary intake history, either a 24-hour food intake or a history of food consumed over a 3- to 5-day period, is also essential. In addition, the child's activity level, perceived food allergies, and dietary restrictions, as well as parental height, should be explored. An assessment of household organization and mealtime behaviours and rituals is important in the collection of pertinent data. Other tests (lead toxicity, anemia, stool-reducing substances, occult blood, ova and parasites, alkaline phosphatase, and zinc levels) are selected only as indicated to rule out organic problems. To prevent the overuse of diagnostic procedures, FTT should be considered early in the differential diagnosis. To avoid the social stigma of FTT during the early investigative phase, many health care workers use the term *growth delay* (or *failure*) until the actual cause is established.

Therapeutic Management

The primary management of FTT is aimed at reversing the cause of the growth failure. If malnutrition is severe, the initial treatment is directed at reversing the malnutrition. The goal is to provide sufficient calories to support "catch-up" growth—a rate of growth greater than the expected rate for age. Any coexisting medical problems are treated.

In most cases of FTT, an interdisciplinary team of physician, nurse, dietitian, child life specialist, occupational therapist, pediatric feeding specialist, and social worker or mental health care provider is needed to deal with the multiple problems. The team may improve the child's nutritional status by providing comprehensive care addressing the biological, psychiatric, and socioeconomic aspects of the child's life (Duggan, Markowitz, & Watkins, 2008). Efforts are made to relieve any additional stresses on the family by offering referrals to welfare agencies or supplemental food programs. In some cases, family therapy may be required; temporary placement in a foster home may relieve the family's stress, protect the child, and allow the child some stability if insurmountable obstacles are preventing appropriate family functioning. Behaviour modification aimed at mealtime rituals (or lack thereof) and family social time may be required. Hospitalization admission is indicated for (1) evidence (anthropometric) of severe acute malnutrition, (2) child abuse or neglect, (3) significant dehydration, (4) caretaker substance use or psychosis, (5) serious intercurrent infection, or (6) outpatient management that does not result in weight gain.

Prognosis

The prognosis for FTT is related to the cause. There are few long-term studies that provide sufficient data for children with FTT; however, some studies indicate that children who had FTT as infants had shorter heights, lower weights, and lower scores on measures of psychomotor development than peers (Rudolf & Logan, 2005). The authors of the analysis caution against widespread generalization based on these findings. Factors related to poor prognosis are severe feeding resistance, lack of awareness in and cooperation from the parent(s), low family income, low maternal educational level, adolescent mother, and early age of onset of FTT. Because later cognitive and motor function is affected by malnourishment in infancy, many of these children may be below normal in intellectual development, have poorer language development and less developed reading skills, attain lower social maturity, and have a higher incidence of behavioural disturbances. Such findings indicate that a long-term plan and follow-up care are needed for the optimum development of these children.

Nursing Care Management

Caring for the child with FTT presents many nursing challenges, whether treatment takes place in the hospital, clinic, or home. Providing a positive feeding environment, teaching the parents successful feeding strategies, and supporting the child and family are essential components of care.

Nurses play a critical role in the diagnosis of FTT through their assessment of the child, parents, and family interactions. Knowledge of the characteristics of children with FTT and their families is essential in helping identify these children and hastening the confirmation of a diagnosis (Box 36-2). Accurate assessment of initial weight and height and daily weight, as well as recording of all food intake, is essential. The nurse needs to document the child's feeding behaviour and the parent–child interaction during feeding, other caregiving activities, and play.

A feature of many children with FTT is their irregularity (low rhythmicity) in activities of daily living. Some children with FTT may typify the "difficult" temperament pattern. However, another type is the passive, sleepy, lethargic infant who does not wake up for feedings. Parents who have been advised to adhere to on-demand feeding schedules may be unsure of whether to wake the child or let the child sleep. Because of their inexperience and lack of guidance, parents may develop a pattern of infrequent feeding that is inadequate to meet the infant's nutritional needs. Such a pattern is particularly detrimental with the breastfeeding infant, for whom frequent nursing is essential to an adequate milk supply.

Some parents are at increased risk for attachment problems because of (1) isolation and social crisis; (2) inadequate support systems, such as for teenage and single mothers; and (3) poor parenting role models as a child. Other factors that

BOX 36-2 Clinical Manifestations of Growth Failure (Failure to Thrive)

- Growth failure (see p. 1005 for definitions)
- Malnutrition
- Developmental delays—social, motor, adaptive, language
- Apathy
- Poor hygiene in some cases
- Withdrawn behaviour
- Feeding or eating disorders, such as vomiting, feeding resistance, anorexia
- No fear of strangers (at age when stranger anxiety is normal)
- Avoidance of eye contact
- Wide-eyed gaze and continual scan of the environment ("radar gaze")
- Stiff and unyielding or flaccid and unresponsive
- Minimal smiling

should be considered are lack of education; physical and mental health problems such as physical and sexual abuse, depression, or drug dependence; immaturity, especially in adolescent parents; and lack of commitment to parenting, such as giving priority to entertainment or employment. Often these parents and their families are under stress and in multiple chronic emotional, social, and financial crises.

Because part of the difficulty between parent and child is dissatisfaction and frustration, the child should have a primary core of nurses (Fig. 36-15). The nurses caring for the child can learn to perceive the child's cues and reverse the cycle of dissatisfaction, especially in the area of feeding. Depending on the cause of FTT, children may be treated on an outpatient basis.

Because many of these children are responding to stimuli that have led to the negative feeding patterns, the first goal is to structure the feeding environment in such a way to encourage eating. Initially staff members and a feeding specialist may need to feed these children to assess thoroughly the difficulties encountered during the feeding process and to devise strategies that eliminate or minimize such problems. General guidelines for the feeding process are outlined in the Guidelines box.

Four primary goals in the nutritional management of FTT are to (1) correct nutritional deficiencies and achieve ideal weight for height, (2) enable catch-up growth, (3) restore optimum body composition, and (4) educate the parents or primary caregivers regarding the child's nutritional requirements and appropriate feeding methods (Corrales & Utter, 2005; Maggioni & Lifshitz, 1995). To increase caloric intake in formula-fed infants, supplements such as Polycose or medium-chain triglycerides may be added slowly. For infants, 24 kcal/30 mL formulas may be provided to increase caloric intake; older children (1 to 6 years) may benefit from a 30 kcal/30 mL formula (AAP, 2009). Other carbohydrate additives include fortified rice cereal and vegetable oil. Because vitamin and mineral deficiencies may be present, multivitamin

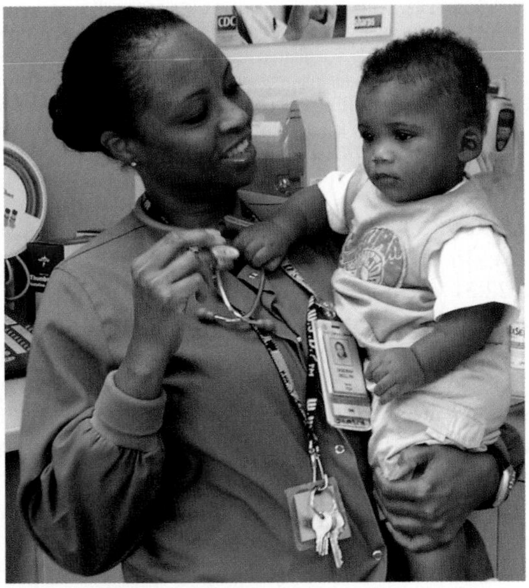

Fig. 36-15 Consistent nursing contact is important in developing trust in infants with failure to thrive.

supplementation, including zinc and iron, is recommended. Usually only in extreme cases of malnourishment are tube feedings or intravenous therapy required.

Besides attending to the physical needs of the child, the interdisciplinary team must plan care for appropriate developmental stimulation. After an approximate **developmental age** is established, a planned program of play is begun. Ideally, a child life specialist is involved to implement and supervise the stimulation program. Every effort should be made to teach the parent how to play and interact with the child.

Nursing care of these children involves a family systems approach. In other words, for the entire family to become healthy, each member must be helped to change. Care of the parents is aimed at helping them increase their feelings of self-esteem through positive, successful parenting skills. Initially this necessitates providing an environment in which they feel

GUIDELINES Feeding Children With Growth Failure (Failure to Thrive)

Provide a primary core of staff to feed the child. The same nurses are able to learn the child's cues and respond consistently.

Provide a quiet, unstimulating atmosphere. A number of these children are very distractible, and their attention is diverted with minimal stimuli. Older children do well at a feeding table; younger children should always be held.

Maintain a calm, even temperament throughout the meal. The child may have a habit of negative outbursts. Limits on eating behaviour definitely need to be provided, but they should be stated in a firm, calm tone. If the nurse is hurried or anxious, the feeding process will not be optimized.

Talk to the child by giving directions about eating. "Take a bite, Lisa" is appropriate and directive. The more distractible the child, the more directive the nurse should be to refocus attention on feeding. Positive comments about feeding need to be actively given.

Be persistent. This is perhaps one of the most important guidelines. Parents often give up when the child begins negative feeding behaviour. Calm perseverance through 10 to 15 minutes of food refusal will eventually diminish negative behaviour. Although forced feeding should be avoided, "strictly encouraged" feeding is essential.

Maintain a face-to-face posture with the child when possible. Encourage eye contact and remain with the child throughout the meal.

Introduce new foods slowly. Often these children have been exclusively bottle-fed. If acceptance of solids is a problem, begin with puréed food and, once accepted, advance to junior and regular solid foods.

Follow the child's rhythm of feeding. The child will set a rhythm when the previous conditions are met.

Develop a structured routine. Disruptions in their other activities of daily living have great impact on feeding responses, so bathing, sleeping, dressing, and playing, as well as feeding, should be structured. The nurse should feed the child in the same way and place as often as possible. The length of the feeding should also be established (usually 30 minutes).

welcomed and accepted. Because these parents are often distrustful of authority figures, it may take some time before they trust the nurse. One approach is to empathize with the parent about the difficulties of childrearing. For example, the nurse may state that many parents find adjusting to parenthood a trying time or that the demands of caring for an infant can become overwhelming.

The nurse teaches infant care techniques to the parents through example and demonstration rather than by lecturing. As the nurse perceives the infant's cues, he or she emphasizes these to the parents. For example, during a feeding the nurse might comment that the infant is still hungry because the child sucks vigorously and looks at the nurse. When the infant is satisfied, the nurse can point out that the infant is signalling this by releasing the strong suck, closing the eyes, and breathing deeply and more slowly.

Plans usually need to be made to implement these interventions at home and may include a home health referral. Social agencies that can provide financial or housing assistance to lessen the stress of everyday life should also be contacted.

Disorders of Unknown Etiology

Sudden Infant Death Syndrome

Sudden infant death syndrome (SIDS) is defined as the sudden death of an infant younger than 1 year of age that remains unexplained after a complete postmortem examination, including an investigation of the death scene and a review of the case history. Since 2002, the data have included another term, *sudden unexplained death in infants* (SUDI). More recently there has been a dramatic decrease in the numbers of SIDS/SUDI cases; this decrease is attributed to the Back to Sleep campaign, initiated in 1999. (See Additional Resources at the end of this chapter for further information on Back to Sleep teaching programs.) SIDS and SUDI combined are the third leading cause of infant deaths (birth to 12 months) and the first leading cause of postneonatal deaths (between 1 and 12 months) (Heron and Smith, 2007). In 2008, SIDS/SUDI claimed the lives of 107 infants in Canada (Statistics Canada, 2011).

Table 36-6 summarizes the major epidemiological characteristics of SIDS.

Table 36-6 Epidemiology of Sudden Infant Death Syndrome (SIDS)

FACTORS	OCCURRENCE
Incidence	107 infants (2008)
Age	Less than 1 year
Sex	Higher percentage of males affected
Time of death	During sleep
Time of year	Increased incidence in winter
Socioeconomic	Increased occurrence in lower socioeconomic class
Birth	Higher incidence in: • Preterm infants, especially infants of extremely and very low birth weight • Multiple births • Neonates with low Apgar scores • Infants with central nervous system disturbances and respiratory disorders such as bronchopulmonary dysplasia • Increasing birth order (subsequent siblings as opposed to firstborn child) • Infants with a recent history of illness
Sleep habits	Highest risk associated with prone position; use of soft bedding; overheating (thermal stress); cosleeping with adult, especially on sofa or noninfant bed
	Infants cosleeping with adult at higher risk if <11 wk old
Feeding habits	Lower incidence in breastfed infants
Pacifier	Lower incidence in infants put to sleep with pacifier
Maternal	Young age; cigarette smoking, especially during pregnancy; poor prenatal care; substance use (heroin, methadone, cocaine); a few studies have shown an increased risk in infants exposed to second-hand environmental tobacco smoke

(Data from American Academy of Pediatrics, Task Force on Infant Sleep Position and Sudden Infant Death Syndrome. [2000]. Changing concepts of sudden infant death syndrome: Implications for infant sleeping environment and sleep position. *Pediatrics, 105*[3], 650–656; American Academy of Pediatrics, Task Force on Sudden Infant Death Syndrome. [2005]. The changing concept of sudden infant death syndrome: Diagnostic coding shifts, controversies regarding the sleeping environment, and new variables to consider in reducing risk. *Pediatrics, 116*[5], 1245–1255; Canadian Paediatric Society, Community Paediatrics Committee. [2004]. Recommendations for safe sleeping environments for infants and children. *Paediatrics and Child Health, 9*[9], 659–663; Statistics Canada. [2011]. *Leading causes of death, infants, by sex, Canada, annual.* Retrieved from http://www5.statcan.gc.ca/cansim/pick-choisir?lang=eng&p2=33&id=1020562.)

Etiology

Numerous theories have been proposed regarding the etiology of SIDS/SUDI; however, the cause remains unknown. One compelling hypothesis is that SIDS/SUDI is related to a **brainstem** abnormality in the neurological regulation of cardiorespiratory control. Abnormalities include prolonged sleep apnea, increased frequency of brief inspiratory pauses, excessive **periodic breathing,** and impaired arousal responsiveness to increased carbon dioxide or decreased oxygen. However, sleep apnea is not the cause of SIDS/SUDI. The vast majority of infants with apnea do not die, and only a minority of SIDS victims have documented apparent life-threatening events (ALTEs) (see Apnea and Apparent Life-Threatening Events, p. 1012). Numerous studies indicate that there is no association between SIDS/SUDI and any childhood vaccine.

A genetic predisposition to SIDS/SUDI has been postulated as a cause. In one study, a genetic mutation on chromosome 6q 22.1-22.31 was positively linked to a syndrome of SIDS and dysgenesis of the testis (Puffenberger et al., 2004). Infants who are male, premature, or of low birth weight, as well infants from socio-economically disadvantaged and Aboriginal populations, have a higher incidence of SIDS (PHAC, 2011b).

Maternal smoking during pregnancy has emerged in numerous epidemiological studies as a major factor in SIDS, and tobacco smoke in the infant's environment after birth has also been shown to have a possible relationship with the incidence of SIDS (AAP, Task Force on Sudden Infant Death Syndrome, 2005). Data show that exposure to tobacco smoke increased an infant's risk for SIDS 1.9 times over that of infants not exposed; 59% of SIDS deaths in smoke-exposed infants were attributed to maternal smoking (Anderson, Johnson, & Batal, 2005). It has been postulated that 12% of all SIDS deaths could be prevented with prenatal maternal smoking cessation (Pollack, 2001). One mechanism proposed as a link between maternal smoking and SIDS is a decrease in the infant's ability to arouse to auditory stimuli in mothers who smoked prenatally (Franco et al., 1999). Increased nicotine concentrations in lung tissue were found in children who died from SIDS compared with a group of control children (McMartin et al., 2002).

Bed sharing refers to a child sharing a bed with an adult or older child on a noninfant bed. Bed sharing has been reported to have an increased association with SIDS. One survey found a high association between infant deaths, use of nonstandard beds (sofa, day bed), and bed sharing; a large percentage of infants were found dead on their backs when bed sharing, which suggests suffocation (Unger et al., 2003). A study from Scotland indicates that, when bed sharing, the risk for SIDS is significantly increased for infants less than 11 weeks of age (Tappin, Ecob, & Brooke, 2005). Other studies have correlated higher incidences of SIDS in the context of infant bed sharing when there is also maternal smoking, bed sharing with multiple family members, maternal overweight, soft bedding, or unintentional asphyxiation resulting from adult intoxication (overlaying) (AAP, Task Force on Sudden Infant Death Syndrome, 2005; CPS, Community Paediatrics Committee, 2004; Carroll-Pankhurst & Mortimer, 2001; Hauck et al., 2003; McGarvey et al., 2003; Person, Lavezzi, & Wolf, 2002). Hauck and colleagues (2003) found that bed sharing and SIDS correlated positively only in cases where the infant was sleeping with someone other than the parent; a high number of SIDS cases involved sleeping on a sofa.

In another report, in which all of the SUDI cases in Québec from 1991 to 2000 were studied, the researchers found that 18% of the 443 cases of sudden death (81 infants) had been in unsafe sleeping environments (Gerez & Côté, 2002). Most often this involved an unaccustomed prone-sleeping situation. An infant lying on an adult bed with a pillow was the next most frequent occurrence; least common was an infant sharing a sofa with another person. In 93% of cases, SUDI occurred in a first-time sleeping arrangement. While there was no control group in this study, the data matched those of other controlgroup studies.

Room sharing refers to a situation in which an infant is sleeping in close proximity to another person in the same room but in a different bed. Room sharing with infants in the age range when most SIDS deaths occur has been shown to be preventive. The term co-sleeping can refer to a range of sleeping practices that include both bed sharing and room sharing. Definitions of this term are not consistent enough to make it universally acceptable (PHAC, 2011b). Co-sleeping occurs in many cultures, and the nurse needs to ensure she asks about this practice to provide appropriate health teaching (see Cultural Awareness box). The latest recommendation for prevention of SIDS from the Public Health Agency of Canada (2011b) is that the infant's crib or bassinette be placed in close proximity to the mother's bed and that the infant be placed in the adult bed only for breastfeeding, then placed to sleep in his or her own crib once the feeding session is completed.

CULTURAL AWARENESS

The Family Bed

Cosleeping, or sharing the "family bed," in which parents allow the children to sleep with them, is a relatively common and accepted practice, especially among populations with African origins, Latin American families, and Asian families, such as the Japanese (Schachter et al., 1989). Although there are no surveys of cosleeping among cultural groups in Canada, one survey in the United States indicates the practice is growing in some areas, especially among young (less than 18 years of age) Black and Asian women in the Southern states; infants in the survey who coslept with an adult were less than 8 weeks old (Willinger et al., 2003). Other groups that practise cosleeping include (1) single parents, whose need for company may encourage this practice; (2) working parents, who desire the closeness at night that was lost during the day; and (3) parents who have had an issue about sleep or separation in their own past (Brazelton, 1990). A study by Coleman (2009) found that Black parents may not value health teaching, particularly related to safe sleep practices. It supported a previous finding that meaningful, culturally beneficial care increases the likelihood that recipients will adhere to health care recommendations.

Other studies have linked sleep position with an increased risk of SIDS. Prone sleeping may cause oropharyngeal obstruction or affect thermal balance or arousal state. One study found that healthy full-term infants had significantly impaired arousal from active and quiet sleep states when sleeping prone (Horne et al., 2001). Rebreathing of carbon dioxide by infants in the prone position is another possible cause for SIDS. Infants sleeping prone and on soft bedding may not be able to move their heads to the side, thus increasing the risk of suffocation and lethal rebreathing. Evidence from other countries and the United States shows an increased incidence of SIDS in infants placed in a side-lying position; these infants are able to turn to a prone position. Thus the side-lying position is no longer recommended for infants sleeping at home or in day cares or hospitals (unless medically indicated); healthy infants be placed to sleep in the supine position (on the back) (PHAC, 2011b). Most preterm infants being discharged from the hospital should be placed in a supine sleeping position unless special factors predispose them to airway obstruction.

Parents need to know that certain sleep environments (prone sleeping, tobacco smoke exposure, soft bedding, noninfant bed surface, use of certain drugs by the individual sharing the bed with the infant, and thermal stress) can increase the risk for SIDS. Soft bedding such as waterbeds, sheepskins, beanbags, pillows, or quilts should be avoided for infant sleeping surfaces. Bedding items such as stuffed animals or toys should be removed from the crib while the infant is asleep (CPS, 2004). Head covering by a blanket has also been found to be a risk factor for SIDS, thus supporting the recommendation to avoid extra bed linens or other items (Mitchell et al., 2008).

Regarding the relation between breastfeeding and SIDS, one study indicated that breastfeeding during the first 16 weeks of life decreased the likelihood of SIDS (Alm et al., 2002). Some studies have found pacifier use in infants to be a protective factor against the occurrence of SIDS; the data for pacifier use in this population of infants (first year of life) are more compelling than data linking pacifier use to the development of dental complications and the inhibition of breastfeeding (Chapman, 2009; Jenik et al., 2009; Jenik & Vain, 2009). Therefore, the Canadian Paediatric Society (2012) has provided a parent guide on the safe use of nonsweetened pacifiers after successful breastfeeding, should parents want to give their infant a pacifier.

Although the etiology of SIDS is ultimately unknown, autopsies have revealed consistent pathological findings, such as pulmonary edema and intrathoracic hemorrhages, that confirm the diagnosis of SIDS. Consequently, autopsies should be performed on all infants suspected of dying of SIDS. The findings should be shared with the parents as soon as possible after the death.

Whether subsequent siblings of an infant who has died of SIDS are at increased risk for SIDS is unclear. Even if the increased risk is correct, families have a 99% chance that their subsequent child will *not* die of SIDS. A review of recurrent sibling deaths attributed to SIDS in England failed to ascertain a precise risk of recurrence; previous studies suggested a recurrence risk range of 1.7 to 10.1, yet the researchers concluded the studies had too many methodological flaws to draw any firm conclusions (Bacon et al., 2008). Others report that recurrence risks for a SIDS death in a family with a previous infant SIDS death range from 2 to 6% (AAP, Task Force on Sudden Infant Death Syndrome, 2005). Home monitoring is not recommended for this group of children, but it is often used by practitioners and may even be requested by parents. Monitoring is best initiated on an individual basis.

evolve **Case Study—Health Problems of Infants**

Nursing Care Management

Nurses have a vital role in preventing SIDS by educating families about practices that may reduce the risk of SIDS, such as avoiding smoking during pregnancy and near the infant; using the supine sleeping position for the infant; avoiding soft, mouldable mattresses, blankets, and pillows; avoiding bed sharing; breastfeeding the infant; and avoiding the infant's overheating during sleep. The infant's head position should be varied to prevent flattening of the skull (positional **plagiocephaly**) (see Patient Teaching box). Parents should be cautioned about the risk of using the prone sleeping position for infants from birth to 6 months of age and the dangers of the infant sleeping on noninfant surfaces along with adults or other children. Postpartum discharge planning, newborn discharges, follow-up home visits, well-baby clinic visits, and immunization visits provide excellent opportunities to educate parents in ways to prevent SIDS.

Additionally, nurses have an important role in modelling behaviours for parents to foster implementation of practices that can decrease the risk of SIDS, such as placing infants in a supine sleeping position in the hospital and limiting pacifier use to naps and bedtime only. In Canada the rate of SIDS decreased by 50% between 1999 and 2004, when prone-sleeping programs were instituted (PHAC, 2008). This decrease may be due to parental behaviour changes, such as placing infants in the prone sleeping position and fewer mothers smoking during pregnancy (Rusen, Sauve, Joseph, & Kramer, 2004). A concern of many health care workers is that infants placed on their back to sleep will aspirate emesis or mucus; studies have failed to show an increase in infant deaths, spitting up during sleep, aspiration, asphyxia, or respiratory failure as a result of supine sleep positioning. It is important that these workers model correct positions for parents (Malloy, 2002; Tablizo et al., 2007).

Loss of a child from SIDS presents several crises for the parents. In addition to grief and mourning the death of their child, the parents must face a tragedy that was sudden, unexpected, and unexplained. The psychological intervention for the family must deal with these additional variables. The discussion here focuses primarily on the objectives of care for families experiencing SIDS, rather than on the process of grief and mourning, which is explored in Chapter 41.

PATIENT TEACHING Safe Sleep for Infants—Reducing the Incidence of Sudden Unexpected Death in Infants

- Always place your baby to sleep on the back. Side and tummy positions are not safe.
- Use a crib that meets current safety standards. The mattress should be firm and fit snugly in the crib. Cover the mattress with only a tight-fitting crib sheet.
- Do not put anything soft, loose, or fluffy in your baby's sleep space. This includes pillows, blankets, comforters, soft or pillow-like bumpers, stuffed animals, and other soft items.
- Use a sleep sack or other type sleeper instead of blankets to keep your baby warm and safe. Make sure your baby doesn't get too warm during sleep.
- Place your baby's separate, safe sleep space near your bed to help you protect her or him and to make breastfeeding easier. This is called room sharing. Bed-sharing is not recommended.
- Never place your baby to sleep on top of any soft surface. This includes adult beds, waterbeds, pillows, cushions, comforters, and sheepskins.
- Do not use anything to prop your baby up or keep him or her on the back.
- Offer your baby a pacifier every time you place her or him down to sleep. If you are breastfeeding, wait until nursing is well established before using a pacifier (usually around 1 month.)
- Avoid smoking
- Educate everyone who cares for your baby about these safe sleep rules!

(Adapted from About Kids Health. [n.d.]. http://www.aboutkidshealth.ca/En/ResourceCentres/PregnancyBabies/NewbornBabies/HealthIssuesinYourNewbornBaby/Pages/Sudden-Infant-Death-Syndrome.aspx; Canadian Paediatric Society, Canadian Foundation for the Study of Infant Deaths, Canadian Institute of Child Health, Health Canada, & Public Health Agency of Canada (2011). *The joint statement on safe sleep: Preventing sudden infant deaths in Canada.* Retrieved from http://www.phac-aspc.gc.ca/hp-ps/dca-dea/stages-etapes/childhood-enfance_0-2/sids/jsss-ecss-eng.php.)

Finding the Infant

Usually it is the mother who finds the child dead in the crib. Typically, the child is in a dishevelled bed, with blankets over the head, and huddled in a corner. Frothy, blood-tinged fluid fills the mouth and nostrils, and the infant may be lying face down in the secretions, suggesting that he or she bled to death. The diaper is wet and full of stool, which is consistent with a cataclysmic type of death. The hands may be clutching the sheets, as if the child were in distress before death. The child's initial appearance, combined with the shock of such an unexpected event, adds to the horror that the parents must face.

Often the mother is alone when she finds the child and must deal with her initial shock, panic, grief, questions of the other siblings, and the decision of where to find help. The first persons to arrive may be the police and ambulance attendants. Ideally, they will handle the situation by asking few questions; giving no indication of wrongdoing, abuse, or neglect; making sensitive judgements concerning any resuscitation efforts for the child; and comforting the members of the family as much as possible. These individuals should be properly informed about SIDS in order to recognize its characteristic signs and tell parents that their child probably died of a disease called *sudden infant death syndrome*. A compassionate, sensitive approach to the family during the first few minutes can help spare them some of the overwhelming guilt and anguish that commonly follow this type of death.

Arriving at the Emergency Department

The first contact that nurses typically have with these families is in the emergency department, when the infant is seen by a physician to be pronounced dead. Usually there is no attempt at resuscitation. During the time in the emergency department several aspects warrant special consideration. Parents should be asked only factual questions, such as when they found the infant, how he or she looked, and whom they called for help. Any remarks that may suggest responsibility, such as why they did not check on the child earlier, why they did not hear the infant cry out, whether the head was buried in a blanket, or whether other siblings were jealous of this child, must be avoided.

The discussion of an autopsy should be presented at this time, emphasizing that a diagnosis cannot be confirmed until the postmortem examination is completed. If the mother was breastfeeding, she needs information about abrupt discontinuation of lactation.

A review of 60 studies indicates that parents experiencing perinatal death perceive health care workers' responses as having a significant impact on the parents' grieving process; many health care workers' behaviours were perceived as thoughtless or insensitive. The findings suggest that nurses and physicians would benefit from more bereavement training (Gold, 2007).

Another important aspect of compassionate care for these parents is allowing them to say good-bye to their child. A debriefing session may help health care workers who dealt with the family and deceased infant to cope with feelings that often arise when a SIDS victim is brought into the acute care facility.

Comprehensive guidelines have been published for health care providers involved in SIDS investigations to assist the family and at the same time to determine that the infant's death was not the result of other factors such as child maltreatment (Canadian Foundation for the Study of Infant Deaths, 2012).

Returning Home

When the parents return home, they should be visited by a competent, qualified professional as soon after the death as possible. Printed material that contains excellent information about SIDS (available from national organizations) should be provided. The Canadian Foundation for the Study of Infant Deaths and Caring for Kids—Back to Sleep are two resources listed in the Additional Resources section at the end of this chapter.

Ideally, the number of visits and plans for subsequent intervention need to be flexible. For example, the siblings may initially appear accepting of the explanation and well adjusted, but may later refuse to go to sleep or ask questions about graves or funerals, indicating their need for further help in dealing with the death. Parents facing the question of a subsequent child will need support. Both the birth of a subsequent child and the survival of that child, especially past the age of death of the previous child, are important transitional stages for parents.

Because the mourning process continues *for at least a year*, and it may be useful to provide referrals to other parents who have lost a child to SIDS.

Positional Plagiocephaly

Since the Back to Sleep campaign began in 1999 in Canada, which advocates nonprone sleeping for infants to prevent SIDS, an increase in the incidence of positional plagiocephaly has been observed (AAP, Task Force on Sudden Infant Death Syndrome, 2005; Littlefield, Saba, & Kelly, 2004). The term *plagiocephaly* connotes an oblique or asymmetrical head; *positional plagiocephaly, deformational plagiocephaly*, or *nonsynostotic plagiocephaly* implies an acquired condition that occurs as a result of cranial **moulding** during infancy (AAP, 2003; Hummel & Fortado, 2005). Because the infant's sutures are not closed, the skull is pliable and, when the infant is placed on the back to sleep, the posterior occiput flattens over time (Fig. 36-16, A); a transient typical bald spot will develop. As a result of prolonged pressure on one side of the skull, that side becomes misshapen; mild facial asymmetry may develop. The sternocleidomastoid muscle may tighten on the preferential side, and torticollis may also develop. Congenital or acquired torticollis may cause plagiocephaly; the discussion here centres only on plagiocephaly caused by the supine sleeping position.

Diagnostic Evaluation

The diagnosis of positional plagiocephaly may be made on physical examination of the infant's head; the infant's head is viewed frontally and from above. The typical infant's head shape will resemble a parallelogram, with unilateral flattening of the occiput, frontal and parietal bossing, a prominent cheekbone, and an anterior ear displacement (AAP, 2003). An evaluation of neck movement and range of motion is also made to determine the presence of torticollis. In most cases,

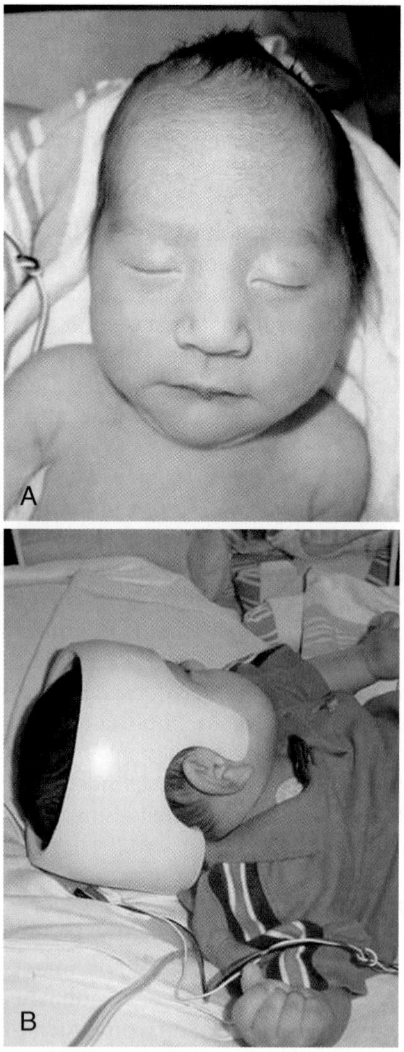

Fig. 36-16 **A:** Plagiocephaly. **B:** Helmet used to correct plagiocephaly. *(Courtesy Dr. Gerardo Cabrera-Meza, Department of Neonatology, Baylor College of Medicine, Houston, TX.)*

skull films and further radiological studies (computed tomographic scan) are used only to rule out **craniosynostosis** or any other cranial deformity that may affect brain growth.

Therapeutic Management

Treatment of torticollis and plagiocephaly initially involves exercises to loosen the tight muscle and changing head position from side to side during feeding, carrying, and sleep. If the plagiocephaly is not resolved within 4 to 8 weeks of physiotherapy, a customized helmet may be worn to decrease the pressure on the affected side of the skull (Biggs, 2003). If no improvement occurs with physiotherapy or a moulded helmet over a given period, the infant may be referred to a pediatric neurosurgeon or craniofacial surgeon (AAP, 2003). In one study, repositioning was not found to be as helpful in reducing plagiocephaly as was the use of an orthotic helmet (see Fig. 36-16, B); those treated with a helmet were older and had a longer treatment period, leading the authors to conclude that early detection and orthotic intervention were likely to be more successful (Graham et al., 2005).

Nursing Care Management

Minor skull flattening is not considered significant, but parents should be taught to prevent plagiocephaly by altering the infant's head position during sleep. Infants should be placed prone on a firm surface during awake time (tummy time), which prevents plagiocephaly and facilitates development of upper shoulder girdle strength; the latter helps in the progressive development of movements such as rolling over and starting to rise up on all fours, which are precursors to crawling and eventually walking. Despite the reported increase in the incidence of positional plagiocephaly, the supine sleeping position is still recommended because it has led to a significant decrease in loss of infant lives from SIDS (CPS, Community Paediatrics Committee, 2004). Additional measures to prevent plagiocephaly include avoiding excessive time spent in car restraint seats or infant seats and bouncers. Alternating the infant's head position during sleep can also prevent unilateral moulding. When a nurse or parent notices plagiocephaly, a consultation with the primary practitioner is recommended to evaluate the head shape and ascertain the need for early intervention.

Nurses are in a unique position in well-child care settings to encourage parents to follow guidelines for preventing plagiocephaly, to demonstrate alternating head placement for sleeping, to demonstrate sternocleidomastoid muscle exercises (as appropriate to the condition), and to encourage tummy time for infants during awake periods. Most important, nurses should continue to encourage parents to place the infant in a supine sleep position despite the development of plagiocephaly. Parents should not become so alarmed by plagiocephaly that they abandon supine sleeping position for the infant; instead they should consult with the practitioner.

Apnea and Apparent Life-Threatening Events

Apnea is defined as a cessation of breathing for 20 seconds. *Apnea of infancy* is defined as an unexplained respiratory pause of 20 seconds or more, or pauses of less than 20 seconds that are accompanied by pallor, cyanosis, bradycardia, or hypotension in the term infant. The latter is a distinct entity from apnea of prematurity. *Apnea of prematurity* is the cessation of breathing longer than 20 seconds, or any period if accompanied by bradycardia and cyanosis; it is not associated with any predisposing conditions (Dudell & Stoll, 2007). An *apparent life-threatening event* (ALTE), formerly referred to as *aborted SIDS death* or *near-miss SIDS*, generally refers to an event that is sudden and frightening to the observer, in which the infant exhibits a combination of apnea, change in colour (pallor, cyanosis, redness), change in muscle tone (usually hypotonia), choking, gagging, or coughing, and which usually involves a significant intervention and even cardiopulmonary resuscitation (CPR) by the caregiver who witnesses the event. The definition of ALTE may include apnea, but ALTE may occur without apnea (Silvestri & Weese-Mayer, 2003).

Apnea during infancy can be a symptom of any one of many disorders: sepsis, seizures or other neurological disorder, upper or lower airway infection or abnormality, gastroesophageal reflux, **hypoglycemia** or other metabolic problems, and impaired regulation of breathing during sleep or feeding. Apnea of infancy may also be a result of intentional harm by an adult caregiver. Delayed ventilatory responses to **hypercapnia** and hypoxia were observed in one study of 69 infants with apnea of infancy (Katz-Salamon, 2004). Abusive head injury has been reported in a small percentage (2.5%) of children with ALTE (Altman et al., 2003). Intentional suffocation and Munchausen syndrome by proxy cases have also been reported with ALTE (Hall & Zalman, 2005). However, in about half the cases no cause is identified. Please see Chapter 39 for more information on this topic.

Infants with a history of ALTEs may be at increased risk for SIDS, but these children constitute only approximately 7 to 12% of all SIDS victims. Most infants with ALTE are less than 6 months of age, and although there has been a significant decrease in SIDS since 1992, the incidence of ALTE has not changed (Hall & Zalman, 2005). A diagnosis of apnea of infancy or idiopathic ALTE is often made when no cause is found.

Results from the Collaborative Home Infant Monitoring study (CHIME) found that apnea and bradycardia occurred at conventional and extreme alarm thresholds in all groups of infants studied: siblings of SIDS infants, infants with ALTEs, symptomatic (of apnea and bradycardia) and asymptomatic preterm infants weighing less than 1750 g at birth, and healthy term infants. The researchers concluded that many infants experience apnea and bradycardia in each of these groups yet do not die (Jobe, 2001; Ramanathan et al., 2001). Furthermore, it was reported that apnea does not appear to be an immediate precursor to SIDS and that cardiorespiratory monitoring is not an effective tool for identifying infants at greater risk for SIDS (AAP, Committee on Fetus and Newborn, 2003). CHIME data indicate that infants with ALTE did not have some of the typical characteristics associated with SIDS infants; these include fewer infants with low birth weight and who are small for gestational age at birth, fewer teenage pregnancies, and a younger infant age at the time of ALTE. The researchers concluded that despite some similar characteristics between ALTE and SIDS, the differences warrant a separate focus on ALTE events (Esani et al., 2008).

Diagnostic Evaluation

An essential component of the diagnostic process includes a detailed description of the event—who witnessed the event, where the infant was during the event, and what, if any, activities were involved (such as during or after a feeding, riding in a car seat restraint, presence of siblings or any minor children, what clothing the infant was wearing). In addition, a prenatal and postnatal history must be obtained. A short period of observation in the emergency department may be appropriate to observe the infant's respiratory pattern and response to feeding. A careful evaluation of the preterm infant in a car restraint is essential; upper airway occlusion and subsequent apnea and cyanosis may occur if the infant is not positioned properly. Reported diagnoses in infants with ALTE include a neurological event such as a seizure (30% of cases seen); gastrointestinal problem, including gastroesophageal reflux (50%); respiratory conditions (20%); and metabolic, cardiac, or child abuse (each less than 5%). In some cases, multiple diagnoses may be made (Hall & Zalman, 2005).

In the event that an underlying diagnosis is not established, home monitoring may be recommended. The most commonly used monitoring is continuous recording of cardiorespiratory patterns (cardiopneumogram, or pneumocardiogram). Four-channel pneumocardiograms (or multichannel pneumogram) monitor heart rate, respirations (chest impedance), nasal airflow, and oxygen saturation. A more sophisticated test, polysomnography (sleep study), also records brain waves, eye and body movements, esophageal manometry, and end-tidal carbon dioxide measurements. However, none of these tests can predict risk. Some children with normal results may still have subsequent apneic episodes.

Therapeutic Management

The treatment of the infant with an ALTE depends on the underlying condition (see above). Treatment of recurrent apnea (without an underlying organic problem) usually involves continuous home monitoring of cardiorespiratory rhythms and in some cases the use of methylxanthines (respiratory stimulant drugs, such as theophylline or caffeine). The decision to discontinue the monitoring is based on the infant's clinical condition. A general guideline for discontinuation is when infants with ALTEs have gone 2 or 3 months without significant numbers of episodes requiring intervention.

Newer home apnea monitors allow downloading of information that assists the practitioner in deciding when to discontinue home monitoring. It is imperative to remember that the home apnea monitor will not predict or prevent SIDS deaths. Furthermore, impedance-based monitors detect chest wall movement and will not detect obstructive apnea unless the episode involves significant bradycardia (see Patient Teaching box).

Nursing Care Management

The diagnosis of an ALTE engenders great anxiety and concern in parents, and the institution of home monitoring presents additional physical and emotional burdens. Parents of infants on home apnea monitors report experiencing emotional distress, especially depression and hostility, during the first few weeks after hospital discharge (Abendroth et al., 1999). For parents of a SIDS victim who have a new infant on home apnea monitoring, the anxiety is compounded by the uncertainty of the future of the living child and grief for the lost child. Home apnea monitoring may offer some predictability and control over the current child's survival through the period of uncertainty.

If monitoring is required, the nurse can be a major source of support to the family in terms of education about the equipment; observation of the infant's status; and immediate intervention during apneic episodes, including CPR. Several reports indicate that the first week to month after discharge is the most stressful for parents, particularly when the rate of false alarms is high (Bennett, 2002). To help the family cope with the numerous procedures they must learn, adequate preparation before discharge and written instructions are essential. In the first few weeks after discharge, parents may benefit by having a practitioner readily available to answer questions regarding false alarms and for other technical assistance (Abendroth et al., 1999).

Several types of home monitors are available and are set up by either a home monitor equipment company or home health

PATIENT TEACHING Using Apnea Monitors or Home Oxygen Saturation Monitors

Use the monitor as instructed by the practitioner.
Do not adjust the monitor to eliminate false alarms. Adjustments could compromise the monitor's effectiveness.
Place the monitor on a firm surface away from the crib and drapes; plug the power cord directly into a wall socket with a three-pronged outlet.
Do not sleep in the same bed as a monitored infant.
Keep pets and children away from the monitor and infant.
Keep the monitor away from possible electrical interferences such as appliances (e.g., electric blankets, televisions, air conditioners, remote telephones [including cellular phones]).
Check the monitor several times a day to be sure that the alarm is working and that it can be heard from room to room. Be certain the caregiver can reach the monitor quickly (in less than 30 seconds).
Periodically check the monitor's breath detection indicator and battery or charger connections.
Be aware that strong signals from nearby radio and television stations, airports, ham radios, cellular phones, or police stations could interfere with the monitor. Check for interference if the monitor is to be operated in these areas.
Read the monitor's user manual carefully; report problems promptly.
Inform community utility and rescue squads of home monitoring as appropriate.
Keep emergency rescue numbers near phones in the home.
Practise safety precautions:

- Remove leads when the infant is not attached to the monitor.
- Unplug the power cord from the electrical outlet when the cord is not plugged into the monitor.
- Use safety covers on electrical outlets to prevent children from inserting objects into a socket.

(Data from U.S. Department of Health and Human Services. [1990]. *FDA safety alert: Important tips for apnea monitor users*. Rockville, MD: Author.)

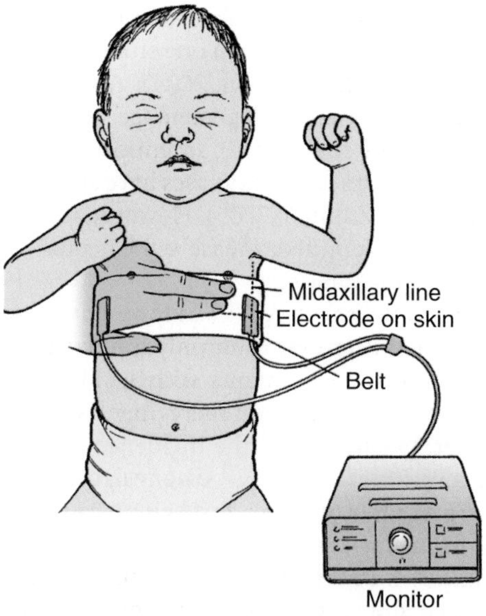

Fig. 36-17 Electrode placement for apnea monitoring. In small infants, one fingerbreadth may be used.

staff. Nurses, especially those involved in the care at home, must become familiar with the equipment, including its advantages and disadvantages. Safety is a major concern because monitors can cause electrical burns and electrocution (see Patient Teaching Box).

Siblings should also be supervised when near the infant and taught that the monitor is not a toy. Other safety practices include informing local utility and rescue squads of the home monitoring in case of an emergency. Telephone numbers for these services should be posted near all telephones in the home.

NURSING ALERT If the infant is apneic, gently stimulate the trunk by patting or rubbing it. If the infant is prone, turn to the back and flick the feet. If there is still no response, begin CPR and activate the emergency medical service—"Call 911!" Never vigorously shake the child. No more than 10 seconds are spent on stimulation before implementing CPR.

Caregivers need detailed information regarding proper attachment of the electrodes to the infant's chest. The electrodes are placed in the midaxillary line, at a space one or two fingerbreadths below the nipple. For home use, electrodes attached to a belt that is positioned around the child's trunk are preferred (Fig. 36-17), so that the electrodes contact the skin in the same area. Monitors may have memory chips that allow for event recording, which can be an effective tool in evaluating the use of the monitor, events immediately before and after the event, and reported frequency of alarms.

Monitors are effective only if they are used. They do not prevent death but alert the caregiver to the ALTE in time to intervene. The need to use the monitor and to respond appropriately to alarms must be stressed. The inability to use the monitor properly can result in the infant's death.

Family Support

Many of the stresses observed during the monitoring period are characteristic of those of families with chronically ill children. The child with an apnea or cardiorespiratory monitor may have additional health care needs such as a gastrostomy, tracheostomy, ostomy, and myriad medications or treatments that exacerbate the parents' stress. Parents report increased stress, including concern for the child's survival, fear of incompetence in assuming home responsibility, inadequate respite care, lack of time for other children and the spouse, social isolation from friends and extended family, constant work, and fatigue. The monitored child is at risk for vulnerable child syndrome, which may lead to lack of parental separation and preferential treatment, causing further family disruption (Bennett, 2002). To deal with these potential effects, nurses need to employ the same interventions as those discussed for children with **chronic illness** and to be aware of the need for referral when difficulties are suspected.

To lessen the continuous responsibility of monitoring, other family members, such as grandparents, should be taught how to manipulate the equipment, read and interpret the signals, and administer CPR. They should be encouraged to stay with the infant for regular periods to allow parents respite. Support groups of other families who have successfully completed monitoring can also be of benefit. Because baby-sitters are difficult to locate, support group members or nursing students may be potential sources of qualified caregivers.

Key Points

- Biological development of the child encompasses proportional changes; sensory changes, including binocularity, depth perception, and visual preference; maturation of biological systems; fine motor development; and gross motor development.
- Erikson's theory of psychosocial development (birth to 1 year) is concerned with acquiring a sense of trust while overcoming a sense of mistrust.
- Piaget's theory of cognitive development, as it applies to the infant, focuses on the sensorimotor phase, which includes the use of reflexes, primary circular reactions, secondary circular reactions, and coordination of secondary schemata and their application to new situations.
- Development of body image begins in infancy; by 1 year of age, infants recognize that they are distinct from their parents.
- Social development of the infant is guided by attachment, language development, personal-social behaviour, and participation in play.
- Temperament influences the type of interaction that occurs between the child and parents and siblings.
- Parents are faced with many concerns, including selecting an appropriate day care, limit-setting and discipline, thumb-sucking and pacifier use, teething, and choice of infant shoes.
- Breast milk provides optimum nutrition for the infant during the first 6 months; gradual introduction of solid food occurs during the second 6 months. Commercial iron-fortified infant formula is an alternative to human milk. Whole milk is not recommended until after 1 year of age.
- Common sleep problems that develop during infancy—and that are easily prevented—are associated with night crying and feeding. Nurses should instruct the parents, after careful assessment, in strategies to deal with the specific problem.
- Cleaning the teeth regularly in early childhood and appropriate dietary intake promote good dental health.
- Recommended routine immunizations include those for HBV, HAV, diphtheria, influenza, tetanus, pertussis, polio, measles, mumps, rubella, pneumococcus, meningococcus, chickenpox, and Hib.
- Recommended immunizations for selected groups of children are rotavirus and HPV vaccines.
- Because injuries are a major cause of death during infancy, parents should be alerted to the possibility of aspiration of foreign objects, suffocation, falls, poisoning, burns, motor vehicle injuries, and bodily damage, as well as preventive actions needed to make the environment safe for infants.
- Treatment of colic may involve change in feeding practices, correction of a stressful environment, behaviour modification, and support of the parent.
- Growth failure, or FTT, may occur in children who have a chronic illness, or it may occur in a family environment in which healthy infant feeding practices are poorly managed or understood. FTT is not always associated with a pattern of a disturbed maternal–infant relationship.
- Factors that place the infant at high risk for SIDS include prone sleeping position, soft bedding, sleeping in a noninfant bed with an adult or older child, poor socioeconomic status, and maternal prenatal smoking.
- Positional plagiocephaly can be easily prevented by allowing the awake infant to have periods of tummy time and by alternating the infant's head position during sleep.
- The primary nursing responsibility in care associated with sudden infant death is educating the newborn's family about the risks for SIDS, modelling appropriate behaviours in the hospital, such as placing the infant in a supine sleep position, and providing emotional support of the family that has experienced a SIDS loss.
- Infants with ALTEs are carefully evaluated for clues to the underlying cause.
- Home apnea or cardiorespiratory monitors do not prevent SIDS.

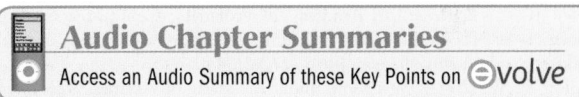

Audio Chapter Summaries

Access an Audio Summary of these Key Points on evolve

References

Abendroth, D., et al. (1999). Do apnea monitors decrease emotional distress in parents of infants at high risk for cardiopulmonary arrest? *Journal of Pediatric Health Care, 13*(2), 50–57.

Alm, B., et al. (2002). Breast-feeding and the sudden infant death syndrome in Scandinavia, 1992–1995. *Archives of Disease in Childhood, 86*(6), 400–402.

Altman, R. L., et al. (2003). Abusive head injury as a cause of apparent life-threatening events in infancy. *Archives of Pediatrics and Adolescent Medicine, 157*(10), 1011–1015.

American Academy of Pediatrics. (2003). Prevention and management of positional skull deformities in infants (clinical report). *Pediatrics, 112*(1), 199–202.

American Academy of Pediatrics. (2009). *Pediatric nutrition handbook* (6th ed.). Elk Grove Village, IL: Author.

American Academy of Pediatrics. (2012). *Fact sheet: Reactive attachment disorder.* Retrieved from http://www.aacap.org/cs/root/facts_for_families/reactive_attachment_disorder.

American Academy of Pediatrics, Committee on Fetus and Newborn. (2003). Apnea, sudden infant death syndrome, and home monitoring. *Pediatrics, 111*(4), 914–917.

American Academy of Pediatrics, Committee on Infectious Diseases & L., Pickering (Ed.) (2009). *2009 Red book: Report of the Committee on Infectious Diseases* (28th ed.). Elk Grove Village, IL: Author.

American Academy of Pediatrics, Task Force on Sudden Infant Death Syndrome. (2005). The changing concept of sudden infant death syndrome: Diagnostic coding shifts, controversies regarding the sleeping environment, and new variables to consider in reducing risk. *Pediatrics, 116*(5), 1245–1255. doi:10.1542/peds.2005-1499

American Dental Association. (2007). For the dental patient ... infants, formula and fluoride. *Journal of the American Dental Association, 138*(1), 132.

American Psychiatric Association. (2000). *Diagnostic and statistical manual of mental disorders* (4th ed.). Washington, DC: Author.

Anderson, J. E. (2004). "Nothing but the tooth": Dispelling myths about teething. *Contemporary Pediatrics, 21*(7), 75–83.

Anderson, M. E., Johnson, D. C., & Batal, H. A. (2005). Sudden infant death syndrome and prenatal maternal smoking: Rising attributed risk in the Back to Sleep era. *BMC Medicine, 3*(1), 4. doi:10.1186/1741-7015-3-4

Arikan, D., et al. (2008). Effectiveness of massage, sucrose solution, herbal tea or hydrolyzed formula in the treatment of infantile colic. *Journal of Clinical Nursing, 17*(13), 1754–1761. doi:10.1111/j.1365-2702.2007.02093.x

Arora, S., et al. (2000). Major factors influencing breastfeeding rates: Mother's perception of father's attitude and milk supply. *Pediatrics, 106*(5), e67.

Bacon, C. J., et al. (2008). How common is repeat sudden infant death syndrome? *Archives of Disease in Childhood, 93*(4), 323–326. doi:10.1136/adc.2006.113969

Barnard, K., et al. (1993). Measurement and meaning of parent–child interaction. In F. Morrison, C. Lord, & D. Keating (Eds.), *Applied developmental psychology* (Vol. 3). New York: Academic Press.

Barnhill, B. J., et al. (1996). Using pressure to decrease the pain of intramuscular injections. *Journal of Pain Symptom Management, 12*(1), 52–58.

Bellemare, S. (2008). Dangers for children in the care of drug users. *Canadian Medical Association Journal, 179*(2), 164. doi:10.1503/cmaj.1080070

Bennett, A. D. (2002). Home apnea monitoring for infants: A discussion of primary care issues. *Advance for Nurse Practitioners, 10*(3), 48–53.

Biggs, W. S. (2003). Diagnosis and management of positional head deformity. *American Family Physician, 67*(9), 1953–1956.

Blackburn, S. T. (2007). *Maternal, fetal, and neonatal physiology: A clinical perspective* (3rd ed.). St. Louis: Saunders.

Block, R. W., Krebs, N. F., & American Academy of Pediatrics, Committee on Child Abuse and Neglect and Committee on Nutrition. (2005). Failure to thrive as a manifestation of child neglect. *Pediatrics, 116*(5), 1234–1237. doi:10.1542/peds.2005-2032

Brady, M. T. (2005). Infectious disease in pediatric out-of-home child care. *American Journal of Infection Control, 33*(5), 276–285. doi:10.1016/j.ajic.2004.11.007

Brazelton, T. (1990). Parent–infant cosleeping revisited. *Brazelton Center Newsletter*, Vol. 2. Boston.

Brenner, R. A., & American Academy of Pediatrics, Committee on Injury, Violence, and Poison Prevention. (2003). Prevention of drowning in infants, children, and adolescents. *Pediatrics, 112*(2), 440–445.

Campion, E. W. (2002). Suspicions about the safety of vaccines. *New England Journal of Medicine, 347*(19), 1474–1475.

Canada Communicable Disease Report. (2010). *Guidelines for the prevention and control of mumps outbreaks in Canada.* 36S1(supplement). Retrieved from http://www.phac-aspc.gc.ca/publicat/ccdr-rmtc/10pdf/36s1-eng.pdf.

Canadian Dental Association. (2010). *Dental care for children.* Retrieved from http://www.cda-adc.ca/en/oral_health/cfyt/dental_care_children/.

Canadian Foundation for the Study of Infant Deaths. (2012). *Resources for public health professionals.* Retrieved from http://www.sidscanada.org/professionalsresearch.html.

Canadian Paediatric Society. (2001). Joint statement on shaken baby syndrome. *Paediatrics and Child Health, 6*(9), 663–667. (Reaffirmed September 2005)

Canadian Paediatric Society. (2003). Recommendations for the use of pacifiers. *Paediatrics and Child Health, 8*(8), 515–519. (Reaffirmed February 2011) Retrieved from http://www.cps.ca/english/statements/cp/cp03-01.htm.

Canadian Paediatric Society. (2006). *Feeding your baby in the first year.* Retrieved from http://www.caringforkids.cps.ca/handouts/feeding_your_baby_in_the_first_year.

Canadian Paediatric Society. (2007). *Healthy bodies: Healthy sleep for your baby and child.* Retrieved from http://www.caringforkids.cps.ca/handouts/healthy_sleep_for_your_baby_and_child.

Canadian Paediatric Society. (2008). Health implications of children in child care centres. Part A. Canadian trends in child care, behaviour and development outcomes. *Paediatrics and Child Health, 13*(2), 863–867. Retrieved from http://www.cps.ca/english/statements/cp/cp08-02.htm.

Canadian Paediatric Society. (2009). Health implications of children in child care centres. Part B. Injuries and infections. *Paediatrics and Child Health, 14*(1), 40–43. Retrieved from http://www.cps.ca/english/statements/cp/cp2009-01.htm.

Canadian Paediatric Society. (2010). *Head injury secondary to suspected child maltreatment—Results of a national surveillance program.* Presented at Safety 2010 World Conference, London, September 2010. Retrieved from http://www.cps.ca/English/Surveillance/CPSP/Publications/Head_injury_Sept2010.pdf.

Canadian Paediatric Society, Community Paediatrics Committee. (2004). Canadian Paediatric Society (CPS) recommendations for safe sleeping environments for infants and children. *Paediatrics and Child Health, 9*(9), 659–663. (Reaffirmed February 2010).

Canadian Paediatric Society, Community Paediatrics Committee. (2012). *Pacifiers (soothers): A user's guide for parents.* Retrieved from http://www.caringforkids.cps.ca/handouts/pacifiers.

Canadian Paediatric Society, First Nations, Inuit and Métis Health Committee. (2007). Vitamin D supplementation: Recommendations for Canadian mothers and infants. *Paediatrics and Child Health, 12*(7), 583–589. (Reaffirmed March 2012).

Canadian Paediatric Society, Infectious Diseases and Immunization Committee. (2010). Recommendations for the use of rotavirus vaccines in infants. *Paediatrics and Child Health, 15*(8), 519–523.

Canadian Paediatric Society, Nutrition and Gastroenterology Committee. (2011). Infantile colic: Is there a role for dietary interventions? *Paediatrics and Child Health, 16*(1), 47–49.

Carey, W. B., & McDevitt, S. C. (1978). Revision of the infant temperament questionnaire. *Pediatrics, 61*(5), 735–739.

Carroll-Pankhurst, C., & Mortimer, E. A. (2001). Sudden infant death syndrome, bed sharing, parental weight, and age of death. *Pediatrics, 107*(3), 530–536.

Centers for Disease Control and Prevention. (2005). Nonfatal motor-vehicle-related backover injuries among children—United States, 2001–2003. *MMWR. Morbidity and Mortality Weekly Report, 54*(06), 144–146.

Centers for Disease Control and Prevention. (2006). Update: Guillain-Barré syndrome among recipients of Menactra meningococcal conjugate vaccine—United States, June 2005–September 2006. *MMWR. Morbidity and Mortality Weekly Report, 55*(41), 1120–1124.

Centers for Disease Control and Prevention. (2009). Recommended immunization schedules for persons aged 0 through 18 years—United States, 2009. *MMWR. Morbidity and Mortality Weekly Report, 57*(51), Q-1–Q-4.

Chapman, D. J. (2009). Does pacifier introduction at 15 days disrupt well-established breastfeeding? *Journal of Human Lactation 25*(4), 466–467. doi:10.1177/0890334409351669

Chung, J. W., Ng, W. M., & Wong, T. K. (2002). An experimental study on the use of manual pressure to reduce pain in intramuscular injections. *Journal of Clinical Nursing, 11*, 457–461.

Cirgin Ellett, M. L. (2003). What is known about colic? *Gastroenterology Nursing, 26*(2), 60–65.

Coleman, J. J. (2009). Culture care meanings of African American parents related to infant mortality and health care. *Journal of Cultural Diversity, 16*(3), 109–120.

Corbett-Dick, P., & Bezek, S. K. (1997). Breastfeeding promotion for the employed mother. *Journal of Pediatric Health Care, 11*(1), 12–19.

Corrales, K. M., & Utter, S. L. (2005). Growth failure. In P. Q. Samour & K. King (Eds.), *Handbook of pediatric nutrition* (3rd ed.). Sudbury, MA: Jones & Bartlett.

Crotteau, C. A., Wright, S. T., & Eglash, A. (2006). What is the best treatment for infants with colic? *Journal of Family Practice, 55*(7), 634–636.

Dahl, R. E. (1998). The development and disorders of sleep. *Advances in Pediatrics, 45*, 73–90.

Dales, L., Hammer, S. J., & Smith, N. J. (2001). Time trends in autism and in MMR immunization coverage in California. *Journal of the American Medical Association, 285*(9), 1183–1185.

Davis, K. F., Parker, K., & Montgomery, G. L. (2004). Sleep in infants and young children, part 2. Common sleep problems. *Journal of Pediatric Health Care, 18*(3), 130–137.

de Los Reyes, E. C. (2010). Autism and immunizations: Separating fact from fiction. *Archives of Neurology, 67*(4), 490–492.

DeStefano, F. (2007). Vaccines and autism: Evidence does not support a causal association. *Clinical Pharmacology and Therapeutics, 82*(6), 756–759.

Dewey, K. G. (2001). Nutrition, growth, and complementary feeding of the breastfed infant. *Pediatric Clinics of North America, 48*(1), 87–104.

Dietitians of Canada, Canadian Paediatric Society, the College of Family Physicians of Canada, and the Community Health Nurses of Canada. (2010). *Promoting optimal monitoring of child growth in Canada: Using the new WHO growth charts.* Retrieved from http://www.cps.ca/english/statements/N/growth-charts-statement-FULL.pdf.

Diggle, L., & Deeks, J. (2000). Effect of needle length on incidence of local reactions to routine immunizations in infants aged 4 months: Randomized controlled trial. *British Medical Journal, 321*(7266), 931–933.

Diggle, L., Deeks, J. J., & Pollard, A. J. (2006). Effect of needle size and immunogenecity and reactogenecity of vaccines in infants: A randomized controlled trial. *British Medical Journal, 333*(7568), 571. doi:10.1136/bmj.38906.704549.7C

Douglass, J. M., Douglass, A. B., & Silk, H. J. (2004). A practical guide to infant oral health. *American Family Physician, 70*(11), 2113–2120.

Drago, D. A. (2005). Kitchen scalds and thermal burns in children five years and younger. *Pediatrics, 115*(1), 10–16. doi:10.1542/peds.2004-0249

Dudell, G. G., & Stoll, B. J. (2007). Respiratory tract disorders. In R. M. Kliegman, et al. (Eds.), *Nelson textbook of pediatrics* (18th ed.). Philadelphia: Saunders.

Duggan, C., Markowitz, R., & Watkins, J. B. (2008). Failure to thrive: Malnutrition in the pediatric outpatient setting. In C. Duggan, J. B. Watkins III, & W. A. Walker (Eds.), *Nutrition in Pediatrics*, (4th ed.). Hamilton, ON: B.C. Decker.

Duro, D., et al. (2002). Association between infantile colic and carbohydrate malabsorption from fruit juices in infancy. *Pediatrics, 109*(5), 797–805.

Ellett, M., Schuff, E., & Davis, J. B. (2005). Parental perceptions of the lasting effects of infant colic. *MCN. American Journal of Maternal Child Nursing, 30*(2), 127–132.

Erikson, E. H. (1963). *Childhood and society* (2nd ed.). New York: Norton.

Esani, N., et al. (2008). Apparent life-threatening events and sudden infant death syndrome: Comparison of risk factors. *Journal of Pediatrics, 152*(3), A2. doi:10.1016/j.jpeds.2007.07.054

Franco, P., et al. (1999). Prenatal exposure to cigarette smoking is associated with a decrease in arousal in infants. *Journal of Pediatrics, 135*(1), 34–38.

Fredrickson, D. D., et al. (2004). Childhood immunization refusal: Provider and parent perceptions. *Family Medicine, 36*(6), 431–438.

Friedman, J., & Saunders, N. (2007). *Canada's baby care book*. Toronto: Robert Rose Publishers.

Gerez, T., & Côté, A. (2002). *Developing a 'reduce-the-risk' campaign for the year 2002 in a low-incidence region*. Presented at the SIDS International 2002 Meeting, Florence, Italy, August 31 to September 4.

Gold, K. J. (2007). Navigating care after a baby dies: A systematic review of parent experiences with health providers. *Journal of Perinatology, 27*(4), 230–237. doi:10.1038/sj.jp.7211676

Graham, J. M., et al. (2005). Management of deformational plagiocephaly: Repositioning versus orthotic therapy. *Journal of Pediatrics, 146*(2), 258–262. doi:10.1016/j.jpeds.2004.10.016

Hall, K. L., & Zalman, B. (2005). Evaluation and management of apparent life-threatening events in children. *American Family Physician, 71*(12), 2301–2308.

Halperin, B. A., et al. (2002). Use of lidocaine-prilocaine patch to decrease intramuscular injection pain does not adversely affect the antibody response to diphtheria–tetanus–acellular pertussis–inactivated poliovirus–*Haemophilus influenzae* type b conjugate and hepatitis B vaccines in infants from birth to 6 months of age. *Pediatric Infectious Diseases Journal, 21*(5), 399–405.

Hanzer, M., Zotter, H., Sauseng, W., Pichler, G., Mulle, W., & Kerbl, R. (2010). Non-nutritive sucking habits in sleeping infants. *Neonatology, 97*(1) 61–66. doi:10.1159/000231518

Harrison, D., Yamada, J., & Stevens, B. (2010). Strategies for the prevention and management of neonatal and infant pain. *Current Pain & Headache Reports, 14*(2):113–123.

Hatfield, L. A. (2008). Sucrose decreases infant neurobehavioural pain response to immunizations: A randomized controlled trial. *Journal of Nursing Scholarship, 40*(3), 219–225. doi:10.1111/j.1547-5069.2008.00229.x

Hauck, F. R., et al. (2003). Sleep environment and the risk of sudden infant death syndrome in an urban population: The Chicago Infant Mortality Study. *Pediatrics, 111*(5 Pt 2), 1207–1214.

Hawkins-Walsh, E. (2003). A behavioural infant sleep intervention resolved sleep problems. *Evidence-Based Nursing, 6*(1), 10–12.

Health Canada. (2005). *Regulatory review and recommendation regarding baby walkers pursuant to the Hazardous Products Act*. Retrieved from http://www.hc-sc.gc.ca/cps-spc/pubs/cons/walker-review-marchette/index-eng.php.

Health Canada. (2010a). *Consumer product safety: Cribs and cradles*. Retrieved from http://hc-sc.gc.ca/cps-spc/child-enfant/equip/_crib-berc/crib-berc-eng.php.

Health Canada. (2010b). *Healthy living: Microwave ovens and food safety*. Retrieved from http://www.hc-sc.gc.ca/hl-vs/iyh-vsv/prod/micro-f-a-eng.php.

Health Canada. (2012). *Food and nutrition: Infant feeding*. Retrieved from http://www.hc-sc.gc.ca/fn-an/nutrition/infant-nourisson/index-eng.php.

Henary, B., et al. (2007). Car safety seats for children: Rear facing for best protection. *Injury Prevention, 13*(6), 398–402. doi:10.1136/ip.2006.015115

Heron, M. P., & Smith, B. L. (2007). Deaths: Leading causes for 2003. *National Vital Statistics Report, 55*(10), 1–92.

Hiscock, H., & Wake, M. (2001). Infant sleep problems and postnatal depression: A community-based study. *Pediatrics, 107*(6), 1317–1322.

Horn, M. I., & McCarthy, A. M. (1999). Children's responses to sequential versus simultaneous immunization injections. *Journal of Pediatric Health Care, 13*(1), 18–23.

Horne, R. S., et al. (2001). The prone sleeping position impairs arousability in term infants. *Journal of Pediatrics, 138*(6), 793–795.

Hornor, G. (2008). Reactive attachment disorder. *Journal of Pediatric Health Care, 22*(4), 234–239. doi:10.1016/j.pedhc.2007.07.003

Hummel, P., & Fortado, D. (2005). Impacting infant head shapes. *Advances in Neonatal Care, 5*(6), 329–342. doi:10.1016/j.adnc.2005.08.009

Hutton, E. K., & Hassan, E. S. (2007). Late vs. early clamping of the umbilical cord in full-term neonates: Systematic review and meta-analysis of controlled trials. *Journal of the American Medical Association, 297*(11), 1241–1252. doi:10.1001/jama.297.11.1241

Hviid, A., et al. (2003). Association between thimerosal-containing vaccine and autism. *Journal of the American Medical Association, 290*(13), 1763–1766.

Institute of Medicine. (2004). *Immunization safety review: Vaccines and autism*. Washington, DC: National Academies Press.

Ize-Ludlow, D., et al. (2004). Neurotoxicities in infants seen with the consumption of star anise tea. *Pediatrics, 114*(5), e653.

Jenik, A., Vain, N., Gorestein, A., & Jocobi, N. E. (2009). Does the recommendation to use a pacifier influence the prevalence of breastfeeding? *Journal of Pediatrics, 155*, 350–354. doi:10.1016/j.jpeds.2009.03.038

Jenik, A., & Vain, N. (2009). The pacifier debate. *Early Human Development, 85*(10 Suppl), 589–591. doi:10.1016/j.earlhumdev.2009.08.025

Jimenez, N., et al. (2006). A comparison of a needle-free injection system for local anesthesia versus EMLA for intravenous catheter insertion in the pediatric patient. *Anesthesia and Analagesia, 102*(2), 411–414. doi:10.1213/01.ane.0000194293.10549.62

Joanna Briggs Institute. (2004). Best practice information sheet: The effectiveness of interventions for infant colic. *Best Practice, 8*(2), 1–6.

Joanna Briggs Institute. (2005). Early childhood pacifier use in relation to breastfeeding, SIDS, infection, and dental occlusion. *Best Practice, 9*(3), 1–6. doi:10.1111/j.1479-6988.2005.00024.x

Jobe, A. H. (2001). What do home monitors contribute to the SIDS problem? (editorial). *Journal of the American Medical Association, 285*(17), 2244–2245.

Kallan, M. J., et al. (2008). Seating patterns and corresponding risk of injury among 0- to 3-year-old children in child safety seats. *Pediatrics, 121*(5), e1342–e1347. doi:10.1542/peds.2007-1512

Katz-Salamon, M. (2004). Delayed chemoreceptor responses in infants with apnoea. *Archives of Disease in Childhood, 89*(3), 261–266.

Koslap-Petraco, M. B., & Parsons, T. (2003). Communicating the benefits of combination vaccines to parents and health care providers. *Journal of Pediatric Health Care, 17*(2), 53–57.

Kotch, J. B., et al. (2007). Hand-washing and diapering equipment reduces disease among children in out-of-home child care centers. *Pediatrics, 120*(1), e29–36. doi:10.1542/peds.2005-0760

Krugman, S. D., & Dubowitz, H. (2003). Failure to thrive. *American Family Physician, 68*(5), 879–886.

Lassman, J. (2002). Water safety. *Journal of Emergency Nursing, 28*(3), 241–243.

Lawrence, R. A., & Lawrence, R. M. (2011). *Breastfeeding: A guide for the medical profession* (7th ed.). St. Louis: Mosby.

Littlefield, T. R., Saba, N. M., & Kelly, K. M. (2004). On the current incidence of deformational plagiocephaly: An estimation based on prospective registration at a single center. *Seminars in Pediatric Neurology, 11*(4), 301–304.

Locklin, M. (2005). The redefinition of failure to thrive from a case study perspective. *Pediatric Nursing, 31*(6), 474–479, 495.

Maggioni, A., & Lifshitz, F. (1995). Nutritional management of failure to thrive. *Pediatric Clinics of North America, 42*(4), 791–810.

Malloy, M. H. (2002). Trends in postneonatal aspiration deaths and reclassification of sudden infant death syndrome: Impact of the "Back to Sleep" program. *Pediatrics, 109*(4), 661–665.

Markowitz, R., & Duggan, C. (2003). Failure to thrive: Malnutrition in the pediatric setting. In W. A. Walker, J. B. Watkins, & C. Duggan (Eds.), *Nutrition in pediatrics* (3rd ed.). Hamilton, ON: Decker.

Martin, J., et al. (2007). Adverse associations of infant and child sleep problems and parent health: An Australian population study. *Pediatrics, 119*(5), 947–955. doi:10.1542/peds.2006-2569

Matteucci, M. J., et al. (2007). Methamphetamine exposures in young children. *Pediatric Emergency Care, 23*(9), 638–640. doi:10.1097/PEC.0b013e31814a6a79

McConnell, M., & Moss, E. (2011). Attachment across the life span: Factors that contribute to stability and change. *Australian Journal of Educational & Developmental Psychology, 11*, 60–77.

McGarvey, C., et al. (2003). Factors relating to the infant's last sleep environment in sudden infant death syndrome in the Republic of Ireland. *Archives of Disease in Childhood, 88*(12), 1058–1064.

McMartin, K. I., et al. (2002). Lung tissue concentrations of nicotine in sudden infant death syndrome. *Journal of Pediatrics, 140*(2), 205–209.

Mecham, N., & Melini, J. (2002). Unintentional victims: Development of a protocol for the care of children exposed to chemicals at methamphetamine laboratories. *Pediatric Emergency Care, 18*(4), 327–332.

Medoff-Cooper, B., Carey, W. B., & McDevitt, S. C. (1993). The Early Infancy Temperament Questionnaire. *Journal of Developmental and Behavioral Pediatrics, 14*(4), 230–235.

Mitchell, E. A., et al. (2008). Head covering and the risk for SIDS: Findings from the New Zealand and German SIDS case-control studies. *Pediatrics, 121*(6), e1478–e1483. doi:10.1542/peds.2007-2749

Morin, K. (2004). Infant nutrition: Solids—when and why. *MCN. American Journal of Maternal Child Nursing, 29*(4), 259.

Morin, K. (2005). Infant nutrition: Preparing baby food at home safely. *MCN. American Journal of Maternal Child Nursing 30*(1), 67.

Mrozek-Budzn, D., Kieltyka, A., & Majewska, R. (2010). Lack of association between measles-mumps-rubella vaccination and autism in children: A case-control study. *Pediatric Infectious Disease Journal, 29*(5), 397–400. doi:10.1097/INF.0b013e3181c40a8a

Neu, M., & Robinson, J. A. (2003). Infants with colic: Their childhood characteristics. *Journal of Pediatric Nursing, 18*(1), 12–20.

Niemela, M., Uhari, M., & Mottonen, M. (1995). A pacifier increases the risk of recurrent acute otitis media in children in day care centers. *Pediatrics, 96*(5 Pt 1), 884–888.

Niemela, M., et al. (2000). Pacifier as a risk factor for acute otitis media: A randomized, controlled trial of parental counseling. *Pediatrics, 106*(3), 483–488.

Person, T. L., Lavezzi, W. A., & Wolf, B. C. (2002). Cosleeping and sudden unexpected death in infancy. *Archives of Pathology and Laboratory Medicine, 126*(3), 343–345.

Piaget, J. (1952). *The origins of intelligence in children.* New York: International Universities Press.

Pinelli, J., & Symington, A. (2000). Non-nutritive sucking for promoting physiologic stability and nutrition in preterm infants. *Cochrane Database of Systemic Reviews, (2)*, CD001071.

Pinelli, J., Symington, A., & Ciliska, D. (2002). Nonnutritive sucking in high-risk infants: Benign intervention or legitimate therapy? *Journal of Obstetric, Gynecologic and Neonatal Nursing, 31*(5), 582–591.

Pollack, H. A. (2001). Sudden infant death syndrome, maternal smoking during pregnancy and effectiveness of smoking cessation intervention. *American Journal of Public Health, 91*(3), 432–436.

Public Health Agency of Canada. (2006). *Canadian immunization guide* (7th ed.). Retrieved from http://www.phac-aspc.gc.ca/publicat/cig-gci/index-eng.php.

Public Health Agency of Canada. (2008). *Canadian perinatal health report,* (2008 ed.). Ottawa: Author.

Public Health Agency of Canada. (2009). *Mumps in Canada, 2007.* Retrieved from http://www.phac-aspc.gc.ca/mumps-oreillons/prof-eng.php.

Public Health Agency of Canada. (2010). *Canadian incidence study of reported child abuse and neglect, 2008.* Retrieved from http://www.phac-aspc.gc.ca/cm-vee/csca-ecve/2008/fs-am/index-eng.php.

Public Health Agency of Canada. (2011a). *Publicly funded immunization programs in Canada—routine schedule for infants and children including special programs and catch-up programs.* Retrieved from http://www.phac-aspc.gc.ca/im/ptimprog-progimpt/table-1-eng.php.

Public Health Agency of Canada. (2011b). *Safe sleep.* Retrieved from http://www.phac-aspc.gc.ca/hp-ps/dca-dea/stages-etapes/childhood-enfance_0-2/sids/index-eng.php.

Public Health Agency of Canada (2011c). *Shaken baby syndrome.* Retrieved from http://www.phac-aspc.gc.ca/hp-ps/dca-dea/stages-etapes/childhood-enfance_0-2/shaken-eng.php.

Public Health Agency of Canada. (2012a). *Canadian adverse events following immunization surveillance system (CAEFISS).* Retrieved from http://www.phac-aspc.gc.ca/im/vs-sv/caefiss-eng.php.

Public Health Agency of Canada. (2012b). *Depression in pregnancy.* Retrieved from http://www.phac-aspc.gc.ca/mh-sm/preg_dep-eng.php.

Puffenberger, E. G., et al. (2004). Mapping of sudden infant death with dysgenesis of the testis syndrome (SIDDT) by a SNP genome scan and identification of TSPYL loss of function. *Proceedings of the National Academy of Sciences USA, 101*(32), 11, 689–691, 694.

Ramanathan, R., et al. (2001). Cardiorespiratory events recorded on home monitors: Comparison of healthy infants with those at increased risk for SIDS. *Journal of the American Medical Association, 285*(17), 2199–2207.

Reis, E. C., & Holubkov, R. (1997). Vapocoolant spray is equally effective as EMLA cream in reducing immunization pain in school-aged children. *Pediatrics, 100*(6), 1025.

Rudolf, M. C., & Logan, S. (2005). What is the long-term outcome for children who fail to thrive? A systematic review. *Archives of Disease in Childhood, 90*(9), 925–931. doi:10.1136/adc.2004.050179

Rusen, I. D., Sauve, R., Joseph, K. S., & Kramer, M. S. (2004). Sudden infant death syndrome in Canada: Trends in rates and risk factors, 1985–1998. *Chronic Diseases in Canada, 25*(1),1–6.

Sacks, D. (Ed.) (2009). *Canadian Paediatric Society guide to caring for your child from birth to age five.* Toronto: Wiley.

Safe Kids Canada. (2006). *Child and youth unintentional injury: 1994–2003, 10 years in review.* Retrieved from http://www.mhp.gov.on.ca/en/prevention/injury-prevention/skc_injuries.pdf.

Safe Kids Canada. (2009). *Media release: Safe Kids Canada unveils startling new data on product safety in the home.* Retrieved from http://www.safekidscanada.ca/professionals/newsroom/media-releases/2009/hidden-comforts-or-hidden-dangers.aspx.

Safe Kids Canada. (2010a). *Safety information: Car seat types.* Retrieved from http://www.safekidscanada.ca/Parents/Safety-Information/Car-Seats/Types/Car-Seat-Types.aspx#rear.

Safe Kids Canada. (2010b). *Safety information: Drowning prevention tips.* Retrieved from http://www.safekidscanada.ca/parents/safety-information/drowning-prevention/index.aspx.

Safe Kids Canada. (2012). *Child passenger safety.* Retrieved from http://www.safekidscanada.ca/professionals/safety-information/child-passenger-safety/index.aspx.

Savino, F., et al. (2007). *Lactobacillus reuteri* (American type culture collection strain 55730) versus simethicone in the treatment of infantile colic: A prospective randomized study. *Pediatrics, 119*(1), e124–e130. doi:10.1542/peds.2006-1222

Schachter, F., et al. (1989). Cosleeping and sleep problems in Hispanic-American urban young children. *Pediatrics 84*(3), 522–530.

Schechter, N. L., et al. (2007). Pain reduction during pediatric immunizations: Evidence-based review and recommendations. *Pediatrics, 119*(5), e1184–e1198. doi:10.1542/peds.2006-1107

Schuval, S. (2003). Avoiding allergic reactions to childhood vaccines (and what to do when they occur). *Contemporary Pediatrics, 22*(4), 29–49, 53.

Silvestri, J. M., & Weese-Mayer, D. (2003). Disorders of respiratory control: Apnea and SIDS. In C. D. Rudolph, A. M. Rudolph, & M. K. Hostetter (Eds.), *Rudolph's pediatrics* (21st ed.). New York: McGraw-Hill.

Spanos, S., et al. (2008). Jet injection of 1% buffered lidocaine versus topical ELA-Max for anesthesia before peripheral intravenous catheterization in children: A randomized controlled trial. *Pediatric Emergency Care, 24*(8), 511–515. doi:10.1097/PEC.0b013e31816a8d5b

Statistics Canada. (2007). 2006 Census: Families, marital status, households and dwelling characteristics. *The Daily, Wednesday, September 12, 2007.* Retrieved from http://www.statcan.gc.ca/daily-quotidien/070912/dq070912a-eng.htm.

Statistics Canada. (2011). *Leading causes of death, infants, by sex, Canada, annual.* Retrieved from http://www5.statcan.gc.ca/cansim/pick-choisir?lang=eng&p2=33&id=1020562.

Stevens, B., Yamada, J., & Ohlsson, A. (2001). Sucrose for analgesia in newborn infants undergoing painful procedures. *Cochrane Database of Systemic Reviews, (4)*, CD001069.

Stevens, B., et al. (1999). The efficacy of developmentally sensitive interventions and sucrose for relieving procedural pain in very low birth weight neonates. *Nursing Research, 48*(1), 35–43.

Tablizo, M. A., et al. (2007). Supine sleeping position does not cause clinical aspiration in neonates in hospital newborn nurseries. *Archives of Pediatrics and Adolescent Medicine, 161*(5), 507–510.

Tappin, D., Ecob, R., & Brooke, H. (2005). Bedsharing, roomsharing, and sudden infant death syndrome in Scotland: A case-control study. *Journal of Pediatrics, 147*(1), 32–37. doi:10.1016/j.jpeds.2005.01.035

Thompson, D. G. (2005). Safe sleep practices for hospitalized infants. *Pediatric Nursing, 31*(5), 400–403, 409.

Touchette, E., et al. (2005). Factors associated with fragmented sleep at night across early childhood. *Archives of Pediatrics and Adolescent Medicine, 159*(3), 242–249.

Unger, B., et al. (2003). Racial disparity and modifiable risk factors among infants dying suddenly and unexpectedly. *Pediatrics, 111*(2), E127–E131.

Weizman, Z., et al. (1993). Efficacy of herbal tea preparation in infantile colic. *Journal of Pediatrics, 122*(4), 650–652.

Wilkerson, R., Northington, L. D., & Fisher, W. (2005). Ingestion of toxic substances by infants and children: What we don't know can hurt. *Critical Care Nursing, 25*(4), 35–44.

Willinger, M., et al. (2003). Trends in infant bed sharing in the United States, 1993–2000: The National Infant Sleep Position Study. *Archives of Pediatrics and Adolescent Medicine, 157*(1), 43–49.

Wilson, M. E., et al. (2000). Family dynamics, parental–fetal attachment and infant temperament. *Journal of Advanced Nursing, 31*(1), 204–210.
Wilson, S. (2001). Attachment disorders: Review and current status. *Journal of Psychology, 135*(1), 37–51.
Wong, D. L. (2003). Topical local anaesthetics: Two products for pain relief during minor procedures. *American Journal of Nursing, 103*(6), 42–45.
Yu, C. Y., Hung, C. H., Chan, T. F., Yeh, C. H., & Lai, C. Y. (2012). Prenatal predictors for father–infant attachment after childbirth. *Journal of Clinical Nursing, 21*, 1577–1583. doi:10.1111/j.1365-2702.2011.04003.x
Zeanah, C. H., & Fox, N. A. (2004). Temperament and attachment disorders. *Journal of Clinical Child and Adolescent Psychology, 33*(1), 82–87.
Zempsky, W. T. (2008). Pharmacologic approaches for reducing venous access pain in children. *Pediatrics, 122*(Suppl 3), S140–S153. doi:10.1542/peds.2008-1055g
Zuckerman, J. (2000). The importance of injecting vaccines into muscle. *British Medical Journal, 321*(7271), 1237–1238.
Zuckerman, J. N., Cockcroft, A., & Zuckerman, A. J. (1992). Site of injection for vaccination. *British Medical Journal, 305*(6862), 1158.

Additional Resources

Attachment Across Cultures: Beliefs, Values, and Practices: http://www.attachmentacrosscultures.org/beliefs/
Canadian Coalition for Immunization Awareness and Promotion: http://www.immunize.cpha.ca/en/default.aspx
Canadian Foundation for the Study of Infant Deaths: http://www.sidscanada.org/backtosleep.html
Caring for Kids—Back to Sleep: http://www.caringforkids.cps.ca/pregnancybabies/safesleepforbaby.htm
Canadian Partnership for Children's Health and Environment (working to protect children from environmental contaminants): http://www.healthyenvironmentforkids.ca/
City of Brampton (Fire and Emergency Services): Is Your Child Safe and Secure (Car seat information and movie)?: http://www.brampton.ca/en/residents/fire-emergency-services/Fire-Safety/Pages/Child-Safe-and-Secure.aspx
Health Canada: Baby Car Seat Carrier Safety Belts Pose Risk of Serious Injury to Infants: http://www.hc-sc.gc.ca/ahc-asc/media/advisories-avis/_2011/2011_126-eng.php
Health Canada: Consumer Product Safety: Childcare Equipment and Children's Furniture: http://www.hc-sc.gc.ca/cps-spc/child-enfant/equip/_crib-berc/storkcraft_video-eng.php
Healthlink BC: Precautions for Sharing a Bed With an Infant: http://www.healthlinkbc.ca/kb/content/special/ta3271.html
Healthy Canadians: Safe Sleep: http://www.healthycanadians.gc.ca/init/kids-enfants/sleep-sommeil/index-eng.php
Public Health Agency of Canada: Child Maltreatment Publications: http://www.phac-aspc.gc.ca/cm-vee/public-eng.php
Resources for parents coping with the loss of their baby: http://www.aboutkidshealth.ca/Pregnancy/Grief-Loss.aspx?articleID=6708&categoryID=PG-nh4-11o
Safe Kids Canada: Safety Information: Car Seats: http://www.safekidscanada.ca/Parents/Safety-Information/Car-Seats/Index.aspx
Transport Canada: Legal Requirements for Children's Motor Vehicle Restraints: http://www.tc.gc.ca/eng/roadsafety/safedrivers-childsafety-programs-index-874.htm
Information for parents on what to consider when selecting a child care facility:
http://www.healthlinkbc.ca/kb/content/special/aa43308.html
http://www.senecac.on.ca/community/KOLTguidetochoosingchildcare.html
http://www.todaysparent.com/lifeasparent/childcare/article.jsp?content=20100302_173310_5996&page=1
http://www.e-laws.gov.on.ca/html/regs/english/elaws_regs_900262_e.htm
http://childcaretoday.ca/index.php

Unit 9

37 The Toddler and Family

Learning Objectives

On completion of this chapter, the reader will be able to:

- Identify the major biological, psychosocial, cognitive, and social developments during the toddler years.
- Relate separation anxiety and negativism to developmental tasks.
- Recognize a child's readiness for toilet training and offer parents guidelines.
- Prepare parents of toddlers for the birth of a sibling.
- Provide parents with guidelines for handling temper tantrums.
- Provide parents with feeding recommendations for the toddler.
- Outline a preventive dental hygiene plan for toddlers.
- Provide anticipatory guidance to parents regarding injury prevention based on the toddler's developmental achievements.

Electronic Resources

Additional information related to the content in Chapter 37 can be found on

evolve the companion Web site at

http://evolve.elsevier.com/Canada/Perry/maternal/

- Examination Review Questions
- Assessment Video Clips
- Case Study—Toilet Training/Toddler Development
- Skill—Car Seat Safety

Promoting Optimum Growth and Development

The term *terrible twos* has often been used to describe the toddler years, the period from 12 to 36 months of age. Although the term may be often used to describe the toddler's *behaviour*, it is not meant to typify or label the child. For children it is a time of intense exploration of the environment as they attempt to figure out how things work and learn how to control others through temper tantrums, negativism, and obstinacy. Although this can be a challenging time for parents and child as each comes to know the other better, it is an extremely important period for developmental achievement and intellectual growth. Toddlers are in fact very lovable at times, but because of their search for autonomy, they may test parents' and caregivers' patience. A developmental screening tool, such as the Canadian Nipissing District Developmental Screening (NDDS), can be used to assess the toddler's rate of **development** and can provide early intervention and guidance for families if there are any delays. The NDDS is for infants and children up to 6 years of age and can be used by nurses, physicians, and other health care providers to assess the level of development (see Additional Resources at the end of this chapter for more information).

Biological Development

Proportional Changes

Growth slows considerably during toddlerhood. The average weight gain is 1.8 to 2.7 kg. The birth weight is quadrupled by 2½ years of age. The rate of increase in height also slows. The usual increment is an addition of 7.5 cm per year and occurs mainly in elongation of the legs rather than the trunk. The average height of a 2-year-old is 86.6 cm. In general, adult height is about twice the 2-year-old child's height. (See Chapter 36 for the formula for height prediction.) Accurate measurement of height and weight during the toddler years should reveal a steady growth curve that is steplike in nature rather than linear (straight), which is characteristic of the growth spurts during the early childhood years. It is important for individual children to have specific measurements taken to accurately track their growth patterns. These measurements need to be done on a regular basis using a growth chart that compares them with the averages of other children. The Dietitians of Canada, Canadian Paediatric Society, College of Family Physicians, and Community Health Nurses of Canada (2010) have put forward a joint recommendation to use the WHO 2006 Child Growth Standards and the 2007 WHO Growth Reference growth charts for Canadian children.

The rate of increase in head circumference slows somewhat by the end of infancy; head circumference is usually equal to chest circumference by 1 to 2 years of age. The usual total increase in head circumference during the second year is 2.5 cm. Then the rate of increase slows until, at age 5 years, the increase is less than 1.25 cm per year. The anterior fontanel closes between 12 and 18 months of age.

Chest circumference continues to increase in size and exceeds head circumference during the toddler years. Its shape also changes as the transverse, or lateral, diameter exceeds the anteroposterior diameter. After the second year the chest circumference exceeds the abdominal measurement; this, in addition to the growth of the lower extremities, gives the child a taller, leaner appearance. However, the toddler still appears relatively squat and "pot-bellied" because of the less well-developed abdominal musculature and short legs. The legs remain slightly bowed or curved during the second year from the weight of the relatively large trunk.

Sensory Changes

Visual acuity of 20/40 is considered acceptable during the toddler years. Full binocular vision is well developed, and any evidence of persistent strabismus requires professional attention as early as possible to prevent **amblyopia**. Depth perception continues to develop but, because of the child's lack of motor coordination, falls from heights are a persistent danger.

The senses of hearing, smell, taste, and touch become increasingly well developed, coordinated with each other, and associated with other experiences. All of the senses are used to explore the environment. Toddlers will visually inspect an object by turning it over; they may taste it, smell it, and touch it several times before they are satisfied with their investigation. They will shake it to see if it makes noise and vigorously test its durability.

Another example of the integrated function of the senses is the toddler's development of specific taste preferences. The toddler is much less likely than an infant to try a new food because of its appearance, texture, or smell, not just its taste.

Maturation of Systems

Most of the physiological systems are relatively mature by the end of toddlerhood. The volume of the respiratory tract and growth of associated structures continue to increase during early childhood, lessening some of the factors that predisposed the child to frequent and serious infections during infancy. The internal structures of the ear and throat continue to be short and straight, and the lymphoid tissue of the tonsils and adenoids continues to be large. As a result, otitis media, tonsillitis, and upper respiratory tract infections are common. The respiratory and heart rates slow, and the blood pressure increases (see Appendix E). Respirations continue to be abdominal.

Under conditions of moderate variation in temperature, the toddler rarely has the difficulties of the young infant in maintaining body temperature. The mature functioning of the renal system serves to conserve fluid under times of **stress**, decreasing the risk of dehydration.

The digestive processes are fairly complete by the beginning of toddlerhood. The acidity of the gastric contents continues to increase and has a protective function, since they are capable of destroying many types of bacteria. Stomach capacity increases to allow for the usual schedule of three meals a day.

One of the more prominent changes of the gastrointestinal system is the voluntary control of elimination. With complete myelination of the spinal cord, control of the anal and urethral sphincters is gradually achieved. The physiological ability to control the sphincters probably occurs somewhere between ages 18 and 24 months. Bladder capacity also increases considerably, and by 14 to 18 months of age the child is able to retain urine for up to 2 hours or longer.

The defence mechanisms of the skin and blood, particularly phagocytosis, are much more efficient in toddlers than in infants. The production of antibodies is well established. However, many young children demonstrate a sudden increase in colds and minor infections when they enter preschool or other group situations, such as day care, because of their exposure to pathogens and the lack of understanding of general hygiene measures such as handwashing.

Gross and Fine Motor Development

The major gross motor skill during the toddler years is the development of locomotion. By 12 to 13 months of age, toddlers walk alone using a wide stance for extra balance, and by 18 months they try to run but fall easily (Fig. 37-1). Between 2 and 3 years of age, refinement of the upright, biped position is evident in improved coordination and equilibrium. At age 2 years, toddlers can walk up and down stairs; by age 2½ years they can jump using both feet, stand on one foot for a second or two, and manage a few steps on tiptoe. By the end of the

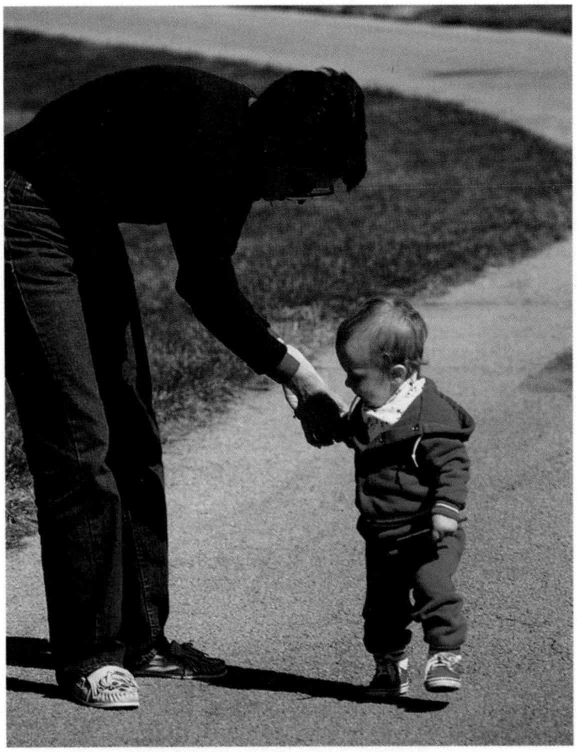

Fig. 37-1 Typical toddling gait.

second year they can stand on one foot, walk on tiptoe, and climb stairs with alternate footing.

Fine motor development is demonstrated in increasingly skilful manual dexterity. For example, by age 12 months toddlers are able to grasp a very small object but are unable to release it at will. At 15 months they can drop a pellet into a narrow-necked bottle. Casting or throwing objects and retrieving them become almost obsessive activities at about 15 months. By 18 months of age, toddlers can throw a ball overhand without losing their balance.

The major features of growth and development for the age groups of 15, 18, 24, and 30 months are summarized in Table 37-1.

Mastery of gross and fine motor skills is evident in all phases of the child's activity, such as play, dressing, language comprehension, response to discipline, social interaction, and propensity for injuries. Activities occur less in isolation and more in conjunction with other physical and mental abilities to produce a purposeful result. For example, the toddler will walk to reach a new location, release a toy to pick it up or to choose a new one, and scribble to look at the image produced. The possibilities of the exploration, investigation, and manipulation of the environment—and its hazards—are endless.

Psychosocial Development

Toddlers are faced with the mastery of several important tasks. If the need for basic **trust** has been satisfied, they are ready to give up dependence for control, independence, and **autonomy**. Some of the specific tasks to be dealt with include the following:

- Differentiation of self from others, particularly the mother
- Toleration of separation from the parent
- Ability to delay gratification
- Control over bodily functions
- Acquisition of socially acceptable behaviour
- Verbal means of communication
- Ability to interact with others in a less egocentric manner

Mastery of these goals is only begun during late infancy and the toddler years, and tasks such as developing interpersonal relationships with others may not be completed until adolescence. However, crucial foundations for successful completion of such **developmental tasks** are established during these early formative years.

Developing a Sense of Autonomy (Erikson)

According to Erikson (1963), the developmental task of toddlerhood is acquiring a sense of autonomy while overcoming a sense of doubt and shame. As infants gain trust in the predictability and reliability of their parents, environment, and interaction with others, they begin to discover that their behaviour is their own and that it has a predictable, reliable effect on others. However, although they realize their will and control over others, they are confronted with the conflict of exerting autonomy and relinquishing the much-enjoyed dependence on others. Exerting their will has definite negative consequences, whereas retaining dependent, submissive behaviour is generally rewarded with affection and approval. At the same time, continued dependency creates a sense of doubt regarding their potential capacity to control their actions. This doubt is compounded by a sense of shame for feeling this urge to revolt against others' will and a fear that they will exceed their own capacity for manipulating the environment.

Just as the infant has the social modalities of grasping and biting, the toddler has the newly gained modality of holding on and letting go. To hold on and let go is evident with the use of the hands, mouth, eyes, and, eventually, the sphincters, when toilet training is begun. These social modalities are expressed constantly in the child's play activities, such as casting or throwing objects; taking objects out of boxes, drawers, or cabinets; holding on tighter when someone says, "No, don't touch"; and spitting out food as taste preferences become strong.

Several characteristics, especially negativism and ritualism, are typical of toddlers in their quest for autonomy. As toddlers attempt to express their will, they often act with *negativism*, the persistent negative response to requests. The words "no" or "me do" can be the sole vocabulary. Emotions are strongly expressed, usually in rapid **mood** swings. One minute, toddlers can be engrossed in an activity, and the next minute they might be extremely frustrated because they are unable to manipulate a toy or open a door. If scolded for doing something wrong, they can have a temper tantrum and almost instantaneously pull at the parent's legs to be picked up and comforted. Understanding and coping with these swift changes in behaviour is often difficult for parents. Many parents find the negativism exasperating and, instead of dealing constructively with it, give in to it, which further threatens children in their search for learning acceptable methods of interacting with others (see Temper Tantrums and Negativism, p. 1031).

In contrast to negativism, which often disrupts the environment, *ritualism*, the need to maintain sameness and reliability, provides a sense of comfort. Toddlers can venture out with security when they know that familiar people, places, and routines still exist. One can easily understand why change, such as hospitalization, represents such a threat to these children. Without the comfortable rituals, there is little opportunity to exert autonomy. Consequently, dependency and **regression** occur (see Regression, p. 1032).

Erikson focused on the development of the *ego*, which may be thought of as reason or common sense, during this phase of psychosocial development. There is a struggle as the child deals with the impulses of the id and attempts to tolerate frustration and learn socially acceptable ways of interacting with the environment. The ego is evident as the child is able to tolerate delayed gratification.

There is also a rudimentary beginning of the *superego*, or conscience, which is the incorporation of the morals of society and the process of acculturation. With the development of the ego, children further differentiate themselves from others and expand their sense of trust within themselves. But as they begin to develop awareness of their own will and capacity to achieve, they also become aware of their ability to fail. This ever-present awareness of potential failure creates doubt and shame. Successful mastery of the task of autonomy necessitates opportunities for self-mastery while withstanding the frustration of necessary limit setting and delayed gratification. Opportunities for self-mastery are present in appropriate play activities, toilet training, the crisis of **sibling rivalry**, and successful interactions with significant others.

Table 37-1 Growth and Development During Toddler Years

AGE (MO)	PHYSICAL	GROSS MOTOR	FINE MOTOR	SENSORY	LANGUAGE	SOCIALIZATION
15	Steady growth in height and weight Head circumference 48 cm Weight 11 kg Height 78.7 cm	Walks without help (usually since age 13 mo) Creeps up stairs Kneels without support Cannot walk around corners or stop suddenly without losing balance Cannot throw ball without falling Runs clumsily; falls often	Constantly casting objects to floor Builds tower of two cubes Holds two cubes in one hand Releases a pellet into a narrow-necked bottle Scribbles spontaneously Uses cup well but rotates spoon before it reaches mouth	Able to identify geometric forms; places round object into appropriate hole Binocular vision well developed Displays an intense and prolonged interest in pictures	Uses expressive jargon Says four to six words, including names "Asks" for objects by pointing Understands simple commands May use head-shaking gesture to denote "no" Uses "no" even while agreeing to the request Uses common repetitive gestures such as putting cup to mouth when empty	Tolerates some separation from parent Less likely to fear strangers Beginning to imitate parents, such as cleaning house (sweeping, dusting), folding clothes May discard bottle Kisses and hugs parents; may kiss pictures in a book
18	Picky eater from decreased growth needs Anterior fontanel closed Physiologically able to control sphincters	Assumes standing position without support Walks up stairs with one hand held Pulls and pushes toys Jumps in place with both feet Seats self on chair Throws ball overhand without falling	Builds tower of three or four cubes Release, prehension, and reach are well developed Turns pages in a book two or three at a time In drawing, makes stroke imitatively Manages spoon without rotation		Says ten or more words Points to a common object, such as a shoe or ball, and to two or three body parts Forms word combinations Forms gesture–word combinations Forms gesture–gesture combinations	Expresses emotions; has temper tantrums Great imitator (domestic mimicry) Takes off gloves, socks, and shoes and unzips Beginning awareness of ownership ("my toy") May develop dependence on transitional objects, such as "security blanket"
24	Head circumference 49–50 cm Chest circumference exceeds head circumference Lateral diameter of chest exceeds anteroposterior diameter Usual weight gain of 1.8–2.7 kg Usual gain in height of 10–12.5 cm May have achieved readiness for beginning daytime control of bowel and bladder Primary dentition of 16 teeth	Goes up and down stairs alone with two feet on each step Runs fairly well, with wide stance Picks up object without falling Kicks ball forward without overbalancing	Builds tower of six or seven cubes Aligns two or more cubes like a train Turns pages of book one at a time In drawing, imitates vertical and circular strokes Turns doorknob; unscrews lid	Accommodation well developed In geometric discrimination, able to insert square block into oblong space	Has vocabulary of approximately 300 words Uses two- or three-word phrases Uses pronouns "I," "me," "you" Understands directional commands Gives first name; refers to self by name Verbalizes need for toileting, food, or drink Talks incessantly	Stage of parallel play Has sustained attention span Temper tantrums decreasing Pulls people to show them something Increased independence from parent Dresses self in simple clothing Develops visual recognition and verbal self-reference ("Me big")
30	Birth weight quadrupled Primary dentition (20 teeth) completed May have daytime bowel and bladder control	Jumps with both feet Jumps from chair or step Stands on one foot momentarily Takes a few steps on tiptoe	Builds tower of eight cubes Adds chimney to train of cubes Good hand–finger coordination; holds crayon with fingers rather than fist Moves fingers independently In drawing, imitates vertical and horizontal strokes; makes two or more strokes for cross		Gives first and last name Refers to self by appropriate pronoun Uses plurals Names one colour	Separates more easily from parent In play, helps put things away; can carry breakable objects; pushes with good steering Begins to notice sex differences; knows own sex May attend to toilet needs without help except for wiping Emotions expand to include pride, shame, guilt, embarrassment

Cognitive Development

Sensorimotor and Preoperational Phase (Piaget)

The period from 12 to 24 months of age is a continuation of the final two stages of Piaget's (1952) sensorimotor phase. During this time, the cognitive processes develop rapidly and at times seem similar to those of mature thinking. However, reasoning skills are still primitive and need to be understood in order to effectively deal with the typical behaviours of a child of this age.

Tertiary Circular Reactions

In the fifth stage of the sensorimotor phase (13 to 18 months of age), the child uses active experimentation to achieve previously unattainable goals. Newly acquired physical skills are increasingly important for the function they serve rather than for the acts themselves. The child incorporates the old learning of secondary circular reactions with new skills and applies the combined knowledge to new situations, with emphasis on the results of the experimentation. In this way, there is the beginning of rational **judgement** and intellectual reasoning. During this stage, there is further differentiation of one's self from objects. This is evident in the child's increasing ability to venture away from the parent and to tolerate longer periods of separation.

The child also starts to develop awareness of a causal relationship between two events. After flipping a light switch, toddlers are aware that a reciprocal response occurs. However, they are not able to transfer that knowledge to new situations. Therefore, every time they see what appears to be a light switch, they must reinvestigate its function. Such behaviour demonstrates the beginning of categorizing data into distinct classes and subclasses. Examples of this type of behaviour are innumerable as toddlers continuously explore the same object each time it appears in a new place.

Because classification of objects is still rudimentary, the appearance of an object denotes its function. For example, if the child's toys are stored in a paper bag or large container, that toy receptacle is no different from the garbage pail or laundry basket. If allowed to turn over the toy receptacle, the child will just as quickly do the same to other similar containers because, in the child's mind, there is no difference. Expecting the child to judge which receptacles are permissible to explore and which are not is inappropriate for this age group. Instead, the forbidden object, such as the garbage pail, should be placed out of reach. This has significance in relation to protecting the toddler from injury; the toddler is not able to differentiate between what is a safe object to play with in any given situation and what is unsafe in another. For example, if the child is allowed to throw a toy ball, he or she does not necessarily understand why a different toy that may harm someone cannot be thrown as well.

The discovery of objects as objects leads to the awareness of their spatial relationships. Children are able to recognize different shapes and their relationship to each other. For example, they can fit slightly smaller boxes into each other (nesting) and can place a round object into a hole, even if the board is turned around, turned upside down, or reversed. Children are also aware of space and the relationship of their body to dimensions such as height. They will stretch, stand on a low stair or stool, and pull a string to reach an object.

Object permanence has also advanced. Although they still cannot find an object that has been invisibly displaced or moved from under one pillow to another without their seeing the change, toddlers are increasingly aware of the existence of objects behind closed doors, in drawers, on countertops, and under tables. Parents are usually acutely aware of this developmental achievement and find high places and locked cabinets the only places inaccessible to toddlers.

Invention of New Means Through Mental Combinations

From ages 19 to 24 months, the child is in the final sensorimotor stage. During this stage, the child completes the more primitive, autistic-like thought processes of infancy and is prepared for the more complex mental operations that occur during the phase of preoperational thought. One of the most dramatic achievements of this stage is in the area of object permanence. Children will now actively search for an object in several potential hiding places. In addition, they can infer a cause when only experiencing the effect. They can infer that an object was hidden in any number of places even if they only saw the original hiding place.

Imitation displays deeper meaning and understanding. There is greater symbolization to imitation. The child is acutely aware of others' actions and attempts to copy them in gestures and in words. Domestic **mimicry** (imitating household activities) and gender-role behaviour become increasingly common during this stage, especially during the second year. Identification with the parent of the same gender becomes apparent by the second year and represents the child's intellectual ability to identify different models of behaviour and to imitate them appropriately (Fig. 37-2).

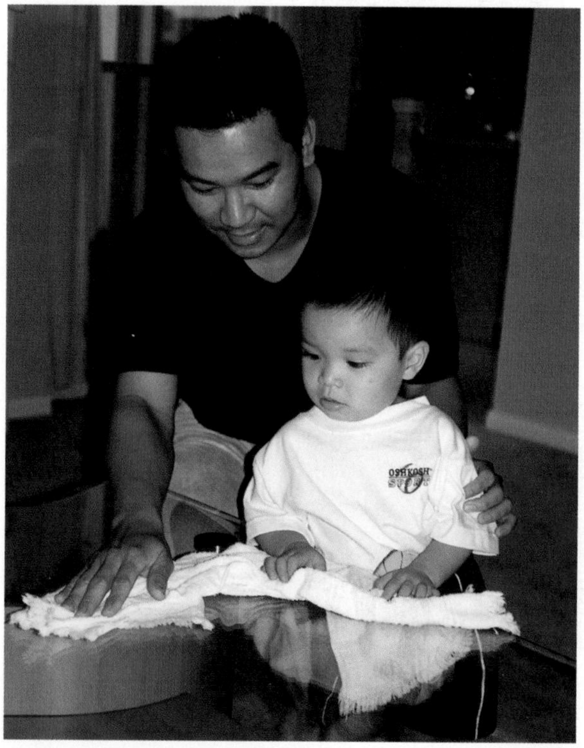

Fig. 37-2 Domestic mimicry and gender-role behaviour are common during toddlerhood.

While the concept of time is still embryonic, children have some sense of timing in terms of anticipation, memory, and a limited ability to wait. They may listen to the command, "Just a minute," and behave appropriately. However, their sense of time is exaggerated—1 minute can seem like an hour. Toddlers' limited attention spans also indicate their sense of immediacy and concern for the present.

Preoperational Phase

At approximately 2 years of age, the child enters the *preconceptual phase* of cognitive development, which lasts until about age 4 years. The preconceptual phase is a subdivision of the *preoperational phase*, which spans ages 2 to 7 years. The preconceptual phase is primarily one of transition that bridges the purely self-satisfying behaviour of infancy and the rudimentary socialized behaviour of latency. *Preoperational thought* implies that children cannot think in terms of operations—the ability to manipulate objects in relation to each other in a logical fashion. Rather, toddlers think primarily on the basis of their perception of an event. Problem solving is based on what they see or hear directly rather than on what they recall about objects and events. Several characteristics are unique to preoperational thought (Box 37-1).

Within the second year, the child increasingly uses language symbolically and is concerned with the "why" and "how" of things. For example, a pencil is "something to write with," and food is "something to eat." However, such mental symbolization is closely associated with prelogical reasoning.

BOX 37-1 Characteristics of Preoperational Thought

Egocentrism—Inability to envision situations from perspectives other than one's own

Example—If a person is positioned between the toddler and another child, the toddler, who is facing the person, will explain that both children can see the middle person's face. The young child is unable to realize that the other person views the middle person from a different perspective, the back.

Implication—Avoid moralizing about "why" something is wrong if it requires an understanding of someone else's feelings or opinion. Telling a child to stop hitting because hitting hurts the other person is often ineffective because, to the aggressor, it feels good to hit someone else. Instead, emphasize that hitting is not allowed.

Transductive reasoning—Reasoning from the particular to the particular

Example—Child refuses to eat a food because something previously eaten did not taste good.

Implication—Accept the child's reasoning; offer refused food at a different time.

Global organization—Reasoning that changing any one part of the whole changes the entire whole

Example—Child refuses to sleep in his or her room because the location of the bed is changed.

Implication—Accept the child's reasoning; use the same bed position or introduce change slowly.

Centration—Focusing on one aspect rather than considering all possible alternatives

Example—Child refuses to eat a food because of its colour, even though its taste and smell are acceptable.

Implication—Accept the child's reasoning.

Animism—Attributing lifelike qualities to inanimate objects

Example—Child scolds stairs for making the child fall down.

Implication—Join the child in the "scolding." Keep frightening objects out of view.

Irreversibility—Inability to undo or reverse the actions initiated physically

Example—When told to stop doing something, such as talking, the child is unable to think of positive activity.

Implication—State requests or instructions positively (e.g., "Be quiet.")

Magical thinking—Believing that thoughts are all-powerful and can cause events

Examples—Child wishes someone died; then if the person dies, the child feels at fault because of the "bad" thought that made the death happen.

- Calling children "bad" because they did something wrong makes children feel as if they are bad.

Implications—Clarify that thoughts do not make things happen and that the child is not responsible.

- Use "I" messages rather than "you" messages to communicate thoughts, feelings, expectations, or beliefs, without imposing blame or criticism. Emphasize that the *act* is bad, not the child.

Inability to conserve—Inability to understand the idea that a mass can be changed in size, shape, volume, or length without losing or adding to the original mass (instead, children judge what they see by the immediate perceptual clues given to them)

Example—If two lines of equal length are presented in such a way that one appears longer than the other, the child will state that one line is longer, even if the child measures both lines with a ruler or yardstick and finds that each has the same length.

Implications—Change the most obvious perceptual clue to reorient the child's view of what is seen. For example, give medicine in a small medicine cup, rather than a large cup, since the child will imagine that the large vessel contains more liquid. If the child refuses the medicine in the small cup, pour it into a large cup, because the liquid will appear to be less in a tall, wide container.

- Give a large, flat cookie rather than a thick, small one, or do the reverse with meat or cheese; the child will usually eat a larger size of favourite food and a smaller size of less favourite food.

For instance, a needle is "something that hurts." Such painful experiences take on new significance because memory is associated with the specific event, and fears are likely to develop, such as resistance to people who wear a uniform or rooms that look like the practitioner's office. Because of the vulnerability of these early years, it is essential to prepare children for any new experience, whether it is a new baby-sitter or a visit to the practitioner or dentist.

Spiritual Development

Spiritual development in children is often discussed in terms of the child's developmental level because the evolution of spirituality often parallels cognitive development (Elkins & Cavendish, 2004). The child's family and environment strongly influence the child's perception of the world around him or her, and this often includes spirituality. Furthermore, family values, beliefs, customs, and expressions of these will influence the child's perception of his or her spiritual self (Elkins & Cavendish, 2004). The relationship between spirituality, illness in childhood, and nursing has been studied in the context of suffering, terminal illness such as cancer, and end-of-life care. In the past two decades there has been increased interest in and focus on spiritual care of adults and children as further understanding of the influence of one's spirituality on health, illness, and well-being has progressed. For instance, the Canadian Virtual Hospice Web site provides information on how to talk to children, including toddlers, about serious illness (see Additional Resources at the end of this chapter).

Toddlers learn about God through the words and the actions of those closest to them. They have only a vague idea of God and religious teachings because of their immature cognitive processes; however, if God is spoken about with reverence, young children associate God with something special. During this period, the designation of powerful religious symbols and images is strongly influenced by the manner in which they are presented; therein lies the potential for the development of guilt and fear or, conversely, love and companionship with religious symbols (Roehlkepartain et al., 2006).

Toddlers begin to assimilate behaviours associated with the divine (folding hands in prayer). Routines such as saying prayers before meals or at bedtime can be important and comforting. Near the end of toddlerhood, when children use preoperational thought, there is some advancement of their understanding of God. Religious teachings, such as reward or fear of punishment (heaven or hell) and moral development (see Chapter 32), may influence their behaviour (Fosarelli, 2003).

Development of Body Image

As in infancy, the development of **body image** closely parallels cognitive development. Developing psychological understanding provides greater self-awareness, and young children learn to answer the question "Who am I?" During their second year, children recognize themselves in a mirror and make verbal references to themselves ("Me big"). With increasing motor ability, toddlers recognize the usefulness of body parts and gradually learn their names. They also learn that certain parts of the body have various meanings; for example, during toilet training the genitalia become significant and cleanliness is emphasized. By 2 years of age there is recognition of gender differences and reference to self by name and then by pronoun. Gender identity is developed by age 3 years. Also by this time, the child begins to remember events with reference to their personal significance, forming an autobiographic memory that helps establish a continuous identity throughout life's events (Thompson, 2001).

Once they begin preoperational thought, toddlers can use symbols to represent objects, but their thinking may lead to inaccuracies. For example, if someone who is pregnant is called "fat," they will describe all "fat" women as having babies. There is a beginning recognition of words used to describe physical appearance, such as "pretty," "handsome," or "big boy." Such expressions eventually influence how children view their own bodies.

Although little research has been done on body-image development in young children, it is evident that body integrity is poorly understood and that intrusive experiences are threatening (Dahlquist et al., 2002). For example, toddlers forcefully resist procedures such as examination of the ear or mouth and taking of an axillary temperature. The procedure itself (e.g., taking vital signs) is not hurting the child, but it represents an intrusion into the child's personal space, which will elicit a strong protest. Toddlers also have unclear body boundaries and may associate nonviable parts, such as feces, with essential body parts. This can be seen in a toddler who is upset by flushing the toilet and watching the stool disappear.

Nurses can assist parents in fostering a positive body image in their child by encouraging them to avoid negative labels, such as "skinny arms" or "chubby legs," self-perceptions that can last a lifetime. Body parts, especially those related to elimination and reproduction, should be called by their correct names. Respect for the body should be practised.

Development of Gender Identity

Just as toddlers explore their environment, they also explore their bodies and find that touching certain body parts is pleasurable. Masturbation can occur and involves manual stimulation of genitalia and posturing movements against objects. If performed in public, the behaviour should be ignored. The child should be taught that it is more acceptable to perform the behaviour in private (Meyer, 2002). Other demonstrations of pleasurable activities include rocking, sucking on fingers, swinging, and hugging people and toys. During the activity the child may perspire, and the activity may be difficult to interrupt.

Children in this age group are learning vocabulary associated with anatomy, elimination, and reproduction. Certain associations between words and functions become significant and can influence future sexual attitudes. For example, if parents refer to the genitalia as dirty, especially in the context of elimination, this association between "genitalia" and "dirty" may be transferred to sexual functions. Gender-role differences become obvious to children and are evident in much of their imitative play. A sense of maleness or femaleness, *gender identity*, is formed by age 3 years. Early attitudes are formed about affectionate behaviours between adults from observing parental and other adult intimate behaviours such as kissing and hugging (see also Chapter 38, Sex Education). The quality of relationships with parents is important to the child's capacity for sexual and emotional relationships later in life (DeLamater & Friedrich, 2002).

Social Development

A major task of the toddler period is differentiation of self from significant others, usually the mother. The differentiation process consists of two phases: *separation*, the child's emergence from a symbiotic fusion with the mother; and *individuation*, those achievements that mark the child's expressions of his or her individual characteristics in the environment. Although the process begins during the latter half of infancy, the major achievements occur during the toddler years (see Table 37-1).

Toddlers have an increased understanding and awareness of object permanence and have some ability to withstand delayed gratification and tolerate moderate frustration. As a result, toddlers react differently to strangers than do infants. The appearance of unfamiliar persons does not represent such a significant threat to their attachment to the mother. They have learned from experience that parents still exist when physically absent. Repetition of events such as going to bed without the parents but waking to find them there again (in the household) reinforces the reliability of such brief separations. Consequently, toddlers are able to venture away from their parents for brief periods.

According to Harpaz-Rotem and Bergman (2006), the separation–individuation phase encompasses the phenomenon of rapprochement; as the toddler separates from the mother and begins to make sense of experiences in the environment, he or she is drawn back to the mother for assistance in verbally articulating the meaning of the experiences. Developmentally the term *rapprochement* means the child moves away and returns for reassurance. If the mother's response to the toddler is inappropriate, the toddler may experience insecurity and confusion.

Transitional objects, such as a favourite blanket or toy, provide security for children, especially when they are separated from parents, dealing with a new stress, or just fatigued (Fig. 37-3). Security objects often become so important to toddlers that they refuse to have them taken away. Such behaviour is normal; there is no need to discourage this tendency. During separations such as day care, hospitalization, or even overnight stays with relatives, transitional objects should be provided to minimize any feelings of fear or loneliness.

Learning to tolerate and master brief periods of separation is an important developmental task of children in this age group. In addition, it is a necessary component of parenting, since brief periods of separation allow parents to regain their energy and patience and to minimize any tendency to direct their irritations and frustrations at the children.

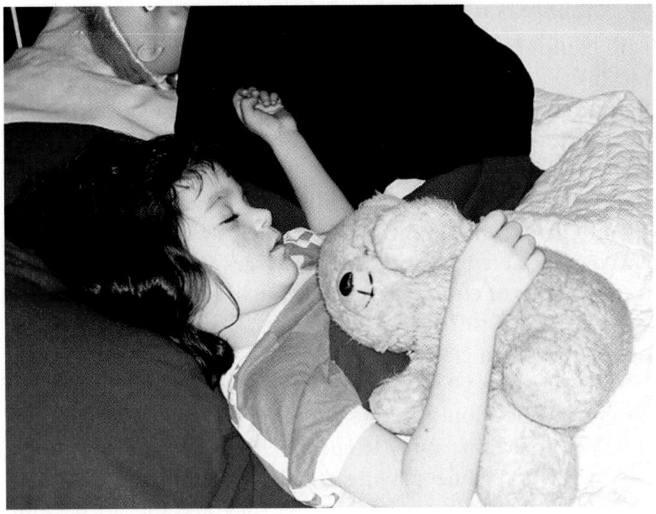

Fig. 37-3 Transitional objects, such as a fuzzy stuffed animal, are sources of security to a toddler.

Language

The most striking characteristic of language development during early childhood is the increasing level of comprehension (see Table 37-1). Although the number of words acquired—from about 4 at 1 year of age to approximately 300 at age 2 years—is notable, the ability to *comprehend and understand speech is much greater than the number of words the child can say*. Bilingual children also achieve their early linguistic milestones in each of the languages at the same time and produce a substantial number of semantically corresponding words in each of their two languages from the very first words or signs (Petitto et al., 2001).

At age 1 year the child uses one-word sentences, or holophrases. The word "up" can mean "pick me up" or "look up there." For the child, the one word conveys the meaning of a sentence, but to others it may mean many things or nothing. At this age about 25% of the vocalizations are intelligible. By the age of 2 years the child uses multiword sentences by stringing together two or three words, such as the phrases "mama go bye-bye" or "all gone," and approximately 65% of the speech is understandable. By 3 years of age the child puts words together into simple sentences, begins to master grammatical rules, and acquires five or six new words daily.

Gestures precede or accompany each of the language milestones up to 30 months of age (putting phone to ear, pointing). Once language is sufficiently mastered, gestures phase out and the pace of word learning increases (Bates & Dick, 2002).

Personal-Social Behaviour

One of the most dramatic aspects of development in the toddler is personal-social interaction. Parents often wonder why their manageable, docile, lovable infant has turned into a determined, strong-willed, volatile little tyrant. In addition, the tyrant of the terrible twos can swiftly and unpredictably revert back to the adorable, cuddly child. All of this is part of growing up and is evident in such areas as dressing, feeding, playing, and establishing self-control.

Toddlers are developing skills of independence, and these are evident in all areas of behaviour. By 15 months children feed themselves, drink well from a covered cup, and manage a spoon with considerable spilling. By 24 months they use a spoon well and by 36 months may be using a fork. Between ages 2 and 3 years they eat with the family and like to help with chores such as setting the table or removing dishes from the dishwasher. However, they lack table manners and may find it difficult to sit through the family's entire meal.

In dressing, toddlers also demonstrate strides in independence. The 15-month-old child helps by putting the arm or foot out for dressing and pulls shoes and socks off. The 18-month-old child removes gloves, helps with pullover shirts, and may be able to unzip. By age 2 years the toddler removes most articles of clothing and puts on socks, shoes, and pants without regard to right or left and back or front. Help is still needed to fasten clothes.

Toddlers also begin to develop concern for the feelings of others and develop an understanding of how adult expectations for behaviour apply to specific situations (e.g., causing a sibling to cry while playing rough) (Thompson, 2001). As parents foster their understanding, they are able to develop control. Age-appropriate discipline contributes to healthy social and emotional development. Positive reinforcement, redirecting, and time-out are appropriate for most toddlers. Social and emotional problems can develop in the youngest children. Early screening and intervention promote more positive developmental outcomes as the young child grows and develops.

Play

Play magnifies the toddler's physical and psychosocial development. Interaction with people becomes increasingly important. The solitary play of infancy progresses to **parallel play**—the toddler plays alongside, not with, other children (see Fig. 33-7). Although sensorimotor play is still prominent, there is much less emphasis on the exclusive use of one sensory modality. The toddler inspects the toy, talks to the toy, tests its strength and durability, and invents several uses for it. Imitation is one of the more distinguishing characteristics of play and enriches the child's opportunity to engage in **fantasy**. With less emphasis on gender-stereotyped toys, play objects such as dolls, carriages, dollhouses, dishes, balls, clay, cooking utensils, child-size furniture, trucks, and dress-up clothes (Fig. 37-4) are suitable for both genders; however,

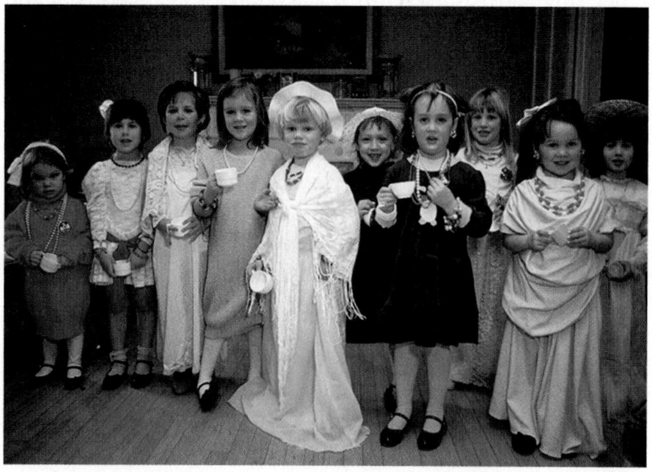

Fig. 37-4 Young children enjoy dressing up.

evolve Case Study—Toilet Training/Toddler Development

boys may be more interested than girls in activities related to trucks, trailers, cars, miniature plastic soldiers or super heroes, and building blocks, whereas girls may prefer doll-related activities.

Increased locomotive skills make push-pull toys, straddle trucks or cycles, a small gym and slide, balls of various sizes, and rocking horses appropriate for the energetic toddler. Finger paints; thick crayons; chalk; a blackboard; paper; and puzzles with large, simple pieces use the child's developing fine motor skills. Interlocking blocks in various sizes and shapes provide hours of fun and, during later years, are useful objects for creative and imaginative play. The most educational toy is the one that fosters the interaction of an adult with a child in supportive, unconditional play. Toys are never substitutes for the attention of devoted caregivers, but toys can enhance these interactions (Glassy, Romano, & Committee on Early Childhood, Adoption, and Dependent Care, 2003).

Certain aspects of play are related to emerging linguistic abilities. Talking is a form of play for toddlers who enjoy musical toys such as age-appropriate MP3 players, "talking" dolls and animals, and toy telephones. Appropriate children's television programs are excellent for children in this age group, who learn to associate words with visual images. However, total media time should be limited to 1 to 2 hours of quality programming per day (Canadian Paediatric Society [CPS], 2003). Toddlers also enjoy "reading" stories from a picture book and imitating the sounds of animals.

Tactile play is also important for the exploring toddler. Water toys, a sandbox with pail and shovel, finger paints, soap bubbles, and clay provide excellent opportunities for creative and manipulative recreation. Adults sometimes forget the fascination of feeling slippery cream, mud, or pudding; catching airy bubbles; squeezing and reshaping clay; or smearing paints. These types of unstructured activities are as important as educational play to allow children freedom of expression.

The selection of appropriate toys must involve safety factors, especially in relation to size and sturdiness. Toddlers' oral activity puts them at risk for aspirating small objects or for ingesting toxic substances. Parents need to be especially vigilant of toys of older siblings or those played with in other children's homes. Toys are a potential source of serious bodily damage to toddlers, who may have the physical strength to manipulate them but not the knowledge to appreciate their danger (see Family-Centred Teaching box, p. 860). Government agencies do not inspect and police all toys on the market. Therefore, adults who purchase play equipment, supervise purchases, or allow children to use play equipment (including toys that are gifts or are purchased by the children themselves) need to evaluate its safety. Adults should also be alert to notices of toys determined to be defective and recalled by the manufacturers. Parents and health care workers can obtain information on a variety of recalled products and can report potentially dangerous toys and child products to the Canadian Toy Testing Council. Printable tips on toy safety are also available from Safe Kids Worldwide (http://www.safekids.org). In addition, Health Canada has a Consumer Product Recall listing, at http://cpsr-rspc.hc-sc.gc.ca/PR-RP/home-accueil-eng.jsp.

Coping With Concerns Related to Normal Growth and Development

Toilet Training

One of the major tasks of toddlerhood is toilet training. Voluntary control of the anal and urethral sphincters is achieved sometime after the child is walking, probably between ages 18 and 24 months. However, complex psychophysiological factors are required for readiness. The child must be able to recognize the urge to let go and hold on and be able to communicate this sensation to the parent. In addition, there may be some necessary motivation in the desire to please the parent by holding on, rather than pleasing oneself by letting go.

Five markers signal a child's readiness to toilet train: motor, language, social milestones, demeanour, and relationship with the parents (CPS, 2010b). According to some experts, physiological and psychological readiness is not complete until ages 22 to 30 months (Schum et al., 2002). However, Schmitt (2004) emphasizes that parents should begin preparing the child for toilet training earlier than 30 months. By this time, the child has mastered the majority of essential gross motor skills, can communicate intelligibly, is in less conflict with parents in terms of self-assertion and **negativism**, and is aware of the ability to control the body and please the parent. On average, girls are developmentally ready to begin toilet training 2 to 2½ months before boys (Schum et al., 2002).

There is no universal right age to begin toilet training or an absolute deadline to complete training. One of the nurse's most important responsibilities is to help parents identify the readiness signs in their child and how to facilitate toilet learning (see Guidelines box). The Canadian Paediatric Society has a helpful parent guide to toilet training (see Additional Resources at the end of this chapter).

Nighttime bladder control normally takes several months to years after daytime training. This is because the sleep cycle needs to mature to the point that the child can awaken in time to urinate. Few children will have night wetting episodes after daytime dryness is achieved; however, those children who do not have nighttime dryness by the age of 6 years are likely to require intervention (Mercer, 2003).

Bowel training is usually accomplished before bladder training because of its greater regularity and predictability. There is a stronger sensation for defecation than for urination, and the sensation of defecation can be brought to the child's attention. A well-balanced diet that includes dietary fibre helps keep stools soft and supports the development and maintenance of regular bowel movements.

A number of techniques can be helpful when initiating training, and cultural differences should be considered in this process. Parents should begin the readiness phase of toilet training by teaching the child how the body functions in relation to voiding and having a stool. Schmitt (2004) suggests that parents talk about how adults and animals perform such functions on a routine basis. Another suggestion is to make toilet training as easy and simple as possible. The selection of the child's clothing is an important consideration, as is the potty chair or use of the toilet. A freestanding potty chair allows children a feeling of security. Planting the feet firmly on the floor also facilitates defecation. Another option is a portable seat attached to the regular toilet, which may ease the transition from potty chair to regular toilet (Fig. 37-5). Placing a small bench under the feet helps stabilize the child's position. It is probably best to keep the potty chair in the bathroom and to let the child observe the excreta being flushed down the toilet to associate these activities with usual practices. If a potty chair is not available, having the child sit facing the toilet tank provides added support.

Practice sessions should be limited to 5 to 8 minutes, and a parent should stay with the child, practising sanitary habits after every session. Children should be praised for their behaviour and successful evacuation. Dressing children in easily removed clothing; using training pants, "pull-on" diapers, or underwear; and encouraging imitation by watching others are other helpful suggestions.

When the child begins to experience regular daytime dryness, parents may experiment with underwear during the day. Daytime accidents are common, particularly during periods of intense activity. Young children become so engrossed in play that, if they are not reminded, they will wait until it is too late to reach the bathroom. Therefore, frequent reminders and trips to the toilet are necessary. Parents often

GUIDELINES Assessing Toilet Training Readiness and How to Facilitate Toilet Learning

Signs of a Child's Toilet Learning Readiness

- Can walk to the potty chair or adapted toilet seat with a footstool
- Can balance while sitting on the potty
- Can remain dry for several hours
- Receptive language skills allow the child to be able to follow simple one- and two-step commands
- Expressive language skills that allow the child to communicate the need to use the potty with word or reproducible gestures

How Parents Can Facilitate a Child's Toilet Learning

- Use an accessible potty chair in the beginning because the child feels more stable and secure and it is the best biomechanical position for the child.
- Sit the child dressed on a potty, then after a soiled diaper has been removed, and then at a regular time schedule.
- Role model use of the toilet.
- Use the same vocabulary.
- Express praise when the child shows an interest in sitting on the potty and is successful.
- Avoid negative comments and punishment.
- Use cotton underpants or training pants after 1 week or more.
- Encourage the child to give a verbal cue when he or she needs to void or have a bowel movement and learn the child's behavioural cues.
- If the child is reluctant at times to have a bowel movement in the potty, try supporting the feet and allow the use of diapers to avoid the pain of constipation, which could delay the learning progress.

(Adapted from Canadian Paediatric Society [2010]. *Toilet learning: Anticipatory guidance with a child-oriented approach*. Retrieved from http://www.cps.ca/english/statements/cp/cp00-02.htm.)

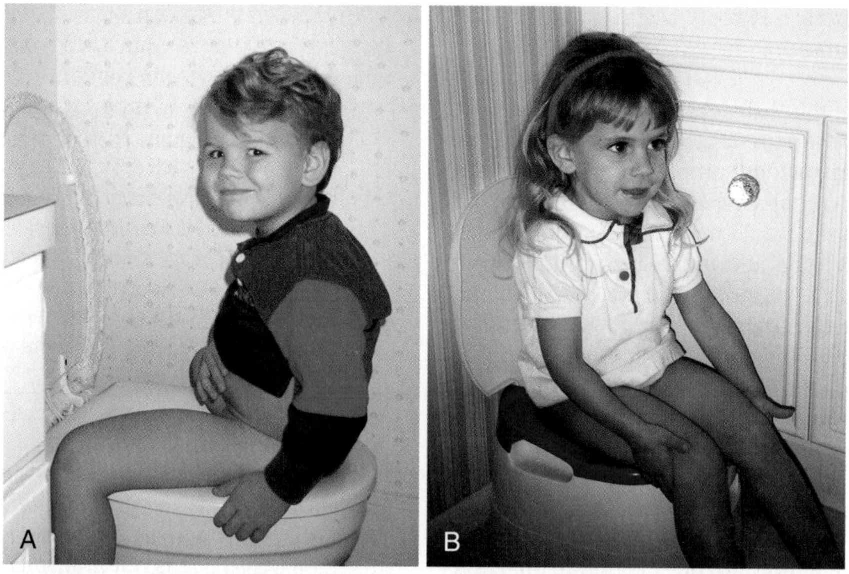

Fig. 37-5 A: Sitting in reverse fashion on a regular toilet provides additional security to a young child. B: Children may begin toilet training sitting on a small potty chair.

forget to plan ahead when the toddler is being toilet trained; before trips outside the house it is important to remind the child to at least try to urinate, to decrease the chance of needing to use the toilet while the car is stuck in traffic.

As the child develops each step of toileting (discussion, undressing, going, wiping, dressing, flushing, and hand washing), he or she gains a sense of accomplishment that parents should reinforce. If the parent–child relationship becomes strained, both may need a break from toilet training to focus on enjoyable activities together. Regression may coincide with a stressful family situation or may occur if the child is being pushed too hard and too fast. Regression is a normal part of toilet training and does not mean failure but should be viewed as a temporary setback to a more comfortable place for the child.

Day care providers also play a role in the support and education of parents regarding toilet-training practices. It is important for parents to inform all caregivers of their individual family values and the child's specific needs when planning for training away from home. Ensuring consistency in care of the toddler and healthy practices in a sanitary environment allows for safe and effective toilet practices in all settings.

Once the child has been successfully toilet trained for bladder control, sudden wetting accidents and frequent urinating urges may require further investigation for a possible urinary tract infection (UTI), especially in girls. Younger children often have a UTI without accompanying fever or painful urination.

Sibling Rivalry

The natural jealousy and resentment of children to a new child in the family is referred to as *sibling rivalry*. The arrival of a new infant represents a crisis for even the best-prepared toddlers. It is not the infant that toddlers resent but the changes that this additional sibling produces, especially the separation from the mother during the birth. The parents now share their love and attention with someone else, the usual routine is disrupted, and toddlers may lose their crib or room, all at a time when they thought they were in control of their world. Sibling rivalry tends to be most pronounced in the firstborn, who experiences *dethronement* (i.e., loss of sole parental attention). It also seems to be most difficult for young children, particularly in terms of mother–child interaction.

While preparation of children for the birth of a sibling is individual, age dictates some important considerations. Time for toddlers is a vague concept. Tomorrow could be yesterday or next week, and a month from now could be never. Preparing children too soon for the birth may lessen their interest by the time the event occurs. A good time to start talking about the new baby is when the toddler becomes aware of the pregnancy and the changes taking place in the home in anticipation of the new member.

Toddlers need to have a realistic idea of what the newborn will be like. Telling them that a new playmate will come home soon sets up unrealistic expectations. Rather, parents should stress the activities that will take place when the baby arrives home, such as diapering, feeding, bathing, and dressing. At the same time, parents should emphasize which routines will stay the same, such as reading stories or going to the park. The disruption of the toddler's routine is significant but can be restored with some effort by the parents. It may be helpful for the father to spend more quality time with the toddler in anticipation of the mother's time being occupied with the new baby. If toddlers have had no contact with an infant, it is a good idea to introduce them to one, if feasible.

A new sibling in the home is stressful, so any additional stresses for the toddler should be avoided or minimized. For example, moving the toddler to a regular bed or to a different room should be done well in advance of the infant's arrival.

Pregnancy is an abstraction for toddlers. They need concrete illustrations of how the baby is growing inside the mother. It is an excellent opportunity for introducing aspects of reproduction and sexuality. Seeing simple pictures of the uterus and fetus and feeling the fetus move help the child feel involved in the experience (see Fig. 10-3). Children also benefit from classes for siblings that may be part of prenatal sessions (see Fig. 10-4).

When the newborn arrives, toddlers keenly feel the changed focus of attention. Visitors may initiate problems when they inadvertently shower the infant with attention and presents while neglecting the older child. Parents can minimize this by alerting visitors to the toddler's needs and by including the child in the visits as much as possible. The toddler can also help with the care of the newborn by getting diapers and doing other small tasks (Fig. 37-6).

How children exhibit jealousy is complex. Some will overtly hit the infant, push the child off the mother's lap, or pull the breast or bottle from the infant's mouth. For this reason, infants must be protected by parental supervision of the interaction between the siblings. More often the expressions of hostility and resentment are more subtle and covert. Toddlers may verbally express a wish that the infant "go back inside mommy," or they will revert to more infantile forms of behaviour, such as demanding a bottle, soiling their underpants, clinging for attention, using baby talk, or aggressively acting out toward others.

Temper Tantrums

Toddlers may assert their independence by violently objecting to discipline. They may lie down on the floor, kick their feet, and scream as loud as possible. Some have learned the effectiveness of holding their breath until the parent relents. Although holding one's breath may cause fainting from lack of oxygen, the accumulation of carbon dioxide will stimulate the respiratory control centre, resulting in no physical harm.

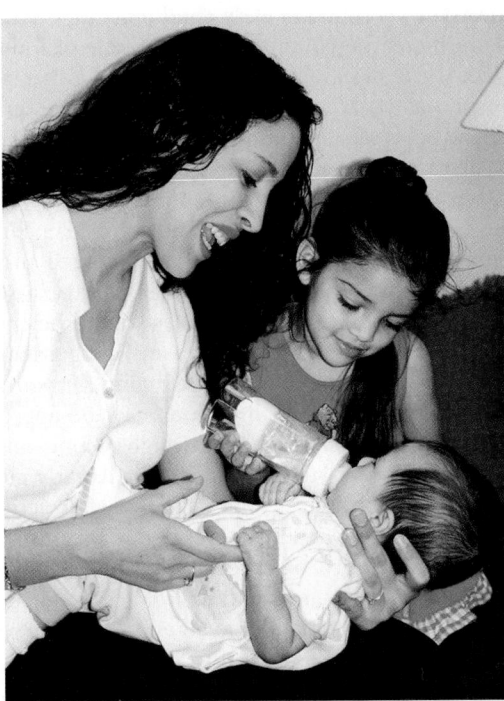

Fig. 37-6 To minimize sibling rivalry, parents should include the toddler during caregiving activities.

Tantrums are an indication of the child's inability to control emotions; toddlers are particularly prone to tantrums because their strong drive for mastery and autonomy is frustrated by adult figures or lack of motor and cognitive skills (Needlman, Howard, & Zuckerman, 1995).

The best approach toward tapering temper tantrums requires consistency and developmentally appropriate expectations and rewards. Ensuring consistency among all caregivers in expectations, prioritizing what rules are important, and developing consequences that are reasonable for the child's level of development can help manage the behaviour (CPS, 2004). For example, a common time for a tantrum is before bed. Active toddlers often have trouble slowing down and, when placed in bed, resist staying there. Parents can reinforce consistency and expectations by stating, "After this story it is bedtime." Starting at 18 months, time-outs work well for managing temper tantrums.

During tantrums parents should ignore the behaviour, provided the behaviour is not injurious to the child, such as violently banging the head on the floor. Parents should continue to be present to provide a feeling of control and security to the child once the tantrum has subsided. At this time, a toy or a favourite activity can be substituted for the request. (See also Limit Setting and Discipline, Chapter 31.) During periods of no tantrums, developmentally appropriate positive reinforcement can be practised.

Other suggestions for handling tantrums include the following (Needlman et al., 1995):

- Offering the child options instead of an "all or none" position
- Picking one's battles carefully and ignoring small skirmishes over unimportant issues
- Giving comfort once the child is able to control emotions but not giving in to the original request
- Praising the child for positive behaviour when he or she is not having a tantrum

Temper tantrums are common during the toddler years and essentially represent normal developmental behaviours. However, temper tantrums can be signs of serious problems. Nurses should be alert to situations that require further evaluation.

Negativism

One of the more difficult aspects of rearing children in this age group is their persistent "no" response to every request. The negativism is not an expression of being stubborn or insolent but a necessary assertion of self-control. One method of dealing with the negativism is to reduce the opportunities for a "no" answer. Asking the child, "Do you want to go to sleep now?" is an almost certain example of a question that will be answered with an emphatic "no." Instead, the parent should tell the child that it is time to go to sleep and proceed accordingly.

In their attempt to exert control, children like to make choices. When confronted with appropriate choices, such as "You may have a peanut-butter-and-jelly sandwich or chicken-noodle soup for lunch," they are more likely to choose one rather than automatically say "no." However, if their response is negative, parents should make the choice for the child.

Regression

The retreat from one's present pattern of functioning to past levels of behaviour is referred to as *regression*. It usually occurs in instances of discomfort or stress when one attempts to conserve psychic energy by reverting to patterns of behaviour that were successful in earlier stages of development. Regression is common in toddlers because almost any additional stress hinders their ability to master present developmental tasks. Any threat to their autonomy, such as illness, hospitalization, separation from parents, or adjustment to a new sibling, represents a need to revert to earlier forms of behaviour, such as increased dependency; refusal to use the potty chair; temper tantrums; demand for the bottle, stroller, or crib; and loss of newly learned motor, language, social, and cognitive skills.

At first, such regression appears acceptable and comfortable for children, but the loss of newly acquired achievements is actually frightening and threatening because children are aware of their helplessness. Parents become concerned about regressive behaviour and often, in their efforts to deal with it, force the child to cope with an additional source of stress—the pressure to live up to expected standards. Brazelton (1999) suggests that these predictable times of regression, or *touchpoints*, are an opportunity to prepare parents for the next step in their child's development.

When regression does occur, the best approach is to ignore it while praising existing patterns of appropriate behaviour. Regression is a child's way of saying, "I can't cope with this present stress and perfect this skill as well, but I will if given patience and understanding." For this reason, it is advisable not to attempt new areas of learning when an additional crisis is present or expected, such as beginning toilet training shortly before a sibling is born or attempting new areas of learning during a brief period of hospitalization.

Promoting Optimum Health During Toddlerhood

Nutrition

During the period from 12 to 18 months of age, the growth rate slows, decreasing the child's need for calories, protein, and fluid. However, the protein (13 g/day) and energy requirements are still relatively high to meet the demands for muscle tissue growth and a high activity level. Estimated energy requirements (EER) for toddlers vary by age, gender, and feeding method; for example, an 18-month-old boy weighing 11.7 kg would have an EER of 961 kcal/day, whereas an 18-month-old girl with a weight of 10.9 kg would have an EER of 899 kcal/day (Institute of Medicine, 2005). The need for minerals such as iron, calcium, and phosphorus may be difficult to meet, considering the characteristic food habits of children in this age group. *Canada's Food Guide* (Health Canada, 2007) gives guidance on how to provide good nutrition for children.

At approximately 18 months of age, most toddlers manifest this decreased nutritional need with a decrease in appetite, a phenomenon known as *physiological anorexia*. They become picky, fussy eaters with strong taste preferences. Toddlers are increasingly aware of the non-nutritive function of food: the pleasure of eating, the social aspect of mealtime, and the control of refusing food. They are influenced by factors other than taste when choosing food. If a family member refuses to eat something, toddlers are likely to imitate that response. If the plate is overfilled, they are likely to push it away, overwhelmed by its size. In essence, mealtime is more closely associated with psychological components than with nutritional ones.

The **ritualism** of this age also dictates certain principles in feeding practices. Toddlers like to have the same dish, cup, or spoon every time they eat. They may reject a favourite food simply because it is served in a different dish. If one food touches another, they often refuse to eat it. Mixed foods, such as stews or casseroles, are rarely favourites. For some children a regular mealtime schedule also contributes to their desire and need for predictability and ritualism.

Many authorities consider this period of picky eating to be a developmental phase and stress that most toddlers will consume the necessary amount of food required for growth (Cathey & Gaylord, 2004).

Developmentally, by 12 months of age most children are eating the same food prepared for the rest of the family. Some may have mastered using a cup, with occasional spilling, although most cannot adeptly use a spoon until 18 months of age or later and generally prefer using their fingers. Because toddlers have unpredictable table manners, it is best to use plastic dishes and cups, for both economic and safety reasons.

Nutritional Counselling

The emphasis on preventing childhood obesity and subsequent cardiovascular disease in Canada has prompted a number of changes in dietary recommendations for children and adults alike. It is now recognized that lifetime eating habits may be established in early childhood, and health care workers are increasingly emphasizing the role of food selection choices, exercise, stress reduction, and other lifestyle choices (such as tobacco and alcohol use) on the quality of adult life and survival. Conditions such as obesity and cardiovascular disease can be prevented by encouraging healthy eating habits in toddlers and their families.

If food is used as a reward or sign of approval, a child may overeat for non-nutritive reasons. If food is forced and mealtime is consistently unpleasant, the usual pleasure associated with eating may not develop. Mealtimes should be enjoyable rather than times for discipline or family arguments. The social aspect of mealtime may be distracting for young children; therefore an earlier feeding hour may be appropriate. Young children are unable to sit through a long meal and become restless and disruptive. This is particularly common when children are brought to the table just after active play. Calling them in from play 15 minutes before mealtime allows them ample opportunity to get ready for eating while settling down their active minds and bodies.

The method of serving food also takes on more importance during this period. Toddlers need to have a sense of control and achievement in their abilities. Giving them large, adult-size portions can be overwhelming. In general, what is eaten is much more significant than how much is consumed. Small amounts of meat and vegetables supply greater food value than a large consumption of bread or potato. Serving sizes need to be appropriate for age (Box 37-2). Substitutions can be provided for foods that they do not enjoy, although this practice should not cater to all of their desires. Frequent nutritious *planned* snacks may provide adequate caloric intake at this age. *Grazing*—nibbling and snacking—is a good way to ensure proper nutrition, provided that appropriate foods are offered; giving the child something to eat merely to pacify is not recommended.

To determine serving size for young children, use the following guidelines:

- A general guide to the serving size of food is 15 mL (1 tablespoon) of solid food per year of age, or one fourth to one third of the adult portion size.
- Use the 15-mL guide for easily measured foods such as vegetables or rice.
- Use the fraction guide for bread or milk.

Mastication skills continue to mature, putting children at risk for choking. Large round foods (hot dogs, grapes, peas, carrots, popcorn, fruit gel snacks) should be avoided. Active play while eating should be discouraged, to prevent choking. Appetite and food preferences are sporadic. Often the interest in food parallels a growth spurt, so that periods of good eating are interspersed with phases of poor eating. If exposed to the same food every day, a young toddler does not learn how to manage the complex sensory information needed to eat new, more difficult foods (vegetables with a different texture versus puréed, slippery fruits). To help prevent "food jags," it is recommended that parents present food in various physical forms. The child may need to progress to eating new foods in a stepwise fashion: visually tolerating the food, interacting with the food, smelling the food, touching the food, tasting, and then eating the food.

This period can be trying for parents and children alike. Because eating habits are established in early life and affect not only the child's future eating habits but also the child's health as an adolescent and adult, it is recommended that toddlers not be forced to eat foods they are reluctant to eat. Evidence indicates that toddlers are able to regulate their hunger and satiety needs internally and that forcing foods during this period may exacerbate or lead to future eating problems (Cathey & Gaylord, 2004). It has also been suggested that parents plan a nutritionally balanced week instead of day because of the way toddlers will restrict food intake in their effort to exert control over their environment (Morin, 2007).

BOX 37-2 Sample Menu for a 2- to 3-Year-Old Based on *Canada's Food Guide*

Breakfast

125 mL 2% milk and
60 mL frozen berries blended into a smoothie
15 g whole grain cereal with
125 mL 2% milk

Snack

½ banana

Lunch

125 mL butternut squash soup
Tuna wrap made with the following:
- ½ of whole-wheat tortilla
- 38 g tuna
- 60 mL green pepper
- 5 mL mayonnaise

125 mL 2% milk

Snack

60 mL cucumber slices with
15 mL dip
125 mL 2% milk

Dinner

Stir fry made with the following:
- 125 mL broccoli, carrots, and cauliflower [frozen medley] and
- 38 g chicken on
- 125 mL cooked brown rice cooked in
- 5 mL oil to cook stir fry

18 g (½) roll with
5 mL nonhydrogenated margarine

Total *Food Guide* Servings for the Day

Vegetable and fruit (vitamin A and C sources): 4 servings a day
Grain: 3 grain servings a day
Milk and alternatives: 2 servings a day
Meat and alternatives: 1 serving a day
Fats and oils: 30 mL

(Adapted from Health Canada. [2011]. *Food and nutrition: Sample one-day menu for Sophie, a three-year-old girl*. Retrieved from http://www.hc-sc.gc.ca/fn-an/food-guide-aliment/choose-choix/advice-conseil/child-enfant_wide-eng.php.)

Dietary Guidelines

Dietary guidelines are necessary to promote adequate energy and nutrient intake to support physical, emotional, psychological, and cognitive development. A number of new dietary guidelines have been developed to address the issue of childhood obesity, sedentary lifestyles, and increase in cardiovascular disease mortality in Canada (see Additional Resources at the end of this chapter). Guidelines such as those outlined on the Health Canada Web site, at http://www.healthycanadians.gc.ca/init/kids-enfants/obesit/index-eng.php, offer suggestions to help children to have healthier lifestyles.

Nutrition during toddlerhood involves a transition as a young toddler is weaned off milk- or formula-based diets. Milk intake, the chief source of calcium and phosphorus, should average two or three servings (700 to 900 mL) a day. However, more than a litre of milk consumption daily considerably limits the intake of solid foods, resulting in a deficiency of dietary iron and other **nutrients**. After 2 years of age, children can be given low-fat milk to reduce daily total fat to less than 30% of calories, saturated fatty acids to less than 10% of calories, and cholesterol to less than 300 mg. Fat restriction of trans fatty acids and of saturated fats is important in the protection of toddlers' cardiovascular health (Allen & Myers, 2006). Other measures to reduce dietary fat include eating lean meats and fat-modified foods (such as low-fat cheese) and cooking with low-fat products. Because less fat in children's diet can also mean fewer calories and nutrients, caregivers must know what kinds of food to choose. *Eating Well With Canada's Food Guide* still recommends using 2% milk in the toddler age group and not restricting nutritious foods because of fat content (Health Canada, 2011).

Iron-fortified cereals and iron-rich foods are recommended for all children beyond 6 months of age. Parents are encouraged to provide an iron-rich diet that includes heme and nonheme iron sources (red meats, poultry, fish, green leafy vegetables, dried fruit, beans) and limit whole-milk consumption. Iron supplementation may be necessary in some cases.

Calcium and vitamin D are essential for healthy bone development. Recent research findings have identified the need for a higher dietary intake of calcium and vitamin D. As well, vitamin D deficiency may play an important role in the development of systemic conditions later in life such as cancer. It is well known that vitamin D deficiency is common in adults and children in Canada. At particular risk are First Nations, Métis, and Inuit populations and others who live in the high Arctic regions where cold-weather clothing and a lack of light decrease the amount of vitamin D produced in the skin. At the same time, these populations have decreased the dietary intake of their traditional vitamin D–rich foods. Children who have high body mass indices (BMIs) and are overweight or obese have lower levels of vitamin D as well (CPS, 2010c).

Research carried out by the U.S. Institute of Medicine on vitamin D and calcium levels has led to new joint recommendations on increased calcium and vitamin D intakes (Health Canada, 2010a). The recommendation for adequate intake of calcium for a child 1 to 3 years of age has increased to 700 mg per day; the tolerable upper intake per day is 2500 mg. Whole milk, cheese, yogourt, legumes (beans), and vegetables (broccoli, collard greens, kale) are good sources of calcium. Popular calcium-fortified foods include waffles, cereals and cereal bars, orange juice, and some white breads. Adequate vitamin D intake is essential to prevent rickets; the new vitamin D recommendation for children aged 1 to 3 years is 600 International Units (IU) (15 mcg) per day, with a tolerable upper level per day at 2500 IU (62.5 mcg). For children under the age of 2 years who live above a northern latitude of 55°, those with dark skin, and those avoiding sunlight, 800 IU (20 mcg) of vitamin D per day should be provided in the winter months (CPS, 2010c). Supplements may be required if food intake is poor or exposure to sunlight is minimal. Sources of vitamin D include fish, fish oils, and egg yolks; additionally, the consumption of 1 litre of vitamin D–fortified milk will provide 400 IU (10 mcg) of vitamin D. Fortified cereals, dairy products, and meat are also good sources of zinc and vitamin E.

Eating Well With Canada's Food Guide (Health Canada, 2007) recommends that children have 4 servings of fruit and vegetables each day. Vitamin C enhances iron absorption. Fruit and vegetables are recommended over fruit juices. Toddlers should consume a maximum of 120 to 180 mL of juice per day. A 180-mL glass of fruit juice equals one fruit serving; however, juices lack the fibre of whole fruit and should not be used as a substitute. High intake of juice can contribute to diarrhea, overnutrition or undernutrition, and the development of caries; thus only 120 to 240 mL of 100% fruit juice per day is recommended (CPS, Nutrition Committee, 2006). Fruit-flavoured drinks advertised as juices may not actually contain 100% juice and should be avoided.

Sleep and Activity

Total sleep decreases only slightly during the second year and averages about 12 hours a day. Most toddlers take one nap a day, and by the end of the second or third year, many relinquish this habit. Children reach an adult pattern of sleep by 3 years of age (Howard & Wong, 2001).

The toddler's activity level is high, and too little physical exercise is rarely a problem as long as inappropriate restrictions are not instituted. With increasing numbers of young children being cared for outside the home, however, attention to the kinds of activity provided is important. For example, children with high activity levels may benefit from an environment in which outdoor play is encouraged.

Sleep problems are common among toddlers, especially going to bed and falling asleep, and are probably related to fears of separation. Bedtime rituals (e.g., same hour of sleep, snack, and quiet activity) are helpful, and transitional objects, such as a favourite stuffed animal or blanket, can help ease the child's insecurity at bedtime (see Fig. 37-3).

As with infants, safe sleeping environments are important at the toddler stage. Many factors affect sleeping arrangements, including parental and cultural values and socioeconomic factors. All of these factors need to be taken into consideration when health care providers are providing guidance on the physical and emotional security of sleeping environments. Although rare, sudden infant death syndrome (SIDS) can occur in children over 1 year of age, as can accidental suffocation or entrapment. Therefore, families need to be educated about the Canadian Paediatric Society's (2010a) recommendations on safe sleeping environments. These recommendations include using cribs that meet the Canadian government's safety regulations, not makeshift temporary beds; dressing the child in sleepers with a thin blanket without pillow-like items and toys for sleep; and preventing exposure to passive smoke (CPS, 2010a). (See Chapter 36 for more information on the relation between a safe sleeping environment and the occurrence of SIDS.)

Dental Health

Regular Dental Examinations

Oral health is an important cornerstone of health for all Canadians. The Health Canada Oral Health Report Card (Canadian Dental Association [CDA], 2010a) indicates that most Canadians have access to professional dental care and have good oral health. However, a minority of the population has difficulty accessing adequate oral health care; these groups include older adults; individuals with low income; people with special needs; some children; and First Nations, Métis, and Inuit peoples. Aboriginal peoples generally have the poorest oral health within Canada and have a lower rate of accessing dental coverage (CDA, 2010a). Poverty, a key social determinant of health, also has an impact on oral health. These groups frequently have poor oral health because of poor diet, such as inappropriate amounts of sweetened juices, milk, and desserts, and lack of good oral hygiene related to disease prevention. Provincial and territorial dental coverage is underused, and the coverage is often limited.

The Canadian Dental Association recommends that dental visits begin during the infant's first year for prevention of dental decay and early diagnosis of dental problems. Families need to have education on how to provide a healthy diet and good oral hygiene for their child. Children at high risk for dental problems should be identified by nurses, nurse practitioners, family doctors, pediatricians, and community health agencies.

Initial visits to the dentist should be nontraumatizing. Because toddlers react negatively to new and potentially frightening experiences, the initial visit can centre around meeting the dentist, seeing the equipment, and sitting in the chair. If the child is cooperative, the dentist may just look at the teeth but reserve a more thorough examination for another visit. *Modelling*, in which the child observes procedures performed on the parent or a cooperative sibling, can also be effective.

Removal of Plaque

Oral hygiene measures should be implemented to remove *plaque*, or soft bacterial deposits that adhere to the teeth and cause dental **caries** (decay or cavities) and periodontal (gum) disease. Poor oral hygiene and poor dietary habits are associated with the development of caries in children. The most effective methods for plaque removal are brushing and flossing. Several brushing techniques exist, although there is no universal agreement regarding the best method. One that is suitable for cleaning the primary teeth is the scrub method. The tips of the bristles are placed firmly at a 45-degree angle against the teeth and gums and moved back and forth in a vibratory motion. The ends of the bristles should be wiggling but not moving forcefully back and forth, as this can damage the gums and enamel. All the surfaces of the teeth should be cleaned in this manner except the lingual (inner) surfaces of the anterior teeth. To clean these surfaces, the toothbrush is placed vertical to the teeth and moved up and down. Only a few teeth are brushed at one time, using six to eight strokes for each section. A systematic approach should be used so that all surfaces are thoroughly cleaned (Fig. 37-7).

For young children, the most effective cleaning is done by parents (Fig. 37-8). Several positions can be used that facilitate access to the mouth and help stabilize the head for comfort:

- Stand with the child's back toward the adult. (When done in front of a bathroom mirror, both the child and adult can see what is being done in the mirror.)
- Sit on a couch or bed with the child's head resting in the adult's lap.
- Sit on the floor or a stool with the child's head resting between the adult's thighs.

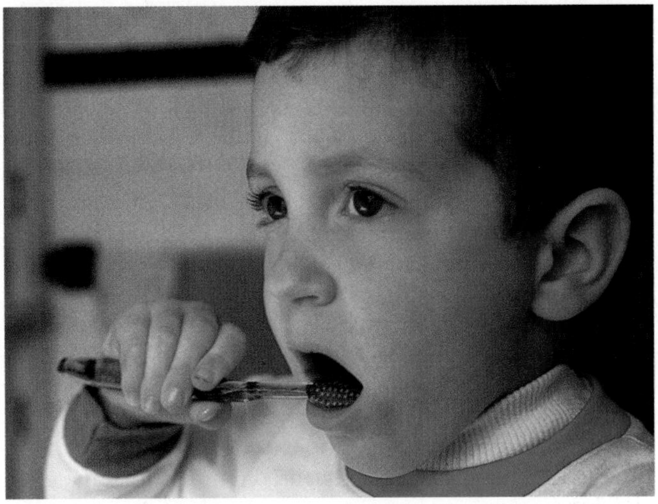

Fig. 37-7 Young children can participate in toothbrushing, but parents need to brush all the child's teeth thoroughly.

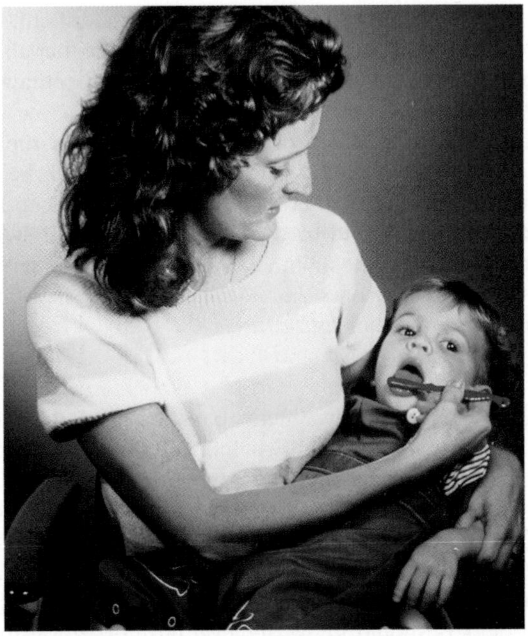

Fig. 37-8 The most effective cleaning of the teeth is done by parents.

With all positions, use one hand to cup the chin and the other to brush the teeth. For easier access to back teeth, hold the mouth partially open.

For effective cleaning, a small toothbrush with soft, rounded, multitufted nylon bristles that are short and uniform in length is recommended. Nylon bristles dry more rapidly after use and retain their shape better than natural bristles. Toothbrushes should be replaced as soon as the bristles are frayed or bent. With young children, brushing may be more easily accomplished using only water, since many children dislike the foam from toothpaste and the foam interferes with visibility.

If a child up to age 3 is identified by a health care provider to be at risk of developing tooth caries, then a minimal amount (the size of a grain of rice) of fluoridated toothpaste should be used (CDA, 2010b). The use of fluoridated toothpaste in this age group is determined by the level of risk of developing tooth caries. Use of fluoridated toothpaste in a small amount has been determined to achieve a balance between the benefits of fluoride and the risk of developing fluorosis. When using toothpaste, children should select the flavour they like, to encourage the brushing habit. If the child is not considered to be at risk, the teeth should be brushed by an adult using a toothbrush moistened only with water.

After the teeth have been cleaned, flossing with dental floss is done to remove plaque and debris from between the teeth and below the gum margin, where brushing is ineffective. Since young children do not have the dexterity to manipulate the floss, parents should be taught the procedure to use in children.

A disclosing agent is helpful in identifying those areas of the teeth where plaque accumulates. It also helps motivate children to clean their teeth because plaque is difficult to see. After cleaning, the mouth is inspected to ensure that all traces of plaque have been removed. Where plaque remains, the teeth are rebrushed.

Ideally, the teeth should be cleaned after each meal and especially before bedtime, and the child should be given nothing to eat or drink after the night brushing, except water. When brushing is impractical, the "swish-and-swallow" method of cleaning the mouth can be taught: with a mouthful of water, the child rinses the mouth and swallows, repeating the procedure three or four times.

Fluoride

In Canada, public water systems have fluoride added to the drinking water. The Federal-Provincial-Territorial Committee on Drinking Water recommends the optimal level of fluoride that is added to public drinking water to prevent tooth decay. The Government of Canada's guideline for fluoride in drinking water indicates a maximum acceptable concentration of 1.5 milligrams per litre (Health Canada, 2010b). All health care providers should know the level of fluoridation in their regional drinking water; this information is available from their public health agency. Fluoride supplementation should be considered for any child after the first permanent tooth eruption on an individual basis when the drinking water is deficient in fluoride. The Canadian Dental Association (2010b) recommends that for young children the total daily fluoride intake from all sources not exceed 0.05 to 0.07 mg fluoride/kg body weight, to minimize the risk of dental fluorosis.

Fluoride, a mineral, is found in water, foods, or drinks in which fluoridated water was used as part of the processing system. Because the water fluoridation process and manufacturing of fluoride toothpaste are almost impossible to standardize in Canada, the dosage of fluoride supplements has been lowered to reduce the incidence of fluorosis. Increased fluoride ingestion, such as when children swallow fluoridated toothpaste, leads to enamel protein retention, hypomineralization of the enamel and dentin, and disturbance of crystal formation. The effects caused by this change range from barely discernible white fibrelike lines or spots to gray-brown stains or pitted areas. Parents should be cautioned against regular use of fluoridated water or beverages such as bottled water containing fluoride if the community water supply already has an adequate amount of fluoride.

When taken, fluoride supplements should remain in the mouth for 30 seconds before swallowing and be taken on an empty stomach. Afterward, the child should not drink or eat for 30 minutes. All fluoride products (toothpaste, supplements, and rinse) need to be stored away from young children to prevent poisoning by accidental ingestion. If the water supply is adequately fluoridated, parents should use tap water to prepare drinks and foods.

Low-Cariogenic Diet

Diet is critical to developing good teeth because carious development depends primarily on fermentable sugars, especially sucrose. Refined table sugar, honey, molasses, corn syrup, and dried fruits such as raisins are highly cariogenic.

Ideally, highly cariogenic foods, especially those containing complex sugars, should be eliminated. However, since this is impractical, some suggestions can be helpful. First, *the frequency with which sugar is consumed is more important than the total amount eaten.* Therefore, when sweets are eaten, they are less damaging if consumed immediately after a meal rather than as a snack between meals. When sweets are served as the dessert, the teeth should be be cleaned afterward, decreasing the amount of time the sugar is in the mouth.

Second, the form of sugar (sucrose) is important. The more cariogenic foods are those that are sticky or hard, since they remain in the mouth longer. Consequently, sucking on lollipops is more cariogenic than eating a chocolate bar. Sometimes the source of the sugar is "hidden," as in numerous prescription and nonprescription medications and in many popular cereals, including the "all-natural" variety. Reading food labels is essential in identifying and eliminating sources of sucrose.

Sugarless gum chewed after eating may actually protect against cavities by stimulating saliva that neutralizes acid. The artificial sweeteners saccharin, aspartame, and Splenda are noncariogenic; sorbitol has low cariogenic potential.

A special form of tooth decay in infants and toddlers is *nursing caries* (also called *nursing bottle caries* or *bottle-mouth caries*); this occurs when the child is routinely given a bottle of milk or juice at naptime or bedtime or uses the bottle as a pacifier while awake. Frequent nocturnal breastfeeding for prolonged periods also leads to extensive destruction of the teeth. The practice of coating pacifiers in honey can also contribute to the development of caries and may be a potential source of botulism poisoning in infants. As the sweet liquid pools in the mouth, the teeth are bathed for several hours in this cariogenic environment. The maxillary (upper) incisors and molars are affected most, since the mandibular (lower) incisors are protected by the lower lip, tongue, and saliva (Fig. 37-9). Severely decayed teeth may require the application of stainless steel bands to preserve the spacing until the permanent teeth erupt.

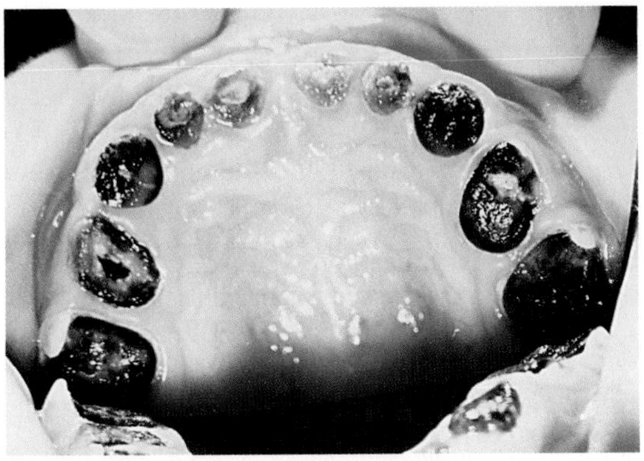

Fig. 37-9 Nursing caries. Note extensive carious involvement of maxillary primary incisors. *(Courtesy Bruce Carter, DDS, Texas Children's Hospital, Houston.)*

Prevention of nursing caries involves eliminating the bedtime bottle completely, feeding the last bottle before bedtime, substituting a bottle of water for milk or juice, not using the bottle as a pacifier, and never coating pacifiers in sweet substances. Juice in bottles, especially commercially available ready-to-use bottles, is discouraged; these beverages are especially damaging because the sugar is more readily converted to acid. Juice should always be offered in a cup to avoid prolonging the bottle-feeding habit. Toddlers should be encouraged to drink from a cup at the first birthday and weaned from a bottle by 14 months of age.

Nurses are in an excellent position to counsel parents regarding the dangers of poor dietary habits and other aspects of dental care.

Injury Prevention

Prevention of injury in children is an important area to address because injuries are the most common cause of death and disability of Canadian children. The most frequent causes of death are drowning, motor vehicle collisions, suffocation, and burns (Pan et al., 2006). Annually, on average, 300 children age 14 years and under are killed in Canada, and over 21,000 children are hospitalized for serious injuries. Overall, the death rates from 2000 to 2005 for injuries in the 0- to 14-year age group dropped by 37% and hospitalization rates by 34% (Public Health Agency of Canada [PHAC], 2009a).

In children 1 to 4 years of age, unintentional injury deaths are caused by drowning (23%) or burns (14%); or as a result of a motor vehicle accident, as a passenger (14%) or pedestrian (14%); or threats to breathing (11%). From 2000 to 2005 this age group represented 10% of unintentional injury deaths in Canada (PHAC, 2009b). The number of intentional injuries (from maltreatment) in children peaks at 1 to 2 years of age as they start to explore their environment (PHAC, 2009a). In 2005, there were 17 homicides per 100,000 children 1 to 9 years of age (PHAC, 2009a) (see Chapter 36, Bodily Damage; Shaken Baby Syndrome).

These children are at high risk of unintentional injuries because of their developmental stage and lack of ability to protect themselves: during early childhood children achieve unrestricted freedom through locomotion and are unaware of danger within their environment. Specific categories of injuries and appropriate prevention are best understood by associating them with the major developmental achievements of young children (Table 37-2). The discussions of injuries in Chapters 29 and 36 are also relevant to safety concerns at this age.

Researchers in Canada have identified a relationship between childhood injuries and determinants of health, including lower income and social status, physical environments with less safe housing and communities, lower education levels, and social environments with higher rates of drug and alcohol use (Gilbride, Wild, Wilson, Svenson, & Spady, 2006).

Motor Vehicle Injuries

Motor vehicle injuries are the second-most frequent cause of accidental deaths and injuries in the 1- to 4-year age group. To reduce the incidence of these injuries, mandatory child car seat legislation was implemented in Canada in 1993, resulting in a decrease of 58% in childhood deaths (PHAC, 2009a). When car seats are installed correctly, the seats decrease the risk of death by 71% in this age group (CPS, 2008b). The seats also decrease the risk of hospitalization by 67% for children age 4 and under. Booster seats provide up to 60% more protection than seat belts (Safe Kids Canada, 2011a). Despite this added protection, however, in Canada, 44 to 81% of car seats and 30 to 50% of booster seats are not installed correctly (CPS, 2008b).

Nurses have a responsibility to educate parents regarding the importance of using car restraints for children under 8 years of age and the proper use of car restraints. Five types of restraints are available: (1) infant-only devices, (2) convertible models for both infants and toddlers, (3) boosters, (4) safety belts, and (5) devices for children with special needs (see Chapter 41). Infant-type restraints are discussed in Chapter 36; convertible restraints and boosters are discussed here. The convertible restraint is suitable for infants in the rear-facing position and for toddlers in the forward-facing position. The transition point for switching to the forward-facing position is defined by the manufacturer but is generally at a body weight of at least 10 kg and a minimum of 1 year of age. Infants who weigh 10 kg before 1 year of age should continue to ride in a rear-facing seat (CPS, 2008a). One study has shown that children from birth to 23 months experienced fewer injuries when riding in rear-facing car restraints (Henary et al., 2007). Another study indicated that children 0 to 3 years of age riding properly restrained in the middle of the back seat had a 43% lower risk of injury than children riding in the outboard (window) seat during a crash (Kallan et al., 2008).

A convertible safety seat is positioned semireclined and facing the rear of the car for a child younger than 1 year weighing less than 10 kg. The seat is positioned upright and facing forward for an older and heavier child (up to 18 kg) or according to the manufacturer's instructions (Fig. 37-10, A). Convertible safety seats should be used until the child weighs at least 13.6 kg or more regardless of age and as long as the child fits properly into the seat (CPS, 2008a). It is important that parents use the rear-facing option as long as the child's age and weight are within the manufacturer's instructions. Convertible restraints have different types of harness systems: a five-point

Table 37-2 Injury Prevention During Early Childhood

DEVELOPMENTAL ABILITIES RELATED TO RISK OF INJURY	INJURY PREVENTION
Motor Vehicles	
Walks, runs, and climbs Able to open doors and gates Can ride tricycle and other toy vehicles Can throw ball and other objects	Use federally approved car restraint. Supervise child while playing outside. Do not allow child to play on curb or behind a parked car. Do not permit child to play in a pile of leaves, snow, or large cardboard container in trafficked area. Supervise tricycle riding. Lock fences and doors if not directly supervising children. Teach child to obey pedestrian safety rules: • Obey traffic regulations; cross only at crosswalks and only when traffic signal indicates it is safe. • Stand back a step from the curb until it is time to cross. • Look left, right, and left again and check for turning cars before crossing the street. • Use sidewalks; when there is no sidewalk, walk on the left, facing traffic. • Wear light colours at night and attach fluorescent material to clothing.
Submersion Injuries	
Able to explore if left unsupervised Has great curiosity Helpless in water; unaware of its danger—may consider "play" in any body of water the same as in the bath; depth of water has no significance	Supervise closely when near any source of water regardless of depth, including buckets. Keep bathroom doors closed and lid down on toilet (or install latch). Have fence around swimming pool and lock gate. Teach swimming and water safety (this is, however, not a substitute for safety).
Burns	
Able to reach heights by climbing, stretching, and standing on toes Pulls objects Explores any holes or opening Can open drawers and closets Unaware of potential sources of heat or fire Plays with mechanical objects	Turn pot handles toward back of stove. Place electrical appliances, such as coffee maker and popcorn machine, toward back of counter. Place guardrails in front of radiators, fireplaces, or other heating elements. Store matches and cigarette lighters in locked or inaccessible area; discard carefully. Place burning candles, incense, hot foods, and cigarettes out of reach. Do not let tablecloth hang within child's reach. Do not let electric cord from iron, curling iron, or other appliance hang within child's reach. Cover electrical outlets with protective plastic caps. Keep electrical wires hidden or out of reach. Do not allow child to play with electrical appliance, wires, or lighters. Stress danger of open flames; teach what "hot" means. Always check bathwater temperature; adjust water heater temperature to 49°C or lower; do not allow children to play with faucets. Apply a sunscreen when child is exposed to sunlight.
Poisoning	
Explores by putting objects in mouth Can open drawers, closets, boxes, and most containers Climbs Cannot read labels Does not know safe dose or amount	Place all potentially toxic agents out of reach or in a locked cabinet. Caution against eating nonedible items, such as plants. Replace medications or poisons immediately in proper storage and out of the child's reach; replace child-guard caps properly. Administer medications as a drug, not as a candy. Do not store surplus toxic agents. Promptly discard empty poison containers; never reuse to store a food item or other poison. Teach child not to play in trash containers. Never remove labels from containers of toxic substances. Do not store toxic liquids in containers not specifically intended for their storage (e.g., an empty pop bottle that the child may drink from, unaware of the difference in contents). Know the number of the nearest poison control centre (http://camponline.org/pdf/poison-control.pdf)

Table 37-2 Injury Prevention During Early Childhood—cont'd

DEVELOPMENTAL ABILITIES RELATED TO RISK OF INJURY	INJURY PREVENTION
Falls	
Able to open doors and some windows Goes up and down stairs Depth perception unrefined Climbs on higher surfaces	Use window guardrail; fasten securely. Place gates at top and bottom of stairs. Keep doors locked or use child-proof doorknob covers at the entry to stairs, high porch, or other elevated area, including laundry chute. Remove unsecured or scatter rugs. Apply nonskid decals in the bathtub or shower. Keep crib rails fully raised and mattress at lowest level. Place carpeting under the crib and in the bathroom. Keep large toys and bumper pads out of the crib or playpen (child can use these as "stairs" to climb out), then move the child to a youth bed when he or she is able to climb out of the crib. Dress in safe clothing (soles that do not "catch" on the floor, tied shoelaces, pant legs that do not touch the floor). Keep child restrained in vehicles; never leave the child unattended in a shopping cart. Supervise the child at playgrounds; select play areas with a soft ground cover and safe equipment.
Choking and Suffocation	
Puts things in mouth May swallow hard or nonedible pieces of food	Avoid large, round chunks of meat, such as whole hot dogs (slice lengthwise into short pieces). Avoid fruit with pits, fish with bones, dried beans, hard candy, chewing gum, nuts, popcorn, grapes, marshmallows. Choose large, sturdy toys without sharp edges or small removable parts. Discard old refrigerators, ovens, and other appliances after removing the door. Select safe toy boxes or chests without heavy, hinged lids. Keep Venetian blind (or shade) cords out of child's reach. Use split cords. Remove drawstrings from clothing.
Bodily Damage	
Still clumsy in many skills Easily distracted from tasks Unaware of potential danger from strangers or other people	Avoid giving the child sharp or pointed objects, such as knives, scissors, or toothpicks, especially when walking or running. Do not allow lollipops or similar objects in the child's mouth when walking or running. Teach safety precautions (e.g., to carry knife or scissors with pointed end away from face). Store all dangerous tools, garden equipment, and firearms in a locked cabinet. Be alert to danger of supervised animals and household pets. Use safety glass and decals on large glassed areas, such as sliding glass doors. Teach the child his or her name, address, and phone number and to ask for help from appropriate people (cashier, security guard, policeman) if lost; have identification on child (sewn in clothes, inside shoe). Teach stranger safety: • Avoid personalized clothing in public places. • Never go with a stranger. • Tell parents if anyone makes the child feel uncomfortable in any way. Always listen to the child's concerns regarding others' behaviour. Teach the child to say "no" when confronted with uncomfortable situations.

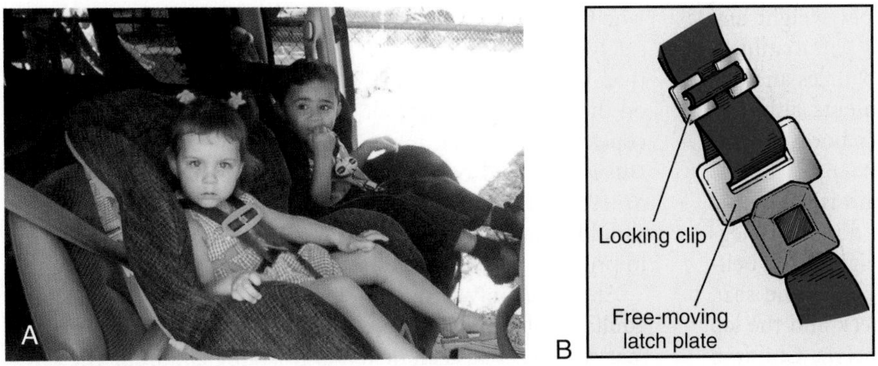

Fig. 37-10 **A:** Convertible car safety seat in forward-facing position. **B:** Use of locking clip.

harness that consists of a strap over each shoulder, one on each side of the pelvis, and one between the legs (all five come together at a common buckle); and a padded shield that uses shoulder straps attached to a shield that is held in place by a crotch strap. With both the infant and toddler restraints, it is important not to add extra blankets, head cushions, or padding between the child and the restraint straps that did not come as original equipment because these "add-ons" create spaces of air between the child and the restraint and decrease support for the back, head, and neck.

The next stage in child restraints is the forward-facing infant/child seats. These can be used for children between 10 kg and at least 22 kg, and up to 122 cm in height, which varies according to the manufacturer's instructions. Some models are a combination of forward-facing infant/child seats that will convert to a child booster seat when the child reaches the appropriate booster weight and height.

Built-in seats are available in some cars and vans. They may be used for children who are at least 1 year of age and weigh at least 10 kg. Built-in seats eliminate installation problems. However, weight and height limits vary. Owners must verify with vehicle manufacturers the details about built-in seats to ensure that the seats will adequately protect their child.

Starting in 2003, the Universal Anchorage System (UAS) (also known as LATCH [Lower Anchors and Tethers for Children]) or ISOFIX (International Standards Organization FIX) universal child safety seat system was implemented as a requirement for all new automobiles and child safety seats. This system provides uniform anchorage consisting of two lower anchorages and one upper anchorage in the rear seat of the vehicle (Fig. 37-11). When used appropriately, the top anchor (tether) strap prevents the child from pitching forward in a crash. If the tether strap is not used, up to 90% of the restraint's protection is lost. Instructions for proper installation of the tether strap and permanent bracket are included with the car restraint. New child safety seats have a hook, buckle, strap, or other connector that attaches to the anchorage. Seat belts are no longer used to anchor child safety seats to newer vehicles.

The third stage in child car restraints is booster car seats. Booster seats are not restraint systems like the convertible devices because they depend on the vehicle belts to hold the child and booster seat in place. These should be used for children who have surpassed the weight or height limits of their forward-facing car seat and weigh at least 18 kg. Booster seats should be used until children are at least 36 kg. Some booster models accommodate children up to 45 kg. It is necessary to always check the label for the lower and upper weight and height limits because they vary depending on the manufacturer. Booster seat legislation varies among provinces and territories; some do not have booster seat requirements, although it is recommended that children stay in their booster seats until they are 8 years old.

A booster seat should be used until the child is able to sit against the back of the seat with feet hanging down and legs bent at the knees (approximately 145 cm in height). The belt-positioning booster model raises a child higher in the seat, moving the shoulder part of the belt off the neck and the lap portion of the belt off the abdomen onto the pelvis. Children

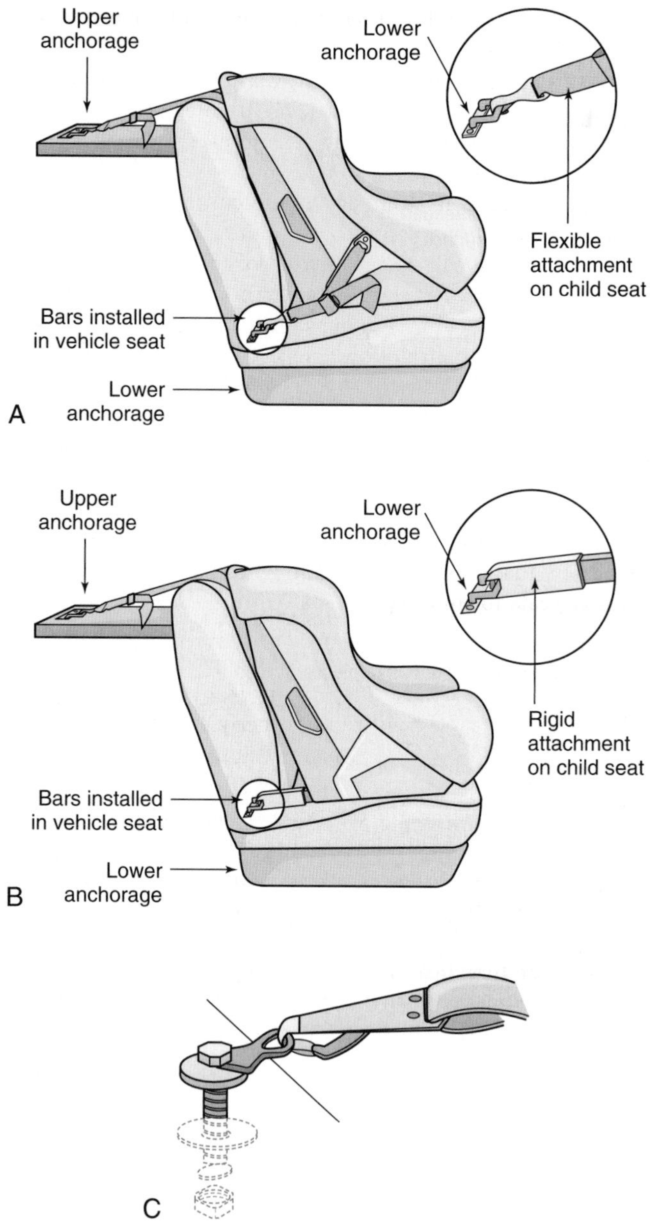

Fig. 37-11 Universal anchorage system (UAS). **A:** Flexible two-point attachment with top tether. **B:** Rigid two-point attachment with top tether. **C:** Top tether. *(Courtesy U.S. Department of Transportation, National Highway Traffic Safety Administration.)*

who outgrow the convertible restraint may still be able to ride safely in a booster seat until the midpoint of the head is higher than the vehicle seat back. Cars with free-sliding latch plates on the lap or shoulder belt require the use of a metal locking clip to keep the belt in a tight-holding position. The locking clip is threaded onto the belt above the latch plate (see Fig. 37-10, B). If parents have newer cars with automatic lap and shoulder belts, they need to have additional lap belts installed to properly secure the restraint.

Shoulder-only automatic belts are designed to protect adults. Children should use the manual shoulder belts in the rear seat. Air bags can be lethal to young children. The safest

Safe Kids Canada. (2011d). *Safety information: Protect your child from flame burns.* Retrieved from http://www.safekidscanada.ca/Parents/Safety-Information/Scalds-and-Burns/Burns/Flame-Burns.aspx.
Safe Kids Canada. (2012a). *Safety information: Carbon monoxide alarms can save your child's life.* Retrieved from http://www.safekidscanada.ca/Parents/Safety-Information/Poison-Prevention/Monoxide-Alarms/Carbon-Monoxide-Alarms.aspx.
Safe Kids Canada. (2012b). *Safety information: Playground safety.* Retrieved from http://www.safekidscanada.ca/Professionals/Safety-Information/Playground-Safety/Index.aspx.
Schmitt, B. D. (2004). Toilet training: Getting it right the first time. *Contemporary Pediatrics, 21*(3), 105–108, 111–112, 115–116.
Schum, T. R., et al. (2002). Sequential acquisition of toilet-training skills: A descriptive study of gender and age differences in normal children. *Pediatrics, 109*(3), e48.
Thompson, R. A. (2001). Caring for infants and toddlers. *The Future of Children, 11*(1), 21–33.

Additional Resources

Attachment Across Cultures: Beliefs, Values, and Practices—Sleeping Practices: http://www.attachmentacrosscultures.org/beliefs/index.html#12
Canadian Dental Association: Dental Care for Children: http://www.cda-adc.ca/en/oral_health/cfyt/dental_care_children
Canadian Hospitals Injury Reporting and Prevention Program (CHIRPP) (national database of circumstances of injuries that require hospital emergency treatment): http://www.phac-aspc.gc.ca/injury-bles/chirpp/index-eng.php
Canadian Paediatric Society—Parent guide to toilet training: http://www.caringforkids.cps.ca/handouts/toilet_learning
Canadian Toy Testing Council: http://www.toy-testing.org (e-mail: cttc@toy-testing.org)
Canadian Virtual Hospice: Talking With Children and Youth About Serious Illness: http://www.virtualhospice.ca/en_US/Main+Site+Navigation/Home/Topics/Topics/Emotional+Health/Talking+with+Children+and+Youth.aspx
Health Canada: Eating Well With Canada's Food Guide: http://www.hc-sc.gc.ca/fn-an/food-guide-aliment/index-eng.php
Health Canada: Healthy Living—Oral Health: http://www.hc-sc.gc.ca/hl-vs/oral-bucco/index-eng.php
Healthy Canadians: Choosing a Car Seat (information on car restraints and government regulations): http://www.healthycanadians.gc.ca/init/kids-enfants/road-routiere/car-re-vehic/choose-choisir/index-eng.php/
Nipissing District Developmental Screen (available at P.O. Box 1493, North Bay, ON, P1B 8K6; 705-752-5081 or 1-888-582-0944; fax 705- 752-4247; e-mail info@ndds.ca): http://www.ndds.ca/language.php
Peel Region Health Department: Car Seat Safety: http://www.peelregion.ca/health/carseat/index.htm
Peel Region Health Department: Toddlers and Preschoolers—Behaviour: Jealousy and Sibling Rivalry: http://www.peelregion.ca/health/family-health/toddlers-and-preschoolers/behaviour/jealousy.htm
Safe Kids Canada (organization providing information on child safety for parents and professionals; educational and advocacy programs originated with the Hospital for Sick Children, Toronto): Suite 2105, 180 Dundas Street West, Toronto, On, M5G 1Z8; tel: 416-813-7288: http://www.safekidscanada.ca/Home/tabid/40/language/en-CA/Default.aspx
Safe Kids Canada: Safety Information—Playground Safety: http://www.safekidscanada.ca/parents/safety-information/playground-safety/index.aspx

References

Allen, R. E., & Myers, A. L. (2006). Nutrition in toddlers. *American Family Physician, 74*(9), 1527–1532, 1533–1534.

Bates, E., & Dick, F. (2002). Language, gesture, and the developing brain. *Developmental Psychobiology, 40*(3), 293–310.

Brazelton, T. B. (1999). How to help parents of young children: The touchpoints model. *Journal of Perinatology, 19*(6 Pt 2), S6–S7.

Canadian Dental Association. (2010a). *A position paper on access to oral health care for Canadians.* Retrieved from http://www.cda-adc.ca/_files/position_statements/CDA_Position_Paper_Access_to_Oral_Health_Care_for_Canadians.pdf.

Canadian Dental Association. (2010b). *CDA position on the use of fluorides in caries prevention.* Retrieved from http://www.cda-adc.ca/_files/position_statements/Fluorides-English-2010-06-08.pdf.

Canadian Paediatric Society. (2002). Preventing playground injuries. *Paediatrics and Child Health, 7*(4), 255–256. (Updated 2007) Retrieved from http://www.cps.ca/english/statements/ip/ip02-01.htm

Canadian Paediatric Society. (2003). Impact of media use on children and youth. *Paediatrics and Child Health, 8*(5), 301–306. (Reaffirmed February 2011)

Canadian Paediatric Society. (2004). Effective discipline for children. *Paediatrics and Child Health, 9*(1), 37–41. (Reaffirmed February 2011)

Canadian Paediatric Society. (2008a). Transportation of infants and children in motor vehicles. *Paediatrics and Child Health, 13(4)*, 313–318.

Canadian Paediatric Society. (2008b). *Car seat safety: Fact sheet.* Retrieved from http://www.cps.ca/English/media/AnnualConference08/fact_sheet.pdf.

Canadian Paediatric Society. (2010a). *Recommendations for safe sleeping environments for infants and children.* Retrieved from http://www.cps.ca/english/statements/cp/cp04-02.htm.

Canadian Paediatric Society. (2010b). *Toilet learning: Anticipatory guidance with a child-oriented approach.* Retrieved from http://www.cps.ca/english/statements/cp/cp00-02.htm.

Canadian Paediatric Society. (2010c). Vitamin D supplementation: Recommendations for Canadian mothers and infants. *Paediatrics and Child Health, 12*(7), 583–589.

Canadian Paediatric Society, Nutrition Committee. (2006). Oral rehydration therapy and early refeeding in the management of childhood gastroenteritis. *Paediatrics and Child Health, 11*(8), 527–531.

Cathey, M., & Gaylord, N. (2004). Picky eating: A toddler's approach to mealtime. *Pediatric Nursing, 30*(2), 101–107.

Centers for Disease Control and Prevention. (2005). Nonfatal motor-vehicle-related backover injuries among children—United States, 2001–2003. *MMWR. Morbidity & Mortality Weekly Report, 54*(06), 144–146.

Dahlquist, L. M., et al. (2002). Distraction for children of different ages who undergo repeated needle sticks. *Journal of Pediatric Oncology Nursing, 19*(1), 22–34.

DeLamater, J., & Friedrich, W. N. (2002). Human sexual development. *Journal of Sex Research, 39*(1), 10–14.

Dietitians of Canada, Canadian Paediatric Society, the College of Family Physicians of Canada, and the Community Health Nurses of Canada. (2010). *Promoting optimal monitoring of child growth in Canada: Using the new WHO growth charts.* Retrieved from http://www.cps.ca/english/statements/N/growth-charts-statement-FULL.pdf.

Elkins, M., & Cavendish, R. (2004). Developing a plan for pediatric spiritual care. *Holistic Nursing Practice, 18*(4), 179–184.

Erikson, E. H. (1963). *Childhood and society* (2nd ed.). New York: Norton.

Fosarelli, P. (2003). Children and the development of faith: Implications for pediatric practice. *Contemporary Pediatrics, 20*(1), 85–98.

Gilbride, S., Wild, C., Wilson, D., Svenson, L., & Spady, D. (2006). Socioeconomic status and types of childhood injury in Alberta: A population-based study. *BioMed Central Pediatrics, 6*, 30. Retrieved from http://www.ncbi.nlm.nih.gov/pmc/articles/PMC1687186/pdf/1471-2431-6-30.pdf.

Glassy, D., Romano, J., & Committee on Early Childhood, Adoption, and Dependent Care. (2003). Selecting appropriate toys for young children: The pediatrician's role. *Pediatrics, 111*(4), 911–913.

Guard, A., & Gallagher, S. S. (2005). Heat related deaths in young children in parked cars: An analysis of 171 fatalities in the United States, 1995–2002. *Injury Prevention, 11*(1), 33–37. doi:10.1136/ip.2003.004044

Harpaz-Rotem, I., & Bergman, A. (2006). On an evolving theory of attachment: Rapprochement—theory of a developing mind. *Psychoanalytic Study of the Child, 61*, 170–189.

Health Canada. (2007). *Eating well with Canada's food guide: How much food you need every day.* Retrieved from http://www.hc-sc.gc.ca/fn-an/food-guide-aliment/basics-base/quantit-eng.php.

Health Canada. (2010a). *Vitamin D and calcium: Updated dietary reference intakes.* Retrieved from http://www.hc-sc.gc.ca/fn-an/nutrition/vitamin/vita-d-eng.php.

Health Canada. (2010b). *Fluoride and human health.* Retrieved from http://www.hc-sc.gc.ca/hl-vs/iyh-vsv/environ/fluor-eng.php.

Health Canada. (2011). *Eating well with Canada's food guide: Children.* Retrieved from http://www.hc-sc.gc.ca/fn-an/food-guide-aliment/choose-choix/advice-conseil/child-enfant-eng.php.

Henary, B., et al. (2007). Car safety for children: Rear facing for best protection. *Injury Prevention, 13*(6), 398–402. doi:10.1136/ip.2006.015115

Howard, B. J., & Wong, J. (2001). Sleep disorders. *Pediatrics in Review, 22*(10), 327–342.

Institute of Medicine. (2005). *Dietary reference intakes for energy, carbohydrate, fiber, fat, fatty acids, cholesterol, protein, and amino acids.* Washington, DC: National Academies Press.

Kallan, M. J., et al. (2008). Seating patterns and corresponding risk of injury among 0- to 3-year-old children in child safety seats. *Pediatrics, 121*(5), e1342–e1347. doi:10.1542/peds.2007-1512

McLaren, C., Null, J., & Quinn, J. (2005). Heat stress from enclosed vehicles: Moderate ambient temperatures cause significant temperature rise in enclosed vehicles. *Pediatrics, 116*(1), e109–e112. doi:10.1542/peds.2004-2368

Mercer, R. (2003). Treating nocturnal enuresis. *Advanced Nursing Practice, 11*(2), 26–31.

Meyer, T. L. (2002). Unveiling the secrecy behind masturbation. *Pediatrics in Review, 23*(4), 148–149.

Morin, K. (2007). Infant nutrition: Toddlers: Start off on the right foot. *MCN: American Journal of Maternal Child Nursing, 32*(2), 122. doi:10.1097/01.NMC.0000264294.79845.2f

Morley, R. E.. Ludemann, J. P., Moxham, J. P., Kozak, F. K., & Riding, K. H. (2004). Foreign body aspiration in infants and toddlers: Recent trends in British Columbia. *Journal of Otolaryngology, 33*(1), 37–41.

Nakamura, S. W., Pollack-Nelson, C., & Chidekel, A. S. (2003). Suction-type suffocation incidents in infants and toddlers. *Pediatrics, 111*(1), e12–e16.

Needlman, R., Howard, B., & Zuckerman, B. (1995). Helping parents get beyond the terrible 2's. *Patient Care, 29*(1), 52–61.

Null, J. (2012). *Hyperthermia deaths of children in vehicles.* San Francisco: San Francisco State University. Retrieved from http://www.ggweather.com/heat

Pan, S., Ugnat, A. M., Semenciw, R., Desmeules, M., Mao, Y., & MacLeod, M. (2006). Trends in childhood injury mortality in Canada, 1979–2002. *Injury Prevention, 12*(30), 155–160.

Petitto, L. A., et al. (2001). Bilingual signed and spoken language acquisition from birth: Implications for the mechanisms underlying early bilingual language acquisition. *Journal of Child Language, 28*(2), 453–496.

Piaget, J. (1952). *The origins of intelligence in children.* New York: International Universities Press.

Public Health Agency of Canada. (2009a). *Injury and child maltreatment analysis of Statistics Canada mortality data and Canadian Institute for Health Information Hospitalization data (2000–2005).* Ottawa, ON: Author.

Public Health Agency of Canada. (2009b). *Child and youth injury in review, 2009 edition—Spotlight on consumer product safety.* Retrieved from http://www.phac-aspc.gc.ca/publicat/cyi-bej/2009/pdf/injrep-rapbles2009_eng.pdf.

Roehlkepartain, E. C., et al. (Eds.). (2006). *The handbook of spiritual development in childhood and adolescence.* Thousand Oaks, CA: Sage.

Safe Kids Canada. (2006). *Child and youth unintentional injury: 1994–2003, 10 years in review.* Retrieved from http://www.mhp.gov.on.ca/en/prevention/injury-prevention/skc_injuries.pdf.

Safe Kids Canada. (2010). *Safety information: Drowning risks.* Retrieved from http://www.safekidscanada.ca/parents/safety-information/drowning-prevention/index.aspx.

Safe Kids Canada. (2011a). *Child passenger safety.* Retrieved from http://www.safekidscanada.ca/Parents/Safety-Information/Car-Seats/Types/Car-Seat-Types.aspx.

Safe Kids Canada. (2011b). *Safety information: How to lower your hot water temperature.* Retrieved from http://www.safekidscanada.ca/Parents/Safety-Information/Scalds-and-Burns/Hot-Liquids/Dangers-of-Hot-Liquids.aspx.

Safe Kids Canada. (2011c). *Safety information: The dangers of hot liquids.* Retrieved from http://www.safekidscanada.ca/Parents/Safety-Information/Scalds-and-Burns/Hot-Liquids/Dangers-of-Hot-Liquids.aspx.

pointed object or by having food or objects such as spoons in their mouths. Preventing such occurrences is the best approach with toddlers. The child should be taught that, when walking with a pointed object such as a knife or scissors, to hold the pointed end away from the face. Dangerous garden or workshop equipment and all firearms should be stored in a locked cabinet. Power lawnmowers are especially dangerous, and young children should not be allowed in an area where a mower is being used, nor should they be taken for a ride on a mower or allowed to operate that device. Toddlers have the dexterity, curiosity, patience, and ability to find hidden items. Safety education for older toddlers should include respect for firearms and their proper and appropriate use, including non-powder guns, such as air guns and rifles, which cause serious penetrating injuries. In addition, the child should be warned of and protected against potential danger from animals (see Animal Bites, Chapter 53).

Toys can be a source of danger, and safety must be a prime consideration when selecting toys (see Family-Centred Teaching box). While most toys have age ranges written on them to designate their safety, this information must be used with knowledge of the specific child's readiness. Please see Additional Resources at the end of this chapter for more information on toy safety and government regulations and recalls for defective toys.

Household safety should be practised and includes the usual precautions recommended for any age group (see Family-Centred Teaching box). An additional safeguard for young children is the use of safety glass in doors, windows, and tabletops; decals can be placed on glassed areas to reduce the likelihood of running through glass. Also, children should not be allowed to run, jump, wrestle, or play ball near glass structures.

Anticipatory Guidance—Care of Families

Understanding toddlers is fundamental to successful childrearing. Nurses, particularly those in ambulatory or child health centres, are in a favourable position to assist parents in facilitating the tasks and meeting the needs of children in this age group. Prevention yields better results than treatment. Anticipatory guidance is paramount to prevent future problems (see Family-Centred Teaching box). Advice, however, is sometimes not the sole answer. Actual assistance, such as being available for telephone consulting, should be part of the nurse's flexible repertoire of interventions. Whether parents are experiencing the childrearing dilemmas of a first or a subsequent child, they benefit from sharing their feelings, frustrations, and satisfactions. They need adult companionship, occasional freedom from childrearing responsibilities, and periodic separations from their children. Part of a nurse's responsibility is to provide opportunities for parents to express their feelings and to meet their physical, mental, and spiritual needs.

Key Points

- The toddler stage, extending from 12 to 36 months, is a period of intense exploration of the environment.
- Biological development during the toddler years is characterized by the acquisition of fine and gross motor skills that allow children to master a wide range of activities.
- Although most of the physiological systems are mature by the end of toddlerhood, development of certain areas of the brain is still occurring, allowing for greater intellectual capacity.
- Locomotion is the major gross motor skill acquired during toddlerhood, followed by increased eye–hand coordination.
- Specific tasks in the psychosocial development of a toddler include differentiating self from others, tolerating separation from parent, coping with delayed gratification, controlling bodily functions, acquiring socially acceptable behaviour, communicating verbally, and interacting with others in a less egocentric manner.
- According to Erikson, the major developmental task of toddlerhood is acquiring a sense of autonomy while overcoming a sense of doubt and shame.
- In Piaget's sensorimotor and preconceptual phases of development, the toddler experiments by incorporating the old learning of secondary circular reactions with new skills and applies this knowledge to new situations. There is the beginning of rational judgement, an understanding of causal relationships, and discovery of objects as objects.
- Preconceptual thought is characterized by egocentrism, centration, global organization of thought processes, animism, and irreversibility.
- Language is the major cognitive achievement in toddlerhood.
- The most striking characteristic of language development during early childhood is the increasing level of comprehension.
- Development of body image occurs with increasing motor ability, at which point toddlers recognize the importance and capacity of body parts.
- The two phases of differentiation of self from significant others are separation and individuation.
- Parental concerns during the toddler years include toilet training; coping with sibling rivalry; limit setting and discipline; and dealing with temper tantrums, negativism, and regression.
- Effective discipline techniques for toddlers include reward, ignoring, and time-out.
- Nutrition is important during the toddler stage because eating habits established in this period have lasting effects in subsequent years.
- Regular dental examinations, fluoride supplementation, removal of plaque, and provision of a low-cariogenic diet promote optimum dental health.
- Because of increased locomotion, toddlers are at high risk for sustaining injuries. Fatal injuries are primarily a result of motor vehicle accidents, drowning, and burns.

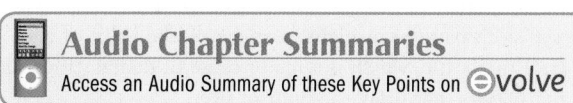

Audio Chapter Summaries
Access an Audio Summary of these Key Points on evolve

it. A Canadian study discovered that the most common foods causing choking were hard and round, and were nuts, raw carrots, and popcorn kernels (Morley, Ludemann, Moxham, Kozak, & Riding, 2004). Therefore, the same precautions as discussed for infants regarding food selection must be used for toddlers (see Chapter 36).

As with infants, play objects for toddlers must be chosen with an awareness of danger from small parts. A toy should not be able to fit into a toilet paper roll, otherwise it could be a choking hazard. Large, sturdy toys without sharp edges or removable parts are safest. Coins, paper clips, pins, bells, button (round) batteries, toy magnets, pull-tabs on cans, thumbtacks, nails, screws, jewellery (especially pierced earrings), and all types of pins are common household objects that can cause significant harm if swallowed or aspirated. Small items such as coloured beads, green peas, pellets, or beans are often placed into the nose by toddlers and may present a danger if aspirated into the airway. Because of the danger of aspiration, parents should be taught emergency procedures for choking (see Airway Obstruction, Chapter 46).

Suffocation from causes seen during infancy is less frequent, but old refrigerators, ovens, and other large appliances are a threat. Toddlers can climb inside these appliances and, if they close the door behind them, can be trapped inside. Removing all doors before discarding or storing old appliances can prevent such tragic deaths. Toddlers may also suffocate when unsafe toy box lids accidentally close on their head or neck. Parents should be advised of this danger and be encouraged to buy storage chests with lightweight, removable covers.

Hollow, semirigid hemispherical or ellipsoidal objects can form suction and cupping around a small child's face, causing complete airway obstruction. Several different types of objects have been involved with choking incidents, including toys, components of toys, and containers (Nakamura, Pollack-Nelson, & Chidekel, 2003).

Bodily Damage

Toddlers are still clumsy in many of their skills and can seriously harm themselves by walking while holding a sharp or

FAMILY-CENTRED TEACHING

Guidance During Toddler Years

Ages 12 to 18 Months

- Prepare parents for expected behavioural changes of the toddler, especially negativism and ritualism.
- Assess present feeding habits and encourage gradual weaning from the bottle and increased intake of solid foods.
- Stress expected feeding changes of picky eating habits, food fads and strong taste preferences, need for scheduled routine at mealtimes, inability to sit through an entire meal, and lack of table manners.
- Prepare parents for potential dangers of the home, particularly those contributing to motor vehicle injuries, poisoning, and falling injuries; give appropriate suggestions for safety proofing the home.
- Discuss the need for firm but gentle discipline and ways to deal with negativism and temper tantrums; stress positive benefits of appropriate discipline.
- Emphasize the importance for both the child and parents of brief, periodic separations.
- Discuss new toys that develop gross and fine motor, language, cognitive, and social skills.
- Emphasize the need for dental supervision, the types of basic dental hygiene at home, and food habits that predispose to caries; stress the importance of supplemental fluoride (according to age [greater than 6 months] and fluoride content of local water supply).

Ages 18 to 24 Months

- Stress the importance of peer companionship in play.
- Explore the need for preparation for an additional sibling (as appropriate); stress the importance of preparing the child for new experiences.
- Assess sleep patterns at night, particularly the habit of a bedtime bottle, which is a major cause of dental caries, and behaviours that delay the hour of sleep.
- Discuss present discipline methods, their effectiveness, and parents' feelings about the child's negativism; stress that negativism is an important aspect of developing self-assertion and independence and is not a sign of spoiling.
- Discuss signs of readiness for toilet training; emphasize the importance of waiting for physical and psychological readiness.
- Discuss development of fears, such as fear of darkness or loud noises, and of habits, such as security blanket or thumb-sucking; stress normalcy of these transient behaviours.
- Prepare parents for signs of regression in time of stress.
- Assess the child's ability to separate easily from parents for brief periods under familiar circumstances.
- Allow parents the opportunity to express their feelings of weariness, frustration, and exasperation; be aware that it is often difficult to love toddlers when they are not asleep!
- Point out some of the expected changes of the next year, such as longer attention span, somewhat less negativism, and increased concern for pleasing others.

Ages 24 to 36 Months

- Discuss the importance of imitation and domestic mimicry and the need to include the child in activities.
- Discuss approaches toward toilet training, particularly realistic expectations and the parents' attitude toward accidents.
- Stress uniqueness of toddlers' thought processes, especially through their use of language, poor understanding of time, view of causal relationships in terms of proximity of events, and inability to see events from another's perspective.
- Stress that discipline still must be structured and concrete and that relying solely on verbal reasoning and explanation leads to injuries, confusion, and misunderstanding.
- Discuss investigation of preschool or a day care centre toward completion of the child's second year.

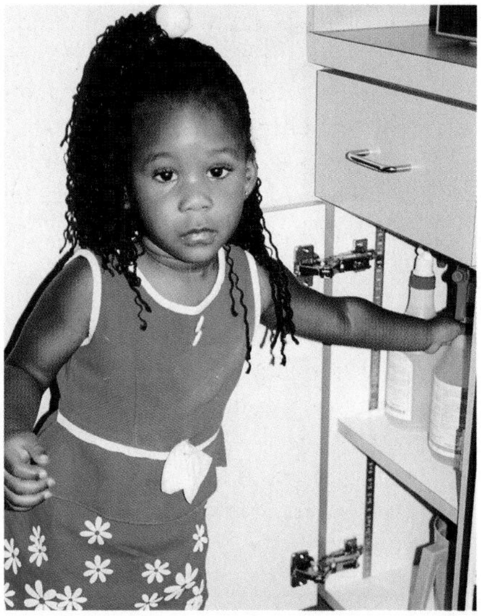

Fig. 37-13 Children are most likely to ingest substances that are on their level, such as cleaning agents stored under sinks, rat poison, plants, or diaper pail deodorants.

NURSING ALERT Parents should have ready access to the telephone number for the local poison control centre. These telephone numbers are in the telephone book under emergency numbers for each individual provincial or territorial poison control centre. They are also available on the Canadian Association of Poison Centres Web site at http://www.capcc.ca/provcentres/nu/nu.html. Parents should be prepared to act on the centre's advice.

Falls

Falls are still a hazard to children in this age group, although by the later part of early childhood, gross and fine motor skills are well developed, decreasing the incidence of falls down stairs or from chairs. Nonetheless, from 1990 to 2007 in Canada, 527,456 (32.7%) children 0 to 4 years of age had injuries that required emergency care. Of these injuries, 56.5% were in boys, 6.7% required observation or admission to the hospital, 14.2% were closed-head injuries, and 12.0% were skull fractures (PHAC, 2009b).

Playground injuries are common and can be serious. These injuries usually are caused by falls and can include fractured bones and brain and spinal injuries. Playground fatalities are rare and almost always caused by strangulation (Safe Kids Canada, 2012b). In children under 5 years of age, head and face injuries are most common (CPS, 2002). Children need to be taught safety at play areas, such as no horseplay on high slides or jungle gyms, *sitting* on swings, and staying away from moving swings. Passive prevention of injury includes placement of grass, sand, or wood chips under play equipment, which lessens injuries. Swing seats should be made of plastic, canvas, or rubber and have smooth or rounded edges. Slides should not exceed an incline of 30 degrees and should have evenly spaced rungs for climbing and protective "tunnels." Please see Additional Resources at the end of the chapter for more information on playground safety.

The climbing and running of the typical toddler are complicated by the child's total lack of appreciation of danger. Gates must be placed at both ends of stairs. Accessible windows that are left open during warm weather must be guarded with a rail. Falling from open windows is a major cause of accidental death in children; parents should be advised that a screened window is not a safety device to prevent falls. Doors leading to stairwells or porches must be locked because preschoolers can easily open them. A convenient type of lock is a sliding bar or hook that can be attached to the door and frame at a level higher than what the child can reach; such locks also have safety clasps or devices that prevent children from opening them.

Cribs and vehicles are other sources of falls. To avoid injury, crib rails should be fully raised, the mattress should be kept at the lowest position, and toys or bumper pads that may be used as steps to climb out should be removed. Once children reach a height of 89 cm, they should sleep in a bed rather than a crib. If a bunk bed is selected, parents should be aware of possible dangers such as falls and head entrapment between the mattress and guardrail or between the supporting mattress slats. If the beds are constructed of tubular metal, parents should check for breaks or cracks in the metal and welds that may lead to collapse and injury. Children who sleep on the top bunk should be 6 years of age or older. Please see Chapter 36 for a discussion on crib safety and the legislative requirements for cribs.

Children can fall from high chairs, shopping carts, carriages, car seats, and strollers if not properly restrained or if the balance changes when the object is weighted down with heavy items. Therefore, proper restraint and adequate supervision are essential. Clothing can also increase the chance of falling. Simple safety measures, such as checking clothing and shoes and keeping shoelaces tied with double knots or using self-adhering closures, can prevent accidents.

Aspiration and Suffocation

Threats to breathing are the third major cause of fatalities in Canadian children. These threats include strangulation, suffocation, choking, and entrapment. For survivors there can be long-term consequences with brain damage due to oxygen deprivation. Each year, approximately 44 Canadian children age 14 years and under die from threats to breathing. Approximately another 380 children have serious injuries and require hospitalization. Most of the Canadian children (80%) who required emergency care for a threat to breathing were under 5 years of age. The majority of these hospitalizations (94%) were from choking on food or other objects and the remainder (6%) were from a mechanical cause, such as strangulation from ropes or blind cords, or suffocating in beds (Safe Kids Canada, 2006).

Small children often put small objects, such as coins, batteries, small toys, and toy parts, into their mouths. Foreign-body aspiration is most common during the second year of life. Usually by 1 year of age children chew well, but they may have difficulty with large pieces of food, such as meat and whole hot dogs, and with hard foods, such as nuts. Young children cannot discard pits from fruit or bones from fish. It takes practice to learn how to chew gum without swallowing be placed in a high area, well out of reach of climbing young children. Hair curling irons may easily burn the hands of curious toddlers when left within easy reach.

Hot objects such as candles, incense, cigarettes, pots of tea or coffee, or irons must be placed away from children. The flame of a candle and the smoke of a cigarette invite investigation. Ashtrays with a centre well are preferred to prevent the cigarette from falling off the rim, and adults should try not to smoke, to cook, or to drink hot liquids when children are physically close. If tablecloths are used, the edges should be placed out of reach to prevent injuries from both burns and falling objects.

Flame burns represent one of the most fatal types of burns and commonly occur when children play with matches and accidentally set themselves (and the home) on fire. In Canada, approximately 19 children aged 14 years and under die from fire or smoke inhalation annually. Another 600 children are hospitalized for serious injuries related to fire exposure (Safe Kids Canada, 2011d). To prevent flame burns, matches and lighters must be stored safely away from children, and parents need to teach children the dangers of playing with such objects. In addition, all homes should have smoke detectors installed to alert the occupants to a fire. Homes without working smoke detectors have three times the risk of fire fatalities compared with homes that have working smoke detectors. Smoke alarms should be installed on every level and near sleeping areas. A safety plan for immediate escape is also essential.

Electrical burns also represent an immediate danger to children. With preschoolers' ability to manipulate small, thin objects, they are able to insert hairpins or other conductive articles into electrical sockets. Young toddlers may explore outlets and wires by mouthing them. Since water is an excellent conductor, the chance for a severe circumoral electrical burn is great. Electrical outlets should have protective guards plugged into them when not in use (Fig. 37-12) or be made inaccessible by having furniture placed in front of them, when feasible. Children should not be allowed to play with electrical cords or appliances, which should be kept out of reach as much as possible.

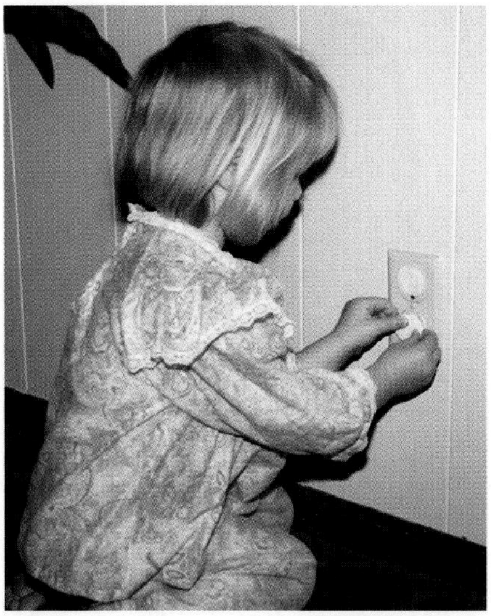

Fig. 37-12 Special plastic caps in electrical sockets prevent young fingers from exploring dangerous areas.

Poisoning

Poisoning is a significant cause of injuries in children. Annually, in Canada approximately 7 children under the age of 14 years die from poisoning; another 1700 children require hospitalization for poison-related injuries. Children ages 1 to 4 years constitute 64% of these poisonings (Safe Kids Canada, 2006).

Toddlers are at the highest risk for poisoning. Mouthing activity continues to be prevalent after 1 year of age, and exploring objects by tasting them is part of children's natural investigation. Many household products, medications, and plants can be poisonous if swallowed, if they come in contact with the skin or eyes, or if inhaled. Although in many instances poisoning does not result in death, it may cause significant morbidity, such as esophageal stricture from lye ingestion. Toddlers are able to climb most heights, open most drawers or closets, and unscrew most lids. By trial and error, younger children also manage to undo tops of bottles, plastic containers, aerosol cans, and jars, including those with child-resistant lids. In addition, toddlers may find medications that have been transferred to regular containers for older adults such as grandparents, who may have difficulty with child-resistant lids. Newer forms of medications, such as transdermal patches and cough-suppressant lozenges, have created additional dangers, since they are not packaged with safety caps and the lozenges look like candy. Unintentional medication ingestion causes 64% of the poisonings in children 14 years and younger. Ingestion of iron pills is of special concern as it is the leading cause of death (Safe Kids Canada, 2006).

The major reason for poisoning is improper storage, particularly when the substance is taken out of the original container (Fig. 37-13). The guidelines suggested in Chapter 36 apply to children in this age group as well (p. 1002). However, unlike the infant, who was confined to certain heights and unable to unlatch inventive locks, young children manage to find access to many high-level, tight-security places. For this age group, only a locked cabinet is safe.

Carbon monoxide is a rare cause of poisoning in children in Canada but is very serious and can cause a coma or death (Safe Kids Canada, 2012a). This toxic gas is colourless and has no odour. Defective appliances, clothes dryers, furnaces, and exhaust fumes from cars in home garages are sources of carbon monoxide poisoning. Unlike smoke detectors, carbon monoxide detectors are not mandatory, but they can save the lives of entire families. The detectors should be installed on every level and near sleeping areas and should be replaced every 5 to 7 years. Fuel-burning appliances should be checked once a year for carbon monoxide leakage (Safe Kids Canada, 2012a).

Emergency and preventive measures for accidental poisoning are discussed in Chapter 36.

Unit 9

38 The Preschooler and Family

Learning Objectives

On completion of this chapter, the reader will be able to:

- Identify the major biological, psychosocial, cognitive, moral, spiritual, and social developments that occur during the preschool years.
- List the benefits of imaginary playmates.
- Prepare preschoolers for preschool or day care experience.
- Provide parents with guidelines for sex education.
- Provide parents with guidelines for dealing with a child's fears, stresses, aggression, and sleep problems.
- Recognize causes of stuttering during preschool years.
- Offer parents suggestions for preventing speech problems.
- Recognize feeding patterns of preschoolers.
- Provide anticipatory guidance to parents regarding injury prevention based on preschoolers' developmental achievements.

Electronic Resources

Additional information related to the content in Chapter 38 can be found on

evolve the companion Web site at

http://evolve.elsevier.com/Canada/Perry/maternal/

- Examination Review Questions
- Assessment Video Clips
- Case Study—Sleep Problems
- Critical Thinking Exercise—Conjunctivitis
- Critical Thinking Exercise—Imitative Play

Promoting Optimum Growth and Development

Combined biological, psychosocial, cognitive, spiritual, and social achievements during the preschool period (3 to 5 years of age) prepare preschoolers for their most significant change in lifestyle: entrance into school. Their control of bodily functions, experience of brief and prolonged periods of separation, ability to interact cooperatively with other children and adults, use of language for mental symbolization, and increased attention span and memory prepare them for the next major period: school years. Successful achievement of previous levels of growth and development is essential for preschoolers in order to refine many of the tasks that were mastered during the toddler years.

Biological Development

The rate of physical growth slows and stabilizes during the preschool years. See Table 38-1 for preschooler heights and weights. The WHO Child Growth Standards 2006 and WHO Growth Reference charts are used to measure and track Canadian preschooler's growth patterns (Dietitians of Canada, Canadian Paediatric Society, College of Family Physicians, and Community Health Nurses of Canada, 2010).

The physical proportions of the preschooler no longer resemble the squat, pot-bellied toddler. The preschooler is slender but sturdy, graceful, agile, and posturally erect. There is little difference in physical characteristics according to gender. Most organ systems can adjust to moderate **stress** and change. During this period, most children are toilet trained. Motor development mainly consists of increases in strength and refinement of previously learned skills. Muscle development and bone growth are still not mature. Excessive activity and overexertion can injure delicate tissues. Good posture, appropriate exercise, and adequate nutrition and rest are essential for optimum development of the musculoskeletal system.

Table 38-1 Growth and Development During Preschool Years

PHYSICAL	GROSS MOTOR	FINE MOTOR	LANGUAGE
Age 3 Yr			
Usual weight gain of 1.8–2.7 kg Average weight of 14.5 kg Usual gain in height of 7.5 cm per year Average height of 95 cm May have achieved nighttime control of bowel and bladder	Rides tricycle Jumps off bottom step Stands on one foot for a few seconds Goes up stairs using alternate feet; may still come down using both feet on step Broad jumps May try to dance, but balance may not be adequate	Builds tower of 9–10 cubes Builds bridge with three cubes Adeptly places small pellets in narrow-necked bottle In drawing, copies a circle, imitates a cross, names what has been drawn; cannot draw stick figure but may make circle with facial features	Has vocabulary of about 900 words Uses primarily telegraphic speech Uses complete sentences of three or four words Talks incessantly regardless of whether anyone is paying attention Repeats sentence of six syllables Asks many questions
Age 4 Yr			
Pulse and respiration rates decrease slightly Growth rate is similar to that of previous year Average weight of 16.7 kg Average height of 103 cm Length at birth is doubled Maximum potential for development of amblyopia	Skips and hops on one foot Catches ball reliably Throws ball overhead Walks down stairs using alternate footing	Uses scissors successfully to cut out picture following outline Can lace shoes but may not be able to tie bow In drawing, copies a square, traces a cross and diamond, adds three parts to stick figure	Has vocabulary of 1500 words or more Uses sentences of four or five words Questioning is at peak Tells exaggerated stories Knows simple songs May be mildly profane if associates with older children Obeys four prepositional phrases, such as *under, on top of, beside, in back of,* or *in front of* Names one or more colours Comprehends analogies, such as, "If ice is cold, fire is ________"
Age 5 Yr			
Pulse and respiration rates decrease slightly Average weight of 18.7 kg Average height of 110 cm Eruption of permanent dentition may begin Handedness is established (about 90% are right-handed)	Skips and hops on alternate feet Throws and catches ball well Jumps rope Skates with good balance Walks backward with heel to toe Jumps from height of 30 cm and lands on toes Balances on alternate feet with eyes closed	Ties shoelaces Uses scissors, simple tools, or pencil very well In drawing, copies a diamond and triangle; adds seven to nine parts to stick figure; prints a few letters, numbers, or words, such as first name	Has vocabulary of about 2100 words Uses sentences of six to eight words, with all parts of speech Names coins (e.g., nickel, dime) Names four or more colours Describes drawing or pictures with much comment and elaboration Knows days of week, months, and other time-associated words Knows composition of objects, such as "A shoe is made of ______." Can follow three commands in succession

It is estimated that with the ambient temperature at 22° to 35.5°C, the vehicle interior temperature rises by 10.5° to 11°C for each 10 minutes, even with a window cracked (Null, 2012). In a study of 171 child fatalities from overheating in a car, 50% of adults who left a child in a car either forgot or were unaware that the child was still in the car. A significant number of those children (32) were left by family members who intended to take the child to day care but forgot the child in the car at the workplace; 22 children were left in the car by a day care worker or driver (Guard & Gallagher, 2005). In addition, leaving children unsupervised in a parked vehicle, especially in a private driveway, provides an opportunity for the child to release the brake or put the car in gear. Parents should be cautioned against leaving children alone in a vehicle *for any reason.*

Prevention of vehicular injuries involves protecting and educating children and adults about the dangers of moving or parked vehicles. Children should never ride in the open back of a truck; the danger of falls can be compounded by another vehicle striking the child or by the truck rolling over. Children in bicycle-towed trailers or bicycle-mounted child seats can also be injured by collisions or falls. Although preschool children are too young to be trusted to always obey, parents should emphasize looking for moving vehicles before crossing the street, recognizing the stop and go colours of traffic lights, and following traffic officers' signals. Physical barriers that limit children from playing near vehicles can help prevent these injuries. Most important, what is preached must be practised. Children learn through imitation, and consistency reinforces learning.

Drowning

Drowning ranks as the second most common cause of fatalities (15%) from unintentional injuries in the 1- to 4-year age group (PHAC, 2009b). With well-developed skills of locomotion, toddlers are able to reach potentially dangerous areas, such as bathtubs, toilets, buckets, swimming pools, hot tubs, and lakes. Their intense drive for exploration and investigation, combined with an unawareness of the danger of water and their helplessness in water, makes drowning always a viable threat. It is also one category of injuries that results in death within minutes, diminishing the chance for rescue and survival. Children under 5 years of age have a small lung capacity; their lungs can fill fast with water and they can drown in 2.5 cm of water. Canadian researchers found that all children under 2 years of age who drowned in bathtubs had been left unsupervised for significant periods of time (Safe Kids Canada, 2010). Adult supervision of children when near any source of water is essential; teaching swimming and water safety can be helpful but cannot be regarded as sufficient protection.

Burns

In Canada approximately 40 children, ages 14 and under, die from fires and other burns every year. Another 770 children are hospitalized for serious burn-related injuries. Fires and flames cause 34% of hospitalizations and fireplaces and woodstoves cause 7.5% (Safe Kids Canada, 2011d). For children under 5 years of age, the causes of hospitalization for burns include scalds (73%), smoke inhalation (2%), appliances and other flame-related injuries (14%), and clothes catching on fire (4%) (Safe Kids Canada, 2006). Because of their thinner skin, children are more vulnerable to burns than adults. Consequently, significant burns can cause permanent scarring with contracting of underlying tissues because of rapid growth and can lead to emotional scarring and physical disabilities (Safe Kids Canada, 2011c). Please see Chapter 53 for information on how to care for a child with a burn.

Toddlers' ability to climb, stretch, and reach objects above their heads makes any hot surface a potential source of danger. Scald burns, the most common type of thermal injury in small children, can result from children pulling hot pots from the stove on top of themselves; of all scald injuries needing hospitalization, 83% were in children under age 5 years (Safe Kids Canada, 2011c). As a precaution, pot handles should be turned toward the back of the stove. Ideally, the knobs for controlling the range burners should be out of reach, not on the front panel where nimble fingers can turn them on and accidentally touch the hot burner. Oven doors should be closed whenever the oven is turned on or when it is cooling. The outside of doors of automatic self-cleaning ovens may become hot and, if touched, could cause a burn. It is also important to keep appliance cords out of reach, to use baby gates, and to keep toddlers seated in the kitchen.

Scald burns are also often caused by exposure to high-temperature tap water. Children come in contact with hot tap water by turning on the hot-water faucet or falling into a bathtub of hot water, or through parental deliberate abuse. Youngsters must always be supervised when they are near tap water, and bathwater temperatures need to be checked. Limiting household water temperatures to 49°C is also recommended for gas or oil-fired heaters and 60°C if using electric heaters. It is not advisable to run the heaters at lower than these temperatures because of the risk of Legionnaire's disease (Safe Kids Canada, 2011b). At 49°C it takes 10 minutes of exposure to the water to cause a full-thickness burn. Conversely, water temperatures of 54°C, a common setting of most water heaters, expose household members to the risk of full-thickness burns within 30 seconds. Nurses can help prevent such burns by advising parents of this common household danger and recommending that they readjust the water heater to a safe temperature. An easy-to-read hot-water gauge that changes colour to show water temperatures between 49° and 60°C is also available; it shows a "hot," "cool," or "OK" water temperature. A special device can be added to the faucet that reduces the water flow once the set temperature is reached, or guards that block access to the faucet can be used. There are also mixing valves available that can be installed in the plumbing to mix hot and cold water. Scalding can also occur when a curious child tries to sip a parent's coffee or tea and spills the boiling liquid down the chin and chest. Thus lidded travelling cups are a safe choice.

Other sources of heat, such as radiators, fireplaces, accessible furnaces, kerosene heaters, or wood-burning stoves, should have a guard placed in front of them. The tops of some of these heaters are designed to become hot enough to boil water to provide humidity; thus they are hazardous if touched or if the pan of water is spilled. Portable electrical heaters must area of the car for children is the back seat. Children who must ride in the passenger side of the front seat with an activated air bag should be positioned as far back as possible. Children should remain in the back seat until the age of 12 years.

An interim order issued by the Minister of Transport in 2007 allowed manufacturers and importers to offer child-restraint systems in Canada that incorporate an internal harness and a tether strap for children up to 30 kg. This arrangement increases the capacity of the restraint systems (the use of children's restraint systems fall under provincial/territorial jurisdiction). This new order changes the definition of "child," where restraint systems are concerned, to mean a person whose weight is not less than 10 kg and not more than 30 kg. It is necessary for all forward-facing seats to be secured to the vehicle with a tether strap, as well as the vehicle seat belt or the UAS (CPS, 2008a).

As of December 2011, the Government of Canada has enacted new safety regulations for motor vehicles and booster seat safety that require manufacturers to modify car seats and booster seats to improve the safety level. These new regulations include an expiration date for car seats; for further information on Canadian regulations regarding child booster seats see Safe Kids Canada (2011a). For any restraint to be effective, it must be used consistently and properly. Examples of misuse include misrouting the vehicle seat belt through the restraint; failing to use the vehicle seat belt to secure the restraint; failing to use a tether strap; failing to use the restraint's harness system; and incorrectly positioning the child, especially by facing infants and toddlers forward instead of rearward. To address these issues, nurses must stress correct use of car restraints and rules that ensure **compliance** (see Family-Centred Teaching box). Children riding in car safety seats are not only better protected but also generally much better behaved than children left unrestrained; this can be important for accident prevention. For additional information about child safety restraints see the Additional Resources section at the end of this chapter.

Children with special needs may require a restraint system that secures them appropriately in the event of a crash. Examples of such devices include car bed restraints for infants who cannot tolerate a semireclining position and specially adapted moulded-plastic chairs for children who have spica casts. The E-Z-On vest is a special safety harness for larger children with poor trunk control. Additional safety restraints and a listing of distributors are available at the SafetyBeltSafe U.S.A. Web site (http://www.carseat.org). The restraints must be approved for use in Canada by the Ministry of Transport. For more information on the Ministry's regulations, please go to http://www.tc.gc.ca/media/documents/roadsafety/TP14772e.pdf.

Injuries to children may also occur during sudden stops when objects are left unrestrained. On sudden impact, a loose toy or package can become a projectile missile. Therefore, all items should be secured or stored in the trunk.

Children over 3 years of age are often involved in pedestrian traffic injuries. Motor vehicle back-over injuries and deaths, along with deaths or serious injury resulting from heat stroke when children were left alone in a car, account for a large number of motor vehicle–related injuries in children (Centers for Disease Control and Prevention, 2005; McLaren, Null, & Quinn, 2005). Given their gross motor skills of walking, running, and climbing, and their fine motor skills of opening doors and fence gates, children are likely to be in hazardous areas when unsupervised. Unaware of danger and unable to approximate the speed of a car, they are often hit by moving vehicles. Running after a ball, riding a tricycle, and playing behind a parked car are common activities that may result in a vehicular tragedy. Toddlers playing in driveways or farmyards are at risk of back-over injury from vehicles in reverse gear. A safety feature that can be used when children are playing in driveways is to attach to the tricycle a pole with a bright-coloured flag that is high enough to be visible through an automobile's back window. Another safeguard is an automatic beeping device installed in many vehicles that beeps loudly when the vehicle is driven in reverse, to alert children to the oncoming car, van, tractor, or truck. Some models now come equipped with rearview motion cameras, enabling the driver to see the driveway clearly while backing out.

Another dangerous situation that has become more commonplace is when children crawl into an open trunk and pull it closed. Asphyxia may occur in such cases; therefore, car trunks should not be left open when children are near and not being supervised. Some cars come equipped with a safety switch that can be activated from inside the trunk to open a closed trunk door.

Overheating (hyperthermia) of toddlers and their subsequent death can occur when they are left in a vehicle in hot weather (more than 27°C). Small children dissipate heat poorly, and an increase in body temperature can cause death in a few hours. In 2011, 33 children died of vehicular hyperthermia in the United States. From 1998 to 2011, more than 50% of the deaths were of children under 2 years of age. During this time period, 23% of the victims were 1 year of age; 20% were 2 years; and 13% were 4 years of age (Null, 2012).

FAMILY-CENTRED TEACHING

Using Car Safety Seats

- Read manufacturer's directions and follow them exactly.
- Anchor the safety seat securely to the car's seat and apply harness snugly to the child.
- Do not start the car until everyone is properly restrained.
- Always use the restraint, even for short trips.
- If the child begins to climb out or undo the harness, firmly say, "No." It may be necessary to stop the car to reinforce the expected behaviour. Use rewards, such as stars or stickers, to encourage appropriate behaviour.
- Encourage the child to help attach buckles, straps, and shields, but always double-check fastenings.
- Decrease boredom on long trips. Keep soft toys in the car for quiet play; talk to the child; point out objects and teach the child about them. Stop periodically. If the child wishes to sleep, make certain the child stays in the restraint.
- Insist that others who transport children also follow these safety rules.

SOCIALIZATION	COGNITION	FAMILY RELATIONSHIPS
Dresses self almost completely if helped with back buttons and told which shoe is right or left Pulls on shoes Has increased attention span Feeds self completely Can prepare simple meals, such as cold cereal and milk Can help to set table; can dry dishes without breaking any May have fears, especially of dark and going to bed Knows own gender and gender of others Play is parallel and associative; begins to learn simple games, but often follows own rules; begins to share	Is in preconceptual phase Is egocentric in thought and behaviour Has beginning understanding of time; uses many time-oriented expressions, talks about past and future as much as about present, pretends to tell time Has improved concept of space, as demonstrated by understanding of prepositions and ability to follow directional command Has beginning ability to view concepts from another perspective	Attempts to please parents and conform to their expectations Is less jealous of younger sibling; may be opportune time for birth of additional sibling Is aware of family relationships and gender-role functions Boys tend to identify more with father or other male figure Has increased ability to separate easily and comfortably from parents for short periods
Very independent Tends to be selfish and impatient Aggressive physically and verbally Takes pride in accomplishments Has mood swings Shows off dramatically, enjoys entertaining others Tells family tales to others with no restraint Still has many fears Play is associative Imaginary playmates are common Uses dramatic, imaginative, and imitative devices Sexual exploration and curiosity demonstrated through play, such as being "doctor" or "nurse"	Is in phase of intuitive thought Causality is still related to proximity of events Understands time better, especially in terms of sequence of daily events Unable to conserve matter Judges everything according to one dimension, such as height, width, or order Immediate perceptual clues dominate judgement Is beginning to develop less egocentrism and more social awareness May count correctly but has poor mathematical concept of numbers Obeys because parents have set limits, not because of understanding of right and wrong	Rebels if parents expect too much, such as impeccable table manners Takes aggression and frustration out on parents or siblings Do's and don'ts become important May have rivalry with older or younger siblings; may resent older sibling's privileges and younger sibling's invasion of privacy and possessions May "run away" from home Identifies strongly with parent of opposite sex Is able to run simple errands outside home
Less rebellious and quarrelsome than at age 4 yr More settled and eager to get down to business Not as open and accessible in thoughts and behaviour as in earlier years Independent but trustworthy, not foolhardy; more responsible Has fewer fears; relies on outer authority to control world Eager to do things right and to please; tries to "live by rules" Has better manners Cares for self totally, occasionally needing supervision in dress or hygiene Not ready for concentrated close work or small print because of slight farsightedness and still unrefined eye-hand coordination Play is associative; tries to follow rules but may cheat to avoid losing	Begins to question what parents think by comparing them with age-mates and other adults May notice prejudice and bias in outside world Is more able to view other's perspective, but tolerates differences rather than understanding them May begin to show understanding of conservation of numbers through counting objects regardless of arrangement Uses time-oriented words with increased understanding Cautious about accepting or believing information	Gets along well with parents May seek out parent more often than at age 4 yr for reassurance and security, especially when entering school Begins to question parents' thinking and principles Strongly identifies with parent of same sex, especially boys with their fathers Enjoys activities such as sports, cooking, and shopping with parent of same sex

Gross and Fine Motor Skills

Walking, running, climbing, and jumping are well established by age 36 months. Refinement in eye–hand and muscle coordination is evident in several areas (Fig. 38-1).

Fine motor development is evident in these children's increasingly skilful manipulation, such as in drawing and dressing. These skills provide readiness for **learning** and independence for entry into school.

Psychosocial Development

Developing a Sense of Initiative (Erikson)

Erikson (1963) maintained that the chief psychosocial task of this preschool period is acquiring a sense of initiative. Children are in a stage of energetic learning. They play, work, and live to the fullest and feel a real sense of accomplishment and satisfaction in their activities. Conflict arises when children overstep the limits of their ability and inquiry and experience a sense of guilt for not having behaved appropriately. Feelings of guilt, anxiety, and fear may also result from thoughts that differ from expected behaviour.

A particularly stressful thought for the preschooler is wishing one's parent dead. A sense of rivalry or development of *superego*, or *conscience*, begins toward the end of the toddler years and is a major task for preschoolers (see Cultural Awareness box). Learning right from wrong and good from bad is the beginning of a sense of morality (see Moral Development section).

Cognitive Development

One task related to the preschool period is readiness for school and scholastic learning. Many thought processes of this period are crucial for achieving this readiness, and because of this prerequisite, children begin school between ages 5 and 6 rather than at an earlier age.

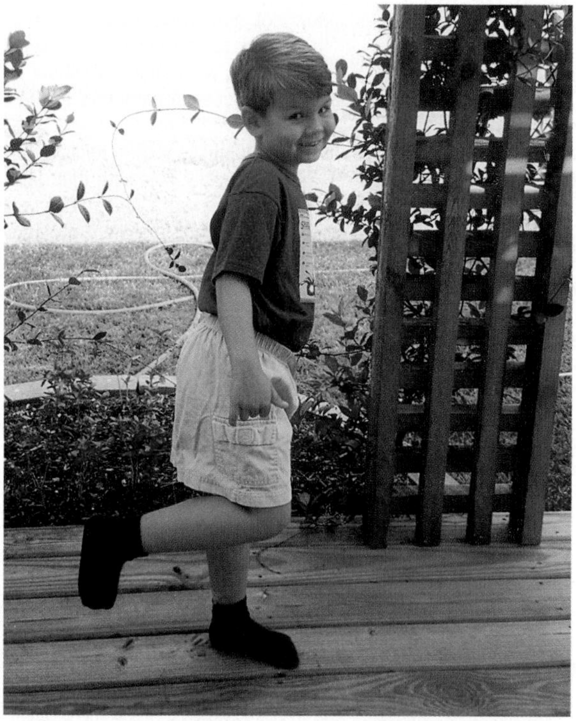

Fig. 38-1 A 4-year-old child has sufficient balance to stand or hop on one foot.

Preoperational Phase (Piaget)

Piaget's cognitive theory (1952) does not include a period specifically for children who are 3 to 5 years old. The *preoperational phase* covers the age span from 2 to 7 years and is divided into two stages: *preconceptual phase*, ages 2 to 4, and the phase of *intuitive thought*, ages 4 to 7. One main transition during these two phases is the shift from totally egocentric thought to social awareness and the ability to consider other viewpoints. Egocentricity is still evident.

Language continues to develop during the preschool stage. Speech remains primarily a vehicle of egocentric communication. Preschoolers assume that everyone thinks as they do and that a brief explanation of their thinking makes the entire thought understood by others. Because of this self-referenced, egocentric verbal communication, it is often necessary to explore and understand a young child's thinking through other, nonverbal approaches. For children in this age group, the most enlightening and effective method is *play*, which becomes the child's way of understanding, adjusting to, and working out life's experiences.

Preschoolers increasingly use language without comprehending the meaning of words, particularly concepts of right and left, causality, and time. Children may use the concepts correctly but only in the circumstances in which they have learned them. For example, they may know how to put on shoes by remembering that the buckle is always on the outside of the foot. If different shoes have no buckles, they cannot reason which shoe fits which foot. In other words, they do not understand the concepts of *right and left*.

Superficially, *causality* resembles logical thought. Preschoolers explain a concept as they heard it described by others, but understanding is limited. An example is the concept of time. Because *time* is still incompletely understood, children interpret it according to their own frame of reference. Consequently, time is best explained in relationship to an event, such as "Your mother will visit you after you finish your lunch." Avoiding words such as *yesterday, tomorrow, next week*, or a named day of the week to express when an event is expected to occur and instead associating time with expected daily events can help children learn about temporal relationships while increasing their trust in others' predictions.

CULTURAL AWARENESS

Learning Sociocultural Mores

Developing a conscience implies learning sociocultural mores of the family's heritage. Depending on the type of attitudes conveyed, children will learn not only appropriate behaviours but also tolerance-based, biased, or prejudicial values concerning their ethnic, religious, and social background and those of other groups. Much of this influence may remain dormant until they associate with children or adults of a different heritage. Depending on the particular group, they may be accepted or ostracized for their attitudes.

Preschoolers' thinking is often described as *magical thinking*. Because of their egocentrism and transductive reasoning, they believe that thoughts are all-powerful. Such thinking places them in the vulnerable position of feeling guilty and responsible for bad thoughts, which may coincide with the occurrence of a wished event. Their inability to logically reason cause and effect of an illness or injury makes it especially difficult for them to understand such events.

Preschoolers believe in the power of words and accept their meaning literally. An example of this type of thinking is when children are called "bad" because they did something wrong: In preschoolers' minds, calling them "bad" means they are a bad person; it is better to say that their actions were bad by saying, for example, "That was a bad thing to do."

Moral Development

Preconventional or Premoral Level (Kohlberg)

Young children's development of moral **judgement** is at the most basic level. They have little, if any, concern about why something is wrong. They behave because of freedom or restriction that is placed on actions. In *punishment and obedience orientation*, children (from about 2 to 4 years) judge whether an action is good or bad depending on whether it results in reward or punishment. If children are punished for it, the action is bad. If they are not punished, the action is good, regardless of the meaning of the act. For example, if parents allow hitting, children will perceive that hitting is good because it is not associated with punishment.

From approximately 4 to 7 years of age, children are in the stage of *naive instrumental orientation*, in which actions are directed toward satisfying their needs and, less frequently, the needs of others. They have a concrete sense of justice and fairness during this period of development.

Spiritual Development

Children's knowledge of faith and religion is learned from significant others in their environment, usually from parents and their religious beliefs and practices (Fosarelli, 2003). Young children's understanding of spirituality is influenced by their cognitive level. Preschoolers have a concrete concept of a God or other deity with physical characteristics, often like an imaginary friend. They understand simple religious stories and memorize short prayers, but their understanding of the meaning of these rituals is limited. Preschoolers benefit from concrete representations of religious practices, such as picture Bible books and small statues. They will imitate religious practices of their parents without fully understanding the significance of these acts.

Development of conscience is strongly linked to spiritual development. At this age, children are learning right from wrong and behaving correctly to avoid punishment. Wrongdoing provokes feelings of guilt, and preschoolers often misinterpret illness as a punishment for real or imagined transgressions. It is important that children view God as one who bestows unconditional love, rather than as a judge of good or bad behaviour. Observing religious traditions and participating in a religious community can help children cope during stressful periods, such as illness, hospitalization, and other traumatic events (Barnes et al., 2000). In many religious faiths, cultural practices and religion are closely intertwined (McEvoy, 2003) and are an important part of the child's and family's life.

Development of Body Image

Preschool years play a significant role in the development of **body image**. With increasing comprehension of language, preschoolers recognize that individuals have undesirable and desirable appearances. They recognize differences in skin colour and racial identity and are vulnerable to learning prejudices and biases. They are aware of the meaning of words such as *pretty* or *ugly*, and they reflect opinions of others regarding their own appearance. By 5 years of age, children compare their size with that of their peers and can become conscious of being large or short, especially if others refer to them as "so big" or "so little" for their age. In one study, negative associations between weight status and self-concept were identified in girls as young as 5 years of age (Davison & Birch, 2001).

Despite advances in body image development, preschoolers have poorly defined body boundaries and little knowledge of their internal anatomy. Intrusive experiences are frightening, especially those that disrupt the integrity of the skin, such as injections and surgery. They fear that if their skin is "broken," all of their blood and "insides" can leak out. Bandages are critical to "keep everything from coming out."

Development of Sexuality

Sexual development during these years is an important phase in the formation of a person's overall sexual identity and beliefs. Preschoolers are forming strong attachments to opposite-sex parents while identifying with same-sex parents. *Sex-typing*, or the process by which an individual develops behaviour, personality, attitudes, and beliefs appropriate for his or her culture and sex, occurs through several mechanisms during this period. As sexual identity develops beyond gender recognition, modesty may become a concern. Gender-role imitation and "dressing up" like Mommy or Daddy are important activities. Attitudes and responses of others to role-playing can condition children to accept the views of others. For example, comments such as "Boys shouldn't play with dolls" can influence a boy's self-concept of masculinity.

Sexual exploration may be more pronounced now than ever before, particularly in terms of exploring and manipulating genitalia. Questions about sexual reproduction may come to the forefront in preschoolers' search for understanding (see Chapters 39 and 40).

Social Development

During the preschool period, the *separation–individuation process* is completed. Preschoolers have overcome much of the anxiety associated with strangers and the fear of separation of earlier years. They relate to unfamiliar people easily and tolerate brief separations from parents with little or no protest, They still need parental security, reassurance, guidance, and approval, especially when entering preschool or elementary school. Prolonged separation, such as that imposed by illness and hospitalization, is difficult, but preschoolers respond to anticipatory preparation and concrete explanation. They can cope with changes in daily routine much better than toddlers, although they may develop more imaginary fears.

Preschoolers gain security and comfort from familiar objects, such as toys, dolls, or photographs of family members **(familiarization play)**. They are able to work through many of their unresolved fears, fantasies, and anxieties through play, especially if guided with appropriate play objects (e.g., dolls, puppets) that represent family members, health care providers, and other children.

Language

During preschool years, language becomes more sophisticated and complex. Both cognitive ability and environment—particularly, consistent role models—influence vocabulary, speech, and comprehension. Language becomes a major mode of communication and social interaction, and its development during the preschool period sets the stage for later success in school (Needlman, 2004) (Fig. 38-2).

By age 6, children can use all parts of speech correctly, except for deviations from the rules. They can define simple things by describing the use, shape, or general category of classification, rather than simply describing their outward appearance. For example, they may define a ball as "round," "something you bounce," or "a toy," rather than only describing its colour. They can give some opposites, such as "If Mommy is a woman, Daddy is a man." They can also describe an object according to its composition, such as "A spoon is made of metal."

Personal-Social Behaviour

evolve Critical Thinking Exercise—Imitative Play

The pervasive **ritualism** and **negativism** of toddlerhood gradually diminish during the preschool years. Although self-assertion is still a major theme, preschoolers demonstrate their sense of autonomy differently. They are able to verbalize their request for independence and perform independently because of their much-refined physical and cognitive development. By 4 or 5 years of age, they need little if any assistance with dressing, eating, or toileting (Fig. 38-3). They can also be trusted to obey warnings of danger, although 3- or 4-year-old children may exceed their boundaries at times.

They are much more sociable and willing to please. They have internalized many standards and values of family and culture. By the end of early childhood they begin to question parental values and compare them with those of their peer group and other authority figures. As a result, they may be less willing to abide by the family's code of conduct. Preschoolers become increasingly aware of their position and role within the family. Although this is a more secure age for experiencing the addition of another sibling, relinquishing the position of only or youngest is still difficult and requires special parental attention to prevent feelings of desertion and resentment (Brazelton & Sparrow, 2001) (see Chapter 37, Sibling Rivalry).

Play

Various types of play are typical of this period, but preschoolers especially enjoy **associative play**—group play in similar or identical activities but without rigid organization or rules (see Fig. 33-8). Play should provide for physical, social, and mental development.

Play activities for physical growth and refinement of motor skills include jumping, running, and climbing. Tricycles, wagons, gym and sports equipment, sandboxes, wading pools, and activities at water parks can help develop muscles and coordination (Fig. 38-4).

Probably the most characteristic and pervasive preschool activity is *imitative, imaginative*, and **dramatic play**. Dress-up clothes, dolls, housekeeping toys, dollhouses, play store toys, telephones, farm animals and equipment, village sets, trains, trucks, cars, planes, hand puppets, and medical kits provide hours of self-expression (Fig. 38-5). Probably at no other time is reproduction of adult behaviour so faithful and absorbing as in 4- and 5-year-old children. Toward the end of the preschool period, children are less satisfied with make-believe or pretend objects and enjoy doing the actual activity, such as cooking and carpentry.

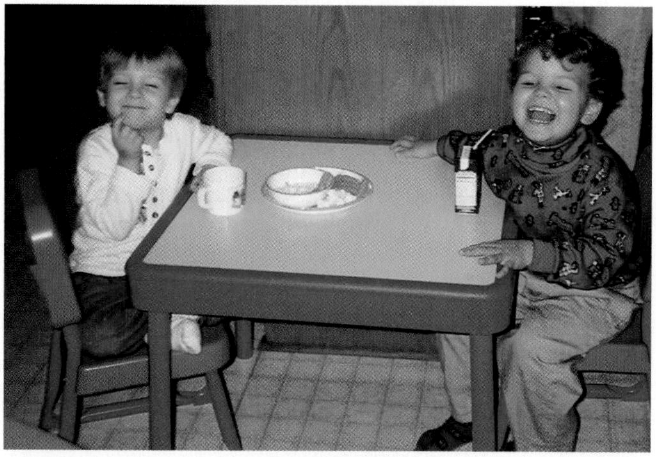

Fig. 38-2 Preschool children enjoy friends and often use nonverbal messages to communicate.

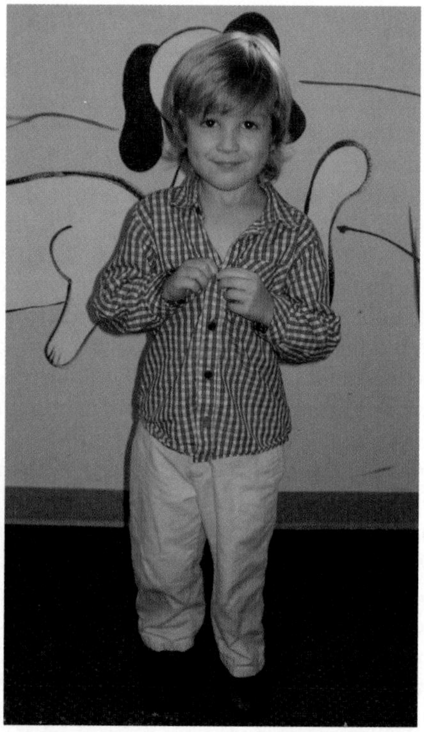

Fig. 38-3 Most preschoolers are able to dress themselves but need help with more difficult items of clothing.

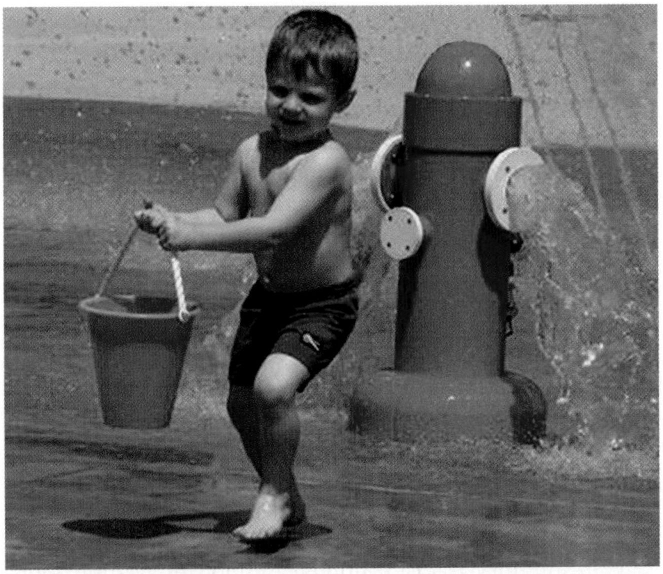

Fig. 38-4 Preschoolers enjoy play activities that promote motor skills such as jumping and running. Water play is an exciting activity for the preschooler.

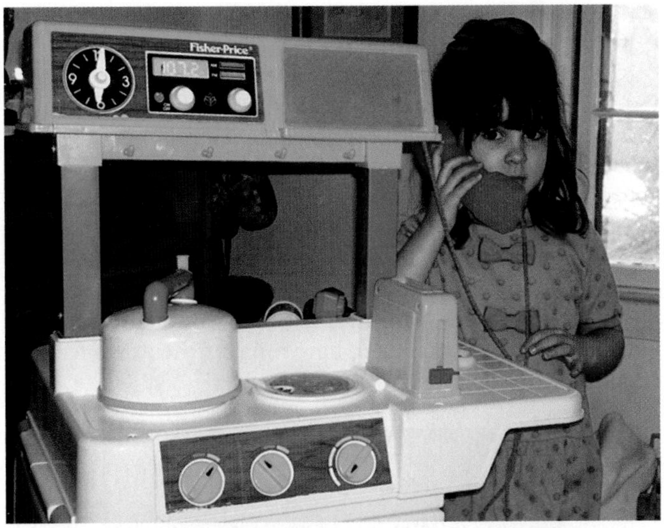

Fig. 38-5 Imaginative and imitative play is typical of preschoolers.

Television and movies also have their place in children's play, although each should be only one part of children's total repertoire of social and recreational activities (see Chapter 33). Parents and other caregivers should supervise the selection of programs, watch and discuss programs with their children, schedule limited time for television viewing, and set a good example of television viewing (Canadian Paediatric Society [CPS], Psychosocial Paediatrics Committee, 2003). Children also enjoy and learn from educational programs. Television viewing, however, may limit time spent in meaningful activities such as reading, story-telling, physical activity, and socialization (CPS, Healthy Active Living and Sports Medicine Committee, 2012).

Television can become an interactive activity when adults view programs with children and discuss program content. In one study, viewing educational programs as preschoolers was associated with higher grades, more book reading, greater emphasis on achievement, increased creativity, and less aggression in adolescent years (Anderson et al., 2001). Researchers emphasize that the content of television viewing appeared more important than the amount viewed.

Play is so much a part of a young child's life that reality and fantasy become blurred. Make-believe is reality during play and only becomes fantasy when toys are put away or dress-up clothes are removed. It is no wonder that imaginary playmates are so much a part of this age period. The appearance of imaginary companions usually occurs between ages 2½ and 3 years, and, for the most part, such playmates are relinquished when the child enters school. Birth order and number of siblings may influence the creation of imaginary companions, with firstborn and only children being more likely to create imaginary playmates (Gleason, Sebanc, & Hartup, 2000).

Imaginary companions serve many purposes: they become friends in times of loneliness, they accomplish what the child is still attempting, and they experience what the child wants to forget or remember. This becomes a way of assuming control and authority in a safe situation. Parents often worry about imaginary playmates, not realizing how normal and useful they are. Parents need to be reassured that the child's fantasy is a sign of health that helps differentiate make-believe and reality. Parents can acknowledge an imaginary companion's presence by calling him or her by name and even agreeing to simple requests such as setting an extra place at the table, but they should not allow the child to use the "playmate" to avoid punishment or responsibility.

Children also benefit from play that occurs between them and a parent. *Mutual play* fosters development from birth through the school years and provides enriched opportunities for learning. Through mutual play, parents can provide tactile and kinesthetic experiences, can maximize verbal and language abilities, and can offer praise and encouragement for exploration of the world. In addition, mutual play encourages positive interactions between parent and child, strengthening their relationship.

Coping With Concerns Related to Normal Growth and Development

Preschool and Kindergarten Experience

While some children are home schooled, many children attend some type of early childhood program, usually preschool or a day care centre. Group care has become commonplace with large number of parents being employed outside home (see Chapter 36, Alternative Child Care Arrangements). Researchers have identified that at least 70% of Canadian children, aged 6 months to 6 years, are in nonparental care (Cleveland, Forer, Hyatt, Japel, & Krashinsky, 2008). Effects of early education and stimulation on children have increasingly gained recognition. (For a discussion of the effects of day care on young children, see Chapter 31, Working Mothers.) Because social development widens to include agemates and other significant adults, preschool provides an excellent vehicle for expanding children's experiences with others. It is also excellent preparation for entrance into elementary school.

In preschool or day care centres, children are exposed to opportunities for learning group cooperation; adjusting to sociocultural differences; and coping with frustration, dissatisfaction, and anger. If activities are tailored to provide mastery and achievement, children increasingly have feelings of success, self-confidence, and personal competence. Whether structured learning is imposed is less important than the social climate, type of guidance, and attitude toward children that is fostered by the teacher or leader. With a teacher who is aware of preschoolers' developmental abilities and needs, children will learn from the activity that is provided. Most programs incorporate a daily schedule of quiet play, active outdoor activity, group activities such as games and projects, creative or free play, and snack and rest periods. Preschool is particularly beneficial for children who lack a peer-group experience, such as only children, and for children from impoverished homes.

One issue that all parents face is their child's readiness for preschool or kindergarten. While there are no absolute indicators for school readiness, the child's social maturity, especially the attention span, is as important as his or her academic readiness. Use of a developmental screening tool such as the Nipissing District Developmental Screen (NDDS) that addresses cognitive (especially language), social, and physical milestones can help identify children who may benefit from diagnostic testing and early intervention programs before they start school (see Chapter 34, p. 929). Also, parents play an integral role in their children's school readiness. They should promote a positive attitude toward learning, read to their children, encourage their children to participate in a variety of activities to explore their talents, and choose appropriate child care or preschool programs (Jellinek, Patel, & Froehle, 2002).

Nurses and other health care workers can guide parents in selecting enriched social and educational early-intervention programs, schools, and child care centres. Careful selection of early-childhood education is an important decision regarding a child's future learning and development. Research indicates multiple influences on school readiness, including family income and the availability of quality child care and early childhood education. To assist with school readiness and child development, innovative programs such as the Human Early Learning Partnership (HELP) have been initiated, which researches the many factors related to child development and makes related program and policy recommendations (see Additional Resources at the end of this chapter).

Licensed and regulated early-childhood programs are mandated to abide by established standards representing minimum requirements and safeguards. Day care centres are regulated in Canada by individual provinces and territories. Such regulation is important to protect children from harm and to promote conditions that are essential for a child's healthy development and learning.

Currently, Canada lacks universal coverage for comprehensive early-childhood development and needs to invest further in this area. Such investment would decrease the need for expensive pediatric remedial programs, and children would stay in school longer, be more employable, and likely have higher incomes as adults (CPS, 2009).

An Aboriginal Head Start preschool program for First Nations, Métis, and Inuit families has demonstrated that locally controlled early-intervention strategies improve the health of these children and help them to grow up healthy and reach their optimum potential. Such strategies include support for physical, personal, and social development (Public Health Agency of Canada [PHAC], 2011a).

When parents are considering an early-childhood development program, areas to evaluate include the facility's daily program, teacher qualifications, staff-to-student ratio, discipline policy, environmental safety precautions, provision of meals, sanitary conditions, whether there is adequate indoor and outdoor space per child, and fee schedule. While references from other parents can help in evaluating a program, personal observation of the facility is recommended. Parents should be encouraged to meet the director and some of the employees at a few facilities so that they can make an informed choice.

Evaluation of a facility's health practices is also important. Children in day care centres have more illnesses than children not in day care centres, especially gastrointestinal tract infections; respiratory tract infections; and hepatitis A, varicella-zoster virus, and cytomegalovirus infections (BC Centre for Disease Control, 2009). Nurses can play an important role here in infection control: They can not only advise parents regarding the evaluation of a facility's sanitary practices but also take an active part in educating staff in measures to minimize transmission of infection (Fig. 38-6).

Children need preparation for the preschool or kindergarten experience. For young children, it represents a change from their usual home environment and a prolonged separation from parents. Before children begin school, parents should present the idea as exciting and pleasurable. Talking to children about activities such as painting, building with blocks, or enjoying swings and outdoor equipment allows children to fantasize about the event in a positive manner. When the first day of school arrives, parents should behave confidently. Such behaviour requires parents to have resolved their own feelings regarding the experience.

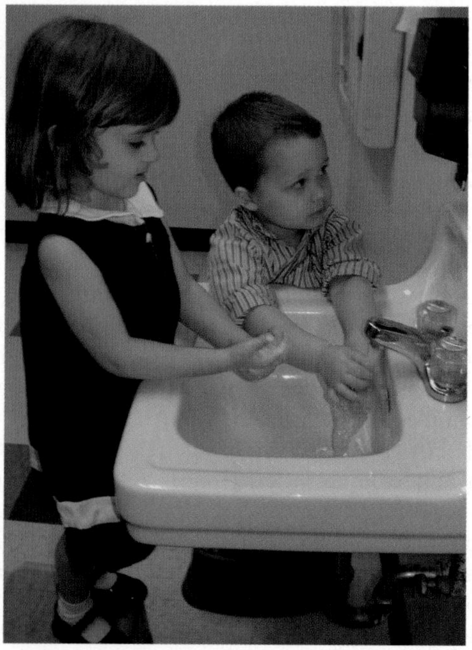

Fig. 38-6 Thorough hand washing is the single most effective method of preventing infection.

Parents should introduce their child to the teacher and the facility. In some instances, it is helpful for parents to remain with the child for at least part of the first day until the child is comfortable and at ease. Other specific actions that can help reduce separation anxiety include providing the school with detailed information about the child's home environment, such as familiar routines, favourite activities, food preferences, names of siblings or pets, and personal habits. Such information helps the teacher to make the child feel familiar in the strange surroundings. When schools automatically request this information, the parent has a valuable clue to the quality of the program—the request represents the staff's awareness of each child's needs. Transitional objects, such as a favourite toy, may also help the child bridge the gap from home to school.

Sex Education

Preschoolers have assimilated a tremendous amount of information during their short lifetimes. Although their thinking may not be mature, they search constantly for explanations and reasons that are logical and reasonable to them. The word "why" seems to supplant the word "no," which was common in toddlerhood. It is only natural that as they learn about "me" they will also want to know "why me" and "how me." Questions such as "Where do babies come from?" are as casual as "What makes it rain?" or "Who is that?" It is the way in which questions about procreation are answered that conditions children, even the youngest, to separate these questions from others about their world.

Two rules govern answering sensitive questions about topics such as sex. The first is to *find out what children know and think.* By investigating the theories that children have produced as a reasonable explanation, parents can give correct information and help children understand why their explanation is inaccurate.

The second rule for giving information is to *be honest.* It is true that the preschooler will forget or misunderstand much of the correct information, but the correct information can be restated until the child absorbs and comprehends the facts. Even though correct anatomical words may be hard to pronounce or even more difficult to remember, they become the foundational content for explaining other concepts later on.

Regardless of whether children are given sex education, they will engage in games of sexual curiosity and exploration. At about 3 years of age, children are aware of anatomical differences between sexes and are concerned with how the other "works." This is not really "sexual" curiosity because many children are still unaware of the reproductive function of genitalia. Their curiosity is for the eliminative function of anatomy. Little boys wonder how girls can urinate without a penis, so they watch girls go to bathroom. Because they cannot see anything but the stream of urine coming out, they want to observe further.

One question that parents often have is how to handle such sexual curiosity. A positive approach is to neither condone nor condemn it but to express that if children have questions, they should ask the parents. Parents should also encourage their child to engage in some other activity. In this way, children can be helped to understand that there are ways to satisfy their sexual curiosity other than through investigative games. This in no way condemns the act but stresses alternate methods to seek solutions and answers. Allowing children unrestricted permissiveness only intensifies their anxiety and concern, since exploring and searching usually yield little evidence to satisfy their curiosity.

There are many variable cultural influences on sex education. Some cultures encourage open discussion and other cultures are more reticent. For example, Aboriginal peoples have generally an open view of sexuality, sexual practices, and sexual orientation. Sex is seen as a way to express an individual's spiritual, emotional, physical, and mental being. (Aboriginal Nurses Association & Planned Parenthood Federation of Canada, 2002). Many excellent books on sex education are available for preschool children at public libraries. The Canadian Federation of Sexual Health's Web site contains information on how to talk about sex with various age groups (see Additional Resources). Parents should read the book themselves *before* giving or reading it to a child.

Another concern for some parents is *masturbation*, or self-stimulation of the genitalia. This occurs at any age for a variety of reasons and, if not excessive, is normal and healthy. It is most common at 4 years of age and during adolescence. For preschoolers, it is a part of sexual curiosity and exploration. If parents are concerned about their children masturbating, it is essential for nurses to investigate circumstances associated with the activity because it may be an expression of anxiety, boredom, or unresolved conflicts. Children who openly and publicly masturbate are inviting a reaction, such as **discipline**, punishment, or criticism. They may be overwhelmed by their sexual feelings and are asking others to help channel them into more constructive outlets. Masturbation, like other forms of sex play, is a private act, and parents should emphasize this to children when teaching them socially acceptable behaviour.

Fears

During the preschool years, a great number and variety of real and imagined fears are present, including fear of the dark, being left alone (especially at bedtime), animals (particularly large dogs), ghosts, sexual matters (castration), and objects or persons associated with pain. The exact cause of children's fears is often unknown. Parents often become perplexed about handling the fears because no amount of logical persuasion, coercion, or ridicule will send away the ghosts, boogeymen, monsters, and devils. Inappropriate television viewing by preschoolers may increase fears and anxieties because of inability to separate reality-based experiences from fantasy portrayed on television.

The concept of *animism*, ascribing lifelike qualities to inanimate objects, helps explain why children fear objects. For example, a child may refuse to use the toilet after watching a television commercial in which the toilet bowel is portrayed as turning into a monster.

Preschoolers also experience fear of annihilation. Because of poorly defined body boundaries and improved cognitive abilities, young children develop concerns related to the loss of body parts. They fear losing body parts with certain medical procedures such as an intravenous insertion or cast application on a limb and may see these procedures as real threats to their existence.

The best way to help children overcome their fears is by actively involving them in finding practical methods to deal with the frightening experience. This may be as simple as keeping a night-light on in child's bedroom for assurance that no monsters lurk in the dark. Exposing children to the feared object in a safe situation also provides a type of conditioning, or *desensitization*. For instance, children who are afraid of dogs should never be forced to approach or touch one, but they may be gradually introduced to the experience by watching other children play with an animal. This type of modelling, with others demonstrating fearlessness, can be effective if the child is allowed to progress at his or her own rate.

Usually by 5 or 6 years of age, children relinquish many fears. Explaining the developmental sequence of fears and their gradual disappearance may help parents feel more secure in handling preschoolers' fears. Sometimes fears do not subside with simple measures or developmental maturation. When children experience severe fears that disrupt family life, professional help is required.

Stress

Although for parents preschool years generally are less troublesome than toddlerhood, this period of life presents children with many unique stresses. Some, such as fears, are innate and stem from preschoolers' unique understanding of the world. Others, such as beginning school, are imposed. Although minimal amounts of stress are beneficial during the early years to help children develop effective coping skills, excessive stress is harmful. Young children are especially vulnerable because of their limited capacity to cope. Expression of frustration, fear, or anxiety is hampered by inadequate expressive language.

To help parents deal with **stress** in their child's life, they must be aware of the signs of stress (see Chapter 33, Stress in Childhood) and be helped to identify the source. Any number of stressors may be present, such as the birth of a sibling, marital discord, divorce and separation, relocation, or illness.

The best approach to dealing with stress is prevention—monitoring the amount of stress in children's lives so that levels do not exceed their coping ability. In many instances, structuring children's schedules to allow rest and preparing them for change, such as entering school, are sufficient measures.

Aggression

The term *aggression* refers to behaviour that attempts to hurt a person or destroy property. Aggression differs from anger, which is a temporary emotional state, but anger may be expressed through aggression. Hyperaggressive behaviour in preschoolers is characterized by unprovoked physical attacks on other children and adults, destruction of others' property, frequent intense temper tantrums, extreme impulsivity, disrespect, and noncompliance. Aggression is influenced by a complex set of biological, sociocultural, and familial variables. Factors that tend to increase aggressive behaviour are gender, frustration, modelling of such behaviour, and reinforcement. Some of the family factors identified as promoting development of aggressive behaviours include low income, low education level, high family stress, lone parenthood, marital discord, maternal depression, and parental drug use (Connors, 2004).

Evidence indicates that boys tend to be more aggressive than girls (Bendersky, Bennett, & Lewis, 2006). *Frustration*, or continual thwarting of self-satisfaction by disapproval, humiliation, punishment, or insults, can lead children to act out against others as a means of release. Especially if they fear their parents, these children will displace their anger on others, particularly peers and other authority figures. This type of aggression often applies to the child who is well behaved at home but is a discipline problem at school or a bully among playmates.

Modelling, or imitating the behaviour of significant others, is a powerful influencing force in preschoolers. Children who see their parents as physically abusive are observing behaviour that they come to know as acceptable, and they may exhibit this behaviour with others (Gershoff, 2002). Another aspect of modelling is the "double standard" for acceptable conduct. For example, in some families, aggression is synonymous with masculinity, and boys are encouraged to defend themselves. Television is also a significant source for modelling at this age. Numerous studies have found a positive correlation between viewing of violent programs and development of aggression. Parents need encouragement to supervise the programs viewed by their preschool children, especially those with aggressive tendencies (Brown & Hamilton-Giachritsis, 2005). *Reinforcement* can also shape aggressive behaviour. Sometimes reward for aggression is negative (e.g., punishment) yet reinforcing because it brings attention. When children exhibit extreme behaviours, such as aggression, parents may be concerned about the need for professional help. Generally, the difference between "normal" and "problematic" behaviour is not behaviour itself but its *quantity* (number of occurrences), *severity* (interference with social or cognitive functioning), *distribution* (different manifestations), *onset* (when behaviour started), and *duration* (at least 4 weeks).

Speech Problems

The most critical period for speech development occurs between 2 and 4 years of age. During this period, children are using their rapidly growing vocabulary faster than they can produce the words. Failure to master sensorimotor integrations results in stuttering or stammering as children try to say the word they are already thinking about. This **dysfluency** in speech pattern is a normal characteristic of language development in children ages 2 to 5 years, affects boys more frequently than girls, and usually resolves during childhood. (Canadian Association of Speech-Language Pathologists and Audiologists, 2012). When parents or other significant persons place undue emphasis on a child's dysfluency, an abnormal speech pattern may develop. The Canadian Association of Speech-Language Pathologists and Audiologists (2012) encourages parents and caregivers of children who stutter to speak slowly, refrain from correcting or criticizing the child's speech, resist the temptation to complete the child's sentences, provide the opportunity for the child to speak frequently, and take time to listen attentively.

The best therapy for speech problems is prevention and early detection. Many provinces and territories have newborn hearing screening, which enables early identification of children with hearing problems; treatment can then begin at birth. Common causes of speech problems are hearing loss, developmental delay, autism, and lack of verbal or psychosocial stimulation (Feldman, 2005). Referral for further evaluation and treatment may be necessary to prevent a problem from interfering with learning. Anticipatory preparation of parents for expected developmental norms may allay caregiver concerns.

Children pressured into producing sounds ahead of their developmental level may develop *dyslalia* (articulation problems) or revert to using infantile speech. Prevention involves educating parents about the usual achievement of speech production during childhood. The Nipissing District Developmental Screen (2011) is an excellent tool for assessing articulation skills in the child and for explaining to parents the expected progression of sounds (see Evolve site and Additional Resources).

Promoting Optimum Health During Preschool Years

Nutrition

Nutritional requirements for preschoolers are fairly similar to those for toddlers (Story, Holt, & Sofka, 2002). The required number of calories per unit of body weight continues to decrease slightly. *Eating Well With Canada's Food Guide* indicates that the active 2- to 3-year-old boy will need 1500 calories and girls of the same age will need 1400 calories. The active male 4- to 5-year-old will need 1650 calories and the active girl of the same age will need 1500 calories (Health Canada, 2007). Fluid requirements may also decrease slightly to approximately 100 mL/kg/day but depend on the activity level, climatic conditions, and state of health. Protein requirements increase with age; the recommended intake for preschoolers is 13 to 19 g/day (Food and Nutrition Board, 2003).

Evidence is increasing that the incidence of coronary heart disease, obesity, and chronic health problems such as diabetes mellitus can be influenced by early eating patterns (Barlow & Expert Committee, 2007). Research supports the efficacy of limiting fat intake, and negative health effects from reducing fat have not been reported (Johnson, 2000). Preschoolers may have decreased fat intake with substitutes such as soy-enriched foods without affecting overall food taste, energy, and nutrient value (Endres et al., 2003). Parents and others who provide soy substitutes should ensure that the products are vitamin enriched and low in fat content (Endres et al., 2003). *Eating Well With Canada's Food Guide*, from Health Canada (2007), supports reducing the amount of saturated fats in children's diets in order to decrease risks of future coronary artery disease. The *Food Guide* recommends that a variety of nutritious foods be offered to children, including some choices that contain fat, such as 2% milk, peanut butter, and avocado, to meet children's nutrient requirements. But children should only have an average saturated fat content of 8 to 9% total energy (Health Canada, 2007). A Health Canada (2004) survey on nutrient intakes of Canadian children aged 1 to 8 years indicated that 47% of 1- to 3-year-olds' diets had total fat intakes below the recommended acceptable macronutrient distribution range (AMDR) levels, in contrast to 4- to 8-year-olds, who had a total fat intake of 88% within the AMDR range.

It is important that all diets contain adequate nutrients such as calcium. The recommendation for daily calcium intake for children 1 to 3 years of age is 700 mg, and the recommendation for children 4 to 8 years of age is 1000 mg (Health Canada, 2010). Milk and dairy products are excellent sources of calcium and vitamin D (fortified). Low-fat milk may be substituted so that the quantity of milk may remain the same while limiting fat intake overall. *Canada's Food Guide* recommends 500 mL of milk daily to meet young children's need for vitamin D (Health Canada, 2007).

Excessive consumption of fruit juices has been associated with adverse health effects such as dental **caries** and gastrointestinal symptoms; *Canada's Food Guide* recommends giving children ages 2 to 4 years four servings of fruit or vegetables and to offer whole fruit instead of fruit juices. Children who are 4 to 8 years of age should have five servings (Health Canada, 2007). Parents should be educated regarding consumption of non-nutritious fruit drinks, which often precludes an adequate intake of milk by the child. While counselling parents about moderation in fruit juice consumption and substituting whole fruit for juice, health care providers should also offer suggestions of more appropriate sources of nutrients such as ascorbic acid, folate, and potassium. Young children's intake of high sugar content or acidic carbonated beverages contributes to the development of dental caries, and consumption of large amounts of non-nutritive calories may displace or preclude intake of nutrients necessary for growth.

In sum, the Health Canada (2004) survey cited earlier indicated that the diets of 1- to 8-year-old Canadian children provided most of their vitamin and mineral needs. Their diets contained acceptable proportions of energy from protein and carbohydrate but lower than recommended levels of potassium and fibre intake.

NURSING ALERT Over the past several decades the level of obesity has increased in young children. Efforts to provide a healthy diet and to encourage physical activity should begin early to help children achieve optimum health (Johnson, 2000; Spear et al., 2007). A Health Canada survey (2004) identified that one in five children had energy intakes that exceeded their energy expenditure. Childhood obesity is an important predictor of adult obesity, so preventing overweight and obesity in childhood is essential (Health Canada, 2010).

The Public Health Agency of Canada has developed a healthy program that is a combination of *Eating Well With Canada's Food Guide* and a physical activity guide. This program has specific guidelines for children and can be found at http://www.phac-aspc.gc.ca/hp-ps/hl-mvs/pa-ap/index-eng.php.

Some preschoolers still have food habits that are typical of toddlers, such as food fads and strong taste preferences. When children reach 4 years of age, they seem to enter another period of finicky eating, which is generally characteristic of the more rebellious behaviour of children in this age group. As with the toddler, small portions should be offered of each item being served. The practice of having the child remain at the table until the "plate is clean" should be avoided because this may contribute to overeating and the development of poor eating habits that contribute to poor health later in life. By age 5 years, children are more agreeable to trying new foods, especially if they are encouraged by an adult who allows them to help with food preparation or experiment with a new taste or different dish (Fig. 38-7). Mealtimes can become battlegrounds if parents expect perfect table manners. Usually the 5-year-old child is ready for the "social" side of eating, but the 3- or 4-year-old child still has difficulty sitting quietly through a long family meal.

The amount and variety of foods consumed by young children vary greatly from day to day. Consequently, parents sometimes worry about the quantity and quality of food that preschoolers consume. Preschoolers can self-regulate their energy intake needs. In general, quality is much more important than quantity, a fact that should be stressed during nutritional counselling.

One way to lessen parental concern about their child's diet is advising parents to keep a weekly record of everything the child eats. In particular, the parents can measure the amount of food, such as setting aside 120 mL of vegetables and serving the child from this premeasured amount, to provide a more accurate estimate of food intake at each meal. When parents look at the food chart at the end of the week, they are usually amazed by how much the child has consumed. In general, preschoolers consume only slightly more than toddlers, or about half an adult's portion.

Sleep and Activity

Sleep patterns vary widely, but the average preschooler sleeps about 12 hours a night and infrequently takes daytime naps. Waking during the night is common throughout early childhood and may be related to social rather than developmental factors (Thiedke, 2001). Motor activity levels continue to be high and allow preschoolers to explore their environment, begin learning physical games and sports, and interact with others. Sedentary activities, such as television and video or computer games, are increasingly appealing and can become an unhealthy substitute for active play.

Preschoolers' increased gross motor abilities and coordination allow them to engage in many physical activities, if only at a novice level. Whether young children should begin formalized training in an activity at this early age is controversial. Training programs must consider the child's physical and psychological immaturity, and readiness to participate in organized sports should be determined individually. The decision to participate should be based on the child's, not the parent's, motivation and enjoyment. The preschooler learns best with egocentric activities and with auditory and visual cues. Activities that should be focused on include running, throwing, catching, and tumbling. Activities need to be fun, encourage exploration and experimentation, and avoid competition (CPS, 2005b).

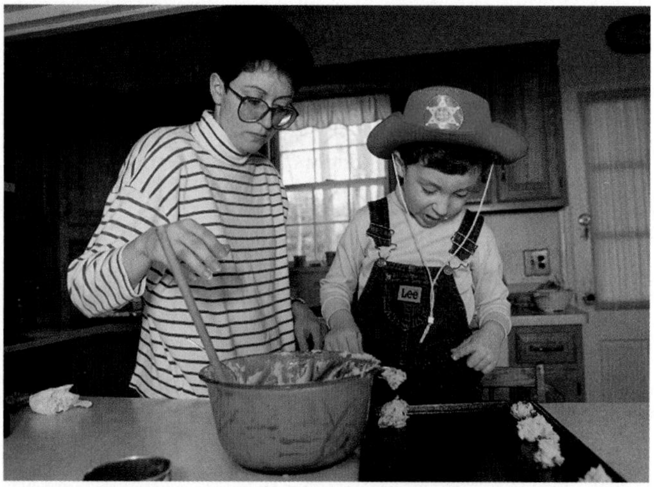

Fig. 38-7 Preschool-age children enjoy helping adults and are more likely to try new foods if they can assist in the preparation.

Sleep Problems

Preschool years are a prime time for sleep disturbances. As toddlers and preschoolers cope with autonomy, separation, and object permanence, they begin to have more sleep problems (Thiedke, 2001). Some have trouble going to sleep, especially after so much activity and stimulation during the day. Others may develop bedtime fears, wake during the night, or have nightmares or sleep terrors. Still others may delay the inevitable through elaborate rituals.

Recommendations for handling a sleep disturbance should be offered only *after* a thorough assessment of the problem. Cultural traditions may dictate sleep practices that are contrary to certain well-accepted professional recommendations; therefore, parents may not perceive a particular sleep practice as a problem (see Cultural Awareness box in Chapter 36, p. 1009). For instance, it is important to explain to parents why infants need to be placed on their back for sleeping and that infants should not share a bed with another person, to potentially prevent the occurrence of sudden infant death syndrome (SIDS). (See Chapter 36 for further information on infant sleeping position.) In the preschooler age group, however, bed sharing is acceptable. See Additional Resources at the end of this chapter for further information on cultural influences on sleep.

Interventions vary greatly; for example, *nightmares* (frightening dreams that are followed by full arousal) and *sleep terrors* (partial arousal from deep, nondreaming sleep) require different approaches. For children who delay going to bed, a recommended approach involves counselling parents about the importance of a consistent bedtime ritual and emphasizing the normalcy of this type of behaviour in young children. Parents should ignore attention-seeking behaviour and not take children into the parents' bed or allow children to stay up past a reasonable hour. Other measures that may be helpful include keeping a light on in the room, providing transitional objects such as a favourite toy, or leaving a drink of water by the bed. Helping children slow down *before* bedtime also reduces the resistance to going to bed. One strategy is to establish limited rituals that signal readiness for bed, such as a bath or story.

Dental Health

By the beginning of the preschool period, the eruption of the deciduous (primary) teeth is complete. Dental care is essential to preserve these temporary teeth and to teach good dental habits (see Chapter 37). Although preschoolers' fine motor control is improved, they still require assistance and supervision with brushing, and parents should floss the teeth. Professional care and prophylaxis, especially fluoride supplements (if needed), should be continued. Routine dental care should be well established during preschool years and is recommended at 6- to 12-month intervals depending on the family history, the child's dental development, and the presence or absence of dental caries (Martof, 2001). For children cared for away from home, parents should be encouraged to monitor the dental care provided by others, including minimizing cariogenic foods.

Trauma to teeth during this period is not uncommon, and prompt evaluation by a dentist is warranted if oral trauma occurs. Preservation of the space previously occupied by an avulsed tooth is necessary for proper eruption of the secondary tooth.

Injury Prevention

Because of improved gross and fine motor skills, coordination, and balance, preschoolers are less prone to falls than toddlers. They tend to be less reckless; listen more to parental rules; and are aware of potential dangers, such as hot objects, sharp instruments, and dangerous heights. Putting objects in the mouth as part of exploration has all but ceased, although accidental poisoning is still a danger. The number of pedestrian motor vehicle injuries among preschoolers tends to increase because they spend a lot of time playing in the parking lot, driveway, or street and riding tricycles, bicycles, and other play vehicles. Preschoolers also run after balls in the street and may forget safety regulations when crossing streets. (See Chapter 37 for more information on childhood injuries and injury prevention.)

In general, the guidelines suggested for injury prevention in Table 37-3 apply to children in this age group as well. However, emphasis is now on *education* concerning safety and potential hazards, in addition to appropriate protection. This is an excellent time to start enforcing the use of safety items such as bicycle helmets to prevent head trauma; children are less likely to warm to the idea later in life because of peer pressure. Because preschoolers are great imitators, it is essential that parents set a good example by "practising what they preach." Children quickly observe discrepancies in what they are told to do and what they see others do. Establishing habits at this time, such as wearing protective equipment, can create long-term safety behaviours.

Anticipatory Guidance—Care of Families

The preschool years present fewer childrearing difficulties than do earlier years. This stage of development is facilitated by appropriate anticipatory guidance in the areas discussed in previous sections (see Family-Centred Teaching box). There is a shift in childrearing practices from protection to education. Whereas injury prevention previously focused on safeguarding the immediate environment, with less emphasis on reasoning, now the protective guardrails or electrical outlet caps may be replaced by verbal explanations of why danger exists and how to avoid it.

During this period, an emotional transition between parent and child occurs. Although children are still attached to their parents and accept all their values and beliefs, they are nearing the period of life when they will question previous teachings and prefer the companionship of peers. Entry into school marks a separation for parents and for children. Parents may need help in adjusting to this change, particularly if one parent has focused his or her daily activities primarily on home responsibilities. All family members must adjust to changes, which is part of the process of growth and development.

FAMILY-CENTRED TEACHING

Guidance During Preschool Years

Age 3 Years

- Prepare parents for child's increasing interest in widening relationships.
- Encourage enrolment in preschool.
- Emphasize the importance of setting limits.
- Prepare parents to expect exaggerated tension-reduction behaviours, such as the need for a "security blanket."
- Encourage parents to offer the child choices.
- Prepare parents to expect marked changes at 3½ years, when the child becomes insecure and exhibits emotional extremes.
- Prepare parents for normal dysfluency in speech and advise them to avoid focusing on the pattern.
- Prepare parents to expect extra demands on their attention as a reflection of the child's emotional insecurity and fear of loss of love.
- Warn parents that the equilibrium of a 3-year-old will change to the aggressive, out-of-bounds behaviour of a 4-year-old.
- Inform parents to anticipate a more stable appetite with more food selections.
- Stress need for protection and education of the child to prevent injury (see Injury Prevention, Chapter 37).

Age 4 Years

- Prepare parents for more aggressive behaviour, including motor activity and offensive language.
- Prepare parents to expect resistance to parental authority.
- Explore parental feelings regarding the child's behaviour.
- Suggest some type of respite for primary caregivers, such as placing the child in preschool for part of the day.
- Prepare parents for the child's increasing sexual curiosity.
- Emphasize the importance of realistic limit setting on behaviour and appropriate disciplinary techniques.
- Prepare parents for the highly imaginative 4-year-old who indulges in "tall tales" (to be differentiated from lies) and develops imaginary playmates.
- Prepare parents to expect nightmares or an increase in them.
- Provide reassurance that a period of calmness begins at about 5 years of age.

Age 5 Years

- Inform parents to expect a tranquil period at around 5 years of age.
- Help parents prepare children for entrance into school environment.
- Make certain that immunizations are up to date before the child enters school.
- Suggest that unemployed parental caregivers consider their own activities when children begin school.
- Suggest swimming lessons for the child.

Infectious Disorders

Communicable Diseases

The incidence of childhood communicable diseases has declined significantly since the advent of immunizations. Serious complications resulting from such infections have been further reduced with the use of antibiotics and antitoxins. However, infectious diseases do occur, and nurses must be familiar with the particular infectious agent to recognize the disease and to institute appropriate preventive and supportive interventions (Table 38-2).

Nursing Care Management

The more common communicable diseases of childhood, their therapeutic management, and specific nursing care are described in Table 38-2. Following is a general discussion of nursing care management for communicable diseases. Identification of the infectious agent is of primary importance to prevent exposure to susceptible individuals. Nurses in ambulatory care settings, child care centres, and schools are often the first persons to see signs of a communicable disease, such as a rash or sore throat. The nurse must operate under a high index of suspicion for common childhood diseases to identify potentially infectious cases and to recognize diseases that require medical intervention. An example is the common symptom of sore throat. Although most often a symptom of a minor viral infection, it can signal diphtheria or a streptococcal infection, such as scarlet fever. Each of these bacterial conditions requires appropriate medical treatment to prevent serious sequelae.

evolve Critical Thinking Exercise–Conjunctivitis

When a communicable disease is suspected, it is important to assess (1) recent exposure to a known case; (2) **prodromal** symptoms (symptoms that occur between early manifestations of the disease and its overt clinical syndrome) or evidence of constitutional symptoms, such as a fever or rash (see Table 38-2); (3) immunization history; and (4) history of having the disease. Immunizations are available for many diseases, and infection usually confers lifelong immunity; therefore, the possibility of many infectious agents can be eliminated on the basis of these two criteria.

Prevent Spread

Prevention consists of two components: prevention of the disease and control of its spread to others. Primary prevention rests almost exclusively on immunization (see Fig. 34-6 for a complete immunization schedule). (The nurse's role in immunization of children is discussed in Chapter 36.)

Control measures to prevent the spread of disease should include techniques to reduce the risk of cross-transmission of infectious organisms between patients and to protect health care workers from organisms harboured by patients. If the child is hospitalized, the facility's policies for infection control should be followed (see Chapter 45). The most important procedure is hand hygiene. Persons directly caring for the child or handling contaminated articles must wash their hands and practise effective standard precautions between care of their patients.

The child should be instructed to practise good handwashing technique after toileting and before eating. For those diseases spread by droplets, the nurse should instruct parents in measures to reduce airborne transmission. The child who is old enough can be taught to cough or sneeze into a sleeve or into a tissue; otherwise, the parent should cover the child's mouth with a tissue and discard it. Usual hygiene measures of not sharing eating and drinking utensils need to be stressed to the family.

NURSING ALERT If a child is admitted to the hospital with an undiagnosed exanthema, strict Tier 2 precautions (contact, airborne, and droplet) and standard precautions are instituted until a diagnosis is confirmed. Childhood communicable diseases requiring these precautions include diphtheria, chickenpox, measles, tuberculosis, adenovirus, *Haemophilus influenzae* type b, influenza, mumps, *Mycoplasma pneumoniae*, pertussis, plague, streptococcal pharyngitis, pneumonia, and scarlet fever (PHAC, 2011b).

Prevent Complications

Although most children recover without difficulty, certain groups are at risk for serious, even fatal, complications from communicable diseases, especially the viral diseases chickenpox and *erythema infectiosum* (EI, fifth disease) caused by human parvovirus B19. Whereas most healthy children are less likely to become infected from either of these viruses, children with immunodeficiency—those receiving steroid or other immunosuppressive therapy, those with a generalized malignancy such as leukemia or lymphoma, or those with an immunological disorder—are at risk for viremia from replication of the varicella-zoster virus (VZV) in the blood. VZV is so named because it causes two distinct diseases: varicella (chickenpox) and zoster (herpes zoster, or shingles). Varicella occurs primarily in children younger than 15 years of age. It leaves the threat of herpes zoster, an intensely painful varicella that is localized to a single dermatome (body area innervated by a particular segment of the spinal cord). In children, the dermatomes most likely affected by herpes zoster are the cervical and sacral dermatomes (Leung, Robson, & Leong, 2006). Immunocompromised patients and healthy infants younger than 1 year of age (who also have reduced immunity) are at a higher risk for reactivation of VZV causing herpes zoster, probably as a result of a deficiency in cellular immunity (Chen et al., 2002). Complications of VZV in children include secondary bacterial infection, depigmentation, and scarring; postherpetic neuralgia in children is uncommon (Leung et al., 2006).

Children with hemolytic disease, such as sickle cell disease, are at risk for aplastic anemia from EI. Parvovirus infects and lyses red blood cell precursors, thus interrupting the production of red blood cells. Thus the virus may precipitate a severe aplastic crisis in patients who need increased red blood cell production to maintain normal red blood cell volumes; thrombocytopenia and neutropenia may also occur as a result of parvovirus B19 infection. The fetus has a relatively high rate of red blood cell production and an immature immune system; it may develop severe anemia and hydrops as a result of maternal HPV infection. Fetal death rates as a result of parvovirus B19 have been estimated to be between 2 and 6% (American Academy of Pediatrics [AAP], Committee on Infectious Diseases, & Pickering, 2009).

The past decade has seen an increase in the incidence of pertussis, particularly in infants less than 6 months old and children 10 to 14 years of age. Early clinical manifestations of pertussis in infants may include gagging, coughing, emesis, and apnea; the typical whooping cough associated with the disease is absent (Hospital for Sick Children, 2010). In older children, the disease may manifest as a common cold (see Table 38-2). It is now recommended that children ages 11 to 18 receive a booster pertussis vaccine (Tdap—tetanus, diphtheria, pertussis) to prevent the disease (see Chapter 36, Immunizations). Because pertussis is very contagious, especially among close household members, pertussis should be identified early and treatment initiated for the child and those who have been exposed. Azithromycin (for infants under 1 month) and erythromycin are administered to infants and children with pertussis (AAP, Committee on Infectious Diseases, & Pickering, 2009).

Prevention of complications from diseases such as diphtheria, pertussis, and scarlet fever requires adherence to antibiotic therapy. With oral preparations, the need to complete the entire course of therapy needs to be stressed (see Chapter 45, Compliance). The use of varicella-zoster immune globulin (VariZIG) or immune globulin intravenous (IGIV) is recommended for children who are immunocompromised, who have no previous history of varicella, and who are likely to contract the disease and have complications as a result (CPS, 2005a). The antiviral agent acyclovir (Zovirax) may be used to treat varicella infections in susceptible immunocompromised persons; it is effective in decreasing the number of lesions; shortening the duration of fever; and decreasing itching, lethargy, and anorexia. The Canadian Paediatric Society (2005a) recommends that oral acyclovir be considered for immunocompromised children who cannot receive VariZIG.

There is evidence that vitamin A supplementation reduces both morbidity and mortality in individuals with measles and that all children with severe measles should be given vitamin A supplements. A single oral dose of 200,000 International Units (6000 mcg) for children at least 1 year old (or half that dose for children 6 to 12 months of age) is recommended. The higher dose may be associated with vomiting and headache for a few hours. The dose should be repeated the next day and only repeated for a third time at 4 weeks if the child has ophthalmological evidence of vitamin A deficiency (Yang, Mao, & Wan, 2005).

NURSING ALERT Although the risk of vitamin A toxicity from these doses (they are 100 to 200 times the recommended dietary allowance) is relatively low, nurses should instruct parents on safe storage of the medication. Ideally, vitamin A should be dispensed in the age-appropriate unit dose, to prevent excessive administration and possible toxicity.

Provide Comfort

Many communicable diseases cause skin manifestations that are bothersome to the child. The chief discomfort from most rashes is itching, and measures such as cool baths (usually without soap) and lotions (e.g., calamine) are helpful.

NURSING ALERT When lotions with active ingredients such as diphenhydramine in Caladryl are used, they should be applied sparingly, especially over open lesions, where excessive absorption can lead to drug toxicity. These lotions should be used with caution in children who are simultaneously receiving an oral antihistamine. Cooling the lotion in the refrigerator beforehand often makes it more soothing on the skin than using it at room temperature.

To avoid overheating, which increases itching, children should wear lightweight, loose, nonirritating clothing and keep out of the sun. If the child persists in scratching, the nails should be kept short and smooth; mittens and clothes with long sleeves or legs may be needed. For severe itching, antipruritic medication, such as diphenhydramine (Benadryl) or hydroxyzine (Atarax), may be required, especially when the child has trouble sleeping because of itching. Loratadine, cetirizine, and fexofenadine do not cause drowsiness and may be preferred for urticaria during the day.

An elevated temperature is common, and both **antipyretic** medicine (acetaminophen or ibuprofen) and environmental manipulation should be implemented (see Chapter 45, Controlling Elevated Temperatures). The acetaminophen is effective in lowering the fever but does not significantly reduce the symptoms of itching, anorexia, abdominal pain, fussiness, or vomiting.

A sore throat, another frequent symptom, is managed with lozenges, saline rinses (if the child is old enough to cooperate), and analgesics. Because most children are anorectic during an illness, bland foods and increased liquids are usually preferred. During the early stages of the disease, children voluntarily curtail their activity, and although bed rest is beneficial, it should not be imposed unless specifically indicated. During periods of irritability, quiet activity (e.g., reading, music, television, video games, puzzles, colouring) helps distract children from the discomfort.

Support Child and Family

Most communicable diseases are benign but may produce considerable concern and anxiety for parents. Often the occurrence of a disease such as chickenpox is the first time the child is acutely uncomfortable. Parents need assistance to cope with manifestations of the illness, such as intense itching.

The family and child need reassurance that recovery is generally rapid. However, visible signs of the dermatosis may be present for some time after the child is well enough to resume usual activities.

NURSING ALERT The occurrence of a communicable disease provides the opportunity to ask parents about the child's immunization status and reinforce the benefits of vaccines for children. The Canadian Paediatric Society (2011) notes the urgent need for a national harmonized immunization schedule for Canada. Although the Public Health Agency of Canada (2006) has a minimum immunization schedule, each province and territory has variable schedules, which can be confusing and put the public at risk.

Text continued on page 1072.

Table 38-2 Communicable Diseases of Childhood

DISEASE

Chickenpox (Varicella) (Fig. 38-8)

Agent—Varicella-zoster virus (VZV)
Source—Primary secretions of respiratory tract of infected persons; to a lesser degree, skin lesions (scabs not infectious)
Transmission—Direct contact, droplet (airborne) spread, and contaminated objects
Incubation period—2-3 wk, usually 14-16 days
Period of communicability—Probably 1 day before eruption of lesions (prodromal period) to 6 days after first crop of vesicles when crusts have formed

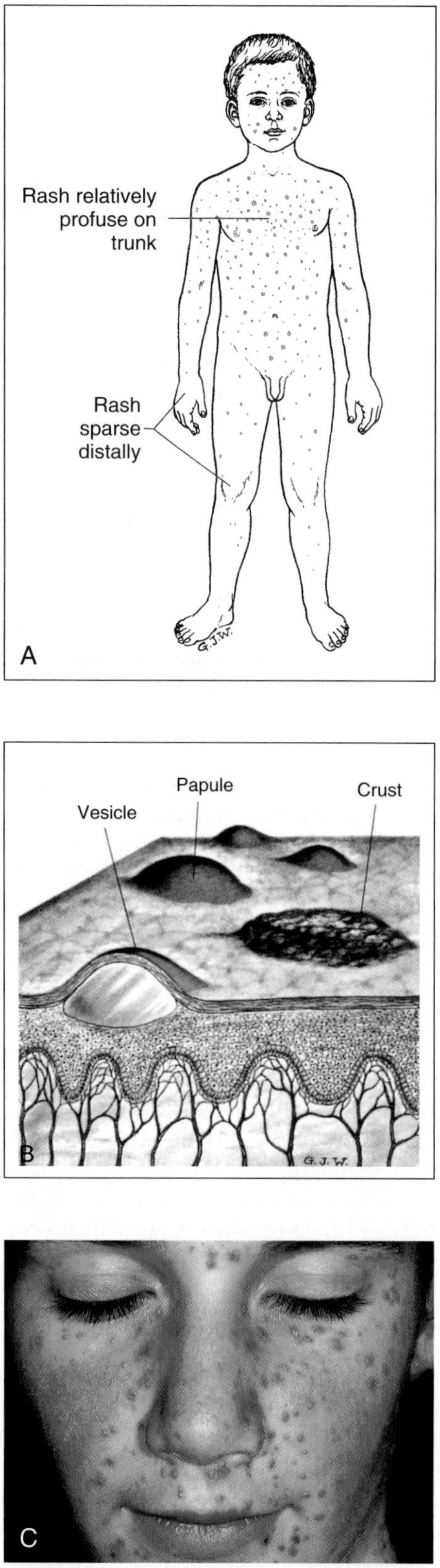

Fig. 38-8 Chickenpox (varicella). **A:** Progression of disease. **B:** Simultaneous stages of lesions. **C:** Clinical view. *(C, From Habif, T. P. [2004].* Clinical dermatology: A color guide to diagnosis and therapy *[4th ed., p. 390, Fig. 12-45]. St. Louis: Mosby.)*

Diphtheria

Agent—*Corynebacterium diphriae*
Source—Discharges from mucous membranes of nose and nasopharynx, skin, and other lesions of infected person
Transmission—Direct contact with infected person, a carrier, or contaminated articles
Incubation period—Usually 2-5 days, possibly longer
Period of communicability—Variable; until virulent bacilli are no longer present (identified by three negative cultures); usually 2 wk but as long as 4 wk

Eryma Infectiosum (Fifth Disease) (Fig. 38-9)

Agent—Human parvovirus B19
Source—Infected persons, mainly school-age children
Transmission—Respiratory secretions, blood, blood products
Incubation period—4-14 days; may be as long as 21 days
Period of communicability—Uncertain but before onset of symptoms in children with aplastic crisis

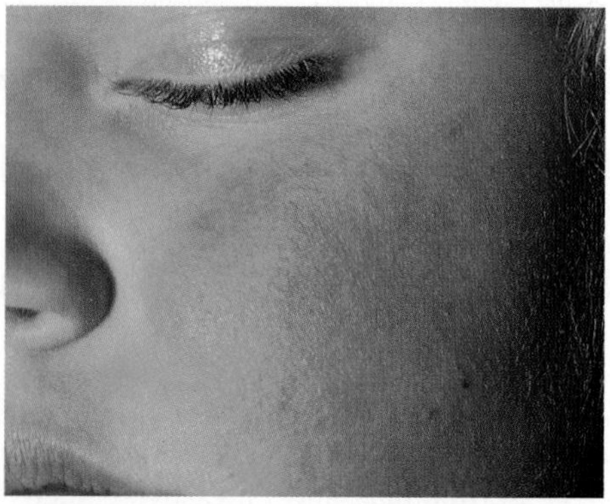

Fig. 38-9 Eryma infectiosum ("Slapped face" appearance). *(From Habif, T. P. [2004].* Clinical dermatology: A color guide to diagnosis and therapy *[4th ed., p. 469, Fig. 14-15]. St. Louis: Mosby.)*

CLINICAL MANIFESTATIONS	THERAPEUTIC MANAGEMENT AND COMPLICATIONS	NURSING CARE MANAGEMENT
Prodromal stage—Slight fever, malaise, and anorexia for first 24 hr; rash highly pruritic; begins as macule, rapidly progresses to papule and then vesicle (surrounded by erythematous base, becomes umbilicated and cloudy, breaks easily and forms crusts); all three stages (papule, vesicle, crust) present in varying degrees at one time **Distribution**—Centripetal, spreading to face and proximal extremities but sparse on distal limbs and less on areas not exposed to heat (i.e., from clothing or sun) **Constitutional signs and symptoms**—Elevated temperature from lymphadenopathy, irritability from pruritus	**Specific**—Antiviral agent acyclovir (Zovirax); varicella-zoster immune globulin (VariZIG) or immune globulin intravenous (IGIV) after exposure in high-risk children **Supportive**—Diphenhydramine hydrochloride or antihistamines to relieve itching; skin care to prevent secondary bacterial infection **Complications**—Secondary bacterial infections (abscesses, cellulitis, necrotizing fasciitis, pneumonia, sepsis) Encephalitis Varicella pneumonia (rare in normal children) Hemorrhagic varicella (tiny hemorrhages in vesicles and numerous petechiae in skin) Chronic or transient thrombocytopenia	Maintain standard, airborne, and contact precautions if hospitalized, until all lesions are crusted; for immunized child with mild breakthrough varicella, isolate until no new lesions are seen. Keep child in home away from susceptible individuals until vesicles have dried (usually 1 wk after onset of disease), and isolate high-risk children from infected children. Administer skin care; give bath and change clothes and linens daily; administer topical calamine lotion; keep child's fingernails short and clean; apply mittens if child scratches. Keep child cool (may decrease number of lesions). Lessen pruritus; keep child occupied. Remove loose crusts that rub and irritate skin. Teach child to apply pressure to pruritic area rather than scratching it. Avoid use of aspirin (possible association with Reye syndrome).
Vary according to anatomical location of pseudomembrane **Nasal**—Resembles common cold, serosanguineous mucopurulent nasal discharge without constitutional symptoms; may be frank epistaxis **Tonsillar/pharyngeal**—Malaise; anorexia; sore throat; low-grade fever; pulse increased above that expected for temperature within 24 hr; smooth, adherent, white or grey membrane; lymphadenitis possibly pronounced ("bull's neck"); in severe cases, toxemia, septic shock, and death within 6–10 days **Laryngeal**—Fever, hoarseness, cough, with or without previous signs listed; potential airway obstruction, apprehensive, dyspneic retractions, cyanosis	Equine antitoxin (usually intravenously); preceded by skin or conjunctival test to rule out sensitivity to horse serum Antibiotics (penicillin G procaine or erythromycin) in addition to equine antitoxin Complete bed rest (prevention of myocarditis) Tracheostomy for airway obstruction Treatment of infected contacts and carriers **Complications**—Toxic cardiomyopathy (second to third week) Toxic neuropathy	Follow standard and droplet precautions until two cultures are negative for *C. diphtheriae*; contact precautions with cutaneous manifestations. Administer antibiotics in timely manner. Participate in sensitivity testing; have epinephrine available. Administer complete care to maintain bed rest. Use suctioning as needed. Observe respiration for signs of obstruction. Administer humidified oxygen as prescribed.
Rash appearing in three stages: **I**—Eryma on face, chiefly on cheeks, "slapped face" appearance; disappears by 1–4 days (Fig. 38-9) **II**—About 1 day after rash appears on face, maculopapular red spots appear, symmetrically distributed on upper and lower extremities; rash progresses from proximal to distal surfaces and may last a week or more **III**—Rash is subsiding but reappears if skin is irritated or traumatized (sun, heat, cold, friction). In children with aplastic crisis, rash is usually absent and prodromal illness includes fever, myalgia, lethargy, nausea, vomiting, and abdominal pain. Child with sickle cell disease may have concurrent vaso-occlusive crisis.	**Symptomatic and supportive**—Antipyretics, analgesics, anti-inflammatory medications Possible blood transfusion for transient aplastic anemia **Complications**—Self-limited arthritis and arthralgia (arthritis may become chronic); more common in adult women May result in serious complications (anemia, hydrops) or fetal death if mother infected during pregnancy (primarily second trimester) Aplastic crisis in children with hemolytic disease or immunodeficiency Myocarditis (rare)	Isolation of child is not necessary, except hospitalized child (immunosuppressed or with aplastic crises) suspected of parvovirus infection is placed on respiratory isolation and standard precautions. Pregnant women need not be excluded from workplace where parvovirus infection is present; they should not care for patients with aplastic crises; explain low risk of fetal death to those in contact with affected children; assist with routine fetal ultrasound for detection of fetal hydrops.

Continued

Table 38-2 Communicable Diseases of Childhood—cont'd

DISEASE

Exanthem Subitum (Roseola) (Fig. 38-10)

Agent–Human herpesvirus type 6 (HHV-6; rarely HHV-7)
Source–Possibly acquired from saliva of healthy adult; entry via nasal, buccal or conjunctival mucosa
Transmission–Year round; no reported contact with infected individual in most cases (virtually limited to children under age 3 yr but peak age is between 6 and 15 mo)
Incubation period–Usually 5-15 days
Period of communicability–Unknown

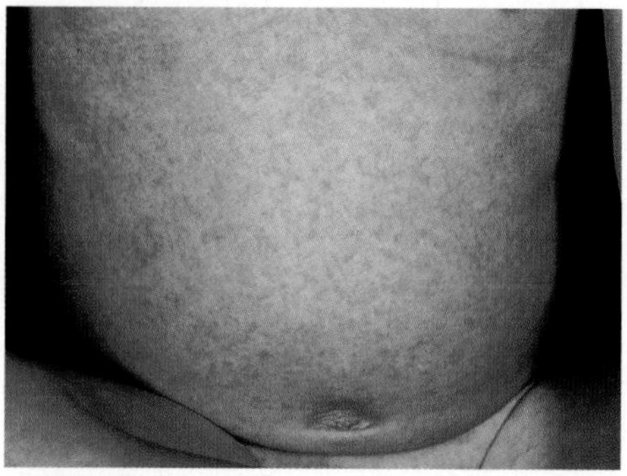

Fig. 38-10 Roseola infantum. *(From Habif, T. P. [2004].* Clinical dermatology: A color guide to diagnosis and therapy *[4th ed., p. 472, Fig. 14-18]. St. Louis: Mosby.)*

Measles (Rubeola) (Fig. 38-11)

Agent–Virus
Source–Respiratory tract secretions, blood, and urine of infected person
Transmission–Usually by direct contact with droplets of infected person; primarily in winter
Incubation period–10-20 days
Period of communicability–From 4 days before to 5 days after rash appears but mainly during prodromal (catarrhal) stage

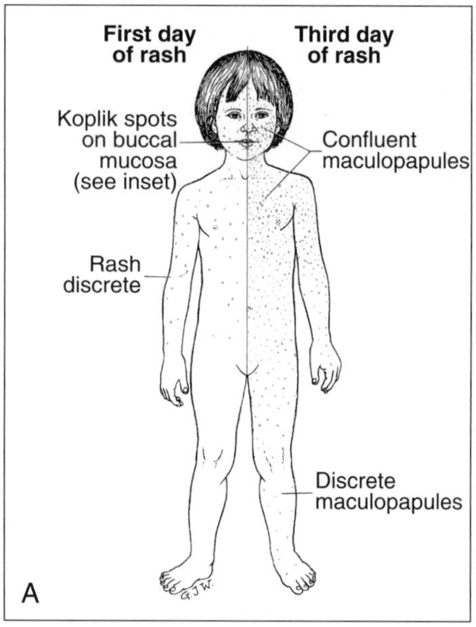

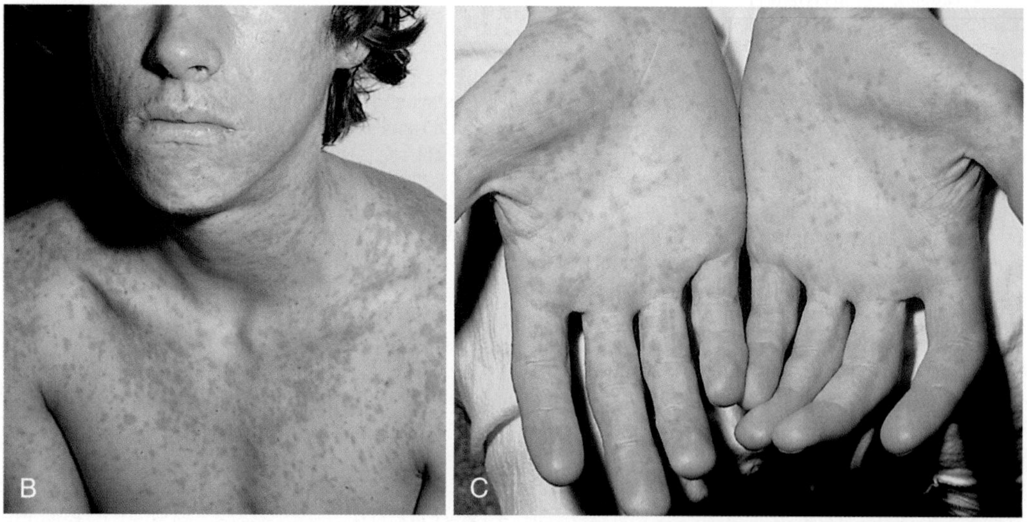

Fig. 38-11 Measles (rubeola). **A:** Progression of disease. **B:** Exanthem first appears at hairline and spreads from head to toe over 3 days. **C:** Measles ultimately involves palms and soles. *(**B** and **C**, From Zitelli, B. J., & Davis, H. W. [2007].* Atlas of pediatric physical diagnosis *[5th ed.]. St. Louis: Mosby; courtesy Michael Sherlock, MD, Lurville, MD.)*

CLINICAL MANIFESTATIONS	THERAPEUTIC MANAGEMENT AND COMPLICATIONS	NURSING CARE MANAGEMENT
Persistent high fever for 3–4 days in child who appears well Precipitous drop in fever to normal with appearance of rash **Rash**—Discrete rose-pink macules or maculopapules appearing first on trunk, then spreading to neck, face, and extremities; nonpruritic, fades on pressure, lasts 1–2 days **Associated signs and symptoms**—Cervical/postauricular lymphadenopathy, inflamed pharynx, cough, coryza	Nonspecific Antipyretics to control fever **Complications**—Recurrent febrile seizures (possibly from latent infection of central nervous system that is reactivated by fever) Encephalitis (rare)	Teach parents measures for lowering temperature (antipyretic medications); ensure adequate parental understanding of specific antipyretic dosage to prevent accidental overdose. If child is prone to seizures, discuss appropriate precautions and possibility of recurrent febrile seizures.
Prodromal (catarrhal) stage—Fever and malaise, followed in 24 hr by coryza, cough, conjunctivitis, Koplik's spots (small, irregular red spots with a minute, bluish white centre first seen on buccal mucosa opposite molars 2 days before rash); symptoms gradually increasing in severity until second day after rash appears, when they begin to subside (Fig. 38-11A) **Rash**—Appears 3–4 days after onset of prodromal stage; begins as erythematous maculopapular eruption on face and gradually spreads downward; more severe in earlier sites (appears confluent) and less intense in later sites (appears discrete); after 3–4 days assumes brownish appearance, and fine desquamation occurs over area of extensive involvement **Constitutional signs and symptoms**—Anorexia, abdominal pain, malaise, generalized lymphadenopathy	Vitamin A supplementation (see p. 1069) **Supportive**—Bed rest during febrile period; antipyretics Antibiotics to prevent secondary bacterial infection in high-risk children **Complications**—Otitis media Pneumonia (bacterial) Obstructive laryngitis and laryngotracheitis Encephalitis (rare but has high mortality)	Isolate until fifth day of rash; if hospitalized, institute droplet precautions. Encourage rest during prodromal stage; provide quiet activity. **Fever**—Instruct parents to administer antipyretics; avoid chilling; if child is prone to seizures, institute appropriate precautions. **Eye care**—Dim lights if photophobia present; clean eyelids with warm saline solution to remove secretions or crusts; keep child from rubbing eyes. **Coryza, cough**—Use cool-mist vaporizer; protect skin around nares with layer of petrolatum; encourage fluids and soft, bland foods. **Skin care**—Keep skin clean; use tepid baths as necessary.

Continued

Table 38-2 Communicable Diseases of Childhood—cont'd

DISEASE
Mumps
Agent–Paramyxovirus **Source**–Saliva of infected persons **Transmission**–Direct contact with other droplet spread from an infected person **Incubation period**–14-21 days **Period of communicability**–Most communicable immediately before and after swelling begins
Pertussis (Whooping Cough)
Agent–*Bordetella pertussis* **Source**–Discharge from respiratory tract of infected person **Transmission**–Direct contact or droplet spread from infected person; indirect contact with freshly contaminated articles **Incubation period**–6-20 days, usually 7-10 days **Period of communicability**–Greatest during catarrhal stage before onset of paroxysms
Poliomyelitis
Agent–Enteroviruses, three types: type 1, most frequent cause of paralysis, both epidemic and endemic; type 2, least frequently associated with paralysis; type 3, second-most frequently associated with paralysis **Source**–Feces and oropharyngeal secretions of infected persons, especially young children **Transmission**–Direct contact with persons with apparent or inapparent active infection; spread is via fecal-oral and pharyngeal-oropharyngeal routes Vaccine-acquired paralytic polio may occur as a result of live oral polio vaccination (no longer available in Canada) **Incubation period**–Usually 7-38 days, with range of 5-35 days **Period of communicability**–Not exactly known; virus present in throat and feces shortly after infection and persists for about 1 wk in throat and 4-6 wk in feces

CLINICAL MANIFESTATIONS	THERAPEUTIC MANAGEMENT AND COMPLICATIONS	NURSING CARE MANAGEMENT
Prodromal stage–Fever, headache, malaise, and anorexia for 24 hr, followed by "earache" that is aggravated by chewing **Parotitis**–Parotid gland(s) (either unilateral or bilateral) enlarges and reaches maximum size in 1-3 days; accompanied by pain and tenderness; or exocrine glands (submandibular) may also be swollen	**Symptomatic and supportive**–Analgesics for pain and antipyretics for fever Intravenous fluid may be necessary for child refusing to drink or child vomiting because of meningoencephalitis **Complications**–Sensorineural deafness Postinfectious encephalitis Myocarditis Arthritis Hepatitis Epididymoorchitis Oophoritis Pancreatitis Sterility (extremely rare in adult males) Meningitis	Isolate during period of communicability; institute droplet and contact precautions during hospitalization. Encourage rest and decreased activity during prodromal phase until swelling subsides. Give analgesics for pain; if child is unwilling to swallow pills or tablets medication, use elixir form. Encourage fluids and soft, bland foods; avoid foods requiring chewing. Apply hot or cold compresses to neck, whichever is more comforting. To relieve orchitis, provide warmth and local support with tight-fitting underpants.
Catarrhal stage–Begins with symptoms of upper respiratory tract infection, such as coryza, sneezing, lacrimation, cough, and low-grade fever; symptoms continue for 1-2 wk, when dry, hacking cough becomes more severe **Paroxysmal stage**–Cough most often occurs at night and consists of short, rapid coughs followed by sudden inspiration associated with a high-pitched crowing sound or "whoop"; during paroxysms, cheeks become flushed or cyanotic, eyes bulge, and tongue protrudes; paroxysm may continue until thick mucous plug is dislodged; vomiting frequently follows attack; stage generally lasts 4-6 wk, followed by convalescent stage. Infants under 6 mo of age may not have characteristic whoop cough, but have difficulty maintaining adequate oxygenation with amount of secretions, frequent vomiting of mucus and formula or breast milk (see also Chapter 36, Immunizations, for discussion of pertussis in adolescents).	Antimicrobial therapy (e.g., erythromycin, clarithromycin, azithromycin) **Supportive treatment**–Hospitalization sometimes required for infants, children who are dehydrated, or those who have complications Increased oxygen intake and humidity Adequate fluids Intensive care and mechanical ventilation may be necessary for infant <6 mo **Complications**–Pneumonia (usual cause of death) Atelectasis Otitis media Seizures Hemorrhage (scleral, conjunctival, epistaxis; pulmonary hemorrhage in neonate) Weight loss and dehydration Hernias (umbilical and inguinal) Prolapsed rectum	Isolate during catarrhal stage; if hospitalized, institute droplet precautions. Obtain nasopharyngeal culture for diagnosis. Encourage oral fluids; offer small amount of fluids frequently. Ensure adequate oxygenation during paroxysms; position infant on side to decrease chance of aspiration with vomiting. Provide high humidity (humidifier or croup tent); suction as needed to prevent choking on secretions. Observe for signs of airway obstruction (increased restlessness, apprehension, retractions, cyanosis). Encourage household contacts to complete antibiotic therapy. Encourage adolescents to obtain pertussis booster (Tdap) (see also Chapter 36, Immunizations). Health care workers should use standard precautions and mask when exposed to children with persistent cough and high suspicion of pertussis.
May be manifested in three different forms: **Abortive or inapparent**–Fever, uneasiness, sore throat, headache, anorexia, vomiting, abdominal pain; lasts a few hours to a few days **Nonparalytic**–Same manifestations as abortive but more severe, with pain and stiffness in neck, back, and legs **Paralytic**–Initial course similar to nonparalytic type, followed by recovery and then signs of central nervous system paralysis	Treatment is supportive Complete bed rest during acute phase Mechanical or assisted ventilation in case of respiratory paralysis Physiotherapy for muscles following acute stage **Complications**–Permanent paralysis Respiratory arrest Hypertension Kidney stones from demineralization of bone during prolonged immobility	Administer mild sedatives as necessary to relieve anxiety and promote rest. Participate in physiotherapy procedures (use of moist hot packs and range-of-motion exercises). Position child to maintain body alignment and prevent contractures or skin breakdown; use footboard or appropriate orthoses to prevent footdrop; use pressure mattress for prolonged immobility. Encourage child to perform activities of daily living to capability; encourage early ambulation with adjuncts; administer analgesics for maximum comfort during physical activity. Provide high-protein diet and bowel management for prolonged immobility. Observe for respiratory paralysis (difficulty in talking, ineffective cough, inability to hold breath, shallow and rapid respirations); report such signs and symptoms to practitioner.

Continued

Table 38-2 Communicable Diseases of Childhood—cont'd

DISEASE

Rubella (German Measles) (Fig. 38-12)

Agent–Rubella virus
Source–Primarily nasopharyngeal secretions of person with apparent or inapparent infection; virus also present in blood, stool, and urine
Incubation period–14-21 days
Period of communicability–7 days before to about 5 days after appearance of rash

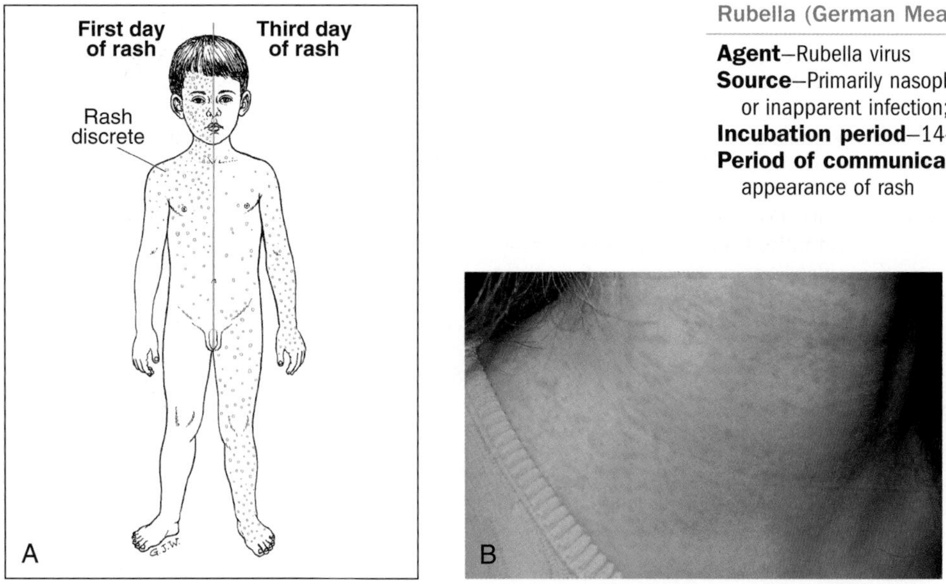

Fig. 38-12 Rubella (German measles). **A**: Progression of rash. **B**: Clinical view. *(**B**, From Zitelli, B. J., & Davis, H. W. [2007].* Atlas of pediatric physical diagnosis *[5th ed.]. St. Louis: Mosby; courtesy Michael Sherlock, MD, Lurville, MD.)*

Scarlet Fever (Fig. 38-13)

Agent–Group A β-hemolytic streptococci
Source–Usually from nasopharyngeal secretions of infected persons and carriers
Transmission–Direct contact with infected person or droplet spread; indirectly by contact with contaminated articles or ingestion of contaminated milk or other food
Incubation period–2-5 days, with range of 1-7 days
Period of communicability–During incubation period and clinical illness, approximately 10 days; during first 2 wk of carrier phase, although may persist for months

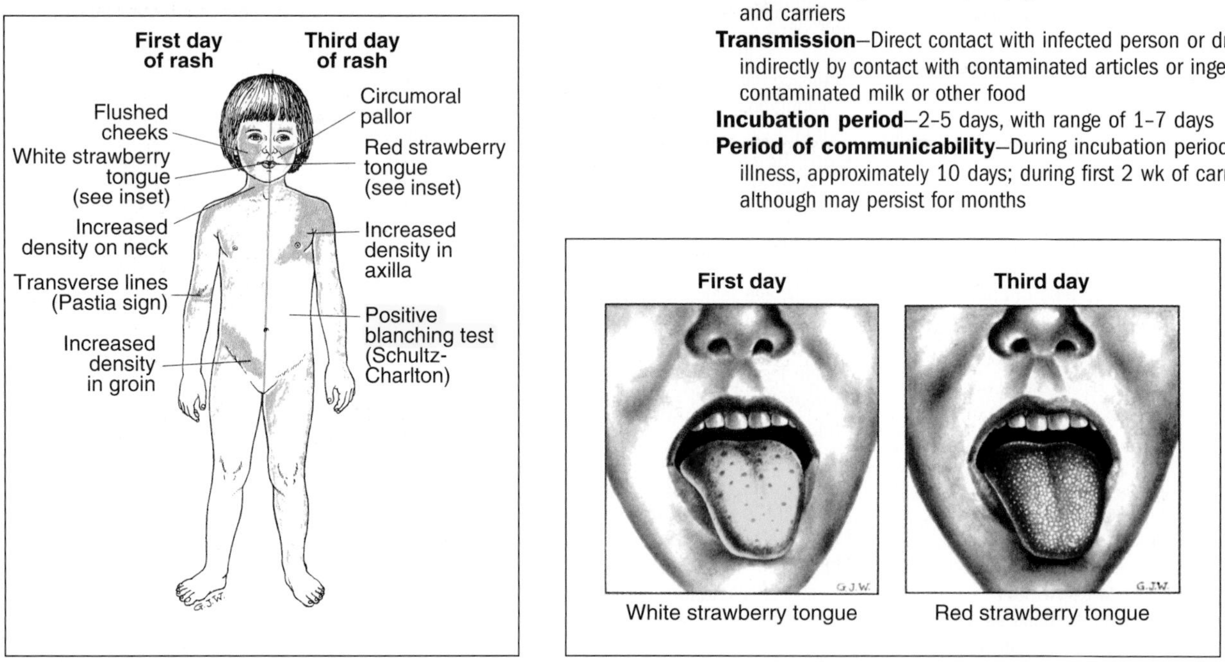

Fig. 38-13 Scarlet fever.

CLINICAL MANIFESTATIONS	THERAPEUTIC MANAGEMENT AND COMPLICATIONS	NURSING CARE MANAGEMENT
Constitutional signs and symptoms—Occasionally low-grade fever, headache, malaise, and lymphadenopathy **Prodromal stage**—Absent in children, present in adults and adolescents; consists of low-grade fever, headache, malaise, anorexia, mild conjunctivitis, coryza, sore throat, cough, and lymphadenopathy; lasts 1-5 days, subsides 1 day after appearance of rash **Rash**—First appears on face and rapidly spreads downward to neck, arms, trunk, and legs; by end of first day, body is covered with discrete, pinkish red maculopapular exanthema; disappears in same order as it began and is usually gone by third day	No treatment necessary other than antipyretics for low-grade fever and analgesics for discomfort **Complications**—Rare (arthritis, encephalitis, or purpura); most benign of all childhood communicable diseases; greatest danger is teratogenic effect on fetus	Reassure parents of benign nature of illness in affected child. Use comfort measures as necessary. Avoid contact with pregnant woman. Monitor rubella titre in pregnant adolescent.
Prodromal stage—Abrupt high fever, pulse increased out of proportion to fever, vomiting, headache, chills, malaise, abdominal pain, halitosis **Enanma**—Tonsils enlarged, edematous, reddened, and covered with patches of exudates; in severe cases appearance resembles membrane seen in diphtheria; pharynx edematous and beefy red; during first 1-2 days tongue coated and papillae become red and swollen (white strawberry tongue); by fourth or fifth day white coat sloughs off, leaving prominent papillae (red strawberry tongue); palate covered with erythematous punctate lesions **Exanthema**—Rash appears within 12 hr after prodromal signs; red pinhead-sized punctate lesions rapidly become generalized but are absent on face, which becomes flushed with striking circumoral pallor; rash more intense in folds of joints; by end of first week desquamation begins (fine, sandpaper-like on torso; sheetlike sloughing on palms and soles), which may be complete by 3 wk or longer	**Treatment of choice**—Full course of penicillin (or erythromycin in penicillin-sensitive children), or oral cephalosporin Antibiotic therapy for newly diagnosed carriers (nose or throat cultures positive for streptococci) **Supportive measures**—Rest during febrile phase, analgesics for sore throat; antipruritics for rash if bothersome **Complications**—Peritonsillar and retropharyngeal abscess Sinusitis Otitis media Acute glomerulonephritis Acute rheumatic fever Polyarthritis (uncommon)	Institute standard and droplet precautions until 24 hr after initiation of treatment. Ensure compliance with oral antibiotic therapy; intramuscular benzathine penicillin G [Bicillin] may be given if parents' reliability in giving oral medications is questionable. Encourage rest during febrile phase; provide quiet activity during convalescent period. Relieve discomfort of sore throat with analgesics, gargles, lozenges, antiseptic throat sprays, and inhalation of cool mist. Encourage fluids during febrile phase; avoid irritating liquids (certain citrus juices) or rough foods (chips); when child is able to eat, begin with soft diet. Advise parents to consult practitioner if fever persists after beginning therapy. Discuss procedures for preventing spread of infection—discard toothbrush; avoid sharing drinking and eating utensils.

Encopresis

Encopresis is repeated voluntary or involuntary passage of feces of normal or near-normal consistency into places not appropriate for that purpose according to an individual's own sociocultural setting. The event must occur at least once a month for at least 3 months, and the child's **chronological** or **developmental age** must be at least 4 years. The fecal incontinence must not be caused by any physiological effect, such as a laxative, or a general medical condition.

Primary encopresis is identified by age 4 when the child has not achieved fecal continence. *Secondary encopresis* is fecal incontinence occurring in a child over 4 years of age after a period of established fecal continence. The disorder is more common in boys than in girls.

One of the most common causes of encopresis is constipation, which may be precipitated by environmental change. Chronic, severe constipation has a tendency to impair the usual movement and contractions of the colon, which can lead to fecal obstruction. Abnormalities in the digestive tract can also lead to encopresis.

Children with encopresis often feel ashamed and may wish to avoid situations that might lead to embarrassment. School performance and attendance are affected as the child's offensive odour becomes a target for scorn and ridicule from classmates. Therapeutic management consists of determining the cause of the soiling and using appropriate interventions to correct the problem. Interventions may involve dietary changes, relief of a fecal impaction, or behavioural therapy. Psychotherapeutic intervention with the child and family is often necessary. Family counselling is directed toward reassurance that most problems resolve successfully, although relapses during periods of stress are possible.

Child Maltreatment

The broad term *child maltreatment* includes intentional physical abuse or neglect, emotional abuse or neglect, and sexual abuse of children, usually by adults. It is one of the most significant social problems affecting children around the world. In 2008, there were an estimated 235,842 Canadian children maltreatment-related investigations by Child Welfare Services. Eighteen percent of these investigations had more than one category of maltreatment. Male and female maltreatment numbers were equal. Of the confirmed cases, 20% suffered physical abuse, 3% were sexual abuse (does not include all nonrelated abusers), 34% showed neglect, and 9% were emotional abuse; 34% had exposure to intimate partner violence. In 2008, two children in Canada died as a result of child maltreatment. First Nations, Métis, and Inuit children were identified as a key at-risk group because they are overrepresented in foster care and have four times the maltreatment rate for non-Aboriginal children (PHAC, 2008). Reported statistics only partially represent the actual incidence of child maltreatment, since many cases likely go unreported.

Child Neglect

Child neglect is the most common form of maltreatment. *Neglect* is generally defined as the failure of a parent or other person legally responsible for the child's welfare to provide for the child's basic needs and an adequate level of care.

Important factors contributing to child neglect are lack of knowledge of child's needs, lack of resources, and caretaker substance use. For example, neglectful parents often demonstrate poor parenting skills. They may be unaware that an infant needs to be fed every 3 to 4 hours, may not know what to feed the child, and may have insufficient funds to buy food. Another serious lack of knowledge is failure to recognize emotional nurturing as an essential need of children. (See also Chapter 36, Growth Failure [Failure to Thrive].)

Types of Neglect

Neglect takes many forms and can be classified broadly as physical or emotional maltreatment. *Physical neglect* involves the deprivation of necessities, such as food, clothing, shelter, supervision, medical care, and education. *Emotional neglect* generally refers to failure to meet the child's needs for affection, attention, and emotional nurturance.

Neglect may also include lack of intervention for or fostering of maladaptive behaviour, such as delinquency or substance use. *Emotional abuse*, an even more difficult aspect of maltreatment to define, refers to the deliberate attempt to destroy or significantly impair a child's self-esteem or competence. Emotional abuse may take the following forms: rejecting, isolating, terrorizing, ignoring, corrupting, verbally assaulting, or overpressuring the child.

Physical Abuse

The Justice Department of Canada defines *child abuse* as violence, mistreatment, or neglect that a child or adolescent may experience while in the care of someone they trust or depend on, such as a parent, sibling, or relative, caregiver, or guardian. Abuse may take place anywhere and may occur, for example, within the child's home or that of someone known to the child (PHAC, 2008). Legal steps to address child abuse in Canada include mandatory reporting laws, creation of child abuse registries, changes to the Criminal Code and the *Canada Evidence Act*, extended time limits for filing charges in child sexual abuse cases, and establishment of child protection agencies run by First Nations, Métis, and Inuit peoples (PHAC, 2008). Minor physical injury is responsible for more reported cases of maltreatment than major physical injury, but major physical abuse causes more deaths.

NURSING ALERT Nurses have a mandatory legal and professional ethical responsibility to report suspected cases of child maltreatment to Child Welfare Services. Every new abuse incident must be reported.

Munchausen Syndrome by Proxy

Munchausen syndrome by proxy (MSBP), also known as factitious disorder by proxy or medical child abuse, is a rare but serious form of child abuse in which caretakers deliberately exaggerate or fabricate histories and symptoms or induce symptoms. It is a form of child maltreatment that may include physical, emotional, and psychological abuse for the gratification of the caretaker. In most cases the perpetrator is the biological mother, with some degree of health care knowledge and training. Health care providers can become easily misled and unknowingly enable the perpetrator (Leider et al., 2005). As a result of the history of symptoms provided by the caretaker, the child endures painful and unnecessary medical testing and procedures. Common symptoms are seizures, nausea and vomiting, diarrhea, and altered mental status; these symptoms are usually witnessed only by the perpetrator. Considerations when determining whether a child is a victim of MSBP include the following:

- Is the child's condition consistent with the reported history?
- Does the diagnostic evidence support the reported history?
- Has anyone other than the caretaker witnessed the symptoms?
- Is treatment being provided primarily because of the caretaker's demands?

Resolution of symptoms after separation from the perpetrator confirms diagnosis.

Factors Predisposing to Physical Abuse

The causes of child abuse are multifaceted. Child maltreatment occurs across all socioeconomic, religious, cultural, racial, and ethnic groups (Goldman et al., 2003). Three risk factors are commonly identified in child abuse: parental characteristics, characteristics of the child, and environmental characteristics. However, no single factor or group of factors is predictive of abuse. Rather, the interaction of these factors is thought to increase the risk of abuse occurring in a particular family.

Parental Characteristics

Certain identified characteristics occur more frequently in parents who abuse their children and are therefore considered risk factors. Younger parents more often are abusers of their children. One-parent families are at higher risk for abuse, and in lone-parent families that include an unrelated partner, the partner is frequently the abuser.

Abusive families are often more socially isolated and have fewer supportive relationships. These parents are often from low-income circumstances, with concurrent undereducation and substance use problems. With little or no available support system and concurrent stressors imposed by the child or environment, these parents are vulnerable to additional crises of any nature and may strike out at the child as a method of releasing their increasing frustration and anxiety.

Other factors identified in abusive parents include low **self-esteem** and little knowledge of appropriate parenting skills. Parenting skills are learned behaviours, and parents who grew up with poor parental role models may have difficulty parenting their own children. Approximately one third of parents who were maltreated as children will subject their children to similar maltreatment (Gara et al., 2000).

Characteristics of the Child

The onus for child abuse is always on the abuser; however, children who are abused have some common characteristics. Children from birth to 3 years of age are at the highest risk for being abused (PHAC, 2010). Infants and small children require constant attention and must have all of their needs met by others. This can result in parental or caretaker fatigue with resultant striking out at the child with physical force, shaking the child, or ignoring the child's needs.

The physical and emotional demands placed on the parents or caretaker of an unwanted, brain-damaged, hyperactive, or physically disabled child may overwhelm them, resulting in abuse. Disabled children may not understand that abusive behaviours are not appropriate so do not tell others or defend themselves. Preterm infants may be at risk for maltreatment because of failure of parent–child bonding during early infancy, increased physical needs, or irritability.

One child in the family may be singled out in an abusive family. Removing that child from the home often places the other siblings at risk for abuse. Therefore, no child is safe if left in the abusive environment unless the parents can be helped to learn new parenting skills and to meet their needs and release their frustration through alternatives other than attacking their children.

Environmental Characteristics

Environment is a significant part of the potentially abusive situation. A typical environment is one of chronic stress, including problems of divorce, poverty, unemployment, poor housing, frequent relocation, and substance use issues. Increased exposure between children and parents, such as that which occurs in crowded living conditions, also increases the likelihood of abuse.

Although most reporting of abuse has been from populations of lower socioeconomic status, as stated before, child abuse is not a problem of any one societal group. Stresses imposed by poverty predispose low-income families to abusive situations, and abuse in these groups is more apt to be reported. However, concealed crises may also be present in upper-income families. Families who have substitute caregivers such as day care providers and baby-sitters may also be at risk for child abuse, especially if the family has not fully evaluated the caregiver. Nurses need to be aware of all these factors to identify the less obvious examples of child abuse and neglect.

Sexual Abuse

Sexual abuse is one of the most devastating types of child maltreatment. Estimates indicate that it has increased significantly during the past decade (PHAC, 2009). Some of the apparent increase can be attributed to increased awareness (Putnam, 2003). One in ten (10%) maltreatment investigations in 1998 involved sexual abuse as the primary reason for investigation. Sexual abuse was confirmed in 38% of abuse cases (PHAC, 2009).

To further protect children from sexual abuse, the Criminal Code has been changed to create new criminal offences relating to child sexual assault, to include female genital mutilation as sexual abuse (see Chapter 4, Cultural Awareness box), and to amend provisions on child sex tourism to make it easier to prosecute offenders. Bill C-15 (Parliament of Canada, 2002), which became law in 2002, aims to protect children from sexual exploitation by criminalizing actions such as luring children via the Internet to meet them somewhere in person; transmitting, making available, or exporting child pornography; or accessing child pornography on the Internet. Sentencing provisions are also strengthened.

As with all forms of child maltreatment, no universal definition for *sexual abuse* exists (Finkel & DeJong, 2001). Sexual abuse and exploitation in Canada involves using a child for sexual purposes. Examples of child sexual abuse include fondling, inviting a child to touch or be touched sexually, intercourse, rape, incest, sodomy, exhibitionism, or involving a child in prostitution or pornography (PHAC, 2009).

Characteristics of Abusers and Victims

Anyone, including siblings and mothers, can be sexual abusers. Offenders come from all levels of society. Adults make up 80% of offenders of sexual abuse, with the remaining 20% being adolescents and preadolescents (Johnson, 2003). Many offenders hold full-time jobs and are active in community affairs, and they may not have prior criminal records (Finkel & DeJong, 2001). Offenders often are employed in or volunteer for positions that will bring them into contact with young girls and boys, such as teachers or coaches (Department of Justice Canada, 2011). Most abusers are male. Approximately 44% of sexual assaults against children and youth were carried out by nonparental family members, 29% of abusers were friends or acquaintances, and only 2% were strangers (PHAC, 2001).

The abusers who were family members were equally likely to be a biological father or step-father and less apt to be a biological mother or foster or adoptive parent (PHAC, 2001). Child sexual abuse may be generational unless discovered and stopped (Johnson, 2003). Offenders may commit many assaults before being caught.

Incestuous relationships between father or stepfather and daughter are generally prolonged, and the victims are usually reluctant to report the situation because of fear of retaliation and fear that they will not be believed. Typically, incestuous relationships begin later than other forms of child abuse. The eldest daughter is usually abused, but in her absence another sister may be substituted. Sibling incest may also occur. Sexual abuse by relatives with a strong emotional bond with the victim is the most devastating to the child.

Boys are also victims of both intrafamilial and extrafamilial abuse. Male victims are much less likely to report abuse, and they may suffer much greater emotional harm from incestuous relationships, especially between mother and son, than female victims. Boys are likely to be subjected to anal penetration and oral–genital contact; to have subtle physical findings; and to be abused by a father, stepfather, or mother's boyfriend.

Children who have a disability or a limiting health condition are at higher risk of sexual assault (CPS, Adolescent Health Committee, 2011). A 2008 British Columbia study reported that these children were three times more likely than non-disabled children to be both physically and sexually abused (Smith et al., 2009).

The number of sexual assaults among First Nations, Métis, and Inuit children is uncertain. There are wide differences in reported statistics, ranging from high to low numbers of assault. Child protection agencies report that the rate of sexual abuse among Aboriginal children and youth is lower than that for the general population, at 0.53 per 1000 versus 0.62 per 1000 (Collin-Vézina, Dion, & Trocmé, 2009). However, there may be significant underreporting in the First Nations, Métis, and Inuit populations, and more research is required.

Initiation and Perpetuation of Sexual Abuse

It is difficult to estimate the number of children in Canada who are sexually abused, as assaults are underreported and there is no nation-wide reporting system. The number of estimated sexual assaults and exploitations, however, is very concerning. Statistics Canada (2004) reported 8800 child and youth sexual assaults in 2002. Family members were responsible for 2863 of these assaults. The forms of substantiated child sexual abuse were touching and fondling of the genitals (68%), attempted and completed intercourse (35%), and an adult exposing genitals to a child (12%). Also reported were sexual exploitation of a child for purposes of financial gain or other profit; 4% of cases involved sexual harassment (including proposition, encouragement, or suggestions of a sexual nature) (PHAC, 2001). The Canadian Incident Study (PHAC, 2001) reported that young girls are most frequently the targets of sexual abuse. The age when children are at highest risk for abuse is 4 to 7 years for girls and 12 to 15 years for boys.

Significant risk factors for child sexual abuse include parental unavailability, lack of emotional closeness, social isolation, emotional deprivation, and communication difficulties. The cycle of sexual abuse often starts insidiously unless it involves an isolated attack, such as rape. Often offenders spend time with the victims to gain their trust before initiating any sexual contact. Most victims are then pressured into being an accessory to the sexual activity through various means (Box 38-1) and may be unaware that sexual activity is part of the offer. Children may not reveal the truth for fear that their parents would not believe them if they told, especially if the offender is a trusted member of the family. Some fear that they will be blamed for the situation, and many young children with limited vocabulary have difficulty describing the activity when they do have the courage or opportunity to reveal the abuse.

Incest most frequently occurs between fathers and daughters, but may be between grandfather and granddaughter or brother and sister. Brother–sister incest has been found to be just as damaging as father–daughter abuse (Cyr et al., 2002). However, not all incestuous relationships follow a pattern of silence. Reports of father–daughter incest during child custody conflicts have become more common and have raised serious concerns regarding the possibility of false accusation. Rather

BOX 38-1 Methods Used to Pressure Children Into Sexual Activity

- Child is offered gifts or privileges.
- Adult misrepresents moral standards by telling the child that what they are doing is "okay to do."
- Isolated and emotionally and socially impoverished children are enticed by adults who meet their needs for warmth and human contact.
- Offender pressures the victim into secrecy regarding the activity by describing it as a "secret between us" that other people may take away if they find out.
- Offender plays on the child's fears, including fear of punishment by the offender, fear of repercussions if the child tells, and fear of abandonment or rejection by the family.

than tolerating or denying the child's sexual abuse, the other parent (usually the mother) is typically the chief accuser.

Nursing Care of the Maltreated Child

A critical responsibility of health care providers is identifying abusive situations as early as possible. The characteristics that may predispose members of some families to commit abuse can serve as a framework for assessing vulnerability but are never predictive of actual abuse. A careful, detailed history and interview combined with a thorough physical examination are the diagnostic tools needed to identify abuse. Nurses have a special role in identifying abuse because they may be the first person to see the child and parent and are the consistent caregivers if the child is hospitalized (see Guidelines box).

During the interview with the child and family, the nurse must be careful to avoid biasing the child's retelling of the events. Some experts suggest that health care providers limit the interview to the child's physical and mental health concerns and leave topics of the family's social, legal, or other problems to the police or Child Protection Services (McClain et al., 2000). If this is not possible, an effort should be made to coordinate the interview process so that all pertinent health care providers can be present.

NURSING ALERT Nurses must be aware of their biases regarding child abuse. Nurses are often less likely to report abuse when the child is a girl and from a middle-income family than if the child is from a lower-income family. Nurses are also significantly less comfortable dealing with sexual abuse, abuse of infants, and fathers as the abusers, and they experience greater discomfort when dealing with abusers of children with disabilities than with abusers of children without disabilities.

Recognition of abuse or neglect necessitates a familiarity with both the physical and behavioural signs that suggest maltreatment (Box 38-2). No one indicator can be used to diagnose maltreatment. It is a pattern or combination of indicators that should arouse suspicion and further investigation. Some situations may be misinterpreted as abuse, such as bleeding disorders, osteogenesis imperfecta, sudden infant death syndrome, and cultural practices such as cupping or coin rubbing that may mimic physical abuse (see Chapter 32, Health Practices). Unintentional injuries, such as burns from metal buckles on car seats, bruising from seat belts, or spiral fractures from a twist and fall injury, may also be wrongly diagnosed as abuse. Normal variants, such as Mongolian spots and congenital anomalies of genitalia, can be mistaken for abuse.

Caregiver–Child Interaction

The nurse can use the initial contact with the family to assess the interaction between the caregiver and the child. Certain behavioural responses of the parents to their child and to the interviewer should alert the nurse to the possibility of maltreatment. Abusive parents may have difficulty showing concern toward their child. They may be unable or unwilling to comfort the child. Abusers may blame the child for the injuries or belittle them for being "clumsy" or "stupid." When interacting with the health care workers the parent may become hostile or uncooperative. During the child's hospitalization they may not participate in the child's care and may show little concern for his or her progress, eventual discharge, or need for follow-up care. Although caregivers and children may vary in responses to a stressful event, an unusual caregiver–child relationship should be noted and factored into the overall evaluation of the child.

Abused children's responses to their parents or the injury may also support the suspicion of abuse. Although no one pattern is typical, extremes of behaviour may be observed. Children may be unresponsive to the parent or excessively

GUIDELINES Talking With Children Who Reveal Abuse

- Provide a private time and place to talk.
- Do not promise not to tell; tell them that you are required by law to report the abuse.
- Do not express shock or criticize their family.
- Use their vocabulary to discuss body parts.
- Avoid using any leading statements that can distort their report.
- Reassure them that they have done the right thing by telling you.
- Tell them that the abuse is not their fault, that they are not bad or to blame.
- Determine their immediate need for safety.
- Let the child know what will happen when you report the incident.

BOX 38-2 Warning Signs of Abuse

- Physical evidence of abuse or neglect, including previous injuries
- Conflicting stories about the "accident" or injury from the parents or others
- Cause of injury blamed on sibling or other party
- An injury inconsistent with the history, such as a concussion and broken arm from falling off a bed
- History inconsistent with child's developmental level, such as a 6-month-old turning on the hot water
- A health concern other than the one associated with signs of abuse (e.g., a chief health concern of a cold when there is evidence of first- and second-degree burns)
- Inappropriate response of caregiver, such as an exaggerated or absent emotional response, refusal to sign for additional tests or to agree to necessary treatment, excessive delay in seeking treatment, or absence of parents for questioning
- Inappropriate response of child, such as little or no response to pain, fear of being touched, excessive or lack of separation anxiety, indiscriminate friendliness to strangers
- Child's report of physical or sexual abuse
- Previous reports of abuse in the family
- Repeated visits to emergency facilities with injuries

clinging and intolerant of separation. They may be overly attached to the abusive parent, possibly in the hope of preventing any upset that may precipitate anger and another attack. During care of the injury, children may be passive and accepting of the discomfort or uncooperative and fearful of any physical contact. They may avoid eye contact. Some children maintain a wary watchfulness of all strangers; some shy away from strangers as if frightened; others are unusually affectionate and outgoing.

History and Interview

Child Physical Abuse

It is often difficult to distinguish child maltreatment from accidental injuries. Caregivers whose history of events may be deceptive or incomplete and children who are nonverbal may make the assessment more complex. A purposeful, skilled history and appropriate interview questions will help the nurse to ensure the right course of action. Knowledge of the mechanism of injury and child development is essential. Cases of abuse are often detected by inconsistencies in child or caregiver history of events compared with physical findings. Children who are verbal can often give a history of the injury. Separating the child from the caregiver may provide a more reliable history. It is important to ask nonleading, open-ended questions. The history should include a narrative of the injury from both the caregiver and child (if verbal). Date, time, and location where injury took place, along with who was present at the time of the injury, are essential questions. Family history for bleeding or bone disorders is important. Areas of the history that can signal abuse are outlined in Box 38-3.

Neglect and Emotional Abuse

Each child may manifest different responses to neglect depending on the situation and the child's developmental age. The goal of the interview is to determine whether the child is in a safe environment and whether the caregiver has the skills and resources to care for the child. It is often difficult to determine whether the circumstances constitute poor parenting skills or true neglect. Warning signals of behaviours to look for are found in Box 38-2.

Sexual Abuse

An essential component to identifying sexual abuse is the interview. Several dynamics may impede the child's revelation of sexual abuse. Child sexual abuse is often perpetrated by someone known to the child, including family members. In some cases, the children may have been sworn to secrecy. They may have been told that no one will believe them or their family would be harmed if they tell someone about the abuse. Small children may imitate behaviours they have had perpetrated on themselves or have seen others do. The nurse must be able to recognize normal, age-related sexual curiosity and self-stimulating behaviours; typically, children do not act out specific details of the sexual act or perform intrusive acts on others unless they have sexual knowledge beyond their normal age-related development (Johnson, 2003).

Children's reports of sexual abuse may vary from contradictory stories to unwavering versions of the experience. Stories that sound contradictory may reflect the child's experiences in several instances of abuse. Also, children who repeatedly tell identical facts may have been prompted to do so. Increasing evidence suggests that the types of interrogation that children are exposed to after reports of sexual abuse shape their thinking. To avoid biasing the interaction, nurses must be very skilful interviewers when questioning children who may be victims of abuse. Medical records should include verbatim statements made by the child and the interviewer that reflect appropriate nonleading questions and statements (Hornor, 2001; McClain et al., 2000).

The child may not be emotionally ready to discuss the abuse. Establishing rapport with the child is essential to gaining his or her trust. Interviews should not be rushed. Engaging the child in play activities while encouraging conversation may help the child discuss the abuse. It may take several interviews or psychological counselling for the child to be forthcoming about the abuse.

Information regarding the last sexual contact is important because it determines the need for a forensic evaluation. Children who have had sexual abuse that has occurred within the past 72 to 96 hours should be considered for forensic testing.

Unfortunately, there is no typical profile of the victim, and there must be a high index of suspicion to identify these children. Physical signs vary and may include any of those listed for sexual abuse. The victim may exhibit various behavioural manifestations, none of which is diagnostic. When abused children exhibit these behaviours, the signs may be incorrectly attributed to the normal stresses of childhood, especially in older school-age children or adolescents. Even signs considered most predictive of sexual abuse, such as certain genital findings, sexually inappropriate behaviour for age, enactment of adult sexual activity, and intense focus on sexual activity (e.g., masturbation), do not always indicate that sexual abuse has occurred. Conversely, abused children may not demonstrate more knowledge of sexual activity than nonabused children. One difference in the abused children's explanation of sexual activity may be unusual affective responses. For example, abused children may have an increased incidence of sleep disorders, temper tantrums, and depression (Calam et al., 1998).

Physical Assessment

Child Physical Abuse

The goal of the physical assessment for child physical abuse is identification of all injuries. A systems approach ensures that the whole body is evaluated. In instances of severe abuse and injuries, the assessment should begin with a rapid assessment of airway, breathing, circulation (ABC), and neurological systems. A systematic head-to-toe examination follows. Attention to areas often overlooked, such as the scalp, behind the ears, and the lingual frenulum, is essential. The child's exterior genitalia and posterior surface should be completely examined.

The location and a detailed description of all injuries should be recorded. Colour, size, and location of all bruising need to be noted. Burn documentation should include location, pattern, demarcation lines, and presence of eschar or blisters. Diagrams of the injuries using a body diagram form are helpful. If available, photographs of the injuries using a measurement tool should be obtained.

Not all forms of physical abuse have obvious signs. Intra-abdominal organ injury from blunt trauma to the abdomen

BOX 38-3 Clinical Manifestations of Potential Child Maltreatment

Physical Neglect

Suggestive Physical Findings

Failure to thrive
Signs of malnutrition, such as thin extremities, abdominal distention, lack of subcutaneous fat
Poor personal hygiene
Unclean or inappropriate dress
Evidence of poor health care, such as delayed immunization, untreated infections, frequent colds
Frequent injuries from lack of supervision

Suggestive Behaviours

Dull and inactive affect; excessively passive or sleepy
Self-stimulatory behaviours, such as finger sucking or rocking
Begging for or stealing food
Absenteeism from school
Child's substance use
Vandalism or shoplifting

Emotional Abuse and Neglect

Suggestive Physical Findings

Failure to thrive
Eating or feeding disorder
Enuresis
Sleep disorder

Suggestive Behaviours

Self-stimulatory behaviours, such as biting, rocking, sucking
During infancy, lack of social smile, and anxiety toward strangers
Withdrawal from environment and people
Unusual fearfulness
Antisocial behaviour, such as destructiveness, stealing, or cruelty toward animals or people
Extremes of behaviour, such as overcompliant and passive, or aggressive and demanding
Lags in emotional and intellectual development, especially language
Suicide attempts

Physical Abuse

Suggestive Physical Findings

Bruises and welts
- On face, lips, mouth, back, buttocks, thighs, or areas of torso
- Regular patterns descriptive of object used, such as belt buckle, hand, wire hanger, chain, wooden spoon; squeeze or pinch marks
- May be present in various stages of healing

Burns
- On soles of feet, palms of hands, back, or buttocks
- Patterns descriptive of object used, such as round cigar or cigarette burns; sharply demarcated areas from immersion in scalding water; rope burns on wrists or ankles from being bound; burns in the shape of an iron, radiator, or electric stove burner
- Absence of "splash" marks and presence of symmetrical burns
- Stun gun injury: lesions circular, fairly uniform (up to 0.5 cm), and paired about 5 cm apart

Fractures and dislocations
- Skull, nose, or facial structures
- Injury denoting type of abuse, such as spiral fracture or dislocation from twisting of an extremity or whiplash from shaking the child
- Multiple new or old fractures in various stages of healing

Lacerations and abrasions
- On backs of arms, legs, torso, face, or external genitalia
- Unusual symptoms, such as abdominal swelling, pain, and vomiting from punching
- Descriptive marks such as from human bites or pulling out of hair

Chemical
- Unexplained repeated poisoning, especially drug overdose
- Unexplained sudden illness, such as hypoglycemia from insulin administration

Suggestive Behaviours

Wary of physical contact with adults
Apparent fear of parents or of going home
Lying very still while surveying environment
Inappropriate reaction to injury, such as failure to cry from pain
Lack of reaction to frightening events
Apprehension when hearing other children cry
Indiscriminate friendliness and displays of affection
Superficial relationships
Acting-out behaviour, such as aggression, to seek attention
Withdrawal behaviour

Sexual Abuse

Suggestive Physical Findings

Bruises, bleeding, lacerations, or irritation of external genitalia, anus, mouth, or throat
Torn, stained, or bloody underclothing
Pain on urination or pain, swelling, and itching of genital area
Penile discharge
Sexually transmitted infection, nonspecific vaginitis, or venereal warts
Difficulty in walking or sitting
Unusual odour in the genital area
Recurrent urinary tract infections
Presence of sperm
Pregnancy in young adolescent

Suggestive Behaviours

Sudden emergence of sexually related problems, including excessive or public masturbation, age-inappropriate sexual play, promiscuity, or overtly seductive behaviour
Withdrawn behaviour, excessive daydreaming
Preoccupation with fantasies, especially in play
Poor relationships with peers
Sudden changes, such as anxiety, weight loss or gain, clinging behaviour
In incestuous relationships, excessive anger at mother for not protecting daughter

Continued

BOX 38-3 Clinical Manifestations of Potential Child Maltreatment—cont'd

Sexual Abuse—cont'd

Suggestive Behaviours—cont'd

Regressive behaviour, such as bed-wetting or thumb-sucking

Sudden onset of phobias or fears, particularly fears of the dark, men, strangers, or particular settings or situations (e.g., undue fear of leaving the house or staying at the day care centre or the baby-sitter's house)

Running away from home

Substance use, particularly of alcohol or mood-elevating drugs

Profound and rapid personality changes, especially extreme depression, hostility, and aggression (often accompanied by social withdrawal)

Rapidly declining school performance

Suicidal attempts or ideation

can occur without signs of external abdominal bruising. Nurses should consider intra-abdominal injury in infants and children who have any other signs of abuse.

NURSING ALERT Incompatibility between the history and the injury is probably the most important criterion on which to base the decision to report suspected abuse.

Neglect and Emotional Abuse

Neglect from deprivation of necessities is easier to identify than emotional neglect or abuse because physical signs are usually evident. Assessment of the child's height, weight, nutritional status, hygiene, and age-appropriate interactions is important for the overall picture of potential neglect. Emotional maltreatment may be readily suspected, but it is difficult to substantiate. Physical signs are often nonspecific, and nurses must rely on behavioural indicators, which range from depression to acting-out behaviour, to help identify a possibly abusive situation. Any persistent and unexplained change in the child's behaviour is an important clue to possible emotional abuse.

Sexual Abuse

Identifying instances of sexual abuse is particularly difficult because, often, few if any obvious physical indications of the activity exist. Physical signs vary and may include any of those listed in Box 38-3 for sexual abuse. The goal of the physical examination is to document genital findings. In most cases the genital examination is normal, which does not mean that sexual abuse did not occur. Fondling or genital-to-genital contact without penetration may leave no physical findings. Forensic-evidence collection should be considered for any child with known or suspected sexual contact within 72 hours. Forensic evidence obtained directly from a prepubertal victim's body diminishes greatly after 24 hours, with the best chance for evidence collection coming from bed linens or the child's underwear (Christian et al., 2000).

The female genital examination should include a description of the vulva, hymen, and surrounding tissue. Abnormal findings of concern are injuries to the posterior vulva or the lower half of the hymenal ring, or abrasions, bruising, or bleeding of the genital or anal tissue. It is often helpful to use a magnifying instrument (colposcope) to detect subtle injuries. There are many variants of normal findings for female genital anatomy, so it is recommended that the examination be done by a practitioner experienced with these types of cases. Contrary to popular myth, the size of the hymenal opening is not predictive of the likelihood of sexual abuse (Christian & Rubin, 2002).

For male victims, presence of swelling, abrasions, or bruising of the genital tissue is of concern for abuse. The anal area should be examined for symmetry, tone, fissures, or scars.

Genital tissue heals quickly and most often without scars. Therefore, unless seen within a few days of injury, the genital tissue may appear normal. In addition, the vaginal and anal mucosa is elastic; therefore penetration without disruption of tissue is possible. This defies another myth that there is always evidence of female virginity.

Nursing Care Management

Protect Child From Further Abuse

Initially, identification of instances of suspected abuse or neglect is essential. The nurse may come in contact with abused children in an emergency department, practitioner's office, home, day care centre, or school.

NURSING ALERT The priority is to remove the child from the abusive situation to prevent further injury.

A court proceeding may be necessary before the child can be placed outside the home or when parental rights are to be terminated. When the courts are involved, they usually require firsthand testimony by the referring parties. Nurses may be subpoenaed to appear in court, or their notes may be introduced as evidence in court hearings. Accurate and factual documentation is essential. Behaviours need to be described, not interpreted, and are recorded daily to establish a progress record (see Guidelines box). Conversations among the nurse, child, and parent should be recorded verbatim as much as possible.

Support Child

Children suspected of being abused are often hospitalized for medical management of their injuries and to allow further assessment of their safety needs. The needs of these children are the same as those of any hospitalized child. The child should be treated as a child with the usual physical needs, **developmental tasks**, and play interests—not as a victim of abuse. The goal of the nurse–child relationship is to provide a role model for the parents in helping them relate positively and constructively to their child and to foster a therapeutic environment for the child in his or her reprieve from the abusing situation.

Support Family

The nurse also needs to encourage the child's relationship with the nonoffending parent. The nurse does not become a substitute parent, but rather acts as a role model for parents

GUIDELINES Recording Assessment Data in Suspected Abuse

History of Injury
- Date, time, and place of occurrence
- Sequence of events with recorded times
- Presence of witnesses, especially person caring for child at time of incident
- Time lapse between occurrence of injury and initiation of treatment
- Interview with child when appropriate, including verbal quotations and information from drawing or other play activities
- Interview with parent, witnesses, or other significant persons, including verbal quotations
- Description of parent–child interactions (verbal interactions, eye contact, touching, parental concern)
- Name, age, and condition of other children in home (if possible)

Physical Examination
- Location, size, shape, and colour of bruises; approximate location, size, and shape on drawing of body outline
- Distinguishing characteristics, such as a bruise in the shape of a hand, or a round burn (possibly caused by cigarette)
- Symmetry or asymmetry of injury; presence of other injuries
- Degree of pain; any bone tenderness
- Evidence of past injuries; general state of health and hygiene
- Developmental level of child; perform screening test (see Developmental Assessment, Chapter 34)

in helping them to relate positively and constructively to their child. When parental ignorance of childrearing practices has played a part in the abuse, the nurse can educate the parent about children's physical and emotional needs. Because of the parents' own childrearing, they may not be aware of nonviolent methods of discipline, such as time-out. They may also need help in dealing with their frustration so that they do not vent anger on the child. Because these parents may be sensitive to criticism or perceptions of domination, teaching is best implemented through demonstration and example rather than through lecturing. Any competent parenting abilities they demonstrate should be praised to promote their sense of parental adequacy.

Family members should be advised to encourage the child to resume normal activities and observe the child for signs of distress. Children express their feelings primarily through behaviour. Parents should be alert for changes in behaviour that indicate distress resulting from the incident, such as remaining in the house, refusing to go to school, changing sleeping patterns, and having more frequent dreams and nightmares. Children should be encouraged to talk about these feelings and nightmares, because the more they talk about the experience, the more they are able to gain control over it.

Referral to appropriate social service agencies is also essential. Many abusive parents live in poverty, and the daily stresses imposed by their circumstances are overwhelming. Resources for financial aid, improved housing, and child care should be sought. Self-help groups can also provide important services. Groups such as Parents Anonymous (a group for parents who have abused or fear that they may abuse their child, but only in terms of physical abuse, not sexual abuse) and Parents United International, Inc. (a group devoted to helping sexually abused families) are accepting and nonjudgemental (see Additional Resources at the end of this chapter).

Plan for Discharge

Discharge planning should begin as soon as the legal disposition for placement has been decided, which may be temporary foster home placement, return to the parents, or permanent termination of parental rights. The latter is the most drastic solution but is necessary in situations of life-threatening abuse. Whenever children are sent to a foster home or juvenile institution, they must be allowed an opportunity to express their feelings. No matter how severe the abuse, they usually mourn the loss of their parents. They need help in understanding why they must not return home and that this new home is in no way a punishment. Whenever possible, foster parents should be encouraged to visit the child in the hospital, and the nurse should take an active role in helping these new parents understand the child.

Some abused children continue to live in torment when they are inadvertently placed in a foster home where they may endure worse circumstances than those in their original home. Being sent from one foster home to another, even if the homes have loving foster parents, can also be distressing to these children. Only through constant evaluation of the placement residence and the child's adjustment to a new environment can the vicious circle of abuse, abandonment, and neglect be stopped.

Prevent Abuse

Prevention of child maltreatment has been an extremely difficult goal. Programs aimed at identifying potential abusers and instituting supportive intervention before the occurrence of an abusive act have met with variable success. However, nurses have played an important role in such programs. For example, home visits by nurses to primiparas who were either teenagers, unmarried, or of low socioeconomic status was noted to be an effective preventive measure (Eckenrode et al., 2000; McMillian, 2000). The nurses provided information on normal child growth and development and routine health care needs, served as informal support persons, and referred families to appropriate services when a need for assistance was identified.

Such programs provide models that can be used to reduce factors that increase the risk of abuse. Nurses in a variety of settings can implement similar activities. For example, nurses in prenatal clinics can prepare expectant families for adjustment to parenthood. Nursery and postpartum nurses can foster the attachment process by encouraging parents to hold and look at their infant and practise skin-to-skin-contact, as well as by teaching **coping** mechanisms for prolonged crying. Nurses in neonatal intensive care units can minimize the effects of separation by encouraging parents to visit the infant and can help parents become comfortable caring for their child. Nurses in ambulatory settings can teach parents appropriate methods of bathing, feeding, toileting, disciplining, and

FAMILY-CENTRED TEACHING

Preventing or Dealing With Sexual Abuse of Children

Sexual assault of children is much more common than most people realize. It may be preventable if children have good preparation. To provide protection and preparation, the following measures can be taken:

- Pay careful attention to who is around children. (Unwanted touch may come from someone liked and trusted.)
- Back up a child's right to say "no."
- Encourage communication by taking seriously what children say.
- Take a second look at signals of potential danger.
- Refuse to leave children in the company of those not trusted.
- Include information about sexual assault when teaching about safety.
- Provide specific definitions and examples of sexual assault.
- Remind children that even "nice" people sometimes do mean things.
- Urge children to tell about anybody who causes them to be uncomfortable.
- Prepare children to deal with bribes, threats, and possible physical force.
- Virtually eliminate secrets between children and parents.
- Teach children how to say "no," ask for help, and control who touches them and how.
- Model self-protective and limit-setting behaviour for children.

Should it ever become necessary to help a child recover from a sexual assault:

- Listen carefully to understand children.
- Support the child for telling through praise, belief, sympathy, and lack of blame.
- Know local resources and choose help carefully.
- Provide opportunities to talk about the assault.
- Provide opportunities for the entire family to go through a recovery process.

Sexual assault affects everyone. To help deal with this social problem:

- Provide care and support to those who have been victimized.
- Recognize that offenders do not change without intervention.
- Organize neighbourhood programs to support each other's efforts to protect children.
- Encourage schools to provide information about sexual assault as a problem of health and safety.
- Organize community groups to support educational treatment and law enforcement programs.

(Modified from Adams, C., & Fay, J. [1981]. *No more secrets: Protecting your child from sexual assault*. San Luis Obispo, CA: Impact.)

preventing injuries, while stressing the normal needs and developmental characteristics of children. Nurses must be sensitive to parental needs for attention, reassurance, and reinforcement, and refer parents to community services and self-help groups.

Unlike preventive efforts for neglect and physical abuse, which are aimed at the potential offender, *prevention of child sexual abuse* centres on education of children to protect themselves. Materials are available for parents that describe sexual abuse and its prevention (see Additional Resources). Supporting parental qualities of respect, affection, empathy, and ability to set boundaries, and providing high-quality child care and education, represent the true preventive approach to sexual abuse. Helpful games such as "What if the baby-sitter wants to wrestle and hug but tells you to keep it a secret?" can be used to explore dangerous situations in advance and help children learn the importance of saying "no." They need reassurance that no matter what the other person says or does, the parents want to know about it and will not punish them. Even if children participate in the activity before telling the parents, they must be reassured that it was not their fault.

It is equally important to teach children safety in terms of potential risk situations. Several suggestions for parents regarding protecting and educating children against possible molestation are presented in the Family-Centred Teaching box. The nurse is frequently in a position to discuss the topic of abuse with parents and to provide guidelines.

Key Points

- The preschool years consist of the period from 3 to 5 years of age, a time considered critical for emotional and psychological development.
- Biological development in the preschool period is characterized by mature body systems and refinement in gross and fine motor behaviour, as evidenced by activities such as running, riding a tricycle, and drawing.
- According to Erikson, acquiring a sense of initiative is the chief psychosocial task of the preschooler. Development of the superego occurs during this period, as conscience begins to emerge.
- According to Piaget, the preschool age is characterized by intuitive (or prelogical) thinking and a move toward logical thought processes through advanced, complex learning; language; and understanding of causality.
- The seeds of moral development are planted during the preschool period. According to Kohlberg, these children are in the stage of naive instrumental orientation, in which they are concerned with satisfying their own needs and, less frequently, the needs of others.
- Social development includes further separation–individuation; more sophisticated language; greater independence; and more complex, imaginative forms of play.
- Areas of special concern to parents during the preschool period are the preschool and kindergarten experience, sex education, fears, stress, and speech problems.
- In selecting an early learning program, parents should inquire about daily activities, teacher qualifications,

accreditation, student–staff ratio, safety, meals, fees, and health practices.

- Two rules that govern how parents answer questions about sex and other sensitive issues are to find out what the children know and to be honest.
- Fears constitute a great part of the preschool period; fear of objects or potential annihilation and parent-induced fears are common.
- Preschool aggression may result from frustration, modelling behaviour, and reinforcement.
- Hesitancy or dysfluency in speech patterns is a normal characteristic of language development. Speech problems can occur when parents express excessive concern over this pattern.
- Health promotion continues to be directed toward proper nutrition, adequate sleep, proper dental care, and injury prevention.
- Child maltreatment may take the form of physical abuse or neglect, emotional abuse or neglect, or sexual abuse.
- Parental, child, and environmental characteristics are criteria that may predispose children to maltreatment.
- Identification of abuse entails securing evidence of maltreatment, taking a history pertaining to the incident, and assessing parental and child behaviours.
- The reported incidence of sexual abuse has increased in the past decade; common forms are incest, molestation, rape, exhibitionism, child pornography, child prostitution, and pedophilia.

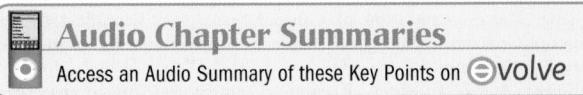

Audio Chapter Summaries
Access an Audio Summary of these Key Points on Evolve

References

Aboriginal Nurses Association & Planned Parenthood Federation of Canada. (2002). *Finding our way: A sexual and reproductive health sourcebook for Aboriginal communities.* Retrieved from http://www.anac.on.ca/sourcebook/part_2_unit_2.htm.

American Academy of Pediatrics, Committee on Infectious Diseases, & Pickering, L. (Ed.). (2009). *2009 red book: Report of the Committee on Infectious Diseases* (28th ed.). Elk Grove Village, IL: Author.

Anderson, D. R., et al. (2001). Early childhood television viewing and adolescent behaviour: The Recontact study. *Monographs of the Society for Research in Child Development, 66*(1), I–VIII, 1–147.

Barlow, S. E., & Expert Committee. (2007). Expert committee recommendations regarding the prevention, assessment, and treatment of child and adolescent overweight and obesity: Summary report. *Pediatrics, 120*(Suppl 4), S164–S192. doi:10.1542/peds.2008-1862

Barnes, L. L., et al. (2000). Spirituality, religion, and pediatrics: Intersecting worlds of healing. *Pediatrics, 104*(6), 899–908.

BC Centre for Disease Control. (2009). *A quick guide to common childhood diseases.* Retrieved from http://www.bccdc.ca/NR/rdonlyres/8061A728-C969-4F38-9082-B0296EF2A128/0/Epid_GF_childhood_quickguide_may_09.pdf.

Bendersky, M., Bennett, D., & Lewis, M. (2006). Aggression at age 5 as a function of prenatal exposure to cocaine, gender, and environmental risk. *Journal of Pediatric Psychology Advance Access, 31*(1), 71–84. doi:10.1093/jpepsy/jsj025

Brazelton, T. B., & Sparrow, J. D. (2001). *Touchpoints 3 to 6: Your child's emotional and behavioural development.* Cambridge, MA: Da Capo Press.

Brown, K. D., & Hamilton-Giachritsis, C. (2005). The influence of violent media on children and adolescents: A public-health approach. *Lancet, 365*(9460), 702–710. doi:10.1016/S0140-6736(05)17952-5

Calam, R., et al. (1998). Psychological disturbances and child sexual abuse: A follow-up study. *Child Abuse & Neglect, 22*(9), 901–913.

Canadian Association of Speech-Language Pathologists and Audiologists. (2012). *Preschool stuttering.* Retrieved from http://www.speechandhearing.ca/en/consumer-info/children/preschool-stuttering.

Canadian Paediatric Society. (2005a). Prevention of varicella in children and adolescents. *Paediatrics and Child Health, 10*(7), 409–412.

Canadian Paediatric Society. (2005b). Sports readiness in children and youth. *Pediatrics and Child Health, 10*(6), 333–334.

Canadian Paediatric Society. (2009). *Early childhood development in Canada: Evidence is there, but dollars are not.* Retrieved from http://www.cps.ca/English/media/NewsReleases/2009/EarlyChildhoodDev.htm.

Canadian Paediatric Society. (2011). A harmonized immunization schedule for Canada: A call for action. *Paediatrics and Child Health, 16*(1), 29–31.

Canadian Paediatric Society, Adolescent Health Committee. (2011). *The sexual abuse of young people with a disability or chronic health condition.* Retrieved from http://www.cps.ca/english/statements/AM/AH11-01.htm#Recommendations.

Canadian Paediatric Society, Healthy Active Living and Sports Medicine Committee. (2012). Healthy active living: Physical activity guidelines for children and adolescents. *Paediatrics and Child Health, 17*(2), 209–210.

Canadian Paediatric Society, Psychosocial Paediatrics Committee. (2003). Impact of media use on children and youth. *Paediatrics and Child Health, 8*(5), 301–306. (Reaffirmed February 2011)

Chen, T. M., et al. (2002). Clinical manifestations of varicella-zoster virus infection. *Dermatology Clinics, 20*(2), 267–282.

Christian, C., et al. (2000). Forensic evidence findings in prepubertal victims of sexual assault. *Pediatrics, 106,* 100–104.

Christian, C. W., & Rubin, D. M. (2002). Sexual abuse. In A. P. Giardino & E. R. Giardino (Eds.), *Recognition of child abuse for the mandated reporter.* St. Louis: GW Medical.

Cleveland, G., Forer, B., Hyatt, D., Japel, C., & Krashinsky, M. (2008). New evidence about child care in Canada: Use patterns, affordability and quality. *IRPP Choices,* 14.

Collin-Vézina, D., Dion, J., & Trocmé, N. (2009) Sexual abuse in Canadian Aboriginal communities: A broad review of conflicting evidence. *Journal of Aboriginal and Indigenous Community Health, 7,* 27–47. Retrieved from http://www.pimatisiwin.com/online/?page_id=609.

Connors, E. A. (2004). Voices from the field—Aggression in young children from a First Nations' perspective. In R. E. Tremblay, R. G. Barr, & R. de V. Peters (Eds.), *Encyclopedia on early childhood development* [online]. Montreal, Québec: Centre of Excellence for Early Childhood Development; 2004, 1–5. Retrieved from http://www.child-encyclopedia.com/documents/ConnorsANGps.pdf.

Cyr, M., et al. (2002). Intrafamilial sexual abuse: Brother–sister incest does not differ from father–daughter incest and stepfather–stepdaughter incest. *Child Abuse and Neglect, 26*(9), 957–973.

Davison, K. K., & Birch, L. L. (2001). Weight status and self-concept in young girls. *Pediatrics, 107*(1), 46–53.

Department of Justice Canada. (2011). *Protecting our children.* Retrieved from http://www.justice.gc.ca/eng/dept-min/pub/dig/prot.html.

Dietitians of Canada, Canadian Paediatric Society, College of Family Physicians of Canada, and Community Health Nurses of Canada. (2010). *Promoting optimal monitoring of child growth in Canada: Using the new WHO growth charts.* Retrieved from http://www.cps.ca/english/statements/N/growth-charts-statement-FULL.pdf.

Eckenrode, J., et al. (2000). Preventing child abuse and neglect with a program of nurse home visitation: The limiting effects of domestic violence. *Journal of the American Medical Association, 284*(11), 1385–1391.

Endres, J., et al. (2003). Soy-enhanced lunch acceptance by preschoolers. *Journal of the American Dietetic Association, 103*(3), 346–351.

Erikson, E. H. (1963). *Childhood and society* (2nd ed.). New York: Norton.

Feldman, H. M. (2005). Evaluation and management of language and speech disorders in preschool children. *Pediatric Reviews, 26*(4), 131–142. doi:10.1542/pir.26-4-131

Finkel, M. A., & DeJong, A. R. (2001). Medical findings in child sexual abuse. In R. M. Reece & S. Ludwig (Eds.), *Child abuse: medical diagnosis and management.* Philadelphia: Lippincott Williams & Wilkins.

Food and Nutrition Board. (2003). *Dietary reference intakes: Guiding principles for nutrition labeling and fortification.* Washington, DC: National Academies Press.

Fosarelli, P. (2003). Children and the development of faith: Implications for pediatric practice. *Contemporary Pediatrics, 20*(1), 85–98.

Gara, M. A., et al. (2000). The abused child as parent: The structure and content of physically abused mothers' perceptions of their babies. *Child Abuse and Neglect, 24*(5), 627–639.

Gershoff, E. T. (2002). Corporal punishment by parents and associated child behaviours and experiences: A meta-analytic and theoretical review. *Psychological Bulletin, 128*(4), 539–579.

Gleason, T. R., Sebanc, A. M., & Hartup, W. W. (2000). Imaginary companions of preschool children. *Developmental Psychology, 36*(4), 419–428.

Goldman, J., et al. (2003). What factors contribute to child abuse and neglect? In J. Goldman, et al. (Eds.), *A coordinated response to child abuse and neglect: The foundation for practice*. Washington, DC: Child Welfare Information. Retrieved from http://www.childwelfare.gov/pubs/usermanuals/foundation/foundatione.cfm.

Health Canada. (2004). *Statistics Canada. Canadian community health survey, cycle 2.2, nutrition—Nutrient intakes from food: Provincial, regional and national data tables*, Vol. 1, 2, & 3 disk. Ottawa: Health Canada Publications. Retrieved from http://www.hc-sc.gc.ca/fn-an/surveill/commun/art-nutr-chil-enf-eng.php#a1.

Health Canada. (2007). *Eating well with Canada's food guide: How much food you need every day*. Retrieved from http://www.hc-sc.gc.ca/fn-an/food-guide-aliment/basics-base/quantit-eng.php.

Health Canada. (2010). *Vitamin D and calcium: Updated dietary reference intakes*. Retrieved from http://www.hc-sc.gc.ca/fn-an/nutrition/vitamin/vita-d-eng.php#t5.

Hornor, G. (2001). Repeated sexual abuse allegations: A problem for primary care providers. *Journal of Pediatric Health Care, 15*(2), 71–76.

Hospital for Sick Children. (2010). *About kids health. Pertussis (whooping cough)*. Retrieved from http://www.aboutkidshealth.ca/En/HealthAZ/ConditionsandDiseases/InfectiousDiseases/Pages/Pertussis(WhoopingCough).aspx.

Jellinek, M., Patel, B. P., & Froehle, M. C. (Eds.). (2002). *Bright futures in practice: Mental health*, Vol. 1. Arlington, VA: National Centre for Education in Maternal and Child Health.

Johnson, M. (2003). Child sexual abuse. In D. O. Thomas, L. M. Bernardo, & B. Herman (Eds.), *Core curriculum for pediatric emergency nursing*. Sudbury, MA: Jones & Bartlett.

Johnson, R. K. (2000). Changing eating and physical activity patterns of U.S. children. *Proceedings of the Nutrition Society, 59*(2), 295–301.

Leider, H. S., et al. (2005). Munchausen syndrome by proxy: A case report. *AACN Clinical Issues 16*(2), 178–184.

Leung, A. K., Robson, W. L., & Leong, A. G. (2006). Herpes zoster in childhood. *Journal of Pediatric Health Care, 20*(5), 300–303.

Martof, A. (2001). Consultation with the specialist: Dental care. *Pediatric Review, 22*(1), 13–15.

McClain, N., et al. (2000). Evaluation of sexual abuse in the pediatric patient. *Journal of Pediatric Health Care, 14*(3), 93–102.

McEvoy, M. (2003). Culture and spirituality as an integrated concept in pediatric care. *MCN. American Journal of Maternal Child Nursing, 28*(1), 39–43.

McMillian, H. (2000). Child maltreatment: What we know in the year 2000. *Canadian Journal of Psychiatry, 45*(8), 702–709.

Needlman, R. (2004). Growth and development: Preschool years. In R. E. Behrman, R. M. Kliegman, & H. B. Jenson (Eds.), *Nelson textbook of pediatrics* (17th ed.). Philadelphia: Saunders.

Nipissing District Developmental Screen. (2011). Retrieved from http://www.ndds.ca/canada.

Parliament of Canada. (2002). *Bill C-15A: An act to amend the criminal code and to amend other acts*. Retrieved from http://www.parl.gc.ca/About/Parliament/LegislativeSummaries/bills_ls.asp?ls=C15A&Parl=37&Ses=1#2.%C2%A0%20Child.

Piaget, J. (1952). *Origins of intelligence in children*. New York: International Universities Press.

Public Health Agency of Canada. (2001). *Child maltreatment in Canada: Canadian incidence study of reported child abuse and neglect: Highlights*. Report prepared by Nico Trocmé and David Wolfe (p. 13). Ottawa: Minister of Public Works and Government Services Canada.

Public Health Agency of Canada. (2006). *Canadian immunization guide* (7th ed.). Retrieved from http://www.phac-aspc.gc.ca/publicat/cig-gci/index-eng.php.

Public Health Agency of Canada. (2008). *Canadian incidence study of reported child abuse and neglect—2008*. Retrieved from http://www.phac-aspc.gc.ca/cm-vee/csca-ecve/2008/fs-am/pdf/csca-2008-fact-sheet.pdf.

Public Health Agency of Canada. (2009). *Child abuse: A fact sheet from the Department of Justice Canada*. Retrieved from http://www.justice.gc.ca/eng/pi/fv-vf/facts-info/child-enf.html.

Public Health Agency of Canada. (2010). *Canadian incidence study of reported child abuse and neglect, 2008*. Retrieved from http://www.phac-aspc.gc.ca/cm-vee/csca-ecve/2008/cis-eci-07-eng.php#c3-3.

Public Health Agency of Canada. (2011a). *Aboriginal Head Start in urban and northern communities*. Retrieved from http://www.hc-sc.gc.ca/fniah-spnia/famil/develop/ahsor-papa_intro-eng.php.

Public Health Agency of Canada. (2011b). *A to z infection diseases*. Retrieved from http://www.phac-aspc.gc.ca/id-mi/az-index-eng.php#varicella.

Putnam, F. W. (2003). Ten year update review: Child sexual abuse. *Journal of the American Academy of Child and Adolescent Psychiatry, 42*(3), 269–278.

Smith, A., Stewart, D., Peled, M., Poon, C., Saewyc, E., & the McCreary Centre Society (2009). *A picture of health: Highlights of the 2008 British Columbia adolescent health survey*. Vancouver, BC: McCreary Centre Society. Retrieved from http://www.mcs.bc.ca/pdf/AHSIV_APictureOfHealth.pdf.

Spear, B. A., et al. (2007). Recommendations for treatment of child and adolescent overweight and obesity. *Pediatrics, 120*(Suppl 4), S254–S288. doi:10.1542/peds.2007-2329F

Statistics Canada. (2004). *Family violence in Canada: A statistical profile* (Cat. no. 85-224-XIE, p. 16). Retrieved from http://www.statcan.ca/english/freepub/85-224-XIE/free.htm.

Story, M., Holt, K., & Sofka, D. (Eds.). (2002). *Bright futures in practice: Nutrition* (2nd ed.). Arlington, VA: National Centre for Education in Maternal and Child Health.

Thiedke, C. C. (2001). Sleep disorders and sleep problems in childhood. *American Family Physician, 63*(2), 277–284.

Yang, H. M., Mao, M., & Wan, C. (2005). Vitamin A for treating measles in children. *Cochrane Database of Systematic Reviews, Issue 4. Art. No. CD001479*. doi:10.1002/14651858.CD001479.pub3

Additional Resources

Aboriginal Nurses Association of Canada: Sexual and Reproductive Health Issues of Concern to Aboriginal People: http://www.anac.on.ca/sourcebook/part_2_unit_2.htm

Attachment Across Cultures: Sleeping, Culture, and Attachment: http://www.attachmentacrosscultures.org/beliefs/sleeping.pdf

Canadian Centre for Child Protection—Family education; has a sexual abuse hotline: http://www.protectchildren.ca/app/en/home

Canadian Federation for Sexual Health: http://www.cfsh.ca/

Canadian Paediatric Society: Chickenpox: http://www.caringforkids.cps.ca/immunization/ChickenpoxFacts.htm

Canadian Society for Exercise Physiology—Recommendations for healthy television viewing: http://www.csep.ca/CMFiles/Guidelines/SBGuidelinesBackgrounder_EY2012_E.pdf

Child Abuse Prevention Web site—Resources for family education on preventing abuse; helpline: http://www.safekidsbc.ca/links.htm

Department of Justice Canada: Age of Sexual Consent: http://www.justice.gc.ca/eng/dept-min/clp/faq.html

Encyclopedia of Early Childhood Development—Information on Canadian child development and behaviour: http://www.child-encyclopedia.com/en-ca/child-aggression/perspectives.html?RId=CA&CId=169

Families Anonymous—For relatives and friends concerned about drug use and related behaviours: http://familiesanonymous.org/

Human Early Learning Partnerships (HELP): http://www.earlylearning.ubc.ca

Kids Help Phone—Phone line that children can call to reach a counsellor, 24 hours a day, across Canada: http://www.kidshelpphone.ca/teens/home/splash.aspx; phone 1-888-668-6868

Nipissing District Developmental Screen—Available at P.O. Box 1493, North Bay, ON, P1B 8K6; 705-752-5081 or 1-888-582-0944; e-mail ndds@xplornet.com: http://www.ndds.ca/canada/

Parents Anonymous: http://www.parentsanonymous.org/

Parents United: http://parents_united.tripod.com/Chapters/canada.htm

Public Health Agency of Canada: Child Maltreatment: http://www.phac-aspc.gc.ca/cm-vee/

Quick and Fun Learning Activities books (suggestions on mutual play), Teacher Created Resources: http://www.teachercreated.com.

Unit 9

39

The School-Age Child and Family

Learning Objectives

On completion of this chapter, the reader will be able to:

- Describe the physical, cognitive, and moral changes that take place during the middle childhood years.
- Describe ways to help a child develop a sense of accomplishment.
- Demonstrate an understanding of the changing interpersonal relationships of school-age children.
- Discuss the role of the peer group in the socialization of the school-age child.
- Discuss the role of schools in the development and socialization of the school-age child.
- Demonstrate an understanding of the types, causes, and prevention of sports injuries in middle childhood.
- Describe the most common causes of growth and maturation failure in later childhood.
- Discuss the manifestations and nursing management of selected emotional and behavioural problems.
- Outline an appropriate health teaching plan for the school-age child.
- Plan a sex education session for a group of school-age children.
- Identify the causes and discuss the preventive aspects of injury in middle childhood.
- Describe health concerns of particular relevance to school-age children of First Nations, Métis, and Inuit background.

Electronic Resources

Additional information related to the content in Chapter 39 can be found on

evolve **the companion Web site at**

http://evolve.elsevier.com/Canada/Perry/maternal/

- Examination Review Questions
- Assessment Video Clips
- Case Study—Attention-Deficit/Hyperactivity Disorder
- Case Study—Injury Prevention
- Critical Thinking Exercise—Turner Syndrome

Promoting Optimum Growth and Development

The segment of the lifespan that extends from age 6 years to approximately 12 years has a variety of labels, each of which describes an important characteristic of the period. These middle years are most often referred to as *school-age* or the *school years*. This period begins with entrance into the school environment, which has a significant impact on children's development and relationships.

While much of this chapter is devoted to the biological, social, emotional, and cognitive changes that occur throughout the school-age years, nurses must also pay attention to other vital factors that influence these children's health and well-being. For example, as is true for younger children, the health of school-age children is strongly related to life circumstances, of which family income remains a strong factor (Raphael, 2010).

While the biological, social, emotional, and cognitive changes discussed throughout the chapter help us understand development during the school-age years, limiting our attention to these aspects of children's lives may divert our attention from vital differences affecting health and well-being. School-age children vary in many ways according to race, gender, ethnicity, and class, and these differences have important implications. In nursing care, failing to account for these differences may lead to well-intentioned but ineffective practices.

Thus, in this chapter, as we discuss **growth** and development in the school-age years, we will do so in the context of these differences and reflect on how nurses can support children and their families in ways that attend to diversity while acknowledging the developmental changes that are ongoing in these children's lives.

Biological Development

Physiologically the middle years begin with the shedding of the first deciduous tooth and end at **puberty** with the acquisition of the final permanent teeth (with the exception of the wisdom teeth). Before 5 or 6 years of age, children have progressed from helpless infants to sturdy, complicated individuals with an ability to communicate, conceptualize in a limited way, and become involved in complex social and motor behaviours. Physical growth is also rapid during the preschool-age years. In contrast, the period of middle childhood, between the rapid growth of early childhood and the prepubescent growth spurt, is a time of gradual growth and development with more even progress in both physical and emotional aspects.

During middle childhood, growth in height and weight assumes a slower but steady pace as compared with that of the earlier years. Between ages 6 and 12, children will grow an average of 5 cm per year to gain 30 to 60 cm in height and will almost double their weight, increasing 2 to 3 kg per year. The average 6-year-old child is about 116 cm tall and weighs about 21 kg; the average 12-year-old child is about 150 cm tall and weighs approximately 40 kg. During this period, girls and boys differ little in size, although boys tend to be slightly taller and heavier than girls. Toward the end of the school-age years, both boys and girls begin to increase in size, although most girls begin to surpass boys in both height and weight.

Proportional Changes

School-age children are more coordinated than they were as preschoolers, and steadier on their feet. Their body proportions take on a slimmer look, with longer legs, varying body proportion, and a lower centre of gravity. Posture improves over that of the preschool period to facilitate locomotion and efficiency in using the arms and trunk. These proportions make climbing, bicycle riding, and other activities easier. Fat gradually diminishes, and its distribution patterns change, contributing to the thinner appearance of the child during the middle years.

Accompanying the skeletal lengthening and fat diminution is an increase in the percentage of body weight represented by muscle tissue. By the end of this age period, both boys and girls double their strength and physical capabilities, and their steady and relatively consistent development of coordination increases their poise and skill. However, this increased strength can be misleading. Although strength increases, muscles are still functionally immature when compared with those of the adolescent, and they are more readily damaged by muscular injury caused by overuse.

The most pronounced changes that indicate increasing maturity in children are a decrease in head circumference in relation to standing height, a decrease in waist circumference in relation to height, and an increase in leg length in relation to height. These observations often provide a clue to a child's degree of physical maturity and have proved useful in predicting readiness for meeting the demands of school. Physical indications of maturity appear to be correlated with success in school.

Specific physiological and anatomical characteristics are typical of children in middle childhood. Facial proportions change as the face grows faster in relation to the remainder of the cranium. The skull and brain grow very slowly during this period and increase little in size. Because all of the primary (deciduous) teeth are lost during this age span, middle childhood is sometimes known as the age of the loose tooth (Fig. 39-1). In the early years of middle childhood, the new secondary (permanent) teeth appear to be too large for the face.

Maturation of Systems

Maturity of the gastrointestinal system is reflected in fewer stomach upsets; better maintenance of blood glucose levels; and an increased stomach capacity, which permits retention of food for longer periods. The school-age child does not need to be fed as carefully, as promptly, or as frequently as the preschool-age child. Caloric needs are less than what they were in the preschool years.

Physical maturation is evident in other body tissues and organs. Bladder capacity, although differing widely among individual children, is generally greater in girls than in boys. The heart grows more slowly during the middle years and is smaller in relation to the rest of the body than at any other period of life. Heart and respiratory rates steadily decrease and blood pressure increases from ages 6 to 12 (see Appendix E).

The immune system becomes more competent in its ability to localize infections and to produce an **antibody–antigen** response. However, children may have several infections in the first 1 to 2 years of school because of increased exposure to other children.

Bones continue to ossify throughout childhood but yield to pressure and muscle pulls more readily than with mature

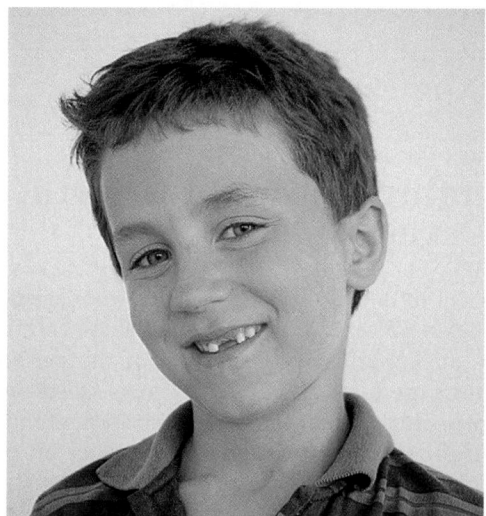

Fig. 39-1 Middle childhood is the stage of development when deciduous teeth are shed.

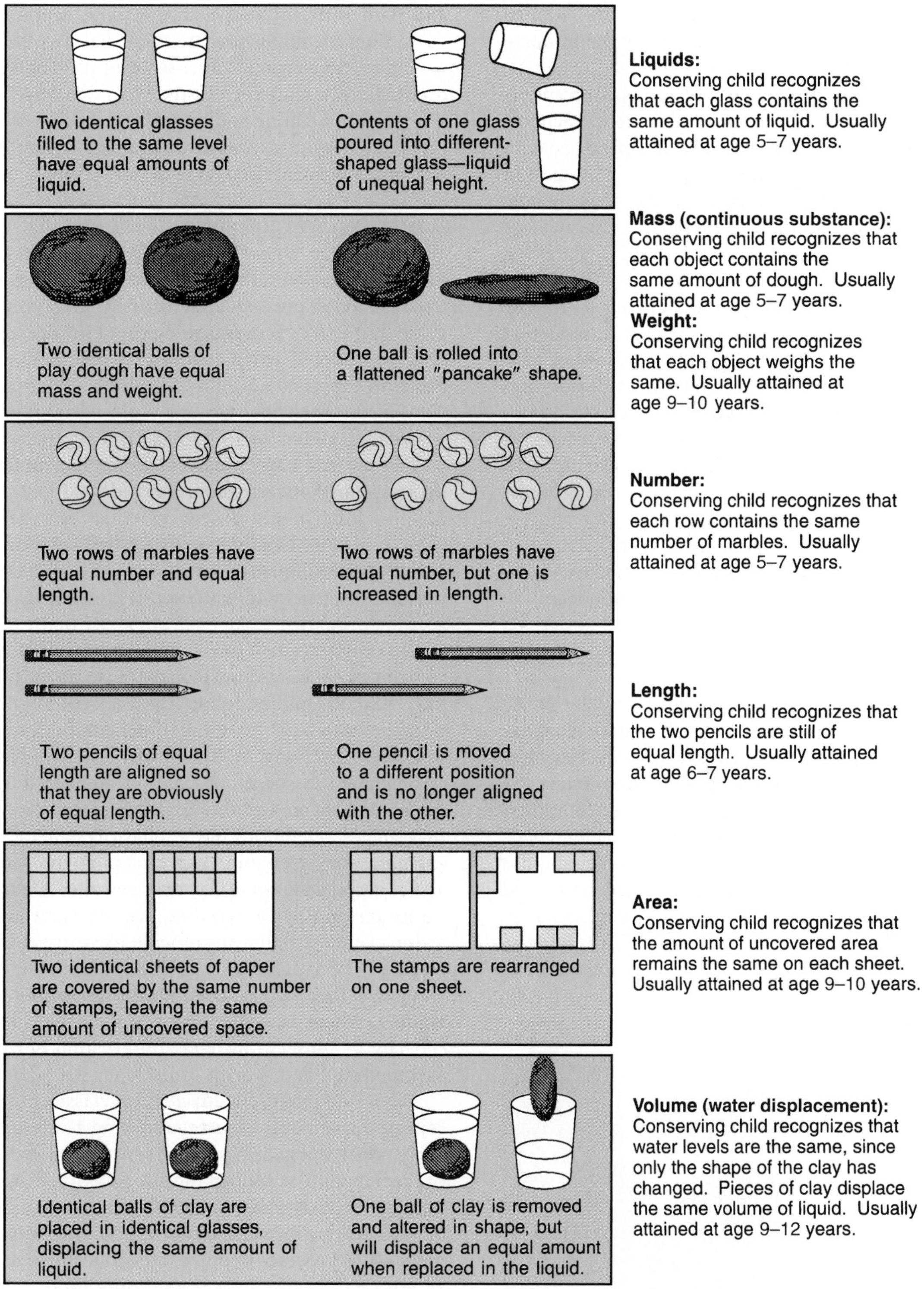
Two identical glasses filled to the same level have equal amounts of liquid.
Contents of one glass poured into different-shaped glass—liquid of unequal height.
Liquids:
Conserving child recognizes that each glass contains the same amount of liquid. Usually attained at age 5–7 years.
Two identical balls of play dough have equal mass and weight.
One ball is rolled into a flattened "pancake" shape.
Mass (continuous substance):
Conserving child recognizes that each object contains the same amount of dough. Usually attained at age 5–7 years.
Weight:
Conserving child recognizes that each object weighs the same. Usually attained at age 9–10 years.
Two rows of marbles have equal number and equal length.
Two rows of marbles have equal number, but one is increased in length.
Number:
Conserving child recognizes that each row contains the same number of marbles. Usually attained at age 5–7 years.
Two pencils of equal length are aligned so that they are obviously of equal length.
One pencil is moved to a different position and is no longer aligned with the other.
Length:
Conserving child recognizes that the two pencils are still of equal length. Usually attained at age 6–7 years.
Two identical sheets of paper are covered by the same number of stamps, leaving the same amount of uncovered space.
The stamps are rearranged on one sheet.
Area:
Conserving child recognizes that the amount of uncovered area remains the same on each sheet. Usually attained at age 9–10 years.
Identical balls of clay are placed in identical glasses, displacing the same amount of liquid.
One ball of clay is removed and altered in shape, but will displace an equal amount when replaced in the liquid.
Volume (water displacement):
Conserving child recognizes that water levels are the same, since only the shape of the clay has changed. Pieces of clay displace the same volume of liquid. Usually attained at age 9–12 years.

Fig. 39-3 Common examples that demonstrate the child's ability to conserve (ages are only approximate).

tell time, to see the relationship of events in time (history) and places in space (geography), and to combine time and space relationships (geology and astronomy).

The ability to read is usually achieved during the school years and becomes the most significant and valuable tool for independent inquiry. Children's capacity to explore, imagine, and expand their knowledge is enhanced by reading.

Moral Development (Kohlberg)

As children move from **egocentrism** to more logical patterns of thought, they also move through stages in the development of conscience and moral standards. According to Kohlberg (1968), young children do not believe that standards of behaviour come from within themselves but that rules are established and set down by others. During the preschool years, family unit. These initial experiences prepared the child to engage in experiences and relationships beyond the intimate family group.

A sense of industry, or a stage of accomplishment, is achieved somewhere between age 6 and adolescence. School-age children are eager to develop skills and participate in meaningful and socially useful work. They acquire a sense of personal and interpersonal competence; receive the systematic instruction prescribed by their individual cultures; and develop the skills needed to become useful, contributing members of their social communities.

Interests expand in the middle years, and with a growing sense of independence, children want to engage in tasks that can be carried through to completion (Fig. 39-2). They gain satisfaction from independent behaviour in exploring and manipulating their environment and from interaction with peers. Often the acquisition of skills provides a way to achieve success in social activities. Reinforcement in the form of grades, material rewards, additional privileges, and recognition provides encouragement and stimulation.

A sense of accomplishment also involves the ability to cooperate, to compete with others, and to cope effectively with people. Middle childhood is the time when children learn the value of doing things with others and the benefits derived from division of labour in the accomplishment of goals. Peer approval is a strong motivating power.

The threat inherent in this period of development is the occurrence of situations that might result in a sense of inferiority. Children with physical and mental limitations may be at a disadvantage in the acquisition of certain skills. When the reward structure is based on evidence of mastery, children who are incapable of developing these skills risk feeling inadequate and inferior. Even children without chronic disabilities may experience feelings of inadequacy in some areas. No child is able to do everything well, and children must learn that they will not be able to master every skill they attempt. All children, even children who usually have positive attitudes toward work and their own abilities, will feel some degree of inferiority when they encounter specific skills that they cannot master.

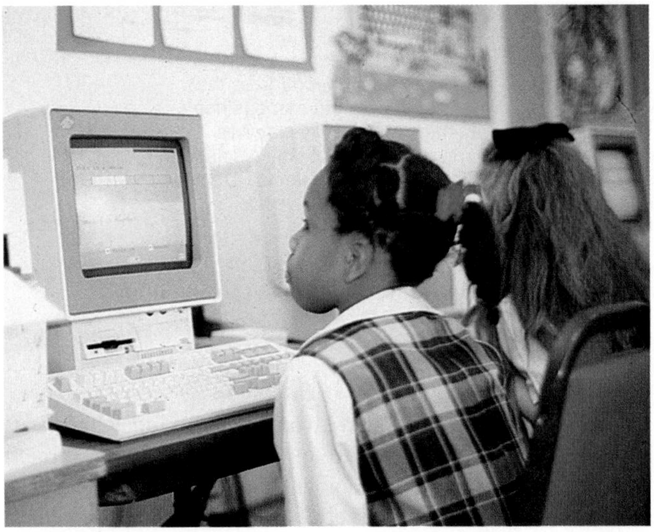

Fig. 39-2 School-age children are motivated to complete tasks working alone.

Children need and want a sense of real achievement. Children achieve a sense of industry when they have access to tasks that need to be done and when they are able to complete the tasks well despite individual differences in their innate capacities and emotional development.

Cognitive Development (Piaget)

When children enter the school years, they begin to acquire the ability to relate a series of events to mental representations that can be expressed both verbally and symbolically (see Table 39-1). This is the stage Piaget (1952) describes as "concrete operations," when children are able to use thought processes to experience events and actions. The rigid, **egocentric** view of the preschool years is replaced by mental processes that allow children to see things from another's point of view.

During this stage, children develop an understanding of relationships between things and ideas. They progress from making **judgements** based on what they see (perceptual thinking) to making judgements based on what they reason (conceptual thinking). They are able to master symbols and to use their memories of past experiences to evaluate and interpret the present.

One cognitive task of school-age children is mastering the concept of conservation (Fig. 39-3). At an early age (about 5 to 7 years), children grasp the concept of reversibility of numbers as a basis for simple mathematics problems (e.g., $2 + 4 = 6$ and $6 - 4 = 2$). They learn that simply altering their arrangement in space does not change certain properties of the environment, and they are able to resist perceptual cues that suggest alterations in the physical state of an object. For example, they recognize that changing the shape of a substance such as a lump of clay does not alter its total mass. They no longer perceive a tall, thin glass of water as containing a greater volume than a short, wide glass; they can distinguish between the weights of items regardless of their size. They recognize that size is not necessarily related to weight or volume. There is a developmental sequence in children's capacity to conserve matter. Conservation of mass usually is accomplished first, weight some time later, and volume last.

School-age children also develop classification skills. They can group and sort objects according to the attributes they share, place things in a sensible and logical order, and hold a concept in mind while making decisions based on that concept. Another characteristic of middle childhood is that children derive enjoyment from classifying and ordering their environment. They become occupied with collections of objects, such as stickers, shells, dolls, cars, cards, and stuffed animals. Depending on their cultural background, they may even begin to order friends and relationships (e.g., best friend, second-best friend).

They also develop the ability to understand relational terms and concepts, such as bigger and smaller; darker and paler; heavier and lighter; to the right of and to the left of; first, last, and intermediate relationships; and more than and less than.

School-age children learn the alphabet and the world of symbols called words, which can be arranged in terms of structure and their relationship to the alphabet. They learn to

Table 39-1 Growth and Development During School-Age Years—cont'd

PHYSICAL AND MOTOR	MENTAL	ADAPTIVE	PERSONAL-SOCIAL
Age 7 Yr			
Begins to grow at least 5 cm in height per year Weight 17.7-30 kg Height 112-130 cm Maxillary central incisors and lateral mandibular incisors erupt More cautious in approaches to new activities Repeats performances to master them Jaw begins to expand to accommodate permanent teeth	Notices that certain items are missing from pictures Can accurately copy a diamond Repeats three numbers backward Develops concept of time; reads ordinary clock or watch correctly to nearest quarter hour; uses clock for practical purposes Attends second grade More mechanical in reading; often does not stop at the end of a sentence; skips words such as "it," "the," and "he"	Uses table knife for cutting meat; may need help with tough or difficult pieces Brushes and combs hair acceptably without help Likes to help and have a choice Is less resistant and stubborn	Is becoming an active member of the family group Takes part in group play Boys prefer playing with boys; girls prefer playing with girls Spends a lot of time alone; does not require a lot of companionship
Ages 8–9 Yr			
Continues to gain 5 cm in height per year Weight 19.5-39.5 kg Height 117-142 cm Lateral incisors (maxillary) and mandibular cuspids erupt Movement is fluid; often graceful and poised Always on the go; jumps, chases, skips Increased smoothness and speed in fine motor control; uses cursive writing Dresses self completely Likely to overdo; hard to quiet down after recess More limber; bones grow faster than ligaments	Gives similarities and differences between two things from memory Counts backward from 20 to 1; understands concept of reversibility Repeats days of the week and months in order; knows the date Describes common objects in detail, not merely their use Makes change out of a quarter Attends third and fourth grades Reads more; may plan to wake up early just to read Reads classic books, but also enjoys comics More aware of time; can be relied on to get to school on time Can grasp concepts of parts and whole (fractions) Understands concepts of space, cause and effect, nesting (puzzles), conservation (permanence of mass and volume) Classifies objects by more than one quality; has collections Produces simple paintings or drawings	Makes use of common tools such as a hammer, saw, screwdriver Uses household and sewing utensils Helps with routine household tasks such as dusting and sweeping Assumes responsibility for share of household chores Looks after all of own needs at the table Buys useful articles; exercises some choice in making purchases Runs useful errands Likes pictorial magazines Likes school; wants to answer all the questions Is afraid of failing a grade; is ashamed of bad grades Is more critical of self Takes music and sport lessons	Is easy to get along with at home Likes the reward system Dramatizes Is more sociable Is better behaved Is interested in boy-girl relationships but will not admit it Goes about home and community freely, alone or with friends Likes to compete and play games Shows preference in friends and groups Plays mostly with groups of own sex but is beginning to mix Develops modesty Compares self with others Enjoys organizations, clubs, and group sports
Ages 10–12 Yr			
Weight 24.5-58 kg Height 127-162.5 cm Posture is more similar to an adult's; will overcome lordosis Remainder of teeth will erupt and tend toward full development (except wisdom teeth) Girls—Pubescent changes may begin to appear; body lines soften and round out Boys—Slow growth in height and rapid weight gain; may become obese in this period	Writes brief stories Attends fifth to seventh grades Writes occasional short letters to friends or relatives on own initiative Uses telephone for practical purposes Responds to magazine, television, or other advertising Reads for practical information or own enjoyment—stories or library books of adventure or romance, animal stories	Makes useful tools or does easy repair work Cooks or sews in small way Raises pets Washes and dries own hair; is responsible for a thorough job of cleaning hair, but may need reminding to do so Is sometimes left alone at home for an hour or so Is successful in looking after own needs or those of other children left in his or her care	Loves friends; talks about them constantly Chooses friends more selectively; may have a "best friend" Enjoys conversation Develops beginning interest in opposite sex (if heterosexual) Is more diplomatic Likes family; family has significant meaning Likes mother and wants to please her in many ways Demonstrates affection Likes father, who is admired and may be idolized Respects parents

bones. Children need ample opportunity to move around and should observe caution in carrying heavy loads. For example, they should shift books or tote bags from one arm to the other or consider backpacks that distribute weight more evenly.

Wider differences between children are observed at the end of middle childhood than at the beginning. These differences become increasingly apparent and, if they are extreme or unique, may create emotional problems. The associated characteristics of height and weight relationships, rapid or slow growth, and other important features of development should be discussed with children and their families. Physical maturity is not necessarily correlated with emotional and social maturity. Seven-year-old children who look like 10-year-old children will, in fact, think and act like 7-year-old children. To expect behaviours appropriate for the older age is unrealistic and can be detrimental to the development of competence and **self-esteem**. Conversely, to treat 10-year-old children who look young physically as though they were younger is an equal disservice to them.

Prepubescence

Preadolescence is the period of approximately 2 years that begins at the end of middle childhood and ends with the thirteenth birthday. Because puberty signals the beginning of the development of secondary sex characteristics, prepubescence typically occurs during preadolescence.

Toward the end of middle childhood, the discrepancies in growth and maturation between boys and girls become apparent. On average, there is a difference of approximately 2 years between girls and boys in the age of onset of **pubescence**. This is a period of rapid growth in height and weight, especially for girls.

There is no universal age at which children assume the characteristics of prepubescence. The first physiological signs appear at about 9 years of age (particularly in girls) and are usually clearly evident in 11- to 12-year-old children. Although preadolescent children do not want to be different, variability in physical growth and physiological changes between children of the same sex and between the two sexes is often striking at this time. This variability, especially in relation to the onset of **secondary sexual characteristics**, is often noticed by the preadolescent. Either early or late appearance of these characteristics can be a source of discomfort to both sexes.

Preadolescence is a period of considerable overlapping of developmental characteristics of both middle childhood and early adolescence. However, several unique characteristics set this period apart from others. Generally, puberty begins at age 10 years in girls and 12 years in boys, but it can be normal for either sex after the age of 8 years. Boys experience little visible sexual maturation during preadolescence.

Table 39-1 summarizes the major developmental achievements of the school-age years.

Psychosocial Development

Freud described middle childhood as the latency period, a time of tranquility between the attachment–separation (Oedipal) phase of early childhood and the eroticism of adolescence. Freud believed that children experience relationships with same-sex peers following the indifference of earlier years and preceding the heterosexual fascination that occurs for many boys and girls in puberty. In today's context Freud's views would be revised to include sexual fascination experienced by children of any sexual orientation (Freud & Fliess, 1954).

Developing a Sense of Industry (Erikson)

Erikson (1963) believed that successful mastery of his first three stages of psychosocial development were important in development of a healthy personality and were related to initial experiences in a loving environment within a stable

Table 39-1 Growth and Development During School-Age Years

PHYSICAL AND MOTOR	MENTAL	ADAPTIVE	PERSONAL-SOCIAL
Age 6 Yr			
Height and weight gain continues slowly Weight 16–26.3 kg Height 106.7–122 cm Central mandibular incisors erupt Loses first tooth Gradual increase in dexterity Active age; constant activity Often returns to finger feeding More aware of hand as a tool Likes to draw, print, colour Vision reaches maturity	Develops concept of numbers Easily counts 13 pennies Knows whether it is morning or afternoon Defines common objects such as fork and chair in terms of their use Obeys three commands in succession Knows right and left hands Says which is pretty and which is ugly of a series of face drawings Describes the objects in a picture rather than simply enumerating them Attends first grade	At the table, uses knife to spread butter or jam on bread At play, cuts, folds, pastes paper; sews crudely if the needle is threaded Takes a bath without supervision; performs bedtime activities alone Reads from memory; enjoys oral spelling game Likes table games, checkers, simple card games Giggles a lot Sometimes steals money or attractive items Has difficulty owning up to misdeeds Tries out own abilities	Can share and cooperate better Has great need for children of own age Will cheat to win Often engages in rough play Often jealous of younger brother or sister Does what adults are seen doing May have occasional temper tantrums Is a boaster Is more independent, probably influenced by school Has own way of doing things Increases socialization

Continued

children adopt and internalize the moral values of their parents. They learn standards for acceptable behaviour, act according to these standards, and feel guilty when they violate them. Although children 6 or 7 years of age know the rules and behaviours expected of them, they do not understand the reasons behind them. Rewards and punishments guide their judgement; a "bad act" is one that breaks a rule or causes harm. This description of moral development includes that young children believe that what other people tell them to do is right and that what they themselves think is wrong. Consequently, children 6 or 7 years old may interpret accidents or misfortunes as punishment for "bad" acts.

Older school-age children are able to judge an act by the intentions that prompted it rather than just its consequences. Rules and judgements become less absolute and authoritarian, and begin to be founded on the needs and desires of others. For older children, a rule violation is likely to be viewed in relation to the total context in which it appears. The situation, as well as the morality of the rule itself, influences reactions. Although younger children judge an act only according to whether it is right or wrong, older children take into account a different point of view. They are able to understand and accept the concept of treating others as they would like to be treated.

Spiritual Development

School-age children begin to learn the difference between the natural and the supernatural but have difficulty understanding symbols. Consequently, religious concepts must be presented to them in concrete terms. Prayer or other religious rituals comfort them, and if these activities are a part of their daily lives, they may help them cope with threatening situations. Their petitions to their god in prayers tend to be for tangible rewards. Although younger children expect their prayers to be answered, as they get older, they begin to recognize that this does not always occur and become less concerned when prayers are not answered. They are able to discuss their feelings about their faith and how it relates to their lives (see Cultural Awareness box).

Social Development

One of the most important socializing agents in the school-age years is the peer group. In addition to parents and the schools, the peer group conveys a substantial amount of information to its members. Peer groups have a culture of their own, with secrets, traditions, and codes of ethics that may promote feelings of solidarity and detachment from adults. Through peer relationships, children often learn how to deal with dominance and hostility, how to relate to persons in positions of leadership and authority, and how to explore ideas and the physical environment.

Peer group identification is an important factor in gaining independence from parents. The aid and support of the group provide the child with enough security to risk the moderate parental rejection brought about by small victories in the development of independence.

A child's concept of the appropriate gender role is also influenced by relationships with peers. During the early school years few gender differences exist in the play experiences of children. Both girls and boys sharse games and other activities. In the later school years the differences in the play of boys and girls may become more marked.

Social Relationships and Cooperation

Daily relationships with peers provide important social interactions for school-age children. For the first time, children join group activities with unrestrained enthusiasm and steady participation. Previous interactions were limited to short periods under considerable adult supervision. With increased skills and wider opportunities, children become involved with one or more peer groups in which they can gain status as respected members.

Valuable lessons are learned from daily interaction with age-mates. First, children learn to appreciate the numerous and varied points of view that are represented in the peer group. As children interact with peers who see the world in ways that are somewhat different from their own, they become aware of the limits of their own point of view. Because age-mates are peers and are not forced to accept each other's ideas as they are expected to accept those of adults, other children have a significant influence on decreasing the egocentric outlook of the child. Consequently, children learn to argue, persuade, bargain, cooperate, and compromise to maintain friendships.

A second lesson that children learn is increasing sensitivity to the social norms and pressures of the peer group. The peer group establishes standards for acceptance and rejection, and children are often willing to modify their behaviour to be accepted by the group. The need for peer approval becomes a powerful influence toward conformity. Children learn to dress, talk, and behave in a manner acceptable to the group. A variety of roles, such as class joker or class hero, may be assumed by individual children to gain approval from the group.

Finally, the interaction among peers leads to the formation of intimate friendships between peers—the school-age period is the time when children may have "best friends" with whom they share secrets, private jokes, and adventures; they come to one another's aid in times of trouble. In the course of these friendships children also fight, threaten each other, break up, and reunite. These relationships, in which the child experiences love and closeness for a peer, may be important as a foundation for relationships in adulthood (Fig. 39-4).

CULTURAL AWARENESS

Religious Orientation

Many schools and communities in Canada have Christian and Jewish orientations toward prayer, holidays, and values. For children of other religious backgrounds, the predominance of these practices and values may result in their feeling conflict and discomfort. It is important that schools and communities exercise sensitivity so as not to offend and confuse children from other religious backgrounds, such as Buddhism, Hinduism, and Islam, or those with no religious background. In Canada, awareness of and openness to the spiritual diversity of First Nations, Métis, and Inuit groups is also important.

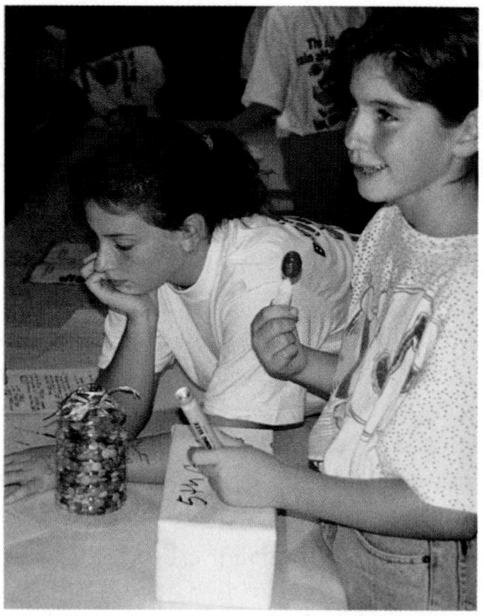

Fig. 39-4 School-age children enjoy engaging in activities with a "best friend."

Clubs and Peer Groups

In contemporary Western society, one of the outstanding characteristics of middle childhood seems to be the formation of formalized groups, or clubs. A prominent feature of these groups is the rigid rules imposed on the members. There is exclusiveness in the selection of persons who have the privilege of joining. Acceptance in the group is often determined on a pass-fail basis according to social or behavioural criteria. Conformity is the core of the group structure. There are often secret codes, shared interests, and special modes of dress, and each child must abide by a standard of behaviour established by the members. Conforming to the rules provides children with feelings of security and relieves them of the responsibility of making decisions. By merging their identities with those of their peers, children are able to move from the family group to an outside group, as a step toward seeking further independence. Peer groups and clubs allow children to substitute conformity to a peer group for conformity to a family at a time when children are still too insecure to function independently.

During the early school years, groups are usually small and loosely organized, with changing membership and no formal structure. The clubs and groups usually do not display elements of cooperation and order that are seen in groups of older children. Although there may be a mixture of both sexes in the early school years, the groups of later school years are composed predominantly of children of the same sex. Common interests are the basis around which the group is structured.

There are dangers in peer-group attachments that become too strong. Peer pressures may force some children to take risks or engage in behaviours that are against their better judgement. For instance, a child's membership in a gang is associated with marked increases in serious delinquent behaviour (Dishion, Nelson, & Yasui, 2005). An integration of family-centred and school-based programs is needed to reduce the influences that may cause children to become affiliated with gangs (Dishion et al., 2005).

Bullying

Peer-group identification and association are essential to a child's socialization. Poor relationships with peers and a lack of group identification can contribute to bullying. *Bullying* is any recurring activity that is intended to harm or bother someone where there is a perceived imbalance of power between the aggressor and the victim (Craig & Pepler, 2007). Bullying often begins between the ages of 4 and 11, when children are forming their own identities at school and through other social activities. Studies have shown that a higher percentage of students engage in bullying behaviours while in middle school and high school than in elementary school, but the percentage of students victimized gradually decreases with age. Boys in elementary school report higher levels of bullying than that for girls in middle and high school. During middle school and high school, boys practise and are the victims of bullying almost twice as much as girls (Health Canada, 2010). Bullying occurs most frequently at school during unstructured times, with recess providing the most common opportunity for bullying, followed by gym classes, lunchrooms, hallways, and buses (Glew et al., 2005).

Bullies may be from any ethnic, racial, or socioeconomic group. They are generally defiant toward adults, antisocial, and likely to break school rules. They have little anxiety, strong self-esteem, and dominant personalities; may come from homes where parental involvement and nurturing are lacking; and may experience or witness violence or abuse at home (Lyznicki, McCaffree, & Robinowitz, 2004). Boys who bully tend to use physical force, whereas girls who bully employ psychological methods such as ostracism or rumours. The use of social media for mass communication has escalated the gravity of many methods of bullying. Bullying by boys is more common than by girls. Children who are targeted for bullying are vulnerable and may have characteristics that are different from the group norm, such as obesity, learning problems, a minority sexual orientation, or different family background (Craig & Pepler, 2007). Children with hidden disabilities such as developmental coordination disorder, specific language impairment, or attention deficit/hyperactivity disorder may receive less protection from their peer group in contrast to a child with a visible disability such as spina bifida (Frederickson, 2010).

Canada does not have a good record of effectively managing bullying. The World Health Organization global survey of health behaviours of school-age children ranks Canada twenty-sixth out of 35 countries for number of bullying incidents (Craig & Harel, 2004). A Canadian federal network, called PrevNET (Promoting Relationships and Eliminating Violence), has been established to prevent bullying, by bridging the gap between research and practice. Bullying needs to be managed directly by adults who will acknowledge the problem and step in to stop it. Children also need empowerment strategies that can give them peer support and that help them in bullying situations (Health Canada, 2010). School personnel can play an important role in implementing anti-bullying interventions in elementary schools, before bullying becomes a part of the school culture (Craig & Pepler, 2007).

The long-term consequences of bullying are significant. Chronic bullies may continue their behaviours into adulthood, negatively influencing their ability to develop and maintain relationships. Victims of bullying often feel socially rejected and can fear school, which can develop into school phobia or long-term problems of depression and low self-esteem (Vreeman & Carroll, 2007).

Relationships With Families

Although the peer group is influential in child development, parents are usually the primary influence in shaping the child's personality, setting standards for behaviour, and establishing value systems. Family values usually take precedence over peer value systems. Although children may appear to reject parental values while testing the new values of the peer group, ultimately they retain and incorporate into their own value systems the parental values they have found to be of worth.

In the middle school years, children want to spend more time in the company of peers and they often prefer peer-group activities to family activities. This can be disturbing to parents. Children may become intolerant and critical of their parents, especially when their parents' ways deviate from those of the group. They discover that parents can be wrong, and they begin to question the knowledge and authority of their parents, who were previously often considered to be all-knowing and all-powerful.

Although increased independence is the goal of middle childhood, children are not prepared to abandon all parental control. They need and want restrictions placed on their behaviour, and they are not prepared to cope with all the problems of their expanding environment. They feel more secure knowing there is an authority figure to implement controls and restrictions. Children may complain loudly about restrictions and try to break down parental barriers, but they are uneasy if they succeed in doing so. They respect adults who prevent them from acting on every urge. Children view this behaviour as an expression of love and concern for their welfare.

Children need stable, secure strength provided by mature adults to whom they can turn during troubled relationships with peers or stressful changes in their world (see Family-Centred Teaching box). With a secure base in a loving family,

FAMILY-CENTRED TEACHING

Guidance for Parents During School Years

Age 6 Years

- Prepare parents for potential strong food preferences and potential refusal of specific food items.
- Prepare parents to expect an increasingly ravenous appetite.
- Prepare parents for emotionality as the child experiences mood changes.
- Help parents anticipate continued susceptibility to illness.
- Review immunization schedule with the parents—if tetanus schedule of 4 initial doses is completed before age 4, a fifth dose of tetanus toxoid is recommended at school entry by age 6 (Public Health Agency of Canada, 2006).
- Teach injury prevention and safety, especially bicycle safety.
- Encourage parents to respect the child's need for privacy and to provide a separate bedroom for the child, if possible.
- Prepare parents for the child's increasing interests outside the home.
- Help parents understand the need to support the child's interactions with peers.

Ages 7 to 10 Years

- Prepare parents to expect an improvement in health with fewer illnesses, although allergies may increase or become apparent.
- Prepare parents to expect an increase in minor injuries.
- Emphasize caution in selecting and maintaining sports equipment, and re-emphasize safety.
- Prepare parents to expect increased involvement with peers and interest in activities outside the home.
- Emphasize the need to encourage independence while maintaining limit-setting and discipline.
- Prepare mothers to expect more demands from the child at age 8 years.
- Prepare fathers to expect increasing admiration from the child at age 10 years; encourage father–child activities.
- Prepare parents for prepubescent changes in girls.

Ages 11 to 12 Years

- Help parents prepare the child for body changes of pubescence.
- Prepare parents to expect a growth spurt in girls.
- Make certain the child's sex education is adequate with accurate information.
- Prepare parents to expect energetic and stormy behaviour at age 11 years, becoming more even-tempered at age 12 years.
- Encourage parents to support the child's desire to "grow up" but to allow regressive behaviour when needed.
- Prepare parents to expect an increase in the child's masturbation.
- Instruct parents that the amount of rest the child needs may increase.
- Help parents educate the child regarding experimentation with potentially harmful activities.

Health Guidance

- Provide information regarding human papilloma virus (HPV) immunization. Health Canada recommends administration to girls and women between ages 9 and 26, preferably before sexual activity has commenced; all provinces have a program to cover this (see Chapter 6) (Public Health Agency of Canada, 2006).
- Help parents understand the importance of regular health and dental care for the child.
- Encourage parents to teach and model sound health practices, including diet, rest, activity, and exercise.
- Stress the need to encourage children to engage in appropriate physical activities.
- Emphasize the importance of providing a safe physical and emotional environment.
- Encourage parents to teach and model safety practices.

it is hoped that children can develop the self-confidence and maturity needed to break loose from the group and stand independently.

Play

Play takes on new dimensions that reflect a new stage of development in the school years (see Table 39-1). Play involves increased physical skill, intellectual ability, and fantasy. In addition, children develop a sense of belonging to a team or club by forming groups and cliques.

Rules and Rituals

The need for conformity in middle childhood is strongly manifested in the activities and games of school-age children. In the preschool years, children's games were either invented for them or played in the company of a friend or an adult. Now children begin to see the need for rules, and their games have fixed and unvarying rules that may be bizarre and extraordinarily rigid. Part of the enjoyment of the game is knowing the rules because knowing means belonging. Conformity and ritual permeate their play and are also evident in their behaviour and language. Childhood is full of chants and taunts, such as "Eeeny, meeny, miney, mo," "Last one is a rotten egg," and "Step on a crack, break your mother's back." Children derive a sense of pleasure and power from such sayings, which have been handed down with few changes through generations.

Team Play

More complex forms of play that evolve from the need for peer interaction are **cooperative play**, team games, and sports. A referee, umpire, or person of authority may be required so that the rules can be followed more accurately. Team play teaches children to modify or exchange personal goals for goals of the group; it also teaches them that division of labour is an effective strategy for attaining a goal. Children learn about competition and the importance of winning—an attribute highly valued in some cultures and by some individuals.

Team play can also contribute to children's social, intellectual, and skill growth. Children work hard to develop the skills needed to become team members, to improve their contribution to the group, and to anticipate the consequences of their behaviour for the group. Team play helps stimulate cognitive growth because children are called on to learn many complex rules, make judgements about those rules, plan strategies, and assess the strengths and weaknesses of members of their own team and members of the opposing team.

Quiet Games and Activities

Although play at this age is highly active, school-age children also enjoy quiet and solitary activities. The middle years are a time for collections, which constitute another ritual. Young school-age children's collections can be an odd assortment of unrelated objects in messy, disorganized piles. Collections of later school years are more orderly, selective, and may be organized in scrapbooks, on shelves, or in boxes.

School-age children become fascinated with complex board, card, video, or computer games that they can play alone, with a best friend, or with a group. As in all games, adherence to the rules is fanatic. Disagreements over rules can cause much discussion and argument, but may be easily resolved by reading the rules of the game.

The newly acquired skill of reading becomes increasingly satisfying as school-age children expand their knowledge of the world through books (Fig. 39-5). School-age children never tire of stories and, as with preschool children, love to have stories read aloud or to read them out loud themselves. Sewing, cooking, carpentry, gardening, and creative activities such as painting, drawing, and playing an instrument are other activities enjoyed. Many creative skills such as those in music, art, and theatre as well as athletic skills such as swimming, karate, dancing, and skating are learned during these years and continue to be enjoyed into adolescence and adulthood (Fig. 39-6).

Ego Mastery

Play affords children the means to acquire mastery over themselves, their environment, and others. Through play, children can feel as big, as powerful, and as skilful as their imaginations will allow. They can also feel in control and attain vicarious mastery and power over whomever and whatever they choose. School-age children still need the opportunity to use large muscles in exuberant outdoor play and the freedom to exert their newfound **autonomy** and initiative. They need space in which to exercise large muscles and to deal with tensions, frustrations, and hostility. Physical skills practised and mastered in play help them to develop a feeling of personal competence, which contributes to a sense of accomplishment and provides status in their peer group.

Developing a Self-Concept

The term *self-concept* refers to a conscious awareness of self-perceptions, such as one's physical characteristics, abilities, values, self-ideals and expectations, and idea of self in relation to others. It also includes one's body image, sexuality, and self-esteem. Although primary caregivers continue to exert influence on children's self-evaluation, the opinions of peers and teachers provide valuable input during middle childhood.

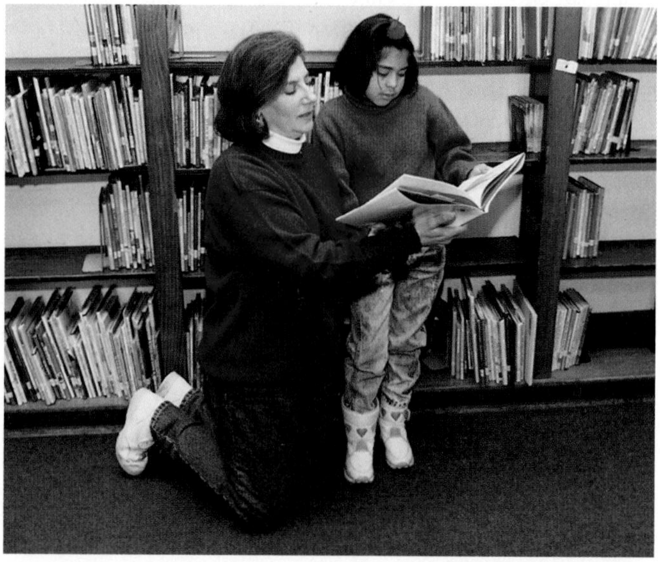

Fig. 39-5 Selecting a book with the assistance of an adult.

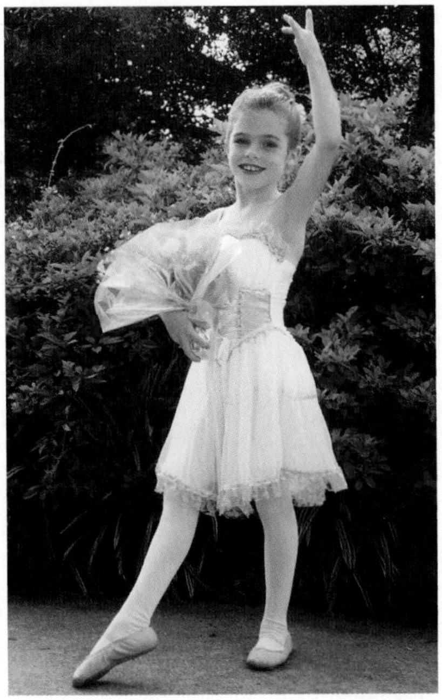

Fig. 39-6 School-age children take pride in learning new skills.

With the emphasis on skill building and broadened social relationships, children are continually engaged in the process of self-evaluation.

Significant adults can often manage to unobtrusively manipulate the environment so that children experience success. Each small success increases a child's self-image. The more positive children feel about themselves, the more confident they will remain in trying for success in the future. All children profit from feeling that they are in some way special to a significant adult. A positive self-concept makes children feel likable, worthwhile, and capable of significant contributions. These feelings lead to self-respect, self-confidence, and happiness. Negative feelings may lead to self-doubt.

Developing a Body Image

School-age children have a relatively accurate and positive perception of their physical selves, but in general they like their physical selves less as they grow older. The head appears to be the most important part of the school-age child's perceived image of self, with hair and eye colour being the characteristics used most frequently to describe the physical self.

Body image is influenced, but not solely determined, by significant others. The number of significant others influencing one's perception of the physical self increases with age. Children are acutely aware of their own body, the bodies of their peers, and those of adults. They are also aware of deviations from the norm. It is important that children learn about bodily functions and that adults provide correct information.

Physical impairments, such as hearing or visual defects, ears that "stick out," or birthmarks, assume great importance during this age span. Increasing awareness of these differences, especially when accompanied by unkind comments and taunts from others, may cause a child to feel inferior and less desirable. This is especially true if the defect interferes with the child's ability to participate in games and activities.

Coping With Concerns Related to Normal Growth and Development

School Experience

School constitutes an important part of the experience of children 6 to 12 years of age. Schools serve as a significant agent in the transmitting of values of society to children. As discussed earlier, school is also a setting for relationships with peers and usually an important socializing agent in the lives of children.

Entrance into school causes a sharp break in the structure of the child's world. For many children, it is their first experience with conforming to a group pattern imposed by an adult who is not a parent and who has responsibility for too many children to be constantly aware of each child as an individual. Most children want to go to school and usually adapt to the new conditions with little difficulty. Successful adjustment is related to the strength of partnerships between the child, the parents, and the school staff. The child's previous experiences, the child's physical and emotional maturity, and the parent's readiness to accept school entrance are also factors in this adjustment.

By the time they enter school, most children have a fairly realistic concept of what school involves. They receive information regarding the role of a student from parents, siblings, playmates, and the media. In addition, most children have had some experience with day care, preschool, or kindergarten. Middle-class children generally have fewer adjustments to make and less to learn about expected behaviour, since schools tend to reflect dominant middle-class customs and values. If the child has attended a preschool program, the focus of the preschool program also affects the child's adjustment. Some preschool programs provide custodial care only, whereas others emphasize emotional, social, and intellectual development.

Classmates have a significant impact on the socialization of children. For some children, school is their first experience of becoming members of a large group of individuals their own age. Peer relationships become increasingly important and influential as children proceed through school (see section Social Relationships and Cooperation, earlier in this chapter). The specific influence exerted by the peer group depends on the individual child's background, interests, and abilities.

Teachers

Children respond best to teachers who possess the characteristics of a warm, loving parent. Teachers in the early grades perform many of the activities formerly assumed by the parent, such as recognizing the child's personal needs (e.g., the need to go to the bathroom, need for help with clothing) and helping to develop their social behaviour (e.g., manners).

Teachers, like parents, are concerned about the child's psychological and emotional welfare. Although the functions of teachers and parents differ, both place constraints on behaviour, and both are in a position to enforce standards of conduct. However, unlike parents, the teacher's primary responsibility involves stimulating and guiding children's intellectual development, not providing for their physical welfare beyond the school setting.

Teachers serve as models that children often try to emulate. Children seek their teachers' approval and avoid their disapproval. The teacher is a significant person in the life of the early schoolchild, and hero worship of a teacher may extend into late childhood and preadolescence. Teachers who make supportive statements that reassure or commend children, use accepting and clarifying statements that help children refine ideas and feelings, and provide assistance that aids children with their own problem solving contribute to the development of a positive self-concept in the school-age child.

Parents

Parents share responsibility for helping children achieve their maximum potential. Parents can supplement the school program in numerous ways (see Patient Teaching box). Cultivating responsibility is the goal of parental assistance. Being responsible for schoolwork helps children learn to keep promises, meet deadlines, and succeed at their jobs as adults. Responsible children may occasionally ask for help (e.g., with a spelling list), but usually they prefer to think through their work by themselves. Excessive pressure or lack of encouragement from parents may inhibit the development of these desirable traits.

Latchkey Children

The term *latchkey children* is used to describe children in elementary school who are left to care for themselves before or after school without the supervision of an adult. The increasing numbers of lone-parent families and families in which both parents work outside the home, together with the lack of available child care, can contribute to this situation.

Inadequate adult supervision after school leaves children at greater risk for injury and delinquent behaviour. In some instances, outside activities are curtailed and relationships with peers may be significantly diminished. Latchkey children may feel more lonely, isolated, and fearful than children who have someone to care for them. To cope with their fears and anxieties while alone, these children may devise strategies such as hiding, playing the television at loud volume, or using pets for comfort. In addition, some latchkey children may have a chronic illness or other health problem that remains improperly treated.

Many communities and persons concerned about the welfare of latchkey children are trying to help these children and their parents deal with this potentially serious problem. Some communities and employers have implemented after-school programs or telephone "hotlines" that provide check-in and reassurance for children. Nurses should be aware of these community services and encourage parents to teach self-help skills to their children.

Limit-Setting and Discipline

Many factors influence the amount and manner of discipline and limit-setting imposed on school-age children. Some of these factors are the parents' psychosocial maturity, the parents' childhood and childrearing experiences, the children's temperament, the context of the children's misconduct, and the children's response to rewards and punishments.

PATIENT TEACHING Helping Children in School

General Guidelines

- Be supportive—Provide companionship; share ideas and thoughts.
- Be positive—Every child should experience some success each day.
- Share an interest in reading—Use the library; discuss books they are reading.
- Support and encourage activity rather than passivity.
- Encourage originality—Help children make their own projects from discarded articles or other available materials.
- Foster the development of hobbies and collections.
- Encourage children to wonder and reflect during free time.
- Encourage family experiences and trips to places of interest.
- Encourage questions—Help children discover sources for information or places to explore and investigate.
- Stimulate creative thinking and problem solving—Help children try out new solutions to problems without fear of making mistakes.
- Use rewards rather than punishment.

Specific Guidelines

- Meet the teacher at the beginning of school and plan to visit the school to see what is taught and expected.
- Send the child to school every day. Teachers are concerned when parents make other plans for their children; it conveys the impression that school is unimportant.
- Demonstrate an interest in what the child is learning.
- Demonstrate an interest in content and growth more than in grades.
- Make it clear to the child that schoolwork is between the child and the teacher; the teacher and child should set goals for better school performance to allow the child to feel responsible for school successes and failures.
- Take advantage of situations that support and reinforce school learning.
- Share information with teachers that will help them understand the child better.
- Communicate with the teacher if there appears to be a problem; avoid waiting for a scheduled conference.
- Provide a quiet, well-lit area for study that is safe from interruption.
- Avoid dictating a study time, but do enforce rules, such as no television until homework is done; accept the child's word that work is complete.
- Help with homework should focus on explaining the question, not giving the answer.
- Teach the child to break large tasks (e.g., a report) down into smaller, manageable tasks spread over the allotted time rather than attempting the entire project the night before it is to be completed.
- Limit home tutoring to special circumstances, such as when the teacher requests parental assistance after a child's prolonged absence.
- Request special help for children with learning problems.
- Support the school staff by showing respect for both the school system and the teacher, especially in the child's presence.

When children develop an ability to see a situation from another's point of view, they are also able to understand the effects of their reactions on others and themselves.

Discipline should take place in a positive, supportive environment with the use of strategies to instruct and guide desired behaviours and eliminate undesired behaviours (Canadian Mental Health Association [CMHA], 2011a). Reasoning is an effective technique for older school-age children. With advancing cognitive skills, they are able to benefit from more complex disciplinary strategies. For example, withholding privileges, requiring compensation, imposing penalties, and contracting can be used with great success. Problem solving is the best approach to limit-setting, and children themselves can be included in the process of determining appropriate disciplinary measures.

Dishonest Behaviour

During middle childhood, children may engage in what is considered to be antisocial behaviour. Previously well-behaved children may engage in lying, stealing, and cheating. Such behaviours are disturbing and challenging to parents.

Lying can occur for a number of reasons. By the time children enter school, they still "tell stories," often exaggerating a story or situation as a means of impressing their family or friends. However, during middle childhood, children become able to distinguish between fact and fantasy. If children do not develop this characteristic, parents need to teach them what is real and what is make-believe.

Young children may lie to escape punishment or to get out of some difficulty even when their misbehaviour is evident. Older children may lie to meet expectations set by others to which they have been unable to measure up. However, most children know that lying and cheating are wrong, and they are concerned when it is observed in their friends. They are quick to tell on others when they detect cheating.

Parents need to be reassured that all children lie occasionally and that sometimes children may have difficulty separating fantasy from reality. Parents should be helped to understand the importance of being truthful in their relationships with children.

Cheating is most common in young children 5 to 6 years of age. They find it difficult to lose at a game or contest, so they may cheat to win. They have not yet realized that this behaviour is wrong, and they do it almost automatically. This behaviour usually disappears as they mature. However, because children model observed behaviours, parents need to be aware of their own behaviour. When parents set examples of honesty, children are more likely to conform to these standards.

As with other ethically related behaviour, stealing is not unexpected in the younger child. Between 5 and 8 years of age, children's sense of property rights is limited, and they tend to take something simply because they are attracted to it or to take money for what it will buy. They are equally likely to give away something valuable that belongs to them. When young children are caught and punished, they are penitent—they "didn't mean to" and "promise to never do it again"—but they are likely to repeat the performance the following day. Often they not only steal but also lie about their behaviour or attempt to justify it with excuses. It is seldom helpful to trap children into admission by asking directly if they committed the offense. Children do not take responsibility for these behaviours until the end of middle childhood.

Children steal for several reasons. Young children may lack a sense of property rights, attempt to acquire a specific object to bribe favours from other children, have a strong desire to own a coveted item, or have a desire for revenge to "get back at someone" (usually a parent for unfair treatment). Older children may steal to supplement an inadequate allowance. Stealing can be an indication that something is seriously wrong or lacking in the child's life. For example, children may steal to make up for love or another satisfaction that they feel is lacking. In most situations it is wise not to attempt to attach a hidden or deep meaning to the stealing. An admonition, together with an appropriate and reasonable punishment, such as having the older child pay back the money or return the stolen items, takes care of most cases. Most children can be taught to respect the property rights of others with little difficulty despite numerous temptations and opportunities. If children's personal rights are respected, they are likely to respect the rights of others. Some children simply need more time to learn the rules regarding private property.

Stress and Fear

Children today experience significant amounts of **stress**, which can cause long-term adjustment and health problems. Stress in childhood comes from a variety of sources such as conflict within the family, interpersonal relationships, poverty, and chronic illness. The school environment and participation in multiple organized activities can be additional sources of stress. The demands from coaches and parents, in addition to school requirements and pressure from teachers to do well on proficiency testing, can place unrealistic expectations on the school-age child (Ryan-Wenger, Sharrer, & Campbell, 2005). In addition, with increasing exposure to sexuality and provocative clothing and behaviours, children of this age group may feel pressured to have a girlfriend or boyfriend, which their maturity level cannot handle and which causes additional stress (Ryan-Wenger et al., 2005).

Increasing **violence** in society has also spilled over into the school setting. In the present information age, in which tragedy is broadcast daily in the media, children come to school knowing more about the latest world events than any previous generation of children. In addition, today's children are often personally aware of violence in their families or communities. Some children know other children who have been killed or children who have brought weapons to school. School-age children can be victims of teasing, bullying, and physical abuse in the school environment (Health Canada, 2011).

To help children cope with stress, parents, teachers, and health care providers need to frequently reassure children that they are safe, have honest and open communication with them, encourage children to express their feelings, and promote a daily routine and reliable limits. It is important to help children build coping strategies to foster self-confidence and overcome fears by providing practical solutions, encouraging a sense of self-control, praising accomplishments, and avoiding criticism (CMHA, 2011b). Adults must recognize signs indicating that a child is undergoing stress, identify the source of the stress promptly, and refer those children who need specialized treatment.

NURSING ALERT The nurse who observes the following signs of stress in a child should explore the situation further:

- Stomach pains or headache
- Changes in sleep patterns or nightmares
- Bed-wetting
- Changes in eating habits
- Aggressive or stubborn behaviour
- Withdrawal or reluctance to participate
- Regression to earlier behaviours (e.g., thumb-sucking)
- Trouble concentrating or changes in academic performance

Children 7 to 12 years of age are capable of identifying their own physiological responses to stress with terms that have meaning to them. They may describe their body's reaction to stress in terms of having tight muscles; being hot or red in the face; tingling; having chills or goose bumps; or experiencing shakiness, heart beating fast, headache, or stomachache (Sharrer & Ryan-Wenger, 2002). Some children may experience headaches or get angry more easily. Children should be taught to recognize these signs as indicators of stress and to use techniques to manage their stress. Children can learn relaxation techniques such as deep-breathing exercises, progressive relaxation of muscle groups, and positive imagery to immediately reduce stress. "Blowing off steam" through physical activity can reduce tension and anxiety. Children can also be encouraged to observe effective coping strategies in others and adopt them for their own use. When an effective strategy has been developed for one situation, parents can show the child how to transfer the coping strategy or technique to other situations (Canadian Psychology Foundation of Canada, 2012).

In addition to stress, school-age children experience a wide variety of fears, including fear of the dark, excessive worry about past behaviour, self-consciousness, social withdrawal, and an excessive need for reassurance. These fears are considered normal for children this age. During the middle range of the school-age years, children become less fearful of body safety than they were as preschoolers, but they still fear being hurt, being kidnapped, or having to undergo surgery. They also fear death and are fascinated by all aspects of death and dying. Fears of noises, darkness, storms, and dogs lessen, while new fears related predominantly to school and family bother children at this age.

Promoting Optimum Health During the School Years

Nutrition

Although caloric needs are diminished in relation to body size during middle childhood, resources are being laid down at this time for the increased growth needs of adolescence. Parents and children need to be aware of the value of a balanced diet toward promoting growth, because children usually eat what their family members eat. The quality of the child's diet depends on the family's pattern of eating.

Likes and dislikes established at an early age tend to continue in middle childhood, although preferences for single foods subside and children develop a taste for a variety of foods. Unfortunately, the easy availability of fast-food restaurants, the influence of the mass media, and the temptation of "junk food" make it easy for children to fill up on empty calories. Foods that do not promote growth, such as sugars, starches, and excess fats, are common in the school-age child's diet. As discussed in Chapter 29, the easy availability of high-calorie foods, combined with the tendency toward more sedentary activities, has contributed to an epidemic of childhood obesity. This problem is discussed further in Chapter 40.

Nutrition education can and should be integrated in the school curriculum throughout the school years. Important aspects of nutrition education include the relationship of nutrition to activity, fitness, and health; elements of a wholesome diet; and how food products are grown, processed, and prepared. A good resource for this is *Eating Well With Canada's Food Guide* (see Additional Resources at the end of this chapter). In addition, some schools are seeking to provide healthy, nutritious meals at school, in the cafeteria. This effort includes the implementation of school policies related to vending machines, corporate sponsorships, and school and sports events. Some schools have initiated "breakfast clubs" for children who do not have access to breakfast at home. Such programs are linked with greater student engagement in the classroom.

The public health nurse can take an active role in nutrition education by working with teachers to plan and implement units on nutrition instruction and by working with parents and children to give nutritional guidance. As previously mentioned, obesity prevention and treatment is currently a health issue in much need of attention.

Sleep and Rest

The amount of sleep and rest required during middle childhood is highly individualized. The amount of sleep depends on the child's age, activity level, and state of health. The growth rate slows in the school-age years, and less energy is expended in growth than during preceding years.

School-age children usually do not require a nap, and they sleep during the night for approximately 11 hours at age 5 years and 9¼ hours at age 12 years (Carno et al., 2003). Although fewer bedtime problems occur during these years, occasional difficulties are still associated with the bedtime ritual. Usually children 6 or 7 years old exhibit few bedtime problems, and encouraging quiet activity before bedtime, such as colouring or reading, facilitates the task of going to bed. However, most children in middle childhood must be reminded frequently to go to bed; 8- to 11-year-old children are particularly resistant. Often these children are unaware that they are tired; if they are allowed to remain up later than usual, they are fatigued the following day. Sometimes, bedtime resistance can be resolved by allowing a later bedtime as the child gets older. Twelve-year-old children usually offer no resistance at bedtime; some even retire early to read a book or listen to music.

Exercise and Activity

Because of the improved capabilities and adaptability of the school-age child, these children have greater speed and exert more effort in motor activities. Larger, stronger muscles enable longer and increasingly strenuous play without exhaustion. While school-age children acquire the coordination, timing, and concentration that are needed to participate in adult-type activities, they may lack the strength, stamina, and control of the adolescent and adult. However, parents, teachers, and coaches must remember that, although children this age are large and appear strong, they may not be ready for strenuous competitive athletics.

All growing children need regular exercise and opportunities for satisfying experiences consistent with individual likes and dislikes. Appropriate activities during the school-age years include running, jumping rope, swimming, skateboarding, roller blading, ice skating, skiing, dancing, and bicycle riding. Positive reinforcement achieved by experiencing increasingly smooth, rhythmic, and efficient use of the body conditions the child toward regular physical activity. Exercise is essential for muscle development and tone, refinement of balance and coordination, increased strength and endurance, and stimulation of body functions and metabolic processes. Children need ample space to run, jump, skip, and climb, in addition to safe indoor and outdoor facilities and equipment. Most children have abundant energy and need little encouragement to engage in physical activity. Children from 5 to 11 years of age require an accumulation of 60 minutes per day of moderate to vigorous activity and vigorous-intensity activities three times a week (Canadian Society for Exercise Physiology, 2012). Children with disabling conditions or those who hesitate to become involved in active play (such as obese children) require special assessment and help so that activities appeal to them and are compatible with their limitations while also meeting their developmental needs.

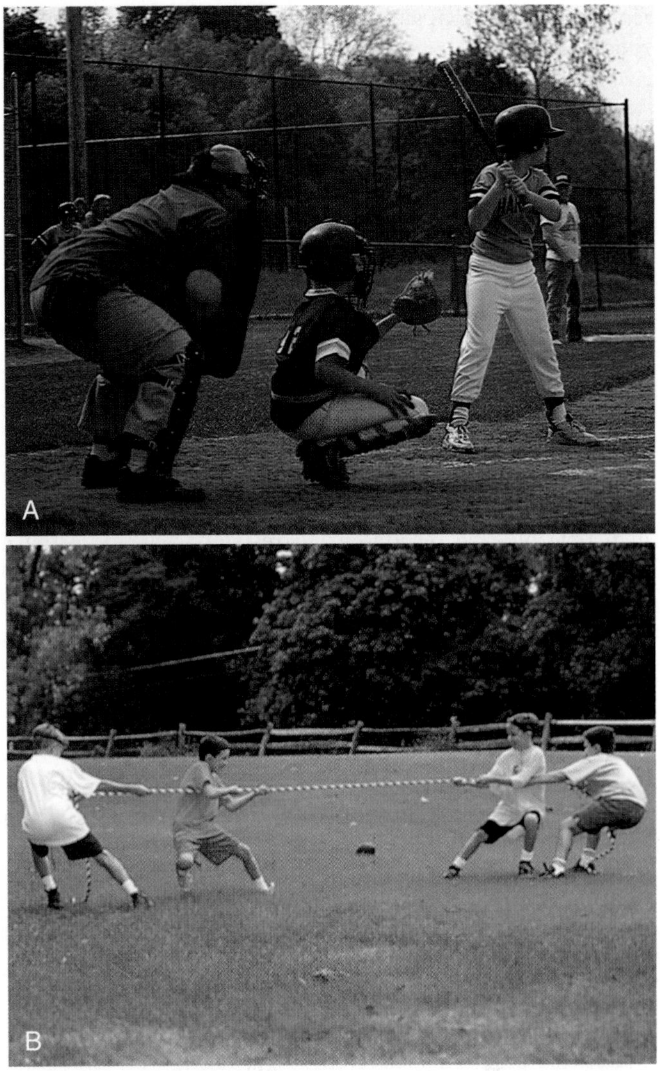

Fig. 39-7 The activities engaged in by school-age children vary according to interest and opportunity. **A:** Little League competitors. **B:** Playing tug-of-war.

Sports

Considerable controversy surrounds the trend toward early participation in competitive athletics and the amount and type of competitive sports that are appropriate for children in the elementary grades. The current view is that virtually every child is suited for some sport, and authorities do not discourage participation if children are matched to the type of sport appropriate to their abilities and to their physical and emotional constitution. School-age children enjoy competition (Fig. 39-7). However, teachers and coaches must understand the physical limitations of children this age and teach them the proper techniques and safety measures needed to avoid injuries. A safe and appropriate sport can be identified for even the most unskilled and uncompetitive child, including children with chronic illnesses and cognitive impairments. Common activities for school-age children include hockey, skiing, softball, soccer, gymnastics, and swimming. Equipment must be maintained in safe condition, and protective apparatus should be worn to prevent serious injury. The Canadian Paediatric Society (CPS) is calling for Canada-wide use of helmets when children are skiing and snowboarding (CPS, Injury Prevention Committee, 2012). The society is also recommending wrist splints as well when children are snowboarding. These activities can lead to significant head and limb injuries and there is evidence that helmets and splints prevent injuries (see Chapter 54, Traumatic Injury).

During the school-age years, girls have the same basic body structure as that of boys and have a similar response to systematic exercise training. However, at puberty, boys become larger and have more muscle mass, and at this stage, it is usually recommended that girls compete only against other girls. Before puberty there is no essential difference in strength and size between girls and boys, making these precautions unnecessary.

Preadolescence is a time to teach fundamental motor skills; develop fitness in a practical, safe, and gradual manner; and promote healthy attitudes and values. Activities should include both practice sessions and unstructured play; the actual game or event should be managed in a manner that stresses mastery of the sport, fun, and enhancement of self-image rather than winning or pleasing others. All children should have an opportunity to participate, and special ceremonies should recognize all participants, not just individuals who excel in sports or athletics.

Acquisition of Skills

School-age children demonstrate increasing fine motor abilities and complex artistic skills. Handedness is well established by the beginning of the school years, and children make great strides in writing and drawing during this period. It is a time of energetic and vibrant creative productivity. With the tools of language and reading, children create poems, stories, and plays. With more advanced fine motor skills, they are able to master an unlimited variety of handicrafts, such as ceramics, needlework, wood carving, and beadwork. They avidly pursue these skills in solitude; with a friend; or through organized groups such as boys' or girls' clubs or special interest groups that use crafts or other activities as a means to occupy, entertain, and educate children.

School-age children are capable of assuming responsibility for their own needs. School-age children can and want to assume their share of household tasks, which may be related to male and female roles defined by their culture. Parents may choose to role model open and flexible gender expectations. Many children also assume responsibility for tasks outside the home, such as baby-sitting, mowing lawns, or paper routes.

Dental Health

The first permanent (secondary) teeth erupt at about 6 years of age, beginning with the 6-year molar, which erupts posterior to the deciduous molars. Other permanent teeth appear in approximately the same order as eruption of the primary teeth and follow shedding of the deciduous teeth (Fig. 39-8). With the appearance of the second permanent (12-year) molar, most permanent teeth are present. Permanent dentition is more advanced in girls than in boys.

Because the permanent teeth erupt during the school-age years, dental hygiene and regular attention to dental caries are important parts of health supervision during this period. Correct brushing techniques should be taught or reinforced, and the role that fermentable carbohydrates play in production of dental caries should be emphasized. It is important to be alert to possible malocclusion problems that may result from irregular eruption of permanent teeth and that may impair function. Regular dental supervision and continued fluoride supplementation are integral parts of the health maintenance program.

The most effective means of preventing dental caries is proper oral hygiene. Children should be taught to perform their own dental care with the supervision and guidance of the parents. Parents should learn the correct brushing technique with their children, and they should monitor their child's efforts until the child can assume full responsibility.

Teeth should be brushed after meals, after snacks, and at bedtime. Children who brush their teeth frequently and become accustomed to the feel of a clean mouth at an early age usually maintain the habit throughout life. For the school-age child with mixed and permanent dentition, the best toothbrush is one with soft nylon bristles and should be comfortable for your child to hold and reach all teeth. Several methods of brushing have been described and recommended for children,

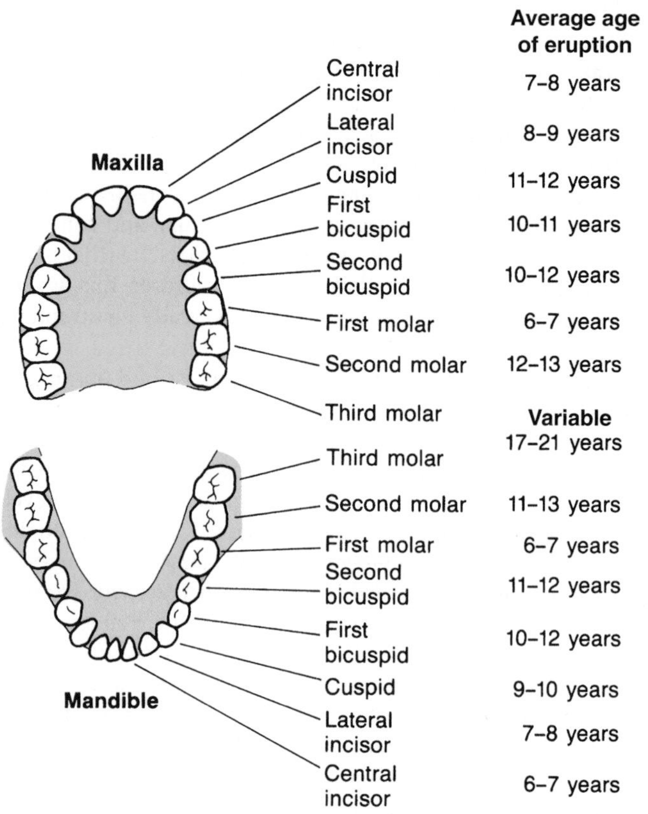

Fig. 39-8 Sequence of eruption of secondary teeth. *(Data from McDonald, R. E., & Avery, D. R. [1994].* Dentistry for the child and adolescent *[6th ed.]. St. Louis: Mosby.)*

but there is no conclusive evidence that one method is superior to another. Thorough cleaning is more important than the specific technique used, and professionals like dentists and dental hygienists should assess factors such as the child's manipulative skills and special needs, and suggest the most appropriate brushing technique and regimen. Flossing follows brushing. Parents should perform the flossing until children acquire the manual dexterity required (usually at about 8 or 9 years of age).

Dental Problems

Limited or inadequate dental care results in the most common dental problems: dental caries, malocclusion, and periodontal disease. **Trauma**, especially tooth avulsion, is another important dental problem. All of these conditions benefit from early intervention to prevent tooth loss.

Dental caries (cavities) is the principal oral problem in children and adolescents. Reducing the incidence and consequences of dental caries is extremely important in childhood. If untreated, dental caries can result in the total destruction of the involved teeth. The prevalence rate of caries increases steadily across the lifespan.

Dental **caries** is a multifactorial disease involving susceptible teeth, cariogenic microflora, and an appropriate oral environment. The incidence of lesions and the likelihood of progressive invasion vary considerably and depend on a number of factors being present in the right combination.

Because many children are exposed to health care but not dental care, oral inspection is an integral part of the physical assessment of every child. Recent research indicates a high incidence of dental caries in baby teeth of First Nations, Métis, and Inuit children; the prevalence of early-childhood caries exceeds 90% in Aboriginal communities (Schroth, Harrison, & Lawrence, 2009). The Canadian Paediatric Society (2011) recommends that action be taken at the first age that caries are observed. If there is any evidence of dental caries or other unhealthy dental state, the child should be referred for dental services. An alarming number of children do not receive regular dental supervision, and a significant number reach adulthood without having undergone dental examinations or treatment by a dentist.

Periodontal disease, an inflammatory and degenerative condition involving the gums and tissues supporting the teeth, often begins in childhood and accounts for a significant amount of tooth loss in adulthood. The more common periodontal problems are *gingivitis* (simple inflammation of the gums) and *periodontitis* (inflammation of the gums and loss of connective tissue and bone in the supporting structures of the teeth).

Gingivitis, the most prevalent periodontal disease, is a reversible inflammatory disease that can begin in early childhood and is most often associated with the buildup of plaque on the teeth. Changes take place in the plaque bacteria, in both the type and number of organisms, causing them to release destructive exotoxins, enzymes, and other noxious agents. These substances produce an inflammatory reaction in the gingival tissues, causing the gums to become red, edematous, tender, and subject to bleeding at the slightest irritation. Management is directed toward prevention by conscientious brushing and flossing, including the use of fluoride. The child should see the dentist at any signs of inflammation or irritation.

Malocclusion occurs when teeth of the upper and lower dental arches do not approximate in the proper relationships. As a result, the physiological function of chewing is less effective and the cosmetic effect is displeasing. Teeth that are uneven, crowded, or overlapping are unable to meet their counterparts in the opposite jaw in the appropriate relationships and may be predisposed to disease in later years.

Orthodontic treatment is most successful when it is started in the late school-age or early teenage years, after the last primary teeth have been shed and before growth ceases. However, referral should be made as soon as malocclusion is evident, since some deformities can be corrected at an earlier age or require treatment in stages over the years.

Dental injury may occur in childhood and includes fractures of varying degrees of severity, chipping, dislocation, or avulsion. All tooth injuries should be treated as a **dental emergency** requiring prompt treatment by a competent dentist to prevent permanent displacement or loss. Delayed examination and diagnosis of tooth damage can result in infection or pulp involvement. Because the loss can affect the remaining teeth, replacement of the lost tooth is needed to maintain normal alignment and position of the other teeth.

A tooth that is avulsed (exarticulated, or "knocked out") should be replanted by the child, parent, or nurse and stabilized as soon as possible so that the blood supply to the tooth can be re-established and the tooth kept alive (see Emergency box). A tooth that is replanted within 15 minutes has a 98% survival rate (Krause-Parello, 2005). Avulsed primary teeth are usually not reimplanted.

As with all injuries to the mouth, an avulsed tooth causes a large amount of bleeding, which is frightening to children and their families. Therefore, the nurse or anyone faced with dental trauma should be prepared to provide support and reassurance during the dental trauma.

Sex Education

Many children experience some form of sex play during or before preadolescence, as a response to normal curiosity, not as a result of love or sexual urges. Children are experimentalists by nature, and sex play is incidental and transitory. Any adverse emotional consequences or guilt feelings depend on how the behaviour is managed by the parents; whether it is discovered; or whether children view their actions as wrong in the eyes of significant persons, particularly the parents.

The child's attitude toward sex is acquired indirectly at an early age. Initial curiosity about differences in body structure between boys and girls and between children and adults arises in the preschool years. Middle childhood is an ideal time for formal sex education, and many authorities believe that the topic is best presented from a lifespan approach. Information about sexual maturation and the process of reproduction minimizes the child's uncertainty, embarrassment, and feelings of isolation that often accompany puberty.

An important component of ongoing sex education is effective communication with parents. If parents either repress the child's sexual curiosity or avoid dealing with it, the sexual information that the child receives may be acquired almost

EMERGENCY

Avulsed Permanent Tooth

Recover the tooth.
Hold tooth by the crown; avoid touching root area.
If the tooth is dirty, rinse it gently under running water or saline; be certain to insert a stopper in the sink or basin (to avoid losing tooth).

To Reimplant Tooth

Insert tooth into the socket; be certain that the lip-side (or convex surface) is facing front.
Have child maintain tooth in place by slowly biting down on a piece of gauze.
Transport child to dentist immediately.
Avoid sudden stops or sharp turns to prevent dislodging the tooth.

If Reluctant to Reimplant Tooth

Place avulsed tooth in a suitable medium for transport:

- Cold milk
- Saliva—under the child's or parent's tongue

If child is holding tooth in the mouth, avoid sudden stops to prevent swallowing of tooth.
DON'T FORGET TO TAKE THE TOOTH.

entirely from peers. Inaccurate information given in secret may result when peers are the primary source of sexual information.

Nurse's Role in Sex Education

No matter where nurses practise, they can provide information on human sexuality to both parents and children. To discuss the topic adequately, nurses must have an understanding of the physiological aspects of sexuality; knowledge of the cultural and societal values; and an awareness of their own attitudes, feelings, and **biases** about sexuality.

When presenting sexual information to school-age children, nurses should treat sex as a normal part of growth and development. They should answer questions honestly, matter-of-factly, and to the same extent as questions about other topics. Answers should be at the child's level of understanding. There may be times when boys and girls should be taught content separately.

Children need help differentiating sex and sexuality. Exercises on clarifying values, identifying role models, engaging in problem-solving skills, and practising responsibility are important to prepare children for early adolescence and puberty. In addition, children need explanations of sexual information provided via the media or jokes. Information concerning pregnancy, contraceptives, and sexually transmitted infections (STIs), including human immunodeficiency virus (HIV) and human papillomavirus (HPV), should be presented in simple, accurate terms.

Preadolescents need precise and concrete information that will allow them to answer questions such as "What if I start my period in the middle of class?" or "How can I keep people from telling I have an erection?" It is important to tell children what they want to know and what they can expect to happen as they become mature sexually.

During interactions with parents, nurses should be open and available for questions and discussion. They can set an example by the language they use in discussing body parts and their function and by the way in which they deal with problems that have emotional overtones, such as exploratory sex play and masturbation. Parents may need help understanding normal behaviours and viewing sexual curiosity in their children as a part of the developmental process. Assessment of the parents' level of knowledge and understanding of sexuality can provide cues to their need for supplemental information that will prepare them for the increasingly complex explanations they will need to provide as their children grow older.

School Health

Child health maintenance is ultimately the responsibility of the parents; however, public schools and health departments in Canada have contributed to the improvement of child health by providing a healthful school environment, health services, and health education that emphasize sound health practices. Varying by province, territory, and school district, most of these functions constitute major components of community health services and involve public funding and health care providers, including nurses. School health programs are involved in ongoing health maintenance through assessment, screening, and referral activities. Health services provided by most schools include health appraisal by consultation, emergency care, safety education, communicable disease control, counselling, and follow-up care. Health education of school-age children is directed toward providing knowledge of health and influencing habits, attitudes, and conduct in relation to health promotion and injury prevention. School districts may allocate their money to programs aimed at improving learning by improving nutrition—for example, some inner city schools in Vancouver and Toronto have breakfast programs for all children.

Traditionally, school nurses were viewed as the individuals who detected diseases in the school, applied bandages, and cared for students who were ill or injured. Although these functions were an important part of the school nurse's job, the role has expanded considerably in recent years. Today, public health and community health nurses may manage and coordinate care required by regular students and students with special health care needs. The term *community health nurse,* used throughout Canada, means the same as or is used instead of the term *public health nurse*. In some parts of Canada *community health nurse* refers to nurses working in the community, of which public health nurses are one group (Canadian Public Health Association, 2010). In many settings, school health services have enlarged into community health centres that meet the needs of not only school-age children but also their families and the community. In these settings, schools provide health care that includes assessment of physical, psychological, emotional, behavioural, and learning problems, as well as comprehensive well-child care (Hackbarth & Gall, 2005).

The level of integration of children with chronic illness or disability into regular classrooms varies among the provinces and territories in Canada. Public or community health nurses are usually available for consultation on integrating the child into the classroom, although the individual parent may need to make arrangements with their local community health nursing organization if their child requires nursing care at school. Public and community health nurses can develop, implement, and evaluate individualized health care plans for these children. Most health jurisdictions aim to provide unregulated care providers such as special education assistants (EAs) to be with all children who require such assistance. Delegation and supervision of unregulated care providers requires skillful nursing assessment, effective communication, and professional judgement (Potter & Grant, 2004).

Injury Prevention

evolve Case Study—Injury Prevention

Currently, data related to accidents in Canada are collected and analyzed by the Canadian Hospitals Injury Reporting and Prevention Program (CHIRPP), a program of the Public Health Agency of Canada (2009). Much of the data relates to children seen in Canada's 10 pediatric hospitals. Nurses and other health care providers can use these data to help prevent injury in children as the details collected relate to the pre-event context of injury.

Because school-age children have developed more refined muscular coordination and control and can apply their cognitive capacities to their behaviour, the number of injuries in middle childhood is less than that in early childhood. In Canada, the leading cause of death for children under 14 years of age is child pedestrian accidents. On average, annually more than 30 child pedestrians under age 14 are killed and 2400 are injured, with most accidents happening between 3 and 6 PM when children are walking home from school and drivers are going home from work (Safe Kids Canada, 2009).

To help reduce the number of child injuries as a passenger in motor vehicle accidents, it is important that nurses emphasize the three automobile safety measures that have been found to reduce the severity of injuries: effective car restraint systems, use of door-lock mechanisms, and appropriate passenger-seating locations in the motor vehicle. The Canadian Paediatric Society's (2008) position statement on motor vehicle safety advises that the rear vehicle seat is the safest place for children under the age of 13 years. Children should use specially designed car restraints until they are 145 cm in height or are 8 to 12 years old, and they should not sit in the front seat until they are 12 years of age (CPS, 2008). Shoulder-lap safety belts should be worn low on the hips, snug, and not on the abdominal area. Children should be taught to sit up straight to allow for proper fit. The shoulder belt is used only if it does not cross the child's neck or face.

The school-age child's desire for riding bicycles increases the risk of injury on streets. Other serious injuries include accidents on skateboards, roller skates, in-line skates, scooters, and other sports equipment. Most injuries occur in or near the home or school. All-terrain vehicles (ATVs), popular with children younger than 16 years of age, are unstable, difficult to handle, and responsible for an increasing number of childhood injuries. In some Canadian jurisdictions, children are not allowed to operate ATVs if they are under 16 years of age. The Canadian Paediatric Society and Safe Kids Canada have advocated for a Canada-wide ban on ATV operation by those under 16 years of age (CPS, 2004).

The most effective means of injury prevention is education of the child and family about the hazards of risk taking and the improper use of equipment. Safety helmets, protective eye and mouth shields, and protective padding are strongly recommended for children engaging in active sports, even though they may not be required equipment. Falls from bicycles, ATVs, and skating devices are the cause of a significant number of head injuries in school-age children. Because head injury is the major cause of bicycle-related fatalities, the most important aspect of bicycle safety is to encourage the rider to wear a protective helmet (Khambalia, MacArthur, & Parkin, 2005). Wearing of a properly fitting helmet can decrease the risk of serious head injury by over 85%; this means that four out of five head injuries could be prevented by the use of helmets (Safe Kids Canada, 2010). British Columbia, Ontario, New Brunswick, Nova Scotia, Alberta, Prince Edward Island, and Manitoba all require cyclists under 18 years of age to wear a bike helmet. Some provinces require helmets for all age groups, as do some municipalities (Safe Kids Canada, 2010). It is also important that children ride bicycles that are the correct size for their bodies (Fig. 39-9).

Physically active school-age children are also highly susceptible to cuts and abrasions; the incidence of childhood fractures, strains, and sprains is high. Trampoline injuries occur most frequently in children ages 5 through 14 years and account for numerous fractures, sprains, and head injuries. Trampolines in the home environment, routine physical education classes, or outdoor playgrounds are not recommended for children of any age (Nysted & Drogset, 2006). Other serious injuries are discussed elsewhere in the book: burns (Chapter 53), eye trauma (Chapter 42), submersion injuries (Chapter 51), and head injuries (Chapter 51). The prevalence of injuries depends on the dangers in the environment, the protection offered by adults, and the children's behaviour patterns. Table 39-2 lists characteristics of school-age children that make them prone to injury and provides suggestions for injury prevention. The Family Centred Teaching boxes provide guidelines for bicycle, skateboard, and in-line skate safety and guidance during the school years.

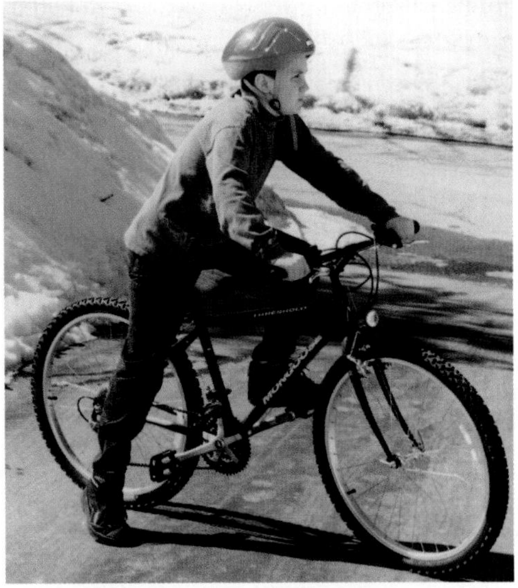

Fig. 39-9 The right-size bike is important; the child should be able to sit on the bike and place the balls of both feet on the ground. The foot should comfortably reach and manipulate the pedal in the down position. Wearing a protective helmet should be mandatory. The helmet should be positioned so it sits low on the forehead and parallel to the ground when the head is held upright. It should not rock back and forth or shift from side to side. The strap should fasten securely under the chin. Courses are available if parents want their children to be exposed to safety information and skills practice on bicycles.

Injury prevention is particularly important in First Nations, Métis, and Inuit communities in Canada, as the leading cause of death for all First Nations people aged 1 to 44 years is injuries. In this group, 26% of all deaths are caused by injuries, compared with 6% for the rest of the Canadian population. The majority of hospital admissions in this population are for falls in all age groups, except 15- to 34-year-olds. School-age First Nations children commonly fall from playground equipment, fences, and trees (Health Canada, 2008).

SPECIAL HEALTH PROBLEMS

Health Problems Related to Sports Participation

Every sport has the potential for injury to the participant—whether the youngster engages in serious competition or participates for enjoyment. Serious injury occurs most often during rough contact sports or to persons who are not physically prepared for the activity. Injuries also occur to children

Table 39-2 Injury Prevention During School-Age Years*

DEVELOPMENTAL ABILITIES RELATED TO RISK OF INJURY	INJURY PREVENTION
Motor Vehicle Accidents	
Is increasingly involved in activities away from home Is excited by speed and motion Is easily distracted by environment Can be reasoned with	Educate child regarding proper use of seat belts while a passenger in a vehicle. Children under 13 years of age should ride in the back seat of a car. Maintain discipline while a passenger in a vehicle (e.g., keep arms inside, do not lean against doors, do not interfere with driver). Remind parents and children that no one should ride in the bed of a pickup truck. Emphasize safe pedestrian behaviour. Insist on child wearing safety apparel (e.g., helmet) when applicable, such as when riding a bicycle, motorcycle, moped, or all-terrain vehicle (see Family Centred Teaching box).
Drowning	
Is apt to overdo May work hard to perfect a skill Has cautious, but not fearful, gross motor actions Likes swimming	Teach child to swim. Teach basic rules of water safety. Select safe and supervised places to swim. Check sufficient water depth for diving. Swim with a companion. Use an approved flotation device. Advocate for legislation requiring fencing around pools. Learn cardiopulmonary resuscitation.
Burns	
Has increasing independence Is adventurous Enjoys trying new things	Make certain the home has smoke detectors. Set water heaters at 49°C to avoid scald burns. Instruct child in behaviour in areas involving contact with potential burn hazards (e.g., gasoline, matches, bonfires or barbecues, lighter fluid, firecrackers, cigarette lighters, cooking utensils, chemistry sets). Instruct child to avoid climbing or flying a kite around high-tension wires. Instruct child in proper behaviour in the event of a fire (e.g., fire drills at home and school). Teach child safe cooking (use low heat; avoid any frying; be careful of steam burns, scalds, or exploding foods, especially from microwaving).
Poisoning	
Adheres to group rules May be easily influenced by peers Has strong allegiance to friends	Educate child regarding hazards of taking nonprescription drugs and chemicals, including aspirin and alcohol. Teach child to say "no" if offered illegal or dangerous drugs or alcohol. Keep potentially dangerous products in properly labelled receptacles, preferably out of reach.
Bodily Damage	
Has increased physical skills Needs strenuous physical activity Is interested in acquiring new skills and perfecting attained skills Is daring and adventurous, especially with peers Frequently plays in hazardous places Confidence often exceeds physical capacity Desires group loyalty and has strong need for friends' approval Attempts hazardous feats Accompanies friends to potentially hazardous facilities Is likely to overdo Growth in height exceeds muscular growth and coordination	Help provide facilities for supervised activities. Encourage playing in safe places. Keep firearms safely locked up except under adult supervision. Teach proper care of, use of, and respect for devices with potential danger (e.g., power tools, firecrackers). Teach children not to tease or surprise dogs, invade their territory, take dogs' toys, or interfere with dogs' feeding. Stress eye, ear, or mouth protection when using potentially hazardous objects or devices or when engaging in potentially hazardous sports. Do not permit use of trampolines except as part of supervised training. Teach safety regarding use of corrective devices (glasses); if the child wears contact lenses, monitor duration of wear to prevent corneal damage. Stress careful selection, use, and maintenance of sports and recreation equipment, such as skateboards and in-line skates (see Family-Centred Teaching box). Emphasize proper conditioning, safe practices, and use of safety equipment for sports or recreational activities. Caution against engaging in hazardous sports. Use safety glass and decals on large glassed areas, such as sliding glass doors. Use window guards to prevent falls. Teach child that he or she should ask for help from appropriate people (e.g., cashier, security guard, police) if lost; have identification on the child (e.g., sewn in clothes, inside shoe). Teach stranger safety: • Avoid personalized clothing in public places. • Caution child to never go with a stranger. • Have child tell parents if anyone makes child feel uncomfortable in any way. • Always listen to child's concerns regarding others' behaviour. • Teach child to say "no" when confronted by uncomfortable situations—practise this with them.

*See also Public Health Agency of Canada. (2011). *Building toward breakthroughs in injury control: A legislative perspective on the prevention of unintentional injuries among children and youth in Canada*. Retrieved from http://www.phac-aspc.gc.ca/hp-ps/dca-dea/publications/break/index-eng.php.

FAMILY-CENTRED TEACHING

Bicycle Safety

- Always wear a properly fitted bicycle helmet that is certified, e.g., by the Canadian Standards Association (CSA); encourage parents to look for the CSA approval sticker on the inside liner of the helmet and to find out if helmet use is legally mandated (legislation varies across provinces) (Public Health Agency of Canada, 2011).
- Replace a helmet every 5 years or sooner if the manufacturer recommends it. Never use a damaged or outgrown helmet.
- Ride bicycles with traffic and away from parked cars.
- Ride single file.
- Walk bicycles through busy intersections only at crosswalks.
- Give hand signals well in advance of turning or stopping.
- Keep as close to the curb as practical.
- Watch for drain grates, potholes, soft shoulders, loose dirt, or gravel.
- Keep both hands on the handlebars, except with signalling.
- Never ride double on a bicycle.
- Do not carry packages that interfere with vision or control; do not drag objects behind the bike.
- Watch for and yield to pedestrians.
- Watch for cars backing up or pulling out of driveways; be especially careful at intersections.
- Look left, right, then left, before turning into traffic or road.
- Never hitch a ride on a truck or other vehicle.
- Learn rules of the road and respect traffic officers.
- Obey all local ordinances.
- Wear shoes that fit securely while riding.
- Wear light colours at night and attach fluorescent material to clothing and the bicycle.
- Equip the bicycle with proper lights and reflectors.
- Be certain the bicycle is the correct size for rider (see Fig. 39-9).
- Have the bicycle inspected to ensure good mechanical condition.
- Children riding as passengers must wear appropriate-size helmets and sit in specially designed protective seats.

(Modified from American Academy of Pediatrics, Committee on Injury and Poison Prevention. [2001]. Bicycle helmets. *Pediatrics, 108*[4], 1030–1032.)

or adolescents when their body is not suited to the sport, when their muscles and body systems (respiratory and cardiovascular) are not conditioned to endure physical stress, or when they lack the insight and judgement to recognize that an activity exceeds their physical abilities. More injuries occur during recreational sports participation than during organized athletic competition.

The environment and the sports or recreational equipment can also present risks. Children who participate in physical

FAMILY-CENTRED TEACHING

Skateboard and In-Line Skate Safety

- Children younger than 5 years of age should not use skateboards or in-line skates because they are not developmentally prepared to protect themselves from injury. Children ages 6 to 8 years should use these only with close adult supervision.
- Children who ride skateboards or in-line skates should wear helmets and other protective equipment, especially on the knees, wrists, and elbows, to prevent injury.
- Skateboards and in-line skates should never be used near traffic. Their use should be prohibited on streets and highways. Activities that bring skateboards together (e.g., "catching a ride") are especially dangerous.
- Some types of use, such as riding homemade ramps on hard surfaces, may be particularly hazardous.

(Data from American Academy of Pediatrics, Committee on Injury and Poison Prevention. [2006]. Skateboard injuries. *Pediatrics, 109*[3], 542–543; American Academy of Pediatrics, Committee on Injury and Poison Prevention. [2006]. In-line skating injuries in children and adolescents. *Pediatrics, 117*[5], 1846–1847; Public Health Agency of Canada. [2002]. *Sports and leisure: Skateboards, scooters, in-line skates.* Retrieved from http://www.phac-aspc.gc.ca/hp-ps/dca-dea/injury/en/sports3-eng.php.)

activity or sports do so in many different environments: indoors and outdoors, on floors, on the ground and snow, on or beneath water surfaces, and sometimes in free air space. Most of these activities also involve equipment.

Acute overload injuries are those that occur suddenly during an activity and produce immediate symptoms. A blow or overstretching, twisting, or sudden stress to tissues can cause these injuries. For descriptions and management of traumatic injuries, see Chapter 54.

Overuse Syndromes

To excel in sports, the young athlete is forced to train longer, harder, and earlier in life than previously. The rewards are an increased level of fitness, better performances, faster times, and the satisfaction of attaining a personal goal. However, the risk of overuse injury is always present and is related to several factors: training errors, muscle–tendon imbalance, anatomical malalignment, incorrect footwear or playing surface, an associated disease state, and growth.

A common feature in overuse injuries is the repetitive microtrauma that occurs to a particular anatomical structure when the same movements are performed over a long period of time. The result is inflammation of the involved structure with symptoms of chronic pain, tenderness, swelling, and disability. Examples of overuse syndromes include "Little League elbow" (tendonitis and osteochondritis from repetitive throwing), "tennis elbow" (lateral epicondylitis from repetitive elbow strain), and Osgood-Schlatter disease (traction apophysitis of the tibial tubercle).

Stress Fractures

Stress fractures occur as a result of repeated muscle contraction and are seen most often in repetitive weight-bearing sports such as running, gymnastics, and basketball. They occur less often in swimmers. The most common symptoms are a sharp, persistent, progressive pain or a deep, persistent, dull ache located over the bone. Sometimes there is pain on impact (heel strike), but the most important clinical sign is pain over the involved bony surface. Diagnosis is established on the basis of clinical observation, but occasionally a bone scan is performed.

Therapeutic Management

Inflammation is common in all overuse syndromes, and management is directed toward rest or alteration of activities, physiotherapy, and medication. Rest is the primary therapy and is usually interpreted as reduced activity and the use of alternative exercise—not bed rest or immobilization with casting. The primary purpose is to alleviate the repetitive stress that initiated the symptoms. It is important to keep the youngster mobile, and training can be continued. Alternative exercise that maintains conditioning without aggravating the injury is selected. For example, pool running (treading water in the deep end of a pool) is an excellent alternative to running. Pool running involves the same movements as running without weight bearing. Other therapies include **cryotherapy**; cold whirlpools; and sometimes taping, bracing, splinting, or other orthoses. Treatment is specific to the injury. Nonsteroidal anti-inflammatory drugs (NSAIDs) are prescribed to reduce pain and inflammation. Topical medications are of questionable value.

Nurse's Role in Sports for Children and Adolescents

Nurses are often involved in sports activities in the areas of preparation and evaluation for activities, prevention of injury, treatment of injuries, and rehabilitation after injury. Selecting an appropriate sport for both recreation and competition is a joint effort of the youngster, parents, and health care providers. The best approach to counselling children and parents regarding sports participation is to encourage activities that are most likely to provide pleasure and physical benefits throughout childhood and into adulthood. Exposure to a variety of activities is better for young children than limiting them to one sport. Parents should be cautioned against overcommitting children to sports activities so that they have time for other activities.

When children sustain athletic injuries, nurses are often responsible for instructions regarding care. Instructions (e.g., schedule for appointments, application of ice, and any restrictions in activity) should be clear and accompanied by written directions. The importance of taking medications as prescribed should also be emphasized, especially if medications are needed for an extended period and if adherence is an issue. Medications given an hour before practice or competition may be advantageous to children who are continuing their activities.

Prevention of sports injuries is the most important aspect of athletic programs. Children should be suited to the activity, and the environment and equipment must be safe. Children should be prepared for the sport, especially if it requires strenuous or continuous physical exertion. Nurses, coaches, and athletic trainers must collaborate to ensure that safety measures are implemented. Stretching exercises, warm-up and cool-down activities, and appropriate training are requirements for safe participation. Protective measures such as pads, taping, and wrapping are also important to prevent injury. Finally, nurses must be aware of environmental safety risks.

Altered Growth and Maturation

The absence of physical or sexual maturation at a time when other children are experiencing positive evidence of sexual development and its associated spurt in growth and physical strength can be a concern to both the parents and their affected child. Fortunately, in most instances, the delay in development is a simple physiological or constitutional delay that represents one end of the normal genetically influenced variation of pubertal growth. These children will go through a delayed but normal puberty and finally catch up, in their late teens, with their more rapidly developing age-mates. Less benign causes of delayed development may be the result of endocrine disorders or chromosomal abnormalities. Delayed development can also be a result of chronic diseases (such as malabsorption or chronic asthma) that are serious enough to slow development or a result of environmental factors (such as stress or poor nutrition).

Rates of maturation are important during the school years, but at puberty it assumes larger proportions to both teens and their parents. Girls or boys who lag behind their peers in physical maturation are painfully aware of their difference in growth. Adolescent girls with delayed maturation feel out of place among companions whose hips and breasts are developing, may feel cheated if they have not yet menstruated, and feel left out when their friends giggle and talk about boys. Adolescent boys with delayed maturation may feel weak and small compared to their more muscular companions, with whom they can no longer compete. Slow-maturing youngsters need support and reassurance that they are not abnormal and that they will develop the physical characteristics they desire.

Serial measurements of growth should be plotted periodically on standard growth charts to determine the pattern of growth and to compare the individual child with the norms for his or her age group. When children are in the extremes of height ranges, it is important to compare their height with that of their parents and siblings.

Tall or Short Stature

Tall Stature

Despite the fact that the average height of boys and girls is steadily increasing, there is a small group of children who, because of some organic disorder or a familial tendency, are excessively tall compared with their peers.

When the rate of height change before puberty suggests the probability of excessive adult height, treatment with hormones may be considered, although there is considerable controversy regarding the use of hormones for this purpose. The use of estrogens is effective in controlling height when therapy is initiated before menarche and before the end of the adolescent growth spurt that normally precedes menarche. The selection of children for hormonal therapy is made on the basis of a careful evaluation of physical, psychological, and social factors.

Short Stature

Short stature is a nonspecific finding that may be the first manifestation of a serious disorder, or it may be of no consequence medically. On a worldwide scale, the most common cause of short stature or delayed development is inadequate nutrition. The major physical disorders that produce delayed development are chronic diseases, endocrine dysfunction, and syndromes of primary **gonad** failure.

Chronic diseases can interfere with growth, but unless the illness is unduly prolonged, catch-up growth occurs. Diseases and disorders that cause some degree of growth delay include asthma, cystic fibrosis, gastrointestinal diseases (such as parasitic infections), malabsorption syndromes, cardiac anomalies, and chronic renal disturbances. The duration of the illness is more significant than the intensity in terms of the effect on growth, although the precise length of time necessary to affect growth permanently has not been determined.

Skeletal disorders that affect growth in stature are those described as dwarfism. Most disorders are caused by congenital defects and disorders, such as achondroplasia, and by inborn errors of metabolism, such as Hurler's syndrome or Hunter's syndrome.

Psychosocial, or deprivation, dwarfism is a stress-induced growth failure. It is defined as growth restriction in children over 2 years of age that is caused by environmental (emotional) stress and is associated with a marked delay in physical growth, delayed developmental skills, and immature behaviour. When these children are removed from the deprived environment, their growth proceeds at a normal or increased rate. (See also Growth Failure [Failure to Thrive], Chapter 36, and Child Maltreatment, Chapter 38.)

Management involves continued medical observation, attention to general health and nutrition, and psychological support. When growth delay is accompanied by poor self-esteem, many authorities recommend hormonal therapy. Testosterone in carefully regulated doses is effective in some cases. Growth hormone is capable of increasing height and is used to treat growth hormone deficiency (see Chapter 52, Hypopituitarism). Its use with children who have constitutional delay is highly controversial.

Nursing Care Management

Deviation from the normal course of puberty is a significant concern for affected adolescents. For some teens, this concern assumes monumental proportions. Most cases of delayed development are caused by simple constitutional delay of puberty, and the child can be assured that normal development will eventually take place.

One difficulty related to size being incongruent with chronological and mental age is the manner in which others relate to the child. People often respond to children with short stature as though they are younger than their age. Consequently, these children may react with babyish or juvenile behaviour, thus establishing a circular pattern of behaviour and response. Conversely, children who are tall or physically advanced for their age are frequently treated as though they are more advanced than their years. They are often considered to be cognitively impaired or immature when they perform according to the normal behavioural expectations for their age.

Listening to distressed adolescents and conveying interest in and concern about them are important interventions. Counselling and therapy need to be individualized for each youth. Encouraging these children to focus on the positive aspects of their bodies and personalities and to adopt sound health practices and practise good grooming fosters a more positive self-image.

Sex Chromosome Abnormalities

Most **sex chromosome** abnormalities are caused by an alteration in sex chromosome number (Table 39-3). Most of these

Table 39-3 Common Sex Chromosome Abnormalities

SYNDROME	CHROMOSOMAL NOMENCLATURE	PHENOTYPE	INCIDENCE (LIVE BIRTHS)	CLINICAL MANIFESTATIONS
Turner's	45,X or 45XO	Female	1:2500 female births*	Short stature; webbed neck; low posterior hairline; shield-shaped chest with widely spaced nipples; sterile; no development of secondary sex characteristics
Triple X, or superfemale	47,XXX (can also be 48,XXXX or 49,XXXXX)	Female	1:850–1250 female births	Normal female characteristics; usually tall; variable mental capacity and behaviour; at risk for impaired language, learning difficulties; fertile
XYY male	47,XYY (can also be 48,XYYY or mosaic)	Male	1:900 male births*	Usually normal sexual development; tendency to be tall with long head; poor coordination; may demonstrate aberrant behaviour
Klinefelter's	47,XXY (48,XXYY, 48,XXXY, 49,XXXXY, and so on, mosaics)	Male	1:850 male births*	Tall with long legs; hypogenitalism; sterile; male secondary sex characteristics may be deficient; may demonstrate aberrant behaviour; learning disabled; possible gynecomastia

*Data from Nora, J. J., & Fraser, F. C. (1989). *Medical genetics: Principles and practice* (3rd ed.). Philadelphia: Lea & Febiger.

conditions are due to nondisjunction. An alteration in the number of sex chromosomes usually does not produce the profound defects associated with the autosomal trisomies. Intelligence may be normal or low normal or the child may have some learning disabilities. Moderate or severe cognitive impairment is less common.

Turner's Syndrome

evolve Critical Thinking Exercise—Turner Syndrome

Turner's syndrome is caused by absence of one of the X chromosomes. Most girls who have this disorder have one X chromosome missing from all cells (45,X). This disorder is often recognized at birth if the newborn has a webbed neck, low posterior hairline, widely spaced nipples, and edema of the hands and feet. It can also be diagnosed at puberty because of three features: short stature, sexual infantilism, and **amenorrhea**. Girls with Turner's syndrome are generally infertile. They may also have difficulty with peer relationships and understanding social cues. They frequently exhibit behavioural problems, especially in relation to their immature, socially isolated behaviour. Diagnosis is confirmed on the basis of a negative sex chromatin test.

Therapy is individualized for these girls and consists primarily of hormone treatment and psychological counselling for both the child and parents. Linear growth can be increased by the administration of growth hormone if therapy is begun early. Estrogen therapy is initiated during the usual time for puberty to promote the development of secondary sex characteristics. Responses to estrogen therapy vary from girl to girl, but gradual feminization is accomplished to some degree in most individuals.

Klinefelter's Syndrome

Klinefelter's syndrome, the most common of all sex chromosome abnormalities, is caused by the presence of one or more additional X chromosomes. Most males with this syndrome have a chromosome complement of 47, XXY. The disorder is seldom recognized before puberty, at which time varying degrees of failure of adolescent virilization occur. Some males are not diagnosed until they appear for evaluation for infertility. All have absence of sperm in the semen (azoospermia), small testes, and defective development of secondary sex characteristics. In 80% of these boys there is a chromatin-positive buccal smear, and the extra chromosome is apparent on chromosome analysis.

Cognitive impairment is a frequent clinical finding and appears to be related to the number of X chromosomes. Boys may also have gross motor skill difficulties, a developmental language delay, poor verbal skills, reduced auditory memory, shyness, passivity, behavioural problems, and school difficulties. Therapy is directed toward enhancing the masculine characteristics through administration of testosterone.

Nursing Care Management

The nursing care of children with Turner's syndrome or Klinefelter's syndrome is primarily supportive. Nurses can assist in diagnosis, explain tests and therapies, and provide support and encouragement to the child and the family. Because both disorders render the individual unable to reproduce, psychological counselling is an important aspect of care. Marriage and sexual relationships are possible, but alternative reproductive options, such as artificial insemination and adoption, should be discussed.

Disorders With Behavioural Components

Attention-Deficit/Hyperactivity Disorder and Learning Disability

evolve Case Study—Attention-Deficit/Hyperactivity Disorder

Attention-deficit/hyperactivity disorder (ADHD) refers to developmentally inappropriate degrees of inattention, impulsiveness, and hyperactivity. ADHD is a psychiatric diagnosis that needs to be made by a psychiatrist, a clinical psychologist, or a physician. It is important to rule out other **behavioural disorders** with similar symptoms. A *learning disability* (LD) refers to a heterogeneous group of disorders manifested by significant difficulties in the acquisition and use of listening, speaking, reading, writing, reasoning, or mathematic skills.

ADHD and LDs affect every aspect of the child's life but are most obvious in the classroom. Early identification of affected children is important because the characteristics of these disorders significantly interfere with the normal course of emotional and psychological development. Many children develop behaviour patterns that impede psychosocial adjustment while they try to cope with cognitive dysfunction. Their behaviour evokes negative responses from others, and repeated exposure to negative feedback adversely affects their self-concept. The characteristics of ADHD can affect the child's written and adaptive skills, social status, and self-esteem (Myers, Eisenhauer, & Ryan, 2003).

Diagnostic Evaluation

The behaviours exhibited by the child with ADHD are not unusual aspects of behaviour. The difference lies in the quality of motor activity and developmentally inappropriate inattention, impulsivity, and hyperactivity that the child displays. The manifestations may be numerous or few, mild or severe, and will vary with the child's developmental level. Any given child will not have every symptom of the condition. A comprehensive battery of tests is needed to confirm a learning disability. These include intelligence tests (many children have normal or above-average intelligence quotients [IQs]); hand–eye coordination tests; and measurements of auditory and visual perception, comprehension, and memory. Often there is a wide gap between verbal and performance scores on IQ tests.

Therapeutic Management

Some controversy exists regarding the management of ADHD—whether to use medications is a big part of this controversy. Management of the child with ADHD usually involves multiple approaches that include family education and counselling, medication, proper classroom placement, environmental manipulation, and sometimes behavioural therapy or psychotherapy for the child. Interventions for children with LDs are primarily educational.

Medication

Stimulant medications are the cornerstone treatment for ADHD and are appropriate for the school-age child with

ADHD. The most frequently prescribed medications are the psychostimulants methylphenidate hydrochloride (Ritalin) and dextroamphetamine sulphate (Dexedrine). These medications increase dopamine and norepinephrine levels, which leads to stimulation of the inhibitory system of the central nervous system. Tricyclic antidepressants, bupropion, and the α_2-adrenergic agonists (clonidine and guanfacine) are second-line medications. In addition, atomoxetine, a presynaptic norepinephrine transport inhibitor, is available for use in children (CPS, 2009). The Canadian Paediatric Society (2009) also recommends the use of extended-release forms of these drugs, if available and affordable, to improve compliance.

Some families prefer to use alternative therapies. The Canadian Paediatric Society (2012) has indicated that essential fatty acids, such as fish oil or primrose oil, may be helpful in the treatment of ADHD, but more research is needed. Biofeedback is still considered to be experimental. The following alternative therapies have little to no evidence that they will help children with ADHD or LDs but are nonetheless used:

- Diet without sugar or additives—May help some children with allergies, food sensitivities, or migraines (little evidence)
- Vitamin supplements (no evidence)
- Valerian, blue-green algae, ginkgo biloba (should not be used in children with clotting conditions)—Herbs that can be calming and may aid memory and thinking but do not alleviate ADHD symptoms. Herbs are not regulated, and pharmacists need to be asked about their strength, safety, and toxicity.
- Antioxidants or antiaging remedies help protect nerve cells but have no proven direct effect on ADHD symptoms. Pyncogenol should not to be used in children with a blood disorder. Melatonin may help with sleep problems but can also cause headaches, fatigue, irritability, and sleepiness, trigger seizures, and possibly delay puberty.
- Hypnotherapy may help with some common ADHD symptoms.
- Homeopathy remedies are a blend of plant, animal, or mineral extracts. No studies have shown that this treatment works for symptoms of ADHD.

Regularly scheduled evaluations with the child and family are essential to assess the effects of medications, behaviour strategies, parent guidance, education programs, and individual and family alternative therapies.

Environmental Manipulation

In ADHD, the child's environment is simplified by decreasing external stimuli and distractions, reducing alternatives, increasing consistency in routines, and encouraging desired patterns of behaviour. Parents need to develop firm but reasonable limits and provide a stable and predictable environment with regular routines of sleeping, eating, working, and playing.

Classroom Education

Special activities are designed to address learning deficits that involve visual perception, auditory perception, and other areas involving integration and coordination. The purpose of programs for children with LDs is to help them move toward more successful achievement and personal adjustment in the regular classroom.

Prognosis

ADHD is relatively stable through early adolescence for most children. Some children experience decreased symptoms during late adolescence and adulthood, but a significant number of these children carry their symptoms into adulthood. The goal for children with LDs is to help them identify their areas of weakness and learn to compensate for them.

Nursing Care Management

Nurses are active participants in all aspects of management of the child with ADHD or LDs. Nurses in the community work with families and school personnel on a long-term basis to help plan and implement therapeutic regimens and to evaluate the effectiveness of therapy. With medication treatment, they should teach parents and affected children to take the stimulant medication in the morning in order to maximize its effectiveness in the classroom and decrease its insomnia-producing potential. If decreased appetite is a concern, the psychostimulant can be given with or after meals rather than before meals. Parents also benefit from practical, specific strategies that help children with ADHD, such as the provision of structure and consistency in dressing, meals, sleep, and discipline.

Nurses must understand which type of LD a child has in order to provide direction for the child, parents, and teachers. Children with an auditory perceptual deficit are often unable to follow directions or to comprehend large amounts of verbal teaching. These children need diagrams, pictures, demonstration, and written lists. Children with visual perceptual deficits may have difficulty reading, lining up numbers for mathematic operations, or judging distance. These children may have dyslexia (letter reversals) and do better with demonstration and a verbal approach. Children with an integrative deficit may have difficulty sequencing data or storing and retrieving sensory data. Multisensory techniques should be used, and comprehension should be checked frequently throughout instruction. Children with dysgraphia often benefit from the use of computers in the classroom, because their handwriting will not improve. They need to find an alternative to physical competition that requires coordination of movement (Learning Disabilities Association of Ontario, 2011).

Enuresis

Enuresis (bed-wetting) is a common and troublesome disorder that is defined as intentional or involuntary passage of urine into bed (usually at night) or into clothes during the day by children who are beyond the age when voluntary bladder control should normally have been acquired. In this disorder, the inappropriate voiding of urine occurs at least twice a week for at least 3 months, and the chronological or developmental age of the child must be at least 5 years. The predominant symptom is urgency that is immediate and accompanied by acute discomfort, restlessness, and urinary frequency. Enuresis is more common in boys; nocturnal bed-wetting usually ceases between 6 and 8 years of age.

Organic causes that may be related to enuresis should be ruled out before psychogenic factors are considered. Organic causes include structural disorders of the urinary tract; urinary tract infection; neurological deficits; disorders that increase the normal output of urine, such as diabetes; and disorders that impair the concentrating ability of the kidneys, such as chronic renal failure or sickle cell disease. A bladder volume of 300 to 350 mL is sufficient to hold a night's urine. (To determine a child's bladder capacity, have the child void in a measuring cup after holding urine for as long as possible. In other cases the enuresis is influenced by emotional factors, although it is doubtful that they are causative factors. Parents report that these children sleep more soundly than other children; however, the depth of sleep has not been identified as the cause of nocturnal enuresis. Enuresis has a strong familial tendency.

Therapeutic techniques used to manage enuresis include medications, bladder training, restriction or elimination of fluids after the evening meal, interruption of sleep to void, and various devices designed to establish a conditioned reflex response to waken the child at the initiation of voiding.

Three types of drugs may be used to treat enuresis: tricyclic antidepressants, antidiuretics, and antispasmodics. The drug used most frequently to inhibit urination is the tricyclic antidepressant imipramine (Tofranil). Another anticholinergic drug, oxybutynin, reduces uninhibited bladder contractions and may be helpful for children with daytime urinary frequency. Desmopressin (DDAVP) nasal spray, an analog of vasopressin, reduces nighttime urine output to a volume less than functional bladder capacity.

Nursing Care Management

No matter what techniques are used, the nurse can help both children and parents to understand the problem of enuresis, the treatment plan, and the difficulties they may encounter in the process. The nurse can also provide consistent support and encouragement to help sustain both the child and the parents through the inconsistent and unpredictable treatment process. Parents need to understand that punishment is contraindicated because of its negative emotional impact and limited success in reducing the behaviour. Children need to believe that they are helping themselves, and they need to sustain feelings of confidence and hope.

Post-Traumatic Stress Disorder

Post-traumatic stress disorder (PTSD) refers to the development of characteristic symptoms after exposure to an extremely traumatic experience or catastrophic event. The traumatic experience is typically life threatening to self or a significant other and may involve grotesque mutilation or death, serious injury, or physical coercion (e.g., an assault, a natural disaster, sexual abuse, or witnessing violence). It is important to note that PSTD is not limited to children who have lived in "wartorn" countries. Events such as automobile, school, or recreational accidents and bullying have been identified as causes of PTSD (Sundelin-Wahlsten, Ahmad, & von Knorring, 2001). The characteristic symptoms are persistent re-experiencing of the traumatic event, avoidance of stimuli associated with the event or trauma, numbing of general responsiveness, and increased arousal.

The response to the event takes place in three stages. The initial response involves intense arousal, which usually lasts for a few minutes to 1 or 2 hours. The stress hormones are at the maximum as the individual prepares for "fight" or "flight." A prolonged arousal phase may indicate **psychosis.**

The second phase, which lasts approximately 2 weeks, is one in which defence mechanisms are mobilized. It is a period of quiescence in which the event appears to have produced no impression. The child feels numb, and stress hormone secretion is absent. Defence mechanisms are less adaptive to specific situations and may not be what the situation demands. Denial that anything is wrong is a frequently observed defence mechanism.

The third phase is one of coping and consciously directed inquiry, which normally extends over 2 to 3 months. The victims want to know what happened and appear to be getting worse, when actually they are getting better. Numerous psychological symptoms, such as depression, phobia, anxiety, and conversion reactions, may be present. Children frequently display repetitive actions. They play out the situation over and over again in an attempt to come to terms with their fear. Flashbacks are common. This phase can be self-perpetuating, and a prolonged reaction can develop into an obsession with the traumatic event. Some traumatic effects remain indefinitely.

Nursing Care Management

Children need to deal with any traumatic event. Their reactions depend heavily on their social environment and the way in which their caretaking adults react to the event. In the second phase of PTSD, the appropriateness of the defence mechanism must be assessed, and children must be assisted in application of their defence. If children do not engage in some catharsis, or if their defence phase is prolonged, they need referral for special psychological help.

Coping is a learned response, and children in the third phase can be helped to deal with their fear. Children usually are willing to accept reasoning. Those who are assisted in their catharsis and allowed expression will survive without serious lasting effects. They should be encouraged to play out the stress and to discuss their feelings about the event. If they are unable to do this, they may become obsessed with the traumatic event and require professional help. Conversion reactions are common obsessive behaviours in children suffering from PTSD.

Children need professional help if any of the phases of PTSD are prolonged. Boys tend to have a prolonged defence phase more often than girls. Occasionally the event will be unrecognized, and the affected child will engage in what is considered to be unusual behaviour. Children exhibiting any sudden change in behaviour need to be assessed for a traumatic event. When the change in behaviour is traced to a traumatic event, treatment can be implemented.

School Phobia

Children, other than beginning students, who resist going to school or who demonstrate extreme reluctance to attend school for a sustained period as a result of severe anxiety or fear of school-related experiences are said to have school phobia. The terms *school refusal* and *school avoidance* are also used to describe this behaviour. School-avoidance behaviours occur in both boys and girls and in children from all socioeconomic levels.

Physical symptoms are prominent and may affect any part of the body (e.g., anorexia, nausea, vomiting, diarrhea, dizziness, headache, leg pains, abdominal pains, or even a low-grade fever). A striking feature of school phobia is the prompt subsidence of symptoms when it is evident that the child can remain at home. Another significant observation is absence of symptoms on weekends and holidays unless they are related to other places such as Sunday school or parties. Occasional mild reluctance is not uncommon among schoolchildren, but if the fear continues for longer than a few days, it must be considered a serious problem.

Nursing Care Management

Treatment for school phobia depends on the cause. The primary goal is to return the child to school. The longer a child is permitted to stay out of school, the more difficult it is for the child to re-enter. Parents must be convinced gently but firmly that immediate return is essential and that it is their responsibility to insist on school attendance.

A school re-entry protocol may be necessary for the child with severe symptoms. In re-entry programs, the child role-plays routines involved in getting ready for school and that occur at school. Relaxation techniques are also used. The child usually goes to school initially for a half-day and then progresses to a full day. Often the school nurse is asked to provide support to the parents and the teacher during the re-entry process. If the problem persists, professional help is recommended.

Recurrent Abdominal Pain

Recurrent abdominal pain (RAP) is a complaint often attributed to a psychogenic etiology, although it can be a symptom of either psychosomatic or organic disease. *RAP* is defined as three or more separate episodes of abdominal pain during a 3-month period, similar to the "spastic" or "irritable" colon syndrome of adulthood. Children with RAP have real pain that is usually located in the periumbilical or epigastric area (or both). On palpation the pain is likely to be experienced in the epigastric area or in the lower right or left quadrant and is accompanied by vague tenderness without muscle guarding. The pain is irregular in time, duration, and intensity and associated with either loose or pellet-formed stools. Other symptoms that may accompany the pain are headache, pallor, dizziness, dysuria, flushing, vomiting, diarrhea, and fatigue.

Children at risk for RAP tend to be high achievers who have extensive personal goals or whose parents have unusually high expectations. They are described as sensitive and overly concerned about what others think of them. They are uncomfortable with expressions of anger or argument, especially in those persons who are significant in their life. School attendance is adversely affected, and these children may exhibit poor learning performance. It is not uncommon for symptoms to be aggravated during school days.

Treatment involves providing reassurance and reducing or eliminating the symptoms. Hospitalization may be necessary, and the child frequently shows improvement in the hospital. Initial efforts are directed toward ruling out organic causes of the pain, relieving discomfort, and attempting to determine the situations that precipitate attacks. A high-fibre diet, psyllium bulk agents, lubricants such as mineral oil, and bowel training are emphasized. Other therapies include cognitive-behavioural therapy, biofeedback, and medications such as famotidine and propantheline bromide (an antispasmodic).

Nursing Care Management

Once the diagnosis has been established, the parents and the child need an explanation of the pain, which can be compared to a skeletal muscle cramp or "charley horse." Reassurance that the symptoms are not unique to their child and that the pain can be expected to subside is helpful in relieving parental fears and anxieties.

The simple measure of having the child rest in a peaceful, quiet environment and providing comfort will often relieve the symptoms in a short time. A heating pad may also help ease the discomfort (see Chapter 35, Nonpharmacological Management). When pain is not relieved by these simple measures, the parents need to be taught how to administer antispasmodics, if prescribed. For example, if pain is precipitated by meals, having the child take the medication 20 to 30 minutes before mealtime may prevent an episode.

The most valuable assistance that the nurse can provide is support and reassurance to the family. When open communication is established and families appreciate the relationship between stress-provoking situations and the child's symptoms, the chance for remedial action is enhanced. Follow-up care and continued support are essential, since the symptoms tend to remit and exacerbate. The availability of a supportive health care provider can be a source of comfort to the child and family.

Eating Disorders

While 13 years is the average age of onset of anorexia nervosa and bulimia, these eating disorders are being identified in children as young as 8 or 9. Epidemiological evidence has shown that the incidence of anorexia nervosa in adolescents has been increasing over the past 50 years; it is now the third most chronic illness affecting adolescent females. A surveillance survey conducted for the Canadian Paediatric Society indicated that 161 children younger than 13 years from across Canada had been diagnosed with an eating disorder, with six girls to every boy. The average age was 11 years (Pinhas, Morris, Crosby, & Katzman, 2011).

Because of the social determinants related to eating disorders, health care professionals must be aware of the current risk status in their area and of the potential development of eating disorders. Prevention is also important; promoting access to information vendors is key for parents and families. Please refer to Chapter 40 for detailed information on eating disorders in children.

Conversion Reaction

Conversion reaction, also known as *hysteria, hysterical conversion reaction*, and *childhood hysteria*, is a psychophysiological disorder with a sudden onset that can usually be traced to a precipitating environmental event. In childhood the disorder is observed with equal frequency in both sexes, although girls outnumber boys during adolescence.

The manifestations involve primarily the voluntary musculature and special senses. Symptoms include abdominal pain, fainting, pseudoseizures, paralysis, headaches, and visual field restriction. The most common symptom is seizure activity, which can be differentiated from symptoms of neurogenic origin by formal tests. A normal electroencephalogram indicates that the origin is not neurogenic. Many children with a conversion reaction have experienced a major family crisis (such as the loss of a parent or other significant person through death, divorce, or moving) before the onset of symptoms.

Nursing Care Management

Nursing care is similar to that for the child with RAP. If significant personality problems are evident, psychiatric consultation is indicated.

Childhood Depression

Depression in childhood is often difficult to detect because children may be unable to express their feelings and tend to act out their problems and concerns. Some states of depression are temporary (e.g., acute depression precipitated by a traumatic event). This might be related to a period of hospitalization; loss of a parent through death or separation; or loss of a significant relationship with something (a pet), someone (a friend or family member), or a place (due to a move from a familiar home, neighbourhood, or city). Children with depression may demonstrate a variety of behaviours (Box 39-1). Most responses in children are not sustained and can be modified with social and family support.

More serious and less common are the depressive responses to chronic stress and loss; these are frequently observed in children with chronic illness or disability when other family members are in denial and often depressed. There is no apparent precipitating event, but there is often a history of frequent disruptions in important relationships. Often, there is also a history of depressive illness in one or both parents. Manifestations in the child are similar to those observed in acute depression, but they occur more frequently and extend over a longer time.

BOX 39-1 Characteristics of Children With Depression

Behaviour

- Predominantly sad facial expression with absence or diminished range of affective response
- Solitary play or work; tendency to be alone; lack of interest in play
- Withdrawal from previously enjoyed activities and relationships
- Lowered grades in school; lack of interest in doing homework or achieving in school
- Diminished motor activity; tiredness
- Tearfulness or crying
- Dependent and clinging or aggressive and disruptive

Internal States

- Utterance of statements reflecting lowered self-esteem, sense of hopelessness, or guilt
- Suicidal ideations

Physiology

- Constipation
- Nonspecific complaints of not feeling well
- Change in appetite resulting in weight loss or gain
- Alterations in sleeping pattern; sleeplessness or hypersomnia

Nursing Care Management

Depressed children are managed by a health team especially prepared in the care of children with mental disorders. Treatment is highly individualized and undertaken in the least restrictive environment. Suicidal children need to be admitted to the hospital for protection if the family is unable to provide constant monitoring. Pharmacotherapy may involve tricyclic antidepressants or serotonin reuptake inhibitors (SSRIs) such as fluoxetine (Prozac), trazodone (Desyrel), sertraline (Zoloft), paroxetine (Paxil), bupropion (Wellbutrin), and venlafaxine (Effexor). Nurses should be aware that depression can easily be overlooked in the child and can interrupt normal growth and development. Recognizing depression and suicidal tendencies in depressed children and making appropriate referrals are important nursing functions. Identification of the depressed child requires a careful history (health, growth and development, social, and family health); interviews with the child; and observations by the nurse, parents, and teachers. (See also Chapter 40, Suicide.)

Social Media

Children are very familiar with different forms of media, and this contact with the media brings benefits as well as risks. Social media sites abound, including Facebook, Twitter, MySpace, blogs, gaming sites, and virtual worlds such as Club Penguin, Second Life, and The Sims. Children also frequent video sites such as YouTube. The benefits of social media and Internet use to children include entertainment as well as development of communication and technical skills. However, there are also risks to children with these media sites, such as cyberbullying. Sexual predators lurk on the Internet and can make dangerous contact with children.

It is recommended that parents talk to their children about their use of the Internet and the dangers that children may face online. Parents also need to address cyberbullying, "sexting," and time management of using social media. Families can create a "family online-use plan" that emphasizes good citizenship and healthy behaviour. Children need parental monitoring with participation and discussion of their online activity (O'Keefe, Clarke-Pearson, & Council on Communications and Media, 2011).

Key Points

- Middle childhood, also known as the school years, is the period of life that extends from 6 to 12 years of age.
- Although growth is slower than in previous years, there is a steady gain in height and weight, with maturation of body systems; primary teeth are lost and replaced by permanent teeth.
- A major task during the middle school years is developing a sense of industry or accomplishment (Erikson).

- Piaget's period of concrete operations refers to the school-age period, when children are able to use their thought processes to experience events and actions and make judgements based on reasoning.
- The child develops a conscience and is able to understand and adhere to rules and standards set by others.
- Entertaining different points of view, becoming sensitive to cultural norms, and forming peer friendships are important features of social development during the school years.
- Cooperative play, team activities, and the acquisition of skills are prime elements of play during the school years; rules and rituals assume greater importance.
- Parental concerns during middle childhood include lying, cheating, stealing, bullying, and school achievement.
- The availability of junk foods, irregular family meals, and schedules of working parents often interfere with optimum nutrition and may lead to obesity.
- Activities involving physical movement should be encouraged; sedentary activities, such as watching television or playing video games for long periods of time, are contributing to health problems in this age group.
- Dental care is important during this time; potential dental problems include caries, periodontal disease, malocclusion, and dental injury.
- Increased socialization and media exposure make the school years an ideal time for sex education.
- Ideally, school health programs include health appraisal, emergency care, safety education, lifestyle support, recommended immunizations, communicable disease control, counselling, guidance, and health education with adjustment to individual student needs.
- Injury prevention is directed toward safety education, provision of safe play areas and equipment, and supervision of sports activities.
- Alterations in growth and maturation may be manifested as short or tall stature, or delayed sexual development.
- Behaviour problems in middle childhood can result from ADHD, enuresis, school phobia, RAP, childhood depression, and conversion reaction.
- Eating disorders are being seen in younger children; an index of suspicion is important to diagnosis.
- Education related to appropriate uses of social media is important.

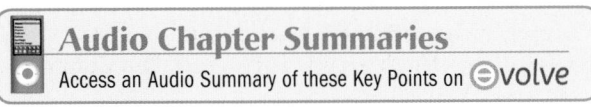

Audio Chapter Summaries
Access an Audio Summary of these Key Points on evolve

References

Canadian Mental Health Association. (2011a). *Children and difficult behaviour.* Retrieved from http://www.cmha.ca/mental_health/children-and-difficult-behaviour/#.T9dYpJhRVAU.

Canadian Mental Health Association. (2011b). *Children and their fears.* Retrieved from http://www.cmha.ca/mental_health/children-and-their-fears/#.T9dSAphRVAU.

Canadian Paediatric Society. (2008). Transportation of infants and children in motor vehicles. *Paediatrics and Child Health, 13*(4), 313–318.

Canadian Paediatric Society. (2009). Extended-release medications for children and adolescents with attention-deficit hyperactivity disorder. *Paediatrics and Child Health, 14*(9), 593–597.

Canadian Paediatric Society. (2011). Early childhood caries in indigenous communities. *Paediatrics and Child Health, 16*(6), 351–357.

Canadian Paediatric Society (2012). *Alternative treatments for attention deficit hyperactivity disorder.* Retrieved from http://www.caringforkids.cps.ca/handouts/alternative_treatments_adhd.

Canadian Paediatric Society, Injury Prevention Committee. (2004). Preventing injuries from all-terrain vehicles. *Paediatrics and Child Health, 9*(5), 337–340.

Canadian Paediatric Society, Injury Prevention Committee. (2012). Skiing and snowboarding injury prevention. *Paediatrics and Child Health, 17*(1), 35–36.

Canadian Psychology Foundation of Canada. (2012). *Kids have stress too.* Retrieved from http://http://www.psychologyfoundation.org/pdf/KHST_yellow2008.pdf.

Canadian Public Health Association. (2010). *Public health–community health nursing practice in Canada: Roles and activities.* Retrieved from http://www.cpha.ca/uploads/pubs/3-1bk04214.pdf.

Canadian Society for Exercise Physiology. (2012). *Canadian physical activity guidelines and Canadian sedentary behaviour guidelines.* Retrieved from http://www.csep.ca/guidelines.

Carno, M. A., et al. (2003). Developmental stages of sleep from birth to adolescence, common childhood sleep disorders: Overview and nursing implications. *Journal of Pediatric Nursing, 18*(4), 274–283.

Craig, W. M., & Harel, Y. (2004). Bullying, physical fighting and victimization. In C. Currie, et al. (Eds.), *Young people's health in context: International report from the HBSC 2001/02 survey. WHO Policy Series: Health policy for children and adolescents* (pp. 133–144) Issue 4. Copenhagen: WHO Regional Office for Europe.

Craig, W. M., & Pepler, D. J. (2007). Understanding bullying from research to practice. *Canadian Psychology, 48*(2), 86–93. doi: 10.1037/cp2007010

Dishion, T. J., Nelson, S. E., & Yasui, M. (2005). Predicting early adolescent gang involvement from middle school adaptation. *Journal of Clinical Child & Adolescent Psychology, 34*(1), 62–73. doi:10.1207/s15374424jccp3401_6

Erikson, E. H. (1963). *Childhood and society* (2nd ed.). New York: Norton.

Frederickson, N. (2010). Bullying or befriending? Children's responses to classmates with special needs. *British Journal of Special Education, 37,* 4–12.

Freud, S., & Fliess, W. (1954). *The origins of psycho-analysis: Letters to Wilhelm Fliess, drafts and notes, 1887–1902.* Edited by M. Bonaparte, A. Freud, & E. Kris; authorized translation by E. Mosbacher & J. Strachey (1st ed.). London: Imago.

Glew, G. M., et al. (2005). Bullying, psychosocial adjustment, and academic performance in elementary school. *Archives of Pediatric & Adolescent Medicine, 159*(11), 1026–1031.

Hackbarth, D., & Gall, G. B. (2005). Evaluation of school-based health center programs and services: The whys and hows of demonstrating program effectiveness. *Nursing Clinics of North America, 40*(4), 711–724. doi:10.1016/j.cnur.2005.07.008

Health Canada. (2008). *First Nations, Inuit, and Aboriginal health: Keeping safe—injury prevention.* Retrieved from http://www.hc-sc.gc.ca/fniah-spnia/promotion/injury-bless/index-eng.php.

Health Canada. (2010). *Bullying.* Retrieved from http://www.healthycanadians.gc.ca/init/kids-enfants/intimidation/index-eng.php.

Health Canada. (2011). *Bullying prevention programs: School-based anti-bullying programs.* Retrieved from http://www.healthycanadians.gc.ca/init/kids-enfants/intimidation/prevention/index-eng.php.

Khambalia, A., MacArthur, C., & Parkin, P. C. (2005). Peer and adult companion helmet use is associated with bicycle helmet use by children. *Pediatrics, 116*(4), 939–942. doi:10.1542/peds.2005-0518

Kohlberg, L. (1968). Moral development. In D. L. Sills (Ed.), *International encyclopedia of the social sciences.* New York: Macmillan.

Krause-Parello, C. A. (2005). Tooth avulsion in the school setting. *Journal of School Nursing, 21*(5), 279–282. doi:10.1177/10598405050210050601

Learning Disabilities of Ontario. (2011). *Dysgraphia: The handwriting learning disability.* Retrieved from http://www.ldao.ca/introduction-to-ldsadhd/ldsadhs-in-depth/articles/about-lds/dysgraphia-the-handwriting-learning-disability/.

Lyznicki, J. M., Mortweet McCaffree, M. A., & Robinowitz, C. B. (2004). Childhood bullying: Implications for physicians. *American Family Physician, 70*(9), 1723–1728.

Myers, S. M., Eisenhauer, N. J., & Ryan, M. E. (2003). ADHD: It is real, and it can be treated. *Clinical Advisor, 6*(3), 15–25.

Nysted, M., & Drogset, J. O. (2006). Trampoline injuries. *British Journal of Sports Medicine, 40*(11), 984–987. doi:10.1136/bjsm.2006.029009

O'Keeffe, G. S., Clarke-Pearson, K., & Council on Communications and Media. (2011). Clinical report—The impact of social media on children, adolescents, and families. *Pediatrics, 127*(4), 800–804. doi:10.1542/peds.2011-0054

Piaget, J. (1952). *The origins of intelligence in children.* New York: International Universities Press.

Pinhas, L., Morris, A., Crosby, R. D., & Katzman, D. K. (2011). Incidence and age-specific presentation of restrictive eating disorders in children. A Canadian Paediatric Surveillance Program study. *Archives of Pediatric Adolescent Medicine, 165*(10), 895–899. doi:10.1001/archpediatrics.2011.145

Potter, P., & Grant, E. (2004). Understanding RN and unlicensed assistive personnel working relationships in designing care delivery strategies. *Journal of Nursing Administration, 34*(1), 19–24.

Public Health Agency of Canada. (2006). *Canadian immunization guide* (7th ed.) Retrieved from http://www.phac-aspc.gc.ca/publicat/cig-gci/index-eng.php.

Public Health Agency of Canada. (2009). *Child and youth injury in review: Spotlight on consumer product safety.* Ottawa, ON: Author.

Public Health Agency of Canada. (2011). *Building toward breakthroughs in injury control: A legislative perspective on the prevention of unintentional injuries among children and youth in Canada.* Retrieved from http://www.phac-aspc.gc.ca/hp-ps/dca-dea/publications/break/index-eng.php.

Raphael, D. (2010). The health of Canada's children. Part II: Health mechanisms and pathways. *Paediatrics and Child Health, 15*(2), 71–76.

Ryan-Wenger, N. A., Sharrer, V. W., & Campbell, K. K. (2005). Changes in children's stressors over the past 30 years. *Pediatric Nursing, 31*(4), 282–288.

Safe Kids Canada. (2009). *Back to school for children means back to safety for drivers and parents, says Safe Kids Canada.* Retrieved from http://www.safekidscanada.ca/professionals/newsroom/media-releases/2009/back-to-school.aspx.

Safe Kids Canada. (2010). *Helmet safety.* Retrieved from http://www.safekidscanada.ca/professionals/advocacy/helmet/index.aspx.

Schroth, R. J., Harrison, R. L., & Moffatt, M. (2009). Oral health of indigenous children and the influence of early childhood caries on childhood health and wellbeing. *Pediatric Clinics of North America, 56,* 1481–1499.

Sharrer, V. W., & Ryan-Wenger, N. A. (2002). School-age children's self-reported stress symptoms. *Pediatric Nursing, 28*(1), 21–27.

Sundelin-Wahlsten, V., Ahmad, A., & von Knorring, A-L. (2001). Traumatic experiences and post-traumatic stress reactions in children from Kurdistan and Sweden. *Acta Paediatrica, 90,* 563–568.

Vreeman, R. C., & Carroll, A. E. (2007). A systematic review of school-based interventions to prevent bullying. *Archives of Pediatric & Adolescent Medicine, 161*(1), 78–88.

Additional Resources

Attention Deficit Hyperactivity Disorder Canada: http://www.adhdCanada.com

Canadian Psychology Foundation of Canada-Kids Have Stress Too: http://www.psychologyfoundation.org/pdf/KHST_yellow2008.pdf

Health Canada: *Eating Well With Canada's Food Guide*: http://www.hc-sc.gc.ca/fn-an/food-guide-aliment/index-eng.php

Health Canada's Office of Natural Health Products: http://www.hc-sc.gc.ca/dhp-mps/prodnatur/index-eng.php

Human Early Learning Partnerships (HELP): http://www.earlylearning.ubc.ca

Learning Disabilities Association of Canada: http://www.ldac-acta.ca/

National Eating Disorder Information Centre: http://www.nedic.ca/

Parenting and Behaviour: How to Foster Your Child's Self-Esteem: http://www.caringforkids.cps.ca/handouts/foster_self_esteem

Public Health Agency of Canada: Injury Prevention: http://www.phac-aspc.gc.ca/inj-bles/index-eng.php

PrevNET (Promoting Relationships and Eliminating Violence): http://www.cmha.ca/mental_health/children-and-depression/

Unit 9

40 The Adolescent and Family

Learning Objectives

On completion of this chapter, the reader will be able to:

- Describe the usual physical changes that occur throughout the adolescent years.
- Discuss typical emotional and cognitive responses of adolescents to the physical changes that take place at puberty.
- Discuss factors that influence an adolescents' developing sense of autonomy and identity.
- Discuss the significance of changing interpersonal relationships and the role of peer groups during adolescence.
- Identify the causes of injuries during adolescence and discuss the possible prevention of injuries.
- Demonstrate an understanding of common disorders of the male and female reproductive systems.
- Demonstrate an understanding of health challenges related to adolescent sexuality.
- Discuss nursing priorities for an adolescent with an eating disorder.
- Describe factors influencing the health of First Nations, Métis, and Inuit youth in Canada.

Electronic Resources

Additional information related to the content in Chapter 40 can be found on

evolve the companion Web site at

http://evolve.elsevier.com/Canada/Perry/maternal/

- Examination Review Questions
- Assessment Video Clips
- Case Study—Behaviours Indicative of Future Child Abuse
- Case Study—Interviewing Adolescents
- Case Study—Teen Smoking
- Critical Thinking Exercise—Depression
- Critical Thinking Exercise—Obesity

Promoting Optimum Growth and Development

Adolescence is a period of transition between childhood and adulthood—a time of rapid physical, cognitive, social, and emotional change. In Canada, social determinants of health, such as family income, education, literacy, ethnicity, and gender, have a profound impact on adolescents' health and help set the stage for adult health. Raphael (2010) has described how these social determinants can bring about health inequalities among Canadian children. See Chapter 32 for more information on the social determinants of health.

Adolescence is generally considered to encompass the time between the onset of **puberty** and full physical maturation. Several terms are used to refer to this stage of growth and development. *Puberty* refers to the maturational, hormonal, and growth process that occurs when the reproductive organs begin to function and the secondary sex characteristics develop. This process is sometimes divided into three stages: *prepubescence*, the period of about 2 years immediately before puberty when the child is developing preliminary physical changes that herald sexual maturity; *puberty*, the point at which sexual maturity is achieved, marked by the first menstrual flow in girls but by less obvious indications in boys; and *postpubescence*, a 1- to 2-year period following puberty during which skeletal growth is completed and reproductive functions become fairly well established. Adolescence, which literally means "to grow into maturity," is generally regarded as the psychological, social, and maturational process initiated by the pubertal changes. It involves three distinct subphases: early adolescence (ages 11 to 14), middle adolescence (ages 15 to 17), and late adolescence (ages 18 to 20). The term *teenage years* is used synonymously with *adolescence* to describe ages 13 through 19. This chapter describes the differences in the stages of adolescence and reflects on how nurses can support youth in ways that attend to these differences while acknowledging the developmental changes that are ongoing.

Biological Development

The physical changes of puberty are primarily the result of hormonal activity under the influence of the central nervous system, although all aspects of physiological functioning are mutually interacting. The obvious physical changes are noted in increased physical growth and in the appearance and development of secondary sex characteristics; less obvious are physiological alterations and neurogonadal maturity, accompanied by the ability to procreate. Physical distinction between the sexes is made on the basis of distinguishing characteristics. **Primary sex characteristics** are the external and internal organs that carry out the reproductive functions (e.g., ovaries, uterus, breasts, penis). **Secondary sex characteristics** are the changes that occur throughout the body as a result of hormonal changes (e.g., voice alterations, development of facial and pubertal hair, fat deposits) but that play no direct part in reproduction.

Hormonal Changes of Puberty

The profound physical changes of puberty are prompted by hormonal influences that are controlled by the anterior pituitary and that occur in response to stimuli from the hypothalamus. Hormonal stimulation of the **gonads** has two effects: (1) production and release of gametes—production of sperm in the male and maturation and release of ova in the female; and (2) secretion of sex-appropriate **hormones**—estrogen and progesterone from the ovaries (female) and testosterone from the testes (male). Testes and adrenals secrete sex hormones. These hormones are produced in varying amounts by both sexes throughout the remainder of the lifespan. The adrenal cortex is responsible for the small amounts secreted before the pubescent years, but the sex hormone production that accompanies maturation of the gonads is responsible for the biological changes observed during puberty.

Estrogen, the feminizing hormone, is found in low quantities during childhood. This hormone is secreted in slowly increasing amounts until about age 11 years. In boys this gradual increase continues through maturation. In girls the onset of estrogen production in the ovary causes a pronounced increase that continues until about 3 years after the onset of menstruation, at which time it reaches a maximum level that continues throughout the reproductive life of the female.

Androgens, the masculinizing hormones, are also secreted in small and gradually increasing amounts up to about 7 or 9 years of age, at which time there is a more rapid increase in both sexes, especially boys, until about age 15 years. These hormones appear to be responsible for most of the rapid growth changes of early adolescence. With the onset of testicular function, the level of androgens (principally testosterone) in boys increases over that in girls and continues to increase until a maximum level is attained at maturity.

Sexual Maturation

The visible evidence of sexual maturation is achieved in an orderly sequence, and the state of maturity can be estimated on the basis of the appearance of these external manifestations. The age at which these changes are observed and the time required to progress from one stage to another vary among children. The time from the appearance of breast buds to full maturity may be 1½ to 6 years for adolescent girls. It may take 2 to 5 years for male genitalia to reach adult size. The stages of development of secondary sex characteristics and genital development have been defined as a guide for estimating sexual maturity and are referred to as the *Tanner stages*. The usual sequence of appearance of maturational changes is presented in Box 40-1.

Sexual Maturation in Girls

In most girls the initial indication of puberty is the appearance of breast buds, an event known as *thelarche*, which occurs between 9 and 13½ years of age (Fig. 40-1). This is followed in approximately 2 to 6 months by the growth of pubic hair on the mons pubis, known as *adrenarche* (Fig. 40-2). In a minority of normally developing girls, however, pubic hair may precede breast development.

The initial appearance of menstruation, or **menarche**, occurs about 2 years after the appearance of the first pubescent changes, approximately 9 months after attainment of peak height velocity and 3 months after attainment of peak weight velocity. Menarche has been related to a critical gain in body fat content (more fat content, earlier menarche), although this association is controversial. The normal age range of menarche is usually 10½ to 15 years, with the average age being 12 years, 9½ months for North American girls. Ovulation and regular menstrual periods usually occur 6 to 14 months after menarche. Girls may be considered to have pubertal delay if breast development has not occurred by age 13 or if menarche has not occurred within 4 years of the onset of breast development.

Sexual Maturation in Boys

The first pubescent changes in boys are testicular enlargement accompanied by thinning, reddening, and increased looseness of the scrotum (Fig. 40-3). These events usually occur between 9½ and 14 years of age. Early puberty is also characterized by the initial appearance of pubic hair. Penile enlargement begins, and testicular enlargement and pubic hair growth continue throughout midpuberty. During this period increasing muscularity, early voice changes, and development of early facial hair also occur. Temporary breast enlargement

BOX 40-1 Usual Sequence of Maturational Changes

Girls

Breast changes
Rapid increase in height and weight
Growth of pubic hair
Appearance of axillary hair
Menstruation (usually begins 2 years after first signs)
Abrupt deceleration of linear growth

Boys

Enlargement of testicles
Growth of pubic hair, axillary hair, hair on upper lip, hair on face and elsewhere on body (facial hair usually appears about 2 years after appearance of pubic hair)
Rapid increase in height
Changes in the larynx and consequently the voice (usually take place along with the growth of the penis)
Nocturnal emissions
Abrupt deceleration of linear growth

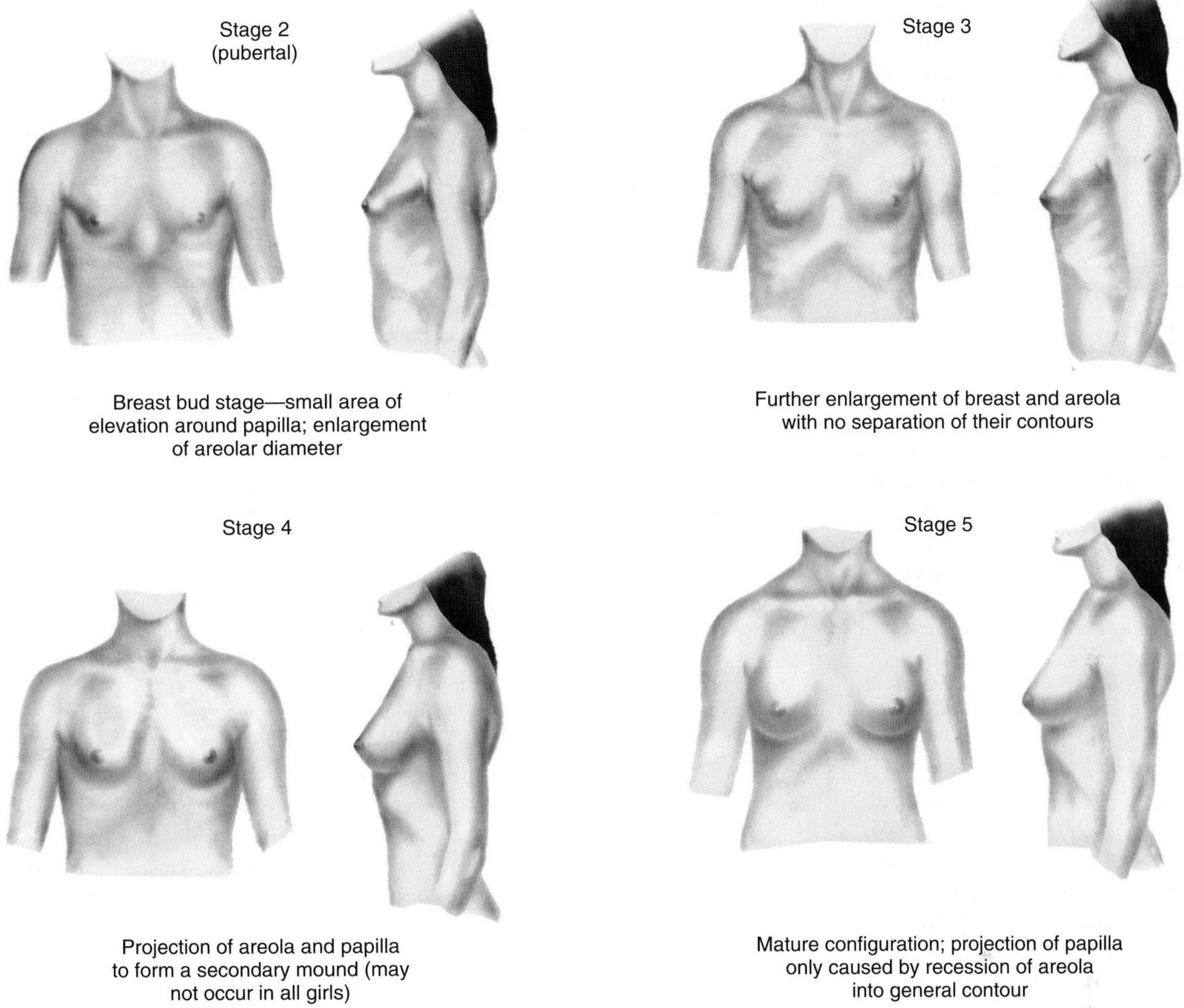

Stage 2
(pubertal)
Breast bud stage—small area of elevation around papilla; enlargement of areolar diameter
Stage 3
Further enlargement of breast and areola with no separation of their contours
Stage 4
Projection of areola and papilla to form a secondary mound (may not occur in all girls)
Stage 5
Mature configuration; projection of papilla only caused by recession of areola into general contour

Fig. 40-1 Development of the breast in girls—average age span: 9 to 13½ years. Stage 1 (prepubertal, elevation of papilla only) is not shown. *(Modified from Marshall, W. A., & Tanner, J. M. [1969]. Variations in pattern of pubertal changes in girls.* Archive of Diseases in Childhood, 44, *291; and Daniel, W. A., & Paulshock, B. Z. [1979]. A physician's guide to sexual maturity.* Patient Care, 13, *122–124.)*

and tenderness, *gynecomastia*, are common during midpuberty, occurring in up to one third of boys. The spurts in height and weight occur concurrently toward the end of midpuberty. For most boys, breast enlargement disappears within 2 years. By late puberty there is a definite increase in the length and width of the penis, testicular enlargement continues, and first **ejaculation** occurs. Axillary hair develops, and facial hair extends to cover the anterior neck. Final voice changes occur secondary to the growth of the larynx. Concerns about pubertal delay should be considered for boys who exhibit no enlargement of the testes or scrotal changes by 13½ to 14 years of age, or if genital growth is not complete 4 years after the testicles begin to enlarge.

Physical Growth

A constant phenomenon associated with sexual maturation is a dramatic increase in growth. The final 20 to 25% of height is achieved during puberty, and most of this growth occurs during a 24- to 36-month period—the adolescent growth spurt. This accelerated growth occurs in all children but, as in other areas of development, is highly variable in age of onset, duration, and extent. The growth spurt begins earlier in girls, usually between ages 9½ and 14½ years; on average it begins between ages 10½ and 16 years in boys. During this period, the average boy gains 10 to 30 cm in height and 7 to 30 kg in weight. The average girl, in whom the growth spurt is slower and less extensive, gains 5 to 20 cm in height and 7 to 25 kg in weight. Growth in height typically ceases 2 to 2½ years after menarche in girls and at age 18 to 20 years in boys.

This increase in size is acquired in a characteristic sequence. Growth in length of the extremities and neck precedes growth in other areas, and since these parts are first to reach adult length, the hands and feet appear larger than normal during adolescence. Increases in hip and chest breadth take place in

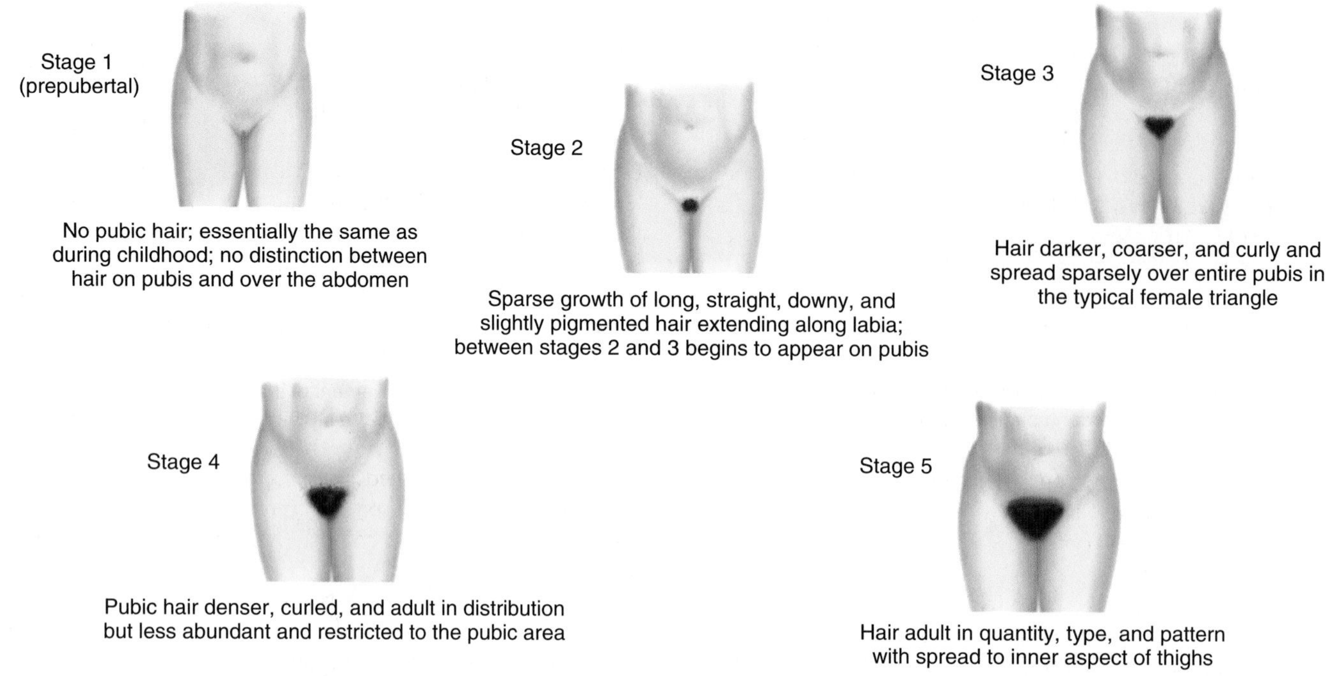
Stage 1
(prepubertal)
No pubic hair; essentially the same as during childhood; no distinction between hair on pubis and over the abdomen
Stage 2
Sparse growth of long, straight, downy, and slightly pigmented hair extending along labia; between stages 2 and 3 begins to appear on pubis
Stage 3
Hair darker, coarser, and curly and spread sparsely over entire pubis in the typical female triangle
Stage 4
Pubic hair denser, curled, and adult in distribution but less abundant and restricted to the pubic area
Stage 5
Hair adult in quantity, type, and pattern with spread to inner aspect of thighs

Fig. 40-2 Growth in pubic hair in girls—average age span for stages 2 through 5: 9 to 13½ years. *(Modified from Marshall, W. A., & Tanner, J. M. [1969]. Variations in pattern of pubertal changes in girls.* Archive of Diseases in Childhood, 44, *291; and Daniel, W. A., & Paulshock, B. Z. [1979]. A physician's guide to sexual maturity.* Patient Care, 13, *122–124.)*

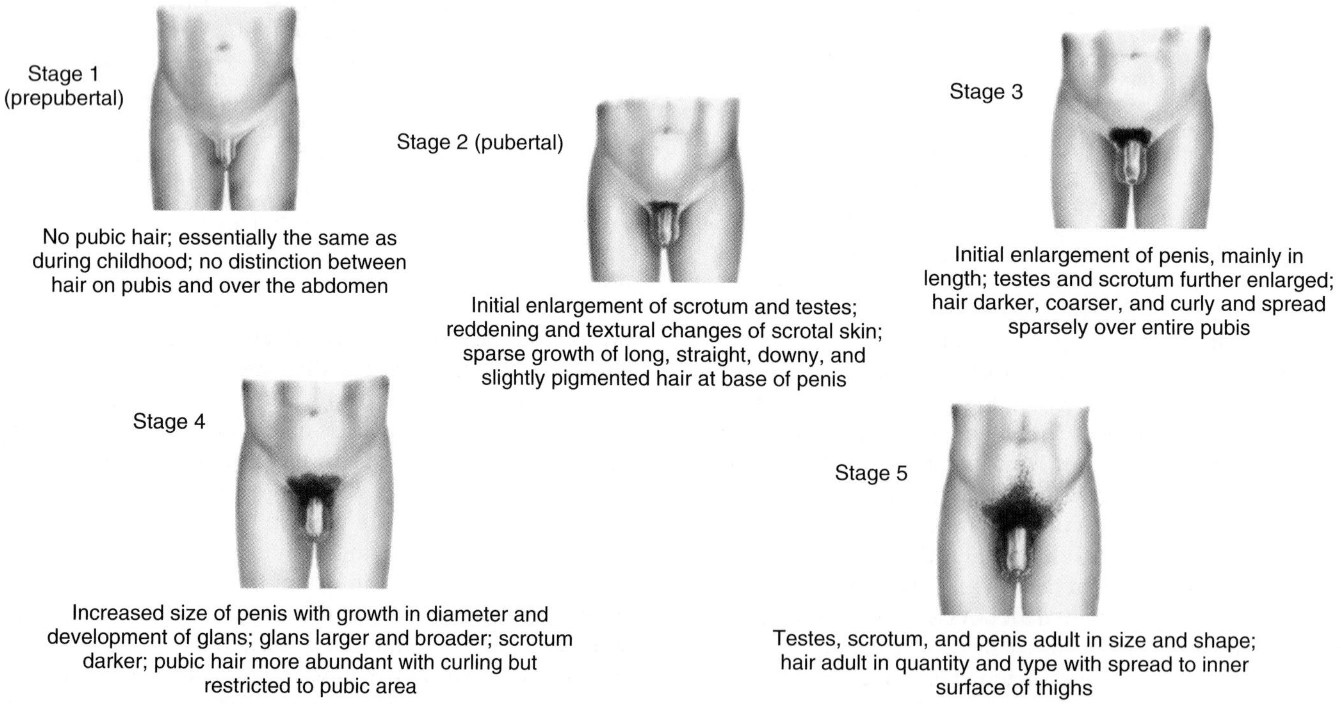
Stage 1
(prepubertal)
No pubic hair; essentially the same as during childhood; no distinction between hair on pubis and over the abdomen
Stage 2 (pubertal)
Initial enlargement of scrotum and testes; reddening and textural changes of scrotal skin; sparse growth of long, straight, downy, and slightly pigmented hair at base of penis
Stage 3
Initial enlargement of penis, mainly in length; testes and scrotum further enlarged; hair darker, coarser, and curly and spread sparsely over entire pubis
Stage 4
Increased size of penis with growth in diameter and development of glans; glans larger and broader; scrotum darker; pubic hair more abundant with curling but restricted to pubic area
Stage 5
Testes, scrotum, and penis adult in size and shape; hair adult in quantity and type with spread to inner surface of thighs

Fig. 40-3 Developmental stages of secondary sex characteristics and genital development in boys—average age span, 9½ to 14 years. *(Modified from Marshall, W. A., & Tanner, J. M. [1969]. Variations in pattern of pubertal changes in girls.* Archive of Diseases in Childhood, 44, *291; and Daniel, W. A., & Paulshock, B. Z. [1979]. A physician's guide to sexual maturity.* Patient Care, 13, *122–124.)*

a few months, followed several months later by an increase in shoulder width. These changes are followed by increases in the length of the trunk and depth of the chest. This sequence of changes is responsible for the characteristic long-legged, gawky appearance of the early adolescent child.

Sex Differences in General Growth Patterns

Sex differences in general growth and distribution patterns are apparent in skeletal growth, muscle mass, adipose tissue, and skin. Skeletal growth differences between boys and girls are apparently a function of hormonal effects at puberty and are evident primarily in limb length. The earlier cessation of growth in girls is caused by epiphyseal unity under the potent effect of estrogen secretion, and the hormonal effect on female bone growth is much stronger than the similar effect of testosterone in boys. In boys the prolonged growth period before puberty and the less rapid epiphyseal closure are reflected in their greater overall height and longer arms and legs. Other skeletal differences are increased shoulder width in boys and broader hip development in girls.

Hypertrophy of the laryngeal mucosa and enlargement of the larynx and vocal cords occur in both boys and girls to produce voice changes. Girls' voices become slightly deeper and considerably fuller. The effect in boys is particularly striking, occurring as boys mature, with the voice often shifting uncontrollably from deep to high tones in the middle of a sentence.

Growth of lean body mass, principally muscle, which tends to occur after the bone growth spurt, takes place steadily during adolescence. Lean body mass is both quantitatively and qualitatively greater in boys than in girls at comparable stages of pubertal development. Muscle development, under the influence of androgenic hormones, increases steadily. Muscles become remarkably well developed in boys, whereas in girls, muscle mass increase is proportionate to general tissue growth.

Nonlean body mass, primarily fat, is also increased but follows a less orderly pattern. There may be a transient increase in subcutaneous fat just before the skeletal growth spurt, especially in boys. This is followed 1 to 2 years later by a modest-to-marked decrease, which is again more notable in boys. Later, variable amounts of fat are deposited to fill out and contour the mature physique in patterns characteristic of the adolescent's sex, particularly in the regions over the thighs, hips, and buttocks and around the breast tissue. Girls with thelarche as the first sign of puberty have earlier menarche and greater body fat and body mass index (BMI) at menarche than girls with adrenarche as the first pubertal sign. This may have long-term effects for increased risk of adult adiposity and obesity (Biro et al., 2003), although the relationship between early **pubescence** and obesity has yet to be fully understood (Kaplowitz, 2008). Obesity can change the timing of puberty, however, and the increased rate of pediatric obesity in Canada (Shields, 2005) may have consequences for many Canadian youth in this regard.

Hormonal influences during puberty cause acceleration in growth and maturation of the skin and its structural appendages. Sebaceous **glands** become extremely active at this time, especially those on the genitalia and in the "flush areas" of the body (i.e., face, neck, shoulders, upper back, and chest). This increased activity and the structural nature of the glands are important in the pathogenesis of a common problem of puberty: acne (see Chapter 53). The eccrine sweat glands, present almost everywhere on the human skin, become fully functional and respond to emotional and thermal stimulation. Heavy sweating appears to be more pronounced in boys than in girls. The apocrine sweat glands, nonfunctional in childhood, reach secretory capacity during puberty. Unlike the eccrine sweat glands, the apocrine glands are limited in distribution and grow in conjunction with hair follicles in the axillae, around the areola of the breast, around the umbilicus, on the external auditory canal, and in the genital and anal regions. Apocrine glands secrete a thick substance as a result of emotional stimulation that, when acted on by surface bacteria, becomes highly odorous.

Body hair assumes very characteristic distribution patterns and changes texture during puberty. Under the influence of gonadal and adrenal androgens, hair coarsens, darkens, and lengthens at sites related to secondary sex characteristics. Pubic and axillary hair appears in both sexes, although pubic hair is more extensive in boys than in girls. Beard, moustache, and body hair on the chest, upward along the linea alba, and sometimes on other areas (e.g., back and shoulders) appears in boys and is androgen dependent. Extremity hair appears in varying amounts in both sexes but is also more prolific in boys.

Physiological Changes

A number of physiological functions are altered in response to some of the pubertal changes. The size and strength of the heart, blood volume, and systolic blood pressure increase, whereas the pulse rate and basal heat production decrease (see Appendix E). Blood volume, which increases steadily during childhood, reaches a higher value in boys than in girls, a fact that may be related to the increased muscle mass in pubertal boys. Adult values are reached for all formed elements of the blood. Respiratory rate and basal metabolic rate, which decrease steadily throughout childhood, reach the adult rate in adolescence. Respiratory volume and vital capacity are increased and to a far greater extent in males than in females. During this period, physiological responses to exercise change drastically: performance improves, especially in boys, and the body is able to make the physiological adjustments needed for normal functioning after exercise is completed. These capabilities are a result of the increased size and strength of muscles and the increased level of cardiac, respiratory, and metabolic functioning.

Norms related to the changes that occur during the early, middle, and late phases of adolescence are summarized in Table 40-1.

Psychosocial Development

Developing a Sense of Identity (Erikson)

Traditional psychosocial theory holds that the developmental crisis of adolescence leads to the formation of a sense of identity (Erikson, 1963). Throughout childhood, individuals go through a continual process of identification as they concentrate on various parts of the body at specific times. During infancy, children identify themselves as being separate from the mother; during early childhood they establish a gender-role identification with the appropriate-sex parent; and in later evolve Case Study—Behaviours Indicative of Future Child Abuse

childhood they establish who they are in relation to others. In adolescence they come to see themselves as distinct individuals, somehow unique and separate from every other individual.

Adolescence begins with the onset of puberty and extends to relative physical and emotional stability at or near graduation from high school. During this time, the adolescent is faced with the crisis of group identity versus alienation. In the period that follows, the individual strives to attain autonomy from the family and develop a sense of personal identity instead of role diffusion. A sense of group identity appears to be essential to developing a sense of personal identity. Young adolescents must resolve questions concerning relationships with a peer group before they are able to resolve questions about who they are in relation to family and society.

Group Identity

During the early stage of adolescence, pressure to belong to a group is intensified. Teenagers find it essential to have a group to which they can belong and that provides them with status. They dress as the group dresses and wear makeup and hairstyles according to group criteria, all of which are different from those of the parental generation. Language, music, and dancing reflect a culture that is exclusive to the adolescent. Adolescent conformity to the peer group and nonconformity to the adult group provides teenagers with a frame of reference in which they can display their own self-assertion while rejecting the identity of their parents' generation. To be different from the group, however, is to be unaccepted and alienated from the group.

Individual Identity

The quest for personal identity is an ongoing process. As adolescents establish identity within a group they also attempt to incorporate multiple body changes into a concept of the self. In addition, as part of their search for identity, adolescents will take stock of their current and past relationships, as well as the directions they hope to take in the future.

Generally, adults who are significant to adolescents have expectations for their behaviour. Often these expectations or demands are persistent enough that adolescents will make decisions that might be made differently if they could be solely responsible for their own **identity formation**. It is all too easy to slip into roles conforming to these external influences without incorporating personal goals or questioning these decisions. Thus an individual may become what parents or others wish them to be, not what might be best for the individual.

Young persons might also form a negative identity when they are perceived negatively for behaving or expressing themselves in ways that are culturally or socially contrary to the values of the community. Labels such as "loser," "juvenile delinquent," "underachiever," "gangster," or "failure" are applied to certain adolescents, who then accept and live up to these labels with behaviours that validate and strengthen them.

The process of evolving a personal identity is time consuming and fraught with periods of confusion, excitement, depression, and discouragement. Determining an identity and a place in the world is a critical feature of adolescence (see Critical Thinking Exercise). However, as the pieces gradually shift and settle into place, a positive identity eventually emerges.

CRITICAL THINKING EXERCISE

Discussing the Future

Jeremy, age 17, will be graduating from high school in the spring. His mother, a lone parent, tells you that she is concerned because graduation is quickly approaching and Jeremy has made no plans for what he will do with his life after graduation. Whenever Jeremy mentions the topic, his mother tells him, "This is what you must do," and begins to outline the steps he must take. Jeremy just walks away. She asks, "What should I do?" What advice should you give Jeremy's mother?

1. Evidence—Is there sufficient evidence to draw any conclusions about what advice the nurse should give Jeremy's mother?
2. Assumptions—Describe an underlying assumption about each of the following issues:
   a. Adolescents and the search for personal identity
   b. The influence of others on the adolescent's search for personal identity
   c. Ways to communicate with adolescents
3. What implications and priorities for nursing care can be drawn at this time?
4. Does the evidence objectively support your argument (conclusion)?
5. Are there alternative perspectives to your arguments? What are they?

Role diffusion results when the individual is unable to formulate a satisfactory identity from the multiplicity of aspirations, roles, and influences.

Gender-Role Identity

Adolescence is the time for consolidation of a gender-role identity. During early adolescence the peer group will begin to communicate expectations regarding heterosexual relationships, although in some circles acceptance of gay relationships may also be expressed. As development progresses, adolescents will encounter expectations for mature gender-role behaviour from both peers and adults. Expectations vary from culture to culture, between geographic areas and socioeconomic groups.

Emotionality

Adolescents vacillate in their emotional states between considerable maturity and childlike behaviour. One minute they are exuberant and enthusiastic; the next minute they are depressed and withdrawn. Unpredictable, but essentially normal, **mood** swings are common during this time. As the tension is relieved, individuals can bring the emotion under control. They may retreat to review what has happened, to master their anger, and to increase their ability to control their emotions and gain from the new experience. Because of these mood swings, adolescents are frequently labelled unstable, inconsistent, and unpredictable. Little things can cause an emotional upheaval and, depending on the teenager's interpretation, can mean a great deal.

Teenagers are generally better able to control their emotions in later adolescence. They can approach problems more calmly and rationally, and although they are still subject to periods of sadness, their feelings are less vulnerable and they begin to demonstrate more mature emotions. Whereas early adolescents react immediately and emotionally, older adolescents can control their emotions until socially acceptable times and places for expression present themselves. They are still subject to heightened emotion, and when it is expressed, their behaviour can reflect feelings of insecurity, tension, and indecision.

Cognitive Development (Piaget)

According to Piaget (1952), cognitive thinking culminates with the capacity for abstract thinking. This stage, the period of formal operations, is Piaget's fourth and last stage. Adolescents are no longer restricted to the real and actual, which was typical of the period of concrete thought. They now have the capacity to think beyond the present. Without having to centre attention on the immediate situation, they can imagine a sequence of events that might occur, such as college and occupational possibilities; how things might change in the future, such as relationships with parents; and the consequences of their actions, such as dropping out of school. At this time their thoughts can be influenced by logical principles rather than just their own perceptions and experiences. They become increasingly capable of scientific reasoning and formal logic.

Adolescents are capable of mentally manipulating more than two categories of variables at the same time. For example, they can consider the relationship between speed, distance, and time in planning a trip. They can detect logical consistency or inconsistency in a set of statements and evaluate a system or set of values in a more analytical manner. For instance, they question the parent who insists on honesty in the teenager but at the same time cheats on an income tax report or expense account.

In adolescence, young people begin to think about both their own thinking and the thinking of others. They wonder what opinion others have of them, and they are able to imagine the thoughts of others. With this capacity comes the ability to differentiate between others' thoughts and their own and to interpret the thoughts of others more accurately. They are able to understand that few concepts are absolute or independent of other influencing factors. As they become aware that other cultures and communities have different norms and standards from their own, it becomes easier for them to accept members of these other cultures, and the decision to behave in their own culture in an accepted manner becomes a more conscious commitment.

Moral Development (Kohlberg)

Although younger children tend to accept the decisions or point of view of adults, adolescents, in their efforts toward autonomy, begin to formulate their own set of morals and values. According to Kohlberg (1968), when old principles are challenged but new independent values have not yet emerged to take their place, young people search for a moral code that preserves their personal integrity and guides their behaviour, especially in the face of strong pressure to violate the old beliefs. Their decisions involving moral dilemmas must be based on an internalized set of moral principles that provides them with the resources to evaluate the demands of the situation and to plan actions that are consistent with their ideals.

Late adolescence is characterized by serious questioning of existing moral values and their relevance to society and the individual. Adolescents can easily take the role of another. They understand duty and obligation based on the reciprocal rights of others, as well as the concept of justice that is founded on making amends for misdeeds and repairing or replacing what has been spoiled by wrong-doing. However, they seriously question established moral codes, often as a result of observing that adults verbally ascribe to a code but do not adhere to it.

Spiritual Development

As adolescents move toward independence from parents and other authorities, some begin to question their families' values and ideals. Others cling to these values as a stable element in their lives as they struggle with the conflicts of this turbulent period. Adolescents need to work out these conflicts for themselves, but they also need support from authority figures and peers for their resolution.

Adolescents are capable of understanding abstract concepts and of interpreting analogies and symbols. They are able to empathize, philosophize, and think logically. Most teens search for ideals and speculate about illogical statements and conflicting ideologies. Their tendency toward introspection and emotional intensity often makes it difficult for others to know what they are thinking. They tend to keep their thoughts private, fearing that no one will understand these feelings that they perceive to be unique and special. However, they may reveal deep spiritual concerns. They need support and encouragement in their struggle for understanding as well as the freedom to question without censure.

Social Development

Adolescents gradually reconfigure their relationship with their families and develop a sense of themselves that allows them to exist separately from their parents. For most adolescents and their parents, this process is fraught with ambivalence as they grapple with the tensions between (a) teenage independence and the responsibilities associated with that independence, and (b) the desire for separateness and the longing to be close to those they love. Feelings of immortality and exemption from the consequences of **risk-taking behaviour**, while usually viewed as negative and unrealistic, can serve an important developmental function at this time. These feelings may give adolescents the courage to separate from their parents and become independent. Part of this emancipation involves developing social relationships outside the family that help teenagers identify their role in society and have a sense of belonging outside of their family bonds. For many, adolescence is a time of intense sociability and often a time of equally intense loneliness. Acceptance by peers, a few close friends, and the secure love of a supportive family support interpersonal maturation.

Relationships With Parents

During adolescence the parent–child relationship changes from one of protection and dependency to one of mutual affection and equality (Table 40-1). The process of achieving independence often involves turmoil and ambiguity as both the parent and adolescent learn to play new roles and work toward this end. Certain behaviours of the adolescent are related to the struggle for independence and the external restrictions and checks that are placed on this maturation process. On the one hand, adolescents are accepted as maturing preadults. They are allowed privileges previously denied, and they are provided with increasing responsibilities. On the other hand, because of their variability in evaluating situations and making sound **judgements**, they are required to adhere to certain regulations and restrictions set by adults. In many families, this state of affairs is exemplified by the struggle between parents and adolescents concerning the use of electronic devices and social networking, and the use of the family car.

With advancing adolescence, teenagers become more competent, and with this competence comes a need for more autonomy. Although they may be psychologically prepared for independence, they are often thwarted in their efforts by lack of money or other barriers. Conflict may arise in relation to the teenager's independent activities as well as the needs of privacy and trust. Parental supervision remains important throughout adolescence and may have a direct influence on adolescent sexual and **substance use** behaviour. Parents should be guided toward an authoritative style of parenting in which authority is used to guide the adolescent while allowing developmentally appropriate levels of freedom and providing clear, consistent messages about expectations. An authoritative style of parenting has been shown to have both immediate and long-term protective effects toward adolescent risk reduction (DeVore & Ginsburg, 2005). However, to gain the trust of adolescents, parents must respect their adolescent's privacy and show an honest and sincere interest in what the adolescent believes and feels (see Family-Centred Teaching box).

Relationships With Peers

Although parents remain the primary influence in their lives, for most teenagers, peers assume a more significant role in adolescence than they did during childhood (see Table 40-1). For many adolescents, the peer group serves as a strong support providing them with a sense of belonging and a feeling of strength and power.

Peer Groups, Diversity, and Identity

Adolescents are usually social, gregarious, and group minded. Thus the peer group has an intense influence on adolescents' self-evaluation and behaviour. To gain acceptance by a group, younger teenagers tend to conform completely in such things as mode of dress, hairstyle, taste in music, and vocabulary. Teenagers use the peer group as a yardstick of what is normal.

The school is psychologically important to adolescents as a focus of social life. Teenagers usually distribute themselves into a relatively predictable social hierarchy. They know to which groups they and others belong. A sense of school connectedness has been found to predict decreased risk-taking behaviours in adolescents (Bond et al., 2007). Such connectedness at school is correlated with caring teachers and the absence of prejudice or discrimination from peers; it is less dependent on class size, attendance, academic preparation, and parental involvement (Maes & Lievens, 2003).

Within the larger peer groups are smaller, distinct, and rather exclusive crowds or cliques of selected close friends who are emotionally attached to each other. The selection tends to follow common tastes, interests, and background. Although cliques may become formalized, most of them remain informal and small. Cliques are usually made up of one gender; girls tend to be more cliquish than boys and to have a greater need for close friendships (Fig. 40-4). Within the intimacy of the group, adolescents gain support in learning

FAMILY-CENTRED TEACHING

Communication With Teens: The Art of Listening

Conflicts between parents and their adolescents are often a result of a natural characteristic of parenthood: the desire to protect one's children from harm or from simply doing something "stupid" or embarrassing or something they may later regret. Teenagers sometimes "bounce" their thoughts and ideas off adults. At times they really want some feedback; at other times they simply want to elicit a reaction.

I found it easy to listen openly, thoughtfully, and without interrupting when my teenagers' friends discussed troublesome topics. However, one day, when one of my own teenagers had a similar conversation with me, the parent part kicked in. I felt responsible and spoke my piece on the spot. This brought communication to a halt and resulted in defensiveness. It was a long time before my child tried to talk to me about anything controversial again. The next time one of my teenagers started a similar conversation, I decided to try to trick myself.

Throughout the entire conversation, I told myself over and over again to act as if this were not my teenager, but rather someone else's child. I found this actually worked quite well, and I was able to listen without interrupting. I continued to use the system, sometimes with more success than at other times.

–Mother of Four

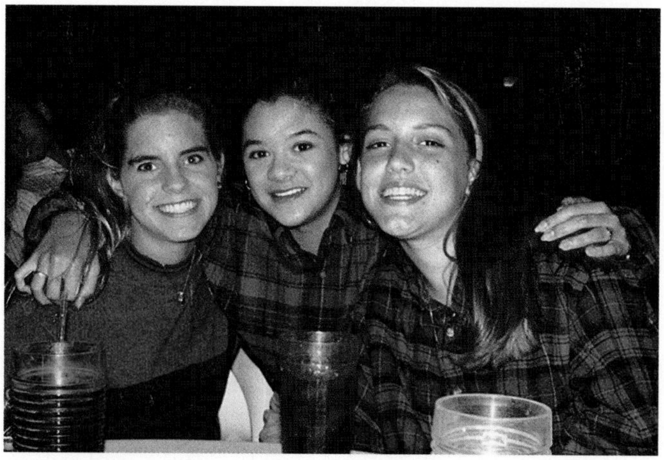

Fig. 40-4 Teenagers often like to gather in small groups.

Table 40-1 Growth and Development During Adolescence

EARLY ADOLESCENCE (11–14 YR)	MIDDLE ADOLESCENCE (15–17 YR)	LATE ADOLESCENCE (18–20 YR)
Growth		
Rapidly accelerating growth Reaches peak velocity Secondary sex characteristics appear	Growth decelerating in girls Stature reaches 95% of adult height Secondary sex characteristics well advanced	Physically mature Structure and reproductive growth almost complete
Cognition		
Explores new-found ability for limited abstract thought Clumsy groping for new values and energies Comparison of "normality" with peers of same sex	Developing capacity for abstract thinking Enjoys intellectual powers, often in idealistic terms Concern with philosophical, political, and social problems	Established abstract thought Can perceive and act on long-range options Able to view problems comprehensively Intellectual and functional identity established
Identity		
Preoccupied with rapid body changes Trying out of various roles Measurement of attractiveness by acceptance or rejection of peers Conformity to group norms	Modifies body image Very self-centred; increased narcissism Tendency toward inner experience and self-discovery Has a rich fantasy life Idealistic Able to perceive future implications of current behaviour and decisions; variable application	Body image and gender-role definition nearly secured Mature sexual identity Phase of consolidation of identity Stability of self-esteem Comfortable with physical growth Social roles defined and articulated
Relationships With Parents		
Defining independence–dependence boundaries Strong desire to remain dependent on parents while trying to detach No major conflicts over parental control	Major conflicts over independence and control Low point in parent–child relationship Greatest push for emancipation; disengagement Final and irreversible emotional detachment from parents; mourning	Emotional and physical separation from parents completed Independence from family with less conflict Emancipation nearly secured
Relationships With Peers		
Seeks peer affiliations to counter instability generated by rapid change Upsurge of close, idealized friendships with members of the same sex Struggle for mastery takes place within peer group	Strong need for identity to affirm self-image Behavioural standards set by peer group Acceptance by peers extremely important—fear of rejection Exploration of ability to attract opposite sex (if heterosexual)	Peer group recedes in importance in favour of individual friendship Testing of romantic relationships against possibility of permanent alliance Relationships characterized by giving and sharing
Sexuality		
Self-exploration and evaluation Limited dating, usually group Limited intimacy	Multiple plural relationships Internal identification of heterosexual, homosexual, or bisexual attractions Exploration of "self appeal" Feeling of "being in love" Tentative establishment of relationships	Forms stable relationships and attachment to another Growing capacity for mutuality and reciprocity Dating as a romantic pair May publicly identify as gay, lesbian, or bisexual Intimacy involves commitment rather than exploration and romanticism
Psychological Health		
Wide mood swings Intense daydreaming Anger outwardly expressed with moodiness, temper outbursts, and verbal insults and name-calling	Tendency toward inner experiences; more introspective Tendency to withdraw when upset or feelings are hurt Vacillation of emotions in time and range Feelings of inadequacy common; difficulty in asking for help	More constancy of emotion Anger more apt to be concealed

about themselves, consideration for the feelings of others, and increased ego development and self-reliance.

To belong is of utmost importance; thus adolescents behave in ways that will ensure their establishment in a group. Adolescents are highly susceptible to social approval, acceptance, and demands. Being ignored or criticized by peers can create feelings of inferiority, inadequacy, and incompetence.

Close Friendships

Personal friendships between individuals usually develop between same-sex and opposite-sex adolescents. These relationships tend to be closer and more stable than those of middle childhood and provide a safe space to test possible roles and identities. Close friends may try a role together, each supporting the other. Since a sense of intimacy grows within a permanent relationship, the stability of this friendship is an important link in the progress toward intimate relationships in young adulthood.

Interests and Activities

Adolescents tend to have busy lives. Some spend a large amount of time engaging in leisure-time activities—sports, video games, parties, and nonstructured time spent with friends. Most adolescents in Canada are connected to others through electronic means: cell phones, gaming consoles, personal tablets, and computers. As teenagers progress through the developmental stages of adolescence, these leisure-time activities move from being mainly family centred toward being peer centred. In addition to providing teenagers with fun and enjoyment, leisure-time activities assist in the development of social, physical, and cognitive skills. These activities also give teenagers the opportunity to learn to set priorities and structure their time (Fig. 40-5).

Today, many adolescents must learn to juggle their time between school, activities, and the responsibilities of a job. Adolescent work experiences provide many benefits, including time management, teamwork skills, and increased income. The advantages to employment may be limited by the time and energy diverted from school and other activities. It is generally recommended that adolescents limit their work to no more than 20 hours per week during the school year.

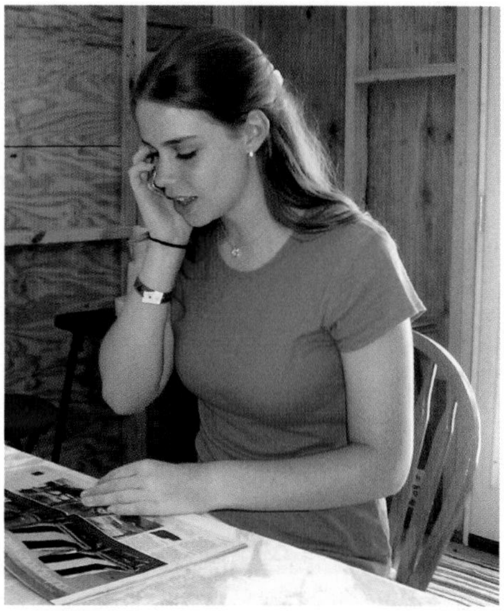

Fig. 40-5 Cell phones and social medial create new ways for adolescents to communicate with peers.

Adolescent Sexuality

Adolescence represents a critical time in the development of sexuality. Hormonal, physical, cognitive, and social changes that occur during adolescence all have an impact on sexual development. Of all the developmental changes that affect adolescent sexuality, none is more obvious than the impact of puberty. Adolescents must come to terms with hormonal influences, physiological manifestations such as menstruation and ejaculation, and physical changes such as breast and genital development. All of these changes have a profound impact on the way in which teenagers perceive their bodies (i.e., **body image**). In addition to transitions in body image, increasing levels of pubertal hormones contribute to increased levels of sexual motivation among both boys and girls.

Developmental theories suggest that changes in sexual motivations and feelings, happening at the same time as shifts in cognitive skills, may contribute to painful conjectures ("Is what I'm feeling normal?"), self-conscious concern ("Am I good looking enough?"), and hypothetical thinking ("What if she wants to have sex?"). The emergence of formal operational thinking also increases adolescents' decision-making capabilities concerning sexual issues. As they mature, teenagers become better able to think through potential risks and benefits of sexual behaviours before they engage in any behaviour. Older adolescents may also be able to conceptualize more long-term consequences of present behaviours. One of the important tasks of adolescence is to incorporate sexuality successfully into close, intimate relationships. This task is made possible by the advanced cognitive abilities that emerge over the course of adolescence (see Table 40-1).

Many teenagers begin to make a shift toward intimate relationships with members of the opposite sex during middle adolescence (Fig. 40-6). Opposite-sex relationships typically begin with peer activities involving both boys and girls, and same-sex relationships may develop in groups of predominantly one gender. Pairing off as couples becomes more common as middle adolescence progresses. The type and degree of seriousness of partner relationships vary. Initial relationships are usually noncommittal, extremely mobile, and seldom characterized by any deep romantic attachments. Sexual activity becomes more common during middle adolescence. The relationship between love and sexual expression is brought into focus during middle adolescence. Most young people oppose exploitation, pressure, or force in sex, as well as sex solely for the sake of physical enjoyment without a personal relationship. Adolescents find it hard to believe that sex can exist without love; therefore, they view each relationship as real love.

An integrated sexual identity often emerges during late adolescence as individuals incorporate sexual experiences, feelings, and knowledge. For most, this identity is consistent with their own physical and mental capacities and with societal limits and expectations. Most older adolescents identify themselves as being predominantly heterosexual or bisexual, with a smaller number self-identifying as homosexual and an

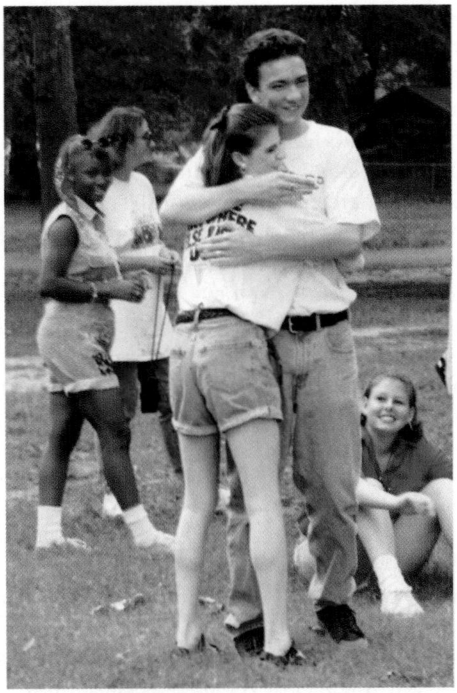

Fig. 40-6 Relationships with peers of both genders are an important part of adolescence.

even smaller group still unsure of their sexual orientation, although this varies somewhat by ethnicity (Canadian Paediatric Society [CPS], 2011; Russell, Seif, & Truong, 2001). Whatever their sexual orientation, many older teenagers possess the capacity to have intimate relationships that satisfy the emotional and sexual needs of both partners.

Sexual orientation encompasses sexual desires, feelings, practices, and identification. A person's sexual orientation may be toward people of the same sex, different sex, or both (same-sex, heterosexual, or bisexual orientation). *Gender identification* refers to how an individual sees himself or herself as a man or a woman and affects one's feelings and behaviours (Johnson & Oliffe, 2012). During adolescence individuals commonly begin to identify their sexual orientation as part of their developing sexual identity. This identification process is generally profoundly influenced by cultural beliefs and values, by societal and family pressures, and by peers. Most adolescents eventually report an orientation toward exclusively heterosexual relationships. For adolescents whose orientation encompasses any same-sex dimensions, the identity process during adolescence can be complicated, especially when community norms disapprove of orientations other than heterosexual. Adolescents who have witnessed harassment or violence directed at gay, lesbian, and bisexual people, for example, may be reluctant to self-identify as belonging to any of these groups, even when their attractions and behaviours are exclusively same-sex or bisexual.

The development of sexual orientation as part of sexual identity includes several developmental milestones during late childhood and throughout adolescence. These milestones do not necessarily occur in the same order for everyone, nor are they completed in the same amount of time. They include (1) the realization of romantic or erotic attraction to people of one or both genders; (2) erotic daydreaming about one or both genders; (3) romantic partners or dates without sexual activity; (4) sexual activity with people of the preferred gender or genders (also, for some teens, sexual activity with a nonpreferred gender, out of curiosity or through social pressure); (5) self-identification of the orientation that best fits one's current circumstances and understanding; (6) publicly self-identifying that orientation, usually to intimate friends and family first, then the wider social group; and (7) an intimate, committed, sexual relationship with a person of the gender appropriate to one's orientation.

There is no evidence that gay, lesbian, or bisexual adults are more or less likely to create long-term, stable relationships than are heterosexual couples. Bisexual adolescents and adults do not generally engage in sexual relationships with both genders concurrently; self-identification as bisexual usually refers to the ability to be attracted to either gender but does not imply that such a person requires partners of both genders, or that one must be equally attracted to and have sexual experience with both genders.

Although the order of these milestones varies greatly among adolescents, adolescents who identify as gay, lesbian, or bisexual tend to publicly self-identify later than heterosexual peers. Without positive gay, lesbian, or bisexual role models or a supportive peer group, sexual-minority teens can feel isolated, and they may not share their orientation with anyone for fear of rejection or violence (see Critical Thinking Exercise). When adolescents who would otherwise identify as bisexual can only find a peer group of gay and lesbian teens, they may focus on their same-gender dimensions of orientation and adopt the label of lesbian or gay; later, they may self-label as bisexual. Likewise, some gay and lesbian adolescents may first identify as heterosexual, then bisexual, before identifying as gay or lesbian.

Development of Self-Concept and Body Image

The sudden growth that takes place in early adolescence creates feelings of confusion. The security of a familiar body

CRITICAL THINKING EXERCISE

Discussing Sexual Orientation With Adolescents

John, a 17-year-old adolescent, comes into the school-based clinic and tells the nurse practitioner that he thinks he is gay. What is the most appropriate response for the nurse practitioner?

1. Evidence—Is there sufficient evidence to draw any conclusions about John's sexual orientation at this time?
2. Assumptions—Describe an underlying assumption about each of the following issues:
   a. Sexual orientation in adolescents
   b. Society's reactions to homosexuality
   c. Health care providers and sexuality
3. What implications and priorities for nursing care can be drawn at this time?
4. Does the evidence support your argument (conclusion)?
5. Are there alternative perspectives to your arguments? What are they?

is lost and the adolescent may feel uncomfortable within their altered body. Consequently, some adolescents may try to either hide their body or advertise it, or they may alternate between the two extremes. Teenagers tend to be acutely aware of their appearance as they begin to acquire images of themselves as adults, but they see discrepancies between their ideal and actual skills and abilities.

Adolescents are continually comparing themselves with their peers and making judgements about their own normality based on these observations. Most youth feel most comfortable when they are just like their friends and age-mates. Perceived defects or deviations from the group average can threaten their idealized image. Any blemish may be magnified out of proportion, and any delay of the visible evidence of maturity is cause for worry. Unfortunately, this is also the time when the hormonal effect of the sebaceous glands produces acne, and even the most insignificant pimple may be viewed as a disfigurement.

The body image that is established during adolescence is the one that individuals retain throughout life. Much of adolescents' search for identity takes a variety of forms. For some, much of this process unfolds in front of a mirror as they try to read from the reflected features just who they are and what they look like to other people. Adolescents may practise facial expressions and postures, try out hair arrangements, worry about a pimple, and in other ways attempt to assess the best means to achieve a maximum effect—to reveal the "true self."

The self-concept becomes more differentiated as adolescents acquire a more complex picture of themselves, one that takes situational factors into account. The self-concept gradually becomes more individualized and more distinct from the concepts of others. Although younger teenagers describe themselves in terms of similarities with peers, as adolescence advances, young people tend to describe themselves in terms of their special characteristics.

Responses to Puberty

The response to the physical changes of pubertal growth and development is manifested differently depending on the stage of development. During early adolescence, young adolescents may be preoccupied with the rapid changes in their body and are interested in the anatomy, physiology, and function of their sexual organs. Boys must also confront the sexual feelings and tensions that accompany puberty, and the appearance of nocturnal emissions may be puzzling, troublesome, or embarrassing. Unless the boy has been prepared in advance, he may find it difficult to discuss his feelings with his parents and may turn to his friends for information and guidance. Many girls also find the rapid changes in their body to be sources of concern. Some girls perceive the increase in weight and associated fat deposition as evidence of obesity and may indulge in fad diets. Although many girls look forward to menstruation and take this event in stride, others may find the first menstrual period a distressing and frightening event. All teenagers, regardless of gender, are concerned with the question, "Am I normal?" To answer this question, they compare their body with those of their peers and with images in the media. This leads to a great deal of uncertainty about their appearance and attractiveness.

If an adolescent does not enter puberty at the same time as his or her peers, considerable inner conflict may occur. Early-maturing girls and boys have higher rates of sexual risk-taking behaviours, delinquency, and substance use than their on-time peers (Costello et al., 2007; Lynne et al., 2007). Nurses who work with adolescents must provide teaching and health care interventions that are appropriate for the adolescent's chronological and cognitive development rather than the stage of physical maturation.

Adolescents strive to achieve the perfect body within their own cultural norms; the "right" clothes and hairstyle become very important. By late adolescence the heightened concern with body image generally subsides and the youth develops a more comfortable relationship with his or her body.

Promoting Optimum Health During Adolescence

The major causes of morbidity and mortality in adolescence are not diseases but health-damaging behaviours. Important sources of morbidity in adolescence include injury, depression, violence, and **sexually transmitted infections** (STIs); obesity may begin in childhood or adolescence, but the health consequences are more evident in early and middle adulthood. Health promotion for this age group often consists mainly of teaching and guidance to avoid risk-taking activities and health-damaging behaviours. Adolescence provides an opportunity for teenagers to learn and incorporate healthy lifestyle behaviours that will benefit them not only during the teenage years but also throughout the lifespan.

Effective health education for adolescents should be guided by a developmentally appropriate, multifaceted approach. Various approaches to engaging with youth regarding health-related issues have been proposed. One of these is motivational interviewing, a collaborative approach intended to improve adherence to health care advice (Gance-Cleveland, 2007). In this process the adolescent is encouraged to introspectively explore feelings of ambivalence and, on the basis of their insights, to develop solutions for effecting change. Education alone, however, is not enough to change behaviour. Effective programs for adolescents must include opportunities to improve communication skills and enhance their social network to make more positive connections (Tuttle, Campbell-Heider, & David, 2006).

As young people progress through adolescence, they assume increasing responsibility for their own health, including maintaining health practices, taking prescribed medications, keeping appointments, and performing procedures, when necessary. Health care providers who work with adolescents should consider the adolescent's increasing independence and responsibility while maintaining privacy and ensuring confidentiality (see Guidelines box and Critical Thinking Exercise). Parents should also respect their teenager's independence and move toward the role of consultant about health issues while also maintaining some level of parental involvement throughout their child's adolescence.

GUIDELINES Interviewing Adolescents

- Ensure confidentiality and privacy; interview the adolescent without the parents.
- Show concern for the adolescent's perspective with statements such as "First, I'd like to talk about your main concerns" and "I'd like to know what you think is happening."
- Offer a nonthreatening explanation for the questions you ask: "I'm going to ask a number of questions to help me better understand your health."
- Maintain objectivity; avoid assumptions, judgements, and lectures.
- Ask open-ended questions when possible; move to more directive questions if necessary.
- Begin with less sensitive issues and proceed to more sensitive ones.
- Use language that both the adolescent and you understand. Clarify terms, such as "having sex."
- Restate: reflect back to adolescents what they have said, along with feelings that may be associated with their descriptions.

CRITICAL THINKING EXERCISE

Respecting Privacy

Jamie, a 17-year-old girl, arrives at the adolescent clinic with her mother, Mrs. S, for a routine history and physical examination with the nurse practitioner. As the nurse practitioner walks with Jamie to an examination room, Mrs. S whispers to the nurse practitioner, "I need to speak with you in private." What principles should guide the nurse practitioner's response to Mrs. S's request?

1. Evidence—Is there sufficient evidence to formulate a response to Jamie's mother?
2. Assumptions—Describe an underlying assumption about each of the following topics:
   a. The role of the adolescent in health care
   b. The role of parents in the health of their adolescent
   c. Adolescents and confidentiality
3. What implications for nursing care should be established at this time?
4. Does the evidence support your conclusion?
5. Are there alternative perspectives that you should consider?

Immunizations

Immunization updates are a significant part of adolescent preventive care and in Canada, most vaccines are included in publicly funded immunizations programs. Immunization schedules vary slightly according to jurisdiction (Public Health Agency of Canada [PHAC, 2011]) (see Fig. 34-6). The following guidelines are based on the recommendations of the National Advisory Committee on Immunization (NACI).

Adolescents 11 to 16 years of age should receive a single tetanus-diphtheria–acellular pertussis (Tdap) vaccine if they have received the recommended childhood series of DTaP immunizations. This vaccine is now required because of the increased incidence of pertussis seen in adolescents and adults who were previously immunized with the DTaP series. Adolescents who have received Td but not Tdap vaccine should also receive a single dose of the Tdap vaccine, provided 5 years have elapsed between the Td and Tdap vaccination (PHAC, 2006).

Meningococcal vaccine (Men-C or Men-C-ACYW, depending on jurisdiction) should be given to preteens (PHAC, 2006).

The human papillomavirus (HPV) vaccine series is recommended only for girls, based on research results at this time. The series may be started as early as 9 years of age, with the second and third doses 2 months and 6 months later, respectively (see Chapter 6, pp. 101–103).

All adolescents who have not previously received two doses of hepatitis B vaccine (HBV) should be vaccinated against hepatitis B virus. The age at which children and youth are offered HBV varies from jurisdiction to jurisdiction (see Chapter 6, p. 105).

In Canada, the hepatitis A vaccine is recommended for individuals of all ages considered to be at risk of exposure.

Annual influenza vaccination with either the live attenuated influenza vaccine or trivalent influenza vaccine is now encouraged for all children and adolescents.

All adolescents should be assessed for previous history of varicella infection or vaccination. Vaccination with the varicella vaccine is recommended for those with no previous history; for those with no previous infection or history of immunization, the varicella vaccine may be given in a single dose (PHAC, 2006).

Any adolescent who has not completed the immunization series for hepatitis A, hepatitis B, poliovirus, and influenza should receive these immunizations according to the latest catch-up schedule (see also Immunizations, Chapter 36).

Nutrition

The rapid and extensive increase in height, weight, muscle mass, and sexual maturity of adolescence is accompanied by increased nutritional requirements. Because nutritional needs are closely related to the increase in body mass, the peak requirements occur in the years of maximum growth, during which the body mass almost doubles. The caloric and protein requirements during this time are higher than at almost any other time of life. The need for proteins as well as for the minerals calcium, iron, and zinc substantially increases during periods of rapid growth: calcium for skeletal growth, iron for expansion of muscle mass and blood volume, and zinc for the generation of both skeletal and bone tissue. Girls with heavy or frequent menses may be especially susceptible to iron deficiency due to blood loss. Calcium intake from food sources is essential during adolescence to assist in the prevention of osteoporosis in adulthood. Eventual bone mass is a balance between the amount of bone laid down during adolescence and the amount later lost with aging. Maximum bone mass is also acquired during adolescence; therefore, the calcium deposited during these years determines the risk of osteoporosis (Ongphiphadhanakul, 2007).

Eating Well With Canada's Food Guide outlines recommended dietary intake for persons throughout the lifespan (Health Canada, 2011a). A recent survey of seventh- to tenth-grade students in Alberta found that a large portion (42%) of adolescents were not meeting the minimum dietary recommendations outlined in *Canada's Food Guide* (Storey et al., 2009). Compared to youth who met the minimum dietary recommendations, these teenagers tended have lower intakes of protein and fibre, higher intakes of carbohydrates and fats, a lower frequency of consuming breakfast, higher numbers of meals eaten away from home, and a lower level of physical activity.

Eating Habits and Behaviour

With adolescence and the move toward independence, family influences on the individual may diminish. Adolescents' interests, attitudes, and routines are altered as an increasing number of meals are eaten away from home. Peers may easily influence the adolescent's eating habits.

Pressure for time and commitments to activities can adversely affect the teenager's eating habits. Omitting breakfast or eating a nutritionally poor breakfast is frequently a problem. Snacks, usually selected on the basis of accessibility rather than nutritional merit, can become a greater part of the habitual eating pattern during adolescence (Fig. 40-7). Excess intake of calories, sugar, fat, cholesterol, and sodium is common among adolescents and is found in all income and racial or ethnic groups and both genders. Inadequate intake of certain vitamins (folic acid, vitamin B_6, vitamin A) and minerals (iron, calcium, zinc) is also evident, particularly among girls and teenagers of low socioeconomic status. In combination with other factors, these dietary patterns could result in increased risk for obesity and chronic diseases such as heart disease, osteoporosis, and some types of cancer later in life.

Overeating or undereating during adolescence presents special problems. When teenage girls experience the normal increase in weight and fat deposition of the growth spurt, they often resort to dieting. The desire for a slim figure and a fear of becoming "fat" can prompt teenage girls to embark on nutritionally inadequate reducing regimens that drain their energy and deprive their growing bodies of essential nutrients. They may resort to diets on their own or with peers in an effort to conform. Many adopt current fad diets and are victims of food misinformation. Boys may be less inclined to undereat; they are more concerned about gaining size and strength. However, they tend to eat foods high in calories but low in other essential nutrients.

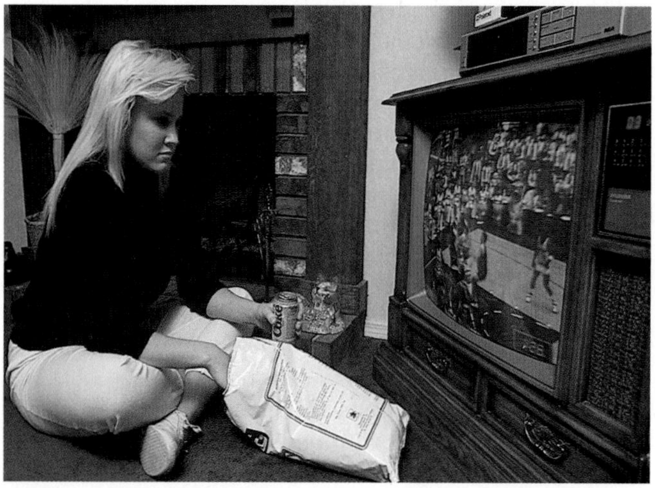

Fig. 40-7 Snacking on empty calories is common among adolescents, especially during inactivity.

Obesity has increased significantly among both children and adolescents in Canada. The obesity currently seen is not a result of metabolic disturbances but of poor dietary habits and sedentary lifestyles. Adolescent obesity poses both immediate and long-term problems for adolescents: obesity is directly linked to the development of cardiovascular disease and other chronic illnesses such as type 2 diabetes.

A contributing factor to the increase in obesity is the fact that over the past two decades, the overall portion size for foods has increased, the largest portions for most foods being found at fast-food restaurants. However, portion sizes for desserts and hamburgers are reportedly largest at home (Nielsen & Popkin, 2003). Lifestyle changes necessary for adolescents to lose weight require the involvement of family members who provide support and encourage active participation.

Anorexia nervosa (AN) and bulimia nervosa (BN) also commonly occur during the adolescent and young-adult years. If left untreated, these disorders, like obesity, can lead to considerable morbidity and mortality (see Chapter 4, p. 50; Chapter 39, Eating Disorders; and discussion later in this chapter).

Nursing Care Management

Adolescents should receive at a minimum an annual assessment of weight, height, and BMI for age, plotted on a standard growth chart (see Appendix C). Healthy dietary habits should be discussed with all adolescents. The frequency of eating at fast-food and other restaurants, consumption of sweetened beverages, and consumption of excessive portion sizes should be identified. A growing concern among children and adolescents is the availability of high-fat, high-carbohydrate snack foods and drinks within the school environment, which may further contribute to obesity; such foods compete with school meals yet are often favourites of adolescents (Story, Nanney, & Schwartz, 2009). In addition to food intake, the nurse should assess the adolescent's level of physical activity and sedentary behaviours. Readiness to change; environmental supports and barriers; and family history of diabetes, heart disease, and early stroke must be considered when planning nutritional education and guidance. Nurses in the school setting can assist in advocating for comprehensive nutritional services for preschool through grade 12 students. Comprehensive nutrition education with access to nutritious meals and snacks and physical activity at school will begin to reverse the trend of childhood obesity (Briggs, Safaii, & Beall, 2003).

To help teenagers select a nutritious diet, it is best to begin with their present diet and actively involve them in the process. Adolescents do not respond well to judgemental attitudes and dislike lectures, but they do respond when their independence is respected and they are given the opportunity to make their own decisions regarding food choices.

In general, adolescents are body conscious and concerned about their appearance. Concrete messages about the relationship between an attractive appearance and the benefits of a healthy lifestyle are most effective. However, helping adolescents arrive at a decision for change is more difficult than providing information. They respond best when the counsellor provides straightforward information, uses instructional methods that actively involve them, talks with them and not at them, and listens to what they have to say.

Sleep and Rest

Adolescents vary in their need for sleep and rest. Rapid physical growth, the tendency toward overexertion, and the overall increased activity of this age contribute to fatigue in adolescents. During growth spurts the need for sleep is increased. Their propensity for staying up late makes it difficult to get up in the morning, and they may sleep late at every opportunity. Adequate sleep and rest at this time are important to a total health regimen.

Exercise and Activity

Although today's youth are said to be less fit than children 20 years ago, adolescents probably spend more time and energy practising and participating in sports activities than members of any other age group. Many adolescents participate in sports within school settings (Fig. 40-8). School-based, health-oriented physical education may provide both immediate effects of the activity and sustained effects through encouragement of lifelong activity patterns. Canadian schools average 170 minutes of physical education per week (grades 11–12). However, the percentage of students taking at least one physical education class per week drops significantly in higher secondary grades (57% among grade 11–12 students) compared to other grades (99% in grades 1–8) (Active Healthy Kids Canada, 2012). To improve health outcomes, school-age children and adolescents should engage in 60 minutes or more of moderate-to-vigorous physical activity daily (Canadian Society for Exercise Physiology, 2012).

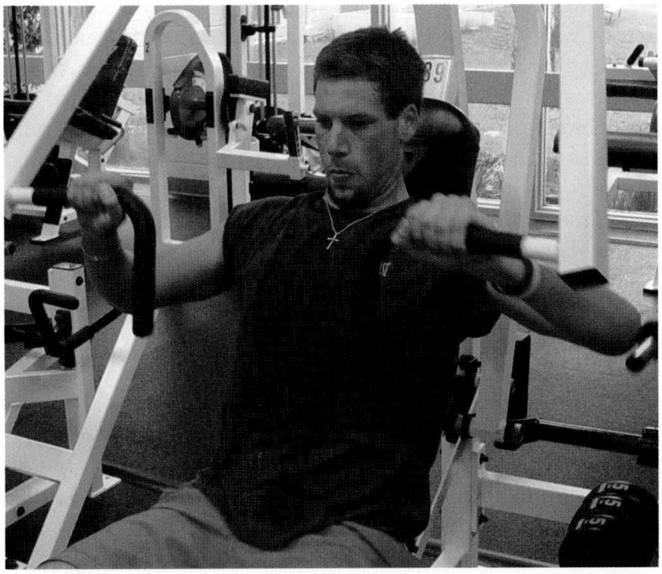

Fig. 40-8 Adolescents should be encouraged to participate in activities that contribute to lifelong physical fitness.

The practice of sports, games, and even dancing contributes significantly to growth and development, the education process, and better health. These activities provide exercise for growing muscles, interactions with peers, and a socially acceptable means of enjoying stimulation and conflict. In addition, competitive activities help teenagers conduct their own self-appraisal and develop self-respect and concern for others. Because physical fitness appears to be a major influence on one's lifelong health status, children and adolescents should be encouraged to participate in activities that contribute to lifelong physical fitness. Nurses can encourage participation as a way to promote health and build self-esteem. However, adolescents should not be encouraged to engage in physical activities that are beyond their physical or emotional capacity (see Health Problems Related to Sports Participation, Chapter 39).

Dental Health

Dental health should not be neglected during adolescence; the rate of caries formation may be significant due to poor nutritional habits (e.g., increased intake of cariogenic substances) and inadequate oral hygiene. Flossing and regular tooth brushing in adolescence serve to remove plaque and prevent periodontal disease. Additional factors that may influence oral health during adolescence include the use of tobacco (particularly chewing tobacco), pregnancy, eating disorders, increased risk for traumatic dental injury and periodontal disease, and increased awareness of appearance (American Academy of Pediatric Dentistry, 2009). Dental care is an aspect of preventive care that substantial proportions of children in Canada do not receive.

Corrective orthodontic appliances (braces) are a fact of life for many teens, particularly during the early adolescent years. These may be a source of embarrassment and concern; however, in some cases these may be considered trendy, depending on the individual's and peers' attitudes toward their cosmetic effects. Reassurance regarding the temporary nature of the annoyance and anticipation of an improved appearance can help make the inconvenience tolerable. It is also important to reinforce the orthodontist's directions regarding use and care of the appliances and to emphasize careful attention to oral hygiene during this time (see also Chapters 37 and 39).

Adequate fluoride remains important throughout the adolescent years. While most teens no longer require oral supplements, the Canadian Dental Association (2010) recommends that adolescents with high caries risk receive oral supplementation—this includes teens who do not brush their teeth or have not brushed with a fluoridated toothpaste twice a day, and those who are assessed as being susceptible to high caries activity because of community or family history.

Personal Care

The body-conscious teenager is highly amenable to discussion and counselling about personal care and hygiene. Body changes associated with puberty bring special needs for cleanliness. The hyperactive sebaceous glands and newly functioning apocrine glands make frequent bathing or showering a necessity, and underarm deodorants and antiperspirants assume an important place in personal care. The adolescent discovers that hair requires more frequent shampooing, and girls often have questions about hair removal, use of cosmetics, and menstrual hygiene. Peer group discussions centre on the advantages of particular products or methods. Adolescents are continually bombarded with messages from the media regarding the best way to enhance their popularity and attractiveness. Nurses are in a position to help them evaluate the relative merits of commercial products.

Vision

Regular vision testing is an important part of health care and supervision during adolescence. During this time, visual refractive difficulties reach a high level that is not exceeded until the fifth decade of life. The increased demands of schoolwork make adequate vision essential for academic success. Consequently, teenagers are more likely to be referred for visual evaluation. The need for corrective lenses can create psychological problems for teenagers if they believe that glasses spoil their appearance or do not fit their body image. Contact lenses may be a preferred solution; a wide variety of lenses are now available at fairly reasonable prices. For some, the impact of a visual defect, no matter how slight, may be stressful.

Hearing

Considerable concern has focused on current teenage practices that cause hearing damage. Cochlear damage from relatively continuous exposure to loud sound levels of music has been documented. The popularity of compact personal music (MP3) players with lightweight earphones is of particular concern to health care providers. When these units are used for extended periods, permanent hearing loss can occur. Although appeals for more judicious use are not always successful, teenagers should be informed of the risk. Efforts directed toward legislating legal limits of the noise exposure that can be achieved through the sets may be another possible solution. (See Chapter 42 for a discussion of noise-related hearing loss.)

Posture

Rapid skeletal growth is often associated with slower muscular growth, and as a result, some teenagers may appear awkward or slump and fail to stand or sit upright. However, some postural defects of adolescence require early medical intervention. Scoliosis is a defect of the spine that occurs frequently in adolescence and is more common in girls than in boys (see Idiopathic Scoliosis, Chapter 54). Most cases are idiopathic, and the defect manifests as a painless curvature of the spine. Fortunately, most of these spinal curvatures will not require treatment. However, because there is no way to predict which curvatures will progress, all curvatures of the spine should be referred for further evaluation.

Body Art

Body art (piercing and tattooing) is generally associated with adolescents' alignment with particular groups, and reflects their shifting sense of identity. The meaning of body art varies by family and individual. The adolescent often seeks body art as an expression of his or her personal identity and style. Tattoos are often obtained to mark significant life events such as new relationships, births, and deaths. Piercing of the ear, nose, nipple, navel, penis, or tongue may sometimes create a health problem. It is a nursing responsibility to caution girls and boys against having piercings performed by friends, mothers, or themselves. Although most cases of piercing are accompanied by few if any serious adverse effects, there is always a danger of complications such as infection, abscess formation, cyst or keloid formation, bleeding, dermatitis, or metal allergy. Using the same unsterilized needle to pierce body parts of multiple teenagers presents the same risk of human immunodeficiency virus (HIV), hepatitis C, and hepatitis B virus transmission as occurs with other needle-sharing activities.

A qualified operator using proper sterile technique should perform the procedure. This is especially important if the adolescent has a history of diabetes, allergies, or skin disorders. Adolescents should be informed about the approximate time for healing after body piercing and the care of the pierced area during and after healing. Some body sites require extra precautions. For example, cartilage (ear, nose) has a poor blood supply and heals slowly and scars easily; nipple piercing puts the adolescent at risk for breast abscess. Penile piercing often penetrates the urethra, requiring the male to sit to void thereafter. Finally, migration of the piercing is common with naval and other flat skin surface piercing. Piercing guns should not be used for piercing anything other than the earlobe because guns place the piercing too deeply.

It is estimated that 3 to 5% of people in Western society have a tattoo. Although there are no recent statistics for body piercing and tattooing among Canadian youth, studies of distinct populations of young adults and adolescents report body art rates as high as 23% (Braverman, 2006). Professionals as well as amateur artists administer tattoos. The risk to the adolescent receiving a tattoo is low. The greatest risk is for the tattoo artist who comes in contact with the patient's blood. Adolescents who are amateur tattoo artists benefit from discussions about **standard precautions (routine practices)** and the hepatitis B vaccination. Many provinces and territories either have no regulations or do not enforce existing regulations for piercing and tattooing facilities. Health Canada (2011b) regulates the dyes used for tattoos or permanent make-up, which are considered to be cosmetic products and must meet the requirements of the Food and Drugs Act and its cosmetics regulations, which are administered by Health Canada. The definition of a cosmetic is "any substance or mixture of substances manufactured, sold, or represented for use in cleansing, improving or altering the complexion, skin, hair or teeth, and includes deodorants and perfumes." The local health department is a source of information about local regulatory requirements. Comprehensive guidelines on tattooing can be found through the Simcoe Muskoka District Health Unit (2011), and the U.S. Centers for Disease Control and Prevention (CDC) has an excellent Web site outlining safety concerns for persons performing and receiving body art (see Additional Resources section at the end of this chapter).

Tanning

The quest for an attractive appearance leads many teenagers to excessive sunbathing and artificial means for tanning. A Canadian Cancer Society study (2007) showed that nearly 65% of Ontario students in grades 7 to 12 tan by one means or another. Seven percent of girls and 4% of boys had used an artificial tanning bed, and the use of artificial tanning among adolescents is rising. This practice has serious long-term risks, and the adolescent should be educated regarding the detrimental effects of sunlight on the skin (see Sunburn, Chapter 53). Long-term effects include premature aging of the skin; increased risk of skin cancer; and, in susceptible individuals, phototoxic reactions.

The long-term effects of tanning machines are similar to those of the sun; dermatologists do not recommend tanning by these means. The Canadian Cancer Society (2006) advocates regulation of the artificial tanning industry, including the banning of marketing artificial tanning to youth. Nova Scotia, New Brunswick, and British Columbia have banned the use of artificial tanning devices by people under the age of 18. Health Canada has asked for voluntary banning for this age group, but it is not being followed by many salons. The Canadian Paediatric Society (2012) has called for a ban for this group as well. Those who insist on using tanning equipment should be warned that goggles must be worn in tanning booths to prevent serious corneal burning. For individuals under 35 years of age there is a 75% increased risk of developing melanoma from exposure to indoor tanning equipment.

Adolescents require education on the use of sunscreens, including hypoallergenic products, with a sun protective factor (SPF) of at least 15 and a nonalcohol base without lanolin, parabens, or fragrance. Broad-spectrum sunscreens that protect against both ultraviolet A and B are most effective. Self-tanning creams safely simulate the appearance of a tan; however, teens using these products should be cautioned that sun protection is still required. Targeting health education messages to adolescents and incorporating educational components relating to sun protection behaviours in school health curricula and in health care visits will increase adolescent knowledge and awareness.

A large cross-sectional study of 12- to 18-year-olds in the United States found that teens are not following these recommendations; 34% had used sunscreen routinely in the past summer and 14% had used a tanning bed at least once (Geller et al., 2002). Cutaneous melanoma, the most common fatal form of skin cancer, is associated with ultraviolet light exposure and affects an increasing number of Canadians (Canadian Dermatologists Association, 2010).

Mental Health

During this time of transition from childhood to becoming an adult, adolescents experience many physiological and emotional changes. This age group often will have a sense of pressure to achieve success at home, school, and in social groups yet lack the experience required to help them realize that these challenges can be overcome as they gain that life experience (Canadian Mental Health Association, 2011). With these changes and pressures, some adolescents may be more vulnerable to developing an **emotional disorder**.

In May 2006, a Senate committee chaired by Senator Michael Kirby released a comprehensive report on mental health and mental illness in Canada: "Out of the Shadows: Report of the Senate Committee on Social Affairs, Science and Technology." It concluded that "children and youth are at a significant disadvantage when compared to other demographic groups affected by mental illness, in that the failings of the mental health system affect them more acutely and severely" (Government of Canada, Standing Senate Committee on Social Affairs, Science and Technology, 2006). Thus, it is especially important for nurses to not only assess the mental health of adolescent patients but also to support those who struggle with mental disorders (see also Serious Health Problems with a Behavioral Component, later in this chapter).

Stress Reduction

The multiple changes occurring in adolescence can result in great stress (Fig. 40-9 and Box 40-2). Adolescents are faced with pressures from peers that often involve flouting adult authority and taking serious health risks, including

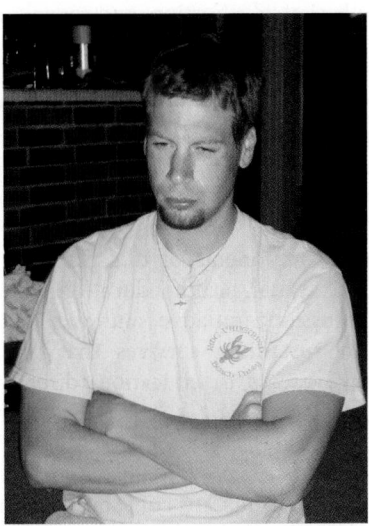

Fig. 40-9 Adolescents may use being alone as a method of coping with stress. Health care providers need to assess whether this indicates clinical depression.

BOX 40-2 Areas of Stress in Adolescence

- Body image
- Sexuality conflicts
- Academic pressures
- Competitive pressures
- Relationships with parents
- Relationships with siblings
- Relationships with peers
- Dating
- Finances
- Decisions about present and future roles
- Career planning
- Ideological conflicts

pressures for sexual experimentation and use of drugs, alcohol, and tobacco, as well as potentially dangerous physical activities.

Early-maturing girls and late-maturing children are especially sensitive to the stresses of being different from their peers. Many feel intense anxiety over their identity. Both early- and late-maturing children can feel out of place among their classmates, but slow-maturing children appear to suffer the most pronounced inner turmoil and may be hesitant to voice their concerns.

Sexual Health

Youth sexual health is a critical consideration for nurses working directly with adolescents and for those involved in creating programs and shaping policy that affects services to youth. The World Health Organization defines sexual health as "a state of physical, mental and social well-being in relation to sexuality [requiring] a positive and respectful approach to sexuality and sexual relationships, as well as the possibility of having pleasurable and safe experiences, free of coercion, discrimination and violence" (World Health Organization, 2011). When we consider the sexual health of youth, topics of STIs, pregnancy, birth control, abortion, and sexual practices come into focus.

The province of Nova Scotia has developed a comprehensive strategy to promote the sexual health of adolescents (Nova Scotia Roundtable on Youth Sexual Health, n.d.). This framework is intended to address youth sexual health on a number of levels, but is particularly directed toward individuals who make decisions affecting youth health. Among the key components of this plan are an emphasis on school-based sexual health education; the involvement of youth in discussion, initiative, and decision making; and developing and sustaining services that will ensure that adolescents have access to education, direct services, and other resources.

Sexuality Education

Contemporary adolescents are constantly exposed to sexual symbolism and erotic stimulation in the media. At the same time, the development of **primary** and **secondary sex characteristics** and the increased sensitivity of the genitalia can produce thoughts and fantasies about sexual relationships. Sexual aspects of interpersonal relationships become particularly important. Societal expectations push adolescents toward dating, and their own inner sex drive urges them toward exploration. This is often exacerbated by peer pressure to be involved in sexual relationships and the adolescent's need to fit in.

North American society continues to do a generally poor job of educating adolescents about pubertal growth and development. Omar, McElderry, and Zakharia (2003) found that 36% of boys and 2% of girls in their study had never been spoken to about pubertal development or sexuality issues. Girls received sex education at a mean age of 13 years and boys at a mean age of 15 years. A large portion of knowledge relating to sex is acquired from adolescents' peers and from television, the Internet, movies, and magazines. In addition, information obtained from their parents may be inaccurate. As a result, the information they accumulate may be incomplete, inaccurate, riddled with cultural and moral judgements, and not very helpful.

The responsibility for providing sexuality education has been assumed by parents; schools; churches; community agencies such as the Canadian Federation for Sexual Health; and health care providers including nurses. Many adolescents perceive nurses, especially school nurses, as individuals who possess important information and who are willing to discuss sex with them. To be able to discuss the topic adequately, nurses must have not only an understanding of the physiological aspects of sexuality and a knowledge of cultural and societal values but also an awareness of their own attitudes, feelings, and biases about sexuality.

Guidelines for sexual health education have been developed by the Public Health Agency of Canada (2008). These guidelines are based on an understanding that sexual health education should be culturally sensitive and respectful of sexual diversity, abilities and choices. Other resources for information about sexuality, sexual health, and sexuality education are the Sex Information and Education Council of Canada (SIECCAN) and Sexualityandu.ca (sponsored by the Society of Obstetricians and Gynaecologists of Canada) (see Additional Resources section at the end of this chapter).

Whether nurses counsel young people on an individual basis, in mixed groups, or in groups segregated by gender makes little difference. Ideally, boys and girls should be able to discuss sexuality objectively with one another and in groups, but this is not always possible. The differences in the rate of maturation between boys and girls and between different members of the same sex often make it desirable to discuss certain aspects of sexuality in segregated groups. As a rule, the need for separate discussion groups diminishes as young people mature.

Sexuality education should consist of instruction concerning normal body functions and should be presented in a straightforward manner using correct terminology. When discussing sex and sexual activities, nurses should use simple but correct language, not street language (although it may be helpful to know), highly scientific terminology, or euphemisms. Once the meanings of biological terms such as *uterus*, *testicles*, and *vagina* are understood, most teenagers prefer to use them in their discussions.

Many girls arrive at menarche with ambivalent attitudes, myths, and illogical beliefs. Even girls adequately prepared for menstruation do not always understand its relationship to the total process of reproduction. Many are under the incorrect impression that the "safe" time for sexual intercourse is midway between menstrual periods.

Teenagers' curiosity and their desire for information extend beyond the need for anatomical and physiological knowledge. They need to know more than the mechanics of conception, pregnancy, and birth. Adolescents, girls in particular, want answers to questions such as "What is it like?" "Does it hurt?" "What happens when ...?" and "Is it all right if you ...?" Boys are often concerned about the fallacy that a relationship exists between penis size and sexual function. They need reassurance that masturbation is a normal and common practice, that some degree of homosexuality is not unusual in early adolescence, and that oral–genital relations can be normal substitutes for intercourse but still carry risks of transmitting STIs.

Teenagers need to discuss intercourse, alternative methods of sexual satisfaction, and how to resist peer pressure. With the increased incidence of STIs, especially HIV infection, the topic of "safer sex," especially abstinence or the use of condoms and abstinence, is essential. Role-playing may help teenagers learn effective approaches to dealing with difficult situations. Sex and sexuality cannot be taught without discussions of mature decision making, sexual responsibility, and values clarification. Adolescents may receive inaccurate and ambiguous messages regarding sexual behaviour; for example, an adolescent may be told that abstinence from vaginal intercourse will prevent transmission of an STI. Accurate and unbiased information about sexual practices should be provided in a setting where the adolescent feels comfortable asking questions without being degraded or made to feel uncomfortable.

Adolescents need role models and life experiences with delayed gratification. Most important, they need problem-solving experience and decision-making skills so that they can anticipate the positive and negative outcomes of a decision. With these types of assistance, teenagers can be sexually responsible young adults.

Pregnancy, Abortion, and Birth Control

The rate of live births to mothers aged 15 to 17 years decreased steadily from 11.0 to 7.4 per 1000 females between 1999 and 2005, and increased to 8.2 per 1000 females in 2008. Similar trends have occurred in teenagers who are 18 and 19 years old (PHAC, 2012). This decreasing rate of pregnancy is likely due to increased access to various forms of contraception (Langille, 2007). Recent research suggests many factors shape the likelihood that a young woman will become pregnant. In research with high school students in Nova Scotia, Langille, Corbett, Wilson, and Schlievert (2010) found that 52.3% of students reported that they were sexually active. Among girls, 84.7% reported using some sort of contraception (hormonal contraception or condoms). Other important findings from this study included the following:

- Many sexually active youth (7.2%) reported reluctance to buy condoms because of feeling embarrassed.
- 35.8% of sexually active youth reported unplanned or unintentional sex as a result of intoxication (drugs or alcohol) in the past year.
- Casual sex was common, with 25.3% of sexually active students reporting having intercourse with someone they did not know particularly well.
- 40.4% of sexually active youth reported having more than one sexual partner within the same time period.
- Clear links exist between alcohol or drug use and sexual risk taking.

While this survey reflects the sexual health of youth in one community in Nova Scotia, the findings alert nurses and other health care providers to the kinds of issues that are important in the development and delivery of services for youth and in the provision of nursing care to adolescents.

Injury Prevention

Physical injuries are the greatest single cause of death among Canadian youth, claiming more lives than all other causes combined. The most vulnerable ages are the years 15 to 24, when accidental injuries account for about 64% of all deaths (PHAC, 2009). In addition, for every youth that dies from trauma, more than 10 have severe injuries (McDonald, 2007). The introduction of a comprehensive staged and graduated driver's licensing system has resulted in some reduction of motor vehicle deaths among youth. Other policies such as banning of cell phone usage and text messaging in some provinces may further reduce rates of motor vehicle injury among youth.

During adolescence, peak physical, sensory, and psychomotor function gives teenagers a feeling of strength and confidence that they have never experienced before, and the physiological changes of puberty give impetus to many basic instinctual forces. One manifestation of this is an increase in energy that simply must be discharged through action, often at the expense of logical thinking and other control mechanisms. The tendency of many adolescents to take chances, act impulsively, overestimate their abilities, or sway to peer pressure make this group vulnerable to severe injury. Injury prevention during adolescence requires a multidimensional approach. To begin, education of youth about potential risks is vital (Box 40-3). Education, however, is not enough; engaging with youth about the motivations for risk-taking behaviour is useful. For such discussions to be effective, the adult must be seen as credible and the tone must be nonjudgemental. Finally, advocating for provincial and federal legislation (such as graduated licensing and banning of cell phones while driving) is another avenue through which nurses can work to reduce injuries among youth in our communities.

Vehicle-Related Injuries

The adolescent's newly acquired ability to drive and the normal developmental need for independence and freedom make the automobile an attractive but potentially dangerous part of many adolescents' lives. In 2005, motor vehicle–related deaths among 15- to 19-year-olds numbered 14.9 per 100,000 persons, compared with a rate of 5.4 per 100,000 persons for all children and youth combined. Within the 15- to 19-year age group, males died from motor vehicle crashes at nearly twice the rate of females: 19.3 per 100,000 boys compared to 10.2 per 100,000 girls (PHAC, 2009). Many factors contribute to the higher rate of crashes among teen drivers: they lack driving experience and maturity, tend to follow the car ahead of them too closely, drive too fast, have other teen passengers in the car, and may consume alcohol before driving (Williams & Ferguson, 2002). Several provinces have enacted graduated driver license laws with restrictions on younger adolescent driving. In British Columbia, for example, at age 14 years, an adolescent may obtain a learner's license by successfully passing a knowledge test. At age 16, upon passing a road test, the teen may drive unsupervised, but with certain imposed conditions (only one other nonfamily member in the car, zero blood alcohol level). The age at which an adolescent can first drive varies among provinces.

In working with teens, nurses have many opportunities to educate teenagers and their parents about the risks of driving

BOX 40-3 Education for Prevention of Adolescent Injury

Motor or Nonmotor Vehicles

Pedestrian—Emphasize and encourage safe pedestrian behaviour.
- At night, walk with a friend.
- If someone is following you, go to the nearest place with people.
- Do not walk in secluded areas; take well-travelled walkways.

Passenger—Promote appropriate behaviour while riding in a motor vehicle.

Driver—Provide competent driver education; encourage judicious use of vehicle; discourage drag racing, "playing chicken"; discourage cell phone usage and text messaging; maintain vehicle in proper condition (brakes, tires, etc.).

Teach and promote safety and maintenance of two-wheeled vehicles.

Encourage wearing of safety apparel such as helmet and long trousers.

Reinforce the dangers of drugs, including alcohol, when operating a motor vehicle.

Falls

Teach and encourage general safety measures in all activities.

Drowning

Teach nonswimmers to swim.

Teach basic rules of water safety:
- Select carefully a place to swim.
- Ensure sufficient water depth for diving.
- Swim with a companion.
- Wear a life vest during water sports (e.g., boating, skiing).
- Avoid swimming, boating, or other water sports after alcohol consumption.

Burns

Reinforce proper behaviour in areas involving contact with burn hazards (gasoline, electric wires, fires).

Advise regarding excessive exposure to natural or artificial sunlight (ultraviolet burn).

Discourage smoking.

Encourage use of sunscreen.

Poisoning

Educate in hazards of drug use, including alcohol.

Other Sources of Physical Harm

Promote proper instruction in sports and use of sports equipment.

Instruct in safe use of and respect for firearms and other devices with potential danger (e.g., power tools, fireworks).

Provide and encourage use of protective equipment when using potentially hazardous devices (e.g., motorcycles, power tools).

Promote access to and provision of safe sports and recreational facilities.

Be alert for signs of depression (potential suicide).

Discourage use and availability of hazardous sports equipment (e.g., trampoline, surfboards).

Instruct in proper use of corrective devices (e.g., glasses, contact lenses, hearing aids).

Encourage judicious application of safety principles and prevention.

while drinking alcohol or when intoxicated and of riding in an automobile with a drunk driver. Many families have developed a plan to arrange a no-questions-asked ride home, to prevent an adolescent from riding with a drunk driver or being tempted to drive after consuming alcohol. The major risk for death in a motor vehicle accident is failure to use a safety restraint. Teenage seat belt use, especially among boys, is lower than adult seat belt usage. An exception to this pattern is recent research findings in British Columbia, which suggest that increasing numbers of adolescents are always wearing seatbelts (66% in 2008 versus 54% in 2003) (Smith et al., 2009). Continued efforts to ensure teenage seat belt use should be focused at the individual educational level and through tough enforcement laws.

Nonautomotive Vehicle Injuries

The increasing use of motorized bicycles, all-terrain vehicles, jet skis, and snowmobiles has caused an increase in injuries among teenagers below the legal age for driving automobiles. In addition, many adolescents ride bicycles without helmets and without lights at night. The overwhelming majority of deaths from bicycle injuries (primarily head injuries) involve teenagers.

Firearms

In Canada, the rate of death from injury involving firearms has steadily declined over the past two decades (Wilkins, 2005). During the same time period, the age gradient for death from injury involving firearms also decreased, and differences among age groups have largely disappeared. Currently, most deaths involving firearms are suicides. The relatively low rates of death from injuries involving firearms can be attributed to Canada's gun laws. A valid license is required to own, borrow, or store a firearm, and many firearms are prohibited or restricted (notably automatic guns and handguns) (Royal Canadian Mounted Police, 2011).

Youth access to firearms is generally through family members and acquaintances. Gun availability in the home is strongly correlated to unintentional death and injury to children and youth (Laws, 2005). In addition, the presence of a gun in the home increases the risk of adolescent suicide and homicide. When guns are in the home, adults must take preventive action to be certain that the guns are never loaded, that they are locked up in a safe place, and that ammunition is stored and locked up separately in a location where only appropriate adults have access to it.

Nonpowder Firearms

Guns that do not use powder (e.g., airguns and airsoft guns), while viewed as toys by many, account for almost as many injuries as powder guns. The regulations regarding use of nonpowder guns are relaxed; they can be purchased legally by adolescents and are labelled as suitable for children as young as 8 years of age. In Canada, some provinces, such as Ontario, restrict the sale of airguns to persons under the age of 18 years. Many cities have bylaws against discharging airguns within city limits.

Nurses are in a good position to advocate for laws regulating the sale of these potentially dangerous "toys."

Sports Injuries

Because the degree of physical maturity, size, coordination, and endurance varies greatly among adolescents of the same age, sports competition can result in predictable and unnecessary injuries for those not fit or suited to particular sports. The matching of adolescent candidates with individual sports should be done relative to physical maturity, height, weight, and physical fitness and skills, particularly in a sport involving rigorous body contact. Age is a less important consideration.

Every sport has some potential for injury, whether one participates in serious competition or for pure enjoyment. Overuse injuries are common in adolescents and result in more time missed from the activity than do fractures. A large number of severe or fatal injuries occur to youths who are not physically prepared for the activity. The increase in strength and vigor in adolescence may tempt adolescents to overextend themselves. The range of injuries sustained in sports or recreational activities can involve any part of the body and extend from relatively minor cuts, bruises, and abrasions to totally incapacitating central nervous system injuries or death. The leading cause of serious sports injuries among boys is participation in football. The increase in girls' competitive sports in high schools in Canada has resulted in an increase in sports-related injuries among this population. Research shows that 48% of grade 10 Canadian girls were injured while playing or training for sports, whereas 10% were injured while running or walking, 1% while biking, 3% while skating, 5% while fighting, 3% while riding in or driving a car, and 2% while doing paid or unpaid work (PHAC, 2012).

Nursing Care Management

Anticipatory guidance with parents and children regarding the expected problems and hazards related to growth and development does not end as children approach maturity. They need education in basic safety precautions and instruction in skills required in the performance of activities such as sports, instruction in handling motor vehicles, proper protective equipment, and instruction in proper maintenance of equipment. During adolescence, however, health and safety education and guidance are more effective when the young people are involved directly. Parents and health care providers can emphasize the importance of safety during performance of activities and the proper conditioning and preparation for sports.

Prevention can occur on a variety of levels. Safety advocacy, changes in public policy, and legislation can help curtail injuries. Examples of such approaches are laws that mandate wearing seat belts, requiring the wearing of a helmet while driving moving vehicles other than automobiles, keeping the legal minimum drinking age (age 18 in Alberta and Québec and age 19 in the rest of the provinces and territories), and instituting curfews for teen drivers. In addition, health education for teenagers and significant adults is essential. Helping adolescents understand their need for engaging in risky behaviour, exploring possible negative outcomes of such behaviour, and weighing possible alternatives are critical components of injury prevention.

Anticipatory Guidance—Care of Families

Both adolescents and their parents are often confused and perplexed about the changes and behaviour of this stage of development. Parents need support and guidance to help them through this trying time. They need to understand the changes taking place in their teenage children and to accept the expected behaviours that accompany the process of detachment. Parents may need help in "letting go" and in promoting the changed relationship from one of dependence to one of mutuality (see Patient Teaching box).

SPECIAL HEALTH PROBLEMS

Disorders Related to the Reproductive System

Amenorrhea

Menarche, or the first menstrual period, occurs relatively late in female pubertal development. Although girls vary in the onset and rate of progression of pubertal development, the sequence and tempo should be the same. When an adolescent girl has no menses, a careful history of the timing of her pubertal development will help determine if there is a need for further evaluation or if reassurance is all that is necessary.

Primary **amenorrhea** is an absence of secondary sex characteristics and no uterine bleeding by 14 to 15 years of age, or absence of uterine bleeding with secondary sex characteristics by 16 years of age (Master-Hunter & Heiman, 2006). No uterine bleeding after attaining **sexual maturity rating** 5 (Tanner; see Figs. 40-1 and 40-2) for 1 year, or after breast development for 4 years, is also considered primary amenorrhea (American Academy of Pediatrics & American College of Obstetricians and Gynecologists, 2006). The cause of primary amenorrhea may be anatomical, hormonal, genetic, or idiopathic. A thorough patient and family history and physical examination will provide clues to the etiology.

Secondary amenorrhea is defined as the absence of menses for 6 months or at least three cycles after menstruation was previously established. Irregular menstrual cycles are common within the first year or two after menarche. These early cycles may be anovulatory, resulting in regular, irregular, or absent bleeding; however, cycle lengths outside the range of 21 to 45 days should be investigated (American Academy of Pediatrics & American College of Obstetricians and Gynecologists, 2006). Girls with a later onset of menarche will take longer to establish regular ovulatory cycles.

PATIENT TEACHING Guidance During Adolescence

Encourage Parents to:

- Accept the adolescent as a unique individual
- Respect the adolescent's ideas, likes and dislikes, and wishes
- Be involved with school functions and attend the adolescent's performances, whether it be a sporting event or a school play
- Listen and try to be open to the teenager's views, even when they disagree with parental views
- Avoid criticism about no-win topics
- Provide an opportunity for choosing options and accept natural consequences of these choices
- Allow the young person to learn by doing, even when choices and methods differ from those of adults
- Provide the adolescent with clear, reasonable limits
- Clarify house rules and consequences for breaking them
- Let society's rules and consequences teach responsibility outside the home
- Allow increasing independence within limitations of safety and well-being
- Be available but avoid pressing the teenager too far
- Respect the adolescent's privacy
- Try to share the adolescent's feelings of joy or sorrow
- Respond to feelings, as well as words
- Be available to answer questions, give information, and provide companionship
- Try to make communication clear
- Avoid comparisons with siblings
- Assist the adolescent in selecting appropriate career goals and preparing for an adult role
- Welcome the adolescent's friends into the home and treat them with respect
- Provide unconditional love
- Be willing to apologize when mistaken

Be Aware That Adolescents:

- Are subject to turbulent, unpredictable behaviour
- Are struggling for independence
- Are extremely sensitive to feelings and behaviour that affect them
- May receive a different message from what was sent
- Consider friends extremely important
- Have a strong need to belong

Pregnancy is the most common cause of secondary amenorrhea and should be ruled out in both types of amenorrhea, even if the adolescent denies sexual activity. Other factors that disturb the hypothalamic–pituitary–gonadal axis and cause secondary amenorrhea include physical or emotional stress; sudden environmental change; hyperthyroidism or hypothyroidism; polycystic ovary disease; chronic illness; extreme weight loss or gain; intensive exercise; AN or BN; ovarian disturbance; and extrinsic pharmacological agents, especially phenothiazines, contraceptive steroids, and heroin. See Chapter 6, p. 84 for further discussion on amenorrhea.

Dysmenorrhea

A certain amount of discomfort during the first day or two of the menstrual flow is extremely common (for more discussion see Chapter 6, pp. 85–87). Most girls experience cramping, abdominal pain, backache, and leg ache, but in a few cases the pain is intolerable and incapacitating. *Primary* **dysmenorrhea** is painful menses not related to any pelvic disease. *Secondary dysmenorrhea* is defined as painful menses with a pathological condition such as endometriosis (Lefebvre et al., 2005). Primary dysmenorrhea usually begins within the first 6 months following menarche. The pain begins with menstrual flow or hours before the onset of bleeding each month, usually continuing for 48 to 72 hours. The exact etiology is widely debated. The pain is clearly related to ovulatory cycles. The overproduction of uterine prostaglandins has been implicated, and women with dysmenorrhea have higher levels of prostaglandins. Overproduction of vasopressin (a hormone that stimulates the contraction of muscular tissue) may also contribute to dysmenorrhea.

Many young women do not seek medical attention for this problem (Lefebvre et al., 2005). Questions related to menstruation and pain associated with it might reasonably be included in all encounters with adolescent girls. A careful history should include the onset of symptoms, the duration, type of pain and relationship to menstrual flow, age at menarche, family history of dysmenorrhea, and sexual history. The nurse should also ask about previous treatment that has been tried, including dosages of medications. Associated symptoms such as nausea, vomiting, diarrhea, and leg and back pain are helpful for diagnosis and treatment. Depending on the results of the history, the physical examination may include a gynecological examination.

Therapeutic Management

First-line treatment for adolescents with dysmenorrhea is the administration of nonsteroidal anti-inflammatory medications (NSAIDs) (see Table 6-1). The girl should begin the medication at the first sign of cramping or bleeding. Girls with vomiting at the time of menstruation benefit from beginning the medication 1 or 2 days before the onset of their menses. NSAIDs should always be taken with food.

Oral contraceptives are also often used to treat primary dysmenorrhea. A variety of other approaches have been effective in reducing the pain some young women experience. These include simple exercises such as pelvic rocking, assuming the knee–chest position, and breathing exercises, and stress reduction measures. Dietary changes, supplements, and herbal medications are often used to treat dysmenorrhea. Randomized controlled clinical trials have demonstrated that vitamin B_1, may be effective in the treatment of dysmenorrhea (Dennehy, 2006). Other complementary and alternative medicine approaches that show some promise include fish oil/vitamin B_{12} combination, vitamin B_6, and magnesium supplements (Lefebvre et al., 2005).

Nursing Care Management

When nurses are asked for advice regarding menstrual problems, they have a valuable opportunity to engage in health teaching concerning menstrual physiology and hygiene, as well as the importance of a well-balanced diet, exercise, and general health maintenance. Health teaching can also help dispel myths about menstruation. When assessment indicates a potential problem and the need for evaluation, referral to an appropriate practitioner, health service, or clinic may be necessary.

Gynecological examinations tend to be stressful experiences for adolescent women. Almost all adolescents are self-conscious about their bodies and the changes taking place. Anticipatory guidance regarding what to expect and suggestions of what to do to relax during the procedure are vital. Most girls favour a semisitting position, which has the additional advantage of allowing eye contact during the procedure. Sometimes a pillow helps the patient feel more comfortable and less vulnerable. The provision of a mirror for the girl to see what is taking place, if she so desires, helps the examiner explain various aspects of anatomy. When possible, it is important to respect the adolescent's request for a female provider.

Vaginitis

Vaginitis is an infection or inflammation of the vagina caused by physical, chemical, or infectious agents. Symptoms usually include itching, irritation, and abnormal vaginal discharge. Physical causes may include a forgotten tampon; chemical irritants include bubble bath, douching, deodorant pads, and tampons. Removing the offending material or discontinuing use of the irritating substance is usually all that is necessary to treat physical or chemical vaginitis. Infectious vaginitis can be caused by *Candida* fungi (yeast), *Trichomonas protozoa* parasites, or bacteria. Some infectious causes of vaginitis can have significant complications, particularly if left untreated. These include gonorrhea, chlamydia, and genital herpes. Diagnosis is confirmed with microscopic evaluation of vaginal secretions. Treatment varies depending on the infectious agent. (See Chapter 6 for further discussion of STIs and treatment of STIs.)

Health teaching is important in the prevention and management of vaginitis. Adolescent girls need reassurance that increased vaginal mucus can occur at the time of ovulation, before menstruation, or with sexual excitement. Teenage girls may mistake these variations as signs of infection. Girls should be taught to wipe from front to back after toileting and to realize that vaginitis can result from irritation, foreign objects, and sexual activity. Nurses should stress the importance of a medical evaluation to determine the exact cause.

Disorders of the Male Reproductive System

For most adolescent boys, structural anomalies of the male reproductive system (hypospadias, hydrocele, phimosis, and cryptorchidism) were identified and corrective measures instituted during early childhood. The most frequent problems related to the reproductive organs in adolescence are (1) infections, such as urethritis (see Urinary Tract Infection, Chapter 50); (2) hematuria; (3) penile problems, such as nonretractable foreskin in uncircumcised males, carcinoma, and trauma; (4) scrotal conditions, such as varicocele (elongation, dilation, and tortuosity of the veins superior to the testicle); and (5) testicular torsion (a condition in which the testicle hangs free from its vascular structures, which can result in partial or complete venous occlusion with rotation).

Although relatively rare, testicular cancer is among the most common cancers in men aged 15 to 34 years (Ellison & Wilkins, 2009). The usual presenting symptom for testicular cancer is a heavy, hard, painless mass (either smooth or nodular) the size of a pea that is palpated on the front or side of the testis. Additional symptoms may include testicular enlargement, groin pain, or sudden accumulation of fluid or blood in the scrotum. Treatment depends on the tumour stage and type and may involve surgical removal of the affected testicle (orchiectomy), often followed by radiation and chemotherapy (Gray & Moore, 2009).

Nursing Care Management

Most adolescent boys are self-conscious about their changing bodies. Preparation is crucial before performing a genital examination. Generally, the most effective approach is to assume a matter-of-fact attitude toward the examination, explain precisely what will take place, and maintain a continuous commentary about what is being done and the findings at each phase of the examination.

The routine health assessment of every adolescent boy should include teaching about testicular cancer. The Canadian Cancer Society (2011) recommends that young men age 15 years and older be taught the signs and symptoms of testicular cancer. They should also know how their testicles normally look and feel. Testicular tumours may be detected by the individual male. There is not enough evidence to recommend regular testicular exams, but it is important for men to know what is normal for them. Young men should be taught to examine their testes while they are in a warm shower or bath, which relaxes the scrotum and helps testes to descend (Canadian Cancer Society, 2011). Any of the following findings should be reported to a health care provider: a lump on the testicle, a painful testicle, a feeling of heaviness or dragging in the lower abdomen or scrotum, or a dull ache in the lower abdomen and groin. This rare malignancy is curable if detected early.

Nurses are in an ideal position to teach adolescents how to examine their testicles in a manner that is respectful and promotes early treatment (see Critical Thinking Exercise).

The normal testicle is a firm organ with a smooth, egg-shaped contour; the epididymis is palpated as a raised swelling on the superior aspect of the testicle and should not be confused with an abnormality.

Gynecomastia

The male breast, although not strictly part of the male reproductive system, responds to hormonal changes. Some degree of bilateral or unilateral breast enlargement occurs frequently in boys during puberty. It is estimated that approximately half of adolescent boys have transient gynecomastia, usually subsiding spontaneously within 1 to 2 years of onset. A careful assessment of the pubertal stage at the onset of gynecomastia; medication history, including anabolic steroids; and the exclusion of renal, liver, thyroid, and endocrine disorders or dysfunction allow the examiner to reassure the adolescent that the changes are pubertal gynecomastia and no further assessment is indicated.

If the condition persists or is extensive enough to cause embarrassment or to produce doubts about gender identity

CRITICAL THINKING EXERCISE

Testicular Self-Examination

At a recent faculty meeting, Paul, the pediatric nurse practitioner who runs the school-based health clinic, presented his plan for a class on testicular self-examination (TSE) to be delivered to the Grade 10 boys. Several teachers questioned the value of providing such a class when time to deliver content relating to "routine academic subjects" is limited. What important issues regarding testicular cancer and TSE should Paul use to justify providing this class to the Grade 10 boys?

1. Evidence—Is there sufficient evidence to justify teaching Grade 10 boys about TSE?
2. Assumptions—Describe the underlying assumption about each of the following:
   a. Detection of testicular cancers in adolescence
   b. Usual presenting symptom of testicular cancer
   c. Knowledge of genital anatomy among adolescent boys
   d. Ways to teach adolescent boys about their anatomy
3. What priorities for nursing care can be drawn at this time?
4. Does the evidence support your nursing intervention?
5. What alternative perspectives might you have?

in the young boy, plastic surgery may be indicated for cosmetic and psychological considerations. Administration of testosterone has no effect on breast development or regression and may aggravate the condition.

Nursing Care Management

Treatment usually consists of assuring the adolescent and his parents that this is a benign and temporary situation. Adolescents who are distressed about physical integrity and masculinity may benefit from the knowledge that this condition occurs in more than 50 to 65% of all adolescent boys.

Eating Disorders

Obesity

Few problems in childhood and adolescence are so obvious to others, are so difficult to treat, and have such effects on current and long-term health as obesity. According to the Public Health Agency of Canada (2010), childhood obesity rates have tripled in Canada over the last 25 years, with rates among First Nations children and youth being two to three times higher than the Canadian average.

The World Health Organization (2011) defines *overweight* as a BMI greater than 25, and *obesity* as a BMI greater than 30. BMI measurements provide the most accurate method for screening children and adolescents for obesity. The new WHO growth charts have recently been adapted for use in Canada and adopted by health authorities in most provinces. These charts include ideal BMI standards according to age and gender (see Table 4-1 for a WHO adult growth chart using BMI). Children and adolescents with a BMI between the eighty-fifth and ninety-seventh percentiles are considered overweight, those between the ninety-fifth and 99.9th percentile are considered obese, and those above the 99.9th percentile are categorized as severely obese (Dietitians of Canada, Canadian Paediatric Society, College of Family Physicians of Canada, & Community Health Nurses of Canada, 2010).

Obesity in childhood and adolescence has been related to elevated blood cholesterol; high blood pressure; respiratory disorders; orthopaedic conditions (Falkner et al., 2006; Taylor et al., 2006); cholelithiasis; some types of cancer, such as non-Hodgkin's lymphoma, leukemia, multiple myeloma, and cancers of the kidney, colon, rectum, breast, pancreas, ovary, and prostate (Pan et al., 2004); nonalcoholic fatty liver disease (Angulo, 2002; Baker et al., 2005); and type 2 diabetes mellitus (Canadian Diabetic Association, 2012). The incidence of metabolic syndrome was 50% in a study group of overweight and obese adolescents (Weiss et al., 2004). Common emotional consequences of obesity include poor body image, low self-esteem, social isolation, and feelings of depression and rejection (Sjöberg, Nilsson, & Leppert, 2005).

evolve Critical Thinking Exercise—Obesity

Etiology and Pathophysiology

A balance between energy intake and energy expenditure is critical to regulating body weight. Factors that raise energy intake or decrease energy expenditure by even small amounts can have a long-term impact on the development of overweight and obesity. For example, a positive balance of one serving of a sweetened juice or soft drink (about 120 kcal) per day would produce a 50 kg increase in body mass over a 10-year period (Hill et al., 2003). The imbalance between level of physical activity and food intake is the obvious explanation of overweight and obesity in childhood and adolescence.

In a small portion of cases (<5%) childhood obesity can be attributed to an underlying disease such as hypothyroidism; adrenal hypercorticoidism; hyperinsulinism; and dysfunction of the central nervous system as a result of tumour, injury, infection, or vascular accident. Obesity is a frequent complication of muscular dystrophy, paraplegia, Down syndrome, spina bifida, and other chronic illnesses that limit mobility.

Inquiry into the causes of childhood obesity has taken several paths. One of these inquiries is related to appetite regulation. Others have explored and found little evidence to support a relationship between obesity and "low metabolism." No differences in basal metabolic rate, sleeping metabolic rate, respiratory quotient, heart rate, or total energy expenditure have been found in normal-weight children with or without a familial predisposition to overweight (Baker et al., 2005).

The tendency toward obesity is manifested whenever environmental conditions are favourable to excessive caloric intake, such as an abundance of food, limited access to low-fat foods, increased availability of high-fat foods, reduced or minimal physical activity, and snacking combined with excessive television viewing. These conditions are exacerbated by commercial pricing strategies that promote unhealthy food choices and overzealous food advertising for high-fat and high-sugar foods that targets children and adolescents.

In addition, a report by the Government of Canada Standing Committee on Health (2007) has drawn attention to the links between childhood obesity and the key determinants of overall health. In particular, family income, education, social support, geographic location, cultural norms and values, biological and genetic factors, accessibility of services for health, and gender are important determinants of body weight among Canadian children and adolescents. Table 40-2 summarizes some of these influences.

Family and cultural eating patterns play a role in whether a child becomes obese; many families and cultures consider fat to be an indication of good health. It is not uncommon for obese children to come from families that provide large meals or admonish children for leaving food on their plates. Parents may have an exaggerated concept of the amount of food children require and expect them to eat more than they need.

Table 40-2 Determinants of Health That Influence Food Intake and Physical Activity in Childhood and Adolescence

Income	Family income determines access to quality food. Family income shapes access to physical activity facilities and organized sports.
Education	Increased education increases resources (i.e., literacy and numeracy) available for decision making related to food and activity choices.
Social environment	Strong communities can strengthen localized food systems. Lack of control over personal lives and communities limits opportunities to promote health (i.e., in many First Nations, Métis, and Inuit communities).
Physical environment/ geographic location	Children and youth living in advantaged neighbourhoods have a far lower risk of becoming obese than those in disadvantaged neighbourhoods. Parental perceptions of public safety influence child and youth physical activity. The cost of food varies widely according to community location, with prices far higher in isolated and northern communities. Access to low-fat, nutritious foods varies by location.
Values and norms	Values and norms vary widely and affect food and physical activity patterns among children and youth.
Biological/genetic factors	First Nations, Métis, Inuit, and South Asian populations have a genetic susceptibility to type 2 diabetes.
Accessibility of services for health	Availability and accessibility of quality health promotion and health intervention services vary. Availability of basic health care services varies.
Culture	Availability of television and video games varies. Family eating patterns vary by culture. Peer group activities and eating patterns vary by culture.
Gender	Adolescent boys, on average, are more active than adolescent girls.

(Adapted from Government of Canada, Standing Committee on Health. [2007]. *Healthy weights for healthy kids.* Ottawa, Canada: Parliament of Canada.)

Lower socioeconomic groups have a greater prevalence of obesity than that of higher-income groups, especially for girls. This difference between groups is often apparent before children are 6 years of age. Children from families with low physical activity levels may adopt these patterns of their parents and other adults. Parental obesity and low levels of physical activity are correlated with decreased physical activity in children. The type and level of adolescents' physical activity may also be influenced by sociocultural factors.

Community factors, such as unsafe neighbourhoods that keep children from playing outside, can influence activity patterns. Many communities lack affordable and accessible areas for low-income youth to be active, thus limiting opportunities for young people to participate in physical activities. In addition, many secondary schools allow students to leave school for lunch. Although well-balanced, nutritious school lunches may be available to students, they will often opt for less nutritious choices available outside of school. School vending machines are also often filled with high-fat and high-calorie foods and soft drinks, although many schools are now banning "junk food."

There is little doubt that, for many adolescents, physical activity levels are far lower than recommended. Research has shown that children who are more active after school and who spend less time watching television are much less likely to be overweight by age 12 than sedentary children (O'Brien et al., 2007). A recent study found that children at age 9 years engaged in approximately 3 hours of daily moderate to vigorous physical activity; by age 15 years, children were only engaging in 49 minutes of moderate to vigorous physical activity. Boys were more active than girls, and the cut-off period for a marked decrease in activity was 13.1 years for girls and 14.7 years for boys (Nader et al., 2008).

Psychological factors also affect eating patterns. In infancy, children experience relief from discomfort through feeding and learn to associate eating with a sense of well-being, security, and the comforting presence of a nurturing person. Eating is soon associated with the feeling of being loved. In addition, the pleasurable oral sensation of sucking provides a connection between emotions and early eating behaviour. Many parents use food as a positive reinforcer for desired behaviours. This practice may become a habit, and the child may continue to use food as a reward, a comfort, and a means of dealing with depression or hostility. Many individuals eat when they are not hungry or in response to boredom, loneliness, sadness, depression, or tiredness. Difficulty determining feelings of satiety can lead to weight problems and may compound the factor of eating in response to emotional rather than physical hunger cues.

Eating behaviours are closely related to memory. Memory and appetite are chemically encoded, with each individual having his or her own circuitry relating to eating behaviours. Like memory, the circuitry can be modified over time (Feldman, Friedman, & Sleisenger, 2002).

Diagnostic Evaluation

A careful history should be obtained regarding the development of obesity and a physical examination performed to differentiate simple obesity from increased fat due to organic causes. A family history of obesity, diabetes, coronary heart disease, and dyslipidemia should be obtained for all children who are overweight or at risk for being overweight. For some, psychological assessment, by interviews and standardized personality tests, may provide insight into the personality and emotional problems that contribute to obesity and that might interfere with therapy.

The history is an important guide to determine the workup. The physical examination should focus on identifying **comorbid** conditions and identifiable causes of obesity. Some areas to focus on include (1) skin for stretch markings and discolourations (e.g., acanthosis nigricans), (2) joints for swelling and evidence of pain, and (3) airway for evidence of obstruction and enlarged tonsils. Basic laboratory studies include a fasting lipid panel; fasting insulin level; fasting glucose hepatic enzymes, including γ-glutamyltransferase; and, in some institutions, hemoglobin A_{1c}. Other studies, such as a sleep study, metabolic studies, and radiographic evaluations, may be added on the basis of the history and physical examination.

It is useful to estimate the degree of obesity to determine the component of body weight that can be modified. All of the following methods have been used to assess obesity: BMI, body weight, weight–height ratios, weight–age ratios, hydrostatic (underwater) weight, skin fold measurements, bioelectrical analysis, computed tomography (CT), magnetic resonance imaging (MRI), and neutron activation. Each of these methods has advantages and disadvantages. Hydrostatic, or underwater, weighing provides the most accurate measurement of lean body weight.

BMI is currently considered the best method to assess weight in children and adolescents. The calculation is based on the individual's height and weight. In adults, BMI definitions are fixed measures without regard for sex and age. The BMI in children and adolescents varies to accommodate age- and gender-specific changes in growth. The formula for BMI calculation is as follows:

$$\text{Weight in kilograms} \div [\text{Height in metres}]^2$$

BMI measures in children and adolescents are plotted on growth charts that enable heath care providers to determine the patient's BMI-for-age (see the Evolve site).

Therapeutic Management

The best approach to the management of obesity is a preventive one. Early recognition and control measures are essential before the child or adolescent reaches an obese state. Health care providers must educate families about the medical complications of obesity, and families should be encouraged to be involved in the treatment plan.

The effectiveness and safety of many treatments of obesity in children and adolescents are unclear (McGovern et al., 2008). Diet modification is an essential part of weight-reduction programs. Dietary counselling is directed toward improving the nutritional quality of the diet rather than dietary restriction. Educating youth about the limits and risks of fad diets is important. *Eating Well With Canada's Food Guide* (Health Canada, 2011a) recommends that for youth ages 14 to 18, daily consumption should include 7 to 8 servings of vegetables and fruit, 6 to 7 servings of grain products, 3 to 4 servings of milk and milk alternatives, and 2 to 3 servings of meat and meat alternatives. Many programs recommend using a food diary as a helpful tool to increase awareness of food choices and eating behaviours. The goal is to encourage the individual to make healthier choices in foods selection and discourage eating food by habit or to appease boredom. The Dieticians of Canada (2010) have published "5 steps to a healthy body weight for teens":

1. Follow the science of *Eating Well With Canada's Food Guide.*
2. Take charge of your lunch.
3. Be a healthy snacker.
4. Eating out? Eat smart.
5. Practise active living.

For adolescents who are severely obese, strict diets may need to be implemented. These include the protein-sparing modified fast, a hypocaloric, ketogenic diet designed to provide enough protein to minimize loss of lean body mass during weight loss. Such diets need to be closely monitored and should be used only with a multidisciplinary team that includes a physician, nutritionist, and behavioural therapist. Generally, the diet consists of 1.5 to 2.5 g of protein per kilogram. The intake of carbohydrates is low enough to induce ketosis. The benefits of the diet are relatively rapid weight loss and anorexia induced by ketosis. Potential complications include protein losses, hypokalemia, hypoglycemia, inadequate calcium intake, and orthostatic hypotension. It is difficult to sustain such diets over a long period of time, and the long-term outcomes of using these diets have not been established.

Medications have been used to promote weight loss in children with certain conditions; examples include metformin in obese adolescents with insulin resistance and hyperinsulinism, octreotide for hypothalamic obesity caused by intracranial tumours, growth hormone in children with Prader-Willi syndrome, and leptin for congenital leptin deficiency. In one study the medication sibutramine, in addition to behavioural therapy, significantly reduced BMI and body weight more than placebo; however, sibutramine was associated with adverse effects (tachycardia and hypertension) (Berkowitz et al., 2006).

Bariatric surgery is increasingly viewed as a reasonable treatment for obese adolescents. In the past, surgery was reserved for those whose attempts to lose or maintain weight loss through conventional nonoperative approaches were unsuccessful and who had serious life-threatening conditions. In 2010, Toronto's Hospital for Sick Children began offering bariatric surgery to patients who a) are between the ages of 12 and 17 years; b) have a BMI greater than the ninety-fifth percentile for their age and gender; and c) have at least one coexisting chronic condition, or for any adolescent between the ages of 12 and 17 years with a BMI above the ninety-ninth percentile. Australian researchers (O'Brien et al., 2010) have found that gastric banding surgery in adolescents can be safe and effective if combined with lifestyle changes and interdisciplinary support.

Nursing Care Management

Nurses play a key role in the compliance and maintenance phases of many weight-reduction programs. Nurses assess, manage, and evaluate the progress of many overweight adolescents. They also play an important role in recognizing potential weight problems and assisting parents and adolescents in preventing obesity. Nursing care of the adolescent who is overweight is outlined in the Nursing Process box.

The presence of obesity may not be obvious from appearance alone. Regular assessment of height and weight and computation of the BMI facilitate early recognition. Children with a BMI greater than or equal to the ninety-fifth percentile for age and sex should receive in-depth medical assessment. Children with a BMI in the eighty-fifth to ninety-fifth percentile range should be evaluated for secondary complications, such as hypertension and hyperlipidemia, and family history (Greaser & Whyte, 2004). Evaluation should include a height and weight history of the adolescent and family members, eating habits, appetite and hunger patterns, and physical activities. A psychosocial history is also helpful in understanding the impact of obesity on the child's life.

Before initiating a treatment plan, it is important to be certain that the family is ready for change. Lack of readiness may result in failure, frustration, and reluctance to address the problem in the future. The nurse should explore with the adolescent the reasons behind the desire to lose weight, since motivation to lose weight is the key to success. Adolescents need to take personal responsibility for their dietary habits and physical activity. Teens who are forced by their parents to seek help are seldom motivated, can become rebellious, and are usually unwilling to control their dietary intake.

Nutritional Counselling

Preventing an increase in body fat during growth is a realistic approach. This is often accomplished by adjusting three aspects of eating:

1. Reducing the quantity eaten, by purchasing, preparing, and serving smaller portions
2. Altering the quality consumed by substituting low-calorie, low-fat foods for high-calorie foods (especially for snacks)
3. Altering situations by severing associations between eating and other stimuli, such as eating while watching television

The most successful diets are those that use ordinary foods in controlled portions rather than diets that require the avoidance of specific foods. Low-carbohydrate diets such as the Atkins diet have been promoted for weight loss in adults and adolescents (Sondike, Copperman, & Jacobson, 2003). However, low-carbohydrate diets can result in ketosis, insulin resistance, and glucose intolerance. More research is needed to evaluate the long-term safety and efficacy of these diets for children and adolescents.

The nurse can teach adolescents and parents how to incorporate favourite foods into their diet and to select satisfying substitutes. The dieting teen should eat what the rest of the family eats, but less of it. When parents buy and prepare smaller amounts, they eliminate tempting second helpings and leftovers. To maintain a healthy diet, it is necessary to encourage the consumption of high-nutrient foods, such as fruits, vegetables, whole grains, and low-fat dairy protein products. Calories and fat should be kept to a healthy level

NURSING PROCESS: THE CHILD OR ADOLESCENT WHO IS OVERWEIGHT

Assessment

The nurse assists in determining the child's or adolescent's body mass index, gathers appropriate anthropometric data, uses standardized growth charts to plot growth, and obtains a comprehensive health history. Further information that is appropriate to obtain in the assessment includes a 24-hour food intake history, family health history, and lifestyle practices that affect the child's or adolescent's well-being. The health interview and nutritional assessment often provide clues and guidelines for further investigation.

Nursing Diagnoses (Problem Identification)

Several nursing diagnoses may be identified after a thorough assessment:

- Situational low self-esteem
- Imbalanced nutrition: more than body requirements
- Risk for injury
- Risk-prone health behaviour
- Disturbed personal identity

Planning

Expected patient outcomes for the adolescent with an eating disorder include the following:

- Child or adolescent will develop a positive self-image
- Adolescent will willingly engage in behaviours to reverse effects of cardiovascular disease
- Healthy personal identity will be achieved
- Healthy eating patterns will be adopted
- Adolescent will assume control for changes in lifestyle designed to lose weight
- Child or adolescent will remain injury free

Implementation

Numerous intervention strategies are discussed on pp. 1138-1141.

Evaluation

The effectiveness of nursing interventions is determined by continual reassessment and evaluation of nursing care based on the following observational guidelines:

- Perform nutritional assessment; measure weight; review diet and nutritional intake (e.g., log); interview adolescent regarding food and eating behaviours; observe eating behaviours
- Interview adolescent regarding self-perceptions; observe behaviour; confer with psychologist and other members of the interdisciplinary team regarding evidence of progress
- Observe adolescent's behaviour; interview him or her regarding attitudes, concerns, and behaviours

without being significantly restricted. To be successful, a dietary program should be nutritionally sound with sufficient satiety value, produce the desired weight loss, and be accompanied by nutrition education and continued support. Children and adolescents should not initiate a reduction diet without health assessment and counselling (Schwimmer, 2004).

Behavioural Therapy

Altering eating behaviour, including reducing inappropriate eating habits, is essential to weight reduction, especially in maintaining long-term weight control. Most behavioural modification programs include the following concepts:

- A description of the behaviour to be controlled, such as eating habits
- Attempts to modify and control the stimuli that govern eating
- Development of eating techniques designed to control the speed of eating
- Positive reinforcement for these modifications through a suitable reward system

Specific strategies to modify eating habits are listed in Box 40-4.

BOX 40-4 Helpful Suggestions to Promote Healthy Eating Habits

Identify current eating patterns and behaviours by keeping a food diary and then look for areas to change. Record everything eaten, including where and when, and associated activities.

Change eating patterns.

- Choose sugar-free beverages or low-fat milk only.
- Limit fast-food consumption to no more than once a week.
- Do not skip meals.
- Eat three meals and one or two snacks per day.
- Try the plate method: one-half plate of vegetables, one-fourth plate of lean meat, and one-fourth plate of starch or starchy vegetables (potatoes, peas).
- Take second helpings of fruits and vegetables (not potatoes) only.
- Avoid low-fat food (these are usually high in sugars).
- Use whole-grain breads, cereals, and pastas.
- Pack your lunch for school.
- Buy healthy foods for snacking.

Change the act of eating.

- Eat meals at the family dinner table.
- Avoid distractions (e.g., television).
- Slow down; meals may last at least 20 to 30 minutes.

Substitute other activities for managing stress, such as hobbies, walking, listening to music, talking to friends on the phone, reading, playing a game.

Provide alternative rewards for reinforcement or accomplishments (e.g., CDs or MP3 downloads, movie, concert, new clothes, new games).

Think positively.

Enlist family involvement and support.

Group Involvement

Commercial groups (e.g., Weight Watchers) or diet workshops composed primarily of adults may be helpful to some teenagers; however, a group of other dieting adolescents is often more effective. Teenage groups include summer camps designed for obese young people and conducted by health care providers school groups organized and led by a school nurse, and groups associated with special clinics.

These groups are concerned not only with weight loss but also with the development of a positive self-image and encouragement of physical activity. Nutrition education, diet planning, and improvement of social skills are essential components of these groups. Improvement is determined by positive changes in all aspects of behaviour.

Family Involvement

There is a definite correlation between family environment, interaction, and obesity. The nurse needs to educate parents in the purposes of the therapeutic measures and their role in supporting such measures. The family needs nutrition education and counselling regarding the reinforcement plan, alterations in the food environment, and ways to maintain helpful attitudes. They can support their child in efforts to change eating behaviours, food intake, and physical activity.

Physical Activity

Regular physical activity is incorporated into all weight-reduction programs. Any form of increased physical activity is beneficial, provided that the activities are age appropriate and enjoyable. In recommendations for physical activity, the current health status and developmental level of the child or adolescent need to be considered. The best choice for exercise is any form that is enjoyable and likely to be sustainable. Aerobic and endurance exercises help oxidize body fats. Light exercise such as walking may provide an opportunity for the family to increase time together and increase caloric expenditure. Walking for 30 minutes each day and decreasing caloric intake by 500 calories per day may significantly reduce the risk of chronic disease. Weight training can increase basal metabolic rate and replace fat mass with muscle mass. However, weight training is not generally recommended for prepubertal children until they have reached physical and skeletal maturity. For prepubertal children, increasing outdoor playtime is likely to be beneficial. Many children find exercise videos and treadmills boring and may not continue with these activities. There are a great variety of physical activities to choose from that are likely to appeal to different people: team sports and individual sports such as dance, bike riding, swimming, tennis, and karate. Limiting sedentary activities such as television viewing (while eating snacks) is the most effective way to encourage physical activity.

Prevention

Weight loss programs do not enjoy the success of therapeutic interventions for other disorders. Gradual accumulation of adipose tissue during childhood establishes a pattern of eating that is difficult to reverse in adolescence. Prevention of obesity should begin in early childhood with the development of healthy eating habits, regular exercise patterns, and a positive relationship between parents and children. Prevention of adolescent obesity is best accomplished by early identification of obesity in the preschool, school-age, and preadolescent periods. Health care providers should encourage frequent health care visits for children who are overweight or obese and should incorporate a dietary history and counselling into each well-infant, well-child, and well-adolescent visit.

Anorexia Nervosa and Bulimia Nervosa

The 2002 Canadian Community Health Survey (CCHS) showed that 0.5% of Canadians over the age of 15 years had been diagnosed with an eating disorder. Anorexia nervosa and bulimia nervosa are most common among adolescent girls, although boys tend to have a substantial incidence of binge eating disorders (Government of Canada, 2006).

Anorexia nervosa (AN) is an eating disorder characterized by an inability to maintain a minimally normal body weight and by severe weight loss in the absence of obvious physical causes. The average age of onset is 13 years, but the disorder can occur as early as 10 years of age and as late as 25 years of age. Individuals with AN are often described as perfectionists, academically high achievers, conforming, and conscientious. Typically, they have high energy levels, even with marked emaciation. Patients with anorexia may eventually develop bulimia (Mehler, 2001).

Adolescents with **bulimia nervosa** (BN) (from the Greek meaning "ox hunger") undertake binge eating and then use compensatory behaviours to prevent weight gain, such as self-induced vomiting; misuse of laxatives, diuretics, or other medications; fasting; or excessive exercise (Government of Canada, 2006). BN is observed more commonly in older adolescent girls and young women; males with bulimia are less common. Patients with BN may be of average or slightly above average weight. The binge-eating behaviour consists of secretive, frenzied consumption of large amounts of high-calorie (or "forbidden") foods during a brief time (usually less than 2 hours). The binge is counteracted by a variety of weight-control methods (purging). These binge–purge cycles are followed by self-deprecating thoughts, a depressed mood, and an awareness that the eating pattern is abnormal.

Although persons with BN have many issues in common with those who have other eating disorders, impulse control and satiety regulation are important problems in BN. Many individuals with BN begin with only occasional binges and purges "just for fun," enjoying the control over their weight while eating amounts of food that would normally produce obesity. As the condition progresses, the frequency of binges increases, the amount of food consumed increases, and they gradually lose control over the binge–purge cycle. The frequency of binging can be anywhere from once per week to seven or eight times per day. Because persons with BN usually binge on high-calorie foods, especially sweets, ice cream, and pastries, insulin production is stimulated to cope with the added carbohydrates. When the food is vomited, the unused insulin stimulates hunger and the desire to eat.

A third eating disorder, identified as eating disorder not otherwise specified (EDNOS), has components of both AN and BN with varying degrees of symptomatology that are not always characteristic of the established diagnostic criteria for AN and BN (National Eating Disorder Information Centre, 2011). Binge eating disorder (BED) is a type of EDNOS. Persons with BED may diet in an attempt to control their weight but without the extreme weight-control compensatory practices of vomiting, laxative use, diuretics, and excessive exercise (Forman, 2012; National Eating Disorder Information Centre, 2011).

Etiology and Pathophysiology

The cause of these disorders remains unclear. There is a distinct psychological component, and the diagnosis is based primarily on psychological and behavioural criteria. Dieting appears to be common to the initiation of both AN and BN. The disorders appear to be caused by a combination of genetic, neurochemical, psychodevelopmental, and sociocultural factors. The dominant aspects of AN are a relentless pursuit of thinness and a fear of fatness, usually preceded by a period of mood disturbances and behaviour changes.

Weight loss may be triggered by a typical adolescent crisis, such as the onset of menstruation or a traumatic interpersonal incident, that precipitates serious, out-of-control dieting. Situations of severe family stress (such as parental separation or divorce) or circumstances in which the adolescent perceives a lack of personal control (such as teasing at school, changing schools, or going to college) may precipitate a desire for control and the decision not to eat. Frequently, there is an exaggerated misinterpretation of the normal fat deposition characteristic of early adolescence or anxiety because of comments that the adolescent is putting on weight.

Many experts have associated the development of an eating disorder with family characteristics such as an adolescent perception of high parental expectations for achievement and appearance, difficulty managing conflict and poor communication styles, enmeshment and occasionally estrangement between family members, devaluation of the mother or the maternal role, and marital tension. Families struggling with an eating disorder have been characterized as often having difficulties responding positively to the adolescent's changing physical and emotional needs. Family stress of any kind may become a significant factor in the development of an eating disorder (Forman, 2012).

Society's emphasis and the media's focus on tall, thin individuals may also play a role. Studies evaluating the possible association of eating disorders and sexual abuse have been conflicting. Childhood sexual abuse may be a factor in some cases of AN.

Patients with eating disorders commonly have psychiatric problems, including affective disorder, anxiety disorder, obsessive-compulsive disorder, and personality disorder. Adult women with eating disorders have been found to have higher than average rates of obsessive-compulsive behaviour traits in their childhood. Patients with eating disorders also tend to have higher than average reported rates of substance use, with alcohol problems being more common in those with BN than in those with AN (Forman, 2012). Many of the clinical findings are directly related to the state of starvation and improve with weight gain.

Many sports and artistic endeavours that emphasize leanness (e.g., ballet and running) and sports in which the scoring is partly subjective (e.g., skating and gymnastics) have been associated with a higher incidence of eating disorders such as AN. The term *female athlete triad*, characterized by disordered eating behaviour, amenorrhea, and osteoporosis, has been applied to young women with restrictive eating disorders and amenorrhea (Female Athlete Triad Coalition, 2011) (see Chapter 6, p. 85).

A genetic role has been postulated for eating disorders; a significant number of young females with a first-degree relative having an eating disorder had a significantly higher rate of eating disorders (Forman, 2012).

Diagnostic Evaluation

Diagnosis of AN is made on the basis of clinical manifestations (Box 40-5) and conformity to the criteria established by the American Psychiatric Association (2000) (Box 40-6).

BOX 40-5 Clinical Manifestations of Anorexia Nervosa

Severe and profound weight loss
Signs of altered metabolic activity:
- Secondary amenorrhea (if menarche attained)
- Primary amenorrhea (if menarche not attained)
- Bradycardia
- Lowered body temperature
- Decreased blood pressure
- Cold intolerance
- Dry skin and brittle nails
- Appearance of lanugo hair

BOX 40-6 Diagnostic Criteria for Anorexia Nervosa

1. Refusal to maintain body weight over a minimal normal weight for age and height (e.g., weight loss leading to maintenance of body weight less than 85% of that expected; or failure to make expected weight gain during period of growth, leading to body weight less than 85% of that expected)
2. Intense fear of gaining weight or becoming fat, even though underweight
3. Disturbance in body image, undue influence of shape or weight on evaluation, or denial of the seriousness of the current low body weight
4. In postmenarcheal females, amenorrhea (i.e., the absence of at least three consecutive menstrual cycles); a woman is considered to have amenorrhea if her periods occur only following hormone (i.e., estrogen) administration

Specify Type

Restricting type—There is no regular binging or purging behaviour (i.e., self-induced vomiting or the misuse of laxatives, diuretics, or enemas).

Binge eating/purging type—During the current episode of anorexia nervosa, the person has regularly engaged in binge eating or purging behaviour (i.e., self-induced vomiting or the misuse of laxatives, diuretics, or enemas).

(Reprinted with permission from the *Diagnostic and Statistical Manual of Mental Disorders,* Fourth Edition, Text Revision [Copyright © 2000]. American Psychiatric Association.)

Diagnosis of BN is confirmed, according to the American Psychiatric Association's *Diagnostic and Statistical Manual of Mental Disorders* (2000) (Box 40-7), by at least two binge-eating episodes per week for the preceding 3 months.

A complete history and physical examination are important for ruling out other causes of weight loss. The medical assessment of an eating disorder should focus on the complications of altered nutritional status and purging. A careful history assesses weight changes, dietary patterns, and the frequency and severity of purging and excessive exercise. The patient's weight and height should be measured and evaluated for appropriateness according to standard weight for height, age, and sex charts, determined according to the percentile of his or her expected body weight or BMI. Box 4-6 provides a screening tool for nurses to use in assessing for eating disorders.

Additional diagnostic measures may include a complete blood count to evaluate for anemia and other hematological abnormalities; erythrocyte sedimentation rate or C-reactive protein to detect evidence of inflammation; electrolytes, calcium, magnesium, phosphorus, blood urea nitrogen, and creatinine; urinalysis, including specific gravity; and bone density studies for osteopenia, which is commonly observed in patients with AN. In patients with prolonged amenorrhea,

BOX 40-7 Diagnostic Criteria for Bulimia

1. Recurrent episodes of binge eating. An episode of binge eating is characterized by both of the following:
   a. Eating, in a discrete period of time (e.g., within any 2-hour period), an amount of food that is definitely larger than most people would eat during a similar period of time and under similar circumstances
   b. A sense of lack of control over eating during the episode (e.g., a feeling that one cannot stop eating or control what or how much one is eating)
2. Recurrent inappropriate compensatory behaviour in order to prevent weight gain, such as self-induced vomiting; misuse of laxatives, diuretics, enemas, or other medications; fasting; or excessive exercise
3. The binge eating and inappropriate compensatory behaviours both occur, on average, at least twice a week for 3 months.
4. Self-evaluation is unduly influenced by body shape and weight.
5. The disturbance does not occur exclusively during episodes of anorexia nervosa.

Specify Type

Purging type—During the current episode of bulimia nervosa, the person has regularly engaged in self-induced vomiting or the misuse of laxatives, diuretics, or enemas.

Nonpurging type—During the current episode of bulimia nervosa, the person has used other inappropriate compensatory behaviours, such as fasting or excessive exercise, but has not regularly engaged in self-induced vomiting or the misuse of laxatives, diuretics, or enemas.

(Reprinted with permission from the *Diagnostic and Statistical Manual of Mental Disorders,* Fourth Edition, Text Revision [Copyright © 2000]. American Psychiatric Association.)

human chorionic gonadotropin is assessed to check for pregnancy. Other tests for patients with amenorrhea include thyroid function tests and measurement of serum prolactin and follicle-stimulating hormone to help rule out prolactinoma (hormone-secreting pituitary tumour), hyperthyroidism, hypothyroidism, or ovarian failure. In addition, a comprehensive cardiac evaluation is often recommended in those with AN. Further diagnostic tests may be required on the basis of the history and findings from the diagnostic tests discussed above.

Therapeutic Management

The treatment of AN involves four major goals:

1. Restoration of a healthy weight
2. Establishment of healthy eating patterns
3. Resolution of disturbed patterns of family interaction
4. Individual psychotherapy to correct deficits and distortions in psychological functioning

Most adolescents are treated on an outpatient basis, but those with problems requiring immediate medical attention, such as severe malnutrition or electrolyte or psychiatric disturbances (severe depression or suicidal ideation), require hospitalization. A multidisciplinary team of dietitians, physicians, nurses, and counsellors should provide the interventions.

Persons with BN may benefit from cognitive-behavioural therapy, other psychotherapy, antidepressant medications, or a combination of antidepressant medication and psychotherapy (Forman, 2012). Nutrition education and meal planning may help the patient with BN maintain an adequate weight and accept foods that are often considered bad or forbidden (Spear, 2005).

Nutrition Therapy

The most important goal is to treat any life-threatening malnutrition and to restore dietary stability and weight gain. This may require the administration of tube feedings or intravenous fluids if the malnutrition is severe. In most cases, it is best to reintroduce food and snacks slowly in a stepwise manner. A reasonable goal is to reach an eventual intake of 2000 to 3000 kcal/day and a weight gain of 0.22 to 0.45 kg per week (American Dietetic Association, 2006). When restoring nutrition, health care providers must avoid the refeeding syndrome, which consists of cardiovascular, neurological, and hematological complications that occur when nutritional replacement is given too rapidly. This syndrome can be avoided with slow refeeding and the addition of phosphorus when total body phosphorus is depleted. Treatment goal weights should be individualized and based on age, height, stage of puberty, premorbid weight, and previous growth charts. In girls who have reached menarche, resumption of menses is an objective measure of return to biological health.

Dietary interventions need to be combined with psychotherapy to improve the underlying psychological misconceptions about weight loss. Another aspect of treatment is to relieve the anxiety related to eating and the depression that accompanies the disorder. The administration of antianxiety or antidepressant medications can be beneficial. However, when these drugs are used, patients should be carefully monitored for cardiovascular adverse effects.

Psychotherapy

Behavioural interventions are often necessary to encourage patients to accomplish the desired caloric intake and weight gain. Weight restoration on an outpatient basis is accomplished with behavioural contracts negotiated between the therapists and the patient. The goal is to increase the patient's feelings of personal control and his or her responsibility for achieving recovery. The contract can stipulate at what weight tube feedings will be implemented, if needed. Individual psychotherapy is aimed at helping the young person resolve the adolescent identity crisis, particularly as it relates to a distorted body image. If the disorder is related to a dysfunctional family situation, therapy is most successful when it is started soon after the onset of illness and directed toward disengagement from and redirection of malfunctioning processes in the family.

Pharmacological Therapy

Pharmacotherapy in the treatment of AN has been disappointing so far. The few studies that have been done have primarily evaluated medications' efficacy in the treatment of comorbid disorders, such as obsessive-compulsive disorders and depression. Anxiolytic medications may be helpful before meals to relieve some patients' anxiety.

Tricyclic antidepressants and fluoxetine belong to a group of medications known as selective serotonin reuptake inhibitors (SSRIs), which have been more successful in association with BN. There is also some evidence that tricyclic antidepressants such as desipramine, imipramine, and amitriptyline; monoamine oxidase inhibitors; and buspirone are more effective than a placebo in decreasing binging and vomiting in patients with BN. Topiramate, an antiepileptic agent, and the selective serotonin antagonist ondansetron may have some benefit in treating BN.

Nursing Care Management

Nurses must maintain a kind and supportive, yet firm, manner in managing the care of the adolescent with an eating disorder, without creating a passive-dependent attitude. The individual requires sustained support and reassurance to cope with ambivalent feelings related to body concept and the desire to be seen as cooperative, reliable, and worthy of receiving kindness. Encouraging the adolescent with education and activities that strengthen self-esteem can facilitate the resocialization process and promote social acceptance among peers.

It is important for nurses to be aware of the physical side effects of AN. Patients frequently limit their fluid intake. Urinary tract problems are common, and ketones and protein may be detected in the urine as a result of breakdown of fat and protein. Vital-sign instability can be severe and can include orthostatic hypotension; the pulse becomes irregular, and the rate decreases markedly. Bradycardia and hypothermia can result in cardiac arrest (see Critical Thinking Exercise).

The health care team responsible for the management of young people with AN should arrange a carefully structured environment. First, there must be consistency. The team needs to decide on an approach and adhere to it. The plan must be structured with reality testing regarding caloric intake and body-image perception. Team members need to provide a

CRITICAL THINKING EXERCISE

Anorexia Nervosa

Jane is a 13-year-old whose grades have been excellent and whom the teachers describe as a "model student." Recently, Jane's teacher told the nurse practitioner that Jane's parents were in the middle of a "messy divorce." In addition, several of Jane's friends told the nurse practitioner that they are concerned about Jane because she runs every day at lunchtime and seldom eats lunch with them. Jane told her friends that she gained weight over the winter months and that she is running because she wants to qualify for the track team this spring. At the time of her routine health interview and sports physical, the nurse practitioner notes that Jane's oral temperature is 36°C and that she weighs 35 kg. Jane has lost 9 kg since her last sports physical. When discussing her menstrual periods with the nurse practitioner, Jane states that she has not had her period for 3 months.

1. Evidence—Is there sufficient evidence to draw any conclusions about Jane's behaviour?
2. Assumptions—Describe some underlying assumptions about the following:
   a. Personality characteristics of individuals with anorexia nervosa (AN)
   b. Factors influencing the development of AN
   c. Clinical manifestations of AN
   d. Treatment of AN
3. What implications for nursing care should be established for Jane at this time?
4. Does the evidence support your conclusion?
5. Are there alternative perspectives that you should consider?

unified front, to avoid any possibility of manipulation or inconsistency.

Second, all team members need to be involved in the treatment; responsibility for the program cannot be left to one person. The role and boundaries of each member must be clearly spelled out. Also, continuity of team members is important; it is helpful to have the same team members all the time.

Another element to successful management of adolescents with AN is open communication among team members. Communication with the patient regarding what is expected is also important. Sometimes the limit-setting may seem unreasonable; if the adolescent does not understand the rationale for the limits, he or she may sabotage the entire program. It is also important to communicate with the family.

Finally, the plan must provide support of the adolescent, the family, and team members. The adolescent's efforts should be supported, and positive feedback should be provided for accomplishments made in normalizing eating habits. Meetings should be held to discuss the feelings and concerns of the patient, immediate caregivers, and team members.

A *behavioural contract*, an agreement that the adolescent makes with others to change a maladaptive behaviour, has proved to be effective in some cases. The written contract is constructed by the therapeutic team and is approved and signed by the adolescent. Unless the adolescent agrees to its terms, the contract can become the source of a power struggle. However, it can be an effective tool that places the responsibility for weight gain or other behavioural change on the adolescent.

Nursing care of the adolescent with BN is similar to care of the patient with AN. Acute care involves careful monitoring of fluid and electrolyte alterations and observation for signs of cardiac complications. Nutritional consultation and follow-up care are essential. The nurse should encourage the adolescent and family members to structure the environment in such a way as to reduce the binging behaviour. Getting rid of binge foods; restricting eating to one room of the house; not engaging in other activities while eating; and substituting exercise, crafts, visualization, and relaxation techniques for binging are helpful interventions.

Health care providers, patients, and families can find assistance and information on the prevention, identification, and treatment of eating disorders from the National Eating Disorder Information Centre in Canada.

Serious Health Problems With a Behavioural Component

Tobacco

Cigarette smoking has continued to decline since the late 1990s, in part because of increased costs, changes in community attitudes about smoking among adults, decreased advertising of cigarettes to children, and increased antismoking advertising as a result of the government lawsuits against tobacco companies (Johnston et al., 2005). In a province-wide survey in 2008, 74% of British Columbian youth reported that they had never smoked a single cigarette (Smith et al., 2009).

Although the number of adult and adolescent smokers has declined in recent years, cigarette smoking is still considered the chief avoidable cause of death. The hazards of smoking at any age are undisputed; a preventive approach to teenage smoking is especially important. Because of its addictive nature, smoking begun in childhood and adolescence can result in a lifetime habit, with increased morbidity and early mortality. Smoking in adolescence has also been related to other risk behaviours: approximately three times as many adolescents who smoke report carrying weapons and drinking alcohol compared with adolescents who do not smoke; other associated risks among Whites include using smokeless tobacco, using marijuana, having multiple sexual partners, not using bicycle helmets, and binge drinking. Research also indicates an association between current use of tobacco and the development of depression (Chaiton, Cohen, O'Loughlin, & Rehm, 2010) and sleep problems (Region of Waterloo, Public Health, 2012) in adolescence. Cigarettes are considered to be a gateway drug; teenagers who smoke are 11.4 times more likely to use illicit drugs (Gordon, 2000).

Youth in the First Nations, Métis, and Inuit populations smoke at a rate of 24.9% compared with 19.7% of non-Aboriginal youth. In one study, Aboriginal adolescents were

evolve Case Study—Teen Smoking

also more likely to have experimented with marijuana and other illicit drugs and to be involved in binge drinking. They were less likely than non-Aboriginal youth to have tried to stop smoking. It is likely that smoking among Aboriginal youth is significantly underreported in the off-reserve population (Elton-Marshall, Leatherdale & Burkhalter, 2011).

The effects of second-hand smoke exposure are also well known and include an increased incidence of low birth weight and subsequent illness in infants, increased incidence of sudden infant death syndrome (if the mother smoked during pregnancy), increased incidence of acute lower respiratory tract infections, and exacerbation of asthma symptoms (wheezing, cough, phlegm, breathlessness) in asthmatic children (Health Canada, 2011c).

Etiology

Teenagers begin smoking for a variety of reasons, including imitation of adult behaviour; peer pressure; a desire to imitate behaviours and lifestyles portrayed in movies and advertisements; and a desire to control weight, especially among females. Teenagers who do not smoke usually have family members and friends who do not smoke or who oppose smoking. Most teens who refrain from smoking have a desire to succeed in academics or athletics (particularly high-performance sports, such as basketball, swimming, and track) and plan to go to college (see Community Focus box). Although smoking among college students has increased in recent years, rates of smoking are highest among adolescents who do not complete high school.

Smokeless Tobacco

The term *smokeless tobacco* refers to tobacco products that are placed in the mouth but not ignited (e.g., chewing tobacco). This substitute for cigarettes continues to pose a hazard to adolescents, although use has declined by about 50% since the peak prevalence in 1995; in 2004 only 16.7% of teens had tried smokeless tobacco by the twelfth grade (Johnston et al., 2005). Many children and adolescents believe that smokeless tobacco is a safe alternative to cigarette smoking and is not addictive, and they believe they can stop using it at any time. However, the number of adolescents who identify it as a health risk has increased since the mid-1990s, with nearly half now agreeing it has health risks (Johnston et al., 2005). These products have also been proved to be carcinogenic, and regular use can cause dental problems, foul-smelling breath, and tooth erosion or loss.

Nursing Care Management

Prevention of regular smoking among teenagers is the most effective way to reduce the overall incidence of smoking. A variety of methods have been employed. Posters, charts, displays, statistics, and the use of examples of actual damaged lungs to communicate the hazards of smoking all have their supporters and doubters. Some schools also use films and demonstrations in science classes.

For the most part, smoking-prevention programs that focus on the negative, long-term effects of smoking on health have been ineffective. Youth-to-youth programs and those emphasizing the immediate consequences are more effective but primarily in improving teenagers' attitudes toward not smoking. Because smoking and smoking-related behaviours are social symbols, antismoking campaigns must address the norms of potential smokers. Anything that ridicules or threatens the social norms of the peer group can be unproductive or counterproductive. Investigators have found that teaching resistance to peer pressure to smoke is effective in early adolescence. Although the effects of these programs may decrease with time, the effects can be enhanced in older adolescents by presenting information in class instead of simply handing out written material to the students (Adelman et al., 2001).

Two areas of focus for antismoking programs are peer-led programs and the use of media in smoking prevention (e.g., television and Internet antismoking ads, and films). Peer-led programs emphasizing the social consequences of smoking have proved most successful. If a significant number of influential peers can "sell" their classmates on the idea that the habit is not popular, the followers will imitate their behaviour. Such programs emphasize short-term rather than long-term consequences (e.g., the effects of smoking on personal

COMMUNITY FOCUS

Early Sexual Maturation, Alcohol, and Cigarettes

Cigarette smoking and alcohol use by adolescents are complex behaviours not explained by any one factor. Some theorists and investigators believe there is a relationship between biological maturation and risk-taking behaviours. For example, girls who are sexually mature at an earlier age than their peers are often attracted to older girls and boys who may engage in risk-taking behaviours. If older teens smoke, drink, and drive while under the influence of alcohol with no adverse consequences (e.g., no motor vehicle accidents), younger teens may believe that they, too, will be safe while smoking, drinking, or riding in an automobile with friends who are drinking.

Although parents and nurses cannot influence the time of biological maturation, they can identify young girls who are at risk for the initiation of risk-taking behaviours because of early puberty. Parents need to understand that an early-maturing daughter might be uncomfortable with her body, and they should take advantage of opportunities to build her self-esteem. Parental sensitivity to the importance of peer-group acceptance and parental support of a teenage daughter who feels left out or different are crucial. School nurses can provide anticipatory guidance to these girls and help them role-play coping strategies for situations that involve offers to smoke and drink. In addition, school nurses can provide information about physical development during puberty and emphasize that not all teenagers mature at the same time or rate.

Teachers, coaches, and community and church leaders can provide opportunities for these girls to "fit in" with their same-age peers through activities that stress mutual goals. For example, an early-maturing girl is typically taller than her age-mates and can be an asset in sports such as basketball and track-and-field events.

appearance, such as unattractive stains on teeth and hands and the unpleasant odour of breath and clothing).

The impact of school-based antismoking programs can be strengthened by expanding these programs to include parents, mass media, youth groups, and community organizations. For example, mass media efforts that involve antismoking radio campaigns have been identified as the most cost-effective mass media intervention. The more effective interventions included young spokespeople, a single message containing information that was previously shown to be effective, and clear language (Pechmann & Reibling, 2000).

Smoking bans in schools accomplish several goals: (1) they discourage students from starting to smoke, (2) they reinforce knowledge of the health hazards of cigarette smoking and exposure to environmental tobacco smoke, and (3) they promote a smoke-free environment as the norm (see Community Focus box).

Substance Use

Although experimentation with drugs during childhood and adolescence is widespread, most children and teens do not become high-risk users. Recent research by the McCreery Centre Society in British Columbia indicates that alcohol and marijuana use has declined throughout the past decade, as has the use of certain drugs, such as cocaine, amphetamines, and mushrooms. The use of other drugs, however, including certain hallucinogens, is on the rise (Smith et al., 2009).

Drug use, misuse, and addiction are culturally defined and are voluntary behaviours. Drug tolerance and physical dependence are involuntary physiological responses to the pharmacological characteristics of the drugs, such as opioids and alcohol. Consequently, an individual can be addicted to a narcotic with or without being physically dependent. A person can also be physically dependent on a narcotic without being addicted (e.g., patients who use opioids to control pain).

First Nations, Métis, and Inuit youth tend to be at particular risk for substance use. Compared with non-Aboriginal youth they have a two to six times greater risk for all alcohol-related problems. They are also more likely to use illicit drugs and use tobacco, alcohol, and cannabis at a younger age than that of non-Aboriginal youth.

Motivation

Most drug use begins with experimentation. The drug may be used only once, may be used occasionally, or may become part of a drug-centred lifestyle. Children and adolescents initiate drug use out of curiosity. Adolescents who use drugs may fall into one of two broad categories—experimenters and compulsive users—or they may fall into a third category somewhere on the continuum between these extremes, as recreational users, principally of drugs such as marijuana, cocaine, alcohol, and prescription medications. For many the goal is peer acceptance; these users fit more closely with the experimenting, intermittent users. For others the goal is intoxication or the sustained intense effects from using a particular drug; these users resemble the compulsive users. They may engage in periodic heavy use, or binges. The groups of greatest concern to health care providers are those whose patterns of use involve high doses or mixed drugs with the danger of overdose, and

COMMUNITY FOCUS

Nonsmoking Strategies

Nurses who work in schools, hospitals, and community agencies can take advantage of all opportunities to provide education about the dangers of smoking, discourage smoking initiation by children and adolescents, encourage smoking cessation, and promote smoke-free environments. In particular, community or school nurses must be alert to the vulnerability of young preteens when they enter junior high or middle school. These nurses are in an ideal position to assess stress, personal conflict, weight concerns, peer pressures, and other factors that place preteens at risk for smoking initiation. Nurses should serve as counsellors to student, teacher, and parent groups and as advocates for antismoking legislative efforts. The following additional strategies are recommended*:

- Provide only brief information about long-term health consequences (e.g., cardiovascular and cancer risks).
- Discuss immediate physiological consequences (e.g., changes in heart rate, blood pressure, respiratory symptoms, and blood carbon monoxide concentrations).
- Mention alternatives to smoking that also establish a self-image that appears independent, mature, or sophisticated (e.g., weight lifting; jogging; dancing; joining a boys' or girls' club; engaging in volunteer work for a hospital, political, religious, or community group).
- Mention the negative effects in detail (e.g., earlier wrinkling of skin; yellow stains on teeth and fingers; tobacco odour on breath, hair, and clothing).
- Mention the increasing ostracism of smokers by nonsmokers, both legal and informal, in the workplace and in public places.
- Mention the increasing evidence that secondhand smoke is injurious to the health of nonsmokers who are regularly exposed, especially small children.
- Acknowledge that many adults, who were enticed to start smoking as teenagers because of its social benefits, now wish they could stop smoking.
- Give adolescents effective arguments to deal with peer pressure (e.g., by not smoking, a teenager demonstrates independence and nonconformity, traits normally prized by youth).
- Request posters or pamphlets from local agencies (e.g., Canadian Cancer Society, Canadian Heart and Stroke Foundation, and Canadian Lung Association) to display in prominent places at school.

*Health Canada has information on the effects of tobacco, smoking cessation, and tobacco control programs at http://www.hc-sc.gc.ca/hc-ps/tobac-tabac/index-eng.php.

those compulsive users vulnerable to dependence, withdrawal syndromes, and altered lifestyle.

Types of Drugs Used

Any drug can be used for nonmedical purposes, and most are potentially harmful to adolescents still going through formative life experiences. Although rarely considered drugs by society, the chemically active substances frequently used are the xanthines and theobromines contained in chocolate, tea, coffee, and colas. Ethyl alcohol and nicotine are other drugs that are legal and socially sanctioned. Any of these substances can produce mild to moderate euphoric or stimulant effects and can lead to physical and psychological dependence.

Drugs with mind-altering abilities that are available on the "street" and are of medical and legal concern are the hallucinogenic, narcotic, hypnotic, and stimulant drugs. In addition, there has been a notable increase in the use of alcohol and volatile substances that are inhaled to achieve an altered sensation (such as gasoline, antifreeze, plastic model airplane cement, typewriter correction fluid, and organic solvents). Nonmedical use of prescription and synthetic medications such as oxycodone, alprazolam (Xanax), and amphetamine-dextroamphetamine (Adderall) has become a concern for professionals who work with children and adolescents. Many of the prescription medications are available at a cheaper cost than that of the more exotic drugs of use and are often found in the medicine cabinet at home. Some Internet Web sites also promote the "safe use" of some psychoactive drugs and supply information on new "designer" drugs that are not detectable on a standard urine drug screening test.

Alcohol

Acute or chronic use of alcohol (ethanol) is responsible for many acts of violence, suicide, accidental injury, and death. Alcohol drinking is likely to begin in the middle-school years and increases with age. By 18 years of age, 80 to 90% of adolescents have tried alcohol. Ethanol is a depressant that reduces inhibitions against aggressive and sexual acting out. Severe physical and psychological symptoms accompany abrupt withdrawal, and long-term use leads to slow tissue destruction, especially of the brain and liver cells. The most noticeable effects of alcohol occur within the central nervous system and include changes in cognitive and autonomic functions such as judgement, memory, learning ability, and other intellectual capacities.

Young alcoholics often drink alone and cannot control their use of alcohol. They often rely on the substance as a defence against depression, anxiety, fear, or anger. Not all of these characteristics are observed in the adolescent who is using alcohol, but if several signs are evident, the child or adolescent should be considered at risk. Referral to a health care provider and detoxification therapy may be necessary. Various groups provide support and counselling for families, including Al-Anon, Ala-Teen, and Alcoholics Anonymous (an organization that has listings in all local telephone directories and via the Internet).

Cocaine

Cocaine is available in two forms: water-soluble cocaine hydrochloride, which is administered by "snorting" or intravenous injection, and nonsoluble alkaloid (freebase) cocaine, which is used primarily for smoking. Crack, or "rock," is a purer, more dangerous form of the drug. It can be produced cheaply and smoked in either water pipes or mentholated cigarettes. The use of cocaine has increased in recent years because of its availability and affordability, its association with persons in glamorous occupations, peer pressure, and its reputation as a sexually enhancing drug.

Cocaine creates a sense of euphoria, or an indefinable high. Withdrawal does not produce the dramatic symptoms observed in withdrawal from other substances. The effects are those commonly seen in depression, including lack of energy and motivation, irritability, appetite changes, psychomotor retardation, and irregular sleep patterns. More serious symptoms include cardiovascular manifestations and seizures. Physical withdrawal should not be confused with the so-called crash after a cocaine high, which consists of a long period of sleep.

Narcotics

Narcotic drugs include **opiates** such as heroin and morphine, and opioids (opiate-like drugs), such as hydromorphone (Dilaudid), hydrocodone, fentanyl, meperidine (Demerol), and codeine. These drugs produce a state of euphoria by removing painful feelings and creating a pleasurable experience and a sense of success accompanied by clouding of the consciousness and a dreamlike state. Physical signs of narcotic use include constricted pupils, respiratory depression, and, often, cyanosis. Needle marks may be visible on the arms or legs of chronic users. Physical withdrawal from opiates is extremely unpleasant unless controlled with supervised tapering doses of the opioid or substitution of methadone.

As important as the physical effects are the indirect consequences related to the illegal status of narcotic use and the problems associated with securing the drug (e.g., the time-consuming searches to obtain the drug and the often illegal methods used to meet the high cost of purchasing it). Health problems also result from self-neglect of physical needs (nutrition, cleanliness, dental care); overdose; contamination; and infection, including HIV and hepatitis B and C infection (see Additional Resources section at the end of this chapter).

Central Nervous System Depressants

Central nervous system depressants include a variety of hypnotic drugs that produce physical dependence and withdrawal symptoms on abrupt discontinuation. They create a feeling of relaxation and sleepiness but impair general functioning. Drugs in this category include barbiturates, nonbarbiturates, and alcohol. Barbiturates combined with alcohol produce a profound depressant effect. Flunitrazepam (Rohypnol), known as the "date rape drug," is a hypnotic drug used by some adolescents. Many women report being raped after unknowingly being given flunitrazepam in a drink. Flunitrazepam is 10 times more powerful than diazepam (Valium). It produces prolonged sedation, a feeling of well-being, and short-term memory loss.

Central Nervous System Stimulants

Amphetamines and cocaine do not produce strong physical dependence and can be withdrawn without much danger. However, psychological dependence is strong, and acute intoxication can lead to violent aggressive behaviour or psychotic episodes characterized by paranoia, uncontrollable agitation, and restlessness. When combined with barbiturates, the euphoric effects are particularly addictive.

Methamphetamine can be snorted, injected, swallowed, or smoked and produces a burst of energy in its users, along with intense, alternating attacks of boldness and paranoia. It provokes excitement far more intense than that caused by cocaine. The drug, with the street names speed, crank, meth, ice, and crystal, is inexpensive and has a longer period of action than that of cocaine. Instead of a short (few minutes) high, as achieved with cocaine, a user can remain "up" for hours on a similar dose of crank.

The use of various volatile substances, or inhalants such as gasoline, model airplane cement, and organic solvents, is also of concern. Adolescents breathe or place these substances into paper or plastic bags or soft drink cans from which they rebreathe the fumes to produce a feeling of euphoria and altered consciousness. These substances contain chemical solvents and are extremely hazardous. Dusters contain Freon, a substance that can cause fatal cardiac arrhythmias. Common inhalant substances are inexpensive and easily obtained, such as gasoline, paint, propane/butane, air fresheners, and formalin (CPS, First Nations, Inuit and Métis Health Committee, 2010). Unfortunately, the use of inhalants is increasing, after nearly a decade of decline (CPS, First Nations, Inuit and Métis Health Committee, 2010). Inhalants are becoming a gateway drug for young children and preteens, who often progress to other harder drugs such as marijuana, heroin, and cocaine. One in five First Nations and Inuit youth reported having used inhalant solvents (1 out of 3 users were under 15 years of age) and over half had started to use solvents before age 11. No research has been done on the Métis population (Chansonneuve, 2007). In response to this danger to Aboriginal youth, the National Youth Solvent Program was established by Health Canada and First Nations communities to promote a stronger cultural identity and cultural healing.

Many young children are unaware of the dangers of "sniffing" or "huffing." In addition to rapid loss of consciousness and respiratory arrest, these substances may cause visual-scanning problems, language deficiencies, motor instability, memory deficits, and attention and concentration problems.

Mind-Altering Drugs

Hallucinogens (psychedelics, psychotomimetics, psychotropics, or illusionogenics) are drugs that produce vivid hallucinations and euphoria. These drugs do not produce physical dependence, and they can be abruptly withdrawn without ill effect. However, the acute and long-term effects are variable, and in some individuals the dissociative behaviour may be prolonged. Cannabis (marijuana, hashish) and lysergic acid diethylamide (LSD) are also included in this category of drugs. According to a recent report from British Columbia, by age 18 years, 15% had tried ecstasy (Stewart et al., 2009).

Nursing Care Management

Nurses who have contact with children and adolescents are in an excellent position to provide information about substance use and to serve as patient advocates (see Additional Resources section at the end of this chapter). The nurse most often encounters young drug users when they are (1) experiencing overdose or withdrawal symptoms, (2) manifesting bizarre behaviour or confusion secondary to drug ingestion, (3) worried that they are or will become addicted, or (4) worried about a friend or family member who is addicted.

Nurses who care for hospitalized adolescents need to know if these youths use drugs compulsively. Drug withdrawal can seriously complicate other illnesses. Nurses should be on the alert for any physical or behavioural clues that indicate the onset of withdrawal or the effects of drugs. Nurses who work in schools or in the community can play an essential role in identifying children, adolescents, and families with substance use problems. These nurses may be the first to identify a child or adolescent who has ingested a particular drug by the child's erratic behaviour in class or on the school grounds. Early identification of those at risk for substance-use problems is an essential aspect of prevention. Pediatric health care providers can also prevent substance use by creating trusting relationships with children and adolescents so that they feel comfortable asking questions about drugs. Health care providers can alert them to Web sites and other aspects of society that may actually encourage experimentation with drugs.

Acute Care

Adolescents experiencing toxic drug effects or withdrawal symptoms are usually seen initially in the emergency department. Experienced emergency department personnel are familiar with the management of acute drug toxicity and the signs, symptoms, and behavioural characteristics associated with a variety of substances. When the drug is questionable or unknown, such expertise can help facilitate management and treatment. Often, observation or a description of the child or adolescent's behaviour is more valuable than reports by patients or their friends.

The treatment for drug toxicity or withdrawal varies according to the drug and the method used. Every effort should be made to determine the type and amount of drug taken, the time of ingestion, the mode of administration, and factors related to the onset of presenting symptoms. It is helpful to know the individual's pattern of use. For example, if two types of drugs are involved, they may require different treatments. Gastric lavage may be employed when the drug has been ingested recently and the cough reflex is intact, but it is of little value when the drug has been administered by the intravenous ("mainlined") or intranasal ("sniffed") route. Because the actual content of most street drugs is highly questionable, other pharmaceutical agents should be administered with caution, except perhaps the narcotic antagonists in cases of suspected opiate overdoses. It is also necessary to assess for possible trauma sustained while the patient was under the influence of the drug.

Long-Term Management

A major factor in the treatment and rehabilitation of young drug users is careful assessment during the nonacute stage to determine the function the drug plays in the adolescent's life. The motivation phase is directed toward exploring the factors that influence drug use. It also involves establishing a feeling of self-worth in the teenager as well as a commitment to self-help.

Rehabilitation begins when adolescents decide that they can and are willing to change. Rehabilitation involves fostering healthy interdependent relationships with caring and supportive adults and exploring alternate mechanisms for problem solving while simultaneously reducing or eliminating drug use. Persons working with troubled youth must be prepared for recidivism, or the tendency to relapse, and maintain a plan for re-entry into the treatment process.

Family Support

Most treatment programs for substance users are based on adult 12-step models such as Alcoholics Anonymous. Research is needed to determine whether these adult models are effective for adolescents. Tough Love is a program based on the premise that parents have the right and responsibility to be the policymakers in the family, to set limits on their children's behaviour, and to take control of the household from out-of-control adolescents. By allowing teenagers to experience the negative consequences of their behaviour, they may become more willing to accept help or to change their behaviour. Another group that provides support and counselling for families affected by a child's substance use is Parents Anonymous. The Government of Canada has a National Anti-Drug Strategy that also provides help for parents seeking to prevent youth substance use. Another source of information is the U.S. National Institute on Drug Abuse. For further information on all of these resources see Additional Resources section at the end of this chapter.

Prevention

Nurses can play an important role in education as well as in individual observation, assessment, and therapy related to substance use. In recent years, a variety of educational programs have been applied with promising results. The most effective prevention strategies are part of a broader, more general effort to promote overall health and success. Health-compromising behaviours are often interconnected and have common antecedents. Prevention efforts that focus on changing only one behaviour (e.g., alcohol, other drug use) are less likely to be successful. Successful programs are those that have promoted parenting skills, social skills among distractible children, academic achievement, and skills to resist peer pressure.

Peer pressure is a powerful tool and can be used effectively in substance use prevention. A group that has had some success in reducing injury from drunk driving is Mothers Against Drunk Driving (MADD). Techniques used by this group include peer counselling, parental guidelines for teenage parties, and community awareness. Nurses should encourage the formation of Students Against Destructive Decision (SADD) chapters in high schools in their communities (see Additional Resources section).

Suicide

Suicide is defined as the deliberate act of self-injury with the intent that the injury results in death. Most experts distinguish between suicidal ideation, suicide attempt (or parasuicide), and suicide. *Suicidal ideation* involves a preoccupation with thoughts about committing suicide and may be a precursor to suicide. Although it is not uncommon for adolescents to experience occasional suicidal thoughts, expressions of preoccupation with suicide should be taken seriously, and an assessment should be conducted for appropriate referral. A *suicide attempt* is intended to cause injury or death. The term *parasuicide* refers to behaviours ranging from gestures to serious attempts to kill oneself. Parasuicide is a preferred term because it makes no reference to intent and because a person's motive may be too difficult or complex to determine. All parasuicidal activity should be taken seriously.

NURSING ALERT A history of a previous suicide attempt is a serious indicator for possible suicide completion in the future. Studies of adolescent suicides have found that as many as half of the adolescents had made previous attempts.

Results from the 2008 British Columbia Adolescent Health Survey indicate that the proportion of youth who seriously consider suicide may be decreasing, at least among certain groups. In 2008, 12% of the youth reported seriously considering suicide, which is a drop from 16% in 1992 (Smith et al., 2009). In Canada, among 15- to 24-year olds, suicide is the cause of death in 24% of all deaths (Canadian Mental Health Association, 2006). Suicide is currently the third leading cause of death in adolescents aged 15 to 19 years, surpassed only by death from motor vehicle crash and homicide (see Chapter 29). On average, 294 Canadian youths die yearly from suicide, and many more attempt suicide. Although the youth suicide rate as a whole is decreasing in Canada, including the rate for male adolescents, the rate for adolescent girls is slightly increasing.

Etiology

Individual, family, and social or environmental factors have all been implicated in suicide. The single most important individual factor is the presence of an active psychiatric disorder (depression, bipolar disorder, **psychosis,** substance use, or conduct disorder). Comorbidity of an affective disorder and substance use also increases the risk for suicide. Approximately 90% of adolescents who completed suicide met criteria for a psychiatric disorder before the suicide (Shain & AAP Committee on Adolescence, 2007). Depression is considered the highest single risk factor for adolescent suicide (Canadian Mental Health Association, 2011). Mental health problems that may predispose to suicide include depression; bipolar disorder; substance use or dependence; panic attacks; post-traumatic stress disorder; and a history of aggression, severe anger, or impulsivity (Shain & AAP Committee on Adolescence, 2007).

Family factors contributing to suicide risk include parental loss; family disruption; a family history of suicide, depression, substance use, or emotional disturbance; child abuse or neglect; unavailable parents; poor communication and isolation within the family; family conflict; and unrealistically high parental expectations or parental indifference with low expectations. Social or environmental factors include incarceration, isolation, acute loss of a boyfriend or girlfriend, lack of future options, and availability of firearms in the home. Cyberbullying and messages on some Internet sites that encourage suicide may also have an impact on suicide rates in the adolescent population (Kirmayer, 2012).

evolve Critical Thinking Exercises—Depression

First Nations, Métis, and Inuit teens and gay and lesbian teens may be at particularly high risk for suicide completion, depending on their own sense of self-esteem and the community in which they reside (Canadian Mental Health Association, 2011) (see Community Focus box). Among First Nations youths the suicide rate is approximately 5 to 7 times and for the Inuit population 11 times that of the non-Aboriginal population (Bhatia, 2010). This is particularly true if they are raised in an environment where they are denied support systems.

Methods

Hanging or suffocation is the most common means of suicide among male and female adolescents. Other methods include firearms, poisoning by gas, and overdose. Adolescents may play a choking game in which there is a temporary cutting off of the airway in order to cause euphoria; some suicides may actually be unintentional deaths but are impossible to differentiate from suicide (Kirmayer, 2012).

COMMUNITY FOCUS

Suicide, Sexual Identity, and Sexual Orientation

A significant number of teenage suicides occur among gay, lesbian, bisexual, and transgender youths. Gay or lesbian adolescents who live in families or communities that do not accept homosexuality are likely to suffer low self-esteem, self-loathing, depression, and hopelessness as a result. Such internalization, without treatment and support, can lead to substance use and, eventually, suicide. Youths most at risk are those who struggle with gender identity issues such as gay identity formation at a young age, intrapersonal conflict regarding sexuality, and nondisclosure of orientation to others.

Supportive parents, friends, or relationships serve as protective factors against suicide. However, many gay, lesbian, bisexual, and transgender adolescents do not feel supported, understood, or accepted by their friends, parents, and families. Nurses who interact with adolescents must be aware of the association between suicide and adolescent homosexuality and gender nonconformity. School nurses may be the first individuals to discuss issues of sexual identity and orientation with adolescents or their families. In their professional capacity, nurses can serve as support persons for these adolescents. Nurses can also provide guidance and resources to families so that they understand how best to nurture and support their child.

Nurses must also capitalize on opportunities or experiences that promote the healthy development of self-esteem in youths who have a nontraditional sexual orientation. Educational programs to raise the level of consciousness about the risk factors for and warning signs of suicide are one example. Another possibility could be programs conducted in or outside of school that are designed to foster peer relationships and competency in social skills among high-risk adolescents and young adults, such as support groups and social organizations for these young people.

NURSING ALERT Parents must be educated on the warning signs of suicide (Box 40-8), especially if their children are depressed, have poor problem-solving skills, or use drugs or alcohol.

Motivation

Suicidal ideation is not uncommon in adolescents. It represents numerous fantasies, such as relief from suffering, a means of gaining comfort and sympathy, or a means of revenge against those who have hurt them. Adolescents have the erroneous perception that the act of suicide will evoke remorse and pity and that they will be able to return and witness the grief. Angry children who are unable to directly punish those who have injured or insulted them may take revenge on those who love them through self-destruction ("They'll be sorry when they find me dead"; "They'll be sorry they were mean to me").

For adolescents who are severely depressed, suicide seems to be the only release from their despair. These adolescents rarely provide evidence of their intent and frequently conceal their suicidal thoughts. Some adolescents, however, tell their peers of their suicidal thoughts or plans but avoid telling adults. Social isolation is a significant factor in distinguishing adolescents who will kill themselves from those who will not. It is also more characteristic of those who complete suicide than of those who make attempts or threats.

The frequency of contagion, or copycat suicides (i.e., an increase in youth suicide that occurs after the suicide of one

BOX 40-8 Warning Signs of Suicide

- Preoccupation with themes of death—focuses on morbid thoughts
- Wants to give away cherished possessions
- Talks of own death, desire to die
- Loss of energy, loss of interest, listlessness
- Exhaustion without obvious cause
- Changes in sleep patterns—too much or too little
- Increased irritability, argumentativeness, or stubbornness
- Physical complaints—recurrent stomach aches, headaches
- Repeated visits to the physician, nurse practitioner, or emergency department for treatment of injuries
- Reckless behaviour
- Antisocial behaviour—engages in drinking, uses drugs, fights, commits acts of vandalism, runs away from home, becomes sexually promiscuous
- Sudden change in school performance—lowered grades, cutting classes, dropping out of activities
- Resists or refuses to go to school
- Remains distant, sad, remote—flat affect, frozen facial expression
- Describes self as worthless
- Sudden cheerfulness following deep depression
- Social withdrawal from friends, activities, interests that were previously enjoyed
- Impaired concentration
- Dramatic change in appetite

teenager is publicized) is disturbing and may indicate that teenagers perceive suicide as glamorous. In addition, young people may not realize the finality of suicide because they have become desensitized from constantly viewing violence and death on television, in video games, or in movies.

Diagnostic Evaluation

Depression is common among adolescents who attempt suicide. It is estimated that in those 15 to 18 years of age, approximately 7.6% had experienced depression and 13.5% had been diagnosed has having suicidal tendencies. Among Canadian female adolescents the rate of depression was 11.1% with 18.4% exhibiting suicidality, and 8.8% of adolescent boys had depression (Cheung & Dewa, 2006). Depression is characterized by both subjective symptoms and objective signs that reflect the adolescent's sadness and despair. Adolescents describe feelings of sadness, despair, helplessness, hopelessness, boredom, loss of interest, and isolation. They may also feel self-reproach, self-deprecation, and guilt. Subjective symptoms of depression or specific changes in behaviour place an adolescent at risk for suicide (Box 40-9).

Therapeutic Management

Threats of suicide should always be taken seriously. There has been a tendency to dismiss a suicide attempt as an impulsive act resulting from a temporary crisis or depression. If a suicide attempt fails to draw attention to their problems or makes them worse, the child or adolescent may conclude that suicide is the only answer. Children and adolescents need to know that someone cares, and they must be provided with swift and efficient crisis intervention. Although ordinary practitioners can manage an acute depressive reaction without difficulty, the adolescent who has made a serious attempt or has a specific plan for suicide should receive immediate attention and competent psychiatric care.

The American Academy of Child and Adolescent Psychiatry (2001) has published a practice parameter for the assessment and treatment of child and adolescent suicide. In addition, the Canadian Mental Health Association (2011) has a youth suicide prevention program.

NURSING ALERT Adolescents who express suicidal feelings and have a specific plan should be monitored at all times. They should not have access to firearms, prescription or over-the-counter medications, belts, scarves, shoestrings, sharp objects, matches, or lighters. If they are intoxicated, they must be restrained or placed in a protective environment until a psychiatrist or psychologist can assess them.

BOX 40-9 Characteristics of Children or Adolescents With Depression

Behaviour

- Predominantly sad facial expression with absence or diminished range of affective response (most of the day)
- Solitary play or work; tendency to be alone; lack of interest in play with friends
- Withdrawal from previously enjoyed activities and relationships
- Lowered grades in school; lack of interest in doing homework or achieving in school; refuses to wake up for school
- Diminished motor activity; tiredness
- Tearfulness or crying
- Inability to concentrate
- Dependent and clinging or aggressive and disruptive
- Recurrent suicidal thoughts or talk

Internal States

- Utterance of statements reflecting lowered self-esteem, sense of hopelessness, or guilt
- Suicidal ideations

Physiology

- Constipation
- Loss of energy; fatigue
- Nonspecific complaints of not feeling well
- Change in appetite resulting in weight loss or gain
- Alterations in sleeping pattern, sleeplessness, or hypersomnia

Nursing Care Management

Nurses play a pivotal role in reducing adolescent suicide. Nurses have the opportunity to provide anticipatory guidance to parents and adolescents. They can teach parents to be supportive and to develop positive communication patterns that help teens feel connected with and loved by their families. To foster healthy development, parents can be encouraged to provide teens with creative outlets and to assist young people in accepting strong emotions—pain, anger, and frustration—as a normal part of the human experience.

Nurses may question parents about signs of depression for young children. At one Canadian hospital adolescents are screened for depression by answering eight yes–no questions; if the adolescent reports five or more signs of depression, the nurse implements a screening for suicidal ideation (Weeks et al., 2004). The depression screening questions consider whether the adolescent reports the following:

- Feeling sad or crying often
- Perceiving that nothing is fun anymore
- Frequently losing his or her temper
- Preferring to be alone instead of with friends
- Sleeping a lot or too little
- Feeling restless or tired much of the time
- Eating infrequently or too often
- Having difficulty making a decision

If the adolescent is considered a suicide risk as a result of the screening, close observation should be implemented by the staff and the primary practitioner notified of the screening results (Weeks et al., 2004).

Care of the suicidal adolescent includes early recognition, management, and prevention. The most important aspect of management is the recognition of warning signs that indicate an adolescent is troubled and might attempt suicide. Health care providers must be alert to the signs of depression, and anyone who exhibits such behaviour should be referred for thorough psychological assessment. Depression is manifested differently in children and adolescents than in adults. In teens it may be masked by impulsive, aggressive behaviours. Defiance, disobedience, behaviour problems, and psychosomatic disturbances can indicate underlying depression, suicidal ideation, and impending suicide attempts.

No threat of suicide should be ignored or challenged. Too often, suicidal threats or minor attempts are confused with bids for attention. It is also a mistake to be lulled into a false sense of security when the adolescent's depression is apparently relieved. The improvement in attitude may mean that the adolescent has made the decision and found the means to carry out the threat. Nurses have an ethical and legal obligation to report attempted or suspected attempted suicides (Canadian Nurses Association, 2008). The mechanism of reporting varies by province and territory, and each nurse must be aware of the appropriate channels for reporting (for example, in British Columbia, nurses and others report to the Ministry for Children and Family Development).

Peers or other confidants are valuable observers and excellent sources of information about **suicide potential**. They may not be able to diagnose depression, but they can sense when a friend has undergone a marked personality change. The peer who detects any changes in a friend is a potential rescuer and should not remain silent about the observations. Friendship does not imply collusion. A peer who believes that a friend may be suicidal should alert someone who can help (e.g., a parent, teacher, guidance counsellor, school nurse), and nurses should be supportive of peers who come forward with such information.

Routine health assessments of adolescents should include questions that assess the presence of suicidal ideation or intent. The following questions can be asked (American Foundation for Suicide Prevention, 2012):

- Do you consider yourself more a happy person, an unhappy person, or somewhere in the middle?
- Have you ever been so unhappy or upset that you felt like being dead?
- Have you ever thought about hurting yourself?
- Have you ever developed a plan to hurt yourself or kill yourself?
- Have you ever attempted to kill yourself?

If children or adolescents express suicidal intent to a nurse, the nurse needs to make a contract, asking them to sign an agreement that they will not attempt suicide during an agreed-on period and that they will call the 24-hour crisis line immediately if they feel that they cannot keep their contract. The amount of time that an adolescent feels comfortable contracting is usually an indication of his or her risk and stability.

Because a suicide attempt is frequently an outgrowth of family distress, it is essential to intervene with the family. It is important to assess family interactions and to recognize disturbed relationships. The most effective approach is recognition of susceptible adolescents during the early stages of family distress so that family counselling can be started. Prevention must be directed toward improving childrearing practices through support and education of parents and changing societal conditions that generate defeat, despair, and maladaptive behaviour.

Although confidentiality is an essential part of adolescent counselling, in the case of self-destructive behaviours, confidentiality cannot be honoured. Suicidal behaviour needs to be reported to the family and other professionals and adolescents informed that this will be done. Such action conveys an important message to the youth: that the professionals understand and care.

Many schools have instituted suicide prevention programs. These programs include services such as drop-in counselling and a peer-counselling telephone line. Information can also be obtained from the Canadian Mental Health Association (see Additional Resources section at the end of this chapter).

Key Points

- The pubescent growth spurt that begins around age 10 in girls and age 12 in boys signals the beginning of adolescence.
- Biological development during puberty is characterized by increased activity of the pituitary gland, which results in sexual maturity and the appearance of secondary sex characteristics.
- Development of body image is closely tied to body changes and social interactions.
- According to Erikson, the major developmental crisis of adolescence is establishing a sense of identity.
- Cognitive development in adolescence includes abstract thought, thinking beyond the present, logical reasoning, and a sense of idealism.
- According to Kohlberg's theory of moral development, adolescents begin to question existing moral values and learn to make their own choices.
- Spiritual development is characterized by the questioning of one's family's values and ideals and a move toward more philosophical thinking.
- Adolescent relationships with parents may be strained; the influence of the peer group increases and intimate relationships assume importance.
- Teenagers demonstrate a wide variety of interests, and their increased physical and cognitive skills allow them to engage in increasingly difficult and complex activities.
- Adolescents' emotions fluctuate.
- Nutritional needs may not be met by teenagers' eating habits, such as snacking and irregular mealtimes.
- Motor vehicle injuries are the primary cause of death from injury in the adolescent years.
- The rapid changes, growth, and stress accompanying the transition to adulthood may predispose adolescents to faulty problem solving.
- The most common health problems related to the female reproductive system during adolescence involve menstrual dysfunction.
- Eating disorders observed in middle and late childhood are obesity, AN, and BN.
- Tobacco smoking is a widespread problem among teenagers. Reasons for smoking include social pressure and mass-media influence.
- The substances used by children and adolescents are alcohol, marijuana, narcotics, central nervous system depressants,

central nervous system stimulants, hydrocarbons and fluorocarbons, and mind-altering drugs.
- Suicide, the deliberate act of self-injury with the intent to kill, may occur because of difficulties coping with stress, disturbed family environment, substance use or dependency, or mental health disorder.
- No threat of suicide by an adolescent should be ignored or challenged.

Audio Chapter Summaries
Access an Audio Summary of these Key Points on Evolve

References

Active Healthy Kids Canada. (2012). *Active Healthy Kids Canada report card on physical activity for children and youth.* Retrieved from http://dvqdas9jty7g6.cloudfront.net/reportcards2012/AHKC%202012%20-%20Report%20Card%20Short%20Form%20-%20FINAL.pdf.

Adelman, W. P., et al. (2001). Effectiveness of a high school smoking cessation program. *Pediatrics, 107*(4), e50.

American Academy of Child and Adolescent Psychiatry. (2001). Practice parameter for the assessment and treatment of children and adolescents with suicidal behavior. *Journal of the American Academy of Child & Adolescent Psychiatry, 40*(7 Suppl), 24S–51S.

American Academy of Pediatric Dentistry. (2009). Adolescent oral health care. *AAPD Reference Manual 2008–2009, 30*(7), 94–101. (Updated 2010) Retrieved from http://guideline.gov/content.aspx?id=24129.

American Academy of Pediatrics & American College of Obstetricians and Gynecologists. (2006). Menstruation in girls and adolescents: Using the menstrual cycle as a vital sign. *Pediatrics, 118*(5), 2245–2250. doi:10.1542/peds.2006-2481

American Dietetic Association. (2006). Position of the American Dietetic Association: Nutrition intervention in the treatment of anorexia nervosa, bulimia nervosa, and other eating disorders. *Journal of the American Dietetic Association, 106*(12), 2073–2082. doi:10.1016/j.jada.2006.09.007

American Foundation for Suicide Prevention. (2012). *When you fear that someone may take their life.* Retrieved from http://www.afsp.org/index.cfm?fuseaction=home.viewPage&page_id=F2F25092-7E90-9BD4-C4658F1D2B5D19A0

American Psychiatric Association. (2000). *Diagnostic and statistical manual of mental disorders* (4th ed.) (DSM-IV TR). Washington, DC: Author.

Angulo, P. (2002). Nonalcoholic fatty liver disease. *New England Journal of Medicine, 346*(16), 1221–1231.

Baker, S., et al. (2005). Overweight children and adolescents: A clinical report of the North American Society for Pediatric Gastroenterology, Hepatology and Nutrition. *Journal of Pediatric Gastroenterology & Nutrition, 40,* 533–543.

Berkowitz, R. I., et al. (2006). Effects of sibutramine treatment in obese adolescents. *Annals of Internal Medicine, 145*(2), 81–90.

Bhatia, J. (2010). Canada: Aboriginal suicides hits crisis rate. *Global Voices,* January 18, 2010. Retrieved from http://globalvoicesonline.org/2010/01/18/.

Biro, F. M., et al. (2003). Pubertal maturation in girls and the relationship to anthropometric changes: Pathways through puberty. *Journal of Pediatrics, 142*(6), 643–646.

Bond, L., et al. (2007). Social and school connectedness in early secondary school as predictors of late teenage substance use, mental health, and academic outcomes. *Journal of Adolescent Health, 40*(4), 357.e9–357.e18. doi:10.1016/j.jadohealth.2006.10.013

Braverman, P. K. (2006). Body art: Piercing, tattooing, and scarification. *Adolescent Medicine, 17,* 505–519. doi:10.1016/j.admecli.2006.06.007

Briggs, M., Safaii, S., & Beall, D. L. (2003). Nutrition services an essential component of comprehensive school health programs. *Journal of the American Dietetic Association, 103*(4), 505–514.

Canadian Cancer Society. (2006). *Facts on skin cancer in Ontario: News and information on ultraviolet radiation.* Retrieved from http://www.cancer.ca/Ontario/Publications/Ontario%20publications/~/media/CCS/Ontario/Files%20List/English%20files%20heading/Library%20PDFs%20-%20English/English_2070595488.ashx.

Canadian Cancer Society. (2007). *Sun bed usage and attitudes among students in Ontario grades 7 to 12: Youthography summary results.* Retrieved from http://www.cancer.ca/~/media/CCS/Ontario/Files%20List/liste%20de%20fichiers/pdf/Youthography%20survey_1856550887.ashx.

Canadian Cancer Society. (2011). *Early detection of testicular cancer.* Retrieved from http://www.cancer.ca/canada-wide/about%20cancer/types%20of%20cancer/early%20detection%20of%20testicular%20cancer.aspx?sc_lang=en.

Canadian Dental Association. (2010). *Fluoride and your child.* Retrieved from http://www.cda-adc.ca/en/oral_health/cfyt/dental_care_children/fluoride.asp?intPrintable=1.

Canadian Dermatologists Association. (2010). *2010 melanoma fact sheet.* Retrieved from http://www.dermatology.ca/patients_public/info_patients/skin_cancer/2010Melanoma-factsheet_e.pdf.

Canadian Diabetic Association. (2012). *Children and type 2 diabetes.* Retrieved from http://www.diabetes.ca/diabetes-and-you/youth/type2/.

Canadian Mental Health Association. (2006). *Suicide statistics.* Retrieved from http://www.ontario.cmha.ca/fact_sheets.asp?cID=3965.

Canadian Mental Health Association. (2011). *Youth and suicide.* Retrieved from http://www.cmha.ca/mental_health/youth-and-suicide/#.T-J2SZFRVAU.

Canadian Nurses Association. (2008). *Code of ethics for registered nurses.* Ottawa, ON: Author.

Canadian Paediatric Society. (2011). *Your teen's sexual orientation.* Retrieved from http://www.caringforkids.cps.ca/handouts/teens_sexual_orientation.

Canadian Paediatric Society, Adolescent Health Committee. (2012). Banning children and youth under the age of 18 years from commercial tanning facilities. *Paediatrics and Child Health, 17*(2), 89.

Canadian Paediatric Society, First Nations, Inuit and Métis Health Committee. (2010). Inhalant abuse. *Paediatrics and Child Health, 15*(7), 443–448.

Canadian Society for Exercise Physiology. (2012). *Canadian physical activity guidelines: For youth 12–17 years.* Retrieved from http://www.csep.ca/CMFiles/Guidelines/CSEP-InfoSheets-youth-ENG.pdf.

Chaiton, M., Cohen, J., McLoughlin, J., & Rehm, J. (2010). Use of cigarettes to improve affect and depressive symptoms in a longitudinal study of adolescents. *Addictive Behaviours, 36*(12), 1054–1064. doi:dx.doi.org/10.1016/j.addbeh.2010.07.002

Chansonneuve, D. (2007). *Addictive behaviours among Aboriginal peoples.* Retrieved from http://www.ahf.ca/downloads/addictive-behaviours.pdf.

Cheung, A. H., & Dewa, C. (2006). Canadian community health survey: Major depressive disorder and suicidality in adolescents. *Healthcare Policy, 2*(2), 76–89.

Costello, E. J., et al. (2007). Pubertal maturation and the development of alcohol use and abuse. *Drug & Alcohol Dependence, 88*(4 Suppl 1), S50–S59. doi:10.1016/j.drugalcdep.2006.12.009

Dennehy, C. E. (2006). The use of herbs and dietary supplements in gynecology: An evidence-based review. *Journal of Midwifery & Women's Health, 51*(6), 402–409. doi:10.1016/j.jmwh.2006.01.004

DeVore, E. R., & Ginsburg, K. R. (2005). The protective effects of good parenting on adolescents. *Current Opinion in Pediatrics, 17*(4), 460–465.

Dietitians of Canada. (2010). *5 steps to a healthy body weight for teens.* Retrieved from http://www.dietitians.ca/Nutrition-Resources-A-Z/Factsheets/Teens/5-Steps-to-a-Healthy-Body-Weight-for-Teens.aspx.

Dietitians of Canada, Canadian Paediatric Society, College of Family Physicians of Canada, & Community Health Nurses of Canada. (2010). *Promoting optimal monitoring of child growth in Canada: Using the new WHO growth charts* [Collaborative statement]. Retrieved from http://www.cps.ca/english/statements/N/growth-charts-statement-FULL.pdf.

Ellison, L. F., & Wilkins, K. (2009). Cancer prevalence in the Canadian population. *Health Reports/Statistics Canada, Canadian Centre for Health Information, 20*(1), 7–19.

Elton-Marshall, T., Leatherdale, S., & Burkhalter, R. (2011). Tobacco, alcohol and illicit drug use among Aboriginal youth living off-reserve: Results from the Youth Smoking Survey. *Canadian Medical Association Journal 183*(8), E480–E486. doi:10.1503/cmaj.101913

Erikson, E. H. (1963). *Childhood and society* (2nd ed.). New York: W. W. Norton.

Falkner, B., et al. (2006). The relationship of body mass index and blood pressure in primary care pediatric patients. *Journal of Pediatrics, 148*(2), 195–200. doi:10.1016/j.jpeds.2005.10.030

Feldman, M., Friedman, L. S., & Sleisenger, M. H. (2002). Obesity: A historical perspective and disease prevalence estimates. In M. Feldman, L. S. Friedman, & M. H. Sleisenger (Eds.), *Sleisenger and Fordtran's gastrointestinal and liver disease* (7th ed.). Philadelphia: Saunders.

Female Athlete Triad Coalition. (2011). *The female triad athlete.* Retrieved from http://www.femaleathletetriad.org/wp-content/uploads/2010/03/FATC_Slideshow_2011.pdf.

Forman, S. F. (2012). *Eating disorders: Epidemiology, pathogenesis, and clinical features.* Retrieved from http://www.uptodate.com/contents/eating-disorders-treatment-and-outcome.

Gance-Cleveland, B. (2007). Motivational interviewing: Improving patient education. *Journal of Pediatric Health, 21*(2), 81–88. doi:10.1016/j.pedhc.2006.05.002

Geller, A. C., et al. (2002). Use of sunscreen, sunburning rates and tanning bed use among more than 10,000 U.S. children and adolescents. *Pediatrics, 109*(6), 1009–1014.

Gordon, S. M. (2000). *Adolescent drug use: Trends in abuse, treatment and prevention.* Wernersville, PA: Caron Foundation.

Government of Canada. (2006). *The human face of mental health and mental illness in Canada, 2006.* Ottawa, ON: Author.

Government of Canada, Standing Committee on Health. (2007). *Healthy weights for healthy kids.* Ottawa, ON: Parliament of Canada.

Government of Canada, Standing Senate Committee on Social Affairs, Science and Technology. (2006). *Out of the shadows at last. Transforming mental health, mental illness and addiction services in Canada.* Ottawa, ON: Parliament of Canada. Retrieved from http://www.parl.gc.ca/Content/SEN/Committee/391/soci/rep/rep02may06-e.htm.

Gray, M., & Moore, K. N. (2009). *Urologic disorders: Adult and pediatric care.* St. Louis: Mosby.

Greaser, J., & Whyte, J. J. (2004). Childhood obesity: Is there effective treatment? *Consultant for Pediatricians, 4*(10), 474–478.

Health Canada. (2011a). *Eating well with Canada's food guide.* Retrieved from http://www.hc-sc.gc.ca/fn-an/food-guide-aliment/index-eng.php.

Health Canada. (2011b). *Information for industry: Tattoo ink.* Retrieved from http://www.hc-sc.gc.ca/cps-spc/cosmet-person/indust/information/tattoo-tatouage-eng.php.

Health Canada. (2011c). *Tobacco: Health concerns.* Retrieved from http://www.hc-sc.gc.ca/hc-ps/tobac-tabac/index-eng.php.

Hill, J. O., et al. (2003). Obesity and the environment: Where do we go from here? *Science, 299*(5608), 853–855.

Johnson, J. L., & Oliffe, J. L. (2012). Gender and community health. In L. L. Stamler & L. Yiu (Eds.), *Community health nursing: A Canadian perspective* (3rd ed., pp. 300–310). Toronto: Pearson.

Johnston, L. D., et al. (2005). *Monitoring the future national results on adolescent drug use: Overview of key findings, 2004* (NIH Pub No 05-5726). Bethesda, MD: National Institute on Drug Abuse.

Kaplowitz, P. B. (2008). Link between body fat and the timing of puberty. *Pediatrics, 121*(Suppl 3), S208–S217. doi:10.1542/peds.2007-1813F

Kirmayer, L. J. (2012). Changing patterns in suicide among young people *Canadian Medical Association Journal, 184,* 1015–1016. doi:10.1503/cmaj.120509

Kohlberg, L. (1968). Moral development. In D. L. Sills (Ed.), *International encyclopedia of the social sciences.* New York: Macmillan.

Langille, D. B. (2007). Teenage pregnancy: Trends, contributing factors and the physician's role. *Canadian Medical Association Journal, 176,* 1601–1602. doi:10.1503/cmaj.070352

Langille, D. B., Corbett, E., Wilson, K., & Schlievert, C. (2010). *Determinants of adolescent pregnancy: Factors influencing youth sexual behaviours in a rural Nova Scotia community.* Halifax, Canada: Dalhousie University Faculty of Medicine.

Laws, C. (2005). Youth and firearms in Canada. *Paediatrics and Child Health, 10*(8), 473–477.

Lefebvre, G., Pinsonneault, O., Antao, V., Black, A., Burnett, M., et al. (2005). Primary dysmenorrhea consensus guideline. *Journal of Obstetrics and Gynaecology Canada, 27*(12), 1117–1146.

Lynne, S. D., et al. (2007). Links between pubertal timing, peer influences and externalizing behaviors among urban students followed through middle school. *Journal of Adolescent Health, 40*(2), 181.e7–181.e13. doi:10.1016/j.jadohealth.2006.09.008

Maes, L., & Lievens, J. (2003). Can the school make a difference? A multilevel analysis of adolescent risk and health behavior. *Social Science Medicine, 56*(3), 517–529.

Master-Hunter, T., & Heiman, D. L. (2006). Amenorrhea: Evaluation and treatment. *American Family Physician, 73*(8), 1374–1382.

McDonald, N. (2007) What's killing and maiming Canada's youth? *Canadian Medical Association Journal, 176*(6), 737. doi:10.1503/cmaj.070172

McGovern, L., Johnson, J. N., Paulo, R., Hettinger, A., Singhal, V., et al. (2008). Treatment of pediatric obesity: A systematic review and meta-analysis of randomized trials. *Journal of Clinical Endocrinology & Metabolism, 93*(12), 4600–4605. doi:10.1210/jc.2006-2409

Mehler, P. S. (2001). Diagnosis and care of patients with anorexia nervosa in primary care settings. *Annals of Internal Medicine, 134,* 1048–1059.

Nader, P. R., et al. (2008). Moderate-to-vigorous activity from ages 9 to 15 years. *Journal of the American Medical Association, 300*(3), 295–305. doi:10.1001/jama.300.3.295

National Eating Disorder Information Centre. (2011). *Definitions.* Retrieved from http://www.nedic.ca/knowthefacts/definitions.shtml.

Nielsen, S. J., & Popkin, B. M. (2003). Patterns and trends in food portion sizes, 1977–1998. *Journal of the American Medical Association, 289*(4), 450–453.

Nova Scotia Roundtable on Youth Sexual Health (n.d.). *Framework for action: Youth sexual health.* Retrieved from http://www.gov.ns.ca/hpp/publications/FINAL_framework_Booklet.pdf.

O'Brien, M., et al. (2007). The ecology of childhood overweight: A 12-year longitudinal analysis. *International Journal of Obesity (London), 31*(9), 1469–1478.

O'Brien, P. E., Sawyer, S. M., Laurie, C., Brown, W. A., Skinner, S., et al. (2010). Laparoscopic adjustable gastric banding in severely obese adolescents. *Journal of the American Medical Association, 303*(6), 519–526.

Omar, H., McElderry, D., & Zakharia, R. (2003). Educating adolescents about puberty: What are we missing? *International Journal of Adolescent Medicine & Health, 15*(1), 79–83.

Ongphiphadhanakul, B. (2007). Osteoporosis: The role of genetics and the environment. *Forum of Nutrition, 60,* 158–167.

Pan S. Y., Johnson, K. C., Ugnat, A. M., Wen, S. W., Mao, Y., for Canadian Cancer Registries Epidemiology Research Group. (2004). Association of obesity and cancer risk in Canada. *American Journal of Epidemiology, 159*(3), 259–268.

Pechmann, C., & Reibling, E. T. (2000). Anti-smoking advertising campaigns targeting youth: Case studies from USA and Canada. *Tobacco Control, 9*(Suppl 2), II18–II131.

Piaget, J. (1952). *The origins of intelligence in children.* New York: International Universities Press.

Public Health Agency of Canada. (2006). *Canadian immunization guide* (7th ed.). Retrieved from http://www.phac-aspc.gc.ca/publicat/cig-gci/index-eng.php.

Public Health Agency of Canada. (2008). *Canadian guidelines for sexual health education.* Retrieved from http://www.phac-aspc.gc.ca/publicat/cgshe-ldnemss/pdf/guidelines-eng.pdf.

Public Health Agency of Canada. (2009). *Child and youth injury in review, 2009 edition—Spotlight on consumer product safety.* Retrieved from http://www.phac-aspc.gc.ca/publicat/cyi-bej/2009/pdf/injrep-rapbles2009_eng.pdf.

Public Health Agency of Canada. (2010). *Backgrounder on the role of the Government of Canada: Childhood obesity.* Retrieved from http://www.phac-aspc.gc.ca/ch-se/obesity/obesitybck-eng.php.

Public Health Agency of Canada. (2011). *Publicly funded immunization programs in Canada—routine schedule for infants and children including special programs and catch-up programs.* Retrieved from http://www.phac-aspc.gc.ca/im/ptimprog-progimpt/table-1-eng.php.

Public Health Agency of Canada. (2012). *Perinatal health indicators for Canada 2011* (Cat. No. HP7-1/2011). Ottawa, ON: Author.

Raphael, D. (2010). The health of Canada's children. Part II: Health mechanisms and pathways. *Paediatrics & Child Health, 15*(2), 71–76.

Region of Waterloo, Public Health. (2012). *Youth and smoking.* Retrieved from http://chd.region.waterloo.on.ca/en/healthylivinghealthprotection/youthsmoking.asp.

Royal Canadian Mounted Police. (2011). *Canadian firearms program.* Retrieved from http://www.rcmp-grc.gc.ca/cfp-pcaf/index-eng.htm.

Russell, S. T., Seif, H., & Truong, N. L. (2001). School outcomes of sexual minority youth in the United States: Evidence from a national study. *Journal of Adolescence, 24*(1), 111–127.

Schwimmer, J. B. (2004). Managing overweight in older children and adolescents. *Pediatric Annals, 33*(1), 39–44.

Shain, B., & American Academy of Pediatrics Committee on Adolescence. (2007). Suicide and suicide attempts in adolescents. *Pediatrics, 120*(3), 669–676. doi:10.1542/peds.2007-1908

Shields, M. (2005). *Measured obesity: Overweight Canadian children and adolescents.* Statistics Canada Cat. No. 82-620-MWE2005001.

Simcoe Muskoka Health Unit. (2011). Tattooing and piercing: Make it safe. Retrieved from http://www.simcoemuskokahealth.org/Topics/SexualHealth/NeedlesSharps/TattooingAndPiercing.aspx.

Sjöberg, R. L., Nilsson, K. W., & Leppert, J. (2005). Obesity, shame, and depression in school-aged children: A population-based study. *Pediatrics, 116*(3), e389–e393. doi:10.1542/peds.2005-0170

Smith, A., Stewart, D., Peled, M., Poon, C., Saewyc, E., & the McCreery Centre Society. (2009). *A picture of health: Highlights from the 2008 BC Adolescent Health Survey.* Vancouver, BC: McCreary Centre Society.

Sondike, S., Copperman, N., & Jacobson, M. S. (2003). Effects of a low-carbohydrate diet on weight loss and cardiovascular risk factors in overweight adolescents. *Journal of Pediatrics, 142*(3), 253–258.

Spear, B. (2005). Weight management: Obesity to eating disorders. In P. Q. Samour & K. King (Eds.), *Handbook of pediatric nutrition* (3rd ed.). Sudbury, MA: Jones & Bartletts.

Stewart, D., et al. (2009). *Adolescent substance use and related harms in British Columbia.* CARBC Bulletin 5. Victoria, Canada: University of Victoria, Centre for Addictions Research of BC.

Storey, K. E., Forbes, L. E., Fraser, S. N., Spence, J. C., Plotnikoff, R. C., et al. (2009). Diet quality, nutrition and physical activity among adolescents: The Web-SPAN (Web-Survey of Physical Activity and Nutrition) project. *Public Health Nutrition, 12*(11), 2009–2017. doi:10.1017/S1368980009990292

Story, M., Nanney, M. S., & Schwartz, M. B. (2009). Schools and obesity prevention: Creating school environments and policies to promote healthy eating and physical activity. *Milbank Quarterly, 87*(1), 71–100.

Taylor, E. D., et al. (2006). Orthopedic complications of overweight in children and adolescents. *Pediatrics, 117*(6), 2167–2173. doi:10.1542/peds.2005-1832

Tuttle, J., Campbell-Heider, N., & David, T. M. (2006). Positive adolescent life skills training for high-risk teens: Results of a group intervention study. *Journal of Pediatric Health, 20*(3), 184–191. doi:10.1016/j.pedhc.2005.10.011

Weeks, S. K., et al. (2004). Getting inside depression and suicide ideation. *Nursing Management, 35*(10), 42–46.

Weiss, R., et al. (2004). Obesity and the metabolic syndrome in children and adolescents. *New England Journal of Medicine, 350*(23), 2362–2374.

Wilkins, K. (2005). Deaths involving firearms. *Health Reports/Statistics Canada, Canadian Centre For Health Information, 16*(4), 37–43.

Williams, A. F., & Ferguson, S. A. (2002). Rationale for graduated licensing and the risks it should address. *Injury Prevention, 8*(Suppl 2), ii9–ii16.

World Health Organization. (2011). *Sexual health.* Retrieved from http://www.who.int/topics/sexual_health/en/.

Additional Resources

Aboriginal Canada Portal: Youth and Youth Organizations and Associations: http://www.aboriginalcanada.gc.ca/acp/site.nsf/eng/ao30911.html

Canadian Cancer Society Encyclopedia: Early Detection of Testicular Cancer: http://info.cancer.ca/cce-ecc/default.aspx?cceid=2056&Lang=E&toc=50

Canadian Federation for Sexual Health: http://www.cfsh.ca/

Canadian Mental Health Association http://www.cmha.ca/mental-health/

Canadian Priorities for Addressing: Obesity as a Cancer and Chronic Disease: Risk Factor: http://www.partnershipagainstcancer.ca/wp-content/uploads/AIA-FINAL-REPORT-NOV-23-3.pdf

Centers for Disease Control and Prevention: NIOSH Science Blog—Body Art: http://blogs.cdc.gov/niosh-science-blog/2008/02/body-art/

Kids Help Phone—Only 24-hour bilingual hotline for children and youth for referral to resources on a variety of issues: Phone: 1-800-668-6868; Web site: http://www.kidshelpphone.ca/Teens/Home.aspx

MADD Canada (Mothers Against Drunk Driving): http://www.madd.ca/madd2/

National Aboriginal Friendship Centres: http://www.nafc.ca/

National Anti-Drug Strategy: Youth Drug Prevention for Parents: http://www.nationalantidrugstrategy.gc.ca/parents/parents.html

National Eating Disorder Information Centre: http://www.nedic.ca/index.shtml

National Institute on Drug Abuse: http://www.nida.nih.gov/NIDAHome.html

National Youth Solvent Program: http://www.hc-sc.gc.ca/fniah-spnia/substan/ads/nysap-pnlasj-eng.php

Parents Anonymous: http://www.parentsanon.org/

Public Health Agency of Canada: The Health of Canada's Young People: A Mental Health Focus: http://www.phac-aspc.gc.ca/hp-ps/dca-dea/publications/health-young-people-sante-jeunes-canadiens/index-eng.php.

SADD (Students Against Destructive Decisions): http://www.sadd.org/

Sex Information and Education Council of Canada (SIECCAN): http://www.sieccan.org

SexualityandU.ca: http://www.sexualityandu.ca/

Tough Love: http://www.toughlove.com

Unit 10

41 Chronic Illness, Disability, and End-of-Life Care

Learning Objectives

On completion of this chapter, the reader will be able to:

- Identify the scope of and changing trends in the care of children with special needs.
- Identify the major reactions of and effects on the family of a child with special needs.
- Define the stages of adjustment to the diagnosis of a chronic condition.
- Recognize the impact of the illness or disability on the developmental stages of childhood.
- Outline nursing interventions that promote the family's optimal adjustment to the child's chronic disorder.
- Outline nursing interventions that support the family at the time of the child's death.
- Define the usual symptoms of grief.

Electronic Resources

Additional information related to the content in Chapter 41 can be found on

evolve the companion Web site at

http://evolve.elsevier.com/Canada/Perry/maternal/

- Examination Review Questions
- Case Study—The Dying Child

Perspectives on the Care of Children With Special Needs

Scope of the Problem

A number of terms and defining characteristics have been used to describe chronic illness and disability in children (Box 41-1). In recent years there have been continuing efforts to develop a definition that better identifies the number of children living with chronic conditions and the impact on health and social services (Jackson, 2000; van Dyck et al., 2004a). Currently, *children with special health care needs* are defined as children who have or are at increased risk for a chronic physical, developmental, behavioural, or emotional condition and who also require health and related services of a type or amount beyond that generally required by children (Msall et al., 2003).

Ongoing progress in medical and technological disease management has contributed to the growing number of children with special health care needs (Martinez & Ercikan, 2009). Technological advances have substantially increased the survival of extremely-low- and very-low-birth-weight infants (Jackson, 2000). Canadian children with chronic illnesses have the highest survival rates of all time, with 98% now living to early adulthood. Children with disabilities are more likely to be in poorer health than children without disabilities (Halfon & Newacheck, 2010). The result of such technological progress is that an estimated 4% of Canadian children aged 5 to 14 years have a physical or cognitive disability (Statistics Canada, 2003). Approximately 30% of school-aged children have a chronic illness (Martinez & Ercikan, 2009). These children require specialized health care of a type or amount beyond that generally required by children with no disability (Perrin, 2004).

The most commonly occurring conditions causing disability are asthma, diabetes, cancer, obesity, unintentional injuries, and mental illness. In Canada, it is estimated that as many as 15% of Canadian children and youth are affected by a mental disorder at any given time. An estimated 29% of First Nations children on reserve aged 0 to 11 years were reported by a parent or guardian as having behavioural or emotional problems (Chief Public Health Officer's Report on the State of Public Health in Canada, 2009).

The impact of chronic illness and disability in children is wide ranging. For some families, the impact is minimal but for many other families, chronic conditions in children present families with additional tasks, responsibilities, and concerns (Ray, 2002). A child's activity level and developmental opportunities can be affected. Days can be lost from school. Children with chronic illness or disability may be at increased risk for behavioural or emotional problems. Parents may lose days from work, experience financial and relationship strains, and be challenged both emotionally and physically as they cope with care of the child.

Siblings are also affected by having a "different" brother or sister and may simultaneously feel guilt and anger or jealousy

BOX 41-1 Common Terms Regarding Children With Special Needs

Chronic illness—A condition that interferes with daily functioning for more than 3 months in a year, causes hospitalization of more than 1 month in a year, or (at time of diagnosis) is likely to do either of these

Congenital disability—A disability that has existed since birth but is not necessarily hereditary

Developmental delay—A maturational lag; an abnormal, slower rate of development in which a child demonstrates a functioning level below that observed in normal children of the same age

Developmental disability—Any mental or physical disability that is manifested before age 22 years and is likely to continue indefinitely

Disability—A temporary, prolonged, or permanent reduction or absence of the ability to perform certain commonplace activities or roles, sometimes referred to as activities of daily living.

Handicap—Handicap refers to the social and environmental consequences of an individual's impairment.

Impairment—Impairment is an abnormality in an organ or in the physical or mental functions of the body that produces disability.

Life-limiting illness—Any illness or condition developed in childhood whereby the child is likely to die before adulthood or with a limited expectation of life thereafter

Technology-dependent child—A child from birth to 21 years with a chronic disability that requires the routine use of a medical device to compensate for the loss of a life-sustaining body function; requires daily ongoing care or monitoring by trained personnel

(Sources: *The Canadian Encyclopedia*, retrieved from http://www.thecanadianencyclopedia.com/PrinterFriendly.cfm?Params=A1ARTA0002310; Danvers, L., et al. [2003]. Providing seamless service for children with life-limiting illness: Experiences and recommendations of professional staff at the Diana Princess of Wales Children's Community Service. *Journal of Clinical Nursing, 12*[3], 351–359.)

toward their ill sibling. Additionally, they suffer secondary losses such as the ability to participate in extracurricular activities or social events because of routines imposed by the affected child's chronic condition.

Trends in Care

Developmental Focus

In focusing on the child's developmental level rather than the **chronological age** or diagnosis, the child's abilities and strengths are emphasized, rather than disabilities. Attention is directed toward normalizing experiences, adapting the environment, and promoting **coping** skills. Nurses often are in vital positions to redirect efforts away from the pathological model, with its focus on weaknesses and problems, and toward the developmental model to meet the unique needs of the child and family.

A developmental focus also considers family development. The life cycle of the family unit reflects changing ages and needs of family members, as well as changing external demands. A family member's serious illness or disability can cause significant stress or crisis at any stage of the family life cycle. Just as with individual development, family development may be interrupted or even regress to an earlier level of functioning. Nurses can use the concept of family development to plan meaningful interventions and to evaluate care.

Family-Centred Care

Children's physical and emotional health, as well as cognitive and social functioning, is strongly influenced by how well their families function (Schor, 2003). The importance of family-centred care—a philosophy that considers the family as the constant in the child's life—is especially evident in the care of children with special needs. As parents learn about the youngster's health care needs, they often become experts in delivering care. Health care providers, including nurses, are adjuncts to the child's care and need to form partnerships with parents. Effective communication and negotiation between parents and nurses are essential to forming trusting and effective partnerships and finding the best ways to meet the needs of the child and family (Corlett & Twycross, 2006). Collaborative relationships are characterized by communication, dialogue, **active listening**, awareness, and acceptance of differences (Schor, 2003).

Family–Health Care Provider Communication

Disclosure of a child's serious, acute, or chronic illness is one of the most stressful aspects of communication between families and health care providers. Often, parents have suspected for some time that something is wrong with their child and believe that their concerns were minimized or ignored by health care providers (Whitehead & Gosling, 2003). Numerous studies have shown that after a diagnosis is made, parents are not always satisfied with the way in which the information is given. The communication may have been flawed by unsympathetic and brief diagnostic interviews, a lack of privacy during diagnostic discussions, and lack of opportunity for the parents to ask questions. Conversely, parents report satisfaction when they perceive the health care providers to be giving information in an open and honest manner with respect for the parents' need for privacy and time to express emotions and ask questions (Davies, Davis, & Sibert, 2003). Similar factors are important in communication of changes in the child's condition throughout the course of the illness.

Providing information to families with a chronically ill child should be a process of repeated discussions to enable the family to process the information and their reactions to that information and allow them to ask for clarification and further information. Nurses play an important role in ensuring that families' needs are met during discussions related to a child's diagnosis, condition, and treatment. The family should be assessed regarding how much information they are comfortable with, what they understand of the information already given to them, and how they are coping with the information, both cognitively and emotionally. Nurses should ensure that the appropriate health care providers address any concerns or further questions that the family may have.

Establishing Therapeutic Relationships

Another important aspect of family-centred care of chronically ill children is establishing a therapeutic relationship with the child and family, which has been shown to predict improved health-related outcomes (Denboba et al., 2006; Trute, Hiebert-Murphy, & Wright, 2008). Families, most often the mother, take on enormous responsibility in providing technical care and symptom management of their child's condition outside the health care institution (Ahmann, 2006; O'Brien & Wegner, 2002; Raina et al., 2005). To build successful therapeutic relationships with families, it is necessary for nurses to recognize parents' expertise in their child's condition and needs. Care conferences, especially multidisciplinary meetings that include family and key health care providers provide an opportunity for sharing ideas and information and expressing feelings or concerns.

The Role of Culture in Family-Centred Care

Issues related to culture, ethnicity, and race can affect access to services, utilization, and follow-through with referrals and recommendations (van Dyck et al., 2004b; Wise et al., 2002; Wood et al., 2002; Zuvekas & Taliaferro, 2003). For some ethnic and minority populations, cultural understandings of illness and disability, structure of family life, social roles for individuals who are disabled, and other factors related to the perception of children may differ from those of mainstream North American culture. These factors may affect family needs and family choices regarding the care of their child with special needs.

Although culture cannot completely explain how an individual will think and act, an understanding of cultural perspectives can help the nurse anticipate and comprehend why families may make certain decisions. Cultural attributes such as values and beliefs regarding illness or disability and its causation, social roles for the ill or disabled, family structure, the role of children, childrearing practices, self versus group orientation, spirituality, and perceptions of time also affect a family's response to illness or disability in a child (Carnevale et al., 2006; Gerlach, 2008; Grossoehme et al., 2010; Marshall et al., 2003; Sterling & Peterson, 2003).

When parents not fluent in the health care provider's language are informed of their child's chronic illness, interpreters familiar with both cultures and languages should be used. Children, family members, and friends of the family should not be used as translators because their presence may prevent parents from openly discussing the issues. When nurses are working with people of cultural backgrounds different from their own, nurses must listen carefully with an initial goal of understanding and articulating the family's perspective. The ability to interpret mainstream medical culture to the family is also important. Furthermore, every effort should be made to incorporate a family's traditional cultural beliefs into the treatment plans. Developing a care plan in conjunction with the family that considers their preferences and priorities is an important first step in formulating a plan that best meets the family's needs (Daudji et al., 2011; Ochieng, 2003).

Shared Decision Making

Shared decision making among the child, family, and health care team can result from open, honest, culturally sensitive communication and the establishment of a therapeutic relationship between the family and health care providers. In a shared decision-making model, the health care providers provide honest, clear information regarding the diagnosis, prognosis, treatment options, and risk–benefit assessment. The patient and family then share information with the health care team about important family values, acceptable levels of discomfort or inconvenience, and the ability to comply with treatments being recommended (Perrin, Lewkowicz, & Young, 2000). This process allows them to discuss all options in terms of the risks and benefits to the child and family, the prognosis or expected course of the illness, and the impact on the family's resources (Box 41-2).

Normalization

Normalization refers to behaviours and intentions of disabled persons to integrate into society by living life as persons without a disability would (Morse, Wilson, & Penrod, 2000). For the chronically ill or disabled child, such behaviours could include attending school, pursuing hobbies and recreational interests, and achieving employment and a level of independence. For their families, it may entail adapting the family routine to accommodate the ill or disabled child's health and physical needs (McDougal, 2002).

Children with chronic illness and disability and their families face numerous challenges in achieving normalization. Families move between the "normal" of living with the experience of chronic childhood illness and the "normal" of the healthy outside world; they often redefine "normal" on the basis of their particular experiences, needs, and circumstances (Nelson, 2002).

Nurses can assist families in normalizing their lives by assessing the family's everyday life, social support systems, coping strategies, family cohesiveness, and family and community resources. Interventions could include encouraging families to reduce stress through delegation of care and family tasks, identifying ways to incorporate care into current routines, structuring the home environment to foster the child's engagement in age-appropriate activities, and ensuring that families have access to appropriate community support services (Jokinen, 2004; Spalding & Salib, 2008). Being supportive of the child's illness and treatment and actively including the family in all aspects of care will improve their self-esteem and promote further development (Shepard & Mahon, 2000).

BOX 41-2 Facilitating Shared Decision Making

- Continually assess the impact of the child's illness and treatment on the family.
- Provide honest, accurate information regarding the **illness trajectory**, anticipated complications, and prognostic information.
- Discuss what the family desires for the child's quality of life.
- Avoid personal opinion or judgement of the family's questions and decisions.

Home care represents the return to a system and set of priorities in which a family's values are as important in the care of a child with a chronic health problem as they are in the care of other children (Spaulding & Salib, 2008).

Goals for Home Care

The goals for home care include the following:

- Normalize the life of a child with special needs, including those with technologically complex care, in a family and community context and setting
- Minimize the disruptive impact of the child's condition on the family
- Foster the child's maximum growth and development

Paralleling normalization and home care is the process of *mainstreaming*, or integrating children with special needs into regular classrooms. Just as the home is the natural environment for children, so school must also be included as an essential component of children's overall physical, intellectual, and social development. Children who attend school have the advantages of learning and socializing with a wide group of peers. There is an increased focus on individualization as plans are made to meet the academic needs of these children along with those of the rest of the students.

A variety of supplemental programs have been designed in school systems to accommodate the special needs of children at school age and younger through *early intervention*, which consists of any sustained and systematic effort to assist children from birth to age 3 years who are disabled and developmentally vulnerable. This change, and increasing opportunities for normalization for children with special needs, has resulted in large part from examination of the *Charter of Rights and Freedoms*. Canada signed the *Convention on the Rights of the Child* on May 28, 1990 and ratified it on December 13, 1991. Examination as to how it is interpreted for children with disabilities is ongoing. Each province and territory may have different legislated policies, laws that govern education and health care for children. It is important for nurses to be aware of the laws within their various jurisdictions and how these laws might affect their patients. Nurses can provide parents with information about the relevant laws and rights and, in some cases, may participate in the development of individualized educational programs or individualized family service plans for children with special needs.

Coordinated Care

It is challenging for parents and other caregivers of children with special health care needs to coordinate the many professionals, programs, and agencies that may be involved with their child's care (Doig, McLennan, & Urichuk, 2009; Trute et al., 2008). The assistance of a knowledgeable case manager or service coordinator can ease the stress of navigating the systems. In Canada, there are three major issues facing children and youth who need home care: 1) a lack of specialized pediatric professionals; 2) a lack of timely access to services that can result in long waits: and 3) integration of these complex services (Hollander & Prince, 2008; Spalding & Salib, 2008). Nurses can play a key role in assisting families to access the appropriate services.

The Family of the Child With Special Needs

A major goal in working with the family of a child with special needs is to support the family's coping and promote their optimal functioning throughout the child's life. Long-term, comprehensive, family-centred approaches extend beyond supporting the child and family during only the critical periods of diagnosis and hospitalization. Rather, comprehensive care involves forming parent–professional partnerships that can support a family's adaptation to the many changes that may be necessary in day-to-day life, determine expectations of and for the child, and provide a long-term perspective.

The impact of a child's medical or developmental condition is often experienced over time, initially as a crisis at the time of diagnosis, which may occur at birth, after a long period of physical or psychological testing, or immediately after a tragic injury. The impact may also be felt before the diagnosis is made, when parents are aware that something is wrong with their child but before medical confirmation (Thomlinson, 2002; Whitehead & Gosling, 2003).

The diagnosis and initial discharge home are critical times for parents (Coffey, 2006). Several factors can make it difficult, including a long duration of uncertainty in the diagnostic process, negative perceptions of chronic illness or disability, insufficient information, and lack of mutual trust between parents and their child's health care team (Nuutila & Salanterä, 2006). Parental feelings of shock, helplessness, isolation, fear, and depression are common (Coffey, 2006; Nuutila & Salanterä, 2006). Throughout the first year, parents may struggle to accept the child's diagnosis and care and the uncertainty of the future (Coffey, 2006). The providing of explicit and uncomplicated information to parents in an empathic way (Nuutila & Salanterä, 2006); assessment of the family's daily routine, living conditions, background knowledge, skills and abilities, and coping behaviours; and evaluation of the family's understanding of the information are components of optimal support at the time of diagnosis and initial discharge home. It is also necessary to reassess parental needs for information and support on a routine basis (Nuutila & Salanterä, 2006).

Impact of the Child's Chronic Illness or Disability

Each member of a family who has a child with special needs is affected by the experience (Sullivan-Bolyai et al., 2003). The effects on the parents and their responses are so critical that they directly influence the other members' reactions and the child's own coping.

Parents

Parents are affected by the stress of grieving for the loss of a perfect child, regardless of whether they receive positive feedback from interactions with their child. Many parents of children with special needs feel satisfaction and fulfillment from the parenting role. For others, parenting may be a series of unrewarding experiences that contribute to feelings of inadequacy and failure (Box 41-3). These responses may be most evident in parents who are responsible for the child's care.

BOX 41-3 Anticipated Parental Stress Points

Diagnosis of the condition—Parents require considerable education while dealing with an emotional response.

Developmental milestones—Times that children normally achieve walking, talking, and self-care are delayed or impossible for the child.

Start of schooling—Particularly stressful are situations in which appropriate schooling will not be in a regular class placement.

Reaching the ultimate attainment—Parents must handle situations such as realizing that ambulation will be impossible or that the child will not learn to read.

Adolescence—Issues such as sexuality and independence become prominent.

Future placement—Decisions about placement must be made when the child becomes an adult or when the parents can no longer care for the child.

Death of the child—Parents coping with the death of a child can suffer enormous stress with physical and psychological effects, including higher levels of depression.

Parents may become preoccupied with their ability to carry out certain procedures, overlooking the child's personal comfort and satisfaction or failing to offer praise for anything less than perfect cooperation or performance. They may pursue a frustrating activity until they achieve "success"—long after the child has become irritable and uncooperative. Parents can become caught in a pattern of interaction that is mutually unrewarding and minimally productive. For these parents, several strategies may be helpful: education regarding what can reasonably be expected of their child, assistance in identifying the child's strengths, praise for a parental job well done, and respite care so that parents can renew their energies.

Parental Roles

Parenting a child with a chronic illness or disability requires much more than raising a typical child. In addition to attending to the routine aspects of parenting, parents of chronically ill children take on the added responsibility of performing complex technical care and symptom management, advocating for their child, and seeking and coordinating health and social services for their ill or disabled child. These responsibilities must then be balanced with the needs of other family members and friends and with personal health and obligations to minimize consequences to the overall functioning of the family (Coffey, 2006; Ray, 2002).

Enormous demands may be placed on parental time, energy, and financial resources. The nurse can assist parents in avoiding role conflicts by providing anticipatory guidance early on. Teaching should address stressors often identified as having an impact on the marriage: (1) the burden of care at home assumed by primarily one parent, (2) the financial burden, (3) the fear of the child dying, (4) pressure from relatives, (5) the hereditary nature of the disease (if applicable), (6) fear that they may become ill and unable to care for their child, and (7) fear of pregnancy. Other causes of tension may centre on the inconveniences associated with care, such as long waits for an appointment, lack of parking near care facilities, or lack of overnight accommodations. Certainly, these last stressors are within health care providers' domain to minimize, if not eliminate.

Mother–Father Differences

Mothers and fathers in the same family often adjust and cope differently as parents of a child with special needs. Some mothers experience a periodic crisis pattern, whereas most fathers tend to experience a steady, gradual recovery. Some research suggests that mothers of children with certain conditions may be more susceptible to psychological distress and fatigue than fathers (Tong et al., 2002). Frequently, mothers are the primary caregivers and are more likely than fathers to give up their job to care for their child, which can result in their social isolation (Coffey, 2006). It can be hard for mothers to get out of the house because of the difficulty in finding alternate caregivers. Also, travelling with the child may require extensive equipment, and there may be physical-access barriers. Some mothers may not have a social network of people who can help with child care, adding to their feelings of isolation (Yantzi, Rosenberg & McKeever, 2007).

Mothers often have greater needs for social support and positive appraisal of the situation, whereas fathers are more likely to use self-controlling behaviours to cope (Goldbeck, 2001).

The father of a child with special needs may struggle with issues that are distinct from those of the mother. He may think that his role of protector is challenged because he does not know how to help and cannot protect the family from the seemingly overwhelming recurring problems. With today's increased emphasis on fathers' involvement in the lives of their children, this vulnerability is felt more profoundly than in the past. Extensive stresses in the family can leave the father feeling depressed, weak, guilty, powerless, isolated, embarrassed, and angry. Fearful that he will lose control or be viewed as weak or ineffectual, the father will often hide feelings and display an outward confidence that may lead others to believe that everything is fine. Fathers may worry about what the future holds for their children, their ability to manage the increasing financial burden, and the daily disruptions of the entire family (Ahmann, 2006; Davies, B., et al., 2004). Some fathers escape in their work as a means of dulling the pain. Common coping strategies tend to be problem oriented and include praying, getting information, looking at options, and weighing choices, in addition to withdrawal (Gerlach, 2008; Marshall et al., 2003).

Lone-Parent Families

Lone-parent families are of special concern. As the only parent of a child who may require extensive, sophisticated, and lifelong care, lone parents may feel an enormous burden. Available financial and emotional resources may already be stretched to the limit. A special effort should be made to assist lone parents in finding financial and support services that can ease the burden of care. Nurses can also assist the lone parent in identifying helping roles that may be acceptable to relatives and friends.

Siblings

Results of studies on how siblings (almost exclusively European Americans) are affected by having a brother or sister with special needs are mixed (Barlow & Ellard, 2006). Generally, the evidence indicates a negative effect on siblings of children with a chronic illness when compared with siblings of healthy children. More recently, this effect has appeared to decrease in significance—most likely because of changes in public attitudes toward the ill and disabled (Sharpe & Rossiter, 2002). Newer research has shown that being a sibling of a child with special needs can have a positive impact on the sibling's life, in being generally more mature and independent and accepting of individual differences (Holland Bloorview Kids Rehabilitation Hospital, 2011).

However, siblings of children with chronic illness or disability also report depression and anxiety more often than their peers (Rossiter & Sharpe, 2001). They can experience guilt at not having their sibling's condition. Most investigators agree that brothers and sisters of children with special needs are no more at risk for severe psychiatric problems than are siblings of children without chronic or disabling conditions. A number of factors increase the risk of negative effects for siblings of ill children. Responsibility for caregiving, differential treatment by parents, and limitations in family resources and recreational time are often the experience of siblings of ill or disabled children (Lobato & Kao, 2002) (Box 41-4).

An important factor in sibling adjustment and coping is information and knowledge regarding their brother or sister's illness or disability. Siblings may be worried about what the disability or condition means and wonder if they can "catch it." They can also worry about how their sibling will fare in the future (Holland Bloorview Kids Rehabilitation Hospital, 2011). While parents are usually in the best position to impart information, they are often overwhelmed with the medical crisis at hand (Fleitas, 2000). Nurses can encourage parents to talk with the siblings about how they perceive their sick brother or sister and to be accepting of the siblings' feelings. Nurses can also be ideal educators and counsellors of siblings during the course of their brother's or sister's illness (Shepard & Mahon, 2000).

Coping With Ongoing Stress and Periodic Crises

Health care providers can help families cope with stress by providing anticipatory guidance and emotional support,

BOX 41-4 Supporting Siblings of Children With Special Needs

Promote Healthy Sibling Relationships

Value each child individually and avoid comparisons. Remind each child of his or her positive qualities and contribution to other family members.

Help siblings see the differences and similarities between themselves and a child with special needs. Create a climate in which children can achieve successes without feeling guilty.

Teach siblings ways to interact with the child.

Seek to be fair in terms of discipline, attention, and resources; require the affected child to do as much for him- or herself as possible.

Let siblings settle their own differences; intervene only to prevent siblings from hurting one another.

Legitimize reasonable anger. Even children with special needs behave badly sometimes.

Respect a sibling's reluctance to be with or to include the child with special needs in activities.

Help Siblings Cope

Listen to siblings to let them know that their thoughts and suggestions are valued.

Praise siblings when they have been patient, have sacrificed, or have been particularly helpful. Do not expect siblings to always act in this manner.

Acknowledge the personal strengths siblings have and their ability to cope with stress successfully.

Provide age-appropriate information about the child's condition, and update when appropriate.

Let teachers know what is happening so they can be understanding and helpful.

Recognize special stress times for siblings and plan to minimize negative effects.

Schedule special time with siblings; have a friend or family member substitute when a parent is unavailable.

Encourage siblings to join or help establish a sibling support group.

Use the services of professionals when needed. If a parent thinks that such a service is necessary for a sibling, it should be provided in as vigorous a manner as a service for the child with special needs.

Involve Siblings

Seek out ways to realistically include siblings in the care and treatment of the child with special needs.

Limit caregiving responsibilities and give recognition when siblings perform them.

Develop a library of children's books on special needs.

Invite siblings to attend meetings to develop plans for the child with special needs (e.g., individualized educational program, individualized family service plan).

Discuss future plans with them.

Solicit their ideas on treatment and service needs.

Have them visit professionals who work with the child.

Help them develop competencies to teach the child new skills.

Provide opportunities for siblings to advocate for the child.

Allow siblings to set their own pace for learning and involvement.

(Data from Carlson, J., Leviton, A., & Mueller, M. [1993]. Services to siblings: An important component of family-centered practice. *ACCH Advocate, 1*[1], 53–56; Powell, T., & Ogle, P. [1985]. *Brothers and sisters—a special part of exceptional families*. Baltimore: Paul H. Brooks; Spokane Washington Deaconess Medical Center, Pediatric Oncology Unit. [1987]. Tips for dealing with siblings. *Candlelighters Childhood Cancer Foundation Quarterly Newsletter, 11*[3,4], 7.)

assisting the family in assessing and identifying specific stressors, aiding the family in developing coping mechanisms and problem-solving strategies, and working collaboratively with parents so that they become empowered in the process.

Concurrent Stresses Within the Family

The ability to deal with the overwhelming stress of a lifelong disability or illness is challenged further when additional stresses are present. Stressors may be situational or developmental. They may be related to marital difficulties, sibling needs, homelessness, or social isolation. Some families may simultaneously be struggling with a family member's alcohol or other substance use issues. Even relatively minor stressors, such as arranging care for siblings, managing the home, and travelling to distant treatment centres, can challenge a family's ability to cope successfully.

Most families, regardless of their income or insurance coverage, have financial concerns. The costs of caring for a child with special needs can be overwhelming. Nurses and social workers can help a family review options for financial assistance, including insurance, and other financial resources; disease-related associations and support groups (Tam & Poon, 2008); and local philanthropic organizations.

Coping Mechanisms

Coping mechanisms are behaviours aimed at reducing the tension caused by a crisis. *Approach behaviours* are coping mechanisms that result in movement toward adjustment and resolution of the crisis. *Avoidance behaviours* result in movement away from adjustment and represent maladaptation to the crisis. Several approach and avoidance behaviours used in coping with a chronic illness or disability are listed in the Guidelines box. Each behaviour must be viewed in the context of all of the variables affecting the family. For example, the observation of several avoidance behaviours in an emotionally healthy family may denote significantly less risk to the successful resolution of the crisis than an equal number of avoidance behaviours in an individual who has few available supports.

Parental Empowerment

Empowerment can be seen as a process of recognizing, promoting, and enhancing competence. For parents of children with chronic conditions, empowerment may occur gradually as strength and capabilities are drawn on to master the child's care, manage family life, and plan for the future. Advocating for the child and developing parent–professional partnerships are part of the promotion of empowerment (Ray, 2002).

Assisting Family Members in Managing Their Feelings

Although previous research has postulated stages of adaptation to a chronic illness or disability, there is a great deal of individual variation in responses to the child's diagnosis, adjustments made, and time frames for coming to terms with a diagnosis. It is important that health care providers recognize and respect a wide range of reactions and coping mechanisms. In fact, members of the family of a child with a chronic illness or disability may experience a number of difficult emotions, including fear, guilt, anger, resentment, and anxiety. Learning to manage these emotions promotes adaptive coping (see Guidelines box). Support from health care providers other family members, and friends can assist family members in managing their feelings. The following discussion examines some common phases of adjustment and emotional reactions.

GUIDELINES Assessing Coping Behaviours

Approach Behaviours

- Asks for information regarding diagnosis and child's present condition
- Seeks help and support from others
- Anticipates future problems; actively seeks guidance and answers
- Endows the illness or disability with meaning
- Shares burden of disorder with others
- Plans realistically for the future
- Acknowledges and accepts child's awareness of diagnosis and prognosis
- Expresses feelings such as sorrow, depression, and anger and realizes reason for the emotional reaction
- Realistically perceives child's condition; adjusts to changes
- Recognizes own growth through passage of time, such as earlier denial and nonacceptance of diagnosis
- Expresses possible loss of child

Avoidance Behaviours

- Fails to recognize seriousness of child's condition despite physical evidence
- Refuses to agree to treatment
- Intellectualizes about the illness, but in areas unrelated to child's condition
- Is angry and hostile to members of the staff, regardless of their attitude or behaviour
- Avoids staff, family members, or child
- Entertains unrealistic future plans for child, with little emphasis on the present
- Is unable to adjust to or accept a change in progression of the disease
- Continually looks for new cures with no perspective toward possible benefit
- Refuses to acknowledge child's understanding of disease and prognosis
- Uses magical thinking and fantasy; may seek "occult" help
- Places complete faith in religion to point of relinquishing own responsibility
- Withdraws from outside world; refuses help
- Punishes self because of guilt and blame
- Makes no change in lifestyle to meet needs of other family members
- Resorts to excessive use of alcohol or drugs to avoid problems
- Expresses suicidal intent
- Is unable to discuss possible loss of child or previous experiences with death

Shock and Denial

The initial diagnosis of a chronic illness or disability is often met with intense emotion and is characterized by shock, disbelief, and sometimes **denial**, especially if the disorder is not obvious, as in chronic illness. Denial as a defence mechanism is necessary to prevent disintegration and is a normal response to grieving for any type of loss. Probably all family members experience various degrees of adaptive denial as they learn of the impact that the diagnosis has and will have on their lives.

In children, the importance of denial has repeatedly been demonstrated as a factor in their positive coping with the diagnosis. Denial allows the child to maintain hope in the face of overwhelming odds and to function adaptively and productively. Like hope, denial may be an adaptive mechanism for dealing with loss that persists until a family or patient is ready for or needs other responses.

Denial is probably the least understood and most poorly dealt-with reaction. Health care providers typically label denial as maladaptive and act inappropriately by attempting to strip it away by giving repeated and sometimes blunt explanations of the prognosis. Denial becomes maladaptive only when it prevents recognition of treatment or rehabilitative goals necessary for the child's optimal survival or development.

Adjustment

For most families, adjustment gradually follows shock and is usually characterized by an open admission that the condition exists. This stage may be accompanied by several responses, which are normal parts of the adaptation process. Probably the most universal of these feelings are guilt and self-accusation. Guilt is often greatest when the cause of the disorder is directly traceable to the parent, as in genetic diseases or accidental injury. It can occur even without any scientific or realistic basis for parental responsibility. Guilt stems from a false assumption that the disability is a result of personal failure or wrongdoing, such as not doing something correctly during pregnancy or the birth. Guilt may also be associated with cultural or religious beliefs. Some parents are convinced that they are being punished for some previous misdeed. Others may see the disorder as a trial sent by God to test their religious strength and faith. With correct information, support, and time, most parents master guilt and self-accusation. The ability to master resentful and self-accusatory feelings of having "caused" the child's disorder is a crucial factor in determining the parents' acceptance of their child.

Other common and normal reactions to a diagnosis are bitterness and anger. Anger directed inward may be evident as self-reproaching or punitive behaviour, such as neglecting one's health and verbally degrading oneself. Anger directed outward may be manifested in either open arguments or withdrawal from communication and may be evident in the person's relationship with the spouse, the child, and siblings. Passive anger toward the ill child may be evident in decreased visiting, refusal to believe how sick the child is, or inability to provide comfort. Among the most common targets for parental anger are members of the staff. Parents may complain about the nursing care, the insufficient time physicians spend with them, or the lack of skill of those who draw blood or start intravenous infusions.

Children are likely to respond with anger as well, and this includes the affected child and the well siblings. Children are aware of the loss engendered by their illness or disability and may react angrily to the restrictions imposed or the feelings of being different. Siblings may also feel anger and resentment toward the ill child and the parents for the loss of routine and parental attention. It is difficult for older children and almost impossible for younger children to comprehend the plight of the affected child. Their perception is of a brother or sister who has the undivided attention of their parents, is showered with cards and gifts, and is the focus of everyone's concern.

During the period of adjustment, four types of parental reactions to the child influence the child's eventual response to the disorder:

1. Overprotection, in which the parents fear letting the child achieve any new skill, avoid all discipline, and cater to every desire to prevent frustration (Box 41-5)
2. Rejection, in which the parents detach themselves emotionally from the child but usually provide adequate physical care or constantly nag and scold the child
3. Denial, in which parents act as if the disorder does not exist or attempt to have the child overcompensate for it
4. Gradual acceptance, in which parents place necessary and realistic restrictions on the child, encourage self-care activities, and promote reasonable physical and social abilities

Reintegration and Acknowledgement

For many families the adjustment process culminates in the development of realistic expectations for the child and reintegration of family life with the illness or disability in a manageable perspective. Because a large portion of this phase is one of grief for a loss, total resolution is not possible until the child

BOX 41-5 Characteristics of Parental Overprotection

- Sacrifices self and rest of family for the child
- Continually helps the child, even when the child is capable
- Is inconsistent with regard to discipline or employs no discipline; frequently applies different rules to the siblings
- Is dictatorial and arbitrary, making decisions without considering the child's wishes, such as keeping the child from attending school
- Hovers and offers suggestions; calls attention to every activity, overdoes praise
- Protects the child from every possible discomfort
- Restricts play, often because of fear that the child will be injured
- Denies the child opportunities for growing up and assuming responsibility, such as learning to give own medications or perform treatments
- Does not understand the child's capabilities and sets goals too high or too low
- Monopolizes the child's time, such as sleeping with the child, permitting few friends, or refusing participation in social or educational activities

dies or leaves home as an independent adult. Therefore, one can regard adjustment as "increased comfort" with everyday living rather than a complete resolution.

This adjustment phase also involves social reintegration in which the family broadens its activities to include relationships outside the home, with the child as an accepted and participating member of the group. This last criterion often differentiates the reaction of gradual acceptance during the adjustment period from total acceptance, or perhaps is more descriptive of the acknowledgement process.

Many parents of children with chronic illnesses experience **chronic sorrow**, feelings of sorrow and loss that recur in waves over time. As the child's condition progresses, parents may experience repeated losses that represent further declines and new caregiving demands. Consequently, families must be assessed on an ongoing basis and offered appropriate support and resources as their needs change over time (Doig et al., 2009).

Establishing a Support System

The diagnosis of a child with a serious health problem or disability is a major **situational crisis** that affects the entire family system. Families can experience positive outcomes as they successfully deal with the many challenges that accompany a child with chronic illness or disability.

One nursing goal is to assess which families are at greater or lesser risk for succumbing to the effects of the crisis. Several variables—available support system, perception of the event, coping mechanisms, reactions to the child, available resources, and concurrent stresses within the family—influence the resolution of a crisis. Although most families cope well, the needs of families at risk are great. If they receive emotional support and guidance early, there is an increased likelihood that they will also cope successfully.

Although it is easy to assume that families of children with the most severe illnesses or disabilities would have the poorest adjustment, the severity of the condition reflects only one part of the overall picture. The level of adjustment is significantly influenced by the *functional burden* on the individual family (Baillargeon & Bernier, 2010; Brehaut et al., 2009; Lach et al., 2009). This concept considers the issues related to caring for and living with the child in relation to the family's resources and ability to cope (Box 41-6). The family of a child with multiple disabilities demanding complex care, yet having many resources and coping skills, may adjust more successfully to the child's situation than the family of a child with a less serious condition and few resources to counterbalance.

Intrafamilial resources, social support from friends and relatives, parent-to-parent support, parent–professional partnerships, and community resources interweave to provide a flexible web of support for the family of a child with a chronic condition.

BOX 41-6 Concept of Functional Burden

Impact of the Child With Special Needs

The child's need for medical and nursing care
The child's fixed deficits
The child's age-appropriate dependency in activities of daily living
The disruptions in the family routine caused by the care
The psychological burden of the prognosis on the family

Family Resources and Ability to Cope

The family's physical resources
The family's emotional resources
The family's educational resources
The family's social supports and available help
The competing demands for family members' time and energy

(Data from Doig, J. L., McLennan, J. D., & Urichuk. [2009]. "Jumping through hoops": Parents' experiences with seeking respite care for children with special needs. *Child: Care, Health and Development, 35*[2], 234–242.)

The Child With Special Needs

The child's reaction to chronic illness or disability depends to a great extent on his or her developmental level, temperament, and available coping mechanisms; on the reactions of family members or significant others; and, to a lesser extent, on the condition itself. A child's conceptual understanding of his or her own illness is based not only on age and developmental level but also on the duration and type of experience accumulated with the disease. Knowledge of these variables is essential in providing the kind of information and support these children need in order to cope with a sometimes overwhelming situation.

Developmental Aspects

The impact of a chronic illness or disability is influenced by the age at onset. While chronic illness affects children of all ages, the developmental aspects of each age group dictate particular stresses and risks for the child. The nurse must also recognize that children need to redefine their condition and its implications as they develop and grow. For example, appearance, skills, and abilities are highly valued by peers (Fig. 41-1); a teenager who is limited in any of these qualities is subject to rejection. This is especially marked when a physical disability interferes with sexual attractiveness. Developmental effects of chronic illness or disability on children are described in Table 41-2 (p. 1171).

Coping Mechanisms

Children with chronic conditions tend to use five distinct patterns of coping (Box 41-7). Children with more positive and accepting attitudes about their chronic illness use a more adaptive coping style characterized by optimism, competence, and compliance. They show fewer behavioural problems at home and at school. The two maladaptive coping patterns—"Feels different and withdraws" and "Is irritable, is moody, and acts out"—are associated with poorer adaptation; children using these strategies have poorer self-concepts, more negative attitudes about their conditions, and more behavioural problems at home and at school.

Well-adapted children gradually learn to accept their physical limitations and find achievement in a variety of

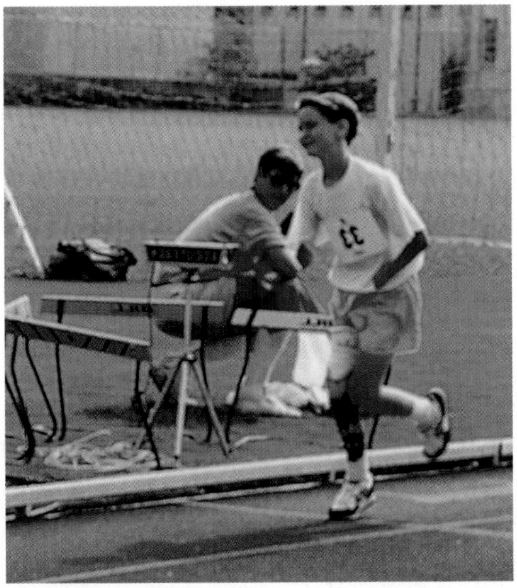

Fig. 41-1 Children with any type of impairment should have the opportunity to develop their skills. *(Courtesy Poyo/Hinton Photography.)*

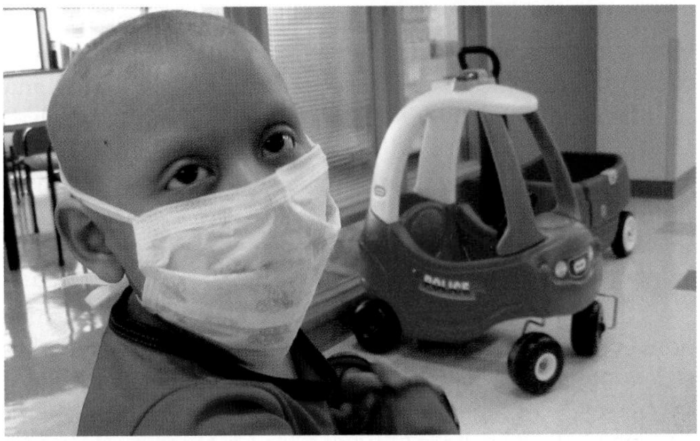

Fig. 41-2 Periods of sadness and anger are appropriate in the child's adjustment to a chronic illness or disability, especially during exacerbations of the disorder.

BOX 41-7 Coping Patterns Used by Children With Special Needs

Develops competence and optimism—Accentuates the positive aspects of the situation and concentrates more on what he or she has or can do than on what is missing or on what he or she cannot do; is as independent as possible

Feels different and withdraws—Sees self as being different from other children because of the chronic health condition; views being different as negative; sees self as less worthy than others; focuses on things he or she cannot do and sometimes over-restricts activities needlessly

Is irritable, is moody, and acts out—Uses proactive and self-initiated coping behaviours, although usually counterproductive in that the behaviours are not ego enhancing or socially responsible and do not result in desired outcomes; acts out irritably, which may or may not be associated with condition's symptoms

Complies with treatment—Takes necessary medications, treatments; adheres to activity restrictions; also uses behaviours that indicate developing independence (e.g., assumes responsibility for taking medication)

Seeks support—Talks with adults, children, physicians, and nurses; develops plans to handle problems as they occur; uses downward comparison (i.e., realizes that others have it worse)

(Modified from Austin, J., Patterson, J., & Huberty, T. [1991]. Development of the Coping Health Inventory for children. *Journal of Pediatric Nursing, 6*[3], 166–174.)

compensatory motor and intellectual pursuits. They function well at home, at school, and with peers. They understand their disorder, which allows them to accept their limitations, assume responsibility for care, and assist in treatment and rehabilitation regimens. They express appropriate emotions, such as sadness, anxiety, and anger, at times of exacerbations, but confidence and guarded optimism during periods of clinical stability (Fig. 41-2). They are able to identify with other similarly affected individuals, promoting positive self-images and displaying pride and self-confidence in their ability to lead a productive, successful life despite the disability.

Hopefulness

Children, particularly adolescents, function well or poorly depending on the presence or absence of hope. Hopefulness is an internal quality that mobilizes humans into goal-directed action that may be satisfying and life sustaining. A sense of hopefulness can produce increased participation in health-seeking behaviours and an improved sense of well-being (Kausar, Jevne, & Sobsey, 2003).

Health Education and Self-Care

Health education is an intervention that promotes better skilled coping. Children need information about their condition, the therapeutic plan, and how the disease or the therapy might affect their particular situation. Children nearing puberty also need to understand the maturation process and how their disability may alter this event. A youngster with Crohn's disease should understand that this disorder is associated with growth failure and delayed puberty; a child with diabetes needs to know that hormonal changes and increased growth needs will alter food and insulin requirements at this time; and a sexually active girl with sickle cell anemia or systemic lupus erythematosus needs to be aware of the risks of pregnancy. The information should not be given all at once but should be timed appropriately to meet the changing needs of the youth, and it should be described and repeated as often as the situation demands.

Responses to Parental Behaviour

Parental behaviour toward the child is one of the more important factors influencing the child's adjustment. In one study, children's perceptions of their mothers' support and maternal perceptions of the psychosocial impact of the child's chronic illness on the family were two of the major predictors of children's psychological adjustment (Immelt, 2006).

Family organization and illness-related support and involvement of parents can influence children's adjustment to chronic illness (Schor, 2003). They often display pride and confidence in their ability to cope successfully with the challenges imposed by their disorder. Anticipatory guidance by the nurse and encouragement of normalizing practices may assist parents in facilitating their child's adjustment.

Type of Illness or Disability

The type of illness or disability also influences the child's emotional response. Interestingly, children with more severe disorders often cope better than those with milder conditions. The presence of multiple conditions may place a child at risk for more behavioural problems (Halfon & Newacheck, 2010). Considering children's cognitive ability and their delay in achieving abstract thinking until adolescence, it is likely that an obvious condition is easier to accept because its limitations are concrete. Children who are blind or physically disabled are constantly reminded of their inability to run. Children with cardiac defects live by rules they do not understand, but also only vaguely and occasionally sense their illness, such as when they try to run and experience dyspnea and fatigue. Therefore, some chronic illnesses pose special threats to children.

The onset of a disabling condition may generate a state of confusion for children, who may have trouble differentiating between actual bodily functions and their image of their bodies. They may also experience problems in identifying themselves and extensions of the self (e.g., wheelchairs, braces, other mechanical or prosthetic devices) and may have difficulty in accepting functional aids.

Nursing Care of the Family and Child With Special Needs

Assessment

Because the nurse may meet a family during any phase of the adjustment process, several assessment areas are important. The family's ability to cope with previous stresses will influence the current situation, and answers to questions about their usual coping skills can provide insight into their ability to cope with having a child with special needs. Knowledge of concurrent stresses, such as financial, marital, and career or unemployment, will help the nurse identify families who may have fewer resources to cope with the child's needs.

Finally, awareness of family members' reactions to the child and the illness or disability is important. Sample questions that the nurse and family can use to evaluate the support system, perception of the illness, coping mechanisms, resources, and concurrent stresses are listed in Table 41-1. Because factors affecting the family's response may change at any point during the illness, assessment must be a continual process.

Special challenges exist in assessing the child's feelings about having a disability. Chapter 34 presents several approaches to encouraging a child to discuss feelings about the condition. The nurse should use a variety of communication techniques, such as drawing and play, as assessment tools rather than relying solely on parental reports. Often, children are neglected partners in their care, and their unique needs are not identified (Young et al., 2003).

The needs of working parents and siblings also should be assessed, a goal that requires flexibility in scheduling appointments to include these important family members. When working parents know that their input is valuable, they will often change their work schedule to meet with a health care provider. Because siblings can be of any age, the use of appropriate communication strategies for assessment must be considered. Nonverbal techniques such as those discussed in Chapter 34 should be considered for these children.

The main objective in working with the family is to help them cope effectively with those stresses imposed by the child's special needs. To achieve this goal, the entire family should be considered in every aspect of the implementation process.

Provide Support at the Time of Diagnosis

The diagnosis is a critical time for parents and can influence how they perceive their health care providers throughout care. Although they may not hear or remember all that is said to them, they can sense the health care provider's attitude, whether it be acceptance, rejection, hope, or despair, and this may influence their ability to absorb the shock and begin adapting to the family's altered future.

Parents may be encouraged to be together when they are informed of their child's condition, thus avoiding the problem of one parent having to interpret or convey complex findings and deal with the initial emotional reaction of the other. The informing session should take place in a private, comfortable setting free of distractions and interruptions, in an atmosphere in which the parents feel free to express their emotions. Their emotional needs need to be acknowledged through acceptance of such expressions as crying, sadness, anger, and disappointment. Emotional support can be offered by having tissues available if a family member cries and demonstrating through facial and body language that this is a difficult and painful period. Although touching is a powerful expression of empathy, it must be used wisely. For example, it can prematurely terminate free expression of feelings, especially when combined with statements such as "Everything will be all right." Nurses should also be aware of cultural issues regarding touching; some individuals of certain cultures may not welcome being touched.

Parents should receive the kind of information they desire. This can be assessed by asking questions such as "Do you prefer to hear detailed information?" Parents or other family members may have different preferences regarding the amount of information they wish to hear. Most parents want a clear, simple explanation of the diagnosis; a prediction of possible futures for the child; advice on what to do next; an opportunity to ask questions; a warm, sympathetic listener; and, most important, time. Understanding of explanations is elicited with such questions as "Do you see what I mean?" or "Is this clear to you?" Technical terms should be clarified with simple, written definitions.

Finally, the informing conference does not end with the presentation of devastating news. Instead, the child's strengths, appealing behaviours, and potential for development need to

Table 41-1 Assessment of Factors Affecting Family Adjustment

FACTORS AFFECTING ADJUSTMENT	ASSESSMENT QUESTIONS
Available Support System	
Status of marital relationship	To whom do you talk when you have something on your mind? (If answer is not the spouse, ask for the reason.)
Alternate support systems	When something is worrying you, what do you do? What helps you most when you are upset?
Ability to communicate	Does talking seem to help when you feel upset?
Perception of the Illness or Disability	
Previous knowledge of disorder	Have you ever heard the word (name of diagnosis) before? Tell me about it (if answer is "yes").
Imagined cause of disorder	What are your thoughts about the causes of the disorder?
Effects of illness or disability on family	How has your child's illness or disability affected you and your family? How has your lifestyle changed?
Coping Mechanisms	
Reactions to previous crises	Tell me one time you've had another crisis (problem, bad time) in your family. How did you solve that problem?
Reactions to the child	Do you find yourself being a little more cautious with this child than with your other children?
Childrearing practices	Do you feel as comfortable disciplining this child as your other children?
Influence of religion	Has your religion or faith been of help to you? Tell me how (if answer is "yes").
Attitudes	How is this child different from the siblings or other children of similar age? Describe your child's personality. Is it easy, difficult, or in between? When you think of your child's future, what thoughts come to mind?
Available Resources	
	What parts of your child's care are causing the most difficulty for you or your family? What services are available to help? What services do you need that currently are not available?
Concurrent Stresses	
	What other problems are you facing now? (Be specific; ask about financial, marital, or sibling stresses, and concerns around extended family or friends.)

be stressed, as well as available rehabilitation efforts or treatment. Parents can be encouraged to view their experiences as a series of challenges that they are capable of handling, particularly with available professional feedback. Parents need to be assured that the nurse will be available to answer questions and provide further assistance. Because of the need for long-term follow-up, the initial informing interview is only one in a series of continuing discussions. In all interactions the family's input needs to be solicited and incorporated into the care plan. Some situations require consideration of special problems.

Support the Family's Coping Methods

For the family to meet the stresses of optimally adjusting to the child's condition, each member must be individually supported so that the family system is strong. Although the family can indefinitely support a member who is in need of assistance, its greatest strength lies in every member supporting each other. The nurse should bear in mind that the family member in greatest need is not necessarily the affected child but may be a parent or sibling who is dealing with stresses.

Parents

The nurse can provide support by being attentive to families' responses to their children. Mothers and fathers need to experience success, joy, and pride in their children in order to give the support they need. Children, too, require support for their interactions, adjustments, and efforts. Their attempts to get to know their care providers and to communicate their needs to them must be reinforced with support.

It is important for nurses to examine their attitudes to determine their ability to engage in parent–professional partnerships. An essential characteristic for this partnership is the belief that parents are equal to professionals and are experts in caring for their child (see Patient Teaching box).

Communication among all family members is also encouraged. Parent group sessions can help parents express thoughts and feelings to each other but often do not take into account siblings' or the child's viewpoint. Therefore, the nurse may need to set up a family session, such as during a home or clinic visit. Although the ideal situation is to have all the members present at one time, often this is not possible. Inviting members to participate at various visits is an appropriate alternative.

PATIENT TEACHING Developing Successful Parent–Professional Partnerships

- Promote primary nursing; in nonhospital settings designate a case manager.
- Acknowledge parents' overall competence and their unique expertise with their child.
- Respect parents' time as having value equal to that of other members of child's health care team.
- Explain or define any medical, technical, or discipline-specific terms.
- Tell families, "I am not sure" or "I don't know," when appropriate.
- Facilitate family's effectiveness in team meetings (e.g., provide parents with same information as other participants).

Parents can be encouraged to discuss their feelings toward the child, the impact of this event on their marriage, and associated stresses such as financial burdens. In addition, the family wage earner may have to sacrifice job opportunities to remain close to a medical facility or to avoid losing insurance benefits.

The nurse needs to regard both parents as able, effective parents, competent and capable of coping with the challenges they face. Every effort should be made to include the parent working outside the home in visits, such as to the nursery, clinic, special school, and stimulation programs. This parent, who is often the father, needs to be included in the assessment process, with specific emphasis on having him describe the child's strengths and difficulties. It is not unusual to find two parents who have differing views of the child's abilities, especially in the area of developmental disabilities (Ahmann, 2006).

Numerous volunteer and community resources are available that provide assistance, rehabilitation, equipment, and funding for a variety of health problems (see Additional Resources at the end of this chapter). National and local disease-oriented organizations may provide needed assistance and support to families that qualify. Provincial and federal departments of health, mental health, social services, and labour may be able to help locate appropriate regional resources. For example, provincial programs for children with special health needs can provide financial assistance for children with many disabling conditions. Local and national sources of respite care and medical day care may also be useful to families. Nurses should become acquainted with these resources in their communities and with vocational programs for special groups.

Parent-to-Parent Support

Just being with another parent who has shared similar experiences can be helpful. It may not need to be a parent of a child with the same diagnosis, since parents in the process of adjusting to a child with special needs—or finding respite services, educational or rehabilitative services, special equipment vendors, and financial counselling—tread a common path.

A parent self-help group can be a means of promoting parent-to-parent support. Group members usually feel less alone and have the opportunity to observe both coping and mastery role-modelling from other members. Parents' groups are also rich resources for information. Even if parents are unable to attend meetings, they can still benefit from group newsletters, blogs, and other resources that often accompany membership.

The nurse can foster parent participation in self-help groups by serving as a referral agent, a group advisory board member, a resource person, a group member, or an assistant in founding a group. Sometimes all that is required to start a group is identifying one or two parents as leaders; sharing with them the names, telephone numbers, and e-mail addresses of other families who have expressed both an interest and a willingness to release this information; and guiding them in how to initiate a first meeting.

Advocate for Empowerment

Nurses can advocate for methods that foster opportunities for parent empowerment. For example, nurses can suggest reimbursement for travel and child care, plus stipends to enable parents' voices to be heard at meetings and conferences. They can encourage parent membership on relevant committees and boards. They can also keep parents informed of pending legislation on child health issues or take action when parents inform them of such initiatives.

The Child

Through ongoing contacts with the child, the nurse will be able to (1) observe the child's responses to the disorder, ability to function, and adaptive behaviours within the environment and with significant others; (2) explore the child's own understanding of his or her illness or condition; and (3) provide support while the child learns to cope with his or her feelings. Children should be encouraged to express their concerns rather than allowing others to express them for them, since open discussions may reduce anxiety.

One of the most important interventions is alleviating the child's feeling of being different and normalizing his or her life as much as possible (see Patient Teaching box, Promoting Normalization). Whenever possible, the nurse should assist the family in assessing the child's daily routine for indications of a need for normalizing practices. For example, the child who remains in a bedroom all day requires a restructured daily routine to provide activities in different parts of the house, such as eating in the kitchen or dining room with the family. Such children may also be deprived of social, recreational, and academic activities that can be better accommodated by applying normalization practices. For example, home and out-of-home health-related treatments should be planned at times that interfere as little as possible with normal daily activities.

Children who are concerned that their condition detracts from their physical attractiveness need attention focused on the normal or conventional aspects of appearance and capabilities. Health care providers can help strengthen and consolidate a child's self-image and help the child fit in with his or her peer group, while allowing the child to express anger, isolation, fear of rejection, feelings of sadness, and loneliness. Children need positive reinforcement for their efforts at

PATIENT TEACHING Promoting Normalization

Preparation—Prepare child in advance for changes that may occur from the illness or disability.
Example—Tell the child in advance the possible adverse effects of medication therapy.

Participation—Include child in as many decisions as possible, especially those relating to his or her care regimen.
Example—The child is responsible for taking medications or scheduling home treatments.

Sharing—Allow family members and the child's peers to be a part of the care regimen whenever possible.
Examples—Give the child his or her medication when the other siblings receive their vitamins.
The parent cooks the same menu for the whole family.
If the child is invited to another's home, the parent advises the family of the child's dietary restrictions.

Control—Identify areas where child can be in control, to decrease feelings of uncertainty, passivity, and helplessness.
Example—The child identifies activities that are appropriate to his or her energy level and chooses to rest when fatigued.

Expectation—Apply the same family rules to the child with a chronic illness or disability as those used with the well siblings or peers.
Example—The child is disciplined, is expected to fulfill household responsibilities, and attends school in accordance with abilities.

enhancing their self-image and for any evidence of improvement. Anything that might improve attractiveness and contribute to a positive self-image should be employed, such as makeup for a teenager with a scar, clothing that disguises a prosthesis, or a hairstyle or wig to cover a deformity or lost hair.

Siblings

The presence of a child with special needs in a family may result in parents paying less attention to the other children. Siblings may respond by developing negative attitudes toward the child or by expressing anger in different forms. The nurse can help by using anticipatory guidance—questioning the parents about what they believe is the best way to have siblings respond to the child and guiding them through ways to meet their other children's needs for attention. This questioning should take place before serious negative effects occur.

Siblings may also experience embarrassment associated with having a brother or sister with an illness or disability. Parents are then faced with the difficulty of responding to this embarrassment in an understanding and appropriate manner without punishing the siblings for how they feel. Parents should be encouraged to talk with the siblings about how they view their affected sibling. For example, siblings of a child who is cognitively impaired may express fears about their ability to bear normal children. Adolescents in particular may not be able to discuss these vital issues with their parents and may prefer to consult with the nurse. Many siblings benefit from sharing their concerns with other young people who are in a similar situation. Support groups for siblings can help decrease isolation, promote expression of feelings, and provide examples of effective coping skills.

The nurse needs to be sensitive to the reactions of siblings and, whenever possible, intervene to promote more positive adjustment. For example, siblings often mention that they are expected to take on additional responsibilities to help the parents care for the child. It is not unusual for them to express a positive reaction to assuming the extra duties but a negative response to feeling unappreciated for doing so. Such feelings can often be minimized by encouraging siblings to discuss this with the parents and by suggesting to parents ways of showing gratitude, such as an increase in allowance, special privileges, and, most significantly, verbal praise.

Educate About the Disorder and General Health Care

Educating the family about the disorder is actually an extension of revealing the diagnosis. Education involves not only supplying technical information but also discussing how the condition will affect the child. Parents may be able to digest only so much information at a time. It may be helpful to provide essential information and then follow by asking, "What else would you like to know about your child's condition?" Responding to parents' questions and concerns ensures that their information needs are met.

Activities of Daily Living

Parents also need guidance in how the condition may interfere with or alter activities of daily living, such as eating, dressing, sleeping, and toileting. One area frequently affected is nutrition. Common problems are undernutrition resulting from food being inappropriately restricted, or loss of appetite, vomiting, or motor deficits that interfere with feeding; overnutrition may also occur, usually because of a caloric intake in excess of energy expenditure or boredom and lack of stimulation in other areas. Although the child requires the same basic nutrients as other children, daily requirements may differ. Special nutritional considerations are discussed as appropriate throughout the text.

Safe Transportation

Modifications may also be needed regarding car safety. Children with conditions such as low birth weight or orthopaedic, neuromuscular, or respiratory problems often cannot safely use conventional car restraints. For example, children with hip spica casts cannot sit properly in child safety seats (see Developmental Dysplasia of the Hip, Chapter 54). Families will need assistance in determining the modifications allowed in their vehicles without affecting safety and insurance coverage (see Chapter 36). Transport Canada strictly limits the amount a car seat can be modified after sale. Safe Kids Canada has valuable information for families on car seat safety (see Additional Resources at the end of this chapter).

If a child requires a wheelchair, the family should consult the wheelchair manufacturer for specific instructions regarding safe transportation by car. Considerations for wheelchairs used with vehicle transportation include securing both the wheelchair and the occupant in the wheelchair. Wheelchairs should be secured facing forward with tie downs at four points. The tie-down system should be dynamically crash tested, as should the occupant securement system that secures the child in the wheelchair. For example, the use of trays would not be recommended for transportation. With children who must travel with additional medical equipment (e.g., oxygen, monitors, or ventilators), this equipment should be anchored to the floor or underneath the vehicle seat or wheelchair. Soft padding should be added around the equipment to reduce movement. A second adult should be present to monitor the condition of a medically fragile child while travelling.

Primary Health Care

Children with special needs require all the usual health care recommended for any child. Attention to injury prevention, immunizations, dental health, and regular physical examinations is essential. Nurses can play an important role in reminding parents of these aspects that are so often neglected when the concern is focused on the child's illness or disability. Specific discussions of nutrition, sleep and activity, dental health, and injury prevention are presented in the chapters on health promotion for specific age groups (see Chapters 36–40). Immunizations are discussed in Chapter 36.

Parents also need to be aware of the importance of communicating the child's condition in the event of a medical emergency. Young children are unable to give information about their disorder, and although older children may be reliable sources, after an accident they may be physically unable to speak. Therefore, all children with any type of chronic condition that may affect medical care should wear some type of identification, such as a MedicAlert bracelet (see Additional Resources), and carry a card from MedicAlert in their wallet that lists the medical condition and a phone number as well as Internet links for accessing emergency medical records and other personal information.

Promote Normal Development

Aside from knowledge of the condition and its effect on the child's abilities, the family must be guided toward fostering appropriate development in their child. Although each stage may take longer to achieve, parents should be guided toward helping the child fully realize his or her potential in preparation for the next developmental stage. Table 41-2 outlines developmental aspects of chronic illness or disability and supportive interventions. With appropriate planning and knowledge of strategies to improve the child's functional abilities, most children can live fulfilling and productive lives.

One important aspect of promoting normal development is to encourage the child's self-care abilities in both activities of daily living and the medical regimen. An assessment of the child's age and physical, emotional, and mental capacities, as well as the support and structure provided by the family, should be considered in determining the appropriate level of self-care in the medical regimen. Even toddlers can be involved in their own care by holding supplies for the parent during a procedure. Over time, children should be encouraged toward greater autonomy in their own self-care.

Early Childhood

During infancy the child is achieving basic trust through a satisfying, intimate, consistent relationship with his or her parents. A special-needs child's early existence may be stressful, chaotic, and unsatisfying. Consequently, he or she may need more parental support and expressions of affection to achieve trust. Likewise, the parents require assistance in finding ways to meet the infant's needs, such as how to hold a rigid or flaccid infant, how to feed a child with tongue thrust or episodes of dyspnea, and how to stimulate a child who seems incapable of achieving any skills.

During early childhood the goal is to achieve separation from parents, autonomy, and initiative. The natural parental response to having a sick child is overprotection. Parents need help in realizing the importance of allowing brief separations of the child from them and from others involved in the child's care and of providing social experiences outside the home whenever possible. Respite care, which provides temporary relief for family members, can be essential in allowing caregivers time away from the daily burdens.

Young children also need the opportunity to develop independence. Frequently the child is able to learn self-help skills, such as holding the bottle, finger feeding, and removing simple articles of clothing, but the parent continues to perform the act. The nurse can guide parents to the usual milestones expected for the child. When a child is unable to perform a skill independently, functional aids should be used. With innovation, many adaptations can be implemented in children's environments to increase their mobility and independence and allow them to play like other children their age. For example, with slight modifications, a child with physical limitations may be able to ride a tricycle (Fig. 41-3).

Another critical component for normal child development is discipline. Discipline and guidance serve several purposes,

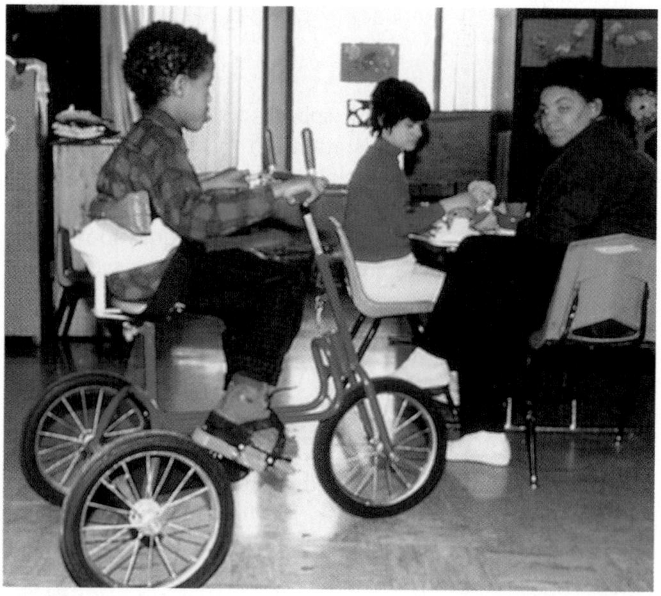

Fig. 41-3 A modified tricycle with block pedals, self-adhesive straps for support, and modified seat and handle bars can help a child with disabilities gain mobility.

Table 41-2 Developmental Effects of Chronic Illness or Disability on Children

DEVELOPMENTAL TASKS	POTENTIAL EFFECTS OF CHRONIC ILLNESS OR DISABILITY	SUPPORTIVE INTERVENTIONS
Infancy		
Develop a sense of trust	Multiple caregivers and frequent separations, especially if hospitalized Deprived of consistent nurturing	Encourage consistent caregivers in hospital or other care settings. Encourage parental presence, "rooming in" during hospitalization, and participation in care.
Bond, or attach, to parent	Delayed because of separation; parental grief for loss of "dream" child; parental inability to accept the condition, especially a visible defect	Emphasize healthy, perfect qualities of infant. Help parents learn special care needs of infant for them to feel competent.
Learn through sensorimotor experiences	More exposure to painful experiences than pleasurable ones Limited contact with environment from restricted movement or confinement	Expose infant to pleasurable experiences through all senses (touch, hearing, sight, taste, movement). Encourage age-appropriate developmental skills (e.g., holding bottle, finger feeding, crawling).
Begin to develop a sense of separateness from parent	Increased dependency on parent for care Overinvolvement of parent in care	Encourage all family members to participate in care to prevent overinvolvement of one member. Encourage periodic respite from demands of care responsibilities.
Toddlerhood		
Develop autonomy	Increased dependency on parent	Encourage independence in as many areas as possible (e.g., toileting, dressing, feeding).
Master locomotor and language skills	Limited opportunity to test own abilities and limits	Provide gross motor skill activity and modification of toys or equipment, such as a modified swing or rocking horse.
Learn through sensorimotor experience; beginning preoperational thought	Increased exposure to painful experiences	Give choices to allow simple feeling of control (e.g., choice of what book to look at, what kind of sandwich to eat). Institute age-appropriate discipline and limit-setting. Recognize that negative and ritualistic behaviours are normal. Provide sensory experiences (e.g., water play, sandbox play, finger painting).
Preschool		
Develop initiative and purpose Master self-care skills	Limited opportunities for success in accomplishing simple tasks or mastering self-care skills	Encourage mastery of self-care skills. Provide devices that make task easier (e.g., self-dressing).
Begin to develop peer relationships	Limited opportunities for socialization with peers; may appear "like a baby" to age-mates Protection within tolerant and secure family causing child to fear criticism and withdraw	Encourage socialization (e.g., inviting friends to play, day care experience, trips to park). Provide age-appropriate play, especially associative play opportunities. Emphasize child's abilities; dress appropriately to enhance desirable appearance.
Develop sense of body image and sexual identification	Awareness of body centring on pain, anxiety, and failure Gender-role identification focused primarily on mothering skills	Encourage relationships with same-sex and opposite-sex peers and adults.
Learn through preoperational thought (magical thinking)	Guilt (thinking he or she caused the illness or disability or is being punished for wrongdoing)	Help child deal with criticisms; realize that too much protection prevents child from learning to cope with realities of the world. Clarify that child's illness or disability is not his or her fault or a punishment.

Continued

Table 41-2 Developmental Effects of Chronic Illness or Disability on Children—Cont'd

DEVELOPMENTAL TASKS	POTENTIAL EFFECTS OF CHRONIC ILLNESS OR DISABILITY	SUPPORTIVE INTERVENTIONS
School Age		
Develop a sense of accomplishment	Limited opportunities to achieve and compete (e.g., many school absences, inability to join regular athletic activities)	Encourage school attendance; schedule medical visits at times other than school; encourage child to make up missed work.
Form peer relationships	Limited opportunities for socialization	Educate teachers and classmates about child's condition, abilities, and special needs. Encourage sports activities (e.g., Special Olympics). Encourage socialization (e.g., Girl Guides, Campfire, Boy Scouts, 4-H Club; having a best friend or club membership).
Learn through concrete operations	Incomplete comprehension of the imposed physical limitations or treatment of the disorder	Provide child with information about his or her condition. Encourage creative activities (e.g., VSA Arts, Ontario and Québec affiliates).
Adolescence		
Develop personal and sexual identity	Increased sense of feeling different from peers and reduced ability to compete with peers in appearance, abilities, special skills	Help child realize that many of the difficulties the teenager is experiencing are part of normal adolescence (rebelliousness, risk taking, lack of cooperation, hostility toward authority).
Achieve independence from family	Increased dependency on family; limited job or career opportunities	Provide instruction on interpersonal and coping skills. Encourage increased responsibility for care and management of the disease or condition (e.g., assuming responsibility for making and keeping appointment [ideally alone], sharing assessment and planning stages of health care delivery, contacting resources). Discuss planning for future and how condition can affect choices.
Form healthy sexual relationships	Limited opportunities for healthy sexual friendships; less opportunity to discuss sexual concerns with peers Increased concern with issues such as why did the teen get this disorder, can he or she have a relationship and have a family	Encourage socialization with peers, including peers with special needs and those without special needs. Encourage activities appropriate for age (e.g., attending mixed-gender parties, sports activities, driving a car). Be alert to cues that signal readiness for information regarding implications of condition on sexuality and reproduction. Emphasize good appearance and wearing stylish clothes, use of makeup. Understand that the adolescent has the same sexual needs and concerns as any other teenager.
Learn through abstract thinking	Decreased opportunity for earlier stages of cognition impeding achievement of level of abstract thinking	Provide instruction on decision making, assertiveness, and other skills necessary to manage personal plans.

such as providing children with boundaries at which to test their behaviour and teaching them socially acceptable behaviour. Resentment and hostility can arise among siblings if different standards are applied to each child. The nurse's responsibility is to help parents learn successful methods of managing a child's behaviours before they become problems.

School Age

For school-age children, the major tasks are entry into school and achieving a sense of industry. Although the importance of school in the life of all children is well known, school absences are significantly higher among children with chronic illness than among their healthy peers. The more school absences the child experiences, the more difficult it is to resume attendance, and school phobia may result. The child should return to school as soon as possible after diagnosis or treatments.

Preparation for entry into or resumption of school is best accomplished through a team approach with the parents, child, teacher, community health nurse, and primary nurse in the hospital. Ideally, this planning should begin before hospital discharge, provided that the child is well enough to resume usual activities. A structured plan should be developed, with attention to those aspects of care that must be continued during school hours, such as administration of medication or other treatments.

Children also need preparation before entering or resuming school. Having a tutor in the hospital or home as soon as children are physically able helps them realize that school will continue and gives them time to consider this prospect (Fig. 41-4). They need to investigate possible answers to the many questions others will ask. One method of anticipatory preparation is to role-play, with the child as the "returned pupil" and the nurse or parent as "other schoolmates." If the child returns to school with some obvious physical change, such as hair loss, amputation, or visible scar, the nurse might also ask questions about these alterations to prompt preparatory responses from the child.

Classroom peers also need preparation, and a joint plan involving the teacher, nurse, and child is best. At a minimum, classmates should be given a description of the child's condition, prepared for any visible changes in the child, and allowed an opportunity to ask questions. The child should have the option of attending this session. As the child's condition changes, particularly if the illness is potentially fatal, school personnel, including the students, need periodic appraisal of the child's status and preparation for what to expect.

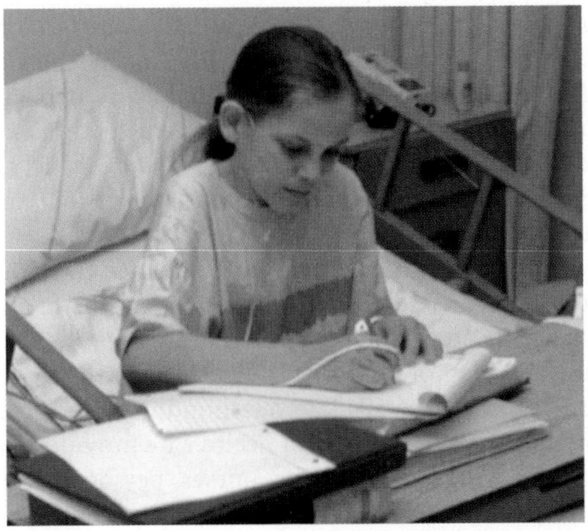

Fig. 41-4 Children with special needs should continue their schooling as soon as their condition permits.

Children with special needs should be encouraged to maintain or re-establish relationships with peers and to participate according to their capabilities in any age-appropriate activities. Alternative activities may be substituted for those that are impossible or that place a strain on the child's condition. Programs such as the Special Olympics offer children an opportunity to compete with their peers and to achieve athletic skill. Summer camps give children with special needs the opportunity to associate with peers and develop a wide variety of skills (see Additional Resources section at the end of this chapter). These children can derive enormous benefits from expressive activities, such as art, music, poetry, dance, and drama. With adaptive equipment and imagination, children can participate in a variety of activities. Organizations such as VSA Arts, Ontario and Québec affiliates, enable children to celebrate and share their accomplishments (see Additional Resources).

Children need the opportunity to interact with healthy peers and to engage in activities with groups or clubs composed of similarly affected age-mates. Such organizations as ostomy clubs, diabetes clubs, and cerebral palsy groups share information and provide support related to the special problems the members face.

Adolescence

Adolescence can be a particularly difficult period for the teenager with special needs and for his or her family. All of the needs discussed previously apply to this age group as well. Developing independence or autonomy is a major task for the adolescent as planning for the future becomes a prominent concern. For these children, the emphasis in the past was on achieving independence from physical assistance; however, recent developments in the fields of special education, adolescent development, and family systems suggest that autonomy be redefined in terms of individuals' capacities to take responsibility for their own behaviour, make decisions regarding their own lives, and maintain supportive social relationships. Given this understanding, even individuals with severe impairment can be viewed as autonomous if they perceive their own needs and take responsibility for meeting them, either directly or by engaging the assistance of others. As adolescents become more autonomous, the nurse can help them articulate their needs, participate in developing their own care plan, and discover and express how others can be of greatest assistance.

Physical symptoms are high on the teenager's list of health-related concerns. Because adolescence is a time of enormous physical and emotional changes, it is important for the nurse to distinguish between body changes related to disability and those that are a result of normal body development. It can be a great comfort for teenagers with disabling conditions to know that many of the changes they experience are normal developmental outcomes.

A sense of feeling different from peers can lead to loneliness, isolation, and depression. Participation in groups of teenagers with chronic conditions or disabilities can help alleviate feelings of isolation and smooth the transition to meaningful relationships in adulthood.

Establish Realistic Future Goals

One of the most difficult adjustments for the child and for those involved in his or her continued care is setting realistic future goals. Sometimes the impact of such planning does not surface until the child finishes school or the parents approach retirement, when a crisis can arise because of disruption of all of the family roles and relationships that maintained stability.

Planning for the future should be a gradual process. All along, the parents should cultivate realistic vocations for the child. For example, if children have physical disabilities, they should be directed toward undertaking intellectual, artistic, or musical pursuits. Children with developmental disabilities need to be taught manual skills. In this way, the child's development proceeds in the direction of self-support through gainful employment.

With prolonged survival, young people with chronic illnesses must deal with new decisions and problems, such as marriage or other long-term relationships, employment, and insurance coverage. With appropriate guidance, individuals with disabilities can attain gainful employment, marriage, and a family. For those whose conditions are genetic, counselling is needed regarding future offspring. Prospective spouses often benefit from an opportunity to discuss their feelings about marriage to an individual with continued health needs and possibly a limited lifespan. Health insurance coverage can be a critical issue if extra health care is needed, such as medications or treatments. Life insurance is another dilemma, especially when children have serious defects, such as congenital heart anomalies.

Perspectives on the Care of Children at the End of Life

Although most childhood illnesses and many injuries and other types of **trauma** respond favourably to treatment, some do not. When a child and family face a prolonged and possibly terminal illness, health care providers must confront the challenge of providing the best possible care to meet the physical, psychological, spiritual, and emotional needs of the child and family during the uncertain course of the illness and at the time of death. When death is sudden and unexpected, nurses are challenged to respond to the grief and shock that families experience and to provide comfort and support in the absence of a prior relationship.

There are many factors contributing to childhood and adolescent death that nurses are likely to encounter: developmental factors, medical advances and technology, and changing social patterns. In infants less than 1 year of age, the leading causes of death are perinatal conditions, congenital malformations, deformations, chromosomal abnormalities, and sudden infant death syndrome. The leading causes of death in children 1 to 4 years of age include accidents (unintentional injuries), **malignant** neoplasms, and **congenital** conditions. In children 5 to 9 years of age, accidents (unintentional injuries), malignant neoplasms, and congenital conditions are the leading causes of death. In children 10 to 14 years of age, accidents (unintentional injuries), malignant neoplasms, and suicide (intentional self-harm) are the most prevalent causes of death. Youths aged 15 to 19 years die most frequently as a result of accidents (unintentional injuries), suicide (intentional self-harm), and malignant neoplasms (Statistics Canada, 2010).

A child who is diagnosed with a life-threatening illness or who is suffering serious, life-threatening trauma needs medical diagnosis and intervention, as well as nursing assessment and care—sometimes for a short time and sometimes over a lengthy period. When cure is no longer possible and life-prolonging measures result in pain and distress to the child, parents need information about available care options to assist them in deciding how they want the health care team to manage the remaining time with their child. It is important to reassure families that, although their child cannot be cured, active care will continue to be provided to maintain the child's comfort. Support is required to assist the child and family during the dying process. As a result, nurses may care for children and families who are making the difficult transition from curative or restorative treatments to palliative care.

Principles of Palliative Care

Palliative care involves a multidisciplinary approach to the management of a terminal illness or the dying process that focuses on symptom control and support rather than on cure or life prolongation in the absence of the possibility of a cure (Field & Behrman, 2004). The World Health Organization (2012a) defines *palliative care* as an approach that improves the quality of life of patients and their families facing the problems associated with life-threatening illness, through the prevention and relief of suffering by means of early identification and assessment and treatment of pain and other problems—physical, psychosocial, and spiritual.

Palliative care interventions do not serve to hasten death; rather, they provide pain and symptom management and address issues faced by the child and family with regard to death and dying. A primary aim of palliative care is to promote optimal functioning and quality of life during the time the child has remaining. The implementation of neonatal and pediatric palliative care consulting services within hospitals has led to enhanced quality of life and end-of-life care for children and their families as well as support for their care providers (Jennings, 2005).

Several principles are hallmarks of palliative care. The child and family are considered the unit of care. The death of a child is an extremely stressful event for a family because it is out of the natural order of things. Children represent health and hope, and their death calls into question the understanding of life. A multidisciplinary team of health care providers consisting of social workers, chaplains, nurses, personal care aides, and physicians skilled in caring for dying patients can assist the family by focusing care on the complex interactions between physical, emotional, social, and spiritual issues.

Palliative care providers seek to create a therapeutic environment that is as homelike as possible, if not in the child's own home. Through education and support of family members, an atmosphere of open communication is established to deal with the child's dying process and its impact on all members of the family.

Decision Making at the End of Life

Discussions concerning the possibility that a child's illness or condition is not curable and that death is an inevitable outcome cause everyone involved a great deal of stress. Physicians, other members of the health care team, and families must consider all information regarding the child's situation in order to make decisions that all parties can agree to, particularly those that will have a profound impact on the child and family.

Ethical Considerations in End-of-Life Decision Making

A number of ethical concerns arise when parents and health care providers are deciding on the best course of care for the dying child. Many parents and health care providers are concerned that not offering treatment that would cause potential pain and suffering, but might extend life, would be considered euthanasia or assisted suicide. To eliminate such concerns, it is necessary to understand the various terms. *Euthanasia* involves an action carried out by a person other than the patient to end the life of the patient suffering from a terminal condition. This action is based on the belief that the act is "putting the patient out of his [or her] misery"; this action has also been called *mercy killing*. *Assisted suicide* is when someone provides the patient with the means to end his or her life and the patient uses that means to do so. The important distinction between these two actions involves who is actually acting to end the person's life.

The Canadian Nurses Association (2008) Code of Ethics for Registered Nurses does not address the active intent on the part of a nurse to end a person's life. It does indicate the nurse's role in maintaining patient dignity by providing interventions to provide comfort and relieve symptoms in the dying patient. When the prognosis for a patient is poor and death is the expected outcome, it is ethically acceptable to withhold or withdraw treatments that may cause pain and suffering and to provide interventions that promote comfort and quality of life.

Physician–Health Care Team Decision Making

Decisions by physicians regarding care are often made on the basis of the progression of the disease or amount of trauma, the availability of treatment options that would provide cure from disease or restoration of health, the impact of such treatments on the child, and the child's overall prognosis. Often the main determinants prompting physicians to discuss end-of-life issues and options for children with critical illnesses include the child's age, premorbid cognitive condition and functional status, pain or discomfort, probability of survival, and quality of life (Masri et al., 2000). When the physician discusses this information openly with families, a shared decision-making process can occur regarding no cardiopulmonary resuscitation (CPR) (also referred to as *do-not-resuscitate [DNR]*) orders and care that is focused on the comfort of the child and family during the dying process (Canadian Paediatric Society, Bioethics Committee, 2008; Fallat & Deschpande, 2004).

Unfortunately, many families are not given the option of terminating treatment and pursuing care focused on comfort and quality of life when cure is unlikely, and staff may be reluctant to raise the question of no CPR orders. The staff may believe that not being able to "save" a child is a "failure." Also, the physician and other members of the health care team may lack knowledge of and experience with the principles of palliative care (Field & Behrman, 2004; Sahler et al., 2000; Sumner, 2003).

Parental Decision Making

Rarely are families prepared to cope with the numerous decisions that must be made when a child is dying. When the death is unexpected, as in the case of an accident or trauma, the confusion of emergency services and possibly a critical care setting presents challenges to parents as they are asked to make difficult choices. If the child has either experienced a life-threatening illness such as cancer or lived with a chronic illness that has now reached its terminal phase, parents are often unprepared for the reality of their child's impending death (see Family-Centred Teaching box). Numerous studies have found that families facing the impending death of a child depend on information provided to them by the health care team, particularly an honest appraisal of the child's prognosis, to make difficult decisions regarding care options for their child (Hinds et al., 2001; Wolfe, Friebert, & Hilden, 2002).

evolve Case Study—The Dying Child

As the group of health care providers who are most involved with families, nurses are in an excellent position to ensure that families are presented with the relevant options available to them. The nurse's first responsibility is to explore the family's wishes. This is best done in concert with the physician, but at times may need to be initiated by the nurse. Statements such as "Tell me about your thoughts for the type of care you want your child to receive when he is dying" or "Have you considered the types of interventions you would like us to use when your child is near death?" can begin discussion of this sensitive but critical aspect of terminal care.

The Dying Child

Children need honest and accurate information about their illness, treatments, and prognosis; this information needs to be given in clear, simple language. In most situations this best occurs as a gradual process over time, characterized by increasingly open dialogue among parents, health care providers, and the child (Young et al., 2003). Providing an atmosphere of open communication early in the course of an illness facilitates answering difficult questions as the child's condition worsens. Providing appropriate literature about the disease and the experience of illness and possible death is also helpful. Exactly how and when to involve children in decisions regarding care during their dying process and death is an individual matter. The child's age or developmental level is an important consideration in the process (Table 41-3). In general, parents should be asked how they would like their child to be told of the prognosis, and they should be included in his or her care. Some parents may request that their child not be told that he

FAMILY-CENTRED TEACHING

Family of the Dying Child

No matter whether you have a PhD or many children, when your child dies, it is a new experience and nothing can prepare you for it. Like so many things in life, experience is the best teacher.

Three of our children have died, and by the time the third was dying, we handled many things differently. We learned a lot about dignity and the rights of the child and family. For example, at first, we didn't know that we had a right to have our child die at home. We also didn't understand pain medications and that if children are taking these medicines and are still in agony, they have not overdosed on the medication.

We learned a lot about case management. With our first two children, lots of different people were making decisions and disagreeing about what was best and what should be done. No one had primary authority. With our third child, one doctor took a primary role. Any questions and problems were handled by one person. I could call him 24 hours a day. It made a lot of difference, and I felt our concerns and needs were better heard and respected.

The nurses caring for our third child at home enabled me to step back and just be his mommy. When I could do this, I realized that we were fighting so hard for his life that we weren't really letting him die. His nurses had worked with him for a long time and really loved him. It was hard for them when we decided to let him die. In his last several days we wanted a lot of family time with our son, and I think the nurses felt left out. Something about their reaction to our increased time with him in the last few days made us feel guilty. If we had all been able to communicate a little more openly, I would have understood that they needed more time with him at the end, too. Everyone's needs could have been met.

–Jeni Stepanek, Mother
Upper Marlboro, MD

or she is dying, even if the child asks. This often places health care providers in a difficult situation. Children, even at a young age, are perceptive. Even if they are not told outright that they are dying, they realize that something is seriously wrong and that it involves them. Often, when parents are helped to understand that honesty and shared decision making between them and their child are important to the child and family's emotional health, the parents may then allow discussion of dying with their child. Parents may require professional support and guidance in this process from a nurse, social worker, or child life specialist who has a good relationship with the child and family.

If given the opportunity, children will tell others how much they want to know. Asking questions such as "If the disease came back, would you want to know?" "Do you want others to tell you everything, even if the news isn't good?" or "If someone were not getting better [or more directly, "were dying"], do you think he would want to know?" helps children set the limits of how much truth they can accept and cope with. Children need time to process many feelings and much information so that they can assimilate, and ideally accept, the inevitable fact of mortality.

Care of the dying adolescent requires the nurse to become knowledgeable about any possible delays or alterations in normal growth and development. Legal and ethical issues, such as informed consent, also come to the forefront with respect to the age at which an adolescent should have autonomy in decision making about care and treatment. Effective communication between the patient, family, and health care team is an important part of optimal care for the dying adolescent (Freyer, 2004).

Treatment Options for Terminally Ill Children

Based on the child and family's decision regarding their wishes for terminal care, they have several options from which to choose.

Hospital Care

Families may choose to remain in the hospital to receive care if the child's illness or condition is unstable and home care is not an option or the family is uncomfortable with providing care at home. If a family chooses to remain at the hospital for terminal care, the setting should be made as homelike as possible. Families should be encouraged to bring familiar items from the child's room at home. In addition, there should be a consistent and coordinated care plan for the child and family's comfort (Johnson, Abernathy, Howell, Brazil, & Scott, 2009; Seow, Barbera, Howell, & Dy, 2010).

Home Care

Some families prefer to take their child home and receive services from a home care agency. Generally, these services entail periodic nursing visits to administer a treatment or provide medications, equipment, or supplies. Many home care agencies can provide nurses and other health care providers who are specially trained in palliative care support for patients and their families. The child's care frequently continues to be directed by the primary physician. Home care is often the option chosen by physicians and families because of the traditional view that a child must be considered to have a life expectancy of less than 6 months to be referred to **hospice care**. Fortunately, a number of hospice organizations are expanding their services to children on the basis of presence of a life-limiting disease process for which cure is not possible, rather than the sole criterion of a limited-time projected prognosis (Seow et al., 2010).

Hospice Care

Parents should be offered the option of caring for their child at home during the final phases of an illness with the assistance of a hospice organization. *Hospice* is a community health care organization that specializes in the care of dying patients by combining the hospice philosophy with the principles of palliative care. *Hospice philosophy* regards dying as a natural process and care of dying patients as including management of the physical, psychological, social, and spiritual needs of the patient and family. Care is provided by a multidisciplinary

Table 41-3 Children's Understanding of and Reactions to Death

CONCEPTS OF DEATH	REACTIONS TO DEATH	NURSING CARE MANAGEMENT
Infants and Toddlers		
Death has least significance to children <6 mo of age. After parent-child attachment and trust are established, the loss, even if temporary, of the significant person is profound. Prolonged separation during the first several years is thought to be more significant in terms of future physical, social, and emotional growth than at any subsequent age. Toddlers are egocentric and can only think about events in terms of their own frame of reference—living. Their egocentricity and vague separation of fact and fantasy make it impossible for them to comprehend absence of life. Instead of understanding death, this age group is affected more by any change in lifestyle.	With the death of someone else, they may continue to act as though the person is alive. As children grow older, they will be increasingly able and willing to let go of the dead person. Ritualism is important; a change in lifestyle could be anxiety producing. This age group reacts more to the pain and discomfort of a serious illness than to the probable fatal prognosis. This age group also reacts to parental anxiety and sadness.	Help parents deal with their feelings, allowing them greater emotional reserves to meet the needs of their children. Encourage parents to remain as near to the child as possible, yet be sensitive to parents' needs. Maintain as normal an environment as possible to retain ritualism. If a parent has died, promote arrangements for a consistent caregiver for the child. Promote primary nursing.
Preschool Children		
Preschoolers believe their thoughts are sufficient to cause death; the consequence is the burden of guilt, shame, and punishment. Their egocentricity implies a tremendous sense of self-power and omnipotence. They usually have some understanding of the meaning of death. Death is seen as a departure, a kind of sleep. They may recognize the fact of physical death but do not separate it from living abilities. Death is seen as temporary and gradual; life and death can change places with one another. They have no understanding of the universality and inevitability of death.	If they become seriously ill, they conceive of the illness as a punishment for their thoughts or actions. They may feel guilty and responsible for the death of a sibling. Their greatest fear concerning death is separation from parents. They may engage in activities that seem strange or abnormal to adults. Because they have fewer defence mechanisms to deal with loss, young children may react to a less significant loss with more outward grief than to the loss of a very significant person. The loss is so deep, painful, and threatening that the child must deny it for a time to survive its overwhelming impact. Behaviour reactions such as giggling, joking, attracting attention, or regressing to earlier developmental skills indicate children's need to distance themselves from tremendous loss.	Help parents deal with their feelings, allowing them greater emotional reserves to meet the needs of their children. Help parents understand their children's behavioural reactions. Encourage parents to remain near the child as much as possible, to minimize the child's great fear of separation from parents. If a parent has died, promote arrangements for a consistent caregiver for the child. Promote primary nursing.

Continued

Table 41-3 Children's Understanding of and Reactions to Death—Cont'd

CONCEPTS OF DEATH	REACTIONS TO DEATH	NURSING CARE MANAGEMENT
School-Age Children		
The children still associate misdeeds or bad thoughts with causing death and feel intense guilt and responsibility for the event. Because of their higher cognitive abilities, they respond well to logical explanations and comprehend the figurative meaning of words. They have a deeper understanding of death in a concrete sense. They particularly fear the mutilation and punishment they associate with death. They personify death as the devil, a monster, or the bogeyman. They may have naturalistic or physiological explanations of death. By age 9–10, children have an adult concept of death, realizing that it is inevitable, universal, and irreversible.	Because of their increased ability to comprehend, they may have more fears, for example: • The reason for the illness • Communicability of the disease to themselves or others • Consequences of the disease • The process of dying and death itself Their fear of the unknown is greater than their fear of the known. The realization of impending death is a tremendous threat to their sense of security and ego strength. They are likely to exhibit fear through verbal uncooperativeness rather than physical aggression. They are interested in postdeath services. They may be inquisitive about what happens to the body.	Help parents deal with their feelings, allowing them greater emotional reserves to meet their children's needs. Encourage parents to remain near the child as much as possible, yet be sensitive to parents' needs. Because of children's fear of the unknown, anticipatory preparation is important. Because the developmental task of this age is industry, interventions of helping children maintain control over their bodies and increasing their understanding can enable them to achieve independence, self-worth, and self-esteem and avoid a sense of inferiority. Encourage children to talk about their feelings, and provide aggressive outlets. Encourage parents to honestly answer questions about dying rather than avoiding the subject or fabricating euphemisms. Encourage parents to share their moments of sorrow with their children. Provide preparation for postdeath services.
Adolescents		
Adolescents have a mature understanding of death. They are still influenced by remnants of magical thinking and are subject to guilt and shame. They are likely to see deviations from accepted behaviour as reasons for their illness.	Adolescents straddle the transition from childhood to adulthood. They have the most difficulty in coping with death. They are least likely to accept cessation of life, particularly if it is their own. Concern is for the present much more than for the past or the future. They may consider themselves alienated from their peers and unable to communicate with their parents for emotional support, feeling alone in their struggle. Adolescents' orientation to the present compels them to worry about physical changes even more than the prognosis. Because of their idealistic view of the world, they may criticize funeral rites as barbaric, money making, and unnecessary.	Help parents deal with their feelings, allowing them greater emotional reserves to meet their children's needs. Avoid alliances with either parent or child. Structure hospital admission to allow for maximum self-control and independence. Answer adolescents' questions honestly, treating them as mature individuals and respecting their needs for privacy, solitude, and personal expressions of emotions. Help parents understand their child's reactions to death and dying, especially that concern for present crises, such as loss of hair, may be much greater than for future ones, including possible death.

group of professionals in the patient's home or an inpatient facility that employs the hospice philosophy. Hospice care for children was introduced in the 1970s, and a number of community hospice organizations now accept children into their care (Davies et al., 2003; Forrester, 2003; Winkler & Mardegian, 2001). Collaboration between the child's primary treatment team and the hospice care team is essential to the success of hospice care. Families may continue to see their primary care physicians as they choose. For more information, refer to Appendix 1 for a list of resources on palliative care and hospice resources.

Hospice care is based on a number of important concepts that significantly set it apart from hospital care:

- Family members are usually the principal caregivers and are supported by a team of professional and volunteer staff.
- The priority of care is comfort. The child's physical, psychological, social, and spiritual needs are considered. Pain and symptom control are primary concerns, and no extraordinary efforts are used to attempt a cure or prolong life.
- The family's needs are considered to be as important as those of the patient.
- Hospice is also concerned with the family's postdeath adjustment, and care may continue for a year or more.

The goal of hospice care is for children to live life to the fullest without pain, with choices and dignity, in the familiar environment of their home, and with the support of their family. Hospice care is covered under provincial health insurance programs and by most insurance plans. The service provides home visits from nurses, social workers, chaplains, and, in some cases, physicians. Medications, medical equipment, and any necessary medical supplies are all provided by the hospice organization providing care.

With children, the home has been the more common environment for implementing the hospice concept; it benefits the family in a variety of ways. Children who are dying are allowed to remain with those they love and with whom they feel secure. Many children who were thought to be in imminent danger of death have gone home and lived longer than expected. Siblings can feel more involved in the child's care and often have more positive perceptions of the death. Parental adaptation is often more favourable, demonstrated by their perceptions of how the experience at home affected their marriage, social reorientation, religious beliefs, and views on the meaning of life and death.

If the home is chosen for hospice care, the child may or may not die in the home. Reasons for final admission to a hospital vary but may be related to the parents' or siblings' wish to have the child die outside the home; exhaustion on the part of the caregivers; and physical problems such as sudden, acute pain or respiratory distress.

Nursing Care of the Child and Family at the End of Life

Regardless of where the child is cared for during the terminal stage of illness, both the child and the family usually experience fear of (1) pain and suffering, (2) dying alone (child) or not being present when the child dies (parent), and (3) actual death. Nurses can help reduce families' fears through attention to the care needs of the child and family.

Fear of Pain and Suffering

The presence of unrelieved pain in a terminally ill child can have detrimental effects on the quality of life experienced by the child and family. Parents believe that having their child in pain is unendurable and results in feelings of helplessness and a sense that they must be present and vigilant to get the necessary pain medications. Persistent pain also creates more stress for the family as a whole. Nurses can alleviate the fear of pain and suffering by providing interventions aimed at treating the pain and symptoms associated with the terminal process in children.

Pain and Symptom Management

Pain control for children in the terminal stages of illness or injury must be given the highest priority. Despite ongoing efforts to educate physicians and nurses on pain management strategies in children, studies have reported that children continue to be undermedicated for their pain (Wolfe et al., 2000). Nearly all children experience some amount of pain in the terminal phase of their illness. The current standard for treating children's pain follows the World Health Organization's (2012b) analgesic pain ladder, which promotes tailoring the pain interventions to the child's level of reported pain. Children's pain should be assessed frequently, and medications adjusted as necessary.

The first step in treating a child in pain is to promptly administer medications such as nonopioids (aspirin and paracetamol). If the pain persists, the second step is to give the child mild opioids (codeine). If the child requires further pain control, the last step, opioid (morphine), should be administered until the child is pain free. These steps are inexpensive and 80 to 90% effective; they need to be followed every 3 to 6 hours on a regular basis. Nerve blocks are available through surgical intervention and may be used if pain medications are not effective or the child is in extreme pain. Techniques such as distraction, relaxation techniques, and guided imagery should be combined with medication therapy to provide the child and family with strategies to control the pain (see Chapter 35 for further discussion of pain management strategies).

In addition to pain, children experience a variety of symptoms during their terminal course as a result of their disease process or as an adverse effect of medicines used to manage pain or other symptoms. These symptoms include fatigue, nausea and vomiting, constipation, anorexia, dyspnea, congestion, seizures, anxiety, depression, restlessness, agitation, and confusion (Hellsten et al., 2000; Wolfe et al., 2002). Each of these symptoms should be aggressively managed with appropriate medications or treatments and with interventions such as repositioning, relaxation, massage, and other measures to maintain the child's comfort and quality of life (see Evidence-Informed Practice box).

EVIDENCE-INFORMED PRACTICE Pediatric Pain and Symptom Management at the End of Life

Ask the Question

In children, what is the pain and symptom experience at the end of life?

Search for Evidence

Search Strategies

Published studies from 2000 to 2005 using the subject terms *child, palliative care, pain,* and *symptoms*; findings dominated by retrospective descriptive studies describing infants and children's end-of-life experiences through the use of medical record reviews and provider and parental surveys

Databases Searched

PubMed, CINAHL

Critically Analyze the Evidence

Children experienced an average of 11 symptoms during their last week of life (Drake, Frost, & Collins, 2003). Pain, dyspnea, and fatigue were the most frequently documented symptoms, experienced by most children at the end of life (Bradshaw et al., 2005; Carter et al., 2004; Drake et al., 2003; Houlahan, Branowicki, Mack, Dinning, & McCabe, 2006). Children and their parents reported high distress with pain and symptoms at the end of life. Parents reported pain and suffering as one of the most important factors in deciding whether to withhold or withdraw life support from their child in the pediatric critical care unit (Meert, Thurston, & Sarnaik, 2000). Some children suffer intractable symptoms that are very difficult to manage (Houlahan et al., 2006).

Documentation was scarce related to symptom management. Morphine was the most commonly prescribed pain medication (Drake et al., 2003; Hongo et al., 2003). Parents reported their children as experiencing high levels of pain near the end of life (Contro et al., 2002). Physicians were more likely than nurses or parents to report that a child's pain and symptoms were well managed at the end of life, whereas the majority of both provider groups believed the child's physical management was difficult (Andresen, Seecharan, & Toce, 2004; Wolfe et al., 2000). A multipronged approach to help relieve physical as well as psychological and spiritual distress is necessary to provide optimum care to this very vulnerable population and their families. To achieve this aim, it is important to engage with patients and families, improving communication and relationships, and involving patients and families in the decision-making process as much as possible about needed services and treatment interventions (Epelman, 2012). Barriers to the adequate provision of pediatric palliative care include developmental issues specific to infants and children; symptoms, their causes, how they are related, and effective treatment strategies; lack of education; and reimbursement issues if the family require services beyond what is covered by their government health plan (Harris, 2004). Physicians reported reliance on trial and error as they learned to care for children at the end of life and the need for specialty consults with palliative care service providers (Jones, 2011). Researchers identified five of the most significant barriers that prevented nursing staff from providing optimal pain management: insufficient physician (MD) orders, insufficient MD orders before procedures, insufficient time to premedicate patients before procedures, the perception of a low priority given to pain management by medical staff, and parents' reluctance to have their child receive pain medication (Czarnecki et al., 2011).

Apply the Evidence: Nursing Implications

Although the philosophy of palliative care encompasses pain and symptom management for infants and children who may not outlive their disease, the provision of that care to ease suffering and provide comfort to those who will die continues to lag. Studies show that children experience significant pain and other distressing symptoms at the end of life that are not well managed. Discrepancies in perceptions of infant and child pain and suffering continue to exist between providers and parents. Barriers to the provision of pediatric palliative care exist. Improvements are needed in the management of pain and symptoms at the end of life for infants and children.

References

Andresen, E. M., Seecharan, G. A., & Toce, S. S. (2004). Provider perceptions of child deaths. *Archives of Pediatric & Adolescent Medicine, 158,* 430–435.

Bradshaw, G., et al. (2005). Cancer-related deaths in children and adolescents. *Journal of Palliative Medicine, 8*(1), 86–95.

Carter, B. S., et al. (2004). Circumstances surrounding the deaths of hospitalized children: Opportunities for pediatric palliative care. *Pediatrics, 114*(3), 361–366.

Contro, N., et al. (2002). Family perspectives on the quality of pediatric palliative care. *Archives of Pediatric & Adolescent Medicine, 156,* 1–29.

Czarnecki, M. L., et al. (2011). Barriers to pediatric pain management: A nursing perspective. *Pain Management Nursing, 12*(3),154–162.

Drake, R., Frost, J., & Collins, J. J. (2003). The symptoms of dying children. *Journal of Pain & Symptom Management, 26*(1), 594–603.

Epelman, C. L. (2012). End of life management in pediatric cancer. *Pediatrics, 129*(4),e975–e982.

Harris, B. (2004). Palliative care in children with cancer: Which child and when? *Journal of the National Cancer Institute Monographs, 32,* 144–149.

Hongo, T., et al. (2003). Analysis of the circumstances at the end of life in children with cancer: Symptoms, suffering and acceptance. *Pediatrics International, 45,* 60–66.

Houlahan, K. M., Branowicki, P. A., Mack, J. W., Dinning, C., & McCabe, M. (2006). Can end of life care for the pediatric patient suffering with escalating and intractable symptoms be improved? *Journal of Pediatric Oncology Nursing, 23*(1), 45–51. doi:10.1177/1043454205283588

Jones, B. W. (2011). The need for increased access to pediatric hospice and palliative care. *Dimensions of Critical Care Nursing, 30*(5), 231–235.

Meert, K. L., Thurston, C. S., & Sarnaik, A. P. (2000). End-of-life decision-making and satisfaction with care: Parental perspectives. *Pediatric Critical Care Medicine, 1*(2), 179–185.

Wolfe, J., et al. (2000). Symptoms and suffering at the end of life in children with cancer. *New England Journal of Medicine, 342*(5), 326–333.

Occasionally, children require very high doses of opioids to control pain. The child on long-term opioid pain management can develop **tolerance** of the medication, meaning that it is necessary to give more drugs to maintain the same level of pain relief. This should not be confused with **addiction**, which is a psychological dependence on the adverse effects of opioids. Addiction is not a factor in managing terminal pain in children. Other obvious reasons for requiring increased doses of opioids include progression of disease and other physiological experiences of pain. It is important to understand that there is no maximum dose that can be given to control pain. Nurses often express concern that administering doses of opioids that exceed what they are familiar with will hasten the child's death. In cases where the child is terminally ill and in severe pain, use of large doses of opioids and sedatives to manage pain is justified when no other treatment options are available that would relieve the pain but make the risk of death less likely (Hawryluck & Harvey, 2000).

Parents' and Siblings' Need for Education and Support

Parents are the primary caregivers when the child is at home, and nurses providing care to the child and family need to teach the family about the medications being given to the child, how to administer medications, and the use of nonpharmacological techniques to control pain. Parents should be kept informed of all medications and treatments given to a child in the hospital and should be encouraged to participate in the child's care to the extent that they desire. This empowers parents and provides a sense of control over the child's comfort and well-being, reducing their fear that their child will be in pain or suffering as he or she is dying. Additionally, better bereavement outcomes (e.g., adaptive coping; family cohesion; less anxiety, stress, and depression) have been reported by parents who were actively involved in their child's care (Goodenough et al., 2004). The grief work of fathers in particular seems to be facilitated when their child dies in the home setting. This pattern may be related to the greater opportunity of working fathers to provide care to and spend time with their child at home than in the hospital setting.

Siblings may feel isolated and displaced while their brother or sister is dying. Parents devote most of their time to the dying child's care and comfort, causing siblings to feel left out of the parent–sick child relationship. Siblings may become resentful of their sick sibling and begin to feel guilty or ashamed about such feelings. Nurses can assist the family by helping the parents identify ways to involve siblings in the caring process, perhaps by bringing some supplies or a favourite toy, game, or food item. Parents should also be encouraged to schedule time to spend with the other children where their focus is on them. Helping parents identify a trusted friend or family member who can sit with the ill child for a short period will allow them to attend to their own needs or those of their other children.

Fear of Dying Alone or of Not Being Present When the Child Dies

When a child is being cared for at home, the burden of care on parents and family members can be great. Often, as the child's condition declines, family members begin the "death vigil." Rarely is a child left alone for any length of time. This can be exhausting for family members, and nurses can assist the family by helping them arrange shifts so that friends or family members can be present with the child and allow others to rest. If the family has limited resources, community organizations such as hospice or churches often have volunteers who are willing to visit and sit with children. It is important that whoever is sitting with the child be aware of when the parent(s) would like to be notified to return to the child's bedside (Fig. 41-5).

When a child is dying in the hospital, parents should be given full access to the child at all times. If parents need to leave, they should be provided with a pager or other means of immediate communication and alerted if staff members note any change in the child that may indicate imminent death. Nurses must advocate for parents' presence in critical care and emergency departments and attend to the parents' needs for food, drinks, comfortable chairs, blankets, and pillows.

Fear of Actual Death

Home Deaths

The majority of children receiving hospice care die at home, often in their own room with family, pets, and other loved possessions around them. The physical process of dying can be distressing to parents because often the child slowly becomes less alert in the days before the actual death. The nurse can assist the family by providing them with information about what changes will occur as the child progresses through the dying process (Box 41-8). During this time, nursing visits often become more frequent and longer in duration to provide the family with additional support as the death nears. The most distressing change for parents to observe is the change in the respiratory pattern. In the final hours of life, the dying patient's respirations may become laboured, with deep breaths and long periods of apnea, referred to as Cheyne-Stokes respirations. Families need to be reassured that this is not distressing to the child and that it is a normal part of the dying process. Use of opioids can slow the respirations to make the child breathe more easily, and scopolamine, usually applied as a topical patch, can help reduce noisy respirations, known as the "death rattle." Noisy respirations are more likely to occur if the child is overhydrated.

All families have the option of admitting their child to the hospital if they feel unable to deal with the death. The child who dies at home must be pronounced dead; hospice programs typically have provisions so that this proceeds smoothly.

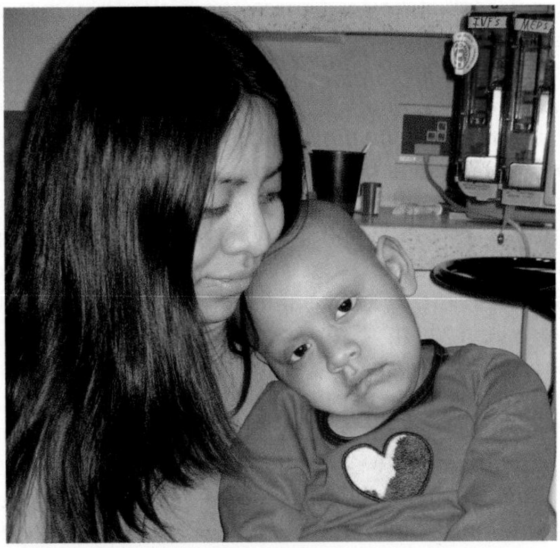

Fig. 41-5 For the dying child there is no greater comfort than the security and closeness of a parent.

BOX 41-8 Physical Signs of Approaching Death

Loss of sensation and movement in the lower extremities, progressing toward the upper body
Sensation of heat, although body feels cool
Loss of senses:
- Tactile sensation decreasing
- Sensitivity to light
- Hearing the last sense to fail

Confusion, loss of consciousness, slurred speech
Muscle weakness
Loss of bowel and bladder control
Decreased appetite and thirst
Difficulty swallowing
Change in respiratory pattern:
- Cheyne-Stokes respirations (waxing and waning of depth of breathing with regular periods of apnea)
- "Death rattle" (noisy chest sounds from accumulation of pulmonary and pharyngeal secretions)

Weak, slow pulse; decreased blood pressure

In some circumstances the police may be notified, with an explanation of the circumstances to prevent unnecessary concern regarding abuse. Providing the police with the number of the responsible practitioner is usually all that is necessary to confirm the cause of death.

Hospital Deaths

Children dying in the hospital of terminal illnesses who are receiving supportive care interventions will experience a similar process. Again, increased nursing presence and attendance to the child and family's needs provide comfort and support for many families.

Death resulting from accident, trauma, or acute illness in settings such as the emergency department or critical care unit often requires the active withdrawal of some form of life-supporting intervention, such as a ventilator or bypass machine. These situations often raise difficult ethical issues (Sine et al., 2001), and parents are often less prepared for the actual moment of death. Nurses can assist these parents by providing detailed information about what will happen as supportive equipment is withdrawn, ensuring that appropriate pain medications are administered to prevent pain during the dying process, and allowing the parents time before the start of the withdrawal to be with and speak to their child. It is important that the nurse attempt to control the environment around the family at this time by providing privacy, asking if they would like to play music, softening lights and monitor noises, and arranging for any religious or cultural rituals that the family may want performed.

After the child's death, the family should be allowed to remain with the body and hold or rock the child if they desire. After the nurse has removed all tubes and equipment from the body, parents should be given the option of assisting with the preparation of the body, such as bathing and dressing. It is important for the nurse to determine whether the family has any specific needs, since many cultures have adopted specific methods for coping with and mourning death, and impeding these practices may interfere with the grieving process (Clements et al., 2003).

At some point the nurse should discuss whether the family has made preparations for the memorial service and whether the staff can help in any way. Parents often have concerns about the funeral, such as siblings' involvement in the death rituals. Although there are no absolute answers to the question of siblings attending the funeral or burial services, the consensus is that the surviving children benefit from being involved in these events. Children need preparation for postdeath services. They should be told what to expect, particularly how the deceased person will look if the coffin is open; allowed their private time to say good-bye; and permitted to stay as long as they wish. Ideally, the parents should prepare the siblings. If the parents' grief prevents this communication, a significant family member or friend should prepare the siblings (see Family-Centred Teaching box).

Organ or Tissue Donation and Autopsy

For some families, organ or tissue donation may be a meaningful act—one that benefits another human being despite the loss of their child. Unfortunately, initiating a discussion about tissue donation is often stressful for staff, and there may be confusion regarding whose responsibility this is. In centres in which transplants are performed, a full-time transplant coordinator is usually available to inform the family about organ donation and to take care of details. If such services are not available, the staff needs to determine which members should discuss this topic with the family. Ideally, the person who knows the family best, knows when the death is expected, or

FAMILY-CENTRED TEACHING

Children Need to Say Good-bye

As a nurse and grief counsellor, I conduct grief workshops with children who have experienced the death of someone special. Children often communicate their feelings of being excluded through drawings. They may draw a picture of the dying person in a hospital bed that is raised too high for them to see the person's face clearly. Sometimes children reveal that they did not get to say good-bye because a family member told them, for example, "You don't want to see your grandma this way. She is too sick for you to visit." If the special person died at home, the children had to stay in their room when the funeral home staff took away the body.

I have learned to never underestimate the importance of allowing children to be involved with the dying person and the significance of a child's loss. Once, when I asked a 6-year-old girl to draw a picture with the theme "This is what I was doing when my __________ died," she drew a picture and completed the sentence with "when my home died." Her grandmother had been like her mother; to the child, her home was gone. We need to give children the choice of being included in the family's activities of saying good-bye.

–Barbara Bilderback, MS, MA, RN, Bereavement Supervisor, Saint Francis Hospice Tulsa, OK

has the opportunity to spend time with the family when the death is unexpected takes this role. Often nurses are in an optimal position to suggest tissue donation after consultation with the attending physician. When possible, the topic should be raised before death occurs. The request should be made in a private and quiet area of the hospital and should be simple and direct, with questions such as "Are you a donor family?" or "Have you ever considered organ donation?"

Some provinces and territories have guidelines concerning requests for organ or tissue donation when a child dies, especially if the patient is brain dead. Written consent from the family is required before donation can proceed. When requests for organ donation are made, health care practitioners must address common misunderstandings families have about brain death and organ donation. Training health care providers on sensitive approaches to requests for organ donation has been shown to increase families' willingness to consent to organ donation (American Academy of Pediatrics, Committee on Hospital Care and Section on Surgery, 2002). The option to donate organs should always be separate from the communication of impending or actual death.

Nurses need to be aware of common questions about organ donation to help families make an informed decision. Healthy children who die unexpectedly are excellent candidates for organ donation. Children with cancer, chronic disease, or infection or those who have suffered prolonged cardiac arrest may not be suitable candidates, although this is individually determined. The nurse should ask whether organ donation was discussed with the child or whether the child ever expressed such a wish. Any number of body tissues or organs can be donated (skin, corneas, bone, kidney, heart, liver, pancreas), and their removal does not mutilate or desecrate the body or cause any suffering. The family may still have an open casket, and there is no delay in the funeral. There is no cost to the donor family, but organ donation does not eliminate funeral or cremation responsibilities. Most religions permit organ donation as long as the recipient benefits from the transplant, although Orthodox Judaism forbids it (see Table 32-1).

In cases of unexplained death, violent death, or suspected suicide, autopsy is required by law. In other instances it may be optional, and parents should be informed of this choice. The procedure, as well as the forms that must be signed, should be explained. The family should know that the child can be in an open casket after an autopsy.

Grief and Mourning

Grief is a process, not an event, of experiencing physiological, psychological, behavioural, social, and spiritual reactions to a personal loss—in this case, the loss of a child. Grief is highly individualized, encompassing a broad range of manifestations from person to person. It is a natural and expected reaction to loss. It is neither orderly nor predictable. Grieving in any form is necessary for healing to occur. When death is the expected or a possible outcome of a disorder, the child and family members may experience anticipatory grief. Anticipatory grief may be manifested in varying behaviours and intensities and may include denial, anger, depression, and other psychological and physical symptoms.

Anticipatory guidance may assist grieving family members. Health care providers should emphasize that grief reactions such as hearing the dead person's voice, feeling distant from others, or seeking reassurance that they did everything possible for the lost person are normal, necessary, and expected. In no way do these reactions signify poor coping, insanity, or an approaching mental breakdown. On the contrary, such behaviours signify that the survivor is working through the acute grief. Anticipatory guidance regarding the mourning process may help families recognize the normalcy of their experiences.

It is important to recognize that some family members may experience complicated grief. *Complicated grief reactions* (more than a year after the loss) include such symptoms as intense intrusive thoughts, pangs of severe emotion, distressing yearnings, feelings of excessive loneliness and emptiness, unusual sleep disturbance, and maladaptive levels of loss of interest in personal activities (Bruce, Gumley, Isham, Fearon, & Phipps, 2011). Bereaved persons experiencing such prolonged and complicated grief should be referred to an expert in grief and bereavement counselling.

Another important aspect of grief is the individual nature of the grief experience. Each member of the family will experience the grief of the child's death in his or her own way based on the particular relationship with that child. This can create potential conflict for families, since each family member can have expectations that the other family members should feel and grieve as they do. Nurses caring for families experiencing grief should be aware of the different grieving styles and help the family learn to recognize and support the uniqueness of each other's grief.

Parental Grief

Parental grief after the death of a child can be the most intense, complex, long-lasting, and fluctuating grief experience compared with that of other bereaved individuals. Although parents experience the primary loss of their child, many secondary losses are felt, such as the loss of part of one's self, hopes and dreams for the child's future, the family unit, prior social and emotional community supports, and often spousal support. It is common for parents of the same child to experience different grief reactions.

Studies of bereaved parents have shown that grieving does not end with the severing of the bond with the deceased child, but rather involves a continuing bond between the parent and the deceased child (Klass, 2001). Parental resolution of grief is a process of integrating the dead child into daily life, where the pain of losing a child is never completely gone, but lessens. There are occasions of brief relapse, but not to the degree experienced when the loss initially occurred. Thus parental grief work is never completed and is a timeless process of accommodating the new reality of being without a child, as it changes over time (Davies, 2004). A child's death can also challenge the marital relationship in several ways. Maternal and paternal reactions often differ (DaSilva, Jacob, & Nascimento, 2010; Reilly, Huws, Hastings, & Vaughan, 2010). Different grieving styles between the couple may hinder communication and support for each other. Differing needs and expectations can place a strain on the marriage.

Sibling Grief

Each child grieves in his or her own way and on his or her own timeline. Children, even adolescents, grieve differently than adults. Adults and children differ more widely in their reactions to death than in their reactions to any other phenomenon. Children of all ages grieve the loss of a loved one, and their understanding and reactions to death depend on their age and developmental level. Children grieve for a longer duration, revisiting their grief as they grow and develop new understandings of death. They do not grieve 100% of the time. They grieve in spurts and can be emotional and sad in one instance and then, just as quickly, off and playing. Children express their grief though play and behaviour. Children can be exquisitely attuned to their parents' grief and will try to protect them by not asking questions or by trying not to upset them. This can set the stage for the sibling to try to become the "perfect child." Children exhibit many of the grief reactions of adults, including physical sensations and illnesses, anger, guilt, sadness, loneliness, withdrawal, acting out, sleep disturbances, isolation, and search for meaning. Again, nurses should be attentive for signs that siblings are struggling with their grief and provide guidance to parents when possible.

At times family members may need assistance in their grieving (see Guidelines box). Communication with the bereaved family is essential, but often nurses do not know what to say and feel helpless in offering words of comfort. The most supportive approach is to avoid judging the family's reactions or offering advice or rationalizations and to focus on feelings. Perhaps the most valuable supportive measure the nurse can perform for families is to listen. Families understand that no words will relieve their pain; all they want is acceptance, understanding, and respect for their grief.

It is important for families to understand that mourning takes a long time. Whereas acute grief may last only weeks or months, resolving the loss is measured in years. Holidays and anniversaries can be particularly difficult, and people who previously had been supportive may now expect the family to have "adjusted." Consequently, prolonged mourning is often silent and lonely.

Many families never receive the support and guidance that could help them resolve the loss. A plan for regular follow-up with bereaved families can be beneficial. At minimum, one follow-up phone call or meeting with the family should be arranged. Families can also be referred to self-help groups. When such groups are not available, nurses can be instrumental in bringing families together or facilitating parent and sibling groups. Formal bereavement programs or bereavement counselling can be helpful as well.

For more information on end-of-life care, refer to Appendix 1.

Nurses' Reactions to Caring for Dying Children

The death of a patient is one of the most stressful aspects of critical care or oncology nursing (see Family-Centred Teaching box). Nurses experience reactions to a fatal illness that are very similar to the responses of family members, including denial, anger, depression, guilt, and ambivalent feelings. It is acceptable to seek support from colleagues and other resources in the workplace. It is important to not use the family of the

GUIDELINES Supporting Grieving Families*

General

- Stay with the family; sit quietly if they prefer not to talk; cry with them if that is acceptable to them.
- Accept the family's grief reactions; avoid judgemental statements (e.g., "You should be feeling better by now").
- Avoid offering rationalizations for the child's death (e.g., "Your child isn't suffering anymore").
- Avoid artificial consolation (e.g., "I know how you feel," or "You are still young enough to have another baby").
- Deal openly with feelings such as guilt, anger, and loss of self-esteem.
- Focus on feelings by using a feeling word in the statement (e.g., "You're still feeling all the pain of losing a child").
- Refer the family to an appropriate self-help group or for professional help, if needed.

At the Time of Death

- Reassure the family that everything possible is being done for the child, if they want lifesaving interventions.
- Do everything possible to ensure the child's comfort, especially relieving pain.
- Provide the child and family with the opportunity to review special experiences or memories in their lives.
- Express personal feelings of loss or frustration (e.g., "We will miss him so much," "We tried everything; we feel so sorry that we couldn't save her").
- Provide information that the family requests, and be honest.
- Respect the emotional needs of family members, such as siblings, who may need brief respites from the dying child.
- Make every effort to arrange for family members, especially parents, to be with the child at the moment of death, if they want to be present.
- Allow the family to stay with the dead child for as long as they wish and to rock, hold, or bathe the child.
- Provide practical help when possible, such as collecting the child's belongings.
- Arrange for spiritual support, based on the family's religious beliefs; pray with the family if no one else can stay with them.

After Death

- Attend the funeral or visitation if there was a special closeness with the family.
- Initiate and maintain contact (e.g., sending cards, telephoning, inviting them back to the unit, making a home visit).
- Refer to the dead child by name; discuss shared memories with the family.
- Discourage the use of drugs or alcohol as a method of escaping grief.
- Encourage all family members to communicate their feelings rather than remaining silent to avoid upsetting another member.
- Emphasize that grieving is a painful process that often takes years to resolve.

**Family* refers to all significant persons involved in the child's life, such as the parents, siblings, grandparents, or other close relatives or friends.

FAMILY-CENTRED TEACHING

A Dying Child: A Nurse's Perspective

Claire was unresponsive with slow, gasping breathing. Her mother asked me what I thought was happening. I replied honestly, "Your baby is dying because of her brain tumour." The mother put her arms around me and cried. We arranged for Claire to be baptized.

Honesty. As painful as the loss of a child is, my job is to assist the family through this experience. Although I usually wait until a private moment, such as driving home, I found tears streaming down my face as family and friends gathered for Claire's baptism. I went into the kitchen to compose myself, only to find several of my colleagues crying as well. Saying good-bye to a dying child will always be a difficult but shared experience.

–Jeanne O'Connor Egan, RN, MSN, Pediatric Clinical Specialist, Children's Hospital Washington, DC

dying child as a source of comfort. Seeking support from the child's family is not acceptable as it puts the therapeutic relationship at risk and crosses professional boundaries for appropriate nurse–patient relationships.

Strategies that can assist the nurse in remaining able to work effectively in these settings include maintaining good general health, developing well-rounded interests, using distancing techniques such as taking time off when needed, developing and using professional and personal support systems, cultivating the capacity for empathy, focusing on the positive aspects of the caregiver role, and basing nursing interventions on sound theory and empirical observations. Attending shared-remembrance rituals assists some nurses in resolving grief (Davis & Eng, 1998). Similarly, attending the funeral services can be a supportive act for both the family and the nurse and in no way detracts from the professionalism of care.

Key Points

- Trends in the treatment of children with chronic illness or disability have focused on developmental age, the child's strengths and uniqueness, family-centred care, normalization, early discharge, home care, mainstreaming, and early intervention.
- Families' reactions to disability or chronic illness are manifested in the following stages: shock and denial, adjustment, reintegration, and acknowledgement.
- The child's reaction to illness or disability depends on the child's developmental level, coping mechanisms, others' reactions, and the illness itself.
- In response to the child with chronic illness or disability, parents may be affected by feelings of inadequacy and failure; excessive demands on time, energy, and financial resources; and strain on the marital relationship.
- Assessment of the family's adjustment to a child's chronic illness, disability, or death includes the availability of a support system, their perception of the event, their coping mechanisms, concurrent stressors, and their response to the child.
- To help parents cope with their child's chronic illness or disability, nurses must offer attentiveness, empathic support, solicitation of suggestions for care, facilitation of communication, an opportunity to express feelings, and referral to volunteer and community agencies.
- Supporting the child involves encouraging self-expression, alleviating feelings of being different, and strengthening the child's self-image.
- Children's concept of death is determined by their cognitive ability and their experience with life-threatening illness.
- Young children see death as temporary and reversible and mainly fear separation.
- School-age children view death as irreversible but not necessarily inevitable and may fear mutilation.
- Children beyond 9 to 10 years of age realize that death is irreversible, universal, and inevitable but may resist the thought of their own death.
- Siblings have special needs, including the need for information, reassurance about their own health status, assurance that they are not responsible for the illness or death, and support for their own grieving process.
- Special needs of the family facing the unexpected death of a child include support while awaiting news of the child's status; a sensitive pronouncement of death; acknowledgement of feelings of denial, guilt, and anger; an opportunity to view the body; and referrals for support.
- Special decisions at the time of dying and death may involve hospital or hospice care, viewing of the body, tissue donation and autopsy, and siblings' attendance at the funeral.
- Acute grief is a syndrome with intense and distressing psychological and somatic symptoms that appear at the time of death.
- Complicated grief is a prolonged, intense grief that can impede an individual's ability to function on a daily basis.
- In dealing with the stress related to a dying young patient, the nurse can cope successfully through self-awareness, consciousness raising, knowledge and practice, an available support system, and maintenance of general good health, and by focusing on the positive rewards of involvement with dying children and their families.

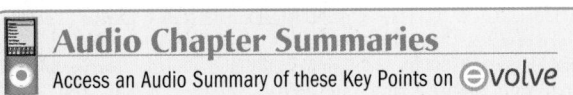

Audio Chapter Summaries

Access an Audio Summary of these Key Points on evolve

References

Ahmann, E. (2006). Supporting fathers' involvement in children's health care. *Pediatric Nursing, 32*(1), 88–90.

American Academy of Pediatrics, Committee on Hospital Care and Section on Surgery. (2002). Pediatric organ donation and transplantation. *Pediatrics, 109*(5), 982–984.

Baillargeon, R. H., & Bernier, J. (2010). The burden of disability in children and youths associated with impairments of psychological functions. *Psychiatry Research, 177*, 199–205. doi:10.1016/j.psychres.2010.03.001

Barlow, J. H., & Ellard, D. R. (2006). The psychosocial well-being of children with chronic disease, their parents and siblings: An overview of the research evidence base. *Child: Care, Health and Development, 32*(1), 19–31. doi:10.1111/j.1365-2214.2006.00591.x

Brehaut, J. C., et al. (2009). Health among caregivers of children with health problems: Findings from a Canadian population-based study. *American Journal of Public Health, 99*(7), 1254–1259. doi:10.2105/AJPH.2007.129817

Bruce, M., Gumley, D., Isham, L., Fearon, P., & Phipps, K. (2011). Post-traumatic stress symptoms in childhood brain tumour survivors and their parents. *Child: Care, Health and Development, 37*(2), 244–251. doi:10.1111/j.1365-2214.2010.01164.x

Canadian Hospice Palliative Care Association and Canadian Network of Palliative Care for Children. (2005). *Pediatric hospice palliative care survey: 2005 highlights*. Retrieved from http://cnpcc.ca/documents/CNPCC_Survey_Presentation_CHPCAConference_Sept05.pdf.

Canadian Hospice Palliative Care Association and Canadian Network of Palliative Care for Children. (2006). *Norms of practice: Pediatric hospice palliative care*. Retrieved from http://www.chpca.net/professionals/standards-and-norms-of-practice.aspx

Canadian Nurses Association. (2008). *Code of ethics for registered nurses*. Retrieved from http://www2.cna-aiic.ca/CNA/documents/pdf/publications/Code_of_Ethics_2008_e.pdf.

Canadian Paediatric Society, Bioethics Committee. (2008). Advance care planning for paediatric patients. *Paediatrics and Child Health, 13*(9), 791–796.

Canuck Place Children's Hospice. (2002). *Policy: Do not resuscitate/Permit natural death*. Retrieved from http://cnpcc.ca/documents/DNAR_PND_CanuckPlace.pdf.

Carnevale, F. A., et al. (2006). Daily living with distress and enrichment: The moral experience of families with ventilator-assisted children at home. *Pediatrics, 117*(1), e48–e60. doi:10.1542/peds.2005-0789

Chief Public Health Officer's Report on The State of Public Health in Canada. (2009). *Chapter 3: The health of Canadian children*. Retrieved from http://www.phac-aspc.gc.ca/cphorsphc-respcacsp/2009/fr-rc/cphorsphc-respcacsp06-eng.php#c3-1.

Clements, P. T., et al. (2003). Cultural perspectives of death, grief, and bereavement. *Journal of Psychosocial Nursing & Mental Health Services, 41*(7), 18–26.

Coffey, J. S. (2006). Parenting a child with chronic illness: A metasynthesis. *Pediatric Nursing, 32*(1), 51–59.

Corlett, J., & Twycross, A. (2006). Negotiation of parental roles within family-centered care: A review of the research. *Journal of Clinical Nursing, 15*(10), 1308–1316. doi:10.1111/j.1365-2702.2006.01407.x

Da Silva, F. M., Jacob, E., & Nascimento, C. (2010). Impact of childhood cancer on parents' relationships: An integrative review. *Journal of Nursing Scholarship, 42*(3), 250–261. doi:10.1111/j.1547-5069.2010.01360.x

Daudji, A., et al. (2011). Perceptions of disability among south Asian immigrant mothers of children with disabilities in Canada: Implications for rehabilitation service delivery. *Disability & Rehabilitation, 33*(6), 511–521. doi:10.3109/09638288.2010.498549

Davies, B., et al. (2004). "Living in the dragon's shadow": Fathers' experiences of a child's life-limiting illness. *Death Studies, 28*(2), 111–135.

Davies, R. (2004). New understandings of parental grief: Literature review. *Journal of Advanced Nursing, 46*(5), 506–513.

Davies, R., Davis, B., & Sibert, J. (2003). Parents' stories of sensitive and insensitive care by paediatricians in the time leading up to and including diagnostic disclosure of a life-limiting condition in their child. *Child: Care, Health and Development, 29*(1), 77–82.

Davis, B., & Eng, B. (1998). Special issues in bereavement and staff support. In D. Doyle, G. W. C. Hanks, & N. MacDonald (Eds.), *Oxford textbook of palliative medicine* (2nd ed.). New York: Oxford University Press.

Denboba, D., et al. (2006). Achieving family and provider partnerships for children with special health care needs. *Pediatrics, 118*(4), 1607–1615. doi:10.1542/peds.2006-0383

Doig, J. L., McLennan, J. D., & Urichuk, L. (2009). "Jumping through hoops": Parents' experiences with seeking respite care for children with special needs. *Child: Care, Health and Development, 35*(2), 234–242. doi:10.1111/j.1365-2214.2008.00922.x.

Dunbrack, J. (2006). *Advance care planning: The Glossary Project—final report*. Retrieved from http://hc-sc.gc.ca/hcs-sss/pubs/palliat/2006-proj-glos/index-eng.php.

Fallat, M. E., & Deshpande, J. K. (2004). Do-not-resuscitate orders for pediatric patients who require anesthesia and surgery. *Pediatrics, 114*(6), 1686–1692.

Field, M. J., & Behrman, R. E. (Eds.). (2004). *When children die: Improving palliative and end-of-life care for children and their families*. Washington, DC: National Academies Press.

Fleitas, J. (2000). When Jack fell down … Jill came tumbling after: Siblings in the web of illness and disability. *MCN: American Journal of Maternal-Child Nursing, 25*, 267–273.

Forrester, L. (2003). One to one care in children's hospice. *Nursing Times, 99*(16), 44–45.

Freyer, D. R. (2004). Care of the dying adolescent: Special considerations. *Pediatrics, 113*(2), 381–388.

Gerlach, A. (2008). "Circle of caring": A First Nations worldview of child rearing. *Canadian Journal of Occupational Therapy, 75*(1), 18–25.

Goldbeck, L. (2001). Parental coping with the diagnosis of childhood cancer: Gender effects, dissimilarity within couples, and quality of life. *Psycho-oncology, 10*, 325–335.

Goodenough, B., et al. (2004). Bereavement outcomes for parents who lose a child to cancer: Are place of death and sex of parent associated with differences in psychological functioning? *Psycho-oncology, 13*(11), 779–791.

Grossoehme, D. H., Ragsdale, J., Cotton, S., Wooldridge, J. L., Grimes, L., & Seid, M. (2010). Parents' religious coping styles in the first year after their child's cystic fibrosis diagnosis. *Journal of Health Care Chaplaincy, 16*(3-4), 109–122. doi:10.1080/08854726.2010.480836

Halfon, N., & Newacheck, P. (2010). Evolving notions of childhood chronic illness. *Journal of the American Medical Association, 2003*(7), 665–666. doi:10.1001/jama.2010.130

Hawryluck, L. A., & Harvey, W. R. (2000). Analgesia, virtue, and the principle of double effect. *Journal of Palliative Care, 16*(Suppl), S24–S30.

Hellsten, M. B., et al. (2000). *End-of-life care for children*. Austin, TX: Texas Cancer Council.

Hinds, P. S., et al. (2001). End-of-life decision making by adolescents, parents, and healthcare providers in pediatric oncology: Research to evidence-based practice guidelines. *Cancer Nursing, 24*, 122–134.

Holland Bloorview Kids Rehabilitation Hospital. (2011). *Common sibling issues*. Retrieved from http://www.hollandbloorview.ca/resourcecentre/family_parenting/siblings/parenting_whataboutme.php.

Hollander, M., & Prince, M. (2008). Organizing healthcare delivery systems for persons with ongoing care needs and their families. *Healthcare Quarterly 11*(1), 44–54.

Hospice House. (2004). *Every child is my child: A report of the workshop—Hospice services for children around the world*. Retrieved from: http://cnpcc.ca/pages/EveryChild.htm.

Immelt, S. (2006). Psychological adjustment in young children with chronic medical conditions. *Journal of Pediatric Nursing, 21*(5), 362–377.

IWK Health Centre. (2003). *Clinical policy/objective manual—Death of a patient*. Retrieved from http://cnpcc.ca/documents/IWK_Policy_DeathOfAPatient.pdf.

Jackson, P. L. (2000). The primary care provider and children with chronic conditions. In P. L. Jackson & P. A. Vessey (Eds.), *Primary care of the child with a chronic condition* (3rd ed.). St. Louis: Mosby.

Jennings, P. D. (2005). Providing pediatric palliative care through a pediatric supportive care team. *Pediatric Nursing, 31*(3), 195–200.

Johnson, A .P., Abernathy, T., Howell, D., Brazil, K., & Scott, S. (2009). Resource utilization and costs of palliative cancer care in an interdisciplinary health care model. *Palliative Medicine, 23*, 448–459. doi:10.1177/0269216309103193

Jokinen, P. (2004). The family life-path theory: A tool for nurses working in partnership with families. *Journal of Child Health Care, 8*(2), 124–133.

Kausar, S., Jevne, R. F., & Sobsey, D. (2003). Hope in families of children with developmental disabilities. *Journal on Developmental Disabilities, 10*(1), 35–46.

Klass, D. (2001). The inner representation of the dead child in the psychic and social narratives of bereaved parents. In R. A. Neimeyer (Ed.), *Meaning reconstruction and the experience of loss*. Washington, DC: American Psychological Association.

Lach, L. M., et al. (2009). The health and psychosocial functioning of caregivers of children with neurodevelopmental disorders. *Disability and Rehabilitation, 31*(8), 607–618.

Lobato, D. J., & Kao, B. T. (2002). Integrated sibling–parent group intervention to improve sibling knowledge and adjustment to chronic illness and disability. *Journal of Pediatric Psychology, 27*, 711–716.

Marshall, E. S., et al. (2003). "This is a spiritual experience": Perspectives of Latter-Day Saint families living with a child with disabilities. *Qualitative Health Research, 13*, 57–76.

Martinez, Y. J., & Ercikan, K., (2009). Chronic illness in Canadian children: What is the effect of illness on academic achievement, and anxiety and emotional disorders? *Child: Care, Health and Development, 35*(3), 391–401.

Masri, C., et al. (2000). Decision making and end-of-life care in critically ill children. *Journal of Palliative Care, 16*(Suppl), S45–S52.

McDougal, J. (2002). Promoting normalization in families with preschool children with type 1 diabetes. *Journal of Specialty Pediatric Nursing, 7*(3), 113–120.

Morse, J. M., Wilson, S., & Penrod, J. (2000). Mothers and their disabled children: Refining the concept of normalization. *Health Care for Women International, 21*(8), 659–676.

Msall, M. E., et al. (2003). Functional disability and school activity limitations in 41,300 school-age children: Relationship to medical impairments. *Pediatrics, 111*, 548–553.

Nelson, A. M. (2002). A metasynthesis: Mothering other-than-normal children. *Qualitative Health Research, 12*, 515–530.

Nuutila, L., & Salanterä, S. (2006). Children with a long-term illness: Parents' experiences of care. *Journal of Pediatric Nursing, 21*(2), 153–160. doi:10.1016/j.pedn.2005.07.005

O'Brien, M. E., & Wegner, C. B. (2002). Rearing the child who is technology dependent: Perceptions of parents and home care nurses. *Journal for Specialists in Pediatric Nursing, 7*, 7–15.

Ochieng, B. M. (2003). Minority ethnic families and family-centered care. *Journal of Child Health Care, 7*(2), 123–132.

Perrin, E. C., Lewkowicz, C., & Young M. H. (2000). Shared vision: Concordance among fathers, mothers, and pediatricians about unmet needs of children with chronic health conditions. *Pediatrics, 105*(1, pt3), 277–285.

Perrin, J. M. (2004). Chronic illness in childhood. In R. E. Behrman, R. M. Kleigman, & H. B. Jensen (Eds), *Nelson textbook of pediatrics* (17th ed.). Philadelphia: Saunders.

Raina, P., et al. (2005). The health and well-being of caregivers of children with cerebral palsy. *Pediatrics, 115*(6), e626–e636. doi:10.1542/peds.2004-1689

Ray, L. D. (2002). Parenting and childhood chronicity: Making visible the invisible work. *Journal of Pediatric Nursing, 17*(6), 424–438.

Reilly, D., Huws, J., Hastings, R., & Vaughan, F. (2010). Life and death of a child with Down syndrome and a congenital heart condition: Experiences of six couples. *Intellectual & Developmental Disabilities, 48*(6), 403–416.

Rossiter, L., & Sharpe, D. (2001). The siblings of individuals with mental retardation: A quantitative integration of the literature. *Journal of Child & Family Studies, 10*(1), 65–84.

Sahler, O., et al. (2000). Medical education about end-of-life care in the pediatric setting: Principles, challenges, and opportunities. *Pediatrics, 105*, 575–584.

Schor, E. L. (2003). Family pediatrics: report of the Task Force on the Family. *Pediatrics, 111*, 1541–1571.

Seow, H., Barbera, L., Howell, D., & Dy, S. (2010). Using more end-of-life homecare services is associated with using fewer acute care services: a population-based cohort study. *Medical Care 48*(2), 118–124. doi:10.1097/MLR.0b013e3181c162ef

Sharpe, D., & Rossiter, L. (2002). Siblings of children with a chronic illness: A meta-analysis. *Journal of Pediatric Psychology, 27*, 699–710.

Shepard, M. P., & Mahon, M. M. (2000). Chronic conditions and the family. In P. L. Jackson & J. A. Vessey (Eds.), *Primary care of the child with a chronic condition* (3rd ed.). St. Louis: Mosby.

Sine, D., et al. (2001). Pediatric extubation: "Pulling the tube." *Journal of Palliative Medicine, 4*, 519–524.

Singh Jassal, S. (Ed.) (2008). *Basic symptom control in paediatric palliative care.* Retrieved from http://cnpcc.ca/documents/2008RainbowHospiceSymptomControlManual.pdf.

Spalding, K., & Salib, D. (2008). *Children and youth home care in Canada. In focus.* Retrieved from http://www.crncc.ca/knowledge/factsheets/pdf/In_Focus_Children_and_Youth_Homecare_FINAL.pdf.

Statistics Canada. (2003). *Educational services and the disabled child.* Retrieved from http://www.statcan.gc.ca/pub/81-004-x/2006005/9588-eng.htm.

Statistics Canada. (2010). *Leading causes of death of children and youth, by age group, 2003 to 2005.* Retrieved from http://www41.statcan.gc.ca/2009/20000/tbl/cybac20000_2009_000_t07-eng.htm.

Sterling, Y. M., & Peterson, J. W. (2003). Characteristics of African American women caregivers of children with asthma. *MCN: American Journal of Maternal-Child Nursing, 28*, 32–38.

Sullivan-Bolyai, S., et al. (2003). Great expectations: A position description for parents as caregivers, part I. *Pediatric Nursing, 29*(6), 52–56.

Sumner, L. H. (2003). Lighting the way: Improving the way children die in America. *Caring, 22*, 14–18.

Tam, C., & Poon, V. (2008) Developing a support group for families with children with disabilities in a Canadian Chinese church community. *Journal of Pastoral Care & Counselling. 62*(4), 343–351.

Thomlinson, E. H. (2002). The lived experience of families of children who are failing to thrive. *Journal of Advanced Nursing, 39*, 537–545.

Tong, H., et al. (2002). Physical functioning in female caregivers of children with physical disabilities compared with female caregivers of children with a chronic medical condition. *Archives of Pediatric & Adolescent Medicine, 156*, 1138–1142.

Trute, B., Hiebert-Murphy, D., & Wright, A. (2008). Family-centered service coordination in childhood health and disability services: The search for meaningful service outcome measures. *Child: Care, Health and Development, 34*(3), 367–372. doi:10.1111/j.1365-2214.2008.00819.x.

van Dyck, P., et al. (2004a). The national survey of children's health: A new data resource. *Maternal & Child Health Journal, 8*(3), 183–188.

van Dyck, P. C., et al. (2004b). Prevalence and characteristics of children with special health care needs. *Archives of Pediatric & Adolescent Medicine, 158*(9), 884–890.

Whitehead, L. C., & Gosling, V. (2003). Parent's perceptions of interactions with health professionals in the pathway to gaining a diagnosis of tuberous sclerosis (TS) and beyond. *Research in Developmental Disabilities, 24*, 109–119.

Winkler, W. D., & Mardegian, C. A. (2001). Completing the continuum of care: The growth of a pediatric hospice program. *Caring, 20*, 22–25.

Wise, P. H., et al. (2002). Chronic illness among poor children enrolled in the temporary assistance for needy families program. *American Journal of Public Health, 92*, 1458–1461.

Wolfe, J., Friebert, S., & Hilden, J. (2002). Caring for children with advanced cancer integrating palliative care. *Pediatric Clinics of North America, 49*(5), 1043–1062.

Wolfe, J., et al. (2000). Symptoms and suffering at the end of life in children with cancer. *New England Journal of Medicine, 342*(5), 326–333.

Wood, P. R., et al. (2002). Relationships between welfare status, health insurance status, and health and medical care among children with asthma. *American Journal of Public Health, 92*, 1446–1452.

World Health Organization. (2012a). *WHO definition of palliative care.* Retrieved from http://www.who.int/cancer/palliative/definition/en/.

World Health Organization. (2012b). *WHO's pain ladder.* Retrieved from http://www.who.int/cancer/palliative/painladder/en/.

Yantzi, N. M., Rosenberg, M. W., & McKeever, P. (2007). Getting out of the house: The challenges mothers face when their children have long-term needs. *Health and Social Care in the Community, 15*(1), 45–55. doi:10.1111/j.1365-2524.2006.00663

Young, B., et al. (2003). Managing communication with young people who have a potentially life threatening chronic illness: Qualitative study of patients and parents. *British Medical Journal, 326*, 1–5.

Zuvekas, S. H., & Taliaferro, G. S. (2003). Pathways to access: Health, insurance, the health care delivery system and racial/ethnic disparities, 1996–1999. *Health Affairs, 22*(2), 139–153.

Additional Resources

Books for Siblings of Children with Special Needs: http://www.parentbooks.ca/Siblings_of_Children_with_Special_Needs.html

Canadian Medic Alert Foundation: http://www.medicalert.ca

Council of Canadians with Disabilities: http://www.ccdonline.ca

Easter Seals Canada: http://easterseals.ca/english/

Holland Bloorview Kids Rehabilitation Hospital: Family Resource Centre: http://www.hollandbloorview.ca/resourcecentre/family_parenting/siblings.php

My Summer Camps—Directory of private, paying camps for children with chronic illnesses or general physical disabilities: http://www.mysummercamps.com/camps/Special_Needs_Camps

Our Kids Go to Camp: http://www.ourkids.net/special-needs-camps.php.

Safe Kids Canada: Safety Information—Car Seats: http://www.safekidscanada.ca/Parents/Safety-Information/Car-Seats/Index.aspx

Special Need Child Canada: http://www.special-need-child-canada.com/special-need-child-blog.html

Special Olympics Canada: http://www.specialolympics.ca

Transport Canada—Information on car safety restraints for children: http://www.tc.gc.ca/eng/roadsafety/safedrivers-childsafety-car-index-873.htm

VSA Arts (has affiliate chapters in Ontario and Québec): http://www.kennedy-center.org/education

World Health Organization: Palliative Care: Symptom Management and End-of-Life Care: http://www.who.int/hiv/pub/imai/genericpalliativecare082004.pdf

Appendix 1

Helpful Resources Related to Children's Palliative and End-of-Life Care

Document Title	Description	Internet Link
Rainbows Children's Hospice Symptom Control Guidelines (Singh Jassal, 2008)	Provides doctors and nursing staff in specialized units and in the community an understanding of the basis of symptom control in palliative care for children	http://cnpcc.ca/documents/2008RainbowHospiceSymptomControlManual.pdf
Advance Care Planning: The Glossary Project—Final Report, developed by J. Dunbrack for Health Canada (2006)	Clarifies the concepts and terms used in advance care planning in Canadian provinces and territories and in the health, social, and legal sectors in order to facilitate pan-Canadian dialogue about advance care planning	http://cnpcc.ca/documents/ACPFinalReport_August22-2006.pdf
CHPCA/CNPCC Norms of Practice: Pediatric Hospice Palliative Care (2006)	The Canadian Hospice Palliative Care Association (CHPCA)'s Canadian Network of Palliative Care for Children (CNPCC) has worked to adapt national principles and norms of practice for children's care; a national consensus process for this was completed in May 2006.	http://www.chpca.net/professionals/standards-and-norms-of-practice.aspx
Presentation on results of survey of Canadian Hospice Palliative Care Services and Canadian Network of Palliative Care for Children Survey (2005)	Preliminary results of completed Canada-wide survey of palliative care services for children; further results to follow	http://cnpcc.ca/documents/CNPCC_Survey_Presentation_CHPCAConference_Sept05.pdf
Together for Short Lives: Downloads and shop	Many helpful resources to assist professionals in palliative and end-of-life care for children	http://www.act.org.uk/shop.asp?section=143&sectionTitle=Resources+and+shop
DNAR/PND policy, Canuck Place Children's Hospice (2002)	Canuck Place Children's Hospice policy on do not attempt resuscitation (DNAR)—permit natural death (PND)	http://cnpcc.ca/documents/DNAR_PND_CanuckPlace.pdf
"Every Child Is My Child": A Report of the Workshop—Hospice services for children around the world, Hospice House, London (2004)	International workshop to recommend building a "virtual network" of national organizations and other groups to facilitate future collaboration, and to encourage WHO to advocate for palliative care	http://cnpcc.ca/pages/EveryChild.htm
IWK Health Centre, Halifax, Nova Scotia Clinical policy/objective manual—Death of a Patient (2003)	Clinical policy and guideline describing provision of support to family and friends, appropriate legal documentation and procedures, and care of the body following the death of a patient	http://cnpcc.ca/documents/IWK_Policy_DeathOfAPatient.pdf

Unit 10

42 Cognitive and Sensory Impairment

Learning Objectives

On completion of this chapter, the reader will be able to:

- Define the classifications of cognitive impairment.
- Outline nursing interventions for the child with cognitive impairment that promote optimum development, including during hospitalization.
- Identify the major biological and cognitive characteristics of the child with Down syndrome.
- Outline nursing interventions for the child with Down syndrome.
- Identify the major characteristics associated with fragile X syndrome.
- List the general classifications of hearing impairment and the effect on speech.
- Outline nursing interventions for the child with hearing impairment, including during hospitalization.
- List the common types of visual disorders in children.
- Outline nursing interventions for the child with visual impairment, including during hospitalization.
- Outline nursing interventions for the child with retinoblastoma.
- Outline nursing interventions for the child with autism spectrum disorder.

Electronic Resources

Additional information related to the content in Chapter 42 can be found on

evolve the companion Web site at

http://evolve.elsevier.com/Canada/Perry/maternal/

- Examination Review Questions
- Case Study—Bacterial Conjunctivitis
- Case Study—Down Syndrome
- Critical Thinking Exercise—Down Syndrome
- Critical Thinking Exercise—Fragile X Syndrome

Cognitive Impairment

General Concepts

Cognitive impairment (CI) is a general term that encompasses any type of mental difficulty or deficiency. This chapter discusses the characteristics and diagnosis of specific types of CI as well as the nursing care required for children with CI. Although the family's needs and concerns are also a primary focus throughout this chapter, the reader is encouraged to review Chapter 41, which details the family's adjustment to disabilities in general.

The definition of intellectual disability in children consists of three components: intellectual functioning, functional strengths and weaknesses, and age younger than 18 years at time of diagnosis. A disability in intellectual functioning is measured by the intelligence quotient (IQ) of 70 to 75 or below. The child with an intellectual disability must demonstrate functional impairment in at least 2 of 10 different adaptive skill areas: communication, self-care, home living, social skills, leisure, health and safety, self-direction, functional academics, community use, and work (American Psychiatric Association, 2000). The classification system by the American Association on Intellectual and Developmental Disabilities provides identification of the individual's specific needs in four established dimensions of care (Box 42-1). In contrast, children with CI have or did have a normal IQ but demonstrate forgetfulness, difficulty concentrating, and confusion, from many causes such as brain injuries. Currently, there is no such classification system in Canada. Careful evaluation to identify the needs of individuals with CI is focused on promoting habilitation for each person. It is anticipated that the functional capabilities of children with CI will improve over time when support is provided.

Diagnosis and Classification

The diagnosis of CI is usually made after a period of suspicion, by professionals or the family, that the child's developmental

BOX 42-1 Dimensions of Care for the Intellectually Disabled

Dimension I—Intellectual functioning and adaptive skills
Dimension II—Psychological and emotional considerations
Dimension III—Physical, health, and etiological considerations
Dimension IV—Environmental considerations

BOX 42-2 Early Behavioural Signs Suggestive of Cognitive Impairment

- Dysmorphic features (e.g., Down syndrome, fragile X syndrome)
- Irritability or unresponsiveness to contact
- Abnormal eye contact during feeding
- Gross motor delay
- Decreased alertness to voice or movement
- Language difficulties or delay
- Feeding difficulties

(From Crocker, A., & Nelson, R. [1999]. Mental retardation. In M. Levine, W. B. Carey, & A. C. Crocker [Eds.], *Developmental-behavioral pediatrics* [3rd ed.]. Philadelphia: Saunders; and Shapiro, B., & Batshaw, M. [2004]. Mental retardation. In R. E. Behrman, R. M. Kliegman, & H. B. Jenson [Eds.], *Nelson textbook of pediatrics* [17th ed.]. Philadelphia: Saunders.)

progress is delayed. In some cases it is confirmed at birth because of recognition of distinct syndromes, such as Down syndrome and **fetal alcohol syndrome**. At the other extreme, the diagnosis is made when problems such as speech delays arouse concern. In all cases a high index of suspicion for developmental delay and behavioural signs (Box 42-2) is necessary for early diagnosis; routine developmental screening can assist in early identification (see Chapter 33). Delays are typically seen in gross and fine motor and speech development, although the latter is most predictive. Developmental delay can be described as any significant lag in a child's physical, cognitive, behavioural, emotional, or social development, when compared against developmental norms. CI is a permanent impairment encompassing cognitive ability and adaptive behaviour that are functioning significantly below average (see Box 42-2). In the absence of clear-cut evidence of CI, it is more appropriate to use a diagnosis of developmental delay (Biasini et al., 1999).

Results of standardized tests are used in making the diagnosis of intellectual disability based on cognitive deficits. Tests for assessing adaptive behaviours include the Vineland Social Maturity Scale and the AAMR Adaptive Behaviour Scale. The Vineland Scale measures the behaviour of individuals with and without disabilities, from birth to adulthood, in four domains: communication, daily living skills, socialization, and motor skills (Doll, 1953). The AAMR Adaptive Scale can be used to assess the behaviour and social adjustment of children ages 6 to 14 years whose adaptive behaviour could potentially mean intellectual disability, emotional disturbance, or other learning problems (Lambert, Nihira, & Leland, 1993). In addition, the Nunavik Adaptive Behavior Scale is available to assess adaptive behaviour in Inuit school-age children and in adults in whom intellectual disability is suspected (Maurice et al., 2007).

A more useful approach for clinical application is classification based on educational potential or symptom severity. For educational purposes the term *educable CI* corresponds to the mildly impaired group, which constitutes about 85% of all people with CI. *Trainable CI* generally applies to children with moderate levels of CI and accounts for about 10% of the intellectually disabled population (American Psychiatric Association, 2000; Walker & Johnson, 2006) (Table 42-1). Although nurses may be familiar with the approximate range of IQ for classifying severity, they should refrain from using numbers as the criterion for assessing or evaluating the child's abilities, since numbers are of little value in counselling parents or training these children.

Etiology

The causes of severe CI are primarily genetic, biochemical, and infectious. Although the etiology is unknown in most cases, familial, social, environmental, and organic causes may predominate. Among individuals with CI, a sizable proportion of the cases are linked to Down syndrome, fragile X syndrome, or fetal alcohol syndrome. General categories of events that may lead to cognitive impairment include the following (Kabra & Gulati, 2003; Walker & Johnson, 2006):

- Infection and intoxication, such as congenital rubella, syphilis, maternal drug consumption (e.g., fetal alcohol syndrome), chronic lead ingestion, or **kernicterus**
- Trauma or physical agent (i.e., injury to the brain suffered during the prenatal, perinatal, or postnatal period)
- Inadequate nutrition and metabolic disorders, such as phenylketonuria or congenital hypothyroidism
- Gross postnatal brain disease, such as neurofibromatosis and tuberous sclerosis
- Unknown prenatal influence, including cerebral and cranial malformations, such as microcephaly and hydrocephalus
- Chromosomal abnormalities resulting from radiation, viruses, chemicals, parental age, and **genetic mutations,** such as Down syndrome and fragile X syndrome
- Gestational disorders, including prematurity, low birth weight, and postmaturity
- Psychiatric disorders that have their onset during the child's developmental period up to age 18 years, such as autism spectrum disorders
- Environmental influences, including evidence of a deprived environment associated with a history of intellectual disability among parents and siblings

Nursing Care of Children With Impaired Cognitive Function

Nurses play a major role in identifying children with CI. In the newborn and early infancy periods, few signs are present, with the exception of Down syndrome (p. 1195). After this age, however, delayed **developmental milestones** are the major clues to CI. In addition, nurses must have a high index of suspicion for early behaviour patterns that may suggest CI

Table 42-1 Classification of Cognitive Impairment

LEVEL (IQ)*	PRESCHOOL (BIRTH–5 YR)—MATURATION AND DEVELOPMENT	SCHOOL AGE (6–21 YR)—TRAINING AND EDUCATION	ADULT (≥21 YR)—SOCIAL AND VOCATIONAL ADEQUACY
Mild—50–55 to approximately 70–75	Often not noticed as delayed by casual observer but is slower to walk, feed self, and talk than most children; follows same sequence in development as normal children	Can acquire practical skills and useful reading and arithmetic to a third- to sixth-grade level with special education; can be guided toward social conformity; achieves mental age of 8–12 yr	Can usually achieve social and vocational skills adequate for self-maintenance; may need occasional guidance and support when under unusual social or economic stress; can adjust to marriage but not childrearing
Moderate—35–40 to 50–55	Noticeable delays in motor development, especially in speech; responds to training in various self-help activities	Can learn simple communication, elementary health and safety habits, and simple manual skills; does not progress in functional reading or arithmetic; achieves mental age of 3–7 yr	Can perform simple tasks under sheltered conditions; participates in simple recreation; travels alone in familiar places; usually incapable of self-maintenance
Severe—20–25 to 35–40	Marked delay in motor development; little or no communication skills; may respond to training in elementary self-care (e.g., self-feeding)	Usually walks, barring specific disability; has some understanding of speech and some response; can profit from systematic habit training; achieves mental age of toddler	Can conform to daily routines and repetitive activities; needs continuing direction and supervision in protective environment
Profound—below 20–25	Gross delay; minimum capacity for functioning in sensorimotor areas; needs total care	Obvious delays in all areas of development; shows basic emotional responses; may respond to skillful training in use of legs, hands, and jaws; needs close supervision; achieves mental age of young infant	May walk; needs complete custodial care; has primitive speech; usually benefits from regular physical activity

*Data from American Psychiatric Association. (2000). *Diagnostic and statistical manual of mental disorders* (4th ed., text revision) (DSM-IV TR). Washington, DC: Author; and Rittey, C. D. (2005). Learning difficulties: What the neurologist needs to know. *Journal of Neurology, Neurosurgery, & Psychiatry, 74*(Suppl 1), 30–36.
IQ, intelligence quotient.

(see Box 42-2). Parental concerns, such as delayed development compared with that of siblings, need to be taken seriously. All children should receive regular developmental assessment, and the nurse is often the person responsible for performing such assessments (see Chapter 33). When delays are found, the nurse must use sensitivity and discretion in revealing this finding to parents.

Nursing Care Management

Educate the Child and Family

In order to teach children with CI, it is necessary to investigate their learning abilities and deficits. This is important for the nurse who may be involved in a home care program or who may be caring for the child in a health care setting. The nurse who understands how these children learn can effectively teach them basic skills or prepare them for various health-related procedures.

Children with CI have a marked deficit in their ability to discriminate between two or more stimuli because of difficulty in recognizing the relevance of specific cues. However, these children can learn to discriminate if the cues are presented in an exaggerated, concrete form and if all extraneous stimuli are eliminated. For example, the use of colours to emphasize visual cues or the use of singing or rhymes to stress auditory cues can help them learn. Their deficit in discrimination also implies that concrete ideas are learned much more effectively than abstract ideas. Therefore, demonstration is preferable to verbal explanation, and learning should be directed toward mastering a skill rather than understanding the scientific principles underlying a procedure.

Another cognitive deficit is in short-term memory. Whereas children of average **intelligence** can remember several words, numbers, or directions at one time, children with CI are less able to do so. Therefore, they need simple, one-step directions. Learning through a step-by-step process requires a task analysis, in which each task is separated into its necessary components and each step is taught completely before proceeding to the next activity.

One critical area of learning that has had a tremendous impact on education for cognitively impaired individuals is motivation. Programs based on the motivational principles of behaviour modification, employing positive reinforcement for specific tasks or behaviours, have demonstrated marked improvement in children's ability to learn. Advances in technology have greatly aided in providing reinforcement, especially in children who are severely disabled and who may have physical disabilities that limit their range of capabilities. For example, with the use of specially designed switches, children can be given control of some event in the environment, such as turning on the television (Fig. 42-1). The television picture becomes reinforcement for activating the switch. Repetitive use of these switches provides an early, simple association with a technical device that may progress to increasingly complex aids.

Early intervention programs comprise a systematic program of therapy, exercises, and activities designed to address developmental delays in disabled children in order to help them achieve their full potential (American Academy of Pediatrics, Committee on Genetics, 2001; Canadian Down Syndrome Society, 2009). There is considerable evidence that

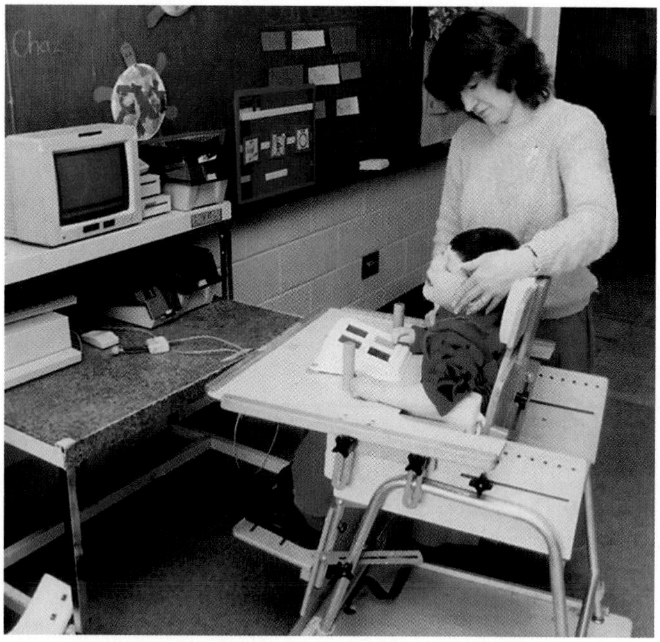

Fig. 42-1 A push panel allows a child with cognitive impairment to turn a computer on and off.

these programs are valuable for cognitively impaired children. Nurses working with these families need to be aware of the types of programs in their community. Under the *Education Act* (1956–1996) and the *Canadian Human Rights Act* (1977), provinces and territories are required to provide educational opportunities for all children with disabilities. Although early intervention programs are available in Canada, Canadian provinces and territories vary widely in their support, thus many expenses may fall to the parents (Parliament of Canada Standing Senate Committee on Social Affairs, Science and Technology, 2006). Services may be provided by private organizations such as the Canadian Down Syndrome Society and Easter Seals Canada (see Additional Resources section at the end of this chapter). Parents should inquire about these programs by contacting the appropriate agencies. The child's education should begin as soon as possible. As children grow older, their education should be directed toward vocational training that prepares them for as independent a lifestyle as possible that is within their scope of abilities.

Teach Child Self-Care Skills

When a child with CI is born, parents need assistance in promoting normal developmental skills that are almost automatically learned by other children. These include self-care skills such as feeding, toileting, dressing, and grooming. In order to teach these skills, a basic knowledge of the developmental sequence in learning the skills demonstrated by children of average intelligence is required. For example, children with subaverage intelligence would not be expected to dress themselves as early as unaffected youngsters.

Teaching self-care skills also necessitates a working knowledge of the individual steps needed to master a skill. For example, before beginning a self-feeding program, the nurse needs to perform a task analysis. After a task analysis, the child is observed in a particular situation, such as eating, to determine what skills are possessed and the child's developmental readiness to learn the task. Family members should be included in this process because their "readiness" is as important as the child's. Numerous self-help aids, such as a plate with suction cups to prevent accidental spills, are available to facilitate independence and can help eliminate some of the difficulties of learning (see Additional Resources).

Promote Child's Optimum Development

Optimum development involves more than achieving independence. It requires appropriate guidance for establishing acceptable social behaviour and personal feelings of self-esteem, worth, and security. These attributes are not simply learned through a stimulation program. Rather, they must arise from the genuine love and caring of family members. However, families need guidance in providing an environment that fosters optimal development. Often it is the nurse who can provide assistance in these areas of childrearing.

Another important area for promoting optimum development and self-esteem is ensuring the child's physical well-being. Any congenital defects, such as cardiac, gastrointestinal, or orthopaedic anomalies, should be repaired. Plastic surgery may be considered when the child's appearance can be substantially improved. Dental health is significant, and orthodontic and restorative procedures can often improve facial appearance immensely.

Encourage Play and Exercise

Children who are cognitively impaired have the same needs for recreation and exercise as other children. However, because of the children's slower development, parents may be less aware of the need to provide such activities (Fig. 42-2). Therefore, the nurse needs to guide parents toward selection of suitable play and exercise activities. Because play for children in each age group has been discussed in earlier chapters (see Chapter 33, Role of Play in Development, and Chapters 36–39), only the exceptions are presented here.

The type of play needs to be based on the child's developmental age, although the need for sensorimotor play may be prolonged for several years. Parents should use every opportunity to expose the child to as many different sounds, sights,

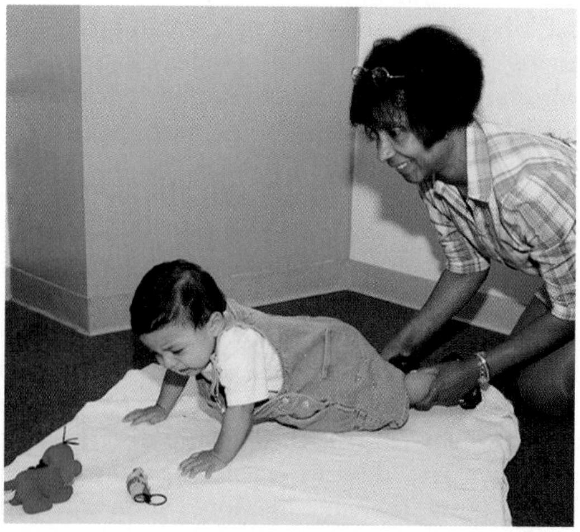

Fig. 42-2 Placing an attractive object outside the child's reach encourages crawling movements. *(Courtesy James DeLeon, Texas Children's Hospital, Houston, TX.)*

and sensations as possible. Appropriate play includes musical mobiles, stuffed toys, water play, floating toys, a rocking chair or horse, a swing, bells, and rattles. The child should be taken on outings, such as trips to the grocery store or shopping centre; other people should be encouraged to visit in the home; and the child should be related to directly, such as by cuddling, holding, and rocking the child; talking to the child in the en face (face-to-face) position; and giving the child "rides" on the parents' shoulders.

Toys should be selected for their recreational and educational value. For example, a large inflatable beach ball is a good water toy; it encourages interactive play and can be used to learn motor skills, such as balance, rocking, kicking, and throwing. A doll with removable clothes and different types of closures can help the child learn dressing skills. Musical toys that mimic animal sounds or respond with social phrases are excellent ways of encouraging speech. Toys should be simple in design so that the child can learn to manipulate them without help. For children with severe cognitive and physical impairment, electronic switches can be used to allow them to operate toys (Fig. 42-3).

Suitable activities for physical activity should be based on the child's size, coordination, physical fitness and maturity, motivation, and health (Fig. 42-4). Some children may have physical problems, such as atlantoaxial instability in children with Down syndrome, that prevent participation in certain sports. These children often have greater success in individual and dual sports than in team sports and enjoy themselves most with children of the same developmental level. The Special Olympics provides these children with a unique competitive opportunity (see Additional Resources section at the end of this chapter).

Safety is a major consideration in selecting recreational and exercise activities. For example, toys that may be appropriate developmentally may present dangers to a child who is strong enough to break them or use them incorrectly.

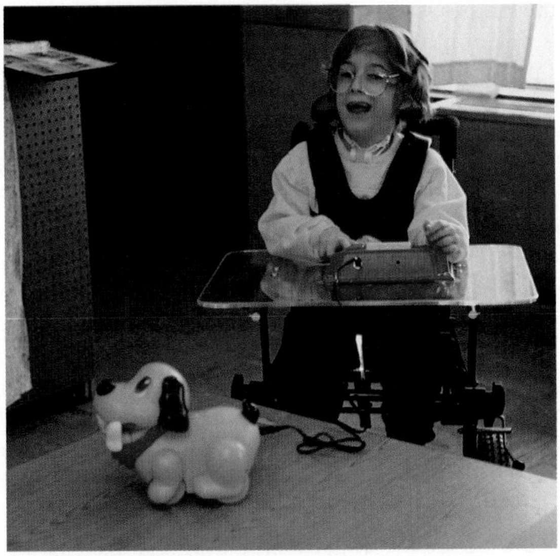

Fig. 42-3 A manual switch allows a child with cognitive impairment to play with a battery-operated toy.

Provide Means of Communication

Verbal skills are typically delayed more than other physical skills. Speech requires hearing and interpretation (receptive skills) and facial muscle coordination (expressive skills). Because both types of skills may be impaired, these children need frequent audiometric testing and should be fitted with hearing aids if indicated. In addition, they may need help in learning to control their facial muscles. For example, some children may need tongue exercises to correct the tongue thrust or gentle reminders to keep the lips closed.

Nonverbal communication may be appropriate for some of these children, and various devices are available. For the child without associated physical disabilities, a talking picture board is helpful. For children with physical limitations, several adaptations or types of communication devices are available to facilitate selection of the appropriate picture or word (Fig. 42-5). Some children may be taught sign language or Blissymbols—a highly stylized system of graphic symbols that

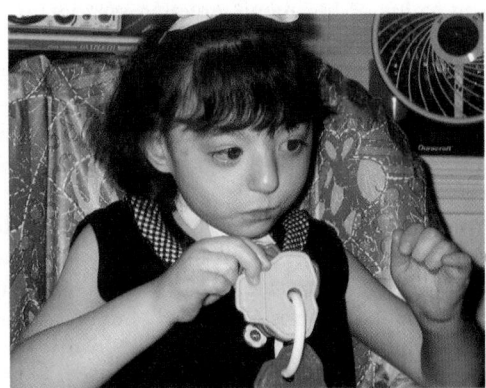

Fig. 42-4 A favourite toy provides stimulation for a young child.

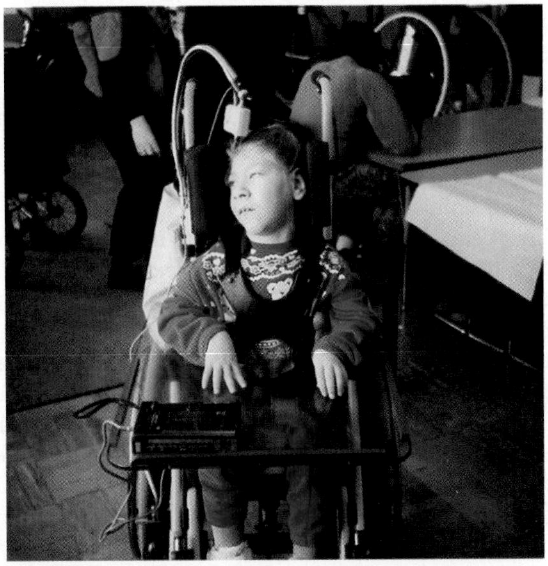

Fig. 42-5 A child with cognitive and physical impairments can activate electronic and communication equipment by moving a device near her head.

represent words, ideas, and concepts. Although the symbols require education to learn their meaning, no reading skill is needed. The symbols are usually arranged on a board, and the person points or uses some type of selector to convey a message.

Establish Discipline

Discipline must begin early. Limit-setting measures need to be simple, consistently applied, and appropriate for the child's mental age. Control measures are based primarily on teaching a specific behaviour rather than on understanding the reasons behind it. Stressing moral lessons is of little value to a child who lacks the cognitive skills to learn from self-criticism or from a lesson based on previous wrong-doing. Behaviour modification, especially reinforcement of desired actions, and time-out are appropriate forms of behaviour control.

Encourage Socialization

Acquiring social skills is a complex task, as is learning self-care procedures. Active rehearsal with role-playing and practice sessions and positive reinforcement for desired behaviour have been the most successful approaches. Parents should be encouraged early to teach their child socially acceptable behaviour: waving goodbye, saying "hello" and "thank you," responding to his or her name, greeting visitors, and sitting modestly. The teaching of socially acceptable sexual behaviour is especially important in order to minimize sexual exploitation. Parents also need to expose the child to strangers so that he or she can practise manners, as there is generally no automatic transfer of learning from one situation to another.

Dressing and grooming are also important aspects of socialization. A child who is dressed in age-appropriate clothing and is well groomed is much more likely to be accepted and to develop good self-esteem. Many attractive outfits can be adapted with self-adhering fasteners and elastic openings to facilitate self-dressing.

As soon as possible, parents should enroll the child in an appropriate preschool program. Not only do these programs provide education and training, but they also offer an opportunity for social experiences among children. As children grow older, they should have peer experiences similar to those of other children, including group outings, sports, and organized activities such as Scouts and Special Olympics. Nurses can assess the child's abilities and encourage others (e.g., parents, teachers) to promote developmentally appropriate peer interaction (Johnson & Walker, 2006; Rehm & Bradley, 2006).

Provide Information on Sexuality

Adolescence may be a particularly difficult time for the family, especially in terms of the child's sexual behaviour, possibility of pregnancy, future plans to marry, and ability to be independent. Frequently, little anticipatory guidance has been offered parents to prepare the child for physical and sexual maturation. The nurse can help in this area by providing parents with information about sexuality education that is geared toward the child's developmental level. For example, the adolescent girl needs a simple explanation of menstruation and instructions on personal hygiene during the menstrual cycle.

These adolescents also need practical sexual information regarding anatomy, physical development, and conception. Because of their easy persuasion and lack of judgement, they need a well-defined, concrete code of conduct. The subtleties of social sexual behaviour are less beneficial than specific instructions for handling certain situations. For example, an adolescent should be firmly told never to go alone anywhere with any person he or she does not know well. To protect him or her from abusive sexual activities, parents must closely observe their teenager's activities and associates. The question of contraceptive protection for these adolescents is often a parental concern.

Parents of these adolescents are often concerned about the advisability of marriage between two individuals with an intellectual disability. There is no conclusive answer; each situation must be judged individually. In some instances marriage is possible, but parenthood may not desirable because of the complexity of childrearing and the potential problem of perpetuating mental deficiency. The nurse should discuss this topic with parents and with the prospective couple, stressing suitable living accommodations and contraceptive methods to prevent pregnancy. If children are conceived, these parents require specialized assistance in learning to meet the needs of their offspring (Johnson & Walker, 2006).

Help Family Adjust to Future Care

Not all families are able to cope with home care of their affected child, especially one who is severely or profoundly impaired or has multiple disabilities. Older parents may not be able to assume care responsibilities after they reach retirement or older age. For these parents, the decision regarding residential placement is a difficult one, and the availability of such facilities varies widely. The nurse working with a family should help them investigate and evaluate various programs, in addition to assisting them in adjusting to the decision for placement.

Care for Child During Hospitalization

Caring for the child during hospitalization can be a special challenge. Frequently, nurses are unfamiliar with children who are cognitively impaired, and they may cope with their feelings of insecurity and fear by ignoring or isolating the child. Not only is this approach nonsupportive, but it may also be destructive for the child's sense of self-esteem and optimum development, and it may hamper the parents' ability to cope with the stress of the experience. One method that successfully avoids this nontherapeutic approach is the use of the mutual participation model in planning the child's care. Parents are encouraged to stay with their child but should not be made to feel as if the responsibility is totally theirs.

When the child is admitted, a detailed history should be taken (see Chapter 34), especially in terms of all self-care activity. During the interview the child's developmental age is assessed. It is best to avoid asking directly about IQ levels, since this may make the parents uncomfortable and often tells little about the child's actual abilities. Questions need to be approached positively. For example, rather than asking, "Is your child toilet trained yet?" the nurse may state, "Tell me about your child's toileting habits." The assessment should also focus on any special devices the child uses, effective measures of limit-setting, unusual or favourite routines, and any behaviours that may require intervention. If the parent states that the child engages in self-injurious activities (such as head banging or self-biting), the nurse should inquire about events that precipitate them and techniques that the parents use to manage them (Bosch & Ringdahl, 2001; Walker & Johnson, 2006).

The nurse also needs to assess the child's functional level of eating and playing; ability to express needs verbally; progress in toilet training; and relationship with objects, toys, and other children. The child should be encouraged to be as independent as possible in the hospital.

Realizing that the child may be lonely in the hospital, the nurse can make certain that toys and other activities are provided. The child should be placed in a room with other children of approximately the same developmental age, preferably a room with only two beds, to avoid overstimulation. The nurse should discuss with the other parents the child's abilities and introduce the parents and children to each other. By the nurse's example of treating the child with dignity and respect, others who may be fearful of what they do not understand are encouraged to accept the child.

Procedures should be explained to the child through methods of communication that are at the appropriate cognitive level. Generally, explanations should be simple, short, and concrete, emphasizing what the child will experience physically. Demonstration either through actual practice or with visual aids is always preferable to verbal explanation. The nurse needs to repeat instructions often and evaluate the child's understanding by asking questions such as "What will it feel like?" "Show me how you must lie," or "Where will the dressing be?" Parents should be included in preprocedural teaching for their own learning and to help the nurse learn effective methods of communicating with the child.

During hospitalization, the nurse should also focus on growth-promoting experiences for the child. For example, hospitalization may be an excellent opportunity to emphasize to parents the abilities that the child does have but has not had the opportunity to practise, such as self-dressing. It may also be an opportunity for social experiences with peers, group play, or new educational and recreational activities. For example, one child who had the habit of screaming and kicking demonstrated a definite decrease in these behaviours after he learned to pound pegs and use a punching bag. Through social services, the parents may become aware of specialized programs for the child. Hospitalization may also offer parents a respite from everyday care responsibilities and an opportunity to discuss their feelings with a concerned professional.

Assist in Measures to Prevent Cognitive Impairment

Besides having a responsibility to families who have a child with CI, nurses also need to be involved in programs aimed at preventing CI. Many of the familial, social, and environmental factors known to cause mild impairment are preventable. Counselling and education can reduce or eliminate such factors (e.g., poor nutrition, cigarette smoking, substance use), which increase the risk of prematurity and intrauterine growth restriction. Interventions should be directed toward improving maternal health by educating women about the dangers of chemicals, including prenatal alcohol exposure, which affects organogenesis, craniofacial development, and cognitive ability (Wilton & Plane, 2006). Other preventive strategies that play an important role include adequate prenatal care; optimal medical care of high-risk newborns; rubella immunization; genetic counselling and prenatal screening, especially for Down or fragile X syndrome (see Chapter 12, p. 279); use of folic acid supplements to prevent neural tube defects during pregnancy and during the childbearing years; newborn screening for treatable inborn errors of metabolism, such as congenital hypothyroidism, phenylketonuria, and galactosemia; and early appropriate therapies and rehabilitation services for children with developmental disabilities.

Down Syndrome

evolve Case Study—Down Syndrome

Down syndrome is the most common chromosomal abnormality of a generalized syndrome, occurring in 1 in every 800 to 1000 live births (Canadian Down Syndrome Society, 2010; Skotko, 2005). It occurs slightly more often in Whites than in Blacks, although the incidence is unchanged in various socio-economic classes.

Etiology

evolve Critical Thinking Exercise—Down Syndrome

While the cause of Down syndrome is not known, evidence from cytogenetic and epidemiological studies supports the concept of multiple causality. Approximately 95% of all cases of Down syndrome are attributable to an extra **chromosome** 21 (group G), thus the name nonfamilial **trisomy** 21 (Canadian Down Syndrome Society, 2009; Walker & Johnson, 2006). Although children with trisomy 21 are born to parents of all ages, there is a statistically greater risk in older women, particularly those older than 35 years of age (see Chapter 8, p. 164). For example, in women 35 years of age, the chance of conceiving a child with Down syndrome is about 1 in 400 live births, but in women age 40 it is about 1 in 110. However, the majority (about 80%) of infants with Down syndrome are born to women younger than age 35. About 3 to 4% of cases may be caused by translocation of chromosomes 15 and 21 or 22. This type of genetic aberration is usually hereditary and is not associated with advanced parental age. From 1 to 2% of affected persons demonstrate *mosaicism*, which refers to the mixture of normal and abnormal cell types. The degree of cognitive and physical impairment is related to the percentage of cells with the abnormal chromosome makeup.

Diagnostic Evaluation

Down syndrome can usually be diagnosed by the clinical manifestations alone (Box 42-3 and Fig. 42-6), but a chromosome analysis should be done to confirm the genetic abnormality.

Several physical problems are associated with Down syndrome. Many of these children have congenital heart malformations, the most common being septal defects. Respiratory tract infections are prevalent and, when combined with cardiac anomalies, are the chief causes of death, particularly during the first year of life. Hypotonicity of chest and abdominal muscles and dysfunction of the immune system probably predispose the child to the development of respiratory tract infections. Other physical problems include thyroid dysfunction, especially congenital hypothyroidism, and an increased incidence of leukemia.

Therapeutic Management

Although no cure exists for Down syndrome, a number of therapies are advocated, such as surgery to correct serious

BOX 42-3 Clinical Manifestations of Down Syndrome

Head and Eyes
*Separated sagittal suture
Brachycephaly
Rounded and small skull
Flat occiput
Enlarged anterior fontanel
*Oblique palpebral fissures (upward, outward slant)
Inner epicanthal folds
Speckling of iris (Brushfield's spots)

Nose and Ears
*Small nose
*Depressed nasal bridge (saddle nose)
Small ears and narrow canals
Short pinna (vertical ear length)
Overlapping upper helices
Conductive hearing loss

Mouth and Neck
*High, arched, narrow palate
Protruding tongue
Hypoplastic mandible
Delayed tooth eruption and microdontia
Abnormal alignment of teeth common
Periodontal disease
*Neck skin excess and laxity
Short and broad neck

Chest and Heart
Shortened rib cage
Twelfth rib anomalies
Pectus excavatum or carinatum
Congenital heart defects common (e.g., atrial septal defect, ventricular septal defect)

Abdomen and Genitalia
Protruding, lax, and flabby abdominal muscles
Diastasis recti abdominis
Umbilical hernia
Small penis
Cryptorchidism
Bulbous vulva

Hands and Feet
Broad, short hands and stubby fingers
Incurved little finger (clinodactyly)
Transverse palmar crease (Simian crease)
*Wide space between big and second toes
*Plantar crease between big and second toes
Broad, short feet and stubby toes

Musculoskeleton and Skin
Short stature
*Hyperflexibility and muscle weakness
Hypotonia
Atlantoaxial instability
Dry, cracked, and frequent fissuring
Cutis marmorata (mottling)

Other
Reduced birth weight
Learning difficulty (average intelligence quotient of 50)
Hypothyroidism common
Impaired immune function
Increased risk of leukemia
Early-onset dementia (in one third)

*Most common findings in modified chart (Pueschel, 1999).

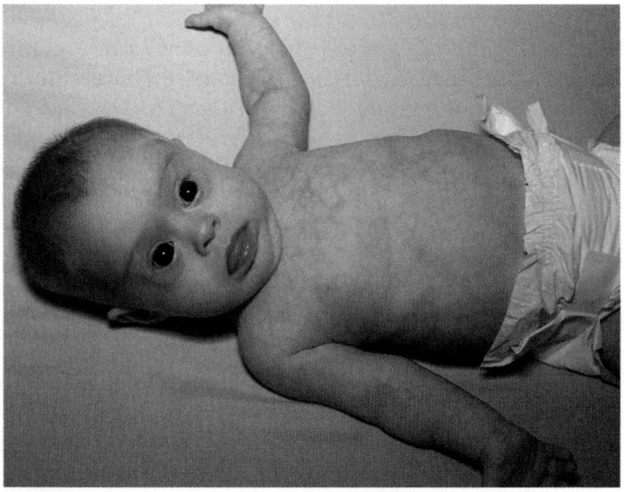

Fig. 42-6 Down syndrome in an infant. Note small, square head with upward slant to eyes, flat nasal bridge, protruding tongue, mottled skin, and hypotonia.

congenital anomalies (e.g., heart defects, strabismus). These children also benefit from an evaluative echocardiogram soon after birth and regular medical care. Evaluation of sight and hearing is essential, and treatment of otitis media is required to prevent auditory loss, which can influence cognitive function. Periodic testing of thyroid function is recommended, especially if growth is severely delayed. Children participating in sports that may involve stress on the head and neck, such as gymnastics, diving, butterfly stroke in swimming, high jump, and soccer, should be evaluated radiologically for atlantoaxial instability. Symptoms of the disorder include neck pain, weakness, and torticollis. Affected children are at risk for spinal cord compression.

NURSING ALERT Report immediately any child with the following signs of spinal cord compression:

- Persistent neck pain
- Loss of established motor skills and bladder or bowel control
- Changes in sensation

Prognosis

Life expectancy for those with Down syndrome has improved in recent years but remains lower than for the general population. More than 80% survive to age 55 years and beyond. As the prognosis continues to improve for these individuals, it will be important to provide for their long-term health care, social, and leisure needs (National Down Syndrome Society, 2006; Van Riper, 2003).

Nursing Care Management

Support the Family at the Time of Diagnosis

Because of the unique physical characteristics, the infant with Down syndrome is usually diagnosed at birth if a prenatal diagnosis had not been established. Parents should be informed of the diagnosis at this time. Parents usually prefer that both of them be present during the informing interview so that they can support one another emotionally. They appreciate receiving reading material about the syndrome and being referred to others for help or advice, such as parent groups or professional counselling (see Additional Resources section at the end of this chapter).

After parents are aware of the diagnosis, they are confronted with the crisis of losing their perfect or dream child and grieving for and accepting their reality child. Consequently, the parents' responses to the child may greatly influence decisions regarding future care. Whereas some families willingly take the child home, others consider immediate residential placement. The nurse must carefully answer questions regarding developmental potential. Institutionalization is no longer an option. For families unable or unready to choose taking the newborn home, specialized foster care or adoption are other options (see Critical Thinking Exercise).

Assist the Family in Preventing Physical Problems

Many of the physical characteristics of Down syndrome can present nursing problems. The hypotonicity of muscles and hyperextensibility of joints complicate positioning. The limp, flaccid extremities resemble the posture of a rag doll; as a result, holding the infant is difficult and cumbersome. Sometimes parents perceive this lack of moulding to their bodies as evidence of inadequate parenting. The extended body position promotes heat loss because more surface area is exposed to the environment. Parents are encouraged to swaddle or wrap the infant tightly in a blanket before picking up the child to provide security and warmth. The nurse also needs to discuss with parents their feelings concerning attachment to the child, emphasizing that the child's lack of clinging or moulding is a physical characteristic, not a sign of detachment or rejection.

Decreased muscle tone compromises respiratory expansion. In addition, the underdeveloped nasal bone causes a chronic problem of inadequate drainage of mucus. The constant stuffy nose forces the child to breathe by mouth, which dries the oropharyngeal membranes, increasing the susceptibility to upper respiratory tract infections. Measures to lessen these problems include clearing the nose with a bulb-type syringe, rinsing the mouth with water after feedings, increasing fluid intake, and using a cool-mist vaporizer to keep the mucous membranes moist and the secretions liquefied. Other helpful measures include changing the child's position frequently, performing postural drainage with percussion if necessary, practising good hand hygiene, and properly disposing of soiled articles such as tissues. If antibiotics are ordered, the nurse needs to stress to the parents the importance of completing the full course of therapy for successful eradication of the infection and the prevention of the growth of resistant organisms.

Inadequate drainage resulting in pooling of mucus in the nose also interferes with feeding. Because the child breathes by mouth, sucking for any length of time is difficult. When eating solids, the child may gag on the food because of mucus in the oropharynx. Parents are advised to clear the nose before each feeding; give small, frequent feedings; and allow opportunities for rest during mealtime.

The protruding tongue also interferes with feeding, especially of solid foods. Parents need to know that the tongue thrust is not an indication of refusal to feed, but a physiological response. Parents are advised to use a small but long, straight-handled spoon to push the food toward the back and side of the mouth. If food is thrust out, it should be refed.

Dietary intake also needs supervision. Decreased muscle tone affects gastric motility, predisposing the child to constipation. Dietary measures such as increased fibre and fluid promote evacuation. The child's eating habits may need careful scrutiny to prevent obesity. Height and weight measurements should be obtained on a serial basis, especially during infancy. Because these children grow more slowly than the general pediatric population's trends, special growth charts developed for these children should be used. The Canadian Dietitians of Canada and Canadian Paediatric Society (2010) recommend that the growth of children with Down syndrome be assessed using the World Health Organization (WHO) 2006 growth chart up to age 5, and then the WHO 2007 growth chart from 5 to 19 years of age, as baseline measurements (see Chapter 36). They also recommend that the Centers for Disease Control and Prevention (CDC) growth chart developed for children with Down syndrome be used to obtain additional information regarding the child's growth patterns (Cronk et al., 1988).

CRITICAL THINKING EXERCISE

Diagnosis of Down Syndrome

The parents of Melissa, a newborn diagnosed as having Down syndrome, ask the nurse, "What are we supposed to do with her?" They further state that they already have three other children at home.

1. Evidence—Is there sufficient evidence to draw conclusions about the parents' concerns regarding their newborn daughter?
2. Assumptions—Describe an underlying assumption about each of the following:
   a. Newborn diagnosed with Down syndrome
   b. Parental care of a newborn with Down syndrome
   c. Newborn with Down syndrome and older siblings
3. What priorities for the nursing response should be established?
4. Does the evidence support your nursing intervention?
5. What alternative perspectives might you have?

During infancy the child's skin is pliable and soft. However, it gradually becomes rough and dry and is prone to cracking and infection. Skin care involves the use of minimal soap and application of lubricants. Lip balm should be applied to the lips, especially when the child is outdoors, to prevent excessive chapping.

Assist in Prenatal Diagnosis and Genetic Counselling

There are now more accurate prenatal screening tests for Down syndrome that are noninvasive. The Society of Obstetricians and Gynaecologists of Canada (SOGC) recommends that all pregnant women in Canada, regardless of age, be offered the choice of a prenatal screening test for the most common clinically significant fetal aneuploidies. The SOGC also recommends that ultrasound be performed in the second semester for dating, assessment of fetal anatomy, and detection of multiple fetuses (SOGC & Canadian College of Medical Geneticists, 2007). If a fetus is identified as having an increased risk for Down syndrome, then more invasive testing, such as **amniocentesis** or **chorionic villus sampling**, should be done. If prenatal testing indicates that the fetus is affected, the nurse should encourage the parents to express their feelings about considering elective abortion and support their decision to terminate or proceed with the pregnancy.

Fragile X Syndrome

Fragile X syndrome is the most common inherited cause of CI and the second most common genetic cause of CI after Down syndrome. It has been described in all ethnic groups and races. The incidence of affected males is 1 in 3600; the incidence of affected females is 1 in 4000 to 6000; the incidence of carrier females is 1 in 100 to 260, and the incidence of carrier males is 1 in 250 to 800 worldwide (Crawford, 2001; National Fragile X Foundation, 2006; Phalen, 2005). It is estimated that 50 to 100 new cases are reported every year in Canada (Canadian Paediatric Society, Canadian Paediatric Surveillance Program, 2012).

The syndrome is caused by an abnormal gene on the lower end of the long arm of the X chromosome. Chromosome analysis may demonstrate a fragile site (a region that fails to condense during mitosis and is characterized by a nonstaining gap or narrowing) in the cells of affected males and females and in carrier females. This fragile site has been determined to be caused by a gene mutation that results in excessive repeats of nucleotide in a specific deoxyribonucleic acid (DNA) segment of the X chromosome. The number of repeats in a normal individual is between 6 and 50. An individual with 50 to 200 base-pair repeats is said to have a permutation and is thus a carrier. When passed from a parent to a child, these base-pair repeats can expand to 200 or more, which is termed a *full mutation*. This expansion occurs only when a carrier mother passes the mutation to her offspring; it does not occur when a carrier father passes the mutation to his daughters. Prenatal diagnosis of the fragile X gene mutation is now possible with direct DNA testing in a family with an established history, using amniocentesis or chorionic villus sampling (Centers for Disease Control and Prevention, 2002; Crawford, 2001). Both affected sexes are fertile and thus capable of transmitting the fragile X disorder.

evolve Critical Thinking Exercise—Fragile X Syndrome

Newborn screening for fragile X syndrome, similar to Down syndrome, is available and being advocated for in the United States to provide early intervention treatment and genetic counselling to the families for future pregnancy planning. The Canadian Paediatric Society and Public Health Agency of Canada are investigating the demographics, clinical features, geographic distribution, and management fragile X syndrome in Canada, as well as determining the potential for newborn screening (Down et al., 2012).

Clinical Manifestations

The classic trend of physical findings in adult men with fragile X syndrome consists of a long face with a prominent jaw (prognathism); large, protruding ears; and large testes (macroorchidism). In prepubertal children, however, these features may be less obvious, and behavioural manifestations may initially suggest the diagnosis (Box 42-4). In carrier females the clinical manifestations are extremely varied.

Therapeutic Management

No cure exists for fragile X syndrome. Medical treatment may include the use of serotonin agents such as carbamazepine (Tegretol) or fluoxetine (Prozac) to control violent temper outbursts and the use of central nervous system stimulants or clonidine (Catapres) to improve attention span and decrease hyperactivity. Protein replacement and gene therapy are treatment options that are being investigated (Phalen, 2005).

All affected children require referral to early intervention programs (speech and language therapy, occupational therapy, and special education assistance) and multidisciplinary assessment, including cardiology (i.e., mitral valve prolapse), neurology (i.e., seizures), and orthopaedic anomalies (Alanay et al., 2007).

Prognosis

Individuals with fragile X syndrome are expected to live a normal lifespan. Their CI may be improved by behavioural and educational interventions.

BOX 42-4 Clinical Manifestations of Fragile X Syndrome

Physical Features

- Increased head circumference
- Long, wide, and protruding ears
- Long, narrow face with prominent jaw
- Strabismus
- Mitral valve prolapse, aortic root dilation
- Hypotonia
- Enlarged testicles (especially postpubertally)

Behavioural Features

- Mild to severe cognitive impairment
- Speech delay; may have rapid speech with stuttering, word repetition
- Short attention span, hyperactivity
- Hypersensitivity to taste, sounds, and touch
- Intolerance to change in routine
- Autistic-like behaviours

Nursing Care Management

Because CI is a fairly consistent finding in individuals with fragile X syndrome, the care given to these families is the same as for any child with CI. Because the disorder is hereditary, genetic counselling is necessary to inform parents and siblings of the risks of transmission. In addition, any male or female with unexplained or nonspecific mental impairment should be referred for genetic testing and, if needed, counselling. Families with a member affected by the disorder should be referred to the Canadian National Fragile X Foundation (see Additional Resources).

Sensory Impairment

Hearing Impairment

In Canada over 23,000 children have some form of hearing impairment, and almost a third of these children have additional disabilities, such as visual or cognitive deficits (Statistics Canada, 2009). Hearing loss is a common major abnormality at birth; approximately 1 to 3 in 1000 normal term infants are profoundly deaf and another 3 in 1000 have serious hearing loss (Canadian Paediatric Society [CPS], 2008).

Definition and Classification

Hearing impairment is a general term indicating disability that may range in severity from mild to profound and includes the subsets of deaf and hard-of-hearing. *Deaf* refers to a person whose hearing disability precludes successful processing of linguistic information through audition, with or without a hearing aid. *Hard-of-hearing* refers to a person who, generally with the use of a hearing aid, has residual hearing sufficient to enable successful processing of linguistic information through audition. Other terms, such as *deaf and dumb*, *mute*, or *deaf-mute*, are unacceptable for describing hearing impairment. Hearing-impaired persons are not dumb and, if mute, have no physical speech defect other than that caused by the inability to hear.

Hearing defects may be classified according to etiology, pathology, or symptom severity. Each is important in terms of treatment, possible prevention, and rehabilitation.

Etiology

Hearing loss may be caused by a number of prenatal and postnatal conditions: a family history of childhood hearing impairment, anatomical malformations of the head or neck, low birth weight, severe perinatal asphyxia, perinatal infection (cytomegalovirus, rubella, herpes, syphilis, toxoplasmosis, bacterial meningitis), chronic ear infection, cerebral palsy, Down syndrome, or administration of ototoxic medications (Gregg, Wiorek, & Arvedson, 2004; Smith, Bale, & White, 2005).

In addition, high-risk neonates who survive formerly fatal prenatal or perinatal conditions may be susceptible to hearing loss from the disorder or its treatment. For example, sensorineural hearing loss may be a result of continuous humming noises or high noise levels associated with incubators, oxygen hoods, or intensive care units, especially when combined with the use of potentially ototoxic antibiotics.

Environmental noise is a special concern. Sounds loud enough to damage sensitive hair cells of the inner ear can produce **irreversible** hearing loss. Very loud, brief noise, such as gunfire, can cause immediate, severe, and permanent loss of hearing. Longer exposure to less intense but still hazardous sounds, such as loud persistent music via headphones, sound systems, concerts, or industrial noises, can also produce hearing loss (Daniel, 2007; Kenna, 2004; Segal et al., 2003). Loud noises combined with the toxic substances of smoking produces a synergistic effect on hearing that causes hearing loss (Mizoue, Miyamoto, & Shimizu, 2003).

Pathology

Disorders of hearing are divided according to the location of the defect. **Conductive** or middle-ear **hearing loss** results from interference of transmission of sound to the middle ear. It is the most common of all types of hearing loss and most frequently a result of recurrent serous otitis media. Conductive hearing impairment involves mainly interference with the loudness of sound.

Sensorineural hearing loss, also called *perceptive* or *nerve deafness*, involves damage to the inner ear structures or the auditory nerve. The most common causes are congenital defects of inner ear structures or consequences of acquired conditions, such as kernicterus, infection, administration of ototoxic medications, or exposure to excessive noise. Sensorineural hearing loss results in distortion of sound and problems in discrimination. Although the child hears some of everything going on around him or her, the sounds are distorted, severely affecting discrimination and comprehension.

Mixed (conductive-sensorineural) **hearing loss** results from interference with the transmission of sound in the middle ear and along neural pathways. It frequently results from recurrent otitis media and its complications.

Central auditory imperception (**central hearing loss**) includes all hearing losses that are not linked to defects in the conductive or sensorineural structures. They are usually divided into organic or functional losses. In the organic type of central auditory imperception, the defect involves the reception of auditory stimuli along the central pathways and the expression of the message into meaningful communication. Examples are *aphasia*, the inability to express ideas in any form, either written or verbal; *agnosia*, the inability to interpret sound correctly; and *dysacusis*, difficulty in processing details or discriminating among sounds. In the functional type of hearing loss, no organic lesion exists to explain a central auditory loss. Examples of functional hearing loss are conversion hysteria (an unconscious withdrawal from hearing to block remembrance of a traumatic event), infantile autism, and childhood schizophrenia.

Symptom Severity

Hearing impairment is expressed in terms of sound intensity in decibels (db), a unit of loudness (Table 42-2); hearing is measured at various frequencies, such as 500, 1000, and 2000 cycles/sec, the critical listening speech range. Hearing impairment can be classified according to hearing threshold level (the measurement of an individual's hearing threshold by means of an audiometer) and the degree of symptom severity as it affects speech (Table 42-3). These classifications offer only general guidelines regarding the effect of the impairment on

Table 42-2 Intensity of Sounds Expressed in Decibels

DECIBELS	REPRESENTATIVE SOUND
0	Softest sound normal ear can hear
10	Heartbeat, rustling of leaves
20	Whisper at 1.5 m
30–45	Normal conversation
60	Noise in average restaurant
70–80	Street noises
80	Loud radio in home
90–100	Train
120	Thunder, loud music (e.g., rock concerts)
140	Jet plane during departure
>140	Pain threshold

Table 42-3 Classification of Hearing Loss Based on Symptom Severity

HEARING LEVEL (db)	EFFECT
Slight—16–25	Has difficulty hearing faint or distant speech Usually is unaware of hearing difficulty Likely to achieve in school but may have problems No speech defects
Mild to moderate—26–55	May have speech difficulties Understands face-to-face conversational speech at 0.9–1.5 m
Moderately severe—56–70 (hard of hearing)	Unable to understand conversational speech unless loud Considerable difficulty with group or classroom discussion Requires special speech training
Severe—71–90 (deaf)	May hear a loud voice if nearby May be able to identify loud environmental noises Can distinguish vowels but not most consonants Requires speech training
Profound—91 (deaf)	May hear only loud sounds Requires extensive speech training

any individual child, since children differ greatly in their ability to use residual hearing.

Therapeutic Management

Conductive Hearing Loss

Treatment of hearing loss depends on the cause and type of hearing impairment. Many conductive hearing defects respond to medical or surgical treatment, such as antibiotic therapy for acute otitis media or insertion of tympanostomy tubes for chronic otitis media. When the conductive loss is permanent, hearing can be improved with the use of a hearing aid to amplify sound.

The nurse should be familiar with the types, basic care, and handling of hearing aids, especially when the child is hospitalized (see Additional Resources). Types of aids include those worn in or behind the ear, models incorporated into an eyeglass frame, or types worn on the body with a wire connection to the ear (Fig. 42-7). One of the most common problems with a hearing aid is acoustic feedback, an annoying whistling sound usually caused by improper fit of the ear mould. Sometimes the whistling may be at a frequency that the child cannot hear but that is annoying to others. In this case, if children are old enough, they can be told of the noise and asked to readjust the aid.

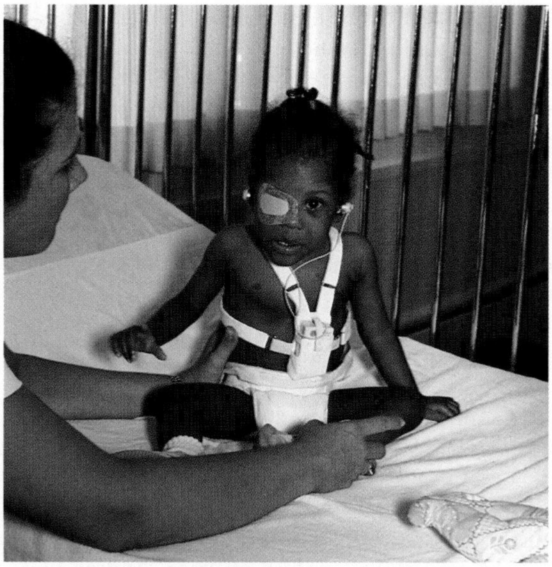

Fig. 42-7 On-the-body hearing aids are convenient for young children, such as this child with severe bilateral hearing loss. Note eye patching for strabismus.

NURSING ALERT To reduce or eliminate whistling from a hearing aid, try reinserting the aid, making certain that no hair is caught between the ear mould and the canal, cleaning the ear mould or ear, or lowering the volume of the aid.

As children grow older, they may become self-conscious about the device. Every effort should be made to make the aid inconspicuous if this is a concern, such as having an appropriate hairstyle to cover behind-the-ear or in-the-ear models; wearing attractive frames for glasses; and placing the on-the-body type where it is not seen, such as under a blouse or sweater. Children should be given responsibility for the care of the device as soon as they are able, since fostering independence is a primary goal of rehabilitation.

NURSING ALERT When parents express concern about their child's hearing and speech development, refer the child for a hearing evaluation. Absence of well-formed syllables (da, na, yaya) by 11 months of age should result in immediate referral.

Sensorineural Hearing Loss

Treatment for sensorineural hearing loss is much less satisfactory. Because the defect is not one of intensity of sound, hearing aids are of less value in this type of defect. The use of cochlear implants (a surgically implanted prosthetic device) provides a sensation of hearing for individuals who have severe or profound hearing loss (Downs & Buchman, 2005; Zeng & Liu, 2006) (see Additional Resources section at the end of this chapter). Children with sensorineural hearing loss have lost or damaged some or all of their hair cells or auditory nerve fibres. Often these children cannot benefit from conventional hearing aids because they only amplify sound that cannot be processed by a damaged inner ear. A cochlear implant bypasses the hair cells to directly stimulate surviving auditory nerve fibres so that they can send signals to the brain. These signals can be interpreted by the brain to produce sound and sensations (Gregg et al., 2004; Zeng & Liu, 2006).

Multichannelled implants are now available. This more sophisticated device stimulates the auditory nerve at a number of locations with differently processed signals. This type of stimulation allows a person to use the pitch information present in speech signals, leading to better understanding of speech. The trend is toward early use of cochlear implants, usually by 18 months of age, to give the child maximum opportunity to develop listening, language, and speaking skills.

Nursing Care Management

Assessment of children for hearing impairment is a critical nursing responsibility. Early detection of hearing loss, preferably within the first 3 to 6 months of life, is essential to improve the language and educational outcomes of those with hearing impairments. Without early intervention, children with hearing impairment have irreversible deficits in communication and in psychosocial skills, cognition, and literacy (Gregg et al., 2004; Kenna, 2004; CPS, Community Paediatrics Committee, 2011). Currently in Canada, some provinces and territories such as Ontario and British Columbia have mandatory newborn hearing screening, and some have partial programs that target at-risk neonates. Usually the screening is done before discharge from the hospital (see Fig. 24-14). The Canadian Paediatric Society (2011) strongly recommends that universal newborn hearing screening be done across Canada.

The discussion here focuses on developmental and behavioural indices associated with hearing impairment. Auditory testing is presented in Chapter 34.

Infancy

At birth the nurse can observe the neonate's response to auditory stimuli, as evidenced by the startle reflex, head turning, eye blinking, and cessation of body movement. The infant may vary in the intensity of the response, depending on the state of alertness. However, a consistent absence of a reaction should lead to suspicion of hearing loss. Box 42-5 summarizes other clinical manifestations of hearing impairment in the infant.

Childhood

The child who is profoundly deaf is much more likely to be diagnosed during infancy than the less severely affected one. If the defect is not detected during early childhood, it likely will become evident during entry into school, when the child has difficulty learning. Unfortunately, some of these children are mistakenly placed in special classes for students with learning disabilities or CI. Therefore, it is essential that the nurse consider a hearing impairment in any child who demonstrates the behaviours listed in Box 42-5.

Of primary importance is the effect of hearing impairment on speech development. A child with a mild conductive hearing loss may speak fairly clearly but in a loud, monotone voice. A child with a sensorineural defect usually has difficulty with articulation. For example, inability to hear higher frequencies may result in the word *spoon* being pronounced "poon." Children with articulation problems need to have their hearing tested.

NURSING ALERT Stress to parents the importance of storing batteries for hearing aids in a safe location and teaching children not to remove the battery from the hearing aid (or supervising young children to prevent the removal). Ingestion of batteries is most often of those from hearing aids, including the child's own aid.

Lipreading

Even though the child may become an expert at lipreading, only about 40% of the spoken word is understood, and less is understood if the speaker has an accent, a moustache, or a beard. Exaggerating pronunciation or speaking in an altered rhythm further reduces comprehension. Parents can help the child understand the spoken word by using the suggestions in

BOX 42-5 Clinical Manifestations of Hearing Impairment

Infants

- Lack of startle or blink reflex to a loud sound
- Failure to be awakened by loud environmental noises
- Failure to localize a source of sound by 6 months of age
- Absence of babble or voice inflections by age 7 months
- Lack of response to the spoken word; failure to follow verbal directions
- Response to loud noises as opposed to the voice

Children

- Use of gestures rather than verbalization to express desires
- Failure to develop intelligible speech by age 24 months
- Monotone and unintelligible speech; lessened laughter
- Vocal play, head banging, or foot stamping for vibratory sensation
- Yelling or screeching to express pleasure, needs, or annoyance (tantrum)
- Asking to have statements repeated or answering them incorrectly
- Greater response to facial expression and gestures than to verbal explanation
- Avoidance of social interaction; preference for playing alone
- Inquiring, sometimes confused facial expression
- Suspicious alertness alternating with cooperation
- Frequently stubbornness because of lack of comprehension
- Irritability at not making themselves understood
- Shy, timid, and withdrawn behaviour
- Often appearing "dreamy," "in a world of their own," or exhibiting inattentiveness

GUIDELINES Facilitating Lipreading

- Attract the child's attention before speaking; use light touch to signal speaker's presence.
- Stand close to the child.
- Face the child directly or move to a 45-degree angle.
- Stand still; do not walk back and forth or turn away to point or look elsewhere.
- Establish eye contact and show interest.
- Speak at eye level and with good lighting on the speaker's face.
- Be certain nothing interferes with speech patterns, such as chewing food or gum.
- Speak clearly and at a slow and even rate.
- Use facial expression to assist in conveying messages.
- Keep sentences short.
- Rephrase message if the child does not understand the words.

the Guidelines box. The child learns to supplement the spoken word with sensitivity to visual cues, primarily body language and facial expression (e.g., tightening the lips, muscle tension, eye contact).

Cued Speech

This method of communication is an adjunct to straight lipreading. Hand signals are used to help the child with a hearing impairment distinguish between words that look alike when formed by the lips (e.g., mat, bat). It is most often used by children with hearing impairments who are using speech, rather than those who are nonverbal.

Sign Language

Sign language, such as American Sign Language (ASL) or British Sign Language (BSL), is a visual gestural language in which hand signals roughly correspond to specific words and concepts in the English language. Family members are encouraged to learn signing because using or watching hands requires much less concentration than lipreading or talking. Also, a symbol method enables some children to learn more and to learn faster. Learning a language promotes cognitive development.

Speech Language Therapy

The most formidable task in the education of a child who is profoundly hearing impaired is learning to speak. Speech is learned through a multisensory approach, using visual, tactile, kinesthetic, and auditory stimulation. Parents should be encouraged to participate fully in the learning process.

Additional Aids

Everyday activities present problems for older children with hearing impairment. For example, they may not be able to hear the telephone, doorbell, or alarm clock. Several commercial devices are available to help them adjust to these dilemmas. A new visual fire alarm is now available as an additional safety device. Flashing lights can be attached to a telephone or doorbell to signal its ringing. Trained hearing ear dogs can provide great assistance because they alert the person to sounds, such as someone approaching, a moving car, a signal to wake up, or a child's cry. Special teletypewriters or telecommunications devices for the deaf (TDD or TTY) help people with impaired hearing communicate with each other over the telephone; the typed message is conveyed via the telephone lines and displayed on a small screen.* Cellular phones and smartphones also offer means of sending text and visual messages.

Any audiovisual medium presents dilemmas for these children, who can see the picture but cannot hear the message. However, with closed captioning a special decoding device is attached to the television, and the audio portion of a program is translated into subtitles that appear on the screen. There are also closed-caption apps available for smartphones and software for computers for closed captioning with video games and online streaming.

The Canadian Hearing Society offers a youth transition program to support career planning.

Socialization

Because socialization is extremely important to the child's development, the nurse should discuss with the family methods of fostering social contact. If children attend a special school for the deaf, they are able to socialize with peers in that setting. Classmates become a potential source of close friendships because they communicate more easily among themselves. Parents should be encouraged to promote these relationships whenever possible.

Children with a hearing impairment may need special help with school or social activities. For children wearing hearing aids, background noise should be kept to a minimum. Because many of these children are able to attend regular classes, the teacher may need assistance in adapting methods of teaching for the child's benefit. The nurse is often in an optimal position to emphasize methods of facilitated communication, such as lipreading (see Guidelines box above). Because group projects and audiovisual teaching aids may hinder the child's learning, these educational methods should be carefully evaluated.

Support the Child and Family

After the diagnosis of hearing impairment is made, parents need extensive support to adjust to the shock of learning about their child's disability and an opportunity to realize the extent of the hearing loss. If the hearing loss occurs during childhood, the child also requires sensitive, supportive care during the long and often difficult adjustment to this sensory loss. Early rehabilitation is one of the best strategies for fostering adjustment. However, progress in learning communication may not always coincide with emotional adjustment. Depression or anger is common, and such feelings are a normal part of the grieving process.

Care for the Child During Hospitalization

The needs of the hospitalized child with impaired hearing are the same as those of any other child, but the disability presents special challenges to the nurse. For example, verbal

*Directory listings stating "TDD or TTY only" before a phone number indicate that regular telephone use is not possible; "TDD or TTY and voice" indicates that both TDD/TYY users and speaking, hearing people can use the telephone number. Information on available electronic aids and new equipment is available on the Canadian Hearing Society Web site. Please see Additional Resources for this address.

explanations must be supplemented by tactile and visual aids, such as books or actual demonstration and practice. Children's understanding of the explanation needs to be constantly reassessed. If their verbal skills are poorly developed, they can answer questions through drawing, writing, or gesturing. For example, if the nurse is attempting to clarify where a spinal tap is done, the child is asked to point to where the procedure will be done on the body. Because these children often need more time to grasp the full meaning of an explanation, the nurse needs to be patient, allowing ample time for understanding.

When communicating with the child, the nurse should use the same principles as those outlined for facilitating lipreading. Ideally, nurses without foreign accents should be assigned to the child. The child's hearing aid should be checked to ensure that it is working properly. If it is necessary to awaken the child at night, the nurse can gently shake the child or turn on the hearing aid before arousing the child. The nurse should always make certain that the child can see him or her before any procedures, even routine ones such as changing a diaper or regulating an infusion. It is important to remember that the child may not be aware of one's presence until alerted through visual or tactile cues.

Ideally, parents should be encouraged to room-in with the child. However, it must be conveyed to them that this is not to serve as a convenience to the nurse but as a benefit to the child. Although the parents' aid can be enlisted in familiarizing the child with the hospital and explaining procedures, the nurse also needs to talk directly to the youngster, encouraging expression of feelings about the experience. If the child's speech is difficult to understand, the nurse should make an effort to become familiar with his or her pronunciation of words. Parents often can be helpful by explaining the child's usual speech habits. Nonverbal communication devices that employ pictures or words that the child can point to are also available. Such boards can be made by drawing pictures or writing the words of common needs on cardboard, such as *parent*, *food*, *water*, or *toilet*.

The nurse has a special role as child advocate and is in a strategic position to alert other health care team members and other patients to the child's special needs regarding communication. For example, the nurse should accompany other practitioners on visits to the child's room to ensure that they speak to the child and that the child understands what is said. Caregivers sometimes forget that the child has the abilities to perceive and learn despite a hearing loss, and consequently they communicate only with the parents. The child's needs and feelings may then remain unrecognized and unmet.

Because children with impaired hearing may have difficulty forming social relationships with other children, the child should be introduced to roommates and encouraged to engage in play activities. The hospital setting can provide growth-promoting opportunities for social relationships. With the assistance of a child life specialist, the child can learn new recreational activities, experiment with group games, and engage in therapeutic play. The use of puppets, dollhouses, role-playing with dress-up clothes, building with a hammer and nails, finger painting, and water play can help the child express feelings that previously were suppressed.

Assist in Measures to Prevent Hearing Impairment

A primary nursing role is to prevent hearing loss. Because the most common cause of impaired hearing is chronic otitis media, it is essential that appropriate measures be instituted to treat existing infections and prevent recurrences. Children with a history of ear or respiratory tract infections or any other condition known to increase the risk of hearing impairment should receive periodic auditory testing.

To prevent the causes of hearing loss that begin prenatally and perinatally, pregnant women need counselling regarding the necessity of early prenatal care, including genetic counselling for known familial disorders; avoidance of all ototoxic medications, especially during the first trimester; tests to rule out syphilis, rubella, or blood incompatibility; medical management of maternal diabetes; strict control of alcohol intake; adequate dietary intake; and avoidance of smoke exposure. The necessity of routine immunization during childhood to eliminate the possibility of acquired sensorineural hearing loss from rubella, mumps, or measles (encephalitis) needs to be stressed.

Excessive noise pollution with or without smoke exposure causes sensorineural hearing loss (Daniel, 2007). The nurse should routinely assess the possibility of environmental pollution (e.g. loud noise and smoking) and advise children and parents of the potential danger of hearing loss. When individuals engage in activities associated with high-intensity noise, such as flying model airplanes, target shooting, or snowmobiling, they should wear ear protection such as earmuffs or earplugs. Even common household equipment, such as lawn mowers, vacuum cleaners, and cordless telephones, may cause noise-induced hearing loss. Parents should be encouraged to monitor children's use of headphones when listening to MP3 players and other portable devices; if the noise can be heard outside the headset it can cause hearing defects.

NURSING ALERT Suspect hazardous noise if the listener experiences (1) difficulty in communication while hearing the sound, (2) ringing in the ears (tinnitus) after exposure to the sound, or (3) muffled hearing after leaving the sound.

Visual Impairment

Visual impairment is a common problem during childhood. In Canada, over 19,000 children have a visual impairment. Seeing disabilities are reported at a rate of 9.1% for males and 10.2% for females aged 5 to 14 years (Statistics Canada, 2009). The nurse's role is clearly one of early assessment and detection, prevention, referral, and, in some instances, rehabilitation.

Definition and Classification

Visual impairment is a general term that refers to visual loss that cannot be corrected with regular prescription lenses. However, more useful definitions for classifying visual impairments exist. *School vision* (also known as *partially sighted*) refers to **visual acuity** between 20/70 and 20/200. The child should be able to obtain an education in the usual public school system with the use of normal-sized print. Near vision is almost always better than distance vision. *Legal blindness*, visual acuity of 20/200 or less and/or a visual field of 20 degrees or less in the better eye, is useful only as a legal definition, not as a medical diagnosis. It allows special considerations with regard to taxes, entrance into special schools, eligibility for aid, and other benefits.

Etiology

Visual impairment can be caused by a number of genetic and prenatal or postnatal conditions. These include perinatal infections (herpes, chlamydia, gonococci, rubella, syphilis, toxoplasmosis); retinopathy of prematurity; trauma; postnatal infections (meningitis); and disorders such as sickle cell disease, juvenile rheumatoid arthritis, Tay-Sachs disease, albinism, and retinoblastoma. In many instances, such as with **refractive errors,** the cause of the defect is unknown.

Refractive errors are the most common types of visual disorders in children. The term *refraction* means bending and refers to the bending of light rays as they pass through the lens of the eye. Normally, light rays enter the lens and fall directly on the retina. However, in refractive disorders the light rays either fall in front of the retina (**myopia**) or beyond it (**hyperopia**). Other eye problems, such as **strabismus**, may or may not include refractive errors, but they are important because, if untreated, they result in blindness from **amblyopia**. These, along with other less frequent visual disorders, are summarized in Box 42-6. In addition to these disorders, other visual problems can be a result of **infection** or **trauma**.

Trauma

Trauma is a common cause of blindness in children. Injuries to the eyeball and adnexa (supporting or accessory structures, such as eyelids, conjunctiva, or lacrimal glands) can be classified as penetrating or nonpenetrating. Penetrating wounds are most often a result of sharp instruments, such as sticks, knives, or scissors; propulsive objects, such as firecrackers, bullets from guns, arrows, or rocks from slingshots; or a powerful contusion by a blunt object, which may occur during a fight or from a serious car accident. Nonpenetrating injuries may be a result of foreign objects in the eyes, lacerations, a blow from a blunt object such as a ball (from baseball, softball, basketball, or racquet sports) or fist, or thermal or chemical burns.

Treatment is aimed at preventing further ocular damage and is primarily the responsibility of the ophthalmologist. It involves adequate examination of the injured eye (with the child sedated or anaesthetized in severe injuries); appropriate immediate intervention, such as removal of the foreign body or suturing of the laceration; and prevention of complications, such as administration of antibiotics or steroids and complete bed rest to allow the eye to heal and blood to reabsorb (see Emergency box). The prognosis varies according to the type

BOX 42-6 Types of Visual Impairment

Refractive Errors

Myopia

Nearsightedness—Ability to see objects clearly at close range but not at a distance

Pathophysiology

Results from eyeball that is too long, causing image to fall in front of retina

Clinical Manifestations

Excessive eye rubbing
Head tilt or forward head thrusts
Difficulty in reading or in doing other close work
Headaches
Dizziness
Clumsiness; walking into objects
Blinking more than usual or irritability when doing close work
Inability to see objects clearly
Poor school performance, especially in subjects that require demonstration, such as arithmetic

Treatment

Corrected with biconcave lenses that focus rays on retina
May be corrected with laser surgery

Hyperopia

Farsightedness—Ability to see objects at a distance

Pathophysiology

Results from eyeball that is too short, causing image to focus beyond retina

Clinical Manifestations

Because of accommodative ability, usually an ability to see objects at all ranges
Most children normally hyperopic until about 7 years of age

Treatment

When required, corrected with convex lenses that focus rays on retina
May be corrected with laser surgery

Astigmatism

Unequal curvatures in refractive apparatus

Pathophysiology

Results from unequal curvatures in cornea or lens that cause light rays to bend in different directions

Clinical Manifestations

Depend on severity of refractive error in each eye
Possible clinical manifestations of myopia

Treatment

Corrected with special lenses that compensate for refractive errors
May be corrected with laser surgery

Anisometropia

Different refractive strength in each eye

Pathophysiology

May develop amblyopia as weaker eye is used less

Clinical Manifestations

Depend on severity of refractive error in each eye
Possible clinical manifestations of myopia

Treatment

Treated with corrective lenses, preferably contact lenses, to improve vision in each eye so the eyes work as a unit
May be corrected with laser surgery

Amblyopia

Lazy eye—Reduced visual acuity in one eye

BOX 42-6 Types of Visual Impairment—cont'd

Pathophysiology
Results when one eye does not receive sufficient stimulation
Each retina receives different images, resulting in diplopia (double vision)
Brain accommodates by suppressing less intense image
Visual cortex eventually does not respond to visual stimulation in that eye, with resultant loss of vision
Clinical Manifestations
Poor vision in affected eye
Treatment
Preventable if treatment of primary visual defect, such as anisometropia or strabismus, begins before 6 years of age

Strabismus
"Squint" or cross-eye—Malalignment of eyes
Estropia—Inward deviation of eye
Exotropia—Outward deviation of eye
Pathophysiology
May result from muscle imbalance or paralysis, poor vision, or congenital defect
Because visual axes are not parallel, brain receives two images, and amblyopia can result
Clinical Manifestations
Squints eyelids together or frowns
Has difficulty focusing from one distance to another
Inaccurate judgement in picking up objects
Unable to see print or moving objects clearly
Closes one eye to see
Tilts head to one side
If combined with refractive errors, may see any of the manifestations listed for refractive errors
Diplopia
Photophobia
Dizziness
Headaches
Crossed eyes
Treatment
Depends on cause of strabismus
May involve occlusion therapy (patching stronger eye) or surgery to increase visual stimulation to weaker eye
Early diagnosis essential to prevent vision loss

Cataracts
Opacity of crystalline lens
Pathophysiology
Prevents light rays from entering eye and refracting on retina
Clinical Manifestations
Gradual decrease in ability to see objects clearly
Possible loss of peripheral vision
Nystagmus (with complete blindness)
Gray opacities of lens
Strabismus
Absence of red reflex
Treatment
Requires surgery to remove cloudy lens and replace lens (with intraocular lens implant, removable contact lens, prescription glasses)
Must be treated early to prevent blindness from amblyopia

Glaucoma
Increased intraocular pressure
Pathophysiology
Congenital type results from defective development of some component related to flow of aqueous humor
Increased pressure on optic nerve causes eventual atrophy and blindness
Clinical Manifestations
Loss of peripheral vision—mostly seen in acquired types
Possible bumping into objects
Perception of halos around objects
Possible complaint of pain or discomfort (pain, nausea, or vomiting if sudden rise in pressure)
Eye redness
Excessive tearing (epiphora)
Photophobia
Spasmodic winking (blepharospasm)
Corneal haziness
Enlargement of eyeball (buphthalmos)
Treatment
Requires surgical treatment (goniotomy) to open outflow tracts
May require more than one procedure

of injury. It is usually guarded in all cases of penetrating wounds because of the high risk of serious complications.

Infections

Infections of the adnexa and structures of the eyeball or globe may occur in children. The most common eye infection is conjunctivitis. Treatment is usually with ophthalmic antibiotics. Severe infections may require systemic antibiotic therapy. Steroids are used with caution because they exacerbate viral infections such as herpes simplex, increasing the risk of damage to the involved structures.

Nursing Care Management

Assessment of children for visual impairment is a critical nursing responsibility. Discovery of a visual impairment as early as possible is essential to prevent social, physical, and psychological damage to the child. Assessment involves (1) identifying those children who by virtue of their history are at risk, (2) observing for behaviours that indicate a vision loss, and (3) screening all children for visual acuity and signs of other ocular disorders such as strabismus. The discussion here focuses on clinical manifestations of various types of visual problems (see Box 42-6). Vision testing is discussed in Chapter 34.

Infancy

At birth, the nurse should observe the neonate's response to visual stimuli, such as following a light or object and cessation of body movement. The infant may vary in the intensity of the response, depending on the state of alertness.

Of special importance in detecting visual impairment during infancy are the parents' concerns regarding visual

EMERGENCY

Eye Injuries

Foreign Object

Examine eye for presence of a foreign body (evert upper lid to examine upper eye).

Remove a freely movable object with the pointed corner of a gauze pad lightly moistened with water.

Do not irrigate the eye or attempt to remove a penetrating object (see following section).

Caution child against rubbing the eye.

Chemical Burns

Irrigate the eye copiously with tap water for 20 minutes.

Evert upper lid to flush thoroughly.

Hold the child's head with the eye under tap of running lukewarm water.

Take child to emergency department.

Have child rest with eyes closed.

Keep the room darkened.

Ultraviolet Burns

If skin is burned, patch both eyes (make certain lids are completely closed); secure dressing with Kling bandages wrapped around the head rather than tape.

Have child rest with eyes closed.

Refer to an ophthalmologist.

Hematoma ("Black Eye")

Use a flashlight to check for gross hyphema (hemorrhage into anterior chamber; visible fluid meniscus across iris; more easily seen in light-coloured than in brown eyes).

Apply ice for the first 24 hours to reduce swelling if no hyphema is present.

Refer to an ophthalmologist immediately if hyphema is present.

Have child rest with eyes closed.

Penetrating Injuries

Take child to emergency department.

Never remove an object that has penetrated the eye.

Follow strict aseptic technique in examining the eye.

Observe for the following:

- Aqueous or vitreous leaks (fluid leaking from point of penetration)
- Hyphema
- Shape and equality of pupils, reaction to light, prolapsed iris (not perfectly circular)

Apply a Fox shield if available (not a regular eye patch) and apply a patch over the unaffected eye to prevent bilateral movement.

Have child maintain bed rest with child in 30-degree Fowler's position.

Caution child against rubbing the eye.

Refer to ophthalmologist.

responsiveness in their child. Their concerns, such as lack of eye contact from the infant, must be taken seriously. During infancy the child should be tested for strabismus. Lack of binocularity after 4 months of age is considered abnormal and must be treated to prevent amblyopia.

<u>NURSING ALERT</u> Suspect blindness if the infant does not react to light or if parents of a child at any age express concern.

Childhood

Because the most common visual impairment during childhood is refractive errors, testing for visual acuity is essential. The public health or community nurse usually assumes major responsibility for vision testing in schoolchildren, but only some provinces and territories have these vision programs in place. Preschool vision screening is important for early detection of amblyopia and to prevent long-term major eye damage, including blindness from this condition. The Public Health Association of Canada recommends universal preschool screening across Canada (Mema, McIntyre & Musto, 2012).

In addition to refractive errors, the nurse should be aware of signs and symptoms that indicate other ocular problems.

Promote Parent–Child Attachment

A crucial time in the life of blind infants is when they and their parents are getting acquainted with each other. Pleasurable patterns of interaction between the infant and parents may be lacking if there is not enough reciprocity. For example, if the parent gazes fondly at the infant's face and seeks eye contact but the infant fails to respond because he or she cannot see the parent, a troubled cycle of responses may occur. The nurse can help parents learn to look for other cues that indicate the infant is responding to them, such as whether the eyelids blink; whether the activity level accelerates or slows; whether respiratory patterns change, such as faster or slower breathing, when the parents come near; and whether the infant makes throaty sounds when they speak to the infant. In time, parents learn that the infant has unique ways of relating to them. They should be encouraged to show affection using nonvisual methods, such as talking or reading, cuddling, and walking the child.

Promote the Child's Optimum Development

Promoting the child's optimum development requires rehabilitation in a number of important areas. These include learning self-help skills and appropriate communication techniques to become independent. Although nurses may not be directly involved in such programs, they can provide direction and guidance to families regarding the availability of programs and the need to promote these activities in their child.

Development and Independence

Motor development depends on sight almost as much as verbal communication depends on hearing. From earliest infancy, parents should be encouraged to expose the infant to as many visual-motor experiences as possible, such as sitting supported in an infant seat or swing. The child should also have ample opportunities to hold up the head, sit unsupported, reach for objects, and crawl.

Despite visual impairment, the child can become independent in all aspects of self-care. The same principles used for promoting independence in sighted children apply, with additional emphasis on nonvisual cues. For example, the child may need help in dressing, such as special arrangement of clothing for style coordination and braille tags to distinguish colours and prints.

The blind child also must learn to become independent in navigational skills. The two main techniques are the tapping method (use of a cane to survey the environment for direction and to avoid obstacles) and guides, such as a sighted human guide or a dog guide, such as a Seeing Eye dog. Children who are partially sighted may benefit from ocular aids, such as a monocular telescope.

Play and Socialization

Blind children do not learn to play automatically. Because they cannot imitate others or actively explore the environment as sighted children do, they depend much more on others to stimulate and teach them how to play. Parents need help in selecting appropriate play materials, especially those that encourage fine and gross motor development and stimulate the senses of hearing, touch, and smell. Toys with educational value are especially useful, such as dolls with various clothing closures.

Blind children have the same needs for socialization as sighted children. Because they have little difficulty in learning verbal skills, they are able to communicate with age-mates and participate in suitable activities. The nurse should discuss with parents opportunities for socialization outside the home, especially regular preschools. The trend is to include these children with sighted children to help them adjust to the outside world for eventual independence.

To compensate for inadequate stimulation, these children may develop blindisms (self-stimulatory activities, such as body rocking, finger flicking, or arm twirling). Such habits restrict the child's social acceptance and are discouraged. Behaviour modification is often successful in reducing or eliminating blindisms.

Education

The main obstacle to the child's learning is the child's total dependence on nonvisual cues. Although the child can learn via verbal lecturing, he or she is unable to read the written word or to write without special education. Therefore, the child must rely on braille, a system that uses raised dots to represent letters and numbers. The child can then read the braille with the fingers and can write a message using a braille writer. However, unless others read braille, this system is not useful for communicating with others. A more portable system for written communication is the use of a braille slate and stylus, or an MP3 player or smartphone with a recording device. A recorder is especially helpful for leaving messages for others and taking notes during classroom lectures. For mathematical calculations, portable calculators with voice synthesizers are available.

MP3 recordings and CDs are significant sources of reading material other than braille books, which are large and cumbersome. The Canadian National Institute for the Blind, Library for the Blind has talking books, braille books, and a special records program, which are available at many local libraries (see Additional Resources section at the end of this chapter). The talking book machine and CD player are provided at no cost to families, and there is no postage fee for returning the materials. Talking watches and clocks are also available.

For written communication children can use a home computer with a voice synthesizer, which "speaks" each letter or word that has been typed.

The child with partial sight can benefit from specialized visual aids that produce a magnified retinal image. The basic devices are accommodation (e.g., bringing the object closer), special plus lenses, handheld and stand magnifiers, telescopes, video projection systems, and large print. E-readers and computer tablets can be easily adjusted to increase the font size. Special equipment is also available to enlarge print. Information about services for the partially sighted is available from the Canadian National Institute for the Blind (CNIB).

Children with diminished vision often prefer to do close work without their glasses and compensate by bringing the object very near to their eyes. This should be allowed. The exception is the child with vision in only one eye, who should always wear glasses for protection.

Care for the Child During Hospitalization

Because nurses are more likely to care for children who are hospitalized for procedures that involve temporary loss of vision than for children who are blind, the following discussion concentrates primarily on the needs of such children. The nursing care objectives in either situation are to (1) reassure the child and family throughout every phase of treatment, (2) orient the child to the surroundings, (3) provide a safe environment, and (4) encourage independence. Whenever possible, the same nurse should care for the child to ensure consistency in the approach.

When sighted children temporarily lose their vision, almost every aspect of the environment becomes bewildering and frightening. They are forced to rely on nonvisual senses for help in adjusting to the blindness without the benefit of any special training. Nurses have a major role in minimizing the effects of temporary loss of vision. They need to talk to the child about everything that is occurring, emphasizing aspects of procedures that are felt or heard. They should approach the child by always identifying themselves as soon as they enter the room. Because unfamiliar sounds are especially frightening, these should be explained. Parents should be encouraged to room with their child and participate in the care. Familiar objects, such as a teddy bear or doll, should be brought from home to help lessen the strangeness of the hospital. As soon as the child is able to be out of bed, he or she can be oriented to the immediate surroundings. If the child is able to see on admission, this opportunity should be taken to point out significant aspects of the room. The child needs to be encouraged to practice ambulation with the eyes closed to become accustomed to this experience.

The room should be arranged with safety in mind. For example, a stool or chair can be placed next to the bed to help the child climb in and out of bed. The furniture should always be placed in the same position to prevent collisions. Cleaning personnel need to be reminded to keep the room in the same order. If the child has difficulty navigating by feeling the walls, a rope can be attached from the bed to the point of destination, such as the bathroom. Attention to details such as well-fitting slippers or robes that do not drag on the floor is important in preventing tripping. Unlike the child who is blind, these children are not familiar with navigating with a cane.

The child should be encouraged to be independent in self-care activities, especially if the visual loss may be prolonged or potentially permanent. For example, during bathing the nurse can set up all the equipment and encourage the child to participate. At mealtime the nurse should explain where each food item is on the tray, open any special containers, prepare cereal or toast, and encourage the child in self-feeding. Favourite finger foods, such as sandwiches, hamburgers, hot dogs, or pizza, may be good selections. The child needs to be praised for his or her efforts at working together and being independent. Any improvements made in self-care, no matter how small, should be stressed.

Appropriate recreational activities should be provided, and if a child life specialist is available, such planning can be done jointly. Because children with temporary blindness have a wide variety of play experiences to draw on, they should be encouraged to select activities. For example, if they like to read, they may enjoy being read to. If they prefer manual activity, they may appreciate playing with clay or building blocks or feeling different textures and naming them. If they need an outlet for aggression, activities such as pounding or banging on a drum can be helpful. Simple board and card games can be played with a "seeing partner" or an opponent who helps with the game. They should have familiar toys from home to play with, since familiar items are more easily manipulated than new ones. If parents want to bring presents, they should be objects that stimulate hearing and touch, such as a radio, music box, or stuffed animal.

Occasionally, children who are blind come to the hospital for procedures to restore their vision. Although this is an extremely happy time, it also requires intervention to help them adjust to sight. They need an opportunity to take in all that they see. They should not be bombarded with visual stimuli. They may need to concentrate on people's faces or their own to become accustomed to this experience. They often need to talk about what they see and to compare the visual images with their mental ones. The children may also go through a period of depression, which must be respected and supported. The nurse or parents should refrain from statements such as "How can you be so sad when you can see again?" Instead, the children should be encouraged to discuss how it feels to see, especially in terms of seeing themselves.

Newly sighted children also need time to adjust to the ability to engage in activities that were impossible before. For example, they may prefer to use braille to read, rather than learning a new "visual approach," because of familiarity with the touch system. Eventually, as they learn to recognize letters and numbers, they will integrate these new skills into reading and writing. However, parents and teachers must be careful not to push them before they are ready. This applies to social relationships and physical activities as well as learning situations.

Assist in Measures to Prevent Visual Impairment

An essential nursing goal is to prevent visual impairment. This involves many of the same interventions discussed under hearing impairments:

- Prenatal screening for pregnant women at risk, such as those with rubella or syphilis infection and family histories of genetic disorders associated with visual loss
- Adequate prenatal and perinatal care to prevent prematurity
- Periodic screening of all children, especially newborns through preschoolers, for congenital blindness and visual impairments caused by refractive errors, strabismus, and other disorders
- Rubella immunization of all children
- Safety counselling regarding the common causes of ocular trauma and safe practices when working with, playing with, or carrying objects such as scissors, knives, and balls

NURSING ALERT A helmet with a face mask should be required for children playing football, hockey, or baseball.

After detection of eye problems, the nurse has a responsibility to prevent further ocular damage by ensuring that corrective treatment is used. For the child with strabismus, occlusion patching of the stronger eye is often needed. Compliance with the procedure is greatest during the early preschool years. It is more difficult to encourage school-age children to wear the occlusive patch because the poor visual acuity of the uncovered weaker eye interferes with school work and the patch sets them apart from their peers. In school they benefit from being positioned favourably (closer to the board or other visual media) and allowed extra time to read or complete an assignment. If treatment of the eye disorder requires instillation of ophthalmic medication, the family should be taught the correct procedure (see Chapter 45).

For the child with refractive errors, the nurse can help the child adjust to wearing glasses. Young children who often pull glasses off benefit from temporal pieces that wrap around the ears or an elastic strap attached to the frames and around the back of the head to hold the glasses on securely. After children appreciate the value of clear vision, they are more likely to wear the corrective lenses.

Glasses should not interfere with any activity. Special protective guards are available during contact sports to prevent accidental injury, and all corrective lenses should be made from safety glass, which is shatterproof. Often, corrective lenses improve visual acuity so dramatically that children are able to compete more effectively in sports. This in itself is a tremendous inducement to continue wearing glasses.

Contact lenses are a popular alternative, especially for adolescents. Several types are available, such as hard lenses, including gas-permeable ones, and soft lenses, which may be designed for daily or extended wear. Contact lenses offer several advantages over glasses, such as greater visual acuity, total corrected field of vision, convenience (especially with the extended-wear type), and optimal cosmetic benefit. Unfortunately, they are usually more expensive and require much more care than glasses, including considerable practice to learn techniques for insertion and removal. If they are prescribed, the nurse can be helpful in teaching parents or older children how to care for the lenses.

Because trauma is the leading cause of blindness in children, the nurse has the major responsibility of preventing further eye injury until specific treatment is instituted. The major principles to follow when caring for an eye injury are outlined in the Emergency box on p. 1206. Because patients with a serious eye injury fear blindness, the nurse should stay with the child and family to provide support and reassurance.

Deaf-Blind Children

The most traumatic sensory impairment is loss of sight and hearing. Obviously, auditory and visual disabilities have profound effects on the child's development. They interfere with the normal sequence of physical, intellectual, and psychosocial growth. Although such children often achieve the usual motor milestones, their rate of development is slower. These children learn communication only with specialized training. Finger spelling is one desirable method often taught to these children. Some deaf-blind children, especially those with residual hearing or sight, can learn to speak. Whenever possible, speech is encouraged because it allows communication with other individuals.

The future prospects for deaf-blind children are, at best, unpredictable. Congenital blindness or deafness may be accompanied by other physical or neurological problems, which further diminish the child's learning potential. The most favourable prognosis is for children who have acquired deafness and blindness and have few, if any, associated disabilities. Their learning capacity is greatly potentiated by their developmental progress before the sensory impairments. Although total independence, including gainful vocational training, is the goal, some deaf-blind children are unable to develop to this level. They may require lifelong parental or residential care. The nurse working with such families needs to help them deal with future goals for the child, including possible alternatives to home care during the parents' advancing years.

Resources for the deaf-blind can be found at Canadian Organizations for Deafblind People, at http://www.deafblind.com/canada.html.

Retinoblastoma

Retinoblastoma, which arises from the retina, is the most common congenital malignant intraocular tumour of childhood. It occurs in approximately 1 in 20,000 babies (Retinoblastoma.ca, 2010). Retinoblastoma is caused by a mutation in a gene and may occur sporadically or be inherited (Hurwitz et al., 2006). Retinoblastoma develops when the mutated gene is unable to produce the natural signals to stop the growth of retinal cells. The majority of cases are nonhereditary and unilateral, with the remainder divided between hereditary and unilateral, and hereditary and bilateral. Hereditary retinoblastomas are transmitted as an autosomal dominant trait with 90% penetrance (Hurwitz et al., 2006).

Diagnostic Evaluation

Retinoblastoma has few grossly obvious signs (Box 42-7). Typically, the most common sign is observed by the parent as a whitish "glow" in the pupil, known as the white reflex or **leukokoria**. Leukokoria represents visualization of the tumour as the light momentarily falls on the mass. The second most common sign of retinoblastoma is acquired strabismus (Hurwitz et al., 2006).

The first step in diagnosis is carefully listening to and recognizing the significance of reports from family members regarding suspected abnormalities within the eye. Eye abnormalities, including white reflex, strabismus, decreased vision, and persistent painful erythematous eyes, should be referred to an ophthalmologist. Definitive diagnosis is usually based on ophthalmoscopic examination with the patient under **general anaesthesia**. Imaging studies, including ultrasonography and computed tomography of the orbit, are done to determine the extent of the disease.

Therapeutic Management

The aim of therapy is to preserve useful vision and eradicate the tumour. Treatment of retinoblastoma depends chiefly on the stage of the tumour at the time of diagnosis. Some of the common focal therapies are (1) plaque brachytherapy (surgical radioactive implant on the sclera until maximum dose has been delivered to the tumour), (2) laser photocoagulation (laser beam to coagulate blood supply to the tumour), (3) cryotherapy (freezing the tumour by destroying the microcirculation to the tumour through microcrystal formation), and (4) thermotherapy (using microwaves or infrared radiation to deliver heat to the tumour) (De Potter, 2002; Melamud, Palekar, & Singh, 2006; Schouten–van Meeteren et al., 2002). Chemoreduction and chemoprevention minimize the use of external beam radiation treatment and thus reduce the risk of radiation-induced malignancies and facial disfigurement.

With advanced tumour growth into the optic nerve, choroid, orbit, and anterior chamber or no hope for useful vision, enucleation (removal) of the affected eye is the treatment of choice. After enucleation, an orbital implant is placed

BOX 42-7 Clinical Manifestations of Retinoblastoma

- White eye reflex (most common sign)
- Strabismus (second most common sign)
- Red, painful eye, often with glaucoma
- Blindness (late sign)

to provide a more natural cosmetic appearance, minimize sinking of the prosthesis, and enable motility of the prosthesis. With bilateral disease, every attempt is made to preserve useful vision in both eyes. Chemotherapy, external beam, radiotherapy, and other treatments (i.e., cryotherapy, laser, plaque brachytherapy, thermotherapy) to both eyes may prevent the need for enucleation.

Prognosis

The overall prognosis for retinoblastoma is favourable, with a survival rate of nearly 90% for both unilateral and bilateral tumours. Retinoblastoma is one of the tumours that may spontaneously regress. Of major concern in long-term survivors is the development of decreased visual acuity; facial disfiguration; and secondary tumours, especially osteogenic sarcoma, other sarcomas, and melanoma. Children with bilateral disease (hereditary form) are more likely to develop secondary cancers than are children with unilateral disease. It is thought that these individuals are predisposed to developing cancer and that radiation increases their risk.

Nursing Care Management

One of the most important nursing goals is to have a high index of suspicion for this rare malignancy. If parents report noticing a strange light in the eye or expression, these concerns must be taken seriously. Families with a history of retinoblastoma require follow-up; the nurse can be instrumental in reminding parents of appointments.

Because the tumour is usually diagnosed in infants or very young children, most of the preparation for diagnostic tests and treatment involves parents. After indirect ophthalmoscopy, the child may not see clearly, or the eyes may be sensitive to light because of pupillary dilation. Parents should be made aware of these normal reactions before the procedure. Screening tests, such as bone surveys and bone marrow aspiration, are rarely performed unless metastatic disease is suspected.

The treatment plan may include focal intraocular therapy with or without chemotherapy, external beam radiation, and, if necessary, enucleation. Enucleation is the treatment of choice if there is extensive disease threatening metastasis or no chance for useful vision. The enucleation procedure and the positive benefits of a prosthesis should be explained to the parents. Showing them pictures of another child with an artificial eye may help them adjust to the thought of disfigurement.

After surgery, the parents should be prepared for the child's facial appearance. An eye patch is in place, and the child's face may be edematous or ecchymotic. Parents often fear seeing the surgical site because they imagine a cavity in the skull. A surgically implanted sphere maintains the shape of the eyeball, and the implant is covered with conjunctiva. When the lids are open, the exposed area resembles the mucosal lining of the mouth. After the child is fitted for a prosthesis, usually within 3 weeks, the facial appearance returns to normal. Initial instructions for care of the prosthesis are given by the ocularist who fits and manufactures the device.

Care of the socket is minimal and easily accomplished. The wound itself is clean and has little or no drainage. If an antibiotic ointment is prescribed, it is applied in a thin line on the surface of the tissues of the socket. To cleanse the site, an irrigating solution may be ordered and is instilled daily or more frequently, before application of the antibiotic ointment. The dressing, consisting of an eye pad taped over the surgical site, needs to be changed daily. After the socket has healed completely, a dressing is no longer necessary, although it is a preventive measure against infection.

Autism Spectrum Disorders

Autism spectrum disorders (ASDs) are complex neurodevelopmental disorders of brain function accompanied by intellectual and social behavioural deficits. ASDs include autistic disorder, Asperger's syndrome, and pervasive developmental disorder not otherwise specified, which are impairments ranging from mild to severe (Croen et al., 2006). ASD is typically noticed during early childhood, primarily from 24 to 48 months of age. It occurs in 1 in 166 children; is about four times more common in males than in females (although females are more severely affected); and is not related to socioeconomic level, race, or parenting style (Courtney-Manning, 2007; Fombonne, 2003a; Schaefer & Lutz, 2006).

Epidemiological studies are still in the early stages in Canada. More surveillance is needed to develop accurate data on the prevalence of autism spectrum disorders (Fombonne, 2003b). The Canadian federal government has recently announced funding for a Chair in Autism Spectrum Disorders in order to research innovative approaches to treat and care for children with ASD (Canadian Institutes of Health Research, 2012).

Etiology

ASD is now recognized as a genetic disorder of prenatal and postnatal brain development (Bloom-DiCicco et al., 2006). Immune and environmental factors (e.g., viral infections) may interact with the genetic susceptibility to increase the incidence of ASD (Bloom-DiCicco et al., 2006). Individuals with ASD may have abnormal electroencephalograms, epileptic seizures, delayed development of hand dominance, persistence of primitive reflexes, metabolic abnormalities (elevated blood serotonin), cerebellar vermal hypoplasia (part of the brain involved in regulating motion and some aspects of memory), and infantile abnormal head enlargement (Bloom-DiCicco et al., 2006; Dawson, 2007).

The strong evidence for a genetic basis in twins is consistent with an autosomal recessive pattern of inheritance. Twin studies demonstrate a high concordance (60 to 96%) for monozygotic (identical) twins and less than 5% concordance for dizygotic (nonidentical) twins. In addition, between 5 and 16% of males with ASD are positive for the fragile X chromosome.

There is a relatively high risk of recurrence of ASD in families with one affected child (Muhle, Trentacoste, & Rapin, 2004; Schaefer & Lutz, 2006). Although several genes have been suggested as possible causative factors in ASD, no specific gene for the disorder has been identified (Dawson, 2007; Kolevzon, Gross, & Reichenberg, 2007; Schanen, 2006).

Contrary to previous reports, autism does not appear to be caused by the measles-mumps-rubella (MMR) and thimerosal-containing vaccines (DeStefano et al., 2004; D'Souza, Fombonne, & Ward, 2006; Muhle et al., 2004) (see Evidence-Informed Practice box). ASD has been reported in association

EVIDENCE-INFORMED PRACTICE Vaccines and Autism Spectrum Disorders

Ask the Question

Is the incidence of autism spectrum disorders (ASDs) or other neurodevelopmental disorders increased in children receiving vaccines containing thimerosal?

Search for Evidence

Search Strategies

English-language publications within the past 15 years, research-based articles (level 3 or lower), and child populations

Databases Searched

PubMed, Cochrane Collaboration, Institute of Medicine, Public Health Agency of Canada, National Advisory Committee on Immunization, American Academy of Pediatrics, Autism Research Institute

Critically Analyze the Evidence

The safety of vaccines administered to children has been a source of controversy for some time. It has been speculated that vaccines can cause some conditions having an unknown etiology, such as autism, sudden infant death syndrome, and multiple sclerosis.

In 1998, a report was published showing that administration of the measles, mumps, and rubella (MMR) vaccine caused a new form of ASD, resulting from chronic inflammatory colonic disease that caused malabsorption of proteins. This condition in turn created autoantibodies that contributed to brain impairment, and ultimately, autism (Canadian Paediatric Society [CPS], Infectious Diseases and Immunization Committee, 2007). This speculation was based on the claims of parents of eight children who developed problems closely after the vaccinations had been given (Wakefield et al., 1998).

In 2007, the Infectious Disease and Immunization Committee of the CPS completed an extensive review of the literature. The committee reviewed large population-based epidemiology studies in Finland (Peltola et al., 1998); Denmark (Madsen et al., 2002); the United States (Dales, Hammer, & Smith, 2001), and England (Kaye, del Mar, & Jick, 2001). These studies showed that there were not enough proven criteria to show any association between the MMR vaccine and autism. The CPS researchers also considered the Institute of Medicine's (2004) review and the Cochrane systematic review (Demicheli, Jefferson, Rivetti, & Price, 2005), which failed to show any association between the MMR vaccine and autism.

In addition, there was speculation that use of a preservative, thimerosal, a mercury ethanyl, in multidose vaccine vials could potentially cause ASD. In Canada, infants under 6 months of age had never received any thimerosal-preserved vaccine. In the United States, thimerosal was removed from vaccines as a safety precaution. A cohort study of 467,450 children in Denmark compared the incidence of ASDs in children vaccinated with thimerosal-containing vaccines with that in children vaccinated with a thimerosal-free formulation of the same vaccine. Results found no relationship between childhood vaccination with thimerosal-containing vaccines and the development of ASDs (Hviid et al., 2003). Subsequent research in other countries and in Canada has not shown any connection between thimerosal and the development of ASD (Fombonne, Zakarian, Bennett, Meng, & McLean-Heywood, 2006).

It is important to note that despite the removal of thimerosal from vaccines, autism rates have continued to rise, and the rate is rising in Canada (Fombonne et al.,2006).

Apply the Evidence: Nursing Implications

Decisions about the total elimination of thimerosal (even traces) from vaccines must balance the potential benefit of no exposure to mercury against the risks of decreased vaccine coverage because of the higher cost of the thimerosal-free vaccine, the risks of sepsis due to the potential bacterial contamination of the preservative-free formulations, and the risk of exposure to alternative preservatives that might replace the thimerosal preservative.

Thimerosal as a preservative has been removed or reduced to trace amounts in all vaccines routinely administered to children except influenza vaccine. The maximum total exposure during the first 6 months of life is less than 3 mcg of mercury. Most vaccines licensed in Canada do not contain thimerosal. The influenza vaccine and most hepatitis B vaccines are multidose vaccines, which do use the preservative thimerosal. In some provinces and territories, parents or guardians have the choice of a thimerosal-free vaccine for immunization of infants against hepatitis B (Public Health Agency of Canada, 2012).

References

Canadian Paediatric Society, Infectious Diseases and Immunization Committee. (2007). Autistic spectrum disorder: No causal relationship with vaccines. *Paediatrics & Child Health, 12*(5), 393–395. (Addendum added 2011)

Dales, L., Hammer, S. J., & Smith, N. J. (2001). Time trends in autism and in MMR immunization coverage in California. *Journal of the American Medical Association, 285*, 1183–1185.

Demicheli, V., Jefferson, T., Rivetti, A., & Price, D. (2005). Vaccines for measles, mumps and rubella in children. *Cochrane Database System Review, 4*, CD004407.

Fombonne, E., Zakarian, R., Bennett, A., Meng, L., & McLean-Heywood, D. (2006). Pervasive developmental disorders in Montreal, Quebec, Canada: Prevalence and links with immunizations. *Pediatrics, 118*, e139–e150.

Hviid, A., et al. (2003). Association between thimerosal-containing vaccine and autism. *Journal of the American Medical Association, 290*(13), 1763–1766.

Institute of Medicine. (2004). *Immunization safety review: Vaccines and autism*. Washington, DC: National Academy Press.

Kaye, J. A., del Mar Melero-Montes, M., & Jick, H. (2001). Mumps, measles and rubella vaccine and the incidence of autism recorded by general practitioners: A time trend analysis. *British Medical Journal, 322*, 460–463.

Madsen, K. M., et al. (2002). A population-based study of measles, mumps, and rubella vaccination and autism. *New England Journal of Medicine, 347*, 1477–1482.

Peltola, H., Patja, A., Leinikki, P., Valle, M., Davidkin, I., & Paunio, M. (1998). No evidence for measles, mumps, and rubella vaccine-associated inflammatory bowel disease or autism in a 14-year prospective study. *Lancet, 351*, 1327–1328.

Public Health Agency of Canada. (2012). *Thimerosal in vaccines and autism*. Retrieved from http://www.phac-aspc.gc.ca/im/q_a_thimerosal-eng.php.

Wakefield, A. J., et al. (1998). Ileal-lymphoidnodular hyperplasia, non-specific colitis, and pervasive developmental disorder in children. *Lancet, 351*(9103), 637–641.

with a number of conditions such as fragile X syndrome, tuberous sclerosis, metabolic disorders, fetal rubella syndrome, *Haemophilus influenzae* meningitis, and structural brain anomalies (Dawson, 2007; Muhle et al., 2004). Recent reports have retrospectively tied ASD to prenatal and perinatal events such as maternal and paternal ages over 40 years (for fathers, 1 in 116 births; for mothers, 1 in 123 births), uterine bleeding during pregnancy, low Apgar score, fetal distress, and neonatal hyperbilirubinemia (Croen et al., 2007; Kolevzon et al., 2007; Muhle et al., 2004). These same researchers, however, urge caution in interpreting these findings.

Clinical Manifestations and Diagnostic Evaluation

Children with ASD demonstrate several peculiar and often seemingly bizarre characteristics, primarily in social interactions, communication, and behaviour. One hallmark characteristic is the inability to maintain eye contact with another person. Parents of autistic children have noted their infants had difficulties with eye contact, avoidance of body contact, and language delay at a very early age (Belschner, 2007; Dawson, 2007). Children with ASD also display limited functional play and may interact with toys in an unusual or odd manner (Belschner, 2007). Children with ASD may have significant gastrointestinal symptoms. Constipation is a common symptom and can be associated with acquired megarectum in children with ASD (Afzal et al., 2003). Other clinical manifestations typically seen in children with autism are described in Box 42-8.

Children with autism do not always have the same manifestations; cases vary from mild forms requiring minimal supervision to severe forms in which self-abusive behaviour is common. The majority (50 to 70%) of children with autism have some degree of CI, with scores typically in the moderate to severe range. More females than males tend to have very low intelligence scores. Despite their relatively moderate to severe disability, some children with autism (known as *savants*) excel in particular areas, such as art, music, memory, mathematics, or perceptual skills such as puzzle building.

Speech and language delays are also common in ASD children. Any child who does not display such language skills as babbling or gesturing by 12 months, single words by 16 months, and two-word phrases by 24 months is recommended for immediate hearing and language evaluation (Grizzle & Simms, 2005). A sudden deterioration in extant expressive speech is also a red-flag event for further evaluation.

Early recognition, referral, diagnosis, and intensive early intervention tend to improve outcomes for children with ASD (Belschner, 2007; Courtney-Manning, 2007). Unfortunately, diagnosis is often not made until 2 to 3 years after symptoms are first recognized. The American Academy of Neurology report has a comprehensive set of suggested diagnostic criteria to be used to either rule out or establish the diagnosis of childhood ASD (Belschner, 2007; Filipek et al., 2000) (see Box 42-8) (see also Additional Resources section at the end of this chapter). At the present time there is no universal screening for autism in Canada. Diagnosis of an autism condition can take 3 to 24 months for preschoolers, and for older children sometimes several years. Increasingly, youth and adults whose ASD was not previously identified are now being diagnosed (Autism Society, 2010).

BOX 42-8 Diagnostic Criteria for Autistic Disorder

A. A total of six (or more) items from (1), (2), and (3), with at least two from (1), and one each from (2) and (3):
   (1) Qualitative impairment in social interaction, as manifested by at least two of the following:
      (a) Marked impairment in the use of multiple nonverbal behaviours such as eye-to-eye gaze, facial expression, body postures, and gestures to regulate social interaction
      (b) Failure to develop peer relationships appropriate to developmental level
      (c) Lack of spontaneous seeking to share enjoyment, interests, or achievements with other people (e.g., by a lack of showing, bringing, pointing out objects of interest)
      (d) Lack of social or emotional reciprocity
   (2) Qualitative impairments in communication as manifested by at least one of the following:
      (a) Delay in, or total lack of, the development of spoken language (not accompanied by an attempt to compensate through alternative modes of communication such as gestures or mime)
      (b) In individuals with adequate speech, marked impairment in the ability to initiate or sustain a conversation with others
      (c) Stereotyped and repetitive use of language or idiosyncratic language
      (d) Lack of varied, spontaneous make-believe play or social imitative play appropriate to developmental level
   (3) Restricted repetitive and stereotyped patterns of behaviour, interests, and activities, as manifested by at least one of the following:
      (a) Encompassing preoccupation with one or more stereotyped and restricted patterns of interest that is abnormal either in intensity or focus
      (b) Apparently inflexible adherence to specific, nonfunctional routines or rituals
      (c) Stereotyped and repetitive motor mannerisms (e.g., hand or finger flapping or twisting, complex whole-body movements)

B. Delays or abnormal functioning in at least one of the following areas, with onset before age 3 years: (1) social interaction, (2) language as used in social communication, or (3) symbolic or imaginative play

C. The disturbance is not better accounted for by Rett's disorder or childhood disintegrative disorder

(From American Psychiatric Association. [2000]. *Diagnostic and statistical manual of mental disorders* [4th ed., text revision] [DSM-IV TR]. Washington, DC: Author.)

Prognosis

ASD is usually a severely disabling condition. However, some children improve with acquisition of language skills and communication with others (Bloom-DiCicco et al., 2006). Some ultimately achieve independence, but most require lifelong adult supervision. Aggravation of psychiatric symptoms occurs in about half of the children during adolescence, with girls having a tendency for continued deterioration.

Early recognition of behaviours associated with ASD is critical to implementing appropriate interventions and family involvement. The prognosis is most favourable for children with communicative speech development by age 6 years and an IQ above 50 at the time of diagnosis.

Nursing Care Management

Therapeutic intervention for the child with ASD is a specialized area involving professionals with advanced training. Although there is no cure for ASD, numerous therapies have been used. The most promising results have been through highly structured and intensive behaviour modification programs. In general, the objective in treatment is to promote positive reinforcement, increase social awareness of others, teach verbal communication skills, and decrease unacceptable behaviour. Providing a structured routine for the child to follow is key in the management of ASD.

When these children are hospitalized, the parents are essential to planning care and, ideally, should stay with the child as much as possible. Nurses should recognize that not all children with ASD are the same; they will require individual assessment and treatment. Decreasing stimulation by using a private room, avoiding extraneous auditory and visual distractions, and encouraging the parents to bring in possessions the child is attached to may lessen the disruptiveness of hospitalization. Because physical contact often upsets these children, minimal holding and eye contact may be necessary to avoid behavioural outbursts. Care must be taken when performing procedures on, administering medicine to, or feeding these children, since they may be either fussy eaters who willfully starve themselves or gag to prevent eating, or indiscriminate hoarders, swallowing any available edible or inedible items, such as a thermometer. Eating habits of ASD children may be particularly problematic for families and may involve food refusal, mouthing objects, eating nonedibles, and smelling and throwing food (Belschner, 2007; Caronna, Augustyn, & Zuckerman, 2007).

Children with ASD need to be introduced slowly to new situations; visits with staff caregivers should be kept short whenever possible. Because these children have difficulty organizing their behaviour and redirecting their energy, they need to be told directly what to do. Communication should be at the child's developmental level, brief, and concrete.

Family Support

As with so many other chronic conditions, ASD involves the entire family and often becomes "a family disease." Nurses can help alleviate the guilt and shame often associated with this disorder by stressing what is known from a biological standpoint and by providing family support. It is imperative to help parents understand that they are not the cause of the child's condition.

Parents need expert counselling early in the course of the disorder and should be referred to the Autism Society of Canada, which provides information about education, treatment programs and techniques, and facilities such as camps and group homes (see Additional Resources).

As much as possible, the family should be encouraged to care for the child in the home. With the help of family support programs in some provinces and territories, families are often able to provide home care and assist with the educational services the child needs. As the child approaches adulthood and parents become older, the family may require assistance in locating a long-term placement facility. Autism groups and parents are lobbying the Canadian government through the courts to provide more financial support to help families pay for the comprehensive treatment costs. Early intervention treatments are critical to improving the child's long-term development (CPS, Psychosocial Paediatrics Committee, 2004).

Key Points

- *Intellectual disabilities* refers to the challenges that some people face in learning and in communication that are usually present from the time they are born or from an early age.
- Causes of severe CI are primarily genetic, biochemical, and infectious. Mild CI is associated primarily with familial, social, and environmental causes, whereas severe CI is more likely to be associated with specific syndromes.
- Education of children with CI emphasizes sensory and verbal discrimination, improvement of short-term memory, motivation, and technological support.
- Optimum development may be promoted through family guidance regarding play, communication, discipline, socialization, and sexuality.
- Prevention of CI focuses on support for the preterm neonate and other high-risk newborns, rubella immunization, genetic counselling, and maternal education regarding the risks of chemical use (e.g., alcohol ingestion) and the importance of adequate nutrition.
- Down syndrome, a chromosomal abnormality, is characterized by mild to moderate CI (most often), physical characteristics, slowed language development, congenital anomalies, sensory problems, and diminished growth and sexual development.
- Fragile X syndrome is characterized by CI and phenotypic findings in affected males. It is considered the most common hereditary cause and the second leading chromosomal cause of CI after Down syndrome.
- Hearing disorders may be classified according to the location of the defect: conductive, sensorineural, mixed conductive-sensorineural, and central auditory imperception.
- Rehabilitation for hearing loss involves parent education and support, hearing aids, lipreading, sign language, speech therapy, and promotion of socialization.
- Prevention of hearing loss includes treatment of infection, universal newborn screening and child auditory testing, immunization, pregnancy and genetic counselling, and reduction of noise pollution.
- Common visual impairments in childhood include refractive errors, amblyopia, strabismus, cataracts, and glaucoma, with trauma and infections being common causes of visual impairment.
- Prevention of visual impairment focuses on prenatal screening, prenatal and perinatal care, periodic vision screening, immunization, and safety counselling.
- Nursing goals in visual rehabilitation include helping the family and child adjust to the child's visual impairment,

promoting parent–child attachment, fostering optimum development and independence, providing for play and socialization, and being aware of educational facilities.

- For the child undergoing ocular surgery, nursing care is aimed at reassuring the child and family throughout treatment, orienting the child to the surroundings, providing a safe environment, and encouraging independence.
- Retinoblastoma is a rare congenital malignant tumour; its most common clinical manifestations are white pupil reflex and strabismus.
- ASDs are a complex neurodevelopmental disorder of brain function accompanied by a broad range and severity of intellectual and behavioural deficits.

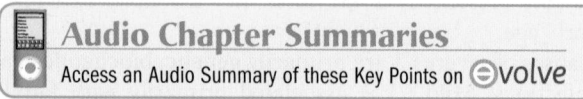

Audio Chapter Summaries

Access an Audio Summary of these Key Points on evolve

References

Afzal, N., et al. (2003). Constipation with acquired megarectum in children with autism. *Pediatrics, 112*(4), 939–942.

Alanay, Y., et al. (2007). Multidisciplinary approach to the management of individuals with fragile X syndrome. *Journal of Intellectual Disability Research, 51,* 151–161. doi:10.1111/j.1365-2788.2006.00942.x

American Academy of Pediatrics, Task Force on Newborn and Infant Hearing. (1999). Newborn and infant hearing loss: Detection and intervention. *Pediatrics, 103*(2), 527–530.

American Psychiatric Association. (2000). *Diagnostic and statistical manual of mental disorders* (4th ed., text revision) (DSM-IV TR). Washington, DC: Author.

Autism Society Canada. (2010). *The right to treatment.* Retrieved from http://www.autismsocietycanada.ca/index.php?option=com_content&view=article&id=30&Itemid=63&lang=en.

Belschner, R. A. (2007). Stop, assess and motivate: The SAM approach to autism spectrum disorder. *American Journal for Nurse Practitioners, 11*(4), 43–50.

Biasini, F. J., et al. (1999). Mental retardation: A symptom and a syndrome. In S. D. Netherton, D. Holmes, & E. Walker (Eds.), *Child and adolescent psychological disorders: A comprehensive textbook,* Vol. 4. New York: Oxford University Press.

Bloom-DiCicco, E., et al. (2006). The developmental neurobiology of autism spectrum disorder. *Journal of Neuroscience, 26*(26), 6897–6906. doi:10.1523/JNEUROSCI.1712-06.2006

Bosch, J. J., & Ringdahl, J. (2001). Functional analysis of problem behavior in children with mental retardation: What is it, and why should pediatric nurses care? *MCN: American Journal of Maternal-Child Nursing, 26*(6), 307–311.

Canadian Dietitians of Canada & Canadian Paediatric Society. (2010). *A health professional's guide for using the new WHO growth charts.* Retrieved from http://www.cps.ca/english/statements/N/DC_HealhProGrowthGuide.pdf.

Canadian Down Syndrome Society. (2009). *Parents helping parents: New parent visiting program.* Retrieved from: http://www.cdss.ca/services/new-parent-programs/parents-helping-parents-new-parent-visiting-program.html.

Canadian Down Syndrome Society. (2010). *What is Down syndrome?* Retrieved from http://www.cdss.ca/images/pdf/brochures/english/celebrate_being_about_down_syndrome_english.pdf.

Canadian Institutes of Health. (2012). *Harper government invests in autism treatment and care.* Newswise, released 3/27/2012. Retrieved from http://www.newswise.com/articles/harper-government-invests-in-autism-treatment-and-care.

Canadian Paediatric Society. (2008). *Your baby's hearing.* Retrieved from http://www.caringforkids.cps.ca/pregnancybabies/BabyHearing.htm.

Canadian Paediatric Society, Community Paediatrics Committee. (2011). Universal newborn screening. *Paediatrics & Child Health, 16*(5), 301–305.

Canadian Paediatric Society, Psychosocial Paediatrics Committee. (2004). Early intervention for children with autism. *Paediatrics & Child Health, 9*(4), 267–270.

Caronna, E. B., Augustyn, M., & Zuckerman, B. (2007). Revisiting parental concerns in the age of autism spectrum disorders. *Archives of Pediatric & Adolescent Medicine, 161,* 406–407.

Centers for Disease Control and Prevention. (2002). Delayed diagnosis of fragile X syndrome—United States, 1990–1999. *MMWR. Morbidity & Mortality Weekly Report, 51*(33), 740–742.

Courtney-Manning, P. (2007). Addressing the crisis in access to autism treatment using health care improvement science. *Archives of Pediatric & Adolescent Medicine, 161,* 414–415.

Crawford, D. C. (2001). fMRI and the fragile X syndrome. *CDC fact sheet.* Retrieved from http://www.cdc.gov/genomics/hugenet/factsheets/FS_FragileX.htm.

Croen, L. A., et al. (2006). A comparison of health care utilization and costs of children with and without autism spectrum disorders in a large group-model health plan. *Pediatrics, 118*(4), 1203–1211.

Croen, L. A., et al. (2007). Maternal and paternal age and the risk of autism spectrum disorders. *Archives of Pediatric & Adolescent Medicine, 161,* 334–340.

Cronk, C., et al. (1988). Growth charts for children with Down syndrome: 1 month to 18 years of age. *Pediatrics, 81*(1), 102–110.

Cunningham, M., Cox, E. O., & Committee on Practice and Ambulatory Medicine and the Section on Otolaryngology and Bronchoesophagology. (2003). Hearing assessment in infants and children: Recommendations beyond neonatal screening. *Pediatrics, 111*(2), 436–440.

Daniel, E. (2007). Noise and hearing loss: A review. *Journal of School Health, 77*(5), 225–231. doi:10.1111/j.1746-1561.2007.00197.x

Dawson, G. (2007). Despite major challenges, autism research continues to offer hope. *Archives of Pediatric & Adolescent Medicine, 161,* 411–412.

De Potter, P. (2002). Current treatment of retinoblastoma. *Current Opinion in Ophthalmology, 13*(5), 331–336.

DeStefano, F., et al. (2004). Age at first measles-mumps-rubella vaccination in children with autism and school-matched control subjects: A population-based study in metropolitan Atlanta. *Pediatrics, 113*(2), 259–266.

Doll, E. A. (1953). *The measurement of social competence: A manual for the Vineland Social Maturity Scale.* Circle Pines, MN: Educational Test Bureau Educational Publishers.

Downs, B. W., & Buchman, C. A. (2005). External auditory canal translocation for cochlear implantation. *Laryngoscope, 115,* 555–556.

D'Souza, Y., Fombonne, E., & Ward, B. J. (2006). No evidence of persisting measles virus in blood mononuclear cells from children with autism spectrum disorder. *Pediatrics, 118,* 1664–1675.

Filipek, P., et al. (2000). Practice parameter: Screening and diagnosis of autism: Report of the Quality Standards Subcommittee of the American Academy of Neurology and the Child Neurology Society. *Neurology, 55*(2 of 2), 468–479.

Fombonne, E. (2003a). The prevalence of autism. *Journal of the American Medical Association, 289,* 87–89.

Fombonne, E. (2003b). Modern views of autism. *Canadian Journal of Psychiatry, 48,* 503–505.

Gregg, R. B., Wiorek, M. A., & Arvedson, J. C. (2004). Pediatric audiology: A review. *Pediatrics in Review, 25*(7), 224–234.

Grizzle, K. L., & Simms, M. D. (2005). Early language development and language learning disabilities. *Pediatrics in Review, 26*(8), 274–283. doi:10.1542/pir.26-8-274

Hall, J. G. (2004). Chromosomal clinical abnormalities. In R. E. Behrman, R. M. Kliegman, & H. B. Jenson (Eds.), *Nelson textbook of pediatrics* (17th ed.). Philadelphia: Saunders.

Hurwitz, R. L., et al. (2006). Retinoblastoma. In P. A. Pizzo & D. G. Poplack (Eds.), *Principles and practice of pediatric oncology* (5th ed.). Philadelphia: Lippincott.

Johnson, C. P., & Walker, W. O. (2006). Mental retardation: Management and prognosis. *Pediatrics in Review, 27*(7), 249–256. doi:10.1542/pir.27-7-249

Kabra, M., & Gulati, S. (2003). Mental retardation. *Indian Journal of Pediatrics, 70*(2), 153–158.

Kenna, M. A. (2004). Medical management of childhood hearing loss. *Pediatric Annals, 33*(12), 822–832.

Kolevzon, A., Gross, R., & Reichenberg, A. (2007). Prenatal and perinatal risk factors for autism: A review and integration of findings. *Archives of Pediatric & Adolescent Medicine, 161,* 326–333.

Lambert, N., Nihira, K., & Leland, H. (1993). *AAMR Adaptive Behavior Scale—School* (2nd ed.). Austin, TX: PRO-ED.

Maurice, P. R., Bouffard, C., Desjardins, S., Michaud. D., Bécu, J., & Clermont, A. (2007). *Nunavik Adaptive Behavior Scale (NABS): Evaluation of adaptive behavior in Inuit population with suspected mental retardation.* Presented at the

19th IUHPE World Conference on Health Promotion and Health Education, Vancouver, BC, June 11, 2007.
Melamud, A., Palekar, R., & Singh, A. (2006). Retinoblastoma. *American Family Physician, 73*(6), 1041–1044.
Mema, S. C., McIntyre, L., & Musto, R. (2012). Childhood vision screening in Canada: Public health evidence and practice. *Canadian Journal of Public Health, 103*(1), 40–45.
Mizoue, T., Miyamoto, R., & Shimizu, T. (2003). Combined effect of smoking and occupational exposure to noise on hearing loss in steel factory workers. *Journal of Occupational & Environmental Medicine, 60*(10), 56–59.
Muhle, E., Trentacoste, S. V., & Rapin, I. (2004). The genetics of autism. *Pediatrics, 113*(5), e472–e486.
National Down Syndrome Society. (2006). *About Down syndrome.* Retrieved from http://www.ndss.org/en/About-Down-Syndrome/Down-Syndrome-Fact-Sheet/.
National Fragile X Foundation. (2006). *Prevalence of fragile X syndrome.* Retrieved from http://www.fragilex.org/fragile-x-associated-disorders.
Parliament of Canada, Standing Senate Committee on Social Affairs, Science and Technology. (2006). *Out of the shadows at last: Transforming mental health, mental illness and addiction services in Canada.* Retrieved from http://www.parl.gc.ca/Content/SEN/Committee/391/soci/rep/rep02may06-e.htm.
Peterson, C. C. (2006). A review of biochemical and ultrasound markers in detection of Down syndrome. *Journal of Perinatal Education, 15*(1), 19–25. doi:10.1097/01.AOG.0000207562.09858.16
Phalen, J. A. (2005). Fragile X syndrome. *Pediatrics in Review, 26*(5), 181–182.
Pueschel, S. M. (1999). The child with Down syndrome. In M. D. Levine, W. B. Carey, & A. C. Crocker (Eds.), *Developmental-behavioral pediatrics* (3rd ed.). Philadelphia: Saunders.
Rehm, R. S., & Bradley, J. F. (2006). Social interactions at school of children who are medically fragile and developmentally delayed. *Journal of Pediatric Nursing, 21*(4), 299–307.
Retinoblastoma.ca. (2010). *What is retinoblastoma?* Retrieved from http://www.retinoblastoma.ca/whatis.htm.
Schaefer, G. B., & Lutz, R. E. (2006). Diagnostic yield in the clinical genetic evaluation of autism spectrum disorders. *Genetics in Medicine, 8*(9), 549–556. doi:10.1097/01.gim.0000237789.98842.f1
Schanen, N. C. (2006). Epigenetics of autism spectrum disorders. *Human Molecular Genetics, 15*(R1-2), R138–R150. doi:10.1093/hmg/ddl213
Schouten–van Meeteren, A. Y., et al. (2002). Overview chemotherapy for retinoblastoma: An expanding area of clinical research. *Medical Pediatrics & Oncology, 38*, 428–438.
Society of Obstetricians and Gynaecologists of Canada, Genetics Committee, & Canadian College of Medical Geneticists, Prenatal Diagnosis Committee. (2007). Clinical Practice Guideline: Screening for fetal aneuploidy in singleton pregnancies. *Journal of Obstetricians and Gynaecologists of Canada, 29* (2), 146–161. Retrieved from http://www.sogc.org/guidelines/documents/gui261CPG1107E.pdf.
Segal, S., et al. (2003). Inner ear damage in children due to noise exposure from toy cap pistols and firecrackers: A retrospective review of 53 cases. *Noise & Health, 5*(18), 13–18.
Skotko, B. (2005). Mothers of children with Down syndrome reflect on their postnatal support. *Pediatrics, 15*, 64–77. doi:10.1542/peds.2004-0928
Smith, R. J., Bale, J. F., & White, K. R. (2005). Sensorineural hearing loss in children. *Lancet, 365*, 879–890. doi:10.1016/S0140-6736(05)71047-3
Statistics Canada. (2009). *Participation and activity limitation study 2006.* Retrieved from http://www.statcan.gc.ca/pub/89-628-x/89-628-x2008009-eng.htm.
Van Riper, M. (2003). A change of plans: The birth of a child with Down syndrome doesn't have to be a negative experience. *American Journal of Nursing, 103*(6), 71–74.
Walker, W. O., & Johnson, C. P. (2006). Mental retardation: Overview and diagnosis. *Pediatrics in Review, 27*(6), 204–212. doi:10.1542/pir.27-6-204
Wilton, G., & Plane, M. B. (2006). The family empowerment network: A service model to address the needs of children and families affected by fetal alcohol spectrum disorders. *Pediatric Nursing, 32*(4), 299–305.
Zeng, F. G., & Liu, S. (2006). Speech perception in individuals with auditory neuropathy. *Journal of Speech, Language, & Hearing Research, 49*, 367–380. doi:10.1044/1092-4388

Additional Resources

Alexander Graham Bell Association for the Deaf and Hard of Hearing: http://www.agbell.org
Autism Canada: http://www.autismcanada.org/
Autism Society of Canada: http://www.autismsocietycanada.ca
Canadian Association of Speech-Language Pathologists and Audiologists: http://www.caslpa.ca
Canadian Down Syndrome Society: http://www.cdss.ca
Canadian Hearing Society—Information on hearing aids and hearing loss: http://www.chs.ca
Canadian National Institute for the Blind (CNIB)—Numerous products available for people with vision problems: http://www.cnib.ca
Canadian Organizations for Deafblind People: http://www.deafblind.com/canada.html
Canadian Radio-Television and Telecommunications Commission: Toll free: 1-877 249 CRTC (2782); Toll free TTY line: 1-877 909 CRTC (2782): http://www.crtc.gc.ca
Down Syndrome Research Foundation: http//www.dsrf.org
Easter Seals Canada: http://www.easterseals.ca
Fragile X Research Foundation of Canada–Support chapters: http://www.fragile-x.ca/Sammons Preston Canada—Resource for a variety of self-help equipment: http://www.sammonspreston.ca
Special Olympics Canada: http://www.specialolympics.ca

Unit 10

43 Family-Centred Home Care

Learning Objectives

On completion of this chapter, the reader will be able to:

- Differentiate home care from hospice care.
- List at least three factors contributing to the increasing emphasis on home care services.
- Describe case management, or care coordination, and its importance in home care.
- List general principles of a family-centred assessment and planning process.
- Identify five key characteristics of collaborative relationships.
- Describe approaches to promoting optimum development, self-care, and education in home care.
- Outline six areas in need of attention for promoting safety in home care.

Electronic Resources

Additional information related to the content in Chapter 43 can be found on

evolve the Companion Web site at

http://evolve.elsevier.com/Canada/Perry/maternal/

- Examination Review Questions
- Case Study—Home Care

General Concepts of Home Care

Definition

Home care has become a routine option for the child patient in today's health care environment. The Canadian Home Care Association (CHCA) (2008) defines *home care* as "an array of services, provided in the home and community setting, that encompass health promotion and teaching, curative intervention, end-of-life care, rehabilitation, support and maintenance, social adaptation and integration, and support for the informal (family) caregiver." With the many advances in medical technology, along with restructuring of the Canadian health system, there has been a rapid increase in the number of children and youth with acute and continuing home care needs across Canada (CHCA, 2008). The growing demand for home care services is in part a result of increasing costs of institutionalized care. More important, however, is that home-based health care acknowledges the family's valuable contribution to the child's overall health in his or her natural environment. Thus home care programs lead to greater parent satisfaction, improved quality of life, and a reduction in the length of hospital stays. There is limited evidence, however, that home care reduces hospital admissions and emergency department visits (Cooper et al., 2006).

Home care is not a new concept in pediatrics. Over the past decades the term has referred to parents caring for mildly ill children at home; to home nursing visits after children are discharged from the hospital; to hospice care; and, more recently, to care at home for children with more serious chronic illness and dependence on medical technology. Providing quality home health care for children generally requires the parents' desire for it and the ability to carry out their part of the care, as well as professional assistance and community preparedness. A natural family environment optimizes growth and development when stress is minimal and support is optimal. The role of the community health or home care nurse in home care is to promote health and prevent disease; collaborate with individuals, families, groups, and communities; build on the capacity of the individual and family; and mobilize resources (Community Health Nurses Association of Canada [CHNA], 2008).

Home care differs from *hospice care*, which is a program of palliative and supportive care services providing physical, psychological, social, and spiritual care for dying persons, their families, and other loved ones. Hospice services are available in both the home and inpatient settings. *End-of-life* care and planning should be considered for any child with a terminal diagnosis. Some patients may be admitted for end-of-life home care services before being ready for admission to hospice services. Many hospice programs have admission criteria that do not permit therapies such as intravenous antibiotics, total **parenteral nutrition**, or enteral feedings that the family may wish to continue. Thus, it is important to discuss early in discharge planning the type of care the family wishes for the child in order to clarify expectations for home care.

Home Care Trends and Needs

The shift toward home-based health care has been propelled by numerous factors. As stated earlier, advances in medical technology have enabled increased survival for children with congenital and acquired illnesses. Preterm infants or children who are ventilator dependent were once cared for indefinitely in a critical care unit or long-term care facility. These children are now able to live with their families in their own home (Feudtner et al., 2005).

Children with conditions such as cancer, kidney disorders, cystic fibrosis, spina bifida, cardiac and respiratory disorders, gastrointestinal disorders, neurodegenerative diseases, and human immunodeficiency virus (HIV) infection may have ongoing health care needs as a result of the disease, its treatment, or adverse effects of treatment (Davis, 2006; Magrabi et al., 2005; Nazer et al., 2006; Stevens et al., 2006). Parents frequently have ongoing stressors after a child's hospitalization for diagnosis and treatment. Subsequent needs may include reinforcing teachings about the disease process, addressing the child's physical care needs and providing emotional support during this change in parental role. For these children, home-based nutrition programs are useful, safe, and well tolerated. There is sufficient evidence that these programs provide a better quality of life, decrease cost of therapy, and improve survival (Daveluy et al., 2006; Howard, 2006).

Improving the quality of life for both the child and the family is one of the driving forces in the effort to move technology-dependent children from the hospital to the home setting. Part of this process involves **normalization**, whereby, over time, families of children with chronic illness begin to perceive the child and their family life as normal (Knafl & Deatrick, 2002) (see Chapter 41). This has important implications for pediatric home care nurses in relation to the assessment of family function and in helping home care nurses gain a better understanding of family dynamics. The normalized family tends to be more flexible with treatments and incorporates the child with a disability or illness into the usual routines of daily living (Knafl & Deatrick, 2002).

Other factors contributing to the increase in home care are the rising cost of institutionalized health care and the shifts in the financing of health care delivery. Inpatient hospital stays have become shorter in part because of the overwhelming cost of lengthy hospitalizations. Children are either not admitted to the hospital at all or are returned home as soon as possible after their illness. Home-based nursing care has decreased the length of hospital stays (Cooper et al., 2006). Likewise, a portion of the financial burden is shifted to the family. Third-party insurance may cover part or all of the costs at home. In some cases, the family may be forced to absorb the costs of certain medications, supplies, transportation, shelter, utilities, food, laundry, housekeeping, and a portion of the nursing care. There is no home care legislation specific to children across the provinces or territories as suggested by an environmental scan report completed in 2006 by the CHCA on home care services for children with special needs. This lack of legislation creates significant differences across jurisdictions in terms of types of home and community care services available to children that are funded (Peter et al., 2007).

Home health care of children is not restricted to children with chronic health care needs. Several short-term, intermittent therapies such as phototherapy, chemotherapy, apnea monitoring, and intravenous antibiotic administration may be successfully delivered in a home setting, where the child may remain with the family, rather than in an acute-care setting. One study found that home health nurses providing asthma education to families of children hospitalized for an asthma exacerbation increased the family's and caregiver's knowledge about asthma symptoms, triggers, and management (Navaie-Waliser et al., 2004). A number of strategies can be implemented in the home setting to reduce the triggers that cause acute asthma exacerbations and often result in hospitalization (see Asthma, Chapter 46).

With the increased demand for nurses in home health and continued, pervasive short supply, there has been an increased focus on the role of the family caregiver in providing home care. Other health care providers that may be needed for home care are also in short supply, such as speech-language pathologists, developmental pediatricians, psychologists, psychiatrists, occupational therapists, and physiotherapists (Williams, Spalding, Deber, & McKeever, 2005). A survey by the National Profile of Family Caregivers in Canada revealed that approximately 4% of adult Canadians (18 years and older) provide care to a family member with a physical or mental disability or chronic illness or who is frail (as quoted by Health Canada, 2002); this represents care above and beyond the daily routine care of the family household.

Sullivan-Bolyai, Knafl, Sadler, and Gilliss (2003) reviewed the literature on family caregivers' responsibilities in the care of an adult or child family member who has a chronic illness. They identified four family-related caregiving responsibilities adapted from the adult literature that may be applied to children's caregivers:

Managing the illness—Providing daily hands-on care, monitoring the child's medical condition, and educating others to care for the child

Identifying, accessing, and coordinating resources—Locating appropriate resources in the community to meet the needs of the child and of the family as the child's caregiver

Maintaining the family unit—Continuing to nurture the family unit: siblings' needs, spousal relationships, and household maintenance

Maintaining self—Grieving the loss of the healthy child; balancing caregiver responsibilities with their own physical, emotional, mental, and personal needs; recognizing stressors and potential caregiver burnout

The researchers developed a multifaceted list of parent caregiving management responsibilities and associated activities that the home health nurse may use to facilitate discussions with parents and families regarding caregiving in the home and its unique requirements (Sullivan-Bolyai et al., 2003). Some of these responsibilities include monitoring the child's condition and behaviour, providing hands-on care and meeting the child's developmental needs, organizing family activities to include the child with a chronic condition, and balancing care of the child and needs of the family (Sullivan-Bolyai et al., 2004).

Nurses can use the results of this research to better understand the magnitude of responsibilities facing the caregiving family and assist them in finding resources to provide some respite from caring for the child to care for each other and maintain self and family integrity.

The Canadian Paediatric Society (CPS) (2008) recommends that physicians advocate for *permanency planning*, through which children and youth with special health care needs obtain placement stability and personal intervention plans. Should the family be unable to support the child, options can include family-based care: adoption, non-relative foster care, kinship foster care, or guardianship foster care. When compared to group residential options, family-based care is the preferred placement option for these children (Farris-Manning & Zandstra, 2003).

Another recommendation is that physicians be aware of community resources available to assist the caregivers of these special-needs children (CPS, 2008). Respite care for caregivers of children with special care needs has been slow in its development and availability, although respite care centres are now common for adults. *Respite care* provides temporary relief to parents and gives them a break from the responsibilities of caring for the child on a daily basis. Such care for ventilator-dependent children and those with skilled technological care requirements is in short supply in some provincial and territorial jurisdictions, given the lack of skilled care providers, early discharge from hospital, and high health needs (Dunbrack, 2003). Nurses can play an important role in advocating for the provision of high-quality respite care so that families and caregivers can maintain appropriate family function, care for themselves, and continue to provide for the care of the child as necessary (Parra, 2003).

Effective Home Care

In providing home-based care for children the nurse has an opportunity to assess and interact with the family in their environment. This assessment can provide the health care team with valuable information about safety, support systems, nutrition, parenting ability, and actual health care practices. Such information will determine future decisions for individualized care and realistic outcomes (Thompson, 2000).

The pediatric home care nurse has two distinct arrangements for implementation of care. Nurses who perform *intermittent skilled nursing* visits may see different types and numbers of patients each day. These nurses typically have an assigned patient caseload and accept responsibility for implementing the care plan. This mode of nursing care is the one most often used today, given the shortage of personnel and decreased reimbursements. Most home visits focus on helping the patient and caregiver achieve independence with care in the home, including home care by therapists, home infusion teaching by nurses, and care management, instead of providing direct physical care. Nurses who perform *private-duty nursing*, or block nursing, are usually assigned individual patients, and they remain in the home for a predetermined time (e.g., an 8- or 12-hour block of time) to provide patient care. The care plan is implemented over the course of the time in the home. Required nursing skills are determined by patient need, parental ability, complexity of family, and the home environment. In both types of home care, the pediatric nurse is responsible for patient and family assessment and evaluating the appropriateness of the care plan (Canadian Public Health Association, 2010) (Box 43-1).

A major issue in providing home care in this era is the lack of qualified pediatric nurses in the home care field. This shortage is particularly true in rural or remote areas (Canadian Research Network for Care in the Community, 2008). Agencies and families are facing much difficulty in staffing required home care services; thus more of the home care must be carried out by family members or other caregivers. According to Page (2001), the lack of pediatric training in some nursing programs, increased acuity of home care patients, and increased pay for nurses working in acute care settings have contributed to a greater than ever nursing shortage in pediatric home health care.

BOX 43-1 Intermittent Skilled Nursing

Health Care Need

Child at risk—Parental substance use; failure to thrive; social or family situation that is potentially detrimental to child's well-being

Chronically ill, but medically stable child with multiple care needs

Education and competency validation of caregiver skills

Skilled procedures—Regularly scheduled injections or infusions, dressing changes, reinforcement of home care teaching; evaluation of caregiver's skills

Technology-dependent child (e.g., ventilator or tracheostomy, home total parenteral nutrition, or enteral feedings by pump)

Chronically ill child with multiple skilled nursing needs

Intervention

Regularly scheduled visits to assess patient status, evaluate home environment, teach care provider skills, determine status of growth and development, set goals with family for positive health outcomes

As-needed home visits during exacerbation of illness to assess physical status and determine appropriate intervention

Assistance with transportation of child to ambulatory centre or practitioner's office for evaluation and diagnostic services

Regular visits of limited duration to perform skilled nursing intervention, assess parental ability and desire to perform procedure, teach procedure technique, supervise parental performance of procedure

Assessment of patient status; evaluation of safety of home environment; teaching, evaluation, and reinforcement of caregivers' skills; determination of status of growth and development; goal setting with family for positive health outcomes

Consideration of the caregiver's willingness and ability to provide care and of his or her limitations is of utmost importance when assessing the appropriateness of the care plan (Box 43-2). It is vital to ensure that patients and families have adequate back-up support and access to resources such as social services. An increasing concern in pediatric home health care is having a managing practitioner to oversee the home care. Shorter hospital stays have increased patients' rapid movement through the continuum of care; a patient may be seen in the emergency department or neonatal intensive care unit, then be discharged to home health without ever seeing a primary care physician. Thus, it is imperative that the provision of care for home patients involve multidisciplinary cooperation and communication among health care workers.

Discharge Planning and Selection of a Home Care Agency

Identification of appropriate local community resources is critical to a successful transfer to home care (Box 43-3). The ultimate goal of discharge planning is for the family to become familiar with the child's needs and to be competent in providing that care. A discharge plan should include emergency management and provision of social and emotional support. The Canadian Paediatric Society (2008) emphasizes that the goal for a home health care program for infants, children, or adolescents with chronic conditions or disabilities is the provision of community-based, culturally effective, comprehensive, and cost-effective health care within a nurturing home environment that maximizes the capabilities of the individual and minimizes the effects of the disabilities.

BOX 43-2 Services That Support Effective Home Care

- Adequate family training and preparation
- Primary care physician willing to oversee medical aspects of home care
- Professional caregivers trained in relevant nursing and communication skills
- Developmental intervention (e.g., physiotherapy, occupational and speech therapy; early intervention)
- Appropriately designed and well-maintained equipment
- Supportive therapies (e.g., respiratory therapy, pharmacy, rehabilitation services, parenteral therapy, physiotherapy, durable medical and infusion supplies, nutritional support)
- Adequate social and psychological support services
- High-quality respite care
- Appropriate home renovation
- Telephone service in the home
- Internet and computer
- Appropriate transportation
- Appropriate locally available emergency facilities
- Competent case management services
- Safe environment (electricity, refrigeration, cleanliness)

(Modified from Office of Technology Assessment [OTA], Congress of the United States. [1987]. *Technology dependent children: Hospital v. home care—a technical memorandum* [OTA-TM-H-38]. Washington, DC: US Government Printing Office; and Bakewell-Sachs, S., & Porth, S. [1995]. Discharge planning and home care of the technology-dependent infant. *Journal of Obstetric, Gynecologic, & Neonatal Nursing 24*[1], 77–83.)

NURSING ALERT If home care equipment is different from hospital equipment, have the portable equipment delivered to the hospital to allow family use before discharge.

Much of the success of home care, particularly for the child who is dependent on medical technology or who has complex medical problems, depends on careful planning and preparation. Discharge planning must begin early; it should be based on the criteria of child and family readiness; it must be a multidisciplinary process, including representatives from acute care, home care, and community settings; and it must involve the family. Predischarge assessment (Box 43-4) and planning should include the following:

- The child's medical, nursing, educational, and other therapeutic needs
- Family members' (including siblings') education and training, coping skills, and adjustment needs
- Community readiness in areas such as availability of equipment, appropriate nursing and other personnel, educational and developmental services, respite care, and emergency plans
- Financial arrangements

Creative financial planning, including negotiating arrangements with the insurance company and public programs, may be required.

Early involvement of the home care agency in the discharge planning process promotes continuity of care and a smooth transition from hospital to home (Box 43-5). Before discharge, a general plan, sometimes called an *individualized home care plan*, should be developed with multidisciplinary input. This care plan should address the range of needs identified as part of the comprehensive predischarge assessment.

NURSING ALERT An excellent method of providing home care instructions is with video recordings. Once the family masters the procedures, consider video recording their performance. Visual learning is most helpful for people who cannot read or who are not fluent in English.

BOX 43-3 Characteristics of a High-Quality Pediatric Home Care Agency

- Fully trained pediatric staff to provide for all aspects of care (nursing, rehabilitation therapies, pharmacy, nutrition, social work, home medical equipment)
- Prompt, responsive staff with 24-hour availability
- Family-centred care
- Comprehensive continuing education programs
- Certification by local, provincial, territorial, and federal regulatory agencies
- Accreditation by Accreditation Canada Home Care Services

(Data from Dittbrenner, H. [1999]. Pediatric home care as a viable new service. *Caring, 18*[2], 12–15; and Lovejoy, D. [1997]. *Making the transition to home health nursing: A practical guide*. New York: Springer.)

BOX 43-4 Example of Predischarge Assessment for Technology-Dependent Infant

The Child's Family

Identification and training of primary caregivers

Identification and training of caregivers for respite and emergency care

Parent employment status while caring for child at home

Family financial picture, especially if one parent must stop working

Sibling preparation

Availability of psychosocial support services

Technical Equipment and Supplies for the Home

Home care company's availability and experience

Home care company's coordination of services with local health care provider and others

24-hour availability and coverage for unexpected situations

Community Nursing and Support Services

Availability, training, and experience

Adequacy of number of personnel to meet needs

Additional training of staff, if needed

24-hour availability of ambulance services and emergency medical services

Physical Environment of the Home

Adequacy of space for equipment and supplies

Heavy equipment (e.g., ventilator, oxygen tanks, compressor) accessibility

Layout of home (e.g., number of floors, stairways, room accessibility, room sizes)

Location and layout of bedrooms

Adequacy of apartment building elevator and fire escape

Telephone access

Type of transportation family uses

Possibility of modifying living space to minimize invasiveness of technology without isolating child

Adequacy of heating and cooling systems

Adequacy of electrical system to accommodate equipment

Emergency Plan

Identification and training of those involved

Written implementation plan: who, what, where, when, how (include telephone numbers)

Notification of utility companies for priority repairs and maintenance

Notification of emergency medical unit (911)

Emergency drill

Primary Care Provider

Identification of local primary provider or pediatrician who is able to assume direct care responsibility and coordinate other care providers

Inclusion of local provider in discharge planning

Information needs of local provider before child's discharge

(From Bakewell-Sachs, S., & Porth, S. [1995]. Discharge planning and home care of the technology-dependent infant. *Journal of Obstetric, Gynecologic, & Neonatal Nursing, 24*[1], 77–83.)

BOX 43-5 Critical Home Care Referral Information

- Scheduled medications
- Durable medical equipment
- Medical supplies
- Transportation needs
- Adaptive equipment
- Rehabilitation therapies (occupational, physical, and speech therapy)
- Psychological counselling
- Social work referral
- Nursing care
- Respite plans
- Key family members
- Demographic information
- Reimbursement information

(Modified from Townsend, J. L. [1997]. Assessment of the child and family. In W. L. Votroubek & J. L. Townsend [Eds.], *Pediatric home care* [2nd ed.]. Gaithersburg, MD: Aspen.)

The plans for transition from hospital to home should include at least two family members learning and demonstrating all aspects of the child's care in the hospital. An in-hospital trial period (such as rooming-in) during which parents provide total care for the child is generally beneficial as well. After a successful trial, the family may benefit from taking the child home on a brief pass before making final discharge plans. The home care nurse plays an important role in assessing this experience with the family. A predischarge home visit allows the home care nurse to meet the family, help them assess their preparedness and the preparedness of the home environment, discuss plans for arranging the child's equipment at home (Fig. 43-1), reinforce prior discharge teaching, and implement any additional teaching that may be necessary (Bakewell-Sachs et al., 2000). Additional factors that should be considered in discharge planning include working parents, extended family, and child care arrangements.

Care Coordination (Case Management)

Traditional definitions of **case management** generally focus on cost control, attainment of desired clinical outcomes, and monitoring and evaluation of care provided. However, for optimum home care of the child who is technology dependent, case management—or care coordination—should be viewed more broadly.

Changes in health care over the past three decades not only have improved survival and decreased morbidity among children with special health care needs but also resulted in higher costs for health care and services provided. Often services are provided by multiple organizations and multiple vendors with different missions and a consistent lack of single systems linking home health care. In addition, eligibility criteria for funding and services are complex and vary from one province or territory to another. As a result, coordination of home care can be challenging, frustrating, and complicated for the family (CPS, 2008).

The concept of *care coordination* is to link children with special home health care needs (and their families) to services

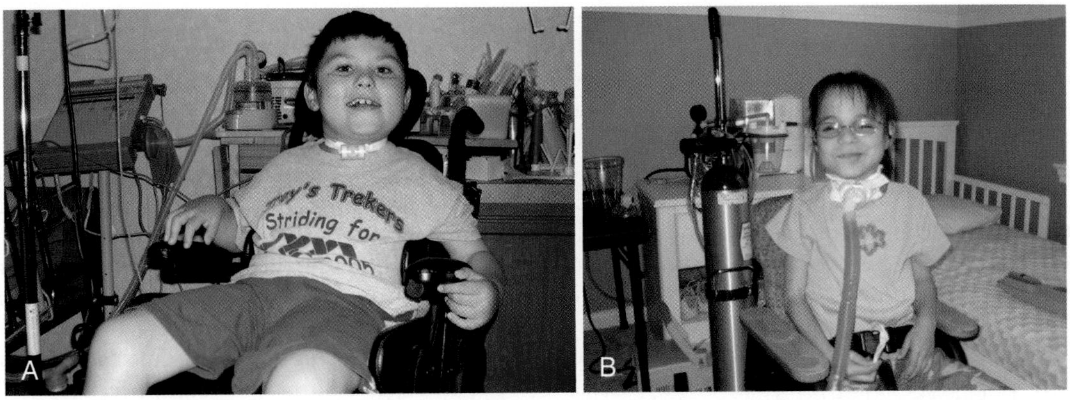

Fig. 43-1 **A:** An essential aspect of preparation for home care is the arrangement of equipment and supplies. **B:** The nurse in the home care setting requires expertise to care for a child who is technology dependent.

and resources in a coordinated effort to provide the child with optimum care. Care coordination has several purposes. Its primary goal is ensuring continuity for the child and family across hospital, home, educational, therapeutic, and other settings. Other goals involve facilitating timely access to services and enhancing child and family well-being (CHCA, 2008). Care should be coordinated among multiple providers to reduce the complexity of care for the child, reduce fragmentation of care, prevent duplication of services, and decrease the burden of care for the family. Case managers from a number of agencies may be involved in the patient's care, which may add to the parents' confusion; the home care nurse should try to coordinate meetings between all case managers and the family and a nurse care coordinator in order to minimize confusion and prevent duplication. Knowing how to access community resources is often confusing for families, given the multiple points of access and provincial or territorial ministries involved (CHCA, 2006). Lindeke and colleagues (2002) have proposed the ideal situation: the family serves as lead care coordinator within the context of family-centred care. Care coordination should ensure that the child's medical, nursing, and health maintenance needs, as well as the financial issues, psychosocial concerns, and educational needs of the child and family, are addressed. The coordinating case manager is often provided by the community care agency to help bring all of the resources together and help with funding information (CHCA, 2008). Care coordination is most effective if a single person works with the family to accomplish the many tasks and responsibilities involved (Box 43-6). The nurse case manager should be knowledgeable about community resources, including primary, secondary, and tertiary health care services; speech, language, hearing, and vision resources; respite care services; financial assistance programs; parent groups; advocacy groups; local, provincial, territorial, and federal public officials; transportation services; and private-sector individuals with an interest in children with disabilities (CHCA, 2008). With a greater focus on outcomes of care in home health care, the nurse case manager is challenged to be resourceful and skilled in communication at a number of levels (Rice, 2006).

Although professionals must always see part of their role as ensuring that integrated, coordinated care is provided, care coordination should promote the family's role as primary decision maker and enhance the family's capability to meet the special needs of the child and the family unit. Families may choose to be involved to varying degrees in coordinating their child's care. Many parents take on increasing responsibility for care coordination over time; they should be encouraged and supported in this role. Home care nurses and case managers should be aware that the termination of private-duty or home care nursing can be a difficult transition for which families may need preparation. A gradual reduction in services allows patients and families to adjust favourably to the changes. Care coordination by office-based nurses for children and youth with special health care needs decreases emergency department visits and periodic office visits, thus significantly decreasing the cost of health care. Increased health care costs are associated with more physician-dependent care coordination activities among such children (Antonelli, Stille, & Antonelli, 2008).

BOX 43-6 Care Coordination for Children With Special Health Care Needs

- Facilitate timely access to services and resources.
- Promote continuity of care.
- Ensure that high-quality care is performed in the home.
- Provide family support and enhance family well-being.
- Improve health, developmental, educational, vocational, psychosocial, and functional outcomes.
- Maximize efficient, effective use of resources.

(Modified from Presler, B. [1998]. Care coordination for children with special health care needs. *Orthopedic Nursing, 17*[25 Suppl], 45–51.)

Role of the Nurse, Training, and Standards of Care

The home care nurse must share a level of technical expertise with the critical care nurse while being able to adapt equipment, procedures, and the nursing process to the home setting. (See Chapter 45 for specific technical skills that may be required in home care practice.) The need for technical expertise must be matched by a knowledge of child development and the ability to work creatively with the child challenged by chronic illness and technology dependence. When caring for patients in the home setting, the nurse must be comfortable making independent nursing judgements and solving problems with no immediate assistance, within the nursing scope of practice. At the same time, the nurse must have excellent interpersonal skills; an ability to work with other professionals and the family; and, most important, an ability to respect family autonomy. Patient outcomes are more readily achievable with a balance of nursing skills that demonstrate clinical excellence; adaptability; accountability; and the development of positive relationships with physicians, patients, and families (Box 43-7).

When working with a home care agency, nurses should expect to receive patient placements appropriate to their expertise. They should also expect to receive orientation to the skills and knowledge base of the home health care nursing specialty and subsequent continuing education to develop as expert practitioners. The minimum initial orientation should include the individual patient's care plan and equipment needs; the agency's policies and procedures, including procedures for addressing any problems that may occur when care is provided in the home; legal liability issues; and documentation procedures. Stronger emphasis should be placed on issues specific to home care.

Supervision of practice, including occasional site visits by a nursing supervisor, should be provided. Mentoring or precepting is ideal. Because of the unique practice environment of home health nurses, it is important for an agency to facilitate sharing among peers to decrease work-related stress, increase job satisfaction, and support high-quality patient care.

Nurses in pediatric home health face increasing demands for providing high-quality care with fewer resources to achieve positive patient outcomes. In doing so, nurses often must refer to the expertise of interdisciplinary team members to ensure that the patient and family receive the necessary care.

The planning, management, and delivery of home health care services in Canada vary among provinces or territories. Currently, nine provinces have legislation related to public home care through various acts and policies (CHCA, 2008). Nursing standards for professional practice and conduct are governed by provincial regulatory bodies. Community health nursing standards of practice have been developed by recognized associate members of the Canadian Nurses Association (CNA). The CNA also offers national certification in community health nursing and hospice palliative care nursing. Despite important differences between pediatric and adult care in the home, as of this writing no national standards specific to pediatric home care practice have been developed. Nursing practice in pediatric home care should be guided by published guidelines, textbooks, peer-reviewed articles, and written standards of care for child patients. An extensive literature review on competencies for home health care is available from the Community Health Care Nurses of Canada (Mildon and Underwood, 2010). Professional nursing organizations such as the CNA, Community Health Nurses of Canada, Canadian Association of Pediatric Nurses (CAPN), provincial colleges of nursing, and others have also published standards of care or nursing Best Practice Guidelines that apply to pediatric home health nursing practice (see Resources on the Evolve Web site).

A quality improvement program is an important component of an effective home care agency. Evidence-informed practice is rapidly becoming an important aspect of home health care, as is benchmarking, in which the product or practice (in this case, patient outcome) is compared with other agencies' outcomes and practices to determine best practice; this allows agencies to see how they measure in comparison to other similar agencies (Wilson, 2003; Yoder-Wise, 2007). In Canada, Accreditation Canada Home Care Services applies sector and service-based standards to home care services, including home nursing care; rehabilitation; and therapies such as physiotherapy, social work, respiratory, dietetics, and speech therapy.

BOX 43-7 Qualities of a Pediatric Home Care Nurse

- Shows competence in skills and case management
- Recognizes that the nurse is a guest in the home
- Respects family culture and adapts appropriately
- Works as a multidisciplinary team member
- Demonstrates expertise in pediatric care (assessment and technical skills)
- Possesses and uses effective communication skills
- Adapts nursing practice in response to the changing health care needs of the child
- Coordinates, facilitates, or advocates for appropriate resource allocation
- Considers the broader determinants of health that influence the health of the child and family

Family-Centred Home Care

Technology dependence, chronic illness, and complex care requirements cross social, cultural, spiritual, and economic boundaries. Regardless of a family's background, the family's values must be respected in the provision of home care services. *The home is the family's domain*, and the child is at home because the family's central role is to nurture and raise their child. The ultimate responsibility for managing the child's health, developmental, and emotional needs lies with the family. Roush and Cox (2000) have developed a framework for helping the home health care nurse understand the significance of the home to the family. The three central concepts of the model are as follows:

Home as familiar—The environment where one is comfortable and at ease because of the familiarity with living arrangements and routines of home

Home as centre—The location of everyday experiences related to time, space, and one's social life

Home as protector—The environment that preserves privacy, safety, and identity

The philosophical basis for family-centred practice is the recognition that the family is the constant in the child's life, whereas the service systems and personnel within those systems fluctuate. The Calgary Family Assessment Model may be helpful to nurses in assessing families and assisting in their management of the complex health care needs of their children (see Chapter 2, p. 19). The model demonstrates tools such as **genograms** to outline a family structure and provide a visual representation of the family and their resources (CNA, 1997; Wright & Leahy, 2005). Families have the most intimate knowledge of the child's strengths and abilities, the challenges of providing care, and the abilities and needs of other family members. Believing that no one knows the child better than the family is critical to the success of any health care plan.

Respect for Diversity

Respect for varied family structures and for racial, ethnic, cultural, spiritual, and socioeconomic diversity among families is essential in home care (see also Chapters 31 and 32). Home care nurses work in close relationship with family members and in the family's own domain. The nurse shares in these relationships, participating in care throughout the course of illness (see Family-Centred Teaching box). Particular attention should be given to communication. The meaning of words used and the way in which they are said may affect individuals from various cultural groups in different ways. Volume of speech and language style must be taken into consideration as part of a family cultural assessment. The home health care nurse must pay particular attention to nonverbal communication. Body language, eye contact, and degree of physical contact have different meanings within particular cultures.

FAMILY-CENTRED TEACHING

Developing Relationships With Culturally Diverse Families

I work in the inner city, and my home care patients come from a variety of racial and ethnic backgrounds. I am White, from Australia. Often, when I first visit a family, there is an initial coolness or apprehension toward me. This is understandable because I am a stranger, and perhaps families think I'll judge them in one way or another. By the end of the first visit, however, there is usually a smile as I leave; by the second visit they often greet me with a smile at the door; and by the third visit, we usually have a friendship, trust, and an ease of communication.

If I'm working on a case for an extended time, I use a holistic nursing approach. This involves being aware of how the child's illness affects the entire family. As I listen over many weeks to their fears and questions, and often as I share faith perspectives, a bond begins to form. I find it a privilege to share in their joys and their pain, and I feel rewarded by the trust that they invest in me.

–Julie Edgerton, RN, Home Care Nurse

(Modified from Ahmann, E. [1994]. Thinking critically about family-centered home care nursing. *Pediatric Nursing, 20*[6], 588–590.)

In 2004, Health Canada researched the First Nation and Inuit populations' home care needs and found that this population was generally younger and received fragmented care. Most caregivers provide a great deal of care each week and about one in three caregivers support two or more persons needing care (Health Canada, 2008).

NURSING ALERT One should not assume that everyone who speaks English can read the language. Colour-coded medication bottles, written schedules, and pillboxes or oral syringes may aid ability to comply with prescription administration. Pictures or special symbols may be helpful when providing instructions for procedures and medication administration.

Families may also differ in their cultural views of children; health care; childrearing practices; and illness, its causes, and its meaning. The family's health care practices and beliefs may influence the level of investment a family will make in the child's care. The family's religion or spirituality can also have a major influence on a family's response to the child's special health care needs. Some families will look for spiritual meaning in and purpose for the illness. Other families may choose to reject past religious ties. In some cultures, religion and beliefs about health care and illness are closely intertwined (McEvoy, 2003); thus it is important that home care nurses assess the relationships among culture, religion, and the family's beliefs about the child's illness (see Community Focus box).

A variety of cultural assessment tools are available, including the Giger and Davidhizar Transcultural Assessment Model (Giger & Davidhizar, 2002). The home care nurse, aware that personal values drive behaviour, must learn about the family's culture, ask questions without implying judgement, interpret the mainstream medical culture, and help families design interventions that meet their preferences (CNA, 2004). When possible, culture-specific teaching materials should be used. Respect for family diversity and awareness of family developmental stages (see Chapter 33) and the stages of a family's adjustment to illness in a child (see Chapter 41) will

COMMUNITY FOCUS

Spiritual Assessment

The mnemonic BELIEF was developed by McEvoy (2003) for pediatric nurses to initiate discussions with parents and children about their faith or religious values and beliefs. The components of the assessment tool are as follows:

Belief system
Ethics or values
Lifestyle
Involvement in a spiritual community (church, synagogue, mosque)
Education
Future events

The tool may be used to develop a culturally sensitive dialogue regarding spiritual matters and practices that affect the child and family.

assist the home care nurse in recognizing and promoting family strengths and in respecting varied coping mechanisms. Use of labels such as "dysfunctional," "difficult," and "noncompliant" can reinforce negative expectations and shape behaviours of both parents and professionals. By contrast, emphasizing, identifying, and building on family strengths and coping mechanisms can promote a central goal in nursing care of the child and family: family empowerment (see Chapter 29).

Parent–Professional Collaboration

Family-centred nursing practice is built on a foundation of parent–professional collaboration, which represents a shift from the traditional unidirectional relationships between health care providers and families. The CNA (2005) supports the principles of family-centred care and interdisciplinary collaboration for the purpose of meeting the health care needs of the community, as outlined in *The Principles and Framework for Interdisciplinary Collaboration in Primary Health Care* (Enhancing Interdisciplinary Collaboration in Primary Health Care [EICP] Steering Committee, 2005). In addition, the Collaborative Family Health Care Association has developed core competencies for health care providers collaborating with families that may also be used as a guide toward family-centred nursing practice (see Additional Resources at the end of this chapter).

Through collaborative caring, the nurse and family can work together and share outcomes in a meaningful way. This approach, essential in the home care setting, is characterized by the following qualities (Kellett & Mannion, 1999):

- Encouraging activities to develop self-confidence and self-esteem
- Displaying increased awareness of and respect for family caregivers
- Recognizing that families vary in defining their role
- Demonstrating an ability to understand the family's approach to caregiving
- Sharing perspectives, not just tasks and functions
- Supporting family members in their primary, irreplaceable role as caregivers
- Exchanging expertise in providing care to the child
- Assisting families in recognizing their contributions as worthwhile
- Identifying strengths and resources of the child and family
- Negotiating options, priorities, and preferences
- Assisting with coping by allowing families to find meaning in caring for the patient at home

Communication with the family should be clear and respectful. The nurse should explain to families the reason for questions, particularly those they may perceive as intrusive, and should tell families who will have access to the information. The nurse must also assure families that they have a right to expect confidentiality in regard to the data collected. When working in the home, the nurse must respect the privacy of family communications that may be overheard.

Communication with family members should include sharing with the family, in a supportive manner, complete and unbiased information about all aspects of the child's condition and care. Parents often feel overwhelming frustration related to obtaining accurate information about their child's illness and its management. Parents want information given slowly and repeated as necessary over time; they want explanations in terms they can understand; and they want the opportunity to ask questions, which should be answered in a straightforward manner. Stating "I don't know" or "I will find out" is better than pretending to know or giving excuses. Unfortunately, the home health care nurse may become a source of added stress on the caregiver or family when the nurse displays unprofessional attitudes or fails to show proper respect for the family's knowledge of the child's needs and care (Harrigan et al., 2002).

A plan can be made with the parents to gather relevant information when necessary (Newton, 2000). Information should be shared with families in a way that has meaning in their cultural context. Many parents report a preference for interactions with health care providers who communicate empathy and concern (Harrigan et al., 2002). Families vary in the amount and delivery of information they can tolerate about their child's status.

NURSING ALERT Home care nurses should restrict their communications with other health care providers to clinically relevant information about the family.

On occasion, disagreements may arise between parents and nurses over proper procedures for the child's care (see Critical Thinking Exercise). Nurses should respect parental preferences in any situation that does not pose danger or risk for the child (see Family-Centred Teaching box). If parents wish to alter a treatment plan that is part of medical orders, the nurse should ask that they negotiate the change with the practitioner because the nurse must follow the written medical orders. If disagreements cannot be resolved, a home care supervisor or case manager (care coordinator) should be contacted to assist with problem solving. Increasingly, home care agencies are developing **ethics** committees and policies for managing difficult situations such as treatment refusal.

The Nursing Process

In the home, the family is a partner in each step of the nursing process. Assessment should address family strengths and resources (Box 43-8). The principles of communication discussed previously need to guide data collection.

All the information gathered as part of the assessment process should be shared with the family. The nurse needs to recognize that the family's perception of their most important need will generally guide their behaviour and consume their attention and energy. Family priorities should guide the planning process.

Both short- and long-term goals should be outlined and agreed on by the child, family, and health care providers involved. The care plan should integrate various disciplines that may be involved with the child to eliminate duplication and coordinate and consolidate care requirements. Cross-training of health care providers and an interdisciplinary mode of treatment can also be useful when a child has multiple and complex care requirements. For example, certain

CRITICAL THINKING EXERCISE

Family-Centred Home Care and Conflicts

A family wants to begin oral feeding with a tracheostomy of their 3-year-old daughter, Sarah, who is ventilator dependent and is being tube fed through a skin-level gastrostomy feeding tube (MIC-KEY). The mother, who has assumed the role of Sarah's primary caregiver, is adamant about starting oral feedings so Sarah can be more like other children her age. One day, the mother asks you, the nurse case manager overseeing the child's home care, to feed Sarah baby food by mouth to see how she tolerates the feeding. The child is alert and sociable yet cannot communicate her wishes except through crying and whining. She has a seizure disorder and has had several episodes of aspiration pneumonia since birth. Sarah appears to have a considerable amount of tongue thrusting and copious amounts of oral mucus that must be suctioned frequently to prevent aspiration; her cough reflex is compromised and usually elicited only with tracheal suctioning.

1. Evidence—Is there sufficient evidence to draw any conclusions about the issue of feeding Sarah at this time?
2. Assumptions—Describe some underlying assumptions about the following:
    a. Sarah's readiness for oral feedings
    b. Sarah's ability to tolerate oral feedings
    c. The mother's request for Sarah to start oral feedings
3. What implications and priorities for nursing care may be drawn at this time?
4. Does the evidence objectively support your argument (conclusion)?
5. Are there alternative perspectives to your arguments? What are they?

physiotherapy or occupational therapy routines may be incorporated into the child's morning nursing procedures, or speech therapy interventions may be conducted by the parent or nurse around eating times so that the entire day is not occupied by procedures. A written schedule of daily routines should be developed and followed by all caregivers.

NURSING ALERT At each home visit, physically handle and look at all medications. Check them against the medical orders and read the labels. There may be discrepancies, duplications, or changes between hospitalizations. Clarify medication purpose, effect, and dosages for the family.

Goals of care and achievement of established outcomes are supported by intervention strategies that reflect normalization (see Chapter 41) and the interests and abilities of the child and family. Nurses can help the family explore a range of alternative strategies, services, and resources so that the family can choose the best match for their situation. Families can participate in evaluating a home care plan on several levels. Families and care providers should regularly review the goals of care and update the care plan as required. The nurse can ask the family open-ended questions at regular intervals to assess their opinions on the effectiveness of care. As part of the evaluation process, families should be acknowledged for their successes and accomplishments. Finally, families should be given an opportunity to evaluate individual home care nurses, the home care agency, and other service providers periodically. The evaluation should address the nurse's knowledge, skills, and respect for the family's choices. The agency should use the evaluations to improve the quality of care (see Family-Centred Teaching box).

FAMILY-CENTRED TEACHING

Knowledgeable Parents

It is not unusual for parents, particularly those whose children have chronic illnesses or complex care regimens, to be more knowledgeable about their child's condition than a nurse who is assigned to the child's care. This can be disconcerting for both the parents and the nurse. It is important to remember and reinforce that, regardless of the condition, parents will always know more about their child than the professional caring for the child. The nurse and parents can set goals for care in an atmosphere of mutual respect. If the parents' goal is respite from prolonged caregiving, they are less likely to want to give long explanations about their child's care, and assistance from an experienced peer may be more appropriate for the nurse to seek. If the parents wish to maintain maximum participation in care delivery, the nurse and the parents can negotiate the collaboration.

When teaching parents to perform complex chronic care regimens at home, include teaching them to expect to know more about their child's care than professionals who may come to assist them, whether that be home health, hospital, or outpatient personnel. At the same time, assure them that what various professionals who work with them will have from working with a multitude of families is a scientific knowledge base and a wealth of options for addressing and solving care problems.

–Teresa L. Hall, MS, RN

BOX 43-8 Sample Family Assessment Questions

- What are the child and family's experiences and expectations of the disease or illness?
- How does that affect the current situation?
- Is the current coping status a reflection of a new condition, the same chronic condition, or a new phase in a chronic condition?
- How can the nurse address family needs and promote health among all family members?
- What specific nursing interventions will facilitate a healthy response to child and family limitations caused by the illness?

(Modified from Gedaly-Duff, V., & Heims, M. L. [1996]. Family child health nursing. In S. M. H. Hanson & S. T. Boyd [Eds.], *Family health care nursing*. Philadelphia: Davis.)

FAMILY-CENTRED TEACHING

What I Learned About Home Care

I learned many things as a result of having home care for four children over a period of 8 years. Two of the major areas I learned about were communication and families' rights. It took a long time to learn some of these things.

Initially I tried very hard to be sensitive to the professionals and often put my own feelings and needs aside. It took a while to learn that I could stand up for myself and my family and that my child could continue to receive good care. One area that was important to me was to have nurses withhold judgement on our parenting style, even if they might have parented differently.

Communication needs to be open and two-way. Families and nurses ought to tell each other what is going well. For example, "Thanks for keeping the room so neat while you're here" can help a nurse see a family's appreciation. There was so little I could do as just "Mommy" that it really meant a lot to me when nurses would say, "That's such a cute outfit you picked out for him today." Communicating about little things, even inconsequential topics such as favourite TV shows, makes it easier to communicate about more important things and about problems. Communication has to be open about problems, too.

–Jeni Stepanek, Mother

In addition to maintaining a sense of control over their child's care, families need to control their home and personal lives. For this reason, nurses should discuss "house rules" with the family and address issues such as the physical environment, private areas in the home, responsibility for maintaining the child's environment, and interactions with siblings (see Guidelines box). One of the more important aspects of the nurse's relationship with the family is maintaining professional boundaries and a therapeutic role that is supportive but not intrusive (McKlindon & Barsteiner, 1999) (see Critical Thinking Exercise).

Technological trends that influence the nursing process in home care include the use of laptop computers (notebooks) and personal tablets to document the home visit; smart phones or small hand-held computers that store large amounts of data, including addresses, appointments, patient tracking systems, textbooks, and pharmacological databases (Government of Canada, 2012); Internet and e-mail services, which increase patient–practitioner accessibility and communication; and telemedicine or telehealth, which has various features, including electronic systems that can transmit physiological data directly to the practitioner via the telephone. The CNA (2007) has developed a position statement on telehealth and the role of the nurse that includes relevant guidelines and standards of practice. Concerns with the increasing use of technology in health care are cost, governmental regulations and patient care standards, liability and malpractice issues, ethics, and confidentiality matters (Rice, 2006).

GUIDELINES Negotiating "House Rules" for Home Care

House Rules

Parking–Identify where to park and community regulations.

Access–State where to enter the home. Is knocking preferred or ringing the bell?

Personal belongings–Where does the nurse store his or her coat, boots, etc.? Does the family prefer slippers to shoes in the home?

Meals–Where may the nurse store his or her food? Note: This is very important given the cultural diversity of patients.

Radio and television–Identify preferences regarding usage. Remember, this may help nurses to remain awake at night.

Patient room–The nurse is responsible for the child's immediate environment. Maintaining a clean working area and cleaning up the room at the end of the shift is the nurse's responsibility.

Telephone–Agency policy may dictate that all personal calls be limited to brief periods and charged to the nurse making them. Note: Many nurses do need to check in with home at some interval during the evening.

Visitors–Identify who may enter the home when the parents are away (e.g., child's friends or grandparents). A list of names should be available.

Privacy–Describe what parts of the home are off-limits to the nurse and at what times.

Child

Routine–Specify times for playtime, bath time, and bedtime. How does the parent want to participate in these routines?

Mealtime–Specify where the family wants the child fed; if tube fed, specify a preference as to how and where it is done.

Clothing–Identify who picks out the child's clothes. Identify where the laundry is and who is responsible for washing the sick child's clothing.

Discipline–Discuss specific guidelines for discipline.

Homework–Discuss when it should be done and who is responsible for it being completed.

Siblings

Discipline–Establish guidelines regarding how parents should be informed of siblings' conflicts and how discipline should be handled. Note: Parents or another caregiver must be in the home when siblings are home.

Patient care–Be specific about how children have helped with the child's care. Discuss any concerns regarding behaviour that may compromise the child's or siblings' safety.

Nursing

Parental notification–Specify what information the family wishes to be aware of immediately and what can wait until they are home.

Limits of responsibility–Specify duties the nurse may not perform, such as transportation of the child to care facilities or babysitting the siblings.

Environment–Discuss the need to have adequate lighting and a comfortable working area.

(Modified from Klug, R. [1993]. Clarifying roles and expectations in home care. *Pediatric Nursing, 19*[4], 375.)

CRITICAL THINKING EXERCISE

Maintaining Therapeutic Boundaries

As the home care nurse who has been working weekly with Derek, a 4-year-old ventilator-dependent child, for about 5 months, you are aware that the parents have become increasingly argumentative with each other. Most of the arguments are about whether Mr. J helps enough with the child's care and the house cleaning. Mr. J works full time at one job, then supplements the family income by working at a part-time job every weekend. Ms. J approaches you to complain about her husband's lack of involvement with the child and his care. Derek requires constant care, and the family has many expenses related to his physical care; the child is severely developmentally impaired and is not expected to improve significantly despite numerous medical interventions. He is the only child, although Ms. J stated at one time they wanted to have many children.

1. Evidence—Is there sufficient evidence to draw any conclusions about the family situation at this time?
2. Assumptions—Describe some underlying assumptions about the following:
   a. Home care of the child with a chronic, terminal condition (see p. 1222)
   b. Impact of the chronic condition, child's prognosis, and required care on the parents
   c. Status of the marriage relationship between Mr. and Ms. J
3. What implications and priorities for nursing care may be drawn at this time?
4. Does the evidence objectively support your argument (conclusion)?
5. Are there alternative perspectives to your arguments? What are they?

BOX 43-9 Incorporating Developmental Support Into the Home Care Plan

Example

A 6-month-old infant with a history of 24-week prematurity and bronchopulmonary dysplasia: currently using cardiorespiratory monitor, oxygen via nasal cannula, and skin-level (MIC-KEY) gastrostomy feedings

Outcome Criteria

Age-appropriate growth and developmental activities promoted with normal parameters achieved

Absence of growth and development deficits for age within limits imposed by illness

Intervention

Assess growth and development with the *Nipissing District Developmental Screening (NDDS)*.

Reassess growth and development every 4 weeks.

Provide a consistent caregiver.

Instruct parents in normal growth and development for the child's age, reasons for delay, and anticipated outcomes.

Inform parents of age-related play and other activities that enhance growth and development and provide stimulation.

Consult with physical, occupational, and speech therapists to incorporate recommendations in daily routines.

Provide visual, auditory, and tactile stimulation, including mobiles with or without colour, music, toys, books, and television.

Hold, rock, pat, and talk to the child.

(Data from Klijanowicz, A. S. [1997]. Care of the high-risk infant. In W. L. Votroubek & J. L. Townsend [Eds.], *Pediatric home care* [2nd ed.]. Gaithersburg, MD: Aspen; Jaffe, M. [1998]. *Pediatric nursing care plans* [2nd ed.]. Englewood, CO: Skidmore-Roth; and Luxner, K., & Jaffe, M. [2004]. *Delmar's pediatric nursing care plans* [3rd ed.]. Clifton Park, NY: Thomson Delmar Learning.)

Promotion of Optimum Development, Self-Care, and Education

There is little question that living at home offers most children with complex medical problems great social and emotional advantages over living in the hospital or other institutional setting. However, in infancy and throughout the developmental stages, a child's medical condition and dependence on medical technology can place constraints on and pose challenges to normal development. For example, the child may have lengthy and repeated hospitalizations; developmental regression can occur in response to stress; fatigue may result from an underlying pathological condition, the exacerbation of an illness, or medication adverse effects; and equipment requirements may impede mobility, exploration, and independence. The challenge of providing support for normal development in a child who is chronically ill and technology dependent requires the best use of opportunities for developmentally appropriate experiences within these constraints.

Home care plans are designed to promote optimum child development through assessment, planning, and referrals, and through interventions that address normalization issues and self-care (Box 43-9). General principles for a family-centred assessment and planning process, addressed earlier in this chapter, are also applied in developmental assessment and planning.

Some parents may not pursue early developmental intervention because they do not believe their child needs the services. In this case, health care providers need to explain the child's developmental needs to parents in ways that are meaningful from the parents' own cultural and socioeconomic perspectives. Only then can parents make truly informed decisions. Once parents have been fully informed of the child's condition, likely developmental sequelae, and the expected benefits of intervention, developmental goals outlined by the child and family should guide planning and intervention.

The impact of chronic illness on development is discussed in Chapter 41. Behaviours that may be observed in children receiving home care that need to be addressed by the nurse include the following:

Infants—Crying, withdrawal, detachment, inability to achieve developmental milestones

Toddlers—Inactivity; sadness; screaming; regressive behaviour; delays in motor, speech, social skills

Preschoolers—Temper tantrums, refusal to comply with routines, refusal to eat or participate in self-care

School-age children—Expression of loneliness, boredom, isolation, depression, and worry about school absences; altered physical growth

Adolescents—Dependency, uncooperativeness, withdrawal, fear of loss of peer status or acceptance at school, altered image

The promotion of coping skills and capability can buffer stress and contribute to good mental health and self-esteem in a child with a chronic illness. The extent to which a child is involved in his or her own care depends on many factors, including parental comfort and support and the child's developmental age, level of interest, and physical ability. Self-care, both in activities of daily living and in regard to the medical condition, is important. The goal for self-care in activities of daily living should be the attainment of age-appropriate competence. Some modifications in the environment, the medical equipment, or the techniques for daily activities are often required to promote and support self-care (Fig. 43-2). Effective teaching for self-care is focused at the child's own level of conceptual understanding and may be augmented by the use of dolls, other models and diagrams, simple explanations, and repetition.

Educational planning is important for the child who has a chronic medical condition. The *Education Act* requires school boards to provide special education programs and services for children with special needs. A child who has difficulty learning qualifies for an individual education plan (IEP) that helps the child succeed in school. Teachers, parents, and other support persons need to collaborate to address the learning needs of the child. Infants, toddlers, and preschool children are eligible for treatment of physical, communication, and developmental needs (physiotherapy, occupational, or speech therapy) at children's treatment centres. The home care nurse should refer the family to local educational and rehabilitation programs.

When a child requiring special medical care is to be placed in an educational setting, the parents, child, school health coordinator, educational evaluation team, and education and administrative staff should meet to determine safe and appropriate placement and the necessary services and personnel to enable the child to attend school in the least restrictive environment. Training of education staff and caregivers is essential to ensuring the child's safety in the educational setting. A thorough discussion of training issues, content, and guidelines for care in the school is provided by Porter and colleagues (1997). Special assistance can also be beneficial in reintegrating previously schooled children, such as those with cancer, into the school setting. The home care nurse may need to assist parents in developing the skills to advocate effectively for their child in the educational system.

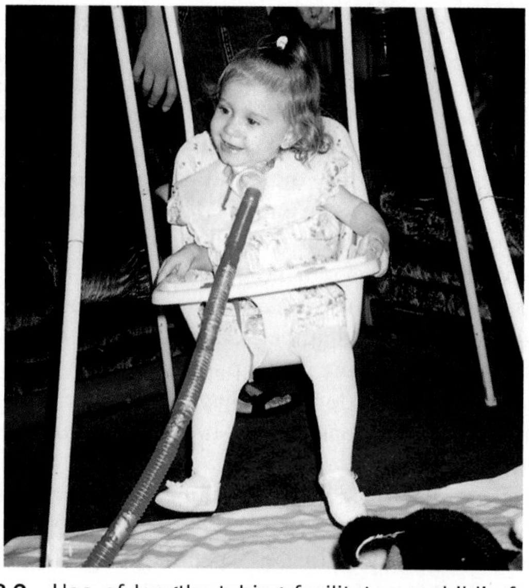

Fig. 43-2 Use of lengthy tubing facilitates a child's freedom of movement.

Safety Issues in the Home

Safety is an important consideration in child home care and should be addressed in the home care plan.

NURSING ALERT Arrangements should be made to ensure that in an emergency the family has adequate methods of communicating with properly trained emergency medical personnel (e.g., a telephone). A cellular phone may be used in place of a landline, but it is advisable to check with the local emergency facilities regarding policies for cell phone use and emergency 911 calls.

The telephone and electric companies (if the use of medical equipment requires electricity) must be notified that the family needs to be placed on a priority service list. In this way the family will learn of any anticipated interruptions in service and will receive priority in reinstatement of interrupted services. Prior contact with rescue squad and local emergency facility personnel can help ensure prompt and appropriate interventions if required. This is especially important if the family lives in a rural location that may not be familiar to local emergency responders. It is recommended that local authorities be given a map marked with key landmarks and intersections for rapid access to the home.

Before hospital discharge, emergency protocols should be developed and reviewed with the parents and professional caregivers. Cardiopulmonary resuscitation guidelines, if appropriate, should be posted near the child's bedside or in another accessible location. A list of emergency telephone numbers can be placed near each home phone and should include those of the rescue squad, emergency department, managing physician(s), nursing agency, and equipment vendor(s) or providers. Additional issues to consider are advance directives and out-of-hospital end-of-life care orders (may vary by province or territory), as indicated. If the patient and family desire enforcement of an advance directive, they must follow specific guidelines, which could prevent undesired lifesaving measures for children with terminal illnesses.

Another aspect of safety relates to the provision of care by appropriately trained individuals. Family members should receive thorough training in the child's care requirements and have the opportunity to demonstrate knowledge and confidence before hospital discharge. Children with complex medical care needs are often admitted to an acute care centre for nonmedical reasons, including lack of parent training and parents' inability to care for a child with complex medical needs (Schanwald, 2005). One study found that although technology-dependent children cared for in the home received adequate care, the time demands of such care had negative effects on the caregiver's school, employment, and social life. Furthermore, a shortage of skilled caregivers often leads to disrupted sleep patterns and increased stress (Heaton et al., 2005). Professional staff caring for the child should have the appropriate background and training for the child's particular care needs. Because of the child's body size, special skill and caution are required in the performance of procedures (e.g., gastrostomy feedings, suctioning) and in monitoring the use of equipment (e.g., ventilator settings, intravenous flow rates, and total fluid volumes).

The activity level and curiosity of young children raise additional safety considerations in the provision of home care. All medications, needles, syringes, and contaminated materials must be securely stored well out of the reach of curious hands. Arrangements for the disposal of sharp items or contaminated materials can be made with the home health agency. Special attention should be given to childproofing the control panels on ventilators, pumps, monitors, and other equipment. The use of clear plastic tape, covers, or panels to cover control knobs or buttons reduces the risk of accidental changes in settings. Much of the medical equipment now in use has special lock-out capabilities that may be used to prevent accidentally altering settings. Electrical cords need to be kept short and out of reach, and safety covers should be used on any open outlets. Equipment should be unplugged when not in use and any wires (e.g., lead wires for an apnea monitor) stored out of reach.

Care at night poses other safety concerns. Parents or other caregivers need to be able to clearly hear monitor, ventilator, or pump alarms at night; an inexpensive intercom system or baby monitor can be used. Steps must be taken to prevent accidental strangulation by apnea, oximeter, or cardiac monitor wires or lengthy intravenous tubing during sleep.

NURSING ALERT Coiling extra tubing and taping it at the exit site, as well as running wires or tubes out the bottoms of pajamas or one-piece infant suits, are precautions against strangulation.

Safe transportation is a vital concern. Wheelchairs and other medical equipment must be properly secured to the vehicle, including vans and buses. Appropriate child restraints must be used. If necessary, an extra adult should be present to monitor the child while in transit. Information on car seat safety and transportation for children with special needs is available from the provincial and territorial ministries of transportation, which provide guidelines for wheelchairs in cars, supine car seats, and equipment transportation. (See also Chapter 37, Motor Vehicle Injuries, for discussion of transportation of children with special needs.)

Family-to-Family Support

Family-to-family support networks can be an important source of emotional and instrumental support and empowerment for families of children with chronic health problems. Family-to-family support does not replace professional sources of support but rather is a unique resource that promotes family strengths through shared experience.

Families will most likely experience increased emotional stress as the result of living with and caring for a child with special needs. A tool that might be helpful to the pediatric home care nurse is the Caregiver Strain Index, a 13-item assessment designed to ascertain caregiver stress and subsequently develop appropriate strategies for individual and family coping (Sullivan, 2003). Other issues that are likely to arise as a result of the child's illness and the constant attention required include labelling the child as being vulnerable, otherwise known as the *vulnerable child syndrome*, in which parents spend too much time preoccupied with the child's welfare while ignoring other family members' needs (Bennett, 2002). As the child with special health care needs develops and grows, parents should impose the same disciplinary rules on the child receiving home care as on siblings to avoid further conflict within the family.

Identification of meaningful sources of support can make a difference in coping abilities. Montagnino and Mauricio (2004) surveyed a group of mothers caring for children in the home who had undergone a tracheostomy and gastrostomy. The researchers found that the mothers experienced significant anxiety, and social interaction within and outside the family was disrupted as a result of the child's condition. The authors recommended that families of children with special health care needs network with other parents in similar conditions through online and local support groups to prevent social disruption and maintain a sense of family normalcy.

Baum (2004) surveyed the caregivers of children with special health care needs about the value of an Internet parent support group, using stress and coping theory as a guide for measuring perceived satisfaction and a number of other characteristics. The survey indicated that parents were satisfied with the information obtained through the Internet support group, with an improved caregiver–child relationship being the strongest outcome factor. Baum suggests that undesirable results may also be obtained via such Internet groups and that parents should carefully evaluate the quality of such support groups.

The nurse can assist the family in their involvement in community social networks. For example, a referral to a parent support group may meet an individual family's needs. The nurse should inform the parents of the group's goals so that they can determine whether they might benefit from this connection. In addition, informal support networks can be extremely beneficial. A link to a family in the same or a similar situation allows the sharing of common experiences. This in itself may decrease the sense of isolation and provide a connection with someone who can truly identify with family struggles.

The nurse should remember that each family member's needs differ. The care plan should acknowledge the needs of each family member (mother, father, siblings, grandparents). Peer support for school-age children and adolescents with complex care needs may be beneficial. These connections can be expanded to include letter writing, e-mails, telephone calls, or specialty camp programs (Johnson, Ravert, & Everton, 2001). Most school-age children and adolescents just want to be accepted by their peers and fit in as a part of the group. Same-age peers may at first be standoffish to children with disabilities, but this is likely out of fear and lack of understanding; helping others see that they have the same dreams, desires, goals, and interests can promote group cohesiveness and understanding.

Key Points

- Effective home care depends on many factors, including the child's medical stability; the family's willingness, training, and ability to accommodate the child's care requirements; and professional, financial, and community support.
- Comprehensive, multidisciplinary discharge planning should begin early and should include the family and a home care coordinator in addition to hospital personnel.
- Thorough education and training of the family or primary caregiver can ease the transition to home.
- Care coordination ensures continuity of care, prevents duplication of services, and reduces fragmentation of services. The family may assume responsibility for varying degrees of care coordination over time.
- The home care nurse must possess a high level of technical expertise while being able to adapt equipment, procedures, and the nursing process to the home setting.
- Accreditation standards apply to agencies that provide home care; standards of practice by the Canadian Nurses Association and other professional nursing organizations can guide nurses in the home setting.
- Family-centred nursing practice is applied in the home setting; diversity in family structures, cultural backgrounds, strengths, and coping mechanisms needs to be respected.
- Collaborative relationships among parents, home care providers, and other health care providers are characterized by communication, dialogue, active listening, awareness and acceptance of differences, and negotiation.
- The nursing process should be adapted to involve the family in each step and to preserve the family's central role in decision making.
- House rules agreed on by the nurse, child, and family enable the family to maintain a feeling of control over their own environment when health care providers are present.
- Individualized home care plans are designed to promote optimum development of the child and to focus on normalization—assessing and incorporating the impact of the child's medical condition and technological requirements on development, self-care, and educational needs.
- Safety in the provision of home care services involves emergency preparations and protocols, appropriate training of family and home care personnel, and the safe use and childproofing of medical equipment.
- Family-to-family support networks can provide emotional and instrumental support and foster family empowerment.

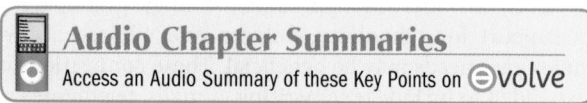

Audio Chapter Summaries
Access an Audio Summary of these Key Points on evolve

References

Antonelli, R. C., Stille, C. J., & Antonelli, D. M. (2008). Care coordination for children and youth with special health care needs: A descriptive, multisite study of activities, personnel, costs, and outcomes. *Pediatrics, 122*(1), e209–e216. doi:10.1542/peds.2007-2254

Bakewell-Sachs, S., et al. (2000). Home care considerations for chronic and vulnerable populations. *Nurse Practitioner Forum, 11*(1), 65–72.

Baum, L. S. (2004). Internet parent support groups for primary caregivers of a child with special health care needs. *Pediatric Nursing, 30*(5), 381–388, 401.

Bennett, A. D. (2002). Home apnea monitoring for infants: A discussion of primary care issues. *Advanced Nursing Practice, 10*(3), 48–53.

Canadian Home Care Association. (2006). *Home care for children with special needs.* Retrieved from http://www.cdnhomecare.ca/media.php?mid=2178.

Canadian Home Care Association. (2008). *Portraits of home care in Canada.* Retrieved from http://www.cdnhomecare.ca/media.php?mid=1877.

Canadian Nurses Association. (1997). *Nursing now: Issues and trends in Canadian nursing (The Family Connection).* Ottawa: Author.

Canadian Nurses Association. (2004). *Position statement: Promoting culturally competent care.* Ottawa: Author.

Canadian Nurses Association. (2005). *Position statement: Interprofessional collaboration.* Ottawa: Author.

Canadian Nurses Association. (2007). *Telehealth: The role of the nurse.* Retrieved from http://www2.cna-aiic.ca/CNA/documents/pdf/publications/PS89_Telehealth_e.pdf.

Canadian Paediatric Society. (2008). Position statement: Special considerations for the health supervision of children and youth in foster care. *Pediatrics and Child Health, 13*(2), 129–132.

Canadian Public Health Association. (2010). *Public health/community nursing practice in Canada: Roles and activities.* Retrieved from http://www.chnc.ca/documents/PublicHealth-CommunityHealthNursinginCanadaRolesandActivities2010.pdf.

Canadian Research Network for Care in the Community. (2008). *Children and youth home care in Canada.* Retrieved from http://www.crncc.ca/knowledge/factsheets/pdf/In_Focus_Children_and_Youth_Homecare_FINAL.pdf.

Community Health Nurses Association of Canada (2008). *Canadian community health nursing standards of practice.* Toronto: Author.

Cooper, C., et al. (2006). Specialist home-based nursing services for children with acute and chronic illnesses. *Cochrane Database of Systematic Reviews, 18*(4), CD004383. doi:10.1007/BF03071208

Daveluy, W., et al. (2006). Dramatic changes in home-based enteral nutrition practices in children during an 11-year period. *Journal of Pediatric Gastroenterology & Nutrition, 43*(2), 240–244. doi:10.1097/01.mpg.0000228095.81831.79

Davis, C. (2006). Safe on the home watch. *Nursing Standard, 20*(34), 20–22.

Dunbrack, J. (2003). *Respite for family caregivers: An environmental scan of publicly funded programs in Canada.* Retrieved from http://www.ccc-ccan.ca/media.php?mid=73.

Enhancing Interdisciplinary Collaboration in Primary Health Care [EICP] Steering Committee. (2005). *The principles and framework for interdisciplinary collaboration in primary health care.* Retrieved from http://eicp.ca/en/principles/documents.asp.

Farris-Manning, C., & Zandstra, M. (2003). *Children in care in Canada: A summary of current issues and trends with recommendations for future research.* Ottawa: Child Welfare League of Canada.

Feudtner, C., et al. (2005). Technology-dependence among patients discharged from a children's hospital: A retrospective cohort study. *BMC Pediatrics, 5*(8), 1–8. doi:10.1186/1471-2431-5-8

Giger, J. N., & Davidhizar, R. (2002). The Giger and Davidhizar Transcultural Assessment Model. *Journal of Transcultural Nursing, 13*(3), 185–188.

Government of Canada. (2012). *E-health technologies: The future is here.* Retrieved from http://investincanada.gc.ca/eng/publications/e-health-canada.aspx.

Harrigan, R. C., et al. (2002). Medically fragile children: An integrative review of the literature and recommendations for future research. *Issues in Comprehensive Pediatric Nursing, 25*(1), 1–20.

Health Canada. (2002). *National profile of family caregivers in Canada—2002: A final report.* Retrieved from http://www.hc-sc.gc.ca/hcs-sss/alt_formats/hpb-dgps/pdf/pubs/2002-caregiv-interven/2002-caregiv-interven-eng.pdf.

Health Canada. (2008). *Continuing care in First Nations and Inuit Communities: Evidence from the research.* Retrieved from http://www.hc-sc.gc.ca/fniah-spnia/pubs/services/_home-domicile/2007_info_contin_care-soins/index-eng.php.

Heaton, J., et al. (2005). Families' experiences of caring for technology-dependent children: A temporal perspective. *Health & Social Care in the Community, 13*(5), 441–450. doi:10.1111/j.1365-2524.2005.00571.x

Howard, L. (2006). Home parenteral nutrition: Survival, cost, and quality of life. *Gastroenterology, 130*(2 Suppl 1), S52–S59. doi:10.1053/j.gastro.2005.09.065

Johnson, K. B., Ravert, R. D., & Everton, A. (2001). Hopkins Teen Central: Assessment of an Internet-based support system for children with cystic fibrosis. *Pediatrics, 107*(2), e24.

Kellett, U. M., & Mannion, J. (1999). Meaning in caring: Reconceptualizing the nurse–family carer relationship in community practice. *Journal of Advanced Nursing, 29*(3), 697–703.

Knafl, K. A., & Deatrick, J. A. (2002). The challenges of normalization for families of children with chronic conditions. *Pediatric Nursing, 28*(1), 49–53, 56.

Lindeke, L. L., et al. (2002). Family-centered care coordination for children with special needs across multiple settings. *Journal of Pediatric Health Care, 16*(6), 290–297.

Magrabi, F., et al. (2005). Designing home telecare: A case study in monitoring cystic fibrosis. *Telemedicine & e-health, 11*(6), 707–719. doi:10.1089/tmj.2005.11.707

McEvoy, M. (2003). Culture and spirituality as an integrated concept in pediatric care. *MCN: American Journal of Maternal/Child Nursing, 28*(1), 39–43.

McKlindon, D., & Barsteiner, J. H. (1999). Therapeutic relationships. *MCN: American Journal of Maternal/Child Nursing, 24*(5), 237–243.

Mildon, B., & Underwood, J. (2010). *Competencies for home health care nursing: A literature review.* Retrieved from http://www.chnc.ca/documents/HomeHealthCompetenciesLiteraturereviewApril122010.pdf.

Montagnino, B. A., & Mauricio, R. V. (2004). The child with a tracheostomy and gastrostomy: Parental stress and coping in the home—a pilot study. *Pediatric Nursing, 30*(5), 373–380, 401.

Navaie-Waliser, M., et al. (2004). Evaluating the needs of children with asthma in home care: The vital role of nurses as caregivers and educators. *Public Health Nursing, 21*(4), 306–315.

Nazer, D., et al. (2006). Home versus hospital intravenous antibiotic therapy for acute pulmonary exacerbations in children with cystic fibrosis. *Pediatric Pulmonology, 41*(8), 744–749. doi: 10.1002/ppul.20433

Newton, M. S. (2000). Family-centered care: Current realities in parent participation. *Pediatric Nursing, 26*(2), 164–168.

Page, D. R. (2001). Pediatric home care: Nursing the shortage. *Caring, 20*(6), 46–47.

Parra, M. M. (2003). Nursing and respite care services for ventilator-assisted children. *Caring, 22*(5), 6–9.

Peter, E., Spalding, K., Kenny, N., Conrad, N., McKeever, P., & Macfarlane, A., (2007). Neither seen nor heard: Children and homecare policy in Canada. *Social Science & Medicine, 64*(8), 1624–1635.

Porter, S., et al. (Eds.), (1997). *Children and youth assisted by medical technology in educational settings: Guidelines for care* (2nd ed.). Baltimore: Paul H. Brookes.

Rice, R. (2006). Case management and leadership strategies for home care nurses. In R. Rice (Ed.), *Home care nursing practice: Concepts and application* (4th ed.). St. Louis: Mosby.

Roush, C. V., & Cox, J. E. (2000). The meaning of home: How it shapes the practice of home and hospice care. *Home Healthcare Nurse, 18*(6), 388–394.

Schanwald, P. R. (2005). Gaps in pediatric care. *Caring, 25*(9), 20–25.

Stevens, B., McKeever, P., Law, M., Booth, M., Greenberg, M., et al. (2006). Children receiving chemotherapy at home: Perceptions of children and parents. *Journal of Pediatric Oncology Nursing, 23*(5), 276–285.

Sullivan, T. (2003). Caregiver Strain Index. *Home Healthcare Nurse, 21*(3), 197–198.

Sullivan-Bolyai, S., Knafl, K. A., Sadler, S., & Gilliss, C. L. (2003). Great expectations: A position description for parents as caregivers: Part I. *Pediatric Nursing, 29*(6), 457–460.

Sullivan-Bolyai, S., Knafl, K.A., Sadler, S., & Gilliss, C. L. (2004). Great expectations: A position description for parents as caregivers: Part II. *Pediatric Nursing, 30*(1), 52–56.

Thompson, J. (2000). Pediatric assessment in the home. *Home Healthcare Nurse, 18*(10), 639–646.

Williams, A. P., Spalding, K., Deber, R. B. & McKeever, P. (2005). *Prescriptions for pediatric home care: Analyzing the impact of the shift from hospital to home and community on children and families.* University of Toronto Department of Health Policy, Management and Evaluation, and From Medicare to Home and Community (M-THAC) Research Unit. Retrieved from http://www.teamgrant.ca/M-THAC%20Greatest%20Hits/M-THAC%20Projects/All%20info/Pediatric%20Home%20Care%20-%20Bonus%20Track/Publications/p8452.pdf.

Wilson, A. (2003). Understanding benchmarks. *Home Healthcare Nurse, 21*(2), 102–107.

Wright, L. M., & Leahey, M. (2005). *Nurses and families: A guide to family assessment and intervention* (4th ed.). Philadelphia: FA Davis.

Yoder-Wise, P. (2007). *Leading and managing in nursing* (4th ed.). St. Louis: Mosby.

Additional Resources

Canadian Home Care Association: http://www.cdnhomecare.ca.
Collaborative Family Healthcare Association: http://www.cfha.net.
Yaldei Developmental Center: Early Intervention: http://www.yaldei.org/?page_id=8.

Unit 10

44 Reaction to Illness and Hospitalization

Learning Objectives

On completion of this chapter, the reader will be able to:

- Identify the stressors of illness and hospitalization for children during each developmental stage.
- List essential priorities of nursing care for a child on admission to the hospital.
- Outline nursing interventions that prevent or minimize the stress of separation during hospitalization.
- Outline nursing interventions that minimize the stress of loss of control during hospitalization.
- Outline nursing interventions that minimize the fear of bodily injury during hospitalization.
- Outline nursing interventions that support parents, siblings, and family during a child's illness and hospitalization.
- Describe nursing interventions needed when children are admitted to special units such as the emergency department.

Electronic Resources

Additional information related to the content in Chapter 44 can be found on

evolve the Companion Web site at

http://evolve.elsevier.com/Canada/Perry/maternal/

- Examination Review Questions
- Critical Thinking Exercise—Discharge Planning
- Skill—Admitting a Child to the Health Care System
- Skill—Preparing the Child for Surgery
- Skill—Therapeutic Play

Stressors of Hospitalization and Children's Reactions

Often, illness and hospitalization are the first crises children must face. Especially during the early years, children are particularly vulnerable to these crises because (1) stress represents a change from the usual state of health and environmental routine and (2) children have a limited number of **coping** mechanisms to resolve stressors (those events that produce stress). Major stressors of hospitalization include separation, loss of control, bodily injury, and **pain**. Children's reactions to these stressors are influenced by their **developmental age**; their previous experience with illness, separation, or hospitalization; their innate and acquired coping skills; the seriousness of the diagnosis; and the support system available.

Separation Anxiety

The major stress from middle infancy throughout the preschool years, especially for children ages 6 to 30 months, is **separation anxiety**, also called *anaclitic depression*. The principal behavioural responses to this stressor during early childhood are summarized in Box 44-1. During the phase of *protest*, children react aggressively to separation from the parent. They cry and scream for their parents, refuse the attention of anyone else, and are inconsolable in their grief (Fig. 44-1). During the phase of *despair*, the crying stops and depression is evident. The child is much less active, is uninterested in play or food, and withdraws from others (Fig. 44-2).

The third stage is *detachment*, also called **denial**. Superficially it appears that the child has finally adjusted to the loss. The child becomes more interested in the surroundings, plays with others, and seems to form new relationships. However, this behaviour is the result of resignation and is not a sign of contentment. The child detaches from the parent in an effort to escape the emotional pain of desiring the parent's presence and copes by forming shallow relationships with others, becoming increasingly self-centred, and attaching primary importance to material objects. This is the most serious stage in that reversal of the potential adverse effects is less likely to occur after detachment is established. However, in most situations, the temporary separations imposed by hospitalization do not cause such prolonged parental absences that the child enters into detachment. In addition, considerable evidence suggests that even with stressors such as separation, children are remarkably adaptable, and permanent ill effects are rare.

Although progression to the stage of detachment is uncommon, the initial stages are frequently observed even with brief separations from either parent. Unless health care team members understand the meaning of each stage of behaviour,

BOX 44-1 Manifestations of Separation Anxiety in Young Children

Phase of Protest

Behaviours observed during later infancy include the following:
- Crying
- Screaming
- Searching for parent with eyes
- Clinging to parent
- Avoiding and rejecting contact with strangers

Additional behaviours observed during toddlerhood include the following:
- Verbally attacking strangers (e.g., "Go away")
- Physically attacking strangers (e.g., kicking, biting, hitting, pinching)
- Attempting to escape to find parent
- Attempting to physically force parent to stay

Behaviours may last from hours to days.

Protest, such as crying, may be continuous, ceasing only with physical exhaustion.

Approach of stranger may precipitate increased protest.

Phase of Despair

Observed behaviours include the following:
- Being inactive
- Withdrawing from others
- Being depressed, sad
- Lacking interest in environment
- Being uncommunicative
- Regressing to earlier behaviour (e.g., thumb sucking, bed-wetting, use of pacifier, use of bottle)

Behaviours may last for a variable length of time.

Child's physical condition may deteriorate from refusal to eat, drink, or move.

Phase of Detachment

Observed behaviours include the following:
- Showing increased interest in surroundings
- Interacting with strangers or familiar caregivers
- Forming new but superficial relationships
- Appearing happy

Detachment usually occurs after prolonged separation from parent; it is rarely seen in hospitalized children.

Behaviours represent a superficial adjustment to loss.

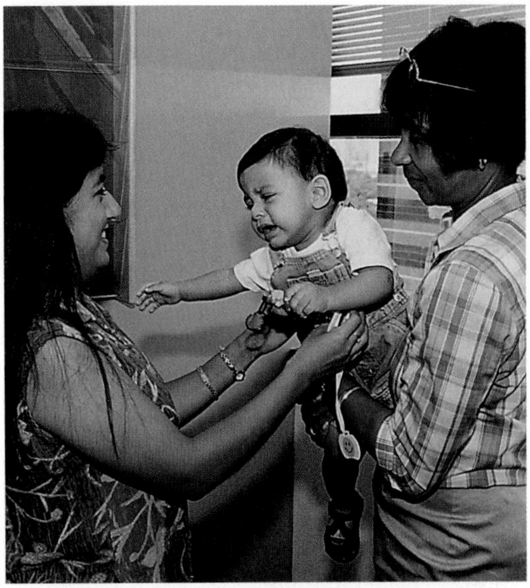

Fig. 44-1 In the protest phase of separation anxiety, children cry loudly and are inconsolable in their grief for the parent. *(Courtesy James DeLeon, Texas Children's Hospital, Houston.)*

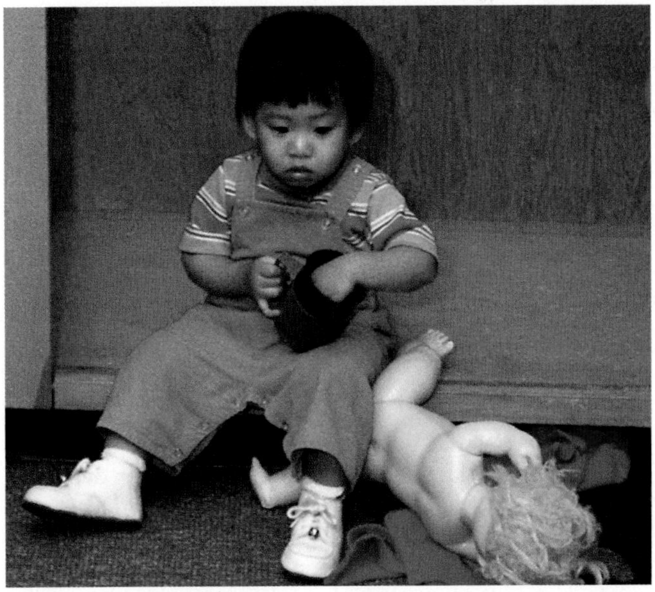

Fig. 44-2 During the despair phase of separation anxiety, children are sad, lonely, and uninterested in food and play.

they may erroneously label the behaviours as positive or negative. For example, they may see the loud crying of the protest phase as "bad" behaviour. Because the protests increase when a stranger approaches the child, they may interpret that reaction as meaning they should stay away. During the quiet, withdrawn phase of despair, health care team members may think that the child is finally "settling in" to the new surroundings, and they may see the detachment behaviours as proof of a "good adjustment." The faster this stage is reached, the more likely it is that the child will be regarded as the "ideal patient."

Because children seem to react "negatively" to visits by their parents, uninformed observers feel justified in restricting parental visiting privileges. For example, during the protest stage, children outwardly do not appear happy to see their parents (Fig. 44-3). In fact, they may even cry louder. If they are depressed, they may reject their parents or begin to protest again. Often they cling to their parents in an effort to ensure their continued presence. Consequently, such reactions may be regarded as "disturbing" the child's adjustment to the new surroundings. If the separation has progressed to the phase of detachment, children will respond no differently to their parents than they would to any other person.

Such reactions are distressing to parents, who are unaware of their meaning. If parents are regarded as intruders, they will see their absence as "beneficial" to the child's adjustment and recovery. They may respond to the child's behaviour by staying

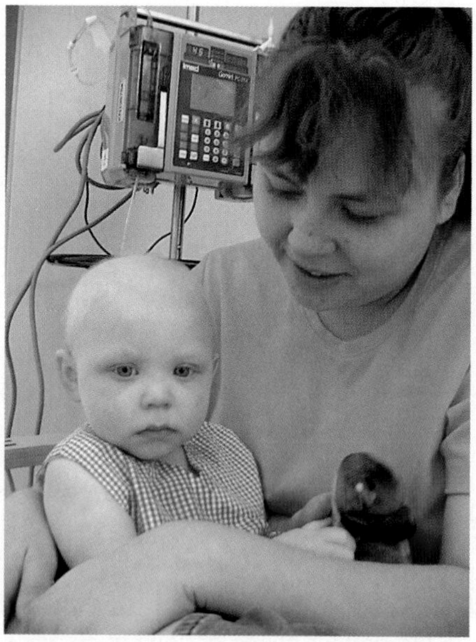

Fig. 44-3 Young children may appear withdrawn and sad even in the presence of a parent. *(Courtesy E. Jacob, Texas Children's Hospital, Houston.)*

for only short periods, visiting less frequently, or deceiving the child when it is time to leave. The result is a destructive cycle of misunderstanding and unmet needs.

Early Childhood

Separation anxiety is the greatest stress imposed by hospitalization during early childhood. If separation is avoided, young children have a tremendous capacity to withstand any other stress. During this period, the typical reactions just described are seen. However, children in the toddler stage demonstrate more goal-directed behaviours. For example, they may plead with the parents to stay and physically try to keep the parents with them or try to find parents who have left. They may demonstrate displeasure on the parents' return or departure by having temper tantrums; refusing to comply with the usual routines of mealtime, bedtime, or toileting; or regressing to more primitive levels of development. However, temper tantrums, bed-wetting, or other behaviours may also be expressions of anger, a physiological response to stress, or symptoms of illness.

Because preschoolers are more secure interpersonally than toddlers, they can tolerate brief periods of separation from their parents and are more inclined to develop substitute trust in other significant adults. However, the stress of illness usually renders preschoolers less able to cope with separation; as a result, they manifest many of the stage behaviours of separation anxiety, although in general the protest behaviours are more subtle and passive than those seen in younger children. Preschoolers may demonstrate separation anxiety by refusing to eat, experiencing difficulty in sleeping, crying quietly for their parents, continually asking when the parents will visit, or withdrawing from others. They may express anger indirectly by breaking their toys, hitting other children, or refusing to cooperate during usual self-care activities. Nurses need to be sensitive to these less obvious signs of separation anxiety in order to intervene appropriately.

Later Childhood and Adolescence

Previous research, usually based on adult recollections, indicated that the family does not play as important a role for school-age children as it does during the toddler and preschool years. However, in a recent study that asked children about their fears when hospitalized, children listed their greatest fears regarding hospitalization as being separated from family and friends, being in an unfamiliar environment, receiving investigations or treatments, and losing self-determination or choices (Coyne, 2006).

Although school-age children are better able to cope with separation in general, the stress and often accompanying **regression** imposed by illness or hospitalization may increase their need for parental security and guidance. This is particularly true for young school-age children who have only recently left the safety of the home and are struggling with the crisis of school adjustment. Middle and late school-age children may react more to the separation from their usual activities and peers than to the absence of their parents. These children have a high level of physical and mental activity that frequently finds no suitable outlets in the hospital environment, and even when they dislike school, they admit to missing its routine and worry that they will not be able to compete or "fit in" with their classmates when they return. Feelings of loneliness, boredom, isolation, and depression are common. Such reactions may occur more as a result of separation than of concern over the illness, treatment, or hospital setting.

School-age children may need and desire parental guidance or support from other adult figures but may be unable or unwilling to ask for it. Because the goal of attaining independence is so important, they are reluctant to seek help directly, fearing that they will appear weak, childish, or dependent. Cultural expectations to "act like a man" or to "be brave and strong" weigh heavily on these children, especially boys, who tend to react to stress with stoicism, withdrawal, or passive acceptance. Often the need to express hostile, angry, or other negative feelings finds outlets in alternate ways, such as irritability and aggression toward parents, withdrawal from hospital personnel, inability to relate to peers, rejection of siblings, or subsequent behavioural problems in school.

For adolescents, separation from home and parents may produce varied emotions, ranging from difficulty coping to welcoming the event. However, loss of peer-group contact may pose a severe emotional threat because of loss of group status, inability to exert group control or leadership, and loss of group acceptance. Deviations within peer groups are poorly tolerated, and although group members may express concern for the adolescent's illness or need for hospitalization, they will continue their group activities, quickly filling the gap of the absent member. During the temporary separation from their usual group, ill adolescents may benefit from group associations with other hospitalized teens.

Loss of Control

One of the factors influencing the amount of stress imposed by hospitalization is the amount of control that patients perceive themselves as having. Lack of control increases the perception of threat and can affect children's coping skills. Many hospital situations decrease the amount of control a child feels. Although the usual sensory stimulations are lacking, the additional hospital stimuli of sight, sound, and smell may be overwhelming. Without insight into the type of environment conducive to children's optimum growth, the hospital experience can at best temporarily slow development and at worst permanently restrict it. Because children's needs vary greatly according to their age, the major areas of loss of control in terms of physical restriction, altered routine or rituals, and dependency are discussed here for each age group.

Infants

Developmentally, infants are in the process of establishing the most important attribute of a healthy personality—trust. Trust is learned through consistent, loving care by a nurturing person. Infants attempt to control their environment through emotional expressions, such as crying or smiling. In the hospital setting, cues may be missed or misinterpreted, and routines may be established to meet the hospital staff's needs instead of the infant's needs. Inconsistent care and deviations from the infant's daily routine may lead to mistrust and a decreased sense of control.

Toddlers

Toddlers are at the developmental stage of striving for autonomy, and this goal is evident in most of their behaviours: motor skills, play, interpersonal relationships, activities of daily living, and communication. When their egocentric pleasures meet with obstacles, toddlers react with negativism, especially temper tantrums. Any restriction or limitation of movement, such as the simple act of making toddlers lie down, can cause forceful resistance and the inability to cooperate.

Loss of control also results from altered routines and rituals. Toddlers rely on the consistency and familiarity of daily rituals to provide a measure of stability and control in their complex world of growing and developing. The experience of hospitalization or illness severely limits their sense of expectation and predictability, since practically every detail of the hospital environment differs from that of the home.

Toddlers' main areas for rituals include eating, sleeping, bathing, toileting, and play. When the routines are disrupted, difficulties can occur in any or all of these areas. The principal reaction to such change is regression. For example, when mealtime and food choices differ from those at home, toddlers often refuse to eat, demand a bottle, or ask others to feed them. Although regression to earlier forms of behaviour may seem to increase toddlers' security and comfort, in reality it is threatening for them to relinquish their most recently acquired achievements.

Enforced dependency is a chief characteristic of the sick role and accounts for the numerous instances of toddler negativism. For example, rigid schedules, different clothes, altered caregiving activities, unfamiliar surroundings, separation from parents, and medical procedures usurp toddlers' control over their world. Although most toddlers initially react negatively and aggressively to such dependency, prolonged loss of autonomy may result in passive withdrawal from interpersonal relationships and regression in all areas of development. Therefore, the effects of the sick role are most severe in instances of chronic, long-term illnesses or in those families who foster the sick role despite the child's improved health.

Preschoolers

Preschoolers also suffer from loss of control caused by physical restriction, altered routines, and enforced dependency. However, their specific cognitive abilities, which make them feel all-powerful, also make them feel out of control. This loss of control in the context of their sense of self-power is a critical influencing factor in their perception of and reaction to separation, pain, illness, and hospitalization.

Preschoolers' egocentric and magical thinking limits their ability to understand events because they view all experiences from their own self-referenced (egocentric) perspective. Without adequate preparation for unfamiliar settings or experiences, preschoolers' fantasy explanations for such events are usually more exaggerated, bizarre, and frightening than the facts. One typical fantasy to explain the illness or hospitalization is that it represents punishment for real or imagined misdeeds. In response to such thinking the child usually feels shame, guilt, and fear.

Preschoolers' preoperational thinking means that they understand explanations only in terms of real events. Purely verbal instructions are often inadequate for them because they are unable to abstract and synthesize beyond what their senses tell them. When combined with their egocentric and magical thinking, this characteristic may lead them to interpret messages according to their particular past experiences. Even with the best preparation for a procedure, they may misconstrue the details.

School-Age Children

Because of their striving for independence and productivity, school-age children are particularly vulnerable to events that may lessen their feeling of control and power. In particular, altered family roles; physical disability; fears of death, abandonment, or permanent injury; loss of peer acceptance; lack of productivity; and inability to cope with stress according to perceived cultural expectation may result in loss of control.

Because of the nature of the patient role, many routine hospital activities usurp individual power and identity. For school-age children, dependent activities such as enforced bed rest, use of a bedpan, inability to choose a menu, lack of privacy, help with a bed bath, or transport by a wheelchair or stretcher can be a direct threat to their security. Although all these procedures seem routine and inconsequential, they allow no freedom of choice to children who want to "act grown-up." However, when children are allowed to exert a measure of control, regardless of how limited it may be, they generally respond well to any procedure. For example, some of the most satisfied and contented patients are school-age children who help make their beds, choose their schedule of activities, and assist in their own care. An increased sense of control usually results from a feeling of usefulness and productivity.

In addition to the hospital environment, illness may also cause a feeling of loss of control. One of the most significant problems of children in this age group is boredom. When physical or enforced limitations curtail their usual ability to care for themselves or to engage in favourite activities, school-age children generally respond with depression, hostility, or frustration. Keeping a normally active child on bed rest is difficult. However, emphasizing areas of control and capitalizing on quiet activities, particularly hobbies such as building models or playing age-appropriate video or board games, promotes their adjustment to physical restriction.

Adolescents

Adolescents' struggle for independence, self-assertion, and liberation centres on the quest for personal identity. Anything that interferes with this poses a threat to their sense of identity and results in a loss of control. Illness, which limits one's physical abilities, and hospitalization, which separates one from one's usual support systems, constitute major situational crises.

The patient role fosters dependency and depersonalization. Adolescents may react to dependency with rejection, uncooperativeness, or withdrawal. They may respond to depersonalization with self-assertion, anger, or frustration. Regardless of the response elicited, hospital personnel often regard them as difficult patients. Parents may not be a source of help because these behaviours serve to isolate them further from understanding the adolescent. Although peers may visit, they may not be able to offer the kind of support and guidance needed. Sick adolescents often voluntarily isolate themselves from agemates until they feel they can compete on an equal basis and meet group expectations. As a result, ill adolescents may be left with virtually no support system.

Loss of control also occurs for many of the reasons discussed for school-age children. However, adolescents are more sensitive to potential instances of loss of control and dependency than are younger children. For example, both groups seek information about their physical status and rely heavily on anticipatory preparation to decrease fear and anxiety. However, adolescents react not only to the kinds of information supplied them but also to the means by which it is conveyed. They may feel threatened by others who relay facts in a condescending manner. Adolescents want to know that others can relate to them on their own level. Thus, a careful assessment of their intellectual abilities, previous knowledge, and present needs is required. The nurse may also need to learn the adolescent's language.

Effects of Hospitalization on the Child

Children may react to the stresses of hospitalization before admission, during hospitalization, and after discharge (Box 44-2). A child's concept of illness is even more important than age and intellectual maturity in predicting the level of anxiety before hospitalization (Clatworthy, Simon, & Tiedeman, 1999). This may or may not be affected by the duration of the condition or prior hospitalizations; therefore, nurses should avoid overestimating the concepts of illness in children who have prior medical experience.

Individual Risk Factors

A number of risk factors make certain children more vulnerable than others to the stresses of hospitalization (Box 44-3).

BOX 44-2 Posthospital Behaviours in Children

Young Children

They show initial aloofness toward parents; this may last from a few minutes (most common) to a few days.

This is frequently followed by dependency behaviours:

- Tendency to cling to parents and demand attention
- Vigorous opposition to any separation (e.g., staying at preschool or with a babysitter)

Other negative behaviours include the following:

- New fears (e.g., nightmares)
- Resistance to going to bed, night waking
- Withdrawal and shyness
- Hyperactivity
- Temper tantrums
- Being finicky with food
- Attachment to a blanket or toy
- Regression in newly learned skills (e.g., self-toileting)

Older Children

Negative behaviours include the following:

- Emotional coldness, followed by intense, demanding dependence on parents
- Anger toward parents
- Jealousy toward others (e.g., siblings)

BOX 44-3 Risk Factors That Increase Children's Vulnerability to the Stresses of Hospitalization

- "Difficult" temperament
- Lack of bonding between child and parent
- Age (especially between 6 months and 5 years)
- Male gender
- Below-average intelligence
- Multiple and continuing stresses (e.g., frequent hospitalizations)

Rural children may exhibit greater degrees of psychological upset than urban children, possibly because urban children have opportunities to become familiar with a local hospital (Strickland, Leeper, Jessee, & Hudson, 1987). Because separation is such an important issue surrounding hospitalization for young children, children who are active and strong willed tend to fare better when hospitalized than youngsters who are passive. Consequently, nurses should be alert to children who passively accept all changes and requests; these children may need more support than the "oppositional" child.

The stressors of hospitalization may cause young children to experience short- and long-term negative outcomes; stressors may be related to the length and number of admissions, multiple invasive procedures, and the parents' anxiety. Common responses include regression, separation anxiety, apathy, fears, and sleep disturbances, especially for children younger than 7 years of age (Melnyk, 2000). Supportive practices, such as family-centred care and frequent family visiting, may lessen the detrimental effects. A child's experience of pain will often determine how the overall hospitalization is experienced (Coyne, 2006). Consequently, nurses should attempt to identify those children at risk for poor coping strategies (Small, 2002).

Children can be prepared for hospitalization through stories and colouring books and a variety of preparation materials. Many hospitals have virtual tours and online materials that parents and children can access to help decrease a child's anxiety. Please see the Additional Resources section at the end of this chapter for materials developed by the Hospital for Sick Children that help prepare children for hospitalization.

Changes in the Pediatric Population

With a growing trend toward shortened hospital stays and outpatient surgery, a greater percentage of the children hospitalized today have more serious and complex problems than those of children hospitalized in the past. Many of these children are fragile newborns and children with severe injuries or disabilities who have survived because of major technological advances, yet have been left with chronic or disabling conditions that require frequent and lengthy hospital stays. The nature of their conditions increases the likelihood that they will experience more invasive and traumatic procedures while they are hospitalized. These factors make them more vulnerable to the emotional consequences of hospitalization and result in their needs being significantly different from those of the short-term patients of the past (see Chapter 41 for further discussion on children with special needs). Most of these children are infants and toddlers, the age group most vulnerable to the effects of hospitalization.

Concern in recent years has focused on the increasing length of hospitalization due to complex medical and nursing care, elusive diagnoses, and complicated psychosocial issues. Without special attention devoted to meeting the child's psychosocial and developmental needs in the hospital environment, the detrimental consequences of prolonged hospitalization may be severe.

Beneficial Effects of Hospitalization

Although hospitalization usually is stressful for children, it can also be beneficial. The most obvious benefit is the recovery from illness, but hospitalization also can present an opportunity for children to master stress and feel competent in their coping abilities. The hospital environment can provide children with new socialization experiences that can broaden their interpersonal relationships. The psychological benefits need to be considered and maximized during hospitalization.

Stressors and Reactions of the Family of the Hospitalized Child

Parental Reactions

The crisis of childhood illness and hospitalization affects every member of the family. Parents' reactions to illness in their child depend on a variety of factors. Although one cannot predict which factors are most likely to influence their response, a number of variables have been identified (Box 44-4).

BOX 44-4 Factors Affecting Parents' Reactions to Their Child's Illness

- Seriousness of the threat to the child
- Previous experience with illness or hospitalization
- Medical procedures involved in diagnosis and treatment
- Available support systems
- Personal ego strengths
- Previous coping abilities
- Additional stresses on the family system
- Cultural and religious beliefs
- Communication patterns among family members

Common themes among parents whose children were hospitalized include feeling an overall sense of helplessness, questioning the skills of staff, accepting the reality of hospitalization, needing to have information explained in simple language, dealing with fear, coping with uncertainty, and seeking reassurance from caregivers. This reassurance involves staff being compassionate, expressing concern for the child, and attending to detail in the child's care (Stranton, 2004).

Sibling Reactions

Siblings' reactions to a sister's or brother's illness or hospitalization, discussed in Chapter 41, differ little from those when a child becomes temporarily ill. Siblings experience loneliness, fear, and worry, as well as anger, resentment, jealousy, and guilt. Various factors have been identified that influence the effects of the child's hospitalization on siblings. Although these factors are similar to those seen when a child has a chronic illness, Commodan (2010) has reported that siblings can feel greater effects from the hospital experience based on the following factors:

- Being younger and experiencing many changes
- Being cared for outside the home by care providers who are not relatives
- Receiving little information about their ill brother or sister
- Perceiving that their parents treat them differently compared with before their sibling's hospitalization

Parents are often unaware of the number of effects that siblings experience during the sick child's hospitalization and the benefit of simple interventions to minimize such effects, such as explicit explanations about the illness and provisions for the siblings to remain at home. Sibling visitation is usually beneficial to the patient, sibling, and parent but should be evaluated on an individual basis. Siblings should be prepared for the visit with developmentally appropriate information and be given the opportunity to ask questions.

Altered Family Roles

In addition to the effects of separation on family roles, loss of parenting, sibling, and offspring roles may affect each family member differently. One of the most common reactions of parents is specialized and intensified attention toward the sick child. The other siblings may regard this as unfair and interpret the parents' attitude toward them as rejection. Although such responses are usually unconscious and unintended, they place unique burdens on ill children. For example, the ill child may feel obligated to play the sick role to meet parents' expectations, especially those children who have had limited physical ability and regain normal health status, such as after corrective heart surgery. Parents may be unable to perceive the child's recovery and thus continue the pattern of overprotection and indulgent attention.

Ill children may also feel jealousy and resentment from other siblings. Because of their singular position in the family, they may be denied the companionship of their brothers and sisters. Rivalry between siblings tends to be greatest for the sibling who is nearest in age to the ill child. Without an understanding of the interpersonal dynamics between siblings, parents are likely to blame the well children for antisocial behaviour. Illness may also result in children's loss of status within either their family or social group. For example, illness in the oldest child may temporarily terminate special privileges as "big" brother or sister.

Nursing Care of the Hospitalized Child

Preparation for Hospitalization

Children and families require individualized care to minimize the potential negative effects of hospitalization. One method that can decrease negative feelings and fear in children is preparing them for hospitalization. The rationale for preparing children for the hospital experience and related procedures is based on the principle that fear of the unknown (fantasy) exceeds fear of the known. When children do not have paralyzing fear to cope with, they are able to direct their energies toward dealing with the other, unavoidable stresses of hospitalization.

Although preparation for hospitalization is a common practice, there is no universal standard or program for all settings. The preparation process may be elaborate with tours, puppet shows, and playtime with miniature hospital equipment; it may involve the use of books, videos, or films; or it may be limited to a brief description of the major aspects of any hospital stay (Stewart, Algren, & Arnold, 1994). No consensus exists on the timing of preparation. Some authorities recommend preparing children 4 to 7 years of age about 1 week in advance so that they can assimilate the information and ask questions. For older children the time may be longer. However, for young children, who may begin to fantasize about what they observed, 1 or 2 days before admission is sufficient time for anticipatory preparation. The length of the session should be tailored to the children's attention span—the younger the child, the shorter the program. The optimal approach is one that is individualized for each child and family.

It is essential for families to prepare for the hospitalization as well as the child. Parents who are unsure or anxious about the hospital will transmit those emotions to the child. Nurses play an important role in helping children and families understand the reason for the hospitalization and what to expect during the admission. The families know their children best and, with the nurses' guidance, can help their children have a sense of mastery of their hospitalization by using their individual coping abilities. The Toronto Hospital for Sick Children's About Kids Web site has good information on the impact of hospitalization on children and families and how to cope positively with it (see Additional Resources section at the end of this chapter).

Regardless of the specific type of program, all children, even those who have been hospitalized before, benefit from an introduction to the environment and routine of the unit. Sometimes it is not possible to prepare the child, as in the event of sudden, acute illness or an accident. However, care should be taken to orient the child and family to hospital routines, establish expectations, and allow for questions.

NURSING ALERT In many hospitals, child life specialists—health care providers with extensive knowledge of child growth and development and of the special psychosocial needs of children who are hospitalized and their families—help prepare children for hospitalization, surgery, and procedures. A collaborative effort between the nurse, child life specialist, and other members of the child's health care team can help ensure the best possible hospital experience for the child and family.

Admission Assessment

The nursing admission history refers to a systematic collection of data about the child and family that allows the nurse to plan individualized care. The nursing admission history presented in Box 44-5 is organized according to the Functional Health Patterns outlined by Gordon (2002). This assessment framework is a guideline for formulating nursing diagnoses. One of the main purposes of the history is to assess the child's usual health habits at home to promote a more normal environment in the hospital. Therefore, questions related to activities of daily living in the nutrition–metabolic, elimination, sleep–rest, and activity–exercise patterns are a major part of the assessment. The questions found under the health perception–health management pattern are directed toward evaluation of the child's preparation for hospitalization and are key factors in determining whether additional preparation is needed. The questions included in the self-perception–self-concept and role–relationship patterns address the child's potential reaction to hospitalization, especially in terms of separation.

The nurse should also inquire about the use of any medications at home, including complementary medicine practices (Box 44-6), as the use of complementary and alternative medicine (CAM) has been increasing in popularity across Canada. A Health Canada (2012) survey identified that 73% of Canadians take natural health products (NHPs) such as vitamins and minerals, herbal products, and homeopathic medicines on a regular basis. The common CAMs in Canada include natural health products, homeopathy, traditional Chinese medicine, and chiropractic treatment. In a Calgary study, Gibbard (2005) found that parents were giving their autistic children CAM to try to decrease autistic symptoms. These CAMs included most commonly vitamins and minerals (63.1%), mind–body therapies (51.7%), and dietary-nutritional

BOX 44-5 Nursing Admission History According to Functional Health Patterns*

Health Perception—Health Management Pattern

Why has your child been admitted?

How has your child's general health been?

What does your child know about this hospitalization?

- Ask the child why he or she came to the hospital.
- If the answer is "For an operation or for tests," ask the child to tell you about what will happen before, during, and after the operation or tests.

Has your child ever been in the hospital before?

- How was that hospital experience?
- What things were important to you and your child during that hospitalization? How can we be most helpful now?

What medications does your child take at home?

- Why or when are they given?
- How are they given (if a liquid, with a spoon; if a tablet, swallowed with water; or other)?
- Does your child have any trouble taking medication? If so, what helps?
- Is your child allergic to any medications?

What, if any, forms of complementary medicine practices are being used?

Nutrition–Metabolic Pattern

What are the family's usual mealtimes?

Do family members eat together or at separate times?

What are your child's favourite foods, beverages, and snacks?

- Average amounts consumed or usual size of portions
- Special cultural practices, such as family eating only ethnic food

What foods and beverages does your child dislike?

What are your child's feeding habits (bottle, cup, spoon, eating by self, needing assistance, any special devices)?

How does your child like the food served (warmed, cold, one item at a time)?

How would you describe your child's usual appetite (hearty eater, picky eater)?

- Has being sick affected your child's appetite? In what ways?

Are there any known or suspected food allergies?

Is your child on a special diet?

Are there any feeding problems (excessive fussiness, spitting up, colic); any dental or gum problems that affect feeding?

- What do you do for these problems?

Elimination Pattern

What are your child's toilet habits (diaper, toilet trained—day only or day and night, use of word to communicate urination or defecation, potty chair, regular toilet, other routines)?

What is your child's usual pattern of elimination (bowel movements)?

Do you have any concerns about elimination (bed-wetting, constipation, diarrhea)?

- What do you do for these problems?

Have you ever noticed that your child sweats a lot?

Sleep–Rest Pattern

What is your child's usual hour of sleep and awakening?

What is your child's type of bed and schedule for naps; length of naps?

Is there a special routine before sleeping (bottle, drink of water, bedtime story, night-light, favourite blanket or toy, prayers)?

Is there a special routine during sleep time, such as waking to go to the bathroom?

Does your child have a separate room or share a room; if shares, with whom?

Does your child sleep with someone or alone (sibling, parent, other person)?

What is your child's favourite sleeping position?

Are there any sleeping problems (falling asleep, waking during night, nightmares, sleep walking)?

Are there any problems in awakening and getting ready in the morning?

- What do you do for these problems?

Activity–Exercise Pattern

What is your child's schedule during the day (preschool, day care centre, regular school, extracurricular activities)?

What are your child's favourite activities or toys (both active and quiet interests)?

What is your child's usual television-viewing schedule and restrictions? Favourite programs at home?

Does your child have any illness or disabilities that limit activity? If so, how?

What are your child's usual habits and schedule for bathing (bath in tub or shower, sponge bath, shampoo)?

What are your child's dental habits (brushing, flossing, fluoride supplements or rinses, favourite toothpaste); schedule of daily dental care?

Does your child need help with dressing or grooming, such as hair combing?

Are there any problems with these patterns (dislike of or refusal to bathe, shampoo hair, or brush teeth) and how do you manage them?

Are there special devices that your child requires help in managing (eyeglasses, contact lenses, hearing aid, orthodontic appliances, artificial elimination appliances, orthopaedic devices)?

Assess functional self-care level for feeding, bathing-hygiene, dressing-grooming, and toileting using the following guidelines: full self-care; requires use of equipment or device; requires assistance or supervision from another person; requires assistance or supervision from another person and equipment or device; is totally dependent and does not participate.

*The focus of the admission history is the child's psychosocial environment. Most of the questions are worded in terms of parental responses. Depending on the child's age, they should be addressed directly to the child when appropriate.

Continued

BOX 44-5 Nursing Admission History According to Functional Health Patterns—cont'd

Cognitive–Perceptual Pattern

Does your child have any hearing difficulty or use a hearing aid?
- Have "tubes" been placed in your child's ears?

Does your child have any vision problems and wear glasses or contact lenses?
Does your child have any learning difficulties?
What is the child's grade in school?

Self-Perception–Self-Concept Pattern

How would you describe your child (e.g., takes time to adjust, settles in easily, shy, friendly, quiet, talkative, serious, playful, stubborn, easygoing)?
What makes your child angry, annoyed, anxious, or sad? What helps when your child feels this way?
How does your child act when annoyed or upset?
What have been your child's experiences with and reactions to temporary separation from you (parent)?
Does your child have any fears (places, objects, animals, people, situations)?
- How do you handle them?

Do you think your child's illness has changed the way he or she thinks about self (e.g., more shy, embarrassed about appearance, less competitive with friends, stays at home more)?

Role–Relationship Pattern

Does your child have a favourite nickname?
What are the names of other family members or others who live in the home (relatives, friends, pets)?
Who usually takes care of your child during the day and night (especially if other than parent, such as babysitter, relative)?
What are the parents' occupations and work schedules?
Are there any special family considerations (adoption, foster child, step-parent, divorce, lone parent)?
Have any major changes in the family occurred lately (death, divorce, separation, birth of a sibling, loss of a job, financial strain, parent beginning a career, other)? Describe child's reaction.
Who are your child's play companions or social groups (peers, younger or older children, adults, prefers to be alone)?
Do things generally go well for your child in school or with friends?
Does your child have "security" objects at home (pacifier, bottle, blanket, stuffed animal, or doll)? Did you bring any of these to the hospital?
How do you handle discipline problems at home? Are these methods always effective?
Does your child have any condition that interferes with communication? If so, what are your suggestions for communicating with your child?
Will your child's hospitalization affect the family's financial support or care of other family members?
What concerns do you have about your child's illness and hospitalization?
Who will be staying with your child while hospitalized?
How can we contact you or another close family member outside the hospital?

Sexuality–Reproductive Pattern

(Answer questions that apply to your child's age group.)
Has your child begun puberty (developing physical sexual characteristics, menstruation)? Have you or your child had any concerns?
How have you approached topics of sexuality with your child?
Do you think you might need some help with some topics?
Has your child's illness affected the way he or she feels about being a boy or a girl? If so, how?
Do you have any concerns about behaviours of your child, such as masturbation, asking many questions or talking about sex, not respecting others' privacy, or wanting too much privacy?
Initiate a conversation about an adolescent's sexual concerns with open-ended to more direct questions and using the terms "friends" or "partners" rather than "girlfriend" or "boyfriend":
- Tell me about your social life.
- Who are your closest friends? (If one friend is identified, the nurse could ask more about that relationship, such as how much time they spend together, how serious they are about each other, if the relationship is going the way the teenager hoped.)
- Might ask about dating and sexual issues, such as the teenager's views on sexuality education, "going steady," "living together," or premarital sex.
- Which friends would you like to have visit in the hospital?

Coping–Stress Tolerance Pattern

(Answer questions that apply to your child's age group.)
What does your child do when tired or upset?
- If upset, does your child want a special person or object?
- If so, explain.

If your child has temper tantrums, what causes them and how do you handle them?
Whom does your child talk to when worried about something?
How does your child usually handle problems or disappointments?
Have there been any big changes or problems in your family recently? If so, how have you handled them?
Has your child ever had a problem with drugs or alcohol or tried to commit suicide?
Do you think your child is "accident prone"? If so, explain.

Value–Belief Pattern

What is your religion?
How is religion or faith important in your child's life?
What religious practices would you like continued in the hospital (e.g., prayers before meals or bedtime; visit by minister, priest, or rabbi; prayer group)?

BOX 44-6 Complementary Medicine Practices and Examples

Nutrition, diet, and lifestyle or behavioural health changes—Macrobiotics, megavitamins, diets, lifestyle modification, health risk reduction and health education, wellness
Mind–body control therapies—Biofeedback, relaxation, prayer therapy, guided imagery, hypnotherapy, music or sound therapy, massage, aromatherapy, education therapy
Traditional and ethnomedicine therapies—Acupuncture, ayurvedic medicine, herbal medicine, homeopathic medicine, Aboriginal medicine, natural products, traditional Asian medicine
Structural manipulation and energetic therapies—Acupressure, chiropractic medicine, massage, reflexology, rolfing, therapeutic touch, Qi Gong
Pharmacological and biological therapies—Antioxidants, cell treatment, chelation therapy, metabolic therapy, oxidizing agents
Bioelectromagnetic therapies—Diagnostic and therapeutic application of electromagnetic fields (e.g., transcranial electrostimulation, neuromagnetic stimulation, electroacupuncture)

therapies (45.5%). While CAM is used more in the adult than the pediatric population, no comprehensive data are available on Canadian usage by adults or children (Canadian Paediatric Society, 2005). The Canadian Paediatric Society (2005) has expressed concern about the lack of research on CAM in Canada in the pediatric population. Furthermore, potential problems with standardization of the products, accurate dosages, and potential drug and herbal interactions have been identified. Any adverse reaction to a natural health product needs to be reported to Health Canada (2011). It is also important that the use of any herbal or complementary therapy be noted in a preoperative assessment because of possible **anaesthesia** or surgical complications related to use of herbal products (Flanagan, 2001). For more information on natural health products, see the Additional Resources section at the end of this chapter.

After collecting the admission data, the nurse must apply the information to the nursing process and communicate it to other staff. Information gathered can offer insight into family dynamics, assist in normalization of the hospital environment, and aid staff members in meeting the child and family's needs. Asking questions and seeking information directly from the child in an age-appropriate manner can yield a wealth of information on his or her understanding of the illness and hospitalization.

Besides completing the nursing admission history, nurses should also perform a physical assessment (see Chapter 34) before planning care. At the very least, the nurse's physical assessment of the child should include observation of the body for any bruises, rashes, signs of neglect, deformities, or physical limitations. The nurse should also listen to the heart and lungs to assess overall physical status to provide baseline data. It is important for nurses to be on alert for any signs of maltreatment, which must be reported to child authorities.

Preparing the Child for Admission

The preparation that children require on the day of admission depends on the kind of prehospital counselling they have received. If they have been prepared in a formalized program, they will usually know what to expect in terms of initial medical procedures, inpatient facilities, and nursing staff. However, prehospital counselling does not preclude the need for support during procedures such as obtaining blood specimens, x-ray tests, or physical examinations. For example, undressing young children before they feel comfortable in their new surroundings can be upsetting to them. Causing needless anxiety and fear during admission may adversely affect the nurse's establishment of trust with these children. Nursing assistance during the admission procedure is vital, regardless of how well prepared any child is for the experience of hospitalization. Spending this time with the child gives the nurse an opportunity to evaluate the child's understanding of subsequent procedures (Fig. 44-4). Ideally, a primary nurse would be assigned, to allow for individualized care and provide a substitute support person for the child.

When a child is admitted, nurses need to follow admission procedures (Box 44-7). One particularly important decision is room assignment. The minimum considerations for room assignment are age, sex, and nature of the illness. No absolute rules govern room selection, but, in general, placing children of the same age group and with similar types of illness in the same room is both psychologically and medically

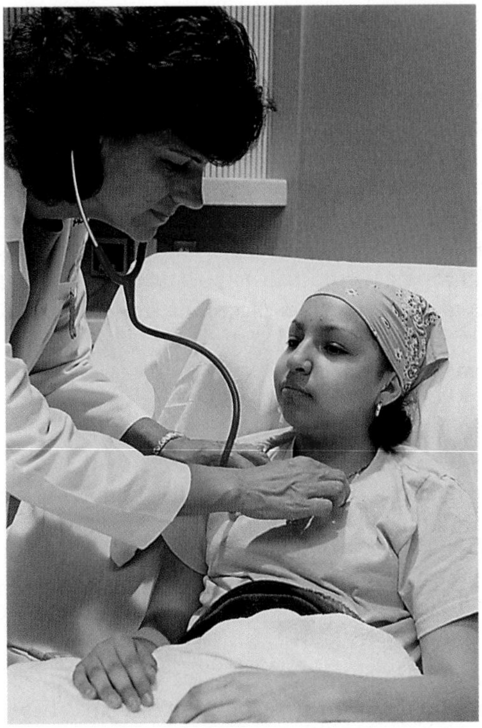

Fig. 44-4 The initial admission procedures give the nurse an opportunity to get to know the child and to assess the child's understanding of the hospital experience.

evolve Skill—Admitting a Child to the Health Care System

BOX 44-7 Guidelines for Admission

Preadmission

Assign a room based on developmental age, seriousness of diagnosis, communicability of illness, and projected length of stay.

Prepare roommate(s) for the arrival of a new patient; when children are too young to benefit from this consideration, prepare parents.

Prepare room for child and family, with admission forms and equipment nearby to eliminate need to leave child.

Admission

Introduce primary nurse to child and family.

Orient child and family to inpatient facilities, especially to the assigned room and unit; emphasize positive areas of pediatric unit.

- **Room**—Explain call light, bed controls, television, bathroom, telephone, etc.
- **Unit**—Direct to playroom, desk, dining area, or other areas.

Introduce family to roommate and his or her parents.

Apply identification band to child's wrist, ankle, or both (if not already done).

Explain hospital regulations and schedules (e.g., visiting hours, mealtimes, bedtime, limitations [give written information if available]).

Perform nursing admission history (see Box 44-5).

Take vital signs, blood pressure, height, and weight.

Obtain specimens as needed and order needed laboratory work.

Support child and assist practitioner with physical examination (for purposes of nursing assessment).

advantageous. However, there are many exceptions. For example, a child who is independent despite physical disabilities may help another child with similar or different limitations, and the parents of the child with disabilities may achieve deeper insight and acceptance of their child's disorder.

Age-grouping is especially important for adolescents. Many hospitals make an effort to place teenagers on their own unit or in a separate, designated section of the pediatric or general unit whenever possible.

Nursing Interventions

Prevent or Minimize Separation

Many hospitals work within a system of family-centred care. This philosophy of care recognizes the integral role of the family in a child's life and acknowledges the family as an essential part of the child's care and illness experience. The family is considered a partner in the child's care (Smith & Conant Rees, 2000) (see Chapter 29). Family-centred care also supports the family by respecting the individual needs of the child and the family and establishing priorities based on the needs and values of the family unit (About Kids Health, 2009; Lewandowski & Tesler, 2003). Consequently, hospitals' policies reflect a changed attitude toward parents; many hospitals no longer consider parents "visitors" and welcome their presence at all times throughout the child's hospitalization. Many hospitals provide facilities such as a chair or bed for at least one person per child, unit kitchen privileges, and other amenities that create a welcoming atmosphere for parents. However, not all hospitals provide such amenities, and parents' own schedules may prevent rooming-in. In such instances, strategies to minimize the effects of separation must be implemented.

A primary nursing goal is to prevent separation anxiety, particularly in children younger than 5 years of age. Nurses must have an appreciation of the child's separation behaviours. The child should be allowed to cry. Even if the child rejects strangers, the nurse can provide support through physical presence. *Presence* is defined as spending time being physically close to the child while using a quiet tone of voice, appropriate choice of words, eye contact, and touch in ways that establish rapport and communicate empathy. If behaviours of detachment are evident, the nurse should maintain the child's contact with the parents by frequently talking about them; encouraging the child to remember them; and stressing the significance of their visits, telephone calls, or letters. The use of cellular phones and personal tablets can increase the contact between the hospitalized child and parents or other significant family members and friends but may not be compatible with medical equipment.

Separation may be equally difficult for parents, especially when they do not understand the behaviours of separation anxiety. To avoid the immediate protest, parents may sneak out or lie to the child about leaving. As a result, instead of learning that absence is associated with a guaranteed return, the child learns that absence means loss of parents. Helping parents recognize that separation behaviours are normal and expected can decrease the parents' anxiety and may ease their fears about leaving their child. Explaining to parents how the child reacts after they leave may also be helpful. Many parents imagine that the child cries for hours after they leave, whereas in reality the child may cry for a few minutes but settle down when comforted by someone else.

Toddlers and preschoolers have a limited concept of time. Time is measured in associations, such as eating dinner "when Daddy comes home." Therefore, when helping parents with children's fears of separation, nurses need to suggest ways of explaining leaving and returning. For example, if parents must leave to go to work or to make meals for other family members, they should tell the child the reason for leaving. They also need to convey the expected time of return in terms of anticipated events. For example, if the parents will return in the morning, they can say to the child, "We'll see you after the sun comes up" or "We'll come back when [a favourite program] is on television."

The young child's ability to tolerate parental absence is limited. Thus parental visits should be frequent (e.g., visiting three times a day for short periods rather than once a day for an extended time). This may necessitate that each parent visit at different times in order to lessen the length of separation. When parents cannot visit, the presence of other significant people can be most comforting for the child (Fig. 44-5).

If parents leave after the child is asleep, they still need to communicate their absence. The parents of a 5-year-old boy

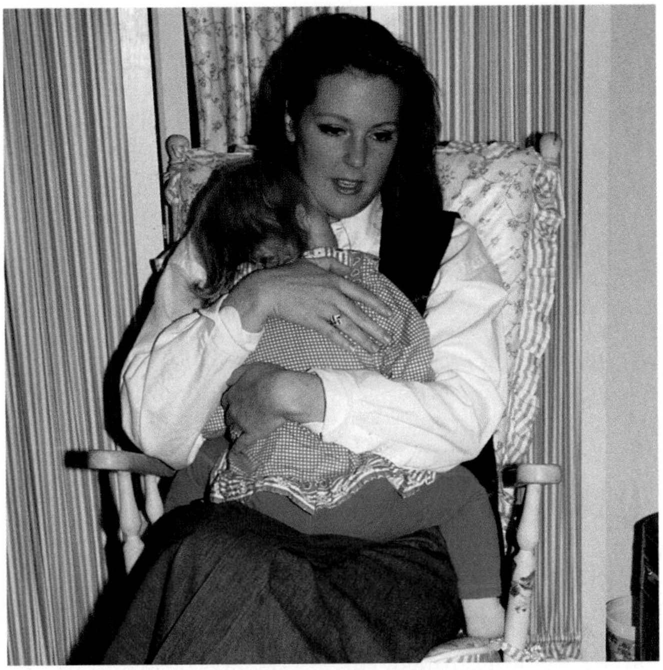

Fig. 44-5 When parents cannot visit, other significant persons can provide comfort to the hospitalized child.

solved this problem by devising a sign; on one side they drew a picture of a telephone, and on the other they drew a hamburger. Before they left, they turned the sign to the appropriate side to tell the child when he awoke that they were out using the telephone or eating.

Older children who know how to tell time may find it helpful to have a clock or watch. However, these children have the same need for honesty from their parents regarding visiting schedules. For adolescents, peer groups are important, thus they often appreciate planning visiting hours with their parents to ensure that they have some private time for friends.

Familiar surroundings also increase the child's adjustment to separation. If parents cannot stay with the child, they should leave favourite articles from home with the child, such as a blanket, toy, bottle, feeding utensil, or article of clothing. Because young children associate such inanimate objects with significant people, they gain comfort and reassurance from these possessions. They make the association that if the parents left this, the parents will surely return. Placing an identification band on the toy lessens the chances of its being misplaced and provides a symbol that the toy is experiencing the same needs as the child. Other mementos of home include photographs, audio or video recordings, or live video online streaming of family members reading a story, singing a song, saying prayers before bedtime, relating events at home, or taking a "talking walk" through the home. The recordings can be played at lonely times, such as on awakening or before sleeping. Some units allow pets to visit, which can have therapeutic benefits for a child. Animals should be carefully screened for medical or behavioural problems, and patients should be screened for allergies.

Older children also appreciate familiar articles from home, particularly photographs, a radio or MP3 player, a favourite toy or game, and their own pyjamas. Often the importance of treasured objects to school-age children is overlooked or criticized. However, many school-age children have a special object to which they formed an attachment in early childhood. Such treasured or transitional objects can help even older children feel more comfortable in a strange environment.

The strange sights, smells, and sounds in the hospital that are commonplace for the nurse can be frightening and confusing for children. It is important for the nurse to try to evaluate stimuli in the environment from the child's point of view (considering also what the child may see or hear happening to other patients) and to make every effort to protect the child from frightening and unfamiliar sights, sounds, and equipment. The nurse should offer explanations or prepare the child for those experiences that are unavoidable. Combining familiar or comforting sights with the unfamiliar can relieve much of the harshness of medical equipment.

Helping children maintain their usual contacts also minimizes the effects of separation imposed by hospitalization. This includes continuing school lessons during the illness and confinement, visiting with friends either directly or through e-mail, text messaging, or telephone calls, and participating in stimulating projects whenever possible (Fig. 44-6). For extended hospitalizations, youngsters enjoy personalizing the hospital room to make it "home" by decorating the walls with posters and cards, rearranging the furniture (when possible), and displaying a collection or hobby.

Minimize Loss of Control

Feelings of loss of control result from separation, physical restriction, changed routines, enforced dependency, and magical thinking. Although some of these cannot be prevented, most can be minimized through individualized planning of nursing care.

Promote Freedom of Movement

Younger children react most strenuously to any type of physical restriction or immobilization. Although temporary

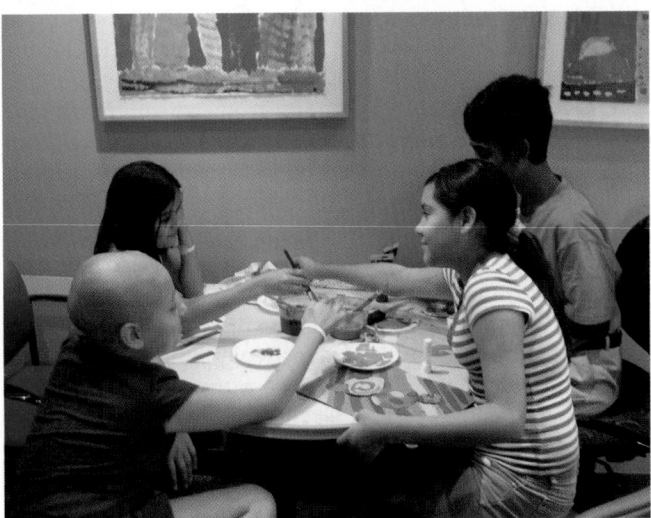

Fig. 44-6 For extended hospitalizations children enjoy having projects with other patients to occupy time.

immobilization may be necessary for some interventions such as maintaining an intravenous line, most physical restriction can be prevented if the nurse and child work together.

For young children, particularly infants and toddlers, preserving parent–child contact is the best means of decreasing the need for or stress of restraint. For example, almost the entire physical examination can be done with the child in a parent's lap, with the parent hugging the child for procedures such as otoscopy. For painful procedures, the nurse should assess the parents' preferences for assisting, observing, or waiting outside the room.

Environmental factors may also restrict movement. Keeping children in cribs or playpens may not represent immobilization in a concrete sense, but it certainly limits sensory stimulation. Increasing mobility by transporting children in carriages, wheelchairs, carts, or wagons provides them with a sense of freedom.

In some cases, physical restraint or isolation is necessary because of the child's medical diagnosis. In these cases, the environment can be altered to increase sensory freedom (e.g., moving the bed toward the window; opening window shades; providing musical, visual, or tactile activities).

Maintain the Child's Routine

Altered daily schedules and loss of rituals are particularly stressful for toddlers and early preschoolers and may increase the stress of separation. The nursing admission history will provide a baseline for planning care around the child's usual home activities. A nonhospitalized child's day, especially during the school years, is structured with specific times for eating, dressing, going to school, playing, and sleeping. However, this time structure vanishes when the child is hospitalized. Although nurses have a set schedule, the child is frequently unaware of it, and the new schedules that are imposed may be rigid. For example, some units have uniform nap times and bedtimes for all children, whereas others allow children to stay up late at night. Many children obtain significantly less sleep in the hospital than at home; the primary causes are delay in sleep onset and early termination of sleep because of hospital routines. Not only are hours of sleep disrupted, but waking hours are spent in passive activities. For example, few institutions impose any limits on the amount of time the child spends watching television, which can delay the onset of sleep.

One technique that can minimize the disruption in the child's routine is establishing a daily schedule. This approach is most suitable for the non–critically ill school-age or adolescent child who has mastered the concept of time. It involves scheduling the child's day to include all those activities that are important to the child and nurse, such as treatment procedures, schoolwork, exercise, television, playroom, and hobbies. Together, the nurse, parent, and child can then plan a daily schedule with times and activities written down (Fig. 44-7) and left in the child's room, with a clock or watch. Whenever possible, a calendar should also be constructed with special events marked, such as favourite television programs, visits by friends or relatives, events in the playroom, and holidays or birthdays. If specific changes in treatment are expected (e.g., "beginning physiotherapy in 2 days"), these can be added.

Eric's Daily Schedule

7:30 AM	– Breakfast, morning bath	3:00 PM	– Tutor (M, W, F)
			– Study time (T, Th)
9:00	– Medications, dressing change	4:00	– Physical therapy
		5:30	– Dinner
11:00	– Physical therapy	9:00	– Medications, dressing change
12:00 PM	– Lunch		
		9:15	– Bedtime

Fig. 44-7 Time structuring is an effective strategy for normalizing the hospital environment and increasing the child's sense of control.

Encourage Independence

The dependent role of the hospitalized patient imposes tremendous feelings of loss on older children. Principal interventions should focus on respect for individuality and the opportunity for decision making. Nurses who are flexible and tolerant can foster patient empowerment.

Enabling children's control involves helping them maintain independence and promoting the concept of self-care. *Self-care* refers to the practice of activities that individuals personally initiate and perform on their own behalf in maintaining life, health, and well-being (Orem, 2001). Although self-care is limited by the child's age and physical condition, most children beyond infancy can perform some activities with little or no help in the hospital. Other approaches include jointly planning care, time structuring, having the child wear street clothes and make choices in food selections and bedtime, continuing school activities, and placing the child in a room with an appropriate age-mate.

Promote Understanding

Loss of control can occur from feelings of having too little influence on one's destiny or from sensing overwhelming control or power over one's fate. Although preschoolers' cognitive abilities predispose them most to magical thinking and delusions of power, all children are vulnerable to misinterpreting causes for stresses such as illness and hospitalization.

Most children feel more in control when they know what to expect, since the element of fear is reduced. Anticipatory preparation and provision of information can help to lessen stress and increase understanding (see Preparation for Diagnostic and Therapeutic Procedures, Chapter 45).

Informing children of their rights while they are hospitalized fosters greater understanding and may relieve some of the feelings of powerlessness they typically experience. Hospitals providing services to children should have a hospital-wide policy on the rights and responsibilities of these patients and of their parents or guardians. The Canadian Institute of Child Health (2002) has developed the Rights of the Child in the Health Care System (Box 44-8).

An increasing number of hospitals and organizations have developed "family rights and responsibilities" that are prominently displayed throughout the hospital or are presented in written form to children and their families on admission (Box 44-9).

evolve Skill–Preparing the Child for Surgery

BOX 44-8 The Rights of the Child in the Health Care System

The Rights of the Child in the Health Care System, which were developed by the Canadian Institute of Child Health, are based on the United Nations Convention on the Rights of the Child and are listed below:

- Right to live and to have my pain and suffering treated, regardless of my age, gender, or income
- Right to be viewed first as a child, then as a patient
- Right to be treated as an unique individual with my own abilities, culture, and language
- Right not be afraid and to cry when I feel hurt
- Right to be safe in an environment that is unfamiliar to me
- Right to ask questions and receive answers that I can understand
- Right to be cared for by people who perceive and meet my needs even though I may be unable to explain what they are
- Right to speak for myself when I am able and to have someone speak on my behalf when I am unable
- Right to have those dear to me close by when I need them
- Right to play and learn even if I am receiving care
- Need to have rights fulfilled

(Adapted from the Canadian Institute of Child Health. [2002]. *The rights of the child in the health care system* [pamphlet]. Retrieved from http://www.sickkids.ca/visitingsickkids/values-and-expectations/index.html.)

Prevent or Minimize Fear of Bodily Injury

Beyond early infancy, all children fear bodily injury from mutilation, bodily intrusion, body-image change, disability, or death. In general, preparation of children for painful procedures decreases their fears and increases the child's ability to cooperate. Manipulating procedural techniques for children in each age group also minimizes the fear of bodily injury. For example, because toddlers and young preschoolers are traumatized by insertion of a rectal thermometer, axillary temperatures or temperatures taken with electronic or tympanic membrane devices can effectively be substituted. Whenever procedures are performed on young children, the most supportive intervention is to do the procedure as quickly as possible while maintaining parent–child contact.

Because of toddler and preschool children's poorly defined body boundaries, the use of bandages may be particularly helpful. For example, telling children that the bleeding will stop after the needle is removed does little to relieve their fears, whereas applying a small Band-Aid usually reassures them. The size of bandages is also significant to children in this age group; the larger the bandage, the more importance is attached to the wound. Watching their surgical dressings become successively smaller is one way young children can measure healing and improvement. Prematurely removing a dressing may cause these children considerable concern for their well-being. Specific pain management strategies are discussed in Chapter 35.

For children who fear mutilation of body parts, it is essential that the nurse repeatedly stress the reason for a procedure and evaluate their understanding. For example, explaining cast removal to preschoolers may seem simple enough, but children's comprehension of the details may vary considerably. Asking them to draw a picture of what they think will happen presents substantial evidence of how they perceive events.

Children may fear bodily injury from a great variety of sources. Imaging machines, strange equipment used for examination, unfamiliar rooms, or awkward positions can be perceived as potentially hazardous. In addition, thoughts and actions can be imagined sources of bodily damage. Therefore, it is important to investigate imagined reasons, particularly of a sexual nature, for illness. Because children may fear revealing such thoughts, using techniques such as drawing or doll play may elicit previously undisclosed misconceptions.

Older children fear bodily injury of both internal and external origins. For example, school-age children are aware of the significance of the heart and may fear the actual operation as much as the pain, the stitches, and the possible scar. Adolescents may express concern about the actual procedure but be much more anxious over the resulting scar.

Children can grasp information only if it is presented on or close to their level of cognitive development. This requires an awareness of the words used to describe events or processes. For example, young children told that they are going to have a CAT (i.e., CT, computed tomography) scan may wonder, "Will there be cats? Or something that scratches?" It is clearer to describe the procedure in simple terms and explain what the letters of the common name stand for. Therefore, to prevent or alleviate fears, nurses must be keenly aware of the medical terminology and vocabulary that they use every day.

When children are upset about their illness, their perception can be changed by (1) providing a somewhat different and less negative account of the disease or (2) offering an explanation that is characteristic of the next stage of cognitive development. An example of the first strategy is reassuring a preschooler who fears that, after a tonsillectomy, another sore throat means a second operation. Explaining that after tonsils are "fixed" they do not need fixing again can help relieve the fear. An example of the latter strategy is to explain that germs made the tonsils sick, and even though germs can cause another sore throat, they cannot cause the tonsils to ever be sick again. This higher-level explanation is based on the school-age child's concept of germs as a cause of disease.

Provide Developmentally Appropriate Activities

A primary goal of nursing care for the child who is hospitalized is to minimize threats to the child's development. Children who experience prolonged or repeated hospitalization are at greater risk for developmental delays or regression. The nurse who provides opportunities for the child to participate in developmentally appropriate activities further normalizes the child's environment and helps reduce interference with the child's development.

Interference with normal development may have long-term implications for the infant and toddler. The nurse can play a primary role in identifying children at risk and helping to plan, implement, and evaluate developmental interventions.

BOX 44-9 What You Value and What You Expect From Us at SickKids

You are important to us, and we remain committed to supporting you as a patient or family member. We will attempt to follow your values and meet your expectations.

Respect:

At SickKids, we value the knowledge you share with us. We take the choices and decisions you make very seriously. We protect your privacy. We are courteous and respectful. We are sensitive and responsive to your beliefs, culture and background.

Understanding:

At SickKids, we treat you as a whole person. We provide comfort and care to support your physical, social, emotional, learning, and developmental needs.

Communication:

At SickKids, we take the time to listen to you. We respond thoughtfully to your concerns. We explain information fully and clearly so you can make informed choices. We take into account your language and special communication needs.

Accountability:

At SickKids, we strive to provide high-quality, safe, child and family-centred care. We engage you as a partner in care. We use publicly funded resources appropriately and effectively.

Flexibility:

At SickKids, we work creatively to accommodate your needs. We try to prevent changes to your schedule and appointments, and we provide an explanation if changes occur.

Transparency:

At SickKids, we identify the members of your healthcare team for you and how they are involved in your care. We provide you with access to your health record. We tell you in advance if you have to pay for any expenses.

What we at SickKids value and what we expect from you:

Engagement:

At SickKids, you continue to provide comfort and support as a family in the special ways that only families can. You strive to attend your appointments, and you inform us of any changes to your schedule. You listen openly to the information provided by your healthcare team.

Speaking up:

At SickKids, you ask questions when you do not understand. You share your concerns with us. You let us know how we can improve the quality of care at SickKids.

Respect:

At SickKids, you treat staff, volunteers, other patients, and families with understanding and dignity. You follow hospital rules, and you treat hospital property with care.

Understanding:

At SickKids, you try to be flexible and understand that not all answers can be provided right away. You acknowledge the important role that SickKids has in research and education. You help contribute to the experiences of students and learners.

(From Hospital for Sick Children. [n.d.] *Values and Expectations.* Toronto, ON: Author. Retrieved from http://www.sickkids.ca/VisitingSickKids/values-and-expectations/index.html.)

School is an integral part of the school-age child's and adolescent's development. Accreditation standards for hospitals serving children consider access to appropriate educational services a key factor in accreditation when a child's treatment requires a significant absence from school (Accreditation Canada, 2010). The nurse can encourage children to resume schoolwork as their condition permits, help them schedule time for studies, and help the family coordinate hospital educational services with their children's schools. Children should have the opportunity to continue art and music classes, as well.

To meet the unique developmental needs of adolescents, special units may be designated that provide both privacy and increased socialization, and appropriate activities. Teenagers should not share space with younger children, who are often perceived as a threat to their maturity.

In caring for the adolescent patient, it is essential to provide flexible routines and activities, such as more group activity, wearing of street clothes, and access to the items so critical to adolescents—telephones (including cellular phones), MP3 players, DVD players, computers, personal tablets, e-mail, video games, and televisions. Because adolescents' food habits are rarely limited to the three traditional meals a day, a ready supply of snacks should be available. However, the most important benefit of these units is increased socialization with peers.

Although regression is expected and normal for all age groups, nurses have the responsibility for fostering the child's growth and development. Hospitalization can become a significant opportunity for learning and advancing. Extended hospitalizations for long-term chronic illness or situations of failure to thrive, abuse, or neglect represent instances in which regression must be seen as an adjustment period, to be followed by plans for promoting appropriate developmental skills.

Provide Opportunities for Play and Expressive Activities

Play is one of the most important aspects of a child's life and an effective tool for managing stress. Because illness and hospitalization constitute crises in a child's life and often involve overwhelming stresses, children need to act out their fears and anxieties as a means of coping with these stresses. As with their other developmental needs, play does not stop when children are ill or in the hospital. On the contrary, play in the hospital serves many functions, including to promote well-being (Box 44-10). Of all hospital facilities, no room alleviates the stressors of hospitalization more than the playroom. In the playroom, children temporarily distance themselves from their illness, hospitalization, and the associated stressors. This room should be a safe haven for children, free from medical or nursing procedures, strange faces, and probing questions. The playroom then becomes a sanctuary in an otherwise frightening environment.

Engaging in play activities also gives children a sense of control. In the hospital environment, most decisions are made for the child; play and other expressive activities offer the child opportunities to make choices for themselves. Even if a child chooses not to participate in a particular activity, the nurse has offered the child a choice, perhaps one of only a few real choices the child has had that day.

A multidisciplinary team often works together to help children and their families adapt and cope with hospitalization. Nurses may play a key role in coordinating the various team member roles. For instance, play therapy can be provided by child life specialists and nurses, with both working together to provide this therapeutic outlet. Art and music therapy are used as well in encouraging creativity and relaxation.

The hospitalized child typically has lower energy levels than those of healthy children of the same age. Hospitalized children may not appear engaged and enthusiastic about an activity, even though they are enjoying the experience. Activities may need to be adjusted or limited according to the child's age, endurance, and special needs.

Diversional Activities

Almost any form of play can be used for diversion and recreation, but the activity should be selected on the basis of the child's age, interests, and limitations (Fig. 44-8). Children do not necessarily need special direction for using play materials. Small children enjoy a variety of small, colourful toys that they can play with in bed or in their room, or more elaborate play equipment, such as playhouses, sandboxes, rhythm instruments, or large boxes and blocks, that may be a part of the hospital playroom.

Games that can be played alone or with another child or an adult are popular with older children, as are puzzles; reading material; quiet, individual activities, such as sewing, stringing beads, and weaving; and Lego blocks and other building materials. Assembling models is an excellent pastime. Well-selected books are of infinite value to the child. Children never tire of stories; having someone read aloud to them gives them much pleasure and is of special value to the child who has limited energy to expend in play. A radio, MP3 player, tablet computer, electronic games, and television are useful tools for entertaining a child. Computers with access to the Internet can provide diversion, educational opportunities, and online support groups.

When supervising play for ill or convalescent children, it is best to select activities that are simpler than would normally be chosen for the child's specific developmental level. These children usually do not have the energy to cope with more challenging activities. Other limitations also influence the type of activities. Special consideration must be given to the child who is confined in terms of movement, has a restricted extremity, or is isolated. Toys for isolated children must be disposable or need to be disinfected after every use. Toys that are not able to be disinfected (e.g., stuffed animals) cannot be used as community toys.

Toys

Parents of hospitalized children often ask nurses about the types of toys that would be best to bring for their child. Although parents often want to buy new toys for the hospitalized child to offer cheer and comfort, it is often better to wait to bring new things, especially in the case of younger children. Small children need the comfort and reassurance of familiar things, such as the stuffed animal that the child hugs and takes to bed at night. These familiar items are a link with home and the world outside the hospital. All toys brought into the hospital should be assessed for safety.

Large numbers of toys often confuse and frustrate a small child. A few small, well-chosen toys are usually preferred to one large, expensive one. Children who are hospitalized for an extended time benefit from changes in toys. Rather than a confusing accumulation of toys, older toys should be replaced periodically as interest wanes.

evolve Skill—Therapeutic Play

BOX 44-10 Functions of Play in the Hospital

- Provides diversion and brings about relaxation
- Helps the child feel more secure in a strange environment
- Lessens the stress of separation and the feeling of homesickness
- Provides a means for release of tension and expression of feelings
- Encourages interaction and development of positive attitudes toward others
- Provides an expressive outlet for creative ideas and interests
- Provides a means for accomplishing therapeutic goals (see Use of Play in Procedures, Chapter 45)
- Places child in active role and provides an opportunity to make choices and be in control

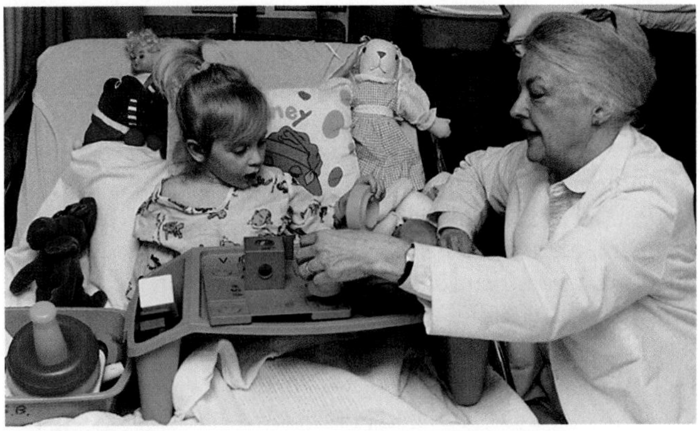

Fig. 44-8 Play materials for children in the hospital need to be appropriate for their age, interests, and limitations.

NURSING ALERT Have parents provide the child with a shoe box, a child's small suitcase, or a backpack to attach to the bed for an easy storage receptacle to prevent small items from becoming lost.

A highly successful diversion for a child who is hospitalized is having the parents bring a box with several small, inexpensive, brightly wrapped items with a different day of the week printed on the outside of each package. The child will eagerly anticipate the time for opening each one. If the parents know when their next visit will be, they can provide the number of packages that corresponds to the time between visits. In this way the child knows that the diminishing packages also represent the anticipated visit from the parent.

Expressive Activities

Play and other expressive activities provide one of the best opportunities for encouraging emotional expression, including the safe release of anger and hostility. Nondirective play that allows children freedom for expression can be tremendously therapeutic. **Therapeutic play** should not be confused with play therapy, a psychological technique reserved for use by trained and qualified therapists as an interpretative method with emotionally disturbed children. Therapeutic play, by contrast, is an effective, nondirective modality for helping children deal with their concerns and fears; at the same time it often helps the nurse gain insights into children's needs and feelings.

Tension release can be facilitated through almost any activity; with younger ambulatory children, large-muscle activity through use of tricycles and wagons is beneficial. Much aggression can be safely directed into pounding and throwing games or activities. Beanbags are often thrown at a target or open receptacle with surprising vigour and hostility. A pounding board can be a favourite item for young children; clay and Play-Doh are beneficial for use at any age.

Creative Expression

Although all children derive physical, social, emotional, and cognitive benefits from engaging in art or other creative activities, children's need for such activities is intensified when they are hospitalized. Drawing and painting are excellent media for expression (Fig. 44-9). Children are more at ease expressing their thoughts and feelings through art, since humans think first in images and later learn to translate these images into words. Children can work individually or work together on a group project, such as a mural painted on a long piece of paper.

Although interpretation of children's drawing requires special training, observing changes in a series of the child's drawings over time can be helpful in assessing psychosocial adjustment and coping. The nurse can use children's drawings, stories, poetry, and other products of creative expression as a springboard for discussion of thoughts, fears, and understanding of concepts or events (see Communication Techniques, Chapter 34). A child's drawing before surgery, for example, may reveal unvoiced concerns about mutilation, body changes, and loss of self-control.

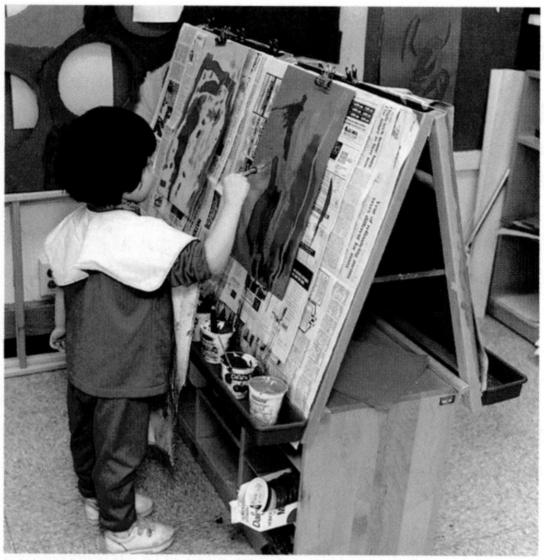

Fig. 44-9 Drawing and painting are excellent media for expression.

Nurses can incorporate opportunities for musical expression into routine nursing care. For example, simple musical instruments, such as bracelets with bells, can be placed on infants' legs for them to shake to accompany mealtime music or dressing changes. The nurse can suggest dance or movement to encourage a child to ambulate.

Holidays provide stimulus and direction for unlimited creative projects. Children can participate in decorating the pediatric unit, giving them a sense of pride and accomplishment, particularly if they are immobilized and isolated. Making gifts for someone at home helps to maintain interpersonal ties.

Dramatic Play

Dramatic play is a well-recognized technique for emotional release, allowing children to re-enact frightening or puzzling hospital experiences. Through the use of puppets, replicas of hospital equipment, or some actual hospital equipment, children can act out the situations that are a part of their hospital experience. Dramatic play enables children to learn about procedures and events that concern them and to assume the roles of the adults in the hospital environment.

Puppets are universally effective for communicating with children. Most children see them as peers and readily communicate with them. Children will tell the puppet feelings that they hesitate to express to adults. Puppets can share children's own experiences and help them find solutions to their problems. Puppets dressed to represent figures in the child's environment—for example, a physician, nurse, child patient, therapist, and members of the child's own family—are especially useful. Small, appropriately attired dolls are equally effective in encouraging the child to play out situations, although puppets are usually best for direct conversation.

NURSING ALERT Make a simple puppet using a large handkerchief. Place some cotton balls in the centre of the cloth and wrap a rubber band over the handkerchief and cotton balls to form a "head." Place the head over the index finger with the rubber band securing it to the finger. Let the cloth drape over the front and back of the hand. The cloth forms four parts of the puppet: the index finger is the head, the thumb and other fingers are the arms, and the draped cloth is the body. Decorate the head by drawing features on it.

When choosing play for a child, medical needs must be considered, but at times a procedure can be postponed briefly to allow the child to complete a special activity (see Critical Thinking Exercise). In addition, any limitations imposed by the child's condition need to be taken into account. At home the play program can be planned around the therapy regimen. Play can be satisfactorily incorporated into the child's care if the nurse and others involved allow some flexibility and use creativity in planning for play.

Maximize Potential Benefits of Hospitalization

Although hospitalization generally represents a stressful time for children and families, it also represents an opportunity for facilitating positive change within the child and among family members. For some families the stress of a child's illness, hospitalization, or both can lead to strengthening of family coping behaviours and the emergence of new coping strategies.

Foster Parent–Child Relationships

The crisis of illness or hospitalization can mobilize parents into more acute awareness of their child's needs. For example, hospitalization provides opportunities for parents to learn more about their children's growth and development. When parents are helped to understand children's usual reactions to stress, such as regression or aggression, they are not only better able to support the child through the hospital experience but also may extend their insights after discharge.

Difficulties in parent–child relationships that existed before hospitalization that are characterized by feeding problems, negative behaviour, and sleep disturbances may decrease during hospitalization. The temporary cessation of such problems sometimes alerts parents to the role they may be playing in promoting the negative behaviour. With assistance from health care providers, parents can restructure ways of relating to their children to foster more positive behaviour.

Hospitalization may also represent a temporary reprieve or refuge from a disturbed home. Typically, abused or neglected children's dramatic physical and social improvement during hospitalization is proof of the benefits and potential growth that can occur during such times. These children temporarily are able to seek support, reassurance, and security from new relationships, particularly with nurses and hospitalized peers.

Provide Educational Opportunities

Illness and hospitalization represent excellent opportunities for children and other family members to learn more about their bodies, each other, and the health professions. For example, during a hospital admission for a diabetic crisis, the child may learn about the disease; the parents may learn about the child's needs for independence, normalcy, and appropriate limits; and each of them may find a new support system in the hospital staff.

Illness or hospitalization can also help older children in choosing a career. Frequently, children have impressions of physicians or nurses that are disproportionately positive or negative. Actual experience with different health care providers can influence their attitude about these professions and even a decision regarding a career in health care.

Promote Self-Mastery

The experience of facing a crisis such as illness or hospitalization, coping successfully with it, and maturing as a result of it constitutes an opportunity for self-mastery. Younger children have the chance to test fantasy versus reality of their fears. They realize that they were not abandoned, mutilated, or punished. In fact, they were loved, cared for, and treated with respect for their individual concerns. It is not unusual for children who have undergone hospitalization or surgery to tell others that "it was nothing" or to display proudly their scars or bandages. For older children, hospitalization may represent an opportunity for decision making, independence, and self-reliance. They are proud of having survived the experience and may feel a genuine self-respect for their achievements. Nurses can facilitate such feelings of self-mastery by emphasizing aspects of personal competence in the child and not focusing on negative behaviour.

Provide Socialization

Hospitalization may offer children a special opportunity for social acceptance. Lonely, asocial, and even delinquent children find a sympathetic environment in the hospital. Children who have a physical handicap or are in some other way "different" from their age-mates may find an accepting social peer group (Fig. 44-10). Although this does not always spontaneously occur, nurses can structure the environment to foster a supportive child group. For example, selection of a compatible

CRITICAL THINKING EXERCISE

Playroom and Hospital Procedures

Hannah, a 7-year-old with cystic fibrosis, has been hospitalized numerous times with complications from the condition. She is playing Candyland with her brother, sister, and several other children in the playroom on the pediatric unit. A pediatric phlebotomist enters the playroom and says, "Hannah, I need to take some blood. I can see that you are playing a game, so I'll just do it while you play. It will just take a minute." Hannah nods her head indicating that she agrees to let the phlebotomist draw the blood at this time. The playroom is usually off-limits for invasive procedures. As Hannah's nurse, you are aware that Dr. Lung wants the results of the laboratory studies as soon as possible to make a decision about her course of therapy.

1. Evidence—Is there sufficient evidence to draw any conclusions about this situation at this time?
2. Assumptions—What are some underlying assumptions about the following?
   a. Children and painful procedures such as venipunctures
   b. The function of play for a hospitalized child
   c. The priority in performing the procedure
   d. Implications of performing the procedure in the playroom
3. What implications and priorities for nursing care can be drawn at this time (i.e., what will you do)?
4. Does the evidence objectively support your argument (conclusion)?
5. Are there alternative perspectives to your conclusions? If so, what are they?

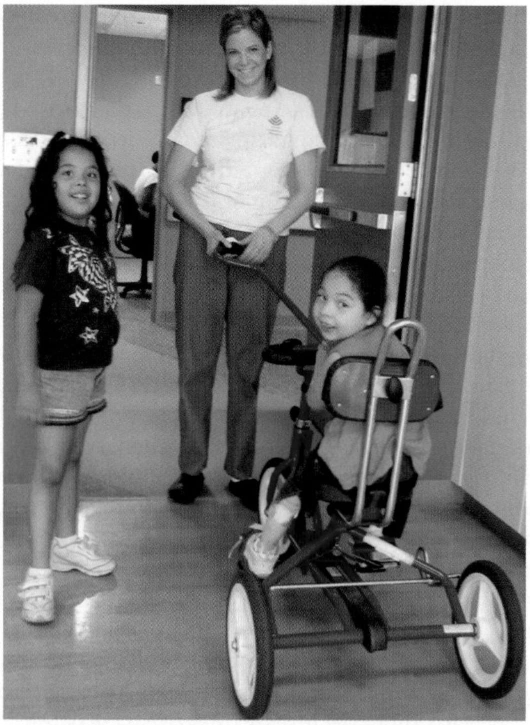

Fig. 44-10 Placing children of the same age group with similar illnesses near each other on the unit is both psychologically and medically supportive. *(Courtesy E. Jacob, Texas Children's Hospital, Houston.)*

roommate can help children gain a new friend and learn more about themselves. Forming relationships with significant members of the health care team, such as the physician, nurse, child life specialist, or social worker, can greatly enhance children's adjustment in many areas of life.

Parents may also encounter a new social group in other parents who have similar problems. The waiting room or hallway "self-help" groups are inherent to every institution. Parents meet while in the hospital or clinic and discuss their children's illnesses and treatments. Nurses can capitalize on this informal gathering by encouraging parents to discuss collectively their concerns and feelings. Nurses can also refer parents to organized parent groups or can use the help and support of parents of recovered hospitalized patients. It is important that nurses emphasize to families that each child responds differently to disease, treatments, and care. Any questions raised during group discussions should be clarified with a nurse or physician.

Nursing Care of the Family

Although it is not possible to predict exactly which factors are most likely to have an effect on the family's reactions, important variables are (1) the seriousness of the child's illness, (2) the family's previous experience with hospitalization, and (3) the medical procedures involved in the diagnosis and treatment. Important information is also obtained in the nursing admission history (see Box 44-5).

Support Family Members

Support involves the willingness to stay and listen to parents' verbal and nonverbal messages. Sometimes the nurse does not give this support directly. For example, the nurse may offer to stay with the child to allow the parents time alone or may discuss with other family members the parents' need for extra relief. Often relatives and friends want to help but do not know how. Suggesting ways to be of assistance, such as babysitting, preparing meals, doing laundry, or transporting the siblings to school, can prompt others to help reduce responsibilities that burden parents.

Support may also be provided through the clergy. Parents with deep religious beliefs may appreciate the counsel of a clergy member, but because of their stress they may not have sufficient energy to initiate the contact. Nurses can be supportive by arranging for clergy to visit, upholding parents' religious beliefs, and respecting the individual meaning and significance of those beliefs (Feudtner, Haney, & Dimmers, 2003).

In offering support it is important to acknowledge the cultural, socioeconomic, and ethnic values of the family. For example, health and illness are defined differently by various ethnic groups. For some, a disorder that has few outward manifestations of illness, such as diabetes, hypertension, or cardiac problems, is not a sickness. Consequently, following a prescribed treatment may be seen as unnecessary. Nurses who appreciate the influences of culture are more likely to intervene therapeutically. (See also Chapter 32, Cultural and Religious Influences on Health Care.)

Parents may need help in accepting their own feelings toward the ill child. If given the opportunity, parents often disclose their feelings of loss of control, anger, and guilt. They often resist admitting to such feelings because they expect others to disapprove of behaviour that is less than perfect. Unfortunately, health personnel, including nurses, sometimes exercise little tolerance for deviation from the expected norm. This only increases the psychological impact of a child's illness on family members. Helping parents identify the specific reason for such feelings and emphasizing that each is a normal and healthy response to stress may reduce the parents' emotional burden.

Family-centred care also addresses the needs of siblings. Support may involve preparing siblings for hospital visits, assessing their adjustment, and providing appropriate interventions or referrals when needed. The Family-Centred Teaching box suggests ways that parents can support siblings during hospitalization.

Provide Information

One of the most important nursing interventions is providing information about (1) the disease, its treatment, the prognosis, and home care; (2) the child's emotional and physical reactions to illness and hospitalization; and (3) the probable emotional reactions of family members to the crisis.

For many families the child's illness is the first contact they have with the hospital experience. Often parents are not prepared for the child's behavioural reactions to hospitalization, such as separation behaviours, regression, aggression, and hostility. Providing the parents with information about these

FAMILY-CENTRED TEACHING

Supporting Siblings During Hospitalization

Trade off staying at the hospital with your spouse or have a surrogate who knows the siblings well stay in the home.

Offer information about the child's condition to young siblings as well as older siblings; respect the sibling who avoids information as a means of coping with the situation.

Arrange for children to visit their brother or sister in the hospital if possible.

Encourage phone visits, mail, e-mail, and text messages between brothers and sisters; provide children with phone numbers, e-mail addresses, writing supplies, and stamps.

Help each sibling identify an extended family member or friend to be their support person and provide extra attention during parental absence.

Make or buy inexpensive toys or trinkets for siblings, one gift for each day the child will be hospitalized.

- Wrap each gift separately and place in a basket, box, or other container at each child's bedside.
- Instruct siblings to open one gift each night at bedtime and to remember that he or she is in the parent's thoughts.

If the child's condition is stable and distance is not prohibitive, plan a special time at home with the siblings or have your spouse or another relative or friend bring the children to meet you at a restaurant or other location near the hospital.

- Have extended family members or friends schedule a visit to the child in the hospital during parental absence.
- Arrange a pass for the child to leave the hospital to join the family if the child's condition permits.

(Data from Craft, M., & Craft, J. [1989]. Perceived changes in siblings of hospitalized children: A comparison of sibling and parent reports. *Child Health Care, 18*[1], 42–48; and Rollins, J. [1992]. *Brothers and sisters: A discussion guide for families*. Landover, MD: Epilepsy Foundation of America.)

normal and expected behavioural responses can lessen the parents' anxiety during the hospitalization. The family is equally unfamiliar with hospital rules, which often compounds their confusion and anxiety. Thus, the family needs clear explanations about what to expect and what is expected of them.

Parents also need to be aware of the effects of illness on the family and of strategies to prevent negative changes. Specifically, parents should keep the family well informed and communicate with everyone as much as possible. They should try to treat all the children equally and in the same way as before the illness occurred. Discipline, which initially may be lessened for the ill child, should be continued to provide a measure of security and predictability. When ill children know that their parents expect certain standards of conduct from them, they feel certain that they will recover. Conversely, when all limits are removed, they fear that something catastrophic will happen.

Helping parents understand the meaning of posthospitalization behaviours of the sick child is necessary for them to tolerate and support such behaviours. In addition, parents should be forewarned of the common reactions following discharge (see Box 44-2). Parents who do not expect such reactions may misinterpret them as evidence of the child's "being spoiled" and demand perfect behaviour at a time when the child is still reacting to the stress of illness and hospitalization. If the behaviours, especially the demand for attention, are dealt with in a supportive manner, most children are able to relinquish them and assume precrisis levels of functioning.

Nurses should also prepare parents for the reactions of siblings—particularly anger, jealousy, and resentment. Older siblings may deny such reactions because they provoke feelings of guilt. However, everyone needs outlets for emotions, and the repressed feelings may surface as problems in school or with age-mates, as psychosomatic illnesses, or in delinquent behaviour.

Probably one of the most neglected areas of communication involves the provision of pertinent, age-appropriate information to siblings. Frequently, age becomes the only factor that leads to an awareness of this problem, since older children may begin to ask questions or request explanations. Even in this situation, however, the information may be seriously inadequate. Children in every age group deserve some explanation of the sibling's illness or hospitalization. Although the exact wording may differ, the explanation should focus on the following concerns: (1) "Will I get sick and have to go to the hospital?" (2) "Did I cause the illness?" (for actual or imagined reasons), and (3) "Will my parents abandon me if my brother or sister doesn't recover?" If parents or nurses address these three questions, the siblings' own fears of illness, guilt, and abandonment are minimized (Melnyk & Alpert-Gillis, 1998).

Encourage Parent Participation

While preventing or minimizing separation is a key nursing goal for the child who is hospitalized, maintaining parent–child contact is also beneficial for the family. One of the best approaches is encouraging parents to stay with their child and to participate in the care whenever possible (Fig. 44-11). Although some health facilities provide special accommodations for parents, the concept of rooming-in can be instituted anywhere. The first requirement is the staff's positive attitude toward parents. A negative attitude toward parent participation can create barriers to collaborative working relationships.

When hospital staff genuinely appreciates the importance of continued parent–child attachment, they foster an environment that encourages parents to stay. When parents are included in the care planning and understand that they are contributing to the child's recovery, they are more inclined to remain with their child and have more emotional reserves to support themselves and the child through the crisis. In an empowerment model of helping, the nurse focuses on parents' strengths and seeks ways to promote growth and family functioning so that the parents can gain more confidence in caring for their child.

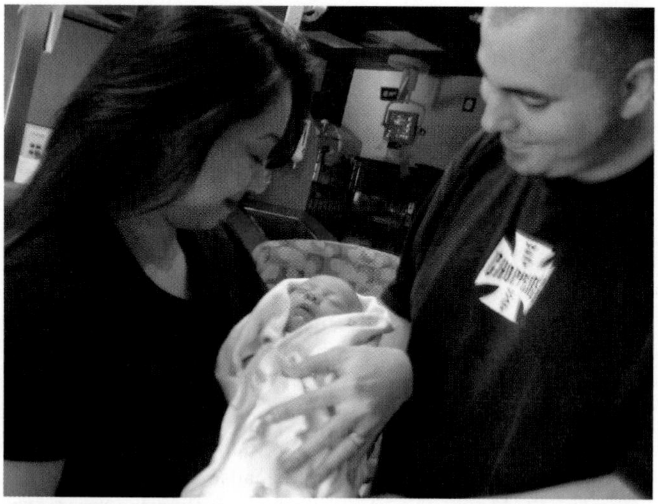

Fig. 44-11 Parental presence during hospitalization provides emotional support for the child and increases the parent's sense of empowerment in the caregiver role. *(Courtesy E. Jacob, Texas Children's Hospital, Houston.)*

Because the mother tends to be the family caregiver, she often spends more time in the hospital than the father. However, not all mothers (or fathers) feel equally comfortable assuming responsibility for their child's care. Some may be under such great emotional stress that they need a temporary reprieve from total participation in caregiving activities. Others may feel insecure in participating in specialized areas of care, such as bathing the child after surgery. By contrast, some mothers may feel a great need to control their child's care. This seems particularly true of young mothers, who have recently established their role as a parent; mothers of children too young to express their needs. Individual assessment of each parent's preferred involvement is necessary to prevent the effects of separation while supporting parents in their needs as well.

With lifestyles and gender roles changing, fathers may assume all or some of the usual "mothering" roles in the household, and it may be the father–child relationship that requires preservation. Fathers need to be included in the care plan and respected for their parental role. For some fathers the child's hospitalization may represent an opportunity to alter their usual caregiving role and increase their involvement. In lone-parent families the caregiver may not be a parent but an extended family member, such as a grandparent or aunt.

One of the potential problems with continuous parent involvement is neglect of the parent's need for sleep, nutrition, and relaxation. Often the sleeping accommodations are limited to a chair, and sleep is disrupted by nursing procedures. Encouraging the parents to leave for brief periods, arranging for sleeping quarters on the unit but outside the child's room, and planning a schedule of alternating visits with another family member can minimize the stresses for the parent.

All too often, nurses respond to parent participation by abandoning their patient responsibilities. Nurses need to restructure their roles to complement and augment the parents' caregiving functions. Even in units structured to provide care by parents, parents frequently feel anxiety in their caregiving responsibilities. Therefore, 24-hour responsibility may be too much for some parents. Assistance and relief by nursing personnel should always be available to these families, and nurses may need to work diligently to establish the strong bond of trust some parents need to take advantage of these opportunities.

Prepare for Discharge and Home Care

Most hospitalizations necessitate some type of discharge preparation. Often this involves education of the family for continued care and follow-up in the home. Depending on the diagnosis, this may be relatively simple or highly complex. Preparing the family for home care demands a high degree of competence in planning and implementing discharge instructions. This usually is best accomplished using an interdisciplinary team approach, which requires a shift from the multidisciplinary team approach used during an acute phase of a child's illness.

Nurses are often key individuals in initiating and carrying out the discharge process. They collaborate with others in the planning and implementation phases to ensure appropriate care after hospitalization. Throughout the hospitalization the nurse should be aware of the need for discharge planning and those assessment factors that affect the family's ability to provide home care. A thorough assessment of the family and home environment should be performed to ensure that the family's emotional and physical resources are sufficient to manage the tasks of home care. In addition to adequate family resources, an investigation of community services, including respite care, is needed to ensure that appropriate support agencies are available, such as emergency facilities, home health agencies, and equipment vendors. Financial resources are also a consideration. To coordinate the immense task of assessment and to plan implementation, a care coordinator or manager should be appointed early in the discharge process.

The preparation for hospital discharge and home care begins during the admission assessment. Short- and long-term goals are established to meet the child's physical and psychosocial needs. For children with complex care needs, discharge planning focuses on obtaining appropriate equipment and health care personnel for the home. Discharge planning is also concerned with those treatments that parents or children are expected to continue at home. In planning appropriate teaching, nurses need to assess (1) the actual and perceived complexity of the skill involved, (2) the parents' or child's ability to learn the skill, and (3) the parents' or child's previous or present experience with such procedures.

The teaching plan incorporates levels of learning, such as observing, participating with assistance, and, finally, acting without help or guidance. Learning of the skill is divided into discrete steps, and each step is taught to the family member until it is learned. Return demonstration of the skill is needed before new skills are introduced. A record of teaching and performance provides an efficient checklist for evaluation. All families need to receive detailed written instructions about home care, with telephone numbers and other contact information for assistance, before they leave the hospital. Communication between the nurse performing discharge planning and home health care is essential for ensuring a smooth transition for the child and family.

After the family is competent in performing the required skills, they are given responsibility for the care. When possible, the family should have a transition or trial period to assume care with minimal health care supervision. This may be arranged on the unit; during a home pass; or in a facility, such as a motel, near the hospital. Such transitions provide a safe practice period for the family, with assistance readily available when needed, and are especially valuable when the family lives far from the hospital.

In many instances parents need only simple instructions and understanding of follow-up care. However, the often overwhelming care assumed by some families, coupled with other stressors they may be experiencing, necessitates continued professional support after discharge. A follow-up home visit or telephone call can give the nurse an opportunity to provide information in perhaps a less stressful learning environment. Appropriate referrals and resources may include visiting nurse or home health agencies, private nurse services, the school system, a physiotherapist, a mental health counsellor, a social worker, and any number of community agencies. Sharing the important issues surrounding the child's and family's needs is essential. Referral summaries should be concise, specific, and factual. When numerous support services are required, periodic collaboration among the professionals involved and the family is an excellent strategy to ensure efficient usage and comprehensive delivery of services.

Care of the Child and Family in Special Hospital Situations

In addition to a general pediatric unit, children may be admitted to special facilities such as an ambulatory or outpatient setting, an isolation room, or critical care.

Ambulatory or Outpatient Setting

The ambulatory or outpatient setting provides needed medical services for the child while eliminating the necessity of overnight admission. Among the benefits of ambulatory care are (1) minimization of the stressors of hospitalization, especially separation from the family; (2) reduced chance of infection; and (3) cost savings. Admission to the ambulatory or outpatient hospital setting usually is for surgical or diagnostic procedures, such as insertion of tympanostomy tubes, hernia repair, adenoidectomy, tonsillectomy, cystoscopy, or bronchoscopy.

In the ambulatory or outpatient setting, adequate preparation is particularly challenging. Ideally, the child and parents should receive preadmission preparation, including a tour of the facility and a review of the day's events. Parents need information in advance to help prepare the child and themselves for surgery and enable them to care for the child at home after the procedure. Parents also appreciate suggestions for items to bring to the hospital, such as blankets or stuffed animals. When preadmission preparation is not possible, time should be allowed on the day of the procedure for children to become acquainted with their surroundings and for nurses to assess, plan, and implement appropriate teaching.

Waiting is usually inevitable in ambulatory settings. Families frequently report waiting to be the most stressful part of the experience. Providing a pager is one way to allow the family (and at times the child) to leave the area and then be paged to return when needed (Ashenberg et al., 1996).

Explicit discharge instructions are important after outpatient surgery (see Family-Centred Teaching box and Prepare for Discharge and Home Care, p. 1252). Parents need guidelines on when to call their practitioner regarding a change in the child's condition. A follow-up telephone call system enables nurses to check on the child's progress within 48 to 72 hours after discharge. It also provides an opportunity for the nurse to review discharge information and answer questions.

Isolation

Admission to an isolation room increases all of the stressors typically associated with hospitalization. There is further separation from familiar persons; additional loss of control; and added environmental changes, such as sensory deprivation and the strange appearance of visitors. Orientation to time and place is affected. These stressors are compounded by children's limited understanding of isolation. Preschool children have difficulty understanding the rationale for isolation because they cannot comprehend the cause-and-effect relationship between germs and illness. They are likely to view isolation as punishment. Older children understand the causality better but still require information to decrease fantasizing or misinterpretation.

When a child is placed in isolation, preparation is essential for the child to feel in control. With young children the best approach is a simple explanation, such as "You need to be in this room to help you get better. This is a special place to make all the germs go away. The germs made you sick, and you could not help that."

All children, but especially younger ones, need preparation in terms of what they will see, hear, or feel in isolation. They should be shown the mask, gloves, and gown and be encouraged to "dress up" in them. Playing with the strange apparel lessens the fear of seeing "ghostlike" people walk into the room. Before entering the room, nurses and other health personnel should introduce themselves and let the child see their face before donning a mask. In this way, the child associates them with significant experiences and gains a sense of familiarity in an otherwise strange and lonely environment.

When the child's condition improves, appropriate play activities should be provided to minimize boredom, stimulate the senses, provide a real or perceived sense of movement, orient the child to time and place, provide social interaction, and reduce depersonalization. For example, the environment can be manipulated to increase sensory freedom by moving the bed toward the door or window. Opening window shades; providing musical, visual, or tactile toys; and increasing interpersonal contact can substitute mental mobility for the limitations of physical movement. Rather than dwelling on the negative aspects of isolation, the child can be encouraged to view this experience as challenging and positive. For example, the nurse can help the child look at isolation as a method of keeping others out and letting only special people in. Children often think of intriguing signs for their doors, such as "Enter

FAMILY-CENTRED TEACHING

Discharge From Ambulatory Settings

Before beginning the discharge, explain that all instructions will also be presented in writing for the family to refer to later.
Provide an overview of the typical trajectory (expected pattern) of recovery.
Discuss expected progression of the child's activity level during the postdischarge period (e.g., "Mary will probably sleep for the rest of the day, feel kind of tired most of tomorrow, but be back to her usual activities the next day").
Explain which activities the child is allowed to do and what is not permitted (e.g., bed rest, bathing).
Discuss dietary restrictions, being very specific and giving examples of "clear fluids" or what is meant by a "full liquid diet."
Discuss nausea and vomiting, if applicable, explaining how much is "normal" and what to do if more occurs (e.g., "Juan may be sick to his stomach and vomit. This is normal. However, if he vomits more than three times, please call us at this number right away.").
Discuss fever and appropriate comfort measures, explaining how much fever is considered "normal," and specifically what to do if the child goes beyond the range.
Explain the amount, location, and kind of pain or discomfort the child may experience.
Send a pain scale home with the family.
Explain how much pain and discomfort is "normal" and what to do if the child surpasses that level or if pain management interventions are unsuccessful.
Discuss pain management, including dosages for pain medications and details on how to administer them.
Describe appropriate nonpharmacological comfort measures, such as holding, rocking, or swaddling. Give any prescribed medication before leaving the facility.
Provide information about each medication that the child will be taking at home.

- Review the details, including dose and route.
- Demonstrate how to administer medications, if necessary (e.g., how to take wrapping off suppositories, how to insert).

Discuss guidelines for requesting other medications.
Request that all prescriptions be filled and given to the family before discharge.
Make certain the family has all of the equipment and supplies (e.g., gauze and tape for dressing changes) they will need at home.
Discuss complications that may occur and the steps to take if they do.
Ensure that appropriate measures are in place for safe transport home.

- Remind the family to use a seat belt or car seat for the child.
- Determine whether there will be one person whose sole responsibility is helping ensure the child's safety and comfort during transport.
- Discuss measures the driver may need to take if this is impossible (e.g., be certain a basin is within the child's reach should vomiting occur; take a route that permits slower traffic and has places along the roadside to stop if necessary).
- Determine the availability of a blanket, pillow, and cup with a lid and straw for the child's use in the car.
- Provide a basin or plastic bag in case of vomiting.

Provide emergency phone numbers for the family to call with any concerns.
Explain that the family will be contacted (give an approximate time) to follow up on the child but that they should not hesitate to call if concerns arise before then.
Ask the family and child, if appropriate, if they have any questions, and problem solve with family members to meet their unique needs.

at your own risk." These signs also encourage people "on the outside" to talk with the child about the ominous greeting.

NURSING ALERT Have the child select a place he or she would like to visit. Help the child decorate the bed and equipment to suit the theme (e.g., truck, circus tent, spaceship, sky). At a set time each day, pretend to go with the child to the special place. Consider including props such as a suitcase or picnic basket.

Emergency Admission

One of the most traumatic hospital experiences for the child and parents is an **emergency** admission. The sudden onset of an illness or the occurrence of an injury leaves little time for preparation and explanation. Sometimes the emergency admission is compounded by admission to a critical care unit (CCU) or the need for immediate surgery. However, even in those instances requiring only outpatient treatment, the child is exposed to a strange, frightening environment and to experiences that may elicit fear or cause pain.

There is a wide discrepancy between what constitutes a medically defined emergency and a patient-defined emergency. A growing concern is the use of major emergency departments for routine primary care health visits. To offset overcrowding in emergency departments, many facilities have minor emergency units or pediatric minor emergency units for after-hours health care. Telephone triage for minor illnesses for patients is also emerging as a health care delivery mode to differentiate illnesses such as a common cold from true life-threatening conditions that require immediate practitioner attention and intervention. Other factors contributing to the overuse of emergency departments (as opposed to the primary practitioner's office) include the increasing number of households in which both parents work full time and cannot afford to take time off during the daytime to take the sick child to a practitioner.

In pediatric populations most visits to an emergency department are for respiratory tract infections; skin conditions, gastrointestinal disorders, and trauma such as poisoning account for most of the remainder of cases. The most common reason parents give for bringing the child to the emergency department is concern about the illness worsening. However, practitioners may not think that the progressive symptoms necessitate immediate or emergency care. One of the nurse's primary goals is to assess the parents' perception of the event and their reasons for considering it serious or life threatening.

Lengthy preparatory admission procedures are often inappropriate for emergency situations. In such instances, nurses must focus their nursing interventions on the essential components of admission counselling (Box 44-11) and complete the process as soon as the child's condition has stabilized.

Unless an emergency is life threatening, children need to participate in their care to maintain a sense of control. Because

BOX 44-11 Guidelines for Special Hospital Admission*

Emergency Admission

Lengthy preparatory admission procedures are often impossible and inappropriate for emergency situations.

Focus assessment on airway, breathing, and circulation; weigh child whenever possible for calculation of drug dosages.

Unless an emergency is life threatening, children need to participate in their care to maintain a sense of control.

Focus on essential components of admission counselling:
- Appropriate introduction to the family
- Use of child's name, not terms such as "honey" or "dear"
- Determination of child's age and some judgement about developmental age (If the child is of school age, asking about the grade level will offer some evidence of intellectual ability.)
- Information about child's general state of health, any problems that may interfere with medical treatment (e.g., allergies), and previous experience with hospital facilities
- Information about the chief concern from both the parents and the child

Admission to Critical Care Unit

Prepare child and parents for elective critical care unit (CCU) admission, such as for postoperative care after cardiac surgery.

Prepare child and parents for unanticipated CCU admission by focusing primarily on the sensory aspects of the experience and on the usual family concerns (e.g., persons in charge of child's care, schedule for visiting, area where family can stay).

Prepare parents for child's appearance and behaviour when they first visit their child in the CCU.

Accompany family to bedside to provide emotional support and answer questions.

Prepare siblings for their visit; plan length of time for sibling visitation; monitor siblings' reactions during visit to prevent them from becoming overwhelmed.

Encourage parents to stay with their child:
- If visiting hours are limited, allow flexibility in the schedule to accommodate parental needs.
- Give family members a written schedule of visiting times.
- If visiting hours are liberal, be aware of family members' needs and suggest periodic respites.
- Assure family that they can call the unit at any time.

Prepare parents for expected role changes and identify ways for parents to participate in the child's care without overwhelming them with responsibilities:
- Help with bath or feeding.
- Touch and talk to the child.
- Help with procedures.

Provide information about the child's condition in understandable language:
- Repeat information often.
- Seek clarification of understanding.
- During bedside conferences, interpret information for family members and the child or, if appropriate, conduct report outside the room.

Prepare child for procedures, even if this involves explanation while the procedure is performed.

Assess and manage pain; recognize that a child who cannot talk, such as an infant or child in a coma or on mechanical ventilation, can be in pain.

Establish a routine that maintains some similarity to daily events in the child's life whenever possible:
- Organize care during normal waking hours.
- Keep regular bedtime schedules, including quiet times when television or radio volume is lowered or turned off.
- Provide uninterrupted sleep cycles (60 minutes for infant, 90 minutes for older child).
- Close and open drapes and dim lights to establish day–night pattern.
- Place curtain around bed for privacy.
- Orient child to day and time; have clocks or calendars in easy view for older children.

Schedule a time when the child is left undisturbed (e.g., during naps, visits with family, playtime, or favourite programs).

Provide opportunities for play.

Reduce stimulation in environment:
- Refrain from loud talking or laughing.
- Keep equipment noise to a minimum:
  - Turn alarms as low as safely possible.
  - Perform treatments requiring equipment at one time.
  - Turn off bedside equipment that is not in use, such as suction and oxygen.
- Avoid loud, abrupt noises.

*See also Box 44-7.

emergency departments are frequently hectic, there is a tendency to rush through procedures to save time. However, the extra few minutes needed to allow children to participate may save many more minutes of useless resistance during subsequent procedures. Other supportive measures include ensuring privacy; accepting various emotional responses to fear or pain; preservation of parent–child contact; explanation of all events before or as they occur; and remaining calm. Pain management strategies are discussed in Chapter 35.

At times, because of the child's physical condition, little or no preparatory counselling for emergency hospitalization can be done. In such situations the implementation of *postvention*, or counselling subsequent to the event, has therapeutic value. The process of postvention involves evaluating children's thoughts regarding admission and related procedures. It is similar to precounselling techniques; however, instead of supplying information, the nurse listens to the explanations offered by the child. Projective techniques such as drawing, doll play, or storytelling are especially effective. The nurse then bases additional information on what has already been understood.

Critical Care Unit

Admission to a critical care unit can be traumatic for both the child and parents. The nature and severity of the illness and the circumstances surrounding the admission are major factors, especially for parents. Parents experience significantly more stress when the admission is unexpected rather than expected. One study found that parental anxiety reached near panic levels initially (Huckabay & Tilem-Kessler, 1999). Stressors for the child and parent are described in Box 44-12. Although several studies have described what parents perceive as most stressful, the most effective strategy may be to simply ask parents what is stressful and implement interventions that will enhance their ability to cope (Board & Ryan-Wenger, 2003; Melnyk & Alpert-Gillis, 1998). Assessment should be repeated periodically to account for changes in perceptions over time.

The family's emotional needs are paramount, and family-centred care is needed when a child is admitted to a critical care unit. Although the same interventions discussed earlier for the stressors of separation and loss of control apply here, additional interventions may also benefit the family and child (see Box 44-12 and Family-Centred Teaching box). In a qualitative study of 19 parents of 10 children in a critical care unit, parents reported that they simply wanted nurses to nurture the child in the same way the family would (Harbaugh, Tomlinson, & Kirschbaum, 2004). Nurse behaviours that exemplified caring and affection were perceived as helpful in decreasing stress. Behaviours perceived as not helpful included separating the child from the parents and communicating poorly with parents. It is important that visiting hours be liberal and flexible enough to accommodate parental needs and involvement (Hazinski, 1999).

Critically ill children become the focus of the parents' lives, and parents' most pressing need is for information (Scott, 1998). They want to know if their child will live and, if so, whether the child will be the same as before. They need to know why various interventions are being done for the child, that the child is being treated for pain or is comfortable, and that the child may be able to hear them even though not awake. When parents first visit the child in the critical care unit, they need preparation regarding the child's appearance. Ideally, the nurse should answer any questions.

Despite the stresses normally associated with CCU admission, a special security develops from being carefully monitored and receiving individualized care. Therefore, planning for transition to the regular unit is essential and should include the following:

- Assignment of a primary nurse on the regular unit
- Continued visits by the CCU staff to assess the child's and parents' adjustment and to act as a temporary liaison with the nursing staff
- Explanation of the differences between the two units and the rationale for the change to less intense monitoring of the child's physical condition
- Selection of an appropriate room, such as one that is close to the nursing station, and a compatible roommate

BOX 44-12 Neonatal or Pediatric Critical Care Unit Stressors for the Child and Family

Physical Stressors

Pain and discomfort (e.g., injections, intubation, suctioning, dressing changes, other invasive procedures)
Immobility (e.g., use of restraints, bed rest)
Sleep deprivation
Inability to eat or drink
Changes in elimination habits

Environmental Stressors

Unfamiliar surroundings (e.g., crowding)
Unfamiliar sounds
- Equipment noise (e.g., monitors, telephone, suctioning, computer printout)
- Human sounds (e.g., talking, laughing, crying, coughing, moaning, retching, walking)

Unfamiliar people (e.g., health care providers, patients, visitors)
Unfamiliar and unpleasant smells (e.g., alcohol, adhesive remover, body odours)
Constant lights (disturb day–night rhythms)
Activity related to other patients
Sense of urgency among staff
Unkind or thoughtless comments from staff

Psychological Stressors

Lack of privacy
Inability to communicate (if intubated)
Inadequate knowledge and understanding of situation
Severity of illness
Parental behaviour (expression of concern)

Social Stressors

Disrupted relationships (especially with family and friends)
Concern with missing school or work
Play deprivation

(Data primarily from Tichy, A. M., et al. [1988]. Stressors in pediatric intensive care units. *Pediatric Nursing, 14*[1], 40–42.)

FAMILY-CENTRED TEACHING

Artists as Partners in Care

A teenage boy with a rare genetic disorder, having made steady progress after awakening from a coma, relapsed and seemed very depressed. When told that a musician was visiting the pediatric critical care unit, he immediately perked up and asked to have his room lights turned on. He whispered endless song requests to the musician. Family members and staff were treated to some of his first smiles in days; his biggest came when the musician held his hand and guided it across the guitar strings while they sang "Born to Be Wild" together at the boy's request. His dad was misty eyed as he thanked the musician for the visit.

A few weeks later the boy's condition worsened and he again lapsed into a coma. There was nothing more to be done. His parents began the necessary preparations to take their son home to die.

We continued to visit our friend and his family, offering a song, a story, or a simple hello. I hold a vivid picture of our final visit. We stood around the boy's bed with his parents singing together songs they remembered from their youth, from more carefree times. Song and laughter filled the boy's room.

Perhaps the boy heard his parents' laughter and knew then that they would be okay. He died a few days later on the morning he was to have been discharged.

–Judy Rollins, MS, RN

(Modified from Rollins, J. [1995]. Placed in our keeping. Unpublished.)

Key Points

- Children are particularly vulnerable to the stressors of illness and hospitalization because stress represents a change from the usual state of health and routine and because they possess limited coping mechanisms.
- The three phases of separation anxiety are protest, despair, and detachment.
- Feelings of loss of control are caused by unfamiliar environmental stimuli, physical restriction, altered routine, and dependency.
- Fear of bodily pain may be manifested in the following ways: infants—facial expressions, body movements; toddlers—intense emotional upset, physical resistance; preschoolers—aggression, verbal expression, dependency; school-age children—precise verbalization of pain, passive requests for support or help, procrastination technique; adolescents—self-control, limited movement.
- Because of their separation from significant people, children who are hospitalized may lack the opportunity to form new attachments in the strange environment of the hospital and exhibit negative behaviours after discharge.
- Nursing care of the child in the hospital is aimed at preventing or minimizing separation, decreasing loss of control, minimizing fear of bodily injury, using play or expressive activities to lessen stress, and maximizing the potential benefits of hospitalization.
- The nurse can maximize potential benefits of hospitalization by fostering parent–child relations, providing educational opportunities, promoting self-mastery, and encouraging socialization.
- Family reactions are influenced by the seriousness of the illness, experience with illness or hospitalization and diagnostic or therapeutic procedures, available support systems, personal ego strengths, coping abilities, presence of additional stressors, cultural and religious beliefs, and family communication patterns.
- Siblings' fear of contracting illness, their younger age, a close relationship with the ill sibling, substitute child care, minimal explanation of the illness, and perceived changes in parenting all increase the deleterious effects of a brother's or sister's illness and hospitalization on siblings.
- Nursing care of the family involves listening to parents' verbal and nonverbal messages; providing clergy support; accepting cultural, socioeconomic, and ethnic values; giving information to families and siblings; and preparing them for discharge and home care.
- Admission to an outpatient setting, emergency department, isolation room, or CCU requires additional intervention strategies to meet the child's and family's needs.

Audio Chapter Summaries

Access an Audio Summary of these Key Points on evolve

References

About Kids Health. (2009). *The health care team.* Retrieved from http://www.aboutkidshealth.ca/en/resourcecentres/congenitalheartConditions/AboutCongenitalHeartConditions/TheHealthCareTeam/Pages/default.aspx.

Accreditation Canada. (2010). *Standards.* Retrieved from http://www.accreditation.ca/accreditation-programs/qmentum/standards/.

Ashenberg, M. D., et al. (1996). Easing the wait: Development of a pager program for families. *Pediatric Nursing, 22*(2), 103–107.

Board, R., & Ryan-Wenger, N. (2003). Stressors and symptoms of mothers with children in the PICU. *Journal of Pediatric Nursing, 18*(3), 195–201.

Canadian Institute of Child Health. (2002). *The rights of the child in the health care system* (pamphlet). Retrieved from http://www.cich.ca/PDFFiles/RightHospitalizedENG.pdf.

Canadian Paediatric Society. (2005). Children and natural products: What a clinician should know. *Paediatrics and Child Health, 10*(4), 227–232. (Reaffirmed 2011) Retrieved from http://www.cps.ca/english/statements/dt/dt05-01.htm.

Clatworthy, S., Simon, K., & Tiedeman, M. E. (1999). Child drawing: Hospital—an instrument designed to measure the emotional status of hospitalized school-aged children. *Journal of Pediatric Nursing, 14*(1), 2–9.

Commodan, E. (2010). Children staying in hospital: A research on psychological stress of caregivers. *Italian Journal of Pediatrics, 36,* 40. doi:10.1186/1824-7288-36-40

Coyne, I. (2006). Children's experiences of hospitalization. *Journal of Child Health Care, 10*(4), 326–336. doi:10.1177/1367493506067884

Feudtner, H. J., Haney, J., & Dimmers, M. A. (2003). Spiritual care needs of hospitalized children and their families: A national survey of pastoral care providers' perceptions. *Pediatrics, 111*(1), e67–e72.

Flanagan, K. (2001). Preoperative assessment: Safety considerations for patients taking herbal products. *Journal of Perianesthesia Nursing, 16*(1), 19–26.

Gibbard, W. B. (2005). *The use of complementary and alternative medicine by children and adolescents with autistic spectrum disorders.* Retrieved from http://dspace.ucalgary.ca/bitstream/1880/44821/1/Gibbard_MSc_2005_Med.pdf.

Gordon, M. (2002). *Manual of nursing diagnosis* (10th ed.). St. Louis: Mosby.
Harbaugh, B. L., Tomlinson, P. S., & Kirschbaum, M. (2004). Parents' perceptions of nurses' caregiving behaviors in the pediatric intensive care unit. *Issues in Comprehensive Pediatric Nursing, 27*(3), 163–178.
Hazinski, M. F. (1999). *Manual of pediatric critical care.* St. Louis: Mosby.
Health Canada. (2011). *Adverse reaction and medical device problem reporting.* Retrieved from http://www.hc-sc.gc.ca/dhp-mps/medeff/report-declaration/index-eng.php.
Health Canada. (2012). *What are natural health products?* Retrieved from http://www.hc-sc.gc.ca/dhp-mps/prodnatur/index-eng.php/.
Huckabay, L. M. D., & Tilem-Kessler, D. (1999). Patterns of parental stress in PICU emergency admission. *Dimensions of Critical Care Nursing, 18*(2), 36–42.
Lewandowski, L. A., & Tesler, M. D. (2003). *Family centered care: Putting it into action.* Washington, DC: American Nurses Association.
Melnyk, B. M. (2000). Intervention studies involving parents of hospitalized young children: An analysis of the past and future recommendations. *Journal of Pediatric Nursing, 15*(1), 4–13.
Melnyk, B. M., & Alpert-Gillis, L. (1998). The COPE Program: A strategy to improve outcomes of critically ill young children and their parents. *Pediatric Nursing, 24*(6), 521–527.
Orem, D. (2001). *Nursing: Concepts of practice* (5th ed.). New York: Mosby.
Scott, L. D. (1998). Perceived needs of parents of critically ill children. *Journal of the Society of Pediatric Nurses, 3*(1), 4–12.
Small, L. (2002). Early predictors of poor coping outcomes in children following intensive care hospitalization and stressful medical encounters. *Pediatric Nursing, 28*(4), 393–401.
Smith, T., & Conant Rees, H. L. (2000). Making family-centered care a reality. *Seminars in Nursing Management, 8*(3), 136–142.
Stewart, E., Algren, C., & Arnold, S. (1994). Preparing children for a surgical experience. *Today's OR Nurse, 16*(2), 9–14.
Stranton, K. M. (2004). Parents' experiences of their child's care during hospitalization. *Journal of Cultural Diversity, 11*(1), 4–11.
Strickland, M. P., Leeper, J. D., Jessee, P., & Hudson, C. (1987). Children's adjustment to the hospital: A rural/urban comparison. *Maternal and Child Nursing Journal, 16*(3), 251–259.

Additional Resources

Health Canada: About Natural Health Products: http://www.hc-sc.gc.ca/dhp-mps/prodnatur/about-apropos/cons-eng.php.
The Hospital for Sick Children: About Kids' Health: http://www.aboutkidshealth.ca/En/HealthAZ/Pages/default.aspx?name=A.

Unit 10

Pediatric Variations of Nursing Interventions

45

Learning Objectives

On completion of this chapter, the reader will be able to:

- Identify those instances in which informed consent is required from parents or guardians and when minors may be considered emancipated and can provide their own informed consent.
- Formulate general guidelines for preparing children for procedures, including surgery.
- Implement play in therapeutic procedures.
- List general strategies for ensuring that children and families make informed choices or are able to follow the treatment plan.
- Outline general hygiene and care procedures for hospitalized children.
- Implement feeding techniques that encourage food and fluid intake.
- Describe methods of reducing the temperature of a child with fever or hyperthermia.
- Describe systems that can be used for infection control.
- Describe safe methods of administering oral, parenteral, rectal, optic, otic, and nasal medications to children.
- Identify nursing responsibilities in maintaining fluid balance.
- Demonstrate correct procedures for postural drainage and tracheostomy care.
- Describe the procedures involved in providing nutrition via gavage, gastrostomy, and parenteral routes.
- Describe the procedures involved in administering an enema and ostomy care to children.

Electronic Resources

Additional information related to the content in Chapter 45 can be found on

evolve **the companion Web site at**

http://evolve.elsevier.com/Canada/Perry/maternal/

- Examination Review Questions
- Animation—Central Venous Access
- Animation—Foley Catheter Insertion
- Animation—IV Line Placement
- Animation—Lumbar Puncture, Infant
- Animation—PICC Line Placement
- Case Study—Pediatric Procedures
- Critical Thinking Exercise—Central Venous Access Device
- Skill—Administering Oral Medications
- Skill—Measuring Oxygen Saturation
- Skill—Preparing the Child for Procedures
- Skill—Urine Specimen Collection

General Concepts Related to Pediatric Procedures

Informed Consent

Before undergoing any invasive procedure, the patient, the patient's legal surrogate, or both must receive sufficient information on which to make an informed health care decision. All decisions should be based on a combination of known facts and personal values. In health care, treatment decisions relate to medical information and personal evaluation of this information. In order to make appropriate decisions, individuals and families must have pertinent information, be able to understand how it applies to themselves or their children, and then make a voluntary decision. These bases of medical decision-making define the three hallmarks of informed choice (Canadian Paediatric Society [CPS], Bioethics Committee, 2004):

1. **Appropriate information:** Appropriate decisions can only be made with sufficient information.
2. **Decision-making capacity:** The person with decision-making capacity must have more than the simple ability to understand. They must be able to realize the purpose of the intervention, the consequences of consent or refusal, the

alternatives, and the magnitude and probabilities of harm and benefit.

3. **Voluntariness:** The decision maker should not be manipulated or coerced, and the option to change one's mind should always be available.

The patient has the right to accept or refuse any health care. If the patient is treated without consent, the hospital or health care provider may be charged with assault and held liable for damages.

Requirements for Obtaining Informed Consent

Written **informed consent** is usually required for medical or surgical treatment, including many diagnostic procedures. One universal consent is not sufficient. Separate informed permissions must be obtained for each surgical or diagnostic procedure, including major or minor surgery, diagnostic tests with an element of risk (e.g., bronchoscopy), and medical treatments with an element of risk (e.g., blood transfusion, radiotherapy).

Children who have partial skills to make decisions should be recognized as having some authority over their own health care. This can be achieved through the concept of *assent*, whereby children are given both information that they can understand and some appropriate choice in their treatment. Assent should include the following elements:

- Helping the patient achieve a developmentally appropriate awareness of the nature of his or her condition
- Telling the patient what he or she can expect
- Making a clinical assessment of the patient's understanding
- Soliciting an expression of the patient's willingness to accept the proposed procedure of care

Multiple methods should be used to provide information, including age-appropriate methods (e.g., DVDs, Internet sources, peer discussion, diagrams, and written materials).

evolve Case Study—Pediatric Procedures

evolve Case Study—Preparing the Child for Procedures

Eligibility for Giving Informed Consent

Informed Consent for Minors

In most parts of Canada, there is no specific legal age for medical consent; instead, the patient's ability to understand and make decisions regarding their own condition, the treatment, and its consequences is more important than their **chronological age.** Québec is the only exception and stipulates an age of consent (14 years) (Canadian Medical Protective Association, 2012). It is important for the nurse to be aware of the procedures and laws that govern informed consent for the province or territory and institution in which they work.

Evidence of Consent

In obtaining informed consent, it is the physician's responsibility to explain the procedure, risks, benefits, and alternatives to the parents or guardians and to the child, if he or she is able to understand this information. The physician needs to convey this information in a way that is fitting to their personal circumstances and ensures their understanding of the treatment and alternatives, including associated risks and benefits. The nurse may reinforce what the patient and parents have been told. A signed consent form is the legal document that signifies that the process of informed consent has occurred. If parents are unavailable to sign consent forms, verbal consent may be obtained via telephone in the presence of two witnesses. Both witnesses record that informed consent was given and by whom. Their signatures indicate that they witnessed the verbal consent.

Informed Consent of Emancipated Minors

Provincial and territorial laws differ with regard to the so-called age of majority, the age at which a person is considered to have all the legal rights and responsibilities of an adult. *Emancipated minors* are those who are no longer dependent on their parents or guardians. They may be supporting themselves or living independently from their families.

Emergency Treatment Without Consent

An emergency exists if the patient is apparently experiencing severe suffering or is at risk of suffering serious bodily harm if treatment is not administered promptly. In cases of emergency when the patient is unable to consent and a substitute decision maker is not readily available, a health practitioner must do what is immediately necessary without consent.

Conflicts in Decision Making for Children

In some situations, conflict may arise if the values and beliefs of the parents differ from those of the health care team or even from each other. Although most conflicts involve a remediable breakdown in communication, sometimes a genuine clash in values exists. Parental decision-making should be accepted by the health care team unless it is obvious to many that the decision is not in the best interest of the child or adolescent. If the health care team feels that the parental decisions are clearly inconsistent with the child or adolescent's best interests and collaboration with other resources, ethics committees, or consultants has not resolved the situation, involvement of local child protection authorities and the legal system may be unavoidable, although this should only be used as a last resort (CPS, Bioethics Committee, 2004).

Consent and Confidentiality

The *Personal Health Information Protection Act* of 2004 (PHIPA) was passed to help protect and safeguard the security and confidentiality of a person's health information. A capable individual, regardless of age, can consent to the collection, use, or disclosure of their own personal health information. If a child is incapable of consenting, a parent may do so on their behalf.

Preparation for Diagnostic and Therapeutic Procedures

Technological advances and changes in health care delivery have resulted in more pediatric procedures being performed in a variety of settings. Many procedures are both stressful and painful experiences. For most procedures the focus of care is on psychological preparation of the child and family. However, some procedures require the administration of sedatives or **analgesics**.

Psychological Preparation

Preparation of children for procedures decreases their anxiety, promotes their assistance, supports their coping skills and may teach them new ones, and facilitates a feeling of mastery in experiencing a potentially stressful event. Many institutions have developed preadmission teaching programs designed to educate the pediatric patient and family by offering hands-on experience with hospital equipment, information about the procedure to be performed, and an overview of departments they may visit (Wright, Stewart, Finley, & Buffet-Jerrott, 2007). Preparatory methods may be formal, such as group preparation for hospitalization. Most preparation strategies used by nurses are informal, focus on providing information about the experience, and are directed at stressful or painful procedures. The most effective preparation is to provide sensory-procedural information and help the child develop coping skills, such as imagery, distraction, or relaxation (Wright et al., 2007).

General guidelines for preparing children for procedures are described in Box 45-1, and age-specific guidelines that consider children's developmental needs and cognitive abilities are presented in Box 45-2. In addition to these suggestions, nurses should consider the child's temperament, existing coping strategies, and previous experiences. Children who are distractible and highly active, as well as those who need more time to adapt may need individualized sessions that are shorter for the active child or more slowly paced for the shy child. Youngsters who tend to cope well may need more emphasis on using their present skills, whereas those who appear to cope less adequately can benefit from more time devoted to simple coping strategies, such as relaxing, breathing, counting, squeezing a hand, or singing.

BOX 45-1 General Guidelines for Preparing Children for Procedures

- Determine details of exact procedure to be performed.
- Review parents' and child's present understanding.
- Base teaching on developmental age and existing knowledge.
- Incorporate parents in the teaching if they desire, especially if they plan to participate in care.
- Inform parents of their supportive role during the procedure, such as standing near the child's head or in the child's line of vision and talking softly to the child.
- Allow for ample discussion to prevent information overload and ensure adequate feedback.
- Use concrete, not abstract, terms and visual aids to describe the procedure. For example, use a simple line drawing of a boy or girl and mark the body part that will be involved in the procedure. Use nonthreatening but realistic models.
- Emphasize that no other body part will be involved.
- If the body part is associated with a specific function, stress the change in or noninvolvement of that ability (e.g., after tonsillectomy, the child can still speak).
- Use words appropriate to the child's level of understanding.
- Avoid words and phrases with dual meanings unless the child understands such words.
- Clarify all unfamiliar words (e.g., "Anaesthesia is a special sleep").
- Emphasize sensory aspects of procedure—what child will feel, see, hear, smell, and touch and what child can do during procedure (e.g., lie still, count out loud, squeeze a hand, hug a doll).
- Allow child to practise procedures that require cooperation (e.g., turning, deep breathing, incentive spirometry).
- Introduce anxiety-laden information last (e.g., starting an intravenous line).
- Be honest with the child about unpleasant aspects of a procedure but avoid creating undue concern. When discussing that a procedure may be uncomfortable, state that it feels differently to different people.
- Emphasize the end of the procedure and any pleasurable events afterward (e.g., going home, seeing parents).
- Stress positive benefits of the procedure (e.g., "After your tonsils are fixed, you won't have as many sore throats").

The exact timing of the preparation for a procedure varies with the child's age and type of procedure. While no exact guidelines govern timing, in general, the younger the child, the closer the explanation should be to the actual procedure in order to prevent undue fantasizing and worrying. With complex procedures, more time may be needed for assimilation of information, especially with older children. For example, the explanation for an injection can immediately precede the procedure for all ages, whereas preparation for surgery may begin the day before for young children and a few days before for older children (although older children's preferences should be elicited).

Establish Trust and Provide Support

The nurse who has spent time with and established a positive relationship with a child will usually find it easier to work together with the child. If the relationship is based on trust, the child will associate the nurse with caregiving activities that give comfort and pleasure most of the time rather than discomfort and stress. If the nurse does not know the child, it is best to be introduced by another staff person whom the child trusts. The first visit with the child should not include any painful procedure and ideally should focus on the child first, then on the explanation of the procedure.

Parental Presence and Support

Children need support during procedures, and for young children the greatest source of support is the parents. They represent security, safety, and comfort. Parental presence is preferable, however, since it can reduce patient and parent anxiety and decrease the need for sedation (Wright et al., 2007). The nurse should assess the parents' preferences for assisting, observing, or waiting outside the room, as well as the child's preference for parental presence. The child's and parents' choice should be respected. Parents who wish to stay should be given an appropriate explanation about the procedure and coached about what to do, where to sit or stand, and what to say in order to help the child through the procedure. Simple instructions such as clarifying where parents can stand or sit in the room and positioning them where they have eye contact with the child can provide support and lessen anxiety. Parents who do not want to be present or participate should be supported in their decision and encouraged to remain close by so that they can be available to console the child immediately after the procedure. Parents should also know that someone will be with their child to provide support. Ideally, this person should inform the parents after the procedure about how the child did.

Provide an Explanation

Age-appropriate explanations are one of the most widely used interventions for reducing anxiety in children

BOX 45-2 Age-Specific Preparation of Children for Procedures, Based on Developmental Characteristics

Infant: Developing a Sense of Trust and Sensorimotor Thought

Attachment to Parent

Involve parent in procedure, if desired.*
Keep parent in infant's line of vision.
If parent is unable to be with infant, place a familiar object with infant (e.g., stuffed toy).

Stranger Anxiety

Have usual caregivers perform or assist with procedure.*
Make advances slowly and in a nonthreatening manner.
Limit number of strangers entering the room during procedure.*

Sensorimotor Phase of Learning

During procedure, use sensory soothing measures (e.g., stroking skin, talking softly, giving pacifier).
Use analgesics (e.g., topical anaesthetic, intravenous opioid) to control discomfort.*
Cuddle and hug infant after stressful procedure; encourage parent to comfort infant.

Increased Muscle Control

Expect an older infant to resist.
Restrain adequately.
Keep harmful objects out of reach.

Memory for Past Experiences

Realize that older infants may associate objects, places, or persons with prior painful experiences and will cry and resist at the sight of them.
Keep frightening objects out of view.*
Perform painful procedures in a separate room, not in crib (or bed).*
Use nonintrusive procedures whenever possible (e.g., axillary temperatures, oral medications).*

Imitation of Gestures

Model desired behaviour (e.g., opening mouth).

Toddler: Developing a Sense of Autonomy and Sensorimotor to Preoperational Thought

Use the same approaches as for an infant, plus the following.

Egocentric Thought

Explain procedure in relation to what the child will see, hear, taste, smell, and feel.
Emphasize those aspects of procedure that require cooperation (e.g., lying still).
Tell child it is okay to cry, yell, or use other means to express discomfort verbally.

Negative Behaviour

Expect treatments to be resisted; the child may try to run away.
Use a firm, direct approach.
Ignore temper tantrums.
Use distraction techniques (e.g., singing a song with the child).
Restrain adequately.

Animism

Keep frightening objects out of view (young children believe objects have lifelike qualities and can harm them).

Limited Language Skills

Communicate using behaviours.
Use a few simple terms familiar to the child.
Give one direction at a time (e.g., "Lie down," then "Hold my hand").
Use small replicas of equipment; allow the child to handle equipment.
Use play; demonstrate on a doll but avoid using the child's favourite doll, since the child may think that the doll is really "feeling" the procedure.
Prepare parents separately to avoid child's misinterpreting of words.

Limited Concept of Time

Prepare the child shortly or immediately before procedure.
Keep teaching sessions short (about 5 to 10 minutes).
Have preparations completed before involving child in procedure.
Have extra equipment nearby (e.g., alcohol swabs, new needle, adhesive bandages) to avoid delays.
Tell the child when procedure is completed.

Striving for Independence

Allow choices whenever possible; the child may still be resistant and negative.
Allow child to participate in care and to help whenever possible (e.g., drink medicine from a cup, hold a dressing).

Preschooler: Developing Initiative and Preoperational Thought

Egocentric

Explain procedure in simple terms and in relation to how it affects the child (as with toddler, stress sensory aspects).
Demonstrate use of equipment.
Allow child to play with miniature or actual equipment.
Encourage "playing out" experience on a doll both before and after procedure to clarify misconceptions.
Use neutral words to describe the procedure.

Increased Language Skills

Use verbal explanation; avoid overestimating comprehension.
Encourage child to express ideas and feelings.

Limited Concept of Time and Frustration Tolerance

Implement the same approaches as for toddlers but may plan longer teaching session (10 to 15 minutes); may divide information into more than one session.

Illness and Hospitalization Viewed as Punishment

Clarify why each procedure is performed; a child will find it difficult to understand how medicine can make him or her feel better and can taste bad at the same time.
Ask child his or her thoughts about why a procedure is performed.

*Applies to any age.

BOX 45-2 Age-Specific Preparation of Children for Procedures, Based on Developmental Characteristics—cont'd

State directly that procedures are never a form of punishment.

Animism

Keep equipment out of sight, except when shown to or used on the child.

Fears of Bodily Harm, Intrusion, and Castration

Point out on drawing, doll, or child where procedure is performed.

Emphasize that no other body part will be involved.

Use nonintrusive procedures whenever possible (e.g., axillary temperature, oral medication).

Apply an adhesive bandage over the puncture site.

Encourage parental presence.

Realize that procedures involving genitalia provoke anxiety.

Allow child to wear underpants with gown.

Explain unfamiliar situations, especially noises or lights.

Striving for Initiative

Involve child in care whenever possible (e.g., holding equipment, removing dressing).

Give choices whenever possible but avoid excessive delays.

Praise child for helping and attempting to cooperate; never shame a child for lack of cooperation.

School-Age Child: Developing Industry and Concrete Thought

Increased Language Skills; Interest in Acquiring Knowledge

Explain procedures using correct scientific or medical terminology.

Explain reason for procedure using simple diagrams.

Explain function and operation of equipment in concrete terms.

Allow child to manipulate equipment; use doll or another person as a model to practise using equipment whenever possible (doll play may be considered childish by older school-age child).

Allow time before and after procedure for questions and discussion.

Improved Concept of Time

Plan for longer teaching sessions (about 20 minutes).

Prepare child before procedure.

Increased Self-Control

Gain child's trust.

Tell child what is expected.

Suggest ways of the child maintaining control (e.g., deep breathing, relaxation, counting).

Striving for Industry

Give the child responsibility for simple tasks (e.g., collecting specimens).

Include child in decision making (e.g., time of day to perform procedure, preferred site).

Encourage active participation (e.g., removing dressings, handling equipment, opening packages).

Developing Relationships With Peers

Prepare two or more children for the same procedure or encourage one peer to help prepare another.

Provide privacy from peers during procedure to maintain self-esteem.

Adolescent: Developing Identity and Abstract Thought

Increasing Abstract Thought and Reasoning

Supplement explanations with reasons why the procedure is necessary or beneficial.

Explain long-term consequences of procedures.

Realize that the adolescent may fear death, disability, or other risks.

Encourage questioning regarding fears, options, and alternatives.

Consciousness of Appearance

Provide privacy.

Discuss how the procedure may affect appearance (e.g., scarring) and what can be done to minimize it.

Emphasize any physical benefits of procedure.

Concern More With Present Than With Future

Realize that immediate effects of the procedure are more significant than future benefits.

Striving for Independence

Involve adolescent in decision making and planning (e.g., time, place, individuals present during procedure, clothing).

Impose as few restrictions as possible.

Suggest methods of maintaining control.

Accept regression to more childish methods of coping.

Realize that the adolescent may have difficulty accepting new authority figures and may resist complying with procedures.

Developing Peer Relationships and Group Identity

This is the same as for school-age children but assumes greater significance.

Allow adolescents to talk with other adolescents who have had the same procedure.

undergoing procedures. Before performing a procedure, it is important to explain what is to be done and what is expected of the child. The explanation should be short, simple, and geared to the child's level of comprehension. Long explanations may increase anxiety in a young child. When explaining the procedure to parents with the child present, the nurse needs to use language appropriate to the child because unfamiliar words can be misunderstood. If the parents need additional preparation, this can be done in an area away from the child. Teaching sessions should be planned at times most conducive to the child's learning (e.g., after a rest period) and for the usual span of attention. Allowing children to handle actual items that will be used in their care, such as a stethoscope, sphygmomanometer, or oxygen mask, helps them develop familiarity with these items and can reduce the threat often associated with their use. Written and illustrated materials are also valuable aids to preparation.

Physical Preparation

One area of special concern is the administration of sedation and analgesia before stressful procedures. Refer to Chapter 35 for information on sedating children.

Performance of the Procedure

Supportive care should continue during the procedure and can be a major factor in a child's ability to cooperate. Ideally, the same nurse who explains the procedure should perform or assist with the procedure. Before beginning, all equipment should be assembled and the room readied to prevent unnecessary delays and interruptions that could increase the child's anxiety.

NURSING ALERT To avoid a delay during a procedure, have extra supplies handy. For example, have tape, bandages, alcohol swabs, and an extra needle when performing an injection or venipuncture.

If possible, procedures should be performed in a special treatment room rather than in the child's hospital room. Traumatic procedures should never be performed in "safe" areas, such as the playroom. If the procedure is lengthy, avoid conversation that could be misinterpreted by the child. As the procedure is nearing completion, inform the child that it is almost over in language the child understands.

Expect Success

Nurses who approach children with confidence and who convey the impression that they expect to be successful are less likely to encounter difficulty. It is best to approach a child as though cooperation is expected. Children sense anxiety and uncertainty in an adult and may respond by striking out or actively resisting. Although it is not possible to eliminate such behaviour in every child, a firm approach with a positive attitude tends to convey a feeling of security to most children.

Involve the Child

Involving children helps to gain their confidence and willingness to work together. When they are given choices they have some measure of control. However, a choice should be given only in situations in which one is available. Asking children, "Do you want to take your medicine now?" leads them to believe they have an option and provides them with the opportunity to legitimately refuse or delay the medication. This places the nurse in an awkward, if not impossible, position. It is much better to state firmly, "It's time to drink your medicine now" and add a choice that they do indeed have (e.g., "Do you want to drink your medicine plain or with a little water?"). Many children respond to tactics that appeal to their maturity or courage. This also gives them a sense of participation and achievement. For example, preschool and school-age children will be proud that they can hold the dressing during the procedure or remove the tape.

Provide Distraction

Distraction is a powerful coping strategy during painful procedures (Algren & Algren, 1997) and is accomplished by focusing the child's attention on something other than the procedure. Singing favourite songs, listening to music, counting out loud, or blowing bubbles to "blow the hurt away" are effective techniques. For other nonpharmacological interventions that may lessen discomfort, see Pain Management, Chapter 35.

Allow Expression of Feelings

The child should be allowed to express feelings of anger, anxiety, fear, frustration, or any other emotion. It is natural for children to strike out in frustration or to try to avoid stress-provoking situations. The child needs to know that it is all right to cry. Behaviour is children's primary means of communication and coping and should be permitted unless it inflicts harm on them or those caring for them.

Postprocedural Support

After the procedure, the child needs reassurance that he or she performed well and is accepted and loved. If the parents did not participate, the child should be united with them as soon as possible so that they can provide comfort.

Encourage Expression of Feelings

Planned activity after the procedure is helpful in encouraging constructive expression of feelings. For verbal children, reviewing the details of the procedure can clarify misconceptions and garner feedback for improving the nurse's preparatory strategies. Play is an excellent activity for all children. Infants and young children should be given the opportunity for gross motor movement. Older children are able to vent their anger and frustration in acceptable pounding or throwing activities. One of the most effective interventions is **therapeutic play**, which includes well-supervised activities such as permitting the child to give an injection to a doll or stuffed toy to reduce the stress of injections (Fig. 45-1).

Provide Positive Reinforcement

Children need to hear from adults that they know the youngsters did the best they could in the situation, no matter how they behaved. It is important for children to know that their worth is not being judged on the basis of their behaviour

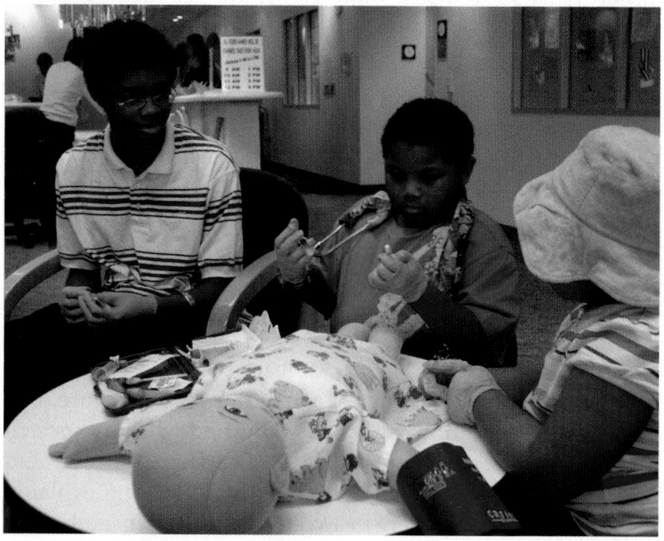

Fig. 45-1 Playing with hospital equipment provides children with the opportunity to play out fears and concerns.

in a stressful situation. Reward systems, such as earning stars, stickers, or a badge of courage, are appealing to children.

Returning to the child a short while after the procedure can help the nurse strengthen a supportive relationship. Relating with the child during a relaxed and nonstressful period allows the child to see the nurse not only as someone associated with stressful situations but as someone with whom to share pleasurable experiences.

Use of Play in Procedures

The use of play is an integral part of relationships with children. As such, its value in specific situations is discussed throughout this book, such as in Chapter 44, in relation to hospitalization. Many institutions have elaborate and well-organized play areas and programs under the direction of child life specialists; other institutions have limited facilities. No matter what the institution provides for children, nurses can include play activities as part of nursing care. Play can be used to teach, express feelings, or achieve a therapeutic goal. Play sessions after procedures can be structured, as directed toward syringe play, or general, with a wide variety of equipment available for children to play with. Routine procedures such as measuring blood pressure and administering oral medication may be of concern to children. Box 45-3 offers suggestions for incorporating play into nursing procedures and activities for the hospitalized child that facilitate learning and adjustment to a new situation.

Surgical Procedures

Preoperative Care

Children experiencing surgical procedures require both psychological and physical preparation. In general, psychological preparation is similar to that previously discussed for any procedure and employs many of the same techniques used in preparing a child for hospitalization, such as films, books, brochures, play, and tours. However, some important differences exist. Even though children are asleep for the actual surgical intervention, they are subjected to numerous preoperative and postoperative procedures. Stress points before and after surgery include the admission process, blood tests, injection of preoperative medication (if prescribed), transport to the operating room, and the stay in the postanaesthesia care unit (PACU).

Surprisingly little research has been conducted on children's perception of the surgical experience and their fears of the event. Although fear of **anaesthesia** is thought to be a major concern among children, little evidence exists to support this. School-age children report few remembered events and even fewer fears. Those events recalled most often were riding to and arriving in the operating room, receiving the preoperative or induction injection, waking up in pain, and not being allowed to eat or drink. The most feared events were the preoperative injection and the mask on the face.

Parental presence during induction of anaesthesia is allowed in some institutions (Fig. 45-2). Potential benefits include minimizing the need for premedication and reducing the struggle that often occurs during separation (Kain, Caldwell-Andrews, & Wang, 2002). Other benefits may include decreasing the child's anxiety during induction (e.g., breath holding and laryngospasm) and decreasing long-term behavioural effects of surgery (Romino et al., 2005). Some institutions endorse the policy, and reports from parents who attend the induction are favourable (Kain et al., 2004). Even though some parents may become anxious, most control their anxiety, do not disrupt the induction, and are able to support the child. Clinical observations show parental presence decreases anxiety in the child and reduces the need for heavy doses of preoperative sedation (Wright et al., 2007).

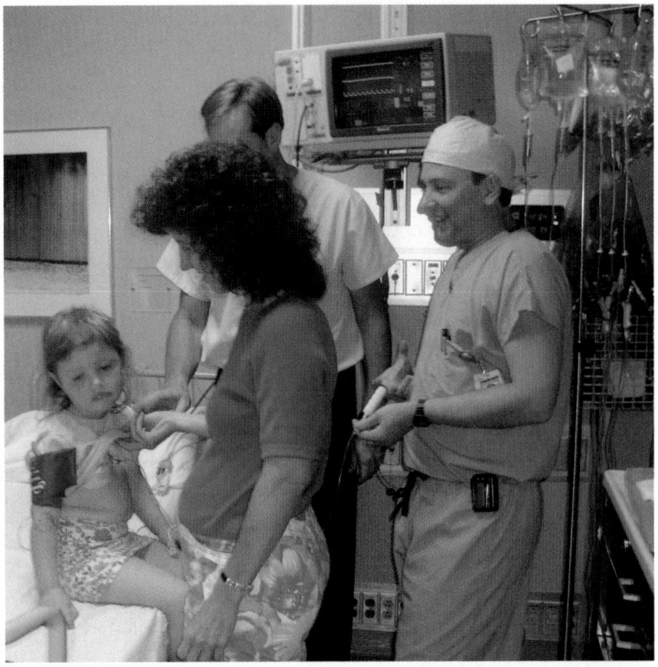

Fig. 45-2 Parental presence during induction of anaesthesia can minimize the child's and parents' anxiety during the preoperative period.

Appropriate education is essential to help parents understand the stages of anaesthesia, what to expect, and how to support their child (Wright et al., 2007). This should be combined with a program that prepares them for what to expect and what is expected of them. When parents choose not to or are not allowed to attend the induction, leaving a favourite possession with the child and uniting the child and parents as soon as possible after surgery (preferably in the PACU) are important actions. During surgery, the family should have a designated place to wait and should be kept informed of the child's progress. They also should know where and when they can visit the child after surgery.

Aside from possibly being separated from the parents before and after surgery, children may be cared for by a number of unfamiliar practitioners, which can instill fear and uncertainty. Although the same supportive nurse should remain with the child through as many of the procedures as possible, the child may have other nurses, especially if he or she returns to a special care unit postoperatively. Many hospitals conduct surgical tours for children and parents in order to familiarize them with the strange environment and introduce them to other individuals who will be involved in their care.

BOX 45-3 Play Activities for Specific Procedures*

Fluid Intake

Make ice pops using the child's favourite juice.
Cut gelatin into fun shapes.
Make a game out of taking a sip when turning the page of a book or in games such as Simon Says.
Use small medicine cups; decorate the cups.
Colour water with food colouring or powdered drink mix.
Have a tea party; pour at a small table.
Let the child fill a syringe and squirt into mouth or use it to fill small cups.
Cut straws in half and place in a small container (much easier for child to suck liquid).
Use a "crazy" straw.
Make a "progress poster"; give rewards for drinking a predetermined quantity.

Deep Breathing

Blow bubbles with a bubble blower.
Blow bubbles with a straw (no soap).
Blow on a pinwheel, feather, whistle, harmonica, balloon, horn, party blower.
Practise band instruments.
Have a blowing contest using boats, cotton balls, feathers, marbles, ping-pong balls, or pieces of paper; blow objects on a table top over a goal line, over water, through an obstacle course, into the air, against an opponent, or up and down a string.*
Suck paper or cloth from one container to another using a straw.
Use blow bottles with coloured water to transfer water from one side to the other.
Dramatize stories such as "I'll huff and puff and blow your house down" from the Three Little Pigs.
Do straw-blowing painting.
Take a deep breath and "blow out the candles" on a birthday cake.
Use a little paint brush to "paint" nails with water and blow nails dry.

Range of Motion and Use of Extremities

Throw beanbags at a fixed or movable target or throw wadded-up paper into a wastebasket.
Touch or kick Mylar balloons held or hung in different positions (if the child is in traction, hang balloon from a trapeze).
Play "tickle toes"; have child wiggle them on request.
Play Twister game or Simon Says.
Play pretend and guessing games (e.g., imitate a bird, butterfly, horse).
Have tricycle or wheelchair races in a safe area.
Play kickball or catch with a soft foam ball in a safe area.
Position bed so that the child must turn to view the television or doorway.
Climb wall like a "spider."
Pretend to teach "aerobic" dancing or exercises; encourage parents to participate.
Encourage swimming, if feasible.
Play video games or pinball (fine motor movement).
Play "hide and seek": hide a toy somewhere in the bed (or room if ambulatory) and have child find it using specified hand or foot.
Provide clay to mould with fingers.
Paint or draw on large sheets of paper placed on the floor or wall.
Encourage combing own hair; play "beauty shop" with the "customer" in different positions.

Soaks

Play with small toys or objects (cups, syringes, soap dishes) in water.
Wash dolls or toys.
Pick up marbles or pennies* from the bottom of a bath container.
Make designs with coins on the bottom of a container.
Pretend a boat is a submarine by keeping it immersed.
During soaks, read to the child; sing with the child; or play a game, such as cards, checkers, or other board game (if both of the child's hands are immersed, move board pieces for the child).
During a sitz bath, when soaking the perineal and rectal area, give the child something to listen to (music, stories) or look at (View-Master, book).
Punch holes in the bottom of a plastic cup, fill with water, and let it "rain" on the child.

Injections

Let child handle the syringe, vial, and alcohol swab and give an injection to a doll or stuffed animal.
Use syringes to decorate cookies with frosting, squirt paint, or target shoot into a container.
Draw a "magic circle" on the area before injection; draw a smiling face in the circle after injection, but avoid drawing on the puncture site.
Allow child to have a "collection" of syringes (without needles); make "wild" creative objects with syringes.
If the child has multiple injections or venipunctures, make a "progress poster"; give rewards for a predetermined number of injections.
Have the child count to 10 or 15 during injection.

Ambulation

Give the child something to push.
- Toddler—Push-pull toy
- School-age child—Wagon or a doll in a stroller or wheelchair
- Adolescent—Decorated intravenous stand

Have a parade; make hats, drums, etc.

Extending Environment (e.g., for Patients in Traction)

Make bed into a pirate ship or an airplane with decorations.
Put up mirrors so that the patient can see around the room.
Move the bed frequently to the playroom, hallway, or outside.

*Small objects such as marbles or coins, as well as latex gloves or balloons, are unsafe for young children because of possible aspiration. Latex products also carry the risk of an allergic reaction.

An important concern is restriction of food and fluids before surgery to avoid aspiration during anaesthesia. Infants require special attention to fluid needs. They should not be without oral fluids for an extended period preoperatively to avoid glycogen depletion and dehydration. Current preoperative fasting guidelines are found in Table 45-1.

Preoperative Sedation

Historically, the most upsetting event for children has been the preoperative injection. Increasingly, more anaesthesiologists are using preoperative sedatives, usually midazolam (Versed), and more parents stay nearby for their children undergoing surgery (Kain et al., 2004). When medications are administered, they should be delivered atraumatically via oral or intravenous (IV) routes. Numerous preanaesthetic medication regimens are used with children, and no consensus exists on the optimal method. The goals for using preoperative medications include (1) anxiety reduction, (2) amnesia, (3) sedation, (4) antiemetic effect, and (5) reduction of secretions (Manworren & Fledderman, 2000). Midazolam provides excellent preoperative anxiety reduction, amnesia, and sedation. It is popular because of its short duration, predictable onset, and rare occurrence of respiratory depression. If children have no preoperative pain, are well prepared psychologically for surgery, and have their parents nearby, preoperative medication may be unnecessary.

Induction of anaesthesia in the pediatric patient is commonly accomplished by administering inhalation agents in combination with nitrous oxide and oxygen by mask. Children may fear induction of anaesthesia by mask. Practices that can minimize anxiety related to the inhalation of anaesthesia are (1) disguising the unpleasant odour of anaesthetic gases by applying a pleasant-smelling substance on the mask; (2) using a transparent plastic mask rather than an opaque black mask and gradually bringing it toward the face; (3) directing a stream of gas toward the child's face from the bare tube until the child becomes drowsy, then using the mask; (4) allowing the child to sit up rather than lie down for anaesthesia induction; and (5) allowing preoperative play with a mask and a doll or manikin.

Table 45-1 Fasting Recommendations to Reduce the Risk of Pulmonary Aspiration*

INGESTED MATERIAL	MINIMUM FASTING PERIOD (HR)†
Clear liquids‡	2
Breast milk	4
Infant formula	6
Nonhuman milk§	6
Light meal¶	6

(From American Society of Anesthesiologists. [1999]. Practice guidelines for preoperative fasting and the use of pharmacological agents to reduce the risk of pulmonary aspiration: Application to healthy patients undergoing elective procedures. *Anesthesiology, 90*[3], 896–905.)

*These recommendations apply to healthy patients who are undergoing elective procedures. They are not intended for women in labour. Following the guidelines does not guarantee that a complete gastric emptying has occurred.

†Fasting periods noted in chart apply to all ages.

‡Examples of clear liquids include water, fruit juices without pulp, carbonated beverages, clear tea, and black coffee.

§Because nonhuman milk is similar to solids in gastric emptying time, the amount ingested must be considered when determining appropriate fasting period.

¶A light meal typically consists of toast and clear liquids. Meals that include fried or fatty foods or meat may prolong gastric emptying time. Both the amount and type of foods ingested must be considered when determining appropriate fasting period.

Postoperative Care

Various psychological and physical interventions and observations are required to prevent or minimize possible untoward effects from anaesthesia and the surgical procedure (see Guidelines box). Although the incidence of serious postoperative complications in healthy children undergoing surgery is less than 1% (Maxwell & Yaster, 2000), continuous monitoring of cardiopulmonary status is essential during the immediate postoperative period. Postanaesthesia complications such as

GUIDELINES Postoperative Care

Ensure that preparations are made to receive the child:
- Bed or crib is ready.
- Intravenous pumps and poles, suction apparatus, and oxygen flow meter are at bedside.

Obtain baseline information:
- Take vital signs, including blood pressure; keep blood pressure cuff in place and deflated to lessen amount of disturbance to child.
- Take and record vital signs more frequently if any value fluctuates.
- Inspect operative area.
- Check dressing, if present: (1) outline any bleeding area on dressing or cast with pen; (2) reinforce, but do not remove, loose dressing; (3) observe areas below surgical site for blood that may have drained toward bed; and (4) assess for bleeding and other symptoms in areas not covered with a dressing, such as throat after tonsillectomy.
- Assess skin colour and characteristics.
- Assess level of consciousness and activity.

Notify physician of any irregularities in the child's condition.

Assess for evidence of pain (see Pain Assessment, Chapter 35).

Review surgeon's orders after completing initial assessment, and check that any preoperative orders, such as seizure or cardiac medications, have been reordered and can be given by available routes (oral preparations may be contraindicated).

Monitor vital signs as ordered and more often if indicated.

Check dressings for bleeding or other abnormalities.

Check bowel sounds.

Observe for signs of shock, abdominal distention, and bleeding.

Assess for bladder distention.

Observe for signs of dehydration.

Detect presence of infection:
- Take vital signs every 2 to 4 hours, as ordered.
- Collect or request needed specimens.
- Inspect wound for signs of infection—redness, swelling, heat, pain, and purulent drainage.

airway obstruction, postextubation croup, laryngospasm, and bronchospasm make maintaining a patent airway and maximum ventilation critical.

Monitoring oxygen saturation and providing supplemental oxygen as needed, maintaining body temperature, and promoting fluid and electrolyte balance are important aspects of immediate postoperative care. Vital signs should be continuously monitored, and each vital sign should be evaluated in terms of adverse effects from anaesthesia, **shock**, or respiratory compromise (Table 45-2).

A change in vital signs that demands immediate attention in the perioperative period is caused by malignant hyperthermia (MH), a potentially fatal genetic myopathy. In susceptible children, anaesthetics such as succinylcholine and halothane can trigger the disorder, producing hypermetabolism, muscle rigidity, and an elevated temperature. Early symptoms of MH include tachycardia and tachyarrhythmias, **tachypnea**, hypercarbia, and metabolic and respiratory acidosis. An elevated temperature is considered by many to be a late sign of the disorder (Redmond, 2001). A family or previous history of sudden high fever associated with a surgical procedure and certain neuromuscular disorders increase the risk for MH; children who have successfully undergone prior surgery without adverse effects may still be considered susceptible. Treatment includes immediate discontinuation of the triggering agent and surgical procedure, hyperventilation with 100% oxygen, and IV dantrolene sodium. Infusions of cool saline, cooling blankets, gastric or peritoneal lavage, packed ice bags in the axillae and groin, and, possibly, cardiopulmonary bypass reduce core temperature (Redmond, 2001). The patient should

Table 45-2 Potential Causes of Postoperative Vital Sign Alterations in Children

ALTERATION	POTENTIAL CAUSE	COMMENTS
Heart Rate		
Increase	Decreased perfusion (shock) Elevated temperature Pain Respiratory distress (early) Medications (atropine, morphine, epinephrine)	Heart rate may increase to maintain cardiac output.
Decrease	Hypoxia Vagal stimulation Increased intracranial pressure Respiratory distress (late) Medications	In the young child, bradycardia is of more concern than tachycardia.
Respiratory Rate		
Increase	Respiratory distress Fluid volume excess Hypothermia Elevated temperature Pain	Body responds to respiratory distress primarily by increasing rate.
Decrease	Anaesthetics, opioids Pain	Decreased respiratory rate from opioids may be compensated for by increase depth of respiration.
Blood Pressure		
Increase	Excess intravascular volume Increased intracranial pressure Carbon dioxide retention Pain Medication (ketamine, epinephrine)	This is serious in preterm infants because it increases risk of intraventricular hemorrhage.
Decrease	Vasodilating anaesthetic agents (halothane, isoflurane, enflurane) Opioids (morphine)	Decreased blood pressure is late sign of shock because of elasticity and constriction of vessels to maintain cardiac output.
Temperature		
Increase	Shock (late sign) Infection Environmental causes (warm room, excess coverings) Malignant hyperthermia	Fever associated with infection usually occurs later than fever of noninfectious origin. Absence of fever does not rule out infection, especially in infants.
Decrease	Vasodilating anaesthetic agents (halothane, isoflurane, enflurane) Muscle relaxants Environmental causes (cool room) Infusion of cool fluids or blood	Malignant hyperthermia requires immediate treatment. Neonates are especially susceptible to hypothermia, with serious or fatal consequences.

(From Smith, D. P. [1991]. *Comprehensive child and family nursing skills*. St. Louis: Mosby.)

be transferred to a critical care unit and closely monitored for stabilization of vital signs, metabolic state, and possible recurrence of symptoms.

Managing pain is a major nursing responsibility after surgery (see Chapter 35). The nurse should assess pain frequently and administer analgesics to provide comfort and facilitate postoperative care routines such as ambulation and deep breathing. **Opioids** are the most commonly used analgesics. Routinely scheduled IV analgesics, patient-controlled analgesia, and epidural infusions, rather than as needed (prn) orders, provide excellent analgesia in postoperative pediatric patients.

Because respiratory infections are a potential complication, every effort should be taken to aerate the lungs and remove secretions. The lungs should be auscultated regularly to identify abnormal sounds or any areas of diminished or absent breath sounds. To prevent hypostatic pneumonia, respiratory movement can be encouraged with incentive spirometers or other motivating activities (see Box 45-3). If these measures are presented as games, the child is more likely to work with the nurse. The child's position needs to be changed every 2 hours and deep breathing encouraged.

Adherence to the Medical Treatment Plan

Adherence, also termed *compliance*, refers to the extent to which the patient's behaviour coincides with the prescribed regimen in terms of taking medication, following diets, or executing other lifestyle changes. In developing strategies to assist with adherence, the nurse must first assess the level of knowledge and understanding. Because many children are too young to assume partial or total responsibility for their care, parents are usually primarily responsible for home management.

Factors relating to the care setting are important in ensuring adherence and should be considered in planning strategies to improve it. Basically, any aspect of the health care environment that increases the family's satisfaction with the physical setting and the relationship with the practitioner positively influences adherence to the treatment regimen. However, the more complex, expensive, inconvenient, and disruptive the treatment protocol, the less likely the family is to comply. Long-term conditions that involve multiple treatments and considerable rearrangement of lifestyle make it more difficult to continue with the proposed plan of care.

Although it is helpful to know those factors that influence adherence, assessing the ability of the child and family to adhere to the plan of care includes more direct measurement techniques. A number of methods exist, each with advantages and disadvantages. The most successful approach includes a combination of at least two of the following methods:

Clinical judgement—This is subject to bias and inaccuracy unless the nurse carefully evaluates the criteria used in assessment.

Self-reporting—Most people overestimate compliance by about 20% even when they admit to lapses.

Direct observation—This is difficult to employ outside the health care setting, and awareness of being observed frequently affects performance.

Monitoring appointments—Keeping appointments indirectly indicates adherence with the prescribed care.

Monitoring therapeutic response—Few treatments yield directly measurable results (e.g., decreased blood pressure, weight loss); record them on a graph or chart.

Pill counts—The nurse counts the number of pills remaining in the original container and compares the number missing with the number of times the medication should have been taken.

Chemical assay—For certain medications, such as digoxin and phenytoin, measurement of plasma drug levels provides information on the amount of medication recently ingested.

Strategies to Promote Adherence to the Treatment Plan

Strategies to assist children and their families to follow the prescribed treatment are composed of various interventions. Some evidence suggests that higher levels of self-esteem and increased autonomy favourably affect adolescent compliance (KyngAs, Kroll, & Duffy, 2000). However, family factors are also important; characteristics associated with following a treatment plan include family support, family reminders, good communication, and expectations for successful completion of the therapeutic regimen (KyngAs et al., 2000). No one approach is always successful, and the best results occur when at least two strategies are used.

Organizational strategies of encouraging treatment adherence have to do with the care setting and the therapeutic plan. The factors listed in Box 45-4 need to be promoted to positively affect adherence to treatment. *Educational strategies*

BOX 45-4 Factors That Positively Influence Following of the Treatment Plan

Individual and Family Factors
High self-esteem
Positive body image
High degree of autonomy (increased locus of control)
Supportive and well-adjusted family
Effective family communication
Family expectation for successful completion of therapy

Care Setting Factors
Perceived satisfaction with care
Positive interactions with practitioners
Continuity of care
Individualized care
Minimum waiting time for appointments
Convenient care setting

Treatment Factors
Simple regimen
Minimum disruption in usual lifestyle
Short duration
Inexpensive
Visible benefits
Tolerable side effects

are used to instruct the family about the treatment plan. Although education is an important factor in enhancing adherence, and patients who are more knowledgeable about their condition are more likely to comply, education alone does not ensure compliant behaviour. The nurse should incorporate teaching principles known to enhance understanding and retention of material. Written materials are essential, especially in any regimen requiring multiple or complex treatments, and they need to be understandable to the average individual, who reads at about the fourth-grade level. *Treatment strategies* relate to the child's refusal or inability to take the prescribed medication. The family may also have difficulty following a prescribed treatment regimen. They may remember and understand the instructions but may not be able to give the medicine as prescribed. Any reason for refusal should be assessed. For example, the child may not be able to swallow pills. In this case, perhaps pills can be crushed or a liquid medication substituted (always review medication to ensure that crushing is acceptable before giving this instruction).

The treatment and medication schedule needs to be assessed to determine if it is reasonable for a home situation. Although an every-6-hour or every-8-hour schedule is reasonable for hospitals, a parent would have difficulty getting up once or twice nightly; instead, a medication could be given during the day at times that would be easy to remember.

Behavioural strategies are designed to modify behaviour directly. Several strategies encouraging the desired behaviour are effective with children. Ideally, positive reinforcement should be employed to strengthen the behaviour and may consist of earning stars or tokens, which gains the child a special privilege or gift. At times, however, disciplinary techniques used by parents (not nurses), such as time-out for young children or withholding privileges for older children, may be needed to improve compliance (see Limit Setting and Discipline, Chapter 31). *Contracting*, a formal process in which exact elements of desired behaviour are explicitly outlined along with rewards or negative consequences, is an effective method with older children.

General Hygiene and Care

Maintaining Healthy Skin

Maintaining an IV line, removing a dressing, positioning a child in bed, changing a diaper, using electrodes, and using restraints have the potential to contribute to skin injury. Skin care must go beyond the daily bath and become a part of each nursing intervention (see Guidelines box). Specific guidelines for skin care of neonates are provided in Sponge Bathing, Cord Care, and Skin Care, Chapter 25.

Assessment of the skin is most easily accomplished during the bath. The nurse should examine the skin for early signs of injury. Risk factors include impaired mobility, protein malnutrition, **edema**, incontinence, sensory loss, anemia, infection, failure to turn the patient, and intubation. Critically ill children often are at high risk of pressure ulcers and skin breakdown, since they often have several risk factors combined. Identification of risk factors helps to determine those children who need a more thorough skin assessment. Assessment should occur within 24 hours of admission so that pressure ulcers and wounds that occurred before admission can be identified (Quigley & Curley, 1996; Registered Nurses' Association of Ontario [RNAO], 2005).

When capillary blood flow is interrupted by pressure, the blood flows back into the tissue when the pressure is relieved. As the body attempts to reoxygenate the area, a bright red flush appears. This reactive **hyperemia**, or flush, is the earliest sign of tissue compromise and pressure-related ischemia. If pressure is prolonged, reactive hyperemia will not be sufficient to revitalize ischemic tissue (RNAO, 2005).

GUIDELINES Skin Care

- Cleanse skin with mild nonalkaline soap or soap-free cleaning agents for routine bathing.
- Provide daily cleansing of eyes, oral, and diaper or perineal areas, and any areas of skin breakdown.
- Apply moisturizing agents during or immediately after bathing.
- Use minimum tape and adhesives. On very sensitive skin, use a protective, pectin-based or hydrocolloid skin barrier between skin and tape or adhesives.
- Use water or adhesive remover (if skin is not fragile) when removing tape or adhesives.
- Place pectin-based or hydrocolloid skin barriers directly over excoriated skin. Leave barrier undisturbed until it begins to peel off, or for 5 to 7 days. With wet, oozing excoriations, place a small amount of stoma powder on site, remove excess powder, and apply skin barrier. Hold barrier in place for several minutes to allow barrier to soften and mould to skin surface.
- Alternate electrode placement and thoroughly assess skin underneath electrodes at least every 24 hours. Alcohol-free skin sealant under leads protects skin from epidermal stripping.
- Be certain fingers or toes are visible whenever extremity is used for an intravenous (IV) or arterial line.
- Keep skin dry (may apply absorbent powder [e.g., cornstarch]) and use soft, smooth bed linen and clothes.
- Use a draw sheet to move a child in bed or onto a gurney; do not drag the child from under the arms.
- Identify children at risk for skin breakdown before it occurs. Employ measures such as pressure-reducing or pressure-relieving devices (e.g., mattress overlay, low-air-loss bed, gel pillows). The Braden Q Scale may be used to assess severity of the ulcer (see Additional Resources section).
- Do not massage reddened bony prominences as this can cause deep tissue damage; provide pressure relief to those areas instead.
- Keep skin free of excess moisture (e.g., urine or fecal incontinence, wound drainage, excessive perspiration).
- Routinely assess the child's nutritional status. A child who is NPO (nothing by mouth) for several days and is receiving only IV fluid is nutritionally at risk, which can also affect the skin's ability to maintain its integrity. Consider parenteral nutrition.

Staging of pressure ulcers is used to classify the amount of tissue damage. Necrotic tissue must be removed so that the tissue depth can be accurately assessed. Accurate documentation of redness or obvious skin breakdown is essential. Colour, size (diameter and depth), location, presence of sinus tracts, odour, exudate, and response to treatment should be observed and recorded at least daily (RNAO, 2005).

Pressure ulcers can develop when the pressure on the skin and underlying tissues is greater than the capillary closing pressure, causing capillary occlusion. If the pressure remains unrelieved, vessels can collapse, resulting in tissue anoxia and cellular death. Pressure ulcers most often occur over bony prominences and are usually very deep, extending into subcutaneous tissue or even deeper into muscle, tendon, or bone. A *pressure-reduction device* reduces pressure but does not prevent pressure from causing capillary closure; thus turning and repositioning the patient are always included when using these devices. Most of these items are overlays that are placed on top of the regular mattress. A *pressure-relief device* maintains pressure below that which would cause capillary closure. These devices are usually high-technology beds that are used for patients who have multiple problems and cannot be turned effectively.

Friction and shear contribute to pressure ulcers. *Friction* occurs when the skin's surface rubs against another surface, such as the bed sheets. Skin damage most often occurs over the elbows, heels, or occiput; is usually limited to the epidermal and upper layers; and may have the appearance of an abrasion. Prevention of friction injury includes the use of protective sheepskin over the elbows or heels; gel pillows under the head of infants and toddlers; moisturizing agents; transparent dressings over susceptible areas; and soft, smooth bed linen and clothing. *Shear* is the result of the force of gravity pushing down on the body and friction of the body against a surface, such as the bed or chair. For example, when a patient is in the semi-Fowler position and begins to slide to the foot of the bed, the skin over the sacral area remains in the same place because of the resistance of the bed surface. The blood vessels in the area are stretched and may cause small-vessel thrombosis and tissue death (RNAO, 2005). Prevention of shear injury includes using lift sheets when repositioning a patient, elevating the bed no more than 30 degrees for short periods, and using the knee gatch to interrupt the pull of gravity on the body toward the foot of the bed.

Epidermal stripping results when the epidermis is unintentionally removed with tape removal. These lesions are usually shallow and irregularly shaped and may blister or weep. Babies are at increased risk for epidermal injury. Prevention of injury includes using no tape when possible and securing dressings with laced binders (Montgomery straps) or stretchy netting (Spandage or stockinette). Use of porous or low-tack tapes (e.g., Medipore, paper, hydrogel) and alcohol-free skin sealants (No Sting Barrier Film) or picture framing wounds with hydrocolloid or wafer barriers (e.g., DuoDERM, Coloplast, Stomahesive) and then taping on top of the barrier will also reduce epidermal stripping.

Tape should be placed so that there is no tension, traction, or wrinkles on the skin. To remove tape, it should be slowly peeled away while stabilizing the underlying skin. Adhesive remover may be used to break the adhesive bond but may be drying to the skin; adhesive removers should be avoided in preterm neonates, since absorption rates vary and toxicity may occur. The adhesive is removed with water to prevent absorption and irritation. Wetting the tape with water or alcohol-based foam hand cleansers may facilitate removal.

Chemical factors can also lead to skin damage. Fecal incontinence, especially when mixed with urine; wound drainage; or gastric drainage around gastrostomy tubes can erode epidermis. The skin can quickly progress from redness to denudement if exposure continues. Moisture barriers, gentle cleansing as soon after exposure as possible, and skin barriers can be used to prevent damage caused by chemical factors (see also Diaper Dermatitis, Chapter 53). In addition, foam dressings that wick moisture away from the skin are helpful around gastrostomy tubes and tracheostomy sites.

Bathing

Most infants and children can be bathed in a basin at the bedside, on the bed, or in a standard bathtub or shower. For infants and young children confined to bed, the towel method can be used. Two towels are immersed in a diluted soap solution and wrung damp. With the child lying supine on a dry towel, one damp towel is placed on top of the child and used to gently clean the body. This towel is discarded, and the child is dried and turned prone. The procedure is repeated using the second damp towel. Commercially available bath cloths may also be used.

Infants and small children should *never* be left unattended in a bathtub, and infants who are unable to sit alone need to be securely held with one hand during the bath. The nurse should securely support the infant's head with one hand, or grasp the farther arm firmly while the head rests comfortably on the nurse's arm. Children who are able to sit without assistance need only close supervision and a pad placed in the bottom of the tub to prevent slipping and loss of balance.

School-age children and adolescents may shower or bathe. Nurses need to use judgement regarding the amount of supervision the child requires. Some can assume this responsibility unaided, whereas others will need someone in constant attendance. Children with cognitive impairments, physical limitations, or suicidal or psychotic problems (who may commit bodily harm) require close supervision.

Children who are ill or debilitated need more extensive assistance with bathing, but should be encouraged to perform as much as they can without overtaxing their energies. Increasing involvement can be expected with improved strength and endurance.

Oral Hygiene

Mouth care is an integral part of daily hygiene and should be continued in the hospital. Infants and debilitated children require the nurse or a family member to perform mouth care. Although young children can manage a toothbrush and should be encouraged to use it, most need assistance to perform satisfactorily. Older children, although capable of brushing and flossing without assistance, sometimes need to be reminded. (See Dental Health, Chapters 36 and 37, for specific oral hygiene techniques; mouth care of children with mucosal ulcers is discussed under nursing care of the child with leukemia in Chapter 49.)

Hair Care

Children should have their hair brushed and combed at least once daily. The hair should be styled for comfort and in a manner pleasing to the child and parents. The hair should not be cut without parental permission, although clipping hair to provide access to a scalp vein for IV insertion may be necessary.

If children are hospitalized for more than a few days, the hair may need shampooing. With infants the hair may be washed during the bath. For most children, washing the hair and scalp once or twice weekly is sufficient unless there is an indication for more frequent washing, such as following a high fever and profuse sweating. Adolescents normally have increased oily sebaceous secretions that require frequent hair care and more frequent shampoos.

Most children can be transported to an accessible sink for shampooing. Those who are unable to be transported can receive a shampoo in their beds with adequate protection, specially adapted equipment or positioning, or dry shampoo caps. When necessary, a shampoo basin may be used or the child may be positioned near the edge of the bed, towels placed under the shoulders, a large plastic garbage bag draped at the edge of the bed with one open end under the shoulders, and the hair placed inside the opening. The other end is opened and placed in a collection container. Water can be transported in a basin.

Feeding the Sick Child

Loss of appetite is a symptom common to most childhood illnesses. Because an acute illness is usually short, the nutritional state is seldom compromised. Urging foods on the sick child may precipitate nausea and vomiting, and in most cases children can be permitted to determine their own need for food.

Refusing to eat may also be one way that children can exert power and control in an otherwise helpless situation. For young children, loss of appetite may be related to the depression caused by separation from their parents. Parents' concern with eating can intensify the problem. Forcing a child to eat can be met with rebellion and reinforces the behaviour as a control mechanism. Parents should be encouraged to relax any pressure during an acute illness. Although it is best to encourage high-quality nutritious foods, the child may desire foods and liquids that contain mostly empty or non-nutritional calories. Some well-tolerated foods include gelatin, diluted clear soups, carbonated drinks, flavoured ice pops, dry toast, and crackers. Even though these substances are not nutritious, they can provide necessary fluid and calories.

Dehydration is always a hazard when children are febrile or anorexic, especially when accompanied by vomiting or diarrhea. Small amounts of flavoured fluids can be offered at frequent intervals and salty foods (which increase thirst) provided, if allowed. If the child has diarrhea, high-carbohydrate liquids (e.g., carbonated beverages, gelatin, flavoured ice pops) should be avoided because they may aggravate the diarrhea by an osmotic effect. Replacing abnormal losses with plain water or undiluted broth may worsen the electrolyte imbalance. Fluids should not be forced, and the child not awakened to take fluids. Forcing fluids may create the same difficulties as with urging unwanted food. Gentle persuasion with preferred beverages will usually meet with success. Using play techniques can also be effective (see Guidelines box).

Once the child is feeling better the appetite usually begins to improve. It is best to take advantage of any hungry period by serving high-quality foods and snacks. If the child still refuses to eat, nutritious fluids, such as prepared breakfast drinks, should be encouraged. Parents can help by bringing in food items from home, especially if the family's cultural eating habits differ from the hospital food. A clinical dietitian may also be consulted for alternative food choices.

When children are placed on special diets, such as clear liquids after surgery or during episodes of diarrhea, assessment of their intake and readiness to advance to more complex foods is essential. Regardless of the type of diet, charting of the amount consumed is an important nursing responsibility. Descriptions need to be detailed and accurate, such as "120 mL of orange juice, one pancake, and 240 mL of milk." Comments such as "ate well" or "ate poorly" are inadequate. Charting the percentage of the meal eaten is also inadequate unless food is measured before serving.

If parents are involved in the child's care, they should be encouraged to keep a list of everything eaten. Use of a premeasured cup for fluids ensures a more accurate estimate of intake. A comparison of the intake at each meal can isolate food deficiencies, such as insufficient intake of meat or vegetables. Behaviours associated with mealtime also may point to possible factors influencing appetite. For example, the observation that "child eats well when with other children but plays with food if left alone in room" can help the nurse plan mealtime activities that stimulate the appetite.

Controlling Elevated Temperatures

An elevated temperature, most frequently from fever but occasionally caused by hyperthermia, is one of the most common symptoms of illness in children. This manifestation is of great concern to parents. To facilitate an understanding of fever, the following terms are defined:

Set point—The temperature around which body temperature is regulated by a thermostat-like mechanism in the hypothalamus

Fever (hyperpyrexia)—An elevation in set point such that body temperature is regulated at a higher level; may be arbitrarily defined as temperature above 38°C

Hyperthermia—Body temperature exceeding the set point, which usually results from the body or external conditions creating more heat than the body can eliminate, as in heat-stroke, aspirin toxicity, seizures, or hyperthyroidism

Body temperature is regulated by a thermostat-like mechanism in the **hypothalamus**. This mechanism receives input from centrally and peripherally located receptors. When temperature changes occur, these receptors relay the information to the thermostat, which either increases or decreases heat production to maintain a constant set point temperature. However, during an infection, **pyrogenic** substances cause an

GUIDELINES Feeding the Sick Child

Take a dietary history (see Chapter 34) and use information to make eating time as much like home as possible.
Encourage parents or other family members to feed the child or to be present at mealtimes.
Make mealtimes pleasant; avoid any procedures immediately before or after eating; make certain the child is rested and pain free.
Serve small, frequent meals rather than three large meals, or serve three meals and nutritious between-meal snacks.
Provide finger foods for young children.
Involve children in food selection and preparation whenever possible.
Serve small portions, and serve each course separately, such as soup first; followed by meat, potatoes, and vegetables; and ending with dessert.

- With young children, camouflage size of food by cutting meat thicker so that less appears on the plate or by folding a cheese slice in half.
- Offer second helpings.

Ensure a variety of foods, textures, and colours.
Provide food selections that are favourites of most children, such as peanut butter and jelly sandwiches, hot dogs, hamburgers, macaroni and cheese, pizza, spaghetti, tacos, fried chicken, corn, and fruit yogourt.
Avoid foods that are highly seasoned, have strong odours, or are all mixed together, unless typical of cultural practices.
Provide fluid selections that are favourites of most children, such as fruit punch, cola, ginger ale, sweetened tea, flavoured ice pops, sherbet, ice cream, milk, milkshakes, eggnog, pudding, gelatin, clear broth, or creamed soups.
Offer nutritious snacks, such as frozen yogourt or pudding, oatmeal, hot cocoa, cheese slices, pieces of raw vegetable or fruit, and dried fruit or cereal.
Make food attractive and different; for example:

- Serve a "picnic lunch" in a paper bag.
- Pack food in a take-out container; decorate the container.
- Put a "face" or a "flower" on a hamburger or sandwich with pieces of vegetable.
- Use a cookie cutter to shape a sandwich.
- Serve pudding, yogourt, or juice frozen as an ice pop.
- Make slurpies or snow cones by pouring flavoured syrup on crushed ice.
- Add food colouring to water or milk.
- Serve fluids through brightly coloured or unusually shaped straws.
- Make "bowtie" sandwiches by cutting them in triangles and placing two points together.
- Slice sandwiches into "fingers."
- Grate mounds of cheese.
- Cut apples horizontally to make circles.
- Put a banana on a hot dog bun and spread with peanut butter.
- Break uncooked spaghetti into toothpick lengths and skewer cheese, cold meat, vegetables, or fruit chunks.

Praise children for what they do eat.
Do not punish children for not eating by removing their dessert or putting them to bed.

increase in the body's normal set point, a process that is mediated by prostaglandins. Consequently, the hypothalamus increases heat production until the core temperature reaches the new set point.

Most fevers in children are of brief duration with limited consequences and are viral in origin. When fever is caused by bacteria, endotoxins are produced that activate the inflammatory process and produce fever (Rote, Huether, & McCance, 2000). Contrary to popular belief, neither the rise in temperature nor its response to antipyretics indicates the severity or cause of infection, which casts doubt on the value of using fever as a diagnostic or prognostic indicator.

Therapeutic management of elevated temperature depends on whether it is due to a fever or hyperthermia. Because the set point is normal in hyperthermia but increased in fever, different approaches must be used to lower body temperature successfully.

Fever

The principal reason for treating fever is the relief of discomfort. Relief measures include pharmacological or environmental intervention. The most effective intervention is the use of antipyretics to lower the set point.

Antipyretic medications include acetaminophen, aspirin, and nonsteroidal anti-inflammatory drugs (NSAIDs). Acetaminophen is the preferred medication; aspirin should not be given to children because of the association between aspirin use in children and Reye's syndrome. One nonprescription NSAID, ibuprofen, is approved for fever reduction in children as young as 6 months of age. Dosage is based on the initial temperature level: 5 mg/kg of body weight for temperatures less than 39.2°C or 10 mg/kg for temperatures greater than 39.2°C. The recommended dosage for pain is 10 mg/kg every 6 to 8 hours, and the recommended maximum daily dose for pain and fever is 40 mg/kg. The duration of fever reduction is generally 6 to 8 hours and is longer with the higher dose. It may be given every 4 hours but no more than five times in 24 hours. Because body temperature normally decreases at night, three or four doses in 24 hours will control most fevers. The nurse should retake the temperature 30 minutes after the antipyretic is given to assess its effect, but temperature should not be repeatedly measured; the child's level of discomfort is the best indication for continued treatment.

Environmental measures to reduce fever may be used if tolerated by the child and if they do not induce shivering. Shivering is the body's way of maintaining the elevated set point by producing heat. Compensatory shivering greatly increases metabolic requirements above those already caused by the fever.

Traditional cooling measures, such as wearing minimum clothing, exposing the skin to the air, reducing room temperature, increasing air circulation, and applying cool, moist compresses to the skin (e.g., the forehead), are effective if employed approximately 1 hour *after* an antipyretic is given so that the set point is lowered. Cooling procedures such as sponging or tepid baths are ineffective in treating febrile children (these measures are effective for hyperthermia) when used either alone or in combination with antipyretics, and they cause considerable discomfort (Sharber, 1997).

Seizures associated with a fever occur in 2 to 5% of all children between the ages of 6 months and 5 years (CPS, 2008a). These febrile seizures usually stop completely by age 5. The older the child is when the first seizure occurs, the lower the chance of further seizures. A family history of febrile seizures is associated with recurring episodes (CPS, 2008a). There is little evidence to support the use of antipyretic medications to prevent febrile seizures; nursing interventions should focus on ways to provide care and comfort during a febrile illness (Purssell, 2000).

Hyperthermia

Although they are helpful in treating fever, antipyretics are of no value in hyperthermia because the set point is already normal. Consequently, cooling measures are used. Cool applications to the skin help reduce the core temperature. Cooled blood from the skin surface is conducted to inner organs and tissues, and warm blood is circulated to the surface, where it is cooled and recirculated. The surface blood vessels dilate as the body attempts to dissipate heat to the environment and facilitate the cooling process.

Commercial cooling devices, such as cooling blankets or mattresses, are available to reduce body temperature. They should be placed on the bed and covered with a sheet or lightweight blanket. Frequent temperature monitoring is essential to prevent excessive cooling of the body.

Traditionally, cool compresses have been used to decrease high temperature. For tepid tub baths it is usually best to start with warm water and gradually add cool water until the desired water temperature of 37°C is reached to accustom the child to the lower water temperature. Generally, the temperature of the water only has to be 1°C less than the child's temperature to be effective. The child should be placed directly in the tub of tepid water for 15 to 20 minutes while water is gently squeezed from a washcloth over the back and chest or gently sprayed over the body from a sprayer. In the bed or crib, cool washcloths or towels are used, exposing only one area of the body at a time. The sponging is continued for approximately 20 minutes. After the tub or sponge bath, the child can be dried and dressed in lightweight pyjamas, a nightgown, or a diaper and placed in a dry bed. The child is dried by gently rubbing the skin surface with a towel to stimulate circulation. The temperature should be retaken 30 minutes after the tub bath or sponge bath. The tub or sponge bath should not be continued or restarted until the skin surface is warm or if the child feels chilled. Chilling causes vasoconstriction, which defeats the purpose of the cool applications. In this condition, little blood is carried to the skin surface; the blood remains primarily in the viscera to become heated.

Whether a temperature elevation in the critically ill child is caused by fever or hyperthermia, it should be treated aggressively. The metabolic rate increases 10% for every 1°C increase in temperature and three to five times during shivering, thus increasing oxygen, fluid, and caloric requirements. If the child's cardiovascular or neurological system is already compromised, these increased needs are especially hazardous. In all children with elevated temperature, attention to adequate hydration is essential. Most children's needs can be met through ingestion of additional oral fluids.

Family Teaching and Home Care

Although most children have learned self-care and hygiene in the home or at school, many have not. For some young children, this is their first introduction to the use of a toothbrush. Much health teaching can be accomplished even when the child is hospitalized for only a short time. The daily bath, hand washing before meals and after bowel and bladder evacuation, and conscientious dental hygiene can be taught during routine care. Positive reinforcement of good hygiene practices helps create a positive body image, enhances self-esteem, and prevents health problems (e.g., teaching girls to wipe the genital area from front to back after toileting).

Although sick children's appetites may be poor and not characteristic of their home eating habits, the hospital stay can provide numerous opportunities for nurses to assess the family's knowledge of good nutrition and to implement teaching as needed to improve nutritional intake.

Fever is one of the most common problems for which parents seek health care. Parental anxiety increases with temperature elevation and its management (Liebman & Barnsteiner, 2001). Parents need to know that sponging is indicated for elevated temperatures from hyperthermia rather than fever and that ice water and alcohol are inappropriate, potentially dangerous solutions (CPS, 2008b). Parents should know how to take the child's temperature and read the thermometer accurately and should have guidelines for seeking professional care (see Patient Teaching box). Some of the newer temperature-measuring devices, such as plastic strips or digital thermometers, may be better suited for home use than hospital use (see Temperature, Chapter 34). If acetaminophen or ibuprofen is indicated, the parents need instruction in administering the medication. Emphasize accuracy in both the amount of medication given and the time intervals at which it is administered.

Safety

While safety is an essential component of any patient's care, children have special characteristics that require an even greater concern for safety. Because small children in the hospital are separated from their usual environment and do not possess the capacity for abstract thinking and reasoning, it is the responsibility of everyone who comes in contact with them to maintain protective measures throughout their hospital stay. Nurses need to understand the age level at which each child is operating and plan for safety accordingly.

Identification bands are particularly important to use with children. Infants and unconscious patients are unable to tell or respond to their names. Toddlers may answer to any name or to a nickname only. Older children may exchange places, give an erroneous name, or choose not to respond to their own names as a form of joke, unaware of the hazards of such practices.

Strangulation Prevention

The hospital environment requires high vigilance by staff to avoid adverse incidents that may stem from the use of products and equipment used in diagnosis, prevention, and treatment. More than a decade ago, Health Canada became concerned about reports of suffocation and death in young children caused by entanglement in IV tubing and monitor leads while being treated in the hospital. In July 2002, Health Canada issued an advisory to hospitals throughout Canada informing them of these risks and providing them with policy recommendations. With the support of the Canadian Association of Paediatric Health Centres, Health Canada revised these recommendations in December 2003 (Health Canada, 2003). The revised recommendations call for hospital policies to consider measures such as the following:

1. Using continuous IV administration only when necessary. For intermittent IV infusion, saline or heparin-locked IV sites should be considered.
2. Providing an appropriate level of supervision for children who have entangled themselves in tubing, including oxygen tubing or leads, or are considered to be at an increased risk of doing so. Factors to be considered might include the following:
   - The child's age and cognitive level
   - The child's mobility and state of agitation
   - The length and number of tubes and leads attached to the patient
3. Using equipment accessories that restrain or stabilize flexible lines to reduce the potential for them to become wrapped around the child's neck or limbs

Environmental Factors

All of the environmental safety measures for the protection of adults apply to children, including good illumination, floors clear of fluid or objects that might contribute to falls, and nonskid surfaces in showers and tubs. All staff members should be familiar with the area-specific fire plan. Staff members should practise proper care and disposal of small objects such as syringe caps, needle covers, and temperature probe covers (Fig. 45-3).

Bathwater should be carefully checked before placing the child in it, and children must never be left alone in a bathtub. Infants are helpless in water, and small children (and some older ones) may turn on the hot water faucet and be severely burned.

Furniture is safest when it is scaled to the child's proportions, is sturdy, and is well balanced to prevent its being easily tipped over. A special hazard for children is the danger of entrapment under an electronically controlled bed when it is activated to descend. Infants and small children must be securely strapped into infant seats, feeding chairs, and strollers. Baby walkers should not be used because they provide

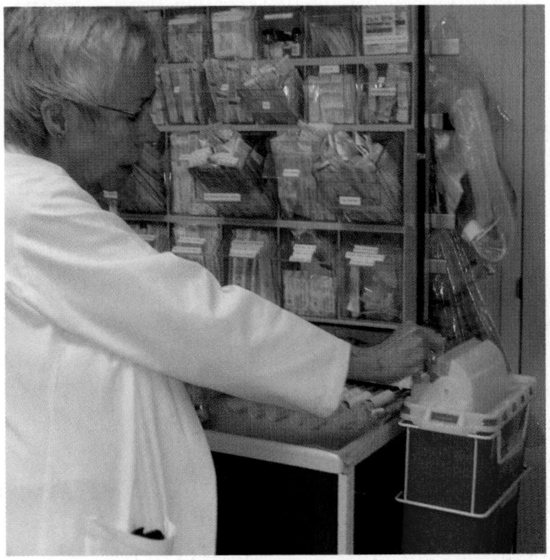

Fig. 45-3 To prevent needlestick injuries, used needles (and other sharp instruments) are not capped or broken and are disposed of in a rigid, puncture-resistant container located near the site of use. Note placement of the container to prevent children's access to the contents.

PATIENT TEACHING The Child With Fever

Call your child's doctor or go to a clinic or emergency department right away if:

- Your child is younger than 3 months old and has a temperature over 38.5°C
- You have recently returned from travelling abroad.
- The fever is over 40°C.
- Your child develops a rash that looks like small purple dots that do not go away when you apply pressure with your fingers (blanching).
- Your child is not able to keep down any fluids and appears dehydrated or the skin looks very pale or grey.
- Your child is having constant pain or is lethargic (very weak) or difficult to wake up.
- Your child has a stiff neck.
- Your child has a seizure associated with fever or seems constantly confused or crying.
- Your child constantly does not use an arm or a leg normally or refuses to stand or put weight on legs.
- Your child has problems breathing.

Call within 24 hours if:

- Your child is between 3 and 6 months old.
- Your child has specific pain, such as ear or throat pain.
- Your child has had a fever for more than 3 days.
- The fever went away for over 24 hours and then came back.
- Your child has a bacterial infection that is being treated with an antibiotic, but the fever is not going away 2 to 3 days after starting the antibiotic.
- Your child cries when going to the bathroom or the urine smells bad.
- You have other questions or concerns.

(Excerpted from AboutKidsHealth. [2009]. *Fever* [by Bruce Minnes, BSc, MD, FRCPC, ABPEM, & Trent Mizzi, MD, BSc, FRCPC]. Retrieved from http://www.aboutkidshealth.ca/En/HealthAZ/ConditionsandDiseases/Symptoms/Pages/Fever.aspx.)

access to hazards and can cause injuries by tipping over. Infants, young children, and those who are weak, paralyzed, agitated, confused, sedated, or cognitively impaired should *never* be left unattended on treatment tables, on scales, or in treatment areas. Even preterm infants are capable of surprising mobility; therefore, portholes in incubators must be securely fastened when not in use. Beds of ambulatory patients should remain locked in place and at a height that allows easy access to the floor.

Crib sides should be kept up and fastened securely unless an adult is at the bedside. It is safer to leave crib sides up, regardless of the child's ability to get out and even when the crib is unoccupied, to remove the child's temptation to climb in. Anyone attending an infant or small child in a crib with the sides down should never turn away without maintaining hand contact with the child; that is, one hand should be kept on the child's back or abdomen to prevent the child from rolling, crawling, or jumping from the open crib (Fig. 45-4). A child who is likely to or has demonstrated the inclination to climb over the sides of the crib is safest when placed in a specially constructed crib with a cover.

Toy Safety

Toys play a vital role in the everyday life of children, and they are no less important in the hospital setting. Nurses are responsible for assessing the safety of toys brought to the hospital by well-meaning parents and friends. Toys should be appropriate to the child's age, condition, and treatment. For example, if the child is receiving oxygen, electrical or friction toys are not safe, since sparks can cause oxygen to ignite. The nurse needs to inspect toys to ensure they are nonallergenic, washable, and unbreakable and have no small, removable parts that can be aspirated or swallowed or in other ways injure a child. All objects within reach of children younger than 3 years should pass the choke tube test. A toilet paper roll is a handy guide. If a toy or object fits into the cylinder (items less than 3 cm across or balls smaller than 4.5 cm), it is a potential choking danger to the child. Broken latex balloons pose a serious aspiration or choking threat to children of all ages if the child puts a piece into the mouth. Latex balloons should *never* be permitted in the hospital setting.

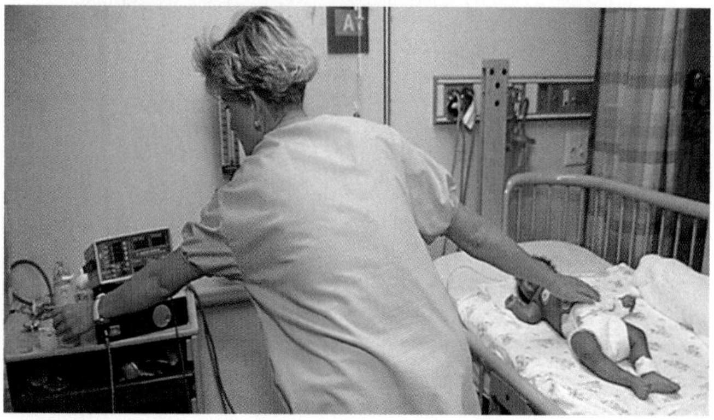

Fig. 45-4 The nurse maintains hand contact when her back is turned.

Preventing Falls

Multiple interventions are needed to minimize pediatric patients' risk of falling. Once individual children are identified as being at risk for falling, visual identification and communication of the risk among all health care providers is essential. The risk of falling can be reduced through patient, family, and staff education.

1. Identify children at risk of falling. Perform a fall risk assessment for patients on admission and throughout hospitalization to identify patients at high risk for falls. Risk factors for hospitalized children include the following:
   - Medication effects—Postanaesthesia or sedation; analgesics or narcotics, especially in those who have never had narcotics in the past and in whom effects are unknown
   - Altered mental status—Secondary to seizures, brain tumours, or medications
   - Altered or limited mobility—Reduced skill at ambulation secondary to developmental age, disease process, tubes, drains, casts, splints, or other appliances; new to ambulation with assistive devices such as walkers or crutches
   - Postoperative children—Risk of hypotension or syncope secondary to large blood loss, a heart condition, or extended bed rest
   - History of falls
   - Infants or toddlers in cribs with side rails down or on the daybed with family members
2. Visually identify patients at risk by doing one or more of the following:
   - Post signs on the door and at the bedside.
   - Apply a special coloured armband labelled "Fall Precautions."
   - Label the chart with a sticker.
   - Document information on the chart.
3. Alter the environment:
   - Keep bed in lowest position, breaks locked, and side rails up.
   - Place call bell within reach.
   - Ensure that all necessary and desired items are within reach (e.g., water, glasses, tissues, snacks).
   - Offer toileting on a regular basis, especially if the patient is taking diuretics or laxatives.
   - Keep lights on at all times, including dim lights while patient is sleeping.
   - Lock wheelchairs before transferring patients.
   - Ensure that the patient has an appropriate-size gown and nonskid footwear. Do not allow gowns or ties to drag on the floor when the patient is ambulating.
   - Keep the floor clean and free of clutter. Post "Wet Floor" sign if the floor is wet.
   - Ensure that the patient has glasses on if he or she normally wears them.
4. Educate patients (as age appropriate):
   - Assist the patient with ambulation even though he or she may have ambulated well before hospitalization.
   - Patients who have been lying in bed will need to get up slowly, sitting on the side of the bed before standing.
5. Educate family members:
   - Call the nursing staff for assistance, and do not allow patients to get up independently.

- Keep the side rails of the crib or bed up whenever the patient is in the crib or bed.
- Do not leave infants on the daybed; put them in the crib with the side rails up.
- When all family members need to leave the bedside, notify staff and ensure that the patient is in the bed or crib with side rails up and that the call bell is within reach (if appropriate).

Infection Control

A Canadian survey identified that 91 children out of 1000 developed hospital-acquired infections (HAIs) (Gravel et al., 2007). These infections occur when there is interaction among patients, health care personnel, equipment, and bacteria (Quality, equipment hold keys to infection control, 2006). HAIs are preventable if caregivers practise meticulous cleaning and disposal techniques. **Routine practices** prevent contact with the blood, body fluids, secretions, and excretions of other people and are used in the care of all patients to reduce the risk of transmission of microorganisms from both recognized and unrecognized sources of infection. Routine practices involve hand hygiene and the use of barrier protection, such as gloves, goggles, gowns, or masks, to prevent contamination from (1) blood; (2) all body fluids, secretions, and excretions *except sweat*, regardless of whether they contain visible blood; (3) nonintact skin; and (4) mucous membranes.

Transmission-based precautions are designed for patients with documented or suspected infection or colonization (presence of microorganism in or on patient but without clinical signs and symptoms of infection) with highly transmissible or epidemiologically important pathogens for which additional precautions beyond routine practices are needed to interrupt transmission in hospitals. There are three types of transmission-based precautions: airborne precautions, droplet precautions, and contact precautions. They may be combined for diseases that have multiple routes of transmission (Box 45-5). They are to be used in addition to routine practices.

The use of *airborne precautions* reduces the risk of the airborne transmission of infectious agents. Airborne transmission occurs by dissemination of either airborne droplet nuclei (small-particle residue [5 mcg or smaller in size] of evaporated droplets that may remain suspended in the air for long periods) or dust particles containing the infectious agent. Microorganisms carried in this manner can be dispersed widely by air currents and may become inhaled by or

BOX 45-5 Types of Precautions and Patients Requiring Them

Routine Practices

Health Canada recommends the term *routine practices* over *standard precautions*, to emphasize that this is the level of care that should be provided for all patients.

Airborne Precautions

In addition to routine practices, use airborne precautions for patients known or suspected to have serious illnesses transmitted by airborne droplet nuclei. Examples of such illnesses include measles, varicella (including disseminated zoster), and pulmonary or laryngeal tuberculosis.

Droplet Precautions

In addition to routine practices, use droplet precautions for patients known or suspected to have serious illnesses transmitted by large-particle droplets. Precautions differ for pediatric patients. Pediatric patients require droplet precautions if they are known or suspected to have any of the following:

- Invasive *Haemophilus influenzae* type b (until 24 hours of appropriate antibiotic received), including meningitis, pneumonia, epiglottitis, and sepsis
- Invasive *Neisseria meningitides* (until 24 hours of appropriate antibiotic received), including meningitis, pneumonia, and sepsis
- Other serious bacterial respiratory tract infections spread by droplet transmission, including diphtheria (pharyngeal), pertussis, streptococcal group A pharyngitis, RSV, parainfluenza and adenovirus. Use droplet precautions for all definite or possible respiratory tract infections until viral infection can be ruled out in pediatric patients.
- Serious viral infections spread by droplet transmission, including adenovirus, influenza, mumps, parvovirus B19, rubella

Contact Precautions

Additional precautions may be indicated for certain organisms when routine practices are not sufficient to control transmission, for instance:

- If the organism has a low infective dose
- If the organism may be transmitted from the source patient's intact skin
- If there is potential for widespread environmental contamination

Precautions differ for pediatric patients. Pediatric patients require contact precautions if they are known or suspected to have any of the following:

- Diarrhea due to *Campylobacter, Rotavirus, Salmonella, Giardia, Shigella, C. difficile, Yersinia,* and pathogenic strains of *E. coli*
- Respiratory tract infections due to adenovirus, parainfluenza virus, rhinovirus, RSV, and influenza (use droplet plus contact precautions)
- Hepatitis A or E, scabies, enteroviral infections, herpes simplex virus: neonatal or disseminated mucocutaneous, antimicrobial-resistant organisms

(From Health Canada. [1999, July]. *Canada communicable disease report supplement: Infection control guidelines: Routine practices and additional precautions for preventing the transmission of infection in health care, 25S4 [pp. 7–10].* Retrieved from http://www.opseu.org/hands/cdr25s4e.pdf.)

deposited on a susceptible host within the same room or over a longer distance from the source patient, depending on environmental factors. Special air handling and ventilation are required to prevent airborne transmission. Airborne precautions apply to patients with known or suspected infection with pathogens transmitted by the airborne route, such as measles, varicella, and tuberculosis.

The use of *droplet precautions* reduces the risk of droplet transmission of infectious agents. Droplet transmission involves contact of the conjunctivae or the mucous membranes of the nose or mouth of a susceptible person with large-particle droplets (larger than 5 mcm in size) containing microorganisms generated from a person who has a clinical disease or who is a carrier of the microorganism. Droplets are generated from the source person primarily during coughing, sneezing, or talking and during procedures such as suctioning and bronchoscopy. Transmission requires close contact between source and recipient persons, since droplets do not remain suspended in the air and generally travel only short distances, usually 1 metre or less, through the air. Because droplets do not remain suspended in the air, special air handling and ventilation are not required to prevent droplet transmission. Droplet precautions apply to any patient with known or suspected infection with pathogens that can be transmitted by infectious droplets (see Box 45-5).

The use of *contact precautions* reduces the risk of transmission of microorganisms by direct or indirect contact. Direct-contact transmission involves a skin-to-skin contact and physical transfer of microorganisms to a susceptible host from an infected or colonized person, such as occurs when turning or bathing patients. Direct-contact transmission also can occur between two patients (e.g., by hand contact). Indirect-contact transmission involves contact of a susceptible host with a contaminated intermediate object, usually inanimate, in the patient's environment. Contact precautions apply to specified patients known or suspected to be infected or colonized with microorganisms that can be transmitted by direct or indirect contact (e.g., wound infections or gastrointestinal infections).

NURSING ALERT The most common piece of medical equipment, the stethoscope, can be a potent source of harmful microorganisms and nosocomial infections. One study found that 80% of 200 stethoscopes were contaminated with at least one microbe (Eckler, 1997).

Nurses caring for young children are frequently in contact with body substances, especially urine, feces, and vomitus. They should exercise judgement concerning those situations when gloves, gowns, or masks are necessary. For example, gloves and possibly gowns should be worn for changing diapers when there are loose or explosive stools. Otherwise, the plastic lining of disposable diapers provides a sufficient barrier between the hands and body substances. The type of diaper may be an important aspect of infection control. Super absorbent disposable diapers with elastic legs contain urine and feces better than cloth diapers.

Antimicrobial-resistant organisms are causing increasing numbers of HAIs. Nearly 70% of HAIs can be attributed to seven pathogens: the gram-positive organisms *Staphylococcus aureus*, coagulase-negative staphylococci, and enterococci; and the gram-negative organisms *Escherichia coli*, *Pseudomonas aeruginosa*, *Enterobacter* organisms, and *Klebsiella pneumoniae*. In hospitals, patients are the most significant sources of methicillin-resistant *S. aureus*, and the main mode of transmission is patient to patient via the hands of a health care provider (Eaton, 2005; Quality, equipment hold keys to infection control, 2006).

NURSING ALERT Hand hygiene is the most critical infection-control practice. Hand hygiene should be followed using the four moments of hand hygiene: (1) before initial contact with the patient or patient environment, (2) before an aseptic procedure, (3) after body-fluid exposure risk, and (4) after contact with a patient or patient environment.

During feedings, gowns should be worn if the child is likely to vomit or spit up, which often occurs during burping. The nurse should wash hands thoroughly after removing the gloves, since gloves fail to provide complete protection. The absence of visible leakage does not indicate gloves are intact.

Another essential practice of infection control is that all needles (uncapped and unbroken) need to be disposed of in a rigid, puncture-resistant container located near the site of use. Consequently, these containers are installed in patients' rooms. Since children are naturally curious, extra attention is needed in selecting a suitable type of container and a location that prevents access to disposed needles (see Fig. 45-3). The use of needleless systems allows secure syringe or IV tubing attachment to vascular access devices without the risk of needlestick injury to the child or nurse.

Transporting Infants and Children

Infants and children usually need to be transported within the unit and to areas outside the pediatric unit. Small infants can be held or carried in the horizontal position with the back supported and the thigh grasped firmly by the carrying arm (Fig. 45-5, A). In the football hold, the infant is carried on the nurse's arm with the head supported by the hand and the body held securely between the nurse's body and elbow (see Fig. 45-5, B). Both of these holds leave the nurse's other arm free for activity. The infant also can be held in the upright position with the buttocks on the nurse's forearm and the front of the body resting against the nurse's chest. The infant's head and shoulders are supported by the nurse's other arm in case the infant moves suddenly (see Fig. 45-5, C). Older infants are able to hold their heads erect but are still subject to sudden movements.

Infants can be transported to other areas, such as the radiology department, in their bassinet or crib. Strollers and wheeled feeding chairs or tables are also convenient transporters in some situations, such as trips to the playroom or nurse's station.

The method of transporting children is determined by their age, condition, and destination. Older children are safe in wheelchairs or on stretchers. Younger children can be transported in a crib, on a stretcher, in a wagon with raised sides, or in a wheelchair with a safety belt. Stretchers should be

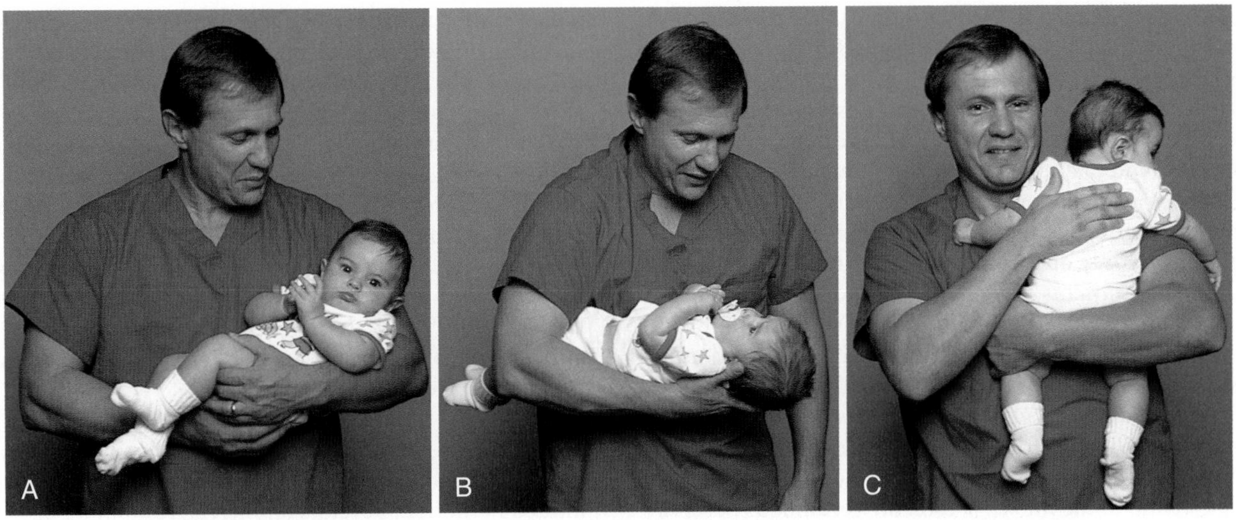

Fig. 45-5 Transporting infants. A: Infant's thigh firmly grasped in nurse's hand. B: Football hold. C: Back supported.

equipped with high sides and a safety belt, both of which are secured during transport.

Restraining Methods and Therapeutic Holding

A *restraint* is any method, physical or mechanical, that restricts a person's movement, physical activity, or normal access to his or her body. Before initiating restraints, the nurse should complete a comprehensive assessment of the patient to determine whether the need for a restraint outweighs the risk of not using one. Restraints can result in loss of dignity, violation of patient rights, psychological harm, physical harm, and even death. Alternative methods should first be considered and documented in the patient's record. The nurse is responsible for selecting the means of least restraint possible. Use of less restrictive restraints is often possible when the child and parents work together with the nurse.

The three types of restraints used with patients include physical, chemical, or environmental restraints (College of Nurses of Ontario, 2009). *Physical restraints* (medical-surgical) are used for children with an artificial airway or airway adjunct for delivery of oxygen, indwelling catheters, tubes, drains, lines, pacemaker wires, or **suture** sites. The physical restraint is used to ensure that safe care is given to the patient. The potential risks of the restraint are offset by the potential benefit of providing safer care. Physical restraints may be instituted for any of the following reasons:

- Risk for interruption of therapy used to maintain oxygenation or airway patency
- Risk of harm if indwelling catheter, tube, drain, line, pacemaker wire, or sutures are removed, dislodged, or ruptured
- Patient confusion, agitation, unconsciousness, or developmental inability to understand direct requests or instructions

Physical restraints can be initiated by an individual order or by protocol; the use of the protocol must be authorized by a physician order. Continued use of restraints must be renewed each day. Patients need to be monitored at least every 2 hours.

Chemical restraints are pharmaceutical interventions administered to keep the individual safe. The *environmental restraint* refers to restraining an individual within a physical space such as in a locked unit in a mental health facility.

Physical restraints can be initiated by an individual order or by protocol; the use of the protocol must be authorized by a physician order. Continued use of restraints must be renewed each day. Patients need to be monitored at least every 2 hours. Children in physical restraints need an in-person evaluation within 1 hour and again every 4 hours until restraints are discontinued. Children in behavioural restraints must be observed and assessed every 15 minutes. Assessment components include signs of injury associated with applying restraint, nutrition and hydration, circulation and range-of-motion of extremities, vital signs, hygiene and elimination, physical and psychological status and comfort, and readiness for discontinuation of restraint. The nurse must use clinical judgement in setting a schedule for when each of these parameters needs to be evaluated because every parameter must be assessed during each 15-minute physical assessment.

Restraints with ties must be secured to the bed or crib frame, not the side rails. Suggestions for increasing safety and comfort while the child is in a restraint include leaving one finger breadth between skin and the device; tying knots that allow for quick release; ensuring that the restraint does not tighten as the child moves; decreasing wrinkles or bulges in the restraint; placing jacket restraints over an article of clothing; placing limb restraints below waist level, below knee level, or distal to the IV; and tucking in dangling straps (Selekman & Snyder, 1997).

An alternative approach for temporary restraint is therapeutic holding. *Therapeutic holding* is the use of a secure, comfortable, temporary holding position that provides close physical contact with the parent or caregiver for 30 minutes or less (Fig. 45-6).

Very little research has been done in this important area of pediatric nursing. Brenner (2007). did an extensive literature review and found that researchers did not focus on the impact of the use of restraint on children or parents. The various researchers suggested that the restraint experience can be very stressful on children and needs to be researched further.

The use of restraints can often be avoided with adequate preparation of the child; parental or staff supervision of the child; or adequate protection of a vulnerable site, such as an infusion device. The nurse needs to assess the child's development, mental status, potential to hurt others or self, and safety. The nurse should carefully consider alternatives to using restraints. Some examples of alternative measures include bringing a child to the nurses' station for continuous observation, providing diversional activities such as music, or encouraging the participation of the parents.

Jacket Restraint

A jacket restraint is sometimes used to keep the child safe in various chairs. The jacket is put on the child with the ties in back so that the child is unable to manipulate them and the long tapes, secured to the understructure of the crib. The jacket restraint is also useful as a means of maintaining the child in a desired horizontal position.

Mummy Restraint or Swaddle

When an infant or small child requires short-term restraint for examination or treatment that involves the head and neck, such as venipuncture, throat examination, and gavage feeding, a papoose board with straps or a mummy wrap effectively controls the child's movements. A blanket or sheet is opened on the bed or crib with one corner folded to the centre. The infant is placed on the blanket with shoulders at the fold and feet toward the opposite corner. With the infant's right arm straight down against the body, the right side of the blanket is pulled firmly across the infant's right shoulder and chest and secured beneath the left side of the body (Fig. 45-7, A). The left arm is placed straight against the infant's side, and the left side of the blanket is brought across the shoulder and chest and locked beneath the body on the right side. The lower corner is folded and brought over the body and tucked or fastened securely with safety pins. Safety pins can be used to fasten the blanket in place at any step in the process.

To modify the mummy restraint for chest examination, the folded edge of the blanket is brought over each arm and under the back, after which the loose edge is folded over and secured at a point below the chest to allow visualization of and access to the chest (see Fig. 45-7, B).

Arm and Leg Restraints

Occasionally, one or more extremities must be restrained or limited in motion. Several commercial restraining devices are available, including disposable wrist and ankle restraints. The restraints must be appropriate to the child's size and padded to prevent undue pressure, constriction, or tissue injury; and the extremity must be observed frequently for signs of irritation or impairment of circulation. The ends of the restraints are never tied to the side rails, since lowering the rail will disturb the extremity, frequently with a jerk that may hurt or injure the child.

Elbow Restraint

Sometimes it is important to prevent the child from reaching the head or face (e.g., after lip surgery, when a scalp vein infusion is in place, or to prevent scratching in skin disorders). Elbow restraints fashioned from a variety of materials function well. Commercial elbow restraints are available. An improvised form of elbow restraint consists of a piece of

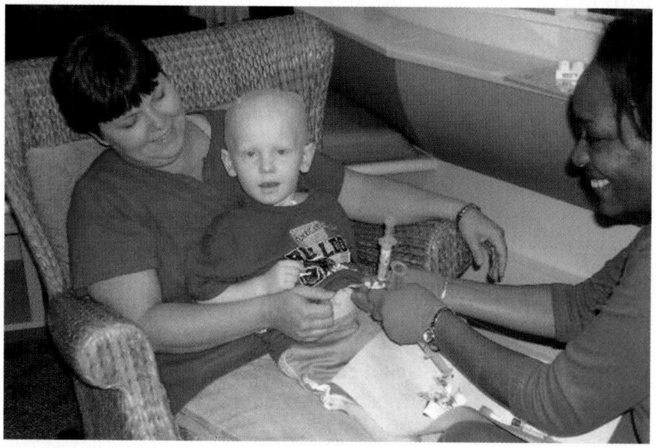

Fig. 45-6 Therapeutic holding of child for extremity venipuncture with parental assistance.

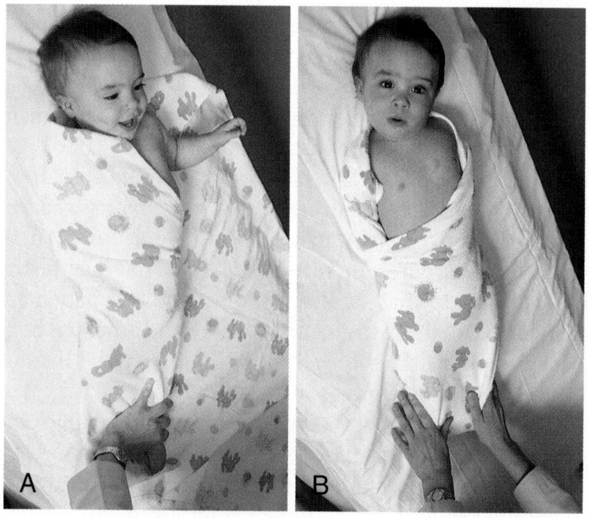

Fig. 45-7 Application of mummy restraint. **A:** Infant is placed on folded corner of blanket and one corner of blanket is brought across the body and secured beneath the body. **B:** The second corner is brought across the body and secured, and the lower corner is folded and tucked or pinned in place; shown here is modified mummy restraint with the chest uncovered.

muslin long enough to reach comfortably from just below the axilla to the wrist with a number of vertical pockets into which tongue depressors are inserted. The restraint is wrapped around the arm and secured with tape or pins. It may be necessary to pin the top of the restraint to the undershirt sleeve to prevent the restraint from slipping.

Positioning for Procedures

Infants and small children are unable to cooperate for many procedures; thus the nurse is responsible for minimizing their movement and discomfort with proper positioning. Older children usually need only minimal, if any, restraint. Careful explanation and preparation beforehand and support and simple guidance during the procedure are usually sufficient. For painful procedures the child should receive adequate analgesia and sedation to minimize pain and the need for excessive restraint. For local **anaesthesia**, buffered lidocaine or a topical anaesthetic can be used to reduce the stinging sensation (see Pain Management, Chapter 35).

Femoral Venipuncture

The nurse places the child supine with the legs in a frog position to provide extensive exposure of the groin area. The infant's legs can be effectively held by the nurse's forearms and hands (Fig. 45-8). Only the side used for the venipuncture is uncovered, so the practitioner is protected should the infant urinate during the procedure. Pressure is applied to the site to prevent oozing from the site.

Extremity Venipuncture

The most common sites of venipuncture are the veins of the extremities, especially the arm and hand. A convenient position is to place the child in the parent's (or assistant's) lap, with the child facing the parent and in the straddle position. Next, the child's arm is placed for venipuncture on a firm surface, such as a treatment table. The child's outstretched arm is partially stabilized by the technician drawing the blood. The parent should hug the child's upper body, preventing movement, and use an arm to immobilize the venipuncture site. This type of restraint also comforts the child because of the close body contact and allows each person to maintain eye contact (see Fig. 45-6).

Lumbar Puncture

Pediatric lumbar puncture (LP) sets contain smaller spinal needles, but sometimes the practitioner will specify a different size or type of needle. The technique for LP in infants and children is similar to that used in the adult, although modifications are suggested in neonates, who have less distress in a side-lying position with modified neck extension than in flexion or a sitting position.

evolve Animation—Lumbar Puncture, Infant

Children are usually controlled best in the side-lying position, with the head flexed and the knees drawn up toward the chest. Even cooperative children need to be held gently to prevent possible trauma from unexpected, involuntary movement. They can be reassured that, although they are trusted, the holding will serve as a reminder to maintain the desired position. It also provides a measure of support and reassurance to them.

The child is placed on the side with the back close to the edge of the examining table on the side from which the practitioner is working. The child's spine is maintained in a flexed position by holding the child with one arm behind the neck and the other behind the thighs (Fig. 45-9). The flexed position enlarges the spaces between the lumbar vertebrae, which facilitates access to the spinal fluid space. It is helpful to wrap the legs before positioning to decrease leg movement.

An alternate position used with small infants and some older children is the sitting position. The child is placed with the buttocks at the edge of the table and with the neck flexed so that the chin rests on the child's chest or the nurse's arm. The infant's arms and legs are immobilized by the nurse's hands.

Specimens and spinal fluid pressure are obtained, measured, and sent for analysis in the same manner as for the adult patient. Vital signs should be taken as ordered, and the child observed for any changes in level of consciousness, motor activity, or other neurological signs. Post-LP headache may

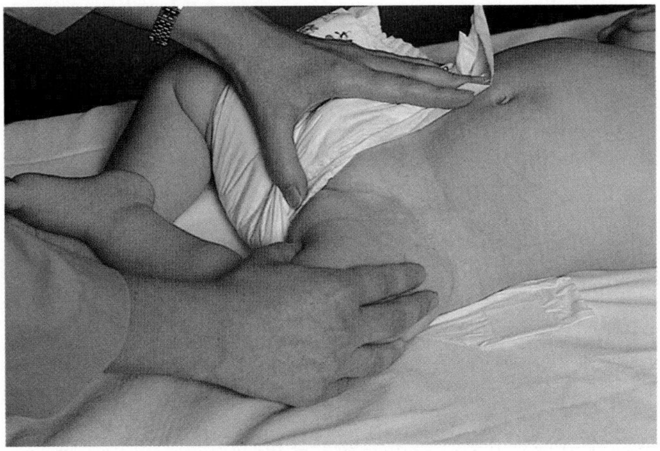

Fig. 45-8 Restraining an infant for femoral venipuncture.

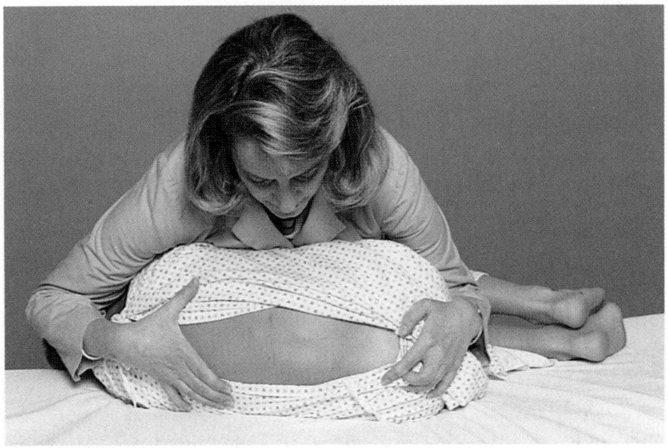

Fig. 45-9 Child in side-lying position for lumbar puncture.

occur and is related to postural changes; this is less severe when the child lies flat. Headache is seen much less frequently in young children than in adolescents.

Bone Marrow Aspiration or Biopsy

The position for a bone marrow aspiration or biopsy depends on the chosen site. In children the posterior or anterior iliac crest is most frequently used, although in infants the tibia may be selected because of easy access to the site and holding of the child. The sternum, which is the most frequent site in adults, is generally avoided in children because the bone is more fragile and adjacent to vital organs.

If the posterior iliac crest is used, the child is positioned prone. Sometimes a small pillow or folded blanket is placed under the hips to facilitate obtaining the bone marrow specimen. Children should receive adequate analgesia or anaesthesia to relieve pain (see Atraumatic Care box). If the child awakens, he or she may need to be held; this is best done with two people—one person to immobilize the upper body and a second person to immobilize the lower extremities.

Collection of Specimens

Urine Specimens

Older children and adolescents can use a bedpan or urinal or can follow directions for collection in the bathroom. However, they may have special needs. School-age children are cooperative but curious. They are concerned about the reasons behind things and are likely to ask questions about the disposition of their specimen and what might be discovered from it. Self-conscious adolescents may be reluctant to carry a specimen through a hallway or waiting room and appreciate a paper bag or other means for disguising the container. The presence of menses may be an embarrassment or a concern to teenage girls; thus, it is a good idea to ask if they are menstruating and to make adjustments as necessary. The specimen can be delayed or a notation made on the laboratory slip to explain the presence of red blood cells.

Preschoolers and toddlers are usually unable to void on request. It is often best to offer them water or other liquids that they enjoy and wait about 30 minutes until they are ready to void voluntarily.

Children will better understand what is expected if the nurse uses familiar terms, such as "pee-pee," "wee-wee," "tee-tee," or "tinkle." Some will have difficulty voiding in an unfamiliar receptacle. Potty chairs or a potty hat placed on the toilet is usually helpful. Toddlers who have recently acquired bladder control may be especially reluctant, since they undoubtedly have been admonished for "going" in places other than those approved by parents. A useful approach is to enlist the help of parents; they are likely to be successful.

For infants and toddlers who are not toilet trained, special urine collection bags with self-adhering material around the opening at the point of attachment are used. To prepare the infant, the genitalia, perineum, and surrounding skin are washed and dried thoroughly because the adhesive will not stick to a moist, powdered, or oily skin surface. The collection bag is easiest to apply if attached first to the perineum, progressing to the symphysis pubis (Fig. 45-10). With girls, the perineum is stretched taut during application to the area to ensure a leak-proof fit. With boys the penis and sometimes the scrotum are placed inside the bag. The adhesive portion of the bag must be firmly applied to the skin all around the genital area to avoid leakage. For low-birth-weight infants, small bags with adhesive that is gentle to the skin are available. Anatomically correct urine collection bags are also available. The diaper is carefully replaced. The bag is checked frequently and removed as soon as the specimen is available, since the moist bag may become loosened on an active child. When urine is

ATRAUMATIC CARE

Lumbar Puncture and Bone Marrow Test

Apply EMLA (a eutectic mixture of lidocaine and prilocaine) to the puncture site at least 60 minutes or LMX cream (lidocaine) at least 30 minutes before the procedure. To identify the lumbar puncture site, draw an imaginary line from the posterior iliac crest across the spine to the opposite iliac crest. The puncture site is intersected by the line at approximately L4. For additional anaesthesia, buffered lidocaine with a 30-gauge needle can be used. Sedation with agents such as propofol (Diprivan) or ketamine is recommended for bone marrow biopsy and aspiration.

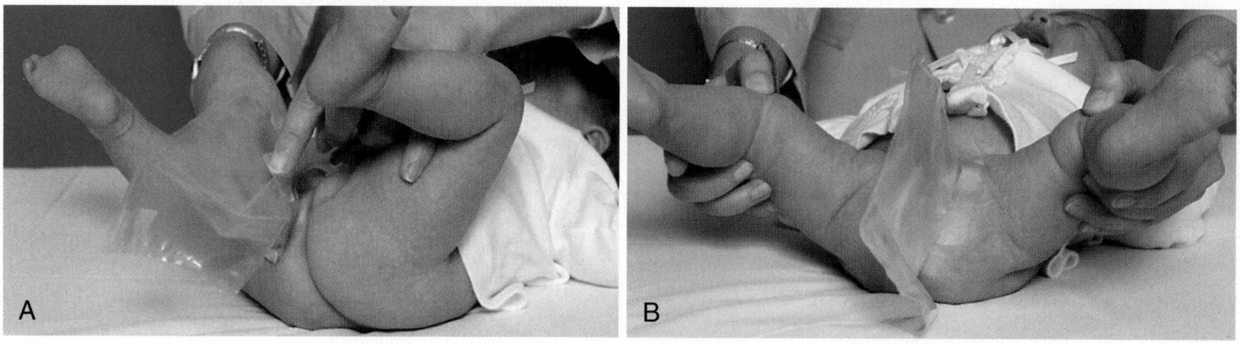

Fig. 45-10 Application of urine collection bag. **A:** On female infants, the adhesive portion is applied to the exposed and dried perineum first. **B:** The bag adheres firmly around the perineal area to prevent urine leakage.

collected for culture, the bag is removed immediately. For some types of urine testing, such as specific gravity, ketones, glucose, and protein, urine can be aspirated directly from the diaper. If the urine is not tested within 30 minutes, the specimen is refrigerated or placed in a sterile container with a preservative.

Urine obtained from disposable diapers can be tested accurately for glucose, ketones, protein, blood, and urea. Superabsorbent disposable diapers may produce a false crystalluria. Specific gravity measurements are accurate for up to 4 hours provided that the disposable diapers are kept folded. Urine samples collected by the cotton ball method were accurate for pH and specific gravity and were atraumatic to the skin of newborns (Burke, 1995).

NURSING ALERT

- When using a urine collection bag, cut a small slit in the diaper and pull the bag through to allow room for urine to collect and to facilitate checking on the contents.
- To obtain small amounts of urine, use a syringe without a needle to aspirate urine directly from the diaper; if diapers with absorbent gelling material that trap urine are used, place a small gauze dressing, some cotton balls, or a urine collection device inside the diaper to collect urine, then aspirate the urine with a syringe.

At times parents may be asked to bring a urine sample to a health care facility for examination, especially when infants are unable to void during an outpatient visit. In this instance parents need instruction on applying the collection device and storing the specimen. Ideally, the specimen should be brought to the designated place as soon as possible; if there is a delay, the sample should be refrigerated and the elapsed time reported to the examiner.

Clean-Catch Specimens

Clean-catch specimens traditionally refer to a urine sample obtained for culture after the urethral meatus is cleaned and the first few millilitres of urine are voided before the urine is collected (*midstream specimen*). In girls, the perineum is wiped with an antiseptic-soaked cotton ball or pad from front to back at least three times, using a new cotton ball or pad each time. In boys, the tip of the penis is cleansed. The area may be wiped with sterile water to prevent accidental contamination of the urine with a solution that may destroy pathogens.

Twenty-Four–Hour Collection

Collection bags are required to collect specimens from infants and small children. Older children require special instruction about notifying someone when they need to void or have a bowel movement so that urine can be collected separately and not discarded. Some older school-age children and adolescents can take responsibility for collection of their own 24-hour specimens and can keep output records and transfer each voiding to the 24-hour collection container.

The collection period always starts and ends with an empty bladder. At the time the collection begins, the child is instructed to void and the specimen is discarded. All urine voided in the subsequent 24 hours is saved in a container with a preservative or is placed on ice. Twenty-four hours from the time the precollection specimen was discarded, the child is again instructed to void, the specimen is added to the container, and the entire collection is taken to the laboratory.

Infants and small children who are bagged for a 24-hour urine collection require a special collection bag. Frequent removal and replacement of adhesive collection devices can produce skin irritation. A thin coating of sealant, such as Skin-Prep, applied to the skin helps to protect it and aids adhesion, unless its use is contraindicated, such as in a preterm infant or a child with irritated skin. Plastic collection bags with collection tubes attached are ideal when the container must be left in place for a time. These can be connected to a collecting device or emptied periodically by aspiration with a syringe. When such devices are not available, a regular bag with a feeding tube inserted through a puncture hole at the top of the bag serves as a satisfactory substitute. However, it is important to empty the bag as soon as the infant urinates to prevent leakage and loss of contents. An indwelling catheter may also be placed for the collection period.

Bladder Catheterization and Other Techniques

Bladder catheterization or suprapubic aspiration is employed when a specimen is urgently needed or when the child is unable to void or otherwise provide an adequate specimen. Catheterization is used to obtain a sterile urine specimen and when urethral obstruction or **anuria** caused by renal failure is believed to be the cause of the child's failure to void. The Canadian Paediatric Society (CPS, Infectious Diseases and Immunization Committee, 2004b) recommends that a diagnosis of urinary tract infection (UTI) that is made with a bag urine specimen in young infants requires confirmation with a suprapubic or urethral catheterization before treatment. A bag urine sample is helpful for dipstick urinalysis and microscopic evaluation. All urine specimens need to be sent to the laboratory for culture as soon as possible. Suprapubic aspiration or catheterization is useful in clarifying the diagnosis of suspected UTI in acutely ill infants.

Preparation for catheterization includes instruction on pelvic muscle relaxation. The toddler, preschooler, or younger child is taught to blow a pinwheel and to press the hips against the bed or procedure table during catheterization to relax the pelvic and periurethral muscles. For the older child or adolescent, the location and function of the pelvic muscles are described. The patient is then taught to contract and relax the pelvic muscles, and the relaxation procedure is repeated during catheter insertion. If the patient vigorously contracts the pelvic muscles when the catheter reaches the striated sphincter (proximal urethra in boys and midurethra in girls), catheter insertion is temporarily stopped. The catheter is neither removed nor advanced; instead, the child is helped to press the hips against the bed or examining table and relax the pelvic muscles. The catheter is then gently advanced into the bladder (Gray, 1996).

Children and adolescents may experience some discomfort and anxiety during this procedure. Assistance and gentle holding may be necessary, especially for the younger child. Most children prefer to have the parents remain with them during the procedure. The parent should be encouraged to talk softly and hold the child's hand as the catheter is inserted. Using distractions such as reading a book, singing a song, or playing with small toys may decrease the child's anxiety. Older children and adolescents may wish to listen to music with headphones. Adolescents should be asked if they would like a parent to remain with them during the procedure. The decision should be made before the perineum is exposed and the sterile field is prepared.

Catheterization is a sterile procedure, and routine practices for body substance protection should be followed. When placing a catheter to obtain a sterile urine specimen or to check for residual urine, the nurse may use a sterile feeding tube if a catheter is unavailable. If the catheter is to remain in place, a Foley catheter is used. Table 45-3 gives guidelines for choosing the appropriately sized catheter and length of insertion. The supplies needed for this procedure include sterile gloves, sterile lubricant anaesthetic, an appropriately sized catheter, povidone-iodine (Betadine) swabs or an alternative cleansing agent and 10 × 10-cm gauze squares, a sterile drape, and a syringe with sterile water if a Foley catheter is used.

NURSING ALERT Identify patients who have allergies to povidone-iodine or latex before using these items in catheterization.

Adolescent boys and children with a history of urethral surgery may be catheterized using a coudé-tipped catheter. The child with myelodysplasia or one who has been identified as being sensitive or allergic to latex is catheterized with a catheter manufactured from an alternative material. When an indwelling catheter is indicated for urinary drainage, a lubricious-coated or silicone catheter is selected because these materials produce less irritation of the urethral mucosa when compared with a Silastic or latex catheter when the catheter is left in place for more than 72 hours.

A 2% lidocaine lubricant jelly with applicator is assembled according to the manufacturer's instructions, and several drops of the lubricant are placed at the meatus. Advise the child that the lubricant is used to reduce discomfort associated with inserting the catheter and that introduction of the lubricant and catheter into the urethra will produce a sensation of pressure and a desire to urinate).

In male patients, insertion of the catheter is done as follows. Grasp the penis with the nondominant hand and retract the foreskin. In uncircumcised newborns and infants the foreskin may be adhered to the shaft; use care when retracting. If the penis is pendulous, place a sterile drape under the penis. Using the sterile hand, swab the glans and meatus three times with povidone-iodine. Gently introduce the tip of the lidocaine jelly applicator into the urethra 1 to 2 cm so that the lubricant flows only into the urethra; insert 5 to 10 mL 2% lidocaine lubricant into the urethra and hold in place for 2 to 3 minutes by gently squeezing the distal penis. Lubricate the catheter and insert into the urethra while gently stretching the penis and lifting it to a 90-degree angle to the body. Resistance may occur when the catheter meets the urethral sphincter. Ask the patient to inhale deeply, and advance the catheter. Do not force a catheter that does not easily enter the meatus, particularly if the child has had corrective surgery. For indwelling catheters, once urine is obtained, advance the catheter to the hub, inflate the balloon with sterile water, pull it back gently to test inflation, and connect it to the closed drainage system. Cleanse the glans and meatus and replace retracted foreskin. If blood is seen at any time during the procedure, discontinue the procedure and notify the practitioner.

For catheter insertion in female patients, place a sterile drape under the buttocks. Use the nondominant hand to gently separate and pull up the labia minora to visualize the meatus. Swab the meatus from front to back three times, using a different povidone-iodine swab each time. Place 1 to 2 mL 2% lidocaine lubricant on the periurethral mucosa, and insert 1 to 2 mL into the urethral meatus. Delay catheterization for 2 to 3 minutes to maximize absorption of the anaesthetic into the periurethral and intraurethral mucosa. Add lubricant to the catheter, and gently insert into the urethra until urine returns, then advance the catheter an additional 2.5 to 5 cm. When using a Foley catheter, inflate the balloon with sterile water and gently pull back, then connect to a closed drainage system. Cleanse the meatus and labia (see Cultural Awareness box). Because the use of lidocaine jelly can increase the volume of intraurethral lubricant, urine return may not be as rapid as when minimal lubrication is used.

Suprapubic aspiration is mainly used when the bladder cannot be accessed through the urethra (such as with some congenital urological birth defects) or to reduce the risk of contamination that may be present when passing a catheter. With the advent of small catheters (5 and 6 French), the need for suprapubic aspiration has decreased. Access to the bladder via the urethra has a much higher success rate than suprapubic aspiration, where success depends on the practitioner's skill at

Table 45-3 Straight Catheter or Foley Catheter*

	SIZE (LENGTH OF INSERTION [CM]) FOR GIRLS	SIZE (LENGTH OF INSERTION [CM]) FOR BOYS
Term neonate	5-6 (5)	5-6 (6)
Infant-3 yr	5-8 (5)	5-8 (6)
4-8 yr	8 (5-6)	8 (6-9)
8 yr-prepubertal	10-12 (6-8)	8-10 (10-15)
Pubertal	12-14 (6-8)	12-14 (13-18)

*Foley catheters are approximately 1 French size larger because of the circumference of the balloon. Example: 10 French Foley = approximately 12 French calibration.

CULTURAL AWARENESS

Bladder Catheterization

Parents may be upset when their child is catheterized. Aside from the trauma the child experiences, some parents may fear that the procedure affects the daughter's virginity. To correct this misconception, the family may benefit from a detailed explanation of the genitourinary anatomy, preferably with a model that shows the separate vaginal and urethral openings. The nurse can also indicate that catheterization has no effect on virginity.

assessing the location of the bladder and the amount of urine in the bladder. Suprapubic aspiration involves aspirating bladder contents by inserting a 20- or 21-gauge needle in the midline approximately 1 cm above the symphysis pubis and directed vertically downward. The skin is prepared as for any needle insertion, and the bladder should contain an adequate volume of urine. This can be assumed if the infant has not voided for at least 1 hour or the bladder can be palpated above the symphysis pubis. This technique is useful for obtaining sterile specimens from young infants, since the bladder is an abdominal organ and is easily accessed. Suprapubic aspiration is painful, thus pain management during the procedure is important.

Stool Specimens

Stool specimens are frequently collected in children to identify parasites and other organisms that cause diarrhea, to assess gastrointestinal function, and to check for occult (hidden) blood. Ideally, stool should be collected without contamination with urine, but in children wearing diapers this is difficult unless a urine bag is applied. Children who are toilet trained should urinate first, flush the toilet, then defecate in the toilet, a bedpan (preferably one that is placed on the toilet to avoid embarrassment), or a commercial potty hat.

NURSING ALERT To obtain a stool specimen, place plastic wrap over the toilet bowl to collect the stool. Use a tongue depressor or disposable spoon or knife to collect the stool.

Stool specimens should be large enough to obtain an ample sampling, not merely a fecal fragment. Specimens should be placed in an appropriate container, which is covered and labelled. If several specimens are needed, the containers are marked with the date and time and kept in a specimen refrigerator. The specimen should be handled carefully to prevent contamination.

Blood Specimens

Whether the specimen is collected by the nurse or others, the nurse is responsible for making certain that specimens, such as serial examinations and fasting specimens, are collected on time and that the proper equipment is available. The collecting, transporting, and storing of specimens can have a major impact on laboratory results.

Venous blood samples can be obtained by venipuncture or by aspiration from a peripheral or central access device. Withdrawing blood specimens through peripheral lock devices in small peripheral veins has met with varying degrees of success. Although it avoids an additional venipuncture for the child, attempting to aspirate blood from the peripheral lock may shorten the life of the device. When using an IV infusion site for specimen collection, consider the type of fluid being infused. For example, a specimen collected for glucose level would be inaccurate if removed from a catheter through which glucose-containing solution was being administered.

NURSING ALERT

- To obtain a blood specimen from a peripheral lock when the infusion solution may interfere with tests results, first aspirate a quantity of blood equal to the volume of fluid in the catheter and discard; then aspirate the blood sample.
- For a blood culture, use the first sample of blood, since organisms are most likely to collect within the catheter itself.

NURSING ALERT On small or anemic children, keep track of the amount drawn over time. Frequent taking of blood specimens can rapidly decrease a child's blood volume. Coordinate blood samples and ask the laboratory to save as much blood as possible to reduce the frequency.

Arterial blood samples are sometimes needed for blood gas measurement, although noninvasive techniques, such as **transcutaneous oxygen monitoring** and pulse oximetry, are used frequently. Arterial samples may be obtained by arterial puncture using the radial, brachial, or femoral arteries; by deep heel puncture; or from indwelling arterial catheters. Adequate circulation should be assessed before arterial puncture by observing capillary refill or performing the *Allen test*, a procedure that assesses the circulation of the radial, ulnar, or brachial arteries. Because unclotted blood is required, only heparinized collection tubes are used. In addition, no air bubbles should enter the tube, since they can alter the blood gas concentration. Crying, fear, and agitation also affect blood gas values; every effort should be made to comfort the child. The nurse should pack the sample in ice to reduce blood cell metabolism and should take it to the laboratory for immediate analysis.

Capillary blood samples are taken from children by a finger stick. A common method for taking peripheral blood samples from infants younger than 6 months of age is by a heel stick. Before the blood sample is taken, the heel is warmed for 3 minutes (see Fig. 25-8). The area is cleansed with alcohol, the infant's foot firmly restrained with the free hand, and the heel punctured with an automatic lancet device. An automatic device delivers a more precise puncture depth and is less painful than using a lance (Vertanen et al., 2001). A surgical blade of any kind is contraindicated. An example of a safe device is the BD Quickheel Safety Lancet. The Tenderfoot Preemie device was compared with the Monolet lancet and was found to be safer than the lancet and required fewer heel punctures, less collection time, and lower recollection rates (Kellam et al., 2001). Shepherd and colleagues (2006) reported the Tenderfoot device to be more effective and safer than a lancet for newborn screening tests. Although obtaining capillary blood gases is a common practice, these measures may not accurately reflect arterial values.

The most serious complications of infant heel puncture are necrotizing osteochondritis from lancet penetration of the underlying calcaneus bone, infection, or abscess (Meehan, 1998). To avoid osteochondritis, the puncture should be no deeper than 2 mm and should be made at the outer aspect of the heel. The boundaries of the calcaneus can be marked by an imaginary line extending posteriorly from a point between the fourth and fifth toes and running parallel to the lateral aspect of the heel and another line extending posteriorly from the middle of the great toe and running parallel to the medial aspect of the heel (Fig. 45-11). Repeated trauma to the walking

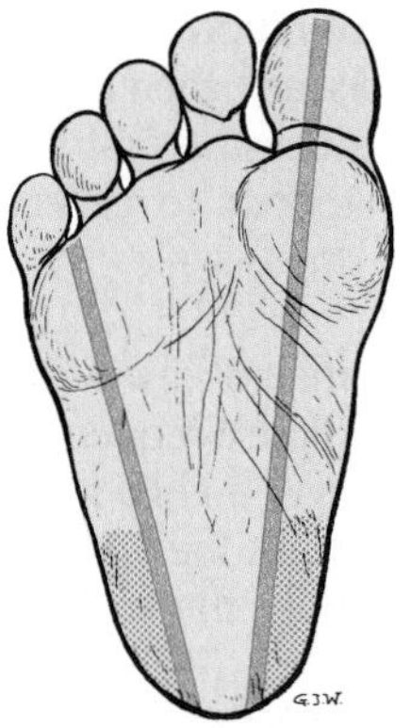

Fig. 45-11 Puncture site (coloured stippled area) on sole of infant's foot.

surface of the heel can cause fibrosis and scarring that may interfere with locomotion.

The specimens should be quickly collected and pressure applied to the puncture site with dry gauze until bleeding stops. The arm is kept extended, not flexed, while pressure is applied for a few minutes after venipuncture in the antecubital fossa to reduce bruising. The site should be covered with an adhesive bandage. In young children, adhesive bandages pose an aspiration hazard; they should be avoided or removed as soon as the bleeding stops. Applying warm compresses to ecchymotic areas increases circulation, helps remove extravasated blood, and decreases pain.

No matter how or by whom the specimen is collected, children, even some older ones, fear the loss of their blood. This is particularly true for children whose condition requires frequent blood specimens. They mistakenly believe that blood removed from their bodies is a threat to their lives. Explaining to them that their body is continuously producing blood can provide them with a measure of reassurance. When the blood is drawn, a comment such as "Just look how red it is. You're really making a lot of nice red blood," confirms this information and affords them an opportunity to express their concern. An adhesive bandage can give added reassurance that the vital fluids will not leak out.

Children have identified venous, arterial, and capillary punctures as the procedures that most frequently cause pain during hospitalization, with arterial punctures being one of the most painful of all procedures experienced (Van Cleve, Johnson, & Pothier, 1996). Children most distressed by venipunctures are toddlers, followed by school-age children and then adolescents. Nurses need to institute pain reduction techniques to lessen the discomfort of these procedures (see Atraumatic Care box).

Respiratory Secretion Specimens

Collection of sputum or nasal discharge is sometimes required for diagnosis of respiratory infections, especially tuberculosis and respiratory syncytial virus (RSV). Older children and adolescents are able to cough and supply sputum specimens when given proper directions. It must be made clear to them that a coughed specimen, not mucus that is cleared from the throat, is needed. It is helpful to demonstrate a deep cough. Infants and small children are unable to follow directions to cough and will swallow any sputum produced; thus gastric washings **(lavage)** may be used to collect a sputum specimen. Sometimes a satisfactory specimen can be obtained using a suction device such as a mucus trap if the catheter is inserted into the trachea and the cough reflex is elicited. A catheter inserted into the back of the throat is not sufficient. For children with a tracheostomy, a specimen is easily aspirated from the trachea or major bronchi by attaching a collecting device to the suction apparatus.

Nasal washings are usually obtained to diagnose an infection of RSV. The child is placed supine, and 1 to 3 mL sterile normal saline is instilled with a sterile syringe (without needle) into one nostril. The contents are aspirated using a small, sterile bulb syringe and are placed in a sterile container. Another method uses a syringe with 5 cm of 18- to 20-gauge tubing. The saline is quickly instilled and then aspirated to recover the nasal specimen. To prevent additional discomfort, all of the equipment should be ready before beginning the procedure.

Other respiratory secretion collection methods include nasopharyngeal swabs to diagnose Bordetella pertussis and throat cultures. The nurse swabs both the tonsils and the posterior pharynx when obtaining a throat culture. The swab stick is inserted into the culture tube. Some culture kits require squeezing an ampule to release the culture medium.

Administration of Medication

Determination of Medication Dosage

Nurses must have an understanding of the safe dosage of medications they administer to children, as well as the expected action, possible adverse effects, and signs of toxicity. Unlike with adult medications, there are few standardized pediatric dosage ranges.

Factors related to growth and maturation significantly alter an individual's capacity to metabolize and excrete drugs. Immaturity or defects in any of the important processes of absorption, distribution, biotransformation, or excretion can significantly alter the effects of a medication. Newborn and preterm infants with immature enzyme systems in the liver (where most drugs are broken down and detoxified), lower plasma concentrations of protein for binding with drugs, and immaturely functioning kidneys (where most drugs are excreted) are particularly vulnerable to the harmful effects of medications. Beyond the newborn period, many drugs are metabolized more rapidly by the liver, necessitating larger doses or more frequent administration. This is particularly important in pain control, since the dosage of analgesics may need to be increased or the interval between doses decreased.

Various formulas involving age, weight, and body surface area (BSA) have been devised to determine children's medication dosage. Because the administration of medication is a nursing responsibility, nurses need knowledge of not only drug action and patient responses but also of some resources for estimating safe dosages for children. The method most often used to determine children's dosage is based on a specific dose per kilogram of body weight, such as 0.1 mg/kg.

ATRAUMATIC CARE

Guidelines for Skin and Vessel Punctures

For Reduction of Pain Associated With Heel, Finger, Venous, or Arterial Punctures

Apply EMLA (an eutectic mixture of lidocaine and prilocaine) topically over the site if time permits (at least 60 minutes). LMX (lidocaine) cream also may be used and requires a shorter application time (30 minutes).

To remove the Tegaderm dressing atraumatically, grasp opposite sides of the film and pull the sides away from each other to stretch and loosen the film. After the film begins to loosen, grasp the other two sides of the film and pull.

Use iontophoresis (Numby Stuff) over the site if time permits (8 to 20 minutes, depending on the amount of current), a vapocoolant spray, or buffered lidocaine (injected intradermally near the vein with a 30-gauge needle) to numb the skin.

Use nonpharmacological methods of pain and anxiety control (e.g., ask child to take a deep breath when the needle is inserted and again when the needle is withdrawn; exhale a large breath or blow bubbles to "blow hurt away"; count slowly and then faster and louder if pain is felt).

Keep all equipment out of sight until used.

Enlist parents' presence or assistance if they wish.

Restrain child *only as needed* to perform the procedure safely; use therapeutic holding (p. 1280).

Allow the skin preparation to dry completely before penetrating the skin.

Use the smallest-gauge needle (e.g., 25 gauge) that permits free flow of blood; a 27-gauge needle can be used for obtaining 1 to 1.5 mL blood and for prominent veins (needle length is only 13 mm).

Emphasize that blood entering the syringe or tube does not hurt, and reassure young children that you did not "take their blood" away and that they have a lot more inside.

Place a small bandage over the puncture site to make removal easy and less painful and to reassure young children that their blood will not "leak out."

Have a "two-try" only policy to reduce excessive insertion attempts—two operators each have two insertion attempts; if insertion is not successful after four punctures, consider alternative venous access, such as a peripherally inserted central catheter (PICC); have a policy for identifying children with difficult access and appropriate interventions (e.g., most experienced operator for the first attempt).*

For Multiple Blood Samples

Use an intermittent infusion device (saline lock) to collect additional samples; consider PICC lines early, not as a last resort.

Coordinate care to allow several tests to be performed on one blood sample using micromethods of testing.

Anticipate tests (e.g., drug levels, chemistry, immunoglobulin levels) and ask the laboratory to save blood for additional testing.

For Heel Lancing in Newborns

Heel lancing has been shown to be more painful than venipuncture (Larsson et al., 1998); consider venipuncture when the amount of blood from the heel would require much squeezing (e.g., genetic screening tests).

EMLA application of 0.5 g for 30 minutes four times a day in preterm infants has been found to be safe (Essink-Tebbes et al., 1999).

Place diapered newborn against the mother's bare chest in skin-to-skin contact 10 to 15 minutes before and during heel lance (Gray, Watt, & Blass, 2000).

During the procedure, allow newborn to suck a pacifier coated with a solution of sucrose. When commercially manufactured 24% sucrose solution is unavailable, add 5 mL of table sugar to 15 mL of sterile water. Use this solution to coat the pacifier, or administer 2 mL to the tongue 2 minutes before the procedure (Blass & Watt, 1999).

*For an example of one hospital's guidelines for reducing excessive IV insertion attempts, see Catudal (1999).

The most reliable method for determining children's dosages is to calculate the proportional amount of BSA to body weight. The ratio of BSA to weight varies inversely with length; the infant who is shorter and weighs less than an older child or adult has relatively more surface area than would be expected from the weight. The usual determination of BSA requires the use of the *West nomogram* or an electronic calculator (widely available on the Internet). The BSA is estimated from the child's height and weight.

Checking Dosage

Administering the correct dosage of a medication is a shared responsibility between the practitioner who orders the medication and the nurse who carries out that order. Children react with unexpected severity to some medications, and ill children are especially sensitive to them. When a dose is ordered that is outside the usual range or when there is some question about the preparation or the route of administration, the nurse should always check with the prescribing practitioner before proceeding with the administration, since the nurse is legally liable for any medication administered.

Even when it has been determined that the dosage is correct for a particular child, many medications are potentially hazardous or lethal. Most facilities have regulations requiring specified medications to be double-checked by another nurse before they are given to the child. Among medications that require such safeguards are antiarrhythmics, anticoagulants, chemotherapeutic agents, electrolytes, and insulin. Others frequently included are epinephrine, opioids, and sedatives. Even if this precaution is not mandatory, nurses are wise to observe it. Errors in decimal point placement may occur and result in a tenfold or greater dosage error.

Identification

Before the administration of any medication, the child must be correctly identified. Two identifiers (e.g., name and medical record number or birth date) are required before medication administration.

Oral Administration

The oral route is preferred for administering medications to children because of the ease of administration. Most are dissolved or suspended in liquid preparations. Although some children are able to swallow or chew solid medications at an early age, solid preparations are not recommended for young children because of the danger of aspiration.

Most pediatric medications come in palatable and colourful preparations for ease of administration. Some have a slightly unpleasant aftertaste, but most children will swallow these liquids with little if any resistance. The nurse can taste a minute amount of an oral preparation to ascertain whether it is palatable or bitter. When the child dislikes the taste it can be camouflaged by various means. Most pediatric units have preparations available for this purpose (see Atraumatic Care box).

Preparation

The devices available to measure medicines are not always sufficiently accurate for measuring the small amounts needed in pediatric nursing practice. Although moulded plastic calibrated cups offer reasonable accuracy in measuring moderate doses of liquids, paper cups are likely to have irregular shapes or crumpled bottoms. Considerable amounts of thick medication may remain in the cup. Measures of less than a teaspoon are impossible to determine accurately with a cup.

The teaspoon is an inaccurate measuring device and is subject to error. Teaspoons vary greatly in capacity, and different persons using the same spoon will pour different amounts. Therefore, a medication ordered in teaspoons should be measured in millilitres; the established standard is 5 mL per teaspoon. A convenient hollow-handled medicine spoon is available to accurately measure and administer the medication. Household measuring spoons can also be used when other devices are not available. A device called the Medibottle has been shown to be more effective in delivering oral medication to infants than the oral syringe (Kraus et al., 2001).

Another unreliable device for measuring liquids is the dropper, which varies to a greater extent than the teaspoon or measuring cup. Droppers are available in numerous sizes, but even with the standard USP dropper, the volume of a drop will vary according to the viscosity (thickness) of the liquid measured; viscous fluids produce much larger drops than thin liquids. Many medications are supplied with caps or droppers designed for measuring each specific preparation. These are accurate when used to measure that specific medication but are not reliable for measuring other liquids. Emptying dropper contents into a medicine cup invites additional error. Because some of the liquid clings to the sides of the cup, a significant amount of the drug can be lost.

The most accurate means for measuring small amounts of medication is the plastic disposable syringe, especially the tuberculin syringe for volumes less than 1 mL. Not only does the syringe provide a reliable measure, but it also serves as a convenient means for transporting and administering the medication. The medication can be placed directly into the child's mouth from the syringe.

Young children and some older children have difficulty swallowing tablets or pills. Because a number of medications are not available in pediatric preparations, the tablet needs to be crushed before it can be given to these children. Commercial devices are available, or simple methods can be employed for crushing tablets. Not all drugs can be crushed (e.g., medication with an enteric or protective coating or formulated for slow release).

Children who must take oral medication for an extended period can be taught to swallow tablets or capsules. Training sessions include verbal instruction, demonstration, reinforcement for swallowing progressively larger candy or capsules, no attention for inappropriate behaviour, and gradual withdrawal of guidance once children can swallow their medication.

Because pediatric doses often require dividing adult preparations of medication, the nurse may be faced with the dilemma of accurate dosage. With tablets, only those that are scored can be halved or quartered accurately. If the medication is soluble, the tablet or contents of a capsule can be mixed in a small, premeasured amount of liquid and the appropriate portion given. For example, if half a dose is required, the tablet is dissolved in 5 mL water or flavoured liquid and 2.5 mL is given.

ATRAUMATIC CARE

Encouraging a Child's Acceptance of Oral Medication

- Give the child a flavoured ice pop or small ice cube to suck to numb the tongue before giving the medication.
- Mix the medication with a small amount (about 5 mL) of sweet-tasting substance, such as honey (except in infants because of the risk of botulism), flavoured syrups, jam, fruit purees, sherbet, or ice cream; avoid essential food items, since the child may later refuse to eat them.
- Give a "chaser" of water, juice, soft drink, ice pop, or frozen juice bar after taking the medication.
- If nausea is a problem, give a carbonated beverage poured over finely crushed ice before or immediately after taking the medication.
- When medication has an unpleasant taste, have child pinch the nose and drink the medicine through a straw. Much of what we taste is associated with smell.
- Flavourings such as apple, banana, and bubble gum can be added at many pharmacies (e.g., FLAVORx) at nominal additional cost. An alternative is to have the pharmacist prepare the medication in a flavoured, chewable troche or lozenge.
- Infants will suck medicine from a needleless syringe or dropper in small increments (0.25 to 0.5 mL) at a time. Use a nipple or special pacifier with a reservoir for the medication.

Administration

Although administering liquids to infants is relatively easy, the nurse must be careful to prevent aspiration. With the infant held in a semireclining position, the medication is placed in the mouth from a spoon, plastic cup, dropper, or syringe (without needle). The dropper or syringe is best placed along the side of the infant's tongue, and the liquid is administered slowly in small amounts, allowing the child to swallow between deposits.

NURSING ALERT In infants up to 11 months of age and children with neurological impairments, blowing a small puff of air in the face frequently elicits a swallow reflex.

Medicine cups can be used effectively for older infants who are able to drink from a cup. Because of the natural outward tongue thrust in infancy, medications may need to be retrieved from the lips or chin and re-fed. Allowing the infant to suck medication that has been placed in an empty nipple or inserting the syringe or dropper into the side of the mouth, parallel to the nipple, while the infant nurses are other convenient methods for giving liquid medications to infants. Medication is not added to the infant's formula feeding because the child may subsequently refuse the formula. Plastic covers on the ends of syringes should be disposed of as these covers are small enough to be aspirated by young children.

The young child who refuses to take medication or resists consistently despite explanation and encouragement may require mild physical restraint. If so, it should be carried out quickly and carefully. Every effort should be made to determine why the child resists, and the reasons for the coercion need to be explained to the child in such a way that the child will know that it is being carried out for his or her well-being and not as a form of punishment. There is always a risk in using even mild forceful techniques. A crying child can aspirate a medication, particularly when lying on the back. If the nurse holds the child in the lap with the child's right arm behind the nurse, the left hand firmly grasped by the nurse's left hand, and the head securely restrained between the nurse's arm and body, the medication can be slowly poured into the mouth (Fig. 45-12).

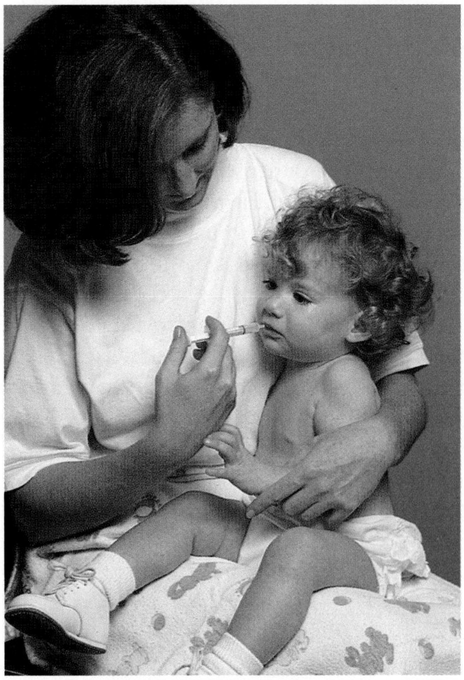

Fig. 45-12 The nurse partially restrains child for easy and comfortable administration of oral medication.

Intramuscular Administration

Selecting the Syringe and Needle

The volume of medication prescribed for small children and the small amount of tissue available for injection require that a syringe be selected that can measure small amounts of solution. For volumes of less than 1 mL, the tuberculin syringe, calibrated in 1/100-mL increments, is appropriate. Minute doses may require the use of a 0.5-mL, low-dose syringe. These syringes, along with specially constructed needles, minimize the possibility of inadvertently administering incorrect amounts of a drug because of dead space, which allows fluid to remain in the syringe and needle after the plunger is pushed completely forward. A minimum of 0.2 mL of the solution remains in a standard needle hub; thus when very small amounts of two drugs are combined in the syringe, such as mixtures of insulin, the ratio of the two drugs can be altered significantly. Measures that minimize the effect of dead space are as follows:

- When two drugs are combined in the syringe, always draw them up in the same order to maintain a consistent ratio between the drugs.
- Use the same brand of syringe (dead space may vary between brands).
- Use one-piece syringe units (needle permanently attached to the syringe).

Dead space is also an important factor to consider when injecting medication, since flushing the syringe with an air bubble adds an additional amount of medication to the prescribed dose. This can be hazardous when very small amounts of a medication are given. Consequently, flushing is not advisable, especially when less than 1 mL of medication is given. Syringes are calibrated to deliver a prescribed drug dose, and the amount of medication left in the hub and needle is not part of the syringe barrel calibrations. Certain drugs such as iron dextran and diphtheria and tetanus toxoid may cause irritation when tracked into the subcutaneous tissue. The Z-track method is recommended for use in infants and children rather than an air bubble. Changing the needle after withdrawing the fluid from the vial is another technique to minimize tracking.

The needle length must be sufficient to penetrate the subcutaneous tissue and deposit the medication into the body of the muscle. The needle gauge should be as small as possible to deliver fluid safely. Smaller-diameter (25- to 30-gauge) needles cause the least discomfort, but larger diameters are needed for viscous medication and prevention of accidental bending of longer needles.

Determining the Site

Older children and adolescents usually pose few problems in selecting a suitable site for intramuscular (IM) injections, but infants, with their small and underdeveloped muscles, have fewer available sites. It is sometimes difficult to assess the amount of fluid that can be safely injected into a single site. Usually 1 mL is the maximum volume that should be administered in a single site to small children and older infants. The muscles of small infants may not tolerate more than 0.5 mL. As the child approaches adult size, volumes approaching those given to adults may be used. However, the larger the amount of solution, the larger the muscle must be into which it is injected.

Major nerves and blood vessels must be avoided. The preferred site for infants is the vastus lateralis (the rectus femoris is not an acceptable site). The ventrogluteal site is relatively free of major nerves and blood vessels, is a relatively large muscle with less subcutaneous tissue than the dorsal site, has well-defined landmarks for safe site location, is less painful than the vastus lateralis, and is easily accessible in several positions. Cook and Murtagh's (2006) research into IM injection sites in children indicates that the ventrogluteal site has not been associated with complications and is the preferred site in children of all ages (Table 45-4). In clinical practice, this site has been safely used in children as young as newborns. The deltoid muscle, a small muscle near the axillary and radial nerves, can be used for small volumes of fluid in children as young as 18 months of age. Its advantages are less pain and fewer adverse effects from the injectate (as observed with immunizations), compared with the vastus lateralis (Ipp et al., 1989). Table 45-4 summarizes the three major injection sites and illustrates the location of the preferred IM injection sites for children.

Table 45-4 Intramuscular Injection Sites in Children

SITE	DISCUSSION
Vastus Lateralis	
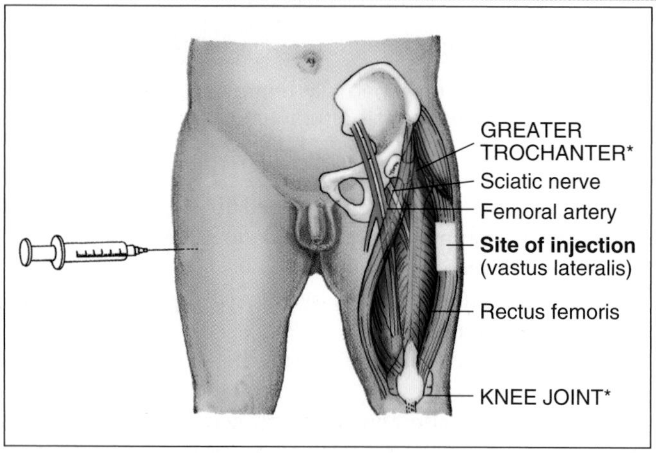	*Location** Palpate to find greater trochanter and knee joints; divide vertical distance between these two landmarks into thirds; inject into middle third. *Needle Insertion and Size* Insert needle perpendicular to knee in infants and young children or perpendicular to thigh or slightly angled toward anterior thigh. 22–25 gauge, 1.6–2.5 cm (5/8–1 inch)† *Advantages* Large, well-developed muscle that can tolerate larger quantities of fluid (0.5 mL [infant] to 2.0 mL [child]) Easily accessible if child is supine, side lying, or sitting *Disadvantages* Thrombosis of femoral artery from injection in midthigh area Sciatic nerve damage from long needle injected posteriorly and medially into small extremity More painful than deltoid or gluteal sites
Ventrogluteal	
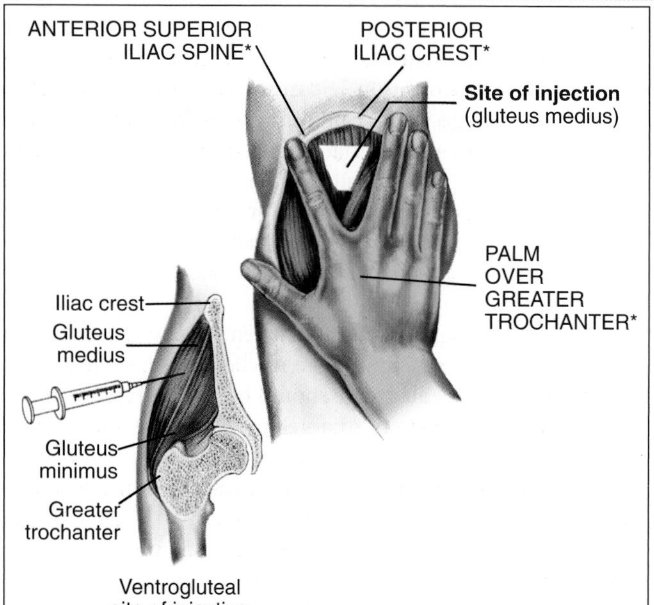 Ventrogluteal site of injection	*Location** Palpate to locate greater trochanter, anterior superior iliac tubercle (found by flexing thigh at hip and measuring up to 1–2 cm above crease formed in groin), and posterior iliac crest; place palm of hand over greater trochanter, index finger over anterior superior iliac tubercle, and middle finger along crest of ileum posteriorly as far as possible; inject into centre of V formed by fingers. *Needle Insertion and Size* Insert needle perpendicular to site but angled slightly toward iliac crest. 22–25 gauge, 1.3–2.5 cm (½–1 inch)† *Advantages* Free of important nerves and vascular structures Easily identified by prominent bony landmarks Thinner layer of subcutaneous tissue than in dorsogluteal site, thus reducing chance of depositing drug subcutaneously rather than intramuscularly Can accommodate larger quantities of fluid (0.5 mL [infant] to 2.0 mL [child]) Easily accessible if child is supine, prone, or side lying Less painful than vastus lateralis *Disadvantages* Health care providers' unfamiliarity with site

Table 45-4 Intramuscular Injection Sites in Children—cont'd

SITE	DISCUSSION
Deltoid	*Location** Locate acromion process; inject only into upper third of muscle that begins about 2 fingerbreadths below acromion. *Needle Insertion and Size* Insert needle perpendicular to site but angled slightly toward shoulder. 22-25 gauge, 1.3-2.5 cm ($\frac{1}{2}$–1 inch) *Advantages* Faster absorption rates than gluteal sites Easily accessible with minimal removal of clothing Less pain and fewer local adverse effects from vaccines as compared with vastus lateralis *Disadvantages* Small muscle mass; can accommodate only limited amounts of medication (0.5-1.0 mL) Small margins of safety with possible damage to radial nerve and axillary nerve (not shown; lies under deltoid at head of humerus)

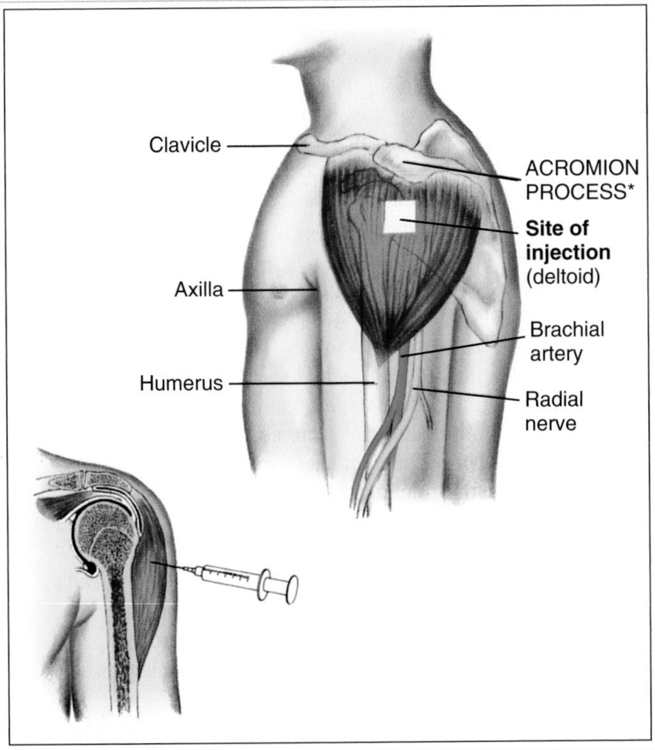

*Locations are indicated by asterisks on illustrations.

†Research has shown that a 2.5 cm (1-inch) needle is needed for adequate muscle penetration in infants 4 months old and possibly in infants as young as 2 months (Cook & Murtagh, 2002).

Administration

Although injections executed with care seldom cause trauma to the child, there have been reports of serious disability related to IM injections in children. Repeated use of a single site has been associated with fibrosis of the muscle with subsequent muscle contracture. Injections close to large nerves, such as the sciatic nerve, have been responsible for permanent disability, especially when potentially neurotoxic medications are administered. There are several reports of tissue damage from penicillin. One of the difficulties in administering the opaque preparations, such as penicillin G, is that aspirated blood cannot be detected at the bottom of the syringe, thus increasing the risk of injecting into a blood vessel. When such drugs are injected, great care must be used in locating the correct site. When aspirating, the nurse should look for blood at the *top* of the syringe near the plunger, since blood may be drawn up through the column of penicillin. One study of IM injection techniques revealed that the straighter the path of needle insertion (e.g., 90-degree angle), the less displacement and shear to tissue, thus reducing discomfort (Katsma & Smith, 1997).

A reported potential hazard with medication in glass ampoules is the presence of glass particles in the ampoule after the container is broken. When the medication is withdrawn into the syringe, the glass particles may also be withdrawn and subsequently injected into the patient. As a precaution, medication from glass ampoules should be drawn up only through a needle with a filter or injected intravenously through a site in the tubing that is distal to an IV filter.

Most children are unpredictable and few can remain still when receiving an injection. Even children who appear to be relaxed and constrained can lose control under the stress of the procedure. It is advisable to have someone available to help hold the child if needed. Because children often jerk or pull away unexpectedly, the nurse should carry an extra needle to exchange for a contaminated one so that the delay is minimal. The child, even a small one, should be told that he or she is receiving an injection (preferably using a phrase such as "putting medicine under the skin"), and then the procedure carried out as quickly and skillfully as possible to avoid prolonging the stressful experience. Invasive procedures such as injections are especially anxiety-provoking in young children. Because injections are painful, the nurse should employ excellent injection technique and effective pain reduction measures to reduce discomfort (see Guidelines box).

Small infants offer little resistance to injections. Although they squirm and may be difficult to hold in position, they can usually be restrained without assistance. The body of a larger infant can be securely held between the nurse's arm and body (Fig. 45-13). To inject into the body of the muscle, the nurse firmly grasps the muscle mass between the thumb and fingers

GUIDELINES Intramuscular Administration of Medication

Use safety precautions in administering medication (e.g., check child's identification).

Apply an eutectic mix of lidocaine and prilocaine (EMLA) topically over site if time permits (at least 60 minutes, preferably 2 to 2½ hours for intramuscular (IM) injection. LMX (lidocaine cream may be applied for a shorter interval (see Pain Management, Chapter 35).

Prepare medication:

- Select needle and syringe appropriate to the following: (1) amount of fluid to be administered (syringe size), (2) viscosity of fluid to be administered (needle gauge), and (3) amount of tissue to be penetrated (needle length).
- Maximum volume to be administered in a single site is 1 mL for older infants and small children.

Determine site of injection (see Table 45-4), making certain that muscle is large enough to accommodate volume and type of medication.

- Acceptable sites for infants and small or debilitated children are the vastus lateralis muscle and the ventrogluteal muscle.
- The dorsogluteal muscle is insufficiently developed to be a safe site for infants and small children.

Administer medication.

- Obtain sufficient help in restraining the child; their behaviour is usually unpredictable.
- Explain briefly what is to be done and, if appropriate, what the child can do to help.
- Expose injection area for unobstructed view of landmarks.
- Select a site where skin is free of irritation and danger of infection; palpate for and avoid sensitive or hardened areas. With multiple injections, rotate sites.
- Place child in a lying or sitting position; the child is not allowed to stand because (1) landmarks are more difficult to assess, (2) restraint is more difficult, and (3) the child may faint and fall.
- Use a new, sharp needle with the smallest diameter that permits free flow of the medication.
- Grasp muscle firmly between the thumb and fingers to isolate and stabilize muscle for deposition of drug in its deepest part; in obese children, spread skin with thumb and index finger to displace subcutaneous tissue and grasp muscle deeply on each side.
- Allow skin preparation to dry completely before skin is penetrated.
- Have medication at room temperature.

Decrease perception of pain.

- Distract the child with conversation.
- Give the child something on which to concentrate (e.g., squeezing a hand or side rail, pinching own nose, humming, counting, yelling "Ouch!").
- Spray vapocoolant (e.g., ethyl chloride or fluorimethane) on site 11 to 15 seconds before injection or place a cold compress or wrapped ice cube on site about a minute before injection, or apply cold to contralateral site.
- Say to the child, "If you feel this, tell me to take it out, please."
- Have the child hold a small adhesive bandage and place it on puncture site after IM injection is given.

Insert needle quickly, using a dartlike motion at a 90-degree angle unless contraindicated.

- Use new needle, not one that has pierced the rubber stopper on vial.

Avoid tracking any medication through superficial tissues:

- Replace needle after withdrawing medication, or wipe medication from needle with sterile gauze.
- If withdrawing medication from an ampoule, use a needle equipped with a filter that removes glass particles; then use a new, nonfilter needle for injection.
- Use the Z-track or air-bubble technique as indicated.
- Avoid depressing the plunger during insertion of the needle.

Aspirate for blood.

- If blood is found, remove syringe from site, change needle, and reinsert into new location.
- If no blood is found, inject into a relaxed muscle:
- **Ventrogluteal**—Place child on side with upper leg flexed and placed in front of lower leg.
- **Vastus lateralis**—Child can be supine, lying on the side, or sitting.

Inject medication slowly.

Remove needle quickly; hold gauze sponge firmly against skin near needle when removing it to avoid pulling on tissue.

Apply firm pressure to the site after injection; massage site to hasten absorption unless contraindicated, as with irritating medications.

Place a small adhesive bandage on puncture site; with young children decorate it by drawing a smiling face or other symbol of acceptance.

Hold and cuddle young child and encourage parents to comfort the child; praise older child.

Allow expression of feelings.

Discard syringe and uncapped, uncut needle in puncture-resistant container located near site of use.

Record time of injection, medication, dose, and injection site.

to isolate and stabilize the site. In obese children, however, it is preferable to first spread the skin with the thumb and index finger to displace subcutaneous tissue and then grasp the muscle deeply on each side.

If the medication is given around the clock, the nurse must wake the child. Although it may seem to be easier to surprise the sleeping child and do it quickly, this can cause the child to fear going back to sleep. When awakened first, children know that nothing will be done unless they are forewarned. See the Guidelines box for techniques that maximize safety and minimize discomfort.

A needleless injection system delivers IM or subcutaneous injections without the use of a needle and eliminates the risk of accidental needle puncture. This needle-free injection

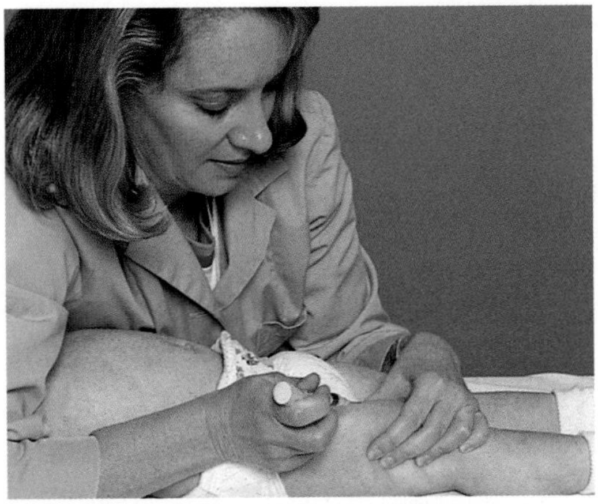

Fig. 45-13 Holding a small child for intramuscular injection. Note how the nurse isolates and stabilizes muscle.

system involves a carbon dioxide cartridge that provides the power to deliver the medication through the skin. Although it is not painless, it may reduce pain and also the anxiety of seeing the needle (Polillio & Killy, 1997).

Subcutaneous and Intradermal Administration

Subcutaneous and intradermal injections are frequently administered to children; the technique differs little from the method used with adults. Examples of subcutaneous injections include insulin, hormone replacement, allergy desensitization, and some vaccines. Tuberculin testing, local anaesthesia, and allergy testing are examples of frequently administered intradermal injections.

Techniques to minimize the pain associated with these injections include changing the needle if it pierced a rubber stopper on a vial, using 26- to 30-gauge needles (only to inject the solution), and injecting small volumes (up to 0.5 mL). The angle of the needle for the subcutaneous injection is typically 90 degrees. In children with little subcutaneous tissue, some practitioners insert the needle at a 45-degree angle. However, the benefit of using the 45-degree angle rather than the 90-degree angle remains controversial.

Although subcutaneous injections can be given anywhere there is subcutaneous tissue, common sites include the centre third of the lateral aspect of the upper arm, the abdomen, and the centre third of the anterior thigh. When giving an intradermal injection into the volar surface of the forearm, the nurse should avoid the medial side of the arm, where the skin is more sensitive.

NURSING ALERT Families often need to learn subcutaneous injection techniques to administer medications, such as insulin, at home. Begin teaching as early as possible to allow the family the maximum amount of practice time possible.

Intravenous Administration

The IV route for administering medications is frequently used in pediatric therapy. For some medications it is the only effective route. This method is used for giving medications to children who have poor absorption as a result of diarrhea, dehydration, or peripheral vascular collapse; who need a high serum concentration of a drug; who have resistant infections that require parenteral medication over an extended time; who need continuous pain relief; and who require emergency treatment.

Insertion sites and observation of the IV infusion are discussed on p. 1299. Several factors need to be considered in relation to IV medication. When a medication is administered intravenously, the effect is almost instantaneous and further control is limited. Most drugs for IV administration require a specified minimum dilution, rate of flow, or both, and many are highly irritating or toxic to tissues outside the vascular system. In addition to the precautions and nursing observations related to IV therapy, factors to consider when preparing and administering medications to infants and children by the IV route include the following:

- Amount of drug to be administered
- Minimum dilution of drug and whether child is fluid restricted
- Type of solution in which drug can be diluted
- Length of time over which drug can be safely administered
- Rate of infusion that child and vessels can tolerate safely
- IV tubing volume capacity
- Time that this or another drug is to be administered
- Compatibility of all drugs that child is receiving intravenously
- Compatibility with infusion fluids

Before any IV infusion, the site of insertion needs to be checked for patency. Medications are never administered with blood products. Only one antibiotic should be administered at a time.

IV infusion is suitable for children who can tolerate the necessary infusion rate and the extra fluid needed to administer the medication. For the very small infant or fluid-restricted child who is not able to tolerate the increased rate of fluids, special delivery systems, such as syringe pumps, are used. Regardless of the technique, the nurse must know the minimum dilutions for safe administration of IV medications to infants and children.

Peripheral Intermittent Infusion Device

The peripheral lock, also known as an **intermittent infusion device** or *saline* or *heparin lock*, is an alternative to a keep-open infusion when extended access to a vein is required without the need for continuous fluid. It is most frequently employed for intermittent infusion of medication into a peripheral venous route. A short, flexible catheter is used as the lock device, and a site is selected where there will be minimal movement, such as the forearm. The catheter is inserted and secured in the same manner as for any IV infusion device, but the hub is occluded with a stopper or injection cap.

The type of device used may vary, and the care and use of the peripheral lock are carried out according to the protocol of the institution or unit. However, the general concept is the same. The catheter remains in place and is flushed with saline after infusion of the medication.

Children may be discharged with a peripheral lock in place to continue receiving medications on a short-term basis without hospitalization. They need to be referred to a home care agency. Those with chronic illnesses who require repeated blood sampling or medications, long-term chemotherapy, or frequent hyperalimentation or antibiotic therapy are best managed with a central venous catheter.

Central Venous Access Device

Central venous access devices (VADs) have several different characteristics. Factors that can influence the type of VAD include the reason for placement of the catheter (diagnosis), length of therapy, risk to the patient in placement of the catheter, and availability of resources to assist the family in maintaining the catheter.

Short-term or nontunneled catheters are used in acute care, emergency, and critical care units. These catheters are made of polyurethane and are placed in large veins such as the subclavian, femoral, or jugular. Insertion is by surgical incision or large percutaneous threading. A chest x-ray film should be taken to verify placement of the catheter tip before administration of fluids or medications.

Peripherally inserted central catheters (PICCs) can be used for short-term to moderate-length therapy. These catheters consist of silicone or polymer material and are placed by specially trained nurses, physicians, or interventional radiologists (Gamulka, Mendoza, & Connolly, 2005). The most common insertion site is above the antecubital area using the median, cephalic, or basilic vein. The catheter is threaded either with or without a guidewire into the superior vena cava. PICCs can be trimmed before insertion, and the decision can be made to insert the catheter midline, which is considered between the insertion site and the axilla. The midline has a dwell time of 2 to 4 weeks. If the catheter is threaded midline, total **parenteral nutrition** (TPN) or any medication known to irritate a peripheral vein (e.g., chemotherapy drugs) should not be administered. The high concentration of glucose in TPN makes it irritating to the vessel; it should be infused through a central catheter.

NURSING ALERT Most PICC lines are not sutured into place, so care is needed when changing the dressing.

Long-term central VADs include tunnelled catheters and implanted infusion ports **(implanted venous access devices)** (Fig. 45-14). They may have single, double, or triple lumens. Several lumens (multilumen) catheters allow more than one therapy to be administered at the same time. Reasons to use multilumen catheters include repeated blood sampling, TPN, administration of blood products or infusion of large quantities or concentrations of fluids, administration of incompatible medications or fluids at the same time (through different lumens), and central venous pressure monitoring.

With any of the central venous catheters, medication is easily instilled through the injection cap. Maintenance of the

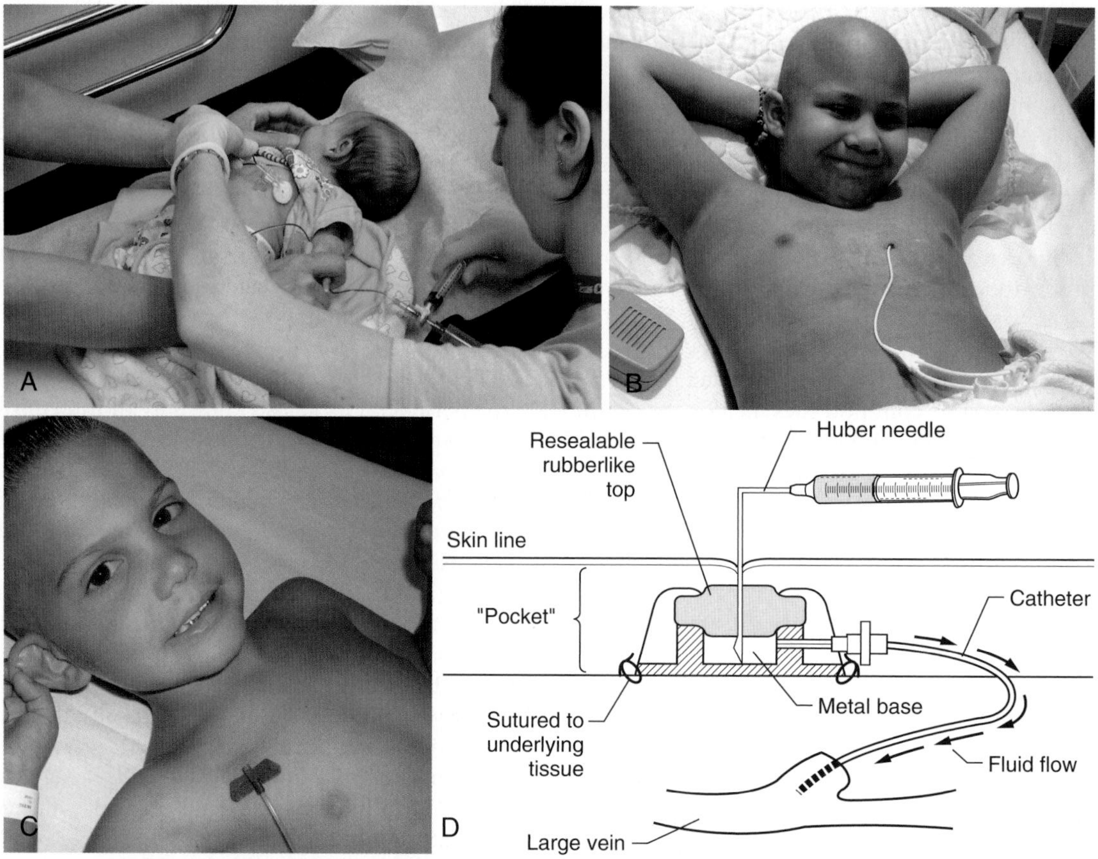

Fig. 45-14 Venous access devices. **A:** Blood being drawn from a central venous catheter. **B:** Child with external central venous catheter. **C:** Child with implanted port with Huber needle in place. **D:** Side view of implanted port.

evolve Animation—Central Venous Access
evolve Critical Thinking Exercise—Central Venous Access Device
evolve Animation—IV Line Placement
evolve Animation—PICC Line Placement

catheter includes dressing changes, flushing to maintain patency, and prevention of occlusion or dislodgment.

NURSING ALERT When working with tunnelled catheters, PICCs, and peripheral intravenous lines (PIVs), avoid using scissors around the tubing or dressing. Removal is best accomplished using fingers and much patience. In the event that a tunnelled catheter is cut, use a padded clamp to clamp the catheter proximal to the exit site to avoid blood loss. Repair kits are available, which may save the catheter and avoid surgery to replace a cut catheter.

With the implanted device the port must be palpated for placement and stabilized, the overlying skin cleansed, and only special noncoring Huber needles used to pierce the port's diaphragm on the top or side, depending on the style. To avoid repeated skin punctures, a special infusion set with a Huber needle and extension tubing with a Luer connection can be used (see Fig. 45-14). With this attached, the injection procedure is the same as for an intermittent infusion device or a central venous catheter. To prevent infection, meticulous aseptic technique must be used any time the devices are entered, including instillation of heparin or saline to prevent clotting (Harris & Maguire, 1999). There should be a protocol stating that the Huber needle needs to be changed at established intervals, usually 5 to 7 days.

Children with a VAD and their parents need to be taught the procedure for care of the VAD before discharge from the hospital, including preparation and injection of the prescribed medication, the flush, and dressing changes. A protective device may be recommended for some active children to prevent accidental dislodgment of the needle. Many children take responsibility for preparing and administering medications. Both verbal and written step-by-step instructions should be provided (Table 45-5).

Infection and catheter occlusion are two of the most common complications of central venous catheters. They require treatment with antibiotics for infection and a fibrinolytic agent, such as alteplase, for clots (Fisher et al., 2004; Shen et al., 2003). Uncapping can be prevented by taping the cap securely to the catheter and the clamped line to the dressing. Leaks can be prevented by using a smooth-edged clamp only. Parents need to keep scissors away from the child to prevent accidental cutting of the catheter. If the catheter leaks, they should be instructed to tape it above the leak and then clamp the catheter at the taped site. The child should be taken to the practitioner as soon as possible to prevent infection or clotting after a catheter leak.

Nasogastric, Orogastric, or Gastrostomy Administration

When a child has an indwelling feeding tube or a gastrostomy, oral medications may be given via that route. The administration of medications via **enteral feeding** tubes is not commonly investigated during drug development and thus is usually considered an "off-label" or unlicensed route of medication administration, so careful consideration must be given to the selection of appropriate formulations that will allow for the safe and effective delivery of medication via enteral feeding tubes. Advantages of this method include the ability to administer oral medications around the clock without disturbing the child and ensuring that the child actually takes the

Table 45-5 Flush Guidelines

Children		
Peripheral lines (Heplock)	**≤24-G CATHETER**	**>24-G CATHETER**
	10 units/mL 2 mL heparin after meds or every 8 hr	5 mL normal saline after meds or every 8 hr
Midline	10 units/mL 3 mL heparin in a 10-mL syringe after meds or every 8 hr	
External central line (nonimplanted, tunneled, or PICC)	10 units/mL 3 mL heparin in a 10-mL syringe after meds or daily	
Implanted port	**INTERMITTENT**	**DORMANT**
	10 units/mL 5 mL heparin after meds	100 units/mL 5 mL heparin every month*
Arterial and central venous pressure continuous monitored lines	1 unit/mL heparin in 55-mL syringes run at 1 mL/hr	
Neonates and Infants		
Peripheral lines (Heplock)	**≤24-G CATHETER**	
	1 unit/mL 2 mL heparin after meds or every 8 hr	
Percutaneous central catheter	1 unit/mL heparin in 20-mL syringe run at 0.2 mL/hr	
Surgically placed CVC ≤5 French	1 unit/mL 2 mL heparin to check for line patency and between meds or TPN known to be compatible or every 8 hr	
Surgically placed CVC >5 French	1 unit/mL 3 mL heparin to check for line patency and between meds or TPN known to be compatible or every 8 hr	

(Modified from Texas Children's Hospital, Houston).
*Patients <6 months of age: 10 units/mL 5 mL every month or 10 units/mL 5 mL every day if accessed.
CVC, Central venous catheter; *PICC*, peripherally inserted central catheter; *TPN*, total parenteral nutrition.

medication. A disadvantage of this method is the risk of occluding or clogging the tube, especially when giving viscous solutions through small-bore feeding tubes. The most important preventive measure is adequate flushing after the medication is instilled (see Guidelines box).

Rectal Administration

The rectal route for administration is less reliable but is sometimes used when the oral route is difficult or contraindicated. It is also used when oral preparations are unsuitable to control vomiting. Some of the medications available in suppository form are acetaminophen, sedatives, analgesics (morphine), and antiemetics. Unless the rectum is empty at the time of insertion, the absorption of the drug may be delayed, diminished, or prevented by the presence of feces. Sometimes the drug is later evacuated, securely surrounded by stool.

To administer a medication rectally, first the wrapping on the suppository is removed and the suppository is lubricated with water-soluble jelly or warm water. Rectal suppositories are traditionally inserted with the apex (pointed end) foremost. Reverse contractions or the pressure gradient of the anal canal may help the suppository slip higher into the canal. Using a glove, the nurse inserts the suppository quickly but gently into the rectum, beyond both of the rectal sphincters. The buttocks are then held together firmly to relieve pressure on the anal sphincter until the urge to expel the suppository has passed—5 to 10 minutes. Sometimes the amount of medication ordered is less than the dosage available. The irregular shape of most suppositories makes the process of dividing them into a desired dose difficult if not dangerous. If the suppository must be halved, it should be cut lengthwise. However, there is no guarantee that the drug is evenly dispersed throughout the petrolatum base.

GUIDELINES Nasogastric, Orogastric, or Gastrostomy Medication Administration in Children

- Use solution, suspension, or dissolvable tablet preparations of medication whenever possible.
- Dilute viscous medication or syrup with a small amount of water if possible.
- If administering tablets, crush tablet to a fine powder and dissolve in a small amount of warm water.
- Never crush enteric-coated or sustained-release tablets or capsules.
- Avoid oily medications because they tend to cling to the side of the tube.
- Do not mix medication with enteral formula unless fluid is restricted. If adding a medication:
  - Check with the pharmacist for compatibility.
  - Shake formula well and observe for any physical reaction (e.g., separation, precipitation).
  - Label formula container with name of medication, dosage, date, and time infusion started.
- Have medication at room temperature.
- Measure medication in a calibrated cup or oral syringe.
- Stop enteral feed or unclamp tubing.
- Check for correct placement of nasogastric or orogastric tube.
- Using an oral syringe, flush tube with water (generally 10 to 30 mL).
- Draw medication into a new oral syringe (if not initially measured into oral syringe).
- Inspect syringe to ensure the contents look appropriate for enteral feeding tube administration (i.e. absence of visible particles that could block feeding tube).
- Push medication into the enteral feeding tube as a bolus dose.
- Flush an equal amount of water down the enteral feeding tube to rinse out the tube and ensure that the total dose was administered.
- With certain drug preparations (e.g., suspensions) more fluid may be needed.
- If administering more than one medication at the same time, flush tube between each medication with clear water.
- Position the patient on the right side (unless contraindicated) to facilitate stomach emptying.
- Restart feed or clamp tube after flushing.

Optic, Otic, and Nasal Administration

There are few differences between administering eye, ear, and nose medication to children and giving them to adults. The major difficulty is in gaining children's cooperation. Older children need only explanation and direction. Although the administration of optic, otic, and nasal medication is not painful, these medications can cause unpleasant sensations that can be eliminated with various techniques.

NURSING ALERT The following steps help reduce unpleasant sensations when administering medications:

Eye—Apply finger pressure to the lacrimal punctum at the inner aspect of the lid for 1 minute to prevent drainage of medication to the nasopharynx and the unpleasant "tasting" of the medication.

Ear—Allow medications stored in the refrigerator to warm to room temperature before instillation.

Nose—Position the child with the head hyperextended to prevent strangling sensations caused by medication trickling into the throat rather than up into the nasal passages.

To instill eye medication, place the child supine or sitting with the head extended, and ask the child to look up. Use one hand to pull the lower lid downward; the hand that holds the dropper rests on the head so that it may move synchronously with the child's head, thus reducing the possibility of trauma to a struggling child or of dropping medication on the child's face (Fig. 45-15). As the lower lid is pulled down, a small conjunctival sac is formed; apply the solution or ointment to this area, never directly on the eyeball. Another effective technique is to pull the lower lid down and out to form a cup effect, into which the medication is dropped. Gently close the lids to prevent expression of the medication, and ask the child to look in all directions to enhance even distribution of the preparation. Wipe excess medication from the inner canthus outward to prevent contamination to the contralateral eye.

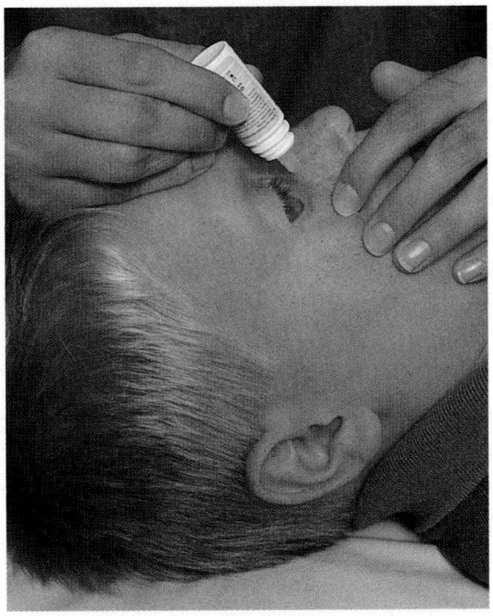

Fig. 45-15 Administering eye drops.

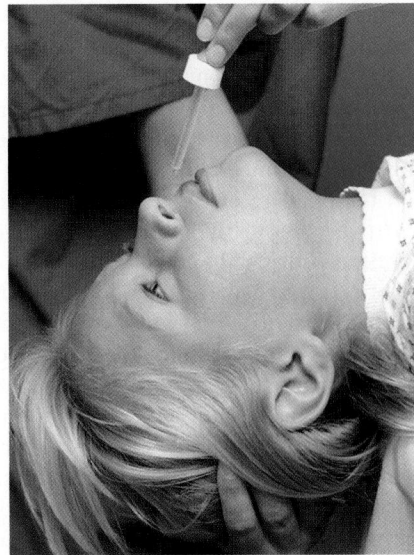

Fig. 45-16 Proper position for instilling nose drops.

Instilling eye drops in infants can be difficult, since they often clench the lids tightly closed. One approach is to place the drops in the nasal corner where the lids meet. The medication pools in this area, and when the infant opens the lids, the medication flows onto the conjunctiva. For young children, playing a game can be helpful, such as instructing the child to keep the eyes closed until the count of three and then open them, at which time the drops are quickly instilled. Ointment can be applied by gently pulling down the lower lid and placing the ointment in the lower conjunctival sac.

NURSING ALERT If both eye ointment and drops are ordered, give drops first, wait 3 minutes, and then apply the ointment to allow each medication to work. When possible, administer eye ointments before bedtime or naptime, since the child's vision will be blurred temporarily.

Ear drops are instilled with the child in the prone or supine position and the head turned to the appropriate side. For children younger than 3 years of age, the external auditory canal is straightened by gently pulling the pinna downward and straight back. The pinna is pulled upward and back in children older than 3 years of age. To place the drops deep in the ear canal without contaminating the tip of the dropper, place a disposable ear speculum in the canal and administer the drops through the speculum. After instillation, the child should remain lying on the unaffected side for a few minutes. Gentle massage of the area immediately anterior to the ear facilitates the entry of drops into the ear canal. The use of cotton balls prevents medication from flowing out of the external canal. However, the pledgets should be loose enough to allow any discharge to exit from the ear. Premoistening the cotton with a few drops of medication prevents the wicking action from absorbing the medication instilled in the ear.

Nose drops are instilled in the same manner as in the adult patient. Unpleasant sensations associated with medicated nose drops can be minimized by positioning the child with the head extended well over the edge of the bed or a pillow (Fig. 45-16). Depending on the infant's size, the infant can be positioned in the football hold (see Fig. 45-5, B); in the nurse's arm with the head extended and stabilized between the nurse's body and elbow, and the arms and hands immobilized with the nurse's hands; or as shown in Figure 45-16. After instillation of the drops, the child should remain in position for 1 minute to allow the drops to come in contact with the nasal surfaces.

Nasal spray dispensers are inserted into the naris vertically and then angled nasally to avoid trauma to the septum and to direct medication toward the inferior turbinate.

Family Teaching and Home Care

The nurse usually assumes the responsibility for preparing families to administer medications at home. The family should understand why the child is receiving the medication and the effects that might be expected, as well as the amount, frequency, and length of time the medication is to be administered. Instruction should be carried out in an unhurried, relaxed manner, preferably in an area away from a busy ward or office.

The caregiver needs to be carefully instructed in the correct dosage. Some persons have difficulty understanding medical terminology from the pharmacy; just because they nod or otherwise indicate an understanding, it cannot be assumed that the message is clear. It is important to ascertain their interpretation of a teaspoon, for example, and to be certain they have accurate measuring devices. The nurse should show or mark the dose point on a dropper or syringe and how to draw up and eliminate bubbles. The parent should be asked to give a return demonstration. This is essential when the medication has potentially serious consequences from incorrect dosage, such as insulin or digoxin, or when more complex administration is required, such as parenteral injections. When teaching a parent to give an injection, the nurse must allot adequate time for instruction and practice.

Home modifications are often necessary because the availability of equipment or assistance can differ from the hospital setting. For example, the parent may need guidance in devising methods that allow for one person to hold the child and safely give the medication (see Patient Teaching box).

The time that the medication is to be administered should be clarified with the parent. For instance, when a medication is prescribed in association with meals, the number of meals that the family is accustomed to eating influences the amount of medication the child receives. Does the child have meals twice a day or five times a day? When a medication is to be given several times during the day, together the nurse and parents can work out a schedule that accommodates the family's routine. This is particularly significant if the medication must be given at equal intervals throughout a 24-hour period. For example, telling parents that the child needs 1 teaspoon of medicine four times a day is subject to misinterpretation, since parents may routinely schedule the doses at incorrect times. Instead, a preplanned schedule based on 6-hour intervals should be set up with the number of days required for therapeutic dosage listed. Written instruction should accompany all medication prescriptions (see Patient Teaching box).

Maintaining Fluid Balance

Measurement of Intake and Output

Accurate measurements of fluid intake and output (I&O) are essential to the assessment of fluid balance. Measurements from all sources—gastrointestinal and parenteral I&O from urine, stools, vomitus, fistulas, nasogastric suction, sweat, and drainage from wounds—must be taken and considered. Although the practitioner usually indicates when I&O measurements are to be recorded, it is a nursing responsibility to keep an accurate I&O record on certain children, including those:

- Receiving IV therapy
- Who underwent major surgery
- Receiving diuretic or corticosteroid therapy
- With severe thermal burns or injuries
- With renal disease or damage
- With congestive heart failure
- With dehydration
- With diabetes mellitus
- With oliguria
- In respiratory distress
- With chronic lung disease

Infants or small children who are unable to use a bedpan or those who have bowel movements with every voiding require the application of a collecting device. If collecting bags are not used, wet diapers or pads are carefully weighed to ascertain the amount of fluid lost. This includes liquid stool, vomitus, and other losses. The volume of fluid in millilitres is equivalent to the weight of the fluid measured in grams. The specific gravity as a measure of osmolality is determined with a refractometer or urine dipsticks and assists in assessing the degree of hydration.

NURSING ALERT 1 g of wet diaper weight = 1 mL urine

In infants with diapers, weigh all dry diapers to be used and note in an indelible marker the dry weight of the diaper; when there is fluid (urine or liquid stool) in the diaper, the amount of output can be approximated by subtracting the weight of the dry diaper from the weight of the wet diaper.

Disadvantages of the weighed-diaper method of fluid measurement include (1) inability to differentiate one type of loss from another because of admixture, (2) loss of urine or liquid stool from leakage or evaporation (especially if the infant is under a radiant warmer), and (3) additional fluid in the diaper (superabsorbent disposable type) from absorption of atmospheric moisture (in high-humidity incubators).

Special Needs When the Child Is NPO

Infants or children who are unable or not permitted to take fluids by mouth (NPO) have special needs. To ensure that they do not receive fluids, a sign can be placed in some obvious place, such as over their beds or on their shirts, to alert others to the NPO status. To prevent the temptation to drink, fluids should not be left at the bedside.

Oral hygiene, a part of routine hygienic care, is especially important when fluids are restricted or withheld. For the young child who cannot brush the teeth or rinse the mouth without swallowing fluid, the mouth and teeth can be cleaned and kept moist by swabbing with saline-moistened gauze.

NURSING ALERT To keep the mouth feeling moist when the child is NPO, give ice chips (if this is permitted by the practitioner) or spray the mouth with an atomizer. To meet the need to suck, the infant can be provided with a safe commercial pacifier.

PATIENT TEACHING Administering Oral, Nasal, or Optic Medication

To administer oral, nasal, or optic medication when only one person is available to hold the child, use the following procedure:

- Place child supine on flat surface (bed, couch, floor).
- Sit facing the child so that the child's head is between the operator's thighs and the child's arms are under the operator's legs.
- Place lower legs over the child's legs to restrain the lower body, if necessary.
- To administer oral medication, place a small pillow under the child's head to reduce risk of aspiration.
- To administer nasal medication, place a small pillow under the child's shoulders to aid flow of liquid through nasal passages.

PATIENT TEACHING Colour-Coded Instructions

If parents have difficulty reading or understanding English, use colours to convey instructions. For example, mark each medication with a colour and place the appropriate colour on a calendar chart or on a drawing of a clock to identify when the medication needs to be given. If a liquid medication and syringe are used, also mark the syringe with colour-coded tape at the place the plunger needs to be.

The child who is fluid restricted presents an equal challenge. Limiting fluids is often more difficult for the child than being NPO, especially when IV fluids are also eliminated. To make certain the child does not drink the entire amount allowed early in the day, the daily allotment is calculated to provide fluids at periodic intervals throughout the child's waking hours. Serving the fluids in small containers gives the illusion of larger servings. No extra liquid should be left at the bedside.

Parenteral Fluid Therapy

Site and Equipment

The site selected for PIV infusion depends on accessibility and convenience. Although it is possible to use any accessible vein in older children, the child's developmental, cognitive, and mobility needs must be considered when selecting a site. Ideally, in older children, the superficial veins of the forearm should be used, leaving the hands free. An older child can help select the site and thereby maintain some measure of control. For veins in the extremities it is best to start with the most distal site and avoid the child's favoured hand to reduce the disability related to the procedure. Restrict the child's movements as little as possible—avoid a site over a joint in an extremity, such as the antecubital space. In small infants a superficial vein of the hand, wrist, forearm, foot, or ankle is usually most convenient and most easily stabilized (Fig. 45-17). Foot veins should be avoided in children learning to walk or already walking. Superficial veins of the scalp have no valves, insertion is easy, and they can be used in infants up to about 9 months of age, but they should be used only when other site attempts have failed. A transilluminator can aid in finding and evaluating veins for access (Fig. 45-18).

Selection of a scalp vein may require clipping the area around the site to better visualize the vein and provide a smoother surface on which to tape the catheter hub and tubing. Clipping a portion of the infant's hair can be upsetting to parents; they should be told what to expect and reassured that the hair will grow in again rapidly (save the hair because parents often wish to keep it). Remove as little as possible, directly over the insertion site and taping surface. A rubber band slipped onto the head from brow to occiput will usually suffice as a tourniquet, although if the vessel is visible, a tourniquet may not be necessary.

<u>**NURSING ALERT**</u> A tab of tape should be placed on the rubber band to help grasp it when removing it from the infant's head. The rubber band should be cut to avoid accidentally dislodging the catheter when moving the rubber band over the IV insertion site. The tape tab will lift the rubber band and allow it to be cut. Hold the rubber band in two places and cut between these areas to prevent the rubber band from snapping on the head.

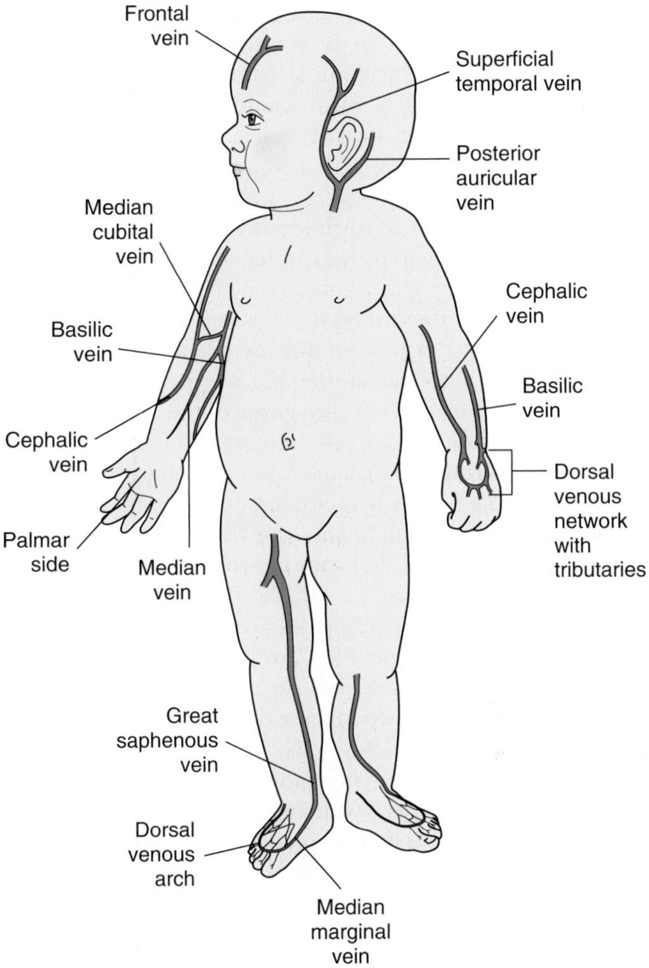

Fig. 45-17 Preferred sites for venous access in infants.

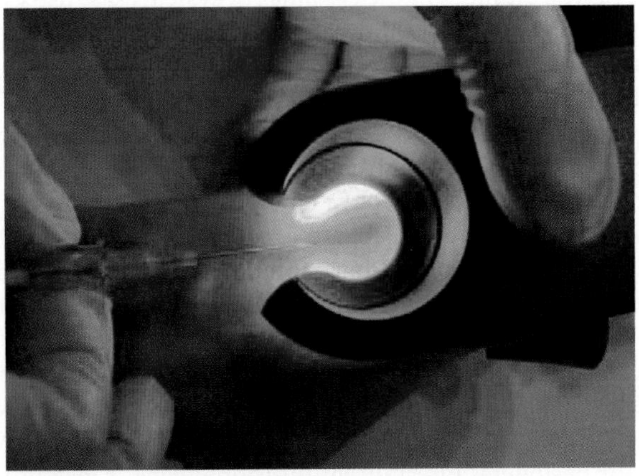

Fig. 45-18 Transilluminator: low-heat light-emitting diode (LED) light placed on the skin to illuminate veins; an opening allows cannulation of the vein.

Situations may occur in which rapid establishment of systemic access is vital, and venous access may be hampered by peripheral circulatory collapse, **hypovolemic shock** (secondary to vomiting or diarrhea, burns, or trauma), cardiopulmonary arrest, or other conditions (Dubick & Holcomb, 2000). *Intraosseous infusion* provides a rapid, safe, and lifesaving alternate route for administration of fluids and medications until intravascular access can be obtained, especially in children who are 6 years of age and younger.

A large-bore needle, such as a bone marrow aspiration needle (e.g., Jamshidi) or an intraosseous needle (e.g., Cook), is inserted into the medullary cavity of a long bone, most often the proximal tibia. This procedure is usually reserved for children who are unconscious or for those who are receiving analgesia, since the procedure is painful. Local anaesthesia should be used for a semiconscious patient. Observe the dependent tissue closely for swelling, since extravasation may be hidden under the leg and compartment syndrome may result.

For most IV infusions in children, a 22- to 24-gauge catheter may be used if therapy is expected to last less than 5 days. The smallest-gauge and shortest-length catheter that will accommodate the prescribed therapy should be chosen. The length of the catheter may be directly related to infection or embolus formation—the shorter the catheter, the fewer the complications (Maki, 1994). The gauge of the catheter should maintain adequate flow of the infusate into the cannulated vein while allowing adequate blood flow around the catheter walls to promote proper hemodilution of the infusate.

Determining the best catheter for the patient early in the therapy provides the best chance of avoiding catheter-related complications (Moureau, 1999). As the length of therapy increases, decisions regarding the type of infusion device (short peripheral, midline, PICC, or central venous catheter) should be explored. Guidelines such as flow charts or algorithms are available to help in these decisions (Catudal, 1999).

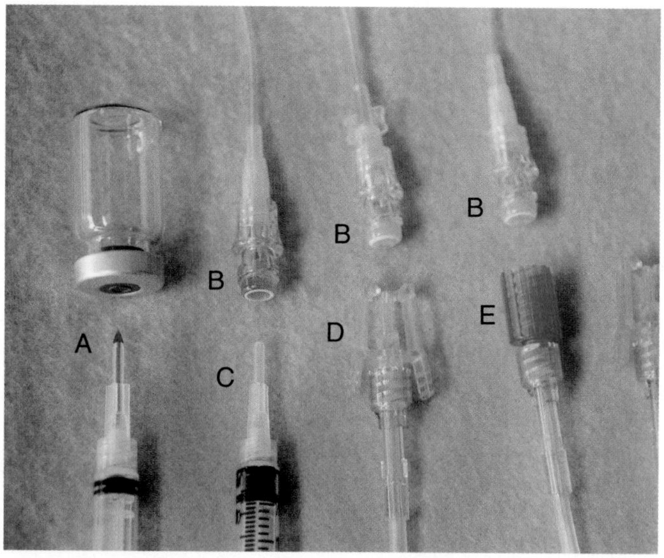

Fig. 45-19 Interlink intravenous access systems. **A:** Blue spike syringe. **B:** Preslit injection port (needleless). **C:** Blunt plastic cannula syringe. **D:** Lever lock cannula. **E:** Threaded lock cannula.

Safety Catheters and Needleless Systems

Intracatheter IV inserters with hollow-bore needles carry a high risk for transmission of blood-borne pathogens from needlestick injuries. Safety catheters with guards can prevent accidental needlesticks. Needleless IV systems are designed to prevent needlestick injuries during administration of IV push medications and IV piggyback medications. Some needleless devices can be used with any tubing, whereas others require the use of the entire IV delivery system for compatibility. Needleless IV systems rely on prepierced septa that are accessed by blunted plastic cannulas or systems that use valves that open and close a fluid path when activated by insertion of a syringe.

Blunt plastic cannulas and preslit injection port sites (Fig. 45-19) eliminate the need for steel needles and conventional injection port sites but remain accessible via hypodermic needles, a drawback except in emergent situations. A syringe with a blue spike is available to access a single-dose vial (see Fig. 45-19, A). The preslit injection port sites are identified by a white ring surrounding the port; this ring alerts users that the system is needleless (see Fig. 45-19, B). Syringes are available with the blunt plastic cannula for accessing these sites (see Fig. 45-19, C). A lever lock (see Fig. 45-19, D) or threaded lock cannula (see Fig. 45-19, E) attaches to an IV line, IV Y site, or peripheral intermittent infusion device. A preslit universal vial adapter (not pictured) provides access to standard multiple-dose vials, and syringe cannulas are then used to access the adapter. Valve technology allows syringes and IV tubing to connect directly in-line without the use of an adapter.

NURSING ALERT Misconnections of tubing have occurred, resulting in patient deaths. Many needleless IV systems allow other types of tubing such as blood pressure and oxygen tubing to connect and instill air directly into the IV line. Before tubing is connected or reconnected to a patient, trace it completely from the patient to the point of origin for verification (Institute for Safe Medication Practices, 2004).

Infusion Pumps

A variety of infusion pumps are available and used in nearly all pediatric infusions to accurately administer medication and minimize the possibility of overloading the circulation. It is important to calculate the amount to be infused in a given length of time, set the infusion rate, and monitor the apparatus frequently (at least every 1 to 2 hours) to make certain that the desired rate is maintained, the integrity of the system remains intact, the site remains intact (free of redness, edema, infiltration, or irritation), and the infusion does not stop. Continuous infusion pumps, although convenient and efficient, are not without risks. Over-reliance on the accuracy of the machine can cause either too much or too little fluid to be infused; its use does not eliminate the need for careful periodic assessment by the nurse. Excess pressure can build up if the machine is set at a rate faster than the vein is able to accommodate (or continues to pump when the needle is out of the lumen).

Securement of a Peripheral Intravenous Line

To maintain the integrity of the IV line, adequate protection of the site is required. The catheter hub should be firmly secured at the puncture site with a transparent dressing and commercial securement device (e.g., StatLock) (Fig. 45-20) or clear, nonallergenic tape. Transparent dressings are ideal because the insertion site is easily observed. Minimal tape should be used at the puncture site and on about 2.5 to 5 cm of skin beyond the site to avoid obscuring the insertion site for early detection of infiltration.

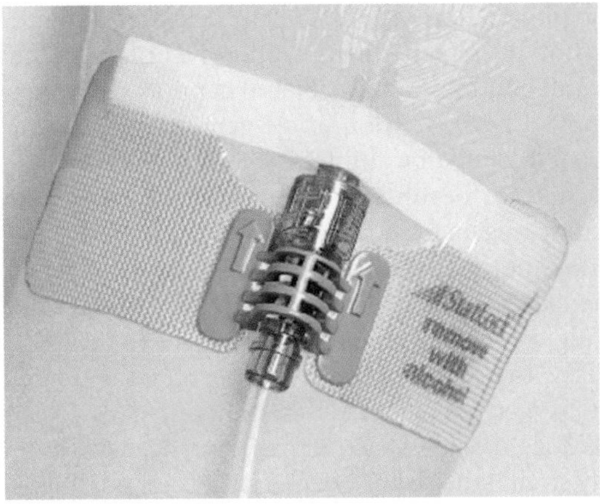

Fig. 45-20 StatLock securement devices enhance peripheral intravenous line dwell time and decrease phlebitis.

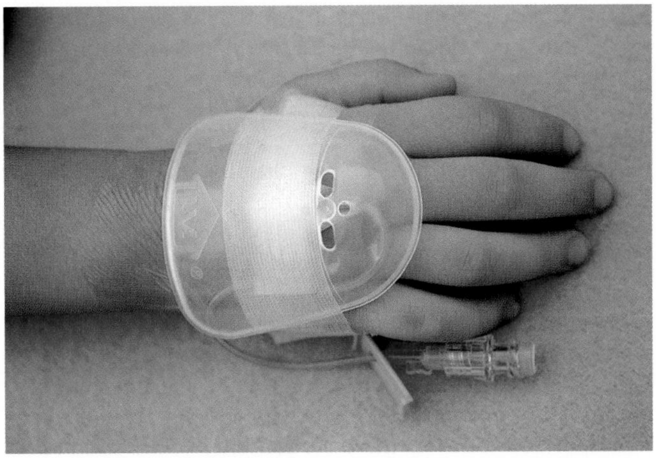

Fig. 45-21 I.V. House used to protect intravenous site.

A protective cover is applied directly over the catheter insertion site to protect the infusion site. Easy access to the IV site for frequent (1- to 2-hour) assessments must be considered. Improvised plastic cups cut in half with the ridged edges covered with tape should not be used as they have injured patients. A commercial site protector, I.V. House, is available in different sizes (Fig. 45-21). Its ventilation holes prevent moisture from accumulating under the dome. This device is designed to protect the IV site; allow for visibility of the site; minimize use of padded boards, splints, or other restraints and tape; and maintain skin integrity. The connector tubing or extension tubing can be looped to make it small enough to fit under the protective cover to prevent accidental snagging of the catheter. It is important to safely secure the IV tubing to prevent infants and children from becoming entangled in the tubing or from accidentally pulling the catheter or needle out. Securing the tubing in this manner also eliminates movement of the catheter hub at the insertion site (mechanical manipulation). A colourful and interesting sticker can be applied to the protecting device to add a positive note to the procedure.

Finger or toe areas should be left unoccluded by dressings or tape to allow for assessment of circulation. The thumb is never immobilized because of the danger of contractures with limited movement later on. An extremity should never be encircled with tape. The use of roll gauze, self-adhering stretch bandages, and Ace bandages can cause the same constriction and hide signs of infiltration (Infusion Nurses Society, 2000a).

Removal of a Peripheral Intravenous Line

When it comes time to discontinue an IV infusion, many children are distressed by the thought of catheter removal. They need a careful explanation of the process and suggestions for helping. Encouraging children to remove or help remove the tape from the site provides them with a measure of control and often fosters their cooperation. The procedure consists of turning off any pump apparatus, occluding the IV tubing, removing the tape, pulling the catheter out of the vessel in the opposite direction of insertion, and exerting firm pressure at the site. A dry dressing (adhesive bandage strip) is placed over the puncture site. The use of adhesive-removal pads can decrease the pain of tape removal, but the skin should be washed after use to avoid irritation. To remove transparent dressings (e.g., OpSite, Tegaderm), pull the opposing edges parallel to the skin to loosen the bond. Inspect the catheter tip to ensure the catheter is intact and that no portion remains in the vein.

NURSING ALERT Consider the child's age, development, neurological status, and predictability (how the child responds to painful treatments) when determining the need for assistance to maintain safety. Manual removal of tape is the preferred method. Only if absolutely necessary should a small cut be made in the tape, using bandage scissors, to facilitate its removal. Before cutting the tape:

- Ensure that all digits are visible.
- Remove any barrier that hinders visibility, such as a protective covering.
- Protect the child's skin and digits by sliding your own finger(s) between the tape and the child's skin so that the scissors do not touch the patient.
- Place a cut on the tape located on the medial aspect (thumb side) of the extremity.

Complications

The same precautions regarding maintenance of asepsis, prevention of infection, and observation for infiltration need to be carried out with patients of any age. However, infiltration is more difficult to detect in infants and small children than in adults. The increased amount of subcutaneous fat and the amount of tape used to secure the catheter often obscure the early signs of infiltration. When the fluid appears to be infusing too slowly or ceases, the usual assessment for obstruction within the apparatus—kinks, screw clamps, shutoff valve, and positioning interference (e.g., a bent elbow)—often locates the difficulty. When these actions fail to detect the problem, it may be necessary to carefully remove some of the dressing to obtain a clear view of the venipuncture site. Dependent areas, such as the palm and undersides of the extremity or the occiput and behind the ears, should be examined.

Whenever possible, the IV infusion should be placed in an extremity to which the identification band (or bracelet) is not attached. Serious circulatory impairment can result from infiltrated solution distal to the band, which acts as a tourniquet, preventing adequate venous return. To check for return blood flow through the catheter, the tubing is removed from the infusion pump, and the bag is lowered below the level of the infusion site. Resistance during flushing or aspiration for blood return also indicates that the IV infusion may have infiltrated surrounding tissue. A good blood return, or lack thereof, is not always an indicator of infiltration in small infants. Flushing the catheter and observing for edema, redness, or streaking along the vein are appropriate for assessment of the IV line.

IV therapy in pediatrics tends to be difficult to maintain because of mechanical factors such as vascular trauma resulting from the catheter, the insertion site, vessel size, vessel fragility, pump pressure, the patient's activity level, operator skill and insertion technique, forceful administration of boluses of fluid, and infusion of irritants or vesicants through a small vessel (Pettit & Hughes, 1999). These factors cause infiltration and extravasation injuries. *Infiltration* is defined as inadvertent administration of a nonvesicant solution or medication into surrounding tissue. *Extravasation* is defined as inadvertent administration of vesicant solution or medication into surrounding tissue (Infusion Nurses Society, 2000a, 2000b). A *vesicant* or *sclerosing agent* causes varying degrees of cellular damage when even minute amounts escape into surrounding tissue. Guidelines are available for determining the severity of tissue injury by staging characteristics, such as the amount of redness, blanching, the amount of swelling, pain, the quality of pulses below infiltration, capillary refill, and warmth or coolness of the area (Infusion Nurses Society, 2000a, 2000b; Montgomery et al., 1999) (see Additional Resources section at the end of this chapter).

Treatment of infiltration or extravasation varies according to the type of vesicant. Guidelines are available outlining the sequence of interventions and specific treatment of infiltration or extravasation with antidotes (Montgomery et al., 1999; Oncology Nursing Society, 1998) (see also Additional Resources).

NURSING ALERT When infiltration or extravasation is observed (signs include erythema, pain, edema, blanching, streaking on the skin along the vein, and darkened area at the insertion site), immediately stop the infusion, elevate the extremity, notify the practitioner, and initiate the ordered treatment as soon as possible. Remove the IV line when it is no longer needed (e.g., after infusing an antidote).

Procedures for Maintaining Respiratory Function

Inhalation Therapy

Oxygen Therapy

Oxygen is administered for **hypoxemia** and may be delivered by mask, nasal cannula, tent, hood, face mask, or ventilator. Oxygen therapy is frequently administered in the hospital, although increasing numbers of children are receiving oxygen in the home. Oxygen delivered to infants is well tolerated by using a plastic hood (Fig. 45-22). The humidified oxygen should not be blown directly into the infant's face. Older infants and children can use a nasal cannula or prongs, which can supply a concentration of oxygen of about 50%. A mask is not well tolerated by children.

For children beyond early infancy, the oxygen tent is a satisfactory means for administration of oxygen (Fig. 45-23). A tent does not require any device to come into direct contact with the face, but the concentration of oxygen within the tent is difficult to control and to maintain above 30 to 50%. A major difficulty with the use of the tent is keeping the tent closed so that the oxygen concentration is maintained.

To reduce oxygen loss, nursing care needs to be planned carefully so that the tent is opened as little as possible. Because oxygen is heavier than air, loss will be greater at the bottom of the tent, so the tent should be tucked in snugly without open edges. The bottom of the tent should be examined more often

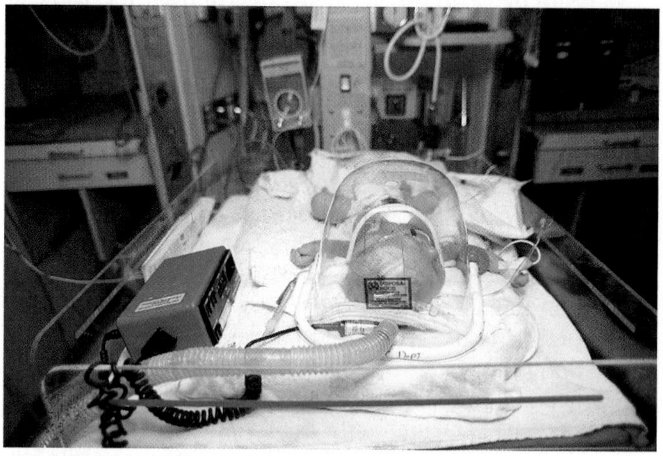

Fig. 45-22 Oxygen administered to infant by means of a plastic hood. Note oxygen analyzer (blue machine).

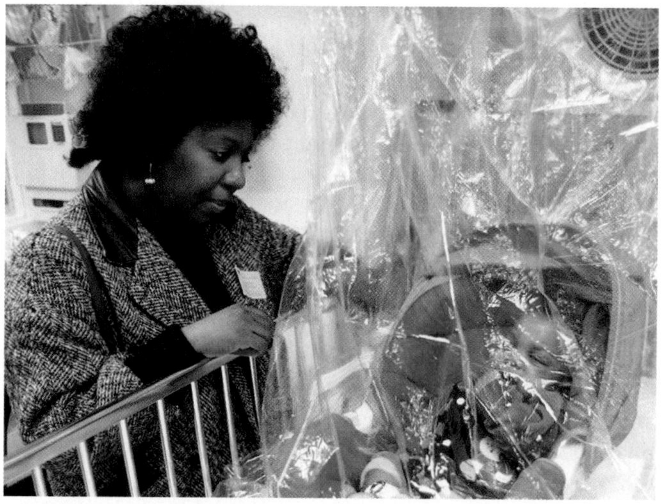

Fig. 45-23 The tent provides a comfortable method for oxygen administration. *(From Hockenberry, M. J. & Wilson, D. [2007]. Wong's nursing care of infants and children [8th ed., p. 1288]. St. Louis, MO: Mosby [Fig. 31-12].)*

when the child is restless and fussy and liable to pull the covers loose. Some tents are even open at the top. Because of the rapidly diffusing qualities of carbon dioxide, the levels of the gas do not build up within these enclosures.

After the tent has been opened for an extended period, it is flushed with oxygen by increasing the flow meter for a few minutes to quickly raise the oxygen and mist concentration. The flow meter is then reset to the prescribed number of litres per minute.

The enclosed tent can become warm; thus some type of cooling mechanism should be provided. The temperature inside the tent must be checked periodically to ensure that it is maintained at the desired level. Although the cool environment can reduce fever and airway inflammation, it can also produce hypothermia and cold stress. It is important to make certain that the child is kept warm and dry. Because oxygen is drying to the tissues, the gas is humidified, which causes moisture to condense on the tent walls.

In some instances the child can be removed from the oxygen tent for activities such as feeding and bathing, whereas in other cases the child is placed in the tent only during periods of rest. Still other children may require oxygen continuously and can be removed from the tent or incubator only if an oxygen source is held close to the child's face. Any change in colour, increased respiratory effort, or restlessness is an indication to return the child to the oxygen tent.

Oxygen Toxicity

Prolonged exposure to high oxygen tensions can damage some body tissues and functions. The organs most vulnerable to the adverse effects of excessive oxygenation are the retina of the extremely preterm infant and the lungs of persons at any age.

Oxygen-induced carbon dioxide narcosis is a physiological hazard of oxygen therapy that may occur in persons with chronic pulmonary disease, such as cystic fibrosis. In these patients the respiratory centre has adapted to the continuously higher arterial carbon dioxide tension ($Paco_2$) levels, and hypoxia becomes the more powerful stimulus for respiration. When the arterial oxygen tension (Pao_2) level is elevated during oxygen administration, the hypoxic drive is removed, causing progressive hypoventilation and increased $Paco_2$ levels, and the child rapidly becomes unconscious. Carbon dioxide narcosis can also be induced by the administration of sedation in these patients.

Monitoring Oxygen Therapy

Pulse oximetry is a continuous, noninvasive method of determining oxygen saturation (Sao_2) to guide oxygen therapy. A sensor composed of a light-emitting diode (LED) and a photodetector is placed in opposition around a foot, hand, finger, toe, or earlobe, with the LED placed on top of the nail when digits are used (Fig. 45-24). The diode emits red and infrared lights that pass through the skin to the photodetector. The photodetector measures the amount of each type of light absorbed by functional hemoglobins. Hemoglobin saturated with oxygen (oxyhemoglobin) absorbs more infrared light than does hemoglobin not saturated with oxygen (deoxyhemoglobin). Pulsatile blood flow is the primary physiological factor that influences accuracy of the pulse oximeter. In

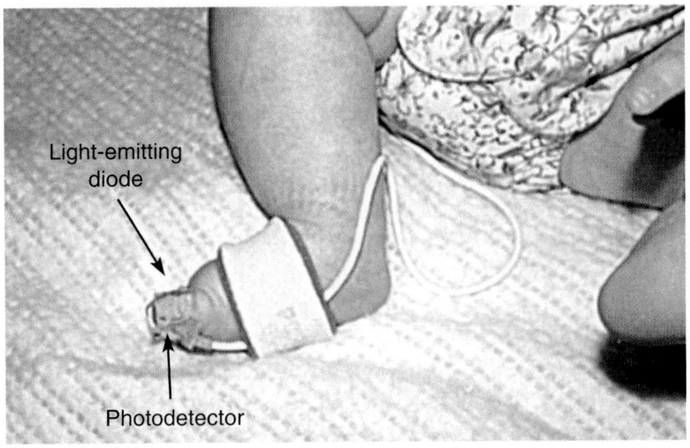

Fig. 45-24 Pulse oximeter sensor. Note that the sensor is positioned with light-emitting diode (LED) opposite the photodetector.

infants, reposition the probe at least every 3 to 4 hours to prevent pressure necrosis; poor perfusion and very sensitive skin may necessitate more frequent repositioning.

Another noninvasive method is *transcutaneous monitoring (TCM)*, which provides continuous monitoring of transcutaneous partial pressure of oxygen in arterial blood ($tcPao_2$) and, with some devices, of carbon dioxide in arterial blood ($tcPaco_2$). An electrode is attached to the warmed skin to facilitate arterialization of cutaneous capillaries. The site of the electrode must be changed every 3 to 4 hours to avoid burning the skin, and the machine must be calibrated with every site change. TCM is used frequently in neonatal intensive care units, but it may not reflect Pao_2 in infants with impaired local circulation or in older infants whose skin is thicker.

Oximetry is insensitive to hyperoxia because hemoglobin approaches 100% saturation for all Pao_2 readings greater than approximately 100 mm Hg, which is a dangerous situation for the preterm infant at risk for developing retinopathy of prematurity (see Chapter 27). Therefore, the preterm infant being monitored with oximetry should have upper limits identified, such as 90 to 95%, and a protocol established for decreasing oxygen when saturations are high.

NURSING ALERT It is important to make certain that sensor connectors and oximeters are compatible. Wiring that is incompatible can generate considerable heat at the tip of the sensor, causing second- and third-degree burns under the sensors. Pressure necrosis can also occur from sensors attached too tightly. Inspect the skin under the sensor frequently.

Correct application of the sensor is essential for accurate Sao_2 measurements. Because the sensor must identify every pulse beat to calculate the Sao_2, movement can interfere with sensing. Some devices synchronize the Sao_2 reading with the heartbeat, thereby reducing the interference caused by motion. Sensors are not placed on extremities used for blood pressure monitoring or with indwelling arterial catheters, since pulsatile blood flow may be affected.

evolve Skill—Measuring Oxygen Saturation

Infant—Secure the sensor to the great toe and tape the wire to the sole of the foot (or use a commercial holder that fastens with a self-adhering closure). Place a snugly fitting sock over the foot, but check the site frequently for colour, temperature, and pulse.

Child—Secure the sensor securely to the index finger and tape the wire to the back of the hand.

Ambient light from ceiling lights and phototherapy, as well as high-intensity heat and light from radiant warmers, can interfere with readings. Thus, the sensor should be covered to block these light sources. IV dyes; green, purple, or black nail polish; nonopaque synthetic nails; and possibly ink used for foot printing can also cause inaccurate Sao_2 measurements. The dyes should be removed or, in the case of porcelain nails, a different area used for the sensor. Skin colour, thickness, and edema do not affect the readings.

Aerosol Therapy

Aerosol therapy can be effective in depositing medication directly into the airway. The value of aerosolized water, or "mist therapy," is controversial in terms of children being able to cooperate enough to correctly inhale all of the medication. This route of administration can be useful in avoiding the systemic adverse effects of certain medications and in reducing the amount of drug necessary to achieve the desired effect. Bronchodilators, steroids, and antibiotics, suspended in particulate form, can be inhaled so that the medication reaches the small airways. Aerosol therapy is particularly challenging in children who are too young to be able to control the rate and depth of breathing. Administration of this therapy requires skill, patience, and creativity.

Medications can be aerosolized or nebulized with air or with oxygen-enriched gas. Handheld nebulizers are the most frequently used equipment. The medicated mist is discharged into a small plastic mask, which the child holds over the nose and mouth. To avoid particle deposition in the nose and pharynx, the child is instructed to take slow, deep breaths through an open mouth during the treatment. For home use an air compressor is necessary to force air through the liquid medication to form the aerosol. Compact, portable units can be obtained from health equipment companies. The **metred-dose inhaler** (MDI) is a self-contained, handheld device that allows for intermittent delivery of a specified amount of medication. Many bronchodilators are available in this form and are successfully used by children with asthma. For children under the age of 5 or 6 years, a spacer device attached to the MDI can help with coordination of breathing and aerosol delivery. It allows the aerosolized particles to remain in suspension longer. (See also Asthma, Chapter 46.)

Assessment of breath sounds and the work of breathing should be done before and after treatments. Young children who become upset by having a mask held close to the face may become fatigued with fighting the procedure and may actually appear worse during and immediately after the therapy. It may be necessary to spend a few minutes calming the child after the procedure and allowing the vital signs to return to baseline to accurately assess changes in breath sounds and the work of breathing.

Bronchial (Postural) Drainage

Bronchial drainage is indicated whenever excessive fluid or mucus in the bronchi is not being removed by normal ciliary activity and cough. Positioning the child to take maximum advantage of gravity facilitates removal of secretions. Postural drainage can be effective in children with chronic lung disease characterized by thick mucus, such as cystic fibrosis.

Postural drainage is carried out three or four times daily and is more effective when it follows other respiratory therapy, such as bronchodilator or nebulization medication. Bronchial drainage is generally performed before meals (or 1 to 1½ hours after meals) to minimize the chance of vomiting and is repeated at bedtime. The duration of treatment depends on the child's condition and tolerance; it usually lasts 20 to 30 minutes. Several positions facilitate drainage from all major lung segments; all positions are not employed at each session. Children will usually cooperate for four to six positions. Older children can tolerate longer periods.

In the hospital an older child can be positioned over an elevated knee rest. Small children and infants can be positioned with pillows or on the therapist's lap and legs. Infants should not be placed in the Trendelenburg position because they do not have an autonomic regulation of blood flow to the head. Special modifications of the techniques are required in children whose conditions, such as head injuries, some types of surgical incisions or burns, and casts, contraindicate the standard positioning.

Chest physical therapy (CPT) usually refers to the use of postural drainage in combination with adjunctive techniques that are thought to enhance the clearance of mucus from the airway. These techniques include manual percussion, vibration, and squeezing of the chest; cough; forceful expiration; and breathing exercises. Special mechanical devices (e.g., ThAIRapy Vest) are also used to perform CPT. Postural drainage in combination with forced expiration has been shown to be beneficial. Noninvasive inspiratory nasal pressure–support ventilation during CPT has demonstrated a significant improvement in respiratory muscle performance and a reduction in oxygen desaturation (Fauroux et al., 1999).

The most common technique used in association with postural drainage is manual percussion of the chest wall. The patient is dressed in a lightweight shirt and placed in a postural drainage position. CPT is contraindicated when patients have pulmonary hemorrhage, pulmonary embolism, end-stage renal disease, increased intracranial pressure, osteogenesis imperfecta, or minimal cardiac reserves.

Artificial Ventilation

Artificial Airways

An artificial airway is usually used in association with mechanical ventilation and in children with upper airway obstruction. Endotracheal intubation can be accomplished via the nasal (nasotracheal), oral (orotracheal), or direct tracheal (tracheostomy) routes. Although it is more difficult to place, nasotracheal intubation is preferred to orotracheal intubation because it facilitates oral hygiene and provides more stable fixation, which reduces the complication of tracheal erosion and the danger of accidental extubation. Only uncuffed endotracheal tubes should be used in children younger than 8 years of age (Curley & Moloney-Harmon, 2001). Air or gas delivered directly to the trachea must be humidified.

Tracheostomy

A *tracheostomy* is a surgical opening in the trachea; the procedure may be done on an emergency basis or may be an elective one, and it may be combined with mechanical ventilation. Pediatric tracheostomy tubes are usually made of plastic or Silastic (Fig. 45-25). The most common types are the Hollinger, Jackson, Aberdeen, and Shiley tubes. These tubes are constructed with a more acute angle than that of adult tubes, and they soften at body temperature, conforming to the contours of the trachea. Because these materials resist the formation of crusted respiratory secretions, they are made without an inner cannula.

Children who have undergone a tracheostomy must be closely monitored for complications such as hemorrhage, edema, aspiration, accidental decannulation, tube obstruction, and the entrance of free air into the pleural cavity. Nursing care focuses on maintaining a patent airway, facilitating the removal of pulmonary secretions, providing humidified air or oxygen, cleansing the stoma, monitoring the child's ability to swallow, and teaching while simultaneously preventing complications.

Because the child may be unable to signal for help, direct observation and use of respiratory and cardiac monitors are essential. Respiratory assessments include breath sounds and the work of breathing, vital signs, tightness of the tracheostomy ties, and the type and amount of secretions. Large amounts of bloody secretions are uncommon and should be considered a sign of hemorrhage. The practitioner should be notified immediately if this occurs.

The child is positioned with the head of the bed raised or in the position most comfortable to the child, with the call light easily available. Suction catheters, suction source, gloves, sterile saline, sterile gauze for wiping away secretions, scissors, an extra tracheostomy tube of the same size with ties already attached, another tracheostomy tube one size smaller, and the obturator are kept at the bedside. A source of humidification is provided because the normal humidification and filtering functions of the airway have been bypassed. IV fluids ensure adequate hydration until the child is able to swallow sufficient amounts of fluids.

Suctioning

The airway must remain patent and requires frequent suctioning during the first few hours after a tracheostomy to remove mucous plugs and excessive secretions. Proper vacuum pressure and suction catheter size are important to prevent atelectasis and decrease hypoxia from the suctioning procedure. Vacuum pressure should range from 60 to 100 mm Hg for infants and children and from 40 to 60 mm Hg for preterm infants. Unless secretions are thick and tenacious, the lower range of negative pressure is recommended. Tracheal suction catheters are available in a variety of sizes. The catheter selected should have a diameter one-half the diameter of the tracheostomy tube. If the catheter is too large, it can block the airway. The catheter is constructed with a side port so that the catheter is introduced without suction and removed while simultaneous intermittent suction is applied by covering the port with the thumb (Fig. 45-26). The catheter is inserted to 0.5 cm beyond or just to the end of the tracheostomy tube. The practice of instilling sterile saline in the tracheostomy tube before suctioning is not supported by research and is no longer recommended (see Evidence-Informed Practice box).

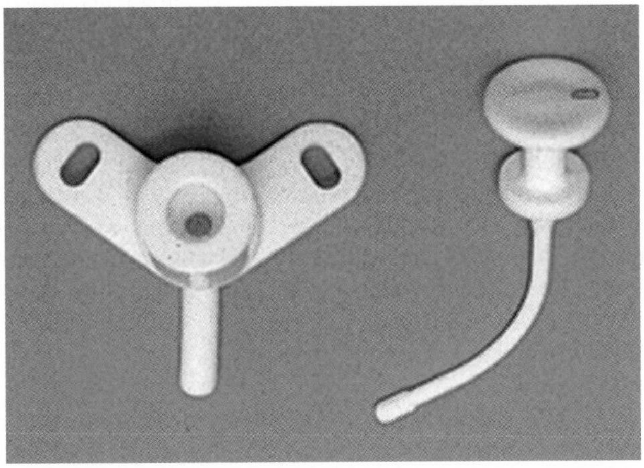

Fig. 45-25 Silastic pediatric tracheostomy tube and obturator.

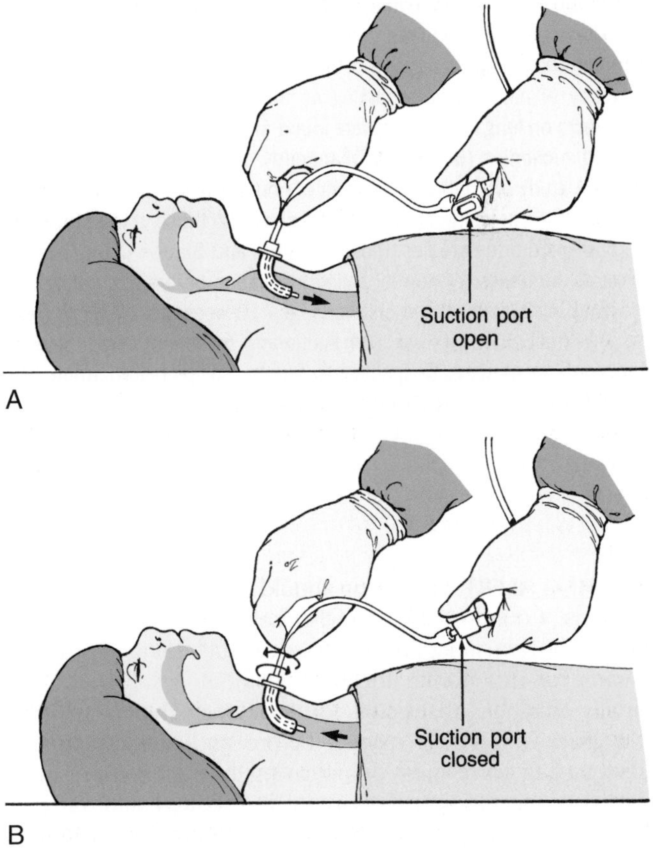

Fig. 45-26 Tracheostomy suctioning. **A:** Insertion, port open. **B:** Withdrawal, port occluded. Note that the catheter is inserted just slightly beyond the end of the tracheostomy tube.

EVIDENCE-INFORMED PRACTICE Normal Saline Instillation Before Suctioning—Helpful or Harmful?

—Marilyn J. Hockenberry

Ask the Question

In intubated children and those with tracheostomy, is normal saline instillation before suctioning helpful or harmful?

Search for Evidence

Search Strategies

English-language publications and research-based articles on suctioning intubated children and those with a tracheostomy

Databases Searched

PubMed, Cochrane Collaboration, MD Consult, BestBETs, PedsCCM

Critically Analyze the Evidence

While instillation of normal saline before endotracheal (ET) tube suctioning has been used for years as a method to loosen and dilute secretions, lubricate the suction catheter, and promote cough, there may be possible adverse effects of this procedure. Adult studies have found decreased oxygen saturation, increased frequency of nosocomial pneumonia, and increased intracranial pressure after instillation of normal saline before suctioning (Ackerman, 1993; Ackerman & Gugerty, 1990; Bostick & Wendelgass, 1987; Hagler & Traver, 1994; Kinlock, 1999; O'Neal et al., 2001; Reynolds et al., 1990).

Two of the first research studies evaluating the effect of normal saline instillation before suctioning in neonates found no deleterious effects. Shorten, Byrne, and Jones (1991) found no significant differences in oxygenation, heart rate, or blood pressure before or after suctioning in a group of 27 intubated neonates. In a second study of nine neonates acting as their own controls, no adverse effects on lung mechanics were found after normal saline instillation and suctioning (Beeram & Dhanireddy, 1992).

A study evaluating the effects of normal saline instillation before suctioning in children found results similar to those in the previously published adult studies. Ridling, Martin, and Bratton (2003) evaluated the effects of normal saline instillation before suctioning in a group of 24 critically ill children, ages 10 weeks to 14 years (level 1 evidence). A total of 104 suctioning episodes were analyzed. Children experienced significantly greater oxygen desaturation after suctioning if normal saline was instilled.

The American Thoracic Society's (2000) official position statement on the care of children with tracheostomies now states that normal saline should not be instilled before suctioning.

Apply the Evidence: Nursing Implications

Studies support that the adverse effects of normal saline instillation before suctioning in children are similar to those found for adults. This technique causes a significant reduction in oxygen saturation that can last up to 2 minutes after suctioning. The evidence does not support the use of normal saline instillation before ET suctioning in children.

References

Ackerman, M. H. (1993). The effect of saline lavage prior to suctioning. *American Journal of Critical Care, 2*(4), 326–330.

Ackerman, M. H., & Gugerty, B. (1990). The effect of normal saline bolus instillation in artificial airways. *Journal: Society of Otorhinolaryngology Head-Neck Nurses, 8*(2), 14–17.

American Thoracic Society. (2000). Care of the child with a chronic tracheostomy. *American Journal of Respiratory Critical Care Medicine, 161*, 297–308. Retrieved from http://www.thoracic.org/statements/resources/respiratory-disease-pediatric/childtrach1-12.pdf.

Beeram, M. R., & Dhanireddy, R. (1992). Effects of saline instillation during tracheal suction on lung mechanics in newborn infants. *Journal of Perinatology, 12*(2), 120–123.

Bostick, J., & Wendelgass, S. T. (1987). Normal saline instillation as part of the suctioning procedure: Effects of PaO_2 and amount of secretions. *Heart & Lung, 16*(5), 532–537.

Hagler, D. A., & Traver, G. A. (1994). Endotracheal saline and suction catheters: Sources of lower airway contamination. *American Journal of Critical Care, 3*(6), 444–447.

Kinlock, D. (1999). Instillation of normal saline during endotracheal suctioning: Effects on mixed venous oxygen saturation. *American Journal of Critical Care, 8*(4), 231–240.

O'Neal, P. V., et al. (2001). Level of dyspnoea experienced in mechanically ventilated adults with and without saline instillation prior to endotracheal suctioning. *Intensive & Critical Care Nursing, 17*(6), 356–363.

Reynolds, P., et al. (1990). Effects of normal saline instillation on secretion volume, dynamic compliance, and oxygen saturation (abstract). *American Review of Respiratory Disease, 141*, A574.

Ridling, D. A., Martin, L. D., & Bratton, S. L. (2003). Endotracheal suctioning with or without instillation of isotonic sodium chloride in critically ill children. *American Journal of Critical Care, 12*(3), 212–219.

Shorten, D. R., Byrne, P. J., & Jones, R. L. (1991). Infant responses to saline instillations and endotracheal suctioning. *Journal of Obstetric, Gynecologic, & Neonatal Nursing, 20*(6), 464–469.

NURSING ALERT Suctioning should require no more than 5 seconds. Counting one one-thousand, two one-thousand, three one-thousand, and so on while suctioning is a simple means for monitoring the time. Without a safeguard, the airway may be obstructed for too long. Hyperventilating the child with 100% oxygen before and after suctioning (using a bag-valve-mask or increasing the fraction of inspired oxygen concentration [FiO_2] ventilator setting) may be performed to prevent hypoxia. Closed tracheal suctioning systems that allow for uninterrupted oxygen delivery may also be used.

In a closed suction system, a suction catheter is directly attached to the ventilator tubing. This system has several advantages. First, there is no need to disconnect the patient from the ventilator, which allows for better oxygenation. Second, the suction catheter is enclosed in a plastic sheath, which reduces the risk of the nurse being exposed to the patient's secretions (Carroll, 1998).

The child should be allowed to rest for 30 to 60 seconds after each aspiration to allow oxygen saturation to return to normal; then the process is repeated until the trachea is clear.

Suctioning should be limited to about three aspirations in one period. Oximetry is used to monitor suctioning and prevent hypoxia.

NURSING ALERT Suctioning is carried out only as often as needed to keep the tube patent. Signs of mucus partially occluding the airway include an increased heart rate, a rise in respiratory effort, a drop in SaO_2, cyanosis, and an increase in the positive inspiratory pressure on the ventilator.

In the acute care setting, aseptic technique is used during care of the tracheostomy. Secondary infection is a major concern, since the air entering the lower airway bypasses the natural defences of the upper airway. Gloves should be worn during the aspiration procedure, although a sterile glove is needed only on the hand touching the catheter. A new tube, gloves, and sterile saline solution should be used each time.

Routine Care

The tracheostomy stoma requires daily care. Assessments of the stoma area include observations for signs of infection and breakdown of the skin. The skin needs to be kept clean and dry, and crusted secretions around the stoma may be gently removed with half-strength hydrogen peroxide. Hydrogen peroxide should not be used with sterling silver tracheostomy tubes because it tends to pit and stain the silver surface. The nurse should be aware of wet tracheostomy dressings, which can predispose the peristomal area to skin breakdown. Several products are available to prevent or treat excoriation. The Allevyn tracheostomy dressing is a hydrophilic sponge with a polyurethane back that is highly absorptive. Other possible barriers to help maintain skin integrity include the use of hydrocolloid wafers (e.g., DuoDERM CGF, Hollister Restore) under the tracheostomy flanges, as well as extra-thin hydrocolloid wafers under the chin.

The tracheostomy tube is held in place with tracheostomy ties made of a durable, nonfraying material. The ties are changed daily and when soiled. New ties are looped through the flanges and tied snugly in a triple knot at the side of the neck before the soiled ties are cut and removed. Some nurses have found that threading the ties through a piece of 6-mm surgical tubing cushions the ties; others have found the tubing irritating to the skin. The ties should be tight enough to allow just a fingertip to be inserted between the ties and the neck (Fig. 45-27). It is easier to ensure a snug fit if the child's head is flexed rather than extended while the ties are being secured. Ties fastened with self-adhering closures are also available. These devices, such as the Dale tracheostomy tube holder, are made of a soft, cushioning, and slightly stretchy material that is very comfortable. They are becoming increasingly popular because of their ease of use and ability to maintain better skin integrity. However, nurses and family members must consider the safety factor and use them only on a child who will not pull and undo the fastener.

Routine tracheostomy tube changes are usually carried out weekly after a tract has been formed to minimize the formation of granulation tissue. The first change is usually performed by the surgeon; subsequent changes are performed by the nurse and, if the child is discharged home with the

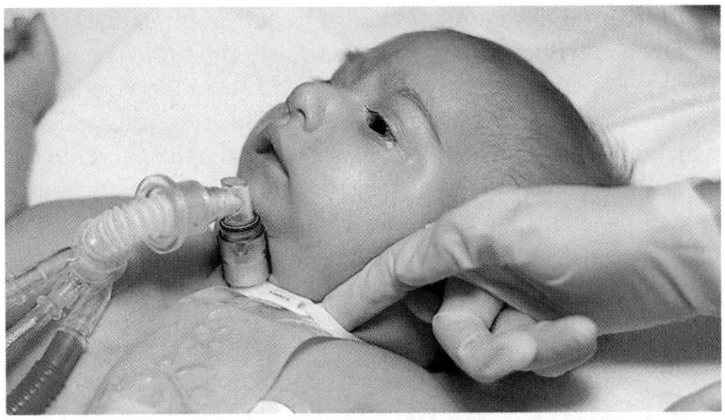

Fig. 45-27 Tracheostomy ties are snug but allow one finger to be inserted.

tracheostomy, by either a parent or a visiting nurse. Ideally, two caregivers participate in the procedure to assist with positioning the child.

Changing the tracheostomy tube is accomplished using sterile technique. Tube changes should occur before meals or 2 hours after the last meal. Continuous feedings should be turned off at least an hour before a tube change. The new, sterile tube is prepared by inserting the obturator and attaching new ties. The child is suctioned before the procedure to minimize secretions, then restrained and positioned with the neck slightly extended. One caregiver cuts the old ties and removes the tube from the stoma. The new tube is inserted gently into the stoma (using a downward and forward motion that follows the curve of the trachea), the obturator is removed, and the ties are secured. The adequacy of ventilation must be assessed after a tube change because the tube can be inserted into the soft tissue surrounding the trachea; breath sounds and respiratory effort should be carefully monitored.

Supplemental oxygen is always delivered with a humidification system to prevent drying of the respiratory mucosa. Humidification of room air for an established tracheostomy can be intermittent if secretions remain thin enough to be coughed or suctioned from the tracheostomy. Direct humidification via a tracheostomy mask can be provided during naps and at night so that the child is able to be up and around unencumbered during much of the day. Room humidifiers are also used successfully.

The inner cannula, if used, should be removed with each suctioning, cleaned with sterile saline and pipe cleaners to remove crusted material, dried thoroughly, and reinserted.

Emergency Care: Tube Occlusion and Accidental Decannulation

Occlusion of the tracheostomy tube is life threatening, and infants and children are at greater risk than adults because of the smaller diameter of the tube. Patency of the tube is maintained with suctioning and routine tube changes to prevent the formation of crusts that can occlude the tube.

NURSING ALERT Life-threatening occlusion is apparent when the child displays signs of respiratory distress and a suction catheter cannot be passed to the end of the tube despite several attempts and instillation of saline. This situation requires an immediate tube change.

Accidental decannulation also requires immediate tube replacement. Some children have a fairly rigid trachea, so the airway remains partially open when the tube is removed. However, others have malformed or flexible tracheal cartilage, which causes the airway to collapse when the tube is removed or dislodged. Because many infants and children with upper airway problems have little airway reserve, if replacement of the dislodged tube is impossible, a smaller-sized tube should be inserted. If the stoma cannot be cannulated with another tracheostomy tube, oral intubation should be performed.

Procedures Related to Alternative Feeding Techniques

Some children are unable to take nourishment by mouth because of anomalies of the throat, esophagus, or bowel; impaired swallowing capacity; severe debilitation; respiratory distress; or unconsciousness. These children are frequently fed by way of a tube inserted orally or nasally into the stomach (*orogastric* or *nasogastric gavage*) or duodenum-jejunum (**enteral** *gavage*), or by a tube inserted directly into the stomach (*gastrostomy*) or jejunum (*jejunostomy*). Such feedings may be intermittent or by continuous drip.

Feeding resistance is a problem that may result from any long-term feeding method that bypasses the mouth. During gavage or gastrostomy feedings, infants are given a pacifier. Non-nutritive sucking has several advantages, such as increased weight gain and decreased crying. However, to prevent the possibility of aspiration, only pacifiers with a safe design may be used (see Fig. 25-19). Using improvised pacifiers made from bottle nipples is not a safe practice.

NURSING ALERT When a child is concurrently receiving continuous-drip gastric or enteral feedings and parenteral (IV) therapy, the potential exists for inadvertent administration of the enteral formula through the circulatory system, especially when the parenteral solution is a fat emulsion, which looks milky. Safeguards to prevent this potentially serious error include the following:

- Use a separate, specifically designed enteral feeding pump mounted on a separate pole for continuous-feeding solutions.
- Label all tubing for continuous enteral feeding with brightly coloured tape or labels.
- Use specifically designed continuous-feeding bags to contain the solutions instead of parenteral equipment, such as a burette.

Gavage Feeding

Infants and children can be fed simply and safely by means of a tube passed into the stomach through either the nares or the mouth. The tube can be left in place or inserted and removed with each feeding. In older children it is usually less traumatic to tape the tube securely in place between feedings. When this alternative is used, the tube should be removed and replaced with a new tube according to hospital policy, specific orders, and the type of tube used. Meticulous hand washing should be practised during the procedure to prevent bacterial contamination of the feeding, especially during continuous-drip feedings (see Atraumatic Care box).

Not all feeding tubes are the same. Polyethylene and polyvinylchloride types lose their flexibility and need to be replaced frequently, usually every 3 or 4 days. The polyurethane and silicone tubes are indwelling and remain flexible, so they can remain in place longer and afford more patient comfort. Use of these small-bore tubes for continuous feeding has reduced the incidence of complications such as pharyngitis, otitis media, and incompetence of the lower esophageal sphincter. Although the increased softness and flexibility of the tubes are advantages, they also have disadvantages such as difficult insertion (may require a stylet or metal guidewire), collapse of the tube during aspiration of gastric contents to test for correct placement, dislodgment during forceful coughing, and unsuitability for thick feedings. Traditional methods for verifying placement are less reliable with the small-bore tubes.

Infants will be easier to control if they are first wrapped in a mummy restraint (see Fig. 45-7). Even tiny infants with random movements can grasp and dislodge the tube. Preterm infants do not ordinarily require restraint, but if they do, a small blanket folded across the chest and secured beneath the shoulders is usually sufficient. Care must be taken so that breathing is not compromised.

Whenever possible, the infant should be held and provided a means of non-nutritive sucking during the procedure to associate the comfort of physical contact with the feeding. When this is not possible, gavage feeding is carried out with the infant or child on the back or toward the right side with the head and chest elevated. Feeding the child in a sitting position helps maintain the placement of the tube in the lowest position, thus increasing the likelihood of correct placement in the stomach (see Guidelines box, Fig. 27-4, and Box 27-4).

ATRAUMATIC CARE

Reducing the Distress of Nasogastric Tube Insertion

Numerous strategies can be used to decrease discomfort during nasogastric (NG) tube insertion. Most important, the nurse performing the procedure should be competent in NG tube placement. The nurse should discuss the procedure with the child in a developmentally appropriate way and give family members the details of what to expect during the procedure. Administration of sedation and analgesia should be considered before NG insertion. The use of topical lidocaine and phenylephrine for the nose and tetracaine and benzocaine spray for the throat before NG insertion has been found to reduce pain and discomfort in a group of adult patients (Singer & Konia, 1999). A smaller-caliber, soft, flexible tube should be used. To prevent the trauma of reinsertion, make certain the NG tube is well secured after placement.

(Data from Maglinte, C. [1999]. Strategies for reducing the pain and discomfort of nasogastric intubation. *Academic Emergency Medicine, 6*[3], 166–168.)

GUIDELINES Nasogastric Tube Feedings in Children

Place child supine with head slightly hyperflexed or in a sniffing position (nose pointed toward ceiling).

Measure tube for approximate length of insertion, and mark the point with a small piece of tape.

Insert a tube that has been lubricated with sterile water or water-soluble lubricant through either the mouth or one of the nares to the predetermined mark. Because most young infants are obligatory nose breathers, insertion through the mouth causes less distress and helps to stimulate sucking. In older infants and children, the tube is passed through the nose and alternated between nostrils. An indwelling tube is almost always placed through the nose.

- When using the nose, slip the tube along the base of the nose and direct it straight back toward the occiput.
- When entering through the mouth, direct the tube toward the back of the throat (see Fig. 45-28, B).
- If the child is able to swallow on command, synchronize passing the tube with swallowing.
- Confirm placement by x-ray examination, if available. Document pH and colour of aspirate (see Evidence-Informed Practice box, p. 1311).

Stabilize tube by holding or taping it to the cheek, not to the forehead, because of possible damage to the nostril. To maintain correct placement, measure and record the amount of tubing extending from the nose or mouth to the distal port when the tube is first positioned. Recheck this measurement before each feeding.

Warm formula to room temperature. Do not microwave! Document pH and colour of aspirate before each feeding to confirm tube placement. Pour formula into the barrel of the syringe attached to the feeding tube. To start the flow, give a gentle push with the plunger, but then remove the plunger and allow the fluid to flow into the stomach by gravity. The rate of flow should not exceed 5 mL every 5 to 10 minutes in preterm and very small infants and 10 mL/min in older infants and children to prevent nausea and regurgitation. The rate is determined by the diameter of the tubing and height of the reservoir containing the feeding and is regulated by adjusting the height of the syringe. A usual feeding may take 15 to 30 minutes to complete.

Flush tube with sterile water (1 or 2 mL for small tubes to 5 to 15 mL or more for large ones), or see discussion of flushing for administering medication through nasogastric tubes in the Guidelines box (p. 1296), to clear it of formula.

Cap or clamp indwelling tubes to prevent loss of feeding. If the tube is to be removed, first pinch it firmly to prevent escape of fluid as the tube is withdrawn. Withdraw the tube quickly.

Position child with the head elevated about 30 degrees and on the right side or abdomen for at least 1 hour in the same manner as after any infant feeding to minimize the possibility of regurgitation and aspiration. If the child's condition permits, burp the youngster after the feeding.

Record the feeding, including the type and amount of residual, the type and amount of formula, and how it was tolerated.

For most infant feedings, any amount of residual fluid aspirated from the stomach is refed to prevent electrolyte imbalance, and the amount is subtracted from the prescribed amount of feeding. For example, if the infant is to receive 30 mL and 10 mL is aspirated from the stomach before the feeding, the 10 mL of aspirated stomach contents is refed along with 20 mL of feeding. Another method can be used in children. If residual fluid is more than one fourth of the last feeding, return the aspirate and recheck in 30 to 60 minutes. When residual fluid is less than one fourth of the last feeding, give the scheduled feeding. If large amounts of aspirated fluid persist and the child is due for another feeding, notify the practitioner.

Two standard methods of measuring tube length for insertion are (1) measuring from the nose to the bottom of the earlobe and then to the end of the xiphoid process or (2) measuring from the nose to the earlobe and then to a point midway between the xiphoid process and the umbilicus (Fig. 45-28, A). For very-low-birth-weight infants, weight can be used to predict insertion length. See Evidence-Informed Practice box on p. 1311 for placement verification techniques.

Gastrostomy Feeding

Feeding by way of a gastrostomy tube is a variation of tube feeding that is often used for children in whom passage of a tube through the mouth, pharynx, esophagus, and cardiac sphincter of the stomach is contraindicated or impossible. It is also used to avoid the constant irritation of a gastric tube in children who require tube feeding over an extended period. Placement of a gastrostomy tube may be performed with the patient under **general anaesthesia** or percutaneously using an endoscope with the patient sedated and under local anaesthesia (percutaneous endoscopic gastrostomy [PEG]). The tube is inserted through the abdominal wall into the stomach about midway along the greater curvature and, when surgically placed, is secured by a purse-string suture. The stomach is anchored to the peritoneum at the operative site. The tube used can be a Foley, wing-tip, or mushroom catheter. Immediately after surgery the catheter is left open and attached to gravity drainage for 24 hours or more.

Postoperative care of the wound site is directed toward prevention of infection and irritation. The area is cleansed at least daily or as often as needed to keep the area free of drainage. After healing takes place, meticulous care is needed to keep the area surrounding the tube clean and dry to prevent excoriation and infection. Daily applications of antibiotic ointment or other preparations may be prescribed to aid in healing and prevent irritation. It is important to prevent excessive pull on the catheter that might cause widening of the opening and subsequent leakage of highly irritating gastric juices. The tube is securely taped to the abdomen, leaving a small loop of tubing at the exit site to prevent tension on the site.

Granulation tissue may grow around a gastrostomy site (Fig. 45-29). This moist, beefy red tissue is not a sign of infection. However, if it continues to grow, the excess moisture can irritate the surrounding skin.

For children receiving long-term gastrostomy feeding, a skin-level device (e.g., MIC-KEY, Bard Button) offers several advantages. The small, flexible silicone device protrudes slightly from the abdomen, is more cosmetically pleasing in appearance, affords increased comfort and mobility to the child, is easy to care for, and is fully immersible in water. The one-way valve at the proximal end minimizes reflux and eliminates the need for clamping. However, the button requires a well-established gastrostomy site and is more expensive than the conventional tube. In addition, the valve may become clogged. When functioning, the valve prevents air from escaping; thus the child may require frequent burping. With some devices, during feedings the child must remain fairly still because the tubing easily disconnects from the opening if the child moves. With other devices, extension tubing can be securely attached to the opening (Fig. 45-30). The feeding is instilled at the other end of the tubing in a manner similar to that for a regular gastrostomy. The extension tubing may also have a separate medication port. Both the feeding and the medication ports have plugs attached. Some skin-level devices require a special tube to decompress the stomach (to check residual or release air).

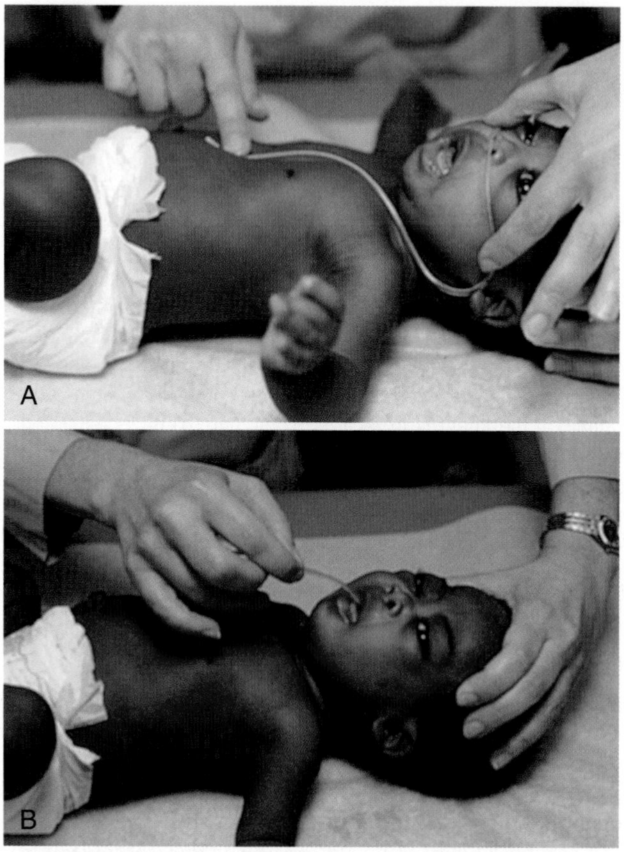

Fig. 45-28 Gavage feeding. **A:** Measuring tube for orogastric feeding from tip of nose to earlobe and to midpoint between end of xiphoid process and umbilicus. **B:** Inserting tube.

Feeding of water, formula, or pureed foods is carried out in the same manner and rate as in gavage feeding. A mechanical pump may be used to regulate the volume and rate of feeding. After feedings, the infant or child is positioned on the right side or in Fowler's position, and the tube may be clamped or left open and suspended between feedings, depending on the child's condition. A clamped tube allows more mobility but is appropriate only if the child can tolerate intermittent feedings without vomiting or prolonged backup of feeding into the tube. Sometimes a Y tube is used to allow for simultaneous decompression during feeding. If a Foley catheter is used as the gastrostomy tube, very slight tension is applied. The tube is securely taped to maintain the balloon at the gastrostomy opening to prevent leakage of gastric contents and to prevent the tube's progression toward the pyloric sphincter, where it may occlude the stomach outlet. As a precaution, the length of the tube should be measured postoperatively and then remeasured each shift to be certain it has not slipped. A mark can be made above the skin level to further ensure its placement. When the gastrostomy tube is no longer needed, it is removed; the skin opening usually closes spontaneously by contracture.

Nasoduodenal and Nasojejunal Tubes

Children at high risk for regurgitation or aspiration, such as those with gastroparesis, mechanical ventilation, or brain injuries, may require placement of a postpyloric feeding tube. Insertion of a nasoduodenal or nasojejunal tube is done by a

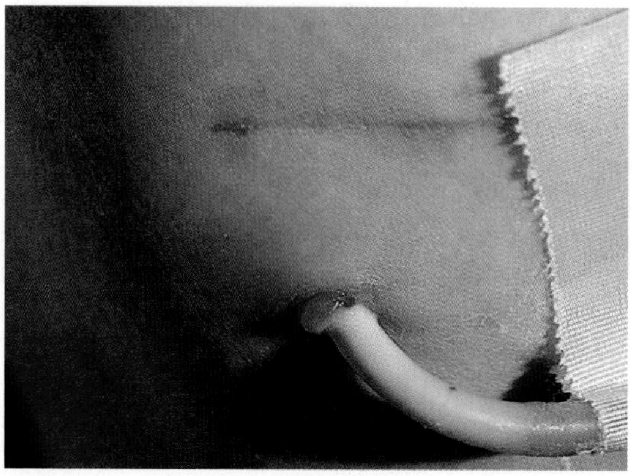

Fig. 45-29 Appearance of healthy granulation tissue around stoma.

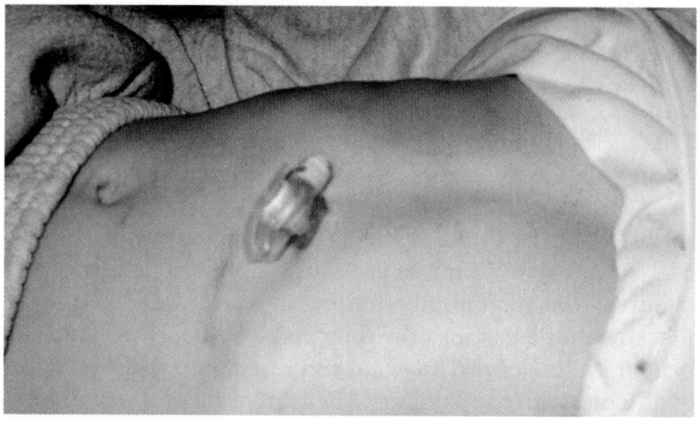

Fig. 45-30 Child with skin-level gastrostomy device (MIC-KEY), which provides for secure attachment of extension tubing to gastrostomy opening.

EVIDENCE-INFORMED PRACTICE Assessing Correct Placement of Nasogastric or Orogastric Tubes in Children

—*Marilyn J. Hockenberry*

Ask the Question

In children, how do we assess for correct placement of nasogastric or orogastric tubes?

Search for Evidence

Search Strategies

English-language publications, research-based articles (level 3 or lower), children or adult populations, comparisons to gold standard (x-ray examination)

Databases Searched

PubMed, Cochrane Collaboration, MD Consult, Joanna Briggs Institute, National Guideline Clearinghouse (AHQR), TRIP Database Plus, PedsCCM, BestBETs

Critically Analyze the Evidence

Studies compared various methods used to evaluate placement of the tube with the gold standard, x-ray examination. Nine articles were found, with five adult and four child sample populations:

- pH-assisted feeding tubes, child (Krafte-Jacobs et al., 1996)
- Bilirubin, adult and child (Metheny et al., 1999; Metheny, Smith, & Stewart, 2000; Westhus, 2004)
- Enzyme tests, child and adult (Metheny et al., 1997; Westhus, 2004)
- Bedside sonography for tube placement, adult (Hernandez-Socorro et al., 1996)
- Aspiration of insufflated air for tube placement, adult (Harrison et al., 1997; Neumann et al., 1995)

The most reliable tests for determining tube placement in the nine published studies (other than the gold standard of x-ray examination) were the combination of:

- pH testing (Gharpure et al., 2000; Huffman et al., 2004; Metheny et al., 2006; Westhus, 2004)
- Visual inspection of aspirate
- Bilirubin and enzyme tests

Bilirubin and enzyme measures are not currently available at the bedside.

Sensitivity and specificity of the bedside tests for children need further evaluation.

Auscultation is an unreliable method to confirm tube placement because of the similarity of sounds produced by air in the bronchus, esophagus, or pleural space.

Apply the Evidence: Nursing Implications

Use x-ray to confirm initial placement. Document pH and colour of aspirate with initial placement.

A pH of 5 or less supports the conclusion that the tip of the tube is in a gastric location.

A pH greater than 5 does not reliably predict the correct distal tip location. It may indicate respiratory or esophageal placement, or the presence of medications to suppress acid secretion.

If pH is greater than 5, use other measures to evaluate tube placement. If bilirubin and enzyme testing is not available, check colour of aspirate. Gastric contents are clear, off-white, or tan; they may be brown tinged if blood is present. Respiratory secretions may look the same. Intestinal contents are often bile stained, light to dark yellow, or greenish brown. It may also be necessary to obtain an x-ray.

A change in pH may indicate tube dislodgment. Check external markings and tube length to ensure that the tube has not moved. If uncertain about placement, obtain an x-ray.

pH and colour of aspirate can be checked before medication or feeding. For continuous feedings, it is recommended that tube placement be checked every 4 hours.

A Visual Bilirubin Scale is effective in determining bilirubin content in feeding tube aspirates (Metheny et al., 2000). Evaluation of the accuracy of the scale is needed with children.

Risk factors for improper tube placement are comatose or semicomatose state, swallowing problems, and recurrent retching or vomiting.

Experience of the individual inserting the tube is always important.

References

Gharpure, V., et al. (2000). Indicators of postpyloric feeding tube placement in children. *Critical Care Medicine, 28*(8), 2962–2966.

Harrison, A. M., et al. (1997). Nonradiographic assessment of enteral feeding tube position. *Critical Care Medicine, 25*(12), 2055–2059.

Hernandez-Socorro, C. R., et al. (1996). Bedside sonographic-guided versus blind nasoenteric feeding tube placement in critically ill patients. *Critical Care Medicine, 24*(10), 1690–1694.

Huffman, S., et al. (2004). Methods to confirm feeding tube placement: Application of research in practice. *Pediatric Nursing, 30*(1), 10–13.

Krafte-Jacobs, B., et al. (1996). Rapid placement of transpyloric feeding tubes: A comparison of pH-assisted and standard insertion techniques in children. *Pediatrics, 98*(2 Pt 1), 242–248.

Metheny, N. A., et al. (1997). pH and concentrations of pepsin and trypsin in feeding tube aspirates as predictors of tube placement. *Journal of Parenteral & Enteral Nutrition, 21*, 279–285.

Metheny, N. A., et al. (1999). pH and concentration of bilirubin in feeding tube aspirates as predictors of tube placement. *Nursing Research, 48*(4), 189–197.

Metheny, N. A., et al. (2006). Tracheobronchial aspiration of gastric contents in critically ill tube-fed patients: Frequency, outcomes, and risk factors. *Critical Care Medicine, 34*(4), 1007–1015.

Metheny, N. A., Smith, L., & Stewart, B. J. (2000). Development of a reliable and valid bedside test for bilirubin and its utility for improving prediction of feeding tube location. *Nursing Research, 49*(6), 302–309.

Neumann, M. J., et al. (1995). Hold that x-ray: Aspirate pH and auscultation prove tube placement. *Journal of Clinical Gastroenterology, 20*(4), 293–295.

Westhus, N. (2004). Methods to test feeding tube placement in children. *MCN: American Journal of Maternal/Child Nursing, 29*(5), 282–291.

trained practitioner because of the risk of misplacement and potential for perforation in tubes requiring a stylet. Accurate placement is verified by radiography. Small-bore tubes may easily clog. The tube needs to be flushed when feeding is interrupted, before and after medication administration, and routinely every 4 hours or as directed by institutional policy. Tube replacement should be considered monthly to ensure optimal tube patency. Continuous feedings are delivered by mechanical pump to regulate volume and rate. Bolus feeds are contraindicated. Tube displacement is suspected in the child showing signs of feeding intolerance such as vomiting. Feedings should be stopped and the practitioner notified.

Total Parenteral Nutrition

TPN provides for the total nutritional needs of infants or children when feeding by the gastrointestinal tract is impossible, inadequate, or hazardous. Some common conditions associated with TPN include chronic intestinal obstruction, inadequate intestinal length, and prophylactically after surgery or during critical illness.

TPN therapy involves IV infusion of highly concentrated solutions of carbohydrates, lipids, amino acids, vitamins, minerals, water, trace elements, and other additives in a single container (Teitelbaum et al., 2005). The highly concentrated solutions require infusion into a vessel with sufficient volume and turbulence to allow for rapid dilution. The wide-diameter vessels selected are the superior vena cava and innominate or intrathoracic subclavian veins approached by way of the external or internal jugular veins. The highly irritating nature of concentrated glucose precludes the use of the small peripheral veins in most instances. However, dilute glucose-protein hydrolysates that are appropriate for infusing into peripheral veins are being used with increasing frequency.

The major nursing responsibilities are the same as for any IV therapy: control of sepsis, monitoring of the infusion rate, and assessment of the patient's tolerance of the solution. The TPN solution must be prepared under sterile conditions. The infusion is maintained at a constant rate by an infusion pump. The TPN infusion rate should not be increased or decreased without the practitioner being informed, since alterations can cause hyperglycemia or hypoglycemia.

General assessments, such as vital signs, I&O measurements, and laboratory tests, facilitate early detection of infection or fluid and electrolyte imbalance. **Hyperglycemia** may occur during the first day or two as the child adapts to the high-glucose load of the hyperalimentation solution. Although hyperglycemia occurs infrequently, insulin may be required to assist the body's adjustment. To prevent **hypoglycemia** at the time the hyperalimentation is disconnected, the rate of the infusion and the amount of insulin are decreased gradually.

Family Teaching and Home Care

When alternative feedings are needed for an extended period, the family may need to learn how to feed the child with a nasogastric, gastrostomy, or TPN feeding regimen. Ample time must be allowed for the family to learn and perform the procedures under supervision before assuming full responsibility for the child's care.

Procedures Related to Elimination

Enema

The procedure for giving an enema to an infant or child does not differ essentially from that for an adult, except for the type and amount of fluid administered and the distance for inserting the tube into the rectum (see Guidelines box). Depending on the volume, a syringe with rubber tubing, an enema bottle, or an enema bag should be used.

An isotonic solution is used in children. Plain water is not used because, being hypotonic, it can cause rapid fluid shift and fluid overload. The Fleet enema (pediatric or adult sized) is not advised for children because of the harsh action of its ingredients (sodium biphosphate and sodium phosphate). Commercial enemas can be dangerous to patients with megacolon and to dehydrated or azotemic children. The osmotic effect of the Fleet enema may produce diarrhea, which can lead to metabolic **acidosis**. Other potential complications are extreme hyperphosphatemia, hypernatremia, and hypocalcemia, which may lead to neuromuscular irritability and coma (Walton et al., 2000).

Because infants and young children are unable to retain the solution after it is administered, the buttocks must be held together for a short time to retain the fluid. The enema is administered and expelled while the child is lying with the buttocks over the bedpan and with the head and back supported by pillows. Older children are usually able to hold the solution if they understand what to do and if they are not expected to hold it for too long. The nurse should have the bedpan handy or, for the ambulatory child, ensure that the bathroom is available before beginning the procedure. An enema is an intrusive procedure and thus threatening to the preschool child; a careful explanation is especially important to ease possible fear.

A preoperative bowel preparation solution given orally or through a nasogastric tube is increasingly being used instead of an enema. The polyethylene glycol–electrolyte lavage solution (GoLYTELY) mechanically flushes the bowel without significant absorption, thereby avoiding potential fluid and electrolyte imbalance. Another effective oral cathartic is magnesium citrate solution.

Ostomies

Children may require stomas for various health problems. The most frequent causes in the infant are necrotizing enterocolitis and imperforate anus (less often, Hirschsprung's disease). In the older child the most frequent causes are inflammatory

GUIDELINES Administration of Enemas to Children

Age	Amount (mL)	Insertion Distance
Infant	120–240	2.5 cm
2–4 yr	240–360	5 cm
4–10 yr	360–480	7.5 cm
11+ yr	480–720	10 cm

bowel disease, especially Crohn's disease (regional enteritis), and ureterostomies for distal ureter or bladder defects.

Care and management of ostomies in the older child differ little from the care of ostomies in the adult patient. The major emphases in pediatric care are preparing the child for the procedure and teaching care of the ostomy to the child and family. The basic principles of preparation are the same as for any procedure (see p. 1261). Simple, straightforward language is most effective, together with the use of illustrations and a replica model (e.g., drawing a picture of a child with a stoma on the abdomen and explaining it as "another opening where bowel movements [or any other term the child uses] will come out"). At another time the nurse can draw a pouch over the opening to demonstrate how the contents are collected. Using a doll to demonstrate the process is an excellent teaching strategy, and special books are available.

Children with ileostomies are fitted immediately after surgery with an appliance to protect the skin from the proteolytic enzymes in the liquid stool. Infants may not be fitted with a pouch in the immediate postoperative period. When stomal drainage is minimal, a gauze dressing will suffice. Parents are usually given a choice of caring for the colostomy with or without an appliance. Pediatric appliances are available in a variety of sizes to ensure an adequate fit.

Ostomy equipment consists of a one- or two-piece system with a hypoallergenic skin barrier to maintain peristomal skin integrity. The pouch should be large enough to contain a moderate amount of stool and flatus but not so large as to overwhelm the infant or child. A backing helps minimize the risk of skin breakdown from moisture trapped between the skin and pouch. Small clips or rubber bands should be avoided to prevent choking in the young child. Granulation tissue may grow around an ostomy site (see Fig. 45-29). This moist, beefy red tissue is not a sign of infection. However, if it continues to grow, the excess moisture can irritate the surrounding skin.

Protection of the peristomal skin is a major aspect of stoma care. Well-fitting appliances are important to prevent leakage of contents. Before the appliance is applied, the skin is prepared with a skin sealant that is allowed to dry. Then stoma paste is applied around the base of the stoma or the back of the wafer. The sealant and paste work together to prevent peristomal breakdown.

In infants with a colostomy left unpouched, skin care is similar to that of any diapered infant. However, the peristomal skin is protected with a wafer barrier, such as a hydrocolloid dressing (e.g., DuoDERM) or a barrier substance (e.g., zinc oxide ointment [Desitin], or a mixture of the zinc oxide ointment and stoma [Stomahesive] powder). A gauze dressing may be applied over the stoma and wafer to absorb stomal drainage. If the skin becomes inflamed, denuded, or infected, the care is similar to the interventions used for diaper dermatitis (see Chapter 53). A product that helps protect healthy skin, heal excoriated skin, and minimize pain associated with skin breakdown is Proshield Plus. The skin protectant adheres to denuded, weeping skin. Proshield Plus can be applied over topical antifungal and antibacterial agents if infection is present. No Sting Barrier Film is a skin sealant that has no alcohol base and can be used on open skin without stinging.

With young children, protecting the pouch from being pulled off is an important consideration. One-piece outfits keep exploring hands from reaching the pouch, and the loose waist prevents any pressure on the appliance. Keeping the child occupied with toys during the pouch change is also helpful. As children mature, their participation in ostomy care should be encouraged. Even preschoolers can assist by holding supplies, pulling paper backings from the appliance, and helping clean the stoma area. Toilet training for bladder control needs to begin at the appropriate time as for any other child.

Older children and adolescents should eventually have total responsibility for ostomy care just as they would for usual bowel function. Adolescents may have concerns about body image and the ostomy's impact on intimacy and sexuality. The nurse should stress to teenagers that the presence of a stoma need not interfere with their activities. These youngsters can choose which ostomy equipment is best suited to their needs. Attractively designed and decorated pouch covers are well liked by teenagers.

An enterostomal therapy nurse specialist is an important member of the health care team and will have additional suggestions and skin care information and ostomy pouching options. Further information may be obtained by contacting the Wound, Ostomy and Continence Nurses Society (see Additional Resources at the end of this chapter).

Family Teaching and Home Care

Because these children are almost always discharged with a functioning colostomy, preparation of the family should begin as early as possible in the hospital. The family needs to be instructed in the application of the device (if used), care of the skin, and appropriate action in case skin problems develop. Early evidence of skin breakdown or stomal complications, such as ribbonlike stools, excessive diarrhea, bleeding, prolapse, or failure to pass flatus or stool, should be brought to the attention of the physician, the nurse, or the stoma specialist. The same principles are applied as discussed earlier in this chapter for adherence, especially in terms of education (p. 1269), and in Chapter 44 for discharge planning and home care.

Key Points

- Before undergoing any invasive procedure, the patient (if old enough to comprehend) and the patient's legal surrogate must receive sufficient information on which to make an informed health care decision (informed consent). In Canada there is no age of consent, except for Québec, where it is 14 years.
- Informed consent is needed for major surgery, minor surgery, and diagnostic tests and medical treatments with an element of risk.
- The major principles in psychological preparation of the child for procedures are to establish trust, provide support, and give an explanation in easy-to-understand terms.
- Preparation for procedures should be based on developmental characteristics of the child and knowledge of the family, emphasizing the importance of the parents' role.

- Most parents and children want to be together during stressful procedures and should be offered this opportunity, with guidance on how the parent can comfort the child.
- In performing a procedure, the nurse should expect success, involve the child when possible in the procedure, provide distraction, and allow for expression of feelings.
- Proper positioning of infants and small children for procedures is essential to minimize movement and discomfort.
- In giving postprocedural support, the nurse should encourage children to express feelings and should give praise for completion of the procedure.
- Stressful times before and after surgery that produce anxiety in children are admission, blood tests, injection of preoperative medication (if used), transportation to the operating room, and return from the PACU.
- Assessment of compliance with a treatment regimen entails measuring factors that affect compliance through clinical judgement, self-reporting, direct observation, monitoring of appointments and therapeutic response, pill counts, and chemical assays.
- Strategies for encouraging treatment adherence may be classified as organizational, educational, and behavioural.
- Knowledge of the ill child's eating habits and favourite foods can help in maintaining adequate nutrition.
- Skin care is essential to prevent skin breakdown.
- Control of fever may be accomplished by administration of antipyretics; hyperthermia is controlled by environmental means (minimum clothing, increased air circulation, hypothermia mattress, or cool compresses).
- Infection control is based on two systems. Routine practices provide protection when the infected person is undiagnosed. Transmission-based precautions add extra interventions for patients diagnosed with or suspected of having an infection.
- Ensuring safety in the hospital setting is a major concern and can be achieved through environmental measures, limit setting, infection control, and safe transportation.
- Restraints should be used cautiously and require a medical order. Use of therapeutic holding can avoid the use of restraints.
- Factors that affect medication dosage determination are growth and maturation, difficulty in evaluating a medication response, and BSA.
- Family teaching regarding medication administration includes telling parents why the child is receiving the medication; its possible effects; and the amount, frequency, and length of time it is to be administered.
- The preferred sites for intramuscular injection in children are the vastus lateralis and ventrogluteal areas.
- Intermittent venous access is accomplished by means of a peripheral intermittent infusion device, a peripherally inserted central catheter, a central venous catheter, or an implanted port.
- Several safety catheters and needleless device systems are available to reduce the risk of needlestick injuries in patients and caregivers.
- Nursing assessment of fluid and electrolyte disturbances entails observation of general appearance, vital signs, and measurement of I&O.
- Oxygen can be administered by hood, mask, nasal cannula, incubator, or oxygen tent.
- Tracheostomy suctioning involves premeasured insertion of the catheter, application of suction for 5 seconds when withdrawing the catheter, and supplemental oxygen before and after suctioning.
- Alternative forms of feeding include gavage feeding, gastrostomy feeding, and TPN.
- In the care of children with ostomies, nurses play an important role in family support and instruction in care of the stoma site.

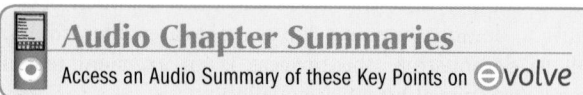

Audio Chapter Summaries
Access an Audio Summary of these Key Points on evolve

References

Algren, C., & Algren, J. (1997). Pediatric sedation essentials for the preoperative nurse. *Nursing Clinics of North America, 32*(1), 17–30.

Blass, E. M., & Watt, L. (1999). Suckling- and sucrose-induced analgesia in human newborns. *Pain, 83*(3), 611–623.

Brenner, M. (2007). Child restraint in the acute care setting of pediatric nursing: An extraordinarily stressful event. *Issues in Comprehensive Pediatric Nursing, 30*(1-2), 29–37, doi:10.1080/01460860701366658

Burke, N. (1995). Alternative methods for newborn urine sample collection. *Pediatric Nursing, 21*(6), 546–549.

Canadian Medical Protective Society. (2012). *Consent: A guide for Canadian physicians.* Retrieved from http://www.cmpa-acpm.ca/cmpapd04/docs/resource_files/ml_guides/consent_guide/com_cg_requirements-e.cfm.

Canadian Paediatric Society. (2008a). *Febrile seizures.* Retrieved from http://www.caringforkids.cps.ca/handouts/febrile_seizures.

Canadian Paediatric Society. (2008b). *Fever and temperature taking.* Retrieved from http://www.caringforkids.cps.ca/handouts/fever_and_temperature_taking.

Canadian Paediatric Society, Bioethics Committee. (2004). Treatment decisions regarding infants, children, and adolescents. *Paediatrics and Child Health, 9*(2), 99–103. Retrieved from http://www.cps/english/statements/B/b904-01.htm.

Canadian Pediatric Society, Infectious Diseases and Immunization Committee. (2004). PID note: Bag urine specimens still not appropriate in diagnosing urinary tract infections in infants. *Pediatrics and Child Health, 9*(6), 377–378. Retrieved from http://www.cps.ca/english/statements/ID/PIDNoteUTI.htm.

Carroll, P. (1998). Closing in on safer suctioning. *RN, 61*(5), 22–27.

Catudal, R. (1999). Pediatric IV therapy: Actual practice. *Journal of Vascular Access Devices, 4*(2), 27–29.

College of Nurses of Ontario. (2009). *Practice standard: Restraints.* Retrieved from http://www.cno.org/Global/docs/prac/41043_Restraints.pdf.

Cook, I. F., & Murtagh, J. (2002). Needle length required for intramuscular vaccination of infants and toddlers: An ultrasonographic study. *Australian Family Physician, 31*(3), 295–297.

Cook, I. F., & Murtagh, J. (2006). Ventrogluteal area: A suitable site for intramuscular vaccination of infants and toddlers. *Vaccine, 24*(13), 2403–2408. doi:10.1016/j.vaccine.2005.11

Curley, M. A. Q., & Moloney-Harmon, P. A. (2001). *Critical care nursing of infants and children* (2nd ed.). Philadelphia: Saunders.

Dubick, M. A., & Holcomb, J. B. (2000). A review of intraosseous vascular access: Current status and military application. *Military Medicine, 165*(7), 552–559.

Eaton, L. (2005). Hand washing is more important than cleaner wards in controlling MRSA. *British Medical Journal, 330*(7497), 922. doi:10.1136/bmj.330.7497.922-b

Eckler, J. (1997). Combating infection. *Nursing, 27*(10), 20.

Essink-Tebbes, C. M., et al. (1999). Safety of lidocaine-prilocaine cream application four times a day in premature neonates: A pilot study. *European Journal of Pediatrics, 158*(5), 421–423.

Fauroux, B., et al. (1999). Chest physiotherapy in cystic fibrosis: Improved tolerance with nasal pressure support ventilation. *Pediatrics, 103*(3), E32.

Fisher, A. A., et al. (2004). The use of alteplase for restoring patency to occluded central venous access devices in infants and children. *Journal of Infusion Nursing, 27*(3), 171–174.
Gamulka, B., Mendoza, C., & Connolly, B. (2005). Evaluation of a unique, nurse-inserted, peripherally inserted central catheter program. *Pediatrics, 115*(6), 1602–1606. doi:10.1542/peds.2004-0542
Gravel, D., et al. (2007). A point prevalence survey of health care–associated infections in pediatric populations in major Canadian acute care hospitals. *American Journal of Infection Control, 35*, 157–162.
Gray, L., Watt, L., & Blass, E. M. (2000). Skin-to-skin contact is analgesic in healthy newborns. *Pediatrics, 105*(1), 110–111. Retrieved from http://www.pediatrics.org/cgi/content/full/105/1/E14.
Gray, M. (1996). Atraumatic urethral catheterization of children. *Pediatric Nursing, 22*(4), 306–310.
Harris, J., & Maguire, D. (1999). Developing a protocol to prevent and treat pediatric central venous catheter occlusions. *Journal of Intravenous Nursing, 22*(4), 194–198.
Health Canada. (2003). *Update: Risk of strangulation of infants by IV tubing and monitor leads – Notice to hospitals.* Retrieved from http://www.hc-sc.gc.ca/dhp-mps/medeff/advisories-avis/prof/_2003/iv_tubes_2_nth-ah-eng.php.
Infusion Nurses Society. (2000a). *Policies and procedures for infusion nursing.* Norwood, MA: The Society.
Infusion Nurses Society. (2000b). Revised infusion nursing standards of practice. *Journal of Intravenous Nursing, 23*(6 Suppl), S17, S39, S41, S45, S49–S50, S60.
Institute for Safe Medication Practices. (2004). Problems persist with life-threatening tubing misconnections. *ISMP Medication Safety Alert,* June 17, 2004. Retrieved from http://www.ismp.org/newsletters/acutecare/articles/20040617.asp.
Ipp, M. M., et al. (1989). Adverse reactions to diphtheria, tetanus, pertussis–polio vaccination at 18 months of age: Effect of injection site and needle length. *Pediatrics, 83*(5), 679–682.
Kain, Z., Caldwell-Andrews, A., & Wang, S. (2002). Psychological preparation of the parent and pediatric surgical patient. *Anesthesia Clinics of North America, 20*(1), 29–44.
Kain, Z. N., et al. (2004). Trends in the practice of parental presence during induction of anesthesia and the use of preoperative sedative premedication in the United States, 1995–2002: Results of a follow-up national survey. *Anesthesia & Analgesia, 98*(5), 1252–1259.
Katsma, D., & Smith, G. (1997). Analysis of needle path during intramuscular injection. *Nursing Research, 46*(5), 288–292.
Kellam, B., et al. (2001). Tenderfoot Preemie vs. a manual lancet: A clinical evaluation. *Neonatal Network, 20*(7), 31–36.
Kraus, D., et al. (2001). Effectiveness and infant acceptance of the Rx Medibottle versus the oral syringe. *Pharmacotherapy, 21*(4), 416–423.
KyngAs, H., Kroll, T., & Duffy, M. (2000). Compliance in adolescents with chronic diseases: A review. *Journal of Adolescent Health, 26*, 379–388.
Larsson, B. A., et al. (1998). Alleviation of the pain of venipuncture in neonates. *Acta Paediatrica, 87*(7), 774–779.
Liebman, M., & Barnsteiner, J. (2001). Fever education: Does it reduce parent fever anxiety? *Pediatric Emergency Care, 17*(1), 47–51.
Maki, D. G. (1994). Infections caused by intravascular devices used for infusion therapy: Pathogenesis, prevention, and management. In A. L. Bisno & F. A. Waldvogel (Eds.), *Infections associated with indwelling medical devices* (2nd ed.). Washington, DC: American Society for Microbiology.
Manworren, R., & Fledderman, M. (2000). Preparation of the child and family for surgery. In B. V. Wise, et al. (Eds.), *Nursing care of the general pediatric surgical patient.* Gaithersburg, MD: Aspen.
Maxwell, L. G., & Yaster, M. (2000). Perioperative management issues in pediatric patients. *Anesthesiology Clinics of North America, 18*(3), 601–632.
Meehan, R. M. (1998). Heelsticks in neonates for capillary blood sampling. *Neonatal Network, 17*(1), 17–24.
Montgomery, L. A., et al. (1999). Guidelines for IV infiltrations in pediatric patients. *Pediatric Nursing, 25*(2), 167–180.
Moureau, N. (1999). Practical access, a back-to-basics review of intravenous therapy. *Journal of Vascular Access Devices, 4*(2 Suppl), 1–4.
Oncology Nursing Society. (1998). *Cancer chemotherapy guidelines and recommendations for practice* (2nd ed.). Pittsburgh: Oncology Nursing Press.
Pettit, J., & Hughes, K. (1999). Neonatal intravenous therapy practices. *Journal of Vascular Access Devices, 4*, 7–16.
Polillio, A. M., & Killy, J. (1997). Does a needleless injection system reduce anxiety in children receiving intramuscular injections? *Pediatric Nursing, 23*(1), 46–49.
Purssell, E. (2000). The use of antipyretic medications in the prevention of febrile convulsions in children. *Journal of Pediatric Nursing, 9*(4), 473–480.
Quality, equipment hold keys to infection control. (2006). *ED Management, 18*(2), 19–21.
Quigley, S. M., & Curley, M. A. Q. (1996). Skin integrity in the pediatric population: Preventing and managing pressure ulcers. *Journal of the Society of Pediatric Nurses, 1*(1), 7.
Redmond, M. C. (2001). Malignant hyperthermia: Perianesthesia recognition, treatment, and care. *Journal of Perianesthesia Nursing, 16*(4), 259–270.
Registered Nurses' Association of Ontario (2005). *Risk assessment and prevention of pressure ulcers.* (Revised 2011) Toronto: Author. Retrieved from http://rnao.ca/sites/rnao-ca/files/Risk_Assessment_and_Prevention_of_Pressure_Ulcers.pdf.
Romino, S. L., et al. (2005). Parental presence during anesthesia induction in children. *AORN Journal, 81*(4), 780–792.
Rote, N., Huether, S., & McCance, K. (2000). Hypersensitivities, infection, and immunodeficiencies. In S. Huether & K. McCance (Eds.), *Understanding pathophysiology* (2nd ed.). St. Louis: Mosby.
Selekman, J., & Snyder, B. (1997). Institutional policies on the use of physical restraints on children. *Pediatric Nursing, 23*(5), 531–537.
Sharber, J. (1997). The efficacy of tepid sponge bathing to reduce fever in young children. *American Journal of Emergency Medicine, 15*(2), 188–192.
Shen, V., et al. (2003). Recombinant tissue plasminogen activator (alteplase) for restoration of function to occluded central venous catheters in pediatric patients. *Journal of Pediatric Hematology & Oncology, 25*(1), 38–45.
Shepherd, A. J., et al. (2006). A Scottish study of heel-prick blood sampling in newborn babies. *Midwifery, 22*(2), 158–168.
Singer, A. J., & Konia, N. (1999). Comparison of topical anesthetics and vasoconstrictors vs. lubricants prior to nasogastric intubation: A randomized, controlled trial. *Academic Emergency Medicine, 6*(3), 184–190.
Teitelbaum, D., et al. (2005). Definition of terms, style, and conventions used in A.S.P.E.N. guidelines and standards. *Nutrition in Clinical Practice, 20*(2), 281–285. doi:10.1177/0148607107031005441
Van Cleve, L., Johnson, L., & Pothier, P. (1996). Pain responses of hospitalized infants and children to venipuncture and intravenous cannulation. *Journal of Pediatric Nursing, 11*, 169–174.
Vertanen, H., et al. (2001). An automatic incision device for obtaining blood samples from the heels of preterm infants causes less damage than a conventional manual lancet. *Archives of Disease in Childhood: Fetal & Neonatal Edition, 84*, F53–F55.
Walton, D. M., et al. (2000). Morbid hypocalcemia associated with phosphate enema in a six-week-old infant. *Pediatrics, 106*(3), e37.
Wright, K. D., Stewart, S. H., Finley, G. A., & Buffett-Jerrott, S. E. (2007). Prevention and intervention strategies to alleviate preoperative anxiety in children. A critical review. *Behavior Modification, 31*(1), 52–79.

Additional Resources

Body Surface Area Calculator for Medication Dosages: http://www.halls.md/body-surface-area/bsa.htm
Braden Q Scale—To assess severity of a pressure ulcer: http://www.health.qld.gov.au/psq/pip/docs/braden.pdf
Canadian Paediatric Society: Preventing Choking and Suffocation in Children: http://www.cps.ca/english/statements/IP/IP12-02.htm
Hospital for Sick Children. Coming for Surgery: http://www.sickkids.ca/visitingsickkids/coming-for-surgery/index.html
Oncology Nursing Society—Guidelines on interventions for infiltration and extravasation: http://www.ons.org
Registered Nurses' Association of Ontario—Best Practice Guideline: Risk Assessment and Prevention of Pressure Ulcers: http://rnao.ca/sites/rnao-ca/files/Risk_Assessment_and_Prevention_of_Pressure_Ulcers.pdf
Wound, Ostomy, and Continence Nurses Society—Staging of pressure ulcers and guidelines for prevention and management of pressure ulcers: http://www.wocn.org

Unit 11

46 Respiratory Dysfunction

Learning Objectives

On completion of this chapter, the reader will be able to:

- Identify the factors leading to respiratory tract infection in the infant or young child.
- Contrast the effects of various respiratory infections observed in infants and children.
- Describe the postoperative nursing care of the child with an adenotonsillectomy.
- Outline a nursing care plan for a child with croup.
- Outline a nursing care plan for a child with acute otitis media.
- Demonstrate an understanding of the ways in which inhalation of noninfectious irritants produce pulmonary dysfunction.
- Describe the ways in which the various therapeutic measures relieve the symptoms of asthma.
- Outline a plan for teaching home care for the child with asthma.
- Describe the physiological effects of cystic fibrosis on the gastrointestinal and pulmonary systems.
- Outline a plan of care for the child with cystic fibrosis.
- List the major signs of respiratory distress in infants and children.
- Describe the nursing care for a child with respiratory failure.

Electronic Resources

Additional information related to the content in Chapter 46 can be found on

evolve **the companion Web site at**

http://evolve.elsevier.com/Canada/Perry/maternal/

- Examination Review Questions
- Anatomy Review—Location of Retractions
- Anatomy Review—Location of Tonsillar Masses
- Animation—Asthma
- Animation—Bag Ventilation
- Animation—Bronchi and Bronchioles
- Animation—Intubation
- Animation—Lung Sounds
- Animation—Respiratory Failure, Infant
- Case Study—Acute Epiglottitis
- Case Study—Bronchiolitis
- Case Study—Cystic Fibrosis
- Case Study—Mononucleosis
- Case Study—Tonsillitis
- Critical Thinking Exercise—Cystic Fibrosis Inheritance Risks
- Critical Thinking Exercise—Ingestion of a Foreign Body

Respiratory Infection

General Aspects of Respiratory Infections

Infections of the respiratory tract are described according to the anatomical area of involvement. The *upper respiratory tract*, or *upper airway*, consists of the oronasopharynx, pharynx, larynx, and upper part of the trachea. The *lower respiratory tract* consists of the lower trachea, mainstem bronchi, segmental bronchi, subsegmental bronchioles, terminal bronchioles, and alveoli. In this discussion, the trachea is considered with lower tract disorders, and infections of the epiglottis and larynx are categorized as croup syndromes. Respiratory infections seldom fall into discrete anatomical areas. Infections often spread from one structure to another because of the contiguous nature of the mucous membrane lining the entire tract. Consequently, respiratory tract infections involve several areas, although the effect on one area may predominate in any given illness.

Etiology and Characteristics

Respiratory infections account for the majority of acute illnesses in children. The etiology and course of these infections are influenced by the age of the child, the season, living conditions, and pre-existing medical problems.

Infectious Agents

The respiratory tract is subject to a wide variety of infective organisms. Most infections are caused by viruses, particularly respiratory syncytial virus (RSV), nonpolio enteroviruses (coxsackieviruses A and B), adenoviruses, parainfluenza viruses, and human meta-pneumoviruses. Other agents involved in primary or secondary invasion include group A β-hemolytic streptococci (GABHS), staphylococci, *Haemophilus influenzae*, *Chlamydia trachomatis*, *Mycoplasma* organisms, and pneumococci.

Age

Infants younger than age 3 months of age have a lower infection rate than that of older children, presumably because of the protective function of maternal **antibodies**. The infection rate increases from 3 to 6 months of age, the time between the disappearance of maternal antibodies and the infant's own antibody production. The viral infection rate remains high during the toddler and preschool years. By 5 years of age, viral respiratory infections are less frequent, but the incidence of *Mycoplasma pneumoniae* and GABHS infections increases.

Some viral agents produce a mild illness in older children but severe lower respiratory tract illness or croup in infants. For example, RSV often causes nothing more than upper respiratory symptoms in older children but can cause severe respiratory compromise in infants.

Size

Anatomical differences influence the response to respiratory tract infections. The diameter of the airways is smaller in young children and subject to considerable narrowing from edematous mucous membranes and increased production of secretions. The distance between structures within the respiratory tract is also shorter in the young child, and organisms may move rapidly down the respiratory tract, causing more extensive involvement. The relatively short and open eustachian tube in infants and young children allows **pathogens** easy access to the middle ear.

Resistance

The ability to resist invading organisms depends on several factors. Deficiencies of the **immune system** place the child at risk for infection. Other conditions that decrease resistance are malnutrition, anemia, fatigue, and chilling of the body. Conditions that weaken defences of the respiratory tract and predispose children to infection include allergies (e.g., allergic rhinitis), preterm birth, bronchopulmonary dysplasia (BPD), asthma, history of RSV infection, cardiac anomalies that cause pulmonary congestion, and cystic fibrosis (CF). Day care attendance, especially if the caregivers smoke, increases the likelihood of infection.

Seasonal Variations

The most common respiratory pathogens appear in epidemics during the winter and spring months. Mycoplasmal infections occur more often in autumn and early winter. Infection-related asthma (e.g., asthmatic bronchitis) occurs more frequently during cold weather, whereas winter and spring are typically the "RSV seasons."

Clinical Manifestations

Infants and young children, especially those between 6 months and 3 years of age, react more severely to acute respiratory tract infection than older children. Young children display a number of generalized signs and symptoms and local manifestations (Box 46-1).

Nursing Care Management

Assessment of the respiratory system follows the guidelines described in Chapter 34 (for assessment of the nose, mouth and throat, chest, and lungs). Special attention should also be given to the components and observations listed in Box 46-2.

Ease Respiratory Efforts

Many acute respiratory infections are mild and cause few symptoms. Although children may feel uncomfortable and have a "stuffy" nose (congestion) and some mucosal swelling, respiratory distress occurs infrequently. Interventions delivered at home are usually sufficient to relieve minor discomfort and ease respiratory efforts. However, children with croup or epiglottitis can develop sufficient swelling to obstruct the airway and may require hospitalization and more complex therapy.

Warm or cool mist is a common therapeutic measure for symptomatic relief of respiratory discomfort. The moisture soothes inflamed membranes and is beneficial when there is hoarseness or laryngeal involvement. However, the use of steam vaporizers in the home is often discouraged because of the hazards related to their use and limited evidence to support their efficacy. Shallow pans with wide surface areas for evaporation increase humidity but should be placed where they do not pose a safety hazard.

A time-honoured method (albeit not evidence informed) of producing warm mist is the shower. Running a shower of hot water into the empty bathtub or open shower stall with the bathroom door closed produces a quick source of steam. Keeping a child in this environment for 10 to 15 minutes provides the same advantages as the mist tent without the fear and restraint associated with the confines of a tent. A small child can be held on the parent's lap. Older children can sit in the bathroom under the supervision of an adult.

Promote Rest

Children who have an acute febrile illness should be placed on bed rest. This is usually not difficult while the temperature is elevated but may become a problem when children begin to feel better. Often children will comply with bed rest if they are allowed to lie quietly on a couch where they can watch television, play a video game, or participate in a quiet activity. If children protest, allowing them to play quietly serves the purpose of rest better than allowing them to cry excessively in bed.

Promote Comfort

Older children are usually able to manage nasal secretions with little difficulty. Parents should be instructed in the correct administration of nose drops and throat irrigations, if ordered (see Chapter 45). For very young infants, who normally breathe through their noses, an infant nasal aspirator or a rubber ear syringe is helpful in removing nasal secretions before feeding. This practice, followed by instillation of saline nose drops, may clear nasal passages and promote feeding. For older infants and children who can tolerate decongestants, vasoconstrictive nose drops may be administered 15 to 20 minutes before feeding and at bedtime. Two drops are instilled; because this shrinks only the anterior mucous membranes, two more drops are instilled 5 to 10 minutes later. Older children often prefer nasal sprays. They can be taught to compress the plastic container at the moment of inspiration. Bottles of nose drops should be used for only one child and one illness because they are easily contaminated with bacteria.

evolve Animation—Lung Sounds

BOX 46-1 Signs and Symptoms Associated With Respiratory Infections in Infants and Small Children

Fever

May be absent in newborn infants
Greatest at ages 6 months to 3 years
Temperature may reach 39.5° to 40.5°C even with mild infections
Often appears as first sign of infection
May be listless and irritable or somewhat euphoric and more active than normal temporarily; some children talk with unaccustomed rapidity
Tendency to develop high temperatures with infection in certain families
May precipitate febrile seizures (see Chapter 51)
Febrile seizures uncommon after 3 or 4 years of age

Meningismus

Meningeal signs without infection of the meninges
Occurs with abrupt onset of fever
Accompanied by the following:

- Headache
- Pain and stiffness in the back and neck
- Presence of Kernig and Brudzinski signs

Subsides as the temperature decreases

Anorexia

Common with most childhood illnesses
Frequently the initial evidence of illness
Persists to a greater or lesser degree throughout febrile stage of illness; often extends into convalescence

Vomiting

Small children vomit readily with illness
Clue to onset of infection
May precede other signs by several hours
Usually short-lived but may persist during the illness
Frequent cause of dehydration if fluid intake is impaired

Diarrhea

Usually mild, transient diarrhea but may become severe
Often accompanies viral respiratory infections
Frequent cause of dehydration

Abdominal Pain

Common complaint
Sometimes indistinguishable from pain of appendicitis
Mesenteric lymphadenitis may be cause
Muscle spasms from vomiting may be a factor, especially in nervous, tense child

Nasal Blockage

Small nasal passages of infants easily blocked by mucosal swelling and exudation
Can interfere with respiration and feeding in infants
May contribute to the development of otitis media and sinusitis

Nasal Discharge

Frequent occurrence
May be thin and watery (rhinorrhea) or thick and purulent
Depends on the type or stage of infection
Associated with itching
May irritate upper lip and skin surrounding the nose

Cough

Common feature
May be evident only during acute phase
May persist several months after a disease

Respiratory Sounds

Sounds associated with respiratory disease:

- Cough
- Hoarseness
- Grunting
- Stridor
- Wheezing

Auscultation:

- Wheezing
- Crackles
- Absence of breath sounds

Sore Throat

Frequent complaint of older children
Young children (unable to describe symptoms) may not complain even when highly inflamed
Child will often refuse to take oral fluids or solids

To avoid rebound congestion, nose drops or sprays should not be administered for more than 3 days.

Hot or cold applications sometimes provide relief for children with painful cervical adenitis. An ice bag or heating pad applied to the neck may decrease the discomfort, but safety precautions must be observed to prevent burns. The ice bag or heating device must be covered, and the heating pad should not be set at high ranges.

Prevent the Spread of Infection

Children and families should be taught to cough or sneeze into their arm (Public Health Agency of Canada [PHAC], 2009), dispose of tissues properly, and wash their hands. Remembering to cover the nose or mouth is often difficult for toddlers; they should be encouraged to wash their hands frequently to prevent the spread of infection. Used tissues should be thrown into the wastebasket immediately, and tissues should not be allowed to accumulate in a pile. Children with respiratory infections should not share drinking cups, washcloths, or towels. To avoid contamination with respiratory viruses, nurses need to wash their hands thoroughly and not touch their eyes or nose.

Efforts should be made to separate affected children from contact with other children. Parents need to keep affected children out of school and day care settings to prevent the spread of infection. Ideally, ill children should be isolated in a separate bedroom at the first sign of illness, but this is difficult

BOX 46-2 Components for Assessing Respiratory Function

Respirations

The pattern of respirations is observed for rate, depth, ease, and rhythm of breathing:

Rate—Rapid (*tachypnea*), normal, or slow for the particular child

Depth—Normal depth, too shallow (*hypopnea*), too deep (*hyperpnea*); usually estimated from the amplitude of thoracic and abdominal excursion

Ease—Effortless; laboured (*dyspnea*); *orthopnea* (difficult breathing except in upright position); associated with intercostal or substernal retractions (inspiratory "sinking in" of soft tissues in relation to the cartilaginous and bony thorax); flaring nares; head bobbing (head of sleeping child with suboccipital area supported on caregiver's forearm bobs forward in synchrony with each inspiration); grunting; or wheezing

Laboured breathing—Continuous, intermittent, becoming steadily worse, sudden onset, at rest or on exertion, associated with wheezing or grunting, associated with pain

Rhythm—Variation in rate and depth of respirations

Other Observations

In addition to respirations, particular attention is addressed to the following:

Evidence of infection—Check for elevated temperature; enlarged cervical lymph nodes; inflamed mucous membranes; and purulent discharges from the nose, ears, or lungs (sputum).

Cough—Observe characteristics of cough (if present): under what circumstances cough is heard (e.g., night only, on arising), nature of cough (paroxysmal with or without wheeze, "croupy" or "brassy"), frequency of cough, associated with swallowing or other activity, character of cough (moist or dry), and productivity.

Wheeze—Note if expiratory or inspiratory, high-pitched or musical, prolonged, slowly progressive or sudden, or associated with laboured breathing.

Cyanosis—Note distribution (peripheral, perioral, facial, trunk, and face), degree, duration, and whether associated with activity.

Abdominal pain—May be a complaint in preschooler and school-age children; it probably represents referred pain from the chest; it may be a complaint in children with pneumonia.

Chest pain—May be a complaint of older children; note location and circumstances: localized or generalized, referred to base of neck or abdomen, dull or sharp, deep or superficial, associated with rapid, shallow respirations or grunting.

Sputum—Older children may provide sputum sample by coughing, whereas young children may need bulb suction to provide a sample; note volume, colour, viscosity, and odour.

Bad breath—May be associated with some lung infections.

to do when living arrangements are crowded and there are several children in the family. Well children should be told to stay away from ill children.

Reduce Temperature

If the child has a significantly elevated temperature, controlling the fever is important. Parents need to know how to take a child's temperature and read the thermometer accurately. Nurses should not assume that all parents can read a thermometer; parents who cannot perform this skill should receive instruction.

If the practitioner prescribes acetaminophen or ibuprofen, parents may need help giving the medication. Most parents can read the label and calculate the desired dose, but some may require careful instruction. It is important to emphasize accuracy in determining both the amount of medication to be given and the time intervals for administration. The child can be given cool liquids to reduce the temperature and minimize the chances of dehydration. (See Controlling Elevated Temperatures, Chapter 45.)

NURSING ALERT Parents should be cautioned about using over-the-counter combination "cold" remedies as these often include acetaminophen. Careful calculation of both the acetaminophen given separately and the acetaminophen in combination medications is necessary to avoid an overdose.

Promote Hydration

Dehydration is a potential complication when children have respiratory tract infections and are febrile or anorexic, especially when vomiting or diarrhea is present. Infants are especially prone to fluid and electrolyte deficits when they have a respiratory illness because a rapid respiratory rate that accompanies such illnesses precludes adequate fluid intake. In addition, the presence of fever increases the total body fluid turnover in infants. If the infant has nasal secretions, this further prevents adequate respiratory effort by blocking the narrow nasal passages when the infant reclines to breastfeed or bottle-feed and ceases the compensatory mouth breathing effort, thus causing the child to limit intake of fluids. Adequate fluid intake is encouraged by offering small amounts of favourite fluids (clear liquids if vomiting) at frequent intervals. High-calorie liquids—such as colas, fruit juice drinks, water flavoured and sweetened with corn syrup, or similar drinks—help prevent **catabolism** and dehydration but should be avoided, especially if diarrhea is present. Oral rehydration solutions such as Infalyte or Pedialyte should be considered for infants; sports drinks such as Gatorade should be considered for older children. Fluids with caffeine (tea, coffee) should be avoided because these may act as a diuretic and promote fluid loss. Breastfeeding infants should continue to be breastfed because human milk confers some degree of protection from infection (see Chapter 26). Fluids should not be forced, and children should not be awakened to take fluids. Forcing fluids creates the same problem as urging unwanted food. Gentle persuasion with preferred beverages or sugar-free popsicles is usually more successful.

To assess their child's level of hydration (see also Chapter 47), parents are advised to observe the frequency of voiding and to notify the nurse or practitioner if there is insufficient voiding. Counting the number of wet diapers in a 24-hour period is a satisfactory method to assess output in infants and toddlers.

Provide Nutrition

Loss of appetite is characteristic of children with acute infections. In most cases children can be permitted to determine their own need for food. Many children show no decrease in appetite, and others respond well to foods such as gelatin, soup, and puddings (see Feeding the Sick Child, Chapter 45). Urging foods on anorexic children may precipitate nausea and vomiting and cause an aversion to feeding that can extend into the convalescent period and beyond.

Encourage Family Support and Home Care

Young children with respiratory tract infections are irritable and difficult to comfort; the family needs support, encouragement, and practical suggestions for comfort measures and administration of medication. In addition to **antipyretics** and nose drops, the child may require antibiotic therapy. Parents of children receiving oral antibiotics must understand the importance of regular administration and continuing the medication for the prescribed length of time, regardless of whether the child appears ill. Parents should be cautioned against giving their child any medications that are not approved by the health practitioner and to avoid giving antibiotics left over from a previous illness or prescribed for another child. Administering unprescribed antibiotics can produce serious adverse effects and reactions (see Chapter 45 for administration of medications and teaching parents).

evolve Anatomy—Location of Retractions

Upper Respiratory Tract Infections

Nasopharyngitis

Acute nasopharyngitis (the equivalent of the "common cold") is caused by rhinovirus, RSV, adenovirus, influenza virus, and parainfluenza virus. Symptoms are more severe in infants and children than in adults. Fever is common in young children, and older children have low-grade fevers, which appear early in the course of the illness. Other clinical manifestations are listed in Box 46-3.

BOX 46-3 Clinical Manifestations of Nasopharyngitis and Pharyngitis

Nasopharyngitis

Younger Child
Fever
Irritability, restlessness
Sneezing
Vomiting or diarrhea

Older Child
Dryness and irritation of nose and throat
Sneezing, chilling sensation
Muscular aches
Cough, sometimes

Physical Signs
Edema and vasodilation of mucosa

Pharyngitis

Younger Child
Fever
General malaise
Anorexia
Moderate sore throat
Headache

Older Child
Fever (may reach 40°C)
Headache
Anorexia
Dysphagia
Abdominal pain
Vomiting

Physical Signs
Younger Child
Mild to moderate hyperemia
Older Child
Mild to fiery red, edematous pharynx
Hyperemia of tonsils and pharynx; may extend to soft palate and uvula
Often abundant follicular exudate that spreads and coalesces to form pseudomembrane on tonsils
Cervical glands enlarged and tender

Therapeutic Management

Children with nasopharyngitis are managed at home. There is no specific treatment, and effective vaccines are not available. Antipyretics are prescribed for mild fever and discomfort (see Chapter 45 for management of fever). Rest is recommended until the child is free of fever for at least 1 day. Decongestants may be prescribed for children older than 5 years of age to shrink swollen nasal passages. The decongestants that exert their effect by vasoconstriction are usually less effective when taken orally than when applied topically as nose drops. Because these medications affect all vascular beds, they should be given with caution to children with diabetes.

Cough suppressants may be prescribed for a dry, hacking cough in older children. However, cough preparations can cause adverse effects such as confusion, hyperexcitability, and sedation; parents should monitor the child carefully for potential adverse effects.

Antihistamines are largely ineffective in the treatment of nasopharyngitis. These medications have a weak atropine-like effect that dries secretions, but they can cause drowsiness or, paradoxically, have a stimulatory effect on children. There is no support for the usefulness of expectorants, and antibiotics are usually not indicated because most infections are viral.

Recent concerns regarding serious adverse effects of cough and cold preparations in young children, particularly infants, and lack of convincing evidence that such medications are effective in reducing symptoms have prompted recommendations by health experts to carefully evaluate the benefits and risks of using such preparations in children under 6 years of age (Canadian Paediatric Society [CPS], 2010d; Ryan, Brewer, & Small, 2008).

NURSING ALERT Parents should be cautioned not to give nonprescription cough and cold remedies to children under 6 years old or if a child has a chronic illness, unless recommended by their health practitioner (CPS, 2010d). The over-the-counter preparations generally are not effective and can increase heart rate and cause sleeplessness.

Prevention

Nasopharyngitis is so widespread in the general population that it is impossible to prevent. Children are more susceptible because they have not yet developed resistance to many viruses. Very young infants are subject to serious complications such as pneumonia, and attempts should be made to protect them from exposure.

Nursing Care Management

A cold is often the parents' first introduction to an illness in their infant. Most discomfort of nasopharyngitis is related to the nasal obstruction, especially in small infants. Elevating the head of the bed or crib mattress assists with drainage of secretions. Nasopharyngeal suctioning and vaporization may also provide relief. Saline nose drops and gentle suctioning with a bulb syringe before feeding are useful.

Maintaining adequate fluid intake is essential. Although a child's appetite for solid foods is usually diminished for several days, it is important to offer favourite fluids to prevent dehydration. Fluids can be cool or warm, depending on individual preference.

Because nasopharyngitis is spread from secretions, the best means for prevention is avoiding contact with affected persons. This goal is difficult to accomplish in family settings, classrooms, and day care centres. Family members with a cold should try to "keep it to themselves" by carefully disposing of tissues; not sharing towels, glasses, or eating utensils; coughing or sneezing into their arms; and washing their hands thoroughly after nose blowing or sneezing. The most frequent carriers of infection are the human hands, which deposit viruses on doorknobs, faucets, toys, and other everyday objects. Children should be taught to wash their hands thoroughly before putting them near their eyes, nose, or mouth.

Family Support

Support and reassurance are important elements of care for families of young children with recurrent upper respiratory infections (URIs). Because URIs are common in children less than 3 years of age, families may feel as if they are on an endless roller coaster of illness. They need reassurance that frequent colds are a normal part of childhood and that by 5 years of age their children will have developed **immunity** to many viruses. Parents who work outside the home should expect to take time off to care for ill children during the fall and winter months. When children spend time routinely in day care centres, their infection rate is usually higher than if they are cared for in the home. Parents should know the signs of respiratory illness complications and should notify a health care provider if complications occur or if the child does not improve within 2 or 3 days (Box 46-4).

BOX 46-4 Early Evidence of Respiratory Complications

Parents should be instructed to notify their regular health care provider if any of the following are noted:

- If the child is less than 3 months of age when a cold starts
- If the child has a fever for more than 5 days
- If the child has a runny nose for more than 10 days
- If the infant's nose cannot be unblocked so that the infant can drink adequate amount of fluids or the child is not eating or drinking
- If the child has pain in the chest
- If the child has any pain in the ear or any fluid draining from it (see p. 1325)
- If the child has a very sore throat
- If the child is vomiting or choking with a cough
- If they have any concerns or need to ask questions

Parents should be instructed to go the nearest emergency department or call 911 if:

- The child is getting more ill.
- The child seems lethargic, very drowsy or irritable.
- The child is having difficulty breathing.
- The child's lips look blue.
- The child has a stiff or painful neck or a headache that is severe.

(Modified from About Kids Health [2009]. *What is a cold?* Retrieved from http://www.aboutkidshealth.ca/En/HealthAZ/ConditionsandDiseases/InfectiousDiseases/Pages/Colds-Viral-Upper-Respiratory-Infections.aspx.)

Acute Streptococcal Pharyngitis

Children who experience GABHS infection of the upper airway (strep throat) are at risk for *rheumatic fever (RF)*, an inflammatory disease of the heart, joints, and central nervous system (see Chapter 48), and *acute glomerulonephritis (AGN)*, an acute kidney infection (see Chapter 50). Permanent damage can result from these sequelae, especially RF.

Clinical Manifestations

GABHS is generally a relatively brief illness that varies in severity from subclinical (no symptoms) to severe toxicity. The onset is often abrupt and characterized by pharyngitis, headache, fever, and abdominal pain (especially in small children). The tonsils and pharynx may be inflamed and covered with exudate (Fig. 46-1), which usually appears by the second day of illness. However, streptococcal infections should be suspected in children older than 2 years of age who have pharyngitis without exudate. Anterior cervical lymphadenopathy (in about 30 to 50% of cases) usually occurs early, and the nodes are often tender. Pain can be relatively mild to severe enough to make swallowing difficult. Clinical manifestations usually subside in 3 to 5 days unless complicated by sinusitis or parapharyngeal, peritonsillar, or retropharyngeal abscess. Nonsuppurative complications may appear after the onset of GABHS (i.e., AGN in about 10 days and RF in an average of 18 days).

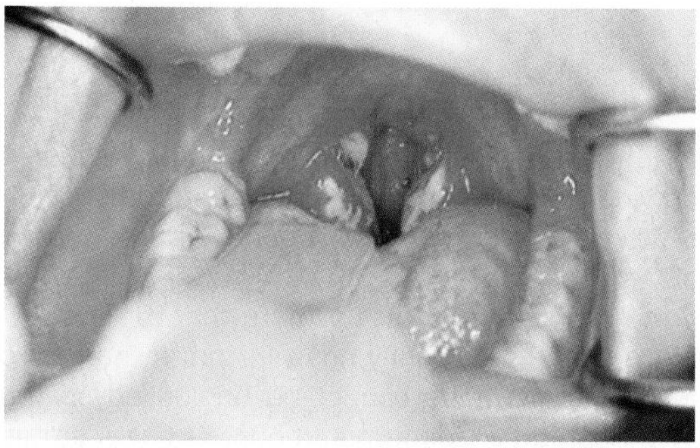

Fig. 46-1 Tonsillitis and pharyngitis. *(Courtesy Dr. Edward L. Applebaum, Head, Department of Otolaryngology, University of Illinois Medical Center, Chicago.)*

evolve Case Study—Tonsillitis
evolve Anatomy Review—Location of Tonsillar Masses

Diagnostic Evaluation

Although 80 to 90% of all cases of acute pharyngitis are viral, a throat culture should be performed to rule out GABHS. Most streptococcal infections are short-term illnesses, and antibody responses appear later than symptoms and are useful only for retrospective diagnosis.

Rapid identification of GABHS with diagnostic test kits (rapid antigen detection test) is possible in the office or clinic setting. Because of the high specificity of these rapid tests, a positive test result generally does not require throat culture confirmation. These rapid kits are not used everywhere in Canada. However, the sensitivities of these kits vary considerably, and a confirmatory throat culture is recommended in patients who have a negative test result (Healthlink BC, 2010).

Therapeutic Management

If streptococcal sore throat infection is present, oral penicillin is prescribed in a dose sufficient to control the acute local manifestations and maintain an adequate level for at least 10 days to eliminate any organisms that might remain to initiate RF symptoms. Penicillin does not prevent the development of AGN in susceptible children; however, it may prevent the spread of a nephrogenic strain of GABHS to others in the family. Penicillin usually produces a prompt response within 24 hours. Patients who have a history of RF or who remain symptomatic after a full course of antibiotics may require a follow-up throat swab.

Intramuscular (IM) benzathine penicillin G is an appropriate therapy, but it is painful and is not the first choice for children. Oral erythromycin is indicated for children allergic to penicillin. Other antibiotics used to treat GABHS are azithromycin, clarithromycin, oral cephalosporins, amoxicillin, and amoxicillin with clavulanic acid (American Academy of Pediatrics [AAP], Committee on Infectious Diseases, & Pickering, 2009).

Nursing Care Management

The nurse often obtains a throat swab for culture and instructs the parents about administering penicillin and **analgesics** as prescribed. Cold or warm compresses to the neck may provide relief. In children who can gargle, warm saline gargles offer relief of throat discomfort. Pain may interfere with oral intake, and children should not be forced to eat. Cool liquids or ice chips are usually more acceptable than solids.

Special emphasis should be placed on correct administration of oral medication and completing the course of antibiotic therapy (see Administration of Medication, Chapter 45). If injections are required, they must be administered deep into a large muscle mass (e.g., vastus lateralis or ventrogluteal muscle). To prevent pain, application of a topical analgesic such as EMLA or LMX 4 over the injection site before the injection is helpful (see Administration of Medication: Intramuscular Administration, Chapter 45). Parents also need to be aware of residual tenderness at the injection site, which may cause the child to limp for a day or two. Local application of heat is helpful in relieving this discomfort.

Nurses play a key role in preventing the spread of disease. Children are considered noninfectious to others 24 hours after initiation of antibiotic therapy, but they should not return to school or day care until they have been taking antibiotics for a full 24-hour period. Nurses should remind the children to discard their toothbrush and replace it with a new one after they have been taking antibiotics for 24 hours. Parents should be cautioned to prevent other household members, especially if immunocompromised, from having close contact with the sick child and avoid sharing drinking or eating items.

Tonsillitis

The tonsils are masses of lymphoid tissue located in the pharyngeal cavity. They filter and protect the respiratory and alimentary tracts from invasion by pathogenic organisms and play a role in antibody formation. Although their size varies, children generally have much larger tonsils than those of adolescents or adults. This difference is thought to be a protective mechanism because young children are especially susceptible to URIs.

Pathophysiology

Several pairs of tonsils are part of a mass of lymphoid tissue encircling the nasal and oral pharynx, known as the *Waldeyer tonsillar ring* (Fig. 46-2). The *palatine* or *faucial tonsils* are located on either side of the oropharynx, behind and below the pillars of the fauces (opening from the mouth). A surface of the palatine tonsils is usually visible during oral examination. The palatine tonsils are those removed during tonsillectomy. The *pharyngeal tonsils*, also known as the *adenoids*, are located above the palatine tonsils on the posterior wall of the nasopharynx. Their proximity to the nares and eustachian tubes causes difficulties in instances of **inflammation**. The *lingual tonsils* are located at the base of the tongue. The *tubal tonsils*, found near the posterior nasopharyngeal opening of the eustachian tubes, are not part of the Waldeyer tonsillar ring.

Etiology

Tonsillitis often occurs with pharyngitis. The causative agent may be viral or bacterial. Because of the abundant lymphoid tissue and the frequency of URIs, tonsillitis is a common cause of morbidity in young children.

Clinical Manifestations

The manifestations of tonsillitis are caused by inflammation. As the palatine tonsils enlarge from **edema**, they may meet in

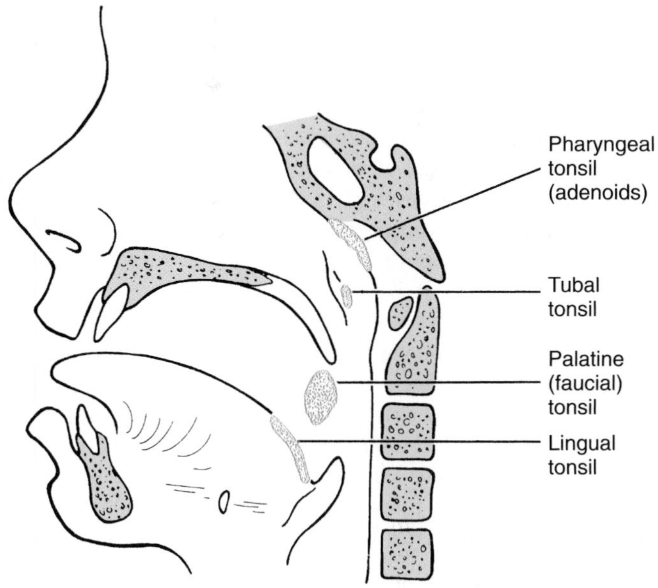

Fig. 46-2 Location of various tonsillar masses.

the midline (kissing tonsils), obstructing the passage of air or food. The child has difficulty swallowing and breathing. When the adenoids enlarge, the space behind the posterior nares becomes blocked, making it difficult or impossible for air to pass from the nose to the throat. As a result, the child breathes through the mouth.

Therapeutic Management

Because tonsillitis is self-limiting, treatment of viral pharyngitis is symptomatic. Throat cultures positive for GABHS infection warrant antibiotic treatment. It is important to differentiate between viral and streptococcal infection in febrile exudative tonsillitis. Because most infections are of viral origin, early rapid tests can eliminate unnecessary antibiotic administration.

Tonsillectomy is the surgical removal of the palatine tonsils. Absolute indications for a tonsillectomy are malignancy, recurrent peritonsillar abscess, and airway obstruction. *Adenoidectomy* (the surgical removal of the adenoids) is recommended for children who have hypertrophied adenoids that obstruct nasal breathing; additional indications for adenoidectomy include recurrent adenoiditis and sinusitis, otitis media (OM) with effusion, airway obstruction and subsequent sleep-disordered breathing, and recurrent rhinorrhea (Benninger & Walner, 2007a). The Canadian Society of Otolaryngology, Head and Neck Surgery (n.d.) lists 6 episodes of tonsillitis per year, missing 20 days of school or work, and or recurrent peritonsillar abcesses as an indication for tonsillectomy or adenotonsillectomy. However, for some children the effectiveness of tonsillectomy or adenoidectomy is modest and may not justify the risk of surgery (van Staaij et al., 2004). In practice, many physicians rely on individualized decision making and do not subscribe to an absolute set of eligibility criteria for these surgical procedures (Paradise et al., 2002). Contraindications to either tonsillectomy or adenoidectomy are (1) cleft palate because tonsils help minimize the escape of air during speech, (2) acute infections at the time of surgery because locally inflamed tissues increase the risk of bleeding, and (3) uncontrolled systemic diseases or blood dyscrasias.

Nursing Care Management

Nursing care involves providing comfort and minimizing activities or interventions that precipitate bleeding. A soft to liquid diet is preferred. A cool-mist vaporizer keeps the mucous membranes moist during periods of mouth breathing. Warm salt-water gargles, throat lozenges, and analgesic-antipyretic medications such as acetaminophen can be used to promote comfort. Often opioids are needed to reduce pain for the child to drink. Combination nonopioid and opioid elixirs or tablets such as acetaminophen with codeine relieve pain and should be given routinely every 4 hours.

If surgery is required, the child requires the same psychological preparation and physical care as for any other surgical procedure (see Chapters 44 and 45). Most tonsillectomy and adenoidectomy (T&A) surgeries now take place in outpatient settings; however, the priorities of preoperative and postoperative care remain the same. The following discussion focuses on postoperative nursing care for T&A, although both procedures may not be performed.

Until they are fully awake, children are placed on their abdomen or side to facilitate drainage of secretions. Routine suctioning is avoided, and, when performed, it is done carefully to avoid trauma to the oropharynx. When alert, children may prefer sitting up. They should be discouraged from coughing frequently, clearing their throat, blowing their nose, or any other activity that may aggravate the operative site.

Some secretions are common, particularly dried blood from surgery. All secretions and vomitus need to be inspected for evidence of fresh bleeding (some blood-tinged mucus is expected). Dark brown (old) blood is usually present in the emesis, in the nose, and between the teeth. If parents do not expect this, they often become frightened at a time when they need to be calm and reassuring.

The throat is sore after surgery. An ice collar provides relief, but many children find it bothersome and refuse to use it. Most children experience moderate pain after a T&A and need pain medication for at least the first 24 hours. Analgesics may be given rectally or intravenously to avoid the oral route. Because pain is continuous, analgesics should be administered at regular intervals. An antiemetic such as ondansetron (Zofran) may be administered postoperatively (see Pain Management, Chapter 35).

Food and fluids should be restricted until children are fully alert and there are no signs of hemorrhage. Cool water, crushed ice, flavoured ice pops, or diluted fruit juice may be given, but fluids with a red or brown colour should be avoided so that fresh or old blood in emesis can be differentiated from the ingested liquid. Raising the head of the bed helps to reduce edema. Citrus juice may cause discomfort and is usually poorly tolerated. Soft foods, particularly gelatin, cooked fruits, sherbet, soup, and mashed potatoes, are started on the first or second postoperative day or as the child tolerates feeding. The pain from surgery often inhibits fluid intake, reinforcing the need for adequate pain control. Milk, ice cream, and pudding are usually not offered, since milk products coat the mouth and throat and may cause the child to clear the throat, which can initiate bleeding.

Postoperative hemorrhage is uncommon but can occur. The nurse needs to observes the throat directly for evidence of bleeding, using a good source of light and, if necessary, carefully inserting a tongue depressor. Other signs of hemorrhage are tachycardia, pallor, frequent clearing of the throat or swallowing by a younger child, and vomiting of bright red blood. Restlessness, an indication of hemorrhage, may be difficult to differentiate from general discomfort after surgery. Decreasing blood pressure is a late sign of shock.

Surgery may be required to cauterize or ligate a bleeding vessel. Airway obstruction may also occur as a result of edema or accumulated secretions and is indicated by signs of respiratory distress, such as stridor, drooling, restlessness, agitation, increasing respiratory rate, and progressive cyanosis. Suction equipment and oxygen should be available after tonsillectomy.

NURSING ALERT The most obvious early sign of bleeding is the child's continuous swallowing of the trickling blood. While the child is sleeping, note the frequency of swallowing. If continuous bleeding is suspected, notify the surgeon immediately.

Family Support and Home Care

Discharge instructions include (1) avoiding irritating or highly seasoned foods; (2) encouraging at least 4 cups of fluid or food with a high fluid content per day (noncitrus products for 7 to 10 days); (3) avoiding gargles or vigorous toothbrushing; (4) avoiding coughing, clearing the throat, or putting objects in the mouth; the child should sneeze with an open mouth; (5) using analgesics (acetaminophen only) or an ice collar for pain; and (6) limiting activity to decrease the potential for bleeding. Objectionable mouth odour and slight ear pain with a low-grade fever are common for a few days postoperatively. Persistent severe earache, fever, very stiff neck, or cough requires medical evaluation. Most children are ready to resume normal activity within 1 to 2 weeks after the operation (About Kids Health, 2009).

Hemorrhage may occur up to 10 days after surgery as a result of tissue sloughing from the healing process. Any sign of bleeding warrants immediate medical attention.

Influenza

Influenza, or flu, is caused by three orthomyxoviruses, which are antigenically distinct: types A and B, which cause epidemic disease, and type C, which is unimportant from an epidemiological standpoint. Influenza is spread from one individual to another by direct contact (large-droplet infection) or by articles recently contaminated by nasopharyngeal secretions. While there is no predilection for a specific age group, attack rates are highest in young children who have had no previous contact with a strain. Influenza is frequently most severe in infants. During epidemics, infection among school-age children is believed to be a major source of transmission in a community. The disease is more common during the winter months and has a 1- to 3-day incubation period. Affected persons are most infectious for 24 hours before and after the onset of symptoms. The virus has a peculiar affinity for epithelial cells of the respiratory tract mucosa, where it destroys ciliated epithelium with metaplastic hyperplasia of the tracheal and bronchial epithelium with associated edema. The alveoli may also become distended with a hyaline-like material. The viruses can be isolated from nasopharyngeal secretions early after the onset of infection, and serological tests identify the type by **complement** fixation or the subgroups by hemagglutination inhibition.

Avian Influenza Virus

Several types of influenza were identified in Asian countries that caused mild to severe disease in adults and children. The avian influenza that has resulted in several deaths in Hong Kong, Vietnam, and Thailand has been identified as subtypes H5 and H7 and has as its **host** chickens and wild ducks, in which the mortality rates range from 90 to 100% (Lee & Krilov, 2005). The virus has also been reported to spread among other animals such as pigs and tigers. In humans the viral manifestations of avian influenza often consist of fever and respiratory symptoms—sore throat, rhinorrhea, and cough—occurring within 3 to 5 days of illness (Chokephaibulkit, 2004). Laboratory findings include leukopenia and thrombocytopenia, and moderately elevated liver transaminases are often identified. Patients may rapidly progress to acute respiratory distress syndrome (ARDS) with acute lung injury. In some children the virus is manifest only as an eye infection (conjunctivitis). For most Canadians, there is a very low risk of contracting the avian flu. It is important to know the risks and how to minimize it when travelling to locations that are affected by this flu (Health Canada, 2011). Treatment is aimed at prompt diagnosis and intervention to reduce the onset of ARDS. The virus may respond to influenza medications such as amantadine, rimantadine, oseltamivir, and zanamivir; cases of avian flu in Southeast Asia were resistant to amantadine and rimantadine (Lee & Krilov, 2005). Rimantadine is not indicated for children.

Pandemic Swine H1N1 and Seasonal Influenza

The pandemic H1N1 influenza virus spread quickly across the world in 2009. It is similar to the seasonal influenza. In Canada, the first wave arrived in the spring and early summer of 2009 and peaked in June with a resurgence in the fall. The incubation period is from 1 to 7 days. It is communicable for about 7 days but can be up to 10 days in children and other individuals that have compromised immune systems. As in the seasonal influenza, the infection can be mild to severe. The viral manifestations often include an acute onset of respiratory illness with fever (except in under 5 and over 65 age groups), cough, sore throat, muscle aches, joint pain, or weakness. In the under-5 age group, gastrointestinal symptoms were present in one third. Two-thirds of hospitalized patients had chronic illnesses, **immunosuppression**, or pregnancy. It can be more severe in those 5 to 64 years of age. Most of the individuals with H1N1 were not hospitalized (PHAC, 2010a). At present, laboratory testing in Canada is done only if a significant exposure has occurred. This exposure includes cases in which an individual has been within 1 metre of a confirmed human case of H1N1 or has had close contact with sick or dead domestic poultry or wild birds (PHAC, 2010a). To obtain updated information on the emergence of and progress in treatment of these and other respiratory viruses, the reader is encouraged to visit the Centers for Disease Control and Prevention (CDC) Web site. A good resource for Canadians is the Public Health Agency of Canada (PHAC) Web site (see Additional Resources section at the end of this chapter).

Clinical Manifestations

The manifestations of influenza may be subclinical, mild, moderate, or severe. Most patients have a dry throat and nasal mucosa, a dry cough, and a tendency toward hoarseness. A flushed face, photophobia, myalgia, hyperesthesia, and sometimes exhaustion and lack of energy accompany a sudden onset of fever and chills. Subglottal croup is common, especially in infants. The symptoms of influenza last for 4 or 5 days. Complications include severe viral pneumonia (often hemorrhagic); encephalitis; and secondary bacterial infections such as OM, sinusitis, or pneumonia. Children need to be closely observed for signs of clinical deterioration including new onset of fever, shortness of breath, unexplained chest or abdominal pain, or lethargy or a change in level of consciousness (CPS, 2010a).

Therapeutic Management

Uncomplicated influenza in children usually requires only symptomatic treatment: acetaminophen or ibuprofen for fever and sufficient fluids to maintain hydration. Zanamivir and rimantadine have been approved for the treatment of flu symptoms in children under 18 years of age. Both medications must also be started within 48 hours of symptom onset. Zanamivir is an inhaled medication effective for type A and B influenza. The drug is taken twice daily for 5 days and is administered by a specially designed oral inhaler (Diskhaler). Zanamivir cannot be used for children younger than 7 years of age. A fourth drug, oseltamivir (Tamiflu), is a neuroaminidase inhibitor that may be administered orally for 5 days to children over 1 year (and adults) to decrease the flu symptoms; as with other antiviral medications, it must be taken within 2 days of the onset of symptoms. It is reported to be effective for types A and B influenza (AAP, Committee on Infectious Diseases, & Pickering, 2009). The Canadian Paediatric Society (2010a) guidelines indicate that oseltamivir generally cannot be used in children under 1 year of age with seasonal influenza but can be used in special circumstances with H1N1 influenza. Bronchospasm and a decline in lung function can occur when zanamivir is used in patients with underlying airway disease such as asthma or chronic obstructive pulmonary disease. Rimantadine is effective only for type A virus; this medication is taken orally by tablet or syrup twice daily for 7 days; it cannot be used for children younger than 1 year of age. Children with influenza (or other similar viruses) should not receive aspirin because of its possible link with Reye syndrome.

FluWatch is part of Canada's national surveillance system that provides information on the spread of influenza and influenza-like illnesses on an on-going basis. Specific information is provided every Friday on influenza viruses that are circulating across Canada (see Additional Resources section at the end of this chapter).

Prevention

The National Advisory Committee in Canada is the national surveillance program that provides information on which viral strains are put into each year's influenza vaccines. Vaccines may be administered to prevent influenza. Four inactivated trivalent influenza viral (TIV) vaccines are available in Canada and are safe and effective provided the **antigens** in the vaccine correlate with the circulating influenza viruses (see Immunizations, Chapter 36). A new intradermal vaccine was approved in Canada in 2010 which is designed for adults and older adults. In the 2010–2011 vaccines, a strain of the H1N1 was added to cover this pandemic concern (PHAC, 2010b). Emphasis in immunization is on providing the influenza vaccine to at-risk populations: children, First Nations, Métis, and Inuit peoples, immunocompromised individuals, chronically ill individuals, older adults, and health care workers. The live-attenuated influenza vaccine (LAIV) is a nasal spray flu vaccine called FluMist and has been approved in Canada for administration in children 2 years of age up to adults age 59 years. However, this preparation contains a live virus and should not be used in individuals who are immunocompromised, have anaphylactic reactions to egg protein, have reactive airway disease, are receiving immunosuppressive therapy, have a chronic respiratory condition, or have a history of Guillain-Barré syndrome. FluMist is available in some pharmacies but the government influenza vaccine program does not provide them. Parents or individuals may purchase them to avoid an injection (CPS, 2010c).

Nursing Care Management

Nursing care is the same as that for any child with a URI, including implementing measures to relieve symptoms. The greatest danger to affected children is development of a secondary infection. Prolonged fever or appearance of fever during early convalescence is a sign of secondary bacterial infection and should be reported to the practitioner for antibiotic therapy.

Otitis Media

OM is one of the 12 most prevalent diseases of early childhood. Its incidence is highest in the winter months. The majority of cases of bacterial OM are preceded by a viral respiratory infection. The two viruses most likely to precipitate OM are RSV and influenza. Most episodes of acute otitis media (AOM) occur in the first 24 months of life, but the incidence decreases with age, except for a small increase at age 5 or 6 years when children enter school. OM occurs infrequently in children older than 7 years of age. Preschool-age boys are affected more frequently than preschool-age girls. Passive smoking increases the risk of persistent middle ear effusion by enhancing attachment of the pathogens that cause otitis to the respiratory epithelium in the middle ear space, prolonging the inflammatory response, and impeding drainage through the eustachian tube (CPS, 2009a). Daycare and a young age are the highest risk factors for OM. The other lesser factors include orofacial abnormalities, household crowding, exposure to cigarette smoke, premature birth, not being breast fed, **immunodeficiency**, and a positive family history of chronic OM (CPS, 2009a). The high rate of chronic suppurative OM among

Aboriginal children is likely due to the fact that First Nations, Métis, and Inuit peoples have 3 times the smoking rates of the general Canadian population (CPS, 2010b).

OM has been defined in a variety of ways. The standard terminology used to define it is outlined in Box 46-5, and AOM treatment guidelines have been published (Canadian Task Force on Preventive Health Care, 2003).

Etiology

Streptococcus pneumoniae, *H. influenzae*, and *Moraxella catarrhalis* are the three most common bacteria causing AOM. The etiology of noninfectious OM is unknown, although OM may occur because of blocked eustachian tubes from the edema of URIs, allergic rhinitis, or hypertrophic adenoids. Chronic OM is frequently an extension of an acute episode.

A relationship has been observed between the incidence of OM and infant feeding methods. Infants fed breast milk have a lower incidence of OM than that of formula-fed infants. Breastfeeding may protect infants against respiratory viruses and allergy because it contains secretory immune globulin A, which limits the exposure of the eustachian tube and middle ear mucosa to microbial pathogens and foreign proteins. Reflux of milk up the eustachian tubes is less likely in breast-fed infants because of the semivertical positioning during breastfeeding compared with positioning during bottle-feeding.

Pathophysiology

OM is primarily a result of malfunctioning eustachian tubes. The eustachian tube is part of a contiguous system composed of the nares, nasopharynx, eustachian tube, middle ear, and mastoid antrum and air cells. Eustachian tubes have three functions relative to the middle ear: (1) protection of the middle ear from nasopharyngeal secretions, (2) drainage of secretions produced in the middle ear into the nasopharynx, and (3) ventilation of the middle ear to equalize air pressure within the middle ear and atmospheric pressure in the external ear canal and to replenish oxygen that has been absorbed.

Mechanical or functional obstruction of the eustachian tube causes accumulation of secretions in the middle ear. Intrinsic obstruction can be caused by infection or allergy; extrinsic obstruction is usually a result of enlarged adenoids or nasopharyngeal tumours. Persistent collapse of the tube during swallowing can cause functional obstruction associated with decreased stiffness or an inefficient opening mechanism. Eustachian tube obstruction results in negative middle ear pressure and, if persistent, produces a transudative middle ear effusion. Drainage is inhibited by sustained negative pressure and impaired ciliary transport within the tube. When the passage is not totally obstructed, contamination of the middle ear can take place by reflux, aspiration, or insufflation during crying, sneezing, nose-blowing, and swallowing when the nose is obstructed.

BOX 46-5 Standard Terminology for Otitis Media

Otitis media (OM)—An inflammation of the middle ear without reference to etiology or pathogenesis

Acute otitis media (AOM)—An inflammation of the middle ear space with a rapid onset of the signs and symptoms of acute infection

- Signs of middle ear effusion with an immobile tympanic membrane with opacification, loss of landmarks, and visible air–fluid level behind the membrane or fluid present in the ear canal from a ruptured tympanic membrane
- Signs of middle ear inflammation with signs with marked discolouration
- Acute onset of symptoms of ear pain or unexpected irritability in a preverbal child

Otitis media with effusion (OME)—Fluid in the middle ear space without symptoms of acute infection

Diagnostic Evaluation

Careful assessment of the tympanic membrane to see if it is immobile with a pneumatic otoscope is essential to differentiate AOM from OM with effusion (OME). Tympanography and acoustic reflectometry are other diagnostic tools; fluid may also be present in the external ear canal from a tympanic membrane rupture. A diagnosis of AOM is made if visual inspection of the tympanic membrane reveals a purulent discoloured effusion; a bulging or full, opacified, or reddened immobile membrane with loss of bony landmarks; and visible air–fluid levels behind the tympanic membrane (CPS, 2009a). Some practitioners also consider the presence of acute onset of less than 48 hours of ear pain with the preceding criteria to be a diagnostic factor in AOM (Powers, 2007). An immobile tympanic membrane or an orange-discoloured membrane indicates OME. Clinical symptoms of otitis are also helpful in making the diagnosis (Box 46-6). In AOM, symptoms such as acute onset of ear pain, fever, and a bulging yellow or red tympanic membrane are usually present. In OME, these symptoms may be absent, and other nonspecific symptoms such as rhinitis, cough, or diarrhea are often present (CPS, 2009a).

Therapeutic Management

Treatment for AOM is one of the most common reasons for antibiotic use in the ambulatory setting. However, concerns about drug-resistant *S. pneumoniae* and other drug resistances have led infectious disease authorities to recommend careful and judicious use of antibiotics for treatment of this illness. Watchful waiting for 48 to 72 hours for spontaneous resolution is safe and appropriate management of AOM in healthy infants over 6 months and in children without craniofacial abnormalities who have mild clinical signs and symptoms and a fever lower than 39°C (CPS, 2009a). It is essential that these children have medical follow-up and that parents be able to recognize a lack of improvement and treat with analgesics. The parents should be given a deferred prescription for antimicrobials if there isn't improvement in the condition. Some reviews of the treatment of AOM show no clear evidence that antibiotics improve outcomes in children younger than 2 years of age with uncomplicated AOM. However, the watchful-waiting approach is not recommended for children younger than 2 years who have persistent acute symptoms of fever and severe

BOX 46-6 Clinical Manifestations of Otitis Media

Acute Otitis Media
Follows an upper respiratory infection
Otalgia (earache)
Fever
Purulent discharge (otorrhea) may or may not be present

Infant or Very Young Child
Crying
Fussy, restless, irritable
Tendency to rub, hold, or pull affected ear
Rolls head from side to side
Difficulty comforting child
Loss of appetite

Older Child
Crying or expressing feelings of discomfort
Irritability
Lethargy
Loss of appetite

Chronic Otitis Media
Hearing loss
Difficulty communicating
Possible feeling of fullness, tinnitus, or vertigo

ear pain (CPS, 2009a). In addition, all cases of AOM in infants younger than 6 months of age should be treated with antibiotics because of the infant's immature immune system and the potential for infection with bacteria other than the three most common organisms found in older infants and children with AOM. Aboriginal children are another group in which watchful waiting is not recommended because of a high incidence of chronic suppurative OM in this group; for them antimicrobials are prescribed (CPS, 2009a).

When antibiotics are warranted, oral amoxicillin in high doses (75 to 90 mg/kg/day, divided twice daily) is the treatment of choice for initial episodes of AOM in children who have not received antibiotics within the past month. The recommendation for the duration of antibiotic therapy is 5 days for most children over 2 years of age and a 10-day course for younger age groups or those with complicated AOM or who have frequent AOM. Second-line antibiotics used to treat OM include amoxicillin, cefprozil, cefuroxime axetil, ceftriaxone IM or IV, azithromycin, and clarithromycin. If initial therapy does not resolve the OM, then amoxicillin-clavulanate or a longer course of ceftriaxone should be given (CPS, 2009a). An important consideration with the use of single-dose IM injections is the pain involved in this therapy. One strategy to minimize pain at the injection site is to reconstitute the cephalosporin with 1% lidocaine. The use of steroids, decongestants, and antihistamines to treat AOM is not recommended.

Supportive care or symptomatic treatment of AOM includes treating the fever and pain. For fever or discomfort associated with OM, analgesic–antipyretic medications such as acetaminophen or ibuprofen may be given. Topical pain relief is recommended by external application of heat or cold, or the practitioner may prescribe topical pain relief drops such as benzocaine drops. Antibiotic ear drops have no value in treating AOM.

Myringotomy, a surgical incision of the eardrum, may be necessary to alleviate the severe pain of AOM. A myringotomy is also performed to provide drainage of infected middle ear fluid in the presence of complications (mastoiditis, labyrinthitis, or facial paralysis) or to allow purulent middle ear fluid to drain into the ear canal for culture. A minimally invasive laser-assisted myringotomy procedure may be performed in outpatient settings.

Tympanostomy tube placement and adenoidectomy are surgical procedures that may be done to treat recurrent OM. Tympanostomy tubes or pressure-equalizer (PE) tubes are grommets that facilitate continued drainage of fluid and allow ventilation of the middle ear. Adenoidectomy is not recommended for treatment of AOM and is performed only in children with recurrent AOM or chronic OME with postnasal obstruction, adenoiditis, or chronic sinusitis.

In some children residual middle ear effusions remain after episodes of AOM. Some children have fluid that persists in the middle ear for weeks or months. Antibiotics are not required for initial treatment of OME but may be indicated for children with persistent effusion for more than 3 months (Gould & Matz, 2010). Placement of tympanostomy tubes is recommended after a total of 4 to 6 months of bilateral effusion with a bilateral hearing deficit (Gould & Matz, 2010). This therapy allows for mechanical drainage of the fluid, which promotes healing of the membrane and prevents scar formation and loss of elasticity. Myringotomy with or without insertion of PE tubes should not be performed for initial management of OME but may be recommended for children who have recurrent episodes of OME with a long cumulative duration (Gould & Matz, 2010). Tonsillectomy either alone or with adenoidectomy is not considered an effective treatment for OME (Gould & Matz, 2010).

OME is frequently associated with mild to moderate impairment of hearing; a hearing test should be performed 3 months after the acute episode of AOM, if OME persists for 3 months or more, or if there is evidence of language or learning delays. Follow-up examinations of children with chronic OME should be maintained on a 3- to 6-month basis until the OME is resolved, a significant hearing loss is identified, or a structural defect of the tympanic membrane or middle ear is identified (Gould & Matz, 2010). Children with hearing loss should be referred to an otolaryngologist and should receive a speech and language evaluation as necessary.

Prevention

In Canada, the pneumococcal conjugate vaccine (PCV7) has limited efficacy in preventing OM because only seven-valent pneumococcal serotypes are in the vaccine (CPS, 2009a). More recently, improved conjugated pneumococcal vaccines with 10-valent and 13-valent serotypes have been developed and approved in Canada. These vaccines will help prevent OM from pneumococci and nontypeable *H. influenza.* Many provinces and territories have incorporated the 13-valent vaccine in their immunization programs (CPS, Infectious Diseases and Immunization Committee, 2011).

evolve Case Study—Mononucleosis

Nursing Care Management

Nursing objectives for the child with AOM include (1) relieving pain, (2) facilitating drainage when possible, (3) preventing complications or recurrence, (4) educating the family in care of the child, and (5) providing emotional support to the child and family.

Analgesic medications such as acetaminophen and ibuprofen are used to treat mild pain. If the ear is draining, the external canal may be cleaned with sterile cotton swabs or cotton balls coupled with topical antibiotic treatment. If ear wicks or lightly rolled sterile gauze packs are placed in the ear after surgical treatment, they should be loose enough to allow accumulated drainage to flow out of the ear; otherwise, infection may be transferred to the mastoid process. The wicks need to stay dry during shampoos or baths. Occasionally, drainage is so profuse that the auricle and the skin surrounding the ear become excoriated from the exudate. This is usually prevented by frequent cleansing and application of various moisture barriers (e.g., Proshield Plus) or petrolatum jelly (e.g., Vaseline).

Tympanostomy tubes may allow water to enter the middle ear, but recommendations for earplugs are inconsistent. Research indicates that swimming without earplugs poses a slightly increased risk of infection (Goldstein et al., 2005). Lake and river water is potentially contaminated, and the wearing of earplugs while swimming in a lake prevents total flooding of the external canal. Bathwater and shampoo water should be kept out of the ear, if possible, because soap reduces the surface tension of water and facilitates entry through the tube. Parents should be aware of the appearance of a grommet (usually a tiny, white, plastic spool-shaped tube) so that they can recognize it if it falls out. They need to be reassured that this is normal and requires no immediate intervention, although they should notify the practitioner.

Prevention of recurrence requires adequate education regarding antibiotic therapy. The symptoms of pain and fever usually subside within 24 to 48 hours, but nurses must emphasize that all of the prescribed medication should be taken. Parents should be aware that potential complications of OM, such as hearing loss, can be prevented with adequate treatment and follow-up care.

Parents also need **anticipatory guidance** regarding methods to reduce the risks of OM, especially in children under 2 years of age. Simple measures, such as good hand and environmental hygiene, sitting or holding an infant upright for feedings, maintaining routine childhood immunizations, and exclusively breastfeeding until at least 3 months of age, can help prevent the occurrence of OM. Propping of bottles should be discouraged, to avoid pooling of milk while the child is in the supine position and to encourage human contact during feeding. Eliminating passive tobacco smoke particularly with preterm infants and known allergens is also recommended. Children under 1 year of age should have limited exposure to daycare (CPS, 2009a).

Early detection of middle ear effusion is essential to prevent complications. Infants and preschool children should be screened for effusion, and all schoolchildren, especially those with learning disabilities, should be tested for middle ear effusion. Frequent audiological evaluations, medical consultation, and education of parents and children are advised when middle ear effusion is detected.

Infectious Mononucleosis

Infectious mononucleosis is an acute, self-limiting infectious disease that is common among adolescents. The illness is characterized by an increase in the mononuclear elements of the blood and by general symptoms of an infectious process. The course is usually mild but occasionally can be severe or, rarely, accompanied by serious complications.

Etiology and Pathophysiology

The herpes-like Epstein-Barr virus (EBV) is the principal cause of infectious mononucleosis. It appears in both sporadic and epidemic forms, but the sporadic cases are more common. The mechanism of spread has not been proved, but it is believed to be transmitted in saliva by direct intimate contact. It is mildly contagious, but the period of communicability is unknown. There is evidence that the virus is spread through sexual contact, especially when multiple partners are involved (Rimsza & Kirk, 2005). The incubation period following exposure is approximately 30 to 50 days (AAP, Committee on Infectious Diseases, & Pickering, 2009).

Diagnostic Tests

The onset of symptoms may be acute or insidious and may appear anywhere from 10 days to 6 weeks after exposure. The presenting symptoms vary greatly in type, severity, and duration (Box 46-7). The clinical manifestations of infectious mononucleosis are usually less severe (often subclinical or unapparent), and the convalescent phase is shorter in younger children than in older children and young adults. The leukocyte count may be normal or low. Usually lymphocytic leukocytosis develops, and there is an increase in atypical leukocytes in the peripheral blood smear. The heterophil antibody test determines the extent to which the patient's serum will agglutinate sheep red blood cells; the response in this test is primarily to immune globulin M, which is present in the first 2 weeks of the illness in adolescents.

BOX 46-7 Clinical Manifestations of Infectious Mononucleosis

Early Signs

Headache
Malaise
Fatigue
Chills
Low-grade fever
Loss of appetite
Puffy eyes

Acute Disease

Cardinal Features

Fever
Sore throat
Cervical adenopathy

Common Features

Splenomegaly (may persist for several months)
Palatine petechiae
Macular eruption (especially on trunk)
Exudative pharyngitis or tonsillitis

The *spot test (Monospot)* is a slide test of venous blood that has high specificity. It is rapid, sensitive, inexpensive, and easy to perform and has an advantage over the heterophil antibody test (i.e., it can detect significant agglutinins at lower levels, thus allowing earlier diagnosis). Blood is usually obtained for the test by finger puncture or venous sampling and is placed on special paper. If the blood agglutinates, forming fragments or clumps, the test is positive for the infection.

Therapeutic Management

No specific treatment exists for infectious mononucleosis. Simple remedies ordinarily relieve the symptoms. A mild analgesic is often sufficient to relieve the headache, fever, and malaise. Rest is encouraged for fatigue but is not imposed for any specific period. Affected persons are instructed to regulate activities according to their own tolerance unless complicating factors are present. Contact sports are discouraged in the presence of splenomegaly.

Antibiotics are contraindicated unless GABHS are present. If sore throat is severe, effective therapies include gargles; hot drinks; anaesthetic troches; or analgesics, including opioids. Corticosteroids have been used to treat respiratory distress from significant tonsillar inflammation, hemolytic anemia, thrombocytopenia, and neurological complications; however, routine use of steroids is not recommended (AAP, Committee on Infectious Diseases, & Pickering, 2009).

Prognosis

The course of this disease is usually self-limiting and uncomplicated. Acute symptoms often disappear within 7 to 10 days, and persistent fatigue subsides within 2 to 4 weeks. Some adolescents may need to restrict vigorous activities for 2 to 3 months, but the disease rarely extends for longer periods. Complications are uncommon but can be serious and require appropriate management.

Nursing Care Management

Nursing responsibilities are directed toward providing comfort measures to relieve symptoms and helping affected adolescents and their families determine appropriate activities for the stage of the disease. The child should be advised to limit exposure to persons outside the family, especially during the acute phase of illness. Children and adolescents may need diet counselling to select foods that contain sufficient calories to meet growth and energy needs but are easy to swallow. It may be more comfortable to limit intake to liquids during the acute phase; milk shakes are a good alternative to solid foods on a temporary basis. Throat pain may be severe enough to require a mild analgesic such as codeine. Careful nursing assessment of swallowing ability is essential because the edema may cause serious airway compromise in some children.

NURSING ALERT Advise the family to seek medical evaluation of the child or adolescent if any of the following occur:

- Breathing becomes difficult.
- Severe abdominal pain develops.
- Sore throat pain is so severe that the child is unable to drink liquids.
- Respiratory stridor is observed.

Croup Syndromes

Croup is a general term applied to a symptom complex characterized by hoarseness, a resonant cough described as "barking" or "brassy" (croupy), varying degrees of inspiratory stridor, and varying degrees of respiratory distress resulting from swelling or obstruction in the region of the larynx. Acute infections of the larynx are important to address in infants and small children because of their increased incidence in these age groups and because the small diameter of the airway in infants and children places them at risk for significant narrowing with inflammation.

Croup syndromes can affect the larynx, trachea, and bronchi. However, laryngeal involvement often dominates the clinical picture because of the severe effects on the voice and breathing. Croup syndromes are described according to the primary anatomical area affected (i.e., epiglottitis [or supraglottitis], laryngitis, laryngotracheobronchitis [LTB], and tracheitis). In general, LTB occurs in very young children, and epiglottitis is more common in older children. A comparison of croup syndromes is provided in Table 46-1.

With widespread immunization programs aimed at preventing *H. influenzae* type B, the cause of most cases of croup in Canada is attributed to viruses (i.e., parainfluenza virus, human meta-pneumovirus, influenza types A and B, adenovirus, and measles).

evolve Case Study—Acute Epiglottitis

Acute Epiglottitis

Acute epiglottitis, or *acute supraglottitis*, is a serious obstructive inflammatory process that occurs predominantly in children 2 to 8 years of age (Rotta & Wiryawan, 2003) but can occur from infancy to adulthood. The disorder requires immediate attention. The obstruction is supraglottic as opposed to the subglottic obstruction of laryngitis. The responsible organism is usually *H. influenzae*. LTB and epiglottitis do not occur together.

Clinical Manifestations

The onset of epiglottitis is abrupt and can rapidly progress to severe respiratory distress. The child usually goes to bed asymptomatic to awaken later with a sore throat and pain on swallowing. The child will have a fever; appear sicker than clinical findings suggest; and insist on sitting upright and leaning forward with the chin thrust out, mouth open, and tongue protruding (*tripod position*). Drooling of saliva is common because of the difficulty or pain on swallowing and excessive secretions.

NURSING ALERT Three clinical observations that have been found to be predictive of epiglottitis are absence of spontaneous cough, presence of drooling, and agitation. When epiglottitis is suspected, the nurse should not attempt to visualize the epiglottis directly with a tongue depressor or take a throat culture but should refer the child for medical evaluation immediately. Throat inspection should be attempted only when immediate endotracheal intubation can be performed, if needed.

The child tends to be irritable and extremely restless and have an anxious, apprehensive, and frightened expression.

Table 46-1 Comparison of Croup Syndromes

	ACUTE EPIGLOTTITIS	ACUTE LTB	ACUTE SPASMODIC LARYNGITIS	ACUTE TRACHEITIS
Age group affected	2–8 yr	Infant or child under 5 yr	1–3 yr	1 mo–6 yr
Etiological agent	Bacterial	Viral	Viral with allergic component	Viral with allergic component
Onset	Rapidly progressive	Slowly progressive	Sudden; at night	Moderately progressive
Major symptoms	Dysphagia Stridor aggravated when supine Drooling High fever Toxic appearance Rapid pulse and respirations	URI Stridor Brassy cough Hoarseness Dyspnea Restlessness Irritability Low-grade fever Nontoxic appearance	URI Croupy cough Stridor Hoarseness Dyspnea Restlessness Symptoms awakening child Symptoms disappearing during day Tendency to recur	URI Croupy cough Purulent secretions High fever No response to LTB therapy
Treatment	Airway protection Racemic epinephrine Corticosteroids Fluids Reassurance	Racemic epinephrine Corticosteroids Fluids Reassurance	Cool mist	Antibiotics Fluids

LTB, laryngotracheobronchitis; *URI,* upper respiratory infection.

The voice is thick and muffled, with a froglike croaking sound on inspiration, but the child is not hoarse. Suprasternal and substernal retractions may be visible. The child will seldom struggle to breathe, and slow, quiet breathing provides better air exchange. The throat will appear red and inflamed, and a distinctive large, cherry-red, edematous epiglottis will be visible on careful throat inspection.

Therapeutic Management

The course of epiglottitis may be fulminant, with respiratory obstruction appearing suddenly. Progressive obstruction leads to hypoxia, **hypercapnia**, and **acidosis** followed by decreased muscle tone; reduced level of consciousness; and, when obstruction becomes more or less complete, a rather sudden death. A presumptive diagnosis of epiglottitis constitutes an **emergency**.

The child who is suspected of having epiglottitis should be examined in a setting where emergency airway equipment is readily available. Examination of the throat with a tongue depressor is contraindicated until experienced personnel and equipment are available to proceed with immediate intubation or tracheostomy in the event that the examination precipitates further or complete obstruction.

If a lateral neck film is indicated, experienced personnel should accompany the child to the radiology department. It is preferable that a young child, who is likely to become more agitated by the procedure, not be transported but remain on the parent's lap in the examination area during portable radiology. Other procedures, such as insertion of an intravenous (IV) line, that are likely to further agitate the child may need to be delayed until an adequate airway is maintained.

Nasotracheal intubation or tracheostomy is usually considered for the child with epiglottitis with severe respiratory distress. It is recommended that the intubation or tracheostomy and any invasive procedure, such as starting an IV infusion, be performed in an area where emergency **airway management** can be easily and quickly accomplished. Humidified oxygen is administered as necessary either via mask in older children or flowby in younger children to avoid further agitation. Whether or not there is an artificial airway, the child requires intensive observation by experienced personnel. The epiglottal swelling usually decreases after 24 hours of antibiotic therapy, and the epiglottis is near normal by the third day. Intubated children are generally extubated at this time. Additional treatment for children with moderate or severe disease includes administration of nebulized epinephrine (racemic epinephrine) or a mixture of helium and oxygen (heliox) to decrease edema. The use of corticosteroids for reducing edema has become a mainstay in the treatment of epiglottitis. Oral corticosteroid is preferred, but other routes of administration include IM, IV, and nebulized (Wright et al., 2005).

Children with suspected bacterial epiglottitis are given antibiotics intravenously, followed by oral administration, to complete a 7- to 10-day course.

Nursing Care Management

Epiglottitis is a serious and frightening disease for the child and family. It is important to act quickly but calmly and to provide support without increasing anxiety. The child should be allowed to remain in the position that provides the most comfort and security, and parents need to be reassured that everything possible is being done to obtain relief for their child.

Acute care of the child is the same as that described later for the child with LTB. Continuous monitoring of respiratory status, including pulse oximetry (and blood gases if the patient is intubated), is an important part of nursing observations, and the IV infusion is maintained as described in Chapter 45.

Acute Laryngitis

Acute infectious laryngitis is a common illness in older children and adolescents. Infants and smaller children experience more generalized involvement (see the following section on LTB). Viruses are the usual causative agents, and the principal complaint is hoarseness, which may be accompanied by other upper respiratory symptoms (e.g., rhinitis, sore throat, nasal congestion) and systemic manifestations (e.g., fever, headache, myalgia, malaise). Associated complaints vary with the infecting virus. Adenoviruses, human meta-pneumoviruses, and influenza viruses are responsible for more systemic involvement; parainfluenza viruses, rhinoviruses, and RSV cause milder illness.

Therapeutic Management and Nursing Care Management

The disease is usually self-limiting without long-term sequelae. Treatment is symptomatic with fluids and humidified air.

Acute Laryngotracheobronchitis

LTB is the most common croup syndrome. It primarily affects children younger than 5 years of age, and the causative organisms are the parainfluenza virus types 2 and 3, human metapneumovirus, RSV, influenza A and B, and *M. pneumoniae*. The disease is usually preceded by a URI, which gradually descends to adjacent structures. It is characterized by gradual onset of low-grade fever, and the parents often report that the child went to bed and later awoke with a barky, brassy cough. Inflammation of the mucosa lining of the larynx and trachea causes a narrowing of the airway. When the airway is significantly narrowed, the child struggles to inhale air past the obstruction and into the lungs, producing the characteristic inspiratory stridor and suprasternal retractions; other classic manifestations include cough and hoarseness. Respiratory distress in infants and toddlers may be manifested by nasal flaring, intercostal retractions, tachypnea, and continuous stridor.

The typical child with LTB is a toddler who develops the classic barking or seal-like cough and acute stridor after several days of rhinitis. When the child is unable to inhale a sufficient volume of air, symptoms of hypoxia become evident. Obstruction that is severe enough to prevent adequate ventilation and exhalation of carbon dioxide can cause respiratory acidosis and eventually respiratory failure. The progression of symptoms is outlined in Box 46-8.

BOX 46-8 Progression of Symptoms in Laryngotracheobronchitis

Stage I
Fear
Hoarseness
Croupy cough
Inspiratory stridor when disturbed

Stage II
Continuous respiratory stridor
Lower rib retraction
Retraction of soft tissue of neck
Use of accessory muscles of respiration
Laboured respiration

Stage III
Signs of anoxia and carbon dioxide retention
Restlessness
Anxiety
Pallor
Sweating
Rapid respirations

Stage IV
Intermittent cyanosis
Permanent cyanosis
Cessation of breathing

(From Walter, E. B., & Shurin, P. A. [1992]. Acute respiratory infections. In S. Krugman, et al. [Eds.], *Infectious diseases of children* [9th ed.]. St. Louis: Mosby.)

Therapeutic Management

The major objective in medical management is maintaining the airway and providing adequate respiratory exchange. Children with mild croup (no stridor at rest) can be managed at home. Parents should be taught the signs of respiratory distress and instructed to summon professional help early if needed. Children who progress to stage II respiratory symptoms should receive medical attention (see Box 46-8).

High humidity with cool mist provides relief for most children. A cool-air vaporizer can be used at home. In the hospital a nebulized mist for older infants and toddlers may be used to provide increased humidity and supplemental oxygen. However, controversy surrounds the use of mist therapy to treat croup; studies have failed to demonstrate any improvement in subglottic edema with mist therapy (Moore & Little, 2006).

Nebulized epinephrine (racemic epinephrine) is often used in children with severe disease, stridor at rest, retractions, or difficulty breathing. The α-adrenergic effects cause mucosal vasoconstriction and subsequently decrease subglottic edema. The onset of action is rapid, and the peak effect is observed in 2 hours. Children may be discharged home following racemic epinephrine after a 2- to 3-hour period of observation for return of acute symptoms.

Oral steroids have proved effective in the treatment of croup; IM dexamethasone may be given to children who are unable to tolerate oral dosing. Nebulized budesonide may be administered in conjunction with IM dexamethasone. A single dose of oral corticosteroid has been shown to decrease hospitalizations and the need for multiple racemic epinephrine treatments in children with mild croup.

In severe cases of LTB, the administration of heliox may serve to reduce the work of breathing and relieve airway obstruction. Because helium has a lower density than that of room air, it forms a respirable gas (with oxygen) that reduces airway turbulence.

evolve Animation—Intubation

Nursing Care Management

The most important nursing function in the care of children with LTB is continuous, vigilant observation and accurate assessment of respiratory status. Pulse oximetry is commonly used for monitoring oxygenation status. Changes in therapy are frequently based on the nurses' observations and assessments and the child's response to therapy and tolerance of procedures. The trend away from early intubation of children with LTB emphasizes the importance of nursing observations and the ability to recognize impending respiratory failure so that intubation can be implemented without delay. Intubation equipment must be readily accessible and taken with the child during transport to other areas (e.g., radiology, operating room).

NURSING ALERT Early signs of impending airway obstruction include increased pulse and respiratory rate; substernal, suprasternal, and intercostal retractions; flaring nares; and increased restlessness.

Infants or small children find that being enclosed in a tent, coughing, having laryngeal spasms, and needing IV therapy are additional sources of distress. In many acute care facilities the mist tent has been abandoned, and the parent is allowed to hold the infant; if cool mist is used in the treatment, it can be administered through a tube held in front of the patient while the child is held on the parent's lap.

Children with mild croup are allowed to drink beverages they like as long as respiratory status is stable, and parents should be encouraged to try whatever comforting measures work best (e.g., holding their child, rocking, singing). If the child is unable to take oral fluids, IV fluids may be required in addition to IV medications (dexamethasone).

The rapid progression of croup, the alarming sound of the cough and stridor, and the child's apprehensive behaviour and ill appearance combine to create a frightening experience for the parents. They need reassurance about their child's progress and an explanation of treatments. The family should be allowed to remain with their child as much as possible.

The nurse should provide the parents with an opportunity to express their feelings and should provide them with referrals as necessary. Parents need frequent reassurance provided in a calm, quiet manner and education regarding what they can do to make their child more comfortable. Home care includes continued humidity, adequate hydration, and nourishment.

Acute Spasmodic Laryngitis

Acute spasmodic laryngitis (spasmodic croup, "midnight croup," or "twilight croup") is distinct from laryngitis and LTB and is characterized by paroxysmal attacks of laryngeal obstruction that occur chiefly at night. Signs of inflammation are absent or mild, and there is often a history of previous attacks lasting 2 to 5 days, followed by uneventful recovery. This condition usually affects children ages 1 to 3 years. Some children appear to be predisposed to the condition; allergies may be implicated in some cases.

The child will go to bed feeling well or with mild respiratory symptoms but awaken suddenly with the characteristic barking, metallic cough; hoarseness; noisy inspirations; and restlessness. The child may appear anxious and frightened. Dyspnea is aggravated by excitement, but there is no fever, the attack subsides in a few hours, and the child will appear well the next day.

Therapeutic Management and Nursing Care Management

Spasmodic croup is usually self-limiting, and most children are managed at home. A cool mist humidifier may be recommended for home treatment. Sometimes the spasm is relieved by sudden exposure to cold air (as when the child is taken out into the night air to see the practitioner). Parents are usually advised to have the child sleep in humidified air until the cough has subsided, to prevent subsequent episodes. Children with moderately severe symptoms may be hospitalized for observation and therapy with cool mist and racemic epinephrine, as for LTB. Some patients respond to corticosteroid therapy.

Bacterial Tracheitis

Bacterial tracheitis, an infection of the mucosa of the upper trachea, is a distinct entity with features of both croup and epiglottitis. The disease occurs more commonly in children under 3 years of age and may be a serious cause of airway obstruction that is severe enough to cause respiratory arrest. It is believed to be a complication of LTB, and although *Staphylococcus aureus* is the most frequent organism responsible, *M. catarrhalis*, *S. pneumonia*, and *H. influenzae* have also been implicated.

Many of the manifestations of bacterial tracheitis are similar to those of LTB but are unresponsive to LTB therapy. There is a history of previous URI with croupy cough, stridor unaffected by position, toxicity, absence of drooling, and high fever. A prominent manifestation is the production of thick, purulent tracheal secretions. Respiratory difficulties are secondary to these copious secretions. Children with this condition may develop a life-threatening upper airway obstruction, respiratory failure, ARDS, and multiple organ dysfunction (Hopkins et al., 2006).

Therapeutic Management and Nursing Care Management

Bacterial tracheitis requires vigorous management with antipyretics and antibiotics. Many children require endotracheal intubation and mechanical ventilation; patients are closely monitored for impending respiratory failure if not intubated. Early recognition to prevent life-threatening airway obstruction is essential.

Lower Respiratory Tract Infections

The *reactive portion* of the lower respiratory tract includes the bronchi and bronchioles in children. Cartilaginous support of the large airways is not fully developed until adolescence. Consequently, the smooth muscle in these structures represents a major factor in the constriction of the airway, particularly in the *bronchioles*, the portion that extends from the bronchi to the alveoli. Table 46-2 compares some of the major features of bronchial and bronchiolar infections.

Bronchitis

Bronchitis (sometimes referred to as *tracheobronchitis*) is inflammation of the large airways (trachea and bronchi), which is frequently associated with a URI. Viral agents are the primary cause of the disease, although *M. pneumoniae* is a common cause in children older than 6 years of age. A dry, hacking, nonproductive cough that worsens at night

Table 46-2 Comparison of Conditions Affecting the Bronchi

	ASTHMA*	BRONCHITIS	BRONCHIOLITIS
Description	Exaggerated response of bronchi to a trigger such as URI, dander, cold air, exercise Bronchospasm, exudation, and edema of bronchi	Usually occurs in association with URI Seldom an isolated entity	Most common infectious disease of lower airways Maximum obstructive impact at bronchiolar level
Age group affected	Infancy to adolescence	First 4 yr of life	Usually children 2–12 mo of age; rare after age 2 yr
Etiological agents	Most often viruses such as RSV in infants but may be any of a variety of URI pathogens	Usually viral Other agents (e.g., bacteria, fungi, allergic disorders, airborne irritants) can trigger symptoms	Peak incidence approximately age 6 mo Viruses, predominantly RSVs; also adenoviruses, parainfluenza viruses, human meta-pneumovirus, and *Mycoplasma pneumoniae*
Predominant characteristics	Wheezing, cough	Persistent dry, hacking cough (worse at night) becoming productive in 2–3 days	Laboured respirations, poor feeding, cough, tachypnea, retractions and flaring nares, emphysema, increased nasal mucus, wheezing, may have fever
Treatment	Inhaled corticosteroids, bronchodilators, leukotriene modifiers, allergen, and control of triggers	Cough suppressants if needed	Provide supplemental oxygen if saturations ≤90%; bronchodilators (optional) Suction nasopharynx Ensure adequate fluid intake Maintain adequate oxygenation

*See Asthma, p. 1344.
RSV, respiratory syncytial virus; *URI,* upper respiratory infection.

and becomes productive in 2 or 3 days characterizes this condition.

Bronchitis is a mild, self-limiting disease that requires only symptomatic treatment, including analgesics, antipyretics, and humidity. Cough suppressants may be useful to allow rest but can interfere with clearance of secretions. Most patients recover uneventfully in 5 to 10 days.

Respiratory Syncytial Virus and Bronchiolitis

Bronchiolitis is an acute viral infection with maximum effect at the bronchiolar level. Although most cases of bronchiolitis are caused by RSV, adenoviruses and parainfluenza viruses are also implicated; recently, human meta-pneumovirus has also been associated with bronchiolitis in children. The infection occurs primarily in winter and spring. By age 2 years most children have been infected at least once. In Canada, RSV infection is the most frequent cause of hospitalization of 12,000 children with bronchiolitis who are less than 2 years old. In northern Canada, Aboriginal children have one of the highest rates of RSV bronchiolitis hospitalizations in the world, with a 1% mortality rate and a 3% mortality rate for children with underlying cardiac or respiratory disease, respectively. In a central northern location, the Inuit children have a bronchiolitis rate of up to 57%. There is a lack of morbidity research in the non-Inuit Aboriginal population. The Canadian RSV season is usually from November to April (CPS, 2009b). In addition, severe RSV infections in the first year of life represent a significant risk factor for the development of asthma up to age 13 (Chávez-Bueno et al., 2005). RSV infection may also occur in children older than 1 year who have a chronic or serious disabling illness.

Risk factors include a birth month of November, December, or January; being in daycare or having siblings in daycare; more than six individuals living in the home; a birth weight less than the tenth percentile for gestational age; male gender; and immediate family history without eczema (CPS, 2009b). A Nunavut study revealed additional factors: maternal smoking during pregnancy, residing in communities outside Iqaluit, being of full Inuit lineage, and overcrowding. Researchers found that breastfeeding appeared to be protective (Banerj, Greenberg, & White, 2009). The risk factors for infants developing severe RSV are being less than 6 weeks old, prematurity under 6 months of age, underlying cardiac or respiratory conditions, and immunocompromise (particularly transplant patients) (CPS, Infectious Diseases and Immunization Committee, 2011).

evolve Case Study–Bronchiolitis

Pathophysiology

RSV affects the epithelial cells of the respiratory tract. The ciliated cells swell, protrude into the lumen, and lose their cilia. RSV produces a fusion of the infected cell membrane with cell membranes of adjacent epithelial cells, thus forming a giant cell with multiple nuclei. At the cellular level this fusion results in multinucleated masses of protoplasm, or *syncytia.*

The bronchiolar mucosa swells, and lumina are subsequently filled with mucus and exudate. The walls of the bronchi and bronchioles are infiltrated with inflammatory cells, and peribronchiolar interstitial pneumonitis is usually present. Because luminal epithelial cells are shed into the bronchioles when they die, the lumina are frequently obstructed, particularly on expiration. The varying degrees of obstruction produced in small air passages lead to hyperinflation, obstructive emphysema resulting from partial obstruction, and patchy areas of atelectasis. Dilation of bronchial passages on inspiration allows sufficient space for intake of air, but narrowing of the passages on expiration prevents air from leaving the lungs.

Thus air is trapped distal to the obstruction and causes progressive overinflation (emphysema).

Clinical Manifestations

The illness usually begins with a URI after an incubation of about 5 to 8 days. Symptoms such as rhinorrhea and low-grade fever often appear first. OM and conjunctivitis may also be present. In time, a cough may develop. If the disease progresses, it becomes a lower respiratory tract infection and manifests typical symptoms (Box 46-9). Infants may have several days of URI symptoms or no symptoms except slight lethargy, poor feeding, or irritability.

Once the lower airway is involved, classic manifestations include signs of altered air exchange, such as wheezing, retractions, crackles, dyspnea, tachypnea, and diminished breath sounds. Apnea may be the first recognized indicator of RSV infection in very young infants.

Diagnostic Evaluation

Identification has been simplified by the development of tests done on nasal or nasopharyngeal secretions, using either rapid immunofluorescent antibody–direct fluorescent antibody staining (DFA), or enzyme-linked immunosorbent assay (ELISA) techniques for RSV antigen detection (see Respiratory Secretion Specimens, Chapter 45).

Therapeutic Management

Bronchiolitis is treated symptomatically with cool humidified oxygen, adequate fluid intake, airway maintenance, and medications. Most children with bronchiolitis can be managed at home. Hospitalization is usually recommended for children with respiratory distress or those who cannot maintain adequate hydration. Other reasons for hospitalization include complicating conditions, such as underlying lung or heart disease or associated debilitated states, or a home environment where adequate management is questionable. The infant who is tachypneic or apneic, has marked retractions, seems listless, or has a history of poor fluid intake should be admitted.

Humidified oxygen is administered in concentrations sufficient to maintain adequate oxygenation (Spo_2) at or above 90% as measured by pulse oximetry. The administration of humidified mist is not fully supported. Routine chest physiotherapy (CPT) is not recommended; infants with abundant nasal secretions benefit from periodic suctioning. Fluids by mouth may be contraindicated because of tachypnea, weakness, and fatigue; thus IV fluids are preferred until the acute stage of the disease has passed.

Clinical assessments and noninvasive oxygen monitoring guide therapy. Medical therapy for bronchiolitis is primarily supportive and aimed at decreasing airway hyperresonance and inflammation and promoting adequate fluid intake. Bronchodilators may provide short-term benefits, yet overall significant improvement in the child's condition is not always appreciable. Racemic epinephrine has been shown to produce modest improvement in ventilation status. Corticosteroids and antihistamines have not been shown to be effective and are not recommended for routine use. Antibiotics are not part of the treatment of RSV unless there is a coexisting bacterial infection such as OM (AAP, 2006). Ribavirin, an antiviral medication (synthetic nucleoside analog), is the only specific therapy approved for hospitalized children; however, use of this drug in infants with RSV is controversial because of concerns about the high cost, aerosol route of administration, potential toxic effects among exposed health care personnel, and conflicting results of efficacy trials (AAP, 2006; Chávez-Bueno et al., 2005; Ventre & Randolph, 2007). This medication is aerosolized and delivered via a small-particle aerosol generator. It may be administered by hood, tent, or mask or through ventilator tubing for 12 to 20 hours daily; average duration of therapy is 3 days.

Prevention of Respiratory Syncytial Virus Infection

The only product available in Canada for prevention of RSV is palivizumab, a monoclonal antibody, which is given monthly in an IM injection during RSV season. According to the Canadian Paediatric Society, candidates for palivizumab include infants at highest risk for a severe RSV infection. The lyophilized powder form of palivizumab should be administered within 6 hours of being reconstituted with sterile water because it is preservative free. The health departments of the provinces and territories direct the use of palivizumab (CPS, Infectious Diseases and Immunization Committee, 2011).

A second-generation monoclonal antibody, motavizumab (Numax), is currently undergoing phase III clinical trials; this medication may be more effective in the prevention of RSV than palivizumab. At the present time, the Canadian Paediatric Society is recommending palivizumab to prevent RSV in high-risk populations (CPS, Infectious Diseases and Immunization Committee, 2011).

Nursing Care Management

Children admitted to the hospital with suspected RSV infection may be assigned separate rooms or grouped with other RSV-infected children. Contact and routine precautions should be used, including hand washing, not touching the nasal mucosa or conjunctiva, and using gloves and gowns

BOX 46-9 Signs and Symptoms of Respiratory Syncytial Virus

Initial

Rhinorrhea
Pharyngitis
Coughing/sneezing
Wheezing
Possible ear or eye drainage
Intermittent fever

With Progression of Illness

Increased coughing and wheezing
Tachypnea and retractions
Cyanosis

Severe Illness

Tachypnea greater than 70 breaths/min
Listlessness
Apneic spells
Poor air exchange; poor breath sounds

when entering the patient's room. Other isolation procedures of potential benefit are those aimed at diminishing the number of hospital personnel, visitors, and uninfected children in contact with the child. Another measure is to make patient assignments so that nurses assigned to children with RSV are not caring for other patients who are considered high risk.

Infants with RSV often have copious nasal secretions, making breathing and nursing or bottle-feeding difficult. The child may lose weight or stop breastfeeding altogether. Encourage breastfeeding mothers to continue feeding the infant, or if feedings are contraindicated because of the acuity of the illness, mothers should pump their milk and store it appropriately for later use (see Chapter 26). Parents should be taught how to instill normal saline drops into the nares and suction the mucus with a bulb syringe before feedings and before bedtime so that the child can eat and rest better. Unfortunately, no medications appropriate for infants can help with these symptoms. To address the issue of decreased fluid intake, parents may offer small amounts of clear fluids, 5 to 10 mL at a time, with a medication syringe every 10 minutes or so to maintain adequate hydration. Infants may cough or vomit as the secretions settle in the stomach.

Additional nursing care is aimed at monitoring oxygenation with pulse oximetry, ensuring that bronchodilator therapy is optimized by using a small mask for delivery, and providing information for the parent regarding the infant's status. The unpredictability of the infant's individual response to the disease can compound parental anxiety when they hear about children who had serious morbidity or died from RSV. However, for the most part, infants recover quickly from the disease and resume normal daily activities, including fluid intake. Such infants are at risk for further episodes of wheezing that may or may not involve an RSV infection; parents may be concerned that the infant has another serious case of RSV. It is important that families receive education on how to prevent RSV infections in young infants, including how to avoid RSV exposure, modes of RSV transmission, no exposure of the infant to smoke, and continuing to breastfeed (see Influenza, p. 1324).

Pneumonias

Pneumonia, inflammation of the pulmonary parenchyma, is common in childhood but occurs more frequently in infancy and early childhood. Clinically, pneumonia may occur either as a primary disease or as a complication of another illness. The various types of pneumonia include the following:

Lobar pneumonia—All or a large segment of one or more pulmonary lobes is involved.

Bronchopneumonia—This begins in the terminal bronchioles, which become clogged with mucopurulent exudate to form consolidated patches in nearby lobules; also called *lobular pneumonia*.

Interstitial pneumonia—The inflammatory process is more or less confined within the alveolar walls (interstitium) and the peribronchial and interlobular tissues.

Although the morphological classification is typically used, the most useful classification of pneumonia is based on the etiological agent (i.e., viral, bacterial, mycoplasmal, or aspiration of foreign substances) (see Aspiration Pneumonia, p. 1341). Histomycosis, coccidioidomycosis, and other fungi also cause pneumonia. The causative agent is identified from the clinical history, the child's age, the general health history, the physical examination, radiography, and the laboratory examination. Other terms that describe pneumonias are hemorrhagic, fibrinous, and necrotizing. *Pneumonitis* is a localized acute inflammation of the lung without the toxemia associated with lobar pneumonia.

The clinical manifestations of pneumonia vary depending on the etiological agent, the child's age, the child's systemic reaction to the infection, the extent of the lesions, and the degree of bronchial and bronchiolar obstruction. The causative agent is identified from the clinical history, the child's age, the general health history, the physical examination, radiography, and the laboratory examination.

Viral Pneumonia

Viral pneumonias, which occur more frequently than bacterial pneumonias, are seen in children of all ages and are often associated with viral URIs. Viruses that cause pneumonia include RSV in infants and parainfluenza, influenza, human meta-pneumovirus, and adenovirus in older children. Few clinical symptoms are unique to a specific virus, and differentiation among viruses is usually made by clinical features such as child's age, past medical history, season of the year, and radiographic and laboratory examination (Box 46-10).

The prognosis is generally good, although viral infections of the respiratory tract render the affected child more susceptible to secondary bacterial invasion, especially when there is denuded bronchial mucosa. Treatment is symptomatic and includes measures to promote oxygenation and comfort, such as oxygen administration with cool mist, CPT and postural drainage, antipyretics for fever management, fluid intake, and family support. Some authorities recommend antimicrobial therapy in the hopes of reducing or preventing secondary bacterial infection, but this therapy should be reserved for

BOX 46-10 General Signs of Pneumonia

Fever—Usually quite high

Respiratory

Cough—Nonproductive to productive with whitish sputum
Tachypnea
Breath sounds—Rhonchi or fine crackles
Dullness with percussion
Chest pain; abdominal pain with lower lobe involvement
Retractions
Nasal flaring
Pallor to cyanosis (depends on severity)
Chest x-ray film—Diffuse or patchy infiltration with peribronchial distribution

Behaviour

Irritable, restless, lethargic

Gastrointestinal

Anorexia, vomiting, diarrhea, abdominal pain

children in whom a bacterial infection is demonstrated by appropriate cultures.

Primary Atypical Pneumonia

Atypical pneumonia refers to pneumonia that is caused by pathogens other than the traditionally most common and readily cultured bacteria (e.g., *S. pneumoniae*). In the category of atypical pneumonias, *M. pneumoniae* and *Chlamydia pneumoniae* are the most common causes of community-acquired pneumonia in children 5 years old or older (Rafei & Lichenstein, 2006). It occurs in the fall and winter months and is more prevalent in crowded living conditions. Most affected persons recover from acute illness in 7 to 10 days with symptomatic treatment followed by a week of convalescence. Hospitalization is rarely necessary.

Bacterial Pneumonia

S. pneumoniae is the most common bacterial pathogen responsible for community-acquired pneumonia in both children and adults (Rafei & Lichenstein, 2006). Other bacteria that cause pneumonia in children are group A streptococcus, *S. aureus*, *M. catarrhalis*, *M. pneumoniae*, and *C. pneumoniae*.

Beyond the neonatal period, bacterial pneumonias display distinct clinical patterns that facilitate their differentiation from other forms of pneumonia. The onset of illness is abrupt and generally follows a viral infection that disturbs the natural defence mechanisms of the upper respiratory tract.

The child with bacterial pneumonia usually appears ill. Symptoms include fever, malaise, rapid and shallow respirations, cough, and chest pain. The pain of pneumonia may be referred to the abdomen and confused with appendicitis. Chills and meningeal symptoms (*meningism*) are common.

Most older children with pneumonia can be treated at home if the condition is recognized and treatment is initiated early. Antibiotic therapy, bed rest, liberal oral intake of fluid, and administration of an antipyretic for fever are the principal therapeutic measures. Follow-up examination is recommended for small infants and toddlers. Hospitalization is indicated when pleural effusion or empyema accompanies the disease, when compliance with therapy is estimated to be poor, in infants less than 1 month old, and when there are chronic illnesses such as heart disease or BPD (Rafei & Lichenstein, 2006). IV fluids may be necessary to ensure adequate hydration, and oxygen is required if the child is in respiratory distress; some children may require initial therapy with parenteral antibiotics because of the severity of illness.

Complications

The classic features and clinical course of pneumonia are seen infrequently because of early and vigorous antibiotic and supportive therapy. However, some children, especially infants, with staphylococcal pneumonia develop empyema, pyopneumothorax, or tension pneumothorax. AOM and pleural effusion are common in children with pneumococcal pneumonia.

Continuous closed-chest drainage may be instituted when purulent fluid is aspirated. If a large amount of purulent drainage is obtained, an appropriate antibiotic is instilled into the pleural space, and active chest drainage is discontinued for approximately 1 hour after the instillation. Closed drainage is continued until drainage fluid is free of pathogens, which rarely requires more than 5 to 7 days. Sometimes, repeated pleural taps are sufficient to remove fluid; however, if the purulent drainage accumulates rapidly and is highly viscous, continuous chest drainage is preferred. Thoracotomy with open debridement of the infected lung tissue may be required; if empyema and pneumothorax tend to recur, a partial thoracoscopic lobectomy may be performed.

Prognosis

The prognosis for pneumonia is generally good, with rapid recovery when symptoms are recognized and treated early. Streptococcal infections vary in duration but usually resolve spontaneously. The course of staphylococcal pneumonia is generally prolonged. The prognosis varies with the length of illness before treatment is begun, although early recognition and treatment are usually effective.

Prevention

The use of the heptavalent pneumococcal conjugate vaccine (PCV; Prevnar) is recommended for infants and children younger than 23 months of age, to be administered at 2, 4, 6, 12, and 15 months of age; studies have demonstrated a decrease in pneumococcal pneumonia in children younger than 24 months. The polyvalent pneumococcal polysaccharide vaccine (PPSV) provides protection from pneumococcal serotypes in children 2 years of age and older (PHAC, 2007a) (see Immunizations, Chapter 36).

Nursing Care Management

For the child being cared for at home, the nurse needs to educate the parents on antibiotic and antipyretic administration, assessment of respiratory status, and oral fluid intake. If the child is ill, solid foods may be rejected; fluid intake should be encouraged until the child feels well enough to eat solids. Parents need to be reassured that the child's appetite will return once the acute phase of the illness has passed. If the cough is disturbing, judicious use of antitussives, especially at bedtime, is often helpful. Most sick children are adept at self-regulation of activity and rest; parents should be encouraged to allow the child appropriate rest and discourage vigorous activities until he or she has been afebrile for 24 hours or more. Return to school or day care is usually permitted according to the type of pneumonia, severity of illness, and practitioner recommendation. It should be emphasized that the infection may be transmitted to other children with close contact.

Nursing care of the hospitalized child with pneumonia is primarily supportive and symptomatic but necessitates thorough respiratory assessment, antibiotics, and evaluation of hydration status; supplemental oxygen may be required if oxygenation status is compromised. The child's respiratory rate and oxygenation status, as well as vital signs, pain level, and general disposition and level of activity, are frequently assessed. Isolation procedures are implemented according to hospital policy, but routine and contact precautions are recommended initially for all children with a URI until the exact cause is known. To prevent dehydration, fluids should be frequently administered intravenously during the acute phase.

Nursing care of the child with a chest tube requires close attention to respiratory status; the chest tube and drainage device used should be monitored for proper function (i.e., drainage is not impeded, vacuum setting is correct, tubing is free of kinks, dressing covering chest tube insertion site is intact, water seal is maintained [if used], and chest tube remains in place). Movement in bed and ambulation with a chest tube should be encouraged according to the child's respiratory status; children often require a mild analgesic such as acetaminophen.

If needed, supplemental oxygen may be administered by nasal cannula or face mask (or face tent [bucket]); small infants may be given humidified oxygen via a plastic head hood or, rarely, via a mist tent. Children are usually more comfortable in a semierect position (Fig. 46-3) but should be allowed to determine the position of comfort. Lying on the affected side (if pneumonia is unilateral) splints the chest on that side and can reduce the pleural rubbing that often causes discomfort. Fever is controlled by the cool environment and administration of antipyretic medications.

Children, especially infants, with ineffectual cough or difficulty handling secretions require suctioning to maintain a patent airway. A simple bulb suction syringe is usually sufficient for clearing the nares and nasopharynx of infants, but mechanical suction should be readily available if needed. A noninvasive suction device may be used to suction the infant's nares without the danger of causing nasal trauma; the device may be connected to mechanical suction for best results. Older children can usually handle secretions without assistance. Postural drainage, CPT, and nebulized bronchodilator treatments may be prescribed, depending on the child's condition.

The hospitalized child may be apprehensive, and the treatments and tests can be frightening and stress producing. Reducing anxiety and apprehension reduces psychological distress, and when the child is more relaxed, the respiratory efforts are lessened. Easing respiratory efforts makes the child less apprehensive; the presence of a caregiver often provides the child with a source of comfort and support. It is important to involve the entire family in the child's care, as appropriate, and to encourage questions and facilitate effective communication. Allowing the child to be involved in regular activities such as quiet play may help reduce the anxiety of hospitalization and separation from friends and family.

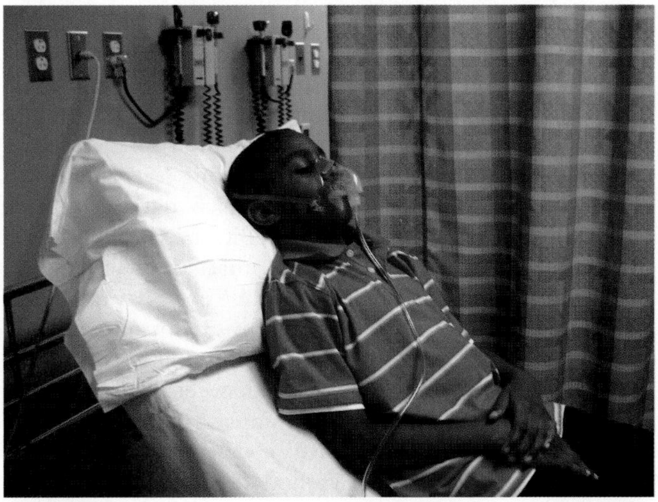

Fig. 46-3 A child placed in a semierect position is often more comfortable, and this position enhances diaphragmatic expansion.

Other Respiratory Tract Infections

Pertussis (Whooping Cough)

Pertussis, or whooping cough, is an acute respiratory tract infection caused by *Bordetella pertussis* that in the past primarily occurred in children younger than 4 years of age who were not immunized. It is highly contagious and is particularly threatening in young infants, who have a higher morbidity and mortality rate. One in three individuals die from pertussis in Canada on an annual basis; young infants who have not completed their pertussis immunization are at the most risk (PHAC, 2007a). Infants less than 6 months of age may not come in to the practitioner with the typical cough; in this age group, apnea is a common presenting manifestation (AAP, Committee on Infectious Diseases, & Pickering, 2009). Likewise, older children are known to manifest the disease with a persistent cough and the absence of the characteristic whoop (see Table 38-2 for clinical manifestations of pertussis and Chapter 36 for immunization). The incidence is highest in the spring and summer months, and a single attack confers lifetime immunity. The resurgence of pertussis in Canada, particularly in older children and adults, is due to weakening immunity from vaccines produced in the mid-1990s. Consequently, two acellular pertussis booster vaccines have been approved in Canada and include one for 2 months to 7 years of age and the other for ages 11 years to 54 years. This older population is a reservoir for pertussis, which can be passed along to the young at-risk infant (PHAC, 2007a).

Tuberculosis

Tuberculosis (TB) is an infectious disease that most Canadians will never develop. In Canada, there are approximately 1600 new cases of reported TB every year. The risk factors for developing TB include the following populations: those with human immunodeficiency virus (HIV) or acquired immune deficiency syndrome (AIDS); those who come in close contact with individuals with known or suspected active TB, with active TB, or who have a past history of TB but did not receive adequate treatment; individuals living in First Nations, Métis, or Inuit communities with high rates of TB; poor, particularly urban homeless individuals; residents of long-term care and correctional facilities; individuals with transplants, diabetes mellitus, or cancer of the head and neck; those with chronic kidney disease who are on dialysis; those who have been infected by TB bacteria within the past 2 years; individuals who have undergone steroid treatments or treatment for **autoimmune disorders;** those who are underweight or were under age 5 when infected with TB; individuals who smoke 1 pack of cigarettes a day or more; and individuals working with any of these groups (Health Canada, 2009a).

TB is caused by *Mycobacterium tuberculosis*, an acid-fast bacillus not readily decolourized by acids after staining. Children are susceptible to the human (*M. tuberculosis*) and the bovine (*Mycobacterium bovis*) organisms. In parts of the world where TB in cattle is not controlled or milk is not pasteurized, the bovine type is a common source of infection.

Although the causative agent for TB is the tubercle bacillus, other factors influence the degree to which the organism produces an altered state in the host. These factors include heredity (resistance to the infection may be genetically transmitted), gender (higher rates in adolescent girls), age (lower resistance in infants, higher incidence during adolescence), stress (emotional or physical), nutritional state, and intercurrent infection (especially HIV, measles, and pertussis). Children with HIV infection have an increased incidence of TB disease, and all children with TB should be tested for HIV.

The source of TB infection in children is usually an infected member of the household or a frequent visitor to the home, such as a babysitter or domestic worker. The lung is the usual portal of entry for the organism. In the lungs, a proliferation of epithelial cells surrounds and encapsulates the multiplying bacilli in an attempt to wall it off, thus forming the typical tubercle. Extension of the primary lesion at the original site causes progressive tissue destruction as it spreads within the lung, discharges material from foci to other areas of the lungs (e.g., bronchi, pleura), or produces pneumonia. Erosion of blood vessels by the primary lesion can cause widespread dissemination of the tubercle bacillus to near and distant sites (miliary TB). Extrapulmonary TB may manifest as superior lymphadenitis, meningitis, and osteoarthritis and may appear in the middle ear and mastoid and on the skin (AAP, Committee on Infectious Diseases, & Pickering, 2009). With the exception of meningitis, treatment for extrapulmonary TB may be with the same medication regimen as for pulmonary TB.

Canada is participating in the World Health Organization's (WHO's) global plan to decrease the rate of TB worldwide by the year 2015. The Canadian government's goal by 2015 is to reduce the Aboriginal TB rate to 3 per 100,000 for on-reserve individuals (Health Canada, 2008a). The rates of TB among First Nations, Métis, and Inuit peoples in 2000 were 8 to 10 times higher than for Canadian-born non-Aboriginals. However, this figure is the lowest rate ever, so some progress has been made in decreasing the tuberculin rate. Aboriginal pediatric and young-adult TB rates are still high, and there is a cycle of transmission that is still present in First Nations, Métis, and Inuit communities. Additional risk factors for this population include substance use; diabetes; HIV; overcrowding, and moving from reserve to reserve (Health Canada, 2006a).

Diagnostic Evaluation

Diagnosis is based on information derived from physical examination, history, tuberculin skin testing, radiographic examinations, and cultures of the organism. The clinical manifestations of the disease are extremely variable (Box 46-11).

The *tuberculin skin test (TST)* is the most important indicator of whether a child has been infected with the tubercle bacillus. The standard dose of purified protein derivative (PPD) is 5 tuberculin units, which is administered using a 27-gauge needle and a 1-mL syringe intradermally into the volar aspect of the forearm. Creation of a visible wheal is crucial to accurate testing. In Canada, the current recommendations are to screen only children who are at high risk for TB infections or who are progressing from latent to active TB disease (Kakkar, Allen, Ling, Pai, & Kitai, 2010).

BOX 46-11 Clinical Manifestations of Tuberculosis

May be asymptomatic or produce a broad range of symptoms:
- Fever
- Malaise
- Anorexia
- Weight loss
- Cough (may or may not be present; progresses slowly over weeks to months)
- Aching pain and tightness in the chest
- Hemoptysis (rare)

With progression:
- Increased respiratory rate
- Poor expansion of lung on the affected side
- Diminished breath sounds and crackles
- Dullness on percussion
- Persistent fever
- Generalized symptoms
- Pallor, anemia, weakness, and weight loss

A *positive reaction* indicates that the individual has been infected and has developed sensitivity to the tubercle bacillus. However, it does not confirm the presence of active disease. Once an individual reacts positively, he or she will always react positively. A previously negative reaction that becomes positive indicates that the person has been infected since the last test. Guidelines for interpreting the TST are listed in Box 46-12. Prompt radiographic evaluation of all children with a positive TST reaction is recommended. The Canadian Paediatric Society recommends that administration of the TST and interpretation of the results be performed and read only by trained health care providers (CPS, Infectious Diseases and Immunization Committee, 2010).

The term *latent tuberculosis infection* (LTBI) is used to indicate infection in a person who has a positive TST, no physical findings of disease, and normal chest radiograph findings. The term *tuberculosis disease* is used when a child has clinical symptoms or radiographic manifestations caused by the *M. tuberculosis* organism. A diagnosis of LTBI or TB disease in a child is a sentinel event usually representing recent transmission of the *M. tuberculosis* organism. New blood tests have been developed to help diagnose LTBI. The two interferon-gamma-release-assay tests (IGRA) that are registered in Canada are QuantiFERON-TB Gold In-Tube assay and the T. Spot-TB test, which provide greater sensitivity and accuracy. The TST is not very sensitive for detecting LTBI and can give a false-positive reading. The Canadian Paediatric Society (CPS, Infectious Diseases and Immunization Committee, 2010) recommends that the IGRA be used as a diagnostic aid in combination with the TST and other radiological and culture tests to help diagnose active TB. IGRA cannot be used to diagnose TB without other positive tests. A negative IGRA test does not mean that a child does not have LTBI.

BOX 46-12 Definition of Positive Tuberculin Skin Test (TST) Results in Infants, Children, and Adolescents*

Induration 5 mm or Greater

Children in close contact with known or suspected contagious cases of tuberculosis (TB) disease

Children suspected of having TB disease:

- Findings on chest x-ray film consistent with active or previously active TB
- Clinical evidence of TB disease†

Children receiving immune suppressive therapy‡ or who have immunosuppressive conditions, including HIV infection

Induration 10 mm or Greater

Children at increased risk of disseminated disease:

- Those younger than 4 years of age
- Those with other medical risk conditions, including Hodgkin's disease, lymphoma, diabetes mellitus, chronic renal failure, or malnutrition

Children at increased risk of exposure to TB disease:

- Those born, or whose parents were born, in high-prevalence (TB) regions of the world
- Those frequently exposed to adults who are HIV infected, homeless, users of illicit drugs, residents of nursing homes, incarcerated or institutionalized, or migrant farm workers
- Those who travel to high-prevalence (TB) regions of the world

Induration 15 mm or Greater

Children 4 years of age or older without any risk factors

(From American Academy of Pediatrics, Committee on Infectious Diseases, & Pickering, L. [Eds.]. [2012]. *Red book: 2012 report of the Committee on Infectious Diseases.* [29th ed.]. Elk Grove Village, IL: The Academy.)

*These definitions apply regardless of previous Bacille Calmette-Guérin (BCG) immunization; erythema at TST site does not indicate a positive test result. TSTs should be read at 48 to 72 hours after placement.

†Evidence by physical examination or laboratory assessment that would include tuberculosis in the working differential diagnosis (e.g., meningitis).

‡Including immunosuppressive doses of corticosteroids.

Therapeutic Management

Medical management of TB disease in children consists of adequate nutrition, pharmacotherapy, general supportive measures, prevention of unnecessary exposure to other infections that would further compromise the body's defences, prevention of reinfection, and sometimes surgical procedures.

The recommended medication regimen for LTBI in children and adolescents includes a daily dose of isoniazid (INH) for 9 months or, alternatively, two or three times per week, with direct observation of therapy (DOT). DOT means that a health care worker or other responsible, mutually agreed-on individual is present when medications are administered to the patient. Rifampin (daily for 6 months; alternatively, DOT twice weekly for 6 months) may be used to treat the child or adolescent who is INH resistant (PHAC, 2008).

For the child with clinically active TB, the goal is to achieve sterilization of the tuberculous lesion. Recommended medication therapy for treating TB disease includes combinations of INH, rifampin, and pyrazinamide (PZA). The American Academy of Pediatrics, Committee on Infectious Diseases, and Pickering (2009) and the Public Health Agency of Canada (2008) recommend a 6-month regimen consisting of INH, rifampin, and PZA given daily for the first 2 months, followed by INH and rifampin given two or three times a week by DOT for the remaining 4 months. DOT decreases the rates of relapse, treatment failures, and drug resistance and is recommended for treatment of children and adolescents with TB in Canada.

If the child is suspected of having multidrug-resistant TB, a fourth medication such as streptomycin (IM injection only) or ethambutol is added. Optimal therapy for TB in children with HIV infection has not been established, and consultation with a specialist is advised. Therapy should always include at least three medications initially and be continued for at least 9 months. INH, rifampin, and PZA, usually with ethambutol or an aminoglycoside, should be given for at least the first 2 months. The three-medication regimen can be used after drug-resistant disease is excluded.

Surgical procedures may be required to remove the source of infection in tissues that are inaccessible to pharmacotherapy or that are destroyed by the disease. Orthopaedic procedures may be performed for correction of bone deformities, and bronchoscopy may be done for removal of a tuberculous granulomatous polyp.

Prognosis

Most children recover from primary TB infection and are often unaware of its presence. However, very young children have a higher incidence of disseminated disease. TB is a serious disease during the first 2 years of life, during adolescence, and in children who are HIV positive. Except in cases of tuberculous meningitis, death seldom occurs in treated children. Antibiotic therapy has decreased the death rate and the hematogenous spread from primary lesions.

Prevention

The only definite means of preventing TB is to avoid contact with the tubercle bacillus. Maintaining an optimal state of health with adequate nutrition and avoiding fatigue and debilitating infections promote natural resistance but do not prevent infection. Pasteurization and routine testing of milk and elimination of diseased cattle have reduced the incidence of bovine TB.

Limited immunity can be produced by the administration of bacille Calmette-Guérin (BCG), a live vaccine containing bovine bacilli with reduced **virulence** (attenuated). In most instances, positive tuberculin reactions develop after inoculation with BCG. The vaccine is not used extensively, even in areas with a high prevalence of disease. BCGs are still used in the provinces and territories that have higher TB rates. In the Northwest Territories, BCGs are given routinely to Aboriginal infants where TB is endemic. They are also available to new immigrants who come from TB-endemic countries. Saskatchewan offers BCGs to all infants in 23 of the 65 communities in the Northern-Inter-Tribal Authority. Manitoba offers BCGs to all infants in most First Nation communities. Nunavut offers BCGs to all infants. Ontario offers BCGs only to infants in the Sioux Lookout Zone. IGRA can be used to help diagnose LTBI in individuals with positive skin tests after BCG vaccines were administered (PHAC, 2010c). However, it may be recommended for long-term protection of infants and children with a negative TST who are not infected with HIV and who (1) are at high risk for continuing exposure to persons with infectious pulmonary TB or (2) are continuously exposed to persons with TB who have bacilli resistant to both INH and rifampin when the child cannot be removed from the environment or given anti-TB medication therapy (AAP, Committee on Infectious Diseases, & Pickering, 2009).

Nursing Care Management

Children with TB receive their nursing care in ambulatory settings, outpatient departments, schools, and public health settings. Most children are not contagious and require only routine precautions. Children with no cough and negative sputum smears can be hospitalized in a regular patient room. However, airborne precautions and a negative-pressure room are required for children who are contagious and hospitalized with active TB disease. Infection control for hospital personnel in contagious cases should include the use of a personally fitted air-purifying N95 or N100 respirator for all patient contacts.

Asymptomatic children with TB can attend school or day care facilities if they are receiving pharmacotherapy. They can return to regular activities as soon as effective therapy has been instituted, adherence to therapy has been documented, and clinical symptoms have diminished. Children receiving pharmacotherapy for TB can receive measles and other age-appropriate live virus vaccines unless they are receiving high-dose corticosteroids, are severely ill, or have specific contraindications to immunization. Children with TB should also receive optimal nutrition and adequate rest.

Nurses assume several roles in management of the disease, including helping the family understand the rationale for diagnostic procedures, assisting with radiographic examinations, performing and interpreting skin tests, and obtaining specimens for laboratory examination.

Skin tests must be carried out correctly to obtain accurate results. The tuberculin is injected intradermally with the bevel of the needle pointing upward. A wheal 6 to 10 mm in diameter should form between the layers of the skin when the solution is injected properly. If the wheal is not formed, the procedure is repeated. The volar or dorsal surface of the forearm is the usual injection site. The reaction to the skin test is determined in 48 to 72 hours; however, reactions occurring after 72 hours should be measured and considered the result (AAP, Committee on Infectious Diseases, & Pickering, 2009). The size of the transverse diameter of induration, not the erythema, is measured. The diameter transverse to the long axis of the forearm is the only one standardized for measurement purposes (AAP, Committee on Infectious Diseases, & Pickering, 2009).

Sputum specimens are difficult or impossible to obtain from an infant or young child because they swallow any mucus coughed from the lower respiratory tract. The best means for obtaining material for smears or culture is by gastric washing (i.e., aspiration of lavaged contents from the fasting stomach). The procedure is carried out and the specimen obtained early in the morning before the customary breakfast time. In some cases, an induced sputum specimen may be obtained by administering aerosolized normal saline for 10 to 15 minutes, followed by CPT and suctioning of the nasopharynx for sputum collection.

Because the success of therapy depends on compliance with the medication regimen, parents need to be instructed about the importance and rationale for DOT. Case finding in the community and follow-up of known contacts—individuals from whom the affected child may have acquired the disease and persons who may have been exposed to the child with the disease—are essential control measures.

Severe Acute Respiratory Syndrome

A severe form of atypical pneumonia identified as severe acute respiratory syndrome (SARS) was first reported in Asia in 2003. SARS is caused by a previously unrecognized coronavirus called SARS-associated coronavirus (SARS Co-V). Additional human coronavirus types have since been identified in Canada, Hong Kong, and the Netherlands. In September 2003, 438 cases of SARS were reported in Canada (Health Canada, 2008b). Clinical manifestations of this disorder include a fever greater than 38°C; headache; cough; shortness of breath; difficulty breathing; and after 2 to 7 days, a dry, nonproductive cough and dyspnea. In some patients the symptoms are severe enough to require intubation and mechanical ventilation. The disease is spread by close contact with a person with SARS. Most cases have involved people who have cared for or lived with someone with SARS or people who have travelled to areas with reported cases of SARS.

In children, two distinct forms of the illness have been observed. Adolescents have malaise, myalgia, chills, and rigor, whereas young children have mainly cough and a runny nose. In younger children the clinical course seems to be milder, and the disease resolves more quickly than in adolescents or adults (Denison, 2005; Stockman et al., 2007).

Laboratory findings include lymphopenia; leukopenia; thrombocytopenia; and elevated lactate dehydrogenase, aspartate aminotransferase, and creatinine kinase levels. The most reliable laboratory diagnostic test is positive antibodies for the SARS Co-V. Chest radiographs in a substantial number of patients reveal focal interstitial infiltrates that progress to more generalized, patchy interstitial infiltrates.

Treatment of SARS involves predominantly supportive care measures. Other therapies such as antibiotics, antiviral medications such as ribavirin, and steroids have been used with mixed results (O'Connor, 2003).

Nursing Care Management

There is an extensive Canadian plan with recommendations on how to provide infection control for individuals with diagnosed or potential SARS or any other potential epidemic of infectious diseases. The recommendations follow the premise that patients with SARS receive the same treatment as any patient with serious community-acquired atypical pneumonia. This includes the use of strict hand washing, contact precautions, and airborne precautions (e.g., an isolation room with negative pressure relative to the surrounding area and the use of an N95 filtering disposable respirator for persons entering the room). Recommendations for stopping the spread of SARS have also been developed. When triaging patients, nurses should place a surgical mask on any patient who has had close contact with someone who has SARS or who has a history of international travel to an area with cases of SARS. Health care workers who have had high-risk, unprotected exposure to SARS should be excluded from duty and should remain home from work to monitor their health for 10 days (Health Canada, 2003).

Pulmonary Dysfunction Caused by Noninfectious Irritants

Foreign Body Aspiration

Small children characteristically explore matter with their mouths and are prone to aspirate a foreign body (FB). They also place objects such as beads, paper clips, small magnets, or food items in the nose, which can easily be aspirated into the trachea. While FB aspiration can occur at any age it is most common in children 1 to 3 years of age. Severity is determined by the location, type of object aspirated, and extent of obstruction. For example, dry vegetable matter, such as a seed, nut, or piece of carrot or popcorn, that does not dissolve and that may swell when wet creates a particularly difficult problem. The high fat content of potato chips and peanuts may cause the added risk of lipoid pneumonia. "Fun foods" are the worst offenders in terms of potential for aspiration. Offending foods in the order of frequency of aspiration are hot dog, round candy, peanut or other nut, grape, cookie or biscuit, other meat, carrot, peas, apple, and peanut butter. Other items include plastic or glass beads, button or disc batteries, and coins. Objects such as small lithium or cadmium batteries may cause esophageal or tracheal corrosion.

Diagnostic Evaluation

The diagnosis of FB aspiration is suspected on the basis of the history and physical signs. Initially, an FB in the air passages produces choking, gagging, wheezing, or coughing. Laryngotracheal obstruction most commonly causes dyspnea, cough, stridor, and hoarseness because of decreased air entry. Up to half of all children with FB ingestion may be asymptomatic (Uyemura, 2005). Cyanosis may occur if the obstruction becomes worse. Bronchial obstruction usually produces cough (frequently paroxysmal), wheezing, asymmetrical breath sounds, decreased airway entry, and dyspnea. When an object is lodged in the larynx, the child is unable to speak or breathe. If the obstruction progresses, the child's face may become livid; if the obstruction is total, the child can become unconscious and die of **asphyxiation**. If obstruction is partial, hours, days, or even weeks may pass without symptoms after the initial period. Secondary symptoms are related to the anatomical area in which the object is lodged and are usually caused by a persistent respiratory tract infection distal to the obstruction. FB aspiration should also be suspected in the presence of acute or chronic pulmonary lesions. Often, by the time secondary symptoms appear, the parents have forgotten the initial episode of coughing and gagging.

Radiographic examination can reveal opaque FBs but is of limited use in localizing nonradiographic matter. Bronchoscopy is required for a definitive diagnosis of objects in the larynx and trachea. Fluoroscopic examination is valuable in detecting FBs in the bronchi. The mainstay of diagnosis and management of FBs is endoscopy. If there is doubt about the presence of an FB, endoscopy can be diagnostic and therapeutic.

Therapeutic Management

FB aspiration may result in life-threatening airway obstruction, especially in infants (because of the small diameter of their airways). Current recommendations for the emergency treatment of the choking child include the use of abdominal thrusts for children older than 1 year of age and back blows and chest thrusts for those younger than 1 year of age (see Airway Obstruction, p. 1368).

An FB is rarely coughed up spontaneously. Most frequently, it must be removed instrumentally by endoscopy. Endoscopy and bronchoscopy require sedation with an agent such as IV propofol or midazolam. The procedure is carried out as quickly as possible because the progressive local inflammatory process triggered by the foreign material hampers removal. A chemical pneumonia soon develops, and vegetable matter begins to macerate within a few days, making it even more difficult to remove. After removal of the FB, the child is usually observed for any complications such as laryngeal edema and discharged home within a matter of hours if vital signs are stable and recovery is satisfactory.

evolve Critical Thinking Exercise—Ingestion of a Foreign Body

Nursing Care Management

A major role of nurses caring for a child who has aspirated an FB is to recognize the signs of FB aspiration and implement immediate measures to relieve the obstruction. All persons working with children must be prepared to deal effectively with aspiration of an FB. Choking on food or other material should not be fatal. Back blows and chest thrusts in infants and abdominal thrusts in children are simple procedures that can be used by both health care providers and laypersons to save lives (see Figs. 46-15 and 46-16). It is the responsibility of nurses to learn these techniques and to teach them to parents and other groups. To aid a child who is choking, nurses must recognize the signs of distress. Not every child who gags or coughs while eating is truly choking.

NURSING ALERT The child in severe distress (1) cannot speak, (2) becomes cyanotic, and (3) collapses. These three signs indicate that the child is truly choking and requires immediate action. The child can die within 4 minutes.

Prevention

Nurses are in a position to teach prevention in a variety of settings. They can educate parents singly or in groups about hazards of aspiration in relation to the developmental level of their children and encourage them to teach their children safety. Parents should be cautioned about behaviours that their children might imitate (e.g., holding foreign objects, such as pins, nails, and toothpicks, in their lips or mouth). (Prevention based on the child's age is discussed in Chapters 36, 37, and 38.)

Aspiration Pneumonia

Aspiration pneumonia occurs when food, secretions, inert materials, volatile compounds, or liquids enter the lung and cause inflammation and a chemical pneumonitis. Aspiration of fluid or foods is a particular hazard in the child who has difficulty swallowing; is unable to swallow because of paralysis, weakness, debility, congenital anomalies, or absent cough reflex; or is force-fed, especially while crying or breathing rapidly. Clinical signs of the aspiration of oral secretions may not be distinguishable from those of other forms of acute bacterial pneumonia. For example, if vegetable matter has been aspirated, manifestations may not appear for several weeks after the event. Classic symptoms include an increasing cough or fever with foul-smelling sputum, deteriorating chest radiographs, and other signs of lower airway involvement. However, these deviations may persist for weeks while the child starts to feel better. Rarely, aspiration causes immediate death from asphyxia; more often the irritated mucous membrane becomes a site for secondary bacterial infection. In addition to fluids, food, vomitus, and nasopharyngeal secretions, other substances that may cause pneumonia are hydrocarbons, lipids, powder, and barium.

Nursing Care Management

Care of the child with aspiration pneumonia is the same as that described for the child with pneumonia from other causes. However, the major focus of nursing care is on the prevention of aspiration. Proper feeding techniques should be carried out for weak, debilitated, and uncooperative children, and preventive measures should be used to prevent aspiration of any material that might enter the nasopharynx. Nasogastric tubes used for feedings should be checked before the initiation of bolus feedings; continuous nasogastric tube feedings also need to be evaluated periodically for proper tube placement. Children who are at risk for swallowing difficulties as a result of illness, physical debilitation, anaesthesia, or sedation should be kept NPO (nothing by mouth) until they can properly swallow fluids effectively. The child who is at risk for vomiting and incapable of protecting the airway should be positioned in a side-lying recovery position (see Fig. 46-17).

Acute Respiratory Distress Syndrome/Acute Lung Injury

ARDS is recognized in children and adults and has been associated with clinical conditions and injuries such as sepsis, **trauma**, viral pneumonia, fat emboli, drug overdose, reperfusion injury after lung transplantation, smoke inhalation, and near-drowning. It is characterized by respiratory distress and hypoxemia that occur within 72 hours of a serious injury or surgery in a person with previously normal lungs. Acute lung injury (ALI) is said to involve a spectrum of inflammatory disease responses to a precipitating event (Frye, 2005). ARDS and ALI cause acute respiratory failure and account for significant morbidity and mortality in critically ill patients (Matthay et al., 2003). Acute pulmonary inflammation with alveolar capillary membrane destruction results in significant hypoxemia, and mechanical ventilation is often required. ARDS is most severe in the spectrum of illnesses in relation to the degree of hypoxemia. Hypoxemia is expressed as the ratio of partial pressure of oxygen (Pao_2) to fraction of inspired oxygen (Fio_2), or P/F ratio, with the P/F ratio for ALI being 300 or less and the P/F ratio for ARDS being 200 or less. Both ALI and ARDS demonstrate radiographic evidence of bilateral alveolar infiltrates without evidence of left-sided heart failure (Rice & Bernard, 2006).

The hallmark of ARDS is increased permeability of the alveolar-capillary membrane that results in pulmonary edema. During the acute phase of ARDS, the alveolocapillary membrane is damaged, with an increasing pulmonary capillary permeability and resulting interstitial edema. Later stages are characterized by pneumocyte and fibrin infiltration of the alveoli, with the start of either the healing process or fibrosis. When fibrosis occurs, the child may demonstrate respiratory distress and the need for mechanical ventilation. In ARDS, the lungs become stiff as a result of surfactant inactivation, gas diffusion is impaired, and eventually bronchiolar mucosal swelling and congestive atelectasis occur. The net effect is decreased functional residual capacity, pulmonary hypertension, and increased intrapulmonary right-to-left shunting of pulmonary blood flow. Surfactant secretion is reduced, and the atelectasis and fluid-filled alveoli provide an excellent medium for bacterial growth.

The criteria for diagnosis of ARDS in children are an acute antecedent illness or injury, acute respiratory distress or failure, no evidence of prior cardiopulmonary disease, and diffuse bilateral infiltrates evidenced on chest radiography. The child with ARDS may first demonstrate only symptoms caused by an injury or infection, but as the condition deteriorates, hyperventilation, tachypnea, increasing respiratory effort, cyanosis, and decreasing oxygen saturation occur. At times, the developing hypoxemia is not responsive to oxygen administration.

Therapeutic Management

Treatment involves supportive measures such as maintenance of adequate oxygenation and pulmonary perfusion, treatment of infection (or the precipitating cause), maintenance of adequate cardiac output and vascular volume, hydration, adequate nutritional support, comfort measures, prevention of complications such as gastrointestinal ulceration and aspiration, and psychological support. Prone positioning may be used to improve oxygenation; this requires close communication and coordination among the health care team (Frye, 2005). Definitive therapy is directed toward improvement of oxygenation. The use of endotracheal intubation, positive end-expiratory pressure, and low tidal volume may be required to ensure maximum oxygen delivery by increasing functional residual capacity, reducing intrapulmonary shunting, and reducing pulmonary fluid. Ventilation with low tidal volume (6 mL/kg of ideal body weight) has been associated with lower mortality rates in children with ALI (Hanson & Flori, 2006).

Additional supportive strategies in the treatment of ARDS in children include the use of permissive hypercapnia, inhaled nitric oxide, exogenous surfactant administration, high-frequency ventilation, partial liquid ventilation, and extracorporeal life support (**extracorporeal membrane oxygenation,** or ECMO). Exogenous surfactant therapy has increased oxygenation status in infants and children with ARDS/ALI and decreased disease severity (Willson, Chess, & Notter, 2008). Once the underlying cause is identified, specific treatment (e.g., antibiotics for infection) is initiated.

Prognosis

In spite of advances in understanding and treating ARDS/ALI, mortality in children ranges from 22% (after severe trauma) to 88% (after bone marrow transplant) (Flori et al., 2005; Frankel & DiCarlo, 2004). The precipitating disorder influences the outcome; the worst prognosis is associated with uncontrolled sepsis, bone marrow transplantation, cancer, and multisystem involvement with hepatic failure. Children who recover may have persistent cough and exertional dyspnea.

Nursing Care Management

The child with ARDS is cared for in a critical care unit during the acute stages of illness. Nursing care involves close monitoring of cardiac output, perfusion, fluid and electrolyte balance, and renal function (urinary output), as well as assessment of oxygenation and respiratory status. Blood gas analysis and pulse oximetry are important evaluation tools. Parenteral and enteral nutritional support is often required because of the length of the acute phase of the illness. Diuretics may be administered to reduce pulmonary fluid, and vasodilators may be administered to decrease pulmonary vascular pressure.

Nursing management also includes managing pain, monitoring the effects of the numerous parenteral fluids and medications used to stabilize the child, and monitoring for changes in the child's hemodynamic status. Most children with ARDS require invasive monitoring via a central venous line and possibly a pulmonary artery catheter to monitor oxygenation and administer medications. The nursing care of the child with ARDS involves close observance of skin condition and prevention of breakdown, passive range of motion for prevention of muscle atrophy and contractures, and nutritional support.

Respiratory distress is a frightening situation for both the child and the parents, and attention to their psychological needs is a major element in the care of these children. The child is often sedated during the acute phase of the illness, and weaning from sedation requires close monitoring for anxiety reduction and comfort.

Smoke Inhalation Injury

A number of noxious substances that may be inhaled are toxic to humans. They are primarily products of incomplete combustion and cause more deaths from fires than flame injuries. The severity of the injury depends on the nature of the substances generated by the material burned, whether the victim is confined in a closed space, and the duration of contact with the smoke. Smoke inhalation results in three types of injury: heat, chemical, and systemic. Three distinct stages occur in the child suffering from inhalation injury:

1. Pulmonary insufficiency, usually during the initial 12 hours
2. Pulmonary edema, usually after 6 to 72 hours, with an increase in the lung fluid and interstitial edema
3. Bronchopneumonia, usually after 72 hours, with a resulting airway obstruction or atelectasis

Heat injury involves thermal injury to the upper airway. Air has low specific heat; thus the injury goes no farther than the upper airway. Reflex closure of the glottis prevents injury to the lower airway.

Chemical injury involves gases that may be generated during the combustion of materials such as clothing, furniture, and floor coverings. Acids, alkalis, and their precursors in smoke can produce chemical burns. These substances can be carried deep into the respiratory tract, including the lower respiratory tract, in the form of insoluble gases. Soluble gases tend to dissolve in the upper respiratory tract.

Synthetic materials are especially toxic, producing gases such as oxides of sulphur and nitrogen, acetaldehyde, formaldehyde, hydrocyanic acid, and chlorine. Heated plastics are the source of extremely toxic vapours, including chlorine and hydrochloric acid from polyvinylchloride and hydrocarbons, aldehydes, ketones, and acids from polyethylene. Irritant gases such as nitrous oxide or carbon dioxide combine with water in the lungs to form corrosive acids; aldehydes cause denaturation of proteins, cellular damage, and edema of pulmonary tissues. Chemical burns to the airways are similar to burns on the skin except that they are painless because the tracheobronchial tree is relatively insensitive to pain.

Inhalation of small amounts of noxious irritants produces alveolar and bronchiolar damage that can lead to obstructive bronchiolitis. Severe exposure causes further injury, including alveolocapillary damage with hemorrhage, necrotizing bronchiolitis, inhibited secretion of surfactant, and formation of hyaline membranes—manifestations of ARDS.

Systemic injury occurs from gases that are nontoxic to the airways (e.g., carbon monoxide [CO], hydrogen cyanide). However, these gases cause injury and death by interfering with or inhibiting cellular respiration. CO is the leading cause of accidental poisonings in Canada. An estimated 414 Canadians died of carbon monoxide poisoning between 2000 and 2007 (Safekids Canada, 2012). It is a colourless, odourless gas with an affinity for hemoglobin 230 times greater than that of oxygen. When it enters the bloodstream, CO combines readily with hemoglobin to form carboxyhemoglobin (COHb). Because it is released less readily, tissue hypoxia reaches dangerous levels before oxygen is available to meet tissue needs.

NURSING ALERT The oxygen saturation (Sa_{O_2}) obtained by pulse oximetry will be normal because the device measures only oxygenated and deoxygenated hemoglobin; it does not measure dysfunctional hemoglobin such as COHb.

Accidental CO poisoning is most often a result of exposure to fumes of heaters or smoke from structural fires, although poorly ventilated recreational vehicles with improperly operated or maintained gas lamps or stoves and cooking in underventilated areas with charcoal grills are also frequent causes. CO is produced by incomplete combustion of carbon or carbonaceous material such as wood or charcoal.

The signs and symptoms of CO poisoning are secondary to tissue hypoxia and vary with the level of COHb. Mild manifestations include headache, visual disturbances, irritability, and nausea, whereas more severe intoxication causes confusion, hallucinations, ataxia, and coma. The bright, cherry-red lips and skin often described are less often observed; pallor and cyanosis are seen more frequently.

Therapeutic Management

Treatment of children with smoke inhalation injury is largely symptomatic. The most widely accepted treatment is placing the child on humidified 100% oxygen as quickly as possible and monitoring for signs of respiratory distress and impending failure. Baseline arterial blood gases (ABGs) and COHb levels need to be obtained. Pa_{O_2} may be within normal limits unless there is marked respiratory depression. If CO poisoning is confirmed, 100% oxygen should be continued until COHb levels fall to the nontoxic range of about 10%. If CO poisoning is severe, the patient may benefit from hyperbaric oxygen therapy; however, the benefits and risks of treatment are debatable (Kao & Nañagas, 2004); there are no published clinical practice guidelines for the therapy, especially in children. Hyperbaric oxygen therapy may be useful in the treatment of neurological complications related to CO poisoning. Please see Additional Resources for more information on medical hyperbaric treatments.

Respiratory distress may occur early in the course of smoke inhalation as a result of hypoxia, or patients who are breathing well on admission may suddenly develop respiratory distress. Therefore, intubation equipment should be readily available. Transient edema of the airways can occur at any level in the tracheobronchial tree. Assessment and localization of the obstruction should be accomplished before severe swelling of the head, neck, or oropharynx occurs. Intubation is often necessary when (1) severe burns in the area of the nose, mouth, and face increase the likelihood of developing oropharyngeal edema and obstruction; (2) vocal cord edema causes obstruction; (3) the patient has difficulty handling secretions; and (4) progressive respiratory distress requires artificial ventilation. Controversy surrounds the use of tracheostomy in this context, but many prefer this procedure when the obstruction is proximal to the larynx and reserve nasotracheal intubation for lower tract involvement.

evolve Animation—Asthma

Nursing Care Management

Nursing care of the child with inhalation injury is the same as that for any child with respiratory distress. Vital signs and other respiratory assessments need to be performed frequently, and the pulmonary status should be carefully observed and maintained. Pulmonary physiotherapy is often part of the therapy, as well as mechanical ventilation, if needed. Fluid requirements for children experiencing inhalation injury are greater than for those with surface burns alone; however, one concern is the development of pulmonary edema. Thus accurate monitoring of intake and output is essential.

In addition to observation and management of the physical aspects of inhalation injury, the nurse will also deal with the psychological needs of a frightened child and distraught parents. As with any accidental injury, the parents may feel overwhelming guilt, even when the injury occurred through no fault of their own. Parents need support, reassurance, and information regarding the child's condition, treatment, and progress.

Environmental Tobacco Smoke Exposure

Numerous investigations indicate that parental smoking is an important cause of morbidity in children. Children exposed to passive or environmental tobacco smoke have an increased number of respiratory illnesses, increased respiratory symptoms (e.g., cough, sputum, and wheezing), and reduced performance on pulmonary function tests. AOM and OME are also increased in children who have smoking parents (see Otitis Media, p. 1325). Indoor exposure to environmental tobacco smoke has been linked to asthma in children. Among children with asthma, there is an association between parental cigarette smoking and asthma exacerbations, trips to the emergency department, medication use, and impaired recovery after hospitalization for acute asthma. Maternal cigarette smoking is associated with increased respiratory symptoms and illnesses in children; decreased fetal growth; increased deliveries of low-birth-weight, preterm, and stillborn infants; and a greater incidence of sudden infant death syndrome (SIDS) (Health Canada, 2006b). Antenatal maternal smoking has also emerged as a significant risk factor for SIDS (AAP, Task Force on Sudden Infant Death Syndrome, 2005). The risk for diagnosis of early-onset asthma in the first 3 years of life is associated with in utero exposure to maternal smoking; grandmaternal smoking was also associated with an increased risk of early-onset asthma in the grandchild even if the mother did not smoke during pregnancy (Li et al., 2005). Exposure to tobacco smoke during childhood may contribute to the development of chronic lung disease in the adult.

Nursing Care Management

Nurses must provide information about the hazards of environmental smoke exposure in all their interactions with children and their family members. This information is especially important for children with respiratory and allergic illnesses. In families in which smokers refuse to or cannot quit, appropriate guidance should be provided for reducing smoke in the child's environment (see Family-Centred Teaching box). Nurses should set an example for children and families and become advocates for "no smoking" ordinances in public places, prohibition of advertising tobacco products in the media, and inclusion of health warnings of sidestream smoke on tobacco products (see Additional Resources section at the end of this chapter). Nurses also have an important role in providing parents with affordable smoking-cessation education resources, including the appropriate use of smoking-cessation pharmacological aids (Sheahan & Free, 2005).

Long-Term Respiratory Dysfunction

Asthma

Asthma is a chronic inflammatory disorder of the airways in which many cells (mast cells, eosinophils, and T lymphocytes) play a role. In susceptible children, inflammation causes recurrent episodes of wheezing, breathlessness, chest tightness, and cough, especially at night or in the early morning. These asthma episodes are associated with airflow limitation or obstruction that is reversible either spontaneously or with treatment. The inflammation also causes an increase in bronchial hyper-responsiveness to a variety of stimuli (National Asthma Education and Prevention Program, 2007). Recognition of the importance of inflammation has made the use of anti-inflammatory agents, especially inhaled steroids, a key component in the treatment of asthma.

Asthma is the most common chronic illness in childhood. It has been diagnosed in 15.6% of Canadian children aged 4 to 11 years. For children 12 years of age and older, the percentage of asthma is 8.3%, and for off-reserve Aboriginal children,

FAMILY-CENTRED TEACHING

Decreasing Childhood Exposure to Environmental Tobacco Smoke

- Maintain a smoke-free home.
- Avoid exposing an infant to environmental smoke.
- Use an air-purifying filter in the home where smoking is unavoidable.
- Encourage exclusive breastfeeding for the first 6 months.
- If smoking cessation is in progress by a breastfeeding mother, suggest she change upper clothing after smoking and before breastfeeding infant.
- Do not smoke around children.
- Change clothing after smoking and before holding an infant in close proximity.
- Restrict smoking to an isolated area of the house where the children do not play or sleep.
- Do not smoke in motor vehicles with children.
- Do not smoke in rooms children use.
- Do not allow visitors to smoke in the home.

the percentage is 11.9%. There are more young boys than girls with asthma, but in the adult population, more women than men have asthma. The number of Canadians with asthma is unfortunately on the rise. Between 1994 and 2005, the number of 35- to 44-year-old women with asthma increased by 60%, and in women 45 to 64 years of age, it was 80%. Asthma increased by 41% in men 34 to 44 years of age (PHAC, 2007b). In terms of determinants of health, asthma appears to be more prevalent in groups with poor socioeconomic status, obesity, and low physical activity levels (Philpott, Houghton, & Luke, 2010).

Asthma is a predominant cause of hospitalization for Canadian children; in 2004, children with asthma who were under 5 years of age had the highest hospitalization rates. Emergency department visits for asthma peak during the third week in September, although occurrence of respiratory tract infections that can trigger asthma peaks in mid-winter. Asthma continues to be a very serious condition and can be life threatening if not controlled. In 2003, 287 Canadians died of asthma. However, children and young adults rarely die from asthma. Fortunately, the number of deaths has been decreasing in all age groups since 1987.

Etiology

Studies of children with asthma indicate that allergy influences both the persistence and the severity of the disease. In fact, *atopy*, or the genetic predisposition for the development of an immune globulin E (IgE)–mediated response to common aeroallergens, is the strongest identifiable predisposing factor for developing asthma (National Asthma Education and Prevention Program, 2007). Although allergens play an important role in asthma, 20 to 40% of children with asthma have no evidence of allergic disease. In addition to allergens, other substances and conditions can serve as triggers that may exacerbate asthma (Box 46-13). It is a complex disorder involving biochemical, genetic, immunological, environmental, infectious, endocrine, and psychological factors. Evidence shows that viral respiratory infections may have a significant role in the development and expression of asthma (National Asthma Education and Prevention Program, 2007).

BOX 46-13 Triggers Tending to Precipitate or Aggravate Asthmatic Exacerbations

Allergens
- Outdoor—Trees, shrubs, weeds, grasses, moulds, pollens, air pollution, spores
- Indoor—Dust or dust mites, mould, cockroach antigen

Irritants—Tobacco smoke, wood smoke, odours, sprays
Exposure to occupational chemicals
Exercise
Cold air
Changes in weather or temperature
Environmental change—Moving to new home, starting new school, etc.
Colds and infections
Animals—Cats, dogs, rodents, horses
Medications—Aspirin, nonsteroidal anti-inflammatory drugs (NSAIDs), antibiotics, β-blockers
Strong emotions—Fear, anger, laughing, crying
Conditions—Gastroesophageal reflux, tracheoesophageal fistula
Food additives—Sulphite preservatives
Foods—Nuts, milk or dairy products
Endocrine factors—Menses, pregnancy, thyroid disease

evolve Animation—Bronchi and Bronchioles

Pathophysiology

There is general agreement that inflammation contributes to heightened airway reactivity in asthma. The mechanisms contributing to airway inflammation are multiple and involve a number of different pathways. It is unlikely that asthma is caused by either a single cell or a single inflammatory mediator; rather, it appears that asthma results from complex interactions among inflammatory cells, mediators, and the cells and tissues present in the airways (National Asthma Education and Prevention Program, 2007). However, recognition of the importance of inflammation has made the use of anti-inflammatory agents a key component of asthma therapy.

Another important component of asthma is bronchospasm and obstruction. The mechanisms responsible for the obstructive symptoms in asthma (Fig. 46-4) include (1) inflammatory response to stimuli; (2) airway edema and accumulation and secretion of mucus; and (3) spasm of the smooth muscle of the bronchi and bronchioles, which decreases the calibre of the bronchioles.

Bronchial constriction is a normal reaction to foreign stimuli, but in the child with asthma it is abnormally severe, producing impaired respiratory function. The smooth muscle arranged in spiral bundles around the airway causes narrowing and shortening of the airway, which significantly increases airway resistance to airflow. Airflow is determined by the size of the airway lumen, degree of bronchial wall edema,

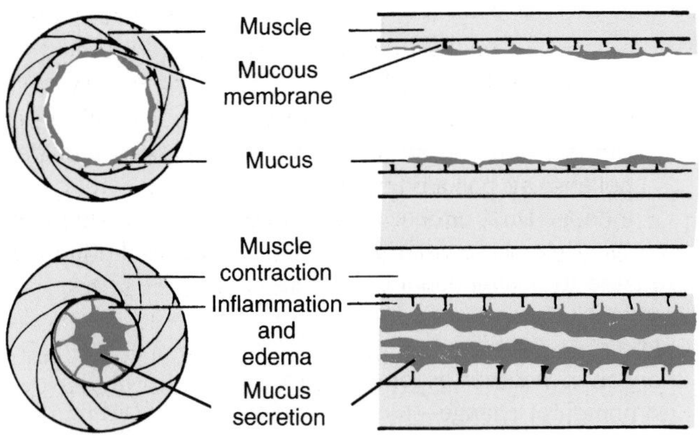

Fig. 46-4 Mechanisms of obstruction in asthma.

mucus production, smooth muscle contraction, and muscle hypertrophy.

Because the bronchi normally dilate and elongate during inspiration and contract and shorten on expiration, the respiratory difficulty is more pronounced during the expiratory phase of respiration.

Increased resistance in the airway causes forced expiration through the narrowed lumen. The volume of air trapped in the lungs increases as airways are functionally closed at a point between the alveoli and the lobar bronchi. This trapping of gas forces the individual to breathe at higher and higher lung volumes. Consequently, the person with asthma fights to inspire sufficient air. This expenditure of effort for breathing causes fatigue, decreased respiratory effectiveness, and increased oxygen consumption. The inspiration occurring at higher lung volumes hyperinflates the alveoli and reduces the effectiveness of the cough. As the severity of obstruction increases, there is reduced alveolar ventilation with carbon dioxide retention, hypoxemia, respiratory acidosis, and, eventually, respiratory failure.

Chronic inflammation may also cause permanent damage (airway remodelling) to airway structures; this remodelling cannot be prevented by and is not responsive to current treatments (National Asthma Education and Prevention Program, 2007).

Diagnostic Evaluation

The classic manifestations of asthma are dyspnea, wheezing, and coughing. However, children may experience symptoms that range from acute episodes of shortness of breath, wheezing, and cough, followed by a quiet period, to a relatively continuous pattern of chronic symptoms that fluctuate in severity (Box 46-14). An attack may develop gradually or appear abruptly and may be preceded by a URI. The age of the child is often a significant factor, since the first attack frequently occurs before the age of 5 years, with some children manifesting clinical signs and symptoms in infancy. In infancy an attack usually follows a respiratory infection. Some children may experience a **prodromal** itching at the front of the neck or over the upper part of the back just before an attack.

NURSING ALERT Shortness of breath with air movement in the chest restricted to the point of absent breath sounds accompanied by a sudden rise in respiratory rate is an ominous sign indicating ventilatory failure and imminent respiratory arrest.

BOX 46-14 Clinical Manifestations of Asthma

Cough

Hacking, paroxysmal, irritative, and nonproductive
Becomes rattling and productive of frothy, clear, gelatinous sputum

Respiratory-Related Signs

Shortness of breath
Prolonged expiratory phase
Audible wheeze
May have a malar flush and red ears
Lips deep, dark red colour
Possible progression to cyanosis of nail beds or circumoral cyanosis
Restlessness
Apprehension
Sweating may be prominent as the attack progresses
Posture—Older children may sit upright with shoulders in a hunched-over position, hands on the bed or chair, and arms braced (tripod position)
Speech—May speak in short, panting, broken phrases

Chest

Hyper-resonance on percussion
Coarse, loud breath sounds
Wheezes throughout the lung fields
Prolonged expiration
Crackles
Generalized inspiratory and expiratory wheezing; increasingly high pitched

With Repeated Episodes

Barrel chest
Elevated shoulders
Use of accessory muscles of respiration
Facial appearance: flattened malar bones, circles beneath the eyes, narrow nose, prominent upper teeth

The diagnosis is determined primarily on the basis of clinical manifestations, history, physical examination, and, to a lesser extent, laboratory tests. Generally, chronic cough in the absence of infection or diffuse wheezing during the expiratory phase of respiration is sufficient to establish a diagnosis.

Pulmonary function tests (PFTs) provide an objective method of evaluating the presence and degree of lung disease and the response to therapy. Spirometry can generally be performed reliably on children by the age of 5 or 6 years and includes either the traditional and simple mechanical spirometer often used in clinics, offices, and the home or new computerized versions. The Asthma Society of Canada, 2012 recommends that spirometry testing be done at the time of initial assessment of asthma, after treatment is initiated and symptoms have stabilized, and at least every 1 to 2 years to assess the maintenance of airway function.

Another key measurement is the *peak expiratory flow rate (PEFR)*, which measures the maximum flow of air that can be forcefully exhaled in 1 second. PEFR is measured in litres per minute using a *peak expiratory flow meter (PEFM)*. Three zones of measurement are typically used to interpret PEFR. The zone system is patterned after a traffic light to make the categories easy to understand and remember (see Guidelines box). Each child needs to establish his or her personal best value. A personal best value should be established during a 2- to 3-week period when the child's asthma is stable. During this period, the child records the PEFR at least twice a day. After the personal best value has been established, the child's current PEFR on any occasion can be compared with the personal best value.

Bronchoprovocation testing (i.e., direct exposure of the mucous membranes to a suspected antigen in increasing concentrations) helps to identify inhaled allergens. Exposure to methacholine, histamine, or cold or dry air may be performed to assess airway responsiveness or reactivity. Exercise challenges may be used to identify children with exercise-induced bronchospasm (Liu et al., 2007). Although these tests are highly specific and sensitive, they place the child at risk for an asthmatic episode and should be done under close observation in a qualified laboratory or clinic.

Skin testing is useful for identifying specific allergens, and those obtained by the puncture technique correlate better than intracutaneous tests with symptoms and measurements of specific IgE antibody. The radioallergosorbent test (RAST) helps identify antigens against various foods and is often useful in determining appropriate therapy. It is recommended that all patients with year-round asthma symptoms be tested with skin tests or laboratory blood analysis to determine sensitization to perennial allergens (e.g., house dust mites, cats, dogs, cockroaches, moulds, and fungus) (CPS, Acute Care Committee, 2012) (see Atraumatic Care box).

In addition to these tests, other important tests include laboratory tests (complete blood count with differential) and chest radiographs. The complete blood count may show a slight elevation in the white blood cell count during acute asthma, but elevations to more than 12,000/mm^3 or an increased percentage of band cells may indicate respiratory tract infection. The presence of eosinophilia greater than 500/mm^3 tends to suggest an allergic or inflammatory disorder.

Frontal and lateral radiographs show infiltrates and hyperexpansion of the airways, with the anteroposterior diameter on physical examination indicating an increased diameter (suggestive of barrel chest). Additional diagnostic tests for conditions such as gastroesophageal reflux may be carried out to determine whether they may contribute to asthma symptoms. Radiography may assist in ruling out a respiratory tract infection.

Therapeutic Management

The overall goals of asthma management are to maintain normal activity levels, maintain normal pulmonary function, prevent chronic symptoms and recurrent exacerbations, provide optimal medication therapy with minimal or no adverse effects, and assist the child in living as normal a life as possible. This includes facilitating the child's social adjustments in the family, school, and community and normal participation in recreational activities and sports. To accomplish these goals, several treatment principles need to be followed (Asthma Society of Canada, 2012):

- A continuous care approach with regular visits (at least every 1 to 6 months) to the health care provider is necessary to control symptoms and prevent exacerbations.
- Prevention of exacerbations includes avoiding triggers, avoiding allergens, and using medications as needed.

GUIDELINES Interpreting Peak Expiratory Flow Rates*

- Green (80 to 100% of personal best) signals all clear. Asthma is under reasonably good control. No symptoms are present, and the routine treatment plan for maintaining control can be followed.
- Yellow (50 to 79% of personal best) signals caution. Asthma is not well controlled. An acute exacerbation may be present. Maintenance therapy may need to be increased. Call the practitioner if the child stays in this zone.
- Red (below 50% of personal best) signals a medical alert. Severe airway narrowing may be occurring. A short-acting bronchodilator should be administered. Notify the practitioner if the peak expiratory flow rate does not return immediately and stay in the yellow or green zones.

*These zones are guidelines only. Specific zones and management should be individualized for each child.

ATRAUMATIC CARE
Skin Testing

To help allay children's fears of skin tests, give them a careful and thorough explanation of what is to be done and how many "pricks" are involved (usually a series of eight on each site, for a total of 30 tests). Very young, anxious patients may benefit from one prick on the arm to demonstrate how it feels. The skin is pierced with a stylet rather than a regular needle and syringe; then a drop of allergen is placed on the site. Another helpful strategy is to have the child count off the number of pricks with the nurse as a distraction. For intradermal skin injection, EMLA or AMETOP Gel(TM) , both topical anaesthetics, reduce or eliminate pain without altering test results. Care must be taken to follow medication package dosages, and application instructions, if these topicals are used. Health Canada (2009b) has put out a warning that some individuals have experienced serious adverse effects such as seizures, irregular heart beat, and difficulty breathing, which has caused death in rare incidents. Usually the complications occur when the topical is applied to large amounts of skin and covered with plastic wrap to increase the effect. Children are more at risk for these adverse effects and some children have experienced them when a close to normal dosage was given.

- Therapy includes efforts to reduce underlying inflammation and relieve or prevent symptomatic airway narrowing.
- Therapy includes patient education, environmental control, pharmacological management, and the use of objective measures to monitor the severity of disease and guide the course of therapy.

Allergen Control

Nonpharmacological therapy is aimed at the prevention and reduction of exposure to airborne allergens and irritants. House dust mites and other components of house dust are frequent agents identified in children allergic to inhalants. The cockroach, another common household inhabitant, is an important allergen in many locations. Exterminating live cockroaches, carefully cleaning kitchen floors and cabinets, putting food away after eating, and taking trash out in the evening are essential measures to control cockroach infestation. The mouse allergen is the most recent allergen to be identified in the homes of urban children with asthma. The role of cat and dog dander in allergen-induced asthma has also been studied. Sensitized persons should carefully evaluate having such pets in the household; there are inconclusive data on cat dander, but there is some evidence that dog dander either has no effect or may be protective (Sharma et al., 2007). Additional sources of pollutants include ozone, particulate matter produced by tobacco smoke, wood-burning stoves, pesticides, lead, mould spores, nitrogen dioxide, and sulphur dioxide; these are believed to contribute to asthma morbidity in children and should be avoided or minimized. As stated earlier, exposure to tobacco smoke is a significant contributing factor in the development of asthma in infants and small children (Sharma et al., 2007). Recommendations for controlling allergens are found in the Patient Teaching box.

Skin testing is used to identify specific allergens so steps can be taken to eliminate or avoid them. Often, simply removing the offending environmental allergens or irritants (e.g., removing carpeting from the home of a child sensitive to mould and dust particles) decreases the frequency of asthma

PATIENT TEACHING “Allergy-Proofing” the Home and Community

- Keep humidity between 30 and 50%; use dehumidifier or air conditioner if available; keep air conditioners clean and free of mould; do not use vaporizers or humidifiers.
- Encase pillows in zippered allergen-impermeable covers or wash pillows in hot water (at least 54.4°C) every week.
- Encase mattress and box springs in zippered allergen-impermeable cover.
- Use foam rubber mattress and pillows or Dacron pillows and synthetic blankets.
- Wash bed linens every 7 to 10 days in hot water (at least 54.4°C).
- Encase polyester comforters in allergen-impermeable covers or wash in hot water (at least 54.4°C) every week; if possible, do not use comforter; use cotton blankets instead.
- Do not use a canopy above the bed; children should not sleep on the bottom bunk of a bunk bed.
- Store nothing under the bed; keep clothing in a closet with the door shut.
- Use washable window shades; avoid heavy curtains; if curtains are used, launder them frequently.
- Remove all carpeting if possible; if not possible, vacuum carpet once or twice a week while the child wears a mask; have child remain out of the room while vacuuming occurs and for 30 minutes after vacuuming.
- If possible, use a central vacuum cleaner with a collecting bag outside of the home or use cleaner filters (e.g., high-efficiency particulate air [HEPA] filters).
- Have air and heating ducts cleaned annually; change or clean filters monthly; cover heating vents with filter material (e.g., cheesecloth) to prevent circulation of dust, especially when heat is turned on after summer.
- Remove unnecessary furniture, rugs, stuffed or real animals, toys, books, upholstered furniture, plants, aquariums, and wall hangings from child's room.
- Use wipeable furniture (wood, plastic, vinyl, or leather) in place of upholstered furniture; avoid rattan or wicker furniture.
- Cover walls with washable paint or wallpaper.
- Limit child's exposure to animals (rabbits, gerbils, hamsters) at school; teach child to stay away from zoos, petting farms, and neighbour's pets.
- Change child's clothes after playing outdoors; wash child's hair nightly if child is outside and pollen count is high.
- Keep child indoors while lawn is being mowed, bushes or trees are being trimmed, or pollen count is high.
- Keep windows and doors closed during pollen season; use air conditioner if possible or go to places that are air conditioned, such as libraries and shopping malls, when the weather is hot.
- Wet-mop bare floors weekly; wet-dust and clean child's room weekly; the child should not be present during cleaning activities.
- Wash showers and shower curtains with bleach or Lysol at least once a month.
- Limit or avoid child's exposure to tobacco and wood smoke; do not allow cigarette smoking in the house or car; select day care centres, play areas, and shopping malls that are smoke free.
- Avoid odours or sprays (e.g., perfumes, talcum powder, room deodorizers, chalk dust at school, fresh paint, cleaning solutions).
- Avoid cellar (basement) as a play area if it is damp and use a dehumidifier in a damp basement.
- Cover all food, including pet food, and put food away in cabinets.
- Store garbage in closed containers.
- Use pesticide sprays, roach bait traps, and boric acid powder to kill cockroaches; if living in an apartment or adjacent housing, encourage neighbours to work together to get rid of cockroaches and mice.
- Repair leaking or dripping faucets; seal cracks and crevices in cabinets and pantry areas.

also been effective in treating acute asthma exacerbation (Blitz et al., 2005).

Antibiotics should not be used to treat acute asthma attacks except when a bacterial infection resulting from another condition such as pneumonia or sinusitis is present (National Asthma Education and Prevention Program, 2007).

A child suspected of having status asthmaticus is usually seen in the emergency department and is often admitted to a pediatric intensive care unit for close observation and continuous cardiorespiratory monitoring. A key component in the prevention of morbidity is helping the child, parents, teachers, coaches, and other adults recognize features of deteriorating respiratory status, use the correct rescue medications effectively, and immediately place the child with deteriorating respiratory status into the care of trained health care providers instead of waiting to see if the asthma gets better on its own. The child going into early status asthmaticus is no different from the adult who is having a myocardial infarction in terms of needing trained medical assistance before the condition deteriorates to irreversible respiratory failure and possible death. Community education regarding asthma recognition and management is an important component of nursing care.

Nursing Care Management

The nursing care of the child with asthma begins with a review of the child's health history; the home, school, and play environment; parent and child attitudes about the child's condition; and a comprehensive physical assessment with focus on the respiratory system. Nursing care of children with asthma involves both acute and long-term care. Nurses who are involved with children in the home, hospital, school, outpatient clinic, or practitioner's office play an important role in helping children and their families learn to live with the condition. The disease can be managed so that it does not require hospitalization or interfere with family life, physical activity, or school attendance. The nursing process in the care of the child with asthma is outlined in the Nursing Care Plan.

Physical assessment of asthma involves the same observations and techniques described in Chapter 34. In addition, the nurse notes and evaluates physical characteristics of chronic respiratory involvement, including chest configuration (e.g., barrel chest), posturing (tripod), and type of breathing. A history of the current and previous episodes and precipitating factors or events provides important information.

Nurses may perform a variety of functions in asthma care, including asthma education in the primary care setting and in schools and other community settings, and care of the child with asthma in the acute care setting, ambulatory care, and critical care. Nurses also obtain information on how asthma affects the child's everyday activities and self-concept, the child's and family's adherence to the prescribed therapy, and their personal treatment goals. Every effort should be made to build a partnership between the child and family and the health care team. Communication is an essential part of this partnership, and health care providers should routinely assess the effectiveness of patient–provider communication. In particular, the child and family's satisfaction with asthma control and with the quality of care should be assessed. The nurse should also assess their perception of the severity of the disease and their level of social support.

One of the major emphases of nursing care is outpatient management by the family. Parents need to be taught how to avoid allergens, recognize and respond to symptoms of bronchospasm, maintain health and prevent complications, and promote normal activities. The nurse should determine any cultural or ethnic beliefs or practices that influence self-management and that may necessitate modifications in educational approaches to meet the family's needs.

Avoid Allergens

One goal of asthma management is avoidance of an exacerbation. Parents need to know how to avoid allergens that precipitate asthma episodes. The nurse can assist the parents in modifying the environment to reduce contact with the offending allergen(s) (see Patient Teaching box, p. 1348). Parents should be cautioned to avoid exposing a sensitive child to excessive cold, wind, or other extremes of weather; smoke; sprays; or other irritants. Foods known to provoke symptoms should be eliminated from the diet.

Approximately 2 to 6% of children with asthma are sensitive to aspirin; thus nurses should caution parents to use other analgesic–antipyretic medications for discomfort or fever and to read package labelling for ingredients. Although aspirin is rarely given to children in Canada, salicylate compounds are in other common medicines such as Pepto-Bismol. Children with aspirin-induced asthma may also be sensitive to NSAIDs and tartrazine (yellow dye number 5, a common food colouring).

NURSING ALERT Parents should be encouraged to avoid administering aspirin to any child unless specifically recommended by and under the supervision of a health practitioner. Acetaminophen is safe for children and is the analgesic of choice.

Relieve Bronchospasm

Parents and older children should be taught to recognize early signs and symptoms of an impending attack so that it can be controlled before symptoms become distressing. Most children can recognize prodromal symptoms well before an attack (about 6 hours) and implement preventive therapy. Objective signs that parents may observe include rhinorrhea, cough, low-grade fever, irritability, itching (especially on the front of the neck and chest), apathy, anxiety, sleep disturbance, abdominal discomfort, and loss of appetite. A variety of easy-to-use, inexpensive PEFMs are available for use in the home and at school to assess changes in pulmonary function (see Patient Teaching box, p. 1354). In general, children 5 years of age and older are able to use a PEFM successfully. However, young children need to be supervised while they are learning to use their PEFM, and their technique should be checked frequently to ensure that it is correct. Children should use the same PEFM over time, and they should bring it for use at every follow-up visit. Using the same brand of meter is recommended because different brands can give significantly different values. The use of a PEFM provides objective monitoring of the severity of asthma and can decrease asthma episodes, of the cough. However, CPT is not recommended during acute, uncomplicated exacerbations of asthma.

Hyposensitization

The role of hyposensitization in childhood asthma has become controversial. In the past, immunotherapy was used for seasonal allergies and when single substances were identified as the offending allergen. It is not recommended for allergens that can be eliminated, such as foods, medications, and animal dander.

The Asthma Society of Canada (2012) recommends immunotherapy for asthma patients in the following situations:

- When there is evidence of a relationship between asthma symptoms and unavoidable exposure to an allergen to which the patient is sensitive
- When symptoms occur all year or at least during a major portion of the year
- When symptom control is difficult with medication therapy because multiple medications are required, the patient is not responsive to available medications, or the patient refuses to take the medications

Injection therapy is usually limited to clinically significant allergens. The initial dose of the offending allergen(s), based on the size of the skin reaction, is injected subcutaneously. The amount is increased at weekly intervals until a maximum tolerance is reached, after which a maintenance dose is given at 4-week intervals. This may be extended to 5- or 6-week intervals during the off-season for seasonal allergens. Successful treatment is continued for a minimum of 3 years and then stopped. If no symptoms appear, acquired immunity is assumed; if symptoms recur, treatment is reinstituted. Hyposensitization injections should be administered only with emergency equipment and medications readily available in the event of an anaphylactic reaction.

Prognosis

The outlook for children with asthma varies widely. Some children's asthma symptoms may improve at puberty, but up to two thirds of children with asthma continue to have symptoms through puberty and into adulthood. The prognosis for control or disappearance of symptoms varies in children, from having rare and infrequent attacks to constantly wheezing or being subject to status asthmaticus. In general, when symptoms are severe and numerous, when symptoms have been present for a long time, and when there is a family history of allergy, there is a greater likelihood of a poor prognosis. Risk factors that may predict persistence of symptoms into childhood (from infancy) include atopy, male gender, exposure to environmental tobacco, and maternal history of asthma (Ross, Mjaanes, & Lemanske, 2003). Many children who outgrow their exacerbations continue to have airway hyper-responsiveness and cough as adults. Furthermore, airway hyper-responsiveness in adults appears to be associated with decreased lung function.

The adolescent age group appears to be most vulnerable, with the greatest increase occurring in children 10 to 14 years of age. No reliable data exist to explain this increase. Factors that have been postulated include exposure of atopic persons to more allergens (particularly in large urban centres), change in severity of the disease, abuse of medication therapy (toxicity), failure of families and practitioners to recognize the severity of asthma, and psychological factors such as denial and refusal to accept the disease.

Risk factors for asthma deaths include early onset, frequent attacks, difficult-to-manage disease, adolescence, history of respiratory failure, psychological problems (refusal to take medications), dependency on or misuse of asthma medications (high use), presence of physical stigmata (barrel chest, intercostal retractions), and abnormal PFTs.

Status Asthmaticus

Status asthmaticus is a medical emergency that can result in respiratory failure and death if unrecognized and untreated. Children who continue to display respiratory distress despite vigorous therapeutic measures, especially the use of sympathomimetics (e.g., albuterol, epinephrine), are considered to be in status asthmaticus. The condition may develop gradually or rapidly, often coincident with complicating conditions, such as pneumonia or a respiratory virus, that can influence the duration and treatment of the exacerbation.

Therapy for status asthmaticus is aimed at improving ventilation, decreasing airway resistance and relieving bronchospasm, correcting dehydration and acidosis, allaying child and parent anxiety related to the severity of the event, and treating any concurrent infection. Humidified oxygen is recommended and should be given to maintain an oxygen saturation greater than 90%. Inhaled aerosolized short-acting β_2-agonists are recommended for all patients. Three treatments of β_2-agonists spaced 20 to 30 minutes apart are usually given as initial therapy, and continuous administration of β_2-agonists may be initiated. A systemic corticosteroid (oral, IV, or IM) may also be given to decrease the effects of inflammation. An anticholinergic such as ipratropium bromide may be added to the aerosolized solution of the β_2-agonist. Anticholinergics have been shown to result in additional bronchodilation in patients with severe airflow obstruction. An IV infusion is often initiated to provide a means for hydration and to administer medications. Correction of dehydration, acidosis, hypoxia, and electrolyte disturbance is guided by frequent determination of arterial pH, blood gases, and serum electrolytes.

Additional therapies in acute asthma attacks include the use of IV magnesium sulphate, a potent muscle relaxant that acts to decrease inflammation and improves pulmonary function and peak flow rate among pediatric patients treated in the emergency department with moderate to severe asthma. Heliox may be administered to decrease airway resistance and thereby decrease the work of breathing; it can be delivered via a nonrebreathing face mask from premixed tanks, which may be blended in a stand-alone unit or within a ventilator. It may be used in acute exacerbations as an adjunct to β_2-agonist and IV corticosteroid therapy to improve pulmonary function until the two latter medications have time to take full effect in decreasing bronchospasm; the effects of heliox are usually seen within 20 minutes of administration, whereas other drugs may take longer to exert the desired effect. Ketamine, a dissociative anaesthetic, is believed to cause smooth muscle relaxation and decrease airway resistance caused by severe bronchospasm in acute asthma (Linzer, 2007); it may be administered as an adjunct to other therapies mentioned previously. Inhaled magnesium sulphate used in addition to a β_2-agonist for acute asthma attacks has cyclic AMP (cAMP). It is believed that the increased cAMP enhances binding of intracellular calcium to the cell membrane, reducing the availability of calcium and thus allowing smooth muscle to relax. Other effects of these medications help stabilize mast cells to prevent the release of mediators. Most β-adrenergics used in asthma therapy affect predominantly the β_2-receptors, which help eliminate bronchospasm and minimize effects such as increased heart rate and gastrointestinal disturbances. These medications can be given via inhalation or as oral or parenteral preparations. The inhaled medication has a more rapid onset of action than the oral form. Inhalation also reduces troublesome systemic adverse effects: irritability, tremor, nervousness, and insomnia. Levalbuterol reportedly causes fewer adverse effects; however, its overall effectiveness in childhood asthma is controversial (Linzer, 2007). The Canadian Paediatric Society (CPS, Acute Care Committee, 2012) recommends the addition of a long-acting β_2-agonist to a low- or medium-dose inhaled corticosteroid to improve lung function and asthma symptoms and decrease the need for a short-acting β_2-agonist. There is some evidence that this combination may actually allow the practitioner to lower the corticosteroid dose and manage asthma symptoms just as effectively (Mintz, 2004). Inhaled β-adrenergic agents should not be taken more than three or four times daily for acute symptoms.

Salmeterol (Serevent) is a long-acting β_2-agonist (bronchodilator) that is used twice a day (no more frequently than every 12 hours). This medication is added to anti-inflammatory therapy and used for long-term prevention of symptoms, especially nighttime symptoms, and exercise-induced bronchospasm. Salmeterol is not used in children younger than 12 years of age, and it is not used to treat acute symptoms or exacerbations.

Theophylline was used for decades to relieve symptoms and prevent asthma attacks; however, it is now used primarily in the emergency department when the child is not responding to maximal therapy (Linzer, 2007). Therapeutic levels should be obtained with this drug because it has a narrow therapeutic window.

Leukotrienes are mediators of inflammation that cause increases in airway hyper-responsiveness. Leukotriene modifiers (such as zafirlukast [Accolate] and montelukast sodium [Singulair]) block inflammatory and bronchospasm effects. These medications are not used to treat acute episodes but are given orally in combination with β-agonists and steroids to provide long-term control and prevent symptoms in mild persistent asthma. Montelukast is approved for children 12 months old and older, whereas zafirlukast is approved for children 7 years and older.

Anticholinergics (atropine and ipratropium [Atrovent]) may also be used for relief of acute bronchospasm. However, these medications have adverse effects that include drying of respiratory secretions, blurred vision, and cardiac and central nervous system stimulation. The primary anticholinergic medication used is ipratropium, which does not cross the blood–brain barrier and therefore elicits no central nervous system effects. Ipratropium, when used in combination with albuterol, has been shown to be effective during acute severe asthma in significantly improving lung function and reducing hospitalizations in children coming to the emergency department (Liu et al., 2007).

Another asthma medication, omalizumab (Xolair), is a monoclonal antibody that blocks the binding of IgE to mast cells. Blocking this interaction eventually inhibits the inflammation that is associated with asthma. Because many patients with asthma are atopic and possess specific IgE antibodies to allergens responsible for airway inflammation, this drug is a promising adjunct to the treatment of asthma. It has been approved for use in children 12 years and older. The medication is administered once or twice a month by subcutaneous injection. Efficacy of omalizumab is not immediate, and clinical trials report that response to the drug was not evident before 12 weeks (Strunk & Bloomberg, 2006). It can be an effective therapy for patients with symptomatic moderate to severe allergic asthma that is poorly controlled with inhaled corticosteroids. However, it is expensive (Courtney, McCarter, & Pollart, 2005), and there have been reported cases of severe anaphylactic reactions.

The use of complementary and alternative medicine (CAM) in children with asthma is reported by several sources; those most commonly used are herbal products, breathing techniques, homeopathy, and acupuncture (Slader et al., 2006). The use of CAM should be evaluated carefully in conjunction with other therapies in the overall management of asthma.

Exercise

Exercise-induced bronchospasm (EIB) is an acute, reversible, usually self-terminating airway obstruction that develops during or after vigorous activity, reaches its peak 5 to 10 minutes after stopping the activity, and usually stops in another 20 to 30 minutes. Patients with EIB have cough, shortness of breath, chest pain or tightness, wheezing, and endurance problems during exercise, but an exercise challenge test in a laboratory is necessary to make the diagnosis.

The problem is rare in activities that require short bursts of energy (e.g., baseball, sprints, gymnastics, skiing) and more common in those that involve endurance exercise (e.g., soccer, basketball, distance running). Swimming is well tolerated by children with EIB because they are breathing air fully saturated with moisture and because of the type of breathing required in swimming.

Children with asthma are often excluded from exercise by parents, teachers, and practitioners, as well as by the children themselves, because they are reluctant to provoke an attack. However, this practice can seriously hamper peer interaction and physical health. Exercise is advantageous for children with asthma, and most children can participate in activities at school and in sports with minimal difficulty, provided their asthma is under control. Participation should be evaluated on an individual basis. Appropriate prophylactic treatment with β-adrenergic agents or cromolyn sodium before exercise usually permits full participation in strenuous exertion.

Chest Physiotherapy

CPT includes breathing exercises and physical training. These therapies help produce physical and mental relaxation, improve posture, strengthen respiratory musculature, and develop more efficient patterns of breathing. For the motivated child, breathing exercises and controlled breathing are of value in preventing overinflation and improving efficiency episodes. Dehumidifiers or air conditioners can be used to control nonspecific factors, such as extremes of temperature, that trigger an episode.

Despite the proven association between the incidence of asthma and exposure to these residential hazards, little evidence-informed research demonstrates an overall reduction in symptoms, even with significant interventions aimed at environmental (housing) modifications such as removal of carpeting, cleaning, and extermination (Sandel et al., 2004; Sharma et al., 2007).

Medication Therapy

Pharmacological therapy is used to prevent and control asthma symptoms, reduce the frequency and severity of asthma exacerbations, and reverse airflow obstruction. A stepwise approach is recommended based on the severity of the child's asthma. Because inflammation is considered an early and persistent feature of asthma, therapy is directed toward long-term suppression of inflammation.

Asthma medications are categorized into two general classes: *long-term control medications (preventer medications)* that decrease airway swelling and prevent asthma episodes to achieve and maintain control of inflammation, and *quick-relief medications (reliever medications)* to treat symptoms and exacerbations quickly (Health Canada, 2010).

Quick-relief and long-term medications are often used in combination. Inhaled corticosteroids, cromolyn sodium and nedocromil, long-acting β_2-agonists, methylxanthines, and leukotriene modifiers are used as long-term control medications. Short-acting β_2-agonists, anticholinergics, and systemic corticosteroids are used as quick-relief or rescue medications. Bronchodilators that relax bronchial smooth muscle and dilate the airways include β_2-agonists, methylxanthines, and anticholinergics that can be used as both quick-relief and long-term medications.

Many asthma medications are given by inhalation with a nebulizer or a **metered-dose inhaler** (MDI). The MDI should always be attached to a spacer when an inhaled corticosteroid is administered to prevent yeast infections in the mouth. Spacers are also important for children who have difficulty coordinating or learning proper inhalation technique (Asthma Society of Canada, 2012). The spacer and holder can be equipped with a mask or a mouthpiece. An alternative propellant to the chlorofluorocarbons (CFCs) is hydrofluoroalkanes; the purported advantages include delivery of more fine particles and less oral deposition (Asthma Society of Canada, 2012). The Canadian government has mandated that MDIs not be manufactured using CFCs (D'Urzo & D'Urzo, 1999). Several currently available CFC-free MDI devices use dry powder (and also called *dry powder inhalers [DPIs]*); these include the Diskus inhaler and the Turbuhaler. These devices are breath activated, and the child needs to inhale as quickly and deeply as possible to use them effectively. The Diskhaler and Aerosolizer are similar, but with the Aerosolizer the medication must be loaded into the inhaler before use. Infants and very young children who have difficulty using MDIs or other inhalers can receive their asthma medications via a nebulizer. When this device is used, the medication is mixed with saline (also available in premixed form) and nebulized with compressed air. Children are instructed to breathe normally with the mouth open to provide a direct route to the trachea.

Corticosteroids are anti-inflammatory drugs used to treat reversible airflow obstruction and control symptoms and reduce bronchial hyper-responsiveness in chronic asthma. A major change in the last two revisions of Canadian national guidelines (Asthma Society of Canada, 2012) is the recommendation that inhaled corticosteroids be used as first-line therapy in children over 5 years of age. Clinical studies of corticosteroids have indicated significant improvement of all asthma parameters, including decreases in symptoms, emergency visits, and medication requirements (CPS, Acute Care Committee, 2012).

Corticosteroids may be administered parenterally, orally, or by inhalation. Oral medications are metabolized slowly, with an onset of action up to 3 hours after administration and peak effectiveness occurring within 6 to 12 hours. Oral systemic steroids may be given for short periods of time (e.g., 3- or 10-day "bursts") to gain prompt control of inadequately controlled persistent asthma or to manage severe persistent asthma. These medications should be given in the lowest effective dose. They have few adverse effects (cough, dysphonia, and oral thrush), and there is strong evidence that they improve the long-term outcomes for children of all ages with mild or moderate persistent asthma. Evidence from clinical trials that monitored children for 6 years indicates that the use of inhaled corticosteroids at recommended doses does not have long-term significant effects on growth, bone mineral density, ocular toxicity, or suppression of the adrenal–pituitary axis (National Asthma Education and Prevention Program, 2007). However, primary care providers should frequently monitor (at least every 3 to 6 months) the growth of children and adolescents taking corticosteroids to assess the systemic effects of these medications and make appropriate reductions in dosages or changes to other types of asthma therapy when necessary. The inhaled corticosteroids include budesonide and fluticasone.

Cromolyn sodium is a nonsteroidal anti-inflammatory drug (NSAID) for asthma. It stabilizes mast cell membranes; inhibits activation and release of mediators from eosinophil and epithelial cells; and inhibits the acute airway narrowing after exposure to exercise, cold dry air, and sulphur dioxide. There is no way to reliably predict whether a child will respond to the drug. Cromolyn sodium has minimal adverse effects (occasional coughing on inhalation of the powder formulation) and may be given via nebulizer or MDI.

Nedocromil sodium inhibits the bronchoconstrictor response to inhaled antigens and inhibits the activity of and release of histamine, leukotrienes, and prostaglandins from inflammatory cells associated with asthma. The drug has few adverse effects and is used for maintenance therapy in asthma; it is not effective for reversal of acute exacerbations and is not used in children under 5 years of age.

β-Adrenergic agonists (short acting) (primarily albuterol, levalbuterol [Xopenex], and terbutaline) are used for treatment of acute exacerbations and for the prevention of exercise-induced bronchospasm. These drugs bind with the β-receptors on the smooth muscle of airways, where they activate adenylate cyclase and convert adenosine monophosphate (AMP) to

NURSING CARE PLAN ● The Child With Asthma

Nursing Diagnosis	Expected Patient Outcomes	Nursing Interventions	Rationale
Risk for suffocation related to interaction between individual and triggering factors (allergens, respiratory tract infection, exercise, irritants, emotions, temperature changes)	Child will have adequate airway exchange.	Assist child and family in recognizing factors such as allergens, irritants, temperature changes, and upper respiratory infections that trigger asthma symptoms.	To avoid asthma exacerbations
	Family and child will assume responsibility for asthma symptom management.	Assist child (according to developmental age) and family in recognizing early signs of an asthmatic episode (use peak expiratory flow meter [PEFM]).	To control symptoms with medication
Child's/Family's Defining Characteristics *(Subjective and Objective Data)*	**The Following NOC Concepts Apply to These Outcomes:**	Educate child and family in the use of inhaled corticosteroids and bronchodilator.	To control symptoms and minimize shortness of breath
Wheezing Dry cough Laboured respirations Dyspnea Intercostal retractions Complaints of tightness in chest, shortness of breath Bronchial inflammation and airway constriction	Asthma Control Anxiety Control Child Development	Educate child and family regarding proper use of rescue medications in case of disease exacerbation.	To prevent illness exacerbations and hospitalization; to prevent adverse effects from improper use of certain asthma medications
		Educate child and family regarding the proper use of metered-dose inhaler with spacer, aerosolized nebulizer, and PEFM (know child's personal best).	To help child and family effectively manage asthma symptoms independently
		The Following NIC Concepts Apply to These Interventions Respiratory Monitoring Administering Inhaled Medications Risk Identification Family Integrity Promotion Energy Management Coping Enhancement Environmental Management	

Nursing Diagnosis	Expected Patient Outcomes	Nursing Interventions	Rationale
Interrupted family processes related to child with a chronic illness	Family will cope with effects of the disease.	Provide family and child (as age appropriate) with explanations about the disease and management.	To provide adequate information To provide realistic expectations
	Family will provide child an appropriate protective environment.	Cooperate with family to develop a written action plan for asthma management.	To provide family and child sense of control
Child's/Family's Defining Characteristics *(Subjective and Objective Data)*	**The Following NOC Concepts Apply to These Outcomes**	Discuss facilitators and barriers to effective asthma management.	To assist family members in understanding their role as being vital in the management of asthma
Anxiety Disruptive family interactions with child and members Family conflicts Inadequate child support Child's health status ignored Family ignoring other members' needs for those of the child with asthma	Family Support Family Normalization	Encourage family and child (as age appropriate) to discuss the impact of the illness on the family's lifestyle.	To provide opportunity to verbalize frustrations and challenges of having a child with a chronic illness
		Evaluate family resources for asthma management in relation to the following: • Access to health care • Medication availability in home and school (or day care as appropriate) • Allergen exposure control and eradication	To enhance family's ability to cope with child's chronic illness
		The Following NIC Concepts Apply to These Interventions Emotional Support Anticipatory Guidance Family Involvement Promotion Financial Resource Assistance Decision-Making Support Mutual Goal Setting	

health care visits, and missed school days (Burkhart et al., 2007).

Children who use a nebulizer, MDI, Diskus, or Turbuhaler to deliver medications need to learn how to use the device correctly. A study of school-age children with asthma indicated that only 7% of these children had effective MDI skills (Winkelstein et al., 2000). The MDI device (Fig. 46-5) delivers medication directly to the airways; thus the child needs to learn to breathe slowly and deeply for better distribution to narrowed airways (see Patient Teaching box).

Young children and those who are unable to manipulate the MDI or coordinate breathing should use spacers. These devices allow the parent or child to deliver the medication from the MDI into the spacer, from which the child then inhales the medication. Spacers also prevent yeast infections in the mouth when corticosteroids are inhaled via an MDI.

The child and parents also need to be cautioned about the adverse effects of prescribed medications and the dangers of overuse of β_2-agonists. They should know that it is important to use these medications when needed but not indiscriminately or as a substitute for avoiding the symptom-provoking allergen. Parents are cautioned against purchasing over-the-counter preparations because these medications can place the children at risk for increased dosage of a drug and toxicity.

PATIENT TEACHING Use of a Peak Expiratory Flow Meter

1. Before each use, make sure the sliding marker or arrow on the peak expiratory flow meter points to zero or is at the bottom of the numbered scale.
2. Stand up straight.
3. Remove gum or any food from your mouth.
4. Close your lips tightly around the mouthpiece. Be sure to keep your tongue away from the mouthpiece.
5. Blow out as hard and as quickly as you can, a "fast hard puff."
6. Note the number by the marker on the numbered scale.
7. Repeat the entire routine three times; wait 30 seconds between each routine.
8. Record the highest of the three readings, not the average.
9. Measure the peak expiratory flow rate (PEFR) close to the same time and same way each day (e.g., morning and evening; before or 15 minutes after taking medication).
10. Keep a chart of your PEFRs.

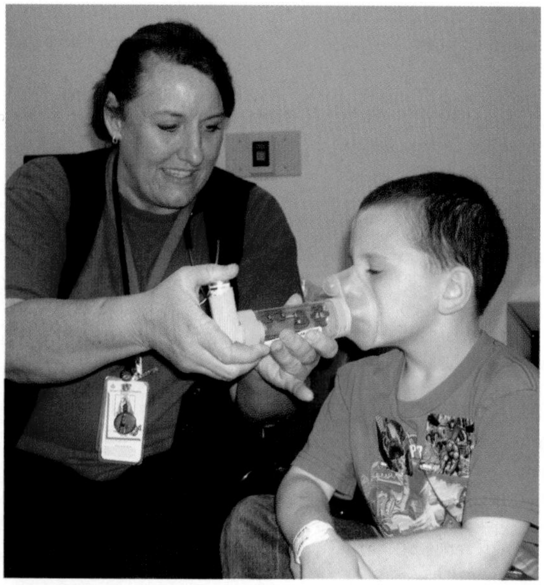

Fig. 46-5 Child using metered-dose inhaler with spacer and face mask.

PATIENT TEACHING Use of a Metered-Dose Inhaler*

Steps for Checking How Much Medicine Is in the Canister

1. If the canister is new, it is full.
2. If the canister has been used repeatedly, it might be empty. (Check product label to see how many inhalations should be in each canister.)
3. The most accurate way to determine how many doses remain in a metered-dose inhaler (MDI) is to count and record each actuation as it is used.
4. Many dry-powder inhalers have a dose-counting device or dose indicator on the canister to let you know when the canister is empty.
5. Placing dry-powder inhalers or MDIs with hydrofluoroalkanes in water will destroy these inhalers.

Steps for Using the Inhaler

1. Remove the cap and hold the inhaler upright.
2. Shake the inhaler.
3. Tilt your head back slightly and breathe out slowly.
4. With the inhaler in an upright position, position the mouthpiece as follows:
   a. About 3 to 4 cm from the mouth or
   b. Insert into an AeroChamber or spacer (this method is recommended for young children and people using corticosteroids)
5. At the end of a normal expiration, depress the top of the inhaler canister firmly to release the medication (into either the AeroChamber or the mouth) and breathe in slowly (about 3 to 5 seconds). Relax the pressure on the top of the canister.
6. Hold the breath for at least 5 to 10 seconds to allow the aerosol medication to reach deeply into the lungs.
7. Remove the inhaler and breathe out slowly through the nose.
8. Wait 1 minute between puffs (if an additional one is needed).

(Adapted from National Asthma Education and Prevention Program. [1997]. *Expert panel report II: Guidelines for the diagnosis and management of asthma* [Pub No 97-4051]. Bethesda, MD: National Heart, Lung, and Blood Institute.)

*Note: Some dry-powder inhalers require a different inhalation technique. To use these dry-powder inhalers, it is important to close the mouth tightly around the mouthpiece of the inhaler and inhale rapidly and deeply.

NURSING ALERT Caution parents of children with asthma and adolescents that long-acting β-adrenergic inhalers (salmeterol) should be used only as directed (usually every 12 hours) and not more frequently. They are not intended to relieve acute asthmatic symptoms.

The family should obtain a PEFM and learn to use this device to monitor the child's asthma. A written asthma action plan that includes the three peak flow metre zones and the child's asthma medications may be obtained from the child's primary care provider. Medications used for asthma exacerbations are also included in the asthma plan. This action plan should be used to make decisions about asthma management at home and at school. The nurse may assist the child and family in preparing this plan, emphasizing that they, and not the health care providers, determine the success of the plan.

Foods known to provoke symptoms should be eliminated from the diet, and parents should be advised to read labels on prepared foods and snacks to determine the presence of allergens.

The child should be protected from a respiratory tract infection that can trigger an attack or aggravate the asthmatic state, especially in young children whose airways are mechanically smaller and more reactive. Annual influenza vaccinations are recommended for children with persistent asthma (PHAC, 2007a). Equipment used for the child, such as nebulizers, must be kept absolutely clean to decrease the chances of contamination with bacteria and fungi.

Breathing exercises and controlled breathing should be taught and encouraged for motivated children, and the nurse should provide information on activities that promote diaphragmatic breathing, side expansion, and improved mobility of the chest wall. Play techniques that can be used for younger children to extend their expiratory time and increase expiratory pressure include blowing cotton balls or a ping-pong ball on a table, blowing a pinwheel, blowing bubbles, or preventing a tissue from falling by blowing it against the wall. Self-care and asthma self-management programs are important in helping the child and family cope with asthma. Most asthma self-management programs for children convey several principles. First, asthma is a common disease that can be controlled with appropriate medication therapy, environmental control, education, and management skills. Second, it is much easier to prevent than to treat an asthma episode; compliance with a therapeutic program is necessary to prevent exacerbations. Third, children with asthma can live full and active lives.

Asthma camps provide an opportunity for children with asthma to engage in physical activity while learning about their disease in a controlled environment with their peers and health care providers. Children who attend asthma camps often demonstrate improved asthma self-management skills.

Self-contained programs and brochures for patient education are available from the Asthma Society of Canada, Canadian Lung Association, and Canadian Allergy, Asthma, and Immunology Foundation. In Canada, the Asthma Society of Canada has educational material available and an innovative Web site that teaches children about asthma. The Asthma Society participates in the Global Initiative for Asthma, which is an asthma network that works with health care providers and public health groups to decrease asthma prevalence, morbidity, and mortality and is. The Canadian Lung Association has educational materials and resources available as well. For all of these resources, see the Additional Resources section at the end of this chapter.

Provide Acute Asthma Care

Children who are admitted to the hospital with acute asthma are ill, anxious, and uncomfortable. The progression or resolution of status asthmaticus is variable. The importance of continual observation and assessment cannot be overemphasized.

When β_2-agonists and corticosteroids are given, the child needs to be monitored closely and continuously for relief of respiratory distress and signs of adverse effects or toxicity. Oral fluid intake may be limited during the acute phase; IV fluid replacement may be required to provide adequate tissue hydration.

Older children may be more comfortable standing (Fig. 46-6), sitting upright, or leaning slightly forward (Fig. 46-7). When possible, the nurse should communicate in such a way that a child can reply in a few words to avoid fatigue. Shortness of breath makes talking difficult.

Children with acute asthma are apprehensive and anxious. The calm, efficient presence of a nurse can help reassure them that they are safe and will be cared for during this stressful period. It is important to assure children that they will not be left alone and that their parents are allowed to remain with them.

Parents need reassurance and want to be informed of their child's condition and therapies. They may believe that they have in some way contributed to the child's condition or could have prevented the episode. Reassurance regarding their efforts expended on the child's behalf and their parenting capabilities can help alleviate their stress. Efforts to reduce parental apprehension also reduce the child's distress, as anxiety is easily communicated to the child from parents and members of the staff.

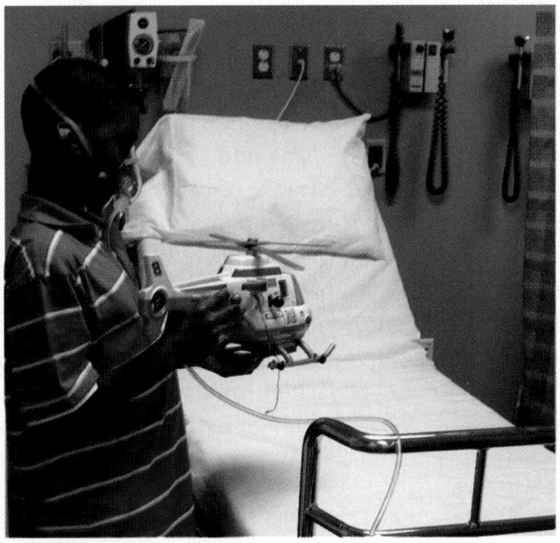

Fig. 46-6 Child with asthma is allowed play activity as tolerated.

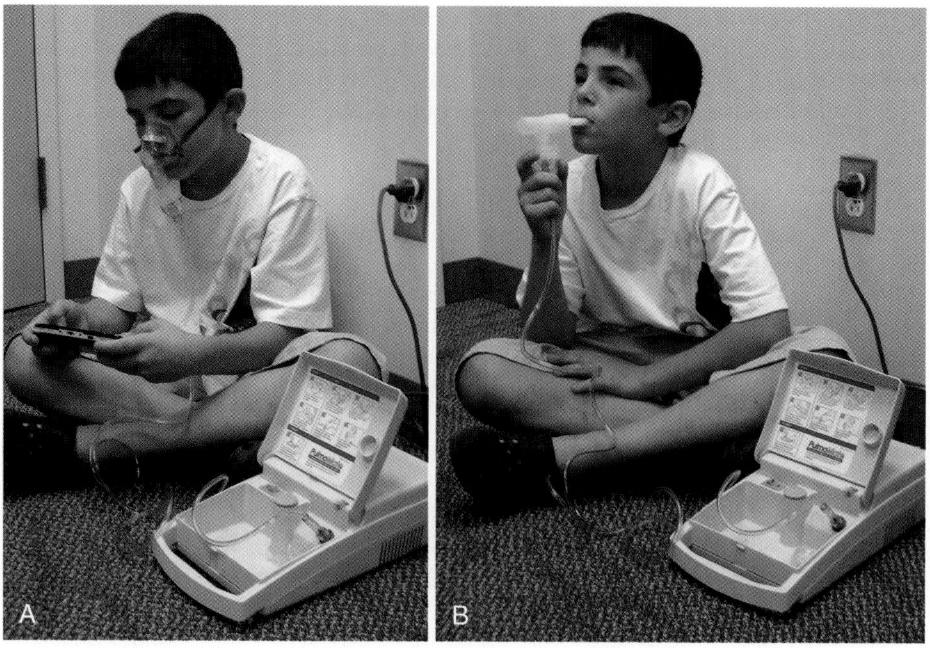

Fig. 46-7 Children with asthma may take a nebulized aerosol treatment with a mask (**A**) or mouthpiece (**B**). *(Courtesy Texas Children's Hospital, Houston.)*

Support the Child or Adolescent and Family

The nurse working with children with asthma can provide support in a number of ways. Many children voice frustration because their exacerbations interfere with their daily activities and social lives. They need education about what to do to prevent an asthma episode. These children also need reassurance from the health team that they can learn to control and cope with their asthma and live a normal life. It is important to be aware of children, especially adolescents, who demonstrate signs of depression and do not comply with therapy as a means of passive suicide.

Children in disruptive family situations (divorce, separation, violence, custodial battles) may disregard daily asthma medication regimen or may be at higher risk as a result of neglect by adults who are in charge of their care. Adolescents struggling with a sense of identity and body image often regard asthma as a condition that will "go away," especially if there is a time lapse between symptoms, and may abandon the therapeutic regimen. In some cases adolescents find themselves in charge of other siblings in blended family situations and may ignore their own health needs. Referral for counselling and guidance is appropriate when the child or adolescent's life is potentially in harm's way and the therapeutic regimen for asthma is abandoned because of other crises.

The short- and long-term adaptation of children with asthma often depends on the family's acceptance of the disorder. The task of living day-to-day with affected children involves the entire family. There are periodic crises and the ever-present threat of a crisis, requiring parental vigilance; sleepless nights; frequent trips to the physician, emergency department, or hospital; and often overwhelming medical expenses. Throughout these stresses, parents should be encouraged to promote as normal a life as possible for their children.

evolve Case Study—Cystic Fibrosis

Cystic Fibrosis

Cystic fibrosis (CF) is inherited as an autosomal recessive trait; the affected child inherits the defective gene from both parents, with an overall incidence of 1 : 4. The mutated gene responsible for CF is located on the long arm of **chromosome** 7. This gene codes a protein of 1480 amino acids called the *cystic fibrosis transmembrane regulator (CFTR)*. The CFTR protein is related to a family of membrane-bound glycoproteins. The glycoproteins constitute a cAMP-activated chloride channel and also regulate other chloride and sodium channels at the surfaces of the epithelial cells.

It is estimated that 1 in every 3600 Canadian children are born with CF. There are currently approximately 4000 children and adults that attend a CF clinic (Cystic Fibrosis Canada, 2010).

Pathophysiology

CF is characterized by several clinical features: increased viscosity of mucous gland secretions, a striking elevation of sweat electrolytes, an increase in several organic and enzymatic constituents of saliva, and abnormalities in autonomic nervous system function. Although both sodium and chloride are affected, the defect appears to be primarily a result of abnormal chloride movement; the CFTR appears to function as a chloride channel. Children with CF demonstrate decreased pancreatic secretion of bicarbonate and chloride and an increase in sodium and chloride in both saliva and sweat. This characteristic is the basis for the sweat chloride diagnostic test. The sweat electrolyte abnormality is present from birth, continues throughout life, and is unrelated to the severity of the disease or the extent to which other organs are involved.

The primary factor, and the one that is responsible for many of the clinical manifestations of the disease, is mechanical obstruction caused by the increased viscosity of mucous gland secretions (Fig. 46-8). Instead of forming a thin, freely flowing secretion, the mucous glands produce a thick mucoprotein that accumulates and dilates them. Small passages in organs such as the pancreas and bronchioles become obstructed as secretions precipitate or coagulate to form concretions in glands and ducts. The earliest postnatal manifestation of CF

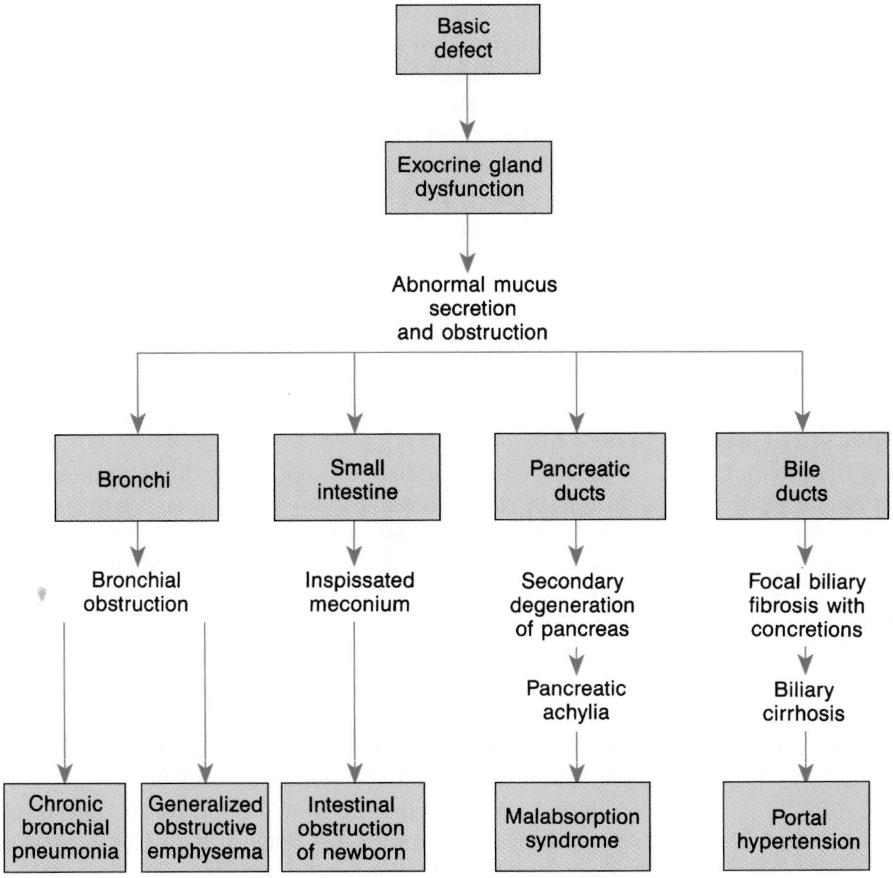

Fig. 46-8 Various effects of exocrine gland dysfunction in cystic fibrosis.

is often meconium ileus in the newborn, in which the small intestine is blocked with thick, puttylike, tenacious, mucilaginous meconium.

In the pancreas the thick secretions block the ducts, eventually causing pancreatic fibrosis. This blockage prevents essential pancreatic enzymes from reaching the duodenum, which causes marked impairment in the digestion and absorption of nutrients. The disturbed function is reflected in bulky stools that are frothy from undigested fat (*steatorrhea*) and foul smelling from putrefied protein (*azotorrhea*). The endocrine function of the pancreas often remains unchanged because the islets of Langerhans are normal but may decrease in number as pancreatic fibrosis progresses. The incidence of diabetes mellitus (cystic fibrosis–related diabetes [CFRD]) is greater in CF children than in the general population (Balinsky & Zhu, 2004), which may be caused by changes in pancreatic architecture and diminished blood supply over time. Consequently, with increased survival and primarily in adolescents and adults, type 1 diabetes is becoming a more frequent finding. There is no relationship between the progression of pulmonary disease and the development of diabetes mellitus in CF. In the liver, localized biliary obstruction and fibrosis are common and become more extensive with time.

A common gastrointestinal complication associated with CF is prolapse of the rectum, which occurs in infancy and childhood and is related to large, bulky stools, malnutrition, and increased intra-abdominal pressure secondary to paroxysmal cough. Affected children of all ages are subject to intestinal obstruction from inspissated or impacted feces. Gumlike masses can obstruct the bowel and produce a partial or complete obstruction, a condition that is referred to as *distal intestinal obstruction syndrome.*

Pulmonary complications are present in almost all children with CF, but the onset and extent of involvement are variable. Symptoms are produced by stagnation of mucus in the airways, with eventual bacterial colonization leading to destruction of lung tissue. The abnormally viscous and tenacious secretions are difficult to expectorate and gradually obstruct the bronchi and bronchioles, causing scattered areas of bronchiectasis, atelectasis, and hyperinflation. The stagnant mucus offers a favourable environment for bacterial growth.

The reproductive systems of both males and females with CF are affected. Females with CF have normal fallopian tubes and ovaries, but fertility can be inhibited by highly viscous cervical secretions, which act as a plug, blocking sperm entry. Women with CF who become pregnant have an increased incidence of premature labour and delivery and low birth weight in the infant. Favourable nutritional status and pulmonary function are positively correlated with favourable pregnancy outcomes. Most adult men (95%) with CF are sterile, which may be caused by blockage of the vas deferens with abnormal secretions or by failure of normal development of the wolffian duct structures (vas deferens, epididymis, and seminal vesicles), resulting in decreased or absent sperm production.

Growth and development are often affected in children with moderate to severe forms of CF. Physical growth may be restricted as a result of decreased absorption of nutrients, including vitamins and fat; increased oxygen demands for pulmonary function; and delayed bone growth. The usual pattern is one of growth failure (failure to thrive), with increased weight loss despite an increased appetite and gradual deterioration of the respiratory system. Clinical manifestations of CF are listed in Box 46-15.

Diagnostic Evaluation

Traditionally the diagnosis of CF was based on a positive sweat chloride test, absence of pancreatic enzymes, radiography, chronic obstructive pulmonary disease, and family history. Newer diagnostic methods make it possible to diagnose CF early in infancy so therapies can be implemented to increase the child's overall survival and quality of life. In addition to the sweat chloride test and factors listed previously, diagnosis may be confirmed by any one of the following: newborn screening, deoxyribonucleic acid (DNA) identification of mutant genes, and abnormal nasal potential difference measurement.

While universal newborn screening for CF has been recommended by Cystic Fibrosis Canada (2011b), it remains controversial. The provinces that do newborn screening are Alberta, Ontario, Saskatchewan, and British Columbia. The newborn screening test consists of an immunoreactive trypsinogen (IRT) analysis performed on a dried spot of blood, which may be followed by direct analysis of DNA for the presence of the ΔF508 mutation or other mutations on the same dried blood spot. Benefits of early screening and detection include earlier nutritional intervention for identified infants (Farrell et al., 2007; Southern et al., 2009); disadvantages include the parental anxiety that false-positive results may generate. Children who are identified and treated early in infancy with aggressive nutritional support have had improved height and weight well into adolescence. An in utero diagnosis of CF is also possible based on detection of two CF mutations in the fetus.

The consistent finding of abnormally high sodium and chloride concentrations in the sweat is a unique characteristic of CF. Parents may report that their infant tastes "salty" when they kiss the infant. The quantitative sweat chloride test (pilocarpine iontophoresis) involves stimulating the production of sweat with a special device (involves stimulation with 3-mA electric current), collecting the sweat on filter paper, and measuring the sweat electrolytes. The quantitative analysis requires a sufficient volume of sweat (more than 75 mg). Two separate samples are collected to ensure the reliability of the test for any individual. Normally, sweat chloride content is less than 40 mmol/L, with a mean of 18 mmol/L. A chloride concentration greater than 60 mmol/L is diagnostic of CF; in infants younger than 3 months a sweat chloride concentration greater than 40 mmol/L is highly suggestive of CF. In some situations DNA testing may be substituted for the sweat test. The presence of a mutation known to cause CF on each *CFTR* gene predicts with a high degree of certainty that the individual has CF; however, multiple *CFTR* mutations may also be present and detected with DNA assay.

Chest radiography reveals characteristic patchy atelectasis and obstructive emphysema. PFTs are sensitive indexes of lung function, providing evidence of abnormal small airway function in CF. Other diagnostic tools that may aid in diagnosis include stool fat or enzyme analysis. Stool analysis requires a 72-hour sample with accurate recording of food intake during that time. Radiographs, including barium enema, are used for diagnosis of meconium ileus.

BOX 46-15 Clinical Manifestations of Cystic Fibrosis

Meconium Ileus*
Abdominal distension
Vomiting
Failure to pass stools
Rapid development of dehydration

Gastrointestinal Manifestations
Large, bulky, loose, frothy, extremely foul-smelling stools
Voracious appetite (early in disease)
Loss of appetite (later in disease)
Weight loss
Marked tissue wasting
Failure to grow
Distended abdomen
Thin extremities
Sallow skin
Evidence of deficiency of fat-soluble vitamins A, D, E, and K
Anemia

Pulmonary Manifestations
Initial signs:
- Wheezing respirations
- Dry, nonproductive cough

Eventually:
- Increased dyspnea
- Paroxysmal cough
- Evidence of obstructive emphysema and patchy areas of atelectasis

Progressive involvement:
- Overinflated, barrel-shaped chest
- Cyanosis
- Clubbing of fingers and toes
- Repeated episodes of bronchitis and bronchopneumonia

*In about 10% of cases.

evolve Critical Thinking Exercise—Cystic Fibrosis Inheritance Risks

Therapeutic Management

Improved survival among patients with CF during the past two decades can be attributed largely to antibiotic therapy and improved nutritional management. Goals of CF therapeutic management are to (1) prevent or minimize pulmonary complications, (2) ensure adequate nutrition for growth, (3) encourage appropriate physical activity, and (4) promote a reasonable quality of life for the child and the family. A multidisciplinary approach to treatment is needed to accomplish these goals.

Management of Pulmonary Problems

Management of pulmonary problems is directed toward prevention and treatment of pulmonary infection by improving ventilation, removing mucopurulent secretions, and administering antimicrobial agents. Many children develop respiratory symptoms by 3 years of age. The large amounts and viscosity of respiratory secretions in children with CF contribute to the likelihood of respiratory tract infections. Recurrent pulmonary infections in the child with CF result in greater damage to the airways; small airways are destroyed, causing bronchiectasis.

The most common pathogens responsible for pulmonary infections are *P. aeruginosa*, *B. cepacia*, *S. aureus*, *H. influenzae*, *E. coli*, and *K. pneumoniae*. *P. aeruginosa* and *B. cepacia* are particularly pathogenic for children with CF, and infections with these organisms are difficult to clear. In addition, children with CF who are chronically colonized with these organisms have poorer survival rates than those of children who are not colonized. Colonization and infection with methicillin-resistant *S. aureus* (MRSA) has emerged as a critical factor in lung infection and pulmonary function in patients with CF. Patients with MRSA required longer hospitalization and multiple antibiotic regimens (Ren et al., 2007). Fungal colonization with *Candida* or *Aspergillus* organisms in the respiratory tract is also common in patients with CF.

Prevention of infection involves a daily routine of CPT to maintain pulmonary hygiene. CPT is usually performed on average twice daily (on rising and in the evening) and more frequently if needed, especially during pulmonary infection. The Flutter mucus clearance device is a small, handheld plastic pipe with a stainless-steel ball on the inside that facilitates removal of mucus (Fig. 46-9). It has the advantage of increasing sputum expectoration and being used without an assistant. Handheld percussors may be used to loosen secretions. Another method to clear mucus is high-frequency chest compression, in which the child temporarily wears a mechanical vest device that provides high-frequency chest wall oscillation. Some children and adolescents with an implantable port may experience localized pain with the vest.

Patients with CF have been found to regress when conventional CPT is discontinued. Therefore, although it is time consuming for the child and family, CPT remains the cornerstone of pulmonary therapy. Forced expiration, or "huffing," with the glottis partially closed helps move secretions from the small airways so that subsequent coughing can move secretions forcefully from the large airways. Several studies indicate that this manoeuvre enhances the pulmonary function of patients with CF. Autogenic drainage involves a variety of breathing techniques, which the older child can use to force mucus in lower lobes up into the airways so it can be successfully expelled. Another mucus-clearing technique involves use of a positive expiratory pressure mask; this technique involves breathing into a mask attached to a one-way valve, which creates resistance—as the patient exhales, the airway is kept open by the pressure, and mucus is forced into the upper airway for expulsion.

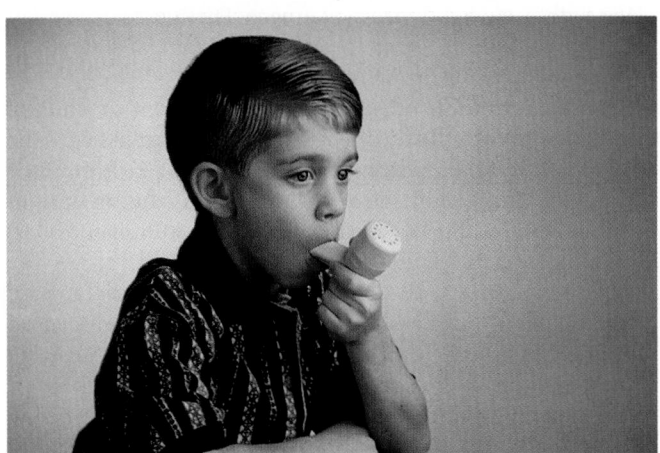

Fig. 46-9 Child using Flutter mucus clearance device. *(Courtesy Scandipharm, Inc.)*

Bronchodilator medication delivered in an aerosol opens bronchi for easier expectoration and is administered before CPT when the patient exhibits evidence of reactive airway disease or wheezing. Another aerosolized medication is recombinant human deoxyribonuclease (DNase, known generically as dornase alfa [Pulmozyme]), which decreases the viscosity of mucus. It is well tolerated and has no major adverse effects; minor reactions are voice alterations and laryngitis. This medication, given daily via nebulization, has resulted in improvements in spirometry, PFTs, dyspnea scores, and perceptions of well-being and has reduced the viscosity of sputum.

Physical exercise is an important adjunct to daily CPT. Exercise stimulates mucus excretion and provides a sense of well-being and increased self-esteem. Any aerobic exercise that the patient enjoys should be encouraged. The ultimate aim of exercise is to increase lung vital capacity, remove secretions, increase pulmonary blood flow, and maintain healthy lung tissue for effective ventilation.

Pulmonary infections need to be treated as soon as they are recognized. In patients with CF characteristic signs of pulmonary infection—fever, tachypnea, and chest pain—may be absent; thus a careful history and physical examination are essential. The presence of **anorexia**, weight loss, and decreased activity should alert the practitioner to pulmonary infection and the need for an antibiotic regimen (Boat & Acton, 2007). Aerosolized antibiotics such as tobramycin, ticarcillin, and gentamicin are beneficial for patients with frequent pulmonary exacerbations. It is not uncommon for the hospitalized child with CF to be placed on as many as two or three antibiotics and one antifungal medication to treat coexisting pulmonary infections.

IV antibiotics may be administered at home as an alternative to hospitalization. The use of peripherally inserted central catheters (PICCs) for the administration of antibiotics in children with CF is a viable option with limited complications and fewer needle punctures to obtain blood specimens and to maintain often lengthy treatment with parenteral antibiotics (Tolomeo & Mackey, 2003). Alternatively, an implanted port offers the advantage of access for blood draws and antibiotic infusion. Patients may receive antibiotic therapy at home and continue daily activities with minimum disruptions. However, when pulmonary function does not improve with outpatient management, hospitalization may be recommended for continued antibiotic therapy and vigorous CPT and postural drainage. Oxygen administration is used for children with acute episodes but must be used cautiously because many children with CF have chronic carbon dioxide retention and the unsupervised use of oxygen can be harmful (see Oxygen

Therapy, Chapter 45). With repeated infection and inflammation, bronchial cysts and emphysema may develop. These cysts may rupture, resulting in a pneumothorax.

NURSING ALERT Signs of a pneumothorax are usually nonspecific and include tachypnea, tachycardia, dyspnea, pallor, and cyanosis. A subtle drop in oxygen saturation (measured by pulse oximetry) may be an early sign of pneumothorax.

Blood streaking of the sputum is usually associated with increased pulmonary infection and often requires no specific treatment. Hemoptysis greater than 250 mL/24 hr for the older child (less for a younger child) indicates a potentially life-threatening event and needs to be treated immediately. Sometimes bleeding can be controlled with bed rest, IV antibiotics, replacement of acute blood loss, IV conjugated estrogens (Premarin) or vasopressin (Pitressin), and correction of any coagulation defects with vitamin K or fresh frozen plasma. If hemoptysis persists, the site of bleeding should be localized via bronchoscopy and cauterized or embolized.

Treatment of nasal polyps includes intranasal corticosteroids, oral antihistamines, and decongestants. If these measures are ineffective, surgical interventions may be necessary.

Because pulmonary damage in patients with CF is believed to be caused by the inflammatory process that occurs with frequent infections, the use of corticosteroids has been studied; however, treatment with corticosteroids for prolonged periods has been associated with linear growth restriction, glucose tolerance abnormalities, and **cataract** formation. Anti-inflammatory medications such as ibuprofen are becoming more important in the treatment of CF, but careful monitoring for adverse effects (gastrointestinal bleeding) is essential.

Management of Gastrointestinal Problems

The principal treatment for pancreatic insufficiency is replacement of pancreatic enzymes, which are administered with meals and snacks to ensure that digestive enzymes are mixed with food in the duodenum. Enteric-coated products prevent the neutralization of enzymes by gastric acids, thus allowing activation to occur in the alkaline environment of the small bowel. The amount of enzymes depends on the severity of the insufficiency, the child's response to enzyme replacement, and the practitioner's philosophy. Usually one to five capsules are administered with a meal, and fewer are taken with snacks. Capsules can be swallowed whole or taken apart, and the contents sprinkled on a small amount of food to be taken at the beginning of the meal. The amount of enzyme is adjusted to achieve normal growth and a decrease in the number of stools to one or two per day. Pancreatic enzymes should be taken within 30 minutes of eating. The enteric-coated beads should not be chewed or crushed, since destroying the enteric coating can lead to inactivation of the enzymes and excoriation of oral mucosa. The powder form should be used cautiously because inhalation of the powder may precipitate acute bronchospasm. Enzymes can be mixed into cereal or fruit such as applesauce. Because the uptake of fat-soluble vitamins is decreased, water-miscible forms of these vitamins (A, D, E, and K) are given, along with multivitamins and the pancreatic enzymes. When high-fat foods are eaten, the child should be encouraged to add extra enzymes.

Children with CF require a well-balanced, high-protein, high-caloric diet (because of the impaired intestinal absorption). In the patient with minimal pulmonary disease, energy requirements up to 5 to 10% above the recommended daily allowances are necessary; for those with severe lung disease, energy requirements may be as high as 20 to 50% or more of the recommended daily allowance (Cystic Fibrosis Canada, n.d.a), Breastfeeding with enzyme supplementation should be continued whenever possible and, when necessary, supplemented with a higher-calorie-per-mL (e.g., 24 kcal/30 mL) formula. For formula-fed infants, commercial cow's milk–based formulas may be adequate to achieve desired growth, but if growth is inadequate, additional caloric intake may be required. In older children with CF, three daily meals and three snacks are recommended to meet energy and growth requirements (Cystic Fibrosis Canada, n.d.a). Growth failure despite adequate nutritional support may indicate deterioration of pulmonary status. Patients with CF may experience frequent anorexia as a result of the copious amounts of mucus produced and expectorated, persistent cough, effect of medications, fatigue, and sleep disruption. They may be placed on nighttime supplemental gastrostomy feedings or parenteral alimentation in an effort to build up nutritional reserves if there has been a history of inability to maintain weight. Enzyme supplementation can be encouraged with gastrostomy feedings; these may be given at the initiation of the infusion, at bedtime, and at the conclusion of the feeding infusion (Cystic Fibrosis Canada, 2012). Meconium ileus and meconium ileus equivalent, or total or partial intestinal obstruction, can occur at any age. Constipation is often the result of a combination of malabsorption (either from inadequate pancreatic enzyme dosage or a failure to take the enzymes), decreased intestinal motility, and abnormally viscous intestinal secretions. These problems usually do not require surgical interventions and may be treated with GoLYTELY or Colyte (osmotic solutions given orally or by nasogastric tubes), other laxatives, stool softeners, or rectal administration of meglumine diatrizoate (Gastrografin).

Rectal prolapse occurs in about 20 to 25% of children with CF (McMullen & Bryson, 2004). The first episode of rectal prolapse is frightening to both parents and the child. Its reduction usually requires immediate guidance and intervention, which is managed by simply guiding the rectum back into place with a gloved, lubricated finger. Further management usually involves attempting to decrease the bulk of daily stools through enzyme replacement.

Children with CF often experience transient or chronic gastroesophageal reflux, which should be treated with the appropriate histamine-receptor antagonist and gastrointestinal motility medication, dietary modifications, and an upright position after feedings or meals (McMullen & Bryson, 2004).

Management of Endocrine Problems

The management of CFRD is critical in the therapeutic treatment of the child with CF. CFRD presents a combination of insulin resistance and insulin deficiency, with unstable glucose homeostasis in the presence of acute lung infection and treatment. Children with CFRD require close monitoring of blood glucose, administration of oral glucose-lowering agents or insulin injections, and diet and exercise management; children with CF may be at increased risk for glucose management problems as a result of decreased nutrient absorption, anorexia, and severity of pulmonary illness. The prevalence of CFRD increases with age, and there is increased morbidity and mortality among children with CFRD compared to those without CFRD (Strausbaugh & Davis, 2007). Microvascular complications such as retinopathy and nephropathy may occur in children and adolescents with CFRD (Schwarzenberg et al., 2007). However, ketoacidosis is rare in individuals with CFRD (Boat & Acton, 2007).

Bone health is of concern in children and adults with CF. The pancreatic insufficiency of CF and chronic steroid use present potential risks for less than optimum bone growth in such children. Assessment of bone health by history and bone mass density evaluation should be considered in assessing the child's (8 years old and older) health status to detect and prevent osteoporosis or osteopenia (Borowitz, Baker, & Stallings, 2002).

The administration of growth hormone (somatropin [Nutropin]) is being investigated as a nutritional adjunct in children with CF to achieve optimum growth; one small study sample suggests an improvement in CF clinical status (Hardin et al., 2005). One randomized study indicates that the drug is well tolerated but does not result in short-term improvement of forced expiratory volume (FEV) in CF patients (Schnabel et al., 2007).

Lung Transplants

Lung transplants have brought new hope to individuals with CF. A patient with CF may require a lung, kidney, pancreas, liver, or heart transplant. The most common transplant is the lungs, which can become damaged by the recurrent infections leading to serious obstructive lung disease. The improved technology and treatment of lung transplantation have improved outcomes for patients with CF. Children with CF and their families who choose transplantation need to be prepared carefully and be fully informed about the procedure, the need for following the strict post-transplant treatment protocols, and the psychological impact of transplantation (Cystic Fibrosis Canada, 2011a).

Double lung transplant recipients with CF indicate that their condition has improved, with less coughing and shortness of breath. They have more energy and strength. The transplanted lungs will not have CF because of the different genetics but the recipient will still have CF in the rest of the body and will need continued CF treatments.

The criteria for acceptance on the transplant list is as follows: forced expiratory volume below 30% or a rapid decline in it, hypoxia <55 mm Hg, hypercapnia >45 mm Hg, life-threatening events such as significant hemoptysis or pneumothoraces, and be a survivable surgical risk (Cystic Fibrosis Canada, 2011a).

Organ donations numbers have increased in Canada but the number waiting for transplants outnumber the available organs. Two living lung donors can donate two lung lobes if they are a tissue match, have good lung function, and are in excellent health. In 2008, there were 40 lung transplants in the Canadian CF population (Cystic Fibrosis Canada, 2011a).

Post-transplant, the recipient stays in the critical care unit on a ventilator for a few days or weeks until the new lungs are working well. Immunosuppressants are given and the recipient must be carefully monitored for signs of organ rejection and infection. Organ rejection can occur mostly within the first 12 months; a chronic rejection or bronchiolitis obliterans can occur over a lengthy period of time, which causes inflammation and lung scarring. If the rejection is very significant, retransplantation may be required (Cystic Fibrosis Canada, 2011a).

Prognosis

The median age of survival for Canadians with CF is currently estimated to be 48.1 years of age. Females with CF have had higher mortality than males with CF (Cystic Fibrosis Canada, 2010). Transplantation has increased survival rates among some patients with CF. Despite considerable progress and a recent surge in new treatment modalities, CF remains a progressive and incurable disease. The pulmonary involvement ultimately determines the patient's outcome because pancreatic enzyme deficiency is less of a problem if adequate nutrition is ensured. With the advances in treatment technology, parents and adolescents are challenged to set future goals that may include college, careers, social relationships, and marriage. Concurrently they are faced with increasing morbidity and higher rates of CF complications as they grow older.

Nursing Care Management

Assessment of the child with CF involves both pulmonary and gastrointestinal observations. Pulmonary assessment is the same as that described for asthma, with special attention to lung sounds, observation of cough, and evidence of decreased activity or fatigue. Gastrointestinal assessment primarily involves observing the frequency and nature of the stools and abdominal distension. Evidence of growth failure (e.g., weight loss, muscle wasting, pallor, anorexia, decreased activity [from baseline norm]) also needs to be noted. Family members should be interviewed to determine the child's eating and eliminating habits and to confirm the child's history of frequent respiratory tract infections or bowel obstruction in infancy.

The nurse should assess the newborn for feeding and stooling patterns, which may indicate a potential problem such as meconium ileus. The nurse should also participate in diagnostic testing, such as the initial newborn screening, IRT, DNA analysis, or sweat chloride test.

Parents are often anxious and puzzled about the diagnostic tests and the possible implications of the test results. They need careful explanations of the disease, how it might affect their family, and what they can do to provide the best possible care for their child. It is crucial to involve the parents in the follow-up for early diagnostic testing; the neonate may require several follow-up visits in the first few weeks of life if initial test results are not conclusive.

The uncertainty, fear, and initial shock associated with the diagnosis can be overwhelming to parents. They must face the impact of the chronic, life-threatening nature of the disease and the prospect of intensive treatment, for which they must assume a major part of the responsibility and are usually ill prepared. They often fear that they will be unable to provide the care that the child needs. One of the most difficult aspects of the diagnosis is the implication inherent in its etiology (i.e., the recognition that each parent contributed the gene responsible for the defect).

Hospital Care

Most patients with CF require hospitalization only for the treatment of pulmonary infection, uncontrolled diabetes, or a coexisting medical problem that cannot be treated on an outpatient basis. When patients with CF are hospitalized, routine precautions with meticulous hand washing should be implemented to decrease the health care–associated spread of organisms to the CF patient and between hospitalized patients with CF (especially when MRSA is prevalent). Contact precautions may be required for specific infections.

When the child with CF is hospitalized for diagnosis or treatment of pulmonary complications, aerosol therapy, chest percussion therapy, and postural drainage need to be instituted or continued. While respiratory therapists often initiate, supervise, and provide these treatments, it is the nurse's responsibility to monitor the patient's tolerance of the procedure and evaluate its effectiveness in relation to treatment goals. The nurse may at times administer aerosol therapy, perform CPT, assist with mucus removal interventions such as the mechanical vest, and teach breathing exercises. CPT should not be performed before or immediately after meals. Planning CPT so that it does not coincide with meals can be difficult in the hospital but is essential to the effectiveness of this treatment.

Supplemental oxygen therapy is administered to the child with mild or moderate respiratory distress, and the child requires frequent assessment of his or her tolerance of the procedure. Noninvasive pulse oximetry provides valuable data about the patient's oxygenation status, and nursing assessments, including observation of respiratory pattern, work of breathing, and lung auscultation, are vital.

One of the nursing challenges in the care of the child with CF is encouraging compliance with the therapeutic medication regimen, which often involves a significant number of medications; pancreatic enzymes; vitamins A, D, E, and K; oral antifungals for *Candida* infection; antihistamines; anti-inflammatory agents; and oral antibiotics. This may be overwhelming to the child. There may also be multiple inhaled bronchodilators, CPT and aerosol treatments, blood glucose monitoring and insulin administration, various other medications, and increased mucus production during the acute phase, thus it is not uncommon for the child with CF to rebel and be noncompliant with this regimen. Gentle coaxing, positive reinforcement, and frank negotiation may be required to encourage the child to adhere to the required medical treatment.

The child's sleep may be disrupted frequently by hospital routines; nursing care should be flexible enough to allow him or her some quiet time without affecting vital care. In some cases a daily schedule of events, including medication administration, CPT, aerosolized therapy, and dressing changes, may need to be mutually developed with the child, nurses, and physician so that the child feels he or she has some control of the care.

The diet for the child with CF represents another challenge; careful planning with a pediatric dietitian and the child may help decrease the loss of appetite and weight loss that are often part of the condition. Patients with CF, especially adolescents, enjoy foods brought from home or an occasional fast food of choice (provided these meet therapeutic requirements). Children in the early stages of CF often have a good appetite. With infection and increased lung involvement, their appetite diminishes, and eventually it becomes a challenge to tempt failing appetites. When dietary intake fails to meet the child's needs for growth, enteral feedings or supplements may need to be considered (Cystic Fibrosis Canada, n.d.b). These feedings may be administered via gastrostomy tube during the night to minimize the disruption of daily activities, including school. A skin-level feeding gastrostomy affords the child few activity restrictions and minimum disruption of body image in comparison to a nasogastric tube or conventional gastrostomy tube. The child and parents should be encouraged to perceive this therapy not as a last-ditch effort but as an adjunct therapy to maintain optimum growth and prevent excessive weight loss (Cystic Fibrosis Canada, n.d.b).

The child needs support during the many treatments and tests that are a part of the hospitalization. IV fluids, IV antibiotics and antifungals, and blood tests are almost always a part of the acute care treatment, and the child may soon associate hospitalization with these stress-provoking procedures.

Depression, anxiety, and disturbed self-image may occur in children and adolescents with CF; young adults with severe symptoms may be especially prone to depression as a result of the realization of the poor prognosis and the reality of unmet life expectations and goals.

Providing support to both the child and the family is essential. The progressive nature of the disease makes each illness requiring hospitalization a potentially life-threatening event. Skilled nursing care and sympathetic attention to the emotional needs of the child and family can help them cope with the stresses associated with repeated respiratory tract infections and hospitalizations.

The child or adolescent who is immobilized as a result of CF requires the same care and attention as the child with immobility from any other chronic or acute illness, including skin care, bowel management, passive range of motion, and positioning.

Home Care

Most children and adolescents with CF can be managed at home. The goals of care include **normalization** and daily activities, including school and peer involvement. The care plan should be flexible so that family activities are disrupted as little as possible. Parents may initially require assistance in finding and contacting durable medical equipment companies that provide home care equipment. They also need opportunities to learn how to use the equipment and to solve problems they may encounter while delivering therapy at home. The many aspects of home care for the child with CF are similar to those of home care for other children and are discussed in Chapter 43.

Patients and family members need education about the preferred diet of nutritious meals with tolerated fat, increased protein and carbohydrate, and the administration of pancreatic enzymes. For infants and young children, the enzymes can be mixed with pureed fruit such as applesauce and fed with a spoon. Capsules are usually suitable for older children. It is important to stress to parents that the enzymes, in the amount regulated to the child's needs, should be administered at the beginning of all meals and snacks.

One of the most important aspects of educating parents for home care is teaching techniques for the removal of mucus (CPT, vest, forced expiration) and breathing exercises. The success of a therapy program depends on conscientious performance of these treatments regularly as prescribed. The number of times these therapies are performed each day is determined on an individual basis, and often parents readily learn to adjust the number and intensity of the treatments to the child's needs. For pulmonary infection, home IV antibiotics may be prescribed. Home IV care may be preferred for willing and competent families, as it reduces tension and usually brings a sense of belonging to the family members. This option depends on a number of factors, including availability of an agency with adequate staff to perform multiple daily home antibiotic infusions. With use of the venous access devices such as PICC lines and implanted ports, the parents and child can be taught the technique of direct administration into the IV line. Around-the-clock administration may be difficult for families and requires certain adjustments, such as waking at least once during the night to give the medication.

Families also need information about medications and possible adverse effects. If a child is receiving ibuprofen, serum drug levels need to be monitored closely to establish therapeutic dosages, and observations for adverse effects such as gastrointestinal irritation are essential.

Children and adolescents with CF should receive routine primary care with special attention to diet, growth and development, and immunizations. Primary care providers should be alert to any weight loss or flattening in the growth curve associated with loss of appetite, which could indicate a pulmonary exacerbation in children with CF (McMullen & Bryson, 2004). In addition to all the recommended routine immunizations, CF patients should be immunized against influenza starting at age 6 months; this should be followed by an annual booster (PHAC, 2007a). Anticipatory guidance concerning issues of discipline, how to incorporate aspects of the treatment regimen into the school environment, and delayed pubertal development are also important considerations for the primary care provider.

Home palliative care for the child or adolescent with CF who is in the terminal stages may be carried out with the assistance of hospice (see Chapter 41).

The nurse can assist the family in contacting resources that provide help to families with affected children. Various special child health services, many local clinics, private agencies, service clubs, and other community groups often offer equipment and medications either free or at reduced rates. Cystic Fibrosis Canada (formerly the Canadian Cystic Fibrosis Foundation) has chapters throughout Canada to provide education and services to families and professionals (see Additional Resources section at the end of this chapter).

Family Support

The most challenging aspect of providing care for the family of a child or adolescent with CF is meeting the emotional needs of the child and family. The diagnosis, treatment, and prognosis for CF are often associated with many problems and frustrations. The diagnosis can evoke feelings of guilt and self-recrimination in parents.

The long-range problems for an infant, child, or adolescent with CF are those encountered in any chronic illness (see Chapter 41). Both the child and the family must make many adjustments, the success of which depends on their ability to cope and also on the quality and quantity of support they receive from outside sources. Combined efforts of a variety of health care providers are needed to provide the most comprehensive services to families. It is often the nurse who assesses the home situation, organizes and coordinates these services, and collects the data needed to evaluate the effectiveness of the services.

The persistent need for treatment several times a day can place tremendous strain on the family. When the child is young, a family member must perform postural drainage and CPT. Children often balk at these treatments, and the parents are placed in the position of insisting on adherence. The stress and anxiety related to this routine may produce feelings of resentment in both the child and the family members. When possible, occasional trusted respite care should be available to allow parents to leave the situation for short periods without undue anxiety about the child's welfare.

The affected child or adolescent may become resentful about the disease, its relentless routine of therapy, and the necessary curtailment it places on activities and relationships. The child's activities are interrupted or built around treatments, medications, and diet. This imposes hardships and influences his or her quality of life. The child should be encouraged to attend school and join age-appropriate peer groups to foster a life that is as normal and productive as possible. Sports are often an important part of the child and adolescent's life; interaction with peers is a valuable life experience, especially to adolescents. The child or adolescent with CF should be encouraged to participate in sports activities as much as physical and pulmonary health allows. Exercise should be encouraged to increase pulmonary vital capacity, promote muscle development, and enhance cardiovascular function.

As the disease progresses, however, family stress should be expected, and the patient may become angry and noncompliant. It is important for the nurse to recognize the family's changing needs and the grief they may experience as the CF worsens. Families should be made aware of sources for counselling. Patients need to be guided into activities that enable them to express anger, sorrow, and fear, without guilt.

Transition to Adulthood

As life expectancy continues to rise for children and adolescents with CF, issues related to marriage, sexuality, childbearing, and career choice have become more pressing. Males must be informed at some point that they may be unable to produce offspring. It is important that the distinction be made between sterility and impotence. Normal sexual relationships can be expected. Female patients may be able to bear children but should be informed of the possible deleterious effects on their respiratory system created by the burden of pregnancy. They also need to know that their children will be carriers of the CF gene. Adolescent females may need counselling concerning the use of oral contraceptives and other contraceptive options (Cystic Fibrosis Canada, 2012).

Adolescents with CF should be encouraged to take responsibility for management of the illness to maximize their life's potential. Many adolescents and young persons with the illness enroll in college or vocational and technical training school and complete degrees by either distance learning or attending a local school. Young people should be encouraged to set life goals and live normal lives to the extent their illness allows.

Life as an independent adult should be encouraged for children with CF. From the time that children can take partial responsibility for their own care (e.g., CPT and taking enzymes), independence and accountability should be fostered. Although the prognosis for these children has improved, many will need continued support as they cope with the demands of surviving with CF.

Anticipatory grief and other aspects related to care of a child with a terminal illness are also part of nursing care. For example, it is important to prepare the child and family members for end-of-life decisions and care.

evolve Animation—Respiratory Failure, Infant

Obstructive Sleep-Disordered Breathing

Pediatric obstructive sleep-disordered breathing reportedly affects between 10 and 12% of children ages 2 to 8 years; obstructive sleep apnea may occur in as many as 2% of all children (Benninger & Walner, 2007b). Obstructive sleep-disordered breathing is said to form a continuum of sleep-disordered breathing ranging from partial obstruction of the upper airway to continuous episodes of complete upper airway obstruction, with the most severe form being obstructive sleep apnea syndrome (OSAS) (Benninger & Walner, 2007b). OSAS is defined by the Canadian Lung Association (2012) as a disorder of breathing during sleep with prolonged partial upper airway obstruction or complete obstruction that disrupts normal respiration during sleep and normal sleep patterns. Common symptoms include nightly snoring, interrupted or disturbed sleep patterns, enuresis, and daytime neurobehavioural problems (AAP, 2002; Chan, Edman, & Koltai, 2004). OSAS is to be distinguished from primary snoring, which is snoring without obstructive apnea, frequent sleep arousals, or abnormalities in gas exchange (AAP, 2002). Interestingly, children with OSAS do not exhibit daytime sleepiness as do adults; the exception may be obese children (Chan et al., 2004). If left untreated, obstructive sleep-disordered breathing may result in complications such as growth failure, cor pulmonale, pulmonary hypertension, poor learning, behavioural problems, attention-deficit/hyperactivity disorder, and death.

The diagnosis of obstructive sleep-disordered breathing is made by a sleep study (*polysomnography*), which provides evidence of sleep disturbance, respiratory pauses, and changes in oxygenation. The six-channel polysomnography can be performed in children of all ages with video or audio recording, and abbreviated (vs. full-night sleep study) polysomnography may be useful; however, this latter method does not predict the severity of OSAS (AAP, 2002).

A common treatment for sleep-disordered breathing in children is adenotonsillectomy, provided there is evidence of adenotonsillar hypertrophy (Benninger & Walner, 2007b). Complications of these surgical interventions are discussed previously in this chapter. Continuous positive airway pressure (CPAP) and bilevel (cycles between high and low pressure) positive airway pressure (BiPAP) may be helpful in older children with sleep-disordered breathing whose condition persists after surgical intervention. CPAP is a long-term therapy with frequent assessments to evaluate the required amount of pressure and the overall effectiveness of the intervention.

Surgical interventions such as tracheotomy may be required for children with craniofacial syndromes such as Goldenhar, Pierre Robin, Apert, and Crouzon, in which there is partial or complete upper airway obstruction (Chan et al., 2004).

Nursing care of the child with sleep-disordered breathing involves early detection by observation of the infant's or child's sleep patterns and active participation in the diagnostic polysomnography. Important nursing roles are insertion of the pH probe into the esophagus, ensuring accurate placement by radiography, and monitoring the sleep study and the patient's response to diagnostic therapy. Counselling families of children with sleep-disordered breathing may involve dietary counselling for exercise programs and weight management, use of the CPAP or BiPAP equipment, and direct postoperative care after the surgical intervention of tonsillectomy or adenoidectomy. The nurse can be instrumental in helping the child and family cope with the chronic illness diagnosis should intervention such as CPAP or BiPAP be required.

Respiratory Emergency

Respiratory Failure

In general, the term *respiratory insufficiency* is applied to two situations: (1) when there is increased work of breathing but gas exchange function is near normal, and (2) when normal blood gas tensions cannot be maintained and hypoxemia and acidosis develop secondary to carbon dioxide retention.

Respiratory failure is defined as the inability of the respiratory apparatus to maintain adequate oxygenation of the blood, with or without carbon dioxide retention. This process involves pulmonary dysfunction that generally results in impaired alveolar gas exchange, which can lead to hypoxemia or hypercapnia. Respiratory failure is the most common cause of cardiopulmonary arrest in children (Rotta & Wiryawan, 2003). *Respiratory arrest* is the cessation of respiration. *Apnea* is the cessation of breathing for more than 20 seconds or for a shorter period when associated with hypoxemia or bradycardia (Curley & Moloney-Harmon, 2001). Apnea can be (1) central, in which respiratory efforts are absent; (2) obstructive, in which respiratory efforts are present; or (3) mixed, in which both central and obstructive components are present.

Effective pulmonary gas exchange requires clear airways, normal lungs and chest wall, and adequate pulmonary circulation. Anything that affects these functions or their relationships can compromise respiration.

Diagnostic Evaluation

Respiratory dysfunction may have an abrupt or an insidious onset. Respiratory failure can occur as an emergency situation or may be preceded by gradual and progressive deterioration of respiratory function. Most clinical manifestations are nonspecific and are affected by variations among individual patients and differences in the severity and duration of inadequate gas exchange.

The diagnosis of respiratory failure is determined by the combined application of three sources of information:

1. Presence or history of a condition that might predispose the patient to respiratory failure
2. Observation of respiratory failure
3. Measurement of arterial blood gases (ABGs) and pH

Nursing observation and judgement are vital to the recognition and early management of respiratory failure. Nurses must be able to assess a situation and initiate appropriate action within moments. Signs of respiratory failure are listed in Box 46-16.

Therapeutic Management

The interventions used in the management of respiratory failure are often dramatic, requiring special skills and emergency procedures. If respiratory arrest occurs, the primary objectives are to recognize the situation and immediately initiate resuscitative measures such as airway positioning, administration of oxygen, cardiopulmonary resuscitation (CPR), suctioning, or intubation. When the situation is not an arrest, the suspicion of respiratory failure is confirmed by assessment; the severity may be defined by ABG analysis. Interventions such as administering supplemental oxygen, positioning, stimulation, suctioning, providing positive pressure ventilation by bag and mask, and early intubation may avert an arrest. When severity is established, an attempt is made to determine the underlying cause by thorough evaluation.

Treatment of respiratory dysfunction involves both specific and nonspecific therapy. Specific therapies are directed toward reversal of the causative factors. However, nonspecific measures are needed to maintain adequate oxygenation and enhance carbon dioxide removal until specific methods take effect. The major reasons for implementing nonspecific treatments are (1) an unknown etiology, (2) lack of specific treatment for a known cause, (3) lack of time for a specific treatment to take effect, and (4) need for specialized personnel or equipment for specific treatment.

The principles of management are to (1) maintain ventilation and maximize oxygen delivery, (2) correct hypoxemia and hypercapnia, (3) treat the underlying cause, (4) minimize extrapulmonary organ failure, (5) apply specific and nonspecific therapy to control oxygen demands, and (6) anticipate complications. Monitoring the patient's condition is critical.

BOX 46-16 Clinical Manifestations of Respiratory Failure

Cardinal Signs

Restlessness
Tachypnea
Tachycardia
Diaphoresis

Early but Less Obvious Signs

Mood changes such as euphoria or depression
Headache
Altered depth and pattern of respirations
Hypertension
Exertional dyspnea
Anorexia
Increased cardiac output and renal output
Central nervous system symptoms (decreased efficiency, impaired judgement, anxiety, confusion, restlessness, irritability, depressed level of consciousness)
Flaring nares
Chest wall retractions
Expiratory grunt
Wheezing or prolonged expiration

Signs of More Severe Hypoxia

Hypotension or hypertension
Dimness of vision
Somnolence
Stupor
Coma
Dyspnea
Depressed respirations
Bradycardia
Cyanosis, peripheral or central

Nursing Care Management

For families whose child has a respiratory arrest, support is aimed at keeping the family informed of the child's status and helping them cope with a near-death experience or an actual death (see Chapter 41). Knowing that their child requires CPR is a frightening and often overwhelming experience for parents. Uncertainty regarding the outcome—both mortality and morbidity—is a primary concern. Traditionally, family members are not allowed to be present during resuscitation efforts in the emergency department. However, studies indicate that family presence during emergencies alleviates the family's anger about being separated from the patient during a crisis, reduces their anxiety, eliminates doubts about what was done to help the patient, and facilitates the grieving process if the patient dies (Mangurten et al., 2006).

Regardless of whether an institution permits parental presence during CPR, nurses must consider the needs, fears, and concerns of family members during an arrest situation. If family presence is not permitted, nurses should arrange for someone to remain with the family during the emergency treatment. After the child's recovery or death, the family will continue to need support and thorough medical information regarding lifesaving measures, the prognosis if the child survives, and the cause of death if the child dies.

Cardiopulmonary Resuscitation

Cardiac arrest in children is less often of cardiac origin than from prolonged hypoxemia secondary to inadequate oxygenation, ventilation, and circulation (shock). Some causes of cardiac arrest include injuries, suffocation (e.g., FB aspiration), smoke inhalation, or infection. In small infants the small size of the airway may easily be compromised by improper positioning with the chin resting on the chest; this can easily be remedied by positioning the infant with the chin elevated (but not hyperextended) so the airway is open. This is common in infants who are not positioned properly in an infant seat or car restraint seat. Respiratory arrest is associated with a better survival rate than cardiac arrest. After cardiac arrest occurs, the outcome of resuscitative efforts is poor.

Complete apnea signals the need for rapid, vigorous action to prevent cardiac arrest. In such situations nurses must initiate action immediately. In the hospital, emergency equipment must be available and easily accessible in all patient care areas. The status of emergency equipment must be checked at least once daily. Regardless of the cause of the arrest, basic procedures need to be carried out and modified according to the child's size.

Optimally, mouth-to-mouth resuscitation should be performed with a barrier device or mask with a one-way valve to prevent infection transmission in both the victim and rescuer. When CPR is anticipated in the workplace or other out-of-hospital settings, rescuers should have access to these devices.

Outside the hospital the first action in an emergency is to quickly assess the extent of any injury and determine whether the child is unconscious. A child who is struggling to breathe but conscious should be transported immediately to an advanced life support (ALS) facility, with the child maintaining whatever position affords the most comfort. Attempting to transport a child by automobile wastes valuable time in obtaining help. Transportation by an emergency medical service (EMS) is recommended. Services in most large communities can institute ALS immediately or en route to a medical facility.

An unconscious child is managed with care to prevent additional trauma if a head or spinal cord injury has been sustained (see Spinal Cord Injuries, Chapter 55). The circumstances in which the child is found offer clues to a possible injury. For example, a child who has been thrown from a bicycle or fallen from a tree is more likely to sustain trauma than a child who is discovered in bed.

Resuscitation Procedure

The 2010 guidelines for **cardiopulmonary resuscitation** (CPR) and emergency cardiac care (ECC) were co-developed by the American Heart Association and the Canadian Heart and Stroke Foundation (American Heart Association [AHA], 2010). These organizations have implemented several changes in CPR guidelines that incorporate the use of the automatic external defibrillator (AED) as part of the treatment of cardiorespiratory arrest in children 1 year of age and older. The new 2010 guidelines recommend using a pediatric-attenuated system first, if one is available; if it is not available the adult AED should be used. For infants less than 1 year of age, a manual defibrillator is the best one to use; if that is not available a pediatric-attenuated defibrillator should be used next, and then the AED (AHA, 2010). The 2010 guidelines indicate that the initial shock should be 2 j/kg, then 4 j/kg strength for all of the following shocks. The AED must not exceed 9 j/kg (AHA, 2010).

The major changes in the 2010 guidelines are intended to simplify CPR for the responders and to encourage bystander response. There is a change in the CPR sequence from Airway-Breathing-Compression (A-B-C) to **Compressions-Airway-Breathing (C-A-B)** in order to make it easier for the bystander to get going and start compressions and defibrillation, which are more critical than respirations. There is still an emphasis on delivering high-quality compressions by pushing hard to at least a 5 cm depth and fast, at least 100/minute, minimizing interruptions, allowing full chest recoil, and avoiding excessive ventilation (AHA, 2010).

The new C-A-B procedure applies to all ages except newborns. The rescuers should continue to provide the A-B-C CPR sequence with a 3 : 1 ratio of compressions to breaths. This stays the same because most newborns with a cardiac arrest started with a respiratory arrest (AHA, 2010).

The EMS process has also changed. The health care provider rescuer needs to check for responsiveness before calling for EMS help (AHA, 2010). The key changes for the health care provider rescuers is to learn teamwork techniques, learn to use waveform capnography, therapeutic hypothermia or cooling, and atropine is no longer recommended for treating asystole (AHA, 2010).

If two rescuers are present, one rescuer should begin CPR while the second rescuer activates the EMS system by calling 911 and obtaining an AED. Pediatric rescuers provide five cycles of basic life support (approximately 2 minutes) before activating EMS; each cycle consists of 30 chest compressions and two ventilations. Because pediatric arrests are most commonly caused by respiratory arrest, maintaining ventilation is primary.

Open the Airway

For effective CPR, the victim is placed on the back on a firm, flat surface, using appropriate precautions. With loss of consciousness the tongue, which is attached to the lower jaw, relaxes and falls back, obstructing the airway. To open the airway, the head is positioned with a head tilt–chin lift manoeuvre by the lay rescuer. Health care providers should open the airway using either a head tilt–chin lift or jaw thrust manoeuvre. A head tilt is accomplished by placing one hand on the victim's forehead and applying firm, backward pressure with the palm to tilt the head back. The fingers of the free hand are placed under the bony portion of the lower jaw near the chin to lift and bring the chin forward (chin lift). This supports the jaw and helps tilt the head back (Fig. 46-10).

The jaw thrust is accomplished by grasping the angles of the victim's lower jaw and lifting with both hands, one on each

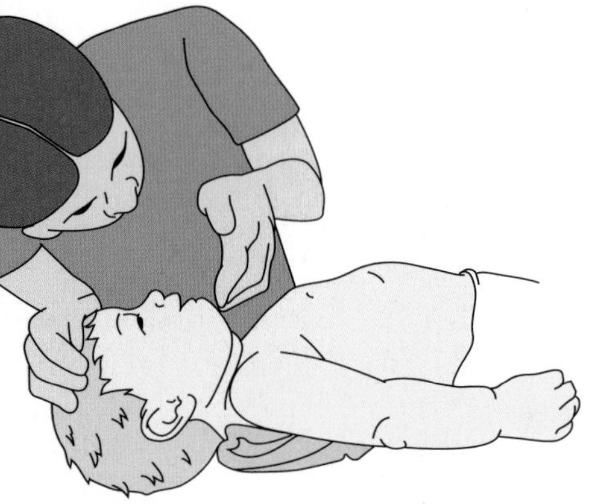

Fig. 46-10 Open airway using the head tilt–chin lift manoeuvre, and check breathing.

side, displacing the mandible upward and outward. *The jaw thrust is recommended for use only by health care workers.* In suspected neck injuries the jaw thrust method should be used while the cervical spine is completely immobilized. After a patent airway has been restored by removal of foreign material and secretions (if indicated) and if the child is not breathing, maintenance of the airway is continued, and rescue breathing is initiated.

Give Breaths

To ventilate the lungs in the infant (from birth to 1 year of age), the bag-valve mask or operator's mouth is placed in such a way that both the mouth and the nostrils are covered (Fig. 46-11). Children (over 1 year of age) are ventilated through the mouth while the nostrils are firmly pinched for airtight contact.

The volume of air in an infant's lungs is small, and the air passages are considerably smaller, with resistance to flow potentially higher than in adults. The rescuer should deliver small puffs of air and assess the rise of the chest to ensure that overinflation does not occur. A gentle rise of the chest is a sufficient indicator of adequate inflation.

The correct volume for each breath is the volume that causes the chest to rise. If air enters freely and the chest rises, the airway is assumed to be clear. Breaths should be given slowly with sufficient volume to make the chest rise.

Check Pulse

After an initial two breaths, the health care provider palpates the pulse to ascertain the presence of a heartbeat. The carotid is the most central and accessible artery in children over 1 year of age. However, the infant's short and often fat neck makes the carotid pulse difficult to palpate. In the infant it is preferable to use the brachial pulse, located on the inner side of the upper arm midway between the elbow and the shoulder (Fig. 46-12). Absence of a carotid or brachial pulse is considered sufficient indication to begin external cardiac massage. *Lay rescuers are not taught to check the pulse but are taught to look for signs of circulation (e.g., normal breathing, coughing, or air movement) in response to rescue breaths.*

Perform Chest Compression

External chest compression consists of serial, rhythmic compressions of the chest to maintain circulation to vital organs until the child achieves spontaneous vital signs or ALS can be provided. *Chest compressions are always interspersed with ventilation of the lungs.* For optimal compressions it is essential that the child's spine be supported on a firm surface during compressions of the sternum and that sternal pressure is forceful but not traumatic. For a small infant, the hard surface can be the rescuer's hand or forearm, with the palm supporting the infant's back. The child's head is positioned for optimal airway opening using the head tilt–chin lift manoeuvre. It is essential to prevent overextension of the head of small infants because this tends to close the flexible trachea.

The placement of the fingers for compression in infants is at a point on the lower sternum just below the intersection of the sternum and an imaginary line drawn between the nipples (Fig. 46-13). Compressions on the child 1 to 8 years of age are applied to the lower half of the sternum (Fig. 46-14). Sternal compression to infants is applied with two fingers on the sternum, exerting a firm downward thrust; chest compression for children is applied with the heel of one hand or two hands, depending on the child's size. Current American Heart Association (2010) guidelines include the addition of the two-thumb technique for chest compressions for infants when two health care providers are present. In the two-thumb technique, one of the two rescuers places both thumbs side by side over the lower half of the infant's sternum; the remaining fingers encircle the infant's chest and support the back. The two-thumb technique is not taught to lay rescuers and is not practical for the health care provider working alone.

The depth of compression needs to be adapted to the child's size. The location, rate, and depth for children older than 8 years of age are the same as for adults.

Lone-rescuer CPR is continued at the ratio of two breaths to 30 compressions for all ages until signs of recovery appear. These signs include palpable peripheral pulses, return of pupils to normal size, the disappearance of mottling and

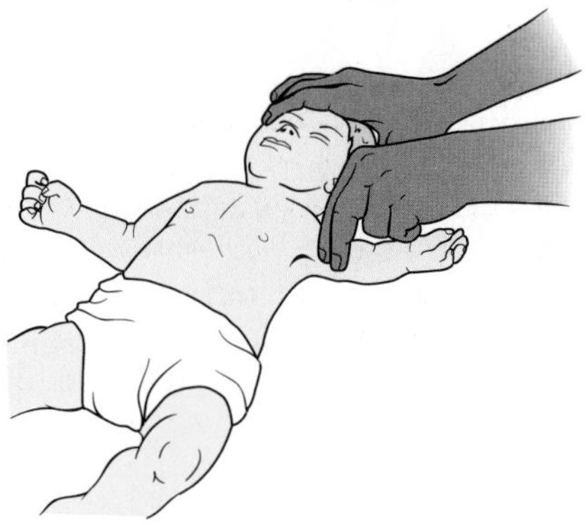

Fig. 46-12 Locating the brachial pulse in an infant.

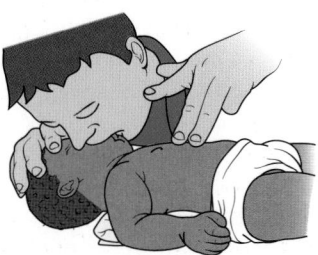

Fig. 46-13 Combining chest compressions with breathing in an infant.

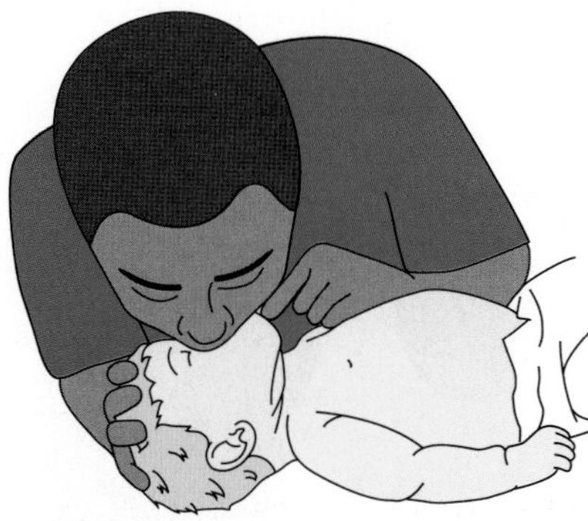

Fig. 46-11 Mouth-to-mouth and nose breathing for an infant.

cyanosis, and possibly return of spontaneous respiration. When two rescuers are present, they should deliver two breaths to each 15 compressions.

Administer Medications

Medications are an important adjunct to CPR, especially cardiac arrest, and are used during and after resuscitation in children. Medications are used to (1) correct hypoxemia, (2) increase perfusion pressure during chest compression, (3) stimulate spontaneous or more forceful myocardial contraction, (4) accelerate cardiac rate, (5) correct metabolic acidosis, and (6) suppress ventricular ectopy. Appropriate fluid therapy is initiated immediately in the hospital or by EMS personnel during transport (see Parenteral Fluid Therapy, Chapter 45, and Shock, Chapter 48). A complete supply of emergency medications is kept and maintained in all EMS vehicles and on all hospital units. The supply should be checked on a regular basis (usually once on each 8- or 12-hour shift). Resuscitation medications are listed in Table 46-3.

When administering medications during CPR (or a "code"), a saline flush is used between medications to prevent drug interactions. The nurse needs to document all medications, dosages, and the time and route of administration.

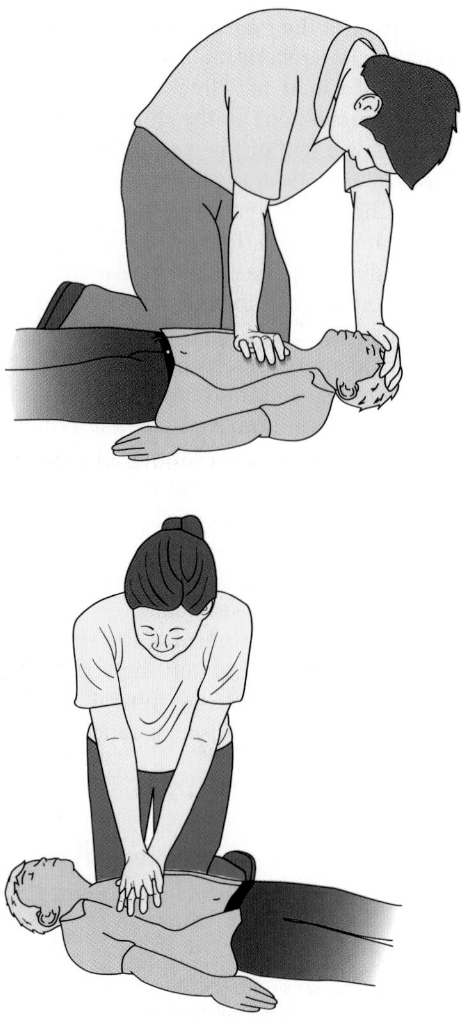

A

B

Fig. 46-14 Chest compressions in a child: one hand for smaller child (**A**) and two hands for larger child (**B**).

Airway Obstruction

Attempts at clearing the airway should be considered for (1) children in whom aspiration of an FB is witnessed or strongly suspected and (2) unconscious, nonbreathing children whose airways remain obstructed despite the usual manoeuvres to open them. When aspiration is strongly suspected, the child should be encouraged to continue coughing as long as the cough remains forceful.

In a conscious choking child, attempt to relieve the obstruction only if:

- The child is unable to make any sounds.
- The cough becomes ineffective.
- There is increasing respiratory difficulty with stridor.

NURSING ALERT Blind finger sweeps should be avoided in infants and children under 8 years old.

Infants

A combination of back blows (over the spine between the shoulder blades) and chest thrusts (on the sternum, same location as for chest compressions) is recommended to relieve the FB obstruction in infants (Fig. 46-15). A choking infant is placed face down over the rescuer's arm with the head supported and lower than the trunk. For additional support, the rescuer should support the arm firmly against the thigh. Up to five quick, sharp, back blows are delivered between the

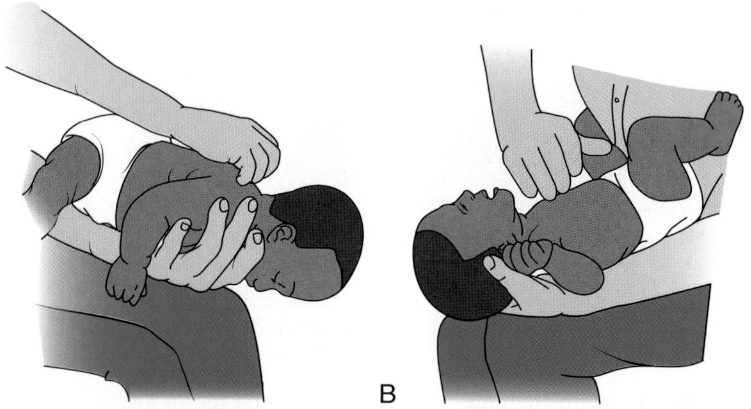

A

B

Fig. 46-15 Relief of foreign body obstruction in an infant: back blows (**A**) and chest thrusts (**B**).

Table 46-3 Medications for Pediatric Cardiopulmonary Resuscitation

MEDICATION AND DOSAGE	ACTION	IMPLICATION
Epinephrine HCl* IV/IO–0.01 mg/kg/dose (1:10,000) ET–0.1 mg/kg/dose (1:1000) Repeat doses–0.1 mg/kg (1:1000)	Adrenergic Acts on both α- and β-receptor sites, especially heart and vascular and other smooth muscle	Most useful drug in cardiac arrest Disappears rapidly from bloodstream after injection; instill 5 mL saline after ET administration May produce renal vessel constriction and decreased urine formation
Sodium bicarbonate IV/IO–1 mmol/kg/dose Newborn–0.5 mmol/mL (4.2%)	Alkalinizer Buffers pH	Infuse slowly and only when ventilation is adequate; flush with saline before and after administration Do not mix with catecholamines or calcium
Atropine sulphate* 0.02 mg/kg/dose Minimum dose–0.1 mg Maximum single dose–infants and children, 0.5 mg; adolescents, 1 mg	Anticholinergic-parasympatholytic Increases cardiac output, heart rate by blocking vagal stimulation in heart	Used to treat bradycardia after ventilatory assessment Always provide adequate ventilation and monitor oxygen saturation Produces pupillary dilation, which constricts with light
Calcium chloride 10% 20 mg/kg IV/IO 0.2 mg/kg/dose q10min	Electrolyte replacement Needed for maintenance of normal cardiac contractility	Used only for hypocalcemia, calcium blocker overdose, hyperkalemia, or hypermagnesemia Administer slowly; very sclerosing; administer in central vein Incompatible with phosphate solutions
Lidocaine HCl* 1 mg/kg/dose	Antidysrhythmic agent Inhibits nerve impulses from sensory nerves	Used for ventricular arrhythmias only
Amiodarone IV–5 mg/kg over 30 min followed by continuous infusion Starting at 5 mcg/kg/min May increase to maximum 10 mcg/kg/min	Antidysrhythmic agent Inhibits adrenergic stimulation; prolongs action potential and refractory period in myocardial tissues; decreases AV conduction and sinus node function	Recommended as first choice for shock-refractory ventricular tachycardia Contraindicated in severe sinus node dysfunction, marked sinus bradycardia, second- and third-degree AV block Monitor electrocardiogram and blood pressure
Adenosine 0.1-0.2 mg/kg as a rapid IV bolus Maximum single initial dose–6-12 mg (given over 1-2 sec) May repeat administration–double initial dose (maximum dose = 12 mg) Follow with ≥5 mL normal saline flush	Antidysrhythmic, for supraventricular tachycardia Causes temporary block through AV node and interrupts reentry circuits	Administer by rapid IV push followed by saline flush May cause transient bradycardia
Naloxone (Narcan)* 0.1 mg/kg/dose† May repeat q2-3 min	Reverses respiratory arrest caused by excessive opiate administration	Evaluate level of pain after administration because analgesic effects of opioids are reversed with large doses of naloxone
Magnesium 25-50 mg/kg/dose Maximum–2 g	Inhibits calcium channels and causes smooth muscle relaxation	Given by rapid IV infusion for suspected hypomagnesemia Have calcium gluconate (IV) available as antidote
Infusions		
Epinephrine HCl infusion 0.05 mcg/kg/min	Adrenergic See Epinephrine above	Titrated to desired hemodynamic effect
Dopamine HCl infusion 2 mcg/kg/min	Agonist Acts on α-receptors, causing vasoconstriction Increases cardiac output	Titrated to desired hemodynamic response
Dobutamine HCl infusion 2 mcg/kg/min	Adrenergic direct-acting β_2-agonist Increases contractility and heart rate	Titrated to desired hemodynamic response Little vasoconstriction, even at high rates
Lidocaine HCl infusion 20-50 mcg/kg/min	Antidysrhythmic Increases electrical stimulation threshold of ventricle	See Lidocaine above Lower infusion dose used in shock

*These medications may be administered via ET tube if IV route is not available.
†Dose of naloxone to reverse respiratory depression without reversing analgesia from opioids is 0.5 mcg/kg in children <40 kg (American Pain Society, 1999).
AV, atrioventricular; *ET,* endotracheal tube; *HCl,* hydrochloride; *IO,* intraosseous; *IV,* intravenous.

infant's shoulder blades with the heel of the rescuer's hand. Less force is required than would be applied to an adult. After delivery of the back blows, the rescuer's free hand is placed flat on the infant's back so that the infant is "sandwiched" between the two hands, making certain the neck and chin are well supported. While the rescuer maintains support with the infant's head lower than the trunk, the infant is turned and placed supine on the rescuer's thigh, where up to five quick downward chest thrusts are applied in rapid succession in the same location as external chest compressions described for CPR. Back blows and chest thrusts are continued until the object is removed or the infant becomes unconscious.

Children

A series of subdiaphragmatic abdominal thrusts (*Heimlich manoeuvre*) is recommended for children older than 1 year of age. The manoeuvre creates an artificial cough that forces air, and with it, the FB, out of the airway. The procedure is carried out with the child in a standing, sitting, or lying position (Fig. 46-16). In the conscious choking child, upward thrusts are delivered to the upper abdomen with the fisted hand at a point just below the rib cage. To prevent damage to the internal organs, the rescuer's hands should not touch the xiphoid process of the sternum or the lower margins of the ribs. Up to five thrusts are repeated in rapid succession until the FB is expelled.

It is neither necessary nor desirable to squeeze or compress the arms during the procedure; it is not a punch or a bear hug. The child may vomit after relief of the obstruction and should be positioned to prevent aspiration. After breathing is restored, the child should receive medical attention and be assessed for complications.

The success of the technique is primarily a result of the obstruction occurring at the end of a maximum respiration. The victim is most likely to choke on food during inspiration; thus the tidal volume plus expiratory reserve volume is present in the lungs. When pressure is exerted on the diaphragm by the manoeuvre, the food bolus is ejected with considerable force by this trapped air.

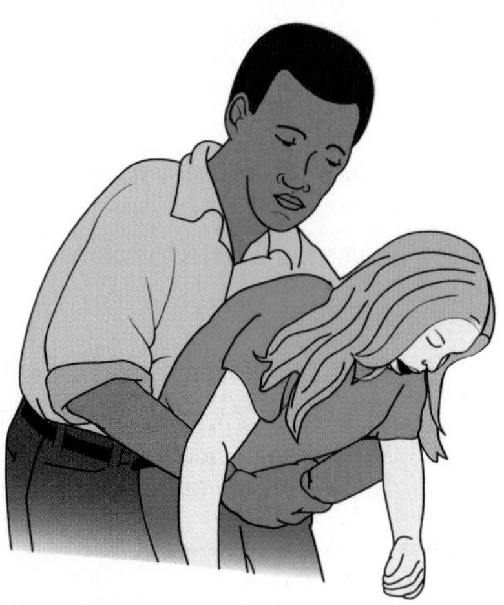

Fig. 46-16 Abdominal thrusts in standing child for relief of foreign body obstruction.

If the child is breathing or resumes effective breathing after emergency interventions, he or she should be placed in the recovery position: the head, shoulders, and torso should be moved simultaneously and the child turned onto the side. The leg not in contact with the ground may be bent and the knee moved forward to stabilize the victim (Fig. 46-17). The child should not be moved in any way if trauma is suspected and should not be placed in the recovery position if rescue breathing or CPR is required.

Key Points

- Acute infection of the respiratory tract is the most common cause of illness in infancy and childhood.
- The incidence and severity of respiratory tract infections are influenced by the infectious agents involved, the child's age, and the child's natural defences.
- Common respiratory tract infections of childhood include nasopharyngitis, pharyngitis (including tonsillitis), influenza, infectious mononucleosis, and OM.
- Croup syndromes involve acute inflammation and variable degrees of obstruction of the epiglottis, larynx, or trachea.
- The primary goals in the care of children with croup are observation for signs of respiratory distress and relief of laryngeal inflammation.
- Common infections of the lower airways are bacterial tracheitis, bronchitis, and RSV-bronchiolitis.
- Pneumonias are classified according to site (lobar, bronchial, or interstitial) or by etiological agent (viral, bacterial, mycoplasmal), or are associated with aspiration of foreign material.
- In TB, susceptibility to the bacillus can be influenced by heredity, age, stress, poor nutrition, and intercurrent infection.
- Second-hand smoke exposure is a major environmental pollutant contributing to respiratory illness in children.
- Asthma is the leading cause of chronic illness in children.
- General therapeutic management of asthma includes assessment of asthma severity, allergen control, medication therapy, symptom management, and sometimes hyposensitization.
- Support for the family of the child with asthma includes education about the disease and its therapy and facilitation of self-management.
- CF is the most common inherited disease in children.
- The diagnosis of CF is based on newborn screening finding of elevated IRT, DNA analysis showing a *CFTR* mutation, and a positive sweat chloride test (increased sweat electrolyte content).
- Choking and respiratory failure are respiratory emergencies that require immediate intervention.

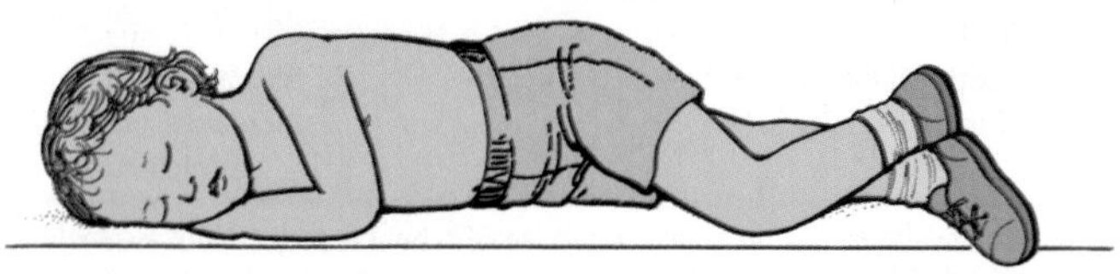

Fig. 46-17 Recovery position for a child after respiratory emergency.

- Abdominal thrusts are used in children in whom FB obstruction is witnessed or strongly suspected. A combination of back blows and chest thrusts is used for infants with FB obstruction.
- In a conscious choking child, attempts to relieve the obstruction are used only if the child is unable to make any sounds, the cough becomes ineffective, or the child has increasing respiratory difficulty with stridor.

Audio Chapter Summaries

Access an Audio Summary of these Key Points on Evolve

References

About Kids Health. (2009). *Tonsil surgery or tonsil and adenoid surgery: Caring for your child after surgery*. Retrieved from http://www.aboutkidshealth.ca/En/HealthAZ/TestsAndTreatments/Procedures/Pages/Tonsil-Surgery-or-Tonsil-and-Adenoid-Surgery-Caring-For-Your-Child-After-the-Operation.aspx.

American Academy of Pediatrics. (2002). Clinical practice guideline: Diagnosis and management of childhood obstructive sleep apnea syndrome. *Pediatrics, 109*(4), 704–712.

American Academy of Pediatrics. (2006). Clinical practice guideline: Diagnosis and management of bronchiolitis. *Pediatrics, 118*(4), 1774–1793. doi:10.1542/peds.2006-2223

American Academy of Pediatrics, Committee on Infectious Diseases, & Pickering, L., (Eds.). (2009). *Red book: 2009 report of the Committee on Infectious Diseases* (28th ed.). Elk Grove Village, IL: Author.

American Academy of Pediatrics, Task Force on Sudden Infant Death Syndrome. (2005). The changing concept of sudden infant death syndrome: Diagnostic coding shifts, controversies regarding the sleeping environment, and new variables to consider in reducing risk. *Pediatrics, 116*(5), 1245–1255. doi:10.1542/peds.2005-1499

American Heart Association. (2010). 2010 American Heart Association Guidelines for cardiopulmonary resuscitation and emergency cardiovascular care science. *Circulation, 122*(18 Suppl 3). doi:10.1161/?CIRCULATION AHA.110.966861

American Pain Society. (1999). *Principles of analgesic use in the treatment of acute pain and chronic cancer pain* (3rd ed.). Glenview, IL: Author.

Asthma Society of Canada. (2012). *About asthma*. Retrieved from http://www.asthma.ca/adults/.

Balinsky, W. & Zhu, C. W. (2004). Pediatric cystic fibrosis: Evaluating costs and genetic testing. *Journal of Pediatric Health Care, 18*, 30–34.

Banerj, A., Greenberg, D., White, L., et al. (2009). Risk factors and viruses associated with hospitalization due to lower respiratory tract infections in Canadian Inuit children: A case control study. *Pediatric Infectious Disease Journal, 28*(8), 102, 697–701. doi:10.1097/INF.0b013e31819f1f89

Benninger, M. & Walner, D. (2007a). Coblation: Improving outcomes for children following adenotonsillectomy. *Clinical Cornerstone, 9*(Suppl 1), S13–S23.

Benninger, M. & Walner, D. (2007b). Obstructive sleep-disordered breathing in children. *Clinical Cornerstone, 9*(Suppl 1), S6–S12.

Blitz, M., et al. (2005). Inhaled magnesium sulfate in the treatment of acute asthma. *Cochrane Database of Systematic Reviews, 20*(3), CD003898.

Boat, T. F., & Acton, J. D. (2007). Cystic fibrosis. In R. M. Kliegman, et al. (Eds.), *Nelson textbook of pediatrics* (18th ed.). Philadelphia: Saunders.

Borowitz, D., Baker, R. D., & Stallings, V. (2002). Consensus report on nutrition for pediatric patients with cystic fibrosis. *Journal of Pediatric Gastroenterology & Nutrition, 35*(3), 246–259.

Burkhart, P. V., et al. (2007). Improved health outcomes with peak flow monitoring for children with asthma. *Journal of Asthma, 44*(2), 137–142. doi:10.1080/02770900601182517

Canadian Lung Association. (2012). *What is sleep apnea*? Retrieved from http://www.lung.ca/diseases-maladies/apnea-apnee/what-quoi/index_e.php.

Canadian Paediatric Society. (2009a). Management of acute otitis media. *Paediatrics & Child Health, 14*(7), 457–460.

Canadian Paediatric Society. (2009b). Prevention of respiratory syncytial virus infection. *Paediatric Child Health, 14*(8), 521–526.

Canadian Paediatric Society. (2010a). *Information on influenza illness for health professionals*. Retrieved from http://www.cps.ca/english/influenza_illnessantiviral.htm.

Canadian Paediatric Society. (2010b). *Use and misuse of tobacco among Aboriginal peoples*. Retrieved from http://www.cps.ca/english/statements/ii/fnih06-01.htm.

Canadian Paediatric Society. (2010c). *FluMist vaccine: Questions and answers*. Retrieved from http://www.cps.ca/english/statements/ID/FluMist.htm#available.

Canadian Paediatric Society. (2010d). *When your child is sick*. Retrieved from http://www.caringforkids.cps.ca/whensick/colds.htm.

Canadian Paediatric Society, Acute Care Committee. (2012). Managing the paediatric patient with an acute asthma exacerbation. *Paediatrics & Child Health, 17*(5), 251–255.

Canadian Paediatric Society, Infectious Diseases and Immunization Committee. (2010). Tuberculosis in children: New diagnostic blood test. *Paediatrics & Child Health 15*(8), 529–533.

Canadian Paediatric Society, Infectious Diseases and Immunization Committee. (2011). Update on the success of the pneumococcal conjugate vaccine. *Paediatrics & Child Health, 16*(4), 233–236.

Canadian Society of Otolaryngology, *Head and Neck Surgery*. (n.d.). Tonsillectomy. Retrieved from http://www.entcanada.org/public2/patient9.asp#bck.

Canadian Task Force on Preventive Health Care. (2003). New grades for recommendations from the Canadian Task Force on Preventive Health Care. *Canadian Medical Association Journal, 169*, 207–208.

Chan, J., Edman, J. C., & Koltai, P. J. (2004). Obstructive sleep apnea in children. *American Family Physician, 69*(5), 1147–1154, 1159–1160.

Chávez-Bueno, S., et al. (2005). Respiratory syncytial virus: Old challenges and new approaches. *Pediatric Annals, 34*(1), 62–68.

Chokephaibulkit, K. (2004). Q&A: Avian influenza virus infection of children in Vietnam and Thailand. *Pediatric Infectious Diseases Journal, 23*(8), 793–794.

Courtney, A. U., McCarter, D. F., & Pollart, S. M. (2005). Childhood asthma: Treatment update. *American Family Physician, 71*(10), 1959–1968.

Curley, M. A. & Moloney-Harmon, P. A. (2001). *Critical care nursing of infants and children*. Philadelphia: Saunders.

Cystic Fibrosis Canada. (2010). *Canadian cystic fibrosis patient data registry report*. Retrieved from http://www.cysticfibrosis.ca/assets/files/pdf/CPDR_ReportE.pdf.

Cystic Fibrosis Canada. (2011a). *Cystic fibrosis and lung transplantation*. Retrieved from http://www.cysticfibrosis.ca/assets/files/pdf/cf&lungtransplantationE.pdf.

Cystic Fibrosis Canada. (2011b). *Newborn screening (NBS)*. Retrieved from http://www.cysticfibrosis.ca/assets/files/pdf/Newborn_Screening_for_cystic_fibrosisE.pdf.

Cystic Fibrosis Canada. (2012). *About cystic fibrosis*. Retrieved from http://www.cysticfibrosis.ca/en/aboutCysticFibrosis/index.php.php.

Cystic Fibrosis Canada. (n.d.a). Nutrition, cystic fibrosis, and the newly diagnosed infant. *CF Health Matters*. Retrieved from http://www.cysticfibrosis.ca/assets/files/pdf/Infants_Diagnosed_with_CF.pdf.

Cystic Fibrosis Canada. (n.d.b). G-tube feeding: Eating without effort. *CF Health Matters*. Retrieved from http://www.cysticfibrosis.ca/assets/files/pdf/G-Tube_Feeding.pdf.

Denison, M. R. (2005). Severe acute respiratory syndrome coronavirus pathogenesis, disease and vaccines: An update. *Pediatric Infectious Disease Journal, 23*(Suppl 11), S207–S214.

D'Urzo, A. D. & D'Urzo, D. K. (1999). Phaseout of chlorofluorocarbons (CFCs) in metered-dose inhalers. Highlights of the Canadian initial transition strategy. *Canadian Family Physician, 45*(7), 1544–1546.

Farrell, P. M., et al. (2007). Evidence on improved outcomes with early diagnosis of cystic fibrosis through neonatal screening: Enough is enough! *Journal of Pediatrics, 147*(Suppl 3), S30–S36. doi:10.1016/j.jpeds.2008.05.005

Flori, H. R., et al. (2005). Pediatric acute lung injury. *American Journal of Respiratory Critical Care Medicine, 171*(9), 995–1001. doi:10.1164/rccm.200404-544OC

Frankel, L. R. & DiCarlo, J. V. (2004). Acute (adult) respiratory distress syndrome (ARDS). In R. E. Behrman, R. M. Kliegman, & H. B. Jenson (Eds.), *Nelson textbook of pediatrics* (17th ed.). Philadelphia: Saunders.

Frye, A. D. (2005). Acute lung injury and acute respiratory distress syndrome in the pediatric patient. *Critical Care Nursing Clinics of North America, 17*(4), 311–318. doi:10.1016/j.ccell.2005.07.008

Goldstein, N. A., et al. (2005). Water precautions and tympanostomy tubes: A randomized, controlled trial. *Laryngoscope, 115*(2), 324–330. doi:10.1097/01.mlg.0000154742.33067.fb

Gould, J. M. & Matz, P. S. (2010). Otitis medis. *Pediatric Review, 31*, 102–116, doi: 10.1542/pir.31-3-102

Hanson, J. H. & Flori, H. (2006). Application of the acute respiratory distress syndrome network low-tidal volume strategy to pediatric acute lung injury. *Respiratory Care Clinics of North America, 12*(3), 349–357.

Hardin, D. S., et al. (2005). Growth hormone treatment enhances nutrition and growth in children with cystic fibrosis receiving enteral nutrition. *Journal of Pediatrics, 146*(3), 324–328. doi:10.1016/j.jpeds.2004.10.037

Health Canada. (2003). *Infection control precautions for respiratory infections transmitted by large droplet and contact. Infection control guidance if there is a SARS outbreak anywhere in the world when an individual presents to a health care institution with a respiratory infection.* Retrieved from http://www.phac-aspc.gc.ca/sars-sras/pdf/sars-icg-outbreakworld_e.pdf.

Health Canada. (2006a). *Tuberculosis in First Nations communities.* Retrieved from http://www.hc-sc.gc.ca/fniah-spnia/diseases-maladies/tuberculos/index-eng.php.

Health Canada. (2006b). *Second-hand smoke.* Retrieved from http://www.hc-sc.gc.ca/hl-vs/iyh-vsv/life-vie/shs-fs-eng.php.

Health Canada (2008a). *Tuberculosis.* Retrieved from http://www.hc-sc.gc.ca/hc-ps/dc-ma/tuberculos-eng.php.

Health Canada. (2008b). *SARS.* Retrieved from http://www.hc-sc.gc.ca/hl-vs/iyh-vsv/diseases-maladies/sars-sras-eng.php.

Health Canada. (2009a). *Tuberculosis.* Retrieved from http://www.hc-sc.gc.ca/hl-vs/iyh-vsv/diseases-maladies/tubercu-eng.php.

Health Canada. (2009b). *Safety information regarding topical anaesthetics and serious adverse events for the public.* Retrieved from http://www.hc-sc.gc.ca/dhp-mps/medeff/advisories-avis/public/_2009/emla_ametop_pc-cp-eng.php.

Health Canada. (2010). *Asthma.* Retrieved http://www.hc-sc.gc.ca/hl-vs/iyh-vsv/diseases-maladies/asthm-eng.php.

Health Canada. (2011). *Avian influence (bird flu).* Retrieved from http://www.hc-sc.gc.ca/hl-vs/iyh-vsv/diseases-maladies/avian-aviare-eng.php.

Healthlink BC. (2010). *Throat culture.* Retrieved from http://www.healthlinkbc.ca/kb/content/medicaltest/hw204006.html.

Hopkins, A., et al. (2006). Changing epidemiology of life-threatening upper airway infections: The re-emergence of bacterial tracheitis. *Pediatrics, 118*(4), 1418–1421. doi:10.1542/peds.2006-0692

Kakkar, F., Allen, U. D., Ling, D., Pai, M., & Kitai, I. C. (2010). Tuberculosis in children: New diagnostic blood tests. *Paediatrics & Child Health, 15*(8), 529–533.

Kao, L. W. & Nañagas, K. A. (2004). Carbon monoxide poisoning. *Emergency Medicine Clinics of North America, 22*(4), 985–1018.

Lee, P. J. & Krilov, L. R. (2005). When animal viruses attack: SARS and avian influenza. *Pediatric Annals, 34*(1), 43–52.

Li, Y. F., et al. (2005). Maternal and grandmaternal smoking patterns are associated with early childhood asthma. *Chest, 127*(4), 1232–1241. doi:10.1378/chest.127.4.1232

Linzer, J. F. (2007). Review of asthma: Pathophysiology and current treatment options. *Clinics in Pediatric Emergency Medicine, 8*(2), 87–95. doi:10.1016/j.cpem.2007.04.003

Liu, A. H., et al. (2007). Childhood asthma. In R. M. Kliegman, et al. (Eds.), *Nelson textbook of pediatrics* (18th ed.). Philadelphia: Saunders.

Mangurten, J., et al. (2006). Effects of family presence during resuscitation and invasive procedures in a pediatric emergency department. *Journal of Emergency Nursing, 32*(3), 225–233. doi:10.1016/j.jen.2006.02.012

Matthay, M. A., et al. (2003). Future research directions in acute lung injury: summary of a NHLBI working group. *American Journal of Respiratory Critical Care Medicine, 167*(7), 1027–1035.

McMullen, A. H. & Bryson, E. A. (2004). Cystic fibrosis. In P. L. Jackson & J. A. Vessey (Eds.), *Primary care of the child with a chronic condition* (4th ed.). St. Louis: Mosby.

Mintz, M. (2004). Asthma update, part II. Medical management. *American Family Physician, 70*(6), 1061–1066.

Moore, M. & Little, P. (2006). Humidified air inhalation for treating croup. *Cochrane Database of Systematic Reviews, 19*(3), CD002870.

National Asthma Education and Prevention Program. (2007). *Guidelines for the diagnosis and management of asthma (EPR-3).* Retrieved from http://www.nhlbi.nih.gov/guidelines/asthma/index.htm.

O'Connor, B. B. (2003). SARS—the latest menacing microbe. *Nursing Spectrum, 13*(12DC), 12–13, April 7.

Paradise, J. L., et al. (2002). Tonsillectomy and adenotonsillectomy for recurrent throat infection in moderately affected children. *Pediatrics, 110*, 7–15.

Philpott, J., Houghton, K., & Luke, A., for Canadian Paediatric Society. (2010). Physical activity recommendations for children with specific chronic health conditions: Juvenile idiopathic arthritis, hemophilia, asthma and cystic fibrosis. *Paediatrics & Child Health, 15*(4), 213–218. Retrieved from http://www.cps.ca/english/statements/HAL/HAL10-01.htm.

Powers, J. H. (2007). Diagnosis and treatment of acute otitis media: Evaluating the evidence. *Infectious Disease Clinics of North America, 21*(2), 409–426. doi:10.1016/j.idc.2007.03.013

Public Health Agency of Canada. (2007a). *Canadian immunization guide 2006* (7th ed.). Retrieved from http://www.phac-aspc.gc.ca/publicat/cig-gci/p04-pneu-eng.php.

Public Health Agency of Canada. (2007b). *Asthma.* Retrieved from http://www.phac-aspc.gc.ca/publicat/2007/lbrdc-vsmrc/asthma-asthme-eng.php.

Public Health Agency of Canada. (2008). Tuberculosis fact sheet. Retrieved from http://www.phac-aspc.gc.ca/tbpc-latb/fa-fi/index-eng.php.

Public Health Agency of Canada. (2009). *Government of Canada launches television advertising on infection prevention in partnership with provinces and territories.* Retrieved from http://www.phac-aspc.gc.ca/media/nr-rp/2009/2009_0921-eng.php.

Public Health Agency of Canada (2010a). *Individual and community based measures to help prevent transmission of influenza-like-illness (ILI), including the pandemic influenza (H1N1) 2009 virus, in the community.* Retrieved from http://www.phac-aspc.gc.ca/alert-alerte/h1n1/hp-ps-info_health-sante-eng.php.

Public Health Agency of Canada. (2010b). *Canada communicable disease report. Statement on seasonal trivalent inactivated influenza vaccine (TIV) for 2010–2011.* Retrieved from http://www.phac-aspc.gc.ca/publicat/ccdr-rmtc/10vol36/acs-6/index-eng.php.

Public Health Agency of Canada. (2010c). *BCG vaccine usage in Canada—Current and historical.* Retrieved from http://www.phac-aspc.gc/tbpc-latb-latb/bcgvac_1206-eng.php.

Rafei, K. & Lichenstein, R. (2006). Airway infectious disease emergencies. *Pediatric Clinics of North America, 53*(2), 215–242. doi:10.1016/j.pcl.2005.10.001

Ren, C. L., et al. (2007). Presence of methicillin-resistant *Staphylococcus aureus* in respiratory cultures from cystic fibrosis patients is associated with lower lung function. *Pediatric Pulmonology, 42*(6), 513–518. doi:10.1002/ppul.20604

Rice, T. W., & Bernard, G. R. (2006). Acute lung injury and acute respiratory distress syndrome: Challenges in clinical trial testing. *Clinics in Chest Medicine, 27*(4), 733–754. doi:10.1016/j.ccm.2006.06.006

Rimsza, M. E., & Kirk, G. M. (2005). Common medical problems of the college student. *Pediatric Clinics of North America, 52*(1), vii, 9–24.

Ross, M. H., Mjaanes, C. M., & Lemanske, R. (2003). Asthma. In C. D. Rudolph, A. M. Rudolph, & M. K. Hostetter (Eds.), *Rudolph's pediatrics* (21st ed.). New York: McGraw-Hill.

Rotta, A. T. & Wiryawan, B. (2003). Respiratory emergencies in children. *Respiratory Care, 48*(3), 248–260.

Ryan, T., Brewer, M., & Small, L. (2008). Over-the-counter cough and cold medication use in young children. *Pediatric Nursing, 34*(2), 174–180, 184.

Safekids Canada. (2012). *Carbon monoxide poisoning.* Retrieved from http://www.safekidscanada.ca/Professionals/Advocacy/Poison/CO-Alarms/Poison-Prevention.aspx.

Sandel, M., et al. (2004). The effects of housing interventions on child health. *Pediatric Annals, 33*(7), 475–481.

Schnabel, D., et al. (2007). A multicenter, randomized, double-blind, placebo-controlled trial to evaluate the metabolic and respiratory effects of growth hormone in children with cystic fibrosis. *Pediatrics, 119*(6), e1230–e1238. doi:10.1542/peds.2006-2783

Schwarzenberg, S. J., et al. (2007). Microvascular complications in cystic fibrosis–related diabetes. *Diabetes Care, 30*(5), 1056–1061. doi:10.1016/j.jcf.2008.05.008

Sharma, H. P., et al. (2007). Indoor environmental influences on children's asthma. *Pediatric Clinics of North America, 54*(1), 103–120. doi:10.1016/j.pcl.2006.11.007

Sheahan, S. L., & Free, T. A. (2005). Counseling parents to quit smoking. *Pediatric Nursing, 31*(2), 98–108.

Slader, C. A., et al. (2006). Complementary and alternative medicine use in asthma: Who is using what? *Respirology, 11*(4), 373–387.

Southern, K. W., et al. (2009). Newborn screening for cystic fibrosis. *Cochrane Database of Systematic Reviews* (*1*), CD001402.

Stockman, L. J., et al. (2007). Severe acute respiratory syndrome in children. *Pediatric Infectious Diseases Journal, 26*(1), 68–74. doi:10.1097/01.inf.0000247136.28950.41

Strausbaugh, S. D., & Davis, P. B. (2007). Cystic fibrosis: A review of epidemiology and pathobiology. *Clinics in Chest Medicine, 28*(2), 279–288. doi:10.1016/j.ccm.2007.02.011

Strunk, R. C. & Bloomberg, G. R. (2006). Omalizumab for asthma. *New England Journal of Medicine, 354*(25), 2689–2695.

Tolomeo, C. & Mackey, W. (2003). Peripherally inserted central catheters (PICCs) in the CF population: One center's experience. *Pediatric Nursing, 29*(5), 355–359.

Uyemura, M. C. (2005). Foreign body ingestion in children. *American Family Physician, 72*(2), 287–291.

van Staaij, B. K., et al. (2004). Effectiveness of adenotonsillectomy in children with mild symptoms of throat infections of adenotonsillar hypertrophy: Open, randomized controlled trial. *British Medical Journal, 329*(7467), 651.

Ventre, K. & Randolph, A. G. (2007). Ribavirin for respiratory syncytial virus infection of the lower respiratory tract in infants and young children. *Cochrane Database of Systematic Reviews, 24*(1), CD000181.

Willson, D. F., Chess, P. R., & Notter, R. H. (2008). Surfactant for pediatric acute lung injury. *Pediatric Clinics of North America, 55*(3), 545–575. doi:10.1016/j.pcl.2008.02.016

Winkelstein, M. L., et al. (2000). Factors associated with medication self-administration in children with asthma. *Clinical Pediatrics, 39*(6), 337–345.

Wright, R. B., et al. (2005). Current pharmacologic options in the treatment of croup. *Expert Opinion in Pharmacotherapy, 6*(2), 255–261. doi:10.1517/14656566.6.2.255

Additional Resources

American Academy of Allergy, Asthma and Immunology: http://www.aaaai.org/home.aspx

American Lung Association: http://www.lung.org

Asthma and Allergy Foundation: http://www.aafa.org

Asthma Society of Canada: Asthma Kids.ca: http://www.asthma.ca/global/kids.php

Canadian Lung Association: http://www.lung.ca

Centers for Disease Control and Prevention: http://www.cdc.gov

Cystic Fibrosis Canada: http://www.cysticfibrosis.ca/en/index.php

Cystic Fibrosis Foundation: What Everyone Should Know About Cystic Fibrosis, and Cystic Fibrosis: A Summary of Symptoms, Diagnosis, and Treatment: http://www.cff.org

Health Canada: Healthy Living—Second-hand Smoke: http://www.hc-sc.gc.ca/hl-vs/iyh-vsv/life-vie/shs-fs-eng.php

Hyperbaric Medical Unit: http://www.uhn.ca/clinics_&_services/services/hyperbaric/professional_information.asp

National Heart, Lung and Blood Institute: http://www.nhlbi.nih.gov

National Lung Health Framework for Canada: http://www.lung.ca/pdf/Lung_Health_Framework_October2008.pdf

Public Health Agency of Canada: http://www.phac-aspc.gc.ca/index-eng.php

Public Health Agency of Canada: FluWatch: http://www.phac-aspc.gc.ca/fluwatch/index-eng.php

Unit 11

47 Gastrointestinal Dysfunction

Learning Objectives

On completion of this chapter, the reader will be able to:

- Identify children at increased risk of developing nutritional disorders.
- Outline a nutritional counselling plan for vitamin or mineral deficiency or excess.
- Describe the characteristics of infants that affect their ability to adapt to fluid loss or gain.
- Formulate a plan of care for the infant with acute diarrhea.
- Compare and contrast the inflammatory bowel diseases.
- Identify the routes of transmission for hepatitis A, B, and C.
- Describe the nursing care of the child with hepatitis.
- Formulate a plan for teaching parents preoperative and postoperative care of the child with a cleft lip or palate.
- Formulate a plan of care for the child with an obstructive gastrointestinal disorder.
- Identify nutritional therapies for the child with a malabsorption syndrome.
- Outline a teaching plan designed to prevent transmission of intestinal parasites.
- Identify the principles in the emergency treatment of poisoning.
- Name four sources of lead in the environment.
- Describe the nursing care of the child with lead poisoning.

Electronic Resources

Additional information related to the content in Chapter 47 can be found on evolve the companion Web site at
http://evolve.elsevier.com/Canada/Perry/maternal/

- Examination Review Questions
- Animation—Appendicitis
- Animation—Digestive Tract, Passage of Food
- Animation—Volvulus, Pediatric
- Case Study—Acute Diarrhea (Gastroenteritis)
- Case Study—Appendicitis
- Case Study—Cleft Lip and Palate
- Case Study—Dehydration and Diarrhea
- Case Study—Heavy Metal Poisoning
- Case Study—Ingestion of an Injurious Agent
- Case Study—Salicylate Ingestion
- Critical Thinking Exercise—Constipation
- Critical Thinking Exercise—Hematemesis
- Critical Thinking Exercise—Home Care for the Adolescent

Nutritional Disturbances

Vitamin Imbalances

While most vitamin deficiencies are rare in North America, vitamin D–deficiency rickets continues to be a problem in Canada, especially among First Nations, Metis and Inuit people. The Canadian Paediatric Society (2007) has identified the following populations at risk:

- Children exclusively breastfed by mothers with an inadequate intake of vitamin D or mothers who had vitamin D deficiency during pregnancy
- Children with dark skin pigmentation
- Children with diets that are low in sources of vitamin D and calcium
- Children who live in northern communities (due to lack of sunlight hours and covering skin during sunlight hours to prevent black fly, mosquito, or other bites)

Health Canada (2010) recommends that term breastfed infants receive 400 International Units (IU)/day (10 mcg), and that this should continue until the infant receives 400 IU of vitamin D from other dietary sources or until 1 year of age. The Canadian Paediatric Society advocates an increase of vitamin intake to 800 IU/day (20 mcg) for children up to 2 years of age in northern Native communities and those with dark skin during the winter months (April to October). Premature infants should receive 200 IU/kg/day to a maximum of 400 IU of vitamin D from all sources beginning shortly after birth, to prevent rickets and vitamin D deficiency (Canadian

Paediatric Society [CPS], 2007). The Canadian Paediatric Society also recommends that children be exposed to short periods of sunlight each day (usually less than 15 minutes) to promote cutaneous production of vitamin D. For children aged 1 year through adolescence, Health Canada (2010) recommends 200 IU of vitamin D per day, although this may be obtained through dietary sources (Health Canada, 2010).

Children may be at risk, secondary to disorders or their treatment. For example, vitamin deficiencies of the fat-soluble vitamins A and D may occur in malabsorptive disorders. Preterm infants may develop rickets in the second month of life as a result of inadequate intake of vitamin D, calcium, and phosphorus. Children receiving high doses of salicylates may have impaired vitamin C storage. Environmental tobacco smoke exposure has been implicated in decreased concentrations of ascorbate in children; thus increased intake of sources of vitamin C should be encouraged even in children minimally exposed to environmental tobacco smoke (Preston et al., 2003; Preston, Rodriguez, & Rivera, 2006). Children with chronic illnesses resulting in **anorexia**, decreased food intake, or possible nutrient malabsorption as a result of multiple medications should be carefully evaluated for adequate vitamin and mineral intake in some form (parenteral or enteral).

Scurvy (caused by a deficiency of vitamin C) is rare in developed countries. Cases have been reported in children who were fed an organic diet deficient in vegetables and fruits (Burk & Molodow, 2007).

An excessive dose of a vitamin is generally defined as 10 or more times the **Recommended Dietary Allowance (RDA)**, although the fat-soluble vitamins, especially A and D, tend to cause toxic reactions at lower doses. With the addition of vitamins to commercially prepared foods, the potential for hypervitaminosis has increased, especially when combined with the excessive use of vitamin supplements. Hypervitaminosis of A and D presents the greatest problems, since these fat-soluble vitamins are stored in the body. High intakes of vitamin A have been linked to physeal growth arrest, which can lead to **osteoporosis**, fracture, and metaphyseal irregularity (Saltzman & King, 2007). Vitamin D is the most likely of all vitamins to cause toxic reactions in relatively small overdoses. The water-soluble vitamins, primarily niacin, B_6, and C, can also cause toxicity. Poor outcomes in infants (e.g., a fatal hypermagnesemia) have been associated with megavitamin therapy with high doses of magnesium oxide (McGuire, Kulkarni, & Baden, 2000), and severe anemia and **thrombocytopenia** have resulted from megadoses of vitamin A (Perrotta et al., 2002).

Deficiencies and excesses of vitamins A, B complex, C, D, E, and K are summarized in Table 47-1. General nursing care management is discussed later in the chapter, and specific interventions are presented in Table 47-1 (see also Chapter 11).

Complementary and Alternative Medicine

The misuse or overuse of vitamins as a part of complementary and alternative medicine (CAM) places some children at risk for health problems. One survey found that a relatively small group of parents routinely gave their children megavitamin therapy; however, the researcher recommends further research to ascertain a more realistic number of children using multivitamin preparations (Loman, 2003). Sawni and colleagues (2007) noted that of persons reportedly using CAM, the most common CAM remedies used in children seen in the emergency department were home or folk remedies (59%), herbs (41%), prayer for healing (14%), and massage therapy (10%). Sick Kids' researchers discovered that more than 30% of adolescent girls who had been diagnosed with an eating disorder had used herbal supplements and other types of alternative medicines to accelerate weight loss (Trigazis, Tennankore, Vohra, & Katzman, 2004).

There is concern among health care workers that terms often used to market supplements such as megavitamins may mislead parents regarding the actual benefits (or harm) of such therapies. The intention here is not to discredit the use of CAM such as vitamin supplements; rather, it is to ensure safety and efficacy in children who may experience inadvertent harm. Parents should be cautioned not to exceed the upper limits of vitamin intake according to the new Dietary Reference Intakes (DRI) (see p. 1380 and the DRI appendix on the Evolve site).

The use of various herbal therapies, or intake of herbs, is also becoming more popular; many of these supplements have been a part of medicine since early days and are beneficial in some cases.

There are reports of an increase in the use of herbs by lactating mothers to increase breast milk supply. The galactogogues fenugreek, blessed thistle, fennel, and chaste tree have been purported to increase maternal milk supply; however, few studies support the efficacy or safety of these herbs in breastfeeding infants. Fenugreek has been the most widely studied, with minimal reported adverse effects in breastfeeding infants (Lawrence & Lawrence, 2011). For a discussion of galactogogues, including those mentioned previously, see Appendix P in Lawrence and Lawrence (2011).

Herbs known to have adverse effects in children include ephedra, comfrey, and pennyroyal; some herbs may not be harmful taken alone but may counteract or potentiate prescription medications when taken concurrently (Loman, 2003). Parents should be fully informed of the use of herbs to ensure that there is more benefit than potential harm in the ingredient being used. Health care workers also need to be knowledgeable about the benefits or potential harm from herbs so that they can appropriately counsel parents and address their concerns. Little research has been performed in children on many over-the-counter herbal medicines, yet some herbs are known to cause harm in children (Kemper & Gardiner, 2007; Lanski et al., 2003; Loman, 2003).

The Canadian Paediatric Society (2005) has outlined their concerns about the use of CAMs, particularly in terms of homeopathic and herbal remedies. The concerns include the lack of research and safety data, particularly in relation to use in the pediatric age group, lack of standardized products, and potential drug interactions. For further information see the Additional Resources section at the end of this chapter.

Mineral Imbalances

A number of minerals are essential nutrients. The *macrominerals* refer to those with daily requirements greater than

Text continued on page 1380.

Table 47-1 Vitamins and Their Nutritional Significance

PHYSIOLOGICAL FUNCTIONS AND SOURCES	RESULTS OF DEFICIENCY OR EXCESS	NURSING CARE MANAGEMENT
Vitamin A (Retinol)*		
Functions Necessary component in formation of pigment rhodopsin (visual purple) Formation and maintenance of epithelial tissue Normal bone growth and tooth development Needed for growth and spermatogenesis Involved in thyroxine formation Antioxidant *Sources* Natural form—Liver, kidney, fish oils, milk and nonskim milk products, egg yolk Provitamin A (carotene)—Carrots, sweet potatoes, squash, apricots, spinach, collards, broccoli, cabbage, artichokes	*Deficiency* Night blindness Keratinization (hardening and scaling) of epithelium Xerophthalmia (hardening and scaling of cornea and conjunctiva) Phrynoderma (toad skin) Drying of respiratory, gastrointestinal, and genitourinary tracts Defective tooth enamel Delayed growth Impaired bone formation Decreased thyroxine formation Decreased resistance to infections *Excess* **Early signs**—Irritability, anorexia, pruritus, fissures at corners of nose and lips, dry skin **Later signs**—Hepatomegaly, jaundice, restricted growth, poor weight gain, thickening of the cortex of long bones with pain and fragility, hard tender lumps in extremities and occiput of the skull Can cause birth defects if excessive maternal intake **NOTE:** Overdose results from ingestion of large quantities of the vitamin only, not the provitamin; large amounts of carotene (carotenemia) cause yellow or orange discolouration of the skin (not the sclera, urine, or feces as in jaundice) but none of the above symptoms.	*Deficiency* Encourage foods rich in vitamin A, such as whole cow's milk (after 12 mo). As milk consumption decreases, encourage foods rich in vitamin A. Ensure adequate intake in preterm infants. Advise parents of safe use of supplements in child with measles. It may play a role in prevention of severity of bronchopulmonary dysplasia in preterm infants (affects growth of respiratory tract epithelial cells). *Excess* Emphasize correct use of vitamin supplements and potential hazards of excess. Evaluate child's dietary habits to calculate approximate intake; if excessive, remove supplemental source (e.g., daily feeding of liver). Advise parents of the benign nature of carotenemia; treatment is avoidance of excess pigmented fruits or vegetables, especially carrots; skin colour returns to normal in 2 to 6 wk.
Vitamin B_1 (Thiamine)†		
Functions Coenzyme (with phosphorus) in carbohydrate metabolism Needed for healthy nervous system Digestion and normal appetite *Sources* Pork, beef, liver, legumes, nuts, whole or enriched grains and cereals, green vegetables, fruits, milk, brown rice	*Deficiency* **Gastrointestinal**—Anorexia, constipation, indigestion **Neurological**—Apathy, fatigue, emotional instability, polyneuritis, tenderness of calf muscles, partial anaesthesia, muscle weakness, paresthesia, hyperesthesia, decreased or absent tendon reflexes, convulsions, coma (in infants) **Cardiovascular**—Palpitations, cardiac failure, peripheral vasodilation, edema *Excess* Headache Irritability Insomnia Weakness	*Deficiency: Vitamin B Complex* Encourage foods rich in B vitamins. Stress proper cooking and storage techniques to preserve potency, such as minimum cooking of vegetables in small amount of liquid and storage of milk in opaque container. Encourage fortified breakfast cereals and soy milk (which have B_{12}) for persons on strict vegetarian diet; dairy products and eggs contain B_{12} if these are allowed; otherwise supplementation may be required. Evaluate need for vitamin supplements when dieting, when using unfortified goat's milk exclusively for infant feeding (deficient in folic acid), or when the breastfeeding mother is a strict vegetarian (vitamin B_{12}). *Excess* Emphasize correct use of vitamin supplements and potential hazards of excess. Individuals with malabsorption syndrome or being treated with hemodialysis or peritoneal dialysis may have increased need for thiamine.

Table 47-1 Vitamins and Their Nutritional Significance—cont'd

PHYSIOLOGICAL FUNCTIONS AND SOURCES	RESULTS OF DEFICIENCY OR EXCESS	NURSING CARE MANAGEMENT
Vitamin B_2 (Riboflavin)†		
Functions Coenzyme (with phosphorus) in carbohydrate, protein, and fat metabolism Maintains healthy skin, especially around mouth, nose, and eyes *Sources* Milk and its products, eggs, organs (liver, kidney, heart), enriched cereals, some green leafy vegetables,‡ legumes	*Deficiency* Ariboflavinosis **Lips**–Cheilosis (fissures at corners of lips), perlèche (inflammation at corners of lips) **Tongue**–Glossitis **Nose**–Irritation and cracks at nasal angle **Eyes**–Burning, itching, tearing, photophobia, blurred vision, corneal vascularization, cataracts **Skin**–Seborrheic dermatitis, delayed wound healing and tissue repair *Excess* Paresthesia, pruritus	Same as vitamin B complex
Niacin (Nicotinic Acid, Nicotinamide)†		
Functions Coenzyme (with riboflavin) in protein and fat metabolism Needed for healthy nervous system and skin and for normal digestion May lower cholesterol *Sources* Meat, poultry, fish, peanuts, beans, peas, whole or enriched grains (except corn and rice) Milk and its products are sources of tryptophan (60 mg tryptophan = 1 mg niacin).	*Deficiency* Pellagra (rash, diarrhea, mental status changes, stomatitis) **Oral**–Stomatitis, glossitis **Cutaneous**–Scaly dermatitis on exposed areas **Gastrointestinal**–Anorexia, weight loss, diarrhea, fatigue **Neurological**–Apathy, anxiety, confusion, depression, dementia *Excess* Release of histamine, a vasodilator (flushing, decreased blood pressure, increased cerebral blood flow; aggravates asthma) Dermatological problems (pruritus, rash, hyperkeratosis, acanthosis nigricans) Increased gastric acidity (aggravates peptic ulcer disease) Hepatotoxicity Increased serum uric acid levels Elevated plasma glucose levels Certain cardiac arrhythmias	Same as vitamin B complex *Excess* If used as hypolipidemic agent, stress safe storage to prevent child's accidental ingestion.
Vitamin B_6 (Pyridoxine)†		
Functions Coenzyme in protein and fat metabolism Needed for formation of antibodies and hemoglobin Needed for utilization of copper and iron Aids in conversion of tryptophan to niacin *Sources* Meats, especially liver and kidney, cereal grains (wheat, corn), yeast, soybeans, peanuts, tuna, chicken, salmon	*Deficiency* Scaly dermatitis Weight loss Anemia Restricted growth Irritability Seizures Peripheral neuritis *Excess* Peripheral nervous system toxicity (unsteady gait, numb feet and hands, clumsiness of hands, sometimes perioral numbness) May cause peptic ulcer disease or seizures	Same as vitamin B complex *Deficiency* Stress proper cooking and storing techniques to preserve potency. Cook food covered in small amount of water. Do not soak food in water. Store in light-resistant container.

*Fat soluble.
†Water soluble.
‡Green leafy vegetables include spinach, broccoli, kale, turnip greens, mustard greens, collards, dandelion greens, and beet greens.

Continued

Table 47-1 Vitamins and Their Nutritional Significance—cont'd

PHYSIOLOGICAL FUNCTIONS AND SOURCES	RESULTS OF DEFICIENCY OR EXCESS	NURSING CARE MANAGEMENT
Folic Acid (Folacin; Reduced Form Called Folinic Acid or Citrovorum Factor)†		
Functions Coenzyme for single-carbon transfer (purines, thymine, hemoglobin) Necessary for formation of red blood cells May prevent neural tube defects (i.e., myelomeningocele) and facial clefts (cleft lip and palate) *Sources* Green leafy vegetables, beets, cabbage, asparagus, liver, kidneys, nuts, eggs, whole grain cereals, legumes, bananas	*Deficiency* Macrocytic anemia Bone marrow depression Glossitis Intestinal malabsorption Growth failure *Excess* Rare because megadoses are not available over the counter May cause insomnia and irritability	Same as vitamin B complex *Deficiency* Stress proper cooking and storing techniques to preserve potency: Cook food covered in small amount of water. Do not soak food in water. Store in light-resistant container. Women of childbearing age should supplement to prevent neural tube defects and orofacial clefts.
Vitamin B_{12} (Cobalamin)†		
Functions Coenzyme in protein synthesis; indirect effect on formation of red blood cells (particularly on formation of nucleic acids and folic acid metabolism) Needed for normal functioning of nervous tissue *Sources* Meat, liver, kidney, fish, shellfish, poultry, milk, eggs, cheese, nutritional yeast, sea vegetables	*Deficiency* Pernicious anemia (one form of deficiency from absence of intrinsic factor in gastric secretions) General signs of severe anemia Lemon-yellow tinge to skin Spinal cord degeneration Delayed brain growth *Excess* Rare	Same as vitamin B complex *Deficiency* Consider fortified foods or supplements in persons over 50 yr of age to meet RDA because malabsorption of food-bound vitamin B_{12} is common.
Vitamin C (Ascorbic Acid)†		
Functions Essential for collagen formation Increases absorption of iron for hemoglobin formation Enhances conversion of folic acid to folinic acid Affects cholesterol synthesis and conversion of proline to hydroxyproline Probably a coenzyme in metabolism of tyrosine and phenylalanine May play role in hydroxylation of adrenal steroids May have stimulating effect on phagocytic activity of leukocytes and formation of antibodies Antioxidant agent (spares other vitamins from oxidation) *Sources* Citrus fruits, strawberries, tomatoes, potatoes, cabbage, broccoli, cauliflower, spinach, papaya, mango, cantaloupe, watermelon, enriched fruit juice	*Deficiency* Scurvy **Skin**–Dry, rough, petechiae; perifollicular hyperkeratotic papules (raised areas around hair follicles) **Musculoskeletal**–Bleeding muscles and joints, pseudoparalysis from pain, swelling of joints, costochondral beading (scorbutic rosary) **Gums**–Spongy, friable, swollen, bleed easily, bluish red or black, teeth loosen and fall out **General disposition**–Irritable, anorexic, apprehensive, in pain, refuses to move, assumes semi-froglike position when supine (scorbutic pose) Signs of anemia Decreased wound healing Increased susceptibility to infection *Excess* Diarrhea Increased excretion of uric acid and acidification of urine (may cause urate precipitation and formation of oxalate stones) **Hemolysis** Impaired leukocytosis activity Damage to β-cells of pancreas and decreased insulin production Reproductive failure "Rebound scurvy" from withdrawal of large amounts	*Deficiency* Encourage foods rich in vitamin C. Evaluate child's diet for sources of vitamin, especially when cow's milk is principal source of nutrition. Tobacco smokers require an additional 35 mg/day; nonsmokers exposed to second-hand smoke should make sure they meet RDA. Stress proper cooking and storage techniques to preserve potency: Wash vegetables quickly; do not soak in water. Cook vegetables in covered pot with minimum water and for short time; avoid copper or cast iron cookware. Do not add baking soda to cooking water. Use fresh fruits and vegetables as soon as possible; store in refrigerator. Store juice in airtight, opaque container. Wrap cut fruit or eat soon after exposing to air. *Excess* Emphasize correct use of vitamin supplements and potential hazards of excess. Identify groups at risk for excessive vitamin C supplements (e.g., those with thalassemia or those receiving anticoagulant or aminoglycoside antibiotic therapy).

Table 47-1 Vitamins and Their Nutritional Significance—cont'd

PHYSIOLOGICAL FUNCTIONS AND SOURCES	RESULTS OF DEFICIENCY OR EXCESS	NURSING CARE MANAGEMENT
Vitamin D_2 (Ergocalciferol) and D_3 (Cholecalciferol)*		
Functions Absorption of calcium and phosphorus and decreased renal excretion of phosphorus *Sources* Direct sunlight Cod liver oil, herring, mackerel, salmon, tuna, sardines Enriched food sources—Milk, milk products, enriched cereals, margarine, breads, many breakfast drinks	*Deficiency* Rickets **Head**—Craniotabes (softening of cranial bones, prominence of frontal bones [bossing]), deformed shape (skull flat and depressed toward middle), delayed closure of fontanels **Chest**—Rachitic rosary (enlargement of costochondral junction of ribs), Harrison groove (horizontal depression in lower portion of rib cage), pigeon chest (sharp protrusion of sternum) **Spine**—Kyphosis, scoliosis, lordosis **Abdomen**—Pot belly, constipation **Extremities**—Bowing of arms and legs, knock knee, sabre shins, instability of hip joints, pelvic deformity, enlargement of epiphyses at ends of long bones **Teeth**—Delayed calcification, especially of permanent teeth **Rachitic tetany**—Seizures *Excess* **Acute**—Vomiting, dehydration, fever, abdominal cramps, bone pain, seizures, coma **Chronic**—Lassitude, mental slowness, anorexia, failure to thrive, thirst, urinary urgency, polyuria, vomiting, diarrhea, abdominal cramps, bone pain, pathological fractures Calcification of soft tissue—Kidneys, lungs, adrenal glands, vessels (hypertension), heart, gastric lining, tympanic membrane (deafness) Osteoporosis of long bones Elevated serum levels of calcium and phosphorus	*Deficiency* Encourage foods rich in vitamin D, especially fortified whole cow's milk (>12 mo of age). Encourage use of vitamin D supplement in all exclusively breastfed infants starting within first 2 wk of life (see text). Observe for possibility of overdose from supplements. If prescribed, supervise proper use of orthoses (splints and braces). *Excess* Same as vitamin A; may include low-calcium diet during initial therapy
Vitamin E (Tocopherol)*		
Functions Production of red blood cells and protection from hemolysis Muscle and liver integrity Coenzyme factor in tissue respiration Minimizes oxidation of polyunsaturated fatty acids and vitamins A and C in intestinal tract and tissues *Sources* Vegetable oils, wheat germ oil, milk, egg yolk, fish, whole grains, nuts, legumes, spinach, broccoli	*Deficiency* Hemolytic anemia from hemolysis caused by shortened life of red blood cells, especially in preterm infants; focal necrosis of tissues *Excess* Little is known; less toxic than other fat-soluble vitamins	*Deficiency* Initiate early feeding in preterm infants; may need supplementation. Potential role as antioxidant in immune function, preventing or limiting the severity of retinopathy and prevention of hemolytic anemia, bronchopulmonary dysplasia, and intracranial hemorrhage
Vitamin K*		
Functions Catalyst for production of prothrombin and blood-clotting factors II, VII, IX, and X by the liver *Sources* Pork, liver, green leafy vegetables, cabbage, tomatoes, egg yolk, cheese	*Deficiency* Hemorrhage *Excess* Hemolytic anemia in individuals who are deficient in glucose 6-phosphate dehydrogenase	*Deficiency* Administer prophylactically to all newborns. Other indications include intestinal disease, lack of bile, prolonged antibiotic therapy; may be used in management of blood-clotting time when anticoagulants such as warfarin (Coumadin) and dicumarol (bishydroxycoumarin), which are vitamin K antagonists, are used.

Table is not intended to be all inclusive.
*Fat soluble.
†Water soluble.
‡Green leafy vegetables include spinach, broccoli, kale, turnip greens, mustard greens, collards, dandelion greens, and beet greens.
RDA, recommended dietary allowance.

100 mg and include calcium, phosphorus, magnesium, sodium, potassium, chloride, and sulphur. *Microminerals*, or trace elements, have daily requirements of less than 100 mg and include several essential minerals and those whose exact role in nutrition is still unclear. The greatest concern with minerals is deficiency, especially of iron, calcium, phosphorus, magnesium, and zinc. Low levels of zinc can cause nutritional growth failure (failure to thrive).

The regulation of mineral balance in the body is complex. Dietary extremes of mineral intake can cause a number of mineral–mineral interactions that could result in unexpected deficiencies or excesses. For example, excessive amounts of one mineral such as zinc can result in a deficiency of another mineral such as copper, even if sufficient amounts of copper are ingested. Thus megadose intake of one mineral may cause deficiency of another essential mineral by blocking its absorption in the blood or intestinal wall or by competing with binding sites on protein carriers needed for metabolism.

Deficiencies can also occur when various substances in the diet interact with minerals. For example, iron, zinc, and calcium can form insoluble complexes with phytates or oxalates (substances found in plant proteins), which impair the bioavailability of the mineral. This type of interaction is important in **vegetarian** diets because plant foods such as soy are high in phytates. Contrary to popular opinion, spinach is not an ideal source of iron or calcium because of its high oxalate content.

Children with certain illnesses are at greater risk for growth failure, especially in relation to bone mineral deficiency as a result of the treatment of the disease, decreased nutrient intake, or decreased absorption of necessary minerals. Those at risk for such deficiencies include children who are receiving or have received radiation and chemotherapy for cancer; children with human immunodeficiency virus (HIV), sickle cell disease, cystic fibrosis, gastrointestinal (GI) malabsorption, or nephrosis; and very low–birth weight preterm infants.

Deficiencies and excesses of the essential macrominerals and microminerals are summarized in Table 47-2. General nursing care management is discussed on this page, and specific nursing interventions are discussed in the table.

Vegetarian Diets

Vegetarian diets have become increasingly popular in North America because people are concerned about hypertension; cholesterol; obesity; cardiovascular disease; the influence of the animal rights movement; and cancer of the stomach, intestine, and colon. The American Dietetic Association and Dietitians of Canada (2003) issued a statement endorsing vegetarian diets for adults and children; the statement further notes that well-planned vegetarian diets are adequate for all stages of the life cycle and promote normal growth. Children and adolescents on vegetarian diets have the potential for lifelong healthy diets and have been shown to have lower intakes of cholesterol, saturated fat, and total fat and higher intakes of fruits, fibre, and vegetables than nonvegetarians (American Dietetic Association and Dietitians of Canada, 2003).

The major types of vegetarianism are as follows:

Lacto-ovo vegetarians, who exclude meat from their diet but consume dairy products and rarely fish

Lactovegetarians, who exclude meat and eggs but drink milk

Pure vegetarians (vegans), who eliminate any food of animal origin, including milk and eggs

Macrobiotics, who are even more restrictive than pure vegetarians, allowing only a few types of fruits, vegetables, and legumes

Semivegetarians, who consume a lacto-ovo vegetarian diet with some fish and poultry (this is an increasingly popular form of vegetarianism and poses little or no nutritional risk to infants unless dietary fat and cholesterol intake is severely restricted).

Many individuals who are concerned about healthy diets subscribe to vegetarian diets that may not be typified by these categories. During nutritional assessment it is necessary to clearly list exactly what the diet includes and excludes (see Additional Resources section at the end of this chapter for further information).

The major deficiencies that may occur in the stricter vegan diets are inadequate protein for growth; inadequate calories for energy and growth; poor digestibility of many of the bulky natural, unprocessed foods, especially for infants; and deficiencies of vitamin B_6, niacin, riboflavin, vitamin D, iron, calcium, and zinc. Strict vegan diets also require supplements of vitamin B_{12} and vitamin D. Vitamin D is essential if a child drinks less than 500 mL of vitamin D–fortified milk daily. Children in this category should receive 400 IU of vitamin D daily. Many of these deficiencies can be avoided in children who are not consuming 100% of the RDA of vitamins and minerals with a multivitamin–mineral supplement (CPS, 2010c; Dunham & Kollar, 2006).

Children on strict vegetarian and macrobiotic diets should be evaluated for iron deficiency anemia and rickets; this may occur as a result of consuming plant foods such as unrefined cereals, which impair the absorption of iron, calcium, and zinc. Other factors that affect iron absorption are listed in Box 47-1 on p. 1384.

Nursing Care Management

Identification of the adequacy of nutrient intake is the initial nursing goal and requires assessment based on a dietary history and physical examination for signs of deficiency or excess. Once assessment data are collected, this information is evaluated against standard intakes to identify areas of concern.

The Dietary Reference Intakes

The **Dietary Reference Intakes** (DRIs) are quantitative estimates of nutrient requirements for planning and evaluating diets for healthy infants and consist of four categories (see Additional Resources section). These include Estimated Average Requirements (EARs) for age and gender categories, tolerable upper-limit (UL) nutrient intakes that are associated with a low risk of adverse effects, adequate intakes (AIs) of nutrients, and new standard RDAs. The guidelines present information about lifestyle factors that may affect nutrient function, such as caffeine intake and exercise, and about how the nutrient may be related to chronic disease. The first DRIs published included calcium, magnesium, phosphorus, vitamin D, and fluoride. Additional groups of nutrients include folate

Table 47-2 Minerals and Their Nutritional Significance

PHYSIOLOGICAL FUNCTIONS AND SOURCES	RESULTS OF DEFICIENCY OR EXCESS	NURSING CARE MANAGEMENT
Calcium*		
Functions Bone and tooth development and maintenance (in combination with phosphorus) Muscle contractions, especially the heart Blood clotting Absorption of vitamin B_{12} Enzyme activation Nerve conduction Integrity of intracellular cement substances and various membranes *Sources* Dairy products, egg yolk, sardines, canned salmon with bones, green leafy vegetables† (except spinach), soybeans, dried beans, peas	*Deficiency* Rickets Tetany Impaired growth, especially of bones and teeth Osteoporosis *Excess* Drowsiness, extreme lethargy Impaired absorption of other minerals (iron, zinc, manganese) Calcium deposits in tissues (renal failure)	*Deficiency* Encourage foods rich in calcium, especially dairy products. Give vitamin D supplements in infants beginning by age 2 mo (see text). Caution that oxalates in leafy vegetables (spinach), oxalates in chocolates, and a high phosphorus intake (especially from carbonated beverages) can decrease calcium absorption. Discourage use of whole cow's milk or other animal milks in newborns and infants under 12 mo because the phosphorus/calcium ratio favours excretion of calcium. Advise against diets that restrict dairy products unless adequate supplementation is followed. *Excess* Emphasize correct use of calcium supplements, especially the possible interaction between megadoses of calcium and resulting deficiency states of other minerals.
Chloride*		
Functions Acid-base and fluid balance Enzyme activation in saliva Component of hydrochloric acid in stomach *Sources* Salt, meat, eggs, dairy products, many prepared and preserved foods	*Deficiency* Acid-base disturbances (hypochloremic alkalosis, dehydration); occurs mostly in combination with sodium loss *Excess* Acid-base disturbance	Deficiency and excess are unusual; most diets supply adequate chloride (usually in combination with sodium). Disease states such as excessive vomiting can necessitate chloride replacement.
Copper‡		
Functions Production of hemoglobin Essential component of several enzyme systems *Sources* Organ meats, oysters, nuts, seeds, legumes, corn oil margarine	*Deficiency* Anemia, leukopenia, neutropenia *Excess* Severe vomiting and diarrhea Hemolytic anemia	*Deficiency* Emphasize the correct use of any vitamin supplement with mineral because deficiency from inadequate food sources is less likely than from excess intake of other minerals, especially zinc and possibly iron. *Excess* Cooking acid foods in unlined copper pots can lead to chronic and toxic accumulation of copper.
Fluoride‡		
Functions Formation of caries-resistant teeth Strong bone development *Sources* Fluoridated water and foods or beverages prepared with fluoridated water, fish, tea	*Deficiency* Increased susceptibility to tooth decay *Excess* Fluorosis (mottling or pitting of enamel) Severe bone deformities	Fluoride has the narrowest range of safe and adequate intake; therefore stress the importance of storing supplements in a safe area. *Deficiency* In areas with optimally fluoridated water, encourage sufficient intake to supply recommended amount of fluoride. In areas of unfluoridated water or when ready-to-use formula, powder formula, bottled water, or breast milk is used, stress the importance of fluoride supplements (age appropriate). *Excess* In areas with excess fluoride in the water, consider the use of bottled water (without fluoride) in drinking and cooking to reduce the fluoride intake to safe levels.

Continued

Table 47-2 Minerals and Their Nutritional Significance—cont'd

PHYSIOLOGICAL FUNCTIONS AND SOURCES	RESULTS OF DEFICIENCY OR EXCESS	NURSING CARE MANAGEMENT
Iodine‡		
Functions Production of thyroid hormone Normal reproduction *Sources* Seafood, kelp, iodized salt, sea salt, enriched bread, milk (from dairy processing); medications, including amiodarone, povidone-iodine, and prenatal vitamins	*Deficiency* Goitre (enlarged thyroid from decreased thyroxine formation) *Excess* Thyrotoxicosis; goitre; hypothyroidism	*Deficiency* Encourage use of iodized salt for individuals living far from the sea. *Excess* If iodine preparations are in the home, stress the importance of safe storage.
Iron		
Functions Formation of hemoglobin and myoglobin Essential part of several enzymes and proteins *Sources* Liver, especially pork, followed by calf, beef, and chicken; kidney, red meat, poultry, shellfish, whole grains, iron-enriched infant formula and cereal, enriched cereals and bread, legumes, nuts, seeds, green leafy vegetables† (except spinach), dried fruits, potatoes, molasses, tofu, prune juice	*Deficiency* Anemia (see Chapter 49) *Excess* Hemosiderosis (excess iron storage in various tissues of the body, especially the spleen, liver, lymph glands, heart, and pancreas) Hemochromatosis (excess iron storage with cellular damage)	*Deficiency* Discourage excessive iron-fortified milk consumption, especially more than 1 L/day (cow's milk is a poor source of iron). If iron supplements are prescribed, teach parents factors that affect absorption. *Excess* Stress the importance of storing iron supplements in a safe area.
Magnesium*		
Functions Bone and tooth formation Production of proteins Nerve conduction to muscles Activation of enzymes needed for carbohydrate and protein metabolism *Sources* Whole grains, nuts, soybeans, meat, green leafy vegetables (uncooked), tea, cocoa, raisins	*Deficiency* Tremors, spasm Irregular heartbeat Muscular weakness Lower extremity cramps Convulsions, delirium *Excess* Nervous system disturbances caused by imbalance in calcium/magnesium ratio	Deficiency and excess are unusual, except in disease states such as prolonged vomiting or diarrhea or kidney dysfunction, where replacement may be needed.
Phosphorus*		
Functions Bone and tooth development (in combination with calcium) Involved in numerous chemical reactions, including protein, carbohydrate, and fat metabolism Acid–base balance *Sources* Dairy products, eggs, meat, poultry, legumes, carbonated beverages	*Deficiency* Weakness, anorexia, malaise, bone pain *Excess* Produces secondary calcium deficiency from imbalanced calcium/phosphorus ratio	*Deficiency* Dietary deficiency is uncommon, although prolonged use of antacids can produce deficiency, in which case supplementation is recommended. To preserve calcium/phosphorus ratio in newborns and infants, discourage use of cow's milk.
Potassium*		
Functions Acid–base and fluid balance (major extracellular fluid areas) Nerve conduction Muscular contraction, especially the heart Release of energy *Sources* Bananas, citrus fruit, dried fruits, meat, fish, bran, legumes, peanut butter, potatoes, coffee, tea, cocoa	*Deficiency* Cardiac arrhythmias Muscular weakness Lethargy Kidney and respiratory failure Heart failure *Excess* Cardiac arrhythmias Respiratory failure Mental confusion Numbness of extremities	Dietary deficiency and excess are unlikely, although disease states such as prolonged nausea and vomiting or the use of certain diuretics can result in hypokalemia; in such instances encourage replacement with supplements of rich food sources such as bananas.

Table 47-2 Minerals and Their Nutritional Significance—cont'd

PHYSIOLOGICAL FUNCTIONS AND SOURCES	RESULTS OF DEFICIENCY OR EXCESS	NURSING CARE MANAGEMENT
Selenium‡		
Functions Antioxidant, especially protective of vitamin E Protects against toxicity of heavy metals Associated with fat metabolism *Sources* Seafood, organs, egg yolk, whole grains, chicken, meat, tomatoes, cabbage, garlic, mushrooms, milk	*Deficiency* Keshan disease (cardiomyopathy in children; found in China) *Excess* Eye, nose, and throat irritation Increased dental caries Liver and kidney degeneration	Deficiency and excess are uncommon in North America, although selenium deficiency can occur in patients receiving prolonged total parenteral alimentation; in these instances supplementation is required.
Sodium*		
Functions Acid–base and fluid balance (major extracellular fluid cation) Cell permeability; absorption of glucose Muscle contraction *Sources* Table salt, seafood, meat, poultry, numerous prepared foods	*Deficiency* Dehydration Hypotension Convulsions Muscle cramps *Excess* Edema Hypertension Intracranial hemorrhage	*Deficiency* Deficient intake is rare, although losses secondary to nausea, vomiting, excessive sweating, and use of diuretics can occur and require replacement. *Excess* Encourage parents to limit excessive use of salt in preparing foods and to limit commercial foods with high sodium content such as smoked meats.
Zinc‡		
Functions Component of about 100 enzymes Synthesis of nucleic acids and protein in immune system and coagulation Release of vitamin A from liver Improved wound healing with vitamin C Normal taste sensitivity *Sources* Seafood (especially oysters), meat, poultry, eggs, wheat, legumes	*Deficiency* Loss of appetite Diminished taste sensation Delayed healing Skin lesions—Erythematous, crusted lesions around body orifices (mouth, nares, anus) Alopecia Diarrhea Growth failure Delayed sexual maturity *Excess* Vomiting and diarrhea Malaise, dizziness Anemia, gastric bleeding Impaired absorption of calcium and copper	Emphasize correct use of zinc supplements and the possible interaction with other minerals. *Deficiency* Encourage food sources rich in zinc, especially protein. Caution that fibre, phytates, oxalates, tannins (in tea or coffee), iron, and calcium adversely affect zinc absorption. Recognize groups at risk for zinc deficiency, such as vegetarians and Hispanics, whose diets may have restricted or low meat content and high fibre and phytate content; and patients with malabsorption syndromes.

Table is not intended to be all inclusive.
*Macrominerals—required intake >100 mg/day.
†Green leafy vegetables include spinach, broccoli, kale, turnip greens, mustard greens, collards, dandelion greens, and beet greens.
‡Microminerals or trace elements—required intake <100 mg/day.

and other B vitamins, dietary antioxidants, micronutrients, macronutrients, trace elements, electrolytes, and food components such as dietary fibre. The comprehensive set of guidelines covers nutrient needs across the lifespan, including infancy. An important factor in the development of the DRIs that affects children, particularly infants 0 to 6 months, is that the AIs are based on the nutrient intake of term, healthy, breastfed infants (by well-nourished mothers), which now represents the gold standard for infant nutrition in this age group.

Eating Well With Canada's Food Guide was developed by Health Canada in 2007 as a guide for adult and childhood nutrition (Fig. 47-1). This guide aims to simplify healthy food choices and provide guidance in both serving sizes and recommended daily servings based on age and sex. The *Food Guide* can be used to ensure that minimal recommendations for all nutrients are met.

Achieving a nutritionally adequate vegetarian diet is not difficult (except with the strictest diets), but it does require careful planning and knowledge of nutrient sources. *Eating Well With Canada's Food Guide* (Health Canada, 2011a) can be adapted to meet the nutrient needs of vegetarians. For children, the lacto-ovo vegetarian diet is nutritionally adequate; however, the vegan diet requires supplementation with vitamins D and B_{12} for children ages 2 to 12 years. Infants should be breastfed for the first 6 months and preferably for 1 year, be introduced to some solid foods at 6 months, and receive iron-fortified cereal for at least 18 months. Vitamin B_{12} supplementation is recommended if the breastfeeding mother's intake of the vitamin is inadequate or if she is not on vitamin supplements (CPS, 2010c). The introduction of solids for vegetarian infants may occur using the same guidelines as for other children (see p. 981). Breast milk from vegetarian mothers can be deficient in vitamin B_{12}; supplementation of

BOX 47-1 Factors That Affect Iron Absorption

Increase

Acidity (low pH)—Administer iron between meals (gastric hydrochloric acid)
Ascorbic acid (vitamin C)—Administer iron with juice, fruit, or multivitamin preparation
Vitamin A
Calcium
Tissue need
Meat, fish, poultry
Cooking in cast iron pots

Decrease

Alkalinity (high pH)—Avoid any antacid preparation
Phosphates—Milk is unfavourable vehicle for iron administration
Phytates—Found in cereals
Oxalates—Found in many fruits and vegetables (plums, currants, green beans, spinach, sweet potatoes, tomatoes)
Tannins—Found in tea, coffee
Tissue saturation
Malabsorptive disorders
Disturbances that cause diarrhea or steatorrhea
Infection

both mother and child is advisable. If human milk or commercial infant formula is not given, fortified soy formula is recommended (American Dietetic Association & Dietitians of Canada, 2003). A variety of foods should be introduced during the early years to ensure a well-balanced intake.

To ensure sufficient protein in the diet, **incomplete protein foods** (those that do not have all the **essential amino acids**) must be eaten at the same meal with other foods that supply the missing amino acids. (**Complete protein foods** have all the essential amino acids.) The three basic combinations of foods consumed by vegetarians that generally provide the appropriate amounts of essential amino acids are as follows:

1. Grains (cereal, rice, pasta) and legumes (beans, peas, lentils, peanuts)
2. Grains and milk products (milk, cheese, yogourt)
3. Seeds (sesame, sunflower) and legumes

Additional dietary considerations for young children are found in Chapters 36 and 37.

Protein-Energy Malnutrition

Malnutrition continues to be a major health problem in the world today, particularly in children under 5 years of age. However, lack of food is not always the primary cause for malnutrition. In many developing and underdeveloped nations, diarrhea (gastroenteritis) is a major factor. Additional factors are bottle-feeding (in poor sanitary conditions), inadequate knowledge of proper child care practices, parental illiteracy, economic and political factors, climate conditions, cultural and religious food preferences, and simply the lack of adequate food. Poverty is an important determinant of health and an underlying cause of malnutrition. The most extreme forms of malnutrition, or *protein-energy malnutrition (PEM)*, are kwashiorkor and marasmus. Both of these conditions are extremely rare in Canada.

PEM may be seen in persons with chronic health problems such as cystic fibrosis, renal dialysis, and GI malabsorption; in older adults who have chronic malnutrition; or in persons with acute illnesses such as prolonged, untreated **anorexia nervosa**.

Food Sensitivity

Food sensitivity is a general term that includes any type of adverse reaction to food or food additives. Food sensitivities can be divided into two broad categories:

1. **Food allergy or hypersensitivity**, which refers to reactions involving immunological mechanisms, usually immune globulin E (IgE); the reactions may be immediate or delayed and mild or severe, such as an anaphylactic reaction.
2. **Food intolerance**, which refers to reactions involving known or unknown nonimmunological mechanisms; lactose intolerance is an example of a reaction that looks like allergy but is caused by deficiency of the enzyme lactase.

However, this classification is not universally accepted; the terms *food sensitivity, hypersensitivity, allergy,* and *intolerance* are often used interchangeably. The American Academy of Allergy, Asthma, and Immunology further suggests defining food-induced reactions according to the following: adverse food reactions, food hypersensitivity (allergy), food anaphylaxis, food intolerance, food idiosyncrasy, food toxicity or poisoning, anaphylactoid reaction to food, pharmacological food reaction, and metabolic food reaction (Health Canada, 2011b).

The clinical manifestations of food hypersensitivity may be divided as follows (Health Canada, 2009a):

Systemic—Anaphylactic, growth failure
Gastrointestinal—Abdominal pain, vomiting, cramping, diarrhea
Respiratory—Cough, wheezing, rhinitis, infiltrates
Cutaneous—Urticaria, rash, atopic dermatitis

Food hypersensitivities usually occur either as an IgE-mediated or non–IgE-mediated immune response; some toxic reactions may occur as a result of a **toxin** found within the food (Health Canada, 2011b). Food allergy is caused by exposure to allergens, usually proteins (but not the smaller amino acids) that are capable of inducing IgE antibody formation (sensitization) when ingested. *Sensitization* refers to the initial exposure of an individual to an allergen, resulting in an immune response; subsequent exposure induces a much stronger response that is clinically apparent. Consequently, food hypersensitivity typically occurs after the food has been ingested one or more times. The most common food allergens are listed in Box 47-2.

Allergies in general demonstrate a genetic component: children who have one parent with allergy have a 50% or greater risk of developing allergy; children who have two parents with allergy have up to a 100% risk of developing allergy. Allergy with a hereditary tendency is referred to as *atopy*. Some infants with atopy can be identified at birth from elevated levels of IgE in cord blood.

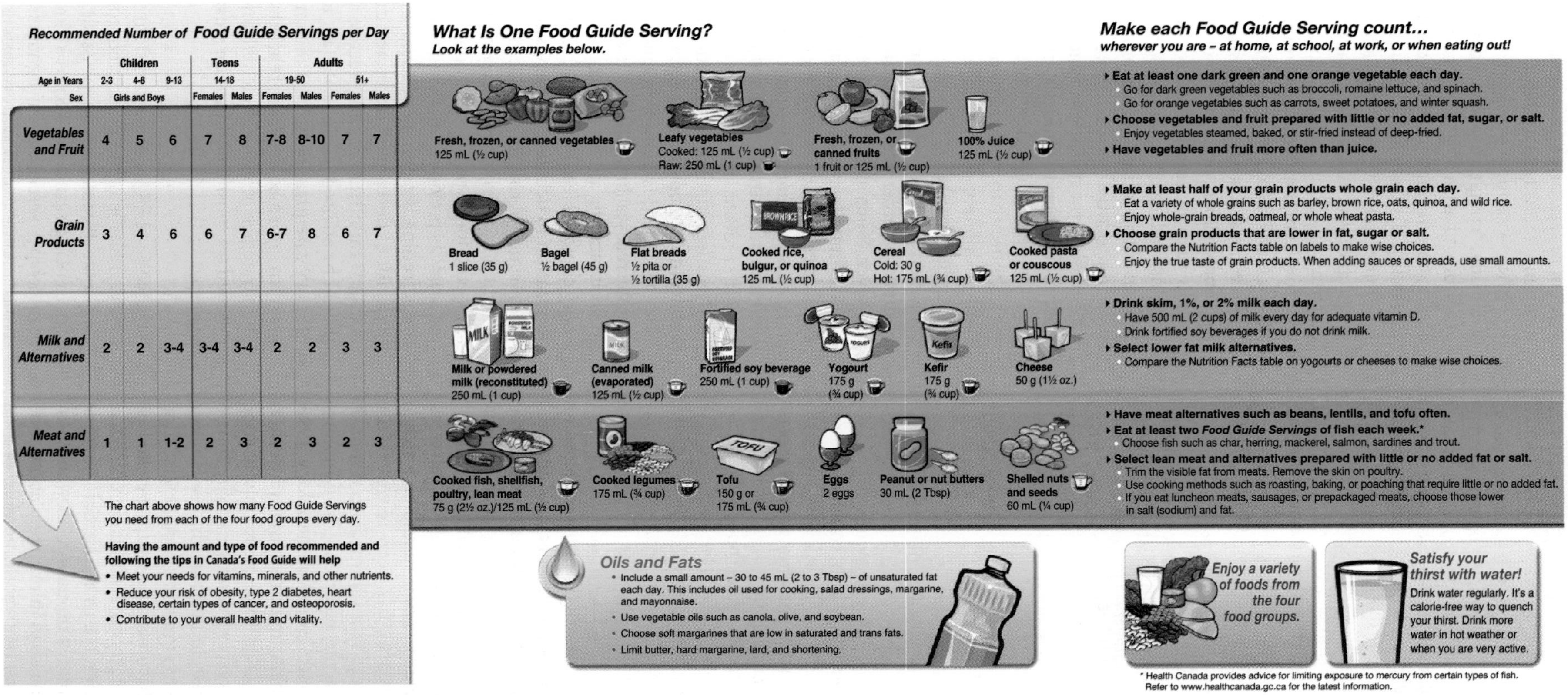

Fig. 47-1 Canada's food guide for healthy eating. *(Canada's Food Guide. Health Canada, 2007 [Revised 2011]. Reproduced with the permission of the Minister of Health, 2011.)*

BOX 47-2 Hyperallergenic Foods and Food Sources

Milk*—Ice cream, butter, margarine (if it contains dairy products), yogourt, cheese, pudding, baked goods, wieners, bologna, canned creamed soups, instant breakfast drinks, powdered milk drinks, milk chocolate
Eggs*—Mayonnaise, creamy salad dressing, baked goods, egg noodles, some cake icing, meringue, custard, pancakes, French toast, root beer
Wheat*—Almost all baked goods, wieners, bologna, pressed or chopped cold cuts, gravy, pasta, some canned soups
Legumes—Peanuts,* peanut butter or oil, beans, peas, lentils
Nuts*—Some chocolates, candy, baked goods, cherry beverages (may be flavoured with a nut extract), walnut oil
Fish or shellfish*—Cod liver oil, pizza with anchovies, Caesar salad dressing, any food fried in same oil as fish
Soy*—Soy sauce, teriyaki or Worcestershire sauce, tofu, baked goods using soy flour or oil, soy nuts, soy infant formulas or milk, soybean paste, tuna packed in vegetable oil, many margarines
Chocolate—Cola beverages, cocoa, chocolate-flavoured drinks
Buckwheat—Some cereals, pancakes
Pork, chicken—Bacon, wieners, sausage, pork fat, chicken broth
Strawberries, melon, pineapple—Gelatin, syrups
Corn—Popcorn, cereal, muffins, cornstarch, corn meal, corn bread, corn tortilla
Citrus fruits—Orange, lemon, lime, grapefruit; any of these in drinks, gelatin, juice, or medicines
Tomatoes—Juice, some vegetable soups, spaghetti, pizza sauce, ketchup
Spices—Chili, pepper, vinegar, cinnamon

*Most common allergens.

Deaths have been reported in children who suffered an anaphylactic reaction to food. Onset of the reactions occurred shortly after ingestion (5 to 30 minutes). In most of the children the reactions did not begin with skin signs, such as hives, red rash, and flushing, but rather mimicked an acute asthma attack (wheezing, decreased air movement in airways, dyspnea). Children with food anaphylaxis should be watched closely because a biphasic response has been recorded in a number of cases in which there is an immediate response, apparent recovery, and then acute recurrence of symptoms (Canadian Society of Allergy and Clinical Immunology, 1995; Sampson, 2003). Parents, teachers, and child day care workers should be educated regarding signs and symptoms of food hypersensitivity reactions. People with food sensitivity should avoid unfamiliar foods and restaurants that do not disclose food ingredients. New labelling guidelines require that food additives such as spices and flavouring be clearly labelled on commercially sold, store-bought foods. Hidden ingredients in prepared foods have been implicated as a potential source of food hypersensitivity. The Allergy Asthma Information Association provides up-to-date Canadian information about food content and labelling, manufacturers' recalls because of food content or labelling errors, and "safe" substitutes for common allergenic foods (see Additional Resources section).

Other symptoms of anaphylaxis to food allergens include wheezing, cough, dyspnea, **urticaria**, abdominal cramps, vomiting, diarrhea, a drop in systemic blood pressure or **shock**, and in small preverbal children, restlessness, urticaria, irritability, listlessness, and unresponsiveness. *Oral allergy syndrome* occurs when a food allergen is ingested (commonly fruits and vegetables) and there is subsequent **edema** and **pruritus** involving the lips, tongue, palate, and throat; recovery from symptoms is usually rapid. *Immediate GI hypersensitivity* is an IgE-mediated reaction to a food allergen; reactions include nausea, abdominal pain, cramping, diarrhea, vomiting, anaphylaxis, or all of these. Additional food hypersensitivities seen in young children include allergic eosinophilic gastritis, allergic eosinophilic gastroenterocolitis, dietary protein enterocolitis (or milk protein intolerance), and dietary protein proctitis.

Although the reason is unknown, many children "outgrow" their food allergies; children may outgrow milk and egg allergies, but peanut allergies may persist. Children who are allergic to more than one food may develop a tolerance to each food at different times. Because of the tendency to lose the hypersensitivity, allergic foods should be reintroduced into the diet after a period of abstinence (usually a year or more) to evaluate whether the food can be safely added to the diet. However, foods associated with severe anaphylactic reactions will continue to present a lifelong risk and must be avoided. Because children with food allergies (usually two or more) are at risk for inadequate nutrient intake and growth failure, it is recommended that they have an annual nutritional assessment to prevent such problems (Christie et al., 2002).

Breastfeeding is now considered to be a primary strategy for avoiding atopy in families with known food sensitivities; however, there is some evidence that cow's milk protein is transferred via breast milk. If supplementation is required, hydrolysated or amino acid formulas, *not soy* formulas, are a good choice (Health Link BC, 2011). An additional recommendation to decrease the incidence of food allergies in children at higher risk for allergies is to begin introducing solid food at 6 months of age. Delaying the introduction of highly allergenic foods past 4 to 6 months may not be as protective for atopy as previously believed (Greer et al., 2008). Exclusive breastfeeding is recommended for 4 to 6 months for infants at high risk of developing atopy, and exclusive breastfeeding for at least 3 months may be protective against wheezing. Parents should be advised to discuss infant feeding practices with the primary care practitioner and obtain adequate information to make an informed decision if there is a family history of atopy. The strategies listed in the Guidelines box are those recommended by most authorities for infants with a family history of atopy.

NURSING ALERT Sampson (2003) suggests that indications for the administration of intramuscular epinephrine in a child with a life-threatening anaphylactic reaction or one who is experiencing severe symptoms include any one of the following: itching sensation or tightness in throat; hoarseness; "barky" cough; difficulty swallowing; dyspnea; wheezing;

GUIDELINES Preventing Atopy in Children

Identify Children at Risk

Family history of allergy

Increased immune globulin E in cord blood and postnatal serum

Dry, flaky skin

Prenatal Precautions (Last Trimester)

Eat healthy; there are no known foods that should be avoided

Postnatal Precautions

Breast milk (preferred for 4 to 6 months), extensively hydrolyzed formula (Nutramigen or Alimentum), or amino acid formula (Neocate or EleCare) exclusively for at least 6 months

No solid food for first 6 months, and then do not delay introducing new food

No whole cow's milk, substitution milks, or soy formula for 12 months

One new food added every few days to identify possible reaction

Read commercial food product labels carefully for ingredients, preservatives

Environmental Control

Limited exposure to dust mites, moulds, furry animals, latex products, and second-hand cigarette smoke

(Data from Health LinkBC, 2011)

cyanosis; respiratory arrest; mild dysrhythmia or mild hypotension; severe bradycardia, hypotension, or cardiac arrest; or loss of consciousness.

Children with extremely sensitive food allergies should wear medical identification such as a Medic Alert bracelet and have an injectable epinephrine cartridge (EpiPen) readily available and know how to use it. It is also helpful for the child to have a copy of the individualized written treatment plan on hand for prompt diagnosis and treatment.

Cow's Milk Allergy

Cow's milk allergy (CMA) (also referred to as cow's milk protein allergy [CMPA] or cow's milk protein intolerance [CMPI]) is a multifaceted disorder representing adverse systemic and local GI reactions to cow's milk protein. (This discussion is centred on cow's milk protein found in commercial infant formulas; whole milk is not recommended for infants younger than the age of 12 months.) The hypersensitivity may be manifested within the first 4 months of life through a variety of signs and symptoms that may appear within 45 minutes of milk ingestion or after a period of several days (Box 47-3). In infants who are highly sensitive to the protein, even a small amount of cow's milk protein may induce an anaphylactic reaction. Cases of contamination of non-cow's milk–based infant formula during the manufacturing process resulting in severe reactions have been documented (Levin, Motala, & Lopata, 2005). The diagnosis may initially be made from the history, although the history alone is not diagnostic; the timing and diversity of clinical manifestations vary greatly.

BOX 47-3 Common Clinical Manifestations of Cow's Milk Sensitivity

Gastrointestinal

Diarrhea

Vomiting

Colic

Abdominal pain

Respiratory

Rhinitis

Bronchitis

Asthma

Wheezing

Sneezing

Coughing

Chronic nasal discharge

Other Signs and Symptoms

Eczema

Excessive crying

Pallor (from anemia secondary to chronic blood loss in gastrointestinal tract)

For example, CMA may be manifested as colic (see p. 1003), diarrhea, vomiting, GI bleeding, gastroesophageal reflux (GER), chronic constipation, or sleeplessness in an otherwise healthy infant.

The incidence of CMA is reported to be approximately 2.5% among infants younger than 1 year of age (CPS, 2009).

Diagnostic Evaluation

A number of diagnostic tests may be performed, including stool analysis for blood (both frank and occult bleeding can occur from the colitis), serum IgE levels, skin-prick or scratch testing, and radioallergosorbent test (measures IgE antibodies to specific allergens in serum by radioimmunoassay). Both skin and radioallergosorbent testing help identify the offending food, but the results are not always conclusive.

The most definitive diagnostic strategy is elimination of milk in the diet, followed by challenge testing after improvement of symptoms. A clinical diagnosis is made when symptoms improve after removal of milk from the diet and two or more challenge tests produce symptoms (Ewing & Allen, 2005). Challenge testing involves reintroducing small quantities of milk in the diet to detect resurgence of symptoms; at times it involves the use of a placebo so that the parent is unaware of (or "blind" to) the timing of allergen ingestion. A double-blind, placebo-controlled food challenge is the gold standard for diagnosing food allergies such as CMA, yet it may not be used very often for diagnosing CMA because of the expense, time involved, and risk for further exposure and anaphylactic reaction (Ewing & Allen, 2005).

Therapeutic Management

Treatment of CMA is elimination of cow's milk–based formula and all other dairy products. For infants fed cow's milk formula, this primarily involves changing the formula to a casein hydrolysate milk formula or extensively hydrolyzed formula (Nutramigen, or Alimentum), in which the protein has been broken down into its amino acids through enzymatic hydrolysis. Although the Canadian Paediatric Society (2009) recommends the use of hydrolyzed formulas for CMA, many practitioners may start a soy formula instead. Approximately 10% of infants who are sensitive to cow's milk protein will also demonstrate sensitivity to soy (Assa'ad, 2006), but soy is less expensive than protein hydrolysate formula. Intolerance to soy is reported to be higher in infants under age 6 months with a family history of atopy and severe GI symptoms (Ewing & Allen, 2005).

Other choices for children who are intolerant to cow's milk–based formula are the amino acid–based formulas Neocate or EleCare, but their cost is a major consideration. Goat's milk is not an acceptable substitute because it cross-reacts with cow's milk protein, is deficient in folic acid, and is unsuitable as the only source of calories. Anaphylactic reaction to goat's milk has been noted in an infant who was also allergic to cow's milk (Pessler & Nejat, 2004). Infants are maintained on the milk-free diet until after 1 year of age, after which time small quantities of milk are reintroduced.

Nursing Care Management

The principal nursing objectives are to prevent and reduce exposure of infants to cow's milk protein by encouraging exclusive breastfeeding in the first 4 to 6 months of life. In addition, nurses have an important role in identifying potential CMA and providing appropriate counselling of parents on the signs and symptoms of CMA and the use of substitute formulas appropriate for infants with diagnosed CMA. Parents need much reassurance regarding the needs of nonverbal infants with such an array of symptoms. Endless nights of lost sleep and a crying infant may promote feelings of parenting inadequacy and role conflict, thus aggravating the situation. Nurses can reassure parents that many of these symptoms are common and the reasons are often never found, yet the child does achieve appropriate growth and development; acute symptoms are reported to the practitioner for further evaluation.

The protein hydrolysate (partially hydrolyzed and extensively hydrolyzed) formulas tend to be less palatable than milk-based formulas so the child may be reluctant to accept the new formula. This can be overcome by adding nonnutritive, hypoallergenic flavour packets or by introducing the formula gradually over a few days, using 30 mL new formula to 210 mL of old formula, then 60 mL to 180 mL, 90 mL to 150 mL, and as needed. Parents also need to be reassured that the infant will receive complete nutrition from the new formula and will suffer no ill effects from the absence of cow's milk. Protein hydrolysate formulas are also expensive; the nurse can play a role in advocating for families to government agencies to assist in paying for the formula.

Once solid foods are started, parents need guidance in avoiding milk products (see Box 47-2), although many children reportedly outgrow cow's milk protein sensitivity by 3 to 4 years of age (Fiocchi & Martelli, 2006).

Lactose Intolerance

Lactose intolerance refers to at least four different entities that involve a deficiency of the enzyme *lactase*, which is needed for the hydrolysis or digestion of lactose in the small intestine; lactose is hydrolyzed into glucose and galactose. **Congenital** *lactase deficiency* occurs soon after birth after the newborn has consumed lactose-containing milk (human milk or commercial formula). This inborn error of metabolism involves the complete absence or severely reduced presence of lactase, is rare, and requires a lifelong lactose-free or extremely reduced lactose diet.

Primary lactase deficiency, sometimes referred to as *late-onset lactase deficiency*, is the most common type of lactose intolerance and occurs usually after 4 or 5 years of age, although the time of onset varies. Ethnic groups with a high incidence of lactase deficiency include Asians, southern Europeans, Arabs, Israelis, and Blacks; Scandinavians tend to have the lowest incidence. Lactose malabsorption manifests as lactose intolerance and is characterized by an imbalance between the ability for lactase to hydrolyze the ingested lactose and the amount of lactose ingested (Heyman & American Academy of Pediatrics Committee on Nutrition, 2006).

Secondary lactase deficiency may occur secondary to damage of the intestinal lumen, which decreases or destroys the enzyme lactase. Cystic fibrosis; sprue; celiac disease; kwashiorkor; or infections such as giardiasis, HIV, or rotavirus may cause temporary or permanent lactose intolerance.

Developmental lactase deficiency refers to the relative lactase deficiency observed in preterm infants of less than 34 weeks of gestation (Heyman & American Academy of Pediatrics Committee on Nutrition, 2006).

The primary symptoms of lactose intolerance include abdominal pain, bloating, flatulence, and diarrhea after the ingestion of lactose. The onset of symptoms occurs within 30 minutes to several hours of lactose consumption. Lactose intolerance is often perceived as an allergy. In several studies with reports of acute GI symptoms ascribed to lactose intolerance, measurement of lactase activity is normal (Goldberg, Folta, & Must, 2002).

Lactose intolerance may be diagnosed on the basis of the history and improvement with a lactose-reduced diet. The breath hydrogen test is used to positively diagnose the condition. Breath samples in lactose-deficient individuals yield a higher percentage of hydrogen (20 ppm [parts per million] or more above baseline). In infants, lactose malabsorption may be diagnosed by evaluating fecal pH and reducing substances; fecal pH in infants is usually lower than in older children, but an acidic pH may indicate malabsorption (Heyman & American Academy of Pediatrics Committee on Nutrition, 2006).

Treatment of lactose intolerance is elimination of offending dairy products; however, some advocate decreasing amounts of dairy products rather than total elimination, especially in small children (Heyman & American Academy of Pediatrics Committee on Nutrition, 2006; Goldberg et al., 2002). In infants, lactose-free or low-lactose formula offers no special advantages over lactose-containing formula, except in the severely malnourished (Heyman & American Academy of Pediatrics Committee on Nutrition, 2006).

One concern is that dairy avoidance in children and adolescents with lactose intolerance contributes to reduced bone mineral density and osteoporosis (Sibley, 2004). There is evidence that dietary lactose enhances calcium absorption and that lactose-free diets may negatively affect bone mineralization (Heyman & American Academy of Pediatrics Committee on Nutrition, 2006). It has been suggested that individuals with lactose maldigestion who do not experience lactose intolerance symptoms continue to consume small amounts of dairy products with meals to prevent reduced bone mass density and subsequent osteoporosis (Sibley, 2004). There is evidence that *probiotics* (food preparations containing microorganisms such as *Lactobacillus*, which alter the GI microflora and thus are beneficial to the host) improve lactose intolerance when live cultures are fermented in dairy products (Zeisel & Erickson, 2003). The positive attributes of probiotics for those with lactose maldigestion include delayed GI transit (slower than milk), positive effects on intestinal and colonic microflora, and a reduction of maldigestion symptoms (de Vrese et al., 2001).

Most people are able to tolerate small amounts of lactose even in the presence of deficient lactase activity (Heyman & American Academy of Pediatrics Committee on Nutrition, 2006; Goldberg et al., 2002) and should be encouraged to continue their intake of dairy products in small amounts to obtain much-needed nutrients. Milk taken at meals may be better tolerated than when taken alone (see Family-Centred Teaching box). Pretreated milk (with microbial-derived lactase) is reported to be effective in improving lactose absorption. Because dairy products are a major source of calcium and vitamin D, supplementation of these nutrients is needed to prevent deficiency. Yogourt contains inactive lactase enzyme, which is activated by the temperature and pH of the duodenum; this lactase activity substitutes for the lack of endogenous lactase. Fresh, plain yogourt may be tolerated better than frozen or flavoured yogourt; hard cheeses, lactase-treated dairy products, and lactase tablets taken with dairy products are also viable options. An important distinction between lactose intolerance and food hypersensitivity is that lactose intolerance does not manifest as an anaphylactic-type reaction.

Nursing Care Management

Nursing care is similar to the interventions discussed for CMA: explaining the dietary restrictions to the family; identifying alternate sources of calcium such as yogourt and calcium supplementation; explaining the importance of supplementation; and discussing sources of lactose, especially hidden sources such as its use as a bulk agent in certain medications, and ways of controlling the symptoms (see Family-Centred Teaching box). Parents should be advised to check with the pharmacist regarding this possibility when obtaining medication.

FAMILY-CENTRED TEACHING

Controlling Symptoms of Lactose Intolerance

- In infants, substitute soy-based formula for cow's milk formula or human milk.
- Limit milk consumption to one glass at a time.
- Drink milk with other foods rather than alone.
- Eat hard cheese, cottage cheese, or yogourt instead of drinking milk.
- Use enzyme tablets (Lactaid, Lactrase) to metabolize the lactose in milk or supplement the body's own lactose (add tablets to milk or sprinkle on dairy products such as ice cream).
- Eat small amounts of dairy foods daily to help colonic bacteria adapt to ingested lactose.

Gastrointestinal Dysfunction

The extensive surface area of the GI tract and its digestive function represent the major means of exchange between the human organism and the environment. Inflammatory and malabsorptive disorders impair the functional integrity of the GI tract. In addition, the infant's intestine is extremely vulnerable to infection. Acute infectious diarrhea causes significant alterations in fluid and electrolyte balance in both infants and children.

Numerous clinical observations provide clues to specific GI problems (Box 47-4). In any disorder that involves GI losses of large amounts of fluid, dehydration poses a serious threat to life and demands immediate attention.

Dehydration

Dehydration is a common body fluid disturbance in infants and children and occurs whenever the total output of fluid exceeds the total intake, regardless of the cause. Dehydration may result from a number of diseases that cause insensible losses through the skin and respiratory tract, through increased renal excretion, and through the GI tract. Although dehydration can result from lack of oral intake (especially in elevated environmental temperatures), more often it is a result of abnormal losses, such as those that occur in vomiting or diarrhea, when oral intake only partially compensates for the abnormal losses. Other significant causes of dehydration are diabetic ketoacidosis and extensive burns.

Water Balance in Infants

Compared with older children and adults, infants and young children have a greater need for water and are more vulnerable to alterations in fluid and electrolyte balance. Infants have a greater fluid intake and output relative to size. Water and electrolyte disturbances occur more frequently and more rapidly, and infants and children adjust less promptly to these alterations.

The fluid compartments in the infant vary significantly from those in the adult, primarily because of an expanded extracellular compartment. The **extracellular fluid** (ECF) compartment constitutes more than half the total body water at birth and has a greater relative content of extracellular sodium and chloride. The infant loses a large amount of fluid at birth and maintains a larger amount of ECF than the adult until about 2 years of age. This contributes to greater and more rapid water loss during this age period.

Fluid losses create compartment deficits that are reflected throughout the duration of dehydration. In general, approximately 60% of fluid lost is from the ECF, and the remaining 40% comes from the **intracellular fluid** (ICF). The amount of fluid lost from the ECF increases with acute illness and decreases with chronic loss.

Fluid losses vary with age and are divided into insensible, urinary, and fecal losses. Approximately two thirds of

evolve Critical Thinking—Hematemesis

BOX 47-4 Clinical Manifestations of Gastrointestinal Dysfunction in Children

Growth failure—Weight consistently below the third percentile, body mass index below the fifth percentile, or a decrease from established growth pattern

Spitting up or regurgitation—Passive transfer of gastric contents into the esophagus or mouth

Vomiting—Forceful ejection of gastric contents; involves a complex process under central nervous system control that causes salivation, pallor, sweating, and tachycardia; usually accompanied by nausea

Projectile vomiting—Vomiting accompanied by vigorous peristaltic waves and typically associated with pyloric stenosis or pylorospasm

Nausea—Unpleasant sensation vaguely referred to the throat or abdomen with an inclination to vomit

Constipation—Delay or difficulty with the passage of stools that is present for 2 weeks or longer; associated with symptoms that may include blood-streaked stools and abdominal discomfort

Encopresis—Involuntary overflow of incontinent stool causing soiling or incontinence secondary to fecal retention or impaction

Diarrhea—Increase in the number of stools with increased water content as a result of alterations of water and electrolyte transport by the gastrointestinal (GI) tract; may be acute or chronic

Hypoactive, hyperactive, or absent bowel sounds—Evidence of intestinal motility problems that may be caused by inflammation or obstruction

Abdominal distension—Protuberant contour of the abdomen that may be caused by delayed gastric emptying, accumulation of gas or stool, inflammation, or obstruction

Abdominal pain—Pain associated with the abdomen that may be localized or diffuse, acute or chronic; often caused by inflammation, obstruction, or hemorrhage

Gastrointestinal bleeding—May be from an upper or lower GI source and may be acute or chronic

- *Hematemesis*—Vomiting of bright red or denatured blood that results from bleeding in the upper GI tract or from swallowed blood from the nose or oropharynx
- *Hematochezia*—Passage of bright red blood per rectum, usually indicating lower GI tract bleeding
- *Melena*—Passage of dark-coloured, "tarry" stools resulting from denatured blood, suggesting upper GI tract bleeding or bleeding from the right colon

Jaundice—Yellow colouration of the skin and sclerae associated with liver dysfunction in infants and children over 2 months of age

Dysphagia—Difficulty swallowing caused by abnormalities in the neuromuscular function of the pharynx or upper esophageal sphincter or by disorders of the esophagus

Dysfunctional swallowing—Impaired swallowing caused by central nervous system defects or structural defects of the oral cavity, pharynx, or esophagus; can cause feeding problems or aspiration

Fever—Common manifestation of illness in children with GI disorders; usually associated with dehydration, infection, or inflammation

insensible losses occur through the skin; the remaining one third is lost through the respiratory tract. Heat and humidity, body temperature, and respiratory rate influence insensible fluid loss. Infants and children have a greater tendency to become highly febrile than do adults. Fever increases insensible water loss approximately 7 mL/kg/24 hr for each degree rise in temperature above 37.2°C. Fever and increased surface area relative to volume are factors that contribute to greater insensible fluid losses in young patients.

Body Surface Area

The infant's relatively greater body surface area (BSA) allows larger quantities of fluid to be lost in insensible losses through the immature skin. It is estimated that the BSA of the preterm neonate is five times greater, and that of the newborn is two to three times greater, than that of the older child or adult. The proportionately longer GI tract in infancy is another source of fluid loss, especially from diarrhea.

Basal Metabolic Rate

The rate of metabolism in infancy is significantly higher than in adulthood because of the larger BSA in relation to the mass of active tissue. Consequently, a greater production of metabolic wastes must be excreted by the kidneys. Any condition that increases metabolism causes greater heat production, insensible fluid loss, and an increased need for water for excretion. The basal metabolic rate in infants and children is higher to support growth and organ function.

Kidney Function

The kidneys of the infant are functionally immature at birth and inefficient in excreting waste products of metabolism. Of particular importance for fluid balance is the inability of the infant's kidneys to efficiently concentrate or dilute urine, conserve or excrete sodium, and acidify urine. The infant is less able to handle large quantities of solute-free water than is the older child, and infants are more likely to become dehydrated when given excessively concentrated commercial formulas or overhydrated when given excessive water or dilute formula.

Fluid Requirements

Infants ingest and excrete a greater amount of fluid per kilogram of body weight than older children. Because electrolytes are excreted with water and the infant has limited ability for conservation, maintenance requirements include both water and electrolytes. The daily exchange of ECF in the infant is greatly increased over that of older children, which leaves the infant little fluid volume reserve in dehydrated states. Fluid requirements depend on hydration status, size, environmental factors, and underlying disease. Box 47-5 lists daily maintenance fluid requirements for children.

Types of Dehydration

The pathophysiology of dehydration is understood by recognizing that the distribution of water between the ECF and ICF spaces depends on active transport of potassium into and sodium out of cells by energy-requiring processes. Sodium is the chief solute in ECF and the primary determinant of ECF volume. Potassium is primarily intracellular. When ECF volume is reduced in acute dehydration, the total body sodium content is almost always reduced as well, regardless of serum sodium measurements. Replacement of fluid volume should therefore be accompanied by sodium replacement as well.

BOX 47-5 Daily Maintenance Fluid Requirements

1. Calculate weight of child in kilograms.
2. Allow 100 mL/kg for first 10 kg.
3. Allow 50 mL/kg for second 10 kg.
4. Allow 20 mL/kg for remainder of weight in kilograms.
5. Divide total amount by 24 hours to obtain rate in millilitres per hour.

Sodium depletion in diarrhea occurs in two ways: out of the body in stool and into the ICF compartment to replace potassium to maintain electrical equilibrium.

Dehydration is classified into three categories on the basis of osmolality and depends primarily on the serum sodium concentration: (1) isotonic, (2) hypotonic, and (3) hypertonic.

Isotonic (*isosmotic* or **isonatremic**) **dehydration,** the primary form of dehydration in children, occurs in conditions in which electrolyte and water deficits are present in approximately balanced proportions. Water and salt are lost in approximately equal amounts. The observable fluid losses are not necessarily isotonic, since losses from other avenues make adjustments so that the sum of all losses, or the net loss, is isotonic. There is no osmotic force between the ICF and the ECF; thus the major loss is sustained from the ECF compartment. This significantly reduces the plasma volume and the circulating blood volume, which affects the skin, muscles, and kidneys. Shock is the greatest threat to life, and the child with isotonic dehydration displays symptoms characteristic of hypovolemic shock. Plasma sodium remains within normal limits, between 138 and 145 mmol/L.

Hypotonic (*hyposmotic* or **hyponatremic**) **dehydration** occurs when the electrolyte deficit exceeds the water deficit, leaving the serum hypotonic. Because ICF is more concentrated than ECF in hypotonic dehydration, water moves from the ECF to the ICF to establish osmotic equilibrium. This movement further increases the ECF volume loss, and shock is a frequent finding. Because there is a greater proportional loss of ECF in hypotonic dehydration, the physical signs tend to be more severe with smaller fluid losses than with isotonic or hypertonic dehydration. Serum sodium concentration is less than 130 mmol/L.

Hypertonic (*hyperosmotic* or **hypernatremic**) **dehydration** results from water loss in excess of electrolyte loss and is usually caused by a proportionately larger loss of water or a larger intake of electrolytes. This type of dehydration is the most dangerous and requires more specific fluid therapy. Hypertonic diarrhea may occur in infants who are given fluids by mouth that contain large amounts of solute or in children who receive high-protein nasogastric (NG) tube feedings that place an excessive solute load on the kidneys. In hypertonic dehydration, fluid shifts from the lesser concentration of the ICF to the ECF. Plasma sodium concentration is greater than 150 mmol/L.

Because the ECF volume is proportionately larger, hypertonic dehydration consists of a greater degree of water loss for the same intensity of physical signs. Shock is less apparent. However, neurological disturbances, including alterations in consciousness, poor ability to focus attention, lethargy, increased muscle tone with hyper-reflexia, and hyperirritability to stimuli, are more likely to occur. Cerebral changes are serious and may result in permanent damage.

Diagnostic Evaluation

Diagnosis of the type and degree of dehydration is necessary to develop an effective plan of therapy. The degree of dehydration has been described as a percentage of body weight dehydrated: mild—less than 3% in older children or less than 5% in infants; moderate—5 to 10% in infants and 3 to 6% in older children; and severe—more than 10% in infants and more than 6% in older children (CPS, 2006; Greenbaum, 2007). Water constitutes only 60 to 70% of the infant's weight. However, adipose tissue contains little water and is highly variable in individual infants and children. A more accurate means of describing dehydration is to reflect acute loss (over a period of 48 hours or less) in millilitres per kilogram of body weight. For example, a loss of 50 mL/kg is considered to be a mild fluid loss, whereas a loss of 100 mL/kg produces severe dehydration. Weight is the most important determinant of the percent of total body fluid loss in infants and younger children. However, often the preillness weight is unknown. Other predictors of fluid loss include a changing level of consciousness (irritability to lethargy), response to stimuli, decreased skin elasticity and turgor, prolonged capillary refill (longer than 2 seconds), increased heart rate, and sunken eyes and fontanels.

Clinical signs provide clues to the extent of dehydration (Table 47-3). Using multiple predictors increases the sensitivity of assessing the fluid deficit, and early studies have shown a reasonably high degree of agreement between experienced observers in assessment of the level of dehydration. Objective signs of dehydration are present at a fluid deficit of less than 5%. Any two of the following signs—capillary refill greater than 2 seconds, abnormal skin turgor, and abnormal respiratory pattern—are predictors of a deficit of at least 5%. Generally, three or more clinical findings are present at a deficit of 5 to 9%, and four or more findings are found with a deficit of 10% or more (Steiner et al., 2004). Shock, tachycardia, and very low blood pressure are common features of severe depletion of ECF volume (see Shock, Chapter 48).

Therapeutic Management

See discussion on therapeutic management of diarrhea, p. 1396.

Nursing Care Management

Nursing observation and intervention are essential for detection and therapeutic management of dehydration. A variety of circumstances cause fluid losses in infants, and changes can take place quickly. An important nursing responsibility is observation for signs of dehydration. Nursing assessment should begin with observation of general appearance and proceed to more specific observations. Conditions in which dehydration may develop quickly include diarrhea; vomiting; sweating; fever; disorders such as diabetes, renal disease, and cardiac anomalies; administration of certain medications (such as diuretics and steroids); and trauma (major surgery,

Table 47-3 Evaluating the Extent of Dehydration

	Level of Dehydration		
CLINICAL SIGNS	**MILD**	**MODERATE**	**SEVERE**
Weight loss—infants	3%–5%	6%–9%	≥10%
Weight loss—children	3%–4%	6%–8%	10%
Pulse	Normal	Slightly increased	Very increased
Respiratory rate	Normal	Slight tachypnea (rapid)	Hyperpnea (deep and rapid)
Blood pressure	Normal	Normal to orthostatic (>10 mm Hg change)	Orthostatic to shock
Behaviour	Normal	Irritable, more thirsty	Hyperirritable to lethargic
Thirst	Slight	Moderate	Intense
Mucous membranes*	Normal	Dry	Parched
Tears	Present	Decreased	Absent, sunken eyes
Anterior fontanel	Normal	Normal to sunken	Sunken
External jugular vein	Visible when supine	Not visible except with supraclavicular pressure	Not visible even with supraclavicular pressure
Skin*	Capillary refill >2 sec	Slowed capillary refill (2–4 sec [decreased turgor])	Very delayed capillary refill (>4 sec) and tenting; skin cool, acrocyanotic or mottled
Urine specific gravity	>1.020	>1.020; oliguria	Oliguria or anuria

(Data from Jospe, N., & Forbes, G. [1996]. Fluids and electrolytes—clinical aspects. *Pediatrics in Review, 17*[11], 395–403; and Steiner, M. J., DeWalt, D. A., & Byerley, J. S. [2004]. Is this child dehydrated? *Journal of the American Medical Association, 291*[22], 2746–2754.)
*These signs are less prominent in patients who have hypernatremia.

evolve Case Study—Acute Diarrhea (Gastroenteritus)

evolve Case Study—Dehydration and Diarrhea

burns, and other extensive injury). In addition, any condition that causes a decrease in oral intake such as herpangina, hand-foot-and-mouth disease, or thrush has the potential to cause dehydration in infants and small children.

Intake and Output

Accurate measurements of fluid intake and output are vital to the assessment of dehydration. This includes oral and parenteral intake and losses from urine, stools, vomiting, fistulas, NG losses, sweat, and wound drainage:

Urine—Frequency, colour, consistency, and volume (when weighing diapers, approximately 1 g wet diaper weight equals 1 mL urine)
Stools—Frequency, volume, and consistency
Vomitus—Volume, frequency, and type
Sweating—Can be only estimated from frequency of clothing and linen changes

In addition to fluid intake and output, the following observations assist in assessment of dehydration:

Vital signs—Temperature (normal, elevated, or lowered depending on degree of dehydration), pulse (tachycardia), respirations (hyperpnea), and blood pressure (hypotension)
Skin—Colour, temperature, turgor, presence or absence of edema, and capillary refill
Mucous membranes—Moisture, colour, and presence and consistency of secretions
Body weight—Decreased in relation to degree of dehydration
Fontanel (infants)—Sunken, soft, or normal
Sensory alterations—Presence of thirst

For nursing interventions, see discussion under specific disorders.

Disorders of Motility

Diarrhea

Diarrhea is a symptom that results from disorders involving digestive, absorptive, and secretory functions. It is caused by abnormal intestinal water and electrolyte transport. Worldwide there are an estimated 1.5 to 2.5 million deaths per year from diarrhea (CPS, 2006). Most children living in developing countries who develop diarrhea have mild forms. However, in the United States approximately 220,000 children younger than age 5 are hospitalized, with comparable rates in Canada (CPS, 2006). Prolonged diarrhea and malnutrition are primary causes of morbidity and mortality in First Nations, Métis, and Inuit populations (CPS, 2006).

Diarrheal disturbances involve the stomach and intestines (gastroenteritis), the small intestine (enteritis), the colon (colitis), or the colon and intestines (enterocolitis). Diarrhea is classified as acute or chronic.

Acute diarrhea, a leading cause of illness in children younger than 5 years of age, is defined as a sudden increase in frequency and a change in consistency of stools, often caused by an infectious agent in the GI tract. It may be associated with upper respiratory or urinary tract infections, antibiotic therapy, or laxative use. Acute diarrhea is usually self-limited (less than 14 days' duration) and subsides without specific treatment if dehydration does not occur. *Acute infectious diarrhea (infectious gastroenteritis)* is caused by a variety of viral, bacterial, and parasitic **pathogens** (Table 47-4).

Chronic diarrhea is defined as an increase in stool frequency and increased water content with a duration of more than 14 days. It is often caused by chronic conditions such as malabsorption syndromes, inflammatory bowel disease (IBD),

Table 47-4 Infectious Causes of Acute Diarrhea

ORGANISM	PATHOLOGY	CHARACTERISTICS	COMMENTS
Viral Agents			
Rotavirus Incubation: 48 hr Diagnosis: enzyme immunoassay (EIA) and latex agglutination assay	Fecal-oral transmission Seven groups (A-G): Most group A virus replicates in mature villus epithelial cells of small intestine; leads to (1) imbalance in ratio of intestinal fluid absorption to secretion and (2) malabsorption of complex carbohydrates	Mild to moderate fever Vomiting followed by the onset of watery stools Fever and vomiting generally abate in approximately 2 days, but diarrhea persists 5–7 days Adult contacts in household may develop symptomatic infection	Most common cause of diarrhea in children <5 yr of age Infants 6–12 mo are most vulnerable Peak occurrences in winter months; important cause of nosocomial infections Affects all ages; usually milder in children >3 yr of age; immune-compromised children at greater risk for complications Virus can live on toys and hard surfaces (sinks, countertops) Vaccine available for infants
Noroviruses (formerly Norwalk-like) Caliciviruses Incubation: 12–48 hr Diagnosis: EIA, reverse-transcriptase polymerase chain reaction (RT-PCR)	Fecal-oral; contaminated food or water Pathology similar to rotavirus Affects villus epithelial cells of small intestine Leads to (1) imbalance in ratio of intestinal fluid absorption to secretion and (2) malabsorption of complex carbohydrates	Abdominal cramps; nausea, vomiting, malaise, low-grade fever, watery diarrhea without blood; duration brief, 2–3 days; tends to resemble so-called food poisoning symptoms with nausea predominating	Affects all ages Multiple strains often named for the location of outbreak (e.g., Norwalk, Sapporo, Snow Mountain, Montgomery) Common in closed populations such as day care and cruise ships
Bacterial Agents			
Escherichia coli Incubation: 3–4 days Variable depending on strain Diagnosis: sorbitol MacConkey agar (SMAC agar) for blood but fecal leukocytes are absent or rare	Five *E. coli* strains produce diarrhea as a result of enterotoxin production, adherence, or invasion; these strains include enterotoxigenic-producing [ETEC], enteroaggregative [EAEC], Shiga toxin-producing [STEC], enteropathogenic [EPEC], and enteroinvasive [EIEC] *E. coli*	Watery diarrhea 1–2 days; then severe abdominal cramping and bloody diarrhea STEC can progress to hemolytic uremic syndrome (HUS) and postdiarrheal thrombotic thrombocytopenia (TTP); 50% require dialysis and 3%–5% die	Food-borne pathogen Traveller's diarrhea Highest incidence in summer Cause of nursery epidemics Symptomatic treatment Antibiotics may worsen course, but meta-analysis shows no harm or benefit from antibiotic therapy (AAP, Committee on Infectious Diseases, & Pickering, 2009) Antimotility agents and opioids should be avoided
Salmonella groups (Nontyphoidal; gram-negative rods, nonencapsulated, nonsporulating) Incubation 6–72 hr Diagnosis: gram-stained stool culture	Invasion of mucosa in the small and large intestine; edema of the lamina propria; focal acute inflammation with disruption of the mucosa and microabscesses	Nausea, vomiting, colicky abdominal pain, bloody diarrhea, fever; symptoms variable: mild to severe May have headache, cerebral manifestations (e.g., drowsiness, confusion, meningismus, seizures) Infants may be afebrile and nontoxic May result in life-threatening septicemia and meningitis Nausea and vomiting typically of short duration; diarrhea may persist as long as 2–3 wk Typically shed virus for average of 5 wk; cases reported up to 1 yr	Incidence highest in warm months: July to November Food-borne outbreaks common Usually transmitted person to person but may transmit via undercooked meats, poultry Poultry and poultry products cause about half the cases In children: pets (e.g., dogs, cats, hamsters, turtles) Communicable as long as organisms are excreted Antibiotics not recommended in uncomplicated cases Antimotility agents also not recommended—prolong transit time and carrier state Incidence decreasing over past 10 yr

Continued

Table 47-4 Infectious Causes of Acute Diarrhea—cont'd

ORGANISM	PATHOLOGY	CHARACTERISTICS	COMMENTS
Salmonella typhi Produces enteric fever–systemic syndrome Incubation usually 7-14 days but could be 3-30 days, depending on size of inoculum Diagnosis: positive blood cultures; also sometimes positive stool and urine Late stage: positive bone marrow culture	Bloodstream invasion; after ingestion, organism attaches to microvilli of ileal brush borders, and bacteria invade the intestinal epithelium via Peyer's patches; is then transported to intestinal lymph nodes and enters bloodstream via thoracic ducts, and circulating organisms reach reticuloendothelial cells causing bacteremia	Manifestations depend on age Abdominal pain; diarrhea; nausea, vomiting, high fever, lethargy Must be treated with antibiotics	Incidence is much lower in developed countries; Ingestion of food, water, or both contaminated with human feces is most common mode of transmission Congenital and intrapartum transmission can occur Three vaccines are available
Shigella species Gram-negative organisms Nonmotile Anaerobic bacilli Incubation: 1-7 days Diagnosis: stool culture Loaded with polymorphonuclear leukocytes	Enterotoxins: invade the epithelium with superficial mucosal ulcerations	Patients appear sick Symptoms begin with fever, fatigue, anorexia Crampy abdominal pain precedes watery or bloody diarrhea Symptoms usually subside in 5-10 days	Most cases in children younger than 9 yr with about one third of cases in children ages 1-4 wk Antibiotics shorten illness and lower mortality risk All patients are at risk for dehydration Acute symptoms may persist for 1 wk or more Antidiarrheal medications not recommended; may predispose to toxic megacolon
Yersinia enterocolitica Incubation period: dose dependent, 1-3 wk Diagnosis: stool culture serology; enzyme-linked immunosorbent assay (ELISA) Patients have leukocytosis; elevated sedimentation rate	Pathology is poorly understood; believe production of enterotoxin	Mucoid diarrhea, sometimes bloody; abdominal pain suggestive of appendicitis; fever, vomiting	Seen more frequently in winter months Transmitted by pets and food Antibiotics usually do not alter the clinical course in uncomplicated cases; they should be used in complicated infections and compromised hosts
Campylobacter jejuni and Campylobacter coli Microaerophilic, motile, gram-negative bacilli Incubation period: 1-7 days Ability to cause illness appears dose related Diagnosis by stool culture, sometimes in the blood Commonly found in gastrointestinal (GI) tract of wild or domestic animals	Not fully understood; possibly (1) adherence to intestinal mucosa by toxin; (2) invasion of the mucosa in the terminal ileum and colon; (3) translocation, in which the organisms penetrate the mucosa and replicate in the lamina propria	Fever, abdominal pain, diarrhea, can be bloody; vomiting Watery, profuse, foul-smelling diarrhea Clinically similar to Salmonella or Shigella Fecal-oral transmission	Most infections in humans relate to consumption of contaminated foods or water; undercooked meats, particularly chicken; unpasteurized milk Also acquired from contaminated household pets (e.g., dogs, cats, hamsters) Bimodal peaks in infants <1 yr and again at ages 15-29 mo Antibiotics do not prolong the carriage of bacteria and may eliminate organism more quickly Erythromycin and azithromycin are medications of choice (5-7 days) Antimotility agents not recommended and tend to prolong symptoms
Vibrio cholerae Gram-negative, motile, curved bacillus living in bodies of salt water Incubation period: 1-3 days Diagnosis by stool culture	Enters via oral route in contaminated food or water; if survives acid stomach environment, travels to the small intestine, adheres to mucosa, and produces toxin	Onset abrupt; vomiting, watery diarrhea without cramping or tenesmus Dehydration can occur quickly	More prevalent in developing countries Rehydration most important treatment Antibiotics can shorten diarrhea Despite continued efforts, still no vaccine

Table 47-4 Infectious Causes of Acute Diarrhea—cont'd

ORGANISM	PATHOLOGY	CHARACTERISTICS	COMMENTS
Clostridium difficile Gram-positive anaerobic bacillus Diagnosis by detecting *C. difficile* toxin in stool culture	Produces two important toxins (A and B) Toxin binds to enterocyte surface receptor, resulting in alteration of permeability, protein synthesis, and direct cytotoxicity	Most cases: mild, watery diarrhea lasting few days Some cases: prolonged diarrhea and illness May cause pseudomembranous colitis Some individuals are extremely ill with high fever, leukocytosis, hypoalbuminemia	Associated with alteration of normal intestinal flora by antibiotics More common in hospitalized persons Adults tend to have more severe symptoms than children Treatment with antibiotics in symptomatic patients—metronidazole Resistant strains have developed Relapse common
Clostridium perfringens Incubation period: 8–24 hr; anaerobic, gram-positive, spore-producing bacilli	Toxins produced in the intestine after ingestion of organism	Acute onset: watery diarrhea, crampy abdominal pain Fever, nausea, and vomiting rare Duration of illness usually 24 hr	Transmitted by contaminated food products, most often meats and poultry Usually self-limiting and medical intervention not needed Oral rehydration usually sufficient Antibiotics serve no purpose and should not be used
Clostridium botulinum Incubation period: 12–26 hr (range, 6 hr to 8 days) Gram-positive, anaerobic, spore-producing bacilli Blood and stool culture should be obtained and transmitted to special laboratory (usually provincial department) to detect toxin	Botulism caused by binding of toxin to the neuromuscular junction	Clinical presentation related to age and the strain of the botulism Abdominal pain, cramping, and diarrhea Other strains: respiratory compromise, central nervous system symptoms	Transmitted in contaminated food products Can be acquired via wound infection Treatment involves supportive care and neutralization of the toxin
Staphylococcus (food poisoning) Incubation period: generally short, 1–8 hr Gram-positive, nonmotile, aerobic, or facultative anaerobic bacteria Diagnosis by identifying organism in food, blood, pus, aspirate	Direct tissue invasion and production of toxin	Clinical presentation depends on site of entry In food poisoning: profuse diarrhea, nausea, and vomiting Low-grade fever and hypothermia may occur	GI illness transmitted in inadequately cooked or refrigerated foods Self-limiting in GI illness Symptomatic treatment Antibiotics not recommended

immunodeficiency, food allergy, lactose intolerance, or chronic nonspecific diarrhea, or it can be the result of inadequate management of acute diarrhea.

Intractable diarrhea of infancy is a syndrome that occurs in the first few months of life, persists for longer than 2 weeks with no recognized pathogens, and is refractory to treatment. The most common cause is acute infectious diarrhea that was not managed adequately.

Chronic nonspecific diarrhea (CNSD), also known as irritable colon or childhood and toddlers' diarrhea, is a common cause of chronic diarrhea in children 6 to 54 months of age. These children have loose stools, often with undigested food particles, and diarrhea greater than 2 weeks' duration. Children with CNSD grow normally and have no evidence of malnutrition, no blood in their stool, and no enteric infection. Dietary indiscretions and food sensitivities have been linked to chronic diarrhea. The excessive intake of juices and artificial sweeteners such as sorbitol, a substance found in many commercially prepared beverages and foods, may be a factor.

Etiology

Most pathogens that cause diarrhea are spread by the fecal–oral route through contaminated food or water or are spread from person to person where there is close contact (e.g., day care centres). Lack of clean water, crowding, poor hygiene, nutritional deficiency, and poor sanitation are major risk factors, especially for bacterial or parasitic pathogens. The increased frequency and severity of diarrheal disease in infants is also related to age-specific alterations in susceptibility to pathogens. For example, the **immune system** of infants has not been exposed to many pathogens and has not acquired protective antibodies; newborns do not have a well-developed GI mucosal barrier to many pathogens, thus increasing the predisposition to gastroenteritis. Worldwide, the most common causes of acute gastroenteritis are infectious agents, viruses, bacteria, and parasites. In developed nations, viruses, primarily rotavirus, cause 70 to 80% of infectious diarrhea.

Rotavirus is the most important cause of serious gastroenteritis among children and a significant hospital-acquired pathogen. Rotavirus disease is most severe in children 3 to 24 months of age. Children younger than 3 months of age have some protection from the disease because of maternally acquired antibodies. Milder disease occurs in breastfeeding infants.

Salmonella, Shigella, and *Campylobacter* organisms are the most frequently isolated bacterial pathogens. *Salmonella* has the highest occurrence in infants; *Giardia* and *Shigella* have the highest incidence among toddlers. *Shigella* infection is uncommon in Canada, accounting for less than 5% of diarrheal illnesses in infants and toddlers. *Campylobacter* infection has a bimodal presentation (highest in children younger than 12 months of age with a second rise in incidence at age 15 to 19 years). *Giardia* and *Cryptosporidium* organisms are parasites. *Cryptosporidium* infection is often associated with outbreaks in young children in day care centres. *Plesiomonas* and *Yersinia* are also parasites that are frequently responsible for causing diarrhea that lasts more than 10 days in a previously healthy adolescent.

Antibiotic administration is frequently associated with diarrhea because antibiotics alter the normal intestinal flora, resulting in an overgrowth of other bacteria such as *Clostridium difficile*. The Public Health Agency of Canada now identifies *C. difficile* as a reportable disease so that rates can be tracked. Antibiotic-associated diarrhea can also be caused by *Salmonella* organisms, *Clostridium porringers* type A, and *Staphylococcus aureus* pathogens (Jabbar & Wright, 2003).

Pathophysiology

Invasion of the GI tract by pathogens results in increased intestinal secretion as a result of enterotoxins, cytotoxic mediators, or decreased intestinal absorption secondary to intestinal damage or **inflammation**. Enteric pathogens attach to the mucosal cells and form a cuplike pedestal on which the bacteria rest. The pathogenesis of the diarrhea depends on whether the organism remains attached to the cell surface, resulting in a secretory toxin (noninvasive, toxin-producing, noninflammatory type diarrhea), or penetrates the mucosa (systemic diarrhea). Noninflammatory diarrhea is the most common diarrheal illness, resulting from the action of enterotoxin that is released after attachment to the mucosa (Ramaswamy & Jacobson, 2001). The most serious and immediate physiological disturbances associated with severe diarrheal disease are (1) dehydration, (2) acid–base imbalance with acidosis, and (3) shock that occurs when dehydration progresses to the point that circulatory status is seriously impaired.

Diagnostic Evaluation

Evaluation of the child with acute gastroenteritis begins with a careful history that seeks to discover the possible cause of diarrhea, assess the severity of symptoms and the risk of complications, and elicit information about current symptoms indicating other treatable illnesses that could be causing the diarrhea. The history should include questions about recent travel, exposure to untreated drinking or washing water sources, contact with animals or birds, day care centre attendance, recent treatment with antibiotics, or recent diet changes. History questions should also explore the presence or absence of other symptoms such as fever and vomiting, frequency and character of stools (e.g., watery, bloody), urinary output, dietary habits, and recent food intake.

Extensive laboratory evaluation is not indicated in children who have uncomplicated diarrhea and no evidence of dehydration because most diarrheal illnesses are self-limiting. Laboratory tests are indicated for children who are severely dehydrated and receiving intravenous (IV) therapy. Watery, explosive stools suggest glucose intolerance; foul-smelling, greasy, bulky stools suggest fat malabsorption. Diarrhea that develops after the introduction of cow's milk, fruits, or cereal may be related to enzyme deficiency or protein intolerance. Neutrophils or red blood cells in the stool indicate bacterial gastroenteritis or IBD. The presence of eosinophils suggests protein intolerance or parasitic infection. Stool cultures should be performed only when blood, mucus, or polymorphonuclear leukocytes are present in the stool; symptoms are severe; there is a history of travel to a developing country; and a specific pathogen is suspected. Gross blood or occult blood may indicate pathogens such as *Shigella, Campylobacter*, or hemorrhagic *Escherichia coli* strains. An enzyme-linked immunosorbent assay (ELISA) may be used to confirm the presence of rotavirus or *Giardia* organisms. If there is a history of recent antibiotic use, the stool should be tested for *C. difficile* toxin. When bacterial and viral cultures are negative and diarrhea persists for more than a few days, stools should be examined for ova and parasites. A stool specimen with a pH of less than 6 and the presence of reducing substances may indicate carbohydrate malabsorption or secondary lactase deficiency. Stool electrolyte measurements may help identify children with secretory diarrhea.

Urine specific gravity should be determined if dehydration is suspected. A complete blood count (CBC), serum electrolytes, creatinine, and blood urea nitrogen (BUN) should be obtained in the child who requires hospitalization. The hemoglobin, hematocrit, creatinine, and BUN levels are usually elevated in acute diarrhea and should normalize with rehydration.

Therapeutic Management

The major goals in the management of acute diarrhea include (1) assessment of fluid and electrolyte imbalance, (2) rehydration, (3) maintenance fluid therapy, and (4) reintroduction of an adequate diet. Infants and children with acute diarrhea and dehydration should be treated first with oral rehydration therapy (ORT). ORT is one of the major worldwide health care advances of the past few decades. It is more effective, safer, less painful, and less costly than IV rehydration. The World Health Organization and the Canadian Paediatric Society recommend ORT as the treatment of choice for most cases of dehydration caused by diarrhea (CPS, 2006). Oral rehydration solutions (ORSs) enhance and promote the reabsorption of sodium and water, and studies indicate that these solutions greatly reduce vomiting, volume loss from diarrhea, and the duration of the illness. ORSs, including reduced osmolarity ORS, are available in Canada as commercially prepared solutions and are successful in treating the majority of infants with dehydration (Fig. 47-2).

After rehydration, children should be placed on an age-appropriate diet (CPS, 2006). Ongoing stool losses should be

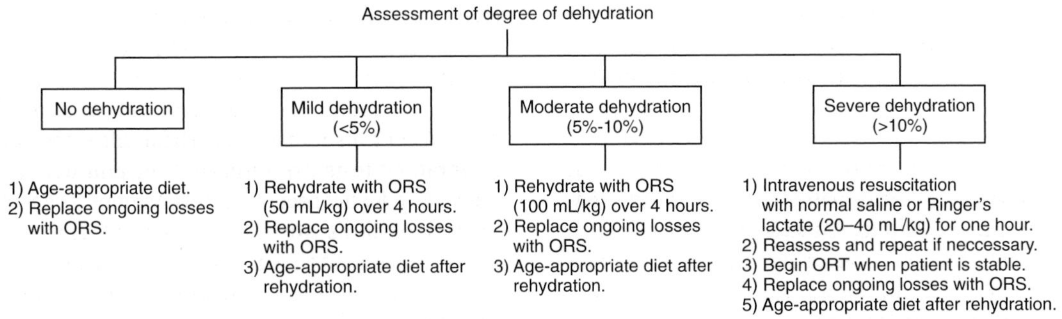

Fig. 47-2 Algorithm for managing acute gastroenteritis in children. *ORS*, oral rehydration solution; *ORT*, oral rehydration therapy. *(From Canadian Paediatric Society. [2006]. Oral rehydration therapy and early refeeding in the management of childhood gastroenteritis.* Journal of Paediatric and Child Health, *11[8], 529.)*

replaced on a 1:1 basis with ORS. If the stool volume is not known, approximately 10 mL/kg of ORS should be given for each diarrheal stool.

Solutions for oral hydration are useful in most cases of dehydration, and vomiting is not a contraindication. A child who is vomiting should be given an ORS at frequent intervals and in small amounts. For young children the caregiver may give the fluid with a spoon or small syringe in 5- to 10-mL increments every 1 to 5 minutes. An ORS may also be given via NG or gastrostomy tube infusion. Infants without clinical signs of dehydration do not need ORT. However, they should receive the same fluids recommended for infants with signs of dehydration in the maintenance phase and for ongoing stool losses. The use of probiotics reduces the risk of antibiotic-associated diarrhea in children by 56% (Szajewska, Ruszczynski, & Radzikowski, 2006). *Lactobacillus* GG, *Saccharomyces boulardii*, and *L. reuteri* have been shown to decrease the duration of watery diarrhea by 1 day, particularly diarrhea as a result of rotavirus (Guandalini, 2008).

Prevention

A human-bovine pentavalent rotavirus vaccine (RotaTeq) became available in 2006, and live-attenuated human rotavirus vaccine (Rotarix) was made available in 2008 for the prevention of rotavirus. Infants should receive three doses of RotaTeq oral vaccine at 2, 4, and 6 months of age. Two doses of Rotarix, given at 2 and 4 months of age, will induce protective immunity (see Immunizations, Chapter 36). The Canadian Pediatric Society (2010a, b) recommends that all babies be vaccinated and is lobbying the government to fund the medication.

NURSING ALERT

- Diarrhea is not managed by encouraging intake of clear fluids by mouth, such as fruit juices, carbonated soft drinks, and gelatin. These fluids usually have high carbohydrate content, very low electrolyte content, and high osmolality.
- Caffeinated soft drinks should be avoided because caffeine is a mild diuretic and may lead to increased loss of water and sodium.
- Chicken or beef broth is not given because it contains excessive sodium and inadequate carbohydrate.
- The BRATT diet (bananas, rice, applesauce, toast, and tea) is now contraindicated for the child and especially for the infant with acute diarrhea because this diet has little nutritional value (low in energy and protein), is high in carbohydrates, and is low in calories. Infants on breast milk should continue to breastfeed, even during the rehydration stage. Other children should start back on their age-appropriate diet as soon as they are rehydrated (CPS, 2006).

Early reintroduction of nutrients is desirable and is gaining more widespread acceptance. Continued feeding or early reintroduction of a normal diet has no adverse effects and actually lessens the severity and duration of the illness and improves weight gain when compared with the gradual reintroduction of foods (CPS, 2006). Infants who are breastfeeding should continue to do so, and ORS should be used to replace ongoing losses in these infants. Formula-fed infants should resume their formula; formula should not be diluted or mixed with additional water. In older children a regular diet, including milk, can generally be offered after rehydration has been achieved. In toddlers there is no contraindication to continuing soft or pureed foods. A diet of easily digestible foods such as cereals, cooked vegetables, and meats is adequate for the older child.

In cases of severe dehydration and shock, IV fluids are initiated whenever the child is unable to ingest sufficient amounts of fluid and electrolytes to (1) meet ongoing daily physiological losses, (2) replace previous deficits, and (3) replace ongoing abnormal losses. Patients who usually require IV fluids are those with severe dehydration, those with uncontrollable vomiting, those who are unable to drink for any reason (e.g., extreme fatigue, coma), and those with severe gastric distension.

The IV solution is selected on the basis of what is known about the probable type and cause of the dehydration—normal saline solution or lactated Ringer's is used to replace volume, after which a saline solution containing 5% dextrose in ¼ normal saline with potassium chloride (20 mmol/L) may be administered as maintenance therapy. Sodium bicarbonate may be added, since acidosis is usually associated with severe dehydration. Although the initial phase of fluid replacement is rapid in both isotonic and hypotonic dehydration, rapid replacement is contraindicated in hypertonic dehydration because of the risk of water intoxication, especially in the brain cells.

After the severe effects of dehydration are under control, specific diagnostic and therapeutic measures are begun to detect and treat the cause of the diarrhea. Because of the self-limiting nature of vomiting and its tendency to improve when dehydration is corrected, anti-emetic agents are often not administered. Ondansetron may be administered to decrease vomiting and increase the effectiveness of oral hydration, thus potentially avoiding IV therapy and hospitalization admissions in children with mild to moderate dehydration (Roslund, Hepps, & McQuillen, 2008). Antidiarrheal medications are not recommended for children. The use of antibiotic therapy in children with acute gastroenteritis is controversial. Antibiotics may shorten the course of some diarrheal illnesses (e.g., those caused by *Shigella* organisms). However, most bacterial diarrheas are self-limiting, and the diarrhea often resolves before the causative organism can be determined. Antibiotics may prolong the carrier period for bacteria such as *Salmonella*. However, antibiotics may be considered in patients with **immunosuppression**, severe symptoms, or persistent disease or in patients who have had transplantation (Jabbar & Wright, 2003).

Nursing Care Management

The management of most cases of acute diarrhea takes place in the home with education of the caregiver. Caregivers are taught to monitor for signs of dehydration (especially the number of wet diapers or voidings) and the amount of fluids taken by mouth and to assess the frequency and amount of stool losses. Education relating to ORT, including the administration of maintenance fluids and replacement of ongoing losses, is important (see Critical Thinking Exercise). ORS should be administered in small quantities at frequent intervals. Vomiting is not a contraindication to ORT unless it is severe. Information about the introduction of a regular diet is essential. Parents need to know that a slightly higher stool output initially occurs with continuation of a normal diet and with ongoing replacement of stool losses. The benefits of a better nutritional outcome with fewer complications and a shorter duration of illness outweigh the potential increase in stool frequency. Parents' concerns should be addressed to ensure compliance with the treatment plan.

If the child with acute diarrhea and dehydration is hospitalized, an accurate weight must be obtained, and intake and output must be carefully monitored. The child may be placed on parenteral fluid therapy with reinstitution of oral fluids and soft foods; keeping the child with gastroenteritis NPO for a long period is usually avoided to prevent changes in intestinal permeability as a result of infection (Centers for Disease Control and Prevention, 2003). Monitoring the IV infusion is an important nursing function. The nurse must ensure that the correct fluid and electrolyte concentration is infused, the flow rate is adjusted to deliver the desired volume in a given time, and the IV site is maintained.

Accurate measurement of output is essential to determine whether renal blood flow is sufficient to permit the addition of potassium to the IV fluids. The nurse is responsible for examination of stools and collection of specimens for laboratory examination (see Collection of Specimens, Chapter 45). Care should be taken when obtaining and transporting stools to prevent possible spread of infection. A clean tongue depressor can be used to obtain specimens for laboratory examination or as an applicator for transfer to a culture medium. Stool specimens should be transported to the laboratory in appropriate containers and media according to hospital policy.

Diarrheal stools are highly irritating to the skin, and extra care is needed to protect the skin of the perianal and perineal region from excoriation (see Diaper Dermatitis, Chapter 53). Rectal temperatures are avoided because they stimulate the bowel, increasing passage of stool.

Support for the child and family involves the same care and consideration given all hospitalized children (see Chapter 44). Parents need to be kept informed of the child's progress and instructed in the use of frequent and proper **hand hygiene** and the disposal of soiled diapers, clothes, and bed linen. If *C. difficile* is the infecting agent, hands must be washed with soap and water and not alcohol-based cleanser. Everyone caring for the child must be aware of "clean" areas and "dirty" areas, especially in the hospital, where the sink in the child's room

CRITICAL THINKING EXERCISE

Diarrhea

A mother brings her 8-month-old infant, Mary, to the primary care clinic. The mother reports that Mary has had a "cold" for about 2 days and this morning she began to vomit and has had diarrhea for the past 8 hours. The mother states that Mary is still breastfeeding but that she is not taking as much fluid as usual and she is having three times as many stools as usual (the stools are watery in consistency). When the nurse practitioner examines Mary, she notes that her temperature is 38.0°C, her pulse and blood pressure are in the normal range, her mucous membranes are moist, and she has tears when she cries. The nurse practitioner also notes that Mary's weight has not changed from when she was seen in the clinic 2 weeks ago for her well-child visit. What interventions should the nurse practitioner include in her initial management of Mary?

1. Evidence—Is there sufficient evidence for the nurse practitioner to draw any conclusions for the initial plan of management?
2. Assumptions—Describe some underlying assumptions about the following:
   a. Clinical manifestations of various levels of dehydration
   b. Management of acute diarrhea
   c. Breastfeeding and the management of acute diarrhea
   d. Use of antidiarrheal medications for acute diarrhea in children
3. What nursing interventions should the nurse practitioner implement at this time?
4. Does the evidence support the nurse practitioner's conclusion?
5. Are there any alternative perspectives that the nurse practitioner should consider?

is used for many purposes. Soiled diapers and linen should be discarded in receptacles close to the bedside. To remind caregivers to keep diapers and other soiled articles away from clean areas, signs can be placed identifying "clean" (e.g., bed table) and "dirty" (e.g., sink, bathroom) areas. The articles that may be stored in each area should be listed on these signs.

Prevention

The best intervention for diarrhea is prevention. The fecal–oral route spreads most infections, and parents need information about preventive measures such as personal hygiene, protection of the water supply from contamination, and careful food preparation.

To reduce the risk of bacteria transmitted via food, parents should be encouraged to do the following (Public Health Agency of Canada [PHAC], 2011):

- **Clean:** Wash hands, utensils, and work areas with hot, soapy water after contact with raw meat to keep bacteria from spreading; wash raw fruits and vegetables with clean, running water before eating.
- **Chill:** Keep cold food cold at or below 4°C; thaw food in the refrigerator; never thaw food on the counter or let it sit out of the refrigerator for more than 2 hours.
- **Separate:** Use one cutting board for raw meat, poultry, and seafood and use a different cutting board for food that is ready-to-eat or cooked; keep raw food away from other food while shopping, and while storing, preparing, and serving foods; place raw meat, poultry and seafood in containers on the bottom shelf of the refrigerator.
- **Cook:** Check ground meat with a fork to make certain no pink is showing before taking a bite; cook all dishes made with ground meat until brown or grey inside or to an internal temperature of 71°C.

Meticulous attention to perianal hygiene, disposal of soiled diapers, proper handwashing, and isolation of infected persons also minimizes the transmission of infection (see Infection Control, Chapter 45).

Parents need information about preventing diarrhea while travelling. They should be cautioned against giving their children adult medications that are used to prevent traveller's diarrhea. Until vaccines or other prophylactic measures are proven to be safe for children, the best measure during travel to areas where water may be contaminated is to allow children to drink only bottled water and carbonated beverages (from the container through a straw supplied from home). Tap water, ice, unpasteurized dairy products, raw vegetables, unpeeled fruits, meats, and seafood should also be avoided. Hand hygiene is an important measure in the prevention of diarrheal disease, particularly in small children with increased hand-to-mouth activity.

The expected outcomes for the child with diarrhea are described in the Nursing Process box.

evolve Critical Thinking Exercise—Constipation

Constipation

Constipation is an alteration in the frequency, consistency, or ease of passing stool. Parents often define constipation as passing less than three stools per week. It may also be defined

NURSING PROCESS: THE CHILD WITH DIARRHEA

Assessment

Observe the infant or child's general appearance and behaviour. Assess for dehydration, such as decreased urinary output; decreased weight; dry mucous membranes; poor skin turgor; sunken fontanel; and pale, cool, dry skin. With severe dehydration, increased pulse and respiration, decreased blood pressure, and a prolonged capillary refill time (longer than 2 seconds) may indicate impending shock (see Table 47-3).

A history provides information about probable etiological agents, such as introduction of a new food, exposure to infectious agents, travel to an area of high susceptibility, contact with foods that might have been contaminated, and contact with pets known to be sources of enteric infections. An allergy, medication, and dietary history may indicate food allergies, use of laxatives or antibiotics, or sources of excess sorbitol and fructose (e.g., apple juice).

Nursing Diagnoses (Problem Identification)

After a thorough assessment, several nursing diagnoses are evident:

Deficient fluid volume related to
– diarrhea (gastrointestinal) losses
– inadequate intake

Risk for infection related to
– microorganisms invading gastrointestinal tract

Impaired skin integrity related to
– irritation caused by frequent loose stools

Planning

Expected patient outcomes include:

- Infant or child will maintain adequate hydration.
- Infant or child will maintain appropriate nutrition for age.
- Infant or child will not spread infection (if etiological agent) to others.
- Family will receive appropriate support and education, especially regarding home care.

Implementation

Numerous intervention strategies are discussed on pp. 1397–1399.

Evaluation

The effectiveness of nursing interventions for the family and the child with diarrhea is determined by continual assessment and evaluation of care based on the following guidelines:

- Monitor fluid losses with careful intake and output measurements and daily weights.
- Monitor food intake, especially calories.
- Observe for evidence of complications from underlying disease (specify) or therapy.
- Observe and interview family to determine extent and effectiveness of care.

as painful bowel movements, which are often blood streaked or include the retention of stool, with or without soiling, even with a stool frequency of more than three stools per week (Loening-Baucke & Pashankar, 2006). However, the frequency of bowel movements is not considered a diagnostic criterion because it varies widely among children. Having extremely long intervals between defecation is termed *obstipation*. Constipation with fecal soiling is referred to as *encopresis*.

Constipation may arise secondary to a variety of organic disorders or in association with a wide range of systemic disorders. Structural disorders of the intestine, such as strictures, ectopic anus, and Hirschsprung disease (HD), may be associated with constipation. Systemic disorders associated with constipation include hypothyroidism, hypercalcemia resulting from hyperparathyroidism or vitamin D excess, and chronic lead poisoning. Constipation may be associated with medications such as antacids, diuretics, anti-epileptics, antihistamines, opioids, and iron supplementation. Spinal cord lesions may be associated with loss of rectal tone and sensation. Affected children are prone to chronic fecal retention and overflow incontinence.

The majority of children have **idiopathic** or *functional constipation* since no underlying cause can be identified. Chronic constipation may occur as a result of environmental or psychosocial factors or a combination of the two. Transient illness, withholding and avoidance secondary to painful or negative experiences with stooling, and dietary intake with decreased fluid and fibre all play a role in the etiology of constipation.

Newborn Period

Normally the newborn infant passes a first meconium stool within 24 to 36 hours of birth. Any infant who does not do so should be assessed for evidence of intestinal atresia or stenosis, HD, hypothyroidism, meconium plugs, or meconium ileus. *Meconium plugs* are caused by meconium that has reduced water content and are usually evacuated after digital examination but may require irrigation with a hypertonic solution or contrast medium.

Meconium ileus, the initial manifestation of cystic fibrosis, is the luminal obstruction of the distal small intestine by abnormal meconium. Treatment is the same as for a meconium plug; early surgical intervention may be needed to evacuate the small intestine.

Infancy

The onset of constipation frequently occurs during infancy and may result from organic causes such as HD, hypothyroidism, and strictures. It is important to differentiate these conditions from functional constipation. Constipation in infancy is often related to dietary practices. It is less common in breastfed infants, who have softer stools than bottle-fed infants. Breastfed infants may also have decreased stools because of more complete use of breast milk with little residue. When constipation occurs with a change from human milk or modified cow's milk to whole cow's milk, simple measures, such as adding or increasing the amount of cereal, vegetables, and fruit in the infant's diet, usually correct the problem. When a bottle-fed infant passes a hard stool that results in an anal fissure, stool-withholding behaviours may develop in response to pain on defecation (see Critical Thinking Exercise).

> **CRITICAL THINKING EXERCISE**
>
> **Constipation**
>
> Jung, an 8-month-old infant, is seen by the pediatric nurse practitioner for his well-child visit. Jung's mother states that he usually has one hard stool every 4 to 5 days, which causes discomfort when the stool is passed. He has also had one episode of diarrhea and two episodes of ribbonlike stools. Abdominal distension and vomiting have not accompanied the constipation, and Jung's growth has been appropriate. Currently his diet consists of cow's milk formula only. Jung's mother reports that the infrequent passage of hard stools began approximately 6 weeks ago when she stopped breastfeeding. Which interventions should the nurse practitioner include in the initial management of Jung's problem?
>
> 1. Evidence—Is there sufficient evidence for the nurse practitioner to draw any conclusions about the management of Jung's problem?
> 2. Assumptions—Describe some underlying assumptions about the following:
>   a. Causes of constipation in infants
>   b. Factors associated with functional constipation in infants
>   c. Management of functional constipation in infants
> 3. What interventions should the nurse practitioner implement at this time?
> 4. Does the evidence support these interventions?
> 5. Are there alternative perspectives that the nurse practitioner should consider? What are they?

Childhood

Most constipation in early childhood is the result of environmental changes or normal development when a child begins to attain control over bodily functions. A child who has experienced discomfort during bowel movements may deliberately try to withhold stool. Over time, the rectum accommodates to the accumulation of stool, and the urge to defecate passes. When the bowel contents are ultimately evacuated, the accumulated feces are passed with pain, thus reinforcing the desire to withhold stool.

Constipation in school-age children may represent an ongoing problem or a first-time event. The onset of constipation at this age is often the result of environmental changes, stresses, and changes in toileting patterns. A common cause of new-onset constipation at school entry is fear of using the school bathrooms, which are noted for their lack of privacy. Early and hurried departure for school immediately after breakfast may also impede bathroom use.

The management of simple constipation consists of a plan to promote regular bowel movements. Often this is as simple as changing the diet to provide more fibre and fluids, eliminating foods known to be constipating, and establishing a bowel routine that allows for regular passage of stool. Stool-softening agents such as docusate or lactulose may also be helpful. Polyethylene glycol (PEG) 3350 without electrolytes is a chemically inert polymer that has been introduced as a new laxative in recent years. It is tolerated well by children because it can be mixed in a beverage of choice (Loening-Baucke & Pashankar, 2006). If other symptoms such as vomiting, abdominal distension, or pain and evidence of growth failure are associated with the constipation, the condition should be investigated further.

Nursing Care Management

Constipation tends to be self-perpetuating. A child who has difficulty or discomfort when attempting to evacuate the bowels has a tendency to retain the bowel contents, and this may initiate a vicious cycle. Nursing assessment begins with an accurate history of bowel habits; diet; events associated with the onset of constipation; medications or other substances that the child may be taking; and the consistency, colour, frequency, and other characteristics of the stool. If there is no evidence of a pathological condition, the major tasks are to educate the parents regarding normal stool patterns and to participate in the education and treatment of the child.

Dietary modifications are essential in preventing constipation. During infancy, simply increasing the carbohydrate (dark corn syrup) in the infant's formula often relieves the problem. During childhood the diet should contain increased amounts of fibre and fluid. Parents benefit from guidance in selecting foods that facilitate bowel movements (Box 47-6). They need reassurance concerning the benign nature of the condition. It is also important to discuss their attitudes and expectations regarding toilet habits.

When constipation persists despite dietary intervention, more aggressive management may be necessary. It is important to differentiate an acute episode of constipation from chronic functional constipation, which can result from chronic stool-withholding behaviour. As the rectal vault becomes distended over time, further complications such as fecal impaction and encopresis may develop (see Chapter 39).

BOX 47-6 High-Fibre Foods

Bread, Grains
- Whole-grain bread or rolls
- Whole-grain cereals
- Bran
- Unrefined (brown) rice

Vegetables
- Raw vegetables, especially broccoli, cabbage, carrots, cauliflower, celery, lettuce, and spinach
- Cooked vegetables, such as those listed previously and asparagus, beans, Brussels sprouts, corn, potatoes, rhubarb, squash, string beans, and turnips

Fruits
- Raw fruits, especially those with skins or seeds, other than ripe banana or avocado
- Raisins, prunes, or other dried fruits

Miscellaneous
- Nuts, seeds, legumes, popcorn
- High-fibre snack bars

Hirschsprung Disease

HD (congenital aganglionic megacolon) is a mechanical obstruction caused by inadequate motility of part of the intestine. It accounts for about one fourth of all cases of neonatal obstruction, although it may not be diagnosed until later in infancy or childhood. The incidence is 1 in 5000 live births (Wyllie, 2007). It is four times more common in males than in females and may follow a familial pattern in about 10% of cases. HD is usually an isolated **birth defect**, but it has been associated with other syndromes, including Down syndrome. Depending on its presentation, it may be an acute, life-threatening, or chronic condition.

Pathophysiology

HD is a developmental disorder of the enteric nervous system that is characterized by the absence of ganglion cells, originating from the neural crest in both the Auerbach myenteric and Meissner submucosal plexuses of the distal intestine. The length of the aganglionic distal bowel depends on the timing of the arrest in craniocaudal migration of ganglion cells. The aganglionic bowel is chronically contracted. This results in absent peristalsis in the affected bowel and the development of a functional intestinal obstruction (Fig. 47-3) (Dasgupta & Langer, 2004). Intestinal distension and ischemia may also occur as a result of distension of the bowel wall, which contributes to the development of *enterocolitis* (inflammation of the small bowel and colon). Enterocolitis is characterized by fever, abdominal distension, and diarrhea that may be severe and lead to life-threatening dehydration or sepsis (Dasgupta & Langer, 2004).

Diagnostic Evaluation

Most children with HD are diagnosed in the first few months of life. Clinical manifestations vary according to the age when symptoms are recognized and the presence of complications such as enterocolitis (Box 47-7). A neonate usually is seen with distended abdomen, feeding intolerance with bilious vomiting, and delay in the passage of meconium. Typically, 95% of normal-term infants pass meconium in the first 24 hours of life, whereas fewer than 10% of infants with HD do so. In older

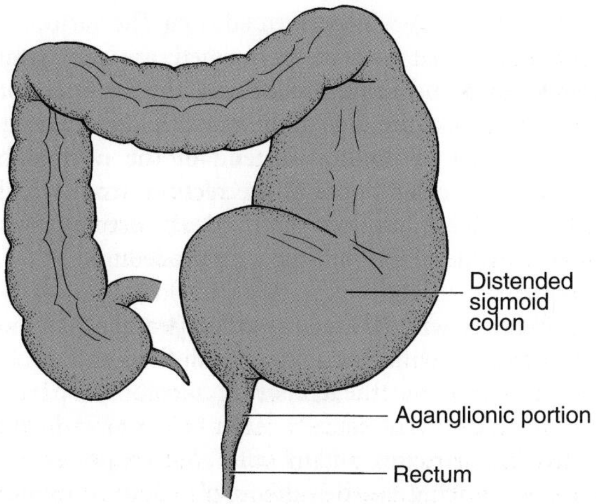

Fig. 47-3 Hirschsprung disease.

BOX 47-7 Clinical Manifestations of Hirschsprung Disease

Newborn Period
- Failure to pass meconium within 24 to 48 hours after birth
- Refusal to feed
- Bilious vomiting
- Abdominal distension

Infancy
- Growth failure
- Constipation
- Abdominal distension
- Episodes of diarrhea and vomiting
- Signs of enterocolitis
- Explosive, watery diarrhea
- Fever
- Appears significantly ill

Childhood (Symptoms Appear More Chronic)
- Constipation
- Ribbonlike, foul-smelling stools
- Abdominal distension
- Visible peristalsis
- Easily palpable fecal mass
- Undernourished, anemic appearance

children a careful history is helpful. Radiographs, an unprepped barium enema, and anorectal manometric examinations assist in the differential diagnosis, which is confirmed by a full-thickness rectal biopsy demonstrating the absence of ganglion cells in the myenteric and submucosal plexuses.

Therapeutic Management

Treatment is primarily surgery to remove the aganglionic portion of the bowel to relieve obstruction and restore normal bowel motility and function of the internal anal sphincter. If the bowel is not significantly distended, this is accomplished in one surgery. However, in most cases two stages are required. First, a temporary ostomy is created proximal to the aganglionic segment to relieve obstruction and allow the normally enervated and dilated bowel to return to its normal size. Complete corrective surgery is performed later. The various surgical procedures that can be performed are the Swenson, Duhamel, Boley, and Soave procedures. The Soave endorectal pull-through procedure, one of the most frequently used procedures, consists of pulling the end of the normal bowel through the muscular sleeve of the rectum, from which the aganglionic mucosa has been removed. The ostomy is usually closed at the time of the pull-through procedure.

Prognosis

Most children with HD require surgery rather than medical therapy. Once the child is stabilized with fluid and electrolyte replacement, if needed, the temporary colostomy is performed and has a high rate of success. After the later pull-through procedure, anal stricture and incontinence are potential complications, requiring further therapy, including dilation or bowel-retraining therapy.

Nursing Care Management

The nursing concerns depend on the child's age and the type of treatment. If the disorder is diagnosed during the neonatal period, the main objectives are to (1) help the parents adjust to a congenital defect in their child, (2) foster infant–parent bonding, (3) prepare them for the medical-surgical intervention, and (4) assist them in colostomy care after discharge.

Preoperative Care

The child's preoperative care depends on the age and clinical condition. A child who is malnourished may not be able to withstand surgery until his or her physical status improves. Often this involves symptomatic treatment with enemas; a low-fibre, high-calorie, and high-protein diet; and, in severe situations, the use of total **parenteral nutrition** (TPN).

Physical preoperative preparation includes the same measures that are common to any surgery (see Surgical Procedures, Chapter 45). In the newborn, whose bowel is sterile, no additional preparation is necessary. However, in other children, preparation for the pull-through procedure involves emptying the bowel with repeated saline enemas and decreasing bacterial flora with oral or systemic antibiotics and colonic irrigations using antibiotic solution. Enterocolitis is the most serious complication of HD. Emergency preoperative care includes frequent monitoring of vital signs and blood pressure for signs of shock; monitoring fluid and electrolyte replacements and plasma or other blood derivatives; and observing for symptoms of bowel perforation, such as fever, increasing abdominal distension, vomiting, increased tenderness, irritability, dyspnea, and cyanosis.

Because progressive distension of the abdomen is a serious sign, the nurse measures abdominal circumference with a paper tape measure, usually at the level of the umbilicus or at the widest part of the abdomen. The point of measurement is marked with a pen to ensure reliability of subsequent measurements. Abdominal measurement can be obtained with the vital sign measurements and is recorded in serial order so that any change is obvious. To reduce stress to the acutely ill child when frequent measurements of abdominal circumference are needed, the tape measure can be left in place beneath the child rather than removed each time.

The child's age dictates the type and extent of psychological preparation. Because a colostomy is usually performed, the child who is of preschool age is told about the procedure in concrete terms with the use of visual aids (see Chapter 44). It is important to time explanations appropriately to prevent the anxiety and confusion that could result from too much information. It is also important to stress to parents and older children that the colostomy for HD is temporary, unless so much bowel is involved that a permanent ileostomy must be performed. In most instances the extent of bowel resection is known before surgery, although the nurse should be aware of cases when doubt exists concerning repair. The nurse should remember that, although a temporary colostomy is favourable in terms of future health and adjustment, it requires additional surgery, which may be stressful to parents and children.

Postoperative Care

Postoperative care is the same as that for any child or infant with abdominal surgery (see Surgical Procedures, Chapter 45). When a colostomy is part of the corrective procedure, stomal care is a major nursing task (see Ostomies, Chapter 45). To prevent contamination of an infant's abdominal wound with urine, the diaper should be pinned below the dressing. Sometimes a Foley catheter is used in the immediate postoperative period to divert the flow of urine away from the abdomen.

Discharge Care

After surgery, parents need instruction concerning colostomy care. Even a preschooler can be included in the care by handing articles to the parent, rolling up the colostomy pouch after it is emptied, or applying barrier preparations to the surrounding skin. Although the diagnosis of HD is less frequent in school-age children or adolescents, children this age can often be involved in colostomy care to the point of total responsibility.

Some institutions and communities have enterostomal therapists who provide expert assistance in planning home care. If families require financial assistance and psychological support, referral to a social worker, home health care agency, or community health nurse can provide continuity of care.

Vomiting

Vomiting is the forceful ejection of gastric contents through the mouth. It is a well-defined, complex, coordinated process that is under central nervous system control and is often accompanied by nausea and retching. Vomiting may be divided into two categories: nonbilious and bilious. Some small intestinal reflux is common in all vomiting. In *nonbilious vomiting*, the majority of bile drains into the more distal portions of the intestine. If an obstruction is present, nonbilious vomiting suggests a more proximal obstruction. *Bilious vomiting* implies a disorder of motility or distal physical blockage. Causes of nonbilious vomiting include infectious, inflammatory, metabolic or endocrinological, neurological, and psychological causes and obstructive lesions. Causes of bilious vomiting include intestinal atresia and stenosis, malrotation with or without volvulus, ileus, intussusceptions, intestinal duplication, mass lesions, incarcerated inguinal hernia, and appendicitis.

Vomiting may also be associated with other processes, including acute infectious diseases, increased intracranial pressure, toxic ingestions, food intolerances and allergies, mechanical obstruction of the GI tract, metabolic disorders, and psychogenic problems. It is common in childhood, is usually self-limiting, and requires no specific treatment. However, complications may occur, including dehydration and electrolyte disturbances, malnutrition, aspiration, and Mallory-Weiss syndrome (small tears in the distal esophageal mucosa).

Therapeutic Management

Management is directed toward detection and treatment of the cause of the vomiting and prevention of complications from the loss of fluid. Fluids are administered in the same manner as and in a similar electrolyte composition to those administered for diarrhea. Although most children respond to these measures, anti-emetic medications may be needed. Antiemetics such as ondansetron (Zofran) and trimethobenzamide (Tigan) block receptors in the chemoreceptor trigger zone; others such as metoclopramide (Reglan) enhance gastroduodenal peristalsis; still others such as promethazine (Phenergan) compete for H_1-receptor sites. For children who are prone to motion sickness, it is helpful to administer an appropriate dose of dimenhydrinate (Gravol) before a trip.

Nursing Care Management

The major focus of nursing care is observing and reporting vomiting behaviour and associated symptoms and implementing measures to reduce the vomiting. Accurate assessment of the type of vomiting, the appearance of the vomitus, and the child's behaviour in association with the vomiting helps to establish a diagnosis.

Nursing interventions are determined by the cause of the vomiting. When the vomiting is a manifestation of improper feeding methods, establishing proper techniques through teaching and example usually corrects the situation. If vomiting is believed to be an indication of obstruction, food is usually withheld, or special feeding techniques are implemented. In situations in which vomiting is related to concurrent infection, dietary indiscretion, or emotional factors, efforts are directed toward maintaining hydration or preventing dehydration.

The thirst mechanism is the most sensitive guide to fluid needs, and ad libitum administration of a glucose-electrolyte solution to an alert child restores water and electrolytes satisfactorily. It is important to include carbohydrate to spare body protein and avoid ketosis resulting from exhaustion of glycogen stores. Small, frequent feedings of fluids or foods are preferred. After vomiting has stopped, more liberal amounts of fluids are offered, followed by gradual resumption of the regular diet.

The vomiting infant or child should be positioned on the side or semireclining to prevent aspiration and observed for evidence of dehydration. It is important to emphasize the need for the child to brush the teeth or rinse the mouth after vomiting to dilute hydrochloric acid that comes in contact with the teeth. A flavoured mouthwash or tooth brushing can freshen the mouth. Careful monitoring of fluid and electrolyte status is necessary to prevent an electrolyte disturbance.

Gastroesophageal Reflux

Gastroesophageal reflux (GER) is defined as the transfer of gastric contents into the esophagus. This phenomenon is physiological, occurring throughout the day, most frequently after meals and at night. It is important to differentiate GER from *gastroesophageal reflux disease (GERD)*, which represents symptoms or tissue damage that results from GER. Approximately 50% of infants younger than 2 months old are reported to have GER (Suwandhi, Ton, & Schwarz, 2006). This "physiological" GER usually resolves spontaneously by 1 year of age. GER becomes a disease when complications such as growth failure, bleeding, or dysphagia develop. GERD is associated with respiratory symptoms, including apnea, bronchospasm, laryngospasm, and pneumonia. Heartburn is also a frequent symptom in children who are able to describe it (Box 47-8). Certain conditions predispose children to a high prevalence of GERD, including neurological impairment, hiatal hernia, repaired esophageal atresia, and morbid obesity (Suwandhi et al., 2006).

BOX 47-8 Clinical Manifestations and Complications of Gastroesophageal Reflux

Symptoms in Infants

Spitting up, regurgitation, vomiting (may be forceful)
Excessive crying, irritability, arching of the back, stiffening
Weight loss, growth failure
Respiratory problems (cough, wheeze, stridor, gagging, choking with feedings)
Hematemesis
Apnea or apparent life-threatening event (ALTE)

Symptoms in Children

Heartburn
Abdominal pain
Noncardiac chest pain
Chronic cough
Dysphagia
Nocturnal asthma
Recurrent pneumonia

Complications

Esophagitis
Esophageal stricture
Laryngitis
Recurrent pneumonia
Anemia
Barrett's esophagus

(Adapted from Rudolph, C. D., et al. [2001]. Guidelines for evaluation and treatment of gastroesophageal reflux in infants and children: Recommendations of the North American Society for Pediatric Gastroenterology and Nutrition. *Journal of Pediatric Gastroenterology & Nutrition, 32*[Suppl 2], S1–S31.)

Sandifer syndrome is an uncommon condition, usually occurring in young children, characterized by repetitive stretching and arching of the head and neck that can be mistaken for a seizure. This manoeuvre likely represents a physiological neuromuscular response attempting to prevent acid refluxate from reaching the upper portion of the esophagus (Cavataio & Guandalini, 2005).

Pathophysiology

Although the pathogenesis of GER is multifactorial, its primary causative mechanism likely involves inappropriate transient relaxation of the lower esophageal sphincter (LES) (Suwandhi et al., 2006). Factors that increase abdominal pressure, such as coughing and sneezing, scoliosis, and overeating, may contribute to GERD. Esophageal symptoms are caused by inflammation from the acid in the gastric refluxate, whereas reactive airway disease may result from stimulation of airway reflexes by the acid refluxate.

Diagnostic Evaluation

The history and physical examination are usually sufficiently reliable to establish the diagnosis of GER. However, the upper GI series is helpful in evaluating the presence of anatomical abnormalities (e.g., pyloric stenosis, malrotation, annular pancreas, hiatal hernia, esophageal stricture). The 24-hour intraesophageal pH monitoring study is the gold standard in the diagnosis of GER (Suwandhi et al., 2006). Endoscopy with biopsy may be helpful to assess the presence and severity of esophagitis, strictures, and Barrett esophagus and to exclude other disorders such as Crohn's disease. Scintigraphy detects radioactive substances in the esophagus after a feeding of the compound and assesses gastric emptying. It can differentiate between aspiration of gastric contents from reflux and aspiration from poor oropharyngeal muscle coordination.

Therapeutic Management

Therapeutic management of GER depends on its severity. No therapy is needed for the infant who is thriving and has no respiratory complications. In symptomatic infants, feeding manoeuvres (e.g., thickened feedings, upright positioning) can improve mild GER symptoms. Thickened feedings do not improve pH scores on 24-hour intraesophageal monitoring but may decrease the number of vomiting episodes. Feedings thickened with 5 to 15 mL of rice cereal per 30 mL of formula may be recommended. This may benefit infants who are underweight as a result of GERD. Constant NG feedings may be necessary for the infant with severe reflux and growth failure until surgery can be performed. Elevating the head of the bed 30 degrees or placing the infant in an infant seat elevated 30 degrees for 1 hour after feedings may decrease GER. Prone positioning of infants also decreases episodes of GER but is recommended only with extreme caution when the risk of GERD complications exceeds the risk of sudden infant death syndrome (Cavataio & Guandalini, 2005). The Canadian Pediatric Society recommends supine positioning for sleep (see Chapter 36). If the prone position is used, parents need to be cautioned to avoid soft bedding. In older children and adolescents, avoidance of certain foods that exacerbate acid reflux (e.g., caffeine, citrus, tomatoes, alcohol, peppermint, spicy or fried foods); lifestyle modifications such as weight control if indicated; small, more frequent meals; and smoking cessation may be helpful in reducing symptoms.

Pharmacological therapy may be used to treat infants and children with GERD. Both H_2-receptor antagonists (cimetidine [Tagamet], ranitidine [Zantac], or famotidine [Pepcid]) and proton pump inhibitors (PPIs; esomeprazole [Nexium], lansoprazole [Prevacid], omeprazole [Prilosec], pantoprazole [Protonix], and rabeprazole [Aciphex]) reduce gastric hydrochloric acid secretion and may stimulate some increase in LES tone. Use of available prokinetic medications (e.g., bethanechol [Urecholine] and metoclopramide) remains controversial. Careful analyses of published data have failed to demonstrate clinical efficacy in modifying the natural history or therapeutic outcomes of GER in childhood (Suwandhi et al., 2006).

Surgical management of GER is reserved for children with severe complications such as recurrent aspiration pneumonia, apnea, severe esophagitis, or growth failure and for children who have failed to respond to medical therapy. The *Nissen fundoplication* (Fig. 47-4) is the most common surgical procedure (Christian & Buyske, 2005). This surgery involves passage of the gastric fundus behind the esophagus to encircle the distal esophagus. The most recent surgical advance for GER is the introduction of the laparoscopic Nissen fundoplication

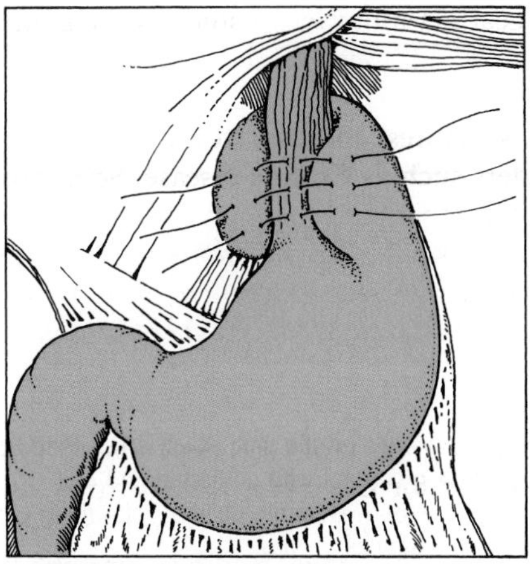

Fig. 47-4 Nissen fundoplication sutures passing through esophageal musculature. *(Redrawn from Campbell, A., & Ferrara, B. [1993].* AORN Journal, *57, 671–679.)*

(Durkin & Shaaban, 2008). Complications following fundoplication include breakdown of the wrap, small bowel obstruction, gas-bloat syndrome, infection, retching, and dumping syndrome (Rudolph et al., 2001).

Nursing Care Management

Nursing care is directed at (1) identifying children with symptoms, (2) educating parents in home care, including feeding, positioning, and medications, and (3) if appropriate, providing care for the child undergoing surgical repair (see Surgical Procedures, Chapter 45). Early in the treatment program, parents should be reassured that most infants and children outgrow GER and often conservative lifestyle changes are sufficient. Parents need support and reassurance to implement lifestyle changes. Although it is not known if lifestyle changes bring additional benefit to patients receiving pharmacological interventions, some changes may be helpful. To help parents cope with the inconvenience of dealing with a child who spits up frequently, simple measures such as using bibs and protective cloths during and after feedings are beneficial.

Older children and adolescents need to know that caffeine, chocolate, and spicy foods may weaken the LES and aggravate symptoms. Exposure to tobacco and alcohol are also associated with GER. Obesity increases abdominal pressure, and weight management may reduce GER symptoms. When medical management is necessary, parents need information about the medications and their potential adverse effects. Prokinetic medications must be given before feedings. Medications for acid control must be timed to provide coverage and given regularly and as ordered.

Intestinal Parasitic Diseases

Intestinal parasitic diseases, including helminths (worms) and protozoa, constitute the most frequent infections in the world. In Canada, the incidence of intestinal parasitic disease, especially giardiasis, has increased among young children who attend day care centres. Young children are especially at risk because of typical hand–mouth activity and uncontrolled fecal activity (About Kids' Health, 2010).

Intestinal parasitic diseases in humans are caused by various infecting organisms. This discussion is limited to the two common parasitic infections among children in Canada: giardiasis and pinworms. Table 47-5 describes the outstanding features of selected helminths that belong to the family of nematodes.

General Nursing Care Management

Nursing responsibilities related to intestinal parasitic infections involve assistance with identification of the parasite, treatment of the infection, and prevention of initial infection or reinfection. Identification of the organism is accomplished by laboratory examination of substances containing the worm, its larvae, or ova. Most are identified by examining fecal smears from the stools of persons suspected of harbouring the parasite. Fresh specimens are best for revealing parasites or larvae; thus collected specimens should be taken directly to the laboratory for examination. If this is not feasible, the specimen is placed in a container with a preservative. Parents need clear instructions on obtaining an adequate sample and the number of samples required (see Stool Specimens, Chapter 45). In most parasitic infections, examination of other family members, especially children, may be carried out to identify those who are similarly affected.

After the diagnosis is confirmed and appropriate treatment is planned, parents need further explanation and reinforcement. Compliance in terms of medication therapy and other measures, such as thorough hand hygiene, is essential for eradication of the parasite. The family needs to understand the nature of transmission and that in some cases the medication must be repeated in 2 weeks to 1 month to kill organisms hatched since initial treatment.

The nurse's most important function is preventive education of children and families regarding hygiene and health habits. Thorough hand washing before eating or handling food and after using the toilet is the most important precautionary method.

Giardiasis

Giardiasis is caused by the protozoan *Giardia lamblia* (also called *Giardia intestinalis, Giardia duodenalis,* and *Lamblia intestinalis*) and is sometimes called "beaver fever." Child care centres and institutions providing care for persons with developmental disabilities are common sites for giardiasis, and the children may pass cysts for months. Children under 5 years and adults 25 to 39 years (usually the parents of these children) are at increased risk of infection. The greatest number of cases are reported in the warmer months of the year, such as July to October (PHAC, 2003). Giardiasis should also be considered in those with a history of recent travel to an endemic area.

The potential for transmission is great, because the *cysts*—the nonmotile stage of the protozoa—can survive in the environment for months. Chief modes of transmission are person to person; contaminated water, food, and animals. Sporadic outbreaks may occur through ingestion of the cysts in fecally

Table 47-5 Selected Intestinal Parasites

CLINICAL MANIFESTATIONS	COMMENTS
Ascariasis—*Ascaris lumbricoides* (Common Roundworm)	
Light infections: asymptomatic Heavy infections: anorexia, irritability, nervousness, enlarged abdomen, weight loss, fever, intestinal colic Severe infections: intestinal obstruction, appendicitis, perforation of intestine with peritonitis, obstructive jaundice, lung involvement—pneumonitis	Transferred to mouth by way of contaminated food, fingers, or toys Largest of the intestinal helminths Affects principally young children 1–4 yr of age Prevalent in warm climates
Hookworm Disease—*Necator americanus*	
Light infections in well-nourished individuals: no problems Heavier infections: mild to severe anemia, malnutrition May be itching and burning followed by erythema and a papular eruption in areas to which the organism migrates	Transmitted by discharging eggs on the soil, which are picked up, causing infection from direct skin contact with contaminated soil Wearing shoes is recommended, although children playing in contaminated soil expose many skin surfaces
Strongyloidiasis—*Strongyloides stercoralis* (Threadworm)	
Light infection: asymptomatic Heavy infection: respiratory signs and symptoms; abdominal pain, distension; nausea and vomiting; diarrhea—large, pale stools, often with mucus Threat to life in children with weakened immunological defenses Elevated eosinophils may be the only manifestation	Transmission is same as for hookworm (direct contact with human skin), except autoinfection (organism can complete its lifecycle in humans) is common Older children and adults affected more often than young children Severe infections may lead to severe nutritional deficiency Prevalent in warm climates
Visceral Larva Migrans—*Toxocara canis* (Dogs); Intestinal Toxocariasis—*Toxocara cati* (Cats)	
Depends on reactivity of infected individual May be asymptomatic except for eosinophilia Specific diagnosis difficult	Transmitted by ingestion of or contact with soil containing eggs from feces of infected dog or cat Dogs and cats should be kept away from areas where children play; sandboxes are especially comment transmission areas More prevalent in hot, humid environments where eggs remain in soil Periodic deworming of diagnosed dogs and cats Control of dog and cat population Continued education and laws to prevent indiscriminate canine and feline defecation
Trichuriasis—*Trichuris trichiura* (Whipworm)	
Light infections: asymptomatic Heavy infections: abdominal pain and distension, diarrhea	Transmitted from contaminated soil or from vegetables grown in soil where eggs are present Most frequent in warm, moist climates Occurs most often in undernourished children living in unsanitary conditions

contaminated water or food. Lakes or streams that are open to human and animal (beaver and other wild and domestic animals) fecal contamination may be sources of infection (PHAC, 2003). In children, person-to-person transmission is the most likely cause. Although individuals infected with giardiasis may be asymptomatic, common symptoms include abdominal cramps and diarrhea (Box 47-9).

Diagnosis of giardiasis may be made by microscopic examination of stool specimens or duodenal fluid or by identification of *G. lamblia* antigens in these specimens by techniques such as enzyme immunoassay (EIA). Because the *Giardia* organisms live in the upper intestine and are excreted in a highly variable pattern, repeated microscopic examination of stool specimens may be required to identify *trophozoites* (active parasites) or cysts. Duodenal specimens are obtained by direct aspiration, biopsy, or the *string* test. In the string test, the child swallows a gelatin capsule with a nylon string attached. Several hours later, the string is withdrawn, and the contents are sent for laboratory analysis. With the availability

BOX 47-9 Clinical Manifestations of Giardiasis

Infants and young children:
- Diarrhea
- Vomiting
- Anorexia
- Growth failure

Children older than 5 years of age:
- Abdominal cramps
- Intermittent loose stools
- Constipation
- Stools may be malodorous, watery, pale, and greasy

Most infections resolve spontaneously in 4 to 6 weeks

Rarely, chronic form occurs:
- Intermittent loose, foul-smelling stools
- Possibility of abdominal bloating, flatulence, sulphur-tasting belches, epigastric pain, vomiting, headache, and weight loss

of EIA techniques to identify *Giardia* antigens in stool specimens, other tests are being used less often.

Therapeutic Management

The medications of choice for treatment of giardiasis are metronidazole (Flagyl), tinidazole (Tindamax), paromomycin (Humatin), and nitazoxanide (Alinia). Metronidazole is said to have an 80 to 95% cure rate (Health Link BC, 2011). Metronidazole and tinidazole have a metallic taste and GI adverse effects, including nausea and vomiting; nitazoxanide has no bitter taste and should be taken with food to avoid GI symptoms. (AAP, Committee on Infectious Diseases, & Pickering, 2009).

Nursing Care Management

The most important nursing consideration is prevention of giardiasis and education of parents, child care centre staff, and those who are entrusted with the daily care of small children. Attention to meticulous sanitary practices, especially during diaper changes, is essential (Fig. 47-5). Nurses can play an important role in educating parents of small children and day care staff regarding appropriate sanitation practices. In addition, young children who are infected or who have diarrhea should be discouraged from swimming in community or private pools until they are infection free. Lakes and streams may contain high numbers of *Giardia* spore cysts, which can be swallowed in the water. When there is a high chance of swallowing water, children should be discouraged from swimming in stagnant bodies of water and in water where children who are known to be infected are swimming. *Giardia* organisms are said to be resistant to chlorine (Hlavsa, Watson, & Beach, 2005). Parents should be encouraged to take small children to the restroom frequently when swimming, to avoid letting children in diapers in swimming areas, and to change diapers away from the water source. After children are infected, family education regarding medication administration is essential.

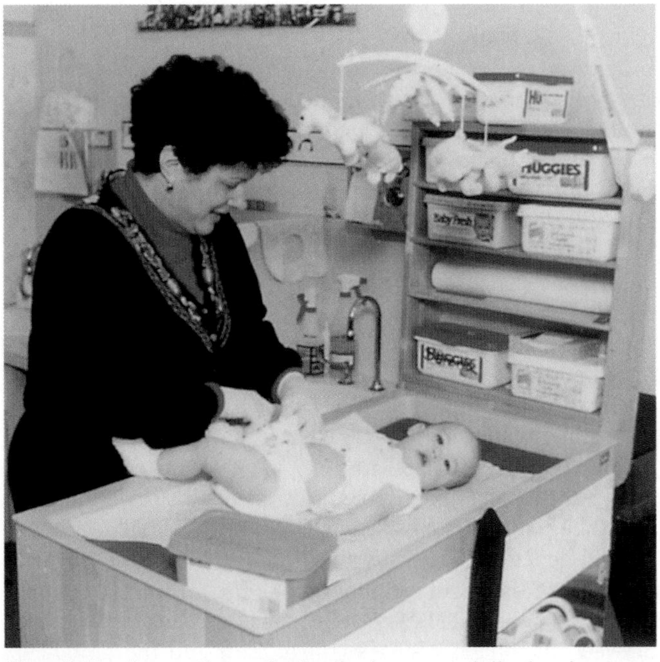

Fig. 47-5 Prevention of giardiasis, especially in day care centres, requires sanitary practices during diaper changes such as discarding paper diapers in a covered receptacle, changing paper covers on the diaper-changing surface, and having facilities for handwashing nearby. Note: Soiled cloth diapers and clothing should be stored in a plastic bag for transport home.

Enterobiasis (Pinworms)

Enterobiasis, or pinworms, caused by the nematode *Enterobius vermicularis*, is a common helminthic infection in Canada. It is universally present in temperate climatic zones and may infect more than 30% of all children at any one time. Crowded conditions such as in classrooms and day care centres favour transmission.

Infection begins when the eggs are ingested or inhaled (they float in the air). The eggs hatch in the upper intestine and then mature and migrate through the intestine. After mating, adult females migrate out the anus and lay eggs (AAP, Committee on Infectious Diseases, & Pickering, 2009). The movement of the worms on skin and mucous membrane surfaces causes intense itching. As the child scratches, eggs are deposited on the hands and underneath the fingernails. The typical hand-to-mouth activity of youngsters makes them especially prone to reinfection. Pinworm eggs persist in the indoor environment for 2 to 3 weeks, contaminating anything they contact, such as toilet seats, doorknobs, bed linen, underwear, and food. Except for the intense rectal itching associated with pinworms, the clinical manifestations are nonspecific (Box 47-10).

Diagnostic Evaluation

Diagnosis is most commonly made from the tape test (see Nursing Care Management). Repeated tests to collect eggs may be necessary, and if there is a possibility that other family members may be infected, a tape test should be performed on them.

Therapeutic Management

The medications available for treatment of pinworms include mebendazole and nonprescription pyrantel pamoate (Combantrin). The medication of choice is mebendazole, which is safe, effective, and convenient, with few adverse effects; however, it is not recommended for children younger than 2 years of age.

BOX 47-10 Clinical Manifestations of Pinworms

Intense perianal itching (principal symptom); evidence of itching in young children includes the following:
- General irritability
- Restlessness
- Poor sleep
- Bed-wetting
- Distractibility
- Short attention span

Perianal dermatitis and excoriation secondary to itching
If worms migrate, possible vaginal and urethral infection

If pyrvinium pamoate is prescribed, parents should be advised that the drug stains stool and vomitus bright red, as well as clothing or skin that comes in contact with it; it is available without prescription and should not be used in children under 2 years without consulting the primary practitioner. Because pinworms are easily transmitted, all household members are treated. The dose of antiparasitic medication should be repeated in 2 weeks to completely eradicate the parasite and prevent reinfection.

evolve Case Study—Appendicitis
evolve Animation—Appendicitis

Nursing Care Management

Nursing care is directed at identifying the parasite, eradicating the organism, and preventing reinfection. Parents need clear, detailed instructions for the tape test. A loop of transparent (not "frosted" or "magic") tape, sticky side out, is placed around the end of a tongue depressor, which is then firmly pressed against the child's perianal area. A convenient, commercially prepared tape is also available for this purpose. Pinworm specimens are collected in the morning as soon as the child awakens and *before* he or she has a bowel movement or bathes. The procedure may need to be performed on 3 or more consecutive days before eggs are collected. Parents should be instructed to place the tongue blade in a glass jar or loosely in a plastic bag so that it can be brought in for microscopic examination. For specimens collected in the hospital, practitioner's office, or clinic, the tape is placed smoothly on a glass slide, sticky side down, for examination.

Compliance with the medication regimen is usually excellent because the duration of treatment is typically only one dose. However, the family should be reminded of the need to take a second dose in 2 weeks to ensure eradication of the eggs.

To prevent reinfection, washing all clothes and bed linens in hot water and vacuuming the house may be recommended. However, there is little documentation on the effectiveness of these measures because pinworms survive on many surfaces. Helpful suggestions include hand hygiene after toileting and before eating, keeping the child's fingernails short to minimize the chance of ova collecting under the nails, dressing children in one-piece sleeping outfits, and daily showering rather than tub bathing. Families should be informed that recurrence is common. Repeated infections should be treated in the same manner as the first one.

Inflammatory Disorders

Acute Appendicitis

Appendicitis, inflammation of the *vermiform appendix* (blind sac at the end of the cecum), is the most common cause of emergency abdominal surgery in childhood. In Canada, the pediatric appendicitis rates have been stable since 1993 at an average rate of 93.2 per 100,000 children (To & Langer, 2010). The average age of children with appendicitis is 10 years, with boys and girls equally affected before puberty. Classically, the first symptom of appendicitis is periumbilical pain, followed by nausea, right lower quadrant pain, and later vomiting with fever (Kwok, Kim, & Gorelick, 2004). Perforation of the appendix can occur within approximately 48 hours of the initial complaint of pain. At the time of initial presentation, about one third of all cases involve an already perforated appendix.

Complications from appendiceal perforation include major abscess, phlegmon, enterocutaneous fistula, peritonitis, and partial bowel obstruction (Kwok et al., 2004). A *phlegmon* is an acute suppurative inflammation of subcutaneous connective tissue that spreads.

Etiology

The cause of appendicitis is obstruction of the lumen of the appendix, usually by hardened fecal material (fecalith). Swollen lymphoid tissue, frequently occurring after a viral infection, can also obstruct the appendix. Another rare cause of obstruction is a parasite such as *Enterobius vermicularis*, or pinworms, which can obstruct the appendiceal lumen.

Pathophysiology

With acute obstruction, the outflow of mucus secretions is blocked, and pressure builds within the lumen, resulting in compression of blood vessels. The resulting ischemia is followed by ulceration of the epithelial lining and bacterial invasion. Subsequent necrosis causes perforation or rupture with fecal and bacterial contamination of the peritoneal cavity. The resulting inflammation spreads rapidly throughout the abdomen (*peritonitis*), especially in young children, who are unable to localize infection. Progressive peritoneal inflammation results in functional intestinal obstruction of the small bowel (*ileus*) because intense GI reflexes severely inhibit bowel motility. Because the peritoneum represents a major portion of total body surface, the loss of ECF to the peritoneal cavity leads to electrolyte imbalance and hypovolemic shock.

Diagnostic Evaluation

Diagnosis is not always straightforward. Fever, vomiting, abdominal pain, and an elevated white blood cell (WBC) count are associated with appendicitis but are also seen in IBD, pelvic inflammatory disease, gastroenteritis, urinary tract infection, right lower lobe pneumonia, mesenteric adenitis, Meckel's diverticulum, and intussusception. Prolonged symptoms and delayed diagnosis often occur in younger children, in whom the risk of perforation is greatest because of their inability to verbalize their complaints. In addition to fever, signs of peritonitis include sudden relief from pain after perforation, subsequent increase in pain (usually diffuse and accompanied by rigid guarding of the abdomen), progressive abdominal distension, tachycardia, rapid shallow breathing, pallor, chills, and irritability.

The diagnosis is based primarily on the history and physical examination (Box 47-11). Pain, the cardinal feature, is initially generalized (usually periumbilical); however, it usually descends to the lower right quadrant. The most intense site of pain may be at *McBurney point*, located at a point midway between the anterior superior iliac crest and the umbilicus. Rebound tenderness is not a reliable sign and is extremely painful to the child. Referred pain, elicited by light percussion around the perimeter of the abdomen, indicates peritoneal irritation. Movement such as riding over bumps in an automobile or on a stretcher, aggravates the pain. In addition to

BOX 47-11 Clinical Manifestations of Appendicitis

- Right lower quadrant abdominal pain
- Fever
- Rigid abdomen
- Decreased or absent bowel sounds
- Vomiting (typically follows onset of pain)
- Constipation or diarrhea may be present
- Anorexia
- Tachycardia; rapid, shallow breathing
- Pallor
- Lethargy
- Irritability
- Stooped posture (guarding)

pain, significant clinical manifestations include fever, a change in behaviour, anorexia, and vomiting.

Laboratory studies usually include a CBC, urinalysis (to rule out a urinary tract infection), and, in adolescent females, serum human chorionic gonadotropin (to rule out an ectopic pregnancy). A WBC count greater than 10×10^6/L and a C-reactive protein (CRP) are common but are not necessarily specific for appendicitis. An elevated percentage of bands (often referred to as "a shift to the left") may indicate an inflammatory process. CRP is an acute-phase reactant that rises within 12 hours of the onset of infection.

Computed tomography (CT) scan has become the imaging technique of choice, although ultrasonography may also be helpful in diagnosing appendicitis. A CT scan is considered positive in the presence of enlarged appendiceal diameter; appendiceal wall thickening; and periappendiceal inflammatory changes, including fat streaks, phlegmon, fluid collection, and extraluminal gas (Aiken & Oldham, 2007).

Therapeutic Management

Treatment of appendicitis before perforation includes rehydration, antibiotics, and surgical removal of the appendix (appendectomy). Laparoscopic surgery is now commonly used to treat nonperforated acute appendicitis. Recovery is rapid, and, if no complications occur, the hospital stay is short.

Ruptured Appendix

Management of the child diagnosed with peritonitis caused by a ruptured appendix often begins preoperatively with IV administration of fluid and electrolytes, systemic antibiotics, and NG suction. Postoperative management includes IV fluids, continued administration of antibiotics, and NG suction for abdominal decompression until intestinal activity returns. Sometimes surgeons close the wound after irrigation of the peritoneal cavity. Other times, they leave the wound open (delayed closure) to prevent wound infection. A Penrose drain may be used to permit transperitoneal drainage. Nonsurgical treatment for ruptured appendix is becoming more common. Treatment with antibiotics and image guided drainage of any abdominal abcesses is now an accepted method of treatment (Whyte, Levin, & Harris, 2008).

Prognosis

Complications are uncommon after a simple appendectomy. The mortality rate for perforating appendicitis has improved from nearly certain death a century ago to less than 1% (0.3%) (Aiken & Oldham, 2007). Early recognition of the illness is essential to prevent complications.

Nursing Care Management

Because abdominal pain is the most common childhood complaint with appendicitis, it is important to assess the severity of pain (see Pain Assessment, Chapter 35). One of the most reliable estimates is the degree of change in behaviour. The younger, nonverbal child will assume a rigid, motionless, side-lying posture with the knees flexed on the abdomen, and there is decreased range of motion of the right hip. Older children may exhibit all of these behaviours while complaining of abdominal pain. They can always indicate a point at which the pain is worse than at any other location.

NURSING ALERT In any instance when appendicitis is suspected, be aware of the danger of administering laxatives or enemas or applying heat to the area. Such measures stimulate bowel motility and increase the risk of perforation.

Postoperative Care

Postoperative care for the nonperforated appendix is the same as for most abdominal procedures. Care of the child with a ruptured appendix and peritonitis is more complex, and the course of recovery is considerably longer (usually 3 to 5 days of hospitalization). The child is maintained on IV fluids, NPO, and the NG tube is kept on low continuous gastric decompression until there is evidence of intestinal activity. Listening for bowel sounds and observing for other signs of bowel activity (e.g., passage of stool) are part of the routine assessment. Management of IV therapy is the same as for any child receiving fluids and parenteral antibiotics. A drain is often placed in the wound during surgery, and frequent dressing changes with meticulous skin care are essential to prevent excoriation of the area surrounding the surgical site. Wound care includes irrigation with antibacterial solution. If the wound is left open, a Montgomery strap may be used to facilitate dressing changes and minimize tape removal and epidermal stripping. Early ambulation with adequate pain management assists in preventing many of the complications associated with prolonged bed rest and immobility (e.g., venous stasis, bowel hypomotility, abdominal pain from intestinal gas).

Management of pain from the incision and repeated dressing changes and irrigations are an essential part of the child's care. Psychological care of the child and parents is similar to that used in other **emergency** situations (see Emergency Admission, Chapter 44). Parents and older children need to express their feelings and concerns regarding the events surrounding the illness and hospitalization. The nurse can provide education and psychosocial support to promote adequate coping and alleviate anxiety for both the child and the family.

Meckel's Diverticulum

Meckel's diverticulum is a remnant of the fetal omphalomesenteric duct that connects the yolk sac with the primitive midgut during fetal life. Normally this structure is obliterated by the fifth to seventh week of gestation, when the placenta replaces the yolk sac as the source of nutrition for the fetus

(Sagar, Kumar, & Shah, 2006). Failure of obliteration may result in an *omphalomesenteric fistula*, a fibrous band connecting the small intestine to the umbilicus, known as Meckel's diverticulum.

Meckel's diverticulum is a true diverticulum because it arises from the antimesenteric border of the small intestine and contains all layers of the intestinal wall with a separate blood supply from the vitelline artery. The diverticulum is usually found within 100 cm of the ileocecal valve and averages 1 to 10 cm in length.

Meckel's diverticulum is the most common congenital malformation of the GI tract and is present in 2 to 4% of the population (Sagar et al., 2006). Its occurrence in males and females is equal, but the incidence of complications is three to four times greater in males. Most symptomatic cases are seen in childhood. Patients requiring surgery are generally younger than 10 years of age, and about 50% are younger than 2 years of age (Sagar et al., 2006).

Pathophysiology

The symptomatic complications of Meckel's diverticulum are ulceration, bleeding, intussusception, intestinal obstruction, diverticulitis, and perforation; bleeding is the most common problem in children. Gastric mucosa is the most common ectopic tissue found in Meckel's diverticulum. Bleeding is caused by peptic ulceration or perforation because of the unbuffered acidic gastric secretion. Several mechanisms can cause obstruction. Intussusception may be led by the diverticulum. Obstruction may also be caused by entanglement of the small intestine around a fibrous cord, trapping of a loop of intestine under the band, incarceration within a hernia sac, or volvulus of the intestinal segment containing the diverticulum. Diverticulitis occurs when peptic ulceration or obstruction leads to inflammation.

Diagnostic Evaluation

Diagnosis is usually based on the history, physical examination, and a specialized radiographic study. The most common clinical presentation in children includes painless rectal bleeding, abdominal pain, or signs of intestinal obstruction (Box 47-12). Bleeding, which may be mild or profuse, often appears as dark red or "currant jelly" stools; it may be significant enough to cause hypotension. The Meckel scan, a technetium-99m pertechnetate scan, detects the presence of gastric mucosa with an overall diagnostic accuracy of 90%. Blood studies are performed to screen for bleeding disorders and anemia.

BOX 47-12 Clinical Manifestations of Meckel's Diverticulum

Abdominal Pain
Similar to appendicitis
May be vague and recurrent

Bloody Stools*
Painless
Bright or dark red with mucus ("currant jelly" stool)
In infants, bleeding may be accompanied by pain

Sometimes
Severe anemia
Shock

*Often an initial sign.

Therapeutic Management

The standard treatment is surgical removal of the diverticulum. When severe hemorrhage increases the surgical risk, interventions to correct hypovolemic shock, such as blood replacement, IV fluids, and oxygen, may be necessary. Antibiotics may be used preoperatively to control infection. If intestinal obstruction has occurred, appropriate preoperative measures are used to reverse electrolyte imbalances and minimize abdominal distension.

Prognosis

If this condition is diagnosed and treated early, full recovery is likely. The mortality rate of untreated Meckel's diverticulum ranges from 2.5 to 15%. Complications of untreated Meckel's diverticulum include GI hemorrhage and bowel obstruction.

Nursing Care Management

Nursing objectives are similar to those for any child undergoing surgery (see Chapter 44). Because the onset of this condition is often rapid, parents require psychological support. The massive intestinal bleeding that can accompany a Meckel's diverticulum is traumatic to both the child and the parents and may significantly affect their emotional reaction to hospitalization and surgery.

Specific preoperative considerations with intestinal bleeding include (1) frequent monitoring of vital signs and blood pressure for shock, (2) keeping the child on bed rest, and (3) recording the approximate amount of blood lost in stools. In the absence of frank hemorrhage, the nurse needs to test the stools for occult blood. Postoperatively, the child requires IV fluids and an NG tube for the decompression and evacuation of gastric contents.

Inflammatory Bowel Disease

Inflammatory bowel disease (IBD) is a term used for two forms of chronic intestinal inflammation: ulcerative colitis (UC) and Crohn's disease (CD). Although UC and CD have similar epidemiological, immunological, and clinical features, there are important differences (Table 47-6).

GI symptoms, extraintestinal and systemic inflammatory responses, and exacerbations and remissions without complete resolution characterize these diseases. Growth failure, particularly common in CD, is an important problem unique to the pediatric population. CD is more disabling, has more serious complications, and has less effective medical and surgical treatment than UC. Because UC is confined to the colon, theoretically it may be cured with a colectomy. Over the past 30 years, the incidence of CD has risen, whereas the incidence of UC in children has remained stable (Silbermintz & Markowitz, 2006). Approximately 0.5% of the Canadian population has IBD, which is one of the highest incidence and prevalence of CD yet reported (Bernstein et al., 2006). Ontario has one of the highest rates of childhood-onset IBD in the

Table 47-6 Clinical Manifestations of Inflammatory Bowel Diseases

CHARACTERISTICS	ULCERATIVE COLITIS	CROHN'S DISEASE
Rectal bleeding	Common	Uncommon
Diarrhea	Often severe	Moderate to severe
Pain	Less frequent	Common
Anorexia	Mild or moderate	May be severe
Weight loss	Moderate	May be severe
Growth delay	Usually mild	May be severe
Anal and perianal lesions	Rare	Common
Fistulas and strictures	Rare	Common
Rashes	Mild	Mild
Joint pain	Mild to moderate	Mild to moderate

world, and there is an accelerated increase in incidence in younger children (Benchimol et al., 2009).

Etiology

Despite decades of research, the etiology of IBD is not completely understood, and there is no known cure. There is evidence to indicate a multifactorial etiology. Research is focused on theories of defective immunoregulation of the inflammatory response to bacteria or viruses in the GI tract in individuals with a genetic predisposition (Silbermintz & Markowitz, 2006). In CD the chronic immune process is characterized by a T helper 1 cytokine profile, whereas in UC the response is more humoral and mediated by T helper 2 cells (Silbermintz & Markowitz, 2006). An epidemiological study by Kugathasan and colleagues (2003) found an equal distribution of IBD among all racial and ethnic groups, contrasting with earlier studies suggesting that IBD typically affects Whites (especially Ashkenazi Jews) more than persons of Asian or African decent. The Kugathasan study also did not demonstrate a higher risk for developing IBD in urban populations, as had been reported in earlier studies.

There is an influence of genetics in the development of CD. Several CD susceptibility genes have been identified, including *NOD2/CARD15* on chromosome 16 associated with ileal disease, *IBD5* on chromosome 5, and *IBD6* on chromosome 6 (Sauer & Kugathasan, 2010). The influence of genetics in UC appears to be smaller than in CD; however, the *MDRI* gene has been associated with UC (Sauer & Kugathasan, 2010).

Environmental factors appear to play a role in the development of IBD. Breastfeeding decreases the risk of developing CD, whereas infantile diarrhea seems to increase the risk. Cigarette smoking also appears to be a risk factor for CD but appears to be protective against UC.

Pathophysiology of Ulcerative Colitis

The inflammation is limited to the colon and rectum, with the distal colon and rectum most severely affected. It affects the mucosa and submucosa and involves continuous segments along the length of the bowel with varying degrees of ulceration, bleeding, and edema. The presentation may be mild, moderate, or severe, depending on the extent of mucosal inflammation and systemic symptoms. Children with UC usually are seen with diarrhea, rectal bleeding, and abdominal pain, often associated with tenesmus and urgency (Silbermintz & Markowitz, 2006). Thickening of the bowel wall and fibrosis are unusual, but long-standing disease can result in shortening of the colon and strictures. Extraintestinal manifestations are less common in UC than in CD. Toxic megacolon is the most dangerous form of severe colitis.

Pathophysiology of Crohn's Disease

The chronic inflammatory process of CD involves any part of the GI tract from the mouth to the anus but most often affects the terminal ileum. The disease involves all layers of the bowel wall (*transmural*) in a discontinuous fashion, meaning that between areas of intact mucosa there are areas of affected mucosa (*skip lesions*). The most common symptoms are abdominal pain, diarrhea, and decrease in appetite resulting in weight loss. Perianal disease, including skin tags, fistulas, and abscesses, occur in CD. Fever, growth delay, and delayed sexual development are seen commonly (Silbermintz & Markowitz, 2006). Mild GI symptoms, poor growth, and extraintestinal manifestations may be present for several years before overt GI symptoms occur. The inflammation may result in ulcerations, fibrosis, adhesions, stiffening of the bowel wall, stricture formation, and fistulas to other loops of bowel, bladder, vagina, or skin. Extraintestinal manifestations include erythema nodosum, pyoderma gangrenosum, arthralgia and arthritis, uveitis and episcleritis, sclerosing cholangitis, autoimmune hepatitis, nephrolithiasis, and pneumonitis (Silbermintz & Markowitz, 2006).

Diagnostic Evaluation

The diagnosis of UC and CD is derived from the history, physical examination, laboratory evaluation, and other diagnostic procedures. Laboratory tests include a CBC to evaluate anemia and an erythrocyte sedimentation rate or CRP to assess the systemic reaction to the inflammatory process. Levels of total protein, albumin, iron, zinc, magnesium, vitamin B_{12}, and fat-soluble vitamins may be low in children with CD. Stools are examined for blood, leukocytes, and infectious organisms. A serological panel is often used in combination with clinical findings to diagnose IBD and to differentiate between CD and UC. In IBD, autoantibodies called antineutrophil cytoplasmic antibodies (ANCAs) may be detected in the blood. The perinuclear antineutrophil cytoplasmic antibody (pANCA) is associated with UC. Approximately 60% of children with UC and 10% of those with CD are pANCA-positive. Anti–*Saccharomyces cerevisiae* antibodies (ASCA) and anti–outer membrane porin of *E. coli* (anti-OmpC) have been found in up to 60% of children with CD (Ruemmele et al., 1998).

In patients with CD, an upper GI series with small bowel follow-through assists in assessing the existence, location, and extent of disease. Upper endoscopy and colonoscopy with biopsies are an integral part of diagnosing IBD. Endoscopy allows direct visualization of the surface of the GI tract so that the extent of inflammation and narrowing can be evaluated. CT and ultrasound also may be used to identify bowel wall inflammation, intra-abdominal abscesses, and fistulas. CD lesions may pierce the walls of the small intestine and colon, creating tracts called *fistulas* between the intestine and adjacent structures such as the bladder, anus, vagina, or skin.

Therapeutic Management

The goals of therapy are to (1) control the inflammatory process to reduce or eliminate the symptoms, (2) obtain long-term remission, (3) promote normal growth and development, and (4) allow as normal a lifestyle as possible. Treatment is individualized and managed according to the type and severity of the disease, its location, and the response to therapy.

Medical Treatment

The goal of any treatment regimen is first to induce remission of acute symptoms and then to maintain remission over time.

5-Aminosalicylates (5-ASAs) are effective in the induction and maintenance of remission in mild to moderate UC. Mesalamine, olsalazine, and balsalazide are now preferred over sulphasalazine because of reduced adverse effects (headache, nausea, vomiting, neutropenia, and oligospermia). Suppository and enema preparations of mesalamine are used to treat left-sided colitis. These medications decrease inflammation by inhibiting prostaglandin synthesis. 5-ASAs can be used to induce remission in mild CD.

Corticosteroids, such as prednisone and prednisolone, are indicated in induction therapy in children with moderate to severe UC and CD. These agents inhibit the production of adhesion molecules, cytokines, and leukotrienes. Although these medications reduce the acute symptoms of IBD, they have adverse effects that relate to long-term use, including growth suppression (adrenal suppression), weight gain, and decreased bone density (Baron, 2002). High doses of IV corticosteroids may be administered in acute episodes and tapered according to clinical response. Budesonide, a synthetic corticosteroid, is designed for controlled release in the ileum and is indicated for ileal and right-sided colitis; budesonide has fewer adverse effects than prednisone and prednisolone (Silbermintz & Markowitz, 2006). Rectal steroid therapy (enemas and foam-based preparations) is available for both induction and maintenance therapy in left-sided colitis.

Immunomodulators, such as azathioprine and its metabolite 6-mercaptopurine (6-MP), are used to induce and maintain remission in children with IBD who are steroid resistant or steroid dependent and in treating chronic draining fistulas. They block the synthesis of purine, thus inhibiting the ability of deoxyribonucleic acid (DNA) and ribonucleic acid (RNA) to hinder **lymphocyte** function, especially that of T cells. Adverse effects include infection, pancreatitis, hepatitis, bone marrow toxicity, arthralgia, and malignancy. Methotrexate has also been shown to be useful in inducing and maintaining remission in CD patients unresponsive to standard therapies. Cyclosporine and tacrolimus have both been shown to be effective in inducing remission in severe steroid-dependent UC. 6-MP or azathioprine is then used to maintain remission. Patients on immunomodulating medications require regular monitoring of their CBC and differential to assess for changes that reflect suppression of the immune system, since many of the adverse effects can be prevented or managed by dose reduction or discontinuation of medication.

Antibiotics, such as metronidazole and ciprofloxacin, may be used as an adjunctive therapy to treat complications such as perianal disease or small bowel bacterial overgrowth in CD. Adverse effects of these medications are peripheral neuropathy, nausea, and a metallic taste.

Biological therapies act to regulate inflammatory and anti-inflammatory cytokines. Tumour necrosis factor-α (TNF-α) is believed to influence active inflammation. With the emergence of the biological agents, specifically the use of antitumour necorosis factor-α (TNF-α) agents, progress has been made in targeting a specific clinical response (Hyams & Markowitc, 2005; Ricart al., 2008). TNF-α is believed to influence active inflammation. Infliximab (Remicade) is a chimeric human-murine monoclonal antibody to TNF-α that is administered intravenously. Children appear to respond to infliximab similarly to adults. Infliximab is approved for the treatment of fistulas in CD and for systemic manifestations of IBD such as ankylosing spondylitis, pyoderma gangrenosum, and chronic uveitis.

Nutritional Support

Nutritional support is important in the treatment of IBD. Growth failure is a common serious complication, especially in CD. It is characterized by weight loss, alteration in body composition, restricted height, and delayed sexual maturation. Malnutrition causes the growth failure, and its etiology is multifactorial. Malnutrition occurs as a result of inadequate dietary intake, excessive GI losses, malabsorption, medication–nutrient interaction, and increased nutritional requirements. Inadequate dietary intake occurs with anorexia and episodes of increased disease activity. Excessive loss of nutrients (protein, blood, electrolytes, and minerals) occurs secondary to intestinal inflammation and diarrhea. Carbohydrate, lactose, fat, vitamin, and mineral malabsorption, as well as vitamin B_{12} and folic acid deficiencies, occur with disease episodes and with medication administration and when the terminal ileum is resected. Finally, nutritional requirements are increased with inflammation, fever, fistulas, and periods of rapid growth (e.g., adolescence).

The goals of nutritional support include (1) correction of nutrient deficits and replacement of ongoing losses, (2) provision of adequate energy and protein for healing, and (3) provision of adequate nutrients to promote normal growth. Nutritional support includes both enteral and parenteral nutrition. A well-balanced, high-protein, high-calorie diet is recommended for children whose symptoms do not prohibit an adequate oral intake. There is little evidence that avoiding specific foods influences the severity of the disease. Supplementation with multivitamins, iron, and folic acid is recommended.

Special enteral formulas, given either by mouth or continuous enteral (NG or gastrostomy) infusion (often at night), may be required. Elemental formulas are completely absorbed in the small intestine with almost no residue. Several studies have demonstrated that a diet consisting only of elemental formula not only improved nutritional status but also induced disease remission, either without steroids or with a diminished dosage of steroids required. An elemental diet is a safe and potentially effective primary therapy for patients with CD. Unfortunately, remission is not sustained when enteral feedings are discontinued unless maintenance medications are added to the treatment regimen.

TPN has also improved nutritional status in patients with IBD. Short-term remissions have been achieved after TPN, although complete bowel rest has not reduced inflammation or added to the benefits of improved nutrition by TPN. Nutritional support is less likely to induce a remission in UC than in CD. However, improvement of nutritional status is important in preventing deterioration of the patient's health status and in preparing the patient for surgery.

Surgical Treatment

Surgery is indicated for UC when medical and nutritional therapies fail to prevent complications. Surgical options include a subtotal colectomy and ileostomy, leaving a rectal stump as a blind pouch. A reservoir pouch is created in the configuration of a J or S to help improve continence postoperatively. An ileoanal pull-through preserves the normal pathway for defecation. *Pouchitis*, an inflammation of the surgically created pouch, is the most common late complication of this procedure and had been reported to occur in up to 50% of cases. Metronidazole and ciprofloxacin are effective in treating pouchitis (Alexander et al., 2003). In many cases UC can be cured with a total colectomy.

Surgery may be required in children with CD when complications cannot be controlled by medical and nutritional therapy. Segmental intestinal resections are performed for small bowel obstructions, strictures, or fistulas. Partial colonic resection is not curative, and the disease often recurs.

Prognosis

IBD is a chronic disease. Relatively long periods of quiescent disease may follow exacerbations. The outcome of the disease is influenced by the regions and severity of involvement, as well as by appropriate therapeutic management. Malnutrition, growth failure, and bleeding are serious complications. The overall prognosis for UC is good.

The development of colorectal cancer (CRC) is a long-term complication of IBD. In UC the cumulative incidence of CRC is 2.5% after 20 years, increasing to 10.8% after 30 years (Rutter et al., 2006). Surveillance colonoscopy with multiple biopsies should begin approximately 10 years after diagnosis of UC or CD and continue every 1 to 2 years (Rubin & Kavitt, 2006). Removal of the diseased colon prevents development of CRC. However, in CD surgical removal of the affected colon does not prevent cancer from developing elsewhere in the GI tract.

Nursing Care Management

The nursing considerations in the management of IBD extend beyond the immediate period of hospitalization. These interventions involve continued guidance of families in terms of (1) managing diet, (2) coping with factors that increase stress and emotional lability, (3) adjusting to a disease of remissions and exacerbations, and (4) when indicated, preparing the child and parents for the possibility of diversionary bowel surgery.

Because nutritional support is an essential part of therapy, encouraging the anorectic child to consume sufficient quantities of food is often a challenge. Successful interventions include involving the child in meal planning; encouraging small, frequent meals or snacks rather than three large meals a day; serving meals around medication schedules when diarrhea, mouth pain, and intestinal spasm are controlled; and preparing high-protein, high-calorie foods such as eggnog, milkshakes, cream soups, puddings, or custard (if lactose is tolerated) (see Feeding the Sick Child, Chapter 45). Foods that are known to aggravate the condition should be avoided. Using bran or a high-fibre diet for active IBD is questionable. Bran, even in small amounts, has been shown to worsen the patient's condition. Occasionally the occurrence of aphthous **stomatitis** (mouth ulcers) further complicates compliance with dietary management. Mouth care before eating and the selection of bland foods can help relieve the discomfort of mouth sores.

When NG feedings or TPN are indicated, nurses play an important role in explaining the purpose and expected outcomes of this therapy. The nurse should acknowledge the anxieties of the child and family members and give them adequate time to demonstrate the skills necessary to continue the therapy at home if needed (see Critical Thinking Exercise).

The importance of continued medication therapy despite remission of symptoms must be stressed to the child and family members. Failure to adhere to the pharmacological regimen can result in exacerbation of the disease (see

CRITICAL THINKING EXERCISE

Inflammatory Bowel Disease

Harpreet, a 13-year-old girl, was admitted to the hospital because of bloody diarrhea, abdominal pain, and weight loss. After a thorough evaluation, including laboratory tests, radiographic studies, and gastrointestinal endoscopy procedures, the diagnosis of Crohn's disease (CD) was made. Medical treatment, including corticosteroid medications and nutritional support, was implemented during this hospitalization.

Harpreet has improved considerably and is to be discharged home this week. Enteral formula administered by continuous nighttime gastrostomy infusion will be continued at home, and both Harpreet and her family are eager to learn how to perform these feedings. You are the nurse who is responsible for Harpreet's discharge planning. Which interventions relating to these feedings should you include in Harpreet's preparations for discharge?

1. Evidence—Are there sufficient data to formulate any specific interventions for discharge?
2. Assumptions—Describe some underlying assumptions about the following:
   a. The goals of nutritional support for children with CD
   b. Teaching required by an adolescent or family member who is administering gastrostomy tube feedings at home
   c. Psychosocial issues related to CD
3. What are the priorities for discharge planning at this time?
4. Does the evidence support your conclusion?
5. Are there alternative perspectives to your conclusion? What are they?

evolve Critical Thinking Exercise—Home Care for the Adolescent

Compliance With Medical Treatment Plan, Chapter 45). Unfortunately, exacerbation of IBD can occur even if the child and family are compliant with the treatment regimen; this is difficult for the child and family to cope with.

Family Support

The nurse should attend to the emotional components of the disease and assess any sources of stress. Frequently, the nurse can help children adjust to problems of growth restriction, delayed sexual maturation, dietary restrictions, feelings of being "different" or "sickly," inability to compete with peers, and necessary absence from school during exacerbations of the illness.

If a permanent colectomy-ileostomy is required, the nurse can teach the child and family how to care for the ileostomy. The nurse can also emphasize the positive aspects of the surgery, particularly accelerated growth and sexual development, permanent recovery, eliminated risk of colon cancer in UC, and normality of life despite bowel diversion. Introducing the child and parents to other ostomy patients, especially those who are the same age, can be effective in fostering eventual acceptance. Whenever possible, continent ostomies should be offered as options to the child.

Because of the chronic and often lifelong nature of the disease, families benefit from the educational services provided by organizations such as the Crohn's and Colitis Foundation of Canada (see Additional Resources at the end of this chapter). Adolescents often benefit by participating in peer-support groups, which are sponsored by the CCFC.

Peptic Ulcer Disease

Peptic ulcers may be classified as acute or chronic, and peptic ulcer disease (PUD) is a chronic condition that affects the stomach or duodenum. Ulcers are described as gastric or duodenal and as primary or secondary. A *gastric ulcer* involves the mucosa of the stomach; a *duodenal ulcer* involves the pylorus or duodenum. Most *primary ulcers* occur in the absence of a predisposing factor and tend to be chronic, occurring more frequently in the duodenum. *Stress ulcers* result from the stress of a severe underlying disease or injury (e.g., severe burns, sepsis, increased intracranial pressure, severe trauma, multisystem organ failure) and are more frequently acute and gastric. About 25% of hospitalized critically ill children have evidence of gastric bleeding (Blanchard & Czinn, 2007).

About 1.7% of children in general pediatric practices have PUD, and the disease represents about 3.4% per 10,000 of pediatric hospital admissions. Primary ulcers are more common in children older than 6 years, and stress ulcers are more common in infants younger than 6 months. Except for very young children, the incidence is two to three times greater in boys than in girls.

Etiology

The exact cause is unknown, although infectious, genetic, and environmental factors are important. There is an increased familial incidence, and the disease is increased in persons with blood group O.

There is a significant relationship between the bacterium *Helicobacter pylori* and ulcers. *H. pylori* is a microaerophilic, gram-negative, slow-growing, spiral-shaped, and flagellated bacterium known to colonize the gastric mucosa in about half of the population of the world (Blanchard & Czinn, 2007; Czinn, 2005). It has been identified in 90 to 100% of adult patients with PUD. *H. pylori* synthesizes the enzyme urease, which hydrolyses urea to form ammonia and carbon dioxide. Ammonia then absorbs acid to form ammonium, thus raising the gastric pH. Also, its flagella allow the bacterium to swim across the viscous gastric mucus and reach the more neutral gastric pH below the mucus (Sgouros & Bergele, 2006). *H. pylori* may cause ulcers by weakening the gastric mucosal barrier and allowing acid to damage the mucosa. It is believed that it is acquired via the fecal–oral route; this hypothesis is supported by finding viable *H. pylori* in feces.

In addition to ulcerogenic medications, both alcohol and smoking contribute to ulcer formation. There is no conclusive evidence to implicate particular foods such as caffeine-containing beverages or spicy foods, but polyunsaturated fats and fibre may play a role in ulcer formation. Psychological factors may play a role in the development of PUD, and stressful life events, dependency, passiveness, and hostility have all been implicated as contributing factors.

Pathophysiology

Most likely, the pathology is due to an imbalance between the destructive (cytotoxic) factors and defensive (cytoprotective) factors in the GI tract. The toxic mechanisms include acid, pepsin, medications such as aspirin and nonsteroidal anti-inflammatory drugs (NSAIDs), bile acids, and infection with *H. pylori*. The defensive factors include the mucus layer, local bicarbonate secretion, epithelial cell renewal, and mucosal blood flow. Prostaglandins play a role in mucosal defense because they stimulate both mucus and alkali secretion. The primary mechanism that prevents the development of peptic ulcer is the secretion of mucus by the epithelial and mucus glands throughout the stomach. The thick mucus layer acts to diffuse acid from the lumen to the gastric mucosal surface, thus protecting the gastric epithelium. The stomach and duodenum produce bicarbonate, decreasing acidity on the epithelial cells and thereby minimizing the effects of the low pH (Chelimsky & Czinn, 2001). When abnormalities in the protective barrier exist, the mucosa is vulnerable to damage by acid and pepsin. Exogenous factors, such as aspirin and NSAIDs, cause gastric ulcers by inhibition of prostaglandin synthesis.

Zollinger-Ellison syndrome may occur in children who have multiple, large, or recurrent ulcers. This syndrome is characterized by hypersecretion of gastric acid, intractable ulcer disease, and intestinal malabsorption caused by a gastrin-secreting tumour of the pancreas.

Diagnostic Evaluation

Diagnosis is based on the history of symptoms, physical examination, and diagnostic testing. The focus is on symptoms such as epigastric abdominal pain, nocturnal pain, oral regurgitation, heartburn, weight loss, hematemesis, and melena (Box 47-13). History should include questions relating to the use of potentially causative substances such as NSAIDs,

BOX 47-13 Characteristics of Peptic Ulcer Disease

Neonates

Usually gastric and secondary to stress or critical illness
Commonly has a history of preterm birth, respiratory distress, sepsis, hypoglycemia, or an intraventricular hemorrhage
Perforation may be first sign that massive bleeding may occur

Infants to 3-Year-Old Children

Most likely to have a secondary ulcer located equally in the stomach or duodenum
Primary ulcers less common and usually located in stomach
Likely to occur in relation to illness, surgery, or trauma
Hematemesis, melena, or perforation

2- to 6-Year-Old Children

Primary or secondary ulcers
Located equally in stomach and duodenum
Perforation more likely in secondary ulcers
Periumbilical pain, poor eating, vomiting, irritability, nighttime waking, hematemesis, melena

Children 6 Years and Older

Usually primary and most often duodenal
More typical of adult type
Chance of recurrence greater
Often associated with *Helicobacter pylori*
Epigastric or vague abdominal pain
Possibly nighttime waking, hematemesis, melena, and anemia

corticosteroids, alcohol, and tobacco. Laboratory studies may include a CBC to detect anemia, stool analysis for occult blood, liver function tests (LFTs), sedimentation rate, or CRP to evaluate IBD; amylase and lipase to evaluate pancreatitis; and gastric acid measurements to identify hypersecretion. A lactose breath test may be performed to detect lactose intolerance.

Radiographic studies such as an upper GI series may be performed to evaluate obstruction or malrotation. An upper endoscopy is the most reliable procedure to diagnose PUD. A biopsy is taken to determine the presence of *H. pylori. H. pylori* can also be diagnosed by a blood test that identifies the presence of the antigen to this organism. The C-urea breath test measures bacterial colonization in the gastric mucosa. This test is used to screen for *H. pylori* in adults and children. Polyclonal and monoclonal stool antigen tests are an accurate noninvasive method for both the initial diagnosis of *H. pylori* and the confirmation of its eradication after treatment (Gisbert, de la Morena, & Abraira, 2006).

Therapeutic Management

The major goals of therapy for children with PUD are to relieve discomfort, promote healing, prevent complications, and prevent recurrence. Management is primarily medical and consists of administration of medications to treat the infection and reduce or neutralize gastric acid secretion. Antacids are beneficial medications to neutralize gastric acid. Histamine (H_2) receptor antagonists (antisecretory medications) act to suppress gastric acid production. Cimetidine (Tagamet), ranitidine (Zantac), and famotidine (Pepcid) are examples of these medications. They have few adverse effects.

PPIs, such as omeprazole and lansoprazole, act to inhibit the hydrogen ion pump in the parietal cells, thus blocking the production of acid. Controlled studies of these drugs have been done in adults, and they are now commonly used to treat ulcers in children. They appear to be well tolerated and have infrequent adverse effects (e.g., headache, diarrhea, nausea and vomiting).

Mucosal protective agents, such as sucralfate and bismuth-containing preparations, may be prescribed for PUD. Sucralfate is an aluminum-containing agent that forms a protective barrier over ulcerated mucosa to protect against acid and pepsin. Sucralfate is available in both pill and liquid forms. Because sucralfate blocks the absorption of other medications, it should be given separately from them.

Bismuth compounds are sometimes prescribed for the relief of ulcers, but they are used less frequently than PPIs. Although these compounds inhibit the growth of microorganisms, the mechanism of their activity is poorly understood. In combination with antibiotics, bismuth is effective against *H. pylori.* Although concern has been expressed about the use of bismuth salts in children because of potential adverse effects, none of these effects has been reported when these compounds have been used in the treatment of *H. pylori* infection.

Triple medication therapy is the recommended treatment regimen for *H. pylori* (O'Connor, Gisbert, & O'Morain, 2009). Combination therapy has demonstrated 90% effectiveness in eradication of *H. pylori* when compared with antibiotic monotherapy. Examples of medication combinations used in triple therapy are (1) bismuth, clarithromycin, and metronidazole, (2) lansoprazole, amoxicillin, and clarithromycin, and (3) metronidazole, clarithromycin, and omeprazole. Common adverse effects of medications include diarrhea, nausea, and vomiting.

In addition to medications, the child with PUD should be given a nutritious diet and advised to avoid caffeine. Adolescents should be warned about gastric irritation associated with alcohol use and smoking.

Children with an acute ulcer who have developed complications, such as massive hemorrhage, require emergency care. The administration of IV fluids, blood, or plasma depends on the amount of blood loss. Replacement with whole blood or packed cells may be necessary for significant loss.

Surgical intervention may be required for complications such as hemorrhage, perforation, or gastric outlet obstruction. Ligation of the source of bleeding or closure of a perforation is performed. A vagotomy and pyloroplasty may be indicated in children with recurring ulcers despite aggressive medical treatment.

Prognosis

The long-term prognosis for PUD is variable. Many ulcers are treated successfully with medical therapy; however, primary duodenal peptic ulcers often recur. Complications such as GI bleeding can occur and extend into adult life. The effect of maintenance medication therapy on long-term morbidity remains to be established with further studies.

Nursing Care Management

The primary nursing goal is to promote healing of the ulcer through compliance with the medication regimen. If an **analgesic–antipyretic** is needed, acetaminophen, not aspirin or an NSAID, is used. Critically ill neonates, infants, and children in critical care units should receive H_2 blockers to prevent stress ulcers. Critically ill children receiving IV H_2 blockers should have their gastric pH values checked at frequent intervals.

The role of stress in ulcer formation should be considered for nonhospitalized children with chronic illnesses. In children, many ulcers occur secondary to other conditions, and the nurse should be aware of family and environmental conditions that may aggravate or precipitate ulcers. Children may benefit from psychological counselling and learning how to cope constructively with stress.

Hepatic Disorders

Acute Hepatitis

Etiology

Hepatitis is an acute or chronic inflammation of the liver that can result from several different causes (e.g., virus, chemical or medication reaction, or other diseases). Nonviral causes of hepatitis include autoimmune hepatitis, Wilson's disease, α_1-antitrypsin deficiency, and steatohepatitis. The following six viruses cause 90% of cases of viral hepatitis (Table 47-7):

1. Hepatitis A virus (HAV)
2. Hepatitis B virus (HBV)
3. Hepatitis C virus (HCV)
4. Hepatitis D virus (HDV)
5. Hepatitis E virus (HEV)
6. Hepatitis G virus (HGV)

Hepatitis A

HAV is the most common form of acute viral hepatitis in most parts of the world. It is a member of the picornavirus family. The virus produces a contagious disease transmitted primarily in contaminated stool spread via the fecal–oral route from person to person. HAV has been associated with miniepidemics in areas of poor hygiene and high population density. There is no chronic or carrier state.

HAV infection affects individuals of all ages, but the highest incidence occurs among preschool- or school-age children younger than 15 years. Children may serve as the source of HAV infection in adults, such as in child care centre exposures. Usually HAV disease in children is mild. It is frequently anicteric and often subclinical. Infected children who show no symptoms may still spread the virus to others. HAV can be severe in children with immunodeficiency disorders. The incubation period is approximately 3 weeks.

Although some cases may be prolonged, the prognosis is excellent. A highly effective vaccine for HAV is available in Canada (see Chapter 36) and is recommended for high-risk patients or persons travelling to a endemic geographical area (Cybulska, Ni, Jimenenez-Rivera, 2011) (see Chapter 6, Hepatitis A).

Hepatitis B

HBV infection can occur as an acute or chronic infection and may range from being asymptomatic and limited to causing fatal fulminant (rapid and severe) hepatitis. HBV varies greatly throughout the world. High-prevalence areas have been identified in Africa and Asia; Canada is considered a low-prevalence area. Transmission is usually via the parenteral route through the exchange of blood or any bodily secretion or fluid. Infections from blood transfusion have been reduced as a result of blood product–screening procedures. Transplantation of organs, intimate physical contact, transmission from mother to infant, and the splashing of contaminated fluids into the mouth or eyes are other sources of infection. Adults whose occupations are associated with exposure to blood or blood products (such as health care workers) are at increased risk for infection and should receive HBV vaccination.

Most HBV infection in children is acquired perinatally. Newborns are at risk for hepatitis if the mother is infected with HBV or was a carrier of HBV during pregnancy. Possible routes of maternal–fetal or maternal–infant transmission include (1) leakage of virus across the placenta late in pregnancy (less than 2% of cases) or during labour, and (2) ingestion of amniotic fluid or maternal blood. Infants who have HBV infection are more than 90% likely to become chronic carriers (Tran, 2009). The incubation period of HBV infection varies from 45 to 160 days.

HBV infection occurs in children and adolescents in the following high-risk groups (see Box 6-6):

- Individuals with hemophilia and others who have received multiple transfusions
- Children and adolescents involved in IV drug use
- Institutionalized children and adolescents
- Preschool-age children in endemic areas
- Individuals engaged in sexual activity with infected partners

Hepatitis C

The number of HCV-positive individuals in Canada is estimated to be 220,000 (Sherman et al., 2007); the highest risk factor is a history of injection drug use. HCV is transmitted through contaminated blood, especially as a result of IV drug use, and from mother to child. Infected HCV mothers transmit between 5 and 20% to children, but the rate varies according to the presence or absence of certain cofactors (particularly maternal coinfection with HIV) and medical conditions (CPS, 2002) (see Chapter 6). One out of 120 mothers in Canada has HCV. Another common route of infection is by percutaneous exposure, which occurs through transfusion of blood or blood products, transplantation of organs or tissues, or sharing of used needles. Transfusion-associated HCV infection is low. The Canadian Paediatric Society (2002) recommends screening the following:

- All infants born to HCV-infected women
- Individuals who received blood products or solid organ transplants before 1992
- Individuals involved in injection drug use

Table 47-7 Comparison of Types A, B, and C Hepatitis

CHARACTERISTICS	TYPE A	TYPE B	TYPE C
Incubation period	15-50 days, average 25-30 days	30-180 days, average 50 days	2 wk-6 mo, average 6-7 wk
Period of communicability	Believed to be later half of incubation period to first week after onset of clinical illness	Variable Virus in blood or other body fluids during late incubation period and acute stage of disease; may persist in carrier state for years to lifetime	Begins before onset of symptoms May persist in carrier state for years
Mode of transmission	Principal route—Fecal-oral Rarely—Parenteral	Principal route—parenteral Less frequent route—oral, sexual, any body fluid Perinatal transfer—transplacental blood (last trimester), at delivery, or during breastfeeding, especially if mother has cracked nipples	Principal route—parenteral Nonparenteral spread possible
Clinical Features			
Onset	Usually rapid, acute	More insidious	Usually insidious
Fever	Common and early	Less frequent	Less frequent
Anorexia	Common	Mild to moderate	Mild to moderate
Nausea and vomiting	Common	Sometimes present	Mild to moderate
Rash	Rare	Common	Sometimes present
Arthralgia	Rare	Common	Rare
Pruritus	Rare	Sometimes present	Sometimes present
Jaundice	Present (many cases anicteric)	Present	Present
Other Features			
Immunity	Present after one attack; no crossover to type B or C	Present after one attack; no crossover to type A or C	Present after one attack; no crossover to type A or B
Carrier state	No	Yes	Yes
Chronic infection	No	Yes	Yes
Prophylaxis			
Immune globulin (Ig)	Passive immunity Successful, especially in early incubation period and pre-exposure prophylaxis	May provide passive immunity Inconsistent benefits; probably of no use	
HAV vaccine	Two inactivated vaccines are approved for children ages 2-18 yr: Havrix and Vaqta; given in a two-dose schedule (6-12 mo between doses)		
HBV Ig (HBIg)	No benefit	Provides passive immunity Postexposure protection possible (for 3-6 months) if given immediately after definite exposure	No benefit
HBV vaccine	No benefit	Provides active immunity Universal vaccination recommended for all children (either newborn or school age, depending on province or territory)	No benefit
Mortality rate			
	0.1%-0.2%	0.5%-2.0% in uncomplicated cases; may be higher in complicated cases	1%-2.0% in uncomplicated cases; may be higher in complicated case

HAV, hepatitis A virus; *HBV*, hepatitis B virus.

- Persons in settings where HCV prevalence is high and risk-factor ascertainment is poor (sexually transmitted disease clinics, correctional facilities)

The clinical course of HCV infection varies. Incubation averages 6 to 7 weeks, with a range of 2 weeks to 6 months. Both acute and chronic HCV infection often produce only mild nonspecific symptoms or no symptoms at all (CPS, 2002). The length of time that maternal antibody is present in infants born to HCV-infected women must be considered, and screening should be done after the infant is 18 months old. However, a routine screening program, such as that for HBV, is not recommended. Current recommendations are to evaluate HCV-infected children at regular intervals to monitor for chronic hepatitis. Most children will be asymptomatic with evidence of chronic hepatitis on liver biopsy. Liver enzyme levels may fluctuate between periods of normal and elevated values.

Hepatitis D

HDV is an important cause of acute and chronic liver disease. HDV is a defective RNA virus that requires the presence of HBV. HDV infection occurs primarily in hemophiliac patients and IV drug users. The incubation period is 2 to 8 weeks. Both acute and chronic forms are more severe than HBV infection and can lead to cirrhosis. Testing for HDV infection is recommended in children with chronic HBV infection or severe liver disease and in children with acute exacerbation of a previously stable liver disease.

Hepatitis E

HEV infection is enterally transmitted. Transmission may occur through the fecal–oral route or from contaminated water. The incubation period is 2 to 9 weeks. This illness is uncommon in children, does not cause chronic liver disease, is not a chronic condition, and has no carrier state. The mortality rate resulting from submassive hepatic necrosis is low except in pregnant women in their third trimester, in whom mortality reaches 20%.

Hepatitis G

HGV is a blood-borne virus that may also be transmitted by organ transplantation. High-risk groups include transfusion recipients, IV drug users, and individuals infected with HCV. Individuals with the virus are often asymptomatic, and most infections are chronic. The incubation period is unknown.

Diagnostic Evaluation

Diagnosis is based on the history (especially regarding possible exposure to a hepatitis virus); physical examination; and serological markers (antibodies or antigens) indicating the presence of active infection with hepatitis A, B, or C or previous infection. Because the liver has a large functional reserve, abnormal laboratory tests may be the only indication of hepatitis. However, LFTs are not specific for the diagnosis of viral hepatitis. Although serum aspartate aminotransferase (AST) and ALT levels are markedly elevated in viral hepatitis, other diseases or conditions may cause their elevation. Serum bilirubin levels peak 5 to 10 days after clinical jaundice appears. When hepatitis is severe, albumin levels are depressed, and prothrombin times are increased.

Diagnosis of viral hepatitis is based on the presence of specific viral markers. Diagnosis of acute HAV infection is based on the presence of anti-HAV immune globulin (immune globulin M [IgM]) antibody in the serum. HBV diagnosis depends on the presence of hepatitis B surface antigen (HBsAg) or anti-HBV core (anti-HBc) IgM antibody. Chronic HBV infection is associated with the persistence of HBsAg and HBV DNA markers. The diagnosis of HCV is based on the detection of anti-HCV antibodies and confirmation by polymerase chain reaction (PCR) for hepatitis C RNA.

An abdominal ultrasound scan provides measurement of liver size, detection of cystic lesions and stones, and imaging of the gallbladder. Cholescintigraphy radionuclide imaging detects abnormalities in liver uptake, concentration, and excretory function. Finally, a liver biopsy aids in assessing the severity of the disease.

Pathophysiology

Pathological changes occur primarily in the parenchymal cells of the liver and result in varying degrees of swelling, infiltration of liver cells by mononuclear cells, subsequent degeneration, necrosis, and fibrosis.

Hepatitis can be self-limited, and complete regeneration of liver cells without scarring may occur. However, some forms of hepatitis do not result in complete return of liver function. These include *fulminant hepatitis*, which is characterized by a severe, acute course and massive destruction of the liver, resulting in liver failure and death in 1 to 2 weeks. *Subacute* or *chronic active hepatitis* is characterized by progressive liver destruction, uncertain regeneration, scarring, and potential cirrhosis.

The initial *anicteric* (absence of jaundice) *phase* usually lasts 5 to 7 days and is often mistaken for influenza. Symptoms include nausea, vomiting, extreme anorexia, malaise, easy fatigability, arthralgia, skin rashes, slight to moderate fever, and epigastric or upper right quadrant abdominal pain. Dark urine is a symptom of the *icteric* (jaundice) *phase*. Pruritus may accompany jaundice and can be bothersome, but many children with acute viral hepatitis do not develop jaundice.

Therapeutic Management

Treatment options for viral hepatitis are limited. The goals of management include early detection, recognition of chronic liver disease, support and monitoring, and prevention of spread of the disease.

HAV infection is an acute disease that resolves with support and management of symptoms. Treatment of HBV and HCV is directed at managing the viral load to prevent further destruction of the liver. Currently, HBV and HCV are treated with interferons, naturally occurring proteins that exert antiviral, antiproliferative, and immunomodulatory effects. An interferon formulation, pegylated interferon, can be administered once a week and has been found to sustain plasma levels and enhance viral suppression (Karnam & Reddy, 2003). Lamivudine and adefovir are two other interferon analogs that suppress the replication of HBV (Yuen & Lai, 2001). A combination of α-interferon and ribavirin has resulted in a sustained response in only 50% of patients with HBV and HCV (Waters & Nelson, 2006).

Another important aspect of the therapeutic management of hepatitis involves hospitalization. Hospitalization is necessary if coagulopathy or fulminant hepatitis is present.

Prevention

Proper hand hygiene and standard isolation precautions can prevent the spread of hepatitis. Prophylactic use of standard immune globulin is effective in preventing HAV infection in situations of pre-exposure (e.g., anticipated travel to areas where HAV is prevalent) or in situations of postexposure during the early part of the incubation period. Hepatitis B immune globulin (HBIg) is effective in preventing HBV infection after exposure. Immune globulin and HBIg must be administered less than 2 weeks after exposure.

Vaccines have been developed to prevent HAV and HBV infection. Since the early 1990s, all provinces and territories have had either a universal school-based hepatitis B vaccination program aimed at children aged 9 to 13 or an infant vaccination program (PHAC, 2006). HBV vaccination is also recommended for high-risk groups. HAV vaccination is recommended for all children beginning at age 12 months and for certain high-risk groups (see Immunizations, Chapter 36). Active immunizations are not available against HCV. It is possible to prevent HDV infection by preventing HBV infection.

Prognosis

The prognosis for children with hepatitis varies and depends on the type of virus. HAV usually causes a mild and brief illness with no carrier state. HBV causes a wide spectrum of acute and chronic illness. Approximately 5% of individuals develop chronic hepatitis B each year, and about half of these develop fulminant liver failure, leading to death in the absence of liver transplantation (Kim et al., 2005). Hepatocellular carcinoma is a potentially fatal complication of HBV infection. HCV causes acute hepatitis that progresses to chronic disease in more than 85% of affected individuals, with approximately 15 to 20% developing cirrhosis or hepatocellular carcinoma (Richmond, Dunning, & Desmond, 2004). HCV infection is a common reason for liver transplantation in adults in Canada (CPS, 2002).

Nursing Care Management

Nursing management depends on the severity of the hepatitis, the medical management, and factors influencing the control and transmission of the disease. Children with benign viral hepatitis are frequently cared for at home, and the clinic or office nurse must explain the medical therapy and control measures. If further assistance is needed for parents to follow through with the therapy, a home health nursing referral may be necessary.

A well-balanced diet and a realistic schedule of rest and activity adjusted to the child's condition should be encouraged. HAV is not infectious within a week after the onset of jaundice, and children may feel well enough to resume school. Parents need to be cautioned about administering any medication to the child, since normal dosages of many medications may become dangerous because of the liver's inability to detoxify and excrete them. Hand hygiene is the single most critical measure in reducing the risk of transmission. The nurse should explain to parents and children the ways in which HAV (oral–fecal route) and HBV (parenteral route) are spread.

Nurses caring for young people with HBV infection and a known or suspected history of illicit IV drug use should help these teens realize the dangers of substance use. Nurses should stress the parenteral mode of transmission of hepatitis and encourage them to seek counselling through a substance use program. HBV and HCV are chronic diseases that require frequent monitoring and management. Many communities have multidisciplinary clinics dedicated to the management of these diseases.

Cirrhosis

Cirrhosis occurs at the end stage of many chronic liver diseases, including biliary atresia (BA) and chronic hepatitis. Cirrhosis can also result from infectious, autoimmune, or toxic factors and from chronic diseases such as hemophilia and cystic fibrosis. A cirrhotic liver is irreversibly damaged.

Clinical manifestations in children are similar to those seen with all chronic liver disorders. Children exhibit jaundice, poor growth, anorexia, muscle weakness, and lethargy. Ascites, edema, GI bleeding, anemia, and abdominal pain may be present with impaired intrahepatic blood flow. Pulmonary function may be impaired because of pressure against the diaphragm from hepatosplenomegaly and ascites. Dyspnea and cyanosis may occur, especially on exertion. Intrapulmonary arteriovenous shunts may develop and cause hypoxemia. Spider angiomas and prominent blood vessels are often present on the upper torso.

Therapeutic Management

Therapy is directed toward (1) frequent assessment of liver status with physical examination and LFTs, and (2) management of specific complications. The only successful treatment for end-stage liver disease and liver failure may be liver transplantation, which has improved the prognosis substantially for many children with cirrhosis. Currently, the 1- and 5-year survival rate for liver transplantation in children is 87% and 77%, respectively; children under 1 year have a poorer 1-year survival (85%) rate than older children (90%) (Hurwitz & Cox, 2007). Increasing numbers of recipients are reaching their second decade after transplant. The increasing lifespan after transplantation is related to advances in surgical techniques and improved preoperative, intraoperative, and postoperative care.

Prognosis

Liver transplantation has revolutionized the approach to liver cirrhosis. Liver failure and cirrhosis are indications for transplantation. Liver transplantation reflects the failure of other medical and surgical measures to prevent or treat cirrhosis. Careful monitoring of the child's condition and quality of life is necessary to evaluate the need for and timing of transplantation (see Family-Centred Teaching box).

Nursing Care Management

Nursing care of the child with cirrhosis is determined by the cause of the cirrhosis, the severity of complications, and the prognosis. The prognosis for life is poor unless successful liver

FAMILY-CENTRED TEACHING

End-Stage Liver Disease

In many cases the child and family must cope with an uncertain progression of the disease. The only hope for long-term survival may be liver transplantation. Transplantation can be very successful, but the waiting period may be long, and there are many more children in need of organs than there are donors. The procedure is performed only at designated medical centres that are often far from the family's home. The nurse should recognize the unique stresses of coping with end-stage liver disease and waiting for transplantation and assist the family in coping with these stressors. The assistance of social workers and support from other parents can be very beneficial.

transplantation occurs. Nursing care of this child is similar to that for any child with a life-threatening illness (see Chapter 41). Hospitalization is usually required when complications occur.

Biliary Atresia

BA is a destructive, idiopathic, inflammatory process that leads to fibrosis and obliteration of the biliary tree (Emerick & Whitington, 2006). BA has been detected in 3.7 in 10,000 live births (Chen et al., 2006). The disorder is more common in girls and preterm infants. The incidence is twice as high in Black as in White infants and more common in Chinese than in either Japanese or White populations.

Etiology and Pathophysiology

The exact cause of BA is unknown. Because it has two distinct forms, postnatal and fetal-embryonic, different pathogenic mechanisms are suggested. Postnatal BA represents 65 to 90% of cases and is probably the result of infection or an immune-mediated mechanism.

Jaundice, manifesting with yellow discolouration of the skin or sclerae, is the most common early symptom of BA. Jaundice, indicating cholestasis (the accumulation of compounds that cannot be excreted because of occlusion or obstruction of the biliary tree), can be visible at a total serum bilirubin concentration as low as 85 mcmol/L. An abnormal direct bilirubin has been designated as greater than17 mcmol/L if the total bilirubin is less than 85 mcmol/L or a value of direct bilirubin that represents more than 20% of the total bilirubin if it is greater than 85 mcmol/L (Emerick &Whitington, 2006). Direct hyperbilirubinemia first appears after the resolution of physiological (neonatal) jaundice. Jaundice is often associated with pale stool and dark urine. Histological study demonstrates bile duct remnants and a progressive inflammatory process.

In the fetal embryonic form of BA, which represents 10 to 35% of cases, there is a congenital absence of biliary ductal patency and an absence of bile duct remnants. Many infants have associated congenital anomalies. Varying degrees of cholestasis occur, resulting in retention of irritants and toxins. Injury to the liver occurs as the result of the inflammation caused by the cholestasis.

Diagnostic Evaluation

Early diagnosis is the key to survival of the child with BA. Infants who undergo surgery in the first 60 days of life have an 80% chance of establishing bile flow. Between 60 and 90 days of life, the chance of re-establishing flow drops to 50%, and after 90 days to 10% (Chen et al., 2006). The typical infant is thriving, appears well, and has only very mild jaundice during the first 6 to 8 weeks (Emerick & Whitington, 2006) but will soon begin failing to grow and thrive.

Several clinical signs may indicate the presence of BA (Box 47-14). Blood tests should include a CBC, electrolytes, bilirubin, and liver enzymes. Additional laboratory analyses, including α_1-antitrypsin level, TORCH titres (see discussion of maternal infections in Chapter 28, p. 748), hepatitis serology, α-fetoprotein, urine cytomegalovirus, and a sweat test, are indicated to rule out other conditions that cause persistent cholestasis and jaundice. Abdominal ultrasonography allows inspection of the liver and biliary system. Hepatobiliary scintigraphy demonstrates biliary patency but does not provide diagnostic certainty. Endoscopic retrograde cholangiopancreatography (ERCP) is performed in very young infants. This procedure, which is done using general anaesthesia, has an 80% reported diagnostic accuracy. Percutaneous liver biopsy is highly reliable when the biopsy contains specimens from a number of portal areas. Definitive diagnosis of BA is obtained during surgical **laparotomy** and an intraoperative cholangiogram.

Therapeutic Management

The primary treatment of BA is *hepatic portoenterostomy (Kasai procedure)*, in which a segment of intestine is anastomosed to the resected porta hepatis to attempt bile drainage. Bile drainage is achieved in approximately 80 to 90% of infants who undergo surgery when younger than 10 weeks of age (Ohi, 2001). However, progressive cirrhosis still occurs in many children, necessitating liver transplantation. Prophylactic antibiotics are given after the Kasai procedure to minimize the risk of ascending cholangitis.

BOX 47-14 Clinical Manifestations of Extrahepatic Biliary Atresia

Jaundice

Earliest manifestation and most striking feature of disorder

First observed in sclera

May be present at birth, but usually not apparent until age 2 to 3 weeks

Urine dark and stains diaper

Stools lighter than expected or white or tan

Hepatomegaly and abdominal distension common

Splenomegaly occurs later

Poor fat metabolism results in:

- Poor weight gain
- General growth failure

Pruritus

Irritability; difficulty comforting infant

Medical management is primarily supportive. It includes nutritional support with infant formulas that contain medium-chain triglycerides and essential fatty acids. Supplementation is usually required with fat-soluble vitamins, a multivitamin, and minerals, including iron, zinc, and selenium. Aggressive nutritional support with continuous tube feedings or TPN is indicated for moderate to severe growth failure (failure to thrive). The enteral solution should be low in sodium. Ursodeoxycholic acid is used to treat pruritus and hypercholesterolemia.

Prognosis

Untreated BA results in progressive cirrhosis and death in most children by 2 years of age. The Kasai procedure improves the prognosis but is not a cure. Biliary drainage can often be achieved if the surgery is done before the intrahepatic bile ducts are destroyed. Long-term survival has been reported in children who receive the Kasai procedure; however, even with successful bile drainage, many children ultimately develop liver failure.

Advances in surgical techniques and the use of immunosuppressive and antifungal medications have improved the success of transplantation. The major obstacle continues to be a shortage of donor livers. Reduced-size, split-liver transplantation, retransplantation, and increased public awareness may improve donor organ availability in the future.

Nursing Care Management

Nursing interventions for the child with BA include support of the family before, during, and after surgical procedures and education regarding the treatment plan. In the postoperative period of a portoenterostomy, nursing care is similar to that after major abdominal surgery. Family members need education relating to the proper administration of medications and nutritional therapy, including special formulas, vitamin and mineral supplements, tube feedings, or parenteral nutrition. Pruritus can often be relieved by medication therapy or comfort measures such as baths; trimming fingernails may help decrease the chance of secondary infection as a result of skin breakdown.

Children and their families also need psychosocial support. The uncertain prognosis, discomfort, and waiting for transplantation produce stress, and hospitalizations, pharmacological therapy, and nutritional therapy impose financial burdens on the family. Families can receive help from the Canadian Liver Foundation, which provides educational materials, programs, and support systems (see Additional Resources section at the end of this chapter).

Structural Defects

Cleft Lip or Cleft Palate

Clefts of the lip (CL) and palate (CP) are facial malformations that occur during embryonic development and are the most common congenital deformities of the head and neck. They may appear separately or, more often, together. CL results from failure of the maxillary and median nasal processes to fuse; CP is a midline fissure of the palate that results from failure of the two sides to fuse.

CL may vary from a small notch to a complete cleft extending into the base of the nose (see Fig. 28-13). Clefts can be unilateral or bilateral. Deformed dental structures are associated with CL. CP alone occurs in the midline and may involve the soft and hard palates. When associated with CL, the defect may involve the midline and extend into the soft palate on one or both sides.

Cleft lip and palate (CL/P) is more common than CP alone and varies by ethnicity. These malformations are two of the most common birth defects in Canada and affect between 400 and 500 newborns every year (Health Canada, 2002). There is a higher incidence in certain ethnic groups, including the First Nations, Métis, and Inuit populations (Health Canada, 2002). Approximately 60 to 80% of children born with CL/P are male. Females have a higher frequency of isolated clefts of the secondary palate. Unilateral clefts are nine times more common than bilateral clefts and occur twice as frequently on the left side. Isolated bilateral CLs are uncommon; approximately 86% of those with bilateral CL also have palatal clefts. Approximately 68% of those with unilateral CLs have an associated palatal cleft (Kirschner & LaRossa, 2000). Although the majority of clefts are nonsyndromic (have no associated identifiable syndrome), associated syndromes occur in varying frequencies according to the specific defect; it is estimated that 10 to 50% of children with CL/P have an associated syndrome (Curtin & Boekelheide, 2004; Merritt, 2005a).

Etiology

Cleft deformities may be an isolated anomaly, or they may occur with a recognized syndrome. CL with or without CP is distinct from isolated CP. Clefts of the secondary palate alone are more likely to be associated with syndromes than is isolated CL or CL/P.

CL/P may be caused by exposure to teratogens such as alcohol, anticonvulsants, steroids, and retinoids. Use of phenytoin during pregnancy is associated with a 10-fold increase in the incidence of CL. The incidence of CL among mothers who smoke during pregnancy is twice as great as the incidence in mothers who do not (Eppley et al., 2005). Alcohol consumption (especially binge drinking) in the first trimester is associated with a higher incidence of oral clefts (DeRoo et al., 2008).

evolve Case Study—Cleft Lip and Palate

Pathophysiology

Cleft deformities represent a genetic defect in cell migration that results in a failure of the maxillary and premaxillary processes to come together between the third and twelfth week of embryonic development. Although often appearing together, CL and CP are distinct malformations embryologically, occurring at different times during the developmental process. Merging of the upper lip at the midline is completed between the seventh and eleventh weeks of gestation. Fusion of the secondary palate (hard and soft palate) takes place later, between the seventh and twelfth weeks of gestation. In the process of migrating to a horizontal position, the palates are separated by the tongue for a short time. If there is delay in this movement or if the tongue fails to descend soon enough, the remainder of development proceeds, but the palate never fuses.

Diagnostic Evaluation

CL with or without CP is apparent at birth. The defect elicits significant emotional reactions in parents. CP is less obvious than CL and may not be detected without a thorough assessment of the mouth. CP is identified when the examiner places a gloved finger directly on the palate. Clefts of the hard palate form a continuous opening between the mouth and the nasal cavity. The severity of the CP has an impact on feeding; the infant is unable to generate negative pressure and create suction in the oral cavity. This impairs feeding, even though in most cases the infant's ability to swallow is normal.

Prenatal diagnosis with fetal ultrasonography is not reliable until the soft tissues of the fetal face can be visualized at 13 to 14 weeks. The sensitivity of fetal ultrasound for facial clefting is almost 100% when CL/P is associated with other structural anomalies. In isolated CP, sensitivity may be 50%; an intact lip is the most difficult to diagnose prenatally (Wilkins-Haug, 2008).

Therapeutic Management

Treatment of the child with isolated CL is surgical and involves no long-term interventions other than possible scar revision. The management of CP involves the cooperative efforts of a multidisciplinary health care team, including pediatrics, plastic surgery, orthodontics, otolaryngology, speech/language pathology, audiology, nursing, and social work. Management is directed toward closure of the cleft(s), prevention of complications, and facilitation of normal growth and development in the child.

Surgical Correction of Cleft Lip

The two most common procedures for repair of CL are the Tennison-Randall triangular flap (Z-plasty) and the Millard rotational advancement technique; Z-plasty is used less frequently. The difference between these two is that the Tennison-Randall procedure crosses the philtral line and the Millard procedure advances a triangle of tissue in the upper third of the lip and does not cross the midline. Surgeons often use a combination of these two techniques to address individual differences. Improved surgical techniques have minimized scar retraction, and in the absence of infection or trauma, healing occurs with little scar formation. However, optimal cosmetic results are difficult to obtain in severe defects. Surgical correction is usually performed at 10 weeks of age (or 4.5 kg). Additional revisions of the lip may be necessary at a later age.

Surgical Correction of Cleft Palate

Previously, CP repair was postponed until a later age than the repair of the CL to take advantage of palatal changes that take place with normal growth. With advanced surgical and anaesthesia techniques, some surgeons are performing palatal repairs in the neonatal period (Merritt, 2005b; Sandberg, Magee, & Denk, 2002); however, the timing of repair remains controversial and may occur at 9 to 15 months to maximize speech production and growth of the midface. Most surgeons prefer to close the cleft before the child develops faulty speech habits. Persistent velopharyngeal insufficiency, manifested by nasal regurgitation and hypernasal speech, may require a posterior pharyngeal flap procedure. Palatal bone grafting may be performed at a later time to build up bone in the alveolus.

Prognosis

Even with good anatomical closure, most children with CL/P have some degree of compensatory speech pattern that requires speech therapy. Physical problems result from inefficient functioning of the muscles of the soft palate and nasopharynx, improper tooth alignment, and varying degrees of hearing loss. Improper drainage of the middle ear as a result of inefficient function of the eustachian tube contributes to recurrent otitis media and otitis media with effusion, which can cause scarring of the tympanic membrane, leading to hearing impairment in many children with CP. Upper respiratory tract infections require immediate and meticulous attention, and extensive orthodontics and prosthodontics may be needed to correct malposition of teeth and maxillary arches.

Long-term problems are related to the child's social adjustment. The better the physical care, the better is the chance for emotional and social adjustment, although the type of the defect and the degree of residual disability are not always directly related to a satisfactory adjustment. Physical defects are a threat to the self-image, and abnormal speech quality is an impediment to social expression.

Nursing Care Management

The immediate nursing problems in the care of an infant with CL and CP deformities are related to feeding the infant and dealing with the parental reaction to the defect. Facial deformities are especially disturbing to parents; CL is a particularly disfiguring, visible defect that may generate a strong negative response in parents. During the initial phase after birth of an infant with CL or CP, it is important for the nurse to address not only the infant's physical needs but also the parents' emotional needs. The concept that infants with CL or CP are at increased risk for failure of maternal attachment has been challenged. In a few studies, maternal–infant attachment was not negatively affected when measured at 1 year (Speltz et al., 1997) and 24 months of age (Coy, Speltz, & Jones, 2002; Maris et al., 2000).

The nurse should encourage expression of parental grief and fears; such expression may promote attachment in the preoperative period. It is especially important to emphasize the positive aspects of the infant's physical appearance and to express optimism regarding surgical correction while acknowledging the parents' concern. The manner of handling the infant should convey to the parents that the infant is indeed a precious human being.

Feeding

Feeding the newborn with CL/P can be difficult, and teaching the parent to successfully feed the child is perhaps one of the most significant and challenging nursing roles. Growth failure in infants with CL, CP, or both has been attributed to preoperative feeding difficulties. After surgical repair most infants with isolated CL or CP and no associated syndrome gain weight successfully or achieve adequate weight and height for age.

Clefts of the lip or palate reduce the infant's ability to suck, which interferes with compression of the areola and renders breastfeeding and bottle-feeding difficult. Liquid taken into the mouth tends to escape via the CP through the nose.

Feeding is best accomplished with the infant's head in an upright position, either held in the caregiver's hand or cradled in the arm. Standard bottle nipples may be unsuitable for these infants, who are unable to generate the suction required; therefore special nipples or other feeding devices are needed.

Breastfeeding the infant with CL/P is a viable option and in some cases more successful than bottle-feeding (Merritt, 2005b). The nipple is positioned and stabilized well back in the oral cavity so that tongue action facilitates milk expression. However, the suction required to stimulate milk let-down may be absent initially; thus a breast pump may be useful before nursing to stimulate the **let-down reflex**. The advantages to breastfeeding include those described in Chapter 26; in addition, there is evidence that breastfeeding infants with CL/P is protective for otitis media (Lawrence & Lawrence, 2011).

A number of special feeding devices are available for feeding the infant with CL/P, and some are more successful than others, depending on a number of factors (Fig. 47-6). One device is the Cleft Lip/Cleft Palate Nurser, which consists of a squeezable plastic bottle and a cross-cut nipple. The Haberman Special Needs Feeder may also be used successfully in infants with a poor or disorganized suck. The Haberman Feeder has a specially designed valve and nipple to adjust the flow of milk to the infant and prevent choking or gagging. A Gravity Flow nipple attached to a squeezable plastic bottle allows formula to be deposited into the mouth of the infant with CL/P. The Pigeon bottle has a nipple with a Y-cut, and the nipple is slightly larger and more bulbous to fit naturally into the oral cavity. A one-way backflow valve prevents milk from flowing retrograde into the bottle to minimize the amount of air the infant swallows. The Pigeon bottle is not a squeezable feeding system.

Using these various types of nipples for feeding also has the advantage of helping to meet the infant's sucking needs. Muscle development is especially important for later development of speech. The nipple is positioned in such a way that it is compressed by the infant's tongue and existing palate. If a single-slit nipple is used, the slit is placed vertically so that the infant will be able to produce and stop the flow of milk by alternately opening and closing the opening. Regardless of which type of nipple is used, gentle, steady pressure on the base of the bottle reduces the chance of choking or coughing, and the person doing the feeding should resist the temptation to remove the nipple because of the noise the infant makes or for fear that the infant will choke. An indication that the infant needs to stop feeding momentarily is the facial signal, which involves elevated eyebrows and a wrinkled forehead; the nipple may be gently removed to allow the infant to swallow formula in the mouth without getting upset. These infants need frequent burping because they have a tendency to swallow excessive amounts of air.

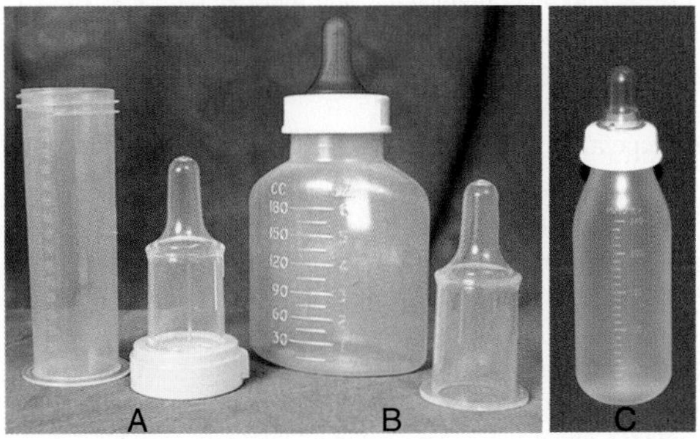

Fig. 47-6 A: Haberman feeder. B: Mead-Johnson bottle used to feed infant with cleft lip and palate. C: Pigeon bottle. *(A and B, Courtesy Texas Children's Hospital, Houston. C, Courtesy Paul Vincent Kuntz, Texas Children's Hospital, Houston.)*

Regardless of the feeding method used, the mother should begin to feed the infant as soon as possible. In this way she is able to help determine the method best suited to her and the infant and to become adept in the technique before discharge.

Preoperative Care

In preparation for surgical repair, parents are frequently taught to accustom the infant to the needs of the early postoperative period, especially if surgery is delayed for several months. The infant must be positioned on the back or side postoperatively. Most infants tolerate these positions well because they are accustomed to being supine for sleeping. It is also helpful to place the infant or child in elbow restraints periodically before admission and to feed the infant with a rubber-tipped Asepto syringe or other device (e.g., soft Sipee cup) that will be used postoperatively.

Postoperative Care for Cleft Lip

The major efforts in the postoperative period are directed toward protecting the operative site. After CL repair (*cheiloplasty*), a metal appliance or adhesive strips are securely taped to the cheeks to relax the surgical site and prevent tension on the suture line caused by crying or other facial movement. Efforts should be made to prevent crying as much as possible to avoid stress on the suture line. Elbow restraints to prevent the infant from rubbing or disturbing the suture line may be applied immediately after surgery. Older infants who roll over require a jacket restraint in addition to restricting arm movement to prevent rolling on the abdomen and rubbing the face on the sheet, especially if the repair involves the lip. It is important to remove the elbow restraints periodically to exercise the arms, provide relief from restrictions, observe the skin for signs of irritation, and provide an opportunity for cuddling and body contact. Sitting the infant in an infant seat provides a change of position and a different view of the environment. Adequate analgesia is required to relieve postoperative pain and to prevent restlessness.

Clear liquids are offered when the infant has fully recovered from the anaesthesia, and feeding is resumed when tolerated. The suture site is carefully cleansed of formula or serosanguineous drainage as needed. A thin layer of antibiotic ointment may be prescribed for application to the suture line after cleansing. Meticulous care of the suture line is essential because inflammation or infection will interfere with optimal healing and the ultimate cosmetic effect of the surgical repair. Gentle aspiration of mouth and nasopharyngeal secretions may be necessary to prevent aspiration and respiratory complications. An upright or infant seat position is helpful in the immediate postoperative period (especially for the infant who has difficulty handling secretions).

Postoperative Care of Cleft Palate

The child with CP repair (*palatoplasty*) is allowed to lie on the abdomen immediately after surgery. The child may resume feeding by breast or cup once the child is fully awake; some surgeons prefer soft Sipee cup or asepto syringe feeding in the postoperative period.

NURSING ALERT Avoid the use of suction or other objects in the mouth, such as tongue depressors, thermometers, pacifiers, spoons, or straws, following a palatoplasty to maintain the integrity of the surgically repaired palate.

Oral packing may be secured to the palate after palatoplasty; this packing is usually removed after 2 to 3 days. Sometimes the infant will have difficulty breathing after surgery because it is often necessary to alter an established pattern of breathing and adjust to breathing through the nose. This is frustrating but seldom requires more than positioning and support. The elbows may be restrained to keep the child's hands away from the mouth. Parents should be instructed to maintain elbow restraints at home until the palate is healed, usually in 4 to 6 weeks. They need to remove the restraints (one at a time) frequently to allow the child to exercise the arms.

The nurse must assess the infant or child's level of postoperative pain. Opioids may be prescribed initially, and acetaminophen may be given as needed thereafter. It is important to manage pain to decrease crying in infants with CL repair.

The older infant or child may be discharged on a blenderized or soft diet, and parents should be instructed to continue the diet until the surgeon directs them otherwise. Parents need to be cautioned against allowing the child to eat hard items (such as toast, hard cookies, and potato chips) that can damage the repaired palate. The expected outcomes are described in the Nursing Process box.

NURSING PROCESS: THE CHILD WITH A CLEFT LIP OR PALATE

Assessment

The lip defect is visible at birth, and assessment involves describing the location and extent of the defect; the cleft palate (CP) is estimated by visualization during crying. CP without cleft lip (CL) is detected by palpating the palate with the gloved finger during the newborn assessment. The emotional impact of the birth of a child with a cosmetic and functional disability is especially traumatic to the family. Consequently, nursing assessment is also concerned with the family's emotional reaction.

Diagnosis (Problem Identification)

After a thorough assessment, several nursing diagnoses are evident:

Imbalanced nutrition: Less than body requirements related to
- oral physical defect
- difficulty eating following surgical procedure

Risk for impaired parenting related to
- infant with a highly visible physical defect

Risk for trauma of the surgical site related to
- infant's developmental need to suck
- increased hand-to-mouth activity

Pain related to
- surgical procedure

Interrupted family processes related to
- child with a physical defect, hospitalization

Planning

The goals of care are related to preoperative care, short-term postoperative care, and long-term management. Goals for the infant and family include the following:

Preoperative Care

Family will cope with the impact of an infant with a defect.
Infant will receive optimal nutrition.
Infant and family will be prepared for surgery.

Postoperative Care

Infant will experience no trauma and minimal or no pain.
Infant will receive optimal nutrition.
Infant will experience no complications.
Infant and family will receive adequate support.
Family will be prepared for care at home and long-term needs of a child with CP.

Implementation

Numerous intervention strategies are discussed on pp. 1421–1425.

Evaluation

The effectiveness of nursing interventions for the family and the child who has CP is determined by continual assessment and evaluation of care based on the following guidelines:

Preoperative Care

Observe and interview family members about their understanding, feelings, and concerns regarding the defect; any anticipated surgery; and their interactions with the infant.
Observe infant during feeding.
Complete preoperative checklist.

Postoperative Care

Inspect operative site, including the protective device.
Observe operative site for evidence of infection, bleeding, sloughing, or irritation.
Observe for behavioural and physiological indicators of pain and response to analgesics.
Observe infant during feeding, measure intake and output, and weigh infant daily.
Observe and interview family regarding their understanding and concerns about the infant, including long-term needs.

Long-Term Care

Children with CL/P often require a variety of services during recovery. Family members need support and encouragement from health care providers and guidance in activities that facilitate a normal outcome for their child. With the combined efforts of the family and the health team, most children achieve a satisfactory outcome. Many children with CL/P have surgical correction that creates a near normal–appearing lip and permits good function. Parents need to understand the function of therapy, the purpose and care of all appliances, and the importance of establishing good mouth care and proper brushing habits.

Throughout the child's development, an important goal is the development of a healthy personality and self-esteem. Many communities have CP parents' groups that offer help and support to families (see Additional Resources section at the end of this chapter).

BOX 47-15 Clinical Manifestations of Tracheoesophageal Fistula

Excessive salivation and drooling
Three C's of tracheoesophageal fistula:
- Coughing
- Choking
- Cyanosis

Apnea
Increased respiratory distress during and after feeding
Abdominal distension

Esophageal Atresia With Tracheoesophageal Fistula

Congenital atresia of the esophagus and tracheoesophageal fistula (TEF) are rare malformations that result from failed separation of the esophagus and trachea by the fourth week of gestation. These defects may occur as separate entities or in combination, and without early diagnosis and treatment they pose a serious threat to the infant's well-being (see Fig. 28-15).

Etiology

Esophageal atresia (EA) with or without an associated TEF is the most common esophageal malformation, occurring in approximately 1 in 3500 live births (Shaw-Smith, 2006). There appears to be an equal sex incidence, but the birth weight of most affected infants is significantly lower than average, and incidence of preterm birth is unusually high. A history of maternal polyhydramnios is present in approximately 50% of infants with the defects. EA/TEF is often present with the VATER or VACTERL syndromes, acronyms for syndromes involving a combination of *V*ertebral, *A*norectal, Cardiovascular, *T*racheo-*E*sophageal, *R*enal, and *L*imb abnormalities. The cardiac and renal anomalies occur most frequently with EA/TEF.

Pathophysiology

The cause of EA/TEF is unknown. In the most frequently encountered form of EA and TEF (80 to 95% of cases), the proximal esophageal segment terminates in a blind pouch, and the distal segment is connected to the trachea or primary bronchus by a short fistula at or near the bifurcation (see Fig. 28-15, C). The second most common variety (8%) consists of a blind pouch at each end, widely separated and with no communication to the trachea (see Fig. 28-15, A). Less frequently, an otherwise normal trachea and esophagus are connected by a common fistula (see Fig. 28-15, E). Extremely rare anomalies involve a fistula from the trachea to the upper esophageal segment (see Fig. 28-15, B) or to both the upper and lower segments (see Fig. 28-15, D).

Diagnostic Evaluation

The disorder is suspected on the basis of clinical manifestations (Box 47-15). EA should also be suspected in cases of maternal polyhydramnios. Although the diagnosis is established on the basis of clinical signs and symptoms, the exact type of anomaly is determined by radiographic studies. A radiopaque catheter is inserted into the hypopharynx and advanced until it encounters an obstruction. Chest films are taken to ascertain esophageal patency or the presence and level of a blind pouch. Sometimes fistulas are not patent, which makes them more difficult to diagnose. The presence of gas in the stomach or small bowel is indicative of a coexisting TEF.

Therapeutic Management

EA is a surgical emergency. The treatment includes maintenance of a patent airway, prevention of pneumonia, gastric or blind pouch decompression, and surgical repair of the anomaly. When EA/TEF is suspected, the infant is immediately taken off oral intake, started on IV fluids, and placed in the position least likely to cause aspiration of either mouth or stomach secretions (usually elevation of the head 30 to 45 degrees, as the infant's condition allows). Removal of secretions from the mouth and upper pouch requires frequent or continuous suction. Because aspiration pneumonia is almost inevitable and appears early, broad-spectrum antibiotic therapy is often instituted.

Primary surgical correction consists of a thoracotomy with division and ligation of the TEF and an end-to-side anastomosis of the esophagus. This may consist of one operation or be staged with two or more procedures. For infants who are preterm, have multiple anomalies, or are in poor condition, a staged procedure is preferred that involves palliative measures, including gastrostomy, ligation of the TEF, and provision of constant drainage of the esophageal pouch. A delayed esophageal anastomosis is usually attempted after several weeks to months when the upper pouch elongates. Further surgical techniques may be performed later to facilitate esophageal lengthening. If an esophageal anastomosis still cannot be accomplished, a cervical esophagostomy (to allow drainage of saliva) and gastrostomy are performed. In some centres, thoracoscopic repair of EA/TEF has been successful, negating the need for a thoracotomy and thus minimizing associated operative complications and morbidities (Achildi & Grewal, 2007; Holcomb et al., 2005).

A primary anastomosis may be impossible because of insufficient length of the two segments of the esophagus. In these cases, an esophageal replacement procedure using a part of the colon, or gastric tube interposition may be necessary to bridge the missing esophageal segment. Many infants with EA (10 to 20%) also have *tracheomalacia*, a weakness in the tracheal wall that occurs when a dilated proximal pouch compresses the trachea in early fetal life or when the trachea does not develop normally because of a loss of intratracheal pressure. Signs of tracheomalacia include barking cough, stridor, wheezing, recurrent respiratory tract infections, cyanosis, and possibly apnea.

Complications of a primary repair include an anastomotic leak, strictures resulting from tension or ischemia, esophageal motility disorders causing dysphagia, and GER.

Prognosis

The prognosis is related to the birth weight, associated congenital anomalies, and time of diagnosis. The survival rate is nearly 100% in full-term infants without severe respiratory distress or other anomalies. In preterm low-birth-weight infants with associated anomalies, the incidence of complications is high.

Nursing Care Management

Nursing responsibility for detection of this malformation begins *immediately* after birth. Ideally, the diagnosis should be made before the initial feeding, but often it is not. If fed, the infant swallows normally but suddenly coughs and struggles, and the fluid is aspirated or returns through the nose and mouth. For this reason, it is customary for the nurse to be present when a parent feeds the child to observe the infant's response. Early breastfeeding should not be prevented unless there is a strong suspicion of EA.

NURSING ALERT Any infant who has an excessive amount of frothy saliva in the mouth or difficulty with secretions and unexplained episodes of cyanosis should be suspected of having an EA/TEF and referred immediately for medical evaluation.

Cyanosis is usually the result of laryngospasm caused by overflow of saliva into the larynx from the proximal esophageal pouch. It normally clears after removal of the secretions from the oropharynx by suctioning. Any suspicion of TEF should be reported immediately. The infant is placed in an incubator or a radiant warmer, and oxygen is administered to help relieve respiratory distress. Intubation and assisted mechanical ventilation may be necessary if the infant is in respiratory distress. When a newborn is suspected of having a TEF, the most desirable position is supine with the head elevated at least 30 degrees. This position minimizes the reflux of gastric secretions up the distal esophagus into the trachea and bronchi.

It is imperative that the source of aspiration be removed at once. Oral fluids need to be withheld and the infant's fluid needs met parenterally. Until surgery, the blind pouch is kept empty by intermittent or continuous suction through an indwelling nasal catheter that extends to the end of the pouch. The catheter needs attention because it has a tendency to become clogged with mucus. It is usually replaced daily. In the event that a staged repair is performed, a gastrostomy tube is inserted and left open so that air entering the stomach through the fistula can escape, thus minimizing the danger that gastric contents will be regurgitated into the trachea. The tube empties by gravity drainage. Feedings through the gastrostomy tube and irrigations with fluid are contraindicated before surgery in the infant with a distal TEF. Nursing interventions include respiratory assessment, airway management, thermoregulation, fluid and electrolyte management, and often nutritional support.

Postoperative Care

Postoperative care is essentially the same as that for any high-risk newborn. The infant is returned to the radiant warmer, and the gastrostomy tube is connected to gravity drainage until the infant can tolerate feedings. At this time, the tube is elevated and secured at a point above the level of the stomach. This allows gastric secretions to pass to the duodenum, and swallowed air can escape through the open tube. Tracheal suction should be done only using a premeasured catheter and with extreme caution to avoid injury to the suture line. If tolerated, gastrostomy feedings may be started and continued until the esophageal anastomosis is healed. Before oral feedings are initiated and the chest tube is removed, a contrast study or esophagram is performed to verify the integrity of the esophageal anastomosis.

The initial attempt at oral feeding must be carefully observed to make certain that the infant can swallow without choking. Oral feedings are begun with sterile water, followed by frequent small feedings of breast milk or formula. Until the infant can take a sufficient amount by mouth, gastrostomy feedings or parenteral nutrition may supplement oral intake. Infants are usually not discharged until they are taking oral fluids well and the gastrostomy tube is removed. However, the infant who has palliative surgery is discharged with the gastrostomy tube in place. The nurse is responsible for making certain that the caregiver is educated and has practised the care of the gastrostomy.

Special Problems

Upper respiratory tract complications are a threat to life in both the preoperative and postoperative periods. In addition to pneumonia, there is a constant danger of respiratory distress resulting from atelectasis, pneumothorax, and laryngeal edema. Any persistent respiratory difficulty after removal of secretions is reported to the surgeon immediately. The infant is monitored for anastomotic leaks, as evidenced by purulent chest tube drainage, increased WBC count, and temperature instability.

Periodic esophageal dilations are often necessary in infants and children to manage strictures; the infant may show signs of choking or inability to swallow, thus indicating necessity for dilation. A significant number of infants develop GER after surgery and are placed on antireflux medications. Additional complications following EA repair include tracheomalacia and recurring TEFs (Naik-Mathuria & Olutoye, 2006).

In the infant awaiting esophageal replacement surgery, the catheter is removed, and the upper esophageal segment is drained through a cervical esophagostomy. An esophagostomy is difficult to care for because the skin becomes irritated by moisture from the continuous discharge of saliva. Frequent removal of drainage and application of a layer of protective ointment may remedy the problem. A dressing or ostomy appliance may be applied to collect the drainage, and an enterostomal therapist can provide additional guidance to prevent or treat skin breakdown.

For the infant who requires esophageal replacement, nonnutritive sucking is provided by a pacifier. Sometimes small amounts of water or formula are given orally; although the liquid drains from the esophagostomy, this process allows the infant to develop mature sucking patterns. Other appropriate oral stimulation prevents feeding aversions. Infants who remain NPO for an extended period or who have not received oral stimulation have difficulty eating by mouth after corrective surgery and may develop oral hypersensitivity and food aversion. They require patient, firm guidance to learn how to take food into the mouth and swallow after repair. A referral to a multidisciplinary feeding behaviour program is often necessary.

As with any congenital anomaly, parents need support in adjusting to the child's condition. One difficulty is the immediate transfer of the sick newborn to the critical care unit and the length of hospitalization. Encouraging parents to visit the infant, participate in care when appropriate, and express their feelings regarding the infant's condition facilitates the attachment process. The nurse in the critical care unit should assume responsibility for ensuring that the parents are kept fully informed of the infant's progress.

Preparing parents for discharge involves teaching them skills they will need at home. They should be taught to observe for behaviours that indicate the need for suctioning and for signs of respiratory distress and constriction of the esophagus (e.g., poor feeding, dysphagia, drooling, regurgitation of undigested food). Discharge planning also includes obtaining the necessary equipment and home nursing services to provide home care.

Hernias

A *hernia* is a protrusion of a portion of an organ or organs through an abnormal opening. The danger from herniation arises when the organ protruding through the opening is constricted to the extent that circulation is impaired or when the protruding organs encroach on and impair the function of other structures. A hernia that cannot be reduced easily is called an *incarcerated hernia*. A *strangulated hernia* is one in which the blood supply to the herniated organ is impaired. The herniations of concern are those that protrude through the diaphragm, the abdominal wall, or the inguinal canal. The other hernias of significance to the pediatric age groups are outlined in Table 47-8.

Obstructive Disorders

Obstruction in the GI tract occurs when the passage of nutrients and secretions is impeded by a constricted or occluded lumen or when there is impaired motility (*paralytic ileus*). Obstructions may be congenital or acquired. Many congenital obstructions such as atresia, imperforate anus, meconium plug, and meconium ileus usually appear in the neonatal period. Other obstructions of congenital etiology such as malrotation, HD, volvulus, incarcerated hernia, and Meckel's diverticulum appear after the first few weeks of life. Intestinal obstruction from acquired causes such as intussusception, pyloric stenosis, and tumours may occur in infancy or childhood. Intestinal obstructions from any cause are characterized by similar signs and symptoms (Box 47-16).

Hypertrophic Pyloric Stenosis

Hypertrophic pyloric stenosis (HPS) occurs when the circumferential muscle of the pyloric sphincter becomes thickened, resulting in elongation and narrowing of the pyloric channel. This produces an outlet obstruction and compensatory dilation, hypertrophy, and hyperperistalsis of the stomach. This condition usually develops in the first 2 to 5 weeks of life, causing projectile nonbilious vomiting, dehydration, metabolic alkalosis, and eventually, growth failure. The precise etiology is unknown. The reported incidence is 1 per 1000 live births in Canada (Goodwin et al., 2008) with a male/female ratio of 6 : 1. There is a genetic predisposition, and siblings and offspring of affected persons are at increased risk of developing HPS. It is more common in full-term than in preterm infants and is seen less frequently in Black and Asian infants than in White infants.

Pathophysiology

The circular muscle of the pylorus thickens as a result of hypertrophy (increased size) and hyperplasia (increased mass). This produces severe narrowing of the pyloric canal between the stomach and the duodenum, causing partial obstruction of the lumen (Fig. 47-7, A). Over time, inflammation and edema further reduce the size of the opening, resulting in complete obstruction. The hypertrophied pylorus may be palpable as an olivelike mass in the upper abdomen. Pyloric stenosis is not a congenital disorder. There is now substantial evidence to support decreased expression of neuronal nitric oxide synthase in the nerve fibres of the pyloric circular muscle in infants with HPS (Huang et al., 2006). In most cases HPS is an isolated lesion; however, it may be associated with intestinal malrotation, esophageal and duodenal atresia, and anorectal anomalies.

evolve Animation–Digestive Tract, Passage of Food

Diagnostic Evaluation

The diagnosis of HPS is often made after the history and physical examination. The olivelike mass is easily palpated when the stomach is empty, the infant is quiet, and the abdominal muscles are relaxed. Vomiting usually occurs 30 to 60 minutes after feeding and becomes projectile as the obstruction progresses. Emesis is nonbilious, usually consisting of stale milk. Often these infants become dehydrated and lethargic and eventually may appear significantly malnourished.

If the diagnosis is inconclusive from the history and physical signs (Box 47-17), ultrasonography will demonstrate an elongated, sausage-shaped mass with an elongated pyloric channel. The widespread availability of diagnostic ultrasonography has made the diagnosis and treatment more expedient. If ultrasound scanning fails to demonstrate a hypertrophied pylorus, upper GI radiography should be done to rule out other causes of vomiting. Laboratory findings reflect the metabolic alterations created by severe depletion of both fluid and electrolytes in the event that vomiting is prolonged and the

Table 47-8 Summary Outline of Hernias

TYPE	MANIFESTATIONS/DIAGNOSTIC EVALUATION	MANAGEMENT
Diaphragmatic (Congenital)		
Protrusion of abdominal organs through opening in diaphragm	**Symptoms:** Mild to severe respiratory distress within a few hours after birth; tachypnea, cyanosis, dyspnea, absent breath sounds in affected area; impaired cardiac output; possible symptoms of shock, severe acidosis **Diagnosis:** Suspected on basis of symptoms—confirmed by radiographic study; often diagnosed prenatally as early as 25th week of gestation	**Therapeutic:** Supportive treatment of respiratory distress and correction of acidosis; possible use of endotracheal intubation, GI decompression, ECMO, high-frequency ventilation and inhaled nitric oxide Surgical reduction of hernia and repair of defect after period of cardiorespiratory stabilization **Nursing:** *Preoperative:* Prompt recognition; resuscitation and stabilization Maintain oxygenation and IV fluids Maintain acid–base balance Administer medications Reduce stimulation—environmental/care activities *Postoperative:* Carry out routine postoperative care and observation Relieve pain and provide comfort Support family because this is a critical illness
Hiatal		
Sliding: Protrusion of an abdominal structure (usually stomach) through esophageal hiatus	**Symptoms:** Dysphagia, growth failure, vomiting, neck contortions, frequent unexplained respiratory problems, bleeding; usually associated with GER; may cause gastric volvulus and obstruction **Diagnosis:** Made by fluoroscopy	**Therapeutic:** Management of GER symptoms; positioning; pharmacological treatment; and dietary management Surgical treatment when complications are related to GER despite medical management **Nursing:** Be alert to significant signs and carry out routine postoperative care
Abdominal		
Umbilical: Weakness in abdominal wall around umbilicus; incomplete closure of abdominal wall, allowing intestinal contents to protrude through opening	**Symptoms:** Noted by inspection and palpation of the abdomen High incidence in preterm and African-American infants Usually closes spontaneously by 1–2 yr of age	**Therapeutic:** No treatment of small defects Operative repair if persists to age 4–6 yr or if defect is >1.5–2.0 cm by age 2 yr Strangulation requires immediate attention **Nursing:** Discourage use of home remedies (e.g., belly bands, coins) Reassure parents
Omphalocele: Protrusion of intra-abdominal viscera into base of umbilical cord; sac is covered with peritoneum without skin **Gastroschisis:** Protrusion of intra-abdominal contents through defect in abdominal wall lateral to umbilical ring; there is never a peritoneal sac covering the intestinal contents	**Symptoms:** Obvious on inspection Observe for other malformations such as bladder exstrophy and hypospadias	**Therapeutic:** Surgical repair of defect *Preoperative:* Large lesions—gradual reduction of defect Prophylactic antibiotic administration **Nursing (preoperative):** Keep sac or viscera moist with saline-soaked pads Use overhead warming unit Routine care of IV fluid administration Nasogastric suction NPO Non-nutritive sucking

ECMO, extracorporeal membrane oxygenation; *GER*, gastroesophageal reflux; *GI*, gastrointestinal; *IV*, intravenous; *NPO*, nothing by mouth.

condition remains undiagnosed. There are decreased serum levels of both sodium and potassium, although these may be masked by the hemoconcentration from ECF depletion. Of greater diagnostic value is a decrease in serum chloride levels and increases in pH and bicarbonate (carbon dioxide content) characteristic of metabolic alkalosis. The BUN level is elevated as evidence of dehydration.

Therapeutic Management

Surgical relief of the pyloric obstruction by pyloromyotomy is the standard treatment for this disorder. The procedure is performed through a right upper quadrant incision (laparotomy) and consists of a longitudinal incision through the circular muscle fibres of the pylorus down to, but not including, the submucosa (see Fig. 47-7, B). The procedure has a high

BOX 47-16 Clinical Manifestations of Mechanical or Paralytic Intestinal Obstruction

Colicky abdominal pain—From peristalsis attempting to overcome the obstruction

Abdominal distension—As a result of accumulation of gas and fluid above the level of the obstruction

Vomiting—Often the earliest sign of a high obstruction; a later sign of lower obstruction (may be bilious or feculent)

Constipation and obstipation—Early signs of low obstructions; later signs of higher obstructions

Dehydration—From losses of large quantities of fluid and electrolytes into the intestine

Rigid and boardlike abdomen—From increased distension

Bowel sounds—Gradually diminish and cease

Respiratory distress—Occurs as the diaphragm is pushed up into the pleural cavity

Shock—Plasma volume diminishes as fluids and electrolytes are lost from the bloodstream into the intestinal lumen (third spacing)

Sepsis—Caused by bacterial proliferation with invasion into the circulation

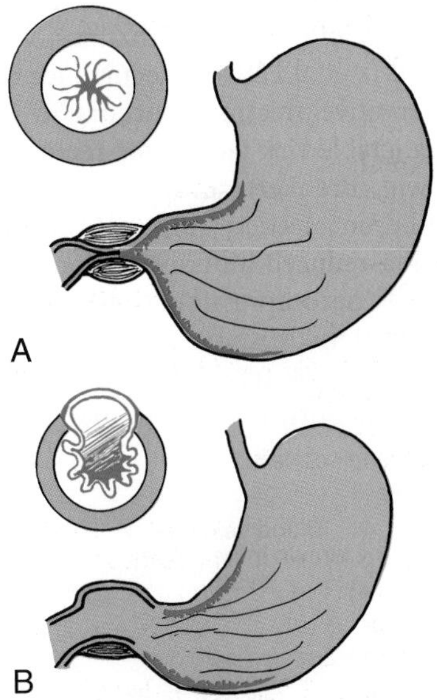

Fig. 47-7 Hypertrophic pyloric stenosis. **A:** Enlarged muscular area nearly obliterates pyloric channel. **B:** Longitudinal surgical division of muscle down to submucosa establishes adequate passageway.

success rate when infants receive careful preoperative preparation to correct fluid and electrolyte imbalances.

Feedings are usually begun 4 to 6 hours postoperatively, beginning with small, frequent feedings of clear liquids followed by formula or breast milk as tolerated. Another procedure, **laparoscopy,** may be performed for infants with HPS. The use of a small incision for the laparoscope results in shorter surgical time, more rapid postoperative feeding, and quicker discharge.

BOX 47-17 Clinical Manifestations of Hypertrophic Pyloric Stenosis

Projectile vomiting
- May be ejected 1 metre from the child when in a side-lying position, 30 cm or more when in a back-lying position
- Occurs shortly after a feeding (may not occur for several hours)
- May follow each feeding or appear intermittently
- Nonbilious vomitus; may be blood tinged

Infant hungry, avid nurser; eagerly accepts a second feeding after vomiting episode

No evidence of pain or discomfort except that of chronic hunger

Weight loss

Signs of dehydration

Distended upper abdomen

Readily palpable olive-shaped tumour in the epigastrium just to the right of the umbilicus

Visible gastric peristaltic waves that move from left to right across the epigastrium

Prognosis

Most infants recover completely and rapidly after pyloromyotomy. Postoperative complications include persistent pyloric obstruction and wound dehiscence. Some infants also have GER.

Nursing Care Management

The diagnosis of HPS is considered in the infant less than 6 to 8 weeks of age who appears alert but often fails to gain weight and has a history of vomiting after milk consumption. Assessment is based on observation of eating behaviours and evidence of other characteristic clinical manifestations.

Preoperative Care

Preoperatively, emphasis is placed on restoring hydration and electrolyte balance; however, often the condition is brought to the practitioner's attention and readily diagnosed before fluid and electrolyte problems occur. Infants are usually given no oral feedings and receive IV fluids with glucose and electrolyte replacement based on laboratory serum electrolyte values. Careful monitoring of the IV infusion and diligent attention to intake, output, and urine specific gravity measurements are important. Vomiting and the number and character of stools need to be observed and recorded accurately.

Observations also include assessment of vital signs, particularly those that might indicate fluid or electrolyte imbalances. These infants may have metabolic alkalosis from loss of hydrogen ions and from potassium, sodium, and chloride depletion if vomiting is prolonged. The skin, mucous membranes, and daily weight are assessed for alterations in hydration status and water gain or loss.

If stomach decompression and gastric lavage are used preoperatively, the nurse is responsible for ensuring that the tube is patent and functioning properly and for measuring and recording the type and amount of drainage. Infants who are receiving IV fluids or have an NG tube for continuous drainage must be observed to prevent the infusion device or tube from becoming dislodged.

General hygienic care, with attention to the skin and mouth in dehydrated infants, is essential. Protection from infection is also important because infants with impaired nutritional status are more susceptible than normal newborns. Parental involvement should be encouraged and promoted.

Postoperative Care

Postoperative vomiting may occur, and most infants, even with successful surgery, exhibit some vomiting during the first 24 to 48 hours because of edema resulting from the surgery. IV fluids are administered until the infant can retain adequate amounts by mouth. Observation of physical signs, monitoring of IV fluids, and careful recording of intake and output are maintained. The infant is also observed for evidence of pain, and appropriate analgesics are given.

Feedings are usually instituted soon after surgery, beginning with clear liquids and advancing to formula or breast milk as tolerated. They are offered slowly, in small amounts, and at frequent intervals as ordered by the practitioner. Observation and recording of feedings and the infant's responses to them are a vital part of postoperative care. Care of the operative site consists of observation for any drainage or signs of inflammation and care of the incision as directed by the surgeon.

Parents should be encouraged to remain with their child and become involved in the child's care. Vomiting of a projectile nature is frightening to parents, and they often believe that they may have done something wrong or that surgery was not successful. Most parents need support and reassurance that the condition is caused by a structural problem and is in no way a reflection on their parenting skills and capacities.

Intussusception

Intussusception is the most common cause of acute intestinal obstruction in children younger than 5 years of age. The peak age is 3 to 9 months (Huppertz et al., 2006). It is more common in boys than in girls and in children with cystic fibrosis. Although specific intestinal lesions can be found in about 3% of these children, the cause is usually not known. More than 90% of intussusceptions do not have a pathological lead point, such as a polyp, lymphoma, or Meckel's diverticulum. The idiopathic cases are most likely a result of hypertrophy of intestinal lymphoid tissue secondary to viral infection. Some cases were associated with administration of the first licensed rotavirus vaccine, the reassortant rhesus-human tetravalent rotavirus vaccine (RRV-IV; RotaShield), which led to its voluntary withdrawal in the late 1990s. No such association has been reported to date from large phase III safety trials with the two new rotavirus vaccines currently being administered in Canada (AAP, Committee on Infectious Diseases, 2009).

Pathophysiology

Intussusception occurs when one portion of bowel invaginates into a more distant portion of the bowel, pulling the mesentery with it. Lymphatic and venous congestion and bowel wall edema can cause obstruction of the intestine, and infarction and perforation of the bowel wall can occur (Huppertz et al., 2006). Venous engorgement also leads to leaking of blood and mucus into the intestinal lumen, forming the classic currant jelly stools. The most common site is the ileocecal valve (ileocolic), where the ileum invaginates into the cecum and colon (Fig. 47-8). Other forms include ileoileal (one part of the ileum invaginates into another section of the ileum) and colocolic (one part of the colon invaginates into another area of the colon, usually in the area of the hepatic or splenic flexure or at some point along the transverse colon).

NURSING ALERT The classic triad of intussusception symptoms (abdominal pain, abdominal mass, bloody stools) is present in 29 to 33% of children (Huppertz et al., 2006). Initially children might also be seen with screaming, irritability, lethargy, vomiting, diarrhea or constipation, fever, dehydration, and shock. Because intussusception is potentially life threatening, the nurse should be aware of alternate presentations, observe these children closely, and refer them for further evaluation.

Diagnostic Evaluation

Frequently subjective findings lead to the diagnosis (Box 47-18), which can be confirmed by ultrasound. Spontaneous reduction occurs in up to 10% of patients.

Therapeutic Management

Conservative treatment consists of radiologist-guided pneumoenema (air enema) with or without water-soluble contrast or ultrasound-guided hydrostatic (saline) enema to reduce the defect; the advantage of the latter is that no ionizing radiation is needed (Huppertz et al., 2006). Recurrence of intussusception after conservative treatment occurs in about 1 in 10 patients; no predictable risk factors for recurrence have been identified. Herwig, Brenkert, and Losek (2009) found that hospitalized children needed minimal interventions after undergoing enema-reduced intussusception.

IV fluids, NG decompression, and antibiotic therapy may be used before hydrostatic reduction is attempted. If these procedures are not successful, the child may require surgical intervention. Surgery involves manually reducing the

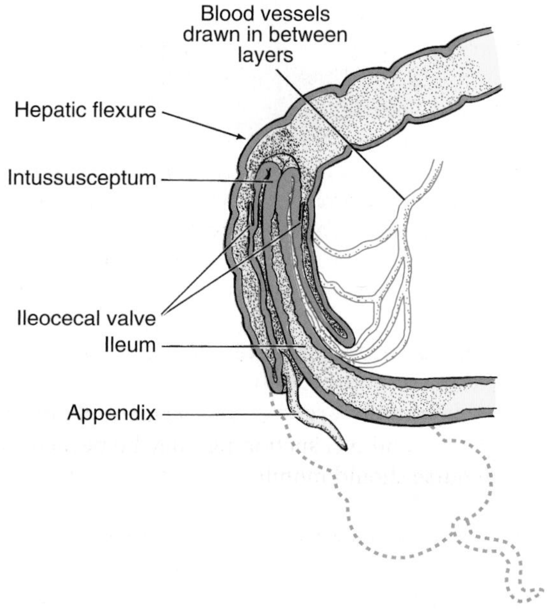

Fig. 47-8 Ileocecal (ileocolic) intussusception.

BOX 47-18 Clinical Manifestations of Intussusception

- Sudden acute abdominal pain
- Child screaming and drawing the knees toward the chest
- Child appearing normal and comfortable during intervals between episodes of pain
- Vomiting
- Lethargy
- Passage of red, currant jelly–like stools (stool mixed with blood and mucus)
- Tender, distended abdomen
- Palpable sausage-shaped mass in upper right quadrant
- Empty lower right quadrant (Dance sign)
- Eventual fever, prostration, and other signs of peritonitis

invagination and, when indicated, resecting any nonviable intestine.

Prognosis

Nonoperative reduction is successful in approximately 80% of cases (Huppertz et al., 2006). Surgery is required for patients in whom the contrast enema is unsuccessful. With early diagnosis and treatment, serious complications and death are uncommon.

Nursing Care Management

The nurse can help establish a diagnosis by listening to the parent's description of the child's physical and behavioural symptoms. It is not unusual for parents to state that they thought something was seriously wrong before others shared their concerns. The description of the child's severe colicky abdominal pain combined with vomiting is a significant sign of intussusception.

As soon as a possible diagnosis of intussusception is made, the nurse should prepare the parents for the immediate need for hospitalization, the nonsurgical technique of hydrostatic reduction, and the possibility of surgery. It is important to explain the basic defect of intussusception. A model of the defect is easily demonstrated by pushing the end of a finger on a rubber glove back into itself or using the example of a telescoping rod. The principle of reduction by hydrostatic pressure can be simulated by filling the glove with water, which pushes the "finger" into a fully extended position.

Physical care of the child does not differ from that for any child undergoing abdominal surgery. Even though nonsurgical intervention may be successful, the usual preoperative procedures, such as maintenance of NPO status, routine laboratory testing (CBC and urinalysis), signed parental consent, and preanaesthetic sedation, are performed. For the child with signs of electrolyte imbalance, hemorrhage, or peritonitis, additional preparation, such as replacement fluids, whole blood or plasma, and NG suctioning, may be needed. Before surgery the nurse should monitor all stools.

NURSING ALERT Passage of a normal brown stool usually indicates that the intussusception has reduced itself. This should be immediately reported to the practitioner, who may choose to alter the diagnostic and therapeutic care plan.

Postprocedural care includes observations of vital signs, blood pressure, intact sutures and dressing, and the return of bowel sounds. After spontaneous or hydrostatic reduction, the nurse should observe for passage of water-soluble contrast material (if used) and the stool patterns, since the intussusception may recur. Children may be admitted to the hospital or monitored on an outpatient basis. A recurrence is treated with the conservative reduction techniques described previously, but a laparotomy is considered for multiple recurrences.

Because hospitalization may be the child's first separation from the parents, it is important to preserve the parent–child relationship by encouraging rooming-in or extended visiting. It may be the parents' first experience with hospitalization, necessitating their preparation for procedures such as IV therapy, frequent vital sign and blood pressure monitoring, dressings, and NPO (see Chapter 44). Because of the rapidity of the onset, diagnosis, and treatment, parents may feel stunned or numb. They may ask few questions, or they may constantly make inquiries, sometimes the same ones several times. If the nurse realizes the circumstances surrounding this condition, the parents' reactions are more likely to be understood and accepted.

evolve Animation—Volvulus

Malrotation and Volvulus

Malrotation of the intestine is caused by the abnormal rotation of the intestine around the superior mesenteric artery during embryological development. Malrotation may manifest in utero or may be asymptomatic throughout life. Infants with malrotation may have intermittent bilious vomiting, recurrent abdominal pain, distension, or lower GI bleeding. Malrotation is the most serious type of intestinal obstruction because, if the intestine undergoes complete volvulus (the intestine twisting around itself), compromise of the blood supply will result in intestinal necrosis, peritonitis, perforation, and death.

Diagnostic Evaluation

It is imperative that malrotation and volvulus be diagnosed promptly and surgical treatment instituted quickly. An upper GI series is the definitive procedure to diagnose this condition.

Therapeutic Management

Surgery is indicated to remove the affected area. Because of the extensive nature of some lesions, short-gut syndrome is a postoperative complication.

Nursing Care Management

Preoperatively, the nursing care is the same as that provided to an infant or child with intestinal obstruction. Postoperatively, the nursing care is similar to that provided to the infant or child who has undergone abdominal surgery.

Anorectal Malformations

Anorectal malformations include a number of anomalies of the genitourinary and pelvic organs. These malformations are among the more common congenital malformations caused by abnormal development, with an incidence of 1 in 5000 to 1 in 15,000 live births (Blackburn, 2007). The anus and rectum originate from an embryological structure called the cloaca. Lateral growth of the cloaca forms the urorectal septum that separates the rectum dorsally from the urinary tract ventrally. The rectum and urinary tract separate completely by the seventh week of gestation. Anomalies that occur reflect the stage of development of these processes.

Imperforate anus includes several forms of malformation without an obvious anal opening (see Fig. 28-17). Many have a fistula from the distal rectum to the perineum or genitourinary system. Anorectal malformations may occur in isolation or as part of the VACTERL or VATER syndromes.

A *persistent cloaca* is a complex anorectal malformation in which the rectum, vagina, and urethra drain into a common channel that opens onto the perineum via the usual urethral site (Chien et al., 2005). *Cloacal exstrophy* is a rare, severe defect in which there is externalization of the bladder and bowel through the abdominal wall. Often the genitalia are indefinite, and chromosome studies are necessary to determine the child's gender, which is almost always female. The exstrophic bladder is separated into two halves by the cecum; other features may include an omphalocele, imperforate anus, and at times a neural tube defect.

Anorectal anomalies are classified according to gender and abnormal anatomical features, including genitourinary and associated pelvic anomalies (Box 47-19). The level of rectal descent is determined by the relationship of the termination of the bowel to the puborectalis sling of the levator ani musculature. About 50% of children with anorectal anomalies have a urological problem.

Diagnostic Evaluation

Checking for patency of the anus and rectum is a routine part of the newborn assessment and should include observations regarding the passage of meconium. Inspection of the perineal area reveals absence of the normal anal opening; however, the appearance of the perineum alone does not accurately predict the level of the lesion. Genitourinary and pelvic anomalies associated with anorectal malformations should be considered.

BOX 47-19 Classification of Anorectal Malformations

Male Defects
- Perineal fistula
- Rectourethral bulbar fistula
- Rectourethral prostatic fistula
- Rectovesicular (bladder neck) fistula
- Imperforate anus without fistula
- Rectal atresia and stenosis

Female Defects
- Perineal fistula
- Vestibular fistula
- Imperforate anus without fistula
- Rectal atresia and stenosis
- Cloaca

(From Peña, A., Hong, A. [2000]. Advances in the management of anorectal malformations. *American Journal of Surgery, 180*[5], 370–376.)

In the newborn, the presence of meconium on the perineum does not always indicate anal patency (particularly in girls) because a fistula may be present and allow evacuation of meconium through the vagina. Fistulas may not be apparent at birth but may become obvious as peristalsis gradually forces the meconium through the fistula. Rectourinary fistulas should be suspected if there is meconium in the urine. Anal stenosis may not be identified until the child is older and comes to the physician with a history of difficult defecation, abdominal distension, and ribbonlike stools.

Abdominal ultrasonography is performed to determine the existence of other malformations. An IV pyelogram and voiding cystourethrogram are recommended for an infant with a high malformation to identify anomalies of the urinary tract. Further examination is also indicated when there is evidence of urinary tract infection or other symptoms. If a syndrome is suspected, cardiac evaluation and spinal films should be obtained.

Therapeutic Management

Successful treatment for anal stenosis is generally accomplished by manual dilations. The procedure is initiated by a physician and repeated on a regular basis by the nurses in the hospital. Parents should be taught to continue the dilations at home. Perineal fistulas are treated by anoplasty during the newborn period. The opening is moved to the centre of the external sphincter, and dilations are begun. More extensive defects are usually managed with a colostomy, and corrective surgical repair is performed later in the first year.

The type of defect, the sacral anatomy, and the quality of muscles influence the long-term prognosis. In general, if the newborn has a deep midline groove, two well-formed buttocks, and an anal dimple, the prognosis for bowel control is better than if the infant has a flat or "rocker" bottom and no midline groove because of associated neurological problems. A functioning interior anal sphincter is important to achieve continence. In its absence, the child may need a bowel program to achieve socially acceptable bowel continence. Other potential complications after surgical treatment include strictures, recurrent rectourinary fistula, mucosal prolapse, and constipation.

Nursing Care Management

The first nursing responsibility is identification of undetected anorectal malformations. A newborn who does not pass a stool within 24 to 48 hours of birth requires further assessment. In addition, meconium that appears at an inappropriate orifice should be reported. Preoperative care includes diagnostic evaluation, GI decompression, and IV fluids.

Nursing care after an anorectoplasty is directed toward healing the surgical site without infection or complications. Care involves keeping the anal area as clean as possible with scrupulous perineal care. A temporary dressing and drain may be placed initially to manage the continuous passage of stool. Protective ointments such as zinc oxide and occlusive dressings such as hydrocolloids decrease skin irritation from frequent loose stools. The preferred position is a side-lying prone position with the hips elevated or a supine position with the legs suspended at a 90-degree angle to the trunk to prevent pressure on perineal sutures.

The infant is given breast milk or formula soon after the repair. Care of the infant with a colostomy involves frequent dressing changes, meticulous skin care, and correct application of a collection device (see Chapter 45).

Family Support, Discharge Planning, and Home Care

Long-term follow-up is important for children with complex malformations. After the definitive pull-through procedure, toilet training is delayed, and complete continence is seldom achieved at the usual age of 2 to 3 years. Prevention of constipation is important, and breastfeeding is encouraged postoperatively. If a cow's milk–based formula is used, a laxative may be prescribed. Bowel habit training, diet modification, and administration of stool softeners or fibre are important aspects of bowel management. Optimum bowel function may not be achieved until late childhood or adolescence. Support and reassurance are important during the slow progression to normal function. Some children never achieve bowel continence and must rely on daily bowel irrigations.

Parents need to be instructed in perineal and wound care or care of the colostomy. Anal dilations may be necessary for some infants. Parents should be advised to observe stooling patterns and notify the physician if there are any signs of anal stricture or complications.

Malabsorption Syndromes

Chronic diarrhea and malabsorption of nutrients characterize malabsorption syndromes. An important complication of malabsorption syndromes in children is growth failure (failure to thrive). Most cases are classified according to the location of the supposed anatomical or biochemical defect. The term *celiac disease* is often used to describe a symptom complex with four characteristics: (1) steatorrhea (fatty, foul, frothy, bulky stools), (2) general malnutrition, (3) abdominal distension, and (4) secondary vitamin deficiencies.

Digestive defects are conditions in which the enzymes necessary for digestion are diminished or absent, such as (1) cystic fibrosis, in which pancreatic enzymes are absent, (2) biliary or liver disease, in which bile flow is affected, or (3) lactase deficiency, in which there is congenital or secondary lactose intolerance.

Absorptive defects are conditions in which the intestinal mucosal transport system is impaired. This may occur because of a primary defect (e.g., celiac disease) or secondary to IBD, resulting in impaired absorption because bowel motility is accelerated (e.g., ulcerative colitis). Obstructive disorders (e.g., HD) also cause secondary malabsorption from enterocolitis.

Anatomical defects, such as extensive resection of the bowel or short-bowel syndrome (SBS), affect digestion by decreasing the transit time of substances and affect absorption by severely compromising the absorptive surface.

Celiac Disease

Celiac disease, also known as *gluten-induced enteropathy, gluten-sensitive enteropathy,* and *celiac sprue*, is an immune-mediated enteropathy of the proximal small intestine triggered by inappropriate immune response to ingested gluten and gluten-related proteins found in wheat, rye, and barley. Celiac disease is one of the most common lifelong disorders affecting approximately 1% of the general population. It is second only to cystic fibrosis as a cause of malabsorption in children. Celiac sprue used to be considered a disease of childhood, but adult presentation is becoming more common. It is seen more frequently in Europe than in North America and is rarely reported in Asians or Blacks. Recent studies suggest the prevalence of celiac disease as being 1 in 322 in children and 1 in 105 adults (Rostom, Murray, & Kagnoff, 2006). The exact cause of celiac disease is unknown, but there appears to be an inherited predisposition with an influence by environmental factors.

Pathophysiology

Genetic predisposition is an essential factor in the development of celiac disease. Membrane receptors involved in preferential antigen presentation to CD4+ T cells play a crucial role in the immune response characteristic of celiac disease. Genes located on the HLA region of chromosome 6 (i.e., HLA-DQ2 or HLA-DQ8) are found in almost 100% of those affected with celiac disease (Murdock & Johnston, 2005). Once the inflammatory reaction is activated by gluten, CD4++ T cells produce cytokines, which are likely to contribute to the intestinal damage. The damage consists of infiltration of the lamina propria, crypt hyperplasia, and villous atrophy and flattening. With sufficient villous atrophy, malabsorption occurs.

Diagnostic Evaluation

Classic symptoms of celiac disease are GI manifestations usually noted several months after the introduction of gluten-containing grains into the diet, usually between the ages of 6 months and 2 years (Box 47-20). Typically, children are seen with impaired growth, chronic diarrhea, abdominal distension, muscle wasting with hypotonia, poor appetite, and lack of energy. The clinical manifestations are usually insidious and chronic. The first evidence may be growth failure and diarrhea. Less typical presentation has been observed in children ages 5 to 7 years who have abdominal pain, nausea, vomiting, bloating, and constipation, or extraintestinal manifestations, including short stature, pubertal delay, iron deficiency, dental enamel defects, and abnormal LFTs. Older children have been found to have osteoporosis. Untreated celiac disease can evolve into celiac crisis, characterized by abdominal distension, explosive watery diarrhea, and dehydration with electrolyte imbalance, leading to hypotensive shock and lethargy.

The diagnosis of celiac disease is based on a biopsy of the small intestine demonstrating the characteristic changes of mucosal inflammation, crypt hyperplasia, and villous atrophy (Sood, 2007). Within a day or two of instituting the gluten-free diet, most children with celiac disease demonstrate a favourable response, including weight gain and improved appetite. Within a few weeks diarrhea and steatorrhea resolve.

Commercially available serological tests for celiac disease include antigliadin antibodies of both the immune globulin A and G classes (IgA and IgG); antiendomysium IgA; and

BOX 47-20 Clinical Manifestations of Celiac Disease

Impaired Fat Absorption
Steatorrhea (excessively large, pale, oily, frothy stools)
Exceedingly foul-smelling stools

Impaired Absorption of Nutrients
Malnutrition
Muscle wasting (especially prominent in legs and buttocks)
Anemia
Anorexia
Abdominal distension

Behavioural Changes
Irritability
Fretfulness
Uncooperativeness
Apathy
Celiac crisis*

Acute, severe episodes of profuse watery diarrhea and vomiting
May be precipitated by:
- Infections (especially gastrointestinal)
- Prolonged fluid and electrolyte depletion
- Emotional disturbance

*In very young children.

antitissue transglutaminase IgA and IgG antibodies for screening first-degree relatives of known celiac disease patients and those with known celiac disease–associated disorders such as type 1 diabetes, thyroiditis, arthritis, primary biliary cirrhosis, Down syndrome, Turner's syndrome, Williams syndrome, and osteopenia or osteoporosis. False-positive results are likely when only one serological test is used, because patients with these disorders can also test positive for these antibodies. Use of more than one test increases diagnostic accuracy (Gelfond & Fasano, 2006). Ruling out total IgA deficiency is necessary to minimize false-negative results.

Therapeutic Management

Treatment of chronic celiac disease is primarily dietary. Although the diet is called *gluten free*, it is actually low in gluten, since it is impossible to remove every source of this protein. Because gluten is found primarily in wheat and rye, but also in smaller quantities in barley and oats, these four foods are eliminated. Corn and rice become substitute grain foods.

Children with untreated celiac disease may have associated lactose intolerance related to intestinal mucosal lesions, which usually improves with gluten withdrawal and intestinal healing. Specific nutritional deficiencies are treated with appropriate supplements, including vitamins, iron, and calories.

Prognosis

Celiac disease is regarded as a chronic disease. The most severe symptoms usually occur in early childhood and again in adult life. Strict dietary avoidance of gluten prevents symptoms and may minimize the risk of developing lymphoma, the most serious complication of the disease.

Nursing Care Management

The main nursing consideration is helping the child adhere to dietary management. Considerable time is involved in explaining to the child and parents the disease process, the specific role of gluten in aggravating the condition, and the foods that must be restricted. Also, a lactose-free diet, which necessitates eliminating all milk products, may be needed initially. It is especially difficult to maintain a diet indefinitely when the child has no symptoms and temporary transgressions result in no difficulties. However, evidence indicates that most individuals who relax their diet experience a relapse of their disease and possibly exhibit growth delay, anemia, or osteomalacia. There is also the risk of developing malignant lymphoma of the small intestine or other GI malignancies.

Although the chief source of gluten is cereal and baked goods, grains are frequently added to processed foods as thickeners or fillers. Gluten is also added to many foods as "hydrolyzed vegetable protein." The nurse must advise parents to read carefully all ingredients on labels to avoid hidden sources of gluten. Many gluten-containing products are easily eliminated from the infant's or young child's diet, but monitoring the diet of a school-age child or adolescent is more difficult. Many "favourite" foods, such as hot dogs, pizza, and spaghetti, are chief offenders. Luncheon preparation away from home is particularly difficult because bread, luncheon meats, and instant soups are not tolerated.

Generally, management includes a diet high in calories and proteins with simple carbohydrates, such as fruits and vegetables, but low in fats. Initially the bowel may be inflamed as a result of the pathological process, so high-fibre foods, such as nuts, raisins, raw vegetables, and raw fruits with skin, should be avoided until inflammation has subsided.

Several organizations and resources are available to help families cope with this condition. The Canadian Celiac Association (http://www.celiac.ca) provides support, guidance, and educational materials to families concerning a gluten-free diet, food sources, recipes, and travel information. Several published cookbooks contain gluten-free recipes.

Short-Bowel Syndrome

Short-bowel syndrome (SBS) is a malabsorptive disorder that occurs when there is decreased mucosal surface area, usually as a result of extensive resection of the small intestine. The most common causes of SBS in children include congenital anomalies (jejunal and ileal atresia, gastroschisis), ischemia (necrotizing enterocolitis), and trauma or vascular injury (volvulus [twisting of bowel on itself]). Other causes include volvulus that results in massive resection, long-segment HD, and omphalocele.

The prognosis for infants and children with SBS has dramatically improved in the past 25 years as a result of advances in parenteral nutrition (PN) and enteral feeding. Both the amount and location of bowel lost are important in determining the severity of the condition. The preservation of the terminal ileum and ileocecal valve influences fluid and nutrient absorption and may avoid problems of bacterial overgrowth by preventing the entrance of bacteria from the colon into the small intestine.

The small intestine has significant capacity for adaptation after resection. During the adaptation process, the villus height increases (villous hyperplasia), and the cell number and absorptive surface area also increase. As villus length and the number of enterocytes available for absorption per centimetre of bowel increase, nutrient absorption increases. Intraluminal enteral feedings stimulate the adaptation process and maintain the structural and functional integrity of the small intestine.

Therapeutic Management

The goals of treatment are to (1) preserve as much length of bowel as possible during surgery, (2) maintain the child's nutritional status, growth, and development while intestinal adaptation occurs, (3) stimulate intestinal adaptation with enteral feeding, and (4) minimize complications related to the disease process and therapy.

Nutritional support is the long-term focus of care. The initial phase of therapy includes PN as the primary source of nutrition. The second phase is the introduction of enteral feeding, which usually begins as soon as possible after surgery. Elemental formulas containing glucose, sucrose and glucose polymers, hydrolyzed proteins, and medium-chain triglycerides facilitate absorption. Usually these formulas are given by continuous infusion through an NG or gastrostomy tube. As the enteral feedings are advanced, the PN solution is decreased in terms of calories, amount of fluid, and total hours of infusion per day. The final phase of nutritional support occurs when growth and development are sustained exclusively by enteral feedings. When PN is discontinued, there is a risk of nutritional deficiency secondary to malabsorption of fat-soluble vitamins (A, D, E, K) and trace minerals (iron, selenium, zinc). Serum vitamin and mineral levels should be obtained, and enteral supplementation of vitamins and minerals may be required. Pharmacological agents have been used to reduce secretory losses. H_2 blockers, PPIs, and octreotide inhibit gastric or pancreatic secretion. Cholestyramine is often prescribed to improve diarrhea that is associated with bile salt malabsorption. Growth factors have also been used to hasten adaptation and enhance mucosal growth, but these uses are still experimental.

Numerous complications are associated with SBS and long-term PN (see Chapter 45). Infectious, metabolic, and technical complications can occur. Catheter sepsis can occur after improper care of the catheter. The GI tract can also be a source of microbial seeding of the catheter. Bowel atrophy may foster increased intestinal permeability of bacteria. A lack of adequate sites for central lines may become a significant problem for the child in need of long-term PN. Hepatic dysfunction, hepatomegaly with abnormal LFTs, and cholestasis may also occur.

Bacterial overgrowth is likely to occur when the ileocecal valve is absent or when stasis exists as a result of a partial obstruction or a dilated segment of bowel with poor motility. Alternating cycles of broad-spectrum antibiotics are used to reduce bacterial overgrowth. This treatment may also decrease the risk of bacterial translocation and subsequent central venous catheter infections. Other complications of bacterial overgrowth and malabsorption include metabolic acidosis and gastric hypersecretion.

Many surgical interventions, including intestinal valves, tapering enteroplasty or stricturoplasty, intestinal lengthening, and interposed segments, have been used to slow intestinal transit, reduce bacterial overgrowth, or increase mucosal surface area. Intestinal transplantation has been performed successfully in children. Only children with a permanent dependence on TPN or severe complications of long-term parenteral nutrition are candidates for transplantation.

Prognosis

The prognosis for infants with SBS has improved with advances in PN and with the understanding of the importance of intraluminal nutrition. Improved surgical techniques for the management of therapy-related problems and the development of more specific immunosuppressive medications for transplantation have all contributed to improved management. The prognosis depends in part on the length of the residual small intestine. An intact ileocecal valve also improves the prognosis. Mortality in infants and children with SBS is usually associated with PN-related problems, such as fulminant sepsis or severe PN cholestasis.

Nursing Care Management

The most important components of nursing care are administration and monitoring of nutritional therapy. During PN therapy, care must be taken to minimize the risk of complications related to the **central venous access device** (i.e., catheter infections, occlusions, dislodgment, or accidental removal). Care of the enteral feeding tubes and monitoring of enteral feeding tolerance are also important nursing responsibilities.

When long-term parenteral nutrition is required, preparing the family for home care is a major nursing responsibility that should be initiated early to prevent a lengthy hospitalization with subsequent problems such as family dysfunction and developmental delays. Many infants and children can be successfully cared for at home with enteral and parenteral nutrition when the family is prepared and provided with adequate support services. Follow-up by a multidisciplinary nutritional support service is essential. The nurse plays an active and important role in the success of a home nutrition program. Home infusion companies provide portable equipment, which enables the child and family to maintain a more normal lifestyle.

When hospitalization is prolonged, the child's developmental and emotional needs must be met. This often requires special planning to promote normal family adjustment and adaptation of the hospital routines. Care of the hospitalized child is discussed in Chapter 44.

Ingestion of Injurious Agents

In Canada there is no national poison centre that monitors and tracks the occurrence of ingestion of injurious agents in the population. Each province and territory has its own regional centre that is responsible for both education and emergency management of these exposures.

Commonly ingested poisons include the following (Bronstein et al., 2008; Franklin & Rodgers, 2008):

- Cosmetics and personal care products (perfume, cologne, aftershave)*
- Cleaning products (hypochlorite ["household"] bleach, pine oil disinfectants)
- Plants (nontoxic GI irritants, oxalates) (Box 47-21)
- Foreign bodies, toys, and miscellaneous substances (desiccants, thermometers, bubble-blowing solutions)

Many poisonings reflect the ready accessibility of the product in the home, where more than 90% of poisonings occur, although a significant number take place elsewhere, such as in a grandparent's or friend's home, a school, or a health care facility.

The following five commonly used and easily available medications (the first four are over-the-counter products) can cause serious or fatal consequences if as little as 1.5 mL or ½ a tablet is ingested: methyl salicylate, camphor, topical imidazolines (sympathomimetics such as those contained in Visine and Clear Eyes), benzocaine, and diphenoxylate-atropine (e.g., Lomotil). Parents must know the importance of keeping such medications away from children. If these agents are ingested, parents need to seek medical treatment immediately. Emesis should not be induced at home. The developmental characteristics of young children predispose them to poisoning by ingestion; infants and toddlers explore their environment through oral experimentation. Because the sense of taste is not discriminating at this age, many unpalatable substances are ingested. In addition, toddlers and preschoolers are developing autonomy and initiative, which increase their curiosity and noncompliant behaviour. Imitation is also a powerful motivator, especially when combined with lack of awareness of danger.

This section is primarily concerned with the immediate emergency treatment of the ingestion of injurious agents. Specific management of corrosive, hydrocarbon, acetaminophen, salicylate, iron, and plant poisoning is summarized in Box 47-22. Because of the importance of lead poisoning among young children, the ingestion of lead is discussed separately. Appropriate suggestions for poisoning prevention are discussed on p. 1441.

Principles of Emergency Treatment

A poisoning may or may not require emergency intervention, but in every instance medical evaluation is necessary to initiate appropriate action. The first action for a caregiver of a child who may have ingested a toxic substance is to consult the local poison control centre (PCC). If the PCC cannot be reached, the child should be taken to the nearest emergency department. Parents are advised to call the (PCC) before initiating any intervention. The local PCC telephone number (usually listed in the front of the telephone directory) should be posted near each phone in the house (see Critical Thinking Exercise and Emergency box).

*The most common substances in each category are in parentheses. Substances ingested are not necessarily the most toxic but often are readily available.

BOX 47-21 Poisonous and Nonpoisonous Plants

Poisonous Plants: Toxic Parts

Apple—Leaves, seeds
Apricot—Leaves, stem, seed pits
Azalea—All parts
Buttercup—All parts
Cherry (wild or cultivated)—Twigs, seeds, foliage
Daffodil—Bulbs
Dumb cane, Dieffenbachia—All parts
Elephant ear—All parts
English ivy—All parts
Foxglove—Leaves, seeds, flowers
Holly—Berries and leaves
Hyacinth—Bulbs
Ivy—Leaves
Mistletoe*—Berries, leaves
Oak tree—Acorn, foliage
Philodendron—All parts
Plum—Pit
Poinsettia†—Leaves, stems, sap
Poison ivy, poison oak—Leaves, fruit, stems, smoke from burning plants
Pothos—All parts
Rhubarb—Leaves
Tulip—Bulbs
Water hemlock—All parts
Wisteria—Seeds, pods
Yew—All parts

Nonpoisonous Plants

African violet
Aluminum plant
Asparagus fern
Begonia
Boston fern
Christmas cactus
Coleus
Gardenia
Grape ivy
Jade plant
Piggyback begonia
Piggyback plant
Prayer plant
Rubber tree
Snake plant
Spider plant
Swedish ivy
Wax plant
Weeping fig
Zebra plant

*Eating one or two berries or leaves is probably nontoxic.
†Mildly toxic if ingested in massive quantities.

NURSING ALERT Each province and territory has its own regional poison control centre, thus it is important to have the emergency number posted near the telephone.

BOX 47-22 Selected Poisonings in Children

Corrosives (Strong Acids or Alkali)

Drain, toilet, or oven cleaners
Electric dishwasher detergent (liquid, because of higher pH, is more hazardous than granular)
Mildew remover
Batteries
Clinitest tablets
Denture cleaners
Bleach

Clinical Manifestations

Severe burning pain in mouth, throat, and stomach
White, swollen mucous membranes; edema of lips, tongue, and pharynx (respiratory obstruction)
Violent vomiting (hemoptysis)
Drooling and inability to clear secretions
Signs of shock
Anxiety and agitation

Comments

Household bleach is a frequently ingested corrosive but rarely causes serious damage.
Liquid corrosives cause more damage than granular preparations.

Treatment

Assess child's breathing and level of consciousness.
Contact regional poison control centre for advice.
Inducing emesis is contraindicated (vomiting redamages the mucosa).
Dilute corrosive with water or milk (usually no more than 120 mL).
Do not neutralize. Neutralization can cause an exothermic reaction (which produces heat and causes increased symptoms or produces a thermal burn in addition to a chemical burn).
Maintain patent airway if needed.
Administer analgesics.
Do not allow oral intake.
Esophageal stricture may require repeated dilations or surgery.

Hydrocarbons

Gasoline
Kerosene
Lamp oil
Mineral seal oil (found in furniture polish)
Lighter fluid
Turpentine
Paint thinner and remover (some types)

Clinical Manifestations

Gagging, choking, and coughing
Nausea
Vomiting
Alterations in sensorium, such as lethargy
Weakness
Respiratory symptoms of pulmonary involvement

- Tachypnea
- Cyanosis
- Retractions
- Grunting

Comments

Immediate danger is aspiration (even small amounts can cause bronchitis and chemical pneumonia).
Gasoline, kerosene, lighter fluid, mineral seal oil, and turpentine cause severe pneumonia.

Treatment

Contact regional poison control centre.
Inducing emesis is generally contraindicated.
Gastric decontamination and emptying are questionable, even when the hydrocarbon contains a heavy metal or pesticide; if gastric lavage must be performed, a cuffed endotracheal tube should be in place before lavage because of a high risk of aspiration.
Symptomatic treatment of chemical pneumonia includes high humidity, oxygen, hydration, and antibiotics for secondary infection.

Acetaminophen

Clinical Manifestations

Occurs in four stages:

1. Initial period (2 to 4 hours after ingestion)
   - Nausea
   - Vomiting
   - Sweating
   - Pallor
2. Latent period (24 to 36 hours)
   - Patient improves
3. Hepatic involvement (may last up to 7 days and be permanent)
   - Pain in right upper quadrant
   - Jaundice
   - Confusion
   - Stupor
   - Coagulation abnormalities
4. Patients who do not die in hepatic stage gradually recover

Comments

It is the most common medication poisoning in children.
It occurs from acute ingestion.
Toxic dose is 150 mg/kg or greater in children.
Because of multiple formulations and concentrations, chronic acetaminophen toxicity is a significant problem.
Parents should be counselled to read product packaging carefully and to consult a health care provider to avoid inappropriate dosing (Abruzzi & Stork, 2002).

Treatment

Antidote N-acetylcysteine (Mucomyst) can usually be given orally but is first diluted in fruit juice or a soft drink because of the antidote's offensive odour.

Continued

BOX 47-22 Selected Poisonings in Children—cont'd

It is given as 1 loading dose and usually 17 maintenance doses in different dosages.
It may be given intravenously, but use is investigational.

Aspirin (Acetylsalicylic Acid [ASA])

Clinical Manifestations

Acute poisoning
- Nausea
- Disorientation
- Vomiting
- Dehydration
- Diaphoresis
- Hyperpnea
- Hyperpyrexia
- Oliguria
- Tinnitus
- Coma
- Convulsions

Chronic poisoning
- Same as for acute poisoning but subtle onset (often mistaken for viral illness)
- Dehydration, coma, and seizures may be more severe
- Bleeding tendencies

Comments

It may be caused by acute ingestion (severe toxicity occurs with 300 to 500 mg/kg).
It may be caused by chronic ingestion (i.e., more than 100 mg/kg/day for 2 or more days) and can be more serious than acute ingestion.
Time to peak serum salicylate level can vary with enteric aspirin or the presence of concretions (bezoars).

Treatment

Hospitalization is required for severe toxicity.
Emesis, lavage, activated charcoal, or cathartic measures may be used.
Lavage will not remove concretions of ASA.
Activated charcoal is important early in ASA toxicity.
Sodium bicarbonate (intravenous) to correct metabolic acidosis and urinary alkalinization may be effective in enhancing elimination; urinary alkalinization is very difficult to achieve.
Be aware of the risk for fluid overload and pulmonary edema.
Prescribe:
- External cooling for hyperpyrexia
- Anticonvulsants
- Oxygen and ventilation for respiratory depression
- Vitamin K for bleeding

In severe cases, hemodialysis (not peritoneal dialysis) may be used.

Iron

Mineral supplement or vitamin containing iron

Clinical Manifestations

Occurs in five stages:
1. Initial period (0.5 to 6 hours after ingestion) (if child does not develop gastrointestinal symptoms in 6 hours, toxicity is unlikely)
   - Vomiting
   - Hematemesis
   - Diarrhea
   - Hematochezia (bloody stools)
   - Gastric pain
2. Latency (2 to 12 hours)
   - Patient improves
3. Systemic toxicity (4 to 24 hours after ingestion)
   - Metabolic acidosis
   - Fever
   - Hyperglycemia
   - Bleeding
   - Shock
   - Death (may occur)
4. Hepatic injury (48 to 96 hours)
   - Seizures
   - Coma
5. Rarely, pyloric stenosis develops at 2 to 5 weeks

Comments

Factors related to frequency of iron poisoning:
- Widespread availability
- Packaging of large quantities in individual containers
- Lack of parental awareness of iron toxicity
- Resemblance of iron tablets to candy (e.g., M&M's)

Toxic dose is based on the amount of elemental iron in various salts (sulphate, gluconate, fumarate), which ranges from 20 to 33%; ingestions of 60 mg/kg are considered dangerous.

Treatment

Emesis or lavage may be used.
For toxic doses lavage may be necessary for all chewable tablets or liquids if spontaneous vomiting has not occurred.
Chelation therapy with deferoxamine is used in severe intoxication (may turn urine a red to orange colour).
If intravenous deferoxamine is given too rapidly, hypotension, facial flushing, rash, urticaria, tachycardia, and shock may occur; stop the infusion, maintain the intravenous line with normal saline, and notify the practitioner immediately.

Plants

See Box 47-21.

Clinical Manifestations

Depends on type of plant ingested
May cause local irritation of oropharynx and entire gastrointestinal tract
May cause respiratory, renal, and central nervous system symptoms
Topical contact with plants can cause dermatitis

Comments

Plants are some of the most frequently ingested substances.
Plant ingestions rarely cause serious problems, although some can be fatal.
Plants can also cause choking and allergic reactions.

Treatment

Induce emesis.
Wash from skin or eyes.
Supportive care as needed.

CRITICAL THINKING EXERCISE

Poisoning

Mrs. B, a neighbour, calls you. She is very upset because her 2-year-old son has eaten several chewable multivitamins with iron. She asks you if she should give her son syrup of ipecac. What should you advise her to do?

1. Evidence—Is there sufficient evidence to formulate an answer for Mrs. B?
2. Assumptions—Answer the following questions and describe some underlying assumptions on which your answers are based:
    a. What is the best initial response when a child ingests a potentially poisonous substance?
    b. What is syrup of ipecac?
    c. What are the dangers involved in the use of syrup of ipecac?
3. What is the priority for nursing care at this time?
4. Does the evidence support your conclusion?
5. What alternative perspectives might you have?

EMERGENCY

Poisoning

1. Assess the victim:
    - Take vital signs; re-evaluate routinely.
    - Initiate cardiorespiratory support if needed.
    - Treat other symptoms, such as seizures.
2. Terminate exposure:
    - Empty mouth of pills, plant parts, or other material.
    - Flush eyes continuously with normal saline (or room-temperature tap water at home) for 15 to 20 minutes.
    - Flush skin and wash with soap and a soft cloth; remove contaminated clothes, especially if a pesticide, acid, alkali, or hydrocarbon is involved.
    - Bring victim of an inhalation poisoning into fresh air.
    - Give one sip of water to dilute ingested poison.
3. Identify the poison:
    - Question the victim and witnesses.
    - Look for environmental cues (empty container, nearby spill, odour on breath) and save all evidence of poison (container, vomitus, urine).
    - Be alert to signs and symptoms of potential poisoning in absence of other evidence, including symptoms of ocular or dermal exposure.
    - Call regional poison control centre or other competent emergency facility for immediate advice regarding treatment.
4. Remove poison and prevent absorption:
    - Place child in side-lying, sitting, or kneeling position with head below chest to prevent aspiration.
    - Administer activated charcoal if ordered (unless used repeatedly, usual dose is 1 g/kg unless amount of toxin is known).

Based on the initial telephone assessment, the PCC will counsel the parents to begin treatment at home or to take the child to an emergency facility. When a call is taken, the name and telephone number of the caller are recorded to re-establish contact if the connection is interrupted. Because most poisonings are managed in the home, expert advice is essential in minimizing adverse effects. When the exact quantity or type of ingested toxin is not known, admission to a health care facility with pediatric emergency treatment services for laboratory evaluation and surveillance is critical after ingestion.

Assessment

The first and most important principle in dealing with a poisoning is to *treat the child first, not the poison.* This requires an immediate concern for life support. Vital signs are taken, and respiratory or circulatory support is instituted as needed. The child's condition is routinely re-evaluated. Because shock is a complication of several types of household poisons, particularly corrosives, measures to reduce the effects of shock, beginning with the CAB (circulation, airway, breathing) of resuscitation, are important. Establishing and maintaining vascular access for rapid intravascular volume expansion is vital in the treatment of pediatric shock.

The emergency department nurse's responsibility is to be prepared for immediate intervention with all of the necessary equipment. Because time and speed are critical factors in recovery from serious poisonings, anticipation of potential problems and complications may mean the difference between life and death.

Gastric Decontamination

Pediatric poisonings are common, yet they rarely result in significant morbidity and mortality (Greene, Harris, & Singer, 2008). The treatment for ingestion of poison will depend on the type of poison ingested. Gastrointestinal decontamination (GID) is used if necessary, depending on the potential toxicity of the poison and the risks versus benefits. GID is needed to remove the ingested poison, by adsorbing the toxin with activated charcoal, performing gastric lavage, or increasing bowel motility (catharsis). Because of continuing controversy regarding the use of these methods, each toxic ingestion should be treated individually (Eldridge, Van Eyk, & Kornegay, 2007; Madden, 2008). Specific antidotes may be administered for certain poisonings.

Syrup of ipecac, an emetic that exerts its action through irritation of the gastric mucosa and by stimulation of the vomiting centre, is no longer recommended for immediate treatment of poison ingestion (AAP, Committee on Environmental Health, 2005; Greene, Harris, & Singer, 2008).

Medications such as calcium channel blockers and benzodiazepines either produce a rapid onset of adverse symptoms (e.g., sedation, seizures, coma) or exaggerate the vagal response induced by gagging, which can lead to significant bradycardia. Under either circumstance, uncontrolled vomiting becomes an undesirable and unsafe event.

No emetic or other substance should be given at home without consultation with a PCC or physician.

A more commonly used method of GI decontamination is the use of *activated charcoal*, an odourless, tasteless, fine black powder that adsorbs many compounds, creating a stable complex. Activated charcoal may replace ipecac as the home remedy of choice, but Eldridge and colleagues (2007) suggest that it is premature to recommend the administration of activated charcoal in the home. Activated charcoal is mixed with water or a saline cathartic to form a slurry. Slurries are neither gritty nor distasteful but resemble black mud. To increase the child's acceptance of activated charcoal, the nurse should mix it with a diet soft drink and serve it through a straw in an opaque container with a cover (such as a disposable coffee cup and lid) or an ordinary cup covered with aluminum foil or placed inside a small paper bag. In one small study, healthy adolescents preferred the taste of activated charcoal mixed with Coca-Cola or chocolate milk mixture instead of water (Cheng & Ratnapalan, 2007). For small children, an NG tube may be required to administer activated charcoal. Because the charcoal solution is thick, a 12-French (or larger) NG tube should be used.

Potential complications from the use of activated charcoal include aspiration (usually in patients with impaired gag reflexes), constipation, and intestinal obstruction (in multiple doses). Superactivated charcoal products for gastric decontamination are reported to be more palatable and just as effective (Criddle, 2007). Cathartics, such as sorbitol, sodium, or magnesium, may be administered to stimulate evacuation of the bowel, thus decreasing systemic absorption of the poison and aiding in the removal of the charcoal. Many commercial preparations of activated charcoal contain cathartics. However, the use of cathartics is controversial, and the American Academy of Clinical Toxicology and European Association of Poisons Centres and Clinical Toxicologists (2004) do not recommend their use in children.

If the child is admitted to an emergency facility, gastric lavage may be performed to empty the stomach of the toxic agent; however, this procedure is associated with serious complications (GI perforation, hypoxia, aspiration), and it is no longer recommended in all cases of ingestion (see Evidence-Informed Practice box). There is no conclusive evidence that gastric lavage decreases morbidity (Criddle, 2007; Greene et al., 2008). In addition, gastric lavage may be of little use if used beyond 1 hour of ingestion (Greene et al., 2008). Conditions that may be appropriate for the use of gastric lavage include presentation within 1 hour of ingestion of a toxin, ingestion in a patient who has decreased GI motility, the ingestion of a toxic amount of a **sustained-release medication,** and a massive or life-threatening amount of poison (Criddle, 2007). When gastric lavage is used, the patient requires a protected airway, possible sedation, and the largest-diameter tube that can be inserted to facilitate passage of gastric contents.

Specific antidotes are available to counteract a minority of poisonings. They are highly effective and should be available in all emergency facilities. The supply of antidotes should be checked routinely and replaced as used or according to expiration dates. Antidotes available to treat toxin ingestion include N-acetylcysteine for acetaminophen poisoning, oxygen for carbon monoxide inhalation, naloxone for opioid overdose, flumazenil for benzodiazepines (diazepam) overdose, digoxin immune Fab (Digibind) for digoxin toxicity, amyl nitrate for cyanide, and antivenin for certain poisonous bites.

Prevention of Recurrence

The ultimate objective is to prevent poisonings from occurring or recurring. Education regarding home safety can be an effective method to prevent poisonings (Kendrick et al., 2008). One effective counselling method is first to discuss the difficulties of constantly watching and safeguarding young children (see Family-Centred Teaching box). In this way, the challenging task of raising children can lead to a discussion of injury prevention as part of the parental role. This approach also incorporates contributory causes for the incident, such as inadequate support systems, marital discord, discipline techniques (especially use of physical punishment), parental distress, or any disruption in the family or family activities, such as vacations, moves, visitors, illnesses, or births.

A visit to the home, especially after repeat poisonings, is recommended as part of the follow-up care to assess hazards, including family factors, and to evaluate appropriate injury-proofing measures. One method of identifying risk areas is to ask specific questions or to have the parent complete a questionnaire designed to isolate factors that predispose children to poisoning. Another approach is to encourage parents to bend down to the child's eye level and survey the home environment for potential hazards. Have the parents try to open cabinets and reach shelves to access poisons.

Passive measures (those that do not require active participation) have been the most successful in preventing poisoning and include using child-resistant closures and limiting the number of tablets in one container. However, these measures alone are not sufficient to prevent poisoning because most toxic agents in the home do not have safety closures. Therefore *active measures* (those that require participation) are essential. Guidelines for preventing the occurrence or recurrence of a poisoning are listed in the Guidelines box.

Heavy Metal Poisoning

Heavy metal poisoning can occur from the ingestion of a variety of substances, the most common being lead. Other sources that are important in terms of children are iron and mercury. *Mercury toxicity*, a rare form of heavy metal poisoning, has occurred in children from a variety of sources, such as broken thermometers or thermostats, broken fluorescent light bulbs, disk batteries, topical medications, gas regulators, cathartics, and interior latex house paint (Clifton, 2007). Elemental mercury (also called *metallic mercury* or *quicksilver*) is nontoxic if ingested and if the GI tract is healthy (e.g., has no fistulas). However, mercury is volatile at room temperature and enters the bloodstream after it is inhaled, causing toxicity (tremors, memory loss, insomnia, gingivitis, diarrhea, anorexia, weight loss). The classic form of mercury poisoning is called *acrodynia* (or "painful extremities").

NURSING ALERT Mercury thermometers are no longer recommended because the inhaled vapours can cause toxicity if the thermometer is broken. To prevent inhalation, spilled mercury must be cleaned up quickly, using disposable towels and rubber gloves and washing the hands well after removing the spill.

Heavy metals have an affinity for certain essential tissue chemicals, which must remain free for adequate cell

EVIDENCE-INFORMED PRACTICE Gastric Lavage in Children

—Curt Roberts and Danna Salinas

Ask the Question

What is the effect of gastric lavage in reducing systemic absorption of toxic substances compared with the administration of activated charcoal or forced emesis?

Search for Evidence

Search Strategies

Keywords included gastric lavage, gastric decontamination, activated charcoal, and toxic ingestion. Searches were limited to English-language articles with human subjects.

Databases Used

PubMed, STAT!Ref, UpToDateOnline, CINAHL, EMBASE, D.A.R.E, Cochrane Library, National Guideline Clearinghouse (AHRQ)

Critically Analyze the Evidence

Eddleston, Juszczak, and Buckley (2003) completed a review of the literature to determine whether gastric lavage pushes poisons beyond the pylorus to assist with faster elimination of toxins from the body. The review examined two studies designed to measure movement of substances through the stomach and into the small intestine after gastric lavage. One study randomized 40 patients to gastric emptying by forced emesis or gastric lavage and maintained a control group of 20 patients in whom gastric emptying was not necessary. Either radiopaque pellets or radiolabelled water was used as a marker. There were no significant differences in the number of pellets in the small bowel between the emesis group and the control group or between the gastric lavage group and the control group. The second study consisted of five volunteers who were subjected to gastric lavage on three occasions. Less poison was found in the small bowel after gastric lavage than after no intervention. The researchers concluded there was no evidence that gastric lavage drives toxins into the small intestine.

Other studies have demonstrated that gastric lavage is equivalent to forced emesis as a method of gastric emptying (American Academy of Clinical Toxicology & European Association of Poisons Centres and Clinical Toxicologists, 2005; Smilkstein, 2002). A randomized crossover study with 12 volunteers who ingested paracetamol 50 mg/kg 1 hour after a standard meal demonstrated that activated charcoal administered within 1 hour of ingestion was more effective than gastric lavage followed by charcoal because there was a delay in administration of the activated charcoal (Christophersen et al., 2002). Forced emesis was superior to gastric lavage when the goal was to remove large particles and fragments. However, the literature supports that gastric emptying has limited benefit in gastrointestinal decontamination because administration of activated charcoal appears to be more effective (American Academy of Clinical Toxicology & European Association of Poisons Centres and Clinical Toxicologists, 2005; Green, Harris, & Singer, 2008; Sheffield & Serwint, 2008; Smilkstein, 2002).

Numerous complications are reported with both gastrointestinal lavage and activated charcoal. Complications of orogastric or nasogastric intubation include esophageal tears or perforation, nasal injury, oropharyngeal injury, gastric perforation, and inadvertent tracheal intubation (American Academy of Clinical Toxicology & European Association of Poisons Centres and Clinical Toxicologists, 2005; Caravati et al., 2001; Eldridge, Van Eyk, & Kornegay, 2007; Smilkstein, 2002). Neither the American Academy of Clinical Toxicology nor the European Association of Poisons Centres and Clinical Toxicologists (2005) has recommended the routine use of gastric lavage in the management of toxic ingestions since 1997. Contraindications to the administration of charcoal also exist, including in patients who have ingested corrosive materials and in those at risk for hemorrhage or perforation due to structural abnormalities or recent surgery.

Apply the Evidence: Nursing Implications

Gastric lavage has little or no effect in reducing absorption, especially when used as an intervention more than 1 hour after ingestion. Single-dose or multidose activated charcoal is most effective when administered within 1 hour of ingestion but may have an effect up to 4 hours after ingestion, depending on the substance. Administration of activated charcoal should not be delayed by the use of forced emesis or gastric lavage.

References

American Academy of Clinical Toxicology, European Association of Poisons Centres and Clinical Toxicologists. (2005). Position paper: Single-dose activated charcoal. *Journal of Toxicology & Clinical Toxicology, 43*, 61–87.

Caravati, E. M., et al. (2001). Esophageal laceration and charcoal mediastinum complicating gastric lavage. *Journal of Emergency Medicine, 20*(3), 273–276.

Christophersen, A. B., et al. (2002). Activated charcoal alone or after gastric lavage: A simulated large paracetamol intoxication. *British Journal of Clinical Pharmacology, 53*(3), 312–317.

Eddleston, M., Juszczak, E., & Buckley, N. (2003). Does gastric lavage really push poisons beyond the pylorus? A systematic review of the evidence. *Annals of Emergency Medicine, 42*(3), 359–364.

Eldridge, D. L., Van Eyk, J., & Kornegay, C. (2007). Pediatric toxicology. *Emergency Medicine Clinics of North America, 25*(2), 283–308.

Greene, S., Harris, C., & Singer, J. (2008). Gastrointestinal decontamination of the poisoned patient. *Pediatric Emergency Care, 24*(3), 176–189.

Sheffield, P., & Serwint, J. R. (2008). Emetics, cathartics and gastric lavage. *Pediatric Review, 29*, 214–215.

Smilkstein, M. J. (2002). Techniques used to prevent gastrointestinal absorption of toxic compounds. In L. R. Goldfrank, et al. (Eds.), *Goldfrank's toxicologic emergencies* (7th ed.). New York: McGraw-Hill.

functioning. When metals are bound to these substances, cellular enzyme systems are inactivated. Treatment involves **chelation**, use of a chemical compound that combines with the metal for rapid and safe excretion.

Lead Poisoning

In North America, lead poisoning emerged as a problem in the early 1900s, when white lead was added to paints and tetraethyl lead was added to gasoline as an antiknock compound. Lead content in paint was decreased in 1975 in Canada; the use of lead in paint and leaded gasoline has since been banned in Canada. Blood lead levels in Canadians aged 6 to 79 years have declined over 70% since the 1970s (PHAC, 2011). Yet because it does not decompose or break down into smaller particles, lead deposited in the past is still present in soil near heavily trafficked areas. Coupled with deteriorating lead-based paint falling from the exterior of nearby houses, soil becomes a significant pathway by which lead poisoning can occur. Today the leading source of lead is from food and drinking water, although other factors, such as whether a home has lead, copper, or plastic service lines, can affect lead exposure level. For infants and toddlers, the ingestion of soil and dust containing lead, along with food and drinking water, are the greatest sources of exposure to lead in the environment (PHAC, 2011).

Cultural practices may also lead to pediatric ingestion of substances containing lead, especially when these are brought in from other countries. Other risk factors for having an elevated blood lead level (BLL) include poverty, age younger than 6 years, dwelling in urban areas, and living in older rental homes where lead decontamination may not be a priority. Children of immigrants and internationally adopted children may have been exposed to sources of lead in their country of origin and should also be carefully evaluated for lead exposure (Woolf, Goldman, & Bellinger, 2007). However, any child is at risk for lead poisoning if hazardous conditions for lead are present in the environment.

FAMILY-CENTRED TEACHING

Poisoning

A poisoning is more than a physical emergency for the child—it usually represents an emotional crisis for the parents, particularly in terms of guilt, self-reproach, and insecurity in the parenting role. The emergency department is no place to admonish the family for negligence, lack of appropriate supervision, or failure to injury-proof the home. Rather, it is a time to calm and support the child and parents while unaccusingly exploring the circumstances of the injury. If the nurse prematurely attempts to discuss ways of preventing such an incident from recurring, the parents' anxiety will block out any suggestions or offered guidance. Therefore it is preferable for the nurse to delay the discussion until the child's condition is stabilized or, if the child is discharged immediately after emergency treatment, to make a public health referral or send a packet of information.

GUIDELINES **Poisoning Prevention**

- Assess possible contributing factors in occurrence of injury, such as discipline, parent–child relationship, developmental ability, environmental factors, and behaviour problems.
- Institute anticipatory guidance for possible future injuries based on child's age and maturational level.
- Refer to visiting nurse agency to evaluate home environment and need for injury-proofing measures.
- Provide assistance with environmental manipulation, such as lead removal, when necessary.
- Educate parents regarding safe storage of toxic substances.
- Advise parents to take medications out of sight of children.
- Teach children the hazards of ingesting nonfood items.
- Advise parents against using plants for teas or medicine.
- Discuss problems of discipline and children's noncompliance and offer strategies for effective discipline.
- Instruct parents regarding correct administration of medications for therapeutic purposes and discontinuation of medication if there is evidence of mild toxicity.
- Advise parents to contact the poison control centre or practitioner immediately when a poisoning occurs.
- Post the phone number of the regional poison control centre with emergency phone list by the telephone.
- Include by the telephone the home address with nearest cross street in case an ambulance is needed. (In an emergency, family members may not remember the house address, and babysitters may not be aware of the information.)

Causes of Lead Poisoning

Although there are numerous sources of lead (Box 47-23), in most instances of acute childhood lead poisoning, the source is food, water, nonintact lead-based paint in an older home, or lead-contaminated bare soil in the yard. Microparticles of lead gain entrance into a child's body through ingestion or

BOX 47-23 Sources of Lead*

Lead-based paint in deteriorating condition
Lead solder
Lead crystal
Battery casings
Lead fishing sinkers
Lead curtain weights
Lead bullets

The following may contain lead:

- Ceramic ware
- Water
- Pottery
- Pewter
- Dyes
- Industrial factories
- Vinyl miniblinds
- Playground equipment
- Collectible toys
- Artists' paints
- Pool cue chalk
- Some imported toys or children's metal jewellery

Occupations and hobbies involving lead:

- Battery and aircraft manufacturing
- Lead smelting
- Brass foundry work
- Radiator repair
- Construction work
- Bridge repair work
- Painting contracting
- Mining
- Ceramics work
- Stained-glass making
- Jewellery making

*Health Canada issues alerts and recalls for products that contain lead and that may unexpectedly pose a hazard to young children.

inhalation and, in the case of an exposed pregnant woman, by placental transfer. When measured, a mother's lead level is nearly the same as that of her unborn child. A level of lead not harmful to an adult woman can be harmful to the fetus.

Inhalation exposure usually occurs during renovation and remodelling activities in the home, whereas ingestion happens during normal day-to-day play and mouthing activities. Sometimes a child will actually swallow loose chips of lead-based paint because it has a sweet taste. Water and food may also be contaminated with lead.

Pathophysiology and Clinical Manifestations

Lead can affect any part of the body, including the renal, hematological, and neurological systems (Fig. 47-9). Of most concern for young children is the developing brain and nervous system, which are more vulnerable than those of an older child or adult. Lead in the body moves via an equilibration process among the blood, the soft tissues and organs, and the bones and teeth. Lead ultimately settles in the bones and teeth, where it remains inert and in storage. This makes up the largest portion of the body burden, approximately 75 to 90%. At the cellular level it competes with molecules of calcium, interfering with the regulating action of calcium.

The neurological system is of most concern when young children are exposed to lead. The developing brain is especially vulnerable. Lead disrupts the biochemical processes and may directly affect the release of neurotransmitters, may cause alterations in the blood–brain barrier, and may interfere with the regulation of synaptic activity (Lidsky & Schneider, 2006).

There is a relationship between anemia and lead poisoning. Children who are iron deficient absorb lead more readily than those with sufficient iron stores. Lead can interfere with the binding of iron onto the **heme** molecule. This sometimes creates a picture of anemia, even though the child is not iron deficient. Lead toxicity to the erythrocytes leads to the release of the enzyme erythrocyte protoporphyrin (EP). Because EP is not sensitive to BLLs of lower lead levels, it is no longer used as a screening test. The BLL test is currently used for screening and diagnosis. However, elevation of the EP level is a good indicator of toxicity from lead and reflects the length of exposure and body burden of lead in the individual child.

Although adults have been shown to suffer adverse renal effects from occupational lead exposure, few studies document renal effects in children at other than extremely high lead levels. One can hypothesize that lead can affect the renal integrity of both children and adults. Thus the renal system of a child is still considered a potential target for its harmful effects.

The lead levels identified in children have declined since the initiation of screening for children at risk for lead

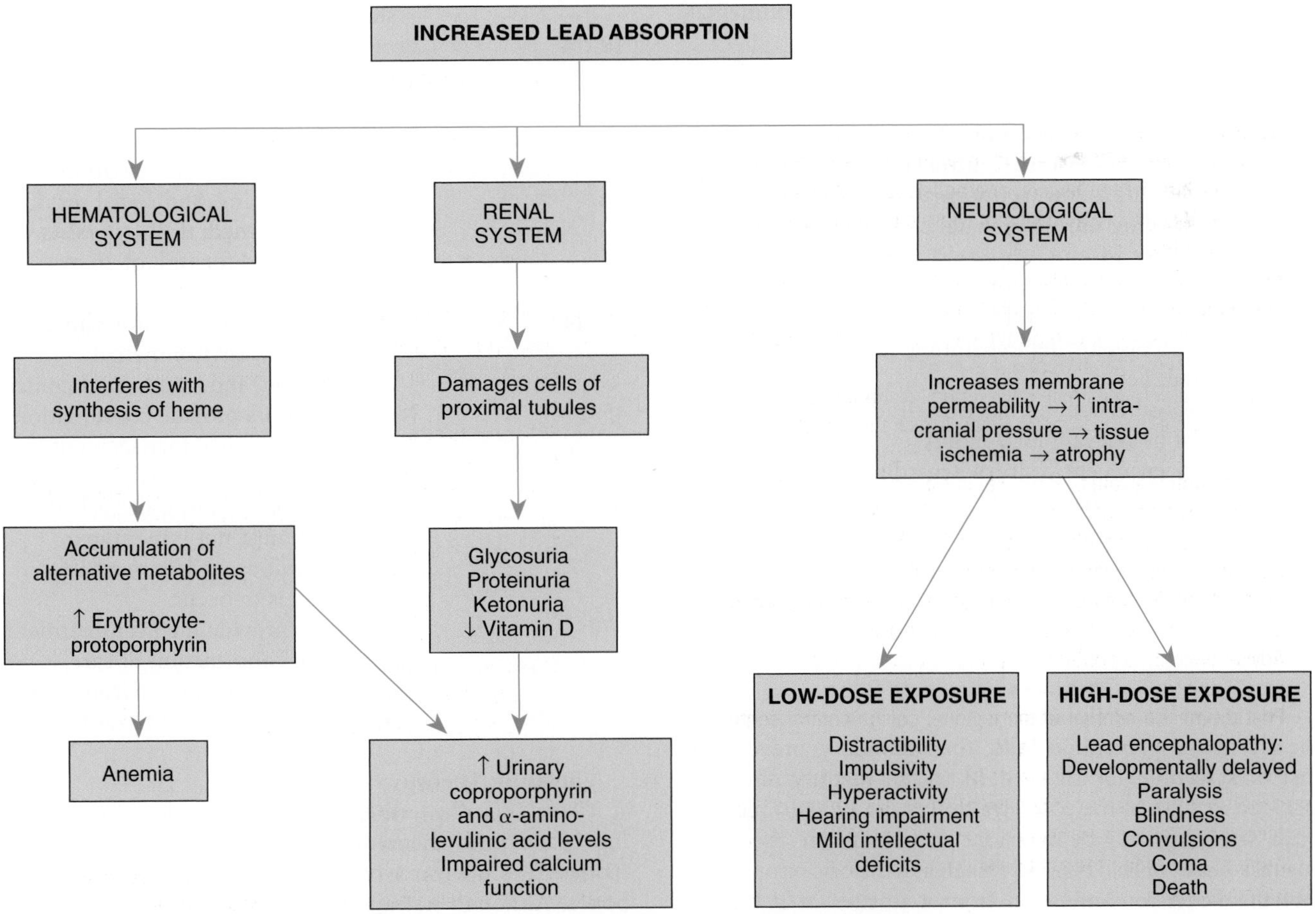

Fig. 47-9 Main effects of lead on body systems.

poisoning. With earlier intervention the most prevalent effects have changed. Since the late 1960s, children have rarely died of lead poisoning, and seizures and cognitive impairment have become less likely. However, even mild and moderate lead poisoning can cause a number of cognitive and behavioural problems in young children, including aggression, hyperactivity, impulsivity, delinquency, disinterest, and withdrawal. Long-term neurocognitive signs of lead poisoning include developmental delays, lowered intelligence quotient (IQ), reading skill deficits, visual–spatial problems, visual–motor problems, learning disabilities, and lower academic success. Physical growth and reproductive efficiency may also be adversely affected by chronic lead toxicity (Woolf et al., 2007).

NURSING ALERT Acute signs of lead poisoning include nausea, vomiting, constipation, anorexia, and abdominal pain. Additional clinical manifestations are hypophosphatemia, glycosuria, and aminoaciduria (Erickson & Thompson, 2005).

Diagnostic Evaluation

Children with lead poisoning rarely have symptoms, even at levels requiring chelation therapy. A diagnosis of lead poisoning is based only on the lead testing of a venous blood specimen from a venipuncture. The collection process is important. Blood must be collected carefully to avoid contamination by lead on the skin. The level of concern for an elevated BLL has dropped from 80 mcg/dL in 1950 to 10 mcg/dL today (American Academy of Pediatrics, Committee on Environmental Health, 2005; Heavey, 2008).

Anticipatory Guidance

Anticipatory guidance lends support to primary prevention efforts. The Centers for Disease Control and Prevention (2005) recommends that the following information be made available to families beginning during prenatal care, at 3 to 6 months, and at 1 year of age:

- Hazards of lead-based paint in older housing
- Ways to control lead hazards safely
- Hazards accompanying repainting and renovation of homes built before 1975
- Other exposure sources, such as traditional remedies, that might be relevant for a family

There has been recent concern regarding toys and other imported play items that have been found to contain lead. Parents should carefully evaluate the source of the toy (manufacturer) or plaything and not assume it is safe. Health Canada (http://www.hc-sc.gc.ca) is an excellent resource for parents and caregivers concerned about the safety of a given toy or product.

Screening for Lead Poisoning

When primary prevention fails, the secondary prevention effort of screening for elevated BLLs can identify children much earlier than in the past. Health Canada (2009b) recommends screening may be necessary in areas where there are unusual sources of lead exposure, such as a historic or ongoing problem of soil contamination from a smelter or if higher blood lead levels have been observed.

Therapeutic Management

The degree of concern, urgency, and need for medical intervention changes as the lead level increases. Education is one of the most important elements of the treatment process. Several areas that the nurse should discuss with the family of every child who has an elevated BLL (10 mcg/dL or higher) include the following (Heavey, 2008):

- The child's BLL and what it means
- Potential adverse health effects of an elevated BLL
- Sources of lead exposure and suggestions on how to reduce exposure, such as importance of wet cleaning to remove lead dust on floors, window sills, and other surfaces
- Importance of good nutrition in reducing the absorption and effects of lead; for persons with poor nutritional patterns, adequate intake of calcium and iron and importance of regular meals
- Need for follow-up testing to monitor the child's BLL
- Results of an environmental investigation if applicable
- Hazards of improper removal of lead paint (dry sanding, scraping, or open-flame burning)

Treatment actions vary depending on the child's BLL. Based on a diagnosis from a venous BLL test, the Centers for Disease Control and Prevention (2002) recommends the following actions:

BLL (MCG/DL)	Action
<10	Reassess or rescreen in 1 year. If exposure status changes, do this sooner.
10–14	Provide family with lead poisoning education, follow-up testing, and social service referral if necessary.
15–19	Provide family with lead poisoning education (dietary and environmental), follow-up testing, and social service referral as needed; if BLL persists, initiate actions for BLL of 20 to 44 mcg/dL.
20–44	Provide coordination of care, clinical management, environmental investigation, and lead hazard control.
45–69	Within 48 hours provide coordination of care and clinical management, including treatment, environmental investigation, and lead hazard control. The child must not remain in a lead-hazardous environment if resolution is to occur.
≥70	*Immediately* provide medical treatment and begin coordination of care, clinical management, environmental investigation, and lead hazard control.

Chelation Therapy

Chelation is the term used for removing lead from circulating blood and, theoretically, some lead from organs and tissues. It is unclear whether chelation affects lead stores in bones. Although not an antidote in the truest sense, it does serve a similar purpose in that the toxic substance or poison is removed from the body. However, chelation does not counteract any effects of the lead.

Historically, two chelating agents have been used consistently: calcium disodium edetate ($CaNa_2EDTA$ or calcium EDTA) and succimer (Chemet, *meso*-2,3 dimercaptosuccinic acid [DMSA]). British anti-Lewisite (BAL, dimercaprol, dimercaptopropanol) is used in conjunction with EDTA. All the agents have potential toxic adverse effects and contraindications. Renal, hepatic, and hematological parameters must be monitored.

Because of the equilibration process among blood, soft tissues, and other sites in the body, there is often a rebound of the BLL after chelation. After the body burden of lead is reduced enough to stabilize the BLL, rebound ceases. Multiple chelation treatments may be necessary. Adequate hydration is essential during therapy because the chelates are excreted via the kidneys.

BAL must not be used in the presence of a glucose 6-phosphate dehydrogenase (G6PD) deficiency or peanut allergy, nor should it be given in conjunction with iron. It is never used as a single-agent therapy, only in conjunction with EDTA. It must be given only at a deep intramuscular site. EDTA should be given intravenously over several hours or, when necessary to restrict fluids, intramuscularly.

Succimer is given orally over a 19-day course of treatment. The capsule is opened and sprinkled on a small amount of food or may be swallowed whole. Adverse effects include nausea, vomiting, diarrhea, loss of appetite, rash, elevated LFTs, and neutropenia. Because the chelates are excreted via the kidneys, adequate hydration is essential.

An oral chelating agent, d-penicillamine, is sometimes used to treat lead poisoning, but low doses should be used in children, and monitoring of renal function and blood counts during administration is essential (Woolf et al., 2007).

Prognosis

Although most of the pathophysiological effects of lead are reversible, the most serious consequences of both high and low lead exposure are the effects on the central nervous system. In children with lead encephalopathy, permanent brain damage can result in cognitive impairment, behaviour changes, possible paralysis, and seizures. However, moderate- to low-dose exposure may also cause permanent neurological deficits. Increased distractibility, short attention span, impulsivity, reading disabilities, and school failure have been associated with lead exposure. There is some evidence that treatment of moderate levels of lead poisoning can result in cognitive improvement (American Academy of Pediatrics, Committee on Environmental Health, 2005).

Nursing Care Management

The primary nursing goal in lead poisoning is to prevent the child's initial or further exposure to lead. For children with low-level exposure, this requires identifying the sources of lead in the environment. Careful history-taking is the most useful and valuable tool and should concentrate on the personal risk questions (see p. 1436). Suggestions for reducing lead in the child's environment are listed in the Community Focus box.

Children who must undergo chelation therapy need to be prepared for the injections, and all efforts should be made to reduce injection pain. Chelating agents are administered deeply into a large muscle mass (see Atraumatic Care box). To lessen the pain from EDTA, the local anaesthetic procaine is injected with the drug. Rotation of sites is essential to prevent the formation of painful areas of fibrotic tissue. Because EDTA and lead are toxic to the kidneys, records of intake and output should be kept, and the results of urinalysis should be assessed to monitor renal functioning.

Extreme caution is required with chelating agents. Incidences of child death from hypocalcemia have been recorded when Na_2EDTA was substituted for $CaNa_2EDTA$ and used as a chelating agent (Centers for Diseases Control and Prevention, 2006).

ATRAUMATIC CARE

Lead Chelation Therapy

To lessen the pain from intramuscular injection of $CaNa_2EDTA$, the local anaesthetic procaine is injected with the drug. Apply eutectic mixture of local anaesthetic (i.e., EMLA) cream over the puncture site 2.5 hours before the injection of EDTA and BAL. Administer intravenous EDTA whenever possible.

NURSING ALERT Calcium EDTA is only administered when there is adequate urinary output. Children receiving the medication intramuscularly must be able to maintain adequate oral intake of fluids.

Discharge planning for children with lead poisoning must include thorough education of families regarding safety from lead hazards, clear instructions regarding medication administration and follow-up, and confirmation that the child will be discharged to a home without lead hazards. Although caution must be used to avoid alarming parents unnecessarily, it is important that they know the risk implications for their child's behaviour and cognitive functions. Nurses should observe the development and behaviour of children who are hospitalized. Any concerns that are identified should be thoroughly evaluated. Referral to a child development or speech and language specialist may be indicated.

As in any situational crisis, parents need support and understanding if their child is treated for lead poisoning. Many families at the highest risk for lead poisoning have the fewest resources to comply with measures such as relocation or removing lead from the environment where the child experiences exposure.

Key Points

- Common nutritional disorders of infancy and early childhood may result from vitamin and mineral deficiency or excess, some types of vegetarian diets, protein-energy malnutrition, and food intolerance.
- Food consumption varies among vegetarians; thus a detailed dietary intake is essential for planning adequate intakes, particularly in children and pregnant and lactating women.

COMMUNITY FOCUS

Reducing Blood Lead Levels

Make sure the child does not have access to peeling paint or chewable surfaces painted with lead-based paint, especially window sills and wells.

If a house was built before 1960 (possibly before 1980) and has hard-surface floors, wet mop them at least once per week. Wipe other hard surfaces (e.g., window sills, baseboards). If there are loose paint chips in an area, such as a window well, use a wet disposable cloth to pick up and discard them. Do not vacuum hard-surfaced floors or window sills or wells, because this spreads dust. Use vacuum cleaners with agitators to remove dust from rugs rather than vacuum cleaners with suction only. If a rug is known to contain lead dust and cannot be washed, it should be discarded.

Wash and dry child's hands and face frequently, especially before eating.

Wash toys and pacifiers frequently.

If soil around the home is or is likely to be contaminated with lead (e.g., if the home was built before 1960 or is near a major highway), plant grass or other ground cover; plant bushes around the outside of the house so that the child cannot play there.

During remodelling of older homes, be sure to follow correct procedures. Be certain children and pregnant women are not in the home, day or night, until the process is completed. After deleading, thoroughly clean house using cleaning solution to damp mop and dust before inhabitants return.

In areas where lead content of water exceeds the drinking water standard and a particular faucet has not been used for 6 hours or more, "flush" the cold-water pipes by running the water until it becomes as cold as it will get (30 seconds to more than 2 minutes). The more time water has been sitting in pipes, the more lead it may contain.*

Use only cold water for consumption (drinking, cooking, and especially for making infant formula).

Hot water dissolves lead more quickly than cold water and thus contains higher levels of lead. First-flush water may be used for nonconsumption uses.

Have water tested by a competent laboratory. This action is especially important for apartment dwellers; flushing may not be effective in high-rise buildings or in other buildings with lead-soldered central piping.

Do not store food in open cans, particularly if cans are imported.

Do not use pottery or ceramic ware that was inadequately fired or is meant for decorative use for food storage or service. Do not store drinks or food in lead crystal.

Avoid traditional remedies or cosmetics that contain lead.

Make sure that home exposure is not occurring from parental occupations or hobbies. Household members employed in occupations such as lead smelting should shower and change into clean clothing before leaving work. Construction and lead abatement workers may also bring home lead contaminants.

Make sure the child eats regular meals, because more lead is absorbed on an empty stomach.

Make sure the child's diet contains sufficient iron and calcium and does not include excessive fat.

(Modified from Centers for Disease Control and Prevention. [2005]. *Preventing lead poisoning in young children*. Atlanta, GA: Author.)

*For more information on quality of drinking water, contact Health Canada: http://www.hc-sc.gc.ca/ewh-semt/water-eau/drink-potab/index-eng.php.

For general information on lead go to Health Canada's lead information page: http://www.hc-sc.gc.ca/ewh-semt/contaminants/lead-plomb/asked_questions-questions_posees-eng.php.

- Protein-energy malnutrition may occur as a complication of underlying disease, lack of parental education about infant nutrition, inappropriate management of food allergy, or incorrect preparation of formula.
- Food intolerance encompasses food allergies and food sensitivities, which can have a number of systemic and local clinical manifestations. CMA and lactose intolerance may occur in some children.
- Infants are subject to fluid depletion because of their greater surface area relative to body mass, high rate of metabolism, and immature kidney function.
- Dehydration can be classified as isotonic, hypotonic, and hypertonic.
- Vomiting and diarrhea account for significant fluid depletion, especially in infants and small children.
- The amount, frequency, and characteristics of stool and vomitus are important nursing observations.
- Diarrhea can be caused by an inflammatory process of infectious origin, a toxic reaction to ingestion of poisonous substances, dietary indiscretions, or infections outside the alimentary tract. The primary treatment of diarrhea is the use of an oral rehydrating solution.
- Intestinal parasitic diseases constitute the most common infections in the world; giardiasis and enterobiasis are the most widespread parasitic infections among children in Canada.
- Structural disorders of the GI tract include CL, CP, EA with TEF, anorectal malformations, and BA.
- CL/P, the most common facial malformation, may involve nutritional, dental, and speech problems.
- Hernias related to the GI tract can be minor (umbilical) or life threatening (diaphragmatic, gastroschisis, omphalocele).
- HD requires surgical removal of aganglionic segments of bowel.
- Postoperative care of the child with abdominal surgery involves assessing the abdomen and providing hydration and nutrition, intravenous fluids, proper positioning, wound care, and psychological support.

- Nursing care of GER is aimed at identifying children with suggestive symptoms, helping parents with home care feeding and positioning, and caring for the child undergoing surgical intervention.
- Although the cause of appendicitis is poorly understood, it is typically a result of obstruction of the lumen, usually by a fecalith. Common signs and symptoms are right lower quadrant abdominal pain, tenderness, and fever.
- Meckel's diverticulum is a congenital malformation of the GI tract characterized by bloody stools.
- IBD refers to UC and CD.
- Peptic ulcers are poorly understood, but contributing factors include interference with the normal protective mechanisms of the mucosal lining and the presence of *Helicobacter pylori.*
- Viral hepatitis is caused by six types of virus: HAV, HBV, HCV, HDV, HEV, and HGV.
- HAV is spread by the fecal–oral route, whereas HBV and HCV are transmitted primarily by the parenteral route. The most effective measure in prevention and control of hepatitis in any setting is hand hygiene.
- BA is a serious disorder, often causing progressive liver failure, which is an indication for liver transplantation.
- General signs of obstruction include colicky abdominal pain, nausea and vomiting, abdominal distension, and decreased stool output.
- HPS is recognized by characteristic projectile vomiting, malnutrition, dehydration, and a palpable mass in the epigastrium and is relieved by pyloromyotomy.
- Intussusception is one of the most common causes of intestinal obstruction during infancy and is characterized by abdominal pain and blood in stools. Treatment is either nonsurgical hydrostatic reduction or surgical reduction.
- Malabsorption syndromes are disorders associated with some degree of impaired digestion or absorption. They include digestive, absorptive, and anatomical defects.
- Celiac disease is characterized by intolerance to gluten. It is thought to be either an inborn error of metabolism or an immunological response.
- SBS is characterized by a loss of intestine resulting in a diminished ability to absorb a regular diet normally. Specialized enteral and parenteral nutrition is a major element of care for these children.
- Although the incidence of poisoning has decreased in the past 30 years as a result of more stringent packaging regulations, childhood poisoning remains a serious health concern.
- The major principles of treatment for poisoning include assessment and the BACs of resuscitation (cardiovascular supportive measures, airway, and breathing), minimization of poison absorption, prevention of complications, family support, and prevention of recurrence.
- Communication with the area poison control centre is essential in the treatment of any poisoning.
- Acetaminophen poisoning is the most common accidental medication poisoning among children and occurs primarily from acute overdose.
- The most important factor contributing to lead poisoning is its availability in the child's environment. Lead-based paint is the most toxic source of lead.
- Because of increasing awareness of the detrimental effects of low levels of lead on the developing nervous system, acceptable BLLs have been decreasing and now are at less than 10 mcg/dL.

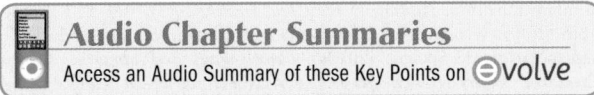

Audio Chapter Summaries

Access an Audio Summary of these Key Points on evolve

References

About Kids' Health. (2010). *Intestinal parasites.* Retrieved from http://www.aboutkidshealth.ca/En/HealthAZ/ConditionsandDiseases/DigestiveSystemDisorders/Pages/Intestinal-Parasites.aspx.

Abruzzi, G., & Stork, C. M. (2002). Pediatric toxicological concerns. *Emergency Medicine Clinics of North America, 20*(1), 223–247.

Achildi, A., & Grewal, H. (2007). Congenital anomalies of the esophagus. *Otolaryngologic Clinics of North America, 40*(1), 219–244.

Aiken, J. J., & Oldham, K. T. (2007). Acute appendicitis. In R. M. Kliegman, et al. (Eds.), *Nelson textbook of pediatrics* (18th ed.). Philadelphia: Saunders.

Alexander, F., et al. (2003). Fate of the pouch in 151 pediatric patients after ileal pouch anal anastomosis. *Journal of Pediatric Surgery, 38*(1), 328–332.

American Academy of Clinical Toxicology, European Association of Poisons Centres and Clinical Toxicologists. (2004). Position paper: Cathartics. *Journal of Toxicology, 42*(3), 243–253.

American Academy of Pediatrics, Committee on Environmental Health. (2005). Lead exposure in children; prevention, detection and management. *Pediatrics, 116*(4), 1036–1046.

American Academy of Pediatrics, Committee on Infectious Diseases. (2009). Prevention of rotavirus disease: updated guidelines for use of rotavirus vaccine. *Pediatrics, 123*(5), 1412–1420.

American Academy of Pediatrics, Committee on Infectious Diseases, & L. Pickering (Ed.). (2009). *Red book: 2009 report of the Committee on Infectious Diseases* (28th ed.). Elk Grove Village, IL: Author.

American Dietetic Association and Dietitians of Canada. (2003). Position of the American Dietetic Association and Dietitians of Canada: Vegetarian diets. *Canadian Journal of Dietetic Practice and Research, 64,* 62–81.

Assa'ad, A. H. (2006). Gastrointestinal food allergy and intolerance. *Pediatric Annals, 35*(10), 718–726.

Baron, M. L. (2002). Crohn's disease in children: This chronic illness can be painful and isolating, but new treatments may help. *American Journal of Nursing, 102*(10), 26–34.

Benchimol, E. I., Guttman, A., Griffiths, A.M., Rabeneck, L., Mack, D.R., Brill, H., Howard, J., Guan, J., & To, T. (2009). Increasing incidence of paediatric inflammatory bowel disease in Ontario, Canada: evidence from health administrative data. *Gut, 58,* 1490–1497. doi:10.1136/gut.2009.188383

Bernstein, C. N., et al. (2006). The epidemiology of inflammatory bowel disease in Canada: A population-based study. *American Journal of Gastroenterology, 101*(7), 1559–1568.

Blackburn, S. (2007). *Maternal, fetal, and neonatal physiology: A clinical perspective* (3rd ed.). St. Louis: Saunders.

Blanchard, S. S., & Czinn, S. J. (2007). Peptic ulcer disease in children. In R. M. Kliegman, et al. (Eds.), *Nelson textbook of pediatrics* (18th ed.). Philadelphia: Saunders.

Bronstein, A. C., et al. (2008). 2007 Annual report of the American Association of Poison Control Center's National Poison Data System (NPDS): 25th annual report. *Clinical Toxicology, 46*(10), 927–1057.

Burk, C. J., & Molodow, R. (2007). Infantile scurvy: An old diagnosis revisited with a modern dietary twist. *American Journal of Clinical Dermatology, 8*(2), 103–106.

Canadian Paediatric Society. (2002). *Canadian paediatric surveillance program hepatitis C virus infection.* Retrieved from http://www.cps.ca/english/surveillance/cpsp/Resources/RHepatitis.htm.

Canadian Paediatric Society. (2005). Children and natural health products: What a clinician should know. *Paediatrics and Child Health, 10*(4), 227–232.

Canadian Paediatric Society. (2006). Oral rehydration therapy and early refeeding in the management of childhood gastroenteritis. *Journal of Paediatric and Child Health, 11*(8), 527–531.

Canadian Paediatric Society. (2007). Vitamin D supplementation: Recommendations for Canadian mothers and infants. *Paediatrics and Child Health, 12*(7), 583–589.

Canadian Paediatric Society. (2009). Concerns for the use of soy-based formula in infant nutrition. *Paediatrics and Child Health, 14*(3), 109–113. Retrieved from http://www.cps.ca/english/statements/N/InfantSoyConcern.htm.

Canadian Paediatric Society. (2010a). *News releases and advisories: Canadian Paediatric Society recommends rotavirus vaccination for all babies.* Retrieved from http://www.cps.ca/English/Media/NewsReleases/2010/Rotavirus.htm.

Canadian Paediatric Society. (2010b). Recommendations for the use of rotavirus vaccines in infants. *Paediatrics & Child Health, 15*(8), 519–523.

Canadian Paediatric Society (2010c). Vegetarian diets in children and adolescents. *Paediatrics & Child Health, 15*(5), 303–314.

Canadian Society of Allergy and Clinical Immunology. (1995). *Anaphalaxis in schools and other child care settings.* Retrieved from http://www.csaci.ca/index.php?page=360.

Cavataio, F., & Guandalini, S. (2005). Gastroesophageal reflux. In S. Guandalini (Ed.), *Essential pediatric gastroenterology and nutrition.* New York: McGraw-Hill.

Centers for Disease Control and Prevention. (2002). *Managing elevated blood lead levels among young children: Recommendations from the Advisory Committee on Childhood Lead Poisoning Prevention.* Atlanta, GA: Author.

Centers for Disease Control and Prevention. (2003). Managing acute gastroenteritis among children: Oral rehydration, maintenance, and nutritional therapy. *MMWR. Moribidity & Mortality Weekly Report, 52*(RR-16), 1–16.

Centers for Disease Control and Prevention. (2005). *Statewide plan for childhood blood lead screening.* Atlanta, GA: Author.

Centers for Disease Control and Prevention. (2006). Deaths associated with hypocalcemia from chelation therapy—Texas, Pennsylvania, and Oregon, 2003–2005. *MMWR. Moribidity & Mortality Weekly Report, 55*(08), 204–207.

Chelimsky, G., & Czinn, S. (2001). Peptic ulcer disease in children. *Pediatrics in Review, 22*(10), 349–355.

Chen, S. M., et al. (2006). Screening for biliary atresia by infant stool color card in Taiwan. *Pediatrics, 117*(4), 1147–1154.

Cheng, A., & Ratnapalan, S. (2007). Improving the palatability of activated charcoal in pediatric patients. *Pediatric Emergency Care, 23*(6), 384–386.

Chien, J. C., et al. (2005). Is urorectal septum malformation sequence a variant of the vertebral defects, anal atresia, tracheo-oesophageal fistula, renal defects and radial dysplasia association? Report of a case and a review of the literature. *European Journal of Pediatrics, 164*(6), 350–354.

Christian, D. J., & Buyske, J. (2005). Current status of antireflux surgery. *Surgical Clinics of North America, 85*(5), 931–947.

Christie, L., et al. (2002). Food allergies in children affect nutrient intake and growth. *Journal of the American Dietetic Association, 102*(11), 1648–1651.

Clifton, J. C. (2007). Mercury exposure and public health. *Pediatric Clinics of North America, 54*(2), 237–269.

Coy, K., Speltz, M. L., & Jones, K. (2002). Facial appearance and attachment in infants with orofacial clefts: A replication. *Cleft-Palate Craniofacial Journal, 39*(1), 66–72.

Criddle, L. M. (2007). An overview of pediatric poisonings. *AACN Advanced Critical Care, 18*(2), 109–118.

Curtin, G., & Boekelheide, A. (2004). Cleft lip and palate. In P. J. Allen & J. A. Vessey (Eds.), *Primary care of the child with a chronic condition.* St. Louis: Mosby.

Cybulska, P., Ni, A., & Jimenez-Rivera, C. (2011). Viral hepatitis: Retrospective review in a Canadian Pediatric Hospital. *IRSN Pediatrics,* Volume 2011, 4 pages. doi:10.5402/2011/182964. Retrieved from http://www.hindawi.com/isrn/pediatrics/2011/182964/.

Czinn, S. J. (2005). *Helicobacter pylori* infection: Detection, investigation, and management. *Journal of Pediatrics, 146*(3 Suppl), S21–S26.

Dasgupta, R., & Langer, J.C. (2004). Hirschsprung disease. *Current Problems in Surgery, 41*(12), 949–988.

DeRoo, L. A., et al. (2008). First-trimester alcohol consumption and the risk of infant oral clefts in Norway: A population-based case-control study. *American Journal of Epidemiology, 168*(6), 638–646.

de Vrese, M., et al. (2001). Probiotics: Compensation for lactase insufficiency. *American Journal of Clinical Nutrition, 73*(2 Suppl), 421S–429S.

Dunham, L., & Kollar, L. (2006). Vegetarian eating for children and adolescents. *Journal of Pediatric Health Care, 20*(1), 27–34.

Durkin, E. T., & Shaaban, A. F. (2008). Recent advances and controversies in pediatric laparoscopic surgery. *Surgical Clinics of North America, 88*(5), 1101–1119.

Eldridge, D. L., Van Eyk, J., & Kornegay, C. (2007). Pediatric toxicology. *Emergency Medicine Clinics of North America, 25*(2), 283–308.

Emerick, K. M., & Whitington, P. F. (2006). Neonatal liver disease. *Pediatric Annals, 35*(4), 281–286.

Eppley, B. L., et al. (2005). The spectrum of orofacial clefting. *Plastic & Reconstructive Surgery, 115*(7), 101e–114e.

Erickson, L., & Thompson, T. (2005). A review of a preventable poison: Pediatric lead poisoning. *Journal of the Society of Pediatric Nurses, 10*(4), 171–182.

Ewing, W. M., & Allen, P. J. (2005). The diagnosis and management of cow's milk protein intolerance in the primary care setting. *Pediatric Nursing, 31*(6), 486–492.

Fiocchi, A., & Martelli, A. (2006). Dietary management of food allergy. *Pediatric Annals, 35*(10), 755–763.

Franklin, R. L., & Rodgers, G. B. (2008). Unintentional child poisonings treated in United States hospital emergency departments: National estimates of incident cases, population-based poisoning rates, and product involvement. *Pediatrics, 122*(6), 1244–1251.

Gelfond, D., & Fasano, A. (2006). Celiac disease in the pediatric population. *Pediatric Annals, 35*(4), 275–279.

Gisbert, J. P., de la Morena, F., & Abraira, V. (2006). Accuracy of monoclonal stool antigen test for the diagnosis of *H. pylori* infection: A systematic review and meta-analysis. *American Journal of Gastroenterology, 101*(8), 1921–1930.

Goldberg, J. P., Folta, S. C., & Must, A. (2002). Milk: Can a "good" food be so bad? *Pediatrics, 110*(4), 826–831.

Goodwin, K. A., et al. (2008). Changes in frequencies of select congenital anomalies since the onset of folic acid fortification in a Canadian birth defect registry. *Canadian Journal of Public Health, 99*(4), 271–275.

Greenbaum, L. (2007). Deficit therapy. In R. M. Kliegman, et al. (Eds.), *Nelson textbook of pediatrics* (18th ed.). Philadelphia: Saunders.

Greene, S., Harris, C., & Singer, J. (2008). Gastrointestinal decontamination of the poisoned patient. *Pediatric Emergency Care, 24*(3), 176–189.

Greer, F. R., et al. (2008). Effects of early nutritional interventions on the development of atopic disease in infants and children: The role of maternal dietary restriction, breastfeeding, timing of introduction of complementary foods, and hydrolyzed formulas. *Pediatrics, 121*(1), 183–191.

Guandalini, S. (2008). Probiotics for children with diarrhea: An update. *Journal of Clinical Gastroenterology, 42*(Suppl 2), S53–S57.

Health Canada. (2002). *Congenital anomalies in Canada—a perinatal health report.* Retrieved from http://www.phac-aspc.gc.ca/publicat/cac-acc02/index-eng.php.

Health Canada. (2009a). *Food allergies: It's your life.* Retrieved from http://www.hc-sc.gc.ca/hl-vs/iyh-vsv/food-aliment/allerg-eng.php.

Health Canada. (2009b). *Lead information package: Some commonly asked questions about lead and human health.* Retrieved from http://www.hc-sc.gc.ca/ewh-semt/contaminants/lead-phomb/exposure-exposition-eng.php#a38.

Health Canada. (2010). *Vitamin D and calcium: Updated dietary reference intakes.* Retrieved from http://www.hc-sc.gc.ca/fn-an/nutrition/vitamin/vita-d-eng.php.

Health Canada. (2011a). *Eating well with Canada's food guide.* Retrieved from http://www.hc-sc.gc.ca/fn-an/food-guide-aliment/index-eng.php/.

Health Canada. (2011b). *Food allergies and intolerances.* Retrieved from http://www.hc-sc.gc.ca/fn-an/securit/allerg/index-eng.php.

Health Link BC. (2011). *Reducing risk of food allergy in your baby: A resource for parents of babies at increased risk of food allergy.* Retrieved from http://www.healthlinkbc.ca/healthyeating/reducing-food-allergy-baby.html.

Heavey, E. (2008). Lead poisoning in children; still a threat. *Nursing, 38*(12), 17–18.

Herwig, K., Brenkert, T., & Losek, J. D. (2009). Enema-reduced intussusception management: Is hospitalization necessary? *Pediatric Emergency Care, 25*(2), 74–77.

Heyman, M. B., & American Academy of Pediatrics Committee on Nutrition. (2006). Lactose intolerance in infants, children, and adolescents. *Pediatrics, 118*(3), 1279–1286.

Hlavsa, M. C., Watson, J. C., & Beach, M. J. (2005). Giardiasis surveillance—United States, 1998–2002. *MMWR. Morbidity & Mortality Weekly Report, 54*(SS1), 9–16.

Holcomb, G. W., III, et al. (2005). Thoracoscopic repair of esophageal atresia and tracheoesophageal fistula: A multi-institutional analysis. *Annals of Surgery, 242*(3), 422–428.

Huang, L.-T., et al. (2006). Low plasma nitrite in infantile hypertrophic pyloric stenosis patients. *Digestive Diseases & Sciences, 51*(5), 869–872.

Huppertz, H. I., et al. (2006). Intussusception among young children in Europe. *Pediatric Infectious Diseases Journal, 25*(1), S22–S29.

Hurwitz, M., & Cox, K. L. (2007). Liver transplantation. In R. M. Kliegman, et al. (Eds.), *Nelson textbook of pediatrics* (18th ed.). Philadelphia: Saunders.

Hyams, J. S., & Markowitz, J. R. (2005). Can we alter the natural history of Crohn disease in children? *Journal of Pediatric Gastroenterology and Nutrition, 40*(3), 262–272.

Jabbar, A., & Wright, R. A. (2003). Gastroenteritis and antibiotic-associated diarrhea. *Primary Care, 30*(1), 63–80.

Karnam, U. S., & Reddy, K. R. (2003). Pegylated interferons. *Clinics in Liver Disease, 7*(1), 139–148.

Kemper, K. J., & Gardiner, P. (2007). Herbal medicines. In R. M. Kliegman, et al. (Eds.), *Nelson textbook of pediatrics* (18th ed.). Philadelphia: Saunders.

Kendrick, D., et al. (2008). Effect of education and safety equipment on poisoning-prevention practices and poisoning: Systematic review, meta-analysis and meta-regression. *Archives of Diseases in Childhood, 93*(7), 599–608.

Kim, W. R., et al. (2005). Mortality and hospitalization for hepatocellular carcinoma in the United States. *Gastroenterology, 129*(2), 486–493.

Kirschner, R. E., & LaRossa, D. (2000). Cleft lip and palate. *Otolaryngology Clinics of North America, 33*(6), 1191–1215.

Kugathasan, S., et al. (2003). Epidemiologic and clinical characteristics of children with newly diagnosed inflammatory bowel disease in Wisconsin: A statewide population-based study. *Journal of Pediatrics, 143*(4), 525–531.

Kwok, M. Y., Kim, M. K., & Gorelick, M. H. (2004). Evidence-based approach to the diagnosis of appendicitis in children. *Pediatric Emergency Care, 20*(10), 690–698.

Lanski, S. L., et al. (2003). Herbal therapy in a pediatric emergency department population: Expect the unexpected. *Pediatrics, 111*(5 pt 1), 981–985.

Lawrence, R. A., & Lawrence, R. M. (2011). *Breastfeeding: A guide for the medical professional* (7th ed.). St. Louis: Mosby.

Levin, M. E., Motala, C., & Lopata, A. L. (2005). Anaphylaxis in a milk-allergic child after ingestion of soy formula cross-contaminated with cow's milk protein. *Pediatrics, 116*(5), 1223–1225.

Lidsky, T. I., & Schneider, J. S. (2006). Adverse effects of childhood lead poisoning: The clinical neuropsychological perspective. *Environmental Research, 100*(1), 284–293.

Loening-Baucke, V., & Pashankar, D. S. (2006). A randomized, prospective, comparison study of polyethylene glycol 3350 without electrolytes and milk of magnesia for children with constipation and fecal incontinence. *Pediatrics, 118*(2), 528–535.

Loman, D. G. (2003). The use of complementary and alternative health care practices among children. *Journal of Pediatric Health Care, 17*(2), 58–63.

Madden, M. A. (2008). Responding to pediatric poisoning. *Nursing, 38*(8), 52–55. doi:10.1097/01.NURSE.0000327496.01064.a9

Maris, C. L., et al. (2000). Are infants with orofacial clefts at risk for insecure mother–child attachments? *Cleft-Palate & Craniofacial Journal, 37*(3), 257–265.

McGuire, J. K., Kulkarni, M. S., & Baden, H. P. (2000). Fatal hypermagnesemia in a child treated with megavitamin/megamineral therapy. *Pediatrics, 105*(2), 414.

Merritt, L. (2005a). Part 1. Understanding the embryology and genetics of cleft lip and palate. *Advances in Neonatal Care, 5*(2), 64–71.

Merritt, L. (2005b). Physical assessment of the infant with cleft lip and/or palate, part II. *Advances in Neonatal Care, 5*(3), 125–134.

Murdock, A. M., & Johnston, S. D. (2005). Diagnostic criteria for coeliac disease: Time for change? *European Journal of Gastroenterology & Hepatology, 17*(1), 41–43.

Naik-Mathuria, B., & Olutoye, O. O. (2006). Foregut abnormalities. *Surgical Clinics of North America, 86*(2), 261–284.

O'Connor, A., Gisbert, J., & O'Morain, C. (2009). Treatment of *Helicobacter pylori* infection. *Helicobacter, 14*(Suppl 1), 46–51.

Ohi, R. (2001). Surgery for biliary atresia. *Liver, 21*(3), 175–182.

Perrotta, S., et al. (2002). Infant hypervitaminosis A causes severe anemia and thrombocytopenia: Evidence of a retinol-dependent bone marrow cell growth inhibition. *Blood, 99*(6), 2017–2022.

Pessler, F., & Nejat, M. (2004). Anaphylactic reaction to goat's milk in a cow's milk-allergic infant. *Pediatric Allergy & Immunology, 15*(2), 183–185.

Preston, A. M., et al. (2003). Influence of environmental tobacco smoke on vitamin C status in children. *American Journal of Clinical Nutrition, 77*(1), 167–172.

Preston, A. M., Rodriguez, C., & Rivera, C. E. (2006). Plasma ascorbate in a population of children: Influence of age, gender, vitamin C intake, and smoke exposure. *Puerto Rico Health Sciences Journal, 25*(2), 137–142.

Public Health Agency of Canada. (2003). *Giardiasis*. Retrieved from http://dsol-smed.phac-aspc.gc.ca/dsol-smed/ndis/diseases/giar-eng.php.

Public Health Agency of Canada. (2006). *Canadian immunization guide* (7th ed.) Retrieved from http://www.phac-aspc.gc.ca/publicat/cig-gci/pdf/cig-gci-2006_e.pdf.

Public Health Agency of Canada. (2011). *Canada's 10 least wanted foodborne pathogens*. Ottawa: Canadian Food Inspection Agency. Retrieved from http://www.inspection.gc.ca/english/fssa/concen/cause/pathogene.pdf.

Ramaswamy, K., & Jacobson, K. (2001). Infectious diarrhea in children. *Gastroenterology Clinics, 30*(3), 611–624.

Ricart, E., et al. (2008). Are we giving biologics too late? The case for early versus late use. *World Journal of Gastroenterology, 14*(36), 5523–5527.

Richmond, J., Dunning, P., & Desmond, P. (2004). Hepatitis C: A medical and social diagnosis. *Australian Nursing Journal, 12*(1), 23–25.

Roslund, G., Hepps, T. S., & McQuillen, K. K. (2008). The role of oral ondansetron in children with vomiting as a result of acute gastritis/gastroenteritis who have failed oral rehydration therapy: A randomized controlled trial. *Annals of Emergency Medicine, 52*(1), 22–29.

Rostom, A., Murray, J. A., & Kagnoff, M. F. (2006). American Gastroenterological Association (AGA) Institute technical review on the diagnosis and management of celiac disease. *Gastroenterology, 131*(6), 1981–2002.

Rubin, D. T., & Kavitt, R. T. (2006). Surveillance for cancer and dysplasia in inflammatory bowel disease. *Gastroenterology Clinics of North America, 35*(3), 581–604.

Rudolph, C. D., et al. (2001). Guidelines for evaluation and treatment of gastroesophageal reflux in infants and children: Recommendations of the North American Society for Pediatric Gastroenterology and Nutrition. *Journal of Pediatric Gastroenterology & Nutrition, 32*(Suppl 2), S1–S31.

Ruemmele, F. M., et al. (1998). Diagnostic accuracy of serological assays in pediatric inflammatory bowel disease. *Gastroenterology, 115*(4), 822–829.

Rutter, M. D., et al. (2006). Thirty-year analysis of colonoscopic surveillance program for neoplasia in ulcerative colitis. *Gastroenterology, 130*(4), 1030–1038.

Sagar, J., Kumar, V., & Shah, D. K. (2006). Meckel's diverticulum: A systematic review. *Journal of the Royal Society of Medicine, 99*(10), 501–505.

Saltzman, M. D., & King, E. C. (2007). Central physeal arrests as a manifestation of hypervitaminosis A. *Journal of Pediatric Orthopedics, 27*(3), 351–353.

Sampson, H. A. (2003). Anaphylaxis and emergency treatment. *Pediatrics, 111*(6 Pt 3), 1601–1608.

Sandberg, S. J., Magee, W. P., & Denk, M. J. (2002). Neonatal cleft lip and cleft palate repair. *AORN Online, 75*(3), 488, 490–499, 501, 503–504, 506–508.

Sauer, C. G., & Kugathasan, S. (2010). Pediatric inflammatory bowel disease: Highlighting pediatric differences in IBD. *Medical Clinics of North America, 94*(1), 35–52.

Sawni, A., et al. (2007). The use of complementary/alternative therapies among children attending an urban pediatric emergency department. *Clinical Pediatrics, 46*(1), 36–41.

Sgouros, S.N., & Bergele, C. (2006). Clinical outcome of patients with *Helicobacter pylori* infection: The bug, the host, or the environment? *Postgraduate Medicine Journal, 82*(967), 338–342.

Shaw-Smith, C. (2006). Oesophageal atresia, tracheo-oesophageal fistula, and the VACTERL association: Review of genetics and epidemiology. *Journal of Medical Genetics, 43*(7), 545–554.

Sherman, M., et al. (2007). Management of chronic hepatitis C: Canadian consensus guidelines. *Canadian Journal of Gastroenterology, 1*(Suppl C), 25C–34C.

Sibley, E. (2004). Carbohydrate intolerance. *Current Opinion in Gastroenterology, 20*(2), 162–167.

Silbermintz, A., & Markowitz, J. (2006). Inflammatory bowel diseases. *Pediatric Annals, 35*(4), 268–274.

Sood, M. R. (2007). Disorders of malabsorption. In R. M. Kliegman, et al. (Eds.), *Nelson textbook of pediatrics* (18th ed.). Philadelphia: Saunders.

Speltz, M. L., et al. (1997). Early predictors of attachment in infants with cleft lip and/or palate. *Child Development, 68*(1), 12–25.

Steiner, M. J., et al. (2004). Is this child dehydrated? *Journal of the American Medical Association, 291*(22), 2746–2754.

Suwandhi, E., Ton, M. N., & Schwarz, S. M. (2006). Gastroesophageal reflux in infancy and childhood. *Pediatric Annals, 35*(4), 259–266.

Szajewska, H., Ruszczynski, M., & Radzikowski, A. (2006). Probiotics in the prevention of antibiotic-associated diarrhea in children: A meta-analysis of randomized controlled trials. *Journal of Pediatrics, 149*(3), 367–372.

To, T. & Langer, J. C. (2010). Does access to care affect outcomes of appendicitis in children? A population-based cohort study. *BMC Health Services Research, 10*, 250.

Tran, T. T. (2009). Management of hepatitis B in pregnancy: Weighing the options. *Cleveland Clinics Journal of Medicine, 76*(Suppl 3), S25–S29.

Trigazis, L., Tennankore, D., Vohra, S., & Katzman, D.K. (2004). The use of herbal remedies by adolescents with eating disorders. *International Journal of Eating Disorders, 35*(2), 223–238.

Waters, L., & Nelson, M. (2006). New therapeutic options for hepatitis C. *Current Opinion in Infectious Diseases, 19*(6), 615–622. doi:10.1097/QCO.0b013e328010a869

Whyte, C., Levin, T., & Harris, B. H. (2008). Early decisions in perforated appendix in children: Lessons from a study of nonoperative management. *Journal of Pediatric Surgery, 43*(8), 1459–1463. doi:10.1016/j.jpedsurg.2007.11.032

Wilkins-Haug, L. (2008). Prenatal diagnosis of orofacial clefts. *Up to Date*, July. Retrieved from http://www.uptodate.com.

Woolf, A. D., Goldman, R., & Bellinger, D. C. (2007). Update on clinical management of childhood lead poisoning. *Pediatric Clinics of North America, 54*(2), 271–294. doi:10.1016/j.pcl.2007.01.008

Wyllie, R. (2007). Motility disorders and Hirschsprung disease. In R. M. Kliegman, et al. (Eds.), *Nelson textbook of pediatrics* (18th ed.). Philadelphia: Saunders.

Yuen, M. F., & Lai, C. L. (2001). Treatment of chronic hepatitis B. *The Lancet Infectious Diseases, 1*(4), 383–393.

Zeisel, S. H., & Erickson, K. E. (2003). Dietary supplements (nutraceuticals). In W. A. Walker, J. B. Watkins, & C. Duggan (Eds.), *Nutrition in pediatrics* (3rd ed.). Hamilton, ON: Decker.

Additional Resources

About Face—Support for cleft lip and palate: http://www.aboutface.ca

Allergy Asthma Information Association: http://www.allergyfoundation.ca/website/allergy-asthma-info-association.htm

Anaphylaxis Canada—Information on food allergies: http://www.anaphylaxis.ca/

Canadian Liver Foundation: www.liver.ca

Crohn's and Colitis Foundation of Canada: http://www.ccfc.ca

Dietitians of Canada—Information on vegetarian diets: http://www.dietitians.ca/

Health Canada: Dietary Reference Intakes: http://www.hc-sc.gc.ca/fn-an/nutrition/reference/dri_rep-rap_anref-list/index-eng.php

National Center for Complementary and Alternative Medicine: http://www.nccam.nih.gov

Public Health Agency of Canada. Hepatitis—A Fact Sheet: http://www.phac-aspc.gc.ca/hcai-iamss/bbp-pts/hepatitis/hep_a-eng.php

United Ostomy Associations of Canada: http://www.ostomycanada.ca

Cardiovascular Dysfunction

Learning Objectives

On completion of this chapter, the reader will be able to:

- Design a plan for assisting a child during a cardiac diagnostic procedure.
- Demonstrate an understanding of the hemodynamics, distinctive manifestations, and therapeutic management of congenital heart disease.
- Outline a care plan for an infant or child with heart failure.
- Describe the care for a child who has hypoxia.
- Describe the care for an infant or a child with a congenital heart defect and its surgical repair.
- Discuss the nurse's role in helping the child and family cope with congenital heart disease.
- Differentiate between rheumatic fever and rheumatic heart disease.
- List the criteria for selected cholesterol screening of children.
- Discuss the assessment and management of hypertension in children and adolescents.
- Outline a care plan for a child with Kawasaki disease.

Electronic Resources

Additional information related to the content in Chapter 48 can be found on

evolve the companion Web site at

http://evolve.elsevier.com/Canada/Perry/maternal/

- Examination Review Questions
- Anatomy Review—Changes in Circulation at Birth
- Anatomy Review—Conduction System of the Heart
- Animation—Cardiac Tamponade, Infant
- Animation—Catheter Placement, Umbilical Vein
- Animation—Heart Sounds
- Animation—Structure of the Heart
- Animation—Subaortic Stenosis
- Case Study—Patent Ductus Arteriosus
- Critical Thinking Exercise—Cardiac Catheterization
- Critical Thinking Exercise—Digoxin Administration
- Critical Thinking Exercise—Patent Ductus Arteriosus

Cardiovascular Dysfunction

Cardiovascular disorders in children are divided into two major groups: **congenital** heart disease and acquired heart disorders. *Congenital heart disease (CHD)* includes primarily anatomical abnormalities present at birth that result in abnormal cardiac function. The clinical consequences of congenital heart defects fall into two broad categories: **heart failure** (HF) and **hypoxemia**. *Acquired cardiac disorders* are disease processes or abnormalities that occur after birth and can be seen in the normal heart or in the presence of congenital heart defects. They result from various factors, including infection, autoimmune responses, environmental factors, and familial tendencies.

History and Physical Examination

Taking an accurate health history is an important first step in assessing an infant or child for possible heart disease. Parents may have specific concerns, such as an infant with poor feeding or fast breathing, or a 7-year-old who can no longer keep up with friends on the soccer field. Others may not realize that their child has a medical problem; their baby has always been pale and fussy.

Asking details about the mother's health history, pregnancy, and birth history are important in assessing infants. Mothers with chronic health conditions, such as diabetes or lupus, are more likely to have infants with heart disease. Some medications, such as phenytoin (Dilantin), are teratogenic to the fetus. Maternal alcohol use or illicit drug use increases the risk of congenital heart defects. Exposures to infections, such as rubella, early in pregnancy may result in congenital anomalies. Infants with low birth weight resulting from intrauterine growth restriction are more likely to have congenital anomalies. High-birth-weight infants have an increased incidence of heart disease.

A detailed family history is also important. There is an increased incidence of congenital cardiac defects if either parent or a sibling has a heart defect. Some diseases, such as **Marfan syndrome**, and some cardiomyopathies are hereditary. A family history of frequent fetal loss, sudden infant death, and sudden death in adults may indicate heart disease. Congenital heart defects are seen in many syndromes such as Down and Turner's syndromes.

The physical assessment of suspected cardiac disease begins with observation of general appearance and proceeds with more specific observations. The following are supplementary

evolve Animation—Heart Sounds

evolve Animation—Structure of the Heart

to the general assessment techniques described for physical examination of the chest and heart in Chapter 34.

Inspection

Nutritional state—Failure to thrive or poor weight gain is associated with heart disease.

Colour—Cyanosis is a common feature of CHD, pallor is associated with poor perfusion.

Chest deformities—An enlarged heart sometimes distorts the chest configuration.

Unusual pulsations—Visible pulsations of the neck veins are seen in some patients.

Respiratory excursion—This refers to the ease or difficulty of respiration (e.g., **tachypnea**, dyspnea, expiratory grunt).

Clubbing of fingers—This is associated with cyanosis.

Palpation and Percussion

Chest—These manoeuvres help discern heart size and other characteristics (e.g., thrills) associated with heart disease.

Abdomen—Hepatomegaly or splenomegaly may be evident.

Peripheral pulses—Rate, regularity, and amplitude (strength) may reveal discrepancies.

Auscultation

Heart rate and rhythm—Listen for fast heart rates (tachycardia), slow heart rates (bradycardia), or irregular rhythms.

Character of heart sounds—Listen for distinct or muffled sounds, murmurs, and additional heart sounds.

Diagnostic Evaluation

A variety of invasive and noninvasive tests may be used in the diagnosis of heart disease (Table 48-1). Some of the more common diagnostic tools that require nursing assessment and intervention are described here.

Electrocardiogram

Bedside cardiac monitoring with the electrocardiogram (ECG) is commonly used in pediatrics, especially in the care of children with heart disease. The bedside monitor provides valuable information about heart rate and rhythm through a graphic display of the ECG tracing and a digital display. An alarm can be set with parameters for individual patient requirements and will sound if the heart rate is above or below the set parameters. Gelfoam electrodes are commonly used and placed on the right side of the chest (above the level of the heart) and the left side of the chest, and a ground electrode is placed on the abdomen. Electrodes should be changed every 1 or 2 days because they irritate the skin. Bedside monitors are an adjunct to patient care and should never be substituted for direct assessment and auscultation of heart sounds. The nurse should assess the patient, not the monitor.

NURSING ALERT Electrodes for cardiac monitoring are often colour coded: white for right, green (or red) for ground, and black for left. Always check to ensure that these colours are placed correctly.

Echocardiography

Echocardiography is one of the most frequently used tests for detecting cardiac dysfunction in children. Recent improvements in echocardiographic techniques have made it increasingly possible to confirm the diagnosis without resorting to

Table 48-1 Procedures for Cardiac Diagnosis

PROCEDURE	DESCRIPTION
Chest radiograph (x-ray)	Provides information on heart size and pulmonary blood flow patterns
Electrocardiography	Graphic measure of electrical activity of heart
Holter monitor	24-hr continuous electrocardiogram (ECG) recording used to assess dysrhythmias
Echocardiography	Use of high-frequency sound waves obtained by a transducer to produce an image of cardiac structures
Transthoracic	Done with transducer on chest
M-mode	One-dimensional graphic view used to estimate ventricular size and function
Two-dimensional	Real-time, cross-sectional views of heart used to identify cardiac structures and cardiac anatomy
Doppler	Identifies blood flow patterns and pressure gradients across structures
Fetal	Imaging fetal heart in utero
Transesophageal (TEE)	Transducer placed in esophagus behind heart to obtain images of posterior heart structures or in patients with poor images from chest approach
Cardiac catheterization	Imaging study using radiopaque catheters placed in a peripheral blood vessel and advanced into heart to measure pressures and oxygen levels in heart chambers and visualize heart structures and blood flow patterns
Hemodynamics	Measures pressures and oxygen saturations in heart chambers
Angiography	Use of contrast material to illuminate heart structures and blood flow patterns
Biopsy	Use of special catheter to remove tiny samples of heart muscle for microscopic evaluation; used in assessing infection, inflammation, or muscle dysfunction disorders and to evaluate for rejection after heart transplant
Electrophysiology (EPS)	Special catheters with electrodes used to record electrical activity from within heart; used to diagnose rhythm disturbances
Exercise stress test	Monitoring of heart rate, blood pressure, ECG, and oxygen consumption at rest and during progressive exercise on a treadmill or bicycle
Cardiac magnetic resonance imaging (MRI)	Noninvasive imaging technique; used in evaluation of vascular anatomy outside of heart (e.g., coarctation of the aorta, vascular rings), estimates of ventricular mass and volume; uses for MRI are expanding

cardiac catheterization. In more and more cases a prenatal diagnosis of CHD can be made by fetal echocardiography.

Echocardiography involves the use of ultrahigh-frequency sound waves to produce an image of the heart's structure. A transducer placed directly on the chest wall delivers repetitive pulses of ultrasound and processes the returned signals (echoes).

Although the test is noninvasive, painless, and associated with no known side effects, it can be stressful for children. The child must lie quietly in the standard echocardiographic positions; crying, nursing, or sitting up often leads to diagnostic errors or omissions. Infants and young children may need a mild sedative; older children benefit from psychological preparation for the test. The distraction of a video or movie is often helpful.

Cardiac Catheterization

Cardiac catheterization is an invasive diagnostic procedure in which a radiopaque catheter is inserted through a peripheral blood vessel into the heart. The catheter is usually introduced through percutaneous technique, in which the catheter is threaded through a large-bore needle that is inserted into the vein. The catheter is guided through the heart with the aid of fluoroscopy. After the tip of the catheter is within a heart chamber, contrast material is injected, and films are taken of the dilution and circulation of the material (angiography). Types of cardiac catheterizations include the following:

Diagnostic catheterizations—These studies are used to diagnose congenital cardiac defects, particularly in symptomatic infants and before surgical repair. They are divided into right-sided catheterizations, in which the catheter is introduced through a vein (usually the femoral vein) and threaded to the right atrium (most common), and left-sided catheterizations, in which the catheter is threaded through an artery into the aorta and then into the heart.

Interventional catheterizations (therapeutic catheterizations)—A balloon catheter or other device is used to alter the cardiac anatomy. Examples include dilating stenotic valves or vessels or closing abnormal connections (Table 48-2).

Electrophysiology studies—Catheters with tiny electrodes that record the impulses of the heart directly from the conduction system are used to evaluate dysrhythmias and sometimes destroy accessory pathways that cause some tachydysrhythmias.

Nursing Care Management

Cardiac catheterization has become a routine diagnostic procedure and may be done on an outpatient basis. However, it is not without risks, especially in neonates and seriously ill infants and children. Possible complications include acute hemorrhage from the entry site (more likely with interventional procedures because larger catheters are used), low-grade fever, nausea, vomiting, loss of pulse in the catheterized extremity (usually transient, resulting from a clot, hematoma, or intimal tear), and transient dysrhythmias (generally catheter induced) (Uzark, 2001). Rare risks include stroke, seizures, tamponade, and death. Researchers from Toronto's Hospital for Sick Kids found a complication rate of 7.3%. Despite significant improvements in technology that have helped decrease the incidence of complications, catheterization complications still occur (Mehta, Lee, Chaturvedi, & Benson, 2008).

Table 48-2 Current Interventional Cardiac Catheterization Procedures in Children

INTERVENTION	DIAGNOSIS
Balloon atrioseptostomy–Use well established in newborns; may also be done under echocardiographic guidance	Transposition of great arteries Some complex single-ventricle defects
Balloon dilation–Treatment of choice	Valvular pulmonic stenosis Branch pulmonary artery stenosis Congenital valvular aortic stenosis Rheumatic mitral stenosis Recurrent coarctation of aorta Further follow-up required in: Native coarctation of aorta in patients over 7 mo old Congenital mitral stenosis
Coil occlusion–Accepted alternative to surgery	Patent ductus arteriosus (<4 mm)
Transcatheter device closure–Several devices used in clinical trials	Atrial septal defect (ASD)
Amplatzer septal occluder–Approved for ASD closure	ASD
Ventricular septal defect devices–Used in clinical trials	Ventricular septal defects
Stent placement	Pulmonary artery stenosis Coarctation of the aorta in adolescents Use to treat other lesions investigational
Radiofrequency ablation	Some tachydysrhythmias

(Data from Allen, H. D., et al. [1998]. Pediatric therapeutic cardiac catheterization: AHA scientific statement. *Circulation, 97,* 609-625; updated data from Rome, J., & Kreutzer, J. [2004]. Pediatric interventional catheterization: Reasonable expectations and outcomes. *Pediatric Clinics of North America, 51,* 1589-1610.)

evolve Animation—Catheter Placement, Umbilical Vein

evolve Critical Thinking Exercise—Cardiac Catheterization

Preprocedural Care

A complete nursing assessment is necessary to ensure a safe procedure with minimum complications. This assessment should include accurate height (essential for correct catheter selection) and weight. Obtaining a history of allergic reactions is important because some of the contrast agents are iodine based. Specific attention to signs and symptoms of infection is crucial. Severe diaper rash may be a reason to cancel the procedure if femoral access is required. Because assessment of pedal pulses is important after catheterization, the nurse should assess and mark pulses (dorsalis pedis, posterior tibial) before the child goes to the catheterization room. The presence and quality of pulses in both feet should be clearly documented. Baseline oxygen saturation using pulse oximetry in children with cyanosis is also recorded.

Preparing the child and family for the procedure is the joint responsibility of the patient care team. School-age children and adolescents benefit from a description of the catheterization laboratory and a chronological explanation of the procedure, emphasizing what they will see, feel, and hear. Older children and adolescents may bring earphones and favourite music so they can listen during the catheterization procedure. Preparation materials such as picture books, videos, or tours of the catheterization laboratory may be helpful. Preparation should be geared to the child's developmental level. The child's caregivers often benefit from the same explanations. Additional information, such as the expected length of the catheterization, description of the child's appearance after catheterization, and usual postprocedure care, should be outlined. (See also Prepare the Child and Family for Invasive Procedures, p. 1478.)

Methods of sedation vary among institutions and may include oral or intravenous (IV) medications (see Chapter 45). The child's age, heart defect, clinical status, and type of catheterization procedure planned are considered when sedation is determined. General anaesthesia may be needed for some interventional procedures. Children are allowed nothing by mouth (NPO) for 4 to 6 hours or more before the procedure, according to institutional guidelines. Infants and patients with polycythemia may need IV fluids to prevent dehydration and hypoglycemia.

Postprocedural Care

Patients may recover from the procedure in a recovery unit, their hospital room, or occasionally critical care. They are placed on a cardiac monitor and a pulse oximeter for the first few hours of recovery. The most important nursing responsibility is observation of the following for signs of complications:

- Pulses, especially below the catheterization site, for equality and symmetry. (Pulse distal to the site may be weaker for the first few hours after catheterization but should gradually increase in strength.)
- Temperature and colour of the affected extremity since coolness or blanching may indicate arterial obstruction
- Vital signs, which are taken as frequently as every 15 minutes, with special emphasis on heart rate, which is counted for 1 full minute for evidence of dysrhythmias or bradycardia
- Blood pressure (BP), especially for hypotension, which may indicate hemorrhage from cardiac perforation or bleeding at the site of initial catheterization
- Dressing, for evidence of bleeding or hematoma formation in the femoral or antecubital area
- Fluid intake, both IV and oral, to ensure adequate hydration. (Blood loss in the catheterization laboratory, the child's NPO status, and diuretic actions of dyes used during the procedure put children at risk for **hypovolemia** and dehydration.)
- Blood glucose levels for hypoglycemia, especially in infants, who should receive dextrose-containing IV fluids

NURSING ALERT If bleeding occurs, direct continuous pressure is applied 2.5 cm above the percutaneous skin site to localize pressure over the vessel puncture.

Depending on hospital policy, the child may be kept in bed with the affected extremity maintained straight for 4 to 6 hours after venous catheterization and 6 to 8 hours after arterial catheterization to facilitate healing of the cannulated vessel. If younger children have difficulty complying, they can be held in the parent's lap with the leg maintained in the correct position. The child's usual diet can be resumed as soon as tolerated, beginning with sips of clear liquids and advancing as the condition allows. The child should be encouraged to void to clear the contrast material from the blood. Generally, there is only slight discomfort at the percutaneous site. To prevent infection, the catheterization area is protected from possible contamination. If the child wears diapers, the dressing can be kept dry by covering it with a piece of plastic film and sealing the edges of the film to the skin with tape. However, the nurse must be careful to continue observing the site for any evidence of bleeding (see Family-Centred Teaching box).

Congenital Heart Disease

The incidence of CHD in children is approximately 5 to 8 per 1000 live births (Park, 2008). About 2 or 3 in 1000 infants will be symptomatic during the first year of life with significant heart disease that will require treatment (Hoffman & Kaplan, 2002). CHD is the major cause of death (other than prematurity) in the first year of life. Although there are more than 35 well-recognized cardiac defects, the most common heart anomaly is ventricular septal defect (VSD).

The exact etiology of most congenital cardiac defects is unknown. Most are thought to be a result of multifactorial inheritance: a complex interaction of **genetic** and environmental factors. The tremendous amount of information being discovered in molecular biology and the Human Genome Project will likely increase our understanding of the genetic causes of congenital heart defects.

FAMILY-CENTRED TEACHING

Care After Cardiac Catheterization

- Remove pressure dressing the day after catheterization. Cover site with an adhesive bandage strip for several days. Put a new bandage on every day for the next 2 days.
- Keep site clean and dry. Avoid tub baths for the first 3 days; older children may shower the first day after catheterization.
- Observe site for redness, swelling, drainage, and bleeding. Monitor for fever. Observe the catheter leg for coolness. Notify practitioner if these occur.
- Avoid strenuous exercise for several days; the child may attend school.
- Resume regular diet without restrictions.
- Use acetaminophen or ibuprofen for pain.
- Keep follow-up appointments per practitioner's instruction.

(Modified from Children's Hospital [Boston] Cardiovascular Program, 2009.)

Some risk factors are known to increase the incidence of congenital heart defects. Maternal factors include chronic illnesses such as diabetes or poorly controlled phenylketonuria, alcohol consumption, and exposure to environmental toxins and infections. Family history of a cardiac defect in a parent or sibling increases the likelihood of a cardiac anomaly. The risk of CHD increases if a first-degree relative (parent or sibling) is affected. The **familial** risk is higher with left-sided obstructive lesions.

Congenital heart anomalies are often associated with **chromosome** abnormalities, syndromes, or congenital defects in other body systems. Down syndrome (**trisomy** 21) and trisomy 13 and 18 are highly correlated with congenital heart defects.

Circulatory Changes at Birth

During fetal life, blood carrying oxygen and nutritive materials from the placenta enters the fetal system through the umbilicus via the large umbilical vein. Oxygenated blood enters the heart by way of the inferior vena cava. Because of the higher pressure of blood entering the right atrium, it is directed posteriorly in a straight pathway across the right atrium and through the *foramen ovale* to the left atrium. In this way, the better-oxygenated blood enters the left atrium and ventricle to be pumped through the aorta to the head and upper extremities. Blood from the head and upper extremities entering the right atrium from the superior vena cava is directed downward through the tricuspid valve into the right ventricle. From here it is pumped through the pulmonary artery, where the major portion is shunted to the descending aorta via the *ductus arteriosus*. Only a small amount flows to and from the nonfunctioning fetal lungs (Fig. 48-1, A).

Before birth the high pulmonary vascular resistance created by the collapsed fetal lung causes greater pressures in the right side of the heart and the pulmonary arteries. At the same time, the free-flowing placental circulation and the ductus arteriosus produce a low vascular resistance in the remainder of the fetal vascular system. With the cessation of placental blood flow from clamping of the umbilical cord and the expansion of the lungs at birth, the hemodynamics of the fetal vascular system undergo pronounced and abrupt changes (see Fig. 48-1, B).

With the first breath, the lungs are expanded, and increased oxygen causes pulmonary vasodilation. With the removal of the placenta, pulmonary pressures start to fall as systemic pressures start to rise. Normally, the foramen ovale closes as the pressure in the left atrium exceeds the pressure in the right atrium. The ductus arteriosus starts to close in the presence of increased oxygen concentration in the blood and other factors.

Altered Hemodynamics

To appreciate the physiology of heart defects, it is necessary to understand the role of pressure gradients, flow, and resistance within the circulation. As with any fluid, blood flows from an area of high pressure to one of lower pressure and toward the path of least resistance in response to the pumping action of the heart. In general, the higher the pressure gradient, the greater the rate of flow; the higher the resistance, the lower the rate of flow.

Normally, the pressure on the right side of the heart is lower than that on the left side, and the resistance in the pulmonary circulation is less than that in the systemic circulation. Vessels entering or exiting these chambers have corresponding pressures. Therefore, if an abnormal connection exists between the

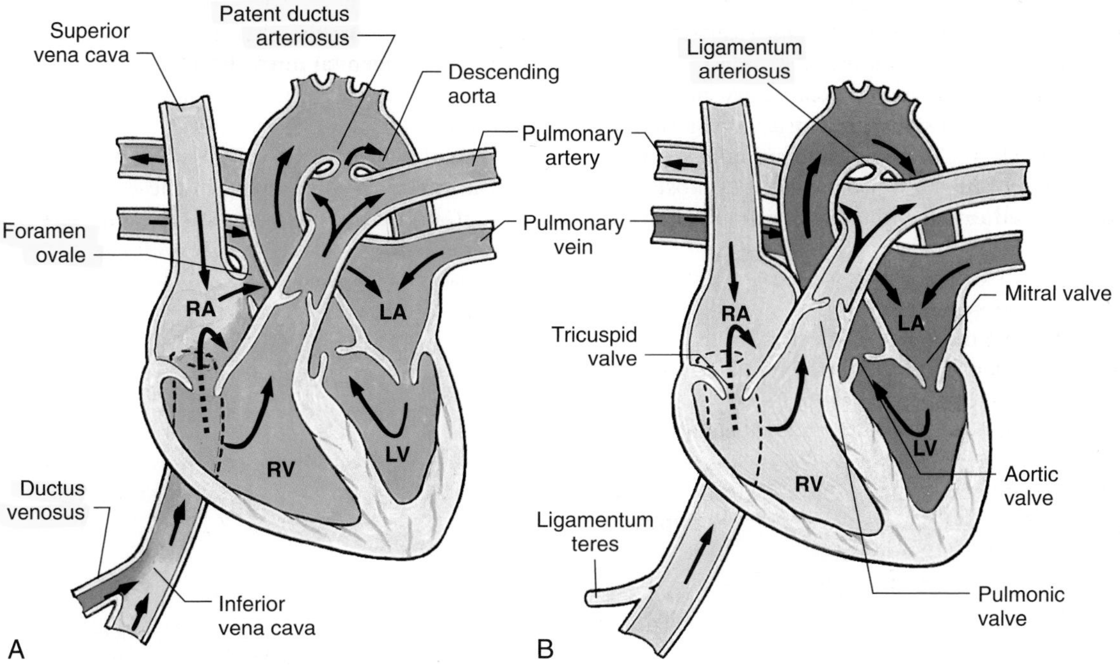

Fig. 48-1 Changes in circulation at birth. **A:** Prenatal circulation. **B:** Postnatal circulation. *Arrows* indicate direction of blood flow. Although four pulmonary veins enter the LA, for simplicity this diagram shows only two. *LA*, Left atrium; *LV*, left ventricle; *RA*, right atrium; *RV*, right ventricle.

evolve Anatomy Review—Conduction System of the Heart
evolve Anatomy Review—Changes in Circulation at Birth

heart chambers (such as a septal defect), blood will necessarily flow from an area of higher pressure (left side) to one of lower pressure (right side). Such a flow of blood is termed a *left-to-right shunt*. Anomalies resulting in cyanosis may result from a change in pressure so that the blood is shunted from the right to the left side of the heart (*right-to-left shunt*) because of either increased pulmonary vascular resistance or obstruction to blood flow through the pulmonic valve and artery. Cyanosis may also result from a defect that allows mixing of oxygenated and deoxygenated blood within the heart chambers or great arteries, such as occurs in truncus arteriosus.

evolve Case Study—Patent Ductus Arteriosus

evolve Critical Thinking Exercise—Patent Ductus Arteriosus

Classification of Defects

Congenital heart defects have been divided into two categories. Traditionally, cyanosis, a physical characteristic, has been used as the distinguishing feature, dividing the anomalies into acyanotic defects and cyanotic defects. In clinical practice, this system is problematic because children with acyanotic defects may develop cyanosis. More often those with cyanotic defects may appear pink and have more clinical signs of HF.

A more useful classification system is based on hemodynamic characteristics (blood flow patterns within the heart). These blood flow patterns are (1) increased pulmonary blood flow; (2) decreased pulmonary blood flow; (3) obstruction to blood flow out of the heart; and (4) mixed blood flow, in which saturated and desaturated blood mix within the heart or great arteries. As a comparison, both classification systems are outlined in Figure 48-2.

With the hemodynamic classification system, the clinical manifestations of each group are more uniform and predictable. Defects that allow blood flow from the higher-pressure left side of the heart to the lower-pressure right side (left-to-right shunt) result in increased pulmonary blood flow and cause HF. Obstructive defects impede blood flow out of the ventricles; obstruction on the left side of the heart results in HF, whereas severe obstruction on the right side causes cyanosis. Defects that cause decreased pulmonary blood flow result in cyanosis. Mixed lesions present a variable clinical picture based on the degree of mixing and amount of pulmonary blood flow; hypoxemia (with or without cyanosis) and HF usually occur together. Using this classification system, the clinical presentation and management of the most common defects are outlined in the following sections and in Box 48-1.

The outcomes of surgical treatment for patients with moderate to severe disease vary. Patient risk factors for increased morbidity and mortality include prematurity or low birth weight, a genetic syndrome, multiple cardiac defects, a non-cardiac congenital anomaly, and age at time of surgery (neonates are a higher risk group). For example, aortic stenosis or coarctation manifesting in the first week of life is more severe and carries a higher mortality than if it becomes apparent at 1 year of age. Outcomes for surgical repair of similar congenital heart defects also vary among treatment centres. In general, the outcomes of surgical procedures have steadily improved in the past decade, with mortality rates for many severe defects below 10%, and the incidence of complications and length of hospital stay have declined (Heart and Stroke Foundation, 2012a).

Defects With Increased Pulmonary Blood Flow

In this group of cardiac defects, intracardiac communications along the septum or an abnormal connection between the great arteries allows blood to flow from the higher-pressure left side of the heart to the lower-pressure right side of the heart (Fig. 48-3). Increased blood volume on the right side of the heart increases pulmonary blood flow at the expense of systemic blood flow. Clinically, patients demonstrate signs and symptoms of HF. Atrial septal defect (ASD), VSD, and patent ductus arteriosus are typical anomalies in this group (see Box 48-1).

Obstructive Defects

Obstructive defects are those in which blood exiting the heart meets an area of anatomical narrowing (*stenosis*), causing obstruction to blood flow. The pressure in the ventricle and great artery before the obstruction is increased, and the pressure in the area beyond the obstruction is decreased. The location of the narrowing is usually near the valve (Fig. 48-4), as follows:

Valvular—At the site of the valve itself

Subvalvular—Narrowing in the ventricle below the valve (also referred to as the *ventricular outflow tract*)

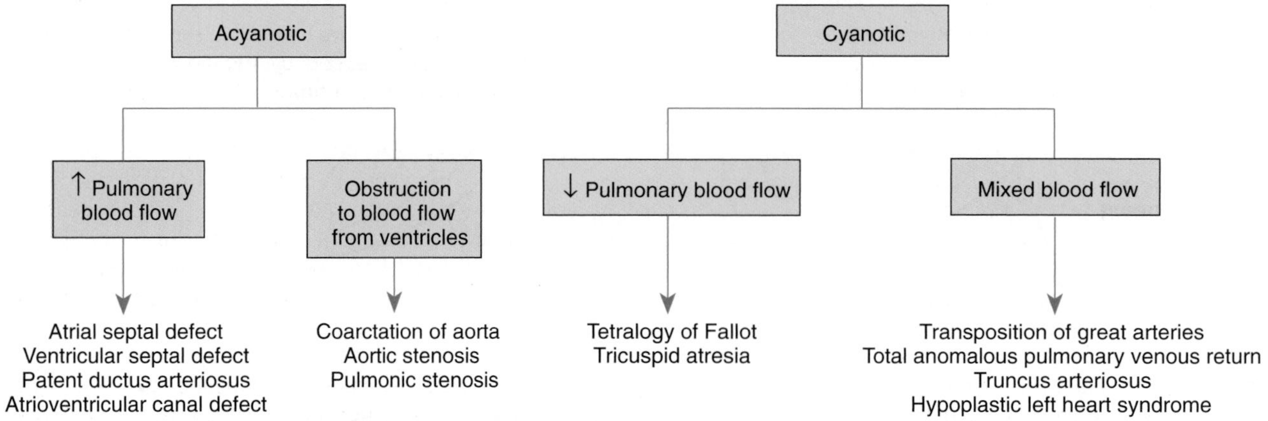

Fig. 48-2 Comparison of acyanotic–cyanotic and hemodynamic classification systems of congenital heart disease.

BOX 48-1 Defects With Increased Pulmonary Blood Flow

Atrial Septal Defect

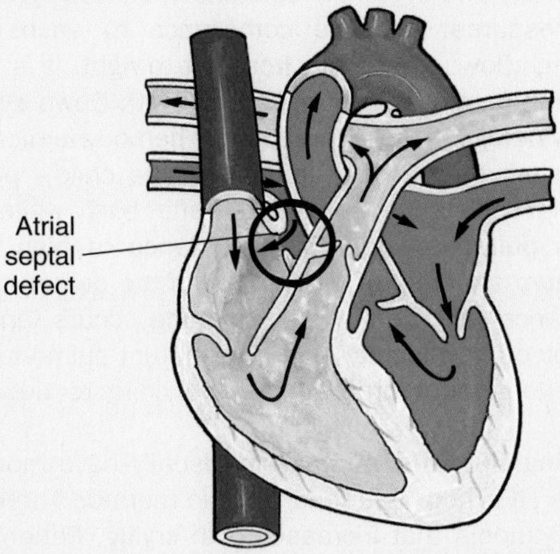

Description—Abnormal opening between the atria, allowing blood from the higher-pressure left atrium to flow into the lower-pressure right atrium. There are three types of atrial septal defects (ASDs):

Ostium primum (ASD 1)—Opening at lower end of septum; may be associated with mitral valve abnormalities

Ostium secundum (ASD 2)—Opening near centre of septum

Sinus venosus defect—Opening near junction of superior vena cava and right atrium; may be associated with partial anomalous pulmonary venous connection

Pathophysiology—Because left atrial pressure slightly exceeds right atrial pressure, blood flows from the left to the right atrium, causing an increased flow of oxygenated blood into the right side of the heart. Despite the low pressure difference, a high rate of flow can still occur because of low pulmonary vascular resistance and the greater distensibility of the right atrium, which further reduces flow resistance. This volume is well tolerated by the right ventricle because it is delivered under much lower pressure than with a ventricular septal defect (VSD). Although there is right atrial and ventricular enlargement, cardiac failure is unusual in an uncomplicated ASD. Pulmonary vascular changes usually occur only after several decades if the defect is left unrepaired.

Clinical manifestations—Patients may be asymptomatic. They may develop heart failure (HF). There is a characteristic systolic murmur with a fixed split second heart sound. There may also be a diastolic murmur. Patients are at risk for atrial dysrhythmias (probably caused by atrial enlargement and stretching of conduction fibres) and pulmonary vascular obstructive disease and emboli formation later in life from chronically increased pulmonary blood flow.

Surgical treatment—Surgical patch closure (pericardial patch or Dacron patch) is done for moderate to large defects. Open repair with cardiopulmonary bypass is usually performed before school age. In addition, the sinus venosus defect requires patch placement, so the anomalous right pulmonary venous return is directed to the left atrium with a baffle. The ASD 1 type may require mitral valve repair or, rarely, replacement of the mitral valve.

Nonsurgical treatment—ASD 2 closure with a device during cardiac catheterization is becoming commonplace and can be done as an outpatient procedure. The Amplatzer Septal Occluder is most commonly used. Smaller defects that have a rim around them for attachment of the device can be closed with a device; large, irregular defects without a rim require surgical closure. Successful closure in appropriately selected patients yields results similar to those from surgery but involves shorter hospital stays and fewer complications. Patients receive low-dose aspirin for 6 months (Rome & Kreutzer, 2004).

Prognosis—Operative mortality is very low (less than 1%). The presence of moderate or severe pulmonary hypertension has a marked adverse effect on survival of patients over 24 years of age at the time of operation (Porter & Edwards, 2008).

Ventricular Septal Defect

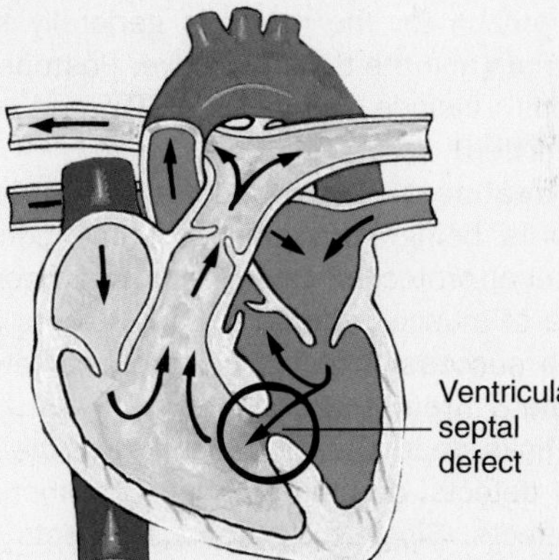

Description—Abnormal opening between the right and left ventricles. May be classified according to location: membranous (accounting for 80%) or muscular. May vary in size from a small pinhole to absence of the septum, which results in a common ventricle. VSDs are frequently associated with other defects, such as pulmonary stenosis, transposition of the great vessels, patent ductus arteriosus (PDA), atrial defects, and coarctation of the aorta. Many VSDs (20 to 60%) close spontaneously. Spontaneous closure is most likely to occur during the first year of life in children having small or moderate defects. A left-to-right shunt is caused by the flow of blood from the higher-pressure left ventricle to the lower-pressure right ventricle.

Pathophysiology—Because of the higher pressure within the left ventricle and because the systemic arterial circulation offers more resistance than the pulmonary circulation, blood flows through the defect into the pulmonary artery. The increased blood volume is pumped into the lungs, which may eventually result in increased pulmonary vascular resistance. Increased pressure in the right ventricle as a result of left-to-right shunting and pulmonary resistance causes the muscle to hypertrophy. If the right ventricle is unable to accommodate the increased workload,

Continued

BOX 48-1 Defects With Increased Pulmonary Blood Flow—cont'd

the right atrium may also enlarge as it attempts to overcome the resistance offered by incomplete right ventricular emptying.

Clinical manifestations—HF is common. A characteristic loud holosystolic murmur is heard best at the left sternal border. Patients are at risk for bacterial endocarditis and pulmonary vascular obstructive disease.

Surgical treatment

Palliative—Pulmonary artery banding (placement of a band around the main pulmonary artery to decrease pulmonary blood flow) may be done in infants with multiple muscular VSDs or complex anatomy. Improvements in surgical techniques and postoperative care make complete repair in infancy the preferred approach.

Complete repair (procedure of choice)—Small defects are repaired with sutures. Large defects usually require that a knitted Dacron patch be sewn over the opening. Cardiopulmonary bypass is used for both procedures. The approach for the repair is generally through the right atrium and the tricuspid valve. Postoperative complications include residual VSD and conduction disturbances.

Nonsurgical treatment—Device closure during cardiac catheterization is being performed in some centres under investigational protocols. One device has been approved for closure of muscular defects. Early results are encouraging, with successful defect closure and few complications (Rome & Kreutzer, 2004).

Prognosis—Risks depend on the location of the defect, the number of defects, and the presence of other associated cardiac defects. Single membranous defects are associated with low mortality (less than 2%); multiple muscular defects can carry a higher risk (Jacobs et al., 2004).

Atrioventricular Canal Defect

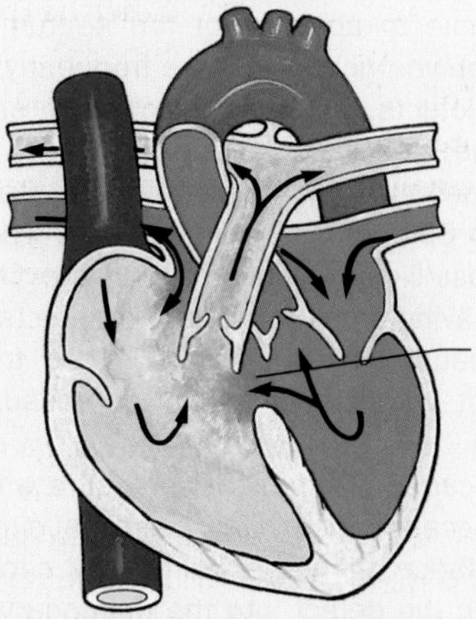

Description—Incomplete fusion of the endocardial cushions. Consists of a low ASD that is continuous with a high VSD and clefts of the mitral and tricuspid valves, which create a large central atrioventricular (AV) valve that allows blood to flow between all four chambers of the heart. The directions and pathways of flow are determined by pulmonary and systemic resistance, left and right ventricular pressures, and the compliance of each chamber, although flow is generally from left to right. It is the most common cardiac defect in children with Down syndrome.

Pathophysiology—The alterations in hemodynamics depend on the severity of the defect and the child's pulmonary vascular resistance. Immediately after birth, while the newborn's pulmonary vascular resistance is high, there is minimum shunting of blood through the defect. Once this resistance falls, left-to-right shunting occurs, and pulmonary blood flow increases. The resultant pulmonary vascular engorgement predisposes the child to development of HF.

Clinical manifestations—Patients usually have moderate to severe HF. There is a loud systolic murmur. There may be mild cyanosis that increases with crying. Patients are at high risk for developing pulmonary vascular obstructive disease.

Surgical treatment

Palliative—Pulmonary artery banding is occasionally done in small infants with severe symptoms. Complete repair in infancy is most common.

Complete repair—Surgical repair consists of patch closure of the septal defects and reconstruction of the AV valve tissue (either repair of the mitral valve cleft or fashioning of two AV valves). Postoperative complications include heart block, HF, mitral regurgitation, dysrhythmias, and pulmonary hypertension.

Prognosis—Operative mortality is less than 5% (Jacobs et al., 2004). A potential later problem is mitral regurgitation, which may require valve replacement.

Patent Ductus Arteriosus

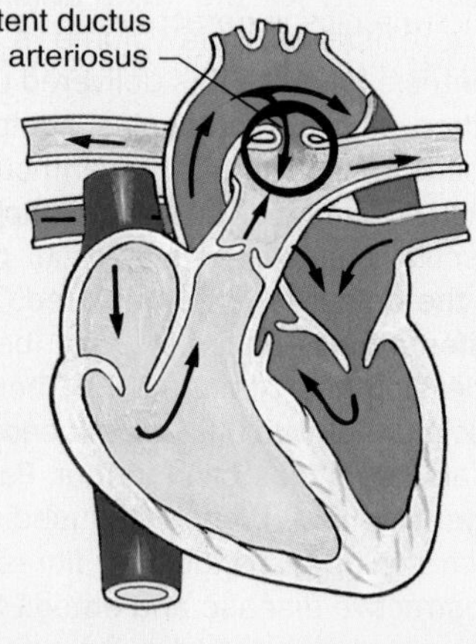

Description—Failure of the fetal ductus arteriosus (artery connecting the aorta and pulmonary artery) to close within the first weeks of life. The continued patency of this vessel allows blood to flow from the higher-pressure aorta to the lower-pressure pulmonary artery, which causes a left-to-right shunt.

Pathophysiology—The hemodynamic consequences of PDA depend on the size of the ductus and the pulmonary

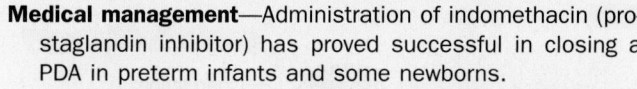

BOX 48-1 Defects With Increased Pulmonary Blood Flow—cont'd

vascular resistance. At birth the resistance in the pulmonary and systemic circulations is almost identical so that the resistance in the aorta and pulmonary artery is equalized. As the systemic pressure comes to exceed the pulmonary pressure, blood begins to shunt from the aorta across the duct to the pulmonary artery (left-to-right shunt). The additional blood is recirculated through the lungs and returned to the left atrium and left ventricle. The effect of this altered circulation is increased workload on the left side of the heart, increased pulmonary vascular congestion and possibly resistance, and potentially increased right ventricular pressure and hypertrophy.

Clinical manifestations—Patients may be asymptomatic or show signs of HF. There is a characteristic machinery-like murmur. A widened pulse pressure and bounding pulses result from runoff of blood from the aorta to the pulmonary artery. Patients are at risk for bacterial endocarditis and pulmonary vascular obstructive disease in later life from chronic excessive pulmonary blood flow.

Medical management—Administration of indomethacin (prostaglandin inhibitor) has proved successful in closing a PDA in preterm infants and some newborns.

Surgical treatment—Surgical division or ligation of the patent vessel is performed via a left thoracotomy. In a newer technique, video-assisted thoracoscopic surgery, a thoracoscope and instruments are inserted through three small incisions on the left side of the chest to place a clip on the ductus. The technique is used in some centres and eliminates the need for a thoracotomy, thereby speeding postoperative recovery.

Nonsurgical treatment—Coils to occlude the PDA are placed in the catheterization laboratory in many centres. Preterm or small infants (with small-diameter femoral arteries) and patients with large or unusual PDAs may require surgery.

Prognosis—Both surgical and nonsurgical procedures can be done at low risk with less than 1% mortality. PDA closure in very preterm infants has a higher mortality rate because of the additional significant medical problems.

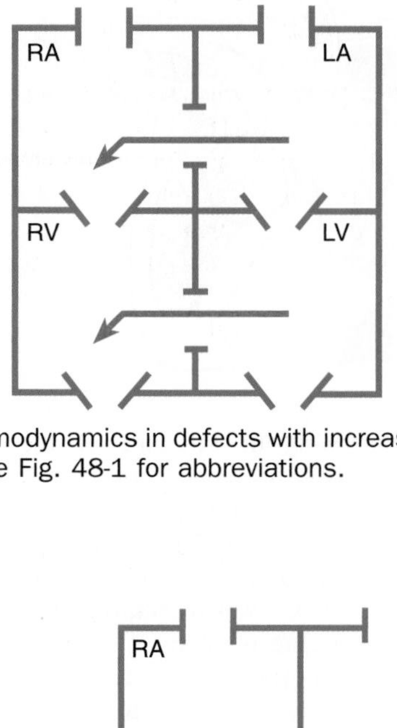

Fig. 48-3 Hemodynamics in defects with increased pulmonary blood flow. See Fig. 48-1 for abbreviations.

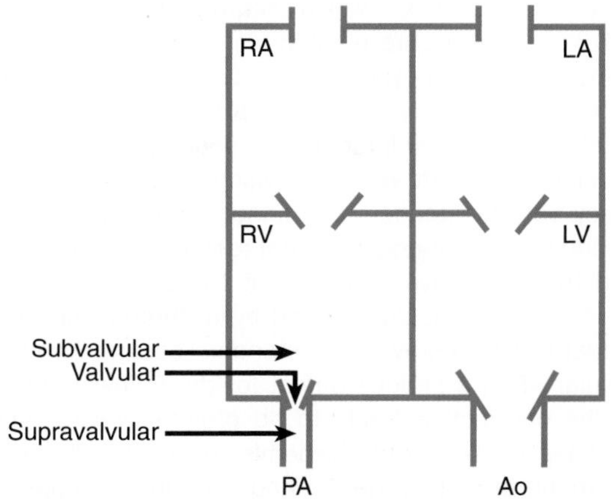

Fig. 48-4 Obstruction to ventricular ejection can occur at the valvular level (shown), below the valve (subvalvular), or above the valve (supravalvular). Pulmonary stenosis is shown here. *Ao*, aorta; *PA*, pulmonary artery. See Fig. 48-1 for additional abbreviations.

Supravalvular—Narrowing in the great artery above the valve

Coarctation of the aorta (narrowing of the aortic arch), aortic stenosis, and pulmonic stenosis are typical defects in this group (Box 48-2). Hemodynamically, there is a pressure load on the ventricle and decreased cardiac output. Clinically, infants and children exhibit signs of HF. Children with mild obstruction may be asymptomatic. Rarely, as in severe pulmonic stenosis, hypoxemia may be seen.

evolve Animation—Subaortic Stenosis

Defects With Decreased Pulmonary Blood Flow

In this group of defects, there is obstruction of pulmonary blood flow and an anatomical defect (ASD or VSD) between the right and left sides of the heart (Fig. 48-5). Because blood has difficulty exiting the right side of the heart via the pulmonary artery, pressure on the right side increases, exceeding left-sided pressure. This allows desaturated blood to shunt right to left, causing desaturation in the left side of the heart and in the systemic circulation. Clinically, these patients are hypoxemic and usually appear cyanotic. Tetralogy of Fallot and tricuspid atresia are the most common defects in this group (Box 48-3).

Mixed Defects

Many complex cardiac anomalies are classified together in the mixed category (Box 48-4) because survival in the postnatal period depends on the mixing of blood from the pulmonary and systemic circulations within the heart chambers. Hemodynamically, fully saturated systemic blood flow mixes with the desaturated pulmonary blood flow, causing a relative desaturation of the systemic blood flow. Pulmonary congestion occurs because the differences in pulmonary artery pressure and aortic pressure favour pulmonary blood flow. Cardiac output decreases because of a volume load on the ventricle. Clinically, these patients have a variable picture that combines some degree of desaturation (although cyanosis is not always

BOX 48-2 Obstructive Defects

Coarctation of the Aorta

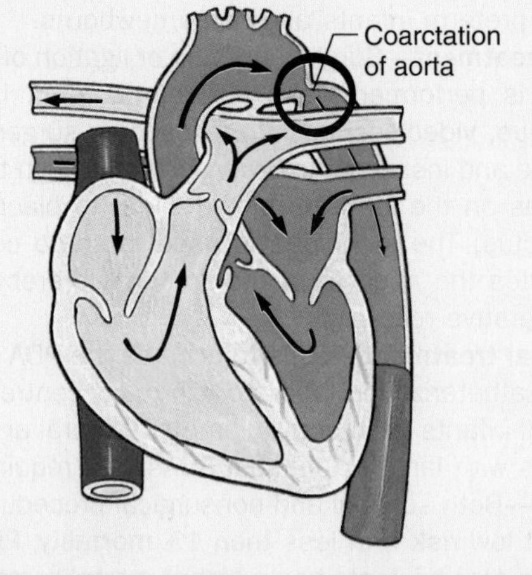

Description—There is localized narrowing near the insertion of the ductus arteriosus, which results in increased pressure proximal to the defect and decreased pressure distal to the obstruction.

Pathophysiology—The effect of a narrowing within the aorta is increased pressure proximal to the defect (upper extremities) and decreased pressure distal to it (lower extremities).

Clinical manifestations—The patient may have high blood pressure and bounding pulses in the arms, weak or absent femoral pulses, and cool lower extremities with lower blood pressure. There are signs of heart failure (HF) in infants. In infants with critical coarctation, the hemodynamic condition may deteriorate rapidly with severe acidosis and hypotension. Mechanical ventilation and inotropic support are often necessary before surgery. Older children may experience dizziness, headaches, fainting, and epistaxis resulting from hypertension. Patients are at risk for hypertension, ruptured aorta, aortic aneurysm, and stroke.

Surgical treatment—Surgical repair is the treatment of choice for infants younger than 6 months of age and for patients with long-segment stenosis or complex anatomy; it may be performed for all patients with coarctation. Repair is by resection of the coarctated portion with an end-to-end anastomosis of the aorta or enlargement of the constricted section using a graft of prosthetic material or a portion of the left subclavian artery. Because this defect is outside the heart and pericardium, cardiopulmonary bypass is not required, and a thoracotomy incision is used. Postoperative hypertension is treated with intravenous sodium nitroprusside, esmolol, or milrinone followed by oral medications, such as angiotensin-converting enzyme inhibitors or β-blockers. Residual permanent hypertension after repair of coarctation of the aorta (COA) seems to be related to age and time of repair. To prevent both hypertension at rest and exercise-provoked systemic hypertension after repair, elective surgery for COA is advised within the first 2 years of life. There is a 15 to 30% risk of recurrence in patients who underwent surgical repair as infants (Beekman, 2008). Percutaneous balloon angioplasty techniques have proved to be effective in relieving residual postoperative coarctation gradients.

Nonsurgical treatment—Balloon angioplasty is being performed as a primary intervention for COA in older infants and children. In adolescents, stents may be placed in the aorta to maintain patency. Recent studies have demonstrated that balloon angioplasty is effective in children and aneurysm formation is rare. The high restenosis rate in young infants limits its application in this group (Rome & Kreutzer, 2004).

Prognosis—Mortality is less than 5% in patients with isolated coarctation; risk is increased in infants with other complex cardiac defects (Jacobs et al., 2004).

Aortic Stenosis

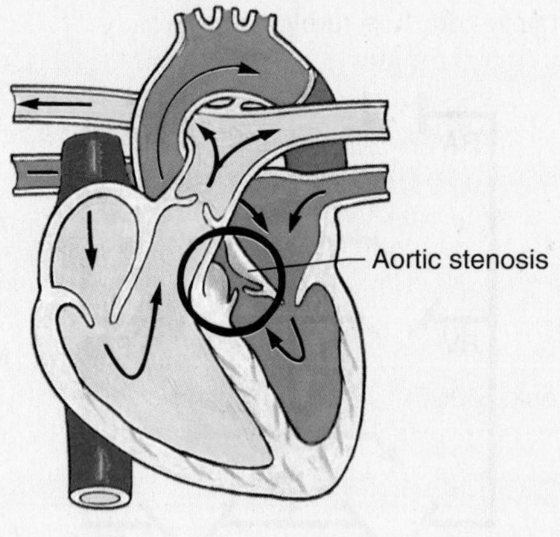

Description—Narrowing or stricture of the aortic valve, causing resistance to blood flow in the left ventricle, decreased cardiac output, left ventricular hypertrophy, and pulmonary vascular congestion. The prominent anatomical consequence of aortic stenosis (AS) is the hypertrophy of the left ventricular wall, which eventually leads to increased end-diastolic pressure resulting in pulmonary venous and pulmonary arterial hypertension. Left ventricular hypertrophy also interferes with coronary artery perfusion and may result in myocardial infarction or scarring of the papillary muscles of the left ventricle, which causes mitral insufficiency. Valvular stenosis, the most common type, is usually caused by malformed cusps that result in a bicuspid rather than tricuspid valve or fusion of the cusps. Subvalvular stenosis is a stricture caused by a fibrous ring below a normal valve; supravalvular stenosis occurs infrequently. Valvular AS is a serious defect for the following reasons: (1) the obstruction tends to be progressive; (2) sudden episodes of myocardial ischemia, or low cardiac output, can result in sudden death; and (3) surgical repair rarely results in a normal valve. This is one of the rare instances

BOX 48-2 Obstructive Defects—cont'd

in which strenuous physical activity may be curtailed because of the cardiac condition.

Pathophysiology—A stricture in the aortic outflow tract causes resistance to ejection of blood from the left ventricle. The extra workload on the left ventricle causes hypertrophy. If left ventricular failure develops, left atrial pressure increases; this causes increased pressure in the pulmonary veins, which results in pulmonary vascular congestion (pulmonary edema).

Clinical manifestations—Newborns with critical AS demonstrate signs of decreased cardiac output with faint pulses, hypotension, tachycardia, and poor feeding. Children show signs of exercise intolerance, chest pain, and dizziness when standing for a long period. A systolic ejection murmur may or may not be present. Patients are at risk for bacterial endocarditis, coronary insufficiency, and ventricular dysfunction.

Valvular Aortic Stenosis

Surgical treatment—Aortic valvotomy is performed under inflow occlusion. It is rarely used because balloon dilation in the catheterization laboratory is the first-line procedure. Newborns with critical AS and small left-sided structures may undergo a stage 1 Norwood procedure (see Hypoplastic Left Heart Syndrome, Box 48-4).

Prognosis—Aortic valve replacement offers a good treatment option and may lead to normalization of left ventricular size and function (Arnold et al., 2008). Results of aortic valvotomy in older children are very good, with mortality and morbidity close to 0% (Shanmugam, MacArthur, & Pollock, 2005). However, aortic valvotomy remains a palliative procedure, and approximately 25% of patients require additional surgery within 10 years for recurrent stenosis. A valve replacement may be required at the second procedure. An aortic homograft with a valve may also be used (extended aortic root replacement), or the pulmonary valve may be moved to the aortic position and replaced with a homograft valve (Ross procedure).

Nonsurgical treatment—The narrowed valve is dilated using balloon angioplasty in the catheterization laboratory. This procedure is usually the first intervention.

Prognosis—Complications include aortic insufficiency or valvular regurgitation, tearing of the valve leaflets, and loss of pulse in the catheterized limb.

Subvalvular Aortic Stenosis

Surgical treatment—Procedure may involve incising a membrane if one exists or cutting the fibromuscular ring. If the obstruction results from narrowing of the left ventricular outflow tract and a small aortic valve annulus, a patch may be required to enlarge the entire left ventricular outflow tract and annulus and replace the aortic valve; this is known as the Konno procedure.

Prognosis—Mortality from surgical repairs of subvalvular AS is less than 5% in major centres; however, about 20% of these patients develop recurrent subaortic stenosis and require additional surgery (Schneider & Moore, 2008).

Pulmonic Stenosis

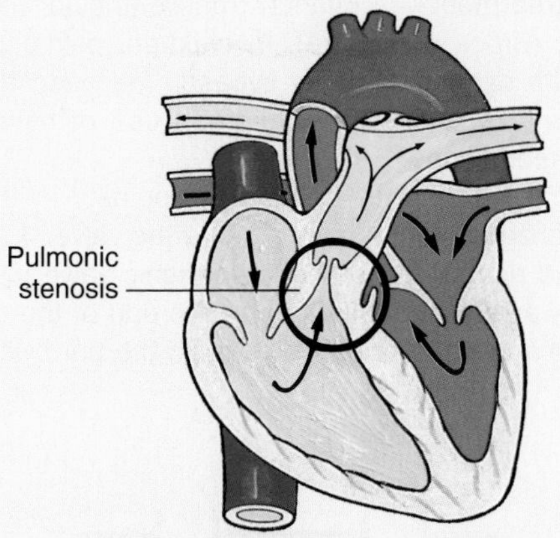

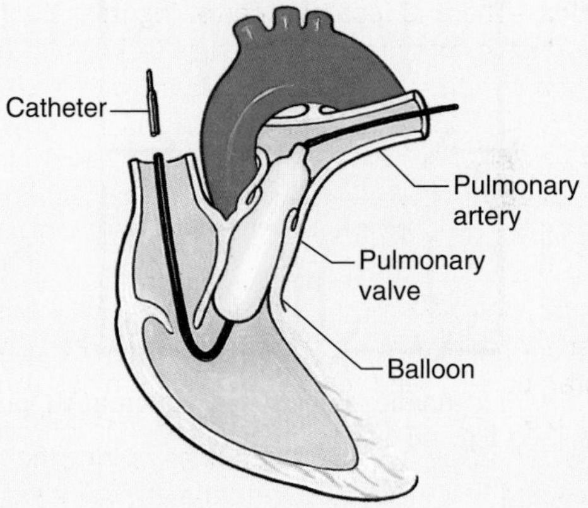

Description—Narrowing at the entrance to the pulmonary artery. Resistance to blood flow causes right ventricular hypertrophy and decreased pulmonary blood flow. Pulmonary atresia is the extreme form of pulmonic stenosis (PS) in that there is total fusion of the commissures and no blood flows to the lungs. The right ventricle may be hypoplastic.

Pathophysiology—When PS is present, resistance to blood flow causes right ventricular hypertrophy. If right ventricular failure develops, right atrial pressure increases; this may result in reopening of the foramen ovale, shunting of unoxygenated blood into the left atrium, and systemic cyanosis. If PS is severe, HF occurs, and systemic venous engorgement is noted. An associated defect such as a patent ductus arteriosus partially compensates for the obstruction by shunting blood from the aorta to the pulmonary artery and into the lungs.

Clinical manifestations—Patients may be asymptomatic; some have mild cyanosis or HF. Progressive narrowing causes increased symptoms. Newborns with severe narrowing will be cyanotic. A loud systolic ejection murmur at the upper left sternal border may be present. However, in severely ill patients the murmur may be much softer due to decreased cardiac output and shunting of blood.

Continued

BOX 48-2 Obstructive Defects—cont'd

Cardiomegaly is evident on chest radiographic films. Patients are at risk for bacterial endocarditis.

Surgical treatment—In infants, transventricular (closed) valvotomy (Brock procedure). In children, pulmonary valvotomy with cardiopulmonary bypass. The need for surgical treatment is rare with widespread use of balloon angioplasty techniques.

Nonsurgical treatment—Balloon angioplasty in the cardiac catheterization laboratory to dilate the valve. A catheter is inserted across the stenotic pulmonic valve into the pulmonary artery, and a balloon at the end of the catheter is inflated and rapidly passed through the narrowed opening (see figure on p. 1461). The procedure is associated with few complications and has proved to be highly effective. It is the treatment of choice for discrete PS in most centres and can be done safely in neonates.

Prognosis—Risk is low for both surgical and nonsurgical procedures; mortality is lower than 1%, slightly higher in neonates. Both balloon dilation and surgical valvotomy leave the pulmonic valve incompetent because they involve opening the fused valve leaflets; however, these patients are clinically asymptomatic. Long-term problems with restenosis or valve incompetence may occur.

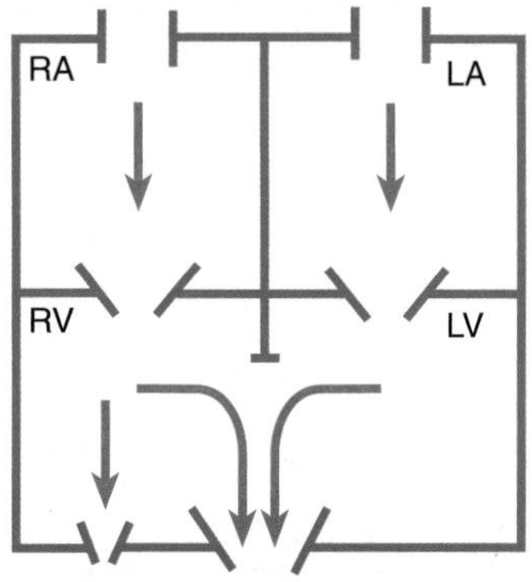

Fig. 48-5 Hemodynamic defects with decreased pulmonary blood flow. See Fig. 48-1 for abbreviations.

visible) and signs of HF. Some defects, such as transposition of the great arteries, cause severe cyanosis in the first days of life and later cause HF. Others, such as truncus arteriosus, cause severe HF in the first weeks of life and mild desaturation.

Clinical Consequences of Congenital Heart Disease

Heart Failure

Heart failure is the inability of the heart to pump an adequate amount of blood to the systemic circulation at normal filling pressures to meet the body's metabolic demands. In children, HF most frequently occurs secondary to structural abnormalities (e.g., septal defects) that result in increased blood volume and pressure within the heart. It can also result from myocardial failure in which the contractility of the ventricle is impaired. This can occur with cardiomyopathy, dysrhythmias, or severe electrolyte disturbances. HF can also occur because of excessive demands on a normal heart muscle, such as sepsis or severe anemia.

Pathophysiology

Heart failure is often separated into two categories: right-sided and left-sided failure. In *right-sided failure*, the right ventricle is unable to pump blood effectively into the pulmonary artery, resulting in increased pressure in the right atrium and systemic venous circulation. Systemic venous hypertension causes hepatosplenomegaly and occasionally **edema**. In *left-sided failure*, the left ventricle is unable to pump blood into the systemic circulation, resulting in increased pressure in the left atrium and pulmonary veins. The lungs become congested with blood, causing elevated pulmonary pressures and pulmonary edema.

Although each type of heart failure produces different signs and symptoms, clinically it is unusual to observe solely right- or left-sided failure in children. Because each side of the heart depends on adequate function of the other side, failure of one chamber causes a reciprocal change in the opposite chamber.

If the abnormalities precipitating HF are not corrected, the heart muscle becomes damaged. Despite compensatory mechanisms, the heart is unable to maintain an adequate cardiac output. Decreased blood flow to the kidneys continues to stimulate sodium and water reabsorption, leading to fluid overload, increased workload on the heart, and congestion in the pulmonary and systemic circulations (Fig. 48-6).

The signs and symptoms of HF can be divided into three groups: (1) impaired myocardial function, (2) pulmonary congestion, and (3) systemic venous congestion (Box 48-5). Because these hemodynamic changes occur from different causes and at differing times, the clinical presentation may vary among children.

Diagnostic Evaluation

Diagnosis is made on the basis of clinical symptoms such as tachypnea and tachycardia at rest, dyspnea, retractions, activity intolerance (especially during feeding in infants), weight gain caused by fluid retention, and hepatomegaly. A chest x-ray film demonstrates cardiomegaly and increased pulmonary blood flow. Ventricular hypertrophy appears on the ECG. An echocardiogram is done to determine the cause of HF, such as a congenital heart defect or poor ventricular function.

Therapeutic Management

The goals of treatment are to (1) improve cardiac function (increase contractility and decrease afterload), (2) remove accumulated fluid and sodium (decrease preload), (3) decrease

BOX 48-3 Defects With Decreased Pulmonary Blood Flow

Tetralogy of Fallot

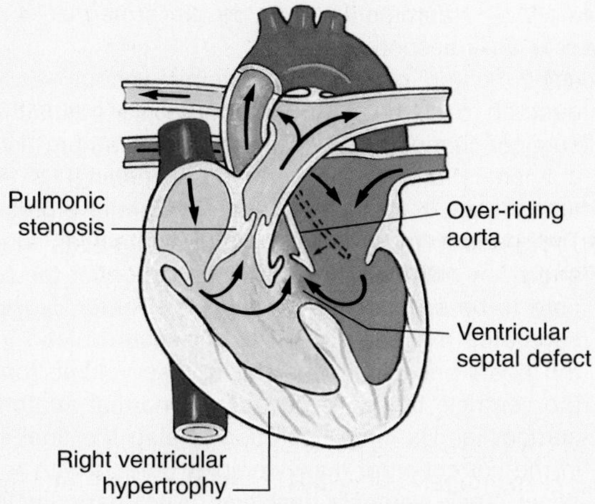

Description—The classic form includes four defects: (1) ventricular septal defect (VSD), (2) pulmonic stenosis (PS), (3) over-riding aorta, and (4) right ventricular hypertrophy.

Pathophysiology—The alteration in hemodynamics varies widely, depending primarily on the degree of PS and also on the size of the VSD and the pulmonary and systemic resistance to flow. Because the VSD is usually large, pressures may be equal in the right and left ventricles. Therefore the shunt direction depends on the difference between pulmonary and systemic vascular resistance. If pulmonary vascular resistance is higher than systemic resistance, the shunt is from right to left. If systemic resistance is higher than pulmonary resistance, the shunt is from left to right. PS decreases blood flow to the lungs and consequently the amount of oxygenated blood that returns to the left side of the heart. Depending on the position of the aorta, blood from both ventricles may be distributed systemically.

Clinical manifestations—Some infants may be acutely cyanotic at birth; others have mild cyanosis that progresses over the first year of life as the PS worsens. There is a characteristic systolic murmur that is often moderate in intensity. There may be acute episodes of cyanosis and hypoxia, called blue spells or tet spells (see p. 1474). Anoxic spells occur when the infant's oxygen requirements exceed the blood supply, usually during crying or after feeding. Patients are at risk for emboli, seizures, and loss of consciousness or sudden death following an anoxic spell.

Surgical treatment

Palliative shunt—In infants who cannot undergo primary repair, a palliative procedure to increase pulmonary blood flow and increase oxygen saturation may be performed. The preferred procedure is a modified Blalock-Taussig shunt operation, which provides blood flow to the pulmonary arteries from the left or right subclavian artery via a tube graft (see Table 48-4). However, in general, shunts are avoided because they may result in pulmonary artery distortion.

Complete repair—Elective repair is usually performed in the first year of life. Indications for repair include increasing cyanosis and the development of hypercyanotic spells. Complete repair involves closure of the VSD and resection of the infundibular stenosis, with placement of a pericardial patch to enlarge the right ventricular outflow tract. In some repairs the patch may extend across the pulmonary valve annulus (transannular patch), making the pulmonary valve incompetent. The procedure requires a median sternotomy and the use of cardiopulmonary bypass.

Prognosis—The operative mortality for total correction of tetralogy of Fallot is less than 3% (Jacobs et al., 2004). With improved surgical techniques there is a lower incidence of dysrhythmias and sudden death; surgical heart block is rare. Heart failure may occur postoperatively.

Tricuspid Atresia

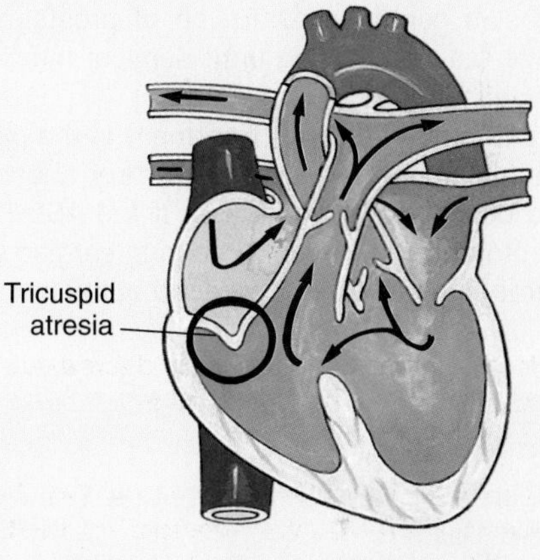

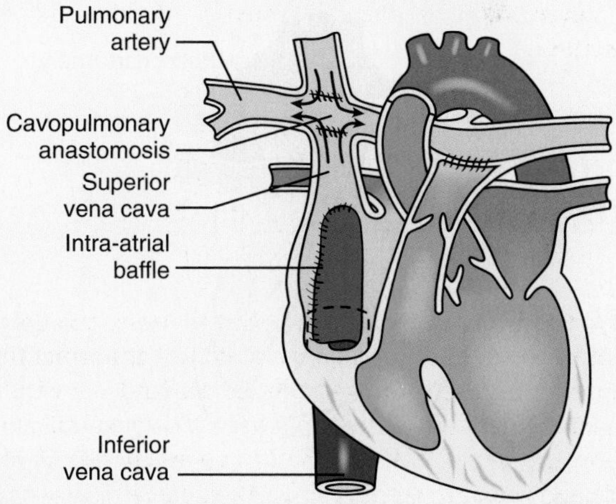

Description—The tricuspid valve fails to develop; consequently there is no communication from the right atrium to the right ventricle. Blood flows through an atrial septal defect (ASD) or a patent foramen ovale to the left side of the heart and through a VSD to the right ventricle and out to the lungs. The condition is often associated with PS

Continued

BOX 48-3 Defects With Decreased Pulmonary Blood Flow—cont'd

and transposition of the great arteries. There is complete mixing of unoxygenated and oxygenated blood in the left side of the heart, which results in systemic desaturation, and varying amounts of pulmonary obstruction, which causes decreased pulmonary blood flow.

Pathophysiology—At birth the presence of a patent foramen ovale (or other atrial septal opening) is required to permit blood flow across the septum into the left atrium; the patent ductus arteriosus allows blood flow to the pulmonary artery into the lungs for oxygenation. A VSD allows a modest amount of blood to enter the right ventricle and pulmonary artery for oxygenation. Pulmonary blood flow usually is diminished.

Clinical manifestations—Cyanosis is usually seen in the newborn period. There may be tachycardia and dyspnea. Older children have signs of chronic hypoxemia with clubbing.

Therapeutic management—For the neonate whose pulmonary blood flow depends on the patency of the ductus arteriosus, a continuous infusion of prostaglandin E_1 is started at 0.1 mg/kg/min until surgical intervention can be arranged.

Surgical treatment—Palliative treatment is the placement of a shunt (pulmonary–to–systemic artery anastomosis) to increase blood flow to the lungs. If the ASD is small, an atrial septostomy is performed during cardiac catheterization. Some children have increased pulmonary blood flow and require pulmonary artery banding to lessen the volume of blood to the lungs. A bidirectional Glenn shunt (cavopulmonary anastomosis) may be performed at 4 to 9 months as a second stage.

Modified Fontan procedure—Systemic venous return is directed to the lungs without a ventricular pump through surgical connections between the right atrium and the pulmonary artery. A fenestration (opening) is sometimes made in the right atrial baffle to relieve pressure. The patient must have normal ventricular function and a low pulmonary vascular resistance for the procedure to be successful. The modified Fontan procedure separates oxygenated and unoxygenated blood inside the heart and eliminates the excess volume load on the ventricle but does not restore normal anatomy or hemodynamics. This operation is also the final stage in the correction of many complex defects with a functional single ventricle, including hypoplastic left heart syndrome.

Prognosis—Surgical mortality is less than 5% (Jacobs et al., 2004); the rate increases when the anatomy is more complex and other risk factors are present. Postoperative complications include dysrhythmias, systemic venous hypertension, pleural and pericardial effusions, and ventricular dysfunction. Long-term concerns are the development of protein-losing enteropathy, atrial dysrhythmias, late ventricular dysfunction, and developmental delays.

BOX 48-4 Mixed Defects

Transposition of the Great Arteries, or Transposition of the Great Vessels

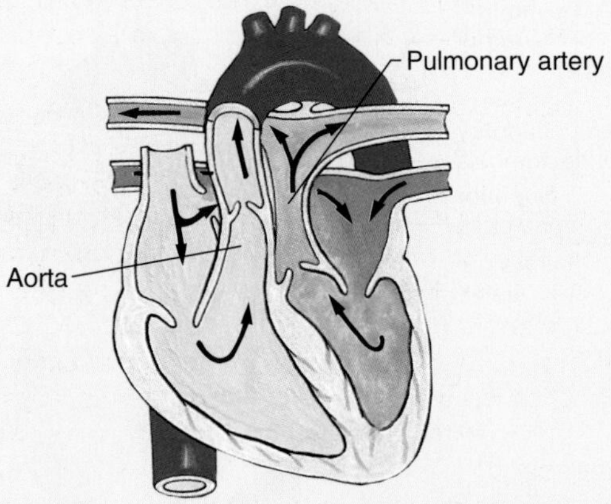

Description—The pulmonary artery leaves the left ventricle, and the aorta exits from the right ventricle, with no communication between the systemic and pulmonary circulations.

Pathophysiology—Associated defects such as septal defects or patent ductus arteriosus must be present to permit blood to enter the systemic circulation or the pulmonary circulation for mixing of saturated and desaturated blood. The most common defect associated with transposition of the great arteries (TGA) is a patent foramen ovale. At birth there is also a patent ductus arteriosus, although in most instances this closes after the neonatal period. Another associated defect may be a ventricular septal defect (VSD). The presence of a VSD increases the risk of heart failure (HF) because it permits blood to flow from the right to the left ventricle, into the pulmonary artery, and finally to the lungs. However, it also produces high pulmonary blood flow under high pressure, which can result in high pulmonary vascular resistance.

Clinical manifestations—Depend on the type and size of the associated defects. Newborns with minimum communication are severely cyanotic and have depressed function at birth. Those with large septal defects or a patent ductus arteriosus may be less cyanotic but have symptoms of HF. Heart sounds vary according to the type of defect present. Cardiomegaly is usually evident a few weeks after birth.

Therapeutic management (to provide intracardiac mixing)—The administration of intravenous prostaglandin E_1 may be initiated to keep the ductus arteriosus open to temporarily increase blood mixing and provide an oxygen saturation of 75% or to maintain cardiac output. During cardiac catheterization or under echocardiographic guidance, a balloon atrial septostomy (Rashkind procedure) may also be performed to increase mixing by opening the atrial septum.

Surgical treatment—An arterial switch procedure is the procedure of choice performed in the first weeks of life. It involves transecting the great arteries, anastomosing the main pulmonary artery to the proximal aorta (just above

BOX 48-4 Mixed Defects—cont'd

the aortic valve), and anastomosing the ascending aorta to the proximal pulmonary artery. The coronary arteries are switched from the proximal aorta to the proximal pulmonary artery to create a new aorta. Reimplantation of the coronary arteries is critical to the infant's survival, and they must be reattached without torsion or kinking to provide the heart with its supply of oxygen. The advantage of the arterial switch procedure is the re-establishment of normal circulation, with the left ventricle acting as the systemic pump. Potential complications of the arterial switch include narrowing at the great artery anastomoses and coronary artery insufficiency.

Intra-atrial baffle repairs—Intra-atrial baffle repairs are rarely performed, although many adolescents and adults survive today with repairs that were done more than 15 years ago. An intra-atrial baffle is created to divert venous blood to the mitral valve and pulmonary venous blood to the tricuspid valve using the patient's atrial septum (Senning procedure) or a prosthetic material (Mustard procedure). A disadvantage is the continuing role of the right ventricle as the systemic pump and the late development of right ventricular failure and rhythm disturbances. Other potential postoperative complications include loss of normal sinus rhythm, baffle leaks, and ventricular dysfunction.

Rastelli procedure—This procedure is the operative choice in infants with TGA, VSD, and severe pulmonic stenosis (PS). It involves closure of the VSD with a baffle, so left ventricular blood is directed through the VSD into the aorta. The pulmonic valve is then closed, and a conduit is placed from the right ventricle to the pulmonary artery to create a physiologically normal circulation. Unfortunately, this procedure requires multiple conduit replacements as the child grows.

Prognosis—Operative mortality is less than 2% (Jacobs et al., 2004). Potential long-term problems include suprapulmonic stenosis and neoaorta dilation and regurgitation.

Total Anomalous Pulmonary Venous Connection

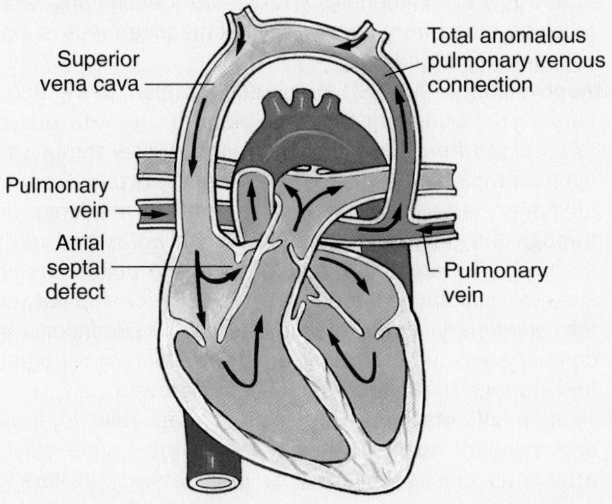

Description—Rare defect characterized by failure of the pulmonary veins to join the left atrium. Instead, the pulmonary veins are abnormally connected to the systemic venous circuit via the right atrium or various veins draining toward the right atrium, such as the superior vena cava. The abnormal attachment results in mixed blood being returned to the right atrium and shunted from the right to the left through an atrial septal defect (ASD). Total anomalous pulmonary venous connection (TAPVC; also called *total anomalous pulmonary venous return* or *total anomalous pulmonary venous drainage*) is classified according to the pulmonary venous point of attachment as follows:

Supracardiac—Attachment above the diaphragm, such as to the superior vena cava (most common form) (see Fig. 48-9)

Cardiac—Direct attachment to the heart, such as to the right atrium or coronary sinus

Infradiaphragmatic—Attachment below the diaphragm, such as to the inferior vena cava (most severe form)

Pathophysiology—The right atrium receives all the blood that normally would flow into the left atrium. As a result, the right side of the heart hypertrophies, whereas the left side, especially the left atrium, may remain small. An associated ASD or patent foramen ovale allows systemic venous blood to shunt from the higher-pressure right atrium to the left atrium and into the left side of the heart. As a result, the oxygen saturation of the blood in both sides of the heart (and ultimately in the systemic arterial circulation) is the same. If the pulmonary blood flow is large, pulmonary venous return is also large, and the amount of saturated blood is relatively high. However, if there is obstruction to pulmonary venous drainage, pulmonary venous return is impeded, pulmonary venous pressure rises, and pulmonary interstitial edema develops and eventually contributes to HF. Infradiaphragmatic TAPVC is often associated with obstruction to pulmonary venous drainage and is a surgical emergency.

Clinical manifestations—Most infants develop cyanosis early in life. The degree of cyanosis is inversely related to the amount of pulmonary blood flow—the more pulmonary blood, the less cyanosis. Children with unobstructed TAPVC may be asymptomatic until pulmonary vascular resistance decreases during infancy, increasing pulmonary blood flow, with resulting signs of HF. Cyanosis becomes worse with pulmonary vein obstruction; once obstruction occurs, the infant's condition usually deteriorates rapidly. Without intervention, cardiac failure will progress to death.

Surgical treatment—Corrective repair is performed in early infancy. The surgical approach varies with the anatomical defect. However, in general, the common pulmonary vein is anastomosed to the back of the left atrium, the ASD is closed, and the anomalous pulmonary venous connection is ligated. The cardiac type is most easily repaired; the infradiaphragmatic type carries the highest morbidity and mortality because of the higher incidence of pulmonary vein obstruction. Potential postoperative complications include reobstruction; bleeding; dysrhythmias, particularly

Continued

BOX 48-4 Mixed Defects—cont'd

heart block; pulmonary artery hypertension; and persistent heart failure.

Prognosis—Mortality for all types is less than 10% (Jacobs et al., 2004) and is lowest for the cardiac type; morbidity increases with the presence of pulmonary vein obstruction.

Truncus Arteriosus

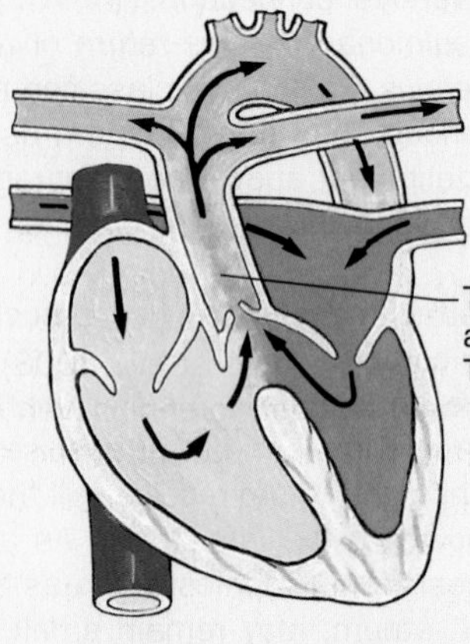

Description—Failure of normal septation and division of the embryonic bulbar trunk into the pulmonary artery and the aorta, which results in development of a single vessel that overrides both ventricles. Blood from both ventricles mixes in the common great artery, which leads to desaturation and hypoxemia. Blood ejected from the heart flows preferentially to the lower-pressure pulmonary arteries, so pulmonary blood flow is increased and systemic blood flow is reduced. There are three types:

Type I—A single pulmonary trunk arises near the base of the truncus and divides into the left and right pulmonary arteries.

Type II—The left and right pulmonary arteries arise separately but in close proximity and at the same level from the back of the truncus.

Type III—The pulmonary arteries arise independently from the sides of the truncus.

Pathophysiology—Blood ejected from the left and right ventricles enters the common trunk so that pulmonary and systemic circulations are mixed. Blood flow is distributed to the pulmonary and systemic circulations according to the relative resistances of each system. The amount of pulmonary blood flow depends on the size of the pulmonary arteries and the pulmonary vascular resistance. Generally, resistance to pulmonary blood flow is less than systemic vascular resistance, which results in preferential blood flow to the lungs. Pulmonary vascular disease develops at an early age in patients with truncus arteriosus.

Clinical manifestations—Most infants are symptomatic with moderate to severe HF and variable cyanosis, poor growth, and activity intolerance. There is a holosystolic murmur at the left sternal border with a diastolic murmur present if truncal regurgitation is present. Thirty-five percent of patients have 22q11 deletions (Goldmuntz and Lin, 2008).

Surgical treatment—Early repair is performed in the first month of life. It involves closing the VSD so that the truncus arteriosus receives the outflow from the left ventricle, excising the pulmonary arteries from the aorta and attaching them to the right ventricle by means of a homograft. Currently homografts (segments of cadaver aorta and pulmonary artery that are treated with antibiotics and cryopreserved) are preferred over synthetic conduits to establish continuity between the right ventricle and pulmonary artery. Homografts are more flexible and easier to use during the procedure and appear less prone to obstruction. Postoperative complications include persistent heart failure, bleeding, pulmonary artery hypertension, dysrhythmias, and residual VSD. Because conduits are not living tissue, they will not grow along with the child and may also become narrowed with calcifications. One or more conduit replacements will be needed in childhood.

Prognosis—Mortality is greater than 10%; future operations are required to replace the conduits.

Hypoplastic Left Heart Syndrome

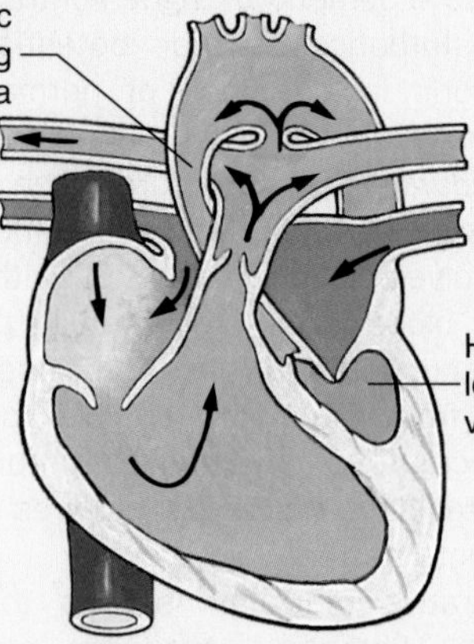

Description—Underdevelopment of the left side of the heart, resulting in a hypoplastic left ventricle and aortic atresia. Most blood from the left atrium flows across the patent foramen ovale to the right atrium, to the right ventricle, and out the pulmonary artery. The descending aorta receives blood from the patent ductus arteriosus supplying systemic blood flow.

Pathophysiology—An ASD or patent foramen ovale allows saturated blood from the left atrium to mix with desaturated blood from the right atrium and to flow through the right ventricle and out into the pulmonary artery. From the pulmonary artery, the blood flows both to the lungs and through the ductus arteriosus into the aorta and out to the body. The amount of blood flow to the pulmonary and systemic circulations depends on the relationship between the pulmonary and systemic vascular resistances. The coronary and cerebral vessels receive blood by retrograde flow through the hypoplastic ascending aorta.

Clinical manifestations—The patient has mild cyanosis and signs of congestive failure until the patent ductus arteriosus closes, followed by progressive deterioration

BOX 48-4 Mixed Defects—cont'd

with cyanosis and decreased cardiac output, leading to cardiovascular collapse. The condition is usually fatal in the first months of life without intervention.

Therapeutic management—Neonates require stabilization with mechanical ventilation and inotropic support preoperatively. A prostaglandin E_1 infusion is needed to maintain ductal patency and ensure adequate systemic blood flow.

Surgical treatment—A multistage approach is used. The first stage is a Norwood procedure, which involves an anastomosis of the main pulmonary artery to the aorta to create a new aorta, shunting to provide pulmonary blood flow (usually with a modified Blalock-Taussig shunt), and creation of a large ASD. Postoperative complications include imbalance of systemic and pulmonary blood flow, bleeding, low cardiac output, and persistent heart failure. A new modification of the first-stage repair is the use of a right ventricle–to–pulmonary artery homograft conduit instead of a shunt to supply pulmonary blood flow (Sano procedure). The second stage is often a bidirectional Glenn shunt procedure (see Fig. 48-9) or a hemi-Fontan operation. Both involve anastomosing the superior vena cava to the right pulmonary artery so superior vena cava flow bypasses the right atrium and flows directly to the lungs. The procedure is usually done at 3 to 6 months of age to relieve cyanosis and reduce the volume load on the right ventricle. The final repair is a modified Fontan procedure (see Tricuspid Atresia, Box 48-3).

Transplantation—Heart transplantation in the newborn period is another option for these infants. Problems include the shortage of newborn organ donors, risk of rejection, long-term problems with chronic immunosuppression, and infection (see Heart Transplantation, p. 1488).

Prognosis—For the first-stage repair, survival rates vary widely in different centres. Some experienced centres are reporting mortality rates of about 5 to 30% (Tweddell et al., 2008). Improved outcomes have been associated with early diagnosis and repair and increased monitoring in the hospital and at home (Tweddel et al., 2008). Long-term problems with repair include worsening ventricular function, tricuspid regurgitation, recurrent aortic arch narrowing, dysrhythmias, and developmental delays. There is a risk of mortality between surgical procedures. The mortality for the later two operations is less than 5%.

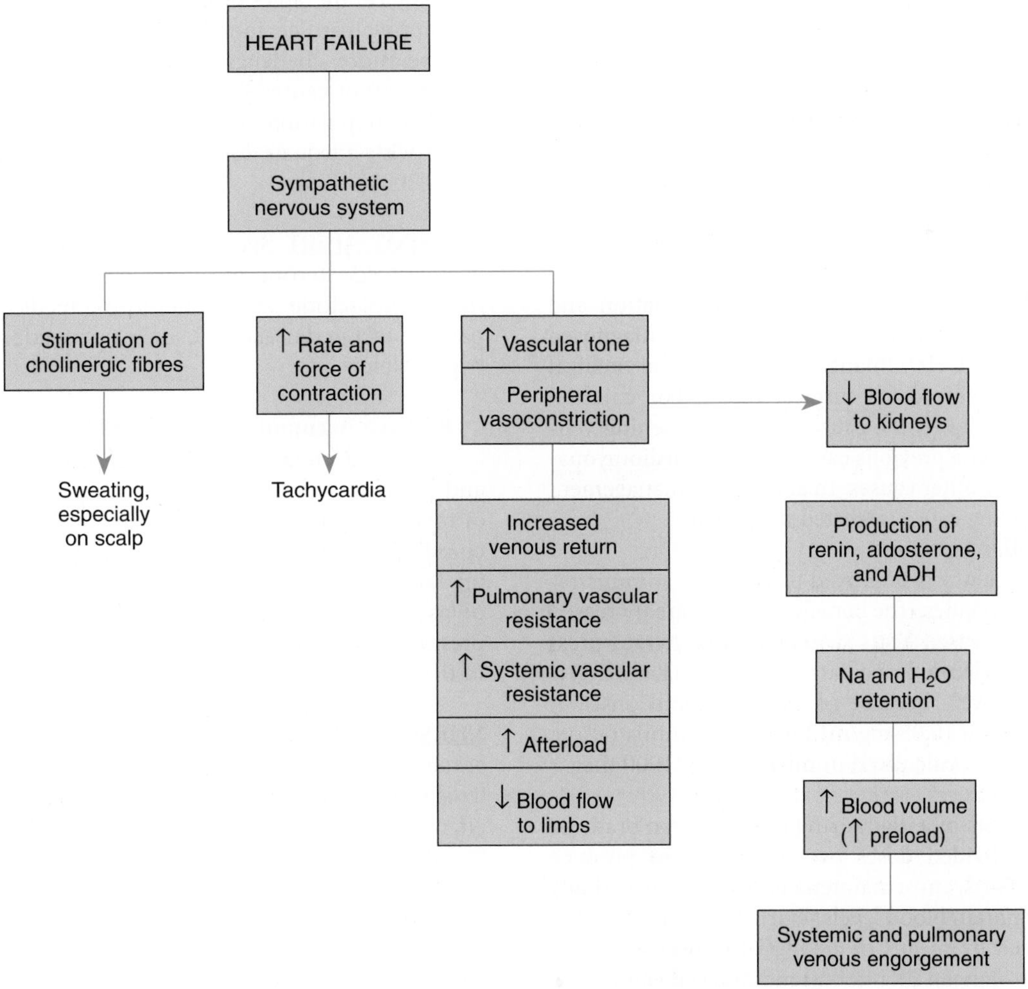

Fig. 48-6 Pathophysiology of heart failure. *ADH*, antidiuretic hormone.

BOX 48-5 Clinical Manifestations of Heart Failure

Impaired Myocardial Function
Tachycardia
Sweating (inappropriate)
Decreased urinary output
Fatigue
Weakness
Restlessness
Anorexia
Pale, cool extremities
Weak peripheral pulses
Decreased blood pressure
Gallop rhythm
Cardiomegaly

Pulmonary Congestion
Tachypnea
Dyspnea
Retractions (infants)
Flaring nares
Exercise intolerance
Orthopnea
Cough, hoarseness
Cyanosis
Wheezing
Grunting

Systemic Venous Congestion
Weight gain
Hepatomegaly
Peripheral edema, especially periorbital
Ascites
Neck vein distension (children)

evolve Critical Thinking Exercise—Digoxin Administration

cardiac demands, and (4) improve tissue oxygenation and decrease oxygen consumption. For most infants diagnosed with HF, the cause is CHD. Infants are stabilized on medical therapy and then referred for surgical repair. For children newly diagnosed with HF, the cause may be worsening ventricular function after a previous cardiac repair, cardiomyopathy, dysrhythmia, or other causes. In addition to management of HF, the underlying cause is treated if possible.

Improve Cardiac Function

Myocardial efficiency is improved through the administration of digitalis glycosides. The beneficial effects are increased cardiac output, decreased heart size, decreased venous pressure, and relief of edema. In pediatrics, digoxin (Lanoxin) is used almost exclusively because of its more rapid onset. It is available as an elixir (0.05 mg/mL) for oral administration. For infants the dose is calculated in micrograms (1000 mcg = 1 mg).

Treatment consists of a digitalizing dosage, given orally or intravenously in divided doses over 24 hours to produce optimal cardiac effects, and a maintenance dosage, given orally twice a day to maintain blood levels. During digitalization the child is monitored by means of an ECG to observe for the desired effects (prolonged PR interval and reduced ventricular rate) and to detect adverse effects, especially dysrhythmias.

A group of medications used in the treatment of HF are the angiotensin-converting enzyme (ACE) inhibitors. As their name implies, these drugs inhibit the normal function of the renin-angiotensin system in the kidney. The ACE inhibitors block the conversion of angiotensin I to angiotensin II so that, instead of vasoconstriction, vasodilation occurs. Vasodilation results in decreased pulmonary and systemic vascular resistance, decreased BP, and a reduction in afterload. Common medications used in pediatrics are captopril (Capoten), enalapril (Vasotec), and lisinopril. The principal adverse effects of ACE inhibitors are hypotension, cough, and renal dysfunction.

Carvedilol, a β-blocker, blocks the α- and β-adrenergic receptors, causing decreased heart rate, decreased BP, and vasodilation. It has been shown to decrease morbidity and mortality in some adults with heart failure and is being used selectively in children. Adverse effects include dizziness, headache, and hypotension.

Severe ventricular dysfunction may also be treated with biventricular pacing, also called *cardiac resynchronization therapy* (CRT). Both ventricles are paced to closely mimic normal ventricular conduction and thereby improve the mechanical function of the heart muscle. This has been used effectively with adult patients with heart failure and is beginning to be applied to the pediatric population. With the pharmacological therapies discussed above, CRT has the potential to improve cardiac function in this group of patients. CRT can be more challenging in pediatric patients because of the variety of causes for heart failure. Initial studies of CRT in this population demonstrate improved outcomes in those with adequate follow-up (Cecchin et al., 2009; Dubin et al., 2005).

NURSING ALERT Because ACE inhibitors also block the action of aldosterone, the addition of potassium supplements or spironolactone (Aldactone) to the medication regimen of patients taking diuretics is usually not needed and may cause hyperkalemia.

Remove Accumulated Fluid and Sodium

Treatment consists of diuretics, possible fluid restriction, and possible sodium restriction. Diuretics are the mainstay of therapy to eliminate excess water and salt to prevent reaccumulation. The most frequently used medications are listed in Table 48-3. Because furosemide and the thiazides are potassium-losing diuretics, potassium supplements may be prescribed, and rich sources of the electrolyte are encouraged in the diet.

NURSING ALERT A fall in the serum potassium level enhances the effects of digitalis, increasing the risk of digoxin toxicity. Increased serum potassium levels diminish digoxin's effect. Therefore, serum potassium levels (normal range 3.5 to 5.5 mmol/L) must be monitored carefully.

Fluid restriction may be required in the acute stages of HF and must be calculated carefully to avoid dehydrating the child, especially if cyanotic CHD and significant polycythemia are present. Infants rarely need fluid restrictions because HF

Table 48-3 Diuretics Used in Heart Failure

ACTIONS	COMMENTS	NURSING CARE MANAGEMENT
Furosemide (Lasix)—Blocks reabsorption of sodium and water in proximal renal tubule and interferes with reabsorption of sodium	Drug of choice in severe heart failure Causes excretion of chloride and potassium (hypokalemia may precipitate digitalis toxicity)	Begin to record output as soon as drug is given. Observe for dehydration caused by profound diuresis. Observe for adverse effects (nausea and vomiting, diarrhea, ototoxicity, hypokalemia, dermatitis, postural hypotension). Encourage foods high in potassium or give potassium supplements. Monitor chloride and acid-base balance with long-term therapy. Observe for signs of digoxin toxicity.
Chlorothiazide (Diuril)—Acts directly on distal tubules to decrease sodium, water, potassium, chloride, and bicarbonate absorption	Less frequently used drug Causes hypokalemia, acidosis from large doses	Observe for adverse effects (nausea, weakness, dizziness, paresthesia, muscle cramps, skin eruptions, hypokalemia, acidosis). Encourage foods high in potassium or give potassium supplements, or both.
Spironolactone (Aldactone)—Blocks action of aldosterone, which promotes retention of sodium and excretion of potassium	Weak diuretic Has potassium-sparing effect; frequently used with thiazides, furosemide Poorly absorbed from gastrointestinal tract Takes several days to achieve maximum actions	Observe for adverse effects (skin rash, drowsiness, ataxia, hyperkalemia). Do not administer potassium supplements.

makes feeding so difficult that they struggle to take maintenance fluids.

Sodium-restricted diets are used less often in children than in adults to control HF because of their potential negative effects on appetite. If salt intake is restricted, additional table salt and highly salted foods are avoided.

Decrease Cardiac Demands

The workload on the heart is reduced when metabolic needs are kept to a minimum. This is accomplished by limiting physical activity (bed rest), maintaining body temperature, treating any infections, reducing the effort of breathing (semi-Fowler position), and using medication to sedate an irritable child.

Improve Tissue Oxygenation

All of the preceding measures serve to increase tissue oxygenation, by either improving myocardial function or lessening tissue oxygen demands. In addition, supplemental cool, humidified oxygen may be administered to increase the amount of available oxygen during inspiration. Oxygen administration is especially helpful in patients with pulmonary edema, intercurrent respiratory tract infections, and increased pulmonary vascular resistance (oxygen is a vasodilator that decreases pulmonary vascular resistance).

NURSING ALERT Oxygen is a drug and is administered only with an appropriate order. In some uncommon circumstances in patients with complex hemodynamics, oxygen can be detrimental.

An oxygen hood, nasal cannula, or face tent is used to deliver oxygen. Nasal cannulas are ideal for long-term oxygen administration because the child can be ambulatory and can easily eat and drink. Cool humidification is necessary to counteract the drying effect of oxygen. The amount of cool humidity needs to be carefully regulated to prevent chilling.

Nursing Care Management

The infant or child with HF may be acutely ill, and some may require critical care until the symptoms improve. Expert nursing care is essential to reduce the cardiac demands that strain the failing heart muscle. During this time, the child and family require emotional support. Although the objectives of nursing care are the same, interventions differ, depending on the child's age (see Nursing Care Plan).

Assist in Measures to Improve Cardiac Function

The nurse's responsibility in administering digoxin includes calculating and administering the correct dosage, observing for signs of toxicity, and instituting parental teaching on medication administration at home. The child's **apical pulse rate** should always be checked before administering digoxin. As a general rule, the drug is not given if the pulse is below 90 to 110 beats/min in infants and young children or below 70 beats/min in older children (the cutoff point for adults is 60 beats/min). However, because the pulse rate varies in children in different age groups, the written medication order should specify at what heart rate the medication is withheld. The nurse should also use judgement in evaluating the pulse rate. If it is significantly lower than the previous recording, the dose should be withheld until the practitioner is notified.

The apical rate is taken because a pulse deficit (radial pulse rate lower than apical) may be present with decreased cardiac output. It is **auscultated** for a full minute to evaluate alterations in rhythm. If the child is monitored by means of an ECG, a rhythm strip is obtained and attached to the chart for rate and rhythm analysis, such as abnormal lengthening of the PR interval (more than 50% increase over predigitalization interval) and dysrhythmias.

Digoxin is a potentially dangerous drug because of its narrow margin of safety of therapeutic, toxic, and lethal doses. Many toxic responses are extensions of its therapeutic effects.

NURSING CARE PLAN ● The Child With Heart Failure (HF)

Nursing Diagnosis Decreased cardiac output related to structural defect, myocardial dysfunction, altered hemodynamics	Expected Patient Outcomes	Nursing Interventions	Rationale
Child's/Family's Defining Characteristics ***(Subjective and Objective Data)*** Tachycardia Tachypnea Ineffective peripheral circulation, cool extremities Hypotension Rapid, weak peripheral pulses Prolonged capillary refill, longer than 2 to 3 seconds Narrow pulse pressure Distended neck veins in older children Cardiomegaly revealed on chest x-ray film Gallop rhythm Edema Rapid weight gain Feeding difficulty Irritability	Child will have adequate cardiac output as evidenced by the following: • Heart rate within acceptable range (state specific range) • Respiratory rate (RR) within acceptable range (state specific range) • Skin warm to touch • Strong and equal peripheral pulses • Blood pressure normal for age • Brisk capillary refill within 2 to 3 seconds • Lack of distended neck veins • Normal sinus rhythm • Lack of edema • Adequate urinary output (state specific; 1 to 2 ml/kg/hr) Child will have age-appropriate weight gain on standardized growth curve. Infant will demonstrate successful feeding. Child, family, or both will be able to state at least four characteristics of HF such as: • Rapid heart rate • Fast breathing • Cool extremities • Puffiness (edema) • Fussiness • Decreased appetite Child, family, or both will be able to state knowledge of care regarding the following: • Medication administration • Elevated head positioning • Sufficient rest periods • Monitoring intake and output • When to contact health care provider **The Following NOC Concepts Apply to These Outcomes** Cardiac Pump Effectiveness Knowledge: Illness Care Tissue Perfusion: Cardiac	Assess and record heart rate, RR, blood pressure, and any signs and symptoms of decreased cardiac output (listed under defining characteristics) every 2 to 4 hours and as needed.	To assess for changes in vital signs and child's physical status that reflect altered cardiac output
		Administer cardiac drugs on schedule. Assess for and record any side effects or any signs or symptoms of toxicity. Follow hospital protocol for administration.	To improve heart function by giving drugs on time and to avoid dangers by giving as prescribed and with careful assessment before administration
		Keep accurate record of intake and output.	To assess for HF, which causes decreased urinary output
		Weigh child or infant on same scale at same time of day. Document results and compare with previous weight.	To observe for weight increase that may indicate excess fluid accumulation
		Administer diuretics on schedule. Assess and record effectiveness and any adverse effects noted.	To prevent fluid retention, which commonly occurs with HF; to eliminate excess water and salt
		Elevate head of bed at a 30- to 45-degree angle.	To promote maximum chest expansion
		Offer small, frequent feedings to infant's or child's tolerance.	To prevent fatigue during feeding and to ensure adequate nutrition since metabolic rate is greater because of poor cardiac function
		Organize nursing care to allow child or infant uninterrupted rest.	To account for decreased energy level and lower tolerance to activity
		Educate child and family about characteristics of HF. Assess and record teaching session.	To provide parent education that can promote measures to improve cardiac function and decrease demands
		Educate child and family about care such as medication administration. Assess and record results and family's participation in care.	To educate on proper medication administration, promote safety, and minimize medication adverse effects
		The Following NIC Concepts Apply to These Interventions Cardiac Care Fluid Management Medication Administration Positioning Vital Signs Monitoring Respiratory Monitoring	

NURSING CARE PLAN ● The Child With Heart Failure (HF)—cont'd

Nursing Diagnosis	Expected Patient Outcomes	Nursing Interventions	Rationale
Ineffective breathing pattern related to pulmonary congestion, decreased cardiac output **Child's/Family's Defining Characteristics** ***(Subjective and Objective Data)*** Tachypnea Dyspnea Retractions Crackles Shortness of breath Cyanosis Pallor Mottling Nasal flaring Grunting Head bobbing Cough Use of accessory muscles Activity intolerance	Child will have effective breathing pattern as evidenced by the following: • RR within acceptable range (state specific range) • Clear and equal breath sounds bilaterally anterior and posterior • Pink or tan colour • Absence of nasal flaring, retractions, cough, and head bobbing • Unlaboured breath sounds • Tolerance of activities appropriate for age	Assess and record RR, breath sounds, and any signs and symptoms of ineffective pattern (listed under characteristics) every 2 to 4 hours and as needed.	To assess for respiratory changes that can be indicators of worsening HF
		Administer humidified oxygen in correct amount, using correct route of delivery. Record percent of oxygen and route of delivery. Assess and record child's response to therapy.	To provide oxygen, which can reduce respiratory distress by easing respiratory effort
		Keep head of bed elevated at a 30- to 45-degree angle.	To promote maximum chest expansion
		Suction if child has ineffective cough or is unable to manage secretions. Assess and record amount and characteristics of secretions.	To maintain patent airway to promote respiratory expansion
	Child, family, or both will be able to state four characteristics of ineffective breathing pattern such as: • Colour change from pink or tan to pale, dusky, or blue colour • Fast breathing • Change in amount or characteristics of secretions, or both • Retractions, head bobbing • Ineffective cough • Decreased or altered activity level	Assess and record oxygen saturation every 2 to 4 hours and as needed.	To evaluate pulmonary effectiveness
		Educate child and family about characteristics of ineffective breathing pattern. Assess and record results.	To provide parent education that can promote measures to improve breathing effort
	Child, family, or both will be able to state knowledge of care regarding: • Positioning to facilitate respiratory effort • Oxygen administration • When to contact health care provider	Educate child and family about care. Assess and record results and family participation in care.	To promote family support
	The Following NOC Concepts Apply to These Outcomes: Activity Tolerance Knowledge: Illness Care Respiratory Status: Gas Exchange Tissue Perfusion: Pulmonary	**The Following NIC Concepts Apply to These Interventions:** Airway Management Airway Suctioning Chest Physiotherapy Family Involvement Promotion Health Education	

NIC, Nursing Interventions Classification; *NOC*, Nursing Outcomes Classification

The nurse must maintain a high index of suspicion for signs of toxicity when administering digoxin (Box 48-6).

Because digoxin toxicity can occur from accidental overdose, great care must be taken in properly calculating and measuring the dosage. When converting milligrams to micrograms to millilitres, the nurse needs to carefully check the placement of the decimal point, since an error causes a significant change in dosage. For example, 0.1 mg is 10 times the dosage of 0.01 mg.

NURSING ALERT Infants rarely receive more than 1 mL (50 mcg, or 0.05 mg) in one dose; a higher dose is an immediate warning of a dosage error. To ensure safety, always compare and check the calculation with another staff member before giving the medication.

These same principles are taught to parents in preparation for discharge, although the correct dose in millilitres is usually specified on the container, thus reducing potential errors in calculation. The nurse needs to watch the parent measure the elixir in the dropper and stress the level mark as the meniscus of the fluid that is observed at eye level. Other instructions for administering digoxin are listed in the Family-Centred Teaching box and Critical Thinking Exercise.

Parents also need to be advised of the signs of toxicity. According to the practitioner's preference, they may be taught to take the pulse before giving the medication. A return demonstration of the procedure from the parents or another principal caregiver should be included as part of the teaching plan. Their level of anxiety in counting the pulse should be assessed, since overconcern about the heart rate may result in excessive withholding of the medication.

Monitor Afterload Reduction

For patients receiving ACE inhibitors for afterload reduction, the nurse should carefully monitor BP before and after dose administration, observe for symptoms of hypotension, and notify the practitioner if BP is low. Numerous medications affecting the kidney can potentiate renal dysfunction; thus children taking multiple diuretics and an ACE inhibitor require careful assessment of serum electrolytes and renal function.

Decrease Cardiac Demands

The infant requires rest and conservation of energy for feeding. Every effort should be made to organize nursing activities to allow for uninterrupted periods of sleep. Whenever possible, parents need to be encouraged to stay with their infant to provide the holding, rocking, and cuddling that help children sleep more soundly. To minimize disturbing the infant, changing bed linen and complete bathing should be done only when necessary. Feeding should be planned to accommodate the infant's sleep and wake patterns. The child is fed at the first sign of hunger, such as when sucking on fists, rather than waiting until he or she cries, because the stress of crying exhausts the limited energy supply. Because infants with HF tire easily and may sleep through feedings, smaller feedings every 3 hours may be helpful. Gavage feedings may be instituted to provide adequate nutrition and allow the infant to rest.

Every effort should be made to minimize unnecessary stress. Older children need an explanation of what is happening to them to decrease anxiety about their illness and necessary treatments such as cardiac monitoring, oxygen administration, and medications. Outlining a plan for the day, preparing the child for tests and procedures, providing quiet activities, and providing adequate rest periods are all helpful

BOX 48-6 Common Signs of Digoxin Toxicity in Children

Gastrointestinal
Nausea
Vomiting
Anorexia

Cardiac
Bradycardia
Dysrhythmias

FAMILY-CENTRED TEACHING

Administering Digoxin

- Give digoxin at regular intervals, usually every 12 hours, such as at 8 AM and 8 PM.
- Administer the drug carefully by slowly directing it to the side and back of the mouth.
- Do not mix the drug with foods or other fluids, since refusal to consume these results in inaccurate intake of the drug.
- If the child has teeth, give water after administering the drug; whenever possible, brush the teeth to prevent tooth decay from the sweetened liquid.
- If a dose is missed, do not give an extra dose or increase the dose. Stay on the same medication schedule.
- If the child vomits, do not give a second dose.
- If more than two consecutive doses have been missed, notify the physician or other designated practitioner.
- Frequent vomiting, poor feeding, or slow heart rate can be signs of toxicity; if they occur, contact the physician.
- If the child becomes ill, notify the physician or other designated practitioner immediately.
- Keep digoxin in a safe place, preferably in a locked cabinet.
- In case of accidental overdose of digoxin, call the nearest poison control centre immediately.

CRITICAL THINKING EXERCISE

Digoxin Toxicity

You are visiting a 3-month-old infant at home who began receiving digoxin and furosemide (Lasix) 5 days ago for management of heart failure (HF). A brief assessment indicates that the infant appears well but is not very active, has a weak suck reflex, and does not exhibit much spontaneous movement during interaction with the mother. The mother mentions that the infant is a good baby and does not cry much except when he is very hungry. She also mentions that he vomited several times yesterday and twice this morning; this was not perceived as unusual because her 3-year-old did the same thing and was diagnosed with gastroesophageal reflux. Further assessment of the infant reveals an irregular heartbeat of 86 to 104 beats/min at rest; the heart rhythm is also noted to be irregular. No murmur or other significant sounds are auscultated.

1. Evidence—Is there sufficient evidence to draw conclusions about this infant?
2. Assumptions—Describe an underlying assumption about each of the following:
   a. Adverse effects of furosemide
   b. Adverse effects of digoxin
   c. Infants with HF
3. What priorities for nursing care should be established for this infant?
4. Does the evidence support your nursing interventions?
5. What alternative perspectives might you have?

interventions with older children. Some infants and children require sedation during the acute phase of illness to allow them to rest.

Temperature needs to be monitored carefully because hyperthermia or hypothermia increases the need for oxygen. Febrile states should be reported to the physician, since infection must be treated promptly. Maintaining body temperature is of special importance in children who are receiving cool, humidified oxygen and in infants, who tend to be diaphoretic and lose heat by way of evaporation.

Skin breakdown from edema is prevented with a change of position every 2 hours (from side to side while in semi-Fowler position) and use of a pressure-relieving mattress or bed. The skin, especially over the sacrum, should be checked for evidence of redness from pressure.

Reduce Respiratory Distress

Careful assessment, positioning, and oxygen administration can reduce respiratory distress. Respirations are counted for 1 full minute during a resting state. Any evidence of increased respiratory distress should be reported, since this may indicate worsening HF.

Infants should be positioned to encourage maximum chest expansion, with the head of the bed elevated; they should sit up in an infant seat or be held at a 45-degree angle. Children prefer to sleep on several pillows and remain in a semi-Fowler or high-Fowler position during waking hours. Safety restraints, such as those used with infant seats, should be applied low on the abdomen and loosely enough to provide both safety and maximum expansion.

The infant or child is often given humidified supplemental oxygen via oxygen hood or tent, nasal cannula, or mask. The child's response to oxygen therapy needs to be carefully evaluated by noting respiratory rate, ease of respiration, colour, and especially oxygen saturation as measured by oximetry.

Respiratory tract infections can exacerbate HF and should be treated appropriately and prevented if possible. The child should be protected from persons with respiratory tract infections and have a noninfectious roommate. For an older child, it is advantageous to choose a roommate who is also confined to bed and relatively quiet to promote a restful environment. Good hand hygiene should be practised before and after caring for any hospitalized child. Antibiotics may be given to combat respiratory tract infection. The nurse needs to ensure that the medication is given at equally divided times over a 24-hour schedule to maintain high blood levels of the antibiotic.

Maintain Nutritional Status

Meeting the nutritional needs of infants with HF or serious cardiac defects is a nursing challenge. The metabolic rate of these infants is greater because of poor cardiac function and increased heart and respiratory rates. Their caloric needs are greater than those of the average infant because of their increased metabolic rate, yet their ability to take in adequate calories is hampered by their fatigue. Feeding for a fragile infant with serious CHD is similar to exercising for an adult, and these infants often do not have the energy or cardiac reserve to do extra work. The nurse needs to seek measures to enable the infant to feed easily without excess fatigue and to increase the caloric density of the formula.

The infant should be well rested before feeding and fed soon after awakening so as not to expend energy on crying. A 3-hour feeding schedule works well for many infants. (Feeding every 2 hours does not provide enough rest between feedings, and a 4-hour schedule requires an increased volume of feeding, which many infants are unable to take.) The feeding schedule should be individualized to the infant's needs. A feeding goal of 150 mL/kg/day and at least 120 kcal/kg/day is common for newborns with significant heart disease (Stetzler, Rudd, & Pick, 2005). Newborns can be breastfed or bottle fed. A soft preemie nipple or a slit in a regular nipple to enlarge the opening decreases the infant's energy expenditure while sucking from a bottle. Infants should be well supported and fed in a semiupright position. The infant may need to rest frequently and may need to have the jaw and cheeks stroked to encourage sucking. Generally, giving an infant about a half hour to complete a feeding is reasonable. Prolonging the feeding time can exhaust the infant and decrease the rest period between feedings.

Infants with feeding difficulties are often gavage fed using a nasogastric tube to supplement their oral intake and ensure adequate calories. If they are very stressed and fatigued, in respiratory distress, or tachypneic to 80 to 100 breaths/min, oral feedings may be withheld and all nutrition given by gavage feedings. Gavage feedings are usually a temporary measure until the infant's medical status improves and nutritional needs can be met through oral feedings. Some infants with severe HF, neurological deficits, or significant gastroesophageal reflux may need placement of a gastrostomy tube to allow adequate nutrition.

The caloric density of formulas is frequently increased by concentration and then adding Polycose, medium-chain triglyceride oil, or corn oil. Infant formulas provide 20 kcal/30 mL, and the use of additives can increase the calories to 30 kcal/30 mL or more. This allows the infant to obtain more calories despite a smaller volume intake of formula. The caloric density of the formula needs to be increased slowly (by 2 kcal/30 mL/day) to prevent diarrhea or formula intolerance. Breastfeeding mothers should be encouraged to provide the infant with alternating feedings of breast milk and high-calorie formulas. Some lactating mothers prefer to feed the child expressed breast milk that has been fortified with Similac or Enfamil powder, Polycose, or corn oil to increase caloric intake. A supplemental nurser may also be helpful. A diet plan specific to the individual infant's needs should be calculated and prescribed by the nutritionist in collaboration with the other health personnel. The nurse needs to reinforce this information with the parents as necessary.

Assist in Measures to Promote Fluid Loss

When diuretics are given, the nurse needs to record fluid intake and output and monitor body weight at the same time each day to evaluate the benefit from the medication. Because profound diuresis may cause dehydration and electrolyte imbalance (loss of sodium, potassium, chloride, bicarbonate), the nurse should observe for signs indicating either complication, as well as signs and symptoms suggesting reactions to the medications. Diuretics should be given early in the day to children who are toilet trained to avoid the need to urinate at night. If potassium-losing diuretics are given, the nurse can encourage foods high in potassium, such as bananas, oranges, whole grains, legumes, and leafy vegetables, and administer prescribed supplements. Serum potassium levels should be checked frequently.

Fluid restriction is rarely necessary in infants because of their difficulty in feeding. However, if fluids are restricted, the nurse can plan fluid intake schedules for a 24-hour period, allowing for most fluids during waking hours. Toddlers and preschoolers should be given small amounts of liquid in small cups so that the containers appear full. Older children can be placed in charge of recording fluid intake.

If salt is limited, the nurse needs to discusses food sources of sodium with the family and discourage their bringing salt-containing treats to the child. At mealtime, the child's tray should be checked to make sure the appropriate diet is being given.

Support the Child and Family

HF is a serious complication of heart disease. Parents and older children are usually acutely aware of the critical nature of the condition. Because stress places additional demands on cardiac function, the nurse should focus on reducing anxiety through anticipatory preparation, frequent communication with the parent regarding the child's progress, and constant reassurance that everything possible is being done.

Home care involves many of the same interventions discussed under Plan for Discharge and Home Care (p. 1481). The nurse needs to teach the family about the medications that need to be administered and alert them to the signs of worsening HF that require medical attention, such as increased sweating, decreased urinary output (noted in fewer wet diapers or infrequent use of the toilet), or poor feeding. Every effort should be made to improve the family's adherence to the medication schedule by adapting the schedule to their usual home routines, avoiding medications during the night, making it as simple as possible, and using charts or visual aids to remember when to give medications (see Chapter 45). Written instructions regarding correct administration of digoxin are essential (see Family-Centred Teaching box, p. 1472), including an explanation of the signs of toxicity.

If HF is the end stage of a severe heart defect, the nurse should care for this child as for any child who is terminally ill, using the principles discussed in Chapter 41.

Hypoxemia

Hypoxemia refers to an arterial oxygen tension (or pressure, Pao_2) that is less than normal and can be identified by a decreased arterial saturation or a decreased Pao_2. **Hypoxia** is a reduction in tissue oxygenation that is caused by low oxygen saturations and Pao_2 and results in impaired cellular processes. *Cyanosis* is a blue discolouration in the mucous membranes, skin, and nail beds of the child with reduced oxygen saturation. It results from the presence of deoxygenated hemoglobin (hemoglobin not bound to oxygen) in a concentration of blood. Cyanosis is usually apparent when arterial oxygen saturations are 80 to 85%. Determination of cyanosis is subjective. It can vary depending on skin pigment, quality of light, colour of the room, or clothing worn by the child. The presence of cyanosis may not accurately reflect arterial hypoxemia because both oxygen saturation and the amount of circulating hemoglobin are involved. Children with severe anemia may not be cyanotic despite severe hypoxemia because the hemoglobin level may be too low to produce the characteristic blue colour. Conversely, patients with polycythemia may appear cyanotic despite a near-normal Pao_2. Heart defects that cause hypoxemia and cyanosis result from desaturated venous blood (blue blood) entering the systemic circulation without passing through the lungs.

Clinical Manifestations

Over time, two physiological changes occur in the body in response to chronic hypoxemia: polycythemia and clubbing. *Polycythemia*, an increased number of red blood cells, increases the oxygen-carrying capacity of the blood. However, anemia may result if iron is not readily available for the formation of hemoglobin. Polycythemia increases the viscosity of the blood and crowds out clotting factors. *Clubbing*, a thickening and flattening of the tips of the fingers and toes, is thought to occur because of chronic tissue hypoxemia and polycythemia (Fig. 48-7). Infants with mild hypoxemia may be asymptomatic except for cyanosis and exhibit near-normal growth and development. Those with more severe hypoxemia may exhibit fatigue with feeding, poor weight gain, tachypnea, and dyspnea. Severe hypoxemia resulting in tissue hypoxia is manifested by clinical deterioration and signs of poor perfusion.

Hypercyanotic spells, also referred to as *blue spells* or *tet spells* because they are often seen in infants with tetralogy of Fallot, may occur in any child whose heart defect includes obstruction to pulmonary blood flow and communication between the ventricles. The infant becomes acutely cyanotic and hyperpneic because a sudden infundibular spasm decreases pulmonary blood flow and increases right-to-left shunting (the proposed mechanism in tetralogy of Fallot). Spells, rarely seen before 2 months of age, occur most frequently in the first year of life. They occur more often in the morning and may be preceded by feeding, crying, defecation, or stressful procedures (see Critical Thinking Exercise). Because profound hypoxemia causes cerebral hypoxia, hypercyanotic spells require prompt assessment and treatment to prevent brain damage or possibly death.

Persistent cyanosis as a result of cyanotic heart defects places the child at risk for significant neurological complications. Cerebrovascular accident (CVA, stroke), brain abscess,

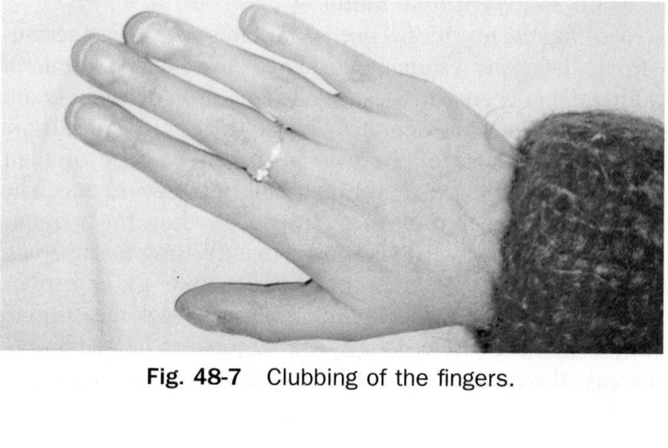

Fig. 48-7 Clubbing of the fingers.

CRITICAL THINKING EXERCISE

Hypercyanotic Spell

A 4-month-old infant known to have tetralogy of Fallot is seen in the emergency department because of a 2-day history of diarrhea, low-grade fever, and poor oral intake. When blood is drawn, he becomes acutely cyanotic with rapid shallow respirations.

1. Evidence—Is there sufficient evidence to draw conclusions about this infant's condition?
2. Assumptions—Describe an underlying assumption about each of the following:
   a. Symptoms associated with tetralogy of Fallot
   b. Diarrhea, low-grade fever, and poor oral intake in a 4-month-old infant
   c. Acute cyanotic episodes in a 4-month-old infant
3. What priorities for nursing care should be established for this infant?
4. Does the evidence support your nursing interventions?
5. What alternative perspectives might you have?

and developmental delays (especially in motor and cognitive development) may result from chronic hypoxia.

Therapeutic Management

Newborns generally exhibit cyanosis within the first few days of life as the ductus arteriosus, which provided pulmonary blood flow, begins to close. Prostaglandin E_1, which causes vasodilation and smooth muscle relaxation, thus increasing dilation and patency of the ductus arteriosus, is administered intravenously to re-establish pulmonary blood flow. The use of prostaglandins has been lifesaving for infants with ductus-dependent cardiac defects. The increase in oxygenation allows the infant to be stabilized and have a complete diagnostic evaluation performed before further treatment is needed.

Hypercyanotic spells occur suddenly, and prompt recognition and treatment are essential. In the hospital setting, spells are often seen during blood drawing or IV insertion, when the child is highly agitated, or after cardiac catheterization. Treatment of a hypercyanotic spell is outlined in the Guidelines box. Placing the infant in the knee–chest position reduces the venous return from the legs (which is desaturated) and increases systemic vascular resistance, which diverts more blood into the pulmonary artery (Fig. 48-8). Morphine, administered subcutaneously or through an existing IV line, helps reduce infundibular spasm. A spell indicates the need for prompt surgical treatment if possible. In infants with defects not amenable to surgical repair, a shunt may be created surgically to increase blood flow to the lungs. Several commonly used shunt procedures are described in Table 48-4 and Figure 48-9. In rare cases, propranolol (Inderal) may be given in the interim to prevent infundibular spasm.

The cyanotic infant and child should be well hydrated to keep the hematocrit and blood viscosity within acceptable limits to reduce the risk of CVAs. Fevers need to be carefully evaluated because bacteremia can result in bacterial endocarditis. The infant should be monitored closely for anemia

GUIDELINES Treating Hypercyanotic Spells

- Place infant in knee–chest position (see Fig. 48-8).
- Use a calm, comforting approach.
- Administer 100% oxygen by blow-by.
- Give morphine subcutaneously or through existing intravenous (IV) line.
- Begin IV fluid replacement and volume expansion if needed.
- Repeat morphine administration.

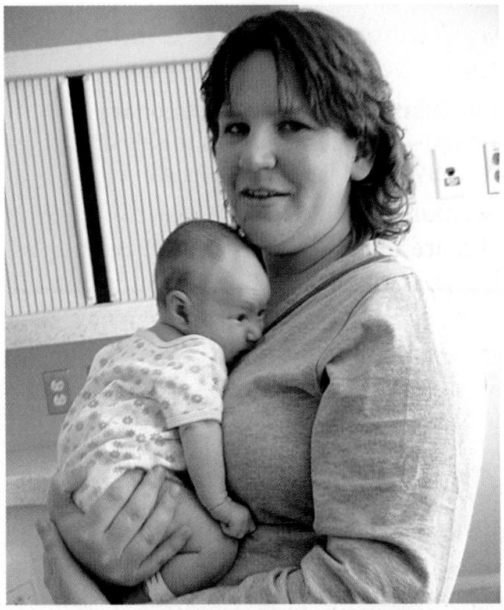

Fig. 48-8 Infant held in knee–chest position.

because of the risk of CVAs and the reduced arterial oxygen-carrying capacity that occurs. Iron supplementation and possibly blood transfusion are used as needed.

Respiratory tract infections or reduced pulmonary function from any cause can worsen hypoxemia in the cyanotic child. Aggressive pulmonary hygiene, chest physical therapy, administration of antibiotics, and use of oxygen to improve arterial saturations are important interventions.

Nursing Care Management

The general appearance of infants and children with significant cyanosis poses unique concerns. Blue lips and fingernails are obvious signs of their hidden cardiac defect. Clubbing and small, thin stature in older children further indicate severe heart disease. Adolescents are especially concerned about their body image; children with cyanosis are often teased about their appearance and singled out as different. When asked what surgery will do, many children reply, "Make me pink." Their joy and excitement after surgery are evident when they see their pink fingers. Parents are often fearful of their child's bluish colour because cyanosis is usually associated with lack of oxygen and severe illness. They also must deal with comments from relatives, friends, and strangers about their child's abnormal colour. They need a simple explanation of hypoxemia and cyanosis and reassurance that cyanosis does not imply a lack of oxygen to the brain. Their questions and fears need to be addressed in a calm, supportive manner, and positive aspects of their child's growth and development

Table 48-4 Selected Shunt Procedures for Children With Cardiac Defects

SHUNT TYPE	COMMENTS
Modified Blalock-Taussig shunt–Subclavian artery to pulmonary artery using Gore-Tex or Impra tube graft	Shunt flow sometimes excessive, requiring use of diuretics Possibility of thrombosis; aspirin usually prescribed postoperatively Easy to ligate at time of definitive correction Shunt size fixed and may become too small as child grows
Sano modification—Right ventricular to pulmonary artery conduit using Gore-Tex	Prevents diastolic runoff of systemic blood into the pulmonary arteries Provides a higher diastolic blood pressure and seemingly better coronary perfusion Used in place of the modified Blalock-Taussig shunt in the Norwood procedure
Central shunt–Ascending aorta to main pulmonary artery using Gore-Tex graft	Length of shunt acts to restrict blood flow; possibility of symptoms of heart failure; diuretic therapy sometimes required Uncommon; used when modified Blalock-Taussig shunt cannot be used Easy to insert and remove at time of repair Possibility of thrombosis; aspirin usually prescribed postoperatively
Bidirectional Glenn shunt (cavopulmonary anastomosis)—Superior vena cava to side of right pulmonary artery; blood flow to both lungs	Done as a second shunt; often used as a staging step to a Fontan procedure Can be incorporated into eventual modified Fontan procedure Relieves severe cyanosis and decreases volume overload on ventricle Carries risk of embolic events (mixing defect); aspirin often prescribed Pulmonary arteriovenous fistulas may occur months or years later, causing desaturation (uncommon finding)

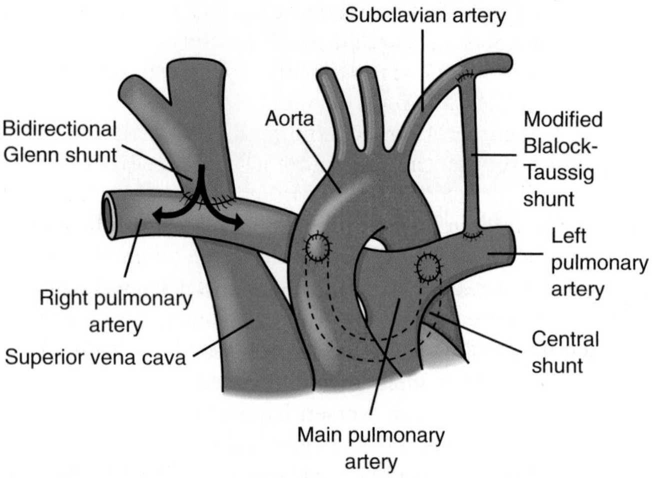

Fig. 48-9 Schematic diagram of cardiac shunts.

should be emphasized. They need to be taught the treatment for hypercyanotic spells (see Guidelines box, p. 1475).

Dehydration must be prevented in hypoxemic children because it potentiates the risk of CVAs. Fluid status should be monitored carefully, with accurate intake and output and daily weight measurements. Maintenance fluid therapy is the minimum requirement, supplemental fluids should be readily available, and gavage feeding or IV hydration is given to children unable to take adequate oral fluids. Fever, vomiting, and diarrhea can cause dehydration and require prompt treatment. Parents need to be instructed in the importance of adequate fluid intake and measures to prevent dehydration. An oral electrolyte solution should be available at home in the event that the infant is unable to tolerate the usual formula. The practitioner should be notified of fever, vomiting, diarrhea, or other problems.

Preventive measures and accurate assessment of respiratory infection are important nursing considerations. Any compromise in pulmonary function will increase the infant's hypoxemia. Good hand hygiene and protection from individuals with an obvious respiratory tract infection are important. Aggressive pulmonary hygiene, treatment with antibiotics or antiviral agents as indicated, and supplemental oxygen to decrease hypoxemia are necessary measures. Infants may need to be gavage fed or given parenteral hydration if respiratory distress prevents oral feeding.

NURSING ALERT Intracardiac shunting of blood from the right side (desaturated) to the left side of the heart allows air in the venous system to go directly to the brain, resulting in an air embolism. Therefore, all IV lines should have filters in place to prevent air from entering the system, the entire tubing should be checked for air, all connections should be taped securely, and any air should be removed.

Nursing Care of the Family and Child With Congenital Heart Disease

When a child is born with a severe cardiac anomaly, the parents are faced with the immense psychological and physical tasks of adjusting to the birth of a child with special needs. Family issues and nursing interventions to support the family are similar to those discussed in Chapter 41. The following discussion is primarily directed (1) toward the family of an infant who has a serious heart defect and requires home care before definitive repair and (2) toward preparation and care of the child and family when invasive procedures (catheterization and surgery) are performed. For nursing care related to the child with hypoxemia and HF, see earlier discussions of these topics.

Nursing care of the child with a congenital heart defect begins as soon as the diagnosis is suspected. Prenatal diagnosis of congenital heart defects is becoming increasingly frequent. New demands are being placed on nurses to counsel and support families as they prepare for the birth of these infants.

Help the Family Adjust to the Disorder

Once parents learn of the heart defect, they are initially in a period of shock, followed by high anxiety and fear that the child will die. The family needs time to grieve before they can assimilate the meaning of the defect. Unfortunately, the demands for medical treatment may not allow this, instead necessitating that the parents immediately give **informed consent** for diagnostic-therapeutic procedures. The nurse can be instrumental in supporting parents in their loss, assessing their level of understanding, supplying information as needed, and helping other members of the health care team understand the parents' reactions (see Family-Centred Teaching box).

Severely ill newborns usually remain in the hospital. Parent–infant attachment is supported by encouraging parents to hold, touch, and look at their child and providing time and privacy for the parents to spend with their newborn.

The effect of a child with a serious heart defect on the family is complex. No member, regardless of the degree of positive adjustment, is unaffected. Mothers frequently feel inadequate in their mothering ability because of the more complex care that infants with congenital heart defects require. They often feel exhausted from the pressures of caring for these children and the other family members. Fathers and siblings may feel neglected and resentful, a reaction similar to the feelings toward family members with other chronic conditions (see Chapter 41). Often, parents do not feel confident leaving the child in another's care. This often sets up a trap for parents, especially mothers, who become locked into the child's care with no relief. Although the fears are justified, they can be minimized by gradually teaching someone (a reliable relative or neighbour) how to care for the child.

The need to maintain discipline and set consistent limits can be difficult for parents. Using behaviour modification techniques in the form of either concrete awards (e.g., a favourite activity) or social reinforcement (e.g., approval) can be effective. However, these techniques are most beneficial if used *before* the child learns to control the family. It is necessary to begin discussions with parents while the child is in infancy regarding the need for discipline to prevent later problems as the child gets older.

Another issue that may develop within family relationships is the child's overdependency. This is often the result of parental fear that the child may die. The nurse can help parents recognize the eventual hazards of continuing dependency and protectiveness as the child grows older and learn ways to foster optimum development. Unless parents are shown what activities the child can do, they may focus on physical limitations and encourage dependency.

The child also needs opportunities for normal social interaction with peers. These children do not need to be prevented from playing with other children because of concern regarding overexertion. Children usually limit their activities if allowed to set their own pace.

A child with CHD may constitute a long-term family crisis. Frequently, the continuing unremitting stresses of care—physical exhaustion, financial costs, emotional upset, fear of death, and concern for the child's future—are not fully appreciated by those caring for the family. Even when the child's condition is stabilized or corrected, the family may need to make adjustments in their lifestyle. Introducing them to other families with similarly affected children can help them adjust to the daily stresses.

FAMILY-CENTRED TEACHING

Diagnosis of Heart Disease

Remember that we don't have your experience. We don't see children every day who have heart disease. We would have been upset finding out our child had to have his tonsils out. How could we ever be prepared for this? Please remember, we only know people who have trivial heart murmurs. How could we ever expect this to happen? And to us, this is the worst problem we've ever heard of.

We still fear most what we don't know and understand. Be honest with us. If you don't know either, tell us. But at least don't leave us wondering about what you know and we don't. Not knowing anything really can be worse than knowing something bad. Be honest, but don't strip us of hope....

Please, remember we are trying to learn complex information in a moment of time. And trying to learn it in a context of great pain and emotional investment. This is our lives you're talking about. Please be thorough, but keep it simple. Tell us again, maybe even again and again, when we can hear better.

(From Schrey, C., & Schrey, M. [1994]. A parent's perspective: Our needs and our message. *Critical Care Nursing Clinics of North America, 6*[1], 113–119.)

Educate the Family About the Disorder

When parents are ready to hear about the heart condition, they require a clear explanation based on their level of understanding. A review of the basic structure and function of the heart is helpful before describing the defect. A simple diagram, pictures, or a model of the heart can help parents visualize the heart and the congenital defect. Parents appreciate receiving written information about the specific condition, and a glossary of frequently used terms is helpful. Parents also require information about prognosis and treatment options.

Increasingly, families are using the Internet as a source of information about heart disease in children (see Additional Resources section at the end of this chapter). They are also finding support through contacts with other parents and parent groups. It is important for parents to realize that not all Web sites offer medically accurate information and that information from other parents might not be applicable to their own situation. Some children with rare, complex heart defects require individualized treatment plans, and general information on the Internet or in books may not apply to their child. Parents should discuss with their health care team, in particular their cardiologist, information they have received from other sources.

Information given to the child must be tailored to his or her developmental age. As the child matures, the level of information should be revised to meet his or her new cognitive level. Preschoolers need basic information about what they will experience more than what is actually occurring physiologically. School-age children benefit from a concrete explanation of the defect. Preadolescents and adolescents often appreciate a more detailed description of how the defect affects their heart. Children of all ages need to express their feelings concerning the diagnosis.

Help the Family Manage the Illness at Home

Parents are the child's principal caregivers and need to develop a positive, supportive working relationship with the health care team. Parents should be aware of the symptoms of their child's cardiac condition and signs of worsening clinical status. Parents of children who may develop HF should be familiar with the symptoms (see Box 48-5) and know when to contact their health care practitioner. Parents of children with cyanosis should be informed about fluid management and hypercyanotic spells. They should have an information sheet with their child's diagnosis, significant treatments such as surgical procedures, allergies, other health care problems, current medications, and health care providers' contact numbers available in case of emergencies and to share with other caregivers such as teachers, babysitters, or day care providers.

The family also needs to be knowledgeable about the therapeutic management of the disorder and the roles that surgery, other procedures, medications, and healthy lifestyle play in maintaining good health. Medications play a critical role in managing some cardiac conditions such as dysrhythmias and severe HF; anticoagulation is used for artificial valves, and antirejection medications are needed after heart transplantation. Some patients must take multiple medications daily for their lifetime. Many medications can be dangerous if taken incorrectly and require close monitoring. Parents need to be taught the correct procedure for giving medications and cautioned to keep them in a safe area to prevent accidental ingestion (see Family-Centred Teaching box, p. 1472).

Another area of parental concern is the child's level of physical activity. Most children do not need to restrict activity, and the best approach is to treat the child normally and allow self-limited activity. Exceptions to self-determined activity primarily involve strenuous recreational and competitive sports in children with specific cardiac problems. Activities and exercise restrictions should be discussed with the child's cardiologist. Deliberately attempting to prevent crying should be avoided because it can establish a maladaptive parental pattern of relating to the infant.

Infants and children with CHD require good nutrition. Breastfeeding should be possible for many infants with CHD. Barbas and Kelleher (2004) found that breastfeeding could be successful with adequate support and education of the mother. Providing adequate nutrition to infants with HF or complex congenital defects is especially difficult because of their high caloric requirements and inability to suck effectively because of fatigue and tachypnea. Instructing parents in feeding methods that decrease the infant's work and giving high-calorie formula are important interventions (see p. 1472 for a discussion on feeding the infant with HF). Children with severe cardiac defects are often anorexic. Encouraging them to eat can be a tremendous challenge. Consultation with a dietitian is often helpful. The child should be given a choice of available high-nutrient foods.

Infants with heart disease should be immunized according to the current guidelines (Public Health Agency of Canada, 2006). Immunization schedules may need to be modified around times of acute illness or surgical procedures (Smith, 2001). Infants and children less than 2 years of age with unrepaired heart defects, cyanotic lesions, pulmonary hypertension, or history of prematurity should receive the vaccine for respiratory syncytial virus (RSV) monthly during RSV season (November to April in North America) (Robinson & Canadian Paediatric Society [CPS], Infectious Diseases and Immunization Committee, 2011).

Infants and children who have serious heart disease are at risk for developmental delays. Multiple factors can influence neurodevelopmental outcomes, including genetics (chromosome abnormalities and microdeletions), family background (parental intelligence quotient [IQ] and socioeconomic status), preoperative factors (including prematurity, cyanosis, shock), intraoperative factors (use of cardiopulmonary bypass, deep hypothermic circulatory arrest), and postoperative factors (hemodynamic instability, hypoxia, **acidosis**, cardiac arrest, stroke, ischemic events). Researchers at the Hospital for Sick Children found that the risk for arterial ischemic stroke/cerebral sinovenous thrombosis was 5.4 strokes per 1000 children undergoing a cardiac surgery (Domi et al., 2008). Efforts to limit the time of deep hypothermic circulatory arrest and provide better neuroprotection during infant surgery may improve outcomes in the future.

Prepare the Child and Family for Invasive Procedures

Chapter 45 provides an extensive discussion of the principles for preparing children for invasive procedures. The American Heart Association (2011) has published information on how to prepare a child for cardiac surgery and addresses issues specific to the child with heart disease. The following discussion highlights some important aspects of preparation for cardiac catheterization and cardiac surgery.

The expected outcomes for preprocedure preparation include reducing anxiety, improving patient collaboration with procedures, enhancing recovery, developing trust with caregivers, and improving long-term emotional and behavioural adjustments after procedures (Maclaren & Cohen, 2007). Important factors to consider in planning preparation strategies are the child's cognitive development, previous hospital experiences, the child's temperament and coping style, timing of preparation, and involvement of the parents. The most beneficial preparation strategies usually combine information giving and coping skills training, such as conscious breathing exercises, distraction techniques, guided imagery, or other behavioural interventions.

Outpatient preoperative and precatheterization workups are common for most elective procedures. Children are then admitted on the morning of the procedure. Preprocedure teaching is often done in the clinic setting or at home and may include a tour of the critical care unit (CCU) and inpatient facilities. Children of different ages and developmental levels require different amounts of information and different approaches. Young children should be prepared close in time to the event, whereas older children and adolescents may benefit from teaching several weeks in advance. Parents should be included in the preparation session to support their child and learn about upcoming events.

A discussion of ways in which the child can cope with the experience should be included. Bringing a familiar stuffed animal or comfort object will help a young child relieve anxiety, whereas advising an older child to bring headphones and favourite music to the catheterization laboratory will help distract him or her during the procedure. Recovery topics after catheterization include lying still to prevent bleeding at the catheter site, advancing diet, controlling pain, and monitoring. After surgery, the nurse should review the importance of ambulation, coughing, deep breathing, drinking, and eating and describe pain management and monitoring routines. Simple coping strategies for use during painful procedures should be reviewed; these include distraction techniques such as counting, blowing, singing, or telling stories.

Children and their families should have a choice about taking a CCU tour. Exposure to the CCU environment can actually increase anxiety in some children, particularly young children, those with previous hospital experiences, and those who are highly anxious (LeRoy et al., 2003). The day before the procedure is usually ample time to allow the child to ask questions and to prevent undue fantasizing about the experience. The child should be protected from the frightening sights in the unit; equipment not in view after surgery, such as equipment located behind or below the bed, needs less attention. The child and parents should be encouraged to ask questions or to explore further any equipment in the room, but they should not be pushed to assimilate more information than they are able.

BOX 48-7 Selected Complications After Cardiac Surgery and Treatment Approaches

Cardiac

Heart failure—Digoxin, diuretics (p. 1462)

Low cardiac output—Intravenous inotropes (Shock, p. 1492)

Dysrhythmias—Identification, drug treatment, possible pacing, cardioversion (p. 1486)

Tamponade (blood or fluid in the pericardial space constricting the heart)—Prompt removal of fluid by pericardiocentesis

Respiratory

Atelectasis—Chest physical therapy, coughing, deep breathing, ambulation

Pulmonary edema—Diuretics

Pleural effusions—Diuretics, possible chest tube drainage

Pneumothorax—Possible chest tube drainage

Neurological

Seizures—Assessment, anti-epileptic drugs

Cerebrovascular accident (stroke), cerebral edema, neurological deficits—Assessment and treatment

Infectious Disease

Infections (especially wound, pneumonia, otitis media, and sepsis)—Antibiotics

Hematological

Anemia—Iron supplementation, possible transfusion

Postoperative bleeding—Initially, clotting factors, blood products; may need repeat surgery to locate and ligate source of bleeding

Other

Postpericardiotomy syndrome (syndrome of fever, leukocytosis, friction rub, pericardial and pleural effusions, and lethargy seen about 7 to 21 days after cardiac surgery; possible viral or autoimmune etiologies)—Antipyretics, diuretics, anti-inflammatory medications

evolve Animation—Cardiac Tamponade, Infant

Provide Postoperative Care

Immediate postoperative care is usually provided by specially trained nurses in critical care units. Many of the procedures, such as arterial pressure and central venous pressure (CVP) monitoring, and the observations related to vital functions require advanced educational training (the reader should refer to critical care texts for further information). However, nurses caring for the child before surgery and during the convalescent period need to be familiar with the major principles of care. Selected complications that may occur postoperatively are described in Box 48-7.

Observe Vital Signs

Vital signs and BP are recorded frequently until stable. Heart rate and respirations are counted for 1 full minute, compared with the ECG monitor, and recorded with activity. The heart rate is normally increased after surgery. Arterial and venous pressures may be monitored. The nurse needs to observe cardiac rhythm and notify the practitioner of any changes in regularity. Dysrhythmias may occur postoperatively secondary to anaesthetics, acid–base and electrolyte imbalance, hypoxia, surgical intervention, or trauma to conduction pathways (p. 1486).

At least hourly, the lungs should be auscultated for breath sounds. Diminished or absent sounds may indicate an area of atelectasis or a pleural effusion or pneumothorax, which necessitates further medical assessment. Temperature changes are typical during the early postoperative period. Hypothermia is expected immediately after surgery from hypothermia procedures, effects of anaesthesia, and loss of body heat to the cool environment. During this period, the child needs to be kept warm to prevent additional heat loss. Infants may be placed under radiant heat warmers. During the next 24 to 48 hours the body temperature may rise to 37.7°C or slightly higher as part of the inflammatory response to tissue trauma. After this period an elevated temperature is most likely a sign of infection and warrants immediate investigation for probable cause.

Intra-arterial monitoring of BP is commonly done after open-heart surgery. A catheter is passed into the radial artery or other artery, and the other end is attached to an electronic monitoring system, which provides a continuous recording of the BP. The intra-arterial line is maintained with a low-rate, constant infusion of heparinized saline to prevent clotting.

Several IV lines are inserted preoperatively: a peripheral IV to give fluids and medications; and a CVP, which is usually inserted in a large vessel in the neck. In addition, intracardiac monitoring lines are sometimes placed intraoperatively in the right atrium, left atrium, or pulmonary artery. Intracardiac lines allow assessment of pressures inside the cardiac chambers, providing vital information about volume status, cardiac output, and ventricular function. All lines must be cared for using strict aseptic technique, and patients must be carefully assessed for bleeding at the time of line removal.

Maintain Respiratory Status

Infants usually require mechanical ventilation in the immediate postoperative period. Early extubation in the operating room or early postoperative period is becoming more common. Children, especially those who did not require cardiopulmonary bypass, may be extubated in the operating room or in the first few postoperative hours. Suctioning is performed only as needed and is performed carefully to avoid vagal stimulation (which can trigger cardiac dysrhythmias) and laryngospasm, especially in infants. Suctioning is intermittent and maintained for no more than 5 seconds at a time to avoid depleting the oxygen supply. Supplemental oxygen is administered with a manual resuscitation bag before and after the procedure to prevent hypoxia. The heart rate is monitored after suctioning to detect changes in rhythm or rate, especially bradycardia. The child should always be positioned facing the nurse to permit assessment of the child's colour and tolerance of the procedure.

NURSING ALERT During suctioning, observe for signs and symptoms of respiratory distress, such as tachypnea, use of accessory muscles for breathing, and restlessness.

When weaning and extubation are completed, humidified oxygen is delivered by mask, hood, or nasal cannula to prevent drying of mucosa. The child should be encouraged to turn and deep breathe at least hourly. Measures such as splinting the operative site and providing analgesics can be used to enhance ventilation and decrease pain. Chest tubes are inserted into the pleural or mediastinal space during surgery or in the immediate postoperative period to remove secretions and air to allow re-expansion of the lung. Drainage should be checked hourly for colour and quantity. Immediately after surgery the drainage may be bright red, but afterward it should be serous. The largest volume of drainage occurs in the first 12 to 24 hours and is greater in extensive heart surgery.

NURSING ALERT Chest tube drainage greater than 3 mL/kg/hr for more than 3 consecutive hours or 5 to 10 mL/kg in any 1 hour is excessive and may indicate postoperative hemorrhage. The surgeon should be notified immediately because cardiac tamponade can develop rapidly and is life threatening.

Chest tubes are usually removed on the first to third postoperative day. Removal of chest tubes is a painful, frightening experience. Analgesics such as morphine sulphate, often combined with midazolam (Versed), should be given before the procedure. Older children should be forewarned that they will feel a sharp, momentary pain. After the suture is cut, the tubes are quickly pulled out at the end of a full inspiration to prevent the intake of air into the pleural cavity. A purse-string suture (placed when the tubes were inserted) is pulled tight to close the opening. A petrolatum-covered gauze dressing is immediately applied over the wound and securely taped on all four sides to the skin so that an airtight seal is formed. It is left on for 1 or 2 days. Breath sounds need to be checked to assess for a pneumothorax.

Monitor Fluids

Intake and output of all fluids must be accurately calculated. Intake is primarily IV fluids; however, a record of fluid used to flush the arterial and CVP lines or to dilute medications is also kept. Output includes hourly recordings of urine (usually a Foley catheter is inserted and attached to a closed collecting device), drainage from chest and nasogastric tubes, and blood drawn for analysis. Urine should be analyzed for specific gravity to assess the concentrating ability of the kidneys and the body's approximate degree of hydration. Renal failure is a potential risk from a transient period of low cardiac output.

NURSING ALERT The signs of renal failure are decreased urinary output (less than 1 mL/kg/hr) and elevated levels of blood urea nitrogen and serum creatinine.

Fluids are restricted during the immediate postoperative period to prevent hypervolemia, which places additional demands on the myocardium, predisposing the patient to cardiac failure. To monitor fluid retention, the child is weighed daily, and the same scale is used at approximately the same time each day to avoid errors in measurement. The child is usually given nothing by mouth for the first 24 hours. If an endotracheal (ET) tube is inserted, oral fluids are usually withheld until the child is extubated. Fluid restriction may be imposed even when oral fluids are given. The nurse needs to calculate the distribution over a 24-hour period based on the child's preoperative weight and drinking habits. The distribution should allow for most fluid to be given during the child's most wakeful and active periods.

Provide Rest and Progressive Activity

After heart surgery, rest should be provided to decrease the workload of the heart and promote healing. The simplest way to ensure individualized, efficient, high-quality care is to plan at the beginning of the shift the nursing procedures to be done, with periods of rest identified. The schedule should be shared with parents to allow them to visit at the most advantageous times, such as after a rest period when no special treatments are anticipated.

A progressive schedule of ambulation and activity is planned, based on the child's preoperative activity patterns and postoperative cardiovascular and pulmonary function. Ambulation is initiated early, usually by the second postoperative day, when chest tubes, arterial lines, and assisted ventilatory equipment may be removed. Activity progresses from sitting on the edge of the bed and dangling the legs to standing up and sitting in a chair. Heart rate and respirations need to be carefully monitored to assess the degree of cardiac demand imposed by each activity. Tachycardia, dyspnea, cyanosis, desaturation, progressive fatigue, or dysrhythmias indicate the need to limit further energy expenditure.

Provide Comfort and Emotional Support

Heart surgery is both painful and frightening for children, and comfort is a primary nursing concern. Several incisions may be used for heart surgery. A median sternotomy is most common, following the sternum down the centre of the chest. A ministernotomy opens the lower sternum. It allows access to the side of the chest through an incision from under the arm around the back to the scapula.

Most patients need IV analgesics for pain control during the immediate postoperative period. Patient-controlled analgesia may be used with children old enough to understand the concept. Nonsteroidal anti-inflammatory drugs (NSAIDs) such as ketorolac (Toradol) may be used intravenously. Paralyzing agents may also be used with the analgesics for children who are agitated or hemodynamically unstable.

After extubation and the removal of lines and tubes, pain can be controlled satisfactorily with oral medications such as ibuprofen, acetaminophen, or codeine. Acetaminophen alone provides adequate pain relief for most children at discharge. Sternotomy incisions are usually well tolerated, with some discomfort when walking and coughing. Thoracotomy incisions are usually more painful because the incision is through muscle; a more aggressive pain management plan with around-the-clock medications for several days is often necessary to allow for adequate rest, ambulation, and pulmonary hygiene.

In addition to pharmacological pain control, every effort should be made to minimize the discomfort of procedures, such as using a firm pillow or favourite stuffed animal placed against the chest incision during movement and when performing treatments *after* pain medication is given, preferably at a time that coincides with the drug's peak effect. Nonpharmacological measures can be used to lessen the perception of pain, and parents should be encouraged to comfort their child as much as possible. (See also Pain Assessment; Pain Management, Chapter 35.)

Children may become depressed after surgery. This is thought to be caused by preoperative anxiety, postoperative psychological and physiological stress, and sensory overstimulation. Typically, the child's disposition improves on leaving the critical care unit. Children may also be angry and uncooperative after surgery as a response to the physical pain and the loss of control imposed by the surgery and treatments. They need an opportunity to express feelings, either verbally or through activity.

Plan for Discharge and Home Care

Ideally, discharge planning begins on admission for cardiac surgery and includes an assessment of the parents' adjustment to the child's altered state of health. Neonates need additional screening tests (such as newborn metabolic screen and hearing tests) and may need immunizations before discharge (Dodds & Merle, 2005). The family needs both verbal and written instructions on medication, nutrition, activity restrictions, subacute bacterial endocarditis, return to school, wound care, and signs and symptoms of infection or complications (see Patient Teaching box). Referrals to community agencies may be warranted to assist parents in the transition from hospital to home and to reinforce the teaching.

The parents also need clear instructions on when to seek medical care for complications and how to contact the health care provider. Follow-up with the cardiologist and primary care provider should be arranged before discharge. Parents should have a summary, including their child's medical condition, medications, and health care providers available for emergencies. Appropriate identification, such as a MedicAlert device, is indicated for children with a pacemaker or heart transplant and for those receiving anticoagulation therapy or antidysrhythmic medication.

Although surgical correction of heart defects has improved dramatically, it is still not possible to completely repair many of the complex anomalies. For many children, repeat procedures are required to replace conduits or grafts or to manage complications such as restenosis. Consequently, the long-term prognosis is uncertain, and full recovery is not always possible. For these families, medical follow-up and continued emotional support are essential. The nurse can often serve as an important primary health care provider and as a resource for referrals when needed.

Acquired Cardiovascular Disorders

Bacterial (Infective) Endocarditis

Bacterial endocarditis (BE), or subacute bacterial endocarditis (SBE), now commonly referred to as *infective endocarditis* (IE), is an infection of the valves and inner lining of the heart. Although it can occur without underlying heart disease, it is most often a sequela of bacteremia in the child with acquired or congenital anomalies of the heart or great vessels.

PATIENT TEACHING Topics to Include in Discharge Teaching After Cardiac Surgery

- Medication teaching (for digoxin, see Family-Centred Teaching box, p. 1472)
- Activity restrictions
- Diet and nutrition
- Wound care (including dressings, if any; suture removal; bathing)
- Infective endocarditis prophylaxis (see Box 48-9)
- Follow-up appointments (cardiologist, primary care provider)
- Community agencies as needed (visiting nurse service, early developmental intervention)
- When to call practitioner; signs and symptoms of postoperative problems
- Review of cardiac defect and surgical repair

It especially affects children with valvular abnormalities, prosthetic valves, shunts, recent cardiac surgery with invasive lines, and rheumatic heart disease with valve involvement. The most common causative agent is *Streptococcus viridans*; other causative agents are *Staphylococcus aureus*, gram-negative bacteria, and fungi such as *Candida albicans*.

Pathophysiology

Organisms may enter the bloodstream from any site of localized infection. In the past, endocarditis was believed to be highly associated with invasive procedures; however, it most likely occurs from routine exposure to bacteremia associated with usual daily activities, although it can also occur after procedures such as dental work (*S. viridans*); after invasive procedures involving the gastrointestinal-genitourinary tract; after cardiac surgery, especially if synthetic material is used (valves, patches, conduits); or from long-term indwelling catheters. The microorganisms grow on the endocardium, forming vegetations (verrucae), deposits of fibrin, and platelet thrombi. The lesion may invade adjacent tissues, such as aortic and mitral valves, and may break off and embolize elsewhere, especially in the spleen, kidney, and central nervous system.

Diagnostic Evaluation

The diagnosis of IE is suspected on the basis of clinical manifestations (Box 48-8). Several laboratory findings may suggest IE (e.g., ECG changes [prolonged PR interval], radiographic evidence of cardiomegaly, anemia, elevated erythrocyte sedimentation rate, leukocytosis, microscopic hematuria). Vegetations on the valve and abnormal valve function can often be visualized by echocardiography. Definitive diagnosis rests on growth and identification of the causative agent in the blood.

Therapeutic Management

Treatment should be instituted immediately and consists of administration of high doses of appropriate antibiotics intravenously for 2 to 8 weeks. Blood cultures are taken periodically to evaluate response to antibiotic therapy.

Prevention involves administration of prophylactic antibiotic therapy 1 hour before procedures known to increase the risk of entry of organisms in very high risk patients. New guidelines only require prophylaxis in patients with the highest risk of poor outcome if they develop endocarditis (Allen & CPS, Infectious Diseases and Immunization Committee, 2010) (Box 48-9). Medications of choice for prophylaxis include amoxicillin, ampicillin, clindamycin, cephalexin, cefadroxil, azithromycin, and clarithromycin.

Nursing Care Management

Ideally, the objective of nursing care is to counsel parents of high-risk children concerning the signs and symptoms of endocarditis and, in certain cases, the need for prophylactic antibiotic therapy before procedures such as dental work. The family's regular dentist should be advised of the child's cardiac diagnosis as an added precaution to ensure preventive treatment. IE prophylaxis is now reserved for very high–risk patients. Many patients who met criteria established in the past may not require prophylaxis under the new guidelines (Wilson et al., 2007) (see Box 48-9). It is important that all children with congenital or acquired heart disease maintain the highest level of oral health to reduce the chance of bacteremia from oral infections.

Parents should also have a high index of suspicion regarding potential infections. Without unduly alarming them, the nurse can stress that any unexplained fever, weight loss, or change in behaviour (lethargy, malaise, anorexia) must be brought to the practitioner's attention. Such symptoms should not be self-diagnosed as a cold or flu. Early diagnosis and treatment are important in preventing further cardiac damage, embolic complications, and growth of resistant organisms.

Treatment of endocarditis requires long-term parenteral medication therapy. In many cases, IV antibiotics may be

BOX 48-8 Clinical Manifestations of Infective Endocarditis

Onset usually insidious
Unexplained fever (low grade and intermittent)
Anorexia
Malaise
Weight loss
Characteristic findings caused by extracardiac emboli formation:
- Splinter hemorrhages (thin black lines) under the nails
- Osler nodes (red, painful intradermal nodes found on pads of phalanges)
- Janeway lesions (painless hemorrhagic areas on palms and soles)
- Petechiae on oral mucous membranes

May be present:
- Heart failure
- Cardiac dysrhythmias
- New murmur or change in previously existing one

BOX 48-9 Patients at High Risk for Endocarditis

Prophylaxis with dental procedures recommended for*
- Previous episode of infective endocarditis
- Prosthetic cardiac valve

Congenital heart disease (CHD), including only
- Unrepaired cyanotic CHD, including palliative shunts and conduits
- Completely repaired congenital heart defect with prosthetic material or device, whether placed by surgery or catheter intervention, during the first 6 months after the procedure

Repaired CHD with residual defects at the site of or adjacent to the site of a prosthetic patch or prosthetic device (which inhibit endothelialization)
Cardiac transplantation recipients who develop cardiac valvulopathy

(Adapted from Wilson, W., et al. [2007]. Prevention of infective endocarditis: Guidelines from the American Heart Association. *Circulation, 116*[15], 1736–1754.)

*Except for the conditions listed, antibiotic prophylaxis is no longer recommended for any other form of CHD.

administered at home with nursing supervision for part of the treatment course. Nursing goals during this period are (1) preparation of the child for IV infusion, usually with an intermittent-infusion device, and several venipunctures for blood cultures; (2) observation for adverse effects of antibiotics, especially inflammation along venipuncture sites; (3) observation for complications, including embolism and HF; and (4) education regarding the importance of follow-up visits for cardiac evaluation, echocardiographic monitoring, and blood cultures.

Rheumatic Fever

Rheumatic fever (RF) is a poorly understood inflammatory disease that occurs after infection with group A β-hemolytic streptococcal (GABHS) pharyngitis. It occurs most often in late school-age children or adolescents and is rare in adults. It is a self-limited illness that involves the joints, skin, brain, serous surfaces, and heart. Cardiac valve damage (referred to as *rheumatic heart disease*) is the most significant complication of RF. The mitral valve is most often affected. In developed countries, RF and rheumatic heart disease have become uncommon. However, RF remains a devastating problem in developing countries and has appeared in Canada but is very rare, with an estimated pediatric incidence of 2.9 per million population per year. Carditis was the most common major manifestation in 59% of cases (CPS, 2007).

Etiology

Strong evidence supports a relationship between upper respiratory tract infection with GABHS and subsequent development of RF (usually within 2 to 6 weeks). Acute RF is the result of an exaggerated immune response to bacteria in a susceptible host (Carapetis, McDonald, & Wilson, 2005). In almost all cases of RF a previous infection with GABHS can be documented by laboratory evidence of rising antibody titres. Prevention or treatment of GABHS infection prevents RF.

Diagnostic Evaluation

Diagnosis is based on a set of guidelines recommended by the Canadian Paediatric Society (Templeton & CPS, 2007). These guidelines, known as *modifications of the Jones criteria*, suggest that the presence of two major manifestations or one major and two minor manifestations, such as fever and arthralgia, with supportive evidence of recent streptococcal infection, indicates a high probability of RF (see Guidelines box).

Children suspected of having RF are tested for streptococcal antibodies. The most reliable and best standardized test is an elevated or rising antistreptolysin O (ASO or ASLO) titre, which occurs in 80% of children with RF.

Therapeutic Management

The goals of medical management are (1) eradication of hemolytic streptococci, (2) prevention of permanent cardiac damage, (3) palliation of the other symptoms, and (4) prevention of recurrences of RF. Penicillin is the medication of choice, either orally or intramuscularly with erythromycin as a substitute in penicillin-sensitive children. Salicylates, naproxen, or prednise are used to control the inflammatory process, especially in the joints, and reduce the fever and discomfort (CPS, 2007). Bed rest is recommended during the acute phase but need not be strict.

The duration of long-term prophylaxis is uncertain, but 5 years since the last episode or age 18, longer with cardiac involvement, is suggested (Gerber et al., 2009).

Children who have had acute RF are susceptible to recurrent RF for the rest of their lives and should be followed medically for at least 5 years. Repeated infections are likely to result in rheumatic heart disease. Children and families must be aware of the need for continuing antibiotic prophylaxis for dental work, infection, and invasive procedures.

GUIDELINES Diagnosis of Initial Attack of Rheumatic Fever (Jones Criteria, 1992 Update)*

Major Manifestations

Carditis
Polyarthritis
Erythema marginatum
Chorea (St. Vitus dance, Sydenham chorea)
Subcutaneous nodes

Minor Manifestations

Clinical Findings

Arthralgia
Fever

Laboratory Findings

Elevated acute-phase reactants
- Erythrocyte sedimentation rate
- C-reactive protein

Supporting Evidence of Antecedent Group A Streptococcal Infection

Positive throat culture or rapid streptococcal antigen test
Elevated or rising streptococcal antibody titre

(From Dajani, A. J., et al. [1992]. Guidelines for the diagnosis of rheumatic fever: Jones criteria, 1992 [update]. *Journal of the American Medical Association, 268,* 2069–2073.)

*If supported by evidence of preceding group A streptococcal infection, the presence of two major manifestations or of one major and two minor manifestations indicates a high probability of acute rheumatic fever.

Nursing Care Management

The objectives of nursing care for the child with RF are to (1) encourage compliance with medication regimens, (2) facilitate recovery from the illness, (3) provide emotional support, and (4) prevent the disease. Because compliance is a major concern in long-term medication therapy, every effort is made to encourage adherence to the therapeutic plan (see Compliance With Treatment, Chapter 45). When treatment compliance is poor, monthly injections may be substituted for daily oral administration of antibiotics, and children need preparation for this often-dreaded procedure.

Interventions during home care are primarily concerned with providing rest and adequate nutrition. Usually, after the febrile stage is over, children can resume moderate activity, and their appetite improves. If carditis is present, the family must be aware of any activity restrictions and may need help in choosing less strenuous activities for the child.

One of the most disturbing and frustrating manifestations of the disease is chorea. The onset is gradual and may occur weeks to months after the illness; it sometimes even occurs in children who have not been diagnosed with RF. It may be mistaken for nervousness, clumsiness, behavioural changes, inattentiveness, and learning disability. It is usually a source of great frustration to the child because the movements, incoordination, and weakness severely limit physical ability. Of utmost importance is stressing to parents and schoolteachers that the sudden movements are involuntary; that the chorea is transitory; and that all manifestations eventually disappear.

Nurses also have a role in prevention, primarily in screening school-age children for sore throats caused by GABHS. This may involve actively participating in throat culture screening programs or referring children with a possible streptococcal infection for testing.

Hyperlipidemia (Hypercholesterolemia)

Hyperlipidemia is a general term for excessive lipids (fat and fatlike substances); *hypercholesterolemia* refers to excessive cholesterol in the blood. High lipid or cholesterol levels play an important role in producing atherosclerosis (fatty plaque on the arteries), which eventually can lead to coronary artery disease, a primary cause of morbidity and mortality in the adult population. A presymptomatic phase of atherosclerosis can begin in childhood. Preventive cardiology is focusing on the screening and management of lipid levels in childhood. The goal is to identify children at high risk and to intervene early.

Cholesterol is part of the lipoprotein complex in plasma that is essential for cellular metabolism. Triglycerides, natural fats synthesized from carbohydrates, are used for energy. Both are major lipids transported on *lipoproteins*, a combination of lipids and proteins, which include the following:

Low-density lipoproteins (LDLs)—These contain low concentrations of triglycerides, high levels of cholesterol, and moderate levels of protein. LDL is the major carrier of cholesterol to the cells. Cells use cholesterol for synthesis of membranes and steroid production. Elevated circulating LDL is a strong risk factor in cardiovascular disease.

High-density lipoproteins (HDLs)—These contain very low concentrations of triglycerides, relatively little cholesterol, and high levels of protein. They transport free cholesterol to the liver for excretion in the bile. High levels of HDL are thought to protect against cardiovascular disease.

Diagnostic Evaluation

Hyperlipidemia is diagnosed on the basis of analysis of blood for a full lipid profile, drawn after a 12-hour fast. A screening thyroid-stimulating hormone (TSH) is useful to rule out hypothyroidism as a cause of secondary hypercholesterolemia. In overweight children, a fasting glucose may be obtained to assess for the potential of metabolic syndrome, which is a combination of multiple symptoms that are associated with increased cardiovascular risk in adults. Blood samples should be collected after having the child sit for 5 minutes, and the tourniquet should be applied immediately before the needle puncture, since posture and vascular stasis may affect results. Diagnostic values for acceptable, borderline, and high total cholesterol and LDL cholesterol levels are listed in Table 48-5.

Screening children for hypercholesterolemia is a controversial issue; some authorities advocate universal screening, and others propose selective screening. Guidelines from the American Academy of Pediatrics' Committee on Nutrition (Daniels, Greer, & Committee on Nutrition, 2008) recommend a strategy that combines two complementary approaches: (1) a *population approach* that aims to lower the average levels of blood cholesterol among all children through population-wide changes in nutrient intake and eating patterns, and (2) an *individualized approach* based on selective screening.

Therapeutic Management

The first step in the treatment of high cholesterol is oriented to lifestyle modification. The Heart and Stroke Foundation (2012b) guidelines advocate a heart-healthy diet for all children. Children with known elevated cholesterol should have individual nutritional counselling by a nutritionist with expertise in pediatric lipids.

Research continues to support the benefit of diets low in saturated fats and trans fats and higher in monounsaturated fats (found in olive and canola oil). Current thinking favours a "Mediterranean"-type diet; whole grains, fruits, and vegetables form the foundation of this diet. In addition, this diet allows the use of monounsaturated fats, such as olive oil and canola oil, which have beneficial effects on HDL cholesterol values. The use of these fats also makes the diet more realistic. Daily aerobic exercise of at least 60 minutes a day is also recommended for children with high cholesterol. In addition, patients and parents should be counselled regarding the negative effects of smoking (both first-hand and second-hand).

For children with severe hypercholesterolemia who fail to respond to dietary modifications (after a 6- to 12-month trial) medication therapy may be necessary. Pharmacological therapy is recommended for children with LDL cholesterol over 4.9 mmol/L with a positive history of early heart disease; over 4.1 L mmol/L in patients with a positive family history and two risk factors; and over 3.4 mmol/L in patients with diabetes. In most situations, medication is reserved for those over 8 years of age (Daniels, Greer, & Committee on Nutrition, 2008).

Bile acid–binding resins act by binding bile acids in the intestinal lumen. Because they are not absorbed by the

Table 48-5 Classification of Cholesterol Levels in Children From Families With a History of Heart Disease

CATEGORY	TOTAL CHOLESTEROL MMOL/L (G/DL)	LDL CHOLESTEROL MMOL/L (G/DL)
Acceptable	<4.39 (170)	<2.8 (110)
Borderline	4.40–5.16 (170–199)	2.8–3.4 (110–129)
High	≥5.17 (200)	≥3.4 (130)

(From the National Cholesterol Education Program. [1992]. Report of the Expert Panel on Blood Cholesterol Levels in Children and Adolescents. *Pediatrics, 89*[3 Pt 2], 527.)
LDL, low-density lipoprotein.

intestine, they do not produce systemic toxicity and are safe for children. Cholestyramine and colestipol are both powders that are mixed with water or juice just before ingestion. Unfortunately, bile acid–binding resins do not adequately reduce LDL cholesterol in the vast majority of patients. Many cannot tolerate the medication because of the taste, gritty texture, and adverse effects, the most significant being constipation, abdominal pain, gastrointestinal bloating, flatulence, and nausea. The most recent findings on lipid abnormalities in children recommend treatment with statins if pharmacological therapy is indicated, using the previously outlined guidelines for treatment (McCrindle et al., 2007). Statins are much more effective at lowering LDL cholesterol and triglycerides and raising HDL cholesterol. They work by inhibiting the enzyme necessary for cholesterol synthesis, are most effective when taken in the evening, and are started at the lowest possible dose in young people. Blood work should be followed closely and should include a fasting lipid profile, liver function tests, and creatinine kinase repeated at 4- and 8-week intervals initially and with dosage changes.

Patients beginning therapy with a statin should be counselled regarding rare but potentially serious adverse effects such as rhabdomyolysis, elevated transaminases, and elevated creatinine kinase. They should discontinue their medication and contact their practitioner if they develop dark urine or new muscle aches. Finally, statin medications are not safe during pregnancy; sexually active adolescents need to take adequate birth control measures. Very long–term studies are unlikely to be available over decades; however, in the shorter-term studies that have been completed, statins seem to have a safety profile for children similar to the one for adults (McCrindle et al., 2007).

A relatively new drug, ezetimibe, works by inhibiting cholesterol absorption. It lowers LDL by preventing intestinal uptake of dietary and biliary cholesterol. Recommended use is in combination therapy with a statin, further lowering LDL values. This medication is currently approved for children older than 10 years of age with extremely severe hyperlipidemia. Several large clinical trials are currently in process regarding this medication to determine the effectiveness (Leiter et al., 2010).

Nursing Care Management

Nurses play an important role in the screening, education, and support of children with hyperlipidemia and their families. When a child is referred to a lipid clinic, it is essential that the family be adequately prepared for the first visit. Generally, the parents are asked to keep a dietary history of the child before this visit. Sometimes they need to complete a questionnaire regarding the child's normal dietary habits during the preceding year. Families should be instructed to keep their child fasting for at least 12 hours before screening. It is important to schedule the blood test early in the morning and arrange for nourishment immediately thereafter. At the visit a full family history should be taken, including the health of both parents and all first-degree relatives. Specific questions should be asked regarding early heart disease, hypertension, strokes (CVAs), sudden death, hyperlipidemia, diabetes, and endocrine abnormalities.

Stringent dietary guidelines may become an issue of control and a source of great stress for many families. Children should not be viewed as having a disease. Rather, the positive aspects of healthy eating, exercising regularly, and avoiding smoking should be emphasized. Basic dietary changes should be encouraged for the whole family so that the affected child is not singled out. Cultural differences must be considered, and recommendations individualized. Substitution rather than elimination needs to be emphasized. Visual aids (e.g., test tubes depicting the amount of fat in a hot dog) are often helpful, especially for children. Diets should be flexible and individually tailored by a nutritionist experienced in combining recommendations that meet both the nutritional demands of the growing child and the lipid modifications. Parents should be encouraged to participate in dietary and educational sessions, ask questions, and share ideas and experiences.

Parents of children who require pharmacological therapy need to understand the purpose, dosage, and possible adverse effects of the various medications. Medication schedules should remain flexible and should not interfere with the child's daily activities. Follow-up phone calls by the nurse between visits allow parents to discuss their concerns and ask any questions that have arisen.

Cardiac Dysrhythmias

Dysrhythmias, or abnormal heart rhythms, can occur in children with structurally normal hearts, as features of some congenital heart defects, and in patients after surgical repair of congenital heart defects. They are also seen in patients with cardiomyopathy and cardiac tumours and can occur secondary to metabolic and electrolyte imbalances. They can be classified in several ways, including by heart rate characteristics (bradycardia and tachycardia) and by the origin of the dysrhythmia in the atria or ventricles. Some dysrhythmias are well tolerated and self-limited. Others may cause decreased cardiac output with associated symptoms, and some can cause sudden death. Treatment depends on the cause of the dysrhythmia and its severity.

In the past decade, many advances have been made in the diagnosis and treatment of pediatric dysrhythmias. Improvements in technology have allowed better diagnosis, the development of ablation techniques, and the expansion of pacemaker capabilities. New antidysrhythmic medications have proved safe and effective in children. Radiofrequency ablation has offered a cure for some dysrhythmias. Pediatric electrophysiology has become a highly specialized field; the reader should consult more detailed sources for an in-depth discussion. The following sections address diagnostic studies and provide a general discussion of the most common tachycardia (supraventricular tachycardia [SVT]) and the most common bradycardia (complete heart block) that require treatment in the pediatric population.

Diagnostic Evaluation

Nurses must be familiar with the standards of normal heart rate for the particular age group. An initial nursing responsibility is recognition of a heartbeat that is abnormal in either rate or rhythm. When a dysrhythmia is suspected, the apical rate is counted for a full minute and compared with the radial rate, which may be lower because not all of the apical beats are felt. Consistently high or low heart rates should be regarded as suspicious. The patient should be placed on a cardiac monitor with recording capabilities. A 12-lead ECG yields more information than the monitor recording and should be done as soon as possible.

The basic diagnostic procedure is the ECG, including 24-hour Holter monitoring. Electrophysiological cardiac catheterization allows for identification of the conduction disturbance and immediate investigation of medications that may control the dysrhythmia. Another procedure that may be used is transesophageal recording. An electrode catheter is passed to the lower esophagus and, when in position at a point proximal to the heart, is used to stimulate and record dysrhythmias.

Dysrhythmias can be classified according to various criteria, such as effect on heart rate and rhythm, as follows:

Bradydysrhythmias—Abnormally slow rate
Tachydysrhythmias—Abnormally rapid rate
Conduction disturbances—Irregular heart rate

Bradydysrhythmias

Sinus bradycardia (slower than normal rate) in children can be caused by the influence of the autonomic nervous system, as with hypervagal tone, or in response to hypoxia and hypotension. Sinus bradycardias are also known to develop after some complex cardiac surgical repairs involving extensive atrial suture lines such as the Fontan procedure.

Complete atrioventricular block (AV block) is also referred to as *complete heart block*. This can be either congenital (occurring in children with structurally normal hearts) or acquired after surgery to repair cardiac defects. AV blocks are most often related to edema around the conduction system and resolve without treatment. Temporary epicardial wires are placed in most patients at surgery; if a rhythm disturbance occurs, temporary pacing can be used. Several days after surgery, the health practitioner removes the wires by pulling slowly and deliberately down on them from the site of insertion.

Some children may need a permanent pacemaker. The pacemaker takes over or assists in the heart's conduction function. The implantation of a pacemaker, in the operating room or possibly the catheterization laboratory, is usually a low risk procedure. The pacemaker is made up of two basic parts: the pulse generator and the lead. The pulse generator is composed of the battery and the electronic circuitry. The lead is an insulated, flexible wire that conducts the electrical impulse from the pulse generator to the heart. Two types of leads are available: transvenous and epicardial. After the lead has been attached to the heart, a small incision is made, and a pocket is formed under the muscle to house and protect the generator. Continuous ECG monitoring is necessary during the recovery phase to assess pacemaker function. The nurse should be aware of the programmed rate and expected individual generator variations. The pacemaker insertion site should be monitored for signs of infection. Analgesics can be given for pain.

Pacemaker functions have become more sophisticated, and some models can adjust heart rate to activity demands or be programmed for overdrive pacing or cardioversion (see Patient Teaching box).

Tachydysrhythmias

Sinus tachycardia (abnormally fast heart rate) secondary to fever, anxiety, pain, anemia, dehydration, or any other etiological factor requiring increased cardiac output should be ruled out before diagnosing an increased heart rate as pathological. SVT is the most common tachydysrhythmia found in children and refers to a rapid regular heart rate of 200 to 300 beats/min. The onset of SVT is often sudden, the duration is variable, and the rhythm may end abruptly and convert back to a normal sinus rhythm. Clinical signs in infants and young children are poor feeding, extreme irritability, and pallor. Children may experience palpitations, dizziness, chest pain, and diaphoresis. If SVT is sustained, signs of HF may be seen.

The treatment of SVT depends on the degree of compromise imposed by the dysrhythmia. In some cases vagal manoeuvres, such as applying ice to the face, massaging the carotid artery (on one side of the neck only), or having an older child perform a Valsalva manoeuvre (e.g., exhaling against a closed glottis, blowing on a thumb as if it were a trumpet for 30 to 60 seconds), have terminated SVT. If vagal manoeuvres fail or the child is hemodynamically unstable, adenosine (a drug that impairs AV conduction) may be used. Adenosine is given by rapid IV push with a saline bolus immediately after the drug because of its very short half-life. If this is unsuccessful or cardiac output is compromised, esophageal overdrive pacing or synchronized cardioversion (delivering an electrical shock to the heart) can be used in the intensive care setting. Sedation is needed for both procedures. Cardioversion should never be done in a conscious patient. More long-term pharmacological treatment includes digoxin or possibly propranolol (Inderal) or amiodarone for severe or recurrent SVT.

A primary focus of nursing care is education of the family regarding the symptoms of SVT and its treatment. SVT may occur again despite therapy. Parents should be taught to take

> **PATIENT TEACHING** Discharge Teaching for the Child With a Pacemaker
>
> Discharge teaching includes information about the signs and symptoms of infection, general wound care, and activity restrictions. Parents and patients, if they are old enough, should be taught to take a pulse and know the settings of the pacemaker. If the patient's low rate is set at 80 beats/min and the heart rate is only 68 beats/min, there is a possible problem with the pacemaker that needs to be investigated. Instructions for telephone transmission of electrogram (ECG) readings are also given. Telephone transmission can be used to transmit ECG strips and also to monitor battery life and pacemaker function. The pacemaker generator will have to be replaced periodically because of battery depletion. Children with pacemakers should wear a medical alert device, and their parents should have a paper identification card with specific pacer data in case of an emergency. Cardiopulmonary resuscitation instruction is suggested for parents.

a radial pulse for a full minute. If medication is prescribed, instructions regarding accurate dosage and the importance of administering the correct dose at specified intervals should be stressed.

Radiofrequency ablation has become first-line therapy for some types of SVT. The procedure is done in the cardiac catheterization laboratory and begins with mapping of the conduction system to identify the dysrhythmia focus. A catheter delivering radiofrequency current is directed at the site, and the area is heated to destroy the tissue in the area. These are lengthy procedures, often 6 to 8 hours, and sedation or general anaesthesia is required. Preparation is similar to that for cardiac catheterization.

A newer procedure, cryoablation, is also used in treatment of SVT. Liquid nitrous oxide is used to cool a catheter to subfreezing temperatures, which then destroys the target tissue by freezing. This procedure is performed in the cardiac electrophysiology catheterization laboratory. This method allows reversible cooling so that the electrophysiologist can test an area first before freezing it to a point where a permanent lesion is formed (Chun & Van Hare, 2004; Hockenberry & Wilson, 2011).

Pulmonary Hypertension

Pulmonary artery hypertension (PAH) describes a group of rare disorders that result in an elevation of pulmonary artery pressure above 25 mm Hg at rest after the neonatal period (Barst, 1999). These disorders are poorly understood, and until recently there was no treatment beyond supportive care. PAH is a progressive, eventually fatal disease for which there is no known cure. It can be difficult to diagnose in the early stages. Often when patients become symptomatic and a diagnosis is made, their disease is rapidly progressing, treatment is unsuccessful, and death occurs within several years. Significant new information about the disease process, genetic links, diagnosis, and treatment has recently been learned that may improve treatments and outcomes for these patients.

PAH affects the small pulmonary arteries and is characterized by vascular narrowing leading to an increase in pulmonary vascular resistance. Why some children develop the disease and others do not is unclear. There are many possible causes of PAH. Cardiac causes occur primarily in patients with a large left-to-right shunt producing increased pulmonary blood flow. If these defects are not repaired early, the high pulmonary flow will cause changes in the pulmonary artery vessels, and the vessels will lose their elasticity. Other causes of PAH include hypoxic lung diseases, thromboembolic diseases causing pulmonary vascular obstruction, collagen vascular diseases, and exposure to toxic substances. Many of the patients have no identifiable cause for PAH and have primary or idiopathic PAH.

Clinical Manifestations

The clinical manifestations include dyspnea with exercise, chest pain, and syncope. Dyspnea is the most common symptom and is caused by impaired oxygen delivery. Chest pain is the result of coronary ischemia in the right ventricle from severe hypertrophy. Syncope reflects a limited cardiac output leading to decreased cerebral blood flow. Right-sided heart dysfunction is steadily progressive; when symptoms of venous congestion and edema are present, prognosis is poor.

Therapeutic Management

Although no cure is known, several therapies have shown promise in slowing the progression of the disease and improving quality of life. In general, situations that may exacerbate the disease and cause hypoxia, such as exercise and high altitudes, are avoided. Supplemental oxygen, especially at night while sleeping, is commonly used to relieve hypoxia. Patients are at risk for thromboembolic events leading to pulmonary **emboli;** thus anticoagulation with warfarin (Coumadin) is often prescribed.

Vasodilator therapy (which relaxes vascular smooth muscle and reduces pulmonary artery pressure) has prolonged the survival of patients with PAH. Oral calcium channel blockers have been successful in some children. Continuous IV prostacyclin has been used with some success in children who did not respond to oral therapy. Although promising, both these therapies have been used in only small numbers of patients and are expensive. Lung transplantation may be another treatment option.

Cardiomyopathy

Cardiomyopathy refers to abnormalities of the myocardium in which the cardiac muscles' ability to contract is impaired. Cardiomyopathies are relatively rare in children. Possible etiological factors include familial or genetic causes, infection, deficiency states, metabolic abnormalities, and collagen vascular diseases. Most cardiomyopathies in children are considered primary or idiopathic, in which the cause is unknown and the cardiac dysfunction is not associated with systemic disease. Some of the known causes of *secondary* cardiomyopathy are anthracycline toxicity (the antineoplastic agents doxorubicin [Adriamycin] and daunomycin), hemochromatosis (from excessive iron storage), Duchenne muscular dystrophy, Kawasaki disease (KD), collagen diseases, and thyroid dysfunction.

Cardiomyopathies can be divided into three broad clinical categories according to the type of abnormal structure and dysfunction present: dilated cardiomyopathy, hypertrophic cardiomyopathy, and restrictive cardiomyopathy.

Dilated cardiomyopathy is characterized by ventricular dilation and greatly decreased contractility resulting in symptoms of HF. This is the most common type of cardiomyopathy in children. Its cause is often unknown. The clinical findings are of HF with tachycardia, dyspnea, hepatosplenomegaly, fatigue, and poor growth. Dysrhythmias may be present and may be more difficult to control with worsening heart failure.

Hypertrophic cardiomyopathy is characterized by an increase in heart muscle mass without an increase in cavity size, usually occurring in the left ventricle and associated with abnormal diastolic filling. It is a familial autosomal dominant genetic abnormality in most cases and is probably the most common genetically transmitted cardiovascular disease. The expression of clinical disease varies greatly among patients. Clinical symptoms usually appear in the school-age period or adolescence and may include anginal chest pain, dysrhythmias, and syncope. Sudden death is possible. Unexplained syncope in children under 18 years of age with known hypertrophic cardiomyopathy had a 60% cumulative risk of sudden death within 5 years of the syncopal event (Spirito et al., 2009). Presentation in infancy includes signs of HF and has a poor prognosis. The ECG demonstrates left ventricular hypertrophy, often with ST-T changes. The echocardiogram is most helpful and demonstrates asymmetrical septal hypertrophy and an increase in left ventricular wall thickness with a small left ventricle cavity.

Restrictive cardiomyopathy, rare in children, describes a restriction to ventricular filling caused by endocardial or myocardial disease or both. It is characterized by diastolic dysfunction and absence of ventricular dilation or hypertrophy. Symptoms are similar to those of HF (see Box 48-5).

Therapeutic Management

Treatment is directed toward correcting the underlying cause whenever feasible. However, in most affected children this is not possible, and treatment is aimed at managing HF and dysrhythmias. Digoxin, diuretics, and aggressive use of afterload reduction agents have been found to be helpful in managing symptoms in those with dilated cardiomyopathy. Practice guidelines for the management of heart failure in children have been outlined and provide an in-depth review of available therapies (Rosenthal et al., 2004). Digoxin and inotropic agents are usually not helpful in the other forms of cardiomyopathy because increasing the force of contraction may exacerbate the muscular obstruction and actually impair ventricular ejection. β-Blockers such as propranolol or calcium channel blockers such as verapamil (Calan) have been used to reduce left ventricular outflow obstruction and improve diastolic filling in those with hypertrophic cardiomyopathy.

Careful monitoring and treatment of dysrhythmias are essential. The placement of an implantable defibrillator (AICD) should be considered for patients at high risk of sudden death from ventricular dysrhythmias. Anticoagulants may be given to reduce the risk of thromboemboli, a complication of the sluggish circulation through the heart. For worsening heart failure and signs of poor perfusion, IV inotropic or vasodilating medications may be needed. Severely ill children may require mechanical ventilation, oxygen administration, and IV medications. Heart transplantation may be a treatment option for patients who have worsening symptoms despite maximum medical therapy.

Nursing Care Management

Because of the poor prognosis in many children with cardiomyopathy, nursing care is consistent with that for any child with a life-threatening disorder (see Chapter 41). One of the most difficult adjustments for the child (especially the normally active youngster with hypertrophic cardiomyopathy) may be the realization of failing health and the need for restricted activity. The child should be included in decisions regarding activity and allowed to discuss his or her feelings, particularly if the disease follows a progressively fatal course. After symptoms of HF or dysrhythmias develop, the same nursing interventions are implemented. If heart transplantation is considered, the needs of the child and family are great in terms of psychological preparation and postoperative care. The nurse plays an important role in assessing the family's understanding of the procedure and long-term consequences. Children of school age and older should be fully informed to give their assent to the procedure (see Informed Consent, Chapter 45).

Heart Transplantation

Heart transplantation has become a treatment option for infants and children with worsening heart failure and a limited life expectancy despite maximum medical and surgical management. Indications for heart transplantation in children are cardiomyopathy and end-stage CHD. It is also an option for patients with some forms of complex congenital cardiac defects, such as hypoplastic left heart syndrome, for whom conventional surgical approaches have a high mortality rate.

Before transplantation, potential recipients undergo a careful cardiac evaluation to determine whether any other medical or surgical options are available to improve the patient's cardiac status. Other organ systems are assessed to identify problems that might increase the risk of or preclude transplantation. A psychosocial evaluation of the patient and family is done to assess family function, support systems, and ability to comply with the complex medical regimen after the transplant. Support services to help the family successfully care for their child are provided when possible.

The number of heart transplants in pediatric patients has been constant for the past decade, at about 400 transplants per year internationally (Boucek et al., 2007). This likely reflects a limit in the number of available donors. Infants are the largest group of pediatric transplant recipients and account for about a fourth of all procedures. The International Society for Heart and Lung Transplantation registry data for all pediatric heart transplant recipients from 1982 to 2005 demonstrated a 1-year actuarial survival rate of 85%. Early rejection within the first year post-transplant is associated with increased late mortality. There is an ongoing risk of death with time from transplant. Infants are associated with higher early mortality and adolescents with higher late mortality. Overall survival was approximately 40% for patients up to 20 years after transplantation (Boucek et al., 2007). Surviving pediatric patients have excellent functional recovery, with less than 10% reporting activity limitations (Boucek et al., 2007).

The post-transplant course is complex. Although heart function is greatly improved or normal after transplantation, the risk of rejection is serious. The leading cause of death in the first 3 years after heart transplantation is rejection, with the greatest risk in the first 6 months (Blume, 2003). Rejection of the heart is diagnosed primarily by endomyocardial biopsy in older children. Serial echocardiograms are often used in infants and young children to reduce the need for invasive biopsies. Immunosuppressants must be taken for life and have many systemic adverse effects. Triple medication therapy for immunosuppression with a calcineurin inhibitor (cyclosporine or tacrolimus), steroids, and azathioprine is most commonly used in pediatric patients, although mycophenolate mofetil is being used more frequently and replacing azathioprine. Steroids are weaned in the first year and may be discontinued in some patients.

Infection is always a risk. Potential long-term problems that may limit survival include chronic rejection, causing coronary artery disease; renal dysfunction and hypertension resulting from cyclosporine administration; lymphoma; and infection. Coronary artery disease is the leading cause of death among late survivors of heart transplantation (Boucek et al., 2007).

Nursing Care Management

Successfully caring for a child after a heart transplant requires the expertise and dedication of many members of the health care team. Nurses play vital roles in assessment, coordination of care, psychosocial support, and patient and family education. The heart transplant recipient must be carefully monitored for signs of rejection, infection, and the adverse effects of the immunosuppressant medications. The patient's and family's psychosocial well-being also needs to be assessed to identify issues such as increased family stress, depression, substance use, and school problems. Noncompliance with an intense medication regimen, especially during adolescence, can lead to serious medical problems and can be fatal. Care of the immunosuppressed child is reviewed in Chapter 49. Psychosocial concerns and appropriate interventions for the child with a life-threatening disorder are presented in Chapter 44.

The first 6 months to 1 year after the transplant are most intense because the risk of complications is greatest and the patient and family are adjusting to a new lifestyle. Patients need to be monitored closely by the health care team, with frequent visits and laboratory tests. Care is usually shared between local health care providers and the transplant centre. Many patients are able to return to school and other age-appropriate activities within 2 to 3 months after the transplant.

Vascular Dysfunction

Systemic Hypertension

Hypertension is defined as the consistent elevation of BP beyond values considered to be the upper limits of normal. The two major categories are *essential hypertension* (no identifiable cause) and *secondary hypertension* (subsequent to an identifiable cause). In recent years, interest in this disorder in adolescents and children has been increasing. Hypertension in children and adolescents is defined as having a systolic or diastolic BP that consistently falls at or over the ninety-fifth percentile. This group is further delineated as follows:

- Stage 1 hypertension includes patients with BP readings between the ninety-fifth and ninety-ninth percentiles.
- Stage 2 hypertension describes patients with BP readings over the ninety-ninth percentile plus 5 mm Hg.

An additional group includes children and adolescents who have prehypertension (or high-normal BP). This prehypertensive group includes those with BP readings that fall consistently between the ninetieth and ninety-fifth percentiles. *The Fourth Report on the Diagnosis, Evaluation, and Treatment of High Blood Pressure in Children and Adolescents* outlines in detail the identification, testing, and treatment recommendations for young people with high BP (National High Blood Pressure Education Program Working Group on High Blood Pressure in Children and Adolescents, 2004).

Etiology

Most instances of hypertension observed in young children occur secondary to a structural abnormality or an underlying pathological process, although this is being challenged by screening programs of relatively healthy children. The most common cause of secondary hypertension is renal disease, followed by cardiovascular, endocrine, and some neurological disorders. As a rule, the younger the child and the more severe the hypertension, the more likely it is to be secondary.

The causes of essential hypertension are undetermined, but evidence indicates that both genetic and environmental factors play a role. The incidence of hypertension has been shown to be higher in children whose parents are hypertensive. Environmental factors that contribute to the risk of developing hypertension include obesity, salt ingestion, smoking, and stress.

Diagnostic Evaluation

From the increasing numbers of hypertensive or potentially hypertensive children and adolescents being identified, a BP determination should be a routine part of annual assessment in healthy children over 3 years old. BP readings should be done in children less than 3 years old who have high risk family histories or those with individual risk factors, including CHD, kidney disease, malignancy, transplant, certain neurological problems, or systemic illnesses known to cause hypertension. Although clinical manifestations associated with hypertension depend largely on the underlying cause, some observations can provide clues to the examiner that an elevated BP may be a factor (Box 48-10). In infants and very young children who cannot communicate symptoms, observation of behaviour provides clues, although gross behavioural changes may not be apparent until complications are present.

No definitive cutoff values are used in the diagnosis of hypertension in the pediatric patient. *The Fourth Report on the Diagnosis, Evaluation, and Treatment of High Blood Pressure in Children and Adolescents* (National High Blood Pressure Education Program Working Group on High Blood Pressure in Children and Adolescents, 2004) provides normative data for children (see Appendix E). BP tables now include

BOX 48-10 Clinical Manifestations of Hypertension

Adolescents and Older Children
Frequent headaches
Dizziness
Changes in vision

Infants or Young Children
Irritability
Head banging or head rubbing
Waking up screaming in the night

the fiftieth, ninetieth, ninety-fifth, and ninety-ninth percentiles for BP readings based on age, gender, and height percentiles. These guidelines are based on auscultatory readings; this is currently the preferred method of assessment. These charts take into account differences in body height. Thus it is important to note that a child who is large for his or her age may normally have a higher BP than a child of average size. Before a diagnosis is made, BP should be measured on at least three separate occasions.

A careful medical and family history should be obtained to screen for other relatives with hypertension or other cardiovascular risk factors. In children with suspected hypertension, initial laboratory data include a urinalysis, renal function studies such as creatinine and blood urea nitrogen, a lipid profile, complete blood count, and electrolytes. Depending on the severity of hypertension, additional testing may be indicated. Testing may include a renal ultrasound to measure kidney size and Doppler flow to detect the possibility of a renal cause, a cardiac echocardiogram to evaluate the presence of end-organ involvement such as left ventricular hypertrophy, and a retinal examination.

Therapeutic Management

Therapy for secondary hypertension involves diagnosis and treatment of the underlying cause. In cases amenable to surgical repair, the nature of the condition, the type of surgery, and the child's age are all important considerations. Children or adolescents with consistently elevated BP readings from no known cause or those with secondary hypertension not amenable to surgical correction may be treated with a combination of nonpharmacological and pharmacological interventions. Dietary practices and lifestyle changes are important in the control of hypertension both for children and for adults. Nonpharmacological measures, such as weight control in overweight patients, increased exercise, limited salt intake, and avoidance of stress and smoking, carry no risk and should be instituted first, except in severe cases. Because the long-term effects of antihypertensive agents on children are not known, medication treatment of asymptomatic children with mild or borderline hypertension is not recommended.

Medication therapy needs to be instituted with caution in children with significant elevations of BP resistant to nonpharmacological intervention. The treatment should begin with one medication; other medications should be added only if control is not obtained. The oral antihypertensive medications used in children include β-blockers, ACE inhibitors, calcium channel blockers, angiotensin-receptor blockers, and diuretics. The goal is to achieve a normotensive state throughout the day without accompanying medication adverse effects.

Nursing Care Management

BP measurement should always be a part of the routine assessment of children over 3 years old and patients under 3 years old who are considered to be at high risk for hypertension. To obtain an accurate reading, it is important to quiet the child or relax the adolescent while the measurement is recorded, to avoid false readings caused by excitement. The chief cause of falsely elevated BP readings is the use of improperly fitting, narrow cuffs. Thus attention to correct measurement technique is essential (see Blood Pressure, Chapter 34).

Nursing counselling and guidance of affected children are challenges. Education aimed at understanding hypertension and its implication over the lifespan is essential in promoting patient and family compliance with both nonpharmacological and pharmacological therapies (see Compliance With Treatment, Chapter 45).

Home BP measurements can facilitate surveillance in youngsters with chronic hypertension and can document effectiveness of therapy. A family member can be instructed in how to take and record accurate BP measurements, thus decreasing the number of trips to a health care facility. This individual needs to understand when to contact the practitioner regarding elevated values. The community nurse can often be a valuable resource in monitoring BP. The nurse plays an important role in assessing individual families and providing targeted information about nonpharmacological modes of intervention, such as diet, weight loss, smoking cessation, and exercise programs. If extensive dietary counselling is required, the child should be referred to a nutritionist with expertise in working with children and adolescents. Exercise regimens should be individualized. Schoolchildren and young adolescents generally prefer team sports rather than individual training, which they may view as a burden rather than an enjoyable activity. If peers and family members can be encouraged to participate in any of the management strategies, the child's compliance with treatment is likely to be greater.

Young hypertensive women should avoid oral contraceptives because of their pressor effects. Other options need to be presented before this form of birth control is discontinued (see Contraception, Chapter 7).

If medication therapy is prescribed, the nurse needs to provide information to the family regarding the reasons for it, how the drug works, and possible adverse effects. General instructions for antihypertensive medications include the following:

- Rise slowly from a horizontal position and avoid sudden position changes.
- Take medication as prescribed.
- Maintain adequate hydration.
- Notify your health practitioner if adverse effects occur, but do not discontinue medication.
- Avoid alcohol and stay on the prescribed diet.

The need for follow-up should be stressed, especially because antihypertensive therapy can sometimes be safely discontinued if BP remains under control over time.

Kawasaki Disease (Mucocutaneous Lymph Node Syndrome)

KD is an acute systemic vasculitis of unknown cause. It is seen in every racial group, and about 75% of the cases occur in children younger than the age of 5 years, with peak incidence in the toddler age group. The acute disease is self-limited. However, without treatment approximately 15 to 25% of children with KD develop coronary artery aneurysms (Belay et al., 2006). Infants younger than 1 year of age are most seriously affected by KD and are at the greatest risk for heart involvement.

Although it is not spread by person-to-person contact, several factors support infectious etiological factors. It is often seen in geographic and seasonal outbreaks, with most cases reported in the late winter and early spring (Newburger et al., 2004).

Pathophysiology

The principal area of involvement is the cardiovascular system. During the initial stage of the illness, extensive inflammation of the arterioles, venules, and capillaries occurs. In addition, segmental damage to the medium-size muscular arteries, mainly the coronary arteries, can occur, causing the formation of coronary artery aneurysms in some children. When death occurs (in less than 0.05% of cases), it is usually the result of myocardial ischemia from coronary thrombosis or, over time, severe scar formation and stenosis in coronary aneurysms (Wilder et al., 2007).

Clinical Manifestations

Because no specific diagnostic test exists for KD, the diagnosis is established on the basis of clinical findings and associated laboratory results (Box 48-11). These criteria should be used as guidelines. Many children with KD do not fulfill standard diagnostic criteria and infants often have an incomplete presentation. Thus it is important to consider KD as a possible diagnosis in any infant or child with prolonged elevated temperature that is unresponsive to antibiotics and not attributable to another cause.

KD manifests in three phases: acute, subacute, and convalescent. The *acute phase* begins with the abrupt onset of high fever that is unresponsive to antibiotics and antipyretics. The child then develops the remaining diagnostic symptoms. During this stage he or she is typically *very* irritable. The *subacute phase* begins with resolution of the fever and lasts until all clinical signs of KD have disappeared. During this phase the child is at greatest risk for the development of coronary artery aneurysms. Echocardiograms are used to monitor myocardial and coronary artery status. A baseline echocardiogram should be obtained at the time of diagnosis for comparison with future studies. Irritability persists during this phase. In the *convalescent phase*, all the clinical signs of KD have resolved, but the laboratory values have not returned to normal. This phase is complete when all blood values are normal (6 to 8 weeks after onset). At the end of this stage the child has regained his or her usual temperament, energy, and appetite.

Cardiac Involvement

Long-term complications of KD include the development of coronary artery aneurysms, disrupting blood flow. In children with aneurysms, there is the potential for myocardial infarction, which can result from thrombotic occlusion of a coronary aneurysm. Over time, as the damaged vessel tries to heal, stenosis of the aneurysm may develop and may lead to myocardial ischemia. Most of the morbidity and mortality occurs in children affected with the largest aneurysms (giant aneurysms larger than 8 mm). Symptoms of acute myocardial infarction in children may include abdominal pain, vomiting, restlessness, inconsolable crying, pallor, and shock.

Therapeutic Management

The current treatment of KD includes high-dose IV gamma-globulin along with salicylate therapy. Gamma-globulin has been demonstrated to be effective at reducing the incidence of coronary artery abnormalities when given within the first 10 days of the illness. A single large infusion of 2 g/kg over 10 to 12 hours is recommended. Retreatment with IV gamma-globulin is indicated in patients who continue with fever after treatment.

Aspirin is given initially in an anti-inflammatory dose (80 to 100 mg/kg/day in divided doses every 6 hours) to control fever and symptoms of inflammation. After fever has subsided, it is continued at an antiplatelet dose (3 to 5 mg/kg/day). Low-dose aspirin is continued in patients without echocardiographic evidence of coronary abnormalities until the platelet count has returned to normal (6 to 8 weeks). If the child develops coronary abnormalities, salicylate therapy is continued indefinitely. Additional anticoagulation (e.g., clopidogrel [Plavix], enoxaparin [Lovenox], or warfarin) may be indicated in children who have medium-size or giant coronary artery aneurysms.

Prognosis

Most children with KD recover fully after treatment. However, when cardiovascular complications occur, serious morbidity may result. Death occurs rarely but almost always results from coronary thrombosis.

Nursing Care Management

In the initial phase the nurse must monitor the child's cardiac status carefully. Intake and output and daily weight measurements are recorded. Although the child may be reluctant to eat and therefore may be partially dehydrated, fluids need to be administered with care because of the usual finding of myocarditis. The child should be assessed frequently for signs

BOX 48-11 Diagnostic Criteria for Kawasaki Disease

Child must have fever for more than 5 days along with four of five clinical criteria (diagnosis may be made on day 4 by an experienced clinician if child has all the clinical criteria):

1. Changes in the extremities: in the acute phase, edema and erythema of the palms and soles, and in the subacute phase, periungual desquamation (peeling) of the hands and feet
2. Bilateral conjunctival injection (inflammation) without exudation
3. Changes in the oral mucous membranes, such as erythema of the lips, oropharyngeal reddening, or "strawberry tongue" (large papillae are exposed)
4. Polymorphous rash
5. Cervical lymphadenopathy (one lymph node larger than 1.5 cm)

Note: Kawasaki disease can be diagnosed with fewer clinical criteria when coronary artery changes are noted.

of HF, including decreased urinary output, gallop rhythm (an additional heart sound), tachycardia, and respiratory distress.

Administration of gamma globulin should follow the same guidelines as for any blood product, with frequent monitoring of vital signs. Patients must be watched for allergic reactions. Cardiac status must be monitored because of the large volume being administered to patients with myocarditis and diminished left ventricular function.

Most nursing care focuses on symptomatic relief. To minimize skin discomfort, cool cloths; unscented lotions; and soft, loose clothing are helpful. During the acute phase, mouth care, including lubricating ointment to the lips, is important for mucosal inflammation. Clear liquids and soft foods can be offered.

Patient irritability is perhaps the most challenging problem. These children need a quiet environment that promotes adequate rest. Their parents need to be supported in their efforts to comfort an often inconsolable child. They may need time away from their child, and nurses can often provide respite care for the family. Parents need to understand that irritability is a hallmark of KD and that they need not feel guilty or embarrassed about their child's behaviour.

Discharge Teaching

Parents need accurate information about the progression of KD, including the importance of follow-up monitoring and when they should contact their practitioner (see Patient Teaching box). Irritability is likely to persist for up to 2 months after the onset of symptoms. Peeling of the hands and feet is painless and occurs primarily in the second and third weeks. Arthritis, especially of the larger weight-bearing joints, may persist for several weeks. Children are typically most stiff in the mornings, during cold weather, and after naps. Passive range-of-motion exercises in the bathtub are often helpful in increasing flexibility. Any live immunizations (e.g., measles-mumps-rubella, varicella) should be deferred for 11 months after the administration of gamma globulin because the body might not produce the appropriate amount of antibodies (American Academy of Pediatrics, Committee on Infectious Diseases, & Pickering, 2009). The decision to give the varicella (chickenpox) vaccine while the child is receiving aspirin therapy is made individually by the practitioner. Temperature should be recorded after discharge until the child has been afebrile for several days.

Shock

Shock, or circulatory failure, is a complex clinical syndrome characterized by inadequate tissue perfusion to meet the metabolic demands of the body, resulting in cellular dysfunction and eventual organ failure. Although the causes are different, the physiological consequences are the same: hypotension, tissue hypoxia, and metabolic acidosis. Circulatory failure in children is a result of hypovolemia, altered peripheral vascular resistance, or pump failure. Types of shock are listed in Table 48-6.

Pathophysiology

A healthy child's circulatory system is able to transport oxygen and metabolic substrates to body tissues, which require a constant source for these essential needs. The cardiac output and distribution to the various body tissues can change rapidly in response to intrinsic (myocardial and intravascular) or extrinsic (neuronal) control mechanisms. In shock states these mechanisms are altered or challenged.

PATIENT TEACHING Concerns for Myocardial Infarction

All parents should understand the unlikely but real possibility of myocardial infarction and the signs and symptoms of cardiac ischemia in a child. At discharge, the ultimate cardiac sequela is generally not known because vessels do not reach their maximum diameter until 4 to 6 weeks after the onset of Kawasaki disease. In addition, the parents of children with known severe coronary artery sequelae may be taught cardiopulmonary resuscitation.

Table 48-6 Types of Shock

CHARACTERISTICS	MOST FREQUENT CAUSES
Hypovolemic	
Reduction in size of vascular compartment Falling blood pressure Poor capillary filling Low central venous pressure	Blood loss (hemorrhagic shock)—Trauma, gastrointestinal bleeding, intracranial hemorrhage Plasma loss—Increased capillary permeability associated with sepsis and acidosis, hypoproteinemia, burns, peritonitis Extracellular fluid loss—Vomiting, diarrhea, glycosuric diuresis, sunstroke
Distributive	
Reduction in peripheral vascular resistance Profound inadequacies in tissue perfusion Increased venous capacity and pooling Acute reduction in return blood flow to the heart Diminished cardiac output	Anaphylaxis (anaphylactic shock)—Extreme allergy or hypersensitivity to a foreign substance Sepsis (septic shock, bacteremic shock, endotoxic shock)—Overwhelming sepsis and circulating bacterial toxins Loss of neuronal control (neurogenic shock)—Interruption of neuronal transmission (spinal cord injury) Myocardial depression and peripheral dilation—Exposure to anaesthesia or ingestion of barbiturates, tranquilizers, opioids, antihypertensive agents, or ganglionic blocking agents
Cardiogenic	
Decreased cardiac output	After surgery for congenital heart disease Primary pump failure—Myocarditis, myocardial trauma, biochemical derangements, heart failure Dysrhythmias—Supraventricular tachycardia, atrioventricular block, and ventricular dysrhythmias; secondary to myocarditis or biochemical abnormalities (occasionally)

Reduced blood flow, as in hypovolemic shock, causes diminished venous return to the heart, low CVP, low cardiac output, and hypotension. Vasomotor centres in the medulla are signalled, causing a compensatory increase in the force and rate of cardiac contraction and constriction of arterioles and veins, thereby increasing peripheral vascular resistance. Simultaneously, the lowered blood volume leads to the release of large amounts of catecholamines, antidiuretic hormone, adrenocorticosteroids, and aldosterone in an effort to conserve body fluids. This causes reduced blood flow to the skin, kidneys, muscles, and viscera to shunt the available blood to the brain and heart. Consequently, the skin feels cold and clammy, there is poor capillary filling, and the glomerular filtration rate and urinary output are significantly reduced.

As a result of impaired perfusion, oxygen is depleted in the tissue cells, causing them to revert to anaerobic metabolism, producing lactic acidosis. The acidosis places an extra burden on the lungs as they attempt to compensate for the metabolic acidosis by increasing respiratory rate to remove excess carbon dioxide. Prolonged vasoconstriction results in fatigue and atony of the peripheral arterioles, which leads to vessel dilation. Venules, less sensitive to vasodilator substances, remain constricted for a time, causing massive pooling in the capillary and venular beds, which further depletes blood volume.

Complications of shock create further hazards. Central nervous system hypoperfusion may eventually lead to cerebral edema, cortical infarction, or intraventricular hemorrhage. Renal hypoperfusion causes renal ischemia with possible tubular or glomerular necrosis and renal vein thrombosis. Reduced blood flow to the lungs can interfere with surfactant secretion and result in acute respiratory distress syndrome (ARDS), characterized by sudden pulmonary congestion and atelectasis with formation of a hyaline membrane. Gastrointestinal tract bleeding and perforation are always a possibility after splanchnic ischemia and necrosis of intestinal mucosa. Metabolic complications of shock may include hypoglycemia, hypocalcemia, and other electrolyte disturbances.

Diagnostic Evaluation

The etiology of shock can be discerned from the history and physical examination. The severity of the shock is determined by measurements of vital signs, including CVP and capillary filling (Box 48-12). Shock can be regarded as a form of compensation for circulatory failure. Because of its progressive nature, it can be divided into the following three stages or phases:

1. **Compensated shock**—Vital organ function is maintained by intrinsic compensatory mechanisms; blood flow is usually normal or increased but generally uneven or maldistributed in the microcirculation.
2. **Decompensated shock**—Efficiency of the cardiovascular system gradually diminishes until perfusion in the microcirculation becomes marginal despite compensatory adjustments. The outcomes of circulatory failure that progress beyond the limits of compensation are tissue hypoxia, metabolic acidosis, and eventual dysfunction of all organ systems.

BOX 48-12 Clinical Manifestations of Shock

Compensated
Apprehensiveness
Irritability
Unexplained tachycardia
Normal blood pressure
Narrowing pulse pressure
Thirst
Pallor
Diminished urinary output
Reduced perfusion of extremities

Decompensated
Confusion and somnolence
Tachypnea
Moderate metabolic acidosis
Oliguria
Cool, pale extremities
Decreased skin turgor
Poor capillary filling

Irreversible
Thready, weak pulse
Hypotension
Periodic breathing or apnea
Anuria
Stupor or coma

3. **Irreversible, or terminal, shock**—Damage to vital organs, such as the heart or brain, is of such magnitude that the entire organism will be disrupted regardless of therapeutic intervention. Death occurs even if cardiovascular measurements return to normal levels with therapy.

At all stages the principal differentiating signs are observed in the (1) degree of tachycardia and perfusion to extremities, (2) level of consciousness, and (3) BP. Additional signs or modifications of these more universal signs may be present, depending on the type and cause of the shock. Initially the child's ability to compensate is effective; thus early signs are subtle. As the shock state advances, signs are more obvious and indicate early decompensation.

In early septic shock there are chills, fever, and vasodilation, with increased cardiac output that results in warm, flushed skin (hyperdynamic, or "hot," shock). A later and ominous development is disseminated intravascular coagulation (see Chapter 49), the major hematological complication of septic shock. Anaphylactic shock is frequently accompanied by urticaria and angioneurotic edema, which is life threatening when it involves the respiratory passages (see Anaphylaxis, p. 1494).

Laboratory tests that assist in assessment are blood gas measurements, pH, and sometimes liver function tests. Coagulation tests are evaluated when there is evidence of bleeding, such as oozing from a venipuncture site, bleeding from any orifice, or petechiae. Cultures of blood and other sites are indicated when there is a high suspicion of sepsis.

Renal function tests are performed when impaired renal function is evident.

Therapeutic Management

Treatment of shock consists of three major interventions: (1) ventilation, (2) fluid administration, and (3) improvement of the pumping action of the heart (vasopressor support). The first priority is to establish an airway and administer oxygen. After the airway is ensured, circulatory stabilization is the major concern. Establishment of adequate IV access, ideally with multilumen central lines, is essential to deliver fluids and medications.

Ventilatory Support

The lung is the organ most sensitive to shock. Decreased distribution or redistribution of blood flow to respiratory muscles plus the increased work of breathing can rapidly lead to respiratory failure. Critically ill patients are unable to maintain an adequate airway. To place the lung at rest and improve ventilation, tracheal intubation is initiated early with positive-pressure ventilation. Supplemental oxygen is always given as soon as possible. Blood gases and pH are monitored frequently.

Increased extravascular lung water caused by edema contributes to the development of respiratory complications. Therapy is directed toward maintaining normal arterial blood gas measurements, normal acid–base balance, and circulation. Efforts are made to remove fluid and prevent its accumulation with the use of diuretics.

Cardiovascular Support

In most cases rapid restoration of blood volume is all that is needed for resuscitation of the child in shock. An isotonic crystalloid solution (normal saline or Ringer's lactate) is the fluid of choice; colloids such as albumin are also used. Successful resuscitation is reflected by an increase in BP and a reduction in heart rate; increased cardiac output results in improved capillary circulation and skin colour. CVP measurements of right atrial pressure help guide fluid therapy, and urinary output measurement is an important indicator of adequacy of circulation. Correction of acidosis, hypoxemia, hypoglycemia, hypothermia, and any metabolic derangements is mandatory.

Temporary pharmacological support may be required to enhance myocardial contractility, reverse metabolic or respiratory acidosis, maintain arterial pressure, or do all of these. The principal agents used to improve cardiac output and circulation are catecholamines, such as dopamine (Intropin) or epinephrine (Adrenalin). Vasodilators that are sometimes used include nitroprusside (Nipride) or milrinone.

Nursing Care Management

The child who is in shock requires intensive observation and care. The *initial action is to ensure adequate tissue oxygenation.* The nurse should be prepared to administer oxygen by the appropriate route and assist with any intubation and ventilatory procedures indicated. Other procedures and activities that require immediate attention are establishing an IV line, weighing the child, obtaining baseline vital signs, placing an indwelling catheter, obtaining blood gases and other measurements, and administering medications as indicated. The child is best positioned flat with the legs elevated. The nurse's responsibilities are to monitor the IV infusion, intake and output, vital signs (including CVP), and general systems assessments on a routine basis. IV medications are titrated according to patient responses, and vital signs are taken every 15 minutes during the critical periods and thereafter as needed. Urinary output is measured hourly; blood gases, hematocrit, pH, and electrolytes are monitored frequently to assess the child's status and the efficacy of therapy. An apnea and cardiac monitor is attached and monitored continuously. In the initial stages of acute shock, more than one nurse is often needed to manage all the necessary activities that must be carried out simultaneously (see Emergency box).

Anaphylaxis

Anaphylaxis is the acute clinical syndrome resulting from the interaction of an allergen and a patient who is hypersensitive to that allergen. When the **antigen** enters the circulatory system, a generalized reaction rapidly takes place. Vasoactive amines (principally histamine or a histamine-like substance) are released and cause vasodilation, bronchoconstriction, and increased capillary permeability.

Severe reactions are immediate in onset; are often life threatening; and frequently involve multiple systems, primarily the cardiovascular, respiratory, gastrointestinal, and

> **EMERGENCY**
>
> **Shock**
>
> **Ventilation**
> Establish airway; be prepared for intubation.
> Administer oxygen, usually 100% by mask.
>
> **Fluid Administration**
> Obtain vascular access (preferably intravenous [IV]; intraosseous in emergency).
> Restore fluid volume as ordered (initial volume resuscitation is 20 mL/kg of isotonic crystalloid [normal saline or Ringer's lactate] over 5 to 20 minutes).
>
> **Cardiovascular Support**
> Administer vasopressors, especially IV epinephrine (dose: 0.01 mg/kg = 0.1 mL/kg of 1:10,000 solution).
> This may be repeated every 3 to 5 minutes for patients in cardiac arrest.
>
> **General Support**
> Provide continuous electrocardiographic monitoring.
> Monitor pulse oximetry.
> Keep child warm and calm.
>
> **In Addition**
> **Septic shock**—Administer broad-spectrum antibiotics intravenously.
> **Anaphylaxis**—Remove allergen if possible; provide intramuscular epinephrine and corticosteroids as ordered.

integumentary systems. Exposure to the antigen can be by ingestion, inhalation, skin contact, or injection. Examples of common allergens associated with anaphylaxis include drugs (e.g., antibiotics, chemotherapeutic agents, radiological contrast media), latex, foods, venom from bees or snakes, and biological agents (antisera, enzymes, hormones, blood products).

NURSING ALERT Penicillin allergy is associated with immediate (within an hour of administration) or accelerated (1 to 72 hours after administration) onset of skin eruption, especially a urticarial rash, or more serious symptoms such as laryngeal edema or anaphylactic shock.

Clinical Manifestations

The onset of clinical symptoms usually occurs within seconds or minutes of exposure to the antigen, and the rapidity of the reaction is directly related to its intensity: the earlier the onset, the more severe the reaction. The reaction may be preceded by symptoms of uneasiness, restlessness, irritability, severe anxiety, headache, dizziness, paresthesia, and disorientation. The patient may lose consciousness. Cutaneous signs of flushing and urticaria are common early signs, followed by angioedema, most notable in the eyelids, lips, tongue, hands, feet, and genitalia.

Bronchiolar constriction may follow, causing narrowing of the airway; pulmonary edema and hemorrhage also may occur. Laryngeal edema with severe acute upper airway obstruction may be life threatening and requires rapid intervention. Shock occurs as a result of mediator-induced vasodilation, which causes capillary permeability and loss of **intravascular fluid** into the interstitial space. Sudden hypotension and impaired cardiac output with poor perfusion are seen.

Therapeutic Management

A successful outcome of anaphylactic reactions depends on rapid recognition and institution of treatment. The goals of treatment are to provide ventilation, restore adequate circulation, and prevent further exposure by identifying and removing the cause when possible.

A mild reaction with no evidence of respiratory distress or cardiovascular compromise can be managed with subcutaneous administration of antihistamines, such as diphenhydramine (Benadryl) and epinephrine.

Moderate or severe distress presents a potentially life-threatening emergency. Establishing an airway is the first concern, as with all shock states. Epinephrine is given subcutaneously or intravenously as an antihistamine and to support the cardiovascular system and increase BP. Other routes for giving epinephrine are intramuscular and via the airway, either nebulized or injected through an ET tube. In severe anaphylaxis, epinephrine by any route is better than none. Fluids are given to restore blood volume. Additional vasopressors may be given to improve cardiac output.

Prevention of a reaction is preferable. Preventing exposure is more easily accomplished in children known to be at risk, including those with (1) a history of previous allergic reaction to a specific antigen; (2) a history of atopy; (3) a history of severe reactions in immediate family members; and (4) a reaction to a skin test, although skin tests are not available for all allergens. Desensitization may be recommended in certain cases.

Nursing Care Management

When an anaphylactic reaction is suspected, both immediate intervention and preparation for medical therapy are nursing responsibilities. Ventilation is ensured by placing the child in a head-elevated position, unless contraindicated by hypotension, to facilitate breathing and administer oxygen. If the child is not breathing, **cardiopulmonary resuscitation** (CPR) is initiated and emergency medical services are summoned.

If the cause can be determined, measures need to be implemented to slow the spread of the offending substance. An IV infusion should be established immediately. Emergency medications should be given intravenously whenever possible; however, epinephrine may be given subcutaneously (see Emergency box). Vital signs and urinary output should be monitored frequently. Medications need to be administered as prescribed, with regular assessment to monitor effectiveness and detect signs of adverse effects of medication and fluid overload.

To prevent an anaphylactic reaction, parents should always be asked about possible allergic responses to foods, latex, medications, and environmental conditions. These need to be displayed prominently on the patient's chart. The specific allergen should be noted, as well as the type and severity of the reaction. Parents are excellent historians, especially when the child has displayed a pronounced reaction to a substance. Medications, including related medications (e.g., penicillin, nafcillin), and other items such as latex that have produced a reaction previously should never be used. If the child is allergic to insect venom, the family should be instructed to purchase an emergency kit to be kept with him or her at all times. If the child is old enough, both the family and the child need to be taught how to use the equipment. The patient should carry medical identification at all times.

Septic Shock

Sepsis and septic shock are caused by an infectious organism (Maar, 2004). Normally an infection triggers an inflammatory response in a local area, which results in vasodilation, increased capillary permeability, and eventually elimination of the infectious agent. The widespread activation and systemic release of inflammatory mediators is called the *systemic inflammatory response syndrome (SIRS)*. Box 48-13 provides the exact definitions for SIRS, infection, sepsis, and severe sepsis. SIRS can occur in response to both infectious and noninfectious (e.g., trauma, burns) causes. When caused by infection, it is called *sepsis*. *Septic shock* is defined as sepsis with organ dysfunction and hypotension.

Most of the physiological effects of shock occur because the exaggerated immune response triggers more than 30 different mediators that result in diffuse vasodilation, increased capillary permeability, and maldistribution of blood flow. This impairs oxygen and nutrient delivery to the cells, resulting in cellular dysfunction. If the process continues, multiple organ dysfunction occurs and may result in death. Table 48-7 includes the age-specific vital signs and laboratory values reflective of septic shock in children.

The incidence of septic shock is increasing in adults and children (Arnal & Stein, 2003), possibly as a result of greater numbers of immunosuppressed patients, more widespread use of invasive devices in the seriously ill, increased awareness of the diagnosis, and a growing number of resistant microorganisms.

Three stages have been identified in septic shock. In early septic shock the patient has chills; fever; and vasodilation with increased cardiac output, which results in warm, flushed skin that reflects vascular tone abnormalities and hyperdynamic, warm, or hyperdynamic-compensated responses. BP and urinary output are normal. The patient has the best chance for survival in this stage. The second stage—the normodynamic, cool, or hyperdynamic-decompensated stage—lasts only a few hours. The skin is cool, but pulses and BP are still normal. Urinary output diminishes, and the mental state becomes depressed. With advancing disease, certain signs of circulatory decompensation that deteriorate to signs of circulatory collapse are indistinguishable from late shock of any cause. In the hypodynamic, or cold, stage of shock, cardiovascular function progressively deteriorates, even with aggressive therapy. The patient has hypothermia, cold extremities, weak pulses, hypotension, and oliguria or anuria. Patients are severely lethargic or comatose. Multiorgan failure is common. This is the most dangerous stage of shock.

Management of septic shock involves measures to provide hemodynamic stability and adequate oxygenation to the tissues and the use of antimicrobials to treat the infectious

BOX 48-13 Definitions of Systemic Inflammatory Response Syndrome, Infection, Sepsis, and Severe Sepsis

Systemic inflammatory response syndrome (SIRS)—The presence of at least two of the following four criteria, one of which must be abnormal temperature or leukocyte count:

1. Core temperature of more than 38.5°C or less than 36°C
2. Tachycardia, defined as a mean heart rate more than 2 SD above normal for age in the absence of external stimulus, chronic drugs, or painful stimuli; or otherwise unexplained persistent elevation over a 0.5- to 4-hour period; or, for children less than 1 year old: bradycardia, defined as a mean heart rate less than the tenth percentile for age in the absence of external vagal stimulus, β-blocker drugs, or congenital heart disease; or otherwise unexplained persistent depression over a 0.5-hour period
3. Mean respiratory rate more than 2 SD above normal for age or mechanical ventilation for an acute process not related to underlying neuromuscular disease or the receipt of general anaesthesia
4. Leukocyte count elevated or depressed for age (not secondary to chemotherapy-induced leukopenia) or more than 10% immature neutrophils

Infection—A suspected or proven (by positive culture, tissue stain, or polymerase chain reaction test) infection caused by any pathogen; or a clinical syndrome associated with a high probability of infection. Evidence of infection includes positive findings on clinical examination, imaging, or laboratory tests (e.g., white blood cells in a normally sterile body fluid, perforated viscus, chest radiograph consistent with pneumonia, petechial or purpuric rash, or purpura fulminans)

Sepsis—SIRS in the presence of or as a result of suspected or proven infection

Severe sepsis—Sepsis plus cardiovascular organ dysfunction or acute respiratory distress syndrome; or two or more other organ dysfunctions

(From Goldstein, B., et al. [2005]. International Pediatric Sepsis Consensus Conference: Definitions for sepsis and organ dysfunction in pediatrics. *Pediatric Critical Care Medicine,* 6[1], 2–8; used with permission. Copyright © 2005, The Society of Critical Care Medicine and the World Federation of Pediatric Intensive and Critical Care Societies.)

Table 48-7 Age-Specific Vital Signs and Laboratory Variables in Septic Shock*

	Heart Rate (beats/min)				
AGE GROUP	TACHYCARDIA	BRADYCARDIA	RESPIRATORY RATE (BREATHS/MIN)	LEUKOCYTE COUNT (LEUKOCYTES × 10^9/L)	SYSTOLIC BLOOD PRESSURE (MM HG)
0 days–1 wk	>180	<100	>60	>34	<65
1 wk–1 mo	>180	<100	>40	>19.5 or <5	<75
1 mo–1 yr	>180	<90	>34	>17.5 or <5	<100
2-5 yr	>140	N/A	>22	>15.5 or <6	<94
6-12 yr	>130	N/A	>8	>13.50 or <4.5	<105
13–<18 yr	>110	N/A	>4	>11 or <4.5	<117

(From Goldstein, B., et al. [2005]. International Pediatric Sepsis Consensus Conference: Definitions for sepsis and organ dysfunction in pediatrics. *Pediatric Critical Care Medicine,* 6[1], 2-8; used with permission.)

*Lower values for heart rate, leukocyte count, and systolic blood pressure are for fifth percentile, and upper values for heart rate, respiratory rate, or leukocyte count are for ninety-fifth percentile.

N/A, not applicable.

organism. As with other forms of shock, hemodynamic stability is achieved with fluid volume resuscitation and inotropic agents as needed. Providing adequate oxygenation often requires intubation and mechanical ventilation, supplemental oxygen, sedation, and paralysis to decrease the work of breathing. Septic shock involves activation of **complement** proteins that promote clumping of the granulocytes in the lung. The granulocytes can release chemicals that can cause direct lung injury to the pulmonary capillary endothelium. This causes a fluid leak into the alveoli, which causes stiff, noncompliant lungs. Disseminated intravascular coagulation and multiorgan dysfunction may also occur and require prompt assessment and management.

Newer therapies are being developed to modify the host immune response by attempting to block various mediators, thereby interrupting the inflammatory cascade.

Early identification of the symptoms of septic shock is critical to patient survival. A high index of suspicion is required in all critically ill patients who are at greater risk for sepsis because of multiple invasive lines and devices, poor nutrition, and impaired immune function. Subtle alterations in tissue perfusion and unexplained tachypnea and tachycardia often are early warning signs. Identification of the infectious agent and prompt treatment are also critical to patient survival. Broad-spectrum antibiotics should be given, and the site of infection should be removed if possible (e.g., drain abscesses, remove indwelling lines). Patients should be managed in a critical care unit, in which continuous monitoring and sophisticated cardiac and respiratory support are available. Multidisciplinary collaboration is essential in managing these critically ill patients.

Key Points

- CHD is the most common form of cardiac disease in children.
- Major categories to investigate in the cardiac history are poor weight gain, poor feeding habits, and fatigue during feeding; frequent respiratory tract infections and difficulties; and evidence of exercise intolerance.
- The most common tests used in assessing cardiac function are radiography, ECG, echocardiography, and cardiac catheterization.
- Cardiac catheterization procedures can be divided into three groups: (1) diagnostic procedures, including angiography, that measure pressures and saturations to establish cardiac diagnosis; (2) interventional procedures, in which catheters or balloon devices are used to correct cardiac defects; and (3) electrophysiology studies, in which catheters with electrodes are used to evaluate dysrhythmias.
- Diagnostic cardiac catheterization provides important information about oxygen saturation of blood within the chambers and great vessels, pressure changes, changes in cardiac output or stroke volume, and anatomical abnormalities.
- Several prenatal factors may predispose children to CHD: maternal rubella during pregnancy, maternal alcoholism, maternal age older than 40 years, and maternal type 1 diabetes.
- Congenital heart defects can be divided into four main groups, as determined by hemodynamic patterns: (1) defects that result in increased pulmonary blood flow, (2) obstructive defects, (3) defects that result in decreased pulmonary blood flow, and (4) mixed defects.
- Clinical consequences of congenital heart defects include HF and hypoxemia. A child can have both hypoxemia and HF, although usually they occur independently.
- Clinical manifestations of HF are impaired myocardial function (tachycardia, cardiomegaly), pulmonary congestion (dyspnea, tachypnea, orthopnea, cyanosis), and systemic congestion (hepatosplenomegaly, edema, distended veins).
- Nursing measures in the care of a child with HF are to assist in improving cardiac function, decrease cardiac demands, reduce respiratory distress, maintain nutritional status, promote fluid loss, and provide family support.
- Clinical manifestations of hypoxemia are cyanosis, polycythemia, clubbing, and delayed growth and development. The child is at increased risk for hypercyanotic spells, CVAs, brain abscess, and bacterial endocarditis.
- Caring for the child with CHD and the family requires helping them to adjust to the disorder and cope with the effects of the defect, as well as fostering growth and promoting family relationships.
- Preoperative care of the child with a congenital heart defect involves introducing the child and family to the hospital and preparing them for preoperative and postoperative procedures.
- Providing postoperative care includes observing vital signs and arterial and venous pressures, maintaining respiratory status, allowing maximum rest, providing comfort, monitoring fluids, planning for progressive activities, giving emotional support, observing for complications of surgery, and planning for discharge and home care.
- Acquired cardiovascular disorders include bacterial endocarditis, RF, hyperlipidemia (hypercholesterolemia), and cardiac dysrhythmias.
- Prevention of infectious endocarditis in certain children with CHD involves administration of prophylactic antibiotics when specific procedures are performed.
- Acute RF is a systemic inflammatory disease that can damage the cardiac valves and is associated with previous GABHS infection.
- Cholesterol screening in children is controversial; currently, children with known risk factors for hyperlipidemia are screened and treated as needed. The influence of childhood cholesterol levels on later development of coronary artery disease is under investigation.
- Common dysrhythmias in children include slow (bradycardias, heart block) and fast (sinus tachycardia, SVT) rhythms.
- Heart transplantation has been extended to infants and children with cardiomyopathy and complex congenital heart defects involving ventricular dysfunction, such as hypoplastic left heart syndrome.
- Education of the child with hypertension and the family focuses on drug therapy, diet control, and appropriate exercise.

- KD is an extensive inflammation of small vessels and capillaries that may progress to involve the coronary arteries, causing aneurysm formation. The administration of γ-globulin is an important aspect of treatment.
- Emergency treatment for shock includes ensuring ventilation; administering vasopressors, fluids, blood, and antibiotics as needed; and providing supportive measures such as correct positioning, warmth, and psychological reassurance to the child and family.
- Persons at risk for anaphylaxis may be identified by a history of previous allergic reaction, history of atopy, history of severe reactions in family, and positive skin test to the allergen.

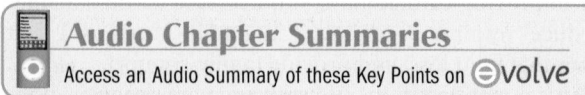

Audio Chapter Summaries

Access an Audio Summary of these Key Points on evolve

References

Allen, U., & Canadian Paediatric Society, Infectious Diseases and Immunization Committee (2010). Infective endocarditis: Updated guidelines. *Paediatrics & Child Health, 15*(4), 205–208.

American Academy of Pediatrics, Committee on Infectious Diseases, & Pickering, L., (Ed.). (2009). *Red book: 2009 report of the Committee on Infectious Diseases* (28th ed.). Elk Grove Village, IL: Author.

American Heart Association. (2011). *Preparing children with surgery.* Retrieved from http://www.heart.org/HEARTORG/Conditions/CongenitalHeartDefects/CareTreatmentforCongenitalHeartDefects/Preparing-Children-for-Surgery_UCM_307732_Article.jsp.

Arnal, L. E., & Stein, F. (2003). Pediatric septic shock: why has mortality decreased? The utility of goal-directed therapy. *Seminars in Pediatric Infectious Diseases, 14*(2), 165–172.

Arnold, R., et al. (2008). Outcome after mechanical aortic valve replacement in children and young adults. *Annals of Thoracic Surgery, 85*(2), 604–610. doi:10.1016/j.athoracsur.2007.10.035

Barbas, K. H., & Kelleher, D. K. (2004). Breastfeeding success among infants with congenital heart disease. *Pediatric Nursing, 30*, 285–289.

Barst, R. J. (1999). Recent advances in the treatment of pediatric pulmonary artery hypertension. *Pediatric Clinics of North America, 46*(2), 333–345.

Beekman, R. H. (2008). Coarctation of the aorta. In H. D. Allen, et al. (Eds.), *Moss and Adams' heart disease in infants, children and adolescents* (7th ed.). Philadelphia: Lippincott Williams & Wilkins.

Belay, E., et al. (2006). Kawasaki syndrome and risk factors for coronary artery abnormalities. *Pediatric Infectious Diseases, 25*(3), 245–249. doi:10.1097/01.inf.0000202068.30956.16

Blume, E. D. (2003). Current status of heart transplantation in children: Update 2003. *Pediatric Clinics of North America, 50*, 1375–1391.

Boucek, M. M., et al. (2007). The Registry of the International Society for Heart and Lung Transplantation: Tenth official pediatric heart transplantation report—2007. *Journal of Heart & Lung Transplantation, 26*(8), 796–807. doi:10.1016/j.healun.2007.06.006

Canadian Paediatric Society. (2007). *Canadian Paediatric Surveillance Program. Acute rheumatic fever.* Retrieved from http://www.web.cps.ca/English/surveillance/cpsp/Studies/rheumatic_fever.htm.

Carapetis, J. R., McDonald, M., & Wilson, N. J. (2005). Acute rheumatic fever. *Lancet, 366*, 155–168. doi:10.1016/S0140-6736(05)66874-2

Cecchin, F., et al. (2009). Cardiac resynchronization therapy (and multisite pacing) in pediatrics and congenital heart disease: Five years experience in a single institution. *Journal of Cardiovascular Electrophysiology, 20*(1), 58–65.

Chun, T. Y. H., & Van Hare, G. H. (2004). Advances in the approach to treament of supraventricular tachycardia in the pediatric population. *Current Cardiology Reports, 6*, 322–326.

Daniels, S. R., Greer, F. R., & the Committee on Nutrition. (2008). Lipid screening and cardiovascular health in childhood. *Pediatrics, 122*, 198–208.

Dodds, K. M., & Merle, C. (2005). Discharging neonates with congenital heart disease after cardiac surgery: A practical approach. *Clinics in Perinatology, 32*, 1031–1042. doi:10.1016/j.clp.2005.09.009

Domi, T., et al. (2008). Frequency, predictors, and neurologic outcomes of vaso-occlusive strokes associated with cardiac surgery in children. *NeoReviews, 122*(6), 1292–1298, doi:10.1542/peds.2007-1459

Dubin, A. M., et al. (2005). Resynchronization therapy in pediatric and congenital heart disease patients. *Journal of the American College of Cardiology, 46*(12), 2277–2283.

Gerber, M. A., et al. (2009). Prevention of rheumatic fever and diagnosis and treatment of acute streptococcal pharyngitis: A scientific statement from the AHA. *Circulation, 119*, 1541–1551.

Goldmuntz, E., & Lin, A. (2008). Genetics of congenital heart defects. In A. D. Allen, D. J. Driscoll, R. E. Shaddy, et al. (Eds). *Moss and Adams' heart disease in infants, children and adolescents.* (7th ed.). Philadelphia: Lippincott Williams & Wilkins.

Heart and Stroke Foundation. (2012a). *Congenital heart disease.* Retrieved from http://www.heartandstroke.com/site/c.ikIQLcMWJtE/b.3484063/k.E84C/Heart_disease__Congenital_heart_disease.htm.

Heart and Stroke Foundation. (2012b). *Healthy kids.* Retrieved from http://www.heartandstroke.com/site/c.ikIQLcMWJtE/b.3479025/k.802B/Healthy_Kids.htm.

Hockenberry, M. J., & Wilson, D. (2011). *Wong's nursing care of infants and children* (9th ed.). St. Louis: Mosby.

Hoffman, J. I. E., & Kaplan, S. (2002). The incidence of congenital heart disease. *Journal of the American College of Cardiology, 39*, 1890–1900.

Jacobs, J. P., et al. (2004). Lessons learned from the data analysis of the second harvest (1998–2001) of the Society of Thoracic Surgeons (STS) Congenital Heart Surgery Database. *Journal of the American College of Cardiology, 26*(1), 18–37.

Leiter, L. A., et al. (2010). Attainment of Canadian and European guidelines' lipid targets with atorvastatin plus ezetimibe vs. doubling the dose of atorvastatin. *International Journal of Clinical Practice, 64*(13), 1765–1772. doi:10.1111/j.1742-1241.2010.02530.x

LeRoy, S., et al. (2003). Recommendations for preparing children and adolescents for invasive cardiac procedures: AHA Scientific Statement. *Circulation, 108*, 2550–2564.

Maar, S. P. (2004). Emergency care in pediatric septic shock. *Pediatric Emergency Care, 20*(9), 617–624.

Maclaren, J., & Cohen, L. L. (2007). Interventions for pediatric procedure-related pain in primary care. *Paediatrics and Child Health, 12*(2), 111–116.

McCrindle, B. W., et al. (2007). Drug therapy of high-risk lipid abnormalities in children and adolescents: A scientific statement from the American Heart Association Atherosclerosis, Hypertension, and Obesity in Youth Committee, Council of Cardiovascular Disease in the Young, with the Council on Cardiovascular Nursing. *Circulation, 115*, 1948–1967. doi:10.1161/CIRCULATIONAHA.107.181946

Mehta R., Lee, K. J., Chaturvedi, R., & Benson, L. (2008). Complications of pediatric cardiac catheterization: A review in the current era. *Catheterization and Cardiovascular Interventions, 72*(2), 278–285.

National High Blood Pressure Education Program Working Group on High Blood Pressure in Children and Adolescents. (2004). The fourth report on the diagnosis, evaluation, and treatment of high blood pressure in children and adolescents. *Pediatrics, 114*(2), 555–576.

Newburger, J. W., et al. (2004). Diagnosis, treatment, and long-term management of Kawasaki disease: A statement for health professionals from the Committee on Rheumatic Fever, Endocarditis and Kawasaki Disease, Council on Cardiovascular Disease in the Young, American Heart Association. *Circulation, 110*(17), 2747–2771.

Park, M. K. (2008). *Pediatric cardiology handbook* (5th ed.). St. Louis: Mosby.

Porter, C. J., & Edwards, W. D. (2008). Atrial septal defects. In H. D. Allen, et al. (Eds.). *Moss and Adams' heart disease in infants, children and adolescents* (7th ed.). Philadelphia: Lippincott Williams & Wilkins.

Public Health Agency of Canada. (2006). *Canadian immunization guide* (7th ed.). Retrieved from http://www.phac-aspc.gc.ca/publicat/cig-gci/index-eng.php.

Robinson, J. L., Canadian Paediatric Society, Infectious Diseases and Immunization Committee. (2011). Preventing respiratory syncytial virus infections (Abridged version). *Paediatrics and Child Health, 16*(8), 488–490.

Rome, J. J., & Kreutzer, J. (2004). Pediatric interventional catheterization: Reasonable expectations and outcomes. *Pediatric Clinics of North America, 51*, 1589–1610.

Rosenthal, D., et al. (2004). International Society for Heart and Lung Transplantation: Practice guidelines for management of heart failure in children. *Journal of Heart & Lung Transplantation, 23*(12), 1313–1333.

Schneider, D. J., & Moore, J. W. (2008). Aortic stenosis. In H. D. Allen, et al. (Eds.). *Moss and Adams' heart disease in infants, children and adolescents* (7th ed.). Philadelphia: Lippincott Williams & Wilkins.

Shanmugam, G., MacArthur, K., & Pollock, J. (2005). Mechanical aortic valve replacement: Long-term outcomes in children. *Journal of Heart Valve Disorders, 14*(2), 166–171.

Smith, P. (2001). Primary care in children with congenital heart disease. *Journal of Pediatric Nursing, 16*(5), 308–319.

Spirito, P., et al. (2009). Syncope and risk of sudden death in hypertrophic cardiomyopathy. *Circulation, 1109*, 1703–1710.

Stetzler, M., Rudd, N., & Pick, B. (2005). Nutrition care for newborns with congenital heart disease. *Clinics in Perinatology, 32*, 1017–1030. doi:10.1016/j.clp.2005.09.010

Templeton, C. G., & Canadian Paediatric Society. (2007). *Canadian Paediatric Surveillance Program: Acute rheumatic fever.* Retrieved from http://www.cps.ca/english/surveillance/cpsp/studies/rheumatic_fever.htm.

Tweddell, J. S., et al., (2008). Hypoplastic left heart syndrome. In A. D. Allen, D. J. Driscoll, R. E. Shaddy, et al. (Eds). *Moss and Adams' heart disease in infants, children and adolescents.* (7th ed.). Philadelphia: Lippincott Williams & Wilkins.

Uzark, K. (2001). Therapeutic cardiac catheterization for congenital heart disease: A new era in pediatric care. *Journal of Pediatric Nursing, 16*(5), 300–307.

Wilder, M., et al. (2007). Delayed diagnosis by physicians contributes to the development of coronary artery aneurysms in children with Kawasaki syndrome. *Pediatric Infectious Diseases, 26*(3), 256–260. doi:10.1097/01.inf.0000256783.57041.66

Wilson, W., et al. (2007). Prevention of infective endocarditis: Guidelines from the American Heart Association. *Circulation, 116*(15), 1736–1754. doi:10.1161/CIRCULATIONAHA.106.183095

Additional Resources

CHASE, The Children's Heart Association For Support and Education, Toronto, Ontario, Canada: http://www.angelfire.com/on/chase

Heart and Stroke Foundation: Heart and Soul: Your Guide to Living With Congenital Heart Disease: http://www.heartandstroke.com/atf/cf/%7B99452D8B-E7F1-4BD6-A57D-B136CE6C95BF%7D/HeartandSoul_English.pdf

Sick Kids Hospital: Congenital Heart Conditions Resource Centre: http://www.aboutkidshealth.ca/En/ResourceCentres/CongenitalHeartConditions/Pages/default.aspx

Western Canadian Children's Heart Network: http://www.westernchildrensheartnetwork.ca/FamilySupport/Default.htm

Unit 11

49 Hematological or Immunological Dysfunction

Learning Objectives

On completion of this chapter, the reader will be able to:

- Distinguish between the various categories of anemia.
- Describe the prevention of iron deficiency anemia and the care of the child with iron deficiency anemia.
- Compare sickle cell anemia and β-thalassemia major in relation to pathophysiology and nursing care.
- Describe the mechanisms of inheritance and nursing care of the child with hemophilia.
- Relate the pathophysiology and clinical manifestations of leukemia.
- Demonstrate an understanding of the rationale of therapies for neoplastic disease.
- Outline a plan of care for the child with neoplastic disease and the family.
- Contrast the pathophysiology and management of the immunodeficiency disorders.
- List nursing precautions and responsibilities during blood transfusion.
- Describe the types of hematopoietic stem cell transplants.

Electronic Resources

Additional information related to the content in Chapter 49 can be found on

evolve the companion Web site at

http://evolve.elsevier.com/Canada/Perry/maternal/

- Examination Review Questions
- Animation—Hemophilia A
- Animation—Platelets and Blood Clotting
- Animation—Sickle Cell Anemia
- Case Study—Acute Lymphoid Leukemia
- Case Study—Sickle Cell Anemia
- Critical Thinking Exercise—Bleeding
- Critical Thinking Exercise—Bone Marrow Test
- Critical Thinking Exercise—HIV Testing in Children

Hematological and Immunological Dysfunction

Several tests can be performed to assess hematological function, including additional procedures to identify the cause of the dysfunction. The following discussion is limited to a description of the most common and one of the most valuable tests, the complete blood cell count (CBC). Other procedures, such as those related to iron, coagulation, and immune status, are discussed throughout the chapter as appropriate. The nurse should be familiar with the significance of the findings from the CBC (Table 49-1) and aware of normal values for age, which are listed in Appendix D.

evolve Animation—Platelets and Blood Clotting

As with any disorder, the history and physical examination are essential to identify hematological dysfunction, and the nurse is often the first person to suspect a problem based on information from these sources. Comments by the parent regarding the child's lack of energy, food diary of poor sources of iron, frequent infections, and bleeding that is difficult to control offer clues to the more common disorders affecting the blood. A careful physical appraisal, especially of the skin, can reveal findings (e.g., pallor, petechiae, bruising) that may indicate minor or serious hematological conditions. Nurses need to be aware of the clinical manifestations of blood diseases to assist in recognizing symptoms and establishing a diagnosis.

Red Blood Cell Disorders

Anemia

The term *anemia* describes a condition in which the number of red blood cells (RBCs) or the hemoglobin (Hgb or Hb) concentration is reduced below normal values for age. This diminishes the oxygen-carrying capacity of the blood, causing a reduction in the oxygen available to the tissues. Anemia is the most common hematological disorder of infancy and childhood and is not a disease itself but an indication or manifestation of an underlying pathological process.

Classification

Anemias are classified in relation to (1) *etiology* or *physiology*, manifested by erythrocyte or Hgb depletion, and

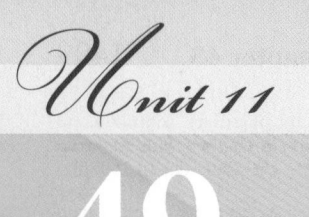

Table 49-1 Tests Performed as Part of the Complete Blood Cell Count

TEST*	DESCRIPTION AND COMMENTS
Red blood cell (RBC) count	Number of RBCs per 10^{12}/L of blood RBCs carry oxygen from the lungs to the rest of the body Indirectly estimates Hgb content of blood Reflects function of bone marrow
Hemoglobin (Hgb) determination	Amount of Hgb (g)/L of whole blood Total blood Hgb primarily dependent on number of circulating RBCs but also on amount of Hgb in each cell
Hematocrit (Hct)	Percent volume of packed RBCs in whole blood Indirectly measures Hgb content
RBC indexes	
Mean corpuscular volume (MCV)	Average or mean volume (size) of a single RBC MCV values are expressed as femtolitres (fL)
Mean corpuscular hemoglobin (MCH)	Average or mean quantity (weight) of Hgb in a single RBC MCH values are expressed as picograms (pg) MCV and MCH depend on accurate counts of RBCs, whereas MCHC does not; thus MCHC is often more reliable All indexes depend on average cell measurements and do not show individual RBC variations (anisocytosis)
Mean corpuscular hemoglobin concentration (MCHC) C)	Average concentration of Hgb in a single RBC MCHC values are expressed as (g)/L
RBC volume distribution width (RDW)	Average size of RBCs Differentiates some types of anemia
Reticulocyte count	Percent reticulocytes in RBCs Index of production of mature RBCs by bone marrow Decreased count indicates depressed bone marrow function Increased count indicates erythrogenesis in response to some stimulus When reticulocyte count is extremely high, other forms of immature RBCs (normoblasts, even erythroblasts) may be present Indirectly estimates hypochromic anemia Usually elevated in patients with chronic hemolytic anemia
White blood cell (WBC) count	Number of WBCs × 10^9/L of blood Total number of WBCs less important than differential count
Differential WBC count	Inspection and quantification of WBC types present in peripheral blood Values are expressed as percentages; to obtain absolute number of any type of WBC, multiply its respective percentage by total number of WBCs
Neutrophils (polys)	Primary defence in bacterial infection; capable of phagocytizing and killing bacteria
Bands	Immature neutrophil Increased numbers in bacterial infection Also capable of phagocytosis and killing
Eosinophils	Named for their staining characteristics with eosin dye Increased in allergic disorders, parasitic diseases, certain neoplasms, and other diseases
Basophils	Named for their characteristic basophilic stippling Contain histamine, heparin, and serotonin; believed to cause increased blood flow to injured tissues while preventing excessive clotting. Can increase in cases of leukemia, chronic inflammation, radiation therapy or hypersensitivity reaction to food
Lymphocytes	Involved in development of antibody and delayed hypersensitivity
Monocytes	Large phagocytic cells that are involved in early stage of inflammatory reaction
Absolute neutrophil count (ANC)	Percent neutrophils/bands times WBC count Indicates capability of body to handle bacterial infections
Platelet count	Number of platelets × 10^9/L of blood Cellular fragments that are necessary for clotting to occur
Stained peripheral blood smear	Visual estimation of amount of Hgb in RBCs and overall size, shape, and structure of RBCs Various staining properties of RBC structures may be evidence of immature forms of erythrocytes Shows variation in size and shape of RBCs: microcytic, macrocytic, poikilocytic (variable shapes)

*See Appendix D for normal values according to ages. Values may vary between Canadian laboratories.

(2) *morphology*, the characteristic changes in RBC size, shape, or colour (Box 49-1). Although the morphological classification is more useful in terms of laboratory evaluation of anemia, the etiological approach provides direction for planning nursing care. For example, anemia with reduced Hgb concentration may be caused by a dietary depletion of iron, and the principal intervention is replenishing iron stores. The classification of anemias is found in Figure 49-1.

Consequences of Anemia

The basic physiological defect caused by anemia is a decrease in the oxygen-carrying capacity of blood and consequently a reduction in the amount of oxygen available to the cells. When the anemia has developed slowly, the child usually adapts to the declining Hgb level.

The effects of anemia on the circulatory system can be profound. Because the viscosity of blood depends almost entirely on the concentration of RBCs, the resulting hemodilution of severe anemia decreases peripheral resistance, causing greater quantities of blood to return to the heart. The increased circulation and turbulence within the heart may produce a murmur. Because the cardiac workload is greatly increased, especially during exercise, infection, or emotional stress, cardiac failure may ensue.

Children seem to have a remarkable ability to function well despite low levels of Hgb. Cyanosis (the result of the quantity of deoxygenated Hgb in arterial blood) is typically not evident. Growth restriction, resulting from decreased cellular metabolism and coexisting anorexia, is a common finding in chronic severe anemia and is frequently accompanied by delayed sexual maturation in the older child.

BOX 49-1 Red Blood Cell Morphology

Size (Cell Size)

Variation in red blood cell (RBC) sizes (anisocytosis)

- Normocytes (normal cell size)
- Microcytes (smaller than normal cell size)
- Macrocytes (larger than normal cell size)

Shape (Cell Shape)

Variation in RBC shapes (poikilocytosis)

- Spherocytes (globular cells)
- Drepanocytes (sickle-shaped cells)
- Numerous other irregularly shaped cells

Colour (Cell Staining Characteristics)

Variation in hemoglobin concentration in the RBCs

- Normochromic (sufficient or normal amount of hemoglobin per RBC)
- Hypochromic (reduced amount of hemoglobin per RBC)
- Hyperchromic (increased amount of hemoglobin per RBC)

Diagnostic Evaluation

In general, anemia may be suspected based on findings in the **history** and physical examination, such as lack of energy, easy fatigability, and pallor; however, unless the anemia is severe, the first clue to the disorder may be alterations in the CBC, such as decreased RBCs, and decreased Hgb and hematocrit (Hct) levels (see Fig. 49-1). Although anemia is sometimes defined as an Hgb level below 100 or 110 g/L, this arbitrary cutoff is inappropriate for all children, because Hgb levels normally vary with age (see Table 49-1 and Appendix D).

Other tests specific to a particular type of anemia are used to determine the underlying cause of anemia. These are discussed in relation to the particular disorder.

Therapeutic Management

The objectives of medical management are to reverse the anemia by treating the underlying cause and to make up for

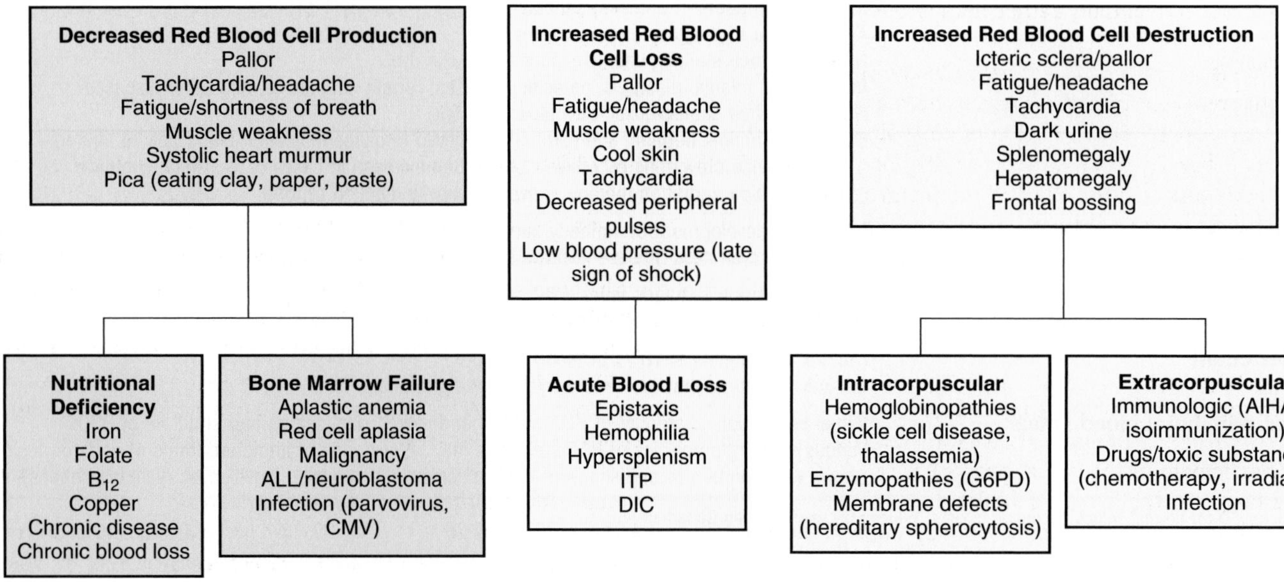

Fig. 49-1 Classifications of anemias. *AIHA*, autoimmune hemolytic anemia; *ALL*, acute lymphoid leukemia; *CMV*, cytomegalovirus; *DIC*, disseminated intravascular coagulation; *G6PD*, glucose-6-phosphate dehydrogenase; *ITP*, idiopathic thrombocytopenic purpura.

any deficiency of blood, blood component, or substance the blood needs for normal functioning. For example, blood or blood cells are replaced after hemorrhage; in nutritional anemias the specific deficiency is replaced.

In patients with severe anemia, supportive medical care may include oxygen therapy, bed rest, and replacement of intravascular volume with intravenous (IV) fluids. The prognosis for anemia depends on the correction of the cause.

Nursing Care Management

The assessment of anemia includes the basic techniques that are applicable to any condition. The age of the infant or child provides some clues regarding the possible etiology of the anemia. For example, iron deficiency anemia occurs more frequently in the toddler between 12 and 36 months of age and during the growth spurt of adolescence.

Racial or ethnic background is also significant. For example, the anemias related to abnormal Hgb levels are found in Southeast Asians and persons of African or Mediterranean ancestry. These same groups may be genetically deficient in the enzyme lactase after the period of infancy. Affected individuals are unable to tolerate lactose in the diet, with consequent intestinal irritation and chronic blood loss.

Special emphasis should be placed on a careful history to elicit any information that might help identify the cause of the anemia. For example, a statement such as "My child drinks lots of milk" is a frequent finding in toddlers with iron deficiency anemia. An episode of diarrhea may have precipitated temporary lactose intolerance in a young child.

Stool examination for occult (microscopic) blood (Hemoccult test) can identify chronic intestinal bleeding that results from a primary or secondary lactase deficiency. It is also important to understand the significance of various blood tests (see Table 49-1).

Prepare the Child and Family for Laboratory Tests

Usually several blood tests are ordered; because they are generally done sequentially rather than at one time, the child is subjected to multiple finger or heel punctures or venipunctures. Laboratory technicians frequently are not aware of the trauma that repeated punctures represent to a child. However, these invasive procedures need not be painful (see Blood Specimens, Chapter 45). For example, the topical application of an eutectic mix of lidocaine and prilocaine (EMLA) before needle punctures can eliminate pain (see Pain Management, Chapter 35). The nurse is responsible for preparing the child and family for the tests by doing the following:

- Explaining the significance of each test, particularly why the tests are not all done at one time
- Encouraging parents or another supportive person to be with the child during the procedure
- Allowing the child to play with the equipment on a doll or participate in the actual procedure (e.g., by cleansing the finger with an alcohol swab)

Older children may appreciate the opportunity to observe the blood cells under a microscope or in photographs. This experience is especially important if a serious blood disorder, such as leukemia, is suspected because it serves as a foundation for explaining the pathophysiology of the disorder.

Bone marrow aspiration is not a routine hematological test but is essential for definitive diagnosis of the leukemias, lymphomas, and certain anemias.

NURSING ALERT The following are suggested explanations for teaching children about blood components:

Red blood cells (RBCs)—Carry the oxygen you breathe from your lungs to all parts of your body
White blood cells (WBCs)—Help keep germs from causing infection
Platelets—Small parts of cells that help make bleeding stop by forming a clot (scab) over the hurt area
Plasma—The liquid portion of blood, which has clotting factors that help make bleeding stop

Decrease Tissue Oxygen Needs

Because the basic pathological process in anemia is a decrease in oxygen-carrying capacity, an important nursing responsibility is to assess the child's energy level and minimize excess demands. The child's level of tolerance for activities of daily living and play needs to be assessed and adjustments made to allow as much self-care as possible without undue exertion. During periods of rest, the nurse can take vital signs and observe behaviour to establish a baseline of nonexertion energy expenditure. During periods of activity, the nurse should repeat these measurements and observations to compare them with resting values.

Prevent Complications

Children who are so severely anemic that they are hospitalized may require oxygen to prevent or reduce tissue hypoxia. Because these children are susceptible to infection, every effort should be made to prevent exposure to infectious agents. All the usual precautions need to be taken to prevent infection, such as practising thorough hand hygiene, selecting an appropriate room in a noninfectious area, restricting visitors or hospital personnel with active infection, and maintaining adequate nutrition. The nurse also needs to observe for signs of infection, particularly temperature elevation and leukocytosis.

Iron Deficiency Anemia

While the rate of iron deficiency anemia (IDA) in Canada is low (3.5 to 10%), there are certain Aboriginal populations in which the rate is high (14 to 50%) (Abdullah et al., 2011). Factors associated with an increased prevalence of IDA in these children include high consumption of evaporated milk and cow's milk after 6 months of age, prolonged exclusive breastfeeding (with limited access to other food sources), and *Helicobacter pylori* infection. Other high-risk groups include children from families of low socioeconomic status, children of Asian background, low-birth-weight infants, and children who drink whole cow's milk before 12 months of age (Abdullah et al., 2011). First Nation, Métis, and Inuit infants and children have a prevalence of iron deficiency of 14 to 24% compared to 4 to 5% for non-Aboriginal children (Zlotkin, 2003). Preterm infants are especially at risk because of their reduced fetal iron supply. Adolescents are at risk because of their rapid growth rate combined with possible poor eating habits.

Nurses can use the *Rourke Baby Record* as a tool for evidenced-informed screening and education related to breastfeeding and nutritional guidelines for infants and children (see Additional Resources section at the end of this chapter).

Pathophysiology

Iron deficiency anemia can be caused by any number of factors that decrease the supply of iron, impair its absorption, increase the body's need for iron, or affect the synthesis of Hgb. Although the clinical manifestations and diagnostic evaluation are similar regardless of the cause, the therapeutic and nursing care management depend on the specific reason for the iron deficiency. The following discussion is limited to iron deficiency anemia resulting from inadequate iron in the diet.

During the last trimester of pregnancy, iron is transferred from mother to fetus. Most of the iron is stored in the circulating erythrocytes of the fetus, with the remainder stored in the fetal liver, spleen, and bone marrow. These iron stores are usually adequate for the first 5 to 6 months in a full-term infant but for only 2 to 3 months in preterm infants or multiple births. If dietary iron is not supplied to meet the infant's growth demands after the fetal iron stores are depleted, iron deficiency anemia results. Physiological anemia should not be confused with iron deficiency anemia resulting from nutritional causes.

Although most toddlers with iron deficiency anemia are underweight, many infants are overweight because of excessive milk ingestion (known as milk babies). These children become anemic for two reasons: milk, a poor source of iron, is given almost to the exclusion of solid foods; and 50% of iron-deficient infants fed cow's milk have an increased fecal loss of blood.

Therapeutic Management

After the diagnosis of iron deficiency anemia is made, therapeutic management focuses on increasing the amount of supplemental iron the child receives. This is usually done through dietary counselling and the administration of oral iron supplements.

In formula-fed infants, the most convenient and best sources of supplemental iron are iron-fortified commercial formula and iron-fortified infant cereal. Iron-fortified formula provides a relatively constant and predictable amount of iron and is not associated with an increased incidence of gastrointestinal (GI) symptoms, such as colic, diarrhea, or constipation. Infants younger than 12 months of age should not be given fresh cow's milk because it may increase the risk of GI blood loss occurring from allergy to the milk protein or from GI mucosal damage resulting from a lack of cytochrome iron (**heme** protein) (Abdullah et al., 2011; Richardson, 2007). If GI bleeding is suspected, the child's stool should be guaiac tested on at least four or five occasions to identify any intermittent blood loss.

Dietary addition of iron-rich foods is usually inadequate as the sole treatment of iron deficiency anemia, since the iron is poorly absorbed and thus provides insufficient supplemental quantities of iron. If dietary sources of iron cannot replace body stores, oral iron supplements are prescribed for approximately 3 months. Ferrous iron, more readily absorbed than ferric iron, results in higher Hgb levels. Ascorbic acid (vitamin C) appears to facilitate the absorption of iron and may be given as vitamin C–enriched foods and juices with the iron preparation.

If the Hgb level fails to rise after 1 month of oral therapy, it is important to assess for persistent bleeding, iron malabsorption, noncompliance, improper iron administration, or other causes for the anemia. Parenteral (IV or intramuscular [IM]) iron administration is safe and effective but painful, expensive, and occasionally associated with regional **lymphadenopathy** or allergic reaction (Andrews et al., 2009; McKenzie, 2004). Thus parenteral iron is reserved for children who have iron malabsorption or chronic hemoglobinuria. Transfusions are indicated for the most severe anemia and in cases of serious infection, cardiac dysfunction, or surgical emergency when anaesthesia is required. Packed RBCs (2 to 3 mL/kg), not whole blood, are used to minimize the chance of circulatory overload. Supplemental oxygen is administered when tissue hypoxia is severe.

Prognosis

The prognosis for a child with this condition is very good. However, there is some evidence that, if the iron deficiency anemia is severe and long-standing, cognitive, behavioural, and motor impairment may result. It is not clear whether these results are irreversible with treatment of iron (Abdulla et al., 2011; Burden et al., 2007).

Nursing Care Management

An essential nursing responsibility is instructing parents in the administration of iron. Oral iron should be given as prescribed in two divided doses between meals, when the presence of free hydrochloric acid is greatest, since more iron is absorbed in the acidic environment of the upper GI tract. Citrus fruit or juice taken with the medication aids in absorption.

NURSING ALERT Cow's milk contains substances that bind the iron and interfere with absorption. Iron supplements should not be administered with milk or milk products (Carley, 2003).

An adequate dosage of oral iron turns the stools a tarry green colour. The nurse needs to advise parents of this normally expected change and inquire about its occurrence on follow-up visits. Absence of the greenish black stool may be a clue to poor administration of iron, in either schedule or dosage. Vomiting or diarrhea can occur with iron therapy. If the parents report these symptoms, the iron can be given with meals and the dosage reduced and then gradually increased until tolerated.

Liquid preparations of iron may temporarily stain the teeth. If possible, the medication should be taken through a straw or given through a syringe or medicine dropper placed toward the back of the mouth. Brushing the teeth after administration of the medication lessens the discolouration.

Diet

A primary nursing objective is to prevent nutritional anemia through family education. Exclusively breastfed infants should receive iron supplements by 6 months of age

(Canadian Paediatric Society [CPS], 2005; Chandran & Gelfer, 2006; Richardson, 2007). Preterm infants fed human milk should begin iron supplements by 1 month of age (Abdullah et al., 2011).

For the formula-fed infant, the nurse should discuss with parents the importance of using iron-fortified formula. For all infants, solid foods should be introduced at the appropriate age during the first year of life. Traditionally, cereals are one of the first semisolid foods to be introduced into the infant's diet at approximately 6 months of age (Abdullah et al., 2011; Chandran & Gelfer, 2006; Glader, 2007). The best solid-food source of iron is commercial iron-fortified cereals. It may be difficult at first to teach the infant to accept foods other than milk. The same principles are applied as those for introducing new foods (see Nutrition, Chapter 36), especially feeding the solid food before the milk. Predominantly milk-fed infants rebel against solid foods, and parents need to be cautioned about this and the need to be firm in not relinquishing control to the child. It may require intense problem solving on the part of both the family and the nurse to overcome the child's resistance.

A difficulty encountered in discouraging the parents from feeding milk to the exclusion of other foods is dispelling the popular myth that milk is a "perfect food." Many parents believe that milk is best for the infant and equate the weight gain with a "healthy child" and "good mothering." The nurse can also stress that overweight is not synonymous with good health.

Sickle Cell Anemia

Sickle cell anemia (SCA) is one of a group of diseases collectively termed *hemoglobinopathies*, in which normal adult Hgb (Hgb A [HbA]) is partly or completely replaced by abnormal sickle HgbS (HbS). Sickle cell disease (SCD) includes all the hereditary disorders with clinical, hematological, and pathological features that are related to the presence of HgbS. Even though the term SCD is sometimes used to refer to SCA, this use is incorrect. Other correct terms for SCA are HgbSS disease and *homozygous sickle cell disease*.

The following are the most common forms of SCD:

SCA, the homozygous form of the disease (HgbSS or SS)

Sickle cell–C disease, a **heterozygous** variant of SCD (HgbSC), including both HgbS and HgbC (SC), in which lysine is substituted for glutamic acid at the sixth position of the β-chain

Sickle thalassemia disease, a combination of sickle cell trait and β-thalassemia trait (Sβ-thal); β+ refers to the ability to still produce some normal HbA; β^0 indicates that there is no ability to produce HbA

Of the SCDs, SCA is the most common form in Blacks, followed by sickle cell–C disease and sickle thalassemia. Numerous other sickle syndromes exist when the HbS is paired with other mutant globins.

SCA is found primarily in 1 in 375 births of Blacks and 1 in 1200 births of Latin Americans, with lower incidence in the other ethnic groups (Driscoll, 2007). The incidence of the disease varies in different geographic locations. Among Blacks, the incidence of sickle cell trait is about 9%. In West Africa the incidence is reported to be as high as 40% among native Africans. The high incidence of sickle cell trait in West Africans is believed by some to be the result of selective protection afforded trait carriers against one type of malaria.

The gene that determines the production of HgbS is situated on an autosome and, when present, is always detectable and therefore dominant. Heterozygous persons who have both normal HgbA and abnormal HgbS are said to have *sickle cell trait*. Persons who are homozygous have predominantly HgbS and have SCA. The inheritance pattern is essentially that of an autosomal recessive disorder. Therefore, when both parents have sickle cell trait, there is a 25% chance with each pregnancy of producing an offspring with SCA.

Although the defect is inherited, the sickling phenomenon is usually not apparent until later in infancy because of the presence of fetal Hbg (HgbF). As long as the child has predominantly HgbF, sickling does not occur because there is less HgbS. The newborn with SCA is generally asymptomatic because of the protective effect of HgbF (60 to 80% HgbF), but this rapidly decreases during the first year; thus the child is at risk for sickle cell–related complications (Driscoll, 2007; Heeney & Dover, 2009).

evolve Animation—Sickle Cell Anemia

evolve Case Study—Sickle Cell Anemia

Pathophysiology

The clinical features of SCA are primarily the result of (1) obstruction caused by the sickled RBCs, and (2) increased RBC destruction (Fig. 49-2). The abnormal adhesion, entanglement, and enmeshing of rigid sickle-shaped cells with one another intermittently block the microcirculation, causing vaso-occlusion. The resultant absence of blood flow to adjacent tissues causes local hypoxia, leading to tissue ischemia and infarction (cellular death). Most of the complications seen in SCA can be traced to this process and its impact on various organs of the body. The effect of sickling and infarction on organ structures occurs in the following sequence (Box 49-2):

1. Stasis with enlargement
2. Infarction with ischemia and repeated destruction
3. Replacement with fibrous tissue (scarring)

Clinical Manifestations

The clinical manifestations of SCA vary greatly in severity and frequency. The most acute symptoms of the disease occur during periods of exacerbation called *crises*. There are several types of episodic crises: vaso-occlusive, acute splenic sequestration, aplastic, hyperhemolytic, cerebrovascular accident (CVA) (stroke), chest syndrome, and infection. The crises may occur individually or concomitantly with one or more other crises. The episode may be a *vaso-occlusive crisis*, preferably called a "painful episode," characterized by distal ischemia and pain; *sequestration crisis*, a pooling of blood in the liver and spleen with decreased blood volume and shock; *aplastic crisis*, diminished RBC production resulting in profound anemia; or *hyperhemolytic crisis*, an accelerated rate of RBC destruction characterized by anemia, jaundice, and reticulocytosis.

Another serious complication is acute chest syndrome (ACS), which is clinically similar to pneumonia. It is the presence of a new pulmonary infiltrate and is associated with chest pain, fever, cough, tachypnea, wheezing, and hypoxia. A CVA (stroke) is a sudden and severe complication, often with no related illnesses. Sickled cells block the major blood vessels in the brain, resulting in cerebral infarction, which causes

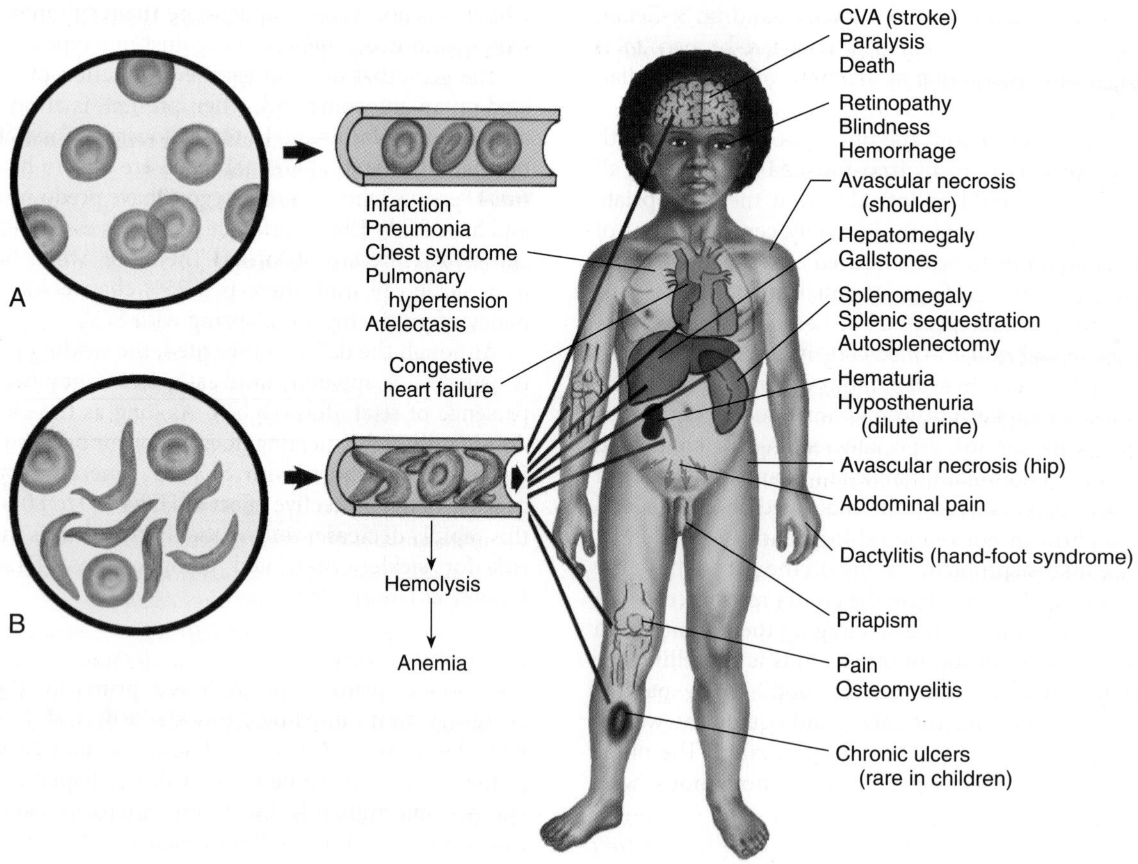

Fig. 49-2 Differences between effects on circulation of normal (**A**) and sickled (**B**) red blood cells with related complications. *CVA*, cerebrovascular accident.

BOX 49-2 Clinical Manifestations of Sickle Cell Anemia

General
Possible growth restriction
Chronic anemia (hemoglobin level of 60 to 90 g/L)
Possible delayed sexual maturation
Marked susceptibility to sepsis

Vaso-Occlusive Crisis
Pain in area(s) of involvement
Manifestations related to ischemia of involved areas
- **Extremities**—Painful swelling of hands and feet (sickle cell dactylitis, or hand-foot syndrome), painful joints
- **Abdomen**—Severe pain resembling acute surgical condition
- **Cerebrum**—Stroke, visual disturbances
- **Chest**—Symptoms resembling pneumonia, protracted episodes of pulmonary disease
- **Liver**—Obstructive jaundice, hepatic coma
- **Kidney**—Hematuria
- **Genitalia**—Priapism (painful, constant penile erection)

Sequestration Crisis
Pooling of large amounts of blood
- Hepatomegaly
- Splenomegaly
- Circulatory collapse

Effects of Chronic Vaso-Occlusive Phenomena
Heart—Cardiomegaly, systolic murmurs
Lungs—Altered pulmonary function, susceptibility to infections, pulmonary insufficiency
Kidneys—Inability to concentrate urine, enuresis, progressive renal failure
Liver—Hepatomegaly, cirrhosis, intrahepatic cholestasis
Spleen—Splenomegaly, susceptibility to infection, functional reduction in splenic activity progressing to autosplenectomy
Eyes—Intraocular abnormalities with visual disturbances; sometimes progressive retinal detachment and blindness
Extremities—Avascular necrosis of hip or shoulder; skeletal deformities, especially lordosis and kyphosis; chronic leg ulcers; susceptibility to osteomyelitis
Central nervous system—Hemiparesis, seizures

variable degrees of neurological impairment. The current treatment for SCD children who have experienced a stroke is chronic transfusion therapy. Repeat CVAs causing progressively greater brain damage occur in approximately 70% of untreated children who have experienced one stroke and do not receive monthly transfusions (Heeney & Dover, 2009).

Diagnostic Evaluation

Ontario is currently the only province offering routine newborn screening for sickle cell disease. At birth the infant has up to 80% of HgbF, which does not carry the defect. Because levels of HgbS are low at birth, Hgb electrophoresis or other tests that measure Hgb concentrations are indicated. Nurses can use antenatal documents to identify populations at risk. Early diagnosis (before 3 months of age) enables initiation of appropriate interventions to minimize complications. The family should be taught to administer prophylactic antibiotics, to identify early signs of infection, and to seek medical therapy as soon as possible.

If SCA is not diagnosed in early infancy, it is likely to manifest symptoms during the toddler and preschool years. SCA is occasionally first diagnosed during a crisis that follows an acute respiratory tract or GI infection. Routine hematological tests are done to evaluate the anemia. Several specific tests detect the presence of the abnormal Hgb in the heterozygote or the homozygote. For screening purposes the sickle-turbidity test (Sickledex) is frequently used because it can be performed on blood from a finger stick and yields accurate results in 3 minutes. However, if the test is positive, Hgb electrophoresis is necessary to distinguish between children with the trait and those with the disease. Hgb electrophoresis ("fingerprinting" of the protein) is an accurate, rapid, and specific test for detecting the homozygous and heterozygous forms of the disease and the percentages of the various types of Hgb.

Therapeutic Management

The aims of therapy are to (1) prevent the sickling phenomena, which are responsible for the pathological sequelae; and (2) treat the medical emergencies of sickle cell crisis. The successful achievement of the aims depends on prompt nursing interventions, medical therapies, patient and family preventive measures, and use of innovative treatments.

Medical management of a crisis is usually directed toward supportive and symptomatic treatment. The main objectives are to provide (1) rest to minimize energy expenditure and oxygen use, (2) hydration through oral and IV therapy, (3) electrolyte replacement because hypoxia results in metabolic acidosis, which also promotes sickling, (4) analgesics for the severe pain from vaso-occlusion, (5) blood replacement to treat anemia and reduce the viscosity of the sickled blood, and (6) antibiotics to treat any existing infection.

Administration of pneumococcal, meningococcal, and *Haemophilus influenzae* type b conjugate vaccines are recommended for these children because of their susceptibility to infection as a result of a functional asplenia. In addition to routine immunizations, the child with SCD should receive an annual influenza vaccination. Oral penicillin prophylaxis is also recommended by 2 months of age to reduce the chance of pneumococcal sepsis (see Evidence-Informed Practice box) (Public Health Agency of Canada [PHAC], 2006a; Redding-Lallinger & Knoll, 2006).

Oxygen therapy is of little therapeutic value unless the patient is hypoxic (Heeney & Dover, 2009). Oxygen is usually not effective in reversing sickling or reducing pain because the oxygen is unable to reach the enmeshed sickled erythrocytes in clogged vessels (Perkins, 2001). In addition, prolonged administration can depress bone marrow, further aggravating the anemia (Heeney & Dover, 2009).

Exchange transfusion, which reduces the number of circulating sickle cells and slows down the vicious circle of hypoxia, thrombosis, tissue ischemia, and injury, has been successful. The procedure is sometimes advocated as a possible preventive technique. A transcranial Doppler (TCD) test identifies the child with SCD who is at high risk for developing a CVA by monitoring the intracranial vascular flow (Driscoll, 2007; Heeney & Dover, 2009). The TCD is performed annually on children from 2 to 16 years of age. If the TCD is abnormal, the recommended treatment is chronic transfusion therapy (Armstrong-Wells et al., 2009; DeBaun & Vichinsky, 2007). However, multiple transfusions carry the risk of transmission of viral infection, hyperviscosity, transfusion reactions, alloimmunization, and hemosiderosis (Driscoll, 2007; Redding-Lallinger & Knoll, 2006). After a CVA, blood transfusions are usually given every 3 to 4 weeks to help prevent a repeat stroke. To reduce iron overload from chronic transfusion therapy, chelation therapy may be started (see p. 1511).

In children with recurrent life-threatening splenic sequestration, splenectomy may be a lifesaving measure. However, the spleen usually atrophies on its own through progressive fibrotic changes (functional asplenia) by 6 years of age. Prophylactic penicillin postsplenectomy and pneumococcal vaccines have decreased the incidence of pneumococcal sepsis. Packed RBC transfusions are recommended for treatment of splenic sequestration and stroke and preoperatively for most surgical procedures in the child with SCD.

The most frequent problem for patients with SCA is vaso-occlusive pain. The chronic nature of this pain can greatly affect the child's development. *Priapism* (continuous or intermittent) is defined as painful erection of the penis. As a vaso-occlusive crisis, the priapism event is caused by sickling in sinusoids of the corpora cavernosa and is treated with aspiration of the corpora cavernosa only when conventional approaches fail (Redding-Lallinger & Knoll, 2006). A multidisciplinary approach is best for vaso-occlusive pain management that includes pharmacological treatment, hydration, physiotherapy, and complementary treatment (e.g., prayer, spiritual healing, massage, herbs, relaxation, acupuncture, and biofeedback) (Redding-Lallinger & Knoll, 2006; Yoon & Black, 2006).

For mild to moderate pain, ibuprofen or acetaminophen (Tylenol) is used initially. If these medications are not effective alone, codeine can be added. The dosages of both medications are titrated (adjusted) to a therapeutic level. Opioids such as immediate- and sustained-release morphine, oxycodone, hydromorphone (Dilaudid), and methadone are administered intravenously or orally for severe pain and given around the clock. Patient-controlled analgesia (PCA) has been used

EVIDENCE-INFORMED PRACTICE Sickle Cell Anemia and Penicillin Prophylaxis

Ask the Question

In children with sickle cell anemia, does prophylaxis with penicillin prevent pneumococcal infection?

Search for Evidence

Search Strategies

Search selection criteria included English-language publication within the past 25 years, research-based articles (level 3 or lower), and child populations.

Databases Used

PubMed, Cochrane Collaboration, MD Consult

Critically Analyze the Evidence

Administration of oral prophylactic penicillin was compared with the 14-valent pneumococcal vaccine in preventing pneumococcal infection in 242 children between the ages of 6 months and 3 years with homozygous sickle cell disease. In the first 5 years of the trial, there were 11 pneumococcal infections in the pneumococcal vaccine group and higher infection rates in those given the vaccine before 1 year of age. No pneumococcal isolates were found in the group receiving penicillin, although four pneumococcal isolates were found in this group within 1 year of stopping the penicillin prophylaxis at age 3 years. This study supported the use of penicillin prophylaxis to prevent pneumococcal infection in children younger than 3 years of age (John et al., 1984).

In a multicentre, randomized, double-blind, placebo-controlled clinical trial, 105 children received penicillin twice daily; a control group of 110 children received a placebo twice daily. The trial was terminated 8 months early when an 84% reduction in the incidence of pneumococcal infections was observed in the group treated with penicillin compared with the placebo group. There were no deaths in the penicillin group, but three deaths from infection occurred in the placebo group. Researchers stressed the importance of screening children during the neonatal period and prescribing prophylactic penicillin to decrease the morbidity and mortality associated with pneumococcal infection (Gaston et al., 1986).

Zarkowsky and colleagues (1986) conducted a retrospective analysis of 178 episodes of bacteremia in children with sickle hemoglobinopathies that occurred during 13,771 patient-years of follow-up ($N = 3451$). The predominant pathogen in patients younger than 6 years of age was *Streptococcus pneumoniae* (66%), and gram-negative organisms were responsible for 50% of the bacteremias in patients 6 years and older. The incidence of pneumococcal bacteremia in children with sickle cell anemia younger than 3 years of age was 6.1 events per 100 patient-years. The results of this study supported prophylactic administration of penicillin for prevention of pneumococcal bacteremia in children younger than 3 years of age.

A cohort study of 315 patients with homozygous sickle cell disease who lived in Jamaica was conducted between June 1973 and December 1981. The patients were divided into three groups to determine whether interventions such as penicillin prophylaxis, parental education in early diagnosis of acute splenic sequestration, and close monitoring in a sickle cell clinic improved survival. A significant decline in deaths from acute splenic sequestration and pneumococcal septicemia and meningitis was found. The research indicated that early detection of sickle cell disease and prophylactic measures could significantly reduce deaths associated with homozygous sickle cell disease (Lee et al., 1995).

In a retrospective longitudinal study conducted from January 1995 through December 1999, 261 children under 4 years of age with sickle cell disease who did not have adequate health insurance were found to have received inadequate refills for antibiotic prophylaxis that placed them at increased risk of developing pneumococcal infection. Study findings showed that an increased number of outpatient visits for preventive care was associated with improved dispensing of prophylactic antibiotic refills (Sox et al., 2003).

Riddington and Owusu-Ofori (2002) conducted a systematic review of randomized controlled trials evaluating the effectiveness of prophylactic antibiotic administration in preventing pneumococcal infection in children with sickle cell disease. The review of published research found that penicillin prophylaxis significantly reduced the risk of pneumococcal infection in children with homozygous sickle cell disease with minimal adverse reactions.

Apply the Evidence: Nursing Implications

The evidence demonstrated that penicillin prophylaxis significantly reduces the risk of pneumococcal infection in children with sickle cell anemia. The epidemiological studies strongly suggest that all children with sickle cell anemia should be started on prophylactic penicillin at 2 months of age. Parents and children with sickle cell anemia should be instructed in the importance of taking the prophylactic penicillin twice daily and seeking medical attention immediately for acute illness, especially if the temperature exceeds 38.3°C, regardless of the use of prophylaxis.

References

Gaston, M. H., et al. (1986). Prophylaxis with oral penicillin in children with sickle cell anemia: A randomized trial. *New England Journal of Medicine, 314*(25), 1593–1599.

John, A. B., et al. (1984). Prevention of pneumococcal infection in children with homozygous sickle cell disease. *British Medical Journal, 288*(6430), 1567–1570.

Lee, A., et al. (1995). Improved survival in homozygous sickle cell disease: Lessons from a cohort study. *British Medical Journal, 311*(7020), 1600–1602.

Riddington, C., & Owusu-Ofori, S. (2002). *Prophylactic antibiotics for preventing pneumococcal infection in children with sickle cell disease.* Retrieved from http://www.cochrane.org/reviews/en/ab003427.html.

Sox, C. M., et al. (2003). Provision of pneumococcal prophylaxis for publicly insured children with sickle cell disease. *Journal of the American Medical Association, 290*(8), 1057–1061.

Zarkowsky, H. S., et al. (1986). Bacteremia in sickle hemoglobinopathies. *Journal of Pediatrics, 109*(4), 579–585.

successfully for sickle cell–related pain. PCA reinforces the patient's role and responsibility in managing the pain and provides flexibility in dealing with pain, which may vary in severity over time (see Pain Management, Chapter 35).

Prognosis

The prognosis varies, but most patients live into the fifth decade. Most of the time, children are without symptoms and participate in normal activities without restrictions. The greatest risk is usually in children younger than 5 years of age, and the majority of deaths in these children are caused by overwhelming infection. Consequently, SCA is a chronic illness with a potentially terminal outcome. Physical and sexual maturation are delayed in adolescents with SCA. Although adults achieve normal height, weight, and sexual function, the delay may present problems to the adolescent (Heeney & Dover, 2009; Redding-Lallinger & Knoll, 2006).

SCD individuals with higher levels of HgbF tend to have a milder disease with fewer complications than those with lower levels (Anderson, 2006; Driscoll, 2007). Hydroxyurea is a Health Canada *Food and Drug Act*–approved medication that increases the production of HgbF, reduces endothelial adhesion of sickle cells, and improves the sickle cell hydration (DeBaun & Vichinsky, 2007; Pack-Mabien & Haynes, 2009). Long-term follow-up of patients taking hydroxyurea alone revealed a 40% reduction in mortality and decreased frequency of vaso-occlusive crisis, ACS, hospital admissions, and need for transfusions, thus making SCD crises milder (Anderson, 2006; Steinberg et al., 2003). Pediatric studies have shown that hydroxyurea can be safely used in children (Miller et al., 2001; Zimmerman et al., 2004).

Hematopoietic stem cell transplantation (HSCT) offers the only cure for some children, although the mortality rate is approximately 8% and graft failures after transplantation range from 9 to 14% (DeBaun & Vichinsky, 2007; Driscoll, 2007) (see p. 1532).

Nursing Care Management

Educate the Family and Child

Family education begins with an explanation of the disease and its consequences. After this explanation, the most important issues to teach the family are to (1) seek early intervention for problems such as fever of 38.5°C or greater, (2) give penicillin as ordered, (3) recognize signs and symptoms of splenic sequestration and respiratory problems that can lead to hypoxia, and (4) treat the child normally. The nurse needs to convey to the family that the child is normal but can get sick in ways that other children cannot.

The nurse should emphasize the importance of adequate hydration to prevent sickling and to delay the adhesion-stasis-thrombosis-ischemia cycle in a crisis. It is not sufficient to advise parents to "force fluids" or "encourage drinking." They need specific instructions on how many daily glasses or bottles of fluid are required. Many foods are also a source of fluid, particularly soups, flavoured ice pops, ice cream, sherbet, gelatin, and puddings.

Increased fluids combined with impaired kidney function result in the problem of enuresis. Parents who are unaware of this fact frequently use the usual measures to discourage bed-wetting, such as limiting fluids at night, and may resort to punishment and shame to force bladder control. Enuresis is treated as a complication of the disease, such as joint pain or some other symptom, to alleviate parental pressure on the child.

Promote Supportive Therapies During Crises

The success of many of the medical therapies relies heavily on nursing implementation. Management of pain is an especially difficult problem and often involves experimenting with various analgesics, including opioids, and schedules before relief is achieved. Unfortunately, these children tend to be undermedicated, resulting in their "clock watching" and demands for additional doses sooner than might be expected. Often this incorrectly raises suspicions of drug addiction, when in fact the problem is one of improper dosage (see Family-Centred Teaching box). In choosing and scheduling analgesics, the goal should be *prevention* of pain.

NURSING ALERT Advise parents to be particularly alert to situations such as hot weather in which dehydration may be a possibility and to recognize early signs of reduced intake such as decreased urinary output (e.g., fewer wet diapers) and increased thirst.

Any pain program should be combined with psychological support to help the child deal with the depression, anxiety, and fear that may accompany the disease. This includes regular visits with the child to discuss any concerns during the hospitalization and positive reinforcement of coping skills, such as successful methods of dealing with the pain and compliance with treatment prescriptions. To reduce the negative connotation associated with the term *crisis*, it is best to say *pain episode*.

Frequently, heat to the affected area is soothing. Cold compresses should not be applied because this enhances sickling and **vasoconstriction**. Bed rest is usually well tolerated during a crisis, although actual rest depends greatly on pain alleviation and organized schedules of nursing care. Some activity, particularly passive range-of-motion exercises, is beneficial to promote circulation. Usually the best course of action is to let children dictate their activity tolerance.

If blood transfusions or exchange transfusions are given, the nurse has the responsibility of observing for signs of transfusion reaction (see Table 49-5). Because hypervolemia from

FAMILY-CENTRED TEACHING

Fear of Addiction

Although the pain during a sickle cell crisis is usually severe and opioids are needed, many families fear that their child will become addicted to the narcotic. Unfortunately, misinformed health care providers may foster this unfounded fear, which results in needless suffering. Very few children who receive opioids for severe pain become behaviourally addicted to the drug (Lynch & Lynch, 2011). Families and older children, especially adolescents, need to be reassured that opioids are medically indicated, high doses may be needed, and children rarely become addicted.

too-rapid transfusion can increase the workload of the heart, the nurse also needs to be alert to signs of cardiac failure.

In splenic sequestration the size of the spleen is gently measured by abdominal palpation (see Abdomen, Chapter 34). The nurse should be aware of spleen size because increasing splenomegaly is an ominous sign. A decreasing spleen size denotes response to therapy. Vital signs and blood pressure are also closely monitored for impending shock. Anemia is typically not a presenting complication in vaso-occlusive crises but is a critical problem in other types of crises. The nurse needs to monitor for evidence of increasing anemia and institute appropriate nursing interventions (see p. 1509). Oxygen is not beneficial in vaso-occlusive episodes unless hypoxemia is present (Heeney & Dover, 2009). It does not reverse sickled RBCs, and if used in the nonhypoxic patient, it decreases **erythropoiesis** (Khoury & Grimsley, 1995). Because prolonged use of oxygen can aggravate the anemia, signs of lack of therapeutic benefit, such as restlessness, increased pallor, and continued pain, are reported.

Intake, especially of IV fluids, and output need to be recorded. The child's weight should be taken on admission to serve as a baseline for evaluating hydration. Because diuresis can result in electrolyte loss, the nurse also should observe for signs of hypokalemia and be familiar with normal serum electrolyte values to report changes.

Recognize Other Complications

Nurses also need to be aware of the signs of ACS and stroke, both potentially fatal complications. It is essential to educate parents about these symptoms.

Support the Family

Families need the opportunity to discuss their feelings about transmitting a potentially fatal, chronic illness to their child. Because of the widely publicized prognosis for children with SCA, many parents express their prevalent fear of the child's death. Three manifestations of SCD that may appear in the first 2 years of life—dactylitis or painful episode, severe anemia (70 g/L), and elevated WBC count—can be predictors of disease severity (DeBaun & Vichinsky, 2007; Ohls & Christensen, 2007). However, nursing care for the family should be the same as for any family with a child with a life-threatening illness. The siblings' reactions, the stress on the marital relationship, and the childrearing attitudes displayed toward the child should be given particular emphasis (see Chapter 31). Several resources are available to the family with a sickling disorder (see Additional Resources section at the end of this chapter).

β-Thalassemia (Cooley Anemia)

The term *thalassemia*, which is derived from the Greek word *thalassa*, meaning "sea," is applied to a variety of inherited blood disorders characterized by deficiencies in the rate of production of specific globin chains in Hgb. The name appropriately refers to descendants of or people living near the Mediterranean Sea, who have the highest incidence of the disease (i.e., Italians, Greeks, and Syrians). Evidence suggests that the high incidence of the disorders among these groups is a result of the selective advantage the trait confers in relation to malaria, as is postulated in SCD. However, the disorder has a wide geographic distribution, probably as a result of genetic migration through intermarriage or possibly as a result of spontaneous mutation.

β-Thalassemia is the most common of the thalassemias and occurs in four forms:

- Two heterozygous forms: *thalassemia minor*, an asymptomatic silent carrier; and *thalassemia trait*, which produces a mild microcytic anemia
- *Thalassemia intermedia*, which is manifested as splenomegaly and moderate to severe anemia
- A homozygous form, *thalassemia major* (also known as *Cooley's anemia*), which results in a severe anemia that would lead to cardiac failure and death in early childhood without transfusion support

Pathophysiology

Normal postnatal Hgb is composed of two α- and two β-polypeptide chains. In β-thalassemia there is a partial or complete deficiency in the synthesis of the β-chain of the Hgb molecule. Consequently, there is a compensatory increase in the synthesis of α-chains, and γ-chain production remains activated, resulting in defective Hgb formation. This unbalanced polypeptide unit is very unstable; when it disintegrates, it damages RBCs, causing severe anemia.

To compensate for the hemolytic process, an overabundance of erythrocytes is formed unless the bone marrow is suppressed by transfusion therapy. Excess iron from **hemolysis** of supplemental RBCs in transfusions and from the rapid destruction of defective cells is stored in various organs (*hemosiderosis*).

Diagnostic Evaluation

The onset of thalassemia major may be insidious and not recognized until the latter half of infancy. The clinical effects of thalassemia major are primarily attributable to (1) defective synthesis of HgbA, (2) structurally impaired RBCs, and (3) the shortened lifespan of erythrocytes (Box 49-3).

Hematological studies reveal the characteristic changes in RBCs (i.e., microcytosis, hypochromia, anisocytosis, poikilocytosis, target cells, and basophilic stippling of various stages). Low Hgb and Hct levels are seen in severe anemia, although they are typically lower than the reduction in RBC count because of the proliferation of immature erythrocytes. Hgb electrophoresis confirms the diagnosis, and radiographs of involved bones reveal characteristic findings.

Therapeutic Management

The objective of supportive therapy is to maintain sufficient Hgb levels to prevent bone marrow expansion and the resulting bony deformities and to provide sufficient RBCs to support normal growth and normal physical activity. Transfusions are the foundation of medical management. Recent studies have evaluated the benefits of maintaining the child's Hgb level above 95 g/L, a goal that may require transfusions as often as every 3 to 5 weeks. The advantages of this therapy include (1) improved physical and psychological well-being because of the ability to participate in normal activities, (2) decreased cardiomegaly and **hepatosplenomegaly,** (3) fewer bone changes, (4) normal or near-normal growth and development until puberty, and (5) fewer infections.

BOX 49-3 Clinical Manifestations of β-Thalassemia

Anemia (Before Diagnosis)
Pallor
Unexplained fever
Poor feeding
Enlarged spleen or liver

Progressive Anemia
Signs of chronic hypoxia
- Headache
- Precordial and bone pain
- Decreased exercise tolerance
- Listlessness
- Anorexia

Other Features
Small stature
Delayed sexual maturation
Bronzed, freckled complexion (if not receiving chelation therapy)

Bone Changes (Older Children If Untreated)
Enlarged head
Prominent frontal and parietal bosses
Prominent malar eminences
Flat or depressed bridge of the nose
Enlarged maxilla
Protrusion of the lip and upper central incisors and eventual malocclusion
Generalized osteoporosis

One of the potential complications of frequent blood transfusions is iron overload. Because the body has no effective means of eliminating the excess iron, the mineral is deposited in body tissues. To minimize the development of hemosiderosis, the oral iron chelator deferasirox has been shown to be equivalent to *deferoxamine (Desferal)*, a parenteral iron-chelating agent, and more tolerable by patients and families (Morris, Singer, & Walters, 2006; Okpala, 2005). Deferoxamine is given intravenously or subcutaneously at home via a portable infusion pump over a period of 8 to 10 hours (usually during sleep) for 5 to 7 days a week. Significant liver fibrosis, cardiac dysfunction, and growth impairment may be prevented if chelation therapy is adequate during childhood (Cunningham et al., 2009).

In some children with severe splenomegaly who demonstrate increased transfusion requirements, a splenectomy may be necessary to decrease the disabling effects of abdominal pressure and to increase the lifespan of supplemental RBCs. Over time, the spleen may accelerate the rate of RBC destruction and thus increase transfusion requirements. After a splenectomy, children generally require fewer transfusions, although the basic defect in Hgb synthesis remains unaffected. A major postsplenectomy complication is severe and overwhelming infection. Therefore, these children continue to receive prophylactic antibiotics with close medical supervision for many years and should receive the pneumococcal and meningococcal vaccines in addition to the regularly scheduled immunizations.

NURSING ALERT Ensure that the family and patient understand the need to notify the health care provider of all fevers of 38.5°C or greater because of the risk of sepsis in a child with asplenia.

Prognosis

Most children treated with blood transfusion and early chelation therapy survive well into adulthood. The most common cause of death is iron-induced heart disease, multiple organ failure, postsplenectomy sepsis, liver disease, and malignancy (Cunningham et al., 2009). HSCT has the best results in the least symptomatic pediatric patients, with an 80% rate of complication-free survival (Lucarelli & Gaziev, 2008; Morris, Singer, & Walters, 2006; Richardson, 2007).

Nursing Care Management

The objectives of nursing care are to (1) promote compliance with transfusion and chelation therapy, (2) assist the child in coping with the anxiety-provoking treatments and the effects of the illness, (3) foster the child's and family's adjustment to a chronic illness, and (4) observe for complications of multiple blood transfusions. Basic to each of these goals is explaining to parents and older children the defect responsible for the disorder, its effect on RBCs, and the potential effects of untreated iron overload (such as diabetes and heart disease). Because the prevalence of this condition is high among families of Mediterranean descent, the nurse also needs to inquire about the family's previous knowledge about thalassemia. All families with a child with thalassemia should be tested for the trait and referred for genetic counselling.

As with any chronic illness, the family's needs must be met for optimal adjustment to the stresses imposed by the disorder (see Chapter 41). Sources of information for the family include the Cooley's Anemia Foundation and the Thalassemia Foundation of Canada (see Additional Resources section at the end of this chapter). Genetic counselling for the parents and fertile offspring is mandatory, and both prenatal diagnosis using amniocentesis at 20 weeks of gestation or fetal blood sampling at 10 weeks and screening for thalassemia trait are available.

Aplastic Anemia

Aplastic anemia (AA) refers to a bone marrow failure condition in which the formed elements of the blood are simultaneously depressed. The peripheral blood smear demonstrates **pancytopenia** or the triad of profound anemia, leukopenia, and thrombocytopenia. *Hypoplastic anemia* is characterized by a profound depression of RBCs but normal or slightly decreased WBCs and platelets.

Etiology

AA can be primary (congenital, or present at birth) or secondary (acquired). The best-known congenital disorder of which AA is an outstanding feature is *Fanconi syndrome*, a rare hereditary disorder characterized by pancytopenia, hypoplasia of the bone marrow, and patchy brown discolouration of the skin resulting from the deposit of melanin and associated with multiple congenital anomalies of the musculoskeletal and genitourinary systems. The syndrome appears to be inherited as an autosomal recessive trait with varying penetrance; thus affected siblings may demonstrate several different combinations of defects.

Several etiological factors contribute to the development of acquired hypoplastic anemia; however, most of the cases are considered idiopathic (Box 49-4). Acquired AA is classified as either severe acquired AA or moderate acquired AA. The following discussion focuses on severe acquired AA, which carries a poorer prognosis and follows a more rapidly fatal course than the primary types.

Diagnostic Evaluation

The onset of clinical manifestations, which include anemia, leukopenia, and decreased platelet count, is usually insidious. Definitive diagnosis is determined from bone marrow aspiration, which demonstrates the conversion of red bone marrow to yellow, fatty bone marrow. *Severe AA* is defined as less than 25% bone marrow cellularity with at least two of the following findings: absolute **granulocyte** count less than 0.5×10^9/L, platelet count less than 20×10^9/L, and absolute **reticulocyte** count less than 1 to 2% (Hord, 2007). *Moderate AA* is defined as more than 25% bone marrow cellularity with the presence of mild or moderate cytopenia (Shimamura & Guinan, 2003).

Therapeutic Management

The objectives of treatment are based on the recognition that the underlying disease process is failure of the bone marrow to carry out its **hematopoietic** functions. Therapy is directed at restoring function to the marrow and involves two main approaches: (1) immunosuppressive therapy to remove the presumed immunological functions that prolong aplasia or (2) replacement of the bone marrow through transplantation. Bone marrow transplantation is the treatment of choice for severe AA when a suitable donor exists (see p. 1532).

Antilymphocyte globulin (ALG) or antithymocyte globulin (ATG) and cyclosporin are the principal medication treatments used for AA. The rationale for using ATG is based on the theory that AA may be a result of autoimmunity. ATG and cyclosporine suppress T cell–dependent autoimmune responses but do not cause bone marrow suppression. Cyclosporine is administered orally for several weeks to months. ATG usually is administrated intravenously over 12 to 16 hours for 4 days, after a test dose to check for hypersensitivity. A course may be repeated, depending on the reduction in circulating **lymphocytes** and the patient's response. Because of the hypersensitivity response associated with ATG (i.e., fever, chills, myalgias), methylprednisolone is given intravenously to prevent these adverse effects. Colony-stimulating factor (CSF) and granulocyte-macrophage colony–stimulating factor (GM-CSF) given parenterally may be used to enhance bone marrow production. Androgens may be used with ATG to stimulate erythropoiesis if the AA is unresponsive to initial therapies.

HSCT should be considered early in the course of the disease if a compatible donor can be found. Transplantation is more successful when performed before multiple transfusions have sensitized the child to leukocyte and human leukocyte antigens (HLAs). HSCT is associated with an 85% survival rate in untransfused patients compared with a 70% survival rate in transfused patients (Marsh, 2005; Young, Calado, & Scheinberg, 2006).

BOX 49-4 Common Causes of Acquired Aplastic Anemia

- Human parvovirus infection, hepatitis, or overwhelming infection
- Irradiation
- Immune disorders such as eosinophilic fasciitis and hypoimmunoglobulinemia
- Medications such as certain chemotherapeutic agents, anticonvulsants, and antibiotics
- Industrial and household chemicals, including benzene and its derivatives, which are found in petroleum products, dyes, paint remover, shellac, and lacquers
- Infiltration and replacement of myeloid elements, such as in leukemia or the lymphomas
- Idiopathic (In most cases no identifiable precipitating cause can be found.)

Nursing Care Management

The care of the child with AA is similar to that of the child with leukemia (see p. 1519)—specifically, preparing the child and family for the diagnostic and therapeutic procedures, preventing complications from the severe pancytopenia, and providing emotional support in the face of a potentially fatal outcome. Information and support are available from the Aplastic Anemia and Myelodysplasia Association of Canada (http://www.aamac.ca).

Because the aspects of nursing care are discussed in the section on leukemia, only the exceptions are presented here. The drug ATG is usually administered by way of a central vein. If not, vigilant care must be directed to the IV infusion to prevent extravasation. Meticulous care of the venous access is essential because of the child's susceptibility to infection. CSFs are usually given by subcutaneous injection over several days. Chemotherapeutic agents have been reported in the treatment of the relapsed patient with AA after ATG and CSF therapy. Many of the adverse effects associated with chemotherapy, such as nausea and vomiting, alopecia, and mucositis, are experienced by children receiving treatment for AA. Specialized care is required for children who have HSCT (see p. 1532).

Defects in Hemostasis

Hemostasis is the process that stops bleeding when a blood vessel is injured. Vascular and plasma clotting factors, as well as platelets, are required. A complex system of clotting, anticlotting, and clot breakdown (*fibrinolysis*) mechanisms exists in equilibrium to ensure clot formation only in the presence of blood vessel injury and to limit the clotting process to the site of vessel wall injury. Dysfunction in these systems leads to bleeding or abnormal clotting. Although the coagulation process is complex, clotting depends on three factors: (1) vascular influence, (2) platelet role, and (3) clotting factors.

Hemophilia

The term *hemophilia* refers to a group of bleeding disorders in which there is a deficiency of one of the factors necessary for coagulation of the blood. Although the symptomatology is similar regardless of which clotting factor is deficient, the identification of specific factor deficiencies allows definitive treatment with replacement agents.

In about 80% of all cases of hemophilia, the inheritance pattern is demonstrated as X-linked recessive. The two most common forms of the disorder are factor VIII deficiency (hemophilia A, or classic hemophilia) and factor IX deficiency (hemophilia B, or Christmas disease). Von Willebrand disease (vWD) is another hereditary bleeding disorder characterized by a deficiency, abnormality, or absence of the protein called von Willebrand factor (vWF) and a deficiency of factor VIII. Unlike hemophilia, vWD affects both males and females. The following discussion is primarily concerned with factor VIII deficiency, which accounts for 80 to 85% of all hemophilia cases.

Pathophysiology

The basic defect of hemophilia A is a deficiency of factor VIII (antihemophilic factor [AHF]). AHF is produced by the liver and is necessary for the formation of thromboplastin in phase I of blood coagulation. The less AHF found in the blood, the more severe the disease. Individuals with hemophilia have two of the three factors required for coagulation: vascular influence and platelets. Therefore, they may bleed for longer periods but not at a faster rate.

Bleeding into subcutaneous and IM tissue is common. *Hemarthrosis*, which is bleeding into a joint space, is the most frequent type of internal bleeding. Bony changes and crippling deformities occur after repeated bleeding episodes over several years. Signs of hemarthrosis are swelling, warmth, redness, pain, and loss of movement. Bleeding in the neck, mouth, or thorax is serious because the airway can become obstructed. Intracranial hemorrhage can have fatal consequences and is one of the major causes of death. Hemorrhage anywhere along the GI tract can lead to anemia, and bleeding into the retroperitoneal cavity is especially hazardous because of the large space for blood to accumulate. Hematomas in the spinal cord can cause paralysis.

Diagnostic Evaluation

Overt, prolonged hemorrhage is readily apparent; bleeding into tissues is less apparent (Box 49-5). The diagnosis is usually made from a history of bleeding episodes, evidence of X-linked inheritance (only one third of the cases are new mutations), and laboratory findings. The tests specific for hemophilia plasma depend on specific factors for a reaction to occur, such as the partial thromboplastin time (PTT). Specific determination of factor deficiencies requires assay procedures normally performed in specialized laboratories. Carrier detection is possible in classic hemophilia using deoxyribonucleic acid (DNA) testing and is an important consideration in families in which female offspring may have inherited the trait.

BOX 49-5 Clinical Manifestations of Hemophilia

- Prolonged bleeding anywhere from or in the body
- Hemorrhage from any trauma—Loss of deciduous teeth, circumcision, cuts, epistaxis, injections
- Excessive bruising, even from a slight injury such as a fall
- Subcutaneous and intramuscular hemorrhages
- Hemarthrosis (bleeding into the joint cavities), especially the knees, ankles, and elbows
- Hematomas—Pain, swelling, and limited motion
- Spontaneous hematuria

evolve Animation—Hemophilia A

Therapeutic Management

The primary therapy for hemophilia is replacement of the missing clotting factor. The products available are factor VIII concentrate from pooled plasma or a genetically engineered recombinant, to be reconstituted with sterile water immediately before use, and DDAVP (1-deamino-8-d-arginine vasopressin), a synthetic form of vasopressin that increases plasma factor VIII and vWF levels and is the treatment of choice in mild hemophilia and vWD if the child shows an appropriate response. DDAVP is not effective in the treatment of severe hemophilia A, severe vWD, or any form of hemophilia B. Vigorous therapy is instituted to prevent chronic crippling effects from joint bleeding.

Other medications may be included in the therapy plan, depending on the source of the hemorrhage. Corticosteroids are given for hematuria, acute hemarthrosis, and chronic synovitis. Nonsteroidal anti-inflammatory drugs (NSAIDs), such as ibuprofen, are effective in relieving pain caused by synovitis; however, they must be used with caution because they inhibit platelet function (Curry, 2004; National Hemophilia Foundation, Bleeding Disorders Information Center, 2006). Oral administration or local application of ε-aminocaproic acid (Amicar) prevents clot destruction; however, its use is limited to mouth or trauma surgery, and a dose of factor concentrate must be given first.

A regular program of exercise and physiotherapy is an important aspect of management. Physical activity within reasonable limits strengthens muscles around joints and may decrease the number of spontaneous bleeding episodes.

Treatment without delay results in more rapid recovery and a decreased likelihood of complications; therefore most children are treated at home. The family needs to be taught the technique of venipuncture and to administer the AHF to children older than 2 to 3 years of age. The child learns the procedure for self-administration at 8 to 12 years of age. Home treatment is highly successful; and the rewards, in addition to the immediacy, are less disruption of family life, fewer school or work days missed, and enhancement of the child's self-esteem and independence.

Primary prophylaxis in hemophilia patients has proved to be effective in preventing bleeding complications by administrating periodic factor replacement. Primary prophylaxis involves the infusion of factor VIII concentrate on a regular basis before the onset of joint damage. Secondary prophylaxis involves the infusion of factor VIII concentrate on a regular basis after the child experiences his or her first joint bleed. The infusions are given three times a week. Aggressive factor replacement may be a cost-effective alternative to primary prophylaxis. This involves the infusion of a high dose of factor VIII concentrate when a joint bleed occurs, followed by 2 days of more standard doses of factor VIII concentrate, with consideration of additional treatment every other day for one week (Scott & Montgomery, 2007).

Prognosis

Although there is no cure for hemophilia, its symptoms can be controlled, and its potentially crippling deformities greatly reduced or even avoided. Today many children with hemophilia function with minimal or no joint damage. They are normal children with an average life expectancy in every respect but one: they have a tendency to bleed, which is a significant inconvenience but not necessarily a life-threatening event.

Gene therapy may prove to be a treatment option in the future. This therapy involves introducing a working copy of the factor VIII gene into a patient who has a flawed copy of the gene. Problems exist with appropriate selection of the **vector,** identification of the cell for gene expression, and control of side effects (Montgomery et al., 2009).

evolve Critical Thinking Exercise—Bleeding

Nursing Care Management

The earlier a bleeding episode is recognized, the more effectively it can be treated. Signs that indicate internal bleeding are especially important to recognize. Children are aware of internal bleeding and are reliable in telling the examiner where an internal bleed is. In addition to the manifestations described (see Box 49-5), the nurse needs to maintain a high level of suspicion when a child with hemophilia demonstrates signs such as headache, slurred speech, loss of consciousness (from cerebral bleeding), and black tarry stools (from GI bleeding).

Prevent Bleeding

The goal of the prevention of bleeding episodes is directed toward decreasing the risk of injury. Prevention of bleeding episodes is geared mostly toward appropriate exercises to strengthen muscles and joints and to allow age-appropriate activity. During infancy and toddlerhood the normal acquisition of motor skills creates innumerable opportunities for falls, bruises, and minor wounds. Restraining the child from mastering motor development can foster more serious long-term problems than allowing the behaviour. However, the environment should be made as safe as possible, with close supervision during playtime to minimize incidental injuries.

The family usually needs assistance in preparing older children for school. A nurse who knows the family can be instrumental in discussing the situation with the teacher and jointly planning an appropriate activity schedule. The physical limitations in regard to active sports may be a difficult adjustment, and activity restrictions must be tempered with sensitivity to the child's emotional and physical needs. Use of protective equipment, such as padding and helmets, is particularly important; noncontact sports, especially swimming, walking, jogging, tennis, golf, fishing, and bowling, should be encouraged (National Hemophilia Foundation, Bleeding Disorders Information Center, 2006).

To prevent oral bleeding, some readjustment in terms of dental hygiene may be needed to minimize trauma to the gums, such as use of a water irrigating device, softening the toothbrush in warm water before brushing, or using a sponge-tipped disposable toothbrush. A regular toothbrush should be small and have soft bristles.

Because any trauma can lead to a bleeding episode, all persons caring for these children must be aware of their disorder. The children should wear medical identification, and older children should be encouraged to recognize situations in which disclosing their condition is important, such as during dental extraction or injections. Health care personnel need to take special precautions to prevent the use of procedures that may cause bleeding, such as IM injections. The subcutaneous route is substituted for IM injections whenever possible. Venipunctures for blood samples are usually preferred for these children. There is usually less bleeding after the venipuncture than after finger or heel punctures. Neither aspirin nor any aspirin-containing compound should be used. Acetaminophen is a suitable aspirin substitute, especially for controlling pain at home.

Recognize and Control Bleeding

As noted, the earlier a bleeding episode is recognized, the more effectively it can be treated. Factor replacement therapy should be instituted according to established medical protocol, and supportive measures—such as *RICE*, which stands for *R*est, *I*ce, *C*ompression, and *E*levation—may be implemented. When parents and older children are taught such measures beforehand, they can be prepared to initiate immediate treatment. Plastic bags of ice or cold packs should be kept in the freezer for such emergencies. However, such measures do not take the place of factor replacement.

Prevent Crippling Effects of Bleeding

As a result of repeated episodes of hemarthrosis, incompletely absorbed blood in the joints, and limitation of motion, bone and muscle changes occur that result in flexion contractures and joint fixation. During bleeding episodes the joint is elevated and immobilized. Active range-of-motion exercises are usually instituted after the acute episode. This allows the child to control the degree of exercise and discomfort. If an exercise program is instituted in the home, a physiotherapist or community health nurse may need to supervise the regimen. Rarely, orthopaedic intervention, such as casting, the application of traction, or the aspiration of blood, may be necessary to preserve joint function. Diet is also an important consideration because excessive body weight can increase the strain on affected joints, especially the knees, and predispose the child to hemarthrosis. Consequently, calories need to be supplied in accordance with energy requirements.

Support the Family and Prepare for Home Care

Genetic counselling is essential as soon as possible after diagnosis. Unlike many other disorders in which both parents carry the trait, the feeling of responsibility for this condition usually rests with the mother. Without an opportunity to discuss her feelings, the marital relationship can suffer. Technology is now available to identify carriers in approximately 80% of cases and may reduce the anxiety regarding childbearing in women who may be at risk of carrying the defective gene, such as sisters or maternal aunts of an affected male. The discovery of factor concentrates has greatly changed the outlook for these children. Bleeding can be minimized, and the child can live a much more normal, unrestricted life. Children are taught to take responsibility for their disease at an early age. They learn their limitations, other preventive measures, and self-administration of the prophylactic AHF.

The needs of families who have children with hemophilia are best met through a comprehensive team approach of physicians (pediatrician, hematologist, orthopedist), nurse practitioner, nurse, social worker, and physiotherapist. Parent-group discussions are beneficial in meeting the needs often best met by similarly affected families. For example, with the improved prognosis for these children, parents and adolescents with hemophilia face vocational and financial problems, in addition to concern over future childbearing. The Canadian Hemophilia Society provides numerous services and publications for both health providers and families (see Additional Resources section at the end of this chapter). Financial support is particularly important. A person with severe hemophilia may require factor replacement therapy and other medical treatments that cost in excess of $70,000 to $90,000 a year.

Idiopathic Thrombocytopenic Purpura

Idiopathic thrombocytopenic purpura (ITP) is an acquired hemorrhagic disorder characterized by (1) *thrombocytopenia*, excessive destruction of platelets, (2) **purpura,** a discolouration caused by petechiae beneath the skin, and (3) normal bone marrow with a normal or increased number of immature platelets (megakaryocytes) and eosinophils. Although the cause is unknown, it is believed to be an autoimmune response to disease-related antigens. It is the most frequently occurring thrombocytopenia of childhood. The greatest frequency of occurrence is between 2 and 10 years of age.

The disease occurs in one of two forms: an acute, self-limited course or a chronic condition (greater than 6 months' duration). The acute form is most often seen after upper respiratory tract infections; after the childhood diseases measles, rubella, mumps, and chickenpox; or after infection with parvovirus B19.

Diagnostic Evaluation

The diagnosis is suspected on the basis of clinical manifestations (Box 49-6). In ITP the platelet count is reduced to below 20×10^9/L; thus tests that depend on platelet function, such as the tourniquet test, bleeding time, and clot retraction, are abnormal. Although there is no definitive test on which to establish a diagnosis of ITP, several are usually performed to rule out other disorders in which thrombocytopenia is a manifestation, such as systemic lupus erythematosus, lymphoma, or leukemia.

Therapeutic Management

Management of ITP is primarily supportive because the course of the disease is self-limited in most cases. Activity is restricted at the onset while the platelet count is low and while active bleeding or progression of lesions is occurring. Treatment for acute presentation is symptomatic and has included prednisone, IV immune globulin (IVIG), and anti-D antibody. These are not curative therapies. Anti-D antibody is a relatively new therapy for ITP. Its infusion causes a transient hemolytic anemia in the patient. Along with the clearance of antibody-coated RBCs, there is prolonged survival of platelets resulting from the blockade of the Fc receptors of the reticuloendothelial cells. The platelet count does not increase until 48 hours after an infusion of anti-D antibody; therefore it is not appropriate therapy for patients who are actively bleeding. The benefits of choosing anti-D antibody therapy over prednisone or IVIG are that anti-D antibody can be given in one dose over 5 to 10 minutes and is significantly less expensive than IVIG. Historically, patients who are treated with prednisone must first undergo a bone marrow examination to rule out leukemia. The use of anti-D antibody alleviates the need for a bone marrow examination. Patients must meet certain criteria before it is administered (Box 49-7). Premedication with acetaminophen 5 to 10 minutes before infusion is recommended.

NURSING ALERT After administration of anti-D antibody, observe the child for a minimum of 1 hour and maintain a patent IV line. Obtain baseline vital signs before the infusion and again 5, 20, and 60 minutes after beginning the infusion. Fever, chills, and headache may occur during or shortly after the infusion. If so, diphenhydramine (Benadryl) and hydrocortisone (Solu-Cortef) should be given, and the patient observed for an additional hour.

BOX 49-6 Clinical Manifestations of Idiopathic Thrombocytopenic Purpura

Easy bruising
- Petechiae
- Ecchymoses
- Most often over bony prominences

Bleeding from mucous membranes
- Epistaxis
- Bleeding gums
- Internal hemorrhage evidenced by hematuria, hematemesis, melena, hemarthrosis, or menorrhagia

Hematomas over lower extremities

BOX 49-7 Criteria for Anti-D Antibody Therapy

- Age between 1 and 19 years; Rh(D)-positive blood type
- Normal white blood count and hemoglobin level for age; platelet count of 20×10^9/L
- No active mucosal bleeding
- No history of reaction to plasma products
- No known immune globulin A deficiency
- No concurrent infection
- Absence of Evans syndrome (characterized by the combination of idiopathic thrombocytopenic purpura and autoimmune hemolytic anemia)
- No suspicion of lupus erythematosus or other collagen-vascular disorder
- No splenectomy

Splenectomy is reserved for patients in whom ITP has persisted for 1 year or longer. It is the only treatment associated with long-term remission for 60 to 90% of children. Splenectomy removes the risk of hemorrhage but increases the risk of septicemia (Buchanan, 2005; Scott & Montgomery, 2007; Wilson, 2009). Before considering splenectomy, it is generally recommended to wait until the child is older than 5 years of age because of the increased risk of bacterial infection. Pneumococcal and meningococcal vaccines are recommended before splenectomy. The child also receives penicillin prophylaxis after splenectomy. The length of prophylactic therapy is controversial, but in general, a minimum of 3 years is recommended.

Prognosis

Most children have a self-limited course without major complications. Some develop chronic ITP and require ongoing therapy. A splenectomy may modify the disease process, and the child will be asymptomatic.

Nursing Care Management

Nursing care is largely supportive and should include teaching regarding possible adverse effects of therapy and limitation in activities while the child's platelet count is 50 to 100 × 10^9/L. Children with ITP should not participate in any contact sports, bike riding, skateboarding, in-line skating, gymnastics, climbing, or running. Parents should be encouraged to engage their children in quiet activities and prevent any injuries to the child's head. The harmful effects of using aspirin and NSAIDs to control pain are critical for these children; salicylate substitutes (such as acetaminophen) are always used. As in any condition with an uncertain outcome, the family needs emotional support.

Disseminated Intravascular Coagulation

Disseminated intravascular coagulation (DIC), also known as *consumption coagulopathy*, is characterized by diffuse fibrin deposition in the microvasculature, consumption of coagulation factors, and endogenous generation of thrombin and plasmin. DIC is a secondary disorder of coagulation that occurs as a complication of a number of pathological processes, such as hypoxia, acidosis, shock, and endothelial damage. It can result from many severe systemic diseases, such as congenital heart disease, necrotizing enterocolitis, gram-negative bacterial sepsis, rickettsial infections, and some severe viral infections.

Pathophysiology

DIC occurs when the first stage of the coagulation process is abnormally stimulated. Although no well-defined sequence of events occurs, two distinct phases can be identified. First, when the clotting mechanism is triggered in the circulation, thrombin is generated in greater amounts than can be neutralized by the body. Consequently, there is rapid conversion of fibrinogen to fibrin, with aggregation and destruction of platelets. If local and widespread fibrin deposition in blood vessels takes place, obstruction and eventual necrosis of tissues occur. Second, the fibrinolytic mechanism is activated, causing extensive destruction of clotting factors. With a deficiency of clotting factors, the child is vulnerable to uncontrollable hemorrhage into vital organs. An additional complication is damage and hemolysis of RBCs (Fig. 49-3).

Diagnostic Evaluation

DIC is suspected when the patient has an increased tendency to bleed (Box 49-8). Hematological findings include prolonged prothrombin time (PT), partial thromboplastin time (PTT), fibrinogen and D-dimer. There is a profoundly depressed platelet count, fragmented RBCs, and depleted fibrinogen.

Therapeutic Management

Treatment of DIC is directed toward control of the underlying or initiating cause, which in most instances stops the coagulation problem spontaneously. Platelets and fresh-frozen plasma may be needed to replace lost plasma components, especially in the child whose underlying disease remains uncontrolled. The extremely ill newborn infant may require exchange transfusion with fresh blood. The IV administration of heparin to inhibit thrombin formation is most often restricted to patients who have not responded to treatment of the underlying disease or replacement of coagulation factors and platelets.

Nursing Care Management

The goals of nursing care are to be aware of the possibility of DIC in the severely ill child and to recognize signs that might

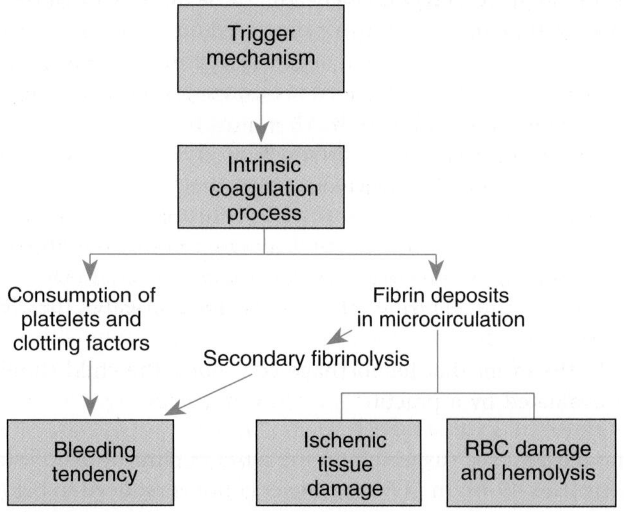

Fig. 49-3 Effects of disseminated intravascular coagulation. *RBC*, red blood cell.

BOX 49-8 Clinical Manifestations of Disseminated Intravascular Coagulation

Petechiae
Purpura
Bleeding from openings in the skin
- Venipuncture site
- Surgical incision

Bleeding from umbilicus, trachea (newborn)
Evidence of gastrointestinal bleeding
Hypotension
Organ dysfunction from infarction and ischemia

indicate its presence. The skills needed to monitor IV infusion and blood transfusions and to administer heparin are the same as for any child receiving these therapies (see p. 1530). (See Chapter 41 for care of the child with a life-threatening illness.)

Epistaxis (Nosebleeding)

Isolated and transient episodes of epistaxis, or nosebleeding, are common in childhood. The nose, especially the septum, is a highly vascular structure, and bleeding usually results from direct trauma, including blows to the nose, foreign bodies, and nose picking, or from mucosal inflammation associated with allergic rhinitis and upper respiratory tract infections. The bleeding ordinarily stops spontaneously or with minimal pressure and requires no medical evaluation or therapy.

Recurrent epistaxis and severe bleeding may indicate an underlying disease, particularly vascular abnormalities, leukemia, thrombocytopenia, and clotting factor deficiency diseases (e.g., hemophilia, vWD). Nosebleeds are sometimes associated with administration of aspirin, even in normal amounts. Persistent episodes of epistaxis require medical evaluation.

Nursing Care Management

In the event of a nosebleed, an essential intervention is to remain calm. Otherwise, the child will become more agitated, the blood pressure will increase, and he or she may resist treatment. Although in most instances a nosebleed is not serious, it can be upsetting to family members as well. They need reassurance that the loss of blood is not serious and that the bleeding usually stops within 10 to 15 minutes.

To control the bleeding, the child is instructed to sit up and lean forward (not lie down) to avoid aspiration of blood. Most nosebleeding originates in the anterior part of the nasal septum and can be controlled by applying pressure to the soft lower portion of the nose with the thumb and forefinger (see Emergency box). During this time, the child breathes through the mouth.

In the event that hemorrhage continues, the child should be evaluated by a practitioner, who may pack the nose with epinephrine-soaked gauze. After a nosebleed, petroleum or water-soluble jelly can be inserted into each nostril to prevent crusting of old blood and to lessen the likelihood of the child's picking at the nose and restarting the hemorrhage. If a child has numerous nosebleeds, factors believed to increase the likelihood of bleeds should be eliminated, such as discouraging nose picking or altering the household humidity by placing a cool-mist humidifier in the child's room. Repeated bleeding episodes lasting longer than 30 minutes may be an indication to refer the child for evaluation for the possibility of a bleeding disorder.

> **EMERGENCY**
>
> **Epistaxis**
>
> - Have child sit up and lean forward (not lie down).
> - Apply continuous pressure to nose with thumb and forefinger for at least 10 minutes.
> - Insert cotton or wadded tissue into each nostril, and apply ice or cold cloth to bridge of nose if bleeding persists.
> - Keep child calm and quiet.

Neoplastic Disorders

Neoplastic disorders are the leading cause of death from disease in children past infancy, and almost half of all childhood cancers involve the blood or blood-forming organs. Leukemias and lymphomas are discussed here. Malignant solid tumours of childhood are discussed elsewhere in relation to the tissues or organs involved.

evolve Case Study—Acute Lymphoid Leukemia

Leukemias

Leukemia, a cancer of the blood-forming tissues, is the most common form of childhood cancer. The annual incidence is 3 to 4 cases per 100,000 Caucasian children younger than 15 years of age (Margolin et al., 2011). It is more common in males and White children, with the peak onset between 2 and 5 years of age (Margolin et al., 2011). It is one of the forms of cancer that has demonstrated dramatic improvements in survival rates. Five-year observed survival proportions for children with acute lymphoid leukemia approaches 90% (whereas acute nonlymphoid leukemia has a nearly 67% survival rate (Canadian Cancer Society/National Cancer Institute of Canada, 2008). (See also Prognosis, p. 1519.)

Classification

Leukemia is a broad term given to a group of malignant diseases of the bone marrow and lymphatic system. Research has revealed that it is a complex disease of varying heterogeneity. Consequently, classification has become increasingly complex, sophisticated, and essential, since identification of the subtype of leukemia has therapeutic and prognostic implications. The following is a brief overview of the major classification systems currently being used.

Morphology

Two forms are generally recognized in children: acute lymphoid leukemia (ALL) and acute nonlymphoid (myelogenous) leukemia (ANLL or AML). Synonyms for ALL include lymphatic, lymphoid, lymphocytic, lymphoblastic, promyelocytic, erythroid, megakaryoblastic, and lymphoblastoid leukemia. Synonyms for the AML type include granulocytic, myelocytic, monocytic, myelogenous, monoblastic, and monomyeloblastic.

Cytochemical markers—Several chemical stains (e.g., terminal deoxynucleotidyl transferase [TdT]) aid in differentiation between ALL and ANLL.

Chromosome studies—Chromosome analysis has become an important tool in the diagnosis of ALL. For example, children with trisomy 21 have 20 times the risk of other children for developing ALL. Children with more than 50 chromosomes on the leukemic cells (hyperdiploid) have the best prognosis (Margolin et al., 2011). Translocations of chromosomes also found on the leukemic cells can denote a good prognosis, as in the trisomies 4 and 10, or a poor prognosis, as in the t(9:22) or Philadelphia chromosome.

Cell-surface immunological markers—Cell-surface antigens have permitted differentiation of ALL into three broad classes: non-T, non-B ALL; B-cell ALL; and T-cell ALL. Children with non-T, non-B ALL have the best prognosis, especially if they have the common ALL antigen, known as CALLA positive (or CD10+), on their cell surfaces (Margolin et al., 2011).

evolve Critical Thinking Exercise—Bone Marrow Test

Pathophysiology

Leukemia is an unrestricted proliferation of immature WBCs in the blood-forming tissues of the body. Although not a "tumour" as such, the leukemic cells demonstrate the same neoplastic properties as solid cancers. The resulting pathological condition and clinical manifestations are caused by infiltration and replacement of any tissue of the body with nonfunctional leukemic cells. Highly vascular organs, such as the spleen and liver, are the most severely affected.

To understand the pathophysiology of the leukemic process, it is important to clarify two common misconceptions. First, although leukemia is an overproduction of WBCs, most often in the acute form the leukocyte count is low (thus the term *leukemia*). Second, these immature cells do not deliberately attack and destroy the normal blood cells or vascular tissues. Cellular destruction takes place by infiltration and subsequent competition for metabolic elements (Table 49-2).

In all types of leukemia the proliferating cells depress the production of formed elements of the blood in bone marrow by competing for and depriving the normal cells of the essential nutrients for metabolism. The most frequent presenting signs and symptoms of leukemia are a result of infiltration of the bone marrow. The three main consequences are (1) anemia from decreased RBCs, (2) infection from **neutropenia,** and (3) bleeding from decreased platelet production. The invasion of the bone marrow with leukemic cells gradually causes a weakening of the bone and a tendency toward fractures. As leukemic cells invade the periosteum, increasing pressure causes severe pain.

Diagnostic Evaluation

Leukemia is usually suspected based on the history, physical manifestations (see Table 49-2), and a peripheral blood smear that contains immature forms of leukocytes, frequently combined with low blood counts. Definitive diagnosis is based on flow cytometry of the cells obtained in the bone marrow aspiration or biopsy. Flow cytometry identifies the specific type of blast cell. Typically, the bone marrow is hypercellular, with primarily **blast cells.** After the diagnosis is confirmed, a lumbar puncture is performed to determine whether there is any central nervous system (CNS) involvement. A few children have CNS involvement at diagnosis, although most are asymptomatic.

Therapeutic Management

Treatment of leukemia involves the use of chemotherapeutic agents, with or without cranial irradiation, in four phases: (1) *induction therapy,* which achieves a complete remission or less than 5% leukemic cells in the bone marrow; (2) *CNS prophylactic therapy,* which prevents leukemic cells from invading the CNS; (3) *intensification therapy* (consolidation), which eradicates residual leukemia cells, followed by delayed intensification, which prevents emergence of resistant leukemic clones; and (4) *maintenance therapy,* which serves to maintain the remission phase. Although the combination of medications and radiation may vary according to institutions, the prognostic or risk characteristics of the patient, and the type of leukemia being treated, the following general principles for each phase are consistently used.

Hematopoietic Stem Cell Transplantation

HSCT has been used successfully for treating children who have ALL and AML. It is not recommended for children with

Table 49-2 Pathology and Related Clinical Manifestations of Leukemia

ORGAN OR TISSUE	CONSEQUENCES	MANIFESTATIONS
Bone marrow dysfunction	Decreased red blood cells—Anemia Neutropenia—Infection Decreased platelets—Bleeding tendencies Invasion of bone marrow—Bone weakness; invasion of periosteum	Pallor, fatigue Fever Hemorrhage (petechiae) Tendency toward fractures Pain
Liver	Infiltration, enlargement, eventual fibrosis	Hepatomegaly
Spleen		Splenomegaly
Lymph glands		Lymphadenopathy
Central nervous system—Meninges	Increased intracranial pressure, ventricular enlargement Meningeal irritation	Severe headache Vomiting Irritability, lethargy Papilledema Eventual coma Pain Stiff neck and back
Hypermetabolism	Cell deprivation of nutrients by invading cells	Muscle wasting Weight loss Anorexia Fatigue

ALL during the first remission because of the excellent results possible with chemotherapy. Because of the poorer prognosis in children with AML, HSCT may be considered during the first remission when a suitable donor is available (Bollard, Krance, & Heslop, 2011) .

HSCT may be not only from antigen-matched related donors but also from matched unrelated or mismatched donors. Peripheral blood stem cell transplants are capable of differentiating into specialized cells of the hematological system and can be obtained from related or unrelated donors or from umbilical cord blood. Regardless of the type of transplant, it is accompanied by significant morbidity and mortality, including graft-versus-host disease (GVHD), overwhelming infection, or severe organ damage.

Prognosis

The most important prognostic factors for determining long-term survival for children with ALL (in addition to treatment) are (1) the initial WBC count, (2) the child's age at the time of diagnosis, (3) the type of cell involved, (4) the sex of the child, and (5) karyotype analysis. Children with a normal or low WBC count and who have non-T, non-B ALL and are CALLA positive have a much better prognosis than those with a high count or other cell types. Children diagnosed between 2 and 9 years of age have consistently demonstrated a better outlook than those diagnosed before 2 or after 10 years of age, and girls appear to have a more favourable prognosis than boys. Children with a DNA index greater than 1.16 (hyperdiploid) and translocation of chromosomes 4 and 10 have a better prognosis (Margolin et al., 2011).

Late Effects of Treatment

Although vigorous treatment of childhood cancers has resulted in dramatically improved survival rates, increasing concern surrounds late effects—adverse changes related to treatment modalities—and recurrence of the disease process. Almost no organ is exempt, and almost every antineoplastic agent, especially irradiation, is responsible for some adverse effect.

The most devastating late effect is development of a second malignancy. Children who received cranial irradiation at age 5 years or younger are most susceptible to developing brain tumours (Bhatia, 2004; Silverman & Sallan, 2003). Treatment with an anthracycline is associated with cardiomyopathy; cranial irradiation and intrathecal chemotherapy are associated with cognitive and neuropsychological deficits, which are just a few of the long-term sequelae. Consequently, close monitoring for late effects is essential, especially with the advent of additional clinical trials.

Nursing Care Management

Nursing care of the child with leukemia is directly related to the therapeutic regimen. The Nursing Care Plan for the child with cancer is found on pp. 1520-1521.

Prepare the Child and Family for Diagnostic and Therapeutic Procedures

From the time before diagnosis to cessation of therapy, children must undergo several tests; the most traumatic are bone marrow aspiration, bone marrow biopsy, and lumbar punctures. Multiple finger sticks and venipunctures for blood analysis and drug infusion are common occurrences. The child needs an explanation of each procedure and what can be expected. In addition, effective pharmacological measures, including conscious and unconscious sedation, and nonpharmacological strategies are used to reduce discomfort associated with these painful procedures.

Relieve Pain

The effective use of analgesia is especially important when the malignant process is uncontrolled and causes acute pain. Dosages of opioids (narcotics) are adjusted, or *titrated*, to the child's needs and administered *around the clock* for optimal pain control. Nonpharmacological strategies should be implemented as needed but are not substitutes for pharmacological management. The reader is encouraged to review the principles of pain assessment and management presented in Chapter 35 and Preparation for Diagnostic and Therapeutic Procedures, Chapter 45, when caring for a child with leukemia.

Prevent Complications of Myelosuppression

The leukemic process and most of the chemotherapeutic agents cause myelosuppression. The reduced numbers of blood cells result in secondary problems of infection, bleeding tendencies, and anemia. Supportive care involves both medical and nursing management. Because these are so closely linked, they are discussed together.

Infection. A frequent complication of treatment for childhood cancer is overwhelming infection secondary to neutropenia. The child is most susceptible to overwhelming infection during three phases of the disease: (1) at the time of diagnosis and relapse when the leukemic process has replaced normal leukocytes; (2) during immunosuppressive therapy; and (3) after prolonged antibiotic therapy, which predisposes the child to the growth of resistant organisms. However, the use of granulocyte colony–stimulating factor (GCSF) has reduced the incidence and duration of infection in children receiving treatment for cancer.

The first defence against infection is prevention. When the child is hospitalized, the nurse needs to use all measures to control transfer of infection. These typically include the use of a private room, restriction of all visitors and health personnel with active infection, and strict hand hygiene technique with an antiseptic solution. In some research centres special germ-free environments are available during complete myelosuppression from intensive chemotherapy or for bone marrow transplant.

NURSING ALERT Live or attenuated viral vaccines are contraindicated in immunosuppressed children and should be deferred until the child's **immune system** function has returned to normal. The administration of an attenuated vaccine (MMR, oral polio) during immunosuppression may result in overwhelming infection. There is no special risk with the administration of inactivated vaccines (Pediacel, Td, Synflorix); however, the child's immune system will likely not respond adequately. Siblings and other family members can receive all routine age-appropriate vaccines except oral polio. Prophylactic measures need only be taken if the vaccinated child develops wild-type varicella infection (Sung et al., 2001).

NURSING CARE PLAN ● The Child With Cancer

Nursing Diagnosis	Expected Patient Outcomes	Nursing Interventions	Rationale
Risk for injury related to chemotherapy treatment	Child will exhibit no complications of chemotherapy.	Administer chemotherapeutic agents using established guidelines.	To minimize inappropriate administration techniques
Child's/Family's Defining Characteristics *(Subjective and Objective Data)*	Child will receive prompt, appropriate treatment of complications.	Assist with procedures for administration of chemotherapeutic agents.	To promote safer cancer treatment
Anaphylaxis—Wheezing, hypotension, urticaria, cyanosis	**The Following NOC Concept Applies to These Outcomes**	Administer medications around the clock to prevent nausea and vomiting before chemotherapy.	To minimize adverse effects of nausea and vomiting
Nausea, vomiting	Risk Control	Administer IV fluid as prescribed.	To maintain hydration
Intravenous (IV) infiltration—Pain, redness, swelling at IV infusion site		Encourage frequent intake of fluids in small amounts.	To promote hydration
		Observe for signs of infiltration of IV site: pain, stinging, swelling, redness.	To prevent infiltration when possible
		Institute policies to treat infiltration if it occurs.	To prevent complications
		Observe child for 30 minutes after infusion of drugs that are associated with risk of anaphylaxis.	To prevent anaphylaxis
		Stop infusion of drug and keep a new normal saline line open if reaction is suspected.	To prevent further reaction
		Have emergency equipment and emergency medications readily available.	To prevent delay in treatment
		The Following NIC Concepts Apply to These Interventions	
		Chemotherapy Management	
		Nausea Management	

Nursing Diagnosis	Expected Patient Outcomes	Nursing Interventions	Rationale
Risk for infection related to depressed body defences	Child will not exhibit signs of infection.	Use good hand hygiene technique.	To minimize exposure to infective organisms
Child's/Family's Defining Characteristics *(Subjective and Objective Data)*	Child will not come in contact with infected persons.	Screen all visitors and staff for signs of infection.	To decrease exposure to possible infective organisms
Fever	**The Following NOC Concepts Apply to These Outcomes**	Use aseptic technique for all invasive procedures.	To decrease chance of infection spread
Altered vital signs	Risk Control	Monitor temperature and blood pressure.	To detect possible infection
Lethargy	Immune Status	Evaluate child for any potential sites of infection: needle puncture sites, mucosa for ulceration, minor abrasions.	To detect signs of possible infection
Change in behaviour	Infection Severity	Provide nutritionally complete diet.	To support body's natural defences
Septic shock		Avoid giving live attenuated virus vaccines.	To prevent overwhelming infection
		Give inactivated virus vaccines.	To prevent specific infections and to avoid placing the child at risk for acquiring the illness
		Administer antibiotics as prescribed.	To treat a specific infection
		Administer granulocyte colony-stimulating factor (G-CSF) as prescribed.	To promote production of infection-fighting cells
		The Following NIC Concepts Apply to These Interventions	
		Infection Protection	
		Infection Control	
		Immunization/Vaccination Management	

The child should be evaluated for potential sites of infection (e.g., mucosal ulcerations, skin abrasions, or skin tears, such as a hangnail) and observed for any elevation in temperature. To identify the source of infection, chest radiographs and blood, stool, urine, and nasopharyngeal cultures are taken. IV antibiotics need to be administered; if this therapy is prolonged, a venous access device, such as a peripherally inserted central catheter or **intermittent infusion device** (saline lock or PRN adaptor), is used to maintain IV access.

Prevention of infection continues to be a priority after discharge from the hospital. Ordinarily, the child is allowed to return to school when the WBC count is at a satisfactory level, usually the absolute neutrophil count (ANC) is $>0.5 \times 10^9$/L. Family members need to be encouraged to practise good hand

NURSING CARE PLAN ● The Child With Cancer—cont'd

Nursing Diagnosis	Expected Patient Outcomes	Nursing Interventions	Rationale
Nursing Diagnosis **Imbalanced nutrition: less than body requirements related to loss of appetite** **Child's/Family's Defining Characteristics** ***(Subjective and Objective Data)*** Weight loss Lack of appetite Nausea	Child's nutritional intake will be adequate. **The Following NOC Concepts Apply to These Outcomes** Nutritional Status: Food and Fluid Intake Nutritional Status: Nutrient Intake	Encourage parents to relax pressure placed on child concerning eating. Allow child any food tolerated; selections can improve once appetite increases. Explain expected increase in appetite if child will be taking steroids. Fortify foods with nutritious supplements. Allow child to be involved in food preparation and selection. Make food appealing. Monitor child's weight. **The Following NIC Concepts Apply to These Interventions** Nutrition Management Nutrition Therapy	To educate that loss of appetite is a consequence of chemotherapy To encourage child to eat To prepare child and family for this change To maximize quality of intake To encourage eating To encourage eating To evaluate for weight change
Nursing Diagnosis **Pain (specify: acute, chronic) related to diagnosis, treatment, physiological effects of cancer** **Child's/Family's Defining Characteristics** ***(Subjective and Objective Data)*** Crying Withdrawal Fear of procedures Reluctance to move Change in vital signs	Child will experience no pain or reduction of pain to level acceptable to the child. **The Following NOC Concepts Apply to These Outcomes** Pain Level Pain: Disruptive Effects Pain Control	Use pharmacological and nonpharmacological interventions before painful procedures. Assess pain with each vital sign measurement. Evaluate effectiveness of pain relief. Administer analgesics as prescribed on preventive schedule (around the clock) when needed. **The Following NIC Concept Applies to These Interventions** Pain Management	To minimize discomfort To determine level of pain To determine effectiveness To prevent pain from recurring
Nursing Diagnosis **Fear related to diagnostic tests, procedures, treatment** **Child's/Family's Defining Characteristics** ***(Subjective and Objective Data)*** Worry and anxiety before procedures Withdrawal Lack of control Outbursts, anger Lack of ability to cooperate	Child will have reduced fear related to diagnostic procedures and treatment. **The Following NOC Concepts Apply to These Outcomes** Fear Self-Control Pain Control	Explain procedures carefully at child's level of understanding. Explain what will take place and what child will feel, see, smell, taste, and hear. Listen to special requests of child when possible. Provide child with some means of involvement with procedures (e.g., holding a piece of equipment, helping put on bandage, counting). Implement distraction techniques and pain reduction interventions. **The Following NIC Concept Applies to These Interventions** Pain Management	To reduce fear of unknown To provide sense of control To provide sense of control To provide sense of control, encourage cooperation, and support child's coping skills To reduce pain

Continued

hygiene at all times to prevent introducing **pathogens** into the home. The child may need to be isolated from school contacts in the event of an outbreak of a childhood disease, especially chickenpox.

Nutrition is another important component of infection prevention. An adequate protein-caloric intake provides the child with better host defences against infection and increased tolerance to chemotherapy and irradiation. However, providing optimal nutrition during periods of anorexia and vomiting from chemotherapy is a tremendous challenge (see Feeding the Sick Child, Chapter 45).

Hemorrhage. Before the use of transfused platelets, hemorrhage was a leading cause of death in patients with leukemia. Now most bleeding episodes can be prevented or controlled with the administration of platelet concentrates or platelet-rich plasma.

NURSING CARE PLAN ● The Child With Cancer—cont'd

Nursing Diagnosis	Expected Patient Outcomes	Nursing Interventions	Rationale
Disturbed body image related to changes caused by cancer and treatment	Child will exhibit positive coping skills.	Encourage child to decide how he or she will cope with hair loss (e.g., wig, cap, scarf, haircut).	To promote early adjustment and preparation for hair loss
Child's/Family's Defining Characteristics	**The Following NOC Concept Applies to These Outcomes**	Provide adequate covering during exposure to sunlight, wind, or cold.	To prevent exposure
(Subjective and Objective Data)	Body Image	Explain that hair begins to regrow in 3 to 6 months and may be a different colour and texture.	Natural hair protection is lost with alopecia
Sadness		Encourage good hygiene and grooming.	To reduce risk of infection
Depression		Encourage rapid return to peer group and friends.	To prepare child for reactions of others
Withdrawal		Encourage visits from friends before discharge.	To support child
Anger		**The Following NIC Concepts Apply to These Interventions**	
		Counselling	
		Body Image Enhancement	

Nursing Diagnosis	Expected Patient Outcomes	Nursing Interventions	Rationale
Interrupted family processes related to having a child with a life-threatening disease	Child and family will demonstrate understanding of the disease and treatment.	Teach parents and child about the disease, and explain all procedures.	To promote understanding
Child's/Family's Defining Characteristics	**The Following NOC Concepts Apply to These Outcomes**	Advise family of expected adverse effects and toxicities; clarify which demand medical evaluation.	To prevent delay in treatment
(Subjective and Objective Data)	Family Functioning	Reassure family that reactions are complications of treatment.	To provide support
Lack of understanding of disease and treatment	Family Coping	Prepare family for what to do when adverse effects occur.	To prevent delay in treatment
• Inability to identify adverse effects of treatment	Family Normalization	Interpret prognostic statistics carefully, realizing family's level of understanding.	To promote understanding
Inability to understand child's treatment plan	Knowledge: Illness Care	Schedule time for family to be together without interruptions.	To encourage communication and expression of feelings
Lack of family support		Help family plan for future.	To promote child's development
		Encourage family to discuss feelings regarding child's disease.	To promote expression of feelings
		The Following NIC Concepts Apply to These Interventions	
		Counselling	
		Family Support*	

*The Canadian Cancer Society has branches in all of the provinces and territories and can provide support to families in a variety of ways, at http://www.cancer.ca/Canada-wide.aspx?sc_lang=encer.

NIC, Nursing Interventions Classification; *NOC,* Nursing Outcomes Classification.

Because infection increases the tendency toward hemorrhage and bleeding sites become more easily infected, skin punctures should be avoided whenever possible. When finger sticks, venipunctures, IM injections, and bone marrow aspirations are performed, aseptic technique must be used, along with continued observation for bleeding. Meticulous mouth care is essential, since gingival bleeding with resultant mucositis is a frequent problem. Because the rectal area is prone to ulceration from various medications, feces and urine are to be removed immediately and the perianal area washed. Use of rectal temperatures should be avoided to prevent trauma. Children should be advised to avoid activities that might cause injury or bleeding, such as riding bicycles or skateboards, climbing trees or playground equipment, and playing contact sports.

Platelet transfusions are generally reserved for a platelet count $<10 \times 10^9$/L, active bleeding episodes that do not respond to local treatment, and those that may occur during induction or relapse therapy. Epistaxis and gingival bleeding are most common. The nurse needs to teach parents and older children measures to control nosebleeding (see p. 1517). Pressure at the site without disturbing clot formation is the general rule.

Anemia. Initially, anemia may be profound from complete replacement of the bone marrow by leukemic cells. During induction therapy, blood transfusions may be necessary. The usual precautions in caring for the child with anemia are instituted (see p. 1503).

Use Precautions in Administering and Handling Chemotherapeutic Agents

In addition to the nurse's many responsibilities in regard to the child and family, nurses must also use safeguards to protect themselves. Handling chemotherapeutic agents may present risks to handlers and their offspring, although the exact degree of risk is not known. Many chemotherapeutic agents are vesicants (sclerosing agents) that can cause severe cellular damage if even minute amounts of the drug infiltrate surrounding tissue. Only nurses experienced with chemotherapeutic agents should administer vesicants. Guidelines are available and must be followed exactly to prevent tissue damage to patients (see Additional Resources section). Interventions for extravasation vary, but each nurse should be aware of the institution's policies and implement them at once.

In addition to extravasation, a potentially fatal complication is anaphylaxis, especially from L-asparaginase, teniposide (VM-26), etoposide (VP-16), bleomycin, and cisplatin. Nursing responsibilities include prevention of, recognition of, and preparation for serious reactions. Prevention begins with a careful history for known allergies.

Most children with cancer have a venous access device, which facilitates administration of IV medications. During treatment and remission, many medications are taken orally at home. Compliance with the medication schedule is essential; nurses play an important role in educating the family about the medications and encouraging adherence to the plan.

NURSING ALERT Chemotherapeutic drugs must be given through a free-flowing IV line. The infusion is stopped immediately if any sign of infiltration (pain, stinging, swelling, or redness at the cannulation site) occurs.

NURSING ALERT When chemotherapeutic and immunological agents are given, the child must be observed for 30 minutes after the infusion for signs of anaphylaxis (cyanosis, hypotension, wheezing, severe urticaria). Emergency equipment (especially a blood pressure monitor and bag-valve-mask) and emergency medications (especially oxygen, epinephrine, antihistamine, aminophylline, corticosteroids, and vasopressors) must be available. If a reaction is suspected, the drug is discontinued, the IV line is flushed with saline, and the child's vital signs and subsequent responses are monitored.

Manage Problems of Drug Toxicity

Chemotherapy presents several nursing challenges. The complexity of the treatment protocols is often overwhelming to families. In addition, each therapy is associated with a number of predictable adverse effects. Nurses must be aware of these effects and use judgement in recognizing reactions and toxicities.

Nausea and Vomiting. The nausea and vomiting that occur shortly after administration of several of the drugs and from cranial or abdominal radiation can be profound. The serotonin-receptor antagonists (e.g., ondansetron, granisetron) are effective in the control of nausea and vomiting occurring after emetogenic chemotherapy and radiotherapy. When combined with dexamethasone, these medications are the treatment of choice in the prevention of delayed emesis (Berde, Billett, & Collins, 2006).

The most beneficial regimen for anti-emetic control has been the administration of the antiemetic before the chemotherapy begins. The goal is to prevent the child from ever experiencing nausea or vomiting, thus preventing development of anticipatory symptoms (the conditioned response of developing nausea and vomiting *before* receiving the medication).

Anorexia. Loss of appetite is a direct consequence of the chemotherapy or irradiation. It is a major problem for parents because it is the one area they feel responsible for, particularly when so many other facets of care are outside their control. There are no universally successful techniques for encouraging a sick child to eat. However, the guidelines in Chapter 45 can be helpful during the anorexic period and can prevent additional problems during the remission.

Some children still do not eat despite these approaches. When loss of appetite and weight persist, the nurse should investigate the family situation to determine whether any factors (e.g., conditioned aversion to food, environmental stress related to eating, controlling behaviour, anger) might be contributing to the problem. Nasogastric tube feedings or total parenteral nutrition may be implemented for children with significant nutritional problems.

Mucosal Ulceration. One of the most distressing adverse effects of several medications is GI mucosal cell damage, which can produce ulcers anywhere along the alimentary tract. Oral ulcers greatly compound anorexia because eating is extremely uncomfortable, but the following interventions may be helpful: (1) provide a bland, moist, soft diet appropriate for the child's age and preferences, (2) use a soft sponge toothbrush (Toothettes) or cotton-tipped applicator, (3) provide frequent mouthwashes with normal saline (using a solution of 5 mL of table salt and 500 mL of water) or sodium bicarbonate mouth rinses (using a solution of 5 mL of baking soda in 1000 mL of water), and (4) use local anaesthetics (e.g., Chloraseptic lozenges) or nonprescription preparations without alcohol (e.g., hydrocortisone dental paste [Orabase], antiseptic mouth rinse [UlcerEase], diphenhydramine [Benadryl], and aluminum and magnesium hydroxide [Maalox] solution). Although local anaesthetics are effective in temporarily relieving the pain, many children dislike the taste and numb feeling they produce.

NURSING ALERT Viscous lidocaine is not recommended for young children; if applied to the pharynx, it may depress the gag reflex, increasing the risk of aspiration. Rarely, seizures have been associated with the use of oral viscous lidocaine (Berde et al., 2006; Cho, Cheng, & Cheng, 2000).

Other preparations that may be used to prevent or treat mucositis include chlorhexidine gluconate (Peridex) because of its dual effectiveness against candidal and bacterial infections, antifungal troches (lozenges) or mouthwash, and lip balm (e.g., Aquaphor) to keep the lips moist. Agents that should not be used include lemon glycerin swabs (which irritate eroded tissue and can decay teeth), hydrogen peroxide (which delays healing by breaking down protein), and milk of magnesia (which dries mucosa).

Stomatitis may cause such difficulty with eating that the child may require hospitalization for hydration, parenteral nutrition, and pain control (often with IV morphine). The child will usually choose the foods that are best tolerated, and the nurse should encourage parents to relax any eating pressures. Because the stomatitis is a temporary condition, the child can resume good food habits after the ulcers heal. Dental hygiene can become a serious problem for children with orthodontic appliances. Sometimes it may be necessary to remove the braces to allow chemotherapy to continue.

Rectal ulcers are managed by meticulous toilet hygiene, warm sitz baths after each bowel movement, and the use of an occlusive ointment or dressing applied to the ulcerated area to promote epithelialization. Stool softeners are necessary to prevent further discomfort. Parents should record bowel movements because the child may voluntarily avoid defecation to prevent discomfort. Rectal thermometers and suppositories are contraindicated because insertion may further traumatize the area.

Neuropathy. Vincristine and, to a lesser extent, vinblastine can cause various neurotoxic effects. Nursing interventions for management of these effects include (1) administering stool softeners or laxatives for severe constipation caused by decreased bowel innervation, (2) maintaining good body alignment and, if patient is on bed rest, using a footboard or high-top shoes to minimize or prevent footdrop, (3) carrying out safety measures during ambulation because of weakness and numbing of the extremities, which may cause difficulty in walking or fine hand movement, and (4) providing a soft or liquid diet for severe jaw pain.

Hemorrhagic Cystitis. Sterile hemorrhagic cystitis, a side effect of chemical irritation to the bladder from cyclophosphamide, can be decreased and often prevented by (1) promoting a liberal fluid intake (at least one and a half times the recommended daily fluid requirement), (2) frequent voiding immediately after feeling the urge, before bed, and after arising, (3) administering the drug early in the day to allow for sufficient oral intake and voiding, and (4) administering mesna (an agent that provides protection to the bladder) as ordered. If oral home administration is prescribed, the family needs specific instructions regarding exactly how much fluid the child must have.

Alopecia. Hair loss is a common side effect of several chemotherapeutic drugs and cranial irradiation, although not all children lose their hair during drug therapy. It is better to warn children and parents of this side effect than to allow them to think that it is only a remote possibility. A soft cotton cap is the most comfortable head wear for children. Polyester increases perspiration and causes itching. Other options include scarves, hats, or a wig.

The nurse should also inform the family that hair regrows in 3 to 6 months and may be of a different colour and texture. Frequently the hair is darker, thicker, and curlier than before. If the child chooses not to wear a wig, attention to some type of head covering, especially in cold climates and during exposure to sun, and scalp hygiene are important. The scalp should be washed like any other body part.

Steroid Effects. Short-term steroid therapy produces no acute toxicities and two beneficial reactions: increased appetite and a sense of well-being. However, it does produce alterations in appearance, which, although not clinically significant, can be distressing to older children. One of these is "moon face," in which the child's face becomes rounded and puffy. It is helpful to reassure the child that, after cessation of the drug, the facial shape will return to normal. Unlike hair loss, little can be done to camouflage this obvious change. If the child resumes activity early in the course of treatment, the change may be less noticeable to peers than after a long absence.

Mood Changes. Shortly after beginning steroid therapy, children experience a number of mood changes that range from feelings of well-being and euphoria to depression and irritability. If parents are unaware of these drug-induced changes, they may become unduly concerned. The nurse should warn them of the reactions and encourage them to discuss the behavioural changes with each other and the child.

Provide Emotional Support

An important aspect of continued emotional support involves the prognosis. Although leukemia is no longer invariably fatal, it must be remembered that survival statistics are only average estimates and apply to children treated with the latest protocols since diagnosis. For the low-risk child the chances may be better, but for the high-risk child they may be significantly poorer. Of those who do survive after discontinuing therapy, some relapse. Only the passage of time is positive confirmation of the child's being ultimately "cured" of the disease. Remission, even in excess of 5 years, cannot be equated with a cure. With increasing concern regarding late effects of treatment, continued surveillance of the child's health status is needed. The nurse working with family members must individualize information regarding the "numbers" and the potential risks. An understanding of each member's emotional needs, as well as competent care of physical ones, is essential to the positive, growth-promoting support of the family. Comprehensive emotional support for the family of the child with a potentially fatal illness is discussed in Chapter 41.

Lymphomas

Pediatric lymphomas are the third most common group of malignancies in children and adolescents. The lymphomas, a group of neoplastic diseases that arise from the lymphoid and hematopoietic systems, are divided into Hodgkin's disease and non-Hodgkin's lymphoma (NHL). These diseases are further subdivided according to tissue type and the extent of disease. NHL is more prevalent in children younger than 14 years of age, whereas Hodgkin's disease is prevalent in adolescence and the young adult period, with a striking increase between ages 15 and 19 years.

Hodgkin's Disease

Hodgkin's disease is a neoplastic disease that originates in the lymphoid system and primarily involves the lymph nodes. It predictably metastasizes to non-nodal or extralymphatic sites, especially the spleen, liver, bone marrow, and lungs, although no tissue is exempt from involvement (Fig. 49-4). It is classified according to four histological types: (1) lymphocytic predominance, (2) nodular sclerosis, (3) mixed cellularity, and (4) lymphocytic depletion. Accurate staging of the extent of disease is the basis for treatment protocols and expected prognoses.

The Ann Arbor staging system assigns a stage based on the number of sites of lymph node involvement, presence of extranodal disease, and history of any symptoms. Patients are classified as A if asymptomatic and as B if they have the following symptoms: temperature of 38°C or higher for 3 consecutive days, drenching night sweats, or unexplained loss of body weight (10% or more) over the preceding 6 months (Hudson, Onciu, & Donaldson, 2011).

Asymptomatic enlarged cervical or supraclavicular lymphadenopathy is the most common presentation of Hodgkin's disease. Other systemic symptoms may be manifested, including fever, weight loss, night sweats, cough, abdominal discomfort, anorexia, nausea, and pruritus. Because multiple organs may be involved, diagnosis is based on several tests and the extent of metastatic disease. Tests include a CBC, erythrocyte sedimentation rate (ESR), serum copper, ferritin level, fibrinogen, immune globulins, uric acid level, liver function tests, T-cell function studies, and urinalysis. Radiographic tests include computed tomography (CT) scans of the neck, chest, abdomen, and pelvis; a positron emission tomography (PET) scan (identifies metastatic or recurrent disease); a chest x-ray film; and, if clinically indicated, a bone scan to identify metastatic disease.

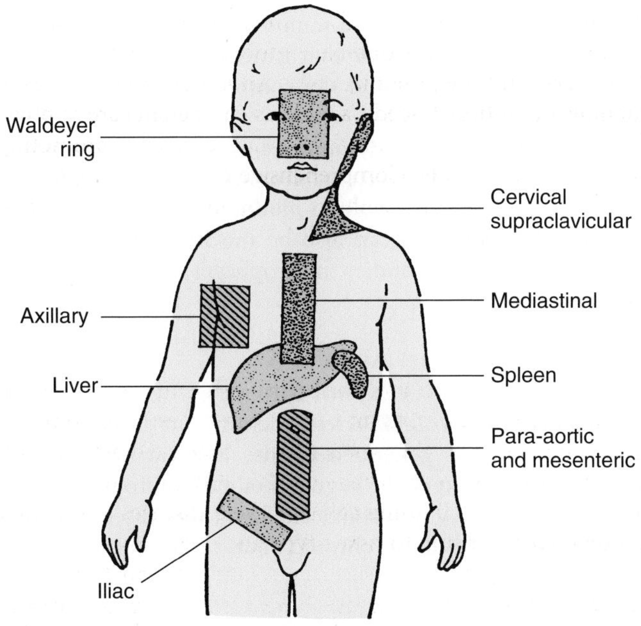

Fig. 49-4 Main areas of lymphadenopathy and organ involvement in Hodgkin's disease.

A lymph node biopsy is essential to establish histological diagnosis and staging. The presence of Reed-Sternberg cells is characteristic of Hodgkin's disease. These large cells, which are multilobed and nucleated with abundant cytoplasm and a typically halolike clear zone around the nucleolus, are often described as having an "owl's eyes" appearance (Hudson et al., 2011). A bone marrow aspiration or biopsy is usually performed. With the advent of CT and PET scans to identify metastatic disease and multiagent chemotherapy to eradicate it, a laparotomy without splenectomy is avoided except in a few selected cases.

Therapeutic Management

The primary modalities of therapy are radiation and chemotherapy. Each may be used alone or in combination based on the clinical staging. Radiation may involve only the involved field (IF), an extended field (EF) (involved areas plus adjacent nodes), or total nodal irradiation (TNI), depending on the extent of involvement.

An effective combination of chemotherapy widely used is MOPP (mechlorethamine, vincristine [Oncovin], procarbazine, prednisone) or ABVD (doxorubicin [Adriamycin], bleomycin, vinblastine, dacarbazine). However, this therapy combination has caused severe late effects, especially secondary malignancies. Other drug combinations such as COPP (cyclophosphamide, vincristine, prednisone, procarbazine) as a substitute for MOPP have minimized late effects.

Follow-up care of children no longer receiving therapy is essential to identify relapse and secondary cancers. In children with splenectomy resulting from laparotomy or splenic irradiation, prophylactic antibiotics are administered for an indefinite period. Immunizations against pneumococci and meningococci are also recommended before the splenectomy.

Prognosis

Long-term survival for all stages of Hodgkin's disease is excellent. Early-stage disease can have survival rates greater than 90%, with advanced stages having rates between 65 and 75%.

Nursing Care Management

Nursing care involves the same objectives as for patients with other types of cancer, specifically (1) preparation for diagnostic and operative procedures, (2) explanation of treatment side effects, and (3) child and family support (see Chapter 41). Because this is most often a disease of adolescents and young adults, the nurse must have an appreciation of their psychological needs and reactions during the diagnostic and treatment phases (see Nursing Care Plan, pp. 1520–1522).

The most common side effect of irradiation is fatigue. This is particularly difficult for active, outgoing school-age children and adolescents because it prevents them from keeping up with their peers. Sometimes adolescents push themselves to the point of physical exhaustion rather than admit and succumb to the decreased activity tolerance. The nurse needs to caution parents to observe for behaviour such as extreme fatigue at the end of the day, falling asleep at the dinner table, inability to concentrate on homework, or an increased susceptibility to infection. A regular bedtime and scheduled rest periods are important for these children, especially during chemotherapy, when myelosuppression increases the risk of infection and debilitation. Before discharge the nurse should discuss a feasible school schedule with the parents and child.

An area of concern for adolescents is the high risk of sterility from irradiation and chemotherapy. Both drugs, particularly procarbazine and alkylating agents, and irradiation to the gonads can lead to infertility. Adolescents should be informed of these adverse effects early in the course of the diagnosis and treatment. Sperm banking is now offered at many cancer centres before the initiation of treatment in adolescent boys. Sexual function is not altered, although the appearance of secondary sexual characteristics and menstruation may be delayed in the pubescent child. Delayed sexual maturation may be an extremely sensitive and stressful issue for children.

Non-Hodgkin's Lymphoma

NHL occurs more frequently in children than Hodgkin's disease. Between 2001 and 2004, approximately 504 lymphoma diagnoses were made in Canadian children between ages 0 and 14. In Canadian adolescents and young adults ages 15 to 29, there were over 6000 new cases of lymphoma between 1992 and 2005 (Canadian Cancer Society's Steering Committee, 2009). Histological classification of childhood NHL is strikingly different from that of Hodgkin's disease:

- The disease is usually diffuse rather than nodular.
- The cell type is either undifferentiated or poorly differentiated.
- Dissemination occurs early, more often, and rapidly.
- Mediastinal involvement and invasion of meninges are common.

NHL exhibits a variety of morphological, cytochemical, and immunological features, not unlike the diversity seen in leukemia. Classification is based on the histological pattern: (1) lymphoblastic, (2) Burkitt or non-Burkitt, or (3) large cell. Immunologically these cells are also classified as T cells; B cells; or non-T, non-B cells (lacking immunological properties). The clinical staging system used in Hodgkin's disease is of little value in NHL, although it has been modified and other systems have been developed.

Diagnostic Evaluation

Because the clinical presentation of most children with NHL is widespread disseminated disease, thorough pathological staging is unnecessary. Clinical manifestations depend on the anatomical site and extent of involvement. These manifestations include many of those seen in Hodgkin's disease and leukemia, as well as organ symptoms related to pressure from enlargement of adjacent lymph nodes, such as intestinal or airway obstruction, cranial nerve palsies, and spinal paralysis.

Recommendations for staging include a surgical biopsy of an enlarged node, histopathological confirmation of disease with cytochemical and immunological evaluation, bone marrow examination, radiographic studies (especially tomograms of the lungs and GI organs), and lumbar puncture.

Therapeutic Management

The treatment protocols for NHL include aggressive use of irradiation and chemotherapy. Similar to leukemic therapy, the protocols include induction, consolidation, and maintenance phases, some with intrathecal chemotherapy. Antineoplastic agents used in the treatment of NHL include vincristine, prednisone, L-asparaginase, methotrexate, 6-mercaptopurine, cytarabine, cyclophosphamide, anthracyclines, and teniposide or etoposide (Gross & Perkins, 2011; Link & Weinstein, 2006).

Prognosis

The prognosis is excellent for children with localized disease, with an almost 100% cure rate; 75 to 90% of children with extensive disease are cured (Gross & Perkins, 2011). Because relapse after 2 years is rare, survival after 24 months is considered a cure.

✱ Nursing Care Management

Nursing care of the child with NHL is similar to that required for children with leukemia. Many of the same medications are used, although the schedules differ. Because of the intense chemotherapy, nursing care is primarily directed toward managing the adverse effects of these agents and providing supportive care to the child and family (see Nursing Care Plan, pp. 1520–1522).

Immunological Deficiency Disorders

A number of disorders can cause profound, often life-threatening alterations within the body's immune system. The most serious are conditions that completely depress immunity, such as severe combined immunodeficiency disease (SCID). However, the one disorder that generates the most anxiety, within both the family and the community at large, is HIV infection/AIDS.

Several classifications of immune dysfunction exist. AIDS, SCID, and Wiskott-Aldrich syndrome (WAS) are syndromes in which the body is unable to mount an immune response. The immune response can also be misdirected. In **autoimmune disorders**, antibodies, macrophages, and lymphocytes attack healthy cells.

HIV Infection and Acquired Immunodeficiency Syndrome

Since the first cases of AIDS were identified in the early 1980s, HIV infection has generated intense medical investigation. Research has led to early diagnosis of and improved medical treatments for HIV infection, changing this disease from a rapidly fatal one to a chronic, but terminal, disease of childhood.

Epidemiology

The overall rate of HIV infection in Canada has remained relatively stable between 2005 and 2008 (PHAC, 2010b).

According to the Canadian Perinatal HIV Surveillance Program, in 2009, 180 children were born to women who were HIV positive, with a rate of transmission of 1% (PHAC, 2010a). This decline occurred despite the fact that the number of infants exposed to HIV has increased (PHAC, 2006b). This trend may be attributed to a result of implementation of recommended HIV counselling and voluntary testing practices, optimal prenatal, antenatal and postpartum care, and the use of antiretroviral therapy (ART) to prevent perinatal transmission. Unsafe sexual activity and IV drug use are major sources of HIV infection in adolescents and young adults. Youth between the ages of 15 and 19 years comprise 26.5% of all reports of HIV-positive status (PHAC, 2010b).

The First Nations, Métis, and Inuit populations are of special concern regarding HIV infection. In 2008, this group represented 66% of all new HIV infections primarily due to street drug injections, compared with a rate of 17% for all other Canadians. From 1998 to 2008, women represented 48.8% of all positive HIV test reports among Aboriginal peoples compared with 20.6% for all other Canadians (PHAC, 2010b).

Etiology

HIV is a retrovirus that is transmitted by lymphocytes and monocytes. It is found in the blood, semen, vaginal secretions, and breast milk. It has an incubation period of months to years (Ezekowitz, 2009). There are different strains of HIV. HIV-2 is prevalent in Africa, whereas HIV-1 subtype B is the dominant strain in Canada. *Horizontal transmission* of HIV occurs through intimate sexual contact or parenteral exposure to blood or body fluids containing visible blood. *Perinatal (vertical) transmission* occurs when an HIV-infected pregnant woman passes the infection to her infant. There is no evidence that casual contact between infected and uninfected individuals can spread the virus.

Pathophysiology

HIV primarily infects a specific subset of T lymphocytes, the CD4 T cells. The virus takes over the machinery of the CD4 lymphocyte, using it to replicate itself, rendering the CD4 cell dysfunctional. The CD4 lymphocyte count gradually decreases over time, leading to progressive immunodeficiency. The count eventually reaches a critical level below which there is substantial risk of opportunistic illnesses, followed by death.

Clinical Manifestations

Common clinical manifestations of HIV infection in children are varied (Box 49-9). The diagnosis of AIDS is associated with certain illnesses or conditions. The most common AIDS-defining conditions observed among Canadian children are listed in Box 49-10. Other problems in these children may include short stature, malnutrition, and cardiomyopathy. CNS abnormalities resulting from HIV infection may include neuropsychological deficits; developmental disabilities; and deficits in motor skills, communication, and behavioural functioning.

Diagnostic Evaluation

For children 18 months of age and older, the HIV enzyme-linked immunosorbent assay (ELISA) and Western blot immunoassay are performed to determine HIV infection. In infants born to HIV-infected mothers, these assays will be positive because of the presence of maternal antibodies derived transplacentally. Maternal antibodies may persist in the infant up to 18 months of age. Thus other diagnostic tests are used, most commonly the HIV polymerase chain reaction (PCR) for detection of proviral DNA. With this technique, more than 95% of infected infants can be diagnosed by 1 to 3 months of age (Ezekowitz, 2009; Goldschmidt & Fogler, 2006).

The Centers for Disease Control and Prevention (1994) has developed a classification system that is still used to describe the spectrum of HIV disease in children (Table 49-3). The system indicates the severity of clinical signs and symptoms and the degree of immunosuppression. Mild signs and symptoms include lymphadenopathy, parotitis, hepatosplenomegaly, and recurrent or persistent sinusitis or otitis media. Moderate signs and symptoms include lymphoid interstitial pneumonitis (LIP) and a variety of organ-specific dysfunctions or infections. Severe signs and symptoms include AIDS-defining illnesses with the exception of LIP. Children with LIP have a better prognosis than those with other AIDS-defining illnesses. In children whose HIV infection is not yet confirmed, the letter *E* (vertically exposed) is placed in front of the classification. The immune categories are based on CD4 lymphocyte counts and percentages. Age adjustment of these numbers is necessary because normal

BOX 49-9 Common Clinical Manifestations of HIV Infection in Children

- Lymphadenopathy
- Hepatosplenomegaly
- Oral candidiasis
- Chronic or recurrent diarrhea
- Failure to thrive
- Developmental delay
- Parotitis

BOX 49-10 Common Defining Conditions for AIDS in Children

- *Pneumocystis carinii* pneumonia
- Lymphoid interstitial pneumonia, pulmonary lymphoid hyperplasia, or both
- Recurrent bacterial infections
- Wasting syndrome
- Candidal esophagitis
- Human immunodeficiency virus encephalopathy
- Cytomegalovirus disease
- *Mycobacterium avium-intracellulare* complex infection
- Pulmonary candidiasis
- Herpes simplex disease
- Cryptosporidiosis

evolve Critical Thinking Exercise—HIV Testing in Children

counts, which are relatively high in infants, decline steadily until 6 years of age, when they reach adult norms (Table 49-4).

Therapeutic Management

The goals of therapy for HIV infection include slowing the growth of the virus, preventing and treating **opportunistic infections,** and providing nutritional support and symptomatic treatment. Antiretroviral medications work at various stages of the HIV life cycle to prevent reproduction of functional new virus particles. Although not a cure, these medications can suppress viral replication, preventing further deterioration of the immune system, thus delaying disease progression. Classes of antiretroviral agents include nucleoside reverse transcriptase inhibitors (e.g., zidovudine, didanosine, stavudine, lamivudine, abacavir), non-nucleoside reverse transcriptase inhibitors (e.g., nevirapine, delavirdine, efavirenz), nucleotide reverse transcriptase inhibitors (e.g., adefovir), protease inhibitors (e.g., indinavir, saquinavir, ritonavir, nelfinavir, amprenavir), and adjunctive antiretrovirals (e.g., hydroxyurea). Combinations of these medications are used to forestall the emergence of drug resistance. ART regimens and guidelines are continually evolving. Therapy is lifelong, making adherence difficult. Laboratory markers (CD4 lymphocyte count, viral load) assist in monitoring both disease progression and response to therapy. The Canadian Paediatric Society (Robinson, CPS, Infectious Diseases and Immunization Committee, 2010) recommends following the U.S. National Institutes of Health (2011) clinical guidelines for the management of HIV. ART is the current standard in Canada for the treatment of HIV-infected pregnant women, and it has significantly reduced the transmission of HIV (Loutfy et al., 2012).

Pneumocystis carinii pneumonia (PCP) is the most common opportunistic infection of children infected with HIV. It occurs most frequently between 3 and 6 months of age. All infants born to HIV-infected women should receive prophylaxis during the first year of life (National Institutes of Health, 2011). Trimethoprim-sulfamethoxazole (TMP-SMZ) is the agent of choice. If adverse effects are experienced with TMP-SMZ, dapsone or pentamidine can be used.

Prophylaxis is often used for other opportunistic infections, such as disseminated *Mycobacterium avium-intracellulare* complex (MAC), candidiasis, or herpes simplex. IVIG has been helpful in preventing recurrent or serious bacterial infections in some HIV-infected children.

Immunization against common childhood illnesses is recommended for all children exposed to and infected with HIV (PHAC, 2006a). Varicella (chickenpox) vaccine and measles-mumps-rubella (MMR) vaccine can be administered if there is no evidence of severe immunocompromise. Because antibody production to vaccines may be poor or decrease over time, immediate prophylaxis after exposure to several vaccine-preventable diseases (e.g., measles, varicella) is warranted. It should be recognized that children receiving IV γ-globulin prophylaxis may not respond to the MMR vaccine (Centers for Disease Control and Prevention, 2003).

HIV infection often leads to marked failure to thrive and multiple nutritional deficiencies. Nutritional management may be difficult because of recurrent illness, diarrhea, and other physical problems. Intensive nutritional interventions

Table 49-3 Pediatric HIV Infection Classification*

IMMUNOLOGICAL CATEGORY	N: NO SIGNS/ SYMPTOMS	A: MILD SIGNS/ SYMPTOMS	B: MODERATE SIGNS/ SYMPTOMS	C: SEVERE SIGNS/ SYMPTOMS
No evidence of suppression	N1	A1	B1	C1
Evidence of moderate suppression	N2	A2	B2	C2
Severe suppression	N3	A3	B3	C3

(From Centers for Disease Control and Prevention. [1994]. 1994 Revised classification system for human immunodeficiency virus infection in children less than 13 years of age. *MMWR: Recommendations & Reports, 43*[RR-12], 1–10.)

*Children whose HIV infection status is not confirmed are classified by using the above table with the letter E (for perinatally exposed) placed before the appropriate classification code (e.g., EN2).

Table 49-4 Immunological Categories Based on Age-Specific CD4 T-Lymphocyte Counts and Percent of Total Lymphocytes

	Age of Child					
	<12 Mo		*1–5 Yr*		*6–12 Yr*	
IMMUNOLOGICAL CATEGORY	mm^3	(%)	mm^3	(%)	mm^3	(%)
No evidence of suppression	≥1500	(≥25)	≥1000	(≥25)	≥500	(≥25)
Evidence of moderate suppression	750-1499	(15–24)	500–999	(15–24)	200–499	(15–24)
Severe suppression	<750	(<15)	<500	(<15)	<200	(<15)

(From Centers for Disease Control and Prevention. [1994]. 1994 Revised classification system for human immunodeficiency virus infection in children less than 13 years of age. *MMWR: Recommendations & Reports, 43*[RR-12], 1–10.)

should be instituted when the child's growth begins to slow or weight begins to decrease.

Prognosis

Early recognition and improved medical care have changed HIV disease from a rapidly fatal illness to a chronic disease. After the introduction of combination ART, the numbers of new AIDS cases and deaths declined substantially. For example, between 1984 and 2003, there were 560 deaths among the 1987 HIV-positive individuals in Southern Alberta. Of these, 436 deaths (78%) occurred during the pre-ART era and 124 (22%) during the current ART era (Krentz, Kliewer, & Gill, 2005). Since 1998, the annual number of AIDS cases among children younger than 13 years of age has remained stable (Klause & Johnson, 2007).

Nursing Care Management

Education concerning transmission and control of infectious diseases, including HIV infection, is essential for children with HIV infection and anyone involved in their care. The basic tenets of routine practices should be presented in an age-appropriate manner, with careful consideration of the educational levels of the individuals (see Infection Control, Chapter 45). Safety issues, including appropriate storage of special medications and equipment (e.g., needles and syringes), need to be emphasized.

Unfortunately, relatives, friends, and the general public may be fearful of contracting HIV infection, and the child and family may be criticized and ostracized. In an effort to protect the child, the family may limit his or her activities outside the home. Although certain precautions are justified in limiting exposure to sources of infections, they must be tempered with concern for the child's normal developmental needs. Both the family and the community need ongoing education about HIV to dispel many of the myths that have been perpetuated by uninformed persons (see Additional Resources at the end of this chapter).

Prevention is a key component of HIV education. Educating adolescents about HIV is essential in preventing HIV infection in this age group. It should include the routes of transmission, the hazards of IV and other recreational drug use, and safer sex practices. Such education should be a part of anticipatory guidance provided to all adolescent patients. Nurses can also encourage adolescents at risk to undergo HIV counselling and testing. In addition to identifying infected teenagers and getting them into care, such counselling affords adolescents an opportunity to learn about, and possibly change, their risky behaviours.

The multiple complications associated with HIV disease are potentially painful (Ezekowitz, 2009). Aggressive pain management is essential for these children to have an acceptable quality of life. Their pain may be caused by infections (e.g., otitis media, dental abscess), encephalopathy (e.g., spasticity), adverse effects of medications (e.g., peripheral neuropathy), or an unknown source (e.g., deep musculoskeletal pain). Sources of pain are related not only to disease processes but also to various treatments these children often undergo, including venipunctures, lumbar punctures, biopsies, and endoscopies. Ongoing assessment of pain is crucial and is most easily accomplished in older children who are able to communicate. Nonverbal and developmentally delayed children are more difficult to assess. The nurse should be alert for signs of pain such as emotional detachment, lack of interactive play, irritability, and depression. Effective pain management depends on the appropriate use of pharmacological agents, including EMLA cream, acetaminophen, NSAIDs, muscle relaxants, and opioids. Tolerance to opioids may indicate increased dosing; monitored use ensures safety. Nonpharmacological interventions (e.g., guided imagery, hypnosis, relaxation, and distraction techniques) are useful adjuncts.

Common psychosocial concerns include disclosing the diagnosis to the child, making custody plans when the parent is infected, and anticipating the loss of a family member. Other stressors may include financial difficulties, HIV-associated stigma, efforts to keep the diagnosis secret, other infected family members, and the multiple losses associated with HIV. Most mothers of these children are single mothers who are also HIV infected. As primary caretakers, they often attend to the needs of their child first, neglecting their own health in the process (see Family-Centred Teaching box). The nurse can encourage the mother to receive regular health care. Family members are often involved in the care of the child, particularly if the mother has symptomatic illness. After the mother's death, a grandparent or other relative typically assumes responsibility for care of the child. The nurse can provide support and encouragement for the new surrogate parent, particularly during the transition phase. Nursing is an integral part of the multidisciplinary team necessary for the successful management of the complex medical and social problems of these families.

Children with HIV infection attend day care centres and schools. It is well established that the risk of HIV transmission in these settings is minimal. These institutions are required to follow Canada's National Workplace Health and Safety (CanOSH) guidelines for infection control measures. Routine practices describing proper management of blood and body

FAMILY-CENTRED TEACHING

Caregivers and the Infant With HIV Infection

Unlike other fatal pediatric diseases, human immunodeficiency virus (HIV) infection is associated with special family alterations. The infant infected in utero faces multiple physical and parental problems. Because the mother is infected, she may be coping with a chronic illness and therefore unable to care for the child. If possible, grandparents or other relatives may assume care. Foster care is often difficult to arrange because of the nature of the disease, especially in relation to the social stigma and the child's multiple medical needs. When these children are hospitalized, the importance of consistent caregivers, especially primary nurses who attend to the youngsters' physical, developmental, and emotional needs, cannot be overemphasized. However, primary nurses may face the risk of over-involvement and must be aware of the boundaries of a therapeutic relationship.

fluids should also be followed. It is recommended that school personnel receive current HIV information and include it in the health education curriculum for kindergarten through twelfth grade (American Academy of Pediatrics, Committee on Pediatric AIDS, 2000). Confidentiality is a major issue in day care or school attendance. Parents and legal guardians have the right to decide whether to inform these agencies of their child's HIV diagnosis. Unfortunately, myths about HIV infection continue to exist, and the family often wishes to avoid any potential criticism or ostracism of the child.

Severe Combined Immunodeficiency Disease

SCID is a defect characterized by the absence of both humoral and cell-mediated immunity. The terms *Swiss-type lymphopenic agammaglobulinemia* (an autosomal recessive form of the disease) and *X-linked lymphopenic agammaglobulinemia* have been used to describe this disorder, which, as the names imply, can follow either mode of inheritance.

Susceptibility to infection occurs early, most often in the first month of life. The child suffers from chronic infection, fails to completely recover from an infection, is frequently reinfected, and is infected with unusual agents. Failure to thrive is a consequence of the persistent illnesses.

Diagnosis is usually based on a history of recurrent, severe infections from early infancy; a familial history of the disorder; and specific laboratory findings, which include lymphopenia, lack of lymphocyte response to antigens, and absence of plasma cells in the bone marrow. Documentation of immune globulin deficiency is difficult during infancy because of the normally delayed response of infants in producing their own immune globulins and material transfer of immune globulin G (IgG).

Therapeutic Management

The definitive treatment for SCID is HSCT from a histocompatible donor, a haplo-identical donor (usually a parent), or a matched unrelated donor. IVIG infusions and PCP prophylaxis are used to augment the humoral immunity until the transplant is performed. Several investigators are attempting gene therapy with some success, but there is a potential complication of insertional mutagenesis (Buckley, 2007).

Nursing Care Management

Nursing care focuses on preventing infection and supporting the child and family. The care is consistent with that needed for HSCT for any condition (see p. 1533). Because the prognosis for SCID is very poor if a compatible bone marrow donor is not available, nursing care is directed at supporting the family in caring for a child with a life-threatening illness (see Chapter 41). Genetic counselling is essential because of the modes of transmission in either form of the disorder.

Wiskott-Aldrich Syndrome

WAS is an X-linked recessive disorder characterized by a triad of abnormalities: (1) thrombocytopenia, (2) eczema, and (3) immunodeficiency of selective functions of B and T lymphocytes. A defective gene has been identified and designated the WAS protein (Bonilla & Geha, 2009; Fleisher, 2006). At birth the presenting symptom may be bloody diarrhea as a result of thrombocytopenia. As the child grows older, recurrent infection and eczema become more severe, and the bleeding becomes less frequent.

Eczema is typical of the allergic type and easily becomes superinfected. Chronic infection with herpes simplex is a frequent problem and may lead to chronic keratitis of the eye with loss of vision. Chronic pulmonary disease, sinusitis, and otitis media result from repeated infections. In children who survive the bleeding episodes and overwhelming infections, malignancy presents an additional risk to survival. Medical treatment involves the following:

- Counteracting the bleeding tendencies with platelet transfusions.
- Using IV γ-globulin to provide passive immunity.
- Administering prophylactic antibiotics to prevent and control infection.

The only curative therapy is HSCT from a matched donor (Buckley, 2007).

Nursing Care Management

Because of the poor prognosis for these children, the main nursing consideration is supporting the family in the care of a fatally ill child (see Chapter 41). Physical care is directed at controlling the problems imposed by the disorder. The measures used to control bleeding are similar to those for hemophilia and vWD (see previous discussions). Another major goal is prevention or control of infection. Because eczema is a troublesome problem, nursing measures specific to this condition are especially important (see Chapter 53). The genetic implications of this X-linked recessive disorder differ little from those of any other X-linked disorder.

Technological Management of Hematological and Immunological Disorders

Blood Transfusion Therapy

Technological advances in blood banking and transfusion medicine enable the administration of only the blood component needed by the child, such as packed RBCs in anemia or platelets for bleeding disorders. However, regardless of the blood component infused, all transfusions have some risks. Nurses need to be aware of the possible complications and the appropriate interventions. Table 49-5 summarizes the major hazards of transfusions, the signs and symptoms typically associated with each, and nursing responsibilities. General guidelines that apply to all transfusions include the following:

- Take vital signs, including blood pressure, *before* administering blood to establish **baseline data** for intra-transfusion and post-transfusion comparison and then every 15 minutes for 1 hour while blood is infusing and on completion of transfusion.
- Check the identification of the recipient with the donor's blood group and type, regardless of the blood product being used.
- Administer the first 50 mL of blood or 20% of the volume (whichever is smaller) *slowly* and stay with the child.

Table 49-5 Nursing Care of the Child Receiving Blood Transfusions

COMPLICATION	SIGNS AND SYMPTOMS	PRECAUTIONS AND NURSING RESPONSIBILITIES
Immediate Reactions		
Hemolytic Reactions		
Most severe type, but rare Incompatible blood Incompatibility in multiple transfusions	Sudden severe headache Chills Shaking Fever Pain at needle site and along venous tract Nausea and vomiting Sensation of tightness in chest Red or black urine Flank pain Progressive signs of shock or renal failure	Identify donor and recipient blood types and groups before transfusion is begun; verify with another nurse or practitioner. Transfuse blood slowly for first 15–20 min and/or initial 20% of blood volume; remain with patient. Stop transfusion immediately in the event signs or symptoms occur, maintain patent intravenous line, and notify practitioner. Save donor blood to re-cross-match with patient's blood. Monitor for evidence of shock. Insert urinary catheter and monitor hourly outputs. Send sample of patient's blood and urine to laboratory for presence of hemoglobin (indicates intravascular hemolysis). Observe for signs of hemorrhage resulting from disseminated intravascular coagulation. Support medical therapies to reverse shock.
Febrile Reactions		
Leukocyte or platelet antibodies Plasma protein antibodies	Fever Chills	Acetaminophen may be given for prophylaxis. Leukocyte-poor red blood cells (RBCs) are less likely to cause reaction. Stop transfusion immediately; report to practitioner for evaluation.
Allergic Reactions		
Recipient reaction to allergens in donor's blood	Urticaria Pruritus Flushing Asthmatic wheezing Laryngeal edema	Give antihistamines for prophylaxis to children with tendency to allergic reactions. Stop transfusion immediately. Administer epinephrine for wheezing or anaphylactic reaction.
Circulatory Overload		
Too rapid transfusion (even a small quantity) Transfusion of excessive quantity of blood (even slowly)	Precordial pain Dyspnea Rales Cyanosis Dry cough Distended neck veins Hypertension	Transfuse blood slowly. Prevent overload by using packed RBCs or administering divided amounts of blood. Use infusion pump to regulate and maintain flow rate. Stop transfusion immediately if there are signs of overload. Place child upright with feet in dependent position to increase venous resistance.
Air Emboli		
May occur when blood is transfused under pressure	Sudden difficulty in breathing Sharp pain in chest Apprehension	Normalize pressure before container is empty when infusing blood under pressure. Clear tubing of air by aspirating it with syringe at nearest Y connector if it is observed in tubing; disconnect tubing and allow blood to flow until air has escaped only if a Y connector is not available.
Hypothermia		
	Chills Low temperature Irregular heart rate Possible cardiac arrest	Allow blood to warm at room temperature (<1 hr). Use approved mechanical blood warmer or electric warming coil to warm blood rapidly; never use microwave oven. Take temperature if patient complains of chills; if subnormal, stop transfusion.
Electrolyte Disturbances		
Hyperkalemia (in massive transfusions or in patients with renal problems)	Nausea, diarrhea Muscle weakness Flaccid paralysis Paresthesia of extremities Bradycardia Apprehension Cardiac arrest	Use washed RBCs or fresh blood if patient is at risk.

Continued

Table 49-5 Nursing Care of the Child Receiving Blood Transfusions—cont'd

COMPLICATION	SIGNS AND SYMPTOMS	PRECAUTIONS AND NURSING RESPONSIBILITIES
Delayed Reactions		
Transmission of Infection		
Hepatitis Human immunodeficiency virus (HIV) infection Malaria Syphilis Other bacterial or viral infection	Signs of infection (e.g., jaundice) Toxic reaction–High fever, severe headache or substernal pain, hypotension, intense flushing, vomiting or diarrhea	Blood is tested for antibodies to HIV, hepatitis C virus, and hepatitis B core antigen; in addition, it is tested for hepatitis B surface antigen and alanine aminotransferase, and a serological test is performed for syphilis; units that test positive are destroyed; individuals at risk for carrying certain viruses are deterred from donation. Report any sign of infection and, if it occurs during transfusion, stop transfusion immediately, send sample for culture and sensitivity testing, and notify practitioner.
Alloimmunization		
Antibody formation Occurs in patients receiving multiple transfusions	Increased risk of hemolytic, febrile, and allergic reactions	Use limited number of donors. Observe carefully for signs of reactions.
Delayed Hemolytic Reaction		
	Destruction of RBCs and fever 5–10 days after transfusion	Observe for post-transfusion anemia and decreasing benefit from successive transfusions.

- Administer with normal saline on a piggyback setup or have normal saline available.
- Administer blood through an appropriate filter to eliminate particles in the blood and prevent the precipitation of formed elements; gently shake the container frequently.
- Use blood within 30 minutes of its arrival from the blood bank; if it is not used, return to the blood bank—do not store in the regular unit refrigerator.
- Infuse a unit of blood (or the specified amount) within 4 hours. If the infusion will exceed this time, the blood should be divided into appropriately sized quantities by the blood bank, and the unused portion refrigerated under controlled conditions.
- If a reaction of any type is suspected, take vital signs, stop the transfusion, maintain a patent IV line with normal saline and new tubing, notify the practitioner, and do not restart the transfusion until the child's condition has been medically evaluated.

Although hemolytic reactions are rare, ABO incompatibility remains the most common cause of death from blood transfusion, and human error is usually responsible (administration of the wrong type to the patient or mislabelling of the blood product) (Bell, 2007; Norville & Bryant, 2002). Hemolysis can also cause the release of large quantities of phospholipids, which are capable of stimulating DIC (see p. 1516). Acute kidney shutdown and eventual renal failure are the results of renal vasoconstriction from antigen–antibody complexes derived from the RBC surface.

Blood is usually administered to children by infusion pump; thus the usual precautions and management related to pumps apply. When the blood is started with a standard transfusion set, the filter chamber is filled to allow the total filter to be used. The drip chamber is partially filled with blood to permit counting of the drops. In adjusting the flow rate, it is important to remember that blood administration sets do not use microdrops (60 drops/mL) but regular drops (usually 10 or 15 drops/mL).

Hematopoietic Stem Cell (Bone Marrow) Transplantation

HSCT is used to establish healthy hemopoiesis in both malignant and nonmalignant disease. Candidates for transplantation are children who have disorders that are unlikely to be cured by other means. Most HSCT patients undergo intensive ablative therapy using high-dose combination chemotherapy with or without total body irradiation (Bollard et al., 2011). After the immune system is suppressed to prevent rejection of the transplanted marrow, the stem cells harvested from the bone marrow, peripheral blood, or umbilical vein of the placenta are given to the patient by IV transfusion. The newly transfused stem cells will begin to repopulate the ablative bone marrow. In essence, a new blood-forming organ will be accepted by the recipient.

The selection process for a suitable donor and the potential complications in transplantation are related to the *HLA system complex*. Some of the major HLAs are A, B, C, D, and DR. There is a wide diversity for each of these HLA loci. There are more than 20 different HLA-As that can be inherited and more than 40 different HLA-Bs.

The genes are inherited as a single unit or *haplotype*. A child inherits one unit from each parent; thus a child and each parent have one identical and one nonidentical haplotype. Because the possible haplotype combinations among siblings follow the laws of Mendelian genetics, there is a one-in-four chance that two siblings have two identical haplotypes and are perfectly matched at the HLA loci.

The importance of HLA matching is to prevent the serious complication known as graft versus host disease, or GVHD. Because the child's immune system is essentially rendered nonfunctional, there is little difficulty with bone marrow rejection by the recipient. However, the donor's marrow may contain antigens not matched to the recipient's antigens, which begin attacking body cells. The more closely the HLA systems match, the less likely GVHD will develop. However, it can occur even with a perfect HLA match because there are as yet unidentified and thus unmatched histocompatibility antigens (Bollard et al., 2011).

Different types of HSCT are now performed in children with cancer. Allogeneic HSCT involves matching a histocompatible donor with the recipient. However, allogeneic HSCT is limited by the presence of a suitable marrow donor.

Because of the limited numbers of patients having HLA-identical siblings, other types of allogeneic transplants have evolved. Umbilical cord blood stem cell transplantation is an established, rich source of hematopoietic stem cells for use in children with cancer. Because stem cells can be found with high frequency in the circulation of newborns, cord blood transplantation has become an alternative for some children. The benefit of using umbilical cord blood is the blood's relative immunodeficiency at birth, allowing for partially matched unrelated cord blood transplants to be successful, with a lower risk of GVHD-related problems (Bollard et al., 2011; Frey et al., 2009).

Autologous HSCTs use the patient's own marrow that was collected from disease-free tissue, frozen, and sometimes treated to remove malignant cells. Children with solid tumours such as neuroblastoma, Hodgkin's disease, NHL, rhabdomyosarcoma, Ewing sarcoma, and Wilms tumour have been treated with autologous HSCTs.

Peripheral stem cell transplants (PSCTs) are also used in children with cancer. PSCT, a type of autologous transplant, differs in the way stem cells are collected from the patient. CSF is first given to stimulate the production of many stem cells (Lanzkowsky, 2005). After the WBC count is high enough, the stem cells are collected by an apheresis machine. This machine filters out peripheral stem cells from whole blood, returning the remainder of the blood cells and plasma to the child. Stem cells have been collected in very small children without problems (Lipton, 2003). The peripheral stem cells are then frozen until the patient is ready for the PSCT.

Nursing Care Management

The care of children undergoing HSCT is similar to that of any child receiving chemotherapy and radiotherapy. The hospitalization is typically 3 to 6 weeks in an isolated environment, during which time the child is subjected to numerous procedures and side effects of therapy. Throughout this long ordeal the family is concerned with successful engraftment and fear of fatal complications (see Family-Centred Teaching box). Consequently, nurses involved with the child and family need to provide sensitive care and maintain a supportive attitude during the many crises that may arise. If the procedure is not successful, the families need care consistent with that required by the family of any child with a life-threatening disorder (see Chapter 41).

Apheresis

Apheresis is the removal of blood from an individual, separation of the blood into its components, retention of one or more of these components, and reinfusion of the remainder of the blood into the individual. It is most often used to remove large quantities of platelets from healthy adult donors. These transfusion products have greatly prolonged the survival of patients with hematological and oncological diseases.

This technique is used to remove peripheral blood stem cells (PBSCs) from children before they receive HSCT or high-dose chemotherapy or radiotherapy, which is severely toxic to the bone marrow. These PBSCs can then be used to restore the child's bone marrow. Apheresis is also used as a therapeutic modality. The blood component that is diseased or toxic is separated from the blood, and the remainder is returned to the individual. Therapeutic apheresis is considered part of standard therapy for many diseases. Plasma is selectively removed from individuals with hyperviscosity, life-threatening complications of myasthenia gravis, Guillain-Barré syndrome, thrombotic thrombocytopenic purpura, and certain drug overdoses. WBCs are removed from individuals with high–WBC count leukemia.

Nursing Care Management

Difficult venous access and small blood volume can limit the ability to use this therapy in the infant and young child. Education of the family and child includes the purposes of the therapy and the technology.

Specially trained individuals perform the apheresis procedure. Attention focuses on the rate of removal, blood component separation, and reinfusion of blood into the child. Vital signs need to be monitored and the child continuously observed for any adverse reactions secondary to the circulatory volume changes and the anticoagulant used.

FAMILY-CENTRED TEACHING

The Decision for a Hematopoietic Stem Cell Transplant

A family's decision for a child to undergo hematopoietic stem cell transplantation (HSCT) may be fraught with challenges. Often the child is facing certain death from the malignancy. The preparation of the child for the transplant also places the patient at great medical risk.

Once the preparatory regimen is begun and the child's immune system is destroyed, there is no turning back. Unlike kidney transplantation, HSCT does not have a "rescue" procedure, such as dialysis, for supportive therapy. If the donor is a sibling, the issue of his or her marrow "saving" the brother or sister can be a concern, especially if the transplant fails. Parents often must leave the home to stay at the transplant centre and encounter additional stressors such as arranging child care, taking a leave from work, and managing finances. The patient faces the greatest stress—fear of HSCT failure or life-threatening complications.

When apheresis components are infused, nursing measures differ depending on whether the product is autologous (blood component from the child) or allogeneic (blood component from another individual). Autologous components are the child's own blood; thus a major precaution is proper identification to ensure the correct component. The rate of infusion should be adjusted to the child's tolerance. If the product is allogeneic, all precautions for blood transfusions apply.

Key Points

- Anemia is defined as the reduction of RBCs or Hgb concentration to levels below normal for age; disorders are classified either by etiology and physiology or by morphology.
- The nurse's role in treatment of anemia is to assist in establishing a diagnosis, prepare the child for laboratory tests, administer prescribed medications, decrease tissue oxygen needs, implement safety precautions, and observe for complications.
- The main nursing goal in prevention of nutritional anemia is parent education regarding correct feeding practices.
- SCA is a hereditary hemoglobinopathy caused by normal adult Hgb (HgbA) being partly or completely replaced by sickle Hgb (HgbS).
- Nursing care of the child with SCA focuses on teaching the family how to prevent and recognize sickle cell problems; managing pain during crises; and helping the child and parents adjust to a lifelong chronic disease.
- Nursing care of the child with β-thalassemia includes observing for complications of multiple blood transfusions, assisting the child in coping with the effects of illness, and fostering parent-child adjustment to long-term illness.
- Causes of acquired AA include irradiation, medications, industrial and household chemicals, infections, and infiltration and replacement of myeloid elements; however, most cases are idiopathic.
- Clotting depends on three processes: vascular spasm, platelet aggregation, and coagulation and clot formation.
- Nursing care of the child with hemophilia involves preventing bleeding by decreasing the risk of injury, recognizing and managing bleeding with factor replacement, preventing the crippling effects of joint degeneration, and preparing and supporting the child and family for home care.
- Goals in the care of the child with leukemia are to prepare the family for diagnostic and therapeutic procedures, prevent complications of myelosuppression, manage problems of irradiation and drug toxicity, and provide continued emotional support.
- The lymphomas include Hodgkin's lymphoma and NHL and are disorders involving the lymphoid system.
- Immunodeficiency disorders render the affected individual unable to fight infectious organisms.
- HIV infection is primarily acquired in infants during pregnancy or birth from an infected mother and in adolescents from engaging in high risk behaviours.
- Blood transfusions supply needed blood components.
- HSCT replaces the diseased or malfunctioning bone marrow with viable blood stem cells.
- Apheresis is the selective removal of a blood component. It can be used to supply cellular elements needed for therapy (i.e., platelets or stem cells) or to remove diseased components.

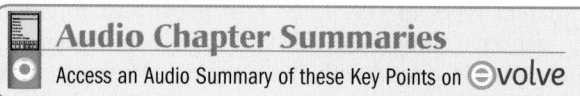

Audio Chapter Summaries
Access an Audio Summary of these Key Points on evolve

References

Abdullah, K., Zlotkin, S., Parkin, P., & Grenier, D. (2011). *Iron-deficiency anemia in children. Canadian Paediatric Surveillance Program.* Retrieved from http://www.cps.ca/english/surveillance/cpsp/resources/Iron-deficiency_anemia.pdf.

American Academy of Pediatrics, Committee on Pediatric AIDS. (2000). Identification and care of HIV-exposed and HIV-infected infants, children, and adolescents in foster care. *Pediatrics, 106*(1), 149–153.

Anderson, N. (2006). Hydroxyurea therapy: Improving the lives of patients with sickle cell disease. *Pediatric Nursing, 32*(6), 541–543.

Andrews, N. C., Ullrich, C. K., & Fleming, M. D. (2009). Disorders of iron metabolism and sideroblastic anemia. In S. H Orkin, et al. (Eds.), *Nathan and Oski's hematology of infancy and childhood* (7th ed.). Philadelphia: Saunders.

Armstrong-Wells, J., et al. (2009). Utilization of TCD screening for primary stroke prevention in children with sickle cell disease. *Neurology, 72,* 1316–1321.

Bell, M. D. (2007). Red blood cell transfusions. *Pediatrics in Review, 28*(8), 299–304. doi:10.1542/pir.28-8-299

Berde, C. B., Billett, A. M., & Collins, J. J. (2006). Symptom management in supportive care. In P. A. Pizzo & D. G. Poplack (Eds.), *Principles and practice of pediatric oncology* (5th ed.). Philadelphia: Lippincott.

Bhatia, S. (2004). Epidemiology. In W. H. B. Wallace & D. M. Green (Eds.), *Late effects of childhood cancer.* London: Arnold.

Bollard, C. M., Krance, R. A., & Heslop, H. E. (2011). Hematopoietic stem cell transplantation in pediatric oncology. In P. A. Pizzo & D. G. Poplack (Eds.), *Principles and practice of pediatric oncology* (6th ed.). Philadelphia: Lippincott.

Bonilla, F. A., & Geha, R. S. (2009). Primary immunodeficiency diseases. In D. Nathan, et al. (Eds.), *Nathan and Oski's hematology of infancy and childhood* (7th ed.). Philadelphia: Saunders.

Buchanan, G. R. (2005). Thrombocytopenia during childhood: What the pediatrician needs to know. *Pediatrics in Review, 26*(11), 401–409. doi:10.1542/pir.26-11-401

Buckley, R. H. (2007). Evaluation of the immune system. In R. F. Behrman, et al. (Eds.), *Nelson textbook of pediatrics* (18th ed.). Philadelphia: Saunders.

Burden, M. J., et al. (2007). An event-related potential study of attention and recognition memory in infants with iron-deficiency anemia. *Pediatrics, 120*(2), 336–345. doi:10.1542/peds.2006-2525

Canadian Cancer Society/National Cancer Institute of Canada (2008). *Canadian cancer statistics 2008.* Toronto: Author.

Canadian Cancer Society, Steering Committee. (2009). *Canadian cancer statistics 2009.* Toronto: Author.

Canadian Paediatric Society. (2005). Exclusive breastfeeding should continue to six months. *Pediatrics and Children's Health, 10*(3), 148.

Carley, A. (2003). Anemia: When is it iron deficiency? *Pediatric Nursing, 29*(2), 127–133.

Centers for Disease Control and Prevention. (1994). 1994 revised classification system for human immunodeficiency virus infection in children less than 13 years of age. *MMWR: Morbidity & Mortality Weekly Report, 43*(RR-12), 1–10.

Centers for Disease Control and Prevention. (2003). Advancing HIV prevention: New strategies for a changing epidemic—United States. *MMWR: Morbidity & Mortality Weekly Report, 52*(15), 329–332.

Chandran, L., & Gelfer, P. (2006). Breastfeeding: The essential principles. *Pediatrics in Review, 27*(11), 409–417. doi:10.1542/pir.27-11-409

Cho, S., Cheng, A. C., & Cheng, M. C. K. (2000). Oral care for children with leukemia. *Hong Kong Medical Journal, 6*(2), 203–208.

Cunningham, M. J., et al. (2009). The thalassemias. In S. H. Orkin, et al. (Eds.), *Nathan and Oski's hematology of infancy and childhood* (7th ed.). Philadelphia: Saunders.

Curry, H. (2004). Bleeding disorder basics. *Pediatric Nursing, 30*(5), 402–405.

DeBaun, M. R., & Vichinsky, E. (2007). Hemoglobinopathies. In R. M. Kliegman, et al. (Eds.), *Nelson textbook of pediatrics* (18th ed.). Philadelphia: Saunders.

Driscoll, M. C. (2007). Sickle cell disease. *Pediatrics in Review, 28*(7), 259–267. doi:10.1542/pir.28-7-259

Ezekowitz, R. A. B. (2009). Hematologic manifestations of systemic diseases. In S. H. Orkin, et al. (Eds.), *Nathan and Oski's hematology of infancy and childhood* (7th ed.). Philadelphia: Saunders.

Fleisher, T. A. (2006). Primary immune deficiencies: Windows into the immune system. *Pediatrics in Review, 27*(10), 363–373. doi:10.1542/pir.27-10-363)

Frey, M. A., et al. (2009). Umbilical cord stem cell transplantation. *Seminars in Oncology Nursing, 25*(2), 115–119.

Glader, B. (2007). Anemias of inadequate production. In R. E. Behrman, et al. (Eds.), *Nelson textbook of pediatrics* (18th ed.). Philadelphia: Saunders.

Goldschmidt, R. H., & Fogler, J. A. (2006). Opportunities to prevent HIV transmission to newborns. *Pediatrics, 117*(1), 208–209. doi:10.1542/peds.2005-0799

Gross, T. G., & Perkins, L. S. (2011). Malignant non-Hodgkin lymphomas in children. In P. A. Pizzo & D. G. Poplack (Eds.), *Principles and practice of pediatric oncology* (6th ed.). Philadelphia: Lippincott.

Heeney, M., & Dover, G. J. (2009). Sickle cell disease. In S. H. Orkin, et al., (Eds.), *Nathan and Oski's hematology of infancy and childhood* (7th ed.). Philadelphia: Saunders.

Hord, J. D. (2007). The acquired pancytopenia. In R. E. Behrman, et al. (Eds.), *Nelson textbook of pediatrics* (18th ed.). Philadelphia: Saunders.

Hudson, M. M., Onciu, M., & Donaldson, S. S. (2011). Hodgkin's disease. In P. A. Pizzo & D. G. Poplack (Eds.), *Principles and practice of pediatric oncology* (6th ed.). Philadelphia: Lippincott.

Khoury, H., & Grimsley, E. (1995). Oxygen inhalation in nonhypoxic sickle cell patients during vaso-occlusive crisis. *Blood, 86*(10), 3998.

Klause, B. D., & Johnson, M. (2007). Paradigm shift: New testing guidelines for HIV. *Advanced Nurse Practitioner, 15*(3), 59–93.

Krentz, H. B., Kliewer, G., & Gill, M. J. (2005). Changing mortality rates and causes of death for HIV-infected individuals living in Southern Alberta, Canada from 1984 to 2003. *HIV Medicine, 6*(2), 99–106, doi:10.1111/j.1468-1293.2005.00271.x

Lanzkowsky, P. (2005). *Manual of pediatric hematology and oncology* (4th ed.). San Diego: Academic Press.

Link, M. P., & Weinstein, H. J. (2006). Malignant non-Hodgkin lymphomas in children. In P. A. Pizzo & D. G. Poplack (Eds.), *Principles and practice of pediatric oncology* (4th ed.). Philadelphia: Lippincott.

Lipton, J. M. (2003). Peripheral blood as a stem cell source for hematopoietic cell transplantation in children: Is the effort in vein? *Pediatric Transplantation, 7*(Suppl 3), 65–70.

Loutfy, M. R., et al. (2012). SOGC clinical practice guideline: Canadian HIV pregnancy planning guidelines. *Journal of Obstetricians and Gynecologists of Canada, 34*(6), 575–590. Retrieved from http://www.sogc.org/guidelines/documents/gui278CPG1206E.pdf.

Lucarelli, G., & Gaziev, J. (2008). Advances in the allogeneic transplantation for thalassemia. *Blood Reviews, 22*, 53–63.

Lynch, M. E., & Lynch, M. (2011). Prescription opioid abuse. What is the real problem and how do we fix it? *Canadian Family Physician, 57*(11), 1241–1242.

Margolin, J. F., Rabin, K. R., & Steuber, C. P. (2011). Acute lymphoblastic leukemia. In P. A. Pizzo & D. G. Poplack (Eds.), *Principles and practice of pediatric oncology* (6th ed.). Philadelphia: Lippincott.

Marsh, J. C. W. (2005). Management of acquired aplastic anemia. *Blood Reviews, 19*, 143–151. doi:10.1016/j.blre.2004.06.002

McKenzie, S. B. (2004). Anemias of disordered iron metabolism and heme synthesis. In S. B. McKenzie (Ed.), *Clinical laboratory hematology*. Upper Saddle River, NJ: Pearson Prentice Hall.

Miller, M., et al. (2001). Hydroxyurea therapy for pediatric patients with hemoglobin SC disease. *Journal of Pediatric Hematology & Oncology, 23*(5), 306–308.

Montgomery, R. R., Gill, J. C., & Di Paola, J. (2009). Hemophilia and von Willebrand disease. In S. H. Orkin, et al. (Eds.) *Nathan and Oski's hematology of infancy and childhood* (7th ed.). Philadelphia: Saunders.

Morris, C. R., Singer, S. T., & Walters, M. C. (2006). Clinical hemoglobinopathies: Iron, lungs and new blood. *Current Opinion in Hematology, 13*, 407–418. doi:10.1097/01.moh.0000245685.24462.4e

National Hemophilia Foundation, Bleeding Disorders Information Center. (2006). *Newly diagnosed: Parent FAQ*. Retrieved from http://www.hemophilia.org/bdi/bdi_newly7c.htm.

National Institutes of Health, Panel on Antiretroviral Therapy and Medical Management of HIV-Infected Children. (2011). *Clinical guidelines portal.* Retrieved from http://www.aidsinfo.nih.gov/Guidelines/.

Norville, R., & Bryant, R. (2002). Blood component deficiencies. In C. R. Baggott, et al. (Eds.), *APON nursing care of children and adolescents with cancer* (3rd ed.). Philadelphia: Saunders.

Ohls, R., & Christensen, R. D. (2007). Hemoglobin disorders. In R. E. Behrman, et al. (Eds.), *Nelson textbook of pediatrics* (18th ed.). Philadelphia: Saunders.

Okpala, I. (2005). New therapies for sickle cell disease. *Hematology & Oncology Clinics of North America, 19*, 975–987. doi:10.1016/j.hoc.2005.08.004

Pack-Mabien, A., & Haynes, J., Jr. (2009). A primary care provider's guide to preventive and acute care management of adults and children with sickle cell disease. *Journal of American Academy of Nurse Practioners, 21*, 250–257.

Pearce, J. M., & Sills, R. H. (2005). Childhood leukemia. *Pediatric Reviews, 26*(3), 96–104.

Perkins, S. (2001). Disorders of hematopoiesis. In R. D. Collins & S. H. Swerdlow (Eds.), *Pediatric hematopathology*. Philadelphia: Churchill Livingstone.

Public Health Agency of Canada. (2006a). *Canadian immunization guide* (7th ed.). Ottawa: Author.

Public Health Agency of Canada. (2006b). *HIV and AIDS in Canada: Surveillance report to December 31, 2005*. Ottawa: HIV/AIDS Clearinghouse.

Public Health Agency of Canada. (2010a). *HIV/AIDS: Surveillance report to December 31, 2007*. Retrieved from http://www.phac-aspc.gc.ca/aids-sida/publication/survreport/index-eng.php.

Public Health Agency of Canada. (2010b). *HIV/AIDS Epi Updates to July 31, 2010*. Retrieved from http://www.phac-aspc.gc.ca/aids-sida/publication/epi/2010/8-eng.php.

Redding-Lallinger, R., & Knoll, C. (2006). Sickle cell disease—pathophysiology and treatment. *Current Problems in Pediatric & Adolescent Health Care, 36*(10), 346–376. doi:10.1016/j.cppeds.2006.07.002

Richardson, M. (2007). Microcytic anemia. *Pediatrics in Review, 28*(1), 5–13. doi:10.1542/pir.28-1-5

Robinson, J. L., Canadian Paediatric Society, Infectious Diseases and Immunization Committee. (2010). Management of HIV-exposed and HIV-infected children. *Paediatrics & Child Health, 15*(6), 379.

Scott, J. P., & Montgomery, R. R. (2007). Platelet and blood vessel disorders. In R. E. Behrman, et al. (Eds.), *Nelson textbook of pediatrics* (18th ed.). Philadelphia: Saunders.

Shimamura, A., & Guinan, E. C. (2003). Acquired aplastic anemia. In D. Nathan, et al. (Eds.), *Nathan and Oski's hematology of infancy and childhood* (6th ed.). Philadelphia: Saunders.

Silverman, L. B., & Sallan, S. E. (2003). Acute lymphoblastic leukemia. In D. Nathan, et al. (Eds.), *Nathan and Oski's hematology of infancy and childhood* (6th ed.). Philadelphia: Saunders.

Steinberg, M. H., et al. (2003). Effect of hydroxyurea on mortality and morbidity in adult sickle cell anemia: Risks and benefits up to 9 years of treatment. *Journal of the American Medical Association, 289*(13), 1645–1651.

Sung, L., et al. (2001). Practical vaccination guidelines for children with cancer. *Pediatrics & Child Health, 6*, 379–383.

Wilson, D. B. (2009). Acquired platelet defects. In S. H. Orkin, et al. (Eds.), *Nathan and Oski's hematology of infancy and childhood* (7th ed.). Philadelphia: Saunders.

Yoon, S. L., & Black, S. (2006). Comprehensive, integrative management of pain for patients with sickle-cell disease. *Journal of Alternative & Complementary Medicine, 12*(10), 995–1001. doi:10.1089/acm.2006.12.995

Young, N. S., Calado, R. T., & Scheinberg, P. (2006). Current concepts in the pathophysiology and treatment of aplastic anemia. *Blood, 108*(8), 2509–2519.

Zimmerman, S., et al. (2004). Sustained long-term hematologic efficacy of hydroxyurea at maximum tolerated dose in children with sickle cell disease. *Blood, 103*(6), 2039–2045.

Zlotkin, S. (2003). Clinical nutrition: 8. The role of nutrition in the prevention of iron deficiency anemia in infants, children and adolescents. *Canadian Medical Association Journal, 168*(1), 59–63.

Additional Resources

Aplastic Anemia and Myelodysplasia Association of Canada: http://www.aamac.ca
BC Cancer Agency—Cancer chemotherapy guidelines: http://www.bccancer.ca
Canadian AIDS Society: http://www.cdnaids.ca/
Canadian Hemophilia Society: http://www.hemophilia.ca
Canadian Paediatric Society: Rourke Baby Record: http://www.cps.ca/english/statements/cp/rourke/rbrnational.pdf
Cooley's Anemia Foundation: http://www.cooleysanemia.org
Oncology Nursing Society—Guideline for cancer chemotherapy: http://www.ons.org
Sickle Cell Association of Ontario: http://www.sicklecellontario.org/
Sickle Cell Disease Association of America: http://www.sicklecelldisease.org/
Thalassemia Foundation of Canada: http://www.thalassemia.ca

50 Genitourinary Dysfunction

Learning Objectives

On completion of this chapter, the reader will be able to:

- Describe the various factors that contribute to urinary tract infections in infants and children.
- Discuss the preoperative preparation of the child and parents when the child has a structural defect of the genitourinary tract.
- Demonstrate an understanding of the causes and mechanisms of edema formation in nephrotic syndrome.
- Outline a nursing care plan for a child with nephrotic syndrome.
- Compare the child with minimal-change nephrotic syndrome and the child with acute glomerulonephritis in terms of clinical manifestations and nursing care.
- Contrast the causes, complications, and management of acute and chronic renal failure.
- List the types of renal dialysis.
- Recognize signs of kidney transplant rejection.

Electronic Resources

Additional information related to the content in Chapter 50 can be found on

evolve **the companion Web site at**

http://evolve.elsevier.com/Canada/Perry/maternal/

- Examination Review Questions
- Animation—Bladder
- Animation—Kidney Function

Genitourinary Dysfunction

Assessment of kidney and urinary tract integrity and diagnosis of renal or urinary tract disease are based on several evaluative tools. Physical examination, **history** taking, and observation of symptoms are the initial procedures. In suspected urinary tract diseases or disorders, further assessment by laboratory, radiological, and other evaluative methods is carried out.

Clinical Manifestations

As in most disorders of childhood, the incidence and type of kidney or urinary tract dysfunction change with the child's age and maturation. In addition, the presenting health concerns and the significance of these concerns vary with maturation. For example, enuresis has greater significance at age 8 years than at age 4. In the newborn, urinary tract disorders are associated with a number of obvious malformations of other body systems, including the curious and unexplained but frequent association between malformed or low-set ears and urinary tract anomalies.

While many of the clinical manifestations of renal disease are common to a variety of childhood disorders, their presence is an indication to obtain further information from the child's history, family history, and laboratory studies as part of a complete physical examination. Suspected renal disease can be further evaluated by means of radiographic studies and renal biopsy (Table 50-1).

evolve Animation—Kidney Function

Laboratory Tests

Both urine and blood studies contribute vital information for the detection of renal problems. The single most important test is probably routine urinalysis. Specific urine and blood tests provide additional information. Because nurses are usually the persons who collect the specimens for examination and who often perform many of the screening tests, they should be familiar with the tests, their functions, and factors that can alter or distort the results of the tests. The major urine and blood tests are outlined in Tables 50-2 and 50-3.

Nursing Care Management

Nursing responsibilities in assessment of genitourinary disorders or diseases begin with observation of the child for any manifestations that might indicate dysfunction. Many conditions have specific characteristics that distinguish them from other disorders. These are discussed throughout the chapter.

The nurse is generally responsible for preparing infants, children, and parents for tests and for collecting urine and (sometimes) blood specimens for observation and laboratory

Table 50-1 Radiological and Other Tests of Urinary System Function

TEST	PROCEDURE	PURPOSE	COMMENTS AND NURSING RESPONSIBILITIES
Urine culture and sensitivity	Collection of sterile specimen	Determines presence of pathogens and the medications to which they are sensitive	Does not require specific parental permission Send specimen to laboratory immediately after collection. Use catheterization, clean-catch, or suprapubic specimen.
Renal and bladder ultrasound	Transmission of ultrasonic waves through renal parenchyma, along ureteral course, and over bladder	Allows visualization of renal parenchyma and renal pelvis without exposure to external beam radiation or radioactive isotopes Visualization of dilated ureters and bladder wall also possible	Noninvasive procedure
Testicular (scrotal) ultrasound	Transmission of ultrasonic waves through scrotal contents and testis	Allows visualization of scrotal contents, including testis Testicular ultrasound is used to identify masses, and Doppler-enhanced ultrasound is used to differentiate hyperemia of epididymo-orchitis from ischemia or torsion	Noninvasive procedure
Scout film	Flat plate roentgenogram of abdomen and pelvis for kidney, ureters, bladder (KUB)	Detects and establishes renal outlines, presence of calculi, or opaque foreign bodies in bladder	Prepare as for routine x-ray film.
Voiding cystourethrography	Contrast medium injected into bladder through urethral catheter until bladder is full; films taken before, during, and after voiding	Visualizes bladder outline and urethra, reveals reflux of urine into ureters, and shows complications of bladder emptying	Prepare child for catheterization.
Radionuclide (nuclear) cystogram	Radionuclide-containing fluid injected through urethral catheter until bladder is full; images generated before, during, and after voiding	Alternative to voiding cystourethrography in children with allergy to intravesical contrast material Allows evaluation of reflux, although visualization of anatomical details is relatively poor	Prepare child for catheterization. Reassure patient and parents that allergic response to contrast materials is avoided by use of radionuclide.
Radioisotope imaging studies	Contrast medium injected intravenously; computer analysis to measure uptake or washout (excretion) for analysis of organ function	DTPA radioisotope used to measure glomerular filtration rate; estimate of differential renal function and renal washout to determine presence and location of upper urinary tract obstruction DMSA radioisotope used to visualize renal scars and differential renal function; does not visualize ureters and bladder MAG3 radioisotope combines features of DTPA (evaluation of upper urinary tract obstruction) with features of DMSA radioisotope (differential renal function)	Insert or assist with insertion of intravenous infusion. Monitor intravenous infusion. Urethral catheterization may accompany DTPA radioisotope scan; prepare child for catheterization when indicated.
Intravenous pyelography (IVP) (intravenous urogram; excretory urogram)	Intravenous injection of a contrast medium Medium secreted and concentrated by tubules X-ray films made 5, 10, and 15 minutes after injection; delayed films (30, 60 minutes, etc.) are obtained if obstruction suspected	Defines urinary tract Provides information about integrity of kidneys, ureters, and bladder Retroperitoneal masses visualized when they shift position of ureters	Preparation for test: **Infants <2 yr of age**—Give no solid food, omit one bottle on morning of examination; perform studies early to avoid withholding of fluids. **Children 2–14 yr of age**—Give cathartic evening before examination, nothing orally after midnight, enema (soapsuds) morning of examination.

Table 50-1 Radiological and Other Tests of Urinary System Function—cont'd

TEST	PROCEDURE	PURPOSE	COMMENTS AND NURSING RESPONSIBILITIES
Computed tomography (CT)	Narrow-beam x-rays and computer analysis providing precise reconstruction of area	Visualizes vertical or horizontal cross section of kidney Especially valuable to distinguish tumours and cysts	Noncontrast scan is noninvasive. Contrast-enhanced CT scan preparation is similar to that for IVP.
Cystoscopy	Direct visualization of bladder and lower urinary tract through small scope inserted via urethra	Investigation of bladder and lower tract lesions; visualizes ureteral openings, bladder wall, trigone, and urethra	Give nothing orally after midnight. Carry out preoperative preparations. Prepare the child for cystoscopy.
Retrograde pyelography	Contrast medium injected through ureteral catheter	Visualizes pelvic calyces, ureters, and bladder	Give cathartic if ordered. Give preoperative medication if ordered. Observe for reaction to contrast medium. Monitor vital signs after procedure.
Renal angiography	Contrast medium injected directly into renal artery via catheter placed in femoral artery (or umbilical artery in newborn) and advanced to renal artery	Visualizes renal vascular system, especially for renal arterial stenosis	Prepare child for insertion of a spinal needle or perfusion catheter in renal pelvis (anaesthetic often required).
Whitaker perfusion test	Injection of contrast material through renal pelvis and ureters Measures pressures in renal pelvis and urinary bladder	Determine presence of obstruction causing upper urinary tract dilation	Give nothing orally 4–6 hr before test. Premedicate as ordered. Prepare setup for procedure. Assist with procedure. Take vital signs. Apply pressure to area with pressure dressing and, if feasible, a sandbag. Place on bed rest for 24 hr. Observe for abdominal pain, tenderness. Monitor input and output; surgical incision may be required in infants.
Renal biopsy	Removal of kidney tissue by open or percutaneous technique for study by light, electron, or immunofluorescent microscopy	Yields histological and microscopic information about glomeruli and tubules; helps distinguish between types of nephritic syndromes Distinguishes other renal disorders	Prepare child for catheterization. Insertion of a rectal tube produces feelings of rectal fullness or pressure. Insertion of needles may be required for sphincter electromyography.
Urodynamics	Set of tests designed to measure bladder filling, storage, and evacuation functions **Uroflowmetry**–Test to determine efficiency of urination **Cystometrogram**–Graphic comparison of bladder pressure as a function of volume **Voiding pressure study**–Comparison of detrusor contraction pressure, sphincter electromyelogram, and urinary flow	Determine characteristic of voiding dysfunction Used to identify type (cause) of incontinence or urinary retention Especially valuable for voiding dysfunction complicated by urinary tract infection, urinary retention, or neurogenic bladder dysfunction	Prepare child for urinary catheterization. The bladder will be filled with saline solution and filling pressures will be recorded; the child may experience fullness, coolness from the saline fluid, and urine leakage during the study.

DMSA, dimercaptosuccinic acid; *DTPA*, diethylenetriamine pentaacetic acid; *MAG3*, mercaptoacetyltriglycine.

Table 50-2 Urine Tests of Renal Function

TEST	NORMAL RANGE	DEVIATIONS	SIGNIFICANCE OF DEVIATIONS
Physical Tests			
Volume	Age-related Infants—<1 mL/kg/hr Children—0.5 mL/kg/hr	Polyuria Oliguria Anuria	Osmotic factors (urinary glucose level in diabetes mellitus) Retention caused by obstructive disease Inadequate bladder emptying caused by neurogenic bladder or obstructive disorder Obstruction of urinary tract; acute renal failure
Specific gravity	With normal fluid intake—1.016-1.022 Newborn—1.001-1.020 Others— 1.001-1.030	High Low	Dehydration Presence of protein or glucose Presence of radiopaque contrast medium after radiological examinations Excessive fluid intake Distal tubular dysfunction Insufficient antidiuretic hormone Diuresis
Osmolality	Newborn— 274-305 mmol/kg H_2O Thereafter—282-300 mmol/kg H_2O	 High or low	Chronic glomerular disease Same as for specific gravity More sensitive index than specific gravity
Appearance	Clear pale yellow to deep gold	Cloudy Cloudy reddish pink to reddish brown Light Dark Red	Contains sediment Blood from trauma or disease Myoglobin after severe muscle destruction Dilute Concentrated Trauma
Chemical Tests			
pH	Newborn—5-7 Thereafter— 4.8-7.8 Average—6	Weak acid or neutral Alkaline	If associated with metabolic acidosis, suggests tubular acidosis If associated with metabolic alkalosis, suggests potassium deficiency Urinary infection Metabolic alkalosis
Protein level	Absent	Present	Abnormal glomerular permeability (e.g., glomerular disease, changes in blood pressure) Most kidney disease Orthostatic in some individuals
Glucose level	Absent	Present	Diabetes mellitus Infusion of concentrated glucose-containing fluids Glomerulonephritis Impaired tubular reabsorption
Ketone levels	Absent	Present	Conditions of acute metabolic demand (stress) Diabetic ketoacidosis
Leukocyte esterase	Absent	Present	Can identify both lysed and intact white blood cells via enzyme detection
Nitrites	Absent	Present	Most species of bacteria convert nitrates to nitrites in the urine

analysis (see Preparation for Diagnostic and Therapeutic Procedures, and Collection of Specimens, Chapter 45). An important nursing responsibility is to maintain careful intake and output and blood pressure measurements on most children with genitourinary dysfunction and those who might be at risk for developing renal complications (e.g., children in **shock**, postoperative patients). For example, any significant degree of renal disease can diminish the glomerular filtration rate, a measure of the amount of plasma from which a given substance is totally cleared in 1 minute. A number of substances can be used, but the most useful clinical estimation of glomerular filtration is the clearance of creatinine, an end product of protein metabolism in muscle and a substance that is freely filtered by the glomerulus and secreted by renal tubular cells. The nurse's responsibility in this test is the collection of urine, usually a 12- or 24-hour specimen.

Table 50-2 Urine Tests of Renal Function—cont'd

TEST	NORMAL RANGE	DEVIATIONS	SIGNIFICANCE OF DEVIATIONS
Microscopic Tests			
White blood cell count	<1 or 2	>5 polymorphonuclear leukocytes/field	Urinary tract inflammatory process
		Lymphocytes	Allograft rejection Malignancy
Red blood cell count	<1 or 2	4-6/field in centrifuged specimen	Trauma Stones Glomerular injury Infection Neoplasms
Presence of bacteria	Absent to a few	>100,000 organisms/mL in centrifuged specimen	Urinary tract infection
Presence of casts	Occasional	Granular casts	Tubular or glomerular disorders Degenerative process in advanced renal disease
		Cellular casts White blood cell Red blood cell Hyaline casts	Pyelonephritis Glomerulonephritis Proteinuria; usually transient

Table 50-3 Blood Tests of Renal Function

TEST	NORMAL RANGE	DEVIATIONS	SIGNIFICANCE OF DEVIATIONS
Urea	Newborn–2.9-10.0 mmol/L Infant, child–2.0-7.1 mmol/L	Elevated	Renal disease–acute or chronic (the higher the urea, the more severe the disease) Increased protein catabolism Dehydration Hemorrhage High protein intake Corticosteroid therapy
Uric acid	Child–120-360 mcmol/L	Increased	Severe renal disease
Creatinine	Infant–10-56 mcmol/L Child–<53 mcmol/L Adolescent–<98 mcmol/L	Increased	Severe renal impairment

Genitourinary Tract Disorders and Defects

Urinary Tract Infection

Infection of the genitourinary tract is one of the most common conditions of childhood. Up to 10% of children will have a febrile urinary tract infection (UTI) during the first 2 years of life (Kanellopoulos et al., 2006). Among febrile males, circumcision status is a consideration in determining risk for UTI. In one study, uncircumcised male infants less than 3 months of age had the highest prevalence of UTI (20.1%) of any group, male or female (Shaikh et al., 2008). Circumcision status should be assessed in male infants with unexplained fever. UTI may involve the urethra and bladder (lower urinary tract) or the ureters, renal pelvis, calyces, and renal parenchyma (upper urinary tract). The Canadian Paediatric Society recommends suprapubic aspiration or urethral catheterization to diagnose urinary tract infections in young infants (see Chapter 45). Urine bagging is frequently inaccurate due to contamination (Canadian Paediatric Society, 2009b). Because it is often impossible to localize the infection, the broad designation *UTI* is applied to the presence of significant numbers of microorganisms anywhere within the urinary tract, except the distal third of the urethra, which is usually colonized with bacteria.

Classification

Infection of the urinary tract may be present with or without clinical symptoms. As a result, the site of infection is often difficult to pinpoint with any degree of accuracy. Various terms used to describe urinary tract disorders include the following:

Bacteriuria—Presence of bacteria in the urine

Asymptomatic bacteriuria—Significant bacteriuria (usually defined as more than 100,000 colony-forming units) with no evidence of clinical infection

Symptomatic bacteriuria—Bacteriuria accompanied by physical signs of UTI (dysuria, suprapubic discomfort, hematuria, fever)

Recurrent UTI—Repeated episode of bacteriuria or symptomatic UTI
Persistent UTI—Persistence of bacteriuria despite antibiotic treatment
Febrile UTI—Bacteriuria accompanied by fever and other physical signs of UTI; presence of a fever typically implies a pyelonephritis
Cystitis—Inflammation of the bladder
Urethritis—Inflammation of the urethra
Pyelonephritis—Inflammation of the upper urinary tract and kidneys
Urosepsis—Febrile UTI coexisting with systemic signs of bacterial illness; blood culture reveals presence of urinary pathogen

Etiology

A variety of organisms can be responsible for UTI. *Escherichia coli* (80% of cases) and other gram-negative enteric organisms are most frequently implicated; these organisms are usually found in the anal and perineal region. Other organisms associated with UTI include *Proteus*, *Pseudomonas*, *Klebsiella*, *Staphylococcus aureus*, *Haemophilus*, and coagulase-negative *Staphylococcus* organisms. Several factors contribute to the development of UTI in childhood including anatomical, physical, and chemical conditions or properties of the child's urinary tract.

Anatomical and Physical Factors

The structure of the lower urinary tract is believed to account for the increased incidence of bacteriuria in females (Rosenthal, 2004). The short urethra, which measures about 2 cm in young girls and 4 cm in mature women, provides a ready pathway for invasion of organisms. In addition, the closure of the urethra at the end of micturition may return contaminated bacteria to the bladder. The longer male urethra (as long as 20 cm in an adult) and the antibacterial properties of prostatic secretions inhibit the entry and growth of pathogens.

NURSING ALERT Considerable evidence suggests there are fewer UTIs among circumcised male infants than among uncircumcised male infants, but the difference is not significant enough to recommend routine circumcision in newborns (Canadian Paediatric Society, 2009a).

The single most important host factor influencing the occurrence of UTI is urinary stasis. Ordinarily, urine is sterile, but at 37°C it provides an excellent culture medium. Under normal conditions the act of completely and repeatedly emptying the bladder flushes away any organisms before they have an opportunity to multiply and invade surrounding tissue. However, urine that remains in the bladder allows bacteria from the urethra to rapidly become established in the rich medium. Incomplete bladder emptying (stasis) may result from reflux (see Vesicoureteral Reflux, p. 1543), anatomical abnormalities (especially those involving the ureters), dysfunction of the voiding mechanism, or extrinsic ureteral or bladder compression that may be caused by constipation. The key to preventing UTI is to maintain adequate blood supply to the bladder wall by avoidance of overdistention and high bladder pressure.

evolve Animation—Bladder

Altered Urine and Bladder Chemistry

Several mechanical and chemical characteristics of the urine and bladder mucosa help maintain urinary sterility. An increased fluid intake promotes flushing of the normal bladder and lowers the concentration of organisms in the infected bladder. Diuresis also seems to enhance the antibacterial properties of the renal medulla.

Most pathogens favour an alkaline medium. Normally, urine is slightly acidic with a median pH of 6.0. A urine pH of about 5 hampers but does not eliminate bacterial multiplication. Much has been reported about the use of cranberry products to increase urine acidity in an effort to prevent UTI. Studies done in adults offer limited evidence for the value of cranberry products in promoting urinary tract health (Bailey et al., 2007; Jepson, Mihaljevic, & Craig, 2004). Further research that controls for the type of cranberry product used, dosing regimens, and patient selection based on age and underlying medical condition is required to clarify unanswered questions before recommendations can be made regarding the use of this supplement, especially in the pediatric population.

Diagnostic Evaluation

The clinical manifestations of UTI depend on the child's age (Box 50-1). Diagnosis of UTI is confirmed by detection of bacteriuria in urine culture, but urine collection is often difficult, especially in infants and very small children. Several factors may alter a urine specimen; contamination of a specimen by organisms from sources other than the urine, such as perineal and perianal flora in bag specimens, is the most frequent cause of false-positive results. Unless the specimen is a first morning sample, a recent high fluid intake may indicate a falsely low organism count. Thus, children should not be encouraged to drink large volumes of water in an attempt to obtain a specimen quickly.

NURSING ALERT A child who exhibits the following should be evaluated for UTI:
- Incontinence in a toilet-trained child
- Strong-smelling urine
- Frequency or urgency

More accurate estimates of bacterial content are obtained from suprapubic aspiration (in children younger than 2 years of age) and properly performed bladder catheterization (as long as the first few millilitres are excluded from collection). The specimen should be taken directly to the laboratory for immediate culture.

Tests to detect bacteriuria are being used with increased frequency in screening for UTI. The dipstick tests for leukocyte esterase or nitrite are quick and inexpensive methods for detecting infection before obtaining final culture results.

Localization of the infection site may involve more specific tests, including percutaneous kidney taps and bladder washout procedures. Other tests such as ultrasonography, voiding cystourethrogram (VCUG), intravenous (IV) pyelogram, and DMSA (dimercaptosuccinic acid) scan may be performed after the infection subsides, to identify anatomical abnormalities contributing to the development of infection and existing kidney changes from recurrent infection.

BOX 50-1 Clinical Manifestations of Urinary Tract Disorders or Disease

Neonatal Period (Birth to 1 Month)
Poor feeding
Vomiting
Failure to gain weight
Rapid respiration (acidosis)
Respiratory distress
Spontaneous pneumothorax or pneumomediastinum
Frequent urination
Screaming on urination
Poor urine stream
Jaundice
Seizures
Dehydration
Other anomalies or stigmata
Enlarged kidneys or bladder

Infancy (1 to 24 Months)
Poor feeding
Vomiting
Failure to gain weight
Excessive thirst
Frequent urination
Straining or screaming on urination
Foul-smelling urine
Pallor
Fever
Persistent diaper rash
Seizures (with or without fever)
Dehydration
Enlarged kidneys or bladder

Childhood (2 to 14 Years)
Poor appetite
Vomiting
Growth failure
Excessive thirst
Enuresis, incontinence, frequent urination
Painful urination
Swelling of face
Seizures
Pallor
Fatigue
Blood in urine
Abdominal or back pain
Edema
Hypertension
Tetany

Therapeutic Management

The objectives of treatment of children with UTI are to (1) eliminate current infection, (2) identify contributing factors to reduce the risk of recurrence, (3) prevent systemic spread of the infection, and (4) preserve renal function. Antibiotic therapy should be initiated on the basis of identification of the pathogen, the child's history of antibiotic use, and the location of the infection. Several antimicrobial medications are available for treating UTI, but all of them can occasionally be ineffective because of resistance of organisms. Common anti-infective agents used for UTI include the penicillins, sulphonamide (including trimethoprim and sulphisoxazole in combination), the cephalosporins, and nitrofurantoin.

If anatomical defects such as primary reflux or bladder neck obstruction are present, surgical correction of these abnormalities may be necessary to prevent recurrent infection. Follow-up study is an important component of medical management, since the relapse rate is high and infection tends to recur 1 to 2 months after termination of treatment. The aim of therapy and careful follow-up is to reduce the chance of renal scarring. However, recurrent infection of the urinary bladder predisposes the individual to transient episodes of vesicoureteral reflux (VUR).

Vesicoureteral Reflux

VUR refers to the abnormal retrograde flow of bladder urine into the ureters. During voiding, urine is swept up the ureters and then flows back into the empty bladder, where it acts as a reservoir for bacterial growth until the next void. *Primary reflux* results from congenitally abnormal insertion of ureters into the bladder; *secondary reflux* occurs as a result of an acquired condition.

It is not clear that reflux necessarily causes infections. What is clear is that reflux is more likely to be associated with recurring kidney infections rather than simple bladder infections (cystitis). In the presence of reflux, infected urine (bacteria) from the bladder has access to the kidney, resulting in kidney infections (pyelonephritis). These children are usually very symptomatic with high fevers, vomiting, and chills. Reflux, when associated with UTI, is the most common cause of renal scarring in children. Renal scarring may occur with the first episode of febrile UTI. Reflux in the presence of sterile urine does not cause renal damage. Therefore, the most important concept in managing VUR is preventing bacteria from reaching the kidneys. VUR is managed conservatively with daily low-dose antibiotic therapy. A urine culture should be done every 2 to 3 months and any time the child has a fever. This method of management requires a motivated, reliable, and cooperative family. Many children will outgrow the reflux over a period of years. An annual VCUG is done to assess the status of the reflux.

For children with mild to moderate reflux, a minimally invasive endoscopic option (subtrigonal injection, or STING) is an alternative to daily antibiotics or open surgical intervention. A bulking agent—dextranomer–hyaluronic acid polymer (Deflux)—is injected into the mucous membrane of the ureter, making retrograde flow of urine more difficult. Overall cure rates relate to the degree of reflux and range from 72 to 96% (Cerwinka, Scherz & Kirsch, 2008; Kirsch, Perez-Brayfield, & Scherz, 2003; Lavelle, Conlin, & Skoog, 2005).

Indications for open surgical intervention include significant anatomical abnormality at the ureterovesical junction, recurrent UTIs, severe forms of VUR, noncompliance with medical therapy, intolerance to antibiotics, and VUR after puberty in females.

Prognosis

With prompt and adequate treatment at the time of diagnosis, the long-term prognosis for UTI is usually excellent. However, the hazard of progressive renal injury is greatest when infection occurs in young children (especially those younger than 2 years of age) and is associated with congenital renal malformations and reflux. Therefore, early diagnosis of children at risk is particularly important.

Nursing Care Management

Nurses should instruct parents to observe regularly for clues suggesting UTI. Unfortunately, the signs of UTI are not as evident as those of upper respiratory tract infection. Many cases go undetected because no one thought to investigate this very common problem.

Because infants and young children often are unable to express their feelings and sensations verbally, it is difficult to detect discomfort they may be experiencing from dysuria. A careful history regarding voiding habits, stooling patterns, and episodes of unexplained irritability may assist in detecting less obvious cases of UTI. Parents should be cautioned to observe for specific clues of UTI in suspected cases.

When infection is suspected, collecting an appropriate specimen is essential. It is the nurse's responsibility to take every precaution to obtain acceptable clean-voided specimens to avoid the use of other, more invasive collecting procedures except when absolutely indicated. Because of the unreliability of a specimen obtained via a urine collection bag, suprapubic aspiration of urine or sterile catheterization should be done in the infant or young child who is seen with fever.

Frequently, additional tests are performed to detect anatomical defects. Children need to be prepared for these tests as appropriate for their age. This includes an explanation of the procedure, its purpose, and what the child will experience (see Preparation for Diagnostic and Therapeutic Procedures, Chapter 45). Sometimes a simple description of the urinary system is helpful. Especially for preschool children, the nurse must clarify that the urinary tract is separate from any sexual function and that the test is for a problem that they did not cause. Children may associate blame for perceived wrongdoing (e.g., masturbation) or unacceptable thoughts with the reason for the illness or the tests. For children younger than 3 to 4 years of age, the procedure can be explained on a doll. For those who are older, a simple drawing of the bladder, urethra, ureters, and kidneys makes the procedure more understandable.

Handling actual equipment, when feasible, can be helpful in allaying anxiety in children of all ages. Anticipatory instruction on distraction techniques such as deep breathing, storytelling, and imagery may help the child relax during the actual procedures. If surgery is indicated, facts and understanding of the procedure will help decrease the child's fear and anxiety concerning more extensive medical-surgical intervention.

Because antibacterial medications are indicated in UTI, the nurse needs to advise parents of proper dosage and administration. When antiseptics such as nitrofurantoin are used for prolonged therapy to maintain urine sterility, parents need an explanation of the medication's continued necessity when no signs of infection are present. For all children an adequate or increased fluid intake should be encouraged.

Prevention

Prevention is the most important goal in both primary and recurrent infection, and most preventive measures are simple hygienic habits that should be a routine part of daily care (see Guidelines box). For example, parents should be taught to cleanse their infant's genital areas from front to back to avoid contaminating the urethral area with fecal organisms. Girls should be taught to wipe from front to back after voiding or defecating. Children should void as soon as they feel the urge (see Critical Thinking Exercise).

Sexually active adolescent girls should be advised to urinate as soon as possible after they have intercourse, to flush out bacteria introduced during the activity. Children who have recurrent UTIs or neurogenic bladder are frequently maintained on daily low-dose antibiotics. Giving the dose at bedtime allows the drug to remain in the bladder overnight.

GUIDELINES Prevention of Urinary Tract Infection

Factors Predisposing to Development

- Short female urethra close to vagina and anus
- Incomplete emptying (reflux) and overdistension of bladder
- Concentrated urine
- Constipation

Measures of Prevention

Practice good perineal hygiene: wipe from front to back.
Avoid tight clothing or diapers; wear cotton panties rather than nylon.
Check for vaginitis or pinworms, especially if child scratches between legs.
Avoid "holding" urine; encourage child to void frequently, especially before long trips or other circumstances in which toilet facilities are not available.
Empty bladder completely with each void. Have the child "double void" (void, wait a few minutes, and void again). Severe cases may require clean, intermittent catheterization or biofeedback instruction.
Avoid straining during defecation and avoid constipation.
Encourage generous fluid intake.

CRITICAL THINKING EXERCISE

Urinary Tract Infection and Constipation

During your assessment of Lisa, a 5-year-old admitted to the hospital for a severe urinary tract infection (UTI), her mother tells you that Lisa has bowel movements every third or fourth day. They are usually large, hard-formed stools, and Lisa sometimes has trouble evacuating the stool.

1. Evidence—Is there sufficient evidence to draw conclusions about Lisa's UTI and constipation?
2. Assumptions—Describe an underlying assumption about each of the following:
   a. UTIs and females
   b. Normal bowel patterns for 5-year-old children
   c. Association between UTIs and constipation
3. What priorities for nursing care should be established for Lisa?
4. Does the evidence support your nursing intervention?
5. What alternative perspectives might you have?

Obstructive Uropathy

Structural or functional abnormalities of the urinary system that obstruct the normal flow of urine can produce renal disorders. When there is interference with urine flow, the backup of urine above the obstruction causes *hydronephrosis* (dilation of the renal pelvis from distention) with eventual pressure destruction of renal parenchyma, although the dilating ureters form a reservoir that reduces the effect on the kidneys for a long time.

Obstruction may be congenital or acquired, unilateral or bilateral, complete or incomplete, with acute or chronic manifestations. The obstruction can occur at any level of the upper or lower urinary tract (Fig. 50-1). Partial obstruction may not be symptomatic unless there is a water or solute diuresis. Boys are affected more frequently than girls, and malformations should be suspected when patients have some other congenital defects (e.g., prune belly syndrome, chromosomal anomalies, anorectal malformations, defects of the pinna of the ear).

Damage to distal nephrons in chronic uropathy alters the ability to concentrate urine, contributing to increased urine flow and metabolic **acidosis** occurring from the decreased excretion of acid secondary to the impaired ability of the distal nephron to secrete hydrogen ions. Partial obstruction results in progressive loss of renal function as a result of irreversible damage to the nephrons. Pooled urine serves as a medium for bacterial growth; therefore UTIs further increase the extent of renal damage.

Early diagnosis and surgical correction or procedures that divert the flow of urine to bypass the obstruction, such as placement of a temporary percutaneous nephrostomy tube or cutaneous ureterostomy, are essential to prevent progressive renal damage. Medical complications of acute or chronic renal failure (CRF) or infection are managed as described for those disorders.

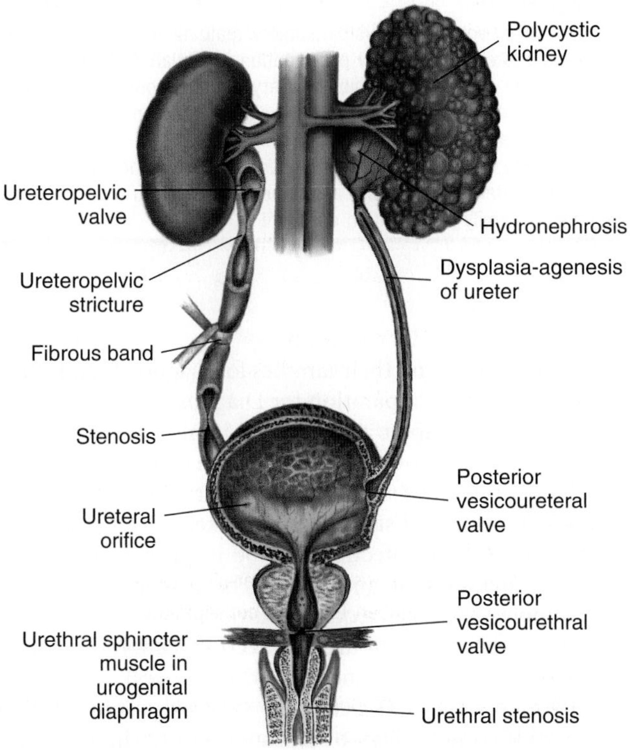

Fig. 50-1 Major sites of urinary tract obstruction.

Nursing Care Management

Nursing goals in urinary tract obstruction include helping to identify cases, assisting with diagnostic procedures, and caring for children with complications. Preparing parents and children for procedures is a major nursing responsibility. Preparation for urinary diversion procedures is of special importance (see Preparation for Diagnostic and Therapeutic Procedures, Chapter 45).

Parents and children need emotional support and counselling during the lengthy management of these disorders. Many children are discharged with ureteral drainage systems in place that must be protected from damage, and the danger of infection is a constant concern. Parents should be taught to care for the equipment and recognize the signs of possible obstruction or infection within the system. Maintaining adequate urine flow is imperative. Fluids should be encouraged. The tube should be observed frequently for indications of obstruction resulting from sediment, small blood clots, or kinking. The physician should inspect any drainage from around the tube.

Children with external diversional systems need psychological support and guidance, especially as they reach adolescence and body image concerns assume more prominence. Peer and family support groups can be helpful. Those with progressive renal deterioration may face the prospect of dialysis or transplantation and the emotions that accompany these procedures.

External Defects

Defects of the external genitourinary tract are serious conditions primarily because of the psychological impact on the child. Satisfactory surgical repair is successful for the more common disorders and is carried out or initiated as early as possible. The major anomalies of the lower genitourinary tract, their description, and their management are outlined in Table 50-4.

Psychological Problems Related to Genital Surgery

Surgery involving sexual organs can be particularly disruptive to children, especially preschoolers fearing punishment, retaliation, body mutilation, or castration. Some of the problems of hospitalization, separation, and anxiety can be eased by hospital practices that are sensitive to the child's needs (see Chapter 44).

A child's **body image** is largely derived as a result of feedback from the primary caregivers, and parental anxiety regarding an acceptable physical appearance and adequate future sexual competency is readily communicated to an affected child. Children with **birth defects** are at risk for developing a distorted body image that reflects the caregiver's subtly communicated evaluation of their bodies. The trend toward repair of visible genital defects is based in large part on these psychological variables. The earlier a repair can be achieved, the more likely it is that the child will develop a healthy body image.

Table 50-4 Defects of the Genitourinary Tract

DEFECT	THERAPEUTIC MANAGEMENT
Inguinal hernia—Protrusion of abdominal contents through inguinal canal into scrotum	Detected as painless inguinal swelling of variable size Surgical closure of inguinal defect
Hydrocele—Fluid in scrotum	Surgical repair indicated if spontaneous resolution not accomplished in 1 yr
Phimosis—Narrowing or stenosis of preputial opening of foreskin	Mild cases—manual retraction of foreskin and proper cleansing of area Severe cases—circumcision or vertical division and transverse suturing of foreskin
Hypospadias—Urethral opening located behind glans penis or anywhere along ventral surface of penile shaft	Objectives of surgical correction: Enable child to void in standing position and direct stream voluntarily in usual manner Improve physical appearance of genitalia Produce a sexually adequate organ
Chordee—Ventral curvature of penis, often associated with hypospadias	Surgical release of fibrous band causing the deformity
Epispadias—Meatal opening located on dorsal surface of penis	Surgical correction, usually including penile and urethral lengthening and bladder neck reconstruction (if necessary)
Cryptorchidism—Failure of one or both testes to descend normally through inguinal canal	Detected by inability to palpate testes within scrotum Medical—Administration of human chorionic gonadotropin (older child) Surgical—Orchiopexy Objectives of therapy: Prevent damage to undescended testicle Decrease incidence of malignant tumour formation Avoid trauma and torsion Close inguinal canal Prevent cosmetic and psychological disability from empty scrotum
Exstrophy of bladder—Eversion of posterior bladder through anterior bladder wall and lower abdominal wall; associated with open pubic arch (a severe defect)	Potential objectives of surgical correction: Preserve renal function Attain urinary control Perform adequate reconstructive repair Improve sexual function (especially in males)
Ambiguous genitalia	
Masculinized female (female pseudohermaphrodite)	Assign gender as female; assign gender while avoiding irreversible surgery, realizing some children may change gender later in life; family participation essential
Incompletely masculinized male (male pseudohermaphrodite)	Assign gender while avoiding irreversible surgery, realizing some children may change gender later in life; family participation essential
True hermaphrodite (both ovaries and testes)	Assign gender while avoiding irreversible surgery, realizing some children may change gender later in life; gender assignment depends on predominant characteristics; family participation essential
Mixed gonadal dysgenesis	Assign gender while avoiding irreversible surgery, realizing some children may change gender later in life; gender assignment depends on predominant characteristics; family participation essential

During the years from 3 to 6, the phallic-oedipal period, children show a strong interest and concern about the genital area, sex differences, and genital normality or its lack. It is also a time when children are frightened of what they perceive to be threats to their body and bodily function. They can view any untoward happening as a punishment for real or imagined wrongdoing or unacceptable sexual feelings, such as masturbation, sex play, or erotic feelings. Surgical repair is recommended before these fears and anxieties develop. After extensive review of the emotional, cognitive, and body-image problems that may occur in children undergoing surgical reconstruction of a genital deformity, Kass (1996) recommended that surgery be accomplished between the ages of 6 and 15 months to minimize the psychological effects of surgery and anaesthesia.

Nursing Care Management

Preparing children and their families for diagnostic and surgical procedures (see Preparation for Diagnostic and Therapeutic Procedures, Chapter 45) and for home care is a major nursing function. Most postoperative care involves care of the surgical site. Tub baths are discouraged for 1 week after simple surgeries. The surgical site needs to be kept clean and otherwise protected from infection and be inspected for signs of infection. Dressings, if any, should be inspected regularly. More complex surgeries require additional care and observation (e.g., catheter care for urethral reconstruction and care of urinary diversion stomas and collection devices).

Some older children's activities, such as pushing, lifting, playing with straddle toys or in sandboxes, swimming, and engaging in rough activities, may be restricted after some types of surgical repairs. Precise restrictions depend on the specific type of surgery. Activities of infants and toddlers are not limited.

In most cases the results of surgery are satisfactory. However, in some of the more severe defects, such as exstrophy and those that require stomas, additional emotional interventions may be needed. A major concern of parents and children is related to surgery affecting the genitalia directly. Concerns about penis size, appearance of the genitalia, potential ability to procreate, and rejection by peers (especially the opposite sex) are potential fears that require psychological adjustment, particularly during adolescence.

Glomerular Disease

Nephrotic Syndrome

Nephrotic syndrome is a clinical state that includes massive **proteinuria, hypoalbuminemia, hyperlipidemia,** and **edema.** The disorder can occur as (1) a primary disease known as *idiopathic nephrosis, childhood nephrosis,* or *minimal-change nephrotic syndrome (MCNS),* (2) a secondary disorder that occurs as a clinical manifestation after or in association with glomerular damage that has a known or presumed cause, or (3) a congenital form inherited as an autosomal recessive disorder. The disorder is characterized by increased glomerular permeability to plasma protein, which results in massive urinary protein loss. The glomerulus is responsible for the initial step in the formation of urine, and the filtration rate depends on an intact glomerular membrane. This discussion is devoted to MCNS because it constitutes 80% of nephrotic syndrome cases.

Pathophysiology

The onset of MCNS can occur at any age but predominantly occurs in children between 2 and 7 years of age. It is rare in children younger than 6 months of age, uncommon in infants younger than 1 year of age, and unusual after the age of 8. Patients with MCNS are twice as likely to be male.

The pathogenesis of MCNS is not understood. There may be a metabolic, biochemical, physiochemical, or immune-mediated disturbance that causes the basement membrane of the glomeruli to become increasingly permeable to protein, but the cause and mechanisms are only speculative.

The glomerular membrane, normally impermeable to albumin and other proteins, becomes permeable to proteins, especially albumin, which leak through the membrane and are lost in urine (*hyperalbuminuria*). This reduces the serum albumin level (*hypoalbuminemia*), decreasing the colloidal osmotic pressure in the capillaries. As a result, the vascular hydrostatic pressure exceeds the pull of the colloidal osmotic pressure, causing fluid to accumulate in the interstitial spaces (*edema*) and body cavities, particularly in the abdominal cavity (*ascites*). The shift of fluid from the plasma to the interstitial spaces reduces the vascular fluid volume (*hypovolemia*), which in turn stimulates the renin-angiotensin system and the secretion of antidiuretic hormone and aldosterone. Tubular reabsorption of sodium and water is increased in an attempt to increase intravascular volume. The elevation of serum lipids is not fully understood. The sequence of events in nephrotic syndrome is diagrammed in Figure 50-2.

Diagnostic Evaluation

The disease is suspected on the basis of clinical manifestations (Box 50-2), especially when weight gain in a previously well child increases slowly over days or weeks. The generalized edema may develop rapidly or gradually but eventually prompts the family to seek medical attention. Parents usually give a history of the child being well but steadily gaining weight; appearing edematous; and then becoming anorexic, irritable, and less active.

The diagnosis of MCNS is suspected on the basis of the history and clinical manifestations (edema, proteinuria, hypoalbuminemia, and hypercholesterolemia in the absence of hematuria and hypertension) in children between the ages of 2 and 8 years. The hallmark of MCNS is massive proteinuria (higher than 3+ on urine dipstick). Hyaline casts, oval fat bodies, and a few red blood cells can be found in the urine of some affected children, although there is seldom gross hematuria. The glomerular filtration rate is usually normal or high.

Total serum protein concentration is low, with the serum albumin significantly reduced and plasma lipids elevated. Hemoglobin and hematocrit are usually normal or elevated as a result of hemoconcentration. The platelet count may be elevated. Serum sodium concentration may be low. If the patient does not respond to a 4- to 8-week course of steroids, a renal biopsy may be needed to distinguish between other types of nephrotic syndrome. The biopsy results of children with MCNS are remarkable for effacement of the foot processes of the epithelial cells lining the basement membrane, but otherwise the kidney tissue is normal.

BOX 50-2 Clinical Manifestations of Nephrotic Syndrome

Weight gain
Puffiness of face (facial edema):
- Especially around the eyes
- Apparent on arising in the morning
- Subsides during the day

Abdominal swelling (ascites)
Pleural effusion
Labial or scrotal swelling
Edema of intestinal mucosa, possibly causing:
- Diarrhea
- Anorexia
- Poor intestinal absorption

Ankle or leg swelling
Irritability
Tendency to fatigue easily
Lethargy
Blood pressure normal or slightly decreased
Susceptibility to infection
Urine alterations:
- Decreased volume
- Frothy

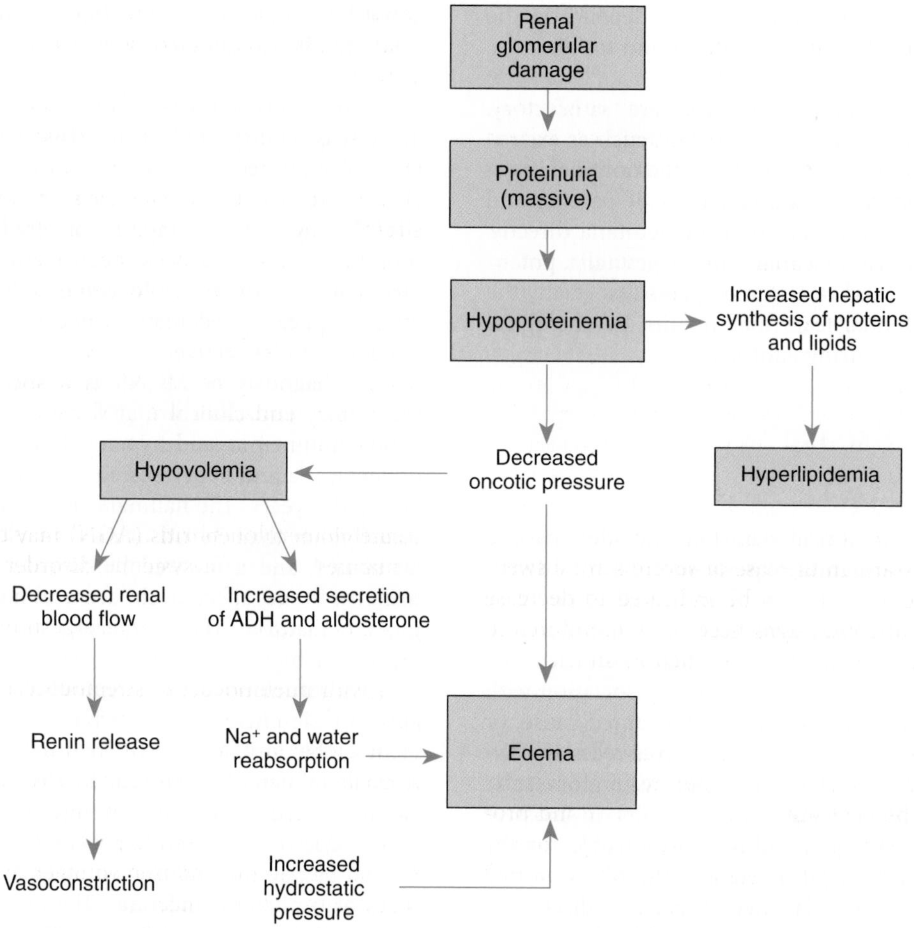

Fig. 50-2 Sequence of events in nephrotic syndrome. *ADH,* antidiuretic hormone.

Therapeutic Management

Objectives of therapeutic management include (1) reducing the excretion of urinary protein, (2) reducing fluid retention in the tissues, (3) preventing infection, and (4) minimizing complications related to therapies. Dietary restrictions include a low-salt diet and, in more severe cases, fluid restriction. If complications of edema develop, diuretic therapy may be initiated to provide temporary relief from edema. Sometimes infusions of 25% albumin are used. Acute infections are treated with appropriate antibiotics.

Corticosteroids are the first line of therapy for MCNS. The starting dosage for prednisone is usually 2 mg/kg body weight/day, in one or more divided doses. Most children respond within 7 to 21 days. The medication is then tapered over a period of several months and eventually stopped if the child remains asymptomatic. About two thirds of children with MCNS have a relapse, heralded first by increased urine protein. Relapses can be diagnosed early if parents are taught routine home monitoring of urine protein by dipstick. Relapses are treated with a repeated course of high-dose steroid therapy. Adverse effects of the steroids include weight gain, rounding of the face, behaviour changes, and increased appetite. Long-term therapy may result in hirsutism, growth restriction, **cataracts**, hypertension, gastrointestinal bleeding, bone demineralization, infection, and **hyperglycemia**. Children who do not respond to steroid therapy, those who have frequent relapses, and those in whom the adverse effects threaten their growth and general health may be considered for a course of therapy using other immunosuppressant medications (cyclophosphamide, chlorambucil, or cyclosporine).

MCNS episodes, both the first episode and the relapse, often happen in conjunction with a viral or bacterial infection. Relapses can also be triggered by allergies and immunizations. Relapses in children with MCNS may continue over many years.

Complications of nephrotic syndrome include infection, circulatory insufficiency secondary to hypovolemia, and thromboembolism. Infections that may be seen in children with nephrotic syndrome include peritonitis, cellulitis, and pneumonia and require prompt recognition and vigorous treatment with appropriate antibiotic therapy.

Prognosis

The prognosis for ultimate recovery in most cases is good. It is a self-limiting disease, and in children who respond to steroid therapy the tendency to relapse decreases with time. With early detection and prompt implementation of therapy to eradicate proteinuria, progressive basement membrane damage is minimized, so that when the tendency to relapse is past, renal function is usually normal or near normal. It is estimated that approximately 80% of affected children have this favourable prognosis.

Nursing Care Management

Continuous monitoring of fluid intake and output is an important nursing function. Strict intake and output records are essential but may be difficult to obtain from very young children. Application of collection bags is irritating to edematous skin that is readily subject to breakdown. Applying diapers or weighing wet pads may be necessary.

NURSING ALERT Another strategy for obtaining a daily urine protein is to place cotton balls in the diaper at night before bedtime and then squeeze them out in the morning.

Other methods of monitoring progress include urine examination for albumin, daily weight, and measurement of abdominal girth. Assessment of edema (e.g., increased or decreased swelling around the eyes and dependent areas), the degree of pitting, and the colour and texture of skin are part of nursing care. Assessing for signs of skin breakdown due to severe edema is necessary. In the case of severe scrotal swelling, the use of a scrotal sling may be indicated to decrease pressure and discomfort. Vital signs need to be monitored to detect any early signs of complications such as shock or an infective process.

Infection is a constant source of danger to edematous children and those receiving corticosteroid therapy. These children are particularly vulnerable to upper respiratory tract infection; they must be kept warm and dry, active, and protected from contact with infected individuals (e.g., roommates, visitors, and personnel). Vital signs should be monitored to detect any early signs of an infective process.

Loss of appetite accompanying active nephrosis can create a perplexing problem for nurses. The combined efforts of nurse, dietitian, parents, and child are needed to formulate a nutritionally adequate and attractive diet. Salt is usually restricted (but not eliminated) during the edema phase and while the child is on steroid therapy. Fluid restriction (if prescribed) is limited to short-term use during massive edema. Every effort should be made to serve attractive meals with preferred foods and a minimum of fuss, but it usually requires considerable ingenuity to entice the child to eat (see Feeding the Sick Child, Chapter 45).

Children usually adjust activities according to their tolerance level. However, they may require guidance in selecting play activities. Suitable recreational and diversional activities are an important part of their care. Irritability and mood swings that accompany steroid therapy are not unusual in these children and may create an additional challenge for the nurse and family.

Family Support and Home Care

Continuous support of the child and family is one of the major nursing considerations. Many children are treated at home during relapses. Parents need to be taught to detect signs of relapse and to call for changes in treatment at the earliest indications. Unless the edema and proteinuria are severe or the parents, for some reason, are unable to care for the ill child, home care is preferred. Parents should be instructed in testing urine for albumin, administering medications, and providing general care. Parents also need to encourage the child to avoid contact with infected playmates, but the child should attend school. Psychological support may be indicated because of body-image changes associated with prolonged and frequent steroid use.

The prolonged course of the relapsing form of nephrotic syndrome is taxing to both the child and the family. The up-and-down course of remissions and exacerbations with periodic disruption of family life by hospitalization places a severe strain on the child and the family, both psychologically and financially. Reassurance regarding this characteristic of the course of the disease, with emphasis on the importance of long-term care, needs to be provided to parents and children to gain their cooperation. A satisfactory response is more likely when relapses are detected and therapy is instituted early, and remissions are prolonged when instructions are carried out faithfully.

Acute Glomerulonephritis

Acute glomerulonephritis (AGN) may be a primary event or a manifestation of a systemic disorder that can range from minimal to severe. Common features include oliguria, edema, hypertension and circulatory congestion, hematuria, and proteinuria. Most cases are postinfectious and have been associated with pneumococcal, streptococcal, and viral infections. *Acute poststreptococcal glomerulonephritis* (APSGN) is the most common of the postinfectious renal diseases in childhood and the one for which a cause can be established in most cases. APSGN can occur at any age but affects primarily early school-age children, with a peak age of onset of 6 to 7 years. It is uncommon in children younger than 2 years of age, and males outnumber females 2 : 1.

Etiology

APSGN is an immune-complex disease that occurs after an antecedent streptococcal infection with certain strains of the group A β-hemolytic streptococcus. Most streptococcal infections *do not* cause APSGN. A latent period of 10 to 21 days occurs between the streptococcal infection and the onset of clinical manifestations. Disease secondary to streptococcal pharyngitis is more common in the winter or spring, but when APSGN is associated with pyoderma (principally impetigo), it may be more prevalent in later summer or early fall, especially in warmer climates. Second episodes of AGN are rare.

Pathophysiology

The pathophysiology of APSGN is still uncertain. Immune complexes are deposited in the glomerular basement membrane. The glomeruli become edematous and infiltrated with polymorphonuclear leukocytes, which occlude the capillary lumen. The resulting decrease in plasma filtration results in an excessive accumulation of water and retention of sodium that expands plasma and interstitial fluid volumes, leading to circulatory congestion and edema. The cause of the hypertension associated with AGN cannot be completely explained by fluid retention. Excess renin may also be produced.

Diagnostic Evaluation

Typically, affected children are in good health until they experience the streptococcal infection. In some instances they have a history of only a mild cold or no previous infection at all.

The onset of nephritis appears after an average latency period of about 10 days (Box 50-3). Because the child appears to be well during the latency period, parents do not recognize the association. The edema is relatively moderate and may not be appreciated by someone unfamiliar with the child's normal appearance.

Urinalysis during the acute phase characteristically shows hematuria and proteinuria. Proteinuria generally parallels the hematuria and may be 3+ or 4+ in the presence of gross hematuria. Gross discolouration of the urine reflects red blood cell and hemoglobin content. Microscopic examination of the sediment shows many red blood cells, leukocytes, epithelial cells, and granular and red blood cell casts. Bacteria are not seen.

Azotemia that results from impaired glomerular filtration is reflected in elevated urea and creatinine levels in at least 50% of cases. Occasionally proteinuria is excessive and the patient may have nephrotic syndrome (i.e., hypoproteinemia and hyperlipidemia).

Cultures of the pharynx are rarely positive for streptococci, since the renal disease occurs weeks after the infection.

Some serological tests are necessary to make the diagnosis of AGN. Circulating serum antibodies to streptococci indicate the presence of a previous infection. The antistreptolysin O (ASO) titre is the most familiar and readily available test for streptococcal infection. Other antibodies that may aid in diagnosis are elevated antihyaluronidase (AHase), antideoxyribonuclease B (ADNase-B), and streptozyme.

All patients with APSGN have reduced serum complement (C3) activity in the early stages of the disease. Rising C3 levels are used as a guide to indicate improvement of the disease and should be normal in almost all patients 8 weeks after the disease onset.

Studies that may be useful include chest x-ray examination, which generally shows cardiac enlargement, pulmonary congestion, or pleural effusion during the edematous phase of acute disease. Renal biopsy for diagnostic purposes is seldom required but may be useful in the diagnosis of atypical cases.

BOX 50-3 Clinical Manifestations of Acute Poststreptococcal Glomerulonephritis

Edema:
- Especially periorbital
- Facial edema more prominent in the morning
- Spreads during the day to involve extremities and abdomen

Anorexia

Urine:
- Cloudy, smoky brown (resembles tea or cola)
- Severely reduced volume

Pallor

Irritability

Lethargy

Child appearing ill

Child seldom expressing specific health concerns

Older children:
- Headaches
- Abdominal discomfort
- Dysuria

Vomiting possible

Mild to moderately elevated blood pressure

Therapeutic Management

Management consists of general supportive measures and early recognition and treatment of complications. Children who have normal blood pressure and a satisfactory urine output can generally be treated at home. Those with substantial edema, hypertension, gross hematuria, or significant oliguria should be hospitalized because of the unpredictability of complications.

Dietary restrictions depend on the stage and severity of the disease, especially the extent of edema. Moderate sodium restriction and even fluid restriction may be instituted for children with hypertension and edema. Foods with substantial amounts of potassium are generally restricted during the period of oliguria.

Regular measurement of vital signs, body weight, and intake and output is essential to monitor the progress of the disease and to detect complications that may appear at any time during the course of the disease. A record of daily weight is the most useful means for assessing fluid balance. Rarely, children with AGN will develop acute renal failure (ARF) with oliguria that significantly alters the fluid and electrolyte balance (resulting in **hyperkalemia**, acidosis, hypocalcemia, and/or hyperphosphatemia). These children require careful management. Peritoneal dialysis or hemodialysis is seldom needed.

Acute hypertension must be anticipated and identified early. Blood pressure measurements should be taken every 4 to 6 hours. A variety of antihypertensive medications and diuretics can be used to control hypertension. Antibiotic therapy is indicated only for those children with evidence of persistent streptococcal infections. It is used to prevent transmission of nephritogenic streptococci to other family members.

Prognosis

Almost all children correctly diagnosed as having APSGN recover completely, and specific immunity is conferred, so that subsequent recurrences are uncommon. Some of these children have been reported to develop chronic disease, but most of these cases are now believed to be different glomerular diseases misdiagnosed as poststreptococcal disease.

Nursing Care Management

Nursing care of the child with glomerulonephritis involves careful assessment of the disease status, with regular monitoring of vital signs (including frequent measurement of blood pressure), fluid balance, and behaviour.

Vital signs provide clues to the severity of the disease and early signs of complications. They need to be carefully measured, and any deviations reported and recorded. The volume and character of urine should be noted and the child weighed daily. Children with restricted fluid intake, especially those who are not severely edematous or those who have lost weight, should be observed for signs of dehydration.

Assessment of the child's appearance for signs of cerebral complications is an important nursing function, since the severity of the acute phase is variable and unpredictable. The child with edema, hypertension, and gross hematuria may be subject to complications, and anticipatory preparations such as seizure precautions and IV equipment should be included in the nursing care plan.

For most children a regular diet is allowed, but it should contain no added salt. Foods high in sodium and salted treats need to be eliminated, and parents and friends should be advised not to bring snacks such as potato chips or pretzels. The total amount of salt ingested is usually less because of poor appetite. Fluid restriction, if prescribed, is more difficult, and the amount permitted should be evenly divided throughout the waking hours. Meal preparation and service require special attention, since the child is indifferent to meals during the acute phase. Again, collaboration with parents and the dietitian and special consideration for food preferences facilitate meal planning.

During the acute phase, children are generally content to lie in bed. As they begin to feel better and their symptoms subside, they will want to be up. Activities should be planned to allow for frequent rest periods. Children who have mild edema and no hypertension, as well as convalescent children who are being treated at home, need follow-up care. Parents need to be instructed regarding general measures, including diet and prevention of infection.

Health supervision is continued, with weekly, followed by monthly, visits for evaluation and urinalysis. Parent education and support is needed to get the child's discharge organized and home care set up. The family needs to learn how to manage the child at home and to have the follow-up care and health supervision arranged.

Miscellaneous Renal Disorders

Hemolytic Uremic Syndrome

Hemolytic uremic syndrome (HUS) is an uncommon, acute renal disease that occurs primarily in infants and small children between the ages of 6 months and 5 years. HUS is one of the most frequent causes of acquired ARF in children (Kliegman et al., 2007). The clinical features of the disease include acquired hemolytic anemia, thrombocytopenia, renal injury, and central nervous system symptoms. The etiology of HUS is thought to be associated with bacterial toxins, chemicals, and viruses. The appearance of the disease has been associated with *Rickettsia* organisms, viruses (especially coxsackievirus, echovirus, and adenovirus), *E. coli*, pneumococci, shigellae, and salmonellae and may represent an unusual response to these infections. Multiple cases of HUS caused by enteric infection of the *E. coli* O157:H7 serotype have been traced to undercooked meat, especially ground beef. Other sources are unpasteurized milk or fruit juice, especially apple; alfalfa sprouts; lettuce; and salami. Drinking or swimming in sewage-contaminated water can also cause infection. The clinical presentation is usually a history of a prodromal illness (most often gastroenteritis or an upper respiratory tract infection) followed by the sudden onset of hemolysis and renal failure.

Pathophysiology

The primary site of injury appears to be the endothelial lining of the small glomerular arterioles, which become swollen and occluded with deposits of platelets and fibrin clots (intravascular coagulation). Red blood cells are damaged as they attempt to move through the partially occluded blood vessels and are removed by the spleen, causing acute hemolytic anemia. The platelet aggregation within the damaged blood vessels or the damage and removal of platelets produce the characteristic thrombocytopenia.

Diagnostic Evaluation

The triad of anemia, thrombocytopenia, and renal failure is sufficient for diagnosis (Box 50-4). Renal involvement is evidenced by proteinuria, hematuria, and urinary casts; blood urea nitrogen (BUN) and serum creatinine levels are elevated. A low hemoglobin and hematocrit and a high reticulocyte count confirm the hemolytic nature of the anemia.

Therapeutic Management

The goals of therapy are early diagnosis and aggressive, supportive care of the ARF and hemolytic anemia. The most consistently effective treatment of HUS is hemodialysis or peritoneal dialysis, which is instituted in any child who has been anuric for 24 hours or who demonstrates oliguria with uremia or hypertension and seizures. Other treatments include use of pharmacological agents, fresh frozen plasma, and plasmapheresis. Blood transfusions with fresh, washed packed cells are administered for severe anemia but are used with caution to prevent circulatory overload from added volume.

Prognosis

With prompt treatment the recovery rate is about 95%, but residual renal impairment ranges from 10 to 50%. Long-term complications include CRF, hypertension, and central nervous system disorders. Death is usually caused by residual renal impairment or central nervous system injury.

Nursing Care Management

Nursing care is the same as that provided in ARF and, for children with continued impairment, includes management of

BOX 50-4 Clinical Manifestations of Hemolytic Uremic Syndrome

Vomiting
Irritability
Lethargy
Marked pallor
Hemorrhagic manifestations:
- Bruising
- Petechiae
- Jaundice
- Bloody diarrhea

Oliguria or anuria
Central nervous system involvement:
- Seizures
- Stupor or coma

Signs of acute heart failure (sometimes)

chronic disease. Because of the sudden and life-threatening nature of the disorder in a previously well child, parents are often ill prepared for the impact of hospitalization and treatment and require support and understanding.

Wilms' Tumour

Wilms' tumour, or nephroblastoma, is the most common malignant renal and intra-abdominal tumour of childhood. Its frequency is estimated to be 7.6 cases per million in White children younger than 15 years (Dome et al., 2006). In North America, Wilms' tumour occurs about three times more often in individuals of African origin than in those of East Asian origin. The peak age at diagnosis is approximately 3 years, and occurrence is slightly more frequent in boys than in girls. Most patients with Wilms' tumour are diagnosed at younger than 5 years of age, with 1 to 2.5% of cases having a familial origin. Unfortunately, there is no method of identifying gene carriers at this time. In Canada, the Canadian Cancer Society reported that between 2001 and 2005, there were 199 cases of Wilms' tumours diagnosed in children 0 to 14 years of age. In addition, there were 27 deaths from Wilms' tumours in children 0 to 14 years of age (Canadian Cancer Society, 2011).

Etiology

Wilms' tumour probably arises from a malignant, undifferentiated cluster of primordial cells capable of initiating the regeneration of an abnormal structure. Its occurrence slightly favours the left kidney, which is advantageous because surgically this kidney is easier to manipulate and remove. In about 10% of cases both kidneys are involved. Studies have shown that development of Wilms' tumour is frequently associated with aniridia, hemihypertrophy, Beckwith-Wiedemann syndrome, or genitourinary anomalies (Dome et al., 2006; Kline & Sevier, 2003).

Diagnostic Evaluation

In a child suspected of having Wilms' tumour, special emphasis is placed on the history and physical examination for the presence of congenital anomalies, a family history of cancer, and signs of malignancy (e.g., weight loss, size of liver and spleen, indications of anemia, lymphadenopathy). Most children with Wilms' tumour are brought to the practitioner because of abdominal swelling or an abdominal mass (Box 50-5). Specific tests include radiographic studies, including abdominal ultrasound and abdominal and chest computed tomography scan; hematological studies; biochemical studies; and urinalysis. Studies to demonstrate the relationship of the tumour to the ipsilateral kidney and the presence of a normal functioning kidney on the contralateral side are essential. If a large tumour is present, an inferior venacavagram is necessary to demonstrate possible tumour involvement adjacent to the vena cava. A bone marrow aspiration may be performed to rule out metastasis, which is rare in children with Wilms' tumour.

NURSING ALERT To reinforce the need for caution, it may be necessary to post a sign on the bed that reads "DO NOT PALPATE ABDOMEN." Careful bathing and handling are also important in preventing trauma to the tumour site.

BOX 50-5 Clinical Manifestations of Wilms' Tumour

Abdominal swelling or mass:
- Firm
- Nontender
- Confined to one side

Hematuria (less than one fourth of cases)
Fatigue and malaise
Hypertension (occasionally)
Weight loss
Fever
Manifestations resulting from compression of tumour mass
Secondary metabolic alterations from tumour or metastasis
If metastasis, symptoms of lung involvement:
- Dyspnea
- Cough
- Shortness of breath
- Chest pain (sometimes)

Therapeutic Management

Combined treatment with surgery and chemotherapy with or without radiation is based on the histological pattern and clinical stage. Surgery is scheduled as soon as possible after confirmation, usually within 24 to 48 hours of admission. A large transabdominal incision is performed for optimal visualization of the abdominal cavity. The tumour, affected kidney, and adjacent adrenal gland are removed. Great care is taken to keep the encapsulated tumour intact, since rupture can seed cancer cells throughout the abdomen, lymph channel, and bloodstream. The contralateral kidney is carefully inspected for evidence of disease or dysfunction. Regional lymph nodes are inspected, and a biopsy is performed when indicated. Any involved structures, such as part of the colon, diaphragm, or vena cava, are removed. Metal clips are placed around the tumour site for exact marking during radiotherapy.

If both kidneys are involved, the child may be treated with radiotherapy or chemotherapy before surgery to decrease the size of the tumour, allowing more conservative surgery. It may be possible to perform a partial nephrectomy on the less affected kidney, with a total nephrectomy on the opposite side. When a transplant is feasible, such as from a twin, sibling, or parent, bilateral nephrectomy is considered as a last resort.

Postoperative radiotherapy is indicated for children with large tumours, metastasis, residual postoperative disease, unfavourable histological characteristics, or recurrence. Chemotherapy is indicated for all stages. The most effective agents for treating Wilms' tumour are actinomycin D (dactinomycin), vincristine, and adriamycin, with the addition of cyclophosphamide for unfavourable histological characteristics or advanced disease (Dome et al., 2006). The duration of therapy ranges from 6 to 15 months.

Prognosis

Survival rates for Wilms' tumour are the highest among all childhood cancers. Children with localized tumour (stages I and II) have a 90% chance of cure with multimodal therapy. Factors that favourably affect the success of further therapy include initial treatment with only vincristine and dactinomycin, relapse to the lungs only, relapse in the abdomen of a patient who received no prior abdominal irradiation, and relapse more than 12 months after diagnosis. Wilms' tumour may recur, especially in the lungs. Both chemotherapy and radiotherapy can induce second malignancies, usually in areas that have been irradiated (Dome et al., 2006).

Nursing Care Management

Nursing care of the child with Wilms' tumour is similar to that of children with other cancers treated with surgery, irradiation, and chemotherapy. However, there are some significant differences; these are discussed for each phase of nursing intervention.

Preoperative Care

The preoperative period is one of swift diagnosis. The nurse faces the challenge of preparing the child and parents for all laboratory and operative procedures within 24 to 48 hours of admission. Explanations should be simple, repetitive, and focused on the child's actual experiences. In addition to the usual preoperative observations, blood pressure is monitored, since hypertension from excess renin production is a possibility.

There are several special preoperative concerns, the most important of which is that the *tumour is not palpated unless absolutely necessary* because manipulation of the mass may cause dissemination of cancer cells to adjacent and distant sites.

Because radiotherapy and chemotherapy are usually begun immediately after surgery, parents need an explanation of what to expect, such as major benefits and adverse effects (see Chapter 49). The timing of the information should be considered to avoid overwhelming the family. Ideally, the nurse should be present during physician–parent conferences to answer questions as they arise. It is usually better to postpone telling the child about these adverse effects until after surgery. **Alopecia**, usually of most concern to older children, does not occur until approximately 2 weeks after the initial treatment regimen. Therefore the child can be prepared for the hair loss postoperatively.

Postoperative Care

Despite the extensive surgical intervention necessary in many children with Wilms' tumour, the recovery is usually rapid. The major nursing responsibilities are the same as those after any abdominal surgery (see Surgical Procedures, Chapter 45). Because these children are at risk for intestinal obstruction from vincristine-induced ileus, radiation-induced edema, and postsurgical adhesion formation, the nurse needs to carefully monitor gastrointestinal activity, such as bowel movements, bowel sounds, distention, vomiting, and pain. The nurse should also monitor blood pressure, urine output, and signs of infection, as well as instituting pulmonary hygiene to prevent postoperative pulmonary complications.

Family Support

The postoperative period is frequently difficult for parents. The shock of seeing their child immediately after surgery may be the first realization of the seriousness of the diagnosis. It also marks the confirmation of the stage of the tumour. During this period, the nurse should be with the parents to assure them of the child's recovery after surgery and to assess their understanding of the total experience. Older children need an opportunity to deal with their feelings concerning the many procedures to which they have been subjected in rapid succession. **Play therapy** with dolls or puppets or through drawing can be extremely beneficial in helping them adjust. It is not unusual for children to feel angry because of the extent of the surgery, the need for additional therapy, or the seriousness of the disorder.

NURSING ALERT Because the child is left with one kidney, certain precautions, such as avoiding contact sports, are recommended to prevent injury to the remaining organ. Prompt detection and treatment of any genitourinary signs or symptoms are mandatory.

Renal Failure

Renal failure is the inability of the kidneys to excrete waste material, concentrate urine, and conserve electrolytes. It can occur suddenly (ARF) in response to inadequate perfusion, kidney disease, or urinary tract obstruction, or it can develop slowly (CRF) as a result of longstanding kidney disease or an anomaly.

Azotemia and *uremia* are terms often used in relation to renal failure. *Azotemia* is the accumulation of nitrogenous waste within the blood. *Uremia* is a more advanced condition in which retention of nitrogenous products produces toxic symptoms. Azotemia is not life threatening, whereas uremia is a serious condition that often involves other body systems.

Acute Renal Failure

ARF is said to exist when the kidneys suddenly are unable to regulate the volume and composition of urine appropriately in response to food and fluid intake and the needs of the organism. The principal feature of ARF is oligoanuria, or reduced urine volume, associated with azotemia, metabolic acidosis, and diverse electrolyte disturbances. ARF is not common in childhood, but the outcome depends on the cause, associated findings, and prompt recognition and treatment.

The pathological conditions that produce ARF caused by glomerulonephritis and HUS are discussed in relation to those disorders. ARF can also develop as a result of a large number of related or unrelated clinical conditions: poor renal perfusion; urinary tract obstruction; acute renal injury; or the final expression of chronic, irreversible renal disease. The most common cause in children is transient renal failure resulting from severe dehydration or other causes of poor perfusion that may respond to restoration of fluid volume.

Pathophysiology

ARF is usually reversible, but the deviations of physiological function can be extreme, and mortality in the pediatric age group remains high. There is severe reduction in the glomerular filtration rate, an elevated urea level, and a significant reduction in renal blood flow.

The clinical course is variable and depends on the cause. In reversible ARF there is a period of severe oliguria, or a low-output phase, followed by an abrupt onset of diuresis, or a high-output phase, and then a gradual return to (or toward) normal urine volumes.

Diagnostic Evaluation

In many instances of ARF the infant or child is already critically ill with the precipitating disorder, and the explanation for development of oliguria may or may not be readily apparent (Box 50-6). When a previously well child develops ARF without obvious cause, a careful history is taken to reveal symptoms that may be related to glomerulonephritis, obstructive uropathy, or exposure to nephrotoxic chemicals (e.g., ingestion of heavy metals, inhalation of carbon tetrachloride or other organic solvents, or medications such as nonsteroidal anti-inflammatory drugs [NSAIDs] (Krause et al., 2005) known to be toxic to the kidneys). Significant laboratory measurements during renal shutdown that serve as a guide for therapy are urea, serum creatinine, pH, sodium, potassium, and calcium.

NURSING ALERT Diminished urine output and lethargy in a child who is dehydrated, is in shock, or has recently undergone surgery should be evaluated for possible ARF.

Therapeutic Management

Treatment of ARF is directed toward (1) treatment of the underlying cause, (2) management of the complications of renal failure, and (3) provision of supportive therapy within the constraints imposed by the renal failure.

Treatment of poor perfusion resulting from dehydration consists of volume restoration, as described in Chapter 47 in the treatment of dehydration. If oliguria persists after restoration of fluid volume or if the renal failure is caused by intrinsic renal damage, the physiological and biochemical abnormalities that have resulted from kidney dysfunction must be corrected or controlled. Initially a Foley catheter is inserted to rule out urine retention, to collect available urine for analysis, and to monitor the results of diuretic administration. The catheter may or may not be removed during the oliguric phase.

The amount of exogenous water provided should not exceed the amount needed to maintain zero water balance. It is calculated on the basis of estimated endogenous water formation and losses from sensible (primarily gastrointestinal) and insensible sources. No allotment is calculated for urine as long as oliguria persists.

When the output begins to increase, either spontaneously or in response to diuretic therapy, the intake of fluid, potassium, and sodium must be monitored and adequate replacement provided to prevent depletion and its consequences. Some patients pass enormous amounts of electrolyte-rich urine.

Complications

The child with ARF has a tendency to develop water intoxication and hyponatremia, which makes it difficult to provide calories in sufficient amounts to meet the child's needs and reduce tissue **catabolism**, metabolic acidosis, hyperkalemia, and uremia. If the child is able to tolerate oral foods, food sources high in concentrated carbohydrate and fat but low in protein, potassium, and sodium may be provided. However, many children have functional disturbances of the gastrointestinal tract, such as nausea and vomiting; thus the IV route is generally preferred and usually consists of essential amino acids or a combination of essential and nonessential amino acids administered by the central venous route.

Control of water balance in these patients requires careful monitoring of feedback information, such as accurate intake and output, body weight, and electrolyte measurements. In general, during the oliguric phase, no sodium, chloride, or potassium is given unless there are other large, ongoing losses. Regular measurement of plasma electrolyte, pH, urea, and creatinine levels is required to assess the adequacy of fluid therapy and to anticipate complications that require specific treatment.

Hyperkalemia is the most immediate threat to the life of the child with ARF. Hyperkalemia can be minimized and sometimes avoided by eliminating potassium from all food and fluid, by reducing tissue catabolism, and by correcting acidosis. Measures to reduce serum potassium levels are oral or rectal administration of an ion-exchange resin such as sodium polystyrene sulphonate (Kayexalate) and peritoneal dialysis or hemodialysis (p. 1559). The resin produces its effect by exchange of its sodium for the potassium, thus binding potassium for removal from the body. This increased sodium concentration may contribute to fluid overload, hypertension, and cardiac failure. Dialysis removes potassium and other waste products from the serum by diffusion through a semipermeable membrane.

NURSING ALERT Any of the following signs of hyperkalemia constitute an emergency and need to be reported immediately:

- Serum potassium concentrations in excess of 7 mmol/L
- Electrocardiographic abnormalities, such as prolonged QRS complex, depressed ST segment, high peaked T waves, bradycardia, or heart block

Hypertension is a frequent and serious complication of ARF, and to detect it early, blood pressure measurements are

BOX 50-6 Clinical Manifestations of Acute Renal Failure

Specific
- Oliguria
- Anuria uncommon (except in obstructive disorders)

Nonspecific (may develop)
- Nausea
- Vomiting
- Drowsiness
- Edema
- Hypertension

Other
- Manifestations of underlying disorder or pathological condition

made every 4 to 6 hours. The most common cause of hypertension in ARF is overexpansion of extracellular fluid and plasma volume together with activation of the renin-angiotensin system. Hypertension is controlled with antihypertensive drugs. Other measures that may be used include limiting fluids and salt.

Anemia is frequently associated with ARF, but transfusion is not recommended unless the hemoglobin drops below 60 g/L. Transfusions, if used, consist of fresh washed, packed red blood cells given slowly to reduce the likelihood of increasing blood volume, hypertension, and hyperkalemia.

Seizures occur often when renal failure progresses to uremia and are also related to hypertension, hyponatremia, and hypocalcemia. Treatment is directed to the specific cause when known. More obscure causes are managed with antiepileptic drugs.

Cardiac failure with pulmonary edema is almost always associated with hypervolemia. Treatment is directed toward reduction of fluid volume, with water and sodium restriction and administration of diuretics.

Prognosis

The prognosis of ARF depends largely on the nature and severity of the causative factor or precipitating event and the promptness and competence of management. The outcome is least favourable in children with rapidly progressive nephritis and cortical necrosis. Children in whom ARF is a result of HUS or AGN recover completely, but residual renal impairment or hypertension is more often the rule. Complete recovery is usually expected in children whose renal failure is a result of dehydration, nephrotoxins, or ischemia. ARF after cardiac surgery is less favourable. It is often impossible to assess the extent of recovery for several months.

Nursing Care Management

Meticulous attention to fluid intake and output is mandatory and includes all of the physical measurements discussed previously in relation to problems of fluid balance. Monitoring fluid balance and vital signs is a continuous process, and nurses need to be constantly on the alert for signs of complications so that appropriate interventions can be implemented. Because these children require intensive observation and often specialized treatment, such as dialysis, they are usually admitted to a critical care unit in which needed equipment and trained personnel are available (see Nursing Care Plan).

Limiting fluid intake requires ingenuity on the part of caregivers to cope with the child who is thirsty. Rationing the daily intake in small amounts of fluid served in containers that give the impression of larger volumes is one strategy. Older children who understand the rationale of fluid limits can help determine how their daily ration should be distributed.

Meeting nutritional needs is sometimes a problem; the child may be nauseated, and encouraging concentrated foods without fluids may be difficult. When nourishment is provided via the IV route, careful monitoring is essential to prevent fluid overload.

The nurse must be continually alert for changes in behaviour that indicate the onset of complications. Infection from reduced resistance, anemia, and general morbidity is a constant threat. Fluid overload and electrolyte disturbances can precipitate cardiovascular complications such as hypertension and cardiac failure. Fluid and electrolyte imbalances, acidosis, and accumulation of nitrogenous waste products can produce neurological involvement manifested by coma, seizures, or alterations in sensorium.

Although children with ARF are usually quite ill and voluntarily diminish their activity, infants may become restless and irritable, and children are often anxious and frightened. Frequent, painful, and stress-producing treatments and tests must be performed. A supportive, empathetic nurse can provide comfort and stability in a threatening and unnatural environment.

Family Support

Providing support and reassurance to parents is among the major nursing responsibilities. The seriousness of ARF and its emergency nature are stressful to parents, and most feel some degree of guilt regarding the child's condition, especially when the illness is a result of ingestion of a toxic substance, dehydration, or a genetic disease. They also need to be kept informed of the child's progress and provided with explanations regarding the therapeutic regimen. The equipment and the child's behaviour are sometimes frightening and anxiety provoking. Nurses can do much to help parents comprehend and deal with the stresses of the situation.

Chronic Renal Failure

The kidneys are able to maintain the chemical composition of fluids within normal limits until more than 50% of functional renal capacity is destroyed by disease or injury. Chronic renal insufficiency or failure begins when the diseased kidneys can no longer maintain the normal chemical structure of body fluids under normal conditions. Progressive deterioration over months or years produces a variety of clinical and biochemical disturbances that culminate in the clinical syndrome known as uremia.

A variety of diseases and disorders can result in CRF. The most frequent causes are congenital renal and urinary tract malformations, VUR associated with recurrent UTI, chronic pyelonephritis, hereditary disorders, chronic glomerulonephritis, and glomerulonephropathy associated with systemic diseases such as anaphylactoid purpura and lupus erythematosus.

Pathophysiology

Early in the course of progressive nephrotic destruction, the child remains asymptomatic with only minimal biochemical abnormalities. Unless the presence of CRF is detected in the process of routine assessment, signs and symptoms that indicate advanced renal damage frequently emerge only late in the course of the disease. Midway in the disease process, as increasing numbers of nephrons are totally destroyed and most others are damaged to varying degrees, the few that remain intact are hypertrophied but functional. These few normal nephrons are able to make sufficient adjustments to stresses to maintain reasonable degrees of fluid and electrolyte balance. Definitive biochemical examination at this time will reveal limited tolerance to excesses or restrictions. As the disease progresses to the end stage, because of a severe reduction in the number of functioning nephrons, the kidneys are

Nursing Care Plan ● The Child With Acute Renal Dysfunction

Nursing Diagnosis	Expected Patient Outcomes	Nursing Interventions	Rationale
Risk for injury related to accumulated electrolytes and waste products	Child will exhibit no evidence of waste product accumulation.	Assist with renal dialysis.	To maintain renal excretory function
Child's/Family's Defining Characteristics *(Subjective and Objective Data)*	**The Following NOC Concept Applies to This Outcome**	Administer sodium polystyrene sulphate (Kayexalate) as ordered.	To reduce serum potassium levels
Excesses in potassium, sodium, and phosphorus	Risk Control	Provide diet low in potassium, sodium, and phosphorus.	To reduce excretory demand on kidneys
Evidence of hyperkalemia, hyperphosphatemia, and uremia		Observe for evidence of accumulated waste products.	To ensure prompt treatment
Excess blood urea nitrogen		Increase water intake.	To increase waste excretion by kidneys
		The Following NIC Concepts Apply to These Interventions Risk Identification Medication Administration Surveillance Teaching: Disease Process	

Nursing Diagnosis	Expected Patient Outcomes	Nursing Interventions	Rationale
Imbalanced nutrition: less than body requirements related to restricted diet	Child will consume an adequate amount of appropriate foods and fluid.	Provide dietary instructions for foods that reduce excretory demands on kidney and provide sufficient calories and protein for growth.	To provide an appropriate diet that can reduce kidney demands
Child's/Family's Defining Characteristics *(Subjective and Objective Data)*	Child will show no evidence of deficiencies or weight loss.	Limit phosphorus, salt, and potassium as prescribed.	To prevent mineral excess
Weight loss	**The Following NOC Concepts Apply to These Outcomes**	Encourage intake of carbohydrates and foods high in calcium.	To provide calories for growth and calcium to prevent bone demineralization
Inadequate growth	Nutritional Status: Nutrient Intake	Arrange for renal dietitian to meet with family to review allowable foods and assist in dietary planning.	To promote understanding of the child's dietary needs and fluid modifications
Poor nutritional intake	Nutritional Status: Food and Fluid Intake	Help hemodialysis patient to fill out menu requests for meals.	To promote appropriate food choice decisions
	Weight Control	**The Following NIC Concepts Apply to These Interventions** Teaching: Prescribed Diet Vital Signs Monitoring Fluid Management Nutrition Management Nutrition Therapy Nutritional Monitoring	

NIC, Nursing Interventions Classification; *NOC*, Nursing Outcomes Classification.

no longer able to maintain fluid and electrolyte balance, and the features of uremic syndrome appear.

The accumulation of various biochemical substances in the blood, those that result from diminished renal function, produces complications such as the following:

Retention of waste products, especially urea and creatinine

Water and sodium retention, which contributes to edema and vascular congestion

Hyperkalemia of dangerous levels

Metabolic acidosis of a sustained nature because of continual hydrogen ion retention and bicarbonate loss

Calcium and phosphorus disturbances, resulting in altered bone metabolism, which in turn causes growth arrest or restriction, bone pain, and deformities known as *renal osteodystrophy*

Anemia caused by hematological dysfunction, including the shortened lifespan of red blood cells, impaired red blood cell production related to decreased production of erythropoietin, prolonged bleeding time, and nutritional anemia

Growth disturbance, probably caused by such factors as renal osteodystrophy, poor nutrition associated with dietary restrictions and loss of appetite, and biochemical abnormalities

Children with CRF seem to be more susceptible to infection, especially pneumonia, UTI, and septicemia, although the reason for this is unclear. These children become extraordinarily sensitive to changes in vascular volume that may cause pulmonary overload, central nervous system symptoms, hypertension, and cardiac failure.

Diagnostic Evaluation

The diagnosis of CRF is usually suspected on the basis of any number of clinical manifestations, a history of prior renal disease, or biochemical findings. The onset is usually gradual, and the initial signs and symptoms are vague and nonspecific (Box 50-7).

Laboratory and other diagnostic tools and tests are of value in assessing the extent of renal damage, biochemical disturbances, and related physical dysfunction (see Tables 50-1 to 50-3). Often they can help establish the nature of the underlying disease and differentiate between other disease processes and the pathological consequences of renal dysfunction.

BOX 50-7 Clinical Manifestations of Chronic Renal Failure

Early Signs
- Loss of normal energy
- Increased fatigue on exertion
- Pallor, subtle (may not be noticed)
- Elevated blood pressure (sometimes)

As the Disease Progresses
- Decreased appetite (especially at breakfast)
- Less interest in normal activities
- Increased or decreased urine output with compensatory intake of fluid
- Pallor more evident
- Sallow, muddy appearance of skin

Child May Develop
- Headache
- Muscle cramps
- Nausea

Other Signs and Symptoms
- Weight loss
- Facial edema
- Malaise
- Bone or joint pain
- Growth restriction
- Dryness or itching of the skin
- Bruised skin
- Sensory or motor loss (sometimes)
- Amenorrhea (common in adolescent girls)

Uremic Syndrome (Untreated)
- Gastrointestinal symptoms: anorexia, nausea and vomiting
- Bleeding tendencies: bruises, bloody diarrheal stools, stomatitis, bleeding from lips and mouth
- Intractable itching
- Uremic frost (deposits of urea crystals on skin)
- Unpleasant "uremic" breath odour
- Deep respirations
- Hypertension
- Heart failure
- Pulmonary edema
- Neurological involvement: progressive confusion, dulled sensorium, coma (ultimately), tremors, muscular twitching, seizures

Therapeutic Management

In irreversible renal failure the goals of medical management are to (1) promote maximum renal function, (2) maintain body fluid and electrolyte balance within safe biochemical limits, (3) treat systemic complications, and (4) promote as active and normal a life as possible for the child for as long as possible. The child is allowed unrestricted activity and is allowed to set his or her own limits. School attendance is encouraged as long as the child is able or home tutoring is arranged.

Diet regulation is the most effective means, short of dialysis, for reducing the quantity of materials that require renal excretion. The goal of diet management in renal failure is to provide sufficient calories and protein for growth while limiting the excretory demands made on the kidney, to minimize metabolic bone disease (*osteodystrophy*), and to minimize fluid and electrolyte disturbances. Dietary protein intake is limited only to the reference daily intake for the child's age. Restriction of protein intake below the Recommended Daily Allowance (RDA) is believed to negatively affect growth and neurodevelopment. Malnutrition may develop in patients with CRF even before they need dialysis (Nailescu, Kaskel, & Kaskel, 2004).

Sodium and water are not usually limited unless there is evidence of edema or hypertension, and potassium is not usually restricted. However, restrictions of any or all three may be imposed in later stages or at any time that abnormal serum concentrations are evident.

Dietary phosphorus is controlled through reduction of protein, milk, and soft-drink intake to prevent or correct the calcium/phosphorus imbalance. Phosphorus levels can be further reduced by oral administration of calcium carbonate preparations or other phosphate-binding agents that combine with the phosphorus to decrease gastrointestinal absorption and thus the serum levels of phosphate. Treatment with 25-OH vitamin D is begun to increase calcium absorption and suppress elevated parathyroid hormone levels.

Metabolic acidosis is alleviated through the administration of alkalizing agents such as sodium bicarbonate or a combination of sodium and potassium citrate.

Growth failure is one major consequence of CRF, especially in the preadolescent. These children grow poorly both before and after the initiation of hemodialysis. The use of recombinant human growth hormone to accelerate growth in children with growth restriction secondary to CRF has been successful (Gorman, Fivush, & Frankenfield, 2005; Mehls et al., 2002; Vimalachandra et al., 2006). Osseous deformities that result from renal osteodystrophy, especially those related to ambulation, are troublesome and require correction if they occur.

Dental defects are common in children with CRF, and the earlier the onset of the disease, the more severe are the dental manifestations (including hypoplasia, hypomineralization, tooth discolouration, alteration in size and shape of teeth, malocclusion, and ulcerative stomatitis). Regular dental care is especially important in these children.

Anemia in children with CRF is related to decreased production of erythropoietin. Recombinant human erythropoietin is offered to these children as thrice-weekly or weekly subcutaneous injections and replaces the need for frequent blood transfusions. The medication corrects the anemia and in turn increases appetite, activity, and general well-being. In addition, a variety of iron preparations are often administered.

Hypertension of advanced renal disease may be managed initially by cautious use of a low-sodium diet, fluid restriction, and perhaps diuretics such as hydrochlorothiazide or furosemide. Severe hypertension requires the use of antihypertensive agents, singly or in combination.

Intercurrent infections are treated with appropriate antimicrobials at the first sign of infection; however, any drug eliminated through the kidneys should be administered with caution. Other complications are treated symptomatically (e.g., central-acting anti-emetics for nausea, anti-epileptics for seizures, and diphenhydramine [Benadryl] for pruritus).

Once evidence of end-stage renal disease (ESRD) appears in a child, the disease runs its relentless course and results in death in a few weeks, unless waste products and toxins are removed from body fluids by dialysis or kidney transplantation. These techniques have been adapted for infants and small children and are implemented in most cases of renal failure after conservative management is no longer effective (see Technologic Management of Renal Failure).

Prognosis

Dialysis and transplantation are the only treatments currently available for children with ESRD. Although children may survive on dialysis, it is not an ideal long-term modality. Complications include infection of access sites, growth failure, and disruption of normal socialization. Many pediatric centres encourage families of children with ESRD to consider kidney transplantation. The North American Renal Transplantation in Children Report of the North American Pediatric Renal Trials and Collaborative Studies (2008) stated a graft survival of 90% at 1 year and 74% at 6 years for living donor kidneys, and 80% at 1 year and 58% at 6 years for cadaver kidneys.

Malignancies, infection, and hypertension are the most life-threatening problems after transplantation (Groothoff, 2005). Long-term graft survival is not guaranteed, and many children require a second or third transplant. Successful kidney transplantation does improve rehabilitation of children with ESRD, both educationally and psychologically. Increasing use of primary or preemptive kidney transplants is becoming the optimal form of renal replacement therapy, leading to substantial improvement in quality of life (Goldstein et al., 2006).

Nursing Care Management

The multiple complications of ESRD are managed according to evidence-informed clinical practice guidelines such as the ESRD Clinical Performance Measures Project (Fadrowski et al., 2007). However, progressive disease places a number of stresses on the child and family, including those of a potentially fatal illness (see Chapter 44). There is a continuing need for repeated examinations that often entail painful procedures, side effects, and frequent hospitalizations. Diet therapy becomes progressively more restricted and intense, and the child is required to take a variety of medications. Ever present in all aspects of the treatment regimen is the agonizing realization that without treatment, death is inevitable.

Some specific stresses related to ESRD and its treatment are predictable. When it first becomes apparent that ESRD is inevitable, both the parents and child experience depression and anxiety. Acceptance is particularly difficult if renal failure progresses rapidly after diagnosis. Denial and disbelief are usually pronounced, especially among the parents. The initiation of dialysis is usually perceived as a positive experience, and after experiencing initial concerns regarding the treatment, the child begins to feel better and parental anxiety is relieved for a time.

Initiating a dialysis regimen is a traumatic and anxiety-provoking experience for most children because it involves surgery for implantation of a vascular access (central venous line, graft, or fistula) for hemodialysis, or a peritoneal catheter for peritoneal dialysis. The initial experience with this procedure is frightening to most children. They need reassurance about the nature of the preparations for dialysis and the conduct of the treatment.

For hemodialysis, the fistula or graft requires needle insertions at each treatment. The goal is to perform pain-free venipuncture. Using buffered lidocaine with a small-gauge needle (30 gauge) to anaesthetize the area before venipuncture of the graft or fistula is one method. Using an anaesthetizing topical preparation such as EMLA (eutectic mixture of local anaesthetics [lidocaine and prilocaine]) 1 hour before venipuncture is another approach (see Pain Management, Chapter 35). Central venous lines eliminate the need for needles but are more prone to infection and other central line complications.

Adolescents, with their increased need for independence and their urge for rebellion, usually adapt less well than younger children. They resent the control and enforced dependence imposed by the rigorous and unrelenting therapy program. They resent being dependent on hemodialysis technology, their parents, and the professional staff. Depression or hostility is common in adolescents undergoing hemodialysis.

The availability of home peritoneal dialysis has offered a greater degree of freedom for persons undergoing long-term dialysis. Independently managing dialysis treatments at home is less disruptive to school and social activities. Patients and their families need to receive an in-depth teaching program to prepare them for assessing, implementing, and monitoring dialysis treatments.

Body changes related to the disease process, including skin discolouration, growth restriction, and lack of sexual maturation, are stress provoking. Dietary and fluid restrictions are particularly burdensome for both children and parents. Children may feel deprived when they are unable to eat foods previously enjoyed and that are unrestricted to other family members. Consequently, they may fail to adhere to their food plan. Patient, supportive, and encouraging nursing care is essential. Children, especially adolescents, should be allowed maximum participation in and responsibility for their own treatment program.

After months or years of dialysis, the parents and child may feel anxiety associated with the prognosis and continued pressures of the treatment. The time spent in transportation to and from the hemodialysis unit and the time spent undergoing dialysis treatments can interfere with the acquisition of developmental and social milestones. Vascular-access and peritoneal dialysis exit site infections may develop and present a common source of aggravation. The possibility of kidney transplantation often provides hope for relief from the rigors of hemodialysis and peritoneal dialysis.

The Kidney Foundation of Canada and other agencies provide a number of services and information for families of children with renal disease (see Additional Resources at the end of this chapter).

Technological Management of Renal Failure

Dialysis

Dialysis is the process of separating colloids and crystalline substances in solution by the difference in their rate of diffusion through a semipermeable membrane. Methods of dialysis currently available for clinical management of renal failure are *peritoneal dialysis*, in which the abdominal cavity acts as a semipermeable membrane through which water and solutes of small molecular size move by osmosis and diffusion according to their respective concentrations on either side of the membrane, and *hemodialysis*, in which blood is circulated outside the body through artificial membranes that permit a similar passage of water and solutes. A third type of dialysis is *hemofiltration*, in which blood filtrate is circulated outside the body by hydrostatic pressure exerted across a semipermeable membrane with simultaneous infusion of a replacement solution. Types of hemofiltration include continuous venovenous hemofiltration, continuous venovenous hemodialysis, and continuous venovenous hemodiafiltration. Hemofiltration is generally reserved for use in ARF, severe fluid overload, inborn errors of metabolism, or after bone marrow transplant (Goldstein, 2003).

Peritoneal dialysis is the preferred form of dialysis for infants, children and parents who wish to remain independent, for families who live a long distance from the medical centre, and for children who prefer fewer dietary restrictions and a gentler form of dialysis. Chronic peritoneal dialysis is most often performed at home. The two types of peritoneal dialysis are continuous ambulatory peritoneal dialysis and continuous cycling peritoneal dialysis. In both methods, commercially available sterile dialysis solution is instilled into the peritoneal cavity through a surgically implanted indwelling catheter which is tunnelled subcutaneously and sutured into place. The warmed solution is allowed to enter the peritoneal cavity by gravity and remains a variable length of time according to the rate of solute removal and glucose absorption in individual patients. The fluid and accumulated toxic wastes are then drained from the peritoneal cavity and a new cycle of fresh dialysis solution is re-instilled. The frequency and timing of the cycles depends on the child's age, fluid balancing needs, and solute removal requirements. Performing this form of dialysis in the home can be empowering for families, especially adolescents. However, the nurse needs to carefully assess for signs of burn out and arrange for respite care as necessary.

NURSING ALERT Observe for changes in the colour of the dialysate draining from the child. The spent solution should be clear. If the colour is cloudy, notify the practitioner immediately (Schaefer, 2003).

Hemodialysis requires the surgical creation of a vascular access and the use of special dialysis equipment—the hemodialyzer, or so-called artificial kidney. Vascular access may be one of three types: fistulas, grafts, or external vascular access devices. An *arteriovenous fistula* is an access in which a vein and artery are connected surgically. The preferred site is the radial artery and a forearm vein that produces dilation and thickening of the superficial vessels of the forearm to provide easy access for repeated venipuncture. An alternative is the creation of a subcutaneous (internal) arteriovenous graft by anastomosing artery and vein, with a synthetic prosthetic graft for circulatory access. The most commonly used material is expanded polytetrafluoroethylene (ePTFE). Both the graft and the fistula require needle insertions with each dialysis treatment.

For external vascular access devices, percutaneous catheters are inserted in the femoral, subclavian, or internal jugular veins, even in very small children. A more permanent form of external access is available via a central catheter inserted surgically into the internal jugular vein. Catheters eliminate the need for skin punctures but require dressing changes and are prone to infection. Home care may need to be arranged to assist the families with caring for their catheter at home, in between hemodialysis treatments.

Hemodialysis is best suited to children who do not have someone in the family who is able to perform peritoneal dialysis and to those who live close to a dialysis centre. The procedure is usually performed three times per week for 4 to 6 hours, depending on the child's size. Hemodialysis achieves rapid correction of fluid and electrolyte abnormalities but can cause side effects in association with this rapid change, such as muscle cramping, headaches, nausea and vomiting, and hypotension. Disadvantages include school absence during hemodialysis treatments and strict fluid and dietary restrictions. Boredom for the child and family is often experienced during the mobility limiting treatments, so planned activities should be introduced (Fig. 50-3).

Most children show rapid clinical improvement with the implementation of dialysis, although it is directly related to the duration of uremia before dialysis and good nutrition. Growth rate and skeletal maturation improve, but recovery of

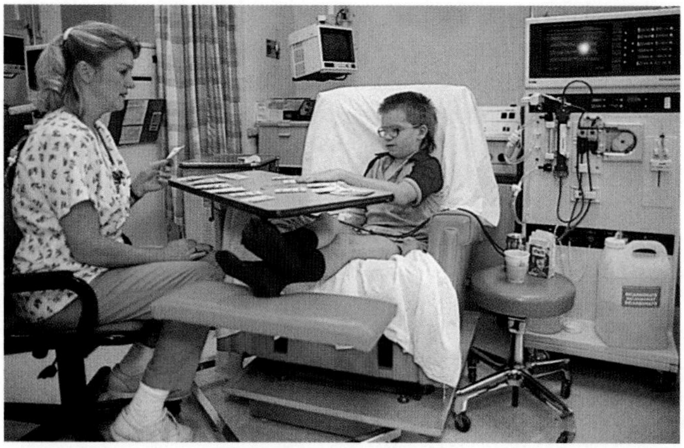

Fig. 50-3 Diversional activities help lessen the boredom children can experience during hemodialysis.

normal growth is infrequent. In many cases, sexual development, although delayed, progresses to completion.

Transplantation

Kidney transplantation is now an acceptable and effective means of therapy in the pediatric age group. Although peritoneal dialysis and hemodialysis are life preserving, both require major alterations in lifestyle. Transplantation offers the opportunity for a relatively normal life and is the preferred form of treatment for children with ESRD. Primary or pre-emptive transplants maintain the greatest amount of normalcy in the family's life.

In terms of wait time for an available kidney for transplantation, discrepancies exist between various populations. Researchers from the Pediatric Renal Outcomes Canada Group found that the time from start of dialysis to the first kidney transplant was longer for First Nations, Métis, and Inuit children than for non-Aboriginal children. Further research is needed to investigate individual and system barriers that contribute to the difference in the wait times (Samuel et al., 2011).

Kidneys for transplant are available from two sources: a *living related donor*, usually a parent or a sibling, or a *cadaver donor*, a dead or brain-dead patient whose family consents to the donation of a healthy kidney. Retransplantation occurs frequently. The primary goal in transplantation is the long-term survival of grafted tissue by securing tissue that is antigenically similar to that of the recipient and by suppressing the recipient's immune mechanism. The immunosuppressant therapy of choice has been corticosteroids (prednisone) in conjunction with cyclosporine or tacrolimus and mycophenolate mofetil. Other therapies include antilymphoblast globulin or monoclonal antibodies. New immunosuppressant medications are rapidly coming into clinical trials and into use in large transplant centres. It is important for the nurse to learn about the medications used in the antirejection protocol(s) and about their adverse effects. Because the immunosuppressant medications are taken indefinitely, transplant patients experience many adverse effects of the medications, including hypertension, growth restriction, cataracts, risk of infection, obesity, characteristics of Cushing's syndrome, and hirsutism (Smith, Nemeth, & McDonald, 2003).

NURSING ALERT The child with a kidney transplant who exhibits any of the following should be evaluated immediately for possible rejection, as this the most common cause of transplant failure:

- Fever
- Swelling and tenderness over graft area
- Diminished urine output
- Elevated blood pressure
- Elevated serum creatinine

Rejection is treated aggressively with immunosuppressant medications and can often be reversed. Some patients do not respond or develop chronic rejection and must eventually return to dialysis or undergo another kidney transplant.

Key Points

- Common inflammatory disorders of the genitourinary tract include UTI, nephrotic syndrome, and AGN.
- Management of UTIs is directed at eliminating infection, detecting and correcting functional or anatomical abnormalities, preventing recurrences, and preserving renal function.
- VUR is the retrograde flow of bladder urine into the ureters.
- Obstructive uropathy is a result of structural or functional abnormalities of the urinary system that obstruct the normal flow of urine.
- The more common defects of the genitourinary tract include phimosis, cryptorchidism, inguinal hernia, hydrocele, and hypospadias.
- Body-image concerns and castration anxiety are particularly intense in children with defects in the genital area.
- Nephrotic syndrome is characterized by increased glomerular permeability to protein, with massive urinary loss of protein resulting in hypoproteinemia and edema.
- Management of nephrotic syndrome is aimed at reducing excretion of protein, reducing or preventing fluid retention by tissues, and preventing infection and other complications.
- Common features of AGN are oliguria, edema, hypertension, circulatory congestion, hematuria, and proteinuria.
- Therapeutic management of AGN involves maintenance of fluid balance, treatment of hypertension, and antibiotic therapy.
- Management of HUS is aimed at control of complications and hematological manifestations of renal failure.
- Wilms' tumour is the most common malignant neoplasm of the kidney in infants and children.
- In ARF, management is directed at determining treatment of the underlying cause, managing complications of renal failure, and providing supportive therapy.
- Abnormalities in CRF are waste product retention, water and sodium retention, hyperkalemia, acidosis, calcium and phosphorus disturbance, anemia, and growth disturbances.
- The types of dialysis used in ESRD are peritoneal dialysis and hemodialysis.
- When the child will need home dialysis, the nurse needs to educate the family about the disease, its implications, the

therapeutic plan, possible psychological effects of the disease, and the treatment and technical aspects of the procedure.

- The major concerns in kidney transplantation are tissue matching and prevention of rejection; psychological concerns involve self-image as related to possible body changes as a result of the effects of corticosteroid therapy.

Audio Chapter Summaries

Access an Audio Summary of these Key Points on evolve

References

Bailey, D. T., et al. (2007). Can a concentrated cranberry extract prevent recurrent urinary tract infections in women? A pilot study. *Phytomedicine, 14*(4), 237–241. doi:10.1016/j.phymed.2007.01.004

Canadian Cancer Society. (2011). *The Canadian cancer encyclopedia.* Retrieved from http://info.cancer.ca/cce-ecc/default.aspx?Lang=E&toc=56.

Canadian Paediatric Society. (2009a). *Neonatal circumcision revisited.* Retrieved from http://www.cps.ca/english/statements/fn/fn96-01.htm.

Canadian Paediatric Society. (2009b). *PID note: Bag urine specimens still not appropriate in diagnosing urinary tract infections in infants.* Retrieved from http://www.cps.ca/english/statements/id/pidnoteuti.htm.

Cerwinka, W. H., Scherz, H. C., & Kirsch, A. J. (2008). Endoscopic treatment of vesicoureteral reflux with dextranomer/hyaluronic acid in children. *Advances in Urology*, 513854. doi:10.1155/2008/513854

Dome, J. S., et al. (2006). Renal tumours. In P. A. Pizzo & D. P. Poplack (Eds.), *Principles and practices of pediatric oncology* (5th ed.). Philadelphia: Lippincott, Williams & Wilkins.

Fadrowski, J. J., et al. (2007). Children on long-term dialysis in the United States: Findings from the 2005 ESRD clinical performance measures project. *American Journal of Kidney Disease, 50*(6), 958–966. doi:10.1053/j.ajkd.2007.09.003

Goldstein, S. L. (2003). Overview of pediatric renal replacement therapy in acute renal failure. *Artificial Organs, 27*(9), 781–785.

Goldstein, S. L., et al. (2006). Health-related quality of life in pediatric patients with ESRD. *Pediatric Nephrology, 21*(6), 846–850. doi:10.1053/j.ajkd.2007.09.021

Gorman, G., Fivush, B., & Frankenfield, D., (2005). Short stature and growth hormone use in pediatric hemodialysis patients. *Journal of Pediatric Nephrology, 20*(12), 794–800.

Groothoff, J. W. (2005). Long-term outcomes of children with end-stage renal disease. *Pediatric Nephrology, 20*(7), 849–853.

Jepson, R. G., Mihaljevic, L., & Craig, J. (2004). Cranberries for preventing urinary tract infections. *Cochrane Database of Systematic Reviews* (*2*), CD001321.

Kanellopoulos, T. A., et al. (2006). First urinary tract infection in neonates, infants and young children: A comparative study. *Pediatric Nephrology, 21*(8), 1131–1137. doi:10.1007/s00467-006-0158-7

Kass, E. (1996). Timing of elective surgery on the genitalia of male children with particular reference to the risks, benefits, and psychological effects of surgery and anaesthesia. *Pediatrics, 97*(4), 590–594.

Kirsch, A. J., Perez-Brayfield, M. R., & Scherz, H. C. (2003). Minimally invasive treatment of vesicoureteral reflux with endoscopic injection of dextranomer/hyaluronic acid copolymer: The Children's Hospital of Atlanta experience. *Journal of Urology, 170*(1), 211–215.

Kliegman, R. M., et al. (2007). Hemolytic-uremic syndrome. In R. M. Kliegman, et al. (Eds.), *Nelson textbook of pediatrics* (18th ed.). Philadelphia: Saunders Elsevier.

Kline, N. E., & Sevier, N. (2003). Solid tumours in children. *Journal of Pediatric Nursing, 18*(2), 96–102.

Krause, I., et al. (2005). Acute renal failure, associated with non-steroidal anti-inflammatory drugs in healthy children. *Pediatric Nephrology, 20*(9), 1295–1298. doi:10.1007/s00467-005-1966-x

Lavelle, M. T., Conlin, M. J., & Skoog, S. J. (2005). Subureteral injection of Defluz for correction of reflux: Analysis of factors predicting success. *Urology, 65*(3), 564–567. doi:10.1016/j.urology.2004.09.068

Mehls, O., et al. (2002). Effectiveness of growth hormone treatment in short children with chronic renal failure. *Journal of Pediatrics, 141*(1), 147–148.

Nailescu, C., Kaskel, P. J., & Kaskel, F. J. (2004). Nutrition and metabolism. In E. D. Avner, W. E. Harmon, & P. Niaudet (Eds.), *Pediatric nephrology* (5th ed.). Philadelphia: Lippincott Williams & Wilkins.

North American Pediatric Renal Trials and Collaborative Studies. (2008). *2008 annual report.* Retrieved from https://web.emmes.com/study/ped/annlrept/Annual%20Report%20-2008.pdf.

Rosenthal, M. (2004). Current concepts in managing UTIs in children. *Infectious Diseases in Childhood, 17*(3), 30–31.

Samuel, S. M., et al., & the Pediatric Renal Outcomes Canada Group. (2011). Dialysis and transplantation among Aboriginal children with kidney failure. *Canadian Medical Association Journal, 188*(10), E665–E672. doi:10.1503/cmaj.101840

Schaefer, F. (2003). Management of peritonitis in children receiving chronic peritoneal dialysis. *Paediatric Drugs, 5*(5), 315–325.

Shaikh, N., et al. (2008). Prevalence of urinary tract infection in childhood: A meta-analysis. *Pediatric Infectious Diseases Journal, 27*(4), 302–308. doi:10.1097/INF.0b013e31815e4122

Smith, J. M., Nemeth, T. L., & McDonald, R. A. (2003). Current immunosuppressive agents: Efficacy, side effects, and utilization. *Pediatric Clinics of North America, 50*(6), 1283–1300. *Cochrane Database of Systematic Reviews*(3), CD003264.

Vimalachandra, D., et al. (2006). Growth hormone for children with chronic kidney disease. *Cochrane Database of Systematic Reviews* (*3*), CD003264.

Additional Resources

Kidney Foundation of Canada: http://www.kidney

PKD Foundation of Canada for Research in Polycystic Kidney Disease (Kidney Failure): http://endpkd.ca/Learn_ARPKD_KidneyFailure_QA.asp

Unit 11

51 Cerebral Dysfunction

Learning Objectives

On completion of this chapter, the reader will be able to:

- Describe the various modalities for assessment of cerebral function.
- Differentiate between the stages of consciousness.
- Formulate a care plan for the unconscious child.
- Distinguish between the types of head injuries and the serious complications.
- Describe the nursing care of a child with a tumour of the central nervous system.
- Outline a care plan for the child with bacterial meningitis.
- Differentiate between the various types of seizure disorders.
- Demonstrate an understanding of the manifestations of a seizure disorder and the management of a child with such a disorder.
- Describe the preoperative and postoperative care of a child with hydrocephalus.

Electronic Resources

Additional information related to the content in Chapter 51 can be found on

evolve the companion Web site at

http://evolve.elsevier.com/Canada/Perry/maternal/

- Examination Review Questions
- Animation—Brain Lobes
- Animation—Seizure, Generalized
- Animation—Subdural Hematoma
- Animation—Ventriculoperitoneal Shunt
- Case Study—Meningitis
- Case Study—Hydrocephalus With Myelomeningocele
- Critical Thinking Exercise—Seizures

Assessment of Cerebral Function

Most of the information about the status of the brain is obtained by indirect measurements. Some of these measurements are discussed elsewhere in relation to numerous aspects of child care (e.g., as part of assessments of health [Chapter 34], newborn status [Chapter 36], cognitive impairment [Chapter 42], hypoxic injury [cerebral palsy, Chapter 55], and attainment of developmental milestones at each stage of development). Since increased intracranial pressure (ICP) and altered states of consciousness have such prominent places in neurological dysfunction, they are described here, followed by techniques for neurological assessment and diagnostic tests.

General Aspects

Children younger than 2 years of age require special evaluation, since they are unable to respond to directions designed to elicit specific neurological responses. Early neurological responses in infants are primarily reflexive; these responses are gradually replaced by meaningful movement in the characteristic **cephalocaudal** direction of development. This evidence of progressive maturation reflects more extensive **myelinization** and changes in neurochemical and electrophysiological properties.

Most information about infants and small children is gained by observing their spontaneous and elicited reflex responses as they develop increasingly complex locomotor and fine motor skills and by eliciting progressively sophisticated communicative and adaptive behaviours. Delay or deviation from expected **critical milestones** helps identify high-risk children. Persistence or reappearance of reflexes that normally disappear indicates a pathological condition. In evaluating the infant or young child, it is also important to obtain the pregnancy and delivery history to determine the possible impact of intrauterine environmental influences known to affect the orderly maturation of the central nervous system (CNS). These influences include maternal **infections**, chemicals, **trauma**, and metabolic insults.

General aspects of assessment that provide clues to the etiology of dysfunction include the following:

Family history—Sometimes offers clues regarding possible genetic disorders with neurological manifestations

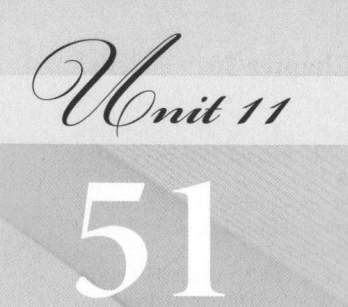

Health history—May provide valuable clues regarding the cause of dysfunction (e.g., an injury, short febrile illness, encounter with an animal or insect, ingestion of neurotoxic substances, inhalation of chemicals, a past illness, or known diabetes mellitus)

Physical evaluation of infants—Includes observation of the following:
- Size and shape of the head
- Spontaneous activity and postural reflex activity
- Sensory responses
- Attitude—normal flexed posture, extreme extension, opisthotonos, hypotonia
- Symmetry in movement of extremities
- Excessive tremulousness or frequent twitching movements
- Altered expiratory cycle—prolonged apnea, ataxic breathing, paradoxic chest movement, and hyperventilation
- Skin and hair texture
- Distinctive facial features
- A high-pitched, piercing cry
- Abnormal eye movements
- Inability to suck or swallow
- Lip smacking
- Asymmetrical contraction of facial muscles
- Yawning (may indicate cranial nerve involvement)
- Muscular activity and coordination
- Level of development

Increased Intracranial Pressure

The brain, tightly enclosed in the solid bony cranium, is well protected but highly vulnerable to pressure that may accumulate within the enclosure. The cranium's total volume—brain (80%), cerebrospinal fluid (CSF) (10%), and blood (10%)—must remain approximately the same at all times. A change in the proportional volume of one of these components (e.g., an increase or decrease in intracranial blood) must be accompanied by a compensatory change in another. In this way, the volume and pressure normally remain constant. Examples of compensatory changes are reduction in blood volume, decrease in CSF production, increase in CSF absorption, or shrinkage of brain mass by displacement of **intracellular fluid** and **extracellular fluid**. Children with open fontanels compensate by skull expansion and widened sutures. However, at any age the capacity for spatial compensation is limited. An increase in ICP may be caused by tumours or other space-occupying lesions, accumulation of fluid within the ventricular system, bleeding, or **edema** of cerebral tissues. Once compensation is exhausted, any further increase in volume will result in a rapid rise in ICP.

Early signs and symptoms of increased ICP are often subtle and assume many patterns (Box 51-1). As pressure increases, signs and symptoms become more pronounced and the level of consciousness (LOC) deteriorates.

BOX 51-1 Clinical Manifestations of Increased Intracranial Pressure in Infants and Children

Infants

Tense, bulging fontanel
Separated cranial sutures
Macewen sign (cracked-pot sound on percussion)
Irritability and restlessness
Drowsiness, increased sleeping
High-pitched cry
Increased fronto-occipital circumference
Distended scalp veins
Poor feeding
Crying when disturbed
Setting-sun sign

Children

Headache
Nausea
Vomiting
Diplopia, blurred vision
Seizures
Indifference, drowsiness
Decline in school performance
Diminished physical activity and motor performance
Increased sleeping
Inability to follow simple commands
Lethargy

Late Signs in Infants and Children

Bradycardia
Decreased motor response to commands
Decreased sensory response to painful stimuli
Alterations in pupil size and reactivity
Flexion or extension posturing
Cheyne-Stokes respirations
Papilledema
Decreased consciousness
Coma

Altered States of Consciousness

Consciousness implies awareness—the ability to respond to sensory stimuli and have subjective experiences. Consciousness has two components: *alertness*, an arousal-waking state, including the ability to respond to stimuli; and *cognitive power*, which includes the ability to process stimuli and produce verbal and motor responses.

An *altered state of consciousness* usually refers to varying states of unconsciousness that may be momentary or may extend for hours, for days, or indefinitely. *Unconsciousness* is depressed cerebral function—the inability to respond to sensory stimuli and have subjective experiences. *Coma* is defined as a state of unconsciousness from which the patient cannot be roused even with powerful stimuli.

evolve Animation—Brain Lobes

Levels of Consciousness

Assessment of LOC remains the earliest indicator of improvement or deterioration in neurological status. LOC is determined by observations of the child's responses to the environment. Other diagnostic tests, such as motor activity, reflexes, and vital signs, are more variable and do not necessarily directly parallel the depth of the comatose state. The most consistently used terms are described in Box 51-2.

Coma Assessment

Several scales have been devised in an attempt to standardize the description and interpretation of the degree of depressed

BOX 51-2 Levels of Consciousness

Full consciousness—Awake and alert; oriented to person, place, and time; behaviour appropriate for age
Confusion—Impaired decision making
Disorientation—Disorientation to time and place, decreased level of consciousness
Lethargy—Limited spontaneous movement, sluggish speech, drowsiness
Obtundation—Arousable with stimulation
Stupor—Remaining in a deep sleep, responsive only to vigorous and repeated stimulation
Coma—No motor or verbal response to noxious (painful) stimuli
Persistent vegetative state (PVS)—The permanently lost function of the cerebral cortex; eyes following objects only by reflex or when attracted to the direction of loud sounds, all four limbs spastic but can withdraw from painful stimuli, hands showing reflexive grasping and groping, face grimacing, some food may be swallowed, groaning or crying but without uttering any words

(Modified from Seidel, H. M., et al. [Eds.]. [2006]. *Mosby's guide to physical examination* [6th ed.]. St. Louis: Mosby.)

NEUROLOGIC ASSESSMENT

Pupils	Right	Size	
		Reaction	
	Left	Size	
		Reaction	

++ = Brisk
\+ = Sluggish
− = No reaction
C = Eye closed by swelling

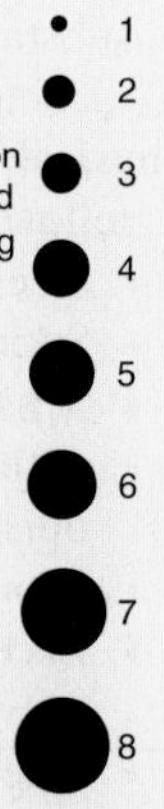

GLASGOW COMA SCALE

Eyes open	Spontaneously	4	
	To speech	3	
	To pain	2	
	None	1	
Best motor response	Obeys commands	6	Usually record best arm or age-appropriate response
	Localizes pain	5	
	Flexion withdrawal	4	
	Flexion abnormal	3	
	Extension	2	
	None	1	

	≥2 years		<2 years
Best response to auditory and/or visual stimulus	Orientation	5	5 Smiles, listens, follows
	Confused	4	4 Cries, consolable
	Inappropriate words	3	3 Inappropriate persistent cry
	Incomprehensible words	2	2 Agitated, restless
	None	1	1 No response
	Endotracheal tube or trach	T	
COMA SCALE TOTAL			

HAND GRIP
Equal
Unequal
R_____L
Weakness

LOC
Alert/oriented × 4
Sleepy
Irritable
Comatose
Disoriented
Combative
Lethargic
Awake
Sleeping
Drowsy
Agitated

MUSCLE TONE
Normal
Arching
Spastic
Flaccid
Weak
Decorticate
Decerebrate
Other _________

EYE MOVEMENT
Normal
Nystagmus
Strabismus
Other _________

FONTANEL/ WINDOW
Soft
Flat
Sunken
Tense
Bulging
Closed
Other _________

MOOD/AFFECT
Happy
Content
Quiet
Withdrawn
Sad
Flat
Hostile

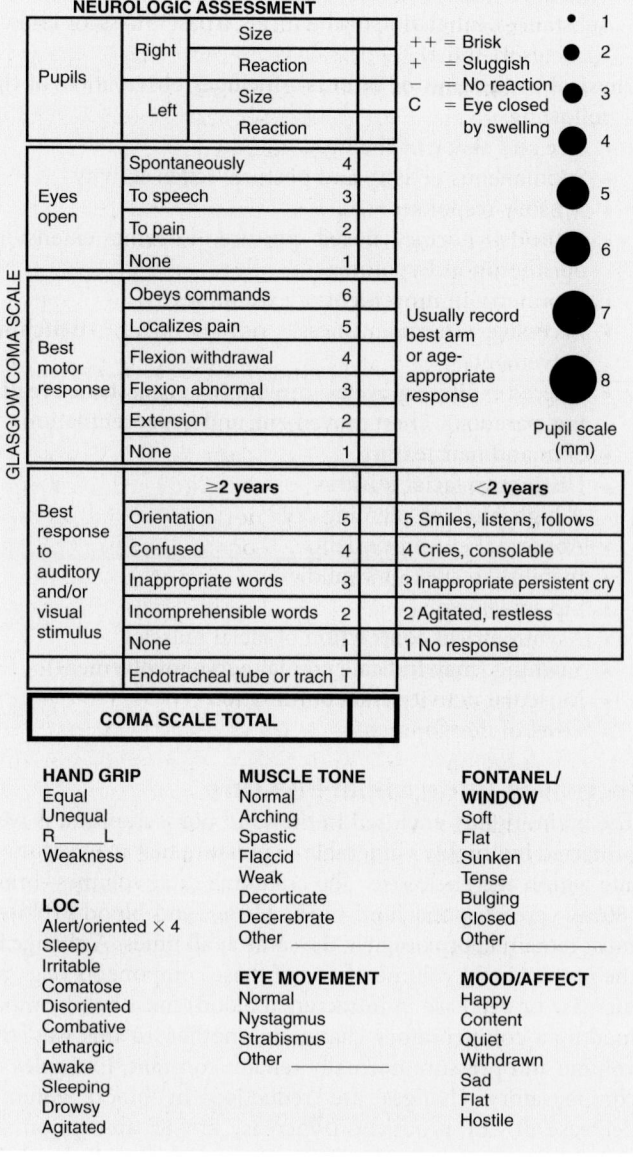

Fig. 51-1 Pediatric coma scale.

consciousness. The most popular of these is the Glasgow Coma Scale (GCS), which consists of a three-part assessment: eye opening, verbal response, and motor response (Fig. 51-1). When LOC is being assessed in young children, it is often useful to have a parent present to help elicit a desired response. An infant or child may not respond in an unfamiliar environment or to unfamiliar voices. Children older than 3 years of age should be able to give their name, although they may not be cognizant of place or time.

Numeric values of 1 through 5 are assigned to the levels of response in each category. The sum of these numeric values provides an objective measure of the patient's LOC. The lower the score, the deeper the coma. A person with an unaltered LOC would score the highest, 15; a score of 8 or below is generally accepted as a definition of coma; the lowest score, 3, indicates deep coma. The legal definition of brain death is according to accepted medical practice in all of the provinces and territories and is largely determined by and varies with individual hospitals or regions. The Canadian Neurocritical Care Group developed guidelines for the diagnosis of brain death in 1999 to establish consistent physical examination criteria for cases of irreversible coma. In 2003, a national forum of Canadian experts made further recommendations to these guidelines (Shemie et al., 2006).

NURSING ALERT Lack of response to painful stimuli is abnormal and should be reported immediately.

Neurological Examination

The purpose of the neurological examination is to establish an accurate, objective baseline of neurological information. It is essential that the neurological examination be documented in a fashion that is able to be reproduced by others. This allows for a comparison of the findings so the observer can detect subtle changes in the neurological status that might not otherwise be evident. Descriptions of behaviours should be simple, objective, and easily interpreted: "Drowsy but awake and conversationally rational/oriented"; "Sleepy but arousable with vigorous physical stimuli. Pressure to nail base of right hand results in upper extremity flexion/lower extremity extension."

Vital Signs

Pulse, respiration, and blood pressure provide information regarding the adequacy of circulation and the possible underlying cause of altered consciousness. Autonomic activity is most intensively disturbed in cases of deep coma or brainstem lesions.

Body temperature is often elevated, and sometimes the elevation may be extreme. High temperature is most frequently a sign of an acute infectious process or heat stroke but may be caused by ingestion of some medications (especially salicylates, alcohol, and barbiturates) or by intracranial bleeding, especially subarachnoid hemorrhage. Hypothalamic involvement may cause elevated or decreased temperature. Coma of a toxic origin may produce **hypothermia**.

The pulse is variable and may be rapid, slow and bounding, or feeble. Blood pressure may be normal, elevated, or at shock levels. **Cushing's response,** or pressor response, which causes a slowing of the pulse and an increase in blood pressure, is uncommon in children; when it occurs, it is a very late sign of ICP. Vital signs are also affected by medications. For assessment purposes, actual changes in pulse and blood pressure are more important than the direction of the change.

Respirations are often slow, deep, and irregular. Slow, deep breathing is often seen in the heavy sleep caused by sedatives, after seizures, or in cerebral infections. Slow, shallow breathing may result from sedatives or **opioids** (narcotics). Hyperventilation (deep and rapid respirations) is usually a result of metabolic acidosis or abnormal stimulation of the respiratory centre in the medulla caused by salicylate poisoning, hepatic coma, or Reye's syndrome (RS).

Breathing patterns have been described with a number of terms (e.g., *apneustic, cluster, ataxic, Cheyne-Stokes*). However, it is better to describe what is being observed rather than placing a label on it because the traditional terms are often used and interpreted incorrectly. Periodic or irregular breathing is an ominous sign of brainstem (especially medullary) dysfunction that often precedes complete apnea. The odour of the breath may provide additional clues (e.g., the fruity, acetone odour of **ketosis**; the foul odour of uremia; the fetid odour of hepatic failure; or the odour of alcohol).

Skin

The skin may offer clues to the cause of unconsciousness. The body surface should be examined for signs of injury, needle marks, petechiae, bites, and ticks. Evidence of toxic substances may be found on the hands, face, mouth, and clothing—especially in small children.

Eyes

Pupil size and reactivity are assessed (Fig. 51-2; see also Fig. 51-1). Pinpoint pupils are commonly observed in poisoning, such as opiate or barbiturate poisoning, or in brainstem dysfunction. Widely dilated and reactive pupils are often seen after seizures and may involve only one side. Dilated pupils may also be caused by eye trauma. Widely dilated and fixed pupils suggest paralysis of cranial nerve III secondary to pressure from herniation of the brain through the tentorium. A unilateral fixed pupil usually suggests a lesion on the same side. If pupils are fixed bilaterally for more than 5 minutes, brainstem damage is usually implied. Dilated and nonreactive pupils are also seen in hypothermia, **anoxia**, ischemia, poisoning with atropine-like substances, or prior instillation of mydriatic medications.

NURSING ALERT The sudden appearance of a fixed and dilated pupil(s) is a neurosurgical emergency.

The description of eye movements should indicate whether one or both eyes are involved and how the reaction was elicited. The parents should be asked about pre-existing **strabismus**, which will cause the eyes to appear normal under compromise. Post-traumatic strabismus indicates cranial nerve VI damage.

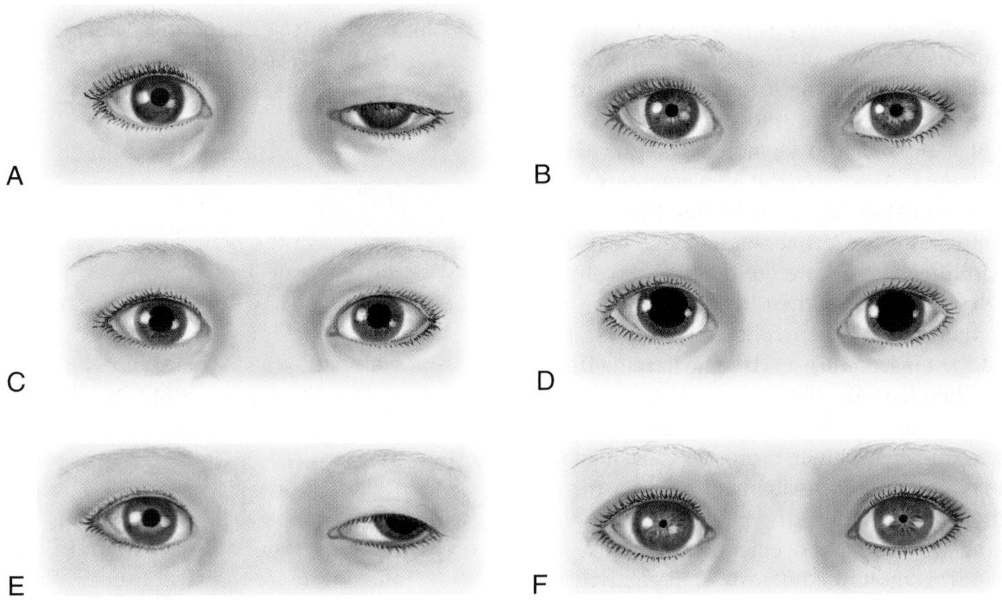

Fig. 51-2 Variations in pupil size with altered states of consciousness. **A:** Ipsilateral pupillary constriction with slight ptosis. **B:** Bilateral small pupils. **C:** Midposition, light fixed to all stimuli. **D:** Bilateral dilated and fixed pupils. **E:** Dilated pupils, left eye abducted with ptosis. **F:** Pinpoint pupils.

Special tests, usually performed by qualified persons, include the following:

Doll's head manoeuvre—Elicited by rotating the child's head quickly to one side and then to the other. Conjugate (paired, or working together) movement of the eyes in the direction opposite to the head rotation is normal. Absence of this response suggests dysfunction of the brainstem or oculomotor nerve (cranial nerve III).

NURSING ALERT Any tests that require head movement should not be attempted until after cervical spine injury has been ruled out.

Caloric test, or oculovestibular response—Elicited with the child's head up (head of bed is elevated 30 degrees) by irrigating the external auditory canal with 10 mL of ice water for 20 seconds, which normally causes conjugate movement of the eyes toward the side of stimulation. This movement is lost when the pontine centres are impaired, thus providing important information in assessment of the comatose patient.

NURSING ALERT The caloric test is painful and is never performed on a child who is awake or on an individual with a ruptured tympanic membrane.

Funduscopic examination—Reveals additional clues. **Papilledema** will not be evident early in the course of unconsciousness because it takes 24 to 48 hours to develop, if it develops at all. Papilledema is characterized by optic disc swelling, indistinct optic disc margins, hemorrhage, tortuosity of vessels, and absence of venous pulsations. The presence of preretinal (subhyaloid) hemorrhages in children is almost invariably a result of acute trauma with intracranial bleeding, usually subarachnoid or subdural hemorrhage.

Motor Function

Observing spontaneous activity, posture, and response to painful stimuli provides clues to the location and extent of cerebral dysfunction. Even subtle movements (e.g., the outward rotation of a hip) should be noted and the child observed for other signs. Asymmetrical movements of the limbs or absence of movement suggests paralysis. In hemiplegia the affected limb lies in external rotation and will fall uncontrollably when lifted and allowed to drop. These observations should be described rather than labelled.

In the deeper comatose states there is little or no spontaneous movement, and the musculature tends to be flaccid. There is considerable variability in the motor behaviour in lesser degrees of coma. For example, the child may be relatively immobile or restless and hyperkinetic; muscle tone may be increased or decreased. Tremors, twitching, and spasms of muscles are common observations. The patient may display purposeless plucking or tossing movements. Combative or negativistic behaviour is not uncommon. Hyperactivity is more common in acute febrile and toxic states than in cases of increased ICP. Seizures are common in children and may be present in coma from any cause. Any repetitive or seizure movements should be described.

Posturing

Primitive postural reflexes emerge as cortical control over motor function is lost in brain dysfunction. These reflexes are evident in posturing and motor movements directly related to the area of the brain involved. Posturing reflects a balance between the lower exciting and the higher inhibiting influences, and strong muscles overcome weaker ones. **Flexion posturing** (Fig. 51-3, A) is seen with severe dysfunction of the **cerebral cortex** or with lesions to corticospinal tracts above the brainstem. Typical flexion posturing includes rigid flexion, with arms held tightly to the body; flexed elbows, wrists, and fingers; plantar flexed feet; legs extended and internally rotated; and possibly fine tremors or intense stiffness. **Extension posturing** (see Fig. 51-3, B) is a sign of dysfunction at the level of the midbrain or lesions to the brainstem. It is characterized by rigid extension and pronation of the arms and legs, flexed wrists and fingers, clenched jaw, extended neck, and possibly an arched back. Unilateral extension posturing is often caused by tentorial herniation.

Posturing may not be evident when the child is quiet but can usually be elicited by applying painful stimuli, such as a blunt object pressed on the base of the nail. Nurses should avoid applying thumb pressure to the supraorbital region of the frontal bone (risk of orbital damage). Noxious stimuli (e.g., suctioning) will elicit a response, as may turning or touching. When the nurse is describing posturing, the stimulus needed to provoke the response is as important as the reaction.

Reflexes

Testing of some reflexes may be of limited value. In general, the corneal, pupillary, muscle-stretch, superficial, and plantar reflexes tend to be absent in deep coma. The state of reflexes is variable in lighter grades of unconsciousness and depends on the underlying pathological process and the location of the lesion. Absence of corneal reflexes and presence of a tonic neck reflex are associated with severe brain damage. The Babinski reflex (see Extremities, Chapter 34) may be of value

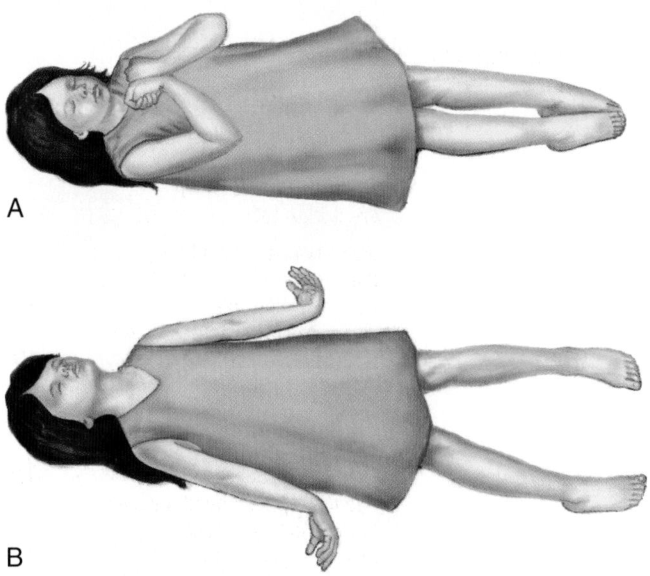

Fig. 51-3 **A:** Flexion posturing. **B:** Extension posturing.

if it is found to be present consistently in children older than 18 months. A positive Babinski reflex is significant in assessment of **pyramidal tract** lesions when it is unilateral and associated with other pyramidal signs.

NURSING ALERT Three key reflexes that demonstrate neurological health in young infants are the Moro, tonic neck, and withdrawal reflexes.

Special Diagnostic Procedures

Numerous diagnostic procedures are used for assessment of cerebral function. Laboratory tests that may help delineate the cause of unconsciousness include blood glucose, urea nitrogen, and electrolyte (pH, sodium, potassium, chloride, calcium, and bicarbonate) tests; clotting studies, hematocrit, and a complete blood count; liver function tests; blood cultures if there is fever; and sometimes studies to detect lead or other toxic substances, such as drugs.

An electroencephalogram (EEG) may provide important information. For example, generalized random, slow activity suggests suppressed cortical function, and localized slow activity suggests a space-occupying lesion. A flat tracing is one of the criteria used as evidence of brain death.

Examination of spinal fluid is carried out when toxic encephalopathy or infection is suspected. Lumbar puncture is ordinarily delayed if intracranial hemorrhage is suspected and is contraindicated in the presence of ICP because of the potential for tentorial herniation.

Auditory and visual evoked potentials are sometimes used in neurological evaluation of very young children. Brainstem auditory evoked potentials are useful for evaluating the continuity of brainstem auditory tracts and are particularly useful for detecting demyelinating disease and neoplasms of the brainstem and distinguishing between brainstem and cortical lesions. For example, a normal evoked potential in a comatose patient suggests involvement of the cerebral hemispheres.

Highly sophisticated tests are carried out with specialized equipment. Two imaging techniques, computed tomography (CT) and magnetic resonance imaging (MRI), assist in diagnosis by scanning both soft tissues and solid matter. Most of these tests are outlined in Table 51-1. Because such tests can be threatening to children, the nurse needs to prepare patients

Table 51-1 Neurological Diagnostic Procedures

TEST	DESCRIPTION	PURPOSE	COMMENTS
Lumbar puncture (LP)	Spinal needle is inserted between L3-L4 or L4-L5 vertebral spaces into subarachnoid space; cerebrospinal fluid (CSF) pressure is measured, and a sample is collected for examination.	*Diagnostic*—Measures spinal fluid pressure, obtains CSF for laboratory analysis *Therapeutic*—Injection of medication	Contraindicated in patients with increased intracranial pressure (ICP) or infected skin over puncture site
Subdural tap	Needle is inserted into anterior fontanel or coronal suture (midline to pupil).	Helps rule out subdural effusions Removes CSF to relieve pressure	Place infant in semi-erect position after subdural tap to minimize leakage from site; prevent child from crying if possible Check site frequently for evidence of leakage
Ventricular puncture	Needle is inserted into lateral ventricle via coronal suture (midline to pupil).	Removes CSF to relieve pressure	Risk of intracerebral or ventricular hemorrhage
Electroencephalography (EEG)	EEG records changes in electrical potential of brain. Electrodes are placed at various points to assess electrical function in a particular area. Impulses are recorded by electromagnetic pen or digitally.	Detects spikes, or bursts of electrical activity that indicate the potential for seizures Used to determine brain death	Patient should remain quiet during procedure; may require sedation Minimize external stimuli during procedure
Nuclear brain scan	Radioisotope is injected intravenously, then counted and recorded after fixed time intervals. Radioisotope accumulates in areas where blood-brain barrier is defective.	Identifies focal brain lesions (e.g., tumours, abscesses) Positive uptake of material with encephalitis and subdural hematoma Visualizes CSF pathways	Requires intravenous (IV) access; patient may require sedation In normal children or noncommunicating hydrocephalus, no retrograde filling of ventricles occurs Areas of concentrated uptake of material are termed hot spots
Endocephalography	Pulses of ultrasonic waves are beamed through head; echoes from reflecting surfaces are recorded graphically.	Identifies shifts in midline structures from their normal positions as a result of intracranial lesions May show ventricular dilation	Simple, safe, rapid procedure Fontanel must be patent

Continued

Table 51-1 Neurological Diagnostic Procedures—cont'd

TEST	DESCRIPTION	PURPOSE	COMMENTS
Real-time ultrasonography (RTUS)	RTUS is similar to CT but uses ultrasound instead of ionizing radiation.	Allows high-resolution anatomical visualization in variety of imaging planes	Produces images similar to CT scan Especially useful in neonatal central nervous system problems Anterior fontanel must be patent
Radiography	Skull films are taken from different views—lateral, posterolateral, axial (submentoventricular), half-axial.	Shows fractures, dislocations, spreading suture lines, craniosynostosis Shows degenerative changes, bone erosion, calcifications	Simple, noninvasive procedure
Computed tomography (CT) scan	Pinpoint x-ray beam is directed on horizontal or vertical plane to provide series of images that are fed into computer and assembled in image displayed on video screen. CT uses ionizing radiation.	Visualizes horizontal and vertical cross section of brain in three planes (axial, coronal, sagittal) Distinguishes density of various intracranial tissues and structures—congenital abnormalities, hemorrhage, tumours, demyelinating and inflammatory processes, calcification	Requires IV access if contrast agent is used Patient may require sedation Rapid
Magnetic resonance imaging (MRI)	MRI produces radiofrequency emissions from elements (e.g., hydrogen, phosphorus), which are converted to visual images by computer.	Permits visualization of morphological feature of target structures Permits tissue discrimination unavailable with many techniques	MRI is a noninvasive procedure except when IV contrast agent is used No exposure to radiation occurs Patient may require sedation Parent or attendant can remain in room with child MRI does not visualize bone detail or calcifications No metal can be present in scanner
Positron emission tomography (PET)	PET involves IV injection of positron-emitting radionucleotide; local concentrations are detected and transformed into visual display by computer.	Detects and measures blood volume and flow in brain, metabolic activity, biochemical changes within tissue	Requires lengthy period of immobility Minimum exposure to radiation occurs Patient may require sedation
Digital subtraction angiography (DSA)	Contrast dye is injected intravenously; computer "subtracts" all tissues without contrast medium, leaving clear image of contrast medium in vessels studied.	Visualizes vasculature of target tissue Visualizes finite vascular abnormalities	Safe alternative to angiography Patient must remain still during procedure; may require sedation
Single-photon emission computed tomography (SPECT)	SPECT involves IV injection of photon-emitting radionuclide; radionuclides are absorbed by healthy tissue at different rate than by diseased or necrotic tissue; data are transferred to computer, which converts image to film.	Provides information regarding blood flow to tissues; analyzing blood flow to organ may help determine how well it is functioning	Requires lengthy period of immobility Minimum exposure to radiation occurs Patient may require sedation

for the tests and provide support and reassurance during the tests (see Preparation for Diagnostic and Therapeutic Procedures, Chapter 45). Children who are old enough to understand require careful explanation of the procedure, why it is being done, what they will experience, and how they can help. School-age children usually appreciate a more detailed description of why contrast material is injected. The importance of lying still for tests, particularly CT, needs to be stressed. Children unfamiliar with the machines can be shown a picture beforehand. Although radiographic examinations are not painful, the machinery is often so frightening in appearance that the child protests because of anxiety.

This is especially true of CT and MRI, both of which require that the child's head be placed within a special immobilizing device. Chin and cheek pads are sometimes used to prevent the slightest head movement, and straps are applied to the body to prevent a slight change in body position. The nurse can explain these events to a frightened child by comparing them to an astronaut's preparation for a space flight. It is important to emphasize to the child that at no time is the procedure painful.

Physical preparation for the diagnostic test may involve administration of a sedative. Many different agents are used for sedation of children undergoing neurological diagnostic procedures. Chloral hydrate or benzodiazepines have been used for decades as short-term sedative agents and remain safe methods of pediatric outpatient sedation (Wetzell, 2007). Chloral hydrate is used alone for sedating children for procedures such as MRI. In recent years other sedative agents have been used safely, alone and in combination, for children in the outpatient setting. These include intravenous (IV) sodium pentobarbital (Nembutal), IV fentanyl (Sublimaze), IV midazolam (Versed) (Wetzell, 2007), and intranasal midazolam (Ljungman et al., 2000; Lloyd, Alredy, & Lloyd, 2000) (see Pain Management, Chapter 35).

Children scheduled to undergo sedation should be helped through the preparation and administration and be assured that someone will remain with them (if possible). Children need continual support and reinforcement during procedures in which they remain conscious. Vital signs and physiological responses to the procedure should be monitored throughout. Many diagnostic procedures performed on an outpatient basis require sedation, and children need recovery time and observation. The nurse should review written instructions with the parents if the child is to be discharged right after a procedure. Children who have undergone a procedure with a general anaesthetic require postanaesthesia care, including positioning to prevent aspiration of secretions and frequent assessment of vital signs and LOC. In addition, other neurological functions such as pupillary responses, motor strength, and movement are tested at regular intervals. Any surgical wound resulting from the test should be checked for bleeding, CSF leakage, and other complications. Children who undergo repeated subdural taps should have their hematocrit level monitored to detect excessive blood loss from the procedure.

Adverse events related to sedation need to be reported. There are differences in terminology and how adverse events are reported in Canada. In order to develop pediatric evidence-informed sedation guidelines, a consensus panel was formed to standardize adverse-event reporting across Canada (Bhatt et al., 2009).

Nursing Care of the Unconscious Child

The unconscious child requires nursing attendance, with observation, recording, and evaluation of changes in objective signs. These observations provide valuable information regarding the patient's progress. Often they serve as a guide to diagnosis and treatment. Careful and detailed observations are essential for the patient's welfare. In addition, vital functions must be maintained and complications prevented through conscientious and meticulous nursing care. The outcome of unconsciousness may be early and complete recovery, death within a few hours or days, persistent and permanent unconsciousness, or recovery with varying degrees of residual mental or physical disability. The outcome and recovery of the unconscious child may depend on the level of nursing care and observational skills.

Emergency measures are directed toward ensuring a patent airway, treatment of shock, and reduction of ICP (if it is increased). Delayed treatment often leads to increased damage. As soon as emergency measures have been implemented—and in many cases concurrently—therapies for specific causes are begun. Because nursing care is closely related to medical management, both are considered here.

Continual observation of LOC, pupillary reaction, and vital signs is essential to manage CNS disorders. Regular assessment of neurological signs is a vital part of nursing comatose children. Vital signs need to be measured and recorded regularly. The frequency depends on the cause of coma, the status, and the progression of cerebral involvement. Intervals may be as short as every 15 minutes or as long as every 2 hours. Significant alterations should be reported immediately. Temperature is taken every 2 to 4 hours, depending on the patient's condition.

An elevated temperature may occur in children with CNS dysfunction; thus a light covering is sufficient. Vigorous efforts, such as tepid sponge baths or application of a hypothermia blanket, are needed to prevent brain damage if temperature exceeds 40°C rectally.

The LOC should be assessed periodically, including size, equality, and reaction of pupils to light. Signs of meningeal irritation such as nuchal rigidity are also assessed. Other aspects of LOC assessment include response to vocal commands, spontaneous behaviour, resistance to care, and response to painful stimuli. Motions of any type, changes in muscle tone or strength, and body position should be noted. Seizure activity should be described according to the type and length of seizure and body areas involved. An anti-epileptic medication such as phenytoin (Dilantin) or phenobarbital can be ordered for control of seizure activity.

Pain management for the comatose child requires astute nursing observation and management. Signs of pain include changes in behaviour (e.g., increased agitation and rigidity, alterations in physiological parameters); increased heart rate, respiratory rate, and blood pressure; and decreased oxygen saturation. Since these findings are not specific for pain, the nurse should observe for their appearance during times of induced or suspected pain and their disappearance after the end of the inciting procedure or the administration of analgesia. A pain assessment record should be used to document indications of pain and the effectiveness of interventions (see Pain Assessment, Chapter 35).

The use of opioids, such as morphine, to relieve pain is controversial because they may mask signs of altered consciousness or depress respirations. However, unrelieved pain activates the stress response, which can elevate ICP. To block the stress response, some authorities advocate the use of **analgesics**, sedatives, and, in some cases such as head injury, paralyzing agents via continuous IV infusion. A frequently used combination is fentanyl, midazolam, and vecuronium (Norcuron). If there are concerns about assessing the LOC or respiratory depression, naloxone (Narcan) can be used to reverse the opioid effects. Acetaminophen (Tylenol) and codeine may also be effective analgesics for mild to moderate pain. Regardless of which medications are used, adequate dosage and regular administration are essential to provide optimal pain relief (see Pain Management, Chapter 35).

Other measures to relieve discomfort include providing a quiet, dimly lit environments; limiting visitors; preventing any sudden, jarring movements, such as banging into the bed; and preventing an increase in ICP. The last is most effectively achieved by proper positioning and prevention of straining, such as during coughing, vomiting, or defecating.

NURSING ALERT When opioids are used, bowel elimination must be closely monitored because of the potential constipating effect. Stool softeners should be given with laxatives as needed to prevent constipation.

Respiratory Management

Respiratory effectiveness is the primary concern in the care of the unconscious child, and establishment of an adequate airway is always the first priority. Carbon dioxide has a potent vasodilating effect and will increase cerebral blood flow (CBF) and ICP. Cerebral hypoxia that lasts longer than 4 minutes nearly always causes irreversible brain damage.

NURSING ALERT Respiratory obstruction and subsequent compromise lead to cardiac arrest. Maintaining an adequate, patent airway is of the utmost importance.

Children in lighter states of coma may be able to cough and swallow, but those in deeper states are unable to handle secretions, which tend to pool in the throat and pharynx. Dysfunction of cranial nerves IX and X places the child at risk for aspiration and cardiac arrest; the child needs to be positioned to prevent aspiration of secretions and the stomach emptied to reduce the likelihood of vomiting. In infants, blockage of air passages from secretions can happen in seconds. In addition, upper airway obstruction from laryngospasm is a frequent complication in comatose children.

An oral airway can be used for the child who is suffering a temporary loss of consciousness, such as after a contusion, seizure, or anaesthesia. For children who remain unconscious for a longer time, a nasotracheal or orotracheal tube is inserted to maintain the open airway and facilitate removal of secretions. A tracheostomy is performed in cases in which laryngoscopy for introduction of an endotracheal tube would be difficult or dangerous. Suctioning is used only as needed to clear the airway, exerting care to prevent increasing ICP. Respiratory status is observed and evaluated regularly. Signs of respiratory embarrassment may be an indication for ventilatory assistance.

When the respiratory centre is involved, mechanical ventilation is usually indicated (see Chapter 46). Blood gas analysis is performed regularly, and oxygen is administered when indicated. Moderately severe hypoxia and respiratory acidosis are often present but are not always evident from clinical manifestations. Hyperventilation frequently accompanies unconsciousness and may lead to respiratory alkalosis, or it may represent the body's attempt to compensate for metabolic acidosis. Thus blood gas and pH determinations are essential guides for electrolyte therapy. Chest physiotherapy is carried out on a regular basis, and the child's position is changed at least every 2 hours to prevent pulmonary complications.

Intracranial Pressure Monitoring

Management of the child with increased ICP is possibly the most formidable task and the most controversial subject in pediatric critical care. It appears that the outcome in pediatric neurological injury may reflect the initial cerebral damage more than the subsequent intracranial hypertension. ICP gives little indication of the severity of the initial insult (Bayir, Kochanek, & Clark, 2003). The Cochrane Group has reviewed research on traumatic encephalopathy and concluded that early detection of raised ICP would improve cerebral perfusion and reduce brain injury. As yet, no studies can provide this evidence, and more research is needed (Forsyth, Wolny, & Rodrigues, 2010). When increased ICP is a result of accumulation of CSF from obstruction of CSF flow, a ventricular tap will provide relief quickly and effectively. Evacuation of a hematoma reduces pressure from this source. Indications for inserting an ICP monitor are as follows:

- GCS evaluation of 8
- GCS evaluation of less than 8 with respiratory assistance
- Deterioration of condition
- Subjective judgement regarding clinical appearance and response (Bhalla, Dewhirst, Sawardekar, Dairo, & Tobias, 2012).

Four major types of ICP monitors are as follows:

1. Intraventricular catheter with fibroscopic sensors attached to a monitoring system
2. Subarachnoid bolt (Richmond screw)
3. Epidural sensor
4. Anterior fontanel pressure monitor

Transducers for both ventricular and subarachnoid monitoring should be set up without the use of a flush device. Direct ventricular pressure measurement remains the gold standard of ICP monitoring.

The catheter method involves introduction of a catheter into the lateral ventricle on the nondominant side, if known, or placement in the subdural space. The catheter has the advantage of providing a means of extraventricular (or continuous) drainage to reduce pressure. A drainage bag attached to the system is kept at the level of the ventricles and can be lowered to decrease ICP (see Critical Thinking Exercise).

NURSING ALERT If the external ventricular drain (EVD) is unclamped for CSF drainage, carefully monitor the level of the collection container. If the container is too low, improper CSF decompression could lower ICP too rapidly, causing bleeding and pain.

With the bolt method, the end of the bolt is placed into the subarachnoid space. The bolt cannot be adequately secured in a small child's pliant skull, although special modifications have been developed for children younger than 6 years of age.

NURSING ALERT The bolt is stabilized with dressings, but these are not changed or disturbed, even to check the site.

The placement of the bolt is not adjusted by anyone except the neurosurgeon who placed the device. The neurosurgeon should be notified if a satisfactory waveform is not observed.

An epidural sensor can be placed between the dura and the skull through a burr hole and connected to a stopcock assembly and a transducer, which provides a readout of the pressure. Correlation of pressure readings is less invasive but may be inconsistent. In infants a fontanel transducer can be used to detect impulses from a pressure sensor and convert them to electrical energy. The electrical energy is then converted to

CRITICAL THINKING EXERCISE

Hydrocephalus

Three-year-old Emma is 5 days postoperative for removal of a posterior fossa tumour. Although an external ventricular drain (EVD) was placed to treat her hydrocephalus, she continues to demonstrate signs of increased intracranial pressure (ICP), including holding the back of her head, anorexia, crying when moved or when strangers enter the room, and intermittent lethargy. On examination, fluid drainage is noted on the mother's clothes, and Emma is experiencing repetitive, rapid eyelid blinking.

1. Evidence—Is there sufficient evidence to draw conclusions about Emma's behaviour, physical assessment findings, and ICP?
2. Assumptions—Describe any underlying assumptions about each of the following:
   a. A preschool-age child who had a posterior fossa tumour removed 5 days ago
   b. A preschool-age child who has an EVD placed to treat the hydrocephalus
   c. A preschool-age child with an EVD who continues to demonstrate physical signs associated with increased ICP after recent surgery
3. What priorities for nursing care should be established?
4. Does the evidence support your nursing intervention?
5. What alternative perspectives might you have?

visible waves or numeric readings on an oscilloscope. ICP measurement from the anterior fontanel is noninvasive but may prove to be inaccurate if the equipment is poorly placed or inconsistently recalibrated. The intraparenchymal pressure monitoring device (e.g., Camino) is a result of fibre-optic technology and performs reliably.

ICP can be increased by instillation of solutions; thus antibiotics are administered systemically if a positive CSF culture is obtained. However, IV ICP monitoring rarely causes infection. Since CSF is a body fluid, routine practices need to be implemented, according to hospital policy (see Infection Control, Chapter 45).

Nurses caring for patients with intracranial monitoring devices must be acquainted with the system, assist with insertion, interpret the monitor readings, and be able to distinguish between danger signals and mechanical dysfunction.

For increased ICP resulting from cerebral edema, several medical measures are available. Osmotic diuretics may provide rapid relief in emergency situations. Although their effect is transient, lasting only about 6 hours, they can be lifesaving in emergencies. These substances are rapidly excreted by the kidneys and carry with them large quantities of sodium and water. Mannitol (or sometimes urea) administered intravenously is the medication most frequently used for rapid reduction. The infusion is generally given slowly but may be pushed rapidly in cases of herniation or impending **cerebral herniation.** Because of the profound diuretic effect of the drug, an indwelling catheter is inserted to ensure bladder emptying. Adrenocorticosteroids are not recommended for cerebral edema secondary to head trauma. $Paco_2$ should be maintained at 25 to 30 mm Hg to produce vasoconstriction, which reduces CSF, thereby decreasing ICP.

Nursing Activities

In cases of high levels of increased ICP, nursing procedures tend to trigger reactive pressure waves in many patients. For example, increased intrathoracic or abdominal pressure will be transmitted to the cranium. Particular care should be taken in positioning these patients to avoid neck vein compression, which may further increase ICP by interfering with venous return.

The child can be propped to one side or the other, and the use of an alternating-pressure mattress reduces the chance of prolonged pressure to vulnerable areas. Frequent clinical assessment of the child cannot be replaced by an ICP monitoring device.

NURSING ALERT The head of the bed is elevated to 15 to 30 degrees, and the child is positioned so that the head is maintained in midline to facilitate venous drainage and avoid jugular compression (Bhalla et al., 2012). Turning side to side is contraindicated because of the risk of jugular compression.

It is important to avoid activities that may increase ICP by causing pain or emotional stress. Gentle range-of-motion exercises can be carried out but should not be performed vigorously. Nontherapeutic touch can cause an increase in ICP. Any disturbing procedures to be performed should be scheduled to take advantage of therapies that reduce ICP, such as osmotherapy and sedation. Environmental noise should be minimized or eliminated to the degree possible. Assessment and intervention to relieve pain are important nursing functions to decrease ICP. Individualizing nursing activities and minimizing environmental stimuli by decreasing noxious procedures can help control ICP (El Bashir, Laundy, & Booy, 2003).

Suctioning and percussion are poorly tolerated and are contraindicated unless concurrent respiratory problems exist. **Hypoxia** and the Valsalva manoeuvre associated with cough both acutely elevate ICP. Vibration, which does not increase ICP, accomplishes excellent results and should be tried first if treatment is needed. If suctioning is necessary, it should be brief and preceded by hyperventilation with 100% oxygen, which can be monitored during suctioning with a pulse oxygen sensor reading to determine oxygen saturation.

Nutrition and Hydration

Fluids and calories are supplied initially via the IV route (see Chapter 45). An IV infusion is started early, and the type of fluid administered is determined by the patient's general condition. Fluid therapy requires careful monitoring and adjustment based on neurological signs and electrolyte determinations. Often, comatose children are unable to cope with the same amounts of fluid they could tolerate at other times, and overhydration must be avoided to prevent fatal cerebral edema.

Hydration is maintained in the same manner (initially by IV and later by feeding tube). When cerebral edema is a threat, fluids may be restricted to reduce the chance of fluid overload. Skin and mucous membranes need to be examined for signs of dehydration. Observation for signs of altered fluid balance related to abnormal pituitary secretions is a part of nursing care.

Altered Pituitary Secretion

An altered ability to handle fluid loads is attributed in part to the syndrome of inappropriate antidiuretic hormone secretion (SIADH) and diabetes insipidus (DI) resulting from hypothalamic dysfunction (see Chapter 52). SIADH frequently accompanies CNS diseases such as head injury, meningitis, encephalitis, brain abscess, brain tumour, and subarachnoid hemorrhage. In the patient with SIADH, scant quantities of urine are excreted, electrolyte analysis reveals hyponatremia and hyposmolality, and manifestations of overhydration are evident. It is important to evaluate all parameters, since the reduced urine output might be erroneously interpreted as a sign of dehydration.

The treatment of SIADH consists of restriction of fluids until serum electrolytes and osmolality return to normal levels. Since SIADH frequently occurs with meningitis in children, fluid restriction is often prescribed. Likewise, DI may occur after intracranial trauma. There is increased urine volume and the accompanying danger of dehydration. Adequate replacement of fluids is essential, and observation of electrolyte balance is necessary to detect signs of hypernatremia and hyperosmolality. Exogenous vasopressin may be administered.

Medications

The cause of unconsciousness determines specific medication therapies. Children with infectious processes are given antibiotics appropriate to the disease and the infecting organism, and corticosteroids are prescribed for inflammatory conditions and edema. Cerebral edema is an indication for osmotherapy with osmotic diuretics. Sedatives or anti-epileptics are prescribed for seizure activity (see p. 1597). Sedation in the combative child provides amnesic and anxiolytic properties in conjunction with a paralytic agent. The combination decreases ICP and allows treatment of cerebral edema. Usual medications include morphine, midazolam, and pancuronium (Pavulon). Midazolam is attractive because of its short half-life.

Deep coma, induced by administration of barbiturates, is controversial in the management of ICP. Barbiturates are currently reserved for the reduction of increased ICP when all else has failed. Barbiturates decrease the cerebral metabolic rate for oxygen and protect the brain during times of reduced **cerebral perfusion pressure**. Barbiturate coma requires extensive monitoring, cardiovascular and respiratory support, and ICP monitoring to assess response to therapy. Paralyzing agents such as pancuronium also may be needed to aid in performing diagnostic tests, improving effectiveness of therapy, and reducing risks of secondary complications. Elevation of ICP or heart rate of patients who are being given paralyzing agents or are under sedation may indicate the need for another dose of either or both medications.

Thermoregulation

Hyperthermia often accompanies cerebral dysfunction; if it is present, measures should be implemented to reduce the temperature to prevent brain damage and to reduce metabolic demands generated by the increased body temperature. Medically induced hypothermia assists in controlling ICP and may result in an improved outcome. **Antipyretics** are the method of choice for fever reduction; cooling devices are used to induce hypothermia. Laboratory tests and other methods can be used in an attempt to determine the cause, if any, of the hyperthermia.

Elimination

A retention catheter is usually inserted in the acute phase, although diapers may be used and weighed to record urine output. The child who formerly had bowel and bladder control is generally incontinent. If the child remains comatose for a long period, the indwelling catheter may be removed and periodic bladder emptying accomplished by intermittent catheterization. Stool softeners are usually sufficient to maintain bowel function, but suppositories or enemas may be needed occasionally for adequate elimination and to prevent an impaction. The passage of liquid stool after a period of no bowel activity is usually a sign of an impaction. To avoid this preventable problem, daily recording of bowel activity is essential.

Hygienic Care

Routine measures for cleansing and maintaining skin integrity are an integral part of nursing care of the unconscious child (see Maintaining Healthy Skin, Chapter 45). The child who is unable to move is prone to develop tissue breakdown. To prevent this the child can be placed on an alternating-pressure or water-filled mattress, which alleviates pressure on vulnerable areas.

Mouth care should be performed at least twice daily, since the mouth tends to become dry or coated with mucus. The teeth should be carefully brushed with a soft toothbrush or cleaned with gauze saturated with saline. Commercially prepared cleansing devices, such as Toothettes, are convenient for cleansing the mouth and teeth. Lips can be coated with ointment or other preparations to protect them from drying, cracking, or blistering. Glycerin swabs should not be used, as they break down tooth enamel.

The deeply comatose child is also prone to eye irritation. The corneal reflexes are absent; thus the eyes are easily irritated or damaged by linen, dust, or other substances that may come in contact with them. There is excessive dryness as a result of incomplete closure of the eyes or decreased secretions, especially if the child is undergoing osmotherapy to reduce or prevent brain edema.

NURSING ALERT The eyes should be examined regularly and carefully for early signs of irritation or **inflammation**. Artificial tears (methylcellulose) are placed in the eyes every 1 to 2 hours. Eye dressings may sometimes be needed to protect the eyes from possible damage.

Positioning and Exercise

The unconscious child is positioned to prevent aspiration of saliva, nasogastric secretions, and vomitus and to minimize

ICP. The head of the bed is elevated, and the child is placed in a side-lying or semiprone position. A small, firm pillow is placed under the head, and the uppermost limbs are flexed and supported with pillows. The weight of the body should not rest on the dependent arm. In the semiprone position, the child lies with the dependent arm at the side behind the body, the opposite side supported on pillows, and the uppermost arm and leg flexed and resting on the pillows. This position prevents undue pressure on the dependent extremities. The dependent position of the face encourages drainage of secretions and prevents the flaccid tongue from obstructing the airway.

Normal range-of-motion exercises help maintain function and prevent contractures of joints. Exercises should be done gently and with full range of motion. A small rolled pad can be placed in the palms to help maintain proper position of the fingers; footboards or boots can be used to help prevent footdrop; and splinting may be needed to prevent severe contractures of the wrist, knee, or ankle in decerebrate children.

Stimulation

Sensory stimulation is important in the care of the unconscious child, just as it is in the care of the alert child. For the temporarily unconscious or semiconscious child, sensory stimulation helps arouse the child to the conscious state and orient the child in terms of time and place. Auditory and tactile stimulation are especially valuable. Tactile stimulation is not appropriate for the child in whom it may elicit an undesirable response. However, for other children, tactile contact often has a relaxing and calming effect. When the child's condition permits, holding or rocking has a soothing effect and provides the body contact needed by young children.

The auditory sense is often present in a state of coma. Hearing is the last sense to be lost and the first one to be regained; thus the child should be spoken to as any other child. Conversation around the child should not include thoughtless or derogatory remarks. A radio playing soft music or a music box or CD or MP3 player is frequently used to provide auditory stimulation. Singing the child's favourite songs or reading a favourite story is a tactic used to maintain the child's contact with a familiar world. Playing songs or stories recorded in the parents' voices can provide a continuous source of familiar stimulation.

Regaining Consciousness

Awakening from a coma is a gradual process; however, sometimes children regain consciousness within a short time. Regaining orientation involves knowing person, place, and time, in that order.

Certain behaviours have been observed when children awaken from the unconscious state. The stress and anxiety they appear to feel in a strange and unfamiliar environment are consistently expressed in silent and withdrawn behaviour. Children respond to basic questioning but usually do not display their prehospitalization personality and social behaviour until they are transferred from the critical care area.

Family Support

Helping parents of an unconscious child cope with the situation is especially difficult. They may demonstrate all the guilt, fear, hostility, and anxiety of any parent of a seriously ill child (see Chapter 44). In addition, these parents are faced with the uncertain outcome of the cerebral dysfunction. The fear of death, intellectual disability, or other permanent disability is present. Nursing intervention with parents depends on the nature of the pathological condition, the parents' personality, and the parent–child relationship before the injury or illness.

If there is little or no residual effect, the child will be dismissed to home care fairly soon. The parents need the most intensive nursing intervention during the period of crisis and uncertainty. During the recovery phase they are given information, information is clarified, and they are encouraged to become involved in the child's care. Often the child's hospitalization is brief; however, some children require extended hospitalization for intensive therapy and rehabilitation.

Like parents who lose a child through death, the parents of the child who is unconscious may attempt to construct a representation of the child. They may bring items that belong to the child, such as favourite toys, music, and other objects cherished by the child. This action is an attempt to provide stimulation for the child in the hope of eliciting a response, to let the hospital staff know the child as the unique individual he or she was before losing consciousness, and to reconstitute an image of the child "lost" to them and for whom they mourn. An awareness of these behaviours and coping mechanisms can provide nurses with the understanding that helps them support the parents in their grief process.

Superimposed on the process of grieving for the "lost" child, parents may be faced with difficult decisions. When the child's brain is so severely damaged that vital functions must be maintained by artificial means, the parents must make the final decision of whether to remove life support systems. Since this decision is so difficult for parents, the practitioner is frequently placed in a position of making the decision indirectly. After providing the parents with all of the information, the practitioner may suggest that the child be removed from the life support to "see if the child can make it without help." While this approach relieves the parents of the decision and can be effective, it must be based on an evaluation of the parents' intellectual level and emotional state. Sometimes parents may even choose to refuse treatment if they believe it to be best for the child and the family (informed dissent). At other times parents request that "everything possible" be done for the child.

When the child has survived the cerebral insult and is not comatose, but physical or mental capacity is limited, either minimally or severely, families must cope with the long and tedious rehabilitation process and the uncertain outcome (see Patient Teaching box). The drain on financial, emotional, and social resources can be enormous.

Cerebral Trauma

Head Injury

Head injury is a pathological process involving the scalp, skull, meninges, or brain as a result of mechanical force. According to Health Canada (2007), injuries are the number one health risk for children and the leading cause of death in children older than 1 year of age in Canada. Tragically, almost 8000

PATIENT TEACHING Preparation for Discharge

- For parents who choose to care for their child at home, planning for home care begins early in the recovery process.
- The family should become involved with the child's care as soon as they indicate an interest and ability to do so.
- They need education and support in learning to care for the child, regular follow-up observation and assessment of the home management, and planning for some respite care of the child.
- Parents need to understand that it is important to plan for periodic relief from the continual care of the child.

children die every year as a result of injuries (Public Health Agency of Canada [PHAC], 2008). It has been estimated that 300 per 100,000 children per year have a **traumatic brain injury** and that 10 per 100,000 children per year die as a result of the brain injury. Studies indicate that as many as three fourths of the childhood deaths caused by mechanical trauma are the direct result of a brain injury. There is evidence to demonstrate that a previous head injury increases a child's risk of having a subsequent head injury (Swaine et al., 2007).

Etiology

The three major causes of brain damage in childhood, in order of importance, are falls, motor vehicle injuries, and bicycle injuries. Neurological injury accounts for the highest mortality rate, with boys affected twice as often as girls. In motor vehicle accidents, children younger than 2 years of age are almost exclusively injured as passengers, whereas older children may also be injured as pedestrians or cyclists. Approximately 75% of bicyclists who die each year, die of brain injuries (Saskatchewan Brain Injury Association, 2010). The majority of deaths from brain trauma caused by bicycle injuries occur in children between the ages of 5 and 19 years. Bicycle helmet laws have been effective in reducing the risk of head injury by 85% and brain injury by 88% (Rivara & Grossman, 2007); however, provincial legislation on the use of bicycle helmets varies from province to province (Think First Canada, 2008).

The exposed nature of the head renders it particularly vulnerable to external violence, and many of the physical characteristics of children predispose them to craniocerebral trauma. For example, infants are frequently left unattended on beds, in high chairs, and in other places from which they can fall. Because the head of an infant or toddler is proportionately larger and heavier in relation to other body parts, it is the most likely to be injured. Incomplete motor development contributes to falls at young ages, and children's natural curiosity and exuberance also increase their risk of injury (see Chapters 37 and 38).

Pathophysiology

The pathology of brain injury is directly related to the force of impact. Intracranial contents (brain, blood, CSF) are damaged because the force is too great to be absorbed by the skull and musculoligamentous support of the head. The elastic, pliable skull of the infant and young child absorbs much of the direct energy of physical impact to the head and affords some protection to intracranial structures. Although nervous tissue is delicate, it usually requires a severe blow to cause significant damage.

A child's response to head injury is different from that of an adult. The larger head size and insufficient musculoskeletal support render the very young child particularly vulnerable to acceleration–deceleration injuries.

Primary head injuries are those that occur at the time of trauma and include skull fracture, contusions, intracranial hematoma, and diffuse injury. Subsequent complications include hypoxic brain damage, increased ICP, infection, and cerebral edema. The predominant feature of a child's brain injury is the amount of diffuse swelling that occurs. Hypoxia and **hypercapnia** threaten the energy requirements of the brain and increase CBF. The added volume across the **blood–brain barrier,** along with the loss of **autoregulation,** exacerbates cerebral edema. Pressure inside the skull that is greater than arterial pressure results in inadequate perfusion.

Cerebral **hyperemia** occurs more often in children than adults, and this volume expansion may account for their tendency to develop intracranial hypertension. However, because the cranium of very young children has the ability to expand and the thin skull is more adherent, they may tolerate increases in ICP better than older children and adults do. Children have a significantly higher percentage of good outcomes, a lower mortality rate, and a lower incidence of surgical mass lesions after severe head trauma. However, their thinner, softer skull may sustain greater long-term damage than previously suggested.

Physical forces act on the head through acceleration, deceleration, or deformation. Acceleration or deceleration is more descriptive of the circumstances responsible for most head injuries. When the stationary head receives a blow, the sudden acceleration causes deformation of the skull and mass movement of the brain. Continued movement of the intracranial contents allows the brain to strike parts of the skull (e.g., the sharp edges of the sphenoid or the irregular surface of the anterior fossa) or the edges of the tentorium.

Although the brain volume remains unchanged, significant distortion takes place as the brain changes shape in response to the force of impact to the skull. This movement can cause bruising at the point of impact (coup) or at a distance as the brain collides with the unyielding surfaces far removed from the point of impact (contrecoup) (Fig. 51-4). Thus a blow to the occipital region can cause severe injury to the frontal and temporal areas of the brain. Sudden deceleration, such as takes place during a fall, causes the greatest cerebral injury at the point of impact. Children with an acceleration–deceleration injury demonstrate diffuse generalized cerebral swelling produced by increased blood volume or a redistribution of cerebral blood volume (cerebral hyperemia) rather than by increased water content (edema), as seen in adults.

Another effect of brain movement is shearing stresses, which may tear small arteries and cause subdural hemorrhages. Damage can also occur when severe compression of the skull forces the brain through the tentorial opening. This can produce irreparable damage to the brainstem (Fig. 51-5).

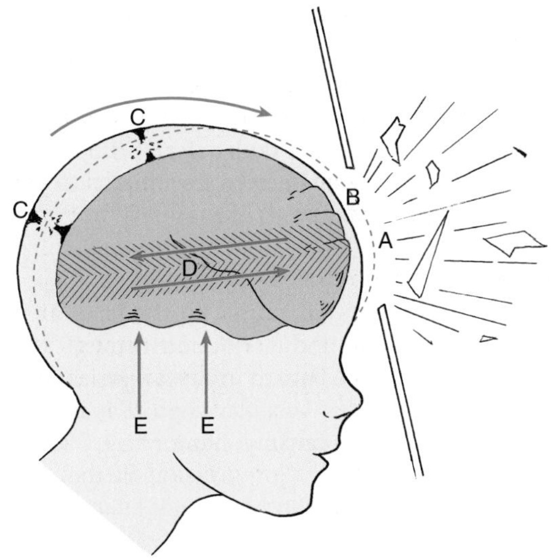

Fig. 51-4 Mechanical distortion of cranium during closed head injury. **A:** Preinjury contour of skull. **B:** Immediate postinjury contour of skull. **C:** Torn subdural vessels. **D:** Shearing forces. **E:** Trauma from contact with floor of cranium. *(Redrawn from Grubb, R. L., & Coxe, W. S. [1974]. Central nervous system trauma: Cranial. In S. G. Eliasson, A. L. Presky, & W. B. Hardin, Jr. [Eds.],* Neurological pathophysiology. *New York: Oxford University Press.)*

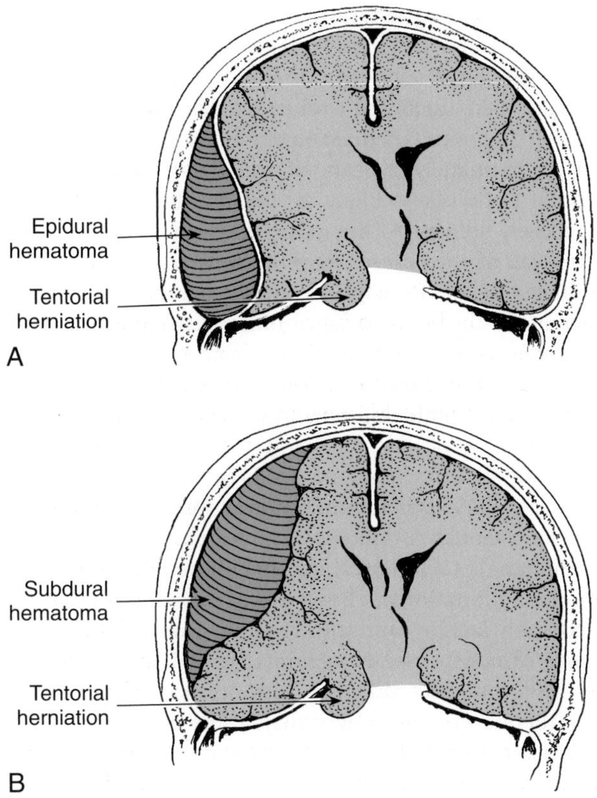

Fig. 51-5 **A:** Epidural (extradural) hematoma and compression of temporal lobe through tentorial hiatus. **B:** Subdural hematoma.

Concussion

The most common head injury is *concussion*, a transient and reversible neuronal dysfunction, with instantaneous loss of awareness and responsiveness, that results from trauma to the head and persists for a relatively short time, usually minutes or hours. It is generally followed by amnesia for the moment of the injury and a variable period after the injury. The common misconception that loss of consciousness is the hallmark of concussion is not true, especially for children. Concussion is correctly defined as a traumatically induced alteration in mental status. Confusion and amnesia following head injury are the hallmarks of concussion.

The pathogenesis of concussion is still unclear but may be a result of shearing forces that cause stretching, compression, and tearing of nerve fibres, particularly in the area of the central brainstem, the seat of the reticular activating system. It has also been suggested that the anatomical alterations of nerve fibres cause the release of large quantities of acetylcholine into the CSF and a reduction in oxygen consumption with increased lactate production.

The majority of concussions that a family physician will see are sports or activity related. Initial concussion management begins with injury recognition and rest until the patient is asymptomatic. Once asymptomatic, a gradual step-wise return to activity should be followed (McCrory et al., 2009).

Contusion and Laceration

The terms *contusion* and *laceration* are used to describe visible bruising and tearing of cerebral tissue. Contusions represent petechial hemorrhages along the superficial aspects of the brain at the site of impact (coup injury) or a lesion remote from the site of direct trauma (contrecoup injury). In serious accidents there may be multiple sites of injury.

The major areas of the brain susceptible to contusion or laceration are the occipital, frontal, and temporal lobes. Also, the irregular surfaces of the anterior and middle fossae at the base of the skull are capable of producing bruises or lacerations on forceful impact. Contusions may cause focal disturbances in strength, sensation, or visual awareness. The degree of brain damage in the contused areas varies according to the extent of vascular injury. Signs will vary from mild, transient weakness of a limb to prolonged unconsciousness and paralysis. However, the signs and symptoms may be clinically indistinguishable from those of concussion.

The lower incidence of cerebral contusion in infancy has been attributed to the infant's pliable skull with less convolutional markings of the inner space between brain tissue and bone. In addition, the infant's brain tissue has a softer consistency, which also reduces surface injury. However, infants who are roughly shaken (shaken baby syndrome) can sustain profound neurological impairment, seizures, retinal hemorrhages, and intracranial subarachnoid or subdural hemorrhages. In addition to these classic injuries, high cervical spinal cord hemorrhages and contusions can occur.

Cerebral lacerations are generally associated with penetrating or depressed skull fractures. However, they may occur without fracture in small children. When brain tissue is actually torn, with bleeding into and around the tear, usually more severe and prolonged unconsciousness and paralysis occur, leaving permanent scarring and some degree of disability.

Fractures

Because of its flexibility, the immature skull is able to sustain a greater degree of deformation than the adult skull before it incurs a fracture. A great deal of force is required to produce a fracture in an infant's skull. However, the undersurface of the skull contains grooves in which the meningeal arteries lie. A fracture that runs through one of these grooves may tear the artery and produce severe and damaging hemorrhage. Hypovolemic hypotension can occur in infants with skull fractures.

The types of fractures that occur are as follows:

Linear fractures are those in which the lines of the fracture are predetermined by the site and velocity of the impact, as well as by the strength of the bone. These are uncommon before 2 to 3 years of age but constitute the majority of childhood skull fractures. Most linear skull fractures are associated with an overlying hematoma or soft-tissue swelling (Schutzman & Greenes, 2001).

Comminuted fractures consist of multiple associated linear fractures. They usually result from intense impact. These types of fractures often result from repeated blows against an object and may suggest child abuse.

Depressed fractures are those in which the bone is locally broken, usually into several irregular fragments that are pushed inward, causing pressure on the brain. The inner portion of the bone is more extensively fragmented than the outer portion, which almost invariably produces tears in the dura. These are uncommon before 2 to 3 years of age. In infants and very young children, the soft, malleable bone may become dented in a peculiar rounded or "ping-pong ball" depression, without laceration of either skin or dura.

Basilar fractures involve the basilar portion of the frontal, ethmoid, sphenoid, temporal, or occipital bones. Because of the proximity of the fracture line to structures surrounding the brainstem, this is a serious head injury. Approximately 80% of the cases may include clinical features such as subcutaneous bleeding in the posterior neck area and over the mastoid process (battle sign). Bleeding around the eyes (raccoon eyes) or bleeding behind the tympanic membrane (hemotympanum) may occur.

Open fractures cause communication between the skull and the scalp or the surfaces of the upper respiratory tract. Open fractures increase the risk of CNS infection. They may have an overlying laceration called a compound fracture. Open fractures can also create an opening in the paranasal sinuses or middle ear that can lead to CSF rhinorrhea or otorrhea. Facial paralysis, vertigo, tinnitus, or hearing loss may develop.

Diastatic fractures are traumatic separations of the cranial sutures. These most frequently affect the lambdoid suture and are rarely seen beyond the first 3 years of life. They require no specific treatment but should be observed for "growing fractures."

Growing fractures are skull fractures with an underlying dural tear that fails to heal properly. The enlargement may be caused by a leptomeningeal cyst, dilated ventricles, or a herniated brain. Neurological symptoms include headache, seizures, and asymmetrical cranial growth. The majority of growing skull fractures occur before 3 years of age (Vignes et al., 2007). Physical examination can reveal the development of a pulsatile mass or enlarging and sunken skull defect. Clinical neurological symptoms may be delayed for months to years after the initial skull fracture.

evolve Animation–Subdural Hematoma

Complications

The major complications of trauma to the head are hemorrhage, infection, edema, and herniation through the tentorium. Infection is always a hazard in open injuries, and edema is related to tissue trauma. Vascular rupture may occur even in minor head injuries, causing hemorrhage between the skull and cerebral surfaces. Compression of the underlying brain produces effects that can be rapidly fatal or insidiously progressive.

NURSING ALERT Post-traumatic meningitis should be suspected in children with increasing drowsiness and fever who also have basilar skull fractures.

Epidural Hemorrhage

The blood accumulates between the dura and the skull to form a hematoma, which, because of the difficulty with which dura is stripped from bone, forces the underlying brain contents downward and inward as the brain expands (see Fig. 51-5, A). Since bleeding is generally arterial, brain compression occurs rapidly. Most often the expanding hematoma is located in the parietotemporal region, forcing the medial portion of the temporal lobe under the edge of the tentorium, where it causes pressure on nerves and blood vessels. The lower incidence of epidural hematoma in childhood has been attributed to the fact that the middle meningeal artery is not embedded in the bone surface of the skull until approximately 2 years of age. Thus a fracture of the temporal bone is less likely to lacerate the artery. Also, the dura closely adheres to the inner table of the skull, especially at the level of the sutures, making separation from bleeding less likely. However, a child's skull can be indented with sufficient force to tear the middle meningeal artery and rebound intact without causing a fracture. Hemorrhage can also derive from dural veins or the dural sinuses, especially in infants and small children, in whom fracture is less likely to occur.

In 20 to 40% of children a skull fracture is not detectable. The classic clinical picture of epidural hemorrhage (momentary unconsciousness followed by a normal period, then lethargy or coma) is seldom evident in children (see Box 51-3 for clinical manifestations). The period of impaired consciousness is frequently lacking, and the symptom-free period is atypical because of nonspecific complaints such as irritability, headache, and vomiting. When it does occur, the symptom-free period frequently lasts longer than 48 hours.

Clinically significant epidural hematomas are uncommon in children younger than 4 years of age. These differences may be caused by the decreased tendency of the resilient skull to fracture; the ability of blood to escape through widened sutures, an open fontanel, or a fracture; bleeding from smaller vessels with less rapid and massive bleeding; lower systolic

BOX 51-3 Clinical Manifestations of Acute Head Injury

Minor Injury
May or may not lose consciousness
Transient period of confusion
Somnolence
Listlessness
Irritability
Pallor
Vomiting

Signs of Progression
Altered mental status (e.g., difficulty rousing child)
Mounting agitation
Development of focal lateral neurological signs
Marked changes in vital signs

Severe Injury
Signs of increased intracranial pressure (see Box 51-1)
Bulging or full fontanel (infant)
Retinal hemorrhage
Extraocular palsies (especially cranial nerve VI)
Hemiparesis
Quadriplegia
Elevated temperature
Unsteady gait (older child)
Papilledema (older child)

Associated Signs
Scalp trauma
Other injuries (e.g., to extremities)

blood pressure in children; and possibly the decreased susceptibility of the child's brain to pressure changes.

Subdural Hemorrhage

A *subdural hemorrhage* is bleeding between the dura and the cerebrum, usually as a result of rupture of cortical veins that bridge the subdural space (see Fig. 51-5, B). Subdural hematomas occur much more frequently than epidural hematomas, most often in infancy, with a peak incidence at 6 months (Myhre et al., 2007).

Unlike epidural hemorrhage, which develops inwardly against the less resistant brain tissue, subdural hemorrhage tends to develop more slowly and spreads thinly and widely until it is limited by the dural barriers—the falx and tentorium. Subdural hematoma is fairly common in infants, frequently as a result of birth trauma, falls, assaults, or violent shaking. The small subdural space and dura firmly attached to the skull in this area are highly vulnerable to increased ICP.

NURSING ALERT Children with a subdural hematoma and retinal hemorrhages should be evaluated for the possibility of child abuse, especially shaken baby syndrome.

Repeated subdural taps often provide relief in the infant, as revealed by follow-up CT scans, improved neurological status, and a flat anterior fontanel. Surgical evacuation of the hematoma is the treatment of choice in the older child and is frequently required in infants.

Cerebral Edema

Some degree of brain edema is expected, especially 24 to 72 hours after craniocerebral trauma. Cerebral edema caused by direct cellular injury or vascular injury induces vascular stasis, anoxia, and further vasodilation. If the progression continues unchecked, ICP exceeds arterial pressure and fatal anoxia ensues, or the pressure causes herniation of a portion of the brain over the edge of the tentorium, compressing the brainstem and occluding the posterior cerebral arteries. Diffuse cerebral swelling and changes in CBF are common patterns after head injury in children.

NURSING ALERT If a child loses consciousness or vomits more than three times following a head injury, medical attention should be sought.

Diagnostic Evaluation

A detailed history, especially a health history, both past and present, is essential in evaluating the child with a craniocerebral trauma. Certain disorders, such as drug allergies, hemophilia, diabetes mellitus, or epilepsy, may produce similar symptoms. Furthermore, even minor traumatic injury can aggravate a pre-existing disease process. Events surrounding the injury often supply significant data. It must be determined whether the infant or child exhibited alterations in consciousness; any other signs and behaviours exhibited by the child must be noted. Since head injuries are frequently accompanied by injuries in other areas, the examination needs to be performed with care to avoid further damage.

NURSING ALERT Stabilize a child's spine after head injury until a spinal cord injury is ruled out.

Initial Assessment

Priorities in the initial stabilization phase of a child with a head injury include assessment of CAB (circulation, airway, breathing); evaluation for shock; a neurological examination, especially LOC; assessment of pupillary symmetry and response to light; and observation for seizures (Bayir et al., 2003). The assessment is carried out quickly in relation to vital signs (see Emergency box). Excited and irritable children may have a rapid pulse, hyperventilate, appear pale, and feel clammy shortly after an injury.

NURSING ALERT Signs of brainstem involvement include deep, rapid, periodic, or intermittent and gasping respirations; wide fluctuations or noticeable slowing of the pulse; and widening pulse pressure or extreme fluctuations in blood pressure. Note that marked hypotension may represent internal injuries.

Ocular signs such as fixed and dilated pupils, fixed and constricted pupils, and pupils that are poorly reactive or nonreactive to light and accommodation indicate increased ICP or brainstem involvement. It is important to remain with the child who demonstrates fixed and dilated pupils, since these are ominous signs, with the probability of respiratory arrest. Dilated, nonpulsating blood vessels indicate increased ICP before the appearance of papilledema. Retinal hemorrhages are seen in acute head injuries.

EMERGENCY

Head Injury

Assess child:
- C—Circulation
- A—Airway (with cervical-spine immobilization)
  - Use jaw thrust to open airway
- B—Bleeding

Clean any abrasions with soap and water.
- Apply clean dressing.
- If bleeding, apply ice to relieve pain and swelling.

Keep NPO (nothing by mouth) until instructed otherwise.

Assess pain, but do not give analgesics or sedatives.

Check pupil reaction every 4 hours (including twice during night) for 48 hours.

Awaken twice during the night to check level of consciousness.

Seek medical attention if any of the following apply:
- Injury sustained:
  - At high speed (e.g., automobile)
  - Fall from a significant distance (e.g., roof, tree, or height greater than that of the child)
  - From great force (e.g., baseball bat)
  - Under suspicious circumstances
- Loss of consciousness
- Amnesia
- Discomfort (crying) more than 10 minutes after injury
- Headache that is severe, worsening, interferes with sleep
- Fluid leak from ears or nose
- Vomiting three or more times
- Swelling in front of or above earlobe or increased swelling
- Confusion or abnormal behaviour
- Difficult to arouse from sleep
- Difficulty speaking
- Blurred vision or seeing double
- Unsteady gait
- Difficulty using extremities
- Neck pain
- Pupils dilated, unequal, or fixed
- Infant with full or bulging fontanel
- Bruising below the eyes

NURSING ALERT Observation of asymmetrical pupils or one dilated, nonreactive pupil in a comatose child is a neurosurgical emergency.

Less urgent but important additional assessments include examination of the scalp for lacerations and palpation for other abnormalities. A significant amount of blood loss can occur from scalp lacerations.

NURSING ALERT Bleeding from the nose or ears needs further evaluation, and a watery discharge from the nose (rhinorrhea) that is positive for glucose (as tested with Dextrostix) suggests leaking of CSF from a skull fracture.

An accurate assessment of clinical signs provides **baseline data.** Serial evaluations, preferably by a single observer, help to detect changes in the neurological status. Alterations in mental status, evidenced by increased difficulty in rousing the child, mounting agitation, development of focal lateral neurological signs, or marked changes in vital signs, usually indicate extension or progression of the basic pathological process.

Special Tests

After a thorough clinical examination, a variety of diagnostic tests are helpful in providing a more definitive diagnosis of the type and extent of the trauma. The severity of a head injury may not be apparent on clinical examination of a child, but it will be detectable on a CT scan. Whenever the child has a history consistent with a serious head injury (e.g., unrestrained occupant in a severe motor vehicle accident or a fall from a significant height), it is important that a scan be performed even if the child initially appears alert and oriented. All children with head injuries who have any alteration of consciousness, headache, vomiting, skull fracture, seizure, or a predisposing medical condition should also undergo CT scanning.

MRI and neurobehavioural assessment after early head injury may be useful in documenting cognitive impairment in relation to structural alterations in the young brain. MRI provides details of soft tissues better than any other noninvasive device. Electroencephalography is not particularly helpful for early diagnosis but is useful for defining seizure activity or focal destructive lesions after the acute phase of illness. Lumbar puncture is rarely used in craniocerebral trauma and is contraindicated in the presence of increased ICP because of the possibility of herniation. In some centres, monitoring ICP is part of the assessment.

Post-Traumatic Syndromes

Post-traumatic syndromes can be clinically manifested because of structural complications resulting from a head injury and through the signs and symptoms demonstrated by the child. Structural complications can include hydrocephalus and focal deficits such as optic atrophy, cranial nerve palsies, motor deficits, DI, aphasia, and seizures. Behavioural disturbances include sleep disturbances, phobias, emotional lability, altered school performance, and changes related to aggressiveness or withdrawal. Postconcussion syndrome is a common sequela to brain injury, with or without loss of consciousness, and can occur within minutes to an hour after a head injury. It is a symptom complex that includes headaches, dizziness, fatigue, irritability, anxiety, insomnia, loss of concentration, and memory impairment (Baandrup & Jensen, 2005; Yeates et al., 2009). Symptoms typically develop within days of the injury and resolve within 3 months. Post-traumatic seizures occur in a number of children who survive a head injury and are more common in younger children than in those over 16 years of age (Baandrup & Jensen, 2005). Seizures are more likely to occur within the first few days of the head injury (Chiaretti et al., 2000). Structural complications (e.g., hydrocephalus) may occur after a head injury. The type of residual effect depends on the location and nature of the disorder.

Therapeutic Management

Most children with mild to moderate concussion who have not lost consciousness can be cared for and observed at home after careful examination reveals no serious intracranial injury.

Nurses should provide parents with clear explanations and instructions and should encourage them to ask questions both before and after leaving the medical facility if clarification is needed (see Family-Centred Teaching box).

The parents should be instructed to check the child every 2 hours to determine any changes in responsiveness. The sleeping child should be wakened to see if he or she can be roused normally. Parents need to maintain contact with the health care provider, who will usually wish to examine the child again in 1 or 2 days. The manifestations of epidural hematoma in children do not generally appear until 24 hours or more after injury.

Children with severe injuries, those who have lost consciousness for more than a few minutes, and those with prolonged and continued seizures or other focal or diffuse neurological signs must be hospitalized until their condition is stable and their neurological signs have diminished.

The child is maintained on nothing by mouth (NPO) or restricted to clear liquids, if able to take fluids by mouth, until it is determined that vomiting will not occur. IV fluids are indicated in the child who is comatose or displays dulled sensorium and in the child with persistent vomiting. Fluid balance is closely monitored by daily weights; accurate intake and output measurements; and serum osmolality to detect early signs of water retention, excessive dehydration, and states of hypertonicity or hypotonicity.

The volume of IV fluid needs to be carefully monitored to avoid aggravating any cerebral edema and to minimize the possibility of overhydration in case of SIADH. However, damage to the hypothalamus or pituitary gland may produce DI with its accompanying hypertonicity and dehydration.

Restlessness can be satisfactorily managed, if necessary, with mild sedation, and headache is usually controlled with acetaminophen. Anti-epileptics are used for seizure control and frequently in cases of suspected contusion or laceration. Antibiotics may be administered if lacerations, CSF leakage, or excessive cerebral tissue damage is present. Prophylactic tetanus toxoid is given as appropriate. Cerebral edema is managed as described for the unconscious child. Hyperthermia is controlled with tepid sponges or a hypothermia blanket.

Surgical Therapy

Scalp lacerations are sutured after the underlying bone is carefully examined. Depressed fractures require surgical reduction and removal of bone fragments. Torn dura is sutured. Ping-pong ball skull fractures in very young infants ordinarily correct themselves within a few weeks and do not require specific treatment, although they can be reduced by pressure against the bone.

Prognosis

The outcome of craniocerebral trauma depends on the extent of injury and complications. However, the outlook is generally more favourable for children than for adults (Masson et al., 2003). More than 90% of children with concussions or simple linear fractures recover without symptoms after the initial period. The incidence of fatalities and neurological sequelae is lower in children than in adults, even in those with severe head injuries. The prognosis for recovery is primarily related to the duration of coma and the degree of injury. The combination of impaired consciousness and skull fracture carries the highest risk of complication.

The concern regarding outcome is increasingly focused on cognitive, emotional, and mental problems. Children experience a higher frequency of psychological disturbances after head injury, whereas adults are more prone to physical complaints. Children may be more vulnerable than adults to long-term cognitive and behavioural dysfunction after diffuse brain injury. Even with recovery, the effects of brain injury on a child's potential can never be known.

True coma (not obeying commands, eyes closed, and not speaking) usually does not last more than 2 weeks. A child's eventual outcome can range from brain death to a persistent vegetative state to complete recovery. However, even the best recovery may be associated with personality changes, including mood lability and loss of confidence; impaired short-term memory; headaches; and subtle cognitive impairments. Many children are left with significant disabilities after a head injury that appear months later as learning difficulties, behavioural changes, or emotional disturbances (Faillace, 2002). Generally, within 6 months to 1 year after the injury, 90% of the long-term neurological outcome has been achieved.

Nursing Care Management

The hospitalized child requires careful neurological assessment and evaluation (including vital signs) repeated at frequent intervals to provide information needed to establish a correct diagnosis, reveal signs and symptoms of increased ICP, determine clinical management, prevent many complications, and provide support to the child and family during the recovery phases.

The child is placed on bed rest, usually with the head of the bed elevated slightly. Appropriate safety measures, such as side rails kept up and seizure precautions for children of all ages, need to be implemented. For the extremely restless child, hard surfaces may have to be padded and restraints used to prevent the possibility of further injury. Care should be individualized according to the child's specific needs. The unconscious child is managed as described in the previous section, but most childhood head injuries are those causing momentary stunning or temporary unconsciousness. Children may be restless and irritable, but more often their reaction is to fall asleep when left undisturbed. A quiet environment helps reduce restlessness and irritability. Shining bright lights directly into the

FAMILY-CENTRED TEACHING

Maintaining Contact

Maintaining contact with parents for continued observation and re-evaluation of the child, when indicated, facilitates early diagnosis and treatment of possible complications from head injury, such as hematoma, hydrocephalus, cysts, and posttraumatic seizures. Children are generally hospitalized for 24 to 48 hours' observation if their family lives far from medical facilities or lacks transportation or a telephone that would provide access to immediate help. Other circumstances such as language or other communication barriers, or even emotional trauma, may hinder learning and make it difficult for families to feel confident in caring for their child at home.

child's face is irritating and often aggravates the child, making assessment of ocular responses difficult.

Frequent examinations of vital signs, neurological signs, and LOC are extremely important nursing observations. When possible, they should be performed by a single observer to better detect subtle changes that may indicate worsening neurological status. Pupils are checked for size, equality, reaction to light, and accommodation. After the initial elevations usually seen following injury, the vital signs generally return to normal unless there is brainstem involvement. An axillary measurement of temperature is the safest method, since seizures are not uncommon and vomiting is a frequent response in children, especially when the child is disturbed.

The most important nursing observation is assessment of the child's LOC. Alterations in consciousness appear earlier in the progression of an injury than alterations of vital signs or focal neurological signs. Some expected responses may be misinterpreted as deviations from the normal. Frequent examinations of alertness are fatiguing to the child; thus the child will often want to fall asleep, which may be confused with depressed consciousness. When left alone, the child will go to sleep. It is not uncommon to observe ocular divergence through the partially closed eyelids.

A key nursing role is to provide sedation and analgesia for the child. The conflict between the need to promote comfort and relieve anxiety in the child versus the need to assess for neurological changes presents a dilemma. However, both goals can be achieved with close observation of the child's LOC and response to analgesics, use of a pain assessment record, and effective communication with the practitioner. To differentiate between sedation from an opioid and sedation from the injury, naloxone can be given slowly to reverse the opioid's sedative effect. Decreasing restlessness after administration of an analgesic most likely reflects pain control rather than a declining LOC.

Observations of position and movement provide additional information. Any abnormal posturing should be noted, as well as whether it occurs continuously or intermittently. The following qualities should be assessed: Are the child's handgrips strong and equal in strength? Are there any signs of flexion-extension posturing? What is the child's response to stimulation? Is movement purposeful, random, or absent? Are movement and sensation equal on both sides or restricted to one side only?

The child may communicate having a headache or other discomfort. The child who is too young to describe a headache will be fussy and resist being handled. The child who suffers from vertigo will often assume a position of comfort and vigorously resist efforts to be moved. Forcible movement causes the child to vomit and display spontaneous **nystagmus**. Seizures, relatively common in children with craniocerebral trauma, may be of any type but are more often generalized, regardless of the type of injury. Any seizure activity should be carefully observed and described in detail. Children in postictal (postseizure) states are lethargic, with sluggish pupils.

Drainage from any orifice should be noted. Bleeding from the ear suggests the possibility of a basal skull fracture. The amount and characteristics of the drainage need to be observed, and since the auditory canal may be a source of infection, dry, sterile cotton can be placed loosely at the orifice and changed when soiled.

Head trauma is frequently accompanied by other undetected injuries; thus any bruises, lacerations, or evidence of internal injuries or fractures of the extremities need to be noted and reported. Associated injuries should be evaluated and treated appropriately.

The child with normal LOC is usually allowed clear liquids unless fluid is restricted. If the child has an IV infusion, it should be maintained as prescribed. The diet is advanced to that appropriate for the child's age as soon as the condition permits. Intake and output need to be measured and recorded, and any incontinence of bowel or bladder noted in the child who has been toilet trained.

The child should be observed for any unusual behaviour, but behaviour should be interpreted in relation to the child's normal behaviour. For example, urinary incontinence during sleep would be of no consequence in a child who routinely wets the bed but would be highly significant for one who is always dry. In addition, a child who is subject to nightmares might cry out and demonstrate agitated behaviour at night. There would be less concern about a child who falls asleep several times during the day if this were consistent with the child's usual behaviour. In this regard, parents are valuable resources. Information obtained from parents at or shortly after admission is helpful in evaluating the child's behaviour (e.g., the ease with which the child is roused normally, the usual sleeping position, how much the child sleeps during the day, motor activity the child is capable of [rolling over, sitting up, climbing], hearing and visual acuity, appetite, and manner of eating [spoon, bottle, cup]).

Family Support

The emotional and educational support of the family of children who have suffered head injury presents a formidable, challenging aspect to nursing care. Witnessing the parents' ordeal of grief and helplessness on seeing their child in an altered state, connected to monitoring equipment in an intensive care unit, evokes empathy. The nurse can encourage the family to be involved in the child's care, to bring in familiar belongings, or to make a tape recording of familiar voices and sounds. Parents may need a demonstration on how to touch or cuddle their child and may want to talk about their grief. The nurse can listen attentively, reinforce what is being done to assist the child, and direct parents toward signs and symptoms of recovery to instill hope without promises. A common phenomenon is for families to seek information from all health care providers, asking, "What will she be like? What do you know?" as they search for some clue that the child is recovering. Honesty and kindness, along with competent care, distinguish excellent nursing abilities.

When the child is discharged, the parents should be advised of probable post-traumatic symptoms that may be expected, such as behavioural changes, sleep disturbances, phobias, and seizures. They should understand observations they need to make and how to contact the physician, nurse, or health facility in case the child develops any unusual signs or symptoms. The importance of follow-up evaluation should be emphasized. It is often advisable to refer the family to a public health agency for home follow-through to be certain that the child receives posthospital evaluation.

Rehabilitation

The rehabilitation and management of the child with permanent brain injury are essential aspects of care. Rehabilitation of brain-injured children is begun as soon as feasible and usually involves the family and a rehabilitation team. Careful assessment of the child's capabilities, limitations, and probable potential needs to be made as early as possible and appropriate interventions implemented to maximize the residual capacities. The Brain Injury Association of Canada provides information and listings of rehabilitation services and support groups throughout the country (see Additional Resources section at the end of this chapter).

Pediatric trauma rehabilitation is a national concern. Coordinating care and services for early rehabilitation involves identifying the child and family's response to the traumatic injury and disability, securing available resources, and recognizing the parental role in the process.

The child with a disability resulting from head trauma requires assessment on a physical, cognitive, emotional, and social level. The child has experienced separation, pain, sensory deprivation and overload, changes in circadian cycle, and fear of the unknown. Recovery and transition require new coping strategies at the same time that regressive and acting-out behaviour may start. Parents and children need honest communication for decision making. A rehabilitation facility or home rehabilitation is advocated when the child has progressed beyond what can be provided in a hospital setting. The Rancho Los Amigos Scale provides a **systematic assessment** of the possible progress a child may achieve after a severe head injury (see Additional Resources).

Prevention

Tremendous strides have been made in the prevention of cerebral damage after head injury in children. New developments requiring research point to the prevention of cellular injury or the primary insult. However, the greatest benefit lies in prevention of head injuries. Nurses can exert a valuable influence on behalf of children through education. The reason injuries remain preventable is that unnecessary risks go unchecked. Inadequate supervision combined with a child's natural sense of indestructibility and exploration can lead to lethal results. Nurses are in the unique position of influencing caregivers in terms of growth and development. Banning the use of infant walkers is an example. This equipment does not help develop motor skills and places infants at risk for head and neck injuries from falls, especially down steps. Public education, coupled with legislative support, can prevent childhood injuries. (For extensive discussions of childhood injuries and prevention, see Chapters 36 to 40. See also Childhood Mortality, Chapter 29.)

Submersion Injuries

Submersion injury is a major cause of accidental death in children. Toddlers aged 1 to 4 years of age are one of the major risk groups (Canadian Red Cross Society, 2006). The term *submersion injury* has replaced the term *near-drowning* and should be used to describe injury occurring up until the time of drowning-related death (American Heart Association, 2005). Most cases of submersion injury involve the following individuals:

- Children who are helpless in water, such as inadequately attended children in or near swimming pools or infants in bathtubs
- Small children who fall into ponds, streams, and flooded excavations, usually near home
- Occupants of pleasure boats who fail to wear life preservers
- Children who have diving accidents
- Children who are able to swim but overestimate their endurance

Accidental drowning occurs five times more often among boys than among girls; almost 40% of children are younger than age 5, and 90% of cases occur in private swimming pools (Canadian Red Cross Society, 2006; Kallas, 2007). New immigrants or visitors to Canada, especially those who have been in Canada for less than 5 years, are four times more likely to be unable to swim than those born in Canada (Lifesaving Society, 2005). Drowning can take place in any body of water, including such unlikely ones as a pail of water. Top-heavy toddlers fall head first into a pail of water, their arms become trapped, and they are unable to free themselves. Hot tubs and whirlpool spas have been implicated in childhood drowning injury. The suction created at the outlet is strong enough to trap even larger children underwater. Drowning as a form of fatal child abuse has also been recognized as a problem. Homicidal drownings are unwitnessed, they usually occur in the home, and the victims are either infants or toddlers. With expeditious treatment many children are being saved.

Pathophysiology

The major pulmonary changes that occur in submersion injury are directly related to the length of submersion (regardless of the type and amount of fluid aspirated), the victim's physiological response, and the development and degree of immersion hypothermia. In addition, cerebral recovery depends on the effectiveness of initial resuscitation and subsequent critical care measures to support cerebral salvage.

Physiological factors that influence the extent of damage from immersion include resistance to asphyxia and anoxia, which shows some individual variation. There is greater resistance with diminishing age; young children can withstand longer periods of submersion. More important is the drowning, or diving, reflex. This neurological response is triggered by immersion of the face in cold water. Blood is shunted away from the periphery, and the flow is concentrated in the brain and heart predominantly.

The problems created by submersion injuries are (1) hypoxia and asphyxiation, (2) aspiration, and (3) hypothermia (except for submersion injuries in hot tubs). Cardiopulmonary arrest is secondary to asphyxiation.

Hypoxia is the primary problem because it results in global cell damage, and different cells tolerate variable lengths of anoxia. Neurons, especially cerebral cells, sustain irreversible damage after 4 to 6 minutes of submersion. The heart and lungs can survive up to 30 minutes. Regardless of the amount of water aspirated, there is arterial hypoxemia (resulting from atelectasis with shunting of blood through the nonventilated alveoli) and a combined respiratory acidosis (resulting from retained carbon dioxide) and metabolic acidosis (caused by buildup of acid metabolites from anaerobic metabolism). The pathological events are directly related to the duration of submersion. The major difficulty is acute ventilatory insufficiency. Approximately 10% of drowning victims die without aspirating fluid but succumb from acute asphyxia as a result of prolonged reflex laryngospasm.

Aspiration of fluid occurs in most drownings. The aspirated fluid results in pulmonary edema, atelectasis, airway spasm, and pneumonitis, which aggravates the hypoxia. It was previously thought that submersion in salt water versus fresh water altered the physiological response to near-drowning. The type of water does not alter the therapy or outcome; the main factors are the duration time of submersion and presence of hypoxia (American Heart Association, 2005).

Hypothermia occurs rapidly in infants and children, partly because of their large surface area relative to body mass and partly as a result of the cold water itself. Water is an excellent heat conductor, and contact with the skin is increased by struggling. Hypothermia may make resumption or maintenance of cardiac function possible if body temperature is less than 30°C. Profound hypothermia is usually evidence of lengthy submersion.

Therapeutic Management

Resuscitative measures should begin at the scene, and the victim should be transported to the hospital with maximal ventilatory and circulatory support. Many victims need care for some time after aspiration of fluid. In the hospital, intensive pulmonary care is implemented and continued according to the patient's needs.

In general, the management of the submersion injury victim is based on the degree of cerebral insult (Box 51-4). The first priority is to restore oxygen delivery to the cells and prevent further hypoxic damage. A spontaneously breathing child will do well in an oxygen-enriched atmosphere; the more severely affected child will require endotracheal intubation and mechanical ventilation. Blood gases and pH are monitored frequently as a guide to oxygen, fluid, and electrolyte therapies.

NURSING ALERT All children who have a submersion injury experience should be admitted to the hospital for observation. Although many patients do not appear to have suffered adverse effects from the event, complications (e.g., respiratory compromise, cerebral edema) may occur 24 hours after the incident.

Aspiration pneumonia is a frequent complication that occurs about 48 to 72 hours after the episode. Bronchospasm, alveolocapillary membrane damage, atelectasis, abscess formation, and acute respiratory distress syndrome are other complications that occur after aspiration of fluid.

Prognosis

Studies report that the best predictors of a good outcome are length of submersion in nonicy water (more than 5°C) for less than 5 minutes and the presence of sinus rhythm, reactive pupils, and neurological responsiveness at the scene.

BOX 51-4 Clinical Manifestations of Submersion Injuries

Category A
Awake, minimal injury
Fully conscious; may have mild hypothermia, mild chest radiograph changes, mild arterial blood gas abnormalities

Category B
Blunted sensorium, moderate injury
Obtund, stuporous, purposeful response to painful stimuli, mild to moderate hypothermia, frequent respiratory distress, abnormal chest radiographs, arterial blood gas abnormalities

Category C
Comatose, severe anoxia
Unarousable, abnormal response to pain, abnormal respiratory pattern, seizures, shock, marked arterial blood gas abnormalities, abnormal chest radiographs, arrhythmias, metabolic acidosis, hyperkalemia, hyperglycemia, disseminated intravascular coagulation
C1—Decorticate posturing, Cheyne-Stokes respirations
C2—Decerebrate posturing, central hyperventilation
C3—Flaccid, apneic, or cluster breathing
C4—Flaccid, apneic, no detectable circulation

The worst prognoses—for death or severe neurological impairment—were in children submerged for more than 10 minutes and not responding to advanced life support within 25 minutes. All children without spontaneous, purposeful movement and normal brainstem function 24 hours after submersion injury suffered severe neurological deficits or death (Kallas, 2007) (see Guidelines box).

Nursing Care Management

Nursing care depends on the child's condition. A child who survives may need intensive respiratory nursing care with attention to vital signs, mechanical ventilation or tracheostomy or both, blood gas determination, chest therapy, and IV infusion. Frequently the child is comatose for an indefinite period and requires the same care as an unconscious child. A difficult aspect in the care of the child victim of near-drowning is helping the parents cope with severe guilt reactions. The magnitude of the event is so great that efforts to provide comfort and support are of only limited success. Parents need to hear that everything possible is being done to treat the child, and this message needs to be repeated often.

The parents of the child who is saved from death are also faced with the anxiety of not knowing what the outcome will be. The situation generates such intense feelings of loneliness, it is important for families to know that they are not alone. They need to be reminded frequently that there are caring people to assist them both during the crisis and later. Additional sources of support that can be recommended are psychiatric and social work consultants, community services, and religious support. Self-help groups are excellent if these are available in the community.

GUIDELINES Establishing Brain Death in Children

1. Coma and apnea must coexist. Child must exhibit complete loss of consciousness, vocalization, and volitional activity.
2. Brainstem function must be absent, as defined by:
   a. Midposition or fully dilated pupils that do not respond to light. Medications may influence and invalidate pupillary assessment.
   b. Absence of spontaneous eye movements and those induced by oculocephalic and caloric (oculovestibular) testing
   c. Absence of movement of bulbar musculature, including facial and oropharyngeal muscles. The corneal, gag, cough, sucking, and rooting reflexes are absent.
   d. Absence of respiratory movements when child is removed from respirator. Apnea testing using standardized methods can be performed but is done after other criteria are met.
3. The child must not be significantly hypothermic or hypotensive for age.
4. Flaccid tone and absence of spontaneous or induced movements, including spinal cord events such as reflex withdrawal or spinal myoclonus, should exist.
5. Examination should remain consistent with brain death throughout the observation and testing period.
6. Observation periods according to age:
   Seven days to 2 months—Two separate examinations and two electroencephalograms (EEGs), separated by at least 48 hours
   Two months to 1 year—Two separate examinations and two EEGs, separated by at least 24 hours
   Over 1 year—Two separate examinations separated by at least 12 hours; if irreversible cause exists, no laboratory testing needed; if difficult to assess extent of reversibility of brain damage, observation indicated for at least 24 hours

(Modified from Task Force for the Determination of Brain Death in Children. [1987]. Guidelines for the determination of brain death in children. *Annals of Neurology, 21,* 616; Janakiraman, N. [1998]. Brain death. *Indian Journal of Pediatrics, 65,* 525–527; and Lutz-Dettinger, N., de Jaeger, A., & Kerremanas, I. [2001]. Care of the potential pediatric organ donor. *Pediatric Clinics of North America, 48,* 715–749.)

Nurses often have difficulty relating to the parents if obvious neglect has precipitated the accident and subsequent problems; it is important for those who care for these children and their families to assess their own feelings about the situation, as well as the family's coping abilities and resources. Caring for submersion victims and their families requires nurses to be sensitive to the needs of the child and family and to recognize their own reactions and emotions.

Prevention

Most drownings, particularly of infants or small children, can be prevented with adequate supervision. Water safety and survival training should be required for all school-age children, and nurses can be active advocates in their communities. Nurses are also in a position to emphasize the importance of adequate adult supervision when children are in the water. Aquatic programs for infants and toddlers do not decrease the risk of drowning; young children should *never* be left unattended when in or near the water (Canadian Red Cross Society, 2006; Kallas, 2007; Safe Kids Canada, 2010). Parents with pools should know **cardiopulmonary resuscitation** techniques. (See also Injury Prevention, Chapters 36 to 40.)

Nervous System Tumours

Brain tumour and neuroblastoma are two major forms of childhood cancer derived from neural tissue. CNS tumours account for approximately 20% of all childhood cancers and occur most often in children under 15 years of age (Blaney et al., 2006; Childhood Cancer Foundation, 2009). Both of these tumours are difficult to treat and have not demonstrated the dramatic improvements in survival seen in other forms of childhood cancer.

Brain Tumours

Brain tumours are the most common solid tumours in children and are the second most common childhood cancer. The majority of tumours (about 60%) are infratentorial (below the tentorium cerebelli), which means that they occur in the posterior third of the brain, primarily in the cerebellum or brainstem. This anatomical distribution accounts for the frequency of symptoms resulting from increased ICP. The other tumours are supratentorial, or within the anterior two thirds of the brain, mainly the cerebrum.

Brain tumours, whether benign or malignant, can arise from any cell within the cranium. Consequently, the cranial cells' origin provides a histological classification for major tumours. For instance, astrocytes (cells that form the supportive tissue for neurons) may form a common glial tumour called an astrocytoma. The major infratentorial tumours are medulloblastomas, cerebellar astrocytomas, brainstem gliomas, and ependymomas, and the major supratentorial tumours are astrocytomas, hypothalamic tumours, optic pathway tumours, and craniopharyngiomas.

Diagnostic Evaluation

The signs and symptoms of brain tumours are directly related to their anatomical location and size and, to some extent, the child's age. In infants, whose cranial sutures are still open, virtually no early detectable symptoms develop. It is not until spinal fluid obstruction causes markedly increased head size that a lesion may be suspected. Even in older children, clinical manifestations are nonspecific. However, the most common symptoms are headache, especially on awakening, and vomiting that is not related to feeding. Vomiting occurs from increased ICP that compresses the brainstem, directly stimulating the vomiting centre in the medulla (Blaney et al., 2006).

Diagnosis of a brain tumour is based subjectively on presenting clinical signs and objectively on neurological tests and histological diagnosis via surgery. Because the signs and symptoms are vague and easily overlooked, early diagnosis relies on a high index of suspicion during history taking.

A number of tests may be used in the neurological evaluation, but the most common diagnostic procedure is MRI, which determines the location and extent of the tumour. Other tests that may be used include CT, angiography, electroencephalography, and lumbar puncture. Lumbar puncture is dangerous in the presence of increased ICP because of the possibility of brainstem herniation following a sudden release of pressure. The definitive diagnosis is based on brain tissue specimens obtained during surgery.

Therapeutic Management

Treatment may involve the use of surgery, radiotherapy, and chemotherapy. All three may be used, depending on the type of tumour. The treatment of choice is total removal of the tumour without residual neurological damage. Patients with the most complete tumour removal have the greatest chance of survival. Radiotherapy is used to treat most tumours and to shrink the size of the tumour before attempting surgical removal. Chemotherapy has emerged in the past decade to delay radiation in children younger than 3 years of age because of the rapid brain development occurring in the first 3 years of life (Blaney et al., 2006; Murray-Ryan & Petriccione, 2002). Chemotherapy is also used as adjunct therapy for residual tumour, nonresectable tumour, or recurrent tumour. Water-soluble agents are able to penetrate the disrupted blood–brain barrier and attack brain tumour cells (Blaney et al., 2006; Murray-Ryan & Petriccione, 2002). Typically, the most commonly used chemotherapy agents are cisplatin, carboplatin, vincristine, cyclophosphamide, lomustine, carmustine, etoposide, ifosfamide, and topotecan. Surgery (biopsy, resection, laser, or stereotactic), radiotherapy (hyperfractionated, fractionated, or stereotactic), and multiagent chemotherapy are all instrumental in the treatment of brain tumours.

Prognosis

The prognosis for the child with a brain tumour depends on the type of brain tumour, the tumour's size, the extent of the disease, and the child's age. Problems associated with treatment and a relatively poor prognosis, primarily in infants and young children, are compounded by serious late effects of therapy. A decline in the incidence of children with medulloblastoma has been significantly linked with a protective effect of maternal folate, iron, and multivitamin supplementation. Along with the recent advances in surgical instrumentation allowing aggressive surgical intervention (e.g., stereotactic surgery, radiosurgery), modifications in radiation (e.g., hyperfractionation, brain mapping) and use of chemotherapy (e.g., intrathecal, intratumoral) have increased the long-term survival rates for many children with brain tumours (Alston et al., 2003; Blaney et al., 2006; Gupta & Berger, 2003).

Nursing Care Management

A brain tumour is often suspected in a child admitted to the hospital with neurological dysfunction, although the actual diagnosis may not yet be confirmed. Establishing a baseline of data with which to compare preoperative and postoperative changes is an essential step toward planning physical care and preventing complications. It also allows the nurse to assess the degree of physical incapacity and the family's emotional reaction to the diagnosis.

Vital signs, including blood pressure and pulse pressure (the difference between systolic and diastolic pressures), need to be taken routinely and more often when any change is noted. Any sudden variations should be reported immediately. It is especially important to note a change in vital signs during or after diagnostic procedures. A routine neurological assessment is also performed at the same time as vital signs, and head circumference is measured on infants and very young children.

The child should be observed for evidence of headache, vomiting, and any seizure activity. The location, severity, and duration of the headache need to be noted, as well as its relationship to activity and time of day. Behaviours such as lying flat and facing away from light or refusing to engage in play are clues to discomfort in the nonverbal child. The child's gait should be observed at least once daily. Head tilt and other changes in posturing are always noted.

Prevent Postoperative Complications

Usually the surgeon will prescribe specific orders for vital signs, neurological checks, positioning, fluid regulation, and medication. These vary somewhat, depending on the location of the craniotomy. The following are general principles of care for infratentorial or supratentorial surgery. Additional aspects of care that are discussed elsewhere may include care of the child with seizures and neurological assessment of the unconscious child.

Vital signs should be taken as frequently as every 15 to 30 minutes until the child is stable. Temperature measurement is particularly important because of hyperthermia resulting from surgical intervention in the hypothalamus or brainstem and from some types of general anaesthesia. To prepare for this reaction, a cooling blanket should be placed on the bed before the child returns to the unit so that it is ready for use when needed. The temperature needs to be monitored carefully when any cooling measures are taken because hypothermia can occur suddenly. Recognizing signs of other complications such as increased ICP, meningitis, and respiratory tract infection is imperative.

Neurological checks are an essential aspect of care and include pupillary reaction to light, LOC, sleep patterns, and response to stimuli. Although children may be comatose for a few days, once they regain consciousness, there should be a steady increase in alertness. Regression to a lethargic, irritable state indicates increasing pressure, possibly caused by meningitis or cerebral edema.

NURSING ALERT Sluggish, dilated, or unequal pupils need to be reported immediately because they may indicate increased ICP and potential brainstem herniation, a medical emergency.

Observations for function are not instituted until the child regains consciousness. However, as soon as possible the nurse should begin testing reflexes, handgrip, and functioning of the cranial nerves. Muscle strength is usually diminished as a result of general weakness after surgery but should improve daily. Ataxia may be significantly worse with cerebellar intervention, but it will slowly improve. Edema near the cranial nerves may depress important functions such as the gag, blink, or swallowing reflex.

Dressings need to be observed for evidence of drainage. If soiled, the dressing is not removed but is reinforced with dry sterile gauze. The approximate amount of drainage should be estimated and recorded. A drain may be placed in the operative site.

NURSING ALERT To keep an accurate account of drainage, the soiled area is circled with a pen every hour or so. In this way, continuous bleeding is easily recognized. The presence of colourless drainage should be reported immediately, since it most likely is CSF from the incisional area. A foul odour from the dressing may indicate an infection. Such a finding should be reported, and a culture is taken.

Correct positioning after surgery is critical to prevent pressure against the operative site, reduce ICP, and avoid the danger of aspiration. If a large tumour was removed, the child should not be placed on the operative side, since the brain may suddenly shift to that cavity, causing trauma to the blood vessels, linings, and the brain itself. The nurse should confer with the surgeon to be certain of the correct position, including degree of neck flexion. The first 24 to 48 hours after brain surgery are critical. If the child's position is restricted, notice of this should be posted above the head of the bed. When the child is turned, any jarring or malalignment must be avoided, to prevent undue strain on the sutures. Two nurses are needed—one supporting the head and the other supporting the body. The use of a turning sheet may facilitate turning a heavy child.

The child with an infratentorial procedure is usually positioned on either side with the bed flat. When a supratentorial craniotomy is performed, the head of the bed is elevated 20 to 30 degrees with the child on either side or on the back. In a supratentorial craniotomy the head elevation facilitates CSF drainage and decreases excessive blood flow to the brain to prevent hemorrhage. Pillows should be placed against the child's back, not head, to maintain the desired position. Ordinarily the head and neck are kept in midline with the body, and the neck should not be flexed (Curley & Moloney-Harmon, 2001).

NURSING ALERT Trendelenburg's position is contraindicated in both infratentorial and supratentorial surgeries because it increases ICP and the risk of hemorrhage. If shock is impending, the practitioner should be notified immediately, before the head is lowered.

With an infratentorial craniotomy, the child is allowed nothing by mouth for at least 24 hours, or longer if the gag and swallowing reflexes are depressed or the child is comatose. With a supratentorial operation, clear fluids may be resumed soon after the child is alert, sometimes within 24 hours. If the child vomits, oral liquids are stopped. Vomiting not only predisposes the child to aspiration, but also increases ICP and the potential for incisional rupture.

The child should be fed to conserve energy and minimize movement. If there is any sign of facial paralysis, the child should be fed slowly to prevent choking or aspiration. Sometimes gavage feeding is necessary when body functions are too depressed to permit safe oral feedings or when the child refuses to eat or drink. IV fluids should be continued until oral fluids are well tolerated. Because of the postoperative cerebral edema and danger of increased ICP, fluids need to be carefully monitored.

Headache may be severe and is largely a result of cerebral edema. Measures to relieve some of the discomfort include providing a quiet, dimly lit environment; restricting visitors; preventing any sudden jarring movements, such as banging into the bed; and preventing an increase in ICP. Avoiding increased ICP is most effectively achieved by proper positioning and prevention of straining, such as during coughing, vomiting, or defecating. As stated earlier, the use of opioids, such as morphine, to relieve pain is controversial because it is thought that they may mask signs of altered consciousness or depress respirations. However, they can be given safely, since naloxone can be used to reverse opioid effects, such as sedation or respiratory depression. Acetaminophen and codeine are also effective analgesics for mild to moderate pain. Regardless of the medications used, adequate dosage and regular administration are essential to providing optimal pain relief (see also Pain Assessment; Pain Management, Chapter 35). Placing an ice bag on the forehead may also provide some headache relief, especially if facial edema is severe.

Support the Child and Family

The family's emotional needs are immense when the diagnosis is a brain tumour, and feelings are influenced by the extent of surgery, any neurological deficits, the expected prognosis, and additional therapy (see Additional Resources section at the end of this chapter). Since few definitive answers can be given before surgery, the surgeon's report is a significant finding that can vary from a completely benign, resected neoplasm to a highly malignant, invasive, and only partially removed tumour. Although parents try to prepare themselves for a potentially fatal diagnosis, it is a shock for them.

Parents should be encouraged to express their feelings about the diagnosis. Often they will express tremendous guilt for viewing the insidious onset of symptoms, such as ataxia, visual difficulty, or headache, as "minor complaints" by the child. Any comments that insinuate that the parents should have sought medical advice sooner should be avoided; such remarks only add to the parents' feelings of guilt and remorse.

During this period, the nurse should also discuss with parents what they plan to tell the child. If the child was prepared honestly, the diagnosis can be expressed in a similar manner. During recovery the child will need additional explanation about the treatment and the reason for any residual neurological effects, such as ataxia or blindness.

Neuroblastoma

Neuroblastomas are the most common malignant extracranial solid tumours in children. In Canada from 2003 to 2007, there were 392 children and youths ages 0 to 19 years who were newly diagnosed with neuroblastoma (Canadian Cancer Society, Steering Committee on Cancer Statistics, 2011). It is rare in adults, and more than 96% of patients diagnosed with neuroblastoma are less than 10 years of age (Mueller & Matthay, 2009). Almost 90% of neuroblastomas are diagnosed in children younger than 5 years of age. Between 2002 and 2006, 71 deaths due to neuroblastoma occurred in children and youths 0 to 19 years of age in Canada (Canadian Cancer Society, Steering Committee on Cancer Statistics, 2011). These tumours originate from embryonic neural crest cells that normally give rise to the adrenal medulla and the sympathetic ganglia. Consequently, the majority of tumours develop in the adrenal gland or the retroperitoneal sympathetic chain. Other sites may be in the head, neck, chest, or pelvis.

Neuroblastoma is a "silent" tumour. In more than 70% of cases, diagnosis is made after metastasis occurs, with the first signs caused by involvement in the nonprimary site, usually the lymph nodes, bone marrow, skeletal system, skin, or liver.

Diagnostic Evaluation

The objective of diagnosis is to locate the primary site and areas of metastasis. The signs and symptoms of neuroblastoma depend on the location and stage of the disease. Most presenting signs are caused by compression of adjacent structures. Skeletal survey; skull, neck, chest, abdominal, and bone CT scans; and bilateral bone marrow aspirations and biopsies are used to locate a tumour mass and metastasis. A metaiodobenzylguanidine (MIBG) scan is used to determine involvement of bone or tissue; however, it is only available at certain centres.

Urinary excretion of catecholamines is detected in approximately 95% of children with adrenal or sympathetic tumours. Analyzing the breakdown products excreted in the urine, namely vanillylmandelic acid, homovanillic acid, dopamine, and norepinephrine, permits detection of suspected tumour before and after medical-surgical intervention (Brodeur & Maris, 2006; Kline & Sevier, 2003). Amplification of proto-oncogene, known as the *N-myc* gene, and chromosomal abnormalities correlates strongly with advanced-stage disease, rapid tumour progression, and a poor prognosis (Brodeur & Maris, 2006).

Therapeutic Management

evolve Case Study–Meningitis

Accurate clinical staging is important for establishing initial treatment. Therefore, surgery is used both to remove as much of the tumour as possible and to obtain biopsies. In early stages, complete surgical removal of the tumour is the treatment of choice. If the tumour is large, partial resection is attempted, with a course of irradiation postoperatively to shrink the tumour in the hope of complete removal at a later date. Surgery is usually limited to biopsy in stages III and IV because of the extensive metastasis, although the use of additional surgery to assess tumour regression or remove a regressed tumour is not unlikely.

Radiotherapy provides emergency management of a massive neuroblastoma causing spinal cord compression (Kline & Sevier, 2003). Radiotherapy also offers palliation for metastatic lesions in the bones, lung, liver, or brain.

Chemotherapy is the mainstay of therapy for extensive local or disseminated disease. Agents used in various combinations include cyclophosphamide, doxorubicin, cisplatin, etoposide, vincristine, ifosfamide, carboplatin, topotecan, and teniposide. In children with high-risk disease or recurrent disease, retinoic acid, radiotherapy, and myeloablative chemotherapy with peripheral stem cell rescue may be used to obtain a longer remission, even though the overall survival rate is poor (Brodeur & Maris, 2006; Kline & Sevier, 2003).

Prognosis

If all stages are grouped together, the 5-year disease-free survival rates range from 88 to 90% for children in the low-risk stage, and from 22 to 30% in children in the high-risk stage (Brodeur & Maris, 2006). Generally, the younger the child at diagnosis (especially younger than 1 year of age), the better the survival rate. Neuroblastoma is one of the few tumours that demonstrate spontaneous regression (especially stage IV-S), possibly as a result of maturity of the embryonic cell or the development of an active immune system.

Nursing Care Management

Nursing considerations are similar to those discussed for leukemia and brain tumours, including psychological and physical preparation for diagnostic and operative procedures; prevention of postoperative complications for abdominal, thoracic, or cranial surgery; and explanation of chemotherapy, radiotherapy, and their side effects.

Since this tumour carries a poor prognosis for many children, every consideration must be given the family in terms of coping with a life-threatening illness (see Chapter 41). Because of the high degree of metastasis at the time of diagnosis, many parents suffer substantial guilt for not having recognized signs earlier. Parents need much support in dealing with these feelings and expressing them to the appropriate people.

Intracranial Infections

The nervous system is subject to infection by the same organisms that affect other organs of the body. However, the nervous system is limited in the ways in which it responds to injury. Laboratory studies are needed to identify the causative agent. The inflammatory process can affect the meninges (meningitis) or brain (encephalitis).

Meningitis can be caused by a variety of organisms, but the three main types are (1) bacterial, or pyogenic, caused by pus-forming bacteria, especially meningococci, pneumococci, and *Haemophilus* organisms, (2) viral, or aseptic, caused by a wide variety of viral agents, and (3) tuberculous, caused by the tuberculin bacillus. Most children with acute febrile encephalopathy have either bacterial meningitis or viral meningitis as the underlying cause.

Bacterial Meningitis

Bacterial meningitis is an acute inflammation of the meninges and CSF. It remains a significant cause of illness in the pediatric age groups because of the residual damage caused by undiagnosed and untreated or inadequately treated cases. Overall, the incidence rate has been highest among children less than 1 year of age and then declines as age increases, except for a smaller peak in the 15- to 19-year age group, with an increased mortality risk in the adolescent and young adult (PHAC, 2008; Saez-Llorens & McCracken, 2003; Sotir et al., 2005).

Bacterial meningitis can be caused by a variety of bacterial agents. Currently, *H. influenzae* type b, *S. pneumoniae*, and *Neisseria meningitidis* (meningococcus) are responsible for bacterial meningitis in 95% of children older than 2 months. Other organisms are β-hemolytic streptococci, *Staphylococcus aureus*, and *Escherichia coli*. The leading causes of neonatal meningitis are group B streptococci, *E. coli*, and *Listeria* monocytogenes. *E. coli* infection is seldom seen beyond infancy.

In Canada, meningococcal outbreaks are almost exclusively due to serogroup C *Neisseria meningitidis*. Immunization campaigns using serogroup C polysaccharide and conjugate vaccines were implemented in some regions during the 1999–2001 outbreak period. Recent data suggest that incidence rates of serogroup C are decreasing; however, more data are needed. An increasing trend in the incidence of serogroup Y disease has been observed in the United States during the past decade, although no such trends have been observed in Canada over this time (PHAC, 2008).

Meningococcal meningitis occurs in epidemic form and is the only type readily transmitted by droplet infection from nasopharyngeal secretions. Although this condition may develop at any age, the risk of meningococcal infection increases with the number of contacts; it occurs predominantly in school-age children and adolescents.

There appear to be some seasonal variations. Meningitis caused by *H. influenzae* primarily occurs in autumn or early winter. Pneumococcal and meningococcal infections can occur at any time but are more common in later winter or early spring.

Pathophysiology

The most common route of infection is vascular dissemination from a focus of infection elsewhere. For example, organisms from the nasopharynx invade the underlying blood vessels and enter the cerebral blood supply or form local thromboemboli that release septic emboli into the bloodstream. Invasion by direct extension from infections in the paranasal and mastoid sinuses is less common. Organisms also gain entry by direct implantation after penetrating wounds, skull fractures that provide an opening into the skin or sinuses, lumbar puncture or surgical procedures, anatomical abnormalities such as spina bifida, or foreign bodies such as an internal ventricular shunt or an external ventricular device. Once implanted, the organisms spread into the CSF, by which the infection spreads throughout the subarachnoid space.

The infective process is like that seen in any bacterial infection: inflammation, exudation, white blood cell accumulation, and varying degrees of tissue damage. The brain becomes hyperemic and edematous, and the entire surface of the brain is covered by a layer of purulent exudate that varies with the type of organism. For example, meningococcal exudate is most marked over the parietal, occipital, and cerebellar regions; the thick, fibrinous exudate of pneumococcal infection is confined chiefly to the surface of the brain, particularly the anterior lobes; and the exudate of streptococcal infections is similar to that of pneumococcal infections, but thinner.

As infection extends to the ventricles, thick pus, fibrin, or adhesions may occlude the narrow passages and obstruct the flow of CSF.

Clinical Manifestations

The clinical manifestations of acute bacterial meningitis depend to a large extent on the child's age. The picture is also influenced to some degree by the type of organism, the effectiveness of therapy for antecedent illness, and whether it occurs as an isolated entity or as a complication of another illness or injury. The onset of illness is likely to be abrupt, with fever, chills, headache, and vomiting that are associated with or quickly followed by alterations in sensorium. See Box 51-5 for clinical manifestations of bacterial meningitis.

NURSING ALERT Any child who is ill and develops a purpuric or petechial rash may have (overwhelming) meningococcemia and must receive medical attention immediately.

Diagnostic Evaluation

A lumbar puncture is the definitive diagnostic test. The fluid pressure is measured, and samples are obtained for culture, Gram stain, blood cell count, and determination of glucose and protein content. The findings are usually diagnostic. Culture and sensitivity testing are needed to identify the causative organism. Spinal fluid pressure is usually elevated, but interpretation is often difficult when the child is crying. Sedation with fentanyl and midazolam can alleviate the child's pain and fear associated with this procedure. If there is evidence or suspicion of increased ICP (papilledema, focal neurological deficits, bulging fontanel), a CT scan of the head may be warranted before the procedure.

The patient generally has an elevated white blood cell count, often predominantly polymorphonuclear leukocytes. The glucose level is reduced, generally in proportion to the duration and severity of the infection. The relationship between the CSF glucose and serum glucose levels is important in evaluating the glucose content of CSF; thus a serum glucose sample is drawn approximately one half hour before the lumbar puncture. Protein concentration is usually increased.

A blood culture is advisable for all children suspected of having meningitis and occasionally will be positive when CSF culture is negative. Nose and throat cultures may provide helpful information in some cases.

Therapeutic Management

Acute bacterial meningitis is a medical emergency that requires early recognition and immediate institution of therapy to prevent death or residual disabilities. The initial therapeutic management includes the following:

- Isolation precautions
- Initiation of antimicrobial therapy: a combination of vancomycin and a third-generation cephalosporin
- Maintenance of hydration
- Maintenance of ventilation
- Reduction of increased ICP
- Management of systemic shock

BOX 51-5 Clinical Manifestations of Bacterial Meningitis

Children and Adolescents

Usually abrupt onset
Fever
Chills
Headache
Vomiting
Alterations in sensorium
Seizures (often the initial sign)
Irritability
Agitation
May develop:
- Photophobia
- Delirium
- Hallucinations
- Aggressive behaviour
- Drowsiness
- Stupor
- Coma

Nuchal rigidity: May progress to opisthotonos
Positive Kernig and Brudzinski signs
Hyperactive but variable reflex responses
Signs and symptoms peculiar to individual organisms:
- Petechial or purpuric rashes (meningococcal infection), especially when associated with a shocklike state
- Joint involvement (meningococcal and *Haemophilus influenzae* infection)
- Chronically draining ear (pneumococcal meningitis)

Infants and Young Children

Classic picture (above) rarely seen in children between 3 months and 2 years of age
Fever
Poor feeding
Vomiting
Marked irritability
Frequent seizures (often accompanied by a high-pitched cry)
Bulging fontanel
Nuchal rigidity (may or may not be present)
Brudzinski and Kernig signs not helpful in diagnosis
Difficult to elicit and evaluate in this age group
Subdural empyema (*H. influenzae* infection)

Neonates: Specific Signs

Extremely difficult to diagnose
Manifestations vague and nonspecific
Well at birth but within a few days begins to look and behave poorly
Refusal of feedings
Poor sucking ability
Vomiting or diarrhea
Poor tone
Lack of movement
Weak cry
Full, tense, and bulging fontanel sometimes appearing late in course of illness
Neck usually supple

Neonates: Nonspecific Signs That May Be Present

Hypothermia or fever (depending on the infant's maturity)
Jaundice
Irritability
Drowsiness
Seizures
Respiratory irregularities or apnea
Cyanosis
Weight loss

- Control of seizures
- Control of temperature
- Treatment of complications

The child should be isolated from other children, usually in a critical care unit for close observation. An IV infusion is started to facilitate the administration of antimicrobial agents, fluids, anti-epileptic medications, and blood, if needed. The child should be placed on a cardiac monitor and in respiratory isolation (Canadian Paediatric Society [CPS], Infectious Diseases and Immunization Committee, 2008)

Medications

Until the causative organism is identified, the choice of antibiotic is based on the known sensitivity of the organism most likely to be the infective agent. After identification of the organism, antimicrobial agents are adjusted accordingly.

Dexamethasone can be used as an adjunctive treatment for children older than 6 weeks of age with suspected bacterial meningitis. It should be given before or within 1 hour of antibiotic administration (CPS, Infectious Diseases and Immunization Committee, 2008; Prober, 2007). It should not be used if aseptic or nonbacterial meningitis is suspected (Bonthius & Karacay, 2002).

Signs of gastrointestinal hemorrhage or secondary infection may complicate steroid administration. Antibiotic treatment with cephalosporins demonstrates superiority for promptly sterilizing the CSF and reducing the incidence of severe hearing impairment.

Nonspecific Measures

Maintaining hydration is a prime concern, and IV fluids and the type and amount of fluid are determined by the patient's condition. The optimum hydration involves correction of any fluid deficits followed by fluid restriction as ordered to prevent cerebral edema. Cerebral edema and electrolyte disturbances are associated with poor neurological outcome following bacterial meningitis (Bonthius & Karacay, 2002). Children with bacterial meningitis must be monitored for signs of increased ICP. If needed, measures to decrease ICP are implemented (see p. 1570).

Complications need to be treated appropriately, such as aspiration of subdural effusion in infants and treatment for disseminated intravascular coagulation syndrome. Shock is managed by restoration of circulating blood volume and maintenance of electrolyte balance. Seizures can occur during the first few days of treatment. These are controlled with the appropriate anti-epileptic medication. Hearing loss is not uncommon. The patient should undergo auditory evaluation 6 months after the illness has resolved.

Lumbar puncture is carried out as needed to determine the effectiveness of therapy. The patient should be evaluated neurologically during the convalescent period.

Prognosis

Approximately 10% of cases of bacterial meningitis are fatal (Health Canada, 2006a). The child's age, duration of illness before antibiotic therapy, rapidity of diagnosis after onset, type of organism, and adequacy of therapy are important in the prognosis for bacterial meningitis. Bacterial meningitis can result in brain damage, hearing loss, or learning disability (Prober, 2007).

Neonatal meningitis carries the highest mortality. However, with the development of new antibiotics and the advent of aggressive supportive care measures, the mortality rate for bacterial meningitis in children caused by *H. influenzae* type b, *S. pneumoniae*, and *N. meningitidis* is less than 10% in most studies (Prober, 2007).

The sequelae of bacterial meningitis are seen most often when the disease occurs in the first 2 months of life and least often in children with meningococcal meningitis. The residual deficits in infants are primarily a result of communicating hydrocephalus and the greater effects of cerebritis on the immature brain. In older children, the residual effects are related to the inflammatory process itself or result from vasculitis associated with the disease. Bacterial meningitis continues to cause substantial morbidity in infants and children. The mortality rate and incidence of poor neurological outcome are highest in patients with pneumococcal meningitis (Prober, 2007).

Hearing impairment is the most common sequela of this disease. Evaluation of cranial nerve VIII is needed for at least a 6-month follow-up period to assess for possible hearing loss.

Prevention

In Canada, meningococcal C conjugate vaccines are recommended for routine immunization of infants, children aged 1 to 4 years, and for adolescent and young adults to prevent the increased risk of serogroup C meningococcal disease in these age groups. The recommended schedule differs depending on the vaccine used. For children at least 5 years of age who have not reached adolescence, immunization with a single dose of MenC-conjugate vaccine may also be considered. A single dose is required for any person at least 1 year of age. Polysaccharide vaccine is not recommended for routine immunization for infants and children in Canada. Routine vaccinations for *H. influenzae* type b and pneumococcal conjugate vaccine are recommended for all children beginning at 2 months of age (CPS, Infectious Diseases and Immunization Committee, 2008; PHAC, 2006) (see Immunizations, Chapter 36).

NURSING ALERT A major priority of nursing care of a child suspected of having meningitis is to administer antibiotics as soon as they are ordered. The child is placed on respiratory isolation for at least 24 hours after initiation of antimicrobial therapy.

Nursing Care Management

The room should be kept as quiet as possible and environmental stimuli kept to a minimum because most children with meningitis are sensitive to noise, bright lights, and other external stimuli. Most children are more comfortable without a pillow and with the head of the bed slightly elevated. A side-lying position is more often assumed because of nuchal rigidity. The nurse should avoid actions that cause pain or increase discomfort, such as lifting the child's head. Evaluating the child for pain and implementing appropriate relief measures are important during the initial 24 to 72 hours. Acetaminophen with codeine is often used. Measures to ensure safety should be observed, because the child is often restless and subject to seizures.

The nursing care of the child with meningitis is determined by the child's symptoms and treatment. Observation of vital signs, neurological signs, LOC, urine output, and other pertinent data needs to be carried out at frequent intervals. The child who is unconscious is managed as described previously (see p. 1569), and all children are observed carefully for signs of the complications just described, especially increased ICP, shock, or respiratory distress. Frequent assessment of the open fontanels is needed in the infant because subdural effusions and obstructive hydrocephalus can develop as a complication of meningitis.

Fluids and nourishment are determined by the child's status. The child with dulled sensorium is usually given nothing by mouth. Other children are allowed clear liquids initially and, if these are tolerated, progress to a diet suitable for their age. Careful monitoring and recording of intake and output are needed to determine deviations that might indicate impending shock or increasing fluid accumulation, such as cerebral edema or subdural effusion.

One of the most difficult problems in the nursing care of children with meningitis is maintaining IV infusion for the length of time needed to provide adequate antimicrobial therapy (usually 10 days). Because continuous IV fluids are usually not necessary, an **intermittent infusion device** is used. In some cases, children who are recovering uneventfully are sent home with the device, and the parents are taught IV medication administration.

Family Support

The sudden nature of the illness makes emotional support of the child and parents extremely important. Parents are upset and concerned about their child's condition and often feel guilty for not having suspected the seriousness of the illness sooner. They need much reassurance that the natural onset of meningitis is sudden and that they acted responsibly in seeking medical assistance when they did. The nurse should encourage the parents to openly discuss their feelings to minimize blame and guilt. They also need to be kept informed of the child's progress and of all procedures, results, and treatments. In the event that the child's condition worsens, they need the same psychological care as parents who face the possible death of their child (see Chapter 41).

Nonbacterial (Aseptic) Meningitis

Aseptic meningitis is caused by many different viruses. The onset may be abrupt or gradual. The initial manifestations are headache, fever, malaise, and gastrointestinal symptoms. Signs of meningeal irritation develop 1 or 2 days after the onset of illness. Onset is more insidious in infants and toddlers. Signs and symptoms are vague and are often thought to be associated with a minor illness.

Diagnosis is based on clinical features and CSF findings. Variations in CSF values in bacterial and viral meningitis are listed in Table 51-2. It is important to differentiate this self-limited disorder from the more serious forms of meningitis.

Treatment is primarily symptomatic, such as acetaminophen for headache and muscle pain, maintenance of hydration, and positioning for comfort. Until a definitive diagnosis is made, antimicrobial agents may be administered and isolation enforced as a precaution against the possibility that the disease might be of bacterial origin. Nursing care is similar to the care of the child with bacterial meningitis.

Encephalitis

Encephalitis is an inflammatory process of the CNS that is caused by a variety of organisms, including bacteria, spirochetes, fungi, protozoa, helminths, and viruses. Most infections are associated with viruses; this discussion is limited to those agents.

Etiology

Encephalitis can occur as a result of (1) direct invasion of the CNS by a virus or (2) postinfectious involvement of the CNS after a viral disease. Often the specific type of encephalitis may not be identified. The cause of more than half the cases reported in Canada is unknown. The majority of cases of known etiology are associated with the childhood diseases of measles, mumps, varicella, and rubella and, less often, with the enteroviruses, herpesviruses, and West Nile virus.

While herpes simplex encephalitis is an uncommon disease, 30% of cases involve children. The initial clinical findings are nonspecific (fever, altered mental status), but most cases evolve to demonstrate focal neurological signs and symptoms. Children may experience focal seizures. The CSF is abnormal in most cases. Because of a rise in the number of children with herpes simplex encephalitis, suspected cases require prompt attention, especially because the diagnosis can be difficult. The clinical diagnosis can be confirmed by the rapid appearance of immunoglobulin M antibody to herpes simplex virus type 1 in CSF and serum. The early use of IV acyclovir reduces mortality and morbidity. Empiric therapy with acyclovir is given before precise virological diagnosis has been established. CSF should be sent for viral titres.

The multiplicity of causes of viral encephalitis makes diagnosis difficult. Most are those involved with arthropod vectors (togaviruses and bunyaviruses) and those associated with hemorrhagic fevers (arenaviruses, filoviruses, and hantaviruses). In Canada, the risk of acquiring West Nile virus is very low, particularly in children; for more information see Additional Resources section at the end of this chapter.

The clinical features of encephalitis are similar regardless of the agent involved. Manifestations can range from a mild benign form that resembles aseptic meningitis, lasts a few days, and is followed by rapid and complete recovery, to a fulminating encephalitis with severe CNS involvement. The onset may be sudden or may be gradual with malaise, fever, headache, dizziness, apathy, nuchal rigidity, nausea and vomiting, ataxia, tremors, hyperactivity, and speech difficulties (Box 51-6). In severe cases the patient has high fever, stupor, seizures, disorientation, spasticity, and coma that may proceed to death. Ocular palsies and paralysis also may occur.

Diagnostic Evaluation

The diagnosis is made on the basis of clinical findings and, where possible, identification of the specific virus. Early in the course of encephalitis, CT scan results may be normal. Later, hemorrhagic areas in the frontotemporal region may be seen. Togaviruses (some of which were formerly labelled arboviruses) are rarely detected in the blood or spinal fluid, but viruses of herpes, mumps, measles, and enteroviruses may be

Table 51-2 Variation of Cerebrospinal Fluid Analysis in Bacterial and Viral Meningitis

MANIFESTATIONS	BACTERIAL*	VIRAL
White blood cell count	Elevated; increased polys	Slightly elevated; increased lymphs
Protein content	Elevated	Normal or slightly increased
Glucose content	Decreased	Normal
Gram stain; bacteria culture	Positive	Turbid or cloudy
Colour	Negative	Clear or slightly cloudy

*Results may vary in the neonate.

BOX 51-6 Clinical Manifestations of Encephalitis

Onset: Sudden or Gradual

Malaise
Fever
Headache
Dizziness
Apathy
Lethargy
Nucal rigidity

Severe Cases

High fever
Stupor
Seizures
Disorientation
Nausea and vomiting
Ataxia
Tremors
Hyperactivity
Speech difficulties—mutism
Altered mental status
Spasticity
Coma (may proceed to death)
Ocular palsies
Paralysis

found in the CSF. Serological testing may be required. The first blood sample should be drawn as soon as possible after onset, with the second sample drawn 2 or 3 weeks later.

Therapeutic Management

Patients suspected of having encephalitis are hospitalized promptly for observation. Treatment is primarily supportive and includes conscientious nursing care, control of cerebral manifestations, and adequate nutrition and hydration, with observation and management as for other cerebral disorders. Viral encephalitis can cause devastating neurological injury. Cerebral hyperemia occurs in severe viral encephalitis, and ICP monitoring to reduce the pressure may be needed (Prober, 2007). Follow-up care with periodic re-evaluation and rehabilitation is important for patients who develop residual effects of the disease.

The prognosis for the child with encephalitis depends on the child's age, the type of organism, and residual neurological damage. Very young children (younger than 2 years of age) may exhibit increased neurological disability, including learning difficulties and seizure disorders.

Nursing Care Management

Nursing care of the child with encephalitis is the same as for any unconscious child and for the child with meningitis. Additional nursing interventions include observation for deterioration in consciousness. Isolation of the child is not necessary; however, good hand hygiene technique must be followed. A main focus of nursing management is the control of rapidly rising ICP. Neurological monitoring, administration of medications, and support of the child and parents are the major aspects of care.

Rabies

Rabies is an acute infection of the nervous system caused by a virus that is almost invariably fatal if left untreated. It is transmitted to humans by the saliva of an infected mammal and is introduced through a bite or skin abrasion. After entry into a new host, the virus multiplies in muscle cells and is spread through neural pathways without stimulating a protective host immune response.

Approximately 85% of rabies cases come from wild animals and 15% from domestic animals. Carnivorous wild animals (skunks, raccoons, and bats) are the animals most often infected with rabies and the cause of most indigenous cases of human rabies in Canada (PHAC, 2006; Toltzis, 2007). The likelihood of human exposure to a rabid domestic animal has decreased greatly due largely to excellent prevention and control programs (PHAC, 2006).

The circumstances of a biting incident are important. An unprovoked attack is more likely than a provoked attack to indicate a rabid animal. Bites inflicted on a child attempting to feed or handle an apparently healthy animal can generally be regarded as provoked. Any child bitten by a wild animal is assumed to be exposed to rabies.

NURSING ALERT Unusual behaviour in an animal is cause for suspicion; children should be warned to beware of wild animals that appear to be friendly.

Although rabies is common among wildlife species, human rabies is rarely acquired. Modern-day prophylaxis is nearly 100% successful. The highest incidence occurs in children under age 15 years. The incubation period usually ranges from 1 to 3 months but may be as short as 10 days or as long as 8 months. Only 10 to 15% of persons bitten develop the disease, but once symptoms are present, rabies progresses to a fatal outcome. In Canada, human fatalities associated with rabies occur in people who fail to seek medical attention, usually because they are unaware of their exposure.

The disease is characterized by a period of general malaise, fever, and sore throat followed by a phase of excitement that features hypersensitivity and increased reaction to external stimuli, convulsions, maniacal behaviour, and choking (Box 51-7). Attempts at swallowing may cause such severe spasm of respiratory muscles that apnea, cyanosis, and anoxia are produced—the characteristics from which the term *hydrophobia* was derived.

Diagnosis is made on the basis of history and clinical features. Treatment is of little avail once symptoms appear, but the long incubation period allows time for the induction of active and passive immunity before the onset of illness.

Therapeutic Management

Two types of immunizing products are available for use in humans: (1) the inactivated rabies vaccines, which induce an active immune response; and (2) the globulins, which contain preformed antibodies. The two types of products should be used concurrently for rabies postexposure treatment when prophylaxis is indicated.

The current therapy for a rabid animal bite consists of thorough cleansing of the wound and passive immunization with human rabies immunoglobulin as soon as possible after exposure to provide rapid, short-term passive immunity (PHAC, 2006; Toltzis, 2007).

Postexposure active immunity is conferred by administration of the human diploid cell rabies vaccine. The first intramuscular injection of the vaccine is given at the same time as the immunoglobulin (day 0) and is followed by injections at 3, 7, 14, and 28 days after the first dose (PHAC, 2006; Toltzis, 2007). Before antirabies prophylaxis is initiated, the local or state health department should be consulted.

Nursing Care Management

Parents and children are frightened by the urgency and seriousness of the situation. They need **anticipatory guidance** for the therapy and support and reassurance regarding the efficacy of the preventive measures for this dreaded disease. The vaccine is well tolerated by children, although they need preparation for the series of injections.

Reye's Syndrome

RS is a disorder defined as toxic encephalopathy associated with other characteristic organ involvement. It is characterized by fever, profoundly impaired consciousness, and disordered hepatic function.

The etiology of RS is not well understood, but most cases follow a common viral illness, most commonly influenza or varicella. RS is a condition characterized pathologically by

BOX 51-7 Clinical Manifestations of Rabies

Initial Signs
General malaise
Fever
Anorexia
Sore throat

Excitement Phase
Hypersensitivity
Increased reaction to external stimuli
Seizures
Fluctuating consciousness
Choking

Severe Spasm of Respiratory Muscles*
Apnea
Cyanosis
Anoxia

*From attempts at swallowing (characteristics from which the term *hydrophobia* was derived).

BOX 51-8 Staging Criteria for Reye's Syndrome

Stage I—Vomiting, lethargy, and drowsiness; liver dysfunction; type I electroencephalogram (EEG); follows commands; pupillary reaction brisk

Stage II—Disorientation, combativeness, delirium, hyperventilation, hyperactive reflexes, appropriate responses to painful stimuli; evidence of liver dysfunction; type I EEG; pupillary reaction sluggish

Stage III—Obtunded, coma, hyperventilation, decorticate rigidity, preservation of pupillary light reaction and oculovestibular reflexes (although sluggish); type II EEG

Stage IV—Deepening coma, decerebrate rigidity, loss of oculocephalic reflexes, large and fixed pupils, loss of doll's eye reflex, loss of corneal reflexes; minimal liver dysfunction; type III or IV EEG; evidence of brainstem dysfunction

Stage V—Seizures, loss of deep tendon reflexes, respiratory arrest, flaccidity; type IV EEG; usually no evidence of liver dysfunction

cerebral edema and fatty changes of the liver. The onset of RS is notable for profuse vomiting and varying degrees of neurological impairment, including personality changes and deterioration in consciousness (Pugliese, Beltramo, & Torre, 2008). The cause of RS is a mitochondrial insult induced by different viruses, drugs, exogenous toxins, and genetic factors. Elevated serum ammonia levels tend to correlate with the clinical manifestations and prognosis.

Definitive diagnosis is established by liver biopsy. The staging criteria for RS are based on liver dysfunction and on neurological signs that range from lethargy to coma (Box 51-8). As a result of improved diagnostic techniques, children who in the past would have been diagnosed with RS are now diagnosed with other illnesses such as viral or metabolic diseases. Cases of unrecognized, drug-induced encephalopathy by anti-emetics given to children during viral illnesses have symptoms similar to those of RS.

The potential association between acetylsalicyclic acid (ASA) therapy for the treatment of fever in children with varicella or influenza and the development of RS precludes its use in these patients. Regulations under the *Food and Drugs Act*, 1985, now require manufacturers to label all over-the-counter products that have ASA with a warning about the dangers of giving ASA to a child or teenager (Health Canada, 2006b).

Therapeutic Management

The most important aspect of successful management of the child with RS is early diagnosis and aggressive therapy. Rapid progression through coma stages and high peak ammonia concentrations are associated with a more serious prognosis. Cerebral edema with increased ICP represents the most immediate threat to life. Recovery from RS is rapid and usually without sequelae if diagnosis is determined early and therapy is initiated promptly.

Prognosis

Although the incidence of RS has markedly decreased, health care providers must remind parents and caregivers to avoid using both aspirin and non-aspirin–containing salicylates during febrile illnesses in children (Bhutta, Van Savell, & Schexnayder, 2003; Kamienski, 2003). Survivors may have subtle neuropsychological deficits. Generally, recovery is good given the gravity of the disease (Bhutta et al., 2003; Kamienski, 2003).

Nursing Care Management

The most important aspect of successful management of the child with RS is early diagnosis and aggressive therapy (Bhutta et al., 2003). Cerebral edema with increased ICP represents the most immediate threat to life. Recovery from RS is rapid and usually without sequelae given early diagnosis and implementation of therapy. In about one third of patients, RS causes death or long-term neurological sequelae (Pugliese et al., 2008).

Care and observations are implemented as for any child with an altered state of consciousness (see p. 1591) and increasing ICP. Accurate and frequent monitoring of intake and output is essential for adjusting fluid volumes to prevent both dehydration and cerebral edema. Because of related liver dysfunction, laboratory studies to determine impaired coagulation, such as prolonged bleeding time, should be monitored.

Parents of children with RS need to be kept informed of the child's progress, to have diagnostic procedures and therapeutic management explained, and to be given concerned and sympathetic support (see Additional Resources at the end of this chapter). Families need to be aware that salicylate, the alleged offending ingredient in aspirin, is contained in other products (e.g., Pepto-Bismol). They should refrain from administering any product for influenza-like symptoms without first checking the label for "hidden" salicylates.

Seizure Disorders

Seizures are caused by excessive and disorderly neuronal discharges in the brain. The manifestation of seizures depends on the region of the brain in which they originate and may include unconsciousness or altered consciousness; involuntary movements; and changes in perception, behaviours, sensations, and posture. Seizures are the most common treatable neurological disorder in children and can occur with a wide variety of conditions involving the CNS.

Epilepsy

Epilepsy is a condition characterized by two or more unprovoked seizures and can be caused by a variety of pathological processes in the brain. Seizures are a symptom of an underlying disease process. A single seizure event should not be classified as epilepsy and is generally not treated with long-term anti-epileptic medications. Some seizures may result from an acute medical or neurological illness and cease once the illness is treated. In other cases, children may have a single seizure without the cause ever being known. Once it is determined that the child has had a seizure, it is important to classify the seizure, according to the Classification of Epileptic Seizures, and assign it to the appropriate epilepsy syndrome, according to the Classification of Epilepsies and Epileptic Syndromes. Optimum treatment and prognosis require an accurate diagnosis and a determination of the cause whenever possible.

Etiology

Seizures in children have many different causes. Seizures are classified according to not only type but also etiology. Acute symptomatic seizures are associated with an acute insult, such as head trauma or meningitis. Remote symptomatic seizures are those without an immediate cause but with an identifiable prior brain injury such as major head trauma, meningitis or encephalitis, hypoxia, stroke, or a static encephalopathy such as intellectual disability or cerebral palsy. Cryptogenic seizures are those occurring with no clear cause. **Idiopathic** seizures are genetic in origin. A partial list of causative factors is presented in Box 51-9.

Pathophysiology

Regardless of the etiological factor or type of seizure, the basic mechanism is the same. Abnormal electrical discharges (1) may arise from central areas in the brain that affect consciousness, (2) may be restricted to one area of the cerebral cortex, producing manifestations characteristic of that particular anatomical focus, or (3) may begin in a localized area of the cortex and spread to other portions of the brain and, if sufficiently extensive, produce generalized seizure activity.

In response to physiological stimuli, such as cellular dehydration, severe hypoglycemia, electrolyte imbalance, sleep deprivation, emotional stress, and endocrine changes, these hyperexcitable cells activate normal cells in surrounding areas and distant, synaptically related cells. A generalized seizure develops when the neuronal excitation from the epileptogenic focus spreads to the brainstem, particularly the midbrain and reticular formation. These centres within the brainstem, known as the *centrencephalic system*, are responsible for the spread of the epileptic potentials. The discharges can originate spontaneously in the centrencephalic system or be triggered by a focal area in the cortex. On the basis of these characteristic neuronal discharges (as recorded by the EEG), seizures are designated as *partial*, *generalized*, and *unclassified* epileptic seizures (Berg et al., 2010). In a large proportion of children, focal seizures spread to other areas, ultimately becoming generalized with loss of consciousness.

BOX 51-9 Etiology of Seizures in Children

Nonrecurrent (Acute)

Febrile episodes
Intracranial infection
Intracranial hemorrhage
Space-occupying lesions (cyst, tumour)
Acute cerebral edema
Anoxia
Toxins
Medications
Tetanus
Lead encephalopathy
Shigella, Salmonella organisms
Metabolic alterations:
- Hypocalcemia
- Hypoglycemia
- Hyponatremia or hypernatremia
- Hypomagnesemia
- Alkalosis
- Disorders of amino acid metabolism
- Deficiency states
- Hyperbilirubinemia

Recurrent (Chronic)

Idiopathic epilepsy
Epilepsy secondary to:
- Trauma
- Hemorrhage
- Anoxia
- Infections
- Toxins
- Degenerative phenomena
- Congenital defects
- Parasitic brain disease
- Hypoglycemia injury

Epilepsy—sensory stimulus
Epilepsy-stimulating states:
- Narcolepsy and catalepsy
- Psychogenic
- Tetany from hypocalcemia, alkalosis

Hypoglycemic states:
- Hyperinsulinism
- Hypopituitarism
- Adrenocortical insufficiency
- Hepatic disorders

Uremia
Allergy
Cardiovascular dysfunction or syncopal episodes
Migraine

evolve Animation—Seizure, Generalized

Seizure Classification and Clinical Manifestations

There are many different types of seizures, and each has unique clinical manifestations. Seizures are classified into three major categories:

1. Partial seizures, which have a local onset and involve a relatively small location in the brain
2. Generalized seizures, which involve both hemispheres of the brain and are without local onset
3. Unclassified epileptic seizures

Descriptions of the different types of seizures are found in Box 51-10 and Table 51-3.

Diagnostic Evaluation

Establishing a diagnosis is critical for establishing a prognosis and planning the proper treatment. The process of diagnosis in a child suspected of having epilepsy includes (1) determining whether epilepsy or seizures exist and not an alternative diagnosis, and (2) defining the underlying cause, if possible. The assessment and diagnosis rely heavily on a thorough history, skilled observation, and several diagnostic tests.

It is especially important to differentiate epilepsy from other brief alterations in consciousness or behaviour. Clinical entities that mimic seizures include migraine headaches, toxic effects of medications, syncope (fainting), breath-holding spells in infants and young children, movement disorders (tics, tremor, chorea), prolonged QT syndrome, sleep disturbances

BOX 51-10 Classification and Clinical Manifestations of Seizures

Partial Seizures

Simple Partial Seizures With Motor Signs

Characterized by:

- Localized motor symptoms
- Somatosensory, psychic, autonomic symptoms
- Combination of these
- Abnormal discharges remaining unilateral

Manifestations:

- Aversive seizure (most common motor seizure in children)—Eye or eyes and head turn away from the side of the focus; awareness of movement or loss of consciousness
- Rolandic (Sylvan) seizure—Tonic-clonic movements involving the face, salivation, arrested speech; most common during sleep
- Jacksonian march (rare in children)—Orderly, sequential progression of clonic movements beginning in a foot, hand, or face and moving, or "marching," to adjacent body parts

Simple Partial Seizures With Sensory Signs

Characterized by various sensations, including the following:

- Numbness, tingling, prickling, paresthesia, or pain originating in one area (e.g., face or extremities) and spreading to other parts of the body
- Visual sensations or formed images
- Motor phenomena such as posturing or hypertonia

Uncommon in children younger than 8 years of age

Complex Partial Seizures (Psychomotor Seizures)

Observed more often in children from 3 years through adolescence

Characterized by the following:

- Period of altered behaviour
- Amnesia for event (no recollection of behaviour)
- Inability to respond to environment
- Impaired consciousness during event
- Drowsiness or sleep usually following seizure
- Confusion and amnesia possibly prolonged
- Complex sensory phenomena (aura)—Most frequent sensation is a strange feeling in the pit of the stomach that rises toward the throat; often accompanied by:
  - Odd or unpleasant odours or tastes
  - Complex auditory or visual hallucinations
  - Ill-defined feelings of elation or strangeness (e.g., déjà vu, a feeling of familiarity in a strange environment)
  - Strong feelings of fear and anxiety; distorted sense of time and self
  - In small children, emission of a cry or attempt to run for help

Patterns of motor behaviour:

- Stereotypic
- Similar with each subsequent seizure
- May suddenly cease activity, appear dazed, stare into space, become confused and apathetic, and become limp or stiff or display some form of posturing
- May be confused
- May perform purposeless, complicated activities in a repetitive manner (automatisms), such as walking, running, kicking, laughing, or speaking incoherently, most often followed by postictal confusion or sleep
- May exhibit oropharyngeal activities, such as smacking, chewing, drooling, swallowing, and nausea or abdominal pain followed by stiffness, a fall, and postictal sleep
- Rarely manifests actions such as rage or temper tantrums; aggressive acts uncommon during seizure

Generalized Seizures

Tonic-Clonic Seizures (Formerly Known as Grand Mal)

Most common and most dramatic of all seizure manifestations

Occur without warning

Tonic Phase

Lasts approximately 10 to 20 seconds

Manifestations:

- Eyes roll upward
- Immediate loss of consciousness
- If standing, falls to floor or ground
- Stiffens in generalized, symmetrical tonic contraction of entire body musculature
- Arms usually flexed
- Legs, head, and neck extended
- May utter a peculiar piercing cry
- Apneic; may become cyanotic
- Increased salivation and loss of swallowing reflex

Clonic Phase

Lasts about 30 seconds but can vary from only a few seconds to a half hour or longer

BOX 51-10 Classification and Clinical Manifestations of Seizures—cont'd

Manifestations:
- Violent jerking movements as the trunk and extremities undergo rhythmic contraction and relaxation
- May foam at the mouth
- May be incontinent of urine and feces

As event ends, movements less intense, occurring at longer intervals, then ceasing entirely

Status Epilepticus

Series of seizures at intervals too brief to allow the child to regain consciousness between the time one event ends and the next begins
- Requires emergency intervention
- Can lead to exhaustion, respiratory failure, and death

Postictal State

Manifestations:
- Appears to relax
- May remain semiconscious and difficult to arouse
- May awaken in a few minutes
- Remains confused for several hours
- Poor coordination
- Mild impairment of fine motor movements
- May have visual and speech difficulties
- May vomit or complain of severe headache
- When left alone, usually sleeps for several hours
- On awakening is fully conscious
- Usually feels tired and complains of sore muscles and headache
- No recollection of entire event

Absence Seizures (Formerly Called Petit Mal or Lapses)

Characterized by:
- Onset usually between 4 and 12 years of age
- More common in girls than in boys
- Usually cease at puberty
- Brief loss of consciousness
- Minimum or no alteration in muscle tone
- May go unrecognized because of little change in child's behaviour
- Abrupt onset; suddenly develops 20 or more attacks daily
- Event often mistaken for inattentiveness or daydreaming
- Events possibly precipitated by hyperventilation, hypoglycemia, stresses (emotional and physiological), fatigue, or sleeplessness

Manifestations:
- Brief loss of consciousness
- Appear without warning or aura
- Usually last about 5 to 10 seconds
- Slight loss of muscle tone may cause child to drop objects
- Ability to maintain postural control; seldom falls
- Minor movements such as lip smacking, twitching of eyelids or face, or slight hand movements
- Not accompanied by incontinence
- Amnesia for episode
- May need to reorient self to previous activity

Atonic and Akinetic Seizures (Also Known as Drop Attacks)

Characterized by:
- Onset usually between 2 and 5 years of age
- Sudden, momentary loss of muscle tone and postural control
- Events recurring frequently during the day, particularly in the morning hours and shortly after awakening

Manifestations:
- Loss of tone causing child to fall to the floor violently; unable to break fall by putting out hand; may incur a serious injury to the face, head, or shoulder
- Loss of consciousness only momentary

Myoclonic Seizures

A variety of seizure episodes

May be isolated as benign essential myoclonus

May occur in association with other seizure forms

Characterized by:
- Sudden, brief contractures of a muscle or group of muscles
- Occur singly or repetitively
- No postictal state
- May or may not be symmetrical
- May or may not include loss of consciousness

Infantile Spasms

Also called infantile myoclonus, massive spasms, hypsarrhythmia, salaam episodes, or infantile myoclonic spasms

Most commonly occur during the first 6 to 8 months of life

Twice as common in boys as in girls

Numerous seizures during the day without postictal drowsiness or sleep

Poor outlook for normal intelligence

Manifestations:
- Possible series of sudden, brief, symmetrical, muscular contractions
- Head flexed, arms extended, and legs drawn up
- Eyes sometimes rolling upward or inward
- May be preceded or followed by a cry or giggling
- May or may not include loss of consciousness
- Sometimes flushing, pallor, or cyanosis

Infants who are able to sit but not stand:
- Sudden dropping forward of the head and neck with trunk flexed forward and knees drawn up—the salaam or jackknife seizure

Less often: alternate clinical forms:
- Extensor spasms rather than flexion of arms, legs, and trunk, and head nodding
- Lightning events involving a single, momentary, shock-like contraction of the entire body

Table 51-3 Comparison of Simple Partial, Complex Partial, and Absence Seizures

CLINICAL MANIFESTATIONS	SIMPLE PARTIAL	COMPLEX PARTIAL	ABSENCE
Age of onset	Any age	Uncommon before age 3 yr	Uncommon before age 3 yr
Frequency (per day)	Variable	Rarely >1–2 times	Multiple
Duration	Usually <30 sec	Usually >60 sec, rarely <10 sec	Usually <10 sec, rarely >30 sec
Aura	May be sole manifestation of seizure	Frequent	Never
Impaired consciousness	Never	Always	Always; brief loss of consciousness
Automatisms	Never	Frequent	Frequent
Clonic movements	Frequent	Occasional	Occasional
Postictal impairment	Rare	Frequent	Never
Mental disorientation	Rare	Common	Unusual

(sleepwalking, night terrors), psychogenic seizures, rage attacks, and transient ischemic attacks (rare in children) (Browne & Holmes, 2004). Cocaine intoxication should be considered in the differential diagnosis of new-onset seizure activity in newborn infants.

The history of the seizure should be equally detailed, including the type of seizure or description of the child's behaviour during the event, the age at onset, and the time at which the seizure occurs (e.g., early morning, before meals, while awake, or during sleep). Any factors that may have precipitated the seizure are important, including fever, infection, head trauma, anxiety, fatigue, sleep deprivation, menstrual cycle, alcohol, and activity (e.g., hyperventilation or exposure to strong stimuli such as bright flashing light or loud noises). If the child can describe any sensory phenomena, these should be recorded. The duration and progression of the seizure (if any) and the postictal feelings and behaviour (e.g., confusion, inability to speak, amnesia, headache, and sleep) should also be recorded. It is important to determine whether more than one seizure type exists. It is often more informative to ask parents to mime the seizure rather than relying on their oral description. Miming often reveals features, such as head turning, that would otherwise go unrecognized. Some seizures are overlooked by parents. For example, some parents may not identify brief head nods or brief single jerks as seizures unless specifically asked whether their child has these symptoms. The family history should include whether other family members have had a seizure, intellectual disability, cerebral palsy, or other neurological disorders. A family history can offer clues to paroxysmal disorders such as migraine headaches, breath-holding spells, febrile seizures, or neurological diseases.

A complete physical and neurological examination, including developmental assessment of language, learning, behaviour, and motor abilities, may provide clues to the cause of the seizures. A number of laboratory and neuroimaging tests may be ordered depending on the child's age, whether this is a new onset seizure, characteristics of the seizure, and the history. Laboratory studies that may prove to be of value include a venous lead level if the history warrants or white blood cell count (for signs of infection). Blood glucose may give evidence of hypoglycemic episodes, and serum electrolytes, blood urea nitrogen, calcium, serum amino acids, lactate, ammonia, and urine organic acids may indicate metabolic disturbances. Blood for chromosomal analysis may also be tested if a genetic etiology is suspected. A toxic screen may be done if alcohol or drug use or withdrawal is suspected. Lumbar puncture can confirm a suspected diagnosis of meningitis. CT may be done to detect a cerebral hemorrhage, infarctions, and gross malformations. MRI provides greater anatomical detail and is used to detect developmental malformations, tumours, and cortical dysplasias (Kuzniecky, 2001).

The EEG is obtained for all children with seizures and is the most useful tool for evaluating a seizure disorder. The EEG confirms the presence of abnormal electrical discharges and provides information on the seizure type and the focus. The EEG is carried out under varying conditions—with the child asleep, awake, awake with provocative stimulation (flashing lights, noise), and hyperventilating. Stimulation may elicit abnormal electrical activity, which is recorded on the EEG. Various seizure types produce characteristic EEG patterns: high-voltage spike discharges are seen in tonic-clonic seizures, with abnormal patterns in the intervals between seizures; a three-per-second spike and wave pattern is observed in an absence seizure; and absence of electrical activity in an area suggests a large lesion, such as an abscess or subdural collection of fluid.

A normal EEG does not rule out seizures because the EEG is only a surface recording that represents approximately 1 hour of time; therefore it may show normal interictal activity. If there is concern about whether a child has seizures or the seizure type cannot be determined, then a long-term video EEG may be done to record the child during wakefulness and sleep. The full body image is recorded on video, with selected EEG channels displayed on the same screen for simultaneous recording and viewing. EEG monitoring is also available in digital EEG and digital video imaging, which allows for greater selection of EEG channels and is available in both routine and long-term EEGs. Polygraph equipment may also be used to monitor physiological data such as respiratory effort, eye movements, heart rate, and systemic blood pressure. These techniques can be used concurrently and are especially valuable in differentiating epileptic activity from paroxysmal behaviour or nonepileptic motor events.

evolve Critical Thinking Exercise—Seizures

Therapeutic Management

The goal of treatment of seizure disorders is to control the seizures or to reduce their frequency and severity, discover and correct the cause when possible, and help the child live as normal a life as possible. If the seizure activity is a manifestation of an infectious, traumatic, or metabolic process, the seizure therapy is instituted as part of the general therapeutic regimen. Management of epilepsy has four treatment options: medication therapy, the ketogenic diet, vagus nerve stimulation, and epilepsy surgery.

Medication Therapy

Persons predisposed to epilepsy have seizures when their basal level of neuronal excitability exceeds a critical point; no event occurs if the excitability is maintained below this threshold. The administration of anti-epileptic medications serves to raise this threshold and prevent seizures. Consequently, the primary therapy for seizure disorders is the administration of the appropriate anti-epileptic medication or combination of medications in a dosage that provides the desired effect without causing undesirable adverse effects or toxic reactions. Anti-epileptic medications are believed to exert their effect primarily by reducing the responsiveness of normal neurons to the sudden, high-frequency nerve impulses that arise in the epileptogenic focus. Thus the seizure is effectively suppressed; however, the abnormal brain waves may or may not be altered. Complete control can be achieved in 80% of children with epilepsy (Curatolo et al., 2009).

Therapy is begun with a single medication known to be effective and to have the lowest toxicity, that is, the safest adverse-effect profile for the child's particular type of seizure. The dosage is gradually increased until the seizures are controlled or the child develops adverse effects. If the medication is effective but does not sufficiently control the seizures, a second medication is added in gradually increasing doses. Once seizures are controlled, the first medication may be tapered to reduce the potential adverse effects of polytherapy. However, this decision is individualized for each child (Browne & Holmes, 2004). Monotherapy remains the treatment method of choice for epilepsy, but polypharmacy may be a viable alternative for children who cannot attain seizure control with only one agent (Leppik, 2000).

Measurement of blood levels of the drug is important if the seizures continue once the child is on a therapeutic dose of medication, to adjust the dosage, and to assist in determining which medication may be causing the adverse effects if the child is on multiple anti-epileptic medications. Some possible causes of low serum blood concentrations are noncompliance, poor absorption, and drug interactions. The dosage needs to be increased as the child grows. Blood cell counts, urinalysis, and liver function tests are obtained at frequent intervals in children receiving particular anti-epileptic medications that can affect organ function.

If complete seizure control is maintained on an anticonvulsant medication for 2 years, it is safe to discontinue the medication for patients with no risk factors. Risk factors include children over 12 years of age at onset, history of neonatal seizures, numerous seizures before control is achieved, and the presence of a neurological dysfunction (e.g., motor handicap or intellectual disability). Up to 25% of children whose medications are discontinued will experience seizure recurrence. Recurrence occurs most frequently within 6 months of discontinuation (Johnston, 2007).

When seizure medications are discontinued, the dosage is decreased gradually over several weeks. Sudden withdrawal of a medication is not recommended because it can cause an increase in the number and severity of seizures.

NURSING ALERT Fosphenytoin is often used to treat seizures instead of IV phenytoin because of possible complications and drug interactions associated with IV phenytoin. If IV phenytoin is used, it should be administered via slow IV push at a rate that does not exceed 50 mg/min. Because phenytoin precipitates when mixed with glucose, only normal saline is used to flush the tubing or catheter. Fosphenytoin may be given in saline or glucose solutions at a rate of up to 150 mg PE (phenytoin equivalent)/min, and it may be given intramuscularly if necessary.

Ketogenic Diet

The ketogenic diet is a high-fat, low-carbohydrate, and adequate-protein diet (Kossoff, Zupec-Kania, & Rho, 2009). Consumption of such a diet forces the body to shift from using glucose as the primary energy source to using fat, and the individual develops a state of ketosis. The diet is rigorous. All foods and liquids the child consumes must be carefully weighed and measured. The diet is deficient in vitamins and minerals; thus, vitamin supplements are necessary. Potential side effects of the diet are constipation, weight loss, lethargy, and kidney stones. It is unknown whether long-term effects such as increased blood lipids will occur (Levy & Cooper, 2003).

The ketogenic diet has been shown to be effective in controlling seizures. In the past decade, four major meta-analyses of the efficacy of the ketogenic diet have shown that the diet reduced seizures by more than 90% in a third of the patients and by more than 50% in half of them (Kossoff et al., 2009).

Vagus Nerve Stimulation

Vagus nerve stimulation uses an implantable device that reduces seizures in individuals who have not had effective control with medication therapy. It is currently indicated as adjunct therapy in patients 12 years and older with partial-onset seizures (with or without secondary generalization). A programmable signal generator is implanted subcutaneously in the chest. Electrodes tunnelled underneath the skin deliver electrical impulses to the left vagus nerve (cranial nerve X). The device is programmed noninvasively to deliver a precise pattern of stimulation to the left vagus nerve. The patient or caregiver can activate the device using a magnet at the onset of a seizure. Studies show a medium reduction in seizures of 35 to 45% after 1 year of therapy (Saillet et al., 2009).

Surgical Therapy

When seizures are determined to be caused by a hematoma, tumour, or other cerebral lesion, surgical removal is the treatment. In children with epilepsy, surgery is reserved for those who suffer from incapacitating, refractory seizures. *Refractory seizures* are usually defined as the persistence of seizures despite adequate trials of three anti-epileptic medications, alone or in combination (Browne & Holmes, 2004).

The epileptogenic area should be in a surgically removable and functionally silent region of the brain. Early removal of the symptomatic area is associated with seizure control and decreased use of anti-epileptic medications (Mathern et al., 1999). An extensive medical (e.g., invasive EEG monitoring), psychosocial, and psychoneurological evaluation is required.

Status Epilepticus

Status epilepticus is a continuous seizure that lasts more than 30 minutes or a series of seizures from which the child does not regain a premorbid LOC (Shorvon & Walker, 2005; Treiman & Walker, 2006). The duration required for seizures to be considered status epilepticus continues to be debated (Chen & Wasterlain, 2006). The initial treatment is directed toward support and maintenance of vital functions, that is, attending to the CAB of life support, administering oxygen, and gaining IV access, immediately followed by IV administration of anti-epileptic agents.

Rectal diazepam is a simple, effective, and safe treatment for home or prehospital management (Pellock & Shinnar, 2005). It is available in a prefilled rectal gel syringe (Diastat) for easy administration. Rectal diazepam is not associated with respiratory depression when used as recommended (Pellock & Shinnar, 2005). Midazolam has been given successfully by intranasal route for treatment of acute epileptic seizures (Ahmad et al., 2006; Fisgin et al., 2000). Intranasal midazolam is not only safe and effective for stopping seizures but is easier to administer than rectal diazepam (Harbord et al., 2004).

For in-hospital management of status epilepticus, IV diazepam or lorazepam (Ativan) is the first-line medication of choice (Browne & Holmes, 2004). Lorazepam may be replacing IV diazepam as the medication of choice. It has a longer duration of action and causes less respiratory depression in children over 2 years of age. Concurrent IV loading with fosphenytoin is usually necessary for sustained control of seizures. Valproic acid has also been reported to be effective in status epilepticus when given rectally or intravenously (Yamamoto & Yim, 2000). The child must be closely monitored during administration to detect early alterations in vital signs that may indicate impending respiratory depression. When diazepam is ineffective, fosphenytoin or phenobarbital is given intravenously as the next line of treatment. This combination of therapy places the child at high risk for apnea, and respiratory support is generally necessary. Children who continue to have seizures despite the above medication treatment may be given anaesthetizing doses of midazolam, propofol, or pentobarbital. In this situation, continuous EEG monitoring is typically done to monitor for and treat electrographic seizures.

NURSING ALERT Diazepam is incompatible with many medications. To give intravenously, inject slowly and directly into the vein or through tubing as close as possible to the vein insertion site.

Nursing care of a child with status epilepticus includes, in addition to the CAB of life support, monitoring blood pressure and body temperature. During the first 30 to 45 minutes of the seizure the blood pressure may be elevated. Thereafter the blood pressure typically returns to normal but may be decreased depending on the medications being administered for seizure control. Hyperthermia requiring treatment may occur as a result of increased motor activity.

Prognosis

Most children who experience a second seizure will experience additional seizures. Therefore, a history of two seizures is sufficient to diagnose epilepsy (Shinnar et al., 2000). Epidemiological studies using population- or community-based cohorts show that the etiology and specific epilepsy syndromes are the most important factors affecting prognosis. Children who have intellectual disability or cerebral palsy are at the highest risk for developing epilepsy. Seizures will remit in more than two thirds of children with childhood onset of seizure. Mortality is increased in children with epilepsy; those with neurological abnormalities or seizures that are refractory to treatment are at the highest risk (Browne & Holmes, 2004).

Nursing Care Management

An important nursing responsibility is to observe the seizure episode and accurately document the events. Any alterations in behaviour preceding the seizure and the characteristics of the episode, such as sensory-hallucinatory phenomena (e.g., an aura), motor effects (e.g., eye movements, muscular contractions), alterations in consciousness, and postictal state, should be noted and recorded (Box 51-11). The nurse should describe only what is observed, rather than trying to label a seizure type. The time that the seizure began and the duration of the seizure should be noted.

The child must be protected from injury during the seizure. Nursing observations made during the event provide valuable information for diagnosis and management of the disorder (see Emergency box). It is impossible to halt a seizure once it has begun, and no attempt should be made to do so. The nurse must remain calm, stay with the child, and prevent the child from sustaining any harm during the seizure. If possible, the child should be isolated from the view of others by closing a door or pulling screens. A seizure can be upsetting to the child, other visitors, and their families. If other persons are present, they should be assured that everything is being done for the child. After the seizure, they can be given a simple explanation about the event as needed.

If the nurse is able to reach the child in time, a child who is standing or seated in a chair (including a wheelchair) should be eased to the floor immediately. During (and sometimes after) the tonic-clonic seizure, the swallowing reflex is lost, salivation increases, and the tongue is hypotonic. Thus, the child is at risk for aspiration and airway occlusion. Placing the child on the side facilitates drainage and helps maintain a patent airway. Suctioning the oral cavity and posterior oropharynx may be necessary. Vital signs should be taken. The child should be allowed to rest if at school or away from home. When feasible, the child should be integrated into the environment as soon as possible. Sending a child with a chronic seizure disorder home from school is not necessary unless requested by the parents.

Seizure precautions are required for children who are known to have seizures or who are under observation for seizures. The extent of these measures depends on the type and frequency of the seizure (Box 51-12).

BOX 51-11 General Observations: The Child During a Seizure

Observations During a Seizure

General Description
Order of events (before, during, and after)
Duration of seizure
- Tonic-clonic—from first signs of event until jerking stops
- Absence—from loss of consciousness until consciousness is regained
- Complex partial—from first sign of unresponsiveness, motor activity, automatisms until there are signs of responsiveness to environment

Onset
Time of onset
Significant precipitating events—missed medication dosage, illness, stress, sleep deprivation, menses

Behaviour
Change in facial expression
Cry or other sound
Stereotypic or automatous movements
Random activity (wandering)
Position of eyes, head, body, extremities
Unilateral or bilateral posturing of one or more extremities

Movement
Change of position, if any
Site of commencement—hand, thumb, mouth, generalized
Tonic phase—length, parts of body involved
Clonic phase—twitching or jerking movements, parts of body involved, sequence of parts involved, generalized, change in character of movements
Lack of movement or muscle tone of body part or entire body

Face
Colour change—pallor, cyanosis, flushing
Perspiration
Mouth—position, deviation to one side, teeth clenched, tongue bitten, frothing at mouth, flecks of blood or bleeding
Lack of expression
Asymmetrical expression

Eyes
Position—straight ahead, deviation upward or outward, conjugate or divergent gaze
Pupils—change in size, equality, reaction to light

Respiratory Effort
Presence and length of apnea

Other
Incontinence

Postictal Observations
Duration of postictal period
State of consciousness
Orientation
Arousability
Motor ability:
- Any change in motor function
- Ability to move all extremities
- Paresis or weakness

Speech
Sensations:
- Complaint of discomfort or pain
- Any sensory impairment

Recollection of preseizure sensations (aura)
Based on a thorough assessment, several nursing diagnoses are identified. The more common diagnoses for the child with a seizure disorder are included in the Nursing Care Plan.

NURSING ALERT Do not move or forcefully restrain the child during a tonic-clonic seizure, and do not place a solid object between the teeth.

Long-Term Care

Care of the child with a recurrent seizure disorder involves physical care and instruction regarding the importance of the medication therapy and, probably more significant, the problems related to the emotional aspects of the disorder. Few diseases generate as much anxiety among relatives as epilepsy. Fears and misconceptions about the disease and its treatment abound in the layperson's mind. For many, it represents the archetype of severe hereditary affliction. Nursing care is directed toward educating the child and family about epilepsy and helping them develop strategies to cope with the psychological and sociological problems related to epilepsy.

Children with epilepsy are prescribed anti-epileptic medications. These medications need to be administered at regular intervals to maintain adequate levels in the blood. The most convenient times for administration seem to be with meals or at bedtime. It is important to impress on the family the necessity of giving the anti-epileptic medication regularly and for as long as required. In general, anti-epileptic medications are continued until the child has been seizure free for 2 years (Johnston, 2007). The medication is then slowly tapered over a period of weeks to avoid the possibility of precipitating a seizure. It is sometimes easy to skip doses or omit them for a variety of reasons, especially when the child is free of seizures most of the time. This is particularly so when the child is older and assumes responsibility for his or her medication. The seizure threshold may be lowered during any illness, but particularly with fever. Parents should be aware that if their child has an illness, he or she is at increased risk for seizures. Parents should contact their health care provider if their child misses medications during an illness because of vomiting.

Rectal preparations of some anti-epileptic medications are highly effective when a child is unable to take oral medications because of repeated vomiting, gastrointestinal surgery, or status epilepticus. Parents can learn to administer rectal anti-epileptic medication for home treatment. Rectal diazepam is a useful adjunctive home treatment for children at risk for prolonged seizures or clusters of seizures. Hospitalization is minimized, and parental confidence is usually enhanced.

EMERGENCY

Seizures

Tonic-Clonic Seizure

During the Seizure

Remain calm.
Time seizure episode.
If child is standing or seated, ease child down to the floor.
Place pillow or folded blanket under child's head.
Loosen restrictive clothing.
Remove eyeglasses.
Clear area of any hazards or hard objects.
Allow seizure to end without interference.
If vomiting occurs, turn child to one side.
Do not:

- Attempt to restrain child or use force
- Put anything in child's mouth
- Give any food or liquids

After the Seizure

Time postictal period.
Check for breathing. Check position of head and tongue.
Reposition if head is hyperextended. If child is not breathing, give rescue breathing and call emergency medical services (EMS).
Keep child on side.
Remain with child.
Do not give food or liquids until child is fully alert and swallowing reflex has returned.
Call EMS when necessary.
Look for medical identification, and determine what factors occurred before onset of seizure that may have been triggering factors.
Check head and body for possible injuries.
Check inside of mouth to see if tongue or lips have been bitten.

Complex Partial Seizure

During the Seizure

Do not restrain child.
Remove harmful objects from area.
Redirect to safe area.
Do not agitate; instead, talk in calm, reassuring manner.
Do not expect child to follow instructions.
Watch to see if seizure generalizes.

After the Seizure

Stay with child and reassure until fully conscious.

Call Emergency Medical Services If

The child stops breathing.
There is evidence of injury or the child is diabetic or pregnant.
The seizure lasts for more than 5 minutes (unless duration of seizure is typically longer than 5 minutes) and written medical order is present.
Status epilepticus occurs.
Pupils are not equal after seizure.
The child vomits continuously 30 minutes after seizure has ended (sign of possible acute problem).
The child cannot be awakened and is unresponsive to pain after seizure has ended.
The seizure occurs in water.
This is the child's first seizure.

(Modified from Epilepsy Foundation. [2001]. *Seizure recognition and first aid.* Retrieved from http://www.epilepsyfoundation.org.)

BOX 51-12 Seizure Precautions

The extent of precautions depends on type, severity, and frequency of seizures. They may include the following:

- Side rails raised when child is sleeping or resting
- Side rails and other hard objects padded
- Waterproof mattress or pad on bed or crib

Appropriate precautions during potentially hazardous activities may include the following:

- Swimming with a companion
- Taking showers; bathing only with close supervision
- Using protective helmet and padding during bicycle riding, skateboarding, in-line skating
- Supervising child during use of hazardous machinery or equipment

Have child carry or wear medical identification.
Alert other caregivers to need for any special precautions.
Child may not drive or operate hazardous machinery or equipment unless seizure free for designated period (varies by state).

NURSING ALERT Children taking phenobarbital or phenytoin should receive adequate vitamin D and folic acid, since deficiencies of both have been associated with these medications. Phenytoin should not be taken with milk.

Nurses should educate the child and parents about the possible adverse reactions to the medications used to treat seizures. Parents need to understand the common adverse effects and be encouraged to report their observations to their health care provider. Parents should understand that the child needs periodic physical assessment and laboratory studies. Possible adverse effects on the hematopoietic system, liver, and kidneys may be reflected in symptoms such as fever, sore throat, enlarged lymph nodes, jaundice, and bleeding (e.g., easy bruising, petechiae, ecchymoses, epistaxis). A common factor in status epilepticus is inadequate blood levels of anti-epileptic medications.

Although children with epilepsy are at increased risk for injury, limitations on activities should be relatively few. The degree to which activities are restricted needs to be individualized for each child and depends on the type, frequency, and

Text continued on p. 1603

NURSING CARE PLAN ● The Child With Seizure Disorder

Nursing Diagnosis	Expected Patient Outcomes	Nursing Interventions	Rationale
Risk for injury related to central nervous system (CNS) dysfunction and inability to control self (motor) secondary to type of seizure	Child will not experience physical injury as a result of seizure activity.	Administer anti-epileptic medication (AED).	To prevent seizure activity
	The Following NOC Concepts Apply to These Outcomes Risk Control Personal Safety Behaviour Safe Home Environment Falls Occurrence	Teach family and child, as appropriate, the purpose of AED medication, action, potential adverse effects, and administration of medications.	To prevent seizure activity and encourage self-care
Child's/Family's Defining Characteristics ***(Subjective and Objective Data)*** Change in level of consciousness (LOC) Disorientation Clonic movements Automatisms Aura Postictal impairment (dependent on the type of seizure)		Monitor for adverse effects of AED and therapeutic levels according to child's growth, illness factors that affect metabolism, and effects of medication.	To prevent secondary effects of AED and prevent seizure from subtherapeutic drug levels
		Stress importance of compliance with medication regimen even if child has no evidence of seizure activity.	To prevent seizure activity
		Advise family and child to avoid situations that are known to precipitate a seizure (e.g., blinking lights, fatigue, excess activity or exercise, physical factors).	To prevent exposure to situations that may cause a seizure
		Assess home care environment for risk factors that may produce childhood physical injury: loose rugs; unprotected stairway; access to water buckets, pool, or standing water.	To prevent physical harm
		Teach parents by anticipatory guidance risk factors for injury in environment based on child's developmental age and type of seizure (e.g., not leaving child in bathtub without adult supervision).	
		Counsel female patients of childbearing age taking AEDs about contraception and birth defects associated with AEDs.	To prevent birth defects in offspring of women taking AEDs
		In the event of a tonic-clonic seizure: • Place child on side. • Time seizure. • Protect child during seizure. • Do not attempt to restrain child or use force. • If child is standing or sitting in wheelchair at beginning of episode, ease child to floor. • Do not put anything in child's mouth. • Place small cushion or blanket under child's head. • Remove child's eyeglasses. • Loosen clothing. • Prevent child from hitting head on objects. • Remove hazards. • Pad objects such as crib, side rails, or wheelchair. • Keep side rails raised when child is sleeping, resting, or having a seizure. • Allow seizure to end without interference.	To prevent injury and trauma To prevent aspiration and maintain a patent airway
		Teach parents or caregiver how to care for child during seizure and in postictal state.	To protect child and caregiver from injury
		Protect child after seizure (postictal period). Time the period. Maintain child in a side-lying or recovery position. Call emergency medical services as necessary or ensure child receives medical evaluation after seizure.	To prevent trauma and implement therapeutic intervention
		The Following NIC Concepts Apply to These Interventions Surveillance: Safety Environmental Management: Safety Medication Administration Teaching: Disease Process Neurological Monitoring Seizure Precautions	

Continued

NURSING CARE PLAN ● The Child With Seizure Disorder—cont'd

Nursing Diagnosis	Expected Patient Outcomes	Nursing Interventions	Rationale
Risk for aspiration and ineffective breathing pattern related to impaired motor activity, loss of consciousness, and loss of airway protection (tonic-clonic seizure)	Child's airway will remain patent. Child will have effective ventilations.	In the event of a seizure, place child in a side-lying position on a flat surface such as floor or bed.	To prevent aspiration and protect airway
		Remain with child.	To determine need for emergency care
	The Following NOC Concepts Apply to These Outcomes	Remove secretions, food, and liquids from mouth when seizure subsides.	To prevent choking, aspiration
Child's/Family's Defining Characteristics ***(Subjective and Objective Data)***	Aspiration Prevention	If child has emesis, place on side.	To prevent choking, aspiration
Reduced LOC	Respiratory Status: Airway Patency	In postictal state monitor oxygenation status.	To determine need for oxygen
Depressed cough reflex	Respiratory Status: Ventilation	Administer oxygen as necessary to maintain pulse oximeter over 89%.	To prevent hypoxia
Apnea		Suction oropharynx once seizure subsides as necessary to clear mucus or food.	To prevent aspiration
Decreased inspiratory pressure		Administer medications intended to stop seizure (rectal diazepam [Diastat], rectal phenytoin, intravenous phenytoin).	To prevent continued seizure activity
		The Following NIC Concepts Apply to These Interventions Risk Identification Aspiration Precautions Oxygen Therapy Medication Administration	

Nursing Diagnosis	Expected Patient Outcomes	Nursing Interventions	Rationale
Risk for injury related to impaired consciousness and automatisms	Child will not experience physical injury and will remain calm.	Time seizure.	To establish duration and possible need for emergency care
	The Following NOC Concepts Apply to These Outcomes	Protect child during seizure. Do not attempt to restrain child or use force.	To prevent injury to child or self
Child's/Family's Defining Characteristics ***(Subjective and Objective Data)***	Risk Control	Remove hazards in immediate environment.	To prevent injury
Immediate loss of consciousness	Safe Home Environment Personal Safety Behaviour	Redirect child to safe area, especially away from windows, stairs, heating elements, or sources of water.	To prevent injury from falls, burns, and drowning
Tonic rigidity replaced by intense jerking movements	Physical Injury Severity	Talk in calm voice and reassuring manner.	To prevent further agitation
May become incontinent of urine and feces	Falls Occurrence	Watch to see whether seizure generalizes into a tonic-clinic seizure.	To determine type of seizure
Postictal impairment Change in vital signs, respiratory status, colour Vomiting		Protect child after seizure (postictal period). Time the period. Stay with child until fully alert.	To provide support, because child may be confused and frightened
		The Following NIC Concepts Apply to These Interventions Risk Identification Environmental Management: Safety Surveillance Seizure Precautions	

NURSING CARE PLAN • The Child With Seizure Disorder—cont'd

Nursing Diagnosis	Expected Patient Outcomes	Nursing Interventions	Rationale
Anxiety/fear (parent), related to child having life-threatening and incapacitating seizure activity*	Parent will cope with child's condition and receive adequate support.	Allow parent(s) to remain with child during seizure.	To decrease fear of unknown and allow parent to see measures taken to protect child
	The Following NOC Concepts Apply to These Outcomes Anxiety Self-Control Coping Fear Self-Control	Instruct parent on proper protection interventions during child's seizure activity: positioning, safety, airway maintenance, reassurance techniques, emergency medication administration.	To promote parent participation and to promote sense of control over situation
Child's/Family's Defining Characteristics ***(Subjective and Objective Data)*** Anguish Fright Feelings of inadequacy and hopelessness Worry, apprehension Panic Excitement		Provide information regarding nature (type) of seizure, therapeutic interventions, and lifestyle modifications.	To promote knowledge of condition, parental intervention, sense of control
		Encourage family involvement in daily care of child, with goal of normalization and promotion of optimal growth and development of child.	To provide hope and promote family functioning and coping
		Involve parents in discussion of fears and anxieties; discuss resource and support options available to family.	To promote family integrity and functioning
		The Following NIC Concepts Apply to These Interventions Support Group Coping Enhancement Anxiety Reduction Family Process Maintenance Active Listening Counselling Decision-Making Support Family Involvement Promotion	

*Nursing diagnosis may also apply to child in the postictal phase, depending on type of seizure and child's understanding and cognitive level.
NIC, Nursing Interventions Classification; *NOC*, Nursing Outcomes Classification.

severity of the seizures; the child's response to therapy; and the length of time the seizures have been controlled. Children with epilepsy are at higher risk for drowning than children without epilepsy. Young children (with or without epilepsy) should *never* be left alone in the bathtub, even for a few seconds. Older children and adolescents should be encouraged to use the shower and reminded not to lock the bathroom door when showering. They should never swim unsupervised.

Because the child is encouraged to attend school, camp, and other normal activities, the school nurse and teachers should be made aware of the child's condition and therapy. They can help ensure regularity of medication administration and provision of any special care the child might need. Teachers, child care providers, camp counsellors, youth organization leaders, coaches, and other adults who assume responsibility for children should be instructed regarding care of the child during a seizure so that they can act calmly for the child's welfare and influence the attitude of the child's peers.

Triggering Factors

Careful and detailed documentation of seizures over time may indicate a pattern. When this occurs, the nurse or responsible adult may intervene to identify the triggering factors and make changes in the environment that may prevent seizures or decrease their frequency. Often the necessary changes are simple but can make an enormous difference in the lives of the child and family.

The most common factors that may trigger seizures in children include emotional stress, sleep deprivation, fatigue, fever, and illness (Frucht et al., 2000; Nakken et al., 2005). Other precipitating factors include sleep, flickering lights, menstrual cycle, alcohol, heat, hyperventilation, and fasting (Frucht et al., 2000). Some individuals have pattern-sensitive epilepsy, that is, seizures precipitated by changes in dark–light patterns, such as those that occur with a flash on a camera, automobile headlights, reflections of light on snow or water, or rotating blades on a fan. A study by Radhakrishnan and colleagues (2005) showed that most of these individuals had absence, myoclonic, or generalized tonic-clonic seizures. Some children have seizures while playing video games. These children are sensitive to intermittent photic stimulation that can trigger an epileptic episode (Shoja et al., 2007). However, the overwhelming majority of children with epilepsy can play video or computer games and watch television without the risk of seizures.

Febrile Seizures

A *febrile seizure* is a seizure related to a febrile illness, in the absence of a central nervous system infection or acute electrolyte imbalance, in children older than 1 month of age without a prior history of afebrile seizures (Ostergaard, 2009). Febrile seizures are one of the most common neurological conditions of childhood, affecting approximately 3 to 8% of children (Sadleir & Scheffer, 2007). Most febrile seizures occur between 6 months and 3 years of age, with the average age of onset between 12 and 30 months. They are unusual after 5 years of age. Boys are affected about twice as often as girls, and there appears to be an increased familial susceptibility.

The cause of febrile seizures is still uncertain. Both animal and human studies demonstrate that there is an age-specific susceptibility to seizures induced by fever and that it is the peak temperature that is important, not the rapidity of the temperature elevation (Ostergaard, 2009). The temperature usually exceeds 38.8°C, and the seizure occurs during the temperature rise rather than after a prolonged elevation. Sometimes it constitutes the dramatic beginning of an illness, often an upper respiratory tract or gastrointestinal infection.

Most febrile seizures have stopped by the time the child is taken to a medical facility. However, if the seizure continues, treatment consists of controlling the seizure with IV or rectal diazepam and reducing the temperature with acetaminophen. Anti-epileptic prophylaxis is not indicated. Parental education and emotional support are important interventions. Parents need reassurance regarding the benign nature of febrile seizures. Parents also need education on how to protect the child from harm and observe exactly what happens to the child during the event. Attempts to lower the temperature will not prevent a seizure. Tepid sponge baths are not recommended for several reasons: they are ineffective in significantly lowering the temperature, the shivering effect further increases metabolic output, and cooling causes discomfort to the child.

Long-term anti-epileptic therapy is usually not required for children with simple febrile seizures. Antipyretic therapy during febrile illness offers symptomatic relief for fever-associated symptoms but appears to be ineffective in preventing a seizure (Ostergaard, 2009; Sadleir & Scheffer, 2007).

NURSING ALERT If a febrile seizure lasts more than 5 minutes, parents should seek medical attention right away. Instruct them to call for emergency assistance (911) and not to place the child who is actively having a seizure in the car.

Cerebral Malformations

evolve Case Study—Hydrocephalus With Myelomeningocele

Cranial Deformities

In the normal newborn the cranial sutures are separated by membranous seams several millimetres wide. For the first few hours to 1 to 2 days after birth, the cranial bones are highly mobile, which allows them to mould and slide over one another, adjusting the circumference of the head to accommodate to the changing shape and character of the birth canal. The principal sutures in the infant's skull are the sagittal, coronal, and lambdoidal sutures, and the major soft areas at the juncture of these sutures are the anterior and posterior fontanels.

After birth, growth of the skull bones occurs in a direction perpendicular to the line of the suture, and normal closure occurs in a regular and predictable order. Although there are wide variations in the age at which closure takes place in individual children, normally all sutures and fontanels are ossified by the following ages:

Eight weeks—Posterior fontanel closed
Six months—Fibrous union of suture lines and interlocking of serrated edges
Eighteen months—Anterior fontanel closed
After 12 years—Sutures unable to be separated by increased ICP

A solid union of all sutures is not completed until late childhood. The closure of a suture before the expected time inhibits the perpendicular growth. Since the normal increase in brain volume requires expansion, the skull is forced to grow in a direction parallel to the fused suture. This alteration in skull growth always produces a distortion of the head shape when the underlying brain growth is normal. The small head with closed and normal shape is a result of deficient brain growth. The suture closure is secondary to this brain growth failure; failure of brain growth is not secondary to suture closure.

Various types of cranial deformities are encountered in early infancy. These include the enlarged head with frontal protrusion (bossing; characteristic of hydrocephalus), the parietal bossing that is seen in chronic subdural hematoma, the small head, and a variety of skull deformities. Some occur during prenatal development; in others, head circumference is usually within normal limits at birth, and the deviation from normal development becomes apparent with advancing age.

Prognosis

The majority of infants with craniosynostosis have normal brain development. The exceptions are those with genetic disorders that involve brain pathological conditions.

Nursing Care Management

Nursing care of families in which there is a child with a cranial defect involves identifying children with deformities and referring them for evaluation. Since no therapy is available for children with microcephaly, nursing care is directed toward helping parents adjust to rearing a child with brain damage (see Chapter 42).

Caring for infants who benefit from surgery requires special emphasis on observation for signs of decreased hematocrit and hemoglobin because of the large blood loss during surgery. A cardiac monitor may demonstrate a resting heart rate of 200 beats/min. Nursing care includes observation for signs of hemorrhage, infection, pain, and swelling, as well as parental education for suture care and safety. Surgical sutures should remain dry and intact. Parents need to observe for any signs of redness, drainage, or swelling and report any temperature greater than 38.4°C.

Early surgical management of craniosynostosis allows proper expansion of the brain and the creation of an acceptable appearance. Parents require special support and education during this time, especially from the health care team.

Hydrocephalus

Hydrocephalus is a condition caused by an imbalance in the production and absorption of CSF in the ventricular system. When production is greater than absorption, CSF accumulates within the ventricular system, usually under increased pressure, producing passive dilation of the ventricles.

Pathophysiology

The causes of hydrocephalus are varied, but the result is either (1) impaired absorption of CSF fluid within the subarachnoid space, obliteration of the subarachnoid cisterns, or malfunction of the arachnoid villi (nonobstructive or communicating hydrocephalus), or (2) obstruction to the flow of CSF through the ventricular system (obstructive or noncommunicating hydrocephalus) (Kinsman & Johnston, 2007). The terms *communicating* and *noncommunicating hydrocephalus* traditionally referred to obstructive and nonobstructive types of hydrocephalus when pneumoencephalography was used to establish the diagnosis; because other diagnostic methods are now used, the terms may be used only as a reference point in the diagnosis. Other authorities suggest that hydrocephalus be classified according to the cause and refer to either congenital or acquired hydrocephalus (Rudy, 2005). Rarely, a tumour of the choroid plexus causes increased CSF secretion. Any imbalance of secretion and absorption causes an increased accumulation of CSF in the ventricles, which become dilated (ventriculomegaly) and compress the brain substance against the surrounding rigid bony cranium. When this occurs before fusion of the cranial sutures, it causes enlargement of the skull and dilation of the ventricles (Fig. 51-6). In children younger than 10 to 12 years of age, partially closed suture lines, especially the sagittal suture, may become diastatic or opened. After 12 years of age the sutures are fused and will not open.

Most cases of noncommunicating hydrocephalus are a result of developmental malformations. Although the defect usually is apparent in early infancy, it may become evident at any time from the prenatal period to late childhood or early adulthood. Other causes include neoplasms, infections, and trauma. An obstruction to the normal flow can occur at any point in the CSF pathway to produce increased pressure and dilation of the pathways proximal to the site of obstruction.

Developmental defects (e.g., Arnold-Chiari malformations, aqueduct stenosis, aqueduct gliosis, and atresia of the foramina of Luschka and Magendie [Dandy-Walker syndrome]) account for most cases of hydrocephalus from birth to 2 years of age. Hydrocephalus is so often associated with myelomeningocele that all infants with this condition should be observed for its development. In the remainder of cases there is a history of intrauterine infection, perinatal hemorrhage, and neonatal meningoencephalitis. In older children hydrocephalus is most often a result of space-occupying lesions, intracranial infections, hemorrhage, or pre-existing developmental defects, such as aqueduct stenosis or the **Arnold-Chiari malformation** (a congenital anomaly in which the cerebellum and medulla oblongata extend down through the foramen magnum).

Diagnostic Evaluation

The two factors that influence the clinical picture in hydrocephalus are the time of onset and pre-existing structural lesions. In infancy, before closure of the cranial sutures, head enlargement is the predominant sign, whereas in older infants and children the lesions responsible for hydrocephalus produce other neurological signs through pressure on adjacent structures before causing CSF obstruction (Box 51-13).

In infancy, the diagnosis of hydrocephalus is based on head circumference that crosses one or more grid lines on the measurement chart within a period of 2 to 4 weeks and on associated neurological signs that are present and progressive. However, other diagnostic studies are needed to localize the site of CSF obstruction. Routine daily head circumference measurements are carried out in infants with myelomeningocele and intracranial infections. In evaluation of a preterm infant, specially adapted head circumference charts are consulted to distinguish abnormal head growth from rapid head growth that takes place normally.

The signs and symptoms in early to late childhood are caused by increased ICP, and specific manifestations are related to the focal lesion. Most commonly resulting from posterior fossa neoplasms and aqueduct stenosis, the clinical manifestations are primarily those associated with space-occupying lesions.

The primary diagnostic tools for detecting hydrocephalus are CT and MRI. Sedation is required, since the child must

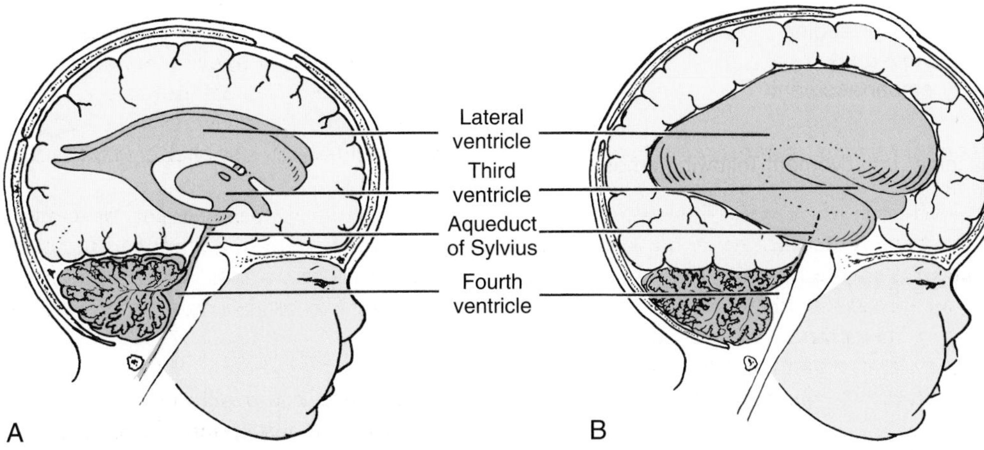

Fig. 51-6 Hydrocephalus: a block in flow of cerebrospinal fluid. **A:** Patent cerebrospinal fluid circulation. **B:** Enlarged lateral and third ventricles caused by obstruction of circulation—stenosis of aqueduct of Sylvius.

remain absolutely still for an accurate picture to be produced. Diagnostic evaluation of children who have symptoms of hydrocephalus after infancy is similar to that used in those with suspected intracranial tumour. In the neonate, echoencephalography is useful in comparing the ratio of lateral ventricle to cortex.

Therapeutic Management

The treatment of hydrocephalus is directed toward relief of the hydrocephalus, treatment of complications, and management of problems related to the effect of the disorder on psychomotor development. The treatment is, with few exceptions, surgical. This is accomplished by direct removal of an obstruction (such as a tumour) or placement of a shunt that provides primary drainage of the CSF from the ventricles to an extracranial compartment, usually the peritoneum (ventriculoperitoneal [VP] shunt) (Fig. 51-7).

Most shunt systems consist of a ventricular catheter, a flush pump, a unidirectional flow valve, and a distal catheter. In all models the valves are designed to open at a predetermined intraventricular pressure and close when the pressure falls below that level, thus preventing backflow of secretions.

The initial shunt is placed when necessary to relieve CSF obstruction, and revisions are needed when signs of malfunction appear. In all mechanisms the initial success rate is relatively high; however, shunts are associated with complications that interfere with continued shunt function or threaten the child's life.

The major complications of VP shunts are infection and malfunction. All shunts are subject to mechanical difficulties, such as kinking, plugging, or separation or migration of the tubing. Malfunction is most often caused by mechanical obstruction either within the ventricles from particulate matter (tissue or exudate) or at the distal end from thrombosis or displacement as a result of growth. The child with a shunt obstruction is often first seen in an emergency department with clinical manifestations of increased ICP, frequently accompanied by worsening neurological status.

The most serious complication, shunt infection, can occur at any time, but the period of greatest risk is 1 to 2 months after placement. The infection is generally a result of intercurrent infections at the time of shunt placement. Infections include septicemia, bacterial endocarditis, wound infection, shunt nephritis, meningitis, and ventriculitis. Meningitis and ventriculitis are of greatest concern, since any complicating CNS infection is a significant predictor of poor intellectual outcome. Infection is treated with massive doses of antibiotics administered by the IV route. A persistent infection requires

evolve Animation—Ventriculoperitoneal Shunt

BOX 51-13 Clinical Manifestations of Hydrocephalus

Infancy (Early)

Abnormally rapid head growth
Bulging fontanels (especially anterior) sometimes without head enlargement:
- Tense
- Nonpulsatile

Dilated scalp veins
Separated sutures
Macewen sign (cracked-pot sound on percussion)
Thinning of skull bones

Infancy (Later)

Frontal enlargement, or bossing
Depressed eyes
Setting-sun sign (sclera visible above the iris)
Pupils sluggish, with unequal response to light

Infancy (General)

Irritability
Lethargy
Infant crying when picked up or rocked and quieting when allowed to lie still
Early infantile reflex acts may persist
Normally expected responses failing to appear
May display:
- Change in level of consciousness
- Opisthotonos (often extreme)
- Lower extremity spasticity
- Vomiting

Advanced cases:
- Difficulty in sucking and feeding
- Shrill, brief, high-pitched cry
- Cardiopulmonary embarrassment

Childhood

Headache on awakening; improvement following emesis or upright posture
Papilledema
Strabismus
Extrapyramidal tract signs (e.g., ataxia)
Irritability
Lethargy
Apathy
Confusion
Incoherence
Vomiting

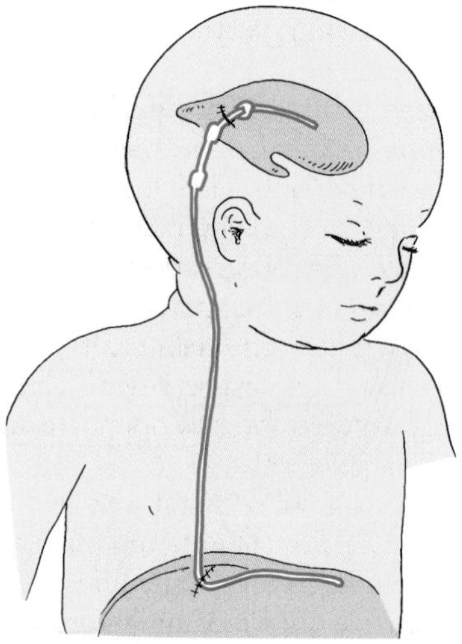

Fig. 51-7 Ventriculoperitoneal shunt. Catheter is threaded beneath the skin.

removal of the shunt until the infection is controlled. External ventricular drainage (EVD) is used until CSF is sterile. The EVD allows for removal of CSF through a tube that is placed in the child's ventricle and flows by gravity into a collection device.

An alternative to shunt placement is the endoscopic third ventriculostomy in children with noncommunicating hydrocephalus. In this procedure, an endoscope is used to make a small opening in the floor of the third ventricle that allows the CSF to flow freely through the previously blocked ventricle. Aldana and colleagues (2003) have shown that endoscopic septal fenestration has an overall patency rate of 81%, which may eliminate the need for a CSF shunt. The complication rate of the endoscopic septal fenestration procedure was 9.3% and included intraventricular hemorrhage, sterile meningitis, and septostomy failure.

Prognosis

The prognosis for children with treated hydrocephalus depends largely on the rate at which hydrocephalus develops, the duration of increased ICP, the frequency of complications, and the cause of the hydrocephalus. For example, malignant tumours may have a high mortality rate regardless of other complicating factors.

Surgically treated hydrocephalus with continued neurosurgical and medical management has a survival rate of about 80%, with the highest incidence of mortality occurring within the first year of treatment. Of the surviving children, approximately one third are both intellectually and neurologically normal, and one half have neurological disabilities.

Nursing Care Management

Preoperatively the infant with diagnosed or suspected hydrocephalus is observed carefully for signs of increasing ICP. In infants the head is measured daily at the largest point, the occipitofrontal circumference (see Head Circumference, Chapter 34, for technique). Fontanels and suture lines are gently palpated for size, signs of bulging, tenseness, and separation. An infant with normal ICP will display bulging under certain circumstances such as straining or crying; therefore such accompanying behaviour should be noted. Irritability, lethargy, or seizure activity, as well as altered vital signs and feeding behaviour, may indicate an advancing pathological condition.

In older children, who are usually admitted to the hospital for elective or emergency shunt revision, the most valuable indicator of increasing ICP is an alteration in the child's LOC and the way in which the child interacts with the environment. Changes are identified by observation and by comparison of present behaviour with customary behaviour, sleep patterns, developmental capabilities, and habits, all obtained through a detailed history and a baseline assessment. This baseline information serves as a guide for postoperative assessment and evaluation of shunt function.

General nursing care of the infant with hydrocephalus may present special problems. Maintaining adequate nutrition often requires flexible feeding schedules to accommodate diagnostic procedures, since feeding before or after handling can precipitate an episode of vomiting. Small feedings at more frequent intervals are often better tolerated than larger ones spaced further apart. These infants are often difficult to feed and require extra time and innovation.

The nurse is responsible for preparing the child for diagnostic tests such as tomography and for assisting the practitioner with procedures such as a ventricular tap, which is often performed to relieve excessive pressure during the preoperative period and for CSF examination. Sedation is required, since the child must remain absolutely still during diagnostic testing. IV pentobarbital or oral chloral hydrate is commonly used for these procedures (see Preparation for Diagnostic and Therapeutic Procedures, Chapter 45).

NURSING ALERT If surgery is anticipated, IV lines should not be placed in a scalp vein on a child with hydrocephalus.

Postoperative Care

Routine postoperative care and observation need to be instituted. In addition, the infant or child should be positioned carefully on the unoperated side to prevent pressure on the shunt valve and pressure areas. The child is kept flat to avoid complications resulting from too-rapid reduction of intracranial fluid. When the ventricular size is reduced too rapidly, the cerebral cortex may pull away from the dura and tear the small interlacing veins, producing a subdural hematoma. This is not a problem in children with elective shunt revision, since their intraventricular size and pressure have been normal. The surgeon will indicate the position to be maintained and the extent of activity allowed. If there is increased ICP, the surgeon will prescribe elevation of the head of the bed and allow the child to sit up to enhance gravity flow through the shunt. Pain management can usually be achieved with acetaminophen with or without codeine for mild to moderate pain and opioids for severe pain (see Pain Management, Chapter 35).

Observation is continued for signs of increased ICP, which indicates obstruction of the shunt. Neurological assessment includes evaluation of pupillary dilation (pressure causes compression or stretching of the oculomotor nerve, producing dilation on the same side as the pressure) and blood pressure (hypoxia to the brainstem causes variability in these vital signs).

NURSING ALERT Arbitrary pumping of the shunt may cause obstruction or other problems and should not be performed unless indicated by the neurosurgeon.

The child should also be observed for abdominal distention, since CSF may cause peritonitis or a postoperative ileus as a complication of distal catheter placement. In addition, intake and output need to be carefully monitored. Children may be placed on fluid restriction with nothing by mouth for 24 hours. The IV infusion should be closely monitored to prevent fluid overload. Routine feeding is resumed after the prescribed NPO period, but the presence of bowel sounds should be determined before feeding a child with a VP shunt.

Since infection is the greatest hazard of the postoperative period, nurses need to be continually on the alert for the usual manifestations of CSF infection, such as elevated vital signs, poor feeding, vomiting, decreased responsiveness, and seizure activity. There may be signs of local inflammation at the operative sites and along the shunt tract. The child's diaper should be kept off the peritoneal dressing site or suture line. Antibiotics are administered by the IV route as ordered, and the nurse may also need to assist the practitioner with intraventricular instillation. The incision site should be inspected for leakage, and any suspected drainage tested for glucose, an indication of CSF.

Meticulous skin care is continued postoperatively, with extra care to prevent tissue damage from pressure. A pressure-reducing mattress or overlay pad underneath the child helps prevent pressure on prominent areas. Skin should be inspected regularly for any signs of pressure, irritation, or infection.

Family Support

Specific needs and concerns of parents during periods of hospitalization are related to the reason for the child's hospitalization (shunt revision, infection, diagnosis) and the diagnostic and surgical procedures to which the child is subjected. Often parents have little understanding of anatomy; they need further exploration and reinforcement of information that was given to them by the physician and neurosurgeon, as well as information about what they can expect. They are especially frightened of any procedure that involves the brain, and the fear of intellectual disability or brain damage is real and pervasive. Nurses can do much to allay their anxiety by explaining the rationale underlying the various nursing and medical activities, such as positioning or testing, and by simply being available and willing to listen to their concerns.

To prepare for the child's discharge and home care, the parents need to be instructed on how to recognize signs that indicate shunt malfunction or infection and how to pump the shunt, if necessary. Active children may have accidents, such as a fall, that can damage the shunt, and the tubing may pull out of the distal insertion site or become disconnected during normal growth.

Safe transportation is an essential issue to discuss with parents. The tendency for the enlarged head to fall forward and to turn to the side, combined with poor head control, influences the type of child restraint system needed. Small infants can be restrained reclining in an approved car-restraint bed.

The management of hydrocephalus in a child is a demanding task for both family and health care providers, and helping a family cope with the child is an important nursing responsibility. It is important to emphasize that hydrocephalus is a lifelong problem and that the child will require evaluation on a regular basis. The overall aim is to establish realistic goals and an appropriate educational program that will help the child to achieve his or her optimal potential.

Families can be referred to community agencies for support and guidance. The Spina Bifida and Hydrocephalus Association of Canada provides information on the condition for families and assist interested groups in establishing local organizations. Helpful booklets are available from this source (see Additional Resources).

Key Points

- LOC is the most important indicator of neurological health; altered levels include full consciousness, confusion, disorientation, lethargy, obtundation, stupor, coma, and persistent vegetative state.
- Complete neurological examination includes LOC; posture; motor, sensory, cranial nerve, and reflex testing; and vital signs.
- Nursing care of the unconscious child focuses on ensuring respiratory management; performing neurological assessment; monitoring ICP; supplying adequate nutrition and hydration; providing medication therapy; promoting elimination, hygienic care, proper positioning, exercise, and stimulation; and providing family support.
- Fractures resulting from head injuries may be classified as depressed, compound, basilar, and diastatic.
- Primary head injury involves features that occur at the time of trauma, including fractured skull, contusions, intracranial hematoma, and diffuse injury. Secondary complications include hypoxic brain damage, increased ICP, infection, cerebral edema, and post-traumatic syndromes.
- The young child's response to head injury is different because of the following features: larger head size; expandable skull; larger blood volume to the brain; small subdural spaces; and thinner, softer brain tissue.
- Problems resulting from near-drowning include hypoxia and asphyxiation, aspiration, and hypothermia.
- Nursing care of the child with a brain tumour includes observing for signs and symptoms related to the tumour, preparing the child and family for diagnostic tests and operative procedures, preventing postoperative complications, planning for discharge, and promoting a return to optimal health.
- Nursing care of the child with meningitis includes administering antibiotics, taking isolation precautions, removing environmental stimuli, ensuring correct positioning, monitoring vital signs, administering IV therapy, promoting adequate fluid and nutritional status, and providing supportive care to the family.
- Routine immunization of infants with *H. influenzae* type b and pneumococcal conjugate vaccines has reduced the incidence of bacterial meningitis.
- Encephalitis may result from direct invasion of the CNS by a virus or from involvement of the CNS after viral disease.
- A seizure is a symptom of an underlying pathological condition and may be manifested by sensory-hallucinatory phenomena, motor effects, sensorimotor effects, or loss of consciousness.
- Partial seizures are categorized as simple (without associated impairment of consciousness) or complex (with impaired consciousness); both types may become generalized.
- Generalized seizures are categorized as tonic-clonic convulsive, absence, atonic and akinetic, myoclonic, and infantile spasms.
- Long-term care of the child with recurrent seizure disorders includes physical care and education regarding the importance of medication therapy and problems related to emotional aspects of the disorder.
- Febrile seizures are the most common type of childhood seizure.
- Many cranial deformities are amenable to surgical correction.

- Hydrocephalus is a symptom of an underlying brain pathological condition demonstrated by impaired absorption of CSF or obstruction to the flow of CSF within the ventricles.
- Therapy for hydrocephalus involves relief of the hydrocephalus, treatment of the underlying brain disorder if possible, prevention or treatment of complications, and management of problems related to psychomotor development.

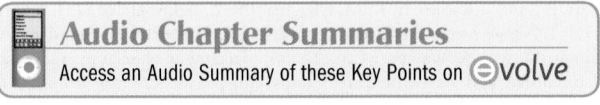

Audio Chapter Summaries

Access an Audio Summary of these Key Points on evolve

References

Ahmad, S., Ellis, J. C., Kamwendo, H., & Molyneux, E. (2006). Efficacy and safety of intranasal lorazepam versus intramuscular paraldehyde for protracted convulsions in children: An open randomised trial. *Lancet, 367*(9522), 1591–1597.

Aldana, P. R., et al. (2003). Results of endoscopic septal fenestration in the treatment of isolated ventricular hydrocephalus. *Pediatric Neurosurgery, 38*(6), 286–294.

Alston, R. D., et al. (2003). Childhood medulloblastoma in northwest England, 1954 to 1977: Incidence and survival. *Developmental Medicine & Child Neurology, 45*(5), 308–314.

American Heart Association. (2005). Part 10.3. Drowning. *Circulation 112*(4), 133–135.

Baandrup, L., & Jensen, R. (2005). Chronic post-traumatic headache: A clinical analysis in relation to the International Headache Classification, 2nd ed. *Cephalalgia, 25*, 132.

Bayir, H., Kochanek, P. M., & Clark, R. S. (2003). Traumatic brain injury in infants and children: Mechanisms of secondary damage and treatment in the intensive care unit. *Critical Care Clinics, 19*(3), 529–549.

Berg, A., et al. (2010). Revised terminology and concepts for organization of seizures and epilepsies: Report of the ILAE Commission on Classification and Terminology, 2005–2009. *Epilepsia, 51*(4), 676–685. doi:10.1111/j.1528-1167.2010.02522.x

Bhalla, T., Dewhirst, E., Sawardekar, A., Dairo, O., & Tobias, J. D. (2012). Perioperative management of the pediatric patient with traumatic brain injury. *Pediatric Anesthesia, 22*(8), 627–640. doi:10.1111/j.1460-9592.2012.03842.x

Bhatt, M., et al. (2009). Consensus-based recommendations for standardizing terminology and reporting adverse events for emergency department procedural sedation and analgesia in children. *Annals of Emergency Medicine, 53*(4), 426–435.

Bhutta, A. T., Van Savell, H., & Schexnayder, S. M. (2003). Reye's syndrome: Down but not out. *Southern Medical Journal, 96*(1), 43–45.

Blaney, S. M., et al. (2006). Tumors of the central nervous system. In P. A. Pizzo & D. G. Pollack (Eds.), *Principles and practice of pediatric oncology* (5th ed.). Philadelphia: Lippincott-Raven.

Bonthius, D. J., & Karacay, B. (2002). Meningitis and encephalitis in children: An update. *Neurologic Clinics, 20*(4), 1013–1038.

Brodeur, G. M., & Maris, J. M. (2006). Neuroblastoma. In P. A. Pizzo & D. G. Pollack (Eds.), *Principles and practice of pediatric oncology* (5th ed.). Philadelphia: Lippincott-Raven.

Browne, T. R., & Holmes, G. L. (2004). *Handbook of epilepsy* (3rd ed.). Philadelphia: Lippincott Williams & Wilkins.

Canadian Cancer Society, Steering Committee on Cancer Statistics. (2011). *Canadian Cancer Statistics 2011*. Toronto: Canadian Cancer Society.

Canadian Neurocritical Care Group. (1999). Guidelines for the diagnosis of brain death. *Canadian Journal of Neurological Science, 26*(1), 4–6.

Canadian Paediatric Society, Infectious Disease and Immunization Committee. (2008). Therapy of suspected bacterial meningitis in Canadian children six weeks of age and older—summary. *Paediatrics & Child Health, 13*(4), 309.

Canadian Red Cross Society. (2006). *Drownings and other water-related injuries in Canada, 10 years of research*. Retrieved from http://www.croixrouge.ca/cmslib/general/drowrep2006overview_en.pdf.

Chen, J. W. Y., & Wasterlain, C. G. (2006). Status epilepticus: pathophysiology and management in adults. *Lancet Neurology, 5*, 246–256. doi:10.1016/S1474-4422(06)70374-X

Chiaretti, A., et al. (2000). Early post-traumatic seizures in children with head injury. *Child's Nervous System, 16*(12), 862–866.

Childhood Cancer Foundation. (2009). *Types of cancer*. Retrieved from http://www.candlelighters.ca/facts/types_of_cancer.html.

Curatolo, P., et al. (2009). Pharmacotherapy of idiopathic generalized epilepsies. *Expert Opinion Pharmacotherapy, 10*(1), 730–734.

Curley, M. A. Q., & Moloney-Harmon, P. A. (2001). *Critical care nursing of infants and children* (2nd ed.). Philadelphia: Saunders.

El Bashir, H., Laundy, M., & Booy, R. (2003). Diagnosis and treatment of bacterial meningitis. *Archive of Diseases in Childhood, 88*(7), 814–819.

Faillace, W. J. (2002). Management of childhood neurotrauma. *Surgical Clinics of North America, 82*(2), 349–363.

Fisgin, T., et al. (2000). Nasal midazolam effects on childhood acute seizures. *Journal of Child Neurology, 15*(12), 833–835.

Forsyth, R., Wolny, S., & Rodrigues, B., & Cochrane Injuries Group. (2010). Routine intracranial pressure monitoring in acute coma. *Cochrane Library, 2*, CD002043. doi:10.1002/14651858.CD002043.pub2

Frucht, M. M., et al. (2000). Distribution of seizure precipitants among epilepsy syndromes. *Epilepsia, 41*(12), 1543–1549.

Gupta, N., & Berger, M. S. (2003). Brain mapping for hemispheric tumors in children. *Pediatric Neurosurgery, 38*(6), 302–306.

Harbord, J. G., et al. (2004). Use of intranasal midazolam to treat acute seizures in paediatric community settings. *Journal of Pediatric Child Health, 40*(9-10), 556–558.

Health Canada. (2006a). *It's your health—meningococcal vaccine*. Retrieved from http://www.hc-sc.gc.ca/hl-vs/iyh-vsv/med/mening-eng.php.

Health Canada. (2006b). *It's your health–Reyes, syndrome*. Retrieved from http://www.hc-sc.gc.ca/hl-vs/iyh-vsv/disease-maladies/reye-eng.php.

Health Canada. (2007). *Safety and injuries*. Retrieved from http://www.hc-sc.gc.ca/hl-vs/securit/index-eng.php.

Johnston, M. V. (2007). Seizures in childhood. In R. M. Kliegman, R. E. Behrman, & H. T. S. Jenson (Eds.), *Nelson textbook of pediatrics* (18th ed.). Philadelphia: Saunders.

Kallas, H. J. (2007). Drowning and submersion injury. In R. M. Kliegman, R. E. Behrman, & H. T. S. Jenson (Eds.), *Nelson textbook of pediatrics* (18th ed.). Philadelphia: Saunders.

Kamienski, M. C. (2003). Reye syndrome. *American Journal of Nursing, 103*(7), 54–57.

Kinsman, S. L., & Johnston, M. V. (2007). Congenital anomalies of the central nervous system. In R. M. Kliegman, R. E. Behrman, & H. T. S. Jenson (Eds.), *Nelson textbook of pediatrics* (18th ed.). Philadelphia: Saunders.

Kline, N. E., & Sevier, N. (2003). Solid tumors in children. *Journal of Pediatric Nursing, 18*(2), 96–102.

Kossoff, E. H., Zupec-Kania, B. A., & Rho, H. M. (2009). Ketogenic diets: An update for child neurologists. *Journal of Child Neurology, 24*(8), 979–988.

Kuzniecky, R. I. (2001). Neuroimaging in pediatric epilepsy. In J. M. Pellock, W. E. Dodson, & B. F. D. Bourgeois (Eds.), *Pediatric epilepsy: Diagnosis and therapy*. New York: Demos Medical Publishing.

Leppik, I. E. (2000). Monotherapy and polypharmacy. *Neurology, 55*(Suppl 3), 525–529.

Levy, R., & Cooper, P. (2003). Ketogenic diet for epilepsy. *Cochrane Database of Systematic Reviews 3*, CD001903. doi:10.1002/14651858.CD001903

Lifesaving Society. (2005). *Study reveals that new Canadians are at higher risk of drowning*. Retrieved from http://www.lifesaving.ca/main.php?lang=english&cat=media&sub=New-Canadians-At-Higher-Risk.

Ljungman, G., et al. (2000). Midazolam nasal spray reduces procedural anxiety in children. *Pediatrics, 105*(1 Pt 1), 73–78.

Lloyd, C. J., Alredy, T., & Lloyd, J. C. (2000). Intranasal midazolam as an alternative to general anaesthesia in the management of children with oral and maxillofacial trauma. *British Journal of Oral & Maxillofacial Surgery, 38*(6), 593–595.

Masson, F., et al. (2003). Epidemiology of traumatic comas: A prospective population-based study. *Brain Injury, 17*(4), 279–293.

Mathern, G. W., et al. (1999). Postoperative seizure control and antiepileptic drug use in pediatric epilepsy surgery patients: The UCLA experience, 1986–1997. *Epilepsia, 40*(12), 1740–1749.

McCrory, P., et al. (2009). Consensus statement on concussion in sport, 3rd International Conference on Concussion in Sport. *Clinical Journal of Sport Medicine, 19*(3), 185–200.

Mueller, S., & Matthay, K. K. (2009). Neuroblastoma: Biology and staging. *Current Oncology Report, 11*(6), 431–438.

Murray-Ryan, J., & Petriccione, M. M. (2002). Central nervous system tumors. In C. R. Baggott, et al. (Eds.), *Nursing care of children and adolescents with cancer* (3rd ed.). Philadelphia: Saunders.

Myhre, S., et al. (2007). Traumatic head injury in infants and toddlers. *Acta Paediatrica, 96*(8), 1159–1163.

Nakken, K. O., et al. (2005). Which seizure-precipitating factors do patients with epilepsy most frequently report? *Epilepsy & Behavior, 6*(1), 85–89. doi:10.1016/j.yebeh.2004.11.003

Ostergaard, J. R. (2009). Febrile seizures. *Acta Paediatrica, 98*(5), 771–773.

Pellock, J. M., & Shinnar, S. (2005). Respiratory adverse events associated with diazepam rectal gel. *Neurology, 64*(10), 1768–1770. doi:10.1212/01.WNL.0000162031.03390.B

Prober, C. G. (2007). Central nervous system infections. In R. M. Kliegman, R. E. Behrman, & H. T. S. Jenson (Eds.), *Nelson textbook of pediatrics* (18th ed.). Philadelphia: Saunders.

Public Health Agency of Canada. (2006). *Canadian immunization guide* (7th ed.). Retrieved from http://www.phac-aspc.sc.ca/publicat/cig-gci/p01-02-eng.php.

Public Health Agency of Canada. (2008). *Leading causes of death and hospitalization in Canada.* Retrieved from http://phac-aspc.gc.ca/publicat/lcd.pcd97/index-eng.php.

Pugliese, A., Beltramo, T., & Torre, D. (2008). Reye's and Reye's-like syndromes. *Cell Biochemistry & Function, 26*(7), 741–746.

Radhakrishnan, K., et al. (2005). Pattern-sensitive epilepsy: Electroclinical characteristics, natural history, and delineation of the epileptic syndrome. *Epilepsia, 46*(1), 48–58. doi:10.1111/j.0013-9580.2005.26604.x

Rivara, F. P., & Grossman, D. (2007). Injury control. In R. M. Kliegman, R. E. Behrman, & H. T. S. Jenson (Eds.), *Nelson textbook of pediatrics* (18th ed.). Philadelphia: Saunders.

Rudy, C. (2005). Hydrocephalus. *Journal of Pediatric Health Care, 19*(2), 111, 127–128. doi:10.1016/j.pedhc.2005.01.002

Sadleir, L. G., & Scheffer, I. E. (2007). Febrile seizures. *British Medical Journal, 334*, 307–311. doi:10.1212/01.wnl.0000344401.02915.00

Safe Kids Canada. (2010). *Drowning prevention.* Retrieved from http://safekidscanada.ca/parents/safety-information/drowning-prevention/index.aspx.

Saez-Llorens, X., & McCracken Jr., G. H. (2003). Bacterial meningitis in children. *Lancet, 361*(9375), 2139–2148.

Saillet, S., et al. (2009). Manipulating the epileptic brain using stimulation: A review of experimental and clinical studies. *Epileptic Disorders, 11*(2), 100–112.

Saskatchewan Brain Injury Association. (2010). *Putting the pieces together: Brain injury.* Retrieved from http://www.sbia.ca/pdf/pieces.pdf.

Schutzman, S. A., & Greenes, D. S. (2001). Pediatric minor head trauma. *Annals of Emergency Medicine, 37*(1), 65–74.

Shemie, S. D., et al., on behalf of the Pediatric Reference Group and the Neonatal Reference Group. (2006). Severe brain injury to neurological determination of death: Canadian forum recommendations. *Canadian Medical Association Journal, 174(6)*, S1–S12. doi:10.1503/cmaj.045142

Shinnar, S., et al. (2000). Predictors of multiple seizures in a cohort of children prospectively followed from the time of their first unprovoked seizure. *Annals of Neurology, 48*(2), 140–147.

Shoji, M. M., et al. (2007). Video game epilepsy in the twentieth century: A review. *Child's Nervous System, 23*(3), 265–267.

Shorvon, S., & Walker, M. (2005). Status epilepticus in idiopathic generalized epilepsy. *Epilepsia, 46*(Suppl 9), 73–79. doi:10.1111/j.1528-1167.2005.00316.x

Sotir, M. J., et al. (2005). Meningococcal disease incidence and mortality in Wisconsin, 1993–2002. *Wisconsin Medical Journal, 104*(3), 38–44.

Swaine, B. R., et al. (2007). Previous head injury is a risk factor for subsequent head injury in children: A longitudinal cohort study. *Pediatrics, 119*(4), 749–758. doi:10.1542/peds.2006-1186

Think First Canada. (2008). *Think First Canada's bicycling injury prevention tips.* Retrieved from http://thinkfirst.ca/documents/BicyclingTips-FINAL.pdf.

Toltzis, P. (2007). Rabies. In R. M. Kliegman, R. E. Behrman, & H. T. S. Jenson (Eds.), *Nelson textbook of pediatrics* (18th ed.). Philadelphia: Saunders.

Treiman, D. M., & Walker, M. C. (2006). Treatment of seizure emergencies: Convulsive and non-convulsive status epilepticus. *Epilepsy Research, 68S*, S77–S82. doi:10.1016/j.eplepsyres.2005.07.020

Vignes, J. R., et al. (2007). Growing skull fracture after minor closed-head injury. *Journal of Pediatrics, 151*(3), 316–318.

Wetzell, R. C. (2007). Anesthesia and perioperative care. In R. M. Kliegman, R. E. Behrman, & H. T. S. Jenson (Eds.), *Nelson textbook of pediatrics* (18th ed.). Philadelphia: Saunders.

Yamamoto, L. G., & Yim, G. K. (2000). The role of intravenous valproic acid in status epilepticus. *Pediatric Emergency Care, 16*(4), 296–298.

Yeates, L. O., et al. (2009). Longitudinal trajectories of postconcussive symptoms in children with mild traumatic brain injuries and their relationship to acute clinical status. *Pediatrics, 123*, 735–743.

Additional Resources

About Kids: Swim for Your Life: http://www.aboutkidshealth.ca/En/News/NewsAndFeatures/Pages/Expert-Opinion-Swim-for-your-life.aspx
Brain Injury Association of Canada: http://biac-aclc.ca/en/
Brain Tumour Foundation of Canada: http://www.braintumour.ca
Canadian Cancer Society: http://www.cancer.ca
Epilepsy Canada: http://www.epilepsy.ca/
Health Canada: http://www.hc-gc.ca
Neurologic Rehabilitation Institute of Ontario: http://www.nrio.com/faq.html
Public Health Agency of Canada: West Nile Virus—Protect Yourself!: http://www.phac-aspc.gc.ca/wn-no/index_e.html
Rancho Los Amigos Rehabilitation Center: The Rancho Levels of Cognitive Functioning: http://www.rancho.org/research_rancholevels.aspx
Safe Kids Canada: http://www.sickkids.ca/Learning/
Spina Bifida and Hydrocephalus Association of Canada: http://www.sbhac.ca
Think First: http://www.thinkfirst.ca

52

Endocrine Dysfunction

Learning Objectives

On completion of this chapter, the reader will be able to:

- Differentiate between the disorders caused by hypopituitary and hyperpituitary dysfunction.
- Describe the manifestations of thyroid hypofunction and hyperfunction and the management of children with the disorders.
- Distinguish between the manifestations of adrenal hypofunction and hyperfunction.
- Differentiate among the various categories of diabetes mellitus.
- Discuss the management and nursing care of the child with diabetes mellitus in the acute care setting.
- Distinguish between a hypoglycemic and a hyperglycemic reaction.
- Design a teaching plan for a child with diabetes mellitus.
- Formulate a teaching plan for the parents of a child with diabetes mellitus.

Electronic Resources

Additional information related to the content in Chapter 52 can be found on

evolve the companion Web site at

http://evolve.elsevier.com/Canada/Perry/maternal/

- Examination Review Questions
- Animation—Adrenal Function
- Case Study—Diabetes Mellitus
- Critical Thinking Exercise—Hypothyroidism

Disorders of Pituitary Function

Deficiencies of the anterior **pituitary hormones** may be due to organic defects or have an **idiopathic** etiology and may occur as a single hormonal problem or in combination with other hormonal deficiencies. The clinical manifestations depend on the hormones involved and the age of onset. If the tropic hormones are involved, the resulting disorder reflects the altered stimulus to the target **gland**. For example, if thyroid-stimulating hormone (TSH) is deficient, thyroid hormone (TH) is also deficient and the child displays the manifestations of hypothyroidism.

An overproduction of the anterior pituitary hormones can result in gigantism (caused by excess growth hormone [GH] production during childhood), hyperthyroidism, hypercortisolism (Cushing's syndrome), and precocious **puberty** from excessive gonadotropins. Overproduction may be caused by hyperplasia of the pituitary cells—which may eventually progress to a tumour (adenoma)—or a primary hypothalamic defect that results in an excess of the hormone's releasing factor. Although the initial clinical manifestations are a result of pituitary oversecretion, eventually pituitary insufficiency occurs, and the signs of panhypopituitarism become evident.

NURSING ALERT Children with panhypopituitarism should wear medical identification, such as a bracelet.

Hypopituitarism

Hypopituitarism is diminished or deficient secretion of pituitary hormones. The consequences of the condition depend on the degree of dysfunction and lead to gonadotropin deficiency with absence or regression of **secondary sex characteristics**; GH deficiency, in which children display restricted somatic growth; TSH deficiency, which produces hypothyroidism; and corticotropin deficiency, which results in manifestations of adrenal hypofunction. Hypopituitarism can result from any of the conditions listed in Box 52-1. The most common organic cause of pituitary undersecretion is tumours in the pituitary or hypothalamic region, especially the craniopharyngiomas.

Constitutional growth delay refers to individuals (usually boys) with delayed linear growth, generally beginning as a toddler, and skeletal and sexual maturation that is behind that of age-mates (Halac & Zimmerman, 2004; Miller & Zimmerman, 2004). Typically these children will reach normal adult height. Often one of the child's parents or another family member has a history of a similar pattern of growth. The untreated child will proceed through normal changes as

BOX 52-1 Clinical Manifestations of Hypopituitarism

Presenting health issue—short stature
- Usually normal growth first year
- Growth during second year drops below established percentile
- Growth measurements below the fifth percentile

Premature aging common in later life
Height may be restricted more than weight
Appear well nourished
Skeletal proportions normal
Tend to be relatively inactive
Less likely to participate in aggressive, sporting-type activities
Bone age nearly always restricted but closely related to height age
Primary teeth usually appear at expected age; eruption of permanent teeth delayed
Teeth overcrowded and malpositioned (because of underdeveloped jaw)
Sexual development usually delayed but normal

expected on the basis of bone age. These changes, although occurring later than in the average child, will appear in normal sequence and manner, and treatment with GH is not usually indicated. However, its use has become controversial, especially in relation to parental and child requests for treatment to accelerate growth.

Diagnostic Evaluation

Only a small number of children with delayed growth or short stature have hypopituitary dwarfism. In most instances the cause is constitutional delay. Diagnostic evaluation is aimed at isolating organic causes, which, in addition to GH deficiency, may include hypothyroidism, oversecretion of cortisol, gonadal aplasia, chronic illness, nutritional inadequacy, Russell-Silver dwarfism, or hypochondroplasia.

A complete diagnostic evaluation should include a family history, a history of the child's growth patterns and previous health status, physical examination, psychosocial evaluation, radiographic surveys, and endocrine studies. Accurate measurement of height (using a calibrated stadiometer) and weight and comparison with standard growth charts are essential. Multiple height measures reflect a more accurate assessment of abnormal growth patterns (Box 52-2) (Hall, 2000).

A skeletal survey in children less than 3 years of age and radiographic examination of the hand-wrist for centres of ossification (bone age) in older children are important in evaluating growth (Box 52-3).

Definitive diagnosis is based on absent or subnormal reserves of pituitary GH. Measuring a single GH level is inaccurate because of the pulsatile secretion of this hormone (Richmond & Rogel, 2008). Because GH levels are normally so low in children that differentiation from abnormal concentrations is unreliable, GH secretion should be stimulated, followed by measurement of blood levels. Exercise is a natural

BOX 52-2 Evaluating the Growth Curve

Ensure reliability of measurements—Accurately obtain and plot height and weight measurements.

Determine absolute height—The child's absolute height bears some relationship to the likelihood of a pathological condition. However, most children who have a height below the lowest percentile (either third or fifth percentile on the height curve) do not have a pathological growth problem.

Assess height velocity—The most important aspect of a growth evaluation is observation of a child's height over time, or height velocity. Accurate determination of height velocity requires at least 4 and preferably 6 months of observation. A substantial deceleration in height velocity (crossing several percentiles) between 3 and 12 or 13 years of age indicates a pathological condition until proven otherwise.

Determine weight-to-height relationship—Determination of the weight-to-height ratio has some diagnostic value in ascertaining the cause of growth restriction in a short child.

Project target height—The height of a child can be judged inappropriately short only in the context of his or her genetic potential. Determine the target height of the child with the formula:

[Father's height (cm) + Mother's height (cm) + 13] /2 for boys

or

[Father's height (cm) + Mother's height (cm) − 13] /2 for girls

Most children achieve an adult stature within approximately 10 cm of the target height.

(Modified from Vogiatzi, M. G., & Copeland, K. C. [1998]. The short child. *Pediatrics in Review, 19*[3], 92–99.)

BOX 52-3 Bone Age for Evaluating Growth Disorders

Bone age refers to a method of assessing skeletal maturity by comparing the appearance of representative epiphyseal centres obtained on x-ray examination with age-appropriate published standards.

Most conditions that cause poor linear growth also cause a delay in skeletal maturation and a restricted bone age. Observation of even a profoundly delayed bone age is never diagnostic or even indicative of a specific diagnosis. A delayed bone age merely indicates that the associated short stature is to some extent "partially reversible," since linear growth will continue until epiphyseal fusion is complete. In comparison, a bone age that is not delayed in a short child is of much greater concern and may, in fact, be of some diagnostic value under certain circumstances.

(Modified from Vogiatzi, M. G., & Copeland, K. C. [1998]. The short child. *Pediatrics in Review, 19*[3], 92–99.)

and benign stimulus for GH release, and elevated levels can be detected after 20 minutes of strenuous exercise in normal children. Also, GH levels are elevated 45 to 90 minutes after the onset of sleep.

Initial assessment of the serum insulin-like growth factor-I (IGF-I) and IGF binding protein 3 (IGFBP3) indicates a need for further evaluation of GH dysfunction if levels are less than −1 standard deviation (SD) below the mean for age. It is recommended that GH stimulation tests be reserved for children with low serum IGF-I and IGFBP3 levels and poor growth who do not have other endocrine or nonendocrine causes for short stature (Richmond & Rogel, 2008).

Studies have shown, however, that traditional GH stimulation tests can yield inaccurate results and be affected by a child's body type or response to stimuli (Hilczer, Smyczynska, & Lewinski, 2006). GH-dependent growth factors may be more sensitive indicators of GH deficiency than GH stimulation tests. Increasingly sensitive radioimmunoassays for GH levels have been developed.

Therapeutic Management

Treatment of GH deficiency caused by organic lesions is directed toward correction of the underlying disease process (e.g., surgical removal or irradiation of a tumour). The definitive treatment of GH deficiency is replacement of GH, which is successful in 80% of affected children. A Cochrane Review concluded that, although GH may improve growth velocity in children, individuals who receive treatment still remain shorter than their peers (Bryant et al. 2007).

The decision to stop GH therapy is made jointly by the child, family, and health care team. Growth rates of less than 2.5 cm/year and a bone age of more than 14 years in girls and more than 16 years in boys are often used as criteria to stop GH therapy (Kliegman et al., 2007). Children with other hormone deficiencies require replacement therapy to correct the specific disorders. This may involve administration of thyroid extract, cortisone, testosterone, or estrogens and progesterone. Treatment with the sex hormones is usually begun during adolescence to promote normal sexual maturation.

Nursing Care Management

The principal nursing consideration in hypothyroidism is identifying children with growth problems. Despite the fact that most growth problems are not a result of organic causes, any delay in normal growth and sexual development poses special emotional adjustments for these children.

The nurse may be a key person in helping establish a diagnosis. For example, if serial height and weight records are not available, the nurse can question parents about the child's growth compared with that of siblings, peers, or relatives. Investigating clothing sizes is often helpful in determining growth at different ages. Parents may comment that the child wears out clothes before growing out of them or that, if the clothing fits the body, it often is too long in the sleeves or legs.

Because the behavioural or physical changes that suggest a tumour are insidious, they are frequently overlooked. It is important to correlate the onset of any positive findings with the initial evidence of growth restriction. For example, visual problems and headache are not uncommon in school-age children and can coincidentally occur after a growth problem is recognized. In fact, headache may represent the emotional trauma caused by short stature rather than be a symptom of a tumour. This line of questioning should be pursued cautiously to avoid alarming parents unduly about the possibility of a brain tumour.

Part of a nurse's role in helping establish a diagnosis is assisting with diagnostic tests. Preparation of the child and family is especially important if a number of tests are being performed, and the child requires particular attention during provocative testing. Blood samples are usually taken every 30 minutes for a 3-hour period. Children also have difficulty overcoming **hypoglycemia** generated by tests with insulin, so they must be observed carefully for signs of hypoglycemia, whereas those receiving glucagon are at risk of nausea and vomiting.

NURSING ALERT Optimum dosing is often achieved when GH is administered at bedtime. Physiological release is more normally stimulated as a result of pituitary release of GH during the first 45 to 90 minutes after the onset of sleep.

Pituitary Hyperfunction

Excess GH before closure of the epiphyseal shafts results in proportional overgrowth of the long bones until the individual reaches a height of 2.4 m or more. Vertical growth is accompanied by rapid and increased development of muscles and viscera. Weight is increased but is usually in proportion to height. Proportional enlargement of head circumference also occurs and may result in delayed closure of the fontanels in young children. Children with a pituitary-secreting tumour may also demonstrate signs of increasing intracranial pressure, especially headache.

If oversecretion of GH occurs after epiphyseal closure, growth is in the transverse direction, producing a condition known as *acromegaly*. Typical facial features include overgrowth of the head, lips, nose, tongue, jaw, and paranasal and mastoid sinuses; separation and **malocclusion** of the teeth in the enlarged jaw; disproportion of the face to the cerebral division of the skull; increased facial hair; thickened, deeply creased skin; and increased tendency toward **hyperglycemia** and diabetes mellitus (DM).

Diagnostic Evaluation

Diagnosis is based on a history of excessive growth during childhood and evidence of increased levels of GH. Radiographic studies may reveal a tumour in an enlarged sella turcica, normal bone age, enlargement of bones (such as the paranasal sinuses), and evidence of joint changes. Endocrine studies to confirm an excess of other hormones, specifically thyroid, cortisol, and sex hormones, should also be included in the differential diagnosis.

Therapeutic Management

If a lesion is present, surgical treatment by cryosurgery or hypophysectomy is performed to remove the tumour when feasible. Other therapies aimed at destroying pituitary tissue include external irradiation and radioactive implants. Depending on the extent of surgical extirpation and degree of pituitary insufficiency, hormone replacement with thyroid extract, cortisone, and sex hormones may be necessary.

Nursing Care Management

The primary nursing consideration is early identification of children with excessive growth rates. Although medical management is unable to reduce growth already attained, further growth can be restricted. The earlier the treatment, the more control there is in predetermining a normal adult height. Nurses in ambulatory settings who are frequently involved in growth screening should refer children who demonstrate excessive linear growth for a medical evaluation. They should also observe for signs of a tumour, especially headache, and evidence of concurrent hormonal excesses, particularly the gonadotropins, which cause sexual precocity.

Children with excessive growth rates require as much emotional support as those with short stature. Children and their parents need an opportunity to express their thoughts. A compassionate nurse can be supportive to these children, especially before adolescence when they are larger than their peers.

Precocious Puberty

Manifestations of sexual development before age 9 years in boys or age 8 years in girls have traditionally been considered precocious development, and these children were recommended for further evaluation (Kaplowitz, 2009). Recent American investigations of the age limit for defining when puberty is precocious showed that the onset of puberty in girls is occurring earlier than previous studies had documented (Biro et al., 2006; Slyper, 2006). Mean onset of puberty was 10.2 and 9.6 years in White and Black girls, respectively. On the basis of these findings, it was recommended that precocious puberty evaluation for a pathological cause be performed for White girls younger than 7 years of age and for Black girls younger than 6 years of age. No change in the guidelines for evaluation of precocious puberty in boys was recommended. However, recent data suggest that boys may be beginning maturation earlier as well (Herman-Giddens, 2006; Slyper, 2006). There are some small cohort studies indicating that Canada is following the same pattern as the U.S. data. There is a concern that early menarche will increase the risk of future breast cancer (Steingraber, 2007).

Normally the hypothalamic-releasing factors stimulate secretion of the **gonadotropic hormones** from the anterior pituitary at the time of puberty. In the male, interstitial cell–stimulating hormone stimulates Leydig's cells of the testes to secrete testosterone; in the female, follicle-stimulating hormone (FSH) and luteinizing hormone stimulate the ovarian follicles to secrete estrogens (Nebesio & Eugster, 2007). This sequence of events is known as the *hypothalamic–pituitary–gonadal axis.* If for some reason the cycle undergoes premature activation, the child will display evidence of advanced or precocious puberty. Causes of precocious puberty are found in Box 52-4.

BOX 52-4 Causes of Precocious Puberty

Central Precocious Puberty

Idiopathic, with or without hypothalamic hamartoma

Secondary

- Congenital anomalies
- Postinflammatory—Encephalitis, meningitis, abscess, granulomatous disease
- Radiotherapy
- Trauma
- Neoplasms

After effective treatment of longstanding pseudoisosexual precocity

Peripheral Precocious Puberty

Familial male-limited precocious puberty

Albright's syndrome

Gonadal or extragonadal tumours

Adrenal

- Congenital adrenal hyperplasia
- Adenoma, carcinoma
- Glucocorticoid resistance

Exogenous sex hormones

Primary hypothyroidism

Incomplete Precocious Puberty

Premature thelarche

Premature menarche

Premature pubarche or adrenarche

(Modified from Root, A. W. [2000]. Precocious puberty. *Pediatrics in Review, 21*[1], 10–19.)

Isosexual precocious puberty is more common among girls than boys. Approximately 50% of children with precocious puberty have *central precocious puberty (CPP)*, in which pubertal development is activated by the hypothalamic gonadotropin-releasing hormone (GnRH). This produces early maturation and development of the gonads with secretion of sex hormones, development of secondary sex characteristics, and sometimes production of mature sperm and ova (Lee, 1999; Root, 2000). CPP occurs more frequently in girls and is usually idiopathic, with 95% demonstrating no causative factor (Carel & Leger, 2008; Greiner & Kerrigan, 2006; Nebesio & Eugster, 2007; Root, 2000). A central nervous system (CNS) insult or structural abnormality is found in more than 90% of boys with CPP (Root, 2000).

Peripheral precocious puberty (PPP) includes early puberty resulting from hormone stimulation other than the hypothalamic GnRH–stimulated pituitary gonadotropin release. Isolated manifestations that are usually associated with puberty may be seen as variations in normal sexual development (Greiner & Kerrigan, 2006). They appear without other signs of **pubescence** and are probably caused by unusual end-organ sensitivity to prepubertal levels of estrogen or androgen. Included are premature thelarche (development of breasts in prepubertal girls), premature pubarche (premature adrenarche, early development of sexual hair), and premature **menarche** (isolated menses without other evidence of sexual development).

Therapeutic Management

Treatment of precocious puberty is directed toward the specific cause, when known. In 50% of cases, precocious pubertal development regresses or stops advancing without any treatment (Carel & Leger, 2008). Precocious puberty of central (hypothalamic–pituitary) origin is managed with monthly injections of a synthetic analogue of luteinizing hormone–releasing hormone, which regulates pituitary secretions (Greiner & Kerrigan, 2006; Muir, 2006). The available preparation, leuprolide acetate (Lupron Depot), is given in a dosage of 0.2 to 0.3 mg/kg intramuscularly once every 4 weeks, although a longer-lasting preparation given every 3 months is also effective in most patients. GnRH analogue (GnRHa) histrelin has been formulated to implant in the subdermal tissue and may be useful for patients who want to avoid injections (Kaplowitz, 2009).

Once treatment is initiated, breast development regresses or does not advance, and growth returns to normal rates, enhancing predicted height. Studies suggest that not all patients attain adult targeted heights. Therapy with GH therapy may be used, or a trial of a nonaromatizable anabolic steroid may be initiated to improve adult height (Carel, & Leger, 2008; Kaplowitz, 2009). Treatment is discontinued at a chronologically appropriate time, allowing pubertal changes to resume. Psychological management of the patient and family is an important aspect of care. Both parents and the affected child should be taught the injection procedure.

Nursing Care Management

Psychological support and guidance of the child and family are the most important aspects of nursing care. Parents need **anticipatory guidance**, support and information resources, and reassurance of the **benign** nature of the condition (Greiner & Kerrigan, 2006; O'Sullivan & O'Sullivan, 2002). Dress and activities for the physically precocious child should be appropriate to the **chronological age**. Sexual interest is not usually advanced beyond the child's chronological age, and parents need to understand that the child's mental age is congruent with the chronological age and that the child's normal, overt manifestations of affection are age appropriate and do not represent sexual advances.

Although the child's sexual behaviour is appropriate for the chronological age, the nurse should emphasize to parents that the child is fertile. Usually no form of contraception is necessary unless the child is sexually active. In this situation, proper counselling is important because hormonal forms of birth control, such as estrogen pills, will prematurely initiate epiphyseal closure, resulting in stunted linear growth.

Diabetes Insipidus

The principal disorder of posterior pituitary hypofunction is diabetes insipidus (DI), also known as neurogenic DI, resulting from undersecretion of antidiuretic hormone (ADH), or vasopressin (Pitressin), and producing a state of uncontrolled diuresis (Makaryus & McFarlane, 2006). This disorder is not to be confused with nephrogenic DI, a rare hereditary disorder affecting primarily males and caused by unresponsiveness of the renal tubules to the hormone.

Neurogenic DI may result from a number of different causes. Primary causes are **familial** or idiopathic; of the total cases, approximately 45 to 50% are idiopathic. Secondary causes include **trauma** (accidental or surgical), tumours, granulomatous disease, **infections** (meningitis or encephalitis), and vascular anomalies (aneurysm). Certain drugs, such as alcohol or phenytoin, can cause a transient polyuria.

The cardinal signs of DI are polyuria and polydipsia. In the older child, signs such as excessive urination accompanied by a compensatory insatiable thirst may be so intense that the child does little more than go to the toilet and drink fluids (Cheetham & Baylis, 2002). Frequently the first sign is enuresis. In the infant the initial symptom is irritability that is relieved with feedings of water but not milk. The infant is also prone to dehydration, electrolyte imbalance, hyperthermia, azotemia, and potential circulatory collapse.

Dehydration is usually not a serious problem in older children, who are able to drink larger quantities of water. However, any period of unconsciousness, such as after trauma or anaesthesia, may be life threatening because the voluntary demand for fluid is absent. During such instances careful monitoring of urine volumes, blood concentration, and intravenous (IV) fluid replacement is essential to prevent dehydration.

NURSING ALERT The child with DI complicated by congenital absence of the thirst centre must be encouraged to drink sufficient quantities of liquid to prevent electrolyte imbalance.

Diagnostic Evaluation

The simplest test used to diagnose this condition is restriction of oral fluids and observation of consequent changes in urine volume and concentration. Normally, reducing fluids results in concentrated urine and diminished volume. In DI, fluid restriction has little or no effect on urine formation but causes weight loss from dehydration. Accurate results from this procedure require strict monitoring of fluid intake and urine output, measurement of urine concentration (specific gravity or osmolality), and frequent weight checks. A weight loss between 3 and 5% indicates significant dehydration and requires termination of the fluid restriction.

NURSING ALERT Small children require close observation during fluid deprivation to prevent them from drinking, even from toilet bowls, flower vases, or other unlikely sources of fluid.

If this test is positive, the child should be given a test dose of injected aqueous vasopressin, which should alleviate the polyuria and polydipsia. Unresponsiveness to exogenous vasopressin usually indicates nephrogenic DI. An important diagnostic consideration is to differentiate DI from other causes of polyuria and polydipsia, especially DM. DI may be the early sign of an evolving cerebral process (De Buyst et al., 2007).

Therapeutic Management

The usual treatment is hormone replacement, either with an intramuscular or subcutaneous injection of vasopressin tannate in peanut oil or with a nasal spray of aqueous lysine vasopressin (Makaryus & McFarlane, 2006; Verbalis, 2003). The injectable form has the advantage of lasting 48 to 72 hours, which affords the child a full night's sleep. However, it has the disadvantage of requiring frequent injections and proper preparation of the drug.

NURSING ALERT To be effective, vasopressin must be thoroughly mixed in the oil by being held under warm running water for 10 to 15 minutes and shaken vigorously before being drawn into the syringe. If this is not done, the oil may be injected minus the ADH. Small brown particles, which indicate drug dispersion, must be seen in the suspension.

Nursing Care Management

The initial objective is identification of the disorder. Because an early sign may be sudden enuresis in a child who is toilet trained, excessive thirst with bed-wetting is an indication for further investigation. Another clue is persistent irritability and crying in an infant that is relieved only by bottle-feedings of water. After head trauma or certain neurosurgical procedures, the development of DI can be anticipated; these patients must be closely monitored.

Assessment includes measurement of body weight, serum electrolytes, blood urea nitrogen, hematocrit, and urine specific gravity taken before surgery and every other day after the procedure. Fluid intake and output should be carefully measured and recorded. Alert patients are able to adjust intake to urine losses, but unconscious or very young patients require closer fluid observation. In children who are not toilet trained, collection of urine specimens may require application of a urine-collecting device.

After confirmation of the diagnosis, parents need a thorough explanation regarding the condition with specific clarification that DI is a different condition from DM. They must realize that treatment is lifelong. If children are to receive the injectable vasopressin, ideally two caregivers should be taught the correct procedure for preparation and administration of the medication. Once children are old enough, they should be encouraged to assume full responsibility for their care.

For emergency purposes, these children should wear medical alert identification. Older children should carry the nasal spray with them for temporary relief of symptoms. School personnel need to be aware of the problem so they can grant children unrestricted use of the lavatory. Failure to permit this may result in embarrassing accidents that often lead to a child's unwillingness to attend school.

Syndrome of Inappropriate Antidiuretic Hormone

The disorder that results from oversecretion of the posterior pituitary hormone, or ADH, is known as syndrome of inappropriate antidiuretic hormone (SIADH). It is observed with increased frequency in a variety of conditions, especially those involving infections, tumours, or other CNS disease or trauma, and is a common cause of hyponatremia in the pediatric population (Lin, Liu, & Lim, 2005; Rivkees, 2008).

The manifestations are directly related to fluid retention and hypotonicity. Excess ADH causes most of the filtered water to be reabsorbed from the kidneys back into central circulation. Serum osmolality is low, and urine osmolality is inappropriately elevated. When serum sodium levels are diminished to 120 mmol/L, affected children display **anorexia**, nausea (and sometimes vomiting), stomach cramps, irritability, and personality changes. With progressive reduction in sodium, other neurological signs, stupor, and convulsions may be evident (Rivkees, 2008). The symptoms usually disappear when the underlying disorder is corrected.

The immediate management consists of restricting fluids. Subsequent management depends on the cause and severity. Fluids continue to be restricted to one-fourth to one-half maintenance. When there are no fluid abnormalities but SIADH can be anticipated, fluids are often restricted expectantly at two-thirds to three-fourths maintenance.

Nursing Care Management

The first goal of nursing management is recognizing the presence of SIADH from symptoms described in patients at risk, especially those in the pediatric intensive care unit.

NURSING ALERT Nausea, vomiting, and malaise may precede the onset of more severe stages such as disorientation, confusion, coma, and seizures (Majzoub & Muglia, 2003).

Accurately measuring intake and output, noting daily weight, and observing for signs of fluid overload are primary nursing functions, especially in the child receiving IV fluids. Seizure precautions should be implemented, and the child and family need education regarding the rationale for fluid restrictions. The rare child with chronic SIADH will be placed on long-term ADH-antagonizing medication, and the child and family will require instructions for its administration.

Disorders of Thyroid Function

The thyroid gland secretes two types of hormones: TH, which consists of the hormones thyroxine (T_4) and triiodothyronine (T_3), and calcitonin. The secretion of thyroid hormones is controlled by TSH from the anterior pituitary, which in turn is regulated by thyrotropin-releasing factor (TRF) from the **hypothalamus** as a negative feedback response. Consequently, hypothyroidism or hyperthyroidism may result from a defect in the target gland or from a disturbance in the secretion of TSH or TRF. Because the functions of T_3 and T_4 are qualitatively the same, the term *TH* is used throughout this discussion.

The synthesis of TH depends on available sources of dietary iodine and tyrosine. The thyroid is the only endocrine gland capable of storing excess amounts of hormones for release as needed. During circulation in the bloodstream, T_4 and T_3 are bound to carrier proteins (thyroxine-binding globulin). They must be unbound before they are able to exert their metabolic effect.

The main physiological action of TH is to regulate the basal metabolic rate and thereby control the processes of growth and tissue differentiation. Unlike GH, TH is involved in many more diverse activities that influence the growth and development of body tissues. Therefore, a deficiency of TH exerts a more profound effect on growth than that seen in hypopituitarism.

Calcitonin helps maintain blood calcium levels by decreasing the calcium concentration. Its effect is the opposite of parathyroid hormone (PTH) in that it inhibits skeletal demineralization and promotes calcium deposition in the bone.

evolve Critical Thinking Exercise—Hypothyroidism

Juvenile Hypothyroidism

Hypothyroidism is one of the most common endocrine problems of childhood. It may be either **congenital** or acquired and represents a deficiency in secretion of TH (Foley, 2001).

Beyond infancy, primary hypothyroidism may be caused by a number of defects. For example, a congenital hypoplastic thyroid gland may provide sufficient amounts of TH during the first year or two but be inadequate when rapid body growth increases demands on the gland. A partial or complete thyroidectomy for cancer or thyrotoxicosis can leave insufficient thyroid tissue to furnish hormones for body requirements. Radiotherapy for Hodgkin's disease or other malignancies may lead to hypothyroidism (Hudson et al., 2011). Infectious processes may cause hypothyroidism. It can also occur when dietary iodine is deficient.

Clinical manifestations depend on the extent of dysfunction and the child's age at onset. Primary congenital hypothyroidism is characterized by low levels of circulating thyroid hormones and raised levels of TSH at birth (Macchia, 2000). The GnRH test and baseline measurement of gonadotropin and sex hormone serum concentrations at 3 months of age are promising options for the assessment of hypothalamic–pituitary–gonadal function in infants with congenital hypothyroidism (van Tijn et al., 2007). The presenting symptoms are decelerated growth from chronic deprivation of TH or thyromegaly. Impaired growth and development are less severe when hypothyroidism is acquired at a later age, and, because brain growth is nearly complete by 2 to 3 years of age, intellectual disability and neurological sequelae are not associated with juvenile hypothyroidism. Other manifestations are myxedematous skin changes (dry skin, puffiness around the eyes, sparse hair), constipation, sleepiness, and mental decline (Box 52-5).

Therapy is TH replacement, the same as for hypothyroidism in the infant, although the prompt treatment needed in the infant is not required in the child. In children with severe symptoms, the restoration of euthyroidism is achieved more gradually with administration of increasing amounts of L-thyroxine over a period of 4 to 8 weeks to avoid symptoms of hyperthyroidism, which can occur with treatment of chronic hypothyroidism. Researchers have found that children treated early continue to have mild delays in reading, comprehension, and arithmetic but catch up by grade six (Rovet & Ehrlich, 2000). However, adolescents may demonstrate problems with memory, attention, and visuospatial processing.

BOX 52-5 Clinical Manifestations of Juvenile Hypothyroidism

Decelerated growth
- Less when acquired at later age

Myxedematous skin changes
- Dry skin
- Puffiness around eyes
- Sparse hair
- Constipation
- Sleepiness
- Mental decline

Nursing Care Management

The importance of early recognition in the infant is discussed in Chapter 28. Growth cessation or restriction in a child whose growth has previously been normal should alert the observer to the possibility of hypothyroidism. After diagnosis and implementation of thyroxine therapy, the importance of compliance and periodic monitoring of response to therapy should be stressed to parents. Children should learn to take responsibility for their own health as soon as they are old enough, at about 9 or 10 years of age.

Goitre

A *goitre* is an enlargement or hypertrophy of the thyroid gland. It may occur with deficient (hypothyroid), excessive (hyperthyroid), or normal (**euthyroid**) TH secretion. It can be congenital or acquired. Congenital disease usually occurs as a result of maternal administration of antithyroid medications or iodides during pregnancy. Acquired disease can result from increased secretion of pituitary TSH in response to decreased circulating levels of TH or from infiltrative neoplastic or inflammatory processes. In areas where dietary iodine (essential for TH production) is deficient, goitre can be endemic.

Enlargement of the thyroid gland may be mild and noticeable only when there is an increased demand for TH (e.g., during periods of rapid growth). Where iodine deficiency is severe, a large percentage of the population displays goitres. Enlargement of the thyroid at birth can be sufficient to cause severe respiratory distress. Sporadic goitre is usually caused by lymphocytic thyroiditis, and intrinsic biochemical defects in synthesis of the hormones are associated with goitres. TH replacement is necessary to treat the hypothyroidism and reverse the TSH effect on the gland.

Nursing Care Management

Large goitres are identified by their obvious appearance. Smaller nodules may be evident only on palpation. Nurses in ambulatory settings need to be aware of the possibility of goitres and report such findings. Benign enlargement of the thyroid gland may occur during adolescence and should not be confused with pathological states. Nodules rarely are caused by a cancerous tumour but always require evaluation. Questions regarding exposure to radiation should be included in the assessment.

NURSING ALERT If an infant is born with a goitre, immediate precautions need to be instituted for emergency ventilation, such as giving supplemental oxygen and having a tracheostomy set nearby. Hyperextension of the neck often facilitates breathing. Immediate surgery to remove part of the gland may be lifesaving in infants born with a goitre.

Lymphocytic Thyroiditis

Lymphocytic thyroiditis (Hashimoto's disease, juvenile autoimmune thyroiditis) is the most common cause of thyroid disease in children and adolescents and is associated with the largest percentage of juvenile hypothyroidism (Szymborska & Staroszczyk, 2000). It accounts for many of the enlarged thyroid glands formerly designated *thyroid hyperplasia of adolescence* or *adolescent goitre*. Although it can develop during the first 3 years of life, it occurs more frequently after age 6. It reaches a peak incidence during adolescence, and there is evidence that the disease is self-limited. The presence of a goitre and elevated thyroglobulin antibody with progressive increase in both thyroid peroxidase antibody and TSH may be predictive factors for future development of hypothyroidism (Radetti et al., 2006).

The presence of an enlarged thyroid gland is usually detected by the practitioner during a routine examination, although it may be noted by parents when the youngster swallows. In most children the entire gland is enlarged symmetrically (though it may be asymmetrical) and is firm, freely movable, and nontender. There may be manifestations of moderate tracheal compression (sense of fullness, hoarseness, and dysphagia), but it is extremely rare for a nontoxic diffuse goitre to enlarge to the extent that it causes mechanical obstruction. Most children are euthyroid, but some display symptoms of hypothyroidism. Other signs suggestive of lymphocytic thyroiditis are found in Box 52-6.

Diagnostic Evaluation

Thyroid function tests are usually normal, although TSH levels may be slightly or moderately elevated. With progressive disease the T_4 decreases, followed by a decrease in T_3 levels and an increase in TSH. A variety of abnormalities in radioactive iodine uptake may be noted. Most affected children have serum antibody titres to thyroid antigens, but fewer children have a positive red blood cell hemagglutination test result. When both tests are used, almost all children with thyroid autoimmunity are detected. However, levels in children are lower than in adults; repeated measurements may be needed in doubtful cases, since titres may increase later in the disease.

Therapeutic Management

In many cases the goitre is transient and asymptomatic and regresses spontaneously within a year or two. Therapy of a nontoxic diffuse goitre is usually simple, uncomplicated, and effective. Oral administration of TH decreases the size of the gland significantly and provides the feedback needed to suppress TSH stimulation, and the hyperplastic thyroid gland gradually regresses in size. Surgery is contraindicated in this disorder. Untreated patients should be evaluated periodically.

Nursing Care Management

Nursing care consists of identifying the youngster with thyroid enlargement, reassuring the child that the condition is probably only temporary, and reinforcing instructions for thyroid therapy.

BOX 52-6 Clinical Manifestations of Lymphocytic Thyroiditis

Enlarged thyroid gland
- Usually symmetrical
- Firm
- Freely movable
- Nontender

Tracheal compression
- Sense of fullness
- Hoarseness
- Dysphagia

Hyperthyroidism (possible)
- Nervousness
- Irritability
- Increased sweating
- Hyperactivity

Hyperthyroidism

The largest percentage of hyperthyroidism in childhood is caused by Graves' disease, which is usually associated with an enlarged thyroid gland and exophthalmos (Ma et al., 2006; Streetman & Khanderia, 2004; Thompson, 2002). Most cases of Graves' disease in children occur between ages 6 and 15, with a peak incidence at 12 to 14 years of age, but the disease may be present at birth in children of thyrotoxic mothers. The incidence is five times higher in girls than in boys.

The hyperthyroidism of Graves' disease is apparently caused by an autoimmune response to TSH receptors, but no specific etiology has been identified. There is definitive evidence for familial association, with a high concordance incidence in twins. Patients with Graves' disease possess the histocompatibility antigens A1, B8, and DR3 (Dallas & Foley, 2003; Simmonds et al., 2005).

The development of manifestations is highly variable. Signs and symptoms develop gradually, with an interval between onset and diagnosis of approximately 6 to 12 months. The principal clinical features are excessive motion—irritability, hyperactivity, short attention span, tremors, insomnia, and emotional lability. Clinical manifestations are presented in Box 52-7.

Exophthalmos (protruding eyeballs), observed in many children, is accompanied by a wide-eyed staring expression, increased blinking, lid lag, lack of convergence, and absence of wrinkling of the forehead when looking upward. As protrusion of the eyeball increases, the child may not be able to completely cover the cornea with the lid. Visual disturbances may include blurred vision and loss of visual acuity. Ophthalmopathy can develop long before or after the onset of hyperthyroidism. A consistent pathogenic link between them has not been identified. It is now thought that Graves' ophthalmopathy is a disorder of autoimmune origin caused by a complex interplay of endogenous and environmental factors (Bartalena et al., 2003).

Diagnostic Evaluation

The presence of a thyroid mass in a child requires a thorough history, including inquiry into prior irradiation to the head and neck and exposure to a goitrogen. The diagnosis is established on the basis of increased levels of T_4 and T_3. TSH is suppressed to unmeasurable levels (Ma et al., 2006). Other tests are rarely indicated.

Therapeutic Management

Therapy for hyperthyroidism is controversial, but all methods are directed toward slowing the rate of hormone secretion.

BOX 52-7 Clinical Manifestations of Hyperthyroidism (Graves' Disease)

Cardinal Signs

Emotional lability
Physical restlessness, characteristically at rest
Decelerated school performance
Voracious appetite with weight loss in 50% of cases
Fatigue

Physical Signs

Tachycardia
Widened pulse pressure
Dyspnea on exertion
Exophthalmos (protruding eyeballs)
Wide-eyed, staring expression with lid lag
Tremor
Goitre (hypertrophy and hyperplasia)
Warm, moist skin
Accelerated linear growth
Heat intolerance (may be severe)
Hair fine and unable to hold a curl
Systolic murmurs

Thyroid Storm

Acute onset:

- Severe irritability and restlessness
- Vomiting
- Diarrhea
- Hyperthermia
- Hypertension
- Severe tachycardia
- Prostration

May progress rapidly to:

- Delirium
- Coma
- Death

The three acceptable modes available are the antithyroid medications, including propylthiouracil (PTU) and methimazole (MTZ, Tapazole), which interfere with the biosynthesis of TH; subtotal thyroidectomy; and ablation with radioiodine (^{131}I iodide) (Rivkees & Cornelius, 2003; Streetman & Khanderia, 2004). Each is effective, but each has advantages and disadvantages.

Thyrotoxicosis (thyroid *crisis* or thyroid *storm*) may occur from the sudden release of the hormone. Although thyrotoxicosis is unusual in children, a crisis can be life threatening. These "storms" are evidenced by the acute onset of severe irritability and restlessness, vomiting, diarrhea, hyperthermia, hypertension, severe tachycardia, and prostration. There may be rapid progression to delirium, coma, and even death. A crisis may be precipitated by acute infection, surgical emergencies, or discontinuation of antithyroid therapy. Treatment, in addition to antithyroid medications, is administration of β-adrenergic blocking agents (propranolol), which provide relief from the adrenergic hyper-responsiveness that produces the disturbing adverse effects of the reaction. Therapy is usually required for 2 to 3 weeks.

The Thyroid Foundation of Canada has extensive information related to the prevention, treatment, and cure of thyroid disease (see Additional Resources section at the end of this chapter).

Nursing Care Management

The initial nursing objective is identification of children with hyperthyroidism. Because the clinical manifestations often appear gradually, the goitre and ophthalmic changes may not be noticed, and the excessive activity may be attributed to behavioural problems. Nurses in ambulatory settings, particularly schools, need to be alert to signs that suggest this disorder, especially weight loss despite an excellent appetite, academic difficulties resulting from a short attention span and inability to sit still, unexplained fatigue and sleeplessness, and difficulty with fine motor skills such as writing. Exophthalmos may develop long before the onset of signs and symptoms of hyperthyroidism and may be the only presenting sign (Thompson, 2002). Exophthalmos is less common in adults than children (Jospe, 2001).

Much of the care of these children is related to treating physical symptoms before a response to medication therapy is achieved. These children need a quiet, unstimulating environment that is conducive to rest. Sometimes hospitalization is necessary during the immediate treatment phase to remove a child from a troubled home. A regular routine is beneficial in providing frequent rest periods, minimizing the stress of coping with unexpected demands, and meeting the children's needs promptly. Physical activity should be restricted. For example, school physical education classes need to be discontinued.

Emotional lability is often manifested by sudden episodes of crying or elation. Such behaviour, coupled with irritability, disrupts interpersonal relationships, creating difficulties within and outside the home. Parents need help in understanding the uncontrollable nature of these outbursts and ways of minimizing them through decreased environmental stimulation, stress, and frustration. The child should be encouraged to express feelings about behaviour and its effect on others. The nurse can encourage the child to concentrate on friendship with one special peer rather than a group until the condition is stabilized.

Heat intolerance may produce considerable family conflict. Preferring a cooler environment than others, the child is likely to open windows, complain about the heat, wear minimum clothing, and remove blankets while sleeping. Although the child should dress in accordance with climatic conditions, the use of light cotton clothing in the home, good ventilation, air conditioning or fans, frequent baths, and adequate hydration is helpful in providing comfort. Hygiene should be stressed because of excessive sweating.

Dietary requirements should be adjusted to meet the child's increased metabolic rate. Although the need for calories is increased, these should be provided in wholesome foods rather than "junk" foods. The child may require vitamin supplements to meet daily requirement. Rather than three large meals, the child's appetite may be better satisfied by five or six moderate meals throughout the day. Family members should refrain from making remarks about the child's appetite because the child may voluntarily restrict his or her eating to avoid such attention.

Once therapy is instituted, the nurse needs to explain the medication regimen, emphasizing the importance of observing for adverse effects of antithyroid medications. Untoward effects of propylthiouracil and related compounds include urticarial rash, fever, arthritis, or arthralgia. There may be enlargement of the salivary and cervical lymph glands, a diminished sense of taste, hepatitis, and **edema** of the lower extremities. Parents should also be aware of the signs of hypothyroidism, which can occur from overdose of the medications. The most common indications are lethargy and somnolence.

NURSING ALERT Children being treated with propylthiouracil or methimazole must be carefully monitored for adverse effects of the medication. Because sore throat and fever accompany the grave complication of leukopenia, these children should be seen by a practitioner if such symptoms occur. Parents and children should be taught to recognize and report symptoms immediately.

Disorders of Parathyroid Function

The parathyroid glands secrete PTH, the main function of which, along with vitamin D and calcitonin, is homeostasis of serum calcium concentration (Perheentupa, 2003). The effect of PTH on calcium is opposite that of calcitonin. The net result of the integrated action of PTH and vitamin D is maintenance of serum calcium levels within a narrow normal range and the mineralization of bone. Secretion of PTH is controlled by a negative feedback system involving the serum calcium ion concentration. Low ionized calcium levels stimulate PTH secretion, causing absorption of calcium by the target tissues; high ionized calcium concentrations suppress PTH.

Hypoparathyroidism

Hypoparathyroidism is a spectrum of disorders that result in deficient PTH. Congenital hypoparathyroidism may be caused by a specific defect in the synthesis or cellular processing of PTH or by aplasia or hypoplasia of the gland (Perheentupa, 2003).

Hypoparathyroidism can also occur secondary to other causes. Postoperative hypoparathyroidism may follow thyroidectomy with acute or gradual onset and be transient or permanent. Two forms of transient hypoparathyroidism may be present in the newborn, both of which are the result of a relative PTH deficiency. One type is caused by maternal hyperparathyroidism or maternal DM. A more common, later form appears almost exclusively in infants fed a milk formula with a high phosphate-to-calcium ratio.

Clinical signs of hypoparathyroidism are found in Box 52-8.

BOX 52-8 Clinical Manifestations of Hypoparathyroidism

Pseudohypoparathyroidism

Short stature
Round face
Short, thick neck
Short, stubby fingers and toes
Dimpling of skin over knuckles
Subcutaneous soft tissue calcifications
Intellectual disability a prominent feature

Idiopathic Hypoparathyroidism

None of the above physical characteristics observed
May include papilledema
May have intellectual disability

Both Types

Dry, scaly, coarse skin with eruptions
Hair often brittle
Nails thin and brittle with characteristic transverse grooves
Dental and enamel hypoplasia
Muscle contractions:
- Tetany
- Carpopedal spasm
- Laryngospasm (laryngeal stridor)
- Muscle cramps and twitching
- Positive Chvostek's sign or Trousseau's sign
- Paresthesias, tingling

Neurological:
- Headache
- Seizures (generalized, absence, or focal)
- Swings of emotion
- Loss of memory
- Depression
- Confusion possible

Gastrointestinal:
- Muscle cramps
- Diarrhea
- Vomiting

Restricted skeletal growth

Diagnostic Evaluation

The diagnosis of hypoparathyroidism is made on the basis of clinical manifestations associated with decreased serum calcium and increased serum phosphorus. Levels of plasma PTH are low in idiopathic hypoparathyroidism but high in pseudohypoparathyroidism. End-organ responsiveness is tested by the administration of PTH with measurement of urinary cyclic adenosine monophosphate (cAMP). Kidney function tests are included in the differential diagnosis to rule out renal insufficiency. Although bone radiographs are usually normal, they may demonstrate increased bone density and suppressed growth.

NURSING ALERT The earliest indication of hypoparathyroidism may be anxiety and mental depression, followed by paresthesia and evidence of heightened neuromuscular excitability:

Chvostek's sign—Facial muscle spasm elicited by tapping the facial nerve in the region of the parotid gland
Trousseau's sign—Carpal spasm elicited by pressure applied to nerves of the upper arm

Tetany–Carpopedal spasm (sharp flexion of wrist and ankle joints), muscle twitching, cramps, seizures, and stridor

Therapeutic Management

The objective of treatment is to maintain normal serum calcium and phosphate levels with minimum complications. Acute or severe tetany is corrected immediately by IV and oral administration of calcium gluconate and follow-up daily doses to achieve normal levels. Twice-daily serum calcium measurements are taken to monitor the efficacy of therapy and prevent hypercalcemia. When diagnosis is confirmed, vitamin D therapy is begun. Vitamin D therapy is somewhat difficult to regulate because the drug has a prolonged onset and a long half-life (see Patient Teaching box).

Long-term management consists of administration of massive doses of vitamin D, and oral calcium supplementation may be useful in maintaining adequate serum calcium levels, although it is not essential. Blood calcium and phosphorus are monitored frequently until the levels have stabilized; they are then monitored monthly and less often until the child is seen at 6-month intervals. Renal function, blood pressure, and serum vitamin D levels are measured every 6 months. Serum magnesium levels are measured every 3 to 6 months to permit detection of hypomagnesemia, which may raise the requirement for vitamin D.

Nursing Care Management

The initial objective is recognition of hypocalcemia. Unexplained convulsions, irritability (especially to external stimuli), gastrointestinal symptoms (diarrhea, vomiting, cramping), and positive signs of tetany should lead the nurse to suspect this disorder. Much of the initial nursing care is related to the physical manifestations and includes institution of seizure and safety precautions; reduction of environmental stimuli (e.g., avoiding sudden or loud noise, bright lights, stimulating activities); and observation for signs of laryngospasm such as stridor, hoarseness, and a feeling of tightness in the throat. A tracheostomy set and injectable calcium gluconate should be located near the bedside for emergency use. The administration of calcium gluconate requires precautions against extravasation of the drug and tissue destruction.

Hyperparathyroidism

Hyperparathyroidism is rare in childhood but can be primary or secondary. The most common cause of primary hyperparathyroidism is adenoma of the gland (Kliegman et al., 2007).

PATIENT TEACHING Vitamin D Toxicity

After initiating treatment for hypoparathyroidism, the nurse should discuss with the parents the need for continuous daily administration of calcium salts and vitamin D. Because vitamin D toxicity can be a serious consequence of therapy, the parents are advised to watch for signs that include weakness, fatigue, lassitude, headache, nausea, vomiting, and diarrhea. Early renal impairment is manifested by polyuria, polydipsia, and nocturia.

The most common causes of secondary hyperparathyroidism are chronic renal disease, renal osteodystrophy, and congenital anomalies of the urinary tract. The common factor is hypercalcemia. The clinical signs of hyperparathyroidism are listed in Box 52-9.

Diagnostic Evaluation

Blood studies to identify elevated calcium and decreased phosphorus levels are routinely performed. Measurement of PTH, as well as several tests to isolate the cause of the hypercalcemia, such as renal function studies, should be included. Other procedures used to substantiate the physiological consequences of the disorder include electrocardiography and radiographic bone surveys.

Therapeutic Management

Treatment depends on the cause of hyperparathyroidism. The treatment of primary hyperparathyroidism is surgical removal of the tumour or hyperplastic tissue. Treatment of secondary hyperparathyroidism is directed at the underlying contributing cause, which subsequently restores the serum calcium balance. However, in some instances, such as in chronic renal failure, the underlying disorder is irreversible. In this case,

BOX 52-9 Clinical Manifestations of Hyperparathyroidism

Gastrointestinal
Nausea
Vomiting
Abdominal discomfort
Constipation

Central Nervous System
Delusions
Confusion
Hallucinations
Impaired memory
Lack of interest and initiative
Depression
Varying levels of consciousness

Neuromuscular
Weakness
Easy fatigability
Muscle atrophy (especially proximal muscles of lower limbs)
Tongue twitching
Paresthesias in extremities

Skeletal
Vague bone pain
Subperiosteal resorption of phalanges
Spontaneous fractures
Absence of lamina dura around teeth

Renal
Polyuria
Polydipsia
Renal colic
Hypertension

treatment is aimed at raising serum calcium levels to inhibit the stimulatory effect of low levels on the parathyroids. This includes oral administration of calcium salts, high doses of vitamin D to enhance calcium absorption, a low-phosphorus diet, and administration of a phosphorus-mobilizing aluminum hydroxide to reduce phosphate absorption.

Nursing Care Management

The initial nursing objective is recognition of the disorder. Because secondary hyperparathyroidism is a consequence of chronic renal failure, the nurse needs to be alert to signs that suggest this complication, especially bone pain and fractures. Because urinary symptoms are the earliest indication, assessment of other body systems for evidence of high calcium levels is indicated when polyuria and polydipsia coexist. Clues to the possibility of hyperparathyroidism include a change in behaviour, especially inactivity; unexplained gastrointestinal symptoms; and cardiac irregularities.

Disorders of Adrenal Function

The adrenal cortex secretes three main groups of hormones collectively called steroids and classified according to their biological activity: (1) glucocorticoids (cortisol, corticosterone), (2) mineralocorticoids (aldosterone), and (3) sex *steroids* (androgens, estrogens, and **progestins**). Alterations in the levels of these hormones produce significant dysfunction in a variety of body tissues and organs. Because the adrenocortical cells are capable of producing any of the steroids, pathological conditions may result in a deficiency or an excess of more than one type of hormone. However, most are rare in children.

The adrenal medulla secretes the catecholamines epinephrine and norepinephrine. Both hormones have essentially the same effects on various organs as those caused by direct sympathetic stimulation, except that the hormonal effects last several times longer. Catecholamine-secreting tumours are the primary cause of adrenal medullary hyperfunction.

Acute Adrenocortical Insufficiency

The acute form of adrenocortical insufficiency (*adrenal crisis*) may have a number of causes during childhood. Although a rare disorder, some of the more common etiological factors include hemorrhage into the gland from trauma, which may be caused by a prolonged, difficult labour; fulminating infections, such as meningococcemia, which result in hemorrhage and necrosis (Waterhouse-Friderichsen syndrome); abrupt withdrawal of exogenous sources of cortisone or failure to increase exogenous supplies during stress; or congenital adrenogenital hyperplasia of the salt-losing type.

Early symptoms of adrenocortical insufficiency include increased irritability, headache, diffuse abdominal pain, weakness, nausea and vomiting, and diarrhea. Other clinical signs are found in Box 52-10. In the newborn, adrenal crisis is accompanied by extreme hyperpyrexia (high temperature), tachypnea, cyanosis, and seizures. Usually there is no evidence of infection or purpura. However, hemorrhage into the adrenal gland may be evident as a palpable retroperitoneal mass.

BOX 52-10 Clinical Manifestations of Acute Adrenocortical Insufficiency

Early Symptoms
Increased irritability
Headache
Diffuse abdominal pain
Weakness
Nausea and vomiting
Diarrhea

Generalized Hemorrhagic Manifestations (Waterhouse-Friderichsen Syndrome)
Fever (increases as condition worsens)
Central nervous system signs:
- Nuchal rigidity
- Seizures
- Stupor
- Coma

Shocklike State
Weak, rapid pulse
Decreased blood pressure
Shallow respirations
Cold, clammy skin
Cyanosis
Circulatory collapse (terminal event)

Newborn
Hyperpyrexia
Tachypnea
Cyanosis
Seizures
Gland evident as palpable retroperitoneal mass (hemorrhagic)

Diagnostic Evaluation

There is no rapid, definitive test for confirmation of acute adrenocortical insufficiency. Routine procedures such as measurement of plasma cortisol levels are too time consuming to be practical. Thus diagnosis is usually made on the basis of clinical presentation, especially when a fulminating sepsis is accompanied by hemorrhagic manifestations and signs of circulatory collapse despite adequate antibiotic therapy. Because there is no real danger in administering a cortisol preparation for a short period, treatment should be instituted immediately. Improvement with cortisol therapy confirms the diagnosis.

Therapeutic Management

Treatment involves replacement of cortisol, replacement of body fluids to combat dehydration and hypovolemia, administration of glucose solutions to correct hypoglycemia, and specific antibiotic therapy in the presence of infection. Initially, IV hydrocortisone (Solu-Cortef) is administered. Normal saline containing 5% glucose is given parenterally to replace lost fluid, electrolytes, and glucose. If hemorrhage has been severe, whole blood may be replaced. In the event that these measures do not reverse the circulatory collapse, vasopressors are used for immediate vasoconstriction and elevation of blood pressure.

Once the child's condition is stabilized, oral doses of cortisone, fluids, and salt are given, similar to the regimen used for chronic adrenal insufficiency. To maintain sodium retention, aldosterone is replaced by synthetic salt-retaining steroids.

Nursing Care Management

Because of the abrupt onset and potentially fatal outcome of this condition, prompt recognition is essential. Vital signs and blood pressure should be taken every 15 minutes to monitor the hyperpyrexia and shocklike state. Seizure precautions need to be instituted, since convulsions from the elevated temperature are not uncommon. As soon as therapy is instituted, the nurse should monitor the child's response to fluid and cortisol replacement. Too-rapid administration of fluids can precipitate cardiac failure, whereas overdosage with cortisol produces hypotension and a sudden fall in temperature.

Once the acute phase is over and the hypovolemia is corrected, the child is given oral fluids, such as small quantities of ginger ale, fruit juice, or salted broth. Too rapid ingestion of oral fluids may induce vomiting, which increases dehydration. Thus the nurse should plan a gradual schedule for reintroducing liquids. For children who refuse to drink, the prospect of having the IV infusion removed once oral fluids are increased is often a motivating factor.

NURSING ALERT Monitor serum electrolyte levels and observe for signs of hypokalemia or hyperkalemia (e.g., weakness, poor muscle control, paralysis, cardiac dysrhythmias, and apnea). The condition is rapidly corrected with IV or oral potassium replacement.

NURSING ALERT When an oral potassium preparation is given, it should be mixed with a small amount of strongly flavoured fruit juice to disguise its bitter taste.

The sudden, severe nature of this disorder necessitates a great deal of emotional support for the child and family. The child may be placed in a critical care unit where the surroundings are strange and frightening. Despite the need for emergency intervention, the nurse must be sensitive to the family's psychological needs and prepare them for each procedure, even if this is a brief statement such as "The intravenous infusion is necessary to replace fluid that the child is losing." Because recovery within 24 hours is often dramatic, the nurse should keep the parents apprised of the child's condition, emphasizing signs of improvement, such as a lowered temperature and elevated blood pressure. If paralysis occurs, the nurse should assure them that this condition is temporary and quickly reversed.

Chronic Adrenocortical Insufficiency (Addison's Disease)

Chronic adrenocortical insufficiency is rare in children. When it does occur, it is usually caused by a destructive lesion of the adrenal gland or neoplasms, or the cause is idiopathic. At one time, generalized tuberculosis was the leading cause of adrenal gland destruction.

Evidence of this disorder is usually gradual in onset, since 90% of adrenal tissue must be nonfunctional before signs of insufficiency are manifested. However, during periods of stress, when demands for additional cortisol are increased, symptoms of acute insufficiency may appear in a previously well child (Box 52-11).

Definitive diagnosis is based on measurements of functional cortisol reserve. The cortisol and urinary 17-hydroxycorticosteroid levels are low and fail to rise, while plasma adrenocorticotropic hormone (ACTH, or corticotropin) levels are elevated with ACTH stimulation, the definitive test for the disease.

Therapeutic Management

Treatment involves replacement of glucocorticoids (cortisol) and mineralocorticoids (aldosterone). Some children are able to be maintained solely on oral supplements of cortisol (cortisone or hydrocortisone preparations) with a liberal intake of salt. During stressful situations, such as fever, infection,

BOX 52-11 Clinical Manifestations of Chronic Adrenocortical Insufficiency

Neurological Symptoms
Muscular weakness
Mental fatigue
Irritability, apathy, and negativism
Increased sleeping, listlessness

Pigmentary Changes
Previous scars
Palmar creases
Mucous membranes
Hair
Hyperpigmentation over pressure points (elbows, knees, or waist)
Less frequently, vitiligo (loss of pigmentation)

Gastrointestinal Symptoms
Dehydration
Anorexia
Weight loss

Circulatory Symptoms
Hypotension
Small heart size
Dizziness
Syncopal (fainting) attacks

Hypoglycemia
Headache
Hunger
Weakness
Trembling
Sweating

Other Signs (Seen in Some Children)
Recurrent, unexplained seizures
Intense craving for salt
Acute abdominal pain
Electrolyte imbalances

emotional upset, or surgery, the dosage must be tripled to accommodate the body's increased need for glucocorticoids. Failure to meet this requirement will precipitate an acute crisis. Overdosage produces the appearance of cushingoid signs.

Children with more severe states of chronic adrenal insufficiency require mineralocorticoid replacement to maintain fluid and electrolyte balance. Other forms of therapy include monthly injections of desoxycorticosterone acetate or implantation of desoxycorticosterone acetate pellets subcutaneously every 9 to 12 months.

Nursing Care Management

Once the disorder is diagnosed, parents need guidance with medication therapy. They must be aware of the continuous need for cortisol replacement. Sudden termination of the medication because of inadequate supplies or inability to ingest the oral form because of vomiting places the child in danger of an acute adrenal crisis. The parents should always have a spare supply of the medication in the home. Ideally they will have a prefilled syringe of hydrocortisone and be instructed in proper technique for intramuscular administration of the medication in case of a crisis. Unnecessary administration of cortisone will not harm the child, but if it is needed, it may be lifesaving. Any evidence of acute insufficiency should be reported to the practitioner immediately.

Parents also need to be aware of adverse effects of the medications. Undesirable effects of cortisone include gastric irritation, which is minimized by ingestion with food or the use of an antacid; increased excitability and sleeplessness; weight gain, which may require dietary management to prevent obesity; and, rarely, behavioural changes, including depression or euphoria. Parents should be aware of signs of overdose and report these to the practitioner. In addition, the medication has a bitter taste, which creates a challenge for nurses and parents in its administration.

Because the body cannot supply endogenous sources of cortical hormones during times of stress, the home environment should be stable and relatively unstressful. Parents need to be aware that during periods of emotional or physical crisis the child requires additional hormone replacement. The child should wear medical identification, such as a bracelet, to permit medical personnel to adjust requirements during emergency care.

Cushing's Syndrome

Cushing's syndrome is a characteristic group of manifestations caused by excessive circulating free cortisol. It can result from a variety of causes, which generally fall under one of five categories (Box 52-12). Cushing's syndrome in young children may be due to an adrenal tumour (Moshang, 2003).

Cushing's syndrome is uncommon in children. When seen, it is often caused by excessive or prolonged steroid therapy that produces a cushingoid appearance (Fig. 52-1). This condition is reversible once the steroids are gradually discontinued. Abrupt withdrawal will precipitate acute adrenal insufficiency. Gradual withdrawal of exogenous supplies is necessary to allow the anterior pituitary an opportunity to secrete increasing amounts of ACTH to stimulate the adrenals to produce cortisol.

BOX 52-12 Etiology of Cushing's Syndrome

Pituitary—Cushing's syndrome with adrenal hyperplasia, usually attributed to an excess of adrenocorticotropic hormone (ACTH)

Adrenal—Cushing's syndrome with hypersecretion of glucocorticoids, generally a result of adrenocortical neoplasms

Ectopic—Cushing's syndrome with autonomous secretion of ACTH, most often caused by extrapituitary neoplasms

Iatrogenic—Cushing's syndrome, frequently a result of administration of large amounts of exogenous corticosteroids

Food dependent—Inappropriate sensitivity of adrenal glands to normal postprandial increases in secretion of gastric inhibitory polypeptide

(Adapted from Magiakou, M. A., et al. [1994]. Cushing's syndrome in children and adolescents: Presentation, diagnosis, and therapy. *New England Journal of Medicine, 331*[10], 629–636.)

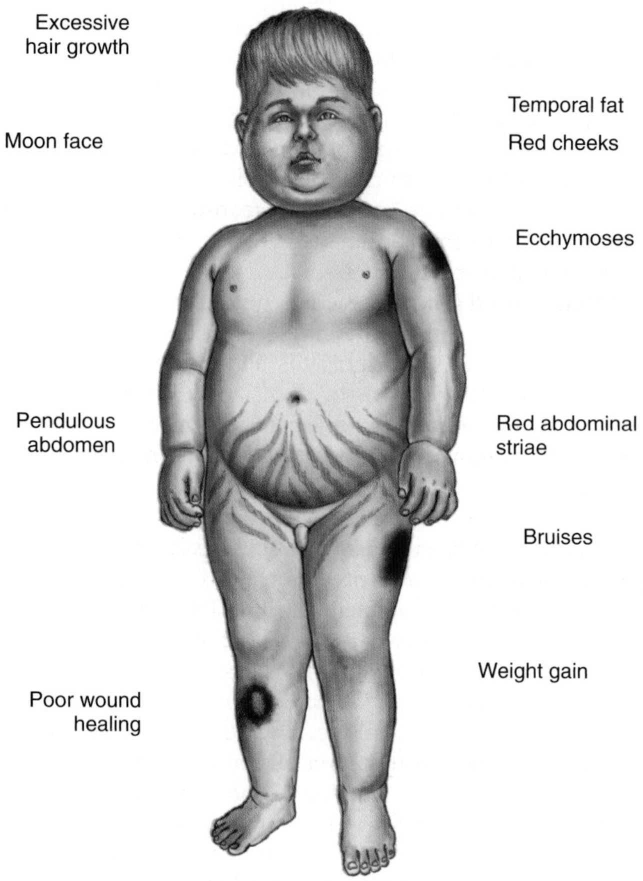

Fig. 52-1 Characteristics of Cushing's syndrome.

Clinical Manifestations

Because the actions of cortisol are widespread, clinical manifestations are equally profound and diverse. Those symptoms that produce changes in physical appearance occur early in the disorder and are of considerable concern to school-age and older children. The physiological disturbances, such as hyperglycemia, susceptibility to infection, hypertension, and hypokalemia, may have life-threatening consequences unless recognized early and treated successfully. Children with short stature may be responding to increased cortisol levels, resulting in Cushing's syndrome. Cortisol inhibits the action of GH.

Diagnostic Evaluation

Several tests are helpful in confirming excess cortisol levels. They include fasting blood glucose levels for hyperglycemia, serum electrolyte levels for hypokalemia and alkalosis, 24-hour urinary levels of elevated 17-hydroxycorticoids and 17-ketosteroids, and radiographic studies of bone for evidence of osteoporosis and of the skull for enlargement of the sella turcica. Another procedure used to establish a more definitive diagnosis is the dexamethasone (cortisone) suppression test (Batista et al., 2007; Nieman & Ilias, 2005). Administration of an exogenous supply of cortisone normally suppresses ACTH production. However, in individuals with Cushing's syndrome, cortisol levels remain elevated. This test is helpful in differentiating between children who are obese and those who appear to have cushingoid features.

Therapeutic Management

Treatment depends on the cause. In most cases surgical intervention involves bilateral adrenalectomy and postoperative replacement of the cortical hormones (the therapy for this is the same as that outlined for chronic adrenal insufficiency). If a pituitary tumour is found, surgical extirpation or irradiation may be chosen. In either of these instances, treatment of panhypopituitarism with replacement of GH, thyroid extract, ADH, gonadotropins, and steroids may be necessary for an indefinite period (Nieman & Ilias, 2005).

Nursing Care Management

Nursing care also depends on the cause. When cushingoid features are caused by steroid therapy, the effects may be lessened with administration of the medication early in the morning and on an alternate-day basis. Giving the medication early in the day maintains the normal diurnal pattern of cortisol secretion. If given during the evening, it is more likely to produce symptoms because endogenous cortisol levels are already low and the additional supply exerts more pronounced effects. An alternate-day schedule allows the anterior pituitary an opportunity to maintain more normal hypothalamic-pituitary-adrenal control mechanisms.

If an organic cause is found, nursing care is related to the treatment regimen. Although a bilateral adrenalectomy permanently solves one condition, it reciprocally produces another syndrome. Before surgery, parents need to be adequately informed of the operative benefits and disadvantages. Postoperative teaching regarding medication replacement is the same as discussed in the previous section.

NURSING ALERT Postoperative complications of adrenalectomy are related to the sudden withdrawal of cortisol. Observe for shocklike symptoms (e.g., hypotension, hyperpyrexia).

Anorexia, nausea, and vomiting are common and may be improved with the use of nasogastric decompression. Muscle and joint pain may be severe, requiring use of analgesics. The psychological depression can be profound and may not improve for months. Parents should be aware of the physiological reasons behind these symptoms in order to be supportive of the child.

Congenital Adrenal Hyperplasia

Congenital adrenal hyperplasia (CAH) is a family of disorders caused by decreased enzyme activity required for cortisol production in the adrenal cortex. The most common defect is 21-hydroxylase deficiency, which is the most common cause of CAH (Stein, Wherrett, & Daneman, 2005). This deficiency occurs in approximately 1 per 12,000 to 15,000 births. In its most severe form it can be life threatening (Glatt, Garzon, & Popovic, 2005).

Excessive androgens cause masculinization of the urogenital system at approximately the tenth week of fetal development. The most pronounced abnormalities occur in the girl, who is born with varying degrees of **ambiguous** genitalia. Masculinization of external genitalia causes the clitoris to enlarge so that it appears as a small phallus. Fusion of the labia produces a saclike structure resembling the scrotum without testes. However, no abnormal changes occur in the internal sexual organs, although the vaginal orifice is usually closed by the fused labia. The label *ambiguous genitalia* should be applied to any infant with hypospadias or micropenis and no palpable gonads, and a diagnostic evaluation for CAH should be contemplated. Boys do not display genital abnormalities at birth, so it may go undetected (New & Ghizzoni, 2003).

Diagnostic Evaluation

Clinical diagnosis is initially based on congenital abnormalities that lead to difficulty in assigning sex to the newborn and on signs and symptoms of adrenal insufficiency or hypertension. Definitive diagnosis is confirmed by evidence of increased 17-ketosteroid levels in most types of CAH (Menon, & Lawson, 2007). Usually the level of 17-hydroxycorticoids is low or near normal. In complete 21-hydroxylase deficiency, blood electrolytes demonstrate loss of sodium and chloride and elevation of potassium. In older children bone age is advanced, and linear growth is increased. Chromosome typing for positive sex determination and to rule out any other genetic abnormality (e.g., Turner's syndrome) is always done in any case of ambiguous genitalia.

Another test that can be used to visualize the presence of pelvic structures is **ultrasonography**, a noninvasive, painless imaging technique that does not require anaesthesia or sedation. It is especially useful in CAH because it readily identifies the absence or presence of female reproductive organs in a newborn or child with ambiguous genitalia. Because ultrasonography yields immediate results, it has the advantage of determining the child's gender long before the more complex laboratory results for chromosome analysis or steroid levels are available.

Therapeutic Management

The initial medical objective is to confirm the diagnosis and assign a sex to the child, usually according to the genotype. In both sexes cortisone is administered to suppress the abnormally high secretions of ACTH. If cortisone is begun early enough, it is very effective. Cortisone depresses the secretion of ACTH by the adenohypophysis, which in turn inhibits the secretion of adrenocorticosteroids and thus stems the progressive virilization. The signs and symptoms of masculinization in the female gradually disappear, and excessive early linear growth is slowed. Puberty occurs normally at the appropriate age.

The recommended oral dosage is divided to simulate the normal diurnal pattern of ACTH secretion. Because these children are unable to produce cortisol in response to stress, it is necessary to increase the dosage during episodes of infection, fever, or other stresses. Acute emergencies require immediate IV or intramuscular administration. Emergency situations include bacterial and viral infections, vomiting, surgery, fractures, major injuries, and sometimes insect stings.

Children with the salt-losing type of CAH require aldosterone replacement, as outlined under chronic adrenal insufficiency, and supplementary dietary salt. Frequent laboratory tests are conducted to assess the effects on electrolytes, hormonal profiles, and renin levels. The frequency of testing needs to be individualized to the child.

Gender assignment and surgical intervention in the newborn with ambiguous genitalia are complex and controversial. It is a significant stress for families who need support from a multidisciplinary team. Early reconstructive surgery should be considered only in the case of severe virilization (Lee et al., 2006). Emphasis is on functional rather than cosmetic outcomes, and surgery can often be delayed. Reports concerning sexual satisfaction after partial clitoridectomy indicate that the capacity for orgasm and sexual gratification is not necessarily impaired.

Unfortunately, not all children with CAH are diagnosed at birth and raised in accordance with their **genetic sex.** Particularly in the case of affected girls, masculinization of the external genitalia may have led to sex assignment as a male. In boys, diagnosis is usually delayed until early childhood, when signs of virilism appear. In these situations it is advisable to continue rearing the child as a male in accordance with assigned sex and phenotype. Hormone replacement may be required to permit linear growth and to initiate male pubertal changes. Surgery is usually indicated to remove the female organs and reconstruct the phallus for satisfactory sexual relations. These individuals are not fertile.

Nursing Care Management

Of major importance is recognition of ambiguous genitalia in newborns. If there is any question regarding assignment of sex, the parents need to be told immediately to prevent the embarrassing situation of informing family members of the child's sex and then having to change the announcement.

As soon as the sex is determined, parents should be informed of the findings and encouraged to choose an appropriate name, and the child should be identified as a male or female, with no reference to ambiguous sex. If the appearance of the enlarged genitalia in a girl concerns the parents, they should be encouraged to discuss their feelings. Suggesting ways to avoid questioning remarks from visitors, such as diapering the child in a separate room, is also helpful. If surgery is anticipated, showing parents before-and-after photographs of reconstruction helps to reinforce the expected cosmetic benefits.

In general, rearing the genetically female child as a girl is preferred because of the success of surgical intervention and the satisfactory results with hormones in reversing virilism and providing a prospect of normal puberty and the ability to conceive. This is in contrast to the choice of rearing the child as a boy, in which case the child is sterile and may never be able to function satisfactorily in heterosexual relationships. If the parents persist in their decision to assign a male sex to a genetically female child, a psychological consultation should be requested to explore their motivations and ensure their understanding of the future consequences for the child.

Nursing care management regarding cortisol and aldosterone replacement is the same as that discussed for chronic adrenocortical insufficiency. Because infants are especially prone to dehydration and salt-losing crises, parents need to be aware of signs of dehydration and the urgency of immediate medical intervention to stabilize the child's condition. Parents should have injectable hydrocortisone available and know how to prepare and administer the intramuscular injection (see Chapter 45).

In the unfortunate situation in which the sex is erroneously assigned and the correct sex determined later, parents need a great deal of help in understanding the reason for the incorrect sex identification and the options for sex reassignment or medical-surgical intervention.

Pheochromocytoma

Pheochromocytoma is a rare tumour characterized by the secretion of catecholamines. The tumour most commonly arises from the chromaffin cells of the adrenal medulla but may occur wherever these cells are found, such as along the paraganglia of the aorta or thoracolumbar sympathetic chain (Pacak et al., 2007). Approximately 10% of these tumours are located in extra-adrenal sites. In children they are frequently bilateral or multiple and are generally benign. Often there is a familial transmission of the condition as an autosomal dominant trait (Kliegman et al., 2007).

The clinical manifestations of pheochromocytoma are caused by an increased production of catecholamines, producing hypertension, tachycardia, headache, decreased gastrointestinal activity with resultant constipation, increased metabolism with anorexia, weight loss, hyperglycemia, polyuria, polydipsia, hyperventilation, nervousness, heat intolerance, and diaphoresis. In severe cases, signs of congestive heart failure are evident.

Diagnostic Evaluation

The clinical manifestations mimic those of other disorders, such as hyperthyroidism or DM.

Therapeutic Management

Definitive treatment consists of surgical removal of the tumour. In children the tumours may be bilateral, requiring a bilateral adrenalectomy and lifelong glucocorticoid and mineralocorticoid therapy.

Nursing Care Management

An initial nursing objective is identification of children with this disorder. Outstanding clues are hypertension and hypertensive attacks. Because of behavioural changes (nervousness, excitability, overactivity, even psychosis), increased cardiac and respiratory activity may appear to be related to an acute anxiety attack. Thus a careful history of the onset of symptoms and association with stressful events is helpful in distinguishing between an organic and a psychological cause for the symptoms.

Preoperative nursing care involves frequent monitoring of vital signs and observation for evidence of hypertensive attacks and congestive heart failure. Therapeutic effects are evidenced by normal vital signs and absence of **glycosuria**. Daily blood glucose levels, urine acetone, and any signs of hyperglycemia need to be noted and reported immediately.

NURSING ALERT Do not palpate the mass. Preoperative palpation of the mass releases catecholamines, which can stimulate severe hypertension and tachyarrhythmias.

The environment should be made conducive to rest and free of emotional stress. This requires adequate preparation during hospital admission and before surgery. Parents should be encouraged to room in with their child and to participate in care. Play activities need to be tailored to the child's energy level without being overly strenuous or challenging because these can increase the metabolic rate and promote frustration and anxiety.

After surgery, the child needs to be observed for signs of shock from the removal of excess catecholamines. If a bilateral adrenalectomy was performed, the nursing interventions are those discussed for chronic adrenocortical insufficiency.

Disorders of Pancreatic Hormone Secretion

DM is a chronic disorder of metabolism characterized by a partial or complete deficiency of the hormone insulin. It is the most common metabolic disease, resulting in metabolic adjustment or physiological change in almost all areas of the body. It is also one of the most common endocrine diseases and chronic conditions in the pediatric population. There are more than 3 million Canadians with diabetes. The different types of DM include type 1, type 2, and a secondary type of diabetes. The characteristics of type 1 DM and type 2 DM are outlined in Table 52-1.

Diabetes Mellitus Type 1

Over 300,000 Canadians have type 1 diabetes. In Canada, there is an annual increase of 3 to 5% with the highest increase in the 5 to 9 years of age group. Canada has the sixth highest incidence of type 1 diabetes in the world for children 14 years

evolve Case Study—Diabetes Mellitus

Table 52-1 Characteristics of Types 1 and 2 Diabetes Mellitus

CHARACTERISTIC	TYPE 1	TYPE 2
Age at onset	<20 yr	Increasingly occurring in younger children
Type of onset	Abrupt	Gradual
Sex ratio	Affects males slightly more than females	Females outnumber males
Percentage of diabetic population	5%-8%	85%-90%
Heredity:		
Family history	Sometimes	Frequently
Human leukocyte antigen	Association	No association
Twin concordance	25%-50%	90%-100%
Ethnic distribution	Primarily Whites	Increased incidence in Aboriginals, Latin Americans, and African origins
Presenting symptoms	Three P's common: polyuria, polydipsia, polyphagia	May be related to long-term complications
Nutritional status	Underweight	Overweight
Insulin (natural):		
Pancreatic content	Usually none	>50% normal
Serum insulin	Low to absent	High or low
Primary resistance	Minimum	Marked
Islet cell antibodies	80%-85%	<5%
Therapy:		
Insulin	Always	20%-30% of patients
Oral agents	Ineffective	Often effective
Diet only	Ineffective	Often effective
Chronic complications	>80%	Variable
Ketoacidosis	Common	Infrequent

of age or younger (Juvenile Diabetes Research Foundation, 2011). DM in children can occur at any age but has a peak incidence between ages 10 and 15 years, with 75% of cases diagnosed before 18 years of age. The incidence in boys is slightly higher than in girls (1 : 1 to 1.2 : 1). In Canada there is still not enough data to determine the incidence of type 1 diabetes in relation to specific ethnic origins.

Type 1 diabetes is characterized by destruction of the pancreatic **β (beta) cells,** which produce insulin; this usually leads to absolute insulin deficiency. Type 1 diabetes has two forms. Immune-mediated DM results from an autoimmune destruction of the β cells; it typically starts in children or young adults who are slim, but it can arise in adults of any age. *Idiopathic type 1* refers to rare forms of the disease that have no known cause.

Diabetes is a great imitator; influenza, gastroenteritis, and appendicitis are the conditions most often diagnosed when it turns out that the disease is really diabetes (Box 52-13).

Pathophysiology

Insulin is needed to support the metabolism of carbohydrates, fats, and proteins, primarily by facilitating the entry of these substances into the cell, with the exception of nerve cells and vascular tissue. With a deficiency of insulin, glucose is unable to enter the cell, and its concentration in the bloodstream increases (*hyperglycemia*). The increased concentration of glucose produces an osmotic gradient that causes the movement of body fluid from the intracellular space to the extracellular space; from there the body fluid is excreted by the kidneys. When the serum glucose level exceeds the renal threshold ±10 mmol/L, glucose "spills" into the urine (*glycosuria*), along with an osmotic diversion of water (*polyuria*), a cardinal sign of diabetes. The urinary fluid losses cause the excessive thirst (*polydipsia*) observed in diabetes. As might be expected, this water washout results in a depletion of other essential chemicals.

Protein is also wasted during insulin deficiency. Because glucose is unable to enter the cells, protein is broken down and converted to glucose by the liver (*glucogenesis*); this glucose then contributes to the hyperglycemia. Without the use of carbohydrates for energy, fat and protein stores are depleted as the body attempts to meet its energy needs. The hunger mechanism is triggered, but the increased food intake (*polyphagia*) enhances the problem by further elevating the blood glucose.

BOX 52-13 Clinical Manifestations of Type 1 Diabetes Mellitus

Polyphagia
Polyuria
Polydipsia
Weight loss
Enuresis or nocturia
Irritability; "not himself" or "herself"
Shortened attention span
Lowered frustration tolerance
Dry skin
Blurred vision
Poor wound healing
Fatigue
Flushed skin
Headache
Frequent infections
Hyperglycemia
- Elevated blood glucose levels
- Glucosuria

Diabetic **ketosis**
- Ketones and glucose in urine
- Dehydration in some cases

Diabetic ketoacidosis
- Dehydration
- Electrolyte imbalance
- Acidosis
- Deep, rapid breathing (Kussmaul's)

Ketoacidosis

When insulin is absent or insulin sensitivity is altered, glucose is unavailable for cellular metabolism, and the body chooses alternate sources of energy, principally fat. Consequently, fats break down into fatty acids, and glycerol in the fat cells is converted by the liver to ketone bodies (β-hydroxybutyric acid, acetoacetic acid, acetone). Any excess is eliminated in the urine (*ketonuria*) or the lungs (*acetone breath*). The ketone bodies in the blood (*ketonemia*) are strong acids that lower serum pH, producing ketoacidosis.

Ketones are organic acids that readily produce excessive quantities of free hydrogen ions, causing a fall in plasma pH. Then chemical buffers in the plasma, principally bicarbonate, combine with the hydrogen ions to form carbonic acid, which readily dissociates into water and carbon dioxide. The respiratory system attempts to eliminate the excess carbon dioxide by increasing the depth and rate of respirations—**Kussmaul's respirations,** or the hyperventilation characteristic of metabolic acidosis. The ketones are buffered by sodium and potassium in the plasma. The kidney attempts to compensate for the increased pH by increasing tubular secretion of hydrogen and ammonium ions in exchange for fixed base, thus depleting the base buffer concentration.

With cellular death, potassium is released from the cell (intracellular fluid) into the bloodstream (extracellular fluid) and excreted by the kidney, where the loss is accelerated by **osmotic diuresis.** The total body potassium is then decreased, even though the serum potassium level may be elevated as a result of the decreased fluid volume in which it circulates. Alteration in serum and tissue potassium can lead to cardiac arrest.

If these conditions are not reversed by insulin therapy in combination with correction of the fluid deficiency and electrolyte imbalance, progressive deterioration occurs, with dehydration, electrolyte imbalance, acidosis, coma, and death. **Diabetic ketoacidosis** (DKA) should be diagnosed promptly in a seriously ill patient and therapy instituted in a critical care unit.

Long-Term Complications

Long-term complications of diabetes involve both the microvasculature and the macrovasculature. The principal microvascular complications are nephropathy, retinopathy, and neuropathy. Microvascular disease develops during the first 30 years of diabetes, beginning in the first 10 to 15 years after puberty, with renal involvement evidenced by proteinuria and clinically apparent retinopathy.

With poor diabetic control, vascular changes can appear as early as 2½ to 3 years after diagnosis; however, with good to excellent control, changes can be postponed for 20 or more years. Intensive insulin therapy appears to delay the onset and slow the progression of clinically important retinopathy, including vision-threatening lesions, nephropathy, and neuropathy. Hypertension and atherosclerotic cardiovascular disease are also major causes of morbidity and mortality in patients with DM (Karnik, Fields, & Shannon, 2007). The postpubertal duration, not the total duration, of type 1 DM is implicated as a risk factor for the development of microvascular disease (Canadian Diabetic Association, 2008). The process appears to be one of glycosylation, in which proteins from the blood become deposited in the walls of small vessels (e.g., glomeruli), where they become trapped by "sticky" glucose compounds (glycosyl radicals). The buildup of these substances over time causes narrowing of the vessels, with subsequent interference with microcirculation to the affected areas (Rosenson & Herman, 2008). Macrovascular disease develops after 25 years of diabetes and creates the predominant problems in patients with type 2 DM.

Other complications have been observed in children with type 1 DM. Hyperglycemia appears to influence thyroid function, and altered function is frequently observed at the time of diagnosis and in poorly controlled diabetes. Limited mobility of small joints of the hand occurs in 30% of 7- to 18-year-old children with type 1 DM and appears to be related to changes in the skin and soft tissues surrounding the joint as a result of glycosylation.

Diagnostic Evaluation

Three groups of children who should be considered as candidates for diabetes are (1) children who have glycosuria, polyuria, and a history of weight loss or failure to gain weight despite a voracious appetite, (2) those with transient or persistent glycosuria, and (3) those who display manifestations of metabolic acidosis, with or without stupor or coma. In every case diabetes must be considered if there is glycosuria, with or without ketonuria, and unexplained hyperglycemia.

Glycosuria by itself is not diagnostic of diabetes. Other sugars, such as galactose, can produce a positive result with certain test strips, and a mild degree of glycosuria can be caused by other conditions, such as infection, trauma, emotional or physical stress, hyperalimentation, and some renal or endocrine diseases.

An 8-hour fasting blood glucose level of ≥7.0 mmol/L or more, a random blood glucose value of >(11.1) mmol/L or more accompanied by classic signs of diabetes, or an oral glucose tolerance test (OGTT) finding of ≥11.1 mmol/L in the 2-hour sample is almost certain to indicate diabetes (Canadian Diabetic Association, 2008). Postprandial blood glucose determinations and the traditional OGTTs have yielded low detection rates in children and are not usually necessary for establishing a diagnosis. Serum insulin levels may be normal or moderately elevated at the onset of diabetes; delayed insulin response to glucose indicates impaired glucose tolerance.

Ketoacidosis must be differentiated from other causes of acidosis or coma, including hypoglycemia, uremia, gastroenteritis with metabolic acidosis, salicylate intoxication encephalitis, and other intracranial lesions. DKA is a state of relative insulin insufficiency and may include the presence of hyperglycemia (blood glucose level, 18.3 mmol/L), ketonemia (strongly positive), acidosis (pH less than 7.30 and bicarbonate less than 15 mmol/L), glycosuria, and ketonuria (Dunning, 2009). Tests used to determine glycosuria and ketonuria are the glucose oxidase tapes (Keto-Diastix).

Therapeutic Management

The management of the child with type 1 DM consists of a multidisciplinary approach involving the family; the child (when appropriate); and professionals, including a pediatric endocrinologist, diabetes nurse educator, nutritionist, and exercise physiologist. Often psychological support from a mental health professional is also needed. Communication among the team members is essential and extends to other individuals in the child's life, such as teachers, the school nurse, the school guidance counsellor, and the coach.

The definitive treatment is replacement of insulin that the child is unable to produce. However, insulin needs are also affected by emotions, nutritional intake, activity, and other life events such as illnesses and puberty. The complexity of the disease and its management requires that the child and family incorporate diabetes needs into their lifestyle. Medical and nutritional guidance are primary, but management also includes continuing diabetes education, family guidance, and emotional support.

Insulin Therapy

Insulin replacement is the cornerstone of management of type 1 DM. Insulin dosage is tailored to each child based on home blood glucose monitoring. The goal of insulin therapy is maintaining near-normal blood glucose values while avoiding too frequent episodes of hypoglycemia. The goals of treatment are to maintain near-normal glucose levels. The recommended glucose levels are listed in Table 52-2. Glycemic control decreases the likelihood of long-term complications in patients with DM (Canadian Diabetic Association, 2008). Insulin is administered as two or more injections per day or as a continuous subcutaneous infusion using a portable insulin pump.

Healthy pancreatic cells secrete insulin at a low but steady basal rate with superimposed bursts of increased secretion that coincide with the intake of nutrients. Consequently, insulin levels in the blood increase and decrease coincidentally with rises and falls in blood glucose levels. In addition, insulin is secreted directly into the portal circulation; thus the liver, which is the major site of glucose disposal, receives the largest concentration of insulin. No matter which method of insulin replacement is used, this normal pattern cannot be duplicated. Subcutaneous injection results in absorption of the drug into the general circulation, thus reducing the concentrations of insulin to which the liver is exposed.

Insulin Preparations. Insulin is available in highly purified pork preparations and in human insulin biosynthesized

Table 52-2 Recommended Glycemic Goals for Children and Adolescents With Type 1 Diabetes

AGE IN YEARS	A_{1C} (%) GLYCATED HEMAGLOBIN	FASTING/PREPRANDIAL (MMOL/L) PLASMA GLUCOSE	2-HOUR POSTPRANDIAL (MMOL/L) PLASMA GLUCOSE	COMMENTS
<6	<8.5	6.0–12.0		Important to minimize hypoglycemia because of potential cognitive impairment
6–12	<8.0	4.0–10.0		Goals should be graduated according to the child's age
13–18	≤7.0	4.0–7.0	5.0–10.0	Appropriate for most adolescents

(Adapted from the Canadian Diabetes Association Clinical Practice Guidelines Expert Committee. [2008]. Canadian Diabetes Association 2008 clinical practice guidelines for the prevention and management of diabetes in Canada [p. S151, Table 1]. *Canadian Journal of Diabetes, 32*[Suppl 1], S1–S201. Retrieved from http://www.diabetes.ca/files/cpg2008/cpg-2008.pdf.)

by and extracted from bacterial or yeast cultures. Most clinicians suggest human insulin as the treatment of choice. Insulin is available in rapid-, intermediate-, and long-acting preparations, and all are packaged in the strength of 100 units/mL. Some insulins are available as premixed insulins, such as 70/30 and 50/50 ratios, the first number indicating the percentage of intermediate-acting and the second number the percentage of rapid-acting insulin. The type of insulin prescribed depends on different factors which include the age, duration of diabetes, socioeconomic factors, family lifestyle, and family, patient, and prescriber preferences. The different types of insulin are listed in Box 52-14 (see also Table 14-2).

NURSING ALERT The human insulins from various manufacturers may be interchangeable, but human insulin and pork insulin or pure pork insulin should never be substituted for one another.

Dosage. Conventional management has consisted of a twice-daily insulin regimen of a combination of rapid-acting and intermediate-acting insulin drawn up into the same syringe and injected before breakfast and before the evening meal. The amount of morning regular insulin is determined by patterns in the late-morning and lunchtime blood glucose values. The morning intermediate-acting dose is determined by patterns in the late afternoon and supper blood glucose values. Fasting blood glucose patterns at breakfast help determine the evening dose of intermediate insulin, and the blood glucose patterns at bedtime help determine the evening dose of rapid-acting (regular) insulin. For some children, better morning glucose control is achieved by a later (bedtime) injection of intermediate-acting insulin.

Regular insulin is best administered at least 30 minutes before meals. This allows sufficient time for absorption and results in a significantly greater reduction in the postprandial rise in blood glucose than if the meal were eaten immediately after the insulin injection. Intensive therapy consists of multiple injections throughout the day with a once- or twice-daily dose of long-acting (Ultralente) insulin to simulate the basal insulin secretion, and injections of rapid-acting insulin before each meal. A multiple daily injection program reduces microvascular complications of diabetes in young, healthy patients who have type 1 DM.

The precise dosage of insulin needed cannot be predicted. Thus the total dosage and percentage of regular- to intermediate-acting insulin should be determined empirically for each child. Usually 60 to 75% of the total daily dose is given before breakfast, and the remainder before the evening meal. Furthermore, insulin requirements do not remain constant but change continuously during growth and development; the need varies according to the child's activity level and pubertal status. For example, less insulin is required during spring and summer months, when the child is more active. Illness also alters insulin requirements. Some children require more frequent insulin administration. This includes children with difficult-to-control diabetes and children during the adolescent growth spurt.

Methods of Administration. Daily insulin is administered subcutaneously by twice-daily injections, by multiple-dose injections, or by means of an insulin infusion pump. The *insulin pump* is an electromechanical device designed to deliver fixed amounts of regular or lispro insulin continuously (basal rate), thereby more closely imitating the release of the hormone by the islet cells (Olohan & Zappitelli, 2003) (see Fig. 14-2). Although the pump delivers a programmed amount of basal insulin, the child or parent must program a dose for the pump to deliver before each meal.

The system consists of a syringe to hold the insulin, a plunger, and a computerized mechanism to drive the plunger. The insulin flows from the syringe through a catheter to a needle inserted into subcutaneous tissue (the abdomen or thigh), and the lightweight device is worn on a belt or a shoulder holster. The needle and catheter are changed every 48 to 72 hours by the child or parent, using aseptic technique, and then taped in place.

Although the pump provides more consistent insulin delivery, it has certain disadvantages. Pump therapy is expensive and requires commitment from the parent and child. A certain level of math skills is required to calculate infusion rates. It should also not be removed for more than 1 hour at a time, which may limit some activities. Skin infections are common; and, as with any other mechanical device, it is subject to malfunction. However, the pumps are equipped with alarms that signal problems, such as a depleted battery, an occluded needle or tubing, or a microprocessor malfunction.

Monitoring

Daily monitoring of blood glucose levels is an essential aspect of appropriate DM management. Plasma blood glucose and hemoglobin A_{1c} goal ranges are found in Table 52-2.

Blood Glucose. Self-monitoring of blood glucose (SMBG) has improved diabetes management and is used successfully by children from the onset of their diabetes. By testing their

BOX 52-14 Types of Insulin

There are four types of insulin, based on the following criteria:

- How soon the insulin starts working (onset)
- When the insulin works the hardest (peak time)
- How long the insulin lasts in the body (duration)

However, each person responds to insulin in his or her own way. That is why onset, peak time, and duration are given as ranges.

Insulin Type (trade name)	Onset	Peak	Duration
Prandial (bolus) Insulin			
Rapid-acting insulin analogues (clear)			
- Insulin aspart (NovoRapid)	10–15 min	1–1.5 hr	3–5 hr
- Insulin lispro (Humalog)	10–15 min	1–2 hr	3–4.75 hr
- Insulin glulisine (Apidra)	10–15 min	1–1.5 hr	3–5 hr
Short-acting insulin (clear)			
- Humulin-R	30 min	2–3 hr	6.5 hr
- Novolin ge Toronto			
Inhaled insulin (approved but not yet available in Canada)	10–20 min	2 hr	6 hr
Basal Insulin			
Intermediate-acting (cloudy)			
- Humulin-N	1–3 hr	5–8 hr	Up to 18 hr
- Novolin ge NPH			
Long-acting basal insulin analogues (clear)			
- Insulin determir (Levemir)	90 min	Not applicable	Up to 24 hr (glargine 24 hr, determir 16–24 hr)
- Insulin glargine (Lantus)			
Premixed Insulin			
Premixed regular insulin–NPH (cloudy)			
- Humulin 30/70			
- Novolin ge 30/70, 40/60/, 50/50			
Premixed analogues (cloudy)			
- Biphasic insulin aspart (NovoMix 30)	A single vial or cartridge contains a fixed ratio of insulin (% of rapid-acting or short-acting insulin to % of intermediate-acting insulin		
- Insulin lispro/lispro protamine (Humalog Mix25 and Mix50)			

(Adapted from the Canadian Diabetes Association Clinical Practice Guidelines Expert Committee. [2008]. Canadian Diabetes Association 2008 clinical practice guidelines for the prevention and management of diabetes in Canada. *Canadian Journal of Diabetes, 32*[Suppl 1], S1–S201. Retrieved from http://www.diabetes.ca/files/cpg2008/cpg-2008.pdf.)

own blood, children are able to change their insulin regimen to maintain their glucose level in the euglycemic (normal) range of 4.4 mmol/L to 6.6 mmol/L. Diabetes management depends to a great extent on SMBG. In general, children tolerate the testing well.

Glycosylated Hemoglobin. The measurement of hemoglobin A_{1c} levels is a satisfactory method for assessing control of the diabetes. As red blood cells circulate in the bloodstream, glucose molecules gradually attach to the hemoglobin A molecules and remain there for the lifetime of the red blood cell, approximately 120 days. The attachment is not reversible; this glycosylated hemoglobin reflects the average blood glucose levels over the previous 2 to 3 months. The test is a satisfactory method for assessing control, detecting incorrect testing, monitoring effectiveness of changes in treatment, defining patients' goals, and detecting noncompliance. Nondiabetic hemoglobin A_{1c} values are generally between 4 and 6% but can vary by laboratory. Diabetes control for children depends on age, with hemoglobin A_{1c} levels of 7 to 8.5% indicating a slightly elevated but acceptable range (Canadian Diabetes Association, 2008). Hemoglobin A_{1c} levels of less than 7% are a well-established goal at most care centres.

Urine. Urine testing for glucose is no longer used for diabetes management; there is poor correlation between simultaneous glycosuria and blood glucose concentrations. However, urine testing can be carried out to detect evidence of ketonuria.

NURSING ALERT It is recommended that urine be tested for ketones every 3 hours during an illness or whenever the blood glucose level is over 13.3 mmol/L or when symptoms of diabetic ketoacidosis are present.

Nutrition

Essentially the nutritional needs of children with diabetes are no different from those of healthy children. Children with diabetes need no special foods or supplements. They need sufficient calories to balance daily expenditure for energy and to satisfy the requirement for growth and development. Unlike the child without diabetes, whose insulin is secreted in response to food intake, insulin injected subcutaneously has a relatively predictable time of onset, peak effect, duration of action, and absorption rate depending on the type of insulin used. Consequently, the timing of food consumption must be regulated to correspond to the timing and action of the insulin prescribed.

Meals and snacks must be eaten according to peak insulin action, and the total number of calories and proportions of basic nutrients must be consistent from day to day. The constant release of insulin into the circulation makes the child prone to hypoglycemia between the three daily meals unless a snack is provided between meals and at bedtime. The distribution of calories should be calculated to fit each child's activity pattern. For example, a child who is more active in the afternoon will need a larger snack at that time. This larger snack might also be split to allow some food at school and some food after school. Food intake should be altered to balance food, insulin, and exercise. Extra food is needed for increased activity.

Concentrated sweets are discouraged, and because of the increased risk for atherosclerosis in persons with DM, fat is reduced to 30% or less of the total caloric requirement. Dietary fibre has become increasingly important in dietary planning because of its influence on digestion, absorption, and metabolism of many nutrients. It has been found to diminish the rise in blood glucose after meals.

Eating Well With Canada's Food Guide provides a flexible, balanced, and easy-to-follow plan that has a specific adaption for First Nations, Métis, and Inuit peoples (Health Canada, 2011b). The plan has been translated into many different languages. Correctly used, the diet allows for flexibility and the incorporation of preferred foods in most instances. For the growing child, food restriction should never be used for diabetes control, although caloric restrictions may be imposed for weight control if the child is overweight. In general, the child's appetite should be the guide for the amount of calories needed, with the total caloric intake adjusted to appetite and activity.

Exercise

Exercise should be encouraged and never restricted unless indicated by other health conditions. Exercise lowers blood glucose levels, depending on the intensity and duration of the activity. An exercise plan should be included as part of diabetes management, and the type and amount of exercise should be planned around the child's interests and capabilities. However, in most instances children's activities are unplanned, and the resulting decrease in blood glucose can be compensated for by providing extra snacks before (and, if the exercise is prolonged, during) the activity. In addition to a feeling of well-being, regular exercise aids in the utilization of food and often results in a reduction of insulin requirements.

Hypoglycemia

Occasional episodes of hypoglycemia are an integral part of insulin therapy, thus an objective of diabetes management is to achieve the best possible glycemic control while minimizing the frequency and severity of hypoglycemia. Even with good control, a child may frequently experience mild symptoms of hypoglycemia. If the signs and symptoms are recognized early and promptly relieved by appropriate therapy, the child's activity should be interrupted for no more than a few minutes. Severe hypoglycemia must be treated with intravenous dextrose and managed in the hospital. Home management with mini-doses of glucagon can prevent or treat hypoglycemia. There is a concern that significant hypoglycemia events can lead to cognitive impairment in children (Strudwick et al., 2005). Decreased cognitive functioning is more apt to occur in children with early onset type 1 diabetes and severe hypoplycemia,

NURSING ALERT Hypoglycemic episodes most commonly occur before meals, or when the insulin effect is peaking.

The signs and symptoms of hypoglycemia are caused by both increased adrenergic activity and impaired brain function. The increased adrenergic nervous system activity plus increased secretion of catecholamines produces nervousness, pallor, tremulousness, palpitations, sweating, and hunger. Weakness, dizziness, headache, drowsiness, irritability, loss of coordination, seizures, and coma are more severe responses and reflect CNS glucose deprivation and the body's attempts to elevate the serum glucose levels.

It is often difficult to distinguish between hyperglycemia and a hypoglycemic reaction (Table 52-3). Because the symptoms are similar and usually begin with changes in behaviour, the simplest way to differentiate between the two is to test the blood glucose level. The blood glucose level is low in hypoglycemia, whereas in hyperglycemia the glucose level is significantly elevated. Urinary ketones may be present after hypoglycemia as a result of starvation ketone production. In doubtful situations it is safer to give the child some simple carbohydrate. This will help alleviate the symptoms in the case of hypoglycemia but will do little harm if the child is hyperglycemic.

Children are usually able to detect the onset of hypoglycemia, but some are too young to implement treatment. Parents should become adept at recognizing the onset of symptoms—for example, a change in a child's behaviour, such as tearfulness or euphoria. In most cases, 10 to 15 g of simple carbohydrate, such as 15 g of table sugar, will elevate the blood glucose level and alleviate the symptoms. The simpler the carbohydrate, the more rapidly it will be absorbed (237 mL of milk equals 15 g of carbohydrate). The rapid-releasing sugar is followed by a complex carbohydrate such as a slice of bread or a cracker and by a protein such as peanut butter or milk.

For a mild reaction, milk or fruit juice is a good food to use in children. Milk supplies them with lactose or milk sugar, as well as a more prolonged action from the protein and fat (aids in decreased absorption). Other glucose sources include different products such as flavoured liquid glucose, carbonated drinks (not sugarless), sherbet, gelatin, or cake icing. All children with diabetes should carry with them glucose tabs, sugar cubes, or sugar-containing candy. A difficulty with candies or icing is that the child may learn to fake a reaction to get the sweets; thus commercial glucose treatment products may be preferred.

Glucagon is sometimes prescribed for home treatment of hypoglycemia. It is available as an emergency kit that must be

Table 52-3 Comparison of Manifestations of Hypoglycemia and Hyperglycemia

VARIABLE	HYPOGLYCEMIA	HYPERGLYCEMIA
Onset	Rapid (minutes)	Gradual (days)
Mood	Labile, irritable, nervous, weepy	Lethargic
Mental status	Difficulty concentrating, speaking, focusing, coordinating Nightmares	Dulled sensorium Confusion
Inward feeling	Shaky feeling Hunger Headache Dizziness	Thirst Weakness Nausea and vomiting Abdominal pain
Skin	Pallor Sweating	Flushed Signs of dehydration
Mucous membranes	Normal	Dry, crusty
Respirations	Shallow, normal	Deep, rapid (Kussmaul's)
Pulse	Tachycardia, palpitations	Less rapid, weak
Breath odour	Normal	Fruity, acetone
Neurological	Tremors	Diminished reflexes Paresthesia
Ominous signs	Late—Hyper-reflexia, dilated pupils, seizure Shock, coma	Acidosis, coma
Blood:		
Glucose		Low: <3.3 mmol/L High: ≥13.8 mmol/L
Ketones	Negative	High, large
Osmolarity	Normal	High
pH	Normal	Low (≤7.25)
Hematocrit	Normal	High
Bicarbonate	Normal	<20 mmol/L
Urine:		
Output	Normal	Polyuria (early) to oliguria (late)
Glucose	Negative	Enuresis, nocturia
Ketones	Negative or trace	High
Vision	Diplopia	Blurred vision

mixed at the time of use and is administered intramuscularly or subcutaneously. Glucagon functions by releasing stored glycogen from the liver and requires about 15 to 20 minutes to elevate the blood glucose level.

NURSING ALERT Vomiting may occur after administration of glucagon; thus precautions against aspiration must be taken (e.g., placing the child on the side), since the child often becomes unconscious.

Once the child is responsive, the lost glycogen stores are replaced by small amounts of sugar-containing fluid administered frequently until the child feels comfortable trying solid foods.

Morning Hyperglycemia

The management of elevated morning blood glucose levels depends on whether the increase is a true dawn phenomenon, insulin waning, or a rebound hyperglycemia (the Somogyi effect). *Insulin waning* is a progressive rise in blood glucose levels from bedtime to morning. It is treated by increasing the nocturnal insulin dose. The *true dawn phenomenon* shows a relatively normal blood glucose level until about 3 AM, when the level begins to rise. The *Somogyi effect* may occur at any time but often entails an elevated blood glucose level at bedtime and a drop at 2 AM with a rebound rise following. The treatment for this phenomenon is decreasing the nocturnal insulin dose to prevent the 2 AM hypoglycemia. The rebound rise in the blood glucose level is a result of counter-regulatory hormones (epinephrine, GH, and corticosteroids), which are stimulated by hypoglycemia. More frequent blood monitoring (especially at times of anticipated peak insulin action) will usually identify these conditions. Trace amounts of urinary ketones aid in identifying undetected hypoglycemia.

Illness Management

Illness alters diabetes management, and maintaining control is usually related to the seriousness of the illness. In a child whose diabetes is well controlled, an illness will run its course as it does in the unaffected child. The goals during an illness are to restore euglycemia, treat urinary ketones, and maintain hydration. Blood glucose levels and urinary ketones should be monitored every 3 hours. Some hyperglycemia and ketonuria are expected in most illnesses, even with diminished food intake, and are an indication for increased insulin. Insulin should never be omitted during an illness, although dosage requirements may increase, decrease, or remain unchanged, depending on the severity of the illness and the child's appetite. Often the child will need supplemental insulin between usual dose times. If the child vomits more than once, if blood glucose levels remain above 13.3 mmol/L, or if urinary ketones remain high, the health care provider should be notified. Simple carbohydrates may be substituted for carbohydrate-containing exchanges in the meal plan. Although insulin and diet are important tools in sick-day care, fluids are the most important intervention. Fluids must be encouraged to prevent dehydration and to flush out ketones.

Therapeutic Management of Diabetic Ketoacidosis

DKA, the most complete state of insulin deficiency, is a life-threatening situation. Management consists of rapid assessment, adequate insulin to reduce the elevated blood glucose level, fluids to overcome dehydration, and electrolyte replacement (especially potassium). The risk factors for cerebral edema include the following: being less than 5 years old; new-onset of diabetes; high initial serum urea; low initial partial pressure of arterial carbon dioxide (pco_2); rapid administration of hypotonic fluids; IV bolus of insulin; early IV insulin infusion (within first hour of administration of fluids); failure of serum sodium to rise during treatment; and use of sodium bicarbonate (Canadian Diabetes Association, 2008).

Because DKA constitutes an emergency situation, the child should be admitted to a critical care facility for management.

The priority is to obtain a venous access for administration of fluids, electrolytes, and insulin. The child should be weighed, measured, and placed on a cardiac monitor. Blood glucose and ketone levels are determined at the bedside, and samples are obtained for laboratory measurement of glucose, electrolytes, blood urea nitrogen, arterial pH, Po_2, Pco_2, hemoglobin, hematocrit, white blood cell count and differential, calcium, and phosphorus.

Oxygen may be administered to patients who are cyanotic and in whom arterial oxygen is less than 80%. Gastric suction is applied to unconscious children to avoid the possibility of pulmonary aspiration. Antibiotics may be administered to febrile children after appropriate specimens are obtained for culture. A Foley catheter may or may not be inserted for urine samples and measurement. Unless the child is unconscious, a collection bag is usually sufficient for accurate assessments.

Fluid and Electrolyte Therapy

All patients with DKA suffer from dehydration (10% of total body weight in severe ketoacidosis) because of the osmotic diuresis, accompanied by depletion of electrolytes, sodium, potassium, chloride, phosphate, and magnesium. Serum pH and bicarbonate reflect the degree of acidosis. Prompt and adequate fluid therapy restores tissue perfusion and suppresses the elevated levels of stress hormones.

The initial hydrating solution is 0.9% saline solution. Current trends suggest more cautious fluid management to reduce the risk of cerebral edema. The fluid deficit is replaced evenly over a period of 36 to 48 hours (Cooke & Plotnick, 2008). While most of the DKA episodes resolve without complications, in a recent Canadian surveillance study, 23% of diabetic children with cerebral edema died and another 15% survived with neurological complications (Lawrence et al., 2005).

Serum potassium levels may be normal on admission, but after fluid and insulin administration the rapid return of potassium to the cells can seriously deplete serum levels, with the attendant risk of cardiac arrhythmias. As soon as the child has established renal function (is voiding at least 25 mL/hr) and insulin has been given, vigorous potassium replacement is implemented. The cardiac monitor is used as a guide to therapy, and configuration of T waves should be observed every 30 to 60 minutes to determine changes that might indicate alterations in potassium concentration (widening of the QT interval and the appearance of a U wave following a flattened T wave indicate hypokalemia; an elevated and spreading T wave and shortening of the QT interval indicate **hyperkalemia**).

Insulin should not be given until urinary ketones and a blood glucose level have been obtained. Continuous IV regular insulin is given at a dosage of 0.1 units/kg/hr. Insulin therapy should be started after the initial rehydration bolus, since serum glucose levels fall rapidly after volume expansion. Blood glucose levels should decrease by 2.8 mmol/L to 5 mmol/L per hour. When blood glucose levels fall to 14 mmol/L to 17 mmol/L, dextrose is added to the IV solution. The goal is to maintain blood glucose levels between 6.7 and 13.3 mmol/L by adding 5 to 10% dextrose (Canadian Diabetes Association, 2008). Sodium bicarbonate is used conservatively; it is used for pH less than 7.0, severe hyperkalemia, or cardiac instability. Because sodium bicarbonate has been associated with increased risk for cerebral edema, children receiving this substance must be carefully monitored for changes in their level of consciousness (Brown, 2004).

When the critical period is over, the task of regulating insulin dosage in relation to diet and activity is started. Children should be actively involved in their own care and given responsibility according to their ability and the guidance of the nurse.

NURSING ALERT Because insulin can chemically bind to plastic tubing and in-line filters, thereby reducing the amount of medication reaching the systemic circulation, an insulin mixture is run through the tubing to saturate the insulin-binding sites before the infusion is started.

Nursing Care Management

Children with DM may be admitted to the hospital at the time of their initial diagnosis; during illness or surgery; or for episodes of ketoacidosis, which may be precipitated by any of a variety of factors. Many children are able to keep the disease under control with periodic assessment and adjustment of insulin, diet, and activity as needed under the supervision of a practitioner. Under most circumstances these children can be managed well at home and require hospitalization only for a serious illness or upset.

However, a small number of children with diabetes exhibit a degree of metabolic lability and have repeated episodes of DKA that require hospitalization, which interferes with education and social development. These children appear to display a characteristic personality structure. They tend to be unusually passive and nonassertive and to come from families that are inclined to smooth over conflicts without resolution. Children in this type of setting experience emotional arousal with little, if any, opportunity or ability to resolve it. Other children from psychosocially dysfunctional families display behavioural and personality problems. This emotional stress causes an increased production of endogenous catecholamines, which stimulate fat breakdown, leading to ketonemia and ketonuria.

Hospital Management

The child with DKA requires intensive nursing care. Vital signs should be observed and recorded frequently. Hypotension caused by the contracted blood volume of the dehydrated state may cause decreased peripheral blood flow, which can be particularly hazardous to the heart, lungs, and kidneys. An elevated temperature may indicate infection and should be reported so that treatment can be implemented immediately.

Careful and accurate records should be maintained, including vital signs (pulse, respiration, temperature, blood pressure), weight, IV fluids, electrolytes, insulin, blood glucose level, and intake and output. A urine collection device or retention catheter is used to obtain the urine measurements, which include volume, specific gravity, and glucose and ketone values. The volume relative to the glucose content is important because 5% glucose in a 300-mL sample is a significantly greater amount than a similar reading from a 75-mL sample. A diabetic flow sheet maintained at the bedside provides an ongoing record of the vital signs, urine and blood tests, amount of insulin given, and intake and output. The level of consciousness needs to be assessed and recorded at frequent intervals. The comatose child generally regains consciousness fairly soon after initiation of therapy but is managed like any unconscious child until then.

When the critical period is over, the task of regulating insulin dosage to diet and activity is begun. The same meticulous records of intake and output, urine glucose and acetone levels, and insulin administration should be maintained. Capable children should be actively involved in their own care and be given responsibility for keeping the intake and output record, testing the blood and urine, and, when appropriate, administering their own insulin—all under the nurse's supervision and guidance (see Patient Teaching box).

Medical Identification

One of the first things the nurse should call to the parents' attention is the need for the child to wear some means of medical identification. Usually recommended is the Medic-Alert identification, a stainless steel or silver- or gold-plated identification bracelet that is visible and immediately recognizable. It contains a collect telephone number that medical personnel can call around the clock for medical records and personal information.

Meal Planning

Normal nutrition is a major aspect of the family education program. Diet instruction is usually conducted by the nutritionist, with reinforcement and guidance from the nurse. The emphasis is on adequate intake for age, consistent menus, complex carbohydrates, and consistent eating times. The family is taught how the meal plan relates to the requirements of growth and development, the disease process, and the insulin regimen. Meals and snacks are modified on the basis of the child's preferences and current menu, preserving cultural patterns and preferences as much as possible. Extensive exchange lists are available that include foods compatible with most lifestyles.

Learning about foods within specific food groups can help in making choices. Weights and measures of foods can be used as eye-training devices for defining serving sizes and should be practised for about 3 months, with gradual progression to estimation of food portions. Even when the child and family become competent in estimating portion sizes, reassessment should take place weekly or monthly and when there is any change of brands.

Family members should also be guided in reading labels for the nutritional value of foods and food content. They need to become familiar with the carbohydrate content of food groups. Substitution with foods of equal carbohydrate content is the skill needed for successful carbohydrate counting. Substitution might be necessary if a food is not available in sufficient quantity or if the teenager wishes to eat fast food with peers. The use of a multiple daily injection program lends flexibility to the timing of meals.

Children should use sugar substitutes in moderation in items such as soft drinks. Artificial sweeteners have been shown to be safe, but if there is any question about amounts, the physician, dietitian, or nurse specialist can provide guidelines based on body weight. Sugar-free chewing gum and candies made with sorbitol may be used in moderation by children with DM. Although sorbitol is less cariogenic than other varieties of sugar substitutes, it is an alcohol sugar that is metabolized to fructose and then to glucose. Furthermore, large amounts can cause osmotic diarrhea. Most dietetic foods contain sorbitol. They are more expensive than regular foods. Also, while a product may be sugar free, it is not necessarily carbohydrate free.

Travelling

Travelling requires planning, especially when a trip involves crossing time zones. Suggestions for travelling encompass what will be needed from the practitioner before leaving, what and how much to take along, needs in transit, what to consider at the destination, and planning for when the child returns home. Planning is needed no matter what type of travel is considered—automobile, plane, bus, or train.

Insulin

Families need to understand the treatment method and the insulin prescribed, including the effective duration, onset, and peak action. They also need to know the characteristics of the various types of insulins, the proper mixing and dilution of insulins, and how to substitute another type when their usual brand is not available (insulin is a nonprescription medication). Insulin need not be refrigerated but should be maintained at a temperature between 15° and 29.5°C. Freezing renders insulin inactive.

Insulin bottles that have been "opened" (i.e., the stopper has been punctured) should be stored at room temperature or refrigerated for up to 28 to 30 days. After 1 month these vials should be discarded. Unopened vials should be refrigerated and are good until the expiration date on the label. Diabetic supplies should not be left in a hot environment.

Injection Procedure

Learning to give insulin injections is a source of anxiety for both parents and children. It is helpful for the learner to know that this important aspect of care will become as routine as brushing the teeth. First, the basic injection technique is taught, using an orange or similar item and sterile normal saline for practice.

Insulin can be injected into any area in which there is adipose (fat) tissue over muscle; the drug is injected at a 90-degree angle. Newly diagnosed children may have lost adipose tissue, and care should be exerted not to inject intramuscularly. The pinch technique is the most effective method for tenting the skin to allow easy entrance of the needle to subcutaneous tissues in children. The site selected will sometimes depend on whether children or parents administer the

PATIENT TEACHING Teaching About Diabetes

The better the parents understand the pathophysiology of diabetes and the function and action of insulin and glucagon in relation to caloric intake and exercise, the better they will understand the disease and its effects on the child. Parents need answers to a number of questions (voiced or unvoiced) to increase their confidence in coping with the disease. For example, they may want to know about the various procedures performed on their child and treatment rationale, such as what is being put in the intravenous bottle and the expected effect.

insulin. The arms, thighs, hips, and abdomen are usual injection sites for insulin. The children can reach the thighs, abdomen, and part of the hip and arm easily but may require help to inject other sites. For example, a parent can pinch a loose fold of skin of the arm while the child injects the insulin.

It is important to remember that the absorption rate varies in different parts of the body (Table 52-4), and insulin absorption is slowed by fat pads that develop in overused injection areas. The methodical use of one anatomical area and then movement to another minimizes variations in absorption rates. The parents and child can be helped to work out a rotation pattern to various areas of the body to enhance absorption. The most efficient rotation plan involves giving about four to six injections in one area (each injection about 2.5 cm apart, or the diameter of the insulin vial from the previous injection) and then moving to another area. Absorption is also altered by vigorous exercise, which enhances absorption from exercised muscles; it is recommended that a site be chosen other than the exercising extremity (e.g., avoiding legs and arms when playing in a tennis tournament).

Injection sites for an entire month can be determined in advance on a simple chart. For example, a "paper doll" (body outline) can be constructed and insulin sites marked by the child. After injection, the child places the date on the appropriate site. To keep in practice, it is a good idea for the parent to give two or three injections a week in areas that are difficult for the child to reach.

The same basic methodology is used when teaching children to give their own insulin injections (Fig. 52-2). They should practise first on an orange or a doll, building confidence gradually. Other devices are available for insulin injection and may offer advantages to some children. Children who do not wish to give themselves injections can be taught to use a syringe-loaded injector (Inject-Ease). With the device, puncture is always automatic. Adolescents respond well to a self-contained and compact device resembling a fountain pen (NovoPen), which eliminates conventional vials and syringes. Preloaded pens may also cause less pain, since the needle is not blunted by piercing the rubber top of the insulin vial.

Continuous Subcutaneous Insulin Infusion. Some children are considered candidates for use of a portable insulin pump, and even some young children with unsatisfactory metabolic control can benefit from its use. The child and the parents need to be taught to operate the device, including the mechanics of the pump, battery changes, and alarm systems. A number of devices are on the market that vary in the basal rates they are able to deliver and in the cost of the equipment.

Table 52-4 Insulin's Onset and Duration of Action Related to Injection Site

	Site of Injection			
	ABDOMEN	ARM	LEG	BUTTOCK
Rate	Very fast	Fast	Slow	Very slow
Duration	Very short	Short	Long	Very long

(From Albisser, A. M., & Sperlich, M. [1992]. Adjusting insulins. *Diabetes Education, 18*[3], 211–218.)

Families can investigate the various devices and select the model that best suits their needs.

Parents and children need to learn (1) the technical aspects of the pump and self-monitoring of blood glucose, (2) prevention and treatment for hyperglycemia, sick-day management, and meal planning, (3) the effects of exercise, stress, and diet on blood glucose levels, and (4) decision-making strategies to evaluate blood glucose patterns and make adjustments in all aspects of the regimen.

Frequent blood glucose measurements (at least four times per day) are an essential part of infusion pump use. Intensive education and supervision are critical to obtaining maximum efficiency and control. This is particularly important if the family has been accustomed to a conventional insulin regimen. They must realize that simply wearing the pump will not normalize blood glucose. The pump is merely an insulin delivery device; frequent, routine blood glucose determinations are necessary to adjust the insulin delivery rate.

The major problem with use of the insulin pump is **inflammation** from irritation or infection at the insertion site. The site should be cleaned thoroughly before the needle is inserted and then covered with a transparent dressing. The site should be changed and rotated every 48 to 72 hours (this may vary) or at the first sign of inflammation. Nurses working where pumps are part of the therapeutic regimen should become familiar with the operation of the specific device being used and the protocol of disease management. Others should be aware of this management technique and be prepared to assist patients using the pump.

Monitoring

Nurses should also be prepared to teach and supervise blood glucose monitoring. SMBG is associated with few complications, and although it does not necessarily lead to improved metabolic control, it provides a more accurate assessment of blood glucose levels than can be obtained with the historical urine testing. Blood glucose monitoring has the added advantage that it can be performed anywhere (see Atraumatic Care box).

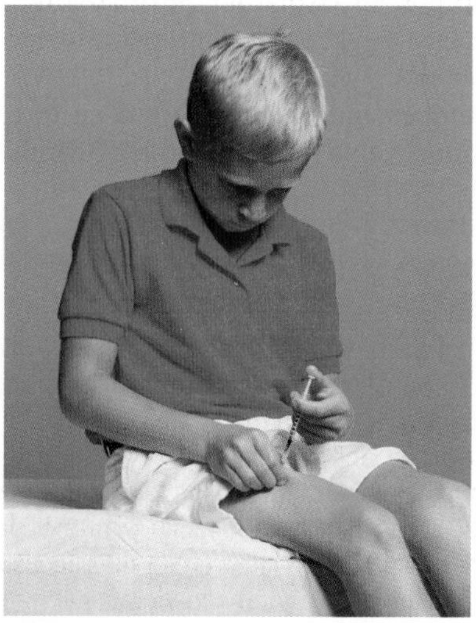

Fig. 52-2 School-age children are able to administer their own insulin.

ATRAUMATIC CARE

Minimizing Pain of Blood Glucose Monitoring

- To enhance blood flow to the finger, hold it under warm water for a few seconds before the puncture.
- When obtaining blood samples, use the ring finger or thumb (blood flows more easily to these areas), and puncture the finger just to the side of the finger pad (more blood vessels and fewer nerve endings).
- To prevent a deep puncture, press the platform of the lancet device lightly against the skin and avoid steadying the finger against a hard surface.
- Use lancet devices with adjustable-depth tips. Begin with the shallowest setting.
- Use glucose monitors that require small blood samples (e.g., Ascensia Elite) to avoid repeated punctures.

Blood for testing can be obtained by two different methods: manually or with a mechanical bloodletting device. A mechanical device is recommended for children, although the child and family should learn to use both methods in the event of mechanical failure. Several lancet devices are available, and each provides a means for obtaining a large drop of blood for testing (Fig. 52-3).

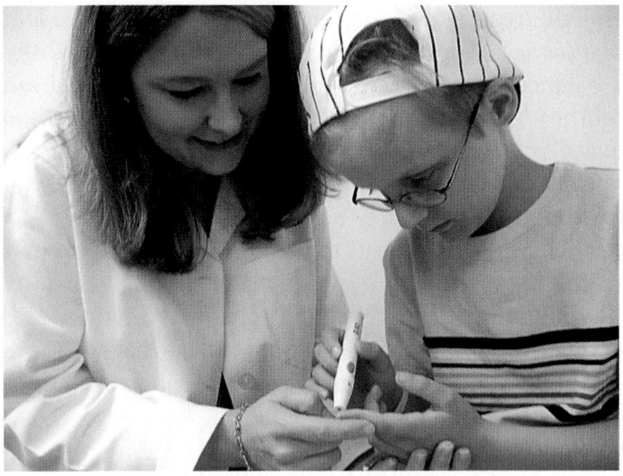

Fig. 52-3 Child using finger-stick device to obtain blood sample.

NURSING ALERT Caution children not to allow anyone else to use their lancet because of the risk of contracting hepatitis B virus or human immunodeficiency virus infection.

The blood sample may be obtained from fingertips or alternate sites such as the forearm. Alternate site testing requires a meter that can test a small volume of blood. Not all meters are capable of this.

Signs of redness and soreness at the site of finger puncture should be examined by the practitioner. It may be evidence of poor technique, poor hygiene, or poor skin healing relative to poor control. Many types of blood-testing meters are available for home use (Fig. 52-4). Newer technology has brought about improvements in meter size and ease of use. The family should be shown features of several meters, including advantages and disadvantages, and allowed to choose equipment that best meets their needs.

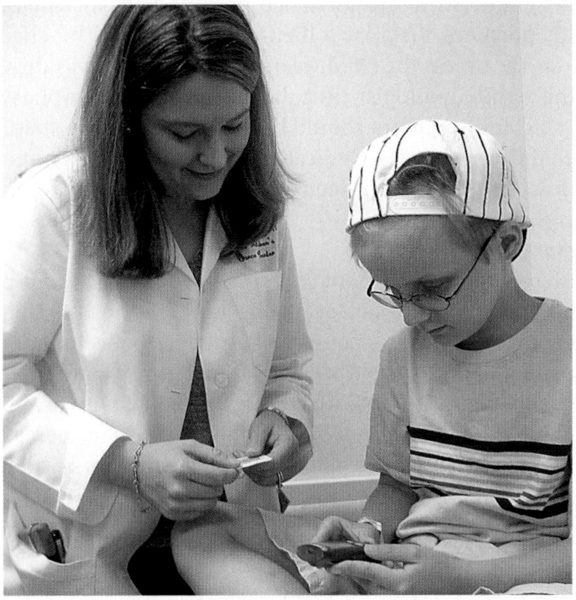

Fig. 52-4 Child using blood glucose monitor and reagent strips to test blood for glucose.

Urine Testing. Testing for urinary ketones is recommended during times of illness or when blood glucose values are elevated. Information on a specific ketone-testing product should include correct procedure, storage, and product expiration. Families need a clear understanding of home management of ketones: using fluids and additional insulin as directed by the health care team.

Signs of Hyperglycemia

Severe hyperglycemia is most often caused by illness, growth, emotional upset, or missed insulin doses. Emotional stress from school examinations or a physical response to immunizations are examples of causes of hyperglycemia. With careful glucose monitoring, any elevation can be managed by adjustment of insulin or food intake. Parents should understand how to adjust food, activity, and insulin at the time of illness or when the child is treated for an illness with a medication known to raise the blood glucose level (e.g., steroids). The hyperglycemia is managed by increasing insulin soon after the increased glucose level is noted. Health care providers should be aware that adolescent girls often become hyperglycemic around the time of their menses and should be advised to increase insulin dosages if necessary.

Signs of Hypoglycemia

Hypoglycemia is caused by imbalances of food intake, insulin, and activity. Ideally, hypoglycemia should be prevented, and parents need to be prepared to prevent, recognize, and treat the problem. They should be familiar with the signs of hypoglycemia and instructed in treatment, including care of the child with seizures. Early signs are adrenergic, including sweating and trembling, which help raise the blood glucose level, much like the reaction when an individual is startled or anxious. The second set of symptoms that follow an untreated adrenergic reaction is neuroglycopenic (also called *brain hypoglycemia*). These symptoms typically include difficulty with balance, memory, attention, or concentration; dizziness or lightheadedness; and slurred speech. Severe and prolonged hypoglycemia leads to seizures, coma, and possible death (Cryer, 2003). Hypoglycemia can be managed effectively, as outlined in the Emergency box.

It is advisable for parents to plan for anticipated excitement or exercise. In addition, gastroenteritis may decrease insulin needs slightly as a result of poor appetite, vomiting, or diarrhea. If the blood glucose level is low but urinary ketones are present, the family should be aware of the increased need for simple carbohydrates and liquids.

Hygiene

All aspects of personal hygiene should be emphasized for the child with diabetes. The child should be cautioned against wearing shoes without socks, wearing sandals, or walking barefoot. Correct nail and extremity care tailored to the individual child (with the guidance of a podiatrist) can begin health practices that last a lifetime. Eyes should be checked once a year unless the child wears glasses, and then as directed by the ophthalmologist. Regular dental care is emphasized, and cuts and scratches should be treated with plain soap and water unless otherwise indicated. Diaper rash in infants and candidal infections in teens may indicate poor diabetes control.

Exercise

Exercise is an important component of the treatment plan. If the child is more active at one time of the day than at another time, food or insulin can be altered to meet that activity pattern. Food should be increased in the summer, when children tend to be more active. Decreased activity on return to school may require a decrease in food intake or increase in insulin dosage. The child who is active in team sports will need a snack about a half hour before the anticipated activity. Races or other competition may call for a slightly higher food intake than at practice times.

Food intake will usually need to be repeated for prolonged activity periods, often as frequently as every 45 minutes to 1 hour. Families should be informed that if increased food is not tolerated, decreased insulin is the next course of action. If the timing of the exercise is changed so that the supper meal is delayed, the insulin in the second or third dose of the day may be moved back to precede the mealtime. Sugar may sometimes be needed during exercise periods for quick response. Elevated blood glucose levels after extreme activity may represent the body's adrenergic response to exercise. If the blood glucose level is elevated (13 mmol/L or higher) before planned exercise, urinary ketones should be checked and the activity may need be postponed until the blood glucose is controlled.

Record Keeping

Home records are an invaluable aid to diabetes self-management. The nurse and family can devise a method to chart insulin administered, blood glucose values, urine ketone results, and other factors and events that affect diabetes control. The child and family should be encouraged to observe for patterns of blood glucose responses to events such as exercise. If lapses in management occur (such as eating a candy bar), the child should be encouraged to note this and not be criticized for the transgression.

Self-Management

Self-management is the key to close control. Being able to make changes when they are needed rather than waiting until the next contact with health care providers is important for self-management and gives the individual and family the feeling they have control over the disease. Psychologically this helps family members feel that they are useful and participating members of the team. Allowing the child to learn to look at records objectively promotes independence in self-management. As children grow and assume more responsibility for self-management, they develop confidence in their ability to manage their disease and confidence in themselves as persons. They learn to respond to the disease and to make more accurate interpretations and changes in treatment when they become adults.

Puberty is associated with decreased sensitivity to insulin that normally would be compensated for by an increased insulin secretion. Health care providers should anticipate that pubertal patients will have more difficulty maintaining glycemic control. Insulin doses commonly need to be increased due to adolescent adjustment issues, psychosocial distress, intentional insulin, and physiological insulin resistance. If there is chronic poor metabolic control with a hemoglobin A_{1C} over 10.0%, then the cause needs to be identified. Possible factors could include depression and eating disorders (Canadian Diabetes Association, 2008). Patients should be taught to give themselves additional doses of rapid-acting insulin (5 to 10% of their daily dose) when their blood glucose levels are increased. For the adolescent, the use of supplemental rapid-acting insulin is preferred to withholding food.

Child and Family Education and Support

For all families, daily compliance with numerous procedures and structured living schedules is difficult. Maintaining

---

EMERGENCY

Hypoglycemia

Mild Reaction—Adrenergic Symptoms

Give child 10 to 15 g of a simple, high-carbohydrate substance (preferably liquid, e.g., 90 mL to 180 mL of orange juice).

Follow with starch-protein snack.

Moderate Reaction—Neuroglycopenic Symptoms

Give child 10 to 15 g of a simple carbohydrate as above.

Repeat in 10 to 15 minutes if symptoms persist.

Follow with larger snack.

Watch child closely.

Severe Reaction—Unresponsive, Unconscious, or Seizures

Administer glucagon as prescribed.

Follow with planned meal or snack when child is able to eat, or add a snack of 10% of daily calories.

Nocturnal Reaction

Give child 10 to 15 g of a simple carbohydrate.

Follow with snack of 10% of daily calories.

good blood glucose control requires ongoing motivation. Nurses can encourage families to adhere to treatment regimens and lifestyle adjustments by emphasizing the benefits of preventing complications such as hypoglycemia. When children are able to accept the difference as a part of life—in other words, that each person is different in some way—then, with adequate parental support, they should be able to adjust well.

Diabetes Mellitus Type 2

Type 2 diabetes arises because of insulin resistance, in which the body fails to use insulin properly, combined with relative (rather than absolute) insulin deficiency leading to predominant insulin resistance. It typically occurs in those who are over 45, overweight, and sedentary and have a family history of diabetes. In North America, the incidence of type 2 diabetes has been increasing over the past 20 years in both the adult and pediatric populations (Canadian Diabetic Association, 2008). Most affected individuals are from high-risk groups, including First Nations, Métis, and Inuit peoples, and persons of African, Latin American, and Asian/Pacific origins. Oster and Toth (2009) researched rural and remote groups in Alberta and found that First Nations individuals had more risk factors for diabetes than Métis and non-Aboriginal individuals, although Métis rates appeared intermediate. Aboriginal people are three to four times more likely to experience type 2 diabetes than non-Aboriginal Canadians (Health Canada, 2011a). The rising rate of type 2 diabetes matches the rising rate of childhood obesity and lack of physical activity; type 2 diabetes is a preventable disease (Canadian Paediatric Society [CPS], 2010).

Four genetic markers have been identified that indicate an increased risk of children developing type 2 diabetes later on in life. These markers are gestational diabetes, obesity, physical inactivity, and a positive family history for type 2 diabetes (CPS, 2010).

Screening and Diagnostic Evaluation

The physical signs of insulin resistance and metabolic syndrome are acanthosis nigricans (AN) (hyperpigmentation and thickening of the skin in the neck and axillary regions), polycystic ovarian syndrome (PCOS), hypertension, dyslipidemia, and steatohepatitis. While these signs do not cause type 2 diabetes they are associated with glucose intolerance and early-onset type 2 diabetes. Although research has not proven that AN is a definitive marker, neck observation for AN is a useful community screening tool that is acceptable to most children (Smith, Gowanlock, Babcock, Collings, & McCarthy, 2004). The at-risk AN group also has impaired glucose tolerance. There may be a type 2 connection because atypical neuropsychiatric medications are used more commonly than in other pediatric populations (Canadian Diabetic Association, 2008).

Screening of fasting plasma glucose is recommended as a routine screening, but an oral glucose tolerance test (OGTT) is more likely to have a higher detection rate for type 2 diabetes. An OGTT test is done when fasting blood glucose is 6.1 to 6.9 mmol/L; it may be done if the level is 5.6 to 6.0 mmol/L and the type 2 diabetes risk is high (Canadian Diabetes Association, 2008).

PCOS is rarely seen in Aboriginal adolescent girls in Canada (CPS, 2010). By contrast, AN was found in 21% of an Ontario First Nations group of children aged 5 to 14 years. Because of their higher risk for type 2 diabetes, Aboriginal children should be screened for type 2 diabetes after age 10. It is also recommended that if additional risk factors are present, physical activity should be increased and greater attention paid to sugar intake (Canadian Agency for Drugs and Technologies in Health, 2010).

Management

The management of type 2 diabetes is similar to that for type 1 diabetes. The pediatric multidisciplinary team needs to address the family about lifestyle, with a focus on healthy eating and physical activity. Psychological issues such as depression and smoking need to be sorted out, with interventions offered. Research has shown that when Aboriginal children receive lifestyle interventions their glycemic control drops to within normal in 2 weeks (Anderson & Dean, 1990). Children with severe metabolic decompensation (DKA, hemoglobin A_{1C} >9.0%) and hyperglycemia who need insulin can be successfully weaned once the glycemic goals are reached, especially if their lifestyle has improved. Metformin has been used safely in adolescents for up to 16 weeks and has halved hemoglobin B_{A1C} levels (Jones et al., 2002).

Short-term complications of type 2 diabetes in children include DKA and a hyperosmolar state. Children who have both at onset have high morbidity and mortality rates. Evidence is building that early-onset type 2 diabetes in adolescents is associated with severe and early-onset microvascularization, which includes retinopathy, neuropathy, and nephropathy; thus these individuals need to be monitored for it. Hypertension is present in 36% of individuals with type 2 diabetes; this also needs monitoring and potential intervention. Other potential complications that require monitoring include dyslipidemia, steatohepatitis, and PCOS (Canadian Diabetes Association, 2008).

Risk Reduction for Type 2 Diabetes

The Canadian Paediatric Society (2010) has recommended the following risk reduction program for decreasing the incidence of type 2 diabetes in the Aboriginal population.

- Culturally based and community-run diabetes prevention programs should be set up in First Nations, Métis, and Inuit communities.
- Aboriginal health care providers should provide type 2 diabetes opportunistic screening.
- In First Nations, Métis, and Inuit communities, traditional values, diets (using Canada's *Food Guide*), activities, and lifestyles should be promoted; group activities with the elders may work most effectively.
- Daily physical activity for at least 60 to 90 minutes, as laid out in *Canada's Physical Activity Guide*, is recommended. Physical activity guidelines are available from the Canadian Society for Exercise Physiology (2011).
- A healthy lifestyle needs to be taught as part of the curriculum at schools, day care, and Head Start programs.

- Community leaders can act as role models and provide appropriate safe environments for physical and other recreational activities.
- Passive activities, such as watching television, working on computers, and playing video games, should be limited to 1.5 to 2 hours per day.

Camping and other special group activities are also useful to children with diabetes. At diabetes camp, children learn that they are not alone. As a result, they become more independent and resourceful in other settings. Useful information about such camps and organizations, as well as resources for children with diabetes, their families, and health care providers, can be obtained from the Canadian Diabetes Association (see Additional Resources).

Several organizations are prepared to assist with education about diabetes and support for individuals with diabetes, including the Juvenile Diabetes Research Foundation Canada and the Canadian Diabetes Educator Certification Board (see Additional Resources).

Key Points

- Pituitary dysfunction is manifested primarily by growth disturbance.
- The main physiological action of TH is to regulate the basal metabolic rate and control the processes of growth and tissue differentiation.
- Disorders of thyroid function include hypothyroidism, autoimmune thyroiditis, goitre, and hyperthyroidism.
- Therapy for hyperthyroidism is directed at slowing the rate of hormone secretion and may include medication therapy, thyroidectomy, or radioiodine therapy.
- Classic forms of hypoparathyroidism in childhood are idiopathic (deficient production of PTH) and pseudohypoparathyroidism (increased PTH production with end-organ unresponsiveness to PTH).
- The adrenal cortex secretes three important groups of hormones: glucocorticoids, mineralocorticoids, and sex steroids.
- Disorders of adrenal function include acute adrenocortical insufficiency, chronic adrenocortical insufficiency, Cushing's syndrome, and CAH.
- Five categories of Cushing's syndrome are pituitary, adrenal, ectopic, iatrogenic, and food dependent.
- Management of CAH includes assignment of a sex according to genotype, administration of cortisone, and, possibly, reconstructive surgery.
- DM is categorized as type 1 diabetes and type 2 diabetes.
- The focus of treatment for type 1 DM is insulin replacement, diet, and exercise.
- Education of families includes explanation of diabetes, meal planning, administering insulin injections, monitoring general hygienic practices, promoting exercise, record keeping, and observing for complications.

Audio Chapter Summaries

Access an Audio Summary of these Key Points on evolve

References

Anderson, K. A., & Dean H. J. (1990). The effect of diet and exercise on a native youth with poorly controlled non-insulin dependent diabetes mellitus. *Beta Release, 14*, 105–106.

Bartalena, L., et al. (2003). Oxidative stress and Graves' ophthalmopathy: In vitro studies and therapeutic implications. *Biofactors, 19*(3-4), 155–163.

Batista, D. L., et al. (2007). Diagnostic tests for children who are referred for the investigation of Cushing syndrome. *Pediatrics, 120*(3), e575–e586.

Biro, F. M., et al. (2006). Pubertal correlates in black and white girls. *Journal of Pediatrics, 148*(2), 234–240. doi:10.1016/j.jpeds.2005.10.020

Brown, T. B. (2004). Cerebral edema in childhood diabetic ketoacidosis: Is treatment a factor? *Emergency Medicine Journal, 21*, 141–144.

Bryant, J., et al. (2007). Recombinant growth hormone for idiopathic short stature in children and adolescents. *Cochrane Database of Systematic Reviews 18*(3), CD004440. doi:10.1002/14651858.CD004440

Canadian Agency for Drugs and Technologies. (2010). *Diabetes in Aboriginal populations: Review of guidelines for screening and treatment.* Retrieved from http://www.cadth.ca/media/pdf/l0205_diabetes_ifirst_nations_population_htis-2.pdf.

Canadian Diabetic Association. (2008). *2008 clinical practice guidelines for prevention and management of diabetes in Canada.* Retrieved from http://www.diabetes.ca/files/cpg2008/cpg-2008.pdf.

Canadian Paediatric Society. (2010). *Risk reduction in Aboriginal children in Canada.* Retrieved from http://www.cps.ca/english/statements/II/FNIH05-01.htm.

Canadian Society for Exercise Physiology. (2011). *Canadian physical activity guidelines.* Retrieved from http://www.csep.ca/english/view.asp?x=804.

Carel, J. C., & Leger, J. (2008). Precocious puberty. *New England Journal of Medicine, 358*, 2366–2377.

Cheetham, T., & Baylis, P. H. (2002). Diabetes insipidus in children: Pathophysiology, diagnoses and management. *Paediatric Drugs, 4*(12), 785–796.

Cooke, D. W., & Plotnik L. (2008). Type I diabetes mellitus in pediatrics. *Pediatric Review, 29*(11), 374–384.

Cryer, P. (2003). Glucose counterregulatory hormones: Physiology, pathophysiology, and relevance to clinical hypoglycemia. In D. Le Roith, S. Taylor, & J. Olefsky (Eds.), *Diabetes mellitus: A fundamental and clinical text* (5th ed.). Philadelphia: Lippincott Williams & Wilkins.

Dallas, J. S., & Foley, T. P. (2003). Hyperthyroidism. In F. Lifshitz (Ed.), *Pediatric endocrinology* (4th ed.). New York: Marcel Dekker.

De Buyst, J., et al. (2007). Clinical, hormonal and imaging findings in 27 children with central diabetes insipidus. *European Journal of Pediatrics, 166*(1), 43–49. doi:10.1007/s00431-006-0206-0

Dunning, T. (2009). *Care of people with diabetes: A manual of nursing practice* (3rd ed.). Oxford: Blackwell.

Foley, T. P. (2001). Hypothyroidism. In R. A. Hoekelman, et al. (Eds.), *Primary pediatric care* (4th ed.). St. Louis: Mosby.

Glatt, K., Garzon, D. L., & Popovic, J. (2005). Congenital adrenal hyperplasia due to 21-hydroxylase deficiency. *Journal for Specialists in Pediatric Nursing, 10*(3), 104–114.

Greiner, M. V., & Kerrigan, J. R. (2006). Puberty: Timing is everything. *Pediatric Annals, 35*(12), 916–922.

Halac, I., & Zimmerman, D. (2004). Evaluating short stature in children. *Pediatric Annals, 33*(3), 171–176.

Hall, D. M. B. (2000). Growth monitoring. *Archives of Disease in Childhood, 82*(1), 10–15.

Health Canada. (2011a). *First Nations, Inuit and Aboriginal Health: Diabetes.* Retrieved from http://www.hc-sc.gc.ca/fniah-spnia/diseases-maladies/diabete/index-eng.php#a7.

Health Canada. (2011b). *Eating well with Canada's food guide.* Retrieved from http://www.hc-sc.gc.ca/fn-an/food-guide-aliment/index-eng.php/.

Herman-Giddens, M. E. (2006). Recent data on pubertal milestones in United States children: The secular trend toward earlier development. *International Journal of Andrology, 29*(1), 241–246. doi:10.1111/j.1365-2605.2005.00575.x

Hilczer, M., Smyczynska, J., & Lewinski, A. (2006). Limitations of clinical utility of growth hormone stimulating tests in diagnosing children with short stature. *Endocrine Regulations, 40*(3), 69–75.

Hudson, M. M., et al. (2011). Hodgkin lymphoma. In P. A. Pizzo & D. G. Poplack (Eds.). *Principles and theories of pediatric oncology.* Philadelphia: Lippincott, Williams & Wilkins.

Jones, K. L., et al. (2002). Effect of metformin in pediatric patients with type 2 diabetes: A randomized controlled trial. *Diabetes Care, 25*, 89–94.

Jospe, N. (2001). Hyperthyroidism. In R. A. Hoekelman, et al. (Eds.), *Primary pediatric care* (4th ed.). St. Louis: Mosby.

Juvenile Diabetes Research Foundation (2011). *Fact sheet. Type 1 diabetes.* Retrieved from http://www.jdrf.ca/index.cfm?fuseaction=home.viewPage&page_id=62495B79-DE19-05A3-5168B63985B9E8B2.

Kaplowitz, P. B. (2009). Treatment of central precocious puberty. *Current Opinions Endocrinology, Diabetes, Obesity, 16*(1), 31–36.

Karnik, A. A., Fields, A. V., & Shannon, R. P. (2007). Diabetic cardiomyopathy. *Current Hypertension Reports, 9*(6), 467–473. doi:10.1007/s11906-007-0086-3

Kliegman, R. M., Behrman, R. E., & Jenson, H. B. (Eds.) (2007). *Nelson textbook of pediatrics* (18th ed.). Philadelphia: Saunders.

Lawrence, S. E., Cummings, E. A., Gaboury I., & Daneman, D. (2005). Population-based study of incidence and risk factors for cerebral edema in pediatric diabetic ketoacidosis. *Journal of Pediatrics, 146* (5), 688–692.

Lee, P. A. (1999). Central precocious puberty: An overview of diagnosis, treatment, and outcome. *Endocrinology Metabolism Clinics of North America, 28*(4), 901–918.

Lee, P. A., et al. (2006). Consensus statement on management of intersex disorders. *Pediatrics, 118*, e488.

Lin, M., Liu, S. J., & Lim, I. T. (2005). Disorders of water imbalance. *Emergency Medicine Clinics of North America, 23*(3), 749–770.

Ma, C., et al. (2006). Radioiodine treatment for pediatric Graves' disease (protocol). *Cochrane Database of Systematic Reviews 4*, CD006294. doi:10.1002/14651858

Macchia, P. E. (2000). Recent advances in understanding the molecular basis of primary congenital hypothyroidism. *Molecular Medicine Today, 6*(1), 36–42.

Majzoub, J. A., & Muglia, L. J. (2003). Disorders of water homeostasis. In F. Lifshitz (Ed.), *Pediatric endocrinology* (4th ed.). New York: Marcel Dekker.

Makaryus, A. N., & McFarlane, S. I. (2006). Diabetes insipidus: Diagnosis and treatment of a complex disease. *Cleveland Clinic Journal of Medicine, 73*(1), 65–71.

Menon, K., & Lawson, M. (2007). Identification of adrenal insufficiency in pediatric critical illness. *Paediatrics & Child Health, 15*(7), 411–412.

Miller, B. S., & Zimmerman, D. (2004). Idiopathic short stature in children. *Pediatric Annals, 33*(3), 177–181.

Moshang, T. (2003). Cushing's disease, 70 years later … and the beat goes on (editorial). *Journal of Clinical Endocrinology & Metabolism, 88*(1), 31–33.

Muir, A. (2006). Precocious puberty. *Pediatrics in Review, 27*(10), 373–381. doi:10.1542/pir.27-10-373

Nebesio, T. D., & Eugster, E. A. (2007). Current concepts in normal and abnormal puberty. *Current Problems in Pediatric & Adolescent Health Care, 37*(2), 50–72.

New, M. I., & Ghizzoni, L. (2003). Update on congenital adrenal hyperplasia. In F. Lifshitz (Ed.), *Pediatric endocrinology* (4th ed.). New York: Marcel Dekker.

Nieman, L. K., & Ilias, I. (2005). Evaluation and treatment of Cushing's syndrome. *American Journal of Medicine, 118*(12), 1340–1346. doi:10.1016/j.amjmed.2005.01.059

Olohan, K., & Zappitelli, D. (2003). The insulin pump. *American Journal of Nursing, 103*(4), 48–56.

Oster, R. T., & Toth, E. L. (2009). Differences in the prevalence of diabetes risk-factors among First Nation, Métis and non-Aboriginal adults attending screening clinics in rural Alberta, Canada. *Rural and Remote Health, 9*(2), 1170. Retrieved from http://www.rrh.org.au.

O'Sullivan, E., & O'Sullivan, M. (2002). Precocious puberty: A parent's perspective. *Archive of Diseases in Childhood, 86*, 320–321.

Pacak, K., et al. (2007). Pheochromocytoma: Recommendations for clinical practice from the First International Symposium. *Nature: Clinical Practice Endocrinology & Metabolism, 3*(2), 92–102. doi:10.1038/ncpendmet0396

Perheentupa, J. (2003). Hypoparathyroidism and mineral homeostasis. In F. Lifshitz (Ed.), *Pediatric endocrinology* (4th ed.). New York: Marcel Dekker.

Radetti, G., et al. (2006). The natural history of euthyroid Hashimoto's thyroiditis in children. *Journal of Pediatrics, 149*(6), 827–832. doi:10.1016/j.jpeds.2006.08.045

Richmond, E. J., & Rogol, A. D. (2008). Growth hormone deficiency in children. *Pituitary, 11*, 115–120.

Rivkees, S. A. (2008). Differentiating appropriate antidiuretic hormone secretion, inappropriate antidiuretic hormone secretion and cerebral salt wasting: The common, uncommon, and misnamed. *Current Opinion in Pediatrics, 20*(4), 448–452.

Root, A. W. (2000). Precocious puberty. *Pediatrics in Review, 21*(1), 10–19.

Rosenson, R. S., & Herman, W. H. (2008). Glycated proteins and cardiovascular disease in glucose intolerance and type II diabetes. *Current Cardiovascular Risk Reports, 2*(1), 43–46.

Rovet, J. F., & Ehrlich, R. (2000). Psychoeducational outcome in children with early-treated congenital hypothyroidism. *Pediatrics, 105*(3), 515–522.

Simmonds, M. J., et al. (2005). Regression mapping of association between the human leukocyte antigen region and Graves disease. *American Journal of Human Genetics, 76*(1), 157–163. doi: 10.1086/426947

Slyper, A. H. (2006). The pubertal timing controversy in the USA, and a review of possible causative factors for the advance in timing of onset of puberty. *Clinical Endocrinology (Oxf), 65*(1), 1–8.

Smith, G. W., Gowanlock, W., Babcock, K., Collings, A., & McCarthy, A. (2004). Prevalence of Acanthosis Nigricans in First Nations children in central Ontario, Canada. *Canadian Journal of Diabetes, 28*(1), 410–414.

Stein, R., Wherrett, D., & Daneman, D., & Canadian Pediatric Endocrine Group. (2005). Management of 21-hydroxylase deficiency congenital adrenal hyperplasia: A survey of Canadian paediatric endocrinologists. *Pediatrics & Child Health, 10*(6), 323–326.

Steingraber, S. (2007). The falling age of puberty in US girls: What we know, what we need to know. *Breast Cancer Fund.* Retrieved from http://www.breastcancerfund.org/assets/pdfs/publications/falling-age-of-puberty.pdf.

Streetman, D. D., & Khanderia, U. (2004). Diagnosis and treatment of Graves disease. *American Journal of Nurse Practitioners, 8*(1), 27–36.

Strudwick, S. K., et al. (2005). Cognitive functioning in children with early onset type 1 diabetes and severe hypoglycemia. *Journal of Pediatrics, 147*, 1431–1437.

Szymborska, M., & Staroszczyk, B. (2000). Thyroiditis in children. *Medycyna Wieku Rozwojowego, IV*(4), 383–391.

Thompson, G. B. (2002). Surgical management in Graves' disease. *Panminerva Medica, 44*(4), 287–293.

van Tijn, D. A., et al. (2007). Early assessment of hypothalamic-pituitary-gonadal function in patients with congenital hypothyroidism of central origin. *Journal of Clinical Endocrinology & Metabolism, 92*(1), 104–109. doi:10.1210/jc.2006-0689

Verbalis, J. G. (2003). Diabetes insipidus. *Reviews in Endocrine & Metabolic Disorders, 4*(2), 177–185.

Additional Resources

American Association of Diabetes Educators: http://www.diabeteseducator.org/
Canadian Diabetes Educator Certification Board: http://cdecb.ca/
Juvenile Diabetes Research Foundation Canada: http://www.jdrf.ca/
National Institute of Diabetes and Digestive and Kidney Diseases: http://www2.niddk.nih.gov/
Thyroid Foundation of Canada: http://www.thyroid.ca/

Unit 11

53 Integumentary Dysfunction

Learning Objectives

On completion of this chapter, the reader will be able to:

- Describe the distribution and configuration of the various skin lesions.
- List the benefits of a moist environment for wound healing.
- Discuss the nursing care related to therapies for skin disorders.
- Contrast the manifestations of and therapies for bacterial, viral, and fungal infections of the skin.
- Compare the skin manifestations related to age in children.
- Outline a care plan to prevent and treat diaper dermatitis.
- Outline a care plan for a child with atopic dermatitis.
- Formulate a teaching plan for an adolescent with acne.
- Describe the methods for assessing a burn wound.
- Discuss the physical and emotional care of a child with a severe burn wound.

Electronic Resources

Additional information related to the content in Chapter 53 can be found on

evolve **the companion Web site at**

http://evolve.elsevier.com/Canada/Perry/maternal/

- Examination Review Questions
- Animation—Burns in Children
- Case Study—Acne Vulgaris
- Case Study—Chickenpox (Varicella)
- Case Study—Burns
- Case Study—Impetigo
- Case Study—Poison Ivy
- Case Study—Varicella in Spite of Vaccine
- Critical Thinking Exercise—Poison Ivy

Integumentary Dysfunction

Skin Lesions

Lesions of the skin result from a variety of etiological factors. Skin lesions originate from (1) contact with injurious agents (infective organisms, toxic chemicals, and physical trauma), (2) hereditary factors, (3) external factors (e.g., allergens), or (4) systemic diseases (e.g., measles, lupus erythematosus, nutritional deficiency diseases). Responses to these agents or factors are highly individualized. An agent that is harmless to one individual may be damaging to another, and a single agent may produce varying degrees of response.

An important factor in the etiology of skin manifestations is the child's age. Infants are subject to "birthmark" malformations and atopic dermatitis (AD) that appear early in life; the school-age child is susceptible to ringworm of the scalp; and acne is a characteristic skin disorder of puberty. Contact dermatitis, such as poison ivy, is seen only when the noxious agent is found in the environment. Tension and anxiety may produce, modify, or prolong skin conditions.

Skin of Younger Children

The major skin layers arise from different embryological origins. Early in the embryonic period, a single layer of epithelium forms from the ectoderm, while simultaneously the corium develops from the mesenchyme. In the infant and small child the epidermis is loosely bound to the dermis. This poor adherence causes the layers to separate easily during an inflammatory process to form blisters. This is especially true in preterm infants, who have a propensity to blister formation and separation of the skin with minor trauma such as the removal of adhesive tape. In contrast, the skin of the older child is thinner, and the cells of all the strata are more compressed.

Pathophysiology of Dermatitis

More than half of the dermatological problems in children are forms of dermatitis. This implies a sequence of inflammatory changes in the skin that are grossly and microscopically similar but diverse in course and causation. Acute responses produce intercellular and intracellular edema, the formation of intradermal vesicles, and an initial infiltration of inflammatory cells into the epidermis. In the dermis there is edema, vascular dilation, and early perivascular cellular infiltration. The location and manner of these reactions produce the lesions characteristic of each disorder. The changes are usually reversible, and the skin ordinarily recovers without blemish unless complicating factors such as ulceration from the primary irritant, scratching, and infection are introduced or underlying vascular disease develops. In chronic conditions permanent effects are seen that vary according to the disorder, the general condition of the affected individual, and the available therapy.

Diagnostic Evaluation

Although this chapter explores the history and subjective symptoms of skin lesions first, the obvious objective characteristics of the lesions are often noted simultaneously. Many skin lesions are easily diagnosed after careful inspection.

History and Subjective Symptoms

Many cutaneous lesions are associated with local symptoms. The most common local symptom is itching (*pruritus*), which varies in intensity. Pain or tenderness often accompanies some skin lesions. Other skin sensations such as burning, prickling, stinging, or crawling are also described. Alterations in local feeling include absence of sensation (*anaesthesia*); excessive sensitiveness (*hyperesthesia*); diminished sensation (*hypesthesia* or *hypoesthesia*); or abnormal sensation, such as burning or prickling (*paresthesia*). These symptoms may remain localized or migrate; may be constant or intermittent; and may be aggravated by a specific activity, such as exposure to sunlight.

It is important to determine whether the child has an allergic condition such as asthma or hay fever or history of a previous skin disease. AD, often associated with allergies, frequently begins in infancy. Important questions for the parent include when the lesion or symptom first appeared; whether it occurred with ingestion of a food or other substance, including any medication; and whether the condition was related to activity such as contact with plants, insects, or chemicals.

Objective Findings

The distribution, size, morphological characteristics, and arrangement of skin lesions provide significant information. Extrinsic causes usually result from physical, chemical, or allergic irritants or from an infectious agent such as bacteria, fungi, viruses, or animal parasites. Skin manifestations are also produced by intrinsic causes such as an infection (measles or chickenpox), drug sensitization, or other allergic phenomena.

Types of Lesions

Skin lesions assume distinct characteristics that are related to the pathological process. Nurses should become familiar with the common terms that are applied to skin lesions because these terms are used in the processes of record keeping and communication. These terms include the following:

Erythema—A reddened area caused by increased amounts of oxygenated blood in the dermal vasculature

Ecchymoses (bruises)—Localized red or purple discolourations caused by extravasation of blood into dermis and subcutaneous tissues

Petechiae—Pinpoint, tiny, and sharp circumscribed spots in the superficial layers of the epidermis

Primary lesions—Skin changes produced by a causative factor; common primary lesions in pediatric skin disorders are macules, papules, and vesicles (Fig. 53-1)

Secondary lesions—Changes that result from alteration in the primary lesions, such as those caused by rubbing, scratching, medication, or involution and healing (Fig. 53-2)

Distribution pattern—The pattern in which lesions are distributed over the body, whether local or generalized, and the specific areas associated with the lesions

Configuration and arrangement—The size, shape, and arrangement of a lesion or groups of lesions (e.g., *discrete, clustered, diffuse,* or *confluent*)

Laboratory Studies

If a skin problem is related to a systemic disease (e.g., collagen or immunodeficiency disease), laboratory studies are performed to identify the condition. Diagnostic techniques include microscopic examination, cultures, skin scrapings or biopsy, cytodiagnosis, patch testing, **Wood light** examination, allergic skin testing, and other laboratory tests such as blood count and sedimentation rate.

Wounds

Wounds are structural or physiological disruptions of the skin that activate normal or abnormal tissue repair responses. Wounds are classified as acute or chronic. *Acute wounds* are those that heal uneventfully within 2 to 3 weeks. *Chronic wounds* are those that do not heal in the expected time frame or are associated with complications. Cofactors that disrupt or delay wound healing include compromised perfusion, malnutrition, and infection. In children, most wounds are acute and can be prevented from becoming chronic wounds through appropriate nursing care. Wounds are also classified as surgical and nonsurgical and then further classified in the same manner as burns: superficial, partial-thickness, or full thickness (complex wounds that include muscle or bone).

Epidermal Injuries

Abrasions are the most common epidermal wounds in children, usually in the form of a skinned knee or elbow. In most injuries the margins of the abraded area are superficial, involving only the outer layers of epidermis, although the central portion may extend into the dermis. Epithelial tissue is composed of labile cells, which are constantly destroyed and replaced throughout the lifespan. Thus epidermal injuries usually result in rapid, uneventful healing and recovery.

Injury to Deeper Tissues

Tissues composed of permanent cells such as muscle and nerve cells are unable to regenerate. These tissues repair themselves by substituting fibrous connective tissue for the injured tissue. This fibrous tissue, or *scar*, serves as a patch to preserve or restore the continuity of the tissue. Wounds involving permanent cells include surgical incisions, lacerations, ulcers, evulsions, and full-thickness burns.

Process of Wound Healing

When the skin is injured, its normal protective barrier function is broken. In the healthy immunocompetent individual,

Macule—flat; nonpalpable; circumscribed; less than 1 cm in diameter; brown, red, purple, white, or tan in colour
Examples: Freckles; flat moles; rubella; rubeola

Plaque—elevated; flat topped; firm; rough; superficial papule greater than 1 cm in diameter; may be coalesced papules
Examples: Psoriasis; seborrheic and actinic keratoses

Patch—flat; nonpalpable; irregular in shape; macule that is greater than 1 cm in diameter
Examples: Vitiligo; port-wine marks

Wheal—elevated, irregularly shaped area of cutaneous edema; solid, transient, changing, variable diameter; pale pink with lighter centre
Examples: Urticaria; insect bites

Papule—elevated; palpable; firm; circumscribed; less than 1 cm in diameter; brown, red, pink, tan, or bluish red in colour
Examples: Warts; drug-related eruptions; pigmented nevi

Nodule—elevated; firm; circumscribed; palpable; deeper in dermis than papule; 1 to 2 cm in diameter
Examples: Erythema nodosum; lipomas

Vesicle—elevated; circumscribed; superficial; filled with serous fluid; less than 1 cm in diameter
Examples: Blister; varicella

Pustule—elevated; superficial; similar to vesicle but filled with purulent fluid
Examples: Impetigo; acne; variola

Bulla—vesicle greater than 1 cm in diameter
Examples: Blister; pemphigus vulgaris

Cyst—elevated; circumscribed; palpable; encapsulated; filled with liquid or semisolid material
Example: Sebaceous cyst

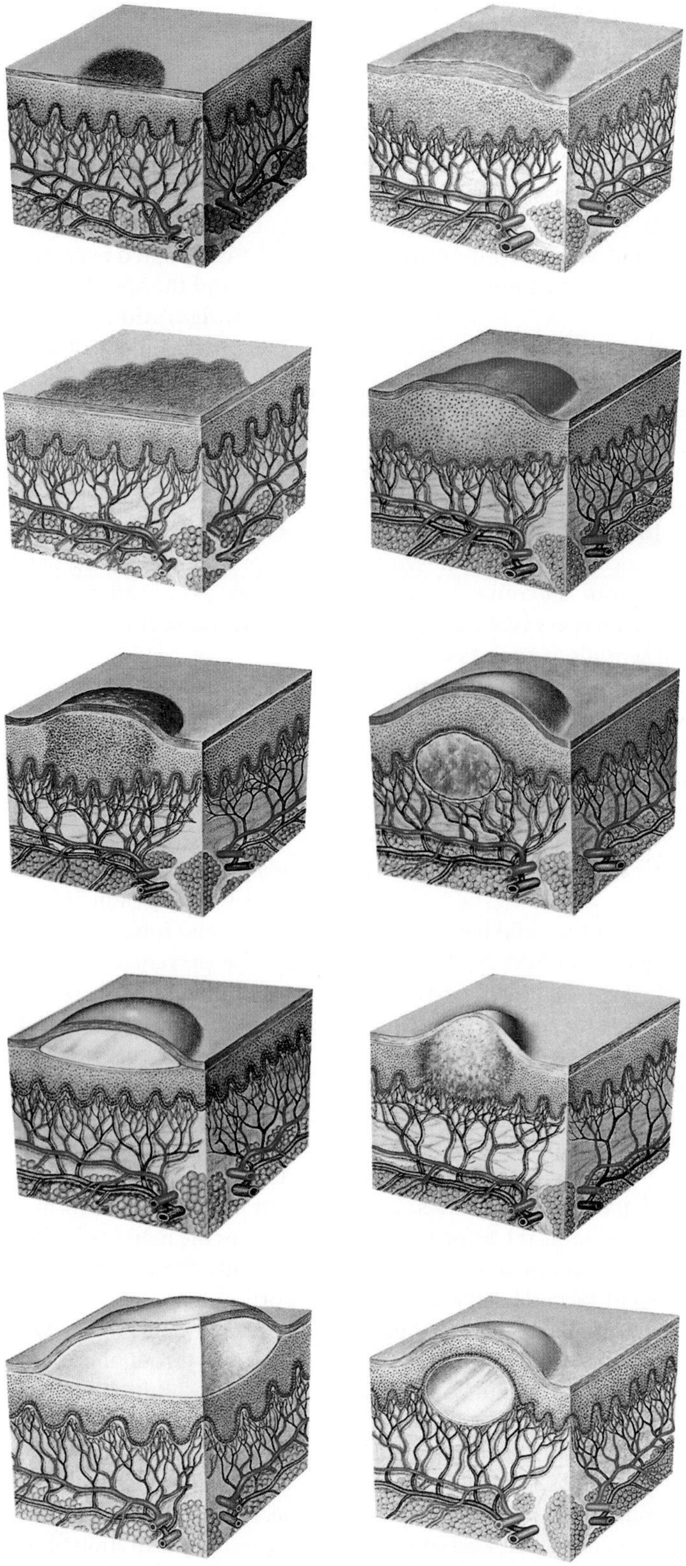

Fig. 53-1 Primary skin lesions. *(From Seidel, H.M., et al. [Eds.]. [2006].* Mosby's guide to physical examination *[6th ed., pp. 183–185]. St. Louis: Mosby [Table 8-4].)*

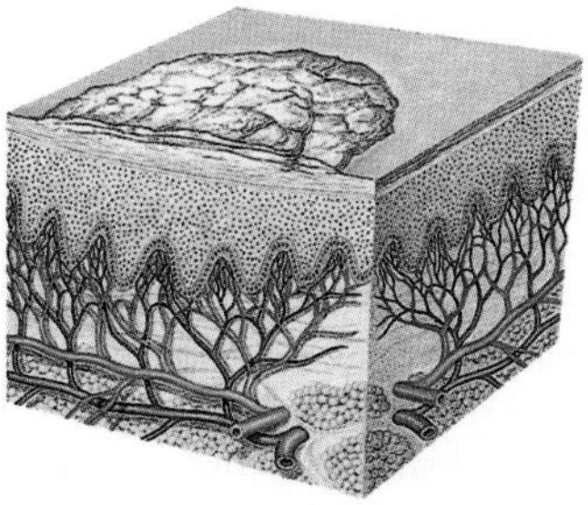

Scale—heaped-up keratinized cells; flaky exfoliation; irregular; thick or thin; dry or oily; varied size; silver, white, or tan in colour
Examples: Psoriasis; exfoliative dermatitis

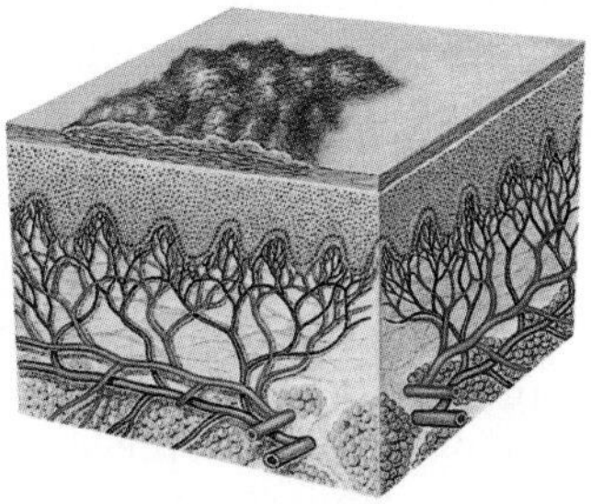

Crust—dried serum, blood, or purulent exudate; slightly elevated; size varies; brown, red, black, tan, or straw in colour
Examples: Scab on abrasion; eczema

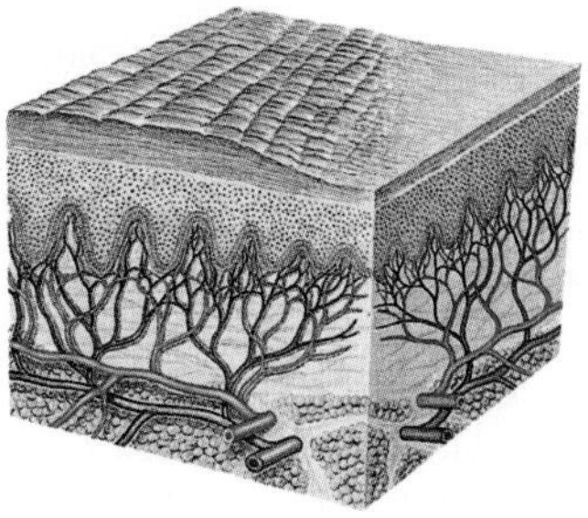

Lichenification—rough, thickened epidermis; accentuated skin markings caused by rubbing or irritation; often involves flexor aspect of extremity
Example: Chronic dermatitis

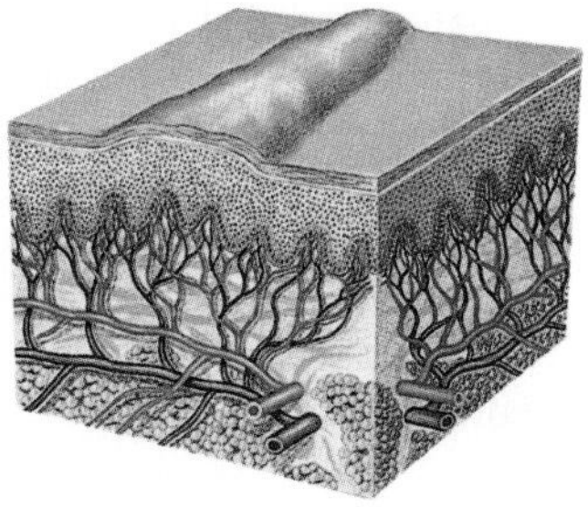

Scar—thin to thick fibrous tissue replacing injured dermis; irregular; pink, red, or white in colour; may be atrophic or hypertrophic
Example: Healed wound or surgical incision

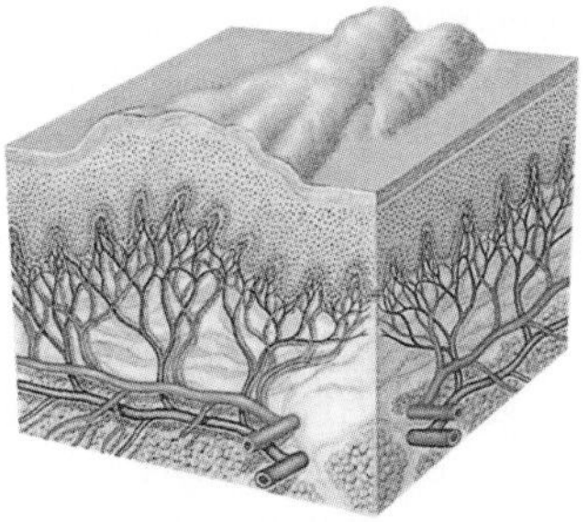

Keloid— irregularly shaped, elevated, progressively enlarging scar; grows beyond boundaries of wound; caused by excessive collagen formation during healing
Example: Keloid from ear piercing or burn scar

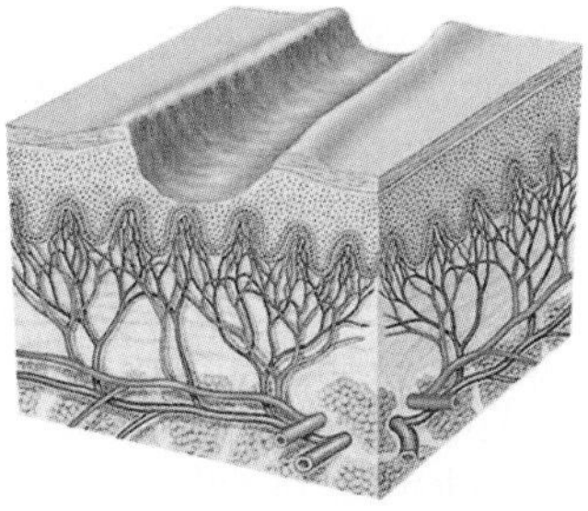

Excoriation—loss of epidermis; linear or hollowed-out crusted area; dermis exposed
Examples: Abrasion; scratch

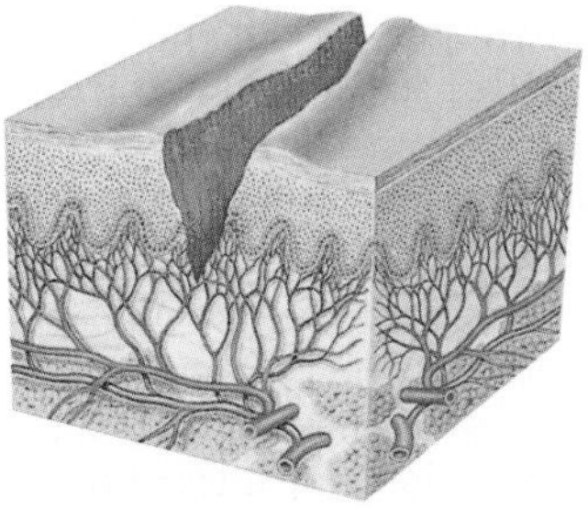

Fissure—linear crack or break from epidermis to dermis; small; deep; red
Examples: Athlete's foot; cheilosis

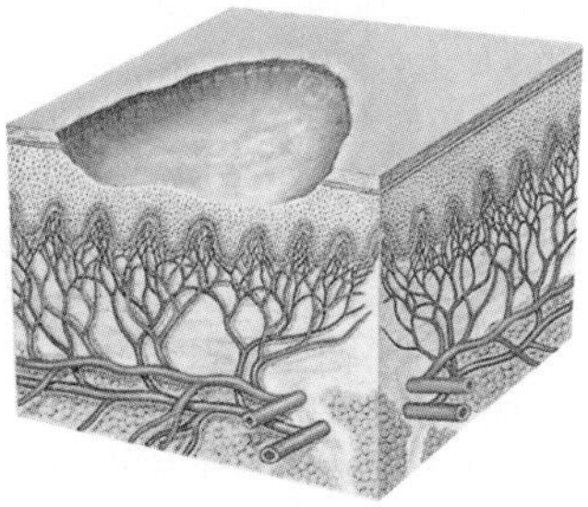

Erosion—loss of all or part of epidermis; depressed; moist; glistening; follows rupture of vesicle or bulla; larger than fissure
Examples: Varicella; variola following rupture

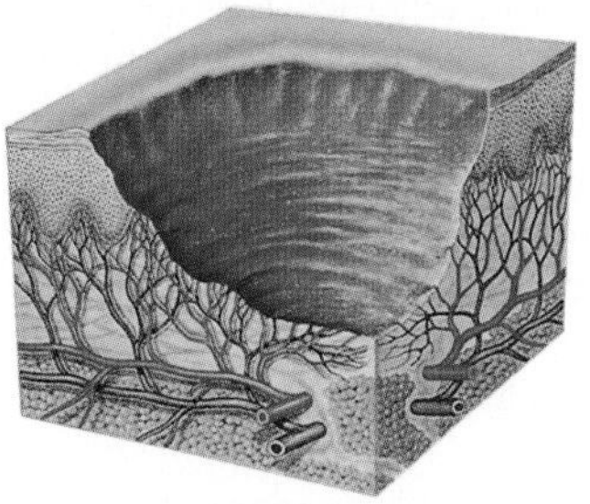

Ulcer—loss of epidermis and dermis; concave; varies in size; exudative; red or reddish blue
Examples: Decubiti; stasis ulcers

Fig. 53-2 Secondary skin lesions. *(From Seidel, H.M., et al. [Eds.]. [2006].* Mosby's guide to physical examination *[6th ed., pp. 186–188]. St. Louis: Mosby [Table 8-5].)*

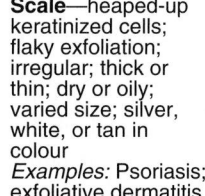

acute traumatic abrasions, lacerations, and superficial skin and soft-tissue injuries heal spontaneously without complications. The healing process is segregated into four phases that are characterized by the particular cells involved and the chemicals produced. The four stages of wound healing are hemostasis, inflammation, proliferation, and remodelling. Some authorities combine the first two phases.

In the *hemostasis* phase, platelets act to seal off the damaged blood vessels and to form a stable clot. Hemostasis occurs within minutes of the initial injury to the skin unless there is an underlying clotting disorder.

Inflammation, the second stage of wound healing, presents a clinical picture that involves erythema, swelling, and warmth, often associated with pain at the wound site. This stage usually lasts up to 4 days after injury. The inflammation phase involves white blood cells such as the neutrophils, monocytes, and macrophages. These cells mount an initial defence against microbial invasion and secrete proteolytic enzymes that destroy nonviable tissue and microorganisms in the wound area.

The *proliferative* phase, which includes *granulation* and *contracture*, is the third stage of healing. This phase lasts from 4 to 21 days in acute wounds, depending on the size of the wound. The phase involves the replacement of dermal tissues and subdermal tissues in deep wounds, as well as the contraction of the wound. The phase is characterized clinically by the presence of granulation tissue, the "beefy," pebbled red tissue in the wound base. Fibroblasts, or immature connective tissue cells, secrete collagen, which provides the foundation for dermal regeneration. Angiocytes regenerate the outer layers of capillaries, and endothelial cells produce the lining in a process called angiogenesis. The formation of granulation tissue, which provides the foundation for the wound, depends on angiogenesis. The keratinocytes are responsible for epithelialization. In the final stage of epithelialization, contracture occurs as the keratinocytes differentiate and form the protective outer layer, or stratum corneum, of the skin.

Remodelling, or *maturation*, is the final phase of the healing process. This phase occurs in the dermis as fibroblasts increase the tissue tensile strength and gradually replace type 3 collagen in the scar tissue with type 1 collagen, thicken the collagen fibres, and reorient the collagen fibres along the lines of tissue tension. Fibroblasts disappear as the wound becomes stronger. The wound edges are brought closer together, and a mature scar is formed. Children heal aggressively with abundant scar tissue, especially during growth spurts. The highly elastic quality of children's skin pulls on the wound, and the wound defends against this pull by forming scar tissue. Remodelling and maturation occur over several months and can take up to 2 years. Thus some wounds that appear to be completely healed can break down suddenly if attention is not paid to the initial causative factors.

The phases of wound healing are complex and may be interrupted by disease conditions, medications, and other systemic and local factors that influence the healing process. When a wound does not follow the "normal wound healing trajectory," it may become stuck in one of the stages and become a chronic wound. It is important that health care providers understand and address the factors that influence wound healing and prevent the development of chronic wounds.

Factors That Influence Wound Healing

The promotion of a moist, crust-free environment that enhances the migration of epithelial cells across the wound and facilitates remodelling is ideal for wound care management. An acute full-thickness wound kept in a moist environment usually re-epithelializes in 12 to 15 days, whereas the same wound when kept open to the air heals in about 25 to 30 days.

Numerous factors can delay healing (Table 53-1). For example, traditional practices, such as the use of antiseptics (hydrogen peroxide and povidone-iodine [Betadine] solutions), which were once thought to prevent infection, are now known to have a cytotoxic effect on healthy cells and minimal effect on controlling infections. Povidone-iodine may also be absorbed through the skin in neonates and young children.

General Therapeutic Management

Some skin disorders demand aggressive therapy, but by and large the major aim of treatment is to prevent further damage, eliminate the cause, prevent complications, and provide relief from discomfort while tissues undergo healing (McCord & Levy, 2006). Factors that contribute to the development of dermatitis and that prolong the course of the disease should be eliminated when possible. The most common causative agents of dermatitis in infants, children, and adolescents are environmental factors (soaps, bubble baths, shampoos, rough or tight clothing, wet diapers, blankets, and toys) and the natural elements (such as dirt, sand, heat, cold, moisture, and wind). Dermatitis may also result from home remedies and medications.

Dressings

The traditional dry gauze dressing should not be used on open wounds, since it allows the wound surface to dry, does little to prevent bacterial invasion, and adheres to the dried scab so that removal disturbs the newly regenerating epithelial cells. In most instances, traditional gauze dressings have been replaced by dressings that promote moist wound healing (Table 53-2). Moist wound healing increases the rate of collagen synthesis and re-epithelialization and decreases pain and inflammation. It also creates an environment for autolytic debridement of necrotic tissue, which creates a clean wound bed and enhances granulation. However, a balance must be achieved between creating a moist wound bed and maintaining a dry periwound area that protects the skin and wound from maceration. The dressing type and frequency of dressing changes help to achieve this balance. The frequency of dressing changes is based on the presence of infection, the type of dressing, the location of the wound, and the amount of drainage. Dressings should always be changed when they are loose or soiled. They should be changed more frequently in areas where contamination is likely (e.g., the sacral area, the buttocks, the tracheal area) or when wound infection is suspected or present.

Topical Therapy

Several agents and methods are available in wound care. In selecting a therapeutic regimen, the practitioner considers (1) the active ingredient, (2) the proper vehicle or base, (3) the cosmetic effect, (4) the cost, and (5) instructions for use.

Table 53-1 Factors That Delay Wound Healing

FACTOR	EFFECT ON HEALING
Dry wound environment	Allows epithelial cells to dry out and die; impairs migration of epithelial cells across wound surface
Nutritional deficiencies	
Vitamin A	Results in inadequate inflammatory response
Vitamin B_1	Results in decreased collagen formation
Vitamin C	Inhibits formation of collagen fibres and capillary development
Protein	Reduces supply of amino acids for tissue repair
Zinc	Impairs epithelialization
Immunocompromise	Results in inadequate or delayed inflammatory response
Impaired circulation	Inhibits inflammatory response and removal of debris from wound area Reduces supply of nutrients to wound area
Stress (pain, poor sleep)	Releases catecholamines that cause vasoconstriction
Antiseptics	
Hydrogen peroxide	Toxic to fibroblasts; can cause subcutaneous gas formation (mimics gas-forming infection)
Povidone-iodine	Toxic to white and red blood cells and fibroblasts
Chlorhexidine	Toxic to white blood cells
Medications	
Corticosteroids	Impair phagocytosis Inhibit fibroblast proliferation Depress formation of granulation tissue Inhibit wound contraction
Chemotherapy	Interrupts the cell cycle; damages DNA or prevents DNA repair
Anti-inflammatory drugs	Decrease the inflammatory phase
Foreign bodies	Increase inflammatory response Inhibit wound closure
Infection	Increases inflammatory response Increases tissue destruction
Mechanical friction	Damages or destroys granulation tissue
Fluid accumulation in area	Inhibits tissues from approximating
Radiation	Inhibits fibroblastic activity and capillary formation May cause tissue necrosis
Diseases	
Diabetes mellitus	Inhibits collagen synthesis Impairs circulation and capillary growth Hyperglycemia impairs phagocytosis
Anemia	Reduces oxygen supply to tissues
Peripheral vascular disease	Reduces oxygen supply to wounds
Uremia	Decreases collagen and granulation tissue

DNA, deoxyribonucleic acid.

Several basic concepts must also be considered. Overtreatment is avoided. For example, when the dermatitis is acute, topical applications should be mild and bland to avoid further irritation. Broken or inflamed skin, especially in children, is more absorbent than intact skin, and chemicals that are nonirritating to intact skin may be quite irritating to inflamed skin.

Topical applications may be applied to treat the disorder, reduce itching, decrease external stimuli, or apply external heat or cold. The emollient action of soaks, baths, and lotions provides a soothing film over the skin surface that reduces external stimuli. Ordinarily, lukewarm, tepid, or cool applications offer the greatest relief.

NURSING ALERT Application of heat tends to aggravate most conditions, and its use is usually reserved for reducing specific inflammatory processes, such as folliculitis and cellulitis.

Ointments in a petrolatum base provide protection from moisture. Therefore, this type of ointment is indicated around gastrostomy tubes, in skin folds, and in the diaper area. Creams are absorbed by the skin and are used for areas where a nongreasy "feel" is desired (e.g., face, hands).

Topical Corticosteroid Therapy

Glucocorticoids are the therapeutic medications used most frequently for skin disorders. Their local anti-inflammatory effects are merely palliative, so the medication must be applied until the condition undergoes a remission or the causative agent is eliminated. Corticosteroids are applied directly to the affected area, are essentially nonsensitizing, and have only minor adverse effects. As with the use of any steroids, their use in large amounts may mask signs of infection, and symptoms may be exacerbated after termination of the medication. Families should be cautioned that the medication cannot be used for all skin disorders. The concentrations available

Table 53-2 Common Wound Care Products

TYPE OF PRODUCT	INDICATIONS	FUNCTION	DRESSING CHANGE FREQUENCY	COMMENTS
Transparent film (e.g., Tegaderm)	Skin tears, IV and tube sites, partial-thickness wounds, primary and secondary dressings	Provides moist wound healing; impermeable to fluid and bacteria; promotes autolytic debridement; nonabsorptive	Daily, up to 7 days	Seals wound from contaminants
Hydrocolloid (e.g., DuoDERM)	Pressure ulcers, partial- and full-thickness wounds, skin tears, tape anchor	Occlusive; impermeable to bacteria and contaminants; promotes autolytic debridement; minimal absorption	Up to 7 days	Do not place over infected or heavily draining wounds
Alginates-hydrofibres—calcium, collagen, and silver (e.g., Aquacel, Fibracol)	Moderate to large drainage, partial- and full-thickness wounds, dehiscence, infection, bleeding	Absorptive	Daily, but depends on amount of drainage; silver impregnated, 3–7 days	Excellent for packing, tunnelling, and undermining; trauma-free removal
Barrier dressings (e.g., Stomahesive wafer, Coloplast wafer)	Protect periwound, tube and tape anchor	Protect skin from drainage or adhesive stripping	Up to once weekly	Excellent around G tube sites; apply around wounds or on skin to attach tape
Barrier cream or ointment (e.g., Sensi-Care, Critic-Aid, Laniseptic)	Perineal and diaper areas	Protects skin from moisture	With each diaper change	Some impregnated with antifungals; choose those formulated to stick to moist lesions
Foam (e.g., Lyofoam, Mepilex, Allevyn, PolyMem)	Moderate to heavy drainage, partial- and full-thickness wounds	More absorptive than gauze	Depends on drainage; up to 7 days	Excellent around leaking tubes and tracheostomies; available with fenestration; comfortable; nonadherent; trauma-free removal
Silver (e.g., SilvaSorb dressing and gel, Arglaes powder)	Infected or colonized full- and partial-thickness wounds	Depends on dressing type; available in foam, hydrocolloid, hydrofibre, alginate, and powder	Depends on dressing type; usually 3–7 days	Consider in wounds recalcitrant to previous treatments; controls odour
Wound gels (e.g., Flaminal)	Dry, partial- and full-thickness wounds and burns	Adds moisture; promotes epithelialization; fills up dead space	Once or twice daily	Easy to use; base frequency on wound moisture
Hydrogel dressing (CarraGauze, CarraDres)	Burns, partial- and full-thickness wounds, painful wounds	Adds moisture; aids autolytic debridement; minimal to moderate absorption	Daily	Nonadherent; trauma- and pain-free removal
Becaplermin gel (Regranex)	Ulcers	Promotes granulation	Daily	Contraindicated in infected and necrotic wounds; refrigerate; expensive
Enzymatic debrider (Accuzyme)	Necrotic wounds in patients who are not surgical candidates	Selectively dissolves necrotic tissue	Once or twice daily	Cross-hatch eschar with a scalpel for enzyme penetration; cover with moist normal saline gauze to activate; avoid use with silver or mercury
Gauze	All wound types	Minor absorption; mild debridement	3–4 times per day	Dries out; poor absorbency; can macerate periwound; increased labour costs and supplies secondary to dressing change frequency

(From McCord, S. S., & Moise, L. [2006]. Practical guide to pediatric wound care. *Seminars in Plastic Surgery, 20*[3], 192–199.)

without prescription are not adequate for stubborn skin conditions (e.g., psoriasis) and may further aggravate inflammation caused by fungus or bacteria. Most parents and children should be counselled that it is both effective and economical to apply only a thin film of topical hydrocortisone and to massage it into the skin. Parents and children should also be advised to use the application for no more than 5 to 7 days because these agents may cause depigmentation and other changes in the skin.

Other Topical Therapies

Other topical treatments include chemical cautery (especially useful for warts), cryosurgery, electrodesiccation (chiefly used for warts, granulomas, and nevi), ultraviolet (UV) therapy (primarily used in psoriasis and acne), laser therapy (especially for birthmarks), and acne therapies such as dermabrasion and chemical peels. New medications called *topical immunomodulators* are effective in reducing the itching of AD (eczema) and preventing "flares."

Systemic Therapy

Systemic medications may be used as an adjunct to topical therapy in some dermatological disorders. The medications most frequently used are corticosteroids, antibiotics, and antifungal medications. Corticosteroids are valuable because of their capacity to inhibit inflammatory and allergic reactions. Dosage is carefully adjusted and gradually tapered to the minimum dosage that is effective and tolerated. In infants and children, the dosage is larger than is usually calculated from body weight ratios. However, prolonged use may temporarily suppress growth.

Antibiotics are used in severe or widespread skin infections. However, because these medications tend to produce hypersensitivity in some patients, they are used with caution. Antifungal medications are the only means for treating systemic fungal infections.

Nursing Care Management

The child's subjective symptoms and the parent's history provide valuable information to help establish a diagnosis. Older children often describe the condition as painful, itching, or tingling or in other descriptive terms. However, much can be determined by also observing the younger child's behaviour. Does the child scratch? Is the child restless or irritable? Does the child favour or avoid using a body part? A careful history provides important clues. Has the child had access to chemicals or been in the woods or around a woodpile? Has the child eaten a new food? Is the child taking medication? Has the child any known allergy? Do siblings or playmates have similar lesions? What soap or bubble bath is used for bathing?

It is important for nurses to not only describe but also assess skin lesions and wounds. The colour, shape, and distribution of lesions and wounds are important. Individual lesions are described according to standard terminology. Sometimes two descriptors are used for a particular characteristic (e.g., maculopapular rash). To confirm or amplify the findings made by inspection, the nurse may gently palpate the skin to detect characteristics such as temperature, moisture, texture, elasticity, and edema. Wounds need to be assessed for depth of tissue damage, evidence of healing, and signs of infection.

NURSING ALERT Signs of wound infection are as follows:

- Increased erythema, especially beyond the wound margin
- Edema
- Purulent exudate
- Pain
- Increased temperature

The frequency of wound assessment depends on the severity and complexity of the wound. For example, simple or chronic wounds are assessed weekly; infected or complex wounds are assessed daily. Wounds are measured at least weekly (height, width, and depth). The wound bed is assessed for colour, drainage, odour, necrosis, granulation tissue, fibrin slough, undermining and condition of the wound edges, and the colour and condition of the surrounding skin.

Therapeutic programs are designed to include general measures such as rest, protection, and relief of discomfort, and specific treatments such as medication and physical techniques. Only a few skin diseases are contagious; thus it is usually not necessary to isolate the affected child, except from persons in danger of acquiring a secondary infection (e.g., a child receiving large doses of corticosteroids or other immunosuppressant medications or a child with an immunological deficiency disorder). However, if the skin manifestation is caused by a viral **exanthema,** such as measles or chickenpox, the child should be prevented from exposing other susceptible children.

Wound Care

Parents can generally manage small skin lesions or wounds at home. The parents should be instructed to wash their hands and then wash the wound gently with mild soap and water or normal saline. They should be cautioned to avoid povidone-iodine, alcohol, and hydrogen peroxide because these products are toxic to wounds.

NURSING ALERT Do not put anything in a wound that you would not put in the eye. The safest solution is normal saline.

Open wounds are covered with a dressing, such as a commercial adhesive bandage, although larger wounds may benefit from the use of occlusive dressings (see Table 53-2). If occlusive dressings are applied, parents should learn how to apply and remove the dressings correctly. For example, hydrocolloid dressings adhere best if a wide margin is left around the wound and the dressing is pressed against intact skin until it adheres. If a dressing needs to be secured, a nonalcohol skin barrier can be applied to protect the skin, or the wound can be "picture framed" with hydrocolloid dressing and dressing tape can be secured to the hydrocolloid. This method of securing the dressing protects the skin when the tape is removed. Montgomery straps or stretch netting can also be used to secure dressings and to avoid the use of tape.

NURSING ALERT Advise parents that the yellow gel forming under hydrocolloid dressings may look like pus and has a distinct odour (somewhat fruity) but is normal leakage.

Dressings need to be removed carefully to protect intact skin and the epithelial surface of the wound. When removing transparent or hydrocolloid dressings, the nurse or parent should raise one edge of the dressing and pull parallel to the skin to loosen the adhesive. The longer the dressings are left on, the easier they are to remove. Less frequent dressing changes decrease wound contamination.

Lacerations present a special challenge. The injured child and family are usually distressed by the bleeding. In particular, scalp lacerations tend to bleed profusely. Parental guilt and shock usually accompany the injury. The initial nursing intervention is to apply pressure to the area and to attempt to calm the child before further examination. Unless there is bleeding from a severed artery, the wound is cleansed with a forced jet of sterile tepid water or saline (via syringe) and examined for extent, depth, and presence of foreign material such as dirt, glass, or fabric fragments.

The location of the wound can facilitate assessment. Wounds over bony areas may contain bone chips, and clear fluid seeping from severe head wounds may indicate cerebrospinal fluid. A pressure dressing is applied for transfer to medical care. After the child is in a medical facility, he or she is prepared for **suturing.**

Puncture wounds that do not require a tetanus booster are soaked in warm water and soap for several minutes. Causing the wound to rebleed may be helpful. An adhesive bandage can be applied if desired. Puncture wounds of the head, chest, or abdomen or those that could still contain a portion of the puncturing object must be evaluated carefully.

Parents should be cautioned against opening blisters or kissing a wound "to make it better." The wound can easily become contaminated from germs in the human mouth. If scabs form, they need to be allowed to slough off without assistance; picking or early removal may cause scarring and secondary infection. Parents should be advised to seek medical help if there is evidence of infection.

Relief of Symptoms

Most therapeutic regimens for skin lesions are directed toward relief of pruritus, the most common complaint. Cooling the affected area and increasing the skin pH with cool baths or compresses and alkaline applications (e.g., baking soda baths) are helpful in reducing the itching. Clothing and bed linen should be soft and lightweight to decrease irritation from friction and stimulation.

During treatment, both the affected and unaffected skin is protected from damage and secondary infection. Preventing scratching is important. Older children can refrain from scratching or rubbing, although they may need to be reminded to do so. Small children may require the use of devices such as mittens (especially during sleep) or special coverings. Keeping fingernails clean, short, and trimmed reduces the risk of secondary infection.

Antipruritic medications, such as diphenhydramine (Benadryl) or hydroxyzine (Atarax), may be prescribed for severe itching, especially if it disturbs the child's rest. Pain and discomfort are usually managed with nonpharmacological measures and mild analgesia. Severe pain requires more potent medication. Occlusive dressings over wounds reduce pain. For suturing wounds a topical anaesthetic or intradermal buffered lidocaine should be used (see Pain Management, Chapter 35).

Topical Therapy

The specific type of topical therapy and the mode of application depend on the nature and location of the lesion. It is especially important to perform proper hand hygiene before and after application of any topical therapy. The skin should be assessed before the application and reassessed after treatment. Any observed changes need to be noted and described.

Wet compresses or dressings cool the skin by evaporation, relieve itching and inflammation, and cleanse the area by loosening and removing crusts and debris. A variety of ingredients, such as plain water or Burow's solution (available without a prescription), can be applied on Kerlix gauze or plain gauze.

Dressings immersed in the desired solution are wrung out slightly and applied to the affected area wet but not dripping. They are applied flat and smooth in such a way that motion is not totally restricted—fingers are wrapped separately, and arms and legs are wrapped so that elbows and knees can bend. Dressings are held in place by Kerlix or other cotton wrap, tubular stockinette, mittens, and socks (two pairs—one to hold the dressings in place, the other to protect from movement). When evaporation begins to dry them, the dressings are removed, rewet in the solution, and reapplied using aseptic technique. The solution is *not* poured or applied with a syringe directly over the dressings. As fluid evaporates, the solution becomes more concentrated, and this could damage sensitive lesions.

Fresh solution at room temperature is applied at 2-, 3-, or 4-hour intervals and allowed to remain on the lesion from 20 to 90 minutes. Wet dressings are seldom continued after about 48 hours. The child needs to be protected against chilling during treatment, and no more than 20% of the body is covered with a dressing at one time, to avoid the risk of hypothermia. After treatment, the skin is dried thoroughly by patting with a towel. Lotion or other medication (if prescribed) is applied at this time.

When the use of wet dressings is not possible, soaks are often used for removal of crusts and for their mild astringent action. The same solutions are used as for wet compresses. Gaining young children's cooperation for hand or foot soaks can be difficult unless the procedure is accompanied by play. Older infants and toddlers delight in playing with brightly coloured objects or poker chips scattered over the bottom of the receptacle, and preschoolers can be challenged to hold a floating item beneath the water's surface. However, these activities require supervision; infants and small children place items in their mouths, and children easily lose control with water play. Washing dishes, cars, dolls, or doll clothes will also occupy time during soaks.

Older children also need something to do during the procedure, such as listening to music or a story or watching television. Placing the solution and the extremity in a plastic sealable bag is an effective method to soak a hand or foot.

Baths are useful in the treatment of widespread dermatitis by evenly distributing the soothing antipruritic and anti-inflammatory effects of the solution, usually oatmeal or mineral oil preparations. The solution is added to a tub of lukewarm water. The temperature of the bath should be tepid, and the treatment usually lasts 15 to 53 minutes. Therapeutic baths are more interesting when toy boats or other items for water play accompany the procedure.

Topical applications are applied to skin lesions to ease discomfort, prevent further injury, and facilitate healing. A thin application of the ointment or cream may be covered with a plastic film and anchored with adhesive, covered with a commercial transparent dressing, or wrapped in Kerlix gauze and held in place by a stretchy net dressing. Topical preparations are applied systematically with the contour of the body surface (not simply up and down). Children love to be "painted," and lotion applications can be fun when an ordinary paintbrush is used. Regardless of the type of preparation used, parents need detailed information on how to apply it and how long the preparation should remain on the skin.

NURSING ALERT Provide written instructions and demonstrate to parents the correct amount of topical medication to apply (e.g., size of a pea; thin film to cover). If more than one preparation is applied, mark the containers with numbers so the parents remember the correct order of application. Stress that more is not necessarily better with some medications, such as steroids.

Home Care and Family Support

Dermatological conditions always involve the family, but few situations require hospitalization and most care is delivered at home. Because the family members must carry out the treatment plan, their cooperation is essential. Regimens that are simple to accomplish in the clinic, hospital, or primary care provider's office may be frustrating and baffling at home. The family may also need assistance in adapting equipment available for home therapy.

It is important that the child and family be given explanations that are as detailed as possible about both the expected and unexpected results of treatment, including any ill effects that might occur. If unexplained reactions develop, the family should be directed to discontinue treatment and report the reactions to the appropriate person. The use of over-the-counter medicines is discouraged unless the preparations have been discussed with the health care provider and have received approval.

Because the skin is the most visible portion of the body, defects in its surface alter its appearance and cause distress for the child. Skin problems may also result in rejection by others. Parents of other children may fear that their children will "catch" the disorder. Occasionally the affected child's own family members reduce their interaction or physical contact with the child. This is seldom a problem with dermatitis of short duration, but chronic conditions can frequently create problems and affect the child's self-esteem.

Infections of the Skin

Bacterial Infections

Normally, the skin harbours a variety of bacterial flora, including the major pathogenic varieties of staphylococci and streptococci. The degree of pathogenicity of the organism depends on its invasiveness and toxicity, the integrity of the skin, and the immune and cellular defences of the host. Children with congenital or acquired immunodeficiency disorders (such as acquired immunodeficiency syndrome [AIDS]), those in a debilitated condition, those receiving immunosuppressant therapy, and those with a generalized malignancy such as leukemia or lymphoma are at risk for developing bacterial infections.

Because of the characteristic "walling-off" process of the inflammatory reaction (abscess formation), staphylococci are more difficult to treat, and the local infected area is associated with an increase in bacteria all over the skin surface that serves as a source of continuing infection. In recent years, the number of community-acquired methicillin-resistant *Staphylococcus aureus* (MRSA) infections has risen (Kaplan, 2006). All of these factors underline the importance of careful hand hygiene when caring for infected children and their lesions to prevent the spread of infection and as an essential prophylactic measure when caring for infants and small children. Common bacterial skin disorders are outlined in Table 53-3.

Nursing Care Management

The major nursing interventions related to bacterial skin infections are to prevent the spread of infection and to prevent complications. Impetigo contagiosa and MRSA infection can easily spread by self-inoculation; thus the child must be cautioned against touching the involved area. Hand hygiene is mandatory before and after contact with an affected child; this practice should be emphasized to all those who care for the child. The Ontario Agency for Health Protection and Promotion (2011) has developed a 4-moment hand hygiene practice, as follows: practise hand hygiene (1) before initial contact with the patient or patient environment, (2) before aseptic procedure, (3) after body fluid exposure risk, and (4) after contact with the patient or patient environment. Many children with AD are colonized with MRSA in the nares and under the fingernails. For many bacterial infections, and for MRSA infection in particular, the child should be provided with washcloths and towels separate from those of other family members. Pyjamas, underwear, and other clothes should be changed daily and washed in hot water. Razors used for shaving should not be shared. To prevent recurrence, some infectious disease specialists recommend bathing in a chlorine bath twice weekly with 5 mL of chlorine per 3.8 L of water (Huang et al., 2009).

Evolve Case Study—Impetigo

Children and parents are often tempted to squeeze follicular lesions. No attempt should be made to puncture the surface of the pustule with a needle or sharp instrument. A child with a sty may waken with the eyelids of the affected eye sealed shut with exudate. The child or the parents should be instructed to gently wipe the lid from the inner to the outer edge with warm water and a clean washcloth until the exudate is removed.

The child with limited cellulitis of an extremity is usually managed at home on a regimen of oral antibiotics and warm compresses. Children with more extensive cellulitis, especially around a joint with lymphadenitis or on the face, are usually admitted to the hospital for parenteral antibiotics, followed by continued treatment at home. Nurses are responsible for teaching the family to administer the medication and apply compresses.

Viral Infections

Viruses are intracellular parasites that produce their effect by using the intracellular substances of the host cells. Composed of only a deoxyribonucleic acid (DNA) or ribonucleic acid (RNA) core enclosed in an antigenic protein shell, viruses are unable to provide for their own metabolic needs or to reproduce themselves. After a virus penetrates a cell of the host organism, it sheds the outer shell and disappears within the cell, where the nucleic acid core stimulates the host cell to

Table 53-3 Bacterial Infections

DISORDER AND ORGANISM	MANIFESTATIONS	MANAGEMENT	COMMENTS
Impetigo contagiosa (Fig. 53-3)—Staphylococci	Begins as a reddish macule Becomes vesicular Ruptures easily, leaving superficial, moist erosion Tends to spread peripherally in sharply marginated irregular outlines Exudate dries to form heavy, honey-coloured crusts Pruritus common Systemic effects—Minimal or asymptomatic	Careful removal of undermined skin, crusts, and debris by softening with 1 : 20 Burow's solution compresses Topical application of bactericidal ointment Systemic administration of oral or parenteral antibiotics (penicillin) in severe or extensive lesions	Tends to heal without scarring unless secondary infection Autoinoculable and contagious Common in toddler, preschooler May be superimposed on eczema
Pyoderma—Staphylococci, streptococci	Deeper extension of infection into dermis Tissue reaction more severe Systemic effects—Fever, lymphangitis	Soap and water cleansing Wet compresses Bathing with antibacterial soap as prescribed Do not share washcloths or towels Mupirocin to nares and lesions as prescribed Systemic antibiotics	Autoinoculable and contagious May heal with or without scarring
Folliculitis (pimple), furuncle (boil), carbuncle (multiple boils)—*Staphylococcus aureus*	Folliculitis—Infection of hair follicle Furuncle—Larger lesion with more redness and swelling at a single follicle Carbuncle—More extensive lesion with widespread inflammation and "pointing" at several follicular orifices Systemic effects—Malaise, if severe	Skin cleanliness Local warm, moist compresses Topical application of antibiotic medications Systemic antibiotics in severe cases Incision and drainage of severe lesions, followed by wound irrigation with antibiotics or suitable drain implantation	Autoinoculable and contagious Furuncle and carbuncle tend to heal with scar formation Never squeeze a lesion
Cellulitis—Streptococci, staphylococci, *Haemophilus influenzae* (Fig. 53-4)	Inflammation of skin and subcutaneous tissues with intense redness, swelling, and firm infiltration Lymphangitis "streaking" frequently seen Involvement of regional lymph nodes common May progress to abscess formation Systemic effects—Fever, malaise	Oral or parenteral antibiotics Rest and immobilization of both affected area and child Hot, moist compresses to area	Hospitalization may be necessary for child with systemic symptoms Otitis media may be associated with facial cellulitis
Staphylococcal scalded skin syndrome—*S. aureus*	Macular erythema with "sandpaper" texture of involved skin Epidermis becoming wrinkled (in 2 days or less), and large bullae appearing	Systemic administration of antibiotics Gentle cleansing with saline, Burow's solution, or 0.25% silver nitrate compresses	Infant subject to fluid loss; impaired body temperature regulation; and secondary infection, such as pneumonia, cellulitis, and septicemia Heals without scarring

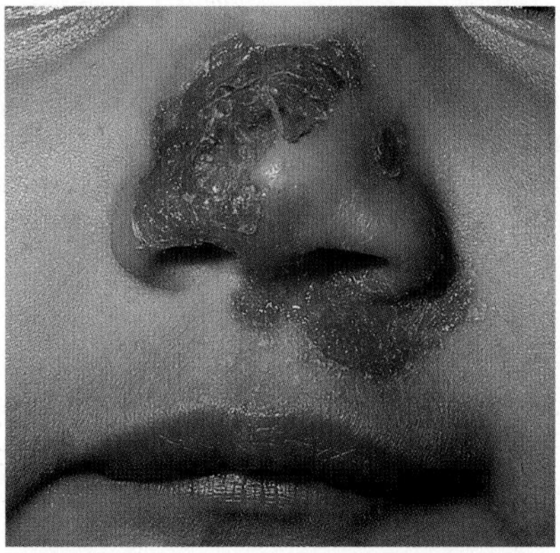

Fig. 53-3 Impetigo contagiosa. *(From Weston, W.L., Lane, A.T., & Morelli, J.G. [2002].* Color textbook of pediatric dermatology *[3rd ed.]. St. Louis: Mosby.)*

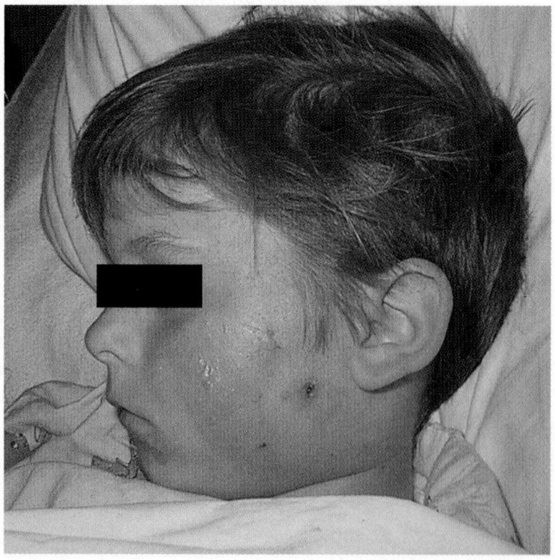

Fig. 53-4 Cellulitis of cheek from puncture wound. *(From Weston, W.L., Lane, A.T., & Morelli, J.G. [2002].* Color textbook of pediatric dermatology *[3rd ed.]. St. Louis: Mosby.)*

form more virus material from its intracellular substance. In a viral infection the epidermal cells react with inflammation and vesiculation (as in herpes simplex) or by proliferating to form growths (warts).

Many of the communicable viral diseases of childhood are associated with rashes, and each rash is characteristic. Other common viral disorders of the skin are outlined in Table 53-4.

Dermatophytoses (Fungal Infections)

The dermatophytoses (ringworm) are infections caused by a group of closely related filamentous fungi that invade primarily the stratum corneum, hair, and nails. These are superficial infections that live on, not in, the skin. They are confined to the dead keratin layers and are unable to survive in the deeper layers. Because the keratin is **desquamated** constantly, the fungus must multiply at a rate that equals the rate of keratin production to maintain itself; otherwise the infection would be shed with the discarded skin cells. Common dermatophytoses are outlined in Table 53-5.

Dermatophytoses are designated by the Latin word *tinea*, with further designation related to the area of the body where they are found (e.g., tinea capitis [ringworm of the scalp]). Dermatophyte infections are most often transmitted from one person to another or from infected animals to humans.

Table 53-4 Viral Infections

INFECTION	MANIFESTATIONS	MANAGEMENT	COMMENTS
Verruca (warts) Human papillomavirus (various types)	Usually well-circumscribed, grey or brown, elevated, firm papules with a roughened, finely papillomatous texture Occur anywhere, but usually appear on exposed areas such as fingers, hands, face, and soles May be single or multiple Asymptomatic	Not uniformly successful Local destructive therapy, individualized according to location, type, and number—surgical removal, electrocautery, curettage, cryotherapy (liquid nitrogen), caustic solutions (lactic acid and salicylic acid in flexible collodion, retinoic acid, salicylic acid plasters), x-ray treatment, laser	Common in children Tend to disappear spontaneously Course unpredictable Most destructive techniques tend to leave scars Autoinoculable Repeated irritation will cause to enlarge Apply topical anaesthetic EMLA
Verruca plantaris (plantar wart)	Located on plantar surface of feet and, because of pressure, is practically flat; may be surrounded by a collar of hyperkeratosis	Apply caustic solution to wart Wear foam insole with hole cut to relieve pressure on wart Soak 20 minutes after 2-3 days; repeat until wart comes out	Destructive techniques tend to leave scars, which may cause problems with walking Apply topical anaesthetic EMLA
Herpes simplex virus Type I (cold sore, fever blister) Type II (genital)	Grouped, burning, and itching vesicles on inflammatory base, usually on or near mucocutaneous junctions (lips, nose, genitalia, buttocks) Vesicles dry, forming a crust, followed by exfoliation and spontaneous healing in 8-10 days May be accompanied by regional lymphadenopathy	Avoidance of secondary infection Burow's solution compresses during weeping stages Topical therapy (penciclovir) to shorten duration of cold sores Oral antiviral (acyclovir) for initial infection or to reduce severity in recurrence Valacyclovir (Valtrex), an oral antiviral, used for episodic treatment of recurrent genital herpes; reduces pain, stops viral shedding, and has a more convenient administration schedule than acyclovir	Heal without scarring unless secondary infection Type I cold sores prevented by using sunscreens protecting against ultraviolet A and ultraviolet B light to prevent lip blisters Aggravated by corticosteroids Positive psychological effect from treatment May be fatal in children with depressed immunity
Varicella-zoster virus (herpes zoster; shingles)	Caused by same virus that causes varicella (chickenpox) Virus has affinity for posterior root ganglia, posterior horn of spinal cord, and skin; crops of vesicles usually confined to dermatome following along course of affected nerve Usually preceded by neuralgic pain, hyperesthesias, or itching May be accompanied by constitutional symptoms	Symptomatic Analgesics for pain Mild sedation sometimes helpful Local moist compresses Drying lotions sometimes helpful Ophthalmic variety: use systemic corticotropin (adrenocorticotropic hormone) or corticosteroids Acyclovir Lidocaine (Lidoderm) topical anaesthetic	Pain in children usually minimal Postherpetic pain does not occur in children Chickenpox may follow exposure; isolate affected child from other children in a hospital or school May occur in children with depressed immunity; can be fatal
Molluscum contagiosum Cause—Pox virus Small, benign tumours	Flesh-coloured papules with a central caseous plug (umbilicated) Usually asymptomatic	Cases in well children resolve spontaneously in about 18 mo Treatment reserved for troublesome cases Apply topical anaesthetic EMLA and remove with curette Use tretinoin gel 0.01% or cantharidin (Cantharone) liquid Curettage or cryotherapy	Common in school-age children Spread by skin-to-skin contact, including autoinoculation and fomite-to-skin contact

EMLA, eutectic mix of lidocaine and prilocaine.

Table 53-5 Dermatophytoses (Fungal Infections)

DISEASE AND ORGANISM	MANIFESTATIONS	MANAGEMENT	COMMENTS
Tinea capitis—*Trichophyton tonsurans, Microsporum audouinii, Microsporum canis* (Fig. 53-5, A)	Lesions in scalp but may extend to hairline or neck Characteristic configuration of scaly, circumscribed patches or patchy, scaling areas of alopecia Generally asymptomatic, but severe, deep inflammatory reaction may occur that manifests as boggy, encrusted lesions (kerions) Pruritic Microscopic examination of scales is diagnostic	Oral griseofulvin Oral ketoconazole for difficult cases Selenium sulphide shampoos Topical antifungal medications (e.g., clotrimazole, haloprogin, miconazole)	Person-to-person transmission Animal-to-person transmission Rarely, permanent loss of hair *M. audouinii* transmitted from one human being to another directly or from personal items; *M. canis* usually contracted from household pets, especially cats Atopic individuals more susceptible
Tinea corporis—*Trichophyton rubrum, Trichophyton mentagrophytes, M. canis, Epidermophyton* organisms (see Fig. 53-5, B)	Generally round or oval, erythematous scaling patch that spreads peripherally and clears centrally; may involve nails (tinea unguium) *Diagnosis*—Direct microscopic examination of scales Usually unilateral	Oral griseofulvin Local application of antifungal preparation such as tolnaftate, haloprogin, miconazole, clotrimazole; apply 1 cm beyond periphery of lesion; continual application 1–2 wk after no sign of lesion	Usually of animal origin from infected pets Majority of infections in children caused by *M. canis* and *M. audouinii*
Tinea cruris ("jock itch")—*Epidermophyton floccosum, T. rubrum, T. mentagrophytes*	Skin response similar to that in tinea corporis Localized to medial proximal aspect of thigh and crural fold; may involve scrotum in males Pruritic *Diagnosis*—Same as for tinea corporis	Local application of tolnaftate liquid Wet compresses or sitz baths may be soothing	Rare in preadolescent children Health education regarding personal hygiene
Tinea pedis ("athlete's foot")—*T. rubrum, Trichophyton interdigitale, E. floccosum*	On intertriginous areas between toes or on plantar surface of feet Lesions vary: Maceration and fissuring between toes Patches with pinhead-sized vesicles on plantar surface Pruritic *Diagnosis*—Direct microscopic examination of scrapings	Oral griseofulvin Local applications of tolnaftate liquid and antifungal powder containing tolnaftate *Acute infections*—Compresses or soaks followed by application of glucocorticoid cream Elimination of conditions of heat and perspiration by clean, light socks and well-ventilated shoes; avoidance of occlusive shoes	Most frequent in adolescents and adults; rare in children, but occurrence increases with wearing of plastic shoes Transmission to other individuals rare, despite general opinion to contrary Ointments not successful
Candidiasis (moniliasis)—*Candida albicans*	Grows in chronically moist areas Inflamed areas with white exudate, peeling, and easy bleeding Pruritic *Diagnosis*—Characteristic appearance	Amphotericin B, nystatin ointment, or other antifungal preparations to affected areas	Common form of diaper dermatitis (see Fig. 53-11) Oral form common in infants Vaginal form in older females May be disseminated in immunosuppressed children

Diagnosis is made from microscopic examination of scrapings taken from the advancing periphery of the lesion, which almost always produces a scale.

Nursing Care Management

When teaching families how to care for ringworm, the nurse should emphasize good health and hygiene. Because of the infectious nature of the disease, affected children should not exchange with other children grooming items, headgear, scarves, or other articles of apparel that have been in proximity to the infected area. Affected children should have their own towels and wear a protective cap at night to avoid transmitting the fungus to bedding, especially if they sleep with another person. Because the infection can be acquired by animal-to-human transmission, all household pets should be examined for the disorder. Other sources of infection are seats with headrests (such as theatre seats), seats in public transportation vehicles, helmets, and gymnasium mats.

Both 2% ketoconazole and 1% selenium sulphide shampoos may reduce colony counts of dermatophytes. These shampoos can be used in combination with oral therapy to reduce the transmission of disease to others. The shampoo should be applied to the scalp for 5 to 10 minutes at least three times per week. The child may return to school once the therapy is initiated.

Alternately, if the child is treated with the drug griseofulvin, the therapy frequently continues for weeks or months, and

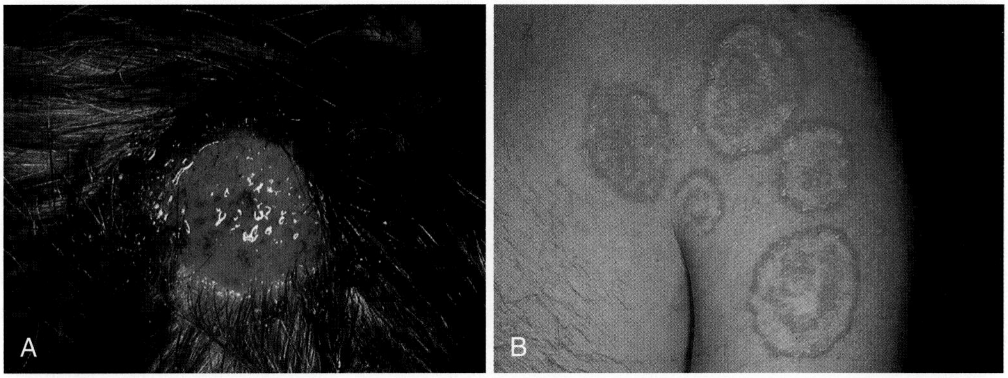

Fig. 53-5 **A:** Tinea capitis. **B:** Tinea corporis. Both infections are caused by *Microsporum canis*, the "kitten" or "puppy" fungus. *(From Habif, T.P. [2004].* Clinical dermatology: A color guide to diagnosis and therapy *[4th ed.]. St. Louis: Mosby.)*

because subjective symptoms subside, children or parents may be tempted to decrease or discontinue the medication. The nurse should emphasize to family members the importance of maintaining the prescribed dosage schedule and of taking the medication with high-fat foods for best absorption. They should also be informed of possible medication adverse effects, such as headache, gastrointestinal upset, fatigue, insomnia, and photosensitivity. For children who take the medication over many months, periodic testing is required to monitor leukopenia and assess liver and renal function. Newer antifungal medications such as terbinafine, itraconazole, and fluconazole may be used when there are adverse reactions to griseofulvin. Currently, these medications are being studied to determine their efficacy and safety in treating tinea capitis in children.

Systemic Mycotic (Fungal) Infections

Mycotic (systemic or deep fungal) infections have the capacity to invade the viscera, as well as the skin. The most common infections are the lung diseases, which are usually acquired by inhalation of fungal spores. These fungi produce a variable spectrum of disease, and some are common in certain geographic areas. They are not transmitted from person to person but appear to reside in the soil, from which their spores are airborne. The cutaneous lesions caused by deep fungal infections are granulomatous and appear as ulcers, plaques, nodules, fungating masses, and abscesses. The course of deep fungal diseases is chronic with slow progression that favours sensitization (Table 53-6).

Skin Disorders Related to Chemical or Physical Contacts

Contact Dermatitis

Contact dermatitis is an inflammatory reaction of the skin to chemical substances, natural or synthetic, that evoke a hypersensitivity response or direct irritation. The initial reaction occurs in an exposed region, most commonly the face and neck, backs of the hands, forearms, male genitalia, and lower legs. Early in the reaction, there is usually a sharp delineation between inflamed and normal skin that ranges from a faint, transient erythema to massive bullae on an erythematous swollen base. Itching is a constant symptom.

The cause may be a primary irritant or a sensitizing agent. A *primary irritant* is one that irritates any skin. A *sensitizing agent* produces an irritation on those individuals who have met the irritant or something chemically related to it, have undergone an immunological change, and have become sensitized. Prior exposure is not necessarily a factor in the reaction. A sensitizer irritates in relatively low concentrations only persons who are allergic to it.

In infants, contact dermatitis occurs on the convex surfaces of the diaper area (see Diaper Dermatitis, p. 1664). Other agents that produce contact dermatitis include plants (poison ivy, oak, or sumac), animal irritants (wool, feathers, and furs), metal (nickel found in jewellery and the snaps on sleepers and denim), vegetable irritants (oleoresins, oils, and turpentine), synthetic fabrics (e.g., shoe components), dyes, cosmetics, perfumes, and soaps (including bubble baths). The major goal in treatment is to prevent further exposure of the skin to the offending substance. Provided there is no further irritation, the skin's normal recuperative powers will often produce healing without treatment. Otherwise, treatment of contact dermatitis is based on severity. Mild cases are treated with topical steroids. Mild to moderately severe cases may require a 2-week course of strong topical corticosteroids. Very severe cases require systemic corticosteroids (Kronemyer, 2003).

Nursing Care Management

Nurses frequently detect evidence of contact dermatitis during routine physical assessments. Skin manifestations in specific areas suggest limited contact, such as around the eyes (mascara), areas of the body covered by clothing but not protected by undergarments (wool), or areas of the body not covered by clothing (UV injury). Generalized involvement is more likely to be caused by bubble bath or soap. Often nurses can determine the offending agent and counsel families regarding management. However, if the lesions persist, are extensive, or show evidence of infection, medical evaluation is indicated.

evolve Case Study—Poison Ivy

Poison Ivy, Oak, and Sumac

Contact with the dry or succulent portions of any of three poisonous plants (ivy, oak, and sumac) produces localized,

Table 53-6 Systemic Mycoses

DISORDER AND ORGANISM	SKIN MANIFESTATIONS	SYSTEMIC MANIFESTATIONS	MANAGEMENT	COMMENTS
North American blastomycosis—*Blastomyces dermatitidis*	Chronic granulomatous lesions and microabscesses in any part of body Initial lesion a papule; undergoes ulceration and peripheral spread	Pulmonary symptoms, such as cough, chest pain, weakness, and weight loss May have skeletal involvement, with bone destruction and formation of cutaneous abscesses	Intravenous (IV) administration of amphotericin B	Usual portal of entry is lungs Source of infection unknown Noninfectious Pulmonary infections may be mild and self-limited and require no treatment Progressive disease often fatal
Cryptococcosis—*Cryptococcus neoformans (Torula histolytica)*	Usually on face; acneiform, firm, nodular, painless eruption	*Central nervous system (CNS) manifestations*—Headache, dizziness, stiff neck, and signs of increased intracranial pressure Low-grade fever, mild cough, lung infiltration	IV amphotericin B; may be administered intrathecally for CNS involvement 5-Fluorocytosine for meningitis Excision and drainage of local lesions	Acquired by inhalation of dust but may enter through skin Prognosis serious Noninfectious Increased incidence in persons receiving corticosteroids with lymphoreticular malignancies, or type 2 diabetes
Histoplasmosis—*Histoplasma capsulatum*	Not distinctive or uniform, but most appear as punched-out or granulomatous ulcers	General systemic symptoms may include pallor, diarrhea, vomiting, irregular spiking temperature, hepatosplenomegaly, and pulmonary symptoms Any tissue of body may be involved with related symptoms	IV amphotericin B for severe cases Oral ketoconazole	Organism cultured from soil, especially where contaminated with fowl droppings Fungus enters through skin or mucous membranes of mouth and respiratory tract Endemic in St. Lawrence Valley region where 20 to 30% of the population test positive on a yearly basis Disseminated diseases most common in infants and children

streaked or spotty, oozing, and painful impetiginous lesions. The offending substance in these plants is an oil, *urushiol*, that is extremely potent. Sensitivity to urushiol is not inborn but is developed after one or two exposures and may change over a lifetime. All parts of the plants contain the oil, including dried leaves and stems. Even smoke from burning brush piles can produce a reaction.

Animals do not seem to be affected by the oil; however, dogs or other animals that have run or played in the plants may carry the sap on their fur, and animals that eat the plants can transfer the oil in their saliva. Shoes, tools, and toys can transfer the oil. Golf balls that have been in the rough are another source of contact.

Urushiol takes effect as soon as it touches the skin. It penetrates through the epidermis and bonds with the dermal layer, where it initiates an immune response. The full-blown reaction is evident after about 2 days, with redness, swelling, and itching at the site of contact. Several days later, streaked or spotty blisters oozing serum from damaged cells produce the characteristic impetiginous lesions (Fig. 53-6). The lesions dry and heal spontaneously, and itching stops by 10 to 14 days.

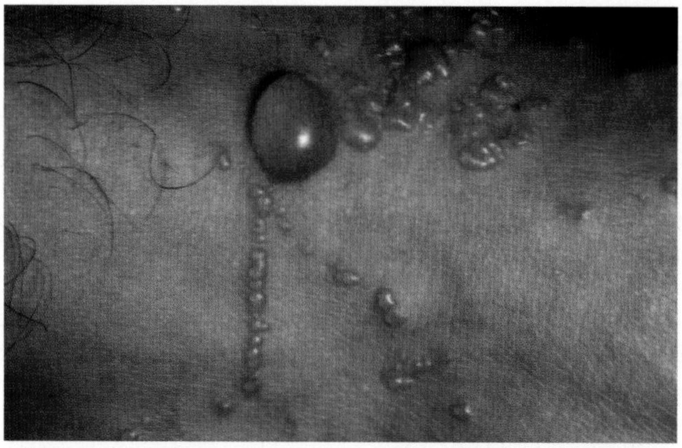

Fig. 53-6 Poison ivy lesions. Note "streaked" blisters surrounding one large blister. *(From Habif, T.P. [2004].* Clinical dermatology: A color guide to diagnosis and therapy *[4th ed.]. St Louis: Mosby.)*

Therapeutic Management

As soon as an exposure is realized, there is no time to waste. The earlier the skin is cleansed, the greater the chance of removing the urushiol before it attaches to the skin. The exposed skin can be cleansed with isopropyl alcohol or vinegar followed by water. A shower with soap and warm water should follow. Clothes, tools, shoes, and any other objects that had contact with the plants should be cleaned with alcohol and then water.

Treatment of the lesions includes calamine lotion, soothing Burow's solution compresses, or Aveeno baths to relieve discomfort. Topical corticosteroid gel is effective for prevention or relief of inflammation, especially when applied before blisters form. Oral corticosteroids may be needed for severe reactions, and a sedative such as diphenhydramine may be ordered.

Nursing Care Management

When it is known that the child has made contact with the plant, the area should be immediately flushed (preferably within 15 minutes) with *cold* running water to neutralize the urushiol not yet bonded to the skin. If there is a stream nearby, an effective method is to have the child enter the water (clothes and all) and allow the water to rinse the oil from both skin and clothing. Harsh soap is contraindicated because it removes protective skin oils and dilutes the urushiol, allowing it to spread; hard scrubbing irritates the skin. All clothing that has come in contact with the plant should be removed with care and thoroughly laundered in hot water and detergent. Every effort needs to be made to prevent the child from scratching the lesions. Although the lesions do not spread by contact with the blister serum or from scratching, they can become secondarily infected.

Prevention

Prevention is best accomplished by avoiding contact and removing the plant from the environment. All children, especially those known to be sensitive, should be taught to recognize the plant. Health Canada (2010) has information on how to eliminate the plants safely. It is important not to burn the plants because the smoke fumes can cause a severe lung reaction in sensitive individuals. The oil on dead plants can cause a reaction for up to 5 years. If poisonous plants are growing in public or community areas, the local authorities should be contacted to remove the plants.

Medication Reactions

Adverse reactions to medications are seen more often in the skin than in any other organ, although any organ of the body can be affected. The reaction may be a result of toxicity related to drug concentration, individual intolerance to the average dosage of the medication, or an allergic or idiosyncratic response. The manifestations may be associated with adverse effects or secondary effects of a medication, either of which are unrelated to its primary pharmacological actions.

Although any medication is capable of producing a reaction in the susceptible individual, some medications have a tendency to produce a particular reaction consistently, and others are more likely to produce an untoward effect. Many are allergenic responses that occur after a previous administration of the medication, even a topical application. Other factors influence a drug response in a particular individual. For example, the incidence increases with the amount and number of medications given.

NURSING ALERT Intravenous (IV) medications are more likely to cause a reaction than oral medications. Stop the medication, but maintain the infusion with normal saline.

Manifestations of medication reactions may be delayed or immediate. A period of 7 days is usually required for a child to develop sensitivity to a medication that has never been administered previously. With prior sensitivity the manifestations appear almost immediately. Rashes are the most common manifestation of adverse medication reactions in children. However, individual medication reactions may vary from a single lesion to extensive, generalized epidermal necrosis such as that seen in Stevens-Johnson syndrome. Cutaneous manifestations can resemble almost any skin disease and can appear in almost any degree of severity. With few exceptions, the distribution of a drug eruption is widespread because it results from a circulating agent; appears as an inflammatory response with itching; is sudden in onset; and may be associated with constitutional symptoms such as fever, malaise, gastrointestinal upsets, anemia, or liver and kidney damage.

In most cases treatment for simple cutaneous reactions consists of discontinuing the medication. Sometimes a decision is made to continue the medication (such as an antibiotic in an infant or small child) until the cause of the rash is clearly indicated. In urticarial-type eruptions antihistamines may be ordered, and for widespread and severe lesions corticosteroids are beneficial. Severe anaphylactic reactions are a medical emergency (see Anaphylaxis, Chapter 48).

Nursing Care Management

The most effective means of management is prevention. Parents always remember a severe reaction. A careful history will elicit evidence of a previous medication reaction. The history should include the drug's name, nature of the reaction, dosage, and how soon after administration the reaction occurred (see Chapter 34).

Nurses who suspect that a rash is caused by a medication should withhold any further dose and report the eruption to the practitioner. Frequent offenders in medication reactions are penicillin and sulphonamides, and nurses must be alert to this possibility. However, even commonplace medications, including aspirin, barbiturates, chemical agents in some foods, flavouring agents, and preservatives, are capable of producing an undesired response. Persons who have severe reactions should wear a medical identification bracelet or necklace in case of emergency or inadvertent administration of the offending medication.

Skin Disorders Related To Animal Contacts

Arthropod Bites and Stings

Bites and stings account for a significant amount of mild to moderate discomfort in children. Most bites and stings are managed by simple symptomatic measures, such as compresses, calamine lotion, and prevention of secondary infection. *Arthropods* include insects and arachnids, such as mites, ticks, spiders, and scorpions. Most arthropods in Canada, including tarantulas, are relatively harmless. Although all spiders produce venom that is injected via fangs, some are unable to pierce the skin and others produce venom that is insufficiently toxic to be harmful. Only scorpions and two spiders—the brown recluse and the black widow—inject venom deadly enough to require immediate attention.

Children bitten by these arachnids must receive medical attention as soon as possible. Major offending creatures, their manifestations, and management are outlined in Table 53-7.

When a hymenopteran (bees in particular) stings, its barbed stinger penetrates the skin. As long as the stinger remains in the skin, the muscles push the stinger deeper and the venom is pumped into the wound. The best approach is to remove the stinger as quickly as possible and to get away from the vicinity of other insects to prevent further injury. Children who have become sensitized to hymenopteran bites may demonstrate a severe systemic response that can be life threatening. One sting can produce generalized urticaria, respiratory difficulty (from laryngeal edema), hypotension, and death. Intramuscular administration of epinephrine provides immediate relief and must be available for emergency use.

Hypersensitive children should wear a medical identification bracelet. They should also have a kit that contains epinephrine and a hypodermic syringe. Families should be reminded to check the expiration date on the kit and to replace an outdated one. They should determine whether someone at the school should be designated to inject the epinephrine in case of an emergency.

Scabies

Scabies is an endemic infestation caused by the scabies mite, *Sarcoptes scabiei*. Lesions are created as the impregnated

Table 53-7 Skin Lesions Caused by Arthropods

MECHANISM AND CHARACTERISTIC	MANIFESTATIONS	MANAGEMENT
Insect Bites—Flies, Gnats, Mosquitoes, Fleas		
Mechanism—Foreign protein in insects' saliva introduced when skin is penetrated for a blood-sucking meal Distribution: Almost everywhere—Fleas, mosquitoes, ants Suburbs and rural areas—Bees Urban areas—Hornets, wasps, yellow jackets	Hypersensitivity reaction Papular urticaria Firm papules; may be capped by vesicles or excoriated Little or no reaction in nonsensitized person	*Treatment:* Use antipruritic medications and baths. Administer antihistamines. Prevent secondary infection. *Prevention:* Avoid contact. Remove focus, such as treating furniture, mattresses, carpets, and pets, where insects may live. Apply insect repellent when exposure is anticipated.
Hymenopterans—Bees, Wasps, Hornets, Yellow Jackets, Fire Ants		
Mechanism: Injection of venom through stinging apparatus Venom contains histamine; allergenic proteins; and often a spreading factor, hyaluronidase Severe reactions caused by hypersensitivity or multiple stings	*Local reaction*—Small red area, wheal, itching, and heat *Systemic reactions*—May be mild to severe, including generalized edema, pain, nausea and vomiting, confusion, respiratory embarrassment, and shock	*Treatment:* Carefully scrape off stinger or pull out stinger as quickly as possible. Cleanse with soap and water. Apply cool compresses. Apply common household product (e.g., lemon juice, paste made with aspirin or baking soda). Administer antihistamines. Severe reactions—Administer epinephrine, corticosteroids; treat for shock. *Prevention:* Teach child to wear shoes; to avoid wearing bright clothing, flowery prints, shiny jewellery, or perfumed grooming products (cologne, scented hairspray), which might attract the insect; and to avoid places where the insect may be contacted. Hypersensitive children should wear medical identification to indicate allergy and therapy needed; family should keep emergency medication and be taught its administration.
Ticks		
Mechanism—In process of sucking blood, head and mouth parts are buried in skin *Characteristics:* Feed on blood of mammals Significant in humans because of pathological organism carried May be vectors of various infectious diseases, such as Rocky Mountain spotted fever, Q fever, tularemia, relapsing fever, Lyme disease Must attach and feed for 1–2 hr to transmit disease Usual habitat is wooded area	Tick usually attached to skin, head embedded Produce firm, discrete, intensely pruritic nodules at site of attachment May cause urticaria or persistent localized edema	*Treatment:* Grasp tick with tweezers (forceps) as close as possible to point of attachment. Pull straight up with steady, even pressure; if bare hands, use a tissue to touch tick during removal; wash hands thoroughly with soap and water. Remove any remaining part (e.g., head) with sterile needle. Cleanse wounds with soap and disinfectant. *Prevention:* Teach children to avoid areas where prevalent. Inspect skin (especially scalp) after being in wooded areas. See discussion on p. 1661.

female burrows into the stratum corneum of the epidermis (never into living tissue) to deposit her eggs and feces. The inflammatory response and intense itching occur after the host becomes sensitized to the mite, approximately 30 to 60 days after initial contact. If the person has been previously sensitized to the mite, the response occurs within 48 hours after exposure. After this time, the areas over which the mite has traveled will begin to itch and develop the characteristic eruption (Box 53-1). Consequently, mites will not necessarily be located at all sites of eruption.

The types of lesions demonstrate great variability. Infants often develop an eczematous eruption; therefore the observer must look for discrete papules, burrows, or vesicles.

Nursing Care Management

The treatment of scabies is the application of a scabicide. Currently, permethrin 5% cream (Elimite) is the medication of choice. Alternative medications are 1% lindane cream or lotion and, 10% crotamiton, or irmectin. Lindane can be neurotoxic and is contraindicated in several age groups. Lindane should be reserved for patients who fail to respond to other therapy (Canadian Paediatric Society [CPS], 2001).

Permethrin is preferred, although its safety has not yet been established in infants less than 2 months of age. Nurses instructing families in the use of scabicides should emphasize the importance of following directions carefully. Lindane should not be used immediately after a bath or shower. Permethrin is applied to all skin surfaces from the neck down to the toes (not just areas with rash, but also areas between the fingers and toes, the umbilicus, and the cleft of the buttocks). The cream should remain on the skin for 8 to 9 hours for children under 6 years and 8 to 14 hours for older children and is then removed by bathing. Lindane should not be used for preterm infants, young infants, people with known seizure disorders, people with hypersensitivity to the product, patients with crusted scabies, or patients with extensive dermatitis. Pregnant women and younger children are often treated with milder scabies medications. Precipitated sulphur (7%) is safe to use alternatively for very young infants, and pregnant and lactating women. Alternatively, isopropyl myristate/cyclomethicone noninsecticide for children 4 years of age or older can be used.

BOX 53-1 Clinical Manifestations of Scabies

Lesion

Children—Minute greyish brown, threadlike (mite burrows), pruritic
- Black dot at end of burrow (mite)

Infants—Eczematous eruption, pruritic

Distribution

Generally in intertriginous areas—Interdigital, axillary-cubital, popliteal, inguinal

Children older than 2 years of age—Primarily hands and wrists

Children younger than 2 years—Primarily feet and ankles

All clothes, bedding, and towels used by the infested person before treatment should be washed in hot water and dried in a hot dryer. Families need to know that although this treatment will kill the mite that causes scabies, it will not eliminate the rash and the itch until the stratum corneum is replaced in approximately 2 to 3 weeks. Oral antihistamines, soothing ointments or lotions can be applied for itching. Antibiotics may be given for secondary infection (CPS, 2001).

Pediculosis Capitis

Pediculosis capitis (head lice) is an infestation of the scalp by *Pediculus humanus capitis*, a common parasite in school-age children. The adult louse lives only about 48 hours when away from a human host, and the lifespan of the average female is 1 month. The female lays her eggs at night at the junction of a hair shaft and close to the skin because the eggs need a warm environment. The *nits*, or eggs, hatch in approximately 7 to 10 days. Itching is usually the only symptom. Common areas involved are the occipital area, behind the ears, and the nape of the neck (Box 53-2).

Diagnostic Evaluation

Diagnosis is made by observation of the white eggs (nits) firmly attached to the hair shafts (Fig. 53-7). Because of their brief lifespan and mobility, adult lice are more difficult to

BOX 53-2 Clinical Manifestations of Pediculosis

Pruritus (caused by crawling insects and insect saliva on skin)
Nits observable on hair shaft (see Fig. 53-7)

Distribution

Occipital area
Behind ears
Nape of neck
Eyebrows and eyelashes (occasionally) (caused by pubic lice)

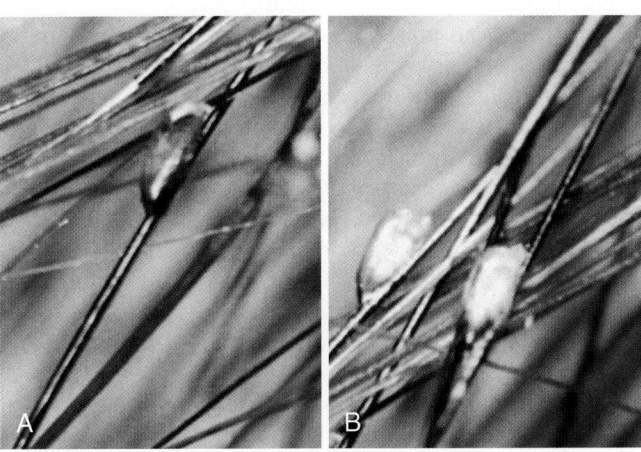

Fig. 53-7 **A:** Empty nit case. **B:** Viable nits. *(From* The contemporary approach to the control of head lice in schools and communities, Pittsburgh *(1991). SmithKline Beecham.)*

locate. Nits must be differentiated from dandruff, lint, hair spray, and other items of similar size and shape. Scratch marks or inflammatory papules, caused by secondary infection, may also be found on the scalp in the vulnerable areas.

Therapeutic Management

Treatment consists of the application of **pediculicides** and manual removal of nit cases. In order to decrease the child's exposure to the pediculicide, the scalp should be well rinsed with cool water and not sitting in the rinse water. The medication of choice for infants and children is permethrin 1% cream rinse (Nix), which kills adult lice and nits. This product and preparations of pyrethrin with piperonyl butoxide (RID or A-200 Pyrinate) can be obtained without a prescription and are more effective and safer than lindane (Strong & Johnstone, 2008). Patients should be treated with these medications when other treatments are not tolerable or have failed. A new non-insecticidal product has been approved by Health Canada for treatment of head lice which contains isopropyl myristate 50% and ST-cyclomethicone 50% for age 4 years and older (CPS, 2008).

Because of concerns that head lice may be developing resistance to chemical shampoos and that repeated exposure of children to strong chemicals on the scalp may be unwise, effective nonchemical control measures are essential. Daily removal of nits from the child's hair with a metal nit comb at least every 2 or 3 days is a control measure after treatment with a pediculicide (Mumcuoglu et al., 2007).

Nursing Care Management

An important nursing role is educating the parents about pediculosis. Nurses should emphasize that *anyone* can get pediculosis; it has no respect for age, socioeconomic level, or cleanliness. The louse does not jump or fly, but it can be transmitted from one person to another on personal items. Lice are more likely to infest White children, those with straight hair, and girls. Children need to be cautioned against sharing combs, hair ornaments, hats, caps, scarves, coats, and other items used on or near the hair. Children who share lockers are more likely to become infested, and slumber parties place children at risk. Lice are not carried or transmitted by pets.

Nurses or parents should carefully inspect children who scratch their head more than usual for bite marks, redness, and nits. The hair is systematically spread with two flat-sided sticks or tongue depressors, and the scalp is observed for any movement that indicates a louse. Nurses should wear gloves when examining the hair. Lice are small and greyish tan, have no wings, and are visible to the naked eye. The nits, or eggs, appear as tiny whitish oval specks adhering to the hair shaft about 6 mm from the scalp. The adherent nature of the nits distinguishes them from dandruff, which falls off readily. Empty nit cases, indicating hatched lice, are translucent rather than white and are located more than 6 mm from the scalp (see Fig. 53-7).

If evidence of infestation is found, it is important to treat the child according to the directions on the label of the pediculicide. Parents should read the directions carefully before beginning treatment. The child should be made as comfortable as possible during the application process because the pediculicide must remain on the scalp and hair for several minutes. Playing "beauty parlour" during the shampoo is a useful strategy. The child lies supine, with the head over a sink or basin, and covers the eyes with a dry towel or washcloth. This prevents medication, which can cause chemical conjunctivitis, from splashing into the eyes. If eye irritation occurs, the eyes must be flushed well with tepid water. It is not necessary to remove the nits after treatment because only live lice cause infestation. However, because none of the pediculicides is 100% effective in killing all the eggs, the makers of some pediculicides recommend manual removal of the nits after treatment (Centers for Disease Control, Division of Parasitic Diseases, 2005). An extra-fine-tooth comb that is included in many commercial pediculicides or is available at community pharmacies facilitates manual removal. If the comb is ineffective in removing the nit cases, the examiner should remove them by scraping them off the strands of hair with his or her fingernails.

Live lice only survive for up to 48 hours away from the host, but nits are shed into the environment and are capable of hatching in 7 to 10 days. Thus parents must take measures to prevent further infestation (see Patient Teaching box). Spraying with insecticide is not recommended because of the danger to children and animals. Families should also be advised that the pediculicide is relatively expensive, especially when several members of the household require treatment. Families may be inclined to try home remedies to treat the lice. A study by Lee and colleagues (2004) showed that home remedies such as petroleum jelly, oils, vinegar, butter, alcohol, and mayonnaise did little to kill louse eggs but increased the risk for skin infection with *S. aureus*. Another study by Pearlman (2004) showed that dry-on pediculicide lotions may effectively treat lice

PATIENT TEACHING Pediculosis Treatment

- Under a good light, check the scalp at the bottom of the neck and behind the ears for lice.
- Use pyrethrin, permethrin, or lindane insecticide to treat lice. Do not to leave the insecticide on any longer than recommended on the label. Do not use lindane on children under 2 years of age. Rinse scalp well with cool water over a sink.
- Alternatively, use isopropyl myristate/cyclomethicone noninsecticide for children 4 years of age or older
- Machine wash all clothing, towels, and bedding in hot water, and dry in a hot dryer for at least 15 minutes. Dry clean other nonwashable items.
- Vacuum all stuffed furniture, pillows, mattresses, carpets, toys, and car seats.
- Store items in airtight plastic bags for 14 days.
- Soak hair combs, brushes, and hair accessories in lice-killing insecticide for 1 hour or in boiling water for 10 minutes.
  - In day care centres, store children's clothing items in separate cubicles.

(Modified from Canadian Paediatric Society. [2008]. *When your child is sick: Head lice*. Retrieved from http://www.caringforkids.cps.ca/handouts/head_lice.).

without the use of current shampoos with neurotoxins, nit removal, or extensive housecleaning. One study (Goates et al., 2006) demonstrated that one 3-minute application of hot air has the potential to eliminate lice infestations.

Prevention

The increasing incidence of pediculosis in schoolchildren is a serious concern for school nurses, parents, and community health agencies. However, school head lice screening programs have not proven to have a significant effect on the incidence of head lice in the school setting; parent education programs may be more helpful in the management of head lice. Children with head lice should be allowed to return to school after proper treatment.

Bed Bugs

Bed bugs, or cimicidae, are small, biting insects that feed off the blood of warm-blooded animals and birds, preferring human blood. Bed bug infestations are becoming increasingly common in Canada due to the increase in travelling (Health Canada, 2011). Cimicidae invade homes by travelling on objects such as clothing, televisions, and mattresses, where they hide in along the folds and on box springs.

Clinical Manifestations

Cimicidae reproduce quickly and travel easily. The insects are 6 mm in length, with wingless, oval bodies which redden with blood intake (Fig. 53-8). The tiny eggs are whitish ovals and are clustered in crevices. They feed at night and bite all over the human body, particularly in the face, neck, and upper body. Cimicidae can survive up to 6 months without feeding. When the insect injects saliva into the skin, it creates localized red, itchy, flat or raised lesions, often linear in a group of three. Some individuals are more sensitive or allergic and react more with welts. Cimicidae do not transmit infection but an infection can develop from scratching the lesions. The bites do not require treatment and disappear quickly. It is important to not scratch and keep the skin clean in order to avoid infection. Antihistamines or creams can help relieve the itchiness and antibiotics can be prescribed if there is secondary infection present (Toronto Public Health Department, 2008).

Cimicidae are very difficult to get rid of (see Patient Teaching box). Various chemicals or nonchemicals are usually needed to eliminate these insects. Available products will usually contain the active ingredients pyrethrin or other pyrethroids or diatomaceous earth. Caution must be used that outdoor products are not used indoors (Health Canada, 2011).

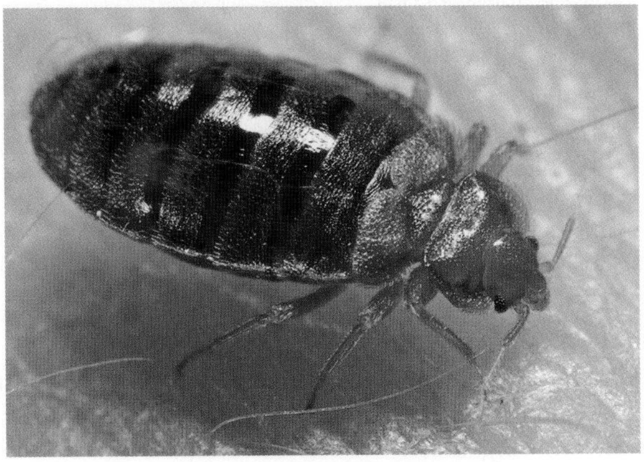

Fig. 53-8 A bed bug biting a human.

Rickettsial Diseases

Rickettsiae, the organisms responsible for a number of disorders (Table 53-8), are transmitted to human beings via arthropods. Mammals become infected only through the bites of infected lice, fleas, ticks, and mites, all of which serve as both infectors and reservoirs. Rickettsiae are intracellular parasites, similar in size to bacteria that inhabit the alimentary tract of a wide range of natural hosts. Rickettsial diseases are more common in temperate and tropical climates where humans live in association with arthropods. Infection in humans is incidental (except epidemic typhus) and not necessary for the survival of the rickettsial species. However, after the organism invades a human, it causes a disease that varies in intensity from a benign, self-limited illness to a disease that is fulminating and fatal.

Lyme Disease

Lyme disease is a tick-borne disease in Canada which is on the increase in incidence although it is still relatively rare (CPS, 2009). It is caused by the spirochete *Borrelia burgdorferi*, which enters the skin and bloodstream through the saliva and feces of ticks, especially the deer tick. Most cases of Lyme disease are reported in parts of southern and southeastern Québec, southern and eastern Ontario, southeastern Manitoba, New Brunswick and Nova Scotia as well as most of southern British Columbia (Public Health Agency of Canada [PHAC], 2010a).

PATIENT TEACHING How to Eliminate Cimicidae in the Home

- Check with the local health department or a pesticide control company to confirm Cimicidae presence.
- Inspect mattress, frame, and underside of beds.
- Vacuum with nozzle daily in your house along any crevices such as baseboards and other crevices and immediately dispose of vacuum contents.
- Wash linens in hottest water possible and cover pillows and mattresses with plastic.
- Remove all unnecessary clutter.
- Seal cracks and crevices.
- Monitor daily, using double-sided carpet sticky tape to catch Cimicidae.
- Inspect any objects coming into the house.
- When travelling, keep luggage off the floor and wrap in plastic. Pull the bed away from the wall, tuck in linen, and keep blankets off the floor.
- Consult professional pesticide services and choose the least risky option to humans and the environment.

(Modified from Toronto Public Health. [2008]. *Bed bugs fact sheet*. Retrieved from http://www.toronto.ca/health/pdf/bedbugs_factsheet.pdf.)

Table 53-8 Eruptions Caused by Rickettsiae

DISORDER, ORGANISM, AND HOST	MANIFESTATIONS	MANAGEMENT	COMMENTS
Rocky Mountain spotted fever—*Rickettsia rickettsii* *Arthropod*—Tick *Transmission*—Tick *Mammal source*—Wild rodents, dogs	*Gradual onset*—Fever, malaise, anorexia, myalgia *Abrupt onset*—Rapid temperature elevation, chills, vomiting, myalgia, severe headache Maculopapular or petechial rash primarily on extremities (ankles and wrists) but may spread to other areas, characteristically on palms and soles	*Control*—Protection from tick bite by wearing proper apparel, tick repellent Tetracycline or chloramphenicol Vigorous supportive therapy	Usually self-limited in children Onset in children may resemble any infectious disease Severe disease rare in children Disease has been reported in Canada, particularly in the southwest, but the overall incidence is unknown Inspect children and dogs regularly if they play in wooded areas See Table 53-7 for management of ticks
Epidemic typhus—*Rickettsia prowazekii* *Arthropod*—Body louse *Transmission*—Infected feces into broken skin *Mammal source*—Humans	Abrupt onset of chills, fever, diffuse myalgia, headache, malaise Maculopapular rash becoming petechial 4-7 days later, spreading from trunk outward	*Control*—Immediate destruction of vectors Tetracycline or chloramphenicol Supportive treatment	Patient should be isolated until deloused See discussion on p. 1659 for management of pediculosis Excreta from infected lice also in dust; disinfect patient's clothing, bedding, and possessions and wash in hot water
Endemic typhus—*Rickettsia typhi* *Arthropod*—Rat fleas or lice *Transmission*—Flea bite; inhaling or ingesting flea excreta *Mammal source*—Rats	Headache, arthralgia, backache followed by fever; may last 9–14 days Maculopapular rash after 1–8 days of fever; begins in trunk and spreads to periphery; rarely involves face, palms, soles	*Control*—Eliminate rat reservoir, insect vectors, or both Tetracycline or chloramphenicol Supportive treatment	Rare in Canada and found mainly in warm climates Shorter duration than epidemic typhus Mild, seldom fatal illness Difficult to distinguish from epidemic typhus
Rickettsialpox—*Rickettsia akari* West Nile Fever *Arthropod*—Mosquitoes *Transmission*—Mosquito bite *Mammal source*—Birds	Maculopapular rash following primary lesion; eschar at site of bite; most don't have symptoms and don't get sick. If illness is present, symptoms appear in 2 to 15 days; fever, headache, and body aches, mild rash, or swollen lymph nodes. If illness is present in person with lower immunity, risk of meningitis and encephalitis	*Control*—Eradication of rodent reservoir and mosquitoes Tetracycline or chloramphenicol Supportive treatment	Self-limited nonfatal disease Found In British Columbia, Manitoba, and Ontario. In 2010, only 3 cases in Canada (Public Health Agency, 2010b)

The disease may initially appear in any of three stages:

1. *Stage 1* consists of the tick bite at the time of inoculation, followed in 3 to 31 days by the development of *erythema migrans* at the site of the bite (Fig. 53-9).
2. *Stage 2*, the most serious stage of the disease, is characterized by systemic involvement of neurological, cardiac, and musculoskeletal systems that appears several weeks after the cutaneous phase is completed.
3. *Stage 3*, or the late stage, includes musculoskeletal pain that involves the tendons, bursae, muscles, and synovia. Arthritis may occur, and late neurological problems include deafness and chronic encephalopathy.

Diagnostic Evaluation

Diagnosis is best made clinically during the early stages by recognizing the characteristic rash, erythema migrans. Serological testing may be used to establish the diagnosis in later stages of the disease.

Therapeutic Management

Early and appropriate treatment is essential to prevent complications. Children older than 8 years of age are treated with oral doxycycline; amoxicillin is recommended for children younger than 8 years of age. The Canadian Paediatric Society recommends following the American Infectious Diseases Society of America's treatment for Lyme disease (Wormser et al., 2006). For patients allergic to penicillin, alternative medications

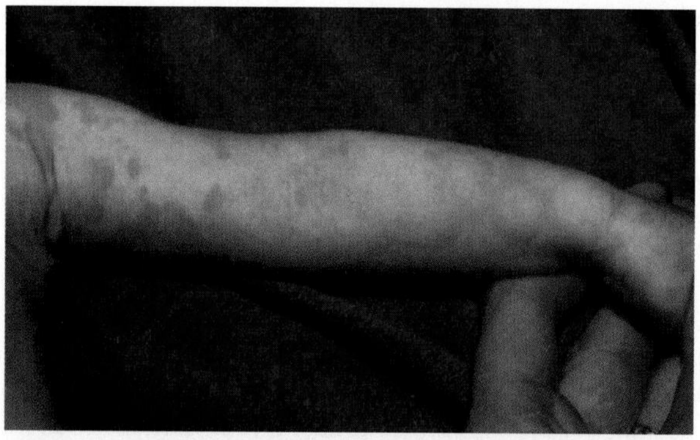

Fig. 53-9 Lyme disease. Note annular red rings in erythema chronicum migrans. *(From Weston, W.L., & Lane, A.T. [2007]. Color textbook of pediatric dermatology [4th ed.]. St Louis: Mosby.)*

include cefuroxime or erythromycin (Wade, 2000). Most experts treat individuals with early Lyme disease for 14 to 21 days. Persons who have removed ticks from themselves should be monitored closely for signs and symptoms of tick-borne diseases for 30 days; in particular they should be monitored for erythema migrans, a red expanding skin lesion at the site of the tick bite that may suggest Lyme disease. People who develop a skin lesion or viral infection–like illness within 1 month of an attached tick should seek prompt medical attention (Wormser et al., 2006). Treatment of erythema migrans most often prevents development of later stages of Lyme disease.

Nursing Care Management

The major thrust of nursing care should be educating parents to protect their children from exposure to ticks. Children should avoid tick-infested areas or wear light-coloured clothing so that ticks can be spotted easily, tuck pant legs into socks, and wear a long-sleeved shirt tucked into pants when in wooded areas. Parents and children need to perform regular tick checks when they are in infested areas (with special attention to the scalp, neck, armpits, and groin areas). Parents should also be alert for signs of the skin lesion, especially if their children have been in tick-infested areas.

Insect repellents containing diethyltoluamide (DEET) and permethrin can protect against ticks, but parents should use these chemicals cautiously. DEET must not be used in children under 6 months. As well, products with citronella or lavender oil should not be used on infants (Safe Kids Canada, 2006). All insecticides should be approved in Canada. Although there have been reports of serious neurological complications in children resulting from frequent and excessive application of DEET repellants, the risk is low when they are used properly. Products with DEET should be applied sparingly according to label instructions and not applied to a child's face or hands or to any areas of irritated skin.

After the child returns indoors, treated skin should be washed with soap and water. If a tick is found, it should be removed carefully with tweezers by gripping the head and mouth parts as closely to the skin as possible and pulling straight out. The tick should be kept in case the child develops Lyme symptoms so the tick can be identified. The area should be washed with soap and disinfected with alcohol or other disinfectant (PHAC, 2010a).

Mammal Bites and Scratches

Pet and Wild Animal Bites

Animal bites are common in childhood. However, children are bitten more often by animals belonging to the family or to neighbours than by stray animals. Most victims of dog bites are boys between the ages of 5 and 9 years (Bernardo et al., 2000; Centers for Disease Control and Prevention, 2003). Most dog or cat injuries are to the upper extremities. Small children are likely to be bitten or scratched on the head, face, and neck because they tend to put their heads near the animal's head and flail their arms rather than protecting their heads. Animal bites are potentially serious because of the likelihood of significant infection. Injuries vary in intensity from small puncture wounds to complete evulsion of tissue that is associated with significant crush injury.

Therapeutic Management

General wound care consists of rinsing the wound with copious amounts of saline or Ringer's lactate under pressure via a large syringe and of washing the surrounding skin with mild soap. A clean pressure dressing is applied, and the extremity is elevated if the wound is bleeding. Medical evaluation is advised because of the danger of tetanus and rabies, although dogs in most urban areas must be immunized against rabies. Bites from wild animals, such as squirrels, bats, raccoons, foxes, and skunks, are also dangerous.

Prophylactic antibiotics are indicated for puncture wounds and wounds in areas that may prove to be cosmetically or functionally impaired if infected. Extensive lacerations are debrided and loosely sutured to allow drainage in the event of infection. Tetanus toxoid is administered according to standard guidelines (see Immunizations, Chapter 36), and rabies protocol is followed (see Rabies, Chapter 51). Injuries to poorly vascularized areas, such as the hands, are more likely to become infected than those in more vascularized areas, such as the face; puncture wounds are more likely to become infected than lacerations.

Nursing Care Management

The most important aspect related to animal bites is prevention. Children should understand animal behaviour and develop respect for animals (see Patient Teaching box).

PATIENT TEACHING Animal Safety

The Humane Society of Canada (2007) offers the following top ten tips to help children avoid dog bites.

- Encourage children to be alert around dogs in their neighbourhood. It is important that children never pet a strange or unfamiliar animal.
- Teach children to never approach a dog that is tied up or confined to a small space; this may lead to fear in the dog and cause the dog to protect its space.
- Never allow children to tease a dog with food or toys; they may become aggravated and attack.
- Approach a dog by offering a closed hand and allowing the dog to smell it first before petting the dog.
- Never allow children to rub a dog along his side or grab his tail, which can cause fear and may lead them to attack.
- Spaying or neutering your dog can lessen any aggressive tendencies and make the dog happier and healthier.
- Never, under any circumstance, leave a family dog alone unsupervised with infants or small children. Children have been maimed and killed this way.
- Dog owners should be responsible and socialize their dogs, which will make them familiar with people and other pets in the neighbourhood.
- If ever confronted by a dog, try to stay calm and do not scream or run away. Try to place an object between you and the dog or throw food or a stick as a distraction to divert the dog's attention.
- It is important to remember that most dogs never bite anyone, but it is always better to be prepared.

Human Bites

Children often acquire lacerations from the teeth of other humans in rough play, during fights, or as victims of child abuse. Many preschool children bite others out of frustration or anger. Because human dental plaque and gingiva harbour pathogenic organisms, all human bites should receive attention. Delayed treatment increases the risk of infection.

If the laceration is less than 6 mm in length, the wound can be treated at home. The wound is washed vigorously with soap and water, and a pressure dressing is applied to stop bleeding. Ice applications minimize discomfort and swelling. Increased pain or redness at the wound site is an indication that the child should receive medical attention for antibiotic therapy. Tetanus toxoid is needed if the child is insufficiently immunized. Wounds larger than 6 mm should receive medical attention.

Cat-Scratch Disease

Cat-scratch disease (*Bartonella henselae*) is the most common cause of regional lymphadenitis in children and adolescents. It usually follows the scratch or bite of an animal (a cat or kitten in 99% of cases). The disease is usually a benign, self-limited illness that resolves spontaneously in about 2 to 4 months. Diagnosis is made on the basis of (1) history of contact with a cat or kitten, (2) the presence of regional lymphadenopathy for several days, and (3) serological identification of the causative organism by indirect fluorescent antibody assay or polymerase chain reaction test. The disease may persist for several months before gradual resolution. In some children, especially those who are immunocompromised, the adenitis may progress to suppuration and serious complications. Treatment is primarily supportive, but antibiotic therapy may hasten the resolution of adenopathy in the disease (PHAC, 2011).

Skin Disorders Associated With Specific Age Groups

Several common dermatological conditions are confined to children in specific age groups. These conditions include diaper, atopic, and seborrheic dermatitis, which occurs predominantly in infants, and acne, which is most common in adolescence.

Diaper Dermatitis

Diaper dermatitis is common in infants and is one of several acute inflammatory skin disorders caused either directly or indirectly by wearing diapers. The peak age of occurrence is 9 to 12 months of age, and the incidence is greater in bottle-fed infants than in breast-fed infants.

Pathophysiology and Clinical Manifestations

Diaper dermatitis is caused by prolonged and repetitive contact with an irritant (e.g., urine, feces, soaps, detergents, ointments, friction). Although the irritant in the majority of cases is urine and feces, a combination of factors contributes to irritation.

Prolonged contact of the skin with diaper wetness produces higher friction, greater abrasion damage, increased transepidermal permeability, and increased microbial counts. Healthy skin is less resistant to potential irritants.

Although ammonia was once thought to cause diaper rash because of its association with the strong odour on diapers and dermatitis, ammonia alone is not sufficient. The irritant quality of urine is related to an increase in pH from the breakdown of urea in the presence of fecal urease. The increased pH promotes the activity of fecal enzymes, principally the proteases and lipases, which act as irritants. Fecal enzymes also increase the permeability of skin to bile salts, another potential irritant in feces. It is believed that the decreased incidence of diaper dermatitis in breastfed infants is related to this interaction between pH and fecal enzymes, since feces from breastfed infants have lower fecal enzyme activity and lower pH.

The eruption of diaper dermatitis is manifested primarily on convex surfaces or in folds. The lesions represent a variety of types and configurations. Eruptions involving the skin in most intimate contact with the diaper (e.g., the convex surfaces of buttocks, inner thighs, mons pubis, scrotum) but sparing the folds are likely to be caused by chemical irritants, especially from urine and feces (Fig. 53-10). Other causes are detergents or soaps from inadequately rinsed cloth diapers or the chemicals in disposable wipes. Perianal involvement is usually the result of chemical irritation from feces, especially diarrheal stools. *Candida albicans* infection produces perianal inflammation and a maculopapular rash with satellite lesions that may cross the inguinal fold (Fig. 53-11). It is seen in up to 90%

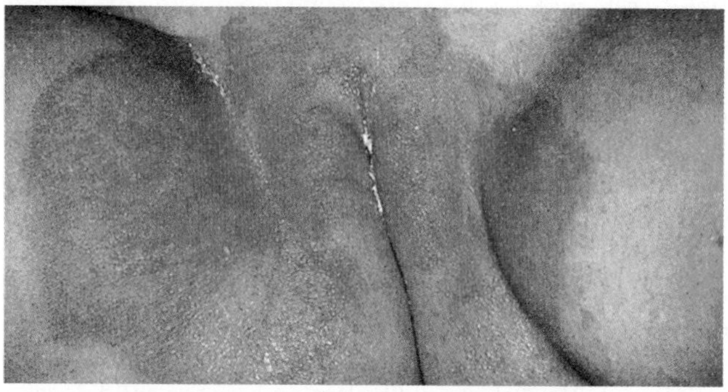

Fig. 53-10 Irritant diaper dermatitis. Note sharply demarcated edges. *(From Habif, T. P. [1996].* Clinical dermatology: A color guide to diagnosis and therapy *[3rd ed.]. St. Louis: Mosby.*

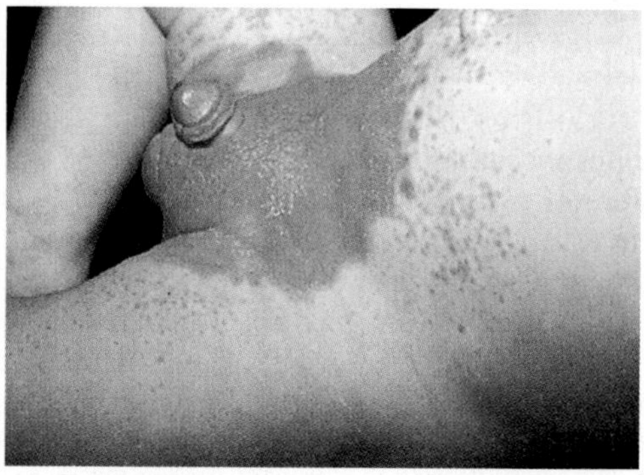

Fig. 53-11 Candidiasis of diaper area. Note beefy red central erythema with satellite pustules. *(From Weston, W.L., Lane, A.T., & Morelli, J.G. [2007].* Color textbook of pediatric dermatology *[4th ed.]. St Louis: Mosby.)*

of infants with chronic diaper dermatitis and should be considered in diaper rashes that are recalcitrant to treatment.

Nursing Care Management

Nursing interventions are aimed at altering the three factors that produce dermatitis: wetness (hydration), pH, and fecal irritants. The most significant factor amenable to intervention is the moist environment created in the diaper area. Changing the diaper as soon as it becomes wet eliminates a large part of the problem, and removing the diaper to expose healthy skin to air facilitates drying. The use of a hair dryer or heat lamp is not recommended because these devices can cause burns.

Guidelines for controlling diaper rash are presented in the Patient Teaching box. A common misconception about using cornstarch on skin is that it promotes the growth of *C. albicans*. Neither cornstarch nor talc promotes the growth of fungi under conditions normally found in the diaper area; however, the use of powders in the hospital is not recommended (Association of Women's Health, Obstetric and Neonatal Nurses, 2007).

Atopic Dermatitis (Eczema)

Eczema or eczematous inflammation of the skin refers to a descriptive category of dermatological diseases and not to a specific etiology. AD is a type of pruritic eczema that usually begins during infancy and is associated with allergy with a hereditary tendency (*atopy*). AD manifests in three forms based on the child's age and the distribution of lesions:

1. *Infantile (infantile eczema)*—Usually begins at 2 to 6 months of age; generally undergoes spontaneous remission by 3 years of age
2. *Childhood*—May follow the infantile form; occurs at 2 to 3 years of age; 90% of children have manifestations by age 5 years
3. *Preadolescent and adolescent*—Begins at about 12 years of age; may continue into the early adult years or indefinitely

The diagnosis of AD is based on a combination of history and morphological findings (Box 53-3). Children with AD have a lower threshold for cutaneous itching than do other children, and many authorities believe the dermatological manifestations appear subsequent to scratching from the intense pruritus. For example, infants rub their faces against bed linen, and their crawling (a form of scratching) results in irritation of knees and elbows. Lesions disappear if the scratching is stopped (Fig. 53-12).

The majority of children with infantile AD have a family history of eczema, asthma, food allergies, or allergic rhinitis, which strongly supports a genetic predisposition. The cause is unknown but appears to be related to abnormal function of the skin, including alterations in perspiration, peripheral vascular function, and heat tolerance. Manifestations of the chronic disease improve in humid climates and get worse in the fall and winter, when homes are heated and environmental humidity is lower. The disorder can be controlled but not cured.

PATIENT TEACHING Controlling Diaper Rash

Keep skin dry.*
- Use superabsorbent disposable diapers to reduce skin wetness.
- If using cloth diapers, use only overwraps that allow air to circulate; avoid rubber pants.
- Change diapers as soon as soiled—especially with stool—whenever possible, preferably once during the night.
- Expose healthy or only slightly irritated skin to air, not heat, to dry completely.

Apply ointment, such as zinc oxide or petrolatum, to protect skin, if skin is very red or has moist, open areas.
- Avoid removing skin barrier cream with each diaper change; remove waste material and reapply skin barrier cream.
- To completely remove ointment, especially zinc oxide, use mineral oil; do not wash vigorously.

Avoid overwashing the skin, especially with perfumed soaps or commercial wipes, which may be irritating.
- You may use a moisturizer or nonsoap cleanser, such as cold cream or Cetaphil, to wipe urine from skin.
- Gently wipe stool from skin using water and mild soap, such as Dove.
- When travelling, fill an old baby wipe container with soft paper towels and warm water.

*Powder helps to keep the skin dry, but talc is dangerous if breathed into the lungs. Plain cornstarch or cornstarch-based powder are safer. When using any powder product, first shake it in to your hand, and then apply to the diaper area. Store the container away from the infant's reach; keep the container closed when not in use.

Therapeutic Management

The major goals of management are to (1) hydrate the skin, (2) relieve pruritus, (3) reduce flare-ups or inflammation by avoiding triggers, and (4) prevent and control secondary infection. The general measures for managing AD focus on reducing pruritus and other aspects of the disease. Management strategies include avoiding exposure to skin irritants or allergens; avoiding overheating; avoiding skin moisture loss and improving skin hydration; and administrating medications such as antihistamines, topical immunomodulators, topical steroids, and (sometimes) mild sedatives as indicated.

Enhancing skin hydration and preventing dry, flaky skin are accomplished in a number of ways, depending on the child's skin characteristics and individual needs. A tepid bath with a mild soap (Dove or Neutrogena), no soap, or an emulsifying oil, followed immediately by application of an emollient (within 3 minutes), assists in trapping moisture and preventing its loss. Bubble baths and harsh soaps should be avoided. The bath may need to be repeated once or twice daily, depending on the child's status; excessive bathing without emollient application only dries out the skin. Some lotions are not effective, and emollients should be chosen carefully to prevent excessive skin drying. Aquaphor, Cetaphil, and Eucerin are acceptable lotions for skin hydration. A nighttime bath, followed by emollient application and dressing in soft cotton pyjamas, may help alleviate most nighttime pruritus.

BOX 53-3 Clinical Manifestations of Atopic Dermatitis

Distribution of Lesions

Infantile form—Generalized, especially cheeks, scalp, trunk, and extensor surfaces of extremities (see Fig. 53-12)

Childhood form—Flexural areas (antecubital and popliteal fossae, neck), wrists, ankles, and feet

Preadolescent and adolescent form—Face, sides of neck, hands, feet, face, and antecubital and popliteal fossae (to a lesser extent)

Appearance of Lesions

Infantile Form

Erythema
Vesicles
Papules
Weeping
Oozing
Crusting
Scaling
Often symmetrical

Childhood Form

Symmetrical involvement
Clusters of small erythematous or flesh-coloured papules or minimally scaling patches
Dry and may be hyperpigmented
Lichenification (thickened skin with accentuation of creases)
Keratosis pilaris (follicular hyperkeratosis) common

Adolescent or Adult Form

Same as childhood manifestations
Dry, thick lesions (lichenified plaques) common
Confluent papules

Other Physical Manifestations

Intense itching
Unaffected skin dry and rough
Children of African descent are likely to exhibit more papular or follicular lesions than are White children
May exhibit one or more of the following:

- Lymphadenopathy, especially near affected sites
- Increased palmar creases (many cases)
- Atopic pleats (extra line or groove of lower eyelid)
- Prone to cold hands
- Pityriasis alba (small, poorly defined areas of hypopigmentation)
- Facial pallor (especially around nose, mouth, and ears)
- Bluish discolouration beneath eyes ("allergic shiners")
- Increased susceptibility to unusual cutaneous infections (especially viral)

Sometimes colloid baths, such as the addition of 2 cups of oatmeal to a tub of warm water, provide temporary relief of itching and may help the child sleep if given before bedtime.

Cool wet compresses are soothing to the skin as well as providing antiseptic protection. Soak a soft cloth with several layers such as cheesecloth in water or Burow's solution. Leave the compress on the skin for 20 to 30 minutes. If the cloth starts to dry, add more fluid to keep it very wet. After the removal of the cloth, pat the skin dry and apply the medicated

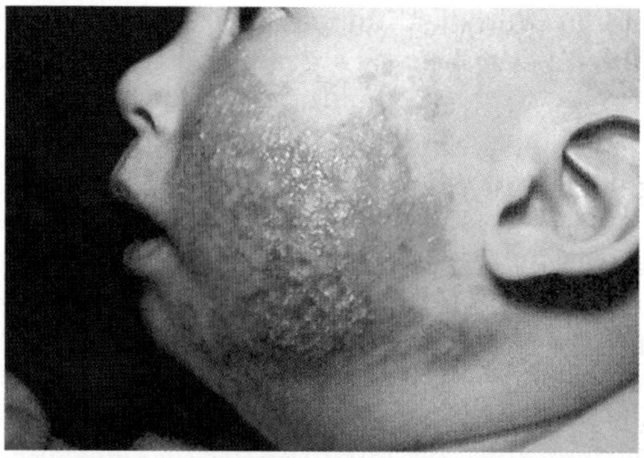

Fig. 53-12 Infantile atopic dermatitis with oozing and crusting of lesions. *(From Weston, W.L., Lane, A.T., & Morelli, J.G. [2002]. Color textbook of pediatric dermatology [4th ed.]. St Louis: Mosby.)*

treatment or emollient (Canadian Dermatology Association, 2009a).

Oral antihistamine medications such as hydroxyzine or diphenhydramine usually relieve moderate or severe pruritus. Nonsedating antihistamines such as loratadine (Claritin) or fexofenadine (Allegra) may be preferred for daytime pruritus relief. Because pruritus increases at night, a mildly sedating antihistamine may be needed.

Occasional flare-ups require the use of topical steroids to diminish inflammation. Low-, moderate-, or high-potency topical corticosteroids are prescribed, depending on the degree of involvement, the area of the body to be treated, the child's age, the potential for local adverse effects (striae, skin atrophy, and pigment changes), and the type of vehicle to be used (e.g., cream, lotion, ointment). Patients receiving topical corticosteroid therapy for chronic conditions should be evaluated for risk factors for suboptimal linear growth and reduced bone density (American Academy of Dermatology, 2003). Topical immunomodulators, a new nonsteroidal treatment for AD, are best used at the beginning of a flare-up just as the skin becomes red and itches. Two immunomodulator medications used in children with AD are tacrolimus and pimecrolimus (Kronemyer, 2003). Tacrolimus is available in two ointment strengths (0.03% and 0.1%); the 0.03% concentration has been approved for use in children 2 years of age and older. Tacrolimus is recommended for intermittent therapy in patients who are not adequately responsive to, or are intolerant of, conventional therapy (Yetman & Parks, 2002). Pimecrolimus is available in a 1% cream that has no systemic accumulation or effects. This medication is approved for use in children with mild to moderate AD. Both medications can be used freely on the face without worrying about steroid adverse effects.

If secondary skin infections occur in children with AD, these infections are managed with appropriate systemic antibiotics.

Nursing Care Management

Assessment of the child with AD includes a family history for evidence of atopy, a history of previous involvement, and any environmental or dietary factors associated with the present and previous exacerbations. The skin lesions are examined for type, distribution, and evidence of secondary infection. Parents should be interviewed regarding the child's behaviour, especially in relation to scratching, irritability, and sleeping patterns. Exploration of the family's feelings and methods of coping is also important.

The nursing care of the child with AD is challenging. Controlling the intense pruritus is imperative if the disorder is to be successfully managed, since scratching leads to new lesions and may cause secondary infection. In addition to the medical regimen, other measures can be taken to prevent or minimize the scratching. Fingernails and toenails need to be cut short, kept clean, and filed frequently to prevent sharp edges. Gloves or cotton stockings can be placed over the hands and pinned to shirtsleeves. One-piece outfits with long sleeves and long pants also decrease direct contact with the skin. If gloves or socks are used, the child needs time to be free from such restrictions. An excellent time to remove gloves, socks, or other protective devices is during the bath or after the child receives sedative or antipruritic medication.

Conditions that increase itching should be eliminated when possible. Woolen clothes or blankets, rough fabrics, and furry stuffed animals should be removed from the child's environment. Because heat and humidity cause perspiration (which intensifies itching), proper dress for climatic conditions is essential. Pruritus is often precipitated by exposure to the irritant effects of certain components of common products such as soaps, detergents, fabric softeners, perfumes, and powders. Most children experience less itching when soft cotton fabrics are worn next to the skin. During cold months, synthetic fabrics (not wool) should be used for overcoats, hats, gloves, and snowsuits. Exposure to latex products, such as gloves and balloons, should also be avoided.

Clothes and sheets should be laundered in a mild detergent and rinsed thoroughly in clear water (without fabric softeners or antistatic chemicals). Putting the clothes through a second complete wash cycle without using detergent reduces the amount of residue remaining in the fabric.

Preventing infection is usually accomplished by preventing scratching. Baths need to be given as prescribed, the water kept tepid, and soaps (except as indicated) and bubble baths avoided, along with oils or powders. Skin folds and diaper areas need frequent cleansing with plain water. A room humidifier or vaporizer may benefit children with extremely dry skin. The skin lesions should be examined for signs of infection—usually honey-coloured crusts or pustules with surrounding erythema. Any signs of infection need to be reported to the practitioner.

NURSING ALERT If the child is being treated with baths for hydration, it is imperative that the emollient preparation be applied immediately after bathing (while the skin is still slightly moist) to prevent drying.

Wet soaks and compresses can be applied and medications for pruritus or infection are administered as directed. The family should be given explicit instructions on the preparation and use of soaks, special baths, and topical medications, including the order of application if more than one is prescribed. It is important to emphasize that one thick application of topical medication is *not* equivalent to several thin applications, and that excessive use of a medication (particularly steroids) can be hazardous. If children have difficulty remaining still for a 10- or 15-minute soak, bath, or dressing application, these can be carried out at naptime or when the child is engrossed in watching television, listening to a story, or playing with tub toys.

Diet modification is another source of frustration to parents. When a hypoallergenic diet is prescribed, parents need help to understand the reason for the diet and the guidelines for avoiding hyperallergenic foods (see p. 1386). Because hypoallergenic diets take time before effects are apparent, parents need reassurance that results may not be seen immediately. If airborne allergens make eczema worse, the family should be counselled about "allergy proofing" the home (see Asthma, Chapter 46).

Family Support

Parents need to be assured that the lesions will not produce scarring (unless secondarily infected) and that the disease is not contagious. However, the child may have repeated exacerbations and remissions. Spontaneous and permanent remission takes place at approximately 2 to 3 years of age in most children with the infantile disorder.

During acute phases, emotional stress can become intense for the family. They need time to discuss negative feelings and to be reassured that these feelings are normal. Stress tends to aggravate the severity of the condition. Thus efforts to relieve anxiety in both the parents and the child have a beneficial emotional and physical effect.

Seborrheic Dermatitis

Seborrheic dermatitis is a chronic, recurrent, inflammatory reaction of the skin. It occurs most commonly on the scalp (cradle cap) but may involve the eyelids (blepharitis), external ear canal (otitis externa), nasolabial folds, and inguinal region. The cause is unknown, although it is more common in early infancy, when sebum production is increased. The lesions are characteristically thick, adherent, yellowish, scaly, oily patches that may or may not be mildly pruritic. Unlike AD, seborrheic dermatitis is not associated with a positive family history for allergy and is common in infants shortly after birth and in adolescents after puberty. Diagnosis is made primarily on the basis of the appearance and the location of the crusts or scales.

Nursing Care Management

Cradle cap may be prevented with adequate scalp hygiene. Not infrequently, parents omit shampooing the infant's hair for fear of damaging the "soft spots," or fontanels. The nurse should discuss how to shampoo the infant's hair and emphasize that the fontanel is like skin anywhere else on the body—it does not puncture or tear with mild pressure.

When seborrheic lesions are present, the treatment is directed at removing the crusts. Parents should be taught the appropriate procedure to clean the scalp. Education may need to include a demonstration. Shampooing should be done daily with a mild soap or commercial baby shampoo; medicated shampoos are not necessary, but an antiseborrheic shampoo containing sulphur and salicylic acid may be used. Shampoo is applied to the scalp and allowed to remain on the scalp until the crusts soften. Then the scalp is thoroughly rinsed. A fine-tooth comb or a soft facial brush helps remove the loosened crusts from the strands of hair after shampooing.

evolve Case Study—Acne Vulgaris

Acne

Acne vulgaris is the most common skin problem treated by physicians during patients' adolescence. Acne is not caused by dirt but by testosterone, a hormone present in males and females that increases during puberty. It stimulates the sebaceous glands of the skin to enlarge and increase in number or produce oil, and plug the pores. Whiteheads, blackheads, and pimples are present in teenage acne. Some research studies have indicated that the earlier the acne is present the worse the acne will be (Canadian Dermatology Association, 2009b.)

One half of the adolescent population experiences acne by the end of the teenage years. Although the disorder can appear before the age of 10 years, the peak incidence occurs in middle to late adolescence (at age 16 to 17 years in girls and 17 to 18 years in boys). It is more common in boys than in girls. The degree to which an individual is affected may range from nothing more than a few isolated comedones to a severe inflammatory reaction. Although the disease is self-limited and not life threatening, it has great significance to the adolescent. Health care providers should not underestimate the impact that acne has on teens.

Numerous factors affect the development and course of acne. Its distribution in families and a high degree of concordance in identical twins suggest hereditary factors. Premenstrual flares of acne occur in nearly 70% of adolescent girls, suggesting a hormonal cause. Studies do not indicate a clear association between stress and acne, but adolescents commonly cite stress as a cause for acne outbreaks. Cosmetics containing lanolin, petrolatum, vegetable oils, lauryl alcohol, butyl stearate, and oleic acid can increase comedone production. Exposure to oils in cooking grease can be a precursor in adolescents who work over fast-food restaurant hot oils. There is no known link between dietary intake and the development or worsening of acne.

Pathophysiology

Acne is a disease that involves the *pilosebaceous follicles* (the hair follicle and sebaceous gland complex) of the face, neck, chest, and upper back. Three pathophysiological factors are involved in the development of acne: excessive sebum production, comedogenesis, and the overgrowth of *Propionibacterium acnes* (Olutunmbi, Paley, & English, 2008).

Comedogenesis (formation of comedones) results in a noninflammatory lesion that may be either an *open comedone* ("blackhead") or a *closed comedone* ("whitehead"). Inflammation occurs with the proliferation of *P. acnes*, which draws in neutrophils, causing inflammatory papules, pustules, nodules, and cysts.

Therapeutic Management

Successful management of acne depends on a cooperative effort between the health care provider, the adolescent, and the parents. Unlike many other dermatological conditions, acne lesions resolve slowly, and improvement may not be apparent for at least 6 weeks. Individual comedones can take several weeks to months to resolve, and papules and pustules usually resolve in about 1 week. The multifactorial causes of acne necessitate a combined approach for successful treatment. Treatment consists of general measures of care and specific treatments determined by the type of lesions involved.

General Measures

Improvement of the adolescent's overall health status is part of the general management. Adequate rest, moderate exercise, a well-balanced diet, reduction of emotional stress, and elimination of any foci of infection are all part of general health promotion.

Cleansing

Dirt or oil on the surface of the skin does not cause acne. Gentle cleansing with a mild cleanser once or twice daily is usually sufficient. Antibacterial soaps are ineffective and may be too drying when used in combination with topical acne medications. For some adolescents hygiene of the hair and scalp appears to be related to the clinical activity of the acne. Acne on the forehead may improve with brushing the hair away from the forehead and more frequent shampooing.

Medications

Treatment success depends on commitment from the adolescent. Before prescribing treatment, the practitioner should determine the adolescent's level of comfort and readiness to begin treatment.

Tretinoin (Retin-A) is the only medication that effectively interrupts the abnormal follicular keratinization that produces microcomedones, the invisible precursors of the visible comedones. Tretinoin alone is usually sufficient for management of comedonal acne (Russell, 2000). Tretinoin is available as a cream, gel, or liquid. This medication can be extremely irritating to the skin and requires careful patient education for optimal usage. The patient should be instructed to begin with a pea-sized dot of medication, which is divided into the three main areas of the face and then gently rubbed into each area. The medication should not be applied for at least 20 to 30 minutes after washing to decrease the burning sensation. The avoidance of sun and the daily use of sunscreen must be emphasized, since sun exposure can result in severe sunburn. Adolescents should be advised to apply the medication at night and to use a sunscreen with a sun protection factor (SPF) of at least 15 in the daytime.

A gel combining 0.25% tretinoin and 1.2% clindamycin phosphate is more effective in treating acne than tretinoin or clindamycin alone (Eichenfield & Wortzman, 2009)

Topical *benzoyl peroxide* is an antibacterial medication that inhibits the growth of *P. acnes* organisms. It is effective against both inflammatory and noninflammatory acne and is an effective first-line agent. This medication is available as a cream, lotion, gel, or wash. The patient should be informed that the medication may have a bleaching effect on sheets, bedclothes, and towels. The adolescent can be reassured that skin bleaching will not occur. Accommodation to the medication can be gained with a gradual increase in the strength and frequency of application.

When inflammatory lesions accompany the comedones, a *topical antibacterial medication* may be prescribed. These agents are used to prevent new lesions and to treat pre-existing acne. Clindamycin, erythromycin-metronidazole, and azelaic acid are all choices for topical antibacterial therapy. Topical antimicrobials combined with benzoyl peroxide are more effective than either product alone.

Systemic antibiotic therapy is used when moderate to severe acne does not respond to topical treatments. Oral antibiotics such as tetracycline, erythromycin, minocycline, and doxycycline are considered safe to use (American Academy of Dermatology, 2006).

Females with mild to moderate acne may respond well to topical treatment and the addition of an *oral contraceptive pill (OCP)*. OCPs reduce the endogenous androgen production and decrease the bioavailability of the woman's circulating androgens. Both of these actions result in decreased acne.

Isotretinoin, 13-cis-retinoic acid (Accutane), is a potent and effective oral medication that is reserved for severe cystic acne that has not responded to other treatments. Isotretinoin is the only agent available that affects factors involved in the development of acne. Only physicians who have taken a comprehensive course about the medication, necessary monitoring of patients, and parameters for pregnancy prevention may manage treatment with istretinoin. Adolescents with multiple, active, deep dermal or subcutaneous cystic and nodular acne lesions are treated for 20 weeks. Multiple adverse effects can occur, including dry skin and mucous membranes, nasal irritation, dry eyes, decreased night vision, photosensitivity, arthralgia, headaches, mood changes, aggressive or violent behaviours, depression, and suicidal ideation. There is some concern that isotretinoin may be associated with increased incidence of depression and suicide despite several findings to the contrary (Webster, 2009). Patients should be monitored for depression, depressive symptoms, and suicidal ideation (Jacobs, Deutsch, & Brewer, 2001). The medication should be given only at the recommended doses for no longer than the recommended duration. The most significant adverse effects of this medication are the teratogenic effects. Isotretinoin is absolutely contraindicated in pregnant women. Sexually active young women must be using an effective contraceptive method during treatment and for 1 month after treatment. Patients receiving isotretinoin should also be monitored for elevated cholesterol and triglyceride levels. Significant elevation may require discontinuation of the medication.

Nursing Care Management

Because acne is so common and its appearance may seem so mild, the health care provider may underestimate the relative importance of the disease to the adolescent. The nurse should assess the individual adolescent's level of distress, current management, and perceived success of any regimen before initiating a referral. If adolescents do not perceive the acne to be a problem, they may lack motivation to follow the treatment plan.

The nurse can provide ongoing support for the adolescent when a treatment plan is initiated. The family is also encouraged to support the adolescent in his or her efforts. Use of medications and basic skin care information should be discussed in detail with the adolescent. Written instructions should accompany the verbal discussion. Information to dispel myths regarding the use of abrasive cleansing products can prevent unnecessary costs and trauma to the skin.

Teenagers need education about the factors that aggravate and damage the skin, such as too vigorous scrubbing. In addition, picking, squeezing, and manual expression with fingernails break down the ductal walls of lesions and cause the acne to worsen. Mechanical irritation, such as vinyl helmet straps that rub areas predisposed to acne, can also cause the development of lesions.

Thermal Injury

Burns

evolve Animation—Burns in Children

Burn injuries are usually attributed to extreme heat sources but may also result from exposure to cold, chemicals, electricity, or radiation. Most burns are relatively minor and do not require definitive medical treatment. However, burns involving a large body surface area, critical body parts, or the older adult or pediatric population often benefit from treatment in specialized burn centres.

In Canada, researchers discovered over a 10-year period (1994 to 2003) that 10,229 children were admitted to Canadian hospitals for burn injuries. Out of that number, 494 children died from their injuries. Children who were aged 1 to 5 years had the highest risk of death. Scalds caused the most thermal injuries and represented 50% of all burn admissions. Boys, and children under 5 years of age had the highest risk of burn injuries. Fortunately, there was a downward trend over that time period with a significant reduction in burn injuries. The decrease is likely due to burn safety programs, and improved burn treatments and hospital admission protocols (Spinks, Wasiak, Clelan, Beben, & Macpherson, 2008). When burns are characterized by patients' age and type of injury, the following patterns become apparent: (1) hot-water scalds are most frequent in toddlers, (2) flame-related burns are more common in older children, (3) 10 to 20% of documented cases of child abuse include burn injuries (Herndon, 2007), and (4) children playing with matches or lighters account for 1 in 10 house fires. In Canada every year, on average, 1300 fires are started by children playing with lighters and matches. These fires caused 150 burn injuries and 20 deaths (Ontario Office of the Fire Marshal, 2010).

The extent of tissue destruction in burns is determined by the intensity of the heat source, the duration of contact or exposure, the conductivity of the tissue involved, and the rate at which the heat energy is dissipated by the skin. A brief exposure to high-intensity heat from a flame can produce burn injuries similar to those induced by long exposure to less intense heat in hot water.

Characteristics of Burn Injury

The physiological responses, therapy, prognosis, and disposition of the injured child are all directly related to the *amount of tissue destroyed*. Thus the severity of the burn injury is assessed on the basis of the percentage of *total body surface area (TBSA)* burned and the *depth* of the burn. Among children in the school-age group or younger age groups, a burn that is 10% of TBSA can be life threatening if not treated correctly. Other important factors in determining the seriousness of the injury are the location of the wounds, the child's age and general health, the causative agent, the presence of respiratory involvement, and any associated injury or condition.

Type of Injury

Most burns result from contact with thermal agents such as a flame, hot surfaces, or hot liquids. Electrical injuries caused by household current have the greatest incidence in young children, who insert conductive objects into electrical outlets and bite or suck on connected electrical cords (Herndon, 2007). These burns occur most commonly during the spring and summer months and are also associated with risk-taking behaviours in boys. Direct contact with high- or low-voltage current, as well as lightning strikes, is the most frequent mechanism of injury. The resistance of the tissue and the path of the electric current are responsible for the damage incurred. Electric current travels through the body following the path of least resistance, which involves the tissues, fluid, blood vessels, and nerves. A more localized burn is produced if skin resistance is high at the area of contact, and a more systemic pattern of injury is produced if skin resistance is low. Often compared with a crush injury, serious electrical trauma results from current passing through vital organs, muscle compartments, and nerve or vascular pathways. Loss of limbs, cardiac fibrillation, respiratory collapse, and burns are common occurrences after exposure to electrical energy. Criteria for admission, as derived from evidence-informed practice for electrical burn injuries, include a history of loss of consciousness, electrocardiographic (ECG) changes, 10% TBSA affected, or the need for monitoring an affected extremity. Cardiac monitoring is thus included in standard burn care when ECG changes are identified on admission (Arnoldo, Klein, & Gibran, 2006).

Chemical burns can cause extensive injury. The severity of injury is related to the chemical agent (acid, alkali, or organic compound) and the duration of contact. The mechanism of injury differs from that in other burns in that there is a chemical disruption and alteration of the physical properties of the exposed body area. Noxious agents exist in many cleaning products commonly found in the home. In addition to concern for localized damage, the potential for systemic toxicity must be addressed. Of particular concern is the exposure of the eyes to chemical agents, the ingestion of caustic substances, and inhalation of toxic gases produced from chemicals.

Extent of Injury

The extent of a burn is expressed as a percentage of the TBSA. This is most accurately estimated by using specially designed age-related charts (Fig. 53-13). It is more efficient to use a chart designed to assign body proportions to children of different ages.

Depth of Injury

A thermal injury is a three-dimensional wound that is also assessed in relation to depth of injury. Traditionally the terms *first-*, *second-*, and *third-degree* have been used to describe the depth of tissue injury. However, with the current emphasis on wound healing, these have been replaced by more descriptive terms based on the extent of destruction to the epithelializing elements of the skin (Fig. 53-14).

Superficial (first-degree) burns are usually of minor significance. With these burns, there is often a latent period followed by erythema. Tissue damage is minimal, the protective functions of the skin remain intact, and systemic effects are rare. Pain is the predominant symptom, and the burn heals in 5 to 10 days without scarring. Mild sunburn is an example of a superficial burn.

Partial-thickness (second-degree) injuries involve the epidermis and varying degrees of the dermis. These wounds are painful, moist, red, and blistered. Superficial partial-thickness burns involve the epidermis and part of the dermis. Dermal elements are intact, and the wound should heal in approximately 14 days with variable amounts of scarring (Fig. 53-15).

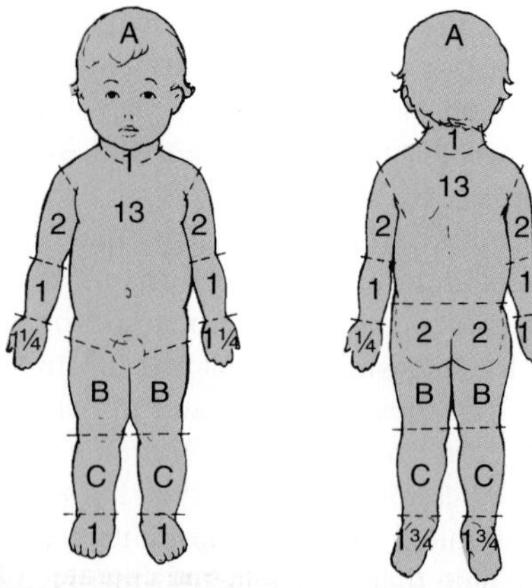

RELATIVE PERCENTAGES OF AREAS AFFECTED BY GROWTH

A

AREA	BIRTH	AGE 1 YR	AGE 5 YR
A = ½ of head	9½	8½	6½
B = ½ of one thigh	2¾	3¼	4
C = ½ of one leg	2½	2½	2¾

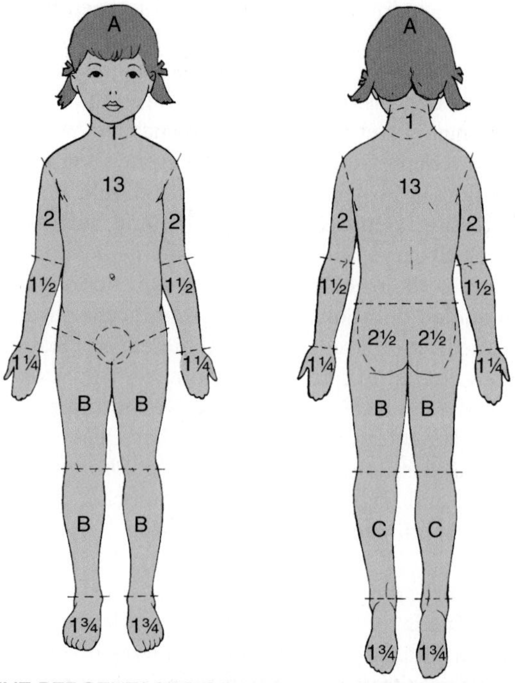

RELATIVE PERCENTAGES OF AREAS AFFECTED BY GROWTH

B

AREA	AGE 10 YR	AGE 15 YR	ADULT
A = ½ of head	5½	4½	3½
B = ½ of one thigh	4½	4½	4¾
C = ½ of one leg	3	3¼	3½

Fig. 53-13 Estimation of distribution of burns in children. **A:** Children from birth to age 5 years. **B:** Older children.

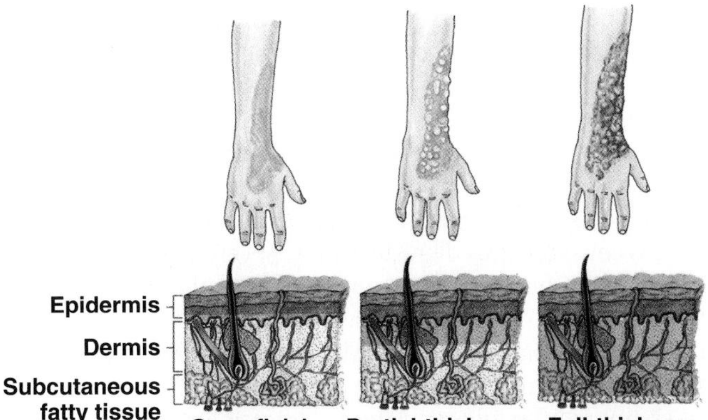

	Superficial (first degree)	Partial-thickness (second degree)	Full-thickness (third degree)
Type of burn	Sunburn; low-intensity flash; brief scald	Scalds; flash flame	Fire; contact with hot objects
Appearance	Dry surface; red; blanches on pressure and refills; minimal or no edema	Blistered; moist; serous drainage; edema; mottled pink or red, reddened; blanches on pressure and refills	Tough, leathery; marbled, pale white, brown, tan, black, or red; does not blanch on pressure; dull, dry; edema
Sensation	Painful; sensitive to touch	Very painful; sensitive to touch	Variable pain, often severe

Fig. 53-14 Classification of burn depth. *(Redrawn from Grant, H.D. & Murray, R.H. [1995]. Emergency care [7th ed.]. Upper Saddle River, NJ: Prentice-Hall.)*

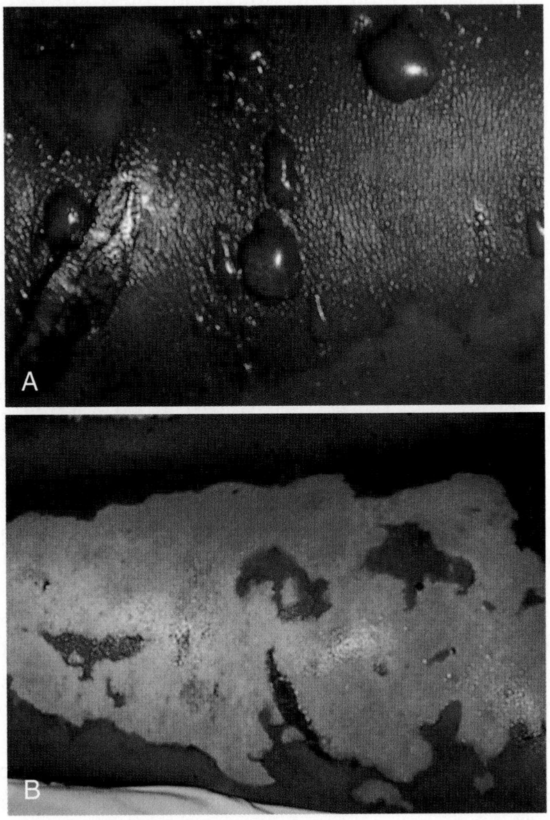

Fig. 53-15 Superficial partial-thickness burns on a Black child. **A:** Blisters intact. **B:** Blisters removed. *(Courtesy Hillcrest Medical Center, Tulsa, OK.)*

The wound is extremely sensitive to temperature changes, exposure to air, and light touch. Although classified as partial-thickness (or second-degree) burns, deep dermal burns resemble full-thickness injuries in many respects. Sweat glands and hair follicles remain intact. The burn may appear mottled, with pink, red, or waxy white areas exhibiting blisters and edema formation. Systemic effects are similar to those encountered with full-thickness burns. Although these wounds heal spontaneously in approximately 21 days, they do so with extensive scarring.

Full-thickness (third-degree) burns are serious injuries that involve the entire epidermis and dermis and extend into subcutaneous tissue (see Fig. 53-14). Nerve endings, sweat glands, and hair follicles are destroyed. The burn varies in colour from red to tan, waxy white, brown, or black and is distinguished by a dry, leathery appearance (Fig. 53-16). Normally, full-thickness burns lack sensation in the area of injury because of the destruction of nerve endings. However, most full-thickness burns have superficial and partial-thickness burned areas at the periphery of the burn, where nerve endings are intact and exposed. Excised **eschar** and donor sites also cause exposed nerve fibres. As the peripheral fibres regenerate, painful sensations return. Consequently, children often experience severe pain related to the size and depth of the burn. Full-thickness wounds are not capable of re-epithelialization and require surgical excision and grafting to close the wound.

Fourth-degree burns are full-thickness injuries that involve underlying structures such as muscle, fascia, and bone. The wound appears dull and dry, and ligaments, tendons, and bone may be exposed (Fig. 53-17).

Severity of Injury

Burns are classified as minor, moderate, or major, which is useful in determining the disposition of the patient for treatment. Burn patients are categorized as (1) those with a *major burn injury*, who require the services and facilities of a specialized burn centre; (2) those with a *moderate burn*, who may be treated in a hospital with expertise in burn care; and (3) those with *minor injuries*, who may be treated on an outpatient basis. The extent and depth of the burn, the causative agent, the body

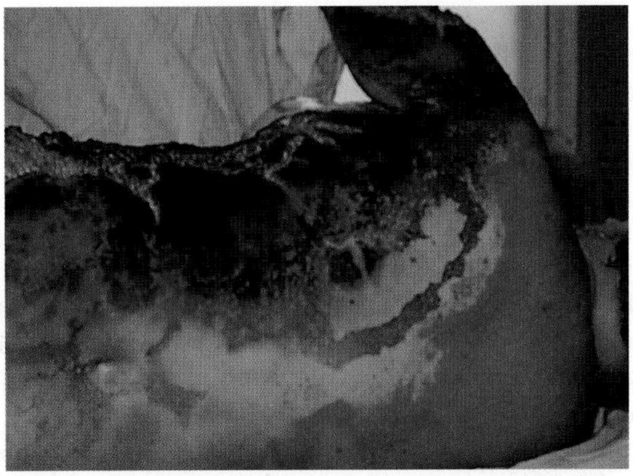

Fig. 53-16 Bottom to top: Deep partial-thickness burn (red area); full-thickness burn (white area); full-thickness burn with eschar (brown area). *(Courtesy Hillcrest Medical Center, Tulsa, OK.)*

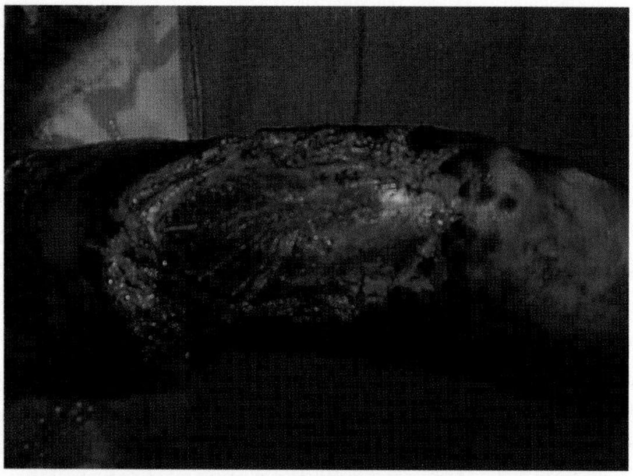

Fig. 53-17 Full-thickness burn with muscle and fascia involved. *(Courtesy Hillcrest Medical Center, Tulsa, OK.)*

evolve Case Study—Burns

area involved, the patient's age, and concomitant injuries and illnesses determine the severity of the injury.

Because the skin of infants is so thin, it is likely to sustain deeper injuries compared with that of older children. Children younger than 2 years of age, especially 6 months or younger, have a significantly higher mortality rate than that of older children with burns of similar magnitude. Acute or chronic illnesses or superimposed injuries also complicate burn care and response to treatment.

Inhalation Injury

Trauma to the tracheobronchial tree often follows inhalation of the heated gases and toxic chemicals produced during combustion. Although direct thermal injury to the upper airway may occur, heat damage below the vocal cords is rare. Inspired heated air is cooled in the upper airway before reaching the trachea. Reflex closure of the cords and laryngospasm also prevent full inhalation. However, evidence of direct thermal injury to the upper airway includes burns of the face and lips, singed nasal hairs, and laryngeal edema. Clinical manifestations may be delayed as long as 24 to 48 hours. Wheezing, increasing secretions, hoarseness, wet crackles, and carbonaceous secretions are signs of respiratory tract involvement. Upper airway obstruction is often associated with burn shock and fluid resuscitation. In such situations, endotracheal intubation may also be necessary to preserve a patent airway.

Inhalation of carbon monoxide is suspected when the injury has occurred in an enclosed space. Mucosal erythema and edema followed by sloughing of the mucosa are manifestations of respiratory tract injury. A mucopurulent membrane replaces the mucosal lining and seriously compromises respiration and ventilation.

Early in the postburn period most pulmonary infections result from nosocomial exposure, immobility, and abdominal distention. The hematogenous variety occurs later and is related to the septic burn wound or other foci, such as phlebitis at the site of an invasive IV line. A significant increase in mortality has been observed when inhalation injury and pneumonia are both present.

Deep burns, especially those circling the thorax, may cause restriction of chest excursion as a result of edema and inelastic eschar formation. Young children are particularly at risk because of the pliability of the skeletal structure. Restriction of the chest is relieved by an escharotomy incision, which allows expansion of the chest wall to facilitate ventilation.

Pathophysiology

Thermal injuries produce both local and systemic effects that are related to the extent of tissue destruction. In superficial burns the tissue damage is minimal. In partial-thickness burns there is considerable edema and more severe capillary damage. With a major burn greater than 30% TBSA, there is a systemic response involving an increase in capillary permeability, allowing plasma proteins, fluids, and electrolytes to be lost. Maximum edema formation in a small wound occurs about 8 to 12 hours after injury. After a larger injury, hypovolemia, associated with this phenomenon, will slow the rate of edema formation, with maximum effect at 18 to 24 hours.

Another systemic response is anemia, caused by direct heat destruction of red blood cells, hemolysis of injured red blood cells, and trapping of red blood cells in the microvascular thrombi of damaged cells. A long-term decrease in the number of red blood cells may occur as a result of increased red blood cell fragility. Initially there is an increased blood flow to the heart, brain, and kidneys, with decreased blood flow to the gastrointestinal tract. There is an increase in metabolism to maintain body heat, providing for the body's increased energy needs.

Complications

Thermally injured children are subject to a number of serious complications, both from the wound and from systemic alterations resulting from the injury. The immediate threat to life is related to airway compromise and profound shock. During healing, infection—both local and systemic sepsis—is the primary complication. Mortality associated with thermal trauma in children increases with the severity of injury and decreases as age advances. In children older than 3 years, the mortality rate is similar to that of adults. Below this age, the survival rate with burns and their associated complications lessens considerably.

A less apparent respiratory tract injury is inhalation of carbon monoxide. Carbon monoxide has a greater affinity for hemoglobin than does oxygen, thereby depriving peripheral tissues and oxygen-dependent organs (such as the heart and brain) of the oxygen needed for survival. Treatment for either of these two problems is 100% oxygen, which reverses the situation rapidly.

Pulmonary problems are a major cause of fatality in children with either thermal burns or complications in the respiratory tract. Respiratory problems include inhalation injuries, aspiration in unconscious patients, bacterial pneumonia, pulmonary edema, pulmonary embolus, post-traumatic pulmonary insufficiency, and atelectasis. The most common cause of respiratory failure in the pediatric age group is bacterial pneumonia, which requires prolonged intubation and sometimes a tracheostomy. Tracheostomies increase the incidence of serious complications and are performed only in extreme cases.

A less common complication is pulmonary edema resulting from fluid overload or acute respiratory distress syndrome (ARDS) in association with gram-negative sepsis. ARDS results from pulmonary capillary damage and leakage of fluid into the interstitial spaces of the lung. A loss of compliance and interference with oxygenation are the consequences of pulmonary insufficiency in conjunction with systemic sepsis.

Wound Sepsis

Sepsis is a critical problem in the treatment of burns and an ever-present threat following the shock phase. Initially, burn wounds are relatively pathogen free unless they are contaminated with potentially infectious material, such as dirt or polluted water. However, dead tissue and exudate provide a fertile field for bacterial growth. On approximately the third postburn day, early colonization of the wound surface by a preponderance of gram-positive organisms (primarily staphylococci) changes to predominantly gram-negative opportunistic organisms, particularly *Pseudomonas aeruginosa*. By the fifth postburn day, bacterial invasion is well under way beneath the surface of the burn wound. Early surgical excision of eschar together with placement of autografts reduces the incidence of sepsis.

Therapeutic Management

Emergency Care

The initial management of the burn patient begins at the scene of injury. The first priority is to stop the burning process (see Emergency box). The child should then be transported immediately to the nearest medical facility for treatment and evaluation. The child and the family are usually extremely frightened and anxious; sensitivity to their emotional state and reassurance should be provided during the transport process.

> **EMERGENCY**
>
> **Burns**
>
> **Minor Burns**
>
> Stop the burning process:
> - Apply cool water to the burn or hold the burned area under cool running water.
> - Do not use ice.
>
> Do not disturb any blisters that form, unless the injury is from a chemical substance.
> Do not apply anything to the wound.
> Cover with a clean cloth if risk of damage or contamination.
> Remove burned clothing and jewellery.
>
> **Major Burns**
>
> Stop the burning process:
> - Flame burns—smother the fire.
> - Place victim in the horizontal position.
> - Roll victim in a blanket or similar object; avoid covering the head.
>
> Assess for an adequate airway and breathing.
> If child is not breathing, begin mouth-to-mouth resuscitation.
> Remove burned clothing and jewellery.
> Cover wound with a clean cloth.
> Keep victim warm.
> Transport to medical aid.
> Begin intravenous and oxygen therapy as prescribed.

Stop the Burning Process. The chief aim of rescue in flame burns is to smother the fire, not fan it. Children tend to panic and run, which spreads the flames and makes assistance more difficult. The injured child should be placed in a horizontal position and rolled in a blanket, rug, or similar article, with care taken not to cover the head and face because of the danger of inhalation of toxic fumes. If nothing is available, the victim should lie down and roll over slowly to extinguish the flames. Remaining in the vertical position may cause the hair to ignite or the inhalation of flames, heat, or smoke.

Major burns with large amounts of denuded skin should not be cooled. Heat is rapidly lost from burned areas, and additional cooling leads to a drop in core body temperature and potential circulatory collapse. Wet dressings also promote vasoconstriction because of cooling, resulting in impaired circulation to the burned area and increased tissue damage. Chemical burns require continuous flushing with large amounts of water before transport to a medical facility. The use of neutralizing agents on the skin is contraindicated, since a chemical reaction is initiated and further injury may result. If the chemical is in powder form, the addition of water may spread the caustic agent. The powder should be brushed off if possible.

Burned clothing is removed to prevent further damage from smouldering fabric and hot beads of melted synthetic materials. Jewellery is removed to eliminate the transfer of heat from the metal and constriction resulting from edema formation. This also provides access to the wound and prevents painful removal later.

Assess the Victim's Condition. As soon as the flames are extinguished, the child is assessed. Circulation, airway, and breathing (CAB) are the primary concerns. Cardiopulmonary complications may result from exposure to electric current, inhalation of toxic fumes and smoke, hypovolemia, and shock. Emergency measures are instituted as appropriate.

Cover the Burn. The burn wound should be covered with a clean cloth to prevent contamination, decrease pain by eliminating air contact, and prevent hypothermia. No attempt should be made to treat the burn. Application of topical ointments, oils, or other home remedies is contraindicated.

Transport the Child to Medical Aid. The child with an extensive burn is not given anything by mouth to avoid aspiration in the presence of paralytic ileus and upper airway edema and to prevent water intoxication. The child is transported to the nearest medical facility. If this cannot be accomplished within a relatively short period, IV access should be established, if possible, with a large-bore catheter. Oxygen is administered, if available, at 100%. A report of the initial assessment and any interventions implemented is given to the medical facility assuming care of the child.

Provide Reassurance. Providing reassurance and psychological support to both the family and the child helps immeasurably during the period of postinjury crisis. Reducing anxiety conserves energy the family and child will need to cope with the physiological and emotional stress of injury.

Minor Burns

Treatment of burns classified as minor can usually be managed adequately on an outpatient basis when it is determined that the parent can be relied on to carry out instructions for care and observation. Patients with less than optimum circumstances may require close follow-up to ensure adherence with treatment.

The wound is cleansed with a mild soap and tepid water. Debridement of the wound includes removal of any embedded debris, chemicals, and devitalized tissue. Removal of intact blisters remains controversial. Some authorities argue that blisters provide a barrier against infection; others maintain that blister fluid is an effective medium for the growth of microorganisms. However, blisters should be broken if the injury is due to a chemical agent to control absorption. Most practitioners favour covering the wound with an antimicrobial ointment to reduce the risk of infection and to provide some form of pain relief. The dressing consists of nonadherent fine-mesh gauze placed over the ointment and a light wrap of gauze dressing that avoids interference with movement. This helps keep the wound clean and protect it from trauma. The caregiver is instructed to wash the wound, reapply the dressing, and return the child to the office or clinic as directed for wound observation. The frequency of dressing changes may vary from every other day to once a day.

Some practitioners prefer an occlusive dressing, such as a hydrocolloid, which is placed over the wound after cleansing. Hydrogel dressings, which are soothing and nonadherent, may also be used. The dressing is changed when leakage occurs—at regular intervals or at least weekly. This method eliminates the discomfort associated with frequent dressing changes but impairs visualization of the wound surface.

If there is a high probability of infection or other complications or if there is doubt about the ability to carry out instructions, the caregiver may be directed to bring the patient in daily for dressing changes and inspection. Another option is to have a nurse make a home visit to inspect the wound and perform the dressing change. Frequent removal of the dressing is an effective mode of debridement. Soaking the dressing in tepid water or normal saline before removal helps loosen the dressing and debris and reduce discomfort. Burns of the face are usually treated by an open method. The wound is washed and debrided in the same manner, and a thin film of antimicrobial ointment is applied.

A tetanus history is obtained on admission. If there is no history of immunization, or if more than 5 years have passed since the last immunization, tetanus prophylaxis is administered. There is no evidence that systemic antibiotic prophylaxis decreases the incidence of infection in small burn wounds (Herndon, 2007). Therefore, antibiotics should be used only when there is evidence of infection. A mild analgesic such as acetaminophen is usually sufficient to relieve discomfort; the antipyretic effect of the medication also alleviates the sensation of heat.

Most minor burns heal without difficulty, but if the wound margin becomes erythematous, gross purulence is noted, or the child develops evidence of systemic reaction, such as fever or tachycardia, hospitalization is indicated. The child should also be evaluated for functional impairment, and the caregiver should be instructed in the exercise and ambulation program. After wound healing, an evaluation of scar maturation and range of motion will indicate any need for further therapy.

Major Burns

The first priority is airway maintenance. Respiratory burns or the inhalation of noxious agents are suggested when there is a history of injury in an enclosed space; edema of the oral and nasal membranes; thermal injury to the face, nares, and upper torso; hyperemia; and blisters or evidence of trauma to the upper respiratory passages. When respiratory involvement is suspected or evident, 100% oxygen is administered and blood gas values, including carbon monoxide levels, are determined.

If the child exhibits changes in sensorium, air hunger, or other signs of respiratory distress, an endotracheal tube is inserted to maintain the airway. When severe edema of the face and neck is anticipated, intubation is performed before swelling makes intubation difficult or impossible. Controlled intubation is preferred to an emergency procedure. Intubation allows for the delivery of humidified oxygen, the removal of secretions from respiratory passages, and the provision of ventilatory support.

When full-thickness burns encircle the chest, constricting eschar may limit chest wall excursion, and ventilation of the child becomes more difficult. Escharotomy of the chest relieves this constriction and improves ventilation.

Fluid Replacement Therapy. The objectives of fluid therapy are to (1) compensate for water and sodium lost to traumatized areas and interstitial spaces, (2) re-establish sodium balance, (3) restore circulating volume, (4) provide adequate perfusion, (5) correct acidosis, and (6) improve renal function.

Fluid replacement is required during the first 24 hours because of fluid shifts that occur after the injury. Various formulas are used to calculate fluid needs, and the one adopted depends on practitioner preference. Crystalloid solutions are used during this initial phase of therapy. Parameters such as vital signs (especially heart rate), urine output, adequacy of capillary filling, and state of sensorium determine adequacy of fluid resuscitation.

After the initial 24-hour period, theoretically there is a capillary seal, and capillary permeability is restored. Colloid solutions such as albumin, Plasma-Lyte, or fresh frozen plasma are useful in maintaining plasma volume. However, children with burn injuries usually require fluids in excess of their calculated maintenance and replacement volume. Reasons for this may include underestimation of burn size (particularly in pediatric patients), pulmonary injury that sequesters resuscitation fluid in the lung, electrical injury with greater tissue destruction than that which is visible, and a delay in the initiation of fluid resuscitation. Irreversible burn shock that persists despite aggressive fluid resuscitation remains a significant cause of death in the immediate postburn period. Fluid balance may continue to be a problem throughout the course of treatment, especially when there is considerable evaporative loss from the wound.

Nutrition. The enhanced metabolic requirements and catabolism in severe burns make nutritional needs of paramount importance and often difficult to satisfy. The diet must provide sufficient calories to meet the increased metabolic needs and enough protein to avoid protein breakdown.

Hypoglycemia can result from the stress of the burn injury because the liver glycogen stores are rapidly depleted.

A high-protein, high-calorie diet is encouraged. Many children have poor appetites and are unable to meet energy requirements solely by oral feeding. Most children with burns in excess of 25% TBSA require supplementation with tube feeding. Early and continued nutritional support is an important part of therapy for seriously burned patients. Enteral feeding provides direct nourishment to the gastrointestinal tract and helps reverse the defective gut barrier that accompanies burn shock (Purdue, 2007).

If nutritional requirements cannot be met entirely by the enteral route, parenteral hyperalimentation is used to supplement intake. However, enteral feeding increases blood flow in the intestinal tract, preserves gastrointestinal function, and minimizes bacterial translocation by decreasing mucosal atrophy of the intestines. These factors make enteral feeding the preferred route of nutritional support (Herndon, 2007).

To facilitate growth and proliferation of epithelial cells, the administration of vitamins A and C is begun early in the postburn period. Zinc is also supplemented because of its important role in wound healing and epithelialization.

Medication. Antibiotics are usually not administered prophylactically. The administration of systemic antibiotics to control wound colonization is not indicated, since decreased circulation to the injured area prevents delivery of the medication to areas of deepest injury. Surveillance cultures and monitoring of the clinical course provide the most reliable indicators of developing infection. Appropriate antibiotics are instituted to treat the specific identified organism. Otitis media should not be overlooked as a source of fever in the pediatric population.

Some form of sedation and analgesia is required in the care of burned children. Morphine sulphate is the medication of choice for severe burn injuries. Morphine has extensive distribution but is metabolized rapidly; continuous infusion or frequent administration is needed for pain management in burns. Morphine is administered intravenously and titrated to individual need. The unstable circulatory status and edema formation preclude intramuscular or subcutaneous administration. When combined, midazolam (Versed) and fentanyl (Sublimaze) also provide excellent IV sedation and analgesia to control procedural pain in children with burns (Herndon, 2007). Dosage monitoring is important because tolerance to opioids may develop. IV analgesics are most effective when they are administered just before the onset of procedural pain.

The use of short-acting anaesthetic agents, such as propofol (Diprivan) and nitrous oxide, has proved beneficial in eliminating procedural pain. Pharyngeal reflexes remain intact, thus ensuring a patent airway. Propofol is an IV sedative hypnotic that produces sedation in less than 1 minute and lasts only a few minutes. Nitrous oxide is a useful short-term analgesic when given in a mixture of gases on a fixed ratio of 50% nitrous oxide and 50% oxygen (Annequin et al., 2000). Initiation of action is approximately 1 minute, with peak effect reached in 3 to 5 minutes. Nitrous oxide is useful to alleviate anxiety and raise the threshold of pain during procedures. The child may self-administer the nitrous oxide mixture with assistance. A major drawback with nitrous oxide is that staff is exposed to the gas because it is self-administered by the patient. For any conscious or unconscious sedation, the child must be monitored continuously during the procedure (see Preoperative Care, Chapter 45; and Pain Assessment and Pain Management, Chapter 35).

Management of the Burn Wound. After the initial period of shock and the restoration of fluid balance, the primary concern is the burn wound. The objectives of wound management include prevention of infection, removal of devitalized tissue, and closure of the wound. The application of dressings and topical antimicrobial therapy reduce pain by minimizing the exposure to air.

Primary Excision. In children with large, full-thickness burn wounds, excision is performed as soon as the patient is hemodynamically stable after initial resuscitation. Because the burn wound precipitates an exaggerated physiological response, many complications do not resolve until the eschar is excised and the wound is closed. Early excision of deep partial- and full-thickness burns reduces the incidence of infection and the threat of sepsis.

Debridement. Partial-thickness wounds require debridement of devitalized tissue to promote healing. Debridement is painful and requires analgesia and a sedative before the procedure. Medications given for pain need to be readily available during this procedure and may need to be titrated upward during the procedure. Hydroxyzine and diphenhydramine are often needed for itching that occurs after whirlpool and debridement. The itching becomes particularly bothersome as the burns heal.

Hydrotherapy is employed to cleanse the wound and involves soaking in a tub or showering at least once a day for no more than 20 minutes. The water loosens and removes sloughing tissue, exudate, and topical medications. Hydrotherapy helps to cleanse not only the wound but the entire body and aids in maintenance of range of motion. Mesh gauze entraps the exudative slough and is readily removed during hydrotherapy. Any loose tissue is carefully trimmed away before the wound is redressed.

Topical Antimicrobial Medications. Methods used for managing the burn wound include the following:

Exposure—Wounds are left open to air; crust forms on partial-thickness wounds, and eschar forms on full-thickness burns.

Open—Topical antimicrobial medication is applied directly to the wound surface and the wound is left uncovered.

Modified—Antimicrobial medication is applied directly or impregnated into thin gauze and applied to the wound; gauze or net secures the area.

Occlusive—Antimicrobial medication is impregnated in gauze or applied directly to the wound; multiple layers of bulky gauze are placed over the primary layer and secured with gauze or net.

All of these methods provide wound coverage and employ some type of topical agent. Topical medications do not eliminate organisms from the wound but can effectively inhibit bacterial growth. To be effective, a topical application must be nontoxic, capable of diffusing through eschar, harmless to viable tissue, inexpensive, and easy to apply. A topical ointment should not encourage the development of resistant strains of bacteria and should produce minimal electrolyte derangement. A comparison of commonly used medications is summarized in Table 53-9.

Biological Skin Coverings. Permanent coverage of extensive burns is a prolonged process that requires repeated operative procedures using general anaesthesia for atraumatic care in debridement and grafting. Early closure shortens the period of metabolic stress and decreases the likelihood of burn wound sepsis. In the acute phase, biological dressings cover and protect the wound from contamination, reduce fluid and protein loss, increase the rate of epithelialization, reduce pain, and facilitate movement of joints to retain range of motion.

Allograft (homograft) skin is obtained from human cadavers that are screened for communicable diseases. Allograft is particularly useful in the coverage of surgically excised deep partial- and full-thickness wounds in extensive burns when available donor sites are limited. Severe immunosuppression occurs in massively burned children, and the allograft becomes adherent. The allograft can remain in place until suitable donor sites become available. Typically, rejection is seen approximately 3 to 4 weeks after application (Herndon, 2007). The insufficient availability of tissue banks and suitable donors limits the use of allografts.

Xenograft from a variety of species, most notably pigs, is commercially available. In large burns, the porcine xenograft is commonly applied when extensive early debridement is indicated to cover a partial-thickness burn; this provides a temporary covering for the wound until an available autograft can be applied to the full-thickness areas (Herndon, 2007). Pigskin dressings are replaced every 1 to 3 days. They are particularly effective in children with partial-thickness scald burns of the hands and face because they allow relatively pain-free movement, which reduces contracture formation and has the added benefit of improving appetite and morale.

When applied early to a superficial partial-thickness injury, biological dressings stimulate epithelial growth and faster wound healing. However, biological dressings must be applied to clean wounds. If the dressing covers areas of heavy microbial contamination, infection occurs beneath the dressing. In the case of partial-thickness burns, such infection may convert the wound to a full-thickness injury.

Synthetic skin coverings are available for the management of partial-thickness burn wounds. Ideally, the dressing should provide the properties of human skin: adherence, elasticity, durability, and hemostasis. Synthetic skin substitutes are readily available, have an indefinite shelf life, and are relatively inexpensive.

Synthetic dressings are composed of a variety of materials and can be used successfully in the management of superficial partial-thickness burns and donor sites. Examples include adherent elastic films; hydroactive materials; or colloidal suspensions that are usually permeable to air, vapour, and fluids.

Biobrane is a flexible silicone-nylon membrane bonded to collagenous peptides of porcine skin. Calcium alginate is another treatment for donor sites. As with biological dressings, it is important that the wound be free of debris before the dressing is applied. Body temperature elevation or evidence of purulence, erythema, or cellulitis around the wound

Table 53-9 Comparison of Common Topical Preparations

AGENT	DRESSINGS	ADVANTAGES	DISADVANTAGES
Silver nitrate 0.5% ($AgNO_3$)	Open, modified or occlusive; impedes joint movement; dressings changed twice daily; keep dressing moist (rewet at least every 2 hr)	Greatly reduces evaporative losses; does not interfere with wound healing; bacteriostatic action against major burn flora, including Pseudomonas and Staphylococcus organisms; inexpensive	Does not penetrate eschar; ineffective on established burn wound infections; little effect on Klebsiella and Aerobacter groups; stains skin, clothing, linens; makes assessment of the wound difficult because of staining; hypotonicity pulls electrolytes from the wound, depleting sodium, potassium, chloride, and magnesium; stings on application
Silver sulphadiazine 1% (AgSD)	Occlusive; motion of joints maintained; applied twice daily; do not use in patients with a history of allergy to sulpha	Little pain on application; bactericidal by altering DNA and cell metabolism; effective against gram-positive and gram-negative bacteria; easy to apply; nontoxic	Transient neutropenia; does not penetrate eschar; forms proteinaceous gel on wound surface that is painful to remove; occasional rashes and pruritus; decreases granulocyte formation
Mafenide acetate 10% (Sulphamylon)	*Cream*—Usually open; do not apply to face; apply twice daily *Solution*—Occlusive; keep dressing moist (rewet at least every 2 hr); protect solution from light	Penetrates eschar and diffuses rapidly into burn wound and underlying tissues; effective in deep flame, electrical, and infected wounds; biostatic against many gram-positive and gram-negative organisms, including Pseudomonas and Clostridium	Difficult and painful to remove cream; pain on application; metabolic acidosis, hypercapnia, and carbonic anhydrase inhibition; inhibits wound healing; hypersensitivity in some patients
Bacitracin	Open, modified; motion of joints maintained; change dressing twice daily	Bactericidal and bacteriostatic against gram-positive organisms; low toxicity; painless application; easy to apply	Limited activity against gram-negative organisms; allergic reaction in sensitive individuals

edges may indicate that the wound has become infected beneath the dressing. If this occurs, prompt discontinuance of the synthetic dressing is indicated. All synthetic dressings are reputed to hasten wound healing and reduce discomfort.

Permanent Skin Coverings. Permanent coverage of deep partial- and full-thickness burns is usually accomplished with a split-thickness skin graft. This graft consists of the epidermis and a portion of the dermis removed from an intact area of skin by a special instrument, the *dermatome* (Fig. 53-18). With extensive burns it is often difficult to find enough viable skin to cover the wounds; therefore available donor sites and special techniques are used. Split-thickness skin grafts may be sheet graft or mesh graft.

Sheet Graft. A sheet of skin, removed from the donor site, is placed intact over the recipient site and sutured in place; this is used in areas where cosmetic results are most visible.

Mesh Graft. A sheet of skin is removed from the donor site and passed through a mesher, which produces tiny slits in the skin that allow the skin to cover 1.5 to 9 times the area of the sheet graft; this results in a less desirable cosmetic and functional outcome (Fig. 53-19).

The donor site is dressed with synthetic wound coverings or fine-mesh gauze until the dressing separates at 10 to 14 days, when the wound is healed. Dressings are not changed on donor sites to avoid damage to newly healed, delicate epithelium. Healed donor sites are available for reharvesting in patients with extensive burns and limited undamaged skin, but the quality of skin is decreased when multiple grafts are taken.

Artificial Skin. The development of Integra, a product that allows the dermis to regenerate, has produced significant improvement in burn wound healing and decreased scar formation. It is applied to partial- and full-thickness burns. The two-layer membrane is made of collagen (a fibrous protein from animal tendons and cartilage) and silicone rubber (i.e., Silastic). The Silastic layer is peeled off after the dermis is formed. The application of artificial skin does not replace the grafting procedure, but it prepares the burn wound to accept an ultrathin autograft. Advantages include faster healing of the burn wound when integrity of the dermis is restored, faster healing of donor sites with the use of ultrathin grafts, and restoration of sweat glands and hair follicles. A disadvantage is its high cost.

Prognosis

Children differ from adults in their responses to thermal injury, and the mortality rates in young children are significantly higher than those in older children and adults. Mortality is greatest for children younger than 48 months of age. Many children who do survive have long-term functional and cosmetic impairments.

Nursing Care Management

Because the care of burned children encompasses a broad range of skills, nursing care has been divided into segments that correspond with the major phases of burn treatment. The acute phase, also referred to as the *emergent* or resuscitative phase, involves the first 24 to 48 hours. The *management phase* extends from the completion of adequate resuscitation through wound coverage. The *rehabilitative phase* begins once the majority of the wounds have healed and rehabilitation has become the predominant focus of the care plan. This phase continues until all reconstructive procedures and corrective measures are accomplished (often a period of months or years).

Acute Phase

The primary emphasis during the emergent phase is the treatment of burn shock and the management of pulmonary status. Monitoring vital signs, output, fluid infusion, and respiratory parameters are ongoing activities in the hours immediately after injury. IV infusion is begun immediately and is regulated to maintain a urine output of at least 1 to 2 mL/kg in children weighing less than 30 kg; an output of 30 to 50 mL/hr is expected in children weighing more than 30 kg. Urine output and specific gravity, vital signs, laboratory data, and objective signs of adequate hydration guide the rate of fluid administration.

Children who are hospitalized with burns require constant observation and assessment for complications. Alterations in

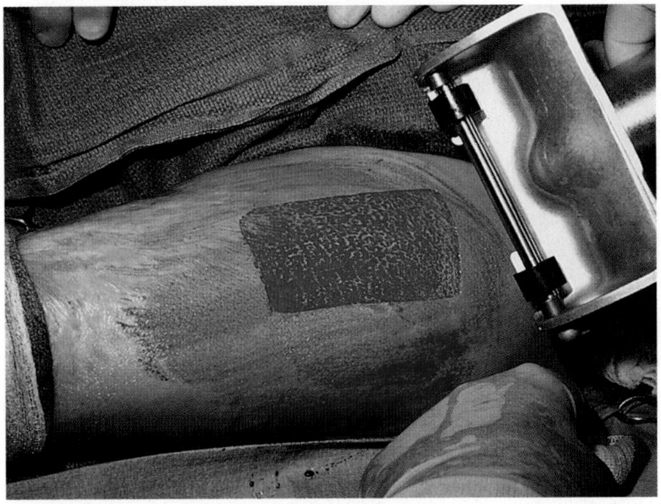

Fig. 53-18 Removal of split-thickness skin graft with a dermatome.

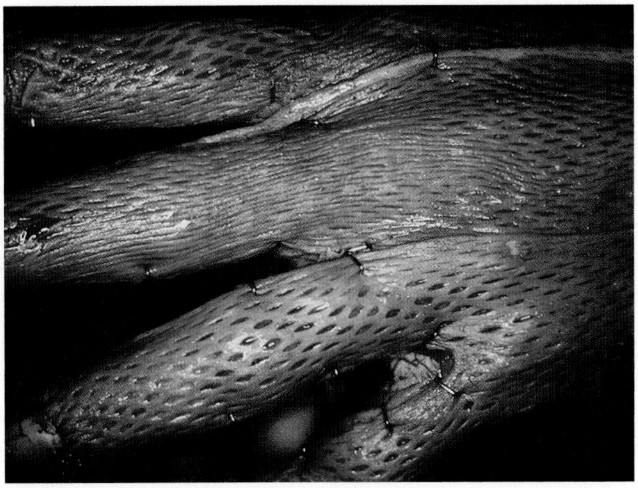

Fig. 53-19 Mesh graft.

electrolyte balance produce clinical symptoms of confusion, weakness, cardiac irregularities, and seizures. Changes in respiratory function and gas exchange are reflected clinically by restlessness, irritability, increased work of breathing, and alterations in blood gas values. The loss of protective function of the skin exposes burned children to increased risk of hypothermia. Edema formation and circulatory impairment result in the loss of sensation and deep throbbing pain.

NURSING ALERT Evaluate the burned extremity and check the pulse every hour. If unable to palpate, use Doppler to ascertain loss of circulation and pulse. If the pulse is lost, escharotomy may be necessary to relieve the edema causing pressure on blood vessels, to restore adequate circulation.

Burn units maintain a pictorial record of the wound to record progress and for legal purposes (if child abuse is suspected). The burn wound is treated according to the protocol of the specific burn facility. The burn team monitors infection control procedures and ensures that staff and visitors comply with established protocols to prevent cross-contamination in the burn unit.

Throughout the acute phase of care, the psychosocial needs of the children and their families should not be overlooked. The child is frightened, uncomfortable, and often confused. Children may be isolated from familiar persons and surroundings; the overwhelming physical needs at this time are the primary focus of the staff and parents. In addition to feeling concern for their child, the family may experience guilt, which may be related to the fact that the parents did not or could not protect their child from injury. Consistency in the information presented and in the staff's attitude can create a sense of familiarity and stability during the acute phase of care. Consistent caregivers can also help decrease the patient and family's anxiety and provide coordination of care. For example, when many teams of consultants and specialists are involved in the child's care, appointing one "spokesperson" decreases the confusion and enhances communication regarding the child's care.

Management and Rehabilitative Phases

After the patient's condition is stabilized, the management phase begins. The multidisciplinary team concentrates on preventing wound infections, closing the wound as quickly as possible, and managing the numerous complications. Although the rehabilitative phase begins when permanent wound closure has been achieved, rehabilitation issues are identified on admission and are included in the care plan throughout the hospital course.

NURSING ALERT Disorientation in the burned patient is one of the first signs of overwhelming sepsis and may indicate inadequate hydration. Assessment of the sensorium is another important indicator of the adequacy of hydration. With inadequate hydration, a spiking fever and diminished bowel sounds accompanied by paralytic ileus are noted and progressively increase over 48 to 72 hours, after which the temperature falls to subnormal limits. At this time the wound deteriorates, the white blood cell count is depressed, and septic shock becomes manifest.

Comfort Management

The severe pain of the wound and resultant therapies, the anxiety generated by these experiences, sleep deprivation, itching related to wound healing, and the conscious and unconscious interpretations of traumatic events contribute to the psychological behaviours commonly observed in children with burns. It is always difficult to deal with a child in pain, and inflicting pain on a helpless child is contrary to the empathic nature of nursing. Interventions to promote comfort may include medications (including IV morphine or midazolam and short-term anaesthetics such as propofol), relaxation techniques, distraction therapy, behavioural techniques, operant conditioning (e.g., tokens, star chart), and family participation.

Children need age-appropriate explanations before all procedures. When children appear to accept pain with little or no response, psychological consultation may be needed. Consistency in caregivers is important. If this is not possible, a carefully developed, multidisciplinary care plan is necessary to provide consistency.

Care of the Burn Wound

The nurse has a major responsibility for cleansing, debriding, and applying topical medications and dressings to the burn wound. Pain medication should be administered so that the peak effect of the drug coincides with the procedure. Children who have an understanding of the procedure to be performed and some perceived control demonstrate less anxious behaviour. Children also respond well to participating in decisions (see Atraumatic Care box).

Outer dressings are removed. Any dressings that have adhered to the wound can be more easily removed by applying tepid water or normal saline. Loose or easily detached tissue is debrided during the cleansing process. In dressing the wound, it is important that all areas be clean, that medication be amply applied, and that no two burned surfaces touch each other (e.g., fingers or toes; ears touching the side of the head). If they are touching, the burned surfaces will heal together, causing deformity or dysfunction.

ATRAUMATIC CARE

Reducing the Stress of Burn Care Procedures

- Have all materials ready before beginning.
- Administer appropriate analgesics and sedatives.
- Remind the child of the impending procedure to allow sufficient time to prepare.
- Allow the child to test and approve the temperature of the water.
- Allow the child to select the area of the body on which to begin.
- Allow the child to request a short rest period during the procedure.
- Allow the child to remove the dressings if desired.
- Provide something constructive for the child to do during the procedure (e.g., holding a package of dressings or a roll of gauze).
- Inform the child when the procedure is near completion.
- Praise the child for cooperation.

Topical medications may be applied directly to the wound with a tongue blade or gloved hand or impregnated into fine-mesh gauze before application. Dressings are then applied to assist in exudate absorption, wound debridement, and increased patient comfort. All dressings applied circumferentially should be wrapped in a distal-to-proximal manner. The dressing is applied with sufficient tension to remain in place but not so tightly as to impair circulation or limit motion. Elastic bandages are applied over dressings to prevent epithelial breakdown, decrease edema, stimulate circulation, and improve mobility. A stable dressing is especially important when the child is ambulatory.

Standard precautions, including the use of protective garb and barrier techniques, should be followed when caring for patients with thermal injuries. Frequent hand hygiene, including the forearm, are the single most important elements of the infection control program. Strict policies for cleaning the environment and patient care equipment should be implemented to minimize the risk of cross-contamination. All visitors and members of other departments should be oriented to the infection control policies, including the importance of hand hygiene and forearm washing and use of protective garb. Visitors should be screened for infection and contagious diseases before patient contact.

Nutrition

Oral feedings are encouraged unless the child is intubated or paralytic ileus persists. Because children with burns often lack an appetite, the child needs encouragement, help, and patience. Consultation between the caregiver and the dietitian helps determine food preferences. Children who are old enough to participate should be included in meal planning. In addition, many children prefer an atmosphere more nearly like that provided at home. Therefore, when possible, many children enjoy sitting at a table and interacting with other children at mealtimes. Painful procedures should not be scheduled near mealtimes, since most children will be too physically exhausted and emotionally upset to eat.

Children who require enteral supplementation must be monitored for feeding intolerance and tube malposition. The nurse should also monitor and report any abdominal distension, diarrhea, or electrolyte and metabolic deviations.

Prevention of Complications

Acute Care

The maintenance of body temperature is important to the child with burns. Core body temperature is supported when energy is conserved with an environmental temperature of 28° to 33°C. Large areas of the body should not be exposed simultaneously during dressing changes. Warmed solutions, linens, occlusive dressings, heat shields, a radiant warmer, and warming blankets assist in preventing hypothermia.

The chief danger during acute care is infection—wound infection, generalized sepsis, or bacterial pneumonia. Accurate and ongoing assessments of all parameters that provide clues to the early diagnosis and treatment of infection are essential. Symptoms of sepsis include a change in the level of consciousness, a rising or falling white blood cell count, hypothermia or hyperthermia, a loss of the progression of wound healing, increasing fluid requirements, hypoactive or absent bowel sounds, a rising or falling blood glucose level, tachycardia, tachypnea, and thrombocytopenia.

Children are reluctant to move if movement causes pain, and they are likely to assume a position of comfort. Unfortunately, the most comfortable position often encourages the formation of contractures and loss of function. Ongoing efforts to prevent contractures include maintaining proper body alignment, positioning and splinting involved extremities in extension, providing active and passive physical therapy, and encouraging spontaneous movement when feasible. Frequent position changes are important to promote adequate bronchopulmonary hygiene and capillary perfusion to common pressure areas. Low–air loss beds are beneficial for the morbidly obese or children with posterior grafts. Special attention should be given to areas at risk for increased pressure, such as the posterior scalp, heels, sacrum, and areas exposed to mechanical irritation from splints and dressings.

Long-Term Care

The rehabilitative phase of care begins once wound coverage is achieved. Scar formation becomes a major problem as burn wounds heal (Fig. 53-20). Contractile properties of the scar tissue can result in disabling contractures, deformity, and disfigurement.

Uniform pressure applied to the scar decreases the blood supply. When pressure is removed, blood supply to the scar is immediately increased; therefore periods without pressure should be brief to avoid nourishment of the hypertrophic tissue. Continuous pressure to areas of scarring can be achieved by elastic bandages or commercially available pressure garments. Because these custom-made garments are often worn for months, revisions may be required as the child grows. It is much easier to prevent scarring and contracture of the wound than to resolve an existing problem. Splints and appliances may also be needed until wound maturation is achieved (Fig. 53-21).

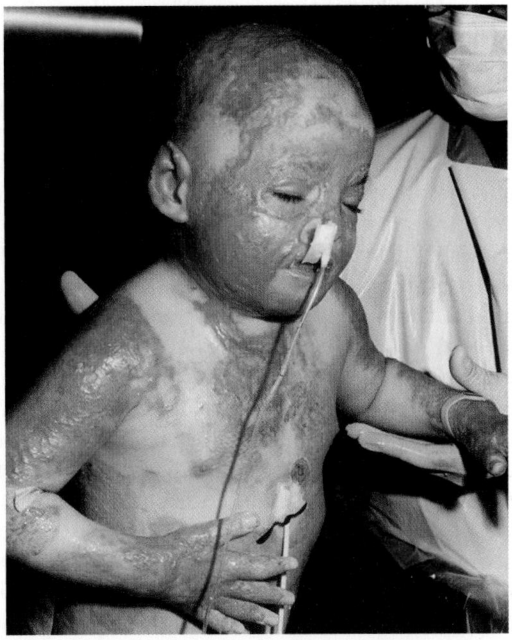

Fig. 53-20 Extensive scars from flame burn. *(Courtesy The Paul and Carol David Foundation Burn Institute, Akron, Ohio.)*

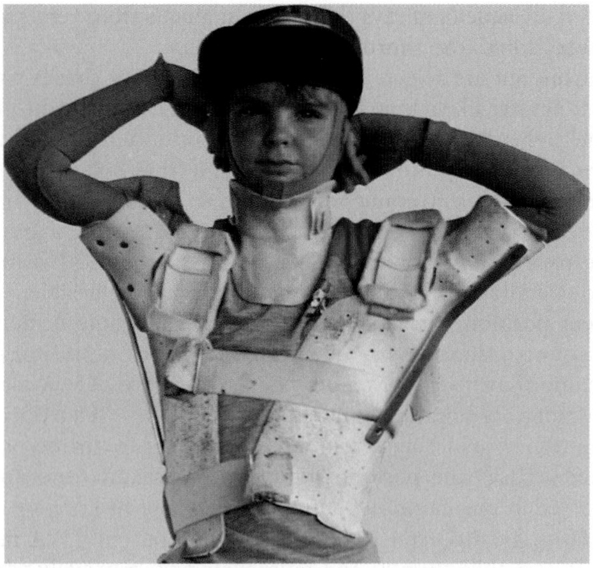

Fig. 53-21 Child in elasticized (Jobst) garment and "airplane" splints.

Scar tissue has certain significant properties, particularly for growing children. Intense itching occurs in healing burn wounds and scar tissue until the scar is no longer active. Itching is usually treated with hydroxyzine (Atarax) or diphenhydramine and frequent applications of a moisturizer, such as Vaseline, Cetaphil, Aquaphor, Eucerin, cocoa butter, or Nivea. Petrolatum-based ointments (Vaseline, Aquaphor) may spread more easily on friable skin than thick creams do. Massage therapy during the application of moisturizers is also beneficial to stretch scar tissue and aid in contracture prevention. Scar tissue has no sweat glands, and children with extensive scarring may experience difficulty during hot weather. Caregivers should be alerted to this possibility and be prepared to institute alternate methods of cooling when necessary.

Scar tissue does not grow and expand, as does normal tissue, which may create difficulties, especially in functional areas such as on the hands and over joints. Additional surgery is sometimes required to allow independent functioning in daily activities, to improve cosmetic appearance, or to restore anatomical integrity.

The nursing activities in the rehabilitative phase of treatment focus on the child and family's adaptation to the burn injury and their ability to reintegrate into the community. The psychological pain and sequelae of severe burn injury are as intense as the physical trauma. The impact of severe burns taxes the coping mechanisms at all ages. Very young children, who suffer acutely from separation anxiety, and adolescents, who are developing an identity, are probably most affected psychologically. Toddlers cannot understand why the parents they love and who have protected them can leave them in such a frightening and unfamiliar place. Adolescents, in the process of achieving independence from the family, find themselves in a dependent role with a damaged body. Being different from others at a time when conformity with peers is so important is difficult to accept.

Anticipation of the return to school can be overwhelming and frightening. It is essential that health care providers recognize the importance of preparing teachers and classmates for the child's return. Teachers need to be provided with information to assist the child and family and to promote the child's optimal adjustment. Hospital-sponsored school re-entry programs use a variety of methods to provide education and information about the implications of the injury, the garments and appliances, and the need for support and acceptance. Telephone calls, videos, information packets, and visits by members of the health care team offer opportunities to help with reintegration into the school environment—a focal point of the child's life.

Psychosocial Support of the Child

Children should begin early to do as much for themselves as possible and to be active participants in their care. Loss of control and perceived helplessness may result in acting-out behaviours. During illness, children regress to a previous developmental level that allows them to deal with stress. As children begin to participate in their care, they gain confidence and self-esteem. Fears and anxieties diminish with accomplishment and self-confidence. If the child will not cooperate in the rehabilitative phase, a behaviour modification program can be initiated to promote or reward the child's accomplishment in care.

Children need to know that their injury and the treatments are not punishment for real or imagined transgressions and that the nurse understands their fear, anger, and discomfort. They also need body contact. This is often difficult to arrange for the child with massive burns. Stroking areas of unburned skin is comforting. Even older children enjoy sitting on the parent's lap and being cuddled and hugged. This can be a reward or a comfort in times of stress, but most of all it should be kept in mind that it is a natural part of childhood.

Psychosocial Support of the Family

Recognizing and respecting each family's strengths, differences, and methods of coping allows the nurse to respond to their unique needs by implementing a family-centred approach to care. In the acute phase, all attention is focused on the child, and the parents feel powerless and ineffectual. Most parents feel overwhelming guilt, whether or not the guilt is justified. They feel responsible for the injury. These feelings may impede the child's rehabilitation. Parents may indulge the child and allow noncompliant behaviours that affect physical and emotional recovery. Parents need to be informed of the child's progress and helped to cope with their feelings while supporting their child. The nurse can help them understand that it is not selfish to look after themselves and their own needs to meet their child's needs. It is important to recognize the parents' need to grieve the change in their child's normal appearance as part of the grieving process. Definitive professional help may be needed for parents whose response to the injury is severe or whose response to stress is manifested in destructive behaviour.

The parents are members of the multidisciplinary team and participate in the development of the care plan. It is important to facilitate their input; to consider all aspects of the physical, emotional, social, and cultural factors affecting the child and family; and to establish a realistic home therapy program.

The family's willingness to assume responsibility for care and their ability to implement the therapeutic regimen are assessed. Home, school, and other environmental factors are explored; financial concerns and available community resources are discussed; and a specific care plan for the child, with an anticipated follow-up program, is developed.

Prevention of Burn Injury

The best intervention is to prevent burns from occurring. Hot liquids in the kitchen and bathroom most commonly injure infants and toddlers. Hot liquids should be kept out of reach; tablecloths and dangling appliance cords are often pulled by toddlers, who spill hot grease and liquids on themselves. Electrical cords and outlets represent a potential risk to small children, who may chew on accessible cords and insert objects into outlets.

Safe Kids Canada (2011) recommends a reduction of water heater thermostats to a maximum of 49°C. The "dial-down" recommendation has been suggested by utility companies, burn treatment centres, medical personnel, and others interested in public safety. However, many water heaters continue to remain set at levels well above the safe level.

Small children are especially at risk for scald injuries from hot tap water because of their decreased reaction time and agility, their curiosity, and the thermal sensitivity of their skin. Caregivers should never leave a child unattended in a bath and without adult supervision. Water should always be tested before a child is placed in the tub or shower.

The increased use of microwave ovens has resulted in burn injuries from the extremely hot internal temperatures generated in heated items. Baby formula, jelly-filled pastries, and hot liquids and dishes may result in cutaneous scalds or the ingestion of overheated liquids. Parents should use caution when removing items from the microwave oven and should always test the food before giving it to children.

As children mature, risk-taking behaviours increase. Matches and lighters are dangerous in the hands of the young. Adults must remember to keep potentially hazardous items out of the reach of children; a lighter, like a match, is a tool for adult use.

Education related to fire safety and survival should begin with the very young. They can practise "stop, drop, and roll" to extinguish a fire. The fire escape route, including a safe meeting place away from the home in case of fire, also should be practised.

Community activities are also helpful in supporting burn survivors and preventing burns. There are different organizations that provide important burn prevention educational programs as well as financial and emotion support to the children with burn injuries and their families (see Additional Resources). An example is TOMA Foundation for Burned Children, which is a Canadian and American organization of firefighters who fundraise and work with interdisciplinary health care providers to provide burn support. There are also burn camps for children in most of the provinces, such as Camp Bucko in Ontario.

Sunburn

Sunburn is a common skin injury caused by overexposure to UV light waves. The sun emits a continuous spectrum of visible and nonvisible light rays that range in length from very short to very long. The shorter, higher-frequency waves are more damaging than longer wavelengths, but much of the light is filtered out as it travels through the atmosphere. Of the light that does filter through, *ultraviolet A (UVA)* waves are the longest and cause only minimum burning, but play a significant role in photosensitive and photoallergic reactions. They are also responsible for premature aging of the skin and potentiate the effects of *ultraviolet B (UVB)* waves. UVB waves are shorter and are responsible for tanning, burning, and most of the harmful effects attributed to sunlight, especially skin cancer.

Numerous factors influence the amount of UVB exposure. Maximum exposure occurs at midday (10 AM to 3 PM), when the distance from the sun to a given spot on the earth is shortest. There is more exposure at higher altitudes and near the equator, and less when the sky is hazy (although the amount of UV radiation that does penetrate is easily underestimated). Window glass effectively screens out UVB but not UVA rays. Fresh snow, water, and sand reflect UV rays, especially when the sun is directly overhead.

Sunburn is usually an epidermal burn, although severe sunburn can be a partial-thickness burn with blister formation. Treatment of sunburn involves stopping the burning process, decreasing the inflammatory response, and rehydrating the skin. Local application of cool tap water soaks, or immersion in a tepid-water bath (temperature slightly below 36.7°C for 20 minutes or until the skin is cool), limits tissue destruction and relieves the discomfort. After the cool applications, a bland oil-in-water moisturizing lotion can be applied. Partial-thickness sunburns are treated the same as those from any heat source (see earlier discussion on burns).

Nursing Care Management

Protection from sunburn is the major goal of management, and the harmful effects of the sun on the delicate skin of infants and children are currently receiving increased attention. To protect skin exposed to the sun for extended periods, skin should be covered with clothing, and Canadian Dermatology Association–approved sun protection agents should be applied.

Two types of products are available for sun protection: *topical sunscreens*, which partially absorb UV light, and *sun blockers*, which block out UV rays by reflecting sunlight. The most frequently recommended sun blockers are zinc oxide and titanium dioxide ointments. Sunscreens are products containing an SPF based on an evaluation of its effectiveness against UV rays. The SPF is a number, such as 15, which indicates that if individuals normally burn in 10 minutes without a sunscreen, use of a sunscreen with SPF 15 allows them to remain in the sun 15 times 10, or 150 minutes ($2\frac{1}{2}$ hours) before acquiring the same degree of burns. The most effective sunscreens against UVB are p-aminobenzoic acid (PABA) and PABA-esters. However, many individuals are allergic to PABA, and sunscreens without PABA are encouraged to prevent these reactions in children. The Canadian Dermatology Association (CDA) provides a sunscreen list on their Web site (http://www.dermatology.ca/programs-resources/programs/recognized-products) that they have approved. The products that have been approved usually have the CDA logo on them.

Sunscreens are applied evenly to all exposed areas, with special attention to skin folds and areas that might become exposed as clothing shifts. Parents need to read labels of sunscreen products carefully for the SPF and follow the manufacturer's directions for application.

NURSING ALERT Sunscreens can be applied to children who are under 1 year of age. Infants should be kept out of the sun or physically shaded from it. Infants should be covered as much as possible with tightly woven fabric, such as cotton, when in the sun. Small amounts of sunscreen can be applied to sun-exposed skin, such as on the back of the hands and face, in small amounts (Canadian Dermatology Association, 2009c). Infants should be kept out of the sun or physically shaded from it. Fabric with a tight weave, such as cotton, offers good protection.

Individuals who work in the community, such as teachers, day care workers, coaches, and youth-group leaders, as well as relatives should all be made aware of sun safety for children. Sunscreens must be applied *liberally*.

Cold Injury

Cold injuries are most commonly seen in very cold regions. The nature of the body's heat-regulating mechanisms is such that the inner portion of the body, or core, produces heat, and the periphery, or outer area, conserves or dissipates heat. When the body attempts to conserve heat, the outer tissues are subjected to low temperatures, and local trauma may result.

Chilblain, redness and swelling of the skin, occurs when extremities, usually the hands, are exposed intermittently to temperatures of −1.1° to 15.5°C. The response may vary but is characterized by intense vasodilation that increases the temperature of involved tissues above that of unaffected tissue and produces edematous, reddish blue patches that itch and burn. As warming takes place, the sensations become more intense, but ordinarily they subside in a few days.

Frostbite is the term used to describe tissue damage caused when excessive heat loss to local tissues allows ice crystals to form in tissues. The frostbitten part appears white or blanched, feels solid, and is without sensation. Rapid rewarming is associated with less tissue necrosis than slow thawing. It restores blood flow and shortens the period of cellular damage. Rewarming produces a flush (sometimes deep purple) and a return of sensation, which is extremely painful. Large blisters may appear in 24 to 48 hours after rewarming and begin to reabsorb within 5 to 10 days, followed by the formation of a hard black eschar. Superficial injury often heals without incident. Rewarming is accomplished by immersing the part in well-agitated water at 37.8° to 42.2°C. Discomfort is managed with analgesics and sedatives. Care of blistered skin is similar to that described for burns. It is seldom possible to estimate the extent of tissue loss until new skin layers are revealed after the eschar layer separates.

Key Points

- A variety of factors can produce lesions of the skin.
- It is important for nurses to be able to describe skin lesions accurately.
- The process of wound healing consists of hemostasis, inflammation, proliferation, and remodelling.
- A moist environment promotes wound healing.
- Bacterial, viral, and fungal infections are common in childhood.
- Some skin diseases are transmitted by arthropod vectors, especially ticks.
- The most common skin infestations of childhood—scabies and pediculosis capitis— affect children of any age and from any social class.
- Contact dermatitis may involve a primary irritant or a sensitizing agent.
- Adverse reactions to medications are manifested more often in the skin than in any other body organ.
- The most common skin disorders of infancy are diaper dermatitis, seborrheic dermatitis, and AD.
- Acne, a disorder affecting many adolescents, is related to hormonal fluctuation, stimulation of the sebaceous glands, excessive sebum production, the formation of comedones, and the overgrowth of the *P. acnes* organism.
- Medication and gentle facial cleansing are the treatments of choice for acne.
- Burns are caused by thermal, chemical, electric, or radioactive agents.
- Burns are assessed on the extent, depth, and severity of the wound.
- Essentials of emergency care of burn injury include stopping the burning process, covering the burn, transporting the injured child to medical aid, and providing reassurance to the child and family.
- Management of minor burns consists of facilitating wound healing, relieving discomfort, and preventing complications.
- Management of major burns consists of facilitating wound healing, relieving discomfort, replacing destroyed skin, preventing or treating complications, and providing rehabilitation.
- Sunscreen is recommended for use when the skin is exposed to the damaging effects of the sun's rays.
- Thermal injuries to the skin can result from exposure to extreme cold.

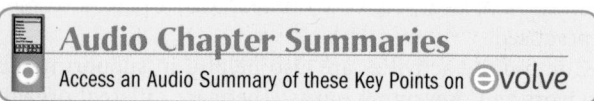

Audio Chapter Summaries
Access an Audio Summary of these Key Points on evolve

References

American Academy of Dermatology. (2003). *Guidelines for the care of atopic dermatitis*. Retrieved from http://www.aad.org/professionals/guidelines/AtopicDermatitis.htm.

American Academy of Dermatology. (2006). *Acne*. Retrieved from http://www.aad.org/public/Publications/pamphlets/Acne.htm.

Annequin, D., et al. (2000). Fixed 50% nitrous oxide oxygen mixture for painful procedures: A French survey. *Pediatrics, 105*(4), E47.

Arnoldo, B., Klein, M., & Gibran, N. S. (2006). Practice guidelines for the management of electrical injuries. *Journal of Burn Care & Research, 27*(4), 439–447.

Association of Women's Health, Obstetric and Neonatal Nurses. (2007). *Neonatal skin care, second edition. Evidence-based clinical practice guideline.*

Retrieved from http://guideline.gov/content.aspx?id=24063&search=baby+powder.
Bernardo, L. M., et al. (2000). Dog bites in children treated in a pediatric emergency department. *Journal of the Society of Pediatric Nurses, 5*(2), 87–95.
Canadian Dermatology Association. (2009a). *Childhood eczema.* Retrieved from http://dermatology.ca/patients_public/info_patients/eczema/eczema_kids.html.
Canadian Dermatology Association. (2009b). *Acne.* Retrieved from http://dermatology.ca/acnepatients_public/info_patients/eczema/eczema_kids.html.
Canadian Dermatology Association. (2009c). *Sun protection for babies.* Retrieved from http://www.dermatology.ca/sap/safety_resources/sun_exposure/babies.html.
Canadian Paediatric Society. (2001). Scabies management. *Paediatrics & Child Health, 6*(110), 775–777. (Reaffirmed 2010) Retrieved from http://www.cps.ca/english/statements/ii/ii01-01.htm.
Canadian Paediatric Society. (2008). Head lice infestations: A clinical update. *Canadian Paediatric Child Health, 12*(8), 692–696.
Canadian Paediatric Society. (2009). Lyme disease in Canada: Q & A for paediatricians. *Paediatrics & Child Health, 14*(3), 103–105.
Centers for Disease Control and Prevention. (2003). Nonfatal dog bite–related injuries treated in hospital emergency departments—United States, 2001. *MMWR: Morbidity & Mortality Weekly Report, 52*(26), 605–610.
Centers for Disease Control and Prevention, Division of Parasitic Diseases. (2005). *Treating head lice infestation.* Retrieved from http://www.cdc.gov/ncidod/dpd/parasites/lice/factsht_head_lice_treating.htm.
Eichenfield, L. F. & Wortzman, M. (2009). A novel gel formulation of 0.25% tretinoin and 1.2% clindamycin phosphate: efficacy in acne vulgaris patients aged 12 to 18 years. *Pediatric Dermatology, 26*(3), 257–261.
Goates, B. M., et al. (2006). An effective nonchemical treatment for head lice: A lot of hot air. *Pediatrics, 188*(5), 1962–1970.
Health Canada. (2010). *Poison ivy pest note.* Retrieved from http://www.hc-sc.gc.ca/cps-spc/pubs/pest/_pnotes/poisonivy-herb.
Health Canada. (2011). *Bed bugs.* Retrieved from http://www.hc-sc.gc.ca/cps-spc/pubs/pest/_pnotes/bedbugs-punaises-lits/index-eng.php.
Herndon, D.N. (Ed.). (2007). *Total burn care* (3rd ed.). London: Saunders.
Huang, J., Abrams, M., Tlougan, B., Rademaker, A., & Paller, A.S. (2009). Treatment of *Staphylococcus aureus* colonization in atopic dermatitis decreases disease severity. *Pediatrics, 123*(5), e808–e814. doi:10.1542/peds.2008-2217
Humane Society of Canada. (2007). *National dog bite awareness campaign.* Retrieved from https://www.humanesociety.com/national-dog-bite-awareness-campaign.
Jacobs, D. G., Deutsch, N. L., & Brewer, M. (2001). Suicide, depression, and isotretinoin: Is there a causal link? *Journal of the American Academy of Dermatology, 45*(5), S168–S175.
Kaplan, S. L. (2006). Community-acquired methicillin-resistant *Staphylococcus aureus* infections in children. *Seminars in Pediatric Infectious Diseases, 17*(3), 113–119.
Kronemyer, B. (2003). Scratching the surface of atopic and contact dermatitis. *Infectious Diseases in Children, 16*(3), 40.
Lee, M. C., et al. (2004). Management and outcome of children with skin and soft tissue abscesses caused by community-acquired methicillin-resistant *Staphylococcus aureus. Pediatric Infectious Diseases Journal, 23*(2), 123–127.
McCord, S. S., & Levy, M. L. (2006). Practical guide to pediatric wound care. *Seminars in Plastic Surgery, 20*(3), 192–199.
Mumcuoglu, K. Y., et al. (2007). International guidelines for effective control of head louse infestations. *Journal of Drugs in Dermatology, 6*(4), 409–414.
Olutunmbi, B. A., Paley, K., & English, J.C. (2008). Adolescent female acne: Etiology and management. *Journal of Pediatric and Adolescence Gynecology, 21*(4), 171–176.
Ontario Agency for Health Protection and Promotion. (2011). *Just clean your hands—your 4 moments for hand hygiene.* Retrieved from http://www.oahpp.ca/services/jcyh/moments.html.
Ontario Office of the Fire Marshal. (2010). *Fire and burn injury.* Retrieved from http://www.ofm.gov.on.ca/en/Fire Safety and Public Education/Risk watch/Fire and Burn Injury/default.asp.
Pearlman, D. L. (2004). A simple treatment for head lice: Dry on, suffocation-based pediculicide. *Pediatrics, 114*(3), e275–e279.
Public Health Agency of Canada. (2010a). *Lyme disease fact sheet.* Retrieved from www.phac-aspc.gc.ca/id-mi/lym-fs-eng.php.
Public Health Agency of Canada. (2010b). *Human West Nile cases in Canada and the United States 2010.* Retrieved from http://www.eidgis.com/wnvmonitor/.
Public Health Agency of Canada. (2011). *Bartonella henselae. Pathogen safety sheet—infectious substances.* Retrieved from http://www.phac-aspc.gc.ca/lab-bio/res/psds-ftss/bartonella-henselae-eng.php.
Purdue, G. F. (2007). American Burn Association presidential address 2006 on nutrition: Yesterday, today, and tomorrow. *Journal of Burn Care & Research, 28*(1), 1–5.
Russell, J. J. (2000). Topical therapy for acne. *American Family Physician, 61*(2), 357–366.
Safe Kids Canada. (2006). *Insect repellents for children.* Retrieved from http://www.caringforkids.cps.ca/keepkidsafe/repellents.htm.
Safe Kids Canada. (2011). *How to lower your hot water temperature: Lower the temperature your hot water heater.* Retrieved from http://www.safekidscanada.ca/Parents/Safety-Information/Scalds-and-Burns/Hot-Water-Temp/Lowering-Hot-Water-Temperature.aspx.
Spinks, A., Wasiak, J., Clelan, H., Beben, N., & Macpherson, A. K. (2008). Ten-year epidemiological study of pediatric burns in Canada. *Journal of Burn Care Research, 29*(3). 482–488.
Strong, M., & Johnstone, P. W. (2008). Interventions for treating scabies. *Cochrane Database of Systematic Reviews, 18*(3), CD000320.
Toronto Public Health Department. (2008). *Bed bugs fact sheet.* Retrieved from http://www.toronto.ca/health/pdf/bedbugs_factsheet.pdf.
Wade, C. F. (2000). Keeping Lyme disease at bay: An integrated approach to prevention. *American Journal of Nursing, 100*(7), 26–31.
Webster, G. F. (2009). Acne: Tips and tricks for the pediatrician. *Pediatrics Annals, 38*(2), 80–83.
Wormser, G. P., et al. (2006). The clinical assessment, treatment, and prevention of Lyme disease, human granulocytic anaplasmosis, and babesiosis: Clinical practice guidelines by the Infectious Diseases Society of America. *Clinics in Infectious Diseases, 43*, 1089–1134.
Yetman, R. J., & Parks, D. (2002). Diagnosis and management of atopic dermatitis. *Journal of Pediatric Health Care, 16*(3), 143–145.

Additional Resources

Canadian Dermatology Association: http://www.dermatology.ca/
CanLyme Canadian Lyme Disease Foundation: http://www.canlyme.com/
Registered Nurses Association of Ontario: Best Practice Guideline. Risk Assessment and Prevention of Pressure Ulcers: http://rnao.ca/bpg/guidelines/risk-assessment-and-prevention-pressure-ulcers
TOMA Foundation for Burned Children: http://www.fondtomafound.org/english/index.htm

Unit 11

54 Musculoskeletal or Articular Dysfunction

Learning Objectives

On completion of this chapter, the reader will be able to:

- Outline a care plan for a child immobilized with an injury or a degenerative disease.
- Formulate a teaching plan for the parents of a child in a cast.
- Explain the functions of the various types of traction.
- Differentiate among the various congenital skeletal defects.
- Design a teaching plan for the parents of a child with a congenital skeletal deformity.
- Describe the therapies and nursing care of a child with scoliosis.
- Outline a care plan for a child with osteomyelitis.
- Differentiate between osteosarcoma and Ewing's sarcoma.
- Describe the nursing care of a child with rheumatoid arthritis.
- Demonstrate an understanding of the management of systemic lupus erythematosus.

Electronic Resources

Additional information related to the content in Chapter 54 can be found on

evolve the companion Web site at

http://evolve.elsevier.com/Canada/Perry/maternal/

- Examination Review Questions
- Animation—Bone Fractures
- Animation—Spine Structure
- Assessment Video
- Case Study—Developmental Dysplasia of the Hip
- Case Study—Fractures
- Case Study—Osteomyelitis
- Critical Thinking Exercise—Osteogenic Sarcoma
- Skill—Monitoring Neurovascular Status

The Immobilized Child

One of the most difficult aspects of illness in children is the immobility it imposes. Children by nature are usually active, and immobility, however temporary, may have lasting effects on the child's developmental progress. The most frequent reasons for immobility are **congenital** defects (e.g., spina bifida); degenerative disorders (e.g., muscular dystrophy); and infections or injuries that impair the integumentary system (severe burns), the musculoskeletal system (e.g., multiple fractures, osteomyelitis), or the neurological system (e.g., spinal cord injury, Guillain-Barré syndrome, traumatic brain injury and coma). At times therapies such as traction and spinal fusion are responsible for prolonged immobilization, although the increasing trends in health care are early mobilization and discharge and outpatient treatment.

Physiological Effects of Immobilization

Many clinical studies, including space program research, have documented predictable consequences that occur after immobilization and the absence of gravitational force. Functional and metabolic responses to restricted movement can be noted in most of the body systems. Each has a direct influence on the child's **growth** and development because homeostatic mechanisms thrive on normal use and need feedback to maintain dynamic equilibrium. Inactivity leads to a decrease in the functional capabilities of the whole body as dramatically as the lack of physical exercise leads to muscle weakness.

Disuse from illness, injury, or a sedentary lifestyle can limit function and potentially delay age-appropriate milestones. Most of the pathological changes that occur during immobilization arise from decreased muscle strength and mass, decreased metabolism, and bone demineralization, which are closely interrelated, with one change leading to or affecting the other. Some results of immobilization are primary and produce a direct effect; other pathophysiological consequences occur frequently but seem to be more indirect and are thus secondary effects. Many pathophysiological changes affect more than one body system, with the primary or secondary effect being demonstrated in both systems.

The major effects of immobilization are outlined briefly in Table 54-1 and are related directly or indirectly to decreased

Table 54-1 Summary of Physical Effects of Immobilization*

PRIMARY EFFECTS	SECONDARY EFFECTS
Muscular System	
Decreased muscle strength, tone, and endurance	Decreased venous return and decreased cardiac output Decreased metabolism and need for oxygen Decreased exercise tolerance Bone demineralization
Disuse atrophy and loss of muscle mass	Catabolism Loss of strength
Loss of joint mobility	Contractures, ankylosis of joints
Weak back muscles	Secondary spinal deformities
Weak abdominal muscles	Impaired respiration
Skeletal System	
Bone demineralization—osteoporosis, hypercalcemia	Negative calcium balance Pathological fractures Calcium deposits Extraosseous bone formation, especially at hip, knee, elbow, and shoulder Renal calculi
Negative calcium balance	Life-threatening electrolyte imbalance
Metabolism	
Decreased metabolic rate	Slowing of all systems Decreased food intake
Negative nitrogen balance	Decline in nutritional state Impaired healing
Hypercalcemia	Electrolyte imbalance
Decreased production of stress hormones	Decreased physical and emotional coping capacity
Cardiovascular System	
Decreased efficiency of orthostatic neurovascular reflexes	Inability to adapt readily to upright position Pooling of blood in extremities in upright posture
Diminished vasopressor mechanism	Orthostatic hypotension (intolerance) with syncope—hypotension, decreased cerebral blood flow, tachycardia
Altered distribution of blood volume	Decreased cardiac workload Decreased exercise tolerance
Venous stasis	Systemic embolus or thrombus development, pulmonary emboli
Dependent edema	Tissue breakdown and susceptibility to infection
Respiratory System	
Decreased need for oxygen	Altered oxygen-carbon dioxide exchange and metabolism
Decreased chest expansion and diminished vital capacity	Diminished oxygen intake Dyspnea and inadequate arterial oxygen saturation; acidosis
Poor abdominal tone and distention	Interference with diaphragmatic excursion Hypostatic pneumonia
Mechanical or biochemical secretion retention	Bacterial and viral pneumonia Atelectasis
Loss of respiratory muscle strength	Poor cough Upper respiratory tract infection
Gastrointestinal System	
Distention caused by poor abdominal muscle tone	Interference with respiratory movements
No specific primary effect	Difficulty in feeding in prone position; gravitation effect on feces through ascending colon, or weakened smooth muscle tone causing constipation Decreased appetite Anorexia

*Not all problems will apply in every situation.

Continued

Table 54-1 Summary of Physical Effects of Immobilization—cont'd

PRIMARY EFFECTS	SECONDARY EFFECTS
Urinary System	
Alteration of gravitational force	Difficulty in voiding in prone position
Impaired ureteral peristalsis	Urinary retention in calyces and bladder Infection Renal calculi
Integumentary System	
No specific primary effect	Decreased circulation and pressure leading to tissue injury and decreased healing capacity Difficulty with personal hygiene

muscle activity, which produces numerous primary changes in the musculoskeletal system with secondary alterations in the cardiovascular, respiratory, metabolic, and renal systems. The musculoskeletal changes that occur during disuse are a result of alterations in gravity and stress on the muscles, joints, and bones. Muscle disuse leads to tissue breakdown and loss of muscle mass (*atrophy*). Muscle atrophy causes decreased strength and endurance, which may take weeks or months to restore.

During immobilization, a joint contracture begins when the arrangement of collagen, the main structural protein of connective tissues, is altered, resulting in a denser tissue that does not glide as easily. Eventually, muscles, tendons, and ligaments can shorten and reduce joint movement, ultimately producing contractures that restrict function. The daily stresses on bone created by motion and weight bearing maintain the balance between bone formation (osteoblastic activity) and bone resorption (osteoclastic activity). During immobilization, more calcium leaves the bone, causing osteopenia (demineralization of the bones), which may predispose bone to pathological fractures. The major musculoskeletal consequences of immobilization are (1) significant decrease in muscle size, strength, and endurance, (2) bone demineralization leading to osteoporosis, and (3) contractures and decreased joint mobility. The larger the portion of the body immobilized and the longer the immobilization, the greater the hazards of immobility.

Prolonged immobilization also causes venous stasis, particularly in the lower extremities; this may lead to thrombus formation, which in turn may obstruct vessels in organs such as the lungs, kidneys, or brain. Pulmonary embolus is a life-threatening complication of immobilization.

Psychological Effects of Immobilization

For children, one of the most difficult aspects of illness is immobilization. Throughout childhood, physical activity is an integral part of daily life and is essential for physical growth and development. The activity helps children deal with a variety of feelings and impulses and provides a mechanism by which they can exert control over inner tensions. Children respond to anxiety with increased activity. Removal of this power deprives them of necessary input and a natural outlet for their feelings and fantasies.

When children are immobilized by disease or as part of a treatment regimen, they experience diminished environmental stimuli with a loss of tactile input and an altered perception of themselves and their environment. Sudden or gradual immobilization narrows the amount and variety of environmental stimuli children receive by means of all of their senses: touch; sight; hearing; taste; smell; and *proprioception*, or the feeling of where they are in their environment. This sensory deprivation commonly leads to feelings of isolation and boredom and of being forgotten, especially by peers.

Physical interference with the activity of young children gives them a feeling of frustration and helplessness. Even speech and language skills require sensorimotor activity and experience. For the toddler, exploration and imitative behaviours are essential to developing a sense of autonomy; the preschooler's expression of initiative is evidenced by the need for vigorous physical activity; the school-age child's development is strongly influenced by physical achievement and competition; and the adolescent relies on mobility to achieve independence. The quest for mastery at every stage of development is related to mobility.

The monotony of immobilization can lead to sluggish intellectual and psychomotor responses, decreased communication skills, increased fantasizing, and even hallucinations and disorientation. Children are likely to become depressed over their loss of ability to function or any marked changes in body image. They may seek the attention of others by reverting to earlier developmental behaviours, such as wanting to be fed or bed-wetting.

Limbs in casts or traction transmit less than normal sensory data. Children who have limited ability to feel others touching them not only experience less tactile stimuli in a physical sense but are also deprived of warm, loving feelings that arise from being touched. The loss of feeling derived from touch can further add to their sense of being isolated and unwanted.

Children may react to immobility by active protest, anger, and aggressive behaviour; or they may become quiet, passive, and submissive. They may believe the immobilization is a justified punishment for misbehaviour. Children should be allowed to express their feelings, but it should be within the limits of safety to their self-esteem and not damaging to the integrity of others. For example, providing an inanimate object to attack rather than a person or a valued possession is safe and therapeutic. When children are unable to express anger and frustration, aggression is often displayed inappropriately through regressive behaviour and outbursts of crying or temper tantrums.

Effect on Families

Even brief periods of immobilization may disrupt family function, and sudden catastrophic illness or chronic disability may severely tax their resources and coping abilities.

The family's needs often must be met by the services of a multidisciplinary team, and nurses play a key role in anticipating the services they will need and in coordinating conferences to plan care. In preparation for discharge, home visits are advisable, and home management is commonly planned weeks in advance of the actual discharge. Such planning includes special considerations for cultural, economic, physical, and psychological needs. A child with a severe disability is very dependent, and caregivers need rest periods to revitalize themselves. Individual and group counselling is beneficial for solving problems in advance and provides an emotional support system. Parent groups may also be helpful and often allow nonthreatening social contact. The families of children with permanent disabilities need long-term resources because some of the most difficult problems arise as they try to sustain high-quality care for many years (see Chapter 41).

Nursing Care Management

Physical assessment of the child who is immobilized as a result of an injury or a degenerative disease focuses not only on the injured part (e.g., fracture or damaged joint) but also on the functioning of other systems that may be affected secondarily (e.g., the circulatory, renal, respiratory, muscular, and gastrointestinal systems). With long-term immobilization there may also be neurological impairment and changes in electrolytes (especially calcium), nitrogen balance, and the general metabolic rate. The psychological impact of immobilization should also be assessed.

Children who require prolonged total immobility and are unable to move themselves in bed should be placed on a special surface to prevent skin breakdown. Frequent position changes also help prevent dependent edema and stimulate circulation, respiratory function, gastrointestinal motility, and neurological sensation. Children at greater risk for skin breakdown include those with prolonged immobilization; orthotic and prosthetic devices, including wheelchairs; and plaster casts. Additional risk factors include poor nutrition, friction (from bed linen with traction), and moist skin (from urine or perspiration). In critically ill children, factors associated with increased skin breakdown included requirement for mechanical ventilation, age less than 2 years, length of stay of 4 days or more, and a respiratory diagnosis on admission (Schindler et al., 2007). In neonates and infants, skin breakdown is more likely to occur on the occiput and on the nasal septum when nasal continuous positive airway pressure devices are used (McCord et al., 2004; Razmus, Roberts, & Curley, 2001).

Nursing care of children at risk includes proactive strategies for preventing skin breakdown when such conditions are present. On admission, each child should have a skin assessment and a score documented in the medical record. The Modified Braden Q Scale for pediatrics is a reliable, objective tool that may be used in the assessment for pressure ulcer development in children who are acutely ill or who are at risk for skin breakdown from neurological conditions and immobilization (Curley et al., 2003). Frequent position changes help prevent dependent edema and stimulate circulation, respiratory function, gastrointestinal motility, and neurological sensations. Anti-embolism stockings or sequential compression devices (SCDs) also help minimize or prevent dependent edema in the lower extremities.

The child should be allowed as much activity as possible within the limitations of the illness or treatment. Most children have an innate ingenuity and natural inclination toward maximizing mobility. They need the opportunity, the materials or objects to stimulate activity, and the encouragement and participation of others. Those who are unable to move need passive exercise and movement, often in consultation with a physiotherapist.

When possible, transporting the child by stretcher, stroller, or wagon outside the confines of the room increases environmental stimuli and provides social contact with others. While hospitalized, children benefit from same-age visitors, computers, personal computer tablets, books, interactive video games, and other items brought from their own room at home, all of which help them function in a more normal way. An activity centre or tray that slants can be particularly helpful for the child with limited mobility to use for drawing, colouring, writing, and playing with small toys such as trucks and cars. A play therapist or child life specialist should be consulted for recreational planning. The use of play (see Chapter 44) and any activity that is tolerated (e.g., turning in bed or changing the location of the bed within the room) help alter the monotony of immobilization and decrease tension and frustration.

Using dolls, stuffed animals, or puppets to illustrate and explain the immobilization is a valuable tool for small children. Placing a cast, tubing, or other restraining equipment on the doll offers the child a nonthreatening opportunity to express, through the doll, feelings concerning the restrictions and feelings toward the nurse and other health care providers.

As soon as possible, hospitalized children should be allowed to wear their own clothes (street clothes, especially for preadolescent and adolescent girls) and resume school and previous activities. A parent or siblings should be allowed to stay overnight and room in with the hospitalized child to minimize the effects of family disruption from hospitalization. Visits from significant persons, such as family members and friends, offer occasions for emotional support and also provide opportunities for learning how to care for the child. If a traumatic incident caused the child's disability, guilt feelings may be displayed overtly or masked behind regressive or aggressive behaviour. The feeling that "I must have been bad for this to happen" is common, and honest feedback stating, "It just happened—it was an accident," needs to be repeated many times.

Some privacy is needed, particularly by the teenager, and most long-term health care facilities recognize that private or semiprivate rooms shared by one or two children are the best environment for rehabilitation. Within the framework of family-centred care, institutions are placing more emphasis on providing a room in which the child's parent may stay overnight and significant others may visit.

High-protein, high-calorie foods should be encouraged, to prevent negative nitrogen balance, which may be difficult to correct by diet, especially if there is **anorexia** as a result of immobility and decreased gastrointestinal function (decreased motility and possibly constipation). Stimulating the appetite with small servings of attractively arranged, preferred foods may be sufficient. Children typically dislike hospital food, which is usually not tailored to their age. In some institutions food services are geared toward children's preferences with child-friendly menus and smaller food portions served. Parents and friends should be allowed to bring in favourite foods from home or other sources such as fast food places, provided they meet necessary requirements for the illness. Allowing such choices enables children to exert more healthy control of their environment and subsequently decreases resistance to treatments and schedules, which is common behaviour evidenced when adults and children are not given any choices in an acute care setting. Sometimes, supplementary nasogastric or gastrostomy feedings or intravenous (IV) fluids may be needed, but these are reserved for serious disability in which oral intake is impossible.

One of the most useful interventions to help children cope with immobility is participation in their own self-care. They can help plan their daily routine; select their diet (when possible); and choose clothes, including innovative adornments such as baseball caps, brightly decorated sunglasses, or brightly coloured stockings, to express their autonomy and individuality. They should be encouraged to do as much as they are able to for themselves to keep muscles active and their interest alive. Most of children's activity of daily living is play; therapies that incorporate play will involve children more in their own care.

With the increased trend toward early mobilization, early discharge, and home health care, many children are discharged home within a few hours or days of hospitalization. Follow-up treatment may take place in the home setting or an outpatient ambulatory facility. Although most of the suggestions discussed in this chapter relate to hospital care, the same consultations (physiotherapist, occupational therapist, child life specialist, and speech therapist) and environment may be considered in the home as well to help the child and family achieve independence and **normalization**.

Family Support and Home Care

The needs of a child with severe or chronic disabilities can be complex, and although the optimal situation is for family members to have time to assimilate the teachings and demonstrations needed to understand the child's situation and care, this is often shortened considerably by moving the child to a rehabilitation facility or even to the home within a matter of days. Even the child who is confined on a short-term basis can be a challenge for the family, which is usually unprepared for the problems imposed by the child's special needs. Home modification is usually needed for facilitating care, especially when it involves traction, large casts, or extended confinement (see Chapter 43). Suitable child care may be needed for times when all family members work.

Just as in the hospital, the child at home should be encouraged to be as independent as possible and to follow a schedule that approximates his or her normal lifestyle as nearly as possible, such as continuing school lessons, regular bedtime, and suitable recreational activities.

Traumatic Injury

Soft-Tissue Injury

Injuries to the muscles, ligaments, and tendons are common in children (Fig. 54-1). In young children, soft-tissue injury usually results from mishaps during play. In older children and adolescents, participation in sports is the more common cause.

Contusions

A *contusion* is damage to the soft tissue, subcutaneous structures, and muscle. The tearing of these tissues and small blood vessels and the inflammatory response lead to hemorrhage, **edema**, and associated pain when the child attempts to move the injured part. The escape of blood into the tissues is observed as *ecchymosis*, a black-and-blue discolouration.

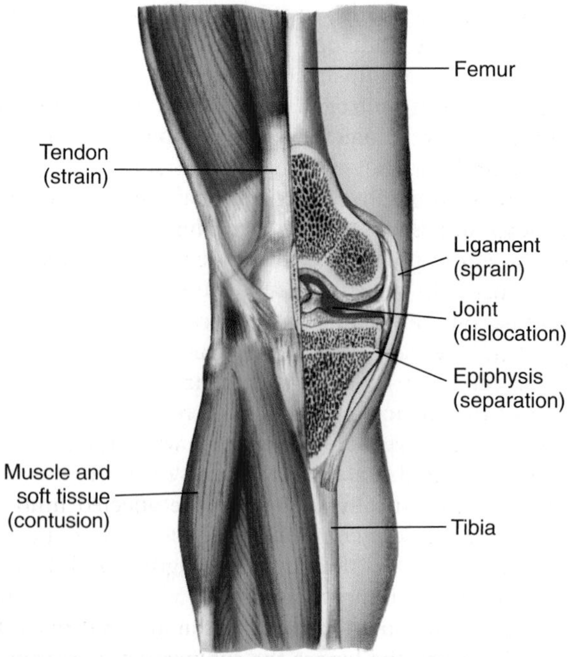

Fig. 54-1 Sites of injuries to bones, joints, and soft tissues.

Large contusions cause gross swelling, pain, and disability, and those sustained while the child is participating in sports usually receive immediate attention from health personnel. Smaller injuries may go unnoticed, allowing continued participation; however, they can become disabling after rest because of pain and muscle spasm. The young athlete is commonly instructed to "walk it off" or disregard the pain. Instead, a qualified health care worker or certified athletic trainer should carry out an assessment of the affected area because further damage to the site may result if the area is severely traumatized. Immediate treatment consists of cold application, as described in the section on sprains (see below). Return to participation is allowed when the strength and range of motion of the affected extremity are equal to those of the opposite extremity. *Myositis ossificans* may occur from deep contusions to the biceps or quadriceps muscles; this condition may result in a restriction of flexibility of the affected limb.

Contusions are crush injuries that occur in children when they slam their fingers (in doors, folding chairs, or equipment) or hit their fingers (as when hammering a nail). A severe crush injury involves the bone, with swelling and bleeding beneath the nail (subungual) and sometimes laceration of the pulp of the distal phalanx. The subungual hematoma can be released by creating a hole at the proximal end of the nail with a battery-operated microcautery device or a heated sterile 18-gauge needle.

Dislocations

Long bones are held in approximation to one another at the joint by ligaments. A dislocation occurs when the force of stress on the ligament is so great as to displace the normal position of the opposing bone ends or to displace the bone end from its socket. The predominant symptom is pain that increases with attempted passive or active movement of the extremity. In dislocations there may be an obvious deformity and inability to move the joint. Dislocation of the phalanges is the most common type seen in children, followed by elbow dislocation.

One of the most common injuries in young children is subluxation of the annular ligament, also called *pulled elbow* or *nursemaids' elbow*. With this injury the annular ligament slips proximally off the radial head into the joint between the radial head and ulna, causing immediate pain and limited supination (Cornwall, 2007). In most cases the injury occurs in a child between the ages of 1 and 3 who receives a sudden longitudinal pull or traction at the wrist while the arm is fully extended and the forearm pronated. It usually occurs when an adult or older sibling who is holding the child by the hand or wrist gives a sudden pull or jerk to prevent a fall or attempts to lift the child by pulling the wrist, or when the child pulls away by dropping to the floor or ground. The child often cries, appears anxious, and refuses to use the affected limb. The practitioner manipulates the arm by applying firm finger pressure to the head of the radius, then supinates and flexes the forearm to return the ligament to its place. A click may be heard or felt, and functional use of the arm returns within minutes. However, the longer the subluxation is present, the longer it takes for the child to recover mobility after treatment. No anaesthetic is usually required but a mild pain reliever such as acetaminophen may be given. In an older child, severe elbow injury or dislocation should be carefully evaluated by a practitioner immediately; likewise, a traumatic elbow injury in the younger child that is not a subluxation should be carefully evaluated.

In children younger than 5 years of age, the hip can be dislocated by a fall. The greatest risk after this injury is the potential loss of blood supply to the head of the femur. Relocation of the hip within 60 minutes after the injury provides the best chance for prevention of damage to the femoral head.

Shoulder dislocations occur most often in older adolescents and are often sports related. In a shoulder dislocation, temporary restriction of the joint, with a sling or bandage that secures the arm to the chest can provide sufficient comfort and immobilization until medical attention is received.

Simple dislocations should be reduced as soon as possible with the child under mild (procedural) sedation and often local anaesthesia. Anaesthetics such as IV ketamine (Ketalar), midazolam (Versed), IV propofol (Diprivan), or fentanyl (Sublimaze) can be used to produce partial or complete analgesia. An unreduced dislocation will be complicated by increased swelling, making reduction difficult and increasing the risk of neurovascular problems. Treatment depends on the severity of the injury.

Sprains

A *sprain* occurs when trauma to a joint is so severe that a ligament is partially or completely torn or stretched by the force created as a joint is twisted or wrenched, often accompanied by damage to associated blood vessels, muscles, tendons, and nerves. Sprains can be graded as follows: grade 1 sprain has minimal pain with damage to the ligaments; grade 2 sprain has more ligament damage and mild joint looseness; and grade 3 has a complete tearing of the ligament with a very loose or unstable joint (About Kids Health, 2004).

The presence of joint laxity is the most valid indicator of the severity of a sprain. In a severe injury the child may describe the joint as "feeling loose" or as if "something is coming apart" and may describe hearing a "snap," "pop," or "tearing." Pain is seldom the principal subjective symptom. There is a rapid onset with swelling (often diffuse), accompanied by immediate disability and appreciable reluctance to use the injured joint.

Strains

A *strain* is a microscopic tear to the musculotendinous unit and has features in common with sprains. The area is painful to touch and swollen. Most strains are incurred over time rather than suddenly, and the rapidity of the appearance provides clues regarding severity. In general, the more rapidly the strain occurs, the more severe the injury. When the strain involves the muscular portion, there is more bleeding, often palpable soon after injury and before edema obscures the hematoma.

Therapeutic Management

The first 6 to12 hours are the most critical period for virtually all soft-tissue injuries. Basic principles of managing sprains and other soft-tissue injuries are summarized in the acronyms *RICE* and *ICES*:

R—Rest	**I**—Ice
I—Ice	**C**—Compression
C—Compression	**E**—Elevation
E—Elevation	**S**—Support

Soft-tissue injuries should be iced immediately. This is best accomplished with crushed ice wrapped in a towel or encased in a screw-top ice bag or resealable storage bag. A plastic bag of frozen vegetables, such as peas, serves as a convenient ice pack for soft-tissue injuries. It is clean, watertight, and easily moulded to the injured part. When available, snow placed in a plastic bag may serve as an ice bag. A wet elastic wrap, which transfers cold better than dry wrap, is applied to provide compression and to keep the ice pack in place. Chemical-activated ice packs are also effective for immediate treatment but are not reusable and must be closely monitored for leakage. A cloth barrier should be used between the ice container and the skin to prevent trauma to the tissues. Ice has a rapid cooling effect on tissues and reduces the pain threshold. Ice therapy should be intermittent and should never be applied for more than 30 minutes at a time because of the body's homeostatic response to cold, which may trigger a decrease in vascularization at the injury site.

Elevating the extremity uses gravity to facilitate venous return and to reduce edema formation in the damaged area. The point of injury should be kept several inches above the level of the heart for therapy to be effective. Several pillows can be used for elevation. Allowing the extremity to be dependent causes excessive fluid accumulation in the area of injury, delaying healing and causing painful swelling.

Torn ligaments, especially those in the knee, are usually treated by immobilization with a knee immobilizer or range-of-motion brace until the child is able to walk without a limp. Crutches are used for mobility to rest the affected extremity. Passive leg exercises, gradually increased to active ones, are begun as soon as sufficient healing has taken place. Parents and children should be cautioned against using any form of liniment or other heat-producing preparation before examination. If the injury requires casting or splinting, the heat generated in the enclosed space can cause extreme discomfort and may even cause tissue damage. In some cases torn knee ligaments are managed with arthroscopy and ligament repair or reconstruction as necessary, depending on the extent of the tear, the ligaments involved, and the child's age. Surgical reconstruction of the anterior cruciate ligament may be performed in young athletes who wish to continue in active sports.

evolve Animation—Bone Fractures
evolve Case Study—Fractures

Fractures

Bone fractures occur when the resistance of bone against the stress being exerted yields to the stress force. Fractures are a common injury at any age but are more likely to occur in children and older adults. Because childhood is a time of rapid bone growth, the pattern of fractures, problems of diagnosis, and methods of treatment differ in the child and the adult. In children fractures heal much faster than in adults. Consequently, children may not require as long a period of immobilization of the affected extremity as an adult with a fracture.

Fracture injuries in children are most often a result of traumatic incidents at home, at school, in a motor vehicle, or in association with recreational activities. Children's everyday activities include vigorous play that predisposes them to injury—climbing, falling down, running into immovable objects, skateboarding, and receiving blows to any part of their bodies.

Aside from automobile accidents or falls from heights, true injuries that cause fractures rarely occur in infancy; thus bone injury in children of that age group warrants further investigation. In any small child, radiographic evidence of fractures at various stages of healing is, with few exceptions, a result of physical abuse. Any investigation of fractures in infants, particularly multiple fractures, should include consideration of osteogenesis imperfecta.

The clavicle is probably the bone most commonly broken in childhood, with approximately half of clavicle fractures occurring in children under 10 years of age. Common mechanisms of injury include a fall with an outstretched hand or direct trauma to the bone.

Fractures in school-age children are often a result of bicycle, automobile, or skateboard injuries. Adolescents are vulnerable to multiple and severe trauma because they are active in sports and mobile on bicycles, all-terrain vehicles, skateboards, skis, snowboards, bicycles, and motorcycles.

Epiphyseal (or Physeal) Injuries

The weakest point of long bones is the cartilage growth plate, or epiphyseal plate. Consequently, this is a common site of damage during trauma. Detection of epiphyseal injuries is sometimes difficult, but it is critical. Fractures involving the epiphysis or epiphyseal plate present special problems in determining whether bone growth will be affected. Treatment of these fractures may include open reduction and internal fixation to prevent or reduce growth disturbances.

Types of Fractures

A fractured bone consists of fragments—the fragment closer to the midline, or the *proximal* fragment; and the fragment farther from the midline, or the *distal* fragment. When fracture fragments are separated, the fracture is *complete*; when fragments remain attached, the fracture is *incomplete*. The fracture line can be any of the following:

Transverse—Crosswise, at right angles to the long axis of the bone

Oblique—Slanting but straight, between a horizontal and a perpendicular direction

Spiral—Slanting and circular, twisting around the bone shaft

The twisting of an extremity while the bone is breaking results in a spiral break. If the fracture does not produce a break in the skin, it is a *simple*, or *closed, fracture*. *Open*, or *compound, fractures* are those with an open wound through which the bone is or has protruded. If the bone fragments cause damage to other organs or tissues (such as the lung or bladder), the injury is said to be a *complicated fracture*. When small fragments of bone are broken from the fractured shaft and lie in the surrounding tissue, the injury is a *comminuted fracture*. This type of fracture is rare in children. The types of fractures seen most often in children are described in Box 54-1 and in Fig. 54-2.

Immediately after a fracture occurs, the muscles contract and physiologically splint the injured area. This phenomenon accounts for the muscle tightness observed over a fracture site and the deformity that is produced as the muscles pull the bone ends out of alignment. This muscle response must be overcome by traction or complete muscle relaxation (e.g., with anaesthesia) in order to realign the distal bone fragment to the proximal bone fragment.

BOX 54-1 Types of Fractures in Children

Plastic deformation—Occurs when the bone is bent but not broken. A child's flexible bone can be bent 45 degrees or more before breaking. However, if bent, the bone will straighten slowly, but not completely, to produce some deformity but without the angulation seen when the bone breaks. Bends occur most commonly in the ulna and fibula, often in association with fractures of the radius and tibia.

Buckle, or torus, fracture—Produced by compression of the porous bone; appears as a raised or bulging projection at the fracture site. These fractures occur in the most porous portion of the bone near the metaphysis (the portion of the bone shaft adjacent to the epiphysis) and are more common in young children.

Greenstick fracture—Occurs when a bone is angulated beyond the limits of bending. The compressed side bends, and the tension side fails, causing an incomplete fracture similar to the break observed when a green stick is broken.

Complete fracture—Divides the bone fragments. These fragments often remain attached by a periosteal hinge, which can aid or hinder reduction.

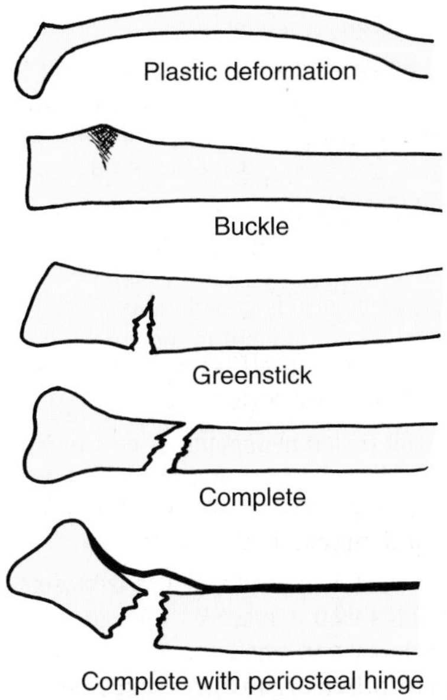

Fig. 54-2 Types of fractures in children.

Bone Healing and Remodelling

Bone healing is characteristically rapid in children because of the thickened periosteum and generous blood supply. When there is a break in the continuity of bone, the osteoblasts are stimulated to maximum activity. New bone cells are formed in immense numbers almost immediately after the injury and, in time, are evidenced by a bulging growth of new bone tissue between the fractured bone fragments. This is followed by deposition of calcium salts to form a callus.

Fractures heal in less time in children than in adults. The approximate healing times for a femoral shaft are as follows:

Neonatal period—2 to 3 weeks
Early childhood—4 weeks
Later childhood—6 to 8 weeks
Adolescence—8 to 12 weeks

Diagnostic Evaluation

A history is often lacking in childhood injuries. Infants are unable to communicate, and older children seldom volunteer information (even under direct questioning) when the injury occurred during suspicious activities. Unless they are witnesses to the injury, parents may misinterpret what the child is trying to say. In cases of child abuse, parents may give false information to protect themselves.

The child may exhibit the same manifestations seen in adults (Box 54-2). However, often a fracture is remarkably stable because of an intact periosteum. The child may even be able to use an affected arm or walk on a fractured leg. In some cases, however, a fracture may not be apparent on radiographs. A fracture should be strongly suspected in a small child who refuses to bear weight or walk.

Radiographic examination is the most useful diagnostic tool for assessing skeletal trauma. The calcium deposits in bone make the entire structure radiopaque. Radiographic films are taken after fracture reduction and, in some cases, may be taken during the healing process to determine satisfactory progress.

Therapeutic Management

The majority of children's fractures heal well, and nonunion is rare. Most fractures are readily reduced by simple traction and

BOX 54-2 Clinical Manifestations of a Fracture

Signs of injury:
- Generalized swelling
- Pain or tenderness
- Diminished functional use of affected part

May be:
- Bruising
- Severe muscular rigidity
- Crepitus (grating sensation at fracture site)

immobilization until healing takes place. However, the position of the bone fragments in relation to one another influences the rapidity of healing and the residual deformity. Healing is prompt and complete with end-to-end apposition, but a gap between fragments delays (or prevents) healing. The goals of fracture management are as follows:

- To regain alignment and length of the bony fragments (reduction)
- To retain alignment and length (immobilization)
- To restore function to the injured parts
- To prevent further injury

In children the bone fragments are usually realigned and immobilized by traction or by closed manipulation and casting until an adequate callus is formed. Weight bearing on lower extremity fractures and active movement for the purpose of regaining function can begin after the fracture site is stable. The child's natural tendency to be active is usually sufficient to restore normal mobility, and physiotherapy is rarely needed. In most cases children's fractures can be managed by closed reduction and cast immobilization, which is most often provided on an outpatient basis with re-evaluation in 7 to 10 days.

Children are most frequently hospitalized for fractures of the femur and the supracondylar area of the distal humerus, which may require internal fixation and pinning; displaced supracondylar fractures in children should be treated surgically (Do & Herrera-Soto, 2003; Shrader, 2008). Fractures of the humerus, which usually result from a fall with the arm in extension, frequently involve the supracondylar portion. These fractures especially place the patient at risk for nerve damage and angulation deformities; thus most children with a fractured humerus are taken to surgery for either a closed or open reduction with a percutaneous pinning of the fractured bone segments. Preoperatively the fracture is reduced with adequate analgesia and a temporary splint for immobilization.

If simple reductions cannot be achieved or if a neurovascular problem is detected after injury, observation in a hospital is indicated. Severe contusions with profound swelling cannot be treated with a cast, which would act as a tourniquet on the extremity. A badly malaligned fracture requires traction for a period before a cast is applied.

Wrist buckle fractures are common in a child who falls and extends the arm forward to break the fall. There are reports of radius or ulna buckle fractures in children treated with a removable splint for 3 to 4 weeks instead of a short arm cast (Plint et al., 2006). The children treated with removable splints had better wrist function, had adequate bone healing, and experienced less inconvenience for bathing compared with the group of children placed in a short arm cast.

The major methods for immobilizing a fracture—casting and traction—are described in the following sections.

Nursing Care Management

Nurses are frequently the persons who make the initial assessment of a child with a suspected fracture (see Emergency box). The child and parents may be frightened and upset, and the child is often in pain. Therefore, if the child is alert and there is no evidence of hemorrhage, the initial nursing interventions are directed toward calming and reassuring the child and parents so that a more extensive assessment can be more easily accomplished.

The child may arrive with the limb supported in some manner; if not, careful support or immobilization may be provided to the affected site. In the event that the limb is supported or immobilized, it may be best not to touch the child but to ask him or her to point to the painful area and to wiggle the fingers or toes. By this time the child may feel relatively safe and will allow someone to gently touch the area just enough to feel the pulse and test for sensation. A child's anxiety is greatly influenced by previous experiences with injury and with health personnel; he or she needs to be told what will happen and what to do to help. The affected limb need not be palpated, and it should not be moved unless properly splinted. If the child is at home or if the practitioner is not present to examine the child, some type of splint should be applied carefully for transport to the medical facility. Parental anxiety may be heightened by the child's pain reaction and fear, and possibly other events surrounding the accident; thus it is important to communicate to the parents that the child will receive the necessary care, including pain management.

The Child in a Cast

The completeness of the fracture, the type of bone involved, and the amount of weight bearing influence how much of the extremity must be included in the cast to immobilize the fracture site completely. In most cases the joints above and below the fracture are immobilized to eliminate the possibility of movement that might cause displacement at the fracture site. Four major categories of casts are used for fractures: *upper*

EMERGENCY

Fracture

Assess the extent of injury and the Five Ps of ischemia assessment
1. **P**ain and point of tenderness
2. **P**ulses present—Distal to the fracture site
3. **P**allor
4. **P**aresthesia—Sensation distal to the fracture site
5. **P**aralysis—Movement distal to the fracture site

Determine the mechanism of injury.
Move the injured part as little as possible.
Cover open wounds with a sterile or clean dressing.
Immobilize the limb, including joints above and below the fracture site; do not attempt to reduce the fracture or push protruding bone under the skin.
- Soft splint (pillow or folded towel)
- Rigid splint (rolled newspaper or magazine)
- Uninjured leg can serve as a splint for a leg fracture if no splint is available

Reassess neurovascular status.
Apply traction if circulatory compromise is present.
Elevate the injured limb if possible.
Apply cold to the injured area.
Call emergency medical services or transport patient to medical facility.

extremity to immobilize the wrist or elbow, *lower extremity* to immobilize the ankle or knee, *spinal* and *cervical* for immobilization of the spine, and *spica* casts to immobilize the hip and knee.

The Cast

Casts are constructed from gauze strips and bandages impregnated with plaster of paris or, more commonly, from synthetic lighter weight and water-resistant materials (e.g., fibreglass and polyurethane resin).

Both types of casting produce heat from the chemical reaction activated by water immediately after application. Plaster casts mould closely to the body part, take several hours to dry, have a smooth exterior, and are inexpensive. The newer synthetic casting material is lighter, dries in 5 to 30 minutes, permits earlier weight bearing, and is water resistant. The disadvantage of synthetic casting is its inability to mould closely to body parts; its rough exterior, which may scratch surfaces; and increased cost.

Synthetic casts have special advantages for children. They come in different colours and with designs (e.g., cartoons, stripes); they are lightweight, durable, easy to clean, and relatively water resistant, depending on the type of inner lining used; only those with a Gore-Tex inner lining may be immersed in water without affecting the cast integrity. Bathing with a synthetic cast may be accomplished by covering the cast with a plastic bag; if the synthetic cast gets wet, it should be dried thoroughly. One drawback to immersion is the time necessary to completely dry the cast. The synthetic casts are difficult to write on. A waterproof marker or colour markers may be used for writing on the cast.

Cast Application

The child's developmental age should be considered before the cast is applied. For preschoolers who fear bodily harm and fantasize about the loss of an extremity, it may be helpful to use a plastic doll or stuffed animal to explain the procedure beforehand. Toddlers and preschoolers do not have easily defined body boundaries; if an extremity is wrapped in a bandage, cast, or splint, to the young child the extremity often ceases to exist. It is also helpful to explain that some synthetic cast material will become warm but will not burn. During the application of the cast various distraction methods can be used, including discussing favourite pets or activities at school, blowing bubbles, and so forth. In this age group explanations such as "This will help your arm get better" are futile because the child has no concept of causality.

Before the cast is applied, the extremities are checked for any abrasions, cuts, or other alterations in the skin surface, and rings or other items that might cause constriction from swelling are removed. The skin may be protected by a cloth stockinette or cotton batting, which is applied liberally to the area to be casted. Particular attention is given to bony prominences, which are padded with extra cotton batting. Some practitioners use a Gore-Tex liner under a hip spica cast to prevent continuous exposure to moisture and possible skin breakdown.

Nursing Care Management

The complete evaporation of the water from a hip spica cast can take 24 to 48 hours when older types of plaster materials are used. Fibreglass cast material dries within minutes. The cast must remain uncovered to allow it to dry from the inside out. Turning the child in a plaster cast at least every 2 hours will help dry a body cast evenly and prevent complications related to immobility. A regular fan or cool-air hair dryer to circulate air may be helpful when the humidity is high.

Heated fans or dryers are not used because they cause the cast to dry on the outside and remain wet beneath or cause burns from heat conduction by way of the cast to the underlying tissue.

A wet plaster cast should be supported by a pillow that is covered with plastic and handled by the palms of the hands to avoid indenting the cast, which can create pressure areas. A dry plaster-of-paris cast produces a hollow sound when it is tapped with the finger. If "hot spots" are felt on the cast surface (usually indicating infection beneath the area), this should be reported so that a window can be made in the cast to observe the site.

During the first few hours after a cast is applied, the chief concern is that the extremity may continue to swell to the extent that the cast becomes a tourniquet, shutting off circulation and producing neurovascular complications. To prevent swelling, elevation of the body part increases venous return. If edema is excessive, casts are bivalved (i.e., cut to make anterior and posterior halves that are held together with an elastic bandage). The cast and the involved extremity need to be observed frequently for neurovascular integrity and any signs of compromise. Permanent muscle and tissue damage can occur within 6 to 8 hours.

NURSING ALERT Observations such as pain (unrelieved by pain medication 1 hour after administration), swelling, discolouration (pallor or cyanosis) of the exposed portions, decreased pulses, decreased temperature, or the inability to move the distal exposed part(s) should be reported immediately.

When an extremity that has sustained an open fracture is casted, a window is often left over the wound area to allow for observation and for dressing of the wound or a splint is used temporarily to allow for observation before casting. For the first few hours after surgery, there may be substantial bleeding that will soak through the cast. Periodically the circumscribed blood-stained area should be outlined with a ball-point pen or pencil and the time indicated to provide a guide for assessing the amount of bleeding.

Usually the child is discharged to home care after a cast is applied in the emergency department or clinic. Parents need instructions on drying and caring for the cast and on checking for signs and symptoms that indicate the cast is too tight or is too loose (see Patient Teaching box). A cast is a badge of honour for the child and serves as visible evidence of an otherwise invisible injury.

Nurses can help families adapt the child's home environment. Home care creates problems especially for children in large casts (e.g., a hip spica). Commonplace situations can become problematic (e.g., transporting a child safely and comfortably in a car). Standard seat belts and car seats may not be readily adapted for use by children in some casts and may

PATIENT TEACHING Cast Care

Keep the casted extremity elevated on pillows or similar support for the first day, or as directed by the health care provider.
Avoid denting the plaster cast with fingertips (use palms of hand to handle) while it is still wet to avoid creating pressure points.
Observe the extremities (fingers or toes) for any evidence of swelling or discolouration (darker or lighter than a comparable extremity), and contact the health care provider if noted.
Check movement and sensation of the visible extremities frequently.
Follow the health care provider's orders regarding any restriction of activities.
Restrict strenuous activities for the first few days.
- Engage in quiet activities but encourage use of muscles.
- Move the joints above and below the cast on the affected extremity.

Encourage frequent rest for a few days, keeping the injured extremity elevated while resting.
Avoid allowing the affected limb to hang in a dependent position for any length of time.
- Keep an injured upper extremity elevated (e.g., in a sling) while upright.
- Elevate a lower limb when sitting and avoid standing for too long.

Do not allow the child to put anything inside the cast. Keep small items that might be placed inside the cast away from small children.
Keep a clear path for ambulation. Remove toys, hazardous floor rugs, pets, or other items the child might stumble over.
Use crutches appropriately if lower limb fracture requires non-weight bearing on affected extremity.
The crutches should fit properly, have a soft rubber tip to prevent slipping, and be well padded at the axilla.
With crutch walking, the child's body weight is supported on the hand grips, not the axilla.

require special seating. The adaptations must meet specific Canadian safety regulations (see Additional Resources at the end of this chapter). Alterations to standard car seats to accommodate the cast are not recommended because the structure may be adversely altered and fail to properly restrain the child.

Parents need to be taught the proper care of the cast (or immobilization device) and helped to devise means for maintaining cleanliness. With a hip spica cast, a superabsorbent disposable diaper (newborn size) may be tucked beneath the entire perineal opening of the cast. A larger (toddler size) diaper can be applied and fastened over the small diaper and cast.

For tightly fitting casts, transparent film dressings can be cut into strips for petalling which keeps the cast dry and prevents crumbling. It allows the observation of skin beneath the dressing. Older infants and small children may stuff bits of food, small toys, or other items under the cast; parents should be alerted to this possibility so that suitable preventive measures can be initiated.

Feeding the infant in a hip spica cast offers problems in positioning. Very young infants can be fed in the supine position with the head elevated; with the infant's hips and legs supported on a pillow at the side, the parent can cuddle the infant in his or her arms during feeding. A somewhat similar position can be used for breastfeeding (i.e., with the infant supported on pillows or held in a "football" hold facing the mother with the legs behind her).

Children in spica casts may find the prone position easier for self-feeding from a small table placed next to the dining table. Small bedpans or other containers offer alternatives to a toilet for elimination. The nurse may suggest waterproofing methods, using plastic wraps that can help with elimination and showers. Baths are possible only if the plaster cast is kept out of the water and covered to prevent it from becoming wet from splashes.

Cast Removal

Cutting the cast to remove it or to relieve tightness is frequently a frightening experience for children. They fear the sound of the cast cutter and are terrified that their flesh, as well as the cast, will be cut. The oscillating blade vibrates rapidly back and forth and will not cut when placed *lightly* on the skin. Children have described it as producing a "tickly" sensation. The vibration also generates heat that may be felt by the child. Both of these feelings should be explained. Many young children come to regard the cast as part of themselves, which intensifies their fear of removal (Fig. 54-3). Preparation for the procedure will help reduce anxiety, especially if a trusting relationship has been established between the child and the nurse. Using the analogy of having fingernails trimmed or a haircut sometimes helps reduce their anxiety. They need continual reassurance that all is going well and they are helping things go well.

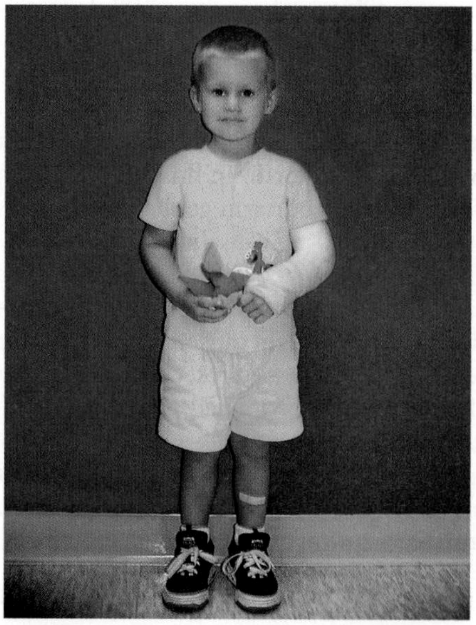

Fig. 54-3 Young children usually adapt well to a cast but often fear the removal.

After the cast is removed, the skin surface will be caked with desquamated skin and sebaceous secretions. Simple soaking in a bathtub is usually sufficient for their removal, but several days may be required to eliminate the accumulation completely. Application of oil or skin lotion may provide comfort. The parents and child should be instructed not to pull or forcibly remove this material with vigorous scrubbing because it may cause excoriation and bleeding.

The Child in Traction

The ever-changing health care arena has witnessed the demise of many long-term treatments involving lengthy hospitalization; one such change is in the area of traction. Most balanced skeletal traction is applied in children after a severe or complex injury to allow physiological stabilization, align bone fragments, and permit closer evaluation of the injured site. Newer technology has produced orthopedic fixation devices that allow partial or full mobility, thus preventing long-term immobilization and its consequences. In many situations, surgical intervention may be carried out within a matter of days; thus skeletal traction devices described here may be used infrequently or only for very short periods.

Purposes of Traction

The three essential components of traction management are traction, countertraction, and friction (Fig. 54-4). To reduce or realign a fracture site, *traction* (forward force) is produced by attaching weight to the distal bone fragment; body weight provides *countertraction* (backward force); and the patient's contact with the bed constitutes the *frictional* force. These forces are used to align the distal and proximal bone fragments by adjusting the line of pull upward or downward and adducting or abducting the extremity.

To attain equilibrium, the amount of forward force is adjusted by adding weight to or subtracting weight from the traction, and countertraction can be increased by elevating the foot of the bed to create a greater gravitational pull to the backward force.

The four primary purposes of traction for reduction of fractures are to do the following:

1. Fatigue the involved muscle and reduce muscle spasm so that bones can be realigned
2. Position the distal and proximal bone ends in desired realignment to promote satisfactory bone healing
3. Immobilize the fracture site until realignment has been achieved and sufficient healing has taken place to permit casting or surgical fixation
4. Allow preoperative or postoperative positioning and alignment, or both

The *all-or-none law*, characteristic of muscle contractibility, influences the complete relaxation. When muscle is stretched, muscle spasm ceases and permits the realignment of the bone ends. The continuous maintenance of traction is important during this phase because releasing the traction allows the normal contracting ability of the muscle to again cause a malpositioning of the bone ends.

The realignment of the fragments is a gradual process that is achieved more rapidly in infants, who have limited muscle tone, than in muscular teenagers. The desired line of pull and callus formation are checked periodically by radiographic examination. The traction pull to some degree immobilizes the fracture site; however, adjunctive immobilizing devices such as splints or casts are sometimes used with skeletal traction. In injuries in which there is severe soft-tissue swelling or vascular and nerve damage, traction may be used until these complications have been resolved and it is safe to apply a cast or to perform surgical fixation. Immobilization with traction will be maintained until the bone ends are in satisfactory realignment, after which a less confining type of immobilization—a cast, pins, or external stabilization device—will be applied.

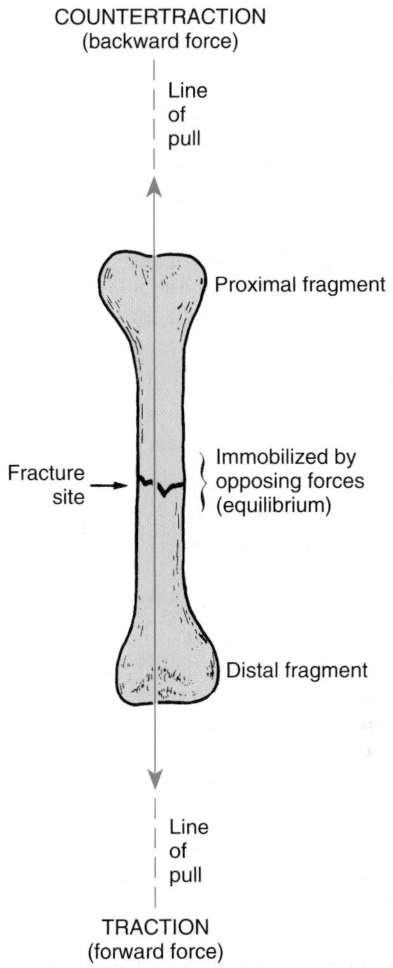

Fig. 54-4 Application of traction for maintaining equilibrium.

Types of Traction (General)

The pull needed for traction can be applied to the distal bone fragment in several ways (Box 54-3). The type of traction applied is determined primarily by the child's age, the condition of the soft tissues, and the type and degree of displacement of the fracture. Fractures most commonly treated by the application of traction are those involving the femur and vertebrae. The major types of traction for specific fractures are discussed in the following sections.

Upper Extremity Traction

The use of upper extremity traction in children is uncommon. Newer surgical techniques allow for early mobilization and optimal results without traction. Nursing care of the child with upper extremity traction is the same as that for lower extremity traction, which is discussed below.

Lower Extremity Traction

The severity of the fracturing force and the ability of the muscles to hold the fracture out of alignment will determine the fracture type and the amount of overriding of the fragments. The periosteum may remain intact, which helps maintain alignment. A fracture in the middle third of the shaft of the femur results in significant overriding but minimal displacement. In a fracture in the lower third of the shaft, the pull of the gastrocnemius muscle causes the distal fragment to become downwardly displaced.

Fractures of the femur can often be reduced with immediate application of a hip spica cast in young children. When traction is required, several types may be used, based on the initial assessment.

Bryant's traction is a type of running traction in which the pull is in only one direction. Skin traction is applied to the legs, which are flexed at a 90-degree angle at the hips. The child's trunk (with the buttocks raised slightly off the bed) provides countertraction.

Buck's extension is a type of skin traction with the legs in an extended position. Except for fracture cases, turning from side to side with care is permitted to maintain the involved leg alignment. Buck's extension is used primarily for short-term immobilization, preoperatively with dislocated hips, for correcting contractures, or for bone deformities such as Legg-Calvé-Perthes disease.

Russell traction uses skin traction on the lower leg and a padded sling under the knee. Two lines of pull, one along the longitudinal line of the lower leg and one perpendicular to the leg, are produced. This combination of pulls allows realignment of the lower extremity and immobilizes the hip and knee in a flexed position. The hip flexion must be kept at the prescribed angle to prevent fracture malalignment, since there is no direct support under the fracture and the skin traction may slip. Special nursing measures include carefully checking the position of the traction so that the amount of desired hip flexion is maintained and damage to the common peroneal nerve under the knee does not produce footdrop.

One of the most common types of skeletal traction is *90-degree–90-degree traction* (90-90 traction) (Fig. 54-5). The lower leg is supported by a boot cast or a calf sling, and a skeletal Steinmann pin or Kirschner's wire is placed in the distal fragment of the femur, resulting in a 90-degree angle at both the hip and the knee. From a nursing standpoint, this traction facilitates position changes, toileting, and prevention of complications related to traction.

Balance suspension traction (Fig. 54-6) may be used with or without skin or skeletal traction. Unless used with another traction, the balanced suspension merely suspends the leg in a desired flexed position to relax the hip and hamstring muscles and does not exert any traction directly on a body part. A *Thomas ring splint* extends from the groin to midair above the foot, and a *Pearson attachment* supports the lower leg. When the child is lifted off the bed, the traction lifts with the child without loss of alignment. This traction requires very careful checking of splints and ropes to make certain that no slippage or fraying has occurred. The traction is of great value in an older and heavier child when it is essential to lift the patient for care.

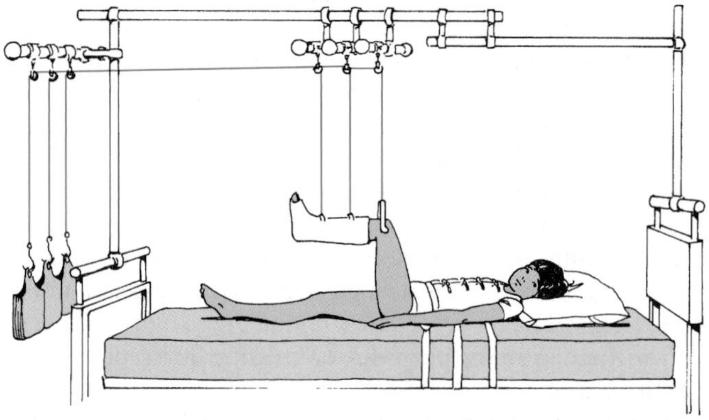

Fig. 54-5 "Ninety-ninety" traction.

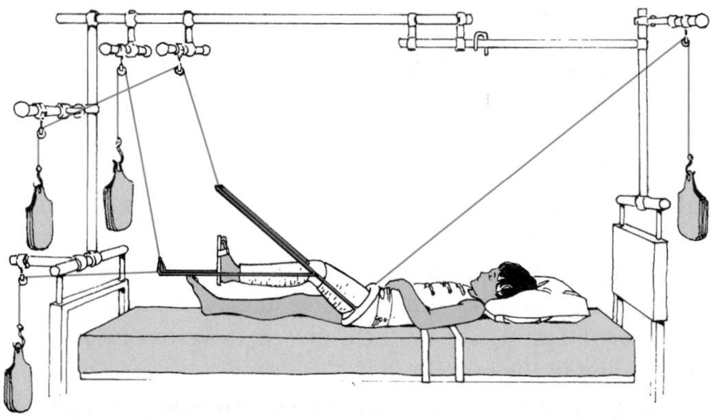

Fig. 54-6 Balance suspension with Thomas ring splint and Pearson attachment.

BOX 54-3 Types of Traction

Manual traction—Applied to the body part by the hands placed distal to the fracture site. Manual traction may be provided during application of a cast but more commonly when a closed reduction is performed.

Skin traction—Applied directly to the skin surface and indirectly to the skeletal structures. The pulling mechanism is attached to the skin with adhesive material or an elastic bandage. Both types are applied over soft, foam-backed traction straps to distribute the traction pull.

Skeletal traction—Applied directly to the skeletal structure by a pin, wire, or tongs inserted into or through the diameter of the bone distal to the fracture.

Cervical Traction

The cervical area is a vulnerable site for flexion or extension injuries to muscle, vertebrae, or the spinal cord. Cervical muscle trauma without other complications is treated with a cervical hard collar to relieve the weight of the head from the fracture site. When a child displaces or fractures a cervical vertebra, it may be necessary to reduce and immobilize the site with cervical skeletal traction. The spinal cord runs through the intravertebral canal, and dislocation or fracture of the vertebrae can also cause spinal cord injury. Nursing assessment of neurological function is essential to prevent further injury during the application and use of cervical skeletal traction.

Most cervical traction is accomplished with the use of a *halo brace* or *halo vest* (Fig. 54-7, A). This device consists of a steel halo attached to the head by four screws inserted into the outer skull; several rigid bars connect the halo to a vest that is worn around the chest, thus providing greater mobility of the rest of the body while avoiding cervical spinal motion altogether. If the injury has been limited to a vertebral fracture without neurological deficit, a halo brace can be applied to permit earlier ambulation.

Cervical traction may also be accomplished by the insertion of *Crutchfield, Barton,* or *Gardner-Wells tongs* through burr holes in the skull and weights attached to the hyperextended head (see Fig. 54-7, B). As the neck muscles fatigue with constant traction pull, the vertebral bodies gradually separate so that the cord is no longer pinched between the vertebrae. Immobilization until fracture healing or surgical fixation can occur is an essential goal of cervical traction.

Nursing Care Management

To assess the child in traction, it is essential to know the purpose for which the traction is applied and to understand the basic principles of traction. Regular assessment of both the child and the traction apparatus is required (see Guidelines box). Many of the nursing problems associated with a child in traction are related to immobility or improper maintenance and care of the traction device, which may lead to complications.

Skeletal traction, when used, should be maintained as originally set by the practitioner. When the child needs to be moved in the bed or the traction needs to be adjusted or released for any other reason, an orthopedist is consulted. For skeletal traction to be effective, the weights need to be hanging freely at all times.

In addition to routine skin observation and care, the child in skeletal traction will need special skin care at the pin site according to hospital policy or practitioner preference. Pin sites should be frequently assessed and cleaned to prevent infection; after the first 48 to 72 hours pin site care may be performed once daily or weekly for mechanically stable pins (Holmes, Brown, & Pin Site Care Expert Panel, 2005). Use of a 2 mg/mL chlorhexidine solution has been recommended as best-practice care for skeletal pin sites by the National Association of Orthopaedic Nurses (Holmes, Brown, & Pin Site Care Expert Panel, 2005). Before the child's discharge, the family needs to be taught pin site care, including how to observe for infection or pin instability, using a return demonstration method. A pressure reduction device, such as a special mattress, decreases the chance of skin breakdown.

When the child is first placed in traction, an increase in discomfort is common as a result of the traction pull fatiguing the muscle. Orthopedic conditions are associated with a higher-than-average number of painful events and a higher percentage of bodily symptoms than other common conditions. IV opioids, including analgesics and muscle relaxants, help during this phase of care and should be administered liberally.

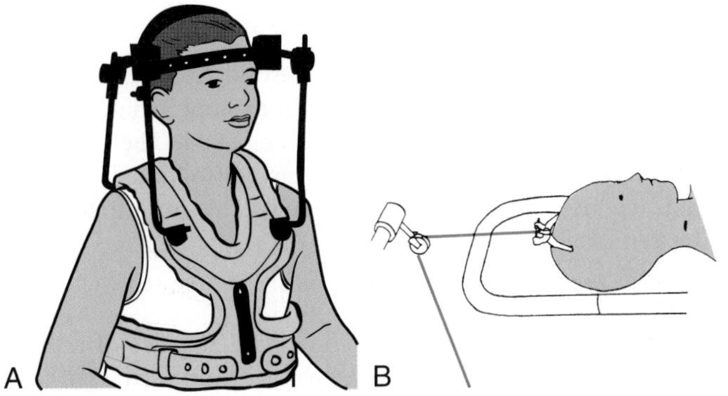

Fig. 54-7 **A:** Halo vest. **B:** Crutchfield tong traction. *(**B**, Redrawn from Hilt, N. E., & Schmitt, E. W. [1975].* Pediatric orthopedic nursing. *St. Louis: Mosby.)*

Distraction

Unlike *traction*, which helps bones realign and fuse properly, *distraction* is the process of separating opposing bone to encourage regeneration of new bone in the created space. Distraction can also be used when limbs are of unequal lengths and new bone is needed to elongate the shorter limb.

External Fixation

The Ilizarov external fixator (IEF) is a common external fixation device. The IEF uses a system of wires, rings, and telescoping rods that permits limb lengthening to occur by manual distraction. In addition to lengthening bones, the device can be used to correct angular or rotational defects or to immobilize fractures. The device is attached surgically by securing a series of external full or half rings to the bone with wires. External telescoping rods connect the rings to each other. Manual distraction is accomplished by manipulating the rods to increase the distance between the rings. A percutaneous osteotomy is performed when the device is applied to create a "false" growth plate. A special osteotomy or corticotomy involves cutting only the cortex of the bone while preserving its blood supply, bone marrow, endosteum, and periosteum. Capillary blood flow to the transected area is essential for proper bone growth. Cut bone ends typically grow at a rate of 1 cm/month. The IEF can result in up to a 15-cm gain in length.

Nursing Care Management

Success of the IEF depends on the child's and family's cooperation; thus before surgery they must be fully informed of the appearance of the device, how it accomplishes bone growth,

evolve **Skill—Monitoring Neurovascular Status**

GUIDELINES Traction Care

Understand Therapy

Understand the purposes of traction.
Understand the function of traction in each specific situation.

Maintain Traction

Check desired line of pull and relationship of distal fragment to proximal fragment. Check whether the fragment is being directed upward, adducted, or abducted.
Check function of each component.

- Position of bandages, frames, splints, specialized boot
- Ropes—In centre track of pulley, taut, no fraying, knots tied securely
- Pulleys—In original position on attachment bar; have not been displaced from original site
- Wheels freely moveable
- Weights—Correct amount of weight, hanging freely, in safe location

Check bed position; the head or foot should be elevated as directed for desired amount of pull and countertraction.
Do not remove skeletal traction or adhesive traction straps on skin traction.

Maintain Alignment

Observe for correct body alignment with emphasis on alignment of shoulder, hip, and leg.
Check after the child has moved.
Maintain correct angles at joints.

Skin Traction

Replace nonadhesive straps or elastic bandage on skin traction *when permitted* or absolutely necessary, but make certain that traction on limb is maintained by someone during procedure.
Assess straps or bandages to ascertain whether they are correctly applied (diagonal or spiral), not too loose or too tight, which could cause slippage and malalignment of traction.
Assess the traction boot to ensure it has not slipped and is not causing compression of the foot, thus impairing the circulation.

Skeletal Traction

Check pin sites frequently for signs of bleeding, inflammation, or infection.
Cleanse and dress pin sites per institution protocol or as ordered.
Apply topical antiseptic or antibiotic to pin sites daily as ordered.
Cover ends of pins with protective rubber or padding to prevent the child's being scratched by the pin.
Note pull of traction on the pin; pull should be even.
Check pin screws to be certain that screws are tight in metal clamp that attaches the traction apparatus to the pin.

Prevent Skin Breakdown

Provide foam overlay or alternating-pressure mattress underneath the hips and back.
Make total-body skin checks for redness or breakdown, especially over areas that receive the greatest pressure.
Wash and dry skin at least daily.
Inspect pressure points daily or more often if risk of breakdown is observed.
Use a skin breakdown assessment scale such as the Modified Braden Q.
Stimulate circulation with gentle massage over pressure areas.
Change position at least every 2 hours to relieve pressure.
Encourage increased intake of oral fluids.
Provide and encourage the patient to eat a balanced diet, including vegetables and fruits.

Prevent Complications

Check pulses in the affected area and compare with pulses in the contralateral site.
Assess circular dressings for excessive tightness.
Assess restrictive bandages or devices used to maintain traction on the affected limb.

- Make certain that they are not too loose or too tight.
- Remove periodically and check for pressure areas.

Encourage deep breathing frequently with maximum inspiratory chest expansion. Note any neurovascular changes, such as:

- Changes in colour in skin and nail beds
- Alterations in sensation, increased pain
- Alterations in motor ability

Take immediate action to correct problem or report to practitioner if neurovascular changes are found.
Record findings of neurovascular changes.
Carry out passive, active, or active-with-resistance exercises of uninvolved joints.
Note if any tightness, weakness, edema, or contractures are developing in uninvolved joints and muscles.
Take measures to correct or prevent further development of weakness, such as applying footboard or foot orthoses to prevent footdrop.

needed alterations in activities, and home and follow-up care. Children need to be involved in learning to adjust the device to accomplish distraction. Children, as well as parents, should be instructed in pin care, including observation for infection and loosening of the pins. Cleaning routines for the pin sites vary among practitioners but should not traumatize the skin.

Children who participate actively in their care report less discomfort. Because the device is external and bulky, the child and family may need to modify clothing for increased comfort and accessibility. Partial weight bearing is allowed (Fig. 54-8), and the child needs to learn to walk with crutches. Alterations in activity include modifications at school and in physical education. Full weight bearing is not allowed until the distraction is completed and bone consolidation has occurred. Follow-up care is essential to maintaining appropriate distraction until the desired leg length is achieved. The device is removed surgically after the bone has consolidated, and the child may need to use crutches or have a cast for 4 to 6 weeks after removal.

Amputation

A child may be born with the congenital absence of a body part, have a traumatic loss of an extremity, or need a surgical amputation for a pathological condition such as osteosarcoma (see p. 1713). With today's surgical technology and the quick thinking of bystanders who save a traumatically amputated

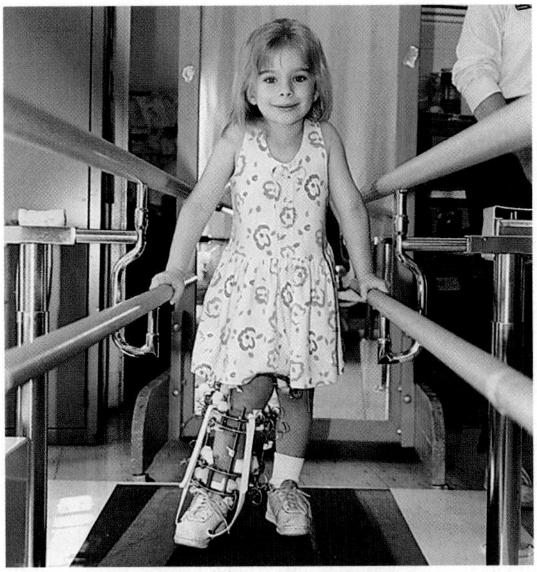

Fig. 54-8 Child with Ilizarov external fixator (right leg) during physiotherapy on parallel bars.

body part, children have had fingers and arms reattached with variable degrees of functional use regained.

NURSING ALERT For an amputated limb or body part that may be reattached, do the following:

1. Rinse limb gently with normal saline.
2. Loosely wrap limb in sterile gauze.
3. Place wrapped limb in a watertight bag.
4. Cool (without freezing) bag in ice water (do not pack in ice because this may harm tissue).
5. Label with child's name, date, and time, and transport with the child to the hospital.

Surgical amputation or the surgical repair of a permanently severed limb focuses on constructing an adequately nourished stump. A smooth, healthy, padded stump, free of nerve endings, is important in prosthesis fitting and subsequent ambulation. In some situations in which there is no vascular or neurological deficit, a cast is applied to the stump immediately after the procedure, and a pylon, metal extension, and artificial foot are attached so that the patient can walk on the temporary prosthesis within a few hours.

Nursing Care Management

Stump shaping is performed postoperatively with special elastic bandaging using a figure-8 bandage, which applies pressure in a cone-shaped fashion. This technique decreases stump edema, controls hemorrhage, and aids in developing the desired contours so that the child will bear weight on the posterior aspect of the skin flap rather than on the end of the stump. Stump elevation may be used during the first 24 hours, but after this time the extremity should not be left in this position because contractures will develop in the proximal joint and seriously hamper ambulation. Monitoring proper body alignment will further decrease the risk of flexion contractures.

For older children and adolescents, arm exercises (as well as parallel bars, which are used in prosthesis-training programs) help build up the arm muscles necessary for walking with crutches. Full range-of-motion exercises of joints above the amputation must be performed several times daily using active and isotonic exercises.

Depending on the child's age, children or their parents will need to learn stump hygiene, including careful soap and water washing every day and checking for skin irritation, breakdown, or infection. A tube of stockinette or powder is used to slide the prosthesis on more easily. Skin must be checked carefully every time the prosthesis is removed, and prosthesis tolerance time must be adjusted to prevent skin breakdown.

For children who have had an amputation, phantom limb sensation is an expected experience because the nerve-brain connections are still present. Gradually these sensations fade, although in many amputees they persist for years. Preoperative discussion of this phenomenon will aid a child in understanding these "unusual feelings" and in not hiding the experiences from others. Limb pain, especially pain that increases with ambulation, should be evaluated for the possibility of a neuroma at the free nerve endings in the stump, or other problems such as a poorly fitting prosthesis or joint instability.

evolve Case Study—Developmental Dysplasia of the Hip

Congenital Defects

Some skeletal defects may be diagnosed at birth or within days, weeks, or months after birth. In other cases the deviation may be difficult to detect without careful inspection. It is imperative that nurses become acquainted with signs of these defects and understand the principles of therapy in order to direct others in the care and management of these children.

Developmental Dysplasia of the Hip

The broad term *developmental dysplasia of the hip (DDH)* describes a spectrum of disorders related to abnormal development of the hip that may develop at any time during fetal life, infancy, or childhood, in which there is a shallow acetabulum, subluxation, or dislocation.

The incidence of hip instability of some kind is approximately 10 per 1000 live births. The incidence of frank dislocation or a dislocatable hip is 1.5 per 1000 live births (Hosalkar et al., 2007), and approximately 16 to 25% of infants with DDH are born breech (Hosalkar et al., 2007). The left hip is involved in 60% of cases, the right hip in 20%, and both hips in 20%. Sixty percent of the patients are girls. White children have a higher incidence of developmental dysplasia than other groups (Maher, Salmond, & Pellino, 2002).

Pathophysiology

The cause of DDH is unknown but certain factors such as gender, birth order, family history, intrauterine position, delivery type, joint laxity, and postnatal positioning are believed to affect the risk of DDH. Predisposing factors associated with DDH may be divided into three broad categories:

1. Physiological factors, which include maternal hormone secretion and intrauterine positioning

CULTURAL AWARENESS

Developmental Dysplasia of the Hip

A striking relationship exists between the development of the dislocation and methods of handling infants. Among the cultures with the highest incidence of dislocation, newly born infants are tightly wrapped in blankets or other swaddling material or are strapped to cradle boards. A Canadian study of a First Nations population showed that there was a 10-fold increase in DDH in tribes that carry babies on a "cradle swaddling board" with the hips strapped in an adducted and extended position (Salter, 1968). It is still a common practice among many Aboriginal mothers (Dezateux & Rosendahl, 2007).

In cultures such as Asian cultures, where some mothers traditionally carry infants on their backs or hips in the widely abducted straddle position, the disorder is virtually unknown. The exception is in Japan, where swaddling boards are still used. When a public education program was initiated in Japan, the practice of swaddling decreased, as well as the DDH rates (Dezateux & Rosendahl, 2007).

BOX 54-4 Clinical Manifestations of Developmental Dysplasia of the Hip

Infant

Shortening of limb on affected side
Restricted abduction of hip on affected side
Unequal gluteal folds (infant prone)
Positive Ortolani test
Positive Barlow test

Older Infant and Child

Affected leg shorter than the other
Telescoping or piston mobility of joint—Head of femur felt to move up and down in buttock when extended thigh is pushed first toward child's head and then pulled distally
Trendelenburg's sign—When child stands first on one foot and then on the other (holding onto a chair, rail, or someone's hands) bearing weight on the affected hip, the pelvis tilts downward on the normal side instead of upward, as it would with normal stability
Greater trochanter prominent and appearing above a line from anterosuperior iliac spine to tuberosity of ischium
Marked lordosis (bilateral dislocations)
Waddling gait (bilateral dislocations)

2. Mechanical factors, which involve breech presentation, multiple fetuses, oligohydramnios, and large infant size. Other mechanical factors may include continued maintenance of the hips in adduction and extension, which will in time cause a dislocation (see Cultural Awareness box).
3. Genetic factors, which entail a higher incidence (6%) of DDH in siblings of affected infants, and an even greater incidence (36%) of recurrence if a sibling and one parent were affected.

Some experts categorize DDH into two major groups: (1) *typical*, in which the infant is neurologically intact; and (2) *teratological*, which involves a neuromuscular defect such as arthrogryposis or myelodysplasia. The teratological forms usually occur in utero and are much less common.

Three degrees of DDH are illustrated in Fig. 28-18 (p. 775). Please see Chapter 28 for further information.

Diagnostic Evaluation

DDH is often not detected at the initial examination after birth; thus all infants should be carefully monitored for hip dysplasia at follow-up visits throughout the first year of life. In the newborn period dysplasia usually appears as hip joint laxity rather than as outright dislocation. The clinical manifestations of DDH are outlined in Box 54-4.

The Ortolani and Barlow tests must be performed by an experienced clinician to prevent further damage to the hip. If these tests are performed too vigorously in the first 2 days of life, when the hip subluxates freely, persistent dislocation may occur (see Fig. 24-10, p. 621).

Radiographic examination in early infancy is not reliable, since ossification of the femoral head does not normally take place until the third to sixth month of life. However, the cartilaginous head can be visualized directly by **ultrasonography**. It is recommended as an adjunct to other diagnostic procedures (American Academy of Pediatrics [AAP], Committee on Quality Improvement and Subcommittee on Developmental Dysplasia of the Hip, 2000). In infants older than age 4 months and in children, radiographic examination is useful in confirming the diagnosis. An upward slope in the roof of the acetabulum (the acetabular angle) greater than 40 degrees with upward and outward displacement of the femoral head is a frequent finding in older children. A computed tomography (CT) scan may be useful to assess the position of the femoral head relative to the acetabulum after closed reduction and casting. The American Academy of Pediatrics (AAP, Committee on Quality Improvement and Subcommittee on Developmental Dysplasia of the Hip, 2000) has published extensive clinical guidelines for the early detection of DDH.

Therapeutic Management

Treatment is begun as soon as the condition is recognized because early intervention is more favourable to the restoration of normal bony architecture and function. The longer treatment is delayed, the more severe the deformity, the more difficult the treatment, and the less favourable the prognosis. The treatment varies with the child's age and the extent of the dysplasia. The goal of treatment is to obtain and maintain a safe, congruent position of the hip joint to promote normal hip joint development.

Newborn to Age 6 Months

The hip joint is maintained by splinting with the proximal femur centred in the acetabulum in an attitude of flexion. Of the numerous devices available, the *Pavlik harness* is the most widely used, and with time, motion, and gravity, the hip works into a more abducted, reduced position (see Fig. 28-19, p. 776). The harness is worn continuously until the hip is clinically and radiographically stable, usually in about 3 to 6 months. After the age of 6 months the Pavlik harness tends to lose its effectiveness because of the child's increasing mobility and strength (Hosalkar et al., 2007).

When adduction contracture is present, skin traction may be used to slowly and gently stretch the hip to full abduction, after which wide abduction is maintained until stability is attained. When maintaining stable reduction is difficult, a hip spica cast is applied and changed periodically to accommodate the child's growth. After 3 to 6 months, sufficient stability is acquired to allow transfer to a removable protective abduction brace. The duration of treatment depends on development of the acetabulum but is usually accomplished within the first year.

Ages 6 to 18 Months

In this age group the dislocation is not recognized until the child begins to stand and walk, when attendant shortening of the limb and contractures of the hip adductor and flexor muscles become apparent (see Fig. 24-10). Gradual reduction by traction is used for approximately 3 weeks. An individualized home traction program may be developed for the child preoperatively to decrease the length of hospitalization and maintain the home environment. The child then undergoes an attempted closed reduction of the hip under general anaesthesia; if the hip is not reducible, an open reduction is performed. After reduction, the child is placed in a hip spica cast for 2 to 4 months until the hip is stable, at which time a flexion-abduction brace is applied.

Older Child

Correction of the hip deformity in older children is inherently more difficult than in the preceding age groups, because secondary adaptive changes and other etiological factors (such as juvenile idiopathic arthritis or nonambulatory cerebral palsy) complicate the condition. Operative closed reduction, which may involve preoperative traction, tenotomy of contracted muscles, and any one of several innominate osteotomy procedures designed to construct an acetabular roof, is usually required. After cast removal and before weight bearing is permitted, range-of-motion exercises help restore movement. Successful reduction and reconstruction become increasingly difficult after the age of 4 years and are usually impossible or inadvisable in children older than 6 years of age because of severe shortening and contracture of muscles and deformity of the femoral and acetabular structures.

Nursing Care Management

Nurses are in a unique position to detect DDH in early infancy. During the infant assessment process and routine nurturing activities, the hips and extremities are inspected for any deviations from normal. These observations should be reported to the attending practitioner, and the ambulatory child who displays a limp or an unusual gait should be referred for evaluation. This may indicate an orthopedic or neurological problem. Nonambulatory children with cerebral palsy should also be assessed for evidence of dislocation.

The major nursing problems in the care of an infant or child in a cast or other device are related to maintenance of the device and adaptation of nurturing activities to meet his or her needs. Generally, treatment and follow-up care of these children are carried out in a clinic, practitioner's office, or outpatient unit. Hospitalization may be necessary for cast application or brace fitting but seldom exceeds 24 to 48 hours. Longer hospitalization is required for open reduction.

The former practice of double- or triple-diapering for DDH is not recommended because it promotes hip extension, thus impeding proper hip development.

The primary nursing goal is teaching parents to apply and maintain the reduction device. The Pavlik harness allows for easy handling of the infant and usually produces less apprehension in the parent than heavy braces and casts. Because of the infant's rapid growth, the straps should be checked in the beginning of therapy every week for possible adjustments (Hart et al., 2006). It is important that parents understand the correct use of the appliance, which may or may not allow for its removal during bathing. Unbuckling or removing the harness is determined individually on the basis of the family's level of understanding and the degree of hip deformity. Parents should be instructed not to adjust the harness without medical supervision. The child should be examined by the practitioner before any adjustment is attempted to make certain the hips are in correct placement before the harness is resecured.

Skin care is an important aspect of the care of an infant in a harness. The following instructions for preventing skin breakdown are stressed:

- Always put an undershirt (or a shirt with extensions that close at the crotch) under the chest straps, and put knee socks under the foot and leg pieces to prevent the straps from rubbing the skin.
- Check frequently (at least two or three times a day) for red areas under the straps and the clothing.
- Gently massage healthy skin under the straps once a day to stimulate circulation. In general, avoid lotions and powders because they can cake and irritate the skin.
- Always place the diaper under the straps.

Parents should be encouraged to hold the infant with a harness and continue care and nurturing activities. The nurse can assist by being available for parents' questions about the necessary adaptations to daily care to decrease the parent's anxiety and possible feelings about the child being hurt by routine caring.

Casts and orthotics devices (harness) offer more challenging nursing problems because they cannot be removed for routine care, although sometimes a brace may be removed for bathing. Care of an infant or small child with a cast requires nursing innovation to reduce skin pressure or friction and to maintain cleanliness of both the child and the cast, particularly in the diaper area.

It is important for nurses, parents, and other caregivers to understand that children in corrective devices need to be involved in all the activities of any child in the same age group. Play and diversion activities should be chosen that can be used in a prone position on the floor or in the seats devised for feeding and other activities.

Congenital Clubfoot

Congenital clubfoot is a complex deformity of the ankle and foot that includes forefoot adduction, midfoot supination, hindfoot varus, and ankle equinus. Deformities of the foot and ankle are described according to the position of the ankle and foot. The more common positions involve the following variations:

Talipes varus—An inversion or a bending inward
Talipes valgus—An eversion or bending outward
Talipes equinus—Plantar flexion, in which the toes are lower than the heel
Talipes calcaneus—Dorsiflexion, in which the toes are higher than the heel

Most cases of clubfoot are a combination of these positions, and the most commonly occurring type of clubfoot (approximately 95%) is the composite deformity *talipes equinovarus (TEV)*, in which the foot is pointed downward and inward in varying degrees of severity (Fig. 54-9). Unilateral clubfoot is somewhat more common than bilateral clubfoot and may occur as an isolated defect or in association with other disorders or syndromes, such as chromosomal defects, arthrogryposis (a generalized immobility of the joints), cerebral palsy, or spina bifida.

The incidence of clubfoot in the general population is 1 to 2 per 1000 live births, with boys affected twice as often as girls. Bilateral clubfeet occur in 50% of the cases (Hosalkar, Spiegel, & Davidson, 2007). The cause of clubfoot is believed to be multifactorial. Some authorities attribute the defect to abnormal positioning and restricted movement in utero, although the evidence is not conclusive. Other experts implicate arrested or abnormal embryonic development.

Classification

The literature describes three major categories of clubfoot: (1) positional clubfoot (also called transitional, mild, or postural clubfoot), which is believed to occur primarily from intrauterine crowding and responds to simple stretching and casting, (2) syndromic (or teratological) clubfoot, which is associated with other congenital anomalies such as myelomeningocele or arthrogryposis and is a more severe form of clubfoot that is often resistant to treatment, and (3) congenital clubfoot, also referred to as idiopathic, which may occur in an otherwise normal child and has a wide range of rigidity and prognosis. The third category may be detected in utero by ultrasonography and is the most common type of TEV seen.

The mild, or postural, clubfoot may correct spontaneously or may require passive exercise or serial casting. There is no bony abnormality, but there may be tightness and shortening of the soft tissues medially and posteriorly. The teratological clubfoot is associated with other congenital anomalies such as myelodysplasia or arthrogryposis. These feet usually require surgical correction and have a high incidence of recurrence. The congenital idiopathic clubfoot, or "true clubfoot," almost always requires surgical intervention because there is bony abnormality.

Diagnostic Evaluation

The deformity is often readily apparent and easily detected prenatally through ultrasonography or at birth. However, it must be differentiated from some positional deformities that can be passively corrected or overcorrected. Radiographic examination is recommended by some clinicians, whereas others may postpone radiographs in infancy (Hosalkar, Spiegel, & Davidson, 2007). Paralytic changes in the lower extremity of children with neuromuscular involvement often produce equinovarus deformity. An increased risk of hip dysplasia is associated with clubfoot deformities.

Therapeutic Management

The goal of treatment for clubfoot is to achieve a painless, plantigrade, and stable foot. Treatment of clubfoot involves three stages: (1) correction of the deformity, (2) maintenance of the correction until normal muscle balance is regained, and (3) follow-up observation to avert possible recurrence of the deformity (see Chapter 28, p. 776). Serial casting is begun shortly after birth, before discharge from the hospital (Fig. 54-10). For more information regarding casting, see Chapter 28. A radiograph or ultrasound is then evaluated to see the relationship of the bones to each other. Failure to achieve normal alignment by 3 months indicates the need for surgical intervention, which may take place between 6 and 12 months

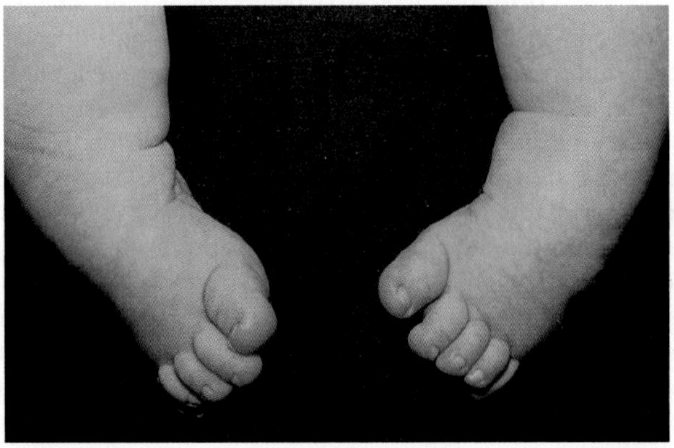

Fig. 54-9 Bilateral congenital talipes equinovarus (congenital clubfoot) in a 2-month-old infant. *(From Zitelli, B. J. & Davis, H. W. [2007]. Atlas of pediatric physical diagnosis [5th ed., p. 8]. St. Louis: Mosby [Fig. 1-12F].)*

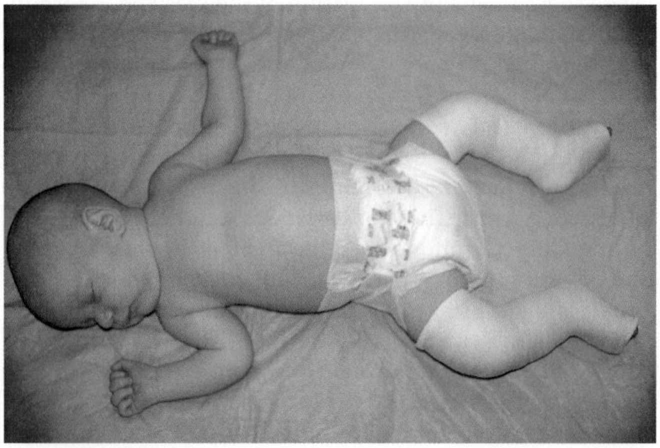

Fig. 54-10 Feet casted for correction of bilateral congenital talipes equinovarus.

of age. The foot (or feet) is immobilized postoperatively for approximately 6 to 12 weeks, and the child is allowed to walk after the cast is removed.

Surgical intervention for clubfoot involves pin fixation and the release of tight joints and tendons. Casting of the affected foot and leg is performed, and after 2 or 3 months, a varus-prevention brace is used to maintain correction. With severe deformities, repeated surgical tendon or joint releases may be necessary.

In recent years several nonsurgical approaches to clubfoot have been reintroduced. These methods involve daily or weekly manipulation and stretching of tissues with either casting (Ponseti's manipulation) or taping and splinting of the affected extremity (French physiotherapy). A percutaneous calcaneal tendon (Achilles tendon) lengthening may be performed before the final casting at 6 to 7 weeks to correct the equinus deformity. With French physiotherapy treatment, a continuous passive motion machine may be used several hours daily to stretch and strengthen muscle groups involved (Faulks & Luther, 2005).

Nursing Care Management

Nursing care of the child with clubfoot is the same as for any child who has a cast (see p. 1692). Because the child will spend considerable time in a corrective device, nursing care plans include both long- and short-term goals. Conscientious observation of the skin and circulation is particularly important in young infants because of their normally rapid growth rate. Because treatment and follow-up care are handled in the orthopedist's office, clinic, or outpatient department, parent education and support are important in nursing care of these children.

Parents need to understand the overall treatment program and the importance of regular cast changes in the long-term effectiveness of the therapy. Reinforcing and clarifying the orthopedist's explanations and instructions, teaching parents about care of the cast or appliance (including vigilant observation for potential problems), and encouraging parents to facilitate normal development within the limitations imposed by the deformity or therapy are all part of nursing responsibilities.

Metatarsus Adductus (Varus)

Metatarsus adductus, or metatarsus varus, is probably the most common congenital foot deformity. In most instances it is a result of abnormal intrauterine positioning, particularly in the firstborn child, and is usually detected at birth. The deformity is characterized by medial adduction of the toes and forefoot, frequently in association with inversion, and by convexity of the lateral border of the foot. Metatarsus adductus may be divided into three categories: type I, in which the forefoot is flexible and corrects easily with manipulation; type II, in which there is only partial flexibility in the forefoot, and it corrects passively past neutral position but only to neutral position with active manipulation; and type III, in which the forefoot is rigid and will not stretch to neutral position with manipulation. Unlike TEV, with which it is often confused, the angulation occurs at the tarsometatarsal joint, whereas the heel and ankle remain in a neutral position. Ankle range of motion is normal. This deformity often causes a pigeon-toed gait in the child.

Therapeutic management depends on the rigidity and type of the deformity. Correction with types I and II can usually be accomplished by gentle manipulation and passive stretching of the foot, which the parent is taught to perform. Repeated and consistent stretching is continued for the first 6 weeks, after which the treatment is based on the flexibility of the foot. With type III, the child will usually require serial manipulation and casting to correct the defect. Casting is performed every 1 to 2 weeks for 6 to 8 weeks, after which a corrective shoe or orthosis may be used. Surgical correction is rarely required for the condition unless there is residual deformity at 4 to 6 years of age, at which time soft-tissue release and serial casting are performed. Older children with deformity may require more extensive surgery (Hosalkar, Spiegel, & Davidson, 2007).

Nursing Care Management

The nursing role primarily involves identifying the defect so that early therapy and instruction of the parents can be initiated. The nurse needs to teach the parents how to hold the heel firmly and to stretch only the forefoot; otherwise, undue force on the heel may produce a valgus deformity. If casting or orthosis is required, the nurse should instruct the parents in cast care and observation of the corrective device (see p. 1694).

Skeletal Limb Deficiency

Congenital limb deficiencies, or reduction malformations (disruption defects), are manifested by a variety of degrees of loss of functional capacity. They are characterized by underdevelopment of skeletal elements of the extremities. The range of malformation can extend from minor defects of the digits to serious abnormalities such as *amelia*, absence of an entire extremity; or *meromelia*, partial absence of an extremity that includes *phocomelia* (seal limbs), interposed deficiency of long bones with relatively good development of hands and feet attached at or near the shoulder or the hips. Most reduction defects are primary defects of development of the limb, but prenatal destruction of the limb can occur, such as the amputation of a limb in utero from constriction of an amniotic band (amniotic band disruption sequence).

Pathophysiology

Limb deficiencies can be attributed to both heredity and environment and can originate at any stage of limb development. Formation of limbs may be suppressed at the time of limb bud formation, or there may be interference in later stages of differentiation and growth. Heredity appears to play a prominent role, and prenatal environmental insults have been implicated in a number of cases. The latter includes the well-publicized thalidomide tragedy of the 1950s and early 1960s, which demonstrated a clear relationship between the time of exposure of the pregnant woman to the anti-emetic medication and the presence and type of limb deformity in the newborn. Many medications may still have similar teratogenic effects in the first trimester of pregnancy; thus medication administration during this period should be carefully evaluated by the practitioner. Unfortunately, during this period, the woman may not realize her pregnant condition unless the event is anticipated, and she may inadvertently consume harmful medications.

Therapeutic Management

Children with congenital limb deficiencies should be fitted with prosthetic devices whenever possible, and the devices should be applied at the earliest possible stage of development in an attempt to match the infant's motor readiness. This favours natural progression of prosthetic use. For example, a young infant with an upper extremity deficiency is fitted with a simple passive device, such as a mitten prosthesis, to encourage limb exploration, sitting (with the extremities needed for support), and bilateral hand activities.

Lower limb prostheses are applied when the infant begins sitting up and can maintain balance. In preparation for prosthetic devices, surgical modification may be necessary to ensure the most favourable use of the device, since severe deformity can interfere with its effective use. Phocomelic digits are preserved for controlling switches of externally powered appliances in upper extremities. Digits (in both upper and lower extremities) provide the child with surfaces for tactile exploration and stimulation. Prostheses are replaced to accommodate the child's growth and increasing capabilities.

Nursing Care Management

Prosthetic application training and habilitation are most successfully carried out in a centre that specializes in meeting the special needs of these children, especially very young children and those with amputations or missing limbs. Therapeutic management involves a prosthetist, who specializes in the development, fitting, and maintenance of prosthetic limbs, and other health care workers such as physiotherapists and occupational therapists. Parents need special attention and support and should be encouraged to assist the child in making age-commensurate adjustments to the environment.

Osteogenesis Imperfecta

Osteogenesis imperfecta (OI) is the most common osteoporosis syndrome in children, characterized by excessive fractures and bone deformity. There are at least seven types of OI, accounting for significant disease variability. Clinical features may include varying degrees of bone fragility, deformity, and fracture, blue sclerae, hearing loss, and dentinogenesis imperfecta (hypoplastic discoloured teeth). The inheritance pattern is autosomal dominant in most cases, although the most severe form demonstrates autosomal recessive inheritance (Box 54-5).

Most types of OI have defects in the *COL1A1* or *COL1A2* genes, which code for polypeptide chains in type 1 procollagen, a precursor of type 1 collagen, a major structural component of bone. The error results in faulty bone mineralization, abnormal bone architecture, and increased susceptibility to fracture.

Classifications for OI are based on clinical features and patterns of inheritance (see Box 54-5). Clinically, type I is the most common, with wide variability of bone fragility; some affected family members have significant deformity and disability, whereas others lead agile, active lives. Type II variants are the most severe and are considered lethal in infancy. Type III OI is characterized by multiple fractures, bone deformity, and severe disability; affected individuals rarely live to 30 years of age. Type IV is similar to type I with blue or white sclerae. Another variant, or type V, has been described in which those affected have a hyperplastic callus, a radiodense metaphyseal band and calcification of the interosseous membrane of the forearm; no collagen **mutations** are noted in this group (Marini, 2007). A type VI has been described with a characteristic mineralization defect, which does not respond to pamidronate therapy as do types I to V (Land et al., 2007). Children affected with this type have no dental involvement and normal sclerae; a bone biopsy is the only way to establish a diagnosis because of the similarities to other types. Type VII follows the autosomal recessive inheritance and was recently described in a consanguinous First Nations community from Northern Québec (Ward, Glorieux, & Rauch, 2002).

BOX 54-5 Classification of Osteogenesis Imperfecta

Type I*
- **A**—Mild bone fragility, blue sclerae, normal teeth, hearing loss (occurs between ages 20 and 30 years), autosomal dominant inheritance
- **B**—Same as A except dentinogenesis imperfecta instead of normal teeth
- **C**—Same as B but no bone fragility

Type II—Lethal; stillborn or die in early infancy; severe bone fragility, multiple fractures at birth; 10% of cases of osteogenesis imperfecta (OI); autosomal recessive inheritance

Type III—Severe bone fragility leading to severe progressive deformities, normal sclerae, marked growth failure, most autosomal recessive inheritance, with a few autosomal dominant inheritance

Type IV
- **A**—Mild to moderate bone fragility; normal sclerae; normal teeth; short stature; variable deformity; autosomal dominant inheritance
- **B**—Same as A except dentinogenesis imperfecta instead of normal teeth; approximately 6% of cases of OI

Type V—Clinically similar to type IV; hyperplastic callus; collagen mutation is negative

Type VI—Sclerae and dentition normal; moderate to severe bone fragility; diagnosis by bone biopsy because of similarities to other types; identified in eight persons to date (Land et al., 2007)

Type VII—Rhizomelia, (shortening of proximal limb segments), coxa vara, along with slightly blue sclera, normal dentition, and moderately severe long bone deformity (Canadian Paediatric Society, n.d.).

*Two thirds of cases are type I.

Therapeutic Management

The treatment for OI is primarily supportive, although patients and families are optimistic about new research advances. Bone marrow transplant for severe OI was first reported in 1999 with positive results; however, this is still considered an experimental treatment. Bisphosphonate therapy with pamidronate, olpadronate, neridronate, or alendronate to promote increased bone density and prevent fractures has become standard therapy for many children with OI. Bisphosphonate therapy reportedly is more beneficial for increasing vertebral bone density but is considered less effective for long bones (Marini, 2007). Bachrach and Ward (2009) suggest data are inadequate to recommend the use of bisphosphonate therapy in children with OI for sole treatment of bone mineral density (BMD) reduction.

The goals of a rehabilitative approach to management are directed toward preventing (1) positional contractures and deformities, (2) muscle weakness and osteoporosis, and (3) malalignment of lower extremity joints prohibiting weight bearing. Lightweight braces and splints help support limbs, prevent fractures, and aid in ambulation. Physiotherapy helps prevent disuse osteoporosis and strengthens muscles, which in turn improves bone density. Surgery is sometimes used to help treat the manifestations of the disease. Surgical techniques are used to correct deformities that interfere with bracing, standing, or walking. For the child with recurrent fractures, inserting an intramedullary rod provides stability to bones.

Because there is a 50% risk of an affected individual passing the gene to an offspring, genetic counselling is recommended.

Nursing Care Management

Infants and children with this disorder require careful handling to prevent fractures. They must be supported when they are being turned, positioned, moved, and held. Even changing a diaper may cause a fracture in severely affected infants. These children should never be held by the ankles when being diapered but should be gently lifted by the buttocks or supported with pillows. Children with current fractures or healing fractures should be screened for osteogenesis imperfecta—the assumption that abuse or neglect is the cause of fractures in children must be carefully evaluated by a multidisciplinary team.

Both parents and the affected child need education regarding the child's limitations and guidelines in planning suitable activities that promote optimum development and protect the child from harm. Realistic occupational planning and genetic counselling are part of the long-term goals of care.

OI is a differential diagnosis that must be ruled out in the event of multiple fractures that may be attributed to nonaccidental injury. A detailed history, no evidence of associated soft-tissue injury, and the presence of other symptoms related to OI help determine the diagnosis.

Acquired Defects

Legg-Calvé-Perthes Disease

Legg-Calvé-Perthes disease, sometimes called *coxa plana* or *osteochondritis deformans juvenilis*, is a self-limited disorder in which there is aseptic necrosis of the femoral head. The disease affects children ages 2 to 12 years, but most cases occur in boys between 4 and 8 years of age as an isolated event. In approximately 10% of cases the involvement is bilateral; most of the affected children have a skeletal age significantly below their chronological age (Hosalkar et al., 2007). The male/female ratio is 4 : 1 or 5 : 1. White children are affected 10 times more frequently than children with African origins.

Pathophysiology

The cause of the disease is unknown, but there is a disturbance of circulation to the femoral capital epiphysis that produces an ischemic aseptic necrosis of the femoral head. During middle childhood, circulation to the femoral epiphysis is more tenuous than at other ages and can become obstructed by trauma, inflammation, coagulation defects, and a variety of other causes. The pathological events seem to take place in four stages (Box 54-6). The entire process may encompass as little as 18 months or continue for several years. The reformed femoral head may be severely altered or appear entirely normal.

Clinical Manifestations and Diagnostic Evaluation

The onset of Legg-Calvé-Perthes disease is usually insidious, and the history may reveal only intermittent appearance of a limp on the affected side or a symptom complex including hip soreness, ache, or stiffness that can be constant or intermittent. The parents may report seeing the child limping, and the limp becomes more pronounced with increased activity. The pain may be experienced in the hip, along the entire thigh, or in the vicinity of the knee joint. The pain and limp are usually most evident on arising and at the end of a long day of activities. The pain is usually accompanied by joint dysfunction and limited range of motion. There may be a vague history of trauma. The diagnosis is established by radiographic examination, with the definitive diagnosis being magnetic resonance imaging (MRI), which demonstrates osteonecrosis.

Therapeutic Management

Because deformity occurs early in the disease process, the aims of treatment are to eliminate hip irritability; restore and

BOX 54-6 Radiographic Stages of Legg-Calvé-Perthes Disease

Stage I: initial or avascular stage—Aseptic necrosis or infarction of the capital femoral epiphysis with degenerative changes producing flattening of the upper surface of the femoral head

Stage II: fragmentation or revascularization stage—Capital bone resorption and revascularization with fragmentation (vascular resorption of the epiphysis) that gives a mottled appearance on radiographs

Stage III: reossification or reparative stage—New bone formation, which is represented on radiographs as calcification and ossification or increased density in the areas of radiolucency. This filling-in process appears to take place from the periphery of the head centrally.

Stage IV: residual or regenerative stage—Gradual reformation of the head of the femur without radiolucency and, it is hoped, to a spherical form maintain adequate range of hip motion; prevent capital femoral epiphyseal collapse, extrusion, or subluxation; and ensure a well-rounded femoral head at the time of healing. Treatment varies according to the child's age at the time of diagnosis and the appearance of the femoral head vasculature and position within the acetabulum. Nonsurgical containment of the femoral head may be accomplished with abduction casts, whereas a pelvic or femoral osteotomy may be used to contain the femoral head. Activity causes microfractures of the soft ischemic epiphysis, which tend to induce synovitis, stiffness, and adductor contracture. The initial therapy is rest and non–weight bearing, which helps reduce inflammation and restore motion. Later, active motion is encouraged. In some cases traction is applied to stretch tight adductor muscles.

Containment can be accomplished in several ways. One is the use of non–weight-bearing devices, such as an abduction brace (e.g., Atlanta Scottish Rite orthosis), leg casts, or a leather harness sling, which prevent weight bearing on the affected limb. Another includes the use of various weight-bearing appliances, such as abduction-ambulation braces or casts after a period of bed rest and traction. A third option consists of surgical reconstruction and containment procedures. Conservative therapy must be continued for 2 to 4 years, although braces constructed from lightweight materials allow the child to maintain a nearly normal activity level. Surgical correction, although subjecting the child to additional risks (e.g., from anaesthesia, infection, blood transfusion), returns the child to normal activities in 3 to 4 months. The use of home traction has also been explored.

Prognosis

The disease is self-limited, but the ultimate outcome of therapy depends on early and efficient treatment and the child's age at the onset of the disorder. Children 5 years and younger, whose epiphyses are more cartilaginous, have the best prognosis for complete recovery. Children over 9 years old have a significant risk for degenerative arthritis, especially with femoral head deformity at the time of diagnosis (Hosalkar et al., 2007). The later the diagnosis is made, the more femoral damage will have occurred before treatment is implemented. In many cases, with good patient compliance, the prognosis is excellent.

Nursing Care Management

Nurses may be the first health care providers to identify affected children and to refer them for medical evaluation. They are also persons on whom the child and the family can rely to help them understand and adjust to the therapeutic measures. Because most of the child's care is conducted on an outpatient basis, the major emphasis of nursing care is teaching the family the care and management of the corrective appliance selected for therapy. The family needs to learn the purpose, function, application, and care of the corrective device and the importance of using it consistently and as instructed, to achieve the desired outcome.

One of the most difficult aspects associated with the disorder is coping with a normally active child who feels well but must remain relatively inactive. Suitable activities must be devised to meet the needs of the child in the process of developing a sense of initiative or industry. Activities that meet the creative urges are usually well received.

Slipped Capital Femoral Epiphysis

Slipped capital femoral epiphysis (SCFE), or coxa vara, refers to the spontaneous displacement of the proximal femoral epiphysis in a posterior and inferior direction. It develops most frequently shortly before or during accelerated growth and the onset of puberty (children between the ages of 10 and 16 years; median age, 13 for boys, 12 for girls) and is most frequently observed in boys and obese children. Bilateral involvement occurs in up to 60% of cases. Osteonecrosis is a common complication of SCFE and is reported to occur in 17 to 47% of all patients (Hosalkar et al., 2007).

Pathophysiology

Most cases of SCFE are idiopathic, although it can be associated with endocrine disorders, renal osteodystrophy, and radiotherapy. The cause of idiopathic SCFE is multifactorial and includes obesity, physeal architecture and orientation, and pubertal hormone changes that affect physeal strength. Approximately 65% of patients with SCFE are above the ninetieth percentile in weight-for-age profiles; obesity is believed to play a significant role in the development of the condition (Hosalkar et al., 2007). Although obesity stresses the physeal plate, SCFE can also occur in children who are not obese. Radiographs show medial displacement of the epiphysis and an uncovered upper portion of the femoral neck adjacent to the physis. There is a widened growth plate and irregular metaphysis. The capital femoral epiphysis remains in the acetabulum, but the femoral neck slips, deforming the femoral head and stretching blood vessels to the epiphysis.

Diagnostic Evaluation

The disorder is suspected when an adolescent or preadolescent displays clinical signs or complains of thigh pain; hip pain may be referred to the knee as a result of the distribution of sensory nerves (Hart, Grottkau, & Albright, 2007) (Box 54-7). The diagnosis is confirmed by radiographic examination.

Therapeutic Management

Treatment goals are to prevent further slippage and provide stability for the epiphysis (Hart et al., 2007). Once the

BOX 54-7 Clinical Manifestations of Slipped Capital Femoral Epiphysis

Limp on affected side
Pain in hip
- Continuous or intermittent
- Frequently referred to groin, anteromedial aspect of thigh, or knee

Restricted internal rotation on adduction with external rotation deformity
Loss of abduction and internal rotation as severity increases
Shortening of lower extremity

diagnosis is established, the child should be made completely non–weight bearing with either crutches or a wheelchair to prevent further slippage. Surgical treatment varies with the degree of displacement. Traditional methods include presurgery bed rest and traction followed by surgical pinning. Surgical pinning involves the placement of a single pin through the femoral neck into the proximal femoral epiphysis to prevent further slippage (Hart et al., 2007). Postsurgical care includes non–weight-bearing crutch ambulation (or wheelchair use if bilateral) for 6 to 8 weeks. SCFE is an emergency and requires early diagnosis and treatment to increase the likelihood of a satisfactory cure. The two most severe complications of SCFE are avascular necrosis of the proximal femoral physis and chondrolysis, which involves the loss of articular cartilage, decreased range of motion, and pain (Hart et al., 2007).

Nursing Care Management

Nursing care is the same as that for a child in a cast or a child in traction, as discussed earlier in this chapter. Postoperative care involves hemodynamic stabilization and assessment for complications. The adolescent needs to be taught the proper use of crutches and the importance of avoiding any weight bearing on the affected hip (if unilateral). The adolescent may be involved in building upper body strength during the convalescent period to increase mobility from bed to wheelchair, as appropriate. Self-care and performance of activities of daily living to capability are encouraged to promote confidence and decrease a sense of helplessness.

Kyphosis and Lordosis

The spine, consisting of numerous segments, can acquire deformity curves of three types: kyphosis, lordosis, and scoliosis (Fig. 54-11).

Kyphosis is an abnormally increased convex angulation in the curvature of the thoracic spine (see Fig. 54-11, B). It can occur secondary to disease processes such as tuberculosis, chronic arthritis, osteodystrophy, or compression fractures of the thoracic spine. The most common form of kyphosis is "postural." Children, especially during the time when skeletal growth outpaces growth of muscle, are prone to exaggeration of a normal kyphosis. They assume abnormal sitting and standing positions. This is particularly common in self-conscious adolescent girls who assume a round-shouldered slouching posture in an attempt to hide their developing breasts. *Scheuermann's kyphosis* is a thoracic curve greater than 45 degrees with wedging greater than 5 degrees of at least three adjacent vertebral bodies and vertebral irregularity.

Postural kyphosis is almost always accompanied by a compensatory postural lordosis, an abnormally exaggerated concave lumbar curvature. Treatment of kyphosis consists of exercises to strengthen shoulder and abdominal muscles and bracing for more marked deformity. With adolescents who are significantly self-conscious about their appearance, the best approach is to emphasize the cosmetic value of corrective therapy and to place the responsibility on the adolescent for carrying out an exercise program at home, with regular visits to and assessments by a therapist. Treatment with a brace may be indicated until skeletal maturity; surgical spinal fusion may be considered for severe, painful, or progressive deforming thoracic curves such as Scheuermann's kyphosis.

Lordosis is an accentuation of the cervical or lumbar curvature beyond physiological limits (see Fig. 54-11, C). It may be a secondary complication of a disease process, a result of trauma, or idiopathic. It is often seen in association with flexion contractures of the hip, scoliosis, obesity, developmental dysplasia of the hip, and slipped capital femoral epiphysis. During the pubertal growth spurt, lordosis of varying degrees is observed in teenagers, especially girls. Unlike kyphosis, severe lordosis is usually accompanied by pain.

Treatment involves management of the predisposing cause when possible, such as weight loss and correction of deformities. Postural exercises or support garments are helpful in relieving symptoms in some cases; however, these do not usually effect a permanent cure.

evolve Animation—Spine Structure

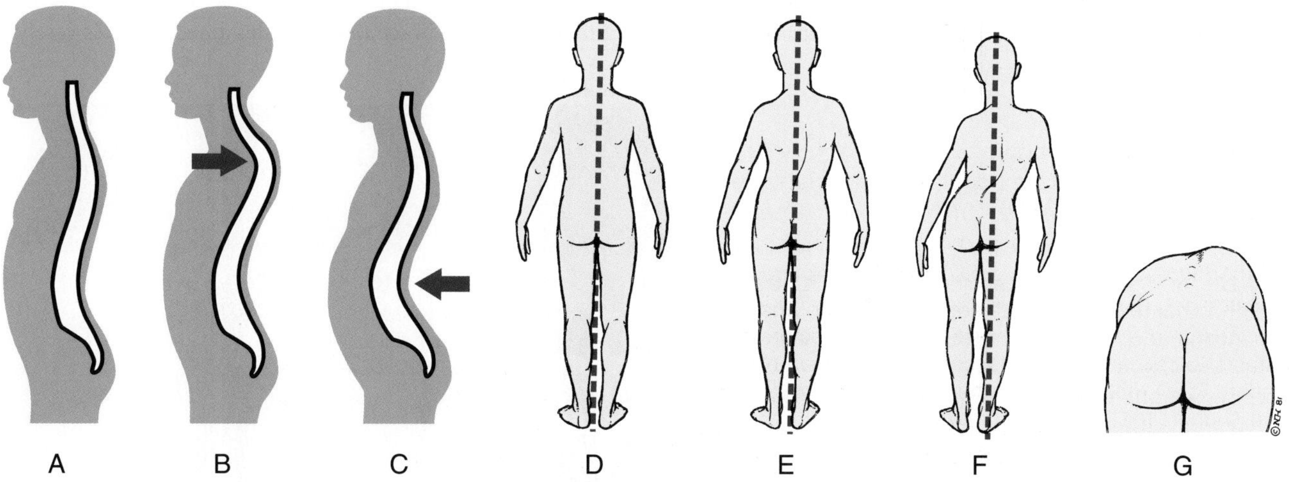

Fig. 54-11 Spinal column curvatures. **A:** Normal spine. **B:** Kyphosis. **C:** Lordosis. **D:** Normal spine in balance. **E:** Mild scoliosis in balance. **F:** Severe scoliosis not in balance. **G:** Rib hump and flank asymmetry seen in flexion caused by rotary component. *(Redrawn from Hilt, N. E., & Schmitt, E. W. [1975].* Pediatric orthopedic nursing. *St. Louis: Mosby.)*

Idiopathic Scoliosis

Scoliosis is a complex spinal deformity in three planes, usually involving lateral curvature, spinal rotation causing rib asymmetry, and thoracic hypokyphosis. It is the most common spinal deformity and can be further classified according to age of onset: *congenital*, during fetal development; *infantile*, at birth or up to 3 years of age; *childhood (juvenile)*, in children 4 to 10 years of age; or *adolescent*, during the growth spurt of early adolescence (the most common type). Scoliosis can be caused by a number of conditions and may occur alone or in association with other diseases, particularly neuromuscular conditions (neuromuscular scoliosis). In most cases, however, there is no apparent cause; thus the name *idiopathic scoliosis*. The following discussion involves the adolescent type, which is often called *adolescent idiopathic scoliosis*. There appears to be a genetic component to the etiology of idiopathic scoliosis; however, the exact relationship has yet to be established.

Idiopathic scoliosis is most noticeable during the preadolescent growth spurt. School screening is somewhat controversial, since there are no controlled studies to demonstrate improved outcomes and a reported number of false positives lead to referrals (Bunnell, 2005). Screenings may cause potential harm in terms of unnecessary medical evaluations and an adverse psychological impact. As a result, the Canadian Paediatric Society (2010) does not recommend screening.

Diagnostic Evaluation

Observation is performed behind an undressed (in undergarments) standing child, noting any asymmetry of shoulder height, scapular or flank shape, or hip height and alignment. When the child bends forward at the waist (the Adams test) with hanging arms, asymmetry of the ribs and flanks may be noted. A scoliometer is also used in the initial screening to measure truncal rotation (also measured by the Adams test). Often a primary curve and a compensatory curve will place the head in alignment with the gluteal cleft. However, in the uncompensated curve the head and hips are not aligned (see Fig. 54-11, E and F). (See Spine, Chapter 34, for additional information.) Definitive diagnosis is made by radiographs of the child in the standing position and use of the Cobb technique (standard measurement of angle curvature), which establishes the degree of curvature. The Risser scale is used to evaluate skeletal maturity on the radiographs; the scale assists in making a determination of the likely progression of the spinal angulature as the child's bones mature. The Tanner maturity rating is also used to evaluate the risk of curve progression in adolescents. Not all spinal curvatures are scoliosis. A curve of less than 10 degrees is considered a postural variation. Curves of less than 20 degrees are mild and, if nonprogressive, do not require treatment.

Intraspinal conditions or other disease processes that can cause scoliosis must be ruled out. The presence of pain, sacral dimpling or hairy patches, cutaneous vascular changes, absent or abnormal reflexes, bowel or bladder incontinence, or left thoracic curve may indicate an intraspinal abnormality such as syringomyelia, diastematomyelia, or tethered cord syndrome. An MRI scan should be obtained for evaluation.

Therapeutic Management

Current management options include observation with regular clinical and radiographic evaluation, orthotic intervention (bracing), and surgical spinal fusion. Treatment decisions are based on the magnitude, location, and type of curve; the age and skeletal maturity of the child or adolescent; and any underlying or contributing disease process. The Canadian Paediatric Society (2010) indicates that there is evidence that individuals with mild clinical scoliosis may not benefit from interventions such as braces and exercises.

Bracing and Exercise

For many curves in the growing child and adolescent, bracing may be the treatment of choice. It is important to realize that *bracing is not curative*, but that it may slow the progression of the curvature to allow skeletal growth and maturity. The two most common types of bracing are (1) the *Boston* and *Wilmington braces*, which are underarm orthoses customized from prefabricated plastic shells, with corrective forces for each patient using lateral pads and decreasing lumbar lordosis, and (2) a *TLSO (thoracolumbosacral orthotic)*, which is an underarm orthosis made of plastic that is custom moulded to the body and then shaped to correct or hold the deformity (Fig. 54-12). The *Milwaukee brace*, which is an individually adapted brace that includes a neck ring, is rarely used

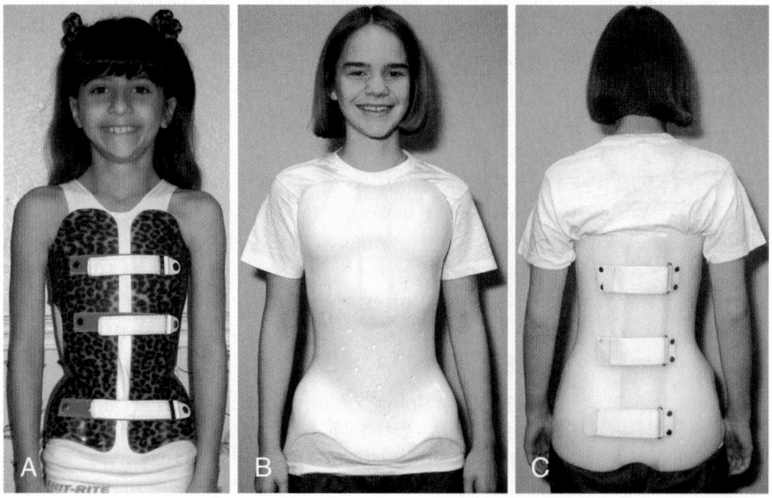

Fig. 54-12 **A:** Standard thoracolumbosacral (TLSO) brace for idiopathic scoliosis. Note the colour and design incorporated into the brace to make it more acceptable to children and adolescents. **B:** Variation of a standard TLSO that fastens in the back **(C)** to provide needed support for the spine curvature.

in scoliosis but is sometimes used in the treatment of kyphosis. The *Charleston nighttime bending brace* is worn only when the child is in bed because it prevents walking because of the severity of the trunk bend. Bracing, although used as the gold standard treatment for mild to moderate curvatures, has not proved to be entirely effective in the treatment of scoliosis (Newton & Wenger, 2001). Compliance in wearing the brace is difficult because of the adolescent's age and preoccupation with body image and appearance. Experts recognize that brace treatment in some children with significant scoliosis may help avoid surgical intervention by slowing curve progression; however, further studies are needed to clarify the effectiveness of bracing (Richards & Vitale, 2008).

Exercises alone and chiropractic treatment are rarely of value in managing scoliosis; transcutaneous electrical nerve stimulation has also proved to be an ineffective treatment for this condition. Exercises are of benefit when used in conjunction with bracing to maintain and increase the strength of spinal and abdominal muscles during treatment.

Surgical Management

Surgical intervention may be required for correction of severe curves (usually 45 degrees or more in skeletally immature patients and 50 to 55 degrees or more in the skeletally mature [Spiegel, Hosalkar, & Dormans, 2007]). The degree of curvature and the cause guide the decision to have surgery. Bracing and exercise have been universally disappointing in curves greater than 40 degrees, and paralytic and congenital curves, which will eventually progress, are best treated with early surgical stabilization if the child's health status will allow major surgery. The child's age and location of the curvature influence the decision for surgery, and any progressive or severe curve that does not respond to more conservative orthotic measures requires surgical correction. Difficulties with balance or seating, respiratory excursion, or pain are also considered.

The surgical technique consists of realignment and straightening with internal fixation and instrumentation combined with bony fusion (*arthrodesis*) of the realigned spine. The goals of surgical intervention are to correct the curvatures on the sagittal and coronal planes and to have a solid, pain-free fusion in a well-balanced torso, with maximum mobility of the remaining spinal segments.

Many instrumentation systems, including Harrington, Dwyer, Zielke, Luque, Cotrel-Dubousset, Isola, TSRH (Texas Scottish Rite Hospital), and Moss Miami, are available. Selection of the system is individualized according to the patient's needs and surgeon's preference. Posterior or anterior surgical approaches can be used.

The Harrington system, the first internal spinal instrumentation device, consists of distraction and compression rods, hooks, and nuts. The posterior elements are decorticated, and bone from the iliac crest or donor bone is placed across the vertebrae to provide fusion. Postoperatively the child is logrolled to prevent spinal motion, and a moulded plastic jacket is used to stabilize the spine until the fusion is solid.

The Luque-rod segmental spinal instrumentation provides segmental stability by the use of wires and L-shaped rods. By way of a posterior approach, the wires are threaded beneath the lamina of each vertebra and tightened around the rods resting along the transverse processes to stabilize the spine. Bone from the iliac crest or donor bone is used to fuse the spine. The advantage of this method is that the patient can be mobile within a few days and requires no postoperative immobilization. The disadvantage is the risk of nerve damage.

The Cotrel-Dubousset instrumentation combines the Harrington and L-rod approaches by using bilateral rods and hooks at many sites. Anterior approaches using the Dwyer or Zielke instrumentation involve screws into the vertebral bodies connected by a cable or rod. These systems require postoperative immobilization with a custom-fitted plastic jacket.

Advances in surgical technology are currently being evaluated, including thoracoscopic spinal fusion and placement of implants; metallic staples may also be placed into the vertebral bodies to achieve spinal fusion and to correct the deformity (Spiegel et al., 2007).

Nursing Care Management

Treatment for scoliosis extends over a significant portion of the affected child's period of growth. In adolescents this period is the one in which their identity, physical and psychological, is formed. The identification of scoliosis as a "deformity," in combination with unattractive appliances and a significant surgical procedure, can have a negative effect on the already fragile adolescent body image. The adolescent and family require excellent nursing care to meet not only physical needs but also psychological needs associated with the diagnosis, surgery, postoperative recovery, and eventual rehabilitation (Slote, 2002). Although these adolescents are encouraged to participate in most peer activities, necessary therapeutic modifications are likely to make them feel different and apart. Nursing care of the adolescent who is facing scoliosis surgery, potential social isolation, pain, and uncertainty, not to mention misunderstood emotions and body image issues, must be evaluated from the adolescent's perspective to be successful in meeting the individual's needs (Napierkowski, 2007). See the Additional Resources section for a patient and family teaching tool for scoliosis.

When a child or adolescent first faces the prospect of a prolonged period in a brace, jacket, or other device, the therapy program and the nature of the device must be explained thoroughly to both the child and the parents so that they will understand the anticipated results, how the appliance corrects the defect, the freedoms and constraints imposed by the device, and what they can do to help achieve the desired goal. The management involves the skills and services of a team of specialists, including an orthopedist, physiotherapist, orthotist (a specialist in fitting orthopedic braces), nurse, social worker, and sometimes a thoracic or pulmonary specialist.

It is difficult for a child to be restricted at any phase of development, but the adolescent needs continual positive reinforcement, encouragement, and as much independence as can be safely assumed during this time. Guidance and assistance regarding anticipated problems, such as selection of clothing and participation in social activities, are appreciated by adolescents. Socialization with peers is strongly encouraged, and every effort should be made to help the adolescent feel attractive and worthwhile.

Preoperative Care

The preoperative workup usually involves a radiographic series, including bending and traction films, pulmonary function studies, and a number of routine laboratory studies (including prothrombin, partial thromboplastin, and bleeding times; blood count; electrolyte levels; urinalysis and urine culture; and blood levels of any medications). Because spinal surgery usually involves considerable blood loss, several options are considered preoperatively to maintain or replace blood volume. These options include autologous blood donations obtained from the patient before the surgery, intraoperative blood salvage, intraoperative hemodilution, erythropoietin administration, and controlled induced hypotension, which must be carefully monitored at all times to prevent physiological instability (Newton & Wenger, 2001).

Surgery for spinal fusion is complex, and often adolescents who require the procedure because of idiopathic scoliosis are not familiar with medical terms, procedures, or experiences. Preoperative teaching is critical for the adolescent to be able to participate in his or her treatment and recovery. Because the surgery is extensive, the patient must be taught how to manage his or her own patient-controlled analgesia (PCA) pump, how to log-roll, and the use and function of other equipment, such as a chest tube (for anterior repair) and Foley catheter. It is recommended that the child or adolescent bring a favourite toy (age dependent) or personal items such as a favourite stuffed animal, laptop computer or personal tablet (for Web surfing and e-mails), movie player, MP3 player, or portable CD player for postoperative use. Meeting with a peer who has undergone a similar surgery is also valuable (Slote, 2002).

Postoperative Care

After surgery, patients are monitored in an acute care setting and log rolled when changing position to prevent damage to the fusion and instrumentation. In some cases an immobilization brace or cast is used postoperatively depending on the type of surgical intervention. Skin care is important, and pressure-relieving mattresses or beds may be needed to prevent pressure wounds (see Maintaining Healthy Skin, Chapter 45).

In addition to the usual postoperative assessments of wound, circulation, and vital signs, the neurological status of the patient's extremities requires special attention. Prompt recognition of any neurological impairment is imperative because delayed paralysis may develop that requires surgical intervention. Common postoperative problems after spinal fusion include neurological injury or spinal cord injury, hypotension from acute blood loss, wound infection, syndrome of inappropriate secretion of antidiuretic hormone, atelectasis, pneumothorax, ileus, delayed neurological injury, and implanted hardware complications (Freeman, 2007; Newton & Wenger, 2001). Superior mesenteric artery (SMA) syndrome may occur several days after spinal surgery; this involves duodenal compression by the aorta and SMA and may result in acute partial or complete duodenal obstruction. Clinical manifestations include epigastric pain, nausea, copious vomiting, and eructation; symptoms are aggravated in the supine position and often relieved with the patient in a left lateral decubitus or prone position.

The adolescent usually has considerable pain for the first few days after surgery and requires frequent administration of pain medication, preferably opioids administered intravenously on a regular schedule. For children able to understand the concept, PCA is recommended (see Pain Assessment; Pain Management, Chapter 35). In most cases the patient begins walking as soon as possible. Depending on the instrumentation used and the surgical approach, most patients are walking by the second or third postoperative day and are discharged by 1 week. In addition to pain management, the patient is evaluated for skin integrity, adequate urine output, fluid and electrolyte balance, and ileus (Slote, 2002). Discharge planning should include a timetable for follow-up with the practitioner and resumption of regular activities.

All patients are started on physiotherapy as soon as they are able, beginning with range-of-motion exercises on the first postoperative day, and many of the activities of daily living in the following days. Self-care, such as washing and eating, is always encouraged. Throughout the hospitalization, age-appropriate activities and contact with family and friends are important parts of nursing care and planning (see The Immobilized Child, p. 1684).

The family needs to be encouraged to become involved in the patient's care in order to facilitate the transition from hospital to home management. An organization that provides education and services to both families and professionals is the National Scoliosis Foundation. The American Academy of Orthopaedic Surgeons and Scoliosis Research Society, an organization of physicians and scientists, have published an excellent book, *Scoliosis*, and the Scoliosis Research Society has educational information available on its Web site. A Canadian scoliosis support association operates from the province of British Columbia.

Infections of Bones and Joints

Osteomyelitis

Osteomyelitis, an infectious process in the bone, can occur at any age but most frequently is seen in children 10 years of age or younger. *Staphylococcus aureus* is the most common causative organism. Acute hematogenous osteomyelitis results when a bloodborne bacterium causes an infection in the bone. Common foci include infected lesions, upper respiratory tract infections, otitis media, tonsillitis, abscessed teeth, pyelonephritis, and infected burns. Exogenous osteomyelitis is acquired from direct inoculation of the bone from a puncture wound, open fracture, surgical contamination, or adjacent tissue infection. Subacute osteomyelitis has a longer course and may be caused by less virulent microbes with a walled-off abscess or Brodie's abscess, typically in the proximal or distal tibia. Chronic osteomyelitis is a progression of acute osteomyelitis and is characterized by dead bone, bone loss, and drainage and sinus tracts.

Generally, healthy bone is not likely to become infected. Factors that contribute to infection include inoculation with a large number of organisms, presence of a foreign body, bone injury, high virulence of an organism, immunosuppression, and malnutrition; certain types and locations of bone are also more vulnerable to infection.

Typically children with acute hematogenous osteomyelitis are seen with a 2- to 7-day history of pain, warmth, tenderness, and decreased range of motion in the affected limb, along with systemic symptoms of fever, irritability, and lethargy (Box 54-8). Symptoms often resemble those observed in other diseases involving bones such as arthritis or leukemia.

Pathophysiology

Osteomyelitis can be acquired exogenously by direct inoculation of bone during trauma or surgery; the hand and foot are common sites. Hematogenous osteomyelitis is seeded by organisms from a pre-existing infection such as tonsillitis or impetigo or from a contiguous source such as an adjacent infected bone or joint. Hematogenous osteomyelitis usually occurs in the metaphyses of long bones such as the femur or tibia. The infecting organism travels from the site of infection to the small end-artery capillary loops in the bone metaphyses, causing obstruction and initiating infection, with complications of bone destruction and abscess formation. In infants the diagnosis is challenging because of the difficulty localizing symptoms and the increased likelihood of multiple bone involvement.

Diagnostic Evaluation

Organism identification and antibiotic susceptibility testing are essential for effective therapy. Cultures of aspirated subperiosteal pus along with cultures of blood, joint fluid, and infected skin samples should be obtained. Bone biopsy is indicated if blood culture results and radiographic findings are not consistent with osteomyelitis. Supporting evidence for osteomyelitis includes leukocytosis and an elevated erythrocyte sedimentation rate. Radiographic signs, except for soft-tissue swelling, are evident only after 2 to 3 weeks. A three-phase technetium bone scan can show areas of increased blood flow, such as occurs in early stages in infected bone, and is useful in locating multiple sites; however, it is not a diagnostic test. CT can detect bone destruction, and MRI provides anatomical details useful in delineating the area of involvement, especially if surgical intervention is planned. Sometimes the osteomyelitis may be unrecognized if it occurs as a complication of a severe toxic and debilitating disease.

BOX 54-8 Clinical Manifestations of Acute Osteomyelitis

General Manifestations

History of trauma to affected bone (frequent)
Child appears very ill
Irritability
Elevated temperature
Restlessness
Rapid pulse
Dehydration

Local Manifestations

Tenderness
Increased warmth
Diffuse swelling over involved bone
Involved extremity painful, especially on movement
Involved extremity held in semiflexion
Surrounding muscles tense and resistant to passive movement

Therapeutic Management

After culture specimens are obtained, empiric therapy is started with IV antibiotics covering the mostly likely organisms. For *S. aureus*, nafcillin or clindamycin is generally used; methicillin-resistant *S. aureus* may require vancomycin. When the infective agent is identified, administration of the appropriate antibiotic is initiated and continued for at least 4 weeks, but the length of therapy is determined by the duration of the symptoms, the response to treatment, and the organism's sensitivity. In selected cases oral antibiotic therapy may follow a shorter IV course. Because of the prolonged duration of high-dose antibiotic therapy, it is important to monitor for hematological, renal, hepatic, ototoxic, and other potential adverse effects.

Surgery may be indicated if there is no response to specific antibiotic therapy, persistent soft-tissue abscess is seen, or the infection spreads to the joint. Opinions differ regarding surgical intervention, but many advocate sequestrectomy and surgical drainage to decompress the metaphyseal space before pus erupts and spreads to the subperiosteal space, forming abscesses that strip the periosteum from bone or form draining sinuses. When these complications occur, a chronic infection usually persists. When surgical drainage is carried out, polyethylene tubes are placed in the wound; one tube instills an antibiotic solution directly into the infected area by gravity, and the other, connected to a suction apparatus, provides drainage.

Nursing Care Management

During the acute phase of illness any movement of the affected limb will cause discomfort; thus the child needs to be positioned comfortably with the affected limb supported. Moving and turning are carried out carefully and gently to minimize pain. The child may require pain medication or sedation. Vital signs should be taken and recorded frequently and measures implemented to reduce a significant temperature elevation.

Antibiotic therapy requires careful observation and monitoring of the IV equipment and site. Because more than one antibiotic is usually administered, the compatibility of the medications needs to be determined and care taken to avoid mixing incompatible medications. For long-term antibiotic therapy, an **intermittent infusion device** or peripherally inserted central catheter is used (see Parenteral Fluid Therapy, Chapter 45). Antibiotic therapy is often continued at home.

Routine practices should be put in effect for children with open wounds, depending on the institution's policies. The wound is managed according to the practitioner's directions. Administration of an antibiotic solution directly into the wound is most efficiently accomplished using a regular infusion setup that is prepared and regulated in the same manner as for any IV infusion. Intake and output should be measured and recorded, and the character of both the wound and drainage noted. The amount and character of drainage on the wound dressing also should be noted.

Casts are sometimes used for immobilization, and, if so, routine cast care needs to be carried out. The extremity should be examined for sensation, circulation, and pain; the area over the inflammation is usually left open for observation. The affected area, casted or uncasted, needs to be assessed for colour, swelling, heat, and tenderness.

The child usually has a poor appetite and may be prone to vomiting. The appetite returns as the acute symptoms recede. During convalescence, adequate nutrition must be maintained to aid healing and formation of new bone.

When the acute stage subsides, children begin to feel better, appetite improves, and they become interested in their surroundings and relationships. Weight bearing on the affected limb is not permitted until healing is well under way in order to avoid pathological fractures. Provision of diversional and constructive activities becomes an important nursing intervention. At this stage the continuous IV infusion may be replaced by a heparin lock system to allow greater freedom.

As the infection subsides, physiotherapy is instituted to ensure restoration of optimum function. The child is usually discharged on a regimen of oral antibiotics, and progress is followed closely for some time.

Septic Arthritis

Septic arthritis is a bacterial infection in the joint. It usually results from hematogenous spread or from direct extension of an adjacent cellulitis or osteomyelitis. Direct inoculation from trauma accounts for 15 to 20% of septic arthritis cases. The most common causative organism is *S. aureus*. Community-acquired methicillin-resistant *S. aureus* is commonly a cause of septic arthritis (Gutierrez, 2005). In addition to *S. aureus*, pathogens seen in neonates include group B streptococci, *Escherichia coli*, and *Candida albicans*. In children 2 months to 5 years of age, *S. aureus*, *Streptococcus pyogenes*, *Streptococcus pneumoniae*, and *Kingella kingae* are the primary organisms causing infection, whereas children older than 5 years are more likely to be infected by *S. aureus* and *S. pyogenes*; sexually active adolescents may be infected by *Neisseria gonorrhoeae* (Gutierrez, 2005).

Knees, hips, ankles, and elbows are the most common joints affected. Clinical manifestations include severe joint pain, swelling, warmth of overlying tissue, and occasionally erythema. The child is resistant to any joint movement. Features of systemic illness such as fever, malaise, headache, nausea, vomiting, and irritability may also be present.

Therapeutic Management and Nursing Care Management

The affected joint is aspirated and the specimen evaluated by Gram stain, culturing (including separate cultures for *Haemophilus influenzae* and *N. gonorrhoeae*), and determination of leukocyte count and glucose, lactate, and protein levels. An infection involving the hip, however, is considered a surgical emergency to prevent compromised blood supply to the head of the femur (Lampe, 2007). In addition, blood culture should be performed, and complete blood count with differential and erythrocyte sedimentation rate or C-reactive protein level should be obtained. Early radiographic findings are limited to soft-tissue swelling but may reveal a foreign body, and such films always provide a baseline for comparison. Technetium scans reveal areas of increased blood flow but will not differentiate between sites. MRI and CT scans provide more detailed images of cartilage loss, joint narrowing, erosions, and ankylosis of progressive disease.

Surgical intervention may also be required if there was a penetrating wound or a possible involvement of a foreign object. Physiotherapy may be initiated for the child who is immobilized in a cast or traction to prevent flexion contractures.

Treatment is IV antibiotic therapy based on Gram stain results and the clinical presentation. The benefits of serial aspirations to demonstrate sterility of synovial fluid and reduce pressure or pain are controversial. Pain management is an important aspect of nursing care, particularly with involvement of a large joint such as the hip. Additional nursing care is the same as for osteomyelitis.

Skeletal Tuberculosis

In children tubercular infection of the bones and joints is acquired by lymphohematogenous spread at the time of primary infection. Occasionally it is from chronic pulmonary tuberculosis. Skeletal tubercular infection is not common in North America but should be considered in communities with high tuberculosis case rates. The infection is most likely to involve the vertebrae, causing tubercular spondylitis. If the infection is progressive, it causes Pott's disease with destruction of the vertebral bodies and results in kyphosis. Symptoms are insidious. The child may report persistent or intermittent pain. Other findings include joint swelling and stiffness; fever and weight loss are not common. Tubercular arthritis can also affect single joints such as a knee or hip and tends to cause severe destruction of adjacent bone. Infection in the fingers causes spina ventosa, a tuberculous dactylitis.

As with pulmonary tuberculosis, the index case should be located. A family and environmental history needs to be obtained and tuberculin skin tests (TSTs) performed. Results of TSTs are positive for the majority of children with tuberculous arthritis; however, the results are not diagnostic, and the clinical and laboratory features do not differentiate tubercular arthritis from a nontubercular septic arthritis. Diagnosis requires isolation of *Mycobacterium tuberculosis* from the site. Patients with the susceptible organism start treatment with combined antituberculosis chemotherapy (isoniazid, rifampin, and pyrazinamide); directly observed therapy is preferred (see also Chapter 46).

Nursing Care Management

Nursing care depends on the site and extent of infection. Tuberculous spondylitis and hip infection may require immobilization, casting, and fusion. Nursing care is the same as for osteomyelitis and septic arthritis.

Bone and Soft-Tissue Tumour

General Concepts: Bone Tumour

Malignant bone tumour represent less than 5% of all malignant neoplasms, but 85% of all primary malignant bone tumours in children are either osteogenic sarcomas or Ewing's sarcomas. The peak ages during childhood are 15 to 19 years. The sexes are affected equally until puberty, at which time the ratio approaches 2 : 1 in favour of males. This propensity for males with a peak incidence during adolescence is thought to result from the accelerated growth rate of osseous tissue.

Neoplastic disease can arise from any tissues involved in bone growth, such as osteoid matrix, bone marrow elements, fat, blood and lymph vessels, nerve sheath, and cartilage. They have several characteristics in common, which are discussed in the following sections, along with specific information about each tumour.

Most malignant bone tumours produce localized pain in the affected site and are often relieved by a flexed position, which relaxes the muscles overlying the stretched periosteum (Box 54-9).

Diagnostic Evaluation

Diagnosis begins with a thorough history and physical examination. A primary objective is to rule out causes such as trauma or infection. Careful questioning regarding pain is essential in determining the duration and rate of tumour growth. Physical assessment focuses on functional status of the affected area, signs of inflammation, size of the mass, involvement of regional lymph nodes, and any systemic indication of generalized malignancy, such as anemia, weight loss, and frequent infection.

Definitive diagnosis is based on radiological studies, such as CT to determine the extent of the lesion; MRI to assess soft tissue, tumour boundaries, and nerve and vessel involvement; radioisotope bone scans to evaluate metastasis; and either needle or surgical bone biopsy to determine the histological pattern. Radiological findings are characteristic for each type of tumour. In osteogenic sarcoma, needlelike new bone formation growing at right angles to the diaphysis (shaft) produces a "sunburst" appearance. In Ewing's sarcoma, the deposits of new bone in layers under the periosteum produce an "onion skin" appearance. In both types of bone tumour, soft-tissue infiltration may be apparent.

At present there is no reliable biochemical test for bone cancers. Elevated alkaline phosphatase levels may occur in osteoid tumour. Several tests may be done for differential diagnosis in terms of secondary bone metastasis from Wilms' tumour, neuroblastoma, retinoblastoma, rhabdomyosarcoma, lymphoma, or leukemia. Lung CT is usually a standard procedure, since pulmonary metastasis is the most common complication of primary bone tumour. Bone marrow aspiration is helpful in diagnosing Ewing's sarcoma in the rare event that the child has bone marrow metastasis.

BOX 54-9 Clinical Manifestations of Bone Tumour

Pain localized at affected site attributed to "growing pains" or trauma
- May be severe or dull
- Often relieved by position of flexion

Frequently brought to attention when the child
- Limps
- Curtails own physical activity
- Is unable to hold heavy objects

Osteosarcoma

Osteosarcoma (osteogenic sarcoma) is the most common bone cancer in children. Its peak incidence is between 10 and 25 years of age (Link, Gebhardt, & Myers, 2006). It presumably arises from bone-forming mesenchyme, which gives rise to malignant osteoid tissue. Most primary tumour sites are in the metaphysis (wider part of the shaft, adjacent to the epiphyseal growth plate) of long bones, especially in the lower extremities. More than half occur in the femur, particularly the distal portion, with the rest involving the humerus, tibia, pelvis, jaw, and phalanges.

Therapeutic Management

Optimum treatment of osteosarcoma is surgery and chemotherapy. The surgical approach consists of surgical biopsy followed by either limb salvage or amputation. Depending on the tumour site, surgery includes amputation of the affected extremity at least 7.5 cm (3 inches) above the proximal tumour margin or above the joint proximal to the involved bone. With tumour of the distal femur, preservation of the hip joint may be possible. Other procedures include an above-the-knee amputation for tumour of the tibia or fibula, a hemipelvectomy for tumour of the innominate (hip) bone, and a forequarter amputation (removal of arm, scapula, and portion of the clavicle on the affected side) for tumour of the upper humerus.

The other surgical approach for selected patients is the *limb salvage procedure*, which involves en bloc resection of the primary tumour with prosthetic replacement of the involved bone. For example, with osteosarcoma of the distal femur, a total femur and joint replacement is performed. Frequently children undergoing a limb salvage procedure will receive preoperative chemotherapy in an attempt to decrease the tumour size and make surgery more manageable (Link et al., 2006).

Chemotherapy plays a vital role in the treatment of osteosarcoma. Antineoplastic medications, such as high-dose methotrexate with citrovorum factor rescue, doxorubicin, bleomycin, actinomycin D, cyclophosphamide, ifosfamide, and cisplatin, may be administered singly or in combination and may be employed both before and after surgery. When pulmonary metastasis is found, thoracotomy and chemotherapy have resulted in prolonged survival and potential cure. These combined-modality approaches have significantly improved the survival rates for osteosarcoma to approximately 60 to 70% in nonmetastatic patients (Heare, Hensley, & Dell'orfano, 2009; Ta et al., 2009). New trials have recently been completed using muramyl tripeptide phosphatidylethanolamine to eradicate micrometastases by stimulating macrophages to kill tumour cells not eliminated by chemotherapy (Link et al., 2006).

Nursing Care Management

Nursing care depends on the type of surgical approach. Obviously the family may have more difficulty adjusting to an amputation than a limb salvage procedure. In either instance, preparation of the child and family is critical. Straightforward honesty is essential in gaining the child's cooperation and trust. The diagnosis of cancer should not be disguised with

evolve Critical Thinking Exercise—Osteogenic Sarcoma

falsehoods such as "infection." To accept the need for radical surgery, the child must be aware of the lack of alternatives for treatment. Although the responsibility of telling the child is generally left to the physician, the nurse should be present at the discussion or be aware of exactly what is said. The child should be told a few days before surgery to allow him or her time to think about the diagnosis and consequent treatment and to ask questions.

Sometimes children have many questions about the prosthesis, limitations on physical ability, and prognosis in terms of cure. At other times they react with silence or with a calm manner that belies their concern and fear. Either response must be accepted, since it is part of the grieving process of a loss. For those who desire information, it may be helpful to introduce them to another amputee before surgery or to show them pictures of the prosthesis. However, the nurse must be careful not to overwhelm children with information. A sound approach is to answer questions without offering additional information. For those who do not pursue additional information, the nurse expresses a willingness to talk.

Before surgery, the child should be informed of the need for chemotherapy, and its adverse effects, but without offering too much information at one time. It is wise to discuss hair loss with an emphasis on positive aspects, such as wearing a wig. Because bone tumours affect adolescents and young adults, it is not unusual for them to become angry over all the radical body alterations.

If an amputation is performed, the child is usually fitted with a temporary prosthesis immediately after surgery, which permits early functioning and fosters psychological adjustment. If this is not done, the child requires stump care, which is the same as for any amputee. A permanent prosthesis is usually fitted within 6 to 8 weeks. During hospitalization the child begins physiotherapy to become proficient in the use and care of the device. There is a unique "Champ Program" in Canada developed by War Amps, which matches mothers and junior counsellors who provide support to children with amputations and their families. This organization provides information, support, financial assistance, and public education programs on child safety (see Additional Resources at the end of this chapter).

Phantom limb pain may develop after amputation. This symptom is characterized by sensations such as tingling, itching, and, more frequently, pain felt in the amputated limb. The child and family need to know that the sensations are real, not imagined. In a Canadian study, adolescent amputees identified the primary triggers of phantom sensation or pain: exercise, objects approaching the stump, cold weather, and "feeling nervous." Forty-percent experienced phantom sensations and pain. Surgical amputation increased the likelihood of phantom manifestations (Wilkins, McGrath, Finley, & Katz, 1998). Amitriptyline (Elavil) has been used successfully in children to decrease the pain (Olsson, 1999).

Discharge planning must begin early in the postoperative period. Once the child has begun physiotherapy, the nurse should consult with the therapist and practitioner to evaluate the child's physical and emotional readiness to re-enter school. It is an opportune time to involve a community nurse in the child's home care. Every effort should be made to promote normalcy and gradual resumption of realistic preamputation activities. Role-playing is beneficial in preparing the child for the inevitable confrontation by others. Environmental barriers, such as stairs, need to be assessed in terms of the accessibility in the school and home, especially because the child may need to use crutches or a wheelchair before complete healing and prosthetic competency are achieved.

The nurse should encourage the child to select clothing that best camouflages the prosthesis, such as pants or long-sleeved shirts. Well-fitted prostheses are so natural looking that girls can usually wear sheer pantyhose without revealing the device. Emphasizing feminine or masculine apparel can help the child regain a feeling of self-identity. Even during the postoperative period, encouraging the child to wear blue jeans and a T-shirt may distract attention from the deformity and focus it on familiar aspects of appearance.

The family and child need much support in adjusting not only to a life-threatening diagnosis but also to alteration in body form and function. Because loss of a limb entails a grieving process, those caring for the child need to recognize that the reactions of anger and depression are normal and necessary. Often parents view the anger as a direct affront to them for allowing the amputation to occur, or they see the depression as rejection. These are not personal attacks but the child's attempts to cope with a loss.

Ewing's Sarcoma (Primitive Neuroectodermal Tumour)

Ewing's sarcoma, classified as a primitive neuroectodermal tumour, is the second most common malignant bone tumour (after osteosarcoma) in childhood. Ewing's sarcoma arises in the marrow spaces of the bone rather than from osseous tissue. The tumour originates in the shaft of long and trunk bones, most often affecting the femur, tibia, fibula, humerus, ulna, vertebrae, scapula, ribs, pelvic bones, and skull (Link et al., 2006). It occurs almost exclusively in individuals under age 30, with the majority being between 4 and 25 years of age.

Therapeutic Management

Surgical amputation is not routinely recommended but may be considered when the results of radiotherapy render the extremity useless or deformed (e.g., from restricted growth in young children). The treatment of choice is intensive irradiation of the involved bone combined with chemotherapy. A widely used drug regimen includes vincristine, actinomycin D, cyclophosphamide or ifosfamide, etoposide, and doxorubicin. The addition of ifosfamide and etoposide has increased the 3-year survival to 80% (Geller & Gorlik, 2010).

Nursing Care Management

The psychological adjustment to Ewing's sarcoma is typically less traumatic than it is to osteosarcoma because of the preservation of the affected limb. Many families accept the diagnosis with relief in knowing that this type of bone cancer does not necessitate amputation, and initially they may not be aware of the damaging effects on the irradiated site. They need preparation for the various diagnostic tests, including bone marrow aspiration and surgical biopsy, and adequate explanation of the treatment regimen. High-dose radiotherapy often causes a skin reaction of dry or moist **desquamation** followed by hyperpigmentation. The child should wear loose-fitting clothes over the irradiated area to minimize additional skin irritation. Because of increased sensitivity, the area should be protected from sunlight and sudden changes in temperature, such as from heating pads or ice packs. The child should be encouraged to use the extremity as tolerated. Occasionally the physiotherapist may plan an active exercise program to preserve maximum function.

The child needs the same considerations for adjusting to the effects of chemotherapy as any other patient with cancer. The drug regimen usually results in hair loss, severe nausea and vomiting, peripheral neuropathy, and possibly cardiotoxicity. Every effort should be made to outline a treatment plan that allows the child maximum resumption of a normal lifestyle and activities (Kline & Sevier, 2003) (see also Nursing Care Plan: The Child With Cancer, Chapter 49).

Rhabdomyosarcoma

Soft-tissue sarcomas are the fourth most common type of solid tumour in children. These malignant neoplasms originate from undifferentiated mesenchymal cells in muscles, tendons, bursae, and fascia, or in fibrous, connective, lymphatic, or vascular tissue. They derive their name from the specific tissue(s) of origin, such as myosarcoma (*myo*, muscle). Rhabdomyosarcoma (*rhabdo*, striated) is the most common soft-tissue sarcoma in children. Striated (skeletal) muscle is found almost anywhere in the body, so these tumours occur in many sites, the most common of which are the head and neck, especially the orbit (eye). Rhabdomyosarcoma arises from embryonic mesenchyme. The disease occurs in children in all age groups but generally affects children between 2 and 6 years of age. In Canada there were 153 new cases of rhabdomyosarcoma from 2003 to 2007 in children aged 0 to 19 years (Canadian Cancer Society, 2012).

The initial signs and symptoms are related to the site of the tumour and compression of adjacent organs (Box 54-10). Some tumour locations, particularly the orbit, produce symptoms early in the course of the illness and contribute to rapid diagnosis and an improved prognosis. Other tumours, such as those of the retroperitoneal area, produce no symptoms until they are large, invasive, and widely metastasized. Unfortunately, many of the signs and symptoms attributable to rhabdomyosarcoma are vague and frequently suggest a common childhood illness, such as "earache" or "runny nose." In some instances a primary tumour site is never identified.

BOX 54-10 Clinical Manifestations of Rhabdomyosarcoma According to Tumour Site

Central Nervous System
Headaches
Morning vomiting
Diplopia

Orbit
Rapidly developing unilateral proptosis
Ecchymosis of conjunctiva
Loss of extraocular movements (strabismus)
Orbital cellulitis

Nasopharynx
Stuffy nose (earliest sign)
Nasal obstruction-dysphagia, nasal voice (obstruction of posterior nasal conchae)
Pain (sore throat and ear)
Epistaxis
Palpable neck nodes
Visible mass in oropharynx (late sign)

Paranasal Sinuses
Nasal obstruction
Local pain, swelling
Discharge (may be unilateral)
Sinusitis
Swelling

Middle Ear
Signs of chronic serous otitis media
Pain, swelling
Mass in external canal
Sanguinopurulent drainage
Facial nerve palsy

Retroperitoneal Area
Usually a "silent" tumour
Abdominal mass
Pain
Signs of intestinal or genitourinary obstruction

Perineum
Visible superficial mass (scrotum, vaginal, or cervical areas)
Bowel or bladder dysfunction (from tumour compression)
Vaginal bleeding or mucosanguineous discharge

Extremity
Pain
Palpable fixed mass
Regional lymph enlargement

Diagnostic Evaluation

Diagnosis begins with a careful examination of the head and neck area, particularly palpation of a nontender, hard mass. The nasopharynx and oropharynx are inspected for any evidence of a visible mass. Radiographic studies to isolate a tumour site are performed, accompanied by chest radiographs, CT, MRI, bone surveys, and bone marrow aspiration to rule out metastasis. A lumbar puncture is indicated for head and neck tumours to examine the cerebrospinal fluid for malignant cells. An excisional biopsy is done to confirm the histological type.

Careful staging is extremely important for planning treatment and determining the prognosis. The Intergroup Rhabdomyosarcoma Study Group has established clinical staging (Wexler, Meyer, & Helman, 2006).

With the change in treatment from radical surgery or radiotherapy to a multimodal approach, survival rates for all stages have increased considerably. Five-year survival rates are approximately 65% (Wexler et al., 2006). Data suggest that children who remain disease free for 2 years are probably cured; however, if relapse occurs, the prognosis for long-term survival is extremely poor.

Therapeutic Management

Because this tumour is highly malignant, with metastasis frequently occurring by the time of diagnosis, aggressive multimodal therapy is recommended. In the past, radical surgical removal of the tumour was the treatment of choice, but with improved survival from combined chemotherapy and irradiation, surgery plays a lesser role. Complete removal of the primary tumour is advocated whenever possible. However, only biopsy is required in certain tumour locations, such as those of the orbit, when followed by irradiation and chemotherapy. This is a fortunate change, since it avoids the devastating effects of enucleation, amputation, or pelvic exenteration.

High-dose irradiation to the primary tumour is recommended, except in group I tumour. Chemotherapy plays a major role in the treatment of all groups. Drugs that are cytotoxic for rhabdomyosarcoma are vincristine, actinomycin D, ifosfamide, cisplatin, carboplatin, etoposide, cyclophosphamide, topotecan, melphalan, and doxorubicin, which are administered for 1 to 2 years, depending on the stage of the disease (Lanzkowsky, 2005).

Nursing Care Management

The nursing responsibilities are similar to those for other types of cancer, especially the solid tumour when surgery is employed. Specific objectives include (1) careful assessment for signs of the tumour, especially during well-child examinations, (2) preparation of the child and family for the multiple diagnostic tests, and (3) supportive care during each stage of multimodal therapy (Kline & Sevier, 2003).

Disorders of Joints

Juvenile Idiopathic Arthritis (Juvenile Rheumatoid Arthritis)

Juvenile idiopathic arthritis (JIA) is a new name replacing *juvenile rheumatoid arthritis (JRA)* in the research literature and in clinical practice. The JRA nomenclature revision to JIA was due in part to the minimally applicable reference to "rheumatoid" in JRA. Only a small percentage of children have a positive rheumatoid factor; furthermore, the JRA classification system focuses more on disease at onset than on disease progression, which is more important (Warren et al., 2001). In 2004 the International League of Associations for Rheumatology further refined the definitions for JIA to provide improved categorization and treatment of the disease (Petty et al., 2004).

JIA is a chronic autoimmune inflammatory disease causing inflammation of joints and other tissue with an unknown cause. JIA starts before age 16 years with peak onset between 1 and 3 years of age. Twice as many girls as boys are affected. The incidence is reported to be approximately 13.9 per 100,000 children per year among White children with an overall prevalence of approximately 113 per 100,000 children (Miller & Cassidy, 2007). The cause is unknown, but two factors are hypothesized: immunogenic susceptibility and an environmental or external trigger such as a virus (e.g., rubella, Epstein-Barr virus, parvovirus B19) (Miller & Cassidy, 2007).

Pathophysiology

The disease process is characterized by chronic inflammation of the synovium with joint effusion and eventual erosion, destruction, and fibrosis of the articular cartilage. Adhesions between joint surfaces and ankylosis of joints occur if the inflammatory process persists.

Clinical Manifestations

The outcome of JIA is variable and unpredictable. The disease, even in severe forms, is rarely life threatening but can cause significant disability. The arthritis tends to wax and wane and eventually becomes inactive in approximately 70% of the cases; however, these children may have severe or minimal joint damage remaining when active arthritis abates. Approximately 30% of the children will have progressive arthritis into adulthood. Their arthritis can cause significant joint deformity and functional disability, requiring medication, physiotherapy, and perhaps future joint replacement. Chronic and acute uveitis, inflammation in the anterior chamber of the eye, can cause permanent vision loss if undiagnosed and not aggressively treated.

Classification of Juvenile Idiopathic Arthritis

JIA is not a single disease, but a heterogeneous group of diseases. The universal Durban classification of JIA, revised and published in 1998, lists several disease categories, each with its own set of criteria and exclusions, which continue to be revised (Petty et al., 1998, 2004):

Systemic arthritis is arthritis in one or more joints associated with at least 2 weeks of fever, rash, lymphadenopathy, hepatosplenomegaly, and serositis.

Oligoarthritis (or pauciarticular arthritis) is arthritis in one to four joints for the first 6 months of disease. It is subdivided to *persistent oligoarthritis* if it remains in four joints or less, and becomes *extended oligoarthritis* if it involves more than four joints after 6 months.

Polyarthritis rheumatoid factor negative affects five or more joints in the first 6 months with a negative rheumatoid factor.

Polyarthritis rheumatoid factor positive also affects five or more joints in first 6 months, but these children have a positive rheumatoid factor.

Psoriatic arthritis is arthritis with psoriasis or an associated dactylitis, nail pitting, or onycholysis or psoriasis in a first-degree relative.

Enthesitis-related arthritis is arthritis, enthesitis (inflammation at the tendon insertion site), or both associated with at least two of the following: sacroiliac or lumbosacral pain, HLA-B27 antigen, arthritis in boys older than 6 years, acute anterior uveitis, inflammatory bowel disease, Reiter's syndrome, or acute anterior uveitis in a first-degree relative.

Diagnostic Evaluation

JIA is a diagnosis of exclusion; there are no definitive tests. Classifications are based on the clinical criteria of age of onset before 16 years, arthritis in one or more joints for 6 weeks or longer, and exclusion of other causes. Laboratory tests may provide supporting evidence of disease.

Sedimentation rate may or may not be elevated. Leukocytosis is frequently present during exacerbations of systemic JIA. Antinuclear antibodies are common in JIA but are not specific for arthritis; however, they help identify children who are at greater risk for uveitis. Plain radiographs are the best initial imaging studies and may show soft-tissue swelling and joint space widening from increased synovial fluid in the joint. Later films can reveal osteoporosis, narrow joint space, erosions, subluxation, and ankylosis. A slit-lamp eye examination is necessary to diagnose uveitis, which is most common in antinuclear antibody–positive young girls with oligoarthritis. Routine examinations are necessary for early diagnosis and treatment to avoid sight-threatening disease (Kump et al., 2006). The Canadian Paediatric Society (2008) is concerned that some children with JIA are not diagnosed early enough and can thus develop long-term complications. The late diagnosis can result in joint contractures, muscle wasting, growth disturbances, impaired functioning, undetected uveitis, and possible sight loss.

Therapeutic Management

There is no cure for JIA. The major goals of therapy are to control pain, preserve joint range of motion and function, minimize effects of inflammation such as joint deformity, and promote normal growth and development. Outpatient care is the mainstay of therapy; lengthy hospitalizations are infrequent. The treatment plan can be exhaustive and intrusive for the child and family, including medication administration, physical and occupational therapy, ophthalmological slit lamp examinations, splints, comfort measures, dietary management, school modifications, and psychosocial support.

Medications

Many arthritis medications are available, and most are effective in suppressing the inflammatory process and relieving pain. These medications may be given alone or in combination and are prescribed in a stepwise manner dependent on disease response to each level.

Nonsteroidal anti-inflammatory drugs (NSAIDs) are the first medications used. Naproxen, ibuprofen, and tolmetin are approved for use in children. They are effective with few common adverse effects other than gastrointestinal irritation and bruising; with naproxen, skin fragility is a possible adverse effect. NSAIDs must be taken with food. There is unofficial use of other NSAIDs approved for arthritis in adults but not yet children. Aspirin, once the medication of choice, has been replaced by NSAIDs because they have fewer adverse effects and easier administration schedules.

Methotrexate is the second-line medication used in children whose symptoms were not relieved with NSAIDS alone. It is started in combination with an NSAID. It is effective, with acceptable toxicity, which requires monitoring of complete blood cell counts and liver function tests. Patient education about possible adverse effects, including discussions with teens about birth defects and avoiding alcohol, is essential. Methotrexate is considered the safest and most effective of the second-line medications for the treatment of JIA (Miller & Cassidy, 2007).

Corticosteroids are potent immunosuppressives used for life-threatening complications, incapacitating arthritis, and uveitis. They are administered at the lowest effective dose for the briefest period and discontinued on a tapering schedule. They may be administered orally, as intra-articular joint injections, as IV pushes, or in eye drop form for uveitis. A single intra-articular injection may provide effective relief for children with pauciarticular disease unresponsive to NSAIDs (Padeh & Passwell, 1998). Prolonged use of systemic steroids is associated with significant adverse effects, including Cushing's syndrome, osteoporosis, increased infection risk, glucose intolerance, **cataracts**, and growth suppression.

Etanercept is a tumour necrosis factor (inhibitor) α-receptor blocker and an effective medication for children with JIA who are nonresponsive to methotrexate (Lovell et al., 2003). It is given twice per week via subcutaneous injections. Possible adverse effects include transient allergic reaction at injection site, increased infection risk, and rare reports of demyelinating disease and pancytopenia. The risk of malignancy is unknown. Parents and patients should be informed that biological medications are new therapies and more will be learned about potential adverse effects in the postmarketing period. Infliximab, a tumour necrosis factor blocker, may also be used but is reported to have more adverse effects than etanercept.

Slow-acting antirheumatic drugs (SAARDs) may require months to be effective and typically work in combination with NSAIDs. SAARDs include sulphasalazine, hydroxychloroquine, gold, and D-penicillamine. SAARDs are used less often because methotrexate has been recognized as the most effective second-line therapy medication.

Physiotherapy and Occupational Therapy

Programs of physical management are individualized for each child and designed to reach the ultimate goal: preserving function or preventing deformity. Physiotherapy is directed toward specific joints, focusing on strengthening muscles, mobilizing restricted joint motion, and preventing or correcting deformities. Occupational therapy assumes responsibility for generalized mobility and performance of activities of daily living.

General treatment or maintenance programs vary; physiotherapists may be involved several times weekly to monthly in the management of a home program, or their visits may be limited to infrequent reviews of the home program for compliance, effectiveness, and need. Normal activities of daily living and the child's natural tendency to be active are usually sufficient to maintain muscle strength and joint mobility.

Exercising in a pool is excellent therapy, since it allows freedom of movement with support and minimal gravitational pull. If there is pain on motion, a hot pack or warm bath before therapy may help.

Practitioners may recommend nighttime splinting to help minimize pain and reduce flexion deformity. Joints most frequently splinted are the knees, wrists, and hands. Positioning during rest is also important. The child rests on a firm mattress with no pillow or a very low one and has no support under the knee. Loss of extension in the knee, hip, and wrist causes special problems and requires vigilance to detect the earliest signs of involvement and vigorous attention to prevent deformity with specialized passive stretching, positioning, and resting splints.

Nursing Care Management

Nursing the child with JIA involves assessment of the child's general health, the status of involved joints, and the child's emotional response to all ramifications of the disease—discomfort, physical restrictions, therapies, and self-concept.

The effects of JIA are manifest in every aspect of the child's life, including physical activities, social experiences, and personality development. Although children with severe disease may have more physical barriers to overcome, studies show that emotional and behavioural functioning is most closely linked with maternal depression and parental distress, not with physical disability. Nursing interventions to support the parents may foster successful adaptation for the entire family. Parental concerns about the disease prognosis, financial and insurance issues, spouse and sibling relationships, and job and schedule conflicts must all be addressed. Referral to social workers, counsellors, or support groups may be needed.

Relieve Pain

The pain of JIA is related to several aspects of the disease: disease severity, functional status, individual pain threshold, family variables, and psychological adjustment. The aim is to provide as much relief as possible with medication and other therapies to help children tolerate the pain and cope as effectively as possible. Nonpharmacological modalities such as behavioural therapy and relaxation techniques have proved effective in modifying pain perception (see Pain Management, Chapter 35) and activities that aggravate pain. Opioid analgesics are typically avoided in juvenile arthritis; however, for children immobilized with refractory pain, short-term opioid analgesics can be part of a comprehensive plan that uses multiple pain relief techniques (Connelly & Schanberg, 2006).

Promote General Health

The child's general health must be considered. A well-balanced diet with sufficient calories to maintain growth is essential. If the child is relatively inactive, caloric intake should match energy needs to avoid excessive weight gain, which places additional stress on affected joints. Sleep and rest are essential for children with JIA. Some children require rest during the day; however, daytime napping that interferes with nighttime sleepiness should be avoided. A bedtime routine that involves comfort measures can help induce sleep. A firm mattress, heated water bed, electric blanket, or sleeping bag helps provide warmth, comfort, and rest. Nighttime splints needed to maintain range of motion might initially be a source of bedtime conflict. The family needs to be instructed on how to use the splint appropriately; the splint should not be painful or impede sleep. Behaviour modification programs that reward splint and exercise compliance may be helpful in reducing compliance barriers.

Well-child care to assess growth, development, and immunization requirements needs to be coordinated between the primary care provider and the rheumatologist. Common childhood illnesses, such as upper respiratory tract infections, may cause arthritis to worsen; consequently, medical attention must be sought quickly for relatively minor illness to prevent arthritis flares. Effective communication between the family, the primary care provider, and the rheumatology team is essential for care coordination.

Children should be encouraged to attend school, even on days when there may be some pain or discomfort. Split days or half days may help a child remain involved in school. Permitting the child to come to school late allows time to gain joint movement and reduces the time at school to avoid exhaustion. It is important that the child attend school to learn skills and engage in social interaction, especially if the JIA continues to limit physical skills. Arranging for two sets of textbooks eliminates the need to carry books to and from school, thus reducing discomfort and difficulty walking. A formal school hearing may be necessary to obtain an individualized education plan, ensured by public law, which includes intensive school modifications.

Facilitate Treatment Compliance

The child and family need to be involved in the therapeutic plan. They need to know the purpose and correct use of any splints and appliances and the medication regimen. The family should be instructed in the administration of medications and the value of a regular schedule of administration to maintain a satisfactory drug level in the body. They need to know that NSAIDs should not be given on an empty stomach and to be alert for signs of medication toxicity. If evidence of drug toxicity is noted, the family should be instructed to notify their health care provider and follow that person's instructions.

Encourage Heat and Exercise

Heat has been shown to be beneficial to children with arthritis. Moist heat is best for relieving pain and stiffness, and the most efficient and practical method is in the bathtub with warm water. In some cases a daily whirlpool bath, paraffin bath, or hot packs may be used as needed for temporary relief of acute swelling and pain. Hot packs are easily applied using a bath towel wrung out after being immersed in hot water or heated in a microwave oven, applied to the area, and covered with plastic for 20 minutes. Commercial pads that warm in only a few minutes in the microwave are also available; electric pads can also be put on a timer. Painful hands or feet can be immersed in a pan of warm water for 10 minutes two or three times daily in addition to tub baths. Pool therapy is the easiest method for exercising a large number of joints. Swimming activities strengthen muscles and maintain mobility in larger joints. Very small children who are frightened of the water can carry out their exercises in the bathtub. Small children love to splash, kick, and throw things in the water. Adult supervision is necessary for all water activities.

Activities of daily living provide satisfactory exercise for older children to maintain maximal mobility with minimal pain. These children should be encouraged in their efforts to be independent and allowed to dress and groom themselves, to assume daily tasks, and to care for their belongings. It is often difficult for children to manipulate buttons, comb or brush hair, and turn faucets, but unless there is an acute flare, parents and other caregivers should not offer assistance. In addition, children should learn and understand why others do not help them. Many helpful devices, such as self-adhering fasteners, tongs for manipulating difficult items, and grab bars installed in bathrooms for safety, can be used to facilitate tasks. A raised (higher) toilet seat often makes the difference between dependent and independent toileting, since weak quadriceps muscles and sore knees inhibit the ability to raise the body from a low sitting position.

A child's natural affinity for play offers many opportunities for incorporating therapeutic exercises. Throwing or kicking a ball and riding a tricycle (with the seat raised to achieve maximum leg extension) are excellent moving and stretching exercises for a very young child whose daily living activities are physically limited.

An effective approach to beginning the day's activities is to awaken children early to give them their medication and then to allow them to sleep for an hour. On arising, children take a hot bath (or shower) and perform a simple ritual of limbering-up exercises, after which they start the day's activities, such as going to school. Exercise, heat, and rest are spaced throughout the remainder of the day according to the child's individual needs and schedule. Parents should be instructed in exercises that meet the child's needs.

In Canada, the Arthritis Society provides many services including education and support groups (see Additional Resources section).

Support the Child and Family

JIA affects every aspect of life for the child and family. Physical limitations may interfere with self-care, school participation, and recreational activities. The intensive treatment plan, including multiple medications, physiotherapy, comfort measures, and medical appointments, is intrusive and disruptive to the parents' work schedule and the family routine. To prevent isolation and foster independence, the family should be encouraged to pursue their normal activities. Unfortunately, the adaptations necessary require resourcefulness and commitment from all family members. At diagnosis and throughout the span of JIA, it is essential to recognize signs of stress and counterproductive coping and provide the necessary support to maximize adaptation. The problems and needs of these families are discussed in Chapter 41; the reader is directed to that chapter for guidance in planning care. (See also Nursing Care Plan, The Child With Arthritis.)

Systemic Lupus Erythematosus

Systemic lupus erythematosus (SLE) is a chronic, multisystem, **autoimmune disease** of the connective tissues and blood vessels characterized by inflammation in potentially any body tissue. Its course and symptoms are variable and unpredictable, with mild to life-threatening complications. In addition to SLE, there are other forms of lupus, such as neonatal lupus, which occurs when maternal autoantibodies cross the placenta and cause transient lupuslike symptoms in the newborn, with the potential serious complication of heart block. The following discussion focuses on SLE.

Reports suggest that survival rates in children with SLE have significantly improved; 5-year survival rates are said to be almost 100%, and 10-year survival rates are close to 90% (Ravelli, Ruperto, & Martini, 2005). SLE is more common in girls, with an approximate 5 : 1 female-to-male ratio, and typically occurs between the ages of 10 and 19 years. There is a familial tendency, although many newly diagnosed patients are unaware of other affected family members. Researchers studied the ethnicity and socioeconomic factors of SLE in Canada and discovered that Asian Canadians and those with Afro-Caribbean origins had a higher frequency of renal involvement and more exposure to immunosuppressives. First Nations, Métis, and Inuit peoples had higher frequencies of antiphospholipid antibodies and **comorbidity**. They also had the least education and the lowest income. Canadians of Asian descent had the youngest onset. The results indicated that there are different lupus phenotypes in ethnic groups but low income was the significant independent predictor for long-term physical damage (Peschken et al., 2009).

The cause of SLE is not known. It appears to result from a complex interaction of genetics with an unidentified trigger that activates the disease. Suspected triggers include exposure to ultraviolet light, estrogen, pregnancy, infections, and medications. Patients with JIA have been known to develop SLE symptoms as a result of the use of tumour necrosis factor medications such as etanercept. Genetic predisposition to SLE is evidenced in an increased concordance rate in twins (tenfold), increased incidence within family members (10 to 16%), and increased frequency of certain gene alleles in population-based studies.

Clinical Manifestations and Diagnostic Evaluation

The child with SLE may have any clinical manifestation with mild to life-threatening severity (Box 54-11). The diagnosis is established when 4 of the 11 diagnostic criteria in Box 54-12 are met; however, children with fewer than 4 criteria who are suspected of having lupus should receive appropriate medical treatment (Klein-Gitelman & Miller, 2007). Kidney involvement heralds progressive disease and the need for rigorous therapeutic management.

Therapeutic Management

The goal of treatment is to ensure the child's health by balancing the medications necessary to avoid exacerbation and complications while preventing or minimizing treatment-associated morbidity. Corticosteroid medications are used to control inflammation; they are administered in doses sufficient to control inflammation, then tapered to the lowest suppressive dose. Other medications include antimalarial preparations, which are useful for rash and arthritis; NSAIDs, which relieve muscle and joint inflammation; and immunosuppressive agents, such as cyclophosphamide, for renal and central nervous system disease. Rituximab, a chimeric anti-CD20 monoclonal antibody, is used to treat SLE in adults and has been shown to be effective in children. The combined use of rituximab and cyclophosphamide has also been shown to be effective for decreasing symptoms in children with SLE (Lehman, 2008). Antihypertensives, aspirin, and antibiotics are just a few of the additional medications that may be necessary to treat or avoid complications.

General supportive care includes sufficient nutrition, sleep and rest, and exercise. Exposure to the sun and ultraviolet B (UVB) light should be limited because of its association with SLE exacerbation.

Nursing Care Management

The principal nursing goal is to help the child and family positively adjust to the disease and therapy. The child and family must learn to recognize subtle signs of disease exacerbation and potential complications of medication therapy. Patient and family education is an ongoing process initiated at diagnosis and individualized. Referral to a social worker, psychologist, or support group may help the child and family make a successful adjustment. Support groups are associated

NURSING CARE PLAN ● The Child With Arthritis

Nursing Diagnosis	Expected Patient Outcome	Nursing Interventions	Rationale
Chronic pain related to joint inflammation **Child's/Family's Defining Characteristics** ***(Subjective and Objective Data)*** Verbal report of pain Guarding behaviour Change in sleep pattern	Child is able to move (joints) and complete activities of daily living with no discomfort or minimal discomfort. **The Following NOC Concepts Apply to These Outcomes** Comfort Level Pain Control Anxiety Self-Control Coping	Use pain rating scale to evaluate pain (discomfort) level.	To provide objective assessment of pain level
		Administer anti-inflammatory medications (nonsteroidal anti-inflammatory drugs [NSAIDs]) promptly on report of pain and around the clock when discomfort is acute.	To manage pain and prevent breakthrough pain
		Administer other rheumatic medications such as methotrexate or slow-acting antirheumatic drugs (SAARDs).	To provided relief from inflammation
		Schedule routine rest periods throughout the day.	
		Encourage child to eat a well-balanced diet and exercise daily.	To prevent obesity and promote wellness
		Help child set up a routine of daily exercise.	To prevent further joint stiffness
		Encourage nonpharmacological pain relief remedies such as the use of a heat pad, moist heat, and pool therapy.	To promote mobility of joints and relieve painful stiff joints To prevent excessive weight gain
		Encourage child to discuss effect of pain on lifestyle and activities.	To provide outlet for emotions such as anger, frustration, depression at having a chronic illness
		The Following NIC Concepts Apply to These Interventions Analgesic Administration Sleep Enhancement Exercise Promotion Medication Management Environmental Management: Comfort	

Nursing Diagnosis	Expected Patient Outcome	Nursing Interventions	Rationale
Impaired physical mobility related to pain and swelling in joints **Child's/Family's Defining Characteristics** ***(Subjective and Objective Data)*** Limited ability to perform fine and gross motor skills Limited range of motion Verbal report of pain Measurable pain on pain scale	Child engages in activities of daily living. **The Following NOC Concepts Apply to These Outcomes** Ambulation Body Mechanics Performance Rest Joint Movement: Ankle Joint Movement: Spine Joint Movement: Wrist Joint Movement: Knee Joint Movement: Hip Joint Movement: Elbow Joint Movement: Fingers	Encourage ambulation and performance of activities of daily living to maximum potential every day.	To keep joints limber and prevent disuse contractures
		Assist with range-of-motion exercises for child who is severely limited.	To promote muscle movement and keep joints limber
		Encourage child to be as active as tolerated.	To promote independence
		Assist with planning and encourage rest periods during the day.	To prevent fatigue
		Encourage taking pain medication such as NSAIDs before ambulation and activity.	To promote activity with minimum pain
		Use nonpharmacological pain adjuncts such as heat pad and hydrotherapy.	To decrease pain and encourage mobility of joints
		Encourage child to be active in self-care activities to maximum potential.	To enhance self-worth and independence
		The Following NIC Concepts Apply to These Interventions Energy Management Exercise Promotion: Stretching Exercise Therapy: Joint Mobility Self-Care Assistance Teaching: Prescribed Activity/Exercise	

NIC, Nursing Interventions Classification; *NOC*, Nursing Outcomes Classification.

BOX 54-11 Clinical Manifestations of Systemic Lupus Erythematosus Related to Tissues Involved

Constitutional—Fever, fatigue, weight loss, anorexia
Cutaneous—Erythematous butterfly rash over bridge of nose and across cheeks, discoid rash, photosensitivity, mucocutaneous ulceration, alopecia, periungual telangiectasias
Musculoskeletal—Arthritis, arthralgia, myositis, myalgia, tenosynovitis
Neurological—Headache, seizure, forgetfulness, behaviour change, change in school performance, psychosis, chorea, stroke, cranial and peripheral neuropathy, pseudotumour cerebri
Pulmonary and cardiac—Pleuritis, basilar pneumonitis, atelectasis, pericarditis, myocarditis, endocarditis
Renal—Glomerulonephritis, nephrotic syndrome, hypertension
Gastrointestinal—Abdominal pain, nausea, vomiting, blood in stool, abdominal crisis, esophageal dysfunction, colitis
Hepatic, splenic, and nodal—Hepatomegaly, splenomegaly, lymphadenopathy
Hematological—Anemia, cytopenia
Ophthalmological—Cotton wool spots, papilledema, retinopathy
Vascular—Raynaud's phenomenon, thrombophlebitis, livedo reticularis

BOX 54-12 Classification Criteria for Systemic Lupus Erythematosus

Four of the following 11 criteria must be met for diagnosis:

1. **Malar rash**—Fixed malar erythema
2. **Discoid rash**—Patchy erythematous lesions
3. **Photosensitivity**—Rash with sun exposure
4. **Oral ulcers**—Painless ulcers in mouth, nose
5. **Arthritis**—Swelling, tenderness, or effusion in two or more peripheral joints (nonerosive)
6. **Serositis**—Pleuritis, pericarditis
7. **Renal disorder**—Proteinuria, casts
8. **Neurological disorder**—Psychosis, seizures
9. **Hematological disorder**—Hemolytic anemia, thrombocytopenia, leukopenia, lymphopenia
10. **Immunological disorder**—Anti-dsDNA, anti-SM, antiphospholipid antibodies, lupus anticoagulant, false-positive syphilis test (RPR)
11. **Antinuclear antibody**

with the Lupus Canada and the Arthritis Society (see Additional Resources).

Key issues include therapy compliance; body-image problems associated with rash, hair loss, and steroid therapy; school attendance; vocational activities; social relationships; sexual activity; and pregnancy. (See Chapter 41 for a discussion on adjusting to a chronic illness.) Specific instructions for avoiding exposure to the sun and UVB light, such as using sunscreens, wearing sun-resistant clothing, and altering outdoor activities, must be provided with great sensitivity to ensure compliance while minimizing the associated feeling of being different from peers (see Sunburn, Chapter 53). Patients need to be instructed to maintain regular medical supervision and seek attention quickly during illness or before elective surgical procedures, such as dental extraction, because of potential needs for increased steroids or prophylactic antibiotics. People with SLE should carry medical identification for their disease and steroid dependence.

Key Points

- Immobility has a profound effect on all aspects of growth and development.
- The major physical consequences of immobilization are loss of muscle strength, endurance, and muscle mass; bone demineralization; loss of joint mobility; and contractures.
- Features of children's fractures not observed in the adult include presence of growth plate, thicker and stronger periosteum, bone porosity, more rapid healing, and less joint stiffness.
- The goals of fracture management are to regain alignment and length of bony fragments, retain alignment and length, and restore function to injured parts.
- The method of fracture reduction is determined by the child's age, degree of displacement, amount of overriding, amount of edema, condition of the skin and soft tissues, sensation, and circulation distal to the fracture.
- The primary purposes of traction are to fatigue involved muscles and reduce muscle spasm, position bone ends in desired realignment, and immobilize the fracture site until realignment has been achieved to permit casting or splinting.
- The etiology of DDH appears to be related to intrauterine, genetic, and cultural factors.
- Treatment of clubfoot consists of manipulation and casting to correct the deformity, maintenance of the correction, and prevention of possible recurrence of the deformity.
- Acquired hip deformities are managed with non–weight-bearing devices (Legg-Calvé-Perthes disease) or surgical stabilization (SCFE).
- Observation for idiopathic scoliosis is an important part of an adolescent's routine physical assessment.
- Idiopathic scoliosis is managed by observation, bracing, and exercise or surgical correction.
- Bone infections are managed with vigorous antibiotic therapy, immobilization of the affected part, and (sometimes) surgical drainage.
- Osteosarcoma is a neoplasm of bone-forming tissues; Ewing's sarcoma is a neoplasm that arises from bone marrow spaces.
- Rhabdomyosarcoma may occur almost anywhere in the body, but the most common sites are the head and neck.
- Nursing care of the child with juvenile arthritis consists of promoting general health, relieving discomfort, preventing deformity, and preserving function.
- SLE is a chronic autoimmune disorder that affects the collagen tissues of the body.

Audio Chapter Summaries
Access an Audio Summary of these Key Points on evolve

References

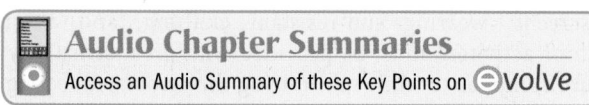

About Kids Health. (2004). *Ankle sprain.* Retrieved from http://. aboutkidshealth.ca/HealthAZ/Ankle-Sprain.aspx?article.

American Academy of Pediatrics, Committee on Quality Improvement and Subcommittee on Developmental Dysplasia of the Hip. (2000). Clinical practice guideline: Early detection of developmental dysplasia of the hip. *Pediatrics, 105*(4), 896–905.

Bachrach, L. K., & Ward, L. M. (2009). Clinical review 1: Bisphosphonate use in childhood osteoporosis. *Journal of Clinical Endocrinology & Metabolism, 94*(2), 400–409. doi:10.1210/jc.2008-1531

Bunnell, W. P. (2005). Selective screening for scoliosis. *Clinics in Orthopedics & Related Research, 434*, 40–45. doi:10.1097/01.blo.0000163242.92733.66

Canadian Cancer Society. (2012). Statistics for childhood soft tissue sarcoma. *Canadian Cancer Encylopedia.* Retrieved from http://info.cancer.ca/cce-ecc/SearchDetails.aspx?Lang=E&lf=sarcoma&cceid=3250.

Canadian Paediatric Society. (2008). Challenge for timely diagnosis of juvenile idiopathic arthritis in children. *Paediatrics & Child Health, 13*(3), 192.

Canadian Paediatric Society. (2010). Preventative health care visits for children and adolescents aged 6 to 17 years: The Greig health record—technical report. *Paediatrics & Child Health, 15*(3), 157–159.

Canadian Paediatric Society. (n.d.) *Osteogenesis imperfecta.* Retrieved from http://www.cps.ca/english/surveillance/cpsp/studies/osteogenesisimperfecta.htm.

Connelly, M., & Schanberg, L. (2006). Opioid therapy for the treatment of refractory pain in children with juvenile rheumatoid arthritis. *Nature: Clinical Practice Rheumatology, 2*(12), 636–637. doi:10.1038/ncprheum0351

Cornwall, R. (2007). Bone and joint disorders: Upper limb. In R. M. Kliegman, et al. (Eds.), *Nelson textbook of pediatrics* (18th ed.). Philadelphia: Saunders.

Curley, M. A., et al. (2003). Predicting pressure ulcer risk in pediatric patients: The Braden Q Scale. *Nursing Research, 52*(1), 22–33.

Dezateux, C., & Rosendahl, R. (2007). Developmental dysplasia of the hip. *Lancet, 369*, 1541–1552. Retrieved from http://ucl.ac.uk/paediatric-epidemiology/pdfs/developmental_dysplasia.pdf.

Do, T., & Herrera-Soto, J. (2003). Elbow injuries in children. *Current Opinion in Pediatrics, 15*(1), 68–73.

Faulks, S., & Luther, B. (2005). Changing paradigm for the treatment of club-feet. *Orthopedic Nursing, 24*(1), 25–30.

Freeman, B. L., III. (2007). Scoliosis and kyphosis. In S. T. Canale & J. H. Beaty, (Eds.), *Campbell's operative orthopaedics* (11th ed.). Philadelphia: Mosby.

Geller, D. S., & Gorlick, R. (2010). Osteosarcoma: A review of diagnosis, management, and treatment strategies. *Clinical Advances in Hematology & Oncology, 8*(10), 705–718.

Glorieux, F. H., Ward, L. M., Rauch F., Lalic L., Roughley, P. J., & Travers, R. (2002). Osteogenesis imperfecta type VI: A form of brittle bone disease with mineralization defect. *Journal of Bone and Mineral Research, 17*(1), 30–38.

Gutierrez, K. (2005). Bone and joint infections in children. *Pediatric Clinics of North America, 52*(3), 779–794. doi:10.1016/j.pcl.2005.02.005

Hart, E. S., Grottkau, B. E., & Albright, M. B. (2007). Slipped capital femoral epiphysis: Don't miss this pediatric hip disorder. *Nurse Practitioner, 32*(3), 14, 16–18, 21. doi:10.1097/01.NPR.0000263076.88826.fa

Hart, E. S., et al. (2006). Developmental dysplasia of the hip: Nursing implications and anticipatory guidance for parents. *Orthopedic Nursing, 25*(2), 100–109.

Heare, T., Hensley, M. A., & Dell'orfano, S. (2009). Bone tumors: Osteosarcoma and Ewing's sarcoma. *Current Opinion in Pediatrics, 21*(3), 365–372. doi:10.1097/MOP.0b013e32832b1111

Holmes, S. B., Brown, S. J., & Pin Site Care Expert Panel. (2005). Skeletal pin site care: National Association of Orthopaedic Nurses guidelines for orthopaedic nursing. *Orthopedic Nursing, 24*(2), 99–107.

Hosalkar, H. S., Spiegel, D. A., & Davidson, R. S. (2007). Bone and joint disorders: The foot and toes. In R. M. Kliegman, et al. (Eds.), *Nelson textbook of pediatrics* (18th ed.). Philadelphia: Saunders.

Hosalkar, H. S., et al. (2007). The hip. In R. M. Kliegman, et al. (Eds.), *Nelson textbook of pediatrics* (18th ed.). Philadelphia: Saunders.

Klein-Gitelman, M. S., & Miller, M. L. (2007). Systemic lupus erythematosus. In R. M. Kliegman, et al. (Eds.), *Nelson textbook of pediatrics* (18th ed.). Philadelphia: Saunders.

Kline, N. E., & Sevier, N. (2003). Solid tumors in children. *Journal of Pediatric Nursing, 18*(2), 96–102.

Kump, L. I., et al. (2006). Visual outcomes in children with juvenile idiopathic arthritis–associated uveitis. *Ophthalmology, 113*(10), 1874–1877. doi:10.1016/j.ophtha.2006.05.016

Lampe, R. M. (2007). Osteomyelitis and suppurative arthritis. In R. M. Kliegman, et al. (Eds.), *Nelson textbook of pediatrics* (18th ed.). Philadelphia: Saunders.

Land, C., et al. (2007). Osteogenesis imperfecta type VI in childhood and adolescence: Effects of cyclical intravenous pamidronate treatment. *Bone, 40*(3), 638–644. doi:10.1016/j.bone.2006.10.010

Lanzkowsky, P. (2005). *Manual of pediatric hematology and oncology* (4th ed.). San Diego: Academic Press.

Lehman, T. J. (2008). Systemic lupus erythematosus in children. *UpToDate.* Retrieved from http://www.uptodate.com.

Link, M. P., Gebhardt, M. C., & Myers, P. A. (2006). Osteosarcoma. In P. A. Pizzo & D. G. Poplack (Eds.), *Principles and practices of pediatric oncology* (5th ed.). Philadelphia: Lippincott.

Lovell, D. J., et al. (2003). Long-term efficacy and safety of etanercept in children with polyarticular-course juvenile rheumatoid arthritis: Interim results from an ongoing multicenter, open-label, extended-treatment trial. *Arthritis & Rheumatism, 48*(1), 218–226.

Maher, A. B., Salmond, S. W., & Pellino, T. A. (2002). *Orthopaedic nursing* (3rd ed.). Philadelphia: Saunders.

Marini, J. C. (2007). Osteogenesis imperfecta. In R. M. Kliegman, et al. (Eds.), *Nelson textbook of pediatrics* (18th ed.). Philadelphia: Saunders.

McCord, S., et al. (2004). Risk factors associated with pressure ulcers in the pediatric intensive care unit. *Journal of Wound, Ostomy and Continence Nursing, 31*(4), 179–183.

Miller, M. L., & Cassidy, J. T. (2007). Juvenile rheumatoid arthritis. In R. M. Kliegman, et al. (Eds.), *Nelson textbook of pediatrics* (18th ed.). Philadelphia: Saunders.

Napierkowski, D. B. (2007). Scoliosis: A case study in an adolescent boy. *Orthopedic Nursing, 26*(3), 147–153. doi:10.1097/01.NOR.0000276963.23270.5c

Newton, P. O., & Wenger, D. R. (2001). Idiopathic and congenital scoliosis. In R. T. Morrissy & S. L. Weinstein (Eds.), *Lovell and Winter's pediatric orthopaedics.* Philadelphia: Williams & Wilkins.

Olsson, G. L. (1999). Neuropathic pain in children. In P. J. McGrath & G. A. Finley (Eds.), *Chronic and recurrent pain in children and adolescents.* Seattle: IASP Press.

Padeh, S., & Passwell, P. (1998). Intraarticular corticosteroid injection in the management of children with chronic arthritis. *Arthritis & Rheumatism, 41*(7), 1210–1214.

Peschken, C., et al. (2009). The 1000 Canadian faces of lupus: Determinants of disease outcome in a large multiethnic cohort. *Journal of Rheumatology, 36*(6), 1200–1208. doi:10.3899/jrheum.080912

Petty, R. E., et al. (1998). Revision of the proposed classification criteria for juvenile idiopathic arthritis: Durban, 1997. *Journal of Rheumatology, 25*(10), 1991–1994.

Petty, R. E., et al. (2004). International League of Associations for Rheumatology classification of juvenile idiopathic arthritis: Second revision, Edmonton, 2001. *Journal of Rheumatology, 31*(2), 390–392.

Plint, A. C., et al. (2006). A randomized, controlled trial of removable splinting versus casting for wrist buckle fractures in children. *Pediatrics, 117*(3), 691–697. doi:10.1542/peds.2005-0801

Ravelli, A., Ruperto, N., & Martini, A. (2005). Outcome in juvenile onset lupus erythematosus. *Current Opinion in Rheumatology, 17*(5), 568–573.

Razmus, I. S., Roberts, K. E., & Curley, M. A. (2001). Pressure ulcers in critically ill children: Incidence and associated factors (abstract). *Critical Care Medicine, 29*(Suppl), A148.

Richards, B. S., & Vitale, M. G. (2008). Screening for idiopathic scoliosis in adolescents: An information statement. *Journal of Bone & Joint Surgery, 90*(1), 195–198. doi:10.2106/JBJS.G.01276

Salter, R. (1968). Etiology, pathogenesis, and possible prevention of congenital dislocation of the hip. *Canadian Medical Association Journal, 98*, 933–945.

Schindler, C. A., et al. (2007). Skin integrity in critically ill and injured children. *American Journal of Critical Care, 16*(6), 568–574.

Shrader, M. W. (2008). Pediatric supracondylar fractures and pediatric physeal elbow fractures. *Orthopedic Clinics of North America, 39*(2), 163–171. doi:10.1016/j.ocl.2007.12.005

Slote, R. J. (2002). Psychological effects of caring for the adolescent undergoing spinal fusion for scoliosis. *Orthopedic Nursing, 21*(6), 19–28.

Spiegel, D. A., Hosalkar, H. S., & Dormans, J. P. (2007). Bone and joint disorders: The spine. In R. M. Kliegman, et al. (Eds.), *Nelson textbook of pediatrics* (18th ed.). Philadelphia: Saunders.

Ta, H. T., et al. (2009). Osteosarcoma treatment: State of the art. *Cancer Metastasis Reviews, 28*(1), 247–263. doi:10.1007/s10555-009-9186-7

Warren, R. W., et al. (2001). Juvenile idiopathic arthritis (juvenile rheumatoid arthritis). In W. J. Koopman (Ed.), *Arthritis and allied conditions.* Philadelphia: Lippincott Williams & Wilkins.

Wexler, L. H., Meyer, W. H., & Helman, L. J. (2006). Rhabdomyosarcoma and the undifferentiated sarcomas. In P. A. Pizzo & D. G. Poplack (Eds.), *Principles and practices of pediatric oncology* (5th ed.). Philadelphia: Lippincott.

Wilkins, L., McGrath, P., Finley, G., & Katz, J. (1998). Phantom limb sensations and phantom limb pain in child and adolescent amputees. *Pain, 78*(1), 7–12.

Additional Resources

About Kids Health—Information on scoliosis: http://www.aboutkidshealth.ca/En/HealthAZ/TestsAndTreatments/MedicalDevices/Pages/Scoliosis-Treatment-with-a-Spinal-Orthosis-Spinal-Brace.aspx

American Academy of Orthopaedic Surgeons and Scoliosis Research Society: http://orthoinfo.aaos.org/main.cfm

Arthritis Society: http://www.arthritis.ca/arthritis%20home/default.asp?s=1&province=ca

Braden Scale for Pediatrics: http://www.therapybc.ca/eLibrary/docs/Resources/Braden%20Q%20scale%20for%20paeds.pdf

Canadian Spine Society: http://www.spinecanada.ca/patients/index.php

Childhood Cancer Foundation Candlelighters Canada—Information about special programs for children with amputations: http://www.childhoodcancer.ca

Health Canada, Car Restraints: http://www.healthycanadians.gc.ca/init/kids-enfants/road-routiere/car-re-vehic/index-eng.php

Lupus Canada: http://www.lupuscanada.org

National Scoliosis Foundation: http://www.scoliosis.org/

Scoliosis: Life, Support and Friends: http://scoliosisnutty.blogspot.com/2009/02/scoliosis-association-of-british.html

Scoliosis Research Society: http://www.srs.org/

War Amps (Child Amputee [CHAMP] Program)—Support group for children undergoing amputation: http://www.waramps.ca/champ/home.html

Unit 11

55 Neuromuscular or Muscular Dysfunction

Learning Objectives

On completion of this chapter, the reader will be able to:

- Discuss the nursing role in helping parents cope with a child with cerebral palsy.
- Formulate a nursing care plan for the preoperative and postoperative care of a child with myelomeningocele.
- Outline a plan of care for a child with Duchenne muscular dystrophy.
- Discuss the prevention and treatment of tetanus.
- Identify the causes of botulism in infants and children.
- List three causes of spinal cord injury in children.

Electronic Resources

Additional information related to the content in Chapter 55 can be found on

evolve the companion Web site at

http://evolve.elsevier.com/Canada/Perry/maternal/

- Examination Review Questions
- Animation—Guillain-Barré Syndrome
- Critical Thinking Exercise—Guillain-Barré Syndrome
- Critical Thinking Exercise—Myelomeningocele

Congenital Neuromuscular or Muscular Disorders

Cerebral Palsy

A definition recently proposed describes cerebral palsy (CP) as a "group of permanent disorders of the development of movement and posture, causing activity limitation, that are attributed to nonprogressive disturbances that occurred in the developing fetal or infant brain" (Rosenbaum et al., 2007). In addition to motor disorders, the condition often involves disturbances of sensation, perception, communication, cognition, and behaviour; secondary musculoskeletal problems; and epilepsy (Rosenbaum et al., 2007). The etiology, clinical features, and course are variable and are characterized by abnormal muscle tone and coordination as the primary disturbances. CP is the most common permanent physical disability of childhood (Hirtz et al., 2007; Yeargin-Allsopp et al., 2008). In the 1960s, the prevalence of CP rose approximately 20%, which most likely reflected the improved survival of extremely-low-birth-weight (ELBW) and very-low-birth-weight (VLBW) infants. However, in the past two decades there has been a decrease in the incidence of CP among ELBW and VLBW infants (Hack & Costello, 2008).

Although the prevalent traditional hypothesis has been that CP results from perinatal problems, especially birth asphyxia, it is now believed that some types of CP result more often from existing prenatal brain abnormalities; the exact cause of these abnormalities remains elusive. It has been estimated that as many as 80% of CP cases are caused by unknown prenatal factors (Krigger, 2006). Intrauterine exposure to maternal chorioamnionitis is associated with an increased risk of CP in infants of normal birth weight and preterm infants (Gibson et al., 2003; Volpe, 2008); however, not all term infants exposed to chorioamnionitis develop CP (Grether et al., 2003; Wu et al., 2003). The prevalence of CP in infants born before 36 weeks of gestation and weighing less than 2000 g has been reported to be 12%. Periventricular leukomalacia and intracerebral hemorrhage in low-birth-weight infants are significant risk factors, as are perinatal stroke and shaken baby syndrome (Golomb et al., 2007).

Additional factors that may contribute to the development of CP postnatally include bacterial meningitis, viral encephalitis, motor vehicle accidents, and child abuse (Krigger, 2006). In summary, as many as 80% of the total cases of CP may be linked to a perinatal or neonatal brain lesion or brain maldevelopment, regardless of the cause (Krageloh-Mann & Cans, 2009). A significant percentage (15 to 60%) of children with CP will also have epilepsy, which makes self-care and progression to normalization more difficult.

Pathophysiology

It is difficult to establish a precise location of neurological lesions based on etiology or clinical signs because no characteristic pathological pattern exists. Some patients have gross malformations of the brain; others may have evidence of vascular occlusion, atrophy, loss of neurons, and degeneration. A few exceptions occur and are related to anatomical areas such as spastic diplegia (associated with preterm birth), caused by hypoxic infarction or hemorrhage in the area adjacent to the lateral ventricles. Ataxic CP may occur in relation to cerebral hypoplasia and, in some cases, severe hypoglycemia (Volpe, 2008). Approximately 70% of cases of neonatal encephalopathy occur as a result of secondary events arising before the onset of labour, such as prenatal stroke, infection, cerebral malformation, and genetic disorders (Menticoglou, 2007).

CP has been classified in several ways. A functional classification is based on the nature and distribution of neuromuscular dysfunction (Box 55-1). Additional classifications describe the area of the brain involved, the degree of motor involvement, accompanying impairments, anatomical distribution, and cause of CP (Rosenbaum et al., 2007).

BOX 55-1 Clinical Classification of Cerebral Palsy

Spastic (Pyramidal)—70 to 80% of All Cases of Cerebral Palsy

Characterized by persistent primitive reflexes, positive Babinski, ankle clonus, exaggerated stretch reflexes, eventual development of contractures

- **Diplegia**—All extremities affected; lower more than upper (30 to 40% of spastic cerebral palsy [CP])
- **Tetraplegia**—All four extremities involved: legs and trunk, mouth, pharynx, and tongue (10 to 15% of spastic CP)
- **Triplegia**—Three limbs involved
- **Monoplegia**—Only one limb involved
- **Hemiplegia**—Motor dysfunction on one side of the body; upper extremity more affected than lower (20 to 30% of spastic CP)

Hypertonicity with poor control of posture, balance, and coordinated motion

Impairment of fine and gross motor skills

Dyskinetic (Nonspastic, Extrapyramidal)

Athetoid—Chorea (involuntary, irregular, jerking movements); characterized by slow, wormlike, writhing movements that usually involve the extremities, trunk, neck, facial muscles, and tongue

Dystonic—Slow, twisting movements of the trunk or extremities; abnormal posture

Involvement of the pharyngeal, laryngeal, and oral muscles causing drooling and dysarthria (imperfect speech articulation)

Ataxic (Nonspastic, Extrapyramidal)

Wide-based gait

Rapid, repetitive movements performed poorly

Disintegration of movements of the upper extremities when the child reaches for objects

Mixed Type

Combination of spastic CP and dyskinetic CP

May be labelled *mixed* when no specific motor pattern is dominant; however, this term is losing favour to more precise descriptions of motor function and affected area of brain involved (Rosenbaum et al., 2007)

(Data from Jones, M. W., et al. [2007]. Cerebral palsy: Introduction and diagnosis, part 1. *Journal of Pediatric Health Care, 21*[3], 146–152; National Institute of Neurological Disorders and Stroke. [2006]. *Cerebral palsy: Hope through research*. Retrieved from http://www.ninds.nih.gov/disorders/cerebral_palsy/detail_cerebral_palsy.htm; and Nehring, W. [2010]. Cerebral palsy. In P. J. Allen J. A. Vessey, & N.A. Schapiro [Eds.], *Primary care of the child with a chronic condition* (5th ed.). St. Louis: Mosby.)

Diagnostic Evaluation

Infants at risk according to known etiological factors associated with CP warrant careful assessment during early infancy to identify the signs of muscular dysfunction as early as possible. The neurological examination and history are the primary modalities for diagnosis. Neuroimaging of the child with suspected brain abnormality and CP is now recommended for diagnostic assessment, with magnetic resonance imaging (MRI) preferred to computed tomography (CT) scan. Metabolic and genetic testing is recommended if no structural abnormality is identified by neuroimaging; laboratory tests are no longer recommended in the diagnostic process for CP (Ashwal et al., 2004).

Early recognition is made more difficult by the lack of reliable neonatal neurological signs. However, infants with known etiological risk factors should be monitored and evaluated closely in the first 2 years of life. The alert observer may be suspicious when a child demonstrates some of the manifestations outlined in Box 55-2. Because cortical control of movement does not occur until later in infancy, motor impairment associated with voluntary control is usually not apparent until after 2 to 4 months of age at the earliest. More often the diagnosis cannot be confirmed until the age of 2 years because motor tone abnormalities may be indicative of another neuromuscular illness.

Diagnosis may also be assisted by identification of persistent primitive reflexes: (1) either the asymmetrical tonic neck reflex or persistent Moro reflex (beyond 4 months of age), and (2) the crossed extensor reflex. The tonic neck reflex normally disappears between 4 and 6 months of age. An "obligatory" response is considered abnormal. Hand preference in the first 2 years of life is reported to be a sign of hemiplegic CP (Berker & Yalçin, 2008). The crossed extensor reflex, which normally disappears by 4 months, is elicited by applying a noxious stimulus to the sole of one foot with the knee extended. Normally the contralateral foot responds with extensor, abduction, and then adduction movements. The possibility of CP is suggested if these reflexes are found after the age at which they should have disappeared.

Therapeutic Management

The goals of therapy for children with CP are early recognition and promotion of optimal development to enable affected children to attain normalization and their potential within the limits of their existing health problems. The disorder is permanent, and therapy is primarily preventive and symptomatic.

Therapy has five broad aims:

1. To establish locomotion, communication, and self-help skills
2. To gain optimal appearance and integration of motor functions
3. To correct associated defects as effectively as possible

4. To provide educational opportunities adapted to the child's needs and capabilities
5. To promote socialization experiences with other affected and unaffected children

Each child is evaluated and managed on an individual basis. The scope of the child's needs requires multidisciplinary planning and care coordination among professionals and the child's family. The goal for the child and family with CP is normalization and promotion of self-care activities that empower the child and family to achieve maximum potential.

Ankle-foot orthoses (AFOs, braces) are worn by many of these children and are used to help prevent or reduce deformity, increase the energy efficiency of gait, and control alignment. Other mobilization devices include wheeled scooter boards that allow children to propel themselves while on the abdomen, wheeled go-carts that provide sitting balance and serve as early "wheelchair" experience for young children, bicycle walkers, and special devices that leave the upper extremities free (Figs. 55-1 and 55-2). Strollers can be equipped with custom seats for dependent mobilization.

Orthopedic surgery may be required to correct contracture or spastic deformities, to provide stability for an uncontrollable joint, and to provide balanced muscle power. This

BOX 55-2 Clinical Signs and Symptoms of Cerebral Palsy

Spastic Type

- Increased muscle tone (hypertonicity)
- Increased deep tendon reflexes and clonus (sudden dorsiflexion of the ankle or rapid distal movement of the patella resulting in alternating spasm and relaxation of the muscles being stretched)
- Flexor, adductor, and internal rotator muscles more involved than extensor, abductor, and external rotator muscles
- Difficulty with fine and gross motor skills
- Most common contracture: that of the heel cord
- Hip adductor contractures leading to progressive subluxation and dislocation
- Knee contractures
- Scoliosis common
- Typical gait crouched, intoeing, scissoring
- Elbow, wrist, and fingers in flexed position with thumb adducted
- Motor weakness of antagonist muscle groups

Dyskinetic Type

- Purposeless, involuntary, uncontrollable movements of face and extremities
- Increased movements with stress and voluntary movements; absent during sleep
- Contractures rare
- Normal deep tendon reflexes

Ataxic Type

- Disturbed coordination
- Lack of equilibrium
- Unsteady gait
- Few orthopedic problems
- Hyporeflexia
- Loss of ability to gauge distance, speed, power of movement
- Muscles hypotonic
- Speech slurred, jerky, explosive
- Nystagmus common

Other Manifestations

- Visual deficits (most common in spastic type)
- Hearing impairment (most common in dyskinetic type)
- Oral motor involvement resulting in drooling and feeding problems
- Developmental delay (40 to 60%; most common in spastic quadriplegia)
- Sensory impairment
- Seizures (approximately 40% of those with spastic hemiplegia affected)

(From Maher, A. B., Salmond, S. W., & Pellino, T. A. [2002]. *Orthopaedic nursing* [3rd ed.]. Philadelphia: Saunders.)

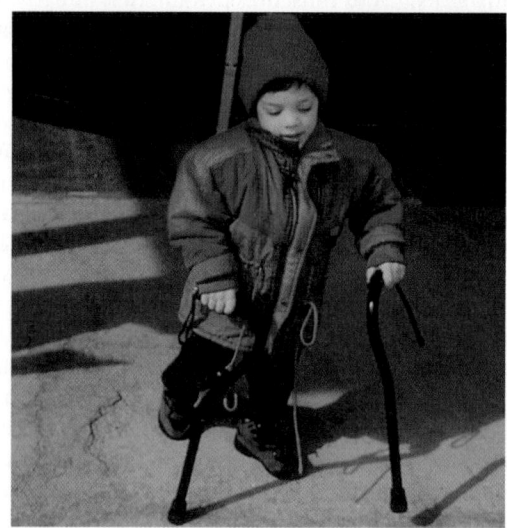

Fig. 55-1 Mobilization device for child.

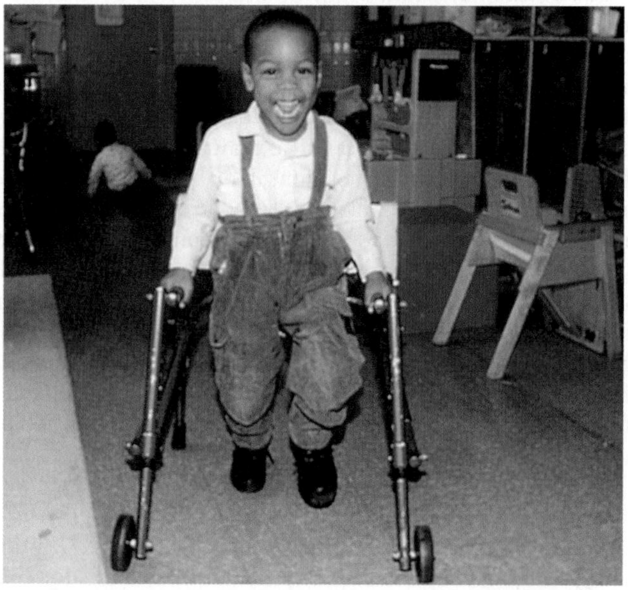

Fig. 55-2 Child ambulating with use of assistive device.

includes tendon-lengthening procedures (especially heel-cord lengthening), release of spastic wrist flexor muscles, and correction of hip and adductor muscle spasticity or contracture to improve locomotion. Orthopedic surgery is generally not performed until after the child is 6 years old (Nehring, 2010). Surgery may also be performed to improve feedings, correct gastroesophageal reflux disease, and correct associated dental problems (Nehring, 2010).

Selective dorsal rhizotomy has provided marked improvement in some children with CP. The procedure involves selectively cutting dorsal column sensory rootlets that have an abnormal response to electrical stimulation. Achieving the benefits from the surgery requires intensive physiotherapy and family commitment. Because the procedure results in flaccid muscles, the child must be retaught to sit, stand, and walk.

Surgical intervention is usually reserved for the child who does not respond to the more conservative measures, but it is also indicated for the child whose spasticity causes progressive deformities. Surgery is primarily used to improve function rather than for cosmetic purposes and is followed by physiotherapy.

Intense pain may occur with muscle spasms in patients with CP. Pharmacological agents given orally (dantrolene sodium, baclofen, and diazepam [Valium]) have had little effectiveness in improving muscle coordination in children with CP; however, they are effective in decreasing overall spasticity. The most common adverse effects of these medications include hepatotoxicity (dantrolene), drowsiness, fatigue, and muscle weakness; less commonly, diaphoresis and constipation may be seen with baclofen. Diazepam is used frequently but should be restricted to older children and adolescents.

Botulinum toxin A (Botox) is also used to reduce spasticity in targeted muscles. Botulinum toxin A is injected into a selected muscle (commonly the quadriceps, gastrocnemius, or medial hamstrings) after a topical anaesthetic or sedation is used. The drug acts to inhibit the release of acetylcholine into a specific muscle group, thereby preventing muscle movement. When it is administered early in the course of the illness, affected muscle contractures may be prevented, particularly in lower extremities, thus avoiding surgical procedures with possible adverse effects. The goal is to allow stretching of the muscle as it relaxes and permit ambulation with an AFO. The major reported adverse effect of botulinum toxin A injection is pain at the injection site (Lukban, Rosales, & Dressler, 2009; Roscigno, 2002). Prime candidates for botulinum toxin A injections are children with spasticity confined to the lower extremities; the drug weakens spasticity so the muscles can be stretched and the child may ambulate with or without orthoses. The onset of action occurs within 24 to 72 hours, with a peak effect observed at 2 weeks and a duration of action of 3 to 6 months (Green, Greenberg, & Hurwitz, 2003).

Children with CP may also experience pain as a result of surgical procedures intended to reduce contracture deformities, position and gastroesophageal reflux, and physiotherapy (McKearnan et al., 2004). Thus pain management is an important aspect of care of the child with CP.

The neurosurgical and pharmacological approach to managing the spasticity associated with CP involves the implantation of a pump to infuse baclofen directly into the intrathecal space surrounding the spinal cord to provide relief of spasticity. Intrathecal baclofen therapy is best suited for children with severe spasticity that interferes with activities of daily living (ADLs) and ambulation. Patients are screened before pump placement by the infusion of a "test dose" of intrathecal baclofen delivered via a lumbar puncture. Close monitoring for adverse effects (hypotonia, somnolence, seizures, nausea, vomiting, headache, and catheter- or pump-related problems [Albright et al., 2003]) and relief of spasticity occurs for several hours after the infusion. If a positive effect is noted, the patient is considered a candidate for pump placement.

The implantation procedure is done in the operating room by a neurosurgeon. The pump, which is approximately the size of a hockey puck, is placed in the subcutaneous space of the midabdomen. An intrathecal catheter is tunneled from the lumbar area to the abdomen and connected to the pump. The pump is filled with baclofen and, using a telemetry wand and a computer, is programmed to provide a set dose. Benefits of intrathecal baclofen include fewer systemic adverse effects than oral medication, dosage titration for maximizing effects, and reversibility of therapy with removal of the pump if so desired (Jacobs, 2001). The patient may remain hospitalized for 3 to 7 days to adjust the dosage and ensure proper healing. Outpatient visits to refill the pump and make dosage adjustments occur about every 4 to 6 weeks, depending on the patient's response to the treatment. This procedure is most suited for a multidisciplinary setting where rehabilitation specialists are readily available and consistently involved in the patient's ongoing care. Abrupt withdrawal of intrathecal baclofen, especially at high doses, may result in adverse effects such as rebound spasticity, pruritus, hyperthermia, rhabdomyolysis, disseminated intravascular coagulation, multiorgan failure, and death. In some cases intrathecal baclofen withdrawal may mimic sepsis.

Anti-epileptic drugs (AEDs) such as carbamazepine (Tegretol) and divalproex (valproate sodium and valproic acid; Depakote) are prescribed routinely for children who have seizures. Gabapentin (Neurontin) has been used in adults with spinal cord injury (SCI) to decrease spasticity with success; no studies are available on the effectiveness of the medication in children. The α_2-adrenergic agonists clonidine (Catapres) and tizanidine (Zanaflex) have been used to decrease spasticity in adults with SCI and multiple sclerosis. The effectiveness of oral tizanidine given in conjunction with botulinum type A has been reported to be more effective than oral baclofen and botulinum type A in one study of children with CP (Dai, Wasay, & Awan, 2008). All medications should be monitored for maintenance of therapeutic levels and avoidance of subtherapeutic or toxic levels.

Dental hygiene is especially important. Regular visits to the dentist and prophylaxis, including brushing, fluoride, and flossing, should be instituted as soon as the teeth erupt. Dental care is important for children being given phenytoin, since they often develop gum hyperplasia. Additional problems common among children with CP include constipation caused by neurological deficits and lack of exercise; poor bladder control and urinary retention; chronic respiratory tract infections and aspiration pneumonia, which occur as a result of gastroesophageal reflux, abnormal muscle tone, immobility, and altered positioning; and skin problems as a result of altered positioning, poor nutrition, and immobility.

A wide variety of technical aids are available to improve the functioning of children with CP. These include electromechanical toys that employ the concept of biofeedback and operate from a head unit. The toy is manipulated only when the head and trunk are in correct alignment. Eye–hand coordination can also be enhanced by computerized toys and games. Microcomputers combined with voice synthesizers help children with speech difficulties to "speak." These and other devices print messages onto screen monitors and paper.

Many other electronic devices allow independent functioning. Sensors can be activated and deactivated by using a headstick or tongue, or other voluntary muscle movement over which the child has control. Voice-activated computer technology may also allow increased mobility and ambulation with specially designed devices such as wheelchairs. The application of this technology makes it possible for persons with CP to function eventually in their own residences and can be extended into the workplace.

Physiotherapy is one of the most frequently used conservative treatment modalities. It requires the specialized skills of a qualified therapist with an extensive repertoire of exercise methods who can design a program to stimulate each child to achieve his or her functional goals. An active therapy program involves the family, the physiotherapist, and often other members of the health team, including the nurse. The most common approach employs traditional types of therapeutic exercises that consist of stretching, passive, active, and resistive movements applied to specific muscle groups or joints to maintain or increase range of motion, strength, and endurance.

Prognosis

In general, the more severe the functional disability, the worse the prognosis. Children with mild to moderate CP have the capability of achieving ambulation between the ages of 2 and 7 years (Berker & Yalçin, 2008). Children with a severe physical disability, cognitive impairment, tube feedings, and severe seizures are known to have a shortened life expectancy. According to available data, approximately 30 to 50% of individuals with CP have cognitive impairment, and an even higher percentage have mild cognitive and learning deficits (Green et al., 2003); however, many children with severe spastic quadriplegic CP have normal intelligence. Growth is affected in children with spastic quadriplegia, and many children remain below the fifth percentile for age and gender. As children with CP transition to adulthood, about 30% remain in the home and are cared for by a parent or caregiver; 50% of individuals with spastic quadriplegia live in independent settings and function at appropriate social levels considering their disability (Green et al., 2003). Vocational rehabilitation and higher education are possible for adults with CP, and one study found that 53% of all persons with CP were able to work outside the home in regular jobs; one third of the severely disabled adults with CP worked outside the home (Murphy, Molnar, & Lankasky, 2000). Survival rates in children and adults with CP are influenced by existing comorbidities (Nehring, 2010).

Nursing Care Management

The nursing process in the care of the child with CP is outlined in the Nursing Process box.

Because children with CP are being identified and treated at an earlier age, parents are participating earlier in treatment programs for their disabled child. They are taught the proper handling and home care of young children with CP and need a carefully planned program so that their change of role from parent to caregiver can be incorporated into the already established relationship. Close work with other multidisciplinary team members is essential. Nurses reinforce the therapeutic plan and assist the family in devising and modifying equipment and activities to continue the therapy program in the home (see the Nursing Care Plan).

Children with CP expend much energy in their efforts to accomplish ADLs, thus more frequent rest periods should be arranged to avoid taxing their limited capabilities. The diet should be tailored to the child's activity and metabolic needs. Gastrostomy feedings may be necessary to supplement regular feedings and ensure adequate weight gain, particularly in the child who is at risk for growth failure and chronic malnutrition. In children with severe CP and subsequent oral feeding difficulties, a feeding gastrostomy should be considered (Rogers, 2004). Gastrostomy feeding as a supplement to oral feeding is often recommended, especially when illness and decreased fluid or medication intake affect the child's well-being (Rogers, 2004). Oral feedings may be continued to maintain oral motor skills. Weight gain is perceived as an important measure of adequate oral feeding efficiency.

Parents may need assistance and advice with medication administration through a gastrostomy tube to prevent clotting of the device. A skin-level gastrostomy is particularly suited for the child with CP.

Because jaw control is often compromised, more normal control can be achieved if the feeder provides stability of the oral mechanism from the side or front of the face. When directed from the front, the middle finger of the nonfeeding hand is placed posterior to the body portion of the chin, the thumb is placed below the bottom lip, and the index finger is placed parallel to the child's mandible (Fig. 55-3). Manual jaw control from the side assists with head control, correction of neck and trunk hyperextension, and jaw stabilization. The middle finger of the nonfeeding hand is placed posterior to the bony portion of the chin, the index finger is placed on the chin below the lower lip, and the thumb is placed obliquely across the cheek to provide lateral jaw stability (Fig. 55-4).

Safety precautions need to be implemented, such as having children wear protective helmets if they are subject to falls or capable of injuring their heads on hard objects. Because the child with CP is at risk for altered proprioception and subsequent falls, the home and play environment should be adapted to the child's needs to prevent bodily harm. Appropriate immunizations should be administered to prevent childhood illnesses and protect against respiratory tract infections such as influenza. Dental problems may be more common in children with CP, thus meticulous attention should be paid to all aspects of dental care.

NURSING PROCESS: CEREBRAL PALSY

Assessment

Nursing assessment includes risk identification of infants with etiological factors that are associated with cerebral palsy (CP). Early recognition of CP is important so early interventions may be implemented (Box 55-3). Ongoing assessment of infants for abnormal muscle tone, inability to achieve developmental milestones, and persistence of neonatal reflexes alerts the nurse to investigate further.

Nursing Diagnoses

After a thorough assessment a number of nursing diagnoses are evident (see the Nursing Care Plan, pp. 1730–1731). Other nursing diagnoses include:

Imbalanced nutrition: less than body requirements related to
- decreased oral intake of nutrients
- uncoordinated oral motor function

Delayed growth and development related to
- inadequate caloric intake
- energy expenditure that exceeds caloric intake

Interrupted family processes related to
- level of care required in caring for the chronically ill child (e.g., medication administration, special feeding methods, physiotherapy, assistive devices [AFOs, wheelchair, braces])

Risk for aspiration related to
- uncoordinated oral motor function resulting in swallowing difficulty
- muscle spasticity

Planning

Expected outcomes for the child with CP include the following:
- Child will receive adequate nutrient intake for body growth (weight gain).
- Child will achieve developmental milestones to maximum potential.
- Family will cope with child's illness and function to maximum potential.
- Child's airway will remain patent.

Implementation

Numerous intervention strategies for the child with CP are found on pp. 1728–1732.

Evaluation

The effectiveness of nursing interventions for the family and child with CP is determined by continual reassessment and evaluation of care based on the following observational guidelines:
- Child's movements and use of mobilization devices
- Child's speech and ability to use communication devices
- Child's activities, especially those related to self-care
- Family perception regarding child's activities and school attendance
- Child's interactions with others and choice of activities; child's feelings and concerns
- Family feelings, concerns, and interaction with the child
- Child's behaviour and responses during hospitalization

BOX 55-3 Early Signs of Cerebral Palsy

Physical Signs
- Persistent primitive reflexes such as Moro, atonic neck past 6 months
- Poor head control (head lag) and clenched hands after 3 months of age
- Stiff or rigid arms or legs; scissoring legs
- Pushing away or arching back; stiff posture
- Floppy or limp body posture
- Inability to sit up without support by 8 months
- Using only one side of the body, or only the arms to crawl
- Hand preference demonstrated before 18 months
- Seizures
- Sensory impairment (hearing, vision)
- After 6 months of age, persistent tongue thrusting

Behavioural Signs
- Feeding difficulties
- Excessive sleeping
- Extreme irritability or crying
- Failure to smile by 3 months
- Lack of interest in surroundings

(Data from Jones, M. W., et al. [2007]. Cerebral palsy: Introduction and diagnosis, part 1. *Journal of Pediatric Health Care, 21*[3], 146–152; and Nehring, W. [2010]. Cerebral palsy. In P. J. Allen, J. A. Vessey, & N.A. Schapiro [Eds.], *Primary care of the child with a chronic condition*. [5th ed.]. St. Louis: Mosby.)

The involvement of physiotherapy, speech therapy, and occupational therapy is particularly important in the establishment and maintenance of muscle function, development of adequate speech and phonation, and identification of modifications necessary for the child's environment so that ADLs can be performed to the child's satisfaction.

As in all aspects of care, educational requirements are determined by the child's needs and potential. Children with mild to moderate involvement are generally able to participate, for varying amounts of time, in regular classes. Resource rooms are available in most schools to provide more individualized attention. Integration of children with CP into regular classrooms should be the initial goal. For those who are unable to benefit from formal education, a vocational training program may be appropriate. At adolescence, prevocational and vocational counselling and guidance can be arranged. At any phase or in any setting, education is geared toward the child's abilities.

Recreational outlets and after-school activities should be considered for the child who is unable to participate in the regular athletic programs and other peer activities. Some children can compete in athletic and artistic endeavours, and many games and pastimes are suited to their capabilities. Competitive sports are also becoming increasingly available to children with disabilities and offer an added dimension to physical activities. The Canadian Cerebral Palsy Sports Association is a national organization that provides sports opportunities for individuals with CP (see Additional Resources section at the end of this chapter). Canada is ranked among the top countries for athletes with CP. The Association

NURSING CARE PLAN ● The Child With Cerebral Palsy

Nursing Diagnosis	Patient Outcomes	Nursing Interventions	Rationale
Impaired physical mobility related to neuromuscular impairment	The infant or toddler will demonstrate active joint movement.	Carry out and teach family to perform stretching exercises on affected joints.	To prevent muscle contractures
	The child will have adequate mobility to perform activities of daily living to maximum potential.	Use assistive devices such as wheelchair, ankle-foot orthoses (AFOs), and wrist splints.	To increase mobility
Child's/Family's Defining Characteristics *(Subjective and Objective Data)*	**The Following NOC Concepts Apply to These Outcomes:**	Administer medications intended to decrease muscle spasticity.	To minimize pain and decrease spasticity
Postural instability during performance of routine activities of daily living	Body Mechanics Performance	Encourage and teach parent(s) to use jaw control during feedings.	To facilitate eating
Limited ability to perform gross motor skills	Ambulation: Wheelchair	Position child semiupright during feedings.	To decrease chance of aspiration and facilitate mobilization of food and fluids through esophagus
Limited range of motion	Joint Movement: Elbow, wrist, neck, knee, hip, ankle	Encourage play exercises that involve joint movement and promote fine and gross motor skill acquisition and repetition.	To promote joint movement; To promote achievement of developmental milestones
Limited ability to perform fine motor skills	Mobility	**The Following NIC Concepts Apply to These Interventions**	
Gait changes		Exercise Therapy: Joint Mobility	
Movement-induced tremor		Exercise Promotion: Stretching	
Persistence of primitive reflexes		Self-Care Assistance	

Nursing Diagnosis	Patient Outcomes	Nursing Interventions	Rationale
Risk for injury related to mobility limitation, neuromuscular impairment, and perception and cognition impairment	Child will remain injury free.	Educate family regarding child's physical limitations that place him or her at greater risk for injury.	To prevent accidental injury during mobilization
	Home physical environment will be safe.	Instruct family in steps to avoid injury: padded furniture, lowered bed or side rails as appropriate, gates on stairs, avoidance of throw rugs and thick carpeting.	To promote family involvement in injury prevention
Child's/Family's Defining Characteristics *(Subjective and Objective Data)*	**The Following NOC Concepts Apply to These Outcomes**	Position child in semiupright position after feedings.	To prevent aspiration
Physical factors: altered mobility	Personal Safety Behaviour	Use jaw support as needed during feedings.	To prevent choking
Neuromuscular factors:	Falls Occurrence	Use appropriate mobilization devices and ensure they are safe for child's age.	To promote personal safety
Limited perception of danger		Encourage mobilization and play activities that stretch muscles.	To prevent muscle contractures
Uncontrollable muscular movements		Teach child which activities of daily living are safe and appropriate to perform without assistance of another person.	To promote self-care
		The Following NIC Concepts Apply to These Interventions	
		Risk Identification	
		Environmental Management: Safety	
		Surveillance: Safety	
		Physical Restraint	
		Parent Education: Childrearing Family	

NURSING CARE PLAN ● The Child With Cerebral Palsy—cont'd

Nursing Diagnosis	Patient Outcomes	Nursing Interventions	Rationale
Pain (chronic) related to involuntary muscle movements (spasticity) and treatments for muscle spasticity **Child's/Family's Defining Characteristics** ***(Subjective and Objective Data)*** Observed evidence of guarded behaviour, grimace, crying, restlessness Atrophy of involved muscle group Altered ability to continue previous activities	Child's optimum comfort level will be maintained. **The Following NOC Concepts Apply to These Outcomes** Comfort Level Pain: Disruptive Effects Depression Level	Administer medications to control spasticity.	To prevent muscle spasm pain
		Perform stretching exercises after pain medication has been administered (60 minutes for oral medications).	To control pain impulses during exercises
		Administer pain medications such as nonsteroidal anti-inflammatory drugs.	To minimize pain
		For treatments such as botulinum toxin A (Botox) injections, apply topical analgesic such as EMLA (an eutectic mix of lidocaine and prilocaine) or LMX4 (4% lidocaine).	To decrease pain of injection at site
		For postoperative pain, administer pain medications on an around-the-clock schedule for 48 to 72 hours; use patient-controlled analgesia pump as child's cognitive and motor skills allow.	To promote personal physical comfort
		Use objective pain scale to assess pain level.	To provide objective measure of pain for intervention
		Encourage child to verbalize effects of pain on activities of daily living.	To provide outlet for frustration related to chronic pain experience
		Use assistive devices such as AFOs.	To decrease muscle spasticity and contractures.
		Teach parent(s) and child appropriate positions to assume while sitting and recumbent to minimize effects of muscle spasticity.	To promote self-care
		The Following NIC Concepts Apply to These Interventions Medication Administration Analgesic Administration Emotional Support Splinting Environmental Management: Comfort Exercise Promotion	

NIC, Nursing Interventions Classification; *NOC*, Nursing Outcomes Classification.

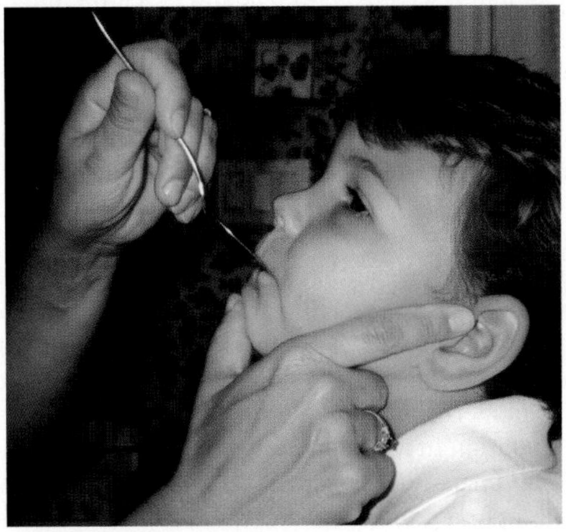

Fig. 55-3 Manual jaw control provided anteriorly.

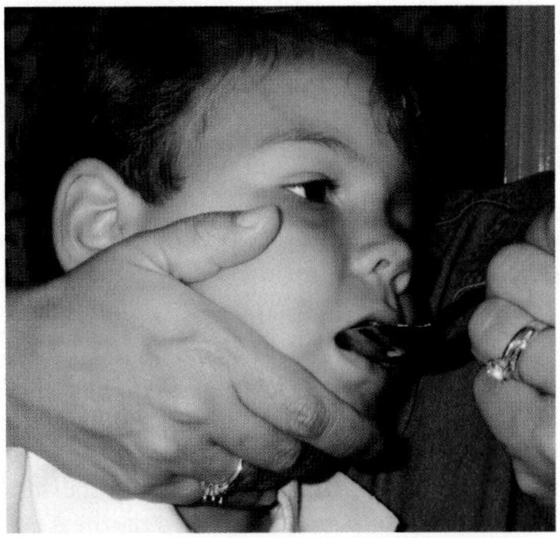

Fig. 55-4 Manual jaw control provided from the side.

supports sports for these individuals at the regional, national, and international levels.

Recreational activities serve to stimulate children's interest and curiosity, help them adjust to their disability, improve their functional abilities, and build self-esteem. Any accomplishment that helps children approach a "normal" way of life enhances their self-concept.

Support the Family

Probably the nursing interventions most valuable to the family are support and help in coping with the emotional aspects of the disorder, many of which are discussed in relation to the child with a disability (see Chapter 41). Initially the parents need supportive counselling directed toward understanding the implications of the diagnosis and all of the feelings that it engenders. Later they need clarification on what they can expect from the child and from health care providers. Educating families in the principles of family-centred care and parent–professional collaboration is essential. The family may require assistance in modifying the home environment for care of the child (see also Chapter 43). Transportation to the practitioner's office and other health care agencies often requires special considerations.

evolve Critical Thinking Exercise—Myelomeningocele

Care management for the child and family with CP is an important nursing role. In many cases the family assumes complete care of the child and becomes adept at meeting his or her individual needs. The home health nurse or care manager has an important role in support and encouragement for families who assume the primary care of a child with CP. Having a child with CP implies numerous problems of daily management and changes in family life, and the nurse can stress principles of normalization.

The nurse needs to support the parents in their frustration, problem solving, concerns, approaches to helping the child, and lack of gratification, as well as the positive approaches they use. All of these aspects must be explored and discussed. Siblings of a child with a disability are also affected and may respond to the child's presence with overt or less evident behavioural problems. The family needs a relationship with nurses who can provide continued contact, support, and encouragement through the long process of habilitation.

Parents may also find help and comfort from parent groups, with whom they can share problems and concerns and from whom they can derive comfort and practical information. Parent support groups are most helpful through sharing experiences and accomplishments. For example, parents can learn from others what it is like to have a child with CP. The national organization Cerebral Palsy Support Foundation of Canada provides support, funding, and aids in locating assistive devices for children and families. This organization also has a resource library for children with CP, families, and health care providers. The Association for the Neurologically Disabled of Canada provides services and support to individuals with neurological disabilities, as well as an extensive list of other resources across Canada. See the Additional Resources section at the end of the chapter for more information.

Support the Hospitalized Child

CP is not a disorder that requires hospitalization; thus when children with CP are hospitalized, they are usually admitted for another reason or for corrective surgery. Nursing care for the child with CP is the same as for any other child with a disability. Children with CP should be approached the same as any child in the hospital. Speech impairment is common in children with CP. To facilitate the care and management of these children, the therapy program should be continued, insofar as their condition allows, during the time they are hospitalized. Encouraging the parent to room in and actively participate in the child's care facilitates a continuation of the home therapy program and helps the child adjust to an unfamiliar environment. However, it is equally important to remember that hospitalization may be the first time a parent can defer care to a nurse and not be the primary caregiver. This respite may be crucial to the parent's well-being.

Spina Bifida (Myelomeningocele)

Abnormalities that derive from the embryonic neural tube (**neural tube defects** [NTDs]) constitute the largest group of congenital anomalies that are consistent with multifactorial inheritance. Normally, the spinal cord and cauda equina are encased in a protective sheath of bone and meninges (Fig. 55-5, A). Failure of neural tube closure produces defects of varying degrees (Box 55-4). They may involve the entire length of the neural tube or may be restricted to a small area.

In Canada, NTDs occur in 1 in every 1000 births. Prenatal supplementation of folic acid and the increased use of prenatal diagnostic techniques and termination of pregnancies have affected the overall incidence of NTDs (see also Prevention, p. 1736).

Myelodysplasia refers broadly to any malformation of the spinal canal and cord. Midline defects involving failure of the osseous (bony) spine to close are called *spina bifida (SB)*, the most common defect of the central nervous system. SB is categorized into two types: spina bifida occulta and spina bifida cystica.

Spina bifida occulta refers to a defect that is not visible externally. It occurs most frequently in the lumbosacral area (L5 and S1) (see Fig. 55-5, B). SB occulta may not be apparent unless there are associated cutaneous manifestations or neuromuscular disturbances.

Spina bifida cystica refers to a visible defect with an external saclike protrusion. The two major forms of SB cystica are meningocele, which encases meninges and spinal fluid but no neural elements (see Fig. 55-5, C), and myelomeningocele (or meningomyelocele), which contains meninges, spinal fluid, and nerves (see Fig. 55-5, D). Meningocele is not associated with neurological deficit, which occurs in varying, often serious, degrees in myelomeningocele. Clinically the term *spina bifida* is used to refer to myelomeningocele.

Pathophysiology

Most authorities believe that the primary defect in NTDs is a failure of neural tube closure during the embryo's early development (the first 3 to 5 weeks). However, evidence also implicates a multifactorial etiology, including medications, radiation, maternal malnutrition, chemicals, and possibly a genetic mutation in folate pathways in some cases, which may result in abnormal development. There is also evidence of a genetic component in the development of SB; myelomeningocele may occur in association with syndromes such as trisomy

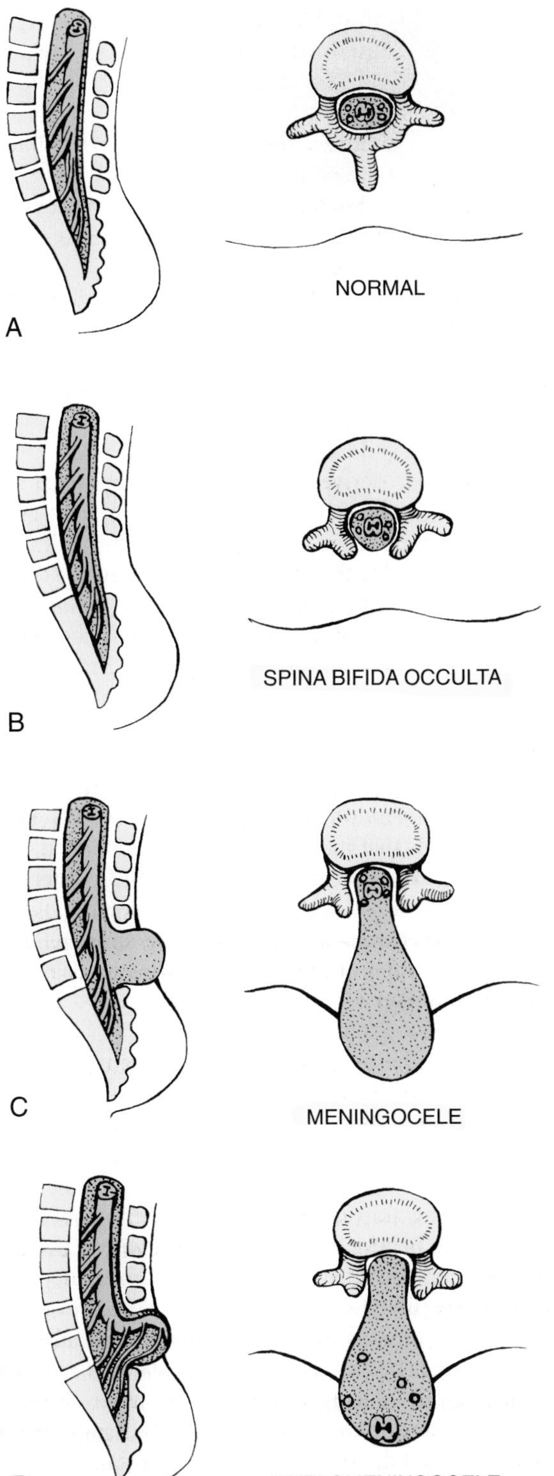

Fig. 55-5 **A** through **D:** Midline defects of osseous spine with varying degrees of neural herniations.

18, PHAVER syndrome, and Meckel-Gruber syndrome (Shaer, Chescheir, & Schulkin, 2007). Additional factors predisposing children to an increased risk of NTDs include prepregnancy maternal obesity, maternal diabetes mellitus, previous NTD pregnancy, low maternal vitamin B_{12} status, maternal hyperthermia, and the use of AEDs (e.g., valproic acid) in pregnancy.

BOX 55-4 Neural Tube Defects

Cranioschisis—A skull defect through which various tissues protrude

Exencephaly—Brain totally exposed or extruded through an associated skull defect; fetus usually aborted

Anencephaly—If fetus with exencephaly survives, degeneration of the brain to a spongiform mass with no bony covering; incompatible with life usually beyond a few days

Encephalocele—Herniation of brain and meninges through a defect in the skull producing a fluid-filled sac

Rachischisis or spina bifida—Fissure in the spinal column that leaves the meninges and spinal cord exposed

Meningocele—Hernial protrusion of a saclike cyst of meninges filled with spinal fluid (see Fig. 55-5, C)

Myelomeningocele (meningomyelocele)—Hernial protrusion of a saclike cyst containing meninges, spinal fluid, and a portion of the spinal cord with its nerves (see Fig. 55-5, D)

The degree of neurological dysfunction depends on where the sac protrudes through the vertebrae, the anatomical level of the defect, and the amount of nerve tissue involved. Most myelomeningoceles involve the lumbar or lumbosacral area (Fig. 55-6). Hydrocephalus with a type II Chiari defect develops in 80% of the children (Kinsman & Johnston, 2007).

Diagnostic Evaluation

The diagnosis of SB is made on the basis of clinical manifestations (Box 55-5) and examination of the meningeal sac. Please see Fig. 55-6, A, to see a normal spinal formation. Diagnostic measures used to evaluate the brain and spinal cord include MRI, ultrasound, CT, and myelography. Laboratory examinations are used primarily to determine causative organisms for common complications associated with myelomeningocele: meningitis and urinary tract infections. Prenatal screening can be done via ultrasound scan of the uterus, testing for elevated maternal concentrations of **alpha-fetoprotein** (AFP, or MS-AFP), and chorionic villus testing (see Chapter 12, p. 286, for further information).

Therapeutic Management

Early surgical closure of the myelomeningocele sac through fetal surgery has been evaluated in relation to prevention of injury to the exposed spinal cord tissue and improvement of neurological and urological outcomes in the affected child. Initial fetal surgical success and survival rates appear to be positive; however, reports vary in relation to the success of fetal surgery in the actual reduction of urological problems, improvement of lower leg function, and prevention of hydrocephalus in the postnatal period. The overall mortality rate from fetal surgery is 4%, and complications include oligohydramnios, preterm delivery, and a smaller birth weight. In addition, elective prelabour Caesarean birth may result in less motor dysfunction (Kaufman, 2004).

Management of the child who has a myelomeningocele requires a multidisciplinary approach involving the specialties

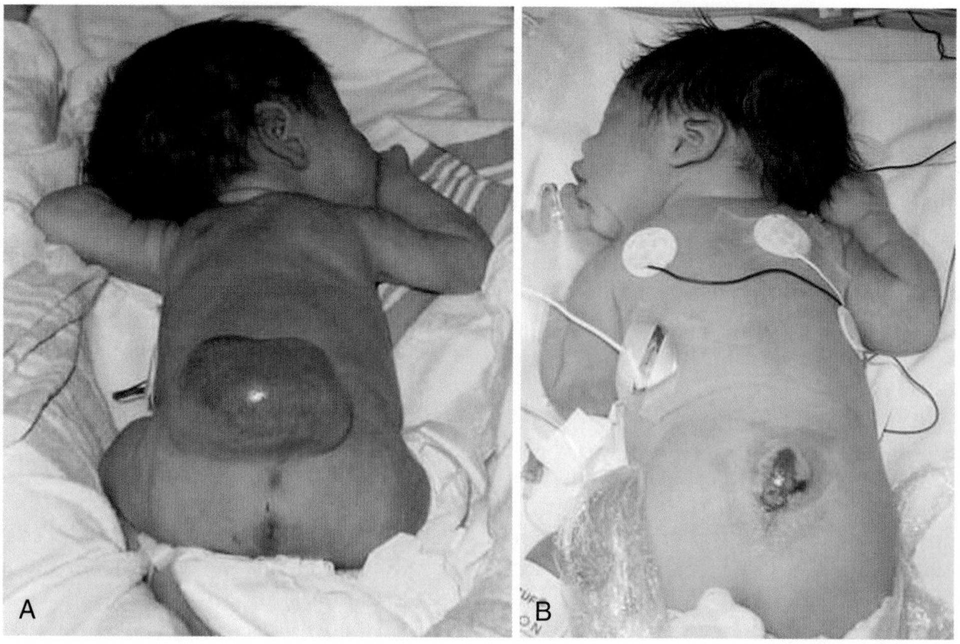

Fig. 55-6 **A:** Myelomeningocele with intact sac. **B:** Myelomeningocele with ruptured sac. *(Courtesy Dr. Robert C. Dauser, Neurosurgery, Baylor College of Medicine, Houston, TX.)*

BOX 55-5 Clinical Manifestations of Spina Bifida

Spina Bifida Cystica

Sensory disturbances usually parallel to motor dysfunction

- Below second lumbar vertebra—Flaccid, partial paralysis of lower extremities, varying degrees of sensory deficit, overflow incontinence with constant dribbling of urine, lack of bowel control, rectal prolapse (sometimes)
- Below third sacral vertebra—No motor impairment, may have saddle anaesthesia with bladder and anal sphincter paralysis

Joint deformities (sometimes produced in utero):

- Talipes valgus or varus contractures
- Kyphosis
- Lumbosacral scoliosis
- Hip dislocation or subluxation

Spina Bifida Occulta

Frequently no observable manifestations

May be associated with one or more cutaneous manifestations:

- Skin depression or dimple
- Port-wine angiomatous nevi
- Dark tufts of hair
- Soft, subcutaneous lipomas

May have neuromuscular disturbances:

- Progressive disturbance of gait with foot weakness
- Bowel and bladder sphincter disturbances

of neurology, neurosurgery, pediatrics, urology, orthopedics, rehabilitation, physiotherapy, and social services, along with intensive nursing care in a variety of specialty areas. The collaborative efforts of these specialists are focused on (1) the myelomeningocele and the problems associated with the defect—hydrocephalus, lower limb paralysis and orthopedic deformities, and genitourinary abnormalities, (2) possible acquired problems that may or may not be associated, such as meningitis, hypoxia, and hemorrhage, and (3) other conditions, such as cardiac or gastrointestinal malformations. Early neurological management of myelomeningocele has demonstrated improved upper urinary tract function and a reduction in the need for surgery (Kessler et al., 2006).

Postnatal Management

Initial care of the newborn involves preventing infection; performing a neurological assessment, including observing for associated anomalies; and dealing with the impact of the anomaly on the family. Although meningoceles are repaired early, especially if there is danger of rupture of the sac, the opinion regarding skin closure of myelomeningocele varies. Most authorities believe that early closure, within the first 24 to 72 hours, offers the most favourable outcome. Early closure, preferably in the first 12 to 18 hours, not only prevents local infection and trauma to the exposed tissues, but also avoids stretching of other nerve roots (which may occur as the meningeal sac expands during the first hours after birth), thus preventing further motor impairment. Broad-spectrum antibiotics are initiated, and neurotoxic substances such as povidone-iodine are avoided at the malformation.

Associated problems are assessed and managed by appropriate surgical and supportive measures. Shunt procedures provide relief from imminent or progressive hydrocephalus (see Chapter 51). Meningitis, urinary tract infection, and ventriculitis are treated with vigorous antibiotic therapy and supportive measures. Surgical intervention for Chiari malformation (a downward herniation of the brain into the brainstem) or for tethered cord (scar tissue binding the spinal cord) is indicated only when the child is symptomatic.

Improved surgical techniques do not alter the major physical disability, spinal defect, or chronic urinary tract infections that affect the quality of life for these children. Superimposed on the physical problems are the effects that the disorder has on family life and finances, including the need for long-term health care services.

Orthopedic Management

Most orthopedists recommend early evaluation and treatment (where indicated) of musculoskeletal problems that will affect later locomotion. Neurological assessment will determine the neurosegmental level of the lesion and enable recognition of spasticity and progressive paralysis, potential for deformity, and functional expectations. Orthopedic management includes prevention of joint contractures, correction of the existing deformity, prevention or minimization of the effects of motor and sensory deficits, prevention of skin breakdown, and acquisition of the best possible function of affected lower extremities. Common orthopedic problems requiring attention in SB include deformities of the knees, hips (subluxation), feet (clubfeet), and spine; fractures and insensate skin further complicate orthopedic care. Other problems that may occur later include kyphosis and scoliosis (Brown, 2001). Because children with this condition often have decreased sensitivity in their lower extremities, preventive skin care is important. A high percentage (60%) of children seen in a wound clinic for skin breakdown had spina bifida (Samaniego, 2003). The status of the neurological deficit remains the most important factor in determining the child's ultimate functional abilities.

With technological advances, a variety of lightweight orthoses, including braces, special "walking" devices, and custom-built wheelchairs, are available to provide mobility to children with spinal cord lesions (see also Chapter 42). Early in infancy, intervention with passive range-of-motion exercises, positioning, and stretching exercises may help decrease the incidence of muscle contractures (Brown, 2001). Corrective surgical procedures, when indicated, are best initiated at an early age so that the child will not lag significantly behind age-mates in developmental progress. Where there is little hope for lower extremity functioning, surgery is seldom recommended unless it will improve sitting position in a wheelchair and function for ADLs and mobility.

Management of Genitourinary Function

Myelomeningocele is one of the most common causes of neuropathic (neurogenic) bladder dysfunction among children. In infants the goal of treatment is to preserve renal function. In older children the goal is to preserve renal function and achieve optimal urinary continence. Urinary incontinence is a chronic, often debilitating problem for the child. In addition, the neuropathic bladder may produce urinary system distress, characterized by symptomatic urinary tract infections, ureterohydronephrosis, and vesicoureteral reflux or renal insufficiency. The characteristics of bladder dysfunction in children vary according to the level of the neurological lesion and the influence of bony growth and development on the spine. Thus ongoing urological monitoring is essential. Evidence is growing that early intervention, based on evaluation during the neonatal period and before complications occur, serves to improve bladder function, reduces the risk of subsequent urinary system distress, and decreases the need for reconstructive surgery of the lower urinary tract (Kessler et al., 2006; Snodgrass & Adams, 2004; Tarcan et al., 2006).

Treatment of renal problems includes (1) regular urological care with prompt and vigorous treatment of urinary tract infections, (2) a method of regular emptying of the bladder, such as clean intermittent catheterization (CIC) taught to and performed by parents and self-catheterization taught to children, (3) medications to improve bladder storage and continence, such as oxybutynin chloride (Ditropan) and tolterodine (Detrol), and (4) surgical procedures such as *vesicostomy* (bladder surgically brought out to the abdominal wall, allowing continuous urinary drainage) and *augmentation enterocystoplasty* (using a segment of bowel or stomach to increase bladder capacity, thereby reducing high bladder pressures).

However, despite the combined efforts of CIC, medication, and surgical intervention, some children with myelodysplasia may continue to experience debilitating urinary incontinence. Many of these children are able to attain social continence with a continent urinary diversion commonly referred to as *Mitrofanoff's procedure*. In this procedure, a catheterizable channel is surgically created from the appendix, ureter, or tapered bowel. The proximal end of the channel is connected to the bladder with the distal end brought out as a small stoma on the abdominal wall, usually at the umbilicus or suprapubic area (Gray & Moore, 2009). The bladder neck may be sutured to prevent urinary leakage from the urethra. CIC through the easily accessible abdominal route fosters greater independence in children, especially in those unable to transfer from a wheelchair to a toilet to perform CIC.

Bowel Control

Some degree of fecal continence can be achieved in most children with myelomeningocele with diet modification, regular toilet habits, and prevention of constipation and impaction. It is frequently a lengthy process. Dietary fibre supplements (recommended 10 g/day), laxatives, stool softeners, suppositories, or enemas aid in producing regular evacuation. Older children and adolescents seeking more independence may attain bowel continence and higher quality of life after undergoing an antegrade continence enema procedure (Doolin, 2006).

In a procedure similar to Mitrofanoff's, the appendix or ileum is used to create a catheterizable channel with attachment of the proximal end to the colon. The distal end of the channel exits through a small abdominal stoma. Every 1 or 2 days, a catheter is passed through the stoma, allowing enema solution to be instilled directly into the colon. After administration of the enema solution, the child sits on the toilet for 30 to 60 minutes as stool is flushed out through the rectum. Frequency of enemas and volume of solution used to completely evacuate the bowel vary among individuals.

Prognosis

The early prognosis for the child with myelomeningocele depends on the neurological deficit present at birth, including motor ability, bladder innervation, and associated neurological anomalies. Early surgical repair of the spinal defect, antibiotic therapy to reduce the incidence of meningitis and ventriculitis, prevention of urinary system dysfunction, and early detection and correction of hydrocephalus have significantly increased the survival rate and quality of life in such children. Overall mortality rate in those children treated aggressively is approximately 10 to 15%, and most deaths occur before age 4, as many as 70% of survivors will have normal intelligence (Kinsman & Johnston, 2007). Multidisciplinary follow-up is required for life. Many children with SB achieve partial independent living and gainful employment. Reports of survival rates vary; many include adults who were born before medical advances and surgical techniques seen in the past 25 years.

Researchers have noted that as adolescents with SB transition to young adulthood, they have increased difficulty obtaining centralized health care for the different health problems associated with SB (Lazzaretti & Pearson, 2010). This chronic condition has an array of associated complications, including hydrocephalus and shunt malfunctions, scoliosis, bowel and bladder management issues, latex allergy, and epilepsy. However, based on current medical knowledge and ethical considerations, aggressive, early management for the child with myelomeningocele improves the prognosis.

Prevention

The widespread use of folic acid among women of childbearing age has significantly decreased the incidence of SB. It has been estimated that a daily intake of 0.4 mg of folic acid in women of childbearing age will prevent 50 to 70% of all cases of NTDs (Centers for Disease Control and Prevention [CDC], 2004). With the 1998 mandate of adding folic acid to cereal products there was a 46% reduction in NTD after the increase in maternal periconceptual intake of folic acid. The greatest reduction was for spina bifida at 53%, anencephaly at 38%, and encephalocele at 31% (De Wals et al., 2007). Before the addition of folic acid to cereal, the NTD rate was higher in the eastern provinces than in the western provinces. After the addition of folic acid, the NTD rates were very similar, Canada-wide (De Wals et al., 2007). Nurses and other health care workers have an important task in disseminating information that may decrease the incidence of birth defects in children by promoting maternal consumption of folic acid. Health Canada, the Canadian Paediatric Society, and Mother Risk all provide information on this topic (see Additional Resources section at the end of this chapter).

In Canada, 39% of pregnancies are unplanned (Statistics Canada, 2003). Adolescent girls and women of childbearing age need to be educated about the necessity of consuming folic acid in order to prevent NTDs. They can take a daily multivitamin supplement containing 0.4 mg folic acid; eat folic acid–fortified breakfast cereal, bread, rice, or pasta; or eat foods naturally rich in folate (green leafy vegetables and citrus fruits) (see Table 11-1). For women who have had a previous pregnancy affected by NTDs, folic acid intake is increased to 4 mg/day under supervision of a practitioner beginning 1 month before a planned pregnancy and continuing during the first trimester. Supplementation of 4 mg of folate should not be given in multivitamin preparations because of the risk of overdose of other vitamins. The only population in which folic acid has not proved to be effective in decreasing the incidence of NTDs is epileptic women taking AEDs during pregnancy.

Nursing Care Management

At birth an examination needs to be performed to assess the intactness of the membranous cyst. During transport to the nursery, every effort should be made to prevent trauma to this protective covering. In addition to the routine assessment of the newborn (see Chapter 24), the infant should be assessed for the level of neurological involvement. Movement of extremities or skin response, especially an anal reflex that might provide clues to the degree of motor or sensory impairment should be noted. It is important to observe the infant's behaviour in conjunction with the stimulus, since limb movements can be induced in response to spinal cord reflex activity that has no connection with the higher centres. Observation of urine output, especially if a diaper remains dry, may indicate urinary retention. Abdominal assessment revealing bladder distension, even with a wet diaper, may indicate urinary overflow in a retentive bladder. The head circumference should be measured daily and the fontanels examined for signs of tension or bulging.

Care of the Myelomeningocele Sac

The infant is usually placed in an incubator or warmer so that temperature can be maintained without clothing or covers that might irritate the spinal defect. When an overhead warmer is used, the dressings over the defect require more frequent moistening because of the dehydrating effect of the radiant heat.

Before surgical closure the myelomeningocele is prevented from drying by the application of a sterile, moist, nonadherent dressing over the defect. The moistening solution is usually sterile normal saline. Dressings are changed frequently (every 2 to 4 hours), and the sac is closely inspected for leaks, abrasions, irritation, or any signs of infection. The sac must be carefully cleansed if it becomes soiled or contaminated. Sometimes the sac ruptures during delivery or transport, and any opening in the sac greatly increases the risk of infection to the central nervous system (see Fig. 55-6, B).

NURSING ALERT Avoid measuring rectal temperatures in infants with SB. Because bowel sphincter function is frequently affected, the thermometer can cause irritation and rectal prolapse.

One of the most important and challenging aspects in the early care of the infant with myelomeningocele is positioning. Before surgery the infant is kept in the prone position to minimize tension on the sac and the risk of trauma. The prone position allows for optimal positioning of the legs, especially in cases of associated hip subluxation. The infant is placed prone with the hips slightly flexed and supported to reduce tension on the defect. The legs are maintained in abduction with a pad between the knees to counteract hip subluxation, and a small roll is placed under the ankles to maintain a neutral foot position. A variety of aids, including diaper rolls, pads, small foam pads, or specially designed frames and appliances, can be used to maintain the desired position.

Prevent Complications

The prone position affects other aspects of the infant's care. For example, in this position the infant is more difficult to keep clean, pressure areas are a constant threat, and feeding becomes a problem. The infant's head is turned to one side for feeding. Fortunately, most defects are repaired early, and the infant can be held for feeding soon after surgery. Special care must be taken to avoid pressure on the operative site.

Diapering the infant may be contraindicated until the defect has been repaired and healing is well advanced or epithelialization has taken place. The padding beneath the diaper area should be changed as needed to keep the skin dry and free of irritation. When urinary retention is detected, CIC is employed. Because the bowel sphincter is frequently affected, there is continual passage of stool, often misinterpreted as diarrhea, which is a constant irritant to the skin and a source of infection to the spinal lesion.

Areas of sensory and motor impairment are subject to skin breakdown and require meticulous care. Placing the infant on a special mattress or mattress overlay reduces pressure on the knees and ankles. Periodic cleansing and gentle massage aid circulation.

Gentle range-of-motion exercises should be carried out to prevent contractures, and stretching of contractures is performed when indicated. However, these exercises may be restricted to the foot, ankle, and knee joint. When the hip joints are unstable, stretching against tight hip flexors or adductor muscles, which act much like bowstrings, may aggravate a tendency toward subluxation. Consultation with a physiotherapist is an important aspect of the short- and long-term management of infants with myelomeningocele.

Infants with unrepaired myelomeningocele may be unable to be held in the arms and cuddled as unaffected infants are; their need for tactile stimulation is met by caressing, stroking, and other comfort measures. One method to protect the sac while the parent is holding the infant is to place a pillow on the parent's lap and lay the infant on its side on the pillow. Individualized developmental care with age-appropriate stimulation is provided (see Developmental Outcome, Chapter 27).

Practitioners need to observe for early signs of infection, such as temperature instability (axillary), irritability, and lethargy, and for signs of increased intracranial pressure, which might indicate developing hydrocephalus.

Provide Postoperative Care

Postoperative care of the infant with myelomeningocele involves the same basic care as that of any postsurgical infant: monitoring vital signs, monitoring intake and output, providing nourishment, observing for signs of infection, and managing pain as needed. Care of the operative site is carried out under the direction of the surgeon and includes close observation for signs of leakage of cerebrospinal fluid (CSF). General care is continued as preoperatively.

The prone position is maintained after surgical closure, although many neurosurgeons allow a side-lying or partial side-lying position unless it aggravates a coexisting hip subluxation or permits undesirable hip flexion. This offers an opportunity for position changes, which reduces the risk of pressure sores and facilitates feeding. If permitted, the infant can be held upright against the body, with care taken to avoid pressure on the operative site. After the effects of anaesthesia have subsided and the infant is alert, feedings may be resumed unless there are other anomalies or associated complications.

Support the Family and Educate Them About Home Care

As soon as the parents are able to cope with the infant's condition, they should be encouraged to become involved in care. They need to learn how to continue at home the care that has been initiated in the hospital—positioning, feeding, skin care, and range-of-motion exercises when appropriate. They need to be taught CIC technique when it is prescribed. Parents also need to know the signs of complications (urinary, neurological, orthopedic) and how to obtain assistance when needed.

The mother who wishes to breastfeed the infant should be encouraged to do so. Shortly after delivery the mother is started on a program of pumping to initiate and maintain milk supply until the infant is stable enough to begin breastfeeding (Hurtekant & Spatz, 2007). This process may require considerable support from nurses, physicians, and family members because of separation from the infant for surgical care and recovery.

The long-range planning with and support of the parents and newborn begin in the hospital and continue throughout childhood and even into young adulthood. The life expectancy of children with SB extends well into adulthood; thus planning should involve long-term goals and plans for optimum function as an adult. Discussion about aspects of adulthood such as receiving educational or vocational training and education, living independently, having a mate, having sexual relationships, and bearing and rearing children is important and should not be overlooked. Advances in care have enabled adolescents to progress into adulthood with fewer concerns; one key factor is the recognition of the subtle signs of neurological deterioration and rapid intervention (Rowe & Jadhav, 2008). Nurses assume an important role as a central member of the health team. As a care manager and coordinator, the nurse reviews information with the family, takes responsibility for family teaching, and acts as a liaison between inpatient and outpatient services. The child will need numerous hospitalizations over the years, and each one will be a source of stress to which the younger child is especially vulnerable (see Chapter 41 for a discussion of care of the child with a disability).

Habilitation involves solving not only problems of self-help and locomotion but also the most distressing problem of urinary or bowel incontinence, which threatens the child's social acceptability. Assistance in preparing the child and the school for the child's special needs helps provide a better initial adjustment to this broader social experience. The Spina Bifida and Hydrocephalus Association Canada is a national centre that provides support and various services for families of children with spinal lesions (see Additional Resources).

Latex Allergy

Latex allergy was identified as a serious health hazard when a report linked intraoperative anaphylaxis with latex in children with SB. The high prevalence of latex allergy (up to 80%) in children with SB has been attributed to the repeated exposure to latex products during surgery and numerous bladder catheterizations and possible disease-associated factors. Some evidence suggests that children with SB are at increased risk for latex allergy as a result of the disease itself rather than repeated latex exposures (Eiwegger et al., 2006). Allergic reactions range from urticaria, wheezing, watery eyes, and rashes to anaphylactic shock. More severe reactions tend to occur when latex comes in contact with mucous membranes, wet skin, the bloodstream, or an airway. There also can be cross-reactions to a number of foods (e.g., banana, avocado, kiwi, chestnut).

Latex allergy has been diagnosed in infants; symptoms include wheezing, facial swelling, facial rash, and anaphylaxis (Kimata, 2004). In addition to patients with SB, high-risk populations include patients with urogenital anomalies or multiple surgeries and health care workers (see Box 55-6 for medical conditions associated with a risk of latex allergy).

The most important goals are prevention of latex allergy and identification of children with a known hypersensitivity (see Guidelines box). High-risk and latex-allergic individuals must be managed in a *latex-free* environment. Care must be taken so that they do not come in direct or secondary contact with products or equipment containing latex *at any time* during medical treatment. Allergy testing has been used to identify latex allergy with varying success. Skin prick testing and provocation testing carry the risk of allergic reaction or anaphylaxis. The radioallergosorbent test (RAST) has been used to measure the serum level of latex-specific immunoglobulin E. The RAST has been shown to be 90 to 95% sensitive (Kellett, 1997). Pretreatment with an antihistamine and steroids (dexamethasone) before and after surgery to reduce the possibility of a serious reaction remains controversial, since it may interfere with healing.

Because children who have SB are prone to develop an allergy to latex, reducing exposure, from birth on, may decrease the chance of allergy development. Many health care facilities are establishing latex-safe environments. Lists have been published of products, such as vinyl gloves, that may be substituted for latex.

NURSING ALERT Ask all patients, not only those at risk, about allergic reactions to latex during the health interview with the parent or child. Be certain that this is a routine part of all preoperative and preprocedural histories. Stress the importance of the allergy history to all personnel (e.g., phlebotomists).

The identification of those sensitive to latex is best accomplished through careful screening of *all* patients (see Guidelines box for questions related to latex allergy). Children with latex allergy should carry or wear some form of medical identification; those who have had serious reactions should also carry an injectable epinephrine pen and a pair of latex-free gloves for emergencies. Education programs regarding latex hypersensitivity are aimed at those who care for high-risk groups, such as children with SB, and may include relatives, school nurses, teachers, child care workers, and babysitters. In addition to educating caregivers about the child's exposure to medical products that contain latex, nurses need to inform them of common nonmedical latex objects. Parents should also be given literature explaining signs and symptoms of latex hypersensitivity and appropriate emergency treatment (see Anaphylaxis, Chapter 48).

BOX 55-6 Medical Conditions Associated With Risk of Latex Allergy

- Spina bifida
- Urogenital anomalies
- Imperforate anus
- Esophageal atresia/tracheoesophageal fistula
- VATER association (vertebral defects, imperforate anus, tracheoesophageal fistula, and radial and renal dysplasia)
- Preterm infants
- Ventriculoperitoneal shunt
- Neurocognitive impairment
- Cerebral palsy
- Tetraplegia
- Multiple surgeries
- Atopy

Spinal Muscular Atrophy

Spinal muscular atrophy (SMA) is a group of disorders characterized by a progressive degeneration of motor neurons, which eventually results in muscle fibre atrophy. The disorder may be manifested early—often at birth—and almost always before 2 years of age; death may occur as a result of respiratory failure by age 2 years (Iannaccone & Burghes, 2002; Lunn & Wang, 2008). The manifestations (Box 55-7) and prognosis are categorized according to the age of onset, severity of weakness, and clinical course; for some children, clinical function may fluctuate between exhibiting symptoms of types 1 and 2, or types 2 and 3 (Sarnat, 2007). A severe rare fetal form of SMA, classified as type 0, is reported to be lethal in the perinatal period (Sarnat, 2007).

Infantile Spinal Muscular Atrophy (Werdnig-Hoffmann Disease)

Progressive infantile SMA (Werdnig-Hoffmann disease), or SMA type 1, is a disorder characterized by progressive weakness and wasting of skeletal muscles caused by degeneration

GUIDELINES Identifying Latex Allergy

- Does your child have any symptoms, such as sneezing, coughing, rashes, or wheezing, when handling rubber products (e.g., balloons, tennis or Koosh balls, adhesive bandage strips) or when in contact with rubber hospital products (e.g., gloves, catheters)?
- Has your child ever had an allergic reaction during surgery?
- Does your child have a history of rashes, asthma, or allergic reactions to medication or foods, especially milk, kiwi, bananas, or chestnuts?
- How would you identify or recognize an allergic reaction in your child?
- What would you do if an allergic reaction occurred?
- Has anyone ever discussed latex or rubber allergy or sensitivity with you?
- Has your child had any allergy testing?
- When did your child last come in contact with any type of rubber product? Were you present?

(Modified from Romanczuk, A. [1993]. Latex use with infants and children: It can cause problems. *MCN: American Journal of Maternal/Child Nursing, 18*[4], 208–212.)

BOX 55-7 Clinical Manifestations of Spinal Muscular Atrophy

Infantile SMA: Type 1 (Werdnig-Hoffmann Disease)

Clinical manifestations within first few weeks or months of life
Onset within 6 months of life
Inactivity the most prominent feature
Infant lying in the frog position with legs externally rotated, abducted, and flexed at knees
Generalized weakness
Absent deep tendon reflexes
Limited movements of shoulder and arm muscles
Active movement usually limited to fingers and toes
Diaphragmatic breathing with intercostal retractions (diaphragmatic paralysis may occur)
Abnormal tongue movements (at rest)
Weak cry and cough
Poor suck reflex
Alert facies
Normal sensation and intellect
Tiring quickly during feedings (if breastfed, may lose weight before noticeable)
Failure to thrive (nutritional)
Affected infants not able to sit alone, roll over, or walk
Early death possible from respiratory failure or infection

Type 2 (Intermediate Spinal Muscular Atrophy)

Onset before 18 months
Early—Weakness confined to arms and legs
Later—Becomes generalized
Legs usually involved to greater extent than arms
Prominent pectus excavatum
Movements absent during complete relaxation or sleep
Some infants able to sit if placed in position, but few can ambulate
Lifespan varies from 7 months to 7 years although may have normal life expectancy

Juvenile SMA: Type 3 (Kugelberg-Welander Disease)

Onset of symptoms after 18 months of age
Normal head control and ability to sit unassisted by 6 to 8 months of age
Thigh and hip muscles weak
Scoliosis common
Failure to walk a common presentation
In those who manage to walk:

- Waddling gait
- Genu recurvatum
- Protuberant abdomen
- Ambulation becomes increasingly difficult
- Confined to a wheelchair by second decade (may vary)

Deep tendon reflexes may be present early but disappear

Note: These classifications are general, and experts suggest there may be variations in lifespan and other characteristics (Iannaccone & Burghes, 2002; Russman et al., 1992).

of anterior horn cells. It is inherited as an autosomal recessive trait and is the most common and most severe paralytic form of the floppy infant syndrome (congenital hypotonia). The sites of the pathological condition are the anterior horn cells of the spinal cord and the motor nuclei of the brainstem, but the primary effect is atrophy of skeletal muscles. The age of onset is variable, but the earlier the onset, the more disseminated and severe the motor weakness.

Diagnostic Evaluation and Therapeutic Management

The diagnosis is based on the molecular genetic marker for the *SMN* (survival motor neuron) gene, which is located on chromosome 5q13. Prenatal diagnosis may be made by genetic analysis of circulating fetal cells in maternal blood (Beroud et al., 2003) or circulating fetal cells in amniotic fluid. The risk of subsequent affected offspring in carriers of the mutant gene or in families with known cases of SMA may also be evaluated genetically. Further diagnostic studies include muscle electromyography (EMG), which demonstrates a denervation pattern, and muscle biopsy; however, genetic analysis has become the gold standard for diagnosis of the condition.

There is no cure for the disease, and treatment is symptomatic and preventive, primarily preventing joint contractures and treating orthopedic problems, the most serious of which is scoliosis. Hip subluxation and dislocation may also occur. Many children benefit from powered chairs, lifts, special pressure-adjustable mattresses, and accessible environmental controls. Muscle and joint contractures require careful attention and care to prevent further complications. Nutritional growth failure (failure to thrive) may occur in infants and toddlers as a result of poor feeding; supplemental gastrostomy feedings may be required to maintain adequate nutritional status and maintain weight gain. The use of lower extremity orthoses may assist with ambulation, but eventually the child may be confined to a wheelchair as muscle atrophy progresses. Sleep-disordered breathing is common in children with SMA and often requires nocturnal mechanical ventilation. Noninvasive ventilation methods such as bilevel positive airway pressure (BiPAP) have decreased the morbidity and increased the survival rate of children with SMA types 1 and 2. Upper respiratory tract infections may occur and are treated with antibiotic therapy.

Prognosis

Prognosis varies according to the age of onset or type as described in Box 55-7. Individuals with progressive infantile SMA may succumb to respiratory tract infections or failure between 1 and 24 months of age (Iannaccone & Burghes, 2002; Lunn & Wang, 2008); however, some may live into their third or fourth decade of life. A significant number of infants with SMA require a tracheotomy, and associated medical conditions in survivors include gastroesophageal reflux, scoliosis, early onset puberty, hip dysplasia, and recurrent oral candidiasis (Bach, 2007).

Nursing Care Management

The infant or small child with progressive muscle weakness requires nursing care similar to that of the immobilized patient (see Chapter 54). However, the underlying goal of treatment should be to assist the child and family in dealing with the illness while progressing toward a life of normalization within the child's capabilities. Special attention should be directed to preventing muscle and joint contractures, promoting independence in performance of ADLs, and incorporating the child into the mainstream of school when possible. In addition, parents need support and resources to be able to provide for the child and remain an intact family. Because children with neuromuscular disease have abnormal breathing patterns that often contribute to early death, it is important to assess adequate oxygenation, especially during the sleep phase when shallow breathing occurs and hypoxemia may develop. Home pulse oximetry may be used to assess the child during sleep and provide noninvasive ventilation as necessary (Bush et al., 2005; Young et al., 2007) (see Duchenne [Pseudohypertrophic] Muscular Dystrophy, p. 1740, for respiratory management). Supportive care also includes management of orthoses and other orthopedic equipment as required.

Because children with SMA are intellectually normal, verbal, tactile, and auditory stimulation are important aspects of developmental care. Supporting them so that they can see the activities around them and transporting them via appropriate means (e.g., wagon, power wheelchair) for a change of environment provide stimulation and a broader scope of contacts.

Children who are able to sit require proper support and attention to alignment to prevent deformities and other complications. Children who survive beyond infancy will need attention to educational needs and opportunities for social interaction with other children. The parents of a child who is chronically ill require much support and encouragement (see Chapter 41) (see Additional Resources). Parents who have not sought genetic counselling should be encouraged to do so to evaluate further risk potential.

Juvenile Spinal Muscular Atrophy (Kugelberg-Welander Disease)

Juvenile SMA (Kugelberg-Welander disease, or SMA type 3, juvenile proximal hereditary muscular atrophy) is a result of anterior horn cell and motor nerve degeneration. The disease is characterized by a pattern of muscular weakness similar to that of infantile SMA (see Box 55-7). Several modes of inheritance have been reported for the disease: autosomal recessive, autosomal dominant, and X-linked recessive.

The onset occurs from younger than 1 year of age into adulthood, with symptoms resembling those of infantile SMA. Proximal muscle weakness (especially of the lower limbs) and muscular atrophy are the predominant features. The disease runs a slowly progressive course. Some children lose the ability to walk 8 to 9 years after the onset of symptoms, but many can still walk after 30 years or more. Many affected persons have a normal life expectancy (Iannaccone, 1998; Lunn & Wang, 2008).

Therapeutic Management and Nursing Care Management

The management is primarily symptomatic and supportive and is related to maintaining mobility as long as possible, preventing complications such as skin breakdown, optimizing and maintaining respiratory function, and providing support to the child and family.

Muscular Dystrophies

Muscular dystrophies (MDs) constitute the largest and most important single group of muscle diseases of childhood. The MDs have a genetic origin in which there is gradual degeneration of muscle fibres, and they are characterized by progressive weakness and wasting of symmetrical groups of skeletal muscles, with increasing disability and deformity. In all forms of MD there is insidious loss of strength, but each type differs in regard to muscle groups affected (Fig. 55-7), age of onset, rate of progression, and inheritance pattern. The most common form, *Duchenne muscular dystrophy (DMD)*, is considered separately in the next section.

Facioscapulohumeral (Landouzy-Dejerine) MD is inherited as an autosomal dominant disorder with onset in early adolescence. It is characterized by difficulty in raising the arms over the head, lack of facial mobility, and a forward slope of the shoulders. The progression is slow, and the lifespan is usually unaffected.

Limb-girdle muscular dystrophy is an autosomal recessive disease of later childhood, adolescence, or early adulthood with variable but usually slow progression. It is characterized by weakness of the proximal muscles of the pelvic and shoulder girdles.

Treatment of the MDs consists mainly of supportive measures, including physiotherapy, orthopedic procedures to minimize deformity, ventilation support, and assistance for the affected child in meeting the demands of daily living.

Duchenne (Pseudohypertrophic) Muscular Dystrophy

DMD is the most severe and the most common MD of childhood. It is inherited as an X-linked recessive trait, and the single-gene defect is located on the short arm of the X chromosome. DMD has a reportedly high mutation rate, with a positive family history in 65% of all cases (Thompson & Berenson, 2001); therefore, genetic counselling is an important aspect of the care of the family.

As in all X-linked disorders, males are affected almost exclusively. At the genetic level, both DMD and Becker's MD (a milder variant) result from mutations of the gene that encodes dystrophin, a protein product in skeletal muscle. Dystrophin is absent from the muscle of children with DMD and is reduced or abnormal in children with Becker's MD. Children with Becker's MD have a later onset of symptoms, which are usually not as severe as those seen in DMD. The incidence is approximately 1 in 3600 male births for the Duchenne form and approximately 1 in 30,000 live births for the Becker type (Sarnat, 2007; Thompson & Berenson, 2001). Box 55-8 describes the characteristics of DMD.

Most children with DMD reach the appropriate developmental milestones early in life, although they may have mild, subtle delays. Evidence of muscle weakness usually appears during the third to seventh year, although there may have been a history of delay in motor development, particularly walking. Difficulties in running, riding a bicycle, and climbing stairs are usually the first symptoms noted. Later, abnormal gait on

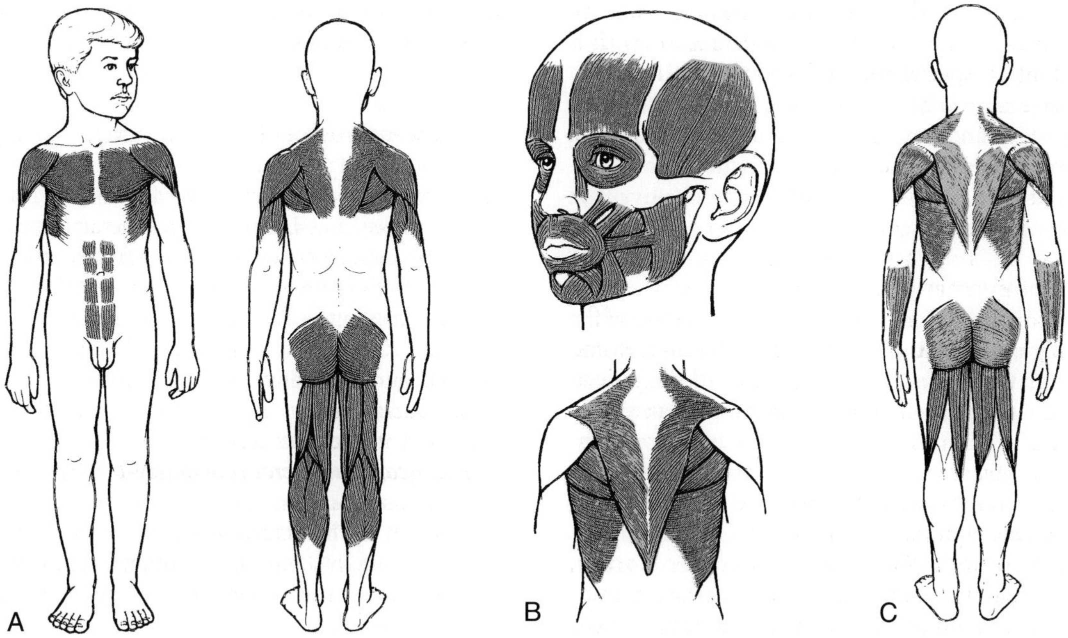

Fig. 55-7 Initial muscle groups involved in muscular dystrophies. **A:** Pseudohypertrophic. **B:** Facioscapulohumeral. **C:** Limb-girdle.

BOX 55-8 Characteristics of Duchenne Muscular Dystrophy

- Early onset, usually between 3 and 5 years of age
- Progressive muscular weakness, wasting, and contractures
- Calf muscle hypertrophy in most patients
- Loss of independent ambulation by 9 to 11 years of age
- Slowly progressive, generalized weakness during teenage years
- Relentless progression until death from respiratory or cardiac failure

BOX 55-9 Clinical Manifestations of Duchenne Muscular Dystrophy

Waddling gait
Lordosis
Frequent falls
Gower sign (child turning onto side or abdomen, flexing knees to assume a kneeling position, then with knees extended gradually pushing torso to an upright position by "walking" the hands up the legs)
Enlarged muscles (especially thighs and upper arms); feel unusually firm or woody on palpation
Later stages: profound muscular atrophy
Cognitive impairment (common)
- Mild (about 20 IQ points below normal)
- Cognitive impairment present in 25 to 30% of patients

Complications:
- Contracture deformities of hips, knees, and ankles
- Disuse atrophy
- Obesity

a level surface becomes apparent. In the early years, rapid developmental gains may mask the progression of the disease. The parents may note that the child has difficulty in rising from a sitting or supine position. Typically, affected boys have a waddling gait and lordosis, fall frequently, and develop a characteristic manner of rising from a squatting or sitting position on the floor (Gower sign). Parents may also notice that the child has enlarged calves (Box 55-9).

Pseudohypertrophy is a term applied to muscular enlargement caused by fatty infiltration. Profound muscular atrophy occurs in later stages, and as the disease progresses, contractures and deformities involving large and small joints are common complications. Ambulation usually becomes impossible by 12 years of age. Facial, oropharyngeal, and respiratory muscles are often spared until the terminal stages of the disease. Ultimately the disease process involves the diaphragm and auxiliary muscles of respiration, and cardiovascular involvement (cardiomyopathy, dysrhythmias, and heart failure) is common. Mild mental delay is common in roughly 30% of all individuals with MD, and many will have permanent learning disabilities; however, children with DMD should be involved in early learning programs and eventually moved into regular classrooms as much as possible. The eventual cause of death is usually respiratory tract infection or cardiac failure; however, much progress has been made in providing ventilatory methods to prolong and maintain quality of life.

Diagnostic Evaluation

The diagnosis of DMD is primarily established by blood polymerase chain reaction (PCR) for the dystrophin gene mutation (Sarnat, 2007). Prenatal diagnosis is also possible as early as 12 weeks of gestation. Serum enzyme measurement, muscle biopsy, and EMG may also be used in establishing the diagnosis. Serum creatine kinase levels are extremely high in the first 2 years of life, before the onset of clinical weakness. If the child demonstrates the usual characteristics, has a positive family history for DMD, and the PCR is positive, the muscle biopsy may be deferred.

Therapeutic Management

No effective treatment exists for childhood MD. The use of the corticosteroids prednisone and deflazacort has been evaluated as a treatment for DMD. Several clinical trials demonstrated increased muscle strength and improved performance and pulmonary function, with significant decrease in the progression of weakness, when prednisone was administered for 6 months. The use of prednisone varies worldwide. Many practitioners are concerned about the adverse effects of steroids but as yet there are no alternatives. Major adverse effects include weight gain and a cushingoid facial appearance. In one study, deflazacort caused less weight gain than prednisone and was effective in decreasing muscle wasting in some children (Angelini, 2007). Currently, an ongoing international study is investigating steroid treatment protocols and seeking to standardize the protocols (Buschby et al., 2010a). The American Academy of Neurology has published a practice parameter for the administration of corticosteroids in the treatment of DMD which is supported by the Canadian Paediatric Society (Manzur et al., 2008; Moxley et al., 2005).

Maintaining optimum function in all muscles for as long as possible is the primary goal; secondary is the prevention of contractures. Children with DMD who remain as active as possible are able to avoid wheelchair confinement for a longer time. Maintenance of function often involves stretching exercises, strength and muscle training, breathing exercises to increase and maintain vital lung capacity, range-of-motion exercises, surgery to release contracture deformities, bracing, and performance of ADLs.

Parents should be involved in making decisions about the child's care; teaching regarding home safety and prevention of falls is important as well. Parents should also be encouraged to have the child keep follow-up appointments for medical care and physical and occupational therapy. Because respiratory tract infections are most troublesome in these children, they should be encouraged to receive influenza and pneumococcal vaccines and to avoid contact with persons with respiratory tract infections.

Eventually respiratory and cardiac problems become the central focus of the debilitating illness. Children with neuromuscular disease have abnormal breathing patterns, particularly during rapid-eye-movement sleep, and hypoxia may occur as a result of inadequate oxygenation (Birnkrant, 2002). The child and parents should be involved in a discussion of long-term ventilation options. Cardiac and respiratory assessment during wake–sleep cycles is imperative. Respiratory care for children with neuromuscular conditions such as SMA and DMD may involve the use of noninvasive ventilation with BiPAP on a temporary or full-time basis, mechanically assisted coughing (MAC), or tracheotomy and relief of airway obstruction with coughing and suctioning devices; the tracheotomy, however, is associated with more complications (Simonds, 2006; Young et al., 2007). Home pulse oximetry may be used to monitor oxygenation during sleep or to aid in decision making regarding the use of MAC to clear the airways.

Several devices are available for children with neuromuscular disease to assist in clearing the airway when the cough reflex is ineffective or diminished. The mechanical cough in-exsufflator (MIE) has been evaluated and found to be safe and effective in the daily management of respiratory function (Kravitz, 2009; Miske et al., 2004). The MIE delivers positive inspiratory pressures at a set rate, followed by negative pressure exsufflation coordinated with the patient's own breathing rhythm; the exsufflation is designed to mimic a cough reflex so mucus can be effectively cleared. Airway suctioning after exsufflation is accomplished as necessary to clear the airways. In children the MIE may be connected directly to a tracheostomy or used with a mouthpiece or face mask.

Survival in individuals with DMD may be prolonged several years with the use of noninvasive ventilation and MAC as alternatives to tracheotomy and airway suctioning (Simonds, 2006). The Canadian Thoracic Society has published extensive guidelines for respiratory monitoring and care of children and adults with DMD (McKim et al., 2011).

Muscular Dystrophy Canada (2012) recommends an extensive cardiac evaluation of the child diagnosed with either DMD or Becker MD. Patients with neuromuscular conditions may not have the typical signs and symptoms of cardiac dysfunction. Thus symptoms such as weight loss, nausea and vomiting, cough, increased fatigue on performance of ADLs, and orthopnea should be carefully evaluated to detect early signs of cardiomyopathy.

Genetic counselling is also recommended for parents, sisters, and maternal aunts and their daughters. Long-term care, end-of-life directives, and palliative care options are issues that must be discussed with the child and family affected by MD. Professional counselling may be required to allow frank discussion of these issues in some cases, and referrals should be made as appropriate (Bushby, 2010b).

Research evaluating a number of treatments for DMD is in progress. These include clinical trials with glutamine and creatine monohydrate to preserve muscle strength; utrophin, a protein that is similar to dystrophin and in large quantities may counteract the effects of the deficiency of dystrophin (Chakkalakal et al., 2005); and the enzyme CT GalNAc transferase, which blocks muscle wasting in mice (Metules, 2002).

Nursing Care Management

The major emphasis of nursing care is to help the child and family cope with a chronic, progressive, incapacitating disease; to help design a program that will afford maximal independence and reduce the predictable and preventable disabilities associated with the disorder; and to help the child and family deal constructively with the limitations the disease imposes on their daily lives. Because of advances in technology, children with MD may live into early adulthood; thus the goals of care should also involve decisions regarding quality of life, achievement of independence, and transition to adulthood.

Working closely with other team members, nurses assist the family in developing the child's self-help skills to give the child the satisfaction of being as independent as possible for as long as possible. This requires continual evaluation of the child's capabilities, which are often difficult to assess. Fortunately, most children with MD instinctively recognize the need to become as independent as possible and strive to do so.

Practical difficulties faced by families are physical limitations of housing and mobility. Some families live in houses or apartments that are unsuited to wheelchairs. Transportation may also be a barrier for families of children with MD. Assisting with these challenges requires team problem solving. Diet, nutritional needs, and nutrition modification should be discussed according to the needs of the individual child and family.

The parents' social activities are also restricted, and the family's activities must be continually modified to accommodate the needs of the affected child. When the child becomes increasingly incapacitated, the family may consider home-based care, an assisted living facility, or respite care. Unless the child is severely incapacitated, he should also be involved in the decisions regarding such care. Nurses can assist with decision making by exploring all available options and resources and supporting the child and family in the decision. Older boys with MD may also need psychiatric or psychological counselling to deal with issues such as depression, anger, and quality of life. Parents also need to be encouraged to become involved in support groups because adequate social support from family, community, and other parents is crucial to appropriate coping in families with children with chronic illness.

Regardless of how successful the program or how well the family adapts to the disorder, superimposed on the physical and emotional problems associated with a child with a long-term disability is the constant knowledge of the ultimate outcome of the disease. All the manifestations seen in the child with a chronic fatal illness are encountered in these families (see Chapter 41).

Nurses are especially valuable health care providers as they come to know the family and the family's problems. Nurses can be alert to the family's problems and needs and make necessary referrals when supplementary services are indicated. Muscular Dystrophy Canada has branches in most communities to assist families in which there is a member with MD (see Additional Resources).

Acquired Neuromuscular Disorders

Guillain-Barré Syndrome (Infectious Polyneuritis)

Guillain-Barré syndrome (GBS), also known as infectious polyneuritis, is an uncommon acute demyelinating polyneuropathy with a progressive, usually ascending flaccid paralysis. Children are affected less often than adults; among children, those between ages 4 and 10 years have higher susceptibility. The male/female ratio is reported to be 1.5 : 1. Two peak time periods have been identified with an increased incidence of GBS: late adolescence and young adulthood.

Congenital GBS is rare yet may be seen in the neonatal period and consists of hypotonia, weakness, and decreased or absent reflexes; maternal neuromuscular disease may or may not be present. Diagnosis is established by the same criteria as in older children, but the symptoms gradually subside over the first few months of life and disappear by 12 months (Sarnat, 2007).

Pathophysiology

GBS is an immune-mediated disease often associated with a number of viral or bacterial infections or the administration of certain vaccines. It has been associated with infectious mononucleosis, measles, mumps, *Campylobacter jejuni* (gastroenteritis), cytomegalovirus, *Borrelia burgdorferi* (Lyme disease), Epstein-Barr virus, *Helicobacter pylori*, and *Mycoplasma* and *Pneumocystis* infections. The onset of GBS symptoms usually occurs within 10 days of the primary infection. Pathological changes in spinal and cranial nerves consist of inflammation and edema with rapid, segmented demyelination and compression of nerve roots within the dural sheath. Nerve conduction is impaired, producing ascending partial or complete paralysis of muscles innervated by the involved nerves. GBS has three phases (Newswanger & Warren, 2004):

1. *Acute or progressive*—Phase starts when symptoms begin and continues until new symptoms stop appearing or deterioration ceases; it may last as long as 4 weeks.
2. *Plateau*—Symptoms remain constant without further deterioration; it may last from days to weeks.
3. *Recovery*—Patient begins to improve and progress to optimum recovery; it usually lasts a few weeks to months depending on the deficits incurred by the illness.

evolve Animation—Guillain-Barre Syndrome

evolve Critical Thinking Exercise—Guillain-Barre Syndrome

Diagnostic Evaluation

Diagnosis of GBS is based on clinical manifestations (Box 55-10), CSF analysis, and EMG findings. CSF analysis reveals an increased protein concentration, and EMG shows evidence of acute muscle denervation; other laboratory studies are usually noncontributory. The symmetrical nature of the paralysis helps differentiate this disorder from spinal paralytic poliomyelitis, which usually affects sporadic muscles.

Therapeutic Management

Treatment of GBS is primarily supportive. In the acute phase patients are hospitalized because respiratory and pharyngeal involvement may require assisted ventilation, sometimes with a temporary tracheotomy. Treatment modalities include aggressive ventilatory support, intravenous administration of immunoglobulin (IVIG), and steroids; plasmapheresis and immunosuppressive medications may also be used. Plasmapheresis has been shown to decrease the length of recovery in patients with severe GBS, yet it is expensive, and adverse effects include hypotension, fever, bleeding disorders, chills, urticaria, and bradycardia. Further evidence reports equal benefits to treatment of GBS with IVIG administration or plasmapheresis; both sped up recovery time in studies reviewed (Hughes & Cornblath, 2005). Children who were treated with IVIG therapy (versus supportive treatment alone) showed significant improvement (Harel & Schoenfeld, 2005; Hughes et al., 2006; Tsai et al., 2007). IVIG therapy is more cost-effective

BOX 55-10 Clinical Manifestations of Guillain-Barré Syndrome

Initial Symptoms

Muscle tenderness
Paresthesia and cramps (sometimes)
Proximal symmetrical muscle weakness

Paralysis

Ascending bilateral paralysis from lower extremities
Frequent involvement of muscles of trunk and upper extremities and those supplied by cranial nerves (especially facial)
Flaccid paralysis with loss of reflexes
May involve facial, extraocular, labial, lingual, pharyngeal, and laryngeal muscles
Intercostal and phrenic nerves:
- Breathlessness in vocalizations
- Shallow, irregular respirations

Other Manifestations

Tendon reflexes depressed or absent
Variable degrees of sensory impairment
Muscle tenderness or sensitivity to slight pressure
Urinary incontinence or retention and constipation

than plasmapheresis. Corticosteroids alone did not decrease the symptoms or shorten the duration of the disease.

Medications that may be administered during the acute phase include a low-molecular-weight heparin to prevent deep vein thrombosis, a mild laxative or stool softener to prevent constipation, pain medication such as acetaminophen, and a histamine-antagonist to prevent stress ulcer formation. Chronic **neuropathic pain** following GBS may be treated with gabapentin, which is reported to be more effective than carbamazepine (Sarnat, 2007).

Course and Prognosis

Better outcomes are associated with younger age, no requirement for mechanical respiratory assistance, slower progression of disease, normal peripheral nerve function on EMG, and treatment with either IVIG or plasmapheresis. Recovery usually begins within 2 to 3 weeks, and most patients regain full muscle strength. The recovery of muscle strength progresses in the reverse order of onset of paralysis, with lower extremity strength being the last to recover. Poor prognosis with subsequent residual effects in children is reportedly associated with cranial nerve involvement, extensive disability at time of presentation, and intubation.

Most deaths associated with GBS are caused by respiratory failure; thus early diagnosis and access to respiratory support are especially important. The rate of recovery is usually related to the degree of involvement and may extend from a few weeks to months. The greater the degree of paralysis, the longer the recovery phase.

Nursing Care Management

Nursing care is essentially supportive and is the same as that required for the child with immobilization and respiratory depression. The emphasis of care is on close observation to assess the extent of paralysis and on prevention of complications, including autonomic dysfunction (hypertension, orthostatic hypotension, syndrome of inappropriate antidiuretic hormone secretion, life-threatening dysrhythmias), respiratory dysfunction, DVT, fear and anxiety, and pain.

During the acute phase of GBS the child's condition should be carefully observed for possible difficulty in swallowing and for respiratory involvement. The child's respiratory function should be closely monitored, and oxygen source, appropriate-sized resuscitation bag and mask, endotracheal intubation and suctioning equipment, tracheotomy tray, and vasoconstrictor medications need to be kept available. Vital signs, including neurological signs and level of consciousness, should be monitored frequently. For the child who develops respiratory impairment, the care is the same as that for any child with respiratory distress requiring mechanical ventilation.

Throughout the recovery phase, special emphasis is placed on the prevention of complications, including proper postural alignment, frequent change of position, assessment of skin at pressure points, and passive range-of-motion exercises. Respiratory care, should intubation be required, requires close monitoring of oxygenation status, usually by pulse oximetry and arterial blood gases; maintenance of an open airway with suctioning; and postural changes to prevent pneumonia. Children with oral and pharyngeal involvement may be fed via a nasogastric tube to ensure adequate feeding. Immobilization, which occurs with GBS, decreases gastrointestinal function; thus problems such as decreased gastric emptying and constipation require nursing assessment and appropriate collaborative interventions.

Prevention of deep vein thrombosis is accomplished with sequential compression (anti-embolism) devices, administration of a low-molecular-weight heparin, and early mobilization and ambulation. Temporary urinary catheterization may be required; urinary retention is not uncommon, and appropriate assessment of urine output is vital. Sensory impairment and paralysis in the lower extremities make the child susceptible to skin breakdown; meticulous skin care must be practised. Although the child may have a generalized paralysis, cognitive function remains intact; thus it is important for nursing care to involve communication with the child regarding procedures and treatments that may be frightening, especially if mechanical ventilation is required. Parents should be encouraged to talk to the child and make eye and physical contact as much as possible to reassure the child during the illness. Psychosocial care of the child with GBS focuses on dealing with the child's anxiety and fear related to the disease itself and the unknown prognosis. In addition, the child's parents should be allowed to express feelings and encouraged to be involved in the child's daily care.

Pain management is essential in the care of children with GBS. Although neuromuscular impairment may make pain perception more difficult to accurately evaluate, objective pain scales should be used. Carbamazepine and gabapentin may be used to manage neuropathic pain in patients with GBS.

Physiotherapy is limited to passive range-of-motion exercises during the evolving phase of the disease. Later, as the disease stabilizes and recovery begins, an active physiotherapy program is implemented to prevent contracture deformities and facilitate muscle recovery. This may include active exercise, gait training, and bracing.

Throughout the course of the illness, support of the child and parents is paramount. The usual rapidity of the paralysis and the long period of recovery greatly tax the emotional reserves of all family members. The parents and child benefit from repeated reassurance that recovery is occurring and from realistic information regarding the possibility of permanent disability. In the event of a residual disability, the family needs assistance in accepting and adjusting to the loss of function (see Chapter 41). The GBS/CIDP Foundation of Canada is a nonprofit organization devoted to support, education, and research. It provides support to families from recovered persons, publishes informational literature and a newsletter, and maintains a list of practitioners experienced with the disease (see Additional Resources).

Tetanus

Tetanus, or lockjaw, is an acute, preventable, but often fatal disease caused by an exotoxin produced by the anaerobic spore-forming, Gram-positive bacillus *Clostridium tetani*. It is characterized by painful muscular rigidity primarily involving the masseter and neck muscles. There are four requirements for the development of tetanus: (1) presence of tetanus spores or vegetative forms of the bacillus, (2) injury to the tissues, (3) wound conditions that encourage multiplication of the organism, and (4) a susceptible host.

Tetanus spores are found in soil; dust; and the intestinal tracts of humans and animals, especially herbivorous animals. The organisms are more prevalent in rural areas but are readily carried to urban areas by the wind. The organisms are not invasive but enter the body by way of wounds, particularly a puncture wound, burn, or crushed area. They may enter through a minor, unnoticed break in the skin, such as a thorn or needle prick, bee sting, or scratch. In the newborn, infection may occur through the umbilical cord, usually in situations in which infants are delivered in severely contaminated surroundings or the mother is not adequately immunized. The disease has the greatest incidence in months when persons are more involved in outdoor activities.

Tetanus is a rare disease in Canada because of tetanus immunizations. However, serosurveys suggest that a significant number of Canadians have nonprotective levels of tetanus antitoxin. The low levels are due to increasing age, birth outside Canada, and absence of immunization records (Public Health Agency of Canada [PHAC], 2007).

Pathophysiology

When prevention efforts are not effective and conditions are favourable, the organisms proliferate and form potent exotoxins, one of which is tetanospasmin. Tetanospasmin affects the central nervous system to produce the clinical manifestations of the disease. The ideal conditions for the organisms' growth are devitalized tissues without access to air, such as wounds that have not been washed or kept clean and those that have crusted over, trapping pus beneath. The exotoxin appears to reach the central nervous system by way of either the neuron axons or the vascular system. The toxin becomes fixed on nerve cells of the anterior horn of the spinal cord and the brainstem. The toxin acts at the myoneural junction to produce muscular stiffness and lower the threshold for reflex excitability.

The incubation period for tetanus varies from 2 days to months and averages 8 days; most cases occur within 14 days. In neonates it is usually 5 to 14 days. Shorter incubation periods have been associated with more heavily contaminated wounds, more severe disease, and a worse prognosis (American Academy of Pediatrics [AAP], Committee on Infectious Diseases, & Pickering, 2009).

The manner of onset varies, but the initial symptoms are usually a progressive stiffness and tenderness of the muscles in the neck and jaw. Eventually all voluntary muscles are affected (Box 55-11). As the child recovers from the disease, the paroxysms become less frequent and gradually subside. Survival beyond 4 days usually indicates recovery, but complete recovery may require weeks.

Therapeutic Management

Preventive measures are based on the child's immune status and the nature of the injury. Specific prophylactic therapy after trauma is administration of tetanus toxoid (see Immunizations, Chapter 36, for age-specific recommendations).

The unprotected or inadequately immunized child who sustains a "tetanus-prone" wound (including wounds contaminated with dirt, feces, soil, and saliva; puncture wounds; avulsions; and wounds resulting from missiles, crushing,

BOX 55-11 Clinical Manifestations of Tetanus

Initial Symptoms

Progressive stiffness and tenderness of muscles in neck and jaw

Characteristic difficulty in opening the mouth (trismus)

Risus sardonicus (sardonic smile) caused by facial muscle spasm

Progressive Involvement

Opisthotonic positioning

Boardlike rigidity of abdominal and limb muscles

Difficulty swallowing

High sensitivity to external stimuli (slight noise, gentle touch, or bright light):

- Trigger paroxysmal muscular contractions that last seconds to minutes
- Contractions recur with increased frequency until almost continuous (sustained tetanic)

Laryngospasm and tetany of respiratory muscles:

- Accumulated secretions
- Respiratory arrest
- Atelectasis
- Pneumonia

Other Aspects

Mentation unaffected; patient alert

Pain and distress are reflected in:

- Rapid pulse
- Sweating
- Anxious expression

Fever usually absent or only mild

burns, and frostbite) should receive tetanus immunoglobulin (TIG). Concurrent administration of both TIG and tetanus toxoid at separate sites is recommended both to provide protection and to initiate the active immune process. Once the individual has received primary tetanus immunization, antitoxin (human) is believed to provide protection for at least 10 years and for a longer period after booster immunization (PHAC, 2007). Completion of active immunization is carried out according to the usual pattern. Antibiotic treatment with oral or intravenous metronidazole (Flagyl) (alternatively parenteral penicillin G) is important in the management of tetanus as an adjunct against vegetative forms of clostridia (AAP, Committee on Infectious Diseases, & Pickering, 2009).

Aggressive supportive care is necessary to treat tetanus in the acute phase. The acutely ill child is best treated in a critical care facility where close and constant observation and equipment for monitoring and respiratory support are readily available. A quiet environment is desirable to reduce the amount of stimuli on the central nervous system.

General supportive care is indicated, including maintaining an adequate airway and fluid and electrolyte balance, managing pain, and ensuring adequate caloric intake. Indwelling oral or nasogastric feedings may be required to maintain adequate fluid and caloric intake; continued laryngospasm may necessitate total parenteral nutrition or gastrostomy feeding. Severe or recurrent laryngospasm or excessive secretions may require advanced **airway management** such as endotracheal intubation.

TIG therapy to neutralize toxins is the most specific therapy for tetanus. Antibiotics are administered to control the proliferation of the vegetative forms of the organism at the site of infection. Local care of the wound by surgical debridement and cleansing helps reduce the numbers of proliferating organisms at the site of injury. The cleansing should be repeated several times during the first 48 hours, and deep, infected lacerations are usually exposed and debrided.

Diazepam is the medication of choice for seizure control and muscle relaxation (Arnon, 2007b), but lorazepam (Ativan) may be used in some cases. Other AEDs may be administered as well. Intrathecal baclofen, magnesium sulphate, dantrolene sodium, and midazolam may also be used in the management of tetanus. Patients with severe tetanus and those who do not respond to other muscle relaxants may require the administration of a neuromuscular blocking agent, such as rocuronium or vecuronium; intrathecal baclofen may be used as a muscle relaxant but only in the critical care unit, since it often induces apnea. Because of their paralytic effect on respiratory muscles, use of these medications requires mechanical ventilation with endotracheal intubation or tracheotomy and constant cardiopulmonary monitoring. Endotracheal tube insertion or tracheostomy should be performed before severe respiratory distress develops. Despite the absence of pain manifestation with these medications, it is important to administer adequate analgesia. The administration of corticosteroids has met with success in some cases.

Nursing Care Management

The care of the child with tetanus requires supportive management with particular attention to airway and breathing. Respiratory status needs to be carefully evaluated for any signs of distress, and appropriate emergency equipment is kept available at all times. The location, extent, and severity of muscle spasms are important nursing observations. Muscle relaxants, opioids, and sedatives that may be prescribed can also cause respiratory depression; the child must be assessed for excessive central nervous system depression. Attention to hydration and nutrition involves monitoring an intravenous infusion, monitoring nasogastric or gastrostomy feedings, and suctioning oropharyngeal secretions when indicated.

In caring for the child with tetanus during the acute phase, the nurse should make every effort to control or eliminate stimulation from sound, light, and touch. Although a darkened room is ideal, sufficient light is essential so that the child can be carefully observed; light appears to be less irritating than vibratory or auditory stimuli. The infant or child should be handled as little as possible and any sudden or loud noise eliminated to prevent seizures.

If a potent muscle relaxant such as vecuronium is used, the total paralysis makes oral communication impossible. The medication is not a sedative, however, and anxiety should be considered in children who are intubated. All of the child's needs must be anticipated and procedures carefully explained beforehand.

Because their mental status is clear, children are aware of what is happening to them and are often extremely anxious. They should not be left alone, and all efforts should be made to reduce anxiety, which can contribute to muscle spasms. Parents should be encouraged to stay with the child to offer security and support. They also need support, information, and reassurance from the nurse.

Botulism

Botulism is an acute flaccid paralysis caused by the preformed toxin produced by the anaerobic bacillus *Clostridium botulinum*. In classic, or foodborne, botulism the most common source of the toxin is a contaminated food source. In addition to foodborne botulism, other forms include wound botulism; infant botulism; and man-made botulism, usually a result of bioterrorism (Arnon, 2007a). In foodborne illness, central nervous system symptoms appear abruptly within a few hours or gradually over several days after ingestion of contaminated food and may not be preceded by acute digestive disturbance (Box 55-12).

Treatment consists of intravenous administration of botulism antitoxin and general supportive measures, primarily respiratory and nutritional. Toxins vary in protein-binding capacity. Some have a relatively short half-life and do not bind to tissues firmly; thus therapy is continued until paralysis abates. Other toxins appear to bind irreversibly to nerve endings and are not amenable to neutralization.

Infant Botulism

Infant botulism, unlike the disease in older persons, is caused by ingestion of spores or vegetative cells of *C. botulinum* and the subsequent release of the toxin from organisms colonizing the gastrointestinal tract. *C. botulinum* types A and B are the most common causative strains of infant botulism. This form of botulism has become more prevalent than any other form.

BOX 55-12 Clinical Manifestations of Botulism

General Signs
Weakness
Dizziness
Headache
Difficulty talking and speaking

Diplopia
Vomiting
Progressive, life-threatening respiratory paralysis

Infant Botulism*
Constipation (a common symptom)
Generalized weakness
Decrease in spontaneous movements
Diminished or absent deep tendon reflexes
Loss of head control
Difficulty feeding
Weak cry
Reduced gag reflex
Progressive respiratory paralysis

*Most commonly diagnosed as a "rule out sepsis" in the acute phase because of clinical presentation.

Many cases of infant botulism occur in breastfed infants who are being introduced to nonhuman milk substances (AAP, Committee on Infectious Diseases, & Pickering, 2009). There appears to be no common food or medication source of the organisms; however, the *C. botulinum* organisms have been found in honey. Botulism may occur in infants as young as 1 week of age up to 12 months of age with peak incidence between 2 and 4 months of age.

The severity of the disease varies widely, from mild constipation to progressive sequential loss of neurological function and respiratory failure (see Box 55-12). The affected infant is usually well before the onset of symptoms. Constipation is a common presenting symptom, and almost all infants exhibit generalized weakness and a decrease in spontaneous movements. Deep tendon reflexes are usually diminished or absent. Cranial nerve deficits are common, as evidenced by loss of head control, difficulty in feeding, weak cry, and reduced gag reflex. SMA type 1 and metabolic disorders are often mistaken for infant botulism in the initial diagnostic phase because of the similarities in clinical manifestations of hypotonia, lethargy, and poor feeding (Francisco & Arnon, 2007). Presenting clinical signs also often mimic those of sepsis in young infants. Botulism toxin exerts its effect by inhibiting the release of acetylcholine at the myoneural junction, thereby impairing motor activity of muscles innervated by affected nerves.

Diagnosis is made on the basis of the clinical history, physical examination, and laboratory detection of the organism in the patient's stool and, less commonly, blood. However, isolation of the organism may take several days; suspicion of botulism by clinical presentation should require emergent treatment (Arnon, 2007a). EMG may be helpful in establishing the diagnosis; however, results may be normal early in the course of the illness.

Treatment consists of immediate administration of botulism immune globulin intravenously without waiting for laboratory diagnosis. In Canada, the botulism antitoxin and immune globulin are not approved for sale and are only available via Health Canada's Special Access Programme (SAP). There are four products available: (1) botulism antitoxin type AB and type E, accessed from the Butantan Institute in Brazil, (2) Novartis trivalent types ABE, (3) botulism immune globulin intravenous (human) (BIG-IV) (BabyBIG®) for pediatric patients under the age of 1 year, and (4) NP-018 (heptavalent) types A to G from Cangene Corporation (PHAC, 2010). Early administration of BIG-IV neutralizes the toxin and stops the progression of the disease. The human-derived botulism antitoxin (BIG-IV) has been evaluated and is now available nationwide for use only in infant botulism. Infants treated with BIG-IV experienced a mean length of hospitalization decrease from 5.7 to 2.6 weeks and spent less time in critical care, had decreased mean duration of mechanical ventilation, and had decreased mean duration of tube or intravenous feeding. In addition, the infants did not experience any adverse events related to BIG-IV. Most infants received BIG-IV treatment within 3 to 18 days of hospitalization for botulism (Arnon et al., 2006).

Approximately 50% of affected infants will require intubation and mechanical ventilation; thus respiratory support is crucial, as is nutritional support, since the infant is unable to feed. Trivalent equine botulinum antitoxin and bivalent antitoxin, used in adults and older children, is not administered to infants. Antibiotic therapy is not part of the management because the botulinum toxin is an intracellular molecule and antibiotics would not be effective; aminoglycosides in particular should not be administered because they may potentiate the blocking effects of the neurotoxin (Arnon, 2007a).

The prognosis is generally good if the patient is adequately treated, although recovery may be slow, requiring a few weeks after severe illness. The average length of stay for infant botulism is 44 days, and the fatality rate is reported to be less than 2%. Untreated patients may require a longer hospitalization.

NURSING ALERT Although the precise source of *C. botulinum* spores has not been identified as originating from honey in many cases of infant botulism, it is still recommended that honey not be given to infants less than 12 months of age because the spores have been found in honey (CDC, 2008).

Nursing Care Management

Nursing responsibilities include observing for and reporting signs of neuromuscular weakness or impairment and providing intensive nursing care when the infant is hospitalized (see Chapter 27). Parental support and reassurance are important. Most infants recover when the disorder is recognized and therapy is implemented. Parents should be aware that, during recovery, patients tire easily when muscular action is sustained. This has important implications for timing the resumption of feedings because of the risk of aspiration. Parents should also be advised that normal bowel activity may not return for several weeks; therefore a stool softener can be beneficial.

Spinal Cord Injuries

SCIs with major neurological involvement traditionally have not been a common cause of physical disability in children. However, a sufficient number of children with these injuries are admitted to major medical centres, and because of the increased survival rate as a result of improved management, nurses are often involved in the care and rehabilitation of children with SCI. Children rarely have spinal injuries and spinal cord injuries. Children who are less than 15 years old account for fewer than 10% of patients who have SCIs (Reilly, 2007).

Mechanisms of Injury

The most common cause of serious spinal cord damage in children is trauma involving motor vehicle crashes (MVCs) (including automobile–bicycle, all-terrain vehicles, and snowmobiles), sports injuries (especially from diving, trampoline activities, gymnastics, and football), birth trauma, and nonaccidental trauma. The increased use of recreational activities involving motorized vehicles such as jet water skis, all-terrain vehicles, and motorcycles has also increased the incidence of SCIs in children. Congenital defects of the spine such as myelomeningocele may in some cases produce the effects of SCI.

Transverse myelitis (inflammation of the spinal cord) has also been reported to develop from inadvertent intra-arterial administration of long-acting penicillin injected into the buttocks. Damage can be extensive enough to result in paraplegia or even lower limb amputation.

In MVCs most SCIs in children are a result of indirect trauma caused by sudden hyperflexion or hyperextension of the neck, often combined with a rotational force. Trauma to the spinal cord without evidence of vertebral fracture or dislocation (SCIWORA) is particularly likely to occur in an MVC when proper safety restraints are not used. An unrestrained child becomes a projectile during sudden deceleration and is subject to injury from contact with a variety of objects inside and outside the vehicle. Individuals who use only a lap seat belt restraint are at greater risk of SCI than those who use a combination lap and shoulder restraint. High cervical spine injuries have been reported in children younger than 2 years of age who are improperly restrained in forward-facing car seats. Infants who are improperly restrained in an infant car seat may experience cervical trauma in a car crash. Small children may also be severely injured by deploying front seat air bags.

Falling from heights occurs less often in children than in adults, but vertebral compression from blows to the head or buttocks can occur in water sports (diving and surfing), falls from horses, or other athletic activities. Birth injuries may occur in breech deliveries from traction force on the spinal cord during delivery of the head and shoulders. When shaken, infants commonly sustain cervical cord damage, as well as subdural hematoma and retinal hemorrhage; cognitive impairment and death may occur subsequent to the traumatic event. Infants have weak neck muscles, and during vigorous shaking their large and heavy heads rapidly wobble back and forth. A significant number of adolescents receive SCIs secondary to gunshot wounds, stabbings, or other violent inflicted injury.

The injury sustained can affect any of the spinal nerves, and the higher the injury, the more extensive the damage. The child can be left with complete or partial paralysis of the lower extremities (*paraplegia*) or with damage at a higher level and without functional use of any of the four extremities (*tetraplegia*). A high cervical cord injury that affects the phrenic nerve paralyzes the diaphragm and leaves the child dependent on mechanical ventilation.

A mild but equally frightening form of cord trauma is *spinal cord compression*, a temporary neural dysfunction without visible damage to the cord. Complete quadriplegia can result but initially may not be differentiated from serious cord injury.

Therapeutic Management

The management of the child with SCI has changed dramatically in the past two decades as a result of improved technology, surgical procedures, and research into the complexity of the spinal cord and its neurological components. Initial care begins at the scene of the accident; education and training of first responder personnel in spinal immobilization, stabilization, and transfer techniques to prevent or reduce the severity of injury are critically important. Because of the complexity of these injuries, it is usually recommended that those with injuries be transported to a spinal injury centre for care by specially trained health care personnel as soon as possible after the injury for appropriate diagnostic evaluation and intervention.

A number of special pediatric immobilization devices are now available that are physiologically appropriate for children's unique characteristics. A large head (proportionately), weak neck musculature, and weak tracheal cartilage predispose small children to airway compromise if placed supine; hence a spinal board with a built-in head drop may serve to protect the child's spine and neck and provide better airway management than the traditional flat board (DeBoer & Seaver, 2004).

Treatment with functional electrical stimulation (an implantable electrical stimulator with leads attached to the paralyzed muscles or nerves) has allowed children with certain SCIs greater mobility and functional use of paralyzed muscles to sit, stand, and walk with the aid of crutches, a walker, or other orthoses. Administration of pharmacological agents such as clonidine hydrochloride may improve ambulation in patients with partial SCI, and exercise therapy through interactive locomotor training has been beneficial in helping some individuals with SCI regain ambulatory function.

In recent years, patients with acute incomplete SCI have benefited from body weight–supported treadmill training, which enhances ambulation and gait training (Barker, 2005). This treatment has enabled some wheelchair-bound SCI patients to walk for short distances.

SCI management guidelines and standards of care have been developed on the basis of research evidence and can be found through the Spinal Cord Injury Rehabilitation Evidence Project (2010). The Rick Hansen Foundation and Accreditation Canada are developing Canadian standards for SCI services. This foundation provides research and resources as well information. The Canadian Paraplegic Association also offers various useful services, such as assistive devices and assistive living (see Additional Resources section at the end of this chapter).

Nursing Care Management

The nursing care of the paraplegic or quadriplegic child is complex and challenging. A multidisciplinary SCI team is equipped to manage the acute phase of the injury, and some members, including the nurse, may follow the patient to eventual recovery. Nursing management is concerned with ensuring adequate initial stabilization of the entire spinal column with a rigid cervical collar with supportive blocks on a rigid backboard. During the acute phase of the injury it is imperative that airway patency be maintained and respiratory function monitored. It is important to evaluate the extent of the neurological damage early to establish a baseline for neurological functioning; continual assessment of function should occur to prevent further deterioration of neurological status as a result of spinal cord edema. The American Spinal Injury Association Impairment Scale may be used to assess neurological function on a routine basis during the patient's recovery (Barker & Saulino, 2002). Once the patient is admitted, further evaluation of the patient's abilities to perform ADLs can be made with the Functional Independence Measure scale; this scale measures the patient's abilities and need for assistance during recovery (Barker & Saulino, 2002).

In any situation in which SCI is suspected or a possibility, the child should be calmed, reassured, and told not to move; no one should be allowed to move the child unless he or she is able to stabilize the entire spine. A rigid cervical collar is used to immobilize the cervical spine, and the child is placed supine on a rigid immobilization board. Infants and small children may be removed in their car seats; no attempt should be made to take them out of the seat.

The nursing care of the child with an SCI is, in most respects, the same as that of any immobilized child (see The Immobilized Child, Chapter 54). Additional aspects of care that should be addressed on an individual basis include hypercalcemia in adolescent males, deep vein thrombosis, latex sensitization, and sleep-disordered breathing (Vogel et al., 2004).

Respiratory care often focuses on maintaining an adequate airway and effective ventilation. The child with a high-level cervical injury (C3 and above) requires continuous ventilatory assistance. In most instances a tracheostomy is the method of choice for greater ease in clearing secretions and for less trauma to tissues during long-term ventilatory dependence. In some children breathing pacemaker devices (phrenic nerve stimulators) are implanted to stimulate the phrenic nerve and produce diaphragmatic contractions and lung expansion without assisted ventilation. In the child who does not require mechanical ventilation, special attention to clearance of secretions is vital because of decreased pulmonary function. In addition to chest physiotherapy, the child may require a cough-assist device to clear secretions effectively (see Duchenne [Pseudohypertrophic] Muscular Dystrophy: Therapeutic Management).

Temperature is often poorly regulated in children with SCI; thus, body temperature must be monitored closely for fluctuations. Response to environmental temperature changes may be slow or absent, and the ability to dissipate heat through the process of shivering may be compromised.

Children with SCI have unique needs in relation to skin care. Because of decreased sensation and impaired mobility, they depend on others to assess and assist in the management of intact skin. Skin care practices are the same as those for any child who is immobilized. A skin score scale such as the Braden Q Scale should be used to objectively evaluate risks for skin breakdown and skin conditions (Curley et al., 2003). An alternating-pressure mattress or other pressure relief or reduction device should be kept underneath the child, and the skin needs to be thoroughly inspected at least once a day (or more often if there is increased risk) for signs of pressure and breakdown, especially over bony prominences.

Bowel and bladder function is often affected in the child with SCI. CIC may be required to regularly empty the neurogenic bladder and prevent urinary tract infections. A regular bowel management program is tailored to the child's needs.

All adaptive devices help children increase their mobility, function, and endurance. The child with some lower extremity function progresses to parallel bars and then to a walker; the child with quadriplegia learns to use a wheelchair—among the most valuable aids available to the child with an SCI (Fig. 55-8). The wheelchair should be selected carefully in relation to where it will be used, the architectural barriers, and the child's functional capacity. For children with severe upper extremity paralysis, a variety of motorized wheelchairs are used; however, the more complex they are, the greater their cost, weight, and tendency to break down. Wheelchair tolerance is gained over time and is accompanied by measures to prevent orthostatic hypotension and pressure ulcers.

A variety of orthoses and other appliances can be adapted for use by many children. The primary purpose of lower

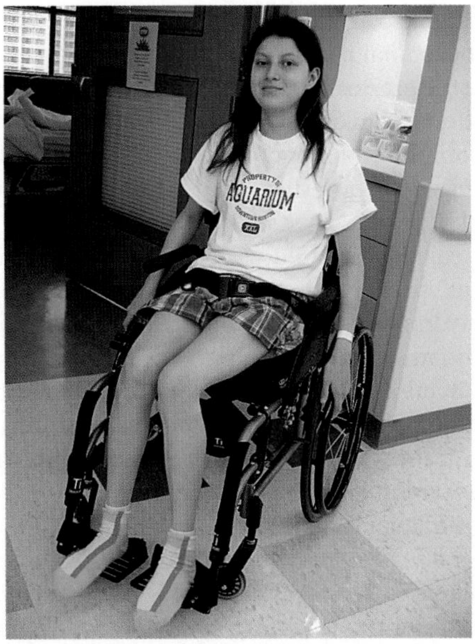

Fig. 55-8 A wheelchair allows adolescent mobility and independence. *(Courtesy Texas Children's Hospital, Houston.)*

extremity bracing in the child with an SCI is for ambulation, although correction of deformities may be attempted.

During the recovery and rehabilitation phase, patients with SCI must be carefully monitored for complications of immobility such as deep vein thrombosis and pulmonary embolus.

The child and family with SCI need to be prepared for the eventual discharge from the acute care facility to a rehabilitation centre. The major aims of physical rehabilitation are to prepare the child and family to achieve normalization and resume life at home and in the community. Additional goals of rehabilitation in children with SCI are to promote independence in mobility and self-care skills, academic achievement, independent living, and employment.

The nurse is a crucial member of the health care team in helping the family cope with the magnitude of the injury and disability, understand the extent of the disability, verbalize expected outcomes, and move toward eventual rehabilitation and normalization within the child's capabilities. The goals of rehabilitation include preparing the child and family to live at home and function as independently as possible.

Key Points

- Clinical manifestations of CP include delayed gross motor development; abnormal motor performance; alterations of muscle tone; abnormal postures; reflex abnormalities; and associated disabilities such as cognitive impairment, seizures, and sensory impairment.
- Therapy for CP takes into account the nature of the physical disability, defects associated with the disorder, and interpersonal and social influences encountered by the affected child.
- Care of the infant and child with myelomeningocele is directed toward protecting the meningeal sac, preventing infection and skin breakdown, observing for signs of urological and bowel complications, and planning appropriate interventions to optimize the child's development.
- SMA is characterized by progressive weakness and wasting of skeletal muscles caused by degeneration of anterior horn cells of the spinal cord.
- MDs are the greatest and most important cause of muscular dysfunction of childhood.
- Major complications of DMD include joint contractures, disuse atrophy, obesity, and respiratory and cardiac problems.
- Nursing care of the child with GBS consists of monitoring vital signs, providing respiratory support and physiotherapy, providing reassurance, and providing support to the child and family.
- Tetanus occurs when tetanus spores or vegetative bacilli enter a wound and multiply in a susceptible host.
- Infant botulism results from the release of toxins from *C. botulinum* colonizing the gastrointestinal tract.
- Therapeutic management of SCI is directed toward immobilizing the entire spinal column at the scene of the traumatic event, safely transporting the patient by health care personnel trained to transport possible spinal trauma victims, evaluating neurological damage, preventing further neurological damage, and implementing an aggressive rehabilitation program designed to help achieve independence and movement.

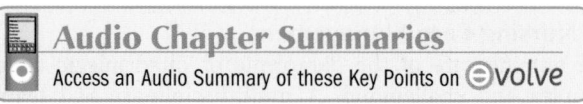

Audio Chapter Summaries
Access an Audio Summary of these Key Points on evolve

References

Albright, A. L., et al. (2003). Long-term intrathecal baclofen therapy for severe spasticity of cerebral origin. *Journal of Neurosurgery, 98*(2), 291–295.

American Academy of Pediatrics, Committee of Infectious Diseases, & Pickering, L. (Ed.) (2009). *Red book: Report of the committee on infectious diseases* (28th ed.). Elk Grove Village, Ill: Author.

Angelini, C. (2007). The role of corticosteroids in muscular dystrophy: A critical appraisal. *Muscle Nerve, 36*(4), 424–435. doi:10.1002/mus.20812

Arnon, S. S. (2007a). Anaerobic bacterial infections: Botulism (*Clostridium botulinum*). In R. M. Kliegman, et al. (Eds.), *Nelson textbook of pediatrics* (18th ed.). Philadelphia: Saunders.

Arnon, S. S. (2007b). Tetanus (*Clostridium tetani*). In R. M. Kliegman, et al. (Eds.), *Nelson textbook of pediatrics* (18th ed.). Philadelphia: Saunders.

Arnon, S. S., et al. (2006). Human botulism immune globulin for the treatment of infant botulism. *New England Journal of Medicine, 354*(5), 462–471.

Ashwal, S., et al. (2004). Practice parameter: Diagnostic assessment of the child with cerebral palsy: Report of the Quality Standards Subcommittee of the American Academy of Neurology and the Practice Committee of the Child Neurology Society. *Neurology, 62*(6), 851–863.

Bach, J. R. (2007). Medical considerations of long-term survival of Werdnig-Hoffmann disease. *American Journal of Physical Medicine & Rehabilitation, 86*(5), 349–355. doi:10.1097/PHM.0b013e31804b1d66

Barker, E. (2005). SCI patients take a big step forward. *RN, 68*(7), 30–34.

Barker, E., & Saulino, M. F. (2002). Special report: First-ever guidelines for spinal cord injuries. *RN, 65*(10), 32–37.

Berker, A. N., & Yalçin, M. S. (2008). Cerebral palsy: Orthopedic aspects and rehabilitation. *Pediatric Clinics of North America, 55*(5), 1209–1225. doi:10.1016/j.pcl.2008.07.011

Beroud, C., et al. (2003). Prenatal diagnosis of spinal muscular atrophy by genetic analysis of circulating fetal cells. *Lancet, 361*(9362), 1013–1014.

Birnkrant, D. J. (2002). The assessment and management of the respiratory complications of pediatric neuromuscular diseases. *Clinical Pediatrics, 41*(5), 301–308.

Brown, J. P. (2001). Orthopaedic care of children with spina bifida: You've come a long way, baby! *Orthopaedic Nursing, 20*(4), 51–58.

Bush, A., et al. (2005). Respiratory management of the infant with type 1 spinal muscular atrophy. *Archive of Diseases in Childhood, 90*(7), 709–711. doi:10.1136/adc.2004.065961

Bushby, K., et al., for the DMD Care Considerations Working Group. (2010a). Diagnosis and management of Duchenne muscular dystrophy, part 1: Diagnosis, and pharmacological and psychosocial management. *Lancet Neurology, 9*, 77–93.

Bushby, K., et al., for the DMD Care Considerations Working Group. (2010b). Diagnosis and management of Duchenne muscular dystrophy, part 2: Implementation of multidisciplinary care. *Lancet Neurology, 9*, 177–189.

Centers for Disease Control and Prevention. (2004). Spina bifida and anencephaly before and after folic acid mandate—United States, 1995–1996 and 1999–2000. *MMWR: Morbidity & Mortality Weekly Report, 53*(17), 362–365.

Centers for Disease Control and Prevention. (2008). *Botulism.* Retrieved from http://www.cdc.gov/nczved/dfbmd/disease_listing/botulism_gi.html.

Chakkalakal, J. V., et al. (2005). Molecular, cellular, and pharmacological therapies for Duchenne/Becker muscular dystrophies. *FASEB Journal, 19*(8), 880–891. doi:10.1096/fj.04-1956rev

Curley, M. A. Q., et al. (2003). Predicting pressure ulcer risk in pediatric patients: The Braden Q Scale. *Nursing Research, 52*(1), 22–33.

Dai, A. I., Wasay, M., & Awan, S. (2008). Botulinum toxin type A with oral baclofen versus oral tizanidine: A randomized pilot comparison in patients with cerebral palsy and equinus foot deformity. *Journal of Child Neurology, 23*(12), 1464–1466. doi:10.1177/0883073808319074

DeBoer, S. L., & Seaver, M. (2004). Pediatric spinal immobilization: C-spines, car seats, and color-coded collars. *Journal of Emergency Nursing, 30*(5), 481–484.

De Wals, P., et al. (2007). Reduction in neural-tube defects after folic acid fortification in Canada. *New England Journal of Medicine, 357*(2). 135–142. doi:10.1056/NEJMoa067103

Doolin, E. (2006). Bowel management for patients with myelodysplasia. *Surgery Clinics of North America, 86*(2), 505–514. doi:10.1016/j.suc.2005.12.009

Eiwegger, T., et al. (2006). Early exposure to latex products mediates latex sensitization in spina bifida but not in other diseases with comparable latex exposure rates. *Clinical & Experimental Allergy, 36*(10), 1242–1246. doi:10.1111/j.1365-2222.2006.02564.x

Francisco, A. M., & Arnon, S. S. (2007). Clinical mimics of infant botulism. *Pediatrics, 119*(4), 826–828.

Gibson, C. S., et al. (2003). Antenatal causes of cerebral palsy: Associations between inherited thrombophilias, viral and bacterial infection, and inherited susceptibility to infection. *Obstetrical & Gynecological Survey, 58*(3), 209–220.

Golomb, M. R., et al. (2007). Association of cerebral palsy with other disabilities in children with perinatal arterial ischemic stroke. *Pediatric Neurology, 37*(4), 245–249.

Gray, M., & Moore, K. N. (2009). *Urologic disorders: Adult and pediatric care.* St. Louis: Mosby.

Green, L., Greenberg, G. M., & Hurwitz, E. (2003). Primary care of children with cerebral palsy. *Clinics in Family Practice, 5*(2), 1–21.

Grether, J. K., et al. (2003). Intrauterine exposure to infection and risk of cerebral palsy in very preterm infants. *Archives of Pediatric & Adolescent Medicine, 157*(1), 26–32.

Hack, M., & Costello, D. W. (2008). Trends in the rates of cerebral palsy associated with neonatal intensive care of preterm children. *Clinical Obstetrics & Gynecology, 51*(4), 763–774.

Harel, M., & Schoenfeld, Y. (2005). Intravenous immunoglobulin and Guillain-Barré syndrome, *Clinical Reviews in Allergy & Immunology, 29*(3), 281–287.

Hirtz, D., et al. (2007). How common are the "common" neurologic disorders? *Neurology, 68*, 326–337.

Hughes, R. A., & Cornblath, D. R. (2005). Guillain-Barré syndrome. *Lancet, 366*(9497), 1653–1666. doi:10.1016/j.vaccine.2007.03.053

Hughes, R. A., et al. (2006). Intravenous immunoglobulin for Guillain-Barré syndrome, *Cochrane Library (1)*, CD002063.

Hurtekant, K. M., & Spatz, D. L. (2007). Special considerations for breastfeeding the infant with spina bifida. *Journal of Perinatal & Neonatal Nursing, 21*(1), 69–75.

Iannaccone, S. T. (1998). Spinal muscular atrophy. *Seminars in Neurology, 18*(1), 19–26.

Iannaccone, S. T., & Burghes, A. (2002). Spinal muscular atrophies. *Advances in Neurology, 88*, 83–98.

Jacobs, J. M. (2001). Management options for the child with spastic cerebral palsy. *Orthopaedic Nursing, 20*(3), 53–59.

Kaufman, B. A. (2004). Neural tube defects. *Pediatric Clinics of North America, 51*(2), 389–419.

Kellett, P. B. (1997). Latex allergy: A review. *Journal of Emergency Nursing, 23*(1), 27–36.

Kessler, T. M., et al. (2006). Early proactive management improves upper urinary tract function and reduces the need for surgery in patients with myelomeningocele. *Neurourology & Urodynamics, 25*(7), 758–762. doi:10.1002/nau.20304

Kimata, H. (2004). Latex allergy in infants younger than 1 year. *Clinical & Experimental Allergy, 34*(12), 1910–1915.

Kinsman, S. L., & Johnston, M. V. (2007). Congenital anomalies of the central nervous system. In R. M. Kliegman, R. E. Behrman, H. B. Jenson, et al., (Eds). *Nelson textbook of pediatrics* (18th ed.). Philadephia: Saunders.

Krageloh-Mann, I., & Cans, C. (2009). Cerebral palsy update. *Brain Development, 31*(7), 537–544.

Kravitz, R. M. (2009). Airway clearance in Duchenne muscular dystrophy. *Pediatrics, 123*(Suppl 4), S231–S235.

Krigger, K. W. (2006). Cerebral palsy: An overview. *American Family Physician, 73*(1), 91–100, 101–102.

Lazzaretti, C. C., & Pearson, C. (2010). Myelodysplasia. In P. J. Allen, J. A. Vessey, & N. A. Schapiro (Eds.), *Primary care of the child with a chronic condition* (5th ed.). St. Louis: Mosby.

Lukban, M. B., Rosales, R. L., & Dressler, D. (2009). Effectiveness of botulinum toxin A for upper and lower limb spasticity in children with cerebral palsy: A summary of evidence. *Journal of Neural Transmission, 116*(3), 319–331.

Lunn, M. R., & Wang, C. H. (2008). Spinal muscular atrophy. *Lancet, 371*(9630), 2120–2133.

Manzur, A. Y., et al. (2008). Glucocorticoid corticosteroids for Duchenne muscular dystrophy. *Cochrane Database Systematic Review, 23*(1), CD003725.

McKearnan, K. A., et al. (2004). Pain in children with cerebral palsy: A review. *Journal of Neuroscience Nursing, 36*(5), 252–259.

McKim, D. A., et al., for the Canadian Thoracic Society Home Mechanical Ventilation Committee. (2011). Home mechanical ventilation: A Canadian Thoracic Society clinical practice guideline. *Canadian Respiratory Journal, 18*(4), 197–215.

Menticoglou, S. M. (2007). How often do perinatal events at full term cause cerebral palsy? *Journal of Obstetrics and Gynecology Canada, 30*(5), 396–403.

Metules, T. (2002). Duchenne muscular dystrophy. *RN, 65*(10), 39–47.

Miske, L. J., et al. (2004). Use of the mechanical in-exsufflator in pediatric patients with neuromuscular disease and impaired cough. *Chest, 125*(4), 1406–1412.

Moxley, R. T., et al. (2005). Practice parameter: Corticosteroid treatment of Duchenne dystrophy. *Neurology, 64*(1), 13–20. doi:10.1212/01.WNL.0000148485.00049.B7

Murphy, K. P., Molnar, G. E., & Lankasky, K. (2000). Employment and social issues in adults with cerebral palsy. *Archives of Physical & Medical Rehabilitation, 81*, 807–811.

Muscular Dystrophy Canada. (2012). *The diagnosis of Duchenne muscular dystrophy: A guide for families.* Retrieved from http://www.muscle.ca/moveit/moveit-may2012/DMDstandardsofcare-E_final_lowres.pdf.

Nehring, W. M. (2010). Cerebral palsy. In P. L. Jackson, J. A. Vessey, & N. A. Schapiro (Eds.), *Primary care of the child with a chronic illness* (5th ed.). St. Louis: Mosby.

Newswanger, D. I., & Warren, C. R. (2004). Guillain-Barré syndrome. *American Family Physician, 69*(10), 2405–2410.

Public Health Agency of Canada. (2007). *Canadian immunization guide* (7th ed.). Retrieved from http://www.phac-aspc.gc.ca/publicat/cig-gci/p04-tet-eng.php.

Public Health Agency of Canada. (2010). *Canada's foodborne illness outbreak response protocol (FIORP) 2010: To guide a multijurisdictional approach.* Retrieved from http://www.phac-aspc.gc.ca/zoono/fiorp-pritioa/ann1-9-eng.php.

Reilly, C. (2007). Pediatric spine trauma. *Journal of Bone and Joint Surgery (American), 89*(Suppl 1), 98–107. doi:10.2106/JBJS.F.00244

Rogers, B. (2004). Feeding method and health outcomes of children with cerebral palsy. *Journal of Pediatrics, 145*(2 Suppl), S28–S32.

Roscigno, C. I. (2002). Addressing spasticity-related pain in children with spastic cerebral palsy. *Journal of Neuroscience Nursing, 34*(3), 123–131.

Rosenbaum, P., et al. (2007). A report: The definition and classification of cerebral palsy, April 2006. *Developmental Medicine & Child Neurology, 49*(S109), 1–44.

Rowe, D. E., & Jadhav, A. L. (2008). Care of the adolescent with spina bifida. *Pediatric Clinics of North America, 55*(6), 1359–1374.

Russman, B. S., et al. (1992). Spinal muscular atrophy: New thoughts on the pathogenesis and classification schema. *Journal of Child Neurology, 7*(4), 347–353.

Samaniego, I. A. (2003). A sore spot in pediatrics: Risk factors for pressure ulcers. *Pediatric Nursing, 29*(4), 278.

Sarnat, H. B. (2007). Neuromuscular disorders. In R. M. Kliegman, et al. (Eds.), *Nelson textbook of pediatrics* (18th ed.). Philadelphia: Saunders.

Shaer, C. M., Chescheir, N., & Schulkin, J. (2007). Myelomeningocele: A review of the epidemiology, genetics, risk factors for conception, prenatal diagnosis, and prognosis for affected individuals. *Obstetric & Gynecological Survey, 62*(7), 471–479. doi:10.1097/01.ogx.0000268628.82123.90

Simonds, A. K. (2006). Recent advances in respiratory care for neuromuscular disease. *Chest, 130*(6), 1879–1886. doi:10.1378/chest.130.6.1879

Snodgrass, W. T., & Adams, R. (2004). Initial urologic management of myelomeningocele. *Urology Clinics of North America, 31*(3), 427–434, viii.

Spinal Cord Injury Rehabilitation Evidence Project. (2010). *Evidence.* Retrieved from http://www.scireproject.com/rehabilitation-evidence.

Statistics Canada. (2003). *Pregnancy outcomes, 2003.* Retrieved from http://www.statcan.gc.ca/start-debut-eng.html.

Tarcan, T., et al. (2006). The timing of primary neurosurgical repair significantly affects neurogenic bladder prognosis in children with myelomeningocele. *Journal of Urology, 176*(3), 1161–1165. doi:10.1016/j.juro.2006.04.042

Thompson, G. H., & Berenson, F. R. (2001). Other neuromuscular disorders. In R. T. Morrissy & S. L. Weinstein (Eds.), *Lovell and Winter's pediatric orthopaedics* (5th ed.). Philadelphia: Lippincott Williams & Wilkins.

Tsai, C. P., et al. (2007). Pharmacoeconomics of therapy for Guillain-Barré syndrome: plasma exchange and intravenous immunoglobulin. *Journal of Clinical Neuroscience, 14*(7), 625–629.

Vogel, L. C., et al. (2004). Unique issues in pediatric spinal cord injury. *Orthopaedic Nursing, 23*(5), 300–308.

Volpe, J. J. (2008). *Neurology of the newborn* (5th ed.). Philadelphia: Saunders.

Wu, Y. W., et al. (2003). Chorioamnionitis and cerebral palsy in term and near-term infants. *Journal of the American Medical Association, 290*(20), 2677–2684.

Yeargin-Allsopp, M., et al. (2008). Prevalence of cerebral palsy in 8-year-old children in three areas of the United States in 2002: A multisite collaboration. *Pediatrics, 121,* 547–554.

Young, H. K., et al. (2007). Outcome of noninvasive ventilation in children with neuromuscular disease. *Neurology, 68*(3), 198–201. doi:10.1212/01.wnl.0000251299.54608.13

Additional Resources

Association for the Neurologically Disabled of Canada: http://www.and.ca/
Canadian Cerebral Palsy Sports Association: http://www.ccpsa.ca/en/default.aspx
Canadian Paediatric Society: http://www.cps.ca/english/index.htm
Canadian Paraplegic Association: https://www.spinalcordinjurycanada.ca/
Cerebral Palsy Support Foundation of Canada: http://www.cpsc.ca/
Families of SMA Canada: http://www.curesma.ca/
GBS/CIDP Foundation of Canada: http://www.gbs-cidp.org/guillain-barre-syndrome-foundation-of-canada-inc/
Health Canada: http://www.hc-sc.gc.ca/index-eng.php/
Motherisk: http://www.motherisk.org
Muscular Dystrophy Canada: http://www.muscle.ca
Rick Hansen Foundation: http://www.rickhansen.com/
Spina Bifida and Hydrocephalus Association Canada: http://www.sbhac.ca/beta/
Spina Bifida and Hydrocephalus Association Canada—List of latex products and alternative products: http://www.sbhac.ca/pdf/Latex_Allergies.pdf

Appendix A

Relationship of Drugs to Breast Milk and Effect on Infant

The drugs listed in this appendix have been categorized by their major use. The ratings given are those listed by Hale (2011). This rating scale labels drugs that transfer into human milk. The ratings are described as follows:

L1 Safest
L2 Safer
L3 Moderately safe
L4 Possibly hazardous
L5 Contraindicated (Not rated)

A comprehensive database (LactMed) is available at http://toxnet.nlm.nih.gov/cgi-bin/sis/htmlgen?LACT.

DRUG	EXCRETED IN MILK	% ADULT DOSE IN MILK	HALE RATING	COMMENTS
Analgesics and Antiinflammatory Drugs (Non-Narcotic)				
Acetaminophen (Abenol, Atasol, Tylenol)	Yes	0.04–1.85	L1	Drug found in milk; drug and metabolite found in infant's urine
Aspirin (Entrophen, Novasen)	Yes	0.5–21	L3	Metabolized in liver
Ibuprofen (Advil, Motrin)	Yes	<0.8	L1	Metabolites are inert; food slows absorption
Indomethacin (Indocid)	Yes	0.07–0.98	L3	Food delays absorption
Ketorolac tromethamine (Toradol)	Yes	0.16–0.4	L2	Food decreases rate but not amount of absorption
Mefenamic acid (Ponstan)	Yes	0.036–0.8	NR	Infant able to excrete via urine
Nalbuphine	Yes	<1	L3	Has active metabolites
Naproxen (Anaprox, Naprosyn)	Yes	0.26–1.1	L3 L4 for chronic use	Food delays absorption
Propoxyphene (Darvon)	Yes	Unknown	L2	Metabolized in liver
Antiinfectives (May Change Intestinal Flora of Infant and Sensitize for Later Allergic Reaction)				
Acyclovir (Zovirax)	Yes	5.6 ± 4.4	L2	Minimal absorption through skin
Amoxicillin	Yes	0.7	L1	Dose-dependent oral availability
Ampicillin	Yes	0.05–0.4	L1	In neonates, up to 12% plasma protein bound; oral availability increases
Carbenicillin (Pyopen, Geopen)	Yes	0.001	L1	Drug is given to neonate; not well absorbed from GI tract
Cefazolin (Ancef)	Yes	0.075	L1	Detected in milk if given intravenously
Cephalexin (Keflex)	Yes	0.85 ± 0.35	L1	Completely gone by 8 hr; absorption less in first few months
Cephalothin	Yes	0.4	L2	Higher volume of distribution in infant
Chloramphenicol (Chloromycetin)	Yes	1.3–7.4	L4	Possible idiosyncratic bone marrow depression
Demeclocycline (Declomycin)	Yes	Unknown	NR	Drug remains in milk 3 days after dose. Drug is given to infants
Erythromycin	Yes	0.1–2.1	L1	Possible jaundice if infant under 1 mo of age
Gentamicin	Yes	Unknown	L2	Appreciable GI absorption in neonate
Isoniazid (Isotamine)	Yes	2.3	L3	Not detected in infant's blood but in urine
Kanamycin	Yes	0.95	L2	Serum half-life in infant is inversely related to age
Metronidazole (Flagyl)	Yes	0.13–36	L2	CPS says to discard milk for 12 to 24 hr if mother takes a high dose*
Nitrofurantoin (Macrodantin)	Yes	0.6	L2	Caution needed in infants with G6PD deficiency
Novobiocin (Albamycin, Cathomycin)	Yes	0.15	NR	Can be given to infant directly

*Canadian Pediatric Society (2006). Maternal infectious diseases, antimicrobial therapy or immunizations: Very few contraindications to breastfeeding. *Pediatrics and Child Heath, 11*(8), 489–491. Retrieved from http://www.cps.ca/english/statements/ID/PIDnote_Oct2006.pdf.

Continued

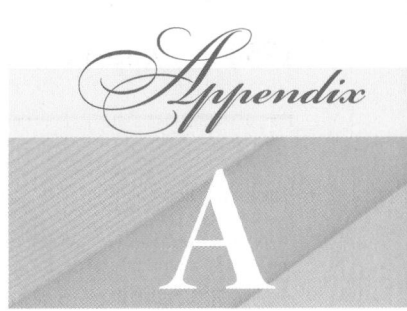

DRUG	EXCRETED IN MILK	% ADULT DOSE IN MILK	HALE RATING	COMMENTS
Nystatin (Nilstat)	No	Not absorbed orally	L1	Can be given to infant directly
Oxacillin	Yes	Trace	NR	Displaces bilirubin from albumin in infants
Penicillin G, benzathine (Bicillin)	Yes	0.8	L1	Best on empty stomach; increased in neonate
Streptomycin	Yes	0.5	L3	
Erythromycin/Sulphisoxazole (Pediazole)	Yes	0.45	L2	Jaundice may develop; avoid in infants with G6PD
Tetracycline HCl	Yes	0.03–4.8	L2	Probably chelated by calcium in milk
Anticoagulants				
Heparin	No	None	L1	Heparin ineffective orally
Warfarin (Coumadin)	Yes	<4.4	L2	Depends on dose mother is taking
Anticonvulsants and Sedatives (Barbiturates May Pass Into Milk But Do Not Sedate Infant)				
Magnesium sulphate	Yes	0.5	L1	
Pentobarbital (Nembutal)	Yes	Traces	L3	Depends on liver for detoxification so may accumulate in newborn
Phenobarbital	Yes	1.5	L3	Sleepiness and decreased sucking possible
Phenytoin (Dilantin)	Yes	1.4–7.2	L2	No problem if mother's plasma concentration is in therapeutic range. Higher doses may cause sleepiness
Antihistamines (May Suppress Lactation; Administer After Breastfeeding; All Pass Into Breast Milk)				
Brompheniramine maleate	Yes	Unknown	NR	Well absorbed from GI tract
Diphenhydramine (Benadryl)	Yes	Unknown	L2	Metabolism shows ethnic variation; volume of distribution is greater in Asians than in Whites
Promethazine (Phenergan, Histantil)	Yes	Unknown	L2	Passage into human milk is expected; increases serum prolactin level
Autonomic Drugs				
Atropine sulphate†	Yes	Unknown	L3	May inhibit lactation
Ergotamine (Cafergot)	Yes	Unknown	L4	May inhibit lactation; vomiting, diarrhea, convulsions in infant
Neostigmine (Prostigmin)	No	None	NR	Poorly absorbed from GI tract
Propantheline bromide	No	Uncontrolled data indicate no measurable levels	NR	Activity of long-acting dose not studied
Propranolol (Inderal)	Yes	0.05–1	L2	Risk of effect almost nonexistent; some Whites are poor absorbers
Cardiovascular Drugs				
Diazoxide (Proglycem)	Unknown	Unknown	NR	Antihypertensive
Digoxin (Lanoxin)	Yes	0.07–14	L2	Not detected in infant's plasma
Hydralazine (Apresoline)	Yes	0.8	L2	Antihypertensive
Methyldopa	Yes	0.02–0.09	L2	Antihypertensive
Nifedipine (Adalat)	Yes	0.00163 ± 0.00125	L2	Calcium channel blocker; minimal amount in milk
Quinidine (Quinate)	Yes	4.1	L2	May suppress prolactin secretion
Diuretics				
Chlorothiazide (Diuril)	Yes	Minimal	L3	Absorption from GI tract is incomplete and dose dependent
Furosemide (Lasix)	Possible	Not found in all samples	L3	Drug is given to neonates under medical management
Spironolactone (Aldactone)	Yes	Unknown	L2	80% of drug is converted to canrenone

†Atropine sulphate is an ingredient in many prescription and nonprescription drugs.

DRUG	EXCRETED IN MILK	% ADULT DOSE IN MILK	HALE RATING	COMMENTS
Gastrointestinal Agents				
Docusate sodium	Yes	Low	NR	Can cause diarrhea and colic in infant
Magnesium hydroxide (Milk of Magnesia)	Yes	Low	L3	May increase bowel activity in infant
Senna (Senokot)	No	None	L3	Older preparations might affect infant's bowel function
Hormones and Contraceptives				
Cortisone	Yes	Unknown	NR	Probably OK to use as replacement therapy in Addison's disease or as one-time dose in a joint
Epinephrine (Adrenalin, EpiPen)	Yes	Unknown	L4	Destroyed in GI tract of infant
Estradiol (Climara, Estraderm)	Yes	0.004–<10	L3	
Estrogen	Yes	0.1	L3	May alter quality and quantity of milk
Insulin	No	None	L1	Not excreted in human milk
Levonorgestrel (Triphasil)	Yes	1.1	L1	Does not affect milk production
Medroxyprogesterone (Depo-Provera, Provera)	Yes	0.86–5	L1 L4 if used first 3 days postpartum	Increased prolactin level before and after sucking; 6-mo injection may affect milk supply; 3-mo injection should not decrease supply
Prednisone (Winpred)	Yes	0.15 ± 0.11	L2 L4 for chronic high doses	
Progesterone	Unknown	Unknown	L3	In low doses, progesterone-only oral contraceptives are OK
Propylthiouracil	Yes	0.03–2.6	NR	Get baseline levels of T_3, T_4, and TSH in infant before and 6 wk after mother starts taking medication
Thyroid and thyroxine (T_4)	Yes	0.3–2.0	L1	Appears to protect breastfed infants of hypothyroid mothers
Tolbutamide	Yes	18	L3	Watch for jaundice
Narcotics				
Cocaine	Yes	Significant levels in milk	L5	No metabolites or drug found in milk after 36 hr or in infant's urine after 60 hr
Codeine	Yes	5 ± 2	L3	Asians metabolize less drug than Whites do
Heroin	Yes	Significant	L4	Level in milk enough to cause addiction in infant
Marijuana (*Cannabis sativa* L.)	Yes	Unknown	L5	Shown in laboratory animals to produce structural changes in nursling's brain cells; infant at risk of inhaling smoke during feeding or when held by person who is smoking
Meperidine (Demerol)	Yes	Unknown	L2 L3 early postpartum	Renal excretion of drug and metabolite is pH dependent. Associated with sedation, poor sucking reflex, and neurobehavioral delay in infants when used during labour and early postpartum.
Methadone	Yes	2.2	L3	No signs in infant if mother getting <20 mg/24 hr; if more than that, withdrawal may be a problem; suggest that mother take daily dose after evening feeding and supplement with formula at next feeding
Morphine	Yes	0.8–1.2	L3	Amounts in breast milk too variable to consider breastfeeding as means of treating withdrawal symptoms; may cause galactorrhea and prolactin increase
Oxycodone	Yes	Unknown	L3	
Psychotropic and Mood-Changing Drugs				
Alcohol (ethanol)	Yes	1–19.5	L3	Milk may smell like alcohol; high amounts may suppress lactation; infant cannot metabolize ethanol
Amitriptyline (Elavil, Levate)	Yes	0.8 ± 0.2	L2	Galactorrhea or prolactin increase
Caffeine	Yes	0.66–2.3	L2	Ability to metabolize it developed by 3–4.5 months

Continued

DRUG	EXCRETED IN MILK	% ADULT DOSE IN MILK	HALE RATING	COMMENTS
Chlordiazepoxide	Yes	Unknown	L3	May contribute to jaundice; may cause drowsiness
Chlorpromazine (Largactil)	Yes	0.07–0.2	L3	May cause drowsiness and lethargy in infants; galactorrhea, increase in prolactin levels reported
Desipramine (Norpramin)	Yes	1	L2	Neither drug nor metabolite recovered from nursing infant's serum or urine; some Whites are poor metabolizers
Diazepam (Valium)	Yes	2–12	L3 L4 if used chronically	Sedation if fed 4 hr but not 8 hr after dose; more in evening milk
Haloperidol (Peridol)	Yes	0.15–2	L2	Causes prolactin increase; in animals, nurslings have behavioral abnormalities; these effects are not seen in humans
Imipramine (Tofranil)	Yes	0.1	L2	Causes galactorrhea and prolactin increase
Lithium carbonate (Carbolith, Duralith)	Yes	1.8	L4	Measurable lithium in infant's serum; inhibits cAMP, which is significant for brain growth; cyanosis, poor muscle tone, and ECG changes seen in breastfeeding infant
Meprobamate	Yes	Unknown	L3	Galactorrhea is seen in some women
Phencyclidine (PCP)	Yes	Unknown	L5	Animal studies show PCP in milk even after drug has been discontinued for 40 days
Theobromine	Yes	20	NR	Chocolate is the most common cause of exposure; if mother consumes >0.5 kg/day, may see irritability or increased bowel activity
Trifluoperazine (Terfluzine)	Yes	Unknown	NR	Excretion into milk not significant after therapeutic doses; galactorrhea reported in some women; increase in serum prolactin levels
Miscellaneous				
DPT	Yes	Minimum	NR	Does not interfere with immunization schedule; breastfeeding may enhance immunization response
Methotrexate	Yes	0.93	L3 (acute) L5 (chronic)	Food delays absorption; peaks at 19 hr in milk
Nicotine	Yes	Unknown	NR Therapeutic Patch L3	May suppress lactation due to a decreased response of prolactin and oxytocin to suckling; smoke exposure may be a risk for SIDS
Poliovirus vaccine	No	None	NR	Live vaccine taken orally; not necessary to withhold breastfeeding; breastfeeding may decrease adverse effects of vaccine
Rh antibodies	Yes	Unknown	NR	Not a contraindication for breastfeeding
Rubella virus vaccine	Yes	Minimum	L2	Will not confer passive immunity
Theophylline (Pulmophylline)	Yes	<1–15	L3	Extremely low clearance in infants <6 mo of age
Tuberculin test	Yes	Unknown	NR	Tuberculin-sensitive mothers can immunize their infants through breast milk; immunity may last several years

(Compiled from Hale, T. W. [2010]. *Medications and mother's milk*. (14th ed.). Amarillo, TX: Hale Publishing; Lawrence, R. A., & Lawrence, R. M. [2011]. *Breastfeeding: A guide for the medical profession* [7th ed.]. St. Louis: Mosby.)

cAMP, cyclic adenosine monophosphate; *DPT*, diphtheria, pertussis, tetanus; *ECG*, electrocardiogram; *GI*, gastrointestinal; *G6PD*, glucose-6-phosphate dehydrogenase; *NR*, not rated; *SIDS*, sudden infant death syndrome; T_3, triiodothyronine; T_4, thyroxine; *TSH*, thyroid-stimulating hormone.

Appendix B

Developmental and Sensory Assessment

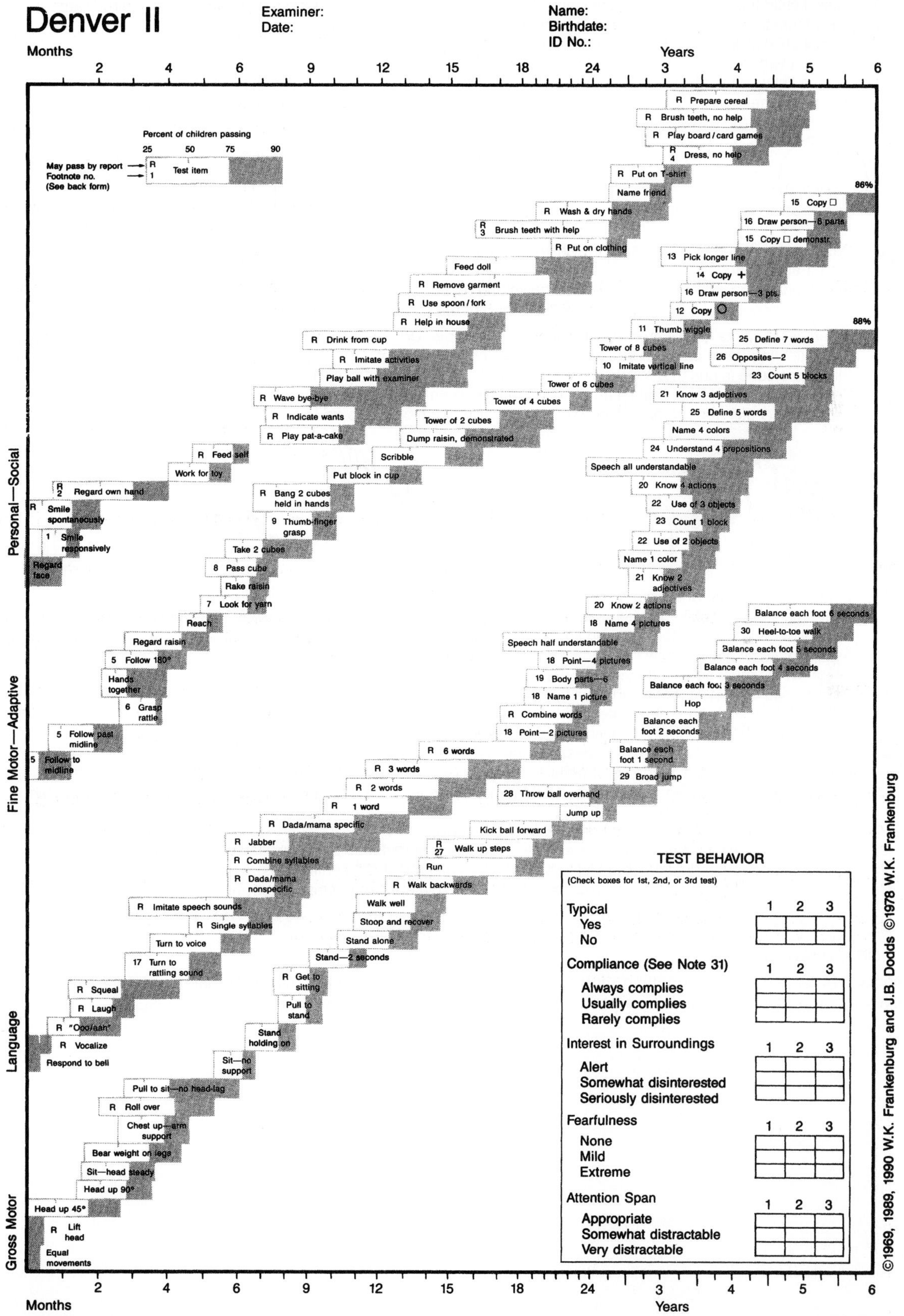
Denver II
Examiner:
Date:
Name:
Birthdate:
ID No.:
Months
Years
2 4 6 9 12 15 18 24 3 4 5 6
Percent of children passing
25 50 75 90
May pass by report
Footnote no.
(See back form)
R
1
Test item
Personal—Social
Fine Motor—Adaptive
Language
Gross Motor
R Prepare cereal
R Brush teeth, no help
R Play board / card games
R 4 Dress, no help
R Put on T-shirt
Name friend
R Wash & dry hands
R 3 Brush teeth with help
R Put on clothing
Feed doll
R Remove garment
R Use spoon / fork
R Help in house
R Drink from cup
R Imitate activities
Play ball with examiner
R Wave bye-bye
R Indicate wants
R Play pat-a-cake
R Feed self
Work for toy
R 2 Regard own hand
R Smile spontaneously
1 Smile responsively
Regard face
86%
15 Copy □
16 Draw person—6 parts
15 Copy □ demonstr.
13 Pick longer line
14 Copy +
16 Draw person—3 pts.
12 Copy ○
11 Thumb wiggle
Tower of 8 cubes
10 Imitate vertical line
Tower of 6 cubes
Tower of 4 cubes
Tower of 2 cubes
Dump raisin, demonstrated
Scribble
Put block in cup
R Bang 2 cubes held in hands
9 Thumb-finger grasp
Take 2 cubes
8 Pass cube
Rake raisin
7 Look for yarn
Reach
Regard raisin
5 Follow 180°
Hands together
6 Grasp rattle
5 Follow past midline
5 Follow to midline
88%
25 Define 7 words
26 Opposites—2
23 Count 5 blocks
21 Know 3 adjectives
25 Define 5 words
Name 4 colors
24 Understand 4 prepositions
Speech all understandable
20 Know 4 actions
22 Use of 3 objects
23 Count 1 block
22 Use of 2 objects
Name 1 color
21 Know 2 adjectives
20 Know 2 actions
18 Name 4 pictures
Speech half understandable
18 Point—4 pictures
19 Body parts—6
18 Name 1 picture
R Combine words
18 Point—2 pictures
R 6 words
R 3 words
R 2 words
R 1 word
R Dada/mama specific
R Jabber
R Combine syllables
R Dada/mama nonspecific
R Imitate speech sounds
R Single syllables
Turn to voice
17 Turn to rattling sound
R Squeal
R Laugh
R "Ooo/aah"
R Vocalize
Respond to bell
Balance each foot 6 seconds
30 Heel-to-toe walk
Balance each foot 5 seconds
Balance each foot 4 seconds
Balance each foot 3 seconds
Hop
Balance each foot 2 seconds
Balance each foot 1 second
29 Broad jump
28 Throw ball overhand
Jump up
Kick ball forward
R 27 Walk up steps
Run
R Walk backwards
Walk well
Stoop and recover
Stand alone
Stand—2 seconds
R Get to sitting
Pull to stand
Stand holding on
Sit—no support
Pull to sit—no head-lag
R Roll over
Chest up—arm support
Bear weight on legs
Sit—head steady
Head up 90°
Head up 45°
R Lift head
Equal movements
TEST BEHAVIOR
(Check boxes for 1st, 2nd, or 3rd test)
Typical
Yes
No
Compliance (See Note 31)
Always complies
Usually complies
Rarely complies
Interest in Surroundings
Alert
Somewhat disinterested
Seriously disinterested
Fearfulness
None
Mild
Extreme
Attention Span
Appropriate
Somewhat distractable
Very distractable
1 2 3
©1969, 1989, 1990 W.K. Frankenburg and J.B. Dodds ©1978 W.K. Frankenburg

A

Fig. B-1 **A:** Denver II.

Continued

DIRECTIONS FOR ADMINISTRATION

1. Try to get child to smile by smile by smiling, talking or waving. Do not touch him/her.
2. Child must stare at hand several seconds.
3. Parent may help guide toothbrush and put toothpaste on brush.
4. Child does not have to be able to tie shoes or button/zip in the back.
5. Move yarn slowly in an arc from one side to the other, about 20 centimetres above child's face.
6. Pass if child grasps rattle when it is touched to the backs or tips of fingers.
7. Pass if child tries to see where yarn went. Yarn should be drooped quickly from sight from tester's hand without arm movement.
8. Child must transfer cube from hand to hand without help of body, mouth, or table.
9. Pass if child picks up raisin with any part of thumb and finger.
10. Line can vary only 30 degrees or less from tester's line.|/
11. Make a fist with thumb pointing upward and wiggle only the thumb. Pass if child initates and does not move any fingers other than the thumb.

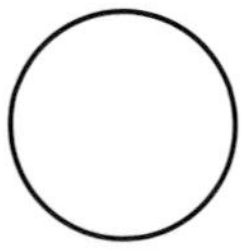

12. Pass any enclosed form. Fail continuous round motions.

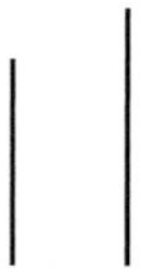

13. Which line is longer? (Not bigger.) Turn paper upside down and repeat. (pass 3 of 3 or 5 of 6)

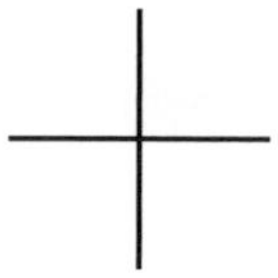

14. Pass any lines crossing near midpoint.

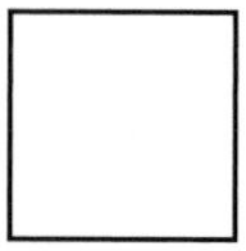

15. Have child copy first. If failed, demonstrate.

When giving items 12, 14, and 15, do not name the forms. Do not demonstrate 12 and 14.

16. When scoring, each pair (2 arms, 2 legs, etc.) counts as one part.
17. Place one cube in cup and shake gently near child's ear, but out of sight. Repeat for other ear.
18. Point to picture and have child name it. (No credit is given for sounds only.) If less than 4 pictures are named correctly, have child point to picture as each is named by tester.

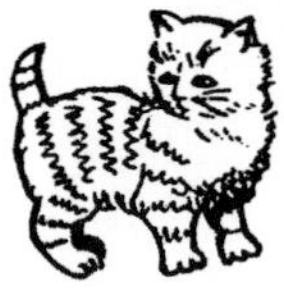
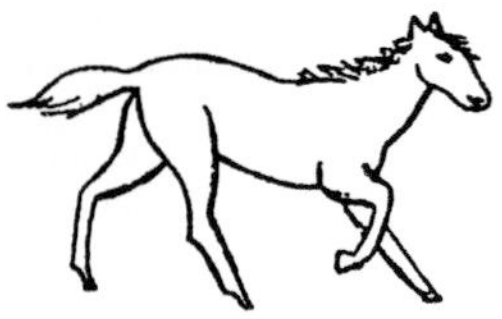
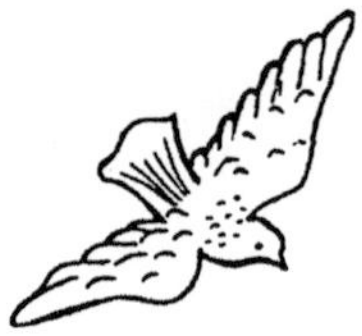
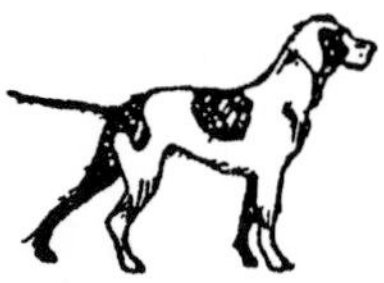
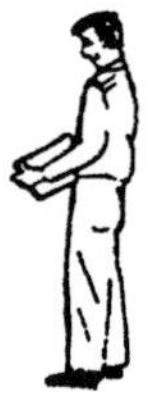

19. Using doll, tell child: Show me the nose, eyes, ears, mouth, hands, feet, tummy, hair, Pass 6 to 8.
20. Using pictures, ask child: Which one files?...says meow?... talks?... barks?... gallops? Pass 2 of 5, 4 of 5.
21. Ask child: What do you do when you are cold?... tired?... hungry? Pass 2 of 3, 3 of 3.
22. Ask child: What do you do with a cup? What is a chair used for? What is a pencil used for? Action words must be included in answers.
23. Pass if child correctly places <u>and</u> says how many blocks are on paper. (1, 5).
24. Tell child: Put block **on** table; **under** table; **in front of** me, **behind** me. Pass 4 of 4. (Do not help child by pointing, moving head or eyes.)
25. Ask child: What is a ball?... lake?... desk?... house?... banana?... curtain?... fence?... ceiling? Pass if defined in terms of use, shape, what it is made of, or general category (such as banana is fruit, not just yellow). Pass 5 of 8, 7 of 8.
26. Ask child: If a horse is big, a mouse is __? If fire is hot, ice is __? If the sun shines during the day, the moon shines during the __? Pass 2 of 3.
27. Child may use wall or rail only, not person. May not crawl.
28. Child must throw ball overhand 1 metre within arm's each of tester.
29. Child must perform standing broad jump over width of test sheet (22 centimetres).
30. Tell child to walk forward, ⊂⊃⊂⊃⊂⊃⊂⊃→ heel within 2.5 centimetres of toe. Tester may demonstrate. Child must walk 4 consecutive steps.
31. In the second year, half of normal children are non-compliant.

B **OBSERVATIONS:**

Fig. B-1, cont'd B: Directions for administration of numbered items on Denver II. *(From Frankenburg, W. K., & Dodds, J. B. [1990].* Denver developmental screening test II—screening manual. *Denver: Denver Developmental Materials.)*

Appendix C

Growth Measurements

WHO GROWTH CHARTS FOR CANADA

BOYS

BIRTH TO 24 MONTHS: BOYS

Length-for-age and Weight-for-age percentiles

NAME: ______

DOB: ______ RECORD # ______

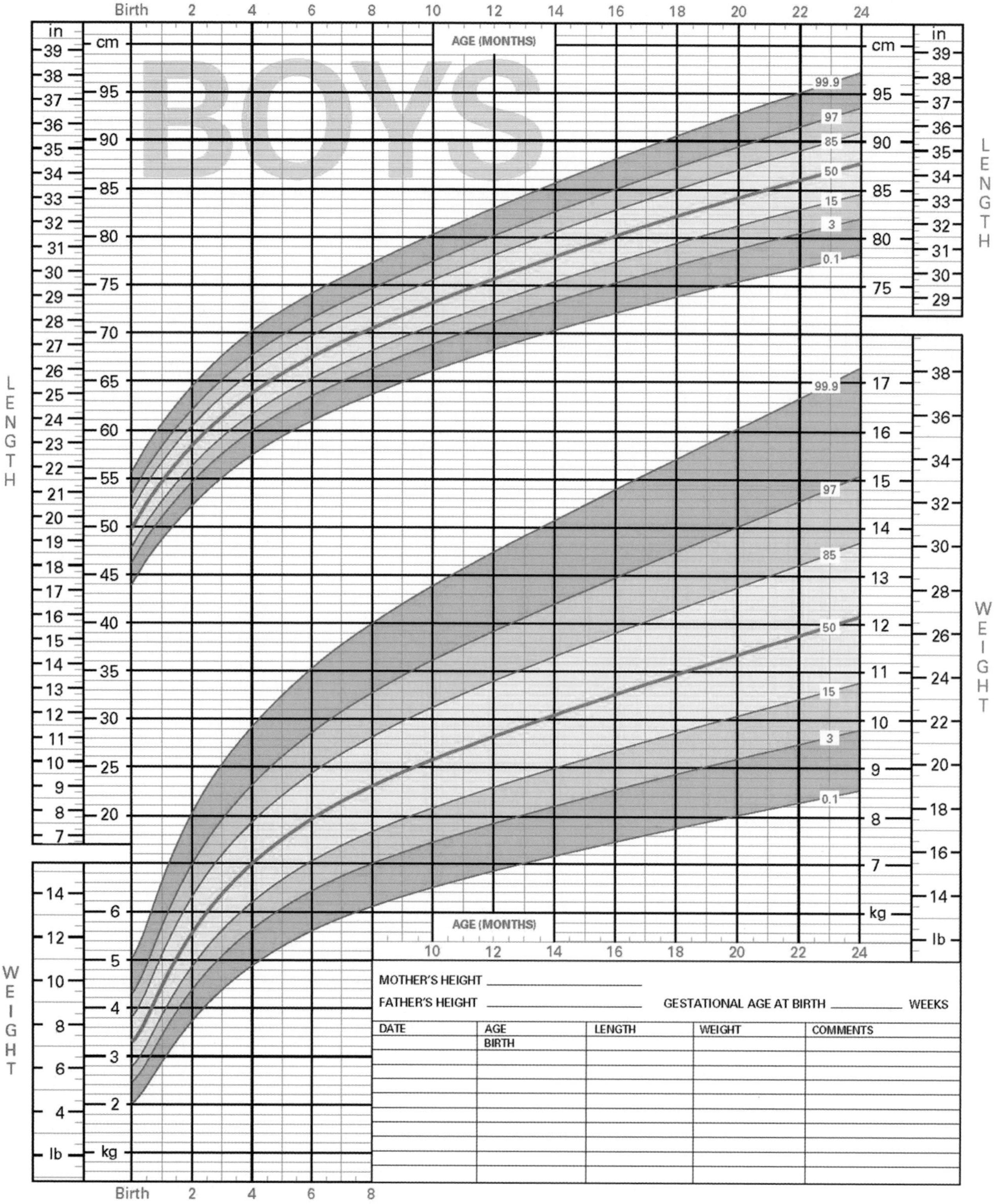

SOURCE: Based on the World Health Organization (WHO) Child Growth Standards (2006) and adapted for Canada by Dietitians of Canada, Canadian Paediatric Society, the College of Family Physicians of Canada and Community Health Nurses of Canada.

WHO GROWTH CHARTS FOR CANADA

BOYS

2 TO 19 YEARS: BOYS

Height-for-age and Weight-for-age percentiles

NAME: ______________________

DOB: ______________ RECORD # __________

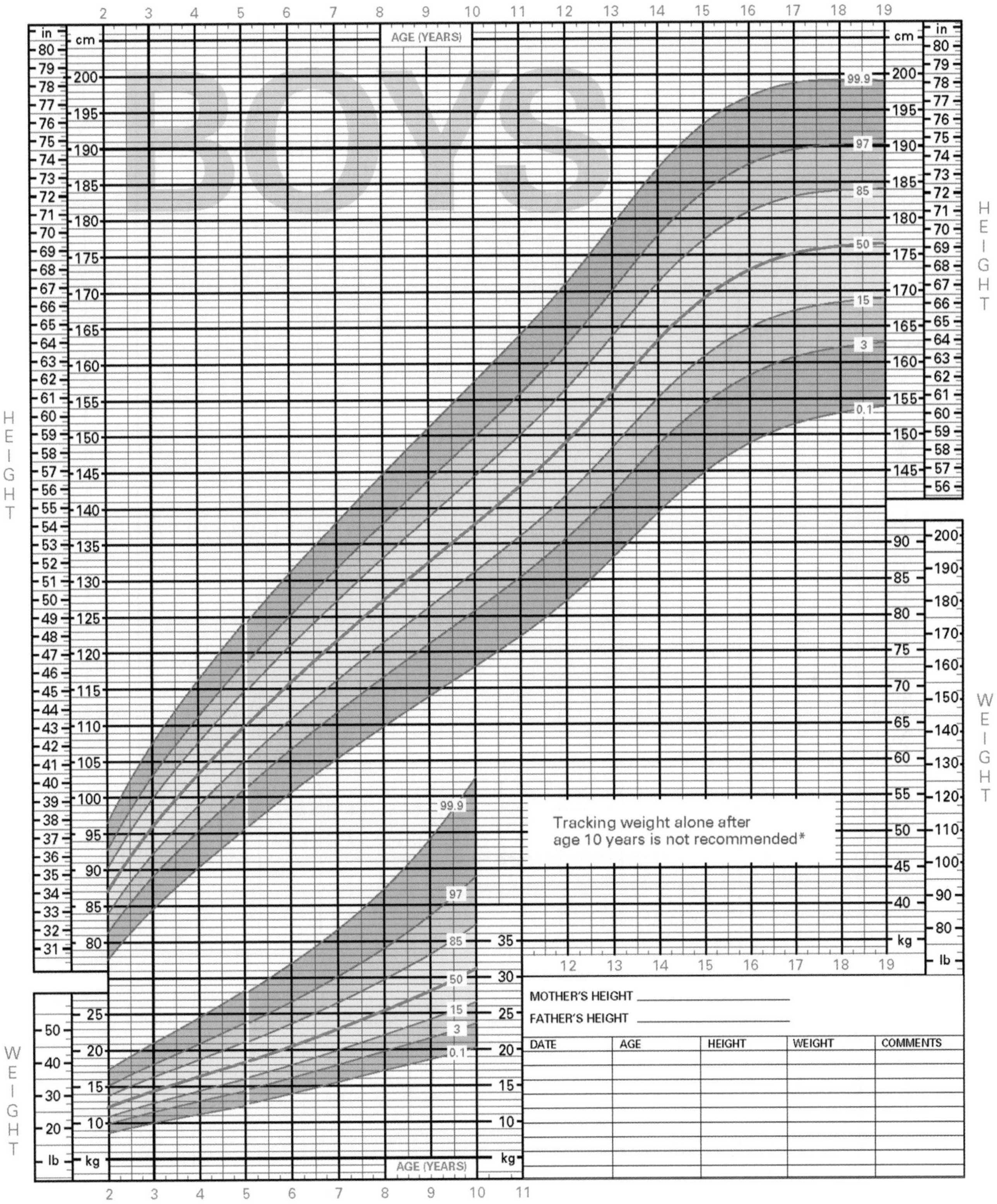

SOURCE: Based on the World Health Organization (WHO) Child Growth Standards (2006) and WHO Reference (2007) adapted for Canada by Dietitians of Canada, Canadian Paediatric Society, the College of Family Physicians of Canada and Community Health Nurses of Canada.

*BMI is a better measure due to variable age of puberty.

WHO GROWTH CHARTS FOR CANADA **GIRLS**

BIRTH TO 24 MONTHS: GIRLS

Length-for-age and Weight-for-age percentiles

NAME: ____________________

DOB: ____________ RECORD # ________

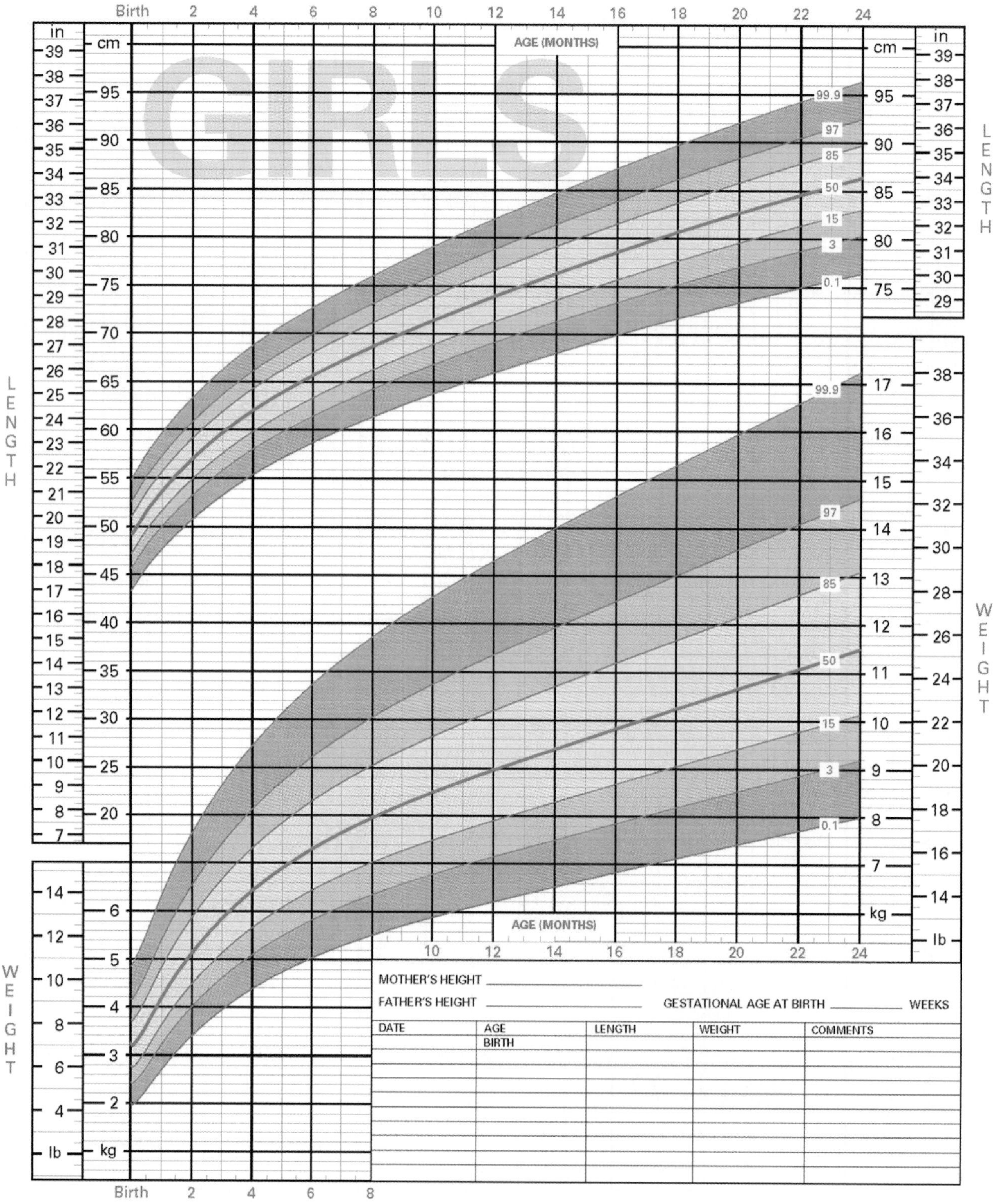

SOURCE: Based on the World Health Organization (WHO) Child Growth Standards (2006) and adapted for Canada by Dietitians of Canada, Canadian Paediatric Society, the College of Family Physicians of Canada and Community Health Nurses of Canada.

WHO GROWTH CHARTS FOR CANADA

GIRLS

2 TO 19 YEARS: GIRLS

Height-for-age and Weight-for-age percentiles

NAME: ______________________

DOB: ______________ RECORD # __________

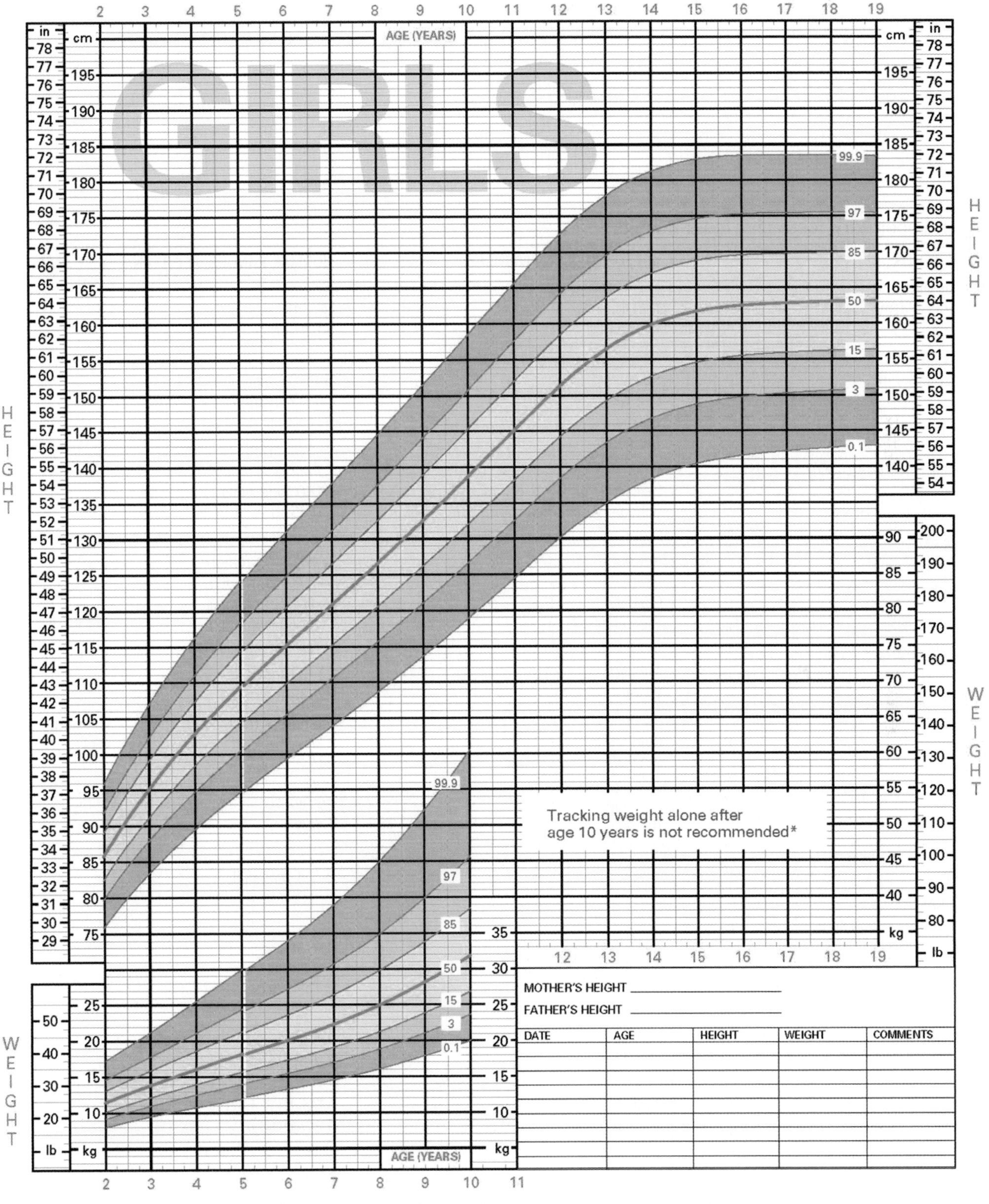

SOURCE: Based on the World Health Organization (WHO) Child Growth Standards (2006) and WHO Reference (2007) adapted for Canada by Dietitians of Canada, Canadian Paediatric Society, the College of Family Physicians of Canada and Community Health Nurses of Canada.

*BMI is a better measure due to variable age of puberty.

Appendix D

Common Laboratory Tests

Common Laboratory Tests and Tests Results*

TEST/SPECIMEN	AGE/GENDER/REFERENCE	NORMAL RANGES IN INTERNATIONAL UNITS (SI)	
Acetaminophen			
Serum or plasma	Therap. conc.	66–200 mcmol/L	
	Toxic conc.	>1300 mcmol/L	
Ammonia nitrogen			
Plasma or serum	Newborn	64–107 mcmol/L	
	0–2 wk	56–92 mcmol/L	
	>1 mo	21–50 mcmol/L	
	Thereafter	0–35.7 mcmol/L	
Antistreptolysin O titre (ASO)			
Serum	2–4 yr	<160 Todd units	
	School-age children	170–330 Todd units	
Base excess			
Whole blood	Newborn	(−10)-(−2) mmol/L	
	Infant	(−7)-(−1) mmol/L	
	Child	(−4)-(+2) mmol/L	
	Thereafter	(−3)-(+3) mmol/L	
Bicarbonate (HCO_3)			
Serum	Arterial	21–28 mmol/L	
	Venous	22–29 mmol/L	
Bilirubin, total		**Premature** (mcmol/L)	**Full term** (mcmol/L)
Serum	Cord	<34	<34
	0–1 day	<137	<103
	1–2 days	<205	<137
	2–5 days	<274	<205
	Thereafter	<340	<171
Bilirubin, direct (conjugated)			
Serum		0–3.4 mcmol/L	
Bleeding time			
Blood from skin puncture			
Ivy	Normal	2–7 min	
	Borderline	7–11 min	
Simplate (G-D)		2.75–8 min	
Blood volume			
Whole blood	Male	0.052–0.083 L/kg	
	Female	0.050–0.075 L/kg	
C-reactive protein (CRP)			
Serum	Cord	0.52–13.3 mg/L	
	2–12 yr	0.67–18 mg/L	
Calcium, ionized			
Serum, plasma, or whole blood	Cord	1.25–1.50 mmol/L	
	Newborn, 3–24 hr	1.07–1.27 mmol/L	
	24–48 hr	1.00–1.17 mmol/L	
	Thereafter	1.12–1.23 mmol/L	

*For a description of abbreviations, see p. 1771.

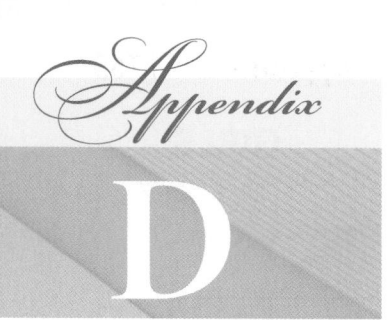

Common Laboratory Tests and Tests Results—cont'd

TEST/SPECIMEN	AGE/GENDER/REFERENCE	NORMAL RANGES IN INTERNATIONAL UNITS (SI)
Calcium, total		
Serum	Cord	2.25-2.88 mmol/L
	Newborn, 3-24 hr	2.3-2.65 mmol/L
	24-48 hr	1.75-3.0 mmol/L
	4-7 days	2.25-2.73 mmol/L
	Child	2.2-2.70 mmol/L
	Thereafter	2.1-2.55 mmol/L
Carbon dioxide, partial pressure (Pco_2)		
Whole blood, arterial	Newborn	27-40 mm Hg
	Infant	27-41 mm Hg
	Thereafter: Male	35-48 mm Hg
	Female	32-45 mm Hg
Carbon dioxide, total (tco_2)		
Serum or plasma	Cord	14-22 mmol/L
	Premature (1 wk)	14-27 mmol/L
	Newborn	13-22 mmol/L
	Infant, child	20-28 mmol/L
	Thereafter	23-30 mmol/L
Cerebrospinal fluid (CSF)		
Pressure		70-180 mm H_2O
Volume		0.06-0.10 L
		0.10-0.16 L
Chloride		
Serum or plasma	Cord	96-104 mmol/L
	Newborn	97-110 mmol/L
	Thereafter	98-106 mmol/L
Sweat	Normal (homozygote)	<40 mmol/L
	Marginal (e.g., asthma, Addison disease, malnutrition)	45-60 mmol/L
	Cystic fibrosis	>60 mmol/L
Cholesterol, total		
Serum or plasma†	Acceptable	<4.4 mmol/L
	Borderline	4.4-5.1 mmol/L
	High	≥5.2 mmol/L
Clotting time (Lee-White)		
Whole blood		5-8 min (glass tubes)
		5-15 min (room temp)
		30 min (silicone tube)
Creatine kinase (CK, CPK)		
Serum	Cord	70-380 U/L
	5-8 hr	214-1175 U/L
	24-33 hr	130-1200 U/L
	72-100 hr	87-725 U/L
	Adult	5-130 U/L
Creatinine		
Serum	Cord	53-106 mcmol/L
	Newborn	27-88 mcmol/L
	Infant	18-35 mcmol/L
	Child	27-62 mcmol/L
	Adolescent	44-88 mcmol/L
	Adult: Male	53-106 mcmol/L
	Female	44-97 mcmol/L
Urine, 24 hr	Premature	72-133 mcmol/kg/24 hr
	Full term	92-174 mcmol/kg/24 hr
	1.5-7 yr	88-133 mcmol/kg/24 hr
	7-15 yr	46-362 mcmol/kg/24 hr
Creatinine clearance (endogenous)		
Serum or plasma and urine	Newborn	0.67-1.09 $mL/sec/m^2$
	Male	1.78-2.32 $mL/sec/m^2$
	Female	1.45-1.78 $mL/sec/m^2$

†From National Cholesterol Education Program. (1992). Report of the expert panel on blood cholesterol levels in children and adolescents. *Pediatrics, 89*(3 pt 2), 527.

Continued

Common Laboratory Tests and Tests Results—cont'd

TEST/SPECIMEN	AGE/GENDER/REFERENCE	NORMAL RANGES IN INTERNATIONAL UNITS (SI)	
Digoxin			
Serum, plasma; collect at least 12 hr after dose	Therap. conc.		
	CHF	1.0-1.9 nmol/L	
	Arrhythmias	1.9-2.6 nmol/L	
	Toxic conc.		
	Child	>3.2 nmol/L	
	Adult	>3.8 nmol/L	
Eosinophil count			
Whole blood, capillary blood		$50\text{-}250 \times 10^6$/L	
Erythrocyte (RBC) count			
Whole blood	Cord	$3.9\text{-}5.5 \times 10^{12}$/L	
	1-3 d	$4.0\text{-}6.6 \times 10^{12}$/L	
	1 wk	$3.9\text{-}6.3 \times 10^{12}$/L	
	2 wk	$3.6\text{-}6.2 \times 10^{12}$/L	
	1 mo	$3.0\text{-}5.4 \times 10^{12}$/L	
	2 mo	$2.7\text{-}4.9 \times 10^{12}$/L	
	3-6 mo	$3.1\text{-}4.5 \times 10^{12}$/L	
	0.5-2 yr	$3.7\text{-}5.3 \times 10^{12}$/L	
	2-6 yr	$3.9\text{-}5.3 \times 10^{12}$/L	
	6-12 yr	$4.0\text{-}5.2 \times 10^{12}$/L	
	12-18 yr: Male	$4.5\text{-}5.3 \times 10^{12}$/L	
	Female	$4.1\text{-}5.1 \times 10^{12}$/L	
Erythrocyte sedimentation rate (ESR)			
Whole blood			
Westergren (modified)	Child	0-10 mm/hr	
	<50 yr: Male	0-15 mm/hr	
	Female	0-20 mm/hr	
Wintrobe	Child	0-13 mm/hr	
	Adult: Male	0-9 mm/hr	
	Female	0-20 mm/hr	
Fibrinogen			
Plasma	Newborn	1.25-3.00 g/L	
	Thereafter	2.00-4.00 g/L	
Galactose			
Serum	Newborn	0-1.11 mmol/L	
	Thereafter	<0.28 mmol/L	
Urine	Newborn	≤3.33 mmol/L	
	Thereafter	<0.08 mmol/day	
Glucose			
Serum	Cord	2.5-5.3 mmol/L	
	Newborn, 1 day	2.2-3.3 mmol/L	
	Newborn, >1 day	2.8-5.0 mmol/L	
	Child	3.3-5.5 mmol/L	
	Thereafter	3.9-5.8 mmol/L	
Whole blood	Adult	3.6-5.3 mmol/L	
CSF	Adult	2.2-3.9 mmol/L	
Urine (quantitative)		<2.8 mmol/day	
Urine (qualitative)		Negative	
Glucose tolerance test (GTT), oral			
Serum			
Dosages		**Normal**	**Diabetic**
Adult: 75 g	Fasting	3.9-5.8 mmol/L	≥7.0 mmol/L
Child: 1.75 g/kg of ideal weight up to maximum of 75 g	60 min	6.7-9.4 mmol/L	≥11 mmol/L
	90 min	5.6-7.8 mmol/L	≥11 mmol/L
	120 min	3.9-6.7 mmol/L	≥11 mmol/L
Growth hormone (GH, somatotropin)			
Plasma	1 day	5-53 mcg/L	
	1 wk	5-27 mcg/L	
	1-12 mo	2-10 mcg/L	
	Fasting child/adult	<0.7-6.0 mcg/L	

Common Laboratory Tests and Tests Results—cont'd

TEST/SPECIMEN	AGE/GENDER/REFERENCE	NORMAL RANGES IN INTERNATIONAL UNITS (SI)
Hematocrit (HCT, Hct)		
Whole blood	1 day (cap)	0.48-0.69 vol fraction
	2 days	0.48-0.75 vol fraction
	3 days	0.44-0.72 vol fraction
	2 mo	0.28-0.42 vol fraction
	6-12 yr	0.35-0.45 vol fraction
	12-18 yr: Male	0.37-0.49 vol fraction
	Female	0.36-0.46 vol fraction
Hemoglobin (Hgb)		
Whole blood	1-3 days (cap)	145-225 g/L
	2 mo	90-140 g/L
	6-12 yr	115-155 g/L
	12-18 yr: Male	130-160 g/L
	Female	120-160 g/L
Hemoglobin A		
Whole blood		>0.95 Hgb fraction
Hemoglobin F		
Whole blood	1 day	0.63-0.92 Hgb fraction
	5 days	0.65-0.88 Hgb fraction
	3 wk	0.55-0.85 Hgb fraction
	6-9 wk	0.31-0.75 Hgb fraction
	3-4 mo	<0.02-0.59 Hgb fraction
	6 mo	<0.02-0.09 Hgb fraction
	Adult	<0.02 Hgb fraction
Immunoglobulin A (IgA)		
Serum	Cord	0.014-0.036 g/L
	1-3 mo	0.013-0.530 g/L
	4-6 mo	0.044-0.84 g/L
	7-12 mo	0.11-1.06 g/L
	2-5 yr	0.14-1.59 g/L
	6-10 yr	0.33-2.36 g/L
	Adult	0.7-3.12 g/L
Immunoglobulin D (IgD)		
Serum	Newborn	None detected
	Thereafter	0-80 mg/L
Immunoglobulin E (IgE)		
Serum		0.1-0.4 mg/L
Immunoglobulin G (IgG)		
Serum	Cord	6.36-16.06 g/L
	1 mo	2.51-9.06 g/L
	2-4 mo	1.76-6.01 g/L
	5-12 mo	1.72-10.69 g/L
	1-5 yr	3.45-12.36 g/L
	6-10 yr	6.08-15.72 g/L
	Adult	6.39-13.49 g/L
Immunoglobulin M (IgM)		
Serum	Cord	0.063-2.50 g/L
	1-4 mo	0.170-1.050 g/L
	5-9 mo	0.33-1.26 g/L
	10-12 mo	0.41-1.73 g/L
	2-8 yr	0.43-2.07 g/L
	9-10 yr	0.52-2.42 g/L
	Adult	0.56-3.52 g/L
Iron		
Serum	Newborn	18-45 mcmol/L
	Infant	7-18 mcmol/L
	Child	9-22 mcmol/L
	Thereafter: Male	12-30 mcmol/L
	Female	9-30 mcmol/L
	Intoxicated child	50.12-456.5 mcmol/L
	Fatally poisoned child	>322.2 mcmol/L

Continued

Common Laboratory Tests and Tests Results—cont'd

TEST/SPECIMEN	AGE/GENDER/REFERENCE	NORMAL RANGES IN INTERNATIONAL UNITS (SI)
Iron-binding capacity, total (TIBC)		
Serum	Infant	17.90–71.60 mcmol/L
	Thereafter	44.75–71.60 mcmol/L
Lead		
Whole blood	Child	<0.48 mcmol/L
Urine, 24 hr		<0.39 mcmol/L
Leukocyte count (WBC count)		
Whole blood	Birth	$9.0–30.0 \times 10^9/L$
	24 hr	9.4–34.0
	1 mo	5.0–19.5
	1–3 yr	6.0–17.5
	4–7 yr	5.5–15.5
	8–13 yr	4.5–13.5
	Adult	4.5–11.0
CSF (cell count)		
	Premature	$0–25 \times 10^6$
	Newborn	$0–20 \times 10^6$
	Neonate	$0–5 \times 10^6$
	Thereafter	$0–5 \times 10^6$
Leukocyte differential count		
Whole blood	Myelocytes	Number fraction 0
	Neutrophils—"bands"	Number fraction $0.03–0.05 \times 10^9$
	Neutrophils—"segs"	Number fraction $0.54–0.62 \times 10^9$
	Lymphocytes	Number fraction $0.25–0.33 \times 10^9$
	Monocytes	Number fraction $0.03–0.07 \times 10^9$
	Eosinophils	Number fraction $0.01–0.03 \times 10^9$
	Basophils	Number fraction $0–0.0075 \times 10^9$
Mean corpuscular hemoglobin (MCH)		
Whole blood	Birth–3 days	31–37 pg
	1 wk–1 mo	28–40 pg
	2 mo	26–34 pg
	3–6 mo	25–35 pg
	0.5–2 yr	28–31 pg
	2–6 yr	24–30 pg
	6–12 yr	25–33 pg
	12–18 yr	25–35 pg
	18–49 yr	26–34 pg
Mean corpuscular hemoglobin concentration (MCHC)		
Whole blood	Birth	300–360 g/L
	1–3 days (cap)	290–370 g/L
	1–2 wk	280–380 g/L
	1–2 mo	290–370 g/L
	3 mo–2 yr	300–360 g/L
	2–18 yr	310–370 g/L
	>18 yr	310–370 g/L
Mean corpuscular volume (MCV)		
Whole blood	1–3 days (cap)	$95–121\ mm^3$
	0.5–2 yr	$70–86\ mm^3$
	6–12 yr	$77–95\ mm^3$
	12–18 yr: Male	$78–98\ mm^3$
	Female	$78–102\ mm^3$
Osmolality		
Serum	Child, adult	275–295 mmol/kg
Urine, random		50–1400 mmol/kg, depending on fluid intake; after 12-hr fluid restriction: >850 mmol/kg
Urine, 24 hr		≅300–900 mmol/kg

Common Laboratory Tests and Tests Results—cont'd

TEST/SPECIMEN	AGE/GENDER/REFERENCE	NORMAL RANGES IN INTERNATIONAL UNITS (SI)
Oxygen, partial pressure (Po_2)		
Whole blood, arterial	Birth	8-24 mm Hg
	5-10 min	33-75 mm Hg
	30 min	31-85 mm Hg
	>1 hr	55-80 mm Hg
	1 day	54-95 mm Hg
	Thereafter (decreased with age)	83-108 mm Hg
Oxygen saturation (Sao_2)		
Whole blood, arterial	Newborn	Fraction saturated 0.85-0.90
	Thereafter	Fraction saturated 0.95-0.99
Partial thromboplastin time (PTT)		
Whole blood (Na citrate)		
Nonactivated		60-85 sec (Platelin)
Activated		25-35 sec
pH		
Whole blood, arterial (must be corrected for body temperature)	Premature (48 hr)	7.35-7.50
	Birth, full term	7.11-7.36
	5-10 min	7.09-7.30
	30 min	7.21-7.38
	>1 hr	7.26-7.49
	1 day	7.29-7.45
	Thereafter	7.35-7.45
Urine, random	Newborn/neonate	5-7
	Thereafter	4.5-8
Stool		7.0-7.5
Phenylalanine		
Serum	Premature	120-450 mcmol/L
	Newborn	70-210 mcmol/L
	Thereafter	50-110 mcmol/L
Urine, 24 hr	10 days-2 wk	6-12 mcmol/day
	3-12 yr	24-110 mcmol/day
	Thereafter	Trace-103 mcmol/day
Plasma volume		
Plasma	Male	0.025-0.043 L/kg
	Female	0.028-0.045 L/kg
Platelet count (thrombocyte count)		
Whole blood (EDTA)	Newborn (after 1 wk, same as adult)	$84\text{-}478 \times 10^9/L$
	Adult	$150\text{-}400 \times 10^9/L$
Potassium		
Serum	Newborn	3.0-6.0 mmol/L
	Thereafter	3.5-5.0 mmol/L
Plasma (heparin)		3.4-4.5 mmol/L
Urine, 24 hr		2.5-125 mmol/day (varies with diet)
Protein		
Serum, total	Premature	43-76 g/L
	Newborn	46-74 g/L
	1-7 yr	61-79 g/L
	8-12 yr	64-81 g/L
	13-19 yr	66-82 g/L
Total		
Urine, 24 hr		10-140 mg/L
		50-80 mg/day
		<250 mg/day (after intense exercise)
CSF		80-320 mg/L
Prothrombin time (PT)		
One-stage (Quick)		
Whole blood (Na citrate)	In general	11-15 sec (varies with type of thromboplastin
	Newborn	Prolonged by 2-3 sec
Two-stage modified (Ware and Seegers)		
Whole blood (sodium citrate)		18-22 sec

Continued

Common Laboratory Tests and Tests Results—cont'd

TEST/SPECIMEN	AGE/GENDER/REFERENCE	NORMAL RANGES IN INTERNATIONAL UNITS (SI)	
RBC count: see Erythrocyte (RBC) count			
Red blood cell volume			
Whole blood	Male	0.020-0.036 L/kg	
	Female	0.019-0.031 L/kg	
Reticulocyte count			
Whole blood	Adults	0.005-0.015 (% of RBC) or 25-75 × 10^9/L	
Capillary	1 day	0.004-0.060 (% of RBC)	
	7 days	<0.001-0.013 (% of RBC)	
	1-4 wk	<0.001-0.012 (% of RBC)	
	5-6 wk	<0.001-0.024 (% of RBC)	
	7-8 wk	0.001-0.029 (% of RBC)	
	9-10 wk	<0.001-0.026 (% of RBC)	
	11-12 wk	0.001-0.013 (% of RBC)	
Salicylates			
Serum, plasma	Therap. conc.	1.1-2.2 mmol/L	
	Toxic conc.	>18.5 mmol/L	
Sedimentation rate: see Erythrocyte sedimentation rate (ESR)			
Sodium			
Serum or plasma	Newborn	134-146 mmol/L	
	Infant	139-146 mmol/L	
	Child	138-145 mmol/L	
	Thereafter	136-146 mmol/L	
Urine, 24 hr		40-220 mmol/day (diet dependent)	
Sweat	Normal	<40 mmol/L	
	Indeterminate	45-60 mmol/L	
	Cystic fibrosis	>60 mmol/L	
Specific gravity			
Urine, random	Adult	1.002-1.030	
	After 12-hr fluid restriction	>1.025	
Urine, 24 hr		1.015-1.025	
Theophylline			
Serum, plasma	Therap. conc.		
	Bronchodilator	56-110 mcmol/L	
	Premature apnea	28-56 mcmol/L	
	Toxic conc.	>110 mcmol/L	
Thrombin time			
Whole blood (Na citrate)		Control time ±2 sec when control is 9-13 sec	
Thyroxine, total (T_4)			
Serum	Cord	103-168 nmol/L	
	Newborn	148-310 nmol/L (lower in low-birth-weight infants)	
	Neonate	116-232 nmol/L	
	Infant	90-194 nmol/L	
	1-5 yr	94-194 nmol/L	
	5-10 yr	83-172 nmol/L	
	Thereafter	65-155 nmol/L	
	Newborn screen (filter paper)	80-284 nmol/L	
Triglycerides (TG)		**Male** (mmol/L)	**Female** (mmol/L)
Serum, after ≥2-hr fast	Cord	0.10-0.98	0.10-0.98
	0-5 yr	0.30-0.86	0.32-0.99
	6-11 yr	0.31-1.08	0.35-1.14
	12-15 yr	0.36-1.38	0.41-1.38
	16-19 yr	0.40-1.63	0.40-1.28
Triiodothyronine (T_3), free			
Serum	Cord	0.3-3.7 pmol/L	
	1-3 day	3.1-9.4 pmol/L	
	6 wk	3.7-8.6 pmol/L	
	Adults (20-50 yr)	3.5-10.0 pmol/L	

Common Laboratory Tests and Tests Results—cont'd

TEST/SPECIMEN	AGE/GENDER/REFERENCE	NORMAL RANGES IN INTERNATIONAL UNITS (SI)
Triiodothyronine, total (T_3-RIA)		
Serum	Cord	0.46-1.08 nmol/L
	Newborn	1.16-4 nmol/L
	1-5 yr	1.54-4 nmol/L
	5-10 yr	1.39-3.70 nmol/L
	10-15 yr	1.23-3.23 nmol/L
	Thereafter	1.77-2.93 nmol/L
Urea nitrogen		
Serum or plasma	Cord	7.5-14.3 mmol/L
	Premature (1 wk)	1.1-9 mmol/L
	Newborn	1.1-4.3 mmol/L
	Infant/child	1.8-6.4 mmol/L
	Thereafter	2.5-6.4 mmol/L
Urine volume		
Urine, 24 hr	Newborn	0.05-0.3 L/day
	Infant	0.35-0.5 L/day
	Child	0.5-1 L/day
	Adolescent	0.7-1.4 L/day
	Thereafter: Male	0.8-1.8 L/day
	Female	0.6-1.6 L/day (varies with intake and other factors)
WBC: see Leukocyte count (WBC count)		

(Modified from Kliegman, R. M., et al. [Eds.]. [2011]. *Nelson textbook of pediatrics* [19th ed.]. Philadelphia: Saunders; Crocetti, M., & Barone, M. A. [Eds.]. [2004]. *Oski's essential pediatrics* [2nd ed.]. Philadelphia: Lippincott Williams & Wilkins; and Fischbach, F., & Dunning, M. B. [2008]. *Manual of laboratory and diagnostic tests* [8th ed.]. Philadelphia: Lippincott Williams & Wilkins.)

Abbreviations Used in Laboratory Tests

ABBREVIATION	TERM	ABBREVIATION	TERM
cap	capillary	mol	mole
CHF	congestive heart failure	Na	sodium
conc.	concentration	Pa	Pascal
CSF	cerebrospinal fluid	RBC	red blood cells
EDTA	ethylenediaminetetraacetate	sec	second
g	gram	temp	temperature
Hgb	hemoglobin	therap.	therapeutic
HgbF	fetal hemoglobin	U	international unit of enzyme activity
hr	hour	vol	volume
IU	International unit	WBC	white blood cells
L	litre	wk	week
M	metre	yr	year
mEq	milliequivalent	$>$	greater than
min	minute	$\geq$	greater than or equal to
mm	millimetre	$<$	less than
mm Hg	millimetres of mercury	$\leq$	less than or equal to
mm H_2O	millimetres of water	$\pm$	plus/minus
mm^3	cubic millimetre	$\cong$	approximately equal to
mo	month		

Prefixes Denoting Decimal Factors

PREFIX	SYMBOL	AMOUNT
Deci	d	one tenth (10^{-1})
Centi	c	one hundredth (10^{-2})
Milli	m	one thousandth (10^{-3})
Micro	mc	one millionth (10^{-6})
Nano	n	one billionth (10^{-9})
Pico	p	one trillionth (10^{-12})
Femto	f	one quadrillionth (10^{-15})

Appendix E

Pediatric Vital Signs and Parameters

Centigrade to Fahrenheit Temperature Conversions

°C	°F	°C	°F	°C	°F
35.0	95.0	37.0	98.6	39.0	102.2
35.2	95.4	37.2	99.0	39.2	102.6
35.4	95.7	37.4	99.3	39.4	102.9
35.6	96.1	37.6	99.7	39.6	103.3
35.8	96.4	37.8	100.0	39.8	103.6
36.0	96.8	38.0	100.4	40.0	104.0
36.2	97.2	38.2	100.8	40.2	104.4
36.4	97.5	38.4	101.1	40.4	104.7
36.6	97.9	38.6	101.5	40.6	105.1
36.8	98.2	38.8	101.8	40.8	105.4
				41.0	105.8

Conversion Formulas

°F = (°C × 9/5) + 32 or (°C × 1.8) + 32
°C = (°F − 32) ÷ 5/9 or (°F − 32) ÷ 0.55

Normal Heart Rates for Infants and Children

	Rate (beats/min)	
AGE		EXERCISE (FEVER)
Newborn	100–180	Up to 220
1 wk to 3 mo	80–160	Up to 220
3 mo to 2 yr	70–150	Up to 200
2 yr to 10 yr	60–110	Up to 200
10 yr to adult	50–100	Up to 200

(From Gillette, P. C. [1989]. Dysrhythmias. In F. H. Adams, G. C. Emmanoulides, & T. A. Riemenschneider [Eds.], *Moss' heart disease in infants, children, and adolescents* [4th ed.]. Baltimore: Williams & Wilkins.

Normal Respiratory Rates for Children

AGE	RATE (BREATHS/MIN)
Newborn	30–60
1–11 mo	20–40
2 yr	20–40
4 yr	20–30
6–12 yr	16–22
13–18 yr	15–20

(From Kliegman, R. M., et al. [Eds.]. [2007]. *Nelson textbook of pediatrics* [18th ed.]. Philadelphia: Saunders.)

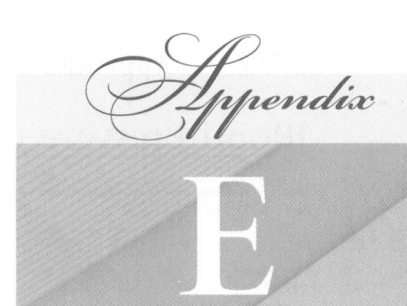

Blood Pressure (BP) Levels for Boys by Age and Height Percentile*

		Systolic BP (mm Hg) Percentile of Height							*Diastolic BP (mm Hg) Percentile of Height*						
AGE (YR)	**BP PERCENTILE**	**5TH**	**10TH**	**25TH**	**50TH**	**75TH**	**90TH**	**95TH**	**5TH**	**10TH**	**25TH**	**50TH**	**75TH**	**90TH**	**95TH**
1	50th	80	81	83	85	87	88	89	34	35	36	37	38	39	39
	90th	94	95	97	99	100	102	103	49	50	51	52	53	53	54
	95th	98	99	101	103	104	106	106	54	54	55	56	57	58	58
	99th	105	106	108	110	112	113	114	61	62	63	64	65	66	66
2	50th	84	85	87	88	90	92	92	39	40	41	42	43	44	44
	90th	97	99	100	102	104	105	106	54	55	56	57	58	58	59
	95th	101	102	104	106	108	109	110	59	59	60	61	62	63	63
	99th	109	110	111	113	115	117	117	66	67	68	69	70	71	71
3	50th	86	87	89	91	93	94	95	44	44	45	46	47	48	48
	90th	100	101	103	105	107	108	109	59	59	60	61	62	63	63
	95th	104	105	107	109	110	112	113	63	63	64	65	66	67	67
	99th	111	112	114	116	118	119	120	71	71	72	73	74	75	75
4	50th	88	89	91	93	95	96	97	47	48	49	50	51	51	52
	90th	102	103	105	107	109	110	111	62	63	64	65	66	66	67
	95th	106	107	109	111	112	114	115	66	67	68	69	70	71	71
	99th	113	114	116	118	120	121	122	74	75	76	77	78	78	79
5	50th	90	91	93	95	96	98	98	50	51	52	53	54	55	55
	90th	104	105	106	108	110	111	112	65	66	67	68	69	69	70
	95th	108	109	110	112	114	115	116	69	70	71	72	73	74	74
	99th	115	116	118	120	121	123	123	77	78	79	80	81	81	82
6	50th	91	92	94	96	98	99	100	53	53	54	55	56	57	57
	90th	105	106	108	110	111	113	113	68	68	69	70	71	72	72
	95th	109	110	112	114	115	117	117	72	72	73	74	75	76	76
	99th	116	117	119	121	123	124	125	80	80	81	82	83	84	84
7	50th	92	94	95	97	99	100	101	55	55	56	57	58	59	59
	90th	106	107	109	111	113	114	115	70	70	71	72	73	74	74
	95th	110	111	113	115	117	118	119	74	74	75	76	77	78	78
	99th	117	118	120	122	124	125	126	82	82	83	84	85	86	86
8	50th	94	95	97	99	100	102	102	56	57	58	59	60	60	61
	90th	107	109	110	112	114	115	116	71	72	72	73	74	75	76
	95th	111	112	114	116	118	119	120	75	76	77	78	79	79	80
	99th	119	120	122	123	125	127	127	83	84	85	86	87	87	88
9	50th	95	96	98	100	102	103	104	57	58	59	60	61	61	62
	90th	109	110	112	114	115	117	118	72	73	74	75	76	76	77
	95th	113	114	116	118	119	121	121	76	77	78	79	80	81	81
	99th	120	121	123	125	127	128	129	84	85	86	87	88	88	89
10	50th	97	98	100	102	103	105	106	58	59	60	61	61	62	63
	90th	111	112	114	115	117	119	119	73	73	74	75	76	77	78
	95th	115	116	117	119	121	122	123	77	78	79	80	81	81	82
	99th	122	123	125	127	128	130	130	85	86	86	88	88	89	90

		Systolic BP (mm Hg) Percentile of Height							Diastolic BP (mm Hg) Percentile of Height						
AGE (YR)	BP PERCENTILE	5TH	10TH	25TH	50TH	75TH	90TH	95TH	5TH	10TH	25TH	50TH	75TH	90TH	95TH
11	50th	99	100	102	104	105	107	107	59	59	60	61	62	63	63
	90th	113	114	115	117	119	120	121	74	74	75	76	77	78	78
	95th	117	118	119	121	123	124	125	78	78	79	80	81	82	82
	99th	124	125	127	129	130	132	132	86	86	87	88	89	90	90
12	50th	101	102	104	106	108	109	110	59	60	61	62	63	63	64
	90th	115	116	118	120	121	123	123	74	75	75	76	77	78	79
	95th	119	120	122	123	125	127	127	78	79	80	81	82	82	83
	99th	126	127	129	131	133	134	135	86	87	88	89	90	90	91
13	50th	104	105	106	108	110	111	112	60	60	61	62	63	64	64
	90th	117	118	120	122	124	125	126	75	75	76	77	78	79	79
	95th	121	122	124	126	128	129	130	79	79	80	81	82	83	83
	99th	128	130	131	133	135	136	137	87	87	88	89	90	91	91
14	50th	106	107	109	111	113	114	115	60	61	62	63	64	65	65
	90th	120	121	123	125	126	128	128	75	76	77	78	79	79	80
	95th	124	125	127	128	130	132	132	80	80	81	82	83	84	84
	99th	131	132	134	136	138	139	140	87	88	89	90	91	92	92
15	50th	109	110	112	113	115	117	117	61	62	63	64	65	66	66
	90th	122	124	125	127	129	130	131	76	77	78	79	80	80	81
	95th	126	127	129	131	133	134	135	81	81	82	83	84	85	85
	99th	134	135	136	138	140	142	142	88	89	90	91	92	93	93
16	50th	111	112	114	116	118	119	120	63	63	64	65	66	67	67
	90th	125	126	128	130	131	133	134	78	78	79	80	81	82	82
	95th	129	130	132	134	135	137	137	82	83	83	84	85	86	87
	99th	136	137	139	141	143	144	145	90	90	91	92	93	94	94
17	50th	114	115	116	118	120	121	122	65	66	66	67	68	69	70
	90th	127	128	130	132	134	135	136	80	80	81	82	83	84	84
	95th	131	132	134	136	138	139	140	84	85	86	87	87	88	89
	99th	139	140	141	143	145	146	147	92	93	93	94	95	96	97

*The 90th percentile is 1.28 standard deviation (SD), the 95th percentile is 1.645 SD, and the 99th percentile is 2.326 SD over the mean.

Blood Pressure (BP) Levels for Girls by Age and Height Percentile*

		Systolic BP (mm Hg) *Percentile of Height*							*Diastolic BP (mm Hg)* *Percentile of Height*						
AGE (YR)	BP PERCENTILE	5TH	10TH	25TH	50TH	75TH	90TH	95TH	5TH	10TH	25TH	50TH	75TH	90TH	95TH
1	50th	83	84	85	86	88	89	90	38	39	39	40	41	41	42
	90th	97	97	98	100	101	102	103	52	53	53	54	55	55	56
	95th	100	101	102	104	105	106	107	56	57	57	58	59	59	60
	99th	108	108	109	111	112	113	114	64	64	65	65	66	67	67
2	50th	85	85	87	88	89	91	91	43	44	44	45	46	46	47
	90th	98	99	100	101	103	104	105	57	58	58	59	60	61	61
	95th	102	103	104	105	107	108	109	61	62	62	63	64	65	65
	99th	109	110	111	112	114	115	116	69	69	70	70	71	72	72
3	50th	86	87	88	89	91	92	93	47	48	48	49	50	50	51
	90th	100	100	102	103	104	106	106	61	62	62	63	64	64	65
	95th	104	104	105	107	108	109	110	65	66	66	67	68	68	69
	99th	111	111	113	114	115	116	117	73	73	74	74	75	76	76
4	50th	88	88	90	91	92	94	94	50	50	51	52	52	53	54
	90th	101	102	103	104	106	107	108	64	64	65	66	67	67	68
	95th	105	106	107	108	110	111	112	68	68	69	70	71	71	72
	99th	112	113	114	115	117	118	119	76	76	76	77	78	79	79
5	50th	89	90	91	93	94	95	96	52	53	53	54	55	55	56
	90th	103	103	105	106	107	109	109	66	67	67	68	69	69	70
	95th	107	107	108	110	111	112	113	70	71	71	72	73	73	74
	99th	114	114	116	117	118	120	120	78	78	79	79	80	81	81
6	50th	91	92	93	94	96	97	98	54	54	55	56	56	57	58
	90th	104	105	106	108	109	110	111	68	68	69	70	70	71	72
	95th	108	109	110	111	113	114	115	72	72	73	74	74	75	76
	99th	115	116	117	119	120	121	122	80	80	80	81	82	83	83
7	50th	93	93	95	96	97	99	99	55	56	56	57	58	58	59
	90th	106	107	108	109	111	112	113	69	70	70	71	72	72	73
	95th	110	111	112	113	115	116	116	73	74	74	75	76	76	77
	99th	117	118	119	120	122	123	124	81	81	82	82	83	84	84
8	50th	95	95	96	98	99	100	101	57	57	57	58	59	60	60
	90th	108	109	110	111	113	114	114	71	71	71	72	73	74	74
	95th	112	112	114	115	116	118	118	75	75	75	76	77	78	78
	99th	119	120	121	122	123	125	125	82	82	83	83	84	85	86
9	50th	96	97	98	100	101	102	103	58	58	58	59	60	61	61
	90th	110	110	112	113	114	116	116	72	72	72	73	74	75	75
	95th	114	114	115	117	118	119	120	76	76	76	77	78	79	79
	99th	121	121	123	124	125	127	127	83	83	84	84	85	86	87
10	50th	98	99	100	102	103	104	105	59	59	59	60	61	62	62
	90th	112	112	114	115	116	118	118	73	73	73	74	75	76	76
	95th	116	116	117	119	120	121	122	77	77	77	78	79	80	80
	99th	123	123	125	126	127	129	129	84	84	85	86	86	87	88
11	50th	100	101	102	103	105	106	107	60	60	60	61	62	63	63
	90th	114	114	116	117	118	119	120	74	74	74	75	76	77	77
	95th	118	118	119	121	122	123	124	78	78	78	79	80	81	81
	99th	125	125	126	128	129	130	131	85	85	86	87	87	88	89

		Systolic BP (mm Hg)							Diastolic BP (mm Hg)						
		Percentile of Height							Percentile of Height						
AGE (YR)	**BP PERCENTILE**	**5TH**	**10TH**	**25TH**	**50TH**	**75TH**	**90TH**	**95TH**	**5TH**	**10TH**	**25TH**	**50TH**	**75TH**	**90TH**	**95TH**
12	50th	102	103	104	105	107	108	109	61	61	61	62	63	64	64
	90th	116	116	117	119	120	121	122	75	75	75	76	77	78	78
	95th	119	120	121	123	124	125	126	79	79	79	80	81	82	82
	99th	127	127	128	130	131	132	133	86	86	87	88	88	89	90
13	50th	104	105	106	107	109	110	110	62	62	62	63	64	65	65
	90th	117	118	119	121	122	123	124	76	76	76	77	78	79	79
	95th	121	122	123	124	126	127	128	80	80	80	81	82	83	83
	99th	128	129	130	132	133	134	135	87	87	88	89	89	90	91
14	50th	106	106	107	109	110	111	112	63	63	63	64	65	66	66
	90th	119	120	121	122	124	125	125	77	77	77	78	79	80	80
	95th	123	123	125	126	127	129	129	81	81	81	82	83	84	84
	99th	130	131	132	133	135	136	136	88	88	89	90	90	91	92
15	50th	107	108	109	110	111	113	113	64	64	64	65	66	67	67
	90th	120	121	122	123	125	126	127	78	78	78	79	80	81	81
	95th	124	125	126	127	129	130	131	82	82	82	83	84	85	85
	99th	131	132	133	134	136	137	138	89	89	90	91	91	92	93
16	50th	108	108	110	111	112	114	114	64	64	65	66	66	67	68
	90th	121	122	123	124	126	127	128	78	78	79	80	81	81	82
	95th	125	126	127	128	130	131	132	82	82	83	84	85	85	86
	99th	132	133	134	135	137	138	139	90	90	90	91	92	93	93
17	50th	108	109	110	111	113	114	115	64	65	65	66	67	67	68
	90th	122	122	123	125	126	127	128	78	79	79	80	81	81	82
	95th	125	126	127	129	130	131	132	82	83	83	84	85	85	86
	99th	133	133	134	136	137	138	139	90	90	91	91	92	93	93

(From U.S. Department of Health and Human Sciences, National Institutes of Health, National Heart, Lung, and Blood Institute. [2005]. *The fourth report on the diagnosis, evaluation, and treatment of high blood pressure in children and adolescents*. Retrieved from http://www.nhlbi.nih.gov/health/prof/heart/hbp/hbp_ped.pdf.)

*The 90th percentile is 1.28 standard deviation (SD), the 95th percentile is 1.645 SD, and the 99th percentile is 2.326 SD over the mean.

Index

A
AAMR Adaptive Behaviour Scale, 1190
Abbreviations used in laboratory tests, 1771t
Abdomen
 blunt trauma during pregnancy, 333–334
 of newborn, 626t–636t, 644
 nutritional status and, 887t–889t
 pediatric examination of, 922–924, 923f
 postpartum changes in, 528–529, 529f
Abdominal breathing, 401, 546f
Abdominal circumference
 of infant, 896f
 ultrasound assessment of, 280–281, 281f
Abdominal hernias, 1428t
Abdominal pain
 during pregnancy, 202
 recurrent, in school-age child, 1109
Abdominal palpation. *See* Leopold's manoeuvres
Abdominal thrusts. *See* Heimlich manoeuvre
Abnormal uterine bleeding (AUB)
 incidence/causes of, 92–93, 93b
 management of, 93–94
 nursing process, 94b
ABO incompatibility in neonate, 767–768
Aborted SIDS death. *See* Apparent life-threatening events (ALTEs)
Abortion
 complications from, 154b
 decriminalization of, 4b
 dilation and evacuation, 154
 emotional considerations, 154–155
 medical, 154
 medical induction of, 154
 overview, 152–153
 surgical, 153–154
Abruptio placentae
 clinical manifestations of, 324t, 326–327, 326f
 collaborative care, 327b, 328
 incidence/etiology of, 326
 maternal/fetal outcomes, 327
Absence seizures, 1594b–1595b, 1596t
Absorptive defects, 1433
Abstract thinking, 1119
Abuse
 child, 1000
  caregiver-child interaction in, 1075–1076
  child neglect in, 1072
Abuse *(Continued)*
  clinical manifestations of, 1077b–1078b
  history/interview in, 1076
  nursing care for, 1075
   discharge plan, 1079
   guidelines for recording data, 1079b
   physical assessment in, 1076–1078
   supporting child/family, 1078–1079
   talking with children who reveal abuse, 1075b
  physical abuse and, 1072–1073
  prevention of, 1079–1080
  protection from further, 1078
  sexual abuse and. *See* Sexual abuse
  warning signs of, 1075b
 of women. *See also* Intimate partner violence (IPV)
  anticipatory guidance for, 56–61, 58f
  prenatal identification of, 215–216
  screening for, 71–72, 72f
Accelerations of fetal heart rate, 433, 433b, 433f
Acceptance of maternal role, 206–207
Accidental decannulation, 1307–1308
Accomplishment, school-age children and, 1085–1087, 1087f
Accreditation Canada Home Care Services, 1222
Acculturation, 21, 829
Acetabular dysplasia, 775
Acetaminophen
 children and, 943, 944t, 947t
 normal test ranges for, 1764t–1771t
 poisoning from, 1437b–1438b
Achilles reflex test, 929f
Acid indigestion during pregnancy, 202
Acid-base balance during pregnancy, 198
Acidemia, 439, 439t
Acknowledgement, with special needs child, 1163–1164
Acne, 1668–1669
Acquired heart disease
 pediatric
  bacterial endocarditis and, 1481–1483, 1482b
  cardiac dysrhythmias and, 1485–1487, 1486b
  cardiomyopathy and, 1487–1488
  hyperlipidemia and, 1484–1485, 1484t
  pulmonary hypertension and, 1487
  rheumatic fever and, 1483–1484, 1483b
Acquired heart disease *(Continued)*
 in pregnancy, 355–356, 356b
Acquired immunodeficiency syndrome (AIDS)
 in children
  clinical manifestations of, 1527, 1527b
  diagnosis of, 1527–1528
  management of, 1528–1529
  nursing care for, 1529–1530
 pregnancy and, 371–373
Acroesthesia, 200–201
Acromegaly, 1613
Across-the-lap position, 684–685, 685f
Activated charcoal, 1439–1440
Activities of daily living, special needs child and, 1169
Activity
 adolescents and, 1127, 1127f
 cognitively impaired children and, 1192–1193
 infants and, 981–983
 preschoolers and, 1060
 school-age children and, 1097–1098
 toddlers and, 1034
Actualizing perinatal loss, 603, 605–606, 606f
Acupressure
 education in, 247
 for labour pain management, 406, 406f
 for nausea and vomiting, 267–268, 268f
Acupuncture, labour pain management and, 406
Acute adrenocortical insufficiency, 1622–1623, 1622b
Acute appendicitis, 1408–1409, 1409b
Acute bacterial meningitis, 1586–1589
Acute chest syndrome (ACS), 1505–1507
Acute diarrhea, 1392, 1393t–1395t
Acute epiglottitis, 1329–1330, 1330t
Acute glomerulonephritis (AGN), 1549–1551, 1550b
Acute hematogenous osteomyelitis, 1710–1712, 1711b
Acute hepatitis, 1416–1419, 1417t
Acute hypertension, 1550
Acute illness, definition of, 793
Acute laryngitis, 1330–1331, 1330t
Acute laryngotracheobronchitis, 1330t, 1331–1332, 1331b
Acute lung injury (ALI), 1342–1343
Acute lymphoid leukemia (ALL), 1517–1518. *See also* Leukemias
Acute nonlymphoid leukemia (ANLL), 1517–1518. *See also* Leukemias
Acute otitis media (AOM), 976, 1325–1328, 1326b–1327b
Acute overload injuries, 1103
Acute poststreptococcal glomerulonephritis (APSGN), 1549–1551, 1550b
Acute renal failure (ARF), 1553–1555, 1554b, 1556b
 dialysis and, 1559–1560
Acute respiratory distress syndrome (ARDS), 1342–1343
Acute spasmodic laryngitis, 1330t, 1332
Acute streptococcal pharyngitis, 1321–1322, 1322f
Acute supraglottitis, 1329–1330
Acute symptomatic seizures, 1593, 1593b
Acute wounds, 1643
Acyanotic heart lesions, 353–354
Acyclovir
 for HSV infection, 104
 for immunocompromised children, 1063
Adams test, 1708
Adaptation to grandparenthood, 572–574, 573f
Adaptation to parenthood, 549. *See also* Parenthood
Adaptation to pregnancy
 grandparent, 210, 212b, 213f
 maternal. *See* Maternal adaptations
 paternal, 208–210, 208b, 209f
 physiological
  breasts, 192–193
  cardiovascular system, 193–195, 194f, 197t
  endocrine system, 203, 203t
  gastrointestinal system, 201–202
  integumentary system, 199–200
  musculoskeletal system, 200, 201f
  neurological system, 200–201
  normal, 298b
  in relation to trauma, 332, 333t
  renal system, 198–199, 199t
  respiratory system, 195–198
  signs of, 188, 189t
  uterus, 188–191
  vagina/vulva, 191–192
 sexual, 207–208
 sibling, 210, 211b–212b, 211f
Addiction, 940b, 952–953, 1509b
Addison's disease, 1623–1624, 1623b
Adenoidectomy, 1323
 for obstructive sleep-disordered breathing, 1364
 for otitis media, 1327
Adenoids, 1322, 1323f
Adequate intake (AI), dietary, 890

Page numbers followed by *f* indicate figures; *t,* tables; and *b,* boxes.

Adherence. *See* Compliance
Adherent retained placenta, 579
Adjustment to diagnosis of special needs child, 1163
Adjuvant analgesics for children, 943, 946t
Adjuvant chemotherapy for breast cancer, 120
Administration of medications
during labour
intramuscular route, 418
intravenous route, 418
nursing care/safety in, 419–420
preparation for, 418–419
signs of complications, 419
spinal/epidural nerve blocks, 419
timing of, 418
pediatric
checking dosage and, 1287–1288
colour-coded instructions, 1298b
determination of dosage and, 1286–1288
immunizations, 992–993
intramuscular, 1289–1293, 1290t–1291t, 1292b, 1293f
intravenous, 1293–1295, 1294f, 1295t
nasogastric/orogastric/gastrostomy, 1295–1296, 1296b
optic/otic/nasal, 1296–1297, 1297f
oral, 1288–1289, 1288b, 1289f
patient/family teaching for, 1297–1298, 1298b
rectal, 1296
subcutaneous/intradermal, 1293
Admission assessment for hospitalization, 1238–1241, 1239b–1241b, 1241f
Admission data, 445–447, 447b
Admission electronic fetal monitor strips, 430
Admission to labour unit, 445, 445f
Adolescence, 845
Adolescent atopic dermatitis, 1665–1667, 1666b
Adolescent idiopathic scoliosis, 1707f–1708f, 1708–1710
Adolescent Pediatric Pain Tool (APPT), 936
Adolescent pregnancy
health risks in, 46
nutritional needs in, 263
parenthood and, 567–568
prenatal care for, 238–240, 238f, 239b
Adolescents, 833f
adopted, 818
alcohol use by, 791–792
amenorrhea and, 1133–1134
anorexia nervosa/bulimia nervosa and
diagnosis of, 1142–1143, 1142b
etiology/pathophysiology of, 1141–1142
incidence of, 1141
Adolescents *(Continued)*
management of, 1143
nursing care for, 1143–1144
anticipatory guidance in parenting, 1133, 1134b
biological development of
hormonal changes during, 1114
physical growth, 1115–1117
physiological changes, 1117
sexual maturation, 1114–1115, 1114b
cigarette smoking and, 1144–1146
cognitive development in, 1119
cognitively impaired, sexuality and, 1194
communicating with, 875–876, 876b, 1120b
dental health for, 1127
dysmenorrhea and, 1134–1135
early sexual maturation and, 1145b
exercise/activity of, 1127, 1127f
growth/development overview, 1121t
gynecomastia and, 1135–1136
health assessment of, 72
health care for, 45–47, 46b
health promotion for, 1124
hospitalization of
loss of control and, 1236
separation anxiety in, 1234
immunizations for, 1125
injury prevention for
education in, 1132b
firearm injuries, 1132–1133
sports injuries, 1133
vehicle-related injuries, 1131–1132
male reproductive system disorders in, 1135
mental health and, 1129
moral development in, 1119
nutrition for, 1125–1127
obesity and
diagnosis of, 1137–1138
etiology/pathophysiology of, 1136–1137, 1137t
incidence of, 1136
management of, 1138
nursing care for, 1138–1139, 1139b
behavioural therapy in, 1140, 1140b
group/family involvement, 1140
nutritional counselling in, 1139–1140
physical activity, 1140
prevention, 1140–1141
personal care and, 1127–1129
preparation for procedures, 1262b–1263b
psychosocial development of, 1117–1119
respecting privacy of, 1125b
responses to puberty, 1124
self-concept/body image development in, 1123–1124
sexual health for
pregnancy/abortion/birth control and, 1131
sex education and, 1130–1131
Adolescents *(Continued)*
sexual history of, 881–882
sexuality and, 1122–1123, 1123f
sleep/rest for, 1127
social development in
interests/activities, 1122
relationships with parents and, 1119–1120
relationships with peers and, 1120–1122, 1120f
with special needs, 1171t–1172t, 1173–1174
spiritual development in, 1119
stress reduction for, 1129–1130, 1129b, 1129f
substance use by, 1146–1149
suicide and
defined/incidence of, 1149
diagnosis/management of, 1151, 1151b
etiology of, 1149–1150
methods of, 1150
motivation for, 1150–1151
nursing care for, 1151–1152
sexual orientation and, 1150b
warning signs of, 1150b
understanding/reactions to death, 1177t–1178t
vaginitis and, 1135
vulnerability of, 33–34
Adoption
cross-racial/international, 818–819
infertility and, 135, 135f
parenting and, 817–819
Adrenal disorders
acute adrenocortical insufficiency, 1622–1623, 1622b
chronic adrenocortical insufficiency, 1623–1624, 1623b
congenital adrenal hyperplasia, 1625–1626
Cushing's syndrome, 1624–1625, 1624f
pheochromocytoma, 1625–1626
Adrenalectomy, 1625b
Adrenalin. *See* Epinephrine
Adrenarche, 1114, 1116f
Advanced cardiac life support (ACLS) protocol, 362
Advanced life support (ALS) facility, 1366
Adventitious sounds, 919–921
Advil. *See* Ibuprofen
Aerosol therapy, 1304
Aerosolizer, 1349
Affect, in sensorimotor development, 965
African ethnicity
breast cancer in, 116f
cosleeping and, 1009b
diabetes mellitus and, 1627t, 1639
health beliefs/practices and, 840t–841t
lactase deficiency and, 834–835, 1503
practices regarding newborns and, 660b
reactions to pain and, 396b
sickle cell anemia in, 216–217, 364, 656t, 1505
Wilms' tumour in, 1552
African ethnicity *(Continued)*
Afterpains, 527
Age
childbirth risks and, 45–47
differences, prenatal care and, 238–240
respiratory infections and, 1317
transition to parenthood and, 567–569
Agent, in epidemiological triangle, 803
Age-specific death rate, 803b
Aggression, in preschoolers, 1058
Agnosia, 1199
Agonal, 920b
Agranulocytosis, 350
Airborne precautions, 1277–1278, 1277b
Airguns, injuries involving, 1133
Airplane splints, 1680f
Airway maintenance
anaphylaxis and, 1495
for CPR, 1366–1367, 1366f
for Duchenne muscular dystrophy, 1742
eclampsia and, 307, 307b
for laryngotracheobronchitis, 1331
for neonates, 644–646, 645f
in unconscious child, 1570
Airway obstruction clearing
in children, 1370, 1370f
in infants, 1368–1370, 1368f
Akinetic seizures, 1594b–1595b
Alaskan Natives, breast cancer and, 116f
Albumin, nephrotic syndrome and, 1547
Alcohol
adolescent use of, 791–792, 1147
childbirth risks with, 47
education about, 229–230
fetal exposure to, 757–759, 758b
interventions for abuse of, 55–56
Alcoholism, 47, 229
Alcohol-related neurodevelopment disorder (ARND), 757–759
Aldactone
breastfeeding and, 1753t–1756t
for congestive heart failure, 1468b, 1469t
Aldosterone, 1623–1624
Alertness, 1563
All fours position, 462b, 462f
Alleles, 163
Allen card test, 910
Allergens
avoidance, asthma and, 1352
control, asthma and, 1348–1349, 1348b
Allergies
breastfeeding and, 676–677
guidelines for, 880b
pediatric health history of, 880
Allergy Asthma Information Association, 1386
Allograft skin coverings, 1676
All-or-none law, 1695
Alopecia, 1524, 1553
Alterations in menstrual cycle, 91–92
Altered states of consciousness, 1563–1564, 1564b

Alternate-cover eye test, 909–910, 910f
Alternative therapies. *See* Complementary and alternative medicine (CAM)
Alveoli, 67, 68f, 176, 610, 710, 716–717
Ambiguous genitalia
 congenital adrenal hyperplasia and, 1625–1626
 in newborns, 626t–636t, 777, 777f
 surgery for, 1546t
Ambivalence, regarding pregnancy, 207
Amblyopia, 909–910, 910f, 1204, 1204b–1205b
Ambulation
 after childbirth, 544–545
 during labour, 458t, 460–461, 461f
 play activities for, 1266b
Ambulatory setting, 1253, 1254b
Amelia, 1703
Amenorrhea
 in adolescents, 1133–1134
 assessment of, 84–85
 hypogonadotropic, 85
American Academy of Allergy, Asthma, and Immunology, 1384
American Dietetic Association, 1380
American Heart Association, 1366
American Sign Language (ASL), 1202
Amitriptyline, 946t
Ammonium nitrogen, 1764t–1771t
Amniocentesis
 fetal rights and, 285b
 monitoring pregnancy risks, 282–284, 282t, 283f
 ultrasound adjunct to, 285b
Amnioinfusion, 438–439
Amnion, development of, 172–173, 172f
Amniotic fluid
 assessment of, 456, 456t
 functions of, 173
 meconium-stained, 476
 smoking/caffeine and, 47
Amniotic fluid embolism (AFE), 523–524, 524b
Amniotic fluid volume (AFV), 289–291
Amniotic infection syndrome, 221
Amniotic membranes, 456
Amniotomy
 for inducing labour, 508
 procedure for, 508b
 purpose of, 456
Amoxicillin
 for chlamydia during pregnancy, 98
 for otitis media, 1327
Amphetamines, 48–49
Amputation, 1698–1699
 osteosarcoma and, 1713–1714
Anaclitic depression. *See* Separation anxiety
Anaesthesia
 fasting recommendations for, 1267t
 for hospitalized children, 1265–1267
Anaesthesia *(Continued)*
 for labour pain management, 407–416, 408b
 maternal hypothermia after, 421
 nerve block, 410–416
 in obese women, 420–421
 preoperative sedation, 1267
Anal reflex, 926
Anal stage of psychosexual development, 851
Analgesia
 breastfeeding and, 1753t–1756t
 after childbirth, 543–544
 for children, 943–944, 944t–946t
  epidural, 947–950
  equianalgesia in, 947t
  evaluating effectiveness of, 953–955
  patient-controlled, 944–947
  routes/methods of administration, 948b–949b
  timing of, 951
  transmucosal/transdermal, 950–951
 defined, 407
 during labour
  maternal hypothermia after, 421
  nerve block analgesia/anaesthesia, 410–416
   combined spinal-epidural, 415
   epidural, 413–415, 414f
   epidural/intrathecal opioids, 415–416
   local infiltration anaesthesia, 410
   nitrous oxide, 416
   postdural puncture headache in, 412–413, 413f
   pudendal nerve block, 410–411, 411f
  nursing care for
   administration of medication, 418–420
   informed consent, 416–418
   safety and general care, 419–420
   signs of potential problems, 419
  systemic, 408–410
   opioid agonist-antagonists, 409, 409b
   opioid agonists, 408–409, 409b
   opioid antagonists, 409–410, 410b
  types of, 408b
 for major burns, 1675
Anaphylactoid syndrome of pregnancy, 523–524, 524b
Anaphylaxis
 in children, 1494–1495
 emergency intervention for, 1494b
 to food allergens, 1386
 during pain management in labour, 419
Anatomical defects, 1433
Androgens, during puberty, 1114
Android pelvis, 383, 384t
Anemia
 in children
  aplastic, 1511–1512, 1512b
  beta-thalassemia, 1510–1511, 1511b
  chronic renal failure and, 1556, 1558
  classification of, 1500–1502, 1502b, 1502f
  consequences of, 1502
  diagnosis of, 1502
  iron deficiency, 1503–1505
  leukemia and, 1522–1523
  management of, 1502–1503
  nursing care for, 1503
  sickle cell, 1505–1510, 1506b, 1506f, 1508b
 in high-risk pregnancy
  folic acid deficiency, 364
  iron deficiency, 364
  overview, 362–364
  sickle cell hemoglobinopathy, 364
  thalassemia, 364–365
Anencephaly, 768–770, 1733b
Aneuploidy, 163–164
Angel dust, 761
Angiomas, 199, 231t–233t, 532
Animal bites, 1000, 1663, 1663b
Animism, 1025b, 1057
Anisometropia, 1204b–1205b
Ankle-foot orthoses, 1726
Anorectal malformations, 774–775, 774f, 1431–1433, 1432b
Anorexia nervosa
 in adolescents, 1126
 amenorrhea and, 85
 chemotherapy and, 1523
 health risks of, 50, 50b
 in school-age children, 1109
Antenatal conditions, fetal risk and, 425t
Antenatal data, for admission, 445–446
Antenatal glucocorticoid therapy, 496–497, 497b
Antepartum care. *See* Prenatal care
Anterior fontanel pressure monitor, 1570
Anthropoid pelvis, 383, 384t
Anthropometry, 890
Antiarrhythmias during pregnancy, 360t
Antibiotics
 cystic fibrosis and, 1359
 for pediatric respiratory infections, 1320
 yeast infections and, 109
Antibody-antigen response, 1084
Anticholinergics, asthma and, 1350
Anticipatory grief, 1183
 cystic fibrosis and, 1364
Anticipatory guidance
 adolescence and, 882b, 1133, 1134b
 health risk prevention and, 56, 56b
 health screening schedule and, 56, 57t
 infants and, 1003, 1003b
 during interviews, 872
 intimate partner violence and, 56–61, 58f
Anticipatory guidance *(Continued)*
 for lead poisoning, 1444
 for otitis media, 1328
 substance use and, 55–56
 toddlers and, 1045b, 1046
Anticoagulants
 breastfeeding and, 1753t–1756t
 contraindicating epidural blocks, 416
 for deep venous thrombosis, 585–586, 586b
 during pregnancy, 355, 359–360, 360t
Anticonvulsants
 breastfeeding and, 1753t–1756t
 for children, 946t
Anti-D antibody therapy, 1515, 1515b
Antidepressants
 children and, 946t
 postpartum depression and, 594, 598
Antiepileptic medications, 1597, 1599–1603
 cerebral palsy and, 1727
Antihemophilic factor (AHF), 1513
Antihistamines, breastfeeding and, 1753t–1756t
Antihypertensive therapy, 305, 306t, 1490
Anti-infectives, breastfeeding and, 1753t–1756t
Anti-inflammatory drugs, breastfeeding and, 1753t–1756t
Antilymphocyte globulin (ALG), 1512
Antimicrobial medications, for burns, 1675–1676, 1676t
Antipsychotic medications for postpartum depression, 596, 596t, 598–599
Antipyretics, 1273, 1572
Antiretroviral therapy (ART), 752–753
 HIV infection in children and, 1528–1529
Antismoking programs, 1145–1146
Antistreptolysin O titre, 1764t–1771t
Antithymocyte globulin (ATG), 1512
Anus
 assessment of newborn, 626t–636t
 examination of pediatric, 926
 imperforate, 774–775, 774f
Anxiolytics, for children, 946t
Aortic valve stenosis, 354, 1460b–1462b
Apgar scoring
 for neonatal assessment, 642–643, 643t
 significance of, 643b
Aphasia, 1199
Apheresis, hematological/immunological disorders and, 1533–1534
Apical impulse
 in infants/children, 901, 920f
 in newborns, 610–611, 637
 in pregnancy, 193

Aplastic anemia (AA), 1511–1512, 1512b
Apnea
  definition of, 1364
  of infancy, 1012–1015, 1014b, 1014f
  of prematurity, 1012
Apparent life-threatening events (ALTEs), 1012–1013
  diagnosis/management of, 1013
  family support for, 1014–1015
  nursing care for, 1013–1014, 1014f
  patient education for, 1014b
Appendicitis, 1408–1409
  in children, 1409b
  during pregnancy, 330
Appendix, displacement of, 202, 202f
Appetite
  after childbirth, 530
  during hospitalization, 1272
  during pregnancy, 201–202
Approach behaviours, 1162, 1162b
Apt test, 285b
Arm circumference, measurement of, 896–897
Arm raises, 546f
Arnold-Chiari malformation, 1605
Aromatase inhibitors, 121
Aromatherapy for pain management, 406–407
Arrangement of skin lesions, 1643
Arterial blood gas (ABG) levels in newborns, 728, 728t
Arterial blood samples, 1285
Arteriovenous fistulas/grafts, 1559
Arthritis
  juvenile idiopathic, 1716–1719, 1720b
  septic, 1712
Arthropod bites/stings, 1657–1663, 1658t
Artificial airways, 1304–1305
Artificial skin, 1677
Artificial sweeteners during pregnancy, 257, 259t
Artificial tanning, 1129
Artificial ventilation, 1304–1308
Ascaris lumbricoides, 1406t
Ascorbic acid, 262, 1376t–1379t
Aseptic meningitis, 1589–1590, 1590t
Ashkenazi Jews, 45, 158, 831, 1411
Asian ethnicity
  breast cancer and, 116f
  cosleeping and, 1009b
  diabetes mellitus and, 1627t, 1639
  health beliefs/practices and, 840t–841t
  lactase deficiency and, 834–835, 1503
  practices regarding newborns and, 660b
  reactions to pain and, 396b
  sickle cell anemia and, 216–217, 656t
ASKED model of cultural competence, 840b
Asphyxia
  fetal responses to, 286
  high-risk infants and, 710
  in newborns, 715
  perinatal, 736
Asphyxiation
  from FB aspiration, 1341
  during infancy, 993–996
  submersion injuries and, 1581–1582
Aspiration abortion, 153–154
Aspiration of fluid, 1582
Aspiration of foreign objects
  during infancy, 993–996
  toddlers and, 1044–1045
Aspiration pneumonia, 1341–1342
Aspirin
  anticoagulant therapy and, 586b
  for children, 947t
  poisoning from, 1437b–1438b
Assent, for pediatric procedures, 1260
Assisted hatching, 134t
Assisted Human Reproduction Act, 133
Assisted reproductive technologies (ARTs)
  complications in, 133–134
  for infertility, 133–134, 133f
  issues regarding, 133b
  list of, 134t
  multiple pregnancies and, 8
Assisted suicide, 1175
Assisted ventilation for respiratory distress, 716t
Association of Women's Health, Obstetric and Neonatal Nurses (AWHONN), 9, 10b
Associative play, 857, 857f, 1054
Asthma
  allergen control for, 1348–1349, 1348b
  avoidance of allergens and, 1352
  care for acute asthma, 1355, 1355f–1356f
  chest physiotherapy for, 1350–1351
  diagnosis/manifestations of, 1346–1347, 1346b–1347b
  etiology of, 1345
  exercise and, 1350
  hyposensitization in, 1351
  incidence of, 1344–1345
  management of, 1347–1352
  medication therapy and, 1349–1350
  nursing care for, 1352–1356, 1353b
  pathophysiology of, 1345–1346, 1346f
  during pregnancy, 365–366
  prognosis in, 1351
  relieving bronchospasms, 1352–1355
    metered-dose inhalers for, 1354b, 1354f
    PEFMs for, 1354b
  severity classification, 365t
  status asthmaticus and, 1351–1352
  supportive care for, 1356
  triggers for, 1345b
Asthma Society of Canada, 1346, 1351, 1355
Astigmatism, 1204b–1205b
Asymmetrical macrosomia, 342
Asymptomatic bacteriuria, 1541–1542
Asynclitism, 389, 390f
Ataxic cerebral palsy, 1725b–1726b
Athetoid movements, 1725b
Atonic seizures, 1594b–1595b
Atopic dermatitis, 1665–1667, 1666b
Atopy
  asthma and, 1345
  food sensitivity and, 1386–1387
  prevention of, 1387b
Atraumatic care in pediatric nursing, 794
Atresia
  biliary, 1419–1420, 1420b
  choanal, 770–771, 771f
  esophageal, 772–773, 773f
Atrial septal defects (ASDs)
  in children, 1457b–1459b
  pregnancy and, 353
Atrioventricular canal defects, 1457b–1459b
Attachment
  assessment of, 558, 559b
  behaviours affecting, 556–560, 557t–558t
  biorhythmicity and, 561
  entrainment and, 561
  infants and, 966
  interventions for, 559t
  parent-infant communication and, 560–562
  parent-infant contact and, 558–560, 560f
  reciprocity/synchrony/habituation and, 561–562
Attention-deficit/hyperactivity disorder (ADHD), 1106–1107
Attitude, fetal, 379, 380f–382f
Atypical pneumonias, 1336
Auditory stimulation
  for infants, 969t
  unconscious child and, 1573
Auditory tests for infants/children, 915, 915t
Augmentation of labour, 511
Aural temperature, 897–901, 899t, 900b–902b
Auscultation
  in cardiovascular assessment, 1452
  pediatric
    of abdomen, 923
    of heart, 921–922, 922t
    of lungs, 919–920, 919b
Authoritarian parenting, 814
Authoritative parenting, 814, 1120
Autism spectrum disorders (ASDs)
  clinical manifestations/diagnosis of, 1212–1213, 1212b
  epidemiology of, 1210
  etiology of, 1210–1212
  nursing care for, 1213
  thimerosal-containing vaccines and, 1211b
Autoimmune disorders, pregnancy and, 369–370
Automobile air bags, 997
Autonomic drugs, breastfeeding and, 1753t–1756t
Autonomy vs. shame/doubt in psychosocial development, 852, 1022
Autopsy
  of children, 1182–1183
  of newborns, 603
Autosomal dominant inheritance disorders, 166–167, 166f
Autosomal recessive inheritance disorders, 167
Avian influenza virus, 1324
Avoidance behaviours, 1162, 1162b
Avulsed permanent tooth, 1099, 1099b
Axillary dissection, for breast cancer, 118
Axillary lymph nodes, 118, 119f
Axillary temperature, 897–901, 899t, 900b–902b
Azithromycin, 98
Azotemia, 1553

B
Babinski reflex, 620, 622t–625t, 624f, 1566–1567
Baby powder, aspiration of, 996
Baby-Friendly Hospital Initiative (BFHI), 11, 699–700
Baby-sitters, 976
Bacille Calmette-Guérin (BCG) vaccine, 1339–1340
Bacitracin, 1676t
Back pain
  during labour, 461, 463b, 464
    fetal malposition and, 499–500
    intradermal sterile water block for, 407, 407f
    transcutaneous electrical nerve stimulation for, 405, 405f
  during pregnancy, 224, 224f
Backs
  of children, 926–927
  of newborns, 626t–636t
Bacterial endocarditis, 1481–1483, 1482b
Bacterial infections
  chlamydia, 98, 755–756
  gonorrhea, 98–99, 221, 750
  group B streptococcus, 221, 446, 755
  neonatal, 755–756
  osteomyelitis and, 1710–1712
  pelvic inflammatory disease and, 100
  in septic arthritis, 1712
  of skin, 1651–1655, 1652t
  syphilis, 99–100, 99f, 750–751, 751f
  tuberculosis, 755
Bacterial pneumonias, 1336
Bacterial tracheitis, 1330t, 1332
Bacterial vaginosis, 108–109, 109t
Bacteriuria, 1541–1542
Balance suspension traction, 1696, 1696f
Balloon atrioseptostomy, 1453, 1453t
Balloon catheters, 508
Ballottement of fetus, 190–191, 192f
Bandl's ring, 384f, 499
Barbiturate coma, 1572
Bariatric surgery, 1138

Bariatric women, pregnancy and. *See* Obesity, maternal
Barlow test, 775
Barrier contraceptives
cervical cap, 143f, 144–147, 147b
contraceptive sponge, 143f, 147
diaphragm, 143–144, 143f, 145b–146b
female condoms, 143, 143f
male condoms, 142–143, 144b
spermicides, 142, 142f
Barton tong traction, 1697, 1697f
Basal body temperature (BBT) method, 138–139, 139b, 139f
Basal metabolic rate (BMR)
changes during pregnancy, 197
fluid loss in infants and, 1390
Base excess, 1764t–1771t
Baseline fetal heart rate, 430–431, 430t, 432f, 432t
Baseline measurements of neonatal physical growth, 626t–636t, 637
Basil insulin, 1631b
Basilar skull fractures, 1576
Bathing
during hospitalization, 1271
during labour, 403–405, 404f
newborns, 670, 671b–672b, 672f
during pregnancy, 222
Battered women. *See* Intimate partner violence (IPV)
Batteries, ingestion of, 998
Battledore placenta, 328, 329f
Bearing-down efforts, 468–478, 469t
Bed bugs, 1661, 1661b, 1661f
Bed rest
adverse effects of, 493b
children's activities during, 494b
preventing preterm labour, 493–494
suggested activities for, 494b
Bed sharing, 1009, 1034
Beds, infant safety and, 996
Bed-wetting, 1107–1108
Behaviour modification theory, 816
Behavioural characteristics
of newborns, 637–641, 637b
additional factors in, 638–639
in Brazelton Neonatal Behavioural Assessment Scale, 637b
response to environmental stimuli, 640–641
sensory behaviours and, 639–640
sleep-wake states, 638
Behavioural contracting, 941b, 1144
Behavioural pain assessment scales for infants/children, 936t
Behavioural repertoires in parent-infant interactions, 566
Behavioural strategies for treatment compliance, 1270
Behavioural therapy for adolescent obesity, 1140, 1140b
BELIEF framework, 837b, 1223b
Bell's Palsy, 369
Bereavement. *See* Grief
Beta-adrenergic agonists, asthma and, 1349–1350
Beta-endorphins, labour pain and, 396
Betamethasone therapy, 496–497, 497b
Beta-thalassemia, 1510–1511, 1511b
Bibliotherapy, 877b–878b
Bicarbonate, 1764t–1771t
Biceps reflex test, 929f
Bicornuate uterus, 129f, 132
Bicycle injuries, 1101, 1101f, 1103b
Bidirectional Glenn shunt, 1476t
Bieri Faces Pain Scale, 935–936, 937t
Bilateral electric breast pumps, 692, 693f
Bile acid–binding resins, 1484–1485
Biliary atresia, 1419–1420, 1420b
Bilious vomiting, 1403
Bilirubin
conjugation of, 652–655
formation/excretion of, 615, 615f
jaundice and, 652–654
normal test ranges for, 1764t–1771t
pregnant vs. nonpregnant values of, 196t–197t
Billings method, 139, 140b
Bimanual palpation, 77–78, 79f
Binge eating. *See* Bulimia nervosa
Biochemical assessment of fetal health
amniocentesis in, 282–284, 283f
chorionic villus sampling in, 284–285, 285f
Coombs' test in, 281–282
overview of, 282t
percutaneous umbilical blood sampling in, 284, 284f
ultrasound as adjunct in, 285
Biochemical markers in preterm labour, 489
Biofeedback
education in, 247
for labour pain management, 406
Biological development
of adolescents
hormonal changes during, 1114
physical growth, 1115–1117
physiological changes, 1117
sexual maturation, 1114–1115, 1114b
childhood
determinants in, 846–848, 847t
external proportions, 846
lymphoid tissues and, 848
neurological maturation, 848
organ systems, 848
physical growth, 846–848, 847t
skeletal growth, 848
of infants
fine motor development, 960
gross motor development, 960–963
Biological development *(Continued)*
maturation of systems, 959–960
proportional changes in, 958–959
of preschoolers, 1049–1052
of school-age children, 1084–1085
of toddlers
gross/fine motor development, 1021–1022
maturation of systems, 1021
proportional changes, 1020–1021
sensory changes, 1021
Biological skin coverings, 1676–1677
Biophysical profile (BPP), 289, 290t
Biopsy
bone marrow, 1282
celiac disease and, 1433
endometrial, 93, 129t
lymph node, 1525
renal, 1538t–1539t
Biorhythmicity, parent-infant bonding and, 561, 562f
Biot respiration, 920b
Biparietal diameter (BPD), 280, 280f
Birth. *See* Childbirth
Birth and death registrations, 8
Birth balls, 461, 463f
Birth canal
bony pelvis, 380–383, 382f
soft tissues, 383–385
Birth centres, 242–243, 243f
Birth control. *See* Contraception
Birth plans, 246, 246b
Birth rates
multiple, 8
as perinatal health indicator, 7b, 8
preterm/postterm, 8
teenage pregnancies and, 46
Birth settings
birth centres, 242–243, 243f
choice of, 11, 11b, 241–242
home birth, 243
labour, delivery, recovery, and postpartum rooms, 242–243, 242f
Birth spacing, 137b
Birth trauma
maternal
cystocele/rectocele, 589–590, 590f
genital fistulas, 590–591, 591f
urinary incontinence, 590, 591f
uterine displacement/prolapse, 589, 589f
neonatal
CNS injuries, 746
nursing care for, 744–746
overview, 743–744
perinatal asphyxia and, 736
physical injuries, 651–652
PNS injuries, 744–746
skeletal injuries, 744–746, 744f
types of, 744t
Birth weight
gestational maturity and, 649f–650f
infant mortality and, 792–793
Birthing beds, 472, 472f
Birthing chairs, 471
Birthing From Within method, 401
Birthing rooms, 474–475, 474f
Birthing stools, 243f, 471
Bisexuality, adolescents and, 1123
Bishop score, 506, 507t
Biting, infants and, 964
Black Canadians. *See* African ethnicity
Black eye, emergency intervention for, 1206b
Bladder
catheterization of
during labour, 458t, 460
pediatric, 1283–1285, 1284t
changes during pregnancy, 193f, 198–199, 199t
exstrophy of, in newborns, 777, 777f
postpartum changes in, 530, 545
preventing distention of, 543
ultrasound of, 1538t–1539t
Blastocyst, 171, 171f
Bleeding disorders. *See* Hemorrhagic disorders in pregnancy
Bleeding time, 1764t–1771t
Blindisms, 1207
Blissymbols, 1193–1194
Blood composition
changes in, 194–195, 196t–197t
after childbirth, 531
Blood glucose
monitoring
in gestational diabetes, 309
in pregestational diabetes, 346–348, 346b
in type 1 DM, 1630–1631, 1630t, 1636–1637, 1637b, 1637f
pregnancy vs. nonpregnancy values of, 196t–197t
Blood lead level (BLL)
reducing, 1446b
treating lead poisoning and, 1444–1445
Blood loss
in abruptio placentae, 324t, 326–327
after childbirth, 541–542, 542f
in placenta previa, 323, 324t
Blood pressure (BP)
maternal
antihypertensive therapy and, 305, 306t
assessment, 300–301, 302b
changes during pregnancy, 194
pediatric
alterations in pediatric surgery, 1268t
for boys, 1774–1775
cuff size for, 902–904, 903f, 903t
for girls, 1776–1777
after heart surgery, 1479–1480

Blood pressure (BP) *(Continued)*
measurement devices for, 901–902, 902t
measurement/interpretation, 904, 904b
of neonates, 611, 626t–636t, 637
orthostatic hypotension and, 904–905
sites for measuring, 903–904, 903f, 904t
systemic hypertension and, 1489–1490
Blood specimens, pediatric
atraumatic care for, 1287b
collection of, 1285–1286, 1286f
heel sticks, 655–659, 657f
venipuncture, 657
Blood tests
during first stage of labour, 456
of renal function, 1541t
Blood transfusions
beta-thalassemia and, 1510–1511
for hematological/immunological disorders
guidelines for, 1530–1532
nursing care for, 1531t–1532t
sickle cell anemia and, 1507
Blood typing, in neonates, 611
Blood volume
changes during pregnancy, 194–195, 196t–197t
after childbirth, 530–531
of neonates, 611
normal test ranges for, 1764t–1771t
Blood-patch therapy, 413, 413f
Blue spells, 1474–1476
Blue spike syringe, 1300, 1300f
Blunt abdominal trauma during pregnancy, 333–334
Blunt plastic cannula syringe, 1300, 1300f
Bodily damage
fear of, hospitalization and, 1245
infants and, 1000
school-age children and, 1102t
toddlers and, 1045–1046
Body art, 1128
Body hair, 1117
Body image
adolescents and, 1123–1124
development of, 855
genital surgery and, 1545
infants and, 965, 965f
preschoolers and, 1053
school-age children and, 1093
toddlers and, 1026
Body mass index (BMI)
ideal weight and, 49, 49t, 252
obesity and, 1136–1138
Body mechanics, education in, 224, 226b, 226f
Body surface area (BSA)
fluid loss in infants and, 1390
medication dosage and, 1286–1288
Body temperature
cerebral dysfunction and, 1564–1565
of children
alterations in pediatric surgery, 1268t
Body temperature *(Continued)*
alternate sites for ill child, 898b
centigrade to fahrenheit conversions, 1773
controlling elevated, 1272–1274
developmental changes in, 849
evidence-informed practice for, 900b–901b
indications of fever, 898b
locations for, 898b, 899t
procedure for, 897–905
reducing in respiratory infections, 1319
types of thermometers for, 902b
of newborns
assessment of, 626t–636t, 636
improved regulation of, 849
parental guidance in, 667
transition to extrauterine life and, 612–613, 612f, 646
of preterm infants, 710–711, 713–714
Bolus insulin, 1631b
Bonding. *See* Attachment
Bone age, 848
growth disorders and, 1612b
Bone marrow aspiration/biopsy
atraumatic care for, 1282b
positioning for, 1282
Bone marrow transplantation. *See* Hematopoietic stem cell transplantation (HSCT)
Bones
distraction for, 1697–1698
fractures of, 1690–1692, 1691b–1692b, 1691f
casting for, 1692–1695, 1694b, 1694f
traction for, 1695–1697, 1695f–1696f, 1696b, 1698b
growth/development of, 848
health of, cystic fibrosis and, 1361
of newborns, 620–621, 620f
osteomyelitis and, 1710–1712, 1711b
of school-age children, 1084–1085, 1085t–1086t
skeletal tuberculosis and, 1712
tumours of, 1712–1713, 1713b
Ewing's sarcoma, 1714–1715
osteosarcoma, 1713–1714
Bony pelvis, 66–67, 66f–67f
labour process and, 380–383, 382f
Booster car seats, 1040
Bordetella pertussis, 1337–1341
Boston braces, 1708–1709
Bottled water during infancy, 979
Bottle-feeding
breastfeeding and, 687–690
with cleft lip/palate, 773f
weaning, 704, 981
Bottle-mouth caries, 1036–1037, 1037f
Botulinum toxin A, cerebral palsy and, 1727
Botulism, 1746–1747, 1747b
Botulism immune globulin, 1747
Boundaries, community, 828–829
Bowel elimination. *See* Elimination
Bowlegs, 927, 927f
Braces, 1127
Brachial plexus injury, 744–745
Brachial pulse, 1367, 1367f
Bracing, scoliosis and, 1708–1709
Bradley method of childbirth, 401
Bradydysrhythmias, 1486
Bradypnea, 920b
Braille, 1207
Brain
aseptic meningitis and, 1589–1590, 1590t
bacterial meningitis and, 1586–1589, 1588b
cerebral trauma and. *See* Head injury
cranial deformities and, 1604
encephalitis and, 1590–1591, 1590b
epilepsy and, 1593–1603, 1593b–1595b, 1596t, 1599b–1603b
febrile seizures and, 1603–1604
fetal, 179
hydrocephalus and, 1604–1608, 1605f–1606f, 1606b
of newborns, 621
rabies and, 1591, 1592b
Reye's syndrome and, 1591–1592, 1592b
submersion injuries and, 1581–1583, 1582b
tumours of, 1583–1585
unconsciousness and. *See* Unconscious child
Brain death, 1564, 1583b
Brain hypoglycemia, 1637–1638
Brain Injury Association of Canada, 1581
Braxton Hicks contractions, 189–190, 388, 490–491
Brazelton Neonatal Behavioural Assessment Scale (BNBAS), 637–638, 637b
Breakthrough bleeding, 91–92
Breast cancer
adjuvant chemotherapy for, 120
breast implants and, 120
breast reconstruction for, 118–120
chemoprevention, 115
chemotherapy for, 121–122
clinical manifestations/diagnosis, 116–117, 116f
etiology of, 114, 115b
genetic testing and, 114–115
hormone therapy for, 120–121, 120b–121b
pathophysiology of, 115–116
postoperative exercises, 123b
pre/postoperative nursing care, 122–124
prognosis, 117–118, 118f
radiation for, 120
screening guidelines, 117t
screening technologies, 117b
surgery for, 118, 119f
Breast Cancer Risk Assessment Tool, 115
Breast implants, 120
Breast milk
banking, 694
expressing/storing, 691–693, 692f
Breast milk *(Continued)*
during first 6 months, 978–979
nutrients provided by, 679–680
unique properties of, 682–683
Breast reconstruction, 118–120
Breast shell, 223, 224f
Breastfeeding. *See also* Lactation
benefits of, 676–677
BFHI support of, 11, 699–700
as birth control method, 141–142
bottles/pacifiers and, 687–690
breast care in, 695
breast examination and, 695
after childbirth, 530, 545
contraindications to, 677
cultural influences on, 678–679
diabetic pregnancy and, 349–350
with donor milk, 694
drugs and, 1753t–1756t
duration of, 687
education in, 223, 223f–224f, 245b
expressing/storing milk, 691–693, 692f, 979
during first 6 months, 978–979
follow-up care, 700
food sensitivity and, 1386–1387
frequency of, 686–687
guidelines for, 689f
insufficient nutrient intake, 699b
jaundice and, 654, 691
latch-on for, 685–686, 685f–686f
maternal care during, 694–698
milk ejection reflex, 686
mother-infant assessment, 683, 684b
newborns with CL/P, 1423
nurse's role in, 698–699
positions for, 684–685, 685f
preterm infants, 718
preventing neonatal infection, 749
rates, in Canada, 8
separation from infant and, 693
SIDS and, 1009–1010
special considerations for, 690–691
supplemental systems for, 681, 681f
supplementation, 687
support for, 547b, 660, 677–679, 678b
twins, 691, 692f
weaning from, 693–694, 981
Breastfeeding Committee for Canada (BCC), 699–700, 700b
Breast(s)
anatomy of, 680–681, 681f
benign breast masses, 114, 114t
care, breastfeeding and, 695
changes during pregnancy, 192–193, 194f
after childbirth, 530
development of, 1114, 1115f
engorgement
abrupt weaning and, 693–694
breastfeeding and, 696–697
examination during pregnancy/lactation, 695
fibroadenomas, 113

Breast(s) *(Continued)*
fibrocystic changes in, 111–113
function/structure of, 67–68, 68f
intraductal papilloma, 114
lipomas, 113
mammary duct ectasia, 113–114
mastitis, 698
neonatal swelling of, 620
nipple discharge, 113
pubertal development of, 918–919
self-examination guidelines, 69b
Breath sounds, 919–920, 920b
Breathing. *See also* Respiration
cerebral dysfunction and, 1565
CPR and, 1367, 1367f
for labour pain management, 399f, 400–401, 400b, 403
Valsalva manoeuvre and, 392
Breech presentation
at birth, 379, 381f
dystocia and, 500–502
external cephalic version with, 501–502, 501f
internal version with, 502
types of, 501f
Brim, 380–383, 382f–383f
British Sign Language (BSL), 1202
Bronchial breath sounds, 920b
Bronchial drainage, 1304
Bronchiolitis, 1333–1337, 1333t
Bronchitis, 1332–1333, 1333t
Bronchodilator medication, cystic fibrosis and, 1359
Bronchopneumonia, 1335
Bronchoprovocation testing, 1347
Bronchopulmonary dysplasia (BPD), 732–733
Bronchospasms, 1352–1355
Bronchovesicular breath sounds, 920b
Brow presentation, 382f, 501
Brown fat, in neonates, 612
Bruising, 651, 651f
Bryant's traction, 1696
Buccal route of drug administration, 948b–949b
Buckle fractures, 1691b, 1691f
Buck's extension, 1696
Buffered lidocaine, 952b
Built-in safety seats, 1040
Bulb syringe, 644–645, 645f
Bulimia nervosa
in adolescents, 1126
in school-age children, 1109
screening for, 50
Bulla, 1644f
Bullying, 1090–1091
Burns
acute care for, 1677–1679
biological skin coverings for, 1676–1677
in children, 789–790, 790f
comfort management and, 1678
complications in, 1672–1673
depth of injury in, 1670–1671, 1671f
education for prevention of, 1132b
extent of injury in, 1670, 1670f
incidence of, 1669
infants and, 999–1000, 999f–1000f
Burns *(Continued)*
inhalation injury in, 1672
long-term care for, 1679–1680, 1679f–1680f
management of
emergency care, 1673, 1673b
major burns and, 1674–1677
minor burns and, 1673–1674
management/rehabilitative phases of care, 1678
nutrition for, 1679
pathophysiology of, 1672–1673
permanent skin coverings for, 1677, 1677f
prevention of, 1681
prognosis for, 1677
psychosocial support and, 1680–1681
school-age children and, 1102t
severity of injury in, 1671–1672
toddlers and, 1042–1043
types of, 1670
wound care, 1675–1676, 1676t, 1678–1679, 1678b
wound sepsis and, 1673
Burping, formula feeding and, 701, 702f
Burping position, 668f
Buttocks, bruising of in newborn, 651, 651f
Buttocks lift, 546f

C
Cadaver donor for kidney transplant, 1560
Caesarean birth
anaesthesia for, 516–517
complications/risks of, 514
definition/incidence of, 513
on demand, 514
fetal malpresentation and, 501
forced, 514–515
health service indicator, 8
home care education, 519, 519b
incisions used in, 513f
indications for, 513–514
intraoperative care during, 517, 517f–518f
measures to reduce, 514b
perimortem, in multisystem trauma, 335
postoperative/postpartum care, 518–519
prenatal preparation for, 515
preoperative care, 515–516
preparation for, 247
scheduled, 515
surgical techniques in, 514
unplanned, 515
Caffeine
breastfeeding and, 696
education in, 229–230
health risks of, 47, 256–257
prenatal exposure to, 762
Calcium
in adolescence, 1125
bone meal for, 261b
laboratory tests for, 1764t–1771t
for maternal nutrition, 260
non-dairy sources, 260b
nutritional significance of, 1381t–1383t
for toddlers, 1034
Calcium-to-phosphorus ratio, infant nutrition and, 680
Calendar rhythm method, 138
Calgary Family Assessment Model, 1223
Calgary Family Assessment Model (CFAM), 19, 19f
Caliciviruses, 1393t–1395t
Caloric intake
for adolescents, 1125
for infants, 679
Caloric test, 1566
Campylobacter coli, 1393t–1395t, 1396
Campylobacter jejuni, 1393t–1395t, 1396
Canada Health Act, 3
Canada Prenatal Nutrition Program (CPNP), 264b
Canada's Food Guide. *See Eating Well With Canada's Food Guide*
Canadian Association of Perinatal and Women's Health Nurses (CAPWHN), 2, 4b
Canadian Dental Association (CDA), 983, 1034–1037, 1127
Canadian Dermatology Association, 1681
Canadian health care
history of, 3–6
maternity services, 3–5, 4b
Millenium Development Goals, 5–6, 5b
Canadian Hearing Society, 1202
Canadian Heart and Stroke Foundation, 1366
Canadian Home Care Association (CHCA), 1216
Canadian Hospitals Injury Reporting and Prevention Program (CHIRPP), 1100
Canadian Human Rights Act, 1191–1192
Canadian Maternity Experiences Survey, 9
Canadian National Institute for the Blind (CNIB), 1207
Canadian Neurocritical Care Group, 1564
Canadian Nurses Association (CNA)
Certification program, 9
Code of Ethics, 796, 796b
Canadian Paediatric Society, 687, 866
Canadian Patient Safety Institute (CPSI), 11, 12b
Canadian Perinatal Surveillance System (CPSS), 7–8, 7b
Canadian Thoracic Society, 1742
Canadian Toy Testing Council, 859, 1028
Cancer
breast. *See* Breast cancer
cervical
genital herpes and, 103
screening for, 29–30, 190
gestational trophoblastic neoplasia, 320
pediatric
bone tumours, 1712–1713, 1713b
Cancer *(Continued)*
Ewing's sarcoma, 1714–1715
osteosarcoma, 1713–1714
brain tumours, 1583–1585
Hodgkin's disease, 1525–1526, 1525f
leukemias. *See* Leukemias
lymphomas, 1524–1526
neuroblastomas, 1585–1586
non-Hodgkin's lymphoma, 1526
rhabdomyosarcoma, 1715–1716, 1715b
Wilms' tumour, 1552–1553, 1552b
skin, 1129
testicular, 1135
Candida albicans, 109
Candidiasis, 1654t
breastfeeding and, 697–698
of diaper area, 1664f
management of, 756
neonatal, 756
vaginal infection and, 109–110, 109t
Capillary blood samples, 1285
Capillary refill time, 921
Caput succedaneum, 617, 618f
Car seats
infants and, 996–997, 997f
newborns and, 669–670, 669f, 738b
toddlers and, 1037–1042, 1039f–1040f, 1041b
Carbamazepine, 946t
Carbohydrates
in breast milk, 682
infant requirements for, 679
newborns and, 614–615
Carbon dioxide partial pressure, 1764t–1771t
Carbon monoxide (CO) poisoning
in children, 1043
smoke inhalation injury and, 1343
Carboprost tromethamine, 583b
Carbuncle, 1652t
Cardiac arrest
in children, 1365–1366
during pregnancy, 362
Cardiac catheterization, 1452t–1453t, 1453, 1454b
Cardiac decompensation, 358b
Cardiac dysrhythmias, 1485–1487, 1486b
Cardiac ischemia, Kawasaki disease and, 1491, 1492b
Cardiac output
changes during pregnancy, 195, 298b
after childbirth, 531
during labour, 386, 391–392, 392b
placenta previa and, 327b
in postpartum hemorrhage, 580b
Cardiac shunts for children, 1475, 1476f, 1476t
Cardinal positions of gaze, 931f
Cardiogenic shock, 1492t
Cardiomyopathy
in IDMs, 736–737
pediatric, 1487–1488
peripartum, 355–356

Cardiopulmonary resuscitation (CPR)
anaphylaxis and, 1495
certification in, 668
parent education in, 727–728
pediatric, 1365–1368, 1366f–1368f, 1369t
of pregnant women, 362, 363b
Cardiovascular drugs, breastfeeding and, 1753t–1756t
Cardiovascular dysfunction
in children
acquired heart disease in. *See* Acquired heart disease, pediatric
anaphylaxis and, 1494–1495
cardiac catheterization in, 1452t–1453t, 1453, 1454b
congenital heart disease in. *See* Congenital heart disease (CHD)
diagnostic evaluation in, 1452–1453, 1452t
heart transplantation and, 1488–1489
history/physical examination, 1451–1452
Kawasaki disease and, 1490–1494, 1491b–1492b
septic shock, 1495–1497, 1496b, 1496t
shock and, 1492, 1492t, 1493b
systemic hypertension and, 1489–1490, 1489b
maternal
abnormal cardiovascular signs, 358t
acquired heart disease and
ischemic heart disease in pregnancy, 355
mitral valve prolapse in, 355
peripartum cardiomyopathy in, 355–356
rheumatic heart disease in, 355
cardiac decompensation in, 358b
cardiopulmonary resuscitation and, 362, 363b
classification of, 352–353, 353b
congenital heart disease and
atrial/ventricular septal defects in, 353–354
coarctation of the aorta in, 354
Marfan syndrome in, 354
mitral/aortic valve stenosis in, 354
patent ductus arteriosus in, 353–354
pulmonic stenosis in, 354
contraindications to pregnancy, 356, 356b
cyanotic heart lesions
Eisenmenger's syndrome in, 354–355
primary pulmonary hypertension in, 355
Tetralogy of Fallot in, 354
Cardiovascular dysfunction *(Continued)*
in intrapartum period, 360–361
medications for, 360t
nursing care for, 356–362, 356b–357b
in postpartum period, 361–362
surgery during pregnancy, 360
Cardiovascular support, in treatment of shock, 1494
Cardiovascular system
maternal
adaptation to pregnancy, 193, 194f, 197t
blood volume/composition, 194–195, 196t–197t
cardiac output, 195
circulation/coagulation times, 195
during labour, 391–392
postpartum adaptation of, 530–531
of newborns, 643b
pediatric
congenital anomalies of, 770
effects of immobilization on, 1685t
nutritional status and, 887t–889t
of preterm infants, 710
transition to extrauterine life, 610–611
Care coordination, home care and, 1220–1221, 1221b
Caregiver Strain Index, 1229
Caregivers
respite care for, 1218
responsibilities of, 1217–1218
Cariogenic foods, 1036–1037
Carpal tunnel syndrome during pregnancy, 200–201, 231t–233t
Caruncle, 908f, 926
Case management, 1220–1221, 1221b
Casting
for bone fractures, 1692–1695, 1694b, 1694f
for clubfoot, 776
for osteomyelitis, 1711–1712
Cataracts, 1204b–1205b
Catecholamines, 1586
Catheterization
cardiac, 1452t–1453t, 1453
during labour, 458t, 460
urinary, 1283–1285, 1284t
Cat-scratch disease, 1664
Causal relationships
preschoolers and, 1052–1053
toddlers and, 1024
Cause-specific death rate, 803b
Cavities. *See* Dental caries
Celiac disease, 1433–1434, 1434b
Cell division process, 168
Cell-surface immunological markers, 1517–1518
Cellulitis, 1652f, 1652t
Centigrade to fahrenheit temperature conversions, 1773
Central auditory imperception, 1199
Central nervous system (CNS). *See also* Neurological system
birth trauma involving, 746
congenital anomalies of
encephalocele/anencephaly, 768–770
hydrocephalus, 769–770
microcephaly, 770
spinal bifida, 768–769, 769f
encephalitis and, 1590–1591, 1590b
of newborns, 643b
of preterm infants, 711
Central nervous system depressants, 1147
Central nervous system stimulants, 1147–1148
Central precocious puberty (CPP), 1614, 1614b
Central shunt procedure, 1476t
Central venous access devices, 1294–1295, 1294f, 1295t
Centration, 1025b
Centrencephalic system, 1593
Centring pregnancy approach, 213b
Cephalhematoma, 617, 618f
Cephalic presentation, 379, 380f
Cephalocaudal development, 845–846
Cephalopelvic disproportion (CPD), 499
Cerebellar function, pediatric assessment of, 928, 928b
Cerebral dysfunction
aseptic meningitis and, 1589–1590, 1590t
assessment of cerebral function in
altered states of consciousness and, 1563–1564, 1564b
general aspects of, 1562–1563
increased intracranial pressure, 1563, 1563b
neurological examination in, 1564–1567, 1565f–1566f
special diagnostic procedures for, 1567–1569, 1567t–1568t
bacterial meningitis and, 1586–1589, 1588b
brain tumours and, 1583–1585
cranial deformities and, 1604
encephalitis and, 1590–1591, 1590b
epilepsy and, 1593–1603, 1593b–1595b, 1596t, 1599b–1603b
febrile seizures and, 1603–1604
head injury and, 1573–1581, 1575f
hydrocephalus and, 1604–1608, 1605f–1606f, 1606b
neuroblastomas and, 1585–1586
rabies and, 1591, 1592b
Reye's syndrome and, 1591–1592, 1592b
submersion injuries and, 1581–1583, 1582b
unconscious child and
elimination and, 1572
family support for, 1573, 1574b
hygienic care for, 1572
Cerebral dysfunction *(Continued)*
intracranial pressure monitoring, 1570–1571
medications for, 1572
nursing care for, 1569
nutrition and hydration for, 1571–1572
positioning/exercise and, 1572–1573
regaining consciousness and, 1573
respiratory management in, 1570
stimulation and, 1573
thermoregulation and, 1572
Cerebral edema, 1577
Cerebral hyperemia, 1574
Cerebral palsy (CP)
defined/factors contributing to, 1724
diagnosis of, 1725, 1726b
early signs of, 1729b
management of, 1725–1728, 1726f
nursing care for, 1728–1732, 1729b–1731b, 1731f
pathophysiology of, 1724–1725, 1725b
prognosis for, 1728
supportive care for, 1732
Cerebrospinal fluid (CSF)
aseptic meningitis and, 1589–1590, 1590t
laboratory tests for, 1764t–1771t
Cervical cancer
genital herpes and, 103
screening for, 29–30, 190
Cervical cap, 143f, 144–147, 147b
Cervical cerclage, 317, 317f
Cervical lacerations, 477
Cervical mucus ovulation-detection method, 139, 140b
Cervical ripening methods
amniotomy, 508, 508b
chemical agents, 507–508, 507b
mechanical agents, 508
overview, 507
oxytocin, 509–511, 509b–510b
Cervical traction, 1697, 1697f
Cervix, 64, 65f
bimanual palpation of, 77–78
changes during pregnancy, 190, 190f, 193f
dilation of, 385f, 386, 455
effacement of, 385, 385f, 455
examination of, 76, 77f
length of, preterm labour and, 490
postpartum changes in, 528
premature dilation of, 316–318
structure of, 64–65, 65f
Chadwick's sign, 191–192
Chalmers, Iain, 10
Changing table, falls from, 998
Charleston nighttime bending braces, 1708–1709
Charter of Rights and Freedom., 1159
Cheating, school-age children and, 1095
Chelation therapy, lead poisoning and, 1444–1445, 1445b
Chemical agents for cervical ripening, 507–508, 507b

Chemical burns, 1670
  emergency intervention for eye injuries and, 1206b
Chemical injury to respiratory tract, 1343
Chemical restraints, 1279
Chemotherapy
  agents, precautions with, 1523
  for brain tumours, 1584
  breast cancer and, 115, 121–122
  gestational trophoblastic neoplasia and, 321
  Hodgkin's disease and, 1525
  leukemia and, 1518–1523
  neuroblastomas and, 1586
  non-Hodgkin's lymphoma and, 1526
  osteosarcoma and, 1713
  rhabdomyosarcoma and, 1716
  Wilms' tumour and, 1552–1553
Chest
  circumference, of toddlers, 1021
  of infants, 959
  of newborns, 610, 626t–636t
  nutritional status and, 887t–889t
  pediatric examination of, 917–919, 918f–919f
  trauma during pregnancy, 334
Chest compression, for CPR, 1367–1368, 1367f–1368f
Chest physiotherapy (CPT), 1304
  for asthma, 1350–1351
  for cystic fibrosis, 1359, 1359f
Chest tube drainage, heart surgery and, 1480
Chest wall stretch, 123b
Cheyne-Stokes respiration, 920b
Chickenpox. *See* Varicella
Chilblain, 1682
Child care arrangement, alternative, 970–976
Child centre-based care, 970–976
Child maltreatment
  caregiver-child interaction in, 1075–1076
  child neglect in, 1072
  clinical manifestations of, 1077b–1078b
  history/interview in, 1076
  incidence of, 1000
  nursing care for, 1075
    discharge plan, 1079
    guidelines for recording data, 1079b
    physical assessment in, 1076–1078
    prevention of abuse, 1079–1080
    supporting child/family, 1078–1079
    talking with children who reveal abuse, 1075b
  physical abuse in, 1072–1073
  protection from further abuse, 1078
  sexual abuse. *See* Sexual abuse, of children
  warning signs of, 1075b
Childbirth
  anaesthesia for, 407–416, 408b
  analgesics for. *See* Analgesia, during labour
  Caesarean. *See* Caesarean birth
Childbirth *(Continued)*
  Canadian Maternity Experiences Survey, 9
  cultural considerations in, 25t–26t
  in delivery room/birthing room, 474–475, 474f
  discomfort during, 394–398
  dystocia and. *See* Dystocia
  emergency, 478, 479b
  estimating date of, 206
  father's preparation for, 209–210
  forceps-assisted, 511–512
  fundal pressure during, 476
  health risks of
    age-related, 45–47
    alcohol and, 47
    environmental hazards, 54–55
    female genital mutilation, 54, 54b
    gynecological conditions, 54
    illicit drugs and, 48–49
    medical conditions, 54
    prescription medications and, 47–48
    substance abuse and, 47
  at home, 243
  impact of, 548
  maternal positions for, 386–388, 387f, 462b
  maternal preparation for, 208
  meconium-stained fluid during, 476
  normal vaginal, 3b, 10–11, 482b–483b
  obstetrical emergencies in
    amniotic fluid embolism, 523–524
    prolapsed umbilical cord, 521–522, 521f–522f, 523b
    rupture of uterus, 522–523
    shoulder dystocia, 520–521, 520f
  pain management for. *See* Pain, during labour/birth
  perineal trauma related to, 476–478
  postterm. *See* Postterm pregnancy
  preterm. *See* Preterm labour and birth
  sequelae of trauma in. *See* Birth trauma, maternal
  settings for, 241–242
  siblings during, 467
  taking history of, 879–881
  vacuum-assisted, 512, 513f
  vertex presentation in, 382f, 389, 475–476, 475f–476f
    external cephalic version for, 501–502, 501f
  water birth, 475, 475f
Childbirth and Postpartum Professional Association (CAPPA), 401
Childbirth education
  in biofeedback, 247
  birth plan development, 246, 246b
  in breastfeeding, 245b
  for Caesarean birth, 247
  classes for, 36–37, 36b
  in conscious breathing, 246–247
Childbirth education *(Continued)*
  current practices in, 244–245
  in energy work/massage/music/acupressure, 247
  in imagery/visualization, 246
  methods of
    Birthing From Within, 401
    Bradley method, 401
    Childbirth and Postpartum Professional Association, 401
    Dick-Read method, 400–401
    evidence-informed education, 402
    HypnoBirthing, 401
    Lamaze method, 401–402, 402b
    outcomes, 402
  outcomes, 247, 402
  overview, 243
  in pain management, 246
  in relaxation, 246
  scope of, 244
Childbirth Without Fear (Dick-Read), 400–401
Childhood atopic dermatitis, 1665–1667, 1666b
Childhood depression, 1110, 1110b
Childhood growth/development. *See* Growth and development
Childhood hysteria, 1109–1110
Childhood injuries, 789–790, 789t
Childhood nephrosis, 1547–1549
Childhood obesity, 788–789, 789f
Children
  characteristics of in child abuse, 1073
  chronic illness/disability in
    common terms for, 1157b
    coordinated care for, 1159
    coping mechanisms for, 1164–1165, 1165b
    cultural issues in, 1158
    developmental aspects of, 1164, 1165f
    establishing realistic goals, 1174
    establishing therapeutic relationships for, 1158
    family education in, 1169–1170
    family issues in
      assisting in managing feelings, 1162–1164
      coping with stress/crises, 1161–1162, 1162b
      establishing support system, 1164
      impact on parents, 1159–1160, 1160b
      impact on siblings, 1160–1161, 1161b
      parental overprotection in, 1163b
    family-centred care for, 1157
    family-health care provider communication, 1157
    impact of type of illness, 1166
    incidence/impact of, 1156–1157
    normalization for, 1158–1159, 1169b
Children *(Continued)*
    nursing care for
      assessment in, 1166, 1167t
      promoting normal development, 1170–1174, 1170f, 1171t–1172t
      support at time of diagnosis, 1166–1167
      support for child, 1168–1169, 1169b
      support for parents, 1167–1168, 1168b
      support for siblings, 1169
    permanency planning for, 1218
    response to parental behaviour, 1165–1166
    shared decision making in, 1158, 1158b
  clearing airway obstruction for, 1370, 1370f
  communicating with, 873–876, 874b, 874f, 877b–878b
  constipation and, 1400–1401
  end-of-life care for
    child's understanding of/reactions to death, 1177t–1178t
    decision making and, 1175–1176
    fear of child dying alone, 1181, 1181f
    grief and mourning, 1183–1184, 1184b
    home deaths, 1181–1182
    hospital deaths, 1182
    nurse's reaction to, 1184–1185, 1185b
    organ/tissue donation/autopsy, 1182–1183
    pain and symptom management, 1179–1181, 1180b
    principles of palliative care in, 1174–1175
    signs of approaching death, 1182b
    treatment options for, 1176–1179
  health care for. *See* Pediatric nursing
  health history for
    features of, 73–74
    history section in, 879
    identifying information for, 876
    outline of, 879b
    present illness, 879
    primary health issue, 876–878
  hospitalization. *See* Hospitalization, pediatric
  impact of divorce on, 819–820, 820b
  manifestations of hearing impairment in, 1201, 1201b
  mental health issues in, 792
  ordinal position of, 811–812, 811b
  pain assessment in
    behavioural measures for, 934, 935f, 936t
    chronic illness/complex pain and, 939–940

Children *(Continued)*
with communication/cognitive impairment, 939
cultural factors in, 939
guidelines for, 880b
multidimensional measures for, 936
physiological measures for, 934–935
self-report measures for, 935–936, 937t
pain management for
nonpharmacologic, 940–955, 941b
pharmacologic. *See* Pharmacological pain management, pediatric
using CAM therapies, 942–943
physical examination of
of abdomen, 922–924
age-specific approaches to, 892t
of anus, 926
back/extremities, 926–928
chest, 917–919
ears, 912–915, 915t
eyes, 907–912, 908f
general appearance, 905
genitalia, 924–926
growth measurements in, 893–897, 896f
guidelines for, 891b
head/neck, 907
heart, 920–922
immunizations, 894f–895f
lungs, 919–920
lymph nodes, 906–907, 907f
mouth/throat, 916–917
neurological system, 928
nose, 915–916
physiological measurements in, 897–905
preparing child for, 890–892, 893f
sequence for, 890
skin/accessory structures, 905–906, 906t
preschool. *See* Preschoolers
school-age. *See* School-age children
substance use in, 791–792
toddlers. *See* Toddlers
unconscious. *See* Unconscious child
violence against, 791
visual impairment in, 1206
Chinese ethnicity
childbearing practices and, 561b
coping with pain and, 396
food patterns of, 269t–270t
health beliefs/practices and, 840t–841t
lactase deficiency and, 45, 158
as visible minority, 5
Chlamydia trachomatis infection
diagnosis/treatment of, 98
neonatal, 755–756
Chloasma, 199
Chloride
laboratory tests for, 1764t–1771t
nutritional significance of, 1381t–1383t
Chlorothiazide
breastfeeding and, 1753t–1756t
for heart failure, 1469t
Choanal atresia, 770–771, 771f
Cholecalciferol. *See* Vitamin D
Cholecystitis, 367, 367b
Cholelithiasis, 367, 367b
Cholesterol
hyperlipidemia and, 1484–1485, 1484t
laboratory tests for, 1764t–1771t
Cholestyramine, hyperlipidemia and, 1484–1485
Chordee, 1546t
Chorea, rheumatic fever and, 1484
Chorioamnionitis, 497
Choriocarcinoma, 320, 321b
Chorion, 172–173, 172f
Chorionic villus sampling (CVS)
fetal rights and, 285b
monitoring pregnancy risks, 284–285, 285f
ultrasound adjunct to, 285b
Chromosomal abnormalities, 163–166, 164f
abnormalities of number, 163–164
Down syndrome. *See* Down syndrome
fragile X syndrome, 1198–1199, 1198b
risk factors for, 276b
of sex chromosomes, 166
structural, 164–166
Chromosomes, 162–163, 1517–1518
Chronic active hepatitis, 1418
Chronic adrenocortical insufficiency, 1623–1624, 1623b
Chronic diarrhea, 1392–1395
Chronic illness
defined, 1157b
pain assessment in, 939–940
Chronic nonspecific diarrhea (CNSD), 1395
Chronic otitis media, 1325–1328, 1327b
Chronic pain syndromes, 955
Chronic renal failure (CRF), 1555–1559, 1557b
dialysis and, 1559–1560
Chronic sorrow, special needs child and, 1164
Chronic wounds, 1643
Chvostek's sign, 1620b–1621b
Cigarette smoking
adolescents and, 1144–1146
breastfeeding and, 696
childbirth risks with, 47
education in, 229–230
interventions for, 55–56, 56b
maternal, SIDS and, 1008–1009
prenatal exposure to, 759
Cimicidae, 1661, 1661b, 1661f
Circulatory system
changes at birth, 1455, 1455f
changes in during pregnancy, 195
fetal development of, 177–178, 177f
Circumcision
care following, 665–667
home care for, 665b
Circumcision *(Continued)*
pain management, 664–665, 666b
procedure, 663–667, 664f–665f
UTIs and, 1541, 1542b
Cirrhosis, 1419–1420
Clarification, in health assessment interview, 70
Classic Caesarean birth, 513f, 514
Classification skills, 1087
Classroom education, learning disabilities and, 1107
Clavicle fractures, birth-related, 744–746, 744f
Clean-catch specimens, 1283
Cleavage, fertilization and, 171, 171f
Cleft lip and palate (CL/P), 772–775, 772f
bottles/nipples for, 773f, 1423, 1423f
in children, 1421–1425, 1424b
Climacteric, 84
Clitoris, 63, 64f
Cloacal exstrophy, 1432
Clonidine, 946t
Closed fracture, 1690–1691
Clostridium botulinum, 1393t–1395t, 1746–1747
Clostridium difficile, 1393t–1395t
Clostridium perfringens, 1393t–1395t
Clothing
for newborns, 669
during pregnancy, 227–228
Clotting disorders. *See* Coagulopathies
Clotting time, laboratory tests for, 1764t–1771t
Clubbing, 1474, 1474f
Clubfoot, 776, 1701–1703, 1702f
Clubs, school-age children and, 1090
Coagulation factors
changes in during pregnancy, 195
after childbirth, 531
in neonates, 615
Coagulopathies
disseminated intravascular coagulation, 329–330, 584–585
idiopathic thrombocytopenic purpura, 584
normal clotting vs., 328–329
postpartum period and, 584–585
von Willebrand's disease, 330, 584
Coanalgesic adjuvant drugs for children, 943, 946t
Coarctation of the aorta, 354, 1460b–1462b
Cobalamin, 262, 1376t–1379t
Cobedding, 725
Cocaine
adolescent use of, 1147
breastfeeding and, 1753t–1756t
childbirth risks with, 48
during pregnancy, 374
prenatal exposure to, 760–761
Cochlear implants, 1200–1201
Cochrane Pregnancy and Childbirth Database, 10
Code of Ethics for Registered Nurses, 796, 796b
Codeine
breastfeeding and, 1753t–1756t
for children, 943, 945t, 947t
Cognitive development
adolescents and, 1119
infants and, 964–965
preschoolers and, 1052–1053
school-age children and, 1087–1088
theories of, 852–853
toddlers and, 1024–1026
Cognitive impairments (CIs)
defined, 1189
diagnosis/classification of, 1189–1190, 1190b, 1191t
dimensions of care for, 1190b
Down syndrome, 1195–1198, 1196b, 1196f
etiology of, 1190
fragile X syndrome, 1198–1199, 1198b
nursing care for
discipline and, 1194
encouraging play/exercise, 1192–1193, 1192f–1193f
encouraging socialization, 1194
future care and, 1194
hospitalization and, 1194–1195
learning skills and, 1191–1192
promoting optimal development, 1192
providing means of communication, 1193–1194, 1193f
self-care skills and, 1192
sexuality and, 1194
prevention of, 1195
Cognitive power, 1563
Cognitive strategies for pain management, 400b
Coitus interruptus, 136–137
Cold applications, for labour pain management, 406
Cold injury, 1682
Cold stress in neonates, 612–613, 613f
Colestipol, 1484–1485
Colic, 1003–1005
incidence/treatment of, 1003–1004
interventions for, 1005b, 1005f
management of, 1004
nursing care for, 1004–1005
Collaboration in pediatric nursing, 795–796
Collaborative Home Infant Monitoring study (CHIME), 1013
Collaborative woman- and family-centred maternity care, 6–7. *See also* Family nursing
Colostrum, 193, 223, 682–683
Colour Tool for pain assessment, 937t
Colour vision testing, 912
Coma, 1563–1564, 1564b, 1564f. *See also* Unconscious child

Combined spinal-epidural analgesia, 415
Comedogenesis, 1668
Comfort measures
for communicable diseases, 1063
for labour pain
nonpharmacologic, 400b, 402–407
pharmacologic, 407–421, 408b
pediatric
CAM therapies for, 942–943
for circumcision, 664–665, 666b
for complications of HIV disease, 1529–1530
after heart surgery, 1481
for leukemia, 1519
nonpharmacologic, 939–940, 941b
pharmacologic. *See* Pharmacological pain management, pediatric
for sickle cell anemia, 1507–1509, 1509b
for terminally ill child, 1179–1181, 1180b
for unconscious child, 1569
postpartum, 543–544
Commercial infant formulas, 701–703
Comminuted bone fractures, 1690–1691
Comminuted skull fractures, 1576
Common-law families, 17
Communicable diseases, 1064t–1070t
assessment of, 1062
comfort measures for, 1063
preventing complications, 1062–1063
preventing spread of, 1062
supportive care for, 1063
Communicating hydrocephalus, 1605
Communication. *See also* Interview process
barriers to, 872, 873b
with children, 873–876, 874b, 877b–878b
cognitively impaired children and, 1193–1194, 1193f
cultural competence in, 22–24, 70b
death of newborn and, 602–604
with language differences, 832–834, 873
parent-infant, 560–562
special needs child and, 1157
technology applications for, 35–36
Community
assets from, 828–829
defined, 801
health assessment of, 30–32, 31f
home care in, 35–40
involvement in perinatal care, 12
vulnerable populations in, 32–35
Community Health Care Nurses of Canada, 1222
Community health nursing. *See also* Community-based health care
overview, 801–802
Community health nursing *(Continued)*
roles/functions of, 802–804
school health and, 1100
Community intervention/evaluation, 806
Community needs assessment, 804–805, 805b–806b
Community planning, 805, 805b–806b
Community resource referrals, 554
Community-based health care
demography and, 802
economics and, 804
epidemiology and, 802–804, 803f
health promotion in, 29–30, 787
needs assessment/diagnosis and, 804–805, 805b–806b
nursing process in, 804–806, 804b
postpartum support with, 11–12
Compensated shock, 1493b, 1494
Competitive sports, 1097–1098
Complementary and alternative medicine (CAM)
ADHD and, 1107
admission assessment and, 1238–1241, 1241b
asthma and, 1350
calcium sources and, 261b
dysmenorrhea and, 87, 88t
nutritional disturbances from, 1375
for pediatric pain management, 942–943
PPMD and, 599, 599b
during pregnancy, 230b
Complete atrioventricular block (AV), 1486
Complete breech, 381f, 454f, 501, 501f
Complete fracture, 1690, 1691b, 1691f
Complete miscarriage, 314, 314f, 315t
Complete rupture of uterus, 522–523
Complex partial seizures, 1594b–1595b, 1596t, 1600b
Compliance
with immunization schedule, 992
with medical treatment plan, 1269–1270, 1269b
Complicated fractures, 1690–1691
Complicated grief reactions, 1183
Complications
from communicable diseases, 1062–1063
postpartum. *See* Postpartum complications
Compound bone fractures, 1690–1691
Compressions-Airway-Breathing (C-A-B) procedure, 1366
Computed tomography (CT)
for assessment of cerebral function, 1567–1568, 1567t–1568t
genitourinary disorders and, 1538t–1539t
for head injury, 1578
for hydrocephalus, 1605–1606
Computer privacy in nursing, 870
Computer-aided detection and diagnosis (CAD), 117b
Conception
cell division and, 168
defined, 168
fertilization and, 170–171, 171f
gametogenesis and, 168, 170f
implantation, 171, 171f
nutritional needs before, 250
ovum and, 168, 170f
sperm and, 168–170, 170f
Conceptual thinking, 1087–1088
Concrete operations stage of cognitive development, 853
Concussion, 1575
Condoms
female, 143, 143f
male, 142–143, 143f, 144b
for STI prevention, 97, 97b
Conduction disturbances, 1486
Conduction heat loss in newborns, 612
Conductive hearing loss, 1199–1200
Condylomata acuminata, 101–103, 102f
Confidentiality
informed consent and, 1260
of interview process, 869–870
Configuration of skin lesions, 1643
Confrontation in health assessment interview, 70
Confusion, 1564b
Congenital adrenal hyperplasia (CAH), 1625–1626
Congenital aganglionic megacolon, 1401–1403, 1401f
Congenital anomalies
cardiovascular, 770
of central nervous system
encephalocele/anencephaly, 768–770
hydrocephalus, 769–770
microcephaly, 770
spina bifida, 768–769, 769f, 1732–1738, 1733b–1734b, 1733f–1734f
evaluation/counselling for, 779
gastrointestinal
anorectal malformation, 774–775, 774f
cleft lip/palate, 772–775, 772f–773f
esophageal atresia/tracheoesophageal fistula, 772–773, 773f
intestinal obstruction, 774
omphalocele/gastroschisis, 773–774, 774f
genetic diagnosis for, 778
genetic evaluation/counselling for, 779
genitourinary
disorders of sex development, 777, 777f
exstrophy of bladder, 777
hypospadias/epispadias, 776–780, 777f
teratoma, 777–778
in IDMs, 735
Congenital anomalies *(Continued)*
musculoskeletal
clubfoot, 776, 1701–1703, 1702f
developmental dysplasia of hip, 775–776, 775f–776f, 1699–1701, 1700b
metatarsus adductus, 1703
osteogenesis imperfecta, 1704–1705, 1704b
polydactyly, 776
skeletal limb deficiency, 1703–1704
nursing care for, 778
respiratory
choanal atresia, 770–771, 771f
congenital diaphragmatic hernia, 771, 771f
screening for, 778–779
supportive care for, 779–780
Congenital clubfoot, 1701–1703
Congenital diaphragmatic hernia (CDH), 771, 771f
Congenital disability, definition of, 1157b
Congenital heart disease (CHD)
acyanotic heart lesions, 353–354
altered hemodynamics and, 1455–1456
categories of, 1451
circulatory changes at birth and, 1455, 1455f
classification of defects in, 1456f
decreased pulmonary blood flow defects, 1459, 1462f, 1463b–1464b
increased pulmonary blood flow defects, 1456, 1457b–1459b, 1459f
mixed defects, 1459–1462, 1464b–1467b
obstructive defects, 1456–1459, 1459f, 1460b–1462b
congestive heart failure in. *See* Congestive heart failure (CHF)
contraindications to pregnancy with, 356, 356b
cyanotic heart lesions, 354–355
discharge/home care in, 1478, 1481, 1481b
etiology of, 1454
family adjustment to, 1477
family education in, 1477–1478, 1477b
hypoxemia in, 1474–1476, 1474f–1475f, 1476t
in newborns, 770
postoperative care for, 1479–1481, 1479b
in pregnancy, 353–355, 353b
preprocedural preparation in, 1478–1479
Congenital lactase deficiency, 1388
Congenital malformations
etiology of, 167b
genetic factors. *See* Genetics
nongenetic factors, 167–168
Congestive heart failure (CHF)
clinical manifestations of, 1468b
diagnosis of, 1462
management of
accumulated fluids/sodium and, 1468–1469, 1469t

Congestive heart failure (CHF) *(Continued)*
cardiac demands and, 1469
improving cardiac function for, 1468
tissue oxygenation and, 1469
nursing care for, 1469–1474, 1470b–1471b
pathophysiology of, 1462, 1467f
Conjunctive stage of spiritual development, 854
Conjunctivitis, chlamydial, 755–756
Conscience, development of, 1052, 1052b
Conscious breathing, 246–247, 403, 403f, 404b
Consciousness, levels of, 1563, 1564b
Conservation, school-age children and, 1087, 1088f
Consolability of newborns, 640
Constipation, 1399–1401
nutritional recommendations for, 268
opioid-induced, 952
pregnancy and, 202
Constitutional growth delay, 1611–1612
Consumer Product Safety Act, 859
Consumption coagulopathy, 1516–1517
Contact dermatitis, 1655–1657
Contact precautions, 1277b, 1278
Continuity of care, support of, 11b
Continuous distending airway pressure, 716t
Continuous epidural block, 414
Continuous positive airway pressure (CPAP), 715, 716f, 716t, 1364
Continuous subcutaneous insulin infusion, 1636
Contraception
abortion as, 152–155
adolescents and, 1131
barrier methods of
cervical cap, 143f, 144–147, 147b
contraceptive sponge, 143f, 147
diaphragm, 143–144, 143f, 145b–146b
female condoms, 143, 143f
male condoms, 142–143, 144b
spermicides, 142, 142f
breastfeeding and, 141–142, 695
after childbirth, 552–553
coitus interruptus method, 136–137
decriminalization of, 4b
defined, 135
effectiveness/failure rate, 135, 135b
emergency, 150
hormonal methods of
combined estrogen-progestin, 147–148
continuous/extended, 150
general classes of, 147t
progestin-only methods, 148
intrauterine devices, 150, 150f, 151b
intrauterine systems, 150–151, 151b
Contraception *(Continued)*
natural methods
basal body temperature, 138–139, 139b, 139f
calendar rhythm, 138
cervical mucus ovulation-detection, 139, 140b
fertility awareness and, 137–138
home predictor test kits for ovulation, 140–141, 142f
standard days, 138, 138f
symptothermal, 139–140, 141f
nursing process for, 135–136, 136b
optimal birth spacing and, 137b
seeking health care for, 42–43, 43b
sterilization as, 151–152
for women with diabetes, 350
Contraceptive sponge, 143f, 147
Contraceptive vaginal ring, 148
Contraceptives, breastfeeding and, 1753t–1756t
Contracting for treatment compliance, 1270
Contraction stress test (CST)
interpretation of, 290t
in third-trimester assessment, 288–289, 289f
Contractions, uterine. *See* Uterine contractions/activity
Contracture, 1646
Contusion, 1575, 1688–1689
Convection heat loss in newborns, 612
Convention on the Rights of the Child, 1159
Conventional level of moral development, 854
Conversion reaction, 1109–1110
Convertible safety seats, 1037–1040, 1039f
Convulsions
eclampsia and, 305–308, 306f, 307b
pre-eclampsia and, 304
Cooley's anemia, 1510–1511
Coombs' test, 281–282, 282t, 767–768
Cooperation in school-age children, 1089–1092
Cooperative play, 857–858, 858f
Coordinated care for special needs children, 1159
Coordination
in pediatric nursing, 795–796
of secondary schematas, 965
Coping
of families with special needs child, 1161–1162, 1162b
supportive care for, 1167–1169, 1168b
of special needs children, 1164–1165, 1165b, 1165f
stress in childhood and, 863–864
Coping with labour algorithm, 398, 399f
Copper, 1381t–1383t
Cord blood collection, 481
Cords, strangulation danger of, 996
Corneal light reflex (Hirschberg) test, 909, 909f
Coronary artery disease (CAD), pregnancy and, 355
Corporal punishment, 816–817
Corpus luteum, 82–84, 83f
Corrosives, poisoning from, 1437b–1438b
Corticosteroids
for asthma, 1349
for children, 946t
for Duchenne muscular dystrophy, 1742
as immunosuppressive therapy, 1560
for inflammatory bowel disease, 1412
for nephrotic syndrome, 1548
for skin disorders, 1647–1649
Cortisol, Addison's disease and, 1623–1624
Cosleeping, 1009, 1009b
Cotrel-Dubousset instrumentation, 1709
Cough etiquette, 109t
Counselling
genetic, 159–161, 159b, 779
HIV, 53–54, 97, 107, 371
nutrition, 267, 367b
pediatric nurse's role in, 795
preconception, 43, 341
sex during pregnancy, 234–235
STI/HIV prevention, 53–54, 97
telephone, 870–871
Counterpressure, for labour pain, 403
Countertraction, 1695, 1695f
Cover eye test, 909
Cow's milk allergy (CMA), 1387–1388, 1387b
Coxa plana, 1705–1706, 1705b
Coxa vara, 1706–1707, 1706b
Cradle cap, 1667
Cradle position for breastfeeding, 684–685, 685f
Cranial deformities, 1604
Cranial nerves, pediatric assessment of, 930t, 931f
Cranioschisis, 1733b
Crawling reflex in newborns, 622t–625t, 623f
C-reactive protein (CRP), 1764t–1771t
Creatine kinase, 1764t–1771t
Creatinine, 1764t–1771t
Creative play, 1248, 1248f
Creativity, through play, 858
Crib safety
accidental falls and, 998
suffocation danger and, 996
toddlers and, 1044
Cricoid pressure, preventing pulmonary aspiration, 516, 516f
CRIES Neonatal Postoperative Pain Scale, 939t
Critical care unit (CCU) admissions, 1255b–1256b, 1256
Critical thinking, 796
Crohn's disease (CD), 1410–1414, 1411t
Cromolyn sodium, asthma and, 1349
Cross-cradle position for breastfeeding, 684–685, 685f
Crossed extension reflex in newborns, 622t–625t, 624f
Cross-racial adoption, 818–819
Croup, 1329
Croup syndromes
acute epiglottitis, 1329–1330
acute laryngitis, 1330–1331
acute laryngotracheobronchitis, 1330t, 1331–1332, 1331b
acute spasmodic laryngitis, 1332
bacterial tracheitis, 1332
comparison of, 1330t
Crude birth rate, 803b
Crude death rate, 803b
Crust, 1645f
Crutchfield tong traction, 1697, 1697f
Crying, communication in, 967
Crying of newborns, 641
Cryoablation, 1487
Cryopreservation of human embryos, 133b
Cryptogenic seizures, 1593
Cryptorchidism, 1546t
Cuddliness of newborns, 640
Cued speech, 1202
Cuffs for pediatric BP measurements, 901–905, 903f, 903t
Cul-de-sac of Douglas, 64
Cultural awareness
bladder catheterization, 1284b
breastfeeding, 678–679
care/disposal of placenta, 480–481
child pain assessment, 939
childbearing expectations, 22, 22b
cosleeping/bed sharing, 1009b, 1034
developmental dysplasia of hip, 1700b
father's participation, 450
food customs, 826, 834–835, 887b
health beliefs/practices, 835–837, 836b, 840t–841t
labour experience, 449–450
learning sociocultural mores, 1052b
maternal nutrition, 268–270, 269t–270t
nursing strategies regarding, 25, 25t–26t
pain of labour/birth, 396, 396b
perinatal care, 5
during postpartum period, 550–552
prenatal care, 236–238, 237b
regarding newborns, 485, 660b
of religious orientations, 1089b
sex education, 1057
special needs child and, 1158
during transition to parenthood, 569–570
Cultural competence
ASKED model of, 840b
fostering, 837–842
guidelines for, 834b
in health care providers, 831–835
integration into care plan, 27
during interviews, 69–70, 70b, 871–872

Cultural competence *(Continued)*
in perinatal care, 22–27, 22b–23b
Cultural diversity
health care and, 44–45
in mother-infant bonding, 561b
perinatal care and, 21–22
respect for in home care nursing, 1223–1224, 1223b
sensitivity to, 831–835
valuing, 22, 23b
Cultural relativism, 832
Cultural safety, 22
Cultural shock, 832
Culture
defined, 21, 825
family and, 21
as health determinant, 44–45, 824–826, 826f
importance of to nursing, 837–842
intimate partner violence and, 59
self-esteem and, 826
social roles and, 825–826
Cunnilingus, 235
Cushing's syndrome, 1624–1625, 1624f
Custody of children, 820–821
Cutaneous disorders. *See* Integumentary disorders
Cutaneous stimulation strategies for pain management, 400b
Cyanosis, 1474–1476
EA/TEF and, 1426
Cyanotic heart lesions, 354–355
CycleBeads necklace, 138, 138f
Cyclic perimenstrual pain and discomfort (CPPD)
dysmenorrhea, 85–87
overview, 85
premenstrual syndrome, 87–89
Cystic fibrosis (CF)
clinical manifestations of, 1358b
diagnosis of, 1358
exocrine gland dysfunction in, 1356–1357, 1357f
genetic factors in, 831
lung transplants and, 1361
management of
for endocrine problems, 1360–1361
for gastrointestinal problems, 1360
for pulmonary problems, 1358–1360
nursing care for, 1361–1364
during pregnancy, 366–367
prognosis for, 1361
transition to adulthood and, 1363–1364
Cystitis, 1541–1542
Cystoceles, 589–590, 590f
Cystoscopy, 1538t–1539t
Cysts, 1644f
Cytochemical markers for leukemia, 1517–1518
Cytomegalovirus (CMV) infection, 753–754, 753f

D

Danazol, endometriosis and, 91
Data collection, community assessment and, 30–32
Day care, 970–976
DDAVP (1-deamino-8-d-arginine vasopressin), 1513
Deaf, definition of, 1199
Deaf-blind children, 1209
Death
of child
child's understanding/reactions to, 1177t–1178t
grief response to, 1183–1184
at home, 1181–1182
in hospital, 1182
nurse's reaction to, 1184–1185, 1185b
signs of approaching, 1182b
child's need to say good-bye, 1182b
maternal, 607
of newborn
communicating/caring techniques for acknowledging/expressing feelings, 604–607
actualizing loss, 603, 604f
care at/after discharge, 606–607
creating memories for parents, 605–606, 606f
decision making and, 603–604
maternal physical needs, 605
postmortem care/documentation, 606
family aspects of, 602
grief responses in, 599–602
nursing care for, 602–607, 602b
parental cultural/spiritual needs, 606
positive coping with, 605
principles of palliative care in, 1174–1175
Debridement of burn wounds, 1675
Decelerations of fetal heart rate
early, 433, 433b, 434f
late, 434, 434f, 435b
prolonged, 435
variable, 434–435, 434f, 435b
Deciduous teeth, 1084, 1084f
Decision making, end-of-life care and, 1175–1176
Decompensated shock, 1493b, 1494
Deep breathing, play activities for, 1266b
Deep tendon reflexes (DTRs)
assessment, 301–302, 302f, 302t
in newborns, 928
Deferasirox, 1511
Dehydration
in diabetic ketoacidosis, 1634
during hospitalization, 1272
pediatric, 1389–1392
evaluating extent of, 1392t
hypoxemic children and, 1476
IV fluids for, 1397–1398
in respiratory infections, 1319–1320
Delayed gratification
infants and, 964
toddlers and, 1022
DeLee-Hillis fetoscope, 425, 425f
Delivery rooms, 474–475, 474f
Deltoid injection site, 1289–1290, 1290t–1291t
Demerol
for children, 947t
for labour pain management, 409
Demography, community health and, 802
Denial
diagnosis of special needs child and, 1163
phase of separation anxiety, 1232
Dental caries
fruit juice and, 1059
school-age children and, 1098–1099
toddlers and, 1036–1037
Dental health
adolescents and, 1127
cerebral palsy and, 1727–1728
for children, 788
education in, 223–224
for infants, 983
preschoolers and, 1060–1061
school-age children and, 1098–1099, 1098f
toddlers and, 1034–1037
Denver II, 1757f–1758f
Depot medroxyprogesterone acetate (DMPA, Depo-Provera), 149–150
Depressed skull fractures, 1576
Depression
nursing care for, 596–598, 597b
postpartum. *See also* Postpartum mood disorder (PPMD)
with psychotic features, 594–596
without psychotic features, 594
risks of, 53
in school-age children, 1110, 1110b
Dermatitis
atopic, 1665–1667, 1666b
contact, 1655–1657
diaper, 756, 1664, 1664f, 1665b
seborrheic, 1667
Dermatological conditions, pregnancy and, 199–200
Dermatological disorders. *See* Integumentary disorders
Dermatome, 1677, 1677f
Dermatophytoses, 1653–1655, 1654t
Descent phase
process of, 389
during second stage of labour, 469–470, 469t
Desensitization, childhood fears and, 1057–1058
Despair phase of separation anxiety, 1232–1234, 1233b, 1233f
Desquamation of skin in newborns, 618
Detachment phase of separation anxiety, 1232–1234, 1233b
Determinants of health
children's health, 786–787, 787t
cultural issues, 44–45, 824–826
environmental safety, 54–55
finances, 44, 827–828
gender, 45
key, 5b
Determinants of health *(Continued)*
nutritional status, 250, 251f
primary social, 824–829
as risk factors, 274, 275b
social status, 45
Dethronement, toddlers and, 1030
Development, growth and. *See* Growth and development
Developmental aspects, 1170–1174, 1171t–1172t
Developmental aspects of chronic illness/disability in children, 1170f
Developmental assessment, 1757f–1758f
Developmental care for preterm infants, 722–726
Developmental delay, 1157b
Developmental disability, 1157b
Developmental dysplasia of hip (DDH)
cultural factors in, 1700b
diagnosis of, 1700, 1700b
management of, 1700–1701
in newborns, 620, 621f, 775–776, 775f–776f
nursing care for, 1701
pathophysiology of, 1699–1700
Developmental lactase deficiency, 1388
Developmental night crying, 982t
Dexamethasone
antenatal glucocorticoid therapy with, 496–497, 497b
for bacterial meningitis, 1588
for children, 946t
Dextroamphetamine sulphate (Dexedrine), 1106–1107
Diabetes insipidus (DI), 1572, 1615–1616
Diabetes mellitus (DM)
genetic factors in, 831
gestational. *See* Gestational diabetes mellitus (GDM)
maternal
breastfeeding and, 696
classification of, 339
metabolic changes of pregnancy, 339–340, 340f
pathogenesis of, 339
pediatric
childhood obesity and, 788–789
type 1
characteristics of, 1627t
clinical manifestations of, 1628b
complications from, 1628–1629
diagnosis of, 1629
exercise and, 1632
hyperglycemia and, 1633, 1633t, 1637
hypoglycemia and, 1632–1633, 1633t, 1637–1638
illness and, 1633
incidence of, 1627–1628
insulin therapy for, 1629–1630, 1631b
ketoacidosis in, 1628–1629, 1633–1634

Diabetes mellitus (DM) *(Continued)*
monitoring blood glucose levels, 1630–1631, 1630t, 1636–1637
nursing care for, 1634–1639
nutrition for, 1631–1632, 1635
pathophysiology of, 1628
self-management and, 1638
supportive care for, 1638–1639
type 2
characteristics of, 1627t
incidence of, 1639
management of, 1639
risk reduction for, 1639–1640
screening for/diagnosis of, 1639
pregestational. *See* Pregestational diabetes mellitus
Diabetic ketoacidosis (DKA)
in diabetic pregnancy, 342
pediatric, 1633–1635
Diagnostic procedures
community health, 805
in health assessment, 79
in prenatal period, 216–218, 217t
Dialysis, 1558–1560, 1560f
Diaper dermatitis, 756, 1664, 1664f, 1665b
Diaper rash, 668–669
Diaphragm
barrier contraceptives, 143–144, 143f
insertion/care of, 145b–146b
Diaphragmatic hernias, 1428t
Diarrhea
pediatric
acute, 1392, 1393t–1395t
diagnosis of, 1396
etiology of, 1395–1396
management of, 1396–1398, 1397f
nursing care for, 1398–1399, 1399b
pathophysiology of, 1396
prevention of, 1399
types of, 1392–1395
Diastasis recti abdominis, 200, 201f, 528–529
Diastatic skull fractures, 1576
Diazepam
for children, 946t
for status epilepticus, 1598
Dick-Read, Dr.Grantly, 400–401
Dietary history
for family/child assessment, 886–887, 886b
maternal nutrition and, 263–267, 265b, 266t
in pediatric health history, 890
Dietary intake
for breastfeeding mothers, 694
chronic renal failure and, 1557
constipation and, 1401, 1401b
cystic fibrosis and, 1362
Down syndrome children, 1197
for gestational diabetes mellitus, 309, 345, 345b
Dietary intake *(Continued)*
guidelines, for toddlers, 1033–1034
hyperlipidemia and, 1484–1485
Dietary Reference Intakes (DRIs)
for infants, 978t
in nutritional assessment, 890
during pregnancy/lactation, 251, 253t–254t
vegetarian diets and, 1380–1384
Diethylstilbestrol (DES), 76b
Dietitians of Canada, 861b, 1138, 1197, 1380
Differentiation
defined, 844
growth pattern, 846
Difficult child, 849–850
Digestion
infants and, 959
neonates and, 614
Digestive defects, 1433
Digestive enzymes in human milk, 682
Digital subtraction angiography (DSA), 1567t–1568t
Digital thermometers for infants/children, 902b
Digoxin
congestive heart failure and, 1469–1472, 1472b
laboratory tests for, 1269, 1764t–1771t
toxicity, 1472b
Dilated cardiomyopathy, 1487
Dilation and curettage (D&C), 315
Dilation and evacuation (D&E)
abortion, 154
after miscarriage, 315
Dilation of cervix during labour, 385f, 386
Dilaudid, 408, 408b
Dinoprostone
cervical ripening with, 507–508
medication guide for, 507b
Diphtheria vaccine, 984–985
contraindications/precautions for, 989t–991t
symptoms/management of, 1064t–1070t
Diplegia, 1725b
Directional trends in growth/development, 845–846, 845f
Disabilities
cognitive. *See* Cognitive impairments (CIs)
defined, 1157b
women with, health assessment for, 70–72
Discharge after birth
Caesarean birth and, 519, 519b
criteria for, 535–536, 536b
dealing with visitors and, 553–554
follow-up care
prescribed medications, 553
routine checkups following, 553
self-management/complications and, 552–554
sexual activity/contraception and, 552–553, 553b
Discipline
cognitively impaired children and, 1194
Discipline *(Continued)*
infants and, 976
in parenting, 814–817, 815b
school-age children and, 1094–1095
special needs children and, 1170–1173
toddlers and, 1028
Disease
distribution of, 803
influencing development, 862
prevention of, 803
Dishonest behaviour, school-age children and, 1095
Diskhaler, asthma and, 1349
Dislocation(s)
in children, 1689
of hip, in newborns, 775. *See also* Developmental dysplasia of hip (DDH)
Disorders of sex development in newborns, 777, 777f
Disorientation, 1564b
Disseminated intravascular coagulation (DIC), 329–330
in children, 1516–1517, 1516b, 1516f
postpartum bleeding and, 584
Distal bone fragment, 1690
Distal intestinal obstruction syndrome, 1357
Distraction, 1697–1698
Distraction during pediatric procedures, 941b
Distress behaviours, 934, 935f
Distribution pattern of skin lesions, 1643
Distributive shock, 1492t
Diuresis, postpartal, 529–530
Diuretics
breastfeeding and, 1753t–1756t
congestive heart failure and, 1468–1469, 1469t, 1473–1474
Diuril
breastfeeding and, 1753t–1756t
for heart failure, 1469t
Divorce, parenting and, 819–821, 820b
Dizygotic (fraternal) twins
characteristics of, 812–813, 812b
formation of, 180, 184f
Documentation in pediatric nursing, 797
Doll's head manoeuvre, 1566
Domestic mimicry, toddlers and, 1024, 1024f
Dominant traits, 163
Donor embryo, 134t
Donor milk banks, 694
Donor oocyte, 134t
Do-not-resuscitate (DNR) orders, 1175
Doppler blood flow analysis
for infant PB measurement, 901–902
ultrasound for, 291, 291f
Doppler ultrasound stethoscope, 220, 221f
Doptone, for IA of fetal heart, 425, 425f
Dorsal rhizotomy, 1727
Double knee roll, 546f
Doulas
functions of, 6
interviewing, 242b
labour support by, 465–466
for perinatal care, 241
Down syndrome
chromosome abnormality, 164
diagnosis of, 1195, 1196b, 1196f
diagnostic procedures for, 220, 278
etiology of, 1195
management of, 1195–1197
nursing care for, 1197–1198
nursing care with diagnosis of, 165b
prenatal diagnosis/genetic counselling for, 1198
preventing physical problems in, 1197–1198
prognosis of, 1197
Drainage following brain tumour surgery, 1585
Dramatic/pretend play, 856–857, 1248–1249
Drawing skills, school-age children and, 1098
Dreams, 877b–878b
Dressing skills
cognitively impaired children and, 1194
preschoolers and, 1054, 1054f
toddlers and, 1028
Drop attacks, 1594b–1595b
Droplet precautions, 1277b, 1278
Drowning
in children, 789–790, 790f
education for prevention of, 1132b
infants and, 1000
school-age children and, 1102t
toddlers and, 1042
Drug therapy
for ADHD, 1106–1107
adjunct to CPR, 1368, 1369t
administration of, 418–420. *See also* Administration of medications
for anorexia nervosa/bulimia nervosa, 1143
antihypertensive, 1490
for asthma, 1349–1350
for bacterial meningitis, 1588
breastfeeding and, 696, 1753t–1756t
for cardiac conditions, 360t
chemotherapeutic agents, 1523
childbirth risks with, 47–48
for congestive heart failure, 1468
as diuretics, 1469t
education in, 229
for enuresis, 1108
for epilepsy, 1597, 1599–1603
history of using, 215, 881
for hyperlipidemia, 1484–1485
immunosuppressants, 1560
infant poisoning and, 998
for infertility, 131–133
for inflammatory bowel disease, 1412
influencing neonatal behaviour, 639
for juvenile idiopathic arthritis, 1717

Drug therapy *(Continued)*
for major burns, 1675
obesity and, 1138
as pain management for terminally ill child, 1179–1181
for peptic ulcer disease, 1415–1416
for PPMD, 596, 596t, 598–599
during pregnancy, 229
prescribed after childbirth, 553
skin reactions to, 1657
toddler poisoning from, 1043
for unconscious child, 1569, 1572
Drug-exposed newborns. *See also* Newborns at risk
nursing care for, 762–765, 764b, 766b
physiological effects of, 756–765, 757t
Dual-earner families, 821–822
Duchenne muscular dystrophy (DMD)
characteristics of, 1740–1741, 1741b
diagnosis of, 1741–1742
management of, 1742
nursing care for, 1742–1743
Ductal carcinoma, 115–116
Ductus arteriosus, failed closure of, 731
Dwarfism, 1105
Dysacusis, 1199
Dysfunctional labour
factors associated with, 498
hypertonic uterine dysfunction, 498–499
hypotonic uterine dysfunction, 499, 500b
Dysfunctional uterine bleeding (DUB), 92–94
Dyskinetic cerebral palsy, 1725b–1726b
Dyslalia, 1059
Dysmenorrhea
in adolescents, 1134–1135
nursing care for, 1134–1135
overview, 85–86
primary, 86–87, 1134
alternative therapies for, 87, 1134
medications for, 87t, 1134
secondary, 87, 1134
Dysplasia
acetabular, 775
bronchopulmonary, 732–733
Dyspnea, 920b
Dysrhythmias, 1485–1487, 1486b
Dyssomnia, 981–982
Dystocia
definition/causes of, 498
dysfunctional labour and, 498–499
fetal causes of, 499–502
maternal position and, 502
nursing care for, 503, 503b
pelvic, 499
psychological responses and, 502–503
shoulder, 520–521, 520f
soft tissue, 499
Dystonic movements, 1725b

E
Ear sensor (LighTouch LTX), 902b
Early childhood
communicative development in, 875, 875f
developmental stage, 845b
Early contact, forming attachment and, 558
Early decelerations of fetal heart rate, 433, 433b, 434f
Early Infancy Temperament Questionnaire, 968
Early intervention for special needs children, 1159
Early pregnancy bleeding, 312–316
Early-childhood education, 1055–1057
Ears
administration of medications to, 1296–1297
auditory tests for infants/children, 915, 915t
external structure, pediatric, 912–913, 912f
internal structure, pediatric, 913–915, 913f–914f
of newborns, 626t–636t, 631f, 643b
nutritional status and, 887t–889t
temperature measurement and, 897–901, 899t, 900b–902b
Easy child, 849
Eating disorders
anorexia nervosa, 1109, 1141–1144, 1142b
bulimia nervosa, 1109, 1141–1144, 1142b
health risks of, 50
obesity, 788–789, 789f, 1136–1141, 1137t, 1139b–1140b
Eating habits of adolescents, 1126, 1126f. *See also* Dietary intake
Eating Well With Canada's Food Guide
dietary recommendations, 257t, 267, 890, 1126, 1385f
guidelines for preschoolers, 1059
guidelines for toddlers, 1033–1034, 1033b
type 1 diabetes and, 1632
vegetarian diets and, 1383–1384
Ecchymoses
in contusions, 1688
defined, 1643
in neonates, 651–652, 651f
Eclampsia, 297–298
in diabetic pregnancy, 341
immediate care, 306–307, 307b
postpartum care, 307–308
symptoms of, 305–306, 306f
Ecomaps, 19, 20f
Economics of health care, 804
Ectoderm, 171f, 172
Ectopic pregnancy
collaborative care for, 318–320
incidence/etiology of, 318, 318f
treatment options, 319
Eczema, 1665–1667, 1666b

Edema
acute glomerulonephritis and, 1550, 1550b
ankle, 231t–233t
carpal tunnel syndrome and, 200–201
cerebral, 1577
leg position for reducing, 228f
nephrotic syndrome and, 1547, 1548f
Edinburgh Postnatal Depression Scale (EPDS), 550, 551f, 596
Educable cognitive impairments, 1190
Education. *See also* Patient/family teaching
apnea/home oxygen saturation monitors, 1014b
bicycle safety, 1103b
Caesarean home care, 519, 519b
car safety seats, 1041b
care for drug-exposed newborns, 765b
child safety, 1002b
childbirth, 400–402
children with cognitive impairment, 1191–1192, 1192f
colicky infant, 1005b
for family of special needs child, 1169–1170
fetal status, 439–440
health, 46, 46b, 795
helping children in school, 1094b
HIV infection, 1529–1530
hospitalized children and, 1246, 1249
introducing solid foods to infants, 981b
jaundice, 663
nutritional, 267
in pain management for terminally ill child, 1181
postpartum depression, 550b, 597b
prenatal
alcohol/smoking/caffeine/drugs, 229–230
breastfeeding, 223, 223f–224f
childbirth, 243–247
dental health, 223–224
employment, 227
immunizations, 229
Kegel exercises, 222–223
medications/herbal preparations, 229
normal discomforts, 230, 231t–233t
nutritional, 222
overview, 222
perinatal, 245–247
personal hygiene, 222
physical activity, 224, 224f
posture/body mechanics, 224, 226f
potential complications, 220b, 230–233
preterm labour, 233–234, 234b, 234f
rest/relaxation, 224–227, 226f, 227b
safety, 227b
travel, 228–229, 229f
UTI prevention, 222

Education *(Continued)*
preterm birth, 497b
prevention of adolescent injury, 1132b
prevention of child sexual abuse, 1080b
safe sleeping for infants, 1010b
sex. *See* Sex education
skateboard/in-line skate safety, 1103b
for special needs children, 1165, 1228
toy safety, 860b–861b
true vs. false labour, 444b
for visually impaired children, 1207
Education Act, 1191–1192, 1228
Educational strategies for treatment compliance, 1269–1270
Effacement of cervix during labour, 385, 385f
Effleurage for labour pain management, 403
Ego mastery, middle childhood play and, 1092
Egocentrism
in preoperational thought, 1025b
toddlers and, 1022
Eisenmenger's syndrome, 354
Ejaculation, 1114–1115
Elbow restraints, 1280–1281
Elbow winging, 123b
Electric breast pumps, 692, 693f
Electric company services, 1228–1229
Electrical burns, 1670
infants and, 999f
toddlers and, 1043, 1043f
Electrical wires/outlets, infants and, 1000, 1000f
Electrocardiogram, 1452, 1452t
Electrocardiography, 1452–1453, 1452t
Electrode placement, monitoring apnea and, 1014, 1014f
Electroencephalography (EEG), 1567, 1567t–1568t
epilepsy and, 1596
Electrolyte balance
acute adrenocortical insufficiency and, 1623b
changes in, 198–199
in neonates, 613
in preterm infants, 719
Electrolyte therapy, diabetic ketoacidosis and, 1634
Electronic continuous thermometers, 901, 902b
Electronic fetal monitoring (EFM)
external, 426–429, 428f
following trauma, 335
history of use, 423
internal, 429, 429f
modes of, 426, 427t, 429f
patient teaching and, 437f, 438b
pattern recognition, 435–440
Electronic intermittent thermometers, 901, 902b
Electronic media, adolescents and, 1122
Electronic medical records, 870
Elimination
after childbirth, 530, 545
during labour, 458t, 460

Elimination *(Continued)*
parental guidance regarding, 667
in preterm infants, 719
spinal bifida and, 1735
toilet training and, 1021, 1029
unconscious child and, 1572
Emancipated minors, 1260
Embolism
amniotic fluid, 523–524, 524b
pulmonary, 585–586
thromboembolism, 585–586, 586b
Embryo adoption, 134t
Embryo cryopreservation, 133b
Embryo hosting, 134t
Embryonic development
amniotic fluid, 173
fetal membranes, 172–173, 172f
milestones in, 181t–183t
overview, 169f, 172
placenta, 174–176, 174f–175f
primary germ layers, 171f, 172
toxic exposures, 176b
umbilical cord, 172f, 173
yolk sac, 171f, 173
Emergency admissions, 1254–1256, 1255b
Emergency childbirth, 478, 479b
Emergency contraception (EC), 150
Emergency department, 23b
Emergency interventions
for amniotic fluid embolism, 524b
for avulsed tooth, 1099b
for burns, 1673, 1673b
cardiopulmonary resuscitation, 363b, 1365–1368, 1366f–1367f
for eclampsia, 307b
for epilepsy, 1600b
for epistaxis, 1517b
for eye injuries, 1206b
during first stage of labour, 467, 467b–468b
for fractures, 1692b
for head injury, 1578b
for hemorrhagic shock, 583b
for hypoglycemia, 1638b
for hypotension with decreased placental perfusion, 413b
for hypovolemic shock, 542b, 583b
induction of labour with oxytocin and, 510b
for poisoning, 1436–1440, 1437b–1439b
for prolapsed cord, 523b
for shock, 1494b
for supine hypotension, 216b
tube occlusion/accidental decannulation, 1307–1308
without consent, 1260
Emergency medical service (EMS), 1366
Emergency protocols, family-centred home care and, 1228
Emotional abuse of children
clinical manifestations of, 1077b–1078b
defined, 1072
history/interview in, 1076
physical assessment in, 1078
types of, 1072
Emotional deprivation, 861–862
Emotional disorders, adolescence and, 1129
Emotional expression through play, 1248
Emotionality, adolescence and, 1118–1119
Emotions during pregnancy, cultural perspectives of, 237
Empathic responses during interviews, 70, 872
Employment Equity Act, 829
Empowerment
from community, 828–829
in family-centred care, 794
of parents of special needs child, 1162
advocacy for, 1168
Encephalitis, 1590–1591, 1590b
Encephalocele, 768–770, 1733b
Encopresis, 1072, 1399–1400
Endemic typhus, 1662t
Endocephalography, 1567t–1568t
Endocervical length predicting preterm labour, 490
Endocrine dysfunction
adrenal disorders and
acute adrenocortical insufficiency, 1622–1623, 1622b
chronic adrenocortical insufficiency, 1623–1624, 1623b
congenital adrenal hyperplasia, 1625–1626
Cushing's syndrome, 1624–1625, 1624f
pheochromocytoma, 1625–1626
insulin secretion disorders and. *See* Diabetes mellitus (DM)
parathyroid disorders and
hyperparathyroidism, 1621–1622, 1621b
hypoparathyroidism, 1620–1621, 1620b
pituitary disorders and
diabetes insipidus, 1615–1616
hypopituitarism, 1611–1613, 1612b
pituitary hyperfunction, 1613–1614
precocious puberty, 1614–1615, 1614b
syndrome of inappropriate antidiuretic hormone secretion, 1616
thyroid disorders and
goitre, 1617
hyperthyroidism, 1618–1620, 1619b
juvenile hypothyroidism, 1617, 1617b
lymphocytic thyroiditis, 1617–1618, 1618b
Endocrine system
adaptations of, 203, 203t
changes during labour, 392
after childbirth, 529
fetal development of, 179
Endoderm, 171f, 172
End-of-life care
child's understanding of/reactions to death, 1177t–1178t
decision making and, 1175–1176
fear of child dying alone, 1181, 1181f
grief and mourning, 1183–1184, 1184b
home deaths, 1181–1182
hospital deaths, 1182
nurse's reaction to, 1184–1185, 1185b
organ/tissue donation/autopsy, 1182–1183
pain and symptom management, 1179–1181, 1180b
principles of palliative care in, 1174–1175
signs of approaching death, 1182b
treatment options for, 1176–1179
Endometrial cycle, 82, 83f
Endometriosis
incidence of, 89–90, 90f
management of, 90–91
Endometritis, 586
Endometrium, 64, 66f
postpartum regeneration of, 527
Endorphins, labour pain and, 396
End-stage liver disease, 1420b
End-stage renal disease (ESRD), 1558–1559
transplantation and, 1560
Enemas, hospitalized children and, 1312, 1312b
Energy drinks during pregnancy, 257
Energy needs
of infants, 679
during pregnancy, 251–256
Energy work, 247, 403
Engagement, birth process and, 380, 389
Engorgement, breast
abrupt weaning and, 693–694
breastfeeding and, 696–697
Enteral feeding, preterm infants and, 718
Enterobiasis, 1407–1408, 1407b
Enterocolitis, 1401
Enthesitis-related arthritis, 1716
Entrainment, parent-infant bonding and, 561
Enuresis, 1107–1108
Environment
for ADHD, 1107
characteristics of, child abuse and, 1073
in epidemiological triangle, 803
for interview process, 869–870, 870f
for labour/childbirth, 398
play activities for extending, 1266b
for preterm infants, 722
Environmental contaminants, breastfeeding and, 696
Environmental hazards influencing development, 862–863
Environmental safety
as health determinant, 54–55
during hospitalization, 1275–1277, 1275f–1276f
Environmental stressors in pediatric/neonatal CCU admission, 1256b
Environmental tobacco smoke exposure, 1344
Enzyme-linked immunosorbent assay (ELISA), 187–188, 1527–1528
Enzymes, pancreatic, 1360
Eosinophil count, 1764t–1771t
Epidemic typhus, 1662t
Epidemiological triangle, 803, 803f
Epidemiology, community health and, 802–804
Epidermal stripping, 1271
Epidural anaesthesia/analgesia
administration of, 419
for children, 947–950
contraindications to, 416
features of, 948b–949b, 950f
for labour pain management, 413–415, 414f
maternal hypotension in, 413b
neonates and, 416
Epidural hematoma, 1575f
Epidural hemorrhage, 1576–1577
Epidural opioids, 415–416
Epidural sensor as ICP monitor, 1570
Epiglottitis, 1329–1330, 1330t
Epilepsy
pediatric
diagnosis of, 1594–1596
emergency intervention for, 1600b
etiology of, 1593, 1593b
management of, 1597–1598
nursing care for, 1598–1603, 1599b, 1601b–1603b
pathophysiology of, 1593
seizure classification/clinical manifestations, 1593–1594, 1594b–1595b, 1596t
seizure precautions, 1600b
status epilepticus and, 1598
during pregnancy, 368
Epinephrine
anaphylactic reactions and, 1386b–1387b, 1387
breastfeeding and, 1753t–1756t
for cardiovascular support, 1494b, 1495
for laryngotracheobronchitis, 1331
Epiphyseal injuries, 1690
Episiotomy
definition/types of, 477–478, 478f
interventions for, 541, 541b
Epispadias, 776–780, 1546t
Epistaxis, 1517, 1517b
Epstein-Barr virus (EBV), 1328
Epulis, 200, 202
Equianalgesia, 944, 947t
Equipment for birthing, 474, 474f
Erb palsy, 744–745, 745f
Ergocalciferol. *See* Vitamin D
Erikson's stages of psychosocial development, 851–852
adolescents and, 1117–1119
infants and, 963–964
preschoolers and, 1052

Erikson's stages of psychosocial development *(Continued)*
  school-age children and, 1085–1087
  toddlers and, 1022
Erosion, 1645f
Erythema, 1643
Erythema infectiosum, 1064f, 1064t–1070t
Erythema migrans, 1662f, 1663–1664
Erythema toxicum, 619, 619f, 651
Erythrocyte sedimentation rate (ESR), 1764t–1771t
Erythromycin
  breastfeeding and, 1753t–1756t
  for chlamydia during pregnancy, 98
  for eye prophylaxis, 647b
Escherichia coli infection, 1393t–1395t
  neonatal, 755
  UTIs and, 1542
Esophageal atresia (EA), 772–773, 773f
Esophageal atresia with tracheoesophageal fistula (EA/TEF), 1425–1427, 1425b
Esophagus during pregnancy, 202
Estimated Average Requirements (EARs), 890, 1380–1384
Estimated date of birth (EDB), 206
Estrogen
  after childbirth, 529
  menstrual cycle and, 82–84
  during puberty, 1114
Estrogen-progestin contraceptives
  oral, 147–148, 148b, 149f
  transdermal contraceptive patch, 148
  vaginal ring, 148
Etanercept, 1717
Ethanol. *See* Alcohol
Ethical issues
  in end-of-life decision making, 1175
  fetal rights and, 285b
  genetic testing and, 162
  in nursing research, 14
  in pediatric nursing, 796, 796b
  in perinatal nursing, 13
  resuscitation of ELBW infants, 708
Ethnicity. *See also* Cultural awareness
  defined, 825, 825f
  food customs and, 834–835
  as health determinant, 45, 826–827
  health problems linked to, 831
  perinatal care and, 5
  respect for, 833
  skin assessments and, 200b
Ethnocentrism, 827
Euglycemia, 343–344, 344t
Euploidy, 163–164
European ethnicity
  breastfeeding and, 660b, 678
  cystic fibrosis and, 45
  lactase deficiency and, 831, 1388
  practices regarding newborns and, 660b
Euthanasia, 1175
Evaporative heat loss in newborns, 612
Evidence of consent, 1260
Evidence-informed practice
  on advanced maternal age, 568b
  on buffered lidocaine during PIV access, 952b
  on childbirth education, 402
  on early discharge after birth, 537b
  on exercise/work in pregnancy, 52b
  on gastric lavage in children, 1441b
  on herbal tea safety, 258b
  on monitoring for neonatal hypoglycemia, 616b
  on optimal birth spacing, 137b
  on pain management for terminally ill child, 1180b
  pediatric nursing and, 796–797
  perinatal nursing and, 9–10, 10b
  on postpartum mood disorder assessment, 595b
  on prenatal breastfeeding education, 245b
  on saline instillation before suctioning, 1306b
  on sickle cell anemia and penicillin, 1508b
  on skin-to-skin contact and, 688b
  on STS contact for preterm infants, 726b
  on temperature measurements in pediatrics, 900b–901b
  thimerosal-containing vaccines and ASDs, 1211b
Ewing's sarcoma, 1714–1715
Exanthem subitum, 1064t–1070t, 1066f
Excision of burn wounds, 1675
Excoriation, 1645f
Exencephaly, 1733b
Exercise
  adolescents and, 1127, 1127f
  asthma and, 1350
  for back pain, 224, 224f
  benefits of, 51, 51f–52f
  after breast surgery, 123b
  breastfeeding and, 694
  after childbirth, 545, 546f
  cognitively impaired children and, 1192–1193
  cultural perspectives, 237–238
  for cystic fibrosis, 1359
  in diabetic pregnancy, 345–346
  education in, 224, 224f
  for GDM, 309
  for juvenile idiopathic arthritis, 1718–1719
  restricted, for pre-eclampsia, 302–303
  school-age children and, 1097–1098
  tips, 225b, 225f
  type 1 diabetes and, 1632, 1638
  unconscious child and, 1572–1573
  weight reduction and, 1140
Exercise-associated amenorrhea, 85
Exercise-induced bronchospasm (EIB), 1350
Exocrine gland dysfunction, 1356–1357, 1357f
Exophthalmos, 1618, 1619b
Experiential history, prenatal care and, 215
Expressive activities for hospitalized children, 1264, 1264f
Expulsion, birth process and, 391
Exstrophy of bladder
  in newborns, 777, 777f
  surgery for, 1546t
Extended contact
  in forming attachment, 560
  in parent-infant bonding, 560f
Extended family, 17, 17f
Extension, birth process and, 391
Extension posturing, 1566, 1566f
External cephalic version (ECV) of fetus, 501–502, 501f
External female genitalia, 63–64, 64f
External fixation, 1697, 1699f
External proportions during growth/development, 846, 847f
External rotation, birth process and, 391
External stimuli, newborn's response to, 640–641
External vascular access devices, 1559
Extracellular fluid (ECF), 960, 1389
Extracorporeal membrane oxygenation (ECMO), 717
Extrapyramidal cerebral palsy, 1725b
Extravasation, 1301–1302
Extremely-low-birth-weight (ELBW) infants
  body temperature in, 713–714
  classification of, 708b
  environmental concerns, 722
  hydration and, 719
  hyperglycemia in, 734–735
  nutrition for, 718
  respiratory distress syndrome and, 728
  respiratory function in, 710
  resuscitation of, 708
  retinopathy of prematurity and, 732
Extremities
  assessment of newborn, 626t–636t
  pediatric examination of, 927
Extremity venipuncture, 1280f, 1281
Eye contact, in parent-infant bonding, 560–561, 561f
Eye prophylaxis
  neonatal care, 646–647, 646f, 647b
  for unconscious child, 1572
Eyes
  administration of medications to, 1296–1297, 1297f
  assessment of newborn, 626t–636t, 630f
  cerebral dysfunction and, 1565–1566, 1565f
  emergency intervention for injuries to, 1206b
Eyes *(Continued)*
  examination guidelines, 911t
  external structure, pediatric, 907–908, 908f
  internal structure, pediatric, 908–909, 908f
  of newborns, 643b
  nutritional status and, 887t–889t
  prenatal assessment of, 301
  vision testing, 909–912
Ezetimibe, 1485

F

Face, of newborns, 626t–636t
FACES Pain Rating Scale, 935–936, 937t
Facial melasma, 199
Facial nerve paralysis, birth process and, 745–746, 745f
Facilitated tucking, 942
Facilitation in nurse interview, 70
Facilitative response, 877b–878b
Facioscapulohumeral muscular dystrophy, 1740, 1741f
Factor VIII concentrate, 1513–1514
Failure to thrive (FTT)
  classification of, 1005
  diagnosis of, 1005–1006, 1006b
  guidelines for feeding, 1007b
  management of, 1006
  nursing care for, 1006–1008, 1007f
  prognosis of, 1006
Fallopian tubes, 65
Falls
  during hospitalization, 1276–1277
  infants and, 997–998
  toddlers and, 1044
False labour, 443, 444b
Family advocacy, 794–795
Family assessment, 18, 882–884, 883b–884b
Family bed. *See* Cosleeping
Family history
  cerebral dysfunction and, 1562–1563
  in health care assessment, 73, 215
Family Life Cycle (Developmental) Theory, 18t
Family Medical Leave Act, 822
Family nursing
  assessment framework, 18
  Calgary Family Assessment Model, 19, 19f
  family systems theory in, 18–19
  overview, 17–18
  as relational inquiry, 20–21, 21b
  theories/models for, 18, 18t
Family planning, 135. *See also* Contraception
Family roles
  adjustment to parenthood and, 550
  cultural sensitivity to, 25
  family size and, 810, 810f
  hospitalized child and, 1237–1238
  learning, 809–813
  multiple births and, 812–813

Family roles *(Continued)*
ordinal position and, 811–812, 811b
Family Stress Theory, 18t
Family teaching. *See* Patient/family teaching
Family-centred care
home care and
central concepts of, 1222
family-to-family support in, 1229–1230
nursing process for, 1224–1226, 1225b–1226b
parent-professional collaboration in, 1224
promoting optimum development in, 1227–1228, 1227b, 1228f
respect for diversity in, 1223–1224, 1223b
safety issues in home for, 1228–1229
key elements of, 793b
philosophy of, 793–794
special needs child and, 1157
Family-Centred Maternity and Newborn Care guidelines, 6, 6b, 6f
Family-controlled analgesia, 948b–949b
Family(ies)
adaptation to pregnancy
by grandparents, 210, 212b, 213f
maternal, 206–210
paternal, 208–210
sibling, 210, 211b–212b, 211f
communicating with, 871–876
contemporary issues in, 822
cultural factors in, 21–22
definitions of, 808
divorce and, 819–821, 820b
dual-earner, 821–822
dynamics, 17
foster parenting and, 822
genograms, 19, 20f, 1223
hospitalized child and
altered family roles and, 1237–1238
parental reactions to, 1237
sibling reactions to, 1237
immobilized child and, 1687–1688
limit setting/discipline in, 814–817, 815b, 817b
lone parenting and, 821
medical history of, 882
multiple births and, 812–813, 812b
in North American culture, 829–831
nursing interventions, 808–809, 809b
ordinal position in, 811–812, 811b
parenting adopted child and, 817–819, 818f
parenting styles and, 814
reconstituted, 821
roles/relationships in, 809–813
same-sex marriages and, 821
school-age children and, 1091–1092
Family(ies) *(Continued)*
parental guidance for, 1091b
sibling interactions in, 810–811, 810f
size/configuration of, 810, 810f
social context for, 16
special needs child and
assisting in managing feelings, 1162–1164
coping with stress/crises, 1161–1162, 1162b
supportive care for, 1167–1169
establishing support system, 1164
family-centred care for, 1157
family-health care provider communication, 1157
impact on parents, 1159–1160, 1160b
impact on siblings, 1160–1161, 1161b
overprotection and, 1163b
structures, 16–17, 882–884
transition to parenthood and, 562–563, 813–814, 813f
for adolescent father, 567–568
for adolescent mother, 567
cultural factors in, 569–570
grandparent adaptation in, 572–574, 573f
for hearing-impaired parent, 571
infant-parent adjustment in, 566–567
maternal adjustment in, 563–564, 563t
nursing care for, 574–575, 574b
for older fathers, 569
for older mothers, 568–569, 568b
parental tasks/responsibilities in, 563
paternal adjustment in, 565–566, 565f–566f, 565t
personal aspirations and, 570
for same-sex couple, 564–565
sibling adaptation in, 571–572, 572f, 573b
social support for, 569
socioeconomic conditions and, 570
for visually impaired parent, 570–571, 571b
Family-to-family support networks, 1229–1230
Fanconi syndrome, 1511–1512
Fat (triglycerides)
in human milk, 682
for infants' nutrition, 679
Fathers
adaptation by. *See* Paternal adaptations
cultural factors and, 833, 833f
of special needs child, 1160
Fatigue, after childbirth, 544
Fat-soluble vitamins, 261–262
Faucial tonsils, 1322, 1323f
Fear(s)
pain of labour/birth and, 396–397, 397f
of preschoolers, 1057–1058
Fear(s) *(Continued)*
of school-age children, 1095–1096
of strangers, 967, 967f, 970
Febrile seizures, 1603–1604
Febrile urinary tract infection, 1541–1542
Feeding
newborns with cleft lip/cleft palate, 1422–1423
sick children, 1272, 1273b
Female athlete triad, 1141–1142
Female condoms, 143, 143f
Female fertility, 126–127, 127b
Female genital mutilation (FGM)
childbirth and, 478
health risks of, 13, 54, 54b
Female genitalia
formation of, 179–180
in neonates, 619
pediatric examination of, 925–926, 926f
Female reproductive system
bony pelvis, 66–67, 66f–67f
breasts, 67–68, 68f
external genitalia, 63–64, 64f
internal structures, 64–65, 65f–66f
life cycle changes in, 68t
neonatal adaptations, 619, 619f
Femoral hernias, 923, 923f
Femoral venipuncture, 1281, 1281f
Fentanyl citrate
for children, 943, 945t, 947t
for labour pain management, 409, 409b
as transdermal patch, 950–951
Ferguson reflex, bearing-down efforts and, 472–473
Fern test
preterm premature rupture of membranes and, 497–498
rupture of membranes and, 446, 447b
Fertility
female, 126–127, 127b
health promotion and, 42–43, 43b
male, 126–127, 128b
Fertility awareness methods (FAMs) of contraception, 137–142
Fertility rates
cultural issues in, 127b
factors affecting, 126–127, 127b–128b
as perinatal health indicator, 7b
trends in, 8
Fertilization process, 168, 170–171, 170f–171f
Fetal alcohol syndrome (FAS), 757–759, 758b, 759f
Fetal bradycardia, 430–431, 431t
Fetal circulation
during labour, 391
PPHN problems, 733–734
Fetal development
assessment of, 219–221, 219f
ballottement and, 190–191, 192f
circulatory system, 177–178, 177f
education on, 222–234
endocrine system, 179
gastrointestinal system, 178
Fetal development *(Continued)*
gestational age, 219–220
health status assessment, 220, 221f, 302
hematopoietic system, 178
immunological system, 180
integumentary system, 180
maternal substance use and, 757f, 757t
milestones in, 181t–183t
musculoskeletal system, 180
neurological system, 179
in relation to trauma, 333
renal system, 178–179
reproductive system, 179–180
respiratory system, 176–177
ultrasound assessment of, 280–281, 280f–281f
viability of, 176
Fetal embryonic biliary atresia, 1420
Fetal fibronectin (FFN) test, 489
Fetal head size, 378–379, 379f
Fetal health assessment
biochemical
amniocentesis for, 282–284, 283f
chorionic villus sampling in, 284–285, 285f
Coombs' test for, 281–282
percutaneous umbilical blood sampling in, 284, 284f
summary of, 282t
nursing role in, 291–292
prenatal screening in
first-trimester screening, 278, 278f
integrated prenatal screening, 278
second-trimester serum screening, 278
recommendations for, 277b
in third-trimester
contraction stress test, 288–289, 289f, 290t
fetal movement counting, 286, 287f
fetal responses to hypoxia/asphyxia, 286
indications for, 285, 286b
nonstress test, 286–288
ultrasound for, 289–291
ultrasound in, 278–281. *See also* Ultrasound
Fetal health surveillance (FHS)
abnormal FHR and, 427f, 428b
admission electronic fetal monitor strips for, 430
amnioinfusion, 438–439
antenatal/intrapartum conditions of risk, 425t
basis for, 423–424, 424b
documentation of, 440, 440f
electronic fetal monitoring in, 423, 426–429
evidence-based practice and, 428b
heart rate patterns in, 430–435
intermittent auscultation for, 425–426, 426b
during labour, overview, 391
nitroglycerine for tachysystole in, 439
normal findings, 425t
nursing care for, 435–440, 436b–437b

Fetal health surveillance (FHS) *(Continued)*
patient teaching with, 439–440
scalp blood sampling, 438
umbilical cord acid-base determination, 439, 439t
Fetal heart rate (FHR)
abnormal, 430t–431t, 436–438
interventions for, 436–438, 438b, 467b–468b
accelerations of, 433, 433f
atypical, 430t–431t, 436–438
interventions for, 436–438, 467b–468b
baseline, 430–431
decelerations of, 433–435, 433b
during first stage of labour, 452–453, 454f
history of using, 423
hypoxia/asphyxia and, 286
during labour, 391
monitoring, 220, 221f, 430t
in nonstress test, 287f–288f
normal, 425t, 430, 430t
periodic/episodic changes in, 431–435
during second stage of labour, 473
ultrasound detection of, 279–280
variability of, 431, 432f, 432t
Fetal hemolytic disease, 283
Fetal lung maturity, 496–497, 497b
Fetal maturity, 283
Fetal membranes, development of, 172–173, 172f
Fetal movement counting, 286, 287f
Fetal nutrition
adolescent pregnancy and, 263
calcium for, 260, 260b–261b
fat-soluble vitamins for, 261–262
fluids for, 256–257, 258b
fluoride for, 261
iron for, 257–260, 260b
magnesium for, 260
maternal weight gain and, 251–256
potassium for, 261
protein for, 256, 257t
sodium for, 261
water-soluble vitamins for, 262
zinc for, 261
Fetal position, 379–380, 380f–381f
Fetal presentation, 379, 380f–381f
Fetal respiration, immediately after birth, 391
Fetal tachycardia, 430, 431t
Fetopelvic disproportion, 499
Fetoscope, 220, 221f
Fetus
adaptation to labour, 391
anomalies of, 499
diabetic pregnancy risks for, 342
labour process and
fetal attitude in, 379
fetal head size and, 378–379, 379f
fetal lie in, 379, 380f
fetal position in, 379–380, 380f
fetal presentation in, 379, 380f–382f
Fetus *(Continued)*
malposition of, 499–500
malpresentation of, 500–502, 501f
maternal relationship to, 208
movement in labour, 378–380, 380f–382f
paternal relationship to, 209, 210b
responses to hypoxia/asphyxia, 286
ultrasound assessment of, 281
Fever
definition of, 1272
pediatric, 898b
controlling, 1273–1274, 1275b
Fibrinogen, 1764t–1771t
Fibrinolysis, 1512–1513
Fibrocystic changes in breasts, 111–113
Fifth disease, 1064f, 1064t–1070t
Filipino ethnicity
food patterns of, 269t–270t
imbalance of forces and, 835
inactivity during pregnancy and, 237–238
Fine motor development
infants and, 960
preschoolers and, 1051t, 1052f
school-age children and, 1098
toddlers and, 1021–1022, 1023t
Finger-to-nose test, 928b
Firearm injuries, adolescents and, 1132–1133
First Nations
breast cancer and, 116f
breastfeeding and, 678
child maltreatment and, 1000
childhood dental caries, 1098–1099
cigarette smoking and, 1144–1145
cleft lip and palate in, 1421
developmental dysplasia of hip in, 1700b
food practices of, 269t–270t, 887b
health beliefs/practices and, 840t–841t
HIV infection in, 1527
home care and, 1223
injury prevention for, 1101
iron deficiency anemia in, 1503
maternity services for, 3–5, 29, 44–45
otitis media in, 1325–1326
preschool program for, 1056
reactions to pain and, 396b
social/economic/health problems of, 830
substance use and, 1146, 1148
suicide and, 792, 1150
traditional postpartum health practices, 552
tuberculosis and, 1338
type 2 DM and, 1639
First stage of labour
admission data, 445–447, 447b
admission to labour unit, 445, 445f
cultural factors in, 449–450
emergency interventions during, 467, 467b–468b
expected maternal progress, 451t
First stage of labour *(Continued)*
laboratory/diagnostic tests, 455–456
nursing care for, 442–443, 443b, 459b–460b
phases of, 389
physical examination in, 450–455, 451f
physical nursing care during, 457–461, 458t
psychosocial factors in, 447–448, 448t
routine precautions during, 451b
signs of complications, 457b
signs of true labour and, 443, 444b, 445
standards of care for, 456–457
stress in, 448–449
supportive care during, 461–467, 464b–465b, 466t
First trimester
abortion in, 153–154
discomforts during, 231t–233t
signs of potential complications in, 220b
First-degree burns. *See* Superficial burns
First-trimester screening (FTS), 278, 278f
Fissures, 1645f
Fistulas, dialysis and, 1559
5-Aminosalicylates (5-ASAs), 1412
Five-digit (GTPAL) system for gravidity/parity, 186–187, 187t
FLACC pain scale, 936t
Flame burns, 1043
Flexion
in mechanism of labour, 389
newborn in position of, 636f
Flexion creases on palm, 906, 906f
Flexion posturing, 1566, 1566f
Fluid balance
acute renal failure and, 1554
changes in, 198–199
in infants, 1389–1390
maintaining for hospitalized child, 1298–1302
in neonates, 613
for preterm infants, 719
Fluid intake
adequate, hypoxemic children and, 1476
during first stage of labour, 457–460, 458t
infant requirements for, 679–680, 1390, 1391b
for maternal nutrition, 256–257
play activities for, 1266b
restriction for CHD, 1473–1474
sickle cell anemia and, 1509
Fluid restriction
for acute renal failure, 1555
for CHD, 1468–1469
Fluid therapy
for diabetic ketoacidosis, 1634
for major burns, 1674
Fluid/blood replacement therapy for postpartum hemorrhage, 584
FluMist vaccine, 1325
Flunitrazepam (Rohypnol), 1147
Fluoride
adolescent supplementation of, 1127
infant supplementation of, 680, 983
for maternal nutrition, 261
nutritional significance of, 1381t–1383t
toddler supplementation of, 1036
Flush guidelines for venous access devices, 1295, 1295t
Flutter mucus clearance device, 1359, 1359f
FluWatch, 1325
Folate (folic acid)
deficiency anemia and, 364
for maternal nutrition, 250
nutritional significance of, 1376t–1379t
periconceptual need for, 250
sources of, 252t
spina bifida prevention and, 1736
Foley catheter, 1284t
Follicle-stimulating hormone (FSH), 82
Folliculitis, 1652t
Follow-up visits in prenatal period, 218–221
Fontanels, 180
Food allergies, 1384–1389, 1386b
cow's milk and, 1387–1388
Food cravings during pregnancy, 262–263
Food customs, 834–835
Food intolerance, 1384
Food sensitivity, 1384–1389
Foodborne illnesses, 267
Foods. *See* Dietary intake
Foot
clubfoot, 776, 1701–1703, 1702f
physical assessment of, 927
Football hold, breastfeeding and, 684–685, 685f
Forced expiration, 1359
Forceps-assisted birth
nursing considerations, 511–512
overview, 511, 511f
prerequisites for, 512b
types of forceps in, 512f
Foreign body (FB) aspiration
infants and, 993–996
respiratory dysfunction and, 1341
toddlers and, 1044–1045
Foreign object, eye injuries and, 1206b
Formal operations stage of cognitive development, 853
Formula feeding
bottles/nipples for, 701
commercial formulas, 701–703
feeding patterns, 701
during first 6 months, 978–979
formula preparation, 702–703, 703b–704b, 979
parent education for, 700
preterm infants, 718–719
rationale for, 700
readiness for, 700
techniques for, 701, 701f–702f
vitamin/mineral supplementation and, 703–704
weaning from, 704

Fornix, 64, 66f
Forward-facing safety seats, 1040
Fosphenytoin, 1597b
Foster care, 822
Fourchette, 63, 64f
The Fourth Report on the Diagnosis, Evaluation, and Treatment of High Blood Pressure in Children and Adolescents, 1489
Fourth stage of labour
  assessment during, 484b
  family-newborn relationship, 485
  overview, 389, 483, 485
  postanaesthesia recovery, 485
Fowler's stages of spiritual development, 854
Fractures, 1690–1692, 1691b–1692b, 1691f
  casting for, 1692–1695, 1694b, 1694f
  skull, 1576
  traction for, 1695–1697, 1695f–1696f, 1696b, 1698b
Fragile X syndrome, 1198–1199, 1198b
French Canadian ethnicity
  maple syrup urine disease and, 656t
  Tay-Sachs disease and, 158, 160f
Freud's stages of psychosexual development, 850–851
Friction, pressure ulcers and, 1271
Friendships, adolescents and, 1122
Frostbite, 1682
Fruit
  for preschoolers, 1059
  for toddlers, 1034
Fruit juices
  excessive consumption of, 1059
  infant nutrition and, 980
  toddler nutrition and, 1034
Frustration, aggression and, 1058
Full consciousness, 1564b
Full mutation, 1198
Full-field digital mammography, 117b
Full-thickness (fourth-degree) burns, 1671, 1672f
Full-thickness (third-degree) burns, 1671, 1671f
Fulminant hepatitis, 1418
Functional burden, special needs child and, 1164, 1164b
Functional health patterns, 1238
Functional hearing loss, 1199
Functional heart murmur, 922
Fundal height
  involution process and, 526
  measuring, 219, 219f
Fundal massage, postpartum, 542–543, 543f
Fundal pressure during childbirth, 476
Fundus
  pediatric examination of, 908–909
  structures of, 908f
Funduscopic examination, 1566
Fungal infections
  cutaneous, 1653–1655, 1654t
  neonatal, 756
Furosemide
  breastfeeding and, 1753t–1756t
  for heart failure, 1469t
Furuncle, 1652t
Fussy infants, breastfeeding and, 690

G
Gabapentin, 946t
Galactorrhea, 113
Galactose, 1764t–1771t
Galactosemia,, 778
Gallbladder, pregnancy and, 202
Games, 857
Gamete intrafallopian transfer (GIFT), 133f, 134t
Gametogenesis, 168, 170f
Gamma-globulin therapy, 1491
Gardnerella, 108–109
Gardner-Wells tong traction, 1697, 1697f
Gastric lavage, 1440, 1441b
Gastroesophageal reflux disease (GERD), 1403
Gastroesophageal reflux (GER), 1403–1405, 1404b
Gastrointestinal agents, breastfeeding and, 1753t–1756t
Gastrointestinal decontamination (GID), 1439–1440
Gastrointestinal dysfunction
  pediatric
    clinical manifestations of, 1390b
    dehydration, 1389–1392, 1392t
    hepatic disorders and
      acute hepatitis, 1416–1419, 1417t
      biliary atresia, 1419–1420, 1420b
      cirrhosis, 1419–1420
    inflammatory disorders
      acute appendicitis, 1408–1409, 1409b
      inflammatory bowel disease, 1410–1414, 1411t
      Meckel's diverticulum, 1409–1410, 1410b
      peptic ulcer disease, 1414–1416, 1415b
    intestinal parasitic diseases, 1405–1408, 1406t
    malabsorption syndromes, 1433–1435
    motility disorders
      constipation, 1399–1401
      diarrhea. *See* Diarrhea
      gastroesophageal reflux, 1403–1405, 1404b
      Hirschsprung disease, 1401–1403, 1401f, 1402b
      vomiting, 1403
    nutritional disturbances and. *See* Nutritional disturbances
    obstructive disorders. *See* Intestinal obstruction
    poisoning and. *See* Poisoning
    structural defects and
      cleft lip and palate, 1421–1425, 1424b
Gastrointestinal dysfunction *(Continued)*
      esophageal atresia with tracheoesophageal fistula, 1425–1427, 1425b
      hernias, 1427, 1428t
  during pregnancy, 367
Gastrointestinal system
  cystic fibrosis and, 1357, 1358b
  fetal development of, 178
  maternal
    adaptation to pregnancy
      abdominal discomfort, 202
      appetite changes, 201–202
      esophagus/stomach/intestines, 202
      gallbladder/liver, 202
      mouth, 202
      teeth, 202
    during labour, 392
    postpartum, 530
  neonatal, transition to extrauterine life and, 613–614
  of newborns, 643b
  pediatric
    congenital anomalies of, 772–775
    effects of immobilization on, 1685t
    review of systems and, 885b
Gastroschisis, 773–774
Gastrostomy administration
  feeding hospitalized children, 1309–1310, 1310f
  feeding preterm infants, 721
  of medications, 1295–1296, 1296b
Gate-control theory of pain, 397
Gavage feeding
  for hospitalized children, 1308–1309, 1309b, 1310f, 1311b
  for preterm infants, 719–721, 720b, 720f
Gender as health determinant, 45
Gender-role identity
  adolescents and, 1118, 1123
  preschoolers and, 1053
  toddlers and, 1024, 1024f, 1026–1027
Gene therapy (gene transfer), 162
General anaesthesia
  for Caesarean birth, 420–421, 516–517, 516f
  for childbirth, 446
General systems assessment during first stage of labour, 450
Generalized seizures, 1593–1594, 1594b–1595b
Genetic counselling, 161, 779, 1198
  Duchenne muscular dystrophy and, 1742
Genetic disorders
  amniocentesis for, 282–284
  evaluation/counselling for, 779
  newborn screening for, 778–779
Genetic testing
  advancements in, 5
  breast cancer risk and, 114–115
  for Down syndrome, 1198
  ethical/legal/social implications, 162
  factors influencing, 162
Genetic testing *(Continued)*
  for fragile X syndrome, 1198
  types of prenatal, 161–162
Genetic transmission
  multifactorial inheritance, 166
  overview, 162, 166
  unifactorial inheritance, 166–167
Genetics
  chromosome abnormalities, 163–166
  clinical, 162–166
  counselling. *See* Genetic counselling
  genes/chromosomes, 162–163
  history taking, 160–161, 160f
  Human Genome Project, 161–162
  impact of genetic disease, 159b
  overview, 157–158
  relevance to nursing, 158–159, 159b
Genital fistulas, 590–591, 591f
Genital stage of psychosexual development, 851
Genital surgery, psychological problems with, 1545–1546
Genital tract infections
  sexually transmitted. *See* Sexually transmitted infections (STIs)
  vaginal infections, 108–110, 109t
Genital tract lacerations, 578–579
Genital warts, 101–103, 102f
Genitalia
  of children
    external defects of, 1545–1547, 1546t
    female, 925–926, 926f
    male, 924–925, 925f
  of newborns, 626t–636t
    ambiguous, 626t–636t, 777, 777f
Genitourinary dysfunction
  acute glomerulonephritis and, 1549–1551, 1550b
  acute renal failure and, 1553–1555, 1554b, 1556b
  chronic renal failure and, 1555–1559, 1557b
  clinical manifestations of, 1537–1540
  dialysis and, 1559–1560
  external defects and, 1545–1547, 1546t
  hemolytic uremic syndrome and, 1551–1552, 1551b
  laboratory tests for, 1538t–1541t
  nephrotic syndrome and, 1547–1549, 1547b, 1548f
  obstructive uropathy and, 1545, 1545f
  spinal bifida and, 1735
  transplantation and, 1560
  urinary tract infection and, 1541–1544, 1543b–1544b
  Wilms' tumour, 1552–1553, 1552b

Genitourinary system
congenital anomalies of, 776–780
of newborns, 643b
Genograms, family, 19, 20f
Genotypes, 163
Genu valgum, 927, 927f
Genu varum, 927, 927f
Geographic location, family medical history and, 882
German measles, 1064t–1070t, 1070f
neonatal, 753
Gestational age
assessment of newborn, 648, 649f–650f, 650b
classification by, 648–651
of fetus, 219–220
influencing neonatal behaviour, 638–639
ultrasound assessment of, 280
Gestational age-related problems
classification of, 708b
large-for-gestational-age infants, 735
nursing care for, 710–733
postterm infants, 733–734
preterm infants, 707–709
small-for-gestational-age infants, 734–735
Gestational conditions
gestational diabetes mellitus. *See* Gestational diabetes mellitus (GDM)
hemorrhagic disorders. *See* Hemorrhagic disorders in pregnancy
hyperemesis gravidarum, 310–312
hypertension in pregnancy, 294–308
nonobstetrical surgery, 330–331
trauma during pregnancy, 331–335
Gestational diabetes mellitus (GDM)
antepartum interventions, 309–310
defined, 339
dietary modifications for, 267
intrapartum interventions, 310
overview, 308
postpartum interventions, 310
risks of, 308
screening for, 308–309, 309f
Gestational trophoblastic disease (GTD), 320–321
Gestational trophoblastic neoplasia (GTN), 320–321
Giardiasis, 1405–1407, 1406b, 1407f
Giger and Davidhizar Transcultural Assessment Model, 1223–1224
Gingival granuloma gravidarum, 200, 202
Gingivitis, 1099
Glascow Coma Scale (GCS), 1563, 1564f
Glaucoma, 1204b–1205b
Global Health eLearning Centre, 13
Global organization in preoperational thought, 1025b
Global perspectives on perinatal care, 12–13, 13f
Glomerular disease
acute glomerulonephritis, 1549–1551, 1550b
nephrotic syndrome, 1547–1549, 1547b, 1548f
Gloves, infection control and, 109t
Glucagon, 1632–1633
Gluconeogenesis, 679
Glucose tolerance test (GIT), 1764t–1771t
Glucosuria, 198–199
Gluten-induced enteropathy, 1433–1434
Glycemic control
maintaining, 343–344, 344t
monitoring blood glucose levels, 346–348, 346b
poor, risks from, 341
preconception counselling for, 341, 341b
Glycosuria
after childbirth, 529
in diabetes mellitus, 339, 1629
Glycosylated hemoglobin, 1631
Goitre, 1617
Gomco clamp, 664, 664f
Gonadotropin-releasing hormone (GnRH)., 82
Gonads, 1114
Gonorrhea
incidence/treatment of, 98–99
neonatal, 750
perinatal complications from, 221
Goodell's sign, 190
Gowns, infection control and, 109t
Graafian follicles, 82, 83f
Graduated extinction, night crying and, 982–983
Grafts, dialysis and, 1559
Grandparents
adaptation to pregnancy, 210, 212b, 213f
adaptation to role of, 572–574, 573f
grief responses of, 602
Grantly Dick-Read method of childbirth preparation, 400–401
Granulation tissue, 1309, 1310f, 1646
Grasp reflex in newborns, 620, 621f, 622t–625t
Graves' disease, 1618–1620, 1619b
Gravida, 186
Gravidity, 186–187
Greenstick fractures, 1691b, 1691f
Grief
comatose child and, 1573
death of child and
for parents, 1183
for siblings, 1184
death of newborn and
acknowledging/expressing feelings, 604–607
actualizing loss, 603, 604f
care at/after discharge, 606–607
communicating/caring techniques for, 602–604
decision making and, 603–604
family aspects of, 602
Grief *(Continued)*
maternal physical needs, 605
memories for parents, 605–606, 606f
nursing care for, 602–607, 602b
parental cultural/spiritual needs, 606
parental grief responses, 599–602
positive coping with, 605
postmortem care/documentation, 606
Gross motor development
infants and
head control, 960–961, 961f
locomotion, 962–963, 963f
rolling over, 961–962
sitting, 962, 962f
play developing, 1054, 1055f
preschoolers and, 1051t, 1052, 1052f
school-age children and, 1097–1098
toddlers and, 1021–1022, 1023t
Group A β-hemolytic streptococcal (GABHS) pharyngitis, 1483
Group B streptococcus (GBS)
neonatal, 755
perinatal complications from, 221
pregnancy and, 446
Group identity, adolescents and, 1118
Growing skull fractures, 1576
Growth and development
of adolescents, 1115–1117, 1121t
biological. *See* Biological development
chronic renal failure and, 1557
cystic fibrosis and, 1357–1358
defined, 844
factors influencing, 859–867
family-centred home care and, 1227–1228, 1227b
growth curve evaluation, 1612b
hospitalized children and, 1245–1246
individual differences in, 846
infants and, 971t–975t
measurement of, 893–897, 896f
height and weight for boys, 1760f–1761f
height and weight for girls, 1762f–1763f
mental, theories of, 852–854
pace of, 846
patterns of, 845–846
personality, theories of, 850–852
physical, 846–848, 847f
physiological changes, 849
potential of preterm infants, 726–728
preschoolers and, 1051t
rates of, 847f
role of play in, 856–859
school-age children and, 1085t–1086t
of self-concept, 855
sex differences in, 1117
stages of, 844–845, 845b
taking history of, 881
temperament and, 849–850
Growth and development *(Continued)*
toddlers and, 1023t
visually impaired children and, 1207
Growth charts, WHO, 893–894, 1136, 1197
Growth failure, 1005–1008
Growth hormone (GH)
deficiency of, 1611–1613, 1612b
excess of, 1613–1614
laboratory tests for, 1764t–1771t
GTPAL (five-digit) system for gravidity/parity, 186–187, 187t
Guidance, anticipatory. *See* Anticipatory guidance
Guillain-Barré syndrome (GBS), 1743–1745, 1744b
Guilt, preschoolers and, 1052–1053
Gums, pregnancy and, 202
Guns, injuries involving, 1132–1133
Gynecoid pelvis, 383, 384t
Gynecological conditions
health risks of, 54
during pregnancy, 331
Gynecological health assessment. *See* Health assessment for women
Gynecological history, 213
Gynecomastia, 1114–1115, 1135–1136

H

H1N1 influenza virus, 1324–1325
Haberman Special Needs Feeder, 1423, 1423f
Habits, history of, 881, 881b
Habitual miscarriage, 314f, 315, 315t
Habituation
environmental stimuli and, 640
in parent-infant bonding, 561–562, 562f
Haemophilus influenzae infection
acute epiglottitis and, 1329
otitis media and, 1326
Haemophilus influenzae type B (Hib) vaccine, 987
Haemophilus vaginitis, 108–109
Hair
assessment of pediatric, 905–906
care during hospitalization, 1272
nutritional status and, 887t–889t
Hair loss, 1524, 1553
Haitian ethnicity
health beliefs/practices and, 840t–841t
practices regarding newborns and, 660b
Hallucinogens, 1148
Halo vest, 1697, 1697f
Hand expression of breast milk, 692, 692f
Hand hygiene, 109t, 1278b
Handicap, definition of, 1157b
Hands-and-knees position, birth process and, 461, 462b, 462f, 472

Hands-poised approach, 476
Haplotypes, 1532
Hard-of-hearing, definition of, 1199
Harrington spinal instrumentation, 1709
Hashimoto's disease, 1617–1618, 1618b
Head
examination of pediatric, 907
nutritional status and, 887t–889t
Head circumference
of fetus, 378–379, 379f
in infants, 959
measuring in pediatric examinations, 897
measuring newborn, 626t–636t, 628f, 637
of school-age children, 1084
in toddlers, 1021
ultrasound assessment of, 280–281, 280f
Head control, infants and, 960–961, 961f
Head injury
clinical manifestations of, 1577b
complications of, 1576–1577
concussion in, 1575
contusion/laceration in, 1575
diagnosis of, 1577–1578
emergency intervention for, 1578b
etiology of, 1574
incidence of, 1573–1574
management of, 1578–1579, 1579b
nursing care for, 1579–1581
pathophysiology of, 1574–1576, 1575f
prevention of, 1581
rehabilitation for, 1581
skull fractures in, 1576
supportive care for, 1580–1581
Head lice, 1659–1661, 1659b, 1659f
Health assessment for women
adolescents and, 72
cultural considerations in, 69–70, 70b
health history for, 73–74
interview in, 69–70, 70f
laboratory/diagnostic procedures for, 79
overview, 68–69
pelvic examination in, 75–77, 75b, 76f–77f
physical examination in, 74–79
vaginal wall examination in, 77–79
women at risk and, 71–72, 72f
women with disabilities and, 70–72, 71f
Health beliefs, cultural/religious influences on, 835–836
Health care
for children. *See* Pediatric nursing
history of Canadian, 3–6
inequities in, 12, 28–29
prenatal. *See* Prenatal care
regionalization of, 274
special needs child and, 1157
well-woman care from, 42
Health care planning, in pediatric nursing, 797–798
Health determinants. *See* Determinants of health
Health education programs, 46, 46b. *See also* Education
Health education, special needs children and, 1165
Health history
cerebral dysfunction and, 1562–1563
pediatric. *See* Pediatric health history
in women's health assessment, 73–74
Health literacy, 12
Health practices, cultural influences on, 836–837, 836b
Health promotion/illness prevention
anticipatory guidance for
health risk prevention, 56, 56b
health screening schedule, 56, 57t
intimate partner violence, 58–61, 58f, 59b–60b, 60t
substance use cessation, 55–56, 56b
cognitive impairment and, 1195
community-based, 29–30
determinants of health and. *See* Determinants of health
in family-centred home care, 1227–1228, 1227b
fertility control/infertility and, 42–43, 43b
hearing impairment, 1203
menopause/perimenopause and, 44
menstrual problems and, 43–44
in pediatric nursing, 787, 795
prenatal/pregnancy interventions in, 43, 44b
visual impairment and, 1206–1209
well-woman care and, 42
Health risk prevention, safety guidelines for, 56, 56b
Health screening
promoting, 56
recommendations for, 57t
Health service indicators, 8
Hearing
of adolescents, 1128
of newborns, 639, 640f
unconscious child and, 1573
Hearing aids, 1200, 1200f
Hearing impairment
additional aids, 1202
with bacterial meningitis, 1589
clinical manifestations of, 1201, 1201b
cued speech and, 1202
definition/classification of, 1199–1200
etiology of, 1199
health assessments for women with, 70–71
hospitalization and, 1202–1203
intensity of sounds and, 1200t
lipreading and, 1201–1202, 1202b
Hearing impairment *(Continued)*
management of, 1200–1201
nursing care for, 1201–1203
parental, 571
parenting with, 571b
pathology of, 1199
prevention of, 1203
sign language and, 1202
socialization and, 1202
speech language therapy for, 1202
speech problems due to, 1058–1059
symptom severity and, 1199–1200, 1200t
testing infants/children for, 912–915, 915t
Heart
pediatric examination of, 920–922
position of, 920f
Heart disease. *See* Cardiovascular dysfunction
Heart failure, 1462. *See also* Congestive heart failure (CHF)
Heart rate
alterations in pediatric surgery, 1268t
fetal. *See* Fetal heart rate (FHR)
of infants, 959, 1773
of newborns, 610–611, 1773
pediatric
dysrhythmias and, 1485–1487
normal, 1773
Heart sounds
differentiating normal, 921–922, 922t
heart murmurs, 922, 922t
of neonates, 611
origin of, 921, 922f
Heart surgery during pregnancy, 360
Heart transplantation in children, 1488–1489
Heartburn, 202, 268
Heat applications
for juvenile idiopathic arthritis, 1718–1719
for labour pain management, 406
Heat injury to respiratory tract, 1343
Heat loss
in neonates, 612, 612f, 646
in SGA infants, 735
Heavy metal poisoning, 1440–1441
Heel punctures/sticks
atraumatic care for, 658b
for blood specimens, 655–659, 657f
Heel-to-shin test, 928b
Hegar sign, 189, 192f
Height
of adolescents, 1115–1117
growth chart for boys, 1760f–1761f
growth chart for girls, 1762f–1763f
growth during childhood, 846–848, 847t
of infants, 958–959
pediatric examination of, 895–896, 896f
Height *(Continued)*
of school-age children, 1084
of toddlers, 1020
Heimlich manoeuvre
in children, 1370, 1370f
in pregnant women, 363f
Helicobacter pylori, 1414
HELLP syndrome
hospital care for, 303–304
in severe pre-eclampsia, 299
Helmets, protective, 1101
Hemarthrosis, 1513
Hematocrit
after childbirth, 531
laboratory tests for, 1764t–1771t
Hematogenous osteomyelitis, 1710–1712
Hematological dysfunction
anemia and, 1500–1503, 1502b, 1502f
apheresis for, 1533–1534
aplastic anemia and, 1511–1512, 1512b
beta-thalassemia and, 1510–1511, 1511b
blood transfusion therapy for, 1530–1532, 1531t–1532t
disseminated intravascular coagulation and, 1516–1517, 1516b, 1516f
epistaxis, 1517, 1517b
hematopoietic stem cell transplantation for, 1532–1533
hemophilia and, 1513–1515, 1513b
Hodgkin's disease and, 1525–1526, 1525f
idiopathic thrombocytopenic purpura and, 1515–1516, 1515b
iron deficiency anemia and, 1503–1505
leukemias and. *See* Leukemias
lymphomas and, 1524–1526
non-Hodgkin's lymphoma, 1526
sickle cell anemia and, 1505–1510, 1506b, 1506f, 1508b
Hematological status of preterm infants, 711
Hematomas
emergency intervention for, 1206b
pelvic, causing PPH, 579
Hematopoietic stem cell transplantation (HSCT)
for aplastic anemia, 1512
for hematological/immunological disorders, 1532–1533, 1533b
for leukemia, 1518–1519
for severe combined immunodeficiency disease, 1530
for sickle cell anemia, 1509
Hematopoietic system
fetal, 178
first year changes in, 959
neonatal adaptations, 611
Hemiplegia, 1725b
Hemodialysis, 1558–1560, 1560f

Hemofiltration, 1559–1560
Hemoglobin
after childbirth, 531
concentrations in neonate, 611
Hemoglobin A, laboratory tests for, 1764t–1771t
Hemoglobin F, laboratory tests for, 1764t–1771t
Hemolytic disease of newborns, 765–768
Hemolytic uremic syndrome (HUS), 1551–1552, 1551b
Hemophilia, 1513–1515, 1513b
Hemorrhage
neonatal, due to birth trauma, 746
pediatric
epidural, 1576–1577
leukemia and, 1521–1522
subdural, 1577
after tonsillectomy, 1324
postpartum. *See* Postpartum hemorrhage (PPH)
Hemorrhagic cystitis, 1524
Hemorrhagic disorders in pregnancy
abruptio placentae, 326–328, 326f
assessment of, 316b
clotting disorders, 328–330
cord insertion/placental variations, 328, 329f
early pregnancy bleeding, 312–316
ectopic pregnancy, 318–320
gestational trophoblastic disease, 320–321, 320f
late pregnancy bleeding, 321–330, 322f
miscarriage, 313–316
placenta previa, 321–326, 323f, 324t
premature dilation of cervix, 316–318
Hemorrhagic shock, 581–584, 583b
Hemorrhoids
postpartum changes in, 528
during pregnancy, 195f, 202
Hemostasis
defects in, 1512–1517
stage of wound healing, 1646
Heparin lock, 1293–1294
Hepatic disorders
acute hepatitis, 1416–1419, 1417t
biliary atresia, 1419–1420, 1420b
cirrhosis, 1419–1420
Hepatic portoenterostomy, 1420
Hepatic system
in fetal development, 178
neonatal adaptations, 614–615
during pregnancy, 202
Hepatitis A virus (HAV) infection, 105, 1416, 1417t
Hepatitis A virus (HAV) vaccine
adolescents and, 1125
contraindications/precautions for, 989t–991t
recommended schedule for, 984
Hepatitis B immune globulin (HBIG), 661, 661b
Hepatitis B vaccine
adolescents and, 1125
contraindications/precautions for, 989t–991t
for neonates, 661, 661b
recommended schedule for, 984
Hepatitis B virus (HBV) infection
breastfeeding and, 698
in children, 1416, 1417t
incidence of, 105
management of, 106
neonatal, 751–752
prevention of, 105–106, 106b
screening/diagnosis of, 105
Hepatitis C virus (HCV) infection, 106
breastfeeding and, 698
in children, 1416–1418, 1417t
Hepatitis D virus (HDV) infection, 1418
Hepatitis E virus (HEV) infection, 1418
Hepatitis G virus (HGV) infection, 1418
Herbal teas, 256–257, 258b
Herbal therapies
breastfeeding and, 696
education in, 229
history of using, 215
for increased milk production, 681
for infertility, 131
for menstrual disorders, 87, 88t, 89
nutritional disturbances from, 1375
for PPH, 580–581, 582t
Heredity
health problems linked to, 831
influencing development, 859
Hernias
in children, 1427, 1428t
pediatric examination of, 923, 923f
Heroin
breastfeeding and, 1753t–1756t
childbirth risks with, 48
prenatal exposure to, 761
Herpes simplex encephalitis, 1590
Herpes simplex virus (HSV)
complications from, 221
incidence/symptoms of, 103, 103f
management of, 104
manifestations/management of, 1653t
in newborns
incidence/symptoms of, 754, 754f
nursing care for, 754
screening for, 446
pregnancy and, 446
screening/diagnosis of, 103–104
Herpes zoster, varicella and, 1062
Hiatal hernias, 202, 1428t
High chairs, falls from, 998
High-density lipoproteins (HDLs), 1484
High-fibre foods, 1401b
High-frequency ventilation, 716t, 717
High-risk infants
birth trauma and. *See* Birth trauma, neonatal
classification of, 708b
High-risk infants *(Continued)*
congenital anomalies in. *See* Congenital anomalies
discharge planning for, 737–738
hemolytic disorders in, 765–767
infants of diabetic mothers. *See* Infants of diabetic mothers (IDMs)
infection and. *See* Neonatal infections
large-for-gestational-age infants, 735
maternal substance use and. *See* Substance use, during pregnancy
nursing care for, 710–733, 729b–730b
postterm infants. *See* Postterm infants
preterm infants. *See* Preterm infants
small-for-gestational-age infants
heat loss in, 735
hypoglycemia/hyperglycemia in, 734–735
perinatal asphyxia in, 734
transport for
to tertiary centre, 738–739, 739b, 739f
from tertiary centre, 739
High-risk pregnancy. *See also* Pregnancy, risk factors in
definition of, 273–274
determinants of health and, 274, 275b
fetal health assessment in. *See* Fetal health assessment
health care regionalization and, 274
hemorrhagic disorders and. *See* Hemorrhagic disorders in pregnancy
maternal health problems and
eclampsia and, 297–298
in diabetic pregnancy, 341
immediate care, 306–307, 307b
postpartum care, 307–308
symptoms of, 305–306, 306f
gestational diabetes mellitus. *See* Gestational diabetes mellitus (GDM)
HELLP syndrome, 299, 303–304
hyperemesis gravidarum, 310–312, 312t
hypertension. *See* Hypertension, in pregnancy
intimate partner violence and, 276
mental health concerns and, 274–276
pre-eclampsia. *See* Pre-eclampsia
nonobstetrical surgery and, 330–331
pre-existing conditions and. *See* Pre-existing conditions
specific risk factors, 276b
trauma and. *See* Trauma, during pregnancy
Hip, developmental dysplasia of, 775–776, 775f
Hirschsprung disease, 1401–1403, 1401f, 1402b
HLA system complex, 1532
Hodgkin's disease, 1525–1526, 1525f
Holding positions for newborns, 668, 668f
Hollister PlastiBell, 664, 665f
Home births, 243
Home care
agency selection for, 1219–1220, 1219b
care coordination in, 1220–1221, 1221b
communication in, 35–36
congenital heart disease and, 1478
cystic fibrosis and, 1362–1363
defined, 1159
definition of, 1216–1217
discharge planning and, 1219–1220, 1220b, 1221f
effective, 1218–1219, 1219b
for end-of-life care, 1176
family-centred
central concepts of, 1222
family-to-family support in, 1229–1230
nursing process for, 1224–1226, 1225b–1226b
parent-professional collaboration in, 1224
promoting optimum development in, 1227–1228, 1227b, 1228f
respect for diversity in, 1223–1224, 1223b
safety issues in home for, 1228–1229
maternal child services, 36–37
in perinatal continuum of care, 35f
role of nurse/training/standards of care, 1221–1222
for special needs children, 1159
trends/needs in, 1217–1218
Home deaths, 1181–1182
Home oxygen saturation monitors, 1013, 1014b
Home uterine activity monitoring (HUAM), 495
Home visits
after discharge, 554
education during, 38–40
first, 37–38
nurse safety and, 40
nursing process, 39b
overview, 37
protocols, 38b
Homeless women
transition to parenthood for, 570
vulnerability of, 34
Homelessness, as health determinant, 827–828
Homograft skin coverings, 1676
Homologous chromosomes, 163
Homozygous sickle cell disease, 1505–1510
Hookworm disease, 1406t
Hopefulness, special needs children and, 1165

Horizontal transmission of HIV, 1527
Hormonal contraception
combined estrogen-progestin, 147–148
continuous/extended, 150
general classes of, 147t
progestin-only methods, 148
Hormonal replacement therapy (HRT), 94
Hormone therapy for breast cancer, 120–121, 120b–121b
Hormones
breastfeeding and, 1753t–1756t
changes during puberty, 1114
after childbirth, 529
effects of changes during pregnancy, 203t
Hospice care
definition of, 1216–1217
for end-of-life care, 1176–1179
Hospital deaths, 1182
Hospitalization
pediatric
admission assessment for, 1238–1241, 1239b–1241b
altered family roles and, 1237–1238
ambulatory/outpatient setting and, 1253, 1254b
bathing and, 1271
beneficial effects of, 1237
changes in population, 1237
cognitively impaired children and, 1194–1195
controlling temperatures and, 1272–1274
critical care unit admission, 1255b–1256b, 1256
for cystic fibrosis, 1362
developmentally appropriate activities and, 1245–1246
emergency admission, 1254–1256, 1255b
end-of-life care and, 1176
family education during, 1274
fear of bodily injury and, 1245
feeding and, 1272, 1273b
hair care and, 1272
hearing impaired children and, 1202–1203
individual risk factors in, 1236–1237, 1236b
infection control during, 1277–1278, 1277b
in isolation, 1253–1254
loss of control in, 1234–1236, 1243–1244
nursing care for
in discharge/home care preparation, 1252–1253
family support in, 1250
parent participation and, 1251–1252
providing information and, 1250–1251
oral hygiene and, 1271–1272
parental reactions to, 1237, 1237b
Hospitalization *(Continued)*
play/expressive activities and, 1246–1249, 1247b, 1247f
posthospital behaviours and, 1236b
potential benefits of, 1249–1250
preparing child for admission, 1241–1242, 1241f
preventing/minimizing separation, 1242–1243, 1243f
restraints/therapeutic holding and, 1279–1281
safety and, 1274–1282
separation anxiety in, 1232–1234, 1233b, 1233f–1234f
sibling reactions to, 1237
skin care and, 1270–1271, 1270b
supporting siblings during, 1251b
transportion and, 1278–1279, 1279f
visually impaired children and, 1207–1208
Host factors in epidemiological triangle, 803
Human bites, 1664
Human chorionic gonadotropin (hCG)
for detecting pregnancy, 187
placenta producing, 174
Human chorionic somatomammotropin (hCS), 174
Human development
beginnings of, 170–171, 171f
critical periods in, 169f
etiology of malformations, 167b
nongenetic factors influencing, 167–168
toxic exposures during, 176b
Human diploid cell rabies vaccine, 1591
Human Early Learning Partnership (HELP), 1056
Human Genome Project, 161–162
Human immunodeficiency virus (HIV)
in children
clinical manifestations of, 1527, 1527b
diagnosis of, 1527–1528, 1528t
management of, 1528–1529
nursing care for, 1529–1530, 1529b
pathophysiology of, 1527
counselling for HIV testing, 107
epidemiology of, 1526–1527
etiology of, 1527
incidence/transmission of, 106–107
management of, 108
neonatal, 752–753
nursing care for, 372–373
obstetrical complications, 372
perinatal transmission, 371–372, 371b
preconception counselling for, 371
Human immunodeficiency virus (HIV) *(Continued)*
pregnancy and, 107–108, 371–372
prenatal screening for, 217–218, 218b
prevention of, 53–54, 53b
screening/diagnosis, 107
Human Milk Banking Association of North America (HMBANA), 694
Human papillomavirus (HPV) infection
incidence/appearance of, 101–102, 102f
management of, 102–103
prevention of, 103
screening/diagnosis, 102
Human papillomavirus (HPV) vaccine, 988
contraindications/precautions for, 989t–991t
for girls, 1125
Human rabies immunoglobulin vaccine, 1591
Husband-Coached Childbirth (Bradley), 401
Hydatidiform mole, 320–321, 320f
Hydramnios in diabetic pregnancy, 342
Hydration
for bacterial meningitis, 1588
for pediatric respiratory infections, 1319–1320
for preterm infants, 719
sickle cell anemia and, 1509
for unconscious child, 1571–1572
Hydrocarbons, poisoning from, 1437b–1438b
Hydrocele, 1546t
Hydrocephalus
diagnosis of, 1605–1606, 1606b
management of, 1606–1607, 1606f
in newborns, 769–770
nursing care for, 1607–1608
pathophysiology of, 1604–1608, 1605f
supportive care for, 1608
Hydrocodone, 945t, 947t
Hydromorphone, 945t, 947t
Hydromorphone hydrochloride, 408, 408b
Hydronephrosis, 1545
Hydrotherapy
for burn wounds, 1675
for labour pain management, 403–405, 404f
Hydroxyurea, 1509
Hygiene care
diabetes mellitus and, 1638
during first stage of labour, 457, 458t
during hospitalization
bathing and, 1271
hair care and, 1272
oral hygiene and, 1271–1272
skin care and, 1270–1271, 1270b
for unconscious child, 1572
Hymen, 63–64, 64f
Hymenopterans, 1657–1663, 1658t
Hyperallergenic foods, 1386b
Hyperbilirubinemia
breastfeeding-associated, 691
causes of, 653t
clinical manifestations of, 652–654
from cold stress, 612–613
education regarding, 663
in IDMs, 737
phototherapy for, 661–663, 662f
Hypercapnia, head injury and, 1574
Hypercholesterolemia, 1484–1485, 1484t
Hypercyanotic spells, 1474–1476
Hyperemesis gravidarum (HG). *See also* Nausea and vomiting of pregnancy (NVP)
clinical manifestations of, 311
collaborative care, 311–312, 312t, 313b
etiology of, 310–311
overview, 310
Hyperemia, 1270
Hyperglycemia
defined, 734–735
diabetes mellitus and, 339, 1633, 1633t, 1637
in diabetic pregnancy, 347, 347b
in high-risk infants, 734–735
total parenteral nutrition and, 1312
Hyperhemolytic crisis, 1505, 1506b
Hyperinsulinemia, 735
Hyperkalemia, 1554, 1556
Hyperlipidemia, 1484–1485, 1484t, 1547, 1548f
Hypermenorrhea, 92
Hyperopia, 1204, 1204b–1205b
Hyperparathyroidism, 1621–1622, 1621b
Hyperpnea, 920b
Hyperpyrexia. *See* Fever
Hypertension
in children, 1489–1490, 1489b
acute glomerulonephritis and, 1550
acute renal failure and, 1554–1555
in pregnancy. *See also* Pre-eclampsia
antihypertensive therapy for, 305, 306t
blood pressure assessment, 300–301
classification of, 295, 295t
defined, 295
eclampsia, 305–308, 306f
monitoring for, 219
morbidity/mortality in, 295
nursing care for, 300–308
pre-eclampsia linked to, 296–308, 296t
significance/incidence of, 294–295
Hyperthermia
cerebral dysfunction and, 1572
children in cars and, 997, 1041–1042
cooling measures for, 1274
definition of, 1272
Hyperthyroidism
in children, 1618–1620, 1619b
during pregnancy, 350–352

Hypertonic dehydration, 1391
Hypertonic uterine dysfunction, 498–499
Hypertrophic cardiomyopathy (HCM), 736–737, 1487–1488
Hypertrophic pyloric stenosis (HPS), 1427–1430, 1429b, 1429f
Hypertrophy of laryngeal mucosa, 1117
Hyperventilation, 920b
Hypervitaminosis, 1375
HypnoBirthing, 401
Hypnosis for labour pain management, 406
Hypoalbuminemia, 1547, 1548f
Hypocalcemia
  in infants of diabetic mothers, 736
  in neonates, 655
Hypoglycemia
  diabetes mellitus and, 340
  in diabetic pregnancy, 342, 345b, 346–347
  emergency intervention for, 1638b
  in high-risk infants, 734–735
  in infants of diabetic mothers, 736
  monitoring for neonatal, 616b
  from neonatal cold stress, 612–613
  in neonates, 654–655
  total parenteral nutrition and, 1312
  type 1 diabetes and, 1632–1633, 1633t, 1637–1638
Hypogonadotropic amenorrhea, 85
Hypomagnesemia, 736
Hypomenorrhea, 91
Hypoparathyroidism, 1620–1621, 1620b
Hypopituitarism, 1611–1613, 1612b
Hypoplastic anemia, 1511
Hypoplastic left heart syndrome, 1464b–1467b
Hyposensitization, asthma and, 1351
Hypospadias, 776–780, 777f, 1546t
Hypothalamic-pituitary cycle, 82, 83f
Hypothalamic–pituitary–gonadal axis, 1614
Hypothalamus, 681
Hypothermia
  after analgesia/anaesthesia, 421
  care for preterm infants with, 714
  due to coma, 1564–1565
  in neonates, 646
  submersion injuries and, 1582
Hypothyroidism
  juvenile, 1617, 1617b
  newborn screening for, 778–779
  during pregnancy, 352
Hypotonic dehydration, 1391
Hypotonic uterine dysfunction
  nursing care for, 500b
  symptoms of, 499
Hypoventilation, 920b
Hypovolemic shock
  characteristics/causes of, 1492t
  emergency interventions for, 542b, 583b
  from PPH, 581–584
  in preterm infants, 710
Hypoxemia, 1474–1476, 1474f–1475f, 1476t
Hypoxia, 1474
  fetal responses to, 286
  head injury and, 1574
  submersion injuries and, 1581–1582
Hysterectomy, 79
Hysteria, school-age children and, 1109–1110
Hysterosalpingography, 132, 132f

I

"I" messages, 877b–878b
Ibuprofen
  breastfeeding and, 1753t–1756t
  for children, 944t
Identical twins
  characteristics of, 812–813, 812b
  formation of, 180–184, 184f
Identification
  with maternal role, 207
  with paternal role, 209
Identity formation in adolescence, 1117–1119
Identity vs. role confusion stage of psychosocial development, 852
Idiopathic hypoparathyroidism, 1620–1621, 1620b
Idiopathic nephrosis, 1547–1549
Idiopathic scoliosis, 1707f–1708f, 1708–1710
Idiopathic seizures, 1593, 1593b
Idiopathic thrombocytopenic purpura (ITP)
  in children, 1515–1516, 1515b
  during postpartum period, 584
Idiopathic type 1 diabetes mellitus, 1628
Ilizarov external fixator (IEF), 1697, 1699f
Illicit drugs. *See also* Substance use
  childbirth risks with, 48–49
  education in, 229–230
  history of using, 215
Illness
  acute, 793
  chronic, 939–940, 1157b
Illocutionary stage of communicative development, 874, 874b
Imagery
  education in, 246
  for labour pain management, 402–403
  during pediatric procedures, 941b
Imaginary companions, 1055
Imaginative/imitative play, 1054, 1055f
Imbalance of forces, 835–836
Imitation in sensorimotor development, 965
Immediate GI hypersensitivity, 1386
Immigrants
  social determinants of health for, 830–831
  vulnerability of, 33
Immobilization
  effect on families, 1687–1688
  family support/home care for, 1688
  nursing care for, 1687–1688
  physiological effects of, 1684–1686, 1685t
  psychological effects of, 1686–1687
Immune globulin intravenous (IGIV)
  idiopathic thrombocytopenic purpura and, 1515
  for immunocompromised children, 1063
Immunizations
  accurate information regarding, 983–984
  administration of, 992–993
  atraumatic care for, 991b–992b
  bacille Calmette-Guérin, 1339–1340
  for children, 788, 894f–895f
  children exposed to HIV/AIDS and, 1528
  compliance with, 992
  congenital heart disease and, 1478
  contraindications/precautions for, 989t–991t
  diphtheria, 984–985
  education in, 229
  Haemophilus influenzae type B, 987
  hepatitis A virus, 984
  hepatitis B virus, 984
  influenza, 987–988, 1325
  leukemia and, 1519b
  measles, 986
  meningococcus, 988, 1589
  mumps, 986
  pertussis, 985
  pneumococcus, 986–987, 1327
  polio, 985
  rabies and, 1591
  reactions to, 988–992
  rotavirus/HPV, 988, 1397
  rubella, 986
  schedule for, 984
  sickle cell anemia and, 1507
  taking history of, 881
  tetanus, 985
  varicella, 987
Immunoglobulin A (IgA), 682, 1764t–1771t
Immunoglobulin D (IgD), 1764t–1771t
Immunoglobulin E (IgE), 1764t–1771t
Immunoglobulin G (IgG), 1764t–1771t
Immunoglobulin M (IgM), 1764t–1771t
Immunological dysfunction
  apheresis for, 1533–1534
  blood transfusion therapy for, 1530–1532, 1531t–1532t
  hematopoietic stem cell transplantation for, 1532–1533
Immunological dysfunction *(Continued)*
  HIV/AIDS and. *See* Human immunodeficiency virus (HIV), in children
  severe combined immunodeficiency disease and, 1530
  Wiskott-Aldrich syndrome, 1530
Immunological system
  after childbirth, 532
  fetal development of, 180
  infants and, 960
  neonatal adaptations, 616
Immunosuppressive therapy
  aplastic anemia and, 1512
  kidney transplant and, 1560
Immunotherapy, asthma and, 1351
Impairment, definition of, 1157b
Imperforate anus, 1432
Impetigo contagiosa, 1652f, 1652t
Implantation process, 171, 171f
Implants, breast, 120
In vitro fertilization, 8
In vitro fertilization-embryo transfer (IVF-ET), 134t
Inability to conserve, preoperational thought and, 1025b
Inappropriate sleep associations, 982t
Inborn errors of metabolism (IEMs), 167, 778–779
Incarcerated hernias, 1427
Incidence of disease, 803
Incompetent cervix, 316–318
Incomplete fracture, 1690
Incomplete miscarriage, 314, 314f, 315t
Incomplete precocious puberty, 1614b
Increased intracranial pressure, 1563, 1563b
Incubators
  light shields for, 722, 722f
  for preterm infants, 713–714
  weaning from, 714
Indicators
  health service, 8
  perinatal health, 7–8, 7b
Individual education plan, special needs children and, 1228
Individual identity, adolescents and, 1118
Individualized home care plan, 1219
Individuating-reflexive stage of spiritual development, 854
Indomethacin
  breastfeeding and, 1753t–1756t
  for suppression of uterine activity, 496, 496b
Induction of labour
  cervical ripening methods, 507–508
  in diabetic pregnancy, 348–349
  indications for, 506, 506b, 507t
  rates of, 8
Industry vs. inferiority stage of psychosocial development, 852
Inevitable miscarriage, 314, 314f, 315t

Infancy. *See also* Infants
communicative development in, 874–875, 874b
of development, 845b
Infant botulism, 1746–1747, 1747b
Infant car seat restraints, 996–997, 997f
Infant formulas. *See* Formula feeding
Infant mortality rates
factors associated with, 3–5, 792–793
as perinatal health indicator, 7, 7b
Infant seats, falls from, 998
Infantile atopic dermatitis, 1665–1667, 1666b, 1666f
Infantile spasms, 1594b–1595b
Infantile spinal muscular atrophy, 1738–1740, 1739b
Infants. *See also* Newborns
activity in, 981
anticipatory guidance for caretakers, 1003, 1003b
apnea/apparent life-threatening events, 1012–1015
biological development of
fine motor development in, 960
gross motor development in, 960–963
maturation of systems in, 959–960
proportional changes in, 958–959
body image development in, 965, 965f
child care arrangements for, 970–976
clearing airway obstruction for, 1368–1370, 1368f
cognitive development in, 964–965
colic in, 1003–1005
congenital anomalies in. *See* Congenital anomalies
constipation and, 1400
death of. *See* Death, of newborn
dental health for, 983
fear of strangers in, 967, 970
growth failure, 1005–1008
growth/development overview, 971t–975t
high-risk. *See* High-risk infants
hospitalization of, 1235. *See also* Hospitalization, pediatric
immunizations for, 983–984
administration of, 992–993
atraumatic care for, 991b–992b
compliance with, 992
contraindications/precautions for, 989t–991t
diphtheria, 984–985
Haemophilus influenzae type B, 987
hepatitis A virus, 984
hepatitis B virus, 984
influenza, 987–988
measles, 986
meningococcus, 988
mumps, 986
pertussis, 985
pneumococcus, 986–987
Infants *(Continued)*
polio, 985
reactions to, 988–992
rotavirus/HPV, 988
rubella, 986
schedule for, 984
tetanus, 985
varicella, 987
infections and. *See* Neonatal infections
injury prevention. *See under* Injury prevention
limit-setting/discipline, 976
manifestations of hearing impairment in, 1201, 1201b
nutrition for. *See also* Breastfeeding
benefits of breastfeeding, 676–677
breastfeeding support, 677–679, 678b
contraindications to breastfeeding, 677
Dietary Reference Intakes in, 978, 978t
during first 6 months, 978–979
formula feeding, 700–704
ineffective breastfeeding and, 699b
introduction of solid foods, 981, 981b
nutrient needs for, 679–680
recommendations for, 676
during second 6 months, 979–980
selection/preparation of solid foods, 980–981
weaning and, 981
positional plagiocephaly, 1011–1012, 1012f
postterm. *See* Postterm infants
preparation for procedures, 1262b–1263b
preterm. *See* Preterm infants
psychosocial development in, 963–964
regurgitation/spitting up, 1003
separation anxiety in, 970
shoes for, 978
sleep problems in, 981–983, 982t
social development of, 966–968
with special needs, 1170–1173, 1171t–1172t
sudden infant death syndrome and, 1008–1011
teething in, 977, 977f
temperament of, 968–970
thumb-sucking/pacifiers and, 976–977
understanding of/reactions to death, 1177t–1178t
visual impairment in, 1205–1206
water balance in, 1389–1390, 1391b
Infants of diabetic mothers (IDMs)
birth trauma/perinatal asphyxia in, 736
cardiomyopathy in, 736–737
congenital anomalies, 735
discharge planning for, 737–738
Infants of diabetic mothers (IDMs) *(Continued)*
hyperbilirubinemia/polycythemia in, 737
hypocalcemia/hypomagnesemia in, 736
hypoglycemia in, 736
macrosomia in, 736, 736f
nursing care for, 737, 737b
pathophysiology of, 735
respiratory distress syndrome, 736
Infection control
day care centres and, 1056, 1056f
in diabetic pregnancy, 342, 344
HIV/AIDS and, 1528
home visits and, 40
after membranes rupture, 456
for neonatal screening, 659–660
pediatric
during hospitalization, 1277–1278, 1277b
leukemia and, 1519–1523
postoperatively, hydrocephalus and, 1607–1608
in postpartum care, 541, 541b
for preterm infants, 711, 712b
routine precautions for, 111, 111b–112b
Infection(s)
emergency interventions for, 467b–468b
in Guillain-Barré syndrome, 1743–1745, 1744b
infants and, 959
intracranial, 1586–1592
neonatal. *See* Neonatal infections
in osteomyelitis, 1710–1712, 1711b
postpartum, 586–588, 587b
preterm labour and, 490
preterm membranes rupture and, 497–498
of respiratory tract, 1316–1317
sepsis, 746–747
in septic arthritis, 1712
in skeletal tuberculosis, 1712
visual impairment and, 1205
Infectious gastroenteritis, 1392
Infectious mononucleosis, 1328–1329, 1328b
Infectious polyneuritis, 1743–1745, 1744b
Infective endocarditis, 1481–1483, 1482b
Inferiority, school-age children and, 1087
Inferiority vs. industry stage of psychosocial development, 852
Infertility
adoption and, 135, 135f
assisted reproductive technologies, 133–134, 133b, 133f
factors associated with, 126–127, 127b–128b
female assessment for, 127–129, 129f, 129t
incidence of, 126
insurance coverage for, 128b
male assessment for, 129, 130b
nonmedical therapies, 131
nursing process, 128b
Infertility *(Continued)*
pharmacological therapies, 131–133
postcoital test, 130
preimplantation genetic diagnosis and, 134–135
psychosocial aspects of, 130–131
seeking health care for, 42–43
surgical procedures for, 132–133
tests/findings for, 129t, 130b
Infiltration, 1301–1302
Inflammation stage of wound healing, 1646
Inflammatory bowel disease (IBD)
in children, 1410–1414, 1411t
during pregnancy, 367
Inflammatory disorders
acute appendicitis, 1408–1409, 1409b
inflammatory bowel disease, 1410–1414, 1411t
Meckel's diverticulum, 1409–1410, 1410b
peptic ulcer disease, 1414–1416, 1415b
Influenza, 1324–1325
Influenza vaccine, 987–988, 1125
Informant, pediatric health history and, 876
Information overload, 872, 873b
Informed consent
for anaesthesia, 418b
for HIV testing, 217, 218b
for pediatric procedures, 1259–1260
eligibility for giving, 1260
requirements for, 1260
for pharmacological pain relief, 416–418
for rubella vaccination, 547b
for screening for drug use, 215b
use of interpreters and, 873
Informed decision making
midwives support of, 11b
promoting, 3b
Infrared thermometers, 901, 902b
Infratentorial brain tumours, 1583–1585
Infusion pumps, 1300
Inguinal hernias, 923, 923f, 1546t
Inhalants, adolescents and, 1148
Inhalation, infant poisoning and, 998
Inhalation burn injury, 1672
Inhalation therapy, 1302–1304, 1302f–1303f
Inhaled nitric oxide (INO) therapy, 717, 948b–949b
Inhalers, asthma and, 1349, 1354, 1354b, 1354f
In-home child care, 970
Initiative vs. guilt stage of psychosocial development, 852, 852f, 1052
Injectable progestins, 149–150
Injections, play activities for, 1266b
Injuries. *See also* Trauma
bone. *See* Fractures
burn. *See* Burns
childhood
causes of, 789t
incidence of, 789–790
vehicle-related, 1131–1132, 1132b

Injuries *(Continued)*
cold, 1682
eye, 1206b
head. *See* Head injury
physical, newborns and, 651–652, 651f
smoke inhalation, 1343–1344
soft-tissue, 1688f
spinal cord, 1748–1750, 1749f
sports, 1101–1104
submersion, 1581–1583, 1582b
Injury prevention
adolescents and
education in, 1132b
firearms, 1132–1133
nursing care for, 1133
sports, 1133
vehicle-related injuries, 1131–1132
infants and, 994b–995b
aspiration of foreign objects, 993–996
bodily damage, 1000
burns, 999–1000, 999f–1000f
drowning, 1000
education in, 1002b
falls, 997–998
motor vehicle injuries, 996–997
nurse's role in, 1001–1003
poisoning, 998–999
shaken baby syndrome, 1001
suffocation, 996
preschoolers and, 1061
school-age children and, 1100–1101, 1102t
toddlers and
aspiration/suffocation, 1044–1045
bodily damage, 1045–1046
burns, 1042–1043
development related to, 1038t–1039t
drowning, 1042
falls, 1044
motor vehicle injuries, 1037–1042
overview, 1037
poisoning, 1043–1044, 1044f
Inlet contracture of pelvis, 499
In-line skate safety
education in, 1103b
school-age children and, 1101
Innocent heart murmur, 922
Insect bites, 1657–1663, 1658t
Inspection in cardiac assessment, 1452
Instruments for birthing, 474, 474f
Insulin
breastfeeding and, 1753t–1756t
changing needs during pregnancy, 339–340, 340f
Insulin deficiency. *See* Diabetes mellitus (DM)
Insulin pump, 348f
Insulin therapy
continuous subcutaneous infusion, 1636
in diabetic pregnancy, 347–348, 348f
for GDM, 310
injection procedure, 1635–1636, 1636f
Insulin therapy *(Continued)*
self-administration guidelines, 347b
site/absorption rate, 1636t
for type 1 diabetes, 1629–1630
types of insulin for, 348t, 1631b
Insulin waning, 1633
Intake and output (I&O) of fluids
acute renal failure and, 1555
dehydration and, 1392
after heart surgery, 1480
measurement of, 1298–1299
nephrotic syndrome and, 1549
sickle cell anemia and, 1510
Integra, 1677
Integrated prenatal screening (IPS), 278
Integrative healing, woman-centred care and, 7
Integumentary disorders
acne and, 1668–1669
arthropod bites/stings and, 1657–1663, 1658t
bed bugs and, 1661, 1661f
Lyme disease and, 1661–1663, 1662f
pediculosis capitis and, 1659–1661, 1659b, 1659f
rickettsial diseases and, 1661, 1662t
scabies and, 1658–1659, 1659b
atopic dermatitis and, 1665–1667, 1666b
burns and. *See* Burns
cold injuries, 1682
contact dermatitis and, 1655–1657
diaper dermatitis and, 1664, 1664f
home care/family support for, 1651
mammal bites/scratches and, 1663
management of
dressings for, 1646, 1648t
systemic therapy for, 1649
topical therapy for, 1646–1651
medication reactions and, 1657
poison ivy/oak/sumac and, 1655–1657, 1656f
during pregnancy, 367–368
seborrheic dermatitis and, 1667
skin infections
bacterial, 1651–1655, 1652t
fungal, 1653–1655, 1654t
systemic mycotic, 1655, 1656t
viral, 1651–1653, 1653t
skin lesions and. *See* Skin lesions
sunburn, 1681–1682
wounds and. *See* Wounds
Integumentary system
changes during labour, 392
changes during pregnancy, 199–200, 199f
after childbirth, 532
ethnic considerations, 200b
fetal development of, 180
transition to extrauterine life and, 616–619
Intellectual development, through play, 858
Intellectual disability. *See* Cognitive impairments (CIs)
Interests of adolescents, 1122, 1122f
Intergroup Rhabdomyosarcoma Study Group, 1715
Interlink intravenous access systems., 1300, 1300f
Intermenstrual bleeding
causes of, 92b
incidence/treatment of, 91–92
Intermittent auscultation (IA)
decision support tool for, 427f
of fetal heart rate, 425–426
frequency of, 426
patient teaching with, 438b
procedure, 426b
Intermittent skilled nursing, 1218, 1218b
Internal female pelvic organs, 64–65, 65f
Internal rotation, birth process and, 390–391
Internal version of fetus, 502
International adoption, 818–819
Internet, child development and, 866–867
Interpersonal relationships, child development and, 861–862, 862f
Interpregnancy interval (IPI), 137b
Interpretation, in nurse interview, 70
Interpreters
for communication assistance, 833–834, 873
use of, 23–24, 24b
guidelines for, 873b
Interstitial pneumonia, 1335
Interview process. *See also* Communication
admission to labour unit, 446–447
with children, 873–876, 874b, 874f, 877b–878b
establishing setting for, 869–870
features of, 69–70, 70f
history taking in, 876–885
during latent phase of labour, 444b
with parents, 871–873
during prenatal period, 218–219
questions for doulas, 242b
Intestinal obstruction
pediatric
anorectal malformations, 1431–1433, 1432b
clinical manifestations of, 1429b
congenital, in newborns, 774
hypertrophic pyloric stenosis, 1427–1430, 1429b, 1429f
intussusception, 1430–1431, 1430f, 1431b
malrotation/volvulus, 1431
during pregnancy, 330–331
Intestinal parasitic diseases
enterobiasis, 1407–1408, 1407b
giardiasis, 1405–1407, 1406b, 1407f
nursing care for, 1405
Intestinal toxocariasis, 1406t
Intestinal transplantation, 1435
Intimate partner violence (IPV). *See also* Abuse, of women
cultural issues, 59
cycle of, 59–61
elements of, 58–61, 58f
interventions, 60b
myths/facts about, 60t
as pregnancy risk factor, 276
prenatal identification of, 215–216
prevention of, 61
safety strategies for, 60b
signs of, 59b
Intracellular fluid (ICF), 1389
Intracranial hemorrhage (ICH), 746
Intracranial infections
aseptic meningitis and, 1589–1590, 1590t
bacterial meningitis and, 1586–1589, 1588b
encephalitis and, 1590–1591, 1590b
rabies and, 1591, 1592b
Reye's syndrome and, 1591–1592, 1592b
Intracranial pressure (ICP)
increase of, 1563, 1563b
monitoring devices for, 1570–1571
Intractable diarrhea of infancy, 1395
Intracytoplasmic sperm injection, 134t
Intradermal analgesia, 948b–949b
Intradermal injections, 1293
Intradermal sterile water block, 407, 407f
Intraductal papilloma, 114
Intramuscular injections
of analgesics, 948b–949b
of medications, 418
administration of, 1291–1293, 1293f
determining site, 1289–1290, 1290t–1291t
guidelines for, 1292b
syringe/needle selection, 1289
for neonates, 661, 662f
Intranasal analgesia, 948b–949b
Intraosseous infusion, 1299
Intrapartum period
cardiac disorders during, 360–361
conditions associated with fetal risk, 425t
in diabetic pregnancy, 349
risks due to obesity, 370
Intrathecal baclofen therapy, 1727
Intrathecal opioids
features of, 948b–949b
for labour pain management, 415–416
Intrauterine devices (IUDs)
complications with, 151b
for contraception, 150, 150f
for emergency contraception, 150
Intrauterine growth restriction (IUGR)
classification of, 708b
common problems of, 734–735
decreased fundal height and, 219
risk factors for, 276b

Intrauterine resuscitation, 436–438, 438b
Intrauterine systems (IUSs)
complications with, 151b
for contraception, 150–151, 150f
Intravenous administration
of analgesics during labour, 418
pediatric
of analgesics, 948b–949b
of antibiotics, CF and, 1359–1360
central venous access device for, 1294–1295, 1294f, 1295t
of medications, 1293–1295
parenteral fluid therapy and complications in, 1301–1302
safety catheters/needleless systems, 1300, 1300f
securing peripheral IV line, 1300–1301, 1301f
site/equipment for, 1299–1300, 1299f
peripheral intermittent infusion device for, 1293–1294
for severe dehydration, 1397–1398
Intravenous antibiotic prophylaxis (IAP), 446
Intravenous fluid intake during labour, 457–460, 458t
Intravenous pyelography (IVP), 1538t–1539t
Intraventricular catheter as ICP monitor, 1570
Introduction during interview, 869
Intuitive thought in preoperational phase, 1052–1053
Intuitive-projective stage of spiritual development, 854
Intussusception, 1430–1431, 1430f, 1431b
Inuit
breast cancer and, 116f
breastfeeding and, 678
bronchiolitis and, 1333
child maltreatment and, 1000
childhood dental caries, 1098–1099
cigarette smoking and, 1144–1145
cleft lip and palate in, 1421
food practices of, 269t–270t, 887b
health beliefs/practices and, 840t–841t
HIV infection in, 1527
home care and, 1223
injury prevention for, 1101
iron deficiency anemia in, 1503
maternity services for, 3–5, 29, 44–45
otitis media in, 1325–1326
preschool program for, 1056
social/economic/health problems of, 830
substance use and, 1146, 1148
suicide and, 792, 1150
traditional postpartum health practices, 552
tuberculosis and, 1338
type 2 DM and, 1639
Invasive ductal carcinoma, 115–116
Invasive meningococcal disease (IMD), 988
Inverted nipples
breast shell for, 224f
pinch test for, 223, 223f
Involuntary uterine contractions, 385–386
Involution of uterus, 526, 527f
Iodine, 1381t–1383t
Iron
in adolescence, 1125
factors affecting absorption of, 1384b
for infant nutrition, 680
laboratory tests for, 1764t–1771t
for maternal nutrition, 257–260
nutritional significance of, 1381t–1383t
poisoning from, 1437b–1438b
storage, in newborns, 614
supplementation, 260, 260b
Iron deficiency anemia (IDA)
in children, 1503–1505
during pregnancy, 364
Iron-fortified cereals, 980, 1034
Irreversibility, preoperational thought and, 1025b
Irreversible shock, 1493b, 1494
Irritability of newborns, 640
Irritant diaper dermatitis, 1664f
Ischemic heart disease during pregnancy, 355
Ischemic phase of menstrual cycle, 82, 83f
Isolation, child placement in, 1253–1254
Isotonic dehydration, 1391
Isotretinoin, 1669
Italian ethnicity
beta-thalassemia and, 1510
child's gender and, 832
food patterns of, 269t–270t
I.V. House site protector, 1301f

J
Jacket restraints, 1280
Japanese ethnicity
communication and, 833–834
cosleeping and, 1009b
food patterns of, 269t–270t
health beliefs/practices and, 840t–841t
Jarish-Herxheimer reaction, 100b
Jaundice
biliary atresia and, 1420, 1420b
breastfeeding and, 654, 691
in neonates, 615, 652–654, 652f, 653t
parent education regarding, 663
phototherapy for, 661–663, 662f
Jet hydrotherapy, 403–405, 404f
Jewish ethnicity. *See also* Ashkenazi Jews
childbirth and, 450
expression of emotion and, 834
food patterns of, 269t–270t
Joanna Briggs Institute (JBI), 10
Joints
juvenile idiopathic arthritis and, 1716–1719
pediatric examination of, 928
septic arthritis and, 1712
skeletal tuberculosis and, 1712
Jones criteria for diagnosis of rheumatic fever, 1483, 1483b
Juvenile autoimmune thyroiditis, 1617–1618, 1618b
Juvenile hypothyroidism, 1617, 1617b
Juvenile idiopathic arthritis (JIA), 1716–1719, 1720b
Juvenile spinal muscular atrophy, 1739b, 1740

K
Kangaroo care. *See* Skin-to-skin (STS) contact
Karyotyping of chromosomes, 163, 164f, 283
Kasai procedure, 1420
Kawasaki disease (KD), 1490–1494, 1491b–1492b
Kegel exercises
after childbirth, 528, 545
education in, 222–223
instructions for, 51, 51b
for uterine displacement, 592–593
Keloid, 1645f
Kernicterus, 653
Ketoacidosis
in diabetic pregnancy, 342
in type 1 diabetes, 1628–1629
Ketogenic diet, epilepsy and, 1597
Ketones, 1628
Ketorolac, 944t
Kidney disease. *See* Renal dysfunction
Kidney Foundation of Canada, 1559
Kidney transplantation, 1560
Kidneys. *See* Renal system
Kindergarten experience of preschoolers, 1055–1057
Kinetic stimulation for infants, 969t
Klinefelter's syndrome, 1105t, 1106
Klumpke palsy, 744–745
Knee jerk reflex test, 929f
Knee-chest position, 1475, 1475f
Knock-knee, 927, 927f
Kohlberg's stages of moral development, 854
adolescents and, 1119
preschoolers and, 1053
school-age children and, 1088–1089
Kugathasan study, 1411
Kugelberg-Welander disease, 1739b, 1740
Kussmaul respiration, 920b, 1628
Kyphosis, 1707, 1707f

L
Labia majora, 63, 64f
Labia minora, 63, 64f
Laboratory tests
abbreviations used in, 1771t
common, 1764t–1771t
during follow-up visits, 220–221
Laboratory tests *(Continued)*
in health assessment, 79
in nutrition assessment, 266–267
in prenatal period, 216–218, 217t
Labour
abnormal patterns in, 503–505, 503t, 504f
abnormally slow. *See* Dystocia
augmentation of, 511
Canadian Maternity Experiences Survey of, 9
cultural practices regarding, 25t–26t
discomfort in, 394–398
father's participation in, 450
fetal adaptation to, 391
fetal health surveillance during. *See* Fetal health surveillance (FHS)
fetal oxygenation in, 424b
first stage of. *See* First stage of labour
fourth stage of. *See* Fourth stage of labour
induction of. *See* Induction of labour
maternal adaptation to, 391–392
maternal positions for, 386–388, 387f
mechanism of, 389–391, 390f
non-English-speaking women in, 450
onset of, 388
pain of. *See* Pain, during labour/birth
passageway in, 380–385
passenger in, 378–380
powers in, 385–386
precipitous, 505
preterm. *See* Preterm labour and birth
process of, 388–391
second stage of. *See* Second stage of labour
siblings during, 467
signs preceding, 388, 388b
stages of, 388–389
third stage of. *See* Third stage of labour
trial of, 505
true vs. false, 443, 444b
Labour, delivery, and recovery (LDR) rooms, 242–243, 242f
Labour, delivery, recovery, and postpartum (LDRP) rooms, 242–243, 242f
Labour induction rates, 8
Labour support
by doulas, 465–466
evidence-based practice and, 464b
by grandparents, 466–467
by nurse, 463–464
overview, 461–462, 466t
by partner, 465, 465b, 465f
Lacerations
care of, 1649–1650
cerebral, 1575
during childbirth, 476–477, 477f
genital tract, 578–579

Lactation. *See also* Breastfeeding
breast anatomy and, 680–681, 681f
milk production, 681, 682f
nutrition during, 270–271
properties of human milk, 682–683
psychotropic medications and, 599
suppression of, 545–547
Lactational amenorrhea method (LAM), 141–142
Lacto-ovo vegetarians, 268–270, 1380
Lactose intolerance, 260, 260b, 1388–1389, 1389b
Lactovegetarians, 1380
Lalonde Report, 3
Lamaze healthy birth practices, 401–402, 402b
Lamaze Institute for Normal Birth (LINB), 401–402
Language
development of, 853–854
infants and, 967
preschoolers and, 1052–1054, 1054f
toddlers and, 1027
Lanugo, 180
Laparoscopy, for female infertility, 132, 132f
Laparotomy, 132, 151, 151f
Large-for-gestational-age (LGA) infants
classification of, 708b
in diabetic pregnancy, 341–342
health issues with, 8
problems associated with, 735
Laryngitis
acute, 1330–1331, 1330t
spasmodic, 1332
Laryngotracheobronchitis (LTB), 1330t, 1331–1332, 1331b
Lasix
breastfeeding and, 1753t–1756t
for heart failure, 1469t
LATCH (Lower Anchors and Tethers for Children) system, 1040, 1040f
LATCH breastfeeding assessment tool, 683
Latchkey children, 1094
Latch-on of infant, 685–686, 685f–686f
Late decelerations of fetal heart rate, 434, 434f, 435b
Late pregnancy bleeding, 321–330, 322f. *See also* Hemorrhagic disorders in pregnancy
Late preterm infants, 649–651
discharge planning for, 737–738, 738b
nursing care for, 710–733, 714b
overview, 708–709
risk factors for, 709t
Late reproductive age, 47
Latency period of psychosexual development, 851
Latent phase of labour, 468–469, 469t
Latent tuberculosis infection (LTBI), 1338
Later childhood, developmental stage, 845b
Lateral position, birthing process and, 461, 461f, 462b, 470f, 471–472
Latex allergy, 1737–1738, 1738b
Latin American ethnicity
breast cancer and, 116f
cosleeping and, 1009b
diabetes mellitus and, 1627t, 1639
expression of emotion and, 834
practices regarding newborns and, 660b
reactions to pain and, 396b
sickle cell anemia and, 1505
sickle cell anemia in, 1505
as visible minority, 829, 830b
Lead, normal test ranges for, 1764t–1771t
Lead poisoning
anticipatory guidance for, 1444
causes of, 1442–1443
diagnosis of, 1444
incidence of, 1441–1442
management of, 1444–1445
pathophysiology/clinical manifestations, 1443–1444, 1443f
prevention of, 1446b
screening for, 1444
sources of, 1442b
Learning disability (LD), 1106–1107
Left-sided heart failure, 1462
Left-to-right shunt, 1455–1456
Leg roll, 546f
Legal blindness, 1203–1204
Legal issues
abortion and, 153b
for abused women, 59–61
adoption and, 817
assisted reproductive technologies, 133
cardiac emergencies and, 360b
in care of mothers/infants, 4b
child maltreatment and, 1072, 1072b
commitment for psychiatric care, 598b
communicable diseases and, 99b
cryopreservation of embryos, 133b
custody arrangements and, 820–821
documentation and, 473b
early discharge after birth and, 536b
fetal monitoring standards, 436b
genetics research and, 162
informed consent for anaesthesia and, 418b
laws regarding live birth and, 604b
midwifery and, 11
reporting attempted suicide and, 1152
rubella vaccination and, 547b
screening for drug use, 215b
standard of care for obstetrical emergencies, 584b
sterilization and, 152
substance use during pregnancy, 373
Legal issues *(Continued)*
Leg/arm restraints, 1280
Legg-Calvé-Perthes disease, 1705–1706, 1705b
Legs
relieving cramps, 228f
resting position for, 228f
Length of newborns, 626t–636t, 628f, 637
Leopold's manoeuvres, 452, 453b, 453f
Lesbian couples, 564–565
Let-down reflex, 681, 686
Lethargy, 1564b
Leukemias
classification of, 1517–1518
diagnosis of, 1518
hemorrhage prevention in, 1521–1522
incidence of, 1517
infection prevention in, 1519–1521
late effects of treatment for, 1519
nursing care for, 1519–1524, 1520b–1522b
pathophysiology of, 1518, 1518t
therapy for, 1518–1519
treatment for
alopecia from, 1524
anemia in, 1522–1523
anorexia from, 1523
hemorrhagic cystitis from, 1524
mood changes from, 1524
mucosal ulceration from, 1523–1524
nausea and vomiting in, 1523
neuropathy from, 1524
steroid effects from, 1524
Leukocyte differential count, 1764t–1771t
Leukocytosis, 611
Leukorrhea, 192
Leukotrienes, 1350
Levels of consciousness, 1563, 1564b
Lever lock cannula, 1300, 1300f
Levonorgestrel intrauterine system, 150–151, 150f
Levorphanol, 945t
Lice, head, 1659–1661, 1659b, 1659f
Lichenification, 1645f
Lidocaine, 950, 950f, 952b
LidoSite Topical System, 951
Lie, fetal, 379, 380f–381f
at birth, 379, 380f–381f
Life-limiting illness, 1157b
Lightening, 189, 190f, 388
Light-headedness, 200–201
Limb deficiency, 1703–1704
Limb salvage procedure, 1713
Limb-girdle muscular dystrophy, 1740, 1741f
Limit-setting
infants and, 976
in parenting, 814–817
school-age children and, 1094–1095
Linea nigra, 199, 199f
Linear skull fractures, 1576
Lingual tonsils, 1322, 1323f
Lipomas, 113
Lipoproteins, hyperlipidemia and, 1484
Lipreading, 1201–1202, 1202b
Liquid crystal skin contact thermometer, 902b
Listening during interviews, 871–872
Listeriosis, 267
Literacy, health, 12
Lithotomy position
for childbirth, 474
for physically disabled women, 71, 71f
during second stage of labour, 472f
supine hypotension and, 216
Live-attenuated influenza vaccine (LAIV), 1325
Liver
changes during pregnancy, 202
disorders of. *See* Hepatic disorders
fetal, 178
palpation of, 924
transplantation, cirrhosis and, 1419, 1420b
Liver biopsy, Reye's syndrome and, 1592
Living related donor for kidney transplant, 1560
LMX anaesthetic cream, 950, 950f
Lobar pneumonia, 1335
Lobular carcinoma, 115–116
Local infiltration anaesthesia, 410
Lochia, 527–528, 528b
Locomotion
infants and, 962–963, 963f
toddlers and, 1021–1022, 1028
Locutionary stage of communicative development, 874, 874b
Lone parenting, 17, 821
special needs child and, 1160
Long-term central venous access devices, 1294, 1294f, 1295t
Lorazepam, 946t
Lordosis, 1707, 1707f
Loss and grief. *See* Grief
Loss of appetite
chemotherapy and, 1523
nephrotic syndrome and, 1549
Loss of control, hospitalization and, 1234–1236
Low health literacy, 34
Low-birth-weight (LBW) infants
nutrition and, 250
preterm infants vs., 488–490
Low-cariogenic diet, 1036–1037
Low-density lipoproteins (LDLs), 1484
Lower extremity traction, 1696
Lower respiratory infections
bronchiolitis/respiratory syncytial virus, 1333–1337, 1334b
bronchitis, 1332–1333
comparison of, 1333t
pneumonias, 1335–1337, 1335b, 1337f
Lower respiratory tract, 1316
Lower-segment Caesarean birth, 513f, 514
Low-lying placenta, 321–322

Lumbar epidural analgesia
for labour pain management, 413–415, 414f
maternal hypotension in, 413b
Lumbar puncture
for assessment of cerebral function, 1567, 1567t–1568t
atraumatic care for, 1282b
for diagnosing bacterial meningitis, 1587
infection control and, 109t
positioning for, 1281–1282, 1281f
Lumpectomy, 118, 119f
Lung(s)
auscultation guidelines, 919b
classification of breath sounds, 920b
pediatric examination of, 919–920, 919f, 920b
transplants, cystic fibrosis and, 1361
Luque-rod segmental spinal instrumentation, 1709
Luteal phase of menstrual cycle, 82, 83f
Lying, school-age children and, 1095
Lymph nodes
Hodgkin's disease and, 1525–1526, 1525f
Kawasaki disease and, 1490–1494, 1491b
location/examination of, 906–907, 907f
Lymphocytic thyroiditis, 1617–1618, 1618b
Lymphoid tissues, 847f, 848
Lymphomas, in children, 1524–1526

M

Macrobiotics, 1380
Macrominerals, 1375–1380
Macrosomia
in diabetic pregnancy, 341–342
in infants of diabetic mothers, 736, 736f
Macules, 1644f
Mafenide acetate, 1676t
Magical thinking
in preoperational thought, 1025b
preschoolers and, 1052–1053
Magnesium
for maternal nutrition, 260
nutritional significance of, 1381t–1383t
Magnesium sulphate
breastfeeding and, 1753t–1756t
for severe pre-eclampsia, 304–305
Magnet reflex in newborns, 622t–625t, 625f
Magnetic resonance imaging (MRI)
for assessment of cerebral function, 1567–1568, 1567t–1568t
for breast cancer screening, 117b
for head injury, 1578
for hydrocephalus, 1605–1606
Mainstreaming, 1159
Major burn injury, 1671–1672, 1674–1677
Malabsorption syndromes
celiac disease, 1433–1434, 1434b
short-bowel syndrome, 1434–1435
Male condoms, 142–143, 143f, 144b
Male fertility, 126–127, 128b
Male genitalia
formation of, 179–180
in neonates, 619–620
pediatric examination of, 924–925, 925f
Male reproductive system
disorders, in adolescents, 1135
neonatal adaptations, 619–620, 619f
Male sterilization, 151f, 152
Malocclusion, 1099
Malpresentation of fetus
dystocia and, 500–501
external cephalic version with, 501–502, 501f
internal version with, 502
Malrotation of intestine, 1431
Mammal bites, 1663–1664
Mammary duct ectasia, 113–114
Mammography, 116f, 117b
Manual breast pumps, 692, 693f
Manual traction, 1696b
Maple syrup urine disease and, 656t
Marfan syndrome, 354
Marginal placenta previa, 321–322
Marijuana
breastfeeding and, 1753t–1756t
childbirth risks with, 48
prenatal exposure to, 760
Masked deprivation, 861–862
Massage
education in, 247
for labour pain management, 403
Mastectomy
for breast cancer, 118, 119f
home care, 122b
postoperative exercises, 123b
Mastery motivation, activities promoting, 850b
Mastitis
breastfeeding and, 698
during postpartum period, 587, 587f
Masturbation
preschoolers and, 1057
toddlers and, 1026
Maternal adaptations
acceptance, 206–207
breastfeeding and, 683
identification with, 207
during labour, 391–392, 392b
overview, 206
postpartum psychosocial needs, 548–552, 549b
postpartum role adjustment, 563–564, 563t
preparing for childbirth, 208
relationship with fetus, 208, 210b
reordering relationships, 207–208, 207f
Maternal child services
advantages of, 36
childbirth education classes, 36–37, 36b
home visits, 37–38, 38b
Maternal death, 607
Maternal glucose levels, 735
Maternal health problems, 274–276, 276b
Maternal hypotension with decreased placental perfusion, 413b, 415
Maternal hypothermia after analgesia/anaesthesia, 421
Maternal mortality rates
global perspective on, 12
as perinatal health indicator, 7b
Maternal nutrition
for adolescent pregnancy, 263
calcium for, 260, 260b–261b
before conception, 250
cultural influences, 268–270, 269t–270t
determinants of health and, 250, 251f
DRIs recommended for, 251, 253t–254t
energy intake and, 251–256
fat-soluble vitamins for, 261–262
fluids for, 256–257, 258b
fluoride for, 261
indicators of risk, 258b
iron for, 257–260, 260b
during lactation, 270–271
magnesium for, 260
medical nutrition therapy, 267
multivitamin/multimineral supplements for, 262
nursing care for, 263–270, 264b
nutrition counselling, 267
nutrition-related discomforts, 267–268
pica/food cravings, 262–263
potassium for, 261
pre-eclampsia, 263
protein for, 256, 257t
safe food preparation and, 267
sodium for, 261
vegetarian diets, 268–270
water-soluble vitamins for, 262
weight gain and, 251–256, 255f, 255t
zinc for, 261
Maternal opioid abstinence symptoms, 409b
Maternal physical status after birth
assessment in fourth stage of labour, 484b
care after placental delivery, 481
rapid changes in, 481
signs of potential problems, 481
Maternal role
infant attachment and, 966
for special needs child, 1160
Maternal serum alpha fetoprotein (MSAFP) levels, 278
Maternal smoking, SIDS and, 1008–1009
Maternal substance use. *See* Substance use, during pregnancy
Maternity nursing. *See* Perinatal nursing
Maternity services
history of, 3–5, 4b
inequities in, 3–6
Maturation, definition of, 844
Maturation of systems
infants and, 959–960
school-age children and, 1084–1085
toddlers and, 1021
Maturation stage of wound healing, 1646
Mazzanti technique for shoulder dystocia, 520, 520f
McGill Model of Nursing, 18t
McRoberts manoeuvre, 520–521, 521f
Mean corpuscular hemoglobin concentration (MCHC), 1764t–1771t
Mean corpuscular hemoglobin (MCH), 1764t–1771t
Mean corpuscular volume (MCV), 1764t–1771t
Measles, 1064t–1070t, 1066f
Measles vaccine, 986
contraindications/precautions for, 989t–991t
Mechanical dilators, 508
Mechanical suffocation in infants, 996
Mechanical ventilation
bronchopulmonary dysplasia and, 732–733
for oxygen therapy, 715–716, 716f, 716t
Mechanism of labour
cardinal movements of, 390f
descent, 389
engagement, 389
expulsion, 391
extension, 391
flexion, 389
internal rotation, 390–391
restitution/external rotation, 391
Meckel's diverticulum, 1409–1410, 1410b
Meconium
amniocentesis for detection of, 283–284
in newborn's stools, 614, 614b, 615f, 1400
Meconium aspiration syndrome (MAS), 733, 733f
Meconium ileus, 1400
Meconium plugs, 1400
Meconium-stained amniotic fluid
abnormal fetal heart rate and, 733, 733f
management of infants with, 476
Media, childhood development and, 864–867
Medical abortion, 154
Medical history
family, 882
in nutrition assessment, 263–264
for prenatal care, 214–215
Medical identification, for type 1 diabetes patients, 1635
Medical induction abortion, 154
Medicare, services covered by, 3
Medication guide
eye prophylaxis, 647b
Hepatitis B immune globulin, 661b
Hepatitis B vaccine, 661b
vitamin K prophylaxis, 647b
Medications. *See* Drug therapy
Mediolateral episiotomy, 478, 478f

Mediterranean ethnicity
beta-thalassemia and, 45, 158, 160f, 364
lactase deficiency and, 1503
Mongolian spots and, 618
sickle cell anemia and, 656t
Mediterranean-type diet, 1484
Meiosis, 168
Menarche, 81, 1114
Meningitis
aseptic, 1589–1590, 1590t
bacterial, 1586–1589, 1588b
Meningocele, 1732, 1733b, 1733f
Meningococcal C vaccine, 988
contraindications/precautions for, 989t–991t
for infants/children, 1589
for preteens, 1125
Menopause
features of, 84
incidence/treatment of, 94
seeking health care for, 44
Menorrhagia, 92
Menstruation
alterations in, 91–92
amenorrhea, 84–85
breastfeeding and, 695
climacteric and, 84
cyclic changes in, 84
disorders, 92–94, 93b–94b
endometriosis, 89–91, 90f
health care for problems in, 43–44
initial appearance of, 1114
menopause, 94
menstrual cycle, 82–84, 83f
overview, 81–82
perimenstrual pain and discomfort, 85–91
prostaglandins and, 84
Mental development theories, 852–854
Mental health issues
in children/youth, 792
as pregnancy risk factor, 274–276
Meperidine hydrochloride
for children, 947t
for labour pain management, 409
Mercury toxicity, 1440
Mercy killing, 1175
Meromelia, 1703
Mesh graft, 1677, 1677f
Mesoderm, 171f, 172
Metabolic disorders
diabetes mellitus. *See* Diabetes mellitus (DM)
hyperthyroidism, 350–352
hypothyroidism, 352
Metabolism
developmental changes in, 849
effects of immobilization on, 1685t
Metatarsus adductus, 1703
Metatarsus varus, 1703
Metered-dose inhalers (MDIs), 1349, 1354, 1354b, 1354f
Methadone
breastfeeding and, 696, 1753t–1756t
for children, 945t, 947t
for opiate use, 374
prenatal exposure to, 761
Methamphetamines
adolescent use of, 1148
childbirth risks with, 48–49
infant exposure to, 999
prenatal exposure to, 761–762
Methimazole, 350, 1620, 1620b
Methotrexate
breastfeeding and, 1753t–1756t
for ectopic pregnancy, 319, 319b–320b
for juvenile idiopathic arthritis, 1717
for medical abortion, 154
Methylergonovine, 583b
Methylphenidate hydrochloride, 1106–1107
Métis
breastfeeding and, 678
child maltreatment and, 1000
childhood dental caries, 1098–1099
cigarette smoking and, 1144–1145
cleft lip and palate in, 1421
food practices of, 269t–270t, 887b
health beliefs/practices and, 840t–841t
HIV infection in, 1527
injury prevention for, 1101
iron deficiency anemia in, 1503
maternity services for, 3–5, 29, 44–45
otitis media in, 1325–1326
preschool program for, 1056
social/economic/health problems of, 830
substance use and, 1146
suicide rate among, 792
traditional postpartum health practices, 552
tuberculosis and, 1338
type 2 DM and, 1639
Metredose inhaler (MDI), 1304
Metrorrhagia
causes of, 92b
incidence/treatment of, 91–92
Mexiletine, 946t
Microcephaly, 770
Microminerals, 1375–1380
Microwave ovens, burn injuries and, 999
Middle adulthood, 46
Middle childhood, 845b. *See also* School-age children
Middle Eastern ethnicity
food patterns of, 269t–270t
practices regarding newborns and, 660b
reactions to pain and, 396b
sickle cell anemia in, 216–217, 364, 656t
Midline episiotomy, 478, 478f
Midpelvis, 380–383, 382f–383f
Midplane contracture of pelvis, 499
Midwifery
legal issues and, 11
perinatal care and, 11, 241
principles of, 11b
Milk ducts, plugged, 698
Milk ejection reflex (let-down), 681, 686
Milk stools, 614b, 615f
Millenium Development Goals (MDGs), 5–6, 5b
Milwaukee braces, 1708–1709
Mind-altering drugs, adolescents and, 1148
Minerals
imbalances in, 1375–1380
for infant nutrition, 680, 703–704
nutritional significance of, 1381t–1383t
during pregnancy/lactation
calcium, 260, 260b–261b
fluoride, 261
iron, 257–260
magnesium, 260
potassium, 261
sodium, 261
zinc, 261
Minilaparotomy, 151, 151f
Minimal-change nephrotic syndrome (MCNS), 1547–1549
Minor burn injury, 1671–1674
Misbehaviour, 815, 815b
Miscarriage
defined, 313
incidence/etiology of, 313–314
nursing care for, 315, 317b
types of, 314–315, 314f, 315t
Misoprostol
for medical abortion, 154
for miscarriage, 316
for postpartum hemorrhage, 583b
Missed miscarriage, 314–315, 314f, 315t
Mitosis, 168
Mitral valve prolapse (MVP), 355
Mitral valve stenosis, 354
Mixed (conductive-sensorineural) hearing loss, 1199
Mobilization devices, 1726, 1726f
Modelling, aggression and, 1058
Moderate burn injury, 1671–1672
Modified Blalock-Taussig shunt, 1476t
Modified radical mastectomy, 118
Molar pregnancy, 320–321, 320f
Molluscum contagiosum, 1653t
Mongan method, 401
Mongolian spots, 618, 618f
Monilial infections, 697–698
Monitoring of apnea/ALTE, 1013–1014, 1014b, 1014f
Monoplegia, 1725b
Monospot, 1329
Monozygotic twins
characteristics of, 812–813, 812b
formation of, 180–184, 184f
Mons pubis, 63, 64f
Montgomery tubercles, 192
Mood stabilizers, 596t
Mood swings
in adolescence, 1118–1119
leukemia treatment and, 1524
Mood-changing drugs, breastfeeding and, 1753t–1756t
Moral development
adolescents and, 1119
premoral level of preschoolers, 1053
Moral development *(Continued)*
stages of, 854
through play, 858
Moraxella catarrhalis, otitis media and, 1326
Morbidity
childhood, 793
statistics/rates, 793, 803, 803b
Morning sickness, 201
Moro reflex
absence of, 745, 745f
in neonates, 622t–625t, 623f
neurological health and, 1567b
Morphine
breastfeeding and, 1753t–1756t
for children, 943, 945t, 947t
for major burns, 1675
Mortality
infant, 792–793
statistics/rates, 792, 803, 803b
Mosaicism, 164
Mothers Against Drunk Driving (MADD), 1149
Mothers of special needs children, 1160
Motility disorders
pediatric
constipation, 1399–1401
diarrhea, 1392–1399, 1393t–1395t, 1397f
gastroesophageal reflux, 1403–1405, 1404b
Hirschsprung disease, 1401–1403, 1401f, 1402b
vomiting, 1403
Motor function, cerebral dysfunction and, 1566
Motor vehicle injuries
in children, 789–790, 790f
infants and, 996–997
school-age children and, 1101, 1102t
toddlers and, 1037–1042
Moulding of newborn's skull, 620, 620f
Mouth
changes during pregnancy, 202
of newborns, 626t–636t
pediatric
internal structures of, 917, 917f
nutritional status and, 887t–889t
pediatric examination of, 916–917, 916f
Mouth care. *See* Oral hygiene
Mouth-to-mouth and nose breathing for CPR, 1367f
Movies, child development and, 864
MP3 players for visually impaired children, 1207
Mucocutaneous lymph node syndrome, 1490–1494, 1491b
Mucosal ulceration, chemotherapy and, 1523–1524
Mucous plug (operculum), 192, 193f
Multiculturalism in Canada, 21
Multidimensional pain assessment tools, 936

Multidisciplinary Collaborative Primary Maternity Care Project (MCP^2), 7
Multifactorial inheritance, genetic transmission and, 166
Multifetal pregnancy, 180–184
adjustment to, 812–813
complications of, 502
prenatal care for, 240–241
rates of, 8
Multigravida, definition of, 186
Multimineral supplements, 262
Multiparous women, 186, 238
Multiple births. *See* Multifetal pregnancy
Multiple sclerosis (MS), pregnancy and, 369
Multivitamin supplements, 262
Mummy restraints, 1280, 1280f
Mumps, 1070f
Mumps vaccine, 986
contraindications/precautions for, 989t–991t
Munchausen syndrome by proxy (MSBP), 1072–1073
Muscle tone, Down syndrome children and, 1197–1198
Muscles
fetal development of, 180
pediatric examination of, 928
Muscular disorders
botulism and, 1746–1747, 1747b
cerebral palsy. *See* Cerebral palsy (CP)
Duchenne muscular dystrophy and, 1740–1743, 1741b, 1741f
Guillain-Barré syndrome and, 1743–1745, 1744b
muscular dystrophies and, 1740, 1741f
spina bifida and, 1732–1738, 1733b–1734b, 1733f–1734f
spinal cord injuries and, 1748–1750, 1749f
spinal muscular atrophy and, 1738–1740, 1739b
tetanus and, 1745–1746, 1745b
Muscular dystrophies, 1740, 1741f
Duchenne muscular dystrophy, 1740–1743, 1741b, 1741f
Muscular Dystrophy Canada, 1742
Musculoskeletal dysfunction
bone tumours and, 1712–1713, 1713b
Ewing's sarcoma, 1714–1715
osteosarcoma, 1713–1714
congenital clubfoot and, 1701–1703, 1702f
developmental dysplasia of hip and, 1699–1701, 1700b
idiopathic scoliosis and, 1707f–1708f, 1708–1710
immobilization and, 1684–1688, 1685t
juvenile idiopathic arthritis and, 1716–1719, 1720b
kyphosis/lordosis and, 1707, 1707f
Musculoskeletal dysfunction *(Continued)*
Legg-Calvé-Perthes disease and, 1705–1706, 1705b
metatarsus adductus and, 1703
osteogenesis imperfecta and, 1704–1705, 1704b
osteomyelitis and, 1710–1712, 1711b
rhabdomyosarcoma and, 1715–1716, 1715b
septic arthritis and, 1712
skeletal limb deficiency and, 1703–1704
skeletal tuberculosis and, 1712
slipped capital femoral epiphysis and, 1706–1707, 1706b
systemic lupus erythematosus and, 1719–1721, 1721b
traumatic injury and
amputation and, 1698–1699
distraction for, 1697–1698, 1699f
fractures and, 1690–1692, 1691b–1692b, 1691f
casting for, 1692–1695, 1694b, 1694f
soft-tissue injury and, 1688–1690, 1688f
traction for, 1695–1697, 1695f–1696f, 1696b, 1698b
Musculoskeletal system
fetal development of, 180
maternal
adaptations to pregnancy, 200, 201f
changes during labour, 392
after childbirth, 532
pediatric
congenital anomalies of, 775–776
effects of immobilization on, 1684–1686, 1685t
nutritional status and, 887t–889t
Music
education in, 247
for labour pain management, 403
Mutual play, 1055
Mutual storytelling, 877b–878b
Myasthenia gravis (MG) during pregnancy, 369–370
Mycobacterium tuberculosis, 1337–1338
Myelodysplasia, 1732
Myelomeningocele. *See* Spina bifida
Myelosuppression, leukemias and, 1519–1523
Myocardial infarction, 1491, 1492b
Myoclonic seizures, 1594b–1595b
Myometrium, 64, 66f
Myopia, 1204, 1204b–1205b
Myositis ossificans, 1689
Myringotomy, 1327
Mythical-literal stage of spiritual development, 854

N

Nägele's rule, 206
Naive instrumental orientation of preschoolers, 1053
Nalbuphine
breastfeeding and, 1753t–1756t
for labour pain management, 409, 409b
Naloxone hydrochloride (Narcan), 409–410, 410b, 761b
Naproxen
breastfeeding and, 1753t–1756t
for children, 944t
Narcotic agonist analgesics, 408–409, 408b
Narcotic agonist-antagonist analgesics, 409, 409b
Narcotic antagonists, 409–410, 410b
Narcotics
adolescent use of, 1147
breastfeeding and, 1753t–1756t
Nasal administration of medications, 1296–1297
Nasal cannula for oxygen therapy, 715, 715f
Nasal washings, 1286
Nasoduodenal tubes, 1310–1312
Nasogastric (NG) tube feeding
atraumatic care for, 1308b
correct placement of, 1311b
for gavage feedings, 719–721, 1308–1309
guidelines for, 1309b
for medication administration, 1295–1296, 1296b
Nasojejunal tubes, 1310–1312
Nasopharyngitis, 1320–1321, 1320b–1321b
National Advisory Committee on Immunization, 984, 1325
Natural family planning (NFP) method of contraception, 137–142
Natural forces, 835
Nausea, chemotherapy and, 1523
Nausea and vomiting of pregnancy (NVP)
coping with, 267–268, 268f
features of, 201
Near-miss SIDS. *See* Apparent life-threatening events (ALTEs)
Nebulizers, 1354, 1354f, 1356f
Necator americanus, 1406t
Neck
of children
nutritional status and, 887t–889t
pediatric examination of, 907
of newborns, 626t–636t
Necrotizing enterocolitis (NEC), 731–732
Nedocromil sodium, 1349
Needleless IV systems, 1300, 1300f
Negativism, toddlers and, 1022, 1031, 1235
Neglect, child
clinical manifestations of, 1077b–1078b
defined, 1072
history/interview in, 1076
physical assessment in, 1078
types of, 1072
Neisseria gonorrhoeae, 98–99
Neonatal abstinence syndrome (NAS)
assessment of, 762–765, 762t
nursing care for, 764–765
scoring system, 763f
Neonatal discharge planning
bathing/cord care/skin care, 670–671, 671b–672b, 672f
body temperature, 667
car seat use, 669–670, 669f
clothing, 669
elimination, 667
follow-up care, 671–672
home care, 673b
non-nutritive sucking, 670
prevention of SIDS, 667–668
rashes, 668–669
respirations, 667
safety/holding, 668, 668f
Neonatal infections
bacterial, 755–756
cytomegalovirus infection, 753–754, 753f
fungal, 756
gonorrhea, 750
hepatitis B virus, 751–752
herpes simplex virus, 754, 754f
human immunodeficiency virus, 752–753
parvovirus B19, 754–755
rubella, 753
sepsis, 746–747, 746t, 748t
syphilis, 750–751, 751f
toxoplasmosis, 749–750
varicella zoster, 751
Neonatal intensive care units (NICUs), 722, 722f
Neonatal sepsis
early-onset, 746–747
late-onset, 747
nursing care for, 747–749, 748b
prevention, 748–749
risk factors for, 746t
signs of, 748t
Neonatal transition to extrauterine life
baseline growth measurements, 637
behavioural characteristics, 637–641, 637b
cardiovascular system, 610–611
gastrointestinal system, 613–614
general appearance, 636, 636f
hematopoietic system, 611
hepatic system, 614–615
immune system, 616
influencing factors, 638–639
integumentary system, 616–619
neurological/neuromuscular system, 621, 622t–625t, 637
physical assessment, 625–637, 626t–636t
renal system, 613
reproductive system, 619–620, 619f
respiratory system, 609–610
response to external stimuli, 640–641
sensory behaviours, 639–640
skeletal system, 620–621
sleep-wake states, 638, 638f
thermogenic system, 612–613
transition period phases, 609

Neoplastic disorders in children, 1517–1524
Nephroblastoma, 1552–1553, 1552b
Nephrotic syndrome, 1547–1549, 1547b, 1548f
Nerve block analgesia/anaesthesia
combined spinal-epidural, 415
epidural, 413–415, 414f
epidural/intrathecal opioids, 415–416
local infiltration, 410
pudendal, 410–411, 411f
spinal, 411–413, 412f
Nerve deafness, 1199
Nervous system tumours
brain tumours, 1583–1585
neuroblastomas, 1585–1586
Neural tube defects (NTDs)
degrees of, 1733b
in neonates, 768–770
screening for, 278
spina bifida. *See* Spina bifida
Neuroblastomas, 1585–1586
Neuroectodermal tumour, 1714–1715
Neuroendocrine factors in child development, 859
Neurogenic diabetes insipidus, 1615–1616
Neurological assessment
of cerebral dysfunction, 1564–1567
of newborn reflexes, 622t–625t, 637
pediatric, 928
Neurological disorders during pregnancy, 368–369
Neurological system
adaptations in, 200–201
changes during labour, 392
after childbirth, 531–532
fetal development of, 179
labour pain origins in, 394–395
maturation of, 847f, 848
nutritional status and, 887t–889t
Neuromuscular disorders
botulism and, 1746–1747, 1747b
cerebral palsy. *See* Cerebral palsy (CP)
Duchenne muscular dystrophy and, 1740–1743, 1741b, 1741f
Guillain-Barré syndrome and, 1743–1745, 1744b
muscular dystrophies and, 1740, 1741f
spina bifida and, 1732–1738, 1733b–1734b, 1733f–1734f
spinal cord injuries and, 1748–1750, 1749f
spinal muscular atrophy and, 1738–1740, 1739b
tetanus and, 1745–1746, 1745b
Neuromuscular system
gestational maturity of, 649f–650f
neonatal adaptations, 621
Neuropathy, chemotherapy-related, 1524
Neutral thermal environment (NTE), 710–711
Nevus flammeus, 619
New Ballard scale for newborn maturity rating, 649f–650f
Newborns. *See also* Infants
behaviours affecting attachment, 557t
biorhythmicity in, 561
breastfeeding assessment for, 683
congenital anomalies in. *See* Congenital anomalies
conjugation of bilirubin in, 652–655
constipation and, 1400
death of. *See* Death, of newborn
discharge planning and. *See* Neonatal discharge planning
effects of epidural block on, 416
entrainment in, 561
high-risk. *See* Newborns at risk
HIV testing of, 218b
hyperbilirubinemia and, 652–654, 653t
parent education regarding, 663
phototherapy for, 661–663, 662f
hypocalcemia in, 655
hypoglycemia and, 654–655
immediate assessment/care of, 481–483
infections and. *See* Neonatal infections
mortality rates, 7b
nursing care of
airway maintenance, 644–646, 645f
from birth through first 2 hours, 642–647
body temperature maintenance, 646
circumcision, 663–667, 664f–665f
classification by gestational age, 648–651
eye prophylaxis, 646–647, 646f, 647b
gestational age assessment, 648, 649f–650f, 650b
hyperbilirubinemia therapy, 661–663
initial physical assessment, 643–644, 643b
intramuscular injections, 661, 662f
laboratory/diagnostic tests, 644, 655b
nursing process, 645b
physical assessment guidelines, 648b
supporting parents in, 660
vitamin K prophylaxis, 647, 647b
nutrition for. *See* Infants, nutrition for
pain assessment in, 938, 938b, 939t
pain management for
alternative therapies for, 942–943
nonpharmacological methods, 940–942, 941b, 942f
pharmacological methods, 943–955
Newborns *(Continued)*
parent-family relationship to, 485
parent-infant interactions, 566–567
physical injuries, 651–652, 651f
physiological jaundice in, 652–654, 652f
reciprocity/synchrony/habituation in, 561–562
reflexes of, 621, 622t–625t
screening of
atraumatic care for, 658b
heel punctures for, 655–659, 657f
for IEMs, 778–779
protective environment for, 659–660
summary of, 656t
urine samples for, 657–659, 659f
venipuncture for, 657
sepsis and. *See* Neonatal sepsis
transition process. *See* Neonatal transition to extrauterine life
Newborns at risk
birth trauma, 743–746
cardiovascular anomalies, 770
CNS anomalies, 768–770
drug-exposed. *See* Substance use, during pregnancy
gastrointestinal system anomalies, 772–775
genetic disorders, 778–779
genitourinary system anomalies, 776–780
gestational age-related problems. *See* Gestational age-related problems
hemolytic disorders, 765–768
infection. *See* Neonatal infections
musculoskeletal system anomalies, 775–776
neonatal abstinence syndrome, 762–765, 762t, 763f
respiratory system anomalies, 770–771
Niacin (nicotinic acid, nicotinamide), 1376t–1379t
Nifedipine
breastfeeding and, 1753t–1756t
for suppression of uterine activity, 495–496, 496b
Nightmares, preschoolers and, 1060
Nighttime fears, 982t
Nighttime feeding, 982t
90-degree–90-degree traction, 1696, 1696f
Nipissing District Developmental Screen (NDDS), 929–931, 931b, 1056
Nipple shields, 697
Nipples
breastfeeding and
preparation for, 223, 223f–224f
soreness due to, 697
discharge from, 113
Nipple-stimulated contraction test, 288–289
Nissen fundoplication, 1404–1405, 1405f
Nitrazine test for pH, 446, 447b
Nitroglycerin
for suppression of uterine activity, 496, 496b
for tachysystole, 439
Nitrous oxide
for analgesia, 416, 948b–949b, 1675
chemical burns from, 1343
Nits, 1659–1661, 1659b, 1659f
Nodules, 1644f
Noise levels in neonatal intensive care units, 722, 722f
Nonadherent retained placenta, 579
Nonautomotive vehicle injuries, 1132
Nonbilious vomiting, 1403
Nonbreastfeeding mothers, 530
Non-Communicating Children's Pain Checklist, 939
Noncommunicating hydrocephalus, 1605
Non-English-speaking women in labour, 450
Nonfamilial trisomy, 1195
Non-Hodgkin's lymphoma (NHL), 1526
Non-hypertrophic cardiomyopathy (non-HCM), 736–737
Noninfectious irritants, pulmonary dysfunction caused by
acute respiratory distress syndrome/acute lung injury, 1342–1343
aspiration pneumonia, 1341–1342
foreign body aspiration, 1341
smoke inhalation injury, 1343–1344
tobacco smoke exposure, 1344
Non-nutritive sucking, 670
gavage feeding and, 1308
infants and, 976–977
during painful procedures, 942, 942f
for preterm infants, 721, 721f
Nonopioids for pediatric pain management, 943, 944t
Nonpharmacological pain management
after childbirth, 541b, 543
during childbirth/labour
acupressure/acupuncture, 406, 406f
application of heat/cold, 406
aromatherapy, 406–407
biofeedback, 406
comfort strategies, 400b, 402–407
conscious breathing, 403, 403f, 404b
effleurage/counterpressure, 403
energy work, 403
hypnosis, 406
imagery/visualization, 402–403
intradermal sterile water block, 407
music, 403
nursing care in, 405b
overview, 398–400
position changes, 407
relaxation, 402, 402f
touch/massage, 403

Nonpharmacological pain management *(Continued)*
transcutaneous electrical nerve stimulation, 405, 405f
water therapy, 403–405, 404f
for infants, 940–942, 941b, 942f
Nonshivering thermogenesis, 612
Nonsmoking strategies, 1145–1146, 1146b
Nonsteroidal anti-inflammatory drugs (NSAIDs)
for asthma, 1349
for children, 943, 944t
for dysmenorrhea, 86, 87t, 1134
for juvenile idiopathic arthritis, 1717
Nonstress test (NST), 286–288, 287f–288f, 288t
Nontunneled catheters, 1294
Nonverbal communication
with children, 876, 878
cognitively impaired children and, 1193–1194
culturally sensitive, 834b
Normal birth process, promotion of, 3b, 10–11
Normal discomforts of pregnancy, 230, 231t–233t
Normalization
for cystic fibrosis patients, 1362–1363
for special needs children, 1158–1159, 1169b, 1217
Noroviruses, 1393t–1395t
North American culture, family life and, 829–831
Nortriptyline, 946t
Nose
of children
administration of medications to, 1296–1297, 1297f
external structures of, 915–916, 916f
internal structures of, 916
nutritional status and, 887t–889t
of newborns, 643b
assessment of, 626t–636t
Nosebleeding, 1517
Not permitted to take fluids by mouth (NPO), 1298–1299
Nubain
breastfeeding and, 1753t–1756t
for labour pain management, 409b
Nuchal cord, 173, 476, 482b–483b
Nuchal translucency (NT) screening, 278, 278f
Nuclear brain scan, 1567t–1568t
Nuclear family, 17, 17f
Nulligravidous women, definition of, 186
Nulliparous women
defined, 186
prenatal care for, 238–240
Numeric Scale for pain assessment, 937t
Nunavik Adaptive Behaviour Scale, 1190
Nurse-activated analgesia, 948b–949b
Nursemaids' elbow, 1689
Nursing
pediatric. *See* Pediatric nursing
perinatal. *See* Perinatal nursing
relevance of genetics and, 158–159, 159b
safety in home visits, 40
vulnerable populations and, 35
Nursing caries, 1036–1037, 1037f
Nutrition
burn injuries and, 1674–1675, 1679
deficiencies in, 49
eating disorders and, 50, 50b
for inflammatory bowel disease, 1412–1413
maternal
cultural perspectives, 238
education in, 222, 267
during lactation, 270–271
for mild pre-eclampsia, 303, 303b
nutrient intake during labour, 457–460, 458t
nutrient needs before conception, 250
nutrient needs during pregnancy, 251–270
obstetrical/gynecological effects on, 263
postpartum care and, 545, 547f
obesity and, 49–50, 49t, 50b
pediatric
adolescents and, 1125–1127
in childhood, 788
congenital heart disease and, 1478
congestive heart failure and, 1473
infants and. *See* Infants, nutrition for
influence on development, 859–861, 861b
leukemia and, 1521
preschoolers and, 1059–1060
in respiratory infections, 1320
school-age children and, 1096
toddlers and, 1032–1034, 1033b
for type 1 diabetes, 1631–1632, 1635
for unconscious child, 1571–1572
for preterm infants
advancing feedings, 721
elimination and, 719
factors involved in, 718
gastrostomy feeding, 721
gavage feeding, 719–721, 720b, 720f
hydration and, 719
non-nutritive sucking and, 721, 721f
oral feeding for, 719
types of, 718–719
Nutrition therapy for anorexia nervosa/bulimia nervosa, 1143
Nutritional assessment
pediatric
clinical examination in, 887–890, 887t–889t
dietary intake in, 886–887, 886b
evaluation of, 890
Nutritional assessment *(Continued)*
during pregnancy, 215
of preterm infants, 711
Nutritional counselling
for adolescent obesity, 1139–1140
for toddlers, 1032–1033
Nutritional disturbances
complementary and alternative medicine and, 1375
food sensitivity and, 1384–1389
mineral imbalances and, 1375–1380, 1381t–1383t
protein-energy malnutrition and, 1384
vegetarian diets and, 1380
vitamin imbalances, 1374–1375, 1376t–1379t

O

Obesity
adolescents and, 1126, 1126f
children and, 788–789, 789f
health risks of, 49–50, 49t, 50b
maternal
anaesthesia and, 420–421
antepartum risks, 370
intrapartum/postpartum risks, 370
nursing care for, 370–371
pregnancy and, 255–256
Object permanence
in sensorimotor development, 964, 964f
toddlers and, 1024
Oblique fracture line, 1690
Obstetrical emergencies
amniotic fluid embolism, 523–524
prolapsed umbilical cord, 521–522, 521f–522f, 523b
rupture of uterus, 522–523
shoulder dystocia, 520–521, 520f
Obstetrical history, 213
Obstipation, 1399–1400
Obstructive sleep apnea syndrome (OSAS), 1364
Obstructive sleep-disordered breathing, 1364
Obstructive uropathy, 1545, 1545f
Obtundation, 1564b
Occiput posterior position of fetus
dystocia and, 499–500
maternal positions for, 461, 463b
Occupational history, 215
Occupational therapy for juvenile idiopathic arthritis, 1717
Ocular alignment testing, 909–910, 909f–910f
Oculovestibular response, 1566
Odour, parent-infant bonding and, 561
Older fathers, 569
Older mothers
childbirth risks for, 47
multiple pregnancies and, 8
perinatal health and, 8
prenatal care for, 238–240
in transition to parenthood, 568–569, 568b
Older women, vulnerability of, 34
Oligoarthritis, 1716
Oligohydramnios, 173, 276b
Oligomenorrhea, 91
Oliguria, 1553–1555, 1554b
Omalizumab, 1350
Omphalocele, 773–774, 774f
Omphalomesenteric fistula, 1409–1410
Onlooker play, 857
On-the-body hearing aids, 1200, 1200f
Oogenesis, 168, 170f
Open bone fractures, 1690–1691
Open skull fractures, 1576
Operculum, 192, 193f
Ophthalmia neonatorum, 646–647, 647b
Ophthalmoscopic examination, 908–912
Opiates, childbirth risks and, 48
Opioid agonist analgesics, 408–409, 408b
Opioid agonist-antagonist analgesics
abstinence symptoms and, 409b
for labour pain management, 409, 409b
Opioid antagonists, 409–410, 410b
Opioids
adolescent use of, 1147
for children, 943–944
adverse effects of, 951b
dosages for, 945t
end-of-life care and, 1180–1181
for leukemia, 1519
for sickle cell anemia, 1507–1509, 1509b
fear of addiction to, 940b, 953
respiratory depression and, 951–952, 953b
Optic administration of medications, 1296–1297
Oral administration of medications, 1288–1289, 1288b, 1289f
Oral allergy syndrome, 1386
Oral contraceptive pills (OCPs)
breakthrough bleeding and, 91–92
combined estrogen-progestin, 147–148, 148b, 149f
for dysmenorrhea, 86
progestin-only, 148–150
Oral feeding for preterm infants, 719
Oral hygiene
during hospitalization, 1271–1272
toddlers and, 1035–1036, 1035f
Oral intake during labour, 457, 458t
Oral rehydration therapy (ORT), 1396
Oral route of drug administration, 948b–949b
Oral sites for temperature measurement, 897–901, 899t, 900b–901b
Oral stage of psychosexual development, 851
Oral stimulation of clitoris, 235
Oral ulcers, chemotherapy-related, 1523–1524

Ordinal position of children, 811–812, 811b
Organ donation, 1182–1183
Organ systems, development of, 848
Organic hearing loss, 1199
Organic heart murmur, 922
Organizational strategies for treatment compliance, 1269–1270, 1269b
Orogastric route
for gavage feedings, 719–721, 720f, 1308–1309, 1310f, 1311b
for medication administration, 1295–1296, 1296b
Orthodontic appliances (braces), 1127
Orthopedic management for spina bifida, 1735
Orthostatic hypotension (OH), 904–905
Oscillometry, 901–904, 902t, 904t
Oseltamivir, 1325
Osmolality, 1764t–1771t
Osmotic diuretics for ICP, 1570, 1572
Osteochondritis, 1285–1286
Osteochondritis deformans juvenilis, 1705–1706, 1705b
Osteogenesis imperfecta (OI), 1704–1705, 1704b
Osteomyelitis, 1710–1712, 1711b
Osteosarcoma, 1713–1714
Ostomies, 1312–1313
Otic administration of medications, 1296–1297
Otitis media (OM), 1325–1328, 1326b–1327b
Otitis media with effusion (OME), 1325–1328, 1326b
Otoscopic examination of ears, pediatric, 915
Ottawa Charter, 3
Oucher Pain Scale, 937t, 939
Outcomes
in abruptio placentae, 327
of childbirth education, 247, 402
in placenta previa, 323–324
Outlet contracture of pelvis, 499
Outlet forceps-assisted birth, 511, 511f
Outpatient setting, 1253
Ovaries, 65, 66f
Overprotection, special needs child and, 1163, 1163b
Overuse syndromes, sports and, 1103–1104
Overweight, definition of, 1136
Ovulation
breastfeeding and, 695
after childbirth, 529
cycle of, 82, 83f
in menstrual cycle, 65, 82–84, 83f
predictor tests, 140–141, 142f
Ovum, 168, 170f
Oxalates, 1380
Oximetry, pulse, 1303–1304, 1303f
Oxycodone
breastfeeding and, 1753t–1756t
for children, 945t, 947t
Oxygen hood, 715, 715f
Oxygen saturation of blood
development of ROP and, 732
fetal, 177–178, 177f
normal test ranges for, 1764t–1771t
Oxygen supply for newborns, 610, 646
Oxygen therapy
pediatric, 1302–1303, 1302f
congestive heart failure and, 1469
monitoring, 1303–1304, 1303f
for preterm infants, 714–718
Oxygen-induced carbon dioxide narcosis, 1303
Oxytocin
indications/contraindications for, 509b
for inducing/augmenting labour, 509–511, 509f
milk production and, 681
postpartum contractions and, 526–527
for postpartum hemorrhage, 583b
protocol for administration of, 510b
Oxytocin-stimulated contraction test, 289

P

Paced breathing. *See* Conscious breathing
Pacemakers, pediatric, 1486, 1486b
Pacific Islanders
breast cancer and, 116f
as visible minority, 829, 830b
Pacifiers
aspiration of, 995–996
infants and, 976–977
non-nutritive sucking and, 670, 670f
recommendations regarding, 687–690
SIDS and, 1009–1010
Pain
developmental changes in response to, 935b
during labour/birth
anxiety/fear and, 396–397, 397f
assessment of coping with, 398, 399f
comfort measures for. *See* Comfort measures, for labour pain
culture and, 396, 396b
distribution of, 395f
environment and, 398
expression of, 395
gate-control theory of, 397
neurological origins, 394–395
perception of, 395
physiological factors in, 396
previous experience with, 397
sociocultural basis of, 447–448, 448t
supportive care for, 398
Pain assessment
in children
behavioural measures for, 934, 935f, 936t
with chronic illness/complex pain, 939–940
with communication/cognitive impairment, 939
cultural factors in, 939
guidelines for, 880b
multidimensional measures for, 936
physiological measures for, 934–935
self-report measures for, 935–936, 937t
in neonates, 938, 938b, 939t
Pain Indicator for Communicatively Impaired Children (PICIC), 939
Pain management
burns injuries and, 1678
for juvenile idiopathic arthritis, 1718
during labour/birth
education in, 246
nonpharmacologic, 398–407, 400b
pharmacologic, 407–421, 408b
pediatric
CAM therapies for, 942–943
for circumcision, 664–665, 666b
for complications of HIV disease, 1529–1530
after heart surgery, 1481
for leukemia, 1519
nonpharmacologic, 939–940, 941b
pharmacologic. *See* Pharmacological pain management, pediatric
for sickle cell anemia, 1507–1509, 1509b
for terminally ill child, 1179–1181, 1180b
for unconscious child, 1569
Palatine tonsils, 1322, 1323f
Palivizumab, 1334
Palliative care
defined, 1174
principles of, 1174–1175
Palmar erythema, 199, 200b
Palpation
of abdomen, 923–924, 924f
Wilms' tumour and, 1552b, 1553
in cardiac assessment, 1452
rectovaginal, 78–79, 79f
Pan-Canadian Health Information Privacy and Confidentiality Framework, 870
Pancreas
cystic fibrosis and, 1356–1357, 1357f
hormone secretion disorders and. *See* Diabetes mellitus (DM)
Pandemic H1N1 influenza virus, 1324–1325
Papanicolaou (Pap) test
function of, 77
procedure, 78b, 78f
Papilledema, 1566
Papules, 1644f
Parachute reflex, 961–962, 962f
Parallel play, 857, 857f, 1028
Paraplegia, 1748
Parasomnias, 981–982
Parasuicide, 1149
Parathyroid disorders
hyperparathyroidism, 1621–1622, 1621b
hypoparathyroidism, 1620–1621, 1620b
Parent education. *See also* Education; Patient/family teaching
on cardiopulmonary resuscitation, 727–728
on formula-feeding, 700–704
on hyperbilirubinemia, 663
on infant care, 559t
Parental attachment. *See* Attachment
Parental characteristics, child abuse and, 1073
Parental decision making, end-of-life care and, 1175
Parental empowerment, 1162
Parental grief. *See also* Grief
acute distress, 600
after death of child, 1183
intense grief, 600–601
overview, 599–600
reorganization, 601–602, 601b
Parent-child relationships, hospitalization and, 1249
Parenteral feeding of preterm infants, 718
Parenteral fluid therapy
complications in, 1301f
infusion pumps and, 1300
safety catheters/needleless systems, 1300, 1300f
securing peripheral IV line, 1300–1301, 1301f
site/equipment for, 1299–1300, 1299f
Parenteral nutrition (PN), short-bowel syndrome and, 1435
Parenthood
adaptation to, 549
adopted children and, 817–819
behaviours, 814
cultural factors in, 569–570
divorce and, 819–821, 820b
in dual-earner families, 821–822
features of, 562–563
hospitalized children and, 1251–1252
infant-parent adjustment, 566–567
limit setting/discipline, 814–817
lone, 821
maternal age and, 567–569
maternal identity establishment, 563–564, 563t
motivation/preparation for, 813
multiple births and, 812–813
newborns and, 660
nursing care for, 574–575, 574b–575b
paternal age and, 567–569
paternal identity establishment, 565–566, 565f–566f, 565t

Parenthood *(Continued)*
personal aspirations and, 570
preterm infants and, 711–713, 712f
supportive care for, 726–727, 727f
in reconstituted families, 821
resuming sexual intimacy, 564
roles of, 809
for same-sex couples, 564–565, 821
social support during, 569
socioeconomic conditions and, 570
special needs child and, 1159–1160, 1160b
overprotection and, 1163, 1163b
supportive care for, 1167–1168, 1168b
tasks/responsibilities of, 563
transition to, 813–814, 813f–814f
visual impairment and, 570–571
Parent-infant relationship
communication and, 560–562
contact and, 558–560, 560f
Parent-professional relationship, 1224
Parents
communicating with, 871–873
helping children in school, 1094, 1094b
loss of child. *See* Parental grief
overprotection by, 1163b
permissive, 814
Parents Anonymous, 1149
Parent-to-parent support, special needs child and, 1168
Parity, 186–187
Parovirus B19 in newborns, 754–755
Paroxysmal abdominal pain, 1003–1005
Partial placenta previa, 321–322
Partial seizures, 1593–1594, 1594b–1595b, 1596t
Partial thromboplastin time (PTT), 1764t–1771t
Partially sighted, 1203–1204
Partial-thickness (second-degree) burns, 1670–1671, 1671f
Passageway (birth canal)
bony pelvis, 380–383, 382f
soft tissues, 383–385
Passenger, labour process and. *See* Fetus, labour process and
Patch, 1644f
Patellar reflex test, 929f
Patent ductus arteriosus (PDA)
in children, 1457b–1459b
during pregnancy, 353–354
in preterm infants, 731
Paternal adaptations
acceptance, 209
identifying with father role, 209
postpartum role adjustment, 565–566, 565f–566f, 565t
preparing for childbirth, 209–210
relationship with fetus, 209, 210b
reordering relationships, 209
styles of, 208b
Paternal role, special needs child and, 1160
Patient safety, risk management and, 11, 12b
Patient-controlled analgesia (PCA), 944–947, 948b–949b, 950f, 950t
Patient/family teaching
administering medications, 1297–1298, 1298b
administration of digoxin, 1472b
allergy-proofing environment, 1348b
alternative feeding techniques, 1312
animal safety, 1663b
cardiac surgery, 1481, 1481b
care after cardiac catheterization, 1454b
care of casts, 1694b
child with head injury and, 1579b
for child with pacemaker, 1486b
congenital heart disease, 1477–1478, 1477b
controlling diaper rash, 1665b
controlling fever, 1275b
controlling lactose intolerance symptoms, 1389b
coping with postpartum blues, 550b
decision for hematopoietic stem cell transplant, 1533b
decreasing exposure to tobacco smoke, 1345b
diabetes and, 1635b
eliminating cimicidae, 1661b
induction of labour with oxytocin, 510b
infant with HIV infection, 1529b
for intermittent ausculation/EFM, 437f, 438b
for ostomies, 1312
pediculosis treatment, 1660b
on pushing/positioning in labour, 439–440
self-care/hygiene and, 1274
sickle cell anemia and, 1509
unconscious child and, 1574b
using peak expiratory flow meter, 1354b
vitamin D toxicity and, 1621b
Pauciarticular arthritis, 1716
Peak expiratory flow meter (PEFM), 1347, 1352–1355, 1354b
Peak expiratory flow rate (PEFR), 1347, 1347b
Pearson attachment, 1696, 1696f
Peau d'orange skin changes, breast cancer and, 116
Pediatric developmental assessment, 928–931
Pediatric health history
features of, 73–74
history section in, 879
identifying information for, 876
outline of, 879b
present illness, 879
primary health issue, 876–878
Pediatric home care nurse, 1221–1222, 1222b
Pediatric nursing
art of, 793–794
atraumatic care in, 794
Pediatric nursing *(Continued)*
childhood health problems, 788–792
critical thinking/nursing process in, 796–798
dental care and, 788
determinants of health and, 786–787, 787t
functions of, 794–796
future trends in, 798
health promotion in, 787
immunizations and, 788
nutrition in, 788
Pediatric Pain Questionnaire (PPQ), 936
Pediatric physical examinations. *See* Physical assessment, pediatric
Pediatric procedures
alternative feeding techniques
family teaching for, 1312
gastrostomy feeding in, 1309–1310, 1310f
gavage feeding in, 1308–1309, 1310f, 1311b
nasoduodenal/nasojejunal tubes in, 1310–1312
total parenteral nutrition in, 1312
artificial ventilation, 1304–1308
bronchial drainage, 1304
compliance with treatment plan, 1269–1270, 1269b
informed consent for, 1259–1260
inhalation therapy, 1302–1304, 1302f
measuring intake and output, 1298–1299
parenteral fluid therapy
complications in, 1301f
infusion pumps and, 1300
safety catheters/needleless systems, 1300, 1300f
securing peripheral IV line, 1300–1301, 1301f
site/equipment for, 1299–1300, 1299f
performance of, 1264
positioning for, 1281–1282
postprocedural support for, 1264
psychological preparation for, 1260–1264, 1261b–1263b
related to elimination
enemas, 1312
ostomies, 1312–1313
specimen collection in
blood, 1285–1286
respiratory secretion, 1286
stool, 1285
urine, 1282, 1282f, 1284t
surgical
postoperative care for, 1267–1269, 1268t
preoperative care for, 1265–1267, 1265f, 1267b
use of play in, 1265, 1266b
Pediatric trauma rehabilitation, 1581
Pediculosis capitis, 1659–1661, 1659b–1660b, 1659f
Peer groups
adolescents and, 1120–1122, 1120f
Peer groups *(Continued)*
as influencing factor, 829
school-age children and, 1089–1092
special needs children and, 1173
Pelvic cavity, 380–383, 382f–383f
Pelvic dystocia, 499
Pelvic examination
collection of specimens, 77
external, 75–76, 76f
after hysterectomy, 79
internal, 76, 77f
overview, 75, 75b, 76f
for physically disabled women, 71, 71f
during pregnancy, 216
vaginal wall examination, 77–79
Pelvic floor
changes in, 192, 193f
in labour process, 385
regaining muscular support, 528
Pelvic hematomas, 579
Pelvic inflammatory disease (PID), 100–101
Pelvic inlet, 380–383, 382f–383f
Pelvic outlet, 380–383, 382f–383f
Pelvic rock, 546f
Pelvis, bony. *See* Bony pelvis
Penetrating injuries to eye, 1206b
Penicillin
acute streptococcal pharyngitis and, 1322
sickle cell anemia and, 1508b
Penile anomalies, 776–780, 777f, 1546t
Penile growth, 1114–1115
Peptic ulcers
in children, 1414–1416, 1415b
pregnancy and, 202
Perceptive hearing loss, 1199
Percutaneous umbilical blood sampling (PUBS)
fetal rights and, 285b
monitoring pregnancy risk factors, 284, 284f
ultrasound adjunct to, 285b
Perimenopause
features of, 84, 94
seeking health care for, 44
Perimortem Caesarean birth, 335
Perinatal asphyxia
in infants of diabetic mothers, 736
in SGA/IUGR infants, 734
Perinatal education, 243–247
Perinatal health indicators, 7–8, 7b
Perinatal loss and grief. *See* Death, of newborn
Perinatal mortality rates, 7b
Perinatal nursing
care provider options, 241–247
choices, 241–247
collaborative woman/family-centred, 6–7
continuum of care, home care in, 35f
cultural competence in, 22–27
current issues in, 10–13
ethical issues in, 13
functions of, 2–3
future goals of, 14, 14b
research in, 13–14
specialization/evidence-informed practice in, 9–10
values/guiding principles for, 2, 3b

Perinatal transmission of HIV, 1527
Perinatally acquired infections
  bacterial, 755–756
  cytomegalovirus infection, 753–754, 753f
  fungal, 756
  gonorrhea, 750
  hepatitis B virus, 751–752
  herpes simplex virus, 754, 754f
  human immunodeficiency virus, 752–753
  overview, 749–756, 749b
  parvovirus B19, 754–755
  rubella, 753
  syphilis, 750–751, 751f
  toxoplasmosis, 749–750
  varicella zoster, 751
Perineum, 64, 64f
  lacerations during birth process, 477, 477f
  postpartum changes in, 528
  trauma, birth process and, 476–478
Periodic breathing, 710
Periodontal disease
  preterm labour and, 490
  school-age children and, 1099
Peripartum cardiomyopathy (PPCM), 355–356
Peripheral blood stem cells (PBSCs), 1533–1534
Peripheral intermittent infusion device, 1293–1294
Peripheral intravenous (PIV) access
  buffered lidocaine during, 952b
  removing, 1301
  securing, 1300–1301, 1301f
Peripheral nervous system injuries, birth process and, 744–746
Peripheral precocious puberty (PPP), 1614, 1614b
Peripheral stem cell transplants (PSCTs), 1533
Peripheral vision testing, 912
Peripherally inserted central catheters (PICCs), 1294, 1359–1360
Peritoneal dialysis, 1559–1560
Periventricular-intraventricular hemorrhage (PV-IVH), 731
Perlocutionary stage of communicative development, 874, 874b
Permanency planning, special needs children and, 1218
Permanent teeth, 1098, 1098f
Permissive parenting, 814
Persistent cloaca, 1432
Persistent pulmonary hypertension of the newborn (PPHN), 733–734
Persistent urinary tract infection, 1541–1542
Persistent vegetative state (PVS), 1564b
Personal aspirations, parenthood and, 570
Personal Health Information Protection Act, 1260
Personal music players, hearing loss and, 1128
Personal protective equipment, 109t
Personal safety behaviours, 40
Personal space, cultural traditions and, 24
Personality development, theories of, 850–852, 851t
Personal-social behaviour
  preschoolers and, 1054, 1054f
  toddlers and, 1027–1028
Pertussis, 1337–1341
  incidence of, 1063
  symptoms/management of, 1064t–1070t, 1337–1341
Pertussis vaccine, 985
  contraindications/precautions for, 989t–991t
Pessaries, 592–593, 592f
Petechiae, 1643
pH, normal test ranges for, 1764t–1771t
Phallic stage of psychosexual development, 851
Pharmacological pain management
  after childbirth, 543–544
  during labour/birth
    analgesia/anaesthesia, 407–416
    nursing care for, 416–421, 417b
    sedatives, 407
    by stage/method, 408b
  pediatric
    coanalgesics, 943, 946t
    epidural analgesia, 947–950
    equianalgesia in, 947t
    evaluation of regimen, 953–955
    after heart surgery, 1481
    monitoring adverse effects in, 951–953, 951b
    nonopioids/NSAIDS, 943, 944t
    opioids, 943–944, 945t
    patient-controlled analgesia, 944–947, 950t
    routes/methods of administration, 948b–949b
    timing of analgesia, 951
    transmucosal/transdermal analgesia, 950–951
Pharmacotherapy. *See* Drug therapy
Pharyngeal tonsils, 1322, 1323f
Pharyngitis, 1320–1321, 1320b–1321b
  acute streptococcal, 1321–1322, 1322f
Phencyclidine (PCP)
  breastfeeding and, 1753t–1756t
  childbirth risks with, 49
  prenatal exposure to, 761
Phenobarbital
  breastfeeding and, 1753t–1756t
  for epilepsy, 1600b
  prenatal exposure to, 762
Phenotype, definition of, 163
Phenylalanine, 1764t–1771t
Phenylalanine deficiency, 778
Phenylketonuria (PKU), 778
Phenytoin
  breastfeeding and, 1753t–1756t
  for epilepsy, 1597b, 1600b
  laboratory tests for, 1269
Pheochromocytoma, 1625–1626
Phocomelia, 1703
Phosphorus
  nutritional significance of, 1381t–1383t
  reduction of in CRF, 1557
Phototherapy, hyperbilirubinemia and, 662–663, 662f, 663b
Phrenic nerve paralysis, birth process and, 746
Phylloquinone. *See* Vitamin K
Physeal injuries, 1690
Physical abuse
  of children
    clinical manifestations of, 1077b–1078b
    defined, 1072–1073
    history/interview in, 1076
    Munchausen syndrome by proxy, 1072–1073
    physical assessment in, 1076–1078
    predisposing factors, 1073
  of women. *See* Abuse, of women; Intimate partner violence (IPV)
Physical assessment
  maternal
    initial, 216–241
    nutrition assessment and, 265–267, 266t
    throughout prenatal period, 219, 219f
  of neonates, 625–637, 626t–636t
  pediatric
    age-specific approaches to, 892t
    cerebral dysfunction and, 1562–1563
    of genitalia, 924–926
    growth measurements in, 893–897, 896f
    guidelines for, 891b
    of head/neck, 907
    of heart, 920–922
    immunizations, 894f–895f
    of lungs, 919–920
    of lymph nodes, 906–907, 907f
    of mouth/throat, 916–917
    of neurological system, 928
    of nose, 915–916
    physiological measurements in, 897–905
    preparing child for, 890–892, 893f
    sequence for, 890
    of skin/accessory structures, 905–906, 906t
  for women
    overview, 74–75
    pelvic examination, 75–77, 75b, 216
    vaginal wall examination, 77–79, 79f
Physical characteristics, ethnicity and, 831
Physical dependence
  defined, 940b
  opiates and, 952–953
Physical fitness. *See* Exercise
Physical restraints, 1279
Physical restriction, hospitalization and, 1243–1244
Physical stressors in pediatric/neonatal CCU admission, 1256b
Physically disabled women, health assessments for, 71, 71f
Physician-health care team decision making, end-of-life care and, 1175
Physicians, perinatal care and, 241
Physiological adaptations
  to labour, 391–392
  of newborn. *See* Neonatal transition to extrauterine life
  postpartum
    abdomen and, 528–529, 529f
    breasts and, 530
    cardiovascular system and, 530–531, 532t
    cervix and, 528
    endocrine system and, 529
    gastrointestinal system and, 530
    integumentary system and, 532
    musculoskeletal system and, 532
    neurological system and, 531–532
    urinary system and, 529–530
    uterus and, 526–528, 527f, 528b
    vagina/perineum and, 528
  to pregnancy
    breasts, 192–193
    cardiovascular system, 193–195, 194f, 197t
    endocrine system, 203, 203t
    gastrointestinal system, 201–202
    integumentary system, 199–200
    musculoskeletal system, 200, 201f
    neurological system, 200–201
    normal, 298b
    in relation to trauma, 332, 333t
    renal system, 198–199, 199t
    respiratory system, 195–198
    signs of, 188, 189t
    uterus, 188–191
    vagina/vulva, 191–192
Physiological anorexia, 1032
Physiological changes in puberty, 1117
Physiological effects of immobilization, 1684–1686, 1685t
Physiotherapy
  for cerebral palsy, 1728
  for juvenile idiopathic arthritis, 1717
Piaget's stages of cognitive development, 852–853
  adolescents and, 1119
  infants and, 964–965
  preschoolers and, 1052–1053
  school-age children and, 1087–1088
  toddlers and, 1024–1026
Pica
  during pregnancy, 201–202, 215
  risks of, 262–263, 263f
Piercing, body, 1128
Pigeon bottle, 1423, 1423f

Pigeon toe, 927
Pinard stethoscope
for fetal heart rate, 220, 221f
for IA of fetal heart, 425
Pincer grasp, 960, 960f
Pinch test for inverted nipples, 223, 223f
Pinocytosis, 175
Pinworms, 1407–1408, 1407b
Pituitary dysfunction
diabetes insipidus and, 1615–1616
hypopituitarism and, 1611–1613, 1612b
pituitary hyperfunction and, 1613–1614
precocious puberty and, 1614–1615, 1614b
syndrome of inappropriate antidiuretic hormone secretion and, 1616
in unconscious child, 1572
Pituitary hormones after childbirth, 529
Placenta
endometrial regeneration at site, 527
examination of expelled, 481f
functions of, 174–176
retained, causing PPH, 579
structure, 174, 174f–175f
Placenta accreta, 328
Placenta increta, 328
Placenta previa
clinical manifestations of, 323, 324t
incidence/etiology of, 323
maternal/fetal outcomes, 323–324
in multifetal pregnancy, 240
nursing care for, 324, 325b
types of, 321–322, 323f
Placental abruption, 326–328, 326f
Placental hormones, postpartum changes in, 529
Placental position, ultrasound assessment of, 281
Placental separation
nursing care after, 481
in third stage of labour, 480–481, 480f
Plantar grasp reflex in newborns, 621f, 622t–625t
Plants, poisonous/nonpoisonous, 1436b–1438b
Plaque, 1644f
removal of, 1035–1036
Plasma volume, 1764t–1771t
Plaster casts, 1693
Plastic bags, suffocation and, 996
Plastic deformation fractures, 1691b, 1691f
Platelet count
laboratory tests for, 1764t–1771t
in neonates, 611
Platypelloid pelvis, 383, 384t
Play
classification of, 856
cognitively impaired children and, 1192–1193, 1192f
content of, 856–857
functions of, 858
hospitalized children and, 1246–1249, 1247b, 1247f
Play *(Continued)*
during infancy, 968, 969t
after pediatric procedures, 1265, 1266b
preschoolers and, 1054–1055
school-age children and, 1092
in sensorimotor development, 965
social character of, 857–858
toddlers and, 1028, 1028f
toy selection for, 858–859
visually impaired children and, 1207
Play therapy, 1248
Playground injuries, 1044
Plexus injury, birth process and, 744–745
Plugged milk ducts, breastfeeding and, 698
Pneumococcal conjugate vaccine (PCV), 986–987
contraindications/precautions for, 989t–991t
for otitis media, 1327
Pneumocystis carinii pneumonia (PCP), 1528
Pneumonias
bacterial, 1336
lower respiratory infections, 1335–1336
nursing care for, 1336–1337, 1337f
primary atypical, 1336
signs of, 1335b
types of, 1335
viral, 1335–1336
Poison ivy, oak, and sumac, 1655–1657, 1656f
Poisoning
assessment of, 1439
children and, 789–790, 790f
common injurious agents, 1435–1436
emergency treatment for, 1436–1440, 1437b–1439b
gastric decontamination, 1439–1440
gastric lavage for, 1440, 1441b
heavy metal, 1440–1441
in infants, 998–999
lead, 1441–1445, 1442b, 1443f
poisonous/nonpoisonous plants and, 1436b–1438b
prevention of, 1440, 1442b
school-age children and, 1102t
toddlers and, 1043–1044, 1044f
Poker Chip Tool for pain assessment, 937t
Poliomyelitis, 1064t–1070t
Poliovirus vaccine, 985
contraindications/precautions for, 989t–991t
Polyarthritis rheumatoid factor negative, 1716
Polyarthritis rheumatoid factor positive, 1716
Polycystic ovarian syndrome (PCOS), 132
Polycythemia, 1474
delayed cord clamping and, 611
in infants of diabetic mothers, 737
Polydactyly, 776
Polyhydramnios, 173
risk factors for, 276b
Polyploidy, 163–164
Polysomnography, 1364
Populations
definition of, 801
vulnerable, 28–29, 32–35
Position, fetal, 379–380, 380f–381f
Positional clubfoot, 1702
Positional plagiocephaly, 1011–1012, 1012f
Positioning
for burping infants, 702f
maternal
for breastfeeding, 684–685, 685f
for epidural block, 414, 414f
for labour/childbirth
changes in, 407
dystocia and, 502
overview, 386–388, 387f
range of, 460–461, 461f–462f, 462b
second stage of labour and, 471–472
throne position, 419–420, 419f
during pregnancy, 439
pediatric
for bone marrow aspiration/biopsy, 1282
for brain tumour surgery, 1585
for ear exam, 913–915, 913f–914f
for extremity venipuncture, 1280f, 1281
for femoral venipuncture, 1281, 1281f
for intramuscular injections, 1291–1292, 1293f
for lumbar puncture, 1281–1282, 1281f
for oral administration of medications, 1289, 1289f
unconscious child and, 1572–1573
Positive reinforcement, 816, 1264–1265
Positive self-talk, 941b
Positive signs of pregnancy, 188, 189t
Positron emission tomography (PET), 1567t–1568t
Postanaesthesia recovery period, 485
Postcoital test (PCT), 130
Postconventional level of moral development, 854
Postdate, definition of, 186
Postdural puncture headache (PDPH)
blood-patch therapy for, 413f
in spinal anaesthesia (block), 412–413
Postoperative care
for brain tumours, 1584–1585
in Caesarean birth, 518–519
cleft lip repair and, 1423
for cleft lip/cleft palate, 1423–1424
for EA/TEF surgery, 1426
for hydrocephalus, 1607–1608
Postoperative care *(Continued)*
myelomeningocele and, 1737
in pediatric surgery, 1267–1269, 1267b, 1268t
for pyloromyotomy, 1430
spinal surgery and, 1710
surgery for Hirschsprung disease and, 1402
Wilms' tumour and, 1553
Postpartum blues, 549–550, 550b. *See also* Postpartum mood disorder (PPMD)
Postpartum care
ambulation in, 544–545
bladder distension prevention, 543
bladder function and, 545
bowel function and, 545
breastfeeding and, 545
in Caesarean birth, 518–519
comfort strategies in, 543–544
discharge education and, 552–554
early discharge criteria and, 535–536, 535b–537b
exercise in, 545, 546f
follow-up after discharge, 553–554
for hypovolemic shock, 542b
infection prevention and, 541, 541b
maintaining uterine tone in, 542–543, 543f
maternal/family teaching checklist and, 538f
nursing care for, 536–547, 539b
nutrition in, 545, 547f
preventing excessive bleeding in, 541–542, 542f
for psychosocial needs, 548–552, 548f, 549b
rest in, 544
Rh immune globulin injection and, 547
routine checkups and, 553
rubella vaccination and, 547
signs of potential problems and, 539b
suppression of lactation and, 545–547
transfer from recovery area in, 534, 535t
for vaginal birth, 540b
Postpartum complications
coagulopathies, 584–585
hemorrhage, 577–584
infections, 586–588, 587b
psychological, 593–599
structural disorders, 588–593
thromboembolic disease, 585–586
Postpartum hemorrhage (PPH)
with contracted uterus, 580
definition/incidence of, 577–578
etiology/risk factors, 578–580, 578b
fluid/blood replacement therapy for, 584
hypotonic uterus and, 580–581
hypovolemic shock from, 581–584
with LGA babies, 8
medication guide for, 583b

Postpartum hemorrhage (PPH) *(Continued)*
  nursing care for, 580–584, 580b–582b
Postpartum mood disorder (PPMD)
  alternative therapies for, 599, 599b
  assessment of, 595b
  depression with psychotic features, 594–596
  depression without psychotic features, 594
  features of, 593, 595
  home visits and, 597–598
  medical management of, 596, 596t
  nursing care for, 596–598, 597b
  providing safety for, 598
  psychiatric hospitalization for, 598
  psychotropic medications for, 598–599
  risk factors for, 594b
Postpartum period
  Canadian Maternity Experiences Survey of, 9
  cardiac disorders during, 361–362
  cardiovascular system during, 530–531
  changes in breasts during, 530
  community-based care during, 11–12
  cultural practices regarding, 25t–26t
  in diabetic pregnancy, 349–350
  endocrine system during, 529
  gastrointestinal system during, 530
  HIV testing during, 218b
  immune system during, 532
  integumentary system during, 532
  interventions for GDM, 310
  musculoskeletal system during, 532
  neurological system during, 531–532
  reproductive system and, 526–529
  risks due to obesity, 370
  stages of maternal, 563, 563t
  urinary system during, 529–530
Postterm birth rates, 8
Postterm infants
  meconium aspiration syndrome, 733, 733f
  overview, 733
  persistent pulmonary hypertension of the newborn in, 733–734
Postterm pregnancy
  definition/incidence of, 505
  home care, 506b
  maternal/fetal risks in, 505
  nursing care for, 505–506
  risk factors for, 276b
Posttraumatic stress disorder (PTSD), school-age children and, 1108
Post-traumatic syndromes, head injuries and, 1578
Postural drainage, 1304
Posture
  adolescents and, 1128
  assessment of newborn, 626t–636t
  education in, 224, 226b, 226f
Posturing, cerebral dysfunction and, 1566, 1566f
Postvention, 1256
Potassium
  laboratory tests for, 1764t–1771t
  for maternal nutrition, 261
  nutritional significance of, 1381t–1383t
Poverty
  health care and, 44
  as health determinant, 827
Powers, birth process and
  primary, 385–386
  secondary, 386
Prandial insulin, 1631b
Preadolescence, 1085
Preadolescent atopic dermatitis, 1665–1667, 1666b
Precipitous labour, 505
Precocious puberty, 1614–1615, 1614b
Preconception care
  components of, 157, 158b
  diabetes mellitus counselling, 341, 341b
  genetic counselling in. *See* Genetics
  seeking health care for, 43
Preconceptual phase in toddlers, 1025–1026
Preconventional level of moral development, 854, 1053
Prednisone, breastfeeding and, 1753t–1756t
Pre-eclampsia. *See also* Hypertension, in pregnancy
  assessing/reporting, 301b
  in diabetic pregnancy, 341
  dietary recommendations, 303, 303b
  etiology of, 298, 298f
  fetal health surveillance, 302
  HELLP syndrome, 299
  hospital care for severe, 303–304, 304b
  hypertension and, 296–308
  magnesium sulphate for severe, 304–305
  maternal nutrition and, 263
  mild, 296–297, 297t
  nursing care for mild, 300b–301b
  pathophysiology of, 298–299, 299f
  prevention of, 298b
  proteinuria and, 296, 297b
  restricted activity for, 302–303
  risk markers for, 296t
  severe, 297, 297t
Pre-existing conditions
  anemia, 362–365
  autoimmune disorders
    myasthenia gravis, 369–370
    systemic lupus erythematosus, 369
  cardiopulmonary resuscitation and, 362, 363b
  cardiovascular disorders, 356b–357b, 359b
Pre-existing conditions *(Continued)*
    acquired heart disease, 353b, 355–356
    congenital heart disease, 353–355, 353b
    contraindications to pregnancy in, 356, 356b
  gastrointestinal disorders
    cholelithiasis/cholecystitis, 367
    inflammatory bowel disease, 367
  HIV/AIDS, 371–373
  integumentary disorders, 367–368
  metabolic disorders
    diabetes mellitus, 339–352, 340f, 343b–344b, 351b
    hyperthyroidism, 350–352
    hypothyroidism, 352
  neurological disorders
    Bell's palsy, 369
    epilepsy, 368
    multiple sclerosis, 369
    restless legs syndrome, 368–369
  obesity, 370–371
  pulmonary disorders
    asthma, 365–366, 365t
    cystic fibrosis, 366–367
  substance use, 373–375
Pre-existing hypertension, 295
Pre-existing hypertension with superimposed pre-eclampsia, 295
Prefixes denoting decimal factors, 1772t
Pregestational diabetes mellitus
  birth date/mode of delivery in, 348–349
  classification of, 339
  complications with, 348
  diet for, 345, 345b
  exercise in, 345–346
  family planning/contraception and, 350
  fetal/neonatal risks, 342
  insulin therapy for, 347–348, 347b, 348t
  intrapartum period, 349
  maternal risks/complications, 341–342
  monitoring blood glucose levels, 346–348, 346b
  nursing care for, 342–350, 343b–344b, 351b
  postpartum period, 349–350
  preconception counselling, 341, 341b
  in pregnancy, 340–342
Pregnancy
  adolescents and, 1131
  alternative therapies during, 230b
  breastfeeding during, 695
  Canadian Maternity Experiences Survey of, 9
  cardiopulmonary resuscitation in, 362, 363b
  confirmation of, 206
  cultural practices regarding, 25t–26t
  depression in, 53
  embryonic/fetal development, 169f, 171–184
Pregnancy *(Continued)*
  exercise in, 51, 52b, 52f
  family adaptation to, *see under* Family(ies)
  gravidity/parity, 186–187, 187t
  heart surgery during, 360
  HIV and, 107–108, 217–218, 218b
  hormonal changes during, 203t
  multifetal, 180–184
  nonobstetrical surgery during, 330–331
  nursing care during. *See* Prenatal care
  nursing care for. *See* Prenatal care
  obesity and, 255–256
  overview, 171–172
  physical adaptations to. *See* Physiological adaptations
  potential complications, 220b
  pre-existing conditions in. *See* Pre-existing conditions
  at risk. *See* Gestational conditions
  risk factors in. *See also* High-risk pregnancy
    amniocentesis for, 282–284, 282t, 283f
    biochemical assessment, 281–285, 282t
    chorionic villus sampling for, 284–285, 285f
    Coombs' test for, 281–282, 282t
    determinants of health as, 274, 275b
    fetal/neonatal health problems, 277–291
    first-/second-trimester screening, 277–281, 277b
    intimate partner violence, 276
    maternal health problems, 274–276, 276b
    mental health issues, 274–276
    nursing role in assessment, 291–292
    percutaneous umbilical blood sampling for, 284, 284f
    psychological considerations, 291–292
    regionalization of health care and, 274
    third-trimester assessment, 285–291, 285b
    ultrasound for, 278–281, 280b
  seeking health care for, 43, 44b
  signs of, 188, 189t
  tests for, 187–188, 187f
  trauma during, 331–335
Pregnancy-Unique Quantification of Emesis (PUQE) Scale, 312t
Preimplantation genetic diagnosis (PGD), 134–135
Prelabour (premature) rupture of membranes (PROM), 497
Preluxation of hip, 775
Premature dilation of cervix
  collaborative care, 317–318, 317f
  etiology of, 317
  overview, 316–317

Premature Infant Pain Profile (PIPP), 938
Premature separation of placenta, 326–328, 326f
Premenstrual dysphoric disorder (PMDD), 88–89
Premenstrual syndrome (PMS), 87–89
Premixed insulin, 1631b
Prenatal care
Centring Pregnancy approach, 213b
confirming pregnancy, 206
cultural influences, 236–238
education and, 222–234
goals of, 44b
interventions, 44b
nursing process for, 210–216, 213f, 214b
overview, 205
preparing for Caesarean, 515
psychosocial support, 235–236
review of systems, 216–241
risks due to obesity, 370
sex counselling, 234–235, 235b
signs of complications, 220b
Prenatal period, 845b
Prenatal screening. *See* Fetal health assessment; Fetal health surveillance (FHS)
Preoperational stage
of cognitive development, 853
preschoolers and, 1052–1053
toddlers and, 1025–1026, 1025b
Preoperative care
Caesarean birth and, 515–516
cleft lip/palate repair and, 1423
ectopic pregnancy and, 319
hypertrophic pyloric stenosis and, 1429–1430
myelomeningocele and, 769
in pediatric surgery, 1265–1267, 1265f, 1267t
spinal surgery and, 1710
surgery during pregnancy and, 331
surgery for Hirschsprung disease and, 1402
Wilms' tumour and, 1553
Prepubescence, 1085
Preschool, 1055–1057
Preschoolers
aggression in, 1058
anticipatory guidance in caring for, 1061, 1061b
biological development of, 1049–1052
body image development, 1053
child maltreatment and
caregiver-child interaction in, 1075–1076
child neglect in, 1072
clinical manifestations of, 1077b–1078b
history/interview in, 1076
nursing care for, 1075, 1078–1080, 1079b
physical abuse in, 1072–1073
physical assessment in, 1076–1078
sexual abuse. *See* Sexual abuse, of children
talking with children who reveal abuse, 1075b
warning signs of, 1075b
Preschoolers *(Continued)*
cognitive development in, 1052–1053
communicable diseases and, 1064t–1070t
assessment of, 1062
preventing complications, 1062–1063
preventing spread of, 1062
providing comfort for, 1063
supportive care for, 1063
dental health for, 1060–1061
encopresis in, 1072
fears of, 1057–1058
growth/development overview, 1051t
hospitalization of
loss of control and, 1235
separation anxiety in, 1234
injury prevention for, 1061
language development in, 1054, 1054f
moral development in, 1053
nutrition and, 1059–1060, 1060f
personal-social behaviour of, 1054, 1054f
play, 1054–1055
preparation for procedures, 1262b–1263b
preschool experience of, 1055–1057
psychosocial development in, 1052
sex education for, 1057
sexual development in, 1053
sleep and activity, 1060
social development in, 1053–1055
with special needs, 1170–1173, 1171t–1172t
speech problems in, 1058–1059
spiritual development in, 1053
stresses for, 1058
understanding of/reactions to death, 1177t–1178t
Prescription medications, 47–48. *See also* Medications
Presence, definition of, 1242
Presentation in labour, fetal. *See* Fetal presentation
Preslit injection port, 1300, 1300f
Pressure ulcers, 1271
Pressure-equalizer (PE) tubes, 1327
Pressure-reduction devices, 1271
Pressure-relief devices, 1271
Presumptive signs of pregnancy
causing concern, 213
overview, 188, 189t
Preterm infants
breastfeeding, 691
bronchopulmonary dysplasia in, 732–733
classification of, 708b
developmental care for, 722–726
discharge planning for, 737–738, 738b
environmental noise and, 722
growth/development potential of, 726–728
late, 708–709
maintaining body temperature, 713–714
necrotizing enterocolitis in, 731–732
Preterm infants *(Continued)*
nursing care for, 710–733, 714b, 729b–730b
nutritional care for, 718–721
oxygen therapy for, 714–718
parental adaptation to, 711–713
patent ductus arteriosus in, 731
periventricular-intraventricular hemorrhage, 731
physical care for, 713
respiratory distress syndrome in, 728–731
retinopathy of prematurity in, 732
skin care for, 721–722, 723b–724b
Preterm labour and birth
accelerating fetal lung maturity, 496–497
bed rest intervention, 493–494
causes of, 490, 490b
defined, 186, 488
early recognition/diagnosis of, 493
home care intervention and, 494–495, 494f
impact of, 497b
incidence of, 8, 707–708
lifestyle modifications, 493
low birth weight vs., 488–490
management of, 497
nursing care for, 490–497, 491b–492b
predicting, 488–490
prevention of, 490–493
risk factors for, 276b, 489b
signs of, 233–234, 234b, 234f, 491b
tocolytic therapy and, 495–496, 495b
Preterm premature rupture of membranes (PPROM)
adverse effects of, 497
definition/incidence of, 497
home vs. hospital care for, 497–498, 498b
Prevalence of disease, 803
Preventive care. *See also* Health promotion/illness prevention
levels of, 29–30, 803
in pediatric nursing, 795
Previous health issues, on pediatric health history, 880
PrevNET (Promoting Relationships and Eliminating Violence), 1090
Priapism, 1507
Primary amenorrhea, 1133
Primary atypical pneumonias, 1336
Primary circular reactions stage in sensorimotor development, 965
Primary dysmenorrhea, 1134
management of, 86–87, 87t
overview, 86
Primary encopresis, 1072
Primary germ layers, 171f, 172
Primary health care, special needs child and, 1170
Primary irritant, 1655
Primary lactase deficiency, 1388
Primary narcissism, 964
Primary powers, birth process and, 385–386, 385f
Primary prevention, 29, 803
Primary pulmonary hypertension, 355
Primary sex characteristics, 1113–1114
Primary skin lesions, 1643, 1644f
Primary vesicoureteral reflux, 1543
Primigravidous women
defined, 186
in latent phase of labour, 444
Primiparous women
defined, 186
prenatal care for, 240
The Principles and Framework for Interdisciplinary Collaboration in Primary Health Care, 1224
Privacy
of electronic medical records, 870
interview process and, 869–870
Private-duty nursing, 1218
Probable signs of pregnancy, 188, 189t
Probiotics, 1388–1389
Progesterone
breastfeeding and, 1753t–1756t
after childbirth, 529
menstrual cycle and, 82–84
Progestin-only contraception
injections, 149–150
oral, 148–150
Prolactin levels
after childbirth, 529
milk production and, 681
Prolapsed umbilical cord
emergency intervention for, 523b
risks/management of, 521–522, 521f–522f
Prolapsed uterus, 589, 589f
Proliferative phase of menstrual cycle, 82, 83f
Proliferative stage of wound healing, 1646
Prolonged decelerations of fetal heart rate, 435
Promoting Relationships and Eliminating Violence (PrevNET), 1090
Prone sleeping, SIDS and, 1009
Propionibacterium acnes, 1668–1669
Proportional changes
in infants, 958–959
in school-age children, 1084
Propylthiouracil (PTU), 350, 1620, 1620b
Prostaglandin E_2
cervical ripening with, 507–508
medication guide for, 507b
Prostaglandins (PGs), 84
Protein
in adolescence, 1125
in human milk, 682
for infant nutrition, 679
for maternal nutrition, 256, 257t
normal test ranges for, 1764t–1771t
Protein-energy malnutrition (PEM), 1384
Proteinuria
after childbirth, 529
nephrotic syndrome and, 1547, 1548f

pre-eclampsia and, 296, 297b
during pregnancy, 199
Protest phase of separation anxiety, 1232–1234, 1233b, 1233f
Prothrombin time (PT), 1764t–1771t
Proximal bone fragment, 1690
Proximodistal trend in growth, 845–846
Pruritic urticarial papules and plaques of pregnancy (PUPPP), 367–368, 368f
Pruritus gravidarum, pregnancy and, 199–200
Pseudohypertrophic muscular dystrophy, 1740–1743, 1741f
Pseudohypoparathyroidism, 1620–1621, 1620b
Pseudostrabismus, 909, 909f
Psoriatic arthritis, 1716
Psychiatric care for PPMD, 598
Psychological considerations
in antenatal assessments, 291–292
in depression, 53
in dystocia, 502–503
in genital surgery, 1545
immobilization and, 1686–1687
preparation for pediatric procedures, 1260–1264, 1261b–1263b
Psychological stressors in pediatric/neonatal CCU admission, 1256b
Psychomotor seizures, 1594b–1595b
Psychosexual development theory, 850–851, 851t
Psychosocial assessments
home visits and, 39b
for pediatric health history, 884–885
Psychosocial development
adolescents and, 1117–1119
infants and, 963–964
school-age children and, 1085–1087
theory of, 851–852, 883b–884b
toddlers and, 1022
Psychosocial support
after childbirth, 548–552, 549b
during pregnancy, 235–236
Psychotherapy for anorexia nervosa/bulimia nervosa, 1143–1144
Psychotropic drugs, breastfeeding and, 1753t–1756t
Puberty
defined, 81
hormonal changes during, 1114
precocious, 1614–1615, 1614b
Pubic hair, 1114, 1116f
Public Health Agency of Canada (PHAC)
core competencies, 802
goals of, 801–802
planning for health emergencies, 3
sexual health education guidelines and, 1130
Pudendal nerve block, 410–411, 411f
Puerperium. *See* Postpartum period
Pulled elbow, 1689
Pulmonary dysfunction. *See* Respiratory dysfunction
Pulmonary function tests (PFTs), 1346
Pulmonary hypertension (PH), 1487
Pulmonary surfactants
fetal respiratory development and, 176–177
lack of, RDS and, 728–731
Pulmonary system
changes in pregnancy, 195–197, 197t
cystic fibrosis and, 1357, 1358b
disorders, during pregnancy, 365–367
Pulmonic stenosis
in children, 1456–1459, 1459f, 1460b–1462b
during pregnancy, 354
Pulse oximetry, 1303–1304, 1303f
Pulse rate
of newborns, 626t–636t, 637
pediatric
cardiopulmonary resuscitation and, 1367, 1367f
cerebral dysfunction and, 1565
in physical assessment, 901, 902t, 921f
Pumping breast milk, 692, 693f
Punctures, skin and vessel, 1287b
Punishment and obedience orientation of preschoolers, 1053
Pupils, cerebral dysfunction and, 1565–1566, 1565f
Pure vegetarians, 1380
Pushing, birth process and, 386
Pustule, 1644f
Pyelonephritis, 1541–1542
Pyloromyotomy, 1428–1429
Pyoderma, 1652t
Pyramidal cerebral palsy, 1725b
Pyridoxine, 262, 1376t–1379t
Pyrosis, 202, 268

Q

Quadrantectomy, 118, 119f
Quadriplegia, 1748
Quickening, 191, 219
Quiet games/activities, 1092, 1092f–1093f
Quinidine, breastfeeding and, 1753t–1756t

R

Rabies, 1591, 1592b
Race. *See also* Ethnicity
definition of, 825
skin colour and, 906t
Rachischisis, 1733b
Radiation heat loss in newborns, 612
Radiation therapy
for brain tumours, 1584
for breast cancer, 120
for Ewing's sarcoma, 1714
for Hodgkin's disease, 1525
for leukemia, 1518–1523
for neuroblastomas, 1586
for non-Hodgkin's lymphoma, 1526
for rhabdomyosarcoma, 1716
for Wilms' tumour, 1552–1553
Radical mastectomy, 118, 119f
Radiofrequency ablation, 1487
Radiography, 1567–1568, 1567t–1568t
Radioisotope imaging studies, 1538t–1539t
Radionuclide cystogram, 1538t–1539t
Raloxifene
breast cancer and, 115, 121
medication guide, 121b
Range of motion
play activities for, 1266b
unconscious child and, 1573
Rapid testing for HIV, 217, 218b
Rapprochement, 1027
Rashes, neonatal, 668–669
Rating game, 877b–878b
Rational judgement, toddlers and, 1024
Reach for knees, 546f
Reactive attachment disorder (RAD), 966
Reading materials, child development and, 864
Reading skills, school-age children and, 1088, 1092, 1092f
Real-time ultrasonography (RTUS), 1567t–1568t
Rear-facing car seats, 996–997, 997f, 1037–1040
Recessive traits, 163
Reciprocity in parent-infant bonding, 561–562, 562f
Recommended dietary allowance (RDA)
of nutrient intake, 890
for vitamins, 1375
Reconstituted families, 821
Reconstructive surgery
breast, 118–120
infertility and, 132
Recovery area, transfer from, 534, 535t
Rectal administration of medications, 1296
Rectal analgesia, 948b–949b
Rectal prolapse, 1360
Rectal sites for temperature measurement, 897–901, 899t, 900b–901b
Rectal ulcers, chemotherapy and, 1524
Rectoceles, 589–590, 590f
Rectovaginal palpation, 78–79, 79f
Recumbent length, 894–895, 896f
Recurrent abdominal pain (RAP), 1109
Recurrent urinary tract infection, 1541–1542
Red blood cell disorders, 1503–1505
anemia in, 1500–1503, 1502b, 1502f
aplastic anemia in, 1511–1512, 1512b
beta-thalassemia in, 1510–1511, 1511b
iron deficiency anemia in, 1503–1505
sickle cell anemia in, 1505–1510, 1506b, 1506f, 1508b
Red blood cells (RBCs)
count, 1501t, 1764t–1771t
levels in neonate, 611
morphology of, 1502b
Reed-Sternberg cells, 1525
Referral to community resources, 554
Reflection in nurse interview, 70
Reflexes
cerebral dysfunction and, 1566–1567
of newborns, 621, 622t–625t
pediatric assessment of, 928, 929f
sensorimotor development and, 965
Refractive errors, visual impairment and, 1204, 1204b–1205b
Refractory seizures, 1597–1598
Refugees, 33
Refusal to sleep, 982t
Regional nerve block, 948b–949b
Registered Nurses' Association of Ontario (RNAO), 550
Regression, toddlers and, 1032, 1235
Regurgitation, 1003
Rehabilitation
burns and, 1677–1678
head injury and, 1581
Reinforcement, aggression and, 1058
Reintegration, special needs child and, 1163–1164
Relational nursing practice, 20–21, 21b
Relationships, child development and, 861–862, 862f
Relaxation
education in, 246
for labour pain management, 402, 402f
during pediatric procedures, 941b
Religious considerations
in child health promotion, 828, 828f, 837–842, 837b, 838t–839t
in contraception, 137–138
in death of newborn, 603b, 606
home care and, 1223b
Remodelling stage of wound healing, 1646
Remote symptomatic seizures, 1593
Renal dysfunction
acute glomerulonephritis and, 1549–1551, 1550b
acute renal failure and, 1553–1555, 1554b, 1556b
chronic renal failure and, 1555–1559, 1557b
in diabetic pregnancy, 342
dialysis and, 1559–1560
hemolytic uremic syndrome and, 1551–1552, 1551b
nephrotic syndrome and, 1547–1549, 1547b, 1548f
transplantation and, 1560
Wilms' tumour, 1552–1553, 1552b
Renal osteodystrophy, 1556–1557
Renal system
fetal development of, 178–179
fluid loss in infants and, 1390
of infants, 960
of newborns, 613

Renal system *(Continued)*
of preterm infants, 711
radiological tests of, 1538t–1539t
testing function of, 1540t–1541t
Renal system adaptations
maternal
anatomical, 198
in fluid/electrolyte balance, 198–199
functional, 198
during labour, 392
overview, 199t
Reproductive system
cystic fibrosis and, 1357
fetal development of, 179–180
neonatal adaptations, 619–620, 619f
postpartum physiological changes, 526–529
Research
in pediatric nursing, 796
in perinatal nursing, 13–14
Research-informed practice. *See* Evidence-informed practice
Respiration
of newborn, 626t–636t
parental guidance regarding, 667
pediatric, 636–637
assessment of, 901, 919–920
breath sounds classification, 920b
bronchial drainage for, 1304
cerebral dysfunction and, 1565
inhalation therapy for, 1302–1304, 1302f–1303f
patterns of, 920b
in unconscious child, 1570
Respiratory arrest, 1364
Respiratory depression, 951–952, 953b
Respiratory distress
congestive heart failure and, 1473
in neonates, 610
Respiratory distress syndrome (RDS)
causes/symptoms/treatment of, 728–731
in infants of diabetic mothers, 736
Respiratory dysfunction. *See also* Respiratory infections
acute respiratory distress syndrome/acute lung injury and, 1342–1343
aspiration pneumonia and, 1341–1342
asthma and, 1344–1356
cystic fibrosis and, 1356–1364
foreign body aspiration and, 1341
obstructive sleep-disordered breathing and, 1364
smoke inhalation injury and, 1343–1344
tobacco smoke exposure and, 1344
Respiratory failure, 1364–1370, 1365b
Respiratory hygiene, 109t
Respiratory infections
clinical manifestations of, 1317, 1318b
croup syndromes and, 1329–1332, 1330t
easing respiratory efforts in, 1317
etiology/characteristics of, 1316–1317
family support in, 1320
lower. *See* Lower respiratory infections
nutrition for, 1320
pertussis, 1337–1341
preventing spread of, 1318–1319
promoting hydration in, 1319–1320
reducing temperature in, 1319
respiratory function assessment in, 1319b
rest and comfort in, 1317–1318
severe acute respiratory syndrome, 1340–1341
tuberculosis, 1337–1340, 1338b–1339b
upper. *See* Upper respiratory tract infections
Respiratory insufficiency, definition of, 1364
Respiratory rate, normal pediatric, 1773
Respiratory secretion specimens, 1286
Respiratory status
pediatric
alterations during surgery, 1268t
after heart surgery, 1480
Respiratory syncytial virus (RSV), 1333–1337, 1333t, 1334b
Respiratory system
of fetus, 176–177
maternal
adaptation to pregnancy
in acid-base balance, 198
in basal metabolic rate, 197
overview, 195
in pulmonary function, 195–197
during labour, 392
of newborns, 643b
pediatric
congenital anomalies of, 770–771
effects of immobilization on, 1685t
of preterm infants, 710
transition to extrauterine life, 609–610
Respite care, 1218
Responsivity in parent-infant interactions, 566–567
Restitution, birth process and, 391
Restless legs syndrome (RLS), 368–369
Restraint systems for infant/child car safety, 1037–1042
Restraints
elbow, 1280–1281
jacket, 1280
leg/arm, 1280
mummy, 1280, 1280f
types of, 1279–1280
Rest/relaxation
adolescents and, 1127
for breastfeeding mothers, 694–695
after childbirth, 544
cultural perspectives, 237–238
education in, 224–227, 226f, 227b, 228f
after pediatric heart surgery, 1480–1481
Restrictive cardiomyopathy, 1488
Resynchronization therapy, 1468
Retained placenta, 579
Reticulocyte count, 1764t–1771t
Retinoblastoma
clinical manifestations of, 1209b
diagnosis of, 1209
management of, 1209–1210
nursing care for, 1210
prognosis of, 1210
Retinol. *See* Vitamin A
Retinopathy, diabetic pregnancy and, 341
Retinopathy of prematurity (ROP), 732
Retrograde pyelography, 1538t–1539t
Review of systems for pediatric health history, 885, 885b
Revised Infant Temperament Questionnaire (RITQ), 968
Reye's syndrome (RS), 1591–1592, 1592b
Rh immune globulin
injection, after childbirth, 547
medication guide for, 548b
Rh incompatibility in neonate
nursing care for, 767–768
pathogenesis of, 765–767
Rho(D) immune globulin for, 4b
Rheumatic fever (RF), 1483–1484, 1483b
Rheumatic heart disease (RHD)
pediatric, 1483
during pregnancy, 355
Rhythm in parent-infant interactions, 566
Ribavirin, 1334
Riboflavin, 1376t–1379t
Rickets, 1374–1375
Rickettsial diseases, 1661, 1662t
Rickettsialpox, 1662t
Rights of the Hospitalized Child, 1244, 1245b
Right-sided heart failure, 1462
Right-to-left shunt, 1455–1456
Rimantadine, 1325
Ringworm, 1653–1655, 1654t
Risk factors in pregnancy. *See* Pregnancy, risk factors in
Ritalin, 1106–1107
Ritgen manoeuvre, 475–476, 476f, 482b–483b
Ritualism, toddlers and, 1022
Rituals, in middle childhood play, 1092
Rocky Mountain spotted fever, 1662t
Rohypnol, 1147
Rolling over, 961–962
Romberg test, 928b
Roseola infantum, 1064t–1070t, 1066f
Rotavirus, 1393t–1395t, 1395–1396
Rotavirus vaccine, 988, 1397
contraindications/precautions for, 989t–991t
Roundworm, 1406t
Routine practices
burn care and, 1679
catheterization and, 1284
during childbirth, 373, 450, 451b, 642
children with HIV infection and, 1529–1530
hospitalization and, 1334–1335, 1362
infection control and, 111b–112b, 541, 1062b, 1277, 1277b
osteomyelitis and, 1711
wound care and, 1711
Routines, hospitalization and, 1244, 1244f
Rubella, 1064t–1070t, 1070f
neonatal, 753
Rubella vaccine
contraindications/precautions for, 989t–991t
during postpartum period, 547
schedule for, 986
Rubeola, 1064t–1070t, 1066f
Rubin technique for shoulder dystocia, 520, 520f
Rules in middle childhood play, 1092
Rupture of membranes
artificial. *See* Amniotomy
infection control after, 456
tests for, 446, 447b
Rupture of uterus, 522–523
Ruptured appendix, 1409
Russell traction, 1696

S

Safe Kids Canada, 1000, 1681
Safety catheters, 1300
Safety issues
administration of medications, 419–420
avoiding dog bites, 1663b
burn injuries and, 1681
car seats, 669–670, 669f
chemotherapeutic agents, 1523
drinking water, 54–55
environmental, 54–55, 862–863, 863b
family-centred home care, 1228–1229
food preparation, 267
holding newborns, 668
home visiting nurse, 40
during hospitalization
environmental factors, 1275–1277, 1275f–1276f
strangulation prevention, 1275
injection practices, 109t
intimate partner violence, 60b
for neonatal screening, 660
PPMD, 598
during pregnancy, 227b
for risk reduction, 56b
toddler sleeping environments, 1034

Safety issues *(Continued)*
with toys, 859, 860b–861b, 1028, 1276
transportation for special needs child, 1169–1170
Salicylates, 1764t–1771t
Saline lock, 1293–1294
Salmeterol, 1350
Salmonella groups, 1393t–1395t, 1396
Salmonella typhi, 1393t–1395t, 1396
Same-sex couples
parent-child attachment in, 966
parenting and, 821
postpartum role adjustment for, 564–565
Sandifer syndrome, 1404
Sano modification shunt procedure, 1476t
Scabies, 1658–1659, 1659b
Scald burns, 999
toddlers and, 1042
Scale, 1645f
Scalp blood sampling, 438
Scalp vein for parenteral fluid therapy, 1299
Scandinavian ethnicity
food patterns of, 269t–270t, 834
lactase deficiency and, 1388
phenylketonuria and, 158
Scarlet fever, 1064t–1070t, 1070f
Scars, 1645f
burn injuries and, 1679–1680, 1679f–1680f
Scheuermann's kyphosis, 1707
School
as influencing factor, 828
in middle childhood, 1093–1094
School health programs, 1100
School phobia
in school-age children, 1108–1109
special needs children and, 1173
School vision, 1203–1204
School-age children
altered growth/maturation in, 1104–1106
attention-deficit/hyperactivity disorder (ADHD) in, 1106–1107
biological development of, 1084–1085
cognitive development in, 1087–1088
communicating with, 875
conversion reaction in, 1109–1110
dental health of, 1098–1099, 1098f
depression in, 1110, 1110b
dishonest behaviour in, 1095
eating disorders in, 1109
enuresis in, 1107–1108
exercise/activity of, 1097–1098
family relationships and, 1091–1092, 1091b
growth/development overview, 1085t–1086t
hospitalization of
loss of control and, 1235–1236
separation anxiety in, 1234
School-age children *(Continued)*
impact of social media on, 1110
injury prevention for, 1100–1101, 1102t
latchkey children, 1094
limit setting/discipline for, 1094–1095
moral development in, 1088–1089
nutrition and, 1096
play and, 1092
posttraumatic stress disorder in, 1108
preparation for procedures, 1262b–1263b
psychosocial development in, 1085–1087, 1087f
recurrent abdominal pain in, 1109
school experiences of, 1093–1094
school health for, 1100
school phobia in, 1108–1109
self-concept development in, 1092–1093
sex chromosome abnormalities in, 1105–1106, 1105t
sex education for, 1099–1100
skills acquired by, 1098
sleep/rest for, 1096
social development in, 1089–1092
with special needs, 1171t–1172t, 1173, 1173f
spiritual development in, 1089
sports and, 1097–1098, 1097f
sports injuries and, 1101–1104
nurse's role in, 1104
stress/fear for, 1095–1096
tall/short stature in, 1104–1105
understanding of/reactions to death, 1177t–1178t
Sclerosing agents, 1302
SCOFF questionnaire, 50b
Scoliosis
idiopathic, 1707f–1708f, 1708–1710
pediatric examination for, 926
Scout film, 1538t–1539t
Screen-film mammography, 117b
Screening
for breast cancer, 117b, 117t
for bulimia nervosa, 50
for cervical cancer, 29–30, 190
community health nursing and, 804
for congenital anomalies, 778–779
for genetic disorders, 778–779
for gestational diabetes mellitus, 308–309, 309f
for hepatitis B, 105
for herpes simplex virus, 103–104
for human immunodeficiency virus, 107, 217–218, 218b
for human papillomavirus, 102
for hypothyroidism, 778–779
for lead poisoning, 1444
for neural tube defects, 278
schedule for, 56, 57t
Scrotum, 1114–1115, 1116f
Seasonal influenza, 1324–1325
Seasonal variations in respiratory infections, 1317
Seborrheic dermatitis, 1667
Second stage of labour
bearing-down efforts, 472–473
duration of, 470
fetal heart rate assessment during, 473
maternal position for, 471–472
nursing care for, 470–471
overview, 389
phases of, 468–470, 469t, 470f
supplies/instruments/equipment, 474
support of partner in, 473–474
Second trimester
abortion in, 154
discomforts during, 231t–233t
fetal heart rate in, 220
serum screening in, 278
signs of potential complications in, 220b
Secondary (permanent) teeth, 1098, 1098f
Secondary amenorrhea, 1133
Secondary circular reactions stage, 965
Secondary encopresis, 1072
Secondary lactase deficiency, 1388
Secondary powers, birth process and, 386
Secondary prevention in community health, 29–30, 803
Secondary sexual characteristics, 1085, 1113–1114
Secondary skin lesions, 1643, 1645f
Secondary vesicoureteral reflux, 1543
Second-hand smoke exposure, 1145
Secretory phase of menstrual cycle, 82, 83f
Sedatives
breastfeeding and, 1753t–1756t
for labour pain management, 407
preoperative, 1267
Seesaw respiration, 920b
Segmental mastectomy, 118, 119f
Seizures
epilepsy and, 1593–1603, 1593b–1595b, 1596t, 1599b–1603b
febrile, 1603–1604
head injury and, 1580
Selenium, 1381t–1383t
Self-care
cognitively impaired children and, 1192
family-centred home care promoting, 1227–1228, 1228f
hospitalization and, 1244, 1274
special needs children and, 1165, 1170
Self-concept
development of, 855
adolescents and, 1123–1124
school-age children and, 1092–1093
through play, 858
maternal, after childbirth, 548–549
Self-esteem
cultural influences on, 826
development of, 855
Self-mastery, hospitalization and, 1249
Semen analysis, male infertility and, 129, 130b
Semirecumbent position during labour/birth, 452f, 461, 462b, 470f, 471–472, 472f
Semivegetarian diet, 268–270, 1380
Sense of industry, school-age children and, 1085–1087, 1087f
Sense of time, toddlers and, 1025
Sense-pleasure play, 856, 856f
Sensitive periods during growth/development, 846
Sensitizing agent, 1655
Sensorimotor phase
in infants, 964–965
in toddlers, 1024–1026
Sensorimotor play, 858
Sensorimotor stage of cognitive development, 853
Sensorineural hearing loss, 1199–1201
Sensory assessment, 1757f–1758f
Sensory awareness of fetus, 179
Sensory development, of toddlers, 1021
Sensory impairments
deaf-blind children, 1209
hearing impairments
additional aids, 1202
clinical manifestations of, 1201, 1201b
cued speech and, 1202
definition/classification of, 1199–1200
etiology of, 1199
hospitalization and, 1202–1203
intensity of sounds and, 1200t
lipreading and, 1201–1202, 1202b
management of, 1200–1201
nursing care for, 1201–1203
pathology of, 1199
prevention of, 1203
sign language and, 1202
socialization and, 1202
speech language therapy for, 1202
symptom severity and, 1199–1200, 1200t
of parents
hearing, 571
visual, 570–571, 571b
visual impairment
definition/classification of, 1203–1204
development/independence and, 1207
education for, 1207
emergency intervention for eye injuries and, 1206b
etiology of, 1204–1205, 1204b–1205b
hospitalization and, 1207–1208

Sensory impairments *(Continued)*
nursing care for, 1205–1209
parent-child attachment and, 1206
play/socialization and, 1207
prevention of, 1208–1209
promoting optimum development and, 1206–1207
retinoblastoma, 1209–1210, 1209b
Sensory stimulation
for pain management, 400b
unconscious child and, 1573
Separation, sensorimotor development and, 964
Separation anxiety
development of, 966–967
hospitalization and
in early childhood, 1234
in late childhood/adolescence, 1234
phases of, 1232–1234, 1233b
preventing/minimizing, 1242–1243, 1243f
in sensorimotor development, 965
Separation-individuation phase
preschoolers and, 1053–1055
toddlers and, 1027
Sepsis, neonatal. *See* Neonatal sepsis
Septic arthritis, 1712
Septic shock, 1495–1497, 1496b, 1496t
Sequential trends in growth/development, 846
Sequestration crisis, 1505, 1506b
Serving sizes of food, toddlers and, 1033
Set point, 1272
Severe acute respiratory syndrome (SARS), 1340–1341
Severe combined immunodeficiency disease (SCID), 1530
Sex chromosome abnormalities, 166
in school-age children, 1105–1106, 1105t
nursing care for, 1106
Sex counselling
alternative behaviours, 235, 236f
countering misinformation, 234
overview, 234, 235b
Sex development disorders in newborns, 777
Sex differences in growth patterns, 1117
Sex education
for adolescents, 1130–1131
for preschoolers, 1057
programs for, 46, 46b
for school-age children, 1099–1100
Sex Information and Education Council of Canada (SIECCAN), 1130
Sex-typing, preschoolers and, 1053
Sexual abuse
of children
abuser/victim characteristics, 1074
clinical manifestations of, 1077b–1078b
history/interview in, 1076
Sexual abuse *(Continued)*
incidence of, 1073
initiation/perpetuation of, 1074–1075, 1074b
physical assessment in, 1078
prevention of, 1080b
memories of during labour, 447–448
prenatal identification of, 215–216
Sexual activity
adolescents and, 1122–1123, 1123f
after childbirth, 552–553, 553b, 564
cognitively impaired children and, 1194
cultural perspectives, 238
during pregnancy, 234–235, 235b
risks of, 53–54
taking history of, 881–882
Sexual development, preschoolers and, 1053
Sexual maturation in adolescents, 1114–1115, 1114b, 1115f–1116f
Sexual orientation
adolescents and, 1122–1123
health care and, 45
suicide and, 1150b
Sexual sensations, breastfeeding and, 695
Sexually transmitted infections (STIs)
bacterial
chlamydia, 98
gonorrhea, 98–99
pelvic inflammatory disease, 100–101
syphilis, 99–100, 99f
home care, 110b
infertility and, 43
prenatal screening for, 217
prevention, 53–54, 53b, 95–98, 95b
range of, 95b
repeated testing for, 221
risk behaviour assessment, 96b
risks of, 53
viral
hepatitis, 105–106
herpes simplex virus, 103–104, 103f
human immunodeficiency virus, 106–108
human papillomavirus, 101–103, 102f
Shaken baby syndrome (SBS), 1001
Shared decision making, special needs child and, 1158, 1158b
Shearing stresses in head injury, 1574–1576, 1575f
Sheet graft, 1677
Shigella species, 1393t–1395t, 1396
Shingles, 1062
Shock
diagnosis of special needs child and, 1163
emergency intervention for, 1494b
pediatric
Shock *(Continued)*
manifestations of, 1492, 1493b
types of, 1492t
in postpartum hemorrhage, 581–584
Shoes for infants, 978
Short stature, school-age children and, 1105
Short-bowel syndrome (SBS), 1434–1435
Short-term catheters, 1294
Short-term memory, cognitive impairment and, 1191
Shoulder blade stretch/squeeze, 123b
Shoulder dystocia
definition/incidence of, 520
fractured clavicle following, 744–746, 744f
nursing care for, 520–521, 520f
Shoulder presentation, birth process and, 379, 381f
Shoulder stretch, 123b
Shunts, cardiac, 1475, 1476f, 1476t
Sibling rivalry in toddlers, 1030–1031, 1031f
Sibling(s)
acceptance of newborn, 571–572, 573b
adaptation to pregnancy, 210, 211b–212b, 211f
grief responses of, 602, 1184
interactions of, 810–811, 810f
interest in newborn, 485, 486f
during labour/childbirth, 467
rivalry, 550, 552f, 571–572
of special needs child, 1161b, 1169
supporting during hospitalization, 1251b
Sickle cell anemia (SCA), 1505–1510, 1506b, 1506f, 1508b
Sickle cell hemoglobinopathy, 364
Sickle cell trait, 1505
Sickle cell-C disease, 1505
Sickle thalassemia disease, 1505
Side bending, 123b
Side-lying position
for breastfeeding, 684–685, 685f
during second stage of labour, 470f, 471–472
Sign language, 1202
Silence during interviews, 872
Silver nitrate, 1676t
Silver sulphadiazine for burns, 1676t
Simcoe Muskoka District Health Unit, 1128
Simple fracture, 1690–1691
Simple mastectomy, 118, 119f
Simple partial seizures, 1594b–1595b, 1596t
Sinciput presentation, 379, 382f
Single knee roll, 546f
Single-gene inheritance disorders
autosomal dominant, 166–167, 166f
autosomal recessive, 167
X-linked dominant, 167
X-linked recessive, 167
Single-photon emission computed tomography (SPECT), 1567t–1568t
Sinus arrhythmia, 959
Sinus bradycardia, 1486
Sitting, infants and, 962, 962f
Skateboard safety
education in, 1103b
school-age children and, 1101
Skeletal injuries, birth process and, 744–746, 744f
Skeletal limb deficiency, 1703–1704
Skeletal system
growth/maturation of, 848
neonatal adaptations, 620–621
sex differences in growth of, 1117
Skeletal traction, 1696b, 1698b
Skeletal tuberculosis, 1712
Skill play, 856, 856f
Skin
changes in puberty, 1117
colour changes of racial groups, 906t
disorders of. *See* Integumentary disorders
of infants, 1642
infections of
bacterial, 1651–1655, 1652t
fungal, 1653–1655, 1654t
systemic mycotic, 1655, 1656t
viral, 1651–1653, 1653t
of newborn, 626t–636t
of newborns, 643b
newborns and, 670
nutritional status and, 887t–889t
pediatric examination of, 905–906, 906f
preterm infants and, 721–722, 723b–724b
unconscious child and, 1565
Skin cancer, tanning and, 1129
Skin fold thickness, 896–897
Skin lesions
care of, 1649–1650
causes of, 1642
diagnosis of, 1643
nursing care for, 1649
pathophysiology of, 1642–1643
relief of symptoms for, 1650
topical therapy for, 1650–1651
Skin punctures, 1287b
Skin testing, asthma and, 1347, 1347b
Skin traction, 1696b, 1698b
Skin-to-skin (STS) contact
to control heat loss, 612
evidence-based practice and, 688b
in forming attachment, 558–560
importance of, 644, 644f
during painful procedures, 942, 943f
for preterm infants, 724–725, 725f, 726b
to stimulate alertness, 690, 690f
Skull fractures
during labour/birth, 744–746
pediatric, 1576
Sleep
adolescents and, 1127
developmental changes in, 849
infancy/early childhood and, 981–983, 982t
preschoolers and, 1060

Sleep *(Continued)*
school-age children and, 1096
toddlers and, 1034
Sleep position, SIDS and, 1009
Sleep study, 1364
Sleep terrors, 1060
Sleep-wake states, 638, 638f
Sleepy infants, breastfeeding and, 690
Slipped capital femoral epiphysis (SCFE), 1706–1707, 1706b
Slow weight gain in newborns, breastfeeding and, 690–691
Slow-acting antirheumatic drugs (SAARDs), 1717
Slow-to-warm-up child, 850
Small-for-gestational-age (SGA) infants
classification of, 708b
common problems of, 8, 734–735
Smelling capacity of newborns, 639
Smoke inhalation injury, 1343–1344
Smokeless tobacco, 1145
Smoking. *See* Cigarette smoking
Soaks, play activities for, 1266b
Social character of play, 857–858
Social determinants of health
community, 828–829
culture, 824–826
ethnicity, 826–827
peer culture, 829
religion, 828
school, 828
socioeconomic status, 827–828
Social development
adolescents and, 1119–1122
infants and
attachment, 966
fear of strangers, 967, 967f, 970
language development, 967
play, 968, 969t
separation anxiety, 966–967
preschoolers and, 1053–1055
school-age children and, 1089–1092
toddlers and, 1027–1028
Social history, prenatal care interview and, 215
Social interactions, parent-infant, 660, 660f
Social media, child development and, 1110
Social roles, cultural factors in, 825–826
Social stressors, pediatric/neonatal CCU admission and, 1256b
Social support during transition to parenthood, 569
Social-affective play, 856
Socialization
cognitively impaired children and, 1194
hearing impaired children and, 1202
hospitalization and, 1249–1250, 1250f
visually impaired children and, 1207
Society, family and, 16
Socioeconomic factors
child development and, 862
as health determinant, 45, 827–828
transition to parenthood and, 570
Sodium
for maternal nutrition, 261
normal test ranges for, 1764t–1771t
nutritional significance of, 1381t–1383t
restriction for CHD, 1468–1469, 1473–1474
Soft bedding, SIDS and, 1009
Soft tissue dystocia, 499
Soft tissues
labour process and, 383–385, 384f
neonatal birth trauma and, 651–652, 651f
pediatric trauma to, 1688–1690, 1688f
rhabdomyosarcoma and, 1715–1716, 1715b
Solid foods
during first 6 months, 979
infant aspiration of, 993–995
introduction of, 980, 981b
during second 6 months, 979–980
selection/preparation of, 980–981
Solitary play, 857
Somatic pain, 394–395
Somogyi effect, 1633
South Asian ethnicity
food patterns of, 269t–270t
as visible minority, 829, 830b
Southeast Asian ethnicity
food patterns of, 269t–270t
lactase deficiency and, 1503
pregnancy and, 545
as visible minority, 829, 830b
Spastic cerebral palsy, 1725b–1726b. *See also* Cerebral palsy (CP)
Spatial relationships, toddlers and, 1024
Special needs children. *See* Children, chronic illness/disability in
Special Olympics, 1173, 1193
Specialization in perinatal nursing, 9
Specific gravity, 1764t–1771t
Specimen collections
blood, 1285–1286
respiratory secretion, 1286
stool, 1285
urine, 1282
24-hour collection of, 1283
bladder catheterization, 1283–1285, 1284t
clean-catch specimens, 1283
procedure for, 1282f
Speech
cognitively impaired children and, 1193–1194
development of, 853–854
problems in preschoolers, 1058–1059
Speech language therapy, hearing impaired children and, 1202
Spermatogenesis, 168, 170f
Spermicides, 142, 142f
Spider nevi. *See* Angiomas
Spina bifida
in newborns, 768–769, 769f
pediatric
bowel control and, 1735
care of myelomeningocele sac, 1736
degrees of, 1732, 1733b, 1733f
diagnosis of, 1733, 1734b, 1734f
family support/home care for, 1737
genitourinary function and, 1735
latex allergy and, 1737–1738
management of, 1733–1736
orthopedic care for, 1735
pathophysiology of, 1732–1733
postnatal care for, 1734–1735
postoperative care for, 1737
preventing complications, 1736–1737
prevention of, 1736
prognosis for, 1735–1736
Spina Bifida and Hydrocephalus Association Canada, 1737
Spina bifida cystica, 1732, 1734b
Spina bifida occulta, 1732, 1733f, 1734b
Spinal anaesthesia (block)
for labour pain management, 411–413, 412f
postdural puncture headache in, 412–413, 413f
Spinal cord compression, 1748
Spinal cord injuries (SPIs), 1748–1750, 1749f
Spinal muscular atrophy (SMA)
infantile (type 1), 1738–1740
juvenile (type 3), 1740
manifestations of, 1739b
Spine, pediatric examination of, 926–927
Spiral fracture line, 1690
Spiritual development, 854
in adolescents, 1119
in preschoolers, 1053
in school-age children, 1089
in toddlers, 1026
Spironolactone
breastfeeding and, 1753t–1756t
for congestive heart failure, 1468b, 1469t
Spitting up, 1003
Splenectomy
beta-thalassemia and, 1511
idiopathic thrombocytopenic purpura and, 1516
Splenic sequestration, 1507, 1510
Spontaneous abortion. *See* Miscarriage
Sports, school-age children and, 1097–1098, 1097f
Sports injuries
adolescents and, 1133
school-age children and, 1101–1104
Spot test, 1329
Sprains, 1689
Squatting, birth process and, 419–420, 420f, 462f, 471, 474–475
Stabilization after trauma
electronic fetal monitoring, 335
perimortem Caesarean birth, 335
primary survey procedures, 334–335
secondary survey procedures, 335
Standard days method (SDM), 138, 138f
Standards of care
for first stage of labour, 456–457
for home care nursing, 1221–1222
for obstetrical emergencies, 584b
Staphylococcal scalded skin syndrome, 1652t
Staphylococcus, 1393t–1395t
Staphylococcus aureus
osteomyelitis and, 1710
septic arthritis and, 1712
Station, fetal, 379–380, 382f
StatLock securement devices, 1301f
Status asthmaticus, 1351–1352
Status epilepticus, 1598
Stealing, school-age children and, 1095
Stepping reflex in newborns, 622t–625t, 623f
Stereotyping, 22, 23b, 833, 833f
Sterilization
female, 151–152, 151f
laws/regulations, 152
male, 151f, 152
nursing care for, 152
Steroid therapy effects, 1524
Stethoscopes, infection transmission and, 1278b
Stillbirths, 7b
Stimulation
of infants, 968, 969t
neonatal behaviour and, 639
Stomach during pregnancy, 202
Stomatitis, chemotherapy and, 1524
Stool specimens, 1285
Stools of newborns, 614, 614b, 615f, 626t–636t
Storage of breast milk, 692–693
Stork bite, 618–619, 619f
Storytelling, 877b–878b
Strabismus, 1204, 1204b–1205b
cerebral dysfunction and, 1565
testing for, 909–910, 910f
Strains, 1689
Stranger anxiety in infants, 967, 970
Strangulated hernias, 1427
Strangulation, precautions against, 1275
Strategic Directions for Nursing and Midwifery Services, 12, 13b
Streptococcus pneumoniae, 1326
Streptococcus viridans, 1481–1482
Stress
adolescents and, 1129–1130, 1129b, 1129f
affecting development, 863–864
concurrent, with special needs child, 1162
health risks of, 51–53
in labour, 448–449
management, 53
in pediatric/neonatal CCU admission, 1256b

Stress *(Continued)*
preschoolers and, 1058
school-age children and, 1095–1096
symptoms of, 53b
Stress fractures, 1103–1104
Striae gravidarum (stretch marks), 192, 199, 199f
Strongyloides stercoralis, 1406t
Structures, family, 16–17, 882–884
Students Against Destructive Decision (SADD), 1149
Stupor, 1564b
Subarachnoid bolt as ICP monitor, 1570
Subarachnoid hemorrhage, 746
Subcultures, 21
Subcutaneous injections, 1293
Subcutaneous route of drug administration, 948b–949b
Subdural hematoma
from birth trauma, 746
head injury and, 1575f
Subdural hemorrhage, 1577
Subdural tap, 1567t–1568t
Subgaleal hemorrhage, 617, 618f
Subinvolution of uterus, 526
Sublimaze. *See* Fentanyl citrate
Sublingual route of drug administration, 948b–949b
Subluxation of hip, 775
Submersion injuries, 1581–1583, 1582b
Subpopulations, definition of, 801
Subpubic arch, angle of, 383, 383f
Substance use
by children/youth, 791–792
history of, 215
during pregnancy, 229–230
alcohol and, 757–759
barriers to treatment, 373
caffeine and, 762
childbirth risks with, 47
cocaine and, 757f, 760–761
drug testing for, 373
heroin and, 761
interventions for, 55–56
legal issues, 373
marijuana and, 760
methadone and, 761
methamphetamine and, 761–762
neonatal effects of, 757t
nursing care for, 373–375
overview, 373, 756–757
perinatal care with, 375b
phencyclidine and, 761
phenobarbital and, 762
tobacco and, 759
Subvalvular aortic stenosis, 1456–1459, 1459f, 1460b–1462b
Succenturiate placenta, 328, 329f
Suctioning, tracheostomy, 1305–1307, 1306b, 1307f
Sudden infant death syndrome (SIDS)
defined/incidence of, 1008
epidemiology of, 1008t
etiology of, 1008–1010
in preterm infants, 727–728
prevention of, 667–668
Sudden unexplained death in infants (SUDI)
arriving at emergency department, 1011
finding infant, 1011
incidence of, 1008
nursing care for, 1010
patient education for, 1010b
returning home, 1011
Sufentanil citrate, 409, 409b
Suffocation
in infants, 789–790, 790f, 996
suicide by, 1150
in toddlers, 1044–1045
Sugarless gum, 1036
Suicidal ideation, 1149–1150
Suicide
adolescents and, 1149–1152, 1150b–1151b
among children/youth, 792
assisted, 1175
Sun blockers, 1681–1682
Sun protection, 863b
Sunburn
in children, 1681–1682
infants and, 999
Superego development
in preschoolers, 1052, 1052b
in toddlers, 1022
Superficial burns, 1670, 1671f
Supernatural forces, 835
Supine hypotension
during first stage of labour, 450–452, 452f
in lithotomy position, 216
during pregnancy, 194
signs/intervention for, 216b
Support groups, for new parents, 554
Supportive care
bacterial meningitis and, 1589
brain tumours and, 1585
burns injuries and, 1680–1681
cerebral palsy and, 1732
community role in, 828–829
for families with special needs child, 1167–1169, 1168b
for head injury, 1580–1581
hydrocephalus and, 1608
immobilized child and, 1688
for juvenile idiopathic arthritis, 1719
during labour and birth
actions and responses to, 466t
benefits of, 461–463, 464b
by doulas, 465–466
guidelines for, 465b
by nurse, 463–464
by partner, 465, 465f
pediatric nursing role of, 795
type 1 diabetes and, 1638–1639
Suprapubic catheterization, 1283–1285, 1284t
Suprapubic pressure, shoulder dystocia and, 520
Supratentorial brain tumours, 1583–1585
Supraventricular tachycardia (SVT), 1486–1487
Surfactant replacement therapy, 716–717
Surgery
for appendicitis, 330
for brain tumours, 1584
for cleft lip, 1422
Surgery *(Continued)*
for cleft palate, 1422
for ectopic pregnancy, 319
for epilepsy, 1597–1598
for esophageal atresia with tracheoesophageal fistula, 1425–1426
for gynecological problems, 331
for head injury, 1579
home care following, 331, 331b
of hydatidiform mole, 321
for hydrocephalus, 1606
for hypertrophic pyloric stenosis, 1428–1429
for inflammatory bowel disease, 1413
for intestinal obstruction, 330–331
for Meckel's diverticulum, 1410
for miscarriage, 315–316
for neuroblastomas, 1586
for osteosarcoma, 1713
postoperative care for, 1267–1269, 1268t
for premature dilation of cervix, 317, 317f
preoperative care for, 1265–1267, 1265f, 1267b
for scoliosis, 1709
for spina bifida, 1733–1736
for Wilms' tumour, 1552–1553
Surgical abortion, 153–154
Surrogate motherhood, 134t
Susceptibility to health problems, 831
Swaddle, 1280, 1280f
Sweat chloride test, 1358
Sweat glands
in adolescents, 1117
in neonates, 617
Swiss-type lymphopenic agammaglobulinemia, 1530
Symbol recognition, infants and, 964
Symptomatic bacteriuria, 1541–1542
Symptothermal method, 139–140, 141f
Synchrony, in parent-infant bonding, 562
Synclitism, 389, 390f
Syndrome of inappropriate antidiuretic hormone secretion (SIADH), 1572, 1616
Syndromic clubfoot, 1702
Synthetic casts, 1693
Synthetic skin coverings, 1676
Synthetic-convention stage of spiritual development, 854
Syphilis
neonatal, 750–751, 751f
symptoms/treatment of, 99–100, 99f
Syringes
for oral administration of medications, 1288
for parental fluid therapy, 1300, 1300f
Systemic arthritis, 1716
Systemic inflammatory response syndrome (SIRS), 1495, 1496b
Systemic injury to respiratory tract, 1343
Systemic lupus erythematosus (SLE)
in children, 1719–1721, 1721b
during pregnancy, 369
Systemic mycoses, 1655, 1656t
Systems theory in family nursing, 18–19

T

Tachydysrhythmias, 1486–1487
Tachypnea, 920b
Tachysystole, oxytocin-induced labour and, 509
Tactile play, 1028
Tactile stimulation
infants and, 964, 969t
unconscious child and, 1573
Talc aspiration, 996
Talipes calcaneus, 1701–1702
Talipes equinovarus (TEV), 1702, 1702f
Talipes equinus, 1701–1702
Talipes valgus, 1701–1702
Talipes varus, 1701–1702
Talking books, 1207
Tall stature, school-age children and, 1104–1105
Tamoxifen
breast cancer and, 115, 120
medication guide, 120b
Tanning, 1129
Tasting capacity of newborns, 639–640
Tattooing, 1128
Tay-Sachs disease, 831
Teachers, child development and, 1093–1094
Team play, school-age children and, 1092
Technology
assisted reproductive, 8
home care and, 1226
for home care communication, 35–36
perinatal care and, 5, 11
Technology-dependent child, 1157b
Teenage pregnancy
perinatal health in, 8
risks in, 46
Teeth
adolescents and, 1127
changes during pregnancy, 202
preschoolers and, 1060–1061
school-age children and, 1084, 1084f
toddlers and, 1034–1037, 1035f
Teething during infancy, 977, 977f
Telangiectatic nevi, 618–619, 619f
Telemedicine, 5
Telephone follow-up, postpartum, 553–554
Telephone services, family-centred home care and, 1228–1229
Telephone triage care management, 870–871, 871b
Telephonic nursing care, 35–36
Television
impact on child development, 864–866, 865b–866b
preschoolers and, 1055

Temper tantrums, toddlers and, 1022, 1031
Temperament
attributes/significance of, 849–850, 850b
childrearing practices related to, 968–970
of infants, 968–970
of newborns, 640
Temperature. *See* Body temperature
Temporal artery temperature (TAT), 897–901, 899t, 900b–901b
Tentorial herniation, 1575f
Teratogens, 167–168, 167b
Teratomas, 777–778
Term, definition of, 186
Terminally ill children. *See* End-of-life care
Tertiary circular reactions, 1024
Tertiary prevention
in community health, 30, 803
for high-risk infants, 738–739, 739b, 739f
Testes, sex hormones and, 1114
Testicular cancer, 1135
Testicular self-examination (TSE), 1135
Testicular ultrasound, 1538t–1539t
Tet spells, 1474–1476
Tetanus, 1745–1746, 1745b
Tetanus immune globulin (TIG), 985, 1745–1746
Tetanus toxoid vaccine, 985
contraindications/precautions for, 989t–991t
Tetanus-diphtheria–acellular pertussis (Tdap) vaccine, 1125
Tetany, 1620b–1621b
Tetracycline ophthalmic ointment, 646–647, 647b
Tetralogy of Fallot, 354, 1459, 1463b–1464b
Tetraplegia, 1725b
Thalassemia, 364–365
Thalassemia intermedia, 1510
Thalassemia major, 1510
Thalassemia minor, 1510
Thalassemia trait, 1510
The Collaborative Partnership approach, 18t
Thelarche, 1114, 1115f
Theophylline
breastfeeding and, 1753t–1756t
normal test ranges for, 1764t–1771t
Therapeutic donor insemination (TDI), 134t
Therapeutic holding, 1279–1280, 1280f
Therapeutic play, 858, 859f, 1248
Therapeutic relationships
in pediatric nursing, 794
special needs child and, 1158
Thermogenic system, 612–613, 612f
Thermometers for children/infants, 901, 902b
Thermoregulation
infants and, 849, 960
in newborns, 612–613, 612f
preterm infants and, 710–711, 713–714
unconscious child and, 1572
Thiamine, 1376t–1379t
Thimerosal-containing vaccines, 1211b
Third stage of labour
assessment/care of newborn, 481–483
cord blood collection, 481
maternal physical status, 481
overview, 389
placental separation in, 478, 480–481, 480f–481f
Third trimester
discomforts during, 231t–233t
fetal well-being assessment in
contraction stress test, 288–289, 289f, 290t
fetal movement counting, 286, 287f
fetal responses to hypoxia/asphyxia, 286
indications for, 285, 286b
nonstress test, 286–288
ultrasound for, 289–291
signs of potential complications in, 220b
Third-person technique, 877b–878b
Thomas ring splint, 1696, 1696f
Thoracic trauma, 334
Thoracolumbosacral orthotic braces, 1708–1709, 1708f
Thought stopping, 941b
Threaded lock cannula, 1300, 1300f
Threadworm, 1406t
Threatened miscarriage, 314, 314f, 315t
Three wishes, 877b–878b
Throat
of newborns, 643b
pediatric examination of, 916–917, 916f–917f
Thrombin time, 1764t–1771t
Thromboembolic disease
medication guide for, 586b
during postpartum period, 585–586
Throne position, birth process and, 419–420, 419f
Thumb-sucking, 976–977
Thyroid disorders
goitre and, 1617
hyperthyroidism and, 350–352, 1618–1620, 1619b
hypothyroidism and, 352
juvenile hypothyroidism and, 1617, 1617b
lymphocytic thyroiditis and, 1617–1618, 1618b
nursing care for, 352
Thyroid Foundation of Canada, 1619
Thyrotoxicosis, 1619, 1619b
Thyroxine, total, 1764t–1771t
Ticks, 1657–1663, 1658t
Time concept, preschoolers and, 1052–1053
Time factor in neonatal behaviour, 639
Time orientation, cultural variations in, 24–25
Time structuring, hospitalization and, 1244, 1244f
Time-out consequence, 816, 817b
Tinea capitis, 1654t, 1655f
Tinea corporis, 1654t, 1655f
Tinea cruris, 1654t
Tinea pedis, 1654t
Tissue donation, 1182–1183
Tissue oxygenation
for anemia, 1503
for heart failure, 1469
for treatment of shock, 1494
Tobacco. *See* Cigarette smoking
Tobacco smoke exposure, 1344, 1345b
Tocolytic therapy
contraindications to, 495b
medication guide for, 496b
nursing care for, 495b
for preterm labour, 331, 495–496
Tocopherol. *See* Vitamin E
Tocotransducer, 426–429, 427t, 428f
Toddlers
anticipatory guidance in caring for, 1046
biological development of
gross/fine motor development, 1021–1022
maturation of systems, 1021
proportional changes, 1020–1021
sensory changes, 1021
body image development, 1026
cognitive development in, 1024–1026
dental health, 1034–1037
gender-identity development, 1026–1027
growth/development overview, 1023t
hospitalization of
loss of control and, 1235
separation anxiety in, 1234
injury prevention for. *See* Injury prevention, toddlers and
invention of new means in, 1024–1025
language development in, 1027
negativism in, 1031
nutrition for, 1032–1034, 1033b
personal-social behaviour of, 1027–1028
play, 1028, 1028f
preconceptual phase in, 1025–1026
thought characteristics, 1025b
preparation for procedures, 1262b–1263b
psychosocial development in, 1022
regression in, 1032
sibling rivalry in, 1030–1031, 1031f
sleep and activity, 1034
social development in, 1027–1028
with special needs, 1170–1173, 1171t–1172t
spiritual development in, 1026
temper tantrums in, 1031
tertiary circular reactions, 1024
toilet training and, 1029–1030, 1029b, 1030f
understanding of/reactions to death, 1177t–1178t
Toeing in, 927
Toilet training
guidelines for, 1029b
toddlers and, 1029–1030, 1030f
Tolerable upper intake level (UL) of nutrients, 890
Tolerance
defined, 940b
opioid, 951b, 953
TOMA Foundation for Burned Children, 1681
Tonic neck reflex, 622f, 622t–625t, 1566–1567
Tonic-clonic seizures, 1594b–1595b, 1600b
Tonsillectomy, 1323
Tonsillitis, 1321–1324, 1322f
Topical antimicrobial medications, 1675–1676, 1676t
Topical corticosteroid therapy, 1647–1648
Topical sunscreens, 1681–1682
Topical/transdermal analgesia, 948b–949b, 950–951
TORCH infections, 749–756, 749b
Torus fractures, 1691b, 1691f
Total anomalous pulmonary venous connection (TAPVC), 1464b–1467b
Total iron-binding capacity, 1764t–1771t
Total life support system, in transporting high-risk infants, 739, 739f
Total mastectomy, 118, 119f
Total parenteral nutrition (TPN), 1312
Total serum bilirubin (TSB), 652–655, 652f
Touch
for labour pain management, 403
in parent-infant communication, 560, 560f
response of newborn to, 640
Tough Love, 1149
Toxic agents
chemotherapy as, 1523–1524
infant poisoning from, 998–999
Toxocara canis, 1406t
Toxoplasmosis, 749–756
Toys
for cognitively impaired children, 1193, 1193f
for infants, 969t
safety of, 859, 860b–861b, 1045, 1276
selection of, 858–859
for toddlers, 1028
Tracheitis, bacterial, 1330t, 1332
Tracheobronchitis, 1332–1333
Tracheoesophageal fistula (TEF), esophageal atresia with, 1425–1427, 1425b
Tracheomalacia, 1425–1426
Tracheostomy, 1305–1308, 1305f
Trachesophageal fistula (TEF), 773–774, 773f
Traction, 1695–1697, 1695f–1696f, 1696b, 1698b
Trainable cognitive impairments, 1190
Trained night crying, 982t
Training for home care, 1221–1222

Transcranial Doppler (TCD) test, 1507, 1509–1510
Transcutaneous electrical nerve stimulation (TENS), 405, 405f
Transcutaneous monitoring (TCM), 1303f
Transdermal analgesia, 948b–949b, 950–951
Transdermal contraceptive patch, 148
Transductive reasoning in preoperational thought, 1025b
Transilluminator, 1299f
Transition phase of labour, 469t, 470
Transition to extrauterine life. *See* Neonatal transition to extrauterine life
Transition to parenthood, 562–563
Transitional objects, toddlers and, 1027
Transitional stools, 614b, 615f
Transmission-based precautions, 1277, 1277b
Transmucosal analgesia, 948b–949b, 950–951
Transplantation
  bone marrow, 1512
  heart, 1488–1489
  intestinal, for SBS, 1435
  kidney, 1560
  liver, cirrhosis and, 1419
  lung, cystic fibrosis and, 1361
Transportation
  of high-risk infants from regional centres, 739
  of high-risk infants to regional centres, 738–739, 739b, 739f
  of hospitalized infants/children, 1278–1279, 1279f
  for special needs child, 1169–1170, 1229
Transposition of great arteries (TGA), 1464b–1467b
Transvaginal ultrasound examination, 279
Transverse fracture line, 1690
Trauma
  newborn, birth-related, 743–744, 744t
    central nervous system injuries and, 746
    peripheral nervous system injuries and, 744–746, 745f
    skeletal injuries and, 744–746, 744f
  pediatric
    blindness and, 1204–1205
    posttraumatic stress disorder and, 1108
    soft-tissue injury, 1688–1690, 1688f
    tooth avulsion and, 1098, 1099b
  during pregnancy
    blunt abdominal, 333–334
    fetal characteristics and, 333
    immediate stabilization for, 334–335
    maternal physiological characteristics and, 333t
Trauma *(Continued)*
    physiological adaptations and, 332
    significance of, 331–332
    thoracic, 334
  visual impairment from, 1204–1205, 1206b
Traumatic brain injury. *See* Head injury
Travel, pregnancy and, 228–229, 229f
Treatment strategies for compliance, 1269–1270
Trendelenburg's position, 1585b
Treponema pallidum. *See* Syphilis
Tretinoin, 1668–1669
Trial of labour (TOL), 505, 519–520
Triceps reflex test, 929f
Trichomoniasis, 109t, 110
Trichuris trichiura, 1406t
Tricuspid atresia, 1459, 1463b–1464b
Triglycerides (TG), 1764t–1771t
Triiodothyronine (T3),, 1764t–1771t
Triiodothyronine, total, 1764t–1771t
Triplegia, 1725b
Trisomal abnormality, 164
Trivalent influenza viral (TIV) vaccines, 1325
Trousseau's sign, 1620b–1621b
True dawn phenomenon, 1633
True labour, 443, 444b
Truncal incurvation reflex, 622t–625t, 625f
Truncus arteriosus, 1464b–1467b
Trust vs. mistrust stage of psychosocial development, 852, 963–964
Tubal ligation, 151–152, 151f, 152b
Tubal occlusion, 151, 151f
Tubal reconstruction
  of tubal ligation, 152
  of vasectomy, 152
Tubal tonsils, 1322, 1323f
Tube occlusion, 1307–1308
Tuberculin skin test (TST), 1338, 1339b
Tuberculosis (TB), 1337–1340
  clinical manifestations of, 1338b
  neonatal, 755
  positive TST results and, 1339b
  skeletal, 1712
Tumours. *See* Cancer
Turner's syndrome, 1105t, 1106
Twenty-four-hour collection of urine specimens, 1283
Twins
  breastfeeding, 691, 692f
  characteristics of, 812–813, 812b
  cobedding of, 725
  formation of, 180–184
  prenatal care for, 240
  weight gain in, 255
Two-digit system, for gravidity/parity, 186, 187t
Tympanostomy, 1327
Type 1 diabetes mellitus. *See also* Diabetes mellitus (DM)
  defined, 339
  diabetic ketoacidosis in, 342
Type 1 diabetes mellitus *(Continued)*
  in pregnancy, 340
  retinopathy in, 341
Type 2 diabetes mellitus. *See also* Diabetes mellitus (DM)
  defined, 339
  in pregnancy, 340
  retinopathy in, 341

U

Ulcerative colitis (UC), 1410–1414, 1411t
Ulcers, 1645f
  peptic, 202, 1414–1416, 1415b
Ultrasound
  adjunct to amniocentesis/CVS/PUBS, 285
  amniotic fluid volume and, 289–291
  biophysical profile and, 289, 290t
  in breast cancer screening, 117b
  Doppler flow analysis and, 291, 291f
  fetal anatomy and, 281
  fetal growth and, 280–281, 280f
  fetal heart activity and, 279–280
  fetal screening and, 220
  in first-trimester screening, 278
  genitourinary disorders and, 1538t–1539t
  gestational age and, 280
  major uses of, 279–281, 280b
  nonmedical use of, 282b
  nursing role in, 281
  placental position/maturation and, 281
  real-time, assessing cerebral function and, 1567t–1568t
  technology of, 278–279, 279f
  transvaginal examination using, 279
Ultrasound stethoscope, 425, 425f
Ultrasound transducer, 426–429, 427t, 428f
Ultraviolet burns, 1206b, 1681–1682
Umbilical cord
  acid-base determination, 439, 439t
  blood collection from, 481
  care of, 671, 671f
  formation of, 172f, 173, 174f
  interventions for prolapse of, 467b–468b
  prolapse of, 521–522, 521f–522f, 523b
Umbilicus, pediatric examination of, 923, 923f
Unclassified seizures, 1593–1594, 1594b–1595b
Unconscious child
  elimination and, 1572
  family support for, 1573
  hygienic care for, 1572
  intracranial pressure monitoring, 1570–1571
  medications for, 1572
  nursing care for, 1569
  nutrition and hydration for, 1571–1572
  positioning/exercise and, 1572–1573
Unconscious child *(Continued)*
  regaining consciousness and, 1573
  respiratory management in, 1570
  stimulation and, 1573
  thermoregulation and, 1572
Unconsciousness, 1563
Undifferentiated stage of spiritual development, 854
Unifactorial inheritance in genetic transmission, 166–167
United Nations Declaration of the Rights of the Child, 795b
Universal Anchorage System (UAS), 1040, 1040f
Universalizing stage of spiritual development, 854
Unoccupied behaviour, in children, 856
Upper extremity traction, 1696
Upper respiratory tract, 1316
Upper respiratory tract infections
  acute streptococcal pharyngitis, 1321–1322, 1322f
  infectious mononucleosis, 1328–1329, 1328b
  influenza, 1324–1325
  nasopharyngitis, 1320–1321, 1320b
    complications with, 1321b
  otitis media, 1325–1328, 1326b
  tonsillitis, 1322–1324, 1322f
Upright position during labour/birth, 460–461, 461f, 462b, 471
Urea nitrogen, 1764t–1771t
Uremia, 1553
Urethra
  after childbirth, 530
  lacerations of, birth process and, 477
Urethritis, 1541–1542
Urinary catheterization, 1283–1285, 1284t
Urinary incontinence (UI), 590, 591f
Urinary system
  after childbirth, 529–530
  pediatric, immobilization and, 1685t
Urinary tract infection (UTI)
  in children
    classification of, 1541–1542
    diagnosis of, 1542, 1543b
    etiology of, 1542
    management of, 1543–1544
    nursing care for, 1544
    prevention of, 1544, 1544b
  during postpartum period, 587
  prevention of, 222
Urine predictor test for ovulation, 140–141, 142f
Urine protein values, 297b
Urine specimens
  collection of, 1282f
  during first stage of labour, 455–456
  monitoring blood glucose levels, 1631, 1637
  for neonatal screening, 657–659, 659f
  procedure for, 1282–1283
  tests for genitourinary disorders, 1538t–1539t

Urine volume, normal test ranges for, 1764t–1771t
Urodynamics, 1538t–1539t
Urosepsis, 1541–1542
Urushiol, 1655–1656
Uterine (fallopian) tubes, 66f
Uterine atony, 578
Uterine contractions/activity
  assessment of, 424
  during breastfeeding, 695
  dysfunctions of. *See* Dysfunctional labour
  during first stage of labour, 451t, 453–455, 454f, 466t
  interventions for inadequate relaxation, 467b–468b
  postpartum, 526–527
  suppression of, 495–496
Uterine displacement/prolapse, 589, 589f
Uterine inversion, 579
Uterine rupture, 522–523
Uterine subinvolution, 579–580
Uteroplacental blood flow, 190
Uterus, 64–65, 65f–66f
  abnormal, infertility and, 128, 129f
  afterpains and, 527
  Braxton Hicks contractions, 189–190
  cervical changes, 190, 190f
  fetal movements and, 190–191, 192f
  hypotonic, 580–581
  involuntary contractions of, 385–386
  involution process, 526, 527f
  in labour process, 384f
  postbirth lochia, 527–528
  restoring tone to, 542–543, 543f
  size/shape/position, changes in, 188–189, 190f–192f
  structural disorders, 588–593, 592b
  uteroplacental blood flow, 190

V

Vaccines. *See* Immunizations
Vacuum-assisted birth, 512, 513f
Vagina, 64
  changes in, 191–192, 193f
  examination, during first stage of labour, 455, 455f
  lacerations, birth-related, 477
  postpartum changes in, 528
  structural disorders, 588–593, 592b
Vaginal birth. *See* Childbirth
Vaginal birth after Caesarean (VBAC)
  education for, 244, 247
  measures to increase, 514b
  overview, 519–520
Vaginal bleeding, 467b–468b. *See also* Hemorrhagic disorders in pregnancy
Vaginal infections
  bacterial vaginosis, 108–109
  candidiasis, 109–110, 109b
  trichomoniasis, 110
  wet smear tests for, 109t
Vaginal wall examination, 77–79
Vaginitis, 108, 1135
Vagus nerve stimulation, 1597
Valsalva manoeuvre, 439–440, 473
Values and Expectations, 1246b
Valvular aortic stenosis, 1456–1459, 1459f, 1460b–1462b
Variable decelerations of fetal heart rate, 434–435, 434f, 435b
Varicella
  complications with, 1062
  symptoms/management of, 1064f, 1064t–1070t
Varicella vaccine, 987
  adolescents and, 1125
  contraindications/precautions for, 989t–991t
Varicella-zoster immune globulin (VariZIG), 1063
Varicella-zoster virus (VZV), 751
  complications with, 1062
  manifestations/management of, 1653t
Varicosities after childbirth, 531
Vasa previa, 328
Vascular spiders, 199
Vasectomy, 151f, 152
Vasoocclusive crisis, 1505, 1507
Vasopressin, 1615–1616, 1616b
Vasopressor support, 1494
Vastus lateralis injection site, 1289–1290, 1290t–1291t
Vegan diets, 268–270, 1380
Vegetarian diets
  DRIs recommended for, 1380–1384
  maternal nutrition and, 268–270
  nutritional disturbances and, 1380
Vehicle-related injuries
  adolescents and, 1131–1132
  education for prevention of, 1132b
Velamentous insertion of the cord, 328, 329f
Venipuncture
  in newborns, 657
  positioning for, 1281, 1281f
Venous access devices (VADs), 1294–1295, 1294f, 1295t
Venous blood samples, 1285
Ventilation of lungs
  for CPR, 1367, 1367f
  for treatment of shock, 1494
Ventilator therapy
  for neonatal respiratory distress, 715–717, 716t
  weaning from, 717–718
Ventricular puncture, 1567t–1568t
Ventricular septal defects (VSDs)
  in children, 1457b–1459b
  during pregnancy, 353
Ventriculoperitoneal shunt, 1606, 1606f
Ventrogluteal injection site, 1289–1290, 1290t–1291t
Verbal communication
  with children, 876, 877b–878b
  cognitively impaired children and, 1193–1194
  culturally sensitive, 834b
Vernix caseosa
  benefits of, 721
  formation of, 180
Verruca, 1653t
Verruca plantaris, 1653t
Vertex presentation
  mechanism of birth with, 475–476, 475f–476f
  occiput presenting in, 379, 380f
Very-low-birth-weight (VLBW) infants
  classification of, 708b
  environmental concerns for, 722
  incidence of, 250
  nutrition for, 718–721
  respiratory distress syndrome in, 728
  retinopathy of prematurity in, 732
  skin-to-skin contact for, 724–725
Vesicants, 1302
Vesicles, 1644f
Vesicoureteral reflux (VUR), 1543
Vesicular breath sounds, 920b
Viability, definition of, 186
Vibrio cholerae, 1393t–1395t
Video games
  child development and, 866
  preschoolers and, 1055
Vietnamese ethnicity
  caring for newborn and, 550b, 569–570
  communication and, 833
  female companion at childbirth and, 450
  health beliefs/practices and, 134t
  sexual activity during pregnancy and, 238
Vineland Social Maturity Scale, 1190
Violence
  against children, 791. *See also* Abuse, child
  intimate partner. *See* Intimate partner violence (IPV)
Viral infections
  hepatitis, 105–106
  herpes simplex virus. *See* Herpes simplex virus (HSV)
  human immunodeficiency virus. *See* Human immunodeficiency virus (HIV)
  human papillomavirus, 101–103
  meningitis, 1589–1590, 1590t
  of skin, 1651–1653, 1653t
Viral pneumonias, 1335–1336
Visceral larva migrans, 1406t
Visceral pain, during labour, 394
Visible minority groups, 829–830, 830b
Vision testing
  of adolescents, 1128
  in children, 910
  guidelines for, 911t
  in infants/difficult-to-test children, 910–912
  in pediatric assessment, 909–912
Visitors, dealing with, 553
Visual acuity
  of infants, 960
  of newborns, 639
  of toddlers, 1021
Visual Analog Scale (VAS) for pain assessment, 937t
Visual impairments
  in children
    definition/classification of, 1203–1204
    development/independence and, 1207
    education for, 1207
    emergency intervention for eye injuries and, 1206b
    etiology of, 1204–1205, 1204b–1205b
    hospitalization and, 1207–1208
    nursing care for, 1205–1209
    parent-child attachment and, 1206
    play/socialization and, 1207
    prevention of, 1208–1209
    promoting optimum development and, 1206–1207
    retinoblastoma, 1209–1210, 1209b
  health assessments for women with, 71
  nursing approaches for parents with, 571b
  parenting with, 570–571
Visual stimulation
  for infants, 969t
  for preterm infants, 722, 722f
Visualization
  education in, 246
  for labour pain management, 402–403
Vital signs
  blood pressure. *See* Blood pressure (BP)
  body temperature. *See* Body temperature
  cerebral dysfunction and, 1564–1565
  during first stage of labour, 450–452
  heart rate. *See* Heart rate
  after heart surgery, 1479–1480
  of newborn, 626t–636t, 636–637
  postpartum, 531, 532t
  respiratory rate, 1773
  septic shock and, 1496t
Vitamin A
  excessive doses of, 1375
  for maternal nutrition, 261
  for measles, 1063
  nutritional significance of, 1376t–1379t
Vitamin B_1, 1376t–1379t
Vitamin B_2, 1376t–1379t
Vitamin B_6, 1376t–1379t
Vitamin B_{12}
  for maternal nutrition, 262
  nutritional significance of, 1376t–1379t
Vitamin C
  for maternal nutrition, 262
  nutritional significance of, 1376t–1379t
Vitamin D
  deficiencies in, 1374–1375
  excessive doses of, 1375
  during first 6 months, 978–979

Vitamin D *(Continued)*
for hypoparathyroidism, 1621, 1621b
for infants' nutrition, 680
for maternal nutrition, 261–262
nutritional significance of, 1376t–1379t
for preschoolers, 1059
for toddlers, 1034
Vitamin E
for maternal nutrition, 262
nutritional significance of, 1376t–1379t
Vitamin K
infant nutrition and, 647, 647b
injection for newborns, 680
maternal nutrition and, 262
nutritional significance of, 1376t–1379t
Vitamins
imbalances in, 1374–1375
for infants' nutrition, 680, 703–704
nutritional significance of, 1376t–1379t
during pregnancy
fat-soluble, 253t–254t, 261–262
water-soluble, 253t–254t, 262
Voice
changes in puberty, 1117
in parent-infant bonding, 561
Voiding cystourethrography, 1538t–1539t
Voiding during labour, 458t, 460
Volvulus of intestine, 1431
Vomiting, 1403
von Willebrand's disease, 330, 584
Vulnerable child syndrome, 1229
Vulnerable populations
overview, 32–35
perinatal care and, 28–29
Vulva, 190f, 191–192
Vulvovaginal candidiasis (VVC), 109–110

W

Waist circumference, 49, 50b
Waldeyer tonsillar ring, 1322, 1323f
Walking surveys, 32, 32b
Wand exercise, 123b
Warfarin, 585–586, 586b
Warm lines, 554
Water birth, 475, 475f
Water intake of infants, 679–680
Water therapy, 403–405, 404f
Waterhouse-Friderichsen syndrome, 1622–1623, 1622b
Water-soluble vitamins, 262
Weaning
from breastfeeding, 693–694
from formula feeding, 704
from opioids, 952–953, 954f
timing of, 981
Weight gain
during childhood, 846–848, 847t
excessive, 255–256
hazards of restricting, 255, 255f
measuring in pediatric examinations, 896, 897f
of newborns, 690–691
pattern of, 252–255
in preterm infants, 719b
recommended, 251–252, 255t
of school-age children, 1084
of toddlers, 1020
Weight loss
in breastfeeding mothers, 694
in preterm infants, 719b
Weight of newborns, 626t–636t, 627f, 637
Well-woman care, 42
Werdnig-Hoffmann disease, 1738–1740, 1739b
West Asian ethnicity, 829, 830b
West Nile fever, 1662t
Western blot immunoassay, 1527–1528
"What if" questions, 877b–878b
Wheals, 1644f
Whipworm, 1406t
Whitaker perfusion test, 1538t–1539t
White blood cell count
after childbirth, 531
during labour, 392b
normal test ranges for, 1764t–1771t
pelvic inflammatory disease and, 100–101
during pregnancy, 195, 197t
Whooping cough. *See* Pertussis
Wilmington braces, 1708–1709
Wilms' tumour, 1552–1553, 1552b
Windows, falls from, 998
Wiskott-Aldrich syndrome, 1530
Withdrawal, 410b
in infants/children
heroin, 761
methadone, 761
opioid, 951b, 952–953. *See also* Neonatal abstinence syndrome (NAS)
maternal, opioid, 409b–410b
Withdrawal method of birth control, 136–137
Withdrawal reflex, 1567b
Woman-centred care, 6–7, 6b
Women
with disabilities, 70–72
at risk for abuse. *See* Abuse, of women
vulnerability of, 33–34
Word association game, 877b–878b
Word-Graphic Rating Scale for pain assessment, 937t
Working mothers, 822
World health Organization (WHO), 893–894
Wound sepsis, 1673
Wounds
care of, 1649–1650
dressings for, 1648t
healing of, 1643–1646, 1647t
management of burn, 1675–1676
nursing care for, 1649
postpartum infection in, 586–587
relief of symptoms for, 1650
topical therapy for, 1650–1651
types of, 1643
Writing skills, school-age children and, 1098

X

Xenograft skin coverings, 1676
X-linked dominant inheritance disorders, 167
X-linked lymphopenic agammaglobulinemia, 1530
X-linked recessive inheritance disorders, 167

Y

Yeast infections, 109–110, 697–698
Yersinia enterocolitica, 1393t–1395t, 1396
Yolk sac, 171f, 173
Young adulthood, 46

Z

Zanamivir, 1325
Zinc
for maternal nutrition, 261
nutritional significance of, 1381t–1383t
Zollinger-Ellison syndrome, 1414
Zygote, 168, 170f
Zygote intrafallopian transfer (ZIFT), 134t

Special Features

ATRAUMATIC CARE

Encouraging Deep Breaths, 920
Encouraging Opening the Mouth for Examination, 916
Encouraging a Child's Acceptance of Oral Medication, 1288
Guidelines for Pain Management During Neonatal Circumcision, 666
Guidelines for Skin and Vessel Punctures, 1287
Heel Punctures, 658
Immunizations, 991
Lead Chelation Therapy, 1445
Lumbar Puncture and Bone Marrow Test, 1282
Minimizing Pain of Blood Glucose Monitoring, 1637
Promoting Relaxation During Abdominal Palpation, 924
Reducing Distress from Otoscopy in Young Children, 913
Reducing Young Children's Fears, 897
Reducing the Distress of Nasogastric Tube Insertion, 1308
Reducing the Stress of Burn Care Procedures, 1678
Skin Testing, 1347

COMMUNITY FOCUS

Accessibility of Diabetes Supplies, 345
Anticipatory Guidance for Health Promotion, 55
Availability of Culturally Appropriate Childbirth Resources, 237
Availability of Maternal Child Services in Your Community, 37
Breastfeeding Support, 547
Canada Prenatal Nutrition Program, 264
Canadian Cancer Society, 123
Community Resources for Loss and Grief, 599
Community Walk-Through, 32
Culturally Appropriate and Adequate Prenatal Care, 12
Culture and Pain, 396
Deciding About a Home Birth, 243
Early Sexual Maturation, Alcohol, and Cigarettes, 1145
Education About Electronic Fetal Monitoring, 439
Healthy Food Choices, 861
Helping Grandparents Bridge the Generation Gap, 573
Home Pregnancy Test Kits, 187
Internet Resources on Genetics, 161
Neonatal Jaundice, 654
Neonatal Transport, 739
Newborn Circumcision, 663
Nonsmoking Strategies, 1146
Preterm and Late-Term Infant Car Seat Evaluation, 738
Prevention of Postpartum Infection, 588
Reducing Blood Lead Levels, 1446
Resources for Alternative and Complementary Methods of Pain Relief, 400
Resources for Families With Children With Genetic Disorders, 159
Resources for Parents Experiencing a High-Risk Pregnancy, 274
Sex Education, Violence Prevention, Sexual Abuse, and Rape Awareness in the Schools, 46
Sexually Transmitted Infections, 95
Spiritual Assessment, 1223
Suicide, Sexual Identity, and Sexual Orientation, 1150
Sun Protection Basics, 863
Support for At-Risk Pregnant Women, 292
Woman With Pre-Eclampsia, 299

CRITICAL THINKING EXCERCISE

Anorexia Nervosa, 1144
Anxiety in a Multipara in Active Labour, 397
Awareness of Physiological Changes of Pregnancy, 188
Caring for an Adolescent Having Her First Pelvic Examination, 73
Constipation, 1400
Contraception for Adolescents, 136
Culturally Competent Care in the Emergency Department, 23
Diagnosis of Down Syndrome, 1197
Diarrhea, 1398
Digoxin Toxicity, 1472
Discussing Sexual Orientation With Adolescents, 1123
Discussing the Future, 1118
Family-Centred Home Care and Conflicts, 1225
Fatigue and Rest After Childbirth, 544
Hydrocephalus, 1571
Hypercyanotic Spell, 1475
Infertility Workup, 131
Inflammatory Bowel Disease, 1413
Intimate Partner Violence, 59
Late Preterm Infant, 713
Late Preterm Infant, Sudden Infant Death Syndrome, and Infant Sleep Position, 669
Maintaining Therapeutic Boundaries, 1227
Maternal Postpartum Blood Loss and Fatigue, 531
Neonatal Breastfeeding, 683
Neonate With Chlamydia, 755
Nutrition and the Overweight Pregnant Woman, 256
Pain Management, 418
Placenta Previa, 323
Playroom and Hospital Procedures, 1249
Poisoning, 1439
Postpartum Adjustment for the Adolescent and the Older Mother, 567
Pregnant Woman Who Is HIV Positive, 372
Premenstrual Syndrome in Adolescents, 88
Preterm Labour, 489
Reducing Cultural Shock, 832
Respecting Privacy, 1125
Smoking Cessation During Pregnancy, 230
Spontaneous vs. Directed Bearing-Down Efforts, 473
Termination of Pregnancy, 153
Testicular Self-Examination, 1136
Ultrasound Dating of Pregnancy, 173
Urinary Tract Infection and Constipation, 1544

CULTURAL AWARENESS

A Clash of Cultures, 550
Bladder Catheterization, 1284
Breast Screening Practices, 117
Communication Variations, 70
Cultural Beliefs and Practices Regarding Newborns, 660
Developmental Dysplasia of the Hip, 1700
Family Bed, 1009
Female Genital Mutilation (FGM), 54
Fertility and Infertility, 127
Food Practices, 887
Fostering Bonding: Women of Varying Ethnic and Cultural Groups, 561
Learning Sociocultural Mores, 1052
Overview of Visible Minority Status in 2006 Canada Census, 830
Religious Orientation, 1089
Some Cultural Beliefs About Pain, 396

EMERGENCY

Amniotic Fluid Embolism (Anaphylactoid Syndrome of Pregnancy), 524
Avulsed Permanent Tooth, 1099
Burns, 1673
Cardiopulmonary Resuscitation of the Pregnant Woman in the Hospital, 363
Eclampsia, 307
Epistaxis, 1517
Eye Injuries, 1206
Fracture, 1692
Head Injury, 1578
Hemorrhagic Shock, 583
Hypoglycemia, 1638
Hypovolemic Shock, 542
Interventions for Emergencies, 467
Maternal Hypotension With Decreased Placental Perfusion, 413

Continued

Special Features—*cont'd*

Poisoning, 1439
Prolapsed Cord, 523
Seizures, 1600
Shock, 1494
Supine Hypotension, 216

EVIDENCE-INFORMED PRACTICE

Assessing Correct Placement of Nasogastric or Orogastric Tubes in Children, 1311
Assessing for Postpartum Mood Disorder, 595
Benefits of Continuous Labour Support, 464
Buffered Lidocaine for Pain Reduction During Peripheral Intravenous Access in Children, 952
Exercise and Work in Pregnancy, 52
Fetal Monitoring and the Machine That Goes "Beep", 428
Gastric Lavage in Children, 1441
Having a Baby Later in Life, 568
How Soon Is Too Soon? Early Discharge After Birth, 537
Monitoring for Hypoglycemia, 616
Normal Saline Instillation Before Suctioning—Helpful or Harmful?, 1306
Optimal Birth Spacing, 137
Pediatric Pain and Symptom Management at the End of Life, 1180
Safety of Herbal Teas During Pregnancy, 258
Searching for and Evaluating the Evidence, 10
Sickle Cell Anemia and Penicillin Prophylaxis, 1508
Skin-to-Skin Contact (Kangaroo Care) for Preterm Infants, 726
Skin-to-Skin Contact for Full-Term Neonates, 688
Temperature Measurement in Pediatrics, 900
Usefulness of Prenatal Breastfeeding Education, 245
Vaccines and Autism Spectrum Disorders, 1211

FAMILY-CENTRED TEACHING

A Dying Child: A Nurse's Perspective, 1185
Activities for Children of Women on Bed Rest, 494
Administering Digoxin, 1472
Artists as Partners in Care, 1257
Bicycle Safety, 1103
Care After Cardiac Catheterization, 1454
Caregivers and the Infant With HIV Infection, 1529
Children Need to Say Good-bye, 1182
Child's Developing Language Skills, 967
Communication With Teens: The Art of Listening, 1120
Controlling Symptoms of Lactose Intolerance, 1389
Decision for a Hematopoietic Stem Cell Transplant, 1533
Decreasing Childhood Exposure to Environmental Tobacco Smoke, 1345
Developing Relationships With Culturally Diverse Families, 1223
Diagnosis of Heart Disease, 1477
Discharge From Ambulatory Settings, 1254
End-Stage Liver Disease, 1420
Family of the Dying Child, 1176
Fear of Addiction, 1509
Fear of Opioid Addiction, 940
Grandparent Adaptation to Pregnancy and Birth, 212
Guidance During Preschool Years, 1061
Guidance During Toddler Years, 1045
Guidance for Parents During School Years, 1091
Impact of Preterm Birth, 497
Implementing Discipline, 815
Knowledgeable Parents, 1225
Maintaining Contact, 1579
Maternal-Paternal-Fetal Relationship, 210
Minimizing Misbehaviour, 815
Newborn Behaviour, 638
Newborn Skin, 617
Paternal Adaptation, 208
Phototherapy and Parent-Infant Interaction, 663
Poisoning, 1442
Preterm Infant, 727
Preventing or Dealing With Sexual Abuse of Children, 1080
Sibling Adaptation to Pregnancy and Birth, 212
Significance of the Apgar Score, 643
Skateboard and In-Line Skate Safety, 1103
Smoking Cessation, 760
Strategies for Facilitating Sibling Acceptance of a New Baby, 573
Supporting Siblings During Hospitalization, 1251
Swelling on the Scalp, 617
Television Viewing, 866
Toy Safety, 860
Using Car Safety Seats, 1041
Using Time-Out, 817
What I Learned About Home Care, 1226

GUIDELINES

Administration of Enemas to Children, 1312
Analyzing the Symptom: Pain, 880
Assessing Coping Behaviours, 1162
Assessing Toilet Training Readiness and How to Facilitate Toilet Learning, 1029
Basal Body Temperature, 139
Cervical Mucus Characteristics, 140
Communicating With Adolescents, 876
Communicating With Children, 874
Culturally Sensitive Interactions, 834
Diagnosis of Initial Attack of Rheumatic Fever (Jones Criteria, 1992 Update), 1483
Effective Auscultation, 919
Establishing Brain Death in Children, 1583
Facilitating Lipreading, 1202
Feeding Children With Growth Failure (Failure to Thrive), 1007
Feeding the Sick Child, 1273
How to Do a Breast Self-Examination, 69
Identifying Latex Allergy, 1738
Initiating a Comprehensive Family Assessment, 883
Interpreting Peak Expiratory Flow Rates, 1347
Interviewing Adolescents, 1125
Intramuscular Administration of Medication, 1292
Managing Opioid-Induced Respiratory Depression, 953
Nasogastric Tube Feedings in Children, 1309
Nasogastric, Orogastric, or Gastrostomy Medication Administration in Children, 1296
Negotiating "House Rules" for Home Care, 1226
Neonatal Skin Care, 723
Nonpharmacological Strategies for Pain Management, 941
Nutrition for Women With Pre-Eclampsia, 303
Performing a Pediatric Physical Examination, 891
Physical Examination of the Newborn, 648
Poisoning Prevention, 1442
Postoperative Care, 1267
Preventing Atopy in Children, 1387
Prevention of Urinary Tract Infection, 1544
Recording Assessment Data in Suspected Abuse, 1079
Review of Systems, 885
Skin Care, 1270
Supporting Grieving Families, 1184
Taking an Allergy History, 880
Talking With Children Who Reveal Abuse, 1075
Traction Care, 1698
Treating Hypercyanotic Spells, 1475
Treatment for Hypoglycemia, 345
Using an Interpreter, 873
Using the Blood Pressure Tables, 904

HOME CARE

After a Mastectomy, 122
Assessing and Reporting Clinical Signs of Pre-Eclampsia, 301
Dietary Management of Diabetic Pregnancy, 345
Exercise Tips for Pregnant Women, 225
Formula Preparation and Feeding, 703
How to Recognize Preterm Labour, 234
Newborn Bath, 671
Newborn Home Care, 673
Nutrition Counselling for the Pregnant Woman With Cholecystitis or Cholelithiasis, 367
Postterm Pregnancy, 506
Posture and Body Mechanics, 226
Resumption of Sexual Intercourse, 553
Sexuality in Pregnancy, 235
Sexually Transmitted Infections, 110